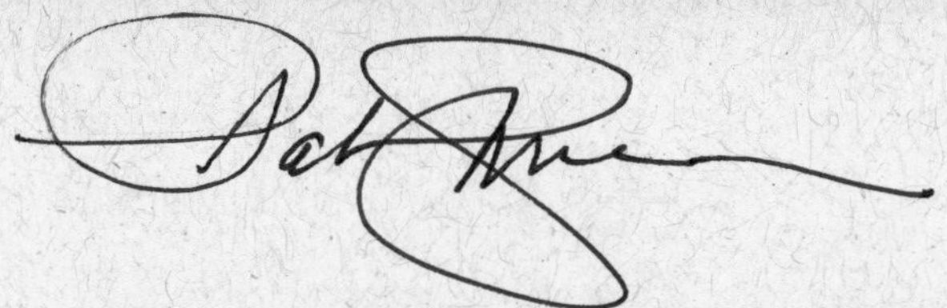

QUICK REFERENCE FOR PEDIATRIC DOSAGES

>2 yr:
4.4 μg/kg 30–60 min before procedure (IM)
Control secretions:
20–100 μg/kg/dose q 4–8 hr (PO)
2–10 μg/kg/dose q 4–8 hr (IM, IV)

Hydrocortisone (Cortef, Solu-Cortef)
Anti-inflammatory/immunosuppressive:
2.5–10 mg/kg/day divided q 6–8 hr (PO)
1–5 mg/kg/day divided q 12–24 hr (IM, IV)

Hydroxyzine hydrochloride (Atarax, Vistaril)
2–4 mg/kg/day divided q 6–8 hr (PO)
0.5–1 mg/kg/dose q 4–6 hr (PO)

Ibuprofen (Advil, Motrin)
Fever:
5–10 mg/kg/dose q 4–6 hr (PO)
Analgesic:
4–10 mg/kg/dose q 6–8 hr (PO)

Imipenem/Cilastatin (Primaxin)
60–100 mg/kg/day divided q 6–8 hr

Ketamine
Procedures:
6–10 mg/kg × 1 dose (PO)
3–7 mg/kg × 1 dose (IM)
0.5–2 mg/kg × 1 dose (IV)
Continuous sedation:
10–15 μg/kg/min (IV)

Lorazepam (Ativan)
Anxiety and sedation:
0.05 mg/kg/dose q 4–8 hr (PO, IV)
Continuous sedation:
0.025–0.2 mg/kg/hr (IV)

Mannitol
ID: 0.5–1 g/kg over 20 min
MD: 0.25 g/kg/hr

Meperidine hydrochloride (Demerol)
Pain:
1–2 mg/kg/dose q 3–4 hr (PO, IM, IV)
For procedures:
0.5–1 mg/kg 2–5 min before procedure

Methylprednisolone (Medrol, Solu-Medrol)
Status asthmaticus:
1 mg/kg/dose q 6 hr (IV)
Anti-inflammatory/immunosuppressive:
0.117–1.66 mg/kg/day divided q 6–12 hr (PO, IM, IV)

Metoclopramide hydrochloride (Reglan)
Gastroesophageal reflux:
0.4–0.8 mg/kg/day in 4 divided doses (PO)
Antiemetic:
1–2 mg/kg/dose q 2–4 hr (IV)

Metronidazole (Flagyl)
Amebiasis:
35–50 mg/kg/day divided q 8 hr (PO)
Anaerobic infections:
30 mg/kg/day divided q 6 hr (PO, IV)

Midazolam hydrochloride (Versed)
Conscious sedation:
0.2–0.5 mg/kg 30–45 min before procedure (PO)
0.05–0.1 mg/kg 3 min before procedure (IV)

Morphine sulfate
0.2–0.5 mg/kg/dose q 4–6 hr (PO)
0.1–0.2 mg/kg/dose q 2–4 hr (IM, IV)

Nafcillin sodium (Unipen)
50–200 mg/kg/day divided q 6 hr (IM, IV)

Nystatin (Mycostatin)
Neonate:
100,000 U 4 times/day (PO)
Infants:
200,000 U 4 times/day (PO)
Children:
500,000 U 4 times/day (PO)

Ondansetron (Zofran)
>3 yr:
0.15 mg/kg/dose (IV)
4–11 yr:
4 mg 3 times/day (PO)
>11 yr:
8 mg 3 times/day (PO)

Penicillin G potassium
100,000–250,000 U/kg/day divided q 4–6 hr (IV)

Penicillin V potassium
<12 yr:
25–50 mg/kg/day divided q 6–8 hr (PO)
≥12 yr:
125–500 mg q 6–8 hr (PO)

Pentobarbital sodium
Hypnotic:
2–6 mg/kg (IM)

Phenobarbital
Anticonvulsant:
LD:
Neonates:
15–20 mg/kg
Infants and children:
15–20 mg/kg
MD:
Neonates:
3–4 mg/kg/day in 1–2 divided doses
Infants:
5–6 mg/kg/day in 1–2 divided doses
1–5 yr:
6–8 mg/kg/day in 1–2 divided doses
5–16 yr:
4–6 mg/kg/day in 1–2 divided doses
>12 yr:
1–3 mg/kg/day in divided doses

Phenytoin (Dilantin)
Anticonvulsant:
LD: 15–20 mg/kg (PO)
MD: 5–10 mg/kg/day (PO)

Piperacillin
200–300 mg/kg/day divided q 4–6 hr (IM, IV)

Prednisone
Anti-inflammatory/immunosuppressive:
0.05–2 mg/kg/day divided 1–4 times/day (PO)
Acute asthma:
1–2 mg/kg/day divided 1–2 times/day

Ranitidine hydrochloride (Zantac)
1.5–2 mg/kg/dose q 12 hr (PO)
0.75–1.5 mg/kg/dose q 6–8 hr (IM, IV)
0.1–0.25 mg/kg/hr (CI)

Rifampin
10–20 mg/kg/day divided q 12–24 hr (PO)

Spironolactone (Aldactone)
1.5–3.5 mg/kg/day divided q 6–24 hr (PO)

Streptomycin sulfate
Infants:
20–30 mg/kg/day divided q 12 hr (IM)
Children:
20–40 mg/kg/day divided q 12–24 hr (IM)

Tetracycline hydrochloride
>8 yr:
25–50 mg/kg/day divided q 6 hr (PO)

Theophylline
6 wk–6 mo:
10 mg/kg/day (PO)
12 mg/kg/day divided q 6–8 hr (IV)
6 mo–1 yr:
12–18 mg/kg/day (PO)
15 mg/kg/day (CI)
1–9 yr:
20–24 mg/kg/day (PO)
1 mg/kg/hr (CI)
9–12 yr:
16 mg/kg/day (PO)
0.9 mg/kg/hr (CI)
12–16 yr:
13 mg/kg/day (PO)
0.7 mg/kg/hr (CI)

Ticarcillin disodium (Ticar)
200–300 mg/kg/day divided q 4–6 hr (IV)

Tobramycin (Tobrex)
2.5mg/kg/dose q 8 hr (IM, IV)

Vancomycin hydrochloride (Vancocin)
>1 mo and children:
40 mg/kg/day divided q 6 hr (IV)

KEY

CI = continuous infusion
ID = initial dose
IM = intramuscular
IV = intravenous
LD = loading dose
MD = maintenance dose
PO = by mouth

Sources: Stringham, D. (Ed.). (1997). *Pediatric drug handbook and formulary*. Orange, CA: Children's Hospital of Orange County.

Lexi-Comp, Inc. (1997). *Formulex program*. Hudson, OH: Lexi-Comp, Inc.

Children and Their Families

THE CONTINUUM OF CARE

Children and Their Families

THE CONTINUUM OF CARE

Vicky R. Bowden, DNSc, RN
Associate Professor
Azusa Pacific University
Azusa, California

Instructor
California State University, Dominguez Hills
Carson, California

Susan B. Dickey, PhD, RN
Associate Professor
Temple University
Philadelphia, Pennsylvania

Cindy Smith Greenberg, DNSc, RN, CPNP
Instructor
University of Phoenix, Southern California Campus
Fountain Valley, California

W.B. SAUNDERS COMPANY
A Division of Harcourt Brace & Company
Philadelphia London Toronto Montreal Sydney Tokyo

W.B. SAUNDERS COMPANY
A Division of Harcourt Brace & Company

The Curtis Center
Independence Square West
Philadelphia, Pennsylvania 19106

Library of Congress Cataloging-in-Publication Data

Bowden, Vicky R.
Children and their families: the continuum of care / Vicky R. Bowden, Susan B. Dickey, Cindy Smith Greenberg.

p. cm.

ISBN 0–7216–5179–8

1. Pediatric nursing. 2. Family nursing. I. Dickey, Susan B. II. Greenberg, Cindy Smith. III. Title.

RJ245.B69 1998 610.73′62—dc21 97–11069

Cover Photograph:
Unique Image Photography
Mullica Hill, New Jersey
Maria Martins, Photographer

CHILDREN AND THEIR FAMILIES: THE CONTINUUM OF CARE ISBN 0–7216–5179–8

Printed in the United States of America.

Last digit is the print number: 9 8 7 6 5 4 3 2 1

Dedication

To my husband and best friend,

Greg

who has been an ever-present source of love, support, and encouragement

To **Christian** *and* **Matthew**

who are our blessings and heritage from the Lord

V.R.B.

To my daughter,

Elizabeth Carla Isaacs

S.B.D.

To my husband,

Jay

who has offered love and support so my dreams could become reality

To **Erin, Jordan,** *and* **Daniel**

who have taught me the joys and trials of parenthood,
and who continually reinforce to me why children are special

C.S.G.

Contributors

Kathleen B. Adlard, BSN, MN
Hematology/Oncology Clinical Nurse Specialist, Children's Hospital of Orange County, Orange, California
Health Challenge: Pediatric Malignancies

Janice Beitz, PhD, RN
Director, Graduate Nursing Program, School of Nursing, LaSalle University, Philadelphia, Pennsylvania
Health Challenge: Alterations in Skin Integrity

Vicky R. Bowden, DNSc, RN
Associate Professor, Azusa Pacific University, Azusa, California; Instructor, California State University, Dominguez Hills, Carson, California
Interdisciplinary Care of the Child and Family; The Child Developing Within the Family; Growth and Development; Promoting Healthy Living; Acute Illness as a Challenge to Health Maintenance; Health Challenge: Alterations in Skin Integrity

Margaret A. Brady, PhD, RN, CPNP
Pediatric Nurse Practitioner, Miller Children's Hospital, Children's Protection Center, Long Beach, California
Health Assessment and Well-Child Care

Vicki L. Brinsko, BA, RN, CIC
Infection Control Practitioner, Manager, Infection Control, Vanderbilt University Medical Center, Nashville, Tennessee
Health Challenge: Pediatric Infections

Natalie Cheffer, MN, RN, CPNP
Lecturer, California State University at Long Beach, Long Beach, California
The Child Developing Within the Family

Brenda Costello-Wells, MSN, RN
Part-time Lecturer, School of Nursing, Indiana University; Care Coordinator, Newborn Intensive Care Unit, Riley Hospital for Children, Indianapolis, Indiana
Health Challenge: Alterations in Children's Mental Health

Susan B. Dickey, PhD, RN
Associate Professor, Temple University, Philadelphia, Pennsylvania
Current Issues in Child and Family Nursing; Unexpected Outcomes of Childbearing

Diane A. DiFazio, MSN, CRNP
Pediatric Nurse Practitioner, Laurel Springs, New Jersey
Health Challenge: Alterations in Endocrine Status

Jennifer A. Disabato, MS, RN, CPNP
Rocky Mountain Pediatric Neurosurgery, Children's Hospital of Denver, Denver, Colorado
Health Challenge: Alterations in Neurologic Status

Catherine Fleischman, MSN, RN
Staff Nurse III, Pediatric Intensive Care Unit, Children's Hospital, Oakland, California
Health Challenge: Alterations in Fluid and Electrolyte Status

Marian B. Fosdal, MA, RN, CPOC
Adjunct Assistant Professor, School of Nursing, Indiana University; Clinical Nurse Specialist/Educator, Riley Hospital for Children, Indianapolis, Indiana
Health Challenge: Alterations in Hematologic Status

Susan D. Foster, BSN, MS
Consultant, Loube Consulting International, Norcross, Georgia
Health Challenge: Inborn Errors of Metabolism

Cyrena M. Gilman, MN, RN, CNN
Manager, Clinical Operations, Pediatric Dialysis, Riley Hospital for Children, Clarian Health Partners, Indianapolis, Indiana
Health Challenge: Alterations in Genitourinary Status

Cindy Smith Greenberg, DNSc, RN, CPNP
Instructor, University of Phoenix, Southern California Campus, Fountain Valley, California
Acute Illness as a Challenge to Health Maintenance; Pain Management in Children; Health Challenge: Alterations in Fluid and Electrolyte Status

Katherine M. Hart, BSN, RN
Clinical Manager, Egleston Children's Hospital at Emory University, Atlanta, Georgia
Health Challenge: Alterations in Musculoskeletal Status

Julie Buerman Herda, MN, RN, CPNP
Pulmonary Nurse Practitioner, Children's Hospital of Orange County, Orange, California
Health Challenge: Alterations in Respiratory Status

Elizabeth F. Hobdell, MSN, PhD, CRNP, CNRN
Clinical Assistant Professor, University of Pennsylvania, School of Nursing; Advanced Practice Nurse, St. Christopher's Hospital for Children, Philadelphia, Pennsylvania
Health Challenge: Alterations in Neurologic Status

Carol Frances Holt, MN, RN
Clinical Instructor, California State University at Long Beach, Long Beach, California
Health Challenge: Alterations in Cardiovascular Status

Lisa Ann Horn, MN, RN
Manager, PCS Education, Emergency Department, Transport and Children's Hospital Community Health Clinic, Children's Hospital of Los Angeles, Los Angeles, California
Health Challenge: The Pediatric Emergency

Christine Hoyler-Grant, MSN, RN, CPNP, CRNP
Nurse Practitioner, Adolescent Gynecology, Planned Parenthood of Southeastern Pennsylvania, Philadelphia, Pennsylvania
Health Challenge: Alterations in Genitourinary Status

Kristine Kirlin Kester, MSN, RN
Clinical Instructor, Nell Hodgson Woodruff School of Nursing at Emory University, Atlanta, Georgia
Health Challenge: Alterations in Musculoskeletal Status

Jeanine Khoury, RN, CPNP
Pediatric Nurse Practitioner, Woodland Pediatrics, Lancaster, South Carolina
Unexpected Outcomes of Childbearing

Robin M. Koeppel, MS, RNC, CPNP
Neonatal Clinical Nurse Specialist/Pediatric Nurse Practitioner, University of California, Irvine Medical Center, Orange, California
Health Challenge: The Neonate

Kathleen Ryan Kuntz, MSN, RN
Clinical Preceptor, University of Pennsylvania School of Nursing and Thomas Jefferson University College of Health Professions; Nursing Faculty, University Affiliated Program of Children's Seashore House, Philadelphia, Pennsylvania; President/Rehabilitation Consultant, Rehab Advantage, Jamison, Pennsylvania; Director of Nursing Education, Children's Seashore House, Philadelphia, Pennsylvania
Rehabilitation, Habilitation, and Home Care: Supporting Health Maintenance

Patricia Kuster, MSN, RN, CPNP
PhD Candidate, University of California, Los Angeles, School of Nursing; Clinical Nurse II, Children's Hospital of Los Angeles, Los Angeles, California
Health Challenge: Alterations in Respiratory Status

Mary Lee Lacy, MSN, RN
Rehabilitation Program Specialist, Children's Hospital of Orange County, Orange, California
Acute Illness as a Challenge to Health Maintenance

Barbara Larson, MEd, RN
Pediatric Educator, Home Care Division, CM HealthCare Resources, Inc., Deerfield, Illinois
Rehabilitation, Habilitation, and Home Care: Supporting Health Maintenance

Terri H. Lipman, PhD, CRNP
Assistant Professor, University of Pennsylvania, School of Nursing; Nurse Practitioner, Section of Diabetes/Endocrinology, St. Christopher's Hospital for Children, Philadelphia, Pennsylvania
Health Challenge: Alterations in Endocrine Status

Elizabeth Jill Mansholt, RN
Chief Operating Officer, CM HealthCare Resources, Inc., Children's Memorial Medical Center, Chicago, Illinois
Promoting Healthy Living

Nancy D. Opie, DNS, RN, FAAN
Professor, Psychiatric Nursing, School of Nursing, Indiana University, Indianapolis, Indiana
Health Challenge: Alterations in Children's Mental Health

Laurie Reyen, MN, RN, CNSN
Assistant Clinical Professor, University of California, Los Angeles; Clinical Nurse Specialist, Parenteral and Enteral Nutrition, Pediatric Gastroenterology, University of California, Los Angeles Children's Hospital, Los Angeles, California
Health Challenge: Alterations in Gastrointestinal Status

Sharon E. Rose, PhD, RNC
Assistant Professor, Department of Family/Community Nursing, College of Nursing, East Tennessee State University, Johnson City, Tennessee
Health Challenge: Alterations in Vision, Hearing, and Communication

Rita L. Secola, MSN, RN
Clinical Nurse Specialist, Oncology/Bone Marrow Transplantation, Children's Hospital of Orange County, Orange, California
Health Challenge: Pediatric Malignancies

Kathryn A. Smith, MN, RN
Assistant Clinical Professor, School of Nursing; University of California, Los Angeles; Adjunct Assistant Professor of Clinical Nursing, Department of Nursing, University of Southern California; Co-Director, ACCESS-MCH, Los Angeles, California
Health Promotion Through Community Care

Jennifer Tiffany-Amaro, MSN, CRNP
Clinical Nurse Specialist, Section of Neurology/PKU, St. Christopher's Hospital for Children, Philadelphia, Pennsylvania
Health Challenge: Alterations in Endocrine Status

Linda Tirabassi, MN, CPNP
Clinical Nurse Specialist, Miller Children's Hospital, Long Beach Memorial Medical Center, Long Beach, California
Health Challenge: Alterations in Respiratory Status

Diane M. Wink, MA, MSN, EdD
Associate Professor, University of Central Florida, School of Nursing, Orlando, Florida
Chronic Conditions as a Challenge to Health Maintenance; The Grieving Family

Consultants and Contributors to Special Sections Within a Chapter

Janice Beitz, PhD, RN
Director, Graduate Nursing Program, School of Nursing, LaSalle University, Philadelphia, Pennsylvania
Health Challenge: Pediatric Infections

Karen Blount, MSN, RN
Children's Hospital of Buffalo, New York
Health Challenge: Alterations in Cardiovascular Status; Health Challenge: Alterations in Musculoskeletal Status; Health Challenge: Pediatric Infections; Health Challenge: Alterations in Skin Integrity

Vicki L. Brinsko, BA, RN, CIC
Infection Control Practitioner, Manager, Infection Control, Vanderbilt University Medical Center, Nashville, Tennessee
Health Challenge: Alterations in Skin Integrity

Lorena Gaskill, MN, RN, CCRN
Gaithersburg, Maryland
Health Challenge: Alterations in Neurologic Status

Jutta Helm, MN, RN
Children's Hospital of Buffalo, Buffalo, New York
Health Challenge: Alterations in Cardiovascular Status; Health Challenge: Alterations in Musculoskeletal Status; Health Challenge: Pediatric Infections; Health Challenge: Alterations in Skin Integrity

Melva Kravitz, PhD, RN
Associate Professor, Yale University School of Nursing; Director, Research and Education, Division of Nursing, Yale–New Haven Hospital, New Haven, Connecticut
Health Challenge: Alterations in Skin Integrity

Kathleen Ryan Kuntz, MSN, RN
Clinical Preceptor, University of Pennsylvania School of Nursing and Thomas Jefferson University College of Health Professions; Nursing Faculty, University Affiliated Program of Children's Seashore House, Philadelphia, Pennsylvania; President/Rehabilitation Consultant, Rehab Advantage, Jamison, Pennsylvania; Director of Nursing Education, Children's Seashore House, Philadelphia, Pennsylvania
Health Challenge: Alterations in Musculoskeletal Status; Health Challenge: Alterations in Neurologic Status

Barbara J. Rondinone, MSN, RN
Nurse Manager, Perioperative Services, Women's and Children's Hospital, Los Angeles County and University of Southern California Medical Center, Los Angeles, California
Acute Illness as a Challenge to Health Maintenance

James W. Sweeney, BSN, RN
Philadelphia Department of Public Health, Immunization Program, Philadelphia, Pennsylvania
Health Assessment and Well-Child Care

Anne E. Winch, MSN, RN, CPNP
Pediatric Clinical Nursing Specialist, Mayo-Eugenio Litta Children's Hospital, Mayo Medical Center, Rochester, Minnesota
Growth and Development; Promoting Healthy Living; Health Assessment and Well-Child Care

Reviewers

Jeanette N. Adams, DrPH, RN, AOCN
Graduate Program Chair, School of Nursing, The University of Texas at Houston, Houston, Texas

Kim Siarkowski Amer, PhDc, RN
Instructor in Nursing, DePaul University, Chicago, Illinois

Janette P. Arblaster, MSN, RN
Tri-County Technical College, Pendleton, South Carolina

Rose Marie Wilcox Arblaster, MSN, RN
Health Consortium, Tri-County Technical College, Pendleton, South Carolina

Kathleen L. Ballenger, MSN, RN
Assistant Professor, Nursing Department, Missouri Western State College, St. Joseph, Missouri

Shirley M. Bass, RN, CFNP/PNP
Assistant Professor, Tennessee State University, Nashville, Tennessee

Peggy H. Batastini, MSN, RNC, MEd
Director, Associate Degree Nursing Program, Columbus College, Columbus, Georgia

Rosalie J. Benchot, MSN, RNC, PhDc
Assistant Professor, Kent State University School of Nursing, Kent, Ohio

Barbara J. Benz, MS, RN
Roswell Park Cancer Institute, State University of New York at Buffalo, Buffalo, New York

Beverly Ruth Bigler, RN, CPNP, EdD
Professor of Nursing, California State University, Los Angeles, California

Clara W. Boyle, RN, EdD
Medical-Surgical Clinical Instructor, Lecturer, Salem State College, Salem, Massachusetts

Robert Maurice Brayden, MD
Assistant Professor of Pediatrics, University of Colorado School of Medicine, Children's Hospital of Denver, Denver, Colorado

Marion E. Broome, PhD, RN, FAAN
Professor, Research Chair, Nursing of Children, University of Wisconsin at Milwaukee, Children's Hospital of Wisconsin, Milwaukee, Wisconsin

Patricia Burgess, MS, RNC
Assistant Professor, Orvis School of Nursing, University of Nevada, Reno, Nevada

Claire M. Chee, RN
Clinical Nurse Specialist, Division of Neurology, Children's Hospital of Philadelphia, Philadelphia, Pennsylvania

Debra Gaddy Cohen, MSN, RN, CPON
North Carolina Baptist Hospital, Winston-Salem, North Carolina

Connie Colter, MS, RN, CPNP
Schneider Children's Hospital, Long Island Jewish Medical Center, New Hyde Park, New York

Alice E. Conway, PhD, RN
Associate Professor, Edinboro University of Pennsylvania, Edinboro, Pennsylvania

Mary Ellen Creighton, RN, CPN
Director of Nursing–Pediatric Services, Children's Hospital of Buffalo, Buffalo, New York

Joetta DeSwarte, MSN, RN, CPON
Clinical Nurse Specialist, Pediatric Hematology, Oncology, Memorial Medical Center, Long Beach, California

Susan Drouin, MSc(A), RN
Lecturer, School of Nursing, McGill University; Nurse Manager, Neonatal Intensive Care Unit, Montreal Children's Hospital, Montreal, Quebec, Canada

Kathryn S. Ewing, RNC + RNCPN
Indiana, Pennsylvania

Salva Failla, RN, DNS
Associate Professor, School of Nursing, Louisiana State University Medical Center, New Orleans, Louisiana

Mary T. Folkerth, MSN, RN, CPNP
Lecturer and Clinical Facilitator, Indiana University East, Richmond, Indiana

Ruth Elizabeth Ford, MSN, RN, OCN
Memorial Sloan-Kettering Cancer Center, New York, New York

Ardella M. Fraley, MN, RN, CPN
Associate Professor, College of Nursing, Montana State University, Missoula, Montana

Margaret Mary Friedhoff, MSN, RN, CPNP
Pediatric Nurse Practitioner, Pediatric Gastroenterology Outpatient Clinic, Medical College of Wisconsin/Children's Hospital of Wisconsin, Milwaukee, Wisconsin

Roberta Pecoraro Gates, MSN, RN, CS
Assistant Professor of Nursing, Darton College, Albany, Georgia

Cherry Anderson Guinn, MSN, RN, EdD
Associate Professor and Coordinator of Family Nursing, University of Tennessee at Chattanooga, Chattanooga, Tennessee

Annette Hallman, MSN, RNC, CNS, CPN
Child Health Nursing Instructor, Methodist Hospital School of Nursing, Lubbock, Texas

Shirley L. Jones, PhDc, RNC
Director of Nursing and Clinical Support Services, Genetics and IVF Institute, Fairfax, Virginia

Beth C. Kurdunowicz, MS, RN, CS
Pediatric Nurse Practitioner, Children's Hospital of Michigan, Detroit, Michigan

Carolyn Jean Lawburgh, BSN, RN, ACLS
Staff Nurse, Intensive Care, Major Hospital, Shelbyville, Indiana

Susan L. Lordi, MS, RN, CPNP
Los Angeles County Office of Education, Downey, California

Linda T. Lowry, MSN, RNCS
Shawnee Community College, ADN Program, Ullin, Illinois

Patricia McCarthy, MSc, RN
Clinical Nurse Specialist, Pediatric Oncology, Children's Hospital of Eastern Ontario, Ontario, Canada

David Kent Miller, BSN, RNC, MSEd
Ivy Tech State College, Columbus, Indiana

Lisa D. Myers, MSN, RN, CPNP
James Whitcomb Riley Hospital for Children, Indianapolis, Indiana

Anita Norton, MSN, RN
Jefferson State Community College, Birmingham, Alabama

Donna Y. Ortega, MS, RN
Professor of Nursing, Community College of Denver, Denver, Colorado

Glenda Jones Pace, BSN, RN
Faculty Member, Edgecombe Community College, Tarboro, North Carolina

Debra Minter Peglow, MN, RNC, CPNP, CDE
Memorial Hospital of South Bend, Indiana University, South Bend Campus, South Bend, Indiana

Elizabeth Jane Piburn, MSN, RN
Cypress College, Cypress, California

Kathleen Simons Piggott, MS, RN
Project Coordinator, South East County Asthma Management Project, Seattle King County Department of Public Health, Renton, Washington

Rebecca Sue Poore, BSN, RN, CCRN
Clinical Nursing Manager and Assistant Director of Nursing, American Transitional Hospital, Tulsa, Oklahoma

Lois H. Rafenski, RN, EdD
Professor, State University of New York at Farmingdale, Farmingdale, New York

Helen L. Redding, MSN, RNC, FNP, BA
Instructor, Tennessee Technological University, Cookeville, Tennessee

Christine M. Rosner, MSN, RN
Assistant Professor, Department of Nursing, Holy Family College, Philadelphia, Pennsylvania

Janice Joy McKiernan Rumfelt, MSN, RNC, EdD
Southern Illinois University at Edwardsville, Edwardsville, Illinois

Deborah DiSchino Ryan, MSN, RN
Assistant Professor, Department of Women and Children, Emory University, Atlanta, Georgia

Kathleen A. Scheller, MSN, RNC
University of Evansville, Evansville, Indiana

Michele Ann Schultze, MSN, RN, PNP
Egleston Children's Hospital at Emory University, Atlanta, Georgia

Gail Zell Serdoz, MSN
Associate Professor, Department of Nursing, College of West Virginia, Beckley, West Virginia

Margaret Anne Shaw, MN, RN, CS, PNP
Egleston Children's Hospital, Atlanta, Georgia

Patricia A. Slater, MSN, RN
Assistant Professor, College of Mount St. Joseph, Cincinnati, Ohio

Dorothy H. Stonebraker, PhD, RN, PNP
Texas Woman's University, Houston, Texas

Mary E. Strickland, MSN, RN
Assistant Professor, Barton College, Wilson, North Carolina

Jane Brocksmith Tiek, MSN, RN
Vincennes University, Good Samaritan Hospital, Vincennes, Indiana

Rosemarie B. Trouton, MSN, RN
Clinical Nurse Educator, General Pediatrics, Penn State University Children's Hospital, Milton S. Hershey Medical Center, Hershey, Pennsylvania

Elias Vasquez, PhD, NNP
Neonatal Nurse Practitioner, Hermann Hospital, K.I.N.D.E.A. Clinic, University of Texas at Houston, Houston, Texas

Kathleen Kelley Walsh, MS, RN
Assistant Professor, Jackson Community College, Jackson, Michigan

Robin L. Watson, MN, RNC
Harbor–UCLA Medical Center, Torrance, California

DeLois Pittman Weekes, MS, RN, DNSc
Boston College School of Nursing, Chestnut Hill, Massachusetts

Janet K. Williams, PhD, RN, CPNP, CGC
Associate Professor, Director of Genetic Counseling, Masters of Nursing Program, University of Iowa, Iowa City, Iowa

Marilyn Kay Witter, BSN, RN, MA (Health Education)
Nursing Instructor, Montcalm Community College, Sidney, Michigan

Gladys M. Word, MSN, EdD
Professor of Nursing, The College of New Jersey, School of Nursing, Ewing, New Jersey

Preface

It is our pleasure to present this text, which offers a fresh approach to pediatric health care. Today's nurse must be well versed in the new technologies, clinical management tools, challenges of cultural diversity, and changing role expectations they will encounter as they interact with children and families seeking health care. The need for *all* nurses to understand and be able to address the health care needs of children and their families has become essential, no longer merely a career option. Community health care settings have expanded their practice domains and are welcoming the influx of children and their families to what have traditionally been adult care arenas. This requires that every student and every nurse be prepared to care for the children they will encounter in their health care practice.

Children and Their Families: The Continuum of Care provides a comprehensive textbook of children's health care that can be used by both students and nurses in a variety of clinical practice settings. In developing this textbook, our goal was to provide the student and nurse with the knowledge base that would enable them to make critical assessments and judgments regarding the child and his or her family in a variety of settings across the continuum of care.

Continuum of Care

Nurses caring for children do so in a system of care that encompasses ambulatory care, hospital care, primary care, rehabilitative services, case management, school health services, and community health services. Nursing faculty have recognized the extension of health care services to a multitude of community-based settings and have intentionally changed nursing curriculums to reflect the need to broaden the scope of student learning experiences to encompass all arenas in which the child's health needs may emerge. This text reflects this new focus, addressing the care of children in a variety of settings, from the home to schools to the medical center. In addition, the text thoroughly covers health promotion, surveillance, and maintenance needs of children from infancy through adolescence. It is recognized that every encounter between the nurse and the family is a teaching encounter. Throughout the duration of the nurse–family relationship will come many opportunities for the nurse to provide the family with strategies to address their current health care needs. In addition, the nurse can act in a proactive manner to give anticipatory guidance that can assist the family as they work to promote their child's growth and development. An extensive discussion of national health care programs and services available for children is presented in Chapter 7, "Health Promotion Through Community Care." The latest national recommendations for health surveillance, anticipatory guidance, and health care practices have been provided, drawing on such resources as the Society of Pediatric Nurses, the American Academy of Pediatrics, *Bright Futures: Guidelines for Health Supervision on Infants, Children, and Adolescents, Healthy People 2000,* and the Agency for Health Care Policy and Research.

Interdisciplinary Approach

This book's unique interdisciplinary perspective highlights the role of the nurse working with *all* members of the health care team to meet the needs of children and their families. The model of nursing care has shifted from one based on a primary care approach to one in which the nurse serves as a vital member of the health care team. Nurses have a primary responsibility to oversee and coordinate the multiplicity of health care services provided to the child and family.

The dynamics of who implements a specific intervention is influenced by nursing practice acts and by the guidelines established by individual health care organizations. In the context of the interdisciplinary team approach, this text highlights the unique role of the nurse by articulating nursing diagnoses, as approved by the North American Nursing Diagnosis Association (NANDA), that are applicable to specific health care challenges. In addition, specific nursing interventions are featured in charts throughout the text. Eighty-one of the nursing interventions classifications (NICs) developed by the Iowa Intervention Project have been incorporated into the text to further delineate the definitive nursing activities that have been identified in research and practice as essential in helping the child and family come to a resolution of the child's actual or potential health care problem.

Use of Care Paths

Care Paths were selected as the clinical tool to present the interdisciplinary plan of care for children with selected diseases and conditions discussed in the text. Although we recognize the need for students to learn and articulate the traditional nursing care plan, we also recognize that in the health care arena the focus is on interdisciplinary collaboration. This agenda is articulated in a plan of care that reflects all of the components of the care for a "typical" child with a particular diagnosis.

The student using this text is likely to already have benefited from the concepts presented in a nursing fundamentals course and a medical-surgical nursing course. This text aims to build on that knowledge and further the student's understanding of collaborative practice and the clinical tools that have been adapted in practice settings to reflect the interdisciplinary care. Through the use of these tools, the student has the opportunity to gain more knowledge about achieving patient outcomes, which in turn will have an effect on the child's length of stay and the optimal use of resources. These issues are defining the delivery of health care and thus must be vital components of any education program for the health professional.

Organization of the Text

The text is divided into four units: Unit 1, Family-Centered Care Throughout the Family Life Cycle; Unit 2, Health Promotion and Illness Prevention; Unit 3, Maintaining Health Across the Continuum of Care; and Unit 4, Managing Health Challenges.

The first three units, containing Chapters 1 to 13, present theories, developmental concepts, and principles of pediatric nursing practice that are germane to each encounter with a child and his or her family regardless of the specific health care concern. These chapters provide a wealth of current knowledge that the student or nurse can draw on to analyze and articulate a child's and family's needs.

Unit 4 builds on the content developed in the first three units to present the health care challenges most commonly seen in the pediatric population. A deliberate effort was made to summarize the health care challenges in a single chapter that reflect pathologies of a particular body system. Thus, the reader looking for information about a specific disease or condition is able to locate the content in an efficient and logical manner.

The content in Chapters 14 to 30 is presented in a consistent format to assist both the instructor and reader in reviewing the assessment, diagnostic, and treatment interventions specific to a particular body system. These chapters are structured as follows:

Assessment of the Child with an Alteration in ____
- Focused Health History
- Focused Physical Assessment
- Nursing Diagnoses and Outcomes
- Developmental and Biological Variances

Diagnostic Criteria for Evaluating Alterations in ____
Treatment Modalities
Alterations in ____________

Each chapter begins with the focused health history and focused physical assessment for conditions that may affect the subject body system. Important developmental and biological variances are highlighted to summarize important physiologic changes occurring as a child grows and develops. A summary chart of nursing diagnoses lists those most likely to apply to many (if not all) of the health challenges covered in the chapter. Also included is a summary of the common treatment modalities used by the interdisciplinary team to manage children facing these health challenges.

Following this introductory content comes coverage of the specific conditions, or "health challenges," commonly seen in children. The discussion of each condition begins with information on incidence, etiology, and pathophysiology. Assessment data, diagnostic test results, and nursing diagnoses unique to the particular condition under discussion are presented. As needed, the reader should refer back to the chapter's introductory section to augment his or her understanding of the general assessment and diagnostic criteria for conditions of the subject body system. The discussion of each condition concludes with presentation of the interdisciplinary care considerations specific to community settings such as the home, school, and daycare facility.

Features of the Text

A variety of pedagogic features have been incorporated into the text to highlight key aspects of care and aid identification of key information.

Chapter Opener

The beginning of each chapter has several features that serve as an introduction or "welcome" to the chapter:

- A brief outline of the chapter contents
- Objectives summarizing what the reader will accomplish or learn from reading this chapter
- Key terms found in the chapter and defined in the Glossary at the end of the text

Drawings and Photographs

More than 400 color photographs and drawings are included to illustrate key points.

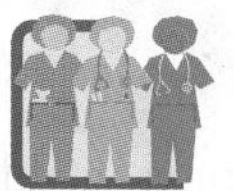

Care Paths

Care paths summarize the interdisciplinary plan of care for a child with a specific condition. Nursing diagnoses are incorporated in each care path to establish the areas of concern that need to be addressed by the health care team. For each nursing diagnosis, patient outcomes are identified as goals to be achieved over a defined time period. The care categories delineate the health care interventions to be performed in each identified time interval to enable achievement of the patient outcomes.

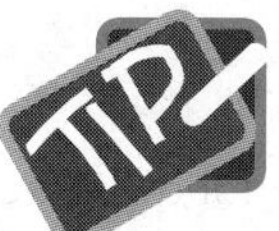

Teaching Intervention Plans (TIPs)

This feature presents an interdisciplinary plan focused on an aspect of care involving patient and/or family education. In each TIP, nursing diagnoses and child/family outcomes define the problem and the desired goals.

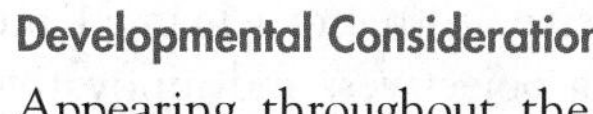

Developmental Considerations

Appearing throughout the text where appropriate, the charts highlight important psychosocial, teaching, physiologic, or pathophysiologic differences between children of various age groups.

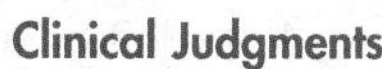

Clinical Judgments

This feature provides a self-check for the reader in evaluating her or his critical thinking skills. Each begins with a clinical situation, or vignette, followed by five questions. These questions follow the format developed by Carnevali and Thomas (1993) in their text *Diagnostic Reasoning and Treatment Decision Making in Nursing:*

1. Question regarding an assessment of the situation.
2. Question in which the student must classify or group related data into patterns.
3. Question in which the student must draw a conclusion or differentiate information.
4. Question regarding the interventions that should now be carried out based on the answers to the three previous questions.
5. Question regarding evaluating the outcomes, evaluating what they should see as outcomes, or, if they do not see certain outcomes, then what referrals or further action should be taken.

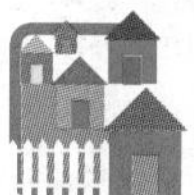

Community Care

These charts present special teaching or clinical information to assist the nurse working with the family in community settings.

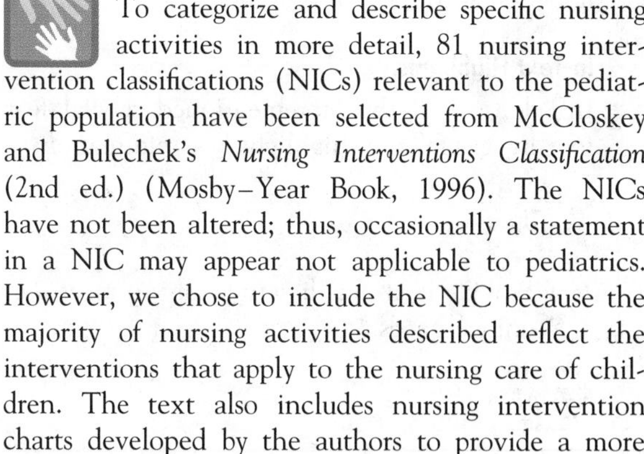

Nursing Interventions

To categorize and describe specific nursing activities in more detail, 81 nursing intervention classifications (NICs) relevant to the pediatric population have been selected from McCloskey and Bulechek's *Nursing Interventions Classification* (2nd ed.) (Mosby–Year Book, 1996). The NICs have not been altered; thus, occasionally a statement in a NIC may appear not applicable to pediatrics. However, we chose to include the NIC because the majority of nursing activities described reflect the interventions that apply to the nursing care of children. The text also includes nursing intervention charts developed by the authors to provide a more in-depth description of particular nursing care activities.

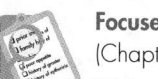

Focused Health History Chart

(Chapters 14–30 only)

This chart summarizes specific health history information the nurse needs to know to assess disorders in a particular body system.

Focused Physical Assessment Chart

(Chapters 14–30 only)

These charts highlight or summarize assessment findings, explaining what would be considered abnormal findings.

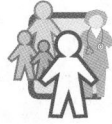

Nursing Diagnoses and Outcomes Chart

These charts summarize the nursing diagnoses and outcomes that are consistently applicable to defined populations of children with specific health challenges. If a clinical condition presents with a unique challenge that has not been adequately defined in the Nursing Diagnoses and Outcomes chart, then more specific nursing diagnoses and outcomes for that particular area of concern are listed where appropriate.

Developmental and Biological Variances Drawing

(Chapters 14–30 only)

This feature highlights important developmental and biological variances to further refine the reader's knowledge of age-appropriate assessment and intervention criteria.

Tests and Procedures Table

(Chapters 14–30 only)

This table describes the tests and procedures used most often in the assessment and diagnosis of conditions affecting a particular system or diagnostic group. The table highlights the health care responsibilities associated with assisting the child in undergoing the test or procedure.

In-Text Highlights

In addition to the aforementioned special features, four in-text features highlight key information:

 Tip

Provide ideas for directing care to meet a child's unique needs.

▽ Alert

Highlight indicators of imminent emergencies or factors to consider that indicate the need for immediate action by the health care provider.

● Worldview

Statements that indicate how cultural, ethnic, or religious practices may influence the perception of an illness, the course of the illness, or the treatment plan.

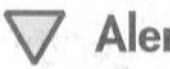

caREminder

A one- to three-sentence reminder of an aspect of care that is especially important for the nurse to remember to ensure safe care.

Chapter Summary

Each chapter ends with the following features:

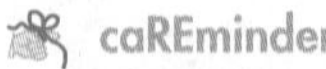

Summary of Key Concepts
A bulleted list summarizing some of the key concepts presented in the chapter.

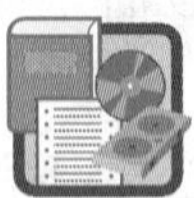

Resources
A list of resources that includes organizations, hotlines, computer resources, and printed materials for the reader to access for additional sources of information. Resources that are particularly directed or developed for children are indicated with an icon. ✏

References
Lists of all references cited in each chapter.

Bibliography
Articles and texts for more extensive review available to the reader.

International Content

Throughout the text, the Worldview features highlight important aspects of transcultural care. In addition, health statistics for Canada are included in appropriate chapters. The Canadian and WHO Immunization schedules are located in Appendix 8. A selected list of Canadian organizations and associations involved in health promotion are presented in Appendix 9. Computer health care resources that can be accessed by all national and international readers are presented at the end of each chapter.

Teaching/Learning Package

For the instructor, we have provided the following teaching tools:

Instructor's Manual

The comprehensive instructor's manual presents chapter outlines, learning objectives, and innovative teaching activities and strategies. The manual also includes copies of all the Care Paths and copy-ready materials to be used as handouts or overheads.

Test Manual

A separate printed test bank includes more than 1000 multiple-choice test questions. The correct answer is identified, and the rationale for the correct answer is provided after each question.

Computerized Test Bank

Available in both IBM and MacIntosh formats, this includes all of the questions and answers from the printed test bank in a form that allows the instructor to select, delete, reorder, and edit questions on the computer, then print out a customized set of test questions for a particular chapter.

Overhead Transparencies

More than 80 full-color transparency acetates reproduce key material from the text, providing an additional teaching tool.

VICKY R. BOWDEN

References

Carnevali, D., & Thomas, M. (1993). Diagnostic reasoning and treatment decision making in nursing. Philadelphia: J.B. Lippincott.

McCloskey, J., & Bulechek, G. (1996). Nursing Interventions Classification (NIC) (2nd ed.). St. Louis: Mosby–Year Book.

Acknowledgments

A book begins as a dream, a tiny seed planted in someone's mind. Before long, others are contacted and asked to share in the vision. As time goes on, the dream begins to take form and shape; it evolves into a product that is far more than the original vision, and in many ways it is always in need of more evolution as the scope, breadth, and depth of nursing knowledge expands.

The seeds for this book were planted by Ilze Rader, former Senior Editor at W. B. Saunders. We are grateful for her inspiration and for her belief in our ability to complete this authorship. As the editorial torch was passed to Barbara Nelson Cullen, we benefited from her ability to set us more firmly to our task and to overcome many deadline hurdles. We are also grateful to the W. B. Saunders production staff, most especially Denise LeMelledo and Arlene Chappelle, for their excellent contributions toward refining the book and moving the production schedule in a timely and efficient manner.

Dreams have to be nourished, tended, and guided to become reality. To Kevin Law, our editor, we owe our deepest gratitude and warmest thanks. Kevin knew when to be silent, when to be strong, when to be kind, and when to be unyielding. Most of all, we appreciate that Kevin knew when to laugh.

We acknowledge and thank the contributors for sharing with us their time and their knowledge. We especially appreciate the tolerance shown by these clinical experts as the book evolved and more work was required to produce a quality text that is a true reflection of the concepts and practices emerging in health care today.

Most of the photographs of children and their families were taken at Children's Hospital of Orange County (CHOC), in Orange, California; many others depict families at the Creekside Christian Fellowship in Irvine, California. Each photograph has a story and each child's life has impressed upon us the preciousness of health, of family love, and of the great blessings that God has given each of us. Our thanks to Rick Williams for his excellent photographic contributions, and to the nursing and administrative personnel at CHOC for assisting us in finding the children and their families to participate in the photographs.

Finally, we want to acknowledge and to thank all of the friends and family members who gave their unfailing support as the book changed from dream to reality. Special thanks to

- Linda Baird, who provided assistance in the preparation of the manuscript, and who was always timely and ready to help, even with midnight requests!
- Cliff Baird, who provided computer rescue service.
- Leo and June Clark and John and Carol Bowden for watching children, for listening, and for giving needed words of encouragement.
- The church family at Creekside Christian Fellowship for prayers, encouragement, and companionship.
- Bill and Barbara Smith, for being a constant source of support and strength.

V.R.B.

Brief Contents

Contents

CHAPTER 3

The Child Developing Within the Family 99

UNIT 2

Health Promotion and Illness Prevention 167

CHAPTER 4

Growth and Development 169

UNIT 3

Maintaining Health Across the Continuum of Care 415

CHAPTER 8

Unexpected Outcomes of Childbearing 417

CHAPTER 9

Acute Illness as a Challenge to Health Maintenance 457

CHAPTER 10

Chronic Conditions as a Challenge to Health Maintenance 527

CHAPTER 17

HEALTH CHALLENGE:

Alterations in Fluid and Electrolyte Status 979

CHAPTER 18

HEALTH CHALLENGE:

Alterations in Gastrointestinal Status 1027

CHAPTER 19

HEALTH CHALLENGE:

Alterations in Genitourinary Status 1111

CHAPTER 20

HEALTH CHALLENGE:

Alterations in Musculoskeletal Status 1217

Key to Special Features

CARE PATHS

An Interdisciplinary Plan of Care for the . . .

TIP LIST

A Teaching Intervention Plan for . . .

NURSING INTERVENTIONS CLASSIFICATION (NIC)

MY CARE PATH

CLINICAL JUDGMENT

NURSING DIAGNOSES AND OUTCOMES

COMMUNITY CARE

DEVELOPMENTAL CONSIDERATIONS

DRUG NOTICE

Family-Centered Care Throughout the Family Life Cycle

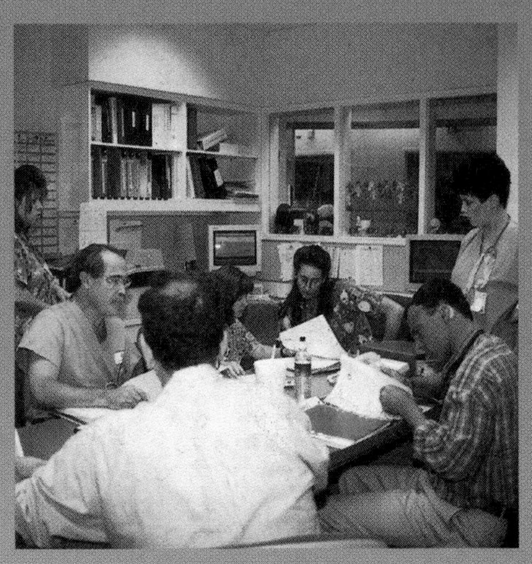

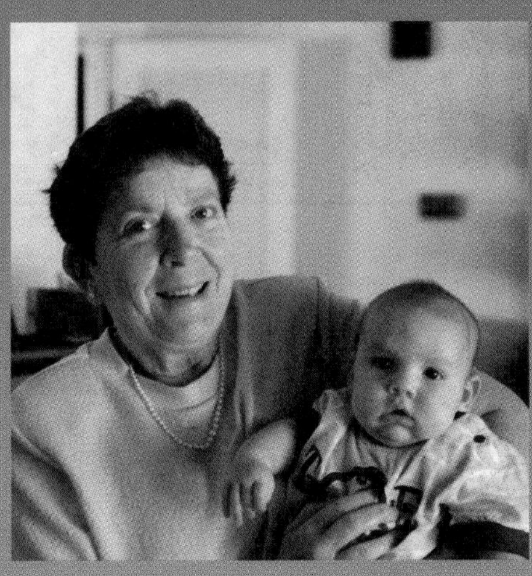

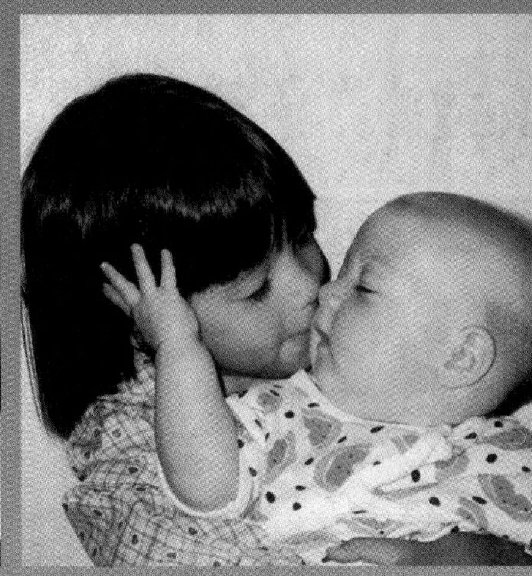

UNIT

1

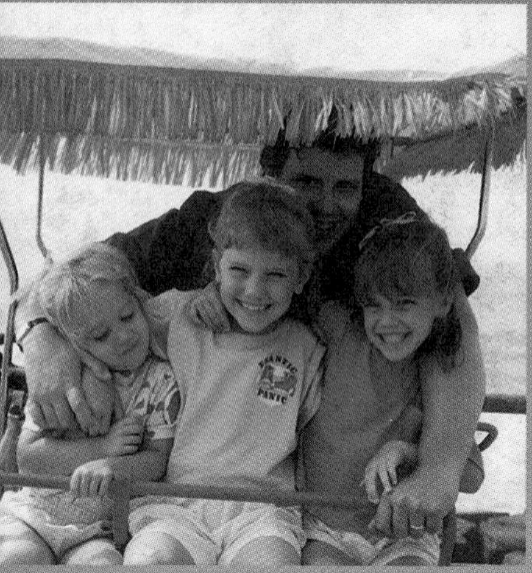

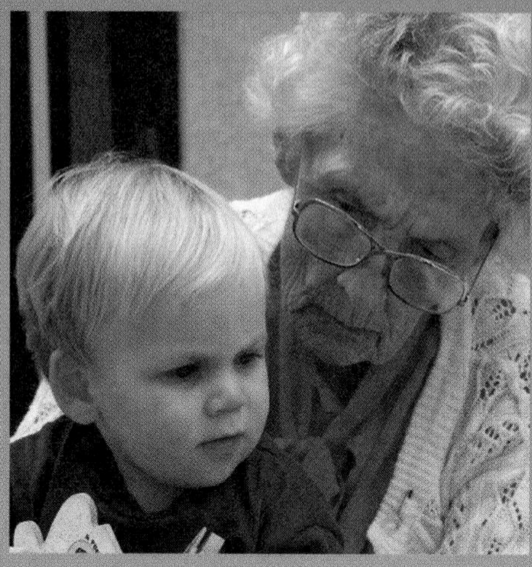

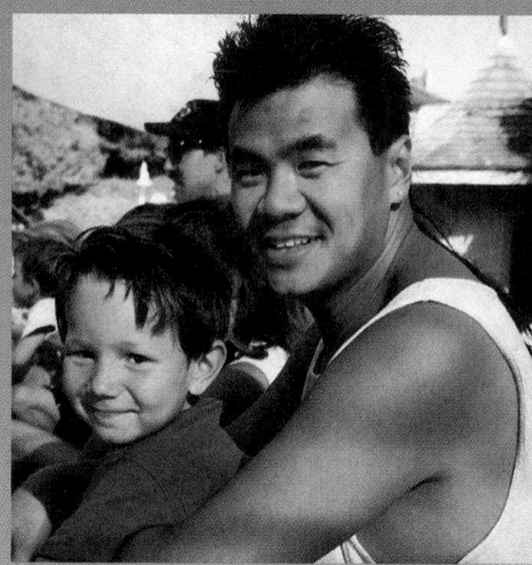

The chapters in Unit 1 present family theories, current issues, and family concerns that affect how child health care is practiced. The text focuses on the interdisciplinary care of children. The nurse is a vital member of a team of professionals who work together to serve the needs of children and their families. In the clinical arena, many new tools have been developed to better manage patient care and to standardize practice. Examples of such tools include care paths, nursing interventions classifications, practice standards, and new publications that summarize health supervision for infants, children, and adolescents. These tools have been woven throughout the text to help the practitioner maintain a family-centered care approach that recognizes current practice concerns as well as the unique needs of children and their families.

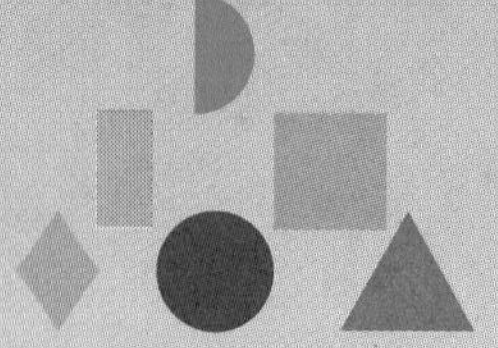

Interdisciplinary Care of the Child and Family

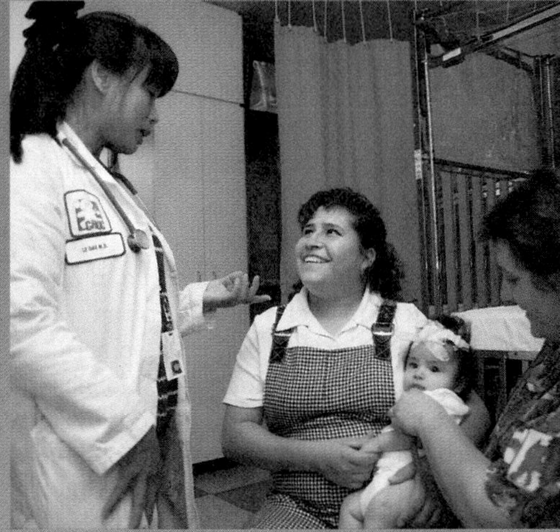

OUTLINE

OBJECTIVES

- Explain the historical and practical basis of the concept of family-centered care.
- Examine the emphasis toward an interdisciplinary approach to family-centered care.
- Describe the various roles the nurse can assume when providing care to the child and the family.
- Understand the specialty certification process.
- Describe the settings in which the nurse caring for children provides family-centered care.
- Discuss the continuing evolution of pediatric health care.

KEY WORDS

aggregate
care path
case management
certification
infant mortality rate
interdisciplinary
managed care
Nursing Interventions Classification (NIC)
settlement nursing
variance

CHAPTER

1

> The two periods of childhood are infancy, which extends from birth to the age of two and a half years, and childhood proper, beginning at that age and lasting until the fourteenth or fifteenth year. The conditions of life during this time are very different from those of mature growth, and the principles upon which adults may be treated will not always apply to children; nor is the same kind of nursing suitable for both adults and children, for a nurse who may be entirely satisfactory for grown people sometimes utterly fails in caring for children. Besides tact and plenty of patience, there must be a certain sympathy that children are always quick to feel, and this, combined with judicious firmness, will make a nurse successful in the management of either well or sick children of any age. When children are sick, the habit of observation on the part of the nurse is of the highest degree of importance, for, since children are helpless and unable to properly understand or explain their own feelings, we have to depend on signs to tell us where the trouble is located, and we may be able to gather facts of much importance from what are apparently quite trivial symptoms.
>
> (Isabel Hampton, 1893, p. 284)

More than 100 hundred years ago, Isabel Adams Hampton, nurse leader, author, and educator, recognized several of the unique elements that have become the enduring principles underlying the care of children today. Hampton's words begin by acknowledging the fundamental differences between children and adults. Hampton recognized that the principles and the practices nurses employ to prevent illness and to promote and maintain the health of children and their families must reflect an understanding of the unique variances between children and adults. Development-specific knowledge must be applied to understand thoroughly the physiologic, psychological, social, and spiritual attributes unique to children of various ages.

Moreover, Hampton emphasized that not all individuals are suited to the care of children and their families. She recognized that caring for children demands a special sensitivity and application of clinical judgment. The health care provider must be able to interact with a population of patients who are often unable to articulate what is wrong with them or where it hurts.

A third principle implied from Hampton's work is that the nurse caring for children must bring a rare combination of interpersonal skills to the practice of this particular branch of nursing. Although caring and nurturing are the essence of this practice, leadership is needed to provide the support, guidance, and discipline that the child and the family often need. The pediatric nurse must be able to shift from tenderly holding a crying, colicky infant to disciplining a 4-year-old having a temper tantrum to supporting the adolescent's choice to not terminate a pregnancy—all the while understanding the developmental, physical, and psychosocial principles that underlie the child's behavior.

Finally, Hampton acknowledged that the health care professional must understand the feelings, signs, and symptoms of children of any age who are well. Pediatrics is a unique, rapidly expanding health care discipline serving a population considered to be among the most vulnerable and disadvantaged in our society (Behrman, Kliegman, & Arvin, 1996). The diversity of age groups (neonates to adolescents), organ systems (e.g., cardiac, nervous, and genitourinary), health care services (well-child, acute illness, and outpatient care), and family systems (single parents, blended families) emphasizes the necessity of providing care to the child and the family by a team of professionals well versed in the principles and practices of pediatrics.

This chapter reviews the fundamental principles and practices upon which the care of children and their families has been built. The chapter begins with an account of the historical roots of child health care, exploring the political, societal, medical, and nursing advances achieved over time, to give the reader a better appreciation of the art and science of child health care as practiced today. It goes on to explore the concepts of family-centered care and an interdisciplinary practice approach and to review the diverse roles, interventions, and settings in which the nurse caring for children functions and practices. Finally, the chapter closes with the future agenda and opportunities for child health care.

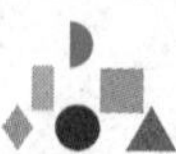

Caring for Children and Their Families: A Historical Perspective

Childhood and adolescence represent a period in the life of a human being that is recognized in industrialized societies as a time for the young person to gradually learn and accept the responsibilities of adulthood. For many decades, scientific inquiry and philosophic and religious discourse ignored the periods of childhood and adolescence. The predominant view held that children came into the world as miniature adults—the *homunculus* theory—innately sinful but potentially redeemable (Aries, 1962). There existed a fear of "spoiling" children and a belief that children left idle would get into mischief and cause misdeeds. Therefore, in all respects, children were treated as small adults and were often severely admonished for their inability to meet adult standards. Children unable physically or mentally to meet the societal demands were viewed as "weak" or "not viable" by a world that emphasized survival of the fittest. Because the life span of many children was relatively short, social investment in the welfare of children was viewed as important only from an economic standpoint.

Children: A Natural Resource

Children have always held a place in world societies as a representation of male virility and female fertility. Throughout time in many cultures, a couple's ability to produce children has been viewed as an omen that the couple had been held in good favor by God. The family unit, through procreation, was meeting its obligation to society to propagate and thus ensure the continuance of the race. In Western civilization, biblical references attest to the sense of shame and disgrace that accompanied those who were "barren." Children were valued for the work they produced and the subsequent additional wealth they were able to bring their parents through their labors. Similarly, children were viewed as "property" of their parents. Children were objects to be used at the parents' discretion to meet religious, financial, and social obligations.

Little is mentioned in early historical writings regarding the health care and general well-being of children. With the beginning of modern science, it became clear that young children had unique characteristics. They were not simply "miniature adults," capable of completing all of the physical and developmental achievement of adults (Cherry & Carty, 1986; Muuss, 1988). In the 19th century, the theory of evolution changed the prevailing thoughts concerning human development. During this time, many theories emerged to explain both the physical and psychological process of development. Distinctive stages or periods of maturation extending from infancy through adulthood were identified and used to define the parameters of pediatric health care. Concurrently, the elevated infant mortality rate and the persistent presence of many childhood illnesses served as motivating forces to implement social, political, and health care reform addressing the physical and social needs of children.

Emergence of Child Health Care

Although gaps exist in the historical literature, archaeologic findings have validated the prevalence of childhood disease and infant demise that plagued society for many centuries. Today it is not uncommon to celebrate the birthday of a great-grandmother. At her side may be her 70-year-old daughter, her 40-year-old grandson, and his three small children. This four-generational celebration of life was unheard of in the 16th, 17th, and 18th centuries. For instance, in Geneva, the average life span in the 16th century was 21.1 years, increasing to 25.67 years in the 17th century and to 33.62 years in the 18th century (Kalisch, 1995). The unhealthy conditions of crowded city slums, child abandonment practices, the poor baby bottle sterilization techniques, and the lack of rational, scientific methods for treating even the most minor of illnesses all were key factors associated with high mortality rates. Infant abandonment was a common practice for families burdened by yet another unwanted child. For example, between 1771 and 1777, nearly 32,000 infants were abandoned and admitted to the Paris Foundling Hospital, at an average rate of 89 children a day. Between 75% and 95% of these children died before reaching the age of 1. In London at this time, it was estimated that 58% of all children died before their fifth birthday, many abandoned at early ages and left in the care of foundling homes (Kalisch, 1995).

District Nursing and Visiting Nursing

Toward the middle of the 19th century, several events laid the groundwork for the emergence of pediatrics as a fledgling branch of scientific medicine and as a health care discipline (Table 1–1). At that time, reliable official lists of live births and of burials indicated that the infant mortality rate (number of deaths occurring during the first year of life per 1000 live births) varied between 250 and 500. The highest rates continued to be among artificially fed babies confined to foundling homes. Poor bottle sterilization and poor general hygiene continued to affect mortality rates of these vulnerable infants. Some metropolitan records showed that in the average community, more than half of the total number of deaths from all causes occurred among children younger than 5 years of age, and three fourths of the total deaths occurred among children younger than the age of 12. The average life span was around 35 to 38 years, with enteric disorders, malnutrition, and the common respiratory and contagious diseases constituting the major causes of death (Kalisch, 1995) (Fig. 1–1).

Poor sanitation was a major contributor to infant mortality and other childhood illnesses. In 1893, the initiation of milk stations in New York City was one of the first public acknowledgments of the relationship between spoiled food supplies and infant health. The milk stations were responsible for the distribution of safe, clean milk offered to the public at a nominal fee. In addition, many cities established ordinances controlling milk production, care, and distribution. By 1910, these and other sanitation efforts that began in New York had expanded to 30 other major cities, resulting in a decreased mortality rate.

Table 1–1
Important Events in Child Health Care

Date	Event
1858	Florence Nightingale establishes district nursing in England.
1870	Abraham Jacobi awarded first professorship in pediatrics in the United States.
1873	Linda Richards, America's first professionally trained nurse, receives diploma from New England Training School for Women and Children.
1877	Visiting nursing begins in New York City with the support of the Women's Branch of the New York Mission.
1879	Mary Eliza Mahoney becomes the first black nurse to graduate in the United States.
1883	Visiting nursing expands to Chicago.
1888	Abraham Jacobi founds the American Pediatric Society, and Harvard University opens the first university department of pediatrics.
1892	Amy Hughes establishes a school of nursing in England.
1893	The first milk station in the United States is established in New York City.
1893	Lillian Wald and Mary Brewster establish the Nurses' Settlement House in New York City on the lower East Side.
1895	Lillian Wald moves Settlement House to Henry Street, and it becomes known as the Henry Street Settlement House.
1902	School nursing is established in the United States by Lillian Wald, with Linda C. Rogers serving as the first school nurse.
1908	New York Division of Child Hygiene established by Lillian Wald and Josephine Baker.
1909	First White House Conference on Children and Youth initiated by President Theodore Roosevelt.
1910	Death of Florence Nightingale.
1912	National Organization for Public Health Nursing formed.
1912	U.S. Children's Bureau created by Congress (in 1953 becomes the Department of Health, Education and Welfare; in 1980 becomes the Department of Health and Human Services).
1915	National Birth Registry established.
1916	Margaret Sanger opens birth control clinics in America.
1919	White House Conference on Child Welfare Standards.
1921	Passage of Sheppard-Towner Act, with establishment of the Division of Maternity and Infancy of the Children's Bureau.
1925	Mary Breckinridge established the Frontier Nursing Service.
1928	May 1—first National Child Health Day.
1929	Sheppard-Towner Act ends.
1929	Establishment of the American Academy of Pediatrics.
1930	White House Conference on Child Health and Protection.
1935	The Emergency Relief Appropriation Act established the Works Progress Administration (WPA).
1935	Social Security Act signed into law by President Franklin D. Roosevelt.
1940	White House Conference on Children in a Democracy.
1943	Emergency Maternity and Infant Care Act (EMIC) made law.
1944	Nursing component of the Henry Street Settlement House becomes the Visiting Nursing Service of New York.
1950	Midcentury White House Conference on Children and Youth.
1953	U.S. Department of Health, Education and Welfare formed.
1960	White House Conference on Children and Youth.
1963	Title V of the Social Security Act amended to create Maternity and Infant Care (MIC) Program.
1965	Titles XVIII and XIX of the Social Security Act establish the Medicare and Medicaid programs.
1965	Establishment of the National Institute of Child Health and Human Development. Head Start programs begin.
1965	Association for the Care of Children's Health is founded.
1966	Child Nutrition Act passed.
1967	Early and Periodic Screening, Diagnosis and Treatment (EPSDT) program started.

Table 1-1
Important Events in Child Health Care *Continued*

Date	Event
1969	Children's Bureau dismantled and parts reformed under the Office of Child Development.
1970	White House Conference on Children.
1970	National Health Service Corps established.
1970	The Nurses' Association of the American College of Obstetricians and Gynecologists (NAACOG) is formed.
1973	National Association of Pediatric Nurses, Associates and Practitioners (NAPNAP) is formed.
1975	Title XX of the Social Security Act is passed: Education for All Handicapped Children Act.
1979	*Healthy People* report by the Surgeon General is published.
1979	United Nations declares 1979 the "Year of the Child."
1981	MCH (Maternal Child Health) Services Block Grant created.
1983	Select Committee on Children, Youth and Families formed in the U.S. House of Representatives.
1985	Crippled Children's Services (CCS) changes name to Program for Children with Special Health Needs (CSHN).
1986	Education of the Handicapped Amendments Act enacted.
1986	National Commission to Prevent Infant Mortality established by Congress.
1990	Society of Pediatric Nurses established.
1991	Publication of *Nursing Agenda for Health Care Reform.*
1993	NAACOG becomes an independent, nonprofit association known as the Association of Women's Health, Obstetric, and Neonatal Nurses (AWHONN).
1994	United Nations declares 1994 the "International Year of the Family."
1994	*Bright Futures: Guidelines for Health Supervision of Infants, Children and Adolescents* is published by the National Center for Education in Maternal and Child Health.
1995	National immunization campaign "Every child by two" started to immunize all 2-year-old children by 1996.

A decline in the instance of diseases such as hypoproteinemic edema, scurvy, rickets, rachitic tetany, vitamin A deficiency, beriberi, pellagra, ariboflavinosis, and iron deficiency anemia was witnessed by health care officials.

Amid these conditions, a growing concern regarding the health and lifestyles of children, especially the children of the poor, began to emerge. The role of the "trained nurse" as promoter and facilitator of child health

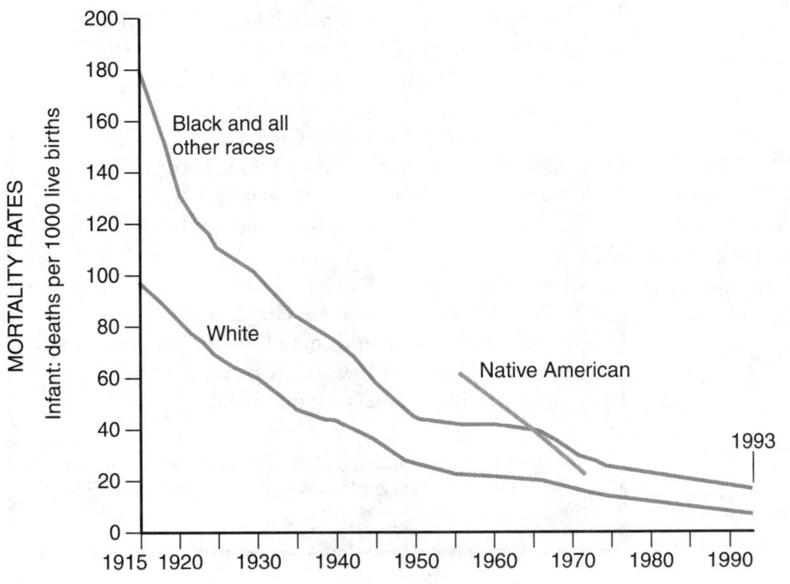

Figure 1-1
United States infant mortality rates, 1915–1993.

care became the model for child care interventions. On October 1, 1873, Linda Richards became America's first professionally trained nurse. She received her diploma from the New England Training School for Women and Children. Mary Eliza Mahoney became the first black nursing school graduate on August 1, 1879. She also attended the New England Training School for Women and Children, completing her course of study in 16 months. These individuals paved the way for many others to follow the path of professional nursing. Using principles from science, psychology, and religion, the trained nurses would become a major force in reducing the rising tide of maternal and child illnesses.

Florence Nightingale, most often thought of in relation to her work in the Crimean War, played an influential role in the development of child health care and preventive health care practices. Nightingale believed that the home environment was more influential than the school for the child; thus, hygienic training at home was necessary to impress upon children the importance of healthful living. In 1858, Nightingale established district nursing in England. The nurses, assigned to specific areas or districts of the city, went to families' homes to teach them about basic health care issues and simple rules for baby care. Nightingale believed that good child care required training and that every mother was really a nurse. Concerning this, Nightingale wrote:

> I look on district nursing . . . as one of the most helpful agencies for raising the poor physically as well as morally, its province being not only nursing the patient but nursing the room, showing the family . . . how to second nurse, and . . . how to nurse health as well as disease (Smith, 1981, p. 1024).

Visiting Nurses in the United States

Following the ideas of Florence Nightingale, visiting nursing began in the United States in 1877 when the Women's Branch of the New York Mission sent its first trained nurses into the homes of the indigent. A little later, the New York Ethical Society placed nurses in several city dispensaries and afterward, in 1883, sent a nurse to Chicago to begin similar work there. Three years later, the Boston Instructive District Nursing Association was organized to promote health education. By 1890, the work of district nursing, or visiting nursing, began to flourish. There were 21 organizations in the United States engaged in the work of visiting nursing, although most employed no more than one nurse each (Kalisch, 1995). The nurses' task was to teach health and hygiene in the home, to ensure the livelihood of the young, and to promote positive parenting practices.

Concurrent with the emergence of visiting nursing, physicians were also taking steps to recognize the special needs of children and their families. In 1870, Abraham Jacobi (1830–1919), who was later to be referred to as the father of pediatrics, was awarded the first professorship in pediatrics in America. With several other physicians he pioneered in the scientific and clinical investigation of childhood diseases. In 1888, he founded the American Pediatric Society, and the first independent university department of pediatrics was organized at Harvard University to teach the specialty of pediatrics (Kalisch, 1995). Thirteen children's hospitals existed in the United States to provide care for the sick child (Chart 1–1), and, in the years to come, nurses and physicians worked together to implement new knowledge and technologies that have enhanced child health care practices (Chart 1–2).

Lillian Wald and Mary Brewster, graduates in 1891 of the New York Hospital for Nursing, were but a mere 2 years out of nursing school when they chose to direct their services to the poor and to the children. In 1893, these two energetic women set up a nurses' settlement house to serve as a focal point for a Visiting Nursing Service. Their primary objectives were to provide nursing care to the sick and to provide health instruction to prevent illness. Their services were rendered regardless of the patient's or family's ability to pay. They treated minor surgical cases, evaluated ailing schoolchildren, and managed caseloads of patients with an assortment of ailments. In modest suits with white blouses and black ties,

Chart 1–1

Early Children's Hospitals in the United States

Hospital	Year Founded
Children's Hospital of Philadelphia	1855
Nursery and Child's Hospital (New York City)	1857
Children's Hospital Medical Center (Boston)	1869
Children's National Medical Center (Washington, DC)	1870
Babies Hospital (New York City)	1870
Children's Hospital of Albany (New York)	1875
Children's Hospital of San Francisco	1875
St. Christopher's Hospital for Children (Philadelphia)	1875
Children's Hospital of Detroit	1877
St. Louis Children's Hospital	1879
Boston Infants' Hospital (Limited to Sick Babies)	1881
Children's Memorial Hospital (Chicago)	1882
Children's Hospital (Cincinnati)	1883

From Barbara Brodie, PhD, RN, FAAN, Professor and Director, Center for Nursing Historical Inquiry, University of Virginia, School of Nursing. Reprinted with permission.

Chart 1–2

Events That Have Affected Child Health Care Practices

1880s	Introduction of silver nitrate solution to cleanse eyes of newborns and prevent ophthalmia neonatorum Thermometer comes into general use by city physicians Use of uterine sutures for cesarean section becomes common practice
1890s	Discovery of X-rays Ten most important drugs were ether, morphine, digitalis, diphtheria antitoxin, smallpox vaccine, iron, quinine, iodine, alcohol, and mercury Introduction of the use of rubber gloves in surgery Thermometer comes into general use by country physicians Bronchoscope was developed
1910s	Margaret Sanger opened first birth control clinic
1920s	Hospitals start adding pediatric facilities Discovery of insulin Advent of sulfonamides
1930s	Premature babies kept alive using "isolettes"
1940s	Introduction of penicillin and corticosteroids Immunization for diphtheria, tetanus, and pertussis Anticonvulsants and antihistamines introduced Research by Spitz and Robertson about detrimental effects of maternal deprivation on institutionalized children
1950s	First testing for phenylketonuria (PKU) First tetralogy of Fallot repair Polio vaccine developed
1960s	Mandatory reporting of child abuse instituted
1970s	Rapid expansion of chemotherapy, electronic fetal monitoring, renal dialysis, open heart surgery, and organ transplants Development of intensive care units
1980s	Introduction of *Haemophilus influenzae* vaccine
1990s	Introduction of hepatitis B and chickenpox vaccines

they made calls where needed and brought health care to the home of anyone who needed their assistance. The visiting nurses focused on attacking the problems of maternal and infant mortality. In the home, mothers were taught nutrition basics, given instruction regarding clothing and supplies for the newborn, and provided with postpartum instruction in well-child care (Kalisch, 1995).

Soon, the visiting nurses were receiving referrals from both families and physicians. Within 2 years, they moved the Nurses' Settlement to larger accommodations at 265 Henry Street, with financial aid provided by banker and philanthropist Jacob H. Schiff and others. The establishment became known as the Henry Street Settlement House. Clearly, a new form of public health nursing, settlement nursing, had arisen to meet the needs of the crowded city districts. Before too long, nine graduate nurses were living in the house, and they were going out each day to make calls on needy families. Lavinia Dock was in the first group of nurses who lived and worked at Henry Street. She would be shaped and molded by her experiences at Henry Street and would later move on to become one of the most prominent leaders in nursing history. By 1909, the Henry Street Settlement House was the headquarters for five administrative nurses and 32 staff nurses providing direct patient care (Fig. 1–2). In 1944, the nursing component of the Henry Street Settlement would become the Visiting Nursing Services of New York.

School Nursing

The nurses at Henry Street kept anecdotal notes about children they encountered who were kept from school because of their illnesses. Time and time again it was

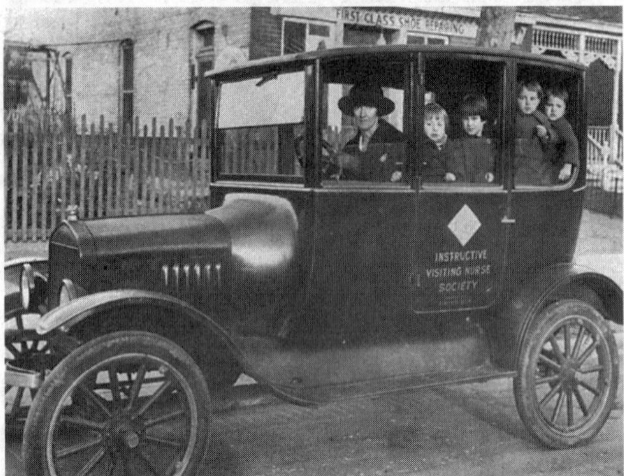

Figure 1–2
A visiting nurse of the 1920s. (Courtesy of the Visiting Nurse Association of Washington, DC.)

evident that children were needlessly kept from school because they had not received adequate health care or because an uninformed and overly cautious teacher refused to allow the child who had been ill (but was no longer contagious) back into the classroom. Attempts to place physicians in the schools had failed. Still, Lillian Wald was convinced that the value of bringing health care and health teaching to the children in their homes was a concept that ideally fit the needs of children in other environments, namely the school. School nursing had already been established in England in 1892 under Amy Hughes. In 1902, Wald approached Dr. Lederle, Commissioner of Health in New York City, about launching school nursing (Wald, 1971). In New York, an average of 15 to 20 children were sent home daily from each school because of health-related issues. The problem climaxed when 300 children were excluded from one school in a single day. Wald believed that nurses could help the children stay healthier, could decrease the number of children excluded from school each day, and could provide effective follow-up care for the children during their periods of exclusion (Kalisch, 1995).

To begin the school nurse program, Wald offered the services of Henry Street nurse Linda L. Rogers for 1 month as a demonstration of what could be done. The experiment was a success. In September 1902, 10,567 children had been sent home from the New York schools for health-related reasons. One year later, with a school nurse in attendance, only 1101 children were sent home. Previously, many children had been sent home for such minor cases as pediculosis, ringworm, scabies, and other problems that were easily treated. The nurse's direct presence and interventions at the school allowed the children to remain in their classes and to benefit from their classroom teachings. The New York Board of Health realized the value of the nursing service and soon appointed dozens of nurses to serve in schools (Fig. 1–3).

Political and Social Agenda

Lillian Wald had clearly begun her lifelong crusade to promote the health and welfare of the young. In 1908, in collaboration with Dr. Josephine Baker, she was instrumental in establishing the New York Division of Child Hygiene. This organization attempted to consolidate public efforts to reduce infant mortality. One of its supported programs included visitations by nurses to new mothers to teach principles of infant feeding and baby care. After the first summer of its operation, the division reported that 1200 fewer infants had died than in the previous summer (Arnold, Brecht, Hockett, Amspacher, & Grad, 1989).

By 1909, the federal government had begun to pay attention to the rising level of concerns regarding children's health and welfare. President Theodore Roosevelt

Figure 1–3
School nurse, New York City, 1905. (From Kalisch, P. A. [1995]. *The advance of American nursing* [3rd ed., p. 179]. Philadelphia: J. B. Lippincott. Reprinted with permission.)

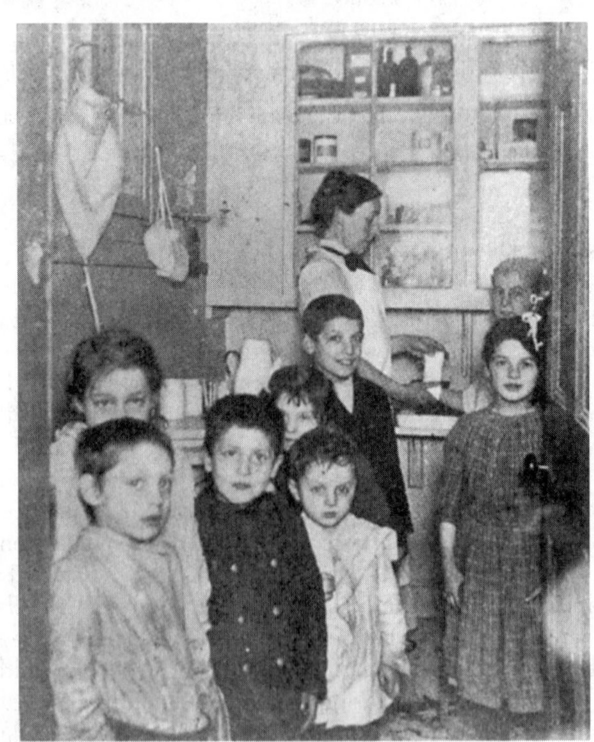

acted to initiate the first White House Conference on Children and Youth. The conference focused on care of dependent children and attempted to address the deplorable working condition of youngsters and the organization of prenatal care services. Similar White House conferences were subsequently held approximately every 10 years, until 1980, to address the welfare, health, education, social, economic, and psychological needs of children.

The Children's Bureau

The 20th century has seen much important legislation and social action regarding the welfare of children. These actions are reflective of a growing, continuing desire by the citizens to meet the needs of children adversely affected by physical, developmental, and social challenges. When, in 1912, Congress created the Children's Bureau as part of the Department of Commerce and Labor, this was only the beginning of an era in which federal programs would play a predominant role in providing for the health of the country's young citizens. The purpose of the bureau was to "investigate and report on all matters pertaining to the welfare of children and child life among all classes of people . . . and shall especially investigate the questions of infant mortality" (U.S. Children's Bureau, 1962, p. 5). Over time, the bureau would be reorganized into the Department of Health, Education and Welfare and eventually the Department of Health and Human Services. Although opponents claimed that formation of the children's bureau represented federal involvement in private issues (the health and well-being of children), the advocates argued that federal coordination of child health initiatives was essential. This argument has forged the path for many other federal programs benefiting children.

Few remember that creating federal programs to support the needs of children was a dream of Lillian Wald's. Several years before the establishment of the Children's Bureau, she had helped found the National Child Labor Committee, a group committed to fighting the ruthless exploitation of child labor. To ensure that all aspects of child health and welfare were promoted, Lillian had repeatedly suggested to the government the need for an agency to orchestrate and implement causes on behalf of the children. In 1905 she was summoned to Washington by President Roosevelt to explain her plan. Four years later, the legislation to establish the Children's Bureau passed, and Julia C. Lathrop, M.D., a resident of the Hull House Settlement in Chicago, was chosen by President Taft to head the new bureau (Pascoe, 1996). Nursing care was an integral part of the services provided under the bureau's functions.

The bureau was responsible for investigating special problems of child health. These investigations fell into three main groups:

- Maternal and infant welfare (including the health and education of the preschool child)
- The care of special groups of children handicapped by physical or mental problems or through delinquency, dependency, or neglect
- Problems related to the child in industry (Kalisch, 1995, p. 281).

Besides conducting research, the bureau compiled, analyzed, and tabulated laws relating to child labor, juvenile courts, illegitimacy, sex offenses against children, mothers' pensions, and interstate placement and adoption of children and actively cooperated with child welfare and children's code commissions in the revision of state laws (Arnold et al., 1989).

The Sheppard-Towner Act

The development of the Children's Bureau heralded the beginning of an era in which many federal programs would be put into place to support women's and children's health and social welfare issues. One of the first major bills passed was the Sheppard-Towner Act in 1921, aimed at providing for the public protection of maternal-child programs. Although the Act was not renewed, its powerful impact on enhancing maternal-child care was significant. The infant death rate declined from 100 per 1000 births in 1915 to 69 per 1000 births in 1928. The greatest decrease was in the death rate from gastrointestinal disease. This was viewed as a direct result of informing the public about proper methods of infant care and feeding. The efforts to renew the Act were well supported by public health nurses, who saw firsthand the positive impact of this legislation on the welfare of their clients. The Act was, however, strongly opposed by the American Medical Association. It was seen as being unsound in policy, wasteful, extravagant, and unproductive of results. In Congress the bill was viewed as "socialistic" and was opposed (Arnold et al., 1989).

The Frontier Nursing Service

During the same period, the Frontier Nursing Service was organized by Mary Breckinridge. This was a nurse midwifery service located in the rural areas of southeastern Kentucky. Although there were no quality nurse midwifery programs in the United States until the early 1930s, the program forged ahead, utilizing midwives who received their training in England or Scotland. The nurse midwives gave antepartal, intrapartal, and postpartal care to women in their districts. They visited their patients at least twice a month until the seventh month of pregnancy and then every week until the time of delivery. Normal deliveries were handled by the nurse midwives; for complicated cases, the physician was called. The Frontier Nursing Service also offered care for infants and children. Babies younger than 1 year of age were examined twice a month, preschool children from 1 to 6 were seen every month, and schoolchildren were examined once every 3 months. During these visits, mothers were taught about diet, cleanliness, health habits, general sanitation, and preventive care. Inoculations against typhoid and diphtheria and vaccinations for smallpox were also given (Kalisch, 1995).

Seven years after its inception, the service was evaluated by Dr. Louis I. Dublin of the Metropolitan Life Insurance Company. Evaluating the first 1000 cases of the Frontier Nursing Service, he found that there were one-third fewer stillborns and one-third fewer deaths among babies in the first year of life than among the general population of Kentucky.

The Social Security Act

The depression years brought drastic cuts in federal services for women and children. By 1934, nine states no longer funded maternal-child health programs and 23 had substantially reduced appropriations (Arnold et al., 1989). However, in 1935 the tide changed again. In this year, President Franklin D. Roosevelt signed the Social Security Act, which established the provision of financial aid to poor families available through the Aid to Families with Dependent Children (AFDC). Title V of the act included the establishment of federal grants-in-all to states that would be matched by state funds to implement three types of programs:

- Maternal and Child Health (MCH)
- Crippled Children's Services (CCS)
- Child Welfare Services

These programs authorized federal grants to states for the provision of prenatal care, well-baby clinics, school health services, immunizations, public health nursing services, and health education (Arnold et al., 1989). Legislation was passed in 1985 to change the name of CCS to the Program for Children with Special Health Needs (CSHN) in order to reflect the broad spectrum of programs involving children who have developmental, behavioral, and educational problems, as well as the home care of medically complex children.

In the ensuing years, several additions would be made to the Social Security Act. In 1963 Title V was amended to create the Emergency Maternity and Infant Care (EMIC) Program to provide comprehensive maternity and infant care for low-income, high-risk patients. By 1966, the Civilian Health Medical Program was established, incorporating the EMIC Program under its jurisdiction.

In 1965, Titles XVIII and XIX of the Social Security program established the Medicare and Medicaid programs. Together, EMIC and Medicaid provided a system that combined clinical maternity care services with a mechanism to finance care. (Chapter 7 provides a detailed discussion of all federal programs supporting child health and welfare issues.) The Omnibus Budget Reconciliation Act of 1981 provided for the continuation of Title V of the Social Security Act as a state-federal partnership and created the MCH Services Block Grant. These block grants consolidated seven existing categorical programs (Maternal and Child Health/Crippled Children's Services, Title V; Social Security Income [SSI]; Hemophilia; Sudden Infant Death Syndrome; Lead-Based Paint Poisoning Prevention; Genetic Diseases; and Adolescent Health Services) into one block, allowing each state to develop its own programs and to establish its own priorities on the basis of state needs.

President John F. Kennedy's interest in mentally retarded citizens would pave the way for further changes in the Social Security Act regarding those mentally or physically challenged. In 1961, the President's Panel on Mental Retardation was appointed with the objective of preparing a national plan to combat mental retardation. The panel found that the prevalence of mental retardation was most closely associated with inadequate prenatal care and premature birth (Arnold et al., 1989). In 1975, Title XX of the Social Security Act, the Education for All Handicapped Children Act, was passed. The legislation provided free appropriate public education to all handicapped children 3 to 21 years of age and provided for the supportive services (speech, counseling, etc.) that ensure the benefits of special education. In 1986, the Education of the Handicapped Amendments Act was enacted to broaden the scope of the earlier law by expanding services for infants and toddlers and their families. A significant aspect of the new law called for development of an Individualized Family Service Plan (IFSP), which required that each infant or toddler and family served receive an interdisciplinary assessment of their particular strengths and needs in order to receive appropriate services (Collin, 1995).

Three other programs authorized in the 1960s were established to provide aid to children: the Early and Periodic Screening, Diagnosis and Treatment program (EPSDT); the Supplemental Food Program for Women, Infants and Children (WIC); and the Comprehensive Neighborhood Health Center and Migrant Health programs (Burns & Thorman, 1993). The Early and Periodic Screening, Diagnosis and Treatment program provided children who were Medicaid recipients with periodic physical and developmental examinations and treatment of certain illnesses. Amendments to this program were contained in the 1989 Omnibus Budget Reconciliation Act (OBRA) to require states to increase access to EPSDT and to expand treatment services to the chronically ill, developmentally disabled, and emotionally disturbed (Smith, 1994). The WIC program provided nutritious food and nutrition education to low-income, pregnant, postpartum, and lactating women and to infants and children up to age 5 years. The Comprehensive Neighborhood Health Center (now known as Community Health Center) and Migrant Health programs were established to provide access to primary health care, prenatal care, and infant care services to low-income and migrant families. (See Chapter 7 for a more in-depth discussion of these programs.)

Healthy People 2000

The national effort to reduce infant mortality, preventable deaths, diseases, and disabilities that began in the 1960s remains a pressing focus of concern of both public and private citizen groups. In 1979, the Surgeon General published a report entitled *Healthy People*, which presented the goals for the health of the American people. Among these goals was the objective that infant health would be improved by 1990, with infant mortality reduced by at least 35% to fewer than 9 deaths per 1000 live births. For school-age children and adolescents, the proposed goals for 1990 included 20% fewer deaths and further investment in programs that would prevent accidents and injuries in this age group. These programs were aimed at accident and injury prevention, prevention of fatal motor vehicle accidents, and alcohol and drug prevention (Igoe, 1990a, 1990b). In 1990, the initiatives of the *Healthy People* publication in 1979 and the *Objectives for the Nation* publication in 1980 were revisited, with new targets established for the year 2000. Two of the objectives for the year 2000 are to reduce the overall infant mortality rate to no more than 7 per 1000 and to reduce the rate among black infants to no more than 11 per 1000.

Social action regarding the welfare of children in the late 19th century and beyond has been highly influenced by economics. Economic barriers to children's health care access have included lack of child service coverage by insurance, the increase in dysfunctional family units, and the rising number of health problems related to indigence faced by many states. It is clear that while costs of health care have continued to rise, the public's ability to deal with the financial burden of preventing illness and promoting and maintaining the health of individual family members has diminished. Health care reform in this century has already raised the social conscience of many citizens to the issues of infant mortality, health care access, quality of life, and health disparities among our citizens. In this time of change, nurses will continue to have an influential voice, as they have in the past. Lillian Wald, Mary Breckinridge, and others may have felt that the tasks before them were overwhelming, yet they forged ahead to bring about changes in national health services offered to infants and children. So, too, can the nurse today work with other health care providers to promote the health and well-being of this vulnerable population of our citizenry.

Influence of Professional Organizations

While legislation empowered state and local governments to provide and support children's health care issues, the formation of several professional organizations also played a major role in this arena (Table 1–2). One of the first organizations founded was the National Organization for Public Health Nursing. The history of pediatric nursing began with the public health nursing movement. A primary focus of the public health nurse was on enhancing the welfare of children in their own homes. The National Organization for Public Health Nursing was an organization of nurses and laypeople engaged in the actual work of public health nursing and in the organization, management, and support of such work. Lillian Wald was the first president. Over the years, this organization and its members would have a pivotal role in demanding more health care services for the young and in ensuring that all children are provided equal access in the community to the health services they need. For instance, in 1920, statistics compiled by the organization showed that 70,000 American babies died in that year because their mothers did not have proper prenatal or postnatal care. Of those deaths, 5000 occurred in New York City.

The first professional organization solely devoted to the care of children was the Association for the Care of Children's Health (ACCH). The organization is devoted to improving ways in which the health care community responds to the unique emotional and developmental needs of children. ACCH members work in hospitals, colleges, schools, clinics, state and provincial agencies, and home care agencies. Membership is interdisciplinary, including those from nursing, social work, and child life services, teachers, and lay personnel. This is the only health care organization in which parents are active members and play a vital role in its mission.

In the 1970s and 1980s, several other organizations were formed to represent specialty interests within the scope of children's health care (Hahn, 1996a, 1996b). These organizations have played a vital role in promoting legislation, developing practice guidelines, and heightening public interest in maternal and child health care issues (see Table 1–2).

Table 1–2
Nursing Organizations with a Focus on Children's Health

Name	Year Established	Purposes and Goals	Journals and Newsletters
Association for the Care of Children's Health (ACCH)	1965	The mission of the ACCH is to ensure that all aspects of children's health are family-centered, psychologically sound, and developmentally appropriate. ACCH believes that health care systems and practices are most effective when they are planned, coordinated, delivered, and evaluated through meaningful collaboration among families and professionals across all disciplines.	*Journal of Children's Health Care* (quarterly) *ACCH News* (bi-monthly newsletter)
Association of Child and Adolescent Psychiatric Nurses (ACAPN)	1971	The purposes of ACAPN are · Promote mental health of infants, children, adolescents, and their families through clinical practice, public policy, and research · Promote excellence in the education of child and adolescent psychiatric nurse practitioners · Promote communication among child and adolescent psychiatric nurses · Foster public awareness and professional recognition of specialty practice in child and adolescent psychiatric nursing The goals of the organization are · Promote public policy, legislation, and funding mechanisms in support of mental health services for infants, children, adolescents, and their families · Ensure access to mental health services for children with serious mental illnesses and their families · Promote the delivery of mental health services that are culturally sensitive and provided in the least restrictive setting · Promote advanced practice in child and adolescent psychiatric nursing · Promote improvements in the clinical care of children and adolescents with mental illness through research and education	*Journal of Child and Adolescent Psychiatric Nursing* (quarterly) *ACAPN News* (quarterly)
Association of Pediatric Oncology Nurses (APON)	1973	APON strives to improve the care given to children who have cancer and their families by · Promoting excellence in the specialty of pediatric oncology nursing · Providing quality publications focusing on pediatric oncology nursing · Promoting communication and collegial exchange among nurses caring for pediatric oncology patients and their families · Encouraging members to contribute to professional and lay literature with regard to nursing care of pediatric oncology patients and their families · Providing national and regional educational programs · Promoting implementation of the scope and standards of pediatric oncology nursing practice developed by APON · Providing liaison with other organizations whose membership may influence the care given to pediatric oncology patients and their families	*Journal of Pediatric Oncology Nursing* (quarterly) *APON Counts* (quarterly newsletter)

Table 1–2
Nursing Organizations with a Focus on Children's Health *Continued*

Name	Year Established	Purposes and Goals	Journals and Newsletters
		· Promoting a positive image of pediatric oncology nursing and its effect on the care of pediatric oncology patients and their families · Supporting local, state, and national legislation affecting the care of pediatric oncology patients and their families and legislation pertaining to the profession of nursing	
Association of Women's Health, Obstetric, and Neonatal Nurses (AWHONN)	1969	AWHONN focuses on four aspects of nursing: education, research, practice, and advocacy. The mission is to promote excellence in nursing practice to improve the health of women and newborns	*Journal of Gynecology and Newborn Nursing* (bimonthly) *AWHONN Voice* (monthly newsletter)
National Association of Neonatal Nurses (NANN)	1984	The mission of this association is to support and promote neonatal nursing. To this end, the association is to 1. Provide a specialty organization that acts as a unified voice to further the work of neonatal nurses in the provision of newborn and family care 2. Facilitate cooperation among nurses in a variety of roles 3. Promote education for neonatal nursing 4. Foster advanced nursing practice 5. Enhance the effectiveness of nursing in the promotion of human well-being 6. Promote ethical and professional conduct 7. Serve as an advocate for the newborn and family 8. Increase public awareness and understanding of the specialty	*Neonatal Network: The Journal of Neonatal Nursing* (bimonthly) *Central Lines* (quarterly newsletter)
National Association of Pediatric Nurse Associates and Practitioners (NAPNAP)	1973	A nonprofit specialty organization devoted to improving the quality of infant and child care. Organizational activities include · Monitor health legislation affecting maternal-child care · Serve in an advisory capacity to state boards of nursing · Produce and distribute materials to educate consumers on child care · Provide opportunities and funding for continuing education for PNPs · Submit testimony on issues affecting child health care and nurse practitioners	*The Journal of Pediatric Nursing* (bimonthly) *The Pediatric Nurse Practitioner* (bimonthly newsletter)
National Association of School Nurses (NASN)	1969	The mission of NASN is to advance the practice of school nursing and provide leadership in the delivery of quality health programs to the school community. Membership is open to registered professional nurses who meet their state's criteria for certification as a school nurse if mandated certification exists; have as their primary assignment school health service, provision, administration, or education; and are eligible for active membership in their state school nurse association if one exists.	*Journal of School Nursing* (five times per year) *NASNewsletter* (five times per year)

Table continued on following page

Table 1–2
Nursing Organizations with a Focus on Children's Health *Continued*

Name	Year Established	Purposes and Goals	Journals and Newsletters
National Organization for Public Health Nursing	1912	Advance public health nursing and standardize public health nursing courses.	*Public Health Nursing*
Society of Pediatric Nurses (SPN)	1990	To improve the nursing care of children and their families and to further the development of pediatric nursing as a subspecialty within the profession of nursing. The mission is to promote the optimal health of children and excellence in nursing care of children and their families. To promote quality health and nursing care of children and their families by · Establishment of position statements and standards of practice · Advancement of the art and science of pediatric nursing through interactive efforts among nurses in clinical practice, research, education, and administration · Advocacy for accessible and affordable comprehensive health care services · Collaboration with other health care professionals, child health advocates, and related organizations	*SPN News* (quarterly newsletter)

The most recent group to form a coalition to improve the care of children and their families, and to further support pediatric nursing as a subspecialty within the profession of nursing, is the Society of Pediatric Nurses (SPN). In 1990, the SPN was established and organized in response to requests and efforts of nurses throughout the country. The purpose of the society is to improve the nursing care of children and their families and to further the development of pediatric nursing as a subspecialty within the profession of nursing. SPN was founded for all nurses who are involved in the care of children and their families, including staff nurses, school and outpatient nurses, clinical nurse specialists, practitioners, administrators, educators, and researchers (Miles, 1996).

Child Health Care in Nursing Education

In the late 1800s and early 1900s, the educational curriculum for the pediatric nurse consisted of "on-the-job" training. Courses in growth and development, discussions about the differences between adults and children, and discussions of the unique psychosocial needs of this vulnerable population were not a part of the nurse's core education. Although Linda Richards, America's first trained nurse, was educated at the New England Hospital for Women and Children, she learned about children and families from the on-site training she received. At that time, there was a certain expectation that women, as nurses, had a natural sense about how to care for the needs of sick children. Antibiotics and immunizations did not exist. The care of children primarily involved infection control, teaching proper hygiene and sanitation, and ensuring that children were provided adequate nutrition and rest.

The first nursing text published in 1893 was *Nursing: Its Principles and Practices*, by Isabel Adams Hampton. This 484-page text had dedicated 28 pages to the nursing care of children. The chapter discussed newborn health and hygiene and specific conditions peculiar to children: thrush, diarrhea, cholera infantum, convulsions, infantile paralysis, chorea, rickets, croup, eczema, and infectious diseases. In 1907, Dr. Robert McCombs wrote a book for nurses about the diseases of children. The diseases of the gastrointestinal tract and respiratory system, as well as disorders of nutrition (rickets and scurvy) and infectious processes, were covered.

During the 1940s and 1950s, the number of nurses serving in advanced practice roles began to grow. The first graduate program in nursing was begun in 1954 by Hildegarde Peplau, educating nurses for the psychiatric clinical nurse specialist's role. The primary focus of nurses in these roles was to serve in acute care settings using advanced assessment, case management, and patient education skills to serve a specific client population. Nurses in this role served as clinical experts at the bedside, providing services directly to the patient as well as acting as a role model for their nurse colleagues (Clancy & Maguire, 1995; Gaedeke & Blount, 1995; Sparacino, Cooper, & Minarik, 1990). By 1964, clinical nurse specialists were the first advanced practice nurses to be consistently prepared at the master's level (American Nurses' Association [ANA], 1994a).

In 1965 at the University of Colorado, nurse Loretta Ford and physician Henry Silver saw the need for the extension of child care services offered by the practicing nurse. This was influenced by the shortage of physicians, especially in rural areas. They began to educate registered nurses to become pediatric nurse practitioners by teaching them to do physical examinations, make diagnoses, and treat patients and assist in family counseling (Brush & Capezuti, 1996). In the 1970s, the neonatal nurse practitioner role evolved (Farah, Breda, & Shiao, 1996). The increasing technology and complexity of neonatal care served as a catalyst to promote the emergence of this autonomous nursing role. Today there are many opportunities for nurses wishing to specialize in child health care to pursue their interests within the structure of a graduate nursing program. The clinical nurse specialist and the nurse practitioner have emerged as highly valued advanced practice roles in both inpatient and outpatient settings.

As the care of children has become more complex, the need to provide a more comprehensive knowledge base in pediatric nursing to nursing students has become more evident. Teaching simple principles of nutrition and hygiene no longer meets the curricular needs of students who are expected to care for the vast range of chronic and acute illnesses they will see in the pediatric population. Yet in educational programs, a real problem exists. As the knowledge base in pediatrics has grown, so has it grown in other specialty areas. Thus, child health care issues must compete with such specialties as psychiatric nursing, medical-surgical nursing, women's health, and geriatric nursing for seminar and clinical hours in the educational program. Given these challenges, the *Standards and Guidelines for Pre-licensure and Professional Education for the Care of Children and Their Families* was published in 1995 with the intent of providing a new vision of education to prepare adequately pre-licensure and new graduates for the complex care of children and their families now and in the future (Pridham, 1995; Selekman, 1995). The standards contain 11 concepts in three domains of knowledge and skills that should be included in every educational program preparing nurses (Chart 1–3). The document does not

Chart 1–3

Standards and Guidelines for Pre-licensure and Early Professional Education for the Nursing Care of Children and Their Families

I. Child, Family, and Societal Factors

1. CONCEPT: Anatomic structures and physiologic, psychologic, and spiritual processes in neonates, infants, children, and adolescents
   Goal: The nurse will integrate knowledge of unique anatomic structures and physiologic, psychologic, and spiritual processes of children from birth through adolescence in the assessments she makes, the care she plans and implements, and her evaluation of care.
2. CONCEPT: Health behavior
   Goal: The nurse will use opportunities to influence positively the health behavior of children and their families.
3. CONCEPT: Separation, loss, and bereavement
   Goal: The nurse will provide supportive care for children and families experiencing separation, loss, and/or death.
4. CONCEPT: Economic, social, and political influences
   Goal: The nurse will use knowledge of how the economic, social, and political environment influences the child's health and the family's care to (a) make assessments, plan strategies, and implement approaches to care of the child that are in accord with the family's economic and social situation and available resources; and (b) work with others in the community to make and implement plans for the health care needs of children.

Chart continued on following page

Chart 1–3

Standards and Guidelines for Pre-licensure and Early Professional Education for the Nursing Care of Children and Their Families *Continued*

II. Clinical Problems or Areas

1. CONCEPT: Safety and injury prevention
   Goal: The nurse will provide and promote safety in order to prevent injury and support the development of the child.

2. CONCEPT: Children with a chronic condition, disability, or special health need and their families
   Goal: The nurse will make assessments, plan strategies of care, and intervene in ways that promote the growth and development of the child with a chronic condition or disability. The nurse will also support the child's and family's management of care, and promote a healthy family life style. Evaluation of nursing care is part of this process.

3. CONCEPT: Children with acute illness or injuries and their families
   Goal: When providing care to children with acute illness or injuries and their families, the nurse will make assessments, plan strategies of care, and intervene in ways that promote the safety, growth, and development of the child and support the child's and family's management of care. Evaluation of care is a part of this process.

III. Care Delivery

1. CONCEPT: Family-centered care
   Goal:
   1. The nurse will use the family-centered approach to:
      A. Assess needs, plan, and implement interventions and evaluate outcomes in partnership with children and their families;
      B. Work with other professionals to support the development of and change in services (health care, educational, and social) relevant to the health of children and their families; and
      C. Advocate for the family and work with other health-care providers and the family to promote coordinated service delivery.
   2. The nurse will participate in developing and working within service delivery systems to support practice that is consistent with principles of a family-centered approach.

2. CONCEPT: Cultural competence
   Goal: The nurse will acknowledge and integrate into health care the beliefs, values, practices and strengths of cultural groups defined by geography, race, ethnicity, religion, or socioeconomic status.

3. CONCEPT: Communication
   Goal: The nurse will communicate effectively with child and family and others who participate in the care and education of the child and the family.

4. CONCEPT: Values and moral and ethical reasoning
   Goal: The nurse will respond to an ethical, moral, or legal dilemma concerning the child's health in ways that promote the development of families and children, assist them in making decisions, and support them in implementing the decisions.

From Pridham, K. (1995). *Standards and guidelines for pre-licensure and early professional education for the nursing care of children and their families.* Washington, DC: Maternal and Child Health Bureau, Health Resources and Services Administration, Public Health Service, U.S. Department of Health and Human Services and the Society of Pediatric Nurses.

produce the curriculum that should be provided within one specific course or set of courses about child health care. Rather, the standards state the goals, process criteria, and outcome criteria for the 11 concepts that can be integrated into all content areas and clinical settings where the needs of children and their families should be discussed. As we move toward the 21st century, this document will serve as a guiding force to direct nursing education for the care of children in our complex society.

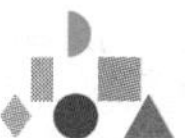

Who We Serve: The Child and the Family

The historical account of pediatrics provides key information to help understand the roles and functions of the child health care provider today. Further understanding of the nurse's role is obtained by clarifying "who" the nurse serves and the philosophy of care that drives child health care practices. Physicians have defined pediatrics as being "concerned with the health of infants, children, and youths, their growth and development, and their opportunity to achieve full potential as adults" (Behrman, et al., 1996, p. 1).

The children seen by pediatric health practitioners range from neonates (younger than 1 month old, including those gestationally premature) to adolescents in their late teens. All health care professionals are now recognizing that care of the child must extend to care of the family and its needs in relation to optimizing the growth and development of the child. The child is an integral entity within the family. The child cannot be viewed as separate and apart from the group of individuals who play such an influential role in molding the child's behavior, emotions, and understanding of the world. Thus, the focus of pediatric nursing is on the child *and* the family. The philosophy of care that has been adopted in pediatric nursing is aptly called "family-centered care" (Chart 1–4).

Chart 1–4

Definitions of Family-Centered Care

- A philosophy, a way of approaching a family rather than a set of procedures (Atkinson, 1976).
- A philosophy of care based on the belief that all families are deeply caring and want to nurture their child (Edelman, 1991).
- Viewing the family not as a collection of individuals but as a discrete entity, as the fundamental unit of medical care delivery (Schwenck & Hughes, 1983).
- Recognizing the individual resources and needs of three partners—the child, the family, and the service providers—in an interactive system (Hanft, 1988).
- The identification of problems and needs of a family and the provision of appropriate service for every family member (Yauger, 1972).
- Designing services in response to needs of the total family including the child with special needs (Friesen, Griesbach, Jacobs, Katz-Leavy, & Olson, 1988).
- A framework for the delivery of nursing care that aims to maximize the effectiveness of the family as the pediatric patient's fundamental source of support. The family includes the child's primary caregivers and significant others designated by the primary caregiver(s) (The Hospital for Sick Children, Toronto, 1989).

Definition of the Family

The traditional configuration of the "nuclear family" has been described as a household in which a man, woman, and children resided, performing four primary functions (Murdock, 1949):

- Socialization
- Protection/safety
- Economic cooperation
- Reproduction/sexual relations

In the American version of this nuclear family, the father worked outside the home (the "breadwinner"), and the mother worked primarily as a homemaker, responsible for maintaining the home and caring for the children. Today, fewer than one third of American families have this traditional structure (Gold, Perrin, Futterman, & Friedman, 1994). More families than ever have mothers who are in the work force. One of every three households in the world has a woman as its sole breadwinner ("The Changing Family Structure," 1993).

The traditional description of a nuclear family is no longer representative of the family units in our society. Single-parent families, couples with no children, blended or step families, adoptive families, and extended family units with a variety of kinship relationships abound, each functioning as a "nuclear family." It is no longer possible to define the family in strict terms of the composition of its members or within the context of its previously defined functions. Therefore, broader definitions have emerged that conceptualize the family without the boundaries previously respected by the law and by societal sanctions (Kavanagh, 1994). In the most general sense, a family today is defined as "two or more people joined together by bonds of sharing and intimacy" (Family Service America, 1984, p. 7). Within this constellation of members, the functions of the family are to provide "for the physical and health needs of its members, serve as a locus of love, intimacy, and motivation, and provide sociologic, cultural and psychologic roots" (Bozett, 1987, p. 4). (See Chapter 3 for a more in-depth discussion of family constellation, structure, and functions.)

caREminder *Although many definitions of family do not fit those stipulated by the law or many religious institutions, when the health and well-being of a loved one is at risk, legal and religious boundaries cannot serve as the sole inclusion criteria for family-centered health care interventions. At the same time, the health care provider's actions cannot overlook the familial connections that are legally sanctioned and need to be recognized when the health care issues related to a child are in question.*

Bozett (1987) suggested that the most workable definition of the family is this: the family is who the patient says it is. This definition frees the nurse from value judgments about the importance of certain familial ties within a given family and allows practices and policies to be instituted that are in the best interest of the child.

Family-Centered Care

Family-centered care is a philosophy of care that acknowledges the importance of the family unit as the fundamental focus of all health care interventions. This model of care recognizes that the family is central in a child's life and should be central in the child's plan of care (Ahmann, 1994b, p. 113). The concept of family-centered care is not new; in fact, it is as old as, if not older than, most of the health professions. In days past, health care providers were family members. Kin served in the roles of medicine man or woman, nurturer, counselor, and even social worker. However, when health care moved to the hospital setting, the individuals became separated from the family, and the focus of care concentrated on the individual alone. In addition, as previously stated, societal changes have made it increasingly difficult to define the family. These factors have added to the challenge to move from a conceptual acceptance of family-centered care to reality-based methods of providing care that focus on both the child and the family.

Ahmann (1994c) noted two significant events in 1987 that have a great impact on the acceptance of a family-centered approach to health care. Two documents published in that year defined the elements of a family-centered approach to health care. The first was a report on children with special needs issued by Surgeon General C. Everett Koop (Department of Health and Human Services, 1987). The second was a document published by the Association for the Care of Children's Health (ACCH), *Family-Centered Care for Children with Special Health Care Needs* (Shelton, Jeppson, & Johnson, 1987). Since then, federal legislation has supported the principles and practices of family-centered health care through such laws as the Individuals with Disabilities Education Act, the Developmental Disabilities Assistance and Bill of Rights Act, and the Mental Health Amendments of 1990.

Elements of Family-Centered Care

The Association for the Care of Children's Health (ACCH) has recognized that the term family-centered care cannot simply be described by a common definition. Rather, family-centered care is best understood by extracting and explaining the elements or compo-

Chart 1–5

Key Elements of Family-Centered Care

- Incorporating into policy and practice the recognition that the *family is the constant* in a child's life, whereas the service systems and support personnel within those systems fluctuate.
- Facilitating *family/professional collaboration* at all levels of hospital, home, and community care:
  - care of an individual child;
  - program development, implementation, evaluation, and evolution; and,
  - policy formation.
- *Exchanging complete and unbiased information* between families and professionals in a supportive manner at all times.
- Incorporating into policy and practice the recognition and *honoring of cultural diversity*, strengths, and individuality within and across all families, including *ethnic, racial, spiritual, social, economic, educational, and geographic diversity.*
- Recognizing and respecting *different methods of coping* and implementing comprehensive policies and programs that provide *developmental, educational, emotional, environmental, and financial supports* to meet the diverse needs of families.
- Encouraging and facilitating *family-to-family support* and networking.
- Ensuring that *hospital, home, and community services and support systems* for children needing special health and developmental care and their families *are flexible, accessible, and comprehensive* in responding to diverse family-identified needs.
- *Appreciating families as families* and children as children, recognizing that they possess a wide range of strengths, concerns, emotions, and aspirations beyond their need for specialized health and developmental services and support.

From Shelton, T. L., & Stepanek, J. S. (1994). *Family-centered care for children needing specialized health and developmental services.* Bethesda, MD: Association for the Care of Children's Health. Reprinted with permission.

nents of this philosophy of care that work together to move an individual or an institution toward providing a family-centered approach. Eight elements have been defined, each serving to reinforce, facilitate, and complement the implementation of the others (Chart 1–5). The elements of family-centered care recognize each family's uniqueness, acknowledge the influence of the family as a constant in the child's life, and emphasize the importance of providing services that demonstrate the value of collaboration between the health care provider, the child, and the family. Family-centered care is based on the premise that a positive adjustment to a child's level of health and well-being requires the involvement of the whole family (Shelton & Stepanek, 1995).

Despite the growing conceptual acceptance of family-centered care, the *practice* of family-centered care has not been fully actualized (Ahmann, 1994a). Technology, economic trends toward downsizing services and staffing, and the presence of a more culturally diverse population of patients are challenges to implementing family-centered care. Health care providers struggle to find the time and energies to reach beyond the procedural boundaries of their work to meet family needs. Barriers have been created by complex organizational structures and policies that separate the child from the family.

Worldview: *Promoting family-centered care can be impeded by the health care provider's limited knowledge and understanding of the cultural issues that affect family life. Within ethnic groups, some families are strongly rooted to their original culture, whereas others are more assimilated to the homogeneous "American" culture. There can be a great range of beliefs, values, and practices among families from the same cultural background. This presents a challenge to clinicians, who must educate themselves about the cultures with which they work, avoiding stereotyping or trying to make the families fit into the clinician's own cultural belief system.*

A growing body of research has further noted the lack of congruence between family needs as perceived by the patient and the family and the same needs as perceived by members of the health care team. Violence in the health care setting has produced additional challenges to providing family-centered care. For instance, concerns regarding infant or child security have tightened visitor policies and forced hospitals to place more monitors on the children's activities and whereabouts in the hospital. A family-centered approach may support liberal visitation of family members for both young and old. The increased number of visitors can lead to increased confusion and security risks within a clinical facility. In addition, there is a concern that increased infection rates and spread of contagious diseases accompany liberal visitation policies. Certainly, these concerns are valid. They can be addressed by security and infection control screening measures that are aimed at safeguarding the child while still supporting family-centered care. (See Chapter 9 for a summary of some of these security and infection control screening measures.)

Family-Centered Care Interventions and Strategies

Family-centered care involves more than merely instituting more liberal visitation rules. A variety of creative strategies can be employed to fulfill the elements of family-centered care (Chart 1–6). Through interdisciplinary interventions that provide education and knowledge to the family, parents and others can be empowered to make informed decisions about their child's care (Dunst & Trivette, 1996; Rushton, 1990a, 1990b). Family-centered care interventions recognize the importance of families in facilitating the growth of their child, especially the child with special health care needs. The needs and resources of each family member and the degree to which the family wants to become involved differ with each family. Yet, the goals remain the same—to optimize the family's ability to interact, intervene, and nurture the child during times of both physical and psychological stress.

Family-centered care is a philosophy of care that must be translated into action. The relevance to the child and the family goes unnoticed unless active measures are taken to ensure that family-centered practices are integrated into every aspect of the health care arena. From legislation supporting family-centered practices to an interdisciplinary team focused upon the needs of the entire family, the elements of family-centered care can be operationalized via a variety of unique strategies. These family-centered strategies need to continue to be described in the health care literature, noting the strategies that have been truly effective in meeting family needs (Collin, 1995). In the same manner, health care providers need to continue to *assess* family needs, *document* how family-centered care has been implemented, *define* factors that facilitate or hinder family-centered care, and *document* the cost-effectiveness of family-centered care.

Implementation of family-centered care interventions has elicited positive feelings from health care staff and reports of increased parent and child satisfaction (DePompei, Whitford, & Beam, 1994; Gill, 1987; Heller & McKlindon, 1996; Johnson, Jeppson, & Redburn, 1992; Stolte & Myers, 1987). Family anxiety is reduced as the family's understanding of and involvement in the child's health care activities are promoted through these interventions.

Chart 1–6

Strategies to Enhance Family-Centered Care

Change visiting policies to promote the presence of the family at the bedside.
Establish family support groups, placing invitations to attend meetings on each child's bed.
Develop activities or programs to support the family as they make the transition from one unit (pediatric intensive care unit) to another (pediatric floor).
Be sure there are an adequate number of sleeping cots for parents.
Establish a sibling hospital visiting policy.
Encourage family visiting in the postanesthesia room.
Use parent questionnaires to better understand family needs.
Involve parents in playroom activities.
Develop mechanisms to support regular contact between the child and out-of-town parents.
Establish a parent committee or family advisory council to advise the hospital on issues of importance.
Create a parent information board containing community resources and information pamphlets.
Create a parent information and orientation program to familiarize parents with the hospital.
Provide a brief parent welcome and orientation program.
Incorporate the family in interdisciplinary conferences regarding the child's care.
Use preoperative videos and tours to ease the child's and family's fear about the pre- and postoperative process.
Establish programs to support the infant or child's transition to home after a lengthy hospitalization.
Encourage parents to chart the child's progress.
Contract with parents to provide care for periods of time during the day.
Provide the family with a copy of the child's care path.
Coordinate and record all of the child's daily activities on a large calendar, visible to everyone.
Provide parking discount for parents.
Establish volunteer child care services for siblings while parents visit the sick child.
Call parents with reports of child's progress or send notes from the child for those hospitalized long term.
Recognize and integrate ethnic, racial, and cultural activities as appropriate into clinical setting (e.g., foods, play items, pictures on wall).
Aim for diversity of health care staff.
Encourage families to bring in culturally significant items such as foods and healing and religious symbols.
Encourage all family members to participate in home care activities.
In the acute care setting, provide support services such as laundry and kitchen facilities to families experiencing long hospitalizations.
Provide activities such as picnics, movies, and special events for children and their families to interact with other families who have children with the same chronic or acute condition.

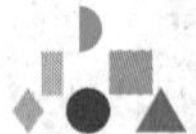

An Interdisciplinary Approach to Health Care

The call for reform within the health care system has had reverberating effects on all aspects of services involved in care of patients. Although many have linked "reform" to a political struggle over limited monetary health care resources, in truth, reform encompasses a much broader perspective of managing, allocating, coordinating, and monitoring the effectiveness of the health care system and its personnel, technologies, and standards. *Nursing's Agenda for Health Care Reform* (1993) embodies the goal of maintaining quality and expanding access to patient care services while controlling and balancing the cost of care. Key concepts of the agenda include the following:

- The call for a restructured health care system that promotes consumer access to services and responsibility for personal health care
- The integration of public and private plans to provide health care services to all citizens and residents
- The provision of essential services to pregnant women and children and "vulnerable" populations
- Steps to reduce health care costs including requiring the use of managed care in the public plan and incentives for consumers and providers to use these plans
- Requiring case management for persons with continuing health needs
- Structuring provisions for long-term care

- Reforms to improve access to insurance coverage (including affordable premiums) and billing procedures

The vehicles driving health care reform include the strategies of *managed care and case management.*

Managed Care and Case Management

Managed care is a system that provides the generalized structure and focus for managing the use, cost, quality, and effectiveness of health care services. Primary and tertiary care settings are implementing managed care initiatives to streamline their processes, become more cost effective, and provide more efficient and effective services for their clients (Haas, 1996; More & Mandell, 1997). Nursing case management is one type of cost containment initiative under the umbrella of managed care.

Managed care systems provide needed services to patients while managing costs and access to the system. The quality of health care is an important outcome measured by the organized health care delivery system. Health maintenance organizations (HMOs) and preferred provider organizations (PPOs) were among the first to use managed care initiatives as an alternative to costly inpatient care. Acute care facilities and physician groups are now collaborating and consolidating to increase enrollees in managed care programs and to provide a broader range of services with less redundancies of costly specialized programs. In years past, it was common practice for the individual physician to hang out a shingle and thereby establish a private practice office. Today, physician groups are the norm, establishing contracts for delivery of patient care with hospitals, making them a partner in managed care organizations.

In a managed care environment, the nursing care delivery system is one initiative that supports cost-effective, patient outcome–oriented care. Managed care can be used with primary, team, functional, case management, and other alternative nursing care delivery systems. The focus is on providing a consistent treatment plan through support of standardized care protocols and by monitoring closely the length of hospitalization for individual patients (Etheredge, 1986; Hampton, 1993). Nursing care is unit based and structurally designed to promote and support care at the patient's bedside.

Case management differs from managed care in that the focus in on a clinical system used for selected patients, who are chosen on the basis of a particular diagnostic category that is considered to involve a high-risk and/or a high-volume population. Case management emphasizes that it is not a strategy used for *all* patients, nor is it a delivery system for one area or one nursing unit. A case management system utilizes an identified individual or group who are accountable for the following:

- Ensuring and facilitating the achievement of quality, clinical, and cost outcomes
- Negotiating, procuring, and coordinating services and resources needed by the patient/family
- Intervening at key points (and/or at significant variances) for individual patients
- Addressing and resolving patterns in group variances that may have a negative quality/cost impact
- Creating opportunities and systems to enhance outcomes (Bower, 1993, p. 1)

Case management systems are used across the continuum of care, over time, and in a variety of settings in which the high-risk patient would benefit from coordination of health care services (Lyon, 1993). The case management movement has been strongly influenced by total quality management (TQM), continuous quality improvement (CQI), and the philosophy of family-centered care (Lumsdon & Hagland, 1993; MacLaren, 1994) (Chart 1–7). To be effective, an organizational philosophy must exist that places the patient and the family at the center of all interactions, with the goal of patient/family satisfaction as the paramount objective.

The New England Medical Center in Boston pioneered the model for nursing case management in 1985, borrowing the term *case management* from the engineering term *project management.* As the model developed, the project team sought to answer four core questions:

- What is required by each discipline to bring patients with similar diagnoses to realistic outcomes?
- What is the best way to produce the work?
- Who is accountable for those outcomes?
- How can we reconstruct care so that this happens more consistently? (Lumsdon & Hagland, 1993, p. 34)

From this process, there have emerged redefined provider roles, distinctive methods for managing services, and tools and techniques for quantifying and monitoring managed care. Through the interventions of a *case manager*, the care provided by multiple disciplines can be coordinated more effectively and in the most cost-effective manner. The case manager follows patients through all settings and stages of their illness, orchestrating services to control the patients' length of stay while maintaining or improving patient outcomes. Case types selected for case management include those that are considered to

- Have high cost (e.g., transplants)
- Be predictably unpredictable or unpatterned patients
- Require chronic repeated admissions

Chart 1–7

The Language of Managed Care

Capitation:	A method of payment for health services in which the provider accepts a fixed amount of payment per subscriber, per period of time, in return for providing specified services.
Case management:	A care delivery system that is multidisciplinary. The purpose is to develop systems of care in which patient outcomes, efficiency, quality, and cost-effectiveness of services are enhanced.
Care path:	A tool that identifies expected patient and/or family outcomes and staff interventions against a time line for certain case types or a particular diagnosis.
CQI:	Continuous quality improvement. A type of ongoing improvement program operationalized in health care settings to ensure that patients are receiving the safest and most effective level of service within the health care environment.
DRG:	Diagnosis Related Group. Instituted in 1983, the Prospective Payment System for Medicare reimburses hospitals and other providers of care at predetermined rates on the basis of the Medicare patient's diagnosis.
HMO:	Health maintenance organization. A type of prepaid insurance option in which enrollees are offered a broad scope of service, are not required to pay a deductible, must pay fixed copayments for services and prescriptions, must choose a physician member of the HMO, and are encouraged to participate in preventive care and health promotion activities offered by the HMO.
Managed care:	Generic term that refers to health insurance plans that offer prepaid or managed fee-for-service health care.
PCP:	Primary care provider: The "gatekeeper" for the enrollee in the managed care plan. Responsible for all primary care for the patient and, in the gatekeeper role, decides when to refer the patient to a specialist.
PPO:	Preferred provider organization. A group of providers (hospitals, physicians, and others) who offer health care services at a discounted fee to their enrollees.
TQM:	Total quality management. A process of continuous improvement through which everyone strives to create and support an environment in which people are committed to serving and addressing the needs and expectations of the patients, the visitors, and the employees.
Variance:	A positive or negative patient outcome that causes patients to deviate from the expectations and patient outcomes identified on the care path.

- Have significant variances in outcomes
- Have high-risk socioeconomic factors
- Involve providers from multiple disciplines

Practice Guidelines

To guide health care practices, practice guidelines have been developed by federal, professional, and agency-based groups. These guidelines are indicators of what a reasonably prudent health care provider(s) practicing in the average situation would do to provide the safe and necessary care to meet the client's needs. Practice guidelines may be disease-specific, patient population–specific, or profession-specific. For instance, critical pathways, or care paths, are disease-specific guidelines. Professional organizations have developed standards of care that are profession-specific, stipulating the type of care involved and the level of provider who should be delivering the care. In addition, in the case of malpractice or negligence, the standard of care is a measuring device to compare how professionals acting in similar situations should conduct themselves. Standards of care are frequently admitted into evidence in litigation as the minimum level of care that is expected in a professional-to-patient interaction.

The Joint Commission on Accreditation of Healthcare Organizations (JCAHO) is the annual publisher of the *Accreditation Manual for Hospitals*, providing standards of care for the various services rendered. Standards are drafted to evaluate health care in a variety of settings and organizations. Interdisciplinary collaboration is one of the primary goals JCAHO expects organizations to reach. The use of practice standards provides a method for promoting interdisciplinary care while ensuring that the child and the family receive optimal health care.

Nursing Classification Systems

Nursing classification systems are a form of practice guidelines that are used to describe, direct, document, study, and demonstrate the effects of nursing care. Two comprehensive classifications to describe nursing exist and are used throughout this text: the classification of nursing diagnosis by the North American Nursing Diagnosis Association (NANDA) and the Nursing Interventions Classification (NIC) (McCloskey & Bulechek, 1996; North American Nursing Diagnosis Association, 1994).

The **NANDA classifications of nursing diagnosis** have evolved since 1973. A nursing diagnosis is a clinical judgment about individual, family, or community responses to actual or potential health problems/life responses. Nursing diagnoses provide the basis for selection of nursing interventions to achieve outcomes for which the nurse is accountable (Carroll-Johnson, 1991).

Gordon (1994) has identified the three structural components of a nursing diagnosis statement as the problem (P), the etiology (E), and the signs and symptoms (S). The problem describes the patient's response to an actual or potential health problem/life process. The etiology describes the cause or causes of the response, most commonly stated using phrases such as "related to," "secondary to," or "due to." The signs and symptoms specify the defining characteristics or observable signs and symptoms that have been demonstrated by the client (Cox et al., 1997).

Throughout this text, nursing diagnoses are presented to assist the student in integrating the nursing process into the interdisciplinary plan of care for the child and the family.

The **Nursing Interventions Classification (NIC)** is a standardized listing of nursing interventions developed by a large research team at the University of Iowa, funded by grants from the National Institute of Nursing (Bowles & Naylor, 1996; Bulechek & McCloskey, 1992; McCloskey, 1995; Tripp-Reimer, Woodworth, McCloskey, & Bulechek, 1996). Each labeled nursing interventions classification includes a definition of the intervention, a set of defining nursing activities, and a short list of background readings (see Charts 1–13, 1–14, and 1–16). In this text, the list of background readings has not been reprinted. The student is encouraged to refer to the McCloskey & Bulechek (1996) text to review these data. NICs are presented throughout the text, where applicable, to assist in delineating the broad scope of nursing actions that can be initiated. The text charts that contain nursing interventions developed by the Iowa Intervention Project are designated as such in the title and source citation.

Care Paths

The key ingredients of a case management system are the designated nurse or core of nurses with expert management and clinical knowledge and skills serving as case managers, a defined case management process for identifying and implementing case management with high-risk populations, and utilization of practice guidelines to direct patient care (Chart 1–8). The practice guidelines are the tools developed by the interdisciplinary team that define expected patient outcomes, appropriate lengths of stay, appropriate utilization of resources, and specific nursing and medical interventions. These practice guidelines or case management plans have been referred to as the "second generation" of nursing care plans. By expanding on the "first generation" of nursing care plans, these guidelines incorporate both nursing and medical diagnoses with specific time frames for attainment of intermediate goals and long-term patient outcomes (Zander, 1988). Today, federal reform measures that encourage more standardization of care, and changes in the JCAHO accreditation guidelines have hastened the emergence of case management guidelines. These guidelines appear in a variety of forms and under a wide range of names

Chart 1–8

Case Management Process

- Identify the patient populations for the case management practice.
  - Establish a method for efficiently linking the case manager with the patients within the identified populations as early in the trajectory as possible.
- Complete or contribute to an assessment or database.
- Define and agree on anticipated outcomes, including time frames.
- Negotiate and/or coordinate a plan between and among the patient, family, and care team members, including brokering required services for the patient or family.
- Implement the plan.
- Monitor and evaluate the patient's status vis-à-vis the plan and anticipated intermediate goals and outcomes in a timely manner.
- Take action.
  - Negotiate activities needed to keep or return the patient to the anticipated path.
  - Adjust the plan to meet the new reality.
  - Negotiate system changes to address patterns identified in aggregate variances.

Chart 1–9

Clinical Management Tools

Anticipated recovery paths
Care maps
Care paths
Care process models
Care tracks
Case care coordination and standard treatment guidelines
Case management
Clinical indicators
Clinical outcomes
Clinical paths or pathways
Clinical progressions
Collaborative care tracks
Collaborative case management plans
Collaborative paths or care paths
Collaborative pathways
Coordinated care
Critical pathways
Expected recovery pathway
Interdisciplinary plan
Key processes
Mercy plans of action for care and treatment (M-PACTS)
Minimum standards
Multidisciplinary plan
Outcome management
Outcomes
Patient pathways
Program evaluation
Quality assurance triggers
Quality improvement—monitoring and evaluation
Recovery routes
Reference guidelines
Service strategies
Standards of care
Standard treatment guidelines
Target tracks
Total quality management and continuous quality improvement
Uniform data system

(Chart 1–9). In the text, they are referred to as "care paths." The critical components of a care path are

- A problem list with expected patient outcomes
- The path of events to occur for each time increment of a care path (Petryshen & Petryshen, 1992)

In many cases, the problem list is written in terms of nursing diagnoses. This text uses this style because nursing diagnoses are extremely well suited to describing patients' problems, which can be the focus of the entire interdisciplinary team. The problem list identifies the actual and potential problems that affect most of the clients within a given case type. For each problem, corresponding desired outcomes are identified. Depending on the setting and case type in which the care path is to be used, outcomes may be defined in terms of hourly, daily, or weekly goals. These are patient-oriented goals that describe what the patient must achieve and/or verbalize to demonstrate that the problem has been resolved.

The list of events to occur on each day, hour, or week specified on the care path designates the tasks and interventions of the interdisciplinary team. These activities represent those tasks that the interdisciplinary team have determined are essential to meet the patient outcomes and reflect normal, usual care of a client with that case type. The listing of events provides a mechanism to hold caregivers accountable for providing the care delineated on the care path. The ability to meet these events serves as an indicator of the patient's progress. The inability to complete the events may indicate a deviation in the client's progress or system problems that are affecting the caregiver's ability to complete the intervention.

Figure 1–4 provides the "shell" of the care path utilized throughout the text. At the top of the care path, the case type is designated. Many facilities also include information such as the primary attending physician, the anticipated length of stay, and the Diagnosis-Related Group (DRG) number. The patient's name plate is stamped on the top of the care path, as this plan of care becomes a permanent part of the patient's record. The patient's problems and corresponding outcomes are listed in accordance with the time frame delineated for the care path. The events of the care path are grouped under like categories. Depending on the events identified, these categories may vary from care path to care path. For instance, the category of "consults" may not be incorporated or needed in all plans of care. In the table, numerous categories of events have been listed. Throughout the text, event categories not used with a particular case type are not presented on that care path.

The generation of a care path is a formalized process requiring the input of representatives from all disciplines that are involved in the treatment of the child

Care Path *An Interdisciplinary Plan of Care for the Child with* ______________

Nursing Diagnosis	Patient/Family Intermediate Outcomes				
	Day:	Day:	Day:	Day:	Day:
#1					
#2					
#3					
#4					
	Care Intervention Categories				
Consults					
Discharge Planning					
Labs					
Medications and IVs					
Monitors					
Nutrition					
Pain Management					
Play Therapy/School					
Procedures (Diagnostics)					
Psychosocial					
Radiology					

Figure 1–4
The care path model that is used throughout this text.

Illustration continued on following page

Rehabilitation				
Safety and Activity				
Self-Care				
Social Service				
Special Considerations				
Visitors				
Teaching				
Tests				
Vital Signs/Baseline Parameters				

Figure 1–4 *Continued*

(Chart 1–10). Generally, the process begins with an exhaustive review of literature to provide a sound theoretical and research base to support the problem list and event categories related to a certain case type. In this manner, care paths are developed on the basis of well-supported care practices rather than a single provider's preferred method or strategy of care. Once the information has been gathered, the interdisciplinary team meets to map out the plan of care. This is an arduous, time-consuming process because interpretation of appropriate intervention strategies can vary from provider to provider, leading to challenging debates among the care path design team. Once the care path is developed, it is tested on a selected number of children. Variances or deviations from the plan of care, either positive or negative, are noted. Positive deviations may indicate that the design team underestimated how quickly a child would be able to resolve a certain problem. Negative deviations may indicate that care paths need to be revised. After the care path has been field tested and any systemic barriers have been resolved, the care path should be instituted with all children who are identified with that case type. The use of care paths does not require that the child is managed under the oversight of a case manager; rather, cases that are considered at high risk are those that may benefit from the coordinating services provided by a case manager.

Traditionally, the health care team has provided documentation of all treatments and patient progress as they occur on a daily basis. Using a care path, such exhaustive documentation is not necessary, because charting often occurs by exception (Petryshen & Petryshen, 1992). This means that, as the patient meets hourly, daily, or weekly outcomes and as the mapped interventions and events are administered, the care path day (hour or week) is simply signed off. However, the critical piece of documentation that must be noted is that of any deviations from the care path. Figure 1–5 provides a format for documenting variances. This information is used by team members to improve the quality of care, to serve as an indicator for areas that may require more focused performance improvement activities (continuous quality improvement), and to provide justification for additional treatment measures or resources and a longer length of hospital stay. Tracking variances over time helps identify patterns within certain case types and may provide information to identify those at greater risk for variances.

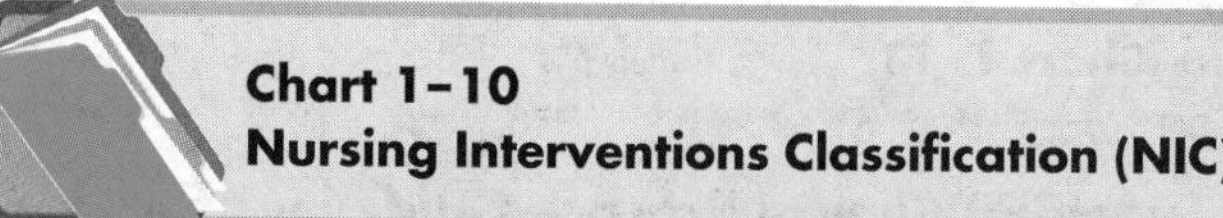

Chart 1–10
Nursing Interventions Classification (NIC)

Critical Path Development

Definition

Constructing and using a timed sequence of patient care activities to enhance desired patient outcomes in a cost efficient manner

Activities

Conduct chart audit to determine current patterns of care for patient population.
Review current standards of practice related to patient population.
Collaborate with other health professionals to develop the critical path.
Identify appropriate intermediate and final outcomes with time frames.
Identify appropriate interventions with time frames.
Share critical path with patient and family, as appropriate.
Evaluate patient progress toward identified outcomes at defined intervals.
Calculate variances and report through appropriate channels.
Document patient progress toward identified outcomes, per agency policy.
Document reason for variances from planned interventions and expected outcomes.
Implement corrective action(s) for variance(s), as appropriate.
Revise critical path, as appropriate.

From McCloskey, J., & Bulechek, G. (1996). *Nursing interventions classification (NIC)* (2nd ed.). St. Louis: Mosby–Year Book. Reprinted with permission.

Figure 1–5
A sample of a variance tracking record.

VARIANCE TRACKING RECORD

Patient: ______________________________

Date of Admission: ______________________________

Care Path Diagnosis: ______________________________

Date	Care Path Day (Hour or Week)	Variance (specify)	Actions Taken	Signature

Other Practice Guidelines

Individual health care organizations, nationally affiliated professional organizations, and federal agencies have also responded to the call for practice guidelines. These practice guidelines can be used to guide the development of care paths, to establish minimum practice standards in a given setting, or to establish policies that specify how treatment interventions should be implemented. In the forefront of these activities has been the Agency for Health Care Policy and Research (AHCPR). The agency was established by Congress in 1989 with the purpose of improving the quality, appropriateness, and effectiveness of health care and improving access to health care services. This mission is completed through agency-sponsored programs that support and conduct health services research and examine the availability, quality, risks, effects, and costs of health care services and technologies. In addition, AHCPR facilitates and promotes the development of clinical practice guidelines (AHCPR, 1996). The AHCPR has an extensive catalog that contains publications describing AHCPR's programs, presenting research findings, assessments of health care technologies, clinical practice guidelines, and research funding opportunities. (See Resources section for the address and toll-free number to obtain this catalog.)

Chart 1–11

AHCPR Clinical Practice Guidelines for Pediatrics*

- Acute pain management in infants, children and adolescents: operative and medicinal procedures
- Sickle cell disease
- Otitis media with effusion in young children
- Evaluation and management of early HIV infection

*Materials include:
- Guideline Overview
- Quick Reference Guide for Clinicians
- Parent Guide
- Spanish Language Parent Guide

The clinical practice guidelines are developed by an interdisciplinary panel of private sector clinicians and other experts whom AHCPR determines would have a valuable contribution to a particular subject area. For instance, a consumer who has dealt with a particular health care problem being addressed through a practice guideline would be considered an expert in that subject and would be invited to participate on the panel. The

Chart 1–12

Available Practice Guidelines for Child Health Care

AWHONN Standards for the Nursing Care of Women and Newborns (1991)
Association of Women's Health, Obstetric, and Neonatal Nursing

Guidelines for the Care of Children with Spina Bifida
Shriners Hospital
1900 Richmond Road
Lexington, KY 40502

Infant and Family-Centered Care Guidelines (1995)
National Association of Neonatal Nurses

Nursing Systems Toward Effective Parenting-Preterm (NSTEP-P)
NCAST Office
University of Washington
Mailstop WJ-10, CDMRC Room 110
Seattle, WA 98195

Outcome Standards of Pediatric Oncology Nursing Practice (1989)
Association of Pediatric Oncology Nurses

Region X Nursing Network Prenatal and Child Health Screening and Assessment Manual
MCH Clearinghouse

Scope and Standards of Advanced Practice Registered Nursing (1996)
American Nurses' Association

Scope of Practice and Outcome Standards of Practice for Pediatric Oncology Nursing (1994)
Association of Pediatric Oncology Nurses

Standards of Care for Neonatal Nursing Practice
National Association of Neonatal Nurses

Standards of Community Health Nursing Practice
American Nurses' Association

Standards of Home Health Nursing Practice (1986)
American Nurses' Association

Standards of Maternal and Child Nursing Practice (1983)
American Nurses' Association Division on Maternal and Child Health Nursing Practice

Standards of Nursing Practice for the Care of Children and Adolescents with Special Health and Developmental Needs
Dr. Gwen Lee, Associate Professor and Director
Division of Parent-Child Nursing, College of Nursing
University of Kentucky Chandler Medical Center
Lexington, KY 40536-0232

Statement on the Scope and Standards of Pediatric Clinical Nursing Practice (1996)
American Nurses' Association and the Society of Pediatric Nurses

panel uses a science-based methodology and their expert clinical judgment to develop the specific guidelines on assessment and management of the clinical condition selected. Extensive literature searches and critical reviews and synthesis of all available empirical evidence are the core activities of the expert panel. Thus, the guidelines reflect a summary of all current research and state-of-the-art knowledge that have proved to be effective in managing a selected clinical problem. The recommendations of each panel are summarized in three formats. The first is a publication that thoroughly shares the scientific information and research findings in a detailed fashion. The second publication is a quick reference guide for clinicians; more concise in its format, this document summarizes the panel's recommendations for assessment and management of the clinical condition. The third publication is a patient's guide. This small brochure explains treatment options and the type of scientifically based care that patients should expect to receive for a certain condition.

Development of these standards is ongoing. To date, 18 standards have been developed, and four of these specifically address children's health issues (Chart 1–11). The guidelines are to be used by health care providers to make better health care decisions and to reduce the delivery of ineffective or inappropriate services. AHCPR guidelines are cited and described throughout this text as appropriate to the discussion topic.

Other organizations and government-supported projects have given rise to standards that are designed for use with specific client populations (Chart 1–12). Standards such as these are intended to define and ensure the quality of care for a selected clientele. Regardless of the practice setting, these standards establish guidelines for practice and include criteria by which to measure achievement of these standards.

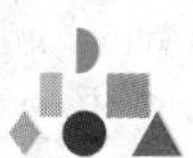

Nursing Roles in Child Health Care

The role and interventions of the nurse are in many ways universal, transcending any client population or care setting. Still, it cannot be disputed that the unique characteristics of children and their families provide stimulating challenges for implementing the nursing role. For some time, pediatric nursing has enjoyed a degree of specialization in health care environments. Special nursing units, clinics, and treatment areas have been designated exclusively as pediatric care areas. Changes in staffing mixes, the declining census of inpatient facilities, and competitiveness among managed care agencies have led to the integration of pediatric health services into adult care areas. The nurse who has adapted interventions to meet the needs of the adult world is challenged to alter health care delivery methods to meet the needs of the pediatric client. A nurse's daily responsibilities are multifaceted, including such roles as health care provider, teacher, advocate, change agent, and utilizer of research. The nurse caring for children must approach these roles with an understanding of the unique features of this client population.

Health Care Provider

In 1980, the American Nurses' Association prepared a social policy statement that included a definition of nursing:

> Nursing is the diagnosis and treatment of human responses to actual or potential health problems (ANA, 1980b).

This brief definition functions as a beginning point to describe the nurse's role as a provider of health care. The nurse uses cognitive, analytic, and psychomotor processes to assess critically and intervene in the care of a human being challenged with a health problem. Through the systematic use of the nursing process, the nurse blends skills and knowledge with a commitment to "care" for the client even when no cure for the patient's health problem is possible, desirable, or necessary (Quinn & Smith, 1987). The nurse works in collaboration with other members of the health care team to meet the needs of the child and the family. Other health team members may include (but are not limited to) physicians, physical therapist, nutritionist, occupational therapist, child life specialist, social worker, and case manager. Each of these individuals has a specific role and function to provide in relation to patient care. The unique aspect of the nurse serving as a health care provider is the manner in which the nurse coordinates the interventions of all other health team members. Nurses' frequent and consistent contacts with the child and the family place them in an excellent position to see the total scope of the patient's needs and to advocate for interventions to be implemented to meet those needs.

Delegation

Within the scope of providing health care to the child and the family, the nurse is involved in delegating certain care activities to unlicensed assistive personnel (UAP). Knowledge regarding *proper* delegation of care activities is essential because the nurse retains the legal liability for the nursing care activities that were delegated. According to the American Nurses' Association (ANA), **delegation** is a partial transfer of authority and responsibility (Chart 1–13). The nurse who delegates continues to be accountable for the completion and outcome of the task (ANA, 1994b). For instance, the nurse

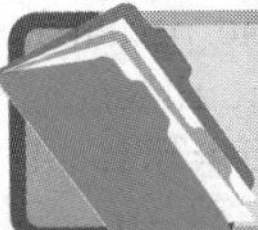

Chart 1–13
Nursing Interventions Classification (NIC)

Delegation

Definition

Transfer of responsibility for the performance of patient care while retaining accountability for the outcome

Activities

Determine the patient care that needs to be completed.
Identify the potential for harm.
Evaluate the complexity of the care to be delegated.
Determine the problem-solving and innovative skills required.
Consider the predictability of the outcome.
Evaluate the competency and training of the health care worker.
Explain task to the health care worker.
Determine the level of supervision needed for the specific delegated intervention or activity (e.g., physically present or immediately available).
Institute controls, so that the nurse can review the interventions or activities of the health care worker and intervene as necessary.
Follow up with health care workers on a regular basis to evaluate their progress in completing the specific tasks.
Evaluate the outcome of the delegated intervention or activity and the performance of the health care worker.
Monitor patient's and family's satisfaction with care.

From McCloskey, J., & Bulechek, G. (1996). *Nursing interventions classification (NIC)* (2nd ed.). St. Louis: Mosby–Year Book. Reprinted with permission.

may delegate to the UAP the task of turning a 3-year-old child who is immobilized in bed with traction to the right femur. However, the nurse is still legally accountable for verifying that correct application of the traction is maintained, the child's circulation to the extremity remains intact, and the family understands the importance of turning to prevent alterations in the integrity of the skin.

The concept of **supervision** is often confused with that of delegation. Supervision encompasses directing, guiding, and influencing the outcome of a person's performance through written or oral mechanisms (Zimmermann, 1996). The individual supervising need not be physically present on site to supervise an activity. For instance, the charge nurse who writes a note in the communication book reminding staff to document the cultural needs of the pediatric patients is performing a supervisory act (ANA, 1994b).

Assignment refers to the shifting of an activity to an individual who retains both responsibility and accountability for the task. Tasks can be assigned to another if the person understands the assignment and has the skill, knowledge, judgment, and legal authority to complete the assignment (Barter & Furmidge, 1994).

As the nurse delegates tasks to assistive personnel, a critical assessment of the child, the family, the task to be completed, and the capabilities of the UAP must be considered. In addition, tasks should not be delegated to UAPs that are outside the scope of their job description, institutional policy, or level of competence (Parkman, 1995). The nurse remains accountable for the outcome of the tasks completed, including documenting the outcomes and sharing relevant outcomes with other members of the interdisciplinary team.

Developmentally Appropriate Care

When caring for the pediatric client, this aspect of the nurse's role demands that the provider have a sound foundation in the basic principles of child health care. As discussed at the beginning of this chapter, pediatric health care encompasses a specialized core of knowledge that is unique to this population. The Society of Pediatric Nurses has collaborated on a project that delineates the standards for pediatric nursing education for pre-licensure students and beginning practitioners (see Chart 1–3).

As there is growing acceptance of these standards, the next most logical step in the practice setting is to ensure that those who care for children are competent to do so as demonstrated by their skills and knowledge in these areas. It is not uncommon for a nurse who is unfamiliar with caring for children to have to "float" to a pediatric care area or to have responsibility for a sick child in a traditionally adult care setting. In this case, the nurse is legally responsible for providing health care that is developmentally appropriate for that child. To fulfill this commitment, the nurse must take whatever steps necessary to ensure that the health care provided is safe, developmentally appropriate, and focused on the distinctive physical differences found in the pediatric population.

Coordinator and Collaborator

The terms "interdisciplinary," "intradisciplinary," "multidisciplinary," and "transdisciplinary" have been creeping into the vocabulary of health care professionals as a sign that a totally different approach to health care is now upon us. Where once health care professionals would operate in their own little worlds, developing diagnostic language, research, and treatment interventions unique to their professional realm, the emphasis has changed to that of creating a more consistent and unified approach by all disciplines to meet the client's health care needs. "Interdisciplinary and intradisciplinary are *in*; rigid application of nursing conceptual perspectives alone is *out*" (Kim & Felton, 1993, p. 118). This new order emphasizes that health team members are respected for their unique contributions, replacing the paternalistic relationships that have dominated professional interactions in the past. The nurse plays an extremely important role in this new era as a coordinator, a collaborator, and a health team member. In most health care settings, the nurse continues to have the most consistent contact with the child, the family, and all members of the health care team. It is imperative that the nurse accept the responsibilities of coordinating the efforts of the health care team. These coordination activities include the following:

- Assisting each discipline to be aware of the patient goals
- Encouraging mechanisms to foster effective communication among all team members
- Identifying interventions of the health team that may be in conflict with identified patient goals
- Ensuring that the child, family, and health team members are communicating effectively with each other
- Monitoring patient care to determine that all services prescribed are appropriately provided to the child and the family

Interdisciplinary care conferences are excellent vehicles for promoting activities that foster collaboration among all team members (Chart 1–14). In the role of coordinator and collaborator, the nurse must be assertive and inquisitive, serving as both a leader and an active participant to ensure that the client's health care needs are met in a positive manner (Chart 1–15).

Advocate

An "advocate" acts to safeguard and to advance the interests of another person, in this case, the patient, in order to enable children and their families to meet their health care needs (Rushton, Armstrong, & McEnhill, 1996). As an advocate, the nurse caring for children can act on two different levels to perform this role. On one level, the nurse serves as a *representative*, a voice for

- The child *and* his or her family to other health care providers
- The child *to* his or her family
- The family *to* the child
- The health care provider *to* the child and the child's family

The health care setting can be an overwhelming environment for the child and the family. In the unfamiliar surroundings of a clinic, a doctor's office, or a hospital unit, it is clear that the family has entered an arena where they are not "at home" and not totally in control of the environment. Mix these feelings of uncertainty with a healthy dose of anxiety, fear of the unknown, weariness, and, often, pain and discomfort, and it becomes easy to recognize why a child and the family may need someone to be their advocate.

In the role of acting as a representative for the child and the family, the nurse may find serving as an advocate for the child *with* the parents or the health care team to be a complex undertaking. The child, viewed as a minor,

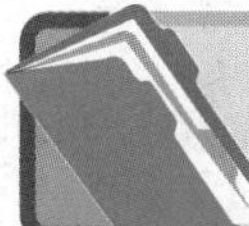

Chart 1–14
Nursing Interventions Classification (NIC)

Multidisciplinary Care Conference

Definition

Planning and evaluating patient care with health professionals from other disciplines

Activities

Summarize health status data pertinent to patient care planning.
Identify current nursing diagnoses.
Describe nursing interventions being implemented.
Describe patient and family response to nursing interventions.
Seek input about effectiveness of nursing interventions.
Discuss progress toward goals.
Revise patient care plan, as necessary.
Solicit input for patient care planning.
Establish mutually agreeable goals.
Review discharge plans.
Discuss referrals, as appropriate.
Recommend changes in treatment plan, as necessary.
Provide data to facilitate evaluation of patient care plan.
Clarify responsibilities related to implementation of patient care plan.

From McCloskey, J., & Bulechek, G. (1996). *Nursing interventions classification (NIC)* (2nd ed.). St. Louis: Mosby–Year Book. Reprinted with permission.

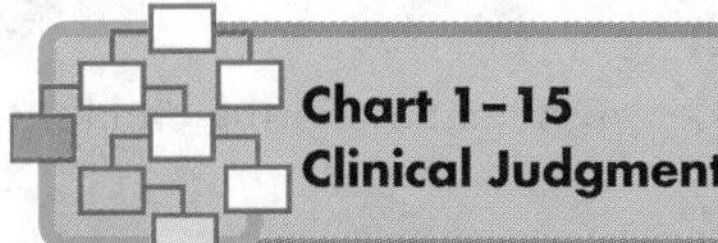

Chart 1–15
Clinical Judgment

Promoting an Interdisciplinary Approach to Care

Matthew is a nurse working on a pediatric unit in a community medical center. Over the past several months Matthew has become concerned regarding the readmission rates of several school-age children with asthma. In particular, he believes that management of the children's asthma in the home and school has not been effective. In addition, he has noted that the children are missing many days of school because of the frequency of the readmissions and the extended length of their stay in the hospital. The physicians who manage these children are members of a private practice group who take turns monitoring the children's progress when they are hospitalized. Parents have verbalized that when their child is hospitalized they do not understand the plan of care and feel the care is fragmented.

Questions:

1. In this situation, what are some of the problems you can identify?
2. Who are the members constituting the interdisciplinary team caring for the children with asthma?
3. What barriers exist in regard to providing an interdisciplinary approach to care of these children?
4. What interventions could Matthew initiate to improve patient care and enhance communication among the members of the interdisciplinary team?
5. How could Matthew determine whether any of these interventions were successful in improving the care provided to this group of children?

Answers:

1. High readmission rate of children with asthma. Potential ineffective home and/or school management of these children. Difficulties in communication and coordination of care among members of the interdisciplinary team. Parent frustration regarding health care services.
2. The members of the physician group, including nurses at the physicians' office; the care providers at the medical center, including nurses and respiratory therapist; the child and the child's family; the child's teacher; and the school nurse.
3. Lack of coordination and communication among team members. Variety of sites in which health care is provided to the child. No identified mechanisms to reduce number of readmissions.
4. Plan a meeting with representatives from the nursing unit, physician group, and school to discuss and analyze the problems. Devise communication mechanism that assists all members of the team in understanding the needs and plan of care for each child. Provide education to school personnel regarding the management of children with asthma.
5. Parents verbalize improved satisfaction with health care services. Readmission rate decreases because of more preventive actions instituted by school personnel and parents. Children attend more days of school.

may not have the right or the cognitive ability to make decisions about his or her own health care. On the other hand, the child can participate in health care decisions and treatment through self-care activities. A study by Perlman and Abramovitch (1987) found that 92% of children were not involved in the communication between their parents and the health care providers. Yet 92% of these children stated they had specific questions relevant to the visit of the health care provider that they wished to ask and have answered. The child is usually not viewed as a consumer and thus may be considered powerless to act to improve her or his access to health care. The nurse can act by empowering children and adolescents to recognize their roles in their own health care. Children are interested in and motivated to learn about themselves and their bodies. The nurse advocate can act to help children to understand their health concerns and assist them in seeking health care assistance when warranted.

The second level of advocacy that exists for the nurse is different from the traditional views of helping or facilitating child and family rights as they work with other health care professionals. At this second level, advocacy is an intervention not directed to the child and the family; rather, the main targets of intervention are the institutional (legal, financial, social) barriers that prevent children and their families from getting the help they need. In this sense "child advocacy" was a term officially developed in 1969 by the Joint Commission on the Mental Health of Children, which recommended the creation of a "National System on Child Advocacy." No such formalized system ever materialized, yet the principles of child advocacy have endured and are practiced by personnel in nursing, medicine, and social and human services. Child advocacy is concerned with identifying and correcting practices and policies that may violate the child's legal and human rights or may seriously harm the child's general welfare or health. As an advocate for the child and the family, the nurse intervenes to protect their health care rights in a variety of ways (Chart 1–16). Child advocacy is also concerned with shaping the social context to create an environment that is supportive of the needs of children and their families.

Within this domain or level of child advocacy there are two types of advocacy responses: *case* and *class* advocacy (Chart 1–17). In case advocacy, the health care provider makes an effort to facilitate an individual child's or family's access to information, to ensure that they have received the benefits to which they are entitled, to ensure that they receive adequate services, and to provide psychosocial support. An example is guiding children into the most appropriate child abuse programs, women's and children's programs, and special support groups. Class advocacy exists when the nurse works on behalf of groups of vulnerable children. Most commonly, this is in the areas of changing delivery service patterns and advancing public policy practices that support child health issues and protect children's rights. Thus, as an advocate, the nurse has responsibilities directed toward the individual (the child), the family, and the community.

Health Educator

Patient education has been described as the process of influencing behavior, producing change in knowledge, attitudes, and skills required to maintain and improve the health of an individual. The education process may begin with the imparting of information, but it also includes interpretation and integration of information in such a manner as to bring about attitudinal or behavioral changes that benefit the person's health status (Rankin & Stallings, 1996).

Florence Nightingale, the nurses on Henry Street, Linda Rogers, and the first public health nurses all have understood the power of providing health education to

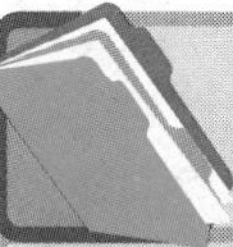

Chart 1–16
Nursing Interventions Classification (NIC)

Patient Rights Protection

Definition

Protection of health care rights of a patient, especially a minor, incapacitated, or incompetent patient unable to make decisions

Activities

Provide patient with "Patient's Bill of Rights."
Provide environment conducive for private conversations between patient, family, and health care professionals.
Protect patient's privacy during activities of hygiene, elimination, and grooming.
Determine whether patient's wishes about health care are known.
Determine who is legally empowered to give consent for treatment or research.
Work with physician and hospital administration to honor patient and family wishes.
Refrain from forcing the treatment.
Note religious preference.
Know the legal status of living wills in the state.
Honor a patient's wishes expressed in a living will or durable power of attorney for health care, as appropriate.
Honor written "Do Not Resuscitate" orders.
Assist the dying person with unfinished business.
Note on medical record any observable facts bearing on the testator's mental competency to make a will.
Intervene in situations involving unsafe or inadequate care.
Be aware of mandatory reporting requirements in the state.
Limit viewing of the patient's record to immediate health care providers.
Maintain confidentiality of patient data.

From McCloskey, J., & Bulechek, G. (1996). *Nursing interventions classification (NIC)* (2nd ed.). St. Louis: Mosby–Year Book. Reprinted with permission.

Chart 1–17

Advocacy: Strategies for Action

Case advocacy	Information sharing to empower the child and the family Matching the child's needs with specialized programs to support those needs Developing an ombudsman program
Class advocacy	Improving legislation to support and strengthen children's rights Pursuing litigation when absolutely necessary on behalf of children Using publicity to create more public awareness of child health issues Developing national standards of care and practice for pediatric health

improve the livelihood, mortality, and general welfare of children. In today's health care arena, skyrocketing health care costs, poor distribution of care, and lack of knowledge on the part of parents often cause families to seek care for their children only when they are sick. Because of budget cuts, there are fewer nurses in the schools, yet there are more children attending them who live in disruptive social situations that make them at higher risk for injury, poor nutrition, abuse, and neglect. In addition, approximately 7.5 million children in the United States have chronic conditions such as developmental disabilities, chronic diseases, and mental health problems (Vessey, 1994, p. 65). Thus, even with regulatory standards in place to encourage discharge planning and patient education, a large population of children and their families are not receiving illness prevention and health promotion education that can defer costly hospitalizations.

Given this milieu, it is imperative that the nurse who comes in contact with the pediatric client and the family *plan* and provide health education opportunities for them. Throughout this text, patient education resources are provided with an emphasis on a developmen-

Chart 1–18

Characteristics of the Health Educator

Confidence	The nurse is an expert about what to teach and is able to identify the main points of information being communicated. The nurse also "speaks the patient's language" and often uses very simple pictures or models. The nurse is very organized and can alleviate the patient's anxiety and instill confidence.
Competence	The nurse decides what is most important and gives clear directions. There exists concern for the patient's safety. The nurse provides good instructions and often gives individualized written instructions about what to do at home, instructing the patient what to do if specific problems should arise. The nurse provides care that is culturally competent.
Communication	The nurse speaks well and listens well. The nurse does not need to be a "long-winded lecturer." The nurse involves the patient by finding out what he or she already knows and uses the patient's problems as examples when teaching. The nurse stops and asks questions to be sure the patient understands instructions. The nurse uses a "show-and-tell" approach. She or he is comfortable talking to the patient's family and involves them in teaching. The nurse teaches the patient whom to call for help after the patient goes home. The nurse reviews what the patient is told by the doctor, dietitian, and physical therapist.
Caring and empathy	The nurse can put himself or herself "in the patient's shoes" and consider how the patient might feel. The nurse understands that patients worry about pain, safety, appearance, and financial costs and addresses these concerns. The nurse is gentle but firm when patients make mistakes as they are learning. The nurse is encouraging and provides enough time for the patient to be successful. Noticing when patients are sad or troubled helps patients confide their concerns to the nurse.

Adapted from Rankin, S., & Stallings, K. (1996). *Patient education: Issues, principles, practices.* Philadelphia: J. B. Lippincott. Used with permission.

tal approach to teaching the child and the family. It is most important that the nurse provide health teaching in collaboration with other members of the interdisciplinary team. In addition, the nurse must be skilled in the health teaching role. Rankin and Stallings (1996) have delineated four characteristics of the excellent nurse-teacher as described by the patients they serve. These characteristics are confidence, competence, communication, and caring (Chart 1–18). The ultimate goal of health teaching is for the nurse and other members of the health care team to use their knowledge and skills to assist the child and the family to prevent illness and promote or maintain optimum levels of health and wellness.

Researcher

Nursing research encompasses three major activities: generation of knowledge, dissemination of knowledge, and utilization of knowledge (Chart 1–19) (Fawcett, 1985). Often, the differences between these activities are not understood by the practicing nurse. Most nurses believe they are not involved in a research role. This belief is based on the presumption that the researcher role primarily involves conducting research projects. In fact, conducting research (generating new knowledge) is but one aspect of a nurse's research role. Equally important to remember is that not all nurses have the same educational preparation to pursue all three types of research activities. The American Nurses' Association Commission on Nursing Research has developed guidelines for research activities appropriate for nurses of associate degree, baccalaureate degree, and master's and doctoral nursing programs. Table 1–3 summarizes the relationship between educational preparation and the types of research activities. This table does not state that nurses prepared at the associate degree level

Chart 1–19

Research Activities

Research Conduct	**Generation of knowledge**
	A systematic, formal, and rigorous process to gain solutions to problems and/or to discover new relationships or facts in the area of clinical practice, nursing education or nursing administation (Waltz & Bausell, 1983) There are three types of research: 1. Basic: A study undertaken to establish new knowledge or facts and develop theories or conceptual frameworks. These findings are not directly and immediately applicable to human beings. 2. Applied: Research that attempts to find solutions to practical problems or to test the practical limits of scientific knowledge developed by basic research. New knowledge developed by applied research can generally be used without delay. 3. Clinical: Research that determines the effects of different ways of applying scientific knowledge in particular practice settings.
Research Dissemination	**Dissemination of knowledge**
	The presentation and interpretation of research findings in various arenas. Examples: • Presentations at conferences • Publication of research reports in books, journals, and monographs • Incorporation of research findings in textbooks, lectures, and seminar discussions • Inservices devoted to discussions of a research report or article
Research Utilization	**Utilization of knowledge**
	Using the findings from one or more research studies to change clinical practice and/or develop the next study in a program of research.

Adapted from Fawcett, J. (1985). A typology of nursing research activities according to educational preparation. *Journal of Professional Nursing, 2,* 75–78. Used with permission.

Table 1–3
Nursing Research Activities by Educational Preparation

Educational Preparation	Generation of Research			Dissemination of Findings	Utilization of Findings
	Basic	Applied	Clinical		
ADN					X
BSN				X	X
MSN			X	X	X
DNSc/PhD		X	X	X	X

From Fawcett, J. (1985). A typology of nursing research activities according to educational preparation. *Journal of Professional Nursing, 2,* 75–78. Reprinted with permission.

(ADN) or baccalaureate level (BSN) cannot conduct research; rather, it emphasizes that, in general, their formal education programs have not prepared them to *design* and *conduct* independent basic, applied, or clinical research.

The dissemination and utilization of research are activities in which all pediatric nurses can be participants. Nurses who conduct research have an obligation to present their work at conferences and through publications such as nursing journals. The nurse caring for children who reads research-based articles and attends conferences has a responsibility to share her interpretations and impressions of the research with her colleagues (Fawcett, 1985). The nurses from BSN programs may have more educational preparation in this area and may feel more comfortable carrying out dissemination activities.

In contrast, all nurses can become involved in using research findings to change and improve clinical practice. Many strategies can be employed to enhance the utilization of research findings (Chart 1–20). Research findings should be used to assist in implementing new practices and in evaluating old practices in regard to their adequacy in meeting patients' needs (Crane, 1985). Three barriers that have been consistently linked to lack of research utilization activities are lack of support from the work environment, lack of availability of research findings, and attitudes of nurses (Champion & Leach, 1989). Lack of support from the work environment exists when such elements as a heavy workload; lack of funds; lack of peer, administrative, and physician support; and patient resistance serve as obstacles to utilizing research in practice. A second major barrier to research utilization is that of availability of findings. Insufficient research, lack of researcher's time to translate studies into "practical terms," and lack of systematic means of sharing research findings all are variables that contribute to this problem. Although such journals as *Nursing Research* and *Advances in Nursing Science* are devoted to publishing current research, they are not read by many practitioners who find the journals costly and complex to read. A third obstacle to research utilization is presented by the negative attitudes held by nurses regarding research. Many nurses view research as irrelevant to their daily practice; thus, little time or energy is devoted to application of research findings.

Chart 1–20

Strategies to Enhance Research Utilization

- Support (time and money) by administrators for nurses to attend nursing conferences
- Availability of libraries with current journals in the medical care setting
- Time for reading made available during the workday for nurses
- Current nursing journals kept on nursing units
- Inservice programs that highlight the findings of nursing research
- Research findings used to update clinical policies and procedures
- Journal clubs that present research findings
- Incentives (positive evaluations and salary increases) provided to nurses who attempt to use research in their clinical practice
- Summaries of current research posted in nursing service areas for staff to read
- Research utilization incorporated in department and individual goals and philosophy
- Poster sessions to have units share their research utilization activities
- Nurses supported and encouraged to be involved in the conduct of research

The child health care provider can participate in several strategies to increase the use of research findings in practice. Using research to guide clinical practice is a fundamental mechanism for elevating the professional status of nurses.

Change Agent

In the Chinese written language the characters used for the word "crisis" are the same as those used for the word "opportunity." As a change agent, the nurse can also view crisis as a opportunity for change. In today's health care arena, it may at times feel as if crisis is the mode in which we continually must work. There are fewer registered nurses at the bedside, patients are more acutely ill by the time they seek health care, the time with a single patient has become shorter, and the resources available to meet patients' needs are fewer and in higher demand. Given this milieu, the nurse caring for children has an opportunity to change the ways in which pediatric health care is practiced and adapted to the needs of the families served.

As an agent of change, the nurse must possess good interpersonal skills, project expertise, the knowledge of how to use available resources, the ability to solve problems, and an understanding of the change process (Kaplan, 1990). The change agent can work in both formal and informal arenas to initiate and direct change for an individual child, a family, a group of colleagues, or an organization. In the selected setting, and for the selected group, the nurse incorporates the nursing process (assessment, diagnosis, planning, intervention, and evaluation) as the model to direct the change process.

The care of children and their families is being integrated into every environment in the health care arena. Standards to improve and provide consistency in the care of children are being developed. Research is helping to break down the old myths about children's needs and what they do or do not understand about their own health. It is an opportune climate for nurses with a strong knowledge base in pediatrics to help children, their families, and the professionals they work with to change their health care practices and their understanding regarding the unique needs of the child.

Consultant

A consultant is characterized as someone who has acknowledged expertise in a specific area and an ability to get things done when not in direct charge of the people concerned (Lange, 1987). The process of consultation involves collaborative problem solving and client decision making that can be viewed or structured in a variety of ways. The consultation event may be conceived of as occurring within a single consulting session or as a series of episodes in an ongoing process.

There are internal and external consultants, who may also be referred to as "generalists" and "specialists" or "affiliated" and "independent." The internal consultant is someone who works within an organization and who is given responsibility to plan and implement constructive change as an identifiable formal or informal function. The external consultant is brought into a situation from outside the organizational setting, that is, as a "hired expert," to perform similar functions. In this case, a more formalized consultant role exists. The definitive definition is spelled out by the Nurse Consultants Association (NCA) in its bylaws as

> An individual who is a currently licensed registered nurse and uses nursing knowledge and experience to promote optimum health care through media other than direct patient care. This individual may be self employed or work for a health related industry. The work medium may be, but is not limited to, education, research, consultation, or product development. The position in which the individual is employed utilizes the knowledge and skill of a professional nurse (NCA, 1984).

Consultation is similar to counseling in that both are facilitating relationships that involve human interactions. Counseling plays a part in consultation in that it helps to create an environment in which problem solutions may be explored and formulated. Counseling is therefore an important skill for the consultant to have. However, counseling never leaves the personal level, whereas consultation is less concerned with interpersonal processes and more concerned with task achievement. Consultation aims to help the client achieve preset goals and uses behavior modifications to achieve those goals. Consultation is a planned, purposeful, and mutually deliberative process in which the consultant and client set goals and objectives on the basis of perceived needs and then develop processes and principles to achieve those goals.

As more and more children with health challenges are examined and treated by those more familiar with adult health issues, nurses with specialty knowledge in pediatrics will be called upon to serve as consultants to these health care providers. The consultative event may be short in nature (starting a difficult intravenous line) or more extensive in scope (developing standards of care). In most cases, nurses with advanced degrees (i.e., clinical nurse specialists, nurse practitioners) serve as the "formal" internal or external consultants. However, nurses of all educational backgrounds with knowledge and experience in child health care may be called upon to consult and assist less experienced nurses in the care of children.

Expanded Roles

The diversity of pediatric health care settings and the challenge to integrate the many roles of the nurse into a defined practice have led to the increased pursuance of advanced practice roles within the profession. These expanded roles are filled by individuals who pursue and demonstrate an increased scope of practice, an in-depth range of knowledge and skills, and a focused domain of service. Most commonly, the path to an advanced practice role is acquired through academic education beyond the entry level of practice for nursing. In most cases this requires that the nurse has completed a master's degree in an area of specialization and is able to apply a broad range of theories and a broad set of postgraduate nursing skills (California Nurses' Association, 1984). This requirement may vary from institution to institution. Expanded roles include the following:

- Nurse practitioner
- Clinical nurse specialist
- Case manager
- Nurse executive
- Nurse educator
- Nurse-midwife
- Nurse anesthetist

(The latter two are not discussed in more detail in this text.) Although traditionally many nurses have advanced to one or more of these roles through longevity and/or demonstrated practical expertise, now the emphasis is on selecting individuals for these roles who are prepared at the master's level. The complexity of the health care system, the drive for third-party reimbursement, and the desire to maintain nursing practice roles on levels consistent with other professions have influenced the move toward advanced education as a prerequisite for moving into the role of educator, administrator, and advanced practitioner.

Nurse Practitioner

The nurse practitioner role evolved in the late 1960s and early 1970s in response to the call for more direct care providers in ambulatory settings who could perform routine preventive and health maintenance services (Brush & Capezuti, 1996). The pediatric nurse practitioner (PNP) is a registered nurse who has completed an organized program of study for nurse practitioner preparation usually offered in schools of nursing and usually as part of the master's in nursing degree program. The PNP employs a wide range of skills, including the following:

- Securing a health and developmental history assessment, laboratory studies, developmental evaluation from the newborn period up to age 21 years
- Discriminating between normal and abnormal findings and evaluating which findings call for treatment, consultation, or referral to collaboration with other health team members
- Providing health maintenance and health promotion services for children and families by including teaching, counseling, advising, treatment, and anticipatory guidance in all health encounters
- Diagnosing and treating selected common acute conditions, illnesses, or minor trauma
- Serving as a consultant to assist others in better understanding the growth and developmental needs of children (ANA, 1973)
- Identifying research issues, interpreting research, and implementing appropriate changes in practice and conducting research

The PNP has historically worked in ambulatory or outpatient settings, focusing on well populations, disease prevention, and minor disease management. Examples of this would include clinics, doctors' offices, schools, and home care settings. Changes in the health care marketplace have created a place for the nurse practitioner in acute care (Callender-Price, 1996). Partnerships with physician groups and positions in HMOs and other managed care organizations have expanded (Cohen & Juszczak, 1997). Role expansion into these arenas has demonstrated several benefits for patient care. The acute care PNP has demonstrated the ability to increase the child's likelihood of adopting more self-care activities, improve the quality and consistency of the patient care, provide cost containment, and provide competent and consistent coverage in areas in which medical staff coverage is unwarranted or unable to fulfill the demand.

PNPs are creating positions for themselves in arenas where economic and societal demands for pediatric health care has increased. These include school-based clinics, private nurse practitioner practices, homeless shelters, and daycare centers. With a background in pediatric nursing and more advanced practice skills, the PNP is ideally prepared to focus on promoting the physical, mental, and emotional development of children served in these health care settings. Typically, PNPs practicing in these settings have less on-site access to physicians for consultation and referrals. Thus, the ability to discriminate between the common, less acute illness and the malady requiring medical intervention is a critical skill. Table 1–4 provides a summary of the health services that a PNP might provide in one of these nontraditional settings.

Funding for the PNP role in a nontraditional setting can be provided through a number of innovative sources. Funding may be provided by the PNP's employer, as would be the case if the PNP was hired by a school district or a daycare corporation. Federal or state funding might be available for full or partial payment through Medicaid, the Early and Periodic Screening, Diagnosis and Treatment program, or Maternal Child Health Block

Table 1–4
Services Provided by the Pediatric Nurse Practitioner (PNP)

Service	PNP Activity
Health Screening/Assessment	· Develop and maintain comprehensive health record · Review health record to evaluate needs (immunization; follow-up) · Provide physical examination and routine laboratory studies (Hct, U/A) as needed—depending on linkage with primary care provider · Perform developmental screening/assessment (DDST, DASE) · Observation of children or early problem identification
First Aid/Emergency Care	· Organize equipment and areas for first-aid activity · Identification and training staff to provide first aid and emergency care as needed · Develop procedure/guidelines for first aid/emergency care
Illness Management/Follow-up	· Assessment of illness to determine disposition · Follow-up of diagnosed and treated illnesses (impetigo, otitis media) · Develop protocols for illness management · Order diagnostic tests to evaluate patient problems · Prescribe medications
Identification/Evaluation of Special-Needs Children	· Communication and collaboration with staff for case finding · In-depth observation of identified child; review health record; obtain comprehensive health history from parent; conference with teacher and parent; evaluation and referral as necessary · Participate on agency interdisciplinary professional team for evaluation and management (conference, consultation, develop care plan) · Liaison with community agencies
Health Education	· Design and/or implement preschool health education program · Resource consultant to teacher · Preceptor for nursing students using site · Role model for positive health behavior
Staff Development	· Conduct needs assessment of staff regarding health-related knowledge · Develop and teach appropriate health-related content (safety, common childhood illnesses)
Community/Parent Education	· Participate in parent-teacher meetings · Develop health newsletter for parents · Develop and/or participate in parenting classes and support groups

From Passarelli, C. (1987). Marketing the PNP to day-care centers. *Pediatric Nursing, 13*(1), 14. Reprinted with permission.

Grants held by individual states for services provided to underserved populations. Foundations and private or public grants may also be a plentiful source of funding, especially if the health care provisions are tied to a research project (Cohen & Juszczak, 1997; Passarelli, 1987). Just as Lillian Wald, creator of the Henry Street Settlement House, demonstrated her ability to perceive the acute needs of the children in her era, so can the creative PNP find a niche in today's diverse community to practice pediatric health care.

Clinical Nurse Specialist

In pediatric medicine there has been a growing awareness of the need for specialization, driven by the rapidly expanding knowledge base in children's health care. The development of specialization in nursing has paralleled this campaign. The increase in knowledge germane to specialization, new technology that requires intellectual competencies and complex skills, and a response to public need have played a major role in the development of the clinical nurse specialist (CNS) role (Peplau, 1965; Sparacino, 1990). The first program designed to prepare nurses at the master's level began in 1954 at Rutgers University with a specialization in psychiatry. Over the past 40 years, great strides have been made to standardize curriculum, clarify entry-level requirements, and define the role of the nurse specialist. Most recently, a debate has occurred regarding the issue of licensing or credentialing the clinical nurse specialist at a national and/or state level. In addition, health care reform, with the consequent downsizing of personnel in health care institutions, has led many experts to support the merger in educational preparation and practice of the CNS and NP roles. Many similarities exist in the core curriculum in nursing schools for these roles. It has been suggested that the CNS-NP be a "case manager," using the five subroles of the CNS (defined later) and the advanced assessment skills of the NP to provide comprehensive care to children and their families (Gaddis, 1996). Many clinical nurse specialists are seeking avenues to combine the two roles by returning to school to gain the knowledge and advanced assessment skills (including ordering tests and prescribing medications) of the nurse practitioner role.

A social policy statement by the American Nurses' Association (1980a) regarding specialization in nursing practice has served as a seminal document to clarify the distinct criteria required to assume the title of clinical nurse specialist and specify the role functions fulfilled by the clinical nurse specialist. The social policy statement defined the nurse specialist as one who "provides an expert approach to health focused on a refined body of knowledge and specialized practice competencies" (ANA, 1980b, p. 19). The clinical nurse specialist role consists of four primary components:

- Expert clinician
- Consultant
- Educator
- Researcher

A fifth role component, that of administrator, may also be an expected function of a clinical nurse specialist in a given institution. Much debate exists over whether or not the CNS can maintain a client-based practice and assume administrative responsibilities at the same time. It is not uncommon for the CNS to find that the administrative role responsibilities are not congruent with the patient-oriented responsibilities (Sparacino et al., 1990).

Pediatric clinical nurse specialists are as diverse in their area of specialization as there exist foci of clinical interests. From the perspective of the neonatal CNS, the pediatric endocrinology CNS, and the child development CNS, the opportunities to utilize an advanced practice role to improve patient outcomes and the practice of nursing care are unlimited.

Case Manager

The fastest emerging role in all practice areas of nursing is that of case manager. As with the roles of nurse executive and nurse educator, no standards have been established that require an advanced degree as a minimal educational standard for practice. A growing number of institutions are recognizing the value of placing an individual in this role who has a grasp of nursing, social, and economic theories that are the foundations of case management systems. Most institutions have selected nurses to fill the case manager positions. However, in some instances, social workers or quality management personnel have held this role. The nurse is optimally suited for this role, as the approach is generally more holistic in nature and the nurse's clinical experiences provide a strong foundation to help coordinate and direct the care delivery by the interdisciplinary team.

Three primary dimensions of the case manager's role have been identified in the literature: the *clinical role*, the *managerial role*, and the *cost containment role* (Cohen & Cesta, 1993; Lephoe, 1996). Chart 1–21 summarizes some of the responsibilities associated with each of these role dimensions. Case management expands on the nursing process to include additional components of case selection, interdisciplinary assessment, collective planning, coordinating, negotiating, evaluating, and documenting the outcomes of cost, quality of care, and client status (More & Mandell, 1997). The caseload of a case manager is influenced by several factors:

- The acuity or complexity of the patient population
- The volume or numbers of patients in the designated patient population
- The case manager's role definition; that is, how much direct care the case manager is expected to provide to the child and the family
- The number and location of geographic areas in which the case manager will be working

The care and management of children in both acute and outpatient settings can benefit greatly from a case management system and the overall coordination activities of a case manager. Developmental differences, dysfunctional family units, inadequate home supervision, and the general vulnerability associated with children who are sick make the provision of care difficult to standardize in the pediatric arena. The case manager is in an optimal position to coordinate the health care team's vision for the child's ultimate well-being with the realities of the individual strengths and weaknesses of the child and her or his support system.

Nurse Executive, Administrator, or Manager

Although all nurses need and use management skills in their daily practice, there is a reluctance among nurses to place themselves in formal management roles. The reasons for this vary. Some have cited the public image of nurses and the historical dependence of nursing on medicine (Ellis & Hartley, 1995). Others believe that nurses simply do not see themselves as leaders and managers in a profession dominated by the call to be "caregivers." Yet another reason may be the extensive time demands

Chart 1–21

Roles of the Case Manager

The Clinical Role

- Assist in the development of protocols that list key tasks or events that should occur when patient problems arise.
- Use practice protocols (care paths) to direct, monitor, and evaluate patient treatment, patient outcome, and responses to treatments.
- Identify variances from the standard protocols.
- Work with other team members to analyze and deal with variances of care.
- Introduce self to child and family, explain the case manager role, and provide them with a business card.
- Conduct patient and family teaching sessions.
- Review the literature about care and management of case types and share findings with peers to improve patient care.
- Manage each patient's transitions from unit to unit within the system.
- Transfer patient accountability to the appropriate person or agency upon patient discharge.

The Cost Containment Role

- Use clinical protocols to ensure that patients do not receive inadequate care because of cost containment measures.
- Use information related to DRGs, the cost of each diagnosis, the allocated length of stay, and the treatments and procedures generally used for each diagnosis to review resources and evaluate the efficiency of care given.
- Assess variances for each DRG and act immediately to control these variances to contain their costs.
- Control for duplication and fragmentation of services provided to the patient.
- Explore strategies to reduce patient length of stay and reduce the number of resources required to manage a patient population while maintaining quality care delivery.
- Maintain a knowledge of the requirements of the payors most frequently used with the client population.

The Managerial Role

- Coordinate care of patients during the course of their hospitalization or outpatient services.
- Establish goals of treatment and length of stay as determined by DRGs.
- Assist in forming the patient's discharge plan.
- Guide the activities, nursing treatments, and interventions of other nursing staff members.
- Serve as teacher and mentor to develop staff and educate them about case management.
- Participate in peer review regarding the management of the caseload.
- Seek peer consultation about cases that are presenting with problems or significant variances.

placed on the nurse administrator. Nurses with young children and an opportunity for a 3-day, 12-hour-shift work week may not have the desire to give up their scheduling freedom to accept 24-hour-a-day patient care responsibilities.

Despite these deterrents, the role of the nurse administrator can be quite fulfilling. Generally, there has been a trend toward graduate preparation as the minimal educational level for nurses pursuing administrative roles (Simms, Price, & Pfoutz, 1985). In the pediatric environment, it is essential that the nurse administrator have a strong clinical background in child health care. For those serving as nurse managers in areas in which children are not the primary focus of care, yet where children are vital recipients of service (e.g., the postanesthesia unit of a university hospital), the manager must still make it her or his responsibility to gain sufficient knowledge about the care and management of children to efficiently direct and supervise the care provided by the staff.

The nurse administrator role spans a broad spectrum of levels in an organization's hierarchy. The nurse may serve as a first-line manager, a supervisor, a department chair, or a top executive. The functions and priorities of the nurse in these roles vary with the organization and with the defined job title and realm of responsibility. The activities of the nurse administrator include serving as a role model, teacher, facilitator, and change agent; managing human and capital resources; participating in self-development and staff and client or community education; participating in research activities; and joining in clinical practice activities as needed. The nurse executive has a major responsibility for the quality of patient care. To achieve this goal, a commitment to family-centered care, a knowledge of the laws and federal regulations that direct health care services to children and their families, and the ability to communicate effectively with this unique population are foundational tools the administrator must use.

Nurse Educator

The role of the nurse as health educator to the child and the family has already been explored in this chapter. Yet another educational role available to the nurse devoted to pediatrics is that of the nurse educator. In this category, an individual can serve in one of two primary settings. The nurse can serve as an educator for students, that is, those entering the professional arena, or the nurse can serve as an educator to nursing staff. Once again, the trend is for those seeking a formal educator role to be prepared at the graduate level (master's or doctoral). In this manner, the person with a master's degree is more likely to come into this role with a knowledge of learning theories, effective teaching strategies, and administrative skills necessary to meet adequately the expectations of the job.

Because more nurses who are not specifically trained in pediatric health care are caring for children, there is a higher demand for child health care nurses to serve in the clinical educator role. Nurses in the clinical setting are required to demonstrate levels of competence regarding the knowledge and skills required to care for the types of patients they are seeing in their daily practice. The child health educator has the opportunity to help others nurses maintain their skills and knowledge regarding pediatric issues of concern. In addition, the educator often plays a pivotal role in providing education to the community to promote the health and welfare of children.

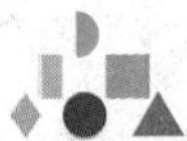

A Note About Certification

Certification is a process in which a voluntary, governing agency validates a registered nurse's qualifications, knowledge, and scope of practice in a defined clinical or functional area of nursing (American Nurses Credentialing Center, 1994). A nurse becomes certified upon meeting eligibility requirements of the certifying agency and upon passing a written examination that tests the nurse's knowledge of current practice standards in a selected area of nursing. Through this process the agency or professional organization acknowledges for the individual and to the general public that the individual has mastered a body of knowledge for a particular specialty (Dickenson-Hazard, 1988b). In some health care institutions the credentialed recipient is entitled to salary increases in recognition of professional achievement. In addition, nurses in advanced practice roles (such as the pediatric nurse practitioner) are frequently required to have met both initial licensure and certification standards to practice in certain states.

There are currently 28 nursing organizations in the United States that provide certification services. The broadest number and scope of certification specialty areas is under the auspices of the American Nurses Credentialing Center. Several other organizations offer certification in specialized areas of child health. In addition, a nurse may pursue certification offered in areas that are not pediatric focused but within whose scope the pediatric patient would be served. Examples of certification in these areas would include services provided by the Na-

Table 1–5
Certification Opportunities

			Qualifications for Certification		Recertification Criteria		
						Methods to Recertify*	
Area	**Credential**	**Certifying Agency**	Current Licensure	Education/Employment	Recertification Interval	*Examination*	*Contact Hours*
Clinical nurse specialist in child and adolescent psychiatric and mental health nursing	RN,CS	ANCC	Unites States or its territories	Master's degree or higher in nursing with specialization in psychiatric or mental health nursing. 800 hours of direct patient contact and 100 hours of individual or group consultation and current practice averaging 4 hr/wk and be currently involved in clinical consultation or supervision and have experience in at least two different treatment modalities.	5 years	Within 5 years	Ongoing consultation/clinical supervision with 1000 practice hours and 75 contact hours of continuing education (CE) courses or 5 academic semester hours and evidence of one published article, book chapter, research project

Table 1–5
Certification Opportunities *Continued*

Area	Credential	Certifying Agency	Qualifications for Certification: Current Licensure	Qualifications for Certification: Education/Employment	Recertification Criteria: Recertification Interval	Methods to Recertify*: *Examination*	Methods to Recertify*: *Contact Hours*
Clinical nurse specialist in community health nursing	RN,CS	ANCC	United States or its territories	Master's degree or higher in nursing with specialization in community/public health nursing practice. 1400 hours postmaster's in area, and 800 of the 1400 hours must be within the last 24 months and current practice to average 12 hr/wk.	5 years	Within 5 years	1500 practice hours and 75 contact hours of CE or 5 academic semester hours and presenter/lecturer in five CE offerings or evidence of publication of one article, book chapter, or research project
Community health nurse	RN,C	ANCC	United States or its territories	BS or higher degree in nursing. 1600 hours within the past 4 years (24 of the last 48 months).	5 years	Within 5 years	1500 practice hours and 75 contact hours of CE or 5 academic semester hours credit within the last 5 years
Developmental disability nurses	RN, CDDN	NLN	United States	4000 hours of developmental disabilities nursing practice within past 5 years.	2 years	At end of 2 years	Documentation of 1000 hours of developmental disabilities nursing practice. 25 contact hours of CE specific to developmental disabilities within past 2 years.
Family nurse practitioner (FNP)	RN,CS	ANCC	United States or its territories	Master's or higher degree in nursing and completed a FNP masters program or postgraduate FNP programs at the graduate level. No minimum hours of care in specialty required.	5 years	Within 5 years	1500 practice hours and 75 contact hours of CE or 5 academic semester hours
Home health nurse	RN,C	ANCC	United States or its territories	BS or higher degree in nursing and practice as RN for a minimum of 2 years. 2000 hours within the last 48 months (300 hours of advanced nursing study may be applied to meet these hours), and current practice minimum of 8 hr/wk.	5 years	Within 5 years	1500 practice hours and 75 contact hours of CE or 5 academic semester hours credit within the last 5 years
Low-risk neonatal nurse	RNC	NCC	United States or Canada	Employed in a specialty area in past 24 months. 2 years, minimum 2000 hours.	3 years	Within 3 years	45 contact hours of CE, 30 of which must be within specific area of concentration
Neonatal intensive care nurse	RNC	NCC	United States or Canada	Employed in a specialty area in past 24 months. 2 years, minimum 2000 hours.	3 years	Within 3 years	45 contact hours of CE, 30 of which must be within specific area of concentration
Neonatal nurse practitioner	RNC	NCC	United States or Canada	Completion of NP certificate or graduate nursing degree in neonatal intensive care. 24 months, 2000 hours.	3 years	Within 3 years	45 contact hours of CE, 30 of which must be within specific area of concentration

Table continued on following page

tional Board of Diabetic Educators, the Enterostomal Therapy Nursing Certification Board, and the National Flight Nurses Association (Dickenson-Hazard, 1988a, 1988b).

Eligibility and recertification requirements for the different agencies vary considerably. Table 1–5 provides a summary of the certification opportunities available for the nurse involved in the care of children. Fee schedules, examination locations, and application information are available upon request from the certifying agency. Addresses for these agencies are printed in the Resources section at the end of this chapter.

Table 1–5
Certification Opportunities *Continued*

			Qualifications for Certification		Recertification Criteria		
						Methods to Recertify*	
Area	Credential	Certifying Agency	Current Licensure	Education/Employment	Recertification Interval	*Examination*	*Contact Hours*
Nursing administration	RN,CNA	ANCC	United States or its territories	BS degree or higher in nursing. 24 months full-time practice within past 5 years, at nurse manager or nurse executive level.	5 years	Within 5 years	Hold middle management or executive-level position, or provide consultive services or education and supervise graduate students for 24 months within the last 5 years, and 150 contact hours of CE or 10 academic semester hours or two of the following: 75 contact hours 5 academic semester hours Evidence of published article or research Participation as lecturer in five CE offerings
Nursing administration advanced	RN, CNAA	ANCC	United States or its territories	Master's or higher degree. 24 months full-time practice within past 5 years, at nurse executive level.	5 years	Within 5 years	Hold executive-level position or provide consultive services or education and supervise graduate students for 24 months within the last 5 years, and 150 contact hours of CE or 10 academic semester hours or two of the following: 75 contact hours 5 academic semester hours Evidence of published article or research Participation as lecturer in five CE offerings
Nursing continuing education/ staff development	RN,C	ANCC	United States or its territories	BS or higher degree in nursing. 4000 hours during past 5 years and current practice 20 hours or more per week.	5 years	Within 5 years	2000 practice hours and minimum of two of the following four categories or double any one: 1. 75 contact hours 2. 5 academic semester hours 3. Evidence of one published article, book chapter, or research project 4. Participation in five CE courses
Pediatric nurse	RN,C	ANCC	United States or its territories	30 contact hours applicable to specialty within last 3 years.	5 years	Within 5 years	1500 practice hours and (two of the following or double any one catagory): 1. 37.5 contact hours 2. 2.5 academic semester hours 3. Presenter or lecturer at five CE offerings. 4. Evidence of published articles, book chapters, or research papers within last 5 years.

Table 1–5
Certification Opportunities *Continued*

Area	Credential	Certifying Agency	Qualifications for Certification: Current Licensure	Qualifications for Certification: Education/Employment	Recertification Criteria: Recertification Interval	Methods to Recertify*: *Examination*	Methods to Recertify*: *Contact Hours*
	RN,CPN	NCB-PNP/N	United States	Graduate with basic nursing education degree or diploma program.	5 years	Within 5 years	One acceptable CE (10 contact hours per year) or academic credit (1 academic credit per year). Documentation must be submitted yearly, beginning the year of the initial certification and continued every year for the 5-year term.
Pediatric nurse practitioner (PNP)	RN,CS	ANCC	United States or its territories	Master's degree in nursing and graduate of a PNP or FNP master's program or formal postgraduate PNP or FNP programs at the graduate level. 600 hours within the past 3 years as PNP or completion of a PNP program within the last 3 years.	5 years	Within 5 years	1500 practice hours and 75 contact hours of CE or 5 academic semester hours
	RN,CS	NCB-PNP/N	United States	Graduate of a program granting a PNP master's degree in nursing or a approved post-master's program. No minimum hours of care in specialty required.	6 years	Within 6 years	Annual self-assessment exercises required by NCBPNP/N for 2 of the 6 years in a recertification cycle—approved for 1 continuing education unit (CEU) (10 contact hours) by NAPNAP. The remaining 4 years may be either self-assessment or completion of 1 CEU (10 contact hours) of approved classes each year.
Pediatric oncology nurse	RN, CPON	CCPON	United States or its territories Foreign applicants can apply	2 years pediatric oncology nursing within past 5 years and supervisor letter verifying candidate has been involved with care of at least 24 encounters with patients per year over past 2 years.	4 years	At end of 4 years	Must meet same qualifications as needed for initial certification process.
School nurse	RN,C	ANCC	United States or its territories	BS or higher degree in nursing and complete a minimum of 15 semester credit hours in selected curriculum areas. a. 200 hours supervised college or university sponsored internship or b. 3600 hours in practice or c. A combination of a and b that totals 3600 hours minimum. (50 hours practice = 900 hours work experience).	5 years	Within 5 years	1500 practice hours and 75 contact hours of CE or 5 academic semester hours credit within the last 5 years
School nurse practitioner	RN,CS	ANCC	United States or its territories	Graduate degree from an approved NLN program and graduate of school nurse practitioner graduate program or formal postgraduate SND program at graduate level. No minimum hours of care in specialty required.	5 years	Within 5 years	1500 practice hours and 75 contact hours of CE or 5 academic semester hours

ANCC, American Nurses Credentialing Center; CCPON, Certification Corporation of Pediatric Oncology Nurses; NCBPNP/N, National Certification Board of Pediatric Nurse Practitioners and Nurses; NCC, National Certification Corporation for the Obstetric, Gynecologic and Neonatal Nurse Specialties; NLN, National League for Nursing.
* The nurse may recertify by examination or contact hours.

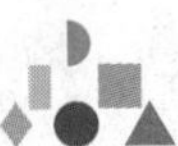

Practice Domains for Care of the Family Unit

Often new graduate nurses are given the impression that there exists but one arena in which their pediatric nursing skills and knowledge can be practiced, and that is the acute care setting. Although this environment might contain a diverse and abundant range of clientele, caring for children and their families in this arena may not be the best match between the nurse's interests, skills, and knowledge and the social milieu of the acute care setting. Providing health promotion, prevention, and maintenance care to the child and the family can be carried out by the nurse in a variety of settings. The clinic, the child's home, a school, a camp, and even the confines of a small plane are environments in which the specialized theoretical and technical knowledge base of the pediatric nurse can be implemented.

Acute Care

The acute care setting provides one of the most rich and diverse arenas for implementing the role of child health care provider. To date, there exist 81 hospitals or medical centers in the United States and four in Canada whose sole focus is on providing acute care or rehabilitative services to the pediatric population. Thousands of additional facilities exist in which pediatric specialty areas (e.g., pediatric units, pediatric intensive care, adolescent units, neonatal intensive care units) are services provided within the arena of a multifocused acute care setting (Fig. 1–6). In addition, because of the changes brought on by managed care and health care reform, nurses in all acute care arenas are likely to have contact with pediatric clients sometime over the course of their nursing practice. It is inevitable, as acute care facilities endeavor to survive in the competitive health care market, that the health care needs of children and their families will transcend nursing units that have been traditionally oriented to adult care. Thus, the opportunities for nurses to serve children and their families in the acute care setting have greatly expanded. In these settings, the nurse must be mindful that interventions and services are provided in a manner consistent with the child's developmental age and current health challenge.

Figure 1–6
A nurse working in a pediatric intensive care unit.

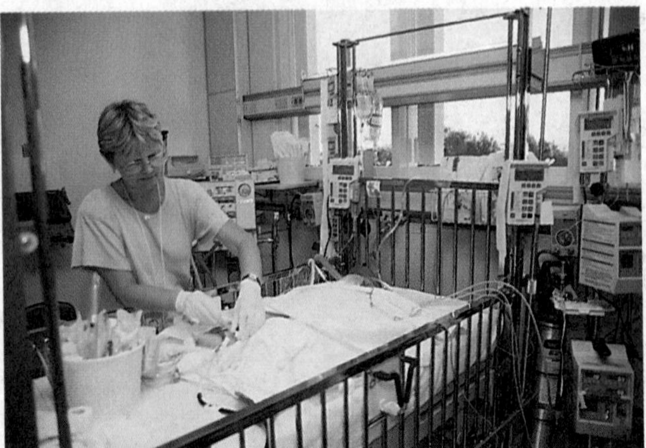

Outpatient Clinics and Offices

For most children and their families, the singular access to and ongoing contact with health care professionals will be through the doors of a clinic or a physician's office. Through long-term, ongoing contact with the family the nurse in this setting has an opportunity to develop a mutually gratifying and therapeutic relationship with the family. The evolving exposure to the well or chronically ill child allows the clinic or office nurse to have a more complete picture of the child's general well-being and ability to achieve developmental milestones. Illness prevention and health promotion activities are the core interventions of the nurse and the nurse's colleagues. For children coping with a chronic illness, the health care team may also focus on maintaining optimum levels of health.

The role of clinic or office nurse is filled with great diversity from day to day. Depending on the size of the medical practice, the nurse may find that her or his work skills and knowledge must extend from bookkeeping to receptionist to laboratory technician. In addition, the clientele may vary extensively. Although the clinic nurse is less likely to encounter the acutely ill or unstable child, the nurse must be prepared at all times for the child who has been managed inappropriately at home and is now in a health crisis.

The clinic or office provides an ideal setting in which to provide health teaching to the child and the caregiver. Several studies have attempted to quantify the amount of time spent by health professionals providing counseling and health teaching during clinic visits. Despite the fact that parents view health teaching as one of their greatest needs, the time spent in this activity is embarrassingly short. One study of pediatricians indicated that the average time for a well-child visit was 10 minutes, with 90 seconds of that time devoted to providing anticipatory health teaching (Reisinger & Bires, 1980). In even the busiest of clinics, the health team can utilize a variety of carefully selected educational media to launch discussions regarding normal developmental milestones, identification and treatment of common childhood illnesses, and therapy regimens applicable to the child's diagnosis. Videos, pamphlets, coloring books, and toys are educational tools the clinic or office nurse can utilize to augment face-to-face discussions with the child and the family.

The clinic or office nurse may also be called upon to participate in research projects directed and approved by the managing health care team. Administering questionnaires, collecting health data, and screening patients for inclusion in the study are but a few ways in which the nurse can utilize research skills. Most important, the ongoing relationship the nurse has established with the child may help to identify any unwarranted side effects of a research protocol.

The nurse working in a specialty pediatric clinic collaborates with an interdisciplinary team to meet the challenges of patients with a chronic or terminal illness. Visits to the clinic by these children often require great coordination to ensure that those in all disciplines who need to see the child are able to do so, to ensure that the family's valuable time is not wasted, and to ascertain that ongoing well-child care is being addressed (Chart 1–22). The nurse serves as a vital link in the communication process between health team members and with the family.

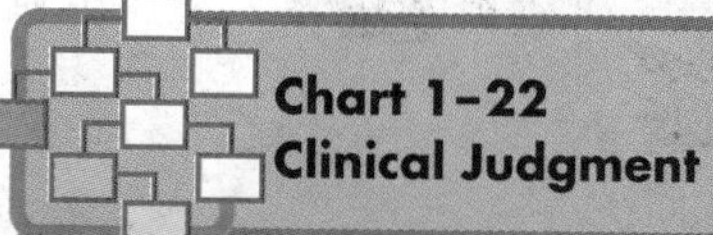

Chart 1–22
Clinical Judgment

Providing Health Care Services in an Outpatient Setting

Tam is a pediatric nurse practitioner practicing in collaboration with a group of family practice physicians. She is responsible for completing all well-child visits and for assessing and intervening in all pediatric minor illnesses that are within her scope of practice. When a child comes to the clinic, vital signs are taken and recorded by a nurse assistant. Tam is responsible for assessing each client, providing the necessary health care interventions, and initiating referral to a physician if indicated. On this particular day, Tam has a very busy schedule.

Questions

1. Tam reviews the vital signs noted on the chart of a 6-month-old being evaluated for a cold. The nurse assistant noted a heart rate of 178, respiratory rate of 62, and temperature of 97°F. Tam enters the room and sees a smiling infant playing in her stroller with no signs of distress noted. What should Tam do?
2. Another child is to receive the varicella vaccine. The nursing assistant has given the family an information sheet about the vaccine. Who is responsible for ensuring that the family understands the information?
3. It is lunchtime and Tam is very hungry. Can she go to lunch and ask one of the physicians to monitor the child in room 3 who was just given a respiratory treatment for an asthma attack?
4. Later in the day, a 5-year-old girl with a hearing impairment is evaluated for her kindergarten physical. What measures should Tam institute to ensure that the child's health needs are attended to in the school setting?
5. Tam has noted that she is seeing more adolescent girls in her practice who are pregnant. She would like to start an educational program for these girls to assist them in adapting to their changing life circumstances. She is not sure which teaching approach might be most effective. How could she acquire this information?

Answers

1. Tam needs to verify the vital signs. She is ultimately accountable for accurate assessment and documentation of the child's status.
2. It is not within the nursing assistant's scope of practice or knowledge base to provide health teaching. Thus, Tam is responsible for all activities related to patient education.
3. It would be appropriate for the physician to monitor and assess the child who has been in distress. It would not be appropriate to assign the same task to a nursing assistant, who lacks the knowledge base and skill to intervene should the child's health condition worsen.
4. After consulting with the child's mother, Tam should call the child's new teacher and school nurse and discuss the child's hearing impairment and strategies to promote the child's success at school.
5. Tam could consult with other nurse practitioners who may have a similar program already established. Tam should review the health care literature and use current research about interventions that have proved to be successful to develop the program.

Community Health Nursing

Historically, public health nursing began in the United States with the work of Lillian Wald and her associates at the Henry Street Settlement House in the 1800s. The health and welfare of subgroups (aggregates) within the population that are at high risk for illness, disability, or death have long been a concern of nursing personnel. Today, two terms, "public health nursing" and "community health nursing," are used synonymously to identify the nursing role and interventions of those who work with families and individuals at the aggregate level. The nurse in the community setting uses skills to study the relationship of environmental, social, and economic factors in a subgroup of patients at risk (Humphrey, 1988). The American Nurses' Association (1980a) has defined community nursing as

> A synthesis of nursing practice and public health practice applied to promoting and preserving the health of populations. The practice is general and comprehensive. It is not limited to a particular age group or diagnosis and is continuing, not episodic. The dominant responsibility is to the population as a whole; nursing directed to individuals, families, or groups contributes to the health of the whole population. Health promotion, health maintenance, health education and management, coordination, and continuity of care are utilized in a holistic approach to the management of the health care of individuals, families, and groups in a community (p. 2).

Within the domain of community health, child health care issues are a dominant area of concern. The nurse with skills and knowledge in child health care can contribute in immeasurable ways to the many child health programs initiated by community health organizations. These programs include efforts to decrease infant mortality and increase prenatal care, decrease the incidence of accidental injuries among children, prevent lead poisoning, provide immunization programs, decrease the incidence of child abuse and neglect, and eliminate adolescent substance use. It has been said that child health status is an important indicator of the health of the nation (Swanson & Albrecht, 1993). Keeping this statement in mind, the nurse with a strong affiliation with children's health issues has the opportunity to affect positively large populations of children and their families through the role of a community health practitioner.

Home Health Care

One of the most rapidly expanding services for provision of health care is the home health care industry (Fig. 1–7). More than 1 million children have chronic conditions that require ongoing health care at home (Kaufman, 1991). Congress has amended federal laws to allow payment for home care services, which are less costly than institutional care. The shift in emphasis and reimbursement from acute institutionalized care to the provision of care in the home or in ancillary clinic settings has advanced home care nursing into a rapidly expanding and constantly changing field of practice (Humphrey, 1988; McClowry, 1993; McClung, 1995). Although home care practices have been shaped by roots in community nursing practice, home care works primarily with ill individuals and their families. Home care requires that the nurse address the environmental, social, and personal factors affecting health, as does community health nursing practice. The emphasis in home care, however, is on working with individuals rather than with population groups.

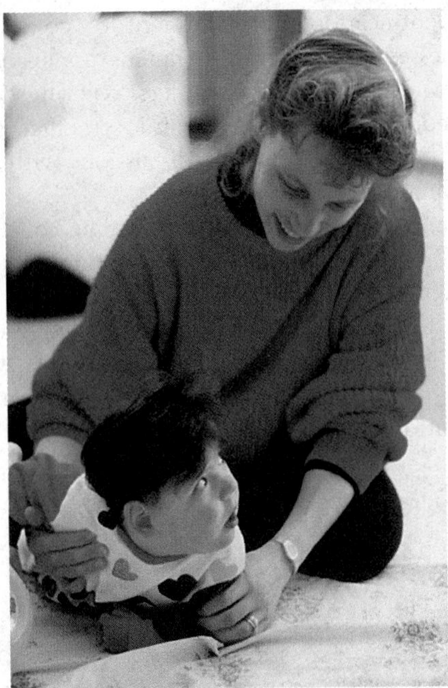

Figure 1–7
The home care nurse works with the child in his familiar home environment to attain his optimal level of functioning.

The National Association for Home Care, an organization that represents home care agencies, hospital home care programs, homemaker or home health aide organizations, and hospices, has defined home care as "services to the recovering, disabled or chronically ill person providing for treatment and/or effective functioning in the home environment." The term "home health agency" refers to a public or private agency that participates in federal insurance programs (Medicaid or Medicare) (Klug, 1992). Home care can assist in the provision of services to adults and children in danger of abuse or neglect. Generally, home care is appropriate whenever a person needs assistance that cannot be easily or effectively provided by family members or friends on an ongoing basis for a short or long period of time (National Association for Home Care, 1987).

Children are referred to a home care agency on the basis of their diagnosis or disease, their need for treatment of a condition, or their need for assistance in working through the end stages of a terminal disease. The focus is on preventing admission to an acute care setting, providing assistance to families, and giving direct treatment in the home (Humphrey, 1988). The environmental, social, psychological, and economic impact on the patient is assessed and included in the treatment plan.

Two of the main differences between hospital care and home care are the environment and the manner in which family-centered care is implemented. In the hospital, there are prescribed standards of practice and a confined area in which to carry them out (Chart 1–23). Hospital treatment plans are well defined. In home care, the standards of care are more ambiguous and the "where, how, and who" aspects of delivering care are less formal. In the home, health care providers have less control over the child's exposure to communicable diseases, hygiene of the home, and equipment available to the child. There may be physical space and financial resource limitations that present unexpected challenges to the health care team.

In addition, it cannot be forgotten that the family's home is their domain. Parents play the central role in implementation of care for the child. Family goals and preferences take priority in the home care plan (Ahmann, 1994d). The need for collaborative practice is critical. Open communication with the family is essential as the nurse works with them to meet the care needs of the affected child. In the home setting, the nurse is challenged to define and maintain a therapeutic relationship with the family. It is not unusual for the home care nurse to develop "family-like" relationships with the child and other family members (Ahmann, 1994d). Close working relationships with the family can make it difficult to distinguish relational boundaries, yet these boundaries are important in order to promote the family's control over the child's care (Ahmann, 1994d). The nurse can facilitate a healthy therapeutic relationship by establishing a contract with the family that outlines the responsibilities of the nurse and the family members. Such items as where to park, the nurse's meals and personal belongings, the child's routine, discipline, how to deal with siblings, and maintaining an adequate work environment are factors to consider and discuss.

Challenges for the nurse in home health care can be boredom, isolation, and a feeling of decreased professional recognition. Supervisory visits to the home, case conferences, and attendance at professional meetings can assist the nurse in overcoming these problems (Klug, 1993).

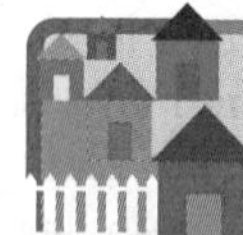

Chart 1–23
Community Care

Contributions of the Community Health Nurse in Pediatric Health Care

The pediatric nurse may be employed by a public or private community health organization to direct and implement federally funded or privately funded programs to improve the health and welfare of children and their families. Some or all of the following responsibilities may be incorporated in this nursing role:

- Advocate for improved individual and community responses to the needs of children.
- Participate in federally funded child health care programs such as Head Start and WIC (Special Supplemental Food Program for Women, Infants and Children).
- Network with other professionals to improve collaboration and coordination of children's health care services.
- Assist school systems to be linked to community health services.
- Act as a catalyst and educator to alert the health professional community, business leaders, religious groups, and voluntary organizations to the needs of children.
- Participate in the development of health care goals and objectives for a community.
- Evaluate the impact of community health programs in meeting the needs of defined populations of children and their families.

Data from Swanson, J., & Albrecht, M. (1993). *Community health nursing: Promoting the health of aggregates.* Philadelphia: W. B. Saunders.

School Nursing

More than 90 years have passed since Linda Rogers was lent to a New York school to intervene on behalf of the health care needs of schoolchildren. Since that time, nurses have become established and required associates of the faculty in both private and public schools. Today's school nurse may be employed by a local school system or by a city, state, or county government agency. The school nurse is required to have obtained a bachelor's degree in nursing and continuing education hours specializing in the role and services of the school nurse.

At one time, a model existed in which a nurse was located at most school sites. Today, with budget cuts presenting continuing challenges to school districts, the school nurse is often found juggling her or his role to meet the needs of several schools for which the nurse is responsible. In these cases, a nurse aide or a health clerk may be responsible for monitoring minor day-to-day health problems at a school's site. The nurse is responsible for overall management and delegation of activities to the aides and for evaluating the appropriateness of interventions provided to ailing children (Chart 1–24).

The newest approach to providing comprehensive health care to young people, especially those from low-income families, is that of school-based health centers, also referred to as **school-based clinics** (Fig. 1–8). These programs are showing great promise for overcoming barriers of income and access to support health-promoting behaviors among students and create healthier student environments. These clinics are located inside the school grounds and are not the same as school-linked clinics, which are off site and thus not as accessible on a day-to-day basis for the students. School-based clinics try to capitalize on many features associated with easy access—convenience, comfort, confidentiality, and cost. One of the greatest strengths of the clinics is the location. Also important are consistency and availability of clinic staff and affordability. Most clinics' services are free, although sometimes a nominal fee is charged (Kirby, 1985; McClowry et al., 1996; Walker, Bowllan, Chevalier, Gullo, & Lawrence, 1996). In many families, both parents work and do not have the time to take the children to the doctor or are not covered by health insurance. In addition, many children have minor problems they do not even tell their parents about (Vessey & Swanson, 1993). The school-based clinic can address these health concerns and provide health education to students of all ages.

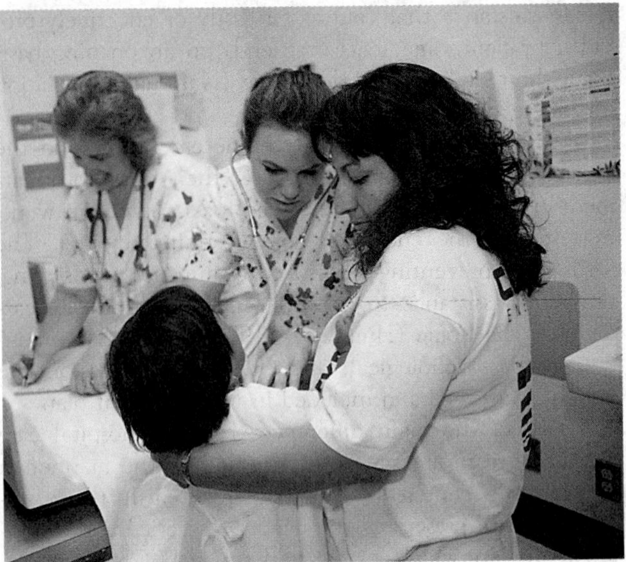

Figure 1-8
School-based clinics are located inside the school to provide accessible and affordable health care services to students.

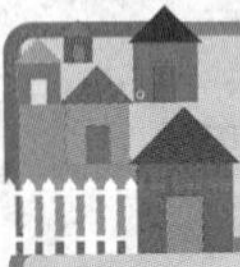

Chart 1-24
Community Care

Interventions of the School Nurse

- Participates in faculty inservice training related to health care issues
- Promotes staff wellness and physical fitness
- Provides classroom instruction regarding health issues
- Coordinates programs focused on particular high-risk topics such as substance use
- Identifies health-related problems that may be affecting a child's school performance
- Links children and their families to available community health resources
- Provides one-on-one health teaching to students who visit the health office
- Works with community officials to identify, control, and ensure treatment in outbreaks of certain illnesses (e.g., tuberculosis, chickenpox)
- Monitors and evaluates illness episodes within a district
- Applies for grants to support health care activities
- Conducts hearing and vision screening
- Conducts scoliosis screening

In general, staffing within the school-based clinics includes a pediatric nurse practitioner or physician's assistant; a clinic assistant/receptionist; and an assortment of health educators, physicians, nutritionists, nurses, and social workers. The staff are trained to deal with the unique growth, social, developmental, and emotional needs of the school-age population they serve. Activities of the clinic may include once-a-year health fairs, ongoing participation in crisis intervention teams, in-class health education, parent education, teacher training, sports medicine clinics, student health clubs, question-and-answer columns in student newspapers, sponsoring immunization programs, involvement in dropout prevention initiatives, and assessing health risk behaviors of their populations (Lear, 1992). The school clinics are able to address a host of health care problems called the "new morbidities" of youth. These problems include teen sexuality, teen pregnancy, sexually transmitted diseases, substance abuse, and violence (Kisker & Brown, 1996; Lear, 1992). The limited research conducted to date has shown that services provided by school-based health clinics have been directly associated with improving student health, lowering birth rates, raising levels of contraceptive use, and improving school attendance (Dryfoos, 1985; General Accounting Office, 1994). Pediatric nurses, nurse practitioners, and public health nurses are the backbone of these clinics, providing the specialty nurse with a rich and diverse clinical setting in which to develop a rewarding career.

Flight Nursing

Technology, urban development, and specialization in pediatrics all have contributed to the growing domain of flight nursing. The first nurses to seek the air were those recruited by nonmilitary airlines to serve as stewardesses. Having a stewardess who was a nurse was a way to instill confidence in passengers using this revolutionary form of transportation (Stevens, 1994). When World War II began, most carriers dropped the registered nurse requirement because of the urgent need for nurses in hospitals and in the armed forces. As United States involvement in World War II increased, so too did the involvement of registered nurses—to such an extent that hospitals and nursing schools had to beg nurses to stay and support the needs at home. In the 1940s, flight nursing officially began with the establishment of the Nursing Division in the Air Surgeon's Office of the United States Air Force (Stevens, 1994). The flight nurses obtained a reputation for dramatically improving the survival rate of the wounded, establishing a record of only five deaths in flight for every 100,000 transported patients (Piemonte & Gurney, 1987).

Over the years, flight nurses have continued to play a major role in serving military needs for medical personnel aboard aircraft during conflicts. In the late 1960s, the flight nurse role expanded with the nurse working on both fixed- and rotary-wing aircraft (Lee, 1991). Further growth came in 1972 when the first civilian flight nursing began at St. Anthony Hospital in Denver. In 1980, a group of four flight nurses met to develop a national organization for flight nurses. One year later the National Flight Nurses Association (NFNA) was founded, and it has grown to a current membership of more than 1700 nurses (Wann, 1994). Members of the organization receive a newsletter, *Across The Board*, and a monthly subscription to the *Journal of Air Medical Transport*.

The first helicopter transport of a premature infant occurred in 1967. The nurse was Sister M. Andre, OSF, a supervisor at what is now Saint Francis Medical Center in Peoria, Illinois. The 3-pound, 7-ounce baby survived the 202-mile flight from Zion, Illinois, but died 3 days later with congenital abnormalities. With no research literature to consult, these early pediatric and neonatal flight teams had to discover new ways to contend with the influence of factors such as the effects of altitude, temperature, motion, and airplane noise on the sick child. With the growing emphasis on pediatric transport, a Pediatric Special Interest Group has been formed within the NFNA. Approximately 40% to 50% of pediatric air transports involve patients younger than 1 year of age, with 20% to 30% of the children 1 to 3 years of age (Fig. 1–9). Many of the infants seen are technologically dependent and are being transferred to a level III neonatal intensive care unit. Many have multiple congenital anomalies or birth complications. Generally the children are transported to a pediatric intensive care unit or a step-down unit. The most frequently encountered illnesses requiring flight transport include respiratory distress (60% to 70%), neurologic problems such as seizures and encephalopathy (20%), trauma (20%,) and an assortment of problems such as bowel obstruction, sickle cell crisis, ingestions, and burns (A.C. Albers, personal communication, September 15, 1994).

Most air ambulance programs today are sponsored by single hospitals. Hospital consortia, public agencies (such as the Highway Patrol), and a handful of freestanding companies account for only about 5% of the programs nationwide (Wann, 1994). The flight team responding to a pediatric health crisis must possess a variety of specialized skills and abilities. Pediatric specialty teams are typically composed of an RN/RN, RN/MD, or RN/MD/respiratory therapist team. Current recommendations by the National Flight Nurses Association for the registered nurse are as follows:

Figure 1–9
The flight nurse works with the air ambulance team to transport critically ill children to specialized acute care facilities.

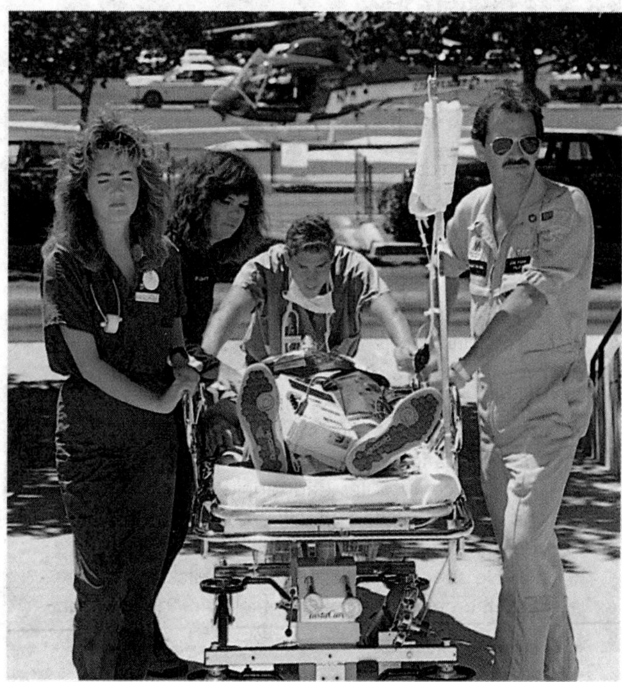

- 3 years intensive care unit or emergency room pediatric experience
- RN with bachelor's in nursing preferred
- Basic life support and pediatric advanced life support validation
- Good physical condition
- Ability to assess physiologic and psychosocial needs of a child rapidly and provide appropriate intervention according to the child's condition
- Ability to evaluate and document the child's response and be prepared to alter the plan of care as needed
- Must feel comfortable working in small spaces and with a limited amount of equipment

Being a flight nurse is a challenging opportunity for the child health care specialist to work with a small team of highly skilled professionals whose job is to always be prepared for the unexpected.

Camp Nursing

For the pediatric nurse who enjoys the challenges of the wilderness, camp nursing can be an exciting respite from other full-time professional responsibilities. There are over 9000 organized camps in the United States attended by approximately 8 million children every year (Pravda, 1988). Camp nurses are licensed personnel responsible for all aspects of health care in a camp setting (Chart 1–25).

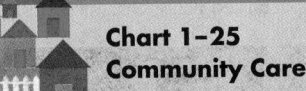

Chart 1–25
Community Care

Responsibilities of the Camp Nurse

- Routine assessment of all campers as they enter the camp (vital signs, retrieval of health cards, evaluation of any identified health concern)
- Dispense medications to campers
- Provide first aid
- Monitor ongoing, nonthreatening ailments
- Assess and triage any major health problems
- Evaluate and reinforce good nutrition and health habits
- Ensure that sanitation requirements are met
- Prepare camp staff prior to arrival of the campers to health center rules and regulations, first-aid and safety tips, and specific information on the campers
- Provide special remedies for homesickness
- Help the children deal with first-time camper fears

Most camps encourage experienced pediatric nurses (2 years or more experience) to apply. Applicants should have basic life support training and basic first-aid training. However, student nurses and nursing faculty can also benefit from the camp nurse experience. For the student, serving as a counselor or nurse assistant can help the individual learn more about normal child growth and development as well as practice technical nursing skills. Clinical placements at specialty camps for the chronically ill offer the student an opportunity to better understand the impact of the illness on the child and the family. Faculty have an opportunity to maintain and upgrade their clinical expertise in a unique setting far from the hospital corridors (Maheady, 1991; Nash, 1987). The camp community also offers an accessible population for nursing research studies.

In addition to the generalized camp setting, there are specialty camps for children with chronic or terminal illnesses. Such camps exist for children with cancer, cystic fibrosis, asthma, and developmental disabilities. One such camp is The Hole in the Wall Gang Camp (THITWGC) founded by Paul Newman, actor, businessman, and philanthropist. The camp was established for children with blood disorders. This camp has an Old West theme, including log cabins, a corral filled with animals, and an old-fashioned dining hall. Newman has added a castle in Ireland as a site for his camps. Another such camp designed especially for technologically dependent children and their families is called SKIP (Special Kids Need Involved People) and is located in Minnesota (Scalise, 1991).

Health facilities at specialty camps permit children in treatment to continue their health care. Because all the children attending the camp are in some phase of a treatment or of a remission cycle, seeing other children undergo various therapies for their condition is not an unusual or unsettling sight. Through the camp experience the children can informally share their concerns or fears with their newfound friends or with counselors specially trained to understand the needs of chronically and terminally ill children.

The primary goal of the specialty camps is to allow the children, who may have had extensive or unpleasant medical treatment and life experiences, to enjoy a real camping experience. The camp programs do not intend to change the children's usual routines or diets, therapies, or resting periods; rather, the children's unique needs are accommodated to enable them to enjoy the experience and leave with pleasant memories (Feeg, 1989). Nursing care is available 24 hours a day, with visits and treatments provided in the child's cabin, if requested (Fig. 1–10).

The safety of the camp setting of group activity for children who may be immunocompromised has come

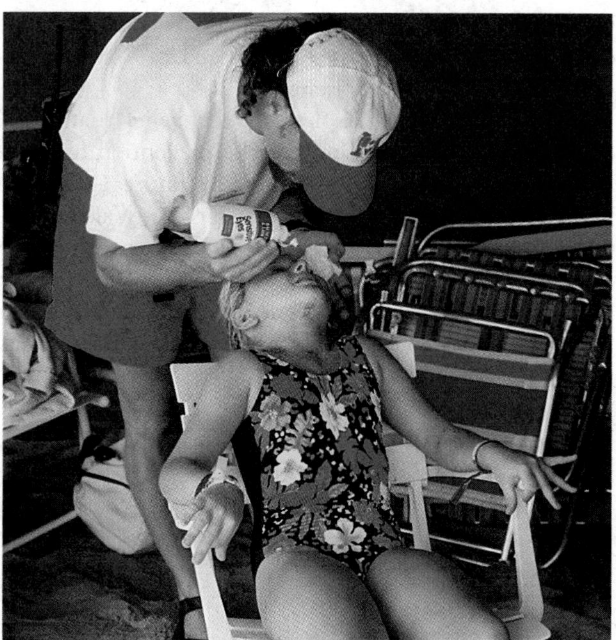

Figure 1–10
A nurse at Camp Ronald McDonald for Good Times applies eye drops to a camper. (Courtesy of Camp Ronald McDonald for Good Times.)

into question. Specifically, those who sponsor cystic fibrosis camps have become concerned that children living in such close quarters, sharing food, clothing, and other articles, may be exposed to one of many antibiotic-resistant respiratory infections that are prevalent among children with cystic fibrosis. Although actions to close these camps have been suggested, a more widely accepted strategy is to increase the vigilant efforts of the health care team to practice and enforce preventive measures to decrease the risk of cross-infection.

Many nurses electing to work as camp nurses do so with the idea that "camp nursing is a nice, relaxing change of pace" or a way to recover from "burnout." Such an idea is misplaced in this environment, where, lacking the technology of the tertiary care setting, the nurse must be quick to assess those who need emergency care, be creative in problem-solving approaches, and always be available with a friendly smile and listening ear. Nurses wishing to participate in these camps must have some experience dealing with the special needs of the children. A variety of books and resources are available to assist the practicing camp nurse (see Resources section). Support for those interested in camp nursing is available through the Association of Camp Nurses. The association seeks to support and develop camp nursing practice by helping to clarify the camp nurse role, facilitate communication among camp nurses, support camp nurse research, and disseminate information developed by camp nurses. Members receive a quarterly newsletter and information about the Camp Nurses Conference.

The camp environment affords an abundance of benefits for the practicing nurse. Some of these benefits are the natural beauty of the camp setting, an opportunity to change one's daily routine, a low-cost way to experience different areas of the country, freedom from the daily chores of cooking and cleaning, the challenge of working as an independent practitioner, time flexibility, and the opportunity to meet and work with children in a healthy environment that promotes their growth and development. Nurses who wish to work in this setting should seek access to the resources provided in this chapter to better prepare themselves for this challenging role.

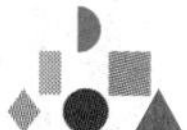

Looking Ahead—The Future of Children's Health Care

The challenges for those providing care to children are many as we face the 21st century. Despite the numerous social, medical, and legal achievements that have been made to secure the health and welfare of the young, several dilemmas continue to confront and jeopardize the health of children. Although the infant mortality rate has dramatically declined since the days of the nurses on Henry Street, infant death rates in the United States ranked 24th among countries or geographic areas with a population of 1 million or more, and the death rate among black infants remains significantly higher than that of white infants (National Center for Health Statistics, 1995). A rising number of adolescents are having children. These infants are often premature or physically challenged in some way. Many are aborted, and some are abandoned within moments of their birth. The challenge to save the lives of infants and children alike remains with us.

How we shall continue to allocate scarce human, financial, and social resources to meet the needs of children and their families is another significant challenge. The focus has long been on providing medical care—high in technology and costs—rather than providing health care. The resources and access to costly medical services are being limited today by the rising cost of services and the growing number of families who do not have health insurance coverage. Decisions regarding allocation of limited health care resources will continue to be a theme in the new century.

These decisions to allocate resources are accompanied by a plethora of moral and ethical concerns. The future of child health care practices will continue to be shaped by the evolution of society's views regarding such issues as the rights of children, abortion, the question of when "life" begins, and the quality of life versus the sanctity of life.

The agenda for our future is being orchestrated by a collaborative effort on the part of all health care professionals. "Interdisciplinary" is not simply a "new age" term, destined to fade away in the years to come. Rather, the concept reflects a vision of health care in which men and women of all disciplines meet on equal footing, sharing their unique skills and knowledge, to provide the most efficient and effective services possible to the child and the family (Kowalski et al., 1996). Health care reform will continue to demand that we work smarter, with less territorial (specialty group) conflict, in a *united* effort to advance child health care practices. To accomplish this, more alliances with the public will be made to ensure the provision of family-centered care and to elevate the health of our citizenry.

Lillian Wald was inspired by the belief that nurses could play a tremendous role in the prevention of illness and the promotion of wellness. The future agenda for health care demands that nurses continue Wald's vision of these services. As we continue to deal with the issues of abuse, adolescent violence, acquired immunodeficiency syndrome, and adolescent pregnancy, a key instrument of intervention the nurse can provide will be the prevention and promotion activities that will put an end to these new morbidities of our young. And, just as Wald became an advocate for children in the political and social arena, so too are we challenged to be voices in our communities to promote the health and welfare of the children and families we serve.

Summary of Key Concepts

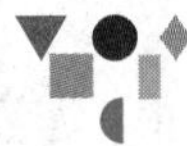

- Family-centered care provided by caring professionals began with Lillian Wald and Mary Brewster at the Henry Street Settlement House.
- Legislation and social policies have been initiated over the past several years that support the health needs of women, infants, and children. These measures have led to a decline in the infant mortality rate and an increase in measures to bring nutrition, schooling, and health services to children faced with social, environmental, or developmental challenges.
- Several specialty nursing organizations exist for the nurse who is interested in working and networking with other professionals to promote health and welfare issues of children and to advance the practice of child health nursing.
- Family-centered care is a philosophy of care that acknowledges the primacy of the family as a unit in the identification, delivery, and evaluation of health care needs.
- In the health care arena, care of the child is orchestrated by an interdisciplinary team of professionals who work together to serve the needs of the child and the family.
- The care path and variance tracking tool are new care plans designed to allow the interdisciplinary team to follow a consistent and planned path of care to better help the child meet selected outcomes in a predetermined time frame.
- Although the roles of the nurse (care provider, teacher, consultant) are similar in different areas of specialization in which the nurse chooses to work, these roles must be adapted to meet the unique developmental needs and health challenges of children whom the nurse may encounter in practice.
- Many opportunities exist for the nurse to specialize in the area of pediatrics. Practice settings for these individuals include the acute care setting, clinics, community health settings, home health care, schools, flight, and camp nurse settings.

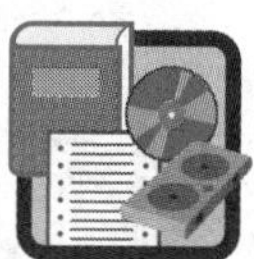

Resources

Organizations

Agency for Health Care Policy and Research
2101 East Jefferson Street
Rockville, MD 20852
(301) 594-1364
Web site: http://www/ahcpr.gov

American Academy of Ambulatory Nurses
North Woodbury Road, Box 56
Pitman, NJ 08071
(609) 582-9617

American Academy of Nurse Practitioners
179 Princeton Boulevard
Lowell, MA 01851
(617) 937-7343

American Association for the History of Nursing
PO Box 90803
Washington, DC 20090-0803
(202) 543-2127
Web site: http://users.aol.com/nursing history.aahn.html

American Association of Office Nurses
109 Kinderkamack Road
Montvale, NJ 07645
(201) 391-2600

American Camping Association
500 State Road 67 North
Martinsville, IN 46151-7902
800-428-CAMP

American Nurses Credentialing Center
600 Maryland Avenue, SW
Suite 100 West
Washington, DC 20024-2571
(800) 274-4262
For ANA membership information and to receive a certification catalog and registration forms

Association for the Care of Children's Health
7910 Woodmont Avenue, Suite 300
Bethesda, MD 20814
(301) 654-6549
(800) 808-ACCH
Web site: http://www.wsd.com/acch.org

Association of Camp Nurses
8504 Thorsonveien NE
Bemidji, MN 56601

Association of Child & Adolescent Psychiatric Nurses, Inc.
1211 Locust Street
Philadelphia, PA 19107
(800) 826-2950

Association of Pediatric Oncology Nurses
4700 West Lake Avenue
Glenview, IL 60025-1485
(847) 375-4724

Association of Women's Health, Obstetric, and Neonatal Nurses
700 14th Street NW, Suite 600
Washington, DC 20005-2019
(202) 662-1600
FAX: (202) 737-0575
(800) 673-8499

Case Management Society of America
8201 Cantrell Road, Suite 230
Little Rock, AR 72207
(501) 225-2229
Web site: http://www.cms.aonline.com

Developmental Disabilities Nurses Association
1720 Willow Creek Circle, Suite 515
Eugene, OR 97402
(800) 888-6733

National Alliance of Nurse Practitioners
PO Box 44707 L'Enfant Plaza SW
Washington, DC 20026

National Association of Childrens' Hospitals and Related Institutions
401 Wythe Street
Alexandria, VA 22314
(703) 684-1355

National Association of Neonatal Nurses
1304 Southpoint Boulevard, Suite 280
Petaluma, CA 94954-6859
(800) 451-3795
Web site: http://www.ajn.org/ajnnet/hrsorgs/nann

National Association of Pediatric Nurse Associates and Practitioners
1101 Kings Highway North, Suite 206
Cherry Hill, NJ 08034
(609) 667-1773

National Association of School Nurses, Inc.
PO Box 1300 Lamplighter Lane
Scarborough, ME 04070
(207) 883-2117
E-mail: nasn@aol.com

National Certification Board of Pediatric Nurse Practitioners and Nurses
416 Hungerford Drive, Suite 222
Rockville, MD 20850-4127
(301) 340-8213
Nationally recognized organization that offers certification to PNPs and pediatric nurses

National Certification Corporation for Obstetric, Gynecologic and Neonatal Nursing Specialists
645 N. Michigan Avenue, Suite 1058
Chicago, IL 60611
1-800-367-5613 or (312) 951-0207
Organization that offers certification for all neonatal nurse and newborn nurse specialty areas

National Flight Nurses Association
216 Higgins Road
Park Ridge, IL 60068
(847) 698-1733
FAX: (847) 698-9407
Web site: www.nfna.org

National Institutes of Health
National Institute of Nursing Research
Mail Stop Code 2178
Building 31, Room 5B03
31 Centre Drive
Bethesda, MD 20892-2178
(301) 496-0207
Web site: http://www.nih.gov/ninr/index.html/

The Society for Nursing History
Nursing Education Department, Box 150
Teachers College,
Columbia University
New York, NY 10027
(212) 678-3946

Society of Pediatric Nurses
2170 South Parker Road
Suite 350
Denver, CO 80231-5711
1-800-723-2902
Web site: http://www/pednurse.org

Visiting Nurses Association of America
3801 East Florida Avenue, Suite 900
Denver, CO 80216
(303) 753-0218

Computer Resources

Center for Nursing Research UT-H
Web site: http://son1.nur.uth.tmc.edu/cnr/cnr.htm/

Midwest Nursing Research Society
Web site: http://www/mnrs.org/

Books and Other Printed Materials

AHCPR Publications Clearinghouse
PO Box 8547
Silver Spring, MD 20907
(800) 358-9295

Provides numerous free publications for people and organizations interested in the quality, appropriateness, effectiveness, and cost-effectiveness of health care in the United States. In addition, individuals may subscribe to the free monthly issue of Research Activities, published by AHCPR, which describes recent findings from research supported by AHCPR and announces grant opportunities, new publications, AHCPR-sponsored conferences, and other information of interest.

Nursing's Agenda for Health Care Reform (1993)
Available from:
American Nurses Publishing
600 Maryland Avenue, SW, Suite 100 West
Washington, DC 20024-2571

Standards and Guidelines for Pediatric Relicensure Nursing Education

National Maternal & Child Health Clearinghouse
(703) 821-8955, extension 254
3201 Greensboro Drive, Suite 600
McLean, VA 22102
Document Inventory Code H112

References

Agency for Health Care Policy and Research. (1996). AHCPR instantFAX contents. Available FAX: 1-301-594-2800.

Ahmann, E. (1994a). Family-centered care: Shifting orientation. *Pediatric Nursing, 20*(2), 113–117.

Ahmann, E. (1994b). Family centered care: The time has come. *Pediatric Nursing, 20*(1), 52–53.

Ahmann, E. (1994c). The United Nations International Year of the Child. *Pediatric Nursing, 20*(5), 529–530.

Ahmann, E. (1994d). Thinking critically about family-centered home care nursing. *Pediatric Nursing, 20*(6), 588–590.

American Nurses' Association. (1973). *Scope of practice for the pediatric nurse practitioner.* Kansas City: Author.

American Nurses' Association. (1980a). *A conceptual model of community health nursing.* Kansas City: Author.

American Nurses' Association. (1980b). *Nursing: A social policy statement.* Kansas City: Author.

American Nurses' Association. (1994a). *Nursing: A social policy statement, 1994 revision.* Kansas City: Author.

American Nurses' Association. (1994b). *Registered professional nurses and unlicensed assistive personnel.* Kansas City: Author.

American Nurses Credentialing Center. (1994). *Certification catalog.* Washington, DC: Author.

Aries, P. (1962). *Centuries of childhood: A social history of family life.* New York: Random House.

Arnold, L., Brecht, M., Hockett, A., Amspacher, K., & Grad, R. (1989). Lessons from the past. *MCN American Journal of Maternal Child Nursing, 14*(2), 75–82.

Atkinson, L. (1976). Is family-centered care a myth? *The American Journal of Maternal Child Nursing, 1*(4), 256–259.

Barter, M., & Furmidge, M. (1994). Unlicensed assistive personnel: Issues related to delegation and supervision. *Journal of Nursing Administration, 24,* 36–40.

Bartlett, E. (1985). At last, a definition. *Patient Education Counselor, 7,* 323–324.

Behrman, R., Kliegman, R., & Arvin, A. (1996). *Nelson textbook of pediatrics* (15th ed.). Philadelphia: W. B. Saunders.

Bower, K. (1993). Case management and critical path systems: Making it real. Paper presented at conference at Harbor-UCLA Medical Center, Los Angeles, CA.

Bowles, K., & Naylor, M. (1996). Nursing intervention classification systems. *IMAGE: Journal of Nursing Scholarship, 28*(4), 303–308.

Bozett, F. (1987). Family nursing and life-threatening illness. In M. Leahey & L. Wright (Eds.), *Families & life-threatening illness* (pp. 2–25). Springhouse, PA: Springhouse.

Brush, B., & Capezuti, E. (1996). Revisiting "a nurse for all settings": The nurse practitioner movement, 1965–1995. *Journal of the American Academy of Nurse Practitioners, 8*(1), 5–11.

Bulechek, G., & McCloskey, J. (1992). Defining and validating nursing interventions. *Nursing Clinics of North America, 27*(2), 289–297.

Burns, M., & Thorman, C. (1993). Broadening the scope of nursing practice: Federal programs for children. *Pediatric Nursing, 19*(6), 546–552.

California Nurses' Association. (1984). *Position statement on specialization in nursing practice.* San Francisco: Author.

Callender-Price, N. (1996). Nurse practitioners move into acute care. *Nurseweek, 9*(15), 1, 7.

Carroll-Johnson, R. (1991). Reflections on the ninth biennial conference. *Nursing Diagnosis, 1,* 50.

Champion, V., & Leach, A. (1989). Variables related to research utilization in nursing: An empirical investigation. *Journal of Advanced Nursing, 14*(9), 705–710.

The changing family structure. (1993). New York: United Nations Department of Public Information.

Cherry, B., & Carty, R. (1986). Changing concepts of childhood in society. *Pediatric Nursing, 12*(6), 421–424, 460.

Clancy, G., & Maguire, D. (1995). Advanced practice nursing in the neonatal intensive care unit. *Critical Care Nursing Clinics of North America, 7*(1), 71–76.

Cohen, E., & Cesta, T. (1993). *Nursing case management*. St. Louis: Mosby–Year Book.

Cohen, S., & Juszczak, L. (1997). Promoting the nurse practitioner role in managed care. *Journal of Pediatric Health Care,* *11*(1), 3–11.

Collin, R. (1995). Nurses in early intervention. *Pediatric Nursing, 21*(6), 524–532.

Cox, H., Hinz, M., Lubno, M., Newfield, S., Ridenour, N., Slater, M., & Sridaromont, K. (1997). *Clinical applications of nursing diagnosis: Adult, child, women's, psychiatric, gerontic, and home health considerations*. Philadelphia: F. A. Davis.

Crane, J. (1985). Research utilization: Theoretical perspectives. *Western Journal of Nursing Research, 7*(2), 261–267.

Department of Health and Human Services. (1987). *Surgeon General's report: Children with special health care needs* (DHHS Publication No. HRS/D/MC 87-2). Washington, DC: U.S. Government Printing Office.

DePompei, P., Whitford, K., & Beam, P. (1994). One institution's effort to implement family-centered care. *Pediatric Nursing, 20*(2), 119–121, 204.

Dickenson-Hazard, N. (1988a). Too many and too much? *Pediatric Nursing, 14*(3), 238–239.

Dickenson-Hazard, N. (1988b). Credentialing mechanisms—what are they? *Pediatric Nursing, 14*(4), 336.

Dryfoos, J. (1985). School-based health clinics: A new approach to preventing adolescent pregnancy? *Family Planning Perspectives, 12*(1), 6–14.

Dunst, C., & Trivette, C. (1996). Empowerment, effective helpgiving practices and family-centered care. *Pediatric Nursing, 22*(4), 334–337, 343.

Edelman, L. (Ed.). (1991). *Getting on board: Training activities to promote the practice of family-centered care*. Bethesda, MD: Association for the Care of Children's Health.

Ellis, J., & Hartley, C. (1995). *Managing and coordinating nursing care*. Philadelphia: J. B. Lippincott.

Etheredge, M. (1986). The maps for managed care. *Definition, 1*(3), 1–3.

Family Service America. (1984). *The state of families, 1984–85*. New York: Author.

Farah, A., Breda, A., & Shiao, S. (1996). The history of the neonatal nurse practitioner in the United States. *Neonatal Network, 15*(5), 11–21.

Fawcett, J. (1985). A typology of nursing research activities according to educational preparation. *Journal of Professional Nursing, 2*, 75–78.

Feeg, V. (1989). A unique setting for pediatrics: The Hole in the Wall Gang Camp. *Pediatric Nursing, 15*(4), 329–332.

Friesen, B. J., Griesbach, J., Jacobs, J. H., Katz-Leavy, J., & Olson, D. (1988). Caring for severely emotionally disturbed children and youth. Improving services for families. *Children Today, 17*(4), 18–22.

Gaddis, M. (1996). Clinical nurse specialist and nurse practitioner role merger. *Central Lines, 12*(1), 14, 17.

Gaedeke, M., & Blount, K. (1995). Advanced practice nursing in pediatric acute care. *Critical Care Nursing Clinics of North America, 7*(1), 61–70.

General Accounting Office. (1994). *School based health centers can expand access for children* (GAO/HEHS Publication No. 95-35). Washington, DC: Author.

Gill, K. (1987). Parent participation with a family health focus: Nurses' attitudes. *Pediatric Nursing, 13*(2), 94–96.

Gold, M., Perrin, E., Futterman, D., & Friedman, S. (1994). Children of gay or lesbian parents. *Pediatrics in Review, 15*(9), 354–358.

Gordon, M. (1994). *Nursing diagnoses: Process and application* (3rd ed). St. Louis: Mosby–Year Book.

Haas, D. (1996). Managed care. *The Journal of the Society of Pediatric Nurses, 1*(2), 95.

Hahn, M. (1996a). Protecting women and children. *Advance for Nurse Practitioners, 4*(2), 53–54.

Hahn, M. (1996b). Spotlight on NAPNAP. *Advance for Nurse Practitioners, 4*(4), 53–55.

Hampton, D. (1993). Implementing a managed care framework through caremaps. *JONA, 23*(5), 21–27.

Hampton, I. (1993). *Nursing: Its principles and practice*. Philadelphia: W. B. Saunders.

Hanft, B. (1988). The changing environment of early intervention services: Implications for practice. *American Journal of Occupational Therapy, 42*(11), 724–731.

Heller, R., & McKlindon, D. (1996). Families as "faculty": Parents educating caregivers about family-centered care. *Pediatric Nursing, 22*(5), 428–431.

Hospital for Sick Children. (1989). *Family centered care philosophy*. Toronto, Canada: Author.

Humphrey, C. (1988). The home as a setting for care. *Nursing Clinics of North America, 23*(2), 305–314.

Igoe, J. (1990a). Beyond green beans and oat bran: A health agenda for the 1990s for school-age youth. *Pediatric Nursing, 16*(3), 289–292.

Igoe, J. (1990b). Healthy people 2000. *Pediatric Nursing, 16*(6), 584–586.

Johnson, B., Jeppson, E., & Redburn, L. (1992). *Caring for children and families: Guidelines for hospitals*. Bethesda, MD: Association for the Care of Children's Health.

Kalisch, P., (1995). *The advance of American nursing* (3rd ed.). Philadelphia: Lippincott–Raven.

Kanter, J. (1989). Clinical case management: Definition, principles and components. *Hospital and Community Psychiatry, 40*(4), 361–368.

Kaplan, S. (1990). The nurse as change agent. *Pediatric Nursing, 16*(6), 603–605.

Kaufman, J. (1991). An overview of public sector financing for pediatric home care: Part 1. *Pediatric Nursing, 17*(3), 280–281.

Kavanagh, K. (1994). Family: Is there anything more diverse? *Pediatric Nursing, 20*(4), 423–426.

Kim, M., & Felton, G. (1993). The current generation of research proposals: Reviewers' viewpoints. *Nursing Research, 42*(2), 118–119.

Kirby, D. (1985). *School-based health clinics: An emerging approach to improving adolescent health and addressing teenage pregnancy*. Washington, DC: Center for Population Options.

Kisker, E., & Brown, R. (1996). Do school-based health centers improve adolescents' access to health care, health status, and risk-taking behavior? *Journal of Adolescent Health, 18*(5), 335–343.

Klug, R. (1992). Selecting a home care agency. *Pediatric Nursing, 18*(5), 504–506.

Klug, R. (1993). Clarifying roles and expectations in home care. *Pediatric Nursing, 19*(4), 374–376.

Kowalski, K., MacMullen, N., Stifter, J., Brundage, J., Slack, J., Strodtbeck, F., & Broome, M. (1996). The high-touch paradigm: A 21st century model for maternal-child nursing. *MCN, 21*, 43–51.

Lange, F. (1987). *The nurse as an individual, group, or community consultant*. Norwalk, CT: Appleton-Century-Crofts.

Lear, J. (1992). Building a health/education partnership: The role of school-based health centers. *Pediatric Nursing, 18*(2), 172–173.

Lee, G. (1991). *Flight nursing: Principles and practices*. St. Louis: Mosby–Year Book.

Lephoe, M. (1996). Managed care brings opportunities for case managers. *Nurseweek*, 9(15), 6.

Lumsdon, K., & Hagland, M. (1993). Mapping care. *Hospitals and Health Networks*, 67, 34–40.

Lyon, J. (1993). Models of nursing care delivery and case management: Clarification of terms. *Nursing Economics*, *11*(3), 163–169.

MacLaren, E. (1994). Basics of managed care. *Nurseweek*, *7*(12), 10–11.

Maheady, D. (1991). Camp nursing practice in review. *Pediatric Nursing*, *17*(3), 247–250.

McCloskey, J. (1995). Help to make nursing visible. *IMAGE: Journal of Nursing Scholarship*, *27*(3), 170, 175.

McCloskey, J., & Bulechek, G. (1996). *Nursing interventions classification (NIC)* (2nd ed.). St. Louis: Mosby–Year Book.

McClowry, S. (1993). Pediatric nursing psychosocial care: A vision beyond hospitalization. *Pediatric Nursing*, *19*(2), 146–148.

McClowry, S., Galehouse, P., Hartnagle, W., Kaufman, H., Just, B., Moed, R., Patterson-Dehn, C. (1996). A comprehensive school-based clinic: University and community partnership. *Journal of the Society of Pediatric Nurses*, *1*(1), 19–26.

McClung, R. (1995). Considerations for the use of a conceptual model in home health nursing. *Pediatric Nursing*, *21*(1), 68–70.

Miles, M. (1996). A historical perspective. *Journal of the Society of Pediatric Nurses*, *1*(1), 46–47.

More, P., & Mandell, S. (1997). *Nursing case management*. New York: McGraw-Hill.

Murdock, G. (1949). *Social structure*. New York: Crowell Collier and Macmillan.

Muuss, R. (1988). *Theories of adolescence*. New York: Random House.

Nash, D. (1987). Summer specialty camps: An overlooked site for student nurses clinical placement. *Journal of Nursing Education*, *28*, 125–127.

National Association for Home Care. (1987). *How to choose a home care agency*. Washington, DC: Author.

National Center for Health Statistics (NCHS). (1995). *Health, United States, 1994* (DHHS Publication No. PHS95-1232). Hyattsville, MD: U.S. Department of Health and Human Services, Public Health Service, CDC.

North American Nursing Diagnosis Association. (1994). *NANDA Nursing diagnoses: Definitions and classification 1995–1996*. Philadelphia: Author.

Nurse Consultants Association. (1984). *By-Laws*. Colorado Springs, CO: Author.

Nursing's agenda for health care reform. (1993). Washington, DC: American Nurses Publishing.

Parkman, C. (1995). Patient care management skills: Delegation and supervision. *Nurseweek*, *8*(26), 12–13.

Pascoe, J. (1996). America's families: Then and now. *Current Problems in Pediatrics*, *26*(5), 159–169.

Passarelli, C. (1987). Marketing the PNP to day-care centers. *Pediatric Nursing*, *13*(1), 11–14, 28.

Peplau, H. (1965). Specialization in professional nursing. *Nursing Science*, *3*(4), 268–287.

Perlman, N., & Abramovitch, R. (1987). Visit to the pediatrician: Children's concerns. *Journal of Pediatrics*, *110*(6), 988–990.

Petryshen, P., & Petryshen, P. (1992). The case management model: An innovative approach to the delivery of patient care. *Journal of Advanced Nursing*, *17*, 1188–1194.

Piemonte, R., & Gurney, C. (1987). *Highlights in the history of the army nurses corps*. Washington, DC: U.S. Army Center of Military History.

Pravda, M. F. (1988). The camp health program and staff orientation. *Pediatric Nursing*, *14*(3), 184–186.

Pridham, K. (1995). *Standards and guidelines for pre-licensure and early professional education for the nursing care of children and their families*. Project MCJ-559327 from the Maternal and Child Health Bureau, Health Resources and Services Administration, Public Health Service, U.S. Department of Health and Human Services.

Quinn, C., & Smith, M. (1987). *The professional commitment: Issues and ethics in nursing*. Philadelphia: W. B. Saunders.

Rankin, S., & Stallings, K. (1996). *Patient education: Issues, principles, practices*. Philadelphia: J. B. Lippincott.

Reisinger, K., & Bires, J. (1980). Anticipatory guidance in pediatric practice. *Pediatrics*, 66, 889–892.

Rushton, C. (1990a). Family-centered care in the critical care setting: Myth or reality. *Children's Health Care*, *19*(2), 68–78.

Rushton, C. (1990b). Strategies for family-centered care in the critical care setting. *Pediatric Nursing*, *16*(2), 195–199.

Rushton, C., Armstrong, L., & McEnhill, M. (1996). Establishing therapeutic boundaries as patient advocates. *Pediatric Nursing*, *22*(3), 185–189.

Scalise, J. (1991). SKIP camp: A summer camp for special kids. *Pediatric Nursing*, *17*(4), 403.

Schwenk, T., & Hughes, C. (1983). The family as a patient in family medicine. *Social Science Medicine*, *17*, 1–16.

Selekman, J. (1995). Standards and guidelines for pediatric prelicensure nursing education published. *Pediatric Nursing*, *21*(6), 541–542.

Shelton, T., & Stepanek, J. (1995). Excerpts from family-centered care for children needing specialized health and developmental services. *Pediatric Nursing*, *21*(4), 362–364.

Shelton, T., Jeppson, E., & Johnson, B. (1987). *Family centered care for children with special health care needs*. Washington, DC: Association for the Care of Children's Health.

Simms, L., Price, S., & Pfoutz, S. (1985). Nurse executives: Functions and priorities. *Nursing Economics*, *3*, 238–244.

Smith, F. (1981). Florence Nightingale: Early feminist. *American Journal of Nursing*, *81*(5), 1021–1024.

Smith, K. (1994). EPSDT and health care reform. *Pediatric Nursing*, *20*(1), 66–67.

Sparacino, P. (1990). A historical perspective on the development of the clinical nurse specialist role. In P. Sparacino, D. Cooper, & P. Minarik (Eds.), *The clinical nurse specialist* (pp. 3–10). Norwalk, CT: Appleton & Lange.

Sparacino, P., Cooper, D. & Minarik, P. (Eds.). (1990). *The clinical nurse specialist*. Norwalk, CT: Appleton & Lange.

Stevens, S. (1994). Aviation pioneers: World War II air evacuation nurses. *Image*, *26*(2), 95–99.

Stolte, K., & Myers, S. (1987). Nurses' responses to changes in maternity care: Part I. Family-centered changes and short hospitalization. *Birth*, *14*(2), 82–86.

Swanson, J., & Albrecht, M. (1993). *Community health nursing: Promoting the health of aggregates*. Philadelphia: W. B. Saunders.

Tripp-Reimer, T., Woodworth, G., McCloskey, J., & Bulechek, G. (1996). The dimensional structure of nursing interventions. *Nursing Research*, *45*(1), 10–17.

U.S. Children's Bureau. (1962). *Five decades of action for children: A history of the children's bureau* (DHEW Publication No. 358). ed. by D. E. Bradbury. Washington, DC: U.S. Government Printing Office.

Vessey, J. (1994). Improving the primary care pediatric nurses provide to children and their families. *Pediatric Nursing*, *20*(1), 64–65.

Vessey, J., & Swanson, M. (1993). School-based clinics and the pediatric nurse: An interview with Surgeon General Designee M. Joyce Elders. *Pediatric Nursing*, *19*(4), 358–362.

Wald, L. (1971). *The house on Henry Street* (reprint of House On Henry Street, New York, Holt and Company, 1915). New York: Dover Publications.

Walker, P., Bowllan, N., Chevalier, N., Gullo, S., & Lawrence, L. (1996). School-based care: Clinical challenges and research opportunities. *The Journal of the Society of Pediatric Nurses, 1*(2), 64–74.

Waltz, C., & Bausell, R. (1983). *Nursing research: Design, statistics and computer analysis.* Philadelphia: F. A. Davis.

Wann, M. (1994). Flight nurses find job satisfaction in the air. *Nurseweek, 7*(14), 1, 8, 21.

Yauger, R. (1972). Does family-centered care make a difference? *Nursing Outlook, 20*(5), 320–323.

Zander, K. (1988). Managed care within acute care settings: Design and implementation via nursing case management. *Health Care Supervisor, 6*(2), 27–43.

Zimmermann, P. (1996). Delegating to assistive personnel. *Journal of Emergency Nursing, 22*(3), 206–212.

Bibliography

Ahmann, E. (1994). Family-centered care: The time has come. *Pediatric Nursing, 24*(1), 52–53.

Buus-Frank, M., Conner-Bronson, J., Mullaney, D., McNamara, L., Laurizo, V., & Edwards, W. (1996). Evaluation of the neonatal nurse practitioner role: The next frontier. *Neonatal Network, 15*(5), 31–40.

Center for Population Options. (1987). *The facts: School-based clinics.* Washington, DC: Author.

Chitty, K. (1993). *Professional nursing: Concepts and challenges.* Philadelphia: W. B. Saunders.

Crane, J. (1985a). Using research in practice: Research utilization; nursing models. *Western Journal of Nursing Research, 7*(4), 494–497.

Crane, J. (1985b). Using research in practice: Research utilization; theoretical perspectives. *Western Journal of Nursing Research, 7*(2), 261–268.

Crumette, B., & Boatwright, D. (1991). Case management in inpatient pediatric nursing. *Pediatric Nursing, 17*(5), 469–473.

Davis, B., & Steele, S. (1991). Case management for young children with special health care needs. *Pediatric Nursing, 17*(1), 15–19.

Dickenson-Hazard, N. (1989). Spotlight on the ANA. *Pediatric Nursing, 15*(1), 72–74.

Edwards-Beckett, J. (1990). The nursing research utilization techniques. *JONA, 20*(11), 25–30.

Ferraro-McDuffie, A., & Booker, K. (1993). Documenting the primary nursing summary note: A leap toward professionalism. *Pediatric Nursing, 19*(2), 189–193.

Gill, K. (1987). Parent participation with a family health focus: Nurses attitudes. *Pediatric Nursing, 13*(2), 94–96.

Giuliano, K., & Poirier, C. (1991). Nursing care management: Critical pathways to desirable outcomes. *Nursing Management, 22*(3), 52–55.

Goodwin, D. (1992). Critical pathways in home health care. *JONA, 22*(2), 35–40.

Hagland, M. (1994). Merger mania? *Hospitals and Health Networks,* 68(10), 46–50.

Hampton, D. (1993). Implementing a managed care framework through care maps. *JONA, 23*(5), 21–27.

Jenkins, J., Covington, C., & Plotnick, J. (1994). Early childhood intervention: The law. *MCN American Journal of Maternal Child Nursing, 19,* 135–142.

Morrison, L., & Fegan, A. (1941). *History of nursing.* Philadelphia: F. A. Davis.

Mosher, C., Cronk, P., Kidd, A., McCormick, P., Stockton, S., & Sulla, C. (1992). Upgrading practice with critical pathways. *American Journal of Nursing, 92*(1), 41–44.

Murphy, M., Gitterman, B., & Silver, H. (1985). Hospital nurse practitioners: A trial approach. *Pediatric Nursing, 11*(4), 269–273, 291.

Muse, V. (1988). Newman's own recipe for giving cheers to kids. *Life,* September, 24–30.

National Organization for Public Health Nursing. (1932). *Manual for public health nursing* (2nd ed.). New York: Macmillan.

Neidig, J., Megel, M., & Koehler, K. (1992). The critical path: An evaluation of the applicability of nursing case management in the NICU. *Neonatal Network, 11*(5), 45–52.

Pittman, K. (1992). Awakening child consumerism in health care. *Pediatric Nursing, 18*(2), 132–136.

Plotnick, J., & Presler, B. (1996). Rugged individualism and compassion: The foundation of public policy. *MCN, 21,* 20–33.

Redick, E., Stroud, A., & Kurack, T. (1994). Expanding the use of critical pathways in critical care. *Dimensions of Critical Care Nursing, 13*(6), 316–324.

Redman, B. (1993). *The process of patient education.* St. Louis: C. V. Mosby.

Ruch, L. (1996). Long-term pediatric care in the managed care environment. *Nursing Management, 27*(4), 40–43.

Rushton, C. (1990a). Family-centered care in the critical care setting: Myth or reality? *Children's Health Care, 19*(2), 68–78.

Rushton, C. (1990b). Strategies for family-centered care in the critical care setting. *Children's Health Care, 16*(2), 195–200.

Ruth-Sanchez, V., Lee, K., & Basque, E. (1996). A descriptive study of current neonatal nurse practitioner practice. *Neonatal Network, 15*(5), 23–29.

Smith, F. (1981). Florence Nightingale: Early feminist. *American Journal of Nursing, 81*(5), 1021–1024.

Sparacino, P., & Cooper, D. (1990). The role components. In P. Sparacino, D. Cooper, & P. Minarik (Eds.), *The clinical nurse specialist* (pp. 11–40). Norwalk, CT: Appleton & Lange.

Steele, S. (1993). Nurse and parent collaborative case management in a rural setting. *Pediatric Nursing, 19*(6), 612–615.

Thompson, D., & Maringer, M. (1995). Using case management to improve care delivery in the NICU. *MCN American Journal of Maternal Child Nursing, 20,* 257–260.

U.S. Children's Bureau. (1924). *Prenatal care* (Publication No. 4). Washington, DC: U.S. Government Printing Office.

U.S. National Commission to Prevent Infant Mortality. (1988). *Death before life: The tragedy of infant mortality.* Washington, DC: Author.

U.S. Public Health Service. (1979). *Healthy people: The surgeon general's report on health promotion and disease prevention* (DHEW Publication No. PHS 79-55071). Washington, DC: U.S. Government Printing Office.

U.S. Public Health Service. (1980). *Promoting health/preventing disease: Objectives for the nation.* Washington, DC: U.S. Government Printing Office.

Vikell, J. (1991). The process of quality management. *Pediatric Nursing, 17*(6), 618–619.

Walizer, E. (1996). Family perspectives on the nurse's nurturing role. *Pediatric Nursing, 22*(6), 537–539.

Weinstein, R. (1991). Hospital case management: The path to empowering nurses. *Pediatric Nursing, 17*(3), 289–294.

Zedelman, L. (Ed.). *Getting on board: Training activities to promote the practice of family-centered care*. Bethesda, MD: Association for the Care of Children's Health.

Current Issues in Child and Family Nursing

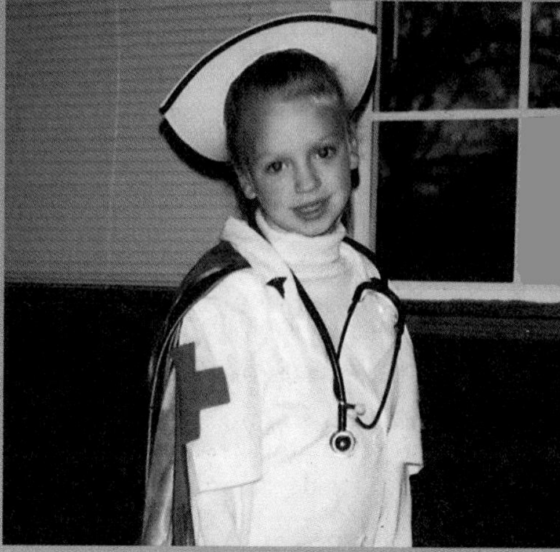

CHAPTER

2

OUTLINE

OBJECTIVES

- Review various factors and issues in the sociopolitical and medical arenas that affect the care of children and their families.
- Render culturally competent and sensitive care.
- Report the available resources for child advocacy groups and child-focused organizations.
- Describe ethical principles that may affect the care of children and their families.
- Review the legal rights of minors and emancipated minors.
- Review the legal rights of parents.
- Examine the issues related to informed consent of minors.
- Examine the difference between the quality and sanctity of life.
- List safety and documentation strategies unique to caring for children.
- Present a summary of research issues to date in family nursing care, specifying design, methods, content focus, and results.
- Identify areas in family nursing care in which more research is needed.

KEY TERMS

advance directives
durable power of attorney
emancipated minor
Healthy Children 2000
informed consent
Patient Self-Determination Act of 1990
Universal Declaration of Human Rights

Poised at the advent of the 21st century, children and their families face problems that challenge their general health and welfare as never before. New or persistent challenges include those related to such trends as rapid technological advancement, steady world population growth, continued environmental decline, and, in the United States specifically, fundamental changes in the health care delivery system.

Nursing care of children and their families must take into account diverse developmental, technological, ethical, and safety issues. Research-based decisions for practice must guide the way, rather than complete reliance on traditional learning styles to which nurses have become accustomed.

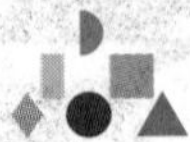

The State of Children's Health

As we enter the 21st century, important trends in child health include the following (Society of Pediatric Nurses, 1995c):

- Increasing numbers of children with no or inadequate medical insurance coverage
- The development of managed care
- Increasing costs and decreasing profits
- Consolidation of community pediatric units in suburban and small town hospitals
- Growth of children's hospitals (especially within hospitals and medical centers)
- A shift to ambulatory care and outpatient care in short procedure units
- An increasing youth market

At the Society of Pediatric Nurses (SPN) national conference in March 1995, a group of nurses caring for children came up with 29 critical issues in child health; see Chart 2–1 (Velsor-Friedrich, 1995).

Major Threats to Children's Health

In the 10 years between 1977 and 1987, a national target set for 1990 was reached with a 21% decline in the rate of overall childhood mortality (U.S. Department of Health and Human Services, 1992). But even as technological advances and improvements in health care delivery continue to lower childhood mortality rates, many factors still threaten the health of children.

Factors Affecting Neonates

Neonates are vulnerable in any society in which barriers to care exist. Such barriers can be related to such factors as inadequate funding of health programs, no health insurance or inadequate insurance, or the perceptions of health care seekers.

Poor Prenatal Care

Approximately 50% of the pregnancies in the United States are unplanned or unintended, mistimed, or totally unwanted (U.S. Department of Health and Human Services, 1992). Unplanned pregnancy is associated with poor prenatal care. When prenatal care is sought in the first trimester, outcomes improve (U.S. Department of Health and Human Services, 1992).

Adequate prenatal care has three basic components (U.S. Department of Health and Human Services, 1992, p. 3):

- Early and continuing risk assessment
- Health promotion
- Medical, nutritional, and psychosocial interventions and follow-up

Nurses and other health care providers need to focus on modifying behaviors and lifestyles that affect birth outcomes of pregnant women. Those behaviors best addressed before pregnancy include smoking, substance abuse, and poor nutrition and those creating psychosocial problems, such as no financial income for the woman

Chart 2–1

Critical Issues in Child Health

- Teenage pregnancies
- Premature and low-birth-weight infants
- Childhood poverty (restructuring of Medicaid)
- Infant mortality
- Child death rates related to unintentional injuries
- Child abuse/neglect
- Teen deaths related to violence (including gang crimes)
- Number of teens not in school and not in labor force
- Homelessness
- Sexual activity and sexually transmitted diseases
- Lack of access to health care
- Lack of health insurance
- Lack of immunizations
- HIV exposure, seropositivity/AIDS
- Restructuring of nursing services

This is a partial list from the March 1995 Society of Pediatric Nurses Conference (Velsor-Friedrich, 1995). Issues included here ranked highest among total of about 29.

and her child. Other areas of concern include family and genetic history, medical problems and chronic illness, and a history of short pregnancy intervals (U.S. Department of Health and Human Services, 1992).

Adolescent Pregnancy

The pregnant adolescent and her offspring are especially vulnerable to lack of prenatal care. Extreme changes in the body that occur during adolescence, largely hormonal and skeletal, often lead to lack of awareness of a pregnancy in the early stages. In addition, the adolescent's lack of knowledge regarding her body and its functions may contribute to this. Further disruptions can occur to family relationships when an unexpected pregnancy occurs. The incidence of prematurity is significantly increased and prognostically poor when the mother is younger than age 15, for physical and psychological reasons.

Neonatal Mortality

The United States can document a steady decline in neonatal mortality rates, including a drop from 29.2 per 1000 live births in 1950 to 10.1 in 1987 (U.S. Department of Health and Human Services, 1992). However, the United States compares poorly with other industrialized countries in providing adequate care for all mothers and infants. The following quotation describes the situation in the United States:

> The continuing disparities between minority and majority populations represent a major health challenge. In 1987, the mortality rate for black infants was still over twice that of whites, and rates for some American Indian tribes and for Puerto Ricans were also considerably higher than for white infants. (U.S. Department of Health and Human Services, 1992, p. 3)

These disparities are related to a myriad of inequities in the United States system of care delivery, including the following:

- Access to prenatal care
- Availability of money, at the individual and institutional levels
- Availability and proximity of services to the underserved, especially urban and rural poor. Cultural beliefs, values, and behaviors surrounding pregnancy and birth influence access to care from both patient and provider perspectives. Improving the health of all mothers and neonates remains a national challenge (U.S. Department of Health and Human Services, 1992).

Preterm and Other High-Risk Neonates

Preterm birth is related to poor long-term outcomes for neonates, including increased mortality. Factors associated with preterm birth include the following (Beachy & Deacon, 1993):

- Low maternal weight before pregnancy
- Low socioeconomic status
- Single marital status
- Use of narcotics and smoked tobacco
- Nulliparity
- Anemia (hemoglobin < 11 g/dL)
- Poor or no prenatal care

Preterm neonates have twice the incidence of congenital anomalies or severe developmental delays than healthy term neonates (U.S. Department of Health and Human Services, 1992). Early intervention in the first 6 months of life can improve outcomes of preterm neonates who have experienced disabling conditions in less than optimal environments (such as neonatal intensive care units) (Parker, Zahr, Cole, & Brecht, 1991).

Rates of human immunodeficiency virus (HIV) infection and cocaine addiction in neonates are on the rise. More than 2000 neonates were born with known HIV infection by 1990 (U.S. Department of Health and Human Services, 1992). Hospitals from some urban communities calculated that 20% of the neonates born in their institutions had cocaine addiction (U.S. Department of Health and Human Services, 1992). This estimate did not include neonates whose mothers had at some point used cocaine or other illegal drugs during the pregnancy but had subsequently quit.

Factors Affecting Children and Adolescents

Major threats to the health of children and adolescents include

- Accidents
- Violence
- Substance abuse
- Sexually transmitted diseases

Other, less urgent but still significant problems affecting health later in life include excessive dietary fat intake and lack of exercise and participation in physical education programs. In addition, the incidences of psychological, emotional, and learning disorders and chronic physical impairments are rising in children (U.S. Department of Health and Human Services, 1992).

Accidents

For people younger than age 25, excluding the first year of life, accidents are the leading cause of death. Approxi-

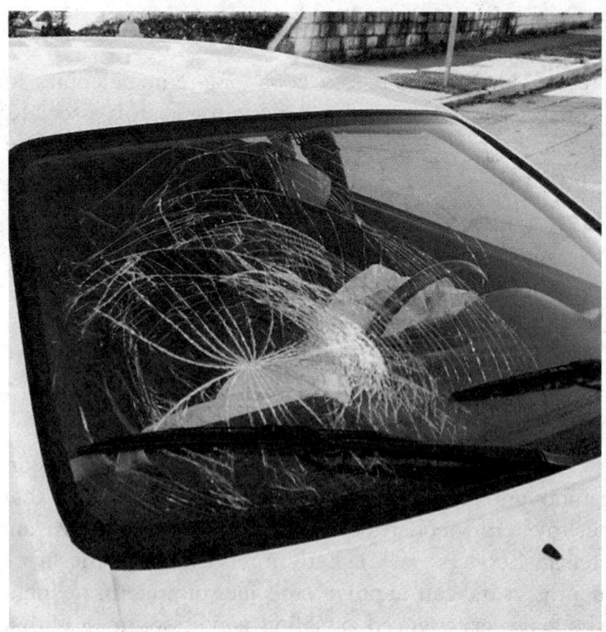

Figure 2–1
Accidents involving motor vehicles are a leading cause of injury and death in children and adolescents. Deployed airbags have resulted in the deaths of more than 35 infants, children, and small adults. All children younger than 12 years of age should ride in the back seat. (Courtesy of Jared Isaacs.)

mately half the deaths in this age group are accidental. Motor vehicle accidents top the list (Fig. 2–1), followed by drowning, fire-related injuries, and burns. More than 50% of the fatalities from motor vehicle accidents in this age group involved the illegal use of alcohol. In the early 1980s, this trend decreased as many states raised the minimum drinking age, but it is on the rise again (U.S. Department of Health and Human Services, 1992).

For infants up to age 1 year, accidents are the fourth ranking cause of death, after certain perinatal conditions, congenital anomalies, and sudden infant death syndrome (SIDS) (National Safety Council, 1995).

The rates of almost all types of injury-related deaths, including those from motor vehicle accidents, drowning, falls, poisoning, and fires, have declined with the increased acceptance of preventive safety measures. The lone major exception is homicide (U.S. Department of Health and Human Services, 1992).

Violence

Today there is an unprecedented epidemic of violence among children and youth. Stories of crime and abuse in the young appear in the media with numbing regularity and present a scientific challenge for outcome measurement of subsequent antisocial behavior (Bower, 1996). The problem is not limited to the United States, although there is an international perception that the United States is a country prone to exceptional amounts of violence involving guns and other weapons. Gang violence is another societal problem involving youths of both genders. There have been many campaigns to decrease youth violence, but all too often this problem is ignored until a tragic incident startles the public.

Family violence is not a new problem, but it becomes new for each generation as it is passed on. Some suggest that the decline of societal mores and the extended family contributes to this problem (Castiglia, 1995). Without a social network available, isolation contributes to inflammatory situations in the home.

Firearms are available to children in rural, suburban, and urban settings—wherever firearms are present. For adolescents, handguns are readily available "on the street" for a modest price. It is estimated that 80% of all deaths attributed to firearms occur in people age 10 to 19 years (Ozmar, 1994). Most handguns in the possession of children or adolescents were taken from their own homes (Benkert et al., 1995). Guns are found in more than 50% of the households in the United States (Benkert et al., 1995). Guns are taken to school, athletic and other public events, and anywhere else that an adolescent is likely to go. They may turn up at the bedside of an adolescent patient. Very young children have been injured by unintentional gunshot wounds inflicted by themselves or a playmate with a gun obtained at home—a gun that may have been mistaken for a realistic-looking toy gun (Fig. 2–2).

The bullet may be perceived as a pathogen, like any other killer disease (Benkert et al., 1995). In the last decade, there has been an increase of more than 20% in death by firearms among minors, with most of these deaths occurring in the home (Chart 2–2). There has

Figure 2–2
A child can easily mistake a real handgun for a very realistic-looking toy gun, with possibly tragic results. Can you identify the real gun? (It's the one on the bottom.)

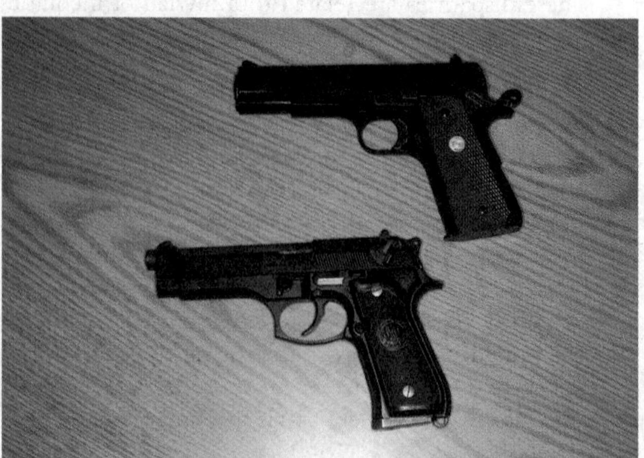

Chart 2–2

Breakdown of Firearm Injuries by Intent of Use

Age 1–9: Half are unintentional and half are homicide.

Age 10–14: One third each for homicide, suicide, and unintentional death.

Age 15–19: Eight percent of firearm deaths are unintentional. Of the remaining deaths, 48% are homicide and 42% are suicide.

Data from Benkert et al., 1995.

been a concomitant rise in the number of juveniles arrested as perpetrators (Fig. 2–3). Sadly, when there is a gun in the house, the risk for suicide increases sixfold (Benkert et al., 1995).

Substance Abuse

Substance abuse, including use of all forms of tobacco, marijuana, common household products as inhalants, traditional narcotics and opiate derivatives, cocaine products, and hallucinogenics, is not a new phenomenon. It remains a major problem; moreover, it has become more common in even younger youths. The current level of illicit drug involvement among the youth of the United States is alarming (Rollins, 1995). (See Chapter 29 for more details.)

The illegal use of tobacco products, while also not a new problem, creates serious damage in the lives of approximately 19% of adolescents (Hardy Havens, 1996). Congress and the President have active plans in progress to reduce the availability and attractiveness of tobacco products to youth.

Sexually Transmitted Diseases

Along with the other "new morbidities of youth" are sexually transmitted diseases (STDs), including HIV infection, the cause of acquired immunodeficiency syndrome (AIDS). STDs are not new; they have been around for thousands of years with periods of quiescence and resurgence. It is beyond the scope of this chapter to discuss each STD fully. However, it is a responsibility of the nurse to possess a working knowledge base about who contracts these diseases and how they are transmitted. STDs find victims even among the very young, through sexual abuse and maternal-to-newborn transmission.

If an STD or sexual abuse is suspected, or if a young person seems concerned that an exposure may have occurred, then appropriate specimens should be collected and diagnostic tests carried out, even if a detailed verbal history renders an unclear picture of the situation.

Factors Affecting Families

Families are under intense pressure in modern society. Factors that threaten the health status of children also often put the integrity of the family unit itself at risk. Such factors include the effects of poverty and inadequate or absent health insurance.

Poverty

In the United States, an estimated 25% to 30% of children live at or below the poverty level (U.S. Department of Health and Human Services, 1992). Yet the United States is currently the richest country in the world. Poverty and the lack of access to health care that often accompanies poverty clearly cause significant damage in children's lives (Bower, 1994).

The link between poverty and disease incidence is clear (U.S. Department of Health and Human Services, 1991). For example, children and adults living in industrial, lower socioeconomic neighborhoods have a higher incidence and more difficult cases of asthma as a result of exposure to the smoke of pollutants. It is documented

Figure 2–3

Increasing numbers of older children and adolescents are involved in serious crimes against persons and property.

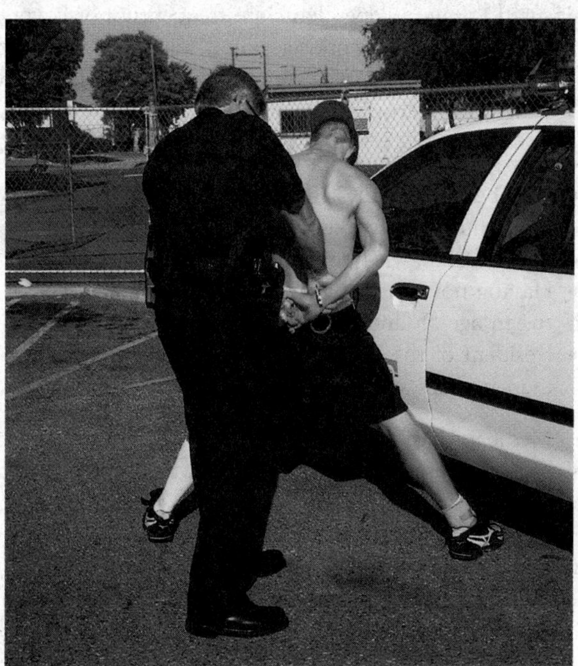

that African Americans have higher asthma-related mortality rates than Caucasians, especially in young age groups. The asthma-related mortality rate in African Americans has increased significantly during the last decade (U.S. Department of Health and Human Services, 1991). Lack of access to medical care is another risk factor for asthma-related deaths, owing to life-threatening delays and complacency (U.S. Department of Health and Human Services, 1991).

Lack of Health Insurance

Almost one in four children in the United States (22.6%) is without health insurance for at least 1 month before age 3 years (News, 1996). The most vulnerable group of children to go without health insurance coverage are those among the working poor (News, 1996). The ever-increasing number of uninsured and underinsured Americans is related to multiple factors, including the following (Society of Pediatric Nurses, 1995c):

- The linkage of health care insurance to employers' ability and willingness to provide coverage, especially to dependents
- The failure of national health care reform legislation to pass
- Inadequacy of coverage by block grants at the state level and increasing costs of health care
- Increasing numbers of persons working in small or self-owned businesses who are unable to provide coverage and have only low socioeconomic job opportunities

Being underinsured has as much an impact as being uninsured, because dependents are frequently not covered at all if there is one working parent with an inadequate policy. The underinsured are most likely to have the following characteristics (Davis, 1994):

- Low socioeconomic status
- Member of a family without a worker or with a minimum wage worker
- Being female with dependent children
- Having nongroup health insurance coverage (between age 55 and 65 in fair or poor health)
- Resident of the Southern United States or outside metropolitan areas

Medicaid has an important role in access to care for uninsured children; however, only one third of poor children are covered. Few states have supplemental funding beyond Medicaid to cover children who are not eligible for Medicaid (Davis, 1994). Another source of concern is increasingly higher turnover in Medicaid enrollment. This is related to changes in employment, with people who were enrolled for a period having been uninsured both before entering and after leaving the program (Davis, 1994). The very poor and unemployed are often covered by public aid programs, whereas the working poor may not qualify for those services. The impact on these families is greater, because they wait longer to seek care and may forgo preventive measures.

With the proposed reform in Medicaid spending, and allocation of federal dollars becoming more and more scarce, it may not matter whether block grants are the "solution." Currently, many legislators assert that the state governments know best how to take care of their own problems. If this becomes a political reality, allocations of health care resources will be distributed according to the value systems of those in power in the state legislature and their political appointees.

Child Health Initiatives

Given the myriad of problems facing children today, setting priorities for child health initiatives is a challenge. Although this challenge was taken up in the early 1990s with the publication of *Healthy People 2000* and *Healthy Children 2000*, the goals set out in these publications have yet to be met (Dunn, 1995; U.S. Department of Health and Human Services, 1996).

Healthy Children 2000

Healthy Children 2000 (U.S. Department of Health and Human Services, 1992) is a special compendium of 170 national health promotion and disease prevention objectives adapted from the full set of 300 objectives published as *Healthy People 2000: National Health Promotion and Disease Prevention Objectives* (U.S. Department of Health and Human Services, 1990). In 1991, the Maternal and Child Health Bureau of the Health Resources and Service Administration, Public Health Service, U.S. Department of Health and Human Services (DHHS) published guidelines that set an agenda to accomplish national health promotion and disease prevention objectives related to mothers, infants, children, adolescents, and youth (U.S. Department of Health and Human Services, 1992, 1996). The family is viewed as the primary unit for the delivery of health services to infants, children, and youth. The family is seen as a principal influence on a child's development and an intermediary between the child and the outside world, including the health care system.

The guidelines in *Healthy Children 2000* are intended for use by policy makers and program managers nationwide, in both public and private sectors. They reflect the three broad goals of *Healthy People 2000*, which are to

- Increase the span of healthy life for Americans
- Reduce health disparities among Americans

- Achieve access to preventive services for all Americans

These ambitious health objectives require collaboration by all invested in the future of the children of our nation in order to achieve the proposed outcomes. The guidelines are a product of a national process. They are deliberately comprehensive in addressing disease prevention and health promotion to allow local communities and states to set priorities for activities from among the recommendations.

As a nation, there is progress being made toward these goals state by state. Each state is free to tailor the opportunities to meet these goals to its own needs. The political climate in the country has changed dramatically since the late 1980s and early 1990s when *Healthy People 2000* and *Healthy Children 2000* were forged. In the latter part of the 1980s and early 1990s, there was Welfare, Medicare, and Medicaid reform. However, the Health Insurance Reform Act of 1996 may help families among the indigent and working poor to achieve greater access for reasonable health insurance options. As we enter the next millennium, there will be juggling and continued stress for vulnerable populations while the implementation of new legislation plays itself out.

Nurses caring for children can work to achieve the goals of *Healthy Children 2000* in a variety of ways. Health status indicators are a reflection of the degree of success. The complex nature of children's health problems occurs at the level of complex sociopolitical forces. Nurses caring for children must be aware that governmental reform in social programs "threatens the safety net for children with special health needs (e.g., Supplemental Security Income [SSI] and children in poverty)" (Dunn, 1995, p. 28A). Education must be structured to include social and political activism. Health promotion and disease prevention should constitute the basis for our health care system (Dunn, 1995).

Child Advocacy Groups and Child-Focused Organizations

Numerous organizations advocate for the health and well-being of children. Some of them are profit- and industry-oriented; however, the majority are nonprofit and have a specific purpose. Most of these organizations are legitimate, with the interests of their intended recipients clearly in mind. They range from unifocal groups that center on one specific condition, such as a specific genetic disorder, to broad and multipurpose organizations like the Easter Seal Society, whose primary focus is the prevention of birth defects. The addresses and telephone numbers of the national offices of these important organizations are included in the Resources List at the end of this chapter. In addition, listings for specialty organizations, such as the Epilepsy Foundation of America, can be found within the appropriate chapters in this book. Specialty and rights organizations arise out of a perceived need in the communities that they serve. These "communities" may be local or national, depending on the numbers of people affected. An example of a smaller organization with a national focus would be the Turner's Syndrome Society of the United States.

Other organizations with broader foci attempt to alleviate the fragmentation of social and health care services that are available to children. The Institute for Child Health Policy (ICHP), an organization within Florida's state university system, was designed to avoid fragmentation of services to children via assistance to federal, state, and local officials and staff. In addition, they help for-profit and nonprofit organizations improve knowledge and skills in child health policy and programs in several ways: development and coordination of policy, training, and applied research (Institute for Child Health Policy, 1995). The Annie E. Casey Foundation (Nelson, 1993), among other children-centered initiatives, seeks rational change through its Child Welfare Reform Initiative. The Initiative seeks to provide more comprehensive, preventive, and cost-effective assistance to families in crisis than currently exists.

National Association of Children's Hospitals and Related Institutions

An important nursing role is putting pediatric patients and their families in touch with organizations that can help them meet their needs. The National Association of Children's Hospitals and Related Institutions (NACHRI) has created a National Agenda for Child Health Care (McAndrews, 1995). Progress is not inevitable for the improvement of children's health care. There are permanent deficits in availability of health and nutrition education. As Medicaid allocations are made, one is reminded of the already unfunded mandates that currently exist. The market cannot reform health care, although this is a belief of many currently holding seats in the legislature. It is up to people interested in the health and well-being of children to help set the priorities in a competitive political climate. NACHRI's diligent integration and setting of national standards helps achieve these goals. With increasing emphasis on block grants to the states, the states will become laboratories for further maltreatment of children whose parents lack the ability to advocate for them (McAndrews, 1995).

Currently, in a worldwide context, the United States is not doing a good job for the nation's children. A preponderance of voters are self-centered rather than other-centered (McAndrews, 1995). Many remain silent and do little to improve needy children's situations. A coalition for America's children has been forged between NACHRI and the American Academy of Pediatrics (McAndrews, 1995). Other organizations, such as SPN, are informally beginning to advance these ideas as well.

Children's Defense Fund

The Children's Defense Fund (CDF) was founded in 1973 by Marian Wright Edelman as an advocacy organization to provide a strong and effective voice for all the children of America, who cannot vote, lobby, or speak out for themselves (Children's Defense Fund, 1996). The organization is especially interested in creative investment in children before the following life-transforming events may occur: getting sick, dropping out of school, suffering family breakdown, or getting into legal trouble (Children's Defense Fund, 1996). Funding for CDF is by private foundations, corporations, and individuals.

World Health Organization and United Nations Children's Fund

In 1990 at a meeting called the World Summit for Children, more than 150 international leaders pledged to meet seven specific major goals in the interest of child survival and development by the year 2000 (United Nations Children's Fund, 1992) (Chart 2–3). The United Nations Children's Fund (UNICEF), in partnership with the World Health Organization (WHO), has pledged to help any nation with its plans by allocating financial resources and expertise. In addition, many industrialized countries have been encouraged to examine ways that they can help, rather than exploit, the survival and health of children in developing nations.

UNICEF has aided in making remarkable progress in developing countries (Igoe, 1990; United Nations Children's Fund, 1992, 1996). UNICEF focuses on a variety of concerns, such as an annual *State of the World Children's Report*, promotion of birth spacing (healthy time intervals between bearing children), life-saving oral rehydration therapy (for diarrheal diseases), and a worldwide immunization campaign.

For nations at peace, UNICEF/WHO initiatives include the following (World Health Organization, 1995):

- Universal child immunization
- Final eradication of polio
- Searching for a "super" (one-shot) vaccine to cover all diseases for which immunizations exist
- Improving birth outcomes by creating opportunities for basic prenatal nutrition (including sources of iodine, iron, vitamin A, and others yet to be identified)
- Creating "baby-friendly" hospitals where breastfeeding is encouraged
- Controlling diarrheal diseases

For children in countries where there are armed conflicts and massive population displacements, planned strategies include emergency relief. Such measures have proven difficult and dangerous for some of the helpers and the recipients involved in United Nations peacekeeping deployments.

Chart 2–3

UNICEF/World Health Organization's Seven Major Goals for the 1990s

- Reduce under-5 child mortality by one third
- Reduce maternal mortality rates by one half
- Reduce under-5 child malnutrition by one half
- Provide access to safe drinking water and sanitation for all
- Provide access to basic education for all children and completion of primary education by 80 percent
- Reduce adult illiteracy rate by one half, with emphasis on female literacy
- Protect children in especially difficult circumstances, particularly in armed conflict

From *UNICEF 1992 report—Review of the year*. Reprinted with permission.

Prevention and Screening Programs

The prevention of unintentional injuries is a major recommendation of *Healthy Children 2000*. Current topics in health promotion include the following (Kimmel, 1994):

- Abnormal patterns of growth
- Childhood nutrition: "from breastmilk to burgers" (Bedinghaus & Doughten, 1994, p. 655)
- Appropriate screening for infants
- Appropriate immunizations
- Injury prevention
- Preventive care for adolescents
- Prevention and appropriate treatment of sports-related injuries for school-age athletes

Specific concerns for well-child care include a variety of newly emerging problems (Kimmel, 1995):

- Office care of the small, premature neonate
- Management of the HIV-positive child
- Assisting with school placement for children with special needs (including the disabled and the gifted)
- The impact of environmental toxins on children
- Common behavioral problems

- Common athletic injuries
- Adolescent contraception

Although these issues have been present in our society—some for many years—many have been largely ignored by providers. Now with mainstreaming medically fragile children into society, more care must be taken to attend to their needs.

The National SAFE KIDS Campaign emerged in response to unintentional injuries being the leading cause of death in children (National Safety Council, 1995). It is a program of the Children's National Medical Center in Washington, DC, but boasts 170 grassroots and local coalitions in 47 states. Injury prevention "saves money because it employs inexpensive, low-tech interventions to avoid the most costly types of care—emergency room treatment and hospitalization" (National SAFE KIDS Campaign, 1994, p. 3). Some of the initiatives being promoted include utilization and implementation of

- Bicycle helmets (to reduce head injury by 85% and brain injury by 90%)
- Smoke detectors (to decrease death in residential fires by 50% with functioning equipment)
- Anti-scald plumbing valves in all home faucets, bathtubs, and showers
- Poisoning prevention (maintaining extant Poison Control Centers at a cost ratio for prevention of $1 to an increase between $4 and $9 for costs of treatment)
- Drowning prevention (water safety education)

The National SAFE KIDS Campaign has already brought some major changes. For every level of the organization, roles have been delineated for the federal government, states, and the local community. The organization's solution to many injury-related problems is incorporated in the "four E's" (Korn, 1995):

- Education
- Enforcement (via public policy such as car seat laws)
- Engineering (of the environment and reinvention of products for safety)
- Evaluation (via statistical data collection through emergency services entry codes to reflect injury frequencies)

The National SAFE KIDS Campaign is an initiative of the private sector. It relies on donations of time, money, and energy by private individuals. The founding sponsor was Johnson & Johnson.

Recommendations for decreasing motor vehicle morbidity and mortality include the use of motorcycle helmets and safety belts (Hardy Havens & Hannan, 1995). Driving under the influence of alcohol or illegal drugs is an increasingly dangerous factor in accidents involving younger drivers (Hardy Havens & Hannan, 1995). The United States Senate has increased the federal role in passing legislation that would require states to lower the allowable blood alcohol content to 0.02% for drivers younger than 21 years (Hardy Havens & Hannan, 1995).

Many other organizations are concerned with injury prevention. The SPN has issued a policy statement on pediatric injury prevention (Society of Pediatric Nurses, 1995a) (Chart 2–4). Many other organizations have been involved in safety campaigns, including Mothers Against Drunk Driving (MADD) and the National Head Injury Foundation.

Nurses caring for children have identified and carried out varied strategies to address the problem of firearm injuries (Benkert et al., 1995):

- Providing gun-safety coloring books for young children
- Making trigger locks available free or at a low cost
- Use of a public health model to increase awareness in the community of this ubiquitous danger
- Changes in rules and regulations in handgun use
- Assistance with programs for safety developed by the National Rifle Association

This is only the beginning. It is essential that additional creative and innovative approaches be initiated by nurses at all levels of practice. All nurses must identify ways that they can reduce this menace in their own communities and take a community-based approach to solving the problem locally.

Other important child health initiatives include reducing the abuse or use of substances such as tobacco (both cigarettes and chewing tobacco), alcohol, and illegal and prescription drugs by children and adolescents. Finally, the overall improvement of nutrition and physical fitness in the young population needs to be a priority.

Screening Controversies

Infant, child, and adolescent screening for a number of disorders is considered in Chapter 7. Developmental screening makes up a major part of the role of nurses working with the young, both on a formal and an informal basis. The National Center for Health Statistics (NCHS) provides sets of normal guidelines for physical growth for children of all ages who are from the United States. These graphs are not norm-referenced and tested for children who are not being raised in the United States. Asian infants and children whose parents have recently immigrated to the United States may not fit in with these norms. Regional differences may exist, so to apply NCHS statistics to children from foreign lands is possibly an unfair comparison. The screening categories addressed in this chapter are discussed because there may

Chart 2–4

SPN Policy Statement on Pediatric Injury Prevention

Injury is the leading cause of death and disability among children in the United States. Annually, more than 10,000 children under the age of fifteen are killed, and another 50,000 are permanently disabled (Wilson et al., 1991). Motor vehicle injuries are the most frequent cause of death, followed by pedestrian/vehicle injuries, burns, falls, drowning, bicycle, and firearm injuries (Children's Safety Network, 1991). The loss or permanent disability of a previously healthy child has an immense impact on the child, the family, and society.

Although the actual medical cost is difficult to determine, the estimated annual total lifetime cost of unintentional injury to children in the United States is $13.8 billion (Rice, McKenzie, & Associates, 1989). There are safety measures and protective equipment that can prevent injury or decrease the severity of the injuries sustained. It is important for nurses and the public to understand that injuries are often preventable. The Society of Pediatric Nurses takes as its mission the promotion of quality health care of children through advocacy for accessible and affordable comprehensive health care, including prevention, acute intervention, and rehabilitative services.

The Society of Pediatric Nurses believes that:

1. Children are our nation's most treasured resource.
2. Many childhood injuries are preventable or can at least be minimized by the use of protective equipment.
3. Preventable injuries utilize a significant amount of resources and health care dollars.
4. The focus of health care providers must shift to primary prevention through education.
5. Pediatric nurses, employed in a variety of settings, have the opportunity to develop and implement injury prevention programs and educate parents and children about the importance of injury prevention.

In an effort to decrease the severity of injuries and the number of injury-related deaths, SPN affirms to:

1. Support pediatric injury prevention programs such as the National SAFE KIDS Campaign.
2. Provide education to SPN members through the newsletter and annual conference, in the area of injury prevention, specifically:
   - Car safety seats/restraints
   - Use of smoke detectors
   - Scald prevention
   - Bicycle helmets
   - Pool safety (i.e., CPR)
   - Firearm safety
   - Poison prevention
3. Encourage members to incorporate injury prevention into their practice.
4. Support injury prevention legislation.
5. Increase public awareness of the importance of injury prevention through active support or national initiatives.

References:
Children's Safety Network. (1991). *A data book of child and adolescent injury.* Washington, DC: National Center for Education in Maternal and Child Health.
Rice, D. P., McKenzie, E. J., & Associates. (1989). *Cost of injury in the United States: A report to Congress.* San Francisco, CA: Institute for Health and Aging, University of California and Injury Prevention Center, The Johns Hopkins University.
Wilson, M., Baker, S., Teret, S., Shock, S., & Garbarino, J. (1991). *Saving children: A guide to injury prevention.* New York: Oxford University Press.
From Society of Pediatric Nurses. (1995). *SPN News, 4*(1), 6. Reprinted with permission.

be controversy as to how the screening is done. In addition, the Early and Periodic Screening, Diagnosis and Treatment (EPSDT) Program for disadvantaged preschool children needs strengthening (Rosen, 1996).

Tuberculosis

There is lack of agreement among experts as to the most appropriate form of tuberculosis (TB) screening for pediatric patients. The tine test was considered effective for many years, but some no longer consider it adequate. Many false negative results occur. The consensus is that the Mantoux test, or the intradermal injection of purified protein derivative (PPD) between layers of dermis and epidermis, is generally considered the most effective. The first screening is generally done between 12 and 15 months of age.

There are many missed opportunities to test for tuberculosis among disadvantaged children (Rosen, 1996).

Taking such opportunities for case finding is important because it is estimated that one third of the world's population is infected with latent disease (Sternberg, 1996). The World Health Organization (1995) calls for urgent action in its policy on drug-resistant diseases. This compelling document urges nurses and others caring for children out of the complacent belief that tuberculosis is an eradicated disease.

Plumbism

Children with elevated blood levels of lead develop behavioral problems and impairment of their intellects. The primary sources for lead poisoning (plumbism) are drinking water, lead-based house paint chips in older houses or the soil around them, air pollution, contaminated dust, and other environmental factors. Lead-based paint is no longer marketed for houses, but children living in houses built before the 1950s live in potentially poisonous environments. Levels of serum lead in affected children are reduced only slightly when loose paint is removed from the environment. The controversy comes with the missed opportunities for detection among disadvantaged children (Rosen, 1996). Testing young children's blood levels should be a routine part of early childhood care. The first screening is generally done at around 9 to 12 months of age in children assumed to be at risk.

Chelation therapy is thought to be more useful, depending on the child's serum lead level (Ruff, Bijur, Markowitz, & Rosen, 1993; Weitzman et al., 1993). See Chapter 30 for a full discussion of plumbism, chelation therapy, and long-term sequelae. The Centers for Disease Control and Prevention (CDC) has recommended that any child with clinical symptoms be treated as an inpatient on an emergent basis (Centers for Disease Control, 1991).

Neonatal Metabolic and Genetic Screening

Many states legally mandate that all neonates born within their boundaries have screening of their blood for any of several inborn errors of metabolism or genetic diseases. This is not controversial by itself. It becomes problematic when early discharge of the neonate precludes accurate assessment of protein breakdown and metabolism, as in phenylketonuria (PKU), or when cost is an issue (for some). Nearly all states in the United States require newborn screening for PKU and congenital hypothyroidism (U.S. Public Health Service, 1995). Some argue that it takes at least 2 to 3 days of ingesting formula or breast milk for phenylalanine levels to rise sufficiently for detection. With 24 hour and earlier discharge, a PKU screening done at that time would be ineffectual. There does not seem to be professional consensus about how screening is handled best in this situation, especially if there is no visiting nurse to the home of an early discharge patient.

National authorities have made the following recommendations for specific conditions (U.S. Public Health Service, 1995):

- Hypothyroidism—before discharge, but no later than day 6 of extrauterine life
- PKU—at time of nursery discharge or transfer whatever the age, but no later than 7 days of age
- Sickle cell disease—universal screening on all infants

Many register surprise at the sickle cell recommendation, but those at risk for sickle cell and other hemoglobinopathies have African, Mediterranean, Asian, Caribbean, and South and Central American genetic backgrounds (U.S. Public Health Service, 1995). Those infants considered at risk for not getting screened are delivered at home, sick at birth, or transferred between hospitals (U.S. Public Health Service, 1995).

Creating new laws mandating detection screening for every disease-producing gene found via the Human Genome Project (HGP) is not practical for state legislative bodies (Bishop & Waldholz, 1990). The HGP is an international collaboration among geneticists to map the entire set of human chromosomes. It is discussed in greater depth in the section on ethical concerns later in this chapter.

Other conditions for which some states require newborn screening include maple syrup urine disease, homocystinuria, biotinidase deficiency, congenital adrenal hyperplasia, cystic fibrosis, and toxoplasmosis (a congenital infection) (U.S. Public Health Service, 1995). Screening the entire population for certain genetic conditions would be very expensive. The objective of identifying "susceptibility genes" allows physiologists to understand the pathophysiology of major illnesses (Bishop & Waldholz, 1990, p. 17). Such screening may be useful when there is a positive family history of the disease. However, for people who carry susceptibility to genetic diseases, this information might be improperly used (e.g., denial of jobs or insurance). Decisions to screen for genetic diseases should be based on obtaining a detailed family history and careful consideration of the family's overall needs.

Some may argue that preventive medical services, such as massive cancer screening programs, create an illusion that if these services were to reach more people, the nation's well-being would be improved. Not all measures for prevention pay for themselves on a population basis (Leutwyler, 1995). However, there are only three strictly medical preventive services evaluated by the Office of Technology Assessment that actually pay for themselves in later cost savings:

- Prenatal care for poor women
- Tests in neonates for some congenital disorders (e.g., PKU and congenital hypothyroidism)
- Most childhood immunizations

With the exception of these maternity and pediatric prevention and screening initiatives, preventing disease is often more expensive than treating it on the aggregate level (Leutwyler, 1995). This idea has not filtered down to the general population, including lawmakers; but as policies evolve, ever more emphasis will be put on the cost-benefit ratio for prevention and screening programs. Mostly, the benefits of prevention and screening are obtained by educated individuals who actively pursue a healthy lifestyle for themselves and their families.

Culturally Sensitive Nursing Care

The *Code for Nurses* of the American Nurses' Association (ANA) specifies that nurses deliver care "without prejudicial behavior . . . transcending all national, ethnic, racial, religious, cultural, political, educational, economic, developmental, personality, role and sexual differences" (American Nurses' Association, 1985, p. 3). This requires nurses to be sensitive to the customs and practices of patients of various cultures, to develop "cultural competency."

Cross-cultural and transcultural studies of child development are very important to the nurse caring for children. The influence of culture on childcare practice, as well as the distribution of knowledge about it, entreats the provider to review his or her own attitudes (Nugent, 1994). Cross-cultural studies provide three important considerations for the nurse caring for children: "challenge our cultural assumptions about the nature of child development . . . controlled studies are not the only source of collecting data about child development . . . appropriateness of program goals and the validity of assessment tools in terms of the cultural backgrounds of the families they serve" (Nugent, 1994, p. 1).

Cultural competency includes the following (Campinha-Bacote, 1994):

- Having an awareness of one's views of different cultures
- Gaining knowledge about cultural groups and their health care practices
- Acquiring skills to be effective in the assessment and implementation of cultural care
- Seeking encounters that will enable the exposure and practice of culturally sensitive care

The idea of including transcultural nursing measures into practice is not new (Leininger, 1981), but many nurses maintain their own limited viewpoints.

What is essential for nurses to be culturally competent? This question is not easily answered, because every provider brings a personal value system and ideological commitment to the practice arena (Capers & Talerico, 1995). Unless a person has undergone extensive self-review of culture of origin and family of origin, self-awareness may be considerably lacking in the behaviors brought to the practice setting.

To improve cultural assessment, dimensions of the child's family must be evaluated, including the following (Grossman, 1996):

- Use of symbolic objects as signals of spiritual belief
- Belief about causation of health problems
- Use of slang terms and linguistic customs
- Non-verbal cultural cues
- Family and kinship structure
- Cooking and dining traditions
- Influence of religion
- Classification of diverse beliefs and practices

See Chart 2–5 for guidelines that nurses caring for children should consider in transcultural assessment.

Worldview: *Non–English speaking children and their parents may need an interpreter to translate medical terms and care instructions. Many state health departments have lists of available interpreters. Other sources of interpreters include Catholic Charity organizations and the American Red Cross Language Bank. Most health care organizations maintain a list of their own employees with foreign language skills.*

Many providers find it especially difficult to deal with differences in opinion that they may have about child-rearing practices and a family's unique practices. Families of children not only seek health care from the professional arena but also incorporate cultural and folk care practices (Capers & Talerico, 1995; Ikeda & Wright, 1996). In addition, seeking out professional help may be a last resort when home and local remedies have not worked or when money and insurance coverage are limited.

By developing cultural competency, nurses can reduce the anxiety, emotional pain, and possible guilt feelings that patients and their parents might be experiencing because of the need to seek professional help. Some families are apt to deny professional care to their children, for example, when parents refuse life-sustaining blood products or immunizations for their children on a religious basis, or when refugees refuse to accept the practices of Western medicine for their children.

Each new wave of immigration brings sets of child-rearing customs that are not well documented for nurses

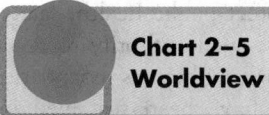

Chart 2–5
Worldview

Guidelines for the Transcultural Interview

The purpose of the transcultural interview is threefold:

- Introduces component parts of cultural assessment
- Allows examination of another culture while examining one's own
- Sharpens interviewing skills

Ethnic Origin	What is the ethnic origin of the family? Do you identify with this ethnic group?
Language	What is the dominant language of the culture? Are there special communication patterns?
Social Organization	What is the type of family structure? Are there ethnic/cultural organizations that these people affiliate with?
Health Practices	What are the cultural factors that affect health seeking behaviors? Who are the health care providers? What folk remedies do these people use for common complaints such as colds, injuries, or menstrual discomfort?
Socioeconomic	What is the general economic status of the group? In what ways is education valued? Have economics affected access to health care for this culture?
Race and Racism	Are there any personal experiences with prejudice or negative stereotyping? What are the common misconceptions of the cultural group? Are there any adverse experiences with the health care system based on these misconceptions or experiences?
Rites of Passage	What are the special customs and costumes associated with weddings, births, holidays, funerals, puberty, and attendance at places of worship?
Values and Beliefs	What are any habits, customs, beliefs, and/or values that affect relationships with members of other populations?
Food	What are the foods most commonly associated with this culture? Are there any food taboos? What foods are associated with special holidays? What foods are associated with healing?

Adapted from M. A. Browning & R. J. Lourie, Department of Nursing, Temple University, Philadelphia. Used with permission.

caring for children in the United States. It is naive to reduce all individuals with similar geographic genetic heritage, such as Asians, to an overall cultural stereotype. This happens when there is lack of knowledge about a distinct cultural group. There may even be vastly different cultural groups that immigrated from the same country or continent of origin, such as the Hmong and Vietnamese. As trust develops, members of these cultural groups may permit study of their beliefs and values, so that providers can work with them in providing health care and child-rearing advice.

Nurses caring for children not only must deliver culturally sensitive care on the individual and family level but also must be politically astute about institutionalized discrimination. Health care reform, on the governmental level (local, state, or national) and in the private sector, has different implications for diverse communities. Some people cannot work or obtain jobs for many reasons. If insurance reform is linked only through the workplace or ability to work, many will be left out—especially dependents such as children (Drayton-Hargrove & Woods, 1995).

Advanced Practice Nursing

A potential solution to the increasing problem of children's limited access to health care is the use of advanced practice nurses (APNs). APNs are able to obtain federal reimbursement for serving the poor. For example, many certified nurse practitioners, certified psychiatric nurse specialists, nurse-midwives, and nurse-anesthetists are directly reimbursed when caring for patients in the Civilian Health and Medical Program of Uniformed Services (CHAMPUS) system. This empowers the profession to improve the circumstances of the poor (Mittelstadt, 1994). Other disciplines are not likely to promote reimbursement opportunities. APNs must be well educated and current on public policy to be equitably reimbursed for services rendered.

Political Advocacy

Nurses caring for children strive to make the world a better place for them. Most people would agree that improving conditions for children is a worthwhile goal, but other issues often seem to carry higher priorities. Many sociopolitical value systems compete for scarce resources, thus challenging efforts to support the needs of children.

One way that a society may be judged is by its treatment of children, elderly, and disabled people. Gradual improvements in the care of these individuals have occurred over the latter half of the 20th century. However, the recent withdrawal of federal health care funding or reallocation of funding to the states as block grants has created regional inequities that threaten continued improvements in care (Mason, Talbott, & Leavitt, 1993). Some contend that these monies are allocated according to political maneuvering. Needy individuals who have a strong advocacy base—including elderly and disabled adults—get better access to funds (Mason et al., 1993). Yet federal entitlement programs, which provide direct reimbursement to recipients with special situations (e.g., kidney failure, disabilities) or care providers, have become an enormous drain on the economy and encourage exploitation. In 1995, 48.7% of federal spending went to entitlement programs (Shays, 1995):

- Social Security (21.8%)
- Medicare (11.6%)
- Medicaid (5.8%)
- Other entitlements (9.5%)

Insurance fraud and severe reimbursement cutbacks by the insurance industry have exacerbated the problem of inadequate resources available for children.

The power of government's role in health care rests on very different constitutional principles at the state and the national levels. Through a state's police powers to enact and enforce laws that protect public health, safety, and general welfare, it has the virtual authority to regulate every aspect of health care within its boundaries (Litman, 1991). These powers have been sustained by the United States Supreme Court—for example, for compulsory immunization against communicable disease (*Jacobsen v. Massachusetts*, 1905).

The role of the federal government in protecting child health is more vague and broad; it rests mainly on judicial interpretation of the Constitution's Welfare Clause (Litman, 1991). In other words, Congress has limited power for carrying out specific changes in the health care system. The United States has an extremely strong tradition and legal base for states' rights; therefore, it is likely that improving access to care for vulnerable populations (such as children) is more likely to occur within individual states. This is a trend that is part of a societal response to the role of big government in earlier parts of the 20th century.

Before 1965, when Congress enacted many legislative changes including Medicare and Medicaid (Titles XVIII and XIX to the Social Security Act), the federal government had a very small role in regulating the country's health care. At the end of the millennium, the pendulum continues to swing in the opposite direction with congressional insurance reform, welfare reform, and reining in the rate of growth for Medicaid.

More changes have occurred in health care reimbursement strategies in the private sector since the early 1990s than in the previous quarter century. This is especially evident in obstetric and neonatal care, where 24-hour (and earlier) discharge policies have been initiated by many insurance companies. Several states, including Maryland, Massachusetts, New Jersey, North Carolina, Pennsylvania, and others, have passed what has been termed anti drive-through delivery legislation. Congress also passed such legislation, which was signed into law by President Clinton in 1996. Each state's laws are different, but they require insurance companies to reimburse for a minimum of 48 hours of inpatient care and neonatal observation after vaginal delivery and 96 hours of coverage after cesarean birth (Gerchufsky, 1996; Pennsylvania Nurses Association, 1996). Similar bills are pending in other states. Such changes are best made at the state level, because the states retain police power for implementation. However, a piece of groundbreaking legislation, The Newborns' and Mothers' Health Protection Act (American Nurses' Association, 1996b), was proposed in the United States Senate in September 1996. It is unusual for the federal government to override states' individual policies on health insurance.

The Health Insurance Reform Act of 1996 created sweeping changes in how health insurance vendors provide their services. This new law brought changes, creating the following provisions (Public Law 104-191, 1996):

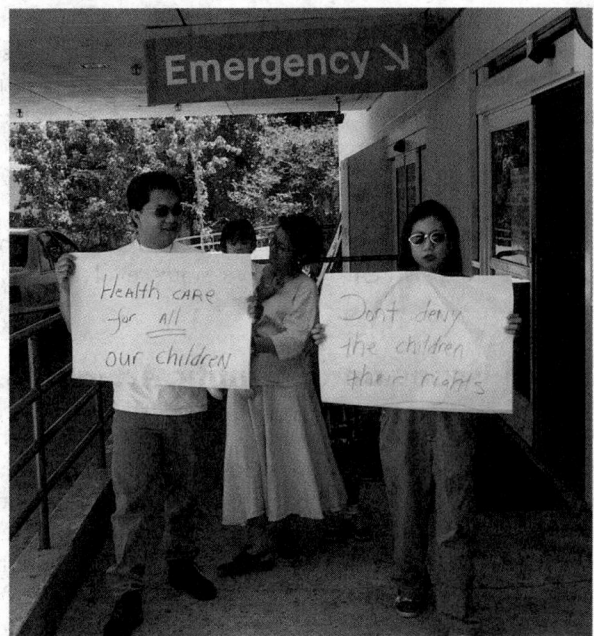

Figure 2–4
Nurses can use the political process to advocate for children's health.

- Improved health care access, portability of insurance coverage (when the insured change jobs), and renewability
- Tax-related health provisions, including an increase in the tax deductions allowed for insurance costs in the self-employed
- Long-term care provisions
- Fraud and abuse prevention measures

States are highly unlikely to give up their roles as providers of care to the indigent, as regulators of the insurance industry and environmental issues within their boundaries, and as monitors of the use of federal funds by local entities (Lipson, 1991). This has particular implications for members of minority and other underserved populations in states where a preponderance of the voting population is conservative and tends to vote for decreases in government spending. Even federal policy has consistently permitted institutionalized bias to occur in United States society (Blendon, Aiken, Freeman, & Corey, 1994; Rice & Winn, 1991; U.S. Department of Health and Human Services, 1992). The underserved are and have been a particularly vulnerable group. It is important that under a block grant approach some federal standards remain to ensure access to safe care.

Nurses have always been politically active in the United States, even though this may not be evident in large numbers (Rogge, 1987). More nurses caring for children need to become political activists so as better to advocate for their patients and the general health of generations to come (Fig. 2–4). This activism must occur at the local, state, and national levels (Mason et al., 1993).

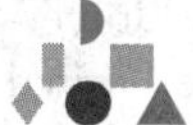

Ethical Issues in the Care of Children

Bioethics is the study of ethics as applied to the life sciences. This includes all forms of life, so preservation of the planet is of concern to bioethicists as well as complex decision-making at the end of life. The application of bioethical principles is very important to nurses caring for children because nurses are able to dispel myths about health in ways that the lay population cannot. For example, AIDS hysteria has led seemingly rational adults to burn down the homes of or deny school access to persons with AIDS (Sterken, 1995). Another situation highlighting the need for ethical knowledge is the case of the Lakeberg twins, which attracted national attention in 1993. Conjoined twins Amy and Angela Lakeberg shared one six-chambered heart and one liver. Only one twin could survive separation surgery, and even the chances for that twin were slim. The medical challenges were great; the ethical challenges, even greater (Thomasma et al., 1996, p. 4). Ethical problems of caring for conjoined twins create true ethical dilemmas when one must be sacrificed so that the other may live. Many felt that the landmark surgery should not have been done, as it created enormous expenses. However, every surgical procedure was experimental at one point in history.

In 1975, an infant born with ectopia cordis (no sternum to keep his heart inside his chest) had a partial repair in the same institution (Children's Hospital of Philadelphia) that did the Lakeberg surgery. He was not expected to live and had an extremely prolonged and unstable course in the intensive care nursery. Today, this young man enjoys swimming, playing basketball, and working at a metal tubing company (Associated Press, 1996). Had the medical and nursing staff given up on him, he would have died in infancy.

Society faces tough decisions about the care and funding of complex situations such as these, and nurses caring for children must participate in this debate. The following sections are concerned with explaining major bioethical challenges for nurses caring for children.

Several sets of ethical standards govern nursing and health care practice. The ANA's Code for Nurses (American Nurses' Association, 1985) is an ethical standard of care. The International Congress of Nursing (ICN) also has a published ethical code. Other disciplines such as medicine have had disciplinary codes since the classical Greek period (the Hippocratic Oath). In modern times, the American Medical Association Code of Ethics has supplanted the Hippocratic Oath. Increasingly, other disciplines are formulating and distributing ethical codes of conduct to their members.

A higher ethical standard of behavior is the Universal Declaration of Human Rights, set forth by the United Nations (UN) on December 10, 1948. The General Assembly of the UN called on all member countries to disseminate, display, and teach the declaration in schools and other institutions.

Ethical Issues in Pediatric Nursing

Family-centered nursing follows a family-centered ethic. Glover (1995) suggests that an ethic of care is too abstract in pediatrics. For example, an ethic of care would pay attention to the context in which a family with a critically ill child is experiencing financial difficulties. Glover (1995) wonders about the limits of what can be done while balancing the obligations to others in a moral community. Provocative situations in pediatric care have always existed. Glover poses no specific solutions, but recommends that providers build a moral community by creating an environment where people can discuss ethical, rather than mere financial or legal, conflicts. Providers can thus begin to set important criteria. For example, what is the ethical obligation to children whose families cannot pay for their care? Glover suggests that nurses do everything possible to bring national attention to questions of justice that the health care community has largely ignored (Glover, 1995). There are many ethical issues besides economic ones, including determining what promotes health or what standards are acceptable for interacting with children.

Individuals involved in pediatric health care may be faced with an overriding value of the sanctity of life on the part of parents, nurses, physicians, relatives, clergy, and others. However, the *sanctity* of life or the idea of right to life at all costs may come in direct conflict with *quality* of life issues, even in pediatric care. Consider the idea that a child with severe congenital anomalies (e.g., anencephaly, or birth without a brain) or burns over extensive parts of the body may be better off if permitted to die without the intervention of major technological advances.

The *quality of life* may be defined as an improvement in ability to function within the activities of daily living as a result of technological advances. This term is often applied to situations where some perceive the quality of life to be lacking. When thought of with regard to self, one usually questions to what extent measures of extraordinary care would be rejected or desired if the person had a conscious choice in the matter (such as being placed on a ventilator permanently). Quality of life issues are hypothetically addressed by individuals who take steps to initiate and write down some form of advance directives.

The *sanctity of life* may also be defined as *the right to life as the highest good.* Sheer existence may be valued without regard for circumstances in the person's existence, or quality of life (Thompson & Thompson, 1985). The sanctity of life, or preserving life for its own sake, is less important as an overriding value for some as the definitions of persistent vegetative states evolve (Wolf, 1988).

Ethical Issues and Scientific Advances

Advances in science and technology require strict attention to the ethical implications of scientific discoveries. An example of this principle in action is the current controversy surrounding genetic engineering. The Human Genome Project, an international collaborative effort to map the entire genome, was begun in the early 1990s. This project aims to discover disease-related genes, with the ultimate goal of alleviating the suffering of countless people of all ages (Bishop & Waldholz, 1990). Because of the work already done, inherited disorders such as cystic fibrosis, PKU, and others soon may be manageable enough to permit affected individuals to live relatively normal lives.

Another example of genetic engineering is the synthetic production of human insulin, or Humulin. In persons with insulin-dependent diabetes mellitus, Humulin precludes the need to use porcine or bovine insulin. Growth hormone is now available through genetic engineering as well. Previously, it had to be extracted from the pituitary glands of sheep or other animals.

Genetic engineering has other beneficial uses besides those of a medical nature. Endangered species can be helped to procreate by genetic "fingerprinting" and identification of less genetically related breeding pairs. Mapping DNA from mummified humans that lived thousands of years ago provides information about the pace at which evolution occurs in humans. Genetic testing can yield precise information in questions of identity, such as missing persons, kidnapped children, or criminal identification (Franklin-Barbajosa, 1992).

Nonetheless, many people worry about the misuse of genetic engineering (Shea, 1995). Germ-line genetic therapy elicits thoughts of eugenics, the abuse of power that new knowledge may bring, and nagging fears of change. This type of genetic "therapy" conjures up the image of transmission of a superior genome from one generation to the next to create a class of persons "superior" to naturally conceived individuals. Some suggest that genetic engineering may ultimately create a "biological underclass" whose members may be discriminated against by employers and insurance carriers (Bishop & Waldholz, 1990). This fear may not be totally unfounded, considering the history of human behavior with regard to misuse of scientific advances and tendencies toward segregation and exploitation of others.

Ethical Principles

The four major ethical principles are autonomy, beneficence, nonmaleficence, and justice. It is beyond the scope of this text to provide more than a rudimentary definition of the principles from which pediatric nursing practice is derived. The student is referred to the many journals, books, and special articles dedicated to the health care of children and their families to broaden an ethical knowledge base.

Some may rank the major bioethical principles in a hierarchical form of importance—for example, that autonomy should override beneficence. This is a value judgment. No one ethical principle necessarily supersedes another. Some even recommend that there is an obligation to maintain a balance between competing ethical principles (Gaylord, 1996). This is also a value judgment, but probably a useful guideline to which nurses caring for children can aspire. Ethical inquiry should provoke the asking of more questions. It is not necessarily a route to quick and easy answers.

Autonomy—Self-Determination

Autonomy is considered to be synonymous with self-determination. In classical ethics, it encompasses independence, self-reliance, and the self-contained ability to decide. It includes a person's right to

- Decide what will be done with his or her person
- Be given information necessary for making informed judgments
- Be told the possible effects of care
- Accept, refuse, or end treatment

This ethical principle has been supported in the United States since 1914, when Judge Cardozo held that "every human being of adult years and sound mind has a right to determine what shall be done with his own body" (*Schloendorff v. the Society of the New York Hospital*, 1914, p. 125). This case precedent has formed the basic societal construct of *informed consent* in 20th century American law (Rosoff, 1981). See the section on informed consent in this chapter for a detailed explanation of the conditional requirements.

Allowing adolescents and parents for less competent, younger children to choose freely and specifically among all care options enables a greater sense of control over individual destiny and greater confidence in the overall direction of care. Protecting and ensuring the autonomy of children and adolescents involve a set of delicate negotiations. Developmental ability and age are the most appropriate guidelines for judging how well those younger than the age of majority may participate in making autonomous decisions (see the later section on informed consent).

Beneficence

Beneficence is the ethical principle of the common good. This concept stands alone as an ethical principle or in relationship to harm, as in the cost-benefit or risk-benefit ratio. The ANA's (1985) Code for Nurses stipulates that acts of beneficence are moral requirements of the profession.

The *risk-benefit ratio* is an analysis of whether or not risks incurred in a treatment modality outweigh the expected benefits. A prime example of applying the risk-benefit ratio to practice is the responsibility to report unethical research protocols such as the one at Willowbrook (Beauchamp & Childress, 1983), in which retarded children who were residents of the facility became unwitting participants in a live hepatitis vaccine trial. Their parents signed a written consent form for their participation. Children who were wards of the state were not enrolled in the study. This research was conducted in the United States in the 1950s after the Nuremberg Code was published as a reaction to atrocious Nazi medical research on humans. It was considered acceptable research by some within the context of that particular era. The ethical justification for conducting this project was that it would benefit future generations.

The *cost-benefit ratio* is similar to the risk-benefit ratio; it is an analysis of whether or not the costs of a treatment or procedure outweigh the expected benefits. Cost may be defined in detriment to the patient and family and/or in monetary units, as for example in the question "What will the cost to the family be if their child is put on life-support for treatment of an end-stage disease process?" This is also called the *benefit-detriment ratio.*

Nonmaleficence/Nonmalfeasance

Nonmaleficence and nonmalfeasance are derived from the Latin word *male,* which means evil; the terms literally mean *do no harm.* To determine whether one is inflicting harm, risk- and detriment-benefit ratios are useful in weighing whether a procedure or policy is more likely to create havoc than provide intended good effects. Mandates to do no harm can be found in all ANA (1985) Code for Nurses statements and originally from the Hippocratic Oath. *Primum non nocere* is the literal translation from Latin, "First (or above all) do no harm." The principle of beneficence is also broader than this, since it also mandates positive actions to help others.

Justice

Justice is a basic principle of bioethics and the life sciences that in health care usually concerns allocation of scarce resources. The principle of justice usually refers to the idea of *distributive justice* in health care.

Justice is an especially important principle for nurses caring for children in the current era of cost containment. Although fiscal responsibility is important, "right sizing" may be a euphemism for permitting uncredentialed or dangerously low levels of staffing to become new norms. Nurses are key decision makers in the allocation of scarce health care resources (Botter & Dickey, 1989). It is important that they "counter the bean counting mentality" when the quality of patient care is in jeopardy (Visintainer-Baranowski, 1995). Unethical business conduct typically "involves the tacit, if not explicit cooperation of others and reflects the values, beliefs, language, and behavioral patterns that define an organization's operating culture" (Paine, 1994, p. 106). Management of potentially unethical situations should be strategized in advance, if possible. In many situations, there are serious, unpleasant consequences for the nurse who speaks out. However, maintaining one's own integrity is usually most important for a long-term sense of well-being. Organizational integrity means that a situation has been created in which managers provide proper leadership and institute systems that promote ethical conduct (Paine, 1994).

Two current issues provide important examples of the application of distributive justice. The *medically fragile child* is a minor with a stabilized medical or health care condition in need of complex health care services to be safely "mainstreamed." Such integration may be into a public school setting or other public activities to meet the provisions of the Individuals with Disabilities Education Act of 1982. Many see mainstreaming as the medically fragile child's just due. In addition, immunizations for *hard-to-reach children* are considered by many to be a right, in addition to protecting the health of the general population at large. Those individuals at risk for not being vaccinated are those from lower income status inner city; minority groups; working poor; those in foster care for abused or neglected children; "new" homeless; and immigrants, refugees, or illegal aliens. See Chapter 7 for a detailed discussion of issues regarding immunizations.

Other Ethical Principles in the Care of Children

Some of the following principles may be derived from the four major bioethical principles described above: autonomy, beneficence, nonmaleficence, and justice. They have specific meaning and importance to the practice of nurses caring for children.

Veracity

Veracity, or truth-telling, is a professional mandate to respect the dignity of another, including children, by avoiding lying or nondisclosure of important information. This is especially important in pediatrics, because the imagination and magical thinking of children can make anticipated procedures seem even worse than they may be. If children are not told the truth, their trust is lost. Health care providers are frequently asked by family members to withhold information from children. The ideal is to present only that information appropriate to the child's developmental level.

A *benevolent deception* is an act of paternalism that, in health care, might be nondisclosure of the grave nature of a patient's condition to the patient or family members. Parents frequently request providers not to tell children when their prognosis is progressive and possibly fatal, although this is not usually in the child's best interest.

Often, parents may feel that benevolent deception is a way to gain their child's cooperation for an anticipated unpleasant medical procedure. This approach has not been useful over time, although it still exists. For example, the child might be told that the family is going some place pleasant on a car trip, rather than to a medical center for day surgery. This type of lying is an ill way of gaining a child's cooperation and sets a precedent for maladaptive coping from the child later in life. It also betrays the child's trust for future health care encounters.

A *placebo* is an inactive substance given to a patient to deceive the patient into a sense of satisfaction or relief because the patient believes the substance to be a specific drug. Parents may tell a child that a piece of candy is a painkilling drug. In a sense, the act of placing a bandage on a scratch is a placebo, because it does little to really alter the condition of the lesion. It is ethically questionable to use placebos as a form of treatment in any setting where health care is provided. Placebos are also used in research trials to evaluate the efficacy of an active drug against no treatment; this use has proven more socially acceptable when a fully informed consent has been obtained from the subject prior to participation in a research protocol.

Paternalism

In health care, paternalism refers to the assumption that the health care professional knows what is "best" for the patient. Acts of paternalism preclude the patient's or family's ability to be a full participant in care owing to nondisclosure of critical information used for autonomous decision-making. This self-centered point of view is tolerated less and less by consumers of health care. Some patients and their families claim that they really do not wish to know what is going on with their care, and they place care in the hands of their providers. In order for this behavior by professionals to be validated ethically, the patient or family must state that they do not wish to have the information. Paternalistic behavior by health care providers is not to be confused with parents acting paternalistically for their children. The connotations are different.

Role Fidelity

Role fidelity is the conduct of oneself as a professional with behavioral loyalty to the standards and ethical codes defined by the overall profession. In pediatric nursing, role fidelity is essential for the maintenance of trust between children and providers. It often makes the difference in whether or not care is sought. Role fidelity may cause taxing emotional conflicts, such as reporting child abuse that results in the separation of a child from a parent. Loyalty to one's ethical role in the practice setting may also mean that the role is strictly delineated to the child and family so that they will know what to expect or not to expect from interdisciplinary plans.

Ethical Decision-Making Models

An ethical decision-making model is a formalized process against which ethical dilemmas may be measured. Many models exist; all follow four basic steps (Thompson & Thompson, 1985):

- Information about the problem is gathered and analyzed.
- Risk-benefit or cost-benefit ratios are weighed against bioethical principles such as nonmaleficence or justice.
- A solution is chosen (with an ethical justification).
- The solution's effectiveness is evaluated.

Ethical dilemmas are inherently perplexing. They are, at bottom, conflicts of values, problems that cannot be resolved solely through analyzing empirical data. Frequently, however, people trained in science try to solve ethical dilemmas by collecting ever more data, thereby avoiding a real solution to the problem (Thompson & Thompson, 1985). Qualities of ethical dilemmas include the following:

- The answer reached will have a far-reaching effect on one's perception of humans, the relationships among humans, and the relationship of humans to society and to the world.
- Such decisions are often precedent setting, having profound relevance to several areas of human concern.

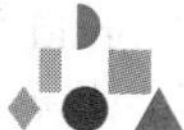

Legal Issues in the Care of Children

This section gives an overview of specific legal concerns associated with the nursing care of children. It does not attempt to explain in detail the legal concepts and constructs as would a law text. Because minors may bring legal action on their own after reaching the age of majority, nurses must be aware of special situations. In addition, with alternative, blended, one-parent, and no-parent families on the increase, the nurse caring for children must be especially astute when in professional situations.

The Patient Self-Determination Act of 1990

The Patient Self-Determination Act of 1990 is part of the Omnibus Budget Reconciliation Act of 1990 (OBRA). It directs that any organization with federal funding providing health care develop a written description for patients of that state's law concerning advance directives regarding withholding or withdrawing life-sustaining treatment. The purpose is so that patients know about advance directives and have a set when they are treated. The Patient Self-Determination Act is relevant to pediatric nursing in many ways, but it is specifically mentioned here because most pediatric institutions are currently nonprofit and draw heavily on federal funding. See Chapter 12 for a discussion on aspects of the dying pediatric patient.

Children are included under coverage for this law, although the implementation for them has not taken on the same set of customs and legal enforcement that review of advance directive for adults has done. For example, if an otherwise usually healthy 3-year-old patient seeks treatment in an emergency department for status asthmaticus, it is assumed that a full measure of pursuit for saving the child's life will be undergone, even if that includes temporary care by extraordinary means, for example, mechanical ventilation. However, another 3-year-old in end-stage liver disease with a history of three previous liver transplants may have very elaborate advance directives created for an emergency.

Advance directives are written, often legal documents that specify an individual's wishes regarding care before contact with a health care provider or agency. Advance directives require witnesses who have reached the age of majority (18 years) and who are not beneficiaries of the will for the person creating the document. Children's parents or legal guardians create advance directives for their children, preferably with participation from the child.

Durable power of attorney is a legal construct thought

of as mainly concerning adults. For minors not considered as being legally emancipated, parents or legal guardians legally assume this role in which someone is identified to make decisions on another's behalf when the person is mentally incapacitated to do so for himself or herself. An example of inability to make decisions for oneself might be a patient with AIDS dementia, where the person recognized the possibility of future incapacitation and identified a proxy to carry durable power of attorney. The person may have clarified wishes concerning a variety of medical and personal situations.

Earlier verbal expressed wishes are sometimes respected by providers as advance directives. Case law acknowledges verbal wishes and remarks (*Cruzan v. Director, Missouri Department of Health*, 1990), but written and appropriately witnessed documents carry much greater weight. With children and adolescents, verbal expressions remembered by their intimates may be the only records, if any, about what their thoughts would be regarding a situation. It is not yet customary even for adults to formalize the process of advance directives. Many people would probably find the prospect of discussing advance directives with their normal children emotionally distressing, because most parents do not expect their children to die before they do. However, the families of children and adolescents with end-stage diseases or situations where there is a high probability risk for death should be actively encouraged to discuss such topics with their offspring before an acute situation arises.

A *living will* is a type of advance directive. It is limited to situations in which the patient's condition is considered terminal or the patient is in some form of end-stage disease. *Terminal* is difficult to define; some say that it describes a condition for which death would be expected within 6 months. Therefore, living wills are not always honored, because they are frequently written when the patient is well and changes may occur as the illness progresses. Family members often override living wills because of grief, guilt, or another emotional reaction. The patient maintains the right to nullify the document. In pediatric nursing, living wills are primarily seen in use with minors who have terminal stages of an illness, when death is imminent and they can express their wishes. Sophisticated health care providers and family members help create a situation in which a living will works best in pediatric practice.

Rights of Minors

An important aspect of health management in nursing of children is protecting the rights of the child under the law. Several legal concerns are very important to the nurse caring for children. These include an understanding of what qualifies as a fully informed consent, assent, or dissent by a minor; child abuse reporting and documentation (see full description later in the chapter); and a full comprehension of parent or guardian access to the child or confidential information regarding that child.

Technically, minors (persons younger than age 18 in most states; 21 in others) have no rights under the United States Constitution. Under Anglo-American customs that eventually became law, a woman and her issue (children) were considered chattel, or property of the man. For these reasons, children were perceived to have no legal rights. Their well-being stemmed largely from the status of the families into which they were born.

Laws regarding the rights of children have been codified mostly at the state level. This has created a "patchwork" of laws across the country, with some states having very liberal laws and others having very conservative ones.

In a classic article, Feshbach and Feshbach (1978) describe historical, social, and developmental perspectives of children's rights. They acknowledge that the "increased awareness of children's rights is a major factor contributing to contemporary ferment regarding public policies for children" (p. 1). The entire issue of the journal in which their article appears is concerned with a number of topics, including the following:

- Ethical issues in the treatment of children
- Alternative family styles
- Child advocacy and family privacy
- Rights and responsibilities in family relationships

These ideas remain germane today.

Rights of Parents

Parents derive some rights from the United States Constitution; the rights to privacy have their roots in the Bill of Rights and later amendments. These rights have been subject to broad interpretation in the United States. Many individuals are unaware that the idea of rights is accompanied by an expectation of responsibilities. Rights typically involve an obligation, usually to others. In the case of parents' rights, the obligation is that the parents provide health and safety for their children. Rights may be interpreted as legal, ethical, or both (Thompson & Thompson, 1985). Ethically related rights are based on fidelity to ethical principles rather than mere legal codes, but they may be enforced by criminal codes. For example, when parents treat their children inhumanely, they can be prosecuted under criminal statutes if the injuries or neglect is severe enough. Another example would be when the courts intervene if the parents withhold medical treatment, such as immunizations (see later discussion of failure to provide treatment).

Stemming from the right to privacy are the rights of parents to raise their children as they wish. This is reminiscent of Thomas Jefferson's statement in the Declaration of Independence with regard to citizens' unalienable rights . . . life, liberty, and the pursuit of happiness. The freedom to parent without interference, especially for minors who were by custom considered chattel, evolved from this document. Although the Declaration of Independence is not a legally governing document as is the Constitution, this is an idea that fostered the Constitution's development and a 200-year evolution of legislative recognition that certain rights are to be protected, among them freedom to parent and privacy.

Alternative parenting styles are recognized as realities in which children live. They may include, but are not limited to, single-parent, two-parent, stepparent, homosexual, blended family, and no-parent family styles. Problems are dealt with by approaches tailored to the family's unique situation. A nonjudgmental approach toward the parent figures is in the best interest of the child, even when steps must be taken to change their behavior in behalf of the child, such as reporting abuse or neglect.

Custody Issues

Recognizing legal custody is important to the practice of pediatric nursing. Failure to follow legal custody guidelines set forth by a judge in a court of law is breaking the law. When the legal custodians (parents, other relatives, or foster parents) entrust health care providers with their children, particularly in overnight stays where they might not always be present, others may arrive to claim custody falsely. If legal custody guidelines are not honored by institutions and persons caring for children or other legal dependents, severe legal liability—not to mention harm to the children—may occur.

When there is an issue regarding with whom a child will live, the legal standard is whatever is in the best interest of the child. Formerly, the presumption of the law was that children were rendered into the custody of their mother. More fathers have sought custody of their children in recent years. All things being equal, judges usually award custody to the mother. However, the judge must explain the rationale for the award. Sometimes, custody is denied to both parents. It may be awarded to other relatives, such as grandparents, aunts and uncles, or cousins. If there is perceived danger to placing a child with relatives, foster care is the next step.

The view that children at times need legal counsel independent of their parents has taken on momentum since the 1970s. A 12-year-old boy in Florida engaged his own attorney to ask the court to permit him to be legally adopted by his third foster family (Landsberg, 1992). The court agreed, despite his biological mother's wish to regain custody. Essentially, the court permitted the minor a "divorce" from his parents.

Visitation Rights

Visitation rights, like custody rights, are granted under the standard of the best interest of the child. If the parents are fighting or cannot manage amicable relations concerning the child, the court may request a psychological evaluation by a licensed professional. The recommendation of the mental health professional is generally followed by the court.

It is mandatory for the people caring for children to establish legal custody circumstances early in a relationship with a child. For example, most formalized pediatric databases for inpatient settings request information regarding legal status during the admission process. Simple questions (such as with whom the child lives) often, but not always, elicit such information. When situations are unclear, more questions must be asked in order best to protect the child from possible harm. If this is not done, and something goes wrong (such as kidnapping), the admitting nurse and the institution may be held legally responsible.

Legal Aspects of Child Abuse Reporting and Documentation

Child abuse reporting is a professional duty imposed by law. The nurse must report suspected child abuse or any living conditions and circumstances that constitute neglect. Neglect includes medical neglect, whereby parents or guardians of an otherwise well-cared-for child for whom adequate food, clothing, and shelter are provided may be held liable when the child's immunization requirements or other health care needs are consistently postponed. Another example may be failure to seek treatment when the child has an obviously life-threatening illness.

When such a report is made with the good faith belief that it is accurate, the nurse cannot be held liable for defamation of character (of the family members or others). The penal codes of almost all 50 states include language that requires professional nurses to report suspected incidents of child abuse or neglect. Such rules and regulations stipulate that professionals who make such reports, when done in good faith, cannot have a lawsuit brought against them for defamation of character or invasion of privacy (Aiken & Catalano, 1994). Chart 2–6 presents some legal considerations associated with reporting child abuse and neglect; Chart 2–7 lists professionals required by law to report suspected child abuse and neglect. See Chapters 29 and 30 for detailed discussions of other aspects of child abuse and neglect.

Chart 2–6

Legal Considerations for Reporting Child Abuse and Neglect

- Privileged communication between the professional person and patient or client (and parents) does not apply.
- Most states have toll-free hotlines for reporting suspected child abuse that are open 24 hours a day.
- Factual documentation without extraneous judgmental information is very important (especially if the case should wind up in court at some future time).
- In most states, the law also includes a stipulation protecting anyone who reports child abuse or who assists in a report. Should such an action be followed by discharge from employment or discrimination in compensation, hire, tenure, terms, conditions, or privileges of employment, the employee may file a cause of action in the Court of Common Pleas.
- Statutes may vary in different states, but in most, the report is processed through the Child Protective Services unit of the Child Welfare Agency after the incident has been centrally reported to the state capital.

Legal Concerns Associated with Failure to Provide Treatment

In the early 1980s, "Baby Doe" bills were introduced in the United States House of Representatives and Senate to expand the definition of child abuse and neglect. This included failure to provide medical treatment or nutrition to infants with life-threatening congenital impairments, and in 1983, The Child Abuse Prevention and Treatment Act was signed into law. One of the most controversial outgrowths of this act was the DHHS's rule requiring hospitals to post notices of a toll-free hotline for reporting infractions of the "failure to treat" law. All neonatal nurseries in institutions receiving any form of federal funding posted such notices, although the interpretation varied from one institution to the next. In some places, the number was readily prominent; whereas, in others, the information was placed on small placards. By June 1984, a compromise statement was drawn up and agreed on by the American Nurses' Association, American Academy of Pediatrics, American Hospital Association, American College of Obstetricians and Gynecologists, and several other organizations. This document is still in force today.

The statement, a proposed amendment to The Child Abuse Prevention and Treatment Act, requires states that participate in the (federally funded) state child abuse grant program to establish procedures for reporting medical neglect (withholding treatment from disabled infants) (American Nurses' Association, 1984). The key clause in the compromise is "withholding of medically indicated treatment," which includes nutrition, medication, and hydration that, in the treating physician's reasonable medical judgment, would improve or correct a disabling condition. The clause continues

> However, the term does not include the failure to provide treatment (other than appropriate nutrition, hydration or medication) to an infant when . . . (a) the infant is chronically and irreversibly comatose . . . (b) the provision of such treatment would merely prolong dying or . . . (c) the provision of such treatment would be virtually futile in terms of the survival of the infant . . . and inhumane (American Nurses' Association, 1984, pp. 1–2).

The country has apparently managed with this compromise, and, therefore, infant cadaver organ donations,

Chart 2–7

Professionals Required to Report Suspected Child Abuse and Neglect

- Chiropractor
- Christian Science practitioner
- Coroner
- Dentist
- Emergency medical technician
- Hospital personnel engaged in the administration, care, and treatment of minor patients
- Intern (medical)
- Law enforcement official
- Licensed physician
- Licensed practical nurse
- Medical examiner
- Mental health professional
- Nurse practitioner
- Occupational therapist
- Optometrist
- Osteopath
- Paramedic
- Peace officer
- Physical therapist
- Podiatrist
- Professional nurse
- School nurse
- Social services worker
- Teacher

This is a partial listing.

especially for liver and heart transplants, have been legally possible in the United States since then.

The courts are most likely to protect the decision-making rights of parents (Rhodes, 1995). The recent case *In re: Baby K* (1993) illustrates the point. Baby K was born anencephalic (without a brain) to a mother who chose not to terminate her pregnancy when she learned of the fetus's futile condition prenatally. The hospital went to court, seeking a declaration that its refusal to provide life-supporting ventilator treatment would not violate any of the following laws: Emergency Medical Treatment and Active Labor Act; Section 504 of the Rehabilitation Act; the Americans with Disabilities Act of 1990; and the Child Abuse Amendments of 1984 (Rhodes, 1995). The court ruled in favor of the mother's decision-making, as do most courts when there is disagreement between parents and caregivers (Rhodes, 1995). Moreover, health care organizations that accept Medicare or Medicaid funding are subject to the Rehabilitation Act (Section 504) that prohibits any program receiving federal financial assistance from discriminating against the disabled (Rhodes, 1995).

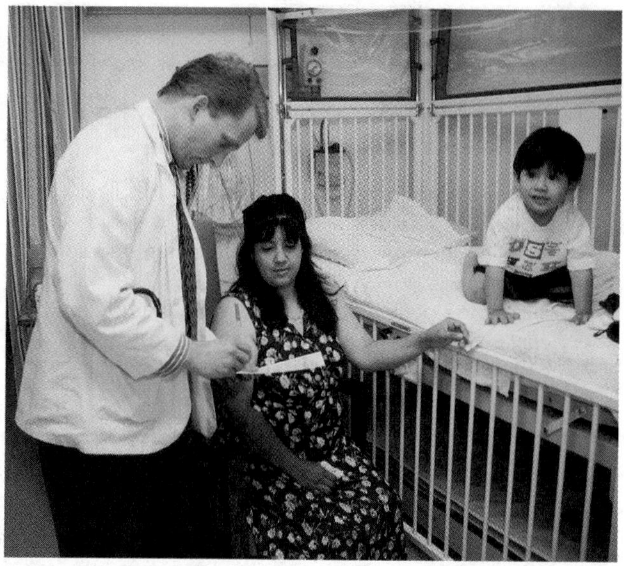

Figure 2–5
Obtaining informed consent from a child's responsible parent is essential before any procedure. A signed form, however, does not mean that full disclosure has occurred.

Confidentiality Issues

Confidentiality, inherent in one's right to privacy and generally recognized by states and the national government, is frequently violated by health care providers or because of the sheer accessibility of patient records in the information age. Contradictions do occur. If the minor is seen by a school nurse for a minor problem, this may not be considered confidential. However, a positive pregnancy test is confidential. There is legally contradictory information that parents may obtain about their children. This varies from state to state. Especially when vulnerable parties, such as children or those at risk to themselves or others (suicidal or violent), are in direct jeopardy, the right to confidentiality may be superseded. The patient and family should be warned that this ethical duty may be overridden. Information of a confidential nature should be protected judiciously.

Informed Consent

Parental consent should be obtained before any treatment or participation in a research study for minors (Fig. 2–5). If the minor is not in the custody of either parent, then consent is obtained from the child's legal guardian. Treatment may be rendered to minors without legal consent in only three general situations (Rhodes & Miller, 1984):

- An emergency in which consent is presumed and failure to treat would lead to permanent damage or death
- A situation in which the consent of a minor is sufficient
- By court order or other form of legal authorization

With abortions, states are changing laws with great enough frequency that the provider is referred to the statutes of the state before participating in this procedure. Each state varies in its requirements regarding inclusion of parents in the decision-making process for abortion in a minor.

The concept of informed consent stems from the ethical principle of autonomy in classical ethics, which on the individual level encompasses independence, self-reliance, and the self-contained ability to decide. This concept has been developing in nursing, biomedical, and legal literature since the early 1970s. It has inspired a multistage process for protecting patient choice in health care. Allowing adolescents and parents to choose freely and specifically among all care options permits a greater sense of control over individual destiny and more confidence in the overall direction of care (Dickey, 1992).

There is consensus in the literature about what constitutes an informed consent. It is generally described as a process that must contain the following six transactions to be considered full disclosure:

- An explanation of the condition
- A fair explanation of the procedures to be used and the consequences
- A description of alternative treatments or procedures
- A description of the benefits to be expected

Chart 2–8

Nursing Considerations in Obtaining a Valid Informed Consent

- Obtain informed consent from the minor patient as well as parents whenever possible to avoid violating the right to self-determination in decision-making.
- Encourage patient trust by respecting the adolescent's maturity. Refusal to acknowledge such maturity may be interpreted as a denial of personhood.
- Know the consent laws in area of practice. Be alert to the sometimes wide variations in such statutes among the various states and commonwealths and the differing situations that they anticipate.
- Avoid witnessing a telephone consent. In cases of withdrawn consent and subsequent legal action, the nurse may be viewed as colluding with the physician to elicit permission from reluctant patients and families. When faced with such a request, suggest that a nonprofessional person witness for the physician instead.

- An offer to answer the patient's inquiries
- Freedom from coercion, unfair persuasions, or inducements

Informed consent is not simply a matter of signing a consent form. Chart 2–8 presents important nursing considerations to keep in mind when obtaining informed consent.

The ANA places the right to self-determination first in its ethical Code for Nurses (American Nurses' Association, 1984). The Code for Nurses alludes to certain developmental and competency considerations. This means that an individual must display cognitive processes indicative of a capacity to make an informed health care decision. To demonstrate the highest degree of respect for persons, some advocate that each patient be individually evaluated for competency to the task at hand (Heath, 1977; Winslow, 1984). Ensurance that a full consent process has taken place is especially important as nurses assume advanced practice roles (Kline, 1995). This empowers children and youth for consumer self-care (Igoe, 1991).

Consent for Minors' Participation in Research

Some believe that children should never be used as human research subjects. It is argued that they are not cognitively and developmentally capable of giving a truly informed consent to participate as a subject. Even proxy consents from parents, they feel, are not good enough to ensure an ethically valid consent. Their objections are not grounded in the theoretical and empirical knowledge bases of development experts, however. Children are asked to participate as subjects in many forms of research (Fig. 2–6). According to federal guidelines, an adolescent may provide consent and a child of younger years may provide assent to participate as a research subject. In addition, a parent must also provide written consent. The law presumes that parents meet the standards of qualified consent for their children (Kline, 1995).

Minors' participation in research without full consent procedures is unlawful. This position was enjoined by the DHHS in final regulations published in the March 3, 1983, *Federal Register*, and effected June 6, 1983. This was reaffirmed by the DHHS Federal Regulations (U.S. Department of Health and Human Services, 1991). They require the permission of parents or legal guardians for all persons younger than age 18 for participation as a research subject. There are a few exceptions, such as minimal risk research or drugs for a life-threatening illness (Holder, 1992). This is reasonable, because participation in a research protocol is rarely an emergency.

Kachoyeanos (1996, p. 205) contends that many institutional review boards (IRBs) suggest obtaining assent from "all developmentally appropriate children over the age of seven" years. This is consistent with federal regulations (U.S. Department of Health and Human Services, 1991). In addition, as for all ages of human subjects, a description of the purpose of the study written at the sixth to eighth grade reading level must be supplied. This includes purpose of the study and the fact that it involves research, risks and discomforts, alternative treatments, and statement that insurance may not cover treatment expenses, because most insurance companies do not fund experimental therapies (U.S. Department of Health and Human Services, 1991). Other requirements include the name and telephone number of an appropriate contact person, a statement of voluntariness of participation, and risks of withdrawing from the study and ending the study treatment.

Developmental Considerations

Professionals concerned about informed consent in children have given many examples of adolescents deciding their own health. Evidence suggests that excluding psychologically or mentally incompetent teens (e.g., the mentally retarded or those using psychotic defense mechanisms), many adolescents have reached the age at which they can make competent decisions when a full consent process takes place (Deatrick, Angst, & Madden, 1994; Dickey, 1992; Weithorn & Campbell, 1982).

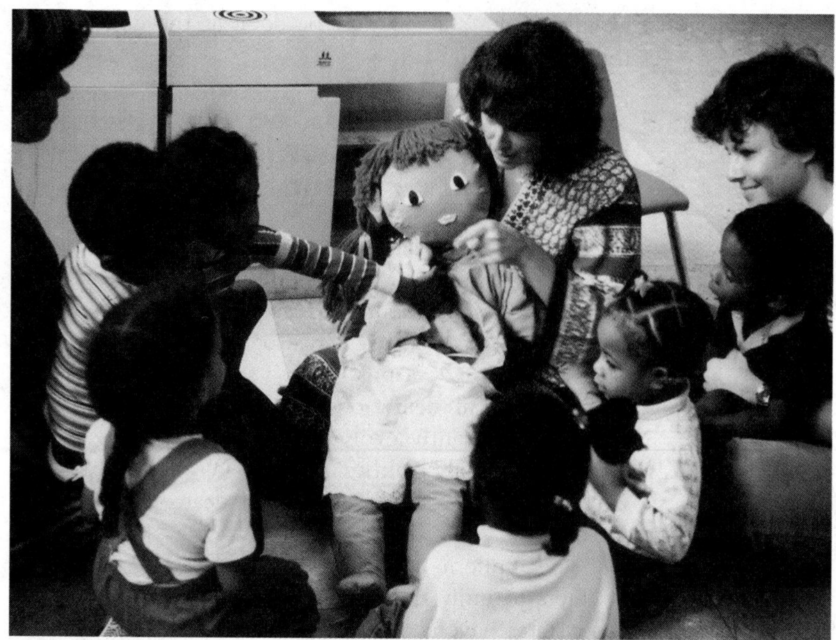

Figure 2–6
Children are often the subjects as well as the focus of research studies. Here a research team uses a doll in a study exploring effective ways to teach children about their bodies. (Courtesy of Judith A. Vessey, Ph.D., C.R.N.P.)

Adolescent Consent

In the professional literature, ethical, moral, and legal aspects of obtaining informed consent from adolescents are often considered together, because in reality, these aspects are frequently intertwined. In most states, the legal age of majority is 18 years, whereas other states establish 21 years of age as the official beginning of adulthood.

Although many health care providers believe that the ability to make reasonable informed consent decisions is based on abstract thinking and formal operations as described by Piaget (1972), there is not a statistically significant contingency relationship (Dickey, 1992). When adolescents of normal and higher intelligence are given all the information to make health care treatment decisions, they probably make them similarly to adults (Dickey, 1992; Weithorn & Campbell, 1982). The key to practice with adolescents, then, is ensuring them full disclosure so that they may participate to the fullest in their own health care.

The law recognizes individuality and differing developmental capabilities of adolescents in a patchwork fashion. Unless an adolescent is considered legally emancipated in the state where care is being provided, and can provide proof, consent signatures of a custodial parent or legal guardian should be obtained. This satisfies the legal requirements of parental consent. The consent signature of the patient should also be obtained whenever possible. Most institutions do not provide for including minors in decision-making, but obtaining such a consent satisfies the thinking adolescent's need to feel a part of crucial health decision-making.

Emancipated Minors

Holder (1977, 1992) defines an emancipated minor as one who is not subject to parental control or regulation in many legal contexts. The law increasingly recognizes that under certain circumstances adolescents will not seek treatment unless confidentiality is guaranteed. Emancipation deals primarily with limited, specific circumstances and specific conditions, such as being married, pregnant, or having a sexually transmitted disease. A minor who is self-sufficient and living away from parent(s) may be considered emancipated. Any minor female who has given birth to a child is usually considered emancipated. Some states have liberalized their laws to permit any minor to consent to the diagnosis and treatment of pregnancy, infectious diseases (especially sexually transmitted), harmful substance use and dependency, and emergency care when life or health is threatened. The legal status of minors regarding emancipation has remained static since the 1970s, although that climate may be changing. Nurses should become aware of the specific statutes, rules, and regulations within each state of practice to avoid unintentionally breaking the law.

Case law for the state where health care is delivered should be consulted when treating any minor without the custodial parent's or legal guardian's knowledge or consent. Most legal cases to date have upheld the following general principles:

- The right to an abortion as an extension of constitutionally guaranteed personal freedoms
- Consultation of a minor's parents or guardian in nonemergency cases

- At least an attempt to consult parents unless dealing with an emancipated minor

Abortion statutes vary from state to state with much greater frequency than the general applications of these laws.

Uncertain Consent

If there is the possibility that a truly informed consent was not obtained before a procedure or protocol, the nurse must notify the attending physician. This is important *even if a consent form has already been signed.* It is an ethical duty of every health care provider to ensure that the patient and appropriate family members have an in-depth picture of clinical eventualities and risks. This helps them deal with unexpected procedural outcomes. Early explanations also leave patients and families the option of obtaining additional opinions, particularly before surgical or invasive procedures. Many lay people are far too intimidated to exercise this right to self-determination on their own. Many individuals do not realize that they can override their insurance carriers to seek additional opinions for care if they are willing to pay for those consultations out-of-pocket. All these measures may ultimately prevent unnecessary pain to the child, unnecessary and traumatic procedures, inaccurate diagnostic opinions from one group of providers, or costly and embarrassing lawsuits.

Telephone Consent

On occasion, the nurse may be asked to witness parental consent obtained by telephone. This is not advisable in most situations, for it can leave the witnessing nurse open to possible legal actions should patient or family expectations remain unfulfilled. The nurse might be considered in collusion with the physician. Nonprofessional support staff can serve as equally valid witnesses at little or no personal risk.

Consent for Autopsy

Obtaining consent for autopsy of a child is a sensitive subject and is solely the physician's responsibility. Nurses, however, frequently become involved in the process when asked to serve as witnesses. Some institutions do not permit nurses to witness any permission request for autopsy, feeling that a court of law may construe such collaboration as an act of "collusion" to "coerce" an unwilling family into granting permission. If a pediatric death meets the criteria for investigation by the medical examiner, the autopsy may be done at the discretion of the medical examiner.

Legal Responsibilities in the Death of a Pediatric Patient

No rules or laws have been addressed specifically for nurses regarding legal responsibilities in a pediatric patient's death. The court system in each state tends to concentrate on the prevailing social policy in decisions involving dying persons. Many state legislatures have arrived at legal definitions of death, but these definitions are constantly evolving as various legal, scientific, and professional realities emerge (Wolf, 1988). (See Chapter 12 for a full discussion of death of a pediatric patient.)

The Uniform Determination of Death Act of 1982 attempts to unify the law on patient death in all states. Most states have adopted some form of this law. The act stipulates that individuals are determined to be dead only when they have sustained either irreversible cessation of circulatory and respiratory functions or irreversible cessation of all functions of the entire brain, including the brain stem.

A determination of death must be made according to accepted standards determined on a state-by-state basis. In some states, registered nurses may legally pronounce death in persons with terminal illnesses when death is the expected outcome of a physical condition. This does not include deaths that occurred in patients as side effects of treatments for the condition. Cardiorespiratory death is determined by the person legally permitted to do so via regulations of a given state. In brain death, the electroencephalogram (EEG) has an isoelectric (flat) readout. There must be complete absence of electrical activity in the brain for death to be declared.

The definition of brain death is evolving (*In re Quinlan*, 1976; Wolf, 1988). It is beyond the scope of this text to include hypothetical situations that may eventually redefine legal brain death. However, whole brain death (legal brain death with all anatomic structures in an irreversible state) is being differentiated from cortical death (higher brain structures) among ethical circles (Emmanuel, 1995; Wolf, 1988). Important questions surrounding pediatric brain death have been raised by Stephenson (1987). The ability of neonates and young children to tolerate long periods of apnea and anoxia has not been substantively researched. The brains of children in these age groups may have an increased resistance to hypoxemia compared with those of adults. Children have impressive abilities to overcome neurologic injuries, especially if the injuries are sustained in a very cold environment, such as near-freezing water. Therefore, care must be taken with the application of adult legal criteria for brain death, especially in children younger than 5 years of age (President's Commission, 1981).

Medical Examiner's Cases

Various local and state laws govern circumstances surrounding a death that must be reported to the medical examiner (coroner). These include deaths with suspicious circumstances of any kind, particularly if a professional error or misjudgment contributed to the death. If a nurse is unsure whether a death occurring in his or her professional sphere is reportable, appropriate individuals should be asked (not necessarily the administration of the institution). A telephone call to the Medical Examiner's office for guidelines and protocols from local and state jurisdictions may be useful.

Professional Liability and Pediatric Cases

Four conditions, called the "four D's," must be met in order to sue for professional malpractice:

- **Duty** owed by the professional to the patient
- **Dereliction of duty** (required act left undone)
- **Damage** suffered (usually physical or developmental)
- **Direct causation** (also known as proximate cause)

In other words, the specific health care provider and the providing organization must have a professional duty to deliver specific forms of care (within reasonably prudent standards). The plaintiff (patient, and for minors, loosely includes family) must then prove that there was dereliction of this duty (failure by the provider or institution to provide care adequately). Unless there is observable damage to the patient and proven by the patient, it is unlikely that a suit will be filed, because an attorney is unlikely to take a case without real merit. In addition, the patient/plaintiff must prove that damage created is of a permanent nature and has been sustained because of the injury (such as inability to participate in sports or manage life similarly to preinjury state). The damage must be proven to prevent a patient/plaintiff's ability to function normally within society.

The most important action to protect against lawsuits, even if a patient was injured permanently, is always to treat the patient and family members politely and respectfully. Avoid lying to patients and family members about circumstances; yet, seek separate legal protection (not the institution's) if involved in an incident with accompanying injury. Nondisclosure and altered records usually become self-evident if the injury is serious enough. Nurses should purchase individual policies for professional liability insurance. If an employee has violated a procedure or policy of an institution, its insurance policy may not cover the act of negligence or malpractice. The relationship between the provider and the patient/family is profoundly important. Many people dislike suing nurses, unless there has been ill will created in the relationship. Nurses enjoy the benefits of positive stereotyping in this way, as the public generally sees them as helpful, informed, and competent advocates of the patient.

Statutes of Limitations

A statute of limitations is the legal amount of time that one has to sue. If filing does not occur within the specific period, the patient loses the right to sue a provider for malpractice or professional negligence. The specific time is defined two ways: from the date of the act or omission of care and treatment; or the date that the patient knew or became aware that some form of malpractice resulted in the injury.

Each state regulates its own statutes of limitations. Some states calculate the time from the date of injury or last treatment by the institution or provider. In the case of minors, other states give the patient/plaintiff until the age of legal majority (usually 18 years, but sometimes 21 years) or the age of majority plus 2 years. Some states are so restrictive as to prevent a person from filing at the age of majority. This protects providers from lawsuits for incidents that occurred many years previously.

In pediatrics, there are major reasons why statutes of limitations may be lengthy. Caring for a damaged child with a normal life expectancy is extremely expensive, especially when the child must attend special programs to optimize development. Charges can be made many years later than they can when an adult statute of limitations is applied, leading to other malpractice or negligence actions. Usually, there is sympathy for a family that is left with the responsibility of caring for the injured or impaired child, whereas there is a tendency to view corporate institutions as having ample insurance coverage to handle the costs of large awards by juries.

The implication for nurses caring for children is that, if involved in some form of practice in which infants and young children are injured, many years can go by before a lawsuit is filed. The statutes of limitations for minors apply even for injury or loss to an adolescent. These legal codes were created to prevent financial devastation to families burdened with the costs of extended and possible lifetime care.

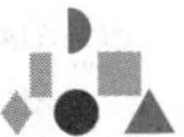

Security Issues in the Care of Children

Nurses are responsible for many aspects of care that require impeccable attention to correct patient identification. Examples include administration of medications, performing and preparing children for a variety of medical and surgical procedures, even transporting to and from various departments. Under any of these circumstances, the consequences of mistaken identity can range from mere embarrassment to personal and professional tragedy. Double-checking the child's identity is a vital part of every nursing procedure, particularly when dealing with preverbal infants or children whose communicative abilities have been precluded by delayed development or impaired by illness or medical treatment. Documentation that these precautions have been taken, such as recording the identification bracelet number of a neonate and later matching it with the birth record and the mother's matching nameband, is very important. Suggestions for the accurate identification of the pediatric patient, both inpatients and outpatients, are presented in Chart 2–9.

Chart 2–9

Pediatric Identification Strategies

- Ensure the presence of a nameband in locations where direct physical care is provided (e.g., the Emergency Department, Day Surgery Unit, or an inpatient setting).
- Always check the child's nameband before performing any nursing procedure. Younger children may answer to any name. Older children may think it is funny to "switch" and trick the nurse.
- Identify and double-check the organ, extremity, or side of the body to be treated.
- Double-check crib and wrist tags before removing or returning infants.
- Be aware of more than one child with the same name. This occurs frequently in newborn nurseries prior to the infant's acquiring a first name.
- Be aware of the child's whereabouts, on or off the unit.
- Check both identification (ID) bands from the delivery setting to match names and numbers in the case of handing a newborn to a mother. It is not realistic to expect newly delivered mothers to recognize their newborns, especially if they are exhausted, sick, or under the influence of mind-impairing medication.
- Ask the mother to keep her own identification band on her wrist when a newborn must remain hospitalized after the mother's discharge. Such ID bands are not removable without cutting them off, and any such handling of the ID band will be readily noticeable.
- Take Polaroid photographs of the parents (especially mother) and infant together in the event of an expected prolonged hospitalization of the newborn. Keep one for the chart, and give them the other one. Have the mother bring her ID band at the time of discharge.

Visitor Identification and Management

Despite how busy any pediatric setting may become, the nurse should be aware of every individual on the premises and also of visitors' or callers' relationships to specific children. Be aware of strangers on the unit and those asking questions about the children. The possibility of unauthorized adults trying to obtain information about a child's condition, or even of kidnapping and abduction, is very real. This is especially true in large and busy settings where visitor flow is difficult to control.

Situations in which children are sick or injured can trigger bizarre, disruptive, or even combative behavior in overstressed relatives or friends. Whether or not such behavior is aimed directly at the nurse, it is the nurse's responsibility to contain the disruption before it disturbs patients, other visitors, or the work of other nursing and medical personnel. If there are threats at gunpoint, polite and respectful compliance, without showing fear if possible, is probably the best approach until law enforcement officials can manage the situation.

All visitors should receive prior parental permission; however, this is not the actuality in most practice settings, especially with short-stay admissions. Information about restrictions should be determined with the initial database. This alerts the nursing staff to situations where custody issues may arise or where there are restraining orders preventing specific individuals from seeing certain children.

Most of the missing children in the United States are abducted by one of their own parents. Some of these abductions occur when the family is experiencing unusual circumstances, such as hospitalization for an acute illness. The abducting parent's emotional needs may even cloud the ability to reason that the child needs acute care. Hundreds of thousands of child abductions by a parent, as opposed to stranger kidnapping, occur each year in the United States. Many families have fingerprinted, blood-typed, and video-printed their children because of such possibilities. Some envision the day when a "DNA fingerprint" of every person will be on file.

Services are available for parents who either are contemplating abducting their own child or have already done so, so that other alternatives may be chosen instead. Mediation and mental health services can provide a great deal of help in these situations, lessening the permanent damage to the family system members, even if such a situation has already occurred. When a health care provider suspects that a child has been abducted, Child Find of America [(800) A-WAY-OUT or (800) 292-9688] and a referral to a competent counseling social service may help. If abduction is in progress or is being contemplated, prior mediation between battling parents and other family members may ease the situation before issues of criminality occur.

These warnings having been heeded, the nurse caring for children strives to maintain as normal an environment as possible for the children. This includes visitations by siblings and other significant relatives; friends, when appropriate; beloved pets, under controlled circumstances and if safe for other persons; and teachers, coaches, clergy, significant baby sitters, or health care providers from other settings.

Documentation Strategies

Accurate and complete documentation is very important to the health maintenance and safety of children. It enables nurses to interpret their role to other disciplines and protect themselves, their patients, and their institutions. Progress toward outcome goals, via the care path (see Chapter 1 for explanation), for example, is as important as information about the child's physical condition. Nurses must explicitly document remaining patient and family teaching needs, including how much patients and their parents have learned about taking responsibility for their own home care, and identify remaining nursing needs. Teaching instructional plans (TIPs), such as those used in this text, ease tracking and documentation of teaching.

Documentation and the Law

Although charts and records are considered the property of the institution, they may be subpoenaed and are admissible evidence in court. Records are considered more reliable than memory, especially because statutes of limitations for pediatric cases are so long (see section earlier in this chapter). Patients and parents (or legal guardians) should have the right to read a child's chart, and it is rarely, if ever, reasonable to withhold information from family members such as parents. Many institutions monitor this by making specific policies, such as requiring the presence of the patient's physician when a chart is read. In some states, records are made accessible to the patient or designee (parents for minors), including a copy if they so wish. Regulations vary from state to state. Withholding information may annoy and alienate patients and their families from a system viewed as unresponsive to their needs.

Nursing Actions for Complete Pediatric Documentation

The following considerations are useful for any setting, but are especially important in the pediatric setting (Chart 2–10). Pediatrics is a subspecialty by its very nature, and thus care of children is not by nature routine. When health care providers leave out information not directly related to a child's immediate condition, much information is lost of the complete picture. For example, how a child tolerates a diet postoperatively is related to a surgical outcome, because blood will be shunted away from the periphery (gastrointestinal tract) if postoperative recovery is compromised. Pulmonary function, skin integrity, and capillary refill are similarly related to a surgical outcome and are part of complete disclosure in record keeping.

A short, but informational, sentence included as a direct quotation from each parent (guardian) helps show family anxiety levels. Words or lack thereof from a previously verbal child demonstrates his or her current degree of interaction with the environment. The notes explain progress in the child's individual plan of care, confirm the presence and level of functioning of each tube or wire, describe the condition of injuries or incisions, and offer a system-by-system assessment of level of functioning. Each body system is assessed to detect any relevant information about that system.

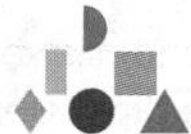

Research in the Care of Children

Research is the avenue by which the scientific knowledge base expands. Many find the knowledge explosion and the information age difficult with which to cope. After all, much research is done with severe sampling problems, even if the premise is respectable. Sampling has everything to do with the provider's ability to use the findings in settings other than that where it was conducted. Sadly, much of the research in health care, especially the smaller projects published in lesser journals, perpetrates findings that are not generalizable. Many federal agencies fund different forms of research on children and families.

A major problem is that no national research agenda for children and families exists (Coughlin & Perry,

Chart 2–10

Guidelines for Pediatric Documentation

- Keep good records—they are a potent defense against malpractice claims with extended statutes of limitations.
- Avoid such clichés as "patient received," "patient appears," or "no complaints."
- Pay extreme attention to accurate detail in describing abuse and trauma-related injuries in the chart for forensic purposes. Take competent photographs of injuries and place them in the chart.
- Be sure that both sides of each page have the child's name stamped at the top.
- Record legibly. Unintelligible and incomplete records may be construed as grounds for negligence.
- Chart all observations and actions. Information that is not charted is considered undone, as in the case of a high-risk child who needs frequent vital signs or treatments.
- Include nursing actions on the patient's behalf. Write the physician's name in the progress notes when reporting a change in the child's condition, e.g., "Dr. Swain notified of temperature elevation to 38.5 degrees C at 1600 [4 P.M.]," not "MD aware."
- Avoid taking verbal orders when possible.
- Abbreviate infrequently, and use only those approved by a committee that represents all patient care disciplines in the institution. Examples of unclear abbreviations are BS, which stands for breath sounds, bowel sounds, or blood sugar, and MS, which stands for multiple sclerosis, magnesium sulfate, or morphine sulfate.
- Describe the family member's or child's behaviors rather than making a valuative comment such as "appropriate," "inappropriate," "manipulative," or "obnoxious" (Kempe & Helfer, 1987). An example of descriptive charting is, "The patient's mother was seen wandering into the intensive care unit down the hall. She was redirected to the parent services lounge, and the nurse manager was able to spend some time with her."
- Include behaviors that evaluate the objectives and outcomes of the written plan of care, such as "Mother was able to demonstrate drawing up the accurate dose [name the amount] of digoxin in an oral syringe." This will exonerate the nurse from claims that teaching was inadequate. This type of charting also demonstrates the amount of time needed for patient/parent teaching and gives a clearer picture of acuity status.
- Perform a detailed system-by-system analysis of children with unusual or potentially critical illnesses or injuries and note physical condition. The frequency of such examination is a matter of nursing judgment; however, each time there is a personnel change, a new assessment should be performed by the professional nurse assuming responsibility.
- Record system-by-system documentation of physical condition. Regardless of the documentation system incorporated at a particular institution, some assessments are important to include (pertinent negatives) in spite of whether the system conveniently permits, as sometimes occurs in computer-based documentation systems. An example of including pertinent negative would be to chart "No dyspnea, grunting, flaring, retracting, pallor or cyanosis; good capillary filling time" when charting a respiratory assessment. Professional judgment guides what to include.
- Include pertinent comments or questions by the patient or family. Record verbatim and enclosed in quotation marks. For example, "How long will Sherry have a sore throat?"—mom. "Will she have to have another transfusion?"—dad. "I can't cough! My throat hurts!"—Sherry.
- Document the level and frequency of professional surveillance (including vital signs).
- Chart the patient's progress with regard to the illness or situation at hand. This avoids temptation to include personality traits or idiosyncrasies that are not germane to the problem at hand (Beachy & Deacon, 1993).
- Be aware of strangers on the unit and those asking questions about the child's chart. Avoid sharing written and spoken information with unknown persons.

1995). Funding for projects from one agency overlaps with another. There is duplication of effort for some topics and neglect of others. There is no central clearinghouse, but even more alarming, no coordinated distribution of findings for taxpayer-funded research on families and children (Coughlin & Perry, 1995). This is wasteful.

Without specific regard to how findings are derived and careful use of the recommendations that researchers make about their findings, the profession encourages a state of "nursing by rumor" rather than sound, scientifically based practice (Vessey, 1994). Nursing is in its infancy with regard to research utilization in practice settings.

A clear example of nursing by rumor is the former nursing practice of teaching parents to place infants on their abdomens after a feeding. The practice was recommended but not research based. Tonkin (1996), who has studied sudden infant death syndrome (SIDS) since the early 1970s, asked parents why they placed their infants prone after feedings. Nurses had told them to do so.

When nurses were asked about this, they stated that they had observed the practice in neonatal units and succumbed to the belief that the infants might vomit and inhale the emesis. Over time, factors related to SIDS were investigated to show four modifiable risk factors that play a large part in the SIDS death rate: prone sleeping, cigarette smoking (by mother), co-sleeping, and not breast-feeding (Mitchell, 1995; Mitchell, Taylor, & Ford, 1992). This is clearly a set of research-based findings that may prevent many deaths by simple behavioral changes.

Few studies have scientifically reported sampling methodology (Beal & Betz, 1993). This is particularly true for pediatric studies. One reason for this is legal and ethical access to enough children to form an adequate sample size. Many study ideas never come to fruition because of some form of obstruction to sample access. There are several deficiencies that devalue the findings of the work (Beal & Betz, 1993):

- Failure to describe the sampling frame and methods
- Small or limited power sample size
- Failure to report number of refusals or lost cases
- Inappropriate generalizations
- Lack of acknowledgment of study limitations

Most of the research reports that Beal and Betz (1993) considered have obsolete findings at this point.

Beal and Betz (1993) reviewed parent-child nursing research published in seven refereed nursing journals throughout the 1980s. The data were based on findings directly from children and their parents. The sampling methodology employed in a preponderance of these studies was amazingly weak. Many samples were acquired while children were in the hospital. There were few targeted studies of prevention and health promotion for children in their early years. Another distressing fact was that it was difficult for the authors to distinguish age groupings of subjects in the reports. Because pediatric nursing has a primarily developmental focus, it is not logical that reported research findings ignore the importance of age. Age is one of the most important foci of studying pre-adult groups.

Recommendations for future pediatric nursing research include the following (Beal & Betz, 1993):

- Moving settings into the community to study issues of health promotion with high-risk groups
- Increasing sample size
- Increasing ethnic heterogeneity (including diverse groups)

These practices will enhance generalizability and relevance to practice (Beal & Betz, 1993).

A pediatric nursing challenge for these times is to convince others of its people-centered orientation. Pediatric nurses at the turn of the millennium will be in a fragile era for adequate and prudent resource allocation and therefore must "form partnerships with those who do not share our vision" of nursing care for children and their families (Visintainer-Baranowski, 1995). One way in which to do this is through competent, outcome-based research. Nurses caring for children must juggle multiple, complex, competing forces to collaborate for the best, research-based, patient care possible.

Maternal and Child Health Bureau Research Priorities

The Research Program of the Maternal and Child Health Bureau (MCHB) of the DHSS has safeguarded and improved health of mothers and children since its establishment in the 1960s. Research grants are awarded to public and private nonprofit institutions of higher learning and to agencies that provide health care. Proposals may be either investigator-initiated (by one or more individuals who have a research background) or program-directed (carried out by people within an institution with a special research focus). Priorities change over time, as do special projects. At the time of this writing, funded research is likely to be in one of these topic areas: poverty, drugs, homelessness, family structure, health outcomes of intervention and treatment, and escalating health care costs. The MCHB promotes dissemination and discussion of findings through conferences and symposia. New policies, statements, and updates are easily obtained via the Internet. The purpose is to bring researchers, providers, policy makers, and program planners together for collaboration on ways to improve health for mothers and children.

Agency for Health Care Policy and Research Priorities

The Agency for Health Care Policy and Research (AHCPR) is the eighth agency within the United States Public Health System, established in 1989. It replaces the National Center for Health Research (NCHR) and the National Center for Health Care Technology Assessment (Hibbard, 1995). The development of research-based practice guidelines is one of AHCPR's primary purposes (Denker, 1995). Periodic suggestions for priority topics are invited. They seek topics related to prevention, diagnosis, treatment, and/or management of common diseases and clinical conditions (American Nurses' Association, 1996a). At the time of this writing, the research priorities related to children and adolescents include acute pain management, cancer pain, depression, sickle cell disease, HIV/AIDS, and otitis media (Denker, 1995). Free copies of current priorities may be obtained from AHCPR (see Resources list at the end of chapter).

Summary of Key Concepts

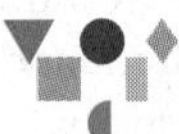

- Pediatric health care issues and concerns are becoming increasingly complex as the next millennium approaches. Major issues include the persistent poor prenatal care that many mothers receive and a relatively high (although declining) infant mortality rate; the continuing toll of accidents, violence, substance abuse, and sexually transmitted disease on our children and adolescents; and the socioeconomic problems of poverty and lack of health insurance, which can restrict access to care for children and their families.
- The role of government in creating access to pediatric care is becoming more and more important. Approaches to culturally competent and culturally sensitive care are also assuming increasing importance as our society becomes more diverse.
- National health concerns and goals for children are delineated in Healthy Children 2000; many of these goals are yet to be attained. Worldwide health concerns of children, with an emphasis on WHO and UNICEF guidelines, projects, and avenues for funding, await implementation. Child advocacy groups and other child-focused organizations, such as NACHRI and the Children's Defense Fund, serve children at the aggregate level.
- The rights of pediatric patients, parents, guardians, and others, custodial and noncustodial, are sometimes complex and must be understood and respected by the nurse and other health care workers.
- Child abuse reporting and documentation are legally required of all professional nurses and many other health care workers. Nurses and other professionals also have legal responsibilities associated with the death of a minor. Security issues, such as visitor identification and management and documentation strategies, also have some aspects unique to the care of children.

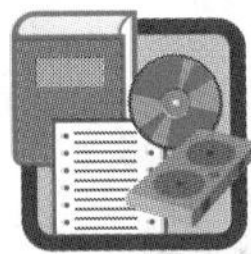

Resources

Organizations

Agency for Health Care Policy and Research (AHCPR)

Center for Research Dissemination and Liaison

AHCPR Publications Clearinghouse
P.O. Box 8547
Silver Spring, MD 20907
(800) 325-9295
(301) 495-3453
For free copies of research priorities: (800) 358-9295
FAX: (301) 594-2800

American Nurses' Association
Department of Governmental Affairs
600 Maryland Avenue, S.W., Suite 100 West
Washington, DC 20024-2571
(202) 651-7000
FAX: (202) 651-7001
Web: http://www.ana.org

American Public Health Association
1015 15th Street, N.W.
Washington, DC 20005
(202) 789-5600

American Red Cross
430 17th Street, N.W.
Washington, DC 20006
(202) 639-3496

Annie E. Casey Foundation
Center for the Study of Social Policy
Washington, DC

Association for the Care of Children's Health (ACCH)
Bethesda, MD
(301) 654-6549

Center to Prevent Handgun Violence
1225 Eye Street, N.W., Suite 1100
Washington, DC 20005

Centers for Disease Control and Prevention
1600 Clifton Road, N.E.
Atlanta, GA 30306
(404) 639-3311
Public Inquiries: (404) 639-3534
AIDS Hotline: (800) 342-AIDS; Spanish (800) 344-SIDA

Child Find of America
(800) A-WAY-OUT
(800) 292-9688

Children's Defense Fund
Washington, DC
(202) 628-8787
Web: http://www.tmn.com/cdf/index.html

The Hastings Center
255 Elm Road
Briarcliff Manor, NY 10510
(914) 762-8500

Institute for Child Health Policy
5700 S.W. 34th Street, Suite 323
Gainesville, FL 32608-5367
(904) 392-5904
FAX: (904) 392-8822
E-mail: ichp@qm.server.ufl.edu

Joint Commission on Accreditation of Healthcare Organizations (JCAHO)
Web: http://www.jcaho.org

Maternal and Child Health Bureau
National Institutes of Health
(301) 443-5720
Chief: Perinatal and Women's Health Branch (301) 443-5720
Communications: (301) 443-3163
Injury prevention program: (301) 443-4026
Publications: National Maternal and Child Health Clearinghouse
8201 Greensboro Drive, Suite 600
McLean, VA 22102
(703) 821-8955, exts. 254 or 265

National Health Council
1730 M Street, N.W., Suite 500
Washington, DC 20036
(202) 785-3910

National Institute of Nursing Research
National Institutes of Health
Bethesda, MD
Web: http://www.ninr.nih.gov
National SAFE KIDS Campaign
1301 Pennsylvania Avenue, N.W., Suite 1000
Washington, DC 20004
(202) 662-0600
FAX: (202) 393-2072

National Safety Council
1121 Spring Lake Drive
Itasca, IL 60143
(800) 621-7619
FAX: (708) 285-0797

U.S. Committee for UNICEF

United Nations Children's Fund
333 E. 38th Street
New York, NY 10016
(212) 686-5522
E-mail: webmaster@unicef.org

U.S. Department of Health and Human Services
Public Health Service
Human Resources and Service Administration
Maternal and Child Health Bureau
Washington, DC 20201

World Health Organization (WHO)
20, Avenue Appia
1211 Geneva 27
Switzerland
(41 22) 791 2111
Telex: 41 54 16
FAX: (41 22) 791 0746
E-mail: postmaster@who.ch
Division of Communicable Diseases: (41 22) 791 2688
FAX: (41 22) 791 4198
Division of Diarrhoeal and Acute Respiratory Disease Control: (41 22) 791 2111
Division of Food and Nutrition: (41 22) 791 3325
Relief Health Advisor: (41 22) 730 4448

Note: Also see Chapter 1 resource list for nursing organizations relevant to children's advocacy. Check World Wide Web to determine existence of Internet access to these agencies. Many have or are developing web pages at press time.

References

Aiken, T. D., & Catalano, J. T. (1994). *Legal, ethical and political issues in nursing.* Philadelphia: F. A. Davis.

American Nurses' Association. (1984). *Capital Update, 2*(6), 1–2.

American Nurses' Association. (1985). *Code for nurses with interpretative statements.* Kansas City, MO: Author.

American Nurses' Association. (1996a). AHCPR seeks research priority topics. *Capital Update, 14*(12), 6.

American Nurses' Association. (1996b). Maternity/Newborn Insurance Bill. *Capital Update, 14*(16), 2.

Associated Press. (1996, August 12). Man born with heart outside body turns 21. *The Bucks County [Pennsylvania] Courier Times*, p. A.

Beachy, P., & Deacon, J. (Eds.). (1993). *Core curriculum for neonatal intensive care nursing.* Philadelphia: W. B. Saunders.

Beal, J. A., & Betz, C. L. (1993). Sampling issues in parent-child nursing research: Implications for nursing practice. *Journal of Pediatric Nursing, 8*(4), 261–262.

Beauchamp, T. L., & Childress, J. F. (1983). *Principles of biomedical ethics* (2nd ed.). New York: Oxford University Press.

Bedinghaus, J., & Doughten, S. (1994). Childhood nutrition: From breastmilk to burgers. *Primary Care, 21*(4), 655–672.

Benkert, M. R., Dianas-Hughes, N., Hazinski, M. F., Moloney-Harmon, P., Rollins, J. A., & Velsor-Friedrich, B. (1995, March). Confronting the epidemic of violence: The pediatric nurse's response. Paper presented at the meeting of the Society of Pediatric Nurses on Nursing Care of Children and Their Families, Washington, DC.

Bishop, J. E., & Waldholz, M. (1990). *Genome.* New York: Touchstone–Simon and Schuster.

Blendon, R. J., Aiken, L. H., Freeman, H. E., & Corey, C. R. (1994). Access to medical care for black and white Americans: A matter of continuing concern. In C. Harrington & C. L. Estes (Eds.), *Health policy and nursing—crisis and reform in the U.S. health care delivery system* (pp. 313–330). Boston: Jones & Bartlett.

Botter, M. L., & Dickey, S. B. (1989). Allocation of resources: Nurses, the key decision makers. *Holistic Nursing Practice, 4*(1), 44–51.

Bower, B. (1994). Growing up poor—poverty packs several punches for child development. *Science News, 146*, 24–25.

Bower, B. (1996). Growing up in harm's way—child victimization develops into a scientific challenge. *Science News, 149*, 332–333.

Campinha-Bacote, J. (1994). Cultural competence in psychiatric mental health nursing: A conceptual model. *Nursing Clinics of North America, 29*(1), 1–8.

Capers, C. F., & Talerico, K. L. (1995). A path to cultural competency in clinical practice. *The Nursing Spectrum, 4*(7), 4.

Castiglia, P. T. (1995). Family violence. *Journal of Pediatric Health Care, 9*, 269–271.

Centers for Disease Control (1991). *Preventing lead poisoning in young children.* Washington, DC: U.S. Department of Health and Human Services.

Child Abuse Prevention and Treatment Act, 42 U.S.C.A.5106a(b)10(c)(1983).

Children's Defense Fund (1996). *Welcome to the Children's Defense Fund* [6 paragraphs]. Available World Wide Web: http://www.tmn.com/cdf/index.html.

Coughlin, P., & Perry, D. (1995). *Statement on child and family health.* Washington, DC: Center for Child Health and Mental Health Policy, Georgetown University Child Development Center. Available World Wide Web: www.ichp@qm.server.ufl.edu.

Cruzan v. Director, Missouri Department of Health, 110 S. Ct. 2841 (1990).

Davis, K. (1994). Inequality and access to health care. In C. Harrington & C. L. Estes (Eds.), *Health policy and nursing—crisis and reform in the U.S. health care delivery system* (pp. 359–375). Boston: Jones & Bartlett.

Deatrick, J., Angst, D. B., & Madden, M. (1994). Promoting self-care with adolescents. *Capsules and Comments in Pediatric Nursing, 1*(2), 11–20.

Denker, A. L. (1995). Closing the research-practice gap. *American Journal of Nursing*, 95(12), 51, 53–55.

Dickey, S. B. (1992). Formal operations, puberty and informed decisions (Doctoral dissertation, University of Pennsylvania, 1992). *Dissertation Abstracts International.* Ann Arbor, MI: University Microfilms (No. DAO 72699).

Drayton-Hargrove, S., & Woods, J. H. (1995, July/August). Ethical analysis of health care reform: Implications for diverse communities. *Journal of Black Nursing Faculty*, 99–103.

Dunn, A. (1995). Priorities for children's health care: How to achieve Healthy People 2000 goals. *Journal of Pediatric Health Care*, 9, 28A.

Emergency Medical Treatment Act, 42 U.S.C.A. 1395dd.

Emmanuel, L. L. (1995). Reexamining death—the asymptotic model and a bounded zone definition. *Hastings Center Report, 25*(4), 27–35.

Feshbach, N. D., & Feshbach, S. (1978). Toward an historical, social, and developmental perspective on children's rights. *Journal of Social Issues, 34*(2), 1–7.

Franklin-Barbajosa, C. (1992, May). DNA profiling—the new science of identity. *National Geographic*, 112–123.

Gaylord, N. (1996, February). Ethical concerns in pediatrics. *Advance for Nurse Practitioners*, 47–48.

Gerchufsky, M. (1996). Are 'drive-through deliveries' putting moms and babies at risk? *Advance for Nurse Practitioners*, 4(2), 22–27.

Glover, J. J. (1995, March). *An ethics of care in the era of cost-containment.* Paper presented at the meeting of the Society of Pediatric Nurses on Nursing Care of Children and Their Families, Washington, DC.

Grossman, D. (1996). Cultural dimensions in home health nursing. *American Journal of Nursing*, 96(7), 33–36.

Hardy Havens, D. M. (1996). Children and tobacco. *Journal of Pediatric Health Care, 10*, 37–40.

Hardy Havens, D. M., & Hannan, C. (1995). The federal role in motor vehicle safety issues. *Journal of Pediatric Health Care*, 9, 279–281.

Health Insurance Reform Act of 1996. U.S. Public Law: 104–191 (8/21/96).

Heath, D. H. (1977). *Maturity and competence.* New York: Gardner Press.

Hibbard, H. (1995). *Outcome based research programs.* Paper presented at the meeting of the Society of Pediatric Nurses on Nursing Care of Children and Their Families, Preconference—Nursing Research and Public Policy: A Partnership for Improving Child Health Care. Washington, DC.

Holder, A. R. (1977). The minor's right to consent to medical treatment. *Connecticut Medicine, 41*, 30–34.

Holder, A. R. (1992). Legal issues in adolescent sexual health. *Adolescent Medicine, 3*(2), 257–267.

Igoe, J. (1990). A blueprint for health promotion: Children's rights and community action. *Pediatric Nursing, 16*(4), 410–411.

Igoe, J. (1991). Empowerment of children and youth for consumer self-care. *American Journal of Health Promotion*, 6(1), 55–65.

Ikeda, J., & Wright, J. (1996). Pediatrics in a culturally diverse society. *Gerber Pediatric Basics, 76*, 10–17.

In re Karen Ann Quinlan, 70 N.J. 10, 355 A.2d 647 (1976).

In re Baby K, 832 F.Supp. 1022 (E.D. Va., 1993).

Institute for Child Health Policy. (1995). *Creative vision in research and service. The mission.* Gainesville, FL: Author. Available Internet: ichp@qm.server.ufl.edu.

Jacobsen v. Massachusetts, 197 U.S. 11 (1905).

Kachoyeanos, M. K. (1996). Elements of informed consent. *MCN, American Journal of Maternal Child Nursing, 21*, 205.

Kempe, C. H., & Helfer, R. (Eds.). (1987). *Helping the battered child and his family* (4th ed.). Chicago: University of Chicago.

Kimmel, S. R. (Ed.). (1994). Well-child care—issues in prevention [Special issue]. *Primary Care, 21*(4).

Kimmel, S. R. (Ed.). (1995). Well-child care—specific clinical concerns [Special issue]. *Primary Care, 22*(1).

Kline, N. E. (1995). A minor's consent to treatment: An ethical dilemma. *Journal of Pediatric Health Care*, 9, 282–284.

Korn, A. R. (1995, March). *National SAFE KIDS Campaign: The politics surrounding initiatives.* Paper presented at the meeting of the Society of Pediatric Nurses on Nursing Care of Children and Their Families, Washington, DC.

Landsberg, M. (1992, September 27). Florida boy divorces parents, sets important precedent. *Bucks County [Pennsylvania] Courier Times*, A-1, A-3.

Leininger, M. M. (1981). Transcultural nursing: Its progress and its future. *Nursing and Health Care*, 365–371.

Leutwyler, K. (1995). The price of prevention. *Scientific American, 272*(4), 124–129.

Lipson, D. J. (1991). An overview of state roles in health care policy. In T. J. Litman & L. S. Robins (Eds.), *Health politics and policy* (2nd ed., pp. 170–189). Albany, NY: Delmar.

Litman, T. J. (1991). Government and health: The political aspects of health care—a sociopolitical overview. In T. J. Litman & L. S. Robins (Eds.), *Health politics and policy* (2nd ed., pp. 3–37). Albany, NY: Delmar.

Mason, D. J., Talbott, S. W., & Leavitt, J. K. (Eds.). (1993). *Policy and politics for nurses: Action and change in the workplace, government, organizations and community* (2nd ed.). Philadelphia: W. B. Saunders.

McAndrews, L. (1995, March). *The national agenda for child health care.* Paper presented at the meeting of the Society of Pediatric Nurses on Nursing Care of Children and Their Families, Preconference—Nursing Research and Public Policy: A Partnership for Improving Child Health Care, Washington, DC.

Mitchell, E. A. (1995). Sleeping position and SIDS. *European Journal of Pediatrics, 154*(Suppl. 1), S27.

Mitchell, E. A., Taylor, B. J., & Ford, R. P. K. (1992). Four modifiable and other major risk factors for cot death: The New Zealand Study. *Journal of Pediatric Child Health*, 28(Suppl. 1), S3–S8.

Mittelstadt, P. C. (1994). Federal reimbursement of advanced practice nurses' services empowers the profession. In C. Harrington & C. L. Estes (Eds.), *Health policy and nursing—crisis and reform in the U.S. health care delivery system* (pp. 341–348). Boston: Jones & Bartlett.

National Safety Council. (1995). *Accident facts, 1995 edition.* Itasca, IL: Author.

National SAFE KIDS Campaign. (1994). *Reform that works: Preventing childhood injuries produces real, documented health care savings.* Washington, DC: Author.

Nelson, D. (1993). Report by Nelson, Executive Director of the Annie E. Casey Foundation. *ABC Focus.* Washington, DC: Annie E. Casey Foundation.

News. (1996). Preschool children face health insurance gaps. *Advance for Nurse Practitioners, 4*(2), 7–8.

Nugent, J. K. (1994). Cross-cultural studies of child development: Implications for clinicians. *Zero to Three, 15*(2), 1, 3–8.

Ozmar, B. (1994). Encountering victims of interpersonal violence. *Critical Care Nursing Clinics of North America, 6,* 515–522.

Paine, L. S. (1994, March-April). Managing for organizational integrity. *Harvard Business Review,* 106–117.

Parker, S., Zahr, L., Cole, J., & Brecht, L. (1991). *Developmental intervention in the NICU for mothers from low SES: Does it improve child outcomes after discharge?* Unpublished manuscript, Department of Pediatrics and Division of Developmental and Behavioral Pediatrics. Boston City Hospital and University School of Medicine and University of California, Los Angeles, School of Nursing.

Pennsylvania Nurses Association. (1996). Mandatory minimum maternity benefits bill signed. *Legislative Bulletin, 15*(3), 3.

Piaget, J. (1972). Intellectual evolution from adolescence to adulthood. *Human Development, 15,* 1–12.

President's Commission for the Study of Ethical Problems in Medical and Biomedical and Behavioral Research. (1981). Guidelines for determination of death. *Journal of the American Medical Association, 246,* 2184.

Rehabilitation Act of 1973, 504; 29 U.S.C.A. 794.

Rhodes, A. M. (1995). In re Baby K. *MCN, American Journal of Maternal Child Nursing, 20,* 251.

Rhodes, A. M., & Miller, R. D. (1984). *Nursing and the law* (4th ed.). Rockville, MD: Aspen.

Rice, M. F., & Winn, M. (1991). Black health care and the American health system: A political perspective. In T. J. Litman & L. S. Robins (Eds.), *Health politics and policy* (2nd ed., pp. 320–334). Albany, NY: Delmar.

Rogge, M. M. (1987). Nursing and politics: A forgotten legacy. *Nursing Research, 36*(1), 26–30.

Rollins, J. A. (1995). *Street drugs: What's hot and what's not.* Paper presented at the meeting of the Society of Pediatric Nurses on Nursing Care of Children and Their Families, Washington, DC.

Rosen, J. F. (1996). Ingredients of urban pediatric health care: Fourth world pediatrics. *Pediatrics, 97*(6), 898–899.

Rosoff, A. J. (1981). *Informed consent: A guide for health care providers.* Rockville, MD: Aspen.

Ruff, H. A., Bijur, P. E., Markowitz, M., & Rosen, J. F. (1993). Declining blood lead levels and cognitive changes in moderately lead poisoned children. *Journal of the American Medical Association, 269,* 1641–1646.

Schloendorff v. the Society of the New York Hospital. 211 N.Y. 125, 105 N.E. 92 (1914).

Shays, C. (1995). *Composition of 1995 federal spending.* Washington, DC: Office of U.S. Representative Christopher Shays.

Shea, J. (1995). Debating the ethics of genetic engineering. *Penn Health Magazine, 1*(3), 7–9.

Society of Pediatric Nurses. (1995a). SPN policy statement on pediatric injury prevention. *SPN News, 4*(1), 6.

Society of Pediatric Nurses. (1995b). SPN policy statement on pediatric firearm injuries. *SPN News, 4*(1), 7.

Society of Pediatric Nurses. (1995c). Report on conference. *SPN News, 4*(2), 2.

Stephenson, C. (1987). Brain death in children—is there a difference? *Focus on Critical Care, 14*(1), 49–56.

Sterken, D. J. (1995). HIV/AIDS in the classroom: Ethical and legal issues surrounding the public education of the HIV infected child. *Journal of Pediatric Health Care, 9*(5), 205–210.

Sternberg, S. (1996). Penetrating the secrets of tuberculosis. *Science News, 149,* 375.

Thomasma, D. C., Muraskas, J., Marshall, P. A., Myers, T., Tomich, P., & O'Neill, J. A. (1996). The ethics of caring for conjoined twins—the Lakeberg twins. *Hastings Center Report, 26*(4), 4–12.

Thompson, J. E., & Thompson, H. O. (1985). *Bioethical decision making for nurses.* Norwalk, CT: Appleton-Century-Crofts.

Tonkin, S. (1996). On listening to parents: The sudden infant death syndrome over 25 years. *Pediatrics, 97*(6), 896–897.

United Nations Children's Fund. (1992). *1992 Report Review of the Year.* New York: Author.

United Nations Children's Fund. (1996). Welcome to the United Nations Children's Fund World Wide Web [9 paragraphs]. Available E-mail: webmaster@unicef.org.

U.S. Department of Health and Human Services. (1990). *Healthy People 2000.* Boston: Jones & Bartlett.

U.S. Department of Health and Human Services. (1991). Protection of human subjects [45 Code of Federal Regulations 46], *Federal Register,* rev. ed., 15–16, 47–48.

U.S. Department of Health and Human Services. (1992). *Healthy Children 2000.* Boston: Jones & Bartlett.

U.S. Department of Health and Human Services. (1996). *Healthy People 2000: Mid-Course Review and 1995 Revision.* Boston: Jones & Bartlett.

U.S. Public Health Service. (1995). Put prevention into practice—newborn screening. *Journal of the American Academy of Nurse Practitioners, 7*(10), 513–517.

Velsor-Friedrich, B. (1995, March). *Prioritizing child health initiatives: A working strategy session.* Paper presented at the meeting of the Society of Pediatric Nurses on Nursing Care of Children and Their Families, Washington, DC.

Vessey, J. A. (1994). Nursing by rumor. *Capsules and Comments in Pediatric Nursing, 1*(3), 1–2.

Visintainer-Baranowski, M. (1995, March). *The specialty of pediatric nursing: The growth of our science and practice.* Paper presented at the meeting of the Society of Pediatric Nurses on Nursing Care of Children and Their Families, Washington, DC.

Weithorn, L. A., & Campbell, S. B. (1982). The competency of children and adolescents to make informed treatment decisions. *Child Development, 53,* 1589–1598.

Weitzman, M., Aschengrau, A., Bellinger, D., Jones, R., Hamlin, J. S., & Beiser, A. (1993). Lead-contaminated soil abatement and urban children's blood lead levels. *Journal of the American Medical Association, 269,* 1647–1654.

Winslow, G. R. (1984). From loyalty to advocacy: A new metaphor for nursing. *Hastings Center Report, 14,* 32–40.

Wolf, S. (1988). The persistent problem of PVS. *Hastings Center Report, 18,* 26–47.

World Health Organization. (1995). WHO calls for action on spread of drug resistant diseases [13 paragraphs]. Available E-mail: postmaster@who.ch.

Bibliography

American Medical Association. (1993). *Adolescent health promotion.* Chicago: Author.

American Nurses' Association. (1993). Summit on Indian health care reform. *Capital Update, 11*(6), 5.

American Nurses' Association. (1996). Children's health coverage declines. *Capital Update, 14*(13), 5.

American Political Network. (1993). Child health gets a grade of C−. *Daily Report Card, 3*(88), 1–2.

Americans with Disabilities Act of 1990. U.S. Public Law 12102(2).

Anderson, A. W. (1991). Health services in the United States: A growth enterprise for a hundred years. In T. J. Litman & L. S. Robins (Eds.), *Health politics and policy* (2nd ed., pp. 38–52). Albany, NY: Delmar.

Annie E. Casey Foundation. (1994). *Kids count data book.* Washington, DC: Annie E. Casey Foundation for the Study of Social Policy.

Bartels, D. M., LeRoy, B. S., & Caplan, A. L. (1993). *Prescribing our future—ethical challenges in genetic counseling.* New York: Aldine de Gruyter.

Battistella, R. M., Begun, J. W., & Buchanan, R. J. (1991). The political economy of health services: A review of major ideological influences. In T. J. Litman & L. S. Robins (Eds.), *Health politics and policy* (2nd ed., pp. 66–92). Albany, NY: Delmar.

Beachy, P., & Deacon, J. (Eds.). (1993). *Core curriculum for neonatal intensive care nursing.* Philadelphia: W. B. Saunders.

Canterbury v. Spence, 464 F.2d 772 (D.C. Cir. 1972).

Children's Defense Fund. (1994). *Child health source book.* Washington, DC: Children's Defense Fund Press.

Curran, W. J., & Shapiro, E. D. (1982). *Law, medicine and forensic science* (3rd ed.). Boston: Little, Brown.

DeMause, L. (1975). Our forebears made childhood a nightmare. *Psychology Today, 8*(4), 85–88.

Dickey, S. B. (1987). *A guide to the nursing of children.* Baltimore: Williams & Wilkins.

Edge, R. S., & Groves, J. R. (1994). *The ethics of health care: A guide for clinical practice.* Albany, NY: Delmar.

Fagin, C. M. (1994). Cost-effectiveness of nursing care revisited: 1981–1990. In C. Harrington & C. L. Estes (Eds.), *Health policy and nursing—crisis and reform in the U.S. health care delivery system* (pp. 313–330). Boston: Jones & Bartlett.

Flarey, D. L. (Ed.). (1995). *Redesigning nursing care delivery: Transforming our future.* Philadelphia: Lippincott.

Hall, J. K. (1994). Understanding the fine line between law and ethics. *The Nursing Institute's C.E. Booklet Series* (pp. 1–5). Springhouse, PA: Springhouse.

Hamilton, D. (1990, February 16). She hopes the baby can be donor. *The Philadelphia Inquirer*, p. 7-A.

Harrington, C., & Estes, C. L. (Eds.). (1994). *Health policy and nursing: Crisis and reform in the U.S. health care delivery system.* Boston: Jones & Bartlett.

Katcher, A., & Haber, J. (1991). The pediatrician and early intervention for the developmentally disabled or handicapped child. *Pediatrics in Review, 10,* 305–311.

Kimmel, S. R. (Ed.). (1994). Well child care: Issues in prevention. *Primary Care, 21*(4).

Kimmel, S. R. (Ed.). (1995). Well child care: Specific clinical concerns. *Primary Care, 22*(1).

Lee, P. C., & Estes, C. L. (Eds.). (1994). *The nation's health* (4th ed.). Boston: Jones & Bartlett.

Leiken, S. L. (1983). Minors' assent or dissent to medical treatment. *Journal of Pediatrics, 102,* 169–176.

Litman, T. J., & Robins, L. S. (Eds.). (1991). *Health politics and policy* (2nd ed.). Albany, NY: Delmar.

Moyer, M. E. (1994). A revised look at the number of uninsured Americans. In C. Harrington & C. L. Estes (Eds.), *Health policy and nursing—crisis and reform in the U.S. health care delivery system* (pp. 352–358). Boston: Jones & Bartlett.

National Center for Children in Poverty. (1995). Number of poor children under six increased from 5 to 6 million 1987–1992. *News and Issues, 5,* 1–2.

Nelms, B. C. (1995). Children first: Is it ever going to happen? *Journal of Pediatric Health Care,* 9, 197–198.

Parens, E. (1996). Taking behavioral genetics seriously. *Hastings Center Report,* 26(4), 13–22.

Raloff, J. (1996). The human numbers crunch—the next half century promises unprecedented challenges. *Science News,* 149, 396–397.

Rifkin, J. (1995). *The end of work.* New York: G. P. Putnam's Sons.

U.S. General Accounting Office (1996). *Health insurance for children: Private insurance coverage continues to deteriorate.* Washington, DC: U.S. Government Printing Office.

Villarruel, A. M. (1996). Medicaid reform. *Journal of the Society of Pediatric Nurses, 1*(1), 43–45.

Zell, E. R. (1994). An analysis of doctor certified medical records of children entering school in 19 urban and one rural area in Arkansas. *Journal of the American Medical Association,* 16, 331–403.

The Child Developing Within the Family

OUTLINE

- **Family Theories**
  - Family Systems Approach
    - Olson Circumplex Model
  - Developmental Approach
    - Family Life Cycle
    - Family Life Spiral
    - Changing Life Cycle
  - Family Stress and Coping Frameworks
    - ABCX and Double ABCX Models
    - Crisis Theory
    - Family Adjustment and Adaptation Response Model
  - Structural-Functional Approach
  - Interactional Approach
  - Institutional Approach
  - Social Exchange Theory
  - Conflict Theory
- **Family Assessment Tools**
- **Family Structure**
  - Nuclear Family
  - Dual-Career Family
  - Extended Family
  - Single-Parent Family
  - Binuclear Family
  - Blended Family
  - Gay and Lesbian Family
  - Communal Family
- **Family Functions**
  - Family Roles
  - The Healthy Family
- **Special Family Issues**
  - Adoption
  - Foster Care
  - Multiple Births
  - Divorce
  - Grandparent Families
  - Teenage Parent Families
  - Homeless Families
- **Cultural and Religious Influences on the Family**
  - Cultural and Religious Concepts
  - Values and Beliefs of Health Care Professionals
  - Health Beliefs and Practices of Culturally Diverse Families
  - Cultural and Spiritual Assessment
  - Health Care Implications

OBJECTIVES

- Discuss selected family theories, delineating their strengths, limitations, and application to nursing practice.
- Explain the family life cycle model as a framework for viewing family development across the life span.
- Identify theory-based family assessment tools that can be utilized in clinical practice.
- Describe different family structures.
- Delineate the functions and roles of family members within the family.
- Examine the impact of selected family issues on the family system.
- Examine the cultural and religious influences that can affect child health care.

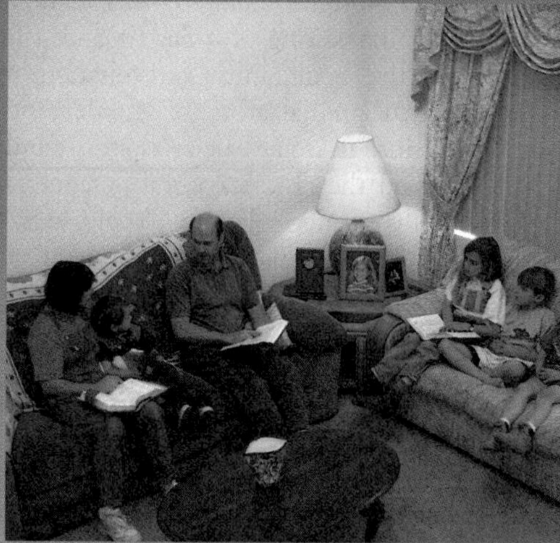

KEY TERMS

acculturation
bicultural
cohesion
crisis
culture
demand
ethnicity
family transition
flexibility
foster care
multiculturality
norms
position
race
religion
role
spirituality

CHAPTER

3

An African proverb states that "it takes a whole village to raise a child." These few, simple words emphasize the significant role of the "community," the "family," in the child-rearing process. The community that surrounds the child affects every aspect of the child's health and general welfare. The quality of life within this community has the greatest effect on the child's ability to achieve developmental tasks and become a functional member of society. For some children, this community is a close-knit group consisting of a parent and a few siblings. For others, the community constellation may include an extended familial group of grandparents, aunts, uncles, and cousins. In some societies, the family unit extends well beyond the child's natural parents to include friends and family members bound closely together as a group that fosters communal living and joint accountability for the rearing of children.

It is not difficult to see that the multiplicity of family configurations in today's society creates a challenge in adhering to one single definition of the term family. As discussed in Chapter 1, traditional descriptions of the nuclear family (mother, father, and children) are no longer representative of the family units in which children are raised in the 20th century. A family as defined by the United States Census Bureau is "a group of people related by blood, marriage, or adoption" (U.S. Bureau of the Census, 1990). This definition does not account for the diversity of functional family forms. A broader, more culturally sensitive definition of the family would be "a group of two or more individuals usually living in close geographic proximity; having close emotional bonds and meeting affectional, socioeconomical, sexual, and socialization needs of the family and wider social system" (Rankin, 1989, p. 174). Gellerstedt and leRoux (1995, p. 68) stated that a family is an emotional system moving together through time. An even broader definition for the nurse to consider is that "family" is anyone the patient says it is (Bozett, 1987; Patterson, 1995) (Chart 3–1).

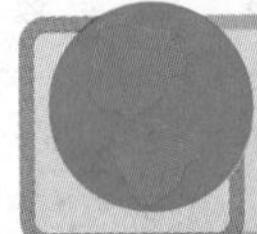

Chart 3–1
Worldview

Family Diversity

The United Nations (UN) designated 1994 as the International Year of the Family, using the motto "Building the smallest democracy at the heart of society." The UN recognized that the family has a variety of forms and functions around the world. Family *diversity* is affected by changing demographics and social and economic patterns.

The various family forms around the world include the following:

Nuclear

Biological
Social
One parent
Adoptive
In vitro

Extended

Three-generation
Kinship
Tribal
Polygamous

Reorganized

Remarried
Community living
Same gender

Not all of these family forms are legally recognized in all societies. The emerging family structures represent the resilience of the family and its ability to evolve to meet the challenges brought about by social change (Ahmann, 1994).

However one chooses to define the child's family, there is no doubt that families in today's society are faced with complex challenges as they try to nurture, develop, and socialize their young. These challenges create stress and often a sense of crisis within the family unit. As the family responds to normal concerns and unusual developmental and situational crises, the children learn adaptive and nonadaptive behaviors to cope with the stressors of life. In response, some children may develop physical illnesses, psychological symptoms, destructive and disruptive behaviors, depression, or anxiety. These can lead to social and academic difficulties when children are unable to cope with stress successfully.

Yet, for many others the family can protect children from the negative outcomes associated with stress by teaching them appropriate mechanisms for coping with the challenges associated with the transitions and changes that accompany the childhood years (Patterson, 1995). It is within the context of the family that the child learns about relationships and behaviors that promote healthy interactions with others. Therefore, to begin to understand the child, it is important first to understand the family, its functions, roles, and structure. Such an understanding is fundamental to providing quality health care (Foster & Phillips, 1992).

This chapter reviews several theories that explain how families develop and interact. The types of families most prevalent in today's society are discussed, and the

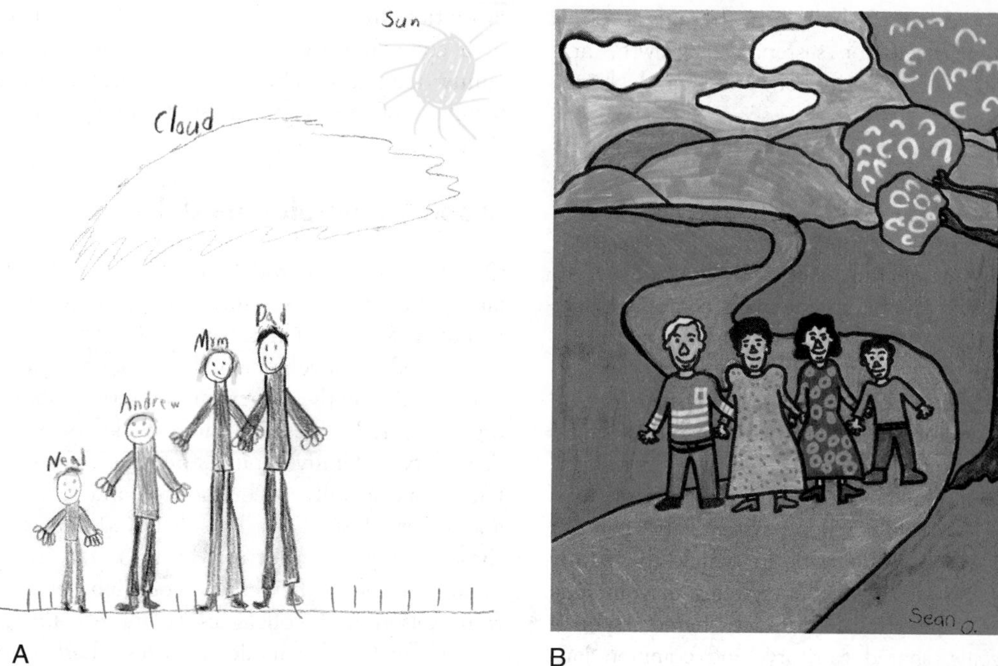

Figure 3–1
A child's drawing of his or her family often provides insight into how the child conceptualizes the family. *A*, A 7-year-old child's drawing of his "traditional" nuclear family. *B*, A 7-year-old child's drawing of his ethnically diverse family. He lives with his grandfather, grandmother, and mother.

impact of divorce, remarriage, and single parenting on these families is described (Fig. 3–1). Family roles, family function, and the healthy family unit are also presented.

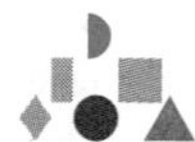

Family Theories

Historically, the family was assessed and analyzed in terms of its individual members. Little emphasis was placed on viewing the members of the family within the context of the familial group with whom they shared a common existence. Since the 1950s, family theorists have attempted to explain and organize conceptual thoughts about the family from a variety of theoretical perspectives. Several approaches have emerged and have been identified as the primary models in terms of which the family has been studied. These models include the following: family systems, developmental, family stress and coping, structural-functional, interactional, institutional, social exchange, and conflict theories (Christensen, 1964; Friedman, 1992; Hill, 1971; Jones & Dimond, 1982; Mercer, 1989; Nye & Bernardo, 1981). Although other frameworks, such as anthropologic, psychoanalytic, Western Christian, legal, and social-psychological, appear in the literature, these have not been as relevant or applicable to nursing science.

This section presents an overview of the theoretical approaches that have contributed the most to nursing practice and our understanding of how families cope with the challenges and stressors of everyday life. From these theories have emerged several tools that the health care professional can use to assess family needs and dynamics. These assessment tools are presented.

Family Systems Approach

Viewing the family as a system is a modification of general systems theory as described by von Bertalanffy in 1968. A system is defined as a goal-directed unit made up of interdependent, interacting parts that endure over a period of time (Friedman, 1992). There are both open and closed systems. An open system is one that receives input from the surrounding environment. That is, the system shares information, materials, and energy with its environment. The functional goal of the system is to ensure survival, continuity, and growth of its components (Friedman, 1992). The open system depends on the interactions with the surrounding environment to achieve growth and change. In contrast, the closed system does not receive input from the environment. In the closed system, the units depend wholly on the relationships within the system itself for sustenance, growth, and change. Therefore, the capacity for growth and change over time is limited.

In this context, the family is viewed as a complex open system consisting of two or more persons tied together by mutual interactions, goals, and needs. Each member of the family influences and is influenced by every other family member, as well as by the other environments with which the family members come into contact. The interrelationships within the family system are so intricately tied together that change by any one person invariably results in changes in all family members.

As an open system, the family is capable of being influenced by and having an impact on the systems adjoining the boundaries. These adjoining systems include other families, the child's school system, the parent's work system, and the community in which the family lives. The interchange with other systems may include sharing of information, physical contact, shared responsibility, mutual goals, shared territory, and common language. For the family to exist as a system among other systems, a certain amount of exchange must take place (Richman, Chapman, & Bowen, 1995). However, among families there are varied degrees of openness depending on the specific reaction of the family to change from the outside. The family with a high degree of openness provides for change. Change is welcomed and considered normal and desirable. Furthermore, communication and rules within the family are related, and individual self-worth is of primary importance. A family that has little exchange with the environment is one that resists change. A closed unit family depends on edict and law and order and operates through force, both physical and psychological. Self-worth is secondary to power and performance.

As a unit, the family has boundaries that separate it from other systems. These boundaries act to filter or translate information that comes into and flows out of the system. Boundaries consist of the rules, sanctions, communication patterns, attitudes, and values that bind the family together and guide their beliefs and practices. The family unit belongs to the many other systems that impinge on its boundaries. It also determines its own degree of interaction with other systems.

The family is a homeostatic system. This implies that, as the family is undergoing a process of continual growth and change, the unit strives to maintain a sense of balance or equilibrium. Parson and Bales (1955, p. 402) referred to this as the "steady state" of an "ongoing system." The family reacts to change in its steady state by attempts to reestablish equilibrium. Adaptation within the family refers to the ability of its members to modify their behavior toward each other and the outer world as the situation demands (Friedman, 1992). Any disruption in the function of one family member results in a compensatory change in the functions of all other family members. Therefore, to restore equilibrium, all members of the system must be involved in the adaptation process.

Olson Circumplex Model

One of the most widely used models to describe the family that uses a systems framework is the Olson Circumplex Model. The goal of the family system is to accommodate developmental and situational change and stress, while at the same time preserving its integrity and organizational cohesion (Cluff, Hicks, & Madsen, 1994). A variety of family coping strategies are used to help the family successfully accommodate and adapt to internal and external stressors. It is believed that the effects of these coping activities can be measured in terms of the family's level of **flexibility**, **cohesion**, and **communication**. Olson and colleagues (Cluff et al., 1994; Olson, 1994) developed a model to assess these three concepts and explain more fully how families react to situational and developmental stressors. The circumplex model is a matrix that identifies 16 types of marital and family systems on the two dimensions of flexibility and cohesion (Fig. 3–2). Family cohesion addresses the degree of emotional bonding that family members have toward one another. Family flexibility is the amount of change in the family's leadership, role relationships, and relationship rules. Family communication is a facilitating dimension; it helps families make changes on the cohesion and flexibility dimensions (Olson, 1993, 1994).

Cohesion and Flexibility. The model illustrates four levels of cohesion and four levels of flexibility. It is hypothesized that the central or balanced levels of these two concepts make for optimal family functioning. The extremes of cohesion (disengaged or enmeshed) and the extremes of flexibility (chaotic or rigid) are generally viewed as problematic to families (Olson, 1988). The family that is evaluated as "too" close and the family that is "too" rigid in its expectations of family members are examples of environments in which the closeness and rigidity are seen as harmful because they do not allow and encourage individual growth within the family unit.

Levels of family functioning change over time and as the family passes through different developmental stages. It is hypothesized that families with the central levels of flexibility and cohesion generally function more adequately across the family life cycle than families with extreme levels (Olson, 1988). This does not imply that balanced families always operate within the central levels of the model. Rather, being balanced signifies that the family system can operate at the extremes for short periods of time and when appropriate because of situational and developmental stressors. In these families extremes

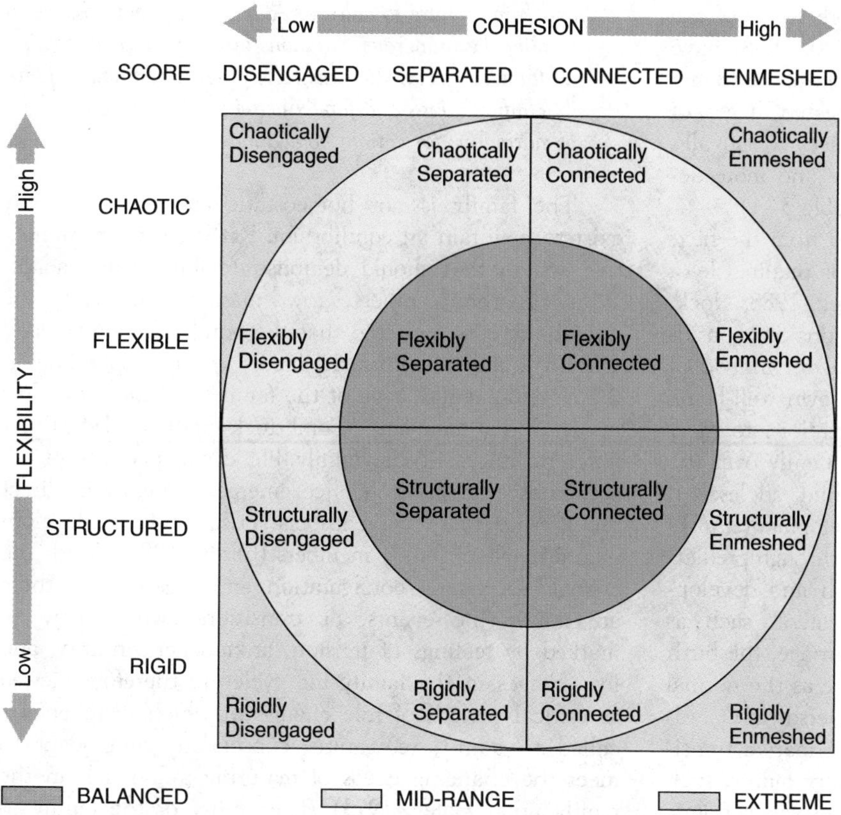

Figure 3–2
The circumplex model identifies 16 family types that vary in their degree of flexibility and cohesion. (Redrawn from Olson, D., Portner, J., & Lavee, Y. [1985]. *FACES III*. St. Paul, MN: Family Social Science. Used with permission.)

are tolerated and even expected, yet the balanced family does not continually operate in that fashion. On the other hand, extreme family types tend to function only at the extremes and strongly discourage any deviation from this pattern of functioning by individual members (Olson, 1988, 1993).

Communication. Communication is the third dimension of the circumplex model and is considered a facilitating dimension. It is considered critical for allowing families to make changes on the other two dimensions (Olson, 1988, 1994). As a facilitating dimension, it is not graphically included on the model with cohesion and flexibility. The indicators of communication can be observed in families using two other instruments, the clinical rating scale and the parent-adolescent communication scale (Olson, 1994). It has been hypothesized that families with central levels of flexibility and cohesion have more positive communication skills than extreme families. In addition, positive family communication enables balanced families to change their levels of flexibility and cohesion more easily than families on the extremes. Thus, positive communication skills enhance family adaptation to situational and developmental stressors (Galvin & Brommel, 1986; Olson, 1988).

The circumplex model builds on family developmental theory and systems theory to hypothesize that families change as they deal with normal transitions in the family life cycle (Olson, 1988). These changes can and should be beneficial to the maintenance and improvement of the family system as the family transforms in composition, role structure, and role functioning.

Developmental Approach

The developmental framework is not considered a unique approach to family theory. Rather, it is a synthesis and logical expansion of several conceptual ideas found in other models, such as the interactional, institutional, structural-functional, and systems theories (Hill, 1971; Hill & Rodgers, 1964; Jones & Dimond, 1982; Mattessich & Hill, 1987). The framework is original in that it focuses on the longitudinal career of the family, often called the **family life cycle** or the **family career**. The central theme of the developmental approach is that the family is a unit that changes over time as a result of the physical and psychosocial transitions of both adult and child members.

Family Life Cycle

Duvall (1962) was among the first to divide the family life cycle into eight stages with developmental tasks at each stage. These stages were based on the criteria of (1) major change in family size, (2) the developmental stage of the oldest child, and (3) the work status of the breadwinner. Carter and McGoldrick (1980, 1988) have conceptualized the family life cycle in a six-phase framework. Several other authors have delineated stages of the family life cycle, primarily adding stages to Duvall's model to account for the childless couple and more detailed transitions in the elderly couple (Table 3–1).

Each developmental stage is separated from the next by the amount of **family transition** that is required by a particular life event (Carter & McGoldrick, 1988; Nock, 1981; Rowe, 1981). These family transitions are considered "normal," and they have implications for individual members who must critically assess their own well-being and alter their role functions and expectations to meet the changing developmental tasks of the family over the life course (Rankin, 1989). Just as the child, adolescent, and adult need to accomplish certain developmental tasks or milestones, the family must also move through predictable transitions for optimal family growth and development. Milestones of individual development, such as starting school, reaching adolescence, marriage, the birth of a new baby, and retirement, often serve as the normal transitions that affect the entire family (Gershwin & Nilsen, 1989). Unexpected events or paranormative transitions are events that do not occur in every family, such as illness, disability, miscarriage, change in socioeconomic status, or divorce, and can result in crisis within the family (Carter & McGoldrick, 1980). These events or transitions can alter the developmental course for all the family members, altering the natural movement of the family (Rolland, 1993).

The developmental theories are based on the assumption that the family is a semiclosed social system made up of interacting personalities (Hill, 1971; Rowe, 1981). Using principles from systems theory, it can be said that the interrelationships within this system are so intricately tied together that change in any one part invariably results in change in the entire system (Friedman, 1992). In the family, each member has specific positions, roles, and normative expectations to fulfill at various points along the family life cycle. *Position* refers to the location of the family member in the family structure, such as husband-father or wife-mother. *Roles* are defined as a set of behaviors that are normatively defined by a culture for a person occupying certain positions. *Norms* are the role behavioral expectations commonly shared by family members (Rowe, 1981). In developmental theory it is assumed that family members change their positions, roles, and norms at various stages in the cycle in order to accommodate the addition and emancipation of children and to maintain family stability.

Worldview: *It should be noted that family positions, roles, and norms often vary greatly from family to family and from culture to culture. Although it is not possible to identify the numerous variations of these concepts within all families, social scientists have observed dominant family configurations and family activities that are identified as normative for certain populations.*

The family is not homeostatic and cannot simply exist to maintain an equilibrium. Rather, it is an interactive system that should demonstrate fluidity and adaptability as the members grow, mature, and leave the household. It is expected that the bonds of cohesion and unity will change within the family system, depending on the developmental stage of the family and the individual needs of its members (Combrinck-Graham, 1985). At different stages in the family life cycle, patterns of togetherness and independence emerge and exist in direct relationship to the psychosocial crises and the developmental goals of family members (Olson, 1988). With the changes in family configuration and organization there are family life events, or transitions, which may be marked by feelings of tension, anxiety, uncertainty, and loss. Stages in the family life cycle are therefore viewed as critical periods of role change in which members are called to adjust, reorganize, consolidate, and adapt to meet the changing needs of maturing individuals in the family unit (Haley, 1973). The ability of the family to adapt, reorganize, and move to the next stage requires changes in boundaries and roles within the family. The family's ability to move through the crisis facilitates their development. If the crisis is not handled adequately, old tensions or new conflicts arise (Rapoport, 1963, 1964). Family therapy is often necessary when families are overwhelmed or caught in a particular stage. Therapy is then directed toward moving the family into the next developmental stage.

Family developmental theory addresses the family from a traditional view of family life. It is difficult to utilize a set sequence of family stages to explain the variety of family transitions that can occur (Aldous, 1990). Its use is limited in the diversity of family forms found in today's society. It does not take into consideration couples who chose not to marry or couples who chose not to have children, as this theory uses children as markers for movement from one stage to the next. Some theorists have developed variations of the traditional family developmental stages for the divorced or remarried family in an attempt to depict the additional stages through which these families are required to move (Carter & McGoldrick, 1988). Other theorists have embraced the concept of critical role transitions to explain differences in the sequencing of stages and a family's approach to a new stage. Other newer approaches to explain the changing dynamics of the family unit include the family life spiral and the changing family unit.

Table 3–1
Theorists' Views of the Developmental Stages of the Family

Duvall (1957)	Feldman (1961)	Rodgers (1964)	Carter & McGoldrick (1980)
			1. Leaving home: single young adults
1. Couple without children	1. Early marriage (childless)	1. Childless couple	2. The joining of families through marriage: the new couple
2. Oldest child less than 30 mo	2. Oldest child an infant	2. All children less than 36 mo	3. Families with young children
3. Oldest child from 2½ to 6 yr	3. Oldest child at preschool	3. Preschool children with oldest 3–6 yr and youngest under 3 yr 4. All children 3–6	
4. Oldest child from 6 to 13 yr	4. All children school age	5. School-age family with infants 6. School-age family with preschoolers 7. All children 6–13 yr	
5. Oldest child from 13 to 20 yr	5. Oldest child a teenager, all others in school	8. Teenage family with infants 9. Teenage family with preschoolers 10. Teenage family with school-agers 11. All children 13–20 yr	4. Families with adolescents
6. When first child leaves until last is gone	6. One or more children at home and one or more children out of the home	12. Young adult family with infants 13. Young adult family with preschoolers 14. Young adult family with school-agers 15. Young adult family with teenagers 16. All children older than 20	5. Launching children and moving on
7. Empty nest to retirement	7. All children out of the home	17. Launching family with infants 18. Launching family with preschoolers 19. Launching family with school-agers 20. Launching family with teenagers 21. Youngest child older than 20	
	8. Elderly couple	22. When all children have been launched until retirement	6. Families in later life
8. Retirement to death of one or both spouses		23. Retirement until death of a spouse 24. Death of first spouse to death of survivor	

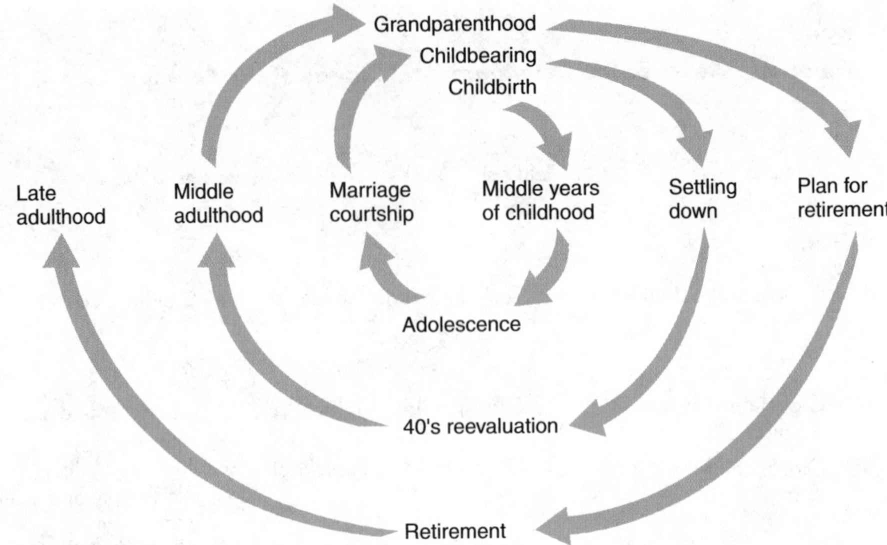

Figure 3–3
The family life spiral shows the overlapping developmental tasks of family members from different generations. (Redrawn from Combrinck-Graham, L. [1985]. A developmental model for family systems. *Family Process, 24*[2], 139–150. Used with permission.)

Family Life Spiral

The family life spiral is a developmental model devised by Combrinck-Graham (1985, 1990) that incorporates overlapping developmental tasks of the individual members of each generation in the family. Erikson's (1963) stage of "generativity" of the adult leads to childbearing and raising of children. The midlife crisis of the adult usually occurs at the period in which the family unit is also dealing with the turmoil of adolescence and the retirement of the grandparents (Fig. 3–3). How the individual works through the individual developmental task has a profound effect on the others who are also trying to move into the next stage of their development. Combrinck-Graham (1990) conceptualized that the family oscillates from periods of closeness, or a *centripetal* family atmosphere, to periods of differentiation, or a *centrifugal* family atmosphere. The child requires constant care and nurturing, whereas the adolescent is moving toward independence. Centripetal forces lead to marriage, sexual intimacy, and childbearing. Centrifugal forces lead to adolescence, retirement, and preparation for death. The family moves between these two forces throughout the family life spiral. The nurse can use this model in attempting to identify what life stages the other family members are in and what impact that has on the family.

Changing Life Cycle

Rankin (1989) developed a developmental family framework that takes into consideration the changing life cycle of American families with respect to their expected transitions (Table 3–2). The *emerging family* is one concerned with the tasks of becoming a family unit. In the traditional life cycle, this would be the stage of beginning families and childbearing families (McGoldrick, Heiman, & Carter, 1993). In this framework, changing emerging families include opposite- or same-sex partners living together with a nonformalized bond. Common, expected transitions encountered by these families include changes in personal relationships, changes in family relationships, and changes in role status. The new couple must establish new roles in their relationship with each other and in their relationship with their families of origin. They must also decide whether or not to move into a parental role. The transition to parenthood is often challenging for the traditional family as well as the non-traditional family. Decisions need to be made defining the role each parent will play in the development of the child.

The *solidifying family* is the family whose primary tasks are to stabilize the bond between the parents and to socialize the children. This stage is consistent with the traditional life cycle with preschool, school-age, and adolescent children. Common transitions that occur in these families require increasingly flexible boundaries to account for the developing independence of children and adolescents (Carter & McGoldrick, 1988).

The *reconstituting family* is one that occurs because of changes in the relationship of its members, such as divorce, death, or separation (Rankin, 1989). The members need to adapt to the loss of the previous family form and adapt to a new type of family, whether it be a single-parent family or a new stepparent family.

The *contracting family* life cycle and the traditional family life cycle are similar in launching children and families in later life. Common transitions encountered in this family type are the changes in the relationships between the children and the new roles that come with these relationships if children are a part of the family. Adaptation to the loss of an adult partner through di-

Table 3–2
Changing Life Cycle: Tasks and Transitions

Family Type	Tasks	Characteristics/Examples	Common Transitions
Emerging	Finding suitable partners	Formalization of marital bond	Change in personal relationships—addition of spouse or significant other. Loss of friends, changes in family relationships
	Constitution of meaningful adult relationships	Decision to live with person of opposite or same sex with non-formalized bond	Changes in roles and status—unmarried to married status, addition of parental role. Possible changes in job, career, related to change in personal relationships
	Decisions related to childbearing and infertility	Traditional or non-traditional family pattern; that is, opposite-sex partners obtain in vitro fertilization or same-sex partners adopt	
	Decision to remain childless	Opposite- or same-sex partners	Change in familiar environment—moving households
Solidifying or reconstituting	Solidification of adult partners' bonds. Child rearing and required interface with schools, health care institutions, and other societal institutions	Stable, non-divorcing families. Child rearing tasks involve nurturance, education, socialization, and provision of climate suitable to development of responsible individuals. Characteristics of families with children are similar whether the family is traditional or not	Change in roles and status—loss or change in marital role through divorce and/or remarriage. Continued career changes Changes in personal relationships—potential loss of significant other, that is, mate, child. Loss of parents in family of origin Changes in physical and mental capacities—major health change
	Reconstitution of family bonds with integration of new family members and loss of old ones	Divorced families and blended families	Changes in possessions—loss or acquisition of loved possessions necessitated by change in income or catastrophic occurrences
Contracting	Launching and release of children to environments separated from family	Traditional nuclear family releases young adult children to armed services, college, marriage, or work	Change in personal relationships—loss of spouse, children, siblings
	Adjusting to loss of adult partner	Death, late-in-life divorce	Change in roles and status—retirement
	Adjusting to loss of work, parental roles	Enforced retirement with consequences of lowered standard of living	Changes in physical and mental capacities—exacerbation of chronic problems, onset of acute episodes
	Integration of leisure time and adjustment to lack of responsibility for children and/or occupation. Development of avocation	Younger, healthy retired couples. Older, healthy workers who choose to continue employment	Changes in familiar environment—moves required by decreased income, loss of spouse, or health problems

From Rankin, S. (1989). Family transitions, expected and unexpected. In C. Gillis, B. Highley, B. Roberts, & I. Martinson (Eds.), *Toward a science of family nursing* (pp. 173–186). Menlo Park, CA: Addison-Wesley. Reprinted with permission.

vorce or death and the changes that come with retirement, such as decreased income and increased leisure time, are also common transitions.

Family Stress and Coping Frameworks

Merging systems and developmental approaches, researchers interested in stress and coping have developed frameworks that explain how families and individuals cope with and adapt to various crisis events. Family stress and coping theories evaluate the impact of acute, unanticipated, and severe external events on the family system. In addition, these theories are used to describe the effects of chronic persistent stressors that may bring long-term hardships on the family. The family experiences normative and non-normative challenges that may undermine family functioning. The challenge for the health care team is to help the family to optimize their resources and coping behaviors for managing the multiple stressors that can affect family life. The child's family may be a source of stress, but, more important, the family should be a resource or refuge protecting the child from the negative effects that are associated with stress (Patterson, 1995; Robinson, 1997). Stress and coping theories can be used to better understand the alterations in family dynamics during times of stress. The ABCX model, crisis theory, and Family Adjustment and Adaptation Response (FAAR) Model, described in the following sections, are examples of models that can be applied to families facing illness, loss, and grief.

A criticism of the stress and coping models has been their inability to explain children's stress coping processes. The models are typically based on using adult-level cognitive and emotional processes to deal with stressful situations (Atkins, 1991).

caREminder: *Children's stressors are not the same as adult stressors. Many of the stressors affecting children are related to situations with parents, teachers, and other family members that are outside the children's control. The stressors children deal with may not be amenable to change by the children themselves; adult assistance is needed.*

The cognitive abilities of children vary considerably from those of adults; thus theories that focus on cognitive appraisal of the situation do not account for these differences. Ryan-Wenger (1992) has noted that a need exists for the development or modification of a stress coping theory that would be specific for children.

ABCX and Double ABCX Models

Hill (1949) was the first to conceptualize a model that describes the processes a family undergoes when a stressor event occurs. The ABCX model described the precrisis variables that accounted for family differences in adaptation to a crisis (Mederer & Hill, 1983, p. 45):

> A (the stressor event)—interacting with B (the family's crisis-meeting resources)—interacting with C (the definition the family makes of the event)—produces X (the crisis).

McCubbin and Patterson (1983) have expanded this model, adding four factors that are believed to influence the family's adaptation over time. The double ABCX model includes postcrisis behaviors as well (Fig. 3–4):

Figure 3–4
The double ABCX model shows how stressors can affect the family over time. (Redrawn from McCubbin, H., & Patterson, J. [1983]. The family stress process: The double ABCX model of adjustment and adaptation. In H. McCubbin, M. Sussman, & J. Patterson [Eds.], *Social stress and the family*. New York: Haworth Press. Used with permission.)

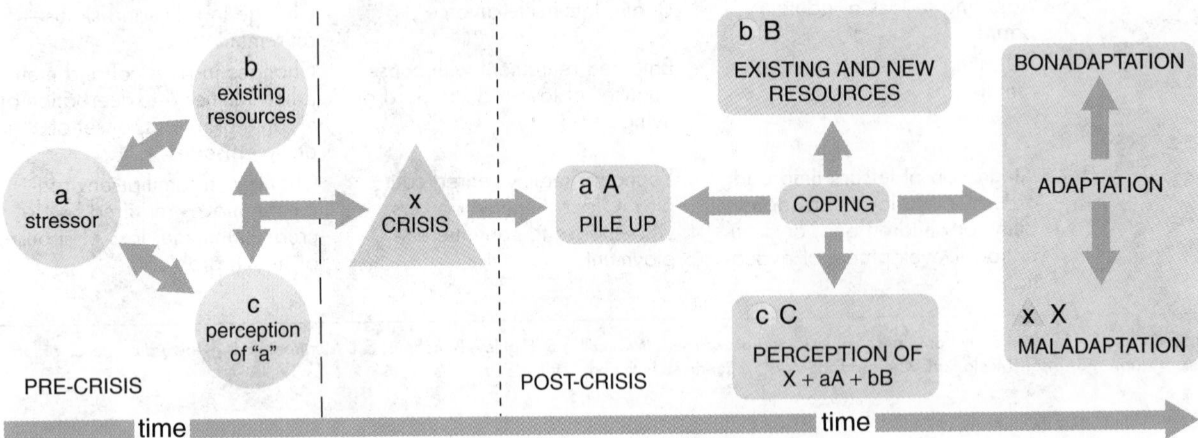

(aA) the accumulation of additional stressors; (bB) family efforts to activate or acquire new coping resources; and (cC) modification by the family of their perception of the total crisis situation. All of the variables relate and contribute to the postcrisis level of family adaptation (xX).

The stressor, or factor, is a life event or transition affecting the family unit that produces, or has the potential to produce, change in the family social system (McCubbin & Patterson, 1983). Family values, boundaries, goals, roles, and interaction patterns are but a few areas of the family life that may change.

The b factor includes the family's resources for meeting the demands of the crisis. Families who are adaptable and capable of making modifications in their actions are able to resist the crisis. Four types of resources used by families are family members' personal resources, the family's internal resources, social support, and coping (Mederer & Hill, 1983).

The c factor refers to how the family defines the stressor and its hardships. This is the subjective meaning the family places on how they feel they are affected by the stressor. Family values, cultural influences, and their previous experiences in dealing with change all affect their definition of the current event.

The a, b, and c factors interact to produce the x factor, or crisis-proneness of the family. In the original model, x, or the crisis, was defined as any sharp or decisive change in the family for which old patterns of interactions and routines were inadequate (Mederer & Hill, 1983). McCubbin and Patterson (1983) have more clearly defined the crisis event as being a family stress or stressor characterized by the inability of the family to restore stability.

The double ABCX model adds factors to the original model that explain how the family adapts over time. The postcrisis variables describe

- Additional life stressors and strains that affect family adaptation
- The critical resources the family employs over time
- The changing definitions the family associates with the stress events
- The coping strategies the family may employ
- The eventual outcomes of the family (McCubbin & Patterson, 1983)

Recognizing that families seldom deal with one stressor at a time, the aA factor refers to the pileup of stressors. This pileup can occur particularly in the aftermath of a major change in the family such as a death or divorce. Additional stressors may emerge from individual family members, the family system, or the community of which the family and its members are a part.

In response to the crisis, the family calls on existing resources and expanded family resources to meet the demands and needs of the crisis. This is the bB factor. The cC factor is the meaning that the family gives to the total crisis situation. This is influenced by the family's belief about what caused the original crisis, the presence of additional stressors, and the old and new resources the family is using to cope with the current situation. Families who are able to redefine the crisis situation as a "challenge" or an "opportunity for growth" are those who are more likely to adapt.

Coping is a bridging concept wherein resources, perception, and behavioral responses interact as families try to adapt and to achieve a balance within the family system. During the coping process, the family may focus energy on one or more of the following areas:

- Eliminating or avoiding stressors and strains
- Managing hardships associated with the situation
- Maintaining the integrity and morale of the family system
- Acquiring new resources
- Implementing any structural changes within the family to accommodate new demands (McCubbin & Patterson, 1983)

The xX factor reflects the interplay between all previous factors. The goal is to reduce or to eliminate disruptions within the family system and to restore a sense of homeostasis. This does not mean that the family returns to its precrisis state of existence; rather, through the crisis process, the family has made changes in roles, relationships, and responsibilities that are reflected in this "new" family system. Failure to resolve the crisis or to allow the crisis to facilitate change and growth in the family system results in maladaptation.

The double ABCX model can be useful for health care professionals in their attempts to better understand families who are responding to a medical crisis among the family members. On the basis of the model, several actions can be employed by the health care team to assist the family in achieving a high degree of adaptation to the current crisis (Chart 3–2).

The model has some weaknesses and may not be the ideal theory to apply to every family. Specifically, the theory has been criticized for its presentation of a crisis as an event-specific stressor, with commentators recognizing that most stressors in family life are not related to a single event. However, the nature of health care issues is such that one can often mark a crisis situation as the period in which a trauma or critical diagnosis involving a family member was made. The model has also been criticized for its attempts to identify the family's perception of the event. It has been questioned whether a family can ever "share" a common definition of the crisis event.

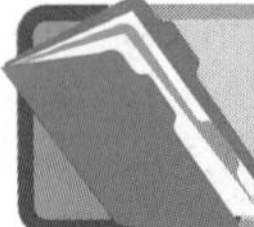

Chart 3–2
Nursing Interventions Classification (NIC)

Crisis Intervention

Definition

Use of short-term counseling to help the patient cope with a crisis and resume a state of functioning comparable to or better than the precrisis state

Activities

Provide atmosphere of support.
Determine whether patient presents safety risk to self or others.
Initiate necessary precautions to safeguard the patient or others at risk for physical harm.
Encourage expression of feelings in a nondestructive manner.
Assist in identification of the precipitants and dynamics of the crisis.
Assist in identification of past/present coping skills and their effectiveness.
Assist in identification of personal strengths and abilities that can be used in resolving the crisis.
Assist in development of new coping and problem-solving skills, as needed.
Assist in identification of available support systems.
Provide guidance about how to develop and maintain support system(s).
Introduce patient to persons (or groups) who have successfully undergone the same experience.
Assist in identification of alternative courses of action to resolve the crisis.
Assist in evaluation of the possible consequences of the various courses of action.
Assist patient to decide on a particular course of action.
Assist in formulating a time frame for implementation of chosen course of action.
Evaluate with patient whether crisis has been resolved by chosen course of action.
Plan with patient how adaptive coping skills can be used to deal with crises in the future.

From McCloskey, J., & Bulechek, G. (1996). *Nursing interventions classification (NIC)* (2nd ed.). St. Louis: Mosby–Year Book. Reprinted with permission.

Lastly, the model has been criticized for omitting the cultural, social, and historical contexts of the family as factors that can influence stress responses in the family (Gilliss, Rose, Hallburg, & Martinson, 1989).

Crisis Theory

A crisis has been defined by Caplan (1961, p. 18) as that occurring

> . . . when a person faces an obstacle to important life goals that is, for a time, insurmountable through the utilization of customary methods of problem solving. A period of disorganization ensues, a period of upset, during which many different abortive attempts at solution are made.

A crisis is generally self-limiting, lasting 4 to 6 weeks. During that time the individual or family experiences four developmental phases (Caplan, 1961). First, there is a rise in tension as the stimulus (crisis event) continues and more discomfort is felt. This is followed by unsuccessful attempts to cope with the situation, leading to more feelings of discomfort. The rise in tension causes the individual or family to move into the third stage, in which internal and external resources are mobilized and emergency problem-solving methods are tried. In the fourth stage, the problem continues and cannot be solved or avoided. Stress and tension increase, leading to major disorganization. Certain balancing factors can influence the return to equilibrium at any time during the phases of the crisis (Fig. 3–5). Health care providers who employ measures to assist families to return to a state of equilibrium can utilize *crisis intervention therapy* as a model for their actions.

Crisis intervention is an extension of short-term psychotherapy. The goal of crisis intervention is to assist the individual or family to resolve the immediate crisis and restore equilibrium to at least the precrisis level. The *ideal* goal would be to improve functioning above the precrisis level (Aguilera, 1994). Crisis intervention is not an appropriate intervention method to use with a family that has a history of dysfunction and problems related to coping with stressors. These families need to undergo more intense long-term therapy and counseling.

A logical, problem-solving approach is the basic framework for effective crisis intervention. The approach begins with the *assessment* phase. The nurse uses this time to assess the individual and family and the circumstances leading to the immediate crisis situation. After an accurate assessment is completed, *therapeutic intervention planning* is initiated to restore the family to the precrisis level of functioning. In the third phase, the *interventions* are carried out. These interventions focus on helping the family gain an understanding of the crisis, garnering more social support and exploring alternative coping mechanisms. In the last phase, resolution of the crisis and anticipatory planning are the areas of focus. Coping strategies that have been beneficial are reinforced and assistance is provided to make realistic plans for the future (Aguilera, 1994; Woolley, 1990).

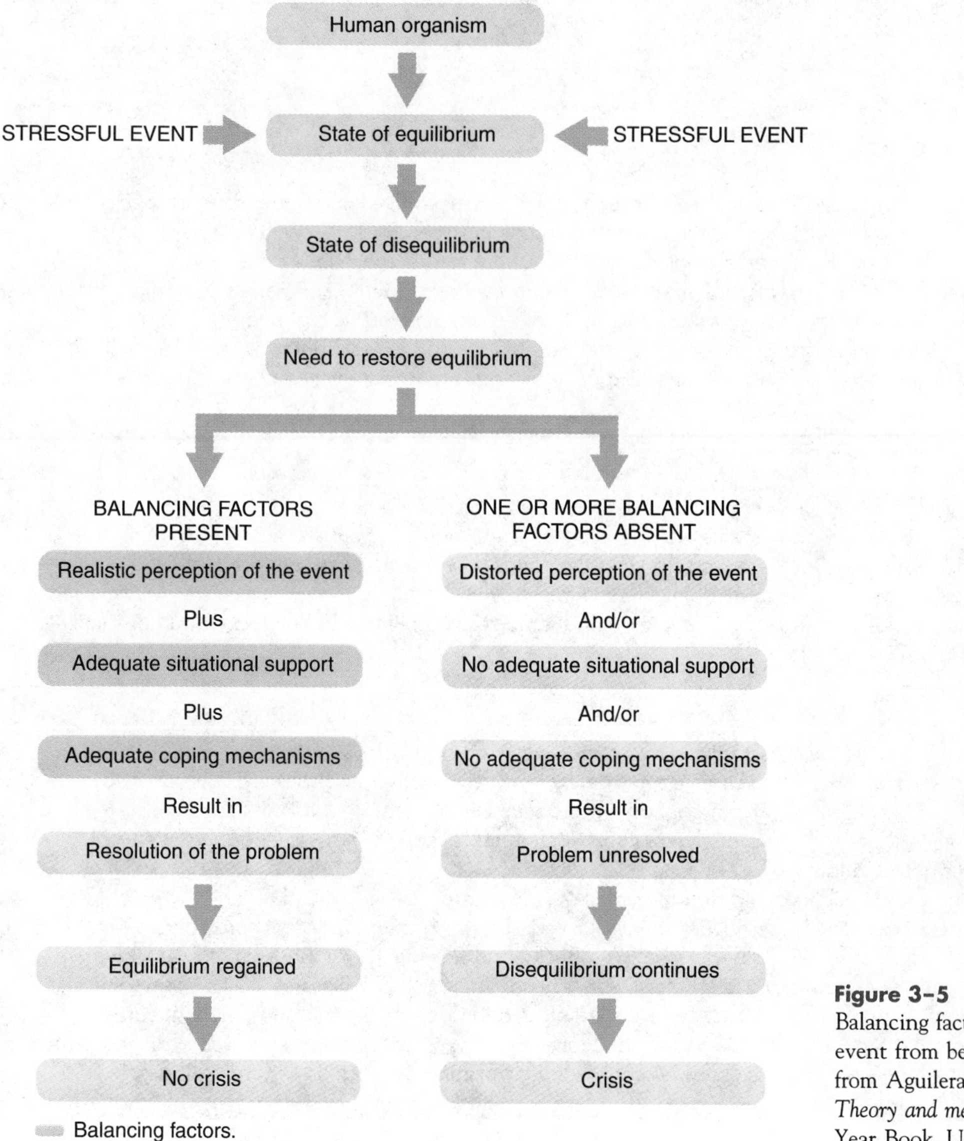

Figure 3–5
Balancing factors can prevent a stressful event from becoming a crisis. (Redrawn from Aguilera, D. [1994]. *Crisis intervention: Theory and methodology*. St. Louis: Mosby–Year Book. Used with permission.)

When using crisis intervention, the nurse should view the family as previously healthy and able to cope with day-to-day stressors. If there is preexisting family dysfunction, a referral to more intensive therapy by a qualified professional would be appropriate at this time. At the point of crisis, the overwhelming nature of the situation may temporarily paralyze the family. If interventions are not employed, damage to family functioning could be permanent. The time frame for nursing intervention is limited because of the self-limiting period of the crisis event. For instance, in the case of a child who is hospitalized after a motor vehicle accident, the nursing assessment would focus on the event that precipitated the crisis and on the problems that have arisen as a result of the crisis. The accident may have been caused by a lack of parental supervision. Now that the child is hospitalized, the parents may be at the bedside all the time, leaving other children at home unattended. A teaching program may be needed to review and institute child safety issues with the family. The nurse must act in an assertive manner with the family, assuming the role of teacher, consultant, change agent, or counselor as needed. The goal of all interventions is to help the family return to the state of functioning at which they were before the crisis (Bozett, 1987).

Crisis intervention is a helpful short-term approach that works nicely within the context of the brief encounters the nurse may have with the child and their family. Using the approach, the nurse may fail to recognize more serious, long-standing problems in the family. Optimizing communication among the family's health care providers, whether they be in the clinic, the school, or the acute

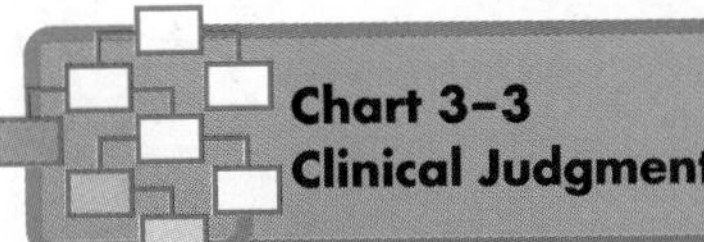

Chart 3–3
Clinical Judgment

A Family in Crisis

Becky is a 16-year-old girl attending public school. She is brought to the nurse's office by her friend Anna. Becky looks pale and sullen and has an unkempt appearance. Although the nurse has not seen Becky recently, she is shocked by her appearance and affect. Becky has always been particular about her appearance and has done well in her classes. A quick review of her student file reveals that she is now getting Ds in four out of six classes. Anna tells the nurse Becky is having family problems. After some discussion with Becky, the nurse learns that Becky is 3 months pregnant. Becky is afraid to tell her parents and her brothers. Her parents are separated right now, and Becky thinks they have enough problems of their own. She states that she does not love the baby's father and she thinks she is too young to be a mother.

Questions

1. To assist Becky to work through this crisis, what further data should the nurse collect?
2. What developmental characteristics of adolescents may have contributed to this current situation?
3. What roles has Becky had in her family? If she were to keep the child, how would those roles change?
4. What three interventions could the nurse employ at this time with Becky?
5. Becky and the nurse agree to meet again next week. How can the nurse determine whether Becky and her family are working through this crisis?

Answers

1. Determine whether Becky has a clear understanding of what has occurred and knows the full range of choices available to her at this time. Determine the level of support Becky may have from friends, family, and the baby's father. Determine how Becky and her family have coped with problems in the past.
2. Egocentrism. Focus on body image. Lack of cognitive maturity. Belief that although she was engaged in sexual activities, *she* would never get pregnant.
3. Becky has had the roles of student, sibling, and daughter. If she keeps the child, she will take on the roles of mother and provider. Becky's family will also have additional roles, such as grandparents and providers.
4. Encourage Becky to speak with her family. Offer to meet with Becky and her family. Put Becky into contact with a support group that deals with teenage pregnancy. Refer Becky to a physician, if she has not already seen one. Provide Becky with information about her choices. Give Becky information about nutrition and personal care.
5. Becky's affect and appearance are improved. Becky says that she has spoken with her parents. Becky arranges for her parents to meet with the nurse. Becky articulates what her choices are in this situation regarding the baby.

care setting, can assist in providing an accurate assessment of the family, their coping abilities, and their eventual resolution of the crisis (Chart 3–3).

Family Adjustment and Adaptation Response Model

The Family Adjustment and Adaptation Response (FAAR) Model is a framework that allows health care providers to assess a family's level of stress on the basis of demands they face and the family's capabilities for meeting those demands (Fig. 3–6). **Demands** are the sources of stress. Demands can emerge from individual members, the family unit, or the community. The three major types of demands are *stressors*, *strains*, and *hassles*. *Stressors* are either normative events (getting married) or non-normative events (a tornado) that happen at a discrete time and produce or call for a change. Death of a family member, acute illness, divorce of parents, and birth of a child are examples of stressors that may affect the family. *Strains* are ongoing tensions resulting from prior stressors or from enacting life's roles. The parent who feels overloaded in caring for a new baby, inability to pay bills after a marital separation, and care of an elderly parent are strains on the family. Daily *hassles* are the minor upsets that can throw off one's schedule and sense of well-being. For instance, losing your car keys, getting a call that your child is ill at school, and running out of diapers are hassles that add to the stress factor in a family (Patterson, 1988, 1995).

Demands create tension or stress and produce or call for a change in individual or family functioning. Families

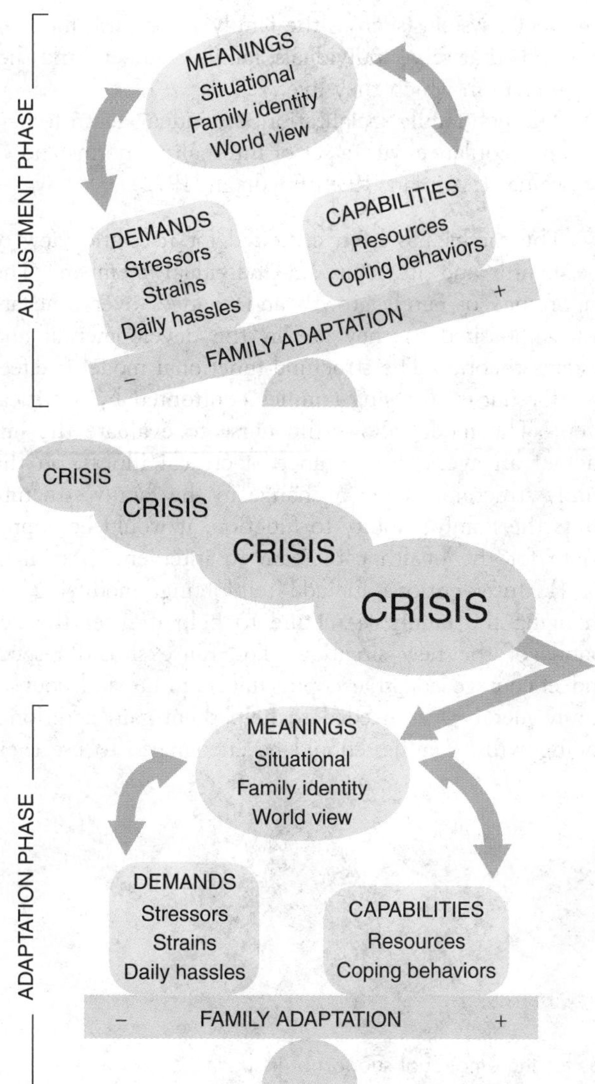

Figure 3–6
During a crisis, the family must learn to adjust the demands placed on them with the capabilities available to them, as illustrated in the Family Adjustment and Adaptation Response (FAAR) Model. (Redrawn from Patterson, J. [1995]. Promoting resilience in families experiencing stress. *Pediatric Clinics of North America, 42*[1], 49. Used with permission.)

never deal with a single demand at one time. Often, the health care professional intervenes solely on the basis of the major stressor affecting the family (an acute illness), when in fact the strains and hassles a family is coping with may be more difficult to manage than the stressor (Patterson, McCubbin, & Warwick, 1990).

The mediators of stress are called **capabilities**. The model emphasizes two types of capabilities, *resources* and *coping behaviors*. The family attempts to balance functioning by using capabilities (resources and coping behaviors) to meet demands (stressors, strains, and hassles). Resources are both tangible (money, health care services, extended family assistance) and intangible (self-esteem, family flexibility, safe neighborhoods). Resources for the family may come from the individual, the family unit, or the community.

Coping is what families do to manage their stress and restore family balance (Patterson, 1995). Families who rely on diverse coping strategies are more successful at achieving a balance in family functioning. Coping behaviors are learned. Children need to be taught how to manage demands and experiment with new behaviors to cope with the variety of demands that affect their development.

The FAAR model also illustrates that the **meaning** the family attributes to their situation is a critical factor in achieving a balance in family functioning. The family's shared meanings include their perception about a *specific stressful event*, their *identity as a family*, and their *view of the world* or world view (Patterson, 1995). When a stressor event occurs, the family begins to construct meanings of the event as they interact with each other and bases them on the meanings they have attributed to their family identity and world view (Patterson & Garwick, 1994).

The outcome of the family's effort to achieve balanced functioning is called **family adjustment** or **family adaptation**. Family adjustment is associated with achieving stability in relation to relatively minor demands (child breaks out with chickenpox). Family adaptation is required when more intense or complex demands are made on the family (newborn child is diagnosed with cerebral palsy). A crisis or state of disequilibrium occurs when a family cannot adjust by using their repertoire of capabilities in relation to the demands they are facing. Family adaptation occurs when, in the presence of a crisis, the family restores homeostasis by acquiring new resources and coping behaviors, reduces the demands it faces, and/or changes the meanings and perceptions associated with the situation (Patterson, 1995).

The health care provider can promote family adjustment and adaptation by focusing on family strengths and teaching family members about their own capabilities. The interdisciplinary team can use this model to understand the family's complex issues and intervene in ways that encourage the family to discover the best solutions to meet their needs and the circumstances of the situation.

Structural-Functional Approach

The structural-functional model focuses on the relationships between the family members and how well the family performs its functions. *Structure* refers to how the family is organized, the manner in which members and their roles are arranged and relate to each other (Friedman, 1992). The structure of the family includes the form it may take, such as a single-parent family, stepfamily, or nuclear family. In addition, the manner in which members relate to one another can be examined in reference to such areas as their communication patterns, the family power structure, and the family roles. The family structure serves to facilitate the achievement of family functions.

Function refers to the outcomes or consequences of the family structure—that is, the goals of the family that are important to the members and to the society. What the family does, or the reason for its existence, is said to be its function. Friedman (1992) has summarized five family functions said to be most germane to assessing the family. These are the affective function, reproductive function, economic function, health care function, and socialization and social placement function (Table 3–3).

Assumptions of the structural-functional approach include the following:

- A family is a social system with functional requirements.
- A family is a small group that has features common to all small groups.
- Social systems such as the family accomplish functions that serve individuals, family members, and the society in which they live.
- Through family socialization, individuals learn to act in accordance with a set of internalized norms and values (Artinian, 1994; Friedman, 1992)

The model has been criticized for its static view of the family and its focus on individual members. The importance of family growth and changes over time are not emphasized as they are in the developmental and systems theories. The structural-functional model is effective for nurses assessing families confronted by a critical event. The model allows the nurse to evaluate the impact of an event, for instance, a critical illness, on the family structure. When a change in the family structure alters the family's ability to function, it would be appropriate for the health care team to intervene (Artinian, 1994). Interventions include reinforcing, modifying, or changing the family's structure to help it meet the demands of the new situation. The nurse should respect and encourage adaptive coping mechanisms and counsel family members as needed to help them gain additional coping skills. Families should be encouraged to use their

Table 3–3
Functions of the Family

Function	Description
Affective function	This function provides for the emotional support of its members through love, encouragement, intimacy, and acceptance. Without the affective function, families would not be able to survive. Children from families who rate high on measures of affective support have higher self-esteem, are better able to cope with stress, and have fewer behavioral problems. During adolescence, they have less delinquency, depression, and drug use.
Reproductive function	The reproductive function provides for the continuation of society as well as the family.
Economic function	This function requires the parents to provide the economic resources to meet the needs of the family financially. Poverty and having insufficient resources are the best predictors of poor health outcomes for children.
Health care function	Through the provision of food, clothing and shelter, and adequate health care, this function is met.
Socialization and social placement function	The family has the responsibility of raising the children to be functional members of society. This occurs through effective parenting, education, and instillation of the family's culture, values, and religion. Parental involvement in the child's school and education has been associated with both better academic performance and improved social maturity.

existing supports to meet their needs, modifying the structure and redistributing responsibilities as necessary to account for the impact of the crisis on individual members.

Interactional Approach

The focus of the interactional approach is on the way in which family members relate to one another. Viewing the family as a set of interacting personalities, this approach highlights internal family dynamics. The processes that are evaluated in the family include role-playing, communication patterns, decision making, coping patterns, and socialization processes (Friedman, 1992). The framework makes no attempt to view the family in relation to its interactions with external social environments. Rather, the focus of this approach is solely on analysis of the internal dynamics of the family.

In the interactional approach, a symbol is defined as a stimulus that has a learned meaning and value for an individual. People learn about symbols through their interactions with other people and in this process come to have shared meanings and values regarding these symbols (Rose, 1980). How family members respond to a situation is determined by the value and meaning each family member and the family as a whole have assigned to aspects (or symbols) of the event.

The approach can be useful to the nurse who wishes to focus attention on how the family functions as its members interact between and among themselves. As the family is affected by a crisis, this model is helpful in identifying and isolating potential or real sources of difficulty among family members as they cope with a new situation. Family members may encounter problems because they do not share the values and meanings of symbols surrounding a particular event. Therefore, members can feel alienated, misunderstood, and in conflict with others who do not understand their feelings and actions.

The interactional approach can be limiting because it does not take into context the interactions between the family and external social systems. Using this model, the family is considered to be a self-contained unit; interactions with other social organizations or individuals outside the family are not analyzed in terms of their impact on family interactions.

Institutional Approach

The institutional approach, or the historical approach, views the family as an institution interacting with other social institutions over a long time. Relationships with other institutions, such as religious, educational, governmental, and economic ones, are evaluated. In particular, the model examines the functions that the family carries out for society and the functions that other institutions provide or carry out for the family. Families in one setting are compared with those in another setting. For instance, families in rural settings would be compared and contrasted with those in urban settings. In addition, changes in the families are evaluated over time and in relation to the impact of changes that have occurred in other societal institutions. Family functions that have changed over time include the following:

- Economic self-sufficiency of the family
- The status of being part of a marital partnership with children
- Education, schooling, or training of children for future work and roles
- Socialization of children
- Care of ill or older family members
- Religious training and practices
- Recreational functions or the presence of family-centered activities
- Reproduction (procreation) functions
- Affective relations and family ties (Friedman, 1992)

This model can be used to compare one type of family system in one era with a family system in another era. For instance, the researcher could use this model to evaluate family function before World War II, when most women did not have jobs outside the home, compared with current times, when working mothers play a major role in the nation's work force.

The approach makes no attempt to study the individual or single family units. A major shortcoming of the institutional approach is that it deals with the model family. No attempt is made to examine the specific relationships in a particular family. The model focuses on the family unit as a whole rather than the internal dynamics of particular family groups. In addition, viewing the family over time and in such a macroscopic fashion is not helpful to the nurse dealing with specific issues regarding a family in distress. However, the institutional approach can be helpful in the assessment, implementation, and evaluation of health care programs and health care legislation that need to be updated on the basis of changing societal and family-based trends.

Social Exchange Theory

The social exchange theory was developed by Homans (1958) and applied to family studies in the 1960s. The theory is based on a model of the social exchange of goods and services between two or more sociopolitical economies. When applied to families, the theory's primary assumption is that interactions between persons are exchanges of skills, goods, commodities, and resources both material and nonmaterial (Mercer, 1989). Equilibrium between persons, or within the family, is based on the premise of reciprocity. That is, through the process of distributive justice, all rewards should be proportionate to the costs and/or efforts. Furthermore, when individuals are involved in a social relationship, they receive certain rewards or benefits from that relationship. In turn, each individual must reciprocate, providing equal rewards or benefits to the other party. If either party fails to reciprocate, the relationship fails because there is no incentive to continue the interactions. Thus, an imbalance can occur when a person does not reciprocate or when one party reciprocates in a greater fashion than the other party. In this case, the one providing the greater rewards or exchanges puts the other person at a disadvantage and therefore controls the relationship. This theory postulates that within the family, behavior is positively reinforced when associated with rewards and negatively reinforced by the use of punishment (Mercer, 1989). The family or the individual makes choices to seek the greatest good or rewards at the least cost. At the same time, the rewards should equal the costs. When this occurs, members feel good and gratified. If rewards are less than costs, anger develops. On the other hand, if received goods are greater than are felt to be deserved, guilt can develop. All individuals and families are unique in how they assign value to certain rewards or costs. For instance, children may be viewed as a reward in one family but viewed as a cost in another.

For nursing, the theory has several limitations that have restricted its broad use in research. Mercer (1989) was unable to find any family research by nurses that had used social exchange theory as a framework. There are no nurse theorists who based a model on this theory. The focus of the theory is on evaluating the complex system of rewards and costs that should explain family interactions. However, the theory does not deal with the underlying psychodynamics of the situation. Thus, an exchange could be taken out of context and viewed objectively, only to have a false assessment made. There is a risk of making judgments about the family on the basis of single interactions rather than the total exchange of services over time.

In addition, the theory does not clearly identify what constitutes a reward or a cost. The nurse using this theory must determine what family members regard as rewards and costs. This analysis is complicated by the different perceptions of the family members and by the simple knowledge that determining what actions actually motivate individuals (and why) is a complex undertaking. The theory has difficulty taking into account altruistic or morally driven rewards that are not weighed by costs incurred to the individual.

Worldview: *The social exchange theory has received some criticism for its cultural bias. Some of its assumptions are based on the premise that when rewards or goods are not received as expected, revenge, anger, and guilt are justifiable outcomes. In cultures in which peace is more highly valued than reward, this theory would not be applicable (Mercer, 1989).*

The strength of social exchange theory lies in its simple application to individuals, family groups, organizations, and societies. The assumptions of the theory transcend history and provide a means of explaining the social exchanges that have led to significant changes in the lives of individuals and societal groups. The theory has been used to answer a broad range of questions related to family violence and family power. The theory is helpful in explaining the interdependence of individuals in a family, especially when they are responding to a major environmental factor or stimulus.

Conflict Theory

Tension and stress are accepted components of our interactions with one another and with social institutions. When tensions grow and the values, beliefs, or actions of an individual, family, or social group become more or less sharply opposed, *conflict* appears. Conflict theory describes and explains the effects of change, conflict, and constraints on social units. The theory is used to determine how and why families remain stable or become unstable during times of conflict. Change and conflict within the family are inevitable. Conflict may have positive and unifying effects on the family, facilitating creativity, innovation, and social change.

The nurse using this theory helps families determine where conflict exists and develop processes to manage or resolve the areas of conflict. Conflict may present in the form of decision-making struggles, the assignment or acceptance of power, and the presence of family violence. In families in which new relationships are being forged because of adoption, marriage, divorce, or remarriage, conflict can be expected. Through negotiation and problem solving, the health care team can help families to identify areas of potential and real conflict and minimize the negative consequences of changes in the family system.

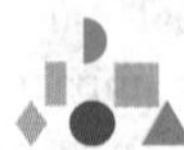

Family Assessment Tools

Assessment of the family can be facilitated by tools that are useful, understandable, and easy to administer. Using theoretical approaches and models of family functioning, several assessment tools have been created that can be used by the health care team to evaluate the family system. Many tools have been developed for clinical and research purposes (Table 3–4). All of the tools have been tested empirically and can be administered and scored by the health care provider. Although most of the tools have been developed by family theorists, nurses have used these measures to better understand the impact of crises, illness, and hospitalization on the family and its individual members.

The Calgary Family Assessment Model (CFAM) is an integrated, multidimensional framework developed by nurses, for health care providers, to assess the family thoroughly and determine whether further intervention is warranted (Wright & Leahey, 1994). The CFAM was based on systems, cybernetics, communication, and change theories. The model is divided into three major categories: structural, developmental, and functional. Each category contains several subcategories (Fig. 3–7).

Figure 3–7
The nurse may use the Calgary Family Assessment Model to assess the family. (Redrawn from Wright, L., & Leahey, M. [1994]. *Nurses and families: A guide to family assessment and intervention.* Philadelphia: F. A. Davis. Used with permission.)

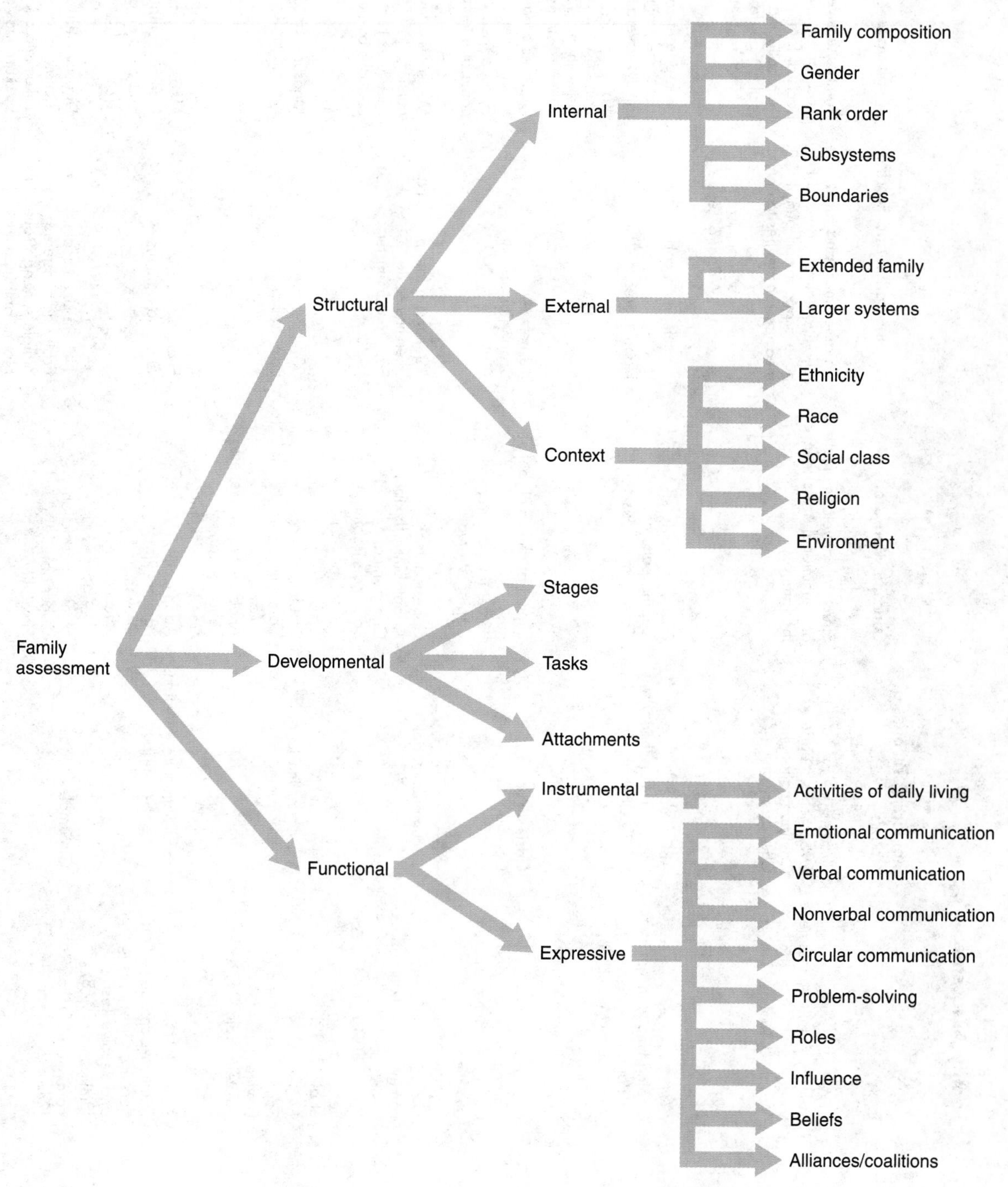

Table 3–4
Family Assessment Tools

Tools	Supporting Theories or Models	Concepts Measured	Administration and Scoring	Advantages	Limitations
CFAM Calgary Family Assessment Model (Wright & Leahey, 1994)	Systems theory Cybernetics theory Communication theory Change theory	Structural, developmental, and functional assessment of the family	An assessment and family intervention model, does not have a paper and pencil measure for families to complete Interview questions are suggested by Wright & Leahey (1994)	Comprehensive assessment model to evaluate multiple aspects of family life Data collected can be used directly to guide and support nursing interventions	Repeated contacts with family are necessary and optimal to obtain comprehensive assessment data
CHIP Coping Health Inventory for Parents (McCubbin, McCubbin, Cauble, & Nevin, 1979)	ABCX model Social support theory Family stress theory Theories of individual psychology of coping	Coping behaviors Coping patterns Coping strategies	45 self-report coping behaviors Hand scored	Each parent can complete the tool to get complete picture of family's overall coping strategy Can be used as pre- and posttest with intervention program aimed at strengthening coping	Not designed to evaluate child members of the family
CICI: PQ Chronicity Impact and Coping Instrument: Parent Questionnaire (Hymovich, 1983)	Crisis theory Coping theory	Impact of child's chronic illness Perceptions of stressors Coping strategies	48 items Scoring unknown	Identifies areas relevant for nursing interventions Can be used to measure outcome of intervention strategies	Only for families with chronically ill child
FACES III/FACES IV Family Adaptation and Cohesion Scale (Olson, 1994; Olson, Portner, & Lavee, 1985; Olson et al., 1982)	Circumplex model	Cohesion Adaptability, flexibility Communication Social desirability	30 items in four-point scale Likert-like scale Easy to administer	Measures relevant for nursing Measures real and ideal perceptions of the family	Family members may be unwilling to assess themselves Assumes family has children
FAD Family Assessment Device (Epstein, Baldwin, & Bishop, 1983)	McMaster model of family functioning	Problem solving Communication Roles Affective responsiveness Behavior control General functioning	53 items Easy to administer	Measures areas nurses could change through care plans	Requires individual to speak for family Not clear if useful with clients of different social and cultural backgrounds or in different life stages
Family APGAR Family Adaptability, Partnership, Growth, Affection and Resolve Test (Smilkstein, 1978)	Family structure, function, and social support	Adaptability Partnership Growth Affection Resolve	Five items Quick to administer	Measures relevant factors Can be completed by adults and children age 10 yr and older	Not to be used to evaluate a family problem in depth
Family Satisfaction (Olson & Wilson, 1982)	Circumplex Model	Family satisfaction Cohesion Flexibility	14-item Likert scale Easily administered Simple scoring procedures Norms obtained	Directly measures family satisfaction Takes into account normative backgrounds and cultural background	None identified

F-Copes Family Crisis Oriented Personal Evaluation Scales (McCubbin, Larsen, & Olson, 1981)	Double ABCX Model	Pile up family resources Meaning and/or perception of a crisis	30-item Likert scale Easily administered Three scales evaluate internal family coping patterns Five scales evaluate external family coping patterns	Identifies family with strong repertoire of coping behaviors	None identified
FES Family Environment Scale (Fuhr, Moos, & Dishotksky, 1981; Moos & Moos, 1976, 1984)	No theoretical position on the nature of families	Relationships Personal growth System maintenance Change	90 items—true-false Scoring is complex Standardized scores; two categories	Short form available Useful for measuring change after interventions Measures real and ideal	A research-oriented tool that does not have a clinical model associated with it; thus clinical utility is unclear
FFI Family Functioning Index (Pless & Satterwhite, 1973)	Family functioning	Communication Togetherness Closeness Decision making Child orientation	15 items Quickly administered Complicated scoring	Identifies families at risk, not level of risk or distress	Not for families without children or with adult children Not sensitive to short- or long-term change, thus does not measure change after a nursing intervention
FFFS Feetham Family Functioning Survey (Roberts & Feetham, 1982)	Ecological systems approach	Three major areas of family relationships: Between family and broader social units such as schools and work Between family and subsystems within the family Between family and individuals within the family	Somewhat complicated scoring	Both parents complete the tool so that discrepant views of family life can be identified. Measures factors nurses could change through care plans Useful with middle-class families	Somewhat difficult to understand
FILE Family Inventory of Life Events and Changes (McCubbin, Patterson, & Wilson, 1981)	Double ABCX Model	Pile up events, aA factor	Seven items Can be hand scored Evaluates life changes on 10 different scales	Can assess stress in a family at a single point in time Examines the multiple stressors a family is experiencing	May be difficult for family members to remember events within the past year
IFF Inventory of Family Feelings (Lowman, 1980)	Families affective structure Patterns of conflict relationships and alliances	Positive or negative feeling toward each member	38 items Three-point Likert-like scale Easily scored	Focuses on a single dimension of interpersonal and family relationship	Limited clinical usefulness because of unidimensionality
SFIS Structural Family Interaction Scale (Perosa, Hansen, & Perosa, 1981)	Minuchin's family functioning theory	Enmeshment and disengagement Neglect or overprotection Rigidity or flexibility Conflict or avoidance Patient management Triangulation of parent-child coalition Detouring	85 items on four-point agreement scale Easy to administer	Useful for family counseling and assessment	Length and complexity of tool make it difficult to use clinically

Additional reference: Spear & Sachs (1985).

Chart 3–4
Nursing Diagnoses and Outcomes

The Family at Risk

Family process alteration related to situational crisis

Outcomes:
Family members agree on roles of each family member.
Family members develop adaptive responses by changing responsibilities to meet the demands of the situation.
Family members identify support systems to assist them and participate in mobilizing those systems.
Family contacts a community support group for continued assistance.
Family members share a realistic perception of the event.
Family members share their feelings about the event with each other.

Coping, family: potential for growth related to impact of current crisis

Outcomes:
Family members discuss impact of current crisis on self.
Family members identify strengths that can be used to assist in coping with crisis event.
Family members identify potential sources of additional stress and make efforts to reduce or eliminate additional stressors.

Ineffective family coping: compromised related to child's behavioral problems

Outcomes:
Family members express their concern about coping with child's behavioral problems.
Family members identify factors that trigger stress and inappropriate behavior.
Family members contact and make use of available sources of support.
Parents meet the developmental needs of their children.
Child meets developmental milestones appropriate for age.

Ineffective family management of therapeutic regimen related to economic difficulties

Outcomes:
Family members cooperate in finding ways to incorporate therapeutic regimen into their lifestyle.
Family members use available support services to ease economic burden of child's care needs.

Parental role conflict related to child's hospitalization

Outcomes:
Parents communicate feelings about present situation.
Parents participate in daily caretaking of their child.
Parents express knowledge of their child's developmental needs.
Parents convey love and warmth to their child.
Parents use available support systems to assist in coping.

High risk for parenting alteration related to ineffective role model

Outcomes:
Parents voice satisfaction with infant or child.
Parents express knowledge of developmental norms.
Parents state plans for well-child care.
Parents provide age-appropriate activities for the infant or child.

As the nurse moves to assess those categories on the right of the branching diagram, the assessment becomes more focused. Data are collected over a series of encounters with the family. The nurse is strongly encouraged not to focus on a single aspect of the model. Rather, all relevant data are collected and integrated to form a clear picture of the family and their needs. From this model, Wright and Leahey (1994) have also developed the Calgary Family Intervention Model (CFIM).

From the assessment, nursing diagnoses can be formulated to articulate the problems identified for a specific family (Chart 3–4). The interdisciplinary team can use these diagnoses to guide interventions to promote family integrity in the presence of developmental and maturational issues faced by the family and its members (Chart 3–5).

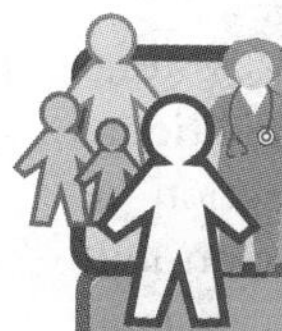

Chart 3–4
Nursing Diagnoses and Outcomes *Continued*

The Family at Risk

Risk for altered parent–infant or parent–child attachment

Outcomes: Parents initiate positive interactions with infant or child, as evidenced by mutual responsiveness and verbal and nonverbal communication.
Parents express confidence in their ability to meet infant's or child's needs.
Parents express confidence in caring for their infant or child at home.
Parents recognize when assistance is needed from others to manage the infant or child.

Role performance alteration related to prolonged family crisis

Outcomes: Family expresses feelings about diminished capacity to perform usual roles in the current crisis situation.
Family recognizes limitations imposed by the crisis and expresses feelings about these limitations.
Family continues to function in usual roles to as great a degree as possible.
Family demonstrates flexibility in altering roles as needed until the crisis is resolved.

Spiritual distress related to situational crisis

Outcomes: Family members express feelings about usual and current religious beliefs.
Family members identify areas of ambivalence and conflict resulting from current situation.
Family members seek appropriate support persons to assist in overcoming spiritual distress.
Family members employ strategies to ease spiritual discomfort.

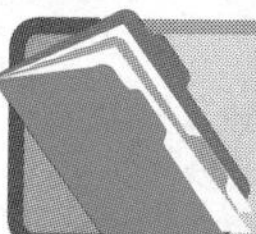

Chart 3–5
Nursing Interventions Classification (NIC)

Family Integrity Promotion

Definition

Promotion of family cohesion and unity

Activities

Be a listener for the family members.
Establish trusting relationship with family members.
Determine family understanding of causes of illness.
Determine guilt family may feel.
Assist family to resolve feelings of guilt.
Determine typical family relationships.
Monitor current family relationships.
Identify typical family coping mechanisms.
Identify conflicting priorities among family members.
Assist family with conflict resolution.
Counsel family members on additional effective coping skills for their own use.
Respect privacy of individual family members.
Provide for family privacy.
Tell family members it is safe and acceptable to use typical expressions of affection.
Facilitate a tone of togetherness within and among the family.
Provide family members with information about the patient's condition regularly, according to patient preference.
Collaborate with family in problem solving.
Assist family to maintain positive relationships.
Facilitate open communications among family members.
Provide for care of patient by family members, as appropriate.
Provide for family visitation.
Refer family to support group of other families dealing with similar problems.
Refer for family therapy, as indicated.

From McCloskey, J., & Bulechek, G. (1996). *Nursing interventions classification (NIC)* (2nd ed.). St. Louis: Mosby–Year Book. Reprinted with permission.

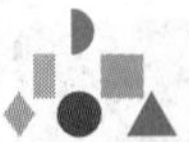

Family Structure

The type of family structure the nurse caring for children may encounter in practice has never been more diverse. The type of family that a child belongs to is less important than the relationships developed or level of cohesion within that family (Hetherington, Law, & O'Connor, 1993). Regardless of the family structure, children need to feel that their family is an acceptable family form (Visher & Visher, 1995a).

The nuclear family—two parents, two or more children, with one parent at home with the children—is a family structure that no longer reflects the diversity and complexity of our contemporary lifestyles. The *postmodern family*, or what Elkind (1996) terms the *permeable family* (dual-earner families, adoptive families, single-parent families, blended families, and the like), is more fluid, flexible, and vulnerable to pressures from outside the family. Several trends in society have significantly altered the composition of the traditional family home. These trends include

- Increase in divorce
- Increase in number of mothers employed outside the home
- Lower birth rate coupled with higher life expectancy
- Number of adults choosing to remain single and never marry or to remain unmarried after divorce or the death of a spouse
- Number of adults delaying marriage and childbearing until later years (Gershwin & Nilsen, 1989)

In addition, the number of alternative family forms has increased. Single-parent families and stepfamilies have become two of the fastest growing family compositions. There has also been a rise in the number of families in which the adults are not the biological parents of the children. These include foster parenting situations and families in which grandparents or other relatives are caretakers of the children.

Nuclear Family

The nuclear family, once considered the traditional family in many industrial societies, consists of a husband, wife, and their immediate children. In the United States, fewer than one third of the families exist in the traditional pattern of a working father, homemaker mother, and one or more children (Gold, Perrin, Futterman, & Friedman, 1994). It is estimated that only 50% of children live with their biological parents until their 18th birthday (Visher & Visher, 1995b).

The nuclear family faces many challenges. At one time the extended family was more of the traditional norm. This structure allowed a greater distribution of responsibilities among family members. These responsibilities included working to obtain finances to manage family needs, child rearing, and maintenance of the home and family daily needs. The trend toward more nuclear family constellations has placed these responsibilities on the shoulders of two adults. Stressful economic circumstances, juggling multiple jobs, the strains of parenting, and the need to maintain a cohesive partnership all place tremendous stress on the nuclear family. Although the standard of living may be higher in a nuclear family than in other family structures, stress levels are often higher. It has been noted that physical punishment and violence are often higher in nuclear families than in extended family households (Bell & Jenkins, 1991; Kavanagh, 1994).

To balance the needs of the family with the internal and external stressors affecting family life, several strategies are being used to "extend" the nuclear family. Many families hire individuals to clean their home and maintain the yard. Couples may live in close proximity to their parents, with parents providing daycare or babysitting services. Many fathers are taking a more active and shared role in parenting responsibilities. Although it has been debated that there is little federal support for the nuclear family, activists are working toward tax laws and access to services that will support the nuclear family rather than be an additional source of stress.

Dual-Career Family

A variation of the traditional family is the dual-career or dual-earner family. In this type of family, both husband and wife have decided to work either for economic reasons or for personal satisfaction. This type of family is becoming more prevalent, as two thirds of all nuclear families have both parents working for pay outside the home (Hayghe, 1990). Most families require the income of two parents to be able to support a middle-class existence (Schor, 1995). Dual-earner families are faced with challenges as they struggle to maintain the family. Dual-earner families must perform at least four jobs: two market jobs for pay and two unpaid jobs in the family (Piotrkowski & Hughes, 1993). The unpaid job is considered "family work" by Pleck (1977). Family work includes household chores and child care tasks performed by the family in order to function effectively (Fig. 3–8). Traditionally, family work was the women's responsibility. However, dual-earner families have been forced to redefine and renegotiate roles and tasks within the family in order to be functional. With both parents working, child care and the completion of household chores have be-

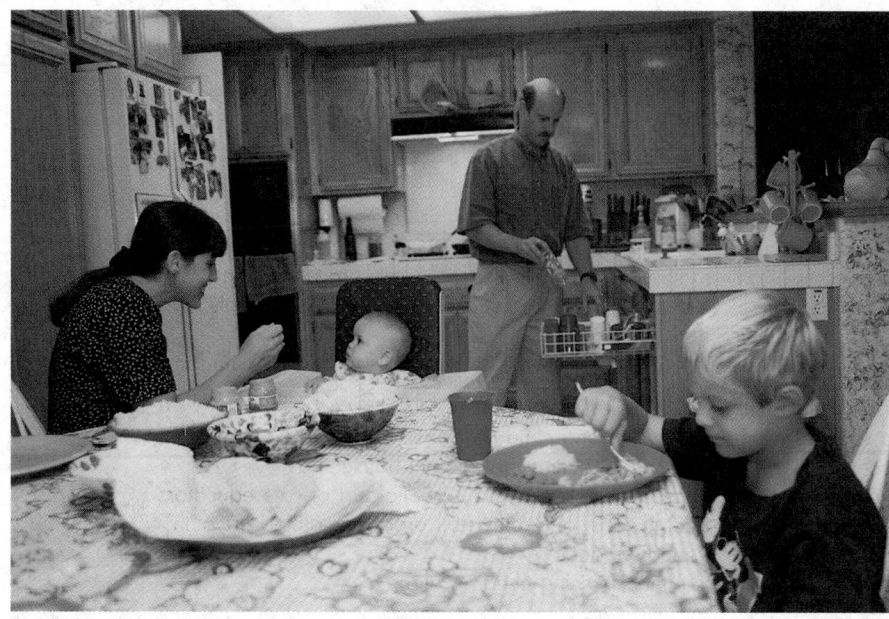

Figure 3–8
In dual-career families, both parents work and share family care duties.

come important issues for the family. It has become increasingly difficult to find affordable, high-quality child care.

The dual-earner family must often find affordable child care services to take care of their children's needs when the parents are not available. Some dual-earner families deal with this situation by arranging alternating work schedules. This is, while one parent is working during the day, the other is at home. In the evening, the "day worker" parent returns home to watch the children while the other parent goes to work. Although this situation eliminates the high cost of child care and maximizes parental contact with the children, it can place stress on the marital relationship, as spousal contact is sacrificed.

Over the past several years, research has focused on alternative family forms such as single parenting and stepfamilies and on the effects of divorce and remarriage. Little attention has been given to the nuclear family or dual-career family and the struggle that numbers of these "traditional" families face in trying to maintain and promote the nuclear family. As more and more legislation and other support systems have arisen to support the non-traditional family, the nuclear family may feel as though they are struggling against governmental, economic, and societal reform to maintain the strength of this type of family system. Raising children in a nuclear family is no guarantee that the children will be healthy and well adjusted. Organizations such as Focus on the Family continue to provide families with resources to deal with developmental and societal challenges in a positive manner (Chart 3–6). See the Resources section at the end of the chapter for an expanded listing of support organizations.

Extended Family

Another more traditional family unit is the extended family. The extended family consists of several generations of the family, including the immediate nuclear family, grandparents, and other relatives such as aunts, uncles, and cousins (Fig. 3–9). Although every nuclear family is part of an extended family unit, few nuclear families elect to live and share resources with members of their extended family. In the past, the rural and agrarian focus of society promoted and often required multigenerational families to cohabitate and share their resources. It was not uncommon for adult children, their spouses, and their children to live with the older parents. The family as a whole engaged in one common occupation such as farming. Thus, family members of all age ranges lived and worked together, benefiting from the sharing of resources and responsibilities.

As society changed to a more mobile, industrialized focus, so, too, has the extended family separated and restructured into smaller family units. In some communities and cultural groups, cohabitation of extended family members continues to be highly valued. But in most cases, the nuclear family forms its own household and members seek a living pursuing their own unique areas of interest. The extended family has not disappeared; rather, it has taken on a new appearance. Many nuclear families continue to rely on members of their extended families as business partners, child care providers, and caretakers of the elderly. In addition, extended family members enjoy socializing together and sharing special family events. In times of stress and crisis, extended family members are likely to offer many resources to support

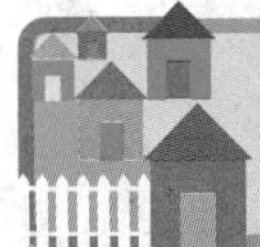

Chart 3–6
Community Care

Resources for the Family

Nurses can direct families to a variety of community resources and groups that can offer support in meeting the challenges confronting them in today's world (see Resources list). One such nonprofit organization is ***Focus on the Family***. Dedicated to strengthening the home, the organization produces several radio programs, magazines, family-oriented books, films, videos, and audiocassettes, all from a Christian perspective. The organization also works to influence public policy to benefit and enhance family life.

Focus on the Family produces several magazines for the family and for professionals who work with families.

Citizen—Update on current events, issues, and public policies that affect families
Focus on the Family—Articles related to all aspects of family life and child rearing
Family Issues Alert—A weekly faxed newsletter regarding current events that impact households
Teachers in Focus—Insight and information on values-based curricula for K–12 public and private educators
Plugged In—Reviews and commentary on the latest music, movies, and television programs aimed at youth
Physician—Information addressing the special needs of medical doctors
Single-Parent Family—Resource to help meet the needs of those raising children alone

In addition, the organization has several journals for children.

To guide families to these resources, they can call Focus on the Family, (719) 531-5181, or access on the Internet at www.fotf.org.

the family even when long distances may separate the households.

This type of family is more common in families experiencing poverty and financial hardships, as it is becoming increasingly difficult to function as a family unit without support from other family members. Grandparents or other relatives living in the household can help with child care when the parents are working.

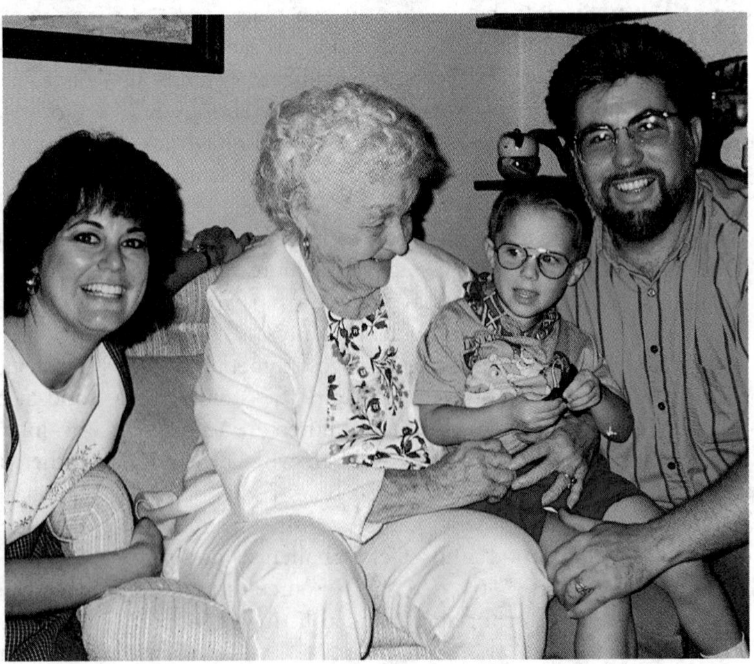

Figure 3–9
The extended family is made up of members from several generations who share resources in order to meet family needs.

Single-Parent Family

Over the past two decades, one of the most dramatic changes in family configurations has been the shift toward more single-parent families or attenuated families. At present, the number of single-parent families in the United States exceeds 10 million (Scanlan, 1994). It is estimated that half of all children younger than 18 years spend some time in a single-parent household (Tanner, 1995), a dramatic rise from the 1960s, when it was estimated that only 8% of all children younger than 18 lived only with their mother.

Single parenting occurs when one parent manages the affairs of a family without a partner (Fig. 3–10). This type of family is formed when the nuclear family unit dissolves through divorce, separation, abandonment, or death of a spouse. The single-parent household is also formed by parental choice when a child lives with his or her unmarried mother or father, when a single person chooses to conceive by either natural or medically supported methods (in vitro fertilization), when a single person accepts the responsibility of raising another family member's child, or when a child is adopted by a single person. In 88% of cases, children in one-parent families live with their mother (Tanner, 1995).

The single-parent family is likely to encounter several challenges because of economic, social, and personal restraints. Economically, single-parent families often have to adjust to a lower level of income. The dual-income family that now finds itself without the financial support of one parent is likely to find it difficult to adjust to a lower standard of living (Bumpass, Sweet, & Martin, 1990). In the same manner, a single person who accepts the responsibility of child rearing quickly learns how expensive children can be. Items such as food, diapers, clothes, and toys can quickly drain a healthy checking account. In addition, most single parents need to work. Thus, the cost of child care can be an added expense.

Single-parent families are generally poorer (Visher & Visher, 1995b). In 1991, the poverty rate of families headed by mothers only was 47% and of those headed by fathers only 20% (Scanlan, 1994). Poverty puts the single-parent family at risk for health problems, early death, and limited educational and employment opportunities (McGoldrick et al., 1993). Single-parent families are affected not only by the high cost of raising children but also by the low salaries obtained by many of the parents. Women continue to lead the majority of single-parent households, with black mothers and teenage mothers having the greatest incidence of single parenthood (Brown & Ferrara, 1992). In the United States, women still make an average of 71 cents for every dollar a man earns for the same job (McGoldrick et al., 1993).

Figure 3–10
A single-parent family may result from divorce, death, or other events.

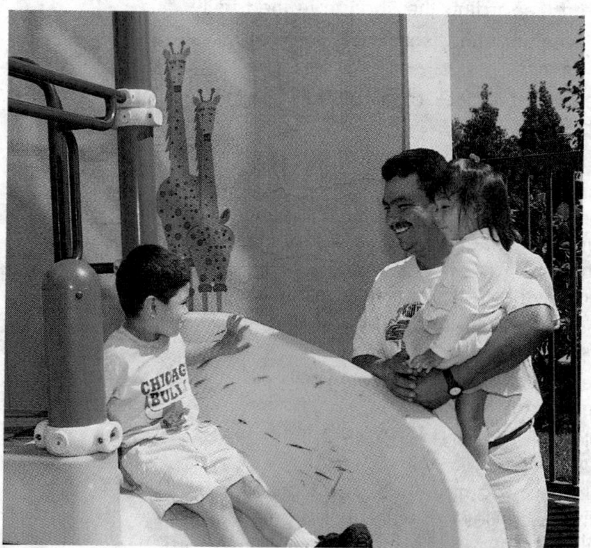

Further undermining the economic basis of the single-parent family is lack of child support from the absent parent. Failure of a parent to pay child support has caused children to overtake the elderly in becoming the single poorest group in the United States. In 1990, it was estimated that $48 billion *should* have been paid in child support to United States children. In actuality, only $14 billion dollars was paid (Scanlan, 1994).

Less than 50% of formerly married mothers receive some financial support from the absent father. For the mothers who never married, this statistic drops to a mere 14%. In many cases, there exists no court order to provide child support. Even when the courts have dictated a support amount, only three of four custodial parents will receive any money. The amount of this support averages about $250 per month. This amount falls far below the actual costs of providing for the child's needs. Failure to keep pace with inflation and with the rising income of the absent parent has also led to inadequacies in court-ordered child support agreements (Scanlan, 1994).

Sources of social support for the single-parent family may also be lacking. The single parent may find it difficult to maintain social relationships as a result of time and economic restraints. Balancing the family, the job, and the details of everyday life leaves little time for the single parent to focus on people and events outside the home. In addition, in cases of divorce, separation, or spousal death, the family's network of social support may erode as previous friends distance themselves from the restructured family. The event that caused the family to restructure into a single-parent household may also lead to the family's seeking a new home, a new community, and a new school for the children. Although the single parent may feel a sense of independence and renewal in making these changes, the child may be overwhelmed by a sense of loss and instability.

The personal or emotional challenges of a single-parent household affect both child and parent. For the child, a major shift in family dynamics occurs as he or she becomes oriented to a single parent serving as the sole (or primary) authority and provider. If the single parent brings a new partner into the home, other relational adjustments must be made.

Single parents are called on to provide most of the emotional support and sustenance for their children. There are few volunteers to give the parent a "break" from the stream of decisions or to serve as the disciplinarian, chauffeur, or cook. The single parent may have to overcome feelings of inadequacy, guilt, anxiety, grief, or loneliness that accompany any major life event, loss, or transition. Attempting to juggle work, maintaining the home, and caring for the children leaves little time for the parent's social or personal needs. In most cases, the single-parent family must accomplish most of the same developmental tasks as do two-parent families but without all of the resources they have to call upon (Wright & Leahey, 1994).

The health care team can assist single-parent families to normalize their lives and smooth out family difficulties. To better serve the family, the nurse needs to seek answers to the following questions:

- How long has the family head been a single parent?
- What circumstances surrounded the organization of the single-parent family?
- What visiting arrangements exist for the noncustodial parent?
- What economic resources does the family have at this time?
- What family and social support systems exist for the single-parent family?
- What other life cycle tasks is the family facing? (Leahey & Wright, 1987)

When confronted with the stressor of a child's illness, these questions help the health care team better understand the current needs of the single-parent family. Specific family concerns can be addressed by demonstrating a sense of empathy, giving credence to the family's problems, and providing specific strategies for intervening therapeutically when necessary (Table 3–5).

Table 3–5
Concerns and Interventions for the Single-Parent Family

Concern	Intervention
Parent feels helpless and overwhelmed	Encourage parent to: Work through own emotions Practice good health habits Keep in touch with family members and friends Socialize with other adults
Single parent feels uncertain regarding parenting and child management practices	Provide parent with information regarding normal growth and development and predictable effects of divorce or death on children
Child exhibits behavioral problems	Teach parent to provide consistent discipline Encourage parent to allow children to express their concerns regarding the change in the family
Child takes on a parent helper role	Determine whether child is still able to have his or her needs met
Child becomes the parent's companion and confidante	Encourage parent to seek other sources of emotional support
Issues related to the absent parent	Openly discuss issues regarding absent parent
Introduction of a new adult into the household	Prepare child ahead of time Discourage parent from casually and frequently having partners of the opposite sex stay the night or move in Define clearly what roles and responsibilities the new adult will have in the household and in regard to child rearing
Making ends meet	Encourage parent to record income and expenses, keeping a budget Plan shopping, using lists to avoid purchasing nonessential items
Managing home responsibilities	Teach children to do many tasks on their own List and divide housework with an assignment for each family member

Binuclear Family

Ahrons and Rodgers (1987) coined the term *binuclear families* to refer to the familial structure of joint custody families. Coparenting or the binuclear family occurs when the child is a member of two nuclear families, after remarriage of both the mother and the father. The responsibility of raising and parenting the child is still considered a joint venture between the two families. Joint physical custody gives both parents legal rights and responsibilities while granting the children equal time with both parents. Joint legal custody, on the other hand, gives both parents legal rights and responsibilities but the children live predominantly with one parent, usually the mother. Research by Wallerstein and Kelly (1980) suggesting that the child benefits from frequent contact with both parents has directed the judicial courts to recognize joint physical custody arrangements as a good answer to custody disputes (Table 3–6). Still other studies have found that children in joint custody were more emotionally troubled than children in single-parent families with limited or no access to the noncustodial parent (Schwartzberg, 1992).

Research has shown that a father's continued involvement with his children is associated with a positive outcome for the children (Friedman, 1992). There is greater paternal contact, involvement, and payment of child support with joint physical custody, and fathers appear more satisfied (Arditti, 1992). Involvement of both parents in a positive parental relationship has been associated with better adjustment in the children (Buchanan, Maccoby, & Dornbusch, 1991). The key to a successful outcome with coparenting is the relationship between the parents. Maccoby and Mnookin (1992) found that couples with joint custody are better educated and have higher incomes than those who received sole custody. In addition, couples that requested joint physical custody seemed less hostile toward each other and the fathers seemed committed to the children before the divorce. When children and parents interact in cocustody arrangements, the children's sense of loss and abandonment is minimized (Kaslow, 1991).

Blended Family

For many years the child's view of stepfamilies has been clouded by such images as the stepmothers of Cinderella, Snow White, and other fairy-tale characters. With the growing rate of divorce and remarriage, more and more children are either part of or know someone who is in a stepfamily. A remarried family consists of a husband and wife maintaining a household, with or without children in the home. One or both of the spouses have previously been in a marital relationship (Glick, 1989). The blended family or stepfamily is defined as "a remarried family with a child under 18 years of age who is the biological child of one of the parents and was born before the remarriage" (Glick, 1989, p. 24).

It is believed that, by the year 2000, the stepfamily will be the most common type of American family (Visher & Visher, 1995b). Between two thirds and three fourths of those who divorce will eventually enter into another marital relationship (Wright & Leahey, 1994). For these restructured families, the redivorce rate is higher than the divorce rate after first marriages. The risk of redivorce increases when children from a prior relationship are present (White & Booth, 1985).

The transitions that accompany remarriage and the formation of the stepfamily present a variety of stressors for the parents and children involved. Even in the most adaptive of families, several developmental issues must

Table 3–6
Joint Custody: Pros and Cons

Pros	Cons
Maintains parent–child relationships	Expects parents who cannot agree during the marriage to make joint decisions after the divorce
Increases likelihood child support will be paid	Has physical impact on the children who must move from one parent's house to the other parent's house on a daily or weekly basis
Gives parents a sense of involvement with children; maintains active participation in parental role	Requires parents to reside within the same community or be at risk of losing job promotion
Allows continued involvement of extended family members: grandparents, aunts, uncles	Children may be involved in lengthy judicial processes to acquire joint custody
Decreases the load of the single parent, resulting in higher quality parenting	

Table 3–7
Developmental Issues in Remarried Families

Steps	Prerequisite Attitude	Developmental Issues
Entering the new relationship	Recovery from loss of first marriage (adequate "emotional divorce")	Recommitment to marriage and to forming a family with readiness to deal with the complexity and ambiguity
Conceptualizing and planning new marriage and family	Accepting one's own fears and those of new spouse and children about remarriage and forming a stepfamily Accepting need for time and patience for adjustment to complexity and ambiguity of Multiple new roles Boundaries: space, time, membership, and authority Affective issues: guilt, loyalty conflicts, desire for mutuality, unresolvable past hurts	Work on openness in the new relationships to avoid pseudomutuality Plan for maintenance of cooperative coparental relationships with ex-spouses Plan to help children deal with fears, loyalty conflicts, and membership in two systems Realignment of relationships with extended family to include new spouse and children Plan maintenance of connections for children with extended family of ex-spouse(s)
Remarriage and reconstitution of family	Final resolution of attachment to previous spouse and ideal of "intact" family Acceptance of a different model of family with permeable boundaries	Restructuring family boundaries to allow for inclusion of new spouse–stepparent Realignment of relationships throughout subsystems to permit interweaving of several systems Making room for relationships of all children with biological (noncustodial) parents, grandparents, and other extended family Sharing memories and histories to enhance stepfamily integration

From McGoldrick, M., & Carter, E. (1980). Forming a remarried family. In E. Carter & M. McGoldrick (Eds.), *The family life cycle: A framework for family therapy* (p. 272). New York: Gardner Press. Reprinted with permission.

be addressed and resolved if the stepfamily is to create its own new identity (Table 3–7). The stepfamily may be subject to several myths regarding the formation of the new family system (Romanczuk, 1987). One common myth is that stepfamilies and nuclear families are the same. The nuclear family originated with two adults and grows with the addition of children and other relatives. The blended family is born of many losses. Coping with these losses takes time and a great deal of emotional energy. Growth of the new family is instantaneous. Adults come with preset patterns of parenting and ideas about how interactions with children should proceed.

Another myth is that the death of a spouse, or the long-term absence of a spouse, makes stepparenting easier. In reality, it is difficult for even the best of stepparents to compete with the idealized image of a dead or absent parent. In addition, the child's feeling of loss and grief can become a difficult barrier to overcome when trying to build new relations with the stepparent.

As the stepfamily forges a new identity, the myth that can be most detrimental is that love happens instantly. Familial affection takes time to develop. False expectations can bring about a sense of failure and resentment between family members. In the same manner, it is also often believed that obedience to the new parent occurs instantaneously. Studies have shown that stepmothers, in their need to provide nurturance and affection, were most often frustrated by the lack of "instant love," whereas fathers have been perceived as more vulnerable to expecting "instant obedience" (Reutter & Strang, 1986). The time it takes to create a new sense of family varies for each family system and is almost always longer than the adults expected. For toddlers and preschoolers, this process takes at least 18 to 24 months; with older children it may take up to 5 to 7 years (Visher & Visher, 1995b).

The other stressors that affect the organization of the new family often include the adjustments that accompany any new marital relationship: difficulties with parenting of stepchildren, adjusting to the children's personalities and habits, and dealing with relationships with former spouses (Visher & Visher, 1995b).

The concerns of the children and adults involved may emerge in several different ways (Chart 3–7). In addition to the stress of a new marital relationship, the stepparent often experiences difficulties with parenting of stepchildren, adjusting to the children's personalities and habits, and gaining acceptance (Visher & Visher, 1992, 1995b). Other stresses experienced by stepparents include relationships with former spouses, adjustment to the new roles of stepparents, and unrealistic expectations in the transition to the new role. This transition is also stressful for the children. Children react to remarriage by experiencing feelings of anger, anxiety, and depression. One study of hospitalized children found that the percentage of children who develop medical or psychiatric problems is higher for children in stepfamilies than for children in first families or in single-parent households (Dickson, Heffron, & Parker, 1990). On the other hand, many researchers are angered by the predominant focus on pathology in the divorce literature and are now trying to focus on the positive attributes of the divorced family.

Gay and Lesbian Family

The lesbian and gay family is another non-traditional family that is becoming more prevalent (Chart 3–8). The gay and lesbian family can be defined by the presence of two or more people who share a same-sex orientation or by the presence of at least one lesbian or gay adult rearing a child (Allen & Demo, 1995). Many couples choose to formalize their relationship with some type of ceremony. These ceremonies can range from an informal exchange of vows to a ceremony in a church similar to the wedding of a heterosexual couple, depending on the couple's belief system.

Increasing numbers of gay men and lesbians are choosing to become parents. It was estimated that there are 1 million to 5 million lesbian mothers, 1 million to 3 million gay fathers, and 6 million to 14 million people in the United States who have one or more lesbian and/or gay parents (Gold et al., 1994). In fact, the 1980s has been called the period of the lesbian baby boom (Zeiden-

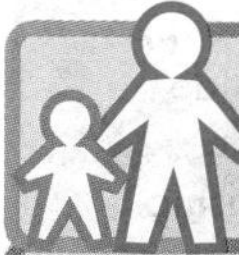

Chart 3–7
Developmental Considerations

Responses to Stepfamilies

	Responses	Health Care Interventions
Toddler or Preschooler	• Clinging to parents • Regressive behaviors such as thumb sucking, bedwetting • Belief that their angry thoughts or behaviors led to family disruption (magical thinking) • Belief that they can magically reunite the family	• Reassure the children that they are not responsible for the dissolution of their parents' marriage. • Include children in family discussions using simple terms. • Praise children for age-appropriate behaviors. • Read age-appropriate books to children about stepfamily situations.
School-age child	• Anger about their powerlessness to stop dissolution of the family • Imagining that they caused the marital breakup • Wishing their parents were together and fantasizing that if they are "good," "bad," or "sick," the parents will come together to help • Acting out anger and guilt by having tantrums, fighting with siblings or classmates, developing psychosomatic symptoms, becoming accident prone, failing in schoolwork, or trying to break up new marriage • Acting "angelic" and, in doing so, hiding their true feelings	• Accept the children's feelings. • Do not force the children to understand the perspective of the adults. • Reassure the children they are not responsible for the dissolution of their parents' marriage. • Encourage the children to communicate with parents and stepparents. • Help the children put feelings into words rather than negative behaviors.

Chart continued on following page

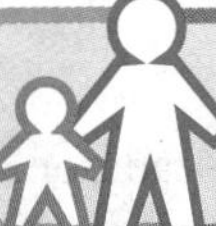

Chart 3–7
Developmental Considerations *Continued*

Responses to Stepfamilies

	Responses	Health Care Interventions
Adolescent	• Frustration and tension as they try to deal with their own identity and sexuality in light of presence of stepsibling or stepparent of the opposite sex • Loss of status of being "in charge" as they make way for new head of household • Divided loyalties that may make them act out in a negative way toward the stepparent • Angered by stepparent who does not view them as mature • Reluctance to become part of stepfamily because of developmental drive for independence and autonomy	• Have family adopt a dress code and make appropriate bedroom arrangements. • Allow adolescents to maintain their independence and integrate at their own pace. • Encourage stepparent to make clear to the adolescent that he or she is not a replacement for a deceased or absent parent. • Emphasize that the adolescent must act in a respectful, if not warm, manner toward the stepparent. • Encourage the adolescent to communicate with parents and stepparents.
Parents	• Loyalty to their children, which predates loyalty to their new spouse, may create conflicts with new spouse • Inability to form solid bond with new spouse because to do so would seem like a betrayal of their relationship with their children • New spouse may feel like an outsider in an established household • Sense of failure and resentment when feelings of love do not happen immediately • Conflict regarding dissimilar parenting styles	• Listen to the parents' concerns. • Provide anticipatory guidance and direct parents to sources of information that provide realistic information about stepfamily life. • Reassure parents that a strong relationship with one another is not a betrayal of their biological children. • Encourage the biological parent to require respect from his or her children toward the new partner as these new relationships develop between the children. • Encourage the biological parent to maintain or become the enforcer of rules for his or her children while the stepparent supports the biological parent in the discipline process. • Encourage the formation of the "parenting coalition" for raising the children. This means that all parents and stepparents cooperate in the parenting experience. • Encourage new spouse to accept that he or she does not have to try to be an "instant" parent. • Recommend that the parents take a parenting course together. • Direct parents to support groups.

stein, 1990). Because of the careful planning involved in conception, the gay or lesbian couple usually has a strong commitment to parenting (Hill, 1987).

Gay men and lesbians become parents in a variety of ways. Lesbians can decide to have children through insemination from a known or unknown donor, heterosexual intercourse, adoption, foster parenting, and coparenting (Martin, 1993; Zeidenstein, 1990). Increasingly, known sperm donors have acknowledged active relationships with the children and their primary parents (Perrin & Kulkin, 1996). Gay men can become parents through the use of a surrogate mother or through adoption and/or foster parenting (Martin, 1993). Some gay and lesbian families are experimenting with three- and four-parent

Chart 3–8

Working with Gay and Lesbian Families: Considerations for the Health Care Provider

- Examine your own attitudes and beliefs toward homosexuality and gay and lesbian parenting.
- Become better informed about the research and misconceptions regarding gay parenting.
- Be supportive of the diversity of family forms in today's society.
- Convey acceptance through the use of gender-neutral terms such as parent or family member when gathering a family history.
- Do not assume all parents are heterosexual.
- Become an advocate for change in social policy and attitudes. Homophobia can lead to decreased self-esteem in children of these functional, caring families.

arrangements. Because some gay men and lesbians have had children in the context of a previous heterosexual relationship, new homosexual relationships may result in a complex of blended or reconstituted families (Perrin & Kulkin, 1996).

Contrary to common misconceptions, children of gay and lesbian parents do not differ from children of heterosexual parents in terms of psychological health and social relationships. Children raised by gay men and lesbians are no more likely to be gay or straight than those raised in heterosexual families (Martin, 1993; Patterson, 1992). Studies have shown that children raised in two-parent homes, regardless of gender, are better adjusted than children raised in single-parent homes (Gold et al., 1994). A common concern is that children of gay and lesbian families will experience the same prejudice that their parents have had to endure. Fortunately, this has not been the case. Children of lesbians and gay men are more aware of the diversity in our society and are better prepared to handle the ignorance and bias of homophobia (Martin, 1993). Laird (1993, p. 316) stated that "children of gay and lesbian parents appear to grow and thrive as well as children in heterosexual families, in spite of the prejudice and discrimination that can and does surround them."

Communal Family

A communal family can be defined as "any group of five or more adults (with or without children) most of whom are unrelated by blood or marriage, who live together without compulsion, primarily for the sake of some ideological goal for which a collective household is deemed essential" (Aidala & Zablocki, 1991, p. 89). Communal living came of age during the late 1960s. Research has shown that most individuals join a commune during times of major social and cultural disjuncture (Zablocki, 1980). Those who join a commune have been found to be college educated and come from intact educated families (Aidala & Zablocki, 1991). People join communes in order to be surrounded by individuals who share common beliefs and practices; in many cases, these are religious beliefs. Principles that guide communal living include collective ownership, the absence of private property accumulation by individual members, and the collective responsibility for all material, cultural, educational, and health needs of the family.

Some communal communities have been described as cults adhering to a set of beliefs or standards that are viewed as deviant by the general society. A charismatic individual is often the source of governance for these communes. Interactions between commune members and outsiders are often discouraged. Thus, health care practices may be neglected or overlooked as commune members rely on internal resources to deal with illness and health promotion issues.

A polygamous family, also referred to as a plural family, is a form of the communal family. The polygamous family consists of one wife with multiple husbands and children or one husband with multiple wives and children. The latter configuration is predominant. In the United States, polygamy is uncommon. However, polygamy continues to be a common practice in many areas in the world (Chaleby, 1985). In 1852, the Mormon religion officially adopted polygamy as a church doctrine and practiced it until the 1890s, when the United States Congress enacted legislation to control polygamy. Today, 30,000 to 50,000 members of fundamentalist Mormon groups in western United States still condone plural marriages on religious grounds (Altman, 1993).

Family Functions

The basic unit in our society is the family. Friedman (1992, p. 4) stated that "the purpose of the family is mediation. The family has to mediate the needs and demands of the family member with those of society." This means that the family is required to meet the basic necessities of society while still meeting the needs of the family members. The family is a medium for the transmission of societal values (Cain, 1980). From a developmental viewpoint, Epstein, Bishop, and Levin (1978) considered that the primary function of the family is to support the development of its members by meeting basic needs such as food and shelter, carrying out developmental tasks for individual growth and family growth through the life cycle, and adapting to hazardous events such as illness and death. From a systems point of view, the main function of family members is to support one another (Minuchin, 1974). Another viewpoint is that the family has two primary functions: to provide material support and supervision (e.g., food, clothing, shelter, safety, health care) and to provide affective and cognitive support, socialization, and education (Schor, 1995). From a structural-functional perspective, the family has affective, reproductive, economic, health care, and socialization functions (see Table 3–3).

These functions not only meet the needs of the family but also, in doing so, meet the needs of the individual and the society. At times, the family may have difficulty in performing some of these functions. For example, providing financially for the family is difficult when a father is laid off from work. He might also have lost the family medical insurance, making it difficult to provide for adequate health care. When these challenges occur, it is important for the nurse to help the family identify additional resources to meet their functional needs.

Family Roles

Family roles and family functions are closely related. A role is defined as a "set of behaviors of an occupant of a particular social position" (Friedman, 1992, p. 233). The family determines the role each family member should play in order to carry out the functions of the family. Roles within the family can be formal or informal. Formal roles are those that must be fulfilled for the family to function smoothly. Some standard parental roles within the family include breadwinner, homemaker, financial manager, child rearer, cook, and chauffeur. The roles of the children may include baby sitter, playmate, and student.

When family members are unable to fulfill their formal roles, other family members must take on those members' roles in order to keep the family functioning. This can lead to role overload. For example, when parents divorce, the single parent must take on the role of the second parent, becoming the breadwinner, the homemaker, and the financial manager. In addition, the older child might have to add the responsibility of becoming the child rearer while the single parent is fulfilling the role of breadwinner. Role overload can also occur when a child family member becomes ill. Roles within the family have to be renegotiated. As the mother or father spends more time at the hospital, the other spouse must fulfill the role of breadwinner while making sure the housework is done. Pediatric nurses need to assess what roles each of the family members plays in order to ensure that role overload does not occur and the functions of the family are fulfilled.

Informal roles in the family are less explicit. Informal roles are the roles family members play in order to meet the emotional needs of the family and help maintain the family's equilibrium (Friedman, 1992). These roles change with the circumstances encountered by the family. Some informal roles include the mediator, the jester, the dominator, the compromiser, the martyr, and the follower (Fig. 3–11). Identification of the family's informal roles can assist the pediatric nurse in assessing the coping mechanisms of the family.

The Healthy Family

What makes a family a "healthy family"? What strengths, coping skills, or other characteristics are found in families that are able to adapt and reorganize when faced with the normal transitions and the unexpected transitions that accompany the family life cycle? Research on healthy families has focused on the coping mechanisms, characteristics, traits, and qualities of healthy families.

Many researchers believe that a healthy family starts with the quality of the couple's relationship. Beavers (1985) identified the attributes of a healthy couple through research on couples that have been successful in maintaining satisfying relationships for many years. He stated that the beliefs and attitudes that are associated with a healthy couple include the following:

- *A modest overt power difference.* Healthy couples are relatively similar in power levels. Roles of the healthy couple are complementary.

Figure 3–11
Siblings can play important roles in the family.

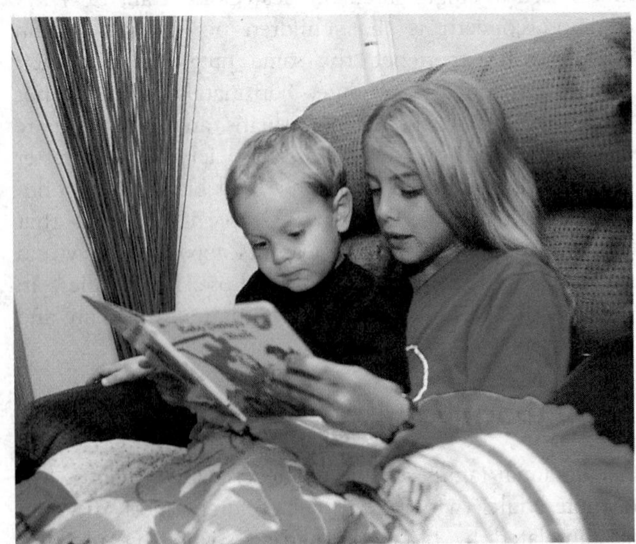

- *The capacity for clear boundaries.* Healthy couples have the ability to tell the difference between one person's feelings and wishes and those of another.
- *The ability to operate mainly in the present.* Healthy couples focus on the present. They look at the past as a guide rather than a directive.
- *A respect for individual choice and autonomy.* Healthy couples encourage expression of personal perceptions and wishes.
- *Skills in negotiating.* Healthy couples have the ability to negotiate solutions that meet the needs of both people.
- *The ability to share positive feelings.* Healthy couples enjoy what they do and express their enjoyment. They find their relationship to be fun, effective, and optimistic.

In the healthy family, honest differences can become opportunities to develop new understandings rather than reasons for struggles and fights to occur. The healthy family believes that family members are not adversaries; they are friends and partners. This allows people to err or disagree without the threat of isolation. Healthy families believe that human encounters can usually be rewarding.

Table 3-8
Critical Family Strengths and Coping Skills over the Family Life Cycle

	Family Stages			
Family Strengths	Couple	Childbearing and School-Age	Teenage and Young Adult	Empty Nest and Retirement
ACCORD: Balanced interrelationship among family members that allows them to resolve conflicts and reduce chronic strain.	X	X		
CELEBRATIONS: Acknowledging birthdays, religious occasions, and other special events.	X	X	X	X
COMMUNICATION: Sharing beliefs and emotions with one another. Emphasis is on how family members exchange information and caring with each other.	X	X		X
FINANCIAL MANAGEMENT: Sound decision-making skills for money management and satisfaction with economic status can contribute to family well-being.	X	X	X	
HARDINESS: A basic strength through which families find the capacity to cope. Emphasizes family members' sense of control over their lives, commitment to the family, confidence that the family will survive no matter what, and the ability to grow, learn, and challenge each other.	X	X	X	X
HEALTH: The physical and psychological well-being of family members can reduce stress and preserve a healthy home atmosphere.	X			X
LEISURE ACTIVITIES: Focuses on similarities and differences of family member preferences for ways to spend free time. Do family members prefer active or passive interests, social or personal activities?	X			
PERSONALITY: Involves acceptance of a partner's traits, behaviors, general outlook, and dependability.	X		X	X
SUPPORT NETWORK: Emphasizes the positive aspects of relationships with in-laws, relatives, and friends.		X	X	
TIME AND ROUTINES: Family meals, chores, togetherness, and other ordinary routines play an important role in creating continuity and stability in family life.	X	X	X	X
TRADITIONS: Honoring holidays and important family experiences carried through generations.	X	X	X	X

From McCubbin, H., & McCubbin, M. (1988). Typologies of resilient families: Emerging roles of social class and ethnicity. *Family Relations, 37,* 247–254. Reprinted with permission.

Trust and cooperation with one another are key components of family interactions. The healthy family is optimistic and hopeful even when human situations are bad. There is meaning to the human enterprise. These families share a belief that there is purpose outside the realm of the family. The healthy family participates in and contributes to the community around them.

Olson (1993) has stated that healthy families are able to balance their level of togetherness versus separateness. Members are able to experience independence from the family while remaining connected to the family unit. The physical and emotional boundaries of the family allow for sharing of family space and a value for time spent together. At the same time, private space is respected. Members are encouraged to participate in friendships outside the family and to share those friendships with the family.

Worldview: *In some ethnic groups (e.g., Hispanic, Southeast Asian) or religious groups (e.g., Amish, Mormon), it may be expected that family members have a higher level of togetherness, with independence and separateness being discouraged. This should not be considered "dysfunctional" if all family members wish the family to be that way. Cultural beliefs are a central part of the family's character and must be considered when evaluating the family dynamics.*

Olson (1993) further asserted that the healthy family has positive communication skills that help the family to balance their levels of flexibility and cohesion in the presence of situational stress or developmental change. Rules exist to guide expectations of family members, yet these rules can be changed when necessary to adapt to family stressors.

Healthy families can be characterized by critical strengths that facilitate efforts to manage the stressors and strains that emerge at different stages of the family life cycle (Table 3–8). In particular, it has been noted that family rituals, characterized by routines and celebrations, are an integral part of a stable family (McCubbin & McCubbin, 1988). Keltner (1992) found that higher levels of family routines and more stimulating family environments were significantly correlated with child health status. Family routines are an important aspect of family life to consider when families encounter illness and hospitalizations that may disrupt their family patterns.

caREminder: *Although a child may be ill or hospitalized for a lengthy period, encourage families to maintain and incorporate as many of their family rituals as possible into the new care routines they establish during this period.*

Healthy families are characterized by parents who have the knowledge, ability, and resources to adjust their child rearing strategies and goals in view of the unique characteristics of the child, their own strengths and weaknesses as parents, and the social and family context in which interactions take place. Parenting goals are clear, supporting the well-being and survival of the children (Gross, 1996).

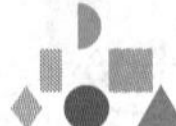

Special Family Issues

Adoption

The adoptive family is considered a variation of the nuclear family, with special needs and considerations related to the expansion and realignment of family boundaries. Adoption has been defined as

> A means of providing some children with security and meeting their developmental needs by legally transferring ongoing parental responsibilities from their birth parents to their adoptive parents; recognizing that in so doing, we have created a new kinship network that forever links those two families together through the child, who is shared by both (Reitz & Watson, 1992, p. 11).

Through the adoption process, a new family system is created (Fig. 3–12). Emotional, social, and physical

Figure 3–12
Through adoption, individuals are joined to become a new family.

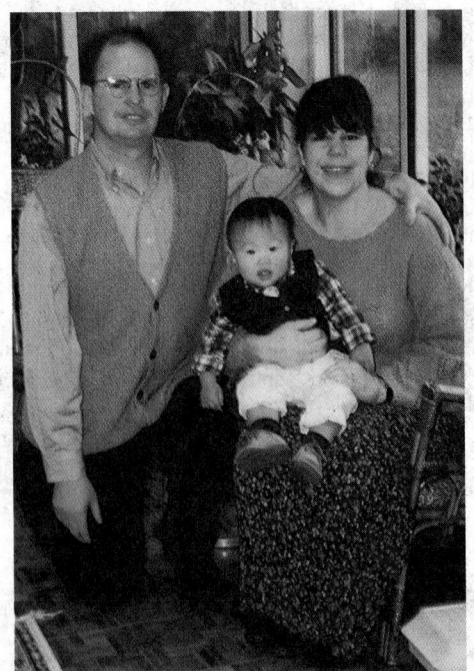

ties may continue to bind the child to his or her family of origin. Even if adoption takes place during infancy and the birth parents choose to sever contact with the child, as the child matures, he or she may wish to reopen relationships with the birth parents. The ties to the family of origin may never be severed completely (Grotevant, McRoy, Elde, & Fravel, 1994).

Adults choose to become adoptive parents for many reasons. Traditional adoptive parents are couples who are unable to conceive their own biological children but still wish to raise a child. For parents who adopt because of infertility, the rate of conception after adopting is 8% to 14% (Roizen, 1995). Lately, preferential adoption has become more common. Preferential adoption takes place when couples have decided to add children to their family for a variety of religious, moral, or personal reasons independent of fertility. Declining social and legal barriers to single-parent adoption have led to an increase in the number of unmarried women and men choosing adoption as a way to start their family (Prowler, 1991).

Approximately 2% of the population is adopted. Of adoptive parents, 52% are nonrelatives of the child and 48% are relatives (Roizen, 1995; Sherry, 1992). The types of children families adopt are changing. There has been a decline in the number of healthy infants available for adoption, as a result of contraception, abortion, and more single women keeping and raising their children (Castiglia, 1994). There has been an increase in the number of children with special needs available for adoption, as a result of parental abuse (including prenatal substance abuse), neglect, abandonment, or death (Brodzinsky & Huffman, 1988). Special needs children also include certain minorities, children older than 6 years, children with chronic illnesses or psychological problems, and children who must be adopted with a sibling (Roizen, 1995). The adoption is at a higher risk for discontinuation when special needs children are involved. If the child is older, has been moved to several different homes, or there is a child of the same age already in the home, difficulties within the family adjustment are likely to occur. Special needs children place more physical and emotional demands on the family. Therefore, families considering adopting a special needs child must spend time critically evaluating their resources and ability to meet the challenges of these special children.

The transition to parenthood for the adoptive parent(s) does not come without its share of challenges. Adoptive parents are burdened by a number of role conflicts that place additional stress on the transition. For instance, the unanticipated crisis of infertility places the couple and individual at risk for psychological problems. Infertile couples often describe feelings of guilt, unworthiness, decreased self-esteem, depression, decreased marital sexual relations, and marital discord. Successful transition to adoptive parenthood requires the couple to mourn and resolve issues related to their infertility. Single people who adopt may feel they must constantly justify to others why they chose adoption and why they feel secure in the knowledge that they can provide a supportive environment for raising a child.

Although the adoption process can be quite long, the suddenness of learning that a child is available "now" for adoption does not allow the parent-to-be much time to prepare emotionally or physically for the actual presence of the wished-for child. Adoptive parents also have fewer role models than biological parents, because adoption is not the norm in Western society. After the adoption, parents may have idealized expectations about the child's behavior that are not realized. If information about the birth parents was sketchy and contact with the birth parents is not possible (closed adoption), adoptive parents may worry about genetic and hereditary traits that may emerge in the child. In an open adoption, birth parents and adoptive parents maintain a degree of ongoing communication. The adoptive parents may initially perceive the openness as a threat to their skills and confidence in establishing a new family structure (Fister & Scholmann, 1995). It is important for the nurse to be aware of these potential concerns and to help the family focus on its strengths and resources during the transition period of the adoption process. Parenting classes specifically for adoptive parents can assist the family in adjusting to their new roles. Content would include the physical aspects of infant care, the emotional aspects of adoption, and a time for sharing so that adoptive parents can gain support and insights from one another (Lobar & Phillips, 1994).

Throughout the life cycle, the adoptive family faces normal transitions associated with child rearing as well as unique transitions related to the adoptive situation. LePere (1987) found the most critical points in the adoptive family life cycle to be

- The application process
- The waiting period after being accepted as adoptive parents (could be as long as 5 to 7 years)
- The time of receiving physical custody of the child
- The waiting period after receiving the child and legalization of the adoption
- Finalization of the adoption by a formal decree of the courts
- School entrance by the adopted child
- Realization by the adopted child of the loss he or she has experienced related to adoption
- The adopted adolescent seeking information about his or her biological family
- Beginning of a family by the adopted child

A particular challenge to the adoptive parents is how the child, and how outsiders, may react to the adoption.

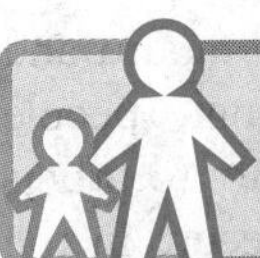

Chart 3–9
Developmental Considerations

Issues Related to Adoption

Age	Issues	Family Interventions
Infant	Separation from interim caregivers and introduction of new adult caregivers Disruption of care routines	If possible, adoptive family should take leave from work to become acquainted with the child. Provide as much consistency as possible regarding who will be caring for the child (including daycare providers and babysitters). Follow infant's previous caregiving routines as much as possible, introducing changes as tolerated by the child. Allow the infant to keep treasured security objects such as a blanket or stuffed animal.
Toddler and preschooler	"Where did I come from?" Generally accepting of being adopted Want reassurance that they are loved Introduction into a new home	Tell the child he or she is adopted. Use books to discuss adoption. Use family photograph album to depict story of adoption. Answer questions about birth parents honestly, yet in simple, positive terms. Establish behavioral expectations for the child and family routines as soon as possible to help child define his or her new boundaries.
School-age child	"Why was I adopted when most people are not?" Worried that their value as a person is less because they are adopted Concerns about being different Aware that they have lost someone who played an extremely important role in their life Imagine birth parents as rich, famous, and more attractive than adoptive parents Adoptive parents may view child's questions about birth parents as a rejection of them	Review the child's adoption story with him or her. Assure the child that he or she is a loved and welcome member of the family. Share letters and pictures of the birth parents with the child, if desired. Reveal who birth parents are, if desired. The health care provider can reassure parents that the child's questioning is part of normal developmental sequence.
Adolescent	Task of developing an identity and discovering how they are different and how they are connected to "their" family Concerns about physical appearance, traits, and family illnesses of their birth family Interest in meeting parents May have idealized picture of birth parents	Give more information about birth parents if available. Provide with pictures and information about traits and family illnesses if possible. Allow adolescent to meet birth parents. If the identity of birth parents is unknown, encourage adolescent to wait until young adulthood to begin search for parents.

The adoptee's understanding of the adoption changes as the child develops (Chart 3–9). As they mature, children should be given every opportunity to learn more about their biological parents if this is their desire. Children who avoid talking about or thinking about adoptive issues are at risk for emotional problems and identity confusion (Bower, 1994). Parents are encouraged to answer questions honestly, giving consideration to the child's age and level of comprehension. As the child gets older, more probing questions are asked. Often, there is limited information available about one or both birth parents. Even so, children should be encouraged to think positively about their birth parents and the circumstances surrounding their adoption (Chart 3–10). People outside the immediate family may express curiosity about the adoption simply because the child looks different from the adoptive parents. In answering these queries, it is important to respect the child's right to privacy regarding the details of the adoption and the birth parents (Peterson, 1997; Roizen, 1995).

Foster Care

Foster care, also known as home care, is a child welfare service in which children are placed in homes away from their parents in an effort to ensure their emotional and physical well-being (Sherry, 1992). The need for foster placement exists when the parents are deemed unwilling or unable to care for their children. In many cases, children are reunited with their parents when the family has demonstrated that interventions to improve the individual, home, or family problems have been instituted. The child in foster care may be placed with relatives (kinship care), in nonrelative family foster care, or in residential group care.

Children placed in foster care are more at risk for emotional, developmental, physical, and behavioral problems (Carlson, 1996; Pronsati, 1996; Sherry, 1992). Several factors contribute to the increased number of problems that foster children may experience. The interplay of factors that led the child to foster care placement is a key issue to consider. The child may have come from an abusive home situation or have been considered to have such severe behavioral problems that the parents felt incapable of caring for the child. Many children in foster care have medical problems. In one study of children enrolled in foster care it was found that 82% had at least one chronic medical condition before placement. Nearly 30% had three or more chronic problems (Pronsati, 1996).

The foster child may experience difficulties related to the transitions from one home or placement setting to another. It may not be easy for the child to establish a trusting relationship with foster caregivers. The child must learn to be flexible and accommodate to new stan-

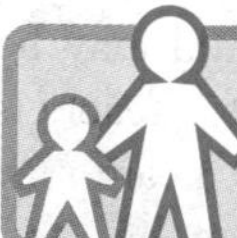

Chart 3–10
Developmental Considerations

Answering Children's Questions About Adoption

As children grow, it is natural for them to want to hear their adoption story and to learn more about their birth parents. The adoption story should be explained at the child's developmental level and include the following elements:

- The adoptive parents' motivation for adoption
- Acknowledgment of the important role of the birth parents in the creation of the child
- The information that the child was conceived, grew inside the birth mother, and was born just like all the other children
- A suggestion that the decision of the birth parents to place him or her for adoption was in no way the fault of the child
- Acknowledgment that there are happy and sad feelings associated with adoption
- A statement of the adoptive parents' love for the child

The specifics of each adoption story will vary according to the circumstances.

As the child matures, more probing questions about the birth parents may be asked:

Why did my mother not want to keep me?
"Your mother chose adoption because she felt unprepared to raise a child, any child, at that time."

Explain that the mother's lack of money, maturity, or resources may have been the reason she felt unprepared to care for the child. Never imply that the reason for the adoption had anything to do with something the child did.

Why don't we know anything about my father? (my mother?)
"Your birth father was most likely overwhelmed by the situation and thought that he was not entitled to be more involved. He probably thinks about you and wonders about how you are doing."

The child should be encouraged to think positively about the birth father or mother.

Did my parents: use drugs, use alcohol, abuse me, have a mental illness?
"Your parents needed help but did not know how to ask for it. So their problem with ________ was a signal that they needed help and needed someone else to care for their child."

Discuss such circumstances with the child in an open and honest fashion.

dards for discipline and "house rules." The child may be placed in a new school, where it takes time for teachers to address any special educational needs. Health care may be discontinuous, as foster children have often had frequent changes in primary care providers (Dubowitz, 1995). Abuse and neglect can occur in the foster care setting. Each of these conditions is an issue that may negatively affect the foster child's health and well-being.

Foster care is intended to serve as a therapeutic and healing intervention to assist children and families in crisis. Health care providers are in a position to support the positive adaptation of the child and the promotion of the child's general health and welfare. Every effort should be made to provide consistent health care to the child to avoid discontinuation of necessary services and exacerbation of chronic problems. The health care provider should be attuned to problems voiced by the child or the foster parents with regard to the foster care experience. Appropriate referrals can be made if the foster parents are not equipped to manage serious problems. Physical and behavioral markers of child maltreatment should be assessed, with appropriate interventions to remove the child from the foster care setting if justified. The health care professional can serve as an advocate for the child in foster care, assisting in monitoring behavioral problems, general health concerns, and the child's ability to meet developmental norms.

Figure 3–13
Identical versus fraternal: characteristics of twins.

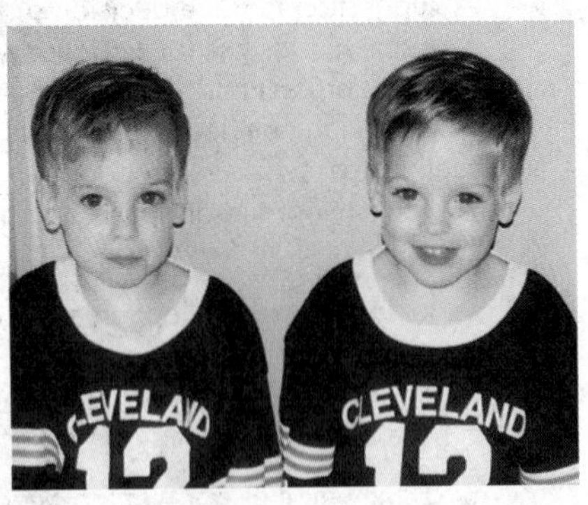

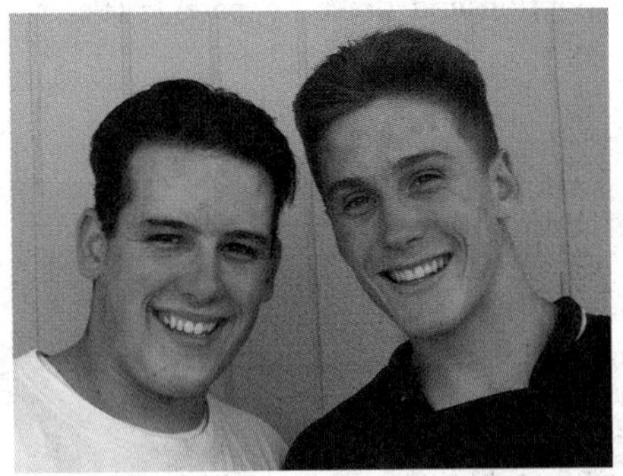

Identical Twins	Fraternal Twins
Monozygotic (Mz)	Dizygotic (Dz)
Fertilization of single ovum by single spermatozoon	Fertilization of two separate ova by two separate spermatozoa (possibly not from the same sexual partner)
Same implantation site, one placenta, one chorion, two amnions	Separate inplantation sites, two placentas, two chorions, two amnions (placentas have been known to fuse)
Same gender	Same or different gender
Same genetic blueprint and physical characteristics	Different genetic blueprint and physical characteristics
High similarity in behaviors that are governed by heredity	Lower rate of similarity for behaviors influenced by heredity
30% of twin births	70% of twin births
Tendency not influenced by familial patterns, maternal age, parity, or ethnicity; may be some relation to therapy for infertility	Tendency affected by familial maternal pattern of inheritance, advanced maternal age, increased parity; more frequent in blacks; increased levels of follicle-stimulating hormone and luteinizing hormone; pregnancy within 1 month of stopping oral contraceptive use, use of infertility drugs (clomiphene citrate and menotropins [Pergonal]), and in vitro fertilization

Multiple Births

To the casual observer, seeing a family with twins, triplets, or even quadruplets is a delight. Strangers stop the family to ask questions about the children's personalities and the parents' ability to "tell them apart" (Fig. 3–13). Multiple births such as twins, triplets, quadruplets, and quintuplets may be the result of one zygote (identical), several zygotes (fraternal), or a combination (some of the children are identical, some fraternal). In the United States, twinning occurs in approximately 1 in 80 to 87 births, triplets in 1 in 6400 (Berkowitz, 1996; Groothuis, 1995).

Worldview: *The incidence of dizygotic twins is positively influenced by ethnicity and socioeconomic class. Dizygotic twins are more likely to occur in the African American population and least likely to occur in the Asian population. Dizygotic twins are more likely in mothers of low socioeconomic class.*

All childbearing families experience similar developmental tasks. The new infant must be integrated into the family, parents must learn new skills and reallocation of tasks, grandparents must adapt to a new role, and the bonds of intimacy that interplayed to create the child must be nurtured and maintained in a new context. For the parents of multiple children, these tasks are complicated by the necessity of managing more than one child with the same amount of support generally afforded the family with a singleton infant. In addition, multiple births are frequently preterm. Twenty percent of infants born before 20 weeks' gestation are twins (Berkowitz, 1996). Multiple births account for 11% of all neonatal deaths (Garcia & Gall, 1990). Surviving children may require lengthy hospitalizations and medical interventions. The infants are likely to be discharged from the hospital at different times, requiring the parents to manage the care of a newborn at home and to monitor and support the activities of the remaining hospitalized children (Mead, Chuffo, Lawlor-Klean, & Meier, 1992).

The family of multiples can expect to undergo many lifestyle changes and have many concerns related to the care of their children (Chart 3–11). The mother is generally homebound after the birth for a longer period of time than the singleton mother. Living space, including size of the car, bedroom, and play areas, and storage places for child supplies and equipment are often found to be inadequate. The physical and emotional energy to support the marital relationship and the relationship with older siblings is tested (Anderson & Anderson, 1987).

Equally challenging for the parent is the task of developing an attachment to and relationship with each child as a unique personality. To promote individuation, parents are encouraged to select different-sounding names for the children and to use individual names when referring to the twins. The children should not be dressed alike all the time and, as they grow, should be encouraged to select clothes that reflect their personalities. Par-

Chart 3–11
Developmental Considerations

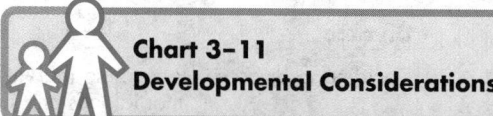

Concerns of Parents with Multiples

Infancy

- Efficient organization of household responsibilities
- Time management skills
- Obtaining, maintaining, and storing stock of baby equipment and supplies (cribs, high chairs, diapers, wipes, formula, baby food)
- Ability to breast-feed or bottle feed babies simultaneously
- Developing same feeding and sleep schedule for all infants
- Ability to respond to babies as separate individuals

Preschoolers

- Delays of verbal and motor skills
- Providing adult stimulation
- Providing activities separate from those of other sibling(s)
- Providing discipline and praise in a consistent and fair manner on the basis of each child's behavior
- Comparing one child with another in terms of behavior
- Higher incidence of delayed toilet training

School-Age and Adolescents

- Entry into school and separation into different classrooms
- Individualizing educational process to meet each child's learning needs
- Discouraging excessive comparisons by teachers and peers
- Promoting independent goals, activities, and peer relationships

Ongoing

- Stress management
- Financial concerns
- Neglecting sibling needs
- Parental self-care needs and personal time
- Parental relations
- Frequent transmission of childhood illnesses among siblings
- Treatment of complications related to preterm birth

Table 3–9
The Family Life Cycle When Divorce Occurs

Stage	Emotional Process of Transition	Developmental Issues
Divorce		
Deciding to divorce	Accepting inability to resolve marital tensions sufficiently to continue relationship	Accepting one's own part in the failure of the marriage
Planning the breakup of the system	Supporting viable arrangements for all parts of the system	Working cooperatively on problems of custody, visitation, and finances Dealing with extended family about the divorce
Separation	Being willing to continue cooperative coparental relationship and joint financial support of children Working on resolution of attachment to spouse	Mourning loss of nuclear family Restructuring marital and parent-child relationships and finances; adaptation to living apart Realigning relationships with extended family; staying connected with spouse's extended family
Divorce	Continued working on emotional divorce: overcoming hurt, anger, guilt, and so forth	Retrieving hopes, dreams, and expectations from the marriage
Postdivorce		
Single-parent (custodial household or primary residence)	Being willing to maintain financial responsibilities, continue parental contact with ex-spouse, and support contact of children with ex-spouse and his or her family	Making flexible visitation arrangements with ex-spouse and his or her family Rebuilding own financial resources Rebuilding own social network
Single-parent (noncustodial)	Being willing to maintain parental contact with ex-spouse and support custodial parent's relationship with children	Finding ways to continue effective parenting relationship with children Maintaining financial responsibilities to ex-spouse and children Rebuilding own social network

From Carter, E., and McGoldrick, M. (1980). The family life cycle and family therapy: An overview. In E. Carter and M. McGoldrick (Eds.) *The family life cycle: A framework for family therapy* (pp. 18–19). New York, Gardner Press. Reprinted with permission.

ents are encouraged to spend quality time with each child separately. Praises and discipline should be merited individually. Siblings should be encouraged to develop their own toy preferences, friendships, special activities, and hobbies. Others who come into contact with the children should be encouraged to treat them as individuals, expecting them to think and behave differently. Several organizations, newsletters, and computer resources are available to connect these special families with others facing the same circumstances (see Resources at the end of the chapter).

Divorce

Most children do not want their parents to get a divorce. Nevertheless, 50% of marriages end in divorce and 60% of those marriages involve children (Hetherington et al., 1993). Annually, divorce rates affect over 1 million

American children (Green, 1995). The steady rise in the divorce rate has affected parents of all age groups, particularly young adults. The average length of a marriage has been estimated to be 6.6 years (Wallerstein, 1992). Many families involved in a divorce have children in the infant, toddler, and preschool age groups. These children can expect to live in a single-parent household for about 5 years before the caretaking parent remarries (Foster & Pascoe, 1995). Because the incidence of divorce is higher in second marriages, children who have coped with one divorce are at risk for experiencing the crisis of divorce a second time.

The frequency with which divorce occurs has forced family theorists to reevaluate the application of the family life cycle model. Carter and McGoldrick (1988) have developed an alternative description of the family life cycle for the family affected by divorce (Table 3–9). They described four phases of the divorce stage and two phases of the postdivorce stage. There are certain prerequisite attitudes that assist family members in making the transition through each phase (column 2) and in working through certain developmental issues (column 3). The impact of divorce affects families differently depending on the stage of the family life cycle at the time of the divorce. For instance, if divorce occurs after the children have been launched from the home, fewer issues regarding custodial arrangements and the economic consequences of the divorce for the children would need to be discussed. The divorcing family usually requires 1 to 3 years to move through the crisis of divorce and to restabilize in its new form (Hetherington, 1982).

Not all children react in the same way when faced with the crisis of divorce. It has been found that most children experience a period of emotional distress after the divorce (Schwartzberg, 1992). The impact of divorce affects children differently depending on their developmental age, gender, and the degree of conflict between the parents (Chart 3–12). The majority return to their normal development within 1 to 2 years without significant long-term psychological problems (Cherlin, 1992). Nursing interventions with families who are experiencing a divorce are aimed at helping the family move through

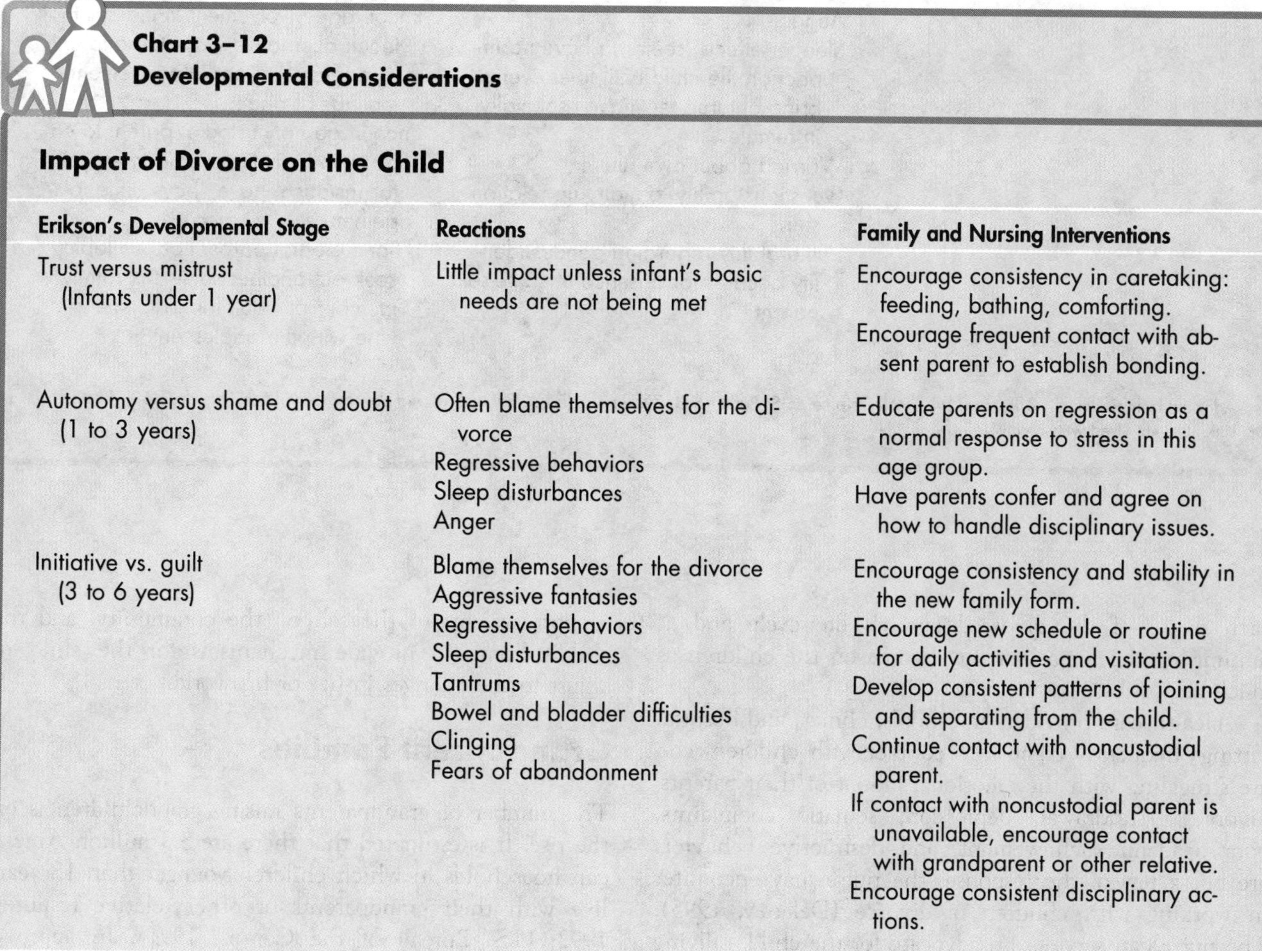

Chart 3–12
Developmental Considerations

Impact of Divorce on the Child

Erikson's Developmental Stage	Reactions	Family and Nursing Interventions
Trust versus mistrust (Infants under 1 year)	Little impact unless infant's basic needs are not being met	Encourage consistency in caretaking: feeding, bathing, comforting. Encourage frequent contact with absent parent to establish bonding.
Autonomy versus shame and doubt (1 to 3 years)	Often blame themselves for the divorce Regressive behaviors Sleep disturbances Anger	Educate parents on regression as a normal response to stress in this age group. Have parents confer and agree on how to handle disciplinary issues.
Initiative vs. guilt (3 to 6 years)	Blame themselves for the divorce Aggressive fantasies Regressive behaviors Sleep disturbances Tantrums Bowel and bladder difficulties Clinging Fears of abandonment	Encourage consistency and stability in the new family form. Encourage new schedule or routine for daily activities and visitation. Develop consistent patterns of joining and separating from the child. Continue contact with noncustodial parent. If contact with noncustodial parent is unavailable, encourage contact with grandparent or other relative. Encourage consistent disciplinary actions.

Chart continued on following page

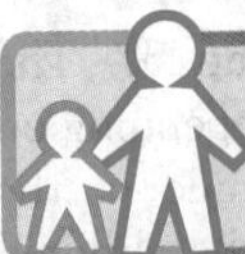

Chart 3–12
Developmental Considerations *Continued*

Impact of Divorce on the Child

Erikson's Developmental Stage	Reactions	Family and Nursing Interventions
Industry vs. inferiority (6 to 12 years)	Feel a sense of responsibility for divorce Fantasize about parental reconciliation Sadness Fearfulness Loyalty conflicts Declining school performance Depression Anger toward one or both parents	Provide regular opportunities for child to talk about feelings. Avoid blaming and speaking in a derogatory manner about other parent (child will want to choose sides). Support child's continuing relationship with both parents. Offer reassurance. Empathize with child's feelings.
Identity vs. role confusion (12 to 18 years)	Engaging in self-destructive behavior: substance abuse, truancy, sexual promiscuity, eating disorders, suicide Declining school performance Feels responsible for taking care of and nurturing their parents Depression Anger Sleeper effects (seems to have no impact on the child until later events bring out true feelings), especially in females Worried about own future Questions ability to maintain relationships Vulnerability regarding gender identity because of absence of same-sex parent	Avoid seeking companionship from adolescents. Provide opportunities for open discussion. Offer appropriate support including other family members, friends, church groups, and peer support groups. Encourage involvement in classes that teach alternative ways to handle disagreements and management of feelings of anger. Encourage noncustodial parent to engage in activities with adolescent, for instance, have "boys' time together." If noncustodial parent not available, seek out another same sex family member or adult friend to spend time with the adolescent.

Adapted from Foster, S., & Pascoe, J. (1995). Divorce. In S. Parker & B. Zuckerman (Eds.). *Behavioral and developmental pediatrics* (p. 360). Boston: Little, Brown. Used with permission.

each phase of the divorced family's life cycle and at minimizing the impact of the divorce on the children as much as possible.

Health care providers in schools, clinics, and hospital settings frequently come into contact with children who are struggling with the emotional fallout of their parents' divorce. Withdrawal, depression, somatic complaints, poor academic achievement, and destructive behaviors are but a few of the responses the nurse may encounter in working with children of divorce (Delaney, 1995). The nurse can serve as an advocate for the child, rallying support systems in the school, the community, and the child's home to provide mechanisms for the child to adjust to the changes in her or his world.

Grandparent Families

The number of grandparents raising grandchildren is on the rise. It is estimated that there are 3.3 million American households in which children younger than 18 years live with their grandparents or other relative (Saluter, 1992; U.S. Bureau of the Census, 1991). In approxi-

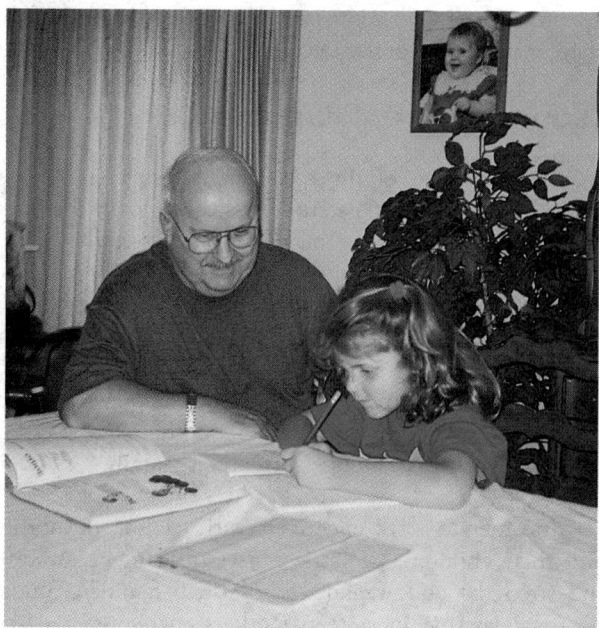

Figure 3–14
Grandparents may assume care of grandchildren because of the parents' death, serious illness, or other problems.

mately one third of these homes neither parent is present to share some of the child rearing responsibilities (U.S. Bureau of the Census, 1991). Although this type of family living arrangement can be found in all cultural groups regardless of socioeconomic level, Saluter (1992) found that black children were much more likely to live in grandparents' homes than were white children or Hispanic children (Fig. 3–14).

Grandparents become the caretakers of their offspring's children for a variety of reasons. The primary reason has been associated with the negative consequences of parental drug or alcohol abuse (Dowell, 1995). These consequences include poverty, homelessness, exposures to the human immunodeficiency virus (HIV) and acquired immunodeficiency syndrome (AIDS), and child abuse and neglect. Other reasons grandparents may become caretakers include death, mental illness, or incarceration of one or both parents. Under any of these conditions, the grandparents may become caregivers through informal arrangements made among family members or through formal arrangements made by the child welfare system (Jendrek, 1994; Kelley & Damato, 1995). When legal or physical custody of the child is removed from the birth parent(s), many grandparents accept responsibility for their grandchildren rather than seeing the children placed in a nonrelative foster care home.

Health care professionals need to be aware of the impact this new family constellation has on the child, the grandparents, and other affected family members. For the younger grandparent, caring for grandchildren may come as an addition to their current parenting role. They may still have young children of their own residing in their household. The addition of more children may lead to financial, emotional, and marital stress. Aunts and uncles (who are still children themselves) may resent the intrusion of the new family members.

Grandparents who are older probably did not expect to be "parents" again. At this point in their lives they may have been looking forward to their retirement years, when they would be freed from the responsibilities of child rearing. Although they may be financially secure and in good physical condition, raising grandchildren leads to increased physical, emotional, and economic vulnerability of the grandparents (Kelley & Damato, 1995). Decreasing energy levels, higher incidence of illness, symptoms of aging, and a tendency to become rigid and controlling are all factors that compete against the growing needs of active young children and rebellious teenagers. In addition, many of the children placed with grandparents have physical as well as emotional problems as a result of the parent's problems that have led to this alternative caregiving situation. Extra medical and financial resources may be needed to support these children. Both the physical health and the financial health of the retired grandparent can be quickly depleted by the constant demands of a medically fragile child.

Raising grandchildren leads to major changes in at least three relationships the grandparent has formed. First, the grandparents may no longer be like their peers. In one study, a grandmother described this experience as feelings of social isolation from her other "senior citizen" friends whose interests and activities were no longer the same as hers (Kelley & Damato, 1995). While these friends may be traveling or volunteering their time to a service organization, the "new parent" grandparent must worry about getting children off to school and to other social events.

The grandparents' role is also changed with respect to the relationship they have with the child's parents. Feelings of anger and resentment may exist as they are forced to take on the responsibilities of parenting. In addition, it may be difficult for the grandparents to witness the deterioration of their own child, who is addicted to drugs and thus unable even to care adequately for him- or herself. For some of these grandparents, caring for their grandchildren may relieve some personal stress as they now know those children are in a safe and secure environment in their home.

Lastly, the grandparents' relationship with the grandchild is altered by their new role as parents. Typically, grandparents can be permissive and generous with their grandchildren. However, in the parenting role, the grandparent now becomes the disciplinarian, and the birth parent (who comes by for occasional visits) may become the more fun-loving adult figure.

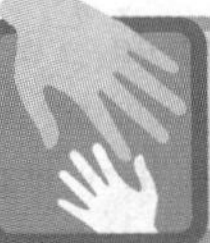

Chart 3–13
Nursing Interventions

Ways to Support Grandparents as Caregivers

- Provide grandparents with information about their state's policies on financial assistance available to kinship caregivers.
- Direct caregivers to apply for Aid to Families of Dependent Children (AFDC) benefits if they are eligible.
- Ensure that grandparents have the same visiting and rooming-in privileges granted to parents in inpatient health care settings.
- Provide parenting classes for updating child care skills.
- Provide education about the special needs of their grandchild, who may be medically fragile or have had prenatal exposure to drugs.
- Encourage grandparents not to neglect their own health care needs.
- Provide transitional care through the use of home nursing visits for newborns or the child with special needs who is discharged to the grandparents' home.
- Refer grandparents to support groups and individual or family counseling when needed.
- Refer grandparents to legal aid agencies or law firms that can assist them in working their way through the complexities of the child welfare system.

There can be many rewarding aspects of caregiving for both the grandparents and their grandchildren. Much joy and love can be shared in these new relationships. For some grandparents, it is an opportunity to enjoy parenting the "second time around" with more confidence and self-assurance. For the grandchildren, being raised in a safe and secure environment is an unmeasurable benefit of this new family constellation.

Health care providers can serve as a resource to grandparent caregivers to connect them with information and services that can assist them in their parenting responsibilities (Chart 3–13). Access to support groups and individual or family counseling have been found to be beneficial in helping grandparents deal with the stressors they may experience (Dowell, 1995). In 1993, the American Association of Retired Persons (AARP) established the Grandparent Information Center to provide information and resources for grandparents who are raising their grandchildren. The names and addresses of this and other resources for grandparents can be found at the end of this chapter in the Resources section.

Teenage Parent Families

At the other end of the spectrum is the family that is headed by adolescent parents, most commonly the teenage mother. In 1990, teenage girls gave birth to almost one of eight infants born in the United States (March of Dimes Birth Defects Foundation, 1993). Although fathers have good intentions before the delivery of supporting both the mother and the child, many fail to do so once the baby is born. In fact, marital rates among adolescent parents are relatively low, as most mothers are choosing to remain single, living with their family of origin (Schor, 1995).

In order to work effectively with adolescent mothers and their children, pediatric nurses need to be aware of the strengths and weaknesses of these families. Studies have shown that most teen mothers encounter both behavioral and developmental difficulties while attempting to raise a child in today's society (Kohlenberg, 1995). Other difficulties include low job status and educational achievement, increased likelihood of living in poverty, less partner involvement, and more time depending on welfare, leading to higher stress and depression. The children of teenage parents are at risk because of such factors as poor prenatal care, nonstimulating environment, lack of preventive health care, poor nutrition, possible low social support, and inadequate supervision (Schor, 1995).

Despite these difficulties, adolescent parents can become independent, successful, productive members of society. Their strengths include physical health as well as energy to care for an active child, optimism and idealism to look into the future, strong support groups made up of peers and extended family, and the developmental readiness for change and advancement (Kohlenberg, 1995). Although teenage parents tend to be more impatient with their children and have low levels of verbal interaction, they demonstrate considerable warmth and love toward their children (Schor, 1995). Nurses need to build on the strengths of these adolescents to increase their chances for success while assisting them in overcoming some of the difficulties. In terms of health outcomes, children of adolescent parents are at high risk for delays in cognitive development, poor academic achievement, and behavioral problems (Schor, 1995). Support from their families of origin and health care professionals can help these adolescent families achieve success.

When most teens are struggling to gain independence from their families of origin, the teenage mother is often forced to rely on her family even more for social and economic support. Many of these mothers choose to stay at home in order to finish high school. If that is the case, communication between the grandparents (especially the grandmother) and the teenage mother regarding the parenting responsibilities for the new infant is essential (Roye & Balk, 1997). Grandparents need to provide support for the adolescent without taking over the teenager's parenting role. If the grandparents become the primary care providers for the new infant, the adolescent fails to develop her own parenting skills (Black & Bentley, 1995). From the infant's perspective, consistent parenting and discipline practices are important in fostering the development of the young child. Toddlerhood can be a challenging time for both the mother and the toddler. Most adolescent parents have high developmental expectations of their toddler. One study found that African American mothers expected their children to achieve developmental milestones such as walking, obedience, and toilet training 3 to 6 months earlier than the norm (Field, Widmayer, Adler, & De Cubas, 1990). Too high expectations, especially for obedience, can lead to the mother's frustration and put the toddler at high risk for abuse. This has profound implications for pediatric nurses. Education on the normal occurrence of developmental milestones as well as appropriate disciplinary techniques is essential for adolescent mothers (Fig. 3–15).

Child rearing practices of adolescent mothers have been found to be quite different from those of older mothers. In a study by Porter (1990), five child rearing characteristics of adolescent mothers were identified. Adolescent mothers tend to discipline their children with physical punishment. Adolescent mothers are unable to read their infant's cues and have a general lack of knowledge regarding the development of their children. The physical environment in teenage homes is not an adequate learning environment for the infant, and the interaction between the adolescent and the infant consists more of nonverbal communication. These findings are consistent with those of Osofsky and Eberhart-Wright (1988), who found that adolescents spend less time holding and talking to their children than older parents. These findings suggest that adolescents can benefit from parenting classes offered by pediatric nurses that discuss discipline, growth and development, infant behavior and cues, and stimulation activities.

Figure 3–15
The adolescent parent faces many challenges as they balance child rearing activities with their own personal and social needs.

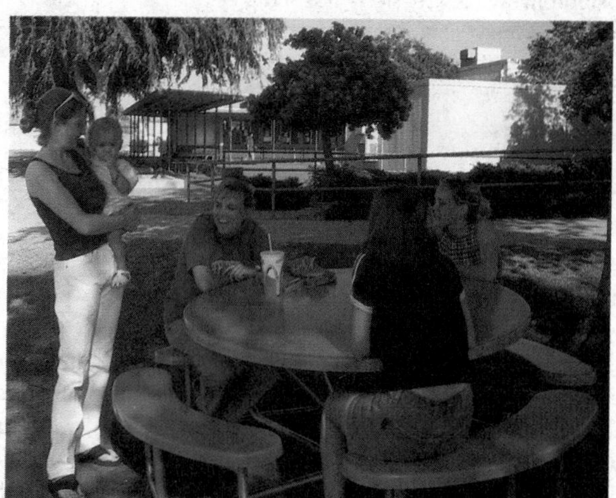

Homeless Families

The estimated homeless population in the United States ranges from as few as 250,000 to nearly 3 million with a projected annual growth rate of 24% (Lissner, 1995). Families with children are the fastest growing homeless population (U.S. Conference of Mayors, 1993). Homeless families that have both a mother and a father usually find themselves homeless because of job loss, insufficient income, or eviction. However, the majority of homeless families are headed by a single female parent. The single mother usually has a limited education and inadequate economic and social supports (Fox, Barrnett, Davis, & Bird, 1990; Wood, Valdez, Hayashi, & Shen, 1990). Many of these women become homeless in attempt to escape a physically abusive relationship with a male. Other women have found themselves in a homeless situation as a result of a family crisis such as parental physical abuse, drug abuse, or mental illness. One fourth of this population has been found to turn to substance abuse as a way of dealing with the stresses of life and homelessness (Axelson & Dail, 1988). The lack of social and emotional support available for these women has been found to increase their likelihood of becoming homeless (Chart 3–14).

Homelessness has an impact on the health and welfare of children and their families. The pediatric nurse needs to be aware of the special health needs of children in homeless families. Children younger than 5 years make up half of the homeless children, and 13% of these children are infants. These infants are at higher risk for low birth weight and prenatal drug exposure, whereas the children are at higher risk for malnutrition and physical delay leading to developmental and behavioral problems such as aggression, dependency, sleep disorders, and speech difficulties (Axelson & Dail, 1988). Many of these children receive inadequate or delayed health care, including immunizations and well-child or ill-child services. In addition, these children live in environments such as crowded shelters, where they are exposed to other children with contagious diseases. School-age children have been noted to show more psychiatric symptoms such as depression, suicidal tendencies, anxiety, and poor school performance (Axelson & Dail, 1988; Bassuk & Rosenburg, 1990; Reimer, Van Cleave, & Galbraith,

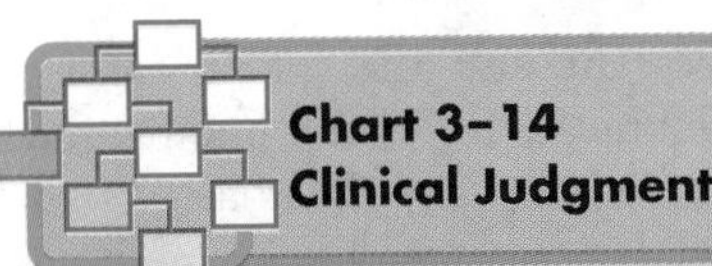

Chart 3–14
Clinical Judgment

The Homeless Family with a Hospitalized Child

Cassie is a 12-month-old white female. She was admitted to the hospital after being seen by a nurse practitioner at a nursing center on the grounds of a homeless shelter. The nurse practitioner had seen the patient on two prior occasions 1 month apart. Cassie has lost weight over the past 2 months despite the education about nutrition and feeding that was provided to the family. After the initial evaluation, Cassie was diagnosed with nonorganic failure to thrive.

Questions

1. What information and observations should be included in the nutritional assessment of the child?
2. Optimally, what members of the health care team should participate in the interdisciplinary care of the child with nonorganic failure to thrive?
3. What are the essential components of the discharge plan for Cassie and her family?
4. When a meal tray is brought for Cassie, you note that she gets little of the food. Instead, the mother tells you Cassie would not eat so she finished up her meal. What interventions should you take with Cassie and her mother?
5. What criteria should be met by Cassie and her family before discharge?

Answers

1. Growth parameters (length, weight, head circumference), child's general appearance, feeding schedule, description of daily nutritional intake, interactions between child and parent during feeding, availability of food and/or competition for limited food among family members, current community services family is using to obtain food (e.g., Special Supplemental Food Program for Women, Infants and Children [WIC], food stamps), interaction, the feeding relationship.
2. Physician—medical evaluation.
   Nurse—assess child–parent interactions during feeding times, coordinate care of interdisciplinary team, discharge planning.
   Dietician—assess nutritional intake and develop meal plan to include required nutritional intake.
   Occupational therapy—conduct developmental assessment including oral-motor feeding skills.
   Social worker or psychologist—assess the family resources and support systems and assist with obtaining necessary resources.
3. Develop feeding strategy with family input and concerns.
   Consult services that would enable the family to met the nutritional, emotional, and developmental needs of Cassie. These services may include WIC, food stamps, local food bank, long-term housing assistance, a parenting program with a nutritional component, possibly supervision by a representative from the Department of Children Services/ Child Protective Services.
4. Remain present when Cassie is to be fed. Determine whether Cassie is truly not eating, and assess the need to change the type of food offered to her. Review with the mother the importance of Cassie's obtaining nutritious food. Discuss with social worker obtaining free meal trays for parents while Cassie is hospitalized.
5. Cassie has demonstrated a weight gain and interest in eating. The family demonstrates understanding of the feeding plan and strategies to enhance their daughter's nutritional intake. Services that will enable the family to have access to food and shelter have been arranged.

1995; Zima, Wells, & Freeman, 1994). These findings demonstrate the need for programs to meet the physical, medical, and educational needs of these at-risk families to prevent negative outcomes for child development and socialization.

Pediatric nurses in multiple settings such as schools, communities, and clinics should be able to identify the children and families at risk and begin to act as an advocate for the family. The nurse should be aware of community resources available for the family, such as public health and education programs, mental health services, free clinics, and shelters. Chapter 7 provides a thorough description of many of these programs that can benefit the homeless family. In addition, the nurse should be aware of the perceived barriers to obtaining well-child care for these families. These barriers include unfamiliarity with health care providers, waiting for appointments and waiting during appointments, and the cost of transportation and/or parking (Reimer et al., 1995).

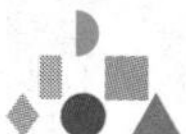

Cultural and Religious Influences on the Family

The cultural composition of North America is changing, with a rise in the numbers of and diversity of minority groups. In the United States from 1980 to 1990, the Asian Pacific, Hispanic, and black populations grew 107%, 53%, and 13%, respectively, whereas the white population increased 6% (Friedman, 1992). By the year 2000, it is projected that one in every three Americans will be a member of an ethnic minority group (Farrell, 1988). This change has required health care professionals to adopt a transcultural and pluralistic perspective in order to work with families with diverse ethnic, religious, and cultural beliefs (Ahmann, 1994; Friedman, 1990).

Cultural and Religious Concepts

Leininger (1991, p. 47) defined culture as "learned, shared, and transmitted values, beliefs, norms and life ways of a particular group that guide their thinking, decisions and actions in patterned ways." Cultural groups can be distinguished by such characteristics as mode of dress, food preferences, values, politics, language, and health care practices (Germain, 1992). **Ethnicity** refers to a common social and cultural heritage of a group that is passed on from one generation to the next. A shared ethnicity is thought to create a sense of identity for a group (Giger and Davidhizar, 1995). **Race** refers to the biophysiologic characteristics of a population group that make it different from others. Not every person in the population group has all of the characteristics, but in general the population group as a whole can be distinguished by these characteristics. **Biculturality** occurs when a person crosses two cultures, lifestyles, and sets of beliefs. For instance, this might occur when an African American child is adopted by a white North American couple. During childhood, the cultural values and beliefs of the couple are transmitted to the child. Yet as the child matures the parents also encourage the child to learn more about and relate to the cultural beliefs of the family of origin. The adolescent grows to understand that she or he is a product of the unique blend of two cultures. **Acculturation** is the process in which a cultural group adapts to or learns how to take on the behaviors of another cultural group. Complete acculturation usually never occurs and is not even necessarily desirable. **Multiculturality** is the concept that although cultural differences exist, there are also many similarities and areas of common ground between cultural groups that have immigrated to America and now claim it as home.

In addition to the cultural similarities and variances among families, it is important to consider the spiritual or religious factors that motivate individual and family beliefs and actions. Spiritual and religious beliefs can directly or indirectly influence the health of children and families (Miller, 1995). **Religion** can be defined as an organized system of commonly held beliefs, rituals, and observances in the worship of God or gods. **Spirituality** is often defined as the basic quality in all humans that involves a belief in something greater than the self and a faith that positively affirms life (Cervantes & Ramirez, 1992). In essence, one can be spiritual without belonging to an organized religion (Miller, 1995).

Values and Beliefs of Health Care Professionals

During the socialization process that occurs as a person enters the health care field, the individual is expected to shed many old thoughts and values and embrace new scientific concepts, ideas, and attitudes. The health care professional comes to accept "modern" medicine as taught and practiced in Western civilization as the answer to meeting the health care needs of families (Boyle & Andrews, 1989). In addition, the health care professional has an array of other values and beliefs about the family, child care practices, and social issues that influence the professional's personal actions and encounters with others. Therefore, when the nurse, enculturated with a certain set of beliefs about health care, encounters a family enculturated with other health care beliefs, the stage is set for a cultural encounter. In most cases, the health care provider and the family share enough common cultural ground to establish a relationship and provide the opportunity for care that respects and appreciates the commonalities and differences in values and beliefs. In some instances, individuals may restrict their view of other worlds and be unable to accept the beliefs and behaviors of other cultural groups. Thus, cultural conflict may occur. It is important for health care professionals to be aware of their own cultural beliefs that affect the health care they provide to others. In addition, professionals should become knowledgeable about the cultural groups represented in their client populations. To provide culturally competent care, nurses must have an understanding of, and respect for, the beliefs and priorities of the families they are serving (Yoos, Kitzman, Olds, & Overacker, 1995). Cultural competence begins when the nurse develops a knowledge base about other cultures and develops strategies to communicate and intervene in ways that support the cultural beliefs and values of others.

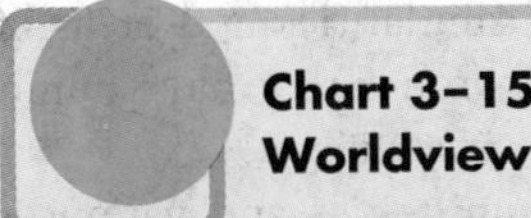

Chart 3–15
Worldview

Home Remedies of Various Cultural Groups

Cultural Group	Malady	Home Remedy
Mexican American	Diarrhea that is green or yellow (cold illness)	Hot tea
	Diarrhea that is white (hot illness)	Cold tea
	Fever	Bundle in blankets
	Caida de la mollera (fallen fontanelle)	Pressing against the palate from inside the mouth or applying eggs to the fontanelle and holding the baby upside down
	Empacho (abdominal pain and cramping)	Massage of abdomen and ingestion of herbal tea
	Cough	Herbal teas
	Skin rash	Apply cornstarch
	Conjunctivitis	Chamomile or breast milk drops in the eyes
	Mal ojo	Limpias (supernatural cleansing or sweeping using herbs and eggs)
African American	Colic	Catnip tea
	Bloody nose	Place keys on a chain around neck to stop bleeding
	Sore throat	Suck yolk out of egg shell, honey and lemon, salt water to gargle, onions around the neck
	Fever	Raw onions placed on the feet and wrapping in warm blankets
	Contraceptive	Nine drops of turpentine 9 days after intercourse
	Cuts and wounds	Salt and pork placed on rag and applied to skin
Asian American	Excess of yang	Acupuncture (puncturing the body with needles at certain points called meridians)
	Excess of yin	Moxibustion (heating pulverized wormwood and applying this to the skin over certain meridians)
	Most common ailments (colic, indigestion, impotence, rheumatism)	Ginseng
	Wounds	Urea
	Excessive mucus	Lime calcium
	Pus boils	Rhinoceros horns
White Protestant American	Common cold	Vaporizer, chicken soup, decongestants, aspirin, rest
	Stomach aches	Eat light and bland foods, Alka Seltzer
	Sore throat	Gargle with salt water, drink tea with lemon and honey
	Insomnia	Glass of wine or warm milk

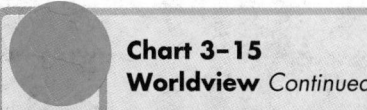

Chart 3–15
Worldview *Continued*

Home Remedies of Various Cultural Groups

Cultural Group	Malady	Home Remedy
Irish American	Prevent flu	Tying bag of camphor around the neck, cleaning out bowels every 8 days with senna
	Earache	Placing heated salt in a sock behind the ear
	Fever	Cool baths and alcohol rubdowns
	Common cold	Tea with toast, a vaporizer, and hot lemonade with a teaspoon of whiskey, hot milk with butter
	Menstrual cramps	Hot milk sprinkled with ginger, hot water bottle on stomach, glass of wine
	Boils	Oatmeal poultice
	Cuts	Boric acid
	Sties	Hot tea bag to area
	Sunburn	Apply vinegar
Italian American	Sore throats	Herb tea, honey, Vicks applied to throat
	Every common ailment	Chicken soup
	Fever	Covering with blankets to sweat
	Boils	Cooked oatmeal wrapped in a cloth (steaming hot) applied to drain pus
	Acne	Apply baby's urine; to draw out pimples, apply hot flaxseed
	Poison ivy	Yellow soap suds
	Toothache	Whiskey applied topically
	Colic	Warm oil on stomach
Native American	Most common disorders	Herbal treatment
	Colic	Mint tea
	Sore throat	Suck yolk out of egg, baking soda, salt water to gargle
	Cuts and wounds	Globe mallow
	Boils	Sand sagebrush
	Snake bites	Bladder pod
	Spider bites	Bath in water soaked with sunflowers
	Digestive disorders	Drink made from boiled water and blue gillia

Health Beliefs and Practices of Culturally Diverse Families

When examining the health and illness beliefs and practices of a different ethnic group, it is important to remember that this information is general and not universal (Spector, 1991). It cannot be applied to every individual in that cultural group. The traditional belief systems of a group are adapted and modified through interactions with other cultures and through the socialization that has taken place within the context of the family (acculturation). Differences within a cultural or ethnic group are related to the social context of the family, the economic class, kinship ties, and geographic location of the family (Kune-Karrer & Taylor, 1995). The goal of the health care provider is to acknowledge cultural differences while underscoring similarities and belonging. A knowledge of traditional beliefs provides a *framework* for the health care professional to begin to assess and intervene in a manner that is safe and effective. As the nurse collects data about the specific cultural and religious practices of a child and its family, care can be further modified to ensure optimum outcomes.

Charts 3–15, 3–16, and 3–17 provide overviews of

Text continued on page 155

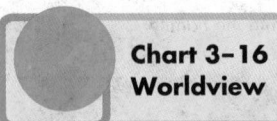

Chart 3–16
Worldview

Cultural Influences on the Family

Cultural Group	Family and Kinship Structure	Communication	Health Beliefs and Practices	Family and Child Care Practices
Hispanics Mexican American	Family is an extensive network composed of nuclear and extended family members. Father is provider and decision maker; mother is family caretaker. Decisions made by father after discussion with older or extended family members. Divorce is uncommon. Out-of-wedlock relationships are common. Children are center of family life.	Eye contact may be considered rude. Looking at or admiring a baby without touching the child can bring about mal ojo (evil eye).	Health represents an equilibrium between hot and cold, wet and dry. An imbalance in these forces causes disease. Cold remedies used to treat hot diseases, and hot remedies used to treat cold diseases. Balance and harmony are accomplished through avoiding some foods and consuming others. Seek curandero, a folk healer, for treatment remedies and spiritual healing ceremonies. May combine advice from curandero with the antibiotics or other therapies from a physician. Resort to prayer or home remedies (remedias caseras) before seeking help from folk practitioner or physician. Often delay seeking medical attention and obtaining screening examinations and immunizations. Tend to have jobs with no health insurance. Mother unlikely to sign consent for child's health care without discussion with the father.	Delay breast-feeding until milk comes in. Feel stress and anger make milk bad and infant can become ill. Neutralize infant bowel when weaning from breast to bottle by feeding only anise tea for 24 hours. More likely to have children without prenatal or postnatal care. Mal ojo or evil eye is an illness that affects children and occurs when someone with special powers looks at or admires a child but does not touch or hold the child. A curandero can treat the child through massage and prayer. Wearing special amulets or charms can protect child from the evil eye. Practice of binding the umbilicus of the newborn is done to prevent bad air from entering the baby. Parent-child relationship is warm and nurturing. Parents are often quite permissive in respect to their childs' behavior.
Puerto Rican	Extended and patriarchial family.	Bilingual—Spanish and English.	Avoid iron supplements because they are considered "hot" medication. Classify foods and medication as hot, cold, and cool. Classify foods as hot and cold.	Children viewed as gift from God. Children taught to obey and respect parents.
Cuban	Strong family ties, which continue as children grow into adulthood.	Bilingual—Spanish and English.	Health promotion important. Belief in biomedical model, although supernatural forces (evil eye) are thought to cause some illnesses that can be cured by ethnic treatments or magic spells. Amulets on a bracelet or necklace may be worn to ward off evil eye. Diet is high in fat, cholesterol, sugar, and fried foods.	Mother primary child caretaker. Plump babies and young children are idealized. School system assumes much of child rearing responsibilities.

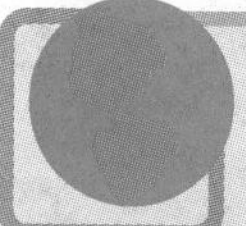

Chart 3–16
Worldview *Continued*

Cultural Influences on the Family

Cultural Group	Family and Kinship Structure	Communication	Health Beliefs and Practices	Family and Child Care Practices
Haitian	Extended family is important as support system. Males are the decision makers and direct caregivers.	Rely on native language.	Believe that God's will must prevail. Rely on folk foods and treatments for illness management. Believe in hot-cold theory. Avoid eggplant, okra, tomatoes, black pepper, cold drinks, milk, rice, bananas, and fish during pregnancy. White foods believed to cause increased vaginal discharge in pregnancy.	Usually breast-feed and believe strong emotions affect quality of milk.
African American	Family of great importance. Many headed by mother in absence of father. In two-parent families egalitarian structure is most prominent. Not uncommon to have extended family living together and older members assisting with child care.		Wife or mother source of advice on medical ailments and when to seek medical treatment. Many believe illness comes from germs. Others believe illness can be due to natural causes (e.g., exposure to wind, rain) or unnatural causes (witchcraft, voodoo, punishment for sin). Poverty and lack of health insurance lead to inadequate health care. Many rely on folk remedies passed on from one generation to next before seeking care from physician. "Granny" or "old lady" is woman in community with knowledge of herbs to treat common illnesses. Spiritualist is someone with special gift from God to heal certain diseases. Prayer is commonly used in response to illness. A diet high in fat and sodium is considered an indication of well-being. Many individuals have lactose intolerance; therefore milk may be inadequate from diets of pregnant women and children.	Begin cereal consumption in infancy at early age. Culture least likely to breast-feed. Strong religious orientation (Baptist predominant). Use belly band or binder to protect newborn's umbilicus from dirt, injury, or hernias. Strict parenting practices are encouraged and meant to develop effective coping abilities in children to prepare them for the presence of racial discrimination they are likely to encounter in society. High respect for authority figures, strong work ethic, and emphasis on achievement. Expression of emotions by males and females is encouraged. Children are expected to use their time wisely, assume responsibilities at an early age, and participate in decision making. Physical forms of discipline often used.

Chart continued on following page

Chart 3–16
Worldview *Continued*

Cultural Influences on the Family

Cultural Group	Family and Kinship Structure	Communication	Health Beliefs and Practices	Family and Child Care Practices
Asian Vietnamese	Patriarchal in structure. Extended families predominant. Primogeniture (first son inherits family's worth).	Avoid confrontations with health care professionals, perhaps answering questions with what they believe the other person wants to hear. May consider health practitioners to be loud and boisterous. Do not touch children on the head. The head is considered sacred because it is where one's consciousness lies. Eye contact may be considered rude. Beckoning with one's hand or finger is the gesture used to beckon dogs and is considered insulting when used with people.	Forces of yang (light, heat, or dryness) and yin (darkness, cold, and wetness) influence the balance and harmony of person's state of health. Seek shaman, a physician-priest, for treatment remedies and spiritual healing ceremonies. Evil spirits enter the body through open orifices such as ears, nose, and mouth, causing infection. If the opening is covered, the bad spirits cannot enter and the illness is cured. Health represents an equilibrium between hot and cold, wet and dry. An imbalance in these forces causes disease.	May delay breast-feeding for 3 days because colostrum is considered "dirty." Breast-feeding low among immigrant Southeast Asians. Breast-feed boys longer than girls. Delay introduction of solid foods up to 18 months. Diet may consist of breast milk and rice water; diet is low in calcium and iron. Excessive consumption of cow's milk (up to eight bottles a day) in the second year of life is common, as is the continual use of the bottle instead of the cup into the third year of life. Avoid praising an infant for fear that a spirit may overhear the praise and be tempted to steal the baby. Parents have an approach to child rearing that is more controlling, achievement oriented, and more encouraging of independence than that of white parents. Balance and harmony are accomplished.
Chinese	Needs of the family come before the needs of the individual. Children repay their parents' love and care by providing for them in their old age. Extended family important, with elderly respected and cared for in the homes of the adult children. Frown upon interracial marriages.	Silence does not necessarily indicate the end of a conversation; it may mean the speaker wishes the listener to consider the content before the speaker continues.	Forces of yang (light, heat, or dryness) and yin (darkness, cold, and wetness) influence the balance and harmony of person's state of health. Health is a state of physical and spiritual harmony with nature. Prevention is key to healthy living. Traditional Chinese medicine is sought first before Western medical services. Use acupuncture, herbal medicines, massage, cupping, skin scraping, and moxibustion as therapies to restore yin and yang. Avoid eating soy sauce during pregnancy because believed to darken baby's skin, shellfish believed to cause allergies in baby, and iron supplements believed to harden bones and lead to difficult delivery.	Primary responsibility for child care belongs to mother. Grandparents may be asked to assist in child care. Cultural healing practices can cause visible bruising or injury to child's skin. Important for children to exhibit self-control. Children socialized not to challenge authority. Pregnancy means woman has "happiness in her body." Many breast-feed until child is 4 to 5 years old. Jade is often worn in form of a charm to keep the child safe.

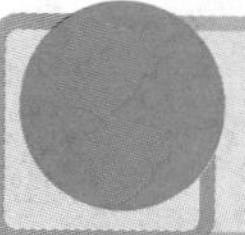

Chart 3–16
Worldview *Continued*

Cultural Influences on the Family

Cultural Group	Family and Kinship Structure	Communication	Health Beliefs and Practices	Family and Child Care Practices
Japanese	Value social group harmony over individual needs and autonomy. Extended and patriarchal family structure. Women traditionally passive.	Silence does not necessarily indicate the end of a conversation; it may mean the speaker wishes the listener to consider the content before the speaker continues. Handshakes are acceptable; pat on the back is not acceptable. Direct eye contact considered a lack of respect.	When in pain, patients stoically withstand discomfort. Women labor in silence. After delivery long periods of rest and recuperation are encouraged. Use natural herbs–Kampō medicine. Use both Western and traditional Oriental healing methods.	Mother has primary responsibility for child rearing and assuring their success in school. Mother may sleep with her child. Colostrum not fed to babies. Only half of all breast-fed babies continue after 1 month of age.
Hmong	Extended family structure.	Do not touch children on the head. The head is considered sacred because it is where one's consciousness lies.	Seek shaman, a physician-priest, for treatment remedies and spiritual healing ceremonies.	Avoid praising an infant for fear that a spirit may overhear the praise and be tempted to steal the baby. Babies may wear colorful hats so that they are disguised as "flowers" and the spirits will not notice them.
European American White Protestant	Nuclear family highly valued. Divorce and remarriage common practice. Goal of individual often seen as more important than goal of the family. Success is measured in terms of financial wealth and status in society.	Pat children on head to show affection or approval. Uncomfortable with periods of silence. Expect people to look you in the eye when they are speaking to you. Avoiding eye contact can be considered an indication that a person is lying.	Rely on modern medicine and health care professionals to treat illness.	Authoritative style of parenting. Children encouraged to value individual differences, the future rather than the present, material well-being, and competition and to consider many options when making decisions. Adults readily praise infant's and child's behavior and appearance Self-reliance is highly valued.
Irish American	Strong family bonds. Emphasis placed on well-being of family, not individual member.	May communicate wing flowery and sometimes exaggerated words. May be overly verbose in descriptions of their condition.	Health comes when person is goal oriented and nurtures a strong religious faith. Health is maintained with a great deal of sleep combined with fresh air, exercise, and balanced diet. Home remedies or treatments are first resort to treat illness. Medical assistance should be sought only in cases of emergency.	Strict followers of the church, typically Protestant or Catholic.

Chart continued on following page

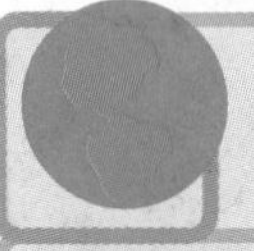

Chart 3–16
Worldview *Continued*

Cultural Influences on the Family

Cultural Group	Family and Kinship Structure	Communication	Health Beliefs and Practices	Family and Child Care Practices
Italian American	Traditional family roles. Father is head of household, and mother is heart of the household, although mother has powerful sway over internal family matters. Children are valued members and are showered with love and affection. Family a source of comfort and pride for individual members. Members maintain close contact or close proximity with nuclear and extended family. Divorce is uncommon in traditional families. Large family size is attributed to adherence to Catholic beliefs and traditions.	Complaining loudly and making demands are often rewarded with attention.	Health is maintained by strong religious influence (Catholic primarily). Faith in God and saints will see them through illness. Beliefs about the cause of illness have been found to include winds and currents that bear diseases, contagion or contamination, heredity, supernatural or human causes, and psychosomatic explanations.	Important to keep child warm in cold weather, stay out of drafts, and not go outside with wet hair. Maintain health with a nutritious diet of fruit, vegetables, pasta, hard cheese, and wine. Children introduced to water-wine mixture at young age.
Native American	Grandparents retain important role in parenting their grandchildren. Extended family network valued. Many Native Americans have married into other tribes and other ethnic groups.	Silence is critical during interactions. Strong need to sit quietly and think before responding to questions. Eye contact may be considered rude. May consider health practitioners to be loud and boisterous.	Wellness exists when there is harmony in body, mind, and spirit. Seek shaman, a physician-priest, for treatment remedies and spiritual healing ceremonies. High incidence of lactose intolerance. Eat nonperishable food items because of lack of refrigeration. Beans main source of protein. Frequent problems with obesity and alcoholism. Often feel that Western medicine places too much emphasis on medications. A holistic approach to healing is valued. Alcoholism is major problem for many families.	High rate of breast-feeding. Mothers retain primary responsibility for child rearing and discipline.

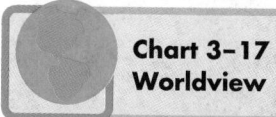

Chart 3–17
Worldview

Examples of Religious Influences on Health Care Beliefs and Practices

Religious Group	Health Care Beliefs and Practices
Catholic	Anoint the sick (called extreme unction or last rites). Do not approve of abortions or contraceptives.
Presbyterian	Blood transfusion acceptable. Believe medical science can be used to cure and prevent suffering. Pastor notified when member ill or hospitalized and prayers given to support ill person.
Jehovah's Witness	Opposed to blood transfusions but may be persuaded in emergency situations. When parents refuse consent to treat a child, a court order may be necessary to obtain necessary care.
Christian Scientist	Diseases of children principally related to the parents' errors of belief impressing themselves upon their offspring.
Jewish	Good health is highly prized. Prayer is an important component of maintaining spiritual and physical well-being. Meat salted to help drain all blood—raw meat needs to be soaked in water before cooking. Milk and meat products must not be mixed (eaten at same time, prepared in same pot, or placed on same plate). In non-kosher kitchens all food should be served on paper plates. Usually breast-feed. Circumcision practiced on eighth day of life by a trained mohel, by child's father, or by physician. Visiting the sick is a religious obligation. Important to observe Jewish holy days.
Muslim	Human body belongs to God, thus organ donations or transplants forbidden. Muslim physician may recommend a blood transfusion to save a life. Autopsy is uncommon because deceased must be buried intact. Cremation is not permitted. Pork, carrion, and blood are forbidden food products.
Buddhists	Preference is for quality rather than quantity of life. Reluctant to have surgery or treatments on holy days. Discourage use of drugs and alcohol.
Hindu	Many dietary restrictions. Illness and injury seen as a result of sins committed in previous life. Will cooperate and accept Western medical practices.

the beliefs and practices of several cultural groups. These groups are defined primarily by race, economic factors, or religious practices. The charts do not represent a comprehensive summary of the practices of all cultural groups. Further discussions of cultural beliefs regarding grief and loss are presented in Chapter 12 and regarding response to pain are presented in Chapter 13 of this text. For a more in-depth discussion of cultural groups the reader should refer to one or more of the textbooks available on transcultural issues.

Cultural and Spiritual Assessment

Health and illness are perceived differently from culture to culture, and these perceptions affect the way a person responds to the health care environment and treatment modalities (Diaz-Gilbert, 1993). Obtaining a person's view of health and illness is an integral component of the health assessment process (Chart 3–18). Understanding cultural perspectives can help the nurse anticipate and understand why families make certain health decisions (Groce & Zola, 1993). Knowledge of a cultural group's characteristics serves as a indicator of the family's background, but it is the nurse's responsibility to clarify what characteristics the family or individuals have chosen to identify and integrate into their lifestyle. Stewart and Bennett (1991) suggested approaching every cross-cultural situation like an experiment. The nurse should have some generalizations about the specific culture to which the family belongs, and by assessing and communicating

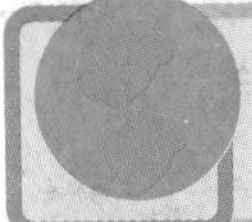

Chart 3–18
Worldview

Components of a Cultural Assessment

Assessment Criteria	Questions
Ethnic or racial identity	Does the family identify itself as belonging to a certain ethnic or racial group? Are the parents both from the same cultural background?
Place of birth	Where were the parents and children born? If born in the United States, where were the parents' parents born? If born out of the United States, how many years have parents lived in the United States?
Geographic mobility	Where have the parents lived? When did they move to their present residence?
Languages spoken	What language(s) is (are) spoken in the home and by whom? What language is preferred when speaking with outsiders?
Family's religion	What is the family's religion? Are both parents from the same religious background? How actively involved is the family in religion-based activities and practices?
Ethnic group affiliation	What are the characteristics of the family's social network? Are friends and associations all from the family's ethnic group? Are recreational, educational, and other social activities within the ethnic reference group or the wider community? To what extent does the family use services and shop within the family's neighborhood or within the wider community?
Neighborhood affiliation	What are the characteristics of the family's neighborhood? Is it ethnically heterogeneous or homogeneous?
Dietary habits and dress	What are the family's dietary habits and dress? Are the family's home decorations, art, and religious objects from the family's ethnic background?
Use of folk systems	To what extent does the family use folk healing practices or practitioners?
Acceptance by community	To what extent is the family affected by discrimination?

From Friedman, M. (1990). Transcultural family nursing. Application to Latino and black families. *Journal of Pediatric Nursing, 5,* 214–222. Reprinted with permission.

with the family, the nurse should be able to clarify what applies and does not apply to the family. This interaction enables the nurse to learn about the family's values, beliefs, and attitudes toward health that influence behavior (Adams-McDarty, 1996). A continuous assessment of the family's perceptions of health care should be incorporated into the ongoing care of the family. These data can provide useful information that can help the nurse modify the plan of care and illuminate areas of patient teaching (Chart 3–19).

Just as it is important for the nurse not to make care decisions solely on the basis of a family's ethnic heritage, it is equally important for the nurse not to make assumptions on the basis of the family's religious affiliation. Individuals and families may have a certain religious affiliation without adhering to all the religion's "official" beliefs and practices (Andrews, 1989). Health care providers tend to ignore the spiritual needs of the child and family because they feel they do not know enough about the particular religion to be of any assistance. The nurse should assess the role of religion and spirituality in the family (Chart 3–20). The role of the nurse is not to offer knowledge but to show the family and the child a willingness to listen and care for them spiritually and to intervene in a manner that supports the family's spiritual needs (Andrews, 1989). When nurses do not know the practices of a particular religion, every attempt should be made to discuss with the family their spiritual needs and develop a plan of care to meet those needs (Chart 3–21).

Health Care Implications

Cultural and religious beliefs and practices of the family can be expected to affect the management of the ill child. The nurse needs to determine whether these practices and beliefs are beneficial for the child. When possible, these beliefs need to be incorporated into the nursing care plan. When these beliefs and practices are detrimental to the health and welfare of the child, compromises need to be made in order to respect the family's beliefs and still maintain the health of the child (Andrews, 1989). When a compromise is not possible, a legal

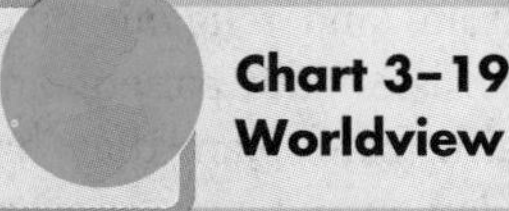

Chart 3–19
Worldview

Questions for Assessing Culture-Related Health Care Perceptions

- Are there times, when someone is ill, that you and your family do not go to the doctor?
- Does the medical staff listen and understand your views and concerns?
- How is our medical practice different from what you or your family have traditionally used?
- Are we doing anything that makes you or anyone in your family uncomfortable?
- How are health and illness talked about, defined, or understood in your culture, community, or family?
- In order to provide better medical care, what do we need to know about your culture or family traditions?
- Who takes care of your child when he or she is ill?
- Do you try to prevent illness by giving your child special foods, herbs, spices, special diets, or food supplements such as vitamins?
- Are any home treatments such as special teas, herbs, honeys, steam, heat, or ice used when the child is ill?
- Do you have any trouble having prescriptions filled? Clarify the reason (e.g., lack of money, do not know location of pharmacy, no transportation).
- Do you have any concerns about reading or understanding the instructions that come on the medicine container? (Use when English is a second language or the parent has stated concerns about comprehending medical terms.)
- Do you or your family ever seek medical help from religious or community leaders or any person other than a medical doctor?

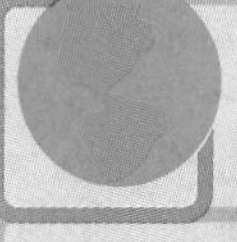

Chart 3–20
Worldview

Questions for Spiritual Assessment

What is your religious preference?
To what extent do you participate in worship and related activities?
Do you have a way of describing God or a deity that is meaningful to you?
Do you have hope?
How do you explain how or why bad things happen to you?
Is there a clergy member or religious leader that you find especially helpful to you?
Do other family members share your spiritual beliefs and practices?
Do you have religious beliefs that relate to your dietary practices?
Do you have religious beliefs that relate to your daily habits and activities?
What events in your life have affected your spiritual beliefs?
What are your spiritual beliefs about God, birth, death, health, and illness?
What are the religious practices that your child ascribes to?

intervention may be necessary in order to ensure that care is provided that is in the best interest of the child's health.

Worldview: *When working with families, the nurse needs to encourage the use of benign or neutral folk practices while discouraging practices or remedies that have a detrimental effect on the child. It is important to share with the family the ill effects some healing practices can have on the child.*

Some religious institutions offer rituals or beliefs that might help an individual prevent illness or offer support should an illness occur. Many religions offer direction on social, moral, and dietary requirements in order to prevent illness. For example, the Mormon religion, as part of its belief system, discourages smoking, excessive alcohol use, and illicit drug use (Miller, 1995). Many people believe that illness is a punishment for breaking a religious code (Spector, 1991, 1995). Many religious institutions have rituals related to having and raising children. Childbearing is an example of an event that is affected by many religious and cultural beliefs and practices. Orthodox Jewish women feel that producing children fulfills the measure of their creation and shows obedience to the ancient rabbinical law to multiply and replenish the earth (Callister, 1995). Male circumcision is another practice with which religious rituals are

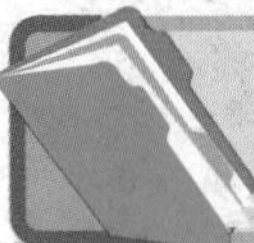

Chart 3–21
Nursing Interventions Classification (NIC)

Spiritual Support

Definition

Assisting the patient to feel balance and connection with a greater power

Activities

Be open to patient's expressions of loneliness and powerlessness.
Encourage chapel service attendance, if desired.
Encourage the use of spiritual resources, if desired.
Provide desired spiritual articles, according to patient preferences.
Refer to spiritual advisor of patient's choice.
Use values clarification techniques to help patient clarify beliefs and values, as appropriate.
Be available to listen to patient's feelings.
Express empathy with patient's feelings.
Facilitate patient's use of meditation, prayer, and other religious traditions and rituals.
Listen carefully to patient's communication, and develop a sense of timing for prayer or spiritual rituals.
Assure patient that nurse will be available to support patient in times of suffering.
Be open to patient's feelings about illness and death.
Assist patient to properly express and relieve anger in appropriate ways.

From McCloskey, J., & Bulechek, G. (1996). *Nursing interventions classification (NIC)* (2nd ed.). St. Louis: Mosby–Year Book. Reprinted with permission.

associated. The ritual of circumcision is practiced on the eighth day of life by a trained mohel, by the child's father, or by a pediatrician (Boyle & Andrews, 1989). These are just a few examples of child rearing practices that are influenced by religious beliefs that should be considered and incorporated into family-centered care practices.

Beliefs about health and illness affect a family's ability to comply with Western medicine and nursing care (Rodriguez-Wargo, 1993). In the health care setting, providers can promote culturally competent care through interventions that bridge or link the health care system with the child and family who are responding from a different cultural context (Chart 3–22). The nurse must use knowledge of traditional cultural and religious practices as a framework in which to assess the patient and build a plan of care. The health care plan that has the most success is the one that demonstrates an appreciation for the cultural variations and similarities of each family.

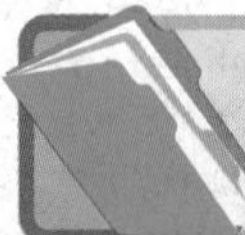

Chart 3–22
Nursing Interventions Classification (NIC)

Culture Brokerage

Definition

Bridging, negotiating, or linking the orthodox health care system with a patient and family of a different culture

Activities

Determine the nature of the conceptual differences that the patient and nurse have of the illness.
Discuss discrepancies openly and clarify conflicts.
Negotiate, when conflicts cannot be resolved, an acceptable compromise of treatment based on biomedical knowledge, knowledge of the patient's point of view, and ethical standards.
Allow the patient more than the usual time to process the information and work through a decision.
Appear relaxed and unhurried in interactions with the patient.
Allow more time for translation, discussion, and explanation.
Use nontechnical language.
Determine the "belief variability ratio"—the degree of distance the patient sees between self and cultural group.
Use a language translator, if necessary (e.g., signing or Spanish).
Include the family, when appropriate, in the plan for adherence with the prescribed regimen.
Translate the patient's symptom terminology into health care language that other professionals can more easily understand.
Provide information to the patient about the orthodox health care system.
Provide information to the health care providers about the patient's culture.

From McCloskey, J., & Bulechek, G. (1996). *Nursing interventions classification (NIC)* (2nd ed.). St. Louis: Mosby–Year Book. Reprinted with permission.

Summary of Key Concepts

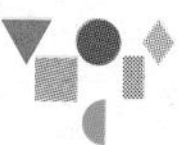

- The family systems approach views the family as an open system. Each family member influences and is influenced by every other family member, as well as by the family's environment. Relationships in the family are tied together; change by any one person invariably results in changes in all family members.
- A developmental approach to the family examines the changes in the family as it experiences certain expected maturational events such as the marriage, the birth of children, and the launching of children. Traditional developmental frameworks do not account for the changing family structure related to divorce, single parenting, and remarriage.
- Maturational and situational events can overwhelm the family's ability to cope and adapt. Stress and coping frameworks such as the double ABCX model can be utilized to assess and intervene for the family experiencing short-term or long-term crises that threaten its integrity.
- The structural-functional approach examines the family in terms of its basic functions. These include affective, reproductive, economic, and health care functions and socialization and social placement functions.
- The interactional approach is useful in determining the value and meanings the family placed on a stressful event. The approach does not evaluate the influence of the external social system on these family perceptions.
- The institutional approach evaluates how families change over time in different societies and in different settings.
- In the social exchange theory, all interactions between persons depend on an exchange of goods, commodities, or resources (both material and nonmaterial). Equilibrium is based on the premise of reciprocity.
- Conflict theory describes and explains the effects of change, conflict, and constraints on the family unit. Change and conflict in the family are inevitable and may have positive and unifying effects on the family.
- A variety of assessment tools have been developed to evaluate family structure, dynamics, and functioning. Some of the tools are clinically useful; most have been developed for research use.
- Although the traditional "nuclear family" was once the predominant type of family structure, many other family forms have developed. These include the extended family, the single-parent family, the binuclear family, the blended family, the gay and lesbian family, and the communal family. Not all of these family structures exist in all societies, nor are they all legally sanctioned.
- Family life is always challenging. Members must learn to change and adapt as they proceed through the stages of the family life cycle. Healthy families embrace the change that accompanies the maturing of the family unit.
- A variety of issues can further challenge the family unit. These issues include divorce, multiple births, adoption, foster care, grandparent families, adolescent families, and homeless families. Each of these cases requires special attention by the health care provider, as these issues cause deviations from the "normal" pattern of family life.
- The nurse must assess the cultural and spiritual framework which surrounds the family's values, beliefs, and actions. Health care interventions that incorporate the unique culture of the family are far more effective in meeting family needs.

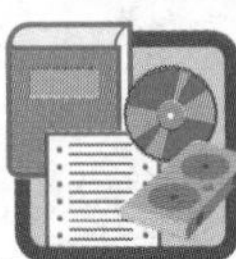

Resources

Organizations

Adoption Resource Exchange for Single Parents
Box 5782
Springfield, VA 22150
(703) 866-5577
Resource for those considering adoption of an older or special needs child

Adoptive Families
3333 Highway 100 N
Minneapolis, MN 55422
(800) 372-3300
Provides a newsletter for adoptive families

Child Welfare League of America
444 First Street, NW
Washington, DC 20001-2085
(202) 638-2952
For information on foster parenting

Children of Lesbians and Gays Everywhere (COLAGE)
2300 Market Street, #165
San Francisco, CA 94114
(415) 861-KIDS (in San Francisco)
(202) 583-8029 (in Washington, DC)
KidsOfGays@aol.com

Committee on Early Childhood, Adoption and Dependent Care
American Academy of Pediatrics
141 Northwest Point Boulevard
PO Box 927
Elk Grove Village, IL 60009-0927
(800) 433-9016

Families Adopting Children Everywhere Inc. (FACE)
P.O. Box 28058
Northwood Station
Baltimore, MD 21239
(410) 488-2656

Focus on the Family
P.O. Box 35500
Colorado Springs, CO 80935-3550
(719) 531-5181
Web: www.fotf.org

Gay and Lesbian Parents Coalition International
PO Box 50360
Washington, DC 20091
(202) 583-8029
GLPCIN@ix.netcom.com

Grandparent Information Center
American Association of Retired Persons (AARP)
601 E Street, NW
Washington, DC 20049
(202) 434-2296
FAX: (202) 434-6474

Grandparents as Parents (GAP)
P.O. Box 964
Lakewood, CA 90714
(310) 924-3996
FAX: (714) 828-1375

Grandparents Who Care
One Rhode Island Street
San Francisco, CA 94103
(415) 865-3000
FAX: (415) 865-3099

National Adoption Center
(800) TOADOPT

National Association of Hispanic Nurses (NAHN)
For information, call (202) 387-2477

National Black Nurses Association (NBNA)
For information, call (202) 393-6870

National Center for Fathering
10200 West 75th Street, Suite 267
Shawnee Mission, KS 66204-2223
(800) 593-DADS
http://www.fathers.com

National Center for Lesbian Rights
1663 Mission Street
San Francisco, CA 94103
(415) 621-0674
NCLRSF@aol.com

National Coalition of Grandparents
137 Larkin Street
Madison, WI 53705
(608) 238-8751
FAX: (608) 238-8751

National Fathers' Network
The Merrywood School
16120 Northeast 8th Street
Bellevue, WA 98008
(206) 747-4004

National Foster Care Resource Center
102 King Hall
Eastern Michigan University
Ypsilanti, MI 48197
(313) 487-0374

National Foster Parent Association
2606 Badger Lane
Madison, WI 53713-2115
(680) 274-9111

National Organization Mother of Twins Club
PO Box 23188
Albuquerque, NM 87192-1188
(505) 275-0955

National Transcultural Nursing Society
College of Nursing
University of Utah
Salt Lake City, UT 84112
(313) 591-8358

Pacific Northwest Coalition of Grandparents Raising Grandchildren
Pierce County Health Department
3629 South D Street
Tacoma, WA 98408
(206) 591-6427
FAX: (206) 627-3943

Parents and Friends of Lesbians and Gays
P.O. Box 27605
Washington, DC 20038-7605
(202)638-4200
http:www.pflag.org

Parents Without Partners
International Headquarters
401 North Michigan Avenue
Chicago, IL 60611-4267
(312) 644-6610

Parents Without Partners International
8807 Colesville Road
Silver Spring, MD 20910-4346
(301) 588-9354

R.O.C.K.I.N.G./Raising Our Children's Kids: An International Network of Grandparents, Inc.
P.O. Box 96
Niles, MI 49120
(616) 683-9038

Second Time Around Parents
Family and Community Service of Delaware County
100 West Front Street
Media, PA 19065
(610) 566-7540
FAX: (610) 566-7677

Stepfamily Association of America
28 Alleghaney Avenue, Suite 1307
Baltimore, MD 21204
(301) 823-7570

Stepfamily Association of America
215 Centennial Mall South, Suite 212
Lincoln, NB 68508
(800) 735-0329

The Stepfamily Foundation
333 West End Avenue
11th Floor
New York, NY 10023
(212) 877-3244

Books and Printed Material

The Adopted Child
PO Box 9362
Moscow, ID 83843
Monthly newsletter for adoptive families

✏ Berman, C. (1982). *What am I doing in a step family?* Secaucus, NJ: Lyle Stuart.

✏ Boshe, S. (1991). *Jenny lives with Eric and Martin.* London: Gay Men's Press.

Double Talk (published bimonthly)
PO Box 412
Amelia, OH 45102
(513) 231-8946
Newsletter for parents of twins

✏ Elwin, R., & Paulse, M. (1990). *Asha's mums.* Toronto: Women's Press.

✏ Evans, M. (1989). *This is me and my two families.* New York: Magination Press.

Gardner, R. (1991). *The parent's book about divorce.* New York: Bantam Books.

✏ Getzoff, A., & McClenahan, C. (1984). *Stepkids: A survival guide for teenagers in step families.* New York: Walker.

Horner, C. T. (1988). *The single-parent family in children's books: An annotated bibliography.* Metuchen, NJ: Scarecrow Press.

Kalter, N. (1990). *Growing up with divorce.* New York: Free Press.

Komar, M. (1991). *Communicating with the adopted child.* New York: Walker Publishing.

✏ Krementz, J. (1988). *How it feels to be adopted.* New York: Knopf.

✏ KIDS Express
PO Box 782
Littleton, CO 80160-0782
Monthly newsletter for children whose parents have divorced or separated

Martin, A. (1993). *The lesbian and gay parenting handbook: Creating and raising our families.* New York: HarperCollins.

Paul, E. (1991). *Adoption choices.* Detroit: Visible Ink Press.
A state-by-state directory of independent adoption facilitators

✏ Newman, L. (1989). *Heather has two mommies.* Boston: Alyson Publications.

Teyber, E. (1992). *Helping children cope with divorce.* New York: Lexington Books.

Today's Father.
Magazine published by National Center for Fathering

Triplet Connection (published bimonthly)
PO Box 99571
Stockton, CA 95209
(209) 474-0885

Twins Magazine (published bimonthly)
PO Box 12045
Overland Park, KS 66212

✏ Resources specifically for children.

References

Adams-McDarty, K. (1996). Perceptions of health and illness in Mexico. *Journal of Multicultural Nursing & Health, 2*(2), 18–22.

Aguilera, D. (1994). *Crisis intervention: Theory and methodology.* St. Louis: Mosby–Year Book.

Ahmann, E. (1994). "Chunky stew": Appreciating cultural diversity while providing health care for children. *Pediatric Nursing, 20*(3), 320–324.

Ahrons, C., & Rodgers, R. (1987). *Divorced families: A multidisciplinary developmental view.* New York: W. W. Norton.

Aidala, A., & Zablocki, B. (1991). The communes of the 1970's: Who joined and why? *Marriage and Family Review, 17*(1–2), 86–116.

Aldous, J. (1990). Family development and the life course: Two perspectives on family change. *Journal of Marriage and the Family, 52,* 571–583.

Allen, K. R., & Demo, D. H. (1995). The families of lesbians and gay men: A new frontier in family research. *Journal of Marriage and the Family, 57,* 111–127.

Altman, I. (1993). Challenges and opportunities of a transactional world view: Case study of contemporary Mormon polygynous families. *American Journal of Community Psychology, 21*(2), 135–163.

Anderson, B., & Anderson, A. (1987). Assessing families with problems attaching to twin infants. In M. Leahey & L. Wright (Eds.), *Families and psychosocial problems* (pp. 64–77). Springhouse, PA: Springhouse.

Andrews, M. (1989). Transcultural perspectives in the nursing care of children and adolescents. In J. S. Boyle and M. M. Andrews (Eds.), *Transcultural concepts in nursing care* (pp. 119–166). Glenview, IL: Scott, Foresman, Little, Brown College Division.

Arditti, J. A. (1992). Differences between fathers with joint custody and noncustodial fathers. *American Journal of Orthopsychiatry, 62,* 186–195.

Artinian, N. T. (1994). Selecting a model to guide family assessment. *Dimensions of Critical Care Nursing, 14*(1), 4–12.

Atkins, F. (1991). Children's perspective of stress and coping: An integrative review. *Issues in Mental Health Nursing, 12*(2), 171–178.

Axelson, L., & Dail, P. (1988). The changing character of homelessness in the United States. *Family Relations, 37*(4), 463–469.

Bassuk, E. L., & Rosenberg, L. (1990). Psychosocial characteristics of homeless children and children with homes. *Pediatrics, 85,* 257–261.

Beavers, W. R. (1985). *Attributes of the healthy couple: Successful systems approach to couples therapy.* New York: W. W. Norton.

Bell, C., & Jenkins, E. (1991). Traumatic stress and children. *Journal of Health Care for the Poor and Underserved, 2*(1), 175–185.

Berkowitz, C. (1996). *Pediatrics: A primary care approach.* Philadelphia: W. B. Saunders.

Black, M. M. & Bentley, M. E. (1995). Adolescent parenthood: A family-centered approach, culturally-based perspective. *Pediatric Basics, 73*(Summer), 2–9.

Bower, B. (1994). Adapting to adoption. *Science News, 146,* 104–106.

Boyle, J. S., & Andrews, M. M. (1989). *Transcultural concepts in nursing care.* Glenview, IL: Scott, Foresman.

Bozett, F. W. (1987). Family nursing and life-threatening illness. In M. Leahey & L. M. Wright (Eds.), *Families and life-threatening illness* (pp. 2–25). Springhouse, PA: Springhouse.

Brodzinsky, D. M., & Huffman, L. (1988). Transition to adoptive parenthood. *Marriage and Family Review, 12*(3–4), 267–286.

Brown, A. L., & Ferrara, R. A. (1992). Diagnosing zones of proximal development. In J. V. Wertsch (Ed.), *Culture communication and cognition* (pp. 273–305). Cambridge: Cambridge University Press.

Buchanan, C. M., Maccoby, E. E., & Dornbusch, S. M. (1991). Caught between parents: Adolescents' experience in divorce homes. *Child Development, 62,* 1008–1029.

Bumpass, L., Sweet, J., & Martin, T. (1990). Changing patterns of remarriage. *Journal of Marriage and the Family, 52,* 747–756.

Cain, A. (1980). Assessment of family structure. In J. Miller & E. Janosik (Eds.), *Family focused care* (pp. 115–131). New York: McGraw-Hill.

Callister, L. (1995). Cultural meanings of childbirth. *JOGNN, 24*(4), 327–331.

Caplan, G. (1961). *An approach to community mental health.* New York: Grune & Stratton.

Carlson, K. (1996). Providing health care for children in foster care: A role for advanced practice nurses. *Pediatric Nursing, 22*(5), 418–422.

Carter, B., & McGoldrick, M. (Eds.) (1980). *The family life cycle: A framework for family therapy.* New York: Gardner Press.

Carter, B., & McGoldrick, M. (Eds.) (1988). *The changing family life cycle: A framework for family therapy.* New York: Gardner Press.

Castiglia, P. (1994). Adoptive families. *Journal of Pediatric Health Care, 8*(4), 181–183.

Cervantes, J., & Ramirez, O. (1992). Spirituality and family dynamics in psychotherapy with Latino children. In L. Vargas & J. Koss-Chioino (Eds.), *Working with culture* (pp. 103–128). San Francisco: Jossey-Bass.

Chaleby, K. (1985). Women of polygamous marriages in an inpatient psychiatric service in Kuwait. *Journal of Nervous and Mental Disease, 173,* 56–58.

Cherlin, A. (1992). *Marriage, divorce and remarriage* (p. 78). Cambridge, MA: Harvard University Press.

Christensen, H. (1964). *Handbook of marriage and the family.* Chicago: Rand McNally.

Cluff, R., Hicks, M., & Madsen, C. (1994). Beyond the circumplex model: I. A moratorium on curvilinearity. *Family Process, 33,* 455–470.

Combrinck-Graham, L. (1985). A developmental model for family systems. *Family Process, 24*(2), 139–150.

Combrinck-Graham, L. (1990). Developments in family systems theory and research. *Journal of the American Academy of Child and Adolescent Psychiatry, 29*(4), 501–512.

Delaney, S. (1995). Divorce mediation and children's adjustment to parental divorce. *Pediatric Nursing, 21*(5), 434–437.

Diaz-Gilbert, M. (1993). Caring for culturally diverse patients. *Nursing, 23*(10), 44–45.

Dickson, L. R., Heffron, W. H., & Parker, C. (1990). Children from disrupted and adoptive homes on an inpatient unit. *American Journal of Orthopsychiatry, 60*(4), 594.

Dowell, E. B. (1995). Caregiver burden; grandmothers raising their high risk grandchildren. *Journal of Psychosocial Nursing, 33*(3), 27–30.

Dubowitz, H. (1995). Foster care. In S. Parker & B. Zuckerman (Eds.), *Behavioral and developmental pediatrics* (pp. 368–370). Boston: Little, Brown.

Duvall, E. (1957). *Family development.* Philadelphia: Lippincott.

Duvall, E. M. (1962). *Family development.* Chicago: Lippincott.

Elkind, D. (1996). On our changing family values. *Educational Leadership, 53*(7), 4–9.

Epstein, N., Baldwin, L., & Bishop, E. (1983). The McMaster family assessment device. *Journal of Marital and Family Therapy,* 9, 171–180.

Erikson, E. (1963). *Childhood and society.* New York: W. W. Norton.

Farrell, J. (1988). The changing pool of candidates for nursing. *Journal of Professional Nursing, 4*(3), 145, 230.

Field, T., Widmayer, S., Adler, S., & De Cubas, M. (1990). Teenage parenting in different cultures, family constellation, and caregiving environments: Effects on infant development. *Infant Mental Health Journal, 11,* 158–174.

Fister, S., & Scholmann, P. (1995). The role of the perinatal nurse in open adoption. *MCN American Journal of Maternal Child Nursing, 20*(1), 9–12.

Foster, M., & Phillips, W. (1992). Family systems theory as a framework for problem solving in pediatric physical therapy. *Pediatric Physical Therapy, 4*(2), 70–73.

Foster, S., & Pascoe, J. (1995). Divorce. In S. Parker & B. Zuckerman (Eds.), *Behavioral and developmental pediatrics* (pp. 359–362). Boston: Little, Brown.

Fox, S. J., Barrnett, R. J., Davies, M., & Bird, H. R. (1990). Psychopathology and developmental delay in homeless children: A pilot study. *Journal of the American Academy of Child and Adolescent Psychiatry, 29,* 732–735.

Friedman, M. (1992). *Family nursing: Theory and practice* (3rd ed.) Norwalk, CT: Appleton & Lange.

Friedman, M. (1990). Transcultural family nursing: Application to Latino and black families. *Journal of Pediatric Nursing, 5*(2), 214–222.

Fuhr, R., Moos, R., & Dishotsky, N. (1981). The use of family assessment and feedback in ongoing family therapy. *American Journal of Family Therapy,* 9(1), 24–36.

Galvin, K., & Brommel, B. (1986). *Family communication: Cohesion and change.* Glenview, IL: Scott, Foresman.

Garcia, P., & Gall, S. (1990). Multiple pregnancy. In D. N. Danforth & J. R. Scott (Eds.), *Danforth's obstetrics and gynecology.* Philadelphia: J. B. Lippincott.

Gellerstedt, M., & leRoux, P. (1995). Beyond anticipatory guidance: Parenting and the family life cycle. *Pediatric Clinics of North America, 42*(1), 65–78.

Germain, C. (1992). Cultural care: A bridge between sickness, illness, and disease. *Holistic Nursing Practice, 6*(3), 1–9.

Gershwin, M., & Nilsen, J. (1989). Healthy families. In C. Gilliss, B. Highley, B. Roberts, & I. Martinson (Eds.), *Toward a science of family nursing* (pp. 77–91). Menlo Park, CA: Addison-Wesley.

Giger, J. N., & Davidhizar, R. E. (1995). *Transcultural nursing.* St. Louis: Mosby–Year Book.

Gilliss, C., Rose, D., Hallburg, J., & Martinson, I. (1989). The family and chronic illness. In C. Gillis, B. Highley, B. Roberts, & I. Martinson (Eds.), *Toward a science of family nursing* (pp. 287–299). Menlo Park, CA: Addison-Wesley.

Glick, P. (1989). Remarried families, step families, and step children: A brief demographic profile. *Family Relations, 38*(1), 24–27.

Gold, M., Perrin, E., Futterman, D., & Friedman, S. (1994). Children of gay or lesbian parents. *Pediatrics in Review, 15*(9), 354–358.

Green, M. (1995). No child is an island. *Pediatric Clinics of North America, 42*(1), 79–87.

Groce, N. E., & Zola, I. K. (1993). Multiculturalism, chronic illness, and disability. *Pediatrics, 91*(5), 1048–1055.

Groothuis, J. (1995). Twins. In S. Parker & B. Zuckerman (Eds.), *Behavioral and developmental pediatrics* (pp. 405–408). Boston: Little, Brown.

Gross, D. (1996). What is a "good" parent? *MCN American Journal of Maternal Child Nursing, 21*(4), 178–182.

Grotevant, H., McRoy, R., Elde, C., & Fravel, D. (1994). Adoptive family system dynamics: Variations by level of openness in adoption. *Family Process, 33*(2), 125–146.

Haley, J. (1973). *Uncommon therapy: The psychiatric techniques of Milton H. Erickson*. New York: W. W. Norton.

Hayghe, H. V. (1990). Family members in the work force. *Monthly Labor Review, 113*(3), 14–19.

Hetherington, E. M. (1982). Modes of adaptation to divorce and single parenthood which enhance family functioning: Implications for a preventive program [Unpublished paper]. Charlottesville, VA: University of Virginia.

Hetherington, E., Law, T., & O'Connor, T. (1993). Divorce: Challenges, changes, and new chances. In F. Walsh (Ed.), *Normal Family Processes* (pp. 208–234). New York: Guilford Press.

Hill, K. (1987). Mothers by insemination: Interviews. In S. Pollack & J. Vaughn (Eds.), *Politics of the heart: A lesbian parenting anthology* (pp. 111–119). Ithaca, NY: Firebrand Books.

Hill, R. (1949). *Families under stress*. New York: Harper & Row.

Hill, R. (1971). Modern systems theory and the family: A confrontation. *Social Science Information, 10*, 7–26.

Hill, R., & Rodgers, K. (1964). The developmental approach. In H. Christensen (Ed.), *Handbook of marriage and the family* (pp. 171–211). Chicago: Rand McNally.

Homans, G. (1958). Social behavior as exchange. *American Journal of Sociology, 63*, 597–606.

Hymovich, D. (1983). The chronicity impact and coping instrument: Parent questionnaire. *Nursing Research, 32*, 275–281.

Jendrek, M. P. (1994). Grandparents who parent their grandchildren: Circumstances and decisions. *Gerontologist, 34*(2), 206–216.

Jones, S., & Dimond, M. (1982). Family theory and family therapy models: Comparative review with implications for nursing practice. *Journal of Psychosocial Nursing and Mental Health Services, 20*(10), 12–19.

Kaslow, F. (1991). The sociocultural context of divorce. *Contemporary Family Therapy: An International Journal, 13*(6), 583–607.

Kavanagh, K. (1994). Family: Is there anything more diverse? *Pediatric Nursing, 20*(4), 423–426.

Kelley, S., & Damato, E. (1995). Grandparents as primary caregivers. *MCN American Journal of Maternal Child Nursing, 20*(6), 326–332.

Keltner, B. (1992). Family influence on child health status. *Pediatric Nursing, 18*(2), 128–131.

Kohlenberg, T. (1995). Teen mothers. In S. Parker & B. Zuckerman (Eds.), *Behavioral and developmental pediatrics* (pp. 396–401). Boston: Little, Brown.

Kune-Karrer, B. M., & Taylor, E. H. (1995). Toward multiculturality: Implications for the pediatrician. *Pediatric Clinics of North America, 42*(1), 21–30.

Laird, J. (1993). Lesbian and gay families. In F. Walsh (Ed.), *Normal family processes* (pp. 282–328). New York: Guilford Press.

Leahey, M., & Wright, L. (1987). *Families and psychosocial problems*. Springhouse, PA: Springhouse.

LePere, D. (1987). Vulnerability to crises during the life cycle of the adoptive family. *Journal of Social Work and Human Sexuality*, 6(1), 73–85.

Leininger, M. (1991). *Cultural care diversity and universality*. New York: National League of Nursing.

Lissner, W. (1995). Homelessness: A complex problem and the federal response. *American Journal of Economics and Sociology, 44*, 385–390.

Lobar, S., & Phillips, S. (1994). The couple choosing private infant adoption. *Pediatric Nursing*, 20(2), 141–145.

Lowman, J. (1980). Measurement of family affective structures. *Journal of Personality Assessment, 44*(2), 130–141.

Maccoby, E. E., & Mnookin, R. H. (1992). *Dividing the child: Social and legal dilemmas of custody*. Cambridge, MA: Harvard University Press.

March of Dimes Birth Defects Foundation. (1993). *March of Dimes statbook*. White Plains, NY: Author.

Martin, A. (1993). *The lesbian and gay parent handbook: Creating and raising our families*. New York: HarperCollins.

Mattessich, P., & Hill, R. (1987). Life cycle and family development. In M. B. Sussman & S. K. Steinmetz (Eds.), *Handbook of marriage and the family* (pp. 437–469). New York: Plenum Publishing.

McCubbin, H., Larsen, A., & Olson, D. (1981). *F-Copes*. Madison, WI: University of Wisconsin.

McCubbin, H., & McCubbin, M. (1988). Typologies of resilient families: Emerging roles of social class and ethnicity. *Family Relations, 37*, 247–254.

McCubbin, H., McCubbin, M., Cauble, A., & Nevin, R. (1979). *Coping health inventory for parents (CHIP)*. St. Paul, MN: Family Social Services, University of Minnesota.

McCubbin, H., & Patterson, J. (1983). Family transitions: Adaptation to stress. In H. McCubbin & C. Figley (Eds.), *Stress and the family: Vol. I. Coping with normative transitions* (pp. 5–25). New York: Brunner/Mazel.

McCubbin, H., Patterson, J., & Wilson, L. (1981). *FILE*. St. Paul, MN: University of Minnesota.

McGoldrick, M., Heiman, M., & Carter, B. (1993). The changing family life cycle. In F. Walsh (Ed.), *Normal family processes* (pp. 405–443). New York: Guilford Press.

Mead, L., Chuffo, R., Lawlor-Klean, P., & Meier, P. (1992). Breastfeeding success with quadruplets. *JOGNN, 21*(5), 221–227.

Mederer, H., & Hill, R. (1983). Critical transitions over the family life span: Theory and research. In H. McCubbin, M. Sussman, & J. Patterson (Eds.), *Social stress and the family: Advances and developments in family stress theory and research* (pp. 39–60). New York: Haworth Press.

Mercer, R. (1989). Theoretical perspectives on the family. In C. Gilliss, B. Highley, B. Roberts, & I. Martinson (Eds.), *Toward a science of family nursing* (pp. 9–36). Menlo Park, CA: Addison-Wesley.

Miller, M. A. (1995). Culture, spirituality and women's health. *JOGNN, 24*(3), 257–263.

Minuchin, S. (1974). *Families and family therapy*. Cambridge, MA: Harvard University Press.

Moos, R. W., & Moos, B. S. (1976). A typology of family social environments. *Family Process, 15*, 357–371.

Moos, R. W., & Moos, B. S. (1984). The process of recovery from alcoholism: III. Comparing functioning in families of alcoholics and matched control families. *Journal of Studies on Alcohol, 45*, 111–118.

Nock, S. (1981). Family life-cycle transitions: Longitudinal effects on family members. *Journal of Marriage and the Family, 43*(3), 703–713.

Nye, F., & Bernardo, F. (1981). *Emerging conceptual frameworks in family analysis.* New York: Praeger.

Olson, D. (1988). Family assessment and intervention: The circumplex model of family systems. *Journal of Psychotherapy and the Family,* 4(½), 7–49.

Olson, D. (1994). Curvilinearity survives: The world is not flat. *Family Process, 33,* 471–478.

Olson, D., & Wilson, M. (1982). *Family satisfaction.* Madison, WI: University of Wisconsin.

Olson, D., McCubbin, H. I., Barnes, H., Larsen, A., Muxen, M., & Wilson, D. (1982). *Family inventories.* St. Paul, MN: University of Minnesota.

Olson, D., Portner, J., & Lavee, Y. (1985). *FACES III.* St. Paul, MN: Family Social Science.

Olson, D. H. (1993). Circumplex model of marital and family systems: Assessing family functioning. In F. Walsh (Ed.), *Normal Family Processes* (pp. 104–137). New York: Guilford Press.

Osofsky, J. D., & Eberhart-Wright, A. (1988). Affective exchanges between high-risk mothers and infants. *International Journal of Psycho-Analysis, 69,* 221–232.

Parson, T. & Bales, R. F. (1955). *Family socialization and interaction process.* New York: Free Press.

Patterson, C. J. (1992). Children of lesbian and gay parents. *Child Development, 63,* 1025–1042.

Patterson, J. M. (1988). Families experiencing stress. The family adjustment and adaptation response model. *Family Systems Medicine,* 5, 202–237.

Patterson, J. M. (1995). Promoting resilience in families experiencing stress. *Pediatric Clinics of North America, 42*(1), 47–63.

Patterson, J., & Garwick, A. (1994). Levels of meaning in family stress theory. *Family Process, 33,* 287–304.

Patterson, J., McCubbin, H., & Warwick, W. (1990). The impact of family functioning on health changes in children with cystic fibrosis. *Social Science Medicine, 31,* 159–164.

Perosa, L., Hansen, J., & Perosa, S. (1981). Development of the structural family interaction scale. *Family Therapy,* 8(2), 77–90.

Perrin, E. C., & Kulkin, H. (1996). Pediatric care for children whose parents are gay or lesbian. *Pediatrics,* 97(5), 629–635.

Peterson, E. (1997). Supporting the adoptive family: A developmental approach. *MCN American Journal of Maternal Child Nursing, 22*(3), 147–152.

Piotrkowski, C., & Hughes, D. (1993). Dual-earner families in context: Managing family and work systems. In F. Walsh (Ed.), *Normal family processes* (pp. 185–207). New York: Guilford Press.

Pleck, J. H. (1977). The work-family role system. *Social Problems, 24,* 417– 427.

Pless, I., & Satterwhite, B. (1973). A measure of family functioning and its application. *Social Science & Medicine, 7,* 613–621.

Porter, C. P. (1990). Clinical and research issues related to teenage mothers' childrearing practices. *Issues in Comprehensive Pediatric Nursing, 13,* 41–58.

Pronsati, M. (1996). Foster children more prone to problems. *Advance for Nurse Practitioners,* 4(8), 20A.

Prowler, M. (1991). *Single parent adoption: What you need to know.* Washington, DC: National Adoption Information Clearinghouse.

Rankin, S. (1989). Family transitions, expected and unexpected. In C. Gillis, B. Highley, B. Roberts, & I. Martinson (Eds.), *Toward a science in family nursing* (pp. 173–186). Menlo Park, CA: Addison-Wesley.

Rapoport, R. (1964). The transition from engagement to marriage. *Acta Sociologica,* 8, 36–55.

Rapoport, R. (1963). Normal crises, family structure and mental health. *Family Process,* 2, 68–79.

Reimer, J., Van Cleave, L., & Galbraith, M. (1995). Barriers to well child care for homeless children under 13. *Public Health Nursing, 12*(1), 61–66.

Reitz, M., & Watson, K. (1992). *Adoption and the family system.* New York: Guilford Press.

Reutter, L., & Strang, V. (1986). Yours, mine and ours: Stepparents and their children. *MCN American Journal of Maternal Child Nursing, 11,* 264–266.

Richman, J., Chapman, M., & Bowen, G. (1995). Recognizing the impact of marital discord and parental depression on children. *Pediatric Clinics of North America, 42*(1), 167–180.

Roberts, C., & Feetham, S. (1982). Assessing family functioning across three areas of relationships. *Nursing Research, 31,* 231–235.

Robinson, D. (1997). Family stress theory: Implications for family health. *Journal of the American Academy of Nurse Practitioners,* 9(1), 17–23.

Rodgers, R. (1964). Toward a theory of family development. *Journal of Marriage and the Family,* 26, 262–270.

Rodriguez-Wargo, T. (1993). Preparing for cultural diversity through education. *Journal of Pediatric Nursing,* 8(4), 272–273.

Roizen, N. (1995). Adoption. In S. Parker & B. Zuckerman (Eds.), *Behavioral and developmental pediatrics* (pp. 339–342). Boston: Little, Brown.

Rolland, J. S. (1993). Mastering family challenges in serious illness and disability. In F. Walsh (Ed.), *Normal family processes* (pp. 444–473). New York: Guilford Press.

Romanczuk, A. N. (1987). Helping the stepparent parent. *MCN American Journal of Maternal Child Nursing, 12,* 106–110.

Rose, A. (1980). A systematic summary of symbolic interaction theory. In J. Riehl & C. Roy (Eds.), *Conceptual models for nursing practice* (pp. 38–50). New York: Appleton-Century-Crofts.

Rowe, G. (1981). The developmental conceptual framework to the study of the family. In F. Nye & F. Bernardo (Eds.), *Emerging conceptual frameworks in family analysis* (pp. 198–222). New York: Praser.

Roye, C., & Balk, S. (1997). Caring for pregnant teens and their mothers, too. *MCN American Journal of Maternal Child Nursing, 22*(3), 153–157.

Ryan-Wenger, N. (1992). A taxonomy of children's coping strategies: A step toward theory development. *American Journal of Orthopsychiatry, 62*(2), 256–263.

Saluter, A. F. (1992). Marital status and living arrangements: March 1991. In *Current population reports, population characteristics* (Series P-20, No. 461). Washington, DC: U.S. Government Printing Office.

Scanlan, C. (1994, February 20). Shortchanging the kids. *Orange County Register,* pp. 1, 12 (Nation section).

Schor, E. (1995). The influence of families on child health. *Pediatric Clinics of North America, 42*(1), 89–103.

Schwartzberg, A. (1992). The impact of divorce on adolescents. *Hospital and Community Psychiatry, 43*(6), 634–637.

Sherry, S. N. (1992). Adoption and foster family care. In M. Levine, W. Carey, & A. Crocker (Eds.), *Developmental-behavioral pediatrics* (pp. 122–127). Philadelphia: W. B. Saunders.

Smilkstein, G. (1978). The family APGAR: A proposal for a family function test and its use by physicians. *Journal of Family Practice,* 6, 1231–1239.

Spear, J., & Sachs, B. (1985). Selecting the appropriate family assessment tool. *Pediatric Nursing, 11,* 349–355.

Spector, R. E. (1991). *Cultural diversity in health and illness* (3rd ed.). East Norwalk, CT: Appleton-Lange.

Spector, R. E. (1995). Cultural concepts of women's health and health-promoting behaviors. *JOGNN, 24*(3), 241–245.

Stewart, E. C., & Bennett, M. J. (1991). *American cultural patterns: A cross-cultural perspective* (pp. 167–168). Yarmouth, ME: Intercultural Press.

Tanner, J. L. (1995). Single parents. In S. Parker & B. Zuckerman (Eds.), *Behavioral and developmental pediatrics* (pp. 387–390). Boston: Little, Brown.

U.S. Bureau of the Census. (1991). *Statistical abstract of the United States: 1991* (111th ed.). Washington, DC: U.S. Government Printing Office.

U.S. Bureau of the Census. (1990). *Statistical abstract of the United States*. Washington, DC: U.S. Government Printing Office.

U.S. Conference of Mayors. (1993). *A status report on hunger and homelessness in America's cities: 1993–A 26 city survey*. Washington, DC.

Visher, J. S., & Visher, E. B. (1992, March). Why stepfamilies need your help. *Contemporary Pediatrics*, 146–164.

Visher, J. S., & Visher, E. B. (1995a). Beyond the nuclear family. *Pediatric Clinics of North America, 42*(1), 31–43.

Visher, J. S., & Visher, E. B. (1995b). Step families. In S. Parker & B. Zuckerman (Eds.), *Behavioral and developmental pediatrics* (pp. 391–395). Boston: Little, Brown.

von Bertalanffy, L. (1968). *General systems theory*. London: Penguin Press.

Wallerstein, J. (1992). Separation, divorce, and remarriage. In M. Levine, W. Carey, & A. Crocker (Eds.), *Developmental-behavioral pediatrics* (pp. 136–146). Philadelphia: W. B. Saunders.

Wallerstein, J. S., & Kelly, J. B. (1980). California's children of divorce. *Psychology Today, 13*(8), 67–76.

White, L., & Booth, A. (1985). The quality and stability of remarriages: The role of stepchildren. *American Sociological Review, 50*, 689–698.

Woolley, N. (1990). Crisis theory: A paradigm of effective intervention with families of critically ill people. *Journal of Advanced Nursing, 15*, 1402–1408.

Wood, D., Valdez, R. B., Hayashi, T., & Shen, A. (1990). Homeless and housed families in Los Angeles: A study comparing demographic, economic and family function characteristics. *American Journal of Public Health, 80*, 1049–1052.

Wright, L., & Leahey, M. (1994). *Nurses and families: A guide to family assessment and intervention*. Philadelphia: F. A. Davis.

Yoos, H., Kitzman, H., Olds, D., & Overaker, I. (1995). Child rearing beliefs in the African-American community: Implications for culturally competent pediatric care. *Journal of Pediatric Nursing, 10*(6), 343–353.

Zablocki, B. (1980). *Alienation and charisma: A study of contemporary communes*. New York: Random House.

Zeidenstein, L. (1990). Gynecological and childbearing needs of lesbians. *Journal of Nurse-Midwifery, 35*(1), 10–18.

Zima, B. T., Wells, K. B., & Freeman, H. E. (1994). Emotional and behavioral problems and severe academic delays among sheltered homeless children in Los Angeles County. *American Journal of Public Health, 84*(2), 260–264.

Bibliography

Ahmann, E. (1994). The United Nations' International Year of the Family. *Pediatric Nursing, 20*(5), 529–530.

Bowen, M. (1991). Italian Americans. In J. N. Giger & R. E. Davidhizar (Eds.), *Transcultural nursing: Assessment and intervention*. St. Louis, MO: Mosby–Year Book.

Campinha-Bacote, J., & Ferguson, S. (1991). Cultural considerations in child rearing practices: A transcultural perspective. *Journal of the National Black Nurses Association, 5*(1), 11–17.

Capers, C. (1992). Teaching cultural content: A nursing education perspective. *Holistic Nursing Practice, 6*(3), 19–28.

Chang, K. (1991). Chinese Americans. In J. Giger & R. Davidhizar (Eds.), *Transcultural nursing: Assessment and intervention* (pp. 395–416). St. Louis: Mosby–Year Book.

Charnes, L., & Moore, P. (1992). Meeting patients' spiritual needs: The Jewish perspective. *Holistic Nursing Practice, 6*(3), 64–72.

Cherry, B., & Giger, J. N. (1995). African Americans. In J. Giger & R. Davidhizar (Eds.), *Transcultural nursing: Assessment and intervention* (pp. 165–204). St. Louis: Mosby–Year Book.

Cluff, R., & Hicks, M. (1994). Superstition also survives: Seeing is not always believing. *Family Process, 33*, 479–482.

de la Flor, L. (1990). Azarcon: A fatal home remedy. *California Coalition Nurse Practitioner News, 3*(1), 3–4.

Eckblad, G. (1993). The "circumplex" and curvilinear functions. *Family Process, 32*, 473–476.

Edelman, M. W. (1988). An advocacy agenda for black families and children. In H.P. McAdoo (Ed.), *Black Families* (2nd ed., pp. 286–295). Newbury Park, CA: Sage.

Fister, S., & Schlomann, P. (1995). The role of the perinatal nurse in open adoption. *MCN American Journal of Maternal Child Nursing, 20*(1), 9–12.

Geissler, E. (1994). *Pocket guide to cultural assessment*. St. Louis: C. V. Mosby.

Gevitz, N. (1991). Christian Science healing and the health care of children. *Perspectives in Biology and Medicine, 34*(3), 421–438.

Glick, P. (1988). Demographic pictures of black families. In H. P. McAdoo (Ed.), *Black families* (2nd ed., pp. 111–132). Newbury Park, CA: Sage.

Grossman, D. (1996). Cultural dimensions in home health nursing. *American Journal of Nursing, 96*(7), 34–38.

Harris, C. C. (1986). Cultural values and the decision to circumcise. *Image: Journal of Nursing Scholarship, 18*(3), 98–104.

Hong, G. K., & Domokos-Cheng Ham, M. (1992). The impact of immigration on the family life cycle: Clinical implications for Chinese Americans. *Journal of Family Psychotherapy, 3*(3), 27–40.

Ikeda, J., & Wright, J. (1996). Pediatrics in a culturally diverse society. *Pediatric Basics, 76*, 10–17.

Julian, T., McKenry, P., & McKelvey, M. (1994). Cultural variations in parenting: Perceptions of Caucasian, African-American, Hispanic, and Asian-American parents. *Family Relations, 43*(1), 30–37.

Koepke, J., Anglin, S., Austin, J., & Delesalle, J. (1991). Becoming parents: Feelings of adoptive mothers. *Pediatric Nursing, 17*(4), 333–336.

Kuipers, J. (1995). Mexican-Americans. In J. N. Giger & R. E. Davidhizar (Eds.), *Transcultural nursing: Assessment and intervention* (pp. 205–236). St. Louis: Mosby–Year Book.

Leininger, M. (1995). *Transcultural nursing concepts, theories, research, and practice*. New York: McGraw-Hill.

Luna, I., Torres de Ardon, E., Lim, Y. M., Cromwell, S. L., Phillips, L. R., & Russell, C. K. (1996). The relevance of familism in cross-cultural studies of family caregiving. *Western Journal of Nursing Research, 18*(3), 267–283.

MacDonald-Clark, N., & Harney-Boffman, J. (1994). Using NCAST and the HOME with a minority population: The Alaska eskimo. *Pediatric Nursing, 20*(5), 481–489.

Mansour, M. (1994). Cultural circles: Application of family systems theory in staff development. *Journal of Nursing Staff Development, 10*(1), 22–26.

Marin, B. (1990). AIDS prevention for non–Puerto Rican Hispanics. In C. Leukefeld, R. Batjes, & Z. Amsel (Eds.), *AIDS and intravenous drug use: Community interventions and prevention* (pp. 35–52). New York: Hemisphere.

Martin, C. (1995). Irish Americans. In J. Giger & R. Davidhizar (Eds.), *Transcultural nursing: Assessment and intervention* (pp. 347–366). St. Louis: Mosby–Year Book.

Massey, J. (1996). Decision making: Traditional Mexican health practices. *Journal of Multicultural Nursing and Health, 2*(2), 39–43.

May, J. (1996). Fathers: The forgotten parent. *Pediatric Nursing, 22*(3), 243–246.

Mazurek Melnyk, B. (1991). Changes in parent-child relationships following divorce. *Pediatric Nursing, 17*(4), 337–341.

McGauhey, P. J., & Starfield, B. (1993). Child health and the social environment of white and black children. *Social Science Medicine*, 36, 867–874.

Mikhail, B. (1994). Hispanic mothers' beliefs and practices regarding selected children's health problems. *Western Journal of Nursing Research, 16*(6), 623–638.

Munoz, E. (1988). Care for the Hispanic poor: A growing segment of American society. *JAMA, 260*, 2711–2712.

Olson, D. (1991). Three-dimensional (3-D) circumplex model and revised scoring of FACES III. *Family Process, 30*, 74–79.

Olson, D., & McCubbin, A. (1983). *Families: What makes them work.* Beverly Hills, CA: Sage.

Rashid, H. (1985). Black research and parent education programs: The need for convergence. *Contemporary Education*, 56, 180–185.

Rotunno, M., & McGoldrick, M. (1982). Italian families. In M. McGoldrick, J. K. Pearce, & J. Giordano (Eds.), *Ethnicity and family therapy.* New York: Guilford Press.

Ruiz, P. (1985). Cultural barriers to effective medical care among Hispanic-American patients. *Annual Review of Medicine, 36*, 63–71.

Russell, K., & Jewel, N. (1992). Cultural impact of health care access: Challenge for improving health of African Americans. *Journal of Community Health Nursing*, 9(3), 161–169.

Taylor, R. J., Chatters, L. M., Tucker, M. B., & Lewis, E. (1990). Development in research on black families: A decade review. *Journal of Marriage and Family, 52*, 993–1014.

White, J., Linhart, J., & Medley, L. (1996). Culture, diet and the maternity patient. *Advance for Nurse Practitioners, 4*(9), 26–29.

Wong, M. G. (1988). The Chinese American family. In C.H. Mindel, R.W. Habenstein, & R. Wright (Eds.), *Ethnic families in America: Patterns and variations* (3rd ed., pp. 230–257). New York: Elsevier Scientific.

Health Promotion and Illness Prevention

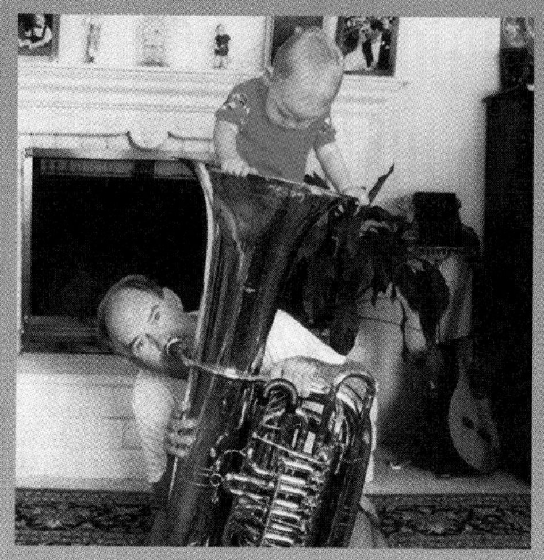

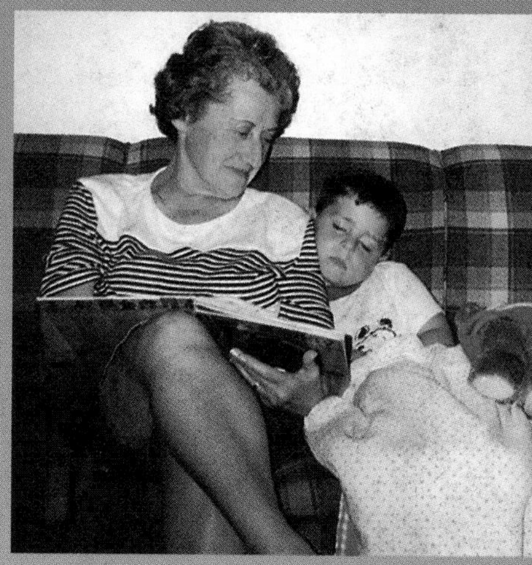

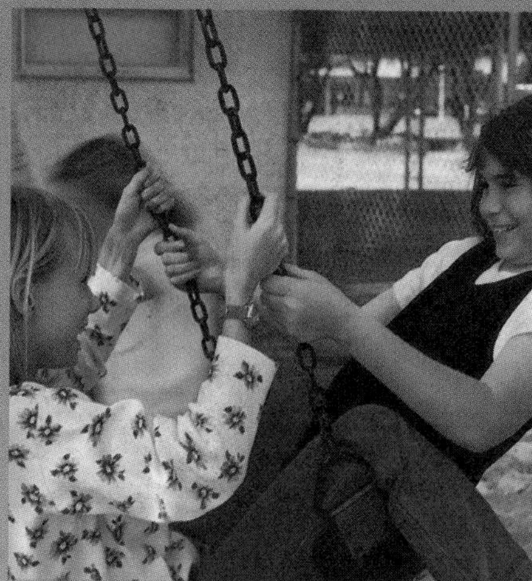

UNIT

2

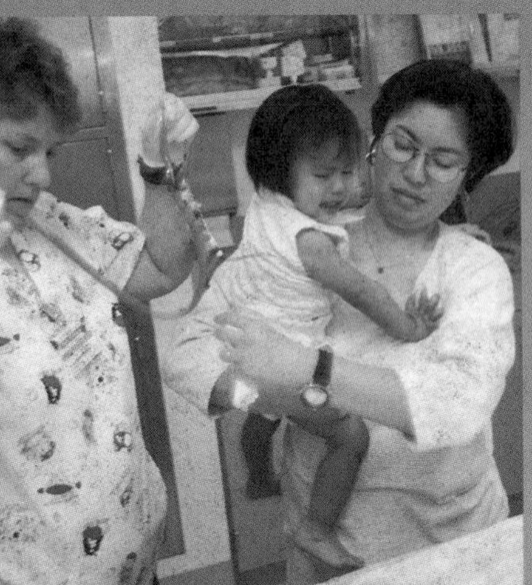

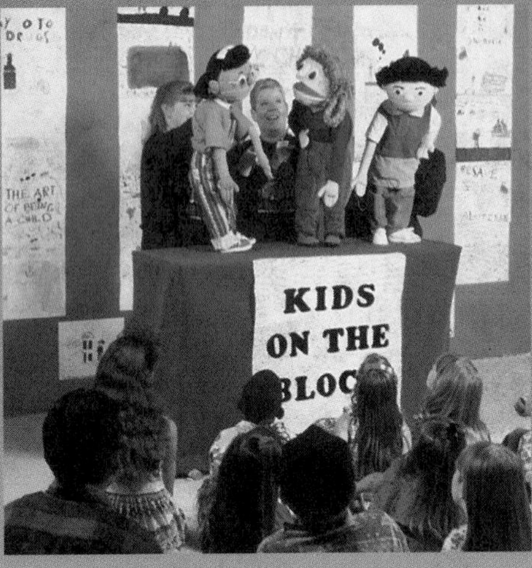

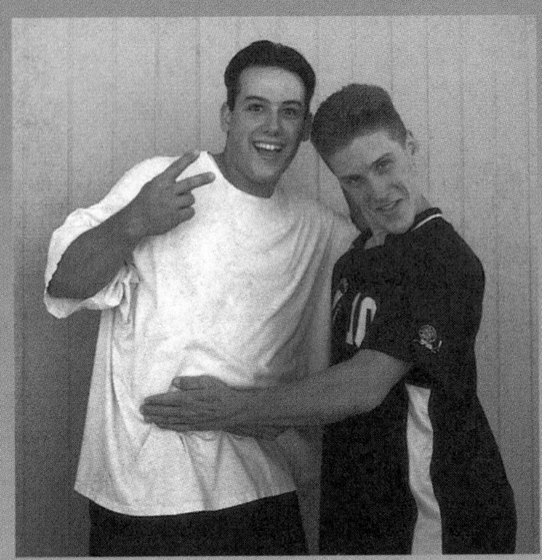

The chapters in this unit address normal patterns of growth and development for infants, children, and adolescents. Various developmental theories are presented and translated into practical ways in which the health care provider and primary caregiver can work together to promote a child's health and prevent illness. Aspects of the physical and developmental assessment are summarized. Special emphasis is given to developmental surveillance—active monitoring of growth and development and early intervention to optimize the child's outcomes even in the presence of developmental challenges.

The care of children is a collaborative process in which family members, health care providers, and community resources are orchestrated to meet a child's health needs. This unit also discusses child health programs that can be assessed in the community to promote the general welfare of children.

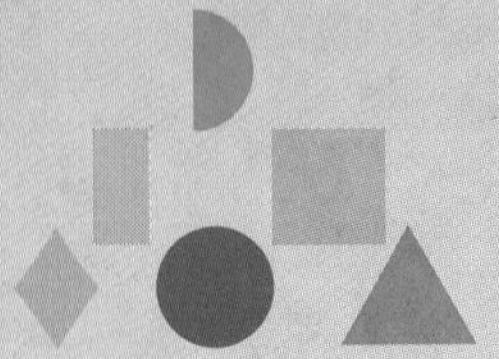

Growth and Development

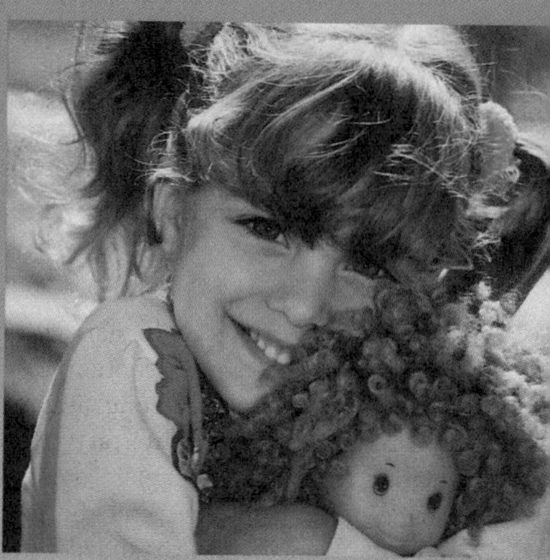

OUTLINE

Principles of Growth and Development
The Study of Growth and Development
- Scientific Methods

Factors Influencing Development
- Biological Factors
  - Heredity
  - Gender
  - Race and Ethnicity
  - Prenatal Exposures
  - Nutrition
- Environmental Factors
  - Temperament
  - The Family
  - The Community

Biological Growth of the Child
- Development of the Fetus
- Changes in General Body Growth
- Musculoskeletal Development
- Neurologic Maturation
- Sensory Organ Development
- Organ Development
  - Cardiovascular System
  - Respiratory System
  - Gastrointestinal System
  - Genitourinary System
- Gender Development
- Endocrine and Metabolic Functions
- Immune Functions

Theories of Development
- Psychosexual Development
- Psychosocial Development
- Cognitive-Intellectual Development
  - Piaget
  - Elkind
  - Information-Processing Theories
  - Multiple Intelligences
- Behavioral Development
  - Classical Conditioning
  - Operant Conditioning
- Social Learning Theories
- Development of Self-Concept
  - Humanistic Theories
- Language Development
- Development of Sexuality
- Moral Development
- Spiritual Development

Developmental Surveillance
- Developmental Assessment Tools
  - Denver Developmental Screening
  - Revised Prescreening Developmental Questionnaire

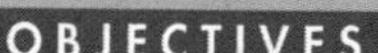

OBJECTIVES

- Explain 10 principles fundamental to understanding the growth and development processes of children.
- Review the scientific methods used to study variables that can impact growth and development.
- Examine the biological and environmental factors that can influence the growth and developmental processes in children.
- Describe the biological development of children from birth through adolescence.
- Articulate selected theories that describe the psychosocial, cognitive, interpersonal, sexual, and moral development of children from birth through adolescence.
- Choose strategies the nurse can use to institute the process of developmental surveillance.

KEY TERMS

behaviorism
catch-up period
classical conditioning
critical period
developmental surveillance
ethnicity
learning theory
multiple intelligences theory
operant conditioning
psychosocial theory
race
teratogen

CHAPTER

4

Every child is an individual and should never be considered a typical boy or girl, one unit of a group who are all alike. Each child has his own *rate of growth*, but the *pattern of growth* shows less variability . . . Although growth and development—physical, mental, social, emotional and spiritual—proceed at different rates, they are so *interrelated* in the majority of children that the result is a progressive development of the whole child, from infancy to adulthood.

Marlow, 1965, p. 12

The study of human growth and development provides explanations of the similarities and differences among us that blend to create our individual physical and social self. Developmental theories help explain the multitude of factors that shape our personalities and the processes that affect our growth. Human growth and development is the process of change. Changes in the physical body occur as tissues form, structures enlarge, and organs and muscles achieve their full degree of strength and function. Changes occur in the individual as cognitive, language, and social skills are achieved.

Principles of Growth and Development

Growth refers to changes in size and function of the whole or any part of the body. These are quantitative changes that can be measured by assessing changes in weight, length, height, and functional output.

Development refers to the qualitative changes that are seen as the individual acquires new skills. Language and thought processes, the capacity to develop social relationships, and the emergence of a unique personality are all products of human development. Developmental assessment tools, cognitive abilities tests, and psychological assessments can measure changes over time in these areas.

Maturation refers to those aspects of development that are genetically influenced. Interaction with the environment has little influence on maturational changes. For instance, toilet training, riding a bike, and reading are skills that cannot be achieved until maturation of neurologic and muscular functions has taken place (Nelms & Mullins, 1982).

Several principles provide the framework for understanding growth and development (Chart 4–1). Although each person emerges at birth as a unique individual, basic patterns and trends are predictable in the growth and development of all humans, in all societies. Growth is systematic and occurs in a sequential pattern. Because of the regularity of the growth processes, stages of growth and development can be differentiated (Chart 4–2). Within these stages, particular growth events and maturational processes are expected to occur. Differentiation and integration of growth tasks evolve. For instance, the child learning to aimlessly extend his or her arm eventually learns to purposefully grasp for an object, bring that object to the mouth, transfer the object to another hand, and throw the object when requested.

Within the sequential patterns of growth each person has his or her own growth trajectory. This trajectory is influenced by environmental factors such as nutrition and sensory stimulation. If these environmental factors are negatively impacted, the growth pattern can be altered. For instance, the child who is acutely malnourished will demonstrate delays in both physical growth and psychosocial development. However, early identification and intervention can prevent potentially irreversible outcomes. The child will undergo a *catch-up period* in

Chart 4–1

Principles of Growth and Development

- Growth is an orderly process, occurring in a systematic fashion.
- Rates and patterns of growth are specific to certain parts of the body.
- Wide individual differences exist in growth rates.
- Growth and development are influenced by multiple factors.
- Development proceeds from the simple to the complex and from the general to the specific.
- Development occurs in a cephalocaudal and a proximodistal progression.
- There are critical periods for growth and development.
- Although gradual and continuous, rates in development vary.
- Humans have an inherent desire to grow and develop.
- Development continues throughout the individual's life span.

Chart 4-2

Stages of Growth and Development

Age	Stages
Prenatal	Germinal—conception until approximately 2 weeks Embryonic—2 to 8 weeks Fetal—8 to 40 weeks
Infancy	Neonatal—birth to 1 month Infancy—1 month to 1 year
Early childhood	Toddler—1 to 3 years Preschooler—3 to 6 years
Middle childhood	School age—6 to 12 years
Late childhood	Adolescent—13 to approximately 18 years

which growth occurs, bringing the child back to his or her own growth trajectory.

Although growth is a systematic process, body systems vary in the rate of development. For instance, the cardiovascular and respiratory systems, although not fully mature at birth, must carry out functions essential for the viability of life outside the womb. In addition, these systems are necessary for the progressive maturation of other systems to complete their development. The lymphatic and genital systems are examples of two systems whose rates and patterns of growth occur over an extended period of time and influence the body at a later point in life—puberty. Early development of these systems, as seen in precocious puberty, is likely to negatively impact other physical and psychosocial developmental patterns for the individual.

Every child has his or her own rate of growth and development, which demonstrates consistency over time. When evaluating a child's growth, it is important to assess the child's patterns of growth over several months or years, rather than base an entire assessment on a single evaluation of the child at a particular time. The terms *normal* or *average* have been used to describe the predictable patterns of growth and development that have been studied and are known to occur within a certain time frame. From this normal or average pattern, each child can be viewed as a *variation of the theme* (Fig. 4–1). That is, given certain expected growth or developmental norms, each child as an individual may grow and mature faster or slower, while still demonstrating adherence to a consistent and predictable pattern of growth and development.

Just as growth trends follow a specific pattern, so do many aspects of development. Development of skills and functions proceeds from the simple to the complex and from the general to the specific. The young child does not progress straight from learning to talk to learning to write. Instead, several other developmental achievements must take place, each building upon the previous accomplishment, to achieve a more specific and higher level skill. Development progresses in a head-to-toe, *cephalocaudal* fashion and in a *proximodistal*, or midline to the periphery, progression (Fig. 4–2). The infant who learns to lift his or her head and then sit, crawl, walk, and run is developing in a cephalocaudal manner. Proximodistal progression is demonstrated as the child develops from

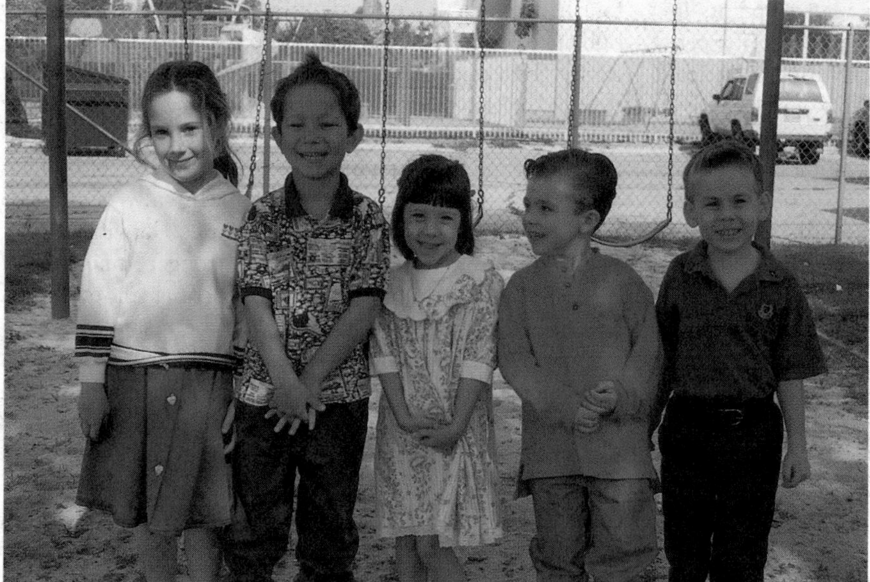

Figure 4–1
The two children on the left are 5 years old; the three on the right are 4 years old. Although the children share the same birth month, the year difference in their ages is significant in respect to their height, shape, and body proportions.

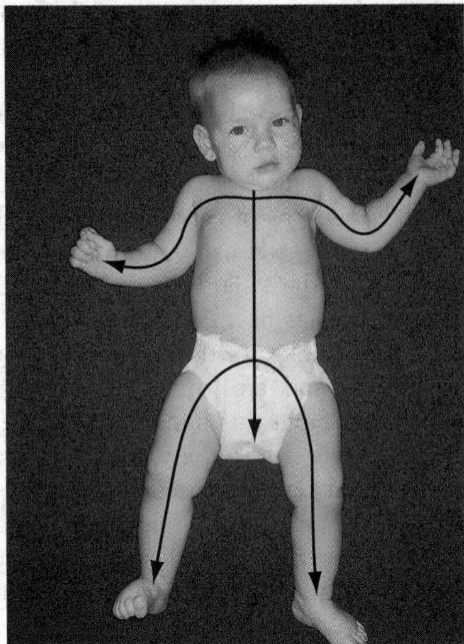

Figure 4–2
The child's pattern of growth is in a head-to-toe direction, or cephalocaudad, and in an inward to outward pattern called proximodistal.

random total body movements toward the use of a specific limb and then on to the use of individual fingers to grasp a small object. Knowledge of the progressive traits helps the nurse to remember and predict the sequential patterns of development. With this knowledge the nurse can provide anticipatory guidance for the parent to enhance the child's achievement of developmental skills (Nelms & Mullins, 1982).

As the child grows and matures, some *critical periods* are known to exist. These time periods refer to points in which the individual is highly sensitive or ready for certain actions (Nelms & Mullins, 1982). During a critical period, the child is vulnerable to positive and negative stimuli that can enhance or defer the achievement of a skill or function. For instance, infants who are born deaf vocalize as all infants do during the first year of life. However, by the age of 1 the deaf child will likely cease these vocalizations and will not progress to other audible verbalizations without active intervention by the caregivers. Sensitive periods appear to exist in regard to the acquisition of certain skills. For example, the child who learns a foreign language in his or her early years will have a much easier time developing these language skills than will the adolescent. Likewise, musical skills are most readily learned in the preschool years. Research regarding "critical periods" continues to grow, providing valuable information regarding times to ensure that opportunities are given for children to acquire specific skills and knowledge.

The individuality of a child's growth and development is highly influenced by factors such as heredity, the environment, nutrition, sensory stimulation, and affection. Although children are raised in the same family, and may even be identical twins, the interactions and experiences each child encounters will be different. Therefore, two children can be expected to respond differently based on their past experiences, stage of development, current disposition, and genetic potential.

All humans have an inherent desire to learn and grow. Abraham Maslow called this "self-actualization," and Carl Rogers called it "directional growth" (Nelms & Mullins, 1982). Children are constantly exploring their environment and testing parameters to seek new information and to acquire new skills. Factors such as illness, sensory deprivation, and physical and mental abuse can negatively impact the child's ability to focus on these inherent desires and to demonstrate progressive developmental achievements. Development is a life-long process. As the child moves through adolescence toward adulthood, changes will continue to occur in the psychosocial, cognitive, physical, and emotional domains of the individual.

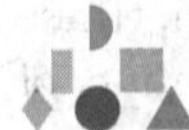

The Study of Growth and Development

The nature and origins of human development have long been a subject of inquiry by philosophers, scientists, psychologists, and medical practitioners. As early as the fourth century BC, Greek philosophers debated whether human actions were guided more by the thymos (emotion), the soma (the body), or the psyche (the soul). *Rationalism*, *empiricism*, *inductive reasoning*, and *deductive reasoning* were terms coined by the early philosophers to represent and to explain the differing views of human behavior. These philosophies were eventually challenged by the 19th century theories of Charles Darwin and Sir Frances Galton. Emphasizing the stronger influence of heredity over environment, their theories of evolution and the "survival of the fittest" were the first to argue for genetic determination of human behaviors. Eventually, psychology emerged as an independent field of study, building upon, but separate from, the heritage of past philosophers. Experimental psychology and descriptive psychology have arisen as the two primary approaches to studying the complexities of human growth and behavior. More recently, *life-span study* has gained favor as a discipline within psychology that focuses on providing information about human change over large segments of the life span in such areas as physical, intellectual, and personality functioning (Freiberg, 1987). As psychologists and others have studied the dynamics of human development, they have done so with an insistence on using scientific methods rather than reasoning processes or opinion as the basis for their explanations, hypotheses, and theories.

Scientific Methods

There are a variety of scientific methods used to study growth and development. *Cross-sectional studies* measure different subjects at the same point in time. For instance, a study would evaluate the cognitive abilities of a large group of 6-year-old children on a particular date. *Longitudinal studies* measure and evaluate changes in the same subjects over a period of time. Some methods to study human development longitudinally include *cohort-sequential, time-sequential,* and *cross-sequential* methods. A *cohort* is a person born at about the same time and in the same society as the group of individuals under study. In *cohort-sequential* research, cohorts are looked at longitudinally for a sequential period of time. The study is usually replicated using cohorts born in different years and continues until the oldest subject in the last study reaches the age of the oldest subject in the first study. *Time-sequential* is a type of cross-sectional research using different times of measurement. The study continues until the oldest subject in the last group reaches the age of the oldest child in the first group. In a *cross-sequential* study several cross sections of cohorts are studied longitudinally with the same times of measurement without regard to age (Freiberg, 1987).

An *experimental study* is one in which the investigator manipulates one or more variables to determine the effect of one variable on another. One group, the *experimental group,* receives the treatment or intervention. This treatment is called the *independent variable.* The changes that occur in the subjects as a result of the independent variable are called the *dependent variables.* To demonstrate that the introduction of a treatment (the independent variable) causes a change (the dependent variables), the second group in the study is the *control group.* Members of the control group do not receive the treatment, but they are observed to see if the same outcomes or dependent variables occur as are found in the experimental group. If the dependent variables are demonstrated by the experimental group and not the control group, the manipulation of the independent variables can be said to have caused the consequences observed in the experimental group.

Observational studies are those in which aspects of the child's growth and development are investigated in the real world. These studies are also called "naturalistic" or "descriptive" studies. The researcher may use equipment such as audiotapes, videotapes, and sound spectrograms to record behaviors as they occur and then analyze segments of these behaviors at a later time. The researchers evaluating the behaviors must be specifically trained to analyze the information collected. If several people analyze the information, they must reach a high level of agreement (interrater reliability) among themselves regarding what they are seeing.

When a researcher is interested in examining the relationship between occurrences of behaviors, he or she would conduct a *correlational study.* The investigator is not trying to prove that one behavior causes another (experimental research) but rather to evaluate the positive and negative relationships that exist between certain variables. In addition, the researcher is trying to observe the strength of a positive or negative influence that particular variables may have on each other. For instance, a positive relationship exists between performance on intelligence tests and school achievement. The higher the child scores on intelligence tests, the higher will be his or her achievement levels in school.

Interviews and *surveys* are used in conjunction with observational or correlational studies to collect information about a person's behavior in the past (*retrospective studies*) or his or her current attitudes about an issue. These methods can be used to collect information from large groups. Surveys and questionnaires are not useful in examining the self-reported behaviors and actions of very young children because they do not have the cognitive and developmental skills to complete the tools. Although parents can be asked to respond for or about the children, or the researcher can ask the child the survey questions and write down the child's answer, these methods may not present a true picture of the child.

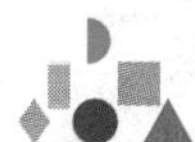

Factors Influencing Development

The research contributions of psychologists and others interested in human development have made it increasingly evident that no single factor can explain the intricacies of growth and change from infancy to old age. Rather, a multiplicity of factors interplay and are so interrelated that it is often difficult to relate an individual's behavior or growth pattern to any specific origin. Heredity, environment, the family, and the community are all major ingredients that interact in different ways to create the uniqueness of each person. Biological factors are those agents that affect patterns of growth by primarily influencing physiologic aspects of the child's development. Subsequent emotional and behavioral patterns or actions in the child may also occur. For instance, nutrition can have an impact on the child's weight gain as well as the development of strong bones and teeth. The child with poor nutrition may also experience irritability and have difficulty concentrating. Environmental factors are the psychological and social extrinsic influences that affect the child's development. Factors such as parenting practices, interactions with peers, and frequent hospitalizations are examples of the extrinsic factors that influence individual development.

Biological Factors

From the moment of conception the role of genetics and prenatal exposures have a tremendous influence on the normal growth and development of the fetus. Throughout the child's life span, several biological factors can impede physical, behavioral, and emotional growth (Chart 4–3). For instance, postnatally, the infant is exposed to an environment that challenges the child's developing immune system. As the child continues to grow, good nutritional practices and health surveillance activities can promote optimum development. On the other hand, physical trauma, ongoing exposures to chemicals, communicable diseases, and the outcomes of natural disasters are all factors that can dramatically change the growth and developmental patterns of the previously healthy child (Chart 4–4). Children "at risk" for developmental problems include those affected by illnesses that impair sensory organs, such as blindness and deafness, and those that contribute to frequent hospitalizations, such as cancer and chronic respiratory conditions (Curry & Duby, 1994). Behavior and emotional maturity can be impacted by the processes encountered when a family is trying to cope with the severe chronic or terminal illness of a young family member. Trauma and illness can cause the child to regress developmentally. These regressive actions and behaviors may be permanent if critical functions of the body have been affected. For example, the ability to walk without an assistive device may no longer be possible for a child who was involved in a motor vehicle accident.

Heredity

Heredity refers to all of the genetic factors that influence who the child is and who he or she will become. A child's biological traits, the determination of gender, and the presence of certain illnesses can be directly linked to genetic inheritance. In addition, studies are being conducted to determine the role of heredity on the presence of certain behavioral traits, such as homosexuality, addictive behaviors, and violent behaviors. The child's genes and chromosomes carry specialized codes that have instructions to determine the child's eye color, height, pre-

Chart 4–3

Biological Risk Factors Affecting Growth and Development

Prenatal and Perinatal Period	Course of Childhood
Genetic or metabolic disorders	Complicated perinatal course
Prematurity	Head injuries
Postmaturity	Lead poisoning
Intrauterine exposures	Failure to thrive
Complicated pregnancy	Malnutrition
Maternal drug/alcohol use during pregnancy	Recurrent otitis media
Congenitally acquired infections	Severe chronic illness
Maternal age <15 yr or >35 yr	Vision and hearing problems
Birth weight less than 1500 g	Physical abuse
O_2 therapy greater than 28 days	Central nervous system infections (meningitis, encephalitis)
Apgar score of 0–3 at 5 minutes	Use of drugs and alcohol
Persistent pulmonary hypertension	Exposure to chemicals
Seizures	Communicable diseases
Symptomatic polycythemia requiring exchange transfusion	Injury related to natural disasters
Presence of congenital anomalies	Temperament
Intrauterine growth retardation	Family history of deafness or blindness
Mother infected with human immunodeficiency virus	Seizure disorder
Anticonvulsants, antineoplastics, or anticoagulants used by mother	Mild to severe mental retardation

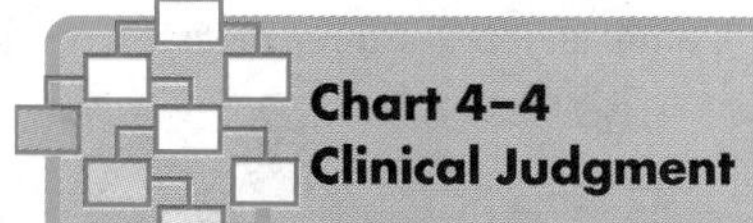

Chart 4–4
Clinical Judgment

Health Promotion During Pregnancy

Leticia is a 17-year-old mother of a 2-year-old girl. She lives in a small apartment with her current boyfriend and her daughter. Although she has not been to see a doctor, she has recently discovered that she is 2 months pregnant. Today Leticia fainted in class and was brought to the health office. She states that she has been so nauseated that she skipped breakfast that morning, "We had no milk for cereal, so I just gave my little girl some cookies, but I did not want any." Her clothes smell of cigarette smoke.

Questions

1. What other information do you need to obtain from Leticia?
2. Of the information she has shared with you, which points will have an effect on your plan of action?
3. What are your major concerns regarding Leticia's health?
4. What interventions should you take at this time?
5. One month later, Leticia stops by the health office to say hello. How would you determine whether Leticia was taking good care of herself as her pregnancy progressed?

Answers

1. Does she have a regular health care provider or know how to access a provider?
   Determine the date of her last menstrual cycle.
   Elicit information regarding her last pregnancy and any complications.
   Assess the dietary patterns of Leticia and her family over the past several days.
   Determine whether Leticia is exposing the fetus to any teratogenic agents.
   Determine whether Leticia is receiving any federal or state assistance to provide for her physical needs or those of her daughter.
2. Leticia is a growing adolescent who is now pregnant. Leticia has not seen a health care provider. Leticia is providing herself and her daughter with inappropriate nutrition.
3. Altered nutrition: Less than body requirements related to poor dietary choices and lack of knowledge regarding dietary needs of the pregnant woman
   Altered health maintenance related to lack of knowledge of her physical needs during pregnancy
   Knowledge deficit: nutritional needs of the toddler
4. Provide Leticia with the telephone number and address of a health care provider.
   Discuss the relationship between nutrition, smoking, other teratogens, and the development of the baby.
   Discuss the dietary needs of pregnant women and how these compare with the needs of small children and adult men.
   Discuss interventions to prevent and manage nausea.
5. Leticia tells you that she saw the nurse midwife and she is now 13 weeks pregnant.
   She states that she has cut down her smoking to two cigarettes a day.
   She states that she is no longer nauseated, but eating crackers before she got up in the morning really helped.
   She is snacking on an apple and drinking milk.

disposition for certain illnesses, and even the triggers that make all of the metabolic pathways work correctly.

The three primary patterns of inheritance are dominant inheritance, recessive inheritance, and X-linked inheritance (Fig. 4–3). These patterns of inheritance influence the transmission of traits such as eye and hair color and the appearance of genetic defects. Several conditions in children can be attributed to genetic abnormalities (Chart 4–5). Through the use of genetic screening techniques such as amniocentesis, chorionic villus sampling, and genetic counseling, many chromosomal aberrations and other disorders can be detected before conception or in the developing fetus. A discussion of these diagnostic techniques is presented in Chapter 8 with a detailed description of some of the genetic abnormalities.

Gender

During the early stages of conception, the child's gender is determined by the joining of the sex chromosomes.

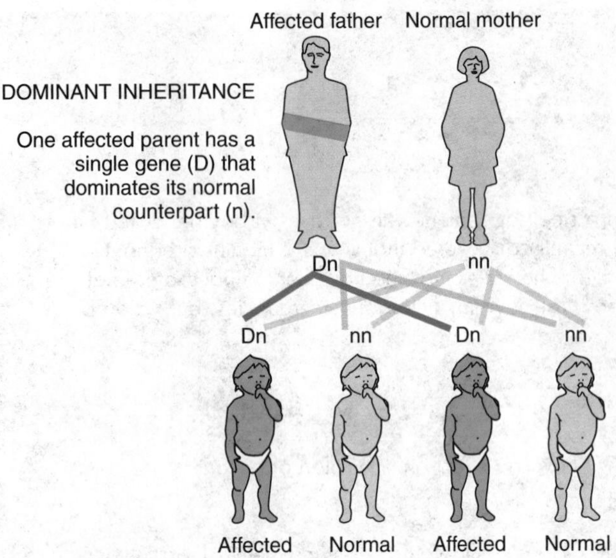
Affected father Normal mother
DOMINANT INHERITANCE
One affected parent has a single gene (D) that dominates its normal counterpart (n).
Dn
nn
Dn
nn
Dn
nn
Affected
Normal
Affected
Normal
Each child has a 50% chance of inheriting either the D or the n from the affected parent.
A

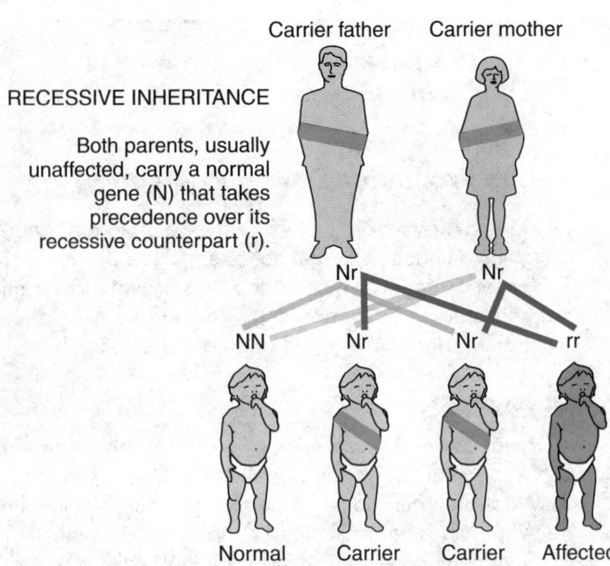
Carrier father Carrier mother
RECESSIVE INHERITANCE
Both parents, usually unaffected, carry a normal gene (N) that takes precedence over its recessive counterpart (r).
Nr
Nr
NN
Nr
Nr
rr
Normal
Carrier
Carrier
Affected
Each child has a 25% chance of inheriting two r genes, which may cause a serious birth defect; a 25% chance of inheriting two Ns, and thus being unaffected; and a 50% chance of being a carrier, like both parents.
B

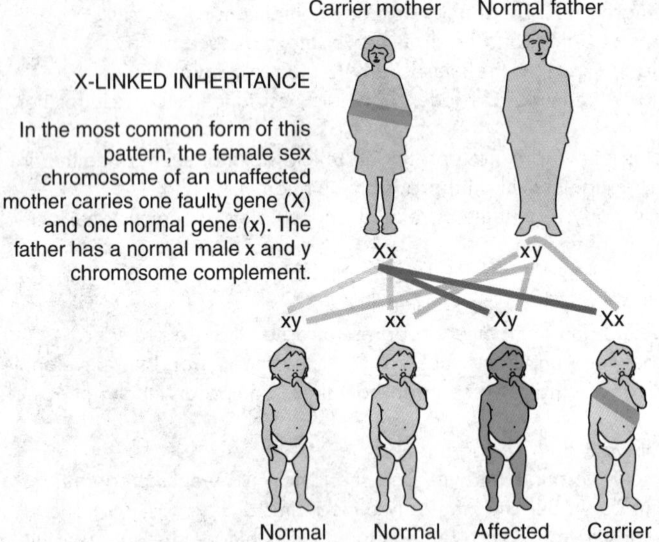
Carrier mother Normal father
X-LINKED INHERITANCE
In the most common form of this pattern, the female sex chromosome of an unaffected mother carries one faulty gene (X) and one normal gene (x). The father has a normal male x and y chromosome complement.
Xx
xy
xy
xx
Xy
Xx
Normal
Normal
Affected
Carrier
Each male child has a 50% chance of inheriting the faulty X and the disorder, and a 50% chance of inheriting the normal x and y. Each female child has a 50% chance of inheriting the faulty X, and thus to be a carrier like the mother, and a 50% chance of *not* inheriting the faulty X.
C

Figure 4–3
Patterns of inheritance. *A*, Dominant inheritance. *B*, Recessive inheritance. *C*, X-linked inheritance.

There are two X chromosomes in females and one X and one Y chromosome in males. From this moment on, the child's gender affects a myriad of physical, personal, and social factors related to the child's growth and development. Internal and external gender-specific biological differences are present at birth and continue to be demonstrated over the course of the person's life. The most obvious biological difference is the presence of either male or female genitalia. Other physical traits influenced by gender include hair distribution, height, and body

Chart 4–5

Examples of the Genetic Origin of Illnesses and Conditions in Children

Down syndrome (trisomy 21)
Klinefelter's syndrome (XXY)
Double Y syndrome (XYY)
Trisomy X (XXX)
Turner's syndrome (XO)
Edwards' syndrome (trisomy 18)
Patau's syndrome (trisomy 13)
Mosaic trisomy 8 (trisomy 8)

physique. Overall health and "survival of the fittest" is also influenced by gender. Some diseases are noted to be more prevalent in one gender over another. Scoliosis is more prevalent in females, and hemophilia, muscular dystrophy, and colorblindness are more common in males. Females, in general, have a longer life span than males. In addition, premature female infants have a higher survival rate than do premature male infants.

Gender identification is the process by which children acquire the attitudes and behaviors deemed by their culture as appropriate for members of their sex (Freiberg, 1987). This process continues throughout the course of the child's development. Gender-based interactions with family members and peers, activities, personal-social attributes, and societal values interplay to influence the way in which children perceive themselves as gender typed.

Race and Ethnicity

The child's race and ethnicity influence patterns of growth and development in both obvious ways and in subtle ways. Race refers to the biophysiologic characteristics of a population group that make it different from others. A child's ethnicity refers to the common social and cultural values, mores, and traditions that are passed on from one generation to the next and that create a sense of identity among members of the ethnic group. Easily visible are the influences of race on physical attributes such as skin color, hair color, body size, and physique. More difficult to describe are the influences of ethnicity on personal mannerisms, social interactions, responses to pain, and the development of one's self-concept. It is known that the incidence of specific malformations varies from race to race (Chart 4–6). In addition, certain physical variations and minor abnormalities may be considered normal findings among children of the same race. For instance, epicanthal folds are normally seen in Asian children and in some non-Asian children. Epicanthal folds are the vertical folds of skin that partially or completely cover the inner canthi of the eye. Epicanthal folds may indicate Down syndrome, glycogen storage disease, or renal agenesis. Similarly, lordosis (excessive backward concavity of the spine) is commonly seen as a normal finding in black females.

Prenatal Exposures

There are a number of drugs, chemicals, and maternal illnesses that have been linked to birth defects in children. The agents that can cause birth defects are called *teratogens*. The effects of prenatal exposures depend on the characteristics of the chemical agent, maternal and fetal physiology, placental factors, and the time during fetal development in which the exposure took place (Kaplan, 1991; Kraemer, 1997) (see Chapter 8 for the schematic illustration of critical periods in prenatal development in which the fetus is highly sensitive to teratogens). It is well known that by the fifth week of embryonic development virtually all chemical agents and drugs will cross the placenta (Kraemer, 1997). Many of these agents will have no harmful effects on the growing fetus. Others are known to have direct and predictable negative effects on fetal development. At the same time it is not always easy to predict why some teratogenic agents may affect one fetus more severely than another. For

Chart 4–6

Common Malformations and Diseases Found in Children of Different Population Groups

Disease	Population group
Cystic fibrosis	Northwestern European
Phenylketonuria	Northwestern European
Sickle cell anemia	African and Mediterranean
Tay-Sachs disease	Ashkenazic Jewish
Clubfoot	Polynesians
Cleft lip and palate	Chinese
Neural tube defects	Whites
Postaxial polydactyly	African
Ellis-van Creveld syndrome	Amish Mennonites
Thalassemia	Quebec, Northern New Brunswick Regions
Umbilical hernias	African
Adrenogenital syndrome	Eskimo
Glucose-6-phosphate dehydrogenase (G-6-PD) deficiency	African and Chinese

instance, a pregnant woman who carefully watches her diet and exercises regularly, yet continues to consume alcohol during her pregnancy may, or may not, be delivered of a healthy child. Intervening variables such as the mother's general health, nutritional status, exercise, anxiety, and the lack of prenatal care are factors that may compound the effects of teratogens on the developing fetus. Research regarding the correlations between teratogens and other intervening variables is continuing in an effort to determine both the short-term and the long-term effects of these elements on the growing child.

Table 4–1 presents a summary of the teratogens most commonly associated with alterations in growth and development. Although many of these agents can cause visible physical deformities of the child, a number of the agents also cause damage to the child's neurologic function or lead to a premature delivery (see Chapter 8 for more discussion on teratogens). The long-term sequelae for children exposed to teratogens in utero and for very-low-birth-weight survivors is a topic of considerable investigation at this time. For example, the number of children exposed to cocaine in utero has dramatically increased in the past decade (Pokorni & Stanga, 1996). Cocaine-exposed infants are at risk for adverse birth outcomes such as prematurity and retarded intrauterine growth. In addition, health problems beyond the newborn period that have been noted by researchers include small stature, hypertonia, higher incidence of sudden infant death syndrome, poor motor performance, and depressed interactive abilities (Bresnahan, Brooks, & Zuck-

Table 4–1
Prenatal Exposures Potentially Harmful to the Developing Fetus

Substance(s)	Possible Resulting Harm to Fetus
Alcohol	Fetal alcohol syndrome Small for gestational age
Illicit drugs (e.g., marijuana, cocaine, heroin, LSD)	Intrauterine growth retardation Prematurity Limb abnormalities Chromosomal abnormalities Malformations of the central nervous system
Amphetamines	Cleft palate Blood vessel transposition
Streptomycin	Cranial nerve damage (deafness) Skeletal abnormalities
Tetracycline	Stains tooth enamel Defective tooth formation Inhibits growth of long bones
Iodides	Thyroid gland enlargement Congenital goiter Hypothyroidism Mental retardation
Methotrexate (found in psoriasis preparations)	Multiple fetal anomalies
Podophyllin (found in laxatives)	Multiple fetal anomalies
Phenytoin and trimethadione (used by epileptics)	Heart abnormalities Cleft lip and palate Microcephaly
Nicotine	Small for gestational age Increased risk for spontaneous abortions Stillbirth Prematurity Increased respiratory problems at birth

erman, 1991; Free, Russell, Mills, & Hathaway, 1990; Kelley, Walsh, & Thompson, 1991; Nolan, 1991). Children who are born at low birth weight are more susceptible to illness and developmental delay in the early months of life. During the school-age years these children score significantly lower on achievement tests than children who had normal birth weights and may encounter school failure (Schraeder, Heverly, O'Brien, & Goodman, 1997).

All health care providers share in the responsibilities of preventing perinatal substance exposure, screening for mothers and children at risk, and providing for the needs of the child experiencing physical or developmental challenges due to in-utero exposures. Families at high risk include the young parent, those with low incomes, mobile families, immigrant families, and those with known alcohol or substance abuse.

Worldview: *Fetuses, infants, young children, and pregnant women in poverty are at a disproportionate risk for teratogenic exposures and their detrimental effects. Sociocultural factors that contribute to this risk include poorly regulated work environments, a higher probability of proximity to hazardous waste, a higher prevalence of nutritional deficiencies, adherence to culturally based practices that have been associated with toxic exposures (e.g., use of pottery for cooking), and drinking water from spent chemical tanks and from local wells (Amaya & Ackall, 1996).*

Many families are unaware of the risk factors associated with intake of certain medications, fluids, and dietary substances that contain agents that are harmful to the fetus. Elements in the environment such as toxic wastes and radiation also pose a threat to the fetus. Nurses can play an instrumental role in providing guidance to the family related to environmental health hazards that can affect the unborn child. The nurse should also integrate assessment of living conditions, including sources of drinking water, dietary practices, and environmental hazards in routine perinatal health assessments (Amaya & Ackall, 1996; Brown, Bellinger, & Matthews, 1990).

Nutrition

Although many factors affecting growth and development cannot be influenced by health care interventions, maintaining a focus on appropriate nutrition from conception throughout the life span will positively affect an individual's health and the quality of life. Nutritional requirements change as the body grows and develops. Nutrition is needed to provide the body with energy to perform several vital functions. Energy is needed for basal metabolism, which keeps the body functioning and maintains body heat. The type of nutrition ingested requires certain amounts of energy to convert the food substances into energy that the body can be used for basal metabolism. Nutrition is needed to replenish the body with energy lost from excreta, from normal processes of growth and development, and from activity requirements. Lastly, nutrition is needed by the body systems when they are threatened or weakened by disease to maintain function and support the healing process.

Poor nutrition accounts for several health and developmental problems seen in children throughout the world. Hunger and malnutrition exists even in developed countries such as the United States and Canada. Malnutrition can be caused by several factors and is known to have adverse, and sometimes, irreversible outcomes on the growing child (Chart 4–7). Pregnant women who are malnourished are at a high risk for miscarriages, stillbirths, and premature delivery. If the newborns are carried to term, they may be poorly nourished and small for gestational age. It has been demonstrated that iron deficiency in utero or during the first 2 years of life can cause permanent damage to brain cell function and to subsequent behavior. Positive correlations between iron status and cognitive functioning as demonstrated by lowered scores on developmental, learning, and school achievement tests have been documented in the literature. In addition, the presence of disruptive behaviors, short attention spans, apathy, and irritability in adolescents have been attributed to anemia in the preschool years (Howard-Teplansky, 1992).

Infants who are born preterm are nutritionally at risk. The last trimester is a period of rapid fetal growth in

Chart 4–7

Factors That May Cause Malnutrition

- Lack of adequate food intake to provide the protein and caloric needs of the body
- Social and cultural differences in food habits that may be nutritionally unsound
- Widespread ease and availability of highly processed and often nutritionally inadequate foods
- Lack of adequate nutrition education in schools and in the home
- Complacency regarding food habits
- Overeating of foods that qualitatively and quantitatively do not meet the needs of the body
- The presence of disease or illness that interferes with the ingestion, digestion, and absorption of food and/or that causes higher nutritional needs
- Failure to adjust nutritional intake based on changing levels of activity and rest and on periods of higher metabolic demands (puberty, pregnancy)

which significant nutritional stores are being established. The premature infant requires nutrition to compensate for the energy no longer provided by the mother, to support the considerable growth that will continue in the ensuing weeks, and to compensate for higher energy demands placed on the infant by stress and illness. Immaturity of the premature infant's digestive system and the inadequacy of sucking and swallowing reflexes compromise the child's ability to receive adequate nutrition. The management and survival of preterm infants has greatly improved due to the understanding and use of parenteral nutrition therapy and specialized formulas.

Infants who are severely undernourished can develop *marasmus*, a condition in which the heart becomes weakened and resistance to illness is very low. *Kwashiorkor* is another nutritional problem often found in children who receive diets low in protein after weaning. These children appear listless, apathetic, and inactive. Their legs and abdomen appear edematous. The child is susceptible to illness because of the severe state of protein deficiency.

In the growing child, inadequate nutrition has been associated with lowered intelligence, poor mental health, increased susceptibility to childhood illnesses, stunted physical growth, and alterations in emotional development. For many children, poor nutrition may be one of several variables affecting the child's overall well-being. Poor housing, poor sanitation, little or no medical care, poor child care practices, and limited educational opportunities for the child can interact to affect the child's growth and development. Malnutrition is more common in children who are experiencing other aspects of poverty. Thus it becomes difficult to isolate the singular effects of poor nutrition on the child's growth and development when so many other intervening factors exist. Children are able to recover from the ill effects of poor nutrition if interventions are provided to prevent recurring or prolonged states of malnutrition.

Protein-calorie deficiencies are just one cause of malnutrition in children. The early introduction of solids in infancy can cause malnutrition. Studies have shown that infants who are consistently given solid foods in the first 3 to 4 months of life have poor nutrition from excessive caloric intakes (Weigley, 1990; Winkelstein, 1984). The risk of obesity is higher in these children. Early introduction of solids interferes with formula feeding and with breastfeeding, may trigger allergies, increases the chance of the infant choking, and can lead to overfeeding. Malnutrition can also be seen in the child who comes to school each day without having had breakfast. This child will have difficulty concentrating and being attentive in school.

In the older child, malnutrition is observed in teens who exist on "fast food" or "junk food" diets. Teens who are left to prepare their own meals may not consistently make nutritious selections. In addition, adolescents coping with anorexia and bulimia are at a very high risk for nutritional deficits, which impact growth and development (see Chapter 29 for a discussion of these two disorders). Hair loss, amenorrhea (cessation of the menstrual cycle), sleep disturbances, bradycardia, cold intolerance, dry skin, and constipation are just a few of the physiologic manifestations of anorexia and bulimia. Preoccupation with food, an obsession with food rituals, and altered family and interpersonal relationships are some of the behavioral manifestations of these illnesses (Muscari, 1988).

Environmental Factors

In addition to the importance of biological factors on development, attention must also be given to the environmental factors that impact individual patterns of growth and development. Although some children may be developmentally disadvantaged because of alterations caused by a biological factor, opportunities to maximize the child's potential can come through the psychosocial, familial, and community assets that enhance development. These include positive relations developed within the family system, exposure to a wide variety of learning opportunities, and a community that socially and politically supports the child and the family.

At the same time, physically healthy children who have limited early social, educational, and environmental experiences are "at risk" for developmental delays. Children who experience parental deprivation, abusive family relationships, or limited social contacts with other children their age will have difficulty achieving developmental norms unless early intervention is provided to alter the child's developmental trajectory (Needlman, 1996). Other vulnerable children include teenage mothers, those who live in poverty, and children who are hospitalized frequently. The family and the community are the environments in which the child will thrive and grow. The relationships and interactions established within these environments will serve as patterns or blueprints for the child's developing social relations and personal life skills. Within these social contexts, many factors interplay to contribute to the child's development (Chart 4–8).

Temperament

The child's characteristic way of thinking, responding, and behaving is referred to as *temperament* (Chess & Thomas, 1992). Temperament is considered to be intrinsic, that is, children are born predisposed to respond to their environment in very different ways (Gross & Conrad, 1995). Temperament becomes an extrinsic factor affecting the child's development because of the interactional patterns that occur between the child and his or

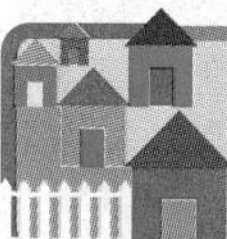

Chart 4–8
Community Care

Environmental Factors Impacting Growth and Development

The Family	The Community
Poor prenatal care*	Lack of adequate social supports
Parents with disabilities*	Poverty*
Parental drug or alcohol use*	Mass media
Maternal deprivation	Political climate
Maternal depression*	Academic resources
Parent and child temperament	Culture
Quality of parent and child interactions	Community violence
Prolonged hospitalization*	Interactions with caregivers
Educational background of parents	School
Financial status	Social acceptance
Child abuse or neglect*	
Homelessness*	
Teenage mother	
Number of children in family	
Family structure	
Relations among siblings	
Relocation	
Influence of spirituality	
Loss of loved one	
Family functioning	
Discipline	
Friends	
Family	
Family travel and recreation	
Position of child in family	
Personal needs and concerns of parents	

* Considered "at risk" factors.

her environment as a result of the child's characteristic way of behaving.

Through the longitudinal research completed by Chess and Thomas, nine temperament categories have been defined (Chess, 1990; Chess & Thomas, 1985, 1986; Thomas & Chess, 1977). The temperament categories are presented in Table 4–2. Individual temperament characteristics are apparent within the first few months of life and are easily identified by the end of the first year. From combinations of the nine characteristics, three temperamental styles or groups have emerged:

- *Easy child*—characterized by regularity, positive approach to new stimuli, very adaptable to change, and predominately has a positive mood.
- *Difficult child*—characterized by irregularity in biological functions, negative approach to new stimuli, slow adaptability, and intense mood expressions that are usually negative.
- *Slow to warm-up child*—characterized by a combination of behaviors that are marked by withdrawal tendencies to the new, slow adaptability, and negative mood expressions of low intensity. Less irregularity is noted in biological functions. This child is often labeled "shy" (Chess, 1990; Chess & Thomas, 1985).

Temperament is believed to have a major impact on behavior and development. The child's temperament influences the dynamic interactions between the child and other people in his or her environment, particularly parents, other family members, teachers, and peers. To explain the healthy or pathologic interactions between the child and the environment, a model of "goodness of fit" and "poorness of fit" was developed by Chess and Thomas (1986). Goodness of fit occurs when the environmental expectations and demands of parents and others are consonant, or in harmony, with the child's temperamental characteristics. When goodness of fit is present, healthy functioning and development can occur. Conversely, poorness of fit is characterized by dissonance between environmental demands and the child's capabilities and temperament style. Poorness of fit is likely to lead to the development of behavior problems and poor parent–child interaction patterns. Thus difficulties can arise when the child's temperament is in conflict with the parent's own behavioral style. For instance, an active child may be quite a challenge for parents who are more low key. A child who has erratic patterns for eating and sleeping may be a behavioral challenge to the grandparents who are very time oriented and orderly in their daily activities.

All of the temperament styles may enhance positive or negative development and behavior (Melvin, 1995). What is more important than the child's particular temperament characteristics is the presence of a good fit in the interactions of the child with the environment.

Parents often think that their biological children should be born with many of their own behavioral characteristics and with a similar disposition. Parents need to learn about their child's temperamental characteristics so that they can be more accepting of the unique qualities in their child.

Several intervention programs have been developed to help parents learn to manage the temperament of

Table 4–2
Temperament Categories

Category	Definition	Examples of Characteristic Behaviors
Activity	Amount of physical energy that drives the child in most situations; includes proportion of active and inactive periods.	Low activity—moves at a slower pace; prefers inactive pastimes such as coloring or playing quietly with toys. High activity—full of energy, fidgety when asked to sit still, restless on days when has to stay inside, and tends to be impulsive (acting before thinking).
Rhythmicity	Predictability or unpredictability of the child's biological patterns such as sleep, hunger, and elimination.	Very rhythmic—regular sleep patterns; will get tired at almost the same time each day; will have a bowel movement every morning around the same time. Arrhythmic—irregular sleep patterns; gets tired at different times each day; bowel movements not predictable.
Approach or withdrawal	Typical initial response of the child to a new stimulus such as a new food, toy, person, or situation.	Approachable—jumps right in to new situations without hesitation. Withdrawn—holds back in a new situation until feels comfortable.
Adaptability	Relative ease or difficulty in negotiating an effective response to a new situation.	Very adaptable—tends to be compliant, cooperative, and go with the flow. Slowly adapts—tends to be stubborn, strong willed, or headstrong.
Threshold of responsiveness	Level of stimulation that evokes a response; how sensitive a child is in each sense—touch, pain, hearing, smell, and vision.	High threshold—does not seem to be sensitive to environmental stimuli that affects the senses (ex. will be able to wear most any clothes, even those that are tight fitting because of high threshold to touch). Low threshold—highly sensitive to stimuli that affects the senses (ex. always likes to smell things and may refuse to wear certain clothes because they feel "funny").
Intensity of reaction	Amount of energy used to express emotions and actions.	Low intensity—expresses emotions quietly and in a low-keyed fashion. High intensity—tends to be loud and dramatic when expressing emotions.
Quality of mood	Amount of pleasant, joyful, and friendly behavior compared with amount of unpleasant and unfriendly behavior.	Positive mood—views the world through rose-colored glasses; tends to miss negative and notice positive things. Negative mood—tends to miss positive and notice negative things.
Distractibility	Degree in which extraneous environmental stimuli can be distracting and interfere with ongoing behavior.	Low distractibility—gets caught up in what he or she is paying attention to and may not notice the things going on in environment High distractibility—tends to shift attention quickly and often; may get easily sidetracked when trying to complete a task.
Attention span and persistence	Length of time and activity is pursued along with the child's capacity to continue the activity despite obstacles.	High persistence—tends to stick with difficult tasks and may not give up even when a task is well beyond his or her skill level. Low persistence—tends to become frustrated and may quickly ask for help, get angry, or simply give up on a difficult task.

Adapted from Chess, S. (1990). Studies in temperament: A paradigm in psychosocial research. *The Yale Journal of Biology and Medicine, 63,* 313–324; and Temperament Intervention for Parents Study (TIPS). (1994). *Temperament dimensions: Definitions.* Tempe, AZ: Author. Used with permission.

their child (Gross & Conrad, 1995; McClowry, 1995; Medoff-Cooper, 1995; Melvin, 1995; Wallace, 1995). The first goal of a temperament-based intervention program is to help parents understand the unique characteristics of their child. Standardized temperament questionnaires are usually used to assist in this process. Next parents are taught how temperament is related to behavior. Lastly, the parents or caregivers are assisted in developing strategies to manage their child based on the child's temperament. When parents verbalize frustration with their child's behavior, the nurse who is informed about temperament-based interventions can offer guidance to families that will foster the child's development and enhance the parent–child interactions.

The Family

The foundation of the growing child's world is built on the environment and exchanges that occur within the family system. The family has a profound effect on every aspect of the child's growth and development. It is within the family that the child learns about gender and social roles, self-acceptance, and self-control. Within the family milieu the child learns ways of interacting with others to meet his or her personal goals and needs. The provisions of food, shelter, and clothing that are provided by the family organization have previously been noted to profoundly affect the growth and development of the maturing child.

It is interesting to note how two children raised in the same family environment can be so different from one another. Genetically, siblings are similar; they share the same parents and the same home environment, yet their experiences in the family are different enough to create very individual and unique personal qualities. Factors that are attributed to the development of these differences include birth order, the age gap between siblings, gender, family size, birthing experience, illnesses of childhood, temperament, sibling behavior, and parenting behavior. Table 4–3 summarizes some of the research findings regarding how these factors influence personal development.

caREminder: *In the assessment of large groups of children and their families, whereas certain correlations may emerge, individual families may not follow the statistical trends. Therefore, it would be inappropriate to tell a person that, because she was the fifth-born female child, separated in age by 10 years from the next older sibling, she will probably not be a high achiever.*

Child-Rearing Practices. Parenting behaviors and child-rearing practices are important factors in determining how children will develop. The quality of interactions among the child, the parents, and the siblings influences the relationships that the child will have with others outside the home. If the parents are overly concerned with their personal needs, their children can perceive this preoccupation as a rejection of themselves. Some of the differences between siblings can be attributed to the functioning of the emotional unit at the time each child was born (Donley, 1993). The variables that affect this emotional unit include the anxiety in the family at the time of each child's birth, characteristics of the child that trigger certain processes in the family, the intensity and direction of relationships, and how the parents relate emotionally to their extended family (Donley, 1993).

Other Family Variables. Several other family variables will influence the development of the child. These include the family structure, family functioning, and family role modeling (discussed in Chapter 3). Family conditions that place the child at risk for school performance problems include divorce, parental unemployment, single-parent households, working mothers, and violence within the home (Reed, McMillan, & McBee, 1995). The influence of relocation, discipline, travel, play, family finances, and loss of a parent or significant other are among the many variables that impact the child as he or she interacts within the family constellation over the course of time.

Family Violence. *Family violence* is defined as a crime committed by a family member or a relative. *Interpersonal violence* is considered the intentional use of physical force against another person that results in injury or death (Ozmar, 1994). Types of interpersonal violence that can occur in the family are child abuse (emotional or physical), sexual assault, spousal abuse, elder abuse, and homicide. Although many cases are detected and reported to the police, it is believed that four times as many cases are unreported (Castiglia, 1995).

A child may be either the direct recipient of violence or a witness to family violence. The child affected by violence against himself or herself will suffer from physical and psychological trauma that impairs normal growth and development. These issues are discussed in more detail in Chapter 29. For the child who is a witness to violence directed toward other family members, physical injury may not impair the child's growth but psychological injury can greatly impact the child's development. It has been estimated that one half of the women and one fourth of the men in psychiatric hospitals are victims of some form of family violence (Eaton, 1994). Children affected by family violence are at risk for low self-esteem, inability to maintain a relationship, and inability to engage in healthy sexual relations as an adult.

The Community

The community encompasses all of the influences provided by interaction with daycare providers, peers, school

Table 4–3
Sample of Factors Within the Family That May Influence Personal Development

Factors	Traits
Birth order	First-borns score higher on IQ tests (Jarman & Oberklaid, 1992). First-borns show greater academic achievement, are more career oriented, and become more successful as adults (Jarman & Oberklaid, 1992). First-born and only children have more advanced language skills than do later-born children (Jarman & Oberklaid, 1992). Fathers tend to talk more to their first-born child than to their later-born child (Jarman & Oberklaid, 1992).
Only children	Only children distinguish themselves in the achievement and intelligence areas when compared with children with siblings (Falbo & Polit-O'Hara, 1985). In personality and adjustment areas, only children are found to be more advantaged than children from medium or large families (Falbo & Polit-O'Hara, 1985).
Spacing between sibling age	Spacing intervals of at least 2 years have been associated with improved verbal ability and academic success of older children (Jarman & Oberklaid, 1992).
Family size	Children from smaller families are generally more intelligent and academically successful and have higher self-esteem than children from large families (Jarman & Oberklaid, 1992).
Gender	Most studies do not find boys more active than girls in the first 3 years of life (Jacklin, 1992). Aggression is slightly higher in boys than in girls (Maccoby & Jacklin, 1980). Tests of intellectual abilities show few differences between boys and girls (Jacklin, 1992). Mothers have been shown to engage in more play with their second-born child if that child differs in sex from the first-born child (Jarman & Oberklaid, 1992).
Temperament	Children with the "difficult child" pattern are more vulnerable to the development of behavioral problems in early and middle childhood (Chess & Thomas, 1992). No differences in "difficult child" temperament are found between girls and boys (Jacklin, 1992). Girls show more timidity than boys (Jacklin, 1992).
Parenting practices	Parents of children who had health problems in infancy have been noted to display parenting disorders ranging from persistent concern about minor infant problems to continued fear that their child may die even after the health problems have been resolved. These parenting concerns have been noted to cause severe emotional disturbances in children (Ladden, 1990). Parents who experienced secure attachments with their parents and saw themselves as having a warm, loving marriage seemed to adapt better to marriage and subsequently to parenting (Belsky & Isabella, 1985).

officials, religious leaders, and social acquaintances. These interactions take place within the context of a social culture that provides boundaries for acceptable and unacceptable patterns of behavior. Role expectations, sex stereotyping, and age-specific norms must be evaluated within the parameters of the community milieu at a given point in time. For instance, encouraging adolescent girls to marry and bear children may be a socially expected developmental task in some communities. However, in the United States, this practice is generally not encouraged, because the adolescent female is not considered to be emotionally, physically, or cognitively ready to accept parenting responsibilities. On the other hand, within the broader community, smaller communities exist that may encourage and foster other developmental expectations of the growing child.

Public priorities and the mass media can have profound effects on children. The political and societal issues that have affected child rearing and child health care practices are discussed in Chapter 2. These include the funding and provision of mandated health service for children identified as "at risk," and the legislation that ensures that the rights of all children are protected. Public priorities are often reflected by the mass media, which in turn can influence a child's perception of socially acceptable behaviors and expectations. The results of research that has examined the effects of viewing violence on television on children's mental health suggest that there may be a causal relationship between television violence and violence in real life. The researchers have noted both psychological and physiologic changes in children who view violence on television (Groer & Howell, 1990). A more thorough discussion of the influences of the media and suggestions regarding how parents and caregivers can monitor and modify these influences are presented in Chapter 5.

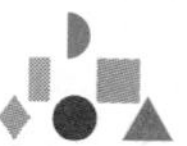

Biological Growth of the Child

As children grow, the most profound changes noted by the casual observer lie in the physical development of the child's body. The annual exchange of holiday pictures among distant friends seems to heighten awareness of how rapidly a child's size and appearance can change in only 1 year (Fig. 4–4). External and internal body structures and functions will undergo changes that are influenced by the child's gender and age, the child's nutritional status, the presence or absence of disease, and the individual genetic attributes of a particular child.

Figure 4–4
Yearly exchange of photographs illustrates how dramatically children change in their appearance over a relatively short period.

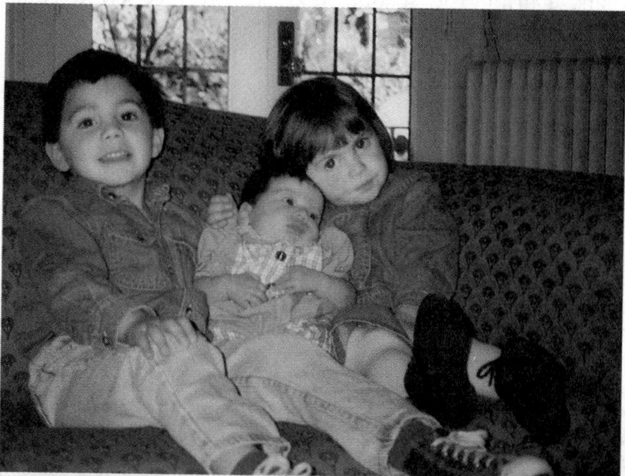

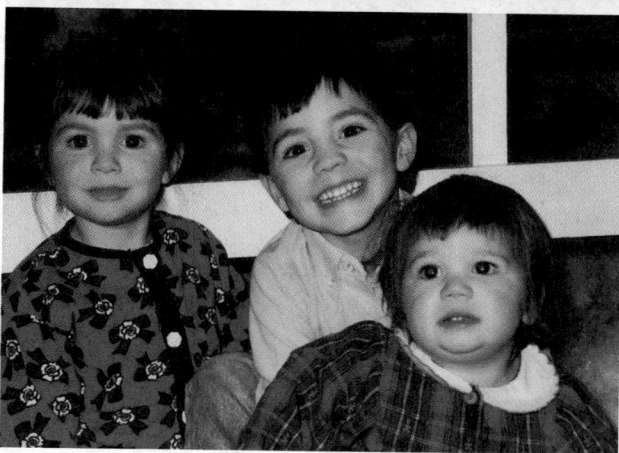

Development of the Fetus

By the time a pregnant woman has missed her menstrual period, the embryo developing within her has implanted in the uterus, uteroplacental circulation has begun, and a primitive neural tube and blood vessels have been formed. This is the *embryo stage,* extending from implantation until the end of the second month. During this period the embryonic disk is composed of three layers that develop into the major organs and tissues. The ectoderm is the rudimentary formation for the nervous system, skin, hair, nails, and sensory organs. The endoderm develops into the mucous membranes of the mouth and anus; the bladder and urethra; endocrine glands such as the thyroid, parathyroid and thymus glands; the tonsils; respiratory tract; and lining of the gastrointestinal system. Major components of the musculoskeletal, genitourinary, reproductive, and cardiac systems arise from the mesoderm. Tendons, muscles, cartilage, bones, connective tissue, kidneys, ureters, heart, circulatory system, blood cells, and all reproductive organs are mesodermic. During the fourth through the eighth weeks, growth of the cranial and caudal ends and the budding of arms and legs produce a human-like shape to the mass of embryonic tissue.

At 9 weeks of gestation, the *fetal period* begins. Over the ensuing weeks, growth of the fetus follows certain predictable patterns (see schematic illustration of critical periods of development in Fig. 8–6). Although cushioned and protected in the mother's womb, the fetus remains susceptible to the influences of many teratogens that can permanently alter the structure and function of various body systems. Organs that are formed from the same layer of the embryonic disk are often affected by the same teratogen. For instance, the heart and kidneys are both formed from the mesoderm. Therefore, if one of these organs is malformed, an assessment should be completed to evaluate whether the other organ arising from the same layer has also been malformed. Some teratogens are so harmful that the fetus may no longer be viable. Spontaneous abortions that occur during the first trimester may result from these negative outcomes. When a teratogen affects the fetus later in the gestational period, the effects may be noted at birth when the infant presents with physical or functional impairments.

By the 10th week, the face of the fetus is recognizably human. External genitalia are clearly distinguishable by the 12th week. At this time ultrasound evaluation of the fetus can be used to help reveal the child's gender to the expectant parents. By the 20th to the 24th week, primitive alveoli have formed and surfactant production has begun in the lungs. If birth occurs from this point on, viability of the fetus is possible. By the third trimester, structural development is complete, while functional development of the systems continues.

Changes in General Body Growth

From the shape of an oval body to the distinctive features of a human fetus, the child in utero grows in weight and length in a progressive and predictable pattern that continues throughout the childhood years. Failure to grow or growth retardation in utero is termed *intrauterine growth retardation*. Depending on the point in pregnancy when intrauterine growth retardation appears, early delivery of the infant by cesarean section may be completed. During the eighth month subcutaneous fat is deposited. This fat changes the wrinkled appearance of the fetus to that of a soft, cuddly infant. The fat also aids in thermoregulation. By the third trimester, fetal weight will triple and length will double as the body stores of protein, fat, iron, and calcium increase.

Growth During Infancy

The child's body proportions undergo many changes before adult proportions are achieved (Fig. 4–5). The newborn's head is approximately one fourth of his or her total body length, and the legs are about one third of the body length. The newborn appears top heavy, with short lower extremities.

After an initial small loss of weight, most newborns regain their birth weight within 10 days of delivery. Weight gain during early infancy is approximately 20 g (⅔ ounce) per day. This gain decreases to about 15 g (½ ounce) per day during the middle and latter half of the first year. Infants double their birth weight by 5 months, although some may double their birth weight by 4 months or earlier. Should this occur, evaluation of the child's nutritional status is warranted. Birth weight is usually tripled by the first birthday. The infant's length increases about 50% during the first year. The crown to rump length, or sitting height, measures the same as the head circumference. Head circumference is equivalent to chest circumference during infancy. Almost no variation in head circumference parameters has been found due to racial, national, or geographic standards. However, head circumference varies significantly in relation to body weight. Median head circumference at 1 year of age is approximately 12 cm (4¾ inches) larger than at birth (Pinyerd, 1992).

Growth of the Young Child

As cephalocaudal and proximodistal growth continues during the childhood years, chest circumference will exceed head circumference and the length of the trunk and extremities will surpass the measurement of the upper portion of the body. The rate of growth continues to decelerate in the toddler years and then remains relatively stable throughout the preschool and school-age years. During the second year the average child gains 2.5 kg (5½ lb), grows in length by 12 cm (4¾ inches), and increases head circumference by less than 2.5 cm (1 inch). As a general guide, adult stature equals the following:

Boys: 2 × height at age 2 years = adult height
5 × weight at age 2 = adult weight

Girls: 2 × height at 1½ years = adult height
5 × weight at 1½ years = adult weight

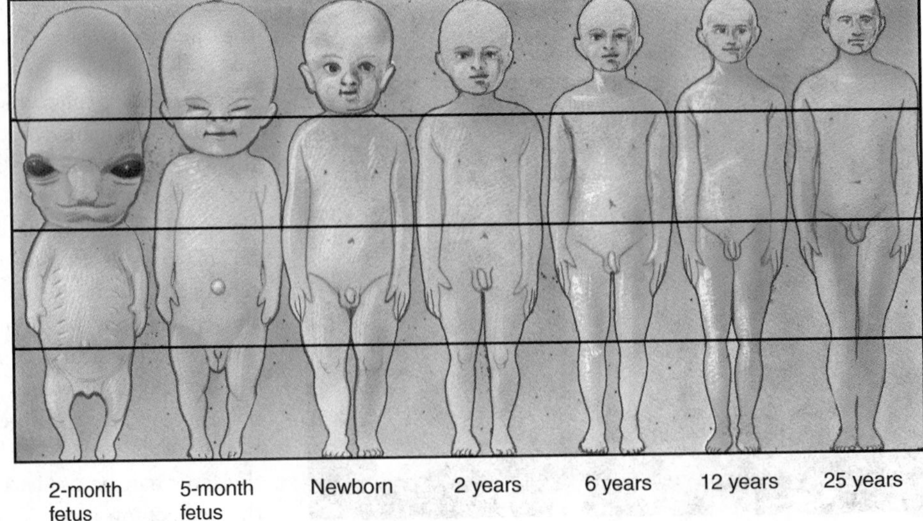

Figure 4–5
Changes in body proportion from the second fetal month to adulthood. (Redrawn from Robbins, W., Brodey S., Hogan, A., et al. [1928]. *Growth*. New Haven, CT: Yale University Press. Used with permission.)

From ages 3 to 7 the average child gains 2 kg (4½ lb) in weight and 7 cm (2¾ inches) in length per year. During the school years, the average weight gain is 3 kg (6½ lb) per year and the average change in stature is an increase of 6 cm (2¼ inches) per year. Accelerated growth changes that are characteristic of the pubertal period may occur as early as 10 years of age in girls and around 12 years of age in boys.

Adolescent Growth

Before puberty, growth in stature predominates in the lower extremities whereas during puberty, truncal growth predominates. The distal extremities reach adult size before the proximal extremities, thus the common complaint among preadolescents that their feet are too big. In association with the hormonal, physical, and emotional changes that occur during puberty the adolescent experiences a period of growth acceleration. Age at onset, peak, and termination vary considerably from one person to another. Females tend to experience the growth spurt and other pubertal changes approximately 2 years ahead of males. Therefore, although previous to this period the mean height of girls was smaller than that of boys, the girls catch up and surpass boys in stature during early adolescence (ages 11 to 13). Girls achieve mature stature sooner than boys. The male growth spurt, although slower to begin, is of a longer duration. By the completion of the adolescent years the boys will surpass the girls in height. During adolescence, boys gain at least 10 cm (4 inches) in height and girls about 8 cm (3 inches). A small amount of growth in stature may occur after age 18, especially in boys. By the end of adolescence, mature stature is about 3.4 times birth length and mature body weight is about 20 times birth weight unless the individual is obese or underweight.

Growth Measurements

Systematic notation of the changes in the child's body proportions is an important aspect of developmental surveillance. Alterations in length, weight, head circumference, and chest circumference from normative standards could indicate the presence of a clinical condition that requires further intervention by the health care team. The most important tools in the evaluation of somatic growth are growth charts constructed by longitudinal, serial measurements of large numbers of children at different ages over a brief period of time. Although physical measurements of a child at a single point in time provide some useful clinical information, serial measurements over months or years provide the most accurate record of the infant's or child's overall general pattern of growth. The physical measurements most often used in assessing children are height and weight, and in infants and young children through age 36 months head circumference is used. All these measurements should be made with care and with the use of a consistent technique.

Of the different growth charts currently available, the most recent were published by the National Center for Health Statistics (NCHS) and provide an important bench marking tool for measuring the growth of children from term birth through adolescence (see Appendix 1). The NCHS charts available for boys and girls cover the following:

- *Birth to 36 months:* recumbent length for age, weight for age, weight for length, and head circumference
- *Two to 18 years:* length for age and weight for age
- *Prepubescence:* age independent, evaluating weight-for-stature percentiles for children before, but not after, the appearance of secondary sex characteristics such as breast development and the presence of pubic or axillary hair.

caREminder: *When using the birth to 36-month interval chart the child should be weighed nude and length should be measured in the recumbent position. For the 2- to 18-year interval charts the child may wear light clothing during weight measurement and upright stature is measured in stocking feet.*

The NCHS tools have been standardized based on following these methods for accurately obtaining the child's weight and length. If recumbent length (used only on the birth to 36-month interval chart) is substituted for stature (standing height) on the 2- to 18-year interval chart, measurement discrepancies up to 2 cm (nearly 1 inch) may be recorded erroneously. Information regarding the clinical methods to assess height, weight, head circumference, and body fat are discussed in Chapter 6.

Each growth chart is composed of seven percentile curves, representing the distribution of weight, length, stature, or head circumference at each age. The percentile lines on these charts indicate the number of normal children expected to fall above and below the index child's measurement. For example, a 6-month-old girl who weighs 7.2 kg is in the 50th percentile for weight; 50% of all healthy 6-month-old female infants will be expected to weigh more and 50% to weigh less. Measurements within the central or intermediate percentiles indicate that growth is within normal limits by current standards. Children who fall either above the 95th or below the 5th percentile require further evaluation, as do children whose height and weight differ by more than two percentile lines or categories. Children who fall off their established pattern for growth for height or weight should be followed more closely for a time with serial measurements and a decision made about the need for further evaluation of growth.

Table 4–4
Causes of Variations in Growth Patterns

	Increase or Accelerated	Decrease or Arrest
Weight	Excessive intake Pregnancy Use of corticosteroids Clinical conditions (e.g., acquired hypothyroidism, Cushing's syndrome) Infants of diabetic mothers	Nutritional deficits Failure to thrive Chronic conditions (e.g., cystic fibrosis, cancer, celiac disease, congenital heart disease) Child abuse (neglect)
Height	Endocrine conditions (e.g., hyperthyroidism, precocious puberty, pituitary gigantism) Klinefelter's syndrome Chromosomal abnormalities (e.g., XXX syndrome in girls) Marfan syndrome	Presence of scoliosis Endocrine disorder (e.g., acquired hypothyroidism, Cushing's syndrome, delayed puberty, Turner's syndrome)
Head circumference	Macrocephaly Hydrocephalus Head trauma	Microcephaly Craniostenosis

For plotting and interpreting growth using a growth chart, it is important to know the age of the child and correct for various factors. In following the growth of an infant born prematurely, subtract the weeks of prematurity from the postnatal age when plotting growth parameters. This correction should continue until 18 months of age for head circumference, 25 months for weight, and 40 months for length, by which times, catch-up growth for the various parameters should be completed.

If growth charts are to be useful assessment tools, their strengths and limitations need to be appreciated. The NCHS data are representative of a population of well-nourished and healthy children in the United States. Although differing from the population in much of the rest of the world, the NCHS charts have been accepted by the World Health Organization (WHO) as the international standard of growth for the first 5 years of life. Disparities in growth between developed and developing countries reflect nutritional rather than genetic differences (Behrman, Kliegman, & Arvine, 1996). The NCHS curves may be less applicable to adolescents as growth during adolescence is linked to the onset of puberty, which can vary widely (Behrman, Kliegman, & Arvin, 1996).

Worldview: *Special challenges may exist in determining the growth standards for internationally adopted children. Correct information regarding the child's gestational age at birth and the child's actual birth date may not be available. Many international adoptees are premature infants. To accurately assess the child, growth and development must be evaluated based on corrected gestational age rather than actual age given by the adoption agency. The age of an older adoptee may not be known. In these cases the physical parameters that may be useful in determining the child's age may be tooth eruption, stage of puberty development, bone age, and, possibly, head circumference.*

The periodic measurement of physical growth may elicit certain findings that should alert the health care provider to the existence of a health problem (Table 4–4). A single significant alteration in height, weight, or head circumference parameters should not cause alarm due to the potential for measurement error. The child who shows a significant change in growth parameters should be monitored closely. The need for growth assessments to be evaluated more frequently than the normal schedule for healthy child visits to the care provider may be warranted.

Musculoskeletal Development

Growth and changes in the musculoskeletal system begin at conception and continue throughout life. Muscular activity is among the primary functions first achieved by the developing fetus. During the fourth to eighth months of gestation, the precursors of skeletal muscle and vertebrae (somites) appear. The back of the forming fetus is bent so the head nearly touches the tail. This tail begins to involute by the eighth week. The presence of arm and leg buds and rudimentary eyes, ears, and nose can be noted. Ossification begins around the eighth week, and the individual assumes a human-like appearance. Fingers, toes, elbows, knees, arms, and legs have all developed. Facial features can now be seen. The first muscle contractions occur, soon followed by lateral flexion movements.

By the end of the first trimester the fetus can move its arms and legs independently of the trunk. By the 17th week, the grasp reflex is present and the fetus can be observed, on ultrasound evaluation, sucking the thumb. By midgestation, the fetus can move its arms and legs just as the newborn can, and, when the mother has periods of rest, is likely to demonstrate a full range of movement inside the womb. This fluttering sensation is called *quickening*. Fetal movements continue in strength and frequency throughout the rest of the pregnancy. By the 29th week, the fetus can kick, suck, and turn, changing positions as needed to find a position of comfort. As the pregnancy nears its completion, these movements can cause discomfort to the mother. During the last 2 months of gestation, further refinement of the musculoskeletal system occurs. Creases in the soles of the feet and an increase in ear cartilage formation occur. The infant born early is missing these features. The neonate at rest will assume the position similar to that maintained in utero. The feet curve inward, the spine is in a rounded position, and the arms remain flexed and close to the body.

The skeleton of the infant and young child is largely made up of preosseous cartilage and physes. The bones are flexible and have a high porosity. The young child's bones can absorb a great deal of energy before breaking and may even bow rather than fracture when a trauma occurs. The young child has an active growth plate at the end of the long bones known as the physeal or epiphyseal plate. Longitudinal growth and alignment of the long bones takes place at the growth plate through the process of endochondral ossification (Fig. 4–6). During this process cartilage becomes ossified, turning it into bone. This process continues until skeletal maturity is complete in adolescence. At that time an increase in androgenic hormones produced during puberty causes the growth plate to gradually stop functioning.

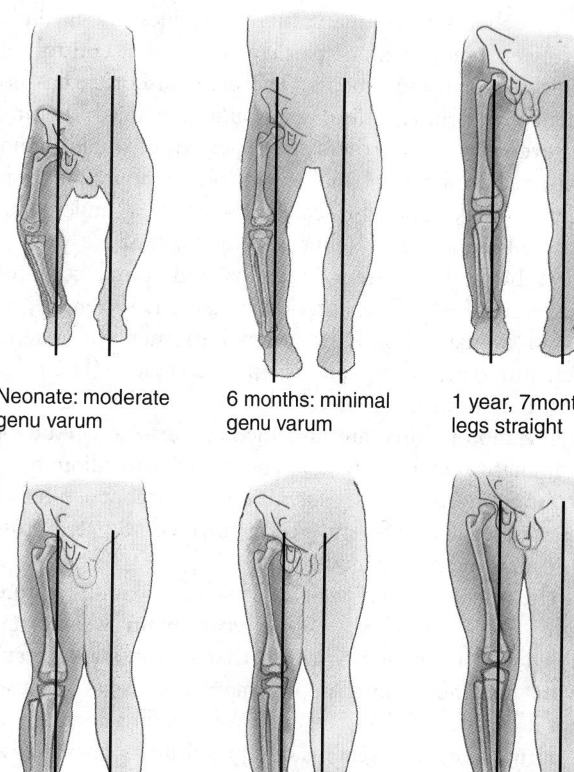

Figure 4–6
The alignment of the child's lower limbs changes throughout the various stages of childhood. (Redrawn from Tachdjian, M. O. [1990]. *Pediatric orthopedics* [2nd ed., vol. 4, p. 2821]. Philadelphia: W. B. Saunders. Used with permission.)

Neurologic Maturation

The neurologic and sensory organs are among the first systems to develop. Functioning of these systems is necessary for the functioning and development of other body systems. The nervous system begins in the first month of gestation as a longitudinal neural plate and neural groove that elongates into a tube with two protrusions at the upper end for the brain. The upper portion will dilate and form the brain, with the remaining portion of the tube forming the spinal cord.

At 8 weeks, the nerves still do not have any anatomic or physiologic connections with either smooth or striated muscle. The embryo is floating freely in the amniotic fluid, with little purposive movement noted. Flexing of the trunk and head extension movements can be elicited in response to tactile stimulation. The hemispheres of the brain become recognizable and cerebellar development is visible.

During the 12th to 14th weeks, the neuromuscular system matures, spreading caudad. By the end of the fourth month the frontal, temporal, parietal, and occipital lobes may be distinguished. Until about the sixth month of gestation, fetal behavior is largely controlled by spinal mechanisms. As maturation continues, the medulla and lower brain centers participate in the control of specific reflexive movements. The cerebral cortex has no influence on behavior until some time after birth. During the seventh month, there is a period of rapid brain growth. Multiplication and expansion of brain function are at a peak, and the cerebral cortex is undergoing additional refinement (Nelms & Mullins, 1982).

At birth, brain stem functions and spinal cord reflexes are present. The autonomic nervous system is intact but immature, and the sympathetic nervous system, which innervates the heart, is still incomplete (Hazinski, 1996). Functions of the cerebral cortex, such as cognition and fine motor skills, are also incomplete. As a result of this immaturity, the infant is able to have cardiorespiratory function and to use reflex movements but is unable to thermoregulate efficiently or to have coordinated gross motor and fine motor movements.

The infant's brain weighs 25% of its adult mature weight (300–350 g). By age 1 year, brain weight has doubled and is about two thirds that of the adult. Brain growth continues until approximately 6 years of age, when it reaches 90% of the adult weight. The increase in size during the early years is due primarily to an increase in nerve fibers and to the development of nerve tracts. At birth, the infant's cranium is not normally fused, allowing for the skull to compress during the birthing process so the head can pass through the narrow birth canal. The sutures of the newborn's skull are easily palpable, with final closure of the cranium not complete until 16 to 18 months of age. The presence of two fontanelles provides a gauge to the processes of cranial fusion. The posterior fontanelle will close at 6 to 8 weeks, with the anterior fontanelle closing at 16 to 18 months.

Neurologic development continues with myelinization and maturation of the neural system becoming complete around age 2. The development of muscle tone, the extinction of reflexes, and the achievement of gross and fine motor skills reflect the continued maturation of the nervous system. The growth of the neuron network permits greater control over large and small muscles that control body movements. Refinement of neural pathways permits the child to have better control and coordination over specific body parts.

Muscle Tone

The mature newborn most often assumes a flexed position of the extremities. It is believed that this flexion pattern is induced by the position of the infant in utero. In infants who are in breech position, flexor positioning of the lower extremities is often absent. The premature infant also demonstrates less motor tone than the term neonate.

The full-term newborn demonstrates increased resistance against gradual stretching (tonic myotactic reflexes) in almost all flexor and in many of the extensor muscles. This can be demonstrated by extending the lower arm of the awake neonate. When released, the arm will recoil to its flexed position. Similarly, a newborn in the standing position has a stepping motion as he or she alternately flexes and extends the lower extremities. Some view this as a reflexive mechanism, whereas other researchers assert that this is a precursor to mature function (Kamm, Thelen, & Jensen, 1990). The demonstration of hypotonia (frog legs) or scissoring with spasticity would be indications that abnormalities in the infant's muscle tone are present.

Reflexes

Reflexive movements that are characteristic of newborn behavior begin to appear by the end of the first trimester. Among the first of the reflexes to appear is the Babinski toe sign (extension of the large toe, with fanning of the small toes on stimulation of the sole of the foot), with later appearance of the swallowing and sucking reflexes.

Reflexive movements of the newborn are indicative of the motor behavior control exerted by the newborn's spinal cord and medulla. Each reflex requires a specific sensory stimulus to generate the stereotyped motor response. As the child matures, motor control expands to different levels of the nervous system. Therefore, many of the reflexes present at birth will normally disappear around the fourth month of age and cannot be elicited by sensory stimulation. These include the Moro reflex, the rooting reflex, and the palmar grasp reflex. Absence of these reflexes or persistence of these reflexes past the period they would normally become extinguished may indicate severe problems of the central nervous system (see Chapter 6).

Gross Motor Development

The acquisition of gross motor skills precedes the development of fine motor skills. Both processes occur in a cephalocaudal fashion, with head control preceding arm and hand control, followed by leg and foot control. All of the extremities move randomly at birth without visible coordination occurring for several months. Movements are symmetrical with no preference shown before 1 year of age for handedness or hemisphere dominance.

Head Control. The newborn has very little head control, and marked head lag is normal. When the infant is pulled by the arms into a semi-Fowler position, the head will be hyperextended and lag behind the alignment of

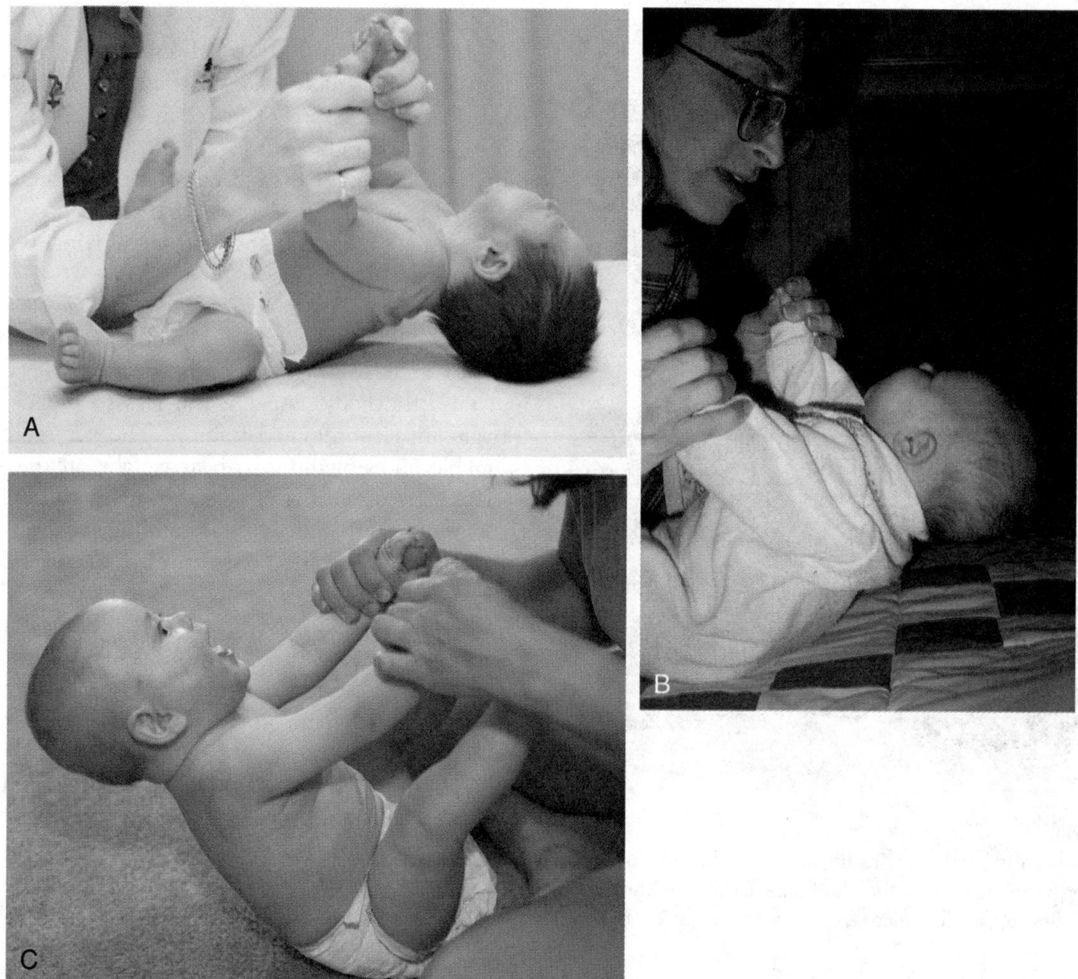

Figure 4–7
A, The newborn has marked head lag when pulled from a lying to a sitting position. B, The 2-month-old demonstrates slight head lag. C, By age 6 months, no head lag is present.

the rest of the body (Fig. 4–7A). In the prone position the infant has the ability to lift the head slightly and move it from side to side (Fig. 4–8A). When placed in a sitting position the infant's head will drop forward onto the chest. Although the infant will attempt to right the head in the correct position, this only serves to make the head flop from one side to another.

At 2 months of age the infant demonstrates slight head lag (see Fig. 4–7B) and is able to hold the head up reasonably well when held in an upright position (Fig. 4–9A). In the prone position the child can turn the head from side to side and can hold the head erect for 20 to 30 seconds at a 45-degree angle.

Between the third and fourth months, the infant achieves the ability to hold the head at 90 degrees and head lag becomes minimal. By the sixth month, head control is well established, as is evidenced by the lack of head lag (see Fig. 4–7C). When prone, the infant lifts the head and upper abdomen off of the surface by weight bearing on the arms (see Fig. 4–8B).

Rolling Over. The newborn is not capable of purposefully rolling the body from one side to the other. When placed in a side-lying position the infant may accidentally roll to a prone or supine position; thus, a blanket roll should be placed behind the infant's back to maintain the infant's body in a stable position. Between 4 and 5 months of age, the infant learns to roll from front to back, then from back to front at between ages 5 and 6 months. Once the child can roll 360 degrees, he or she can then learn to pull to a sitting position and eventually learn to roll from the back to a knee-chest position to a standing position in one fluid movement.

Sitting Up. The development of head control must precede the ability to sit. At 1 month of age, when the infant lacks substantial head control, the entire back is uniformly rounded and both features prohibit a sitting

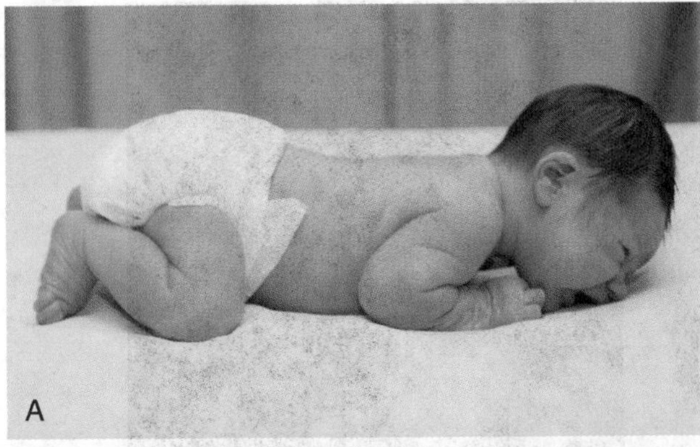

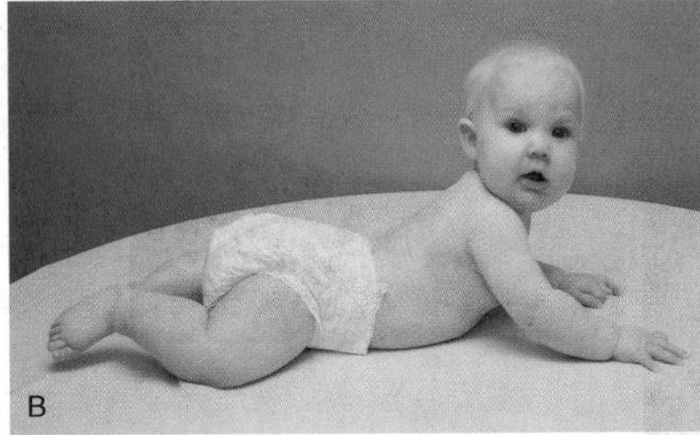

Figure 4–8
A, The newborn is barely able to lift his or her head while lying prone. *B*, By age 6 months, the infant easily lifts the head, chest, and upper abdomen and can bear weight on the hands.

posture. At 2 months of age, the infant still requires adult assistance to maintain a sitting position (see Fig. 4–9A). Therefore, to be upright the infant must be supported in an angled seat, which provides full head, back, and posterior support. Between 5 and 6 months of age, the spinal column has straightened enough and head control is sufficient to allow the infant to sit in a tripod position. The legs are extended in a wide V-based fashion, and the hands are used to provide support and stability (see Fig. 4–9*B*). By 8 months of age the infant can sit upright for long periods of time (see Fig. 4–9C). The child can also easily change from a lying to a sitting position and vice versa.

Locomotion. The development of locomotion involves several different but related capabilities. The child must be able to bear weight, use the arms to support, push, and raise the body, and use the legs to propel the body forward in a coordinated fashion. The very young infant is unable and unwilling to bear weight on the legs (Fig. 4–10A). By 6 months of age, the infant can bear weight fairly well when pulled to a standing position (see Fig. 4–10*B*). Although the infant can use the arms to lift the upper chest off a flat surface, no attempt is yet made to use the arms to pull or push the body. Some infants may begin crawling as early as 7 months. This involves moving the body forward using the arms and legs while keeping the belly on the floor. This pattern of movement progresses to creeping when the child is able to raise the belly off the floor and support his or her body weight with the hands and knees. The child can usually maneuver from the sitting position to the creeping position easily (see Fig. 4–10C). At 9 months the child may also be able to pull into a standing position by holding onto something. The infant may continue to creep and pull to a standing position for quite some time without displaying further interest in walking. Creeping is a very efficient method of locomotion. Even once walking is well established in the second year it is not uncommon for the child to use the hands and knees to move from one

Figure 4–9
A, At age 2 months, the infant needs assistance to maintain an upright position. *B*, At age 6 months, the infant can sit alone in the tripod position, using the hands for support and stability. C, By age 8 months, the infant can sit without support and focus on play activities.

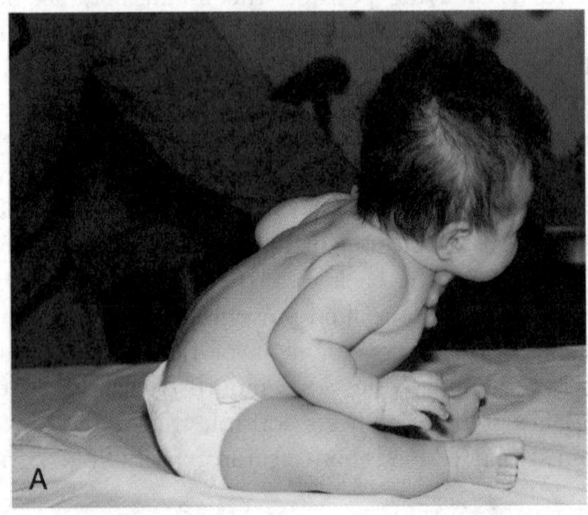

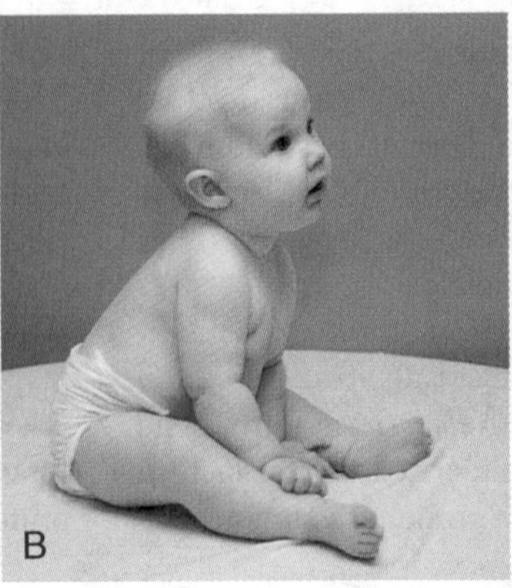

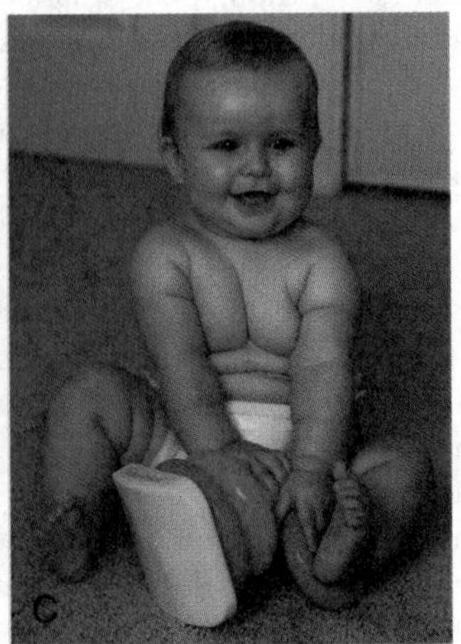

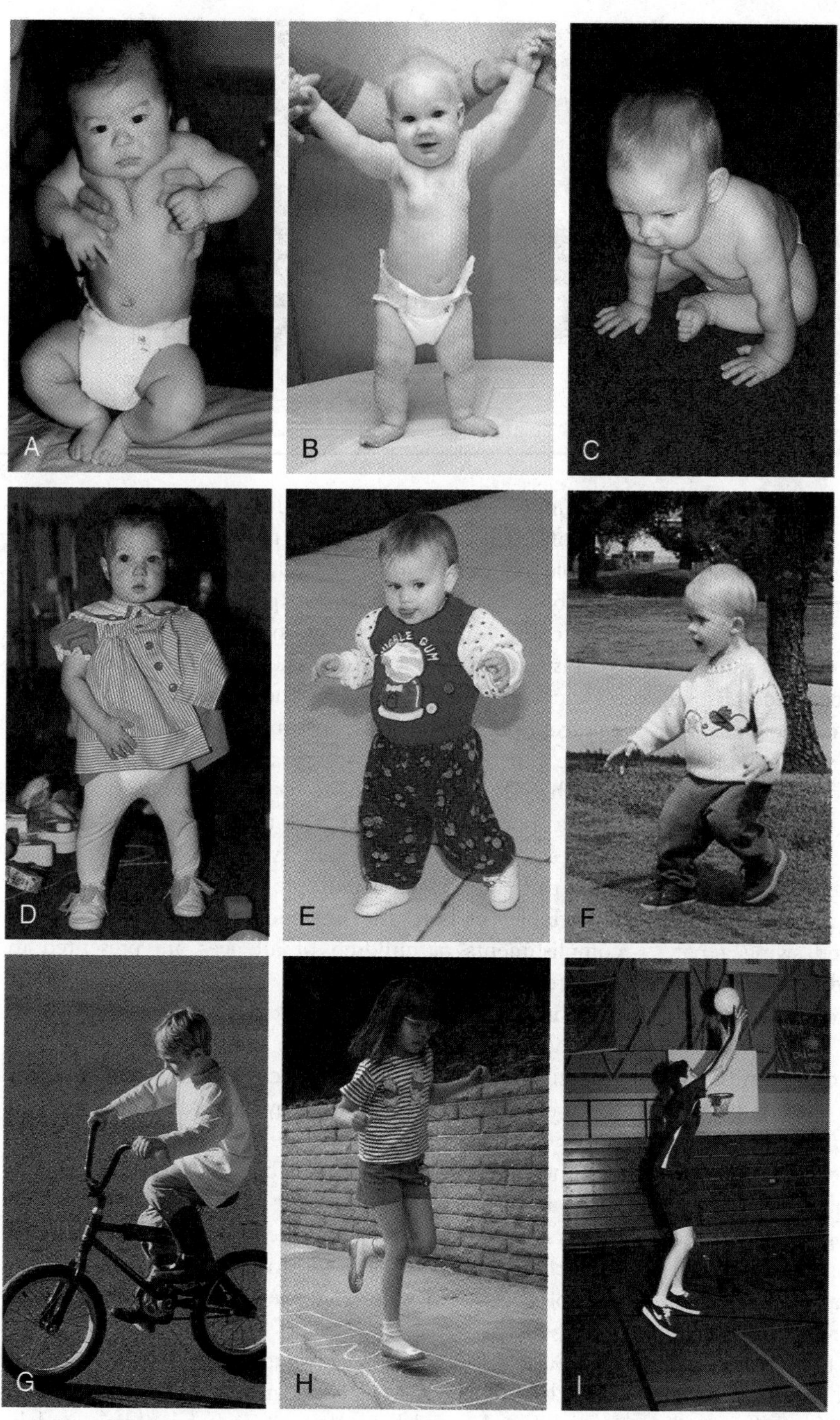

Figure 4–10
A, The 2-month-old is unable to bear weight on the legs. *B*, By age 6 months, the infant bears full weight on the legs. *C*, At 9 months, the infant is able to maneuver into a position for crawling in which the arms and knees bear weight. *D*, By 1 year, the child is able to stand independently from a crouched position. *E*, At 13 months, the child walks and toddles quickly. When moving fast, the child brings the arms to the upper chest area to maintain stability. *F*, By 15 months, the child can run with arms extended outward. *G*, The 5-year-old is able to ride a bike. *H*, The 7-year-old can easily hop on one foot. *I*, The high school student uses multiple locomotion skills to play basketball.

place to the next, especially if the child has been playing on the floor.

Once the child is able to pull into a standing position he or she next learns to stand independently and bend the knees to change from a crouching position to a standing position (see Fig. 4–10*D*). The cautious child is likely to stay close to a support mechanism (such as a piece of furniture) as he or she learns how to maneuver upright. Most likely, the first steps will be taken as the child moves from one piece of furniture to the next or from the support of one parent's arms to those of another. Some infants may begin walking as early as 10 months of age. Ninety-five percent of children walk independently by 18 months of age (see Fig. 4–10*E*). Within 15 months of the initiation of independent walking the child's gait will be mature. Until that time the walk is wide-based, marked by frequent stumbling. In the initial stages of walking the toddler maintains the arms flexed

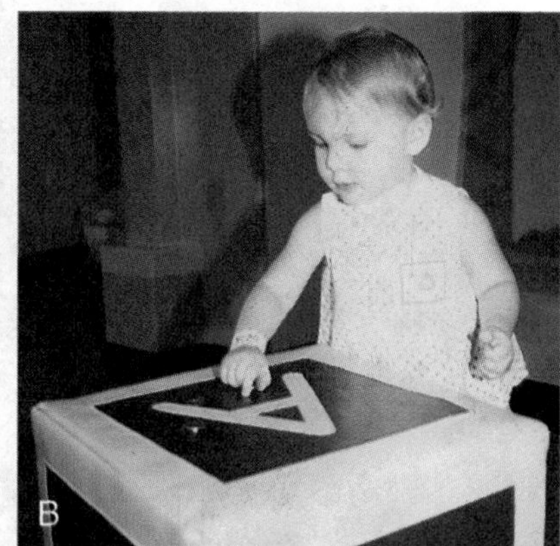

Figure 4–11
A, Palmar grasp. The 6-month-old uses the entire hand to pick up an object. *B*, Pincer grasp. The 12-month-old uses the thumb and index finger to pick up small objects.

and close to the sides of the body. The line of the body while ambulating has a forward lunge to it. As the child becomes more steady on the feet a more upright position is assumed and the arms relax and move freely as the child walks (see Fig. 4–10*F*).

By 2 years of age the pace of the child's gait has steadily improved such that running can be accomplished without stumbling. The 2-year-old can kick a ball, climb well, and maneuver up and down stairs one at a time. The 3-year-old can go up and down the stairs using alternating feet, can stand on one foot momentarily, and can ride a tricycle. Locomotion continues as the 4-year-old learns to hop and walk down the stairs on alternating feet. The arms, no longer needed to propel the body, can now throw a ball overhead and swing a bat. By 5 years of age the preschooler can ride a bike, stand on one foot for 10 seconds, and learn to skip (see Fig. 10–4G).

Once the child enters school many opportunities to learn new locomotion skills are presented through participation in organized games and sports activities (see Fig. 4–10*H* and *I*). Refinement of gross motor skills such as balancing, throwing, and complex combined activities (run–turn–jump–throw) continue through adolescence. As the child experiences growth changes during puberty, clumsy movements may be noted. The rapidity of physical changes in height, in length of extremities, and in distribution of body weight may impact the adolescent's perception of body image and proportion, requiring some mental adjustments to develop a sense of comfort with his or her changing shape.

Fine Motor Development

The newborn has very little control over fine motor movement. Actions made with the hands consist of broad sweeping actions and bringing the hand to the mouth. Objects placed in the newborn's hand will be involuntarily grasped and then dropped without notice by the infant. During the second month the child's ability to hold an object improves. Over the ensuing months, the ability to reach and grasp progresses from the gross hand control of the palmar grasp to a more refined ability to grasp smaller objects using the thumb and forefinger in a pincer grasp (Fig. 4–11). The pincer grasp begins to emerge around the eighth to ninth month. With mastery of the pincer grasp the infant can learn to hold a cup with handles, pick up small pieces of food, and crudely hold a spoon. By 1 year of age, use of the pincer grasp is well established, as is the ability to transfer objects from hand to hand and hold multiple objects in a hand. Summary tables of both the fine motor and gross motor accomplishments of children of all ages are presented in Chapter 5.

Refinement of fine motor skills continues throughout childhood (Fig. 4–12). By age 2 the child can hold a crayon and color using a vertical stroking motion. The pages of a book can be turned by the toddler and a tower of six blocks can be built. In the third year the child uses his fine motor skills to copy a circle and a cross and to build using very small blocks. The 4-year-old can use scissors, and the ability to color becomes more refined (the child is able to color within certain borders). The 5-year-old begins to write some letters and draws a person with body parts.

During the school-age years, writing skills improve. The child advances to cursive writing. Fine motor coordination is enhanced by such activities as building models, sewing, playing a musical instrument, and painting. Fine motor work generally requires focused periods of concentration to complete. Girls demonstrate more interest in these quiet, intense activities than do boys. The school-age years are an opportune time to introduce typing skills, which can be transferred to activities on the computer. Both boys and girls are likely to show interest in technology because these skills are being used more extensively in the classroom.

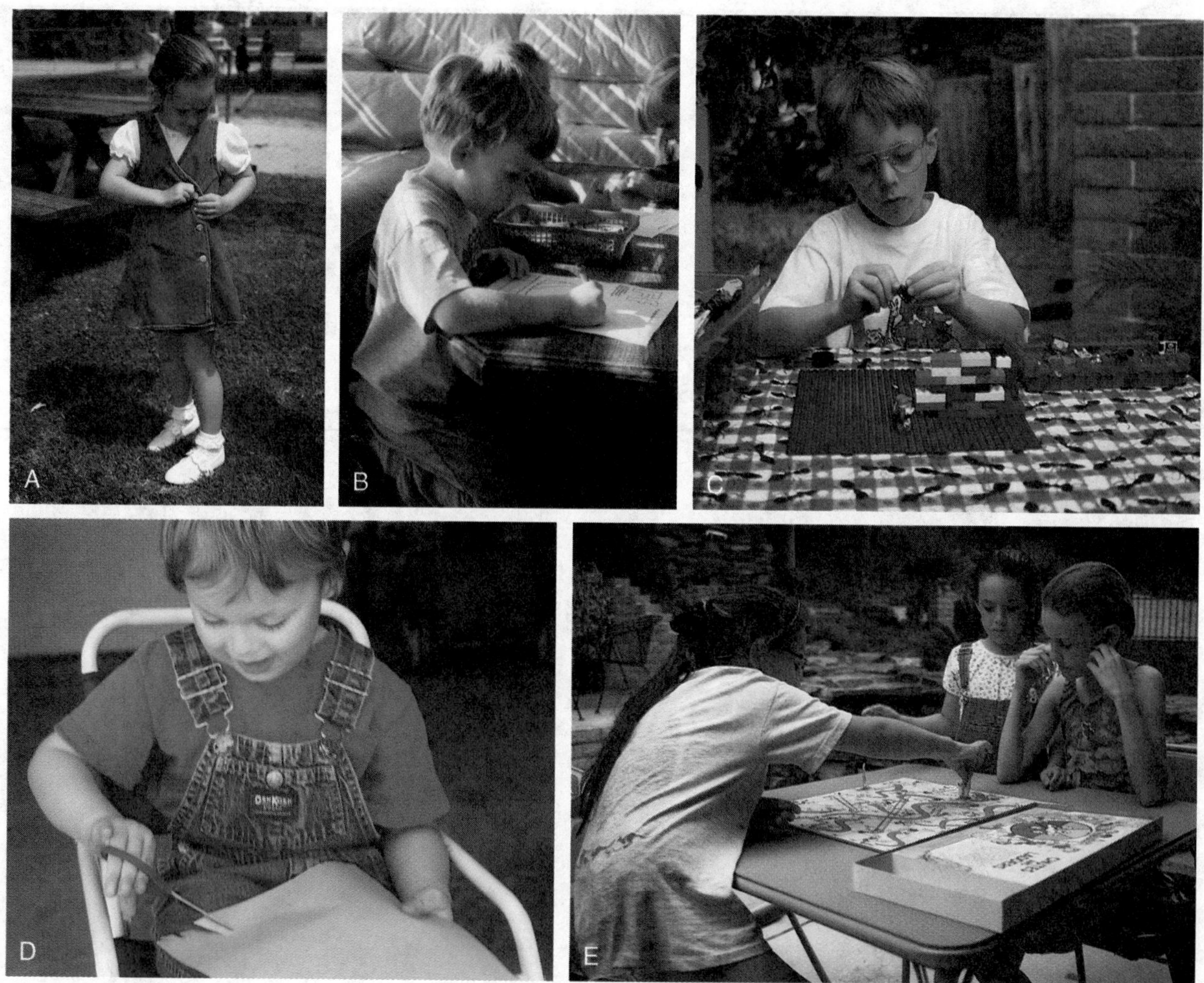

Figure 4–12
The child progressively achieves mastery of fine motor skills and cognitive abilities, such as *(A)* buttoning clothes, *(B)* holding a crayon, *(C)* building with small blocks, *(D)* using scissors, and *(E)* playing a board game.

Sensory Organ Development

Eyes

At the end of the first trimester the eyes are set far to the side of the head, and the neural connections to the eyes begin to develop. Eyebrows and eyelashes do not form until the sixth month. A thin membrane keeps the eyes fused until the end of the 28th week when the eyes begin to open and the pupils respond to light.

Visual function at birth is limited, improving rapidly over the next few years as the structure develops (Chart 4–9). The blink reflex is present in normal newborns. Tear glands begin to secrete within the first 2 weeks of life. Transient strabismus is a normal finding in the first few months. By 5 to 6 weeks of age the infant is able to fixate on an object and follow a bright toy or light. At 3 to 4 months the infant is able to reach for objects at varying distances from them. The ability to fuse two retinal images together in the brain begins to mature at about 9 months of age but is not fully mature until around age 6. The macula will mature by the end of the first year. Also by the end of the first year, mature adult functioning of eye muscles will be attained. Full anatomic maturity of the eye will not be reached until about 3 years of age. Visual acuity, approximately 20/300 at birth, will not reach 20/20 until the child is about 4 years of age (Reed & Davidhizar, 1997). Full visual maturity is attained by the sixth year. The interpretation of visual experiences begins during the first year and will

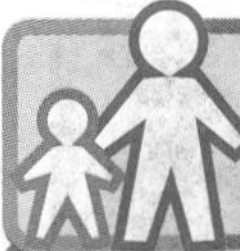

Chart 4–9
Developmental Considerations

Development of Vision

Birth–2 Weeks

Central acuity is 20/300.
Nystagmus is present.
Alertness is noted to visual stimulus 8 to 12 inches from eyes.
Pupils begin to enlarge.
Tear glands begin to secrete.

2–4 Weeks

Head and eye follow objects up to 90-degree arc.
Very little attention is given to stimuli beyond 2 feet.
Blinking is evident at approaching objects.

6–12 Weeks

Alertness is noted to moving objects, although convergence and following are jerky and inexact.
Head and eyes follow objects through 180-degree arc.
Fascination is evident for bright objects.
Tear glands begin to display response to emotion.
Newborn regards own hands.
Visual-motor coordination begins.

16–20 Weeks

Central acuity is 20/200.
Interest is shown in stimuli more than 3 feet away.

20–28 Weeks

Color preference for bright reds and yellows develops.
Ciliary muscle function begins.
Accommodation and convergence reflexes begin.
Hand-eye coordination begins to develop.
True blinking appears.
Ultimate color of the iris can be determined.

36–44 Weeks

Central acuity exceeds 20/200.
Depth perception is developing.
Visual regard for object with movement of the eyes horizontally and vertically to follow the object is present.

continue to mature for the duration of life. A discussion of conditions that can alter vision is presented in Chapter 28.

Ears

Ear formation begins around the fifth week in utero and remains susceptible to teratogenic influences until approximately the 16th week. These teratogens include ototoxic drugs, radiation, and infection. By the end of the first trimester, ear formation is complete and the ears are located in the appropriate position relative to other facial structures. In children younger than 3 years of age the ear canal is directed upward. In the older child the ear canal is directed downward and forward. The ears of the term neonate lie flat against the head and are well formed with firm cartilage. The top of the ear is in alignment with the inner and outer canthi of the eyes. Low-set ears may indicate the presence of a chromosomal aberration.

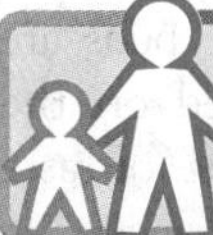

Chart 4-9
Developmental Considerations *Continued*

Development of Vision

1 Year

Pupils have enlarged to midposition and their diameter continues to increase.
Cornea is adult size (12 mm).
Central acuity is 20/100.
Fusion is present, although of poor quality and readily interrupted.
Ability to discriminate geometric forms is present.
Infant stacks blocks and places peg in small round hole.

2 Years

Central acuity is 20/40.

3 Years

Central acuity is 20/30.
Convergence is smoother.
Amblyopia can occur from disuse.
Attention span is fair.
Fixation on small pictures or toys is approximately 50 seconds.
Afterimages can be described by the child.

4 Years

Acuity is nearly 20/20.
Child is distinguishing letters and shapes.
Lacrimal glands are fully developed.

6 Years

Central acuity is established.
Physiologic hyperopia decreases.
Gross attention span is approximately 20 minutes.
Detailed attention span is approximately 2 minutes.
Color shading can be differentiated.

Data from Johnson, T., Moore, W., & Jeffries, J. (Eds.) (1978). *Children are different.* Columbus, OH: Ross Laboratories.

Hearing. The fetus responds to sounds as early as the 26th week of gestation (Coplan, 1995). The newborn is capable of sound discrimination at birth and will fix his or her gaze on the source of the mother's voice when she speaks in preference of other human voices within 12 hours of birth. The neonate responds more readily to high-pitched sound and is startled by loud noises (Philbin, 1996). Mucus in the eustachian tube or vernix caseosa in the external ear canal may limit hearing at birth but resolves quickly.

Over the next few months the infant begins to cease activity when sound is presented at a conversational level. By 5 to 6 months the infant is able to localize to sounds presented on a horizontal plane and begins to imitate selected sounds vocalized by an adult. In the 7- to 12-month period the infant is able to localize to sound presented in any plane and responds to his or her name even when spoken quietly. After the first birthday the child is able to point to familiar objects or people when asked. By 18 months the child can hear and follow a simple command without gestures or other visual cues. At this point, children who have difficulty attaining language milestones must be evaluated for hearing loss (see Language Development later in this chapter for more information regarding language milestones).

Congenital hearing loss is strongly linked to genetic

influences. Between 46% and 60% of severe childhood hearing loss is attributed to genetics. Of these cases, 20% are the result of autosomal dominant genes, 80% are a result of autosomal recessive genes, and less than 2% are attributed to sex-linked inheritance. One third of genetic-linked hearing loss occurs in association with some type of congenital syndrome. Five to 10 percent of deaf children are the product of deaf parents (Schlesinger, 1995).

Hearing loss can also be attributed to postnatal conditions and illnesses that occur in childhood. These include hyperbilirubinemia, use of ototoxic medications, meningitis, and otitis media with effusion. A thorough discussion of hearing disorders in children is provided in Chapter 28.

Nose

The newborn will react to strong odors such as ammonia and fresh onion. Infants are able to detect the smell of their mother's breasts as early as 6 to 10 days after birth. The ability to smell and differentiate smells continues to improve as the child matures. Discrimination of smell is influenced by the child's attentiveness to this particular sense. For instance, the child whose temperament style is characterized by a low threshold to stimulus is likely to be highly sensitive to the smells in the environment.

The structure of the nose may influence smell only in the sense that a blockage or malformation may impair the ability to smell. The nose of the newborn should be placed midline on the face. A malformed or misshapen nose may occur in the presence of chromosomal problems, choanal atresia, or perforation or deviation of the septum. Infants have a small nasal bridge and are obligate nose breathers until 1 month of age.

Mouth

Oral Cavity. Formation of the palate occurs during the seventh and eighth week of gestation, at which time the fetus is sensitive to teratogens that can impact development of the oral cavity. The most common abnormalities seen are cleft lip and cleft palate. Cleft lip is a result of incomplete fusion of embryonic structures surrounding the primitive oral cavity. Cleft palate represents failure of the primary and secondary palatine plates to fuse.

In healthy newborns the hard and soft palates are intact, the uvula is midline, the tongue freely moves in the mouth, and lips and lip movement are symmetrical. The oral cavity and structures within it continue to grow in proportion to other facial structures as the child matures.

Taste. The sense of taste is immature in newborns, although they can distinguish between sugar, lemon, salt, and quinine. Sensitivity to strong tastes becomes heightened at 2 to 3 months. At this time the taste buds are maturing, and they are more widely distributed on the tongue than are those of older infants. The sense of taste is not fully intact until approximately 2 years of age.

Teeth. Tooth formation begins approximately the 7th week in utero with the differentiation of specialized oral epithelial cells. Calcification of teeth begins at 4 months' gestation and is not completed until young adulthood. Eruption of teeth occurs about the sixth month of life. Some children may experience the appearance of the first tooth before this time; in others this does not occur until the latter months of the first year. There are 20 deciduous teeth, with eruption completed by age 2½. The first permanent molar and lower incisor teeth erupt around age 6, and most are present by age 12 (Fig. 4–13).

Tonsils. The tonsils are located in the pharyngeal cavity and are part of the lymphatic system. Tonsillar tissue is usually not evident in the newborn. The tonsils in toddlers and preschool children are generally larger than in adults, usually extending beyond the palatine arch until the age of 11 or 12 years.

Skin

The back and the arms of the developing fetus are covered with fine hair called *lanugo*. This hair begins to form at 16 weeks, covers the fetus in utero, and begins to recede around the 36th week. Presence of lanugo will most likely be noted on the infant born prematurely, and, to some degree, on the full-term baby. As the infant continues to mature outside the womb, the lanugo continues to recede.

Another protective covering that can be found on the developing fetus is the *vernix caseosa*. This cheese-like coating on the skin develops around the 24th week, remaining until the fetus is full term. On delivery, the newborn may have varying amounts of vernix caseosa. The substance can be easily washed off the infant's skin during the first bath.

The newborn's skin is soft and smooth and has a translucent appearance. Superficial vessels are prominent, giving the skin a red color. Sweat and sebaceous glands are present in the newborn but do not become functional until 2 months of age. Some do not become functional until the onset of puberty. At this time considerable development of sweat and sebaceous glands is evident and associated with the development of acne vulgaris and body odor.

Mongolian spots, which are blue irregular flat-shaped areas found on the sacral and buttocks area, usually disappear by the first or second year. In some children they may persist for a longer time. More information regarding skin alterations that are common in the childhood years, such as dermatitis, acne, and sunburn, is provided in Chapter 25.

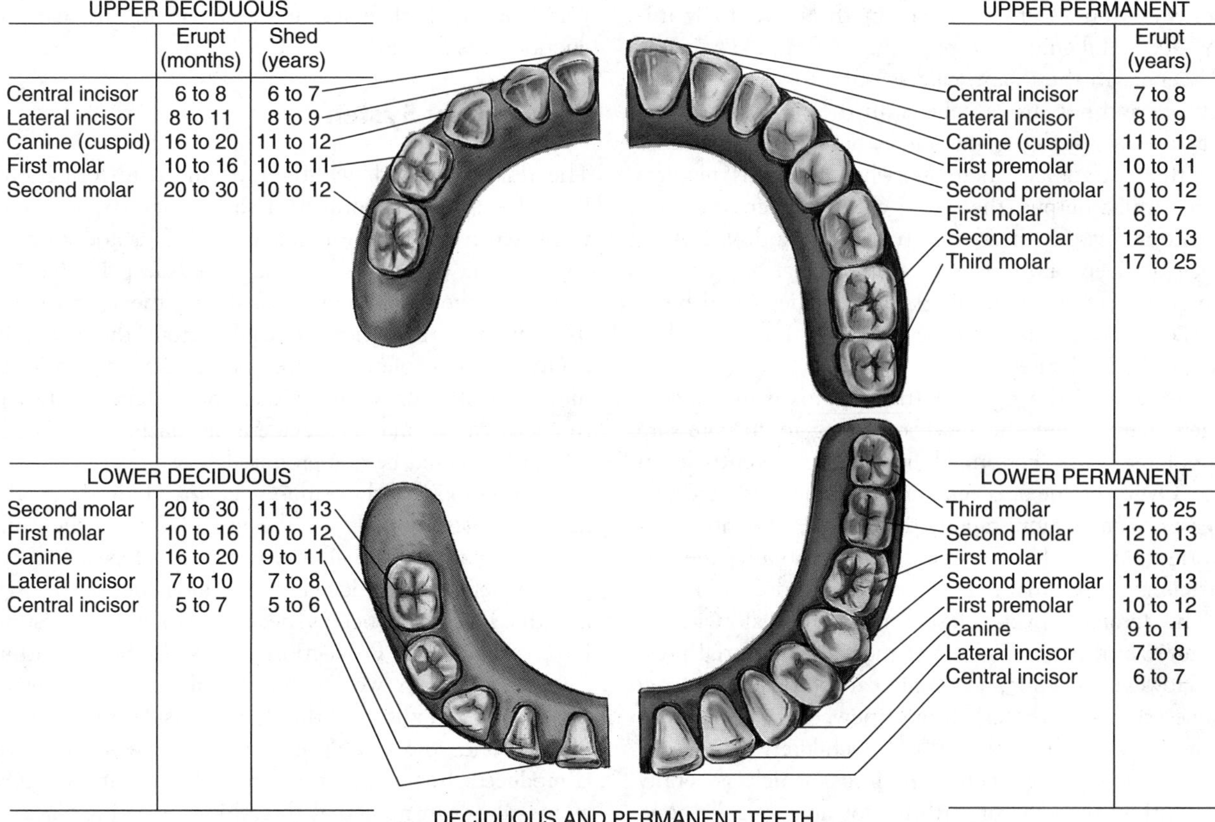

UPPER DECIDUOUS
Erupt (months)
Shed (years)
Central incisor 6 to 8 6 to 7
Lateral incisor 8 to 11 8 to 9
Canine (cuspid) 16 to 20 11 to 12
First molar 10 to 16 10 to 11
Second molar 20 to 30 10 to 12
UPPER PERMANENT
Erupt (years)
Central incisor 7 to 8
Lateral incisor 8 to 9
Canine (cuspid) 11 to 12
First premolar 10 to 11
Second premolar 10 to 12
First molar 6 to 7
Second molar 12 to 13
Third molar 17 to 25
LOWER DECIDUOUS
Second molar 20 to 30 11 to 13
First molar 10 to 16 10 to 12
Canine 16 to 20 9 to 11
Lateral incisor 7 to 10 7 to 8
Central incisor 5 to 7 5 to 6
LOWER PERMANENT
Third molar 17 to 25
Second molar 12 to 13
First molar 6 to 7
Second premolar 11 to 13
First premolar 10 to 12
Canine 9 to 11
Lateral incisor 7 to 8
Central incisor 6 to 7
DECIDUOUS AND PERMANENT TEETH

Figure 4–13
Sequence of eruption of primary (deciduous) and secondary (permanent) teeth. (From Jarvis, C. [1996]. *Physical examination and health assessment* [2nd ed., p. 390]. Philadelphia: W. B. Saunders. Reprinted with permission.)

During the first year there is an increase in subcutaneous fat. When the child becomes ambulatory the proportion of subcutaneous fat begins to diminish. By age 3 most children have a leaner appearance than has been noticed in previous years. During puberty, subcutaneous fat becomes more abundant in certain body areas, especially in females.

The fingernails and toenails began forming at the end of the first trimester. At birth, nailbeds are fully formed on the normal newborn. Those infants born prematurely have incomplete formation of their nails.

Organ Development

During the third and fourth weeks of gestation, the main organs begin to form in a cephalocaudal direction. By the eighth week, basic organ development is complete. Although the organs are in place and functioning in a primitive fashion, the organs will not be able to work to sustain life until about the 20th week of development. Further functional development of many organs continues with transition of the fetus to extrauterine life. In addition, other functional and structural changes continue as the child physically grows and matures in the ensuing years.

Cardiovascular System

Formation of the heart begins by the 16th day of gestation. Blood cells join to the yolk sac's wall, and the system of blood vessels and a single heart tube begins to take shape. The heart appears as a bulge on the anterior surface of the developing fetus. By the sixth or seventh week the septum and then the valves begin to develop. The rhythmic beat of the heart has begun by the eighth week and can be heard with a stethoscope by the 16th week beating at 120 to 160 beats per minute. Fetal circulation develops slowly, providing blood to the brain, liver, heart, and kidneys. At birth, changes in circulation occur that allow the heart and lungs to work in a coordinated effort to sustain circulation once supported by the placenta (discussed in more detail in Chapter 15).

Thus, at birth, the heart of the normal infant is simply a smaller version of the adult heart with a few minor variations. Cardiac output in the newborn is initially 400 mL/kg/min, dropping to 200 mL/kg/min by adolescence. In the infant, cardiac output is a function of heart rate and not stroke volume. In the young child, the heart rate is usually higher and the stroke volume is lower than in adults. Therefore, when the body requires higher cardiac output, the young child compensates by a correlate increase in heart rate (i.e., tachycardia). During periods of sleep or persistent vagal stimulation (by suctioning, defecation, or feeding) transient decreased heart rate (i.e., bradycardia) can be found in infants and is generally well tolerated.

The mass of the right ventricle approximates that of the left ventricle in the newborn owing to the pressure and volume work performed by the right ventricle in utero. Over the next several months the left ventricle increases in mass more rapidly than the right ventricle as it works to pump both systemically. Eventually, the left ventricle is predominant, as is seen in the adult heart.

The foramen ovale closes in the normal newborn soon after birth as a result of changes in interatrial pressure. However, the foramen ovale can be reopened using a probe (cardiac catheter) in most newborns and remains patent in approximately 50% of children at age 5 (Yeager, 1988). The ductus arteriosus, which generally closes within 18 hours of birth, is not anatomically gone until approximately 2 weeks of age.

During infancy the heart is more horizontally placed and has a larger diameter in relation to the diameter of the total chest than is apparent in the adult. The apex of the heart is one or two intercostal spaces higher than in the adult. Therefore, the apical pulse, or point of maximum impulse (PMI), is auscultated at the fourth intercostal space in children younger than 7 years of age and in the fifth intercostal space in the child older than 7. The PMI becomes more lateral as the child grows and as heart diameter decreases in relation to chest diameter.

Healthy premature infants are prone to having a high frequency of arrhythmias. This is most likely due to the immaturity of the autonomic nervous system. Sinus arrhythmias are a normal finding in infants, although they would be considered an abnormal finding in the older child and adolescent. Innocent systolic murmurs are common in infants and young children. Diastolic murmurs at any age are considered pathologic (Gessner, 1997).

Hematopoiesis. During fetal development the main site of hematopoiesis is the liver. By birth, hematopoietic activity will primarily occur in the bone marrow. In the early childhood years, most of the child's bones contain active hematopoietic activity. As the child matures, this tissue in the long bones is gradually replaced with fat. During periods of extreme hematopoietic stress the long bones can resume active blood production. During later childhood and into adulthood the pelvis, sternum, ribs, vertebrae, skull, clavicles, and scapulae are the main production sites for blood.

Respiratory System

The respiratory and digestive system begin formation at the same time and form as a single tube. By the fourth week, separation of the two systems begins and lung buds appear. The lung buds may be seated deep in the abdomen until the diaphragm closes during the seventh week, thus dividing the thoracic cavity from the abdominal cavity. If incomplete closures occur, diaphragmatic hernias with abdominal organ contents extending into the thoracic cavity may be evident at birth. In this case, respiration would be compromised.

Formation of the sinuses begins during the third month of gestation. Until the age of 2 to 3 the child's sinuses remain very small and poorly developed.

Surfactant is produced by the lungs during the sixth month. This substance is necessary to aid in postnatal lung expansion. Production of surfactant continues through the 28th week, and the alveoli are formed at this time. Viability of the fetus outside the womb is possible once the alveoli are formed and some surfactant is produced. In the womb the fetus has respiratory movements, although no actual "breathing" is taking place.

At birth the most dramatic respiratory changes take place when the infant draws his or her first breath. The intake of oxygen pushes amniotic fluid out of the alveoli, allowing for the expansion of the pulmonary bed. Approximately 50 million alveoli are present at birth, and 250 million more are added by 2 years of age, at which time most alveolar formation is complete (Snapp, 1996).

The infant and young child's respiratory system is notably different from that of the older child and adult. During the childhood years, changes in the structure and function of the respiratory system occur. The alveoli and airways grow, changing in size and configuration. The child has fewer alveoli than the adult. The collateral pathways of ventilation are not completely developed during infancy; therefore, airway obstruction can have more severe effects in the young child. By later childhood and adolescence, the terminal airways are larger and collateral ventilation is improved (Hazinski, 1996). The infant's sternum and ribs are primarily cartilaginous, resulting in a soft chest wall. The ribs are horizontally oriented, and intercostal muscles are poorly developed at this time (Hazinski, 1996). This is in contrast to the adult's rib cage, which is more rigid and where the bones are angled more vertically.

The adult uses his or her accessory muscles to aid in the respiratory process. Poor development of these muscles requires the infant and young child to be more dependent on diaphragmatic function to contribute to the movement of the chest wall during respiration.

Infants are obligatory nose breathers for approximately 1 month after birth. The cartilage in the infant's larynx is very soft and can easily be compressed if the child's neck is flexed or hyperextended. The narrowest part of the child's airway is the cricoid cartilage, and, as a whole, the larynx is proportionately smaller in diameter and straighter than the larynx in the older child and adult.

Gastrointestinal System

Once the digestive system separates from the respiratory system, it begins a period of rapid growth. Because the abdominal cavity is small, from the 6th to the 10th weeks a part of the abdominal contents will extend into the base of the umbilical cord. As the abdominal cavity grows, the intestines should once again move into the abdomen. This occurs around the 13th week. Failure to do so leads to a variety of disorders, including omphalocele (a condition in which the child is born with the intestines outside the abdominal cavity) and susceptibility to intussusception and bowel obstruction.

During the second month of fetal life, the intestines begin to produce meconium as a result of fetal metabolism. The pancreas develops during the 12th week. The development of the swallowing reflex at 16 weeks allows the fetus to swallow amniotic fluid. If the fetus becomes stressed, hypoxia can cause vagal stimulation, an increase in bowel motility, and a lack of sphincter tone. The meconium may leave the bowel and move into the amniotic fluid, making it likely that the fetus will swallow some of the meconium. This is not a problem until the point of delivery when the newborn is ready to take his or her first breaths. Further aspiration of the meconium into the newborn's respiratory passages can cause deleterious effects if not noted and treated on delivery of the newborn.

The terminal segment of the anal canal, the anus, arises from a pit invagination of the skin. The anus is supplied by somatic sensory nerves and is sensitive to touch even at birth. As myelinization of the spinal cord becomes complete and the musculature of the anus develops more fully the child will be able to have voluntary control over defecation. This generally occurs between 2 to 5 years of age.

At birth the child's gastrointestinal system remains immature and will not maintain full maturity until approximately 2 years of age. Until full maturity is reached, many variations exist in the child's digestive tract and in digestion compared with that of the adult. In the first 3 to 4 months of life the sucking reflex and extrusion reflex are present. The extrusion reflex protects the infant from ingesting food substances that the gastrointestinal system is too immature to digest. The production of saliva in large enough quantities to begin the process of digestion in the oral cavity does not occur until approximately age 4 months. The infant is prone to frequent spit-ups after feeding owing to the immature muscle tone of the lower esophageal sphincter. Intestinal peristalsis is faster in young children, with emptying times being 2½ to 3 hours in the newborn and extending to 3 to 6 hours in older infants and children. Faster gastric emptying time affects the ability of the digestive tract to break down and absorb the child's oral intake. For instance, it is not uncommon for the infant to eat corn and defecate corn that has undergone no physical changes in appearance after having traveled the digestive system. The frequent output of undigested food particles is further influenced by the gastrocolic reflex, which rapidly moves contents toward the colon. The newborn's stomach capacity is 10 to 20 mL, increasing to 100 to 200 mL in a 2-month-old, 1500 mL in an adolescent, and 2000 to 3000 mL in the adult (Engel, 1997).

The infant's stomach is round and lies horizontally until about 2 years of age when the angle becomes more vertical and upright. The intestines undergo a growth spurt when the child is 1 to 3 years of age and again in the later teen years. The liver is generally palpable 1 to 2 cm below the right costal margin in the first year of life. The spleen is normally palpable 1 to 2 cm below the left costal margin in the first few weeks of life. Thereafter, the ability to palpate these organs becomes more difficult as the trunk elongates and the child acquires additional subcutaneous fat.

The diameter of the abdomen is larger than the diameter of the chest in children younger than the age of 4 and has a "pot-bellied" appearance in both sitting and standing positions owing to poorly developed abdominal musculature (Fig. 4–14). Up to the age of 13, the child continues to have a pot belly in the standing position. A superficial venous pattern is readily visible on the infant's abdomen, remaining observable until adolescence. The omentum is poorly developed in early childhood, and thus localization of intra-abdominal infection or an inflammatory reaction is less likely to occur than in the older child and adolescent.

Genitourinary System

At 4 weeks of gestation, the kidneys are present in a rudimentary form. Urine forms between the 11th and 12th weeks of development. In utero the placenta serves as a pseudokidney, regulating fetal fluid and electrolyte balance. The kidneys do not function independently until after birth.

In the first 1 to 2 years of life, the kidneys reach full functional maturity. Until maturity is reached the infant is predisposed to dehydration during periods of fluid loss such as those caused by diarrhea, fever, fluid restrictions, and reduced fluid intake. In the early years, renal blood

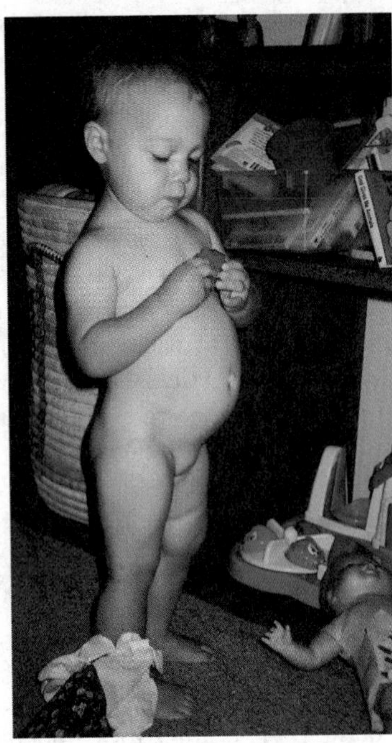

Figure 4–14
The toddler's physique is characterized by a pot-bellied, bow-legged appearance.

flow is slow, the reabsorption of amino acids is limited, autoregulation is not fully developed, and the ability to concentrate urine is minimal. As the kidneys mature and systemically there is increased cardiac output and increased plasma proteins, renal function improves.

The newborn's bladder capacity is approximately 30 mL, increasing to 150 mL at 3 years, 270 mL at 7 years, and up to 600 to 800 mL in the adult. Although the kidneys do not reach maximal size until age 35 to 40, the kidneys of infants and children have a larger diameter compared with the size of the abdominal cavity that is present in the adult. The child's kidneys are more vulnerable to trauma owing to their size in proportion to the abdomen and because they are less protected by the ribs and have less fat padding.

Gender Development

External genitalia are present at 8 weeks, the beginning of the fetal stage. However, the ability to distinguish between male and female genitalia is not possible until further formation takes place. During early embryonic development, male and female genital structures are similar. It is during the third month that primitive urogenital structures enlarge and fuse to form the male's penis and scrotum or shrink and have minimal fusion to form the female's labia and clitoris. These external changes can be detected on ultrasound. The internal sex organs are also developing at this time. The male's testes do not descend into the scrotum until about 36 weeks' gestation. An indirect hernia is produced if the tube that precedes the descent of the testes fails to close.

At birth the external female genitalia have increased pigmentation because of hormonal influences. The clitoris and labia majora are likely to be edematous. Both the edema and increased pigmentation recede within the next month. The scrotum of the full-term male is pink or dark brown, depending on the child's complexion, and rugae are present. Both testes should be descended. Penile erections occur when the penis is stimulated or when the infant is voiding. The foreskin on the penis is not retractable if the child is not circumcised. The foreskin remains adherent until approximately age 3.

Both female and male reproductive organs remain relatively unchanged until early adolescence. The beginning of puberty marks the onset of significant changes in the development of the gonads, reproductive organs, and secondary sex characteristics. The length of time pubertal changes require and the age at which they begin vary from person to person. In general, puberty begins earlier in females (as early as age 10) and is of a shorter duration than that which occurs in boys.

Pubertal events are characterized by several other physical changes in addition to those that affect reproductive organs. Skeletal growth and body composition changes occur, increased strength and endurance is attained, and anatomic and biochemical alterations in the central nervous system and the endocrine system are made. Figures 4–15 and 4–16 summarize the typical progression of female and male development during puberty. Early or delayed onset of pubertal signs is a cause for concern because either can indicate endocrine dysfunction and be a source of personal distress for the child (Chart 4–10).

Endocrine and Metabolic Functions

The thyroid, thymus, and pancreas develop around the 12th week of gestation. Endocrine functions are immature at birth. For example, infants have a high metabolic rate that correlates with higher glucose needs. However, the infant also has low glycogen stores; therefore, the child can rapidly become hypoglycemic during periods of stress. As the youth approaches the adult years, these processes change. Under stress, the adult generally becomes hyperglycemic because epinephrine and glycogen secretion stimulate glycogen breakdown, resulting in increased blood glucose level (Hazinski, 1996).

Stress in the infant also stimulates the secretion of growth hormone, which then increases calcium deposi-

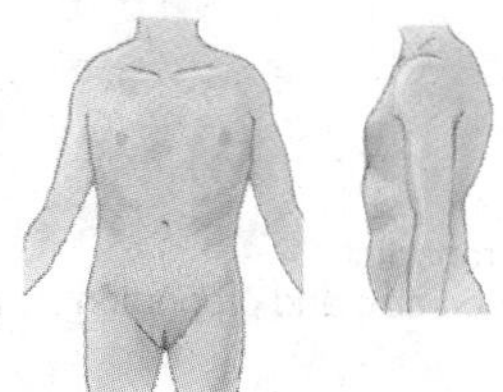

Stage I
Breasts: Preadolescent; elevation of the papilla only
Pubic hair: None

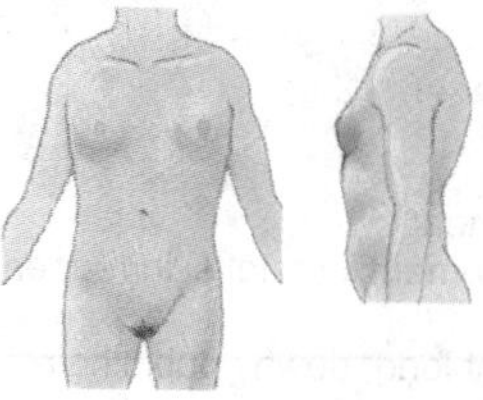

Stage II
Breasts: Breast budding (thelarche); small mound formed by elevation of the breast and papilla, with enlargement of the areolar diameter
Pubic hair: Sparse growth of long, downy pubic hair over mons veneris or labia majora; may occur with breast budding or several weeks or months later (pubarche)

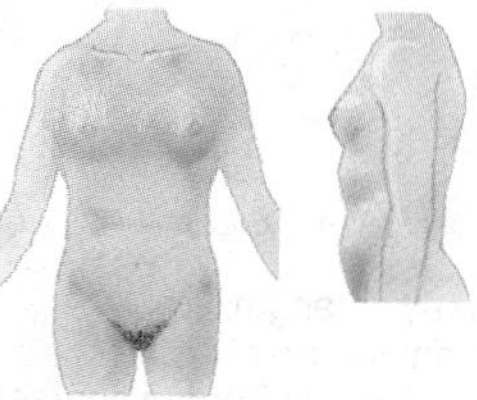

Stage III
Breasts: Further enlargement of breast tissue and areola with no separation of their contours
Pubic hair: Increased amount of hair and changes in the character of the hair (darker, coarser, and more curly), spread sparsely over junction of pubes

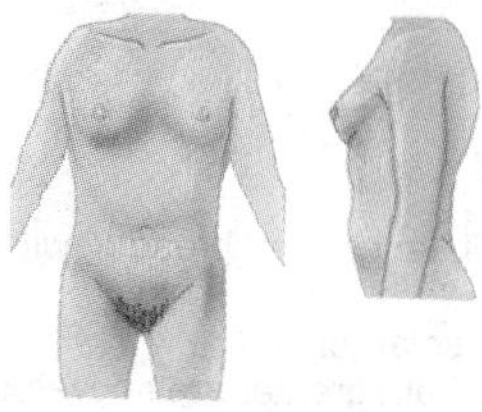

Stage IV
Breasts: Double contour form: projection of areola and papilla form a secondary mound on top of breast tissue
Pubic hair: Adult appearance but less area covered; no spread to medial aspects of thighs

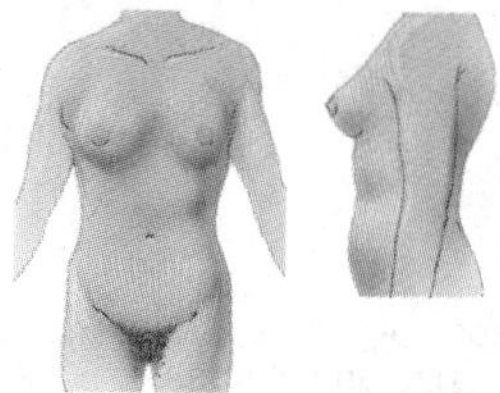

Stage V
Breasts: Larger, more mature breast with single contour form
Pubic hair: Adult distribution and quantity, with spread to medial aspect of thighs

Figure 4–15
Development of secondary sex characteristics in girls.

tion in the bone, causing hypocalcemia. The infant has immature regulation of growth hormone production. Thus, in cases of severe stress, the infant needs to be monitored for hypocalcemia (Hazinski, 1996).

Metabolic functions are established in utero as genetic information is transferred to the developing cells. At birth, metabolic functions should be intact and functioning. Mutational events in utero can lead to the development of biochemical disorders that impact the child's metabolic function. The affected genes result in either a structurally altered enzyme that is not capable of normal catalytic activity or causes an inhibition of enzyme synthesis. In most cases the neonate appears normal at birth; however, signs and symptoms develop rapidly as the infant's metabolic functions begin to respond to the intake of human milk or formula and the demands of extrauterine life. Some alterations do not make themselves known until later childhood. Rarely do problems in metabolic function appear as late as adulthood. The inborn errors of metabolism most commonly seen in the pediatric population are discussed in Chapter 27.

Immune Functions

The lymphoid system performs the same function in children as in adults; however, the maturity of the system

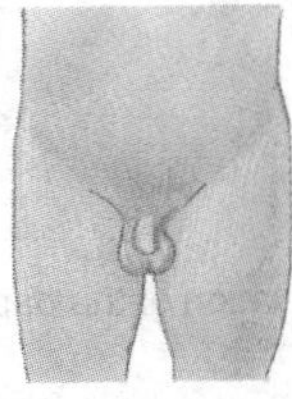

Stage I
Penis: Childhood size and proportion
Testes and scrotum: Childhood size and proportion
Pubic hair: None

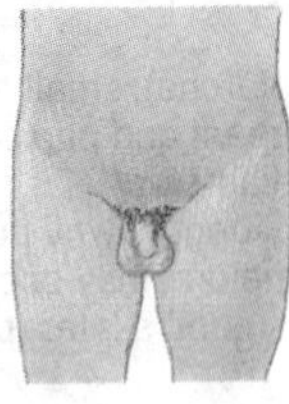

Stage II
Penis: Slight or no enlargement
Testes and scrotum: Enlargement; scrotal skin reddens, changes in texture
Pubic hair: Sparse growth of long, downy pubic hair mainly at the base of the penis

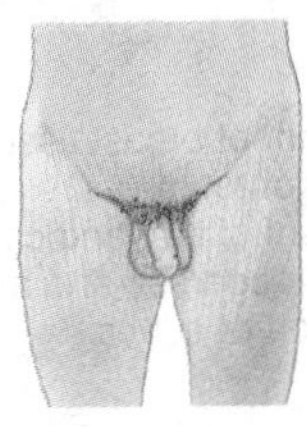

Stage III
Penis: Enlargement, particularly in length
Testes and scrotum: Further enlargement
Pubic hair: Darker, coarser, curlier hair spread sparsely over the pubic symphysis

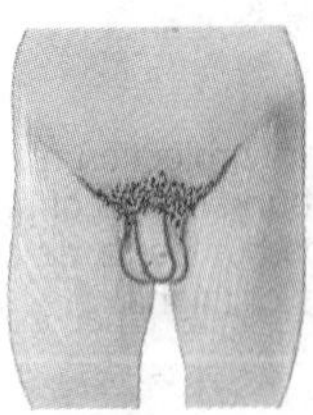

Stage IV
Penis: Further enlargement in length and breadth, with development of the glans
Testes and scrotum: Further enlargement
Pubic hair: Coarse and curly hair; greater area covered than in Stage III, but still less than in an adult, with no spread to thighs

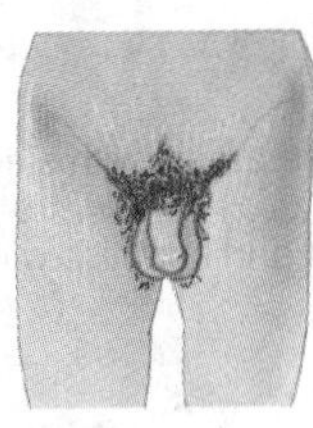

Stage V
Penis: Adult in size and shape
Testes and scrotum: Adult in size and shape
Pubic hair: Adult distribution and quantity, with spread to thighs but not to abdomen

Figure 4–16
Development of secondary sex characteristics in boys.

varies at different ages. For instance, the fetus passively acquires antibodies from the mother during the sixth month of gestation. Immunoglobulins G, A, and M (IgG, IgA, IgM) are almost completely derived by transfer to the developing fetus from the mother. This allows temporary protection against such diseases as measles, mumps, poliomyelitis, and rubella (Nelms & Mullins, 1982). At birth, the infant has the immunologic reactivity to respond to a large variety of antigens. At the same time this exogenous source of immunoglobulins suppresses the infant's own ability to synthesize the immunoglobulins. Therefore, as maternal stores in the infant catabolize the child experiences a period in which immunoglobulin levels are low because the child's own system is not fully activated to create the antibodies that are needed. This usually occurs around the sixth month. Adult levels of IgM are attained at approximately 1 year of age, with levels of IgG reached at 5 years of age and those of IgA at 10 years of age.

Several other factors make the infant and young child more at risk for infection. The newborn's immune system is not as efficient as that of an adult. Cell-mediated immunity is less well developed than the adult; as a result, recovery from congenital infections may be de-

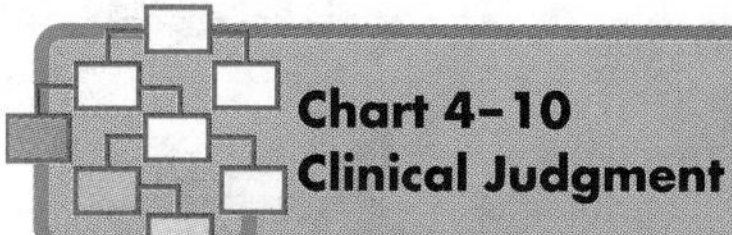

Chart 4–10
Clinical Judgment

Assessment of Changes During Puberty

Tom Yee is a nurse and a father of a 12-year-old who plays on a junior-high soccer team. Mr. Yee was asked to talk to the team about ways to stay healthy during their adolescent years. After the presentation, Mr. Yee asks if there are any questions. One boy shouts out, "How come my bratty little sister is now taller than I am?"; another boy interjects, "Yeah, my 11-year-old sister is starting to get a big chest, too!"

Questions

1. From the comments of the boys, what do you think is at the heart of their concerns?
2. For this preadolescent age group, what are some of the topics Mr. Yee should have covered in his "keeping healthy" presentation?
3. Should Mr. Yee start a discussion about the physical and reproductive changes that occur during puberty at this time?
4. How should Mr. Yee intervene to address the concerns of these boys?
5. What are some of the physical changes Mr. Yee should tell them will occur during puberty?

Answers

1. They see other kids around them going through lots of physical changes and they are concerned whether they are abnormal or will they, too, be growing bigger and taller.
2. Nutrition, sports safety, car safety, and hazards of smoking and substance use.
3. Mr. Yee can discuss some of the physical changes that will occur during puberty. However, a detailed discussion of male and female reproduction and changes in the reproductive system would not be appropriate at this time because of the setting (not because of their age). Plan another session to discuss these other topics.
4. Briefly discuss the physical changes between boys and girls that is occurring in this age group. Determine whether there is a need for another presentation that would present more detailed information about adolescent sexuality. Obtain consent from parents to have a second presentation, and ask fathers to attend with their sons.
5. Pubertal changes begin in girls as early as age 10. Boys develop secondary sex characteristics later and may not begin these changes for up to 2 years after girls. This development in boys includes an increase in height. The physique changes, with more muscle mass added. Genitalia enlarge, and their shape changes. Hair growth increases in certain body areas such as under the arms and in the pubic area. Hair line on the forehead may recede a little. The voice deepens. Acne may begin to appear.

layed and the effects of the condition more devastating for the newborn.

Lymph nodes in children have the same distribution patterns as adults. However, the nodes are more predominant in the young child until the time of puberty. The amount of lymphoid tissue is considerable during infancy and continues to increase at a steady rate until after puberty. During early childhood, lymphoid tissue responds to infection by excessive swelling and hyperplasia. These clinical signs may persist long after the primary infection has diminished. The lymph nodes can harbor infection, posing a liability for the child. Swelling of the lymph glands and spleen can lead to other health care problems because swollen nodes can block the airway. A swollen and enlarged spleen is more at risk for traumatic injury because the child's abdominal structures have little subcutaneous fat to protect the internal organs from injury.

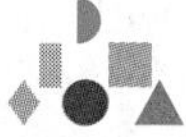

Theories of Development

Psychosexual Development

The work of Sigmund Freud is one of the most familiar psychoanalytic theories. Freud believed that humans are driven by a need to resolve certain biologically determined drives that center around sexual urges. Although Freud did not believe that children experienced adult sexual feelings, he did believe that children had certain sensual and pleasurable urges that they acted on through their behaviors and in their interactions with others. The sexual instinct is called *eros*. The energy created by the sexual instinct is called *libido*. According to Freud's the-

Table 4–5
Freud's Stages of Psychosexual Development

Psychosexual Stage	Body Area of Focus	Description	Results of Trauma or Fixation
Oral—birth to 1 year	Mouth	Enjoys sucking, chewing, biting on things such as mother's breast, rubber nipple, thumb, blanket, or bottle	Oral fixations such as nail biting, cigarette smoking, gum chewing, excessive eating
Anal—1 to 3 years	Anus	Libido centered on gaining mastery in using anal muscles. Toilet training accomplished at this time.	Anal fixations such as parsimony, orderliness, punctiliousness, obstinacy, possessiveness; difficulty controlling anger, aggressive feelings, and impulses
Phallic—3 to 6 years	Genitalia (penis, clitoris, and vagina)	Resolution of the Oedipus and Electra complex. Sex roles and moral development take place.	Boy will remain overly attached to his mother, fearing father may castrate him; may resent father and authority figures. Girl will remain overly attached to father and has "penis envy"—wishing to be a man.
Latency—6 to 12 years	Sex drives repressed; no area of focus	Nonsexual urges. Children focus on learning to control their impulses and find appropriate outlets for their drives. Energies shift to physical and intellectual activities.	Prolonged or exaggerated Oedipal or Electra complex
Genital—12 years to adulthood	Genitalia	Interest in peers as sexual partners. Task is to learn mature patterns of heterosexual behavior.	Failure to develop mature, acceptable methods of obtaining sexual gratification

ory, beginning with the newborn, the developing human is focused on a core need to satisfy a sensual drive (Table 4–5).

In each stage of development a different region of the body becomes the focus of sensual pleasure. The goal of the child is to proceed through each stage without trauma so that he or she will emerge as a "well-adjusted" adult. Freud believed that trauma in any given stage would result in some *fixation* or alteration in psychosexual development. Each stage builds on the next. As the focus of sensual pleasure shifts from one body region to another, the child must be willing to let go of the previous focus and to move on to another stage of development. If conflict has occurred at a certain stage, resolution of that sensual pleasure may not be complete and the child may be reluctant to move on to the next stage. Even if the child does move onward, psychosocial adjustment may be impaired, with fixations becoming apparent as the child continues to mature.

Freud's childhood stages were derived entirely from his experiences with adults. His theory was built on his work with neurotic personalities who sought psychiatric treatment. His theories have been criticized for his views on male supremacy and gender differences. Critics of Freud's work posit that many of the sexual conflicts he believed were developmental are more likely attributable to the responses of children growing up under the mores and values of late 19th century European society. Freud's theory also did not take into account any cultural differences among individuals. Although the areas of body focus seem appropriately correlated to the behaviors seen in children of specific age groups (sucking during infancy, gaining bowel control during toddlerhood), focus on these body parts can also be attributed to the natural acquisition of, and expected changes in, the functional abilities of these body structures.

Psychosocial Development

The most widely accepted and clinically relevant theories of personality development were developed by Erik Erikson in the 1960s. Erikson met Freud and studied psychoanalysis under Freud's daughter Anna. Erikson agreed with the idea that, at certain biological maturation points, the child was faced with crises or conflicts that needed to be resolved. Unlike Freud, however, Erikson did not believe these conflicts were sexual in their orientation. Rather, he believed that social and cultural factors influenced central issues that are germane to determining behaviors and actions at given time periods in the child's life. Erikson's theory of psychosocial development is based on the *epigenetic principle:* personality develops according to predetermined steps that are maturational and set by the growing person's readiness to be a part of a widening social radius and that society is structured to encourage the challenges that arise during these stages and to safeguard and encourage the proper rate and sequence of their unfolding (Erikson, 1963). The critical steps are turning points, or moments of decision between progress and regression, integration, and retardation (Erikson, 1963). Erikson called his stages or critical points the *Eight Ages of Man* (Table 4–6). Each stage is denoted by an emphasis on two opposing outcomes that are possible. During each stage, the individual is presented with a crisis. If a particular crisis is handled well, then a positive outcome prevails. If the crisis is not handled well, a negative outcome results. Thus, each stage is characterized and named after the opposing outcomes that emerge as maturation through that age is achieved. The theory also asserts that each psychosocial strength is related to all others, that each strength is dependent on the proper development in the proper sequence, and that each strength exists in some form before its critical time of emphasis normally arrives. As the child matures, a certain strength becomes more predominant, meets its crisis, and finds its lasting solution during the stage indicated (Erikson, 1963). Each stage lays the foundation for negotiating the challenges of the stages that follow.

Erikson emphasizes that the effects of culture, social-

Table 4–6
Erikson's Psychosocial Stages of Development

Stage	Characteristics	Outcomes
Trust vs. mistrust Birth–1 year	Caregiver responds in warm, caring manner to child's needs to create trusting environment. If care is inconsistent and unreliable, mistrust develops.	*Positive:* hope, tolerates frustration, can delay gratification, sense of trust *Negative:* suspicion, withdrawal, focus on negative aspect of people's behavior
Autonomy vs. shame and doubt 1–3 years	Child practices and attains new physical skills developing autonomy. If not allowed to do things he or she can do, or pushed into doing something when not ready, child may develop sense of shame or doubt.	*Positive:* will, self-control, positive self-esteem, self-confidence *Negative:* compulsion, impulsivity
Initiative vs. guilt 3–6 years	Initiative is demonstrated when the child is able to formulate a plan of action and carry it out. Believes that desires and actions are basically sound. If the child is punished for expressing his or her desires, then child will develop a sense of guilt.	*Positive:* purpose, enjoys accomplishments, self-starters *Negative:* inhibition, afraid to accept new challenges, guilt over one's actions
Industry vs. inferiority 6–12 years	Child acquires skills such as reading, writing, and mathematics and social skills. Through acquisition of these skills he or she develops a sense of industry. If always compared to others, or made to believe he or she is inadequate, child will develop sense of inferiority.	*Positive:* competence, enjoys learning about new things, perseverance, takes criticism well *Negative:* inadequacy, inferiority, gives up easily
Identity vs. role confusion 12–19 years	The adolescent investigates and identifies alternatives regarding his or her vocational and personal future. Premature choices, or the inability to make these choices, will lead to role confusion.	*Positive:* fidelity, confidence in self-identity, optimism, control of one's destiny *Negative:* diffidence, defiance, socially unacceptable identity, sense of purposelessness

Table continued on following page

Table 4–6
Erikson's Psychosocial Stages of Development *Continued*

Stage	Characteristics	Outcomes
Intimacy vs. isolation 19–25 years	Love relationships are developed. Fear of intimate relationships will lead to a sense of isolation.	*Positive:* love, development of deep interpersonal relationships *Negative:* exclusivity, avoidance of commitment, avoidance of relationships
Generativity vs. stagnation 25–50 years	Parenting, nurturing others, and fulfilling civic responsibilities are the tasks. The adult finds ways to be productive and of help to others in order to grow personally.	*Positive:* care, concern for future generations of the society, desire to help others *Negative:* stagnated, rejection of others, self-indulgence, self-absorbed, highly critical of others
Ego integrity vs. despair 50 and older	Reflection on one's life and one's achievements. A sense of pride or despair is developed regarding the accomplishments in life that have been made or were lost.	*Positive:* wisdom, self-satisfaction *Negative:* disdain, disgust, bitterness concerning lost opportunities

ization, and the historical moment will impact identity development. Therefore, his theory cannot be used as a blueprint to describe a single personality type. Children from different cultures develop and achieve the developmental tasks through a variety of socially acceptable mechanisms. For instance, achieving the stage of industry in United States' society is somewhat dependent on formal school achievements, whereas in other societies, the ability to farm or to catch animals for food is evidence of industry during middle childhood. Erikson's theory has been criticized for being overly broad and general and for being difficult to evaluate in an experimental setting (Kaplan, 1991).

Several other theorists have contributed to an understanding of personality development (Table 4–7). Their nonstage theories uniformly disagree with Freudian theory regarding the factors that motivate the development of different personality types. The theories of Jung, Adler,

Table 4–7
Contributions of Psychosocial Theorists

Theorist	Summary of Concepts
Carl Jung	The concepts of extraversion and introversion are associated with Jung's theory. The extravert directs interest to others, rather than to self. The extravert is adaptable, social, and governed by objective reality. The introvert directs energies toward the self, has obsessive-compulsive tendencies, is self-centered and rigid, and is governed by subjective feelings.
Alfred Adler	Developed theory of individual psychology. He believed that people are motivated to move from a position of inferiority or inadequacy toward feelings of security, power, worth, and superiority. He wrote extensively about inferiority complexes and mechanisms of compensation and overcompensation people use to hide their feelings of inadequacy.
Karen Horney	The primary motivator of behavior is basic anxiety, which begins with birth as the child enters a frightening world. People develop defense mechanisms to cope with this basic anxiety. Those who do not develop coping strategies will have one of these neurotic trends: moving toward people, moving away from people, or moving against people.
Harry Stack Sullivan	Believed interpersonal relationships in society were motivators of behavior. Fear of social disapproval or poor interpersonal relationships highly influence the child's actions.

Horney, and Sullivan can be useful in explaining variations in personality development and as a theoretical basis to focus on solutions to specific behavioral problems.

Cognitive-Intellectual Development

The cognitive theories of development explore how an individual comes to think, to perceive, to process, and to understand information about himself or herself and the environment. Some of the approaches evaluate cognition in relation to the child's specific developmental age (Piaget, Elkind), whereas others focus on explaining the processes of cognition that occur regardless of age-specific considerations (information-processing theories).

Piaget

Since the 1930s, Jean Piaget has been a leader in the exploration of cognitive development. He has outlined a complex four-stage theory to explain the assimilation and accommodation of information. *Assimilation* refers to the process of taking in information from the environment and incorporating this into one's existing knowledge structure, or *schema*. When this information changes the person's existing schema to include the new information, this process is called *accommodation*. Each stage is characterized by a different way of thinking, or of assimilating and accommodating information. Progress through each stage is gradual and orderly, varying in pace from child to child. Piaget's stages of cognitive development are summarized in Table 4–8. Piaget coined many terms to explain the concepts in his theory. Definitions of these terms are found in Table 4–9.

The original work of Piaget has been criticized for its weak scientific approach. Piaget used his own two children as subjects to develop his theory. His experiments were not controlled. He presented the children with a problem and observed how they reasoned and how they tried to solve that problem. Therefore, he may have underestimated the influence of formal learning on the development of cognitive processes (Hauck, 1991). For instance, Piaget believed that the child's display of magical thinking was a result of a lack of differentiation between mental fantasy and physical reality phenomena in a child's mind. Current research would support the existence of magical thinking, or "control by thinking," but would suggest that it is a result of, or follows from, an ability to differentiate between mental and physical phenomena. The child is learning to control by doing or by acting through calculating and anticipating outcomes (Vikan & Clausen, 1994). Piaget was able to articulate the sequences of development that lead a child to the point of adult understanding of such concepts as mathematics, time, and space. His theory does point to the importance of active experience in a child's development. Parents are encouraged to seek activities and to provide play experiences for their children that give them the opportunity to solve problems and reason in a logical manner. Piaget's theories are of particular importance to health care personnel to better understand how children think about health-related events (Chart 4–11). The nurse who is able to articulate the developmental differences in the cognitive abilities of children is better able to implement the nursing process in an age-appropriate individualized manner (Green, 1991; Hauck, 1991).

Elkind

Piagetian theory has been analyzed and expanded by numerous individuals. David Elkind, a psychologist, has focused some of his work on explaining the nature of egocentrism in children. Egocentrism refers to the lack of differentiation in some area of interaction. At each stage in development, this lack of differentiation takes a unique form and is manifested in unique ways (Elkind, 1967, 1986). Children view reality quite differently at different age levels. Children's view of reality can be distorted to the degree that egocentric thought affects their behavior and actions. During infancy, the child experiences a lack of differentiation between the object and the "experiences of the object" (Elkind, 1967). The young child is unable to differentiate between words and their referents and between self-created play, dream symbols, and reality. As the child matures, the school-age years are characterized by an inability to differentiate between mental constructs and perceptual givens. Adolescents are able to conceptualize the thoughts of both themselves and others; however, they are unable to differentiate between what others are thinking about and their own mental preoccupations (Elkind, 1967, 1984).

A primary focus of Elkind's work has been focused on adolescent thinking. Because of the emerging ability to think abstractly, adolescents become preoccupied with ideological issues (social, political, and religious). Concepts like metaphor and simile can be grasped, as well as can contradictions in belief systems. On the other hand, the egocentrism of adolescence creates a situation in which the adolescent does not make totally rational choices because he or she is so caught up and consumed by thoughts of self and self-needs. Elkind described four behaviors that typify adolescent egocentric thought processes. *Pseudostupidity* occurs when the adolescent asks apparently "dumb" questions indicating difficulty reconciling concrete and formal operations. For instance, a trumpet player who has a band concert that evening may ask the band director if he needs to take his instrument. The *imaginary audience* is characterized by super self-consciousness. For example, an adolescent may believe that everybody is watching him and evaluating his actions

Table 4-8
Piaget's Stages of Cognitive Development

Stage	Characteristics
Sensorimotor stage (birth–2 years)	
Substage 1: use of reflexes (birth–1 month)	Reflex responses to external stimuli Random body movements Genuinely intelligent behavior absent
Substage 2: primary circular reactions (1–4 months)	Active effort to reproduce behavior that was first performed by chance Accidentally acquired behavior becomes a new sensorimotor habit
Substage 3: secondary circular reactions (4–8 months)	Greater awareness of environment Increased interest in results of actions Begins to understand causality by recognizing that certain actions have certain results Dim awareness of before and after Achievement of hand–eye coordination Beginning development of object permanence
Substage 4: coordination of secondary circular reactions (8–12 months)	Solution of simple problems possible Demonstrates anticipatory behavior More highly developed object permanence
Substage 5: tertiary circular reactions (12–18 months)	Rudimentary trial and error activities present Beginning of reasoning Evident object permanence
Substage 6: invention of new meanings through deduction (18–24 months)	Well-developed understanding of the nature of objects Understands basic concept of causality Well-developed object permanence View of self as separate from others Ability to use symbols mentally
Preoperational stage (2–7 years)	
Stage 1: preconceptual stage (2–4 years)	Forms symbolic thought Is egocentric in thoughts, feelings, and experiences Is egocentric in perception of objects and events Displays deferred imitation Understands instructions literally
Stage 2: perceptual or intuitive stage (4–7 years)	Prelogical reasoning appears Experiences and objects are judged by outside appearances and results Can concentrate on only one characteristic of an object at a time (centration) Uses words to express thoughts Demonstrates illogical reasoning (transductive reasoning) Play becomes more socialized
Concrete operations (7–11 years)	Acquisition of conceptual skills that permit logical manipulation of symbols Thinking is still limited by reliance on what is observed, on tangible concrete events or objects Able to shift attention from one perceptual attribute to another (decentration) Able to reverse thinking (reversibility) Acquires conservation skills Enjoys collecting and classifying objects Able to appreciate a joke
Formal operations (11 years–death)	Able to logically manipulate abstract and unobservable concepts Uses scientific approach to solve problems Able to conceive the distant future concretely and set realistic long-term goals Can solve complex verbal problems

Table 4-9
Piaget's Terminology

Term	Stage Present or Attained	Definition
Object permanence	Sensorimotor	Knowledge that objects still exist even when not in sight
Symbolic thought	Sensorimotor	Ability to represent internally certain events that are not currently affecting the child's sense organs
Deferred imitation	Sensorimotor	Ability to imitate an action in the absence of the model demonstrating that action
Egocentrism and "omnipotence"	Preoperational	Inability to distinguish between own perception and that of someone else
Transductive reasoning	Preoperational	From a particular event to another event
Animism	Preoperational	Anthropomorphism. The child attributes human traits to inanimate objects or to animals.
Realism	Preoperational	Child's tendency to attribute real physical properties to mental events
Phantasm or magical thinking	Preoperational	A perception of things that have no physical reality such as an imaginary playmate
Morality of restraint	Preoperational	Belief that rules are sacred and unalterable (yet unable to follow the rules)
Syncretism	Preoperational	Belief that co-occurring events belong together (e.g., mom gets out her Bible, we must be going to church)
Artificialism	Preoperational	Belief that all objects and events exist to serve the needs of humans, especially the self
Irreversibility	Preoperational	Inability to mentally reverse in thinking and cannot backtrack steps in a thinking pattern
Centration	Preoperational	Inability to consider several aspects of the situation simultaneously. The child tends to focus his or her attention on one detail or aspect of an event.
Decentration	Concrete operational	The ability to shift attention from one perceptual attribute to another
Reversibility	Concrete operational	Can reverse actions or thinking (e.g., 10 = 10)
Conservation	Concrete operational	Comprehends that amount, weight, physical properties, and volume of substances are not changed by physical movement (e.g., the volume of water poured from a cup to a glass is the same)
Class intention and class extension	Concrete operational	Ability to define a class and list all of the members of that class
Relativism	Concrete operational	Two or more aspects of a problem may be operated (manipulated) simultaneously
Serialization	Concrete operational	Masters the ordinal number line; can group and sort/place in logical order

and behaviors. In a sense he believes he is on stage and everyone is focused on his activity. What he fails to perceive is that all adolescents have the same sense of super self-consciousness; thus, as individuals, they are all focused on their own actions and what others may think and spend little time concerned about the actions of others. *Personal fable* occurs because the adolescent thinks he or she is more special than anyone else and not subject to the natural laws. For instance, although a friend might get pregnant, although she, too, is having

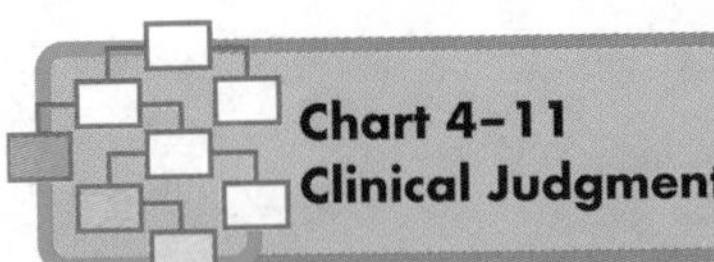

Chart 4–11
Clinical Judgment

Assessment of Cognitive and Psychosocial Development

Jordan (age 7) and Daniel (age 4) are brothers admitted to the hospital because of injuries obtained in a motor vehicle accident. They share a hospital room. They will be discharged later in the day after teaching has been completed regarding care of their wounds. As you enter the room they are yelling at each other, fighting over which television show to watch. The parents left to eat breakfast. Jordan has a set of small blocks on his bedside table, Daniel has six small race cars on the bed beside him. An unopened model for a plane is located at the end of Daniel's bed.

Questions

1. Based on your quick assessment of the situation, what will be the focus of your interactions with the boys today?
2. According to their ages what stages of cognitive and psychosocial development would you place the boys in as a beginning point for your assessment?
3. Do you think the boys are acting in an age-appropriate fashion?
4. After you get the boys to calm down, you tell them that you will be teaching them how to care for their injuries at home. What aspects of this would be appropriate to teach each boy?
5. When the boys are being discharged, how would you determine whether your teaching was effective?

Answers

1. Providing age-appropriate diversionary activities, explaining the rules of conduct while in the hospital, and providing discharge teaching regarding wound care
2. Jordan:
    School-age
    Latency stage (Freud)
    Industry versus inferiority (Erikson)
    Concrete operations (Piaget)

   Daniel:
    Preschooler
    Phallic stage (Freud)
    Initiative versus guilt (Erikson)
    Preoperational stage (Piaget)
3. Yes. Sibling fighting would be expected at these ages. The toys they are playing with are appropriate for their age. The airplane model is too advanced for Daniel's level of fine motor skills; however, this is probably why it remains unopened on his bed.
4. Teach the boys separately because your approach needs to be different with each child. Daniel should be taught first. Terminology needs to be very simple. He can assist in his care by taking off the tape, opening packages, and helping to put the new dressing back on the wound. He can practice these activities on a doll. These activities promote feelings of accomplishment within Daniel's developmental skill level. Jordan can watch Daniel but should be asked not to intervene. When it is Jordan's turn, he can participate by gathering the necessary equipment, removing the bandage, completing the first cleaning of the wound (parents do the second), and placing a new bandage on his wound. He should also clean up after the task is finished.
5. Jordan is able to tell his parents what they will need to clean his wounds and can demonstrate on a doll how to complete the dressing change. Daniel states he is the helper. His job is to be still and help his mother change his bandage.

unprotected sexual relations, the adolescent believes she would never get pregnant. Lastly, the adolescent is characterized by *apparent hypocrisy*. The adolescent expresses an idea and believes that such expression is the same as having worked for and achieved an action. Or the adolescent will claim a certain ideology and yet take actions that are in direct contrast to his or her stated beliefs. For example, the adolescent will criticize the horrible conditions caused by environmental pollutants and then be seen dropping trash from the window of a car. No correlation is made between expressed ideologies and practical action.

Information-Processing Theories

The information processing approach can be used to explain the steps an individual goes through to take in, process, and act on information. It is not a single consistent theory developed by one person. Rather, information-processing theories are based on programs of research by many people analyzing different aspects of cognition, each with a slightly different focus (Hauck, 1991). Unlike Piaget, the information-processing theorists believe that many of the basic processes for registering, storing, and processing information do not change with age. Rather what does change is the person's capacity, speed, and efficiency to process information (Siegler, 1983, 1986). Information-processing theories view cognition as a process on a continuum, rather than a pattern of development that occurs in specific stages.

In information-processing theories the computer is used as an analogy to the human mind. From the moment the person receives an input, an array of subprocesses must occur before an action can take place. Just as one types on the computer keyboard (the input), a range of technological processes occur in rapid succession to display the words on the screen, save them as requested, and recall them when needed. For the human to accomplish a similar task, operations such as attention to the object (encoding), perception, short-term and long-term memory, retrieval, and storage processes must all be intact and must all be completed for cognition to occur.

Information-processing theories have been especially helpful in analyzing the effects of hearing, vision, and communication deficits on the learning process. Injuries or congenital insults that cause sensory handicaps or mental retardation directly affect information processing. This approach to cognitive development is fairly new and requires more investigation as technologies are developed to explore the functions of the brain.

Multiple Intelligences

Students of psychology and education have begun to embrace a new theory of human intelligence that is broader and more comprehensive in its approach than previously accepted cognitive theories. The study of *multiple intelligences* addresses the concept that humans possess different talents, or multiple capacities, ranging from musical intelligence to the intelligence involved in understanding oneself (Table 4–10) (Gardner, 1993). This widespread interest in the theory of multiple intelligences was launched in 1983 by Howard Gardner, a developmental

Table 4–10
The Eight Intelligences

Intelligence	Skill	Application
Linguistic	The gift of language	Poets, authors, writers
Logical-mathematical	Problem-solving abilities	Mathematicians, accountants, scientists, cashiers
Spatial	Ability to form a mental model of a spatial world and be able to maneuver and operate using that model	Sailors, engineers, surgeons, sculptors, painters
Musical	Ability to play an instrument, sing, create music	Musicians, composers
Body-kinesthetic	Ability to solve problems or to fashion products using one's whole body or parts of the body	Dancers, athletes, surgeons, craftspeople
Naturalist	Ability to distinguish between different kinds of plants and animals	Zoologists, botanists, microbiologists
Interpersonal	Ability to understand other people, what motivates them, how they work, how to cooperate with them	Successful salespeople, politicians, teachers, clinicians, religious leaders
Intrapersonal	Capacity to form an accurate understanding of oneself and be able to use that understanding to operate effectively in life. Allows one to understand and work with oneself.	Evidence in any life experiences in which it is clear that the person truly understands his or her feelings and emotions and uses this knowledge to understand and guide personal behavior

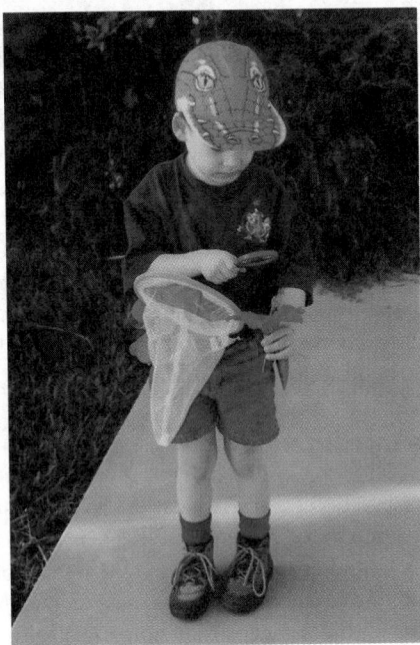

Figure 4–17
Multiple intelligence theory asserts that a young child's interest in certain activities and skills should be nurtured, because this may represent a high level of intelligence in that area.

psychologist at the Harvard Graduate School of Education. Gardner's publication of the *Frames of Mind*, a book that outlined seven intelligences, quickly became a work embraced by professional educators, parents, and educated lay persons who were interested in transforming approaches to educating children and adolescents and in stimulating change in the current educational system. Since that time, Gardner has suggested that there may be an eighth intelligence, that of the naturalist (Fig. 4–17) (Viadero, 1996).

Gardner's theory specifically challenges the prevalent notion that intelligence is tied to the ability to provide succinct answers in a speedy fashion to problems primarily involving linguistic and logical skills (Gardner, 1993). In particular, the theory of multiple intelligences steps beyond the definitions of cognitive development asserted by theorists such as Jean Piaget. Gardner believes that Piaget and others have measured and developed their theories based primarily on a single dimension of cognition—the development of logical-mathematical intelligence. Multiple intelligences theory takes a more pluralistic view, recognizing that there are many different and discrete facets of cognition. The theory acknowledges that different people have different cognitive strengths and contrasting cognitive styles (Gardner, 1993). The theory challenges the dependence on the linguistic mode of instruction utilized by most educators and educational systems as the primary and most effective manner in which to help children learn. Gardner believes that all of the intelligences are unevenly distributed, coexist, and can change over time. The responsibility of educators is to capitalize on the student's individual intellectual strengths.

The theory of multiple intelligences stems from the premise that there is a natural developmental trajectory of learning that begins with *raw patterning ability*. The "raw" intelligence is predominant during the first year of life. In subsequent stages, the intelligences are grasped through a *symbol system*. These symbols include learning sentences through stories, learning music through singing and playing songs, and experiencing body-kinesthetic development through dance. Children demonstrate their abilities in the various intelligences through their grasp of the various symbol systems. As development progresses, each intelligence with its accompanying symbol system is represented in a *notational system*. For instance, mathematics, reading, musical notation, and mapping are second-order notational systems. The marks on the paper come to stand for symbols. In our culture, mastery of these symbols is typically acquired in a formal educational system. During adolescence and adulthood, the mastery of an intelligence is expressed through vocational and professional pursuits.

In each of the intelligence domains, it is possible to have *at-promise individuals*. These are people who are highly endowed with the core abilities and skills of that intelligence. For example, Babe Ruth, the famous baseball player, was outstanding in body-kinesthetic intelligence. With each intelligence, the particular developmental trajectory of an individual "at promise" varies. For instance, some young children with mathematics and musical intelligence are able to perform at, or near, adult-level expectations. In contrast, the interpersonal and intrapersonal intelligences appear to develop more gradually, and child prodigies in these areas are rare. In addition, mature performance in one area does not imply mature performance in another area.

Knowledge of these intelligence categories can be used by parents, teachers, and health care professionals to provide activities to enhance development of the child's intelligences. Parents can assist children in their choice of activities and assist adolescents in their choice of careers within the context of their dominant intelligence. Teachers and the educational system can create individual-centered schools where student profiles, goals, and interests are matched to particular curricula and particular styles of teaching and learning. There is a need to create and use "intelligence fair" instruments to assess all forms of intelligence, not merely linguistic or logical-mathematical (i.e., IQ, SAT). In the community, children and adolescents need assistance in complementing their formal academic learning with opportunities involving the full spectrum of their intelligences.

Behavioral Development

The behavioral approach is structured on the interactions that occur between a child and his or her environment, which in turn determines the behavior of the child. Behaviorists believe that the roots of a person's behavior are tied to his or her experiences. If experience (the environment) is altered, then behavior change follows. This approach has been very successful in modifying the behaviors of some people in certain circumstances. The two most prevalent behavioral techniques are classical conditioning and operant conditioning. The behavioral theories have been criticized for their mechanical approach to human interactions. The effects of the consciousness and thought processes on individual action are not well accounted for by the theories. Human behavior is afforded little qualitative difference from the behavior and expected responses in animals. The theories are well tested in the laboratory setting, with an emphasis on the effects of the environment on human behavior. However, translation of these findings to real-life settings where other mental processes may come into play demonstrates that classical and operant conditioning can only partially explain a person's behavior.

Classical Conditioning

Classical conditioning was first introduced by Ivan Pavlov and was further explored by John Watson. The approach to learning involves pairing a neutral stimulus with an unconditioned stimulus to elicit an unconditioned response. This process is continued until the neutral stimulus is able to elicit a response without being paired with the original stimulus. The stimulus that elicits the response before conditioning is called the *unconditional stimulus*. The subsequent response is the *unconditioned response*. The *conditioned stimulus* is a neutral stimulus that, when paired with the unconditioned stimulus, eventually elicits the desired response by itself. The learned response is the *conditioned response*. In a similar circumstance, the individual learns stimulus generalization, that is, to apply the association of a certain behavior with a stimulus to circumstances that feature similar stimuli. The individual eventually learns *discrimination*, the process of differentiating among stimuli, and *extinction*, the weakening and disappearance of a learned response.

Classical conditioning has been thoroughly evaluated in laboratory settings in which the environment and exposure to stimuli can be highly monitored. It is a useful theory in understanding acquired emotional responses in children (e.g., unusual fears about dogs). The theory does not take into account the higher mental capacities of humans to utilize thinking and information-processing abilities to determine response patterns.

Operant Conditioning

Operant conditioning holds that behaviors are repeated or are reduced in frequency based on the environmental consequences of reinforcement or punishment. B. F. Skinner popularized this concept of *stimulus-response learning*. In operant conditioning, the child's behavior is followed by a negative or positive reinforcer that decreases or increases the likelihood of that behavior being repeated. A *positive reinforcer* is a pleasant stimulus that follows a behavior and that increases the frequency of that behavior. For instance, giving a child a piece of candy each time he sits still during a haircut is a positive reinforcer that rewards the child and encourages him to sit still the next time he has a haircut as he anticipates receiving more candy. A *negative reinforcer* is activated when an unpleasant stimulus is removed after a behavior has occurred and results in an increase in frequency of that behavior. For instance, in a laboratory a rat is placed in a box with an electrical floor grid that delivers a shock to the rat. Each time the rat presses a lever there is a cessation in the shocks. Thus the rat is reinforced to press the lever and remove the unpleasant stimuli. *Punishment* is the process in which an unpleasant stimulus is introduced after a response has been made and the response decreases. The child who receives a spanking for biting a sibling would be expected not to repeat the biting behavior. Skinner and his associates also believed that behavior could be shaped. *Shaping* is the process in which a new behavior is acquired by taking a known behavior and continually reinforcing it to bring it closer and closer to the desired behavior. These principles have been applied successfully as behavior modification techniques to change parenting responses to a child's actions and vice versa.

Social Learning Theories

The social learning theories explain human behavior based on the processes of imitation, observation learning, and reinforcement. Although the behavioral theories stress the importance of structuring stimulus and reinforcements to create certain behavioral responses, social learning theorists acknowledge that a child does not have to be reinforced or punished to change his or her behavior. Children learn by observing and imitating. They watch and monitor the consequences of the behavior of others. Therefore, others, especially parents, siblings, and peers, serve as models for the child's behavior. Simply observing another person may be sufficient to lead to a learned response. Reinforcement, particularly parental reinforcement, may not be needed to elicit the learned response.

Models who hold a high status in the child's eye are seen as especially credible. For example, a child may watch a cartoon show and see characters interacting and fighting in a certain manner. If he is not familiar with the show, the child will most likely not imitate what he has seen. However, when the child goes to daycare and observes several of the other children pretending to be the same cartoon characters, he will be more inclined to imitate the behaviors of his respected friends. Social-learning theories are helpful in explaining the powerful influence that social groups and the media can have on children's behavior. Although parents may choose not to exhibit or to expose their children to certain behaviors in the home, children may be influenced by modeling that is occurring in their play group or by other influential adults, such as grandparents or family friends.

One of the primary authors of social-learning theory, Albert Bandura, suggested that there is a four-step process that occurs between the observed modeled event and its acquisition. The first step is paying *attention* to the model. Attention is influenced by the characteristics of the model, the value of the model's behavior, and the characteristics of the observer (Kaplan, 1991). A model that holds high prestige or is in favorable status with the observer will gain more attention. Furthermore, the behaviors must be those which the observer values or considers important. Lastly, characteristics of the observer, such as his or her arousal state, interest, and present and past performance, influence the attention stage.

Once the child has attended to the behavior, *retention* must occur. During this step the information is encoded and stored in the child's memory. During the *motor reproduction* step, the retained information is retrieved and the child executes the behavior he or she has seen modeled. The child's developmental abilities influence his or her ability to replicate the behaviors. On the other hand, the child may have seen a behavior modeled, may store that information, but may never exhibit that behavior. The child may witness a murder on television, yet never attempt to repeat those actions, because he or she has inhibitions, morals, and values that prevent him or her from acting on every behavior witnessed.

During the final step, *motivational processes* occur in which reinforcement of the behavior must be made available to the child. The three types of reinforcement that motivate the child's behavior are *direct reinforcement*, *vicarious reinforcement*, and *self-reinforcement*. During direct reinforcement the person observing the child's behavior (which he or she has modeled from another) may provide positive or negative feedback regarding the child's actions. This feedback may make the child realize that he or she should not model that behavior again. Vicarious reinforcement is provided when the child sees others reinforced for their actions. If a child sees someone else rewarded for certain behaviors, it would encourage such behaviors on the part of the observer. Observing others being punished for their actions is likely to convey information about behaviors that are not well tolerated. Self-reinforcement occurs when an individual reinforces himself or herself for performing a particular act (Kaplan, 1991).

Bandura believes that learning involves a complex relationship that occurs between the person, the behavior, and the environment; each affects the other's actions and reactions. The person shapes the environment and the behavior, the environment shapes the person and the behavior, and the behavior shapes the person and the environment. For instance, children may watch what is considered to be a "violent" cartoon on television. The children respond to this environmental stimuli by modeling the violent behaviors. If enough children continue to watch the program, the show (the environment) will continue to be televised. If enough parents are frustrated by the behaviors from the show that they see their child modeling, they may petition to have the show canceled. If the show is no longer viewed, the child may then quit modeling the violent behaviors performed by the cartoon "buddies."

Robert Sears is another theorist who has utilized social-learning theories to explain the socialization process of children. Sears and his colleagues proposed three phases of the social-learning process. The earliest stage, *rudimentary behaviors*, occurs in infancy. The infant is motivated to act to avoid pain and reduce displeasures associated with his or her basic needs (hunger, elimination, temperature regulation). The infant learns which behaviors will produce the most rapid response to have his or her needs met. Thus, the child learns to associate the behaviors (crying, kicking, smiling, cooing) with the responses elicited from the parent.

As the child matures, *secondary behavioral systems* develop. In these systems, dyadic interactions (between two people) lead to the fulfillment of certain expected behaviors on the part of both participants. For instance, during the rudimentary phase, crying may have initiated feeding. During the secondary phase, asking for food brings mother and food and a whole repertoire of other discrete behaviors that are linked to mealtime. This includes washing hands, praise for washing hands, sitting at a particular location, saying prayers, reinforcement for saying prayers, eating with the mouth closed, politely asking for seconds, and so on. The complex social behaviors are being reinforced during these dyadic interactions. In addition, social learning by *identification* is taking place. The child learns to imitate the influential and powerful model presented by the mother and father. As the child imitates these behaviors they are reinforced. In the absence of the parent, the child still demonstrates identification if he or she continues to display those same gestures and actions of the loved parent.

The final phase of learning occurs when the child moves beyond the family boundaries, seeking other sources for reinforcements of behavior. School friends, church groups, interactive clubs, and gangs can all become potential sources of reinforcement of behavior. The child uses members of these groups to reinforce his or her actions and may also use self-reinforcement in the process of maturing and becoming more self-reliant.

The social learning theories have been criticized for their lack of a developmental framework. The process of imitation is viewed as the same, regardless of the child's developmental age and cognitive maturation. Therefore, the theories do not explain age-related changes that can occur in the learning process. The theories are useful to help understand the presence of certain behaviors in children, such as altruism and aggression. Parents should be encouraged to look at the models in their children's environment and to be aware of the powerful influence others can have on the child's behavior.

Development of Self-Concept

Humanistic Theories

The humanistic theories of development are also called the *phenomenological theories*. As a recognized psychological framework, humanism has existed for approximately the past 30 years. The theories emphasize and value the meanings associated with the human experience itself and postulate that what a person perceives the world to be is more important than external reality (Freiberg, 1987). From the humanistic viewpoint, all people are seen as basically good, with a desire to become all that they are capable of being. The experiences a person has within the family and the environment either hinder or foster potential for growth. The humanistic theories are build on the tenet that people cannot love others unless they love themselves. Everyone is unique, and the major focus in psychology should be to emphasize this uniqueness rather than try to fit actions and behaviors into universal laws and behaviors. Thus, a major goal of parenting is to foster an environment in which the individual child feels loved and accepted for what he or she is, even if that differs from parental hopes or expectations. Child rearing should involve few rules, roles, and expectations of what constitutes a "good child." Feelings of guilt and punishment are seen as counterproductive to fostering acceptance and self-actualization. Some of the major theorists who have contributed to the humanistic approach are Abraham Maslow, Carl Rogers, and Albert Ellis (Table 4–11). Their theories help to explain how people achieve and maintain a healthy personality. The humanistic theorists do not spend a lot of time trying to explain or to understand a person's past experiences as they relate to current behavior. Rather, their emphasis is on the "here and now" and on the belief that all people have the potential to enhance their emotional lives and psychological well-being.

Table 4–11
Humanistic Theories

Theorist	Major Tenets
Abraham Maslow—hierarchy of needs	Basic human needs are organized into a hierarchy of relative potency from lower-order requirements such as physiologic needs and safety to higher-order needs such as love, esteem, and self-actualization.
Carl Rogers	We all shape our own personalities. To change we must acknowledge to ourselves what we are. People should not impose their negative opinions, their directions, and their value systems on others.
Albert Ellis	There are four human life goals: to survive, to be happy, to get along with members of a social group, and to relate intimately with a few select members of this group. People make assumptions about how to meet these goals and evaluate meanings attached to these goals. Belief systems that are based on irrational assumptions and meanings lead to disturbed emotional reactions.

Language Development

Although the word *infant* means "without language," language acquisition is rooted in infancy through the many verbal and nonverbal exchanges children have with their caregivers. Language is the symbol system used for the storage and exchange of information (Coplan, 1995). Language is a basic tool used for interpersonal relationships. It is also a primary indicator of a child's developmental level. Speech acquisition is tied to the achievement of other physiologic and social factors such as neurologic maturation, musculoskeletal development, and the innate desire to communicate with others. The child's ability to read and write are manifestations of language development. The presence of a speech or language disorder can have a profound impact on the child's ability to develop social relations, attain success in school, and feel confident when communicating with others (see Chapter 28 for a complete discussion of communication disorders). Although language development proceeds in certain predictable patterns, some children learn to speak sooner than others their age, whereas some children may acquire language much later. Albert Einstein and Winston Churchill are two famous individuals who are known to have been slow to speak in childhood (Freiberg, 1987).

Language is conveyed through the use of three different symbol systems. One is *auditory expressive language*, the utterances of sound and eventually words. The earliest forms of auditory expressive language include open vowel sounds such as crying, cooing, and gurgling. By 5 months of age, laughing and the use of monosyllabic utterances appears, such as "ba" and "ga." Between 6 and 8 months of age, polysyllabic vocalizations can be made by the infant such as "lalalalala" and "dadadada." By 12 months of age, the infant has acquired one or two words. At 24 months of age the toddler is acquiring one or two new words per day and is well on the way to developing a full repertoire of words to verbally express his or her needs and desires (Chart 4–12).

Humans also use *auditory receptive language*, which is the ability to listen and comprehend. The auditory receptive language skills of the young child are much more

Chart 4–12
Developmental Considerations

Development of Language

Age	Auditory Expressive Language	Auditory Receptive Language	Visual Language
Newborn	Cooing Crying	Responds to vocal stimuli by eye widening or changes in respiratory rate or suck rate	Gives alert visual fixation to caregiver's verbal stimuli Links mother's voice with her face and when crying is comforted by her voice
4–5 months	Laughing Monosyllables (ba, ga) Razzing	Turns head to locate source of a voice or bell	Social smile Visual localization of auditory stimuli (turning to a voice or a bell)
6–8 months	Polysyllabic babbling (lalalala)	Attends selectively to his or her own name when uttered by an adult Responds to tones of voice	Attends to common gesture games like patty cake and peek-a-boo
9–12 months	Sporadically utters "mama," "dada"; then learns to spontaneously say "mama" and "dada" and label the correct parent Shakes head "no"	Comprehends the words "no" and "stop" Listens selectively to familiar words	Reciprocates and initiates gesture games Waves bye-bye Expresses desires by pointing to object and making sounds or crying
12 months	Says one or two words other than "mama" or "dada" Begins to acquire one new word per week	Responds to one-step commands (give it to me) unaccompanied by a gestural cue Can bring familiar object from another room on request	Uses index finger pointing and single-word naming to signify desired object
18–24 months	Uses 10–20 words	Has receptive vocabulary of more than 100 words	Points to body parts
24 months	Acquires one or more new words per day Has vocabulary of 50 words Begins to produce jargon and two-word phrases ("me down") Begins to use pronouns Speech is one-half intelligible	Can follow simple novel two-step commands (put your shoes away, then go sit down) Names simple objects on command Has receptive vocabulary of more than 300 words	Points to objects on command

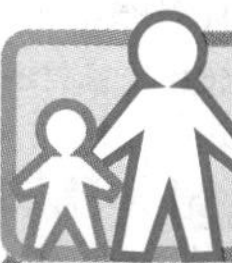

Chart 4–12
Developmental Considerations *Continued*

Development of Language

Age	Auditory Expressive Language	Auditory Receptive Language	Visual Language
30 months	Beginning of telegraphic speech—three- to five-word sentences containing a recognizable subject and predicate but lacking conjunctions, articles, the verb "to be," and other small connecting words ("Me want bear.")	Points to objects described by use (give me the one we drink with) Follows prepositional commands (put the napkin under the cup)	Uses fingers to count one–two
3 years	Acquires several new words a day Uses three- to four-word sentences Uses regular plurals Uses pronouns (I, me, you) Can count three objects Can tell age, sex, and full name Speech is three-fourths intelligible	Has receptive vocabulary of 800 words Knows function of common objects Understands spatial relationships (on, in, under)	Uses fingers to count or show age
4 years	Speaks four- to five-word sentences Can tell a story Uses past tense Names one color Can count four objects Speech is completely intelligible Normal dysfluency (stuttering)	Understands same/different	Begins to make letters and numbers
5–6 years	Speaks sentences of more than five words Uses future tense Names four colors Can count 10 or more objects Dysfluencies resolve Uses nouns, plurals, possessives Narrative has cause-and-effect sequence	Recalls part of a story Follows three-part commands Receptive language between 1500 and 2000 words Able to follow three- and four-step commands Understands "where," "when," and "why"	Matches identical shapes or figures Discriminates left versus right Copies square, circle, and cross Begins to write words Begins to read
7–9 years	Uses temporal prepositions (before, after) Uses past and future tenses Narrative has proper sequence	Understands passive verb forms (the cat was hit by a car)	No reversals of "b" and "d" persist Sight word vocabulary increases
10–12 years	Changes style of language (formal versus informal) to fit different contexts and different listeners (parents versus peers)	Understands multiple meanings of words Knows meanings of figurative language (simile, metaphor, analogy)	Attempts three-dimensional shapes in artwork Copies complex shapes and figures Begins to understand maps and geography Good sight word vocabulary
13+ years	Complex sentence structure Can speak and write about abstract concepts	Understands linguistic explanations of abstract concepts Understands how to "play on words" (Call me a cab. Okay, hi cab)	Understands architectural plans Understands complex spatial relationships Uses and creates maps and schematic drawings

extensive than their auditory expressive language system. As early as the 26th week of gestation, fetuses can respond to sound (Coplan, 1995). The newborn responds to verbal stimuli by eye widening, an increase in respiratory rate, or an increase in sucking rate. By 2 to 3 months of age, the infant listens and watches the adult speaking. When the adult becomes silent the infant interjects with his or her own vocalizations. By 4 months of age the infant turns the head and attends to the sound of a bell ringing in a certain direction. Between 7 and 9 months the child selectively attends to his or her name being spoken by an adult. The words "no" and "stop" are understood by the mischievous infant. At 2 years of age, although the toddler can utter only about 50 words, the child can follow simple commands. Parents may believe that the young child does not understand their words because the child is not able to vocalize. This is incorrect. By 36 months, a child comprehends about 800 words. It is important for parents to understand that if they use simple, clear language when speaking to the young child, effective communication can take place even if the child utters no words.

caREminder: *Health care providers need to be careful about the topics they discuss in the presence of the young child. The child may comprehend several of the key points of the dialogue, yet misinterpret their full meaning based on their cognitive development.*

Language is also conveyed *visually*. Gestures and hand signals are used to convey a broad scope of expressive meaning. The American Sign Language system is based on visual language skills. Prelinguistic visual milestones begin with the newborn who attends to language with alert visual fixation (Coplan, 1995). As the child acquires verbal language skills, he or she will be using a broad scope of visual language skills to communicate with others. For instance, the social smile indicates that the child is happy or pleased with the actions of another person. The young child learns to wave bye-bye, blow a kiss, and point to the ground when he or she wants out of a high chair. The child will point to objects he or she wants and screams out if the parent does not understand this communication. Deaf infants exposed to American Sign Language use their visual and receptive language skills to acquire language that parallels the stages of oral language development in the child who can hear (Petitto & Marentette, 1991).

Theories of Language Acquisition

There are four primary approaches used to describe how language is developed. The *empirical approach* is supported by the theorist B. F. Skinner, who popularized the concept of stimulus-response learning. Using this approach, language is a verbal behavior that is acquired in the same fashion as all other new behaviors. Consequences (rewards and punishments) are used in everyday life to teach the child language skills. For instance, the child points to a cookie. Parents respond "say cookie," and the child says something that approximates the word "cookie" and receives a cookie from the parent. A new word is acquired. Although there is little doubt that reinforcement impacts language development, this approach does not explain how children can do and say things that they have never heard before.

Another approach is the nativist or rationalist approach advocated by Noam Chomsky (1968). Chomsky asserted that humans are born with an innate tendency to acquire language. He maintained that all languages share certain basic structural characteristics. Although the words and order of words may vary from culture to culture, there is a common universal grammar that consists of rules and principles that are used to generate sentences and meanings. Humans have inherited the biological structure (the central nervous system) to process these common linguistic features. The mental blueprint for acquiring language is called the *language acquisition device (LAD)*. The LAD is the inborn capacity that permits the acquisition of grammatical rules that allow the child to translate words and sentences and later produce words and sentences.

Interactionists reject the idea that language is acquired empirically by imitation and practice (Berko, 1958; Brown, 1973). In this approach, there is an agreement that language acquisition is innate and that a biological system like the LAD may guide language development. However, this approach also emphasizes that language development is equally influenced by the ways in which children learn though experience to attach concepts and meanings to words.

A fourth view of language acquisition is supported by Piaget (1926) and called the *cognitive approach*. The child has the capability to learn language in concert with the development of other cognitive capabilities. The development of thought parallels the development of speech and language. As the child is able to create a mental scheme, the child has a corresponding ability to apply a linguistic label to it. Piaget asserted that the ability to symbolically represent events emerged at around 1½ to 2 years in age, the same time that the child is able to master language skills. Vygotsky (1962) agreed that language acquisition was a cognitive process; however, he did not believe that language developed from the same origin as thought processes. He believed that thought and language originated from two separate roots, a preintellectual stage and a prelinguistic stage. At around age 2 these two lines of development meet and merge so that what the child thinks now influences what is said. This theory helps to explain why children rapidly acquire new language at a time when they are also demonstrating a great deal of interest and curiosity about their environment.

Factors That Influence Language Development

Girls are generally more advanced than boys in verbal acquisition. The speech control center of the brain is located in the dominant cerebral hemisphere, which for most individuals is on the left side. During infancy and early childhood, girls demonstrate advanced development of their left cerebral hemisphere that would accelerate verbal fluency. First-born and only children have more advanced language skills than do later-born children. This is because younger siblings do not receive as much direct verbal input from adults as did the first-born child. In addition, the linguistic input from older siblings is not as optimal as that received from an adult in regard to learning correct language rules and structure (Jarman & Oberklaid, 1992).

Worldview: *It was once thought that children who were exposed to two languages at the same time had delays in language acquisition. Peal and Lambert (1962) found this not to be true. Bilingual children who acquired their second language at an early age have demonstrated more flexibility in their use of labels and words. Bilingual children demonstrated higher cognitive capabilities than monolingual children. In addition, bilingual children learn to see the world from two different perspectives and from two different cultures.*

A primary influence on impaired auditory expressive language development is the presence of some degree of hearing loss. One infant per thousand is born with bilateral severe-to-profound hearing loss (Coplan, 1995). The cause of congenital deafness can be genetic or can be acquired from intrauterine conditions such as infections (cytomegalovirus, rubella, syphilis) or anomalies. Hearing loss is also higher in premature children who have corresponding postnatal complications (e.g., poor Apgar score, need for mechanical ventilation, hyperbilirubinemia). Permanent partial hearing loss is associated with bacterial meningitis, certain infectious diseases (mumps, measles, Epstein-Barr virus), the use of ototoxic drugs, and head trauma. Mild to moderate transient hearing loss can also be associated with otitis media with effusion.

Alert: *Approximately 15% of infants experience 90 or more days of otitis media with effusion in the first year of life (Finitzo, Gunnarson, & Clark, 1990). The child who experiences an increased incidence of this disorder should be evaluated for hearing loss, and delays in speech development should be monitored carefully as the child's clinical condition improves. If speech development remains delayed or impaired, referral to a speech therapist is warranted.*

The presence of a developmental disorder may impact language acquisition. For instance, children who are mentally retarded have language delay in all areas: auditory expressive, auditory receptive, and visual. The child with a developmental language disorder will have variable degrees of expressive and receptive language impairment. Visual language skills are usually normal. Children who are autistic display delayed and deviant language (Coplan, 1995).

Development of Sexuality

The child's sexual development is influenced by biological, social, and psychological factors. The biological factors include the child's chromosomal sex, the external sexual organs, and the internal reproductive structures. Biological problems can occur in which the child's gender is difficult to determine at birth owing to the presence of ambiguous genitalia or chromosomal abnormalities. In these cases, the sexual identification that is assigned and the subsequent style of child rearing may not be consistent with the hormonal and structural factors that were present at birth.

The social and psychological factors of sexual development interact to create a person's gender identity. Throughout the child's life, interactions with significant adults and peers impact the self-perception, the preferences, and the gender-associated behaviors that are culturally attributed to males or females.

Gender identification and the awareness of one's sexuality begin in the toddler years. The foundation for this process has already been laid with the development of trust and consistency of need fulfillment obtained during infancy. As the child's cognitive processes and language skills increase, opportunities arise that reinforce gender identification. The child quickly learns to imitate gender behavior and pretend to be mommy or daddy. The toddler learns to name and to draw body parts. Body orifices are explored, and questions about mother's or father's body may arise. Parents are encouraged to use correct terminology when referring to body parts and not to overact if the child is seen exploring his or her body parts.

In the preschool years, parents may note a definite focus by the child on their genitalia and "private" parts. Name calling using words associated with the genitalia or the elimination processes is common. The child continues to explore the body through masturbation and exploration of other children's genitalia. Parents should be teaching about personal privacy and the social appropriateness of actions. Facts about reproduction should be given.

caREminder: *Children at this stage should be taught about who can, and under what conditions someone can, touch their genitalia or "private" parts, and what to do if someone touches them inappropriately.*

The school-age years mark a change from focusing primarily on the parents for gender identification toward a focus on peers for identity development. Children at this age may engage in kissing, hugging, and other forms of physical contact with members of the opposite sex. Expressions of sexuality are primarily a response of cognitive and emotional factors, rather than physical desire. The child develops close relationships with boys and girls in his or her age group. Within the context of these relationships, sexual stereotyping and role-playing is reinforced. Parents and other significant adults should offer basic information about the changes that occur in the body with adolescence. In addition, discussions regarding reproduction and sexual activity should take place. Both the school-age child and the adolescent will seek out this information from other "sources" to answer their queries. These other sources may provide inaccurate and misleading information to the young person.

The adolescent experiences tremendous changes in his or her sexual development as he or she deals with the physical maturation of the sexual organs. (Refer to the section on gender development for a complete description of the physical changes that occur during this time.) Throughout puberty, the adolescent explores the changes in his or her body and the way it functions. Physical sexual desire may emerge, or responses to physical stimuli may be associated more with the need for emotional gratification rather than physical needs (Fig. 4–18). During this period, adults should encourage the adolescent to express his or her feelings regarding his or her changing body and corresponding emotions. Parents can assist in clarifying values and in making decisions regarding gender-related activities. Information regarding sexually transmitted diseases, contraception, and pregnancy should be readily available for the adolescent. Many health care providers are directing their efforts toward encouraging adolescents to delay the start of intercourse. The increasing number of boys and girls having intercourse at earlier ages means that there is likely to be a variety of partners over time with a corresponding rise in the incidence of sexually transmitted diseases and teenage pregnancies (Howard, 1992).

Figure 4–18
During adolescence, emerging sexuality is expressed in the development of intimate relationships.

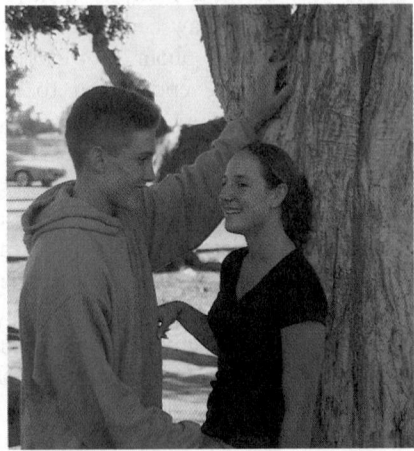

Moral Development

Moral development is thought to be significantly correlated with intellectual reasoning and age. Psychologists differ in their beliefs regarding how a child's moral reasoning and subsequent moral behaviors develop. Proponents of Freudian psychology believe that it is the *superego,* the inner conscience of the child, that influences moral behavior. According to this theory, the child seeks to identify and internalize the ideals and values of adults around them, creating an ego ideal. The child's conscience will cause a sense of guilt when misbehavior occurs. Thus, morality is an outcome of the ego ideal and the conscience acting together to regulate thoughts and actions within the superego.

Giving another view of the process, the behaviorist believes that moral behavior is learned like any other behavior (Kaplan, 1991). Sharing, giving, lying, and stealing are actions that are reinforced (positively or negatively) by authority figures and are therefore incorporated into the child's repertoire of acceptable behaviors. Social learning theorists add that these actions are influenced by watching and imitating others. None of these theories has been widely accepted as a way to explain all of the variations found in moral development.

The cognitive developmental theories are most frequently utilized to explain the processes of moral reasoning, that is, how individuals gain their ideas about right and wrong and justice and injustice. Piaget outlined two stages of moral development (Duska & Whelan, 1975). In the stage of *moral realism,* rules are viewed as sacred, literal, and inflexible. Justice is whatever the law or authority commands. Children in this stage cannot take into account the view of other people and can think of only one thing, or aspect of a thing, at a time. Children will evaluate their own acts based on the consequences and the desire to avoid punishment, not the intent or motivation (Killen, 1991).

At age 7 to 8 years, interaction with peers begins to be influenced by a sense of give and take. "Fairness" becomes a prominent issue. The stage called *moral relativ-*

ism emerges around age 11 or 12. In this stage, children learn to evaluate the intentions of others before judging their answers as right or wrong. Thinking is no longer egocentric. Motives and circumstances can be taken into account when making a moral judgment. Rules are more flexible and can be elaborated and applied to several different situations and scenarios.

Piaget's theories have been criticized for presenting too narrow an approach to moral development. His belief that the essence of all morality is in the respect one holds for the rules and obeying authority does not account for individual or situational nuances (Duska & Whelan, 1975). Additional research has demonstrated that children as young as 6 years of age evaluate moral transgressions using the basis of fairness, welfare, and the intentions of the act (Killen, 1991). The sequence of moral development can be more fully understood by evaluating the works of Lawrence Kohlberg and Carol Gilligan.

Kohlberg (1981) identified three levels of moral reasoning, with two stages at each level (Table 4–12). Kohlberg's theory has been the most widely tested and successfully applied to many cultures. In this stage theory, sequential development must occur to attain the next

Table 4–12
Kohlberg's Six Stages of Moral Reasoning

Stage	Moral Outlook	Reasons for Moral Actions
Pre-Conventional Morality		
Stage 1: Punishment and Obedience Orientation Ages 5–8	Avoid breaking rules.	Avoidance of punishment
Stage 2: Instrumental Relativist Orientation Ages 7–10	Right actions satisfy one's own needs and only sometimes the needs of others.	Desire to serve one's own interests in a world where everyone has his own interests If you help others, they will owe you something, which is a debt to be collected later.
Conventional Morality		
Stage 3: Interpersonal Concordance of "Good Boy–Nice Girl" Orientation Ages 10–12	Good behavior is that which pleases or helps others and is approved by them.	Need to see oneself as a good person Belief in the Golden Rule Desire to maintain rules and follow authority to support stereotypical good behavior Need to gain approval of others
Stage 4: Law and Order Orientation Ages 12–25	Orientation toward authority, fixed rules, and the maintenance of the social order	Need to do one's duty and to show respect for authority and the social order
Post-Conventional Morality		
Stage 5: Social Contract Legalistic Orientation Ages 25–35 (if reached)	Aware that people hold a variety of values and opinions, although there are also rights and rules that have been constitutionally and democratically agreed on.	Obligation to law because of one's social contract with society Good is done because it serves the greatest number of people.
Stage 6: Universal Ethical Principle Orientation Ages 25–35 (if reached)	Self-chosen ethical principles based on abstract principles are the foundation for action. Laws or social agreements are considered valid because they are consistent with one's ethical principles.	A belief and commitment to the validity of universal moral principles. Desire to uphold abstract principles that define right behavior for self Unjust laws may be broken when they conflict with broad moral principles.

Table 4–13
Gilligan's Stages of Moral Development

Stage	Description
Stage 1: Survival Orientation	Egocentric perspective describes a great concern for self and a lack of awareness of other's needs. Being moral is surviving by being submissive to authority and the moral sanctions imposed by society.
Transition from selfishness to responsibility	*Responsibility for and to others is more important than survival and submission.*
Stage 2: Conventional Care	There is a lack of distinction between what others want and what is right. The right, or moral, action is whatever pleases others best. Being moral involves not hurting others, with no thought of the hurt to self that might be done.
Transition from goodness to truth	*Move from not simply hurting others, but also not hurting self through one's moral actions.*
Stage 3: Integrated Care	The needs of self and others becomes integrated. Moral actions take into account equally self-beliefs as well as other's beliefs.

higher stage of moral reasoning. Levels of development correlate with the reasoning behind moral decisions, not the decisions or acts themselves. Testing of Kohlberg's theory has demonstrated an apparent end of moral development for most women at level II, stage 3 (Omery, 1986). The higher stages of reasoning place an emphasis on justice, individual rights, and the rights of others.

Carol Gilligan (1982) has challenged this view, asserting instead that women have a different orientation to moral questions. Gilligan feels that females view moral questions in terms of how the issues affect interpersonal relationships, whereas the male emphasis is on individual rights and self-fulfillment (Kaplan, 1991). Gilligan does not believe that Kohlberg's model reflects these gender-based responses to morality. In her view, the differences in moral reasoning can be traced to the differences in child-rearing practices of boys and girls. Boys are more likely to be encouraged to be independent, assertive, and achievement oriented. Duty and fairness are highly emphasized. In contrast, girls are more likely to be encouraged to nurture, to take responsibility for others, and to learn to be sensitive and caring. Moral decisions can cause internal conflict between the female's perception of her personal needs and the needs of others. In many cases, a female's decisions are made to maintain or solidify the relationship with others rather than assert her individual rights. Gilligan developed a model of the development of moral reasoning with three levels and two transitional stages to explain how feminine moral development is neither deviant nor arrested but simply different (Omery, 1986) (Table 4–13).

Spiritual Development

The spiritual dimension of the child encompasses the need to find satisfactory answers to the meaning of life, illness, and death (Highfield & Cason, 1983). Although the need to find meaning and purpose for one's life does not generally begin to develop until early adolescence, all children experience a need for love, relatedness, and forgiveness. Throughout the child's life, questions regarding birth, suffering, death, hope, and forgiveness will be introduced and explored within the context of everyday experiences. The child's approach and response to these inquiries will be based on his or her corresponding level of cognitive and moral development.

Little research has been completed regarding spiritual development in children. It is known that faith, or the confidence or trust in a higher power, person, or thing, can be a driving force supporting the child and family through difficult times. Faith is most often associated with religious belief and the attitudes, observances of tenets, and values that are a part of a particular religious group (Betz, 1981). Fowler (1974) has identified stages in the development of faith in children and adults (Table

Figure 4–19
Religious practices and traditions guide adolescents in developing their own concept of spirituality. (Courtesy of Lou Metzger.)

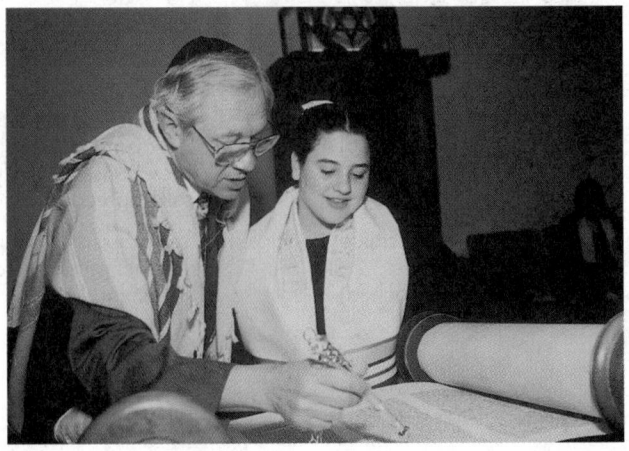

Table 4–14
Stages of Faith Development

Stage	Description	Nursing Interventions
Stage 0: Undifferentiated (infancy)	Feelings of trust, warmth, security, mistrust, and shame are incorporated into the child's conceptual ideas about himself or herself and his or her caretaker. These feelings are the foundation for subsequent faith development.	Focus is on supporting caregivers. Reassure parents about the adequacy of their parenting skills. Reassure parents that child's illness is not a result of supernatural powers punishing them. Provide for trust and security needs of infant in parents' absence.
Stage I: Intuitive-Projective (toddlerhood)	Parents and other significant others provide primary knowledge of faith. Child learns to imitate religious gestures and behaviors. Egocentrism and magical thinking affect perceptions of transcendental beings. Child does not understand differences between natural and supernatural.	Minimize magical beliefs that are negative and destructive by focusing on reality. Help child to realize illness is not a result of "being bad." Promote the continuance of religious rituals during illness and crises.
Stage II: Mythical-Literal (school-age)	Learns to distinguish religious fact from fantasy. Heavily influenced by attitudes of family and authority figures such as priest, minister, or rabbi. Uses fantasies to explain events or facts that cannot be understood. Begins to learn to differentiate between natural and supernatural. Faith beliefs are concrete and literal. God is perceived as having human qualities and characteristics. Able to articulate their faith.	Clarify magical and fantastical beliefs through teaching. Explain all events and procedures that are unfamiliar in the health care setting. Promote use of prayer and other religious rituals. Allow child to talk about his or her faith.
Stage III: Synthetic-Convention (preadolescent)	Begins to reflect and question religious beliefs and practices as exposed to more varied opinions. Relies on authority figures for answers to questions of faith. Begins to perceive God as a spirit and understand spiritual component of others. More clearly understands differences between natural and supernatural.	Assure child that illness is not a result of punishment by a supernatural being. Clarify conflicting and confusing information to the child. Encourage visits by respected authority figures. Promote incorporation of religious rituals and articles into hospital environment as desired by the child.
Stage IV: Individuating-Reflexive (adolescence to young adulthood)	Seeks to come to terms with own beliefs and personalize these. In the process may reject previous religious training, revert to a previous stage of religious belief and practices, or adopt some other extreme hedonistic attitude. Faith is a blended application of self-expression and beliefs and practices learned in the past.	Provide open and accepting attitude of child's beliefs. Engage in active listing as child "tries out" his or her emerging belief system. Offer support of authority figures, though these may be rejected at this time. Encourage use of religious rituals and articles as the child feels comfortable doing so.

4–14). Interventions can be provided that help the child meet his or her spiritual needs. These include encouraging children to read stories regarding faith and religious figures, encouraging the use of prayer, and promoting activities with other children that have a religious or spiritual focus (Fig. 4–19). Chapter 12 contains further discussion regarding meeting the spiritual needs of children experiencing grief and loss.

Developmental Surveillance

Developmental, behavioral, and emotional problems can be difficult to detect in young children. Accurate assessments of the child's growth and development may be hindered by infrequent access to the child to establish a developmental baseline assessment and to evaluate progress over time. Many problems may present very subtly. Therefore, the uncooperative child may elicit inconclusive or false-positive findings when attempts at direct assessment are being made by the practitioner. In addition, parents may not have accurate knowledge of the developmental milestones that their child should be achieving at any given point in time. The astute health care practitioner can utilize every contact with the child as an opportunity to employ *developmental surveillance*, the active and intentional evaluation of the child and the family to identify those who may be at risk for developmental variation. Developmental surveillance is a flexible, continuous process in which both informal and formal assessment techniques are used to evaluate the child's developmental progress from birth onward (Curry & Duby, 1994; Dworkin, 1989). The techniques include identification of parental concerns, child observations, screening, immunizations, and anticipatory guidance (Frankenburg, 1994).

Valid assessment of children requires a perspective that encompasses quantitative as well as qualitative changes of developmental processes. Although the importance of early intervention for children with developmental problems is widely recognized, the identification of children who require intervention, particularly those with subtle deficits or delays, has been fraught with complications. At issue is the need for identification procedures that are specific and sensitive enough to detect significant variations in development and are valid for the population being screened, yet are relatively simple and user-friendly in a variety of clinical settings. Use of developmental screening tests has constituted the major approach to identification of children with developmental problems. Accurate screening contributes to parental well-being, helps distribute limited diagnostic services and health care dollars in a effective manner, and helps ensure that those children who need intervention are identified as early as possible.

Parental concerns are the primary and the most helpful measure to identify children in need of formal developmental assessment. Approximately 80% of children who demonstrate developmental delay during formal testing have parents who shared concerns regarding their child's abilities. On the other hand, 20% to 25% of parents do not raise questions when they need to or are overly concerned when there is no evidence to support these concerns (Glascoe, 1995). The developmental surveillance process should utilize parental concerns and informal clinical observation of the child as the basis for early detection of developmental delays. Additionally, nurses providing direct patient care should have a knowledge of the clinical conditions (i.e., low birth weight, birth asphyxia, infection) and the behaviors (i.e., irritability, head positioning, abnormal reflexes) that make the child at risk for the presence of developmental problems (Collin, 1995). Figure 4–20 depicts the process that should be used to employ developmental surveillance techniques and for determining when to administer formal screening tests. Chapter 6 presents a summary of parental information and health care provider observations that can be elicited during contacts with the child and the family as part of the developmental surveillance process. Guidelines for developmental surveillance have been articulated by the Maternal and Child Health Bureau and several maternal child professional organizations in a resource book entitled *Bright Futures: Guidelines for Health Supervision of Infants, Children, and Adolescents* (see Resources).

Developmental Assessment Tools

A variety of developmental screening tests are available to assist the health care provider assess children suspected of delayed development. Assessment tools can utilize both direct and indirect measures to evaluate the child. *Direct screening measures* involve actual observations of the child by the evaluator or caregiver. In a clinical setting, direct observation of the child's abilities may be difficult because the child's fear and anxiety may inhibit normal developmental responses. Creating a trusting, warm atmosphere is essential to the administration of any developmental screening test. Direct measures may rely on the caregiver's observations. The findings of these measures may be adversely influenced by the caregiver's biased perception of the child's abilities. *Indirect screening measures* are tools that identify factors that may place a child at risk for developmental delay. Such factors include the environment, the child's temperament, and emotional and behavioral functioning.

It is important that developmental screening tests not be used to predict later developmental status in children (Frankenburg, Chen, & Thorton, 1988). A common misconception is that a developmental screening test can identify all children who will later be "normal" and all those who will later exhibit delays in development. Nurses and other health care professionals should be aware that a developmental screening test evaluates a child's development only at the current time, much like a snapshot captures the child's image at a certain point in time. Attempting to predict later normal development

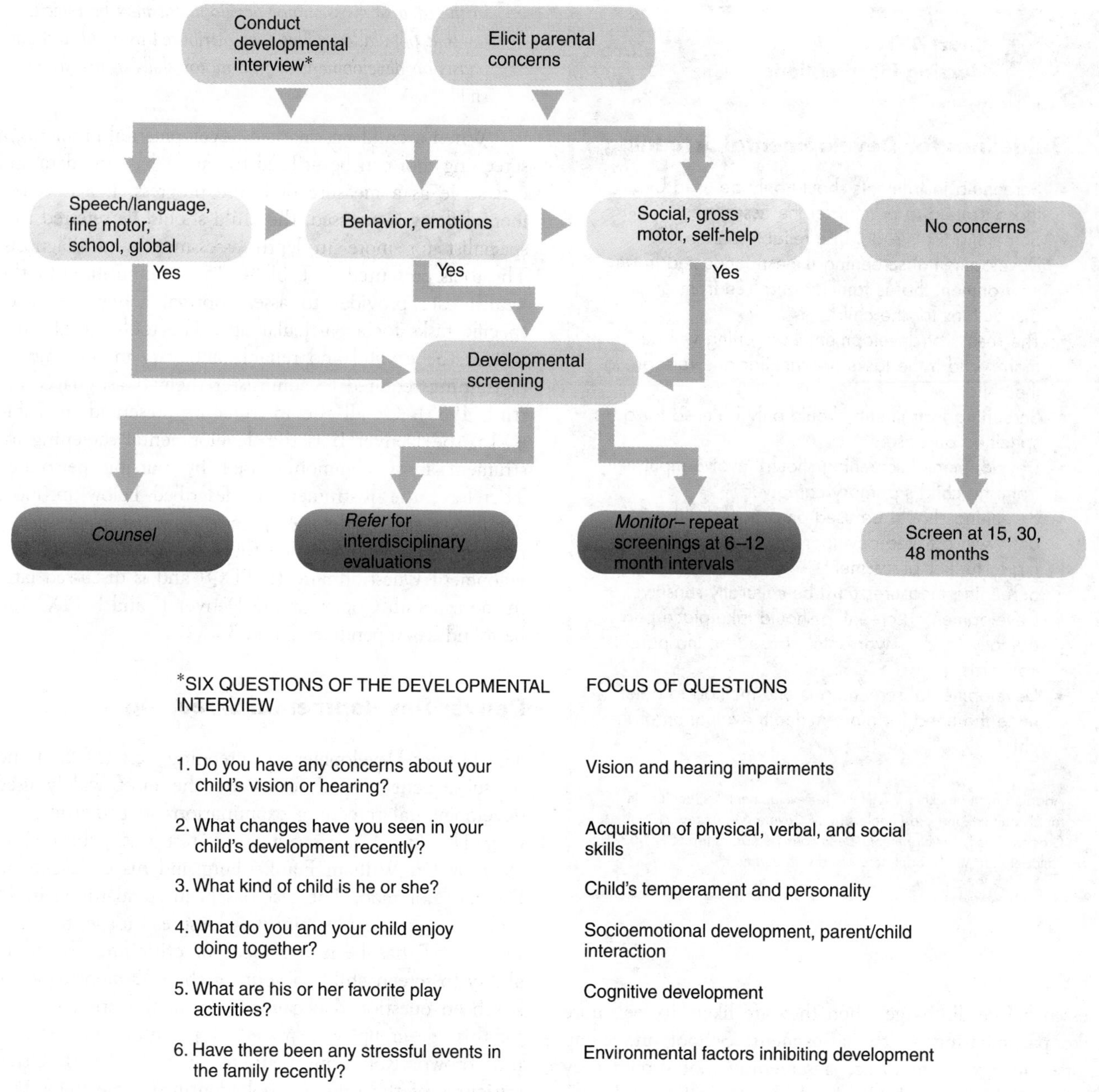

*SIX QUESTIONS OF THE DEVELOPMENTAL INTERVIEW	FOCUS OF QUESTIONS
1. Do you have any concerns about your child's vision or hearing?	Vision and hearing impairments
2. What changes have you seen in your child's development recently?	Acquisition of physical, verbal, and social skills
3. What kind of child is he or she?	Child's temperament and personality
4. What do you and your child enjoy doing together?	Socioemotional development, parent/child interaction
5. What are his or her favorite play activities?	Cognitive development
6. Have there been any stressful events in the family recently?	Environmental factors inhibiting development

Figure 4–20
Developmental surveillance: the decision-making process.

on the basis of the results of a developmental screen is dangerous, as an array of environmental factors may subsequently intervene, influencing a child's development. Individual variations from developmental norms may be transient and may indicate the need for more comprehensive evaluation. However, if a child exhibits major developmental delays early in life, predicting later developmental problems can be made with a somewhat greater degree of confidence, underscoring the importance of early intervention for children with developmental problems. The passage of Public Law 99-457, the Education of the Handicapped Act Amendments of 1986, has also served to emphasize the importance of developmental assessment and early identification and intervention for children experiencing developmental problems.

Developmental screening should be performed routinely on children to evaluate achievement of developmental milestones. Chart 4–13 presents a set of guidelines that should be used during all screening procedures. Well-child health care visits are an opportune time to complete the screening. Hospitalized children can be as-

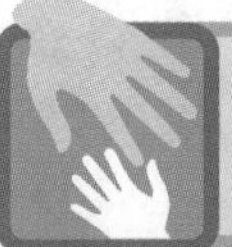

Chart 4-13
Nursing Interventions

Guidelines for Developmental Screening

- Screening instruments should only be used by those trained to administer the assessment.
- Screening tools should be reliable and valid.
- Developmental screening is best conducted in an environment that is familiar and free from other distractions for the child.
- The results of developmental screening will be more valid if the tasks are familiar and relevant to the child.
- Screening instruments should only be used for a specified purpose.
- Developmental screening should involve input from the child's primary caregiver.
- Screening should be used on a pass/fail basis only with a failed developmental screening leading to further assessment.
- Screening measures must be culturally sensitive.
- Developmental screening should take place periodically, and as warranted, based on the parents' concerns.
- Developmental screening is one method to determine the need for more in-depth evaluation of the child.

Adapted from Blackman, T. (1992). Developmental screening: Infants, toddlers and preschoolers. In M. Levine, W. Carey, & A. Crocker (Eds.), *Developmental-behavioral pediatrics* (pp. 617–623). Philadelphia: W. B. Saunders. Used with permission.

sessed before discharge when they are likely to feel more like participating in the assessment. School and camp nurses may wish to utilize a screening tool should they suspect delays in a child's development or if a teacher or caregiver shares concerns regarding an aspect of the child's development.

For parents, the data collected during such a screening provide information that can be used to guide activities with the child. If areas existed in which the child fell below age-specific achievements, instructions can be provided to assist the parents to enhance their child's skills in that area. Often, a child may demonstrate a specific delay simply because that task has not been emphasized in the home environment.

Worldview: *Culture may highly influence a child's developmental achievements. For instance, in cultural environments in which fine motor skills are emphasized, delays in the area of gross motor development may be typical for that population. This was attributed to a cultural emphasis on development of fine motor skills in the young child.*

When a child has marked developmental problems, a screening tool can be utilized to gather baseline data and can serve as a measure of future progress. If a developmental delay is assessed, the child should be referred to a specialist for more in-depth assessment and diagnosis. The tools presented in Table 4–15 can be utilized by the health care provider to assess normal achievements or specific tasks for a particular age. The tools are all considered to be valid and reliable and vary in the amount of training required to administer them (Castiglia & Petrini, 1985). Of all the instruments presented in Table 4–15, the Denver II is the developmental screening instrument most commonly used by nursing personnel. Therefore, the instrument is described below in more detail for the reader. A parent-answered prescreening form is also available called the revised Prescreening Development Questionnaire (R-PDQ) and is discussed later in more detail. Copies of the Denver II and R-PDQ can be found in Appendixes 2 and 3.

Denver Developmental Screening

The Denver Developmental Screening Test (DDST) and its subsequent revised forms are the most widely used developmental screening examinations in pediatric practice. The first Denver Screening test was published in 1967 by Dr. William Frankenburg and his colleagues in Denver, Colorado. The test has been standardized in 15 different countries. Despite its widespread usage, the original DDST has been the focus of criticism. The tool's ability to screen children younger than 30 months of age has been questioned because many of the original items for this age group were passed by parental report (Sciarillo, Brown, Robinson, Bennett, & Sells, 1986). Other criticisms of the original tool identified some items that were difficult to administer and/or interpret; considerable variation in the ability of the DDST to identify children with developmental delays; limitations in the assessment of developing language skills; and cultural biases (Borowitz & Glascoe, 1986; Lynn, 1987; Meisels, 1989; Meisels & Margolis, 1988; Sciarillo et al., 1986). The authors of the original tool were also concerned about the applicability of the 1967 norms to the 1990s (Frankenburg et al., 1990). As a result, in 1989, the test was substantially revised, restandardized, and renamed; the Denver II has been available since 1990 for developmental screening of children from birth to 6 years (see Appendix 2) (Frankenburg et al., 1990). With the development of the Denver II, the DDST and the DDST-R are no longer being published and should not be utilized in clinical practice.

The Denver II provides an overall assessment of development as well as specific data in four domains retained from the previous DDST and DDST-R: Personal-Social, Fine Motor-Adaptive, Language, and Gross Motor. The Denver II differs from the original DDST and DDST-R in several ways. The number of items included has increased from 105 to 125; most of the 20 new items were designed to assess expressive language and articulation skills. The new test form reflects an age scale that conforms to the American Academy of Pediatrics Health Supervision Visit Schedule. The norms have been updated and restandardized, and ratings of behavioral characteristics such as interest in surroundings or fearfulness are now included. The Denver II also allows identification of significant subpopulation differences attributable to race, sex, maternal education, and place of residence (rural, semirural, urban). Many items previously tested by parental report now require observation by the examiner.

Originally, the DDST was designed for easy administration by individuals with a minimum of formal training. Many individuals were prepared by reviewing the manual and then testing children; this method of preparation led to additional criticisms and questioning of the DDST's accuracy (Thorpe & Werner, 1974). A major goal of the revision was to correct this problem. A 2-day training course for *master instructors* is now offered in Denver, Colorado, and in other selected sites around the country. This course prepares master instructors in the use of specific instructional methods to teach individuals how to perform the screening test. A new screening manual, technical manual, and video program supplement the learning experience. Successful completion of a written, as well as an observational, proficiency test prepares participants to screen infants and children using the Denver II. Screening results by individuals who have not received this specialized instruction are questionable (Wade, 1992).

The Denver II can be administered in a 15- to 20-minute period (Fig. 4–21). The vertical axis of the test form lists the four domains assessed: Personal-Social, Fine Motor-Adaptive, Language, and Gross Motor; the horizontal axis lists the age divisions monthly until 24 months and then every 3 months until 6 years of age. The test form also contains a place in the bottom right corner to rate the child's behavioral characteristics during the assessment. Using the age scale that appears across the top and bottom of the test form, a vertical line is drawn to indicate the child's age at the time of testing. Each test item is designated by a bar that represents the ages at which 25%, 50%, 75%, and 90% of the tested population could perform the particular item. Test items

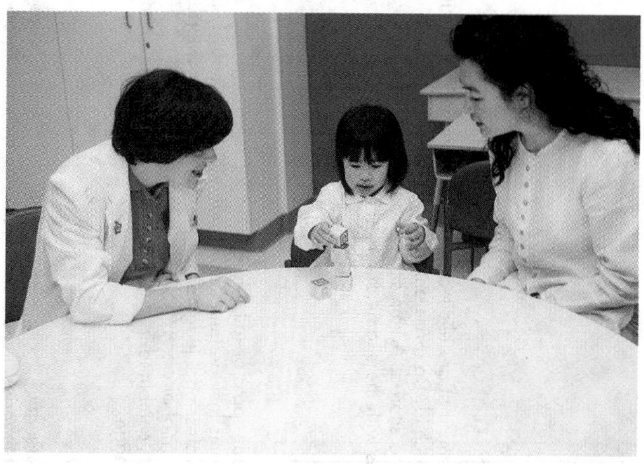

Figure 4–21
During developmental screening tests, parents are encouraged to stay near the child and promote a sense of comfort and security. Parents are instructed not to prompt the child or ask questions during the screening. After the screening procedures, the evaluator will review the results with the parent.

to both the left and right of the line are administered, as well as the test items intersected by the line. The kits for testing include a red skein of wool; raisins; a small clear bottle with a ⅝-inch opening; a rattle with a narrow handle; eight 1-inch square blocks in red, blue, yellow, and green colors; a small bell; a tennis ball; and a pencil. Three new items have been added to the testing materials used in administering the test: a doll, a feeding bottle, and a cup.

Pass, fail, or refusal scores are assigned to all items. Evaluation of each item to determine if significant differences exist on the basis of sex, ethnic group, maternal education, and place of residence allows the examiner to evaluate children delayed on specific items against norms for the subpopulations. This enables the examiner to view the delay with respect to sociocultural or environmental differences. Item performance is interpreted in relation to children's ages, as delay, caution, no opportunity, normal, or advanced performance. Two or more delays produce an abnormal overall test score, whereas one delay and/or two or more cautions result in a suspect score. Caution must be used in interpretation of success or failure on tasks. Parents tend to regard screening tests as a definitive indicator of their child's intelligence or other skill levels. If the child is not passing on most skills found under each domain, further, more detailed developmental testing is indicated.

caREminder: *If the child is ill, the Denver II may not be an accurate assessment of the child's skills and abilities. The child's weakness, anxiety, and physical restrictions could affect the outcome of the assessment. For instance,*

Text continued on page 234

Table 4–15
Developmental Screening Tools

Tool	Purpose	Screening Value	Administration	Scoring
Battelle Developmental Inventory Screening Test (6 months to 8 years)	Uses combination of direct elicitation, parental description, and observation to provide cutoffs and age-equivalent scores for developmental domains of gross/fine motor, personal, adaptive, expressive/receptive, language and cognitive.	Can be used to meet criteria for participation in early intervention programs.	Child interview/assessment. Takes about 30 minutes, longer with older children.	96 items that are elicited from observations/questioning of the child. Data are entered on a record sheet, which is hand scored. Administration and scoring manual comes with the examination.
Boyd Developmental (birth to 8 years)	Visually portrays significant aspects of growth and development in three areas: motor, communication, and self-sufficiency skill.	Provides a framework for anticipatory guidance and the design of treatment programs.	Parent interview—open-ended questions and child observation. No estimates of time required; should be administered in a relaxed manner. Instruction manual available. Administer at 6-month intervals until age 2, then yearly until age 8.	Scored—pass or fail. No criteria for referral given. Testing items include tennis ball, bell, etc. Relies heavily on the professional judgment of the screener. No criteria for normal or abnormal performance. Results combined in one visual report pictorialized on one page.
Carey Infant Temperament Questionnaire (4 to 8 months) (also known as Carey-McDevitt)	Determines the mother's general impression of her infant's temperament, her comparison with other infants of the same age, and the baby's temperament. Designed to assess infant's emotional reaction or behavioral responses in the early months of life.	Identifies infants at risk for poor mother–infant interaction. Parental guidance can be developed. One value is that many mothers' stated perceptions of infants were sharpened from completing the questionnaire.	Takes 25 minutes for the mother, and 10 to 15 minutes for scoring. No training required.	Questionnaire completed by mother: 97 items. Score in ten categories: temperament, activity, rhythmicity, approach, adaptability, intensity, mood, persistence, distractibility, and threshold. Several general areas of questioning: sleep, feeding, soiling and wetting, diapering, dressing, bathing, responses to people, responses to new situations. Second part is questionnaire about mother's general impressions of the infant's temperament, including activity level, positive and negative moods, and sociability. Scoring yields one of five diagnostic clusters: difficult, slow to warm up, intermediate, high or low, or easy. Infants of different temperaments develop at different rates.
Denver II (birth to 6 years)	Provides overall assessment of development as well as specific data in the four domains of Personal-social, Fine Motor-Adaptive, Language, and Gross Motor.	Most widely used measure to screen children for possible developmental delays. Examiner can evaluate delays on a specific item against norms for subpopulations related to the child's gender, ethnic group, maternal education, and place of residence.	Takes 15–20 minutes. Person administering test should receive instruction from a "master instructor" to perform the test in the correct manner. A screening manual, technical manual, and video program supplement the teaching from the master instructor.	To evaluate developmental milestones 125 items are arranged on an age scale that conforms to the American Academy of Pediatrics (AAP) Health Supervision Visit Schedule for newborns to children age 6. Pass, fail, or refusal scores are assigned to an item. Two or more delays produce an abnormal overall test score, whereas one delay and/or two or more cautions result in a suspect score.
Developmental Profile II (birth to 9 years)	An interview guide administered to a parent, teacher, or any other person who knows the child well for the purpose of screening general development.	Lacks referral criteria but is useful as a comprehensive test of general development. Tool covers five development areas: physical, self-help, social, academic, and communication.	Takes 20 to 40 minutes. Requires skill in interviewing; administration and scoring is easily taught to persons with basic interviewer skills. Manual gives step-by-step instructions.	Parent interview gives information about physical/motor, self-help, social, academic, and communication skills. There are 168 items arranged into categories at 6-month intervals from birth to age 4, then yearly to age 9. Scored as pass or fail. Scoring is clearly defined in manual.

Draw-A-Person: A Quantitative Scoring System (DAP) (4 to 17 years)	Assesses intellectual development and provides a baseline of a child's drawing abilities based on elements in the child's drawing of a person.	Studies of children's drawings have demonstrated a developmental sequence for those younger than 6 years of age. Drawings of children older than 6 often reflect ethnic and geographic variations. This test should not be used as an intelligence test in the absence of other accepted measures.	Child is given a paper and pencil with an eraser and asked to "draw a person." No further directions are offered. Child is given whatever time is needed to finish the picture. Time required is usually 15–30 minutes.	Sixty-four items are scored for 14 different criteria (e.g., arms, mouth, trunk, attachment of body parts, clothing, hair). Points are earned by the presence of each item, detail, and proportion. Scoring is not affected by the child's artistic ability. Validity and reliability studies indicated that the test remains a relatively consistent, culture-free way of assessing cognitive maturity.
Dubowitz (1 to 5 days)	Identifies neurologic signs and external characteristics, the gestational age of newborns.	Facilitates the differentiation of developmental expectations based on age.	Once interviewer is skilled, takes approximately 10 minutes. Requires instruction manual and practice.	Observation of infant's external characteristics and neurologic reflexes. External criteria include skin texture, presence or absence of plantar creases, lanugo, genital development, position and mobility of ears. Neurologic criteria and reflexes to be observed. Score each category.
Early Screening Inventory (ESI) (4 to 6 years)	Identifies children needing special educational services.	Assesses perceptual motor and language functioning.	Takes 10–15 minutes. Minimal instructions. Easy to understand.	Composite score obtained. Although each section is designed to stand alone, no section is meant to stand alone. Any conclusions drawn from ESI results are based on overall performance.
Home Observation for Measurement of the Environment (HOME) (birth to 3 years; 3 to 6 years)	Inventories various types of home stimulation for the child.	Best used with selected developmental assessment tools. Designed to evaluate the environment from the child's point of view. The HOME has eight subscales: stimulation through toys, games, and reading material; positive social responsiveness; physical environment (safe, clean, and conducive to development); pride, affection, and warmth; stimulation of academic behavior; modeling and encouragement of social maturity; variety of stimulation; and physical punishment.	Takes approximately 30 minutes to administer and 15 minutes to score. Relies on beginning interrater reliability (works in pairs for first 12 home visits).	Nurse observes mother/child interaction. Interviews mother in the home when the child is awake. The assessor determines the frequency of contacts between caregivers and children; the responsiveness of the environment to the child's needs; the emotional climate; the types of sensory experience; and the types of discipline used. This expanded database is used for parental guidance as well as alerting the assessor to potential problem areas and identifying guidelines for intervention.
Kansas Infant Development Screen (KIDS) (birth to 24 months)	Gives a general indication of the developmental level of the child.	Measures quantitative development in relation to commonly accepted pediatric milestones. Gives a general indication of the developmental level of the child in just one test. The items measure quantities of development and do not measure the skill a child has in relation to any milestone.	Average time: 4–5 minutes. Minimal instructions. Easy to understand.	Physical examination and interview with parents. Graph plots milestones on a vertical axis and age on the horizontal axis. Boxes are shaded opposite the items currently applying to the child. Referral for diagnostic examination is made if delays are evident on two consecutive testings.

Table continued on following page

Table 4–15
Developmental Screening Tools *Continued*

Tool	Purpose	Screening Value	Administration	Scoring
McCarthy Scales of Children's Abilities (MCSA) (2.5 to 8 years)	Assesses intellectual and motor development.	Identifies children with learning disabilities or with auditory, visual, or speech defects. May identify gifted children.	Takes 45 minutes to test children younger than age 5. Takes 1 hour with older children. Administering individual is self-trained and uses a scoring manual.	Separate scores for verbal, memory, quantitative, perceptual-performance, motor, and general cognitive. Index—an indicator of the child's present level of intellectual functioning.
McCarthy Screening Tests (MST) (4 to 6.5 years)	Identifies children "at risk" for learning problems.	Measures cognitive and sensorimotor functions that are central to the successful performance of school tasks (verbal memory, right/left orientation, leg coordination, draw-a-design, numerical memory, and conceptual grouping).	Takes 20 minutes. Self-train with manual, training material, and practice.	Tests child's ability to repeat words and sentences. Child's cognitive knowledge of laterality with regard to own body and with reference to picture of a boy. Evaluates drawings made by examiner and copies drawings from a model. Ability to repeat sequences of digits in the order presented and reverse order. Blocks of several shapes, sizes, and colors to measure child's ability to deal logically with objects, to classify, and to generalize.
Minnesota Child Development Inventory (MCDI) (1 to 6 years)	Assists in the diagnosis of those children whose development is the subject of concern.	The tool assesses general development, gross motor, fine motor, expressive language, comprehension conceptual, situation-comprehension, self-help, and personal-social areas.	Takes 10 to 15 minutes. Mother reports concerns regarding her child.	Has 150 statements describing children's behavior: 87 describe development between 4.5 and 5.5 years; 63 items describe adjustment problems and symptoms. Scoring is a clerical task. Results are interpreted in percentile norms for the developmental and adjustment scales and in terms of frequency of occurrence for the symptom items. A child is considered to be potentially at risk if (1) the child's mother reports a handicap or special problems, (2) scores on any of the developmental scales are in the bottom 5% of the age group, (3) scores on any of the adjustment scales are in the extreme 5%, and (4) symptom items are reported.
NCAST Parent–Infant Interaction Feeding Scale (birth to 1 year)	Assesses caregiver–infant interaction during feeding.	Provides data regarding parent–child interaction. The validity of this scale in predicting later IQ has been established in several studies.	Requires observation of an entire feeding episode, which can include breast, bottle, or solid feeding. The length of the feeding varies with the age of the child and type of feeding.	A 76-item binary scale is divided into six subscales of sensitivity to cues, response to distress, social-emotional growth fostering, cognitive growth fostering, clarity of cues, and responsiveness to parent. Use of the instrument and scoring requires training.
Neonatal Behavioral Assessment Scale (NBAS) (birth to 2 months)	Assess the interactive behavior of infants with their environment and their parents. Gives behavioral "portrait" of the infant, describing the newborn's strengths, adaptive responses, and possible vulnerabilities.	Detection of abnormalities as well as developing insight about infant's repertoire of behavior. Examiner can share data with parents to develop appropriate caregiving strategies to enhance parent–infant relationship.	Takes about 25 minutes to administer. NABS requires training to be able to administer the exam effectively and reliably. For training information call Brazelton Institute (see Resources).	Contains 28 behavioral and 18 reflex items. Scale does not yield a single score but instead assesses the newborn's capabilities across different developmental areas and describes how the newborn integrates these areas as they interact with the environment.

Neonatal Perception Inventory (NPI) (administered in first week of life and 1 month later)	Measures mother's perception of the average infant in relation to her own infant.	Identifies mother who shows few attachment behaviors and who will require additional assessment or immediate interventions. Determines effect of specific interventions.	Takes a short time (approximately 5 minutes) to answer only 6 questions. No training required.	Observation. Check response by mother for six questions that look for degree of dissonance. Reassess 1 month later, and look for reduced dissonance.
Preschool Development Inventory (PDI) (3 to 5 years)	Brief screening inventory measures child's general developmental status, including language comprehension, expressive language, fine motor, self-help, personal-social, situation-comprehension, and gross motor. Symptoms and behavior problems list includes items pertaining to sensory-motor, language, somatic problems, immaturity, hyperactivity, and behavioral and emotional problems.	Identifies children with special educational needs.	Time required varies, parent report. No training required. Can be administered over the telephone, completed in waiting rooms, or sent home before a second visit devoted to scoring and interpretation.	Parent completes 60 items. Describes child in own words, reports special problems or handicaps, and raises questions or expresses concerns about child.
Prescreening Developmental Questionnaire (R-PDQ) (3 months to 6 years)	Identifies children requiring further screening with the Denver Developmental Screening Test.	Early identification of children with developmental problems. It may also be used as a systematic method to follow a child's developmental progress.	Takes 3–6 minutes. Requires information sheet for health care provider. Parents respond and need no training.	Select 10 questions appropriate to child's age. Scored—pass or fail. Score of 8 or less is positive, and test should be repeated in a few weeks. If still positive, then do complete DDST.
Revised Developmental Screening Inventory (RDSI) (4 weeks to 36 months)	Assesses the five fields of behavior: adaptive, gross motor, fine motor, language, personal-social.	Determines if the infant has retarded development. No established referral criteria.	Takes 20–30 minutes. Instructions and scoring on sheets. Requires history and observation. Recommended for general practitioners and well-baby clinic nurses.	For each age, there are 1 to 5 items in each of the five areas being screened. A maturity level is assigned, and the child is then categorized as A—definitely normal; B—borderline or questionably abnormal; or N—normal advanced. Acceptable referral guidelines must be established with the professional who would receive the referrals.
Revised Parent Developmental Questionnaire (4 weeks to 36 months)	Assesses five fields of the Revised Developmental Screening Inventory (see above).	Determines by parent response if the older infant has retarded development. Effective over wide educational and social strata.	Time not determined. Minimal time for explanation. No training required. Completed by parents in homes or waiting rooms.	Parental observation scored yes or no to one item in each of five areas of RDSI. Grouping of questions allows for assessment of developmental quotients. Questions provide basis for referral.
Vineland Adaptive Behavior Scales (birth to 18 years, 11 months)	Assesses acquisition of personal and social skills of children in five domains of communication, daily living skills, socialization, motor skills, and maladaptive behavior.	Based on Orem's nursing model; is useful in measuring individual differences in child's rate of growth and change in acquiring social skills.	Takes 20–60 minutes to administer. Semistructured interview of parent or primary caregiver guided by standard questions.	Average ages for acquisition of certain behaviors are placed in order on a scoring sheet, with symbols used to indicate the child's performance of the behavior and the frequency of the behavior. Deficits in each area are identified and can be assessed further to identify specific problems.

if a child has an intravenous line in his or her dominant right hand, then testing of fine motor skills may not accurately reflect the child's dexterity.

It is not the intent of this discussion to explain in detail the instructions for administration of the Denver II. However, Chart 4–14 summarizes interventions that should be utilized to ensure success during the testing process and validity of the findings.

The authors of the Denver II contend that its validity, like that of any test, is determined by the extent to which it measures what it purports to measure. The test's

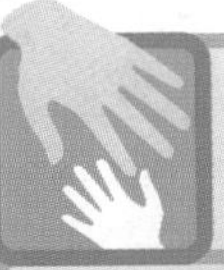

Chart 4–14
Nursing Interventions

Administering and Interpreting the Denver II Screening Test

Before administration, the nurse should be trained to administer the Denver II Screening Test.

Before Assessment

- Determine whether the child was born prematurely, and calculate the age adjustment. (Up to 24 months of age, allowances are made for prematurity by subtracting the number of weeks of missed gestation from the current age to arrive at the adjusted age.)
- Find the child's adjusted or actual age on the top and bottom of the chart, and draw a line connecting these two points. (Items that cross the line are to be tested. In addition, those that immediately precede and follow the line should also be evaluated.)

Preparation of the Parent

- Emphasize that this is not an intelligence test but rather is a method to determine what developmental skills the child can now achieve.
- Tell the parent that the child is not expected to perform all items on the test that you will be evaluating today.
- Ask parents not to interrupt the testing and state that you will answer their questions and explain all findings at the end of the assessment.

Preparation of the Child

- Present the assessment as a game.
- If a child will not cooperate on one item, move on to another and come back to the missed item at a later time.
- Keep all test items out of sight of the child until they are needed, so as not to distract the child.
- Complete each item as quickly as possible.
- After completing an item, return the toy used back to a location out of sight of the child so the toy will not distract the child's attention during testing of other items.
- Allow the child to sit or be near the parent during the examination, if so desired.

After the Screening

- Ask parents whether the child's performance was typical of his or her usual behaviors.
- If typical behaviors were displayed, explain the results beginning with those the child passed, then those the child was not expected to pass, and finally those items the child failed.
- If the child's behavior was not typical, the examiner should explore the reasons for this with the parent (e.g., child's fear, tiredness, hunger, sickness). The screening should be rescheduled to be completed at another time. The examiner should share positive findings.
- Use the screening to direct parents to activities they should be focusing on with their child. Review activities that are beyond the child's current level of achievement, and direct parents to activities that can enhance their child's skills.
- When explaining delays, explore with the parents the possible reasons for these delays. Sometimes children are not able to complete a task because they have never been exposed to that task (e.g., using scissors).
- Respond honestly to parents' concerns and questions. Emphasizing the necessity of further developmental testing is more helpful to the parent than offering false reassurance.

validity is therefore established by the precision with which ages corresponding to 25%, 50%, 75%, and 90% passing each item have been determined. The manner in which the test was standardized on more than 2000 children ensures a hig degree of face validity. The test form is therefore analogous to a growth curve (Dworkin, 1989) and is not determined by its agreement with a myriad of tests, many of which do not agree with each other. However, Adesman (1992) and Glascoe et al. (1992) suggest that the Denver II lacks validity because it did not agree with their findings of children with or without problems. It has also been suggested that the tool is not as accurate as an instrument that evaluates only one or two domains in a narrower age range (Adesman, 1992). Some of the cultural bias of the original tool has been addressed, as have the limitations inherent in the original sample. The Denver II has value as an aid in developmental surveillance, when used in combination with parental concerns, child observations, immunizations, and anticipatory guidance to promote the child's growth and development (Frankenburg, 1994).

Revised Prescreening Developmental Questionnaire (R-PDQ)

Because developmental assessment is a collaborative effort among parents and health care professionals, Dr. William Frankenburg and his colleagues in Denver, Colorado, developed an instrument for parents to complete as part of the DDST, and later revised it as well (Frankenburg, Fandal, & Thornton, 1987). The revised Prescreening Developmental Questionnaire (R-PDQ) is the result of their work (see Appendix 3). The R-PDQ consists of 150 questions from the Denver II with parents asked to answer a subset of these questions based on their child's age. Four different forms are available based on age and are color-coded: orange (birth to 9 months), purple (9 to 24 months), gold (2 to 4 years), and white (4 to 6 years). The parent or caregiver answers the questions until one of the following criteria is met: three "No's" are circled (No items do not have to be consecutive) or all of the questions on both sides of the form have been answered. In reviewing the R-PDQ, attention is focused on the number of delays. A child with no delays is viewed as developing normally. If a child has one delay, age-appropriate developmental activities are discussed with the parent or caregiver and plans made to repeat the R-PDQ screen in 1 month. On rescreening, detection of one or more delays prompts administration of the Denver II as soon as possible. If on the first screening with R-PDQ, a child is assessed to have two or more delays, the recommendation is to proceed with assessment with the Denver II.

The Denver II and R-PDQ should be considered valuable tools for nurses to assess children's development and discuss the findings with their parents. Pediatric nurses are in a prime position to screen for developmental problems. With appropriate training and practice, they can easily and effectively use the Denver II and R-PDQ in their practice.

Summary of Key Concepts

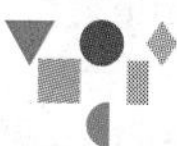

- Growth and development are influenced by multiple factors. Although the patterns and rates of growth are specific to certain parts of the body, variations in growth rates differ among children.
- Development proceeds from the simple to complex and from the general to the specific. Development occurs in a cephalocaudal and a proximodistal progression.
- Biological factors that are known to influence growth and development include heredity, gender, race, prenatal exposures, and nutrition.
- A child's interactions with environmental forces such as family, friends, the community, and social milieu are unique to that individual. Extrinsic factors interact with biological factors to influence the child's development in a manner that is likely to be different than how the same variables affect another child.
- No single developmental theory can be used to explain or interpret a child's behavior.
- Freud believed that in each stage of development there is a different region of the body that becomes the focus of sensual pleasure. Children must satisfy their sensual drives as they proceed through each stage to emerge as well-adjusted adults.

- Erikson's theory of psychosocial development consists of eight stages in which a developmental crisis is presented. If a particular crisis is handled well, then a positive outcome prevails. If the crisis is not handled well, then developmental maturation is arrested.
- Piaget described a four-stage cognitive developmental theory to explain how children mature in their assimilation and accommodation of information processing.
- Elkind believes that adolescent behavior is highly influenced by the adolescent's inability to differentiate between what others are thinking about and his or her own mental preoccupations.
- Information-processing theories can be used to explain the steps an individual goes through to take in, process, and act on information.
- The theory of multiple intelligences addresses the concept that people possess different talents, or multiple capacities or intelligences, that should be nurtured to capitalize on an individual's intellectual strengths.
- Behaviorists believe that the roots of a person's behavior are tied to experiences. Classical conditioning and operant conditioning are two of the most familiar theories used to explain how individuals learn behavior from interactions with stimuli in their environment.
- Social learning theories are used to explain how children learn through the processes of imitation, observational learning, and reinforcement.
- The humanist views all people as basically good, with an innate desire to become all that they are capable of being. Using this developmental approach as a basis for child rearing the family should focus on optimizing opportunities for the child to develop as a unique individual striving to reach his or her highest potential. Feelings of guilt and punishment should be downplayed so as not to inhibit personal growth.
- Language is composed of three symbol systems. Auditory expressive language consists of the vocalizations that a child begins to utter within the first few months of life. Expressive language expands as the child progresses from monosyllabic sounds to the use of words and sentences. Auditory receptive language is the child's ability to comprehend verbal communication and act on what he or she comprehends. Visual language skills also begin during the newborn period. The infant demonstrates attentiveness to verbal stimuli and responds with a fixed gaze, a smile, and eventually gestures.
- The development of sexuality is influenced by biological gender assignment, interactions with significant adults and peers that emphasize gender-associated behaviors and gender identification, and the physical and psychosocial changes that occur as the adolescent goes through puberty.
- A child's level of moral development is best determined based on the reasoning behind the moral decision, not the decision itself.
- The development of faith is influenced by the child's cognitive and emotional stage of development. Nurses can support the child's spiritual development by providing a nonjudgmental environment supportive of self-expressions of faith.
- The nurse should utilize every contact with the child and the family as an opportunity to employ developmental surveillance. Through intentional informal and formal evaluation techniques the nurse can identify those children who may be at risk for developmental variation.
- Developmental screening tools should be utilized by trained professionals to assess the child's ability to achieve normal developmental achievements and tasks.

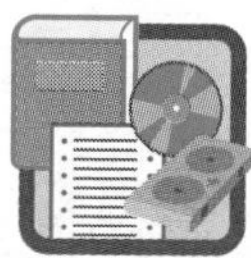

Resources

Organizations

National Center for Perinatal Addiction Research and Education (NAPARE)
11 East Hubbard Street, Suite 200
Chicago, IL 60611
(312) 329-2512

Books and Printed Materials

American Guidance Service
P.O. Box 99
Publisher's Building
Circle Pines, MN 55014-1796
(612) 786-4343
Vineland Adaptive Behavior Scales

Behavior Science Systems, Inc.
P.O. Box 580274
Minneapolis, MN 55440
(612) 929-6220
Minnesota Child Development Inventory (MCDI)
Preschool Development Inventory (PDI)

Brazelton Institute
1295 Boylston Street, Suite 320
Boston, MA 02215
(617) 355-4959
Neonatal Behavioral Assessment Scale

Center on Human Development
901 East 18th Street
University of Oregon
Eugene, OR 97403
Infant Monitoring Questionnaires

Denver Developmental Materials, Inc.
P.O. Box 6919
Denver, CO 80206-9019
(303) 355-4729
Denver II
Denver Prescreening Developmental Questionnaire
Home Screening Questionnaire

Developmental Disabilities Nurses Association
1720 Willow Creek Circle, Suite 515
Eugene, OR 97402
(800) 888-6733

Developmental Evaluation Materials
P.O. Box 27391
Houston, TX 77277
Revised Developmental Screening Inventory (DSI)
Revised Parental Developmental Questionnaire

Home Inventory LLC
13 Saxony Circle
Little Rock, AR 72209
(501) 569-3423
Home Observation for Measurement of the Environment (HOME)

Human Growth Foundation
7777 Leesburg Pike, Suite 202S
Falls Church, VA 22043
(800) 451-6434

National Genetics Foundation
250 West 57th Street
New York, NY 10019

National Maternal and Child Health Clearinghouse
8201 Greensboro Drive, Suite 600
McLean, VA 22102
(703) 821-8955 ext. 254 or 265
FAX: (703) 821-2098
Bright Futures: Guidelines for Health Supervision of Infants, Children, and Adolescents

NCAST
University of Washington
Box 357920
Seattle, WA 98195-7920
(206) 543-8528
E-mail: ncast@u.washington.edu
Parent-Infant Interaction Feeding Scale

Psychology Corporation
555 Academic Court
San Antonio, TX 78204-2498
(800) 228-0752
Draw-A-Person: A Quantitative Scoring System
McCarthy Scales of Children's Abilities (MSCA)

Riverside Publishing
8420 Bryn Mawr Avenue
Chicago, IL 60631
(800) 767-8378
Battelle Developmental Inventory Screening Test

Teachers College Press
1234 Amsterdam Avenue
New York, NY 10027
Early Screening Inventory (ESI)

Western Psychological Services
12031 Wilshire Boulevard
Los Angeles, CA 90025
Goodenough-Harris Drawing Test
Developmental Profile II

Computer Resources

Pascoe@vms.macc.Wisc.Edu (Internet) or Pascoe@wiscmacc (Bitnet)
To gain access to the Ambulatory Pediatric Association on-line handouts for parents on developmental, behavioral, and social skills development and discipline.

Interfaith Health Program
http://www.interaccess.com/ihpnet/

References

Adesman, A. (1992). Is the Denver II developmental test worthwhile? *Pediatrics, 90*(6), 1009–1010.

Amaya, M., & Ackall, G. (1996). Perinatal lead exposure. *Reflections, 22*(3), 18–19.

Belsky, J., & Isabella, R. (1985). Marital and parent-child relationships in family of origin and marital change following the birth of a baby: A retrospective analysis. *Child Development,* 56, 342–349.

Berko, J. (1958). The child's learning of English morphology. *Word, 14,* 150–177.

Betz, C. (1981). Faith development in children. *Pediatric Nursing, 7*(2), 22–25.

Borowitz, K., & Glascoe, F. (1986). Sensitivity of the Denver Developmental Screening Test in speech and language screening. *Pediatrics, 78,* 1075–1078.

Bresnahan, K., Brooks, C., & Zuckerman, B. (1991). Prenatal cocaine use: Impact on infants and mothers. *Pediatric Nursing, 17,* 123–129.

Brown, R. (1973). Development of the first language in the human species. *American Psychologist,* 28, 97–106.

Brown, M., Bellinger, D., & Matthews, J. (1990). In utero lead exposure. MCN, *15*(2), 94–96.

Castiglia, P. (1995). Family violence. *Journal of Pediatric Health Care,* 9, 269–271.

Castiglia, P., & Patrini, M. (1985). Selecting a developmental screening tool. *Pediatric Nursing, 11*(1), 8–17.

Chess, S. (1990). Studies in temperament: A paradigm in psychosocial research. *Yale Journal of Biology and Medicine,* 63, 313–324.

Chess, S., & Thomas, A. (1985). Temperamental differences: A critical concept in child health care. *Pediatric Nursing, 11,* 167–171.

Chess, S., & Thomas, A. (1986). *Temperament in clinical practice.* New York: Guilford.

Chess, S., & Thomas, A. (1992). Dynamics of individual behavioral development. In M. Levine, W. Carey, & A. Crocker (Eds.). *Developmental-behavioral pediatrics* (pp. 84–94). Philadelphia: W. B. Saunders.

Chomsky, N. (1968). *Language and mind.* New York: Harcourt.

Collin, R. (1995). Nurses in early intervention. *Pediatric Nursing, 21,* 529–532.

Coplan, J. (1995). Normal speech and language development: An overview. *Pediatrics in Review, 16*(3), 91–100.

Curry, D., & Duby, J. (1994). Developmental surveillance by pediatric nurses. *Pediatric Nursing,* 20, 40–44.

Donley, M. (1993). Attachment and the emotional unit. *Family Process, 32,* 3–20.

Duska, R., & Whelan, M. (1975). *Moral development: A guide to Piaget and Kohlberg.* New York: Paulist Press.

Dworkin, P. (1989). British and American recommendations for developmental monitoring: The role of surveillance. *Pediatrics,* 84, 1000–1010.

Eaton, L. (1994). Childhood memories. *Nursing Times,* 90, 14–15.

Elkind, D. (1967). Egocentrism in adolescence. *Child Development,* 38, 1025–1034.

Elkind, D. (1984). Teenage thinking: Implications for health care. *Pediatric Nursing, 10,* 383–385.

Elkind, D. (1986). David Elkind discusses parental pressures. *Pediatric Nursing, 12,* 417–418.

Engel, J. (1997). *Pocket guide to pediatric assessment.* St. Louis: Mosby–Year Book.

Erikson, E. (1963). *Childhood and society.* New York: W. W. Norton and Company.

Falbo, T., & Polit-O'Hara, D. (1985). Only children: What do we know about them. *Pediatric Nursing, 11,* 356–360.

Finitzo, T., Gunnarson, A., & Clark, J. (1990). Auditory deprivation and early conductive loss from otitis media. *Topics in Language Disorders, 11,* 29–42.

Fowler, J. (1974). Toward a developmental perspective on faith. *Religious Education,* 69, 207–219.

Frankenburg, W. (1994). Preventing developmental delays: Is developmental screening sufficient? *Pediatrics,* 93, 586–593.

Frankenburg, W., Chen, J., & Thorton, S. (1988). Common pitfalls in the evaluation of developmental screening tests. *The Journal of Pediatrics, 113,* 1110–1113.

Frankenburg, W., Dodds, J., Archer, P., Bresnick, B., Maschka, P., Edelman, N., & Shapiro, H. (1990). *Denver II screening manual.* Denver, CO: Denver Developmental Materials, Incorporated.

Frankenburg, W., Fandal, A., & Thornton, S. (1987). Revision of Denver Prescreening Developmental Questionnaire. *Journal of Pediatrics, 110,* 653–657.

Free, T., Russell, F., Mills, B., & Hathaway, D. (1990). A descriptive study of infants and toddlers exposed prenatally to substance abuse. *MCN, 15,* 245–249.

Freiberg, K. (1987). *Human development: A life-span approach.* Boston: Jones and Barlett.

Gardner, H. (1993). *Multiple intelligences: The theory in practice.* New York: Basic Books.

Gessner, I. (1997). What makes a heart murmur innocent? *Pediatric Annals,* 26, 83–87.

Gilligan, C. (1982). *In a different voice.* Cambridge, MA: Harvard University Press.

Glascoe, F. (1995). Developmental screening. In S. Parker & B. Zuckerman (Eds.), *Behavioral and developmental pediatrics* (pp. 25–29). Boston: Little, Brown, & Company.

Glascoe, F., Byrne, K., Ashford, L., Johnson, K., Chang, B., & Strickland, B. (1992). Accuracy of the Denver II in developmental screening. *Pediatrics,* 86, 1221–1225.

Green, A. (1991). Application of Jean Piaget's theory of human development for nursing children in an adult intensive therapy unit. *Intensive Care Nursing,* 7, 236–239.

Groer, M., & Howell, M. (1990). Autonomic and cardiovascular responses of preschool children to television programs. *JCPN,* 3, 134–138.

Gross, D., & Conrad, B. (1995). Temperament in toddlerhood. *Journal of Pediatric Nursing, 10,* 146–151.

Hauck, M. (1991). Cognitive abilities of preschool children: Implications for nurses working with young children. *Journal of Pediatric Nursing,* 6, 230–235.

Hazinski, M. F. (1996). *Nursing care of the critically ill child.* St. Louis: C. V. Mosby.

Highfield, M., & Cason, C. (1983). Spiritual needs of patients: Are they recognized? *Cancer Nursing,* 6, 187–192.

Howard, M. (1992). Delaying the start of intercourse among adolescents. *Adolescent Medicine,* 3, 181–193.

Howard-Teplansky, R. (1992). Nutrition and development. In M. Levine, W. Carey, & A. Crocker (Eds.), *Developmental-behavioral pediatrics* (pp. 276–284). Philadelphia: W. B. Saunders.

Jacklin, C. (1992). *Gender.* In M. Levine, W. Carey, & A. Crocker (Eds.). *Developmental-behavioral pediatrics* (pp. 95–100). Philadelphia: W. B. Saunders.

Jarman, F., & Oberklaid, F. (1992). Brothers and sisters. In M. Levine, W. Carey, & A. Crocker (Eds.). *Developmental-behavioral pediatrics* (pp. 117–121). Philadelphia: W. B. Saunders.

Kamm, K., Thelen, E., & Jensen, J. (1990). A dynamical system approach to motor development. *Physical Therapy,* 70, 763–774.

Kaplan, P. (1991). *A child's odyssey: Child and adolescent development.* St. Paul: West Publishing.

Kelley, S., Walsh, J., & Thompson, K. (1991). Birth outcomes, health problems, and neglect with prenatal exposure to cocaine. *Pediatric Nursing, 17,* 130–136.

Killen, M. (1991). Children's evaluations of morality in the context of peer, teacher-child, and familial relations. *The Journal of Genetic Psychology, 151*(3), 395–410.

Kohlberg, L. (1981). *The philosophy of moral development: Moral stages and the idea of justice.* New York: Harper & Row.

Kraemer, K. (1997). Placental transfer of drugs. *Neonatal Network, 16*(2), 65–67.

Ladden, M. (1990). The impact of preterm birth on the family and society. *Pediatric Nursing, 16,* 515–518.

Lynn, M. (1987). Update: Denver Developmental Screening Test. *Journal of Pediatric Nursing, 2,* 348–351.

Maccoby, E., & Jacklin, C. (1980). Sex differences in aggression: A rejoinder & reprise. *Child Development, 51,* 563.

Marlow, D. (1965). *Textbook of pediatric nursing.* Philadelphia: W. B. Saunders.

McClowry, S. (1995). The influence of temperament on development during middle childhood. *Journal of Pediatric Nursing, 10,* 160–165.

Medoff-Cooper, B. (1995). Infant temperament: Implications for parenting from birth through 1 year. *Journal of Pediatric Nursing, 10,* 141–145.

Meisels, S. (1989). Can developmental screening tests identify children who are developmentally at-risk? *Pediatrics, 83,* 578.

Meisels, S., & Margolis, L. (1988). Is the early and periodic screening, diagnosis and treatment program effective with developmentally disabled children? *Pediatrics, 81,* 262–271.

Melvin, N. (1995). Children's temperament: Intervention for parents. *Journal of Pediatric Nursing, 10,* 152–159.

Muscari, M. (1988). Effective nursing strategies for adolescents with anorexia nervosa and bulimia nervosa. *Pediatric Nursing, 14,* 475–482.

Needlman, R. (1996). Growth and development. In R. Behrman, R. Kliegman, & A. Arvin (Eds.), *Nelson textbook of pediatrics* (pp. 30–72). Philadelphia: W. B. Saunders.

Nelms, B., & Mullins, R. (1982). *Growth and development: A primary health care approach.* Englewood Cliffs, NJ: Prentice-Hall.

Nolan, E. (1991). Infants at risk: A time for action. *Pediatric Nursing, 17,* 175–178.

Omery, A. (1986). Moral development: A differential evaluation of dominant models. In P. Chinn (Ed.), *Ethical issues in nursing* (pp. 37–53). Rockville, MD: Aspen.

Ozmar, B. (1994). Encountering victims of interpersonal violence. *Critical Care Nursing Clinics of North America, 6,* 515–522.

Peal, E., & Lambert, W. (1962). The relation of bilingualism to intelligence. *Psychological Monographs, 76*(546), 1–23.

Petitto, L., & Marentette, P. (1991). Babbling in the manual mode: Evidence for the ontogeny of language. *Science, 251,* 1493–1496.

Philbin, M. (1996). Some implications of early auditory development for the environment of hospitalized preterm infants. *Neonatal Network, 15*(8), 71–73.

Piaget, J. (1926). *The language of the child.* New York: Harcourt.

Pinyerd, B. (1992). Assessment of infant growth. *Journal of Pediatric Health Care, 6,* 302–308.

Pokorni, J. & Stanga, T. (1996). Serving infants and families affected by maternal cocaine abuse: Part I. *Pediatric Nursing, 22,* 439–442.

Reed, B., & Davidhizar, R. (1997). Setting their sights: Visual development in newborns. *Advance for Nurse Practitioners, 5,* 67–70.

Reed, D., McMillan, J., & McBee, R. (1995). Defying the odds: Middle schoolers in high risk circumstances who succeed. *Middle School Journal, 27,* 3–10.

Schlesinger, H. (1995). Hearing Loss. In S. Parker & B. Zuckerman (Eds.), *Behavioral and Developmental Pediatrics* (pp. 174–179). Boston: Little, Brown, & Company.

Schraeder, B., Heverly, M., O'Brien, C., & Goodman, R. (1997). Academic achievement and educational resource use of very low birth weight survivors. *Pediatric Nursing, 23,* 21–25 & 44.

Sciarillo, W., Brown, M., Robinson, N., Bennett, F., & Sells, C. (1986). Effectiveness of the DDST with biologically vulnerable infants. *Developmental and Behavioral Pediatrics, 7,* 77–83.

Siegler, R. (1983). Information processing approaches to development. In W. Kessen (Ed.), *Handbook of child psychology, Vol. 1: History, theory and methods.* New York: Wiley.

Siegler, R. (1986). *Children's thinking.* Englewood Cliffs, NJ: Prentice-Hall.

Snapp, B. (1996). Lung physiology: Clinical applications. *Central Lines, 12*(2), 1–5.

Thomas, A., & Chess, S. (1977). *Temperament and development.* New York: Brunner-Mazel.

Thorpe, H., & Werner, E. (1974). Developmental screening of preschool children: A critical review of inventories used in health and educational programs. *Pediatrics, 53,* 362–369.

Viadero, D. (1996). Expert testimony. *Teacher Magazine, 7*(4), 24–25.

Vikan, A., & Clausen, S. (1994). Freud, Piaget, or neither? Beliefs in controlling others by wishful thinking and magical behavior in young children. *The Journal of Genetic Psychology, 154*(3), 297–314.

Vygotsky, L. (1962). *Thought and language.* Cambridge, MA: MIT Press.

Wade, G. (1992). Update on the Denver II. *Pediatric Nursing, 18,* 140–141.

Wallace, M. (1995). Temperament and the hospitalized child. *Journal of Pediatric Nursing, 10*(3), 173–180.

Weigley, E. (1990). Changing patterns in offering solids to infants. *Pediatric Nursing, 16,* 439–441.

Winkelstein, M. (1984). Overfeeding in infancy: The early introduction of solid foods. *Pediatric Nursing, 10,* 205–208.

Yeager, S. (1988). Pediatric cardiology. In J. Crapo, M. Hamilton, & S. Edgman (Eds.), *Medicine & pediatrics in one book* (pp. 60–94). St. Louis: C. V. Mosby.

Bibliography

Boyce, W., Barr, R., & Zeltzer, L. (1992). Temperament and the psychobiology of childhood stress. *Pediatrics, 90,* 483–486.

Calhoun, J. (1997). Eye examinations in infants and children. *Pediatrics in Review, 18,* 28–31.

Dempster, J. (1996). Fetal alcohol syndrome: The nurse practitioner perspective. *Journal of the American Academy of Nurse Practitioners, 8,* 343–349.

Donley, S. R. (1991). Spiritual dimensions of health care: Nursing's mission. *Nursing & Health Care, 12,* 178–183.

Elkind, D. The teenager's reality. *Pediatric Dentistry, 9,* 337–341.

Gardner, H. (1991). *The unschooled mind: How children think and how schools should teach.* New York: Basic Books.

Koniak-Griffin, D., & Ludington-Hoe, S. (1988). Developmental and temperament outcomes of sensory stimulation in healthy infants. *Nursing Research, 37*, 70–75.

McClowry, S. (1990). The relationship of temperament to pre- and posthospitalization behavioral responses of school-age children. *Nursing Research*, 39, 30–35.

McCown, D. (1984). *Moral development in children. Pediatric Nursing*, 10, 42–44.

Melvin, N., & McClowry, S. (1985). Clinical applications of children's temperament. *Journal of Pediatric Nursing, 10*, 139–140.

Ricchini, W. (1997). Tips for communicating with children. *Advances for Nurse Practitioners*, 5, 83–85.

Schraeder, B., Heverly, M., O'Brien, C., & McEvoy-Shields, K. (1992). Vulnerability and temperament in very low birth weight school-aged children. *Nursing Research, 41*, 161–165.

Schraeder, B., Heverley, M., & Rappaport, J. (1990). The value of early home assessment in identifying risk in children who were very low birth weight. *Pediatric Nursing, 16*, 268–272.

Still, J. (1984). How to assess spiritual needs of children and their families. *Journal of Christian Nursing*, Spring, 4–6.

Warner-Robbins, C., & Christiana, N. (1989). The spiritual needs of persons with AIDS. *Family & Community Health, 12*(2), 43–51.

Promoting Healthy Living

CHAPTER

5

OUTLINE

Infants
- Nutrition
- Oral Health
- Infant Care
- Promotion of Social Competence
- Injury and Illness Prevention

Toddlers
- Nutrition
- Oral Health
- Hygiene and Personal Care
- Promotion of Social Competence
- Injury and Illness Prevention

Preschoolers
- Nutrition
- Oral Health
- Hygiene and Personal Care
- Promotion of Social Competence
- Injury and Illness Prevention

School-Age Children
- Nutrition
- Oral Health
- Hygiene and Personal Care
- Promotion of Social Competence
- Injury and Illness Prevention

Adolescents
- Nutrition
- Oral Health
- Hygiene and Personal Care
- Promotion of Social Competence
- Injury and Illness Prevention

OBJECTIVES

- Discuss the needs of the child related to nutrition, elimination, hygiene, and personal care.
- Select age-appropriate interventions to promote healthy personal and social development of the child.
- State the developmental surveillance and milestone concerns of children from infancy through adolescence.
- Identify aspects of the physical examination and screening procedures that would be completed during age-specific health care evaluations.
- Select interventions to promote illness and injury prevention for the child and the family.

KEY TERM

Developmental surveillance

A primary goal of the health care community is to work in collaboration with families to promote the growth, development, adaptation, and functioning of children. Most parents invest considerable time, personal resources, and finances to meet the needs of their children. Many parents seek the knowledge and assistance of health care professionals and others who work with children to provide them with guidance regarding child-rearing issues. Health care personnel are responsible for serving as an assessable support to the parents as they strive to nurture, protect, and socialize their child. The interdisciplinary health care team plays a critical role in promoting healthy development of the child. Although the focus of health care is often directed toward the assessment, diagnosis, and treatment of illness, the initiation of interventions that promote child health and wellness is an important, if not the primary, focus in pediatrics. Over the course of the childhood years the interdisciplinary team is likely to have many contacts with the child and the family for both routine health appraisals and urgent care needs. Each encounter with the family is an opportunity to assess family functioning and address specific developmental issues of the child and family members. Initiating interventions to deal with identified problems and providing anticipatory guidance are two of the primary actions that should be employed to support the child-rearing family. To fulfill these responsibilities, the nurse and other members of the health care team must have a thorough understanding of age-appropriate milestones and the practical methods to support achievement of these developmental goals. Building upon the information presented in Chapter 4, Growth and Development, the discussion in this chapter includes a variety of issues related to promoting healthy development from infancy through adolescence.

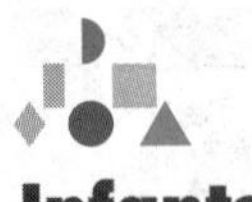

Infants

When parents bring their newborn home for the first time, it is one of the most exhilarating, exciting, and frightening events that they will ever experience. Over the course of the next year, they will be faced with a multitude of changes. For at no other point in life will a person move through so many developmental milestones as are covered in the first 12 months of life. Most first-time parents are unprepared for the rapidity with which they must adjust to their infant's changing needs. Just when they become accustomed to a 3-hour feeding schedule, their child now requires solid food. One moment the child cannot even roll from side to side, the next he or she is crawling after the family cat. With each subtle behavioral adjustment, the caregivers must learn to adapt themselves and the child's environment to provide a safe, nurturing, and secure arena for the child to grow and develop.

Nutrition

Breast-Feeding

After the child is born, the optimal nutritional support comes in the form of human milk (Corbett-Dick & Bezek, 1997). Ideally, the decision to breast-feed should be made before the child's birth. Today, breast-feeding is the feeding method most encouraged by health care providers, owing to the composition of the milk, the additional immunity it provides the infant in the form of antibodies, and the fact that it has the most easily digestible form of protein. Human milk is readily available, is inexpensive, and encourages bonding between the mother and infant.

Many new mothers have a disappointing experience with breast-feeding because they lack the knowledge, resources, and support to deal successfully with the situation when problems occur. Difficulties can arise when the mother does not have the support or instruction she needs when first attempting to breast-feed. She may not have adequate knowledge to prevent problems such as sore nipples and engorgement or know the correct interventions to implement when a problem does occur (TIP 5–1). In her frustration, she may give up trying to breast-feed. The nurse plays an important role in providing the mother with the education she needs to have a successful breast-feeding experience (Chart 5–1). Community resources such as the La Leche League are also available for the mother to use if she is having difficulty with breast-feeding. Before discharge from the hospital or birthing center the nurse should provide the family with a list of resources that can be used if the need arises (see Resources).

The newborn's first feeding optimally occurs in the delivery room. The first "milk" that is let down is colostrum. The colostrum contains more protein, salt, and antibodies than regular milk but less fat and calories. This is produced for several days until the mother starts producing milk.

Positioning

Proper positioning while breast-feeding enables the newborn to latch on properly and effectively and promotes the mother's comfort during feeding. Poor positioning can lead to sore nipples and a frustrated and hungry infant who is not able to suckle and get enough milk (Munson, 1996; Peters, 1997). The newborn should have the entire areola in his or her mouth, not just the nipple.

TIP 5–1 A Teaching Intervention Plan for Common Breast-Feeding Problems

Nursing Diagnosis and Family Outcomes

- Ineffective breast-feeding related to difficulty with breast-feeding process
  Outcomes: Mother expresses physical and psychological comfort with breast-feeding.
  Mother reports she is able to effectively initiate actions to relieve breast-feeding problems when they occur.
  Neonate feeds successfully on both breasts and appears to be satisfied after feeding.

Prevention and Intervention Measures

Painful Nipples

Prevention

- This is most commonly caused by improper care of breasts, poor latching-on technique, or excessive moisture created by leakage of milk.
- Avoid soaps, oils, lotions, or self-prescribed treatments.
- Position infant properly at breast, ensuring that entire areola is grasped.
- Instruct mother to hold the breast with the thumb above the areola and fingers and palm underneath it and to gently compress the breast and direct it into the infant's mouth; a scissors grasp may also be used, compressing the areola between two fingers and supporting the breast to facilitate the infant's ability to grasp the areola properly.
- Apply small amount of breast milk to areola after a feeding and let it dry.
- Change nursing pads frequently; use of plastic-backed pads traps moisture and should be avoided.
- Expose nipples to air as much as possible; use of hair dryer on low setting may be helpful.
- Approximately 10 minutes at each breast provides 90% of the available milk.

Interventions

- Nurse infant on less affected breast first and affected breast second.
- Ensure proper positioning of infant at breast with entire areola grasped.
- Allow let-down reflex before putting infant to breast.
- Change infant's position at breast.
- Taking aspirin or acetaminophen 30 minutes before a feeding may relieve excessive discomfort.
- Applying ice to nipples after feeding may decrease discomfort.

Engorgement

Prevention

- Frequent nursing (every 2 to 4 hours) on both breasts promotes complete emptying of ducts.
- Provide proper support of breasts with well-fitting nursing bra, worn 24 hours a day.
- Divide feeding time relatively evenly between both breasts.
- Alternate from feeding to feeding the breast that infant nurses at first; some mothers find it helpful to place a safety pin on their bra strap or an extra nursing pad on the side where the infant last nursed as a reminder.

Interventions

- Manually express milk before putting infant to breast to nurse.
- Apply warm compresses or take a warm shower 10 to 15 minutes before feeding.
- If breasts are severely engorged, use of cold compresses may help to decrease vascularity after a feeding.
- Massage breasts to promote emptying.
- If discomfort is excessive, consider taking aspirin or acetaminophen 30 minutes before feeding.

TIP continued on following page

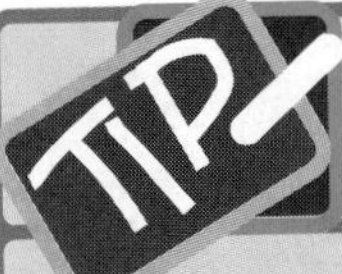

TIP 5–1 A Teaching Intervention Plan for Common Breast-Feeding Problems *Continued*

Let-Down Reflex

Prevention

- The "let-down" reflex, controlled primarily by the hormones prolactin and oxytocin, allows delivery of milk from the alveoli and smaller milk ducts for the breast into the large lactiferous ducts and sinuses.
- Encourage infant to nurse at both breasts.
- Observe infant to see if he or she is swallowing every few sucks at the start of the feeding.
- Expose the opposite breast while nursing and see if milk flows from it as infant sucks.
- Slide a finger into the corner of the infant's mouth, breaking his or her suction to see if there is flow from that breast.

Interventions

- RELAX! Sit in a comfortable chair with good support for your back and arms.
- Listen to soothing music.
- Minimize distractions by finding a quiet corner.
- Gently massage the breast.
- Apply warmth to breast. Take a warm shower.
- Avoid alcohol, illegal drugs, and smoking because all contain substances that can interfere with let-down and affect the contents of breast milk.

Latching-On

Prevention

- Proper latching-on involves the infant taking the whole breast in his or her mouth, jaws closing around the areola, gums forming a circular seal, and creation of a vacuum effect; as the tongue strokes upward pressing the nipple against the palate, the milk ducts are emptied.
- Avoid bottles or pacifiers until breast-feeding is well established.
- Observe feeding with the mother–baby couple, intervening to promote proper latching-on.

Interventions

- Make sure infant's tongue is down with the nipple directly on top of it during the feeding.
- Make sure infant is awake and alert when feeding; unwrap infant from blankets as needed.
- If nipples are partially inverted, use a nipple shield to draw out the nipple.
- Sprinkle glucose water on nipples before feeding. When the infant opens his or her mouth and tastes the glucose, the mouth can be directed and attached to the nipple in the correct fashion.

Inadequate Milk Supply

Interventions

- Milk production depends on supply and demand.

Three comfortable positions can be used to achieve this goal. In the side-lying position the mother lies on her side in the recumbent position. Pillows can be used to support the mother's back. The infant is placed in a side-lying position with the mouth parallel to the mother's nipple and the feet toward the mother's waist. Many mothers prefer to sit in a chair or up in bed while breast-feeding. The mother's back and her arms should be well supported to prevent strain. A pillow under the knees or a stool to place her feet on provides additional support.

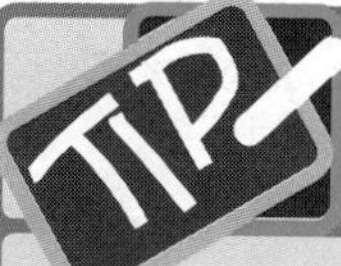

TIP 5-1 A Teaching Intervention Plan for Common Breast-Feeding Problems *Continued*

- Reassure mother in her efforts to breast-feed, reinforcing that milk supply will be adequate and is dependent on frequent nursing.
- Encourage nursing at both breasts, six to eight times daily.
- Encourage adequate rest, nutrition, and fluids.
- Avoid use of supplemental formula feedings until breast-feeding is well established (usually 3 to 4 weeks after delivery).
- Monitor infant's growth.
- Supplementation with formula may be indicated. Consider use of a nursing trainer worn around the mother's neck. The trainer consists of a small plastic bag that holds formula and a thin, flexible tube that is held or taped along the breast to the nipple; while providing supplementation, the infant's desire to nurse at the breast is reinforced, stimulating milk production.

Mastitis

Prevention

- Breast-feed every 2 to 4 hours to prevent inflammation of the mammary glands due to inadequate emptying of the ducts.
- Massage breasts before beginning a feeding.
- Ice compresses applied to breasts and removed 10 to 15 minutes before a feeding and followed by application of warm compresses may promote complete emptying.
- Position infant at the breast with infant's chin toward obstructed area to prevent the development of sore nipples and cracking of the skin around the nipples.

Interventions

- Treat with antibiotics for 10 days.
- Continue breast-feeding to keep breasts well drained.
- Continue all preventive efforts listed here.

Fussy or Gassy Infant

Prevention

- Choose diet with care. What a mother eats and drinks may have some impact on breast milk volume and nutritional content.
- Drink caffeinated beverages in moderation.
- If a mother suspects that the infant is intolerant of something she has eaten, she can try to eliminate the suspected food and follow the infant's response.

Contact Health Care Provider if

- Mother has a fever.
- Infant refuses to eat.
- Infant remains fussy and irritable during 2-hour time increments between feedings.
- Infant is difficult to arouse or appears listless.

The infant is cradled across the mother's abdomen in a stomach-to-stomach alignment, with the infant's head slightly elevated. While in the sitting position, the mother can also use the football hold to cradle the infant's body such that the newborn is positioned at the mother's side with the feet extending toward her back. A pillow or blanket can be used to support the infant as the mother uses her arm and hand to support the baby's head and neck area as he or she nurses. This technique is often used when twins are nursed simultaneously.

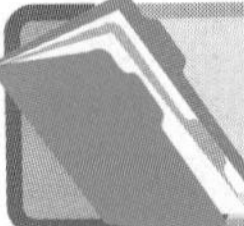

Chart 5–1
Nursing Interventions Classification (NIC)

Breast-Feeding Assistance

Definition

Preparing a new mother to breast-feed her infant

Activities

Provide early mother/infant contact opportunity to breast-feed within 2 hours after birth.
Assist parents in identifying infant arousal cues as opportunities to practice breast-feeding.
Monitor infant's ability to suck.
Encourage mother to ask for assistance with early attempts to nurse, accomplishing 8 to 10 feedings in 24 hours.
Monitor infant's ability to grasp the nipple correctly (e.g., "latch-on" skills).
Encourage comfort and privacy in early attempts to breast-feed.
Encourage mother not to restrict infant sucking time.
Instruct mother on proper positioning.
Instruct proper technique to break suction of nursing infant.
Monitor skin integrity of nipples.
Instruct on nipple care, including how to prevent nipple soreness.
Discuss the use of a breast pump, if newborn is unable to breast-feed initially.
Monitor increased filling of breasts in response to nursing and/or pumping.
Inform mother of pump options available, if needed to maintain lactation.
Instruct on how to control breast congestion with timely emptying by nursing or pumping.
Instruct on storage and warming of breast milk.
Provide formula supplementation only when necessary.
Instruct mother on how to burp newborn.
Instruct mother on normal characteristics of infant voiding and stooling.
Monitor letdown reflex.
Instruct mother on well-balanced diet during lactation.
Encourage mother to drink fluids to satisfy thirst.
Encourage mother to avoid use of cigarettes and birth control pills until lactation is well established.
Instruct mother about infant growth spurts.
Encourage use of comfortable, cotton, supportive nursing bra.
Instruct to avoid using plastic-lined nursing pads.
Encourage mother to contact health care practitioner before taking any medication while nursing.
Identify maternal support system for maintaining lactation.
Encourage frequent rest periods.
Encourage continued lactation on return to work or school.
Provide written material to reinforce instruction at home.
Refer mother to a lactation consultant, as appropriate.

From McCloskey, J., & Bulechek, G. (1996). *Nursing interventions classification (NIC)* (2nd ed.). St. Louis: Mosby–Year Book. Reprinted with permission.

Fathers may feel left out of the feeding process because they are not able to provide the newborn with the nutrition or able to hold the infant during the feeding. One way to encourage father participation is to have the father be the "helper." He can get the child while the mother finds a position of comfort. He can also observe the feeding to note whether the child is properly latching onto the breast (Munson, 1996). He may also participate by feeding water or juice between feedings when the newborn is older.

Breast-Feeding Routine

The mother should nurse the infant for 20 to 30 minutes each feeding, starting with 10 minutes on the first breast, burping the infant well, and then alternating to the second breast. The infant will be much more energetic and will empty the first breast faster than the second, so it is important with each feeding to alternate which breast the newborn nurses from first. If the infant becomes sleepy after nursing on the first breast, he or she can be stimulated with a diaper change, burping, or talking, so as to be alert enough to finish nursing on the second breast. To help a mother remember which breast to begin the next feeding, she can place a safety pin on the bra strap of the side that should be used next time. The mother can also wear a ring that is switched from hand to hand to indicate which side to start the next feeding.

Breast-feeding newborns do not routinely need water offered between feedings. Ingestion of water may unintentionally cause a decrease in milk production because the infant will not feel as hungry and will not nurse as vigorously. The well-nourished breast-fed infant does not need any supplemental vitamins or minerals, with the exception of iron and vitamin D. Iron supplements should be started at 4 to 6 months of age to infants who are exclusively breast-fed. It is during this period that fetal iron stores will be depleted. If the infant is not being given any iron-fortified formula or iron-fortified cereal on a regular basis, iron supplements will need to be administered orally to the child.

caREminder: *Oral ferrous sulfate can stain the teeth and will cause the infant's stools to be dark green or black. Parents should be advised to rinse the infant's mouth with a small amount of water after administering the iron supplement and to be aware of the changes in their child's stool color.*

The breast-fed infant who has deeply pigmented skin or who does not receive enough sunlight should be given 400 IU of vitamin D daily.

Pumping the Breast

If the mother is planning to be away from the infant during feeding times because of work or other activities, she may elect to pump her breast to provide milk for her child in her absence. In preparation for a return to work, the mother should start pumping the breast about 2 weeks before her return to work. The ideal time to begin pumping is between the infant's first two feedings of the day. It has been demonstrated that a mother's milk diminishes during the day, and this will enable the mother to produce a good amount. Pumping can be completed at the workplace as long as the mother has a block of time (10 to 30 minutes, one to four times per day) to pump, a place to refrigerate the milk, and privacy (Corbett-Dick & Bezek, 1997). Many women find breast pumps easier to use than expressing breast milk by hand. Many different pumps are available, and a certified lactation consultant can assist the mother in making a choice. It is recommended that a mother who needs to use a breast pump do so on a regular basis to stimulate her milk supply as long as she wishes to continue to breast-feed. Once the breast milk has been expressed, it can be refrigerated up to 48 hours and frozen for as long as 3 months. Freezing the milk does not harm it, but it does destroy some of the antibodies.

Bottle-Feeding

If the mother is unable or unwilling to breast-feed, the infant's nutrition can come from commercial formula. By the age of 2 months, almost 60% of infants are bottle-fed (Snow & Fry, 1990). The mother who chooses to bottle-feed her infant will require teaching regarding the preparation and administration of fluids with this method. Chart 5–2 provides a summary of the activities that should take place to ensure safe and effective bottle-feeding.

The breast-feeding mother may elect to introduce the bottle to use as supplemental feedings when she is at work or engaged in other activities that take her away from the infant during feedings. The best time to introduce the bottle to the breast-fed child is at 3 to 4 weeks of age. The mother may begin offering the infant a bottle to replace one or more of the feedings from the breast. These bottles can contain breast milk, water, or formula. It may take several tries for the infant to accept a rubber nipple, particularly if the infant has never been exposed to a pacifier.

Tip: *If the infant has been breast-fed and balks at taking the bottle, try to have someone other than the mother offer the bottle (an ideal time for the father to become involved). Also, try bottle-feeding when the infant is sleepy, distracted, or very hungry. Use expressed milk at first as the infant is used to the taste, spreading a little on the rubber nipple. Experiment with different-shaped nipples, and warm the nipple to about body temperature. If the problem seems to be the acceptance of an alternate caregiver, have the alternate caregiver use the same perfume as the mother or a receiving blanket the mother has used so the infant gets the same scents as when mother is feeding him or her.*

Once the infant has accepted the bottle (and this may just be 1 or 2 oz at first), a bottle should be offered at least once a week (or more often) to keep up the infant's skill in using the nipple. Three primary types of nipples are available commercially for the normal newborn. The regular nipple is elongated and teat shaped. The NUK nipple has a wide, flat tip that fits below the hard palate. The Playtex nipple is short and has a square shape. If the infant is premature and has a weak suck, the use of premature or special care nipples is not recommended. Use of these nipples does not promote development of the muscles needed to suck, and infants using these nipples have a greater risk for aspiration.

The choice of expressing breast milk or using formula is up to the mother. She may not be able to pump at her place of work or, owing to the environment, may not be able to relax enough to "let her milk down."

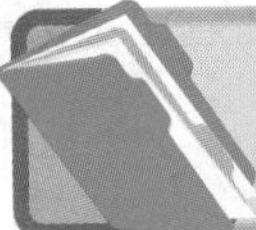

Chart 5–2
Nursing Interventions Classification (NIC)

Bottle-Feeding

Definition

Preparation and administration of fluids to an infant via a bottle

Activities

Determine infant state before initiating feeding.
Give initial feeding of sterile water to determine infant's suck, gag, and swallow reflex, as well as esophageal patency, as appropriate.
Warm formula to room temperature before feeding.
Hold infant during feeding.
Position infant in a semi-Fowler's position for feeding.
Burp the infant frequently during and after the feeding.
Place nipple on top of tongue.
Control fluid intake by regulating softness of nipple, size of the hole, and size of the bottle.
Increase infant alertness by loosening infant's clothes, rubbing hands and feet, or talking to infant.
Encourage sucking by stimulating the rooting reflex, if appropriate.
Increase effectiveness of suck by compressing cheeks in unison with suck, if appropriate.
Provide chin support to decrease leaking of formula and improve lip closure.
Monitor fluid intake.
Monitor infant weight, as appropriate.
Boil unpasteurized milk.
Boil water used for preparing formula, if indicated.
Instruct parent or caregiver on sterilization techniques for feeding equipment.
Instruct parent or caregiver on proper dilution of concentrated formula.
Instruct parent on proper storage of formula.
Determine water source used to dilute concentrated or powdered formula.
Determine fluoride content of water used to dilute concentrated or powdered formula and refer for fluoride supplementation, if indicated.
Caution parent or caregiver about using microwave oven to warm formula.
Instruct and demonstrate to parent oral hygiene techniques appropriate to infant's dentition to be used after each feeding.
Instruct parents to use water in any bottle given to the infant to feed self in bed.

From McCloskey, J., & Bulechek, G. (1996). *Nursing interventions classification (NIC)* (2nd ed.). St. Louis: Mosby–Year Book. Reprinted with permission.

Using formula is a supplemental alternative that can be highly successful. As with breast milk, formula will meet the nutritional needs of the infant for the first 4 to 6 months of life (Table 5–1).

Commercial formulas provide easily digestible protein, calories for energy, fat, iron, vitamins, and minerals necessary for growth and development. Most formulas are cow's milk based. It is important to discuss with the parents the type of formula to use (Table 5–2). Most infants are started on an iron-fortified formula that provides 20 kcal/oz. Low-iron formulas should be avoided because most infants tolerate the regular iron-fortified formulas well, without any constipation, gastrointestinal disturbances, or toxic effect. If there is a history of lactose intolerance in the family, the pediatrician may recommend a soy formula.

Formula Preparation

Many of the commercial formulas come pre-made and ready-to-feed and simply need to be poured into a sterilized bottle. Concentrated or powdered formulas should be prepared by carefully following the manufacturer's directions.

Alert: *Parents should be instructed to not alter the composition of the formula by adding more or less water than is directed in the instructions. Overdiluted formulas can cause water intoxication and lead to malnutrition. Feeding a too-concentrated formula can cause renal problems.*

Formulas should not be prepared any more than 24 hours in advance and should be refrigerated. Any formula left over after 24 hours should be discarded because of the potential for bacterial growth. The temperature of the formula for feeding should be room or body temperature, although some infants do not mind cold (from the refrigerator) formula, particularly in hot weather. Formula should not be heated in a microwave oven because this often heats formula unevenly and could cause portions of the formula to be exceptionally hot and cause burns. As with breast-fed infants, there should be no need for supplemental water during the first 6 months, unless the child has a fever or is having diarrhea or the weather is very hot. The use of supplemental vitamins and minerals is generally not necessary for the first 6 months. After the sixth month, fluoride supplements are recommended if local water supplies are not fluoridated or if the infant is given ready-to-eat cereals in which fluoridated water is not added.

Parents should not offer unmodified whole cow's milk (or goat's milk) to their child until the child is at least 12 months old. Whole cow's milk (or goat's milk) can contribute to anemia because it is deficient in iron and has a much more complex structure to digest. By the time the infant is a year old, his or her body is more physiologically ready to digest whole milk because the

Table 5–1
Nutritional Needs of Infants

Age	Formula or Breast Milk	Solid Foods	Total Caloric Needs
Newborn–2 mo	2–4 oz every 2–4 hr	No solid foods should be introduced.	120 cal/kg/day
2–4 mo	3–6 oz every 3–4 hr	No solid foods should be introduced.	120 cal/kg/day
4–6 mo	6–8 oz every 4½–6 hr	Introduce solid foods beginning with cereal products. Breast-fed infant can be sustained on mother's milk alone.	120 cal/kg/day
6–12 mo	6–8 oz every 6–8 hours (with maximum of 32 oz per day)	Introduce solid foods. Introduce the cup. Offer finger foods.	100 cal/kg/day

gastrointestinal tract is more mature and there is less tendency toward allergic reactions. Infants should never receive low-fat or nonfat milk because it does not have the fat, calories, and nutrients needed for digestion of proteins and for the rapid growth and development at this age.

Positioning

Positioning is as important in bottle-feeding as it is in breast-feeding. The infant's head should be elevated, and the infant should be held close to the mother. The bottle should be tilted so the formula fills the nipple. The hole in the nipple should allow the milk to drop slowly from the bottle, not "stream" out or need to be "squeezed" out. About halfway through the feeding, the bottle should be removed from the infant's mouth and the infant is burped. The infant will "burp" up a little air and possibly a little formula. This is very common and is known as a "wet" burp. As long as the volume returned is small and this only occurs when air is passing the vocal cords, it is normal.

Bottles should never be "propped," that is, the infant should not be laid down with a bottle positioned on a pillow or blanket to hold the bottle to the baby's mouth. When the infant is fed by propping the bottle, there is a significant risk for aspiration of the formula and an increased potential for development of otitis media, owing to the pooling of milk in the eustachian tubes. Furthermore, this method does not encourage bonding with the infant and may cause the child to become uninterested in feeding.

Schedule

Whether breast- or bottle-fed, the infant will want to feed about every 2½ hours for the first 2 to 3 weeks, taking about 2 to 3 oz. In the first month of life, infants should be awakened to eat if sleeping for more than 4 hours. In the second month, the infant usually develops a more sustained schedule, lasting 4 to 5 hours between feedings and taking about 4 oz until 3 to 4 months old. At 5 to 6 months of age, the infant is usually taking 7 to 8 oz per feeding. When the infant is able to go longer than 4 hours between feedings, one of the nighttime feedings should be eliminated. Some infants do this naturally as they increase the length of time they sleep at night. Other infants may get into a habit of waking frequently in the night to be fed. In this case, when the infant awakes and indicates he or she wants to be fed, rather than feeding, the infant should be "patted" and calmed or should be offered a pacifier. After a few nights of not receiving a midnight feeding, the infant may arouse but will learn not to expect food and thus will go back to sleep.

Starting Solid Foods

By 4 to 6 months of age, the infant should be developmentally ready for the introduction of solid foods. Before this time, breast milk or formula can meet all the nutritional needs of the infant. The infant's chronological age is not as meaningful as whether the infant demonstrates the necessary skills to be able to handle spoon feeding (Chart 5–3).

Progression of Food Introduction

The first solid food should be rice cereal mixed with a little breast milk or formula. Rice cereal is very bland, is easily digestible, and has a low incidence of allergic reactions. During the first attempts, a semi-liquid consistency allows the infant to use the "suck" and then swallow reflex while adjusting to the modification of food delivery

Table 5–2
Common Formulas for Infants and Young Children

Type	Formula (Manufacturer)	Kilocalories/oz.
Premature formulas	Enfamil Human Milk Fortifier (3.8 g) Added to 100 mL Preterm Milk (Mead Johnson)	24
	Enfamil Premature (Mead Johnson)	24
	Similac NeoCare (Ross)	22
	Similac Natural Care Human Milk Fortifier (Ross)	24
	Similac Special Care (Ross)	24
	SMA-Preemie (Wyeth Ayerst)	24
Cow's milk–based formulas	Bonamil (Wyeth-Ayerst)	20
	Enfamil (Mead Johnson)	20
	Gerber (Gerber)	20
	Lactofree (Mead Johnson)	20
	Similac (Ross)	20
	Similac PM/60/40 (Ross)	20
	SMA (Wyeth Ayerst)	20
Hydrolyzed whey–based formulas	Good Start (Carnation)	20
Nutrient-dense cow's milk–based formulas	SMA (Wyeth-Ayerst)	24
	SMA (Wyeth-Ayerst)	27
	Enfamil (Mead Johnson)	24
	Similac (Ross)	24
	Similac (Ross)	27
Soy-based formulas	Alsoy (Carnation)	20

Table 5-2
Common Formulas for Infants and Young Children *Continued*

Type	Formula (Manufacturer)	Kilocalories/oz.
Soy-based formulas (*Continued*)	Gerber (Gerber)	20
	Isomil (Ross)	20
	Isomil DF (Ross)	20
	Isomil SF (Ross)	20
	Nursoy (Wyeth-Ayerst)	20
	Prosobee (Mead Johnson)	20
Casein hydrolysate (hypoallergenic) formulas	Alimentum (Ross)	20
	Nutramigen (Mead Johnson)	20
	Pregestimil (Mead Johnson)	20
For special feeding problems	Portagen (Mead Johnson)	20
	Monodisaccharide-free diet powder Product 3232A (Mead Johnson)	13 Using 81.0-g powder and water to make one quart
	Protein-Vitamin-Mineral Formula Component (Ross)	Add 30 g powder, CHO, and fat to 900 mL water
	RCF CHO-Free Formula Base (Ross)	12 Dilute 1 : 1 without added CHO
For feeding beyond 4–6 mo of age with solid foods added to the diet	Follow-Up (Carnation)	20
	Follow-Up Soy (Carnation)	20
For feeding beyond 1 yr	Whole cow's milk	20
	Next Step (Mead Johnson)	20
	Next Step Soy (Mead Johnson)	20
	Similac Toddler's Best (Ross)	20
Nutrient-dense formulas for feeding beyond 1 yr	Kindercal (Mead Johnson)	30
	PediaSure (Ross)	30
	PediaSure with Fiber (Ross)	30

Chart 5–3

Assessing Readiness to Begin Introduction of Solid Foods to the Infant

- The tongue-thrust reflex must be extinguished.
- Drooling must be present
- The infant must be able to sit fairly upright.
- A fairly organized suck-swallow reflex must be present.
- Sensory readiness cues such as mouthing of toys and objects are demonstrated.
- The infant is easily distracted from the bottle or breast-feeding.
- The infant must have doubled his or her birth weight and weigh about 13 lb
- The infant demonstrates an interest in table food by reaching for food or eating utensils or protesting when he or she sees others eat food.

with the spoon. Introduction of the spoon may cause some turning away, spitting out, and batting away with the hands, but with patience and perseverance, the infant will eventually accept the spoon. It is important not to introduce the spoon when the infant is extremely hungry, tired, or ill. The best time to start solids is at the noon or early evening feeding when the infant is not sleepy and more interested in participating in a new activity. An infant spoon, coated with a pliable plastic and properly sized for the infant's mouth, is used because this is softer than the feel of metal. If one of these is not available, any spoon smaller than a teaspoon will work.

Cereals should not be mixed in the bottle with the formula or breast milk for the infant to drink. This only serves to increase the calories ingested without allowing the infant to learn the process of meal taking and experience the various consistencies of solid foods. When rice cereal is introduced to the infant, a small amount of breast milk or formula is given to drink before offering the cereal mixed with formula or breast milk. A small amount of cereal is placed toward the middle to the back of the tongue. The infant will most likely not know what to do with the cereal in his or her mouth and may spit it out or make a face expressing displeasure. Most of the first feedings will not be swallowed; rather, the food usually ends up everywhere on the child. Once the infant grows accustomed to the cereal and is having no difficulty swallowing, the amount of cereal offered can be increased. After about a week, if feeding is going well, another type of cereal may be introduced. Cereals should be introduced in the order of rice, oats, barley, and wheat once a careful assessment of family allergies and siblings' allergies has been done. Before adding another kind of solid food, one should wait for 4 to 7 days to ensure no allergic or adverse reactions have occurred. Wheat cereals have the highest incidence of allergic reactions in infants. Cereal products can sustain the child's needs for solid food up until age 6 months.

After the introduction of cereal products and given the child's increasing nutritional needs, other solid foods are introduced. These foods are introduced very slowly, no more than one per week, again to prevent allergic reactions. The order of introduction should be cereals, fruits, vegetables, and meats. The food should be pureed and of a very thin consistency to begin. As teeth erupt and the child gains skills in swallowing and chewing, the texture of the food can be varied and become thicker and chunkier. Foods that are easily aspirated or choked on should be avoided. Also, the infant should always be supervised by an adult while he or she is eating to reduce the high risk of choking or other accident. At 6 months of age, solid foods are served two to three times per day at family mealtimes. By 9 months, the infant is offered solid foods three to four times a day.

caREminder: *When an infant is hospitalized or in any situation that caregivers change, it is important to assess which foods have already been introduced to the child and to not introduce new foods during the course of the illness. Every effort must be made to ensure that an allergic reaction to a food is not triggered during an illness event, because it then becomes difficult to ascertain the true cause of symptoms such as a rash, vomiting, or diarrhea.*

Certain foods are avoided until late in the first year because they are considered significant allergens or the infant's gastrointestinal system is not adequately mature to handle the food. These include eggs, corn syrup solids, citrus fruits and juices, tomatoes, strawberries, seafood, spices, and chocolate. When introducing vegetables such as peas, beans, or beets, it is common to find some green or red particles in the stool for the first day or so after the food is first given. Because the intestinal tract has not totally matured, it must adapt to a new food, and some of it may be passed undigested.

Alert: *To prevent botulism, the infant should not be given honey until after the first birthday. Also, foods with low acid content such as home-canned fruits and vegetables should not be offered.*

Introduction of the Cup

At 6 months of age, use of the cup to drink fluids may be started by placing a small amount of juice or water in a cup. Or instead of giving a bottle, a small amount of formula or breast milk can be placed in a cup to help the child become accustomed to the idea of using a cup. Until the infant is proficient at using the cup (meaning he or she is taking most from the cup), bottle- or breast-feeding remains the primary method by which the infant receives formula or human milk.

Cups with specialized covers can be used to prevent spills and to regulate the rapidity and amount of fluid that flows at a time. In some cases, a specialized top may cause the liquid to flow too fast and may frighten the child, causing regression and putting off this developmental step. Handles on the cups allow easy grasping of the cup and stability as the infant tries to bring it to the mouth. In the early use of the cup, it is filled approximately one-fourth full because this cuts down on the amount that is lost if any should spill.

With the introduction of the cup comes the introduction of fruit juices. The amount of juice served is limited to 4 to 6 oz/day so as not to suppress the child's desire to have breast milk or formula. In addition, consumption of 12 or more fluid oz a day of fruit juice by young children has been associated with short stature and obesity (Dennison, Rockwell, & Baker, 1997). The first fruit juice is usually low acidity and may be diluted to half strength with water. Low acidity juices include apple juice and white grape juice; orange juice, grapefruit juice, and pineapple juice should be avoided until the infant's bowel is more mature.

Weaning

Once the infant is able to drink a sufficient amount of fluids from the cup, it is an opportune time for weaning from the bottle or breast. The breast-fed infant who is comfortable using the cup may be weaned directly from breast to cup. Although the infant may tolerate this well, weaning from the breast may make the mother feel depressed and saddened as she stops producing milk and feels no longer "needed" for her nutritional support. Supporting the mother through this time is essential because these feelings may severely impact her perceptions of her relationship with the infant.

The infant who is bottle-feeding can be weaned by changing the fluid that is placed in the bottle. Formula should only be offered in the cup, and water should only be offered in the bottle. The infant will be attracted to the cup because it contains the more palatable liquid. Weaning can also be completed gradually by eliminating all except the nighttime bottle. If the bottle is not in sight and accessible during the day, the infant quickly learns that the bottle will only be offered at bedtime.

Elimination

The first bowel movement a newborn has after birth is passing the meconium. If the delivery was without complications, this was not passed while the newborn was still in utero. If the infant experienced fetal distress (an indication that an infant in utero is experiencing lack of oxygen or fetal blood supply), the first indication is "meconium staining" or release of meconium stool into the amniotic fluid. The meconium is a sticky, thick, greenish-black, tarry stool that is made up of epithelial cells, salts, bile, and mucus and usually is without a strong odor. This stool appears within the first 24 hours and may persist for up to 3 days.

The stools of the breast-fed infant are usually yellow and very soft to thick liquid in consistency with an aromatic and little or no unpleasant smell. There is less amount of stool from breast-fed infants. The bottle-fed infant may have pale yellow-brown almost liquid stools to stools that are greenish-brown and pasty. Once the infant starts feeding, the stools take on a consistency determined by the food ingested. The newborn generally has a bowel movement every time he or she is fed; but if the infant does not have a bowel movement for several days, this, too, is normal. As the child develops, elimination patterns become more rhythmic and individualized for that child. Some infants have two or three bowel movements a day, some have only one, and both are perfectly normal depending on the particular child. Infants usually bear down, grunt, and appear to "strain" when having a bowel movement. This is not necessarily a sign of difficulty in having a bowel movement.

The infant's first urination occurs within the first 24 hours of life. Production of urine is 200 to 300 mL/day, increasing as the infant matures, which can translate into 6 to 10 diapers per day. The child voids when the bladder is filled beyond 15 mL and could void as frequently as every hour. Healthy urine is clear, colorless to a very pale yellow, and does not have a strong odor. If an infant is dehydrated, there will be no wet diaper for a period of several hours and/or the urine will appear darker in color and may have a stronger odor, indicating concentration of the urine. Although this is not the only indication of dehydration, the nurse should be alerted to the possibility and check other potential signs.

Constipation

Constipation is present when an infant has very hard stools or the lack of stool beyond his or her normal schedule. The appearance of hard stools usually occurs more in formula-fed infants, in infants who are starting solid foods, and in infants who are ill. This is usually due to a change in the amount of water or fluids they are receiving while eating solids or the lack of water taken when an infant is feeling ill. Also, if the weather is very hot, the child may need extra water to increase the water in the stool.

When constipation occurs, offering low-acidic fruit

juices (such as apple or white grape juice) to infants younger than 4 months up to twice a day can be very effective. Enemas or suppositories are not recommended for small infants. If the child is taking solids, increasing the amount of high-fiber baby foods such as cereals, prunes, and peaches may assist in elimination; bananas and carrots should be avoided because they may increase the constipation (see Chapter 18 for more information on constipation and diarrhea).

Diarrhea

Although the infant normally has very soft to liquid stools, he or she should not be having severe watery stools. Diarrhea is usually a sign of illness or intolerance to a specific food or type of formula. It is important to monitor the infant closely if he or she is having frequent watery diarrhea because this could lead to dehydration (see Chapter 17). It is imperative that the infant continue to ingest formula or human milk to correct the fluid loss. Breast-fed and bottle-fed infants may need to be offered extra water (or electrolyte solutions) between feedings. When a formula intolerance is suspected, the infant should be given clear liquids for 4 to 6 hours and then offered a soy-based formula. The health care provider should be contacted immediately if the infant refuses to accept the bottle or the breast, cries without tears, does not have a wet diaper for over 8 hours, or has a dry mouth, or if any blood is seen in the diarrhea. The infant with diarrhea is at risk for diaper rash. Thus, meticulous perineal care, frequent diaper changes, and the use of a barrier agent should be employed to prevent skin breakdown (see Chapter 25 for a detailed discussion of diaper dermatitis).

Oral Health

Sequence of Tooth Eruption

Teething can be one of the most difficult and exasperating times for new parents because it is usually associated with some discomfort on the child's part. The first teeth, usually the lower central incisors, erupt between 6 and 10 months of age, although it is not uncommon for this to be delayed until the child is a year old. The next teeth to appear are the four upper incisors (central first then lateral), which are evident at between 8 and 13 months of age, followed by the two lower lateral incisors, and then the first four molars (both upper and lower). By the time the child is a year old, approximately 10 teeth will have erupted. This is an average, and it is not uncommon for some children to have more and for some children to just be starting to develop teeth. Figure 4–13 depicts the sequence of tooth eruption for primary and secondary teeth.

Teething

Gum care should be started soon after birth. A soft washcloth should be used to massage the gums with plain water or a small dab of infant gum cleaner. This soothes the gum area and allows the teething process to be less painful. It also allows the infant to become used to the daily ritual of dental hygiene.

After the tooth breaks through, a soft washcloth can continue to be used, or an infant finger toothbrush or small soft toothbrush can be used. Many parents believe that teething elicits signs of illness, including fever, excessive drooling, and crankiness. In most cases, these problems are due to other sources (Brazelton, 1992). Rubbing the gums where the eruptions are occurring with a clean finger for about 2 minutes reduces the swelling and provides comfort. The use of topical anesthetics or analgesics is not usually very helpful because they "wash" away quickly. Additionally, the infant touches the area with the tongue and causes the tongue to be numb rather than the affected tooth area. Teething rings that are cold, not frozen, also reduce the swelling and the discomfort of teething.

caREminder: *Frozen teething rings can cause frostbite on the gums and are so hard as to cause trauma to the gums. Alcohol spirits (such as whiskey) should never be used on the gums.*

Teething biscuits and small bagels are also good for teething infants depending on the infant's age. The child should not be given anything that cannot be easily chewed or that could break off into large pieces and cause choking.

Oral Care

Performing good oral hygiene at least twice daily prevents oral infections, soothes the gums, and comforts the child while the teething process is occurring. The child from the time of infancy should have the mouth cleaned at least twice a day. The infant's erupting teeth can be brushed with a soft toothbrush or rubbed lightly with the corner of a soft washcloth.

caREminder: *Parents should be strongly encouraged not to put the child to bed with a bottle at any time. One of the leading causes of tooth decay in young children is baby bottle tooth decay (BBTD), also known as nursing bottle caries, nursing caries, and nursing bottle syndrome (Von Burg, Sanders, & Weddell, 1995).*

Baby bottle tooth decay occurs when carbohydrates in the formula, breast milk, and fruit juice are allowed to remain on the teeth for a prolonged period of time. There is also the increased incidence of otitis media in children who are allowed to go to bed with a bottle of milk or juice. It is believed the otitis media is caused from the contents of the bottle pooling in the eustachian tubes and contributing to bacterial growth. Prevention is the key to good dental health. If the child must have a bedtime bottle, it should contain water.

Fluoride is important for teeth protection and growth. It is generally provided in sufficient amounts through the community water supply. If this is not the case, the physician can prescribe fluoride by means of oral drops. Children who receive too much fluoride can develop mottled or "speckled" teeth.

Infant Care

Bathing

The infant does not actually need much bathing the first few weeks of life. It is important to keep the diaper area meticulously clean to avoid diaper rash, but until the cord falls off, the infant should be only receiving sponge baths. All of the articles needed for the bath should be collected before bathing. Supplies needed include a basin of lukewarm water, two to three towels, a washcloth, cotton balls, mild soap, baby shampoo, baby powder, cornstarch, lotion (optional), fresh diaper, and clean clothes.

For the sponge bath, the infant can be placed on a padded flat area near a sink or on a changing table. During the bathing, only the parts of the body that are being cleansed should be exposed so as to avoid chilling the infant. The bath begins with a cleansing of the eyes from inner to outer areas, rinsing the cloth and proceeding to the rest of the face. The perineal area should be cleansed last. Each body part should be dried before moving on to wash another part of the body. All body crease areas should be washed and dried carefully, particularly the folds in the neck and perineal area. These areas are particularly prone to rashes because they are warm and moist. The hair can be washed about twice a week with a very mild tear-free baby shampoo. Hair washing can be done immediately after washing the infant's face and neck.

The umbilical cord should be dried well and have rubbing alcohol applied to the stump with a cotton-tipped applicator until it falls off. To prevent infection and improper healing, the cord area should not be submerged in water until the stump has fallen off. Once the stump has fallen off, tub bathing may begin. This may occur in a sink or plastic tub. It is best to line the basin with a towel to reduce the slippage and make the surface more comfortable for the infant. The basin should be filled with about 2 inches of water that is warm, not hot, to the inside of the wrist or elbow. The first few baths should be short. If the infant protests too much, sponge baths can be continued for 1 or 2 weeks before trying tub bathing again.

Parents should use bath time as bonding time by talking, cooing, and singing to the infant. The bath should be unhurried and nonstressful. If the infant is enjoying the experience, then extra play time in the water should be permitted (Chart 5–4).

When the child is able to sit upright without much support, a tub ring or tub seat can be used to stabilize the infant as he or she plays in the bath. The older infant is likely to begin moving around quite a bit in the bathtub. The water level should remain low enough so that if the older infant were to lie on his or her abdomen in the tub, his or her face would not easily be immersed in the water.

caREminder: *An infant should never be left alone when bathing, whether in a tub of water or on a counter. Instruct parents to prepare for any interruptions by taking the phone off the hook or engaging the answering machine; if the door bell rings or a sibling screams, the infant should be wrapped up and taken with the parent.*

Skin Care

Infants do not generally need any lotions or talcum on their skin. Many parents like to use lotions because it gives them an opportunity to massage the infant, increasing the sense of bonding and togetherness. If lotions or powders are used, they should be hypoallergenic. Lotions should be put on the parent's hands first to warm the cream before applying it to the infant's skin. Powder should always be placed on the hand first to reduce the powder in the air and prevent the infant from inhaling the powder.

Several normal alterations in the infant's skin can be noted during the first few months. Erythema toxicum, a rash of red splotches with yellowish-white bumps in their center, commonly appears only during the first few days after birth and requires no treatment. Sucking blisters look like water blisters and are common in newborns who have been sucking a body part when in utero. These are most commonly found on the hands, wrist, and forearm. Milia are tiny white or yellow spots on the cheeks, nose, or chin, caused by immature sweat and oil glands. They also require no treatment and usually disappear within the first 2 to 3 weeks of life. Newborn acne, which is pimples on the cheeks, chin, and forehead, is caused by maternal hormones still circulating in the infant that stimulate the sebaceous glands. The acne usually disappears within the first few months of life. Parents should not treat the acne except by washing the infant's face two to three times per day with water. Chapter 25 presents a detailed discussion of both normal and abnormal skin lesions commonly seen in the infant and child.

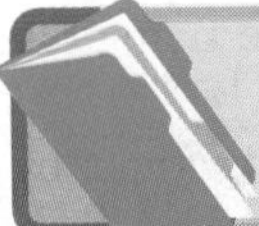

Chart 5–4
Nursing Interventions Classification (NIC)

Teaching: Infant Care

Definition

Instruction on nurturing and physical care needed during the first year of life

Activities

Demonstrate reflexes to parents and explain their significance to infant care.
Provide anticipatory guidance about developmental changes during the first year of life.
Give information about adding solid foods to diet during the first year.
Give information about weaning from breast or bottle to the cup.
Instruct parents on formula preparation and selection.
Give parents information about pacifiers.
Instruct parents on appropriate fluoride supplementation.
Give information about developing dentition and oral hygiene during the first year.
Discuss alternatives to a bedtime bottle to prevent nursing bottle caries.
Encourage parents to talk and read to infant.
Assist parents in interpreting infant cues, nonverbal cues, crying, and vocalizations.
Provide anticipatory guidance about changing sleep patterns during the first year.
Provide anticipatory guidance about changing elimination patterns during the first year.
Instruct parents on how to treat and prevent diaper rash.
Encourage parents to hold, cuddle, massage, and touch infant.
Encourage parents to provide pleasurable auditory and visual stimulation to promote growth.
Encourage parents to play with infant.
Give examples of safe toys or available things in home that can be used as toys.
Demonstrate ways in which parents can stimulate infant's development.
Inform parents of the importance of regular child health care and immunizations.
Assist parents in learning to take infant's temperature.
Inform parents of physical symptoms that require professional attention.
Assist parents in anticipating safety hazards in home environment and how these change as child develops mobility during the first year.
Provide information about safety needs of infant while in a motor vehicle.
Assist parents in describing infant's temperament and planning care and activities that complement infant's behavioral style.
Assist parents in articulating ways to integrate infant into family system.
Provide parents with written materials appropriate to identified knowledge needs.

From McCloskey, J., & Bulechek, G. (1996). *Nursing interventions classification (NIC)* (2nd ed.). St. Louis: Mosby–Year Book. Reprinted with permission.

The infant should not be overexposed to the sun because the skin is quite sensitive and can be easily burned.

Alert: *Before 6 months of age, sunscreens should not be applied to the infant's skin because the ingredients in the lotions may cause an allergic skin reaction.*

After 1 year of age, sunscreens should always be applied before the infant plays in the sun (see Chapter 25 for more information regarding application of sunscreens).

Thumb Sucking or the Pacifier

The infant receives a great deal of comfort and gratification by sucking. In addition to sucking the mother's nipple or the bottle nipple, the young infant can often be seen sucking parts of the hand. For some infants this urge to suck is very strong. It is most often noted when the infant is hungry or tired. Parents generally foster the need for oral stimulation during times of distress by offering a pacifier whenever the infant cries.

The choice of thumb sucking versus a pacifier is

often one a parent cannot make. Although parents may offer the pacifier frequently and remove the infant's thumb from the mouth, the infant will ultimately be the one to select the form of non-nutritive sucking that is most desirable.

The thumb is readily available to the infant. The child does not have to have hand-eye coordination to get the thumb to the mouth. Therefore, in the early months, use of the thumb keeps parents from having to constantly assist the child by putting a pacifier in his or her mouth. Thumb sucking reaches its height at 15 to 18 months of age. There are no indications that thumb sucking can damage the alignment of the teeth unless the sucking persists past age 5. The thumb tends to be dirty when the child places the thumb in the mouth. Wash the hands of the child with water before the child's nap to ensure that the thumb that goes in the mouth is clean. When it is not convenient to have soap and water available, cleansing wipes can be kept available to clean the child's hands; even though the cleansing wipes are alcohol based and contain perfume, it is better for the thumb to be clean. It is generally more difficult to wean the child from the thumb than the pacifier because it is harder for parents to regulate the presence of the thumb. If the older child is unable to break the habit of thumb sucking, the dentist may suggest the use of an intraoral appliance that interferes with placement of the finger or thumb in the mouth and has been demonstrated to be successful in stopping thumb sucking in preschoolers and school-age children.

Pacifiers come in a variety of shapes. If the infant is bottle-feeding, the shape of the pacifier should be similar to the shape of the nipple used during feedings.

caREminder: *Nipples intended for use with prepared formula bottles should never be used as pacifiers because they can be aspirated when not attached to a bottle base.*

Studies have indicated that the use of pacifiers may lead to early weaning from the breast (Victora, Tomasi, Olinto, & Barros, 1993). It is believed that the pacifier allows the infant to become lazy regarding feeding and produce less intense stimulation of the nipples, which in turn causes decreased production of milk. During the early months, the pacifier must be placed in the infant's mouth by an adult. As the infant matures, he or she will be able to find the pacifier in the crib and place it in the mouth. Pacifiers can be equally as dirty as using the thumb. Pacifier clips can be used to attach the pacifier to the infant's shirt and prevent the pacifier from constantly falling on the ground. Weaning from the pacifier is somewhat easier than from thumb sucking. As with weaning from the bottle, use of the pacifier can be limited to sleep time. Then as pacifiers fall apart the toddler is encouraged to throw that one away and say "bye-bye" to it, until all pacifiers have met the same fate. Another method of weaning is to cut the tip off the pacifier. When the child uses the pacifier, no sucking action is possible. The "broken" pacifier can be placed in the trash by the youngster until all pacifiers have been thrown away.

Sleep

In the first month of life, the average sleeping time for an infant is 16 to 20 hours. This takes into account the fact that some infants sleep as little as 10 hours a day and others as much as 23 hours a day. Not surprisingly, the infant who sleeps very little tends to grow into the child who sleeps very little and eventually into the adult who requires little sleep. As in all aspects of development, the sleep needs of children vary from infant to infant. As the child develops within the first year, hours spent sleeping decrease to an average of 14¼ per day at 6 months and 13¾ per day by 1 year of age.

For many parents, a primary goal within the first few months is to have the infant achieve a pattern in which he or she sleeps for a 7- to 8-hour period through the night. For the tired and bleary-eyed caregiver, this extended sleep pattern is a welcome developmental milestone. To achieve this goal, the stabilization of hunger metabolism and sleep/wake cycles must first be established. From birth through the eighth week, the daily routine for most infants is a continual repeat of a 2½- to 3-hour cycle that starts with the beginning of one feeding and ends with the beginning of the next feeding. Within this cycle the caregiver should be promoting a daytime pattern of eating, followed by wake time, preceded by a nap time of approximately 1½ hours in length. During the late evening and nighttime hours, the cycle would only consist of eating and sleeping activities. Between the third and the fourth month, the infant will extend the nighttime sleep to 10 to 12 hours, continuing this pattern for the rest of the first year.

Concurrently, daytime naps increase in length to approximately 2 hours; and the infant subsequently drops the number of naps and feedings per day, thereby elongating the periods of wakefulness. The newborn who requires six to eight naps a day tapers off to three to four naps a day at 3 months and to two naps at 6 months. The need for both a morning and afternoon nap, lasting about 2 hours each, continues until the child is approximately 16 months of age (Chart 5–5).

Parents can follow several guidelines that help foster good sleep habits in children at an early age. The most important guideline is to promote the activities of eating, wake time, and nap time, in that order. Often the first two activities are reversed. This creates a situation in which the infant must have a bottle or be breast-fed to go to sleep. For some parents, this has meant letting the child fall asleep in the crib with a bottle of milk hanging

Chart 5–5
Developmental Considerations

Childhood Sleep Patterns

Age	Hours of Sleep 2 ¦ 4 ¦ 6 ¦ 8 ¦ 10 ¦ 12 ¦ 14 ¦ 16 ¦ 18	Average Total Hours of Sleep/Day
1 wk	#########*****/*****/****	16½
1 mo	#########*****/****/***	15½
3 mo	##########****/***/***	15
6 mo	##############***/***	14¼
9 mo	##############**/**	14
12 mo	############**/***	13¾
18 mo	############****	13
2–3 yr	############*****	12–13
4–5 yr	##############	11
6–7 yr	#############	10½
8–9 yr	############	10
10–14 yr	###########	9–9¾
15–18 yr	#########	8–8½

/, Naps during day; #####, night sleep.

from the mouth. It is important for an infant to learn how to soothe himself or herself by thumb sucking, rooting around in bed, head shaking, or listening to soft music or the sound of a parent's voice. The parent may want to cuddle the infant and then place him or her in the crib while he or she is still awake and continue to talk or sing to him or her until the infant falls asleep. This "teaches" the infant how to soothe himself or herself and fall asleep without a bottle or breast.

caREminder: *The American Academy of Pediatrics has recommended that all infants without respiratory problems or reflux be placed on the side or back to sleep, because sleeping in the prone position has been linked to sudden infant death syndrome (SIDS) (Lerner, 1993) (Fig. 5–1).*

Parents may believe the infant is more comfortable sleeping on his or her stomach, but this is not so, nor should an infant have a pillow placed under the head.

There are two types of sleep: active and quiet (Chart 5–6). Active sleep is also known as rapid eye movement (REM) sleep and is the time the infant is in a light sleep and may cry out or fuss. It is easy to awaken the infant during this time. The infant can find a blanket, pacifier, or thumb to quiet himself or herself if left alone. Swaddling and nesting are also helpful to some infants. Some infants like to sleep tightly swaddled, whereas others prefer to sleep loosely swaddled. Some infants have a difficult time settling back down after they awaken in the middle of the night. If the infant is older than 4 months, the parents should not immediately respond to the infant if he or she starts to fuss. By the time the infant is 3 months old, the amount of quiet sleep time has nearly doubled. If the infant has been sleeping longer during the day and wakes frequently at night, the daytime naps can be shortened and the child will usually be more tired at night. When the infant does wake during the night, deal with the reason in as brief a time as possible with love but without sustained cuddling, which may tend to encourage the infant to repeat the activity.

Clothing

Baby showers provide many new mothers with all sorts of adorable outfits for the expected arrival. Many of these outfits may rarely be used because they are either too small or because the child is growing so rapidly that he or she passes through the smaller sizes rather quickly. For instance, a newborn outfit sized for a 6-lb infant may not fit the 10-lb baby boy that arrived. A general rule of thumb is to encourage parents and friends to buy big and to limit the amount of clothes that are sized for 3 months and younger.

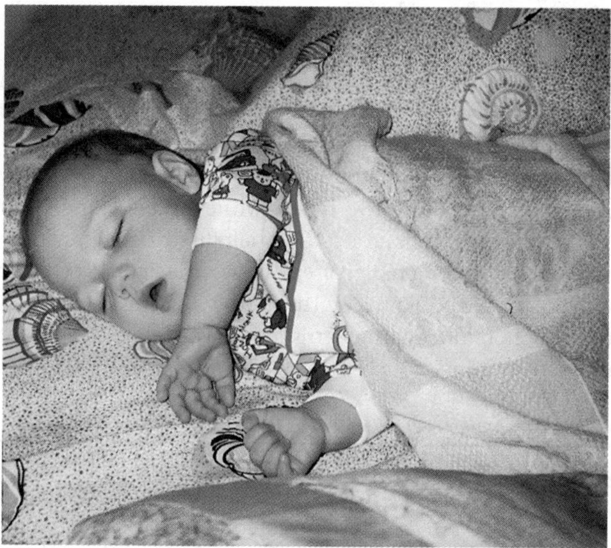

Figure 5–1
The infant should be placed on the side or back to sleep. A pillow or bedroll can be used to keep the baby on his or her side.

Clothing should be loose enough to allow no constriction of the child's extremities. Garments that have "feet" in them should be checked periodically for loose threads to prevent the possibility of a thread constricting the toes. Clothing should be avoided that is tight around the neck, arms, or legs, because these could be potential safety hazards, as well as being uncomfortable. Clothing should be durable, easily washable, and machine dryable. Washing instructions located on the clothing should be followed to maintain the safety and integrity of the garment. For example, flame-retardant chemicals are removed if garments are washed in soap and not detergent. Choosing items that have snap openers down the legs makes dressing and diaper changing much easier. Items with oval rather than round necks are easier to fit over the large round heads of infants. All sleepwear should be flame retardant.

A common misconception is that infants are cold and need to be kept warmer than adults. Therefore, parents often overdress the infant and the child becomes overheated and uncomfortable and fussy. Although newborns do need to be dressed more warmly than toddlers, by the time they are 3 months old they are fairly able to stabilize their temperature and can usually be dressed as normally as adults. In the winter, layers of clothing offer more warmth than single layers. A general rule is to put one more layer of clothes on the infant than the mother is wearing in the same environment. One area that is an exception is the necessity of providing infants with hats, both in the winter and the summer—in the winter to minimize heat loss (90% of the heat loss occurs through the uncovered head) and in the summer to prevent sunburn and overheating.

Promotion of Social Competence

Temperament

Temperament is defined as the combination of intellectual, emotional, ethical, and physical characteristics of an individual. It is the natural inborn style of behavior of each individual. Every child has his or her own set of temperament traits or characteristics (Turecki, 1995).

Chart 5–6

Infant States

The states of arousal that are not good times for interacting with an infant are

- Quiet or active sleep
- Drowsy
  - Opens and closes eyes
  - Eyes glazed, with heavy-lidded look
  - Delayed responsiveness
  - May occur when arousing from a sleep state
- Crying
  - Irregular respirations
  - Facial grimaces
  - Cries
  - Color changes
  - Sensitive to stimuli and may respond with crying
  - Uses self-consoling behaviors

The awake state that is the best time for the child to interact with the infant is

- Quiet alert
  - Minimal body activity
  - Regular respirations
  - Face has bright shiny look
  - Eyes wide and bright
  - Most attentive to stimuli

The child can also interact with the infant during an active alert stage. However, the infant may become fussy and require a change in stimuli, a need to be fed, or a need to pursue some consoling behaviors.

- Active alert
  - Much body activity
  - Irregular respirations
  - Facial movement
  - Eyes open, but not bright
  - Fussiness

There are nine temperament traits that can be used to classify a child from being very easy to raise to being very difficult. The traits are activity level, distractibility, intensity, regularity, persistence, sensory threshold, approach/withdrawal, adaptability, and mood (see Chapter 4). By assessing a child for these traits, a professional or a parent can determine to what extent the resulting behaviors may be expected (Turecki, 1995).

Brazelton identified three types of temperaments of infants. These are the average child, the quiet child, and the active child. Each is a totally normal developmental type consistent with specific characteristics that "categorize" the infant. Many times these characteristics are strictly parental perceptions of what the child is like, and many parents link the personality type to use of drugs during delivery or parenting skills.

The average child is usually easy going and is predictable in his or her responses to environmental stimulations. The quiet child is unusually quiet, does not cry as much as the average child, yet does not appear developmentally delayed in any way. The active child can often be referred to as a "difficult" child. These are the children that even as infants are restless, are irritable, cry inconsolably, and often have unpredictable schedules for feeding and sleeping (Turecki, 1995).

The Colicky Baby

The colicky infant is very difficult to deal with. The fact that there always appears to be nothing that a parent can do to alleviate the crying and discomfort that the infant is experiencing produces stress and strain on the relationships as well as a feeling of inadequacy as a new parent. It is quite common for an infant to have a normal "fussy" period during the day (usually around 6 P.M. to midnight), but if the crying does not stop and continues around the clock, or the infant appears inconsolable, often pulling up legs and passing gas, this may be colic. Sometimes, in breast-fed infants this is a reaction to something the mother has eaten, but rarely is it a sensitivity to milk or milk products. Colic may also indicate a medical problem, but again this is very rare. Colic episodes generally peak at about 6 weeks of age and stop at about 3 months of age (Froese-Fretz & Keefe, 1997; Shelov, 1993).

Several interventions can be implemented to alleviate this problem. If the mother is breast-feeding the infant, she should eliminate foods from her diet that produce gas (e.g., cabbage, onions, broccoli) and reduce her caffeine intake. Particularly if there are family histories of milk intolerance or other allergies, the mother should eliminate milk products from her diet. If the infant is bottle-feeding, a formula that is not based on cow's milk can be tried. Usually the colic will be better in 1 to 2 days if it is due to a food intolerance.

Other strategies are to use a baby carrier to keep the infant close to the body and in motion or to place the infant near a steady rhythmic sound such as a vacuum cleaner or clothes dryer. Laying the infant on his or her stomach across the parent's knees, often utilizing a pacifier, while rocking on the knees, often helps relieve any discomfort. Cuddling the infant while in a rocking chair or rocking the infant is often helpful. Rocking with a wind-up swing or cradle often allows the infant to relax and go to sleep. Some of the new vibrating chair seats are also helpful. Warm baths may also relax the infant and soothe him or her into sleep or a comfortable state (Chart 5–7).

Interventions can be based on the "REST regimen." Regulate the infant's state by preventing overarousal. Infant states should be learned by parents and modulated (see Chart 5–6). Use environmental cues such as light and dark, noise and quiet to help synchronize the infant's behavior. Provide structure and repetition so that events become predictable and recurrent for the infant. Use touch (chest-to-chest or skin-to-skin) to soothe the child and diminish stimulation (Froese-Fretz & Keefe, 1997; Keefe, Froese-Fretz, & Kotzer, 1996).

Parenting during this time is extremely challenging. It is important for the parents to occasionally get away from the crying of the infant just to clear their minds. A trusted sitter or friend can stay with the child for a few hours at least once each week. If this is not available, the parents may alternate caregiving activities to give each other a breather. Parents should also be provided with

Chart 5–7

Strategies for Calming a Colicky Infant

- Check with the health care provider to be sure the fussiness is due to colic and not another medical cause.
- Evaluate the mother's diet. Eliminate foods that may produce gas, such as onions and cabbage.
- Evaluate whether the infant has a milk allergy. Have mother stop consuming cow's milk and try a formula that has no cow's milk in it.
- Have the mother eliminate caffeine from her diet.
- Use "Snugli" type baby carrier to keep the infant close to the body, and walk to allow the motion and body contact to soothe the infant.
- Use wind-up or battery-powered swing.
- Run the vacuum or place the infant near the washing machine for the steady rhythmic sound.
- Introduce a pacifier—even to breast-fed infants.
- Rock infant on caregiver's knees with infant turned on his or her stomach and possibly using a pacifier.

support and empathy as they cope with this stressful experience.

Relationships

Bonding and Attachment

Bonding is a process that occurs between the parent and the newborn that includes an exchange of visual eye contacts, sounds, touches, and exploration. Bonding is an important foundation between the parent (usually the mother) and the infant. It encourages a protectiveness that is part of the attachment process. It is important for the health care professional to do as much as possible to encourage this bonding and attachment process. It is not uncommon for a mother not to immediately bond with her infant after a particularly difficult delivery.

Certain identifiable characteristics indicate that bonding is occurring. These include eye-to-eye contact, physical contact, and communication. Some of these characteristics may be difficult to observe, particularly if the delivery was a cesarean section and the mother is recovering from anesthesia. There may also be cultural issues to be considered that do not allow certain behaviors to take place. Bonding may be delayed during the process if the parent has medical problems, is ill, or the infant is removed from the mother immediately after birth owing to illness or frailty. If there is family discord, or an ineffective support system, it may contribute to poor or inadequate bonding (Smith, 1991).

To promote bonding, the mother and infant should have time together as soon as possible, where the mother can cuddle, view, talk to, and examine the infant. Although it is ideal for this to occur within the first hour after delivery, it may occur later without any problem (Smith, 1991). The bonding should occur even if the child is in an intensive care unit—it may be difficult, but the mother should be allowed to at least view the infant and touch the infant's hand or foot. The parent should be encouraged to be close and display normal modes of affection.

Sibling Adjustment to the Newborn

The arrival of the new family member affects all aspects of family life and impacts all relationships in the family. Not only are the parents welcoming a new child into the home, other children will welcome and need to adjust to a new brother or sister. Having a sibling has been described as the single most beneficial way in which children can learn how to relate and interact appropriately with others. Within sibling relationships feelings of love, loyalty, frustration, and jealousy all emerge at some point or another (Fig. 5–2). The goal as a parent is to promote interactions that support the development of healthy sibling relationships.

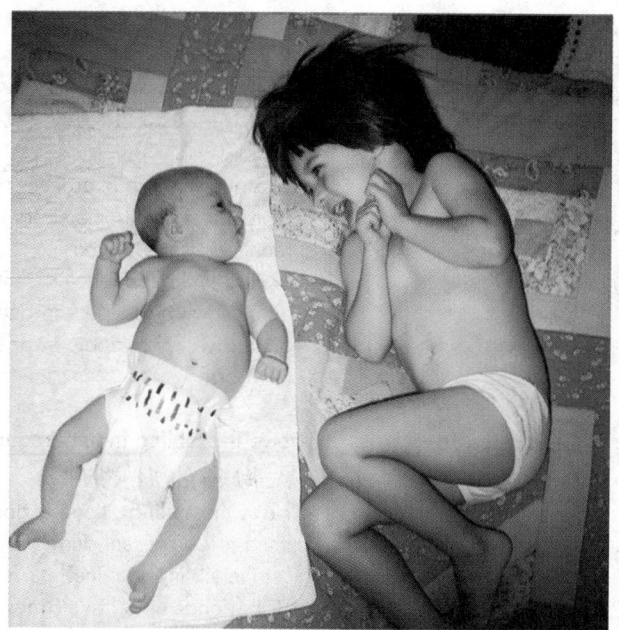

Figure 5–2
Children learn to relate and interact appropriately with others through the sibling relationship.

Some degree of stress over the birth of a younger sibling can be expected. The degree of stress or upset after the birth of the sibling does not predict the quality of future sibling relationships. Many older siblings have demonstrated significant developmental gains after the birth of their sibling. For instance, the child who reverts to sucking the thumb may also begin to start dressing himself or herself. Siblings spaced about 2 years apart are likely to experience the highest degree of stress regarding the arrival of a new brother or sister. This is because they must deal with increased separation from the mother at a time when separation and the decreased lack of attention is especially difficult to deal with. In addition, the younger child may not have the cognitive and verbal skills to express complex emotions.

There is no "best time" for telling siblings about the pregnancy and birth. The timing depends on the age of the older children. Younger children do not need much lead time because they are not able to measure time in terms of weeks or months. The beginning of the second trimester is a good time to share the news with children, or at the point at which the mother's protruding abdomen would be evident to the child. School-age children should hear the news as soon as the family plans to tell friends and other family members. Older siblings should learn the news before it is shared with grandparents or others so that they do not accidentally hear the information from someone besides the parents (TIP 5–2).

The news of the pregnancy may not be greeted with joy by the older sibling. The older child may struggle

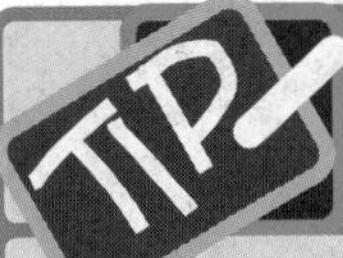

TIP 5–2 A Teaching Intervention Plan to Prepare Siblings for the Arrival of the Newborn

Nursing Diagnosis and Family Outcomes

- Alteration in family process related to addition of new members
  Outcomes: Family members will voice realistic expectation of sibling's behavior and reaction to the newborn.
  Sibling will experience feelings of support, love, and nurturance from parents.
  Sibling will participate in activities to prepare for the arrival of the newborn
  Sibling will participate in age-appropriate care activities and social interactions with the newborn.

Guidance for Family Members

Involve the Sibling in the Pregnancy

Activities for the Child

- Have the sibling attend a doctor's appointment with the mother. If possible, allow the child to be present during the ultrasound examination.
- Let the sibling feel the fetus's movements.
- Visit friends who have a newborn in their home. Discuss what it will be like to have "our baby" at home.
- See if the hospital provides sibling classes in which the older child can learn about newborns.
- Read books together about what happens during pregnancy, what it is like after the newborn is born, and what it is like to be a big brother or sister.
- Male and female toddlers and preschoolers can benefit from having a doll to teach the sibling about the care of the newborn and to allow the child expression of his or her feelings regarding the arrival of the sibling.

Preparation for the Newcomer

- Encourage the older child to help prepare and decorate the infant's room. Let the sibling be involved in selecting and purchasing clothes for the newborn.
- Encourage the older child to help select the newborn's name.
- Place a picture of the older sibling in the newborn's room.
- Let the older sibling pick the outfit the newborn will wear home from the hospital.

Avoid Pursuing New Developmental Challenges

Changes in the Child's Environment and Routines

- Changes in the older child's environment or routine should be made several months before the birth so that the child will not feel pushed out or shoved aside for the newborn.
- If the child will be starting a new daycare or nursery school, do this well in advance of the delivery.
- Do not make any demands for new skills such as toilet training and bottle weaning during the months just preceding the delivery. Even if the child appears ready, wait until after he or she has adjusted to the arrival of the newcomer.

Increase Father's Participation

- Have the father get more involved in the daily activities of the child. The sibling will better tolerate less motherly attention during the mother's hospitalization and after the newborn's arrival if the father or another significant family member has become more involved in the child's care.

The Time of Delivery

Siblings at the Birth

- Some hospitals and birthing centers permit siblings to be included in the birthing process. These children must be prepared in advance for the sights and sounds they will encounter.

TIP continued on following page

TIP 5–2 A Teaching Intervention Plan to Prepare Siblings for the Arrival of the Newborn *Continued*

- An adult who is emotionally close to the child should be assigned the responsibility of monitoring the child during the birthing process.
- In general, studies have shown that children younger than the age of 4 have difficulty attending the birth. At these ages they are still quite dependent on their mother for emotional support and can become overly concerned and distressed by the mother's physical exertion during the birthing process.

Care of the Sibling Left at Home

- Tell the child where the mother is going and who will care for the child while the mother is at the hospital. Optimally, the child should know the "baby sitter" well and the sitter should have been thoroughly prepared to step in at any time.
- Prepare in advance written instructions of the older children's routines for the baby sitter to follow.
- Encourage the father, grandparents, or special friends to take the child on a special outing while the mother is in the hospital.

Visiting Mother in the Hospital

- Try to have the older child visit the mother each day.
- If the older sibling cannot visit, send along a picture of mother and baby.
- Call the older children daily from the hospital.
- Take a special gift to the hospital to give to the older child as a present from his or her new sibling.

Welcoming the Newborn Home

- Have the older sibling come to the hospital and join the new family on the trip home.
- When entering the home, spend the first moments with the older sibling. Let someone else carry the newborn into the house and get the newborn settled.
- Do not give the sibling the impression of always being tired and haggard. The child may think that the mother was hurt by the newborn's birth.
- Have a special party to welcome the infant home. Some suggest doing this 1 week after the newborn comes home. Give the sibling "gifts" from the newborn. Have a cake and make it a real celebration.
- Refer to the newborn as "our baby" or "your brother or sister."
- Ask visitors to give some extra attention to the older sibling.
- Allow the older sibling to unwrap the newborn's gifts.

Promoting Positive Sibling Encounters

Encourage Interactions

- Encourage the older sibling to touch and play with the newborn in the presence of an adult. Allow him or her to hold the infant while sitting in a chair or on the ground.
- Encourage the sibling to talk or to tell stories to the newborn.
- Teach the sibling to attract the newborn's attention with bright toys.
- Teach the sibling when are the best times to interact with the newborn. This depends on the newborn's states of arousal.

Parents' Reactions

- At certain times the older child's need for parental support may be more important than the needs of the newborn.
- Let the sibling play a game of "pretend baby" if his or her desire to be a baby is apparent. A few minutes of being treated like a baby are generally enough, because the child must understand that being the baby means no going outside to play or walking or eating snacks or other "big boy or girl" activities.

TIP continued on following page

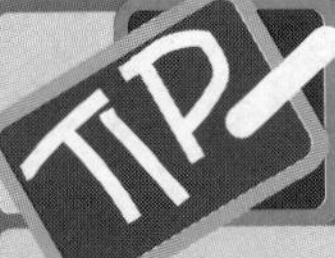

TIP 5–2 A Teaching Intervention Plan to Prepare Siblings for the Arrival of the Newborn *Continued*

- Do not always tell the older sibling to "be quiet" because of the newborn. Most newborns will learn to sleep through all sorts of noises. Constant silencing of the older child can cause resentment.
- Intervene promptly if the older sibling shows aggressive behavior toward the newborn, such as physical or verbal attacks.
- Teach civil behaviors. Promote sharing, respect for property, and the right to privacy. Teach children to be loyal to one another regardless of the anger they may feel at times.
- Avoid comparing and labeling the siblings.

Enlisting the Older Sibling as a Helper

- As the older child feels comfortable, let him or her help wash to newborn or feed the newborn or find toys or the pacifier for the newborn. Emphasize how much the newborn "likes" the older sibling and how it makes the newborn happy to have his or her brother or sister help.
- On the other hand, do not expect the older sibling to shoulder adult responsibilities.

Regressive Behaviors

- Do not criticize the older sibling if he or she begins to display regressive behaviors such as thumb sucking or bedwetting. Rather, praise and reward grown-up behaviors in siblings. Be tolerant of regressive behaviors and realize that these symptoms will resolve over time.
- If the child is old enough, encourage him or her to talk about his or her feelings about the newborn.
- Explain why the "rules" or what is considered acceptable behaviors are not the same for every child in the family.

Providing the Older Sibling with Extra Attention

- Try to give at least 30 minutes a day of special time or "our time" with just the mother and the older child.
- In the evening, have father or another family relative or close friend participate in a special activity with the older sibling each day while mother is feeding the newborn.
- Spend some time with the older sibling looking through his or her baby album.

with the new role, especially if he or she has been an only child for a long period of time. The sibling may worry about the changes that will occur in the family (Smith, 1991). Providing loving support and developmentally appropriate discussions can help the child to adapt to the changes.

The older child may also feel frustrated because he or she has already noted changes in the home environment during the mother's pregnancy. Many physical and psychological changes occur to the mother during the pregnancy. Although the mother may feel physically well, the child may be deprived of the mother's attention as she focuses inward on her pregnancy and the fetus growing inside her. The normal physiologic changes of pregnancy may cause the mother to be more tired, irritable, and moody. In addition, as her abdomen grows it may be increasingly more difficult to pick up and carry younger siblings or to even sit with them on her lap.

How a child experiences the mother's pregnancy and subsequent arrival of a new sibling is affected by three factors:

1. The child's state of emotional and social development
2. The child's cognitive abilities, such as the child's ability to reason and solve problems
3. The child's level of separation and independence from the mother

The need of the sibling at this time is to continue to feel loved, wanted, and valued. This is important regardless of the child's age and how he or she may show his or her feelings. TIP 5–2 summarizes several interventions that can be helpful in alleviating sibling jealousy and promoting bonding between siblings. To promote successful sibling relationships, a parent should anticipate and know that the impact on the older child begins during the pregnancy and will continue through the first several months of the newborn's arrival at home. Older siblings need to actively participate in the pregnancy and the preparation for the newborn. Changes in the older child's environment or routine should be made several months before the arrival of the new sibling.

When an Infant Cannot Come Home from the Hospital Immediately. The newborn may experience some health problems that require him or her to stay in the hospital after the mother has been discharged. It may be just a few days or, if the newborn was born premature, several weeks before the infant can come home. During the pregnancy, older siblings have been told that their mother would go to the hospital and then *mother and baby* would come home from the hospital. The sibling may have difficulty understanding why the newborn cannot come home.

Parents need to provide explanations that are age appropriate as to why the child needs to be cared for at the hospital by the doctors and nurses. If hospital policy allows, siblings should be encouraged to go see the newborn. If the infant is in a newborn intensive care unit, the older child may only be allowed to look through a window at their younger sibling. If the newborn is on a ventilator, parents need to determine whether the older sibling will do well seeing the newborn with all of that equipment. In all cases, children should be prepared by their parents regarding all that they might see in the hospital and what the newborn will look like.

The older sibling can be provided with pictures of the newborn. And if the sibling does visit the newborn in the hospital, a picture of the family can be taped to the baby's bassinet or incubator. The sibling can be told that the newborn likes to look at his or her family and is excited about coming home.

Notes can be written from the newborn to the sibling, and the sibling can write notes or color pictures to be given to the newborn. The older sibling can be updated as to the infant's progress. If the newborn is not doing well, the sibling should be told. The older child will see the parent's stress and be concerned.

When an Infant Has a Noticeable Physical Defect. The sibling must be prepared for how the child may look or act differently than other newborns. The parents should openly discuss how "our baby" is different. With consideration of the sibling's developmental age, the questions he or she may have can be answered as to why the newborn is different and how this may have occurred. Books about "special" babies and "special" children are available to be read to older children. Although the parents may be experiencing a sense of grief or loss regarding a newborn's health, the young sibling may not have had a set of expectations regarding what the newborn would be like. Children can be very tolerant and accepting of how others look. The sibling will most likely react to the newborn in response to the parents' reactions to the newborn. Modeling a gentle approach and a loving acceptance of the infant will highly influence the sibling's acceptance of the "special" child.

Child–Father Bonding

Fathers should be brought into the bonding process as soon as possible. After the infant is born, many fathers feel left out—not needed for feeding (particularly in breast-fed infants) or other care. Fathers can become involved, and should, with all aspects of the infant's care and cuddling. Fathers can bathe, massage, cuddle, diaper, and carry infants. Fathers need to have private time to bond with the infant as well. This should be encouraged but not pushed.

Play

During the first few weeks of life, neither the exhausted parent nor the newborn is very interested in play time. During the periods of wakefulness, the newborn is bonding with the new parents, eating, and developing a sense of the surrounding environment. At this time the infant is very egocentric; everything revolves around him or her. The ideal play activities are adjusted to the infant's developmental age. At 1 month, hanging brightly colored objects for him or her to watch and using musical mobiles over the bed that are either brightly colored or have highly contrasting black and white motifs provide good "toys." Being able to watch himself or herself in a mirror or watch other people's faces is an activity that will absorb an infant's attention. Infants prefer to gaze at bright colors over pale colors and human faces to any other patterns. During the early months, activities that include cuddling, rocking, massaging, and singing are the most nurturing for the infant. The infant is extraordinarily sensitive to touch and movement. The use of an infant carrier that keeps the infant close to the carrier's body is an excellent method of providing soothing movement for the child. The newborn is also very responsive to soft sounds of music and the human voice. A very fussy newborn may become quiet by just hearing soft music or a caregiver's voice. The infant should also be given the opportunity to have "floor time" (Fig. 5–3). The infant is placed supine or prone on a blanket on the floor, preferably a carpeted area. The infant is free to move all body parts without being confined by an infant seat or car seat. Placing the child on his or her abdomen

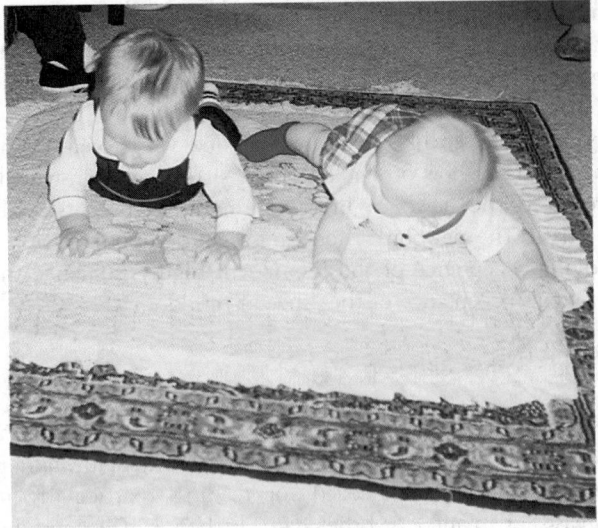

Figure 5–3
During floor time, an infant should be placed on the abdomen and allowed to move the body freely.

is especially important in giving the infant an opportunity to develop head control as he or she lifts the head up and off the blanket. Toys placed close to the child aid in stimulating eye movement and gross motor movement as the child attempts to reach the toys.

As the infant matures and developmental milestones are progressing, he or she will become more sociable, appearing to interact more with surroundings. At about 3 months of age, the child begins to reach for toys and attempt to grasp, but that skill does not mature until about age 6 months. The infant loves sitting up and watching the activities in the environment. Mobiles and mirrors can be continued, "busy boxes" in the crib are begun, and play gyms are used during floor time. This is also a good age to start reading to the infant if this has not been started already. Many parents believe they can increase the child's IQ if they encourage reading at an early age and instruct the infant to read by the time he or she is 3 years old. Research regarding this claim is not as yet conclusive, but there are many claims fostered by popular books regarding this belief.

By 6 months, the child is able to grasp large toys, loves to play peek-a-boo, likes to listen to stories, and usually loves water and water play. In the bath, the infant loves to pour the water in and out of cups, swatting and dunking floating objects, squirting sponges, and so on. Imitating and repetition skills are becoming more defined, and he or she loves games that allow him or her to copy what is being done (e.g., making funny faces or noises, clapping, laughing) and repeating it over and over. The infant is experimenting with the environment—banging pots and pans may seem annoying, but the 6-month-old is fascinated with the sounds he or she can produce.

At 8 to 9 months, the infant's manual dexterity is improving and he or she is able to grasp large toys, turn large book pages, and shake a rattle. A large box set up with lots of objects (not always toys) is ideal. The objects can be items such as balls, oatmeal boxes, plastic margarine containers, wooden spoons, and old plastic bowls. During this time, the infant loves to imitate the parent's activities, such as cooking and cleaning. Care must be taken to ensure that play objects are not too small or have parts that can come apart and be easily lodged in the throat, nose, or ears or have sharp edges or be made of toxic substances. The infant is also usually crawling by now and may be very fast and curious about his or her surroundings. If the house has not been "childproofed" before, it is now an absolute necessity.

By 1 year, the infant has developed enough motor control to coordinate both hands at once, which allows him or her to bang things together and operate simple mechanisms. He or she loves to sit in a highchair and drop items off to the floor—although it seems as though the infant is doing this to be mischievous, he or she is discovering gravity and is amazed that the objects always move in the same direction. The infant is experimenting with different types of objects, sizes, textures, and shapes to see if they all do the same thing—hit the floor. This is usually a favorite game. His or her manual dexterity has matured enough that the infant can pick up small objects from a plate, table, or off the floor.

Daycare and Baby Sitters

An estimated 30% of all preschool children in the United States are enrolled in some form of part-time or full-time organized daycare (Lombardi, 1992). The number of children in daycare services has substantially increased over the past 25 years. Economic changes, the increased number of single parents and very young parents, and the expansion of opportunities for women in the workplace are a few of the factors that have influenced the need for families to make alternative child care arrangements. Most parents would agree that selecting a safe and competent daycare facility is a very difficult and stressful task. The decisions made must take into account such issues as the distance of the center from the parents' place of employment or from the child's home, the hours daycare services are provided, the numbers and ages of other children being served, and the cost of the services provided. Nursing personnel can help parents select suitable daycare facilities and provide families with suggestions to help all involved parties adjust to the child care arrangements. In addition, child health care providers can play a key role in educating daycare staff to ensure a safe environment and help prevent and reduce the transmission of infectious diseases.

Types of Daycare Services

There are two basic types of daycare services: in-home care and center-based care. In-home care refers to services provided in either the child's home, the home of a caregiver, or the home of one of the children within the daycare group. Caregivers may live in the home with the family, come to the child's home, or have the children come to their home. Care provided through in-home arrangements may be offered by personnel who are authorized by a state licensing board, in which case the licensing board defines the number and ages of children who can be cared for at any one time. In addition, the board establishes certain environmental and safety criteria that must be adhered to by the caregiver. In-home daycare may also be provided by individuals who are not licensed, such as family members, friends, baby sitters, or au pairs.

Center-based care is provided in a licensed daycare facility that may be privately owned, federally funded, or associated with a neighborhood project or workplace facility (Wong, 1986). In these settings, six or more children receive care for several hours a day. The ratio of caregivers to children is determined by the ages of the child; younger children may be at a 1:3 ratio and older children (about 5 years old) at a 1:8, 9, or 10 ratio. All ages of children may be served, with children of similar ages generally grouped together.

Choosing a Daycare Provider

Selecting a daycare provider is one of the more complex tasks facing new parents. The considerations that must be addressed when choosing a child care provider are location, hours of service, cost, religious or cultural beliefs, and characteristics of the individual care provider. Are both parents working full-time, or is this a single parent family? Is it better to have the child care provider closer to a workplace or closer to home? What hours are needed for the child care provider? How much can the family afford for child care? Are there religious or cultural beliefs that need to be taken into consideration? Once these questions are answered, there is the next choice of in-home or center-based care (Table 5–3).

When the decision has been made to use an in-home provider, the parents will need to advertise and interview prospective care providers unless they utilize an agency placement service. In either case, an interview should be conducted face to face, preferably with the child available to ascertain the potential caregiver's interaction and the child's acceptance of the caregiver. A list of interview questions is provided in Chart 5–8 as a guideline to assist new parents with what to evaluate when selecting a daycare setting.

Baby Sitters

Selecting the infant's first baby sitter (usually done within the first few weeks of life for some respite) can be a difficult and sometimes scary task. This person may be a teenager within the neighborhood or a relative or close friend. Many of the same guidelines can be used to choose a good baby sitter as were discussed earlier to hire any daycare provider. The baby sitter should be left with a list of emergency phone numbers and the name and phone number of the nearest available neighbor should an emergency arise (Chart 5–9). Parents should notify the sitter where they will be, how they can be contacted, and how long they will be gone. Separation anxiety is common for a child around 9 months of age. Parents should not attempt to just sneak out the door when the sitter arrives so as to avoid a crying scene with the infant. The child needs to learn that the parents may leave but that they do come back. It is better to create some ritual behaviors surrounding a parents' good-bye than to have the child worry that his or her parents will simply disappear when a certain individual comes to the home.

Daycare for Sick or Medically Fragile Children

When the infant or child is sick, the parent may be unable to stay home and be with that child. Yet, few daycare providers appreciate having the sick child brought to them with the potential of infecting other children. To assist parents coping with this type of situation, daycare centers for sick children have emerged. Some of these centers may have a "spots" room where they accept children with chickenpox or rashes, fevers, and other potentially contagious diseases as well as children recuperating from surgeries or with noncontagious illness. It is wise to investigate the availability of such services before they are needed because often there is a registration fee and processing procedure that must take place before placing the child with this center.

For those infants and toddlers with handicaps or long-term medical conditions requiring specialized care, daycare centers for the medically fragile child may be available. Because these children need nursing care, developmental stimulation, physical, occupational, or speech therapy, and special feeding or routine care, the staff consists of registered nurses and other allied health care personnel, along with childhood educators. Admission to these programs is generally reserved for children who cannot be served by other "regular" daycare programs, preschools, or specialized health care services.

Table 5–3
Types of Care Providers: Advantages and Disadvantages

Type	Advantages	Disadvantages
In-Home Care Providers		
Sitter (non–family member hired to come to house) Family member Au pair (young person sponsored from foreign country)	Very convenient location One-to-one attention for the child Secure comfortable surroundings for child When the child is ill, care continues to be provided. Consistent care provided by one person Caregiver knows child's moods, habits, and likes/dislikes. Meals are prepared for the child's specific tastes. Some sitters and au pairs will do laundry and light housework. Cultural and religious beliefs are easier to implement. Less frequent exposure to illness	When caregiver is ill, replacement is needed or parent must remain at home. No group or social interaction between peer groups Could be expensive Rivalry could develop between caregiver and parent. Privacy may be invaded by caregiver (particularly live-in caregivers). Caregiver may leave suddenly, leaving parents without any care provider. Parents must do interviewing/reference checks of potential applicants. If care is provided by family member, this could cause tension within the family. May lack wide variety of age-appropriate toys and activities
Center-Based Care Providers		
Institutional, community based, family home based	Regulated and inspected by licensing agency Required to follow specific regulations regarding provider ratio, cleanliness, and qualifications of staff Often teachers have degrees or the corporation provides training in early childhood education. Children get to interact with peers and develop peer relationships. Usually have structured programs designed to meet developmental needs of children Exposed to wide variety of age-appropriate toys, educational materials, and activities If a teacher is sick, off, or on vacation, the child still receives care (may not be true in family home–based care). If center-based care is provided by a parent's workplace, location is usually convenient and hours are usually flexible to the parent's schedule. Usually less expensive than in-home care	May not be conveniently located Hours may be rigid. Children are exposed to illness. Potential for less individual attention May not respect individual religious or cultural beliefs Meals are prepared for large groups and are not altered for specific tastes (although allergies are considered).

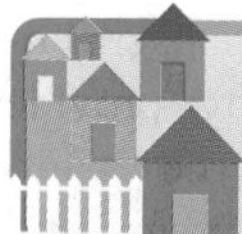

Chart 5–8
Community Care

Interview Questions for Evaluating Daycare Options

- Is the program licensed or registered?
- What are the hours?
- Is the location convenient?
- What is the cost (or for in home—what is the rate)?
- What days of the year is service not provided? Is tuition paid for these days?
- What meals will be provided and at what times?
- Will the child leave the facility on field trips or other excursions with the care provider?
- Staffing:
  - What is the ratio of staff to child?
  - What is the education of the staff?
  - How often does the staff turn over?
- Tour the facility to observe the following:
  - Watch the interaction of the children and the teachers.
  - What sort of toys and activities are you observing? Are there enough? Are they age appropriate? Are the teachers using the instruments creatively?
  - Count staff to children—is there an appropriate number?
  - Look at the characteristics of the environment—is it friendly or sterile, is it cluttered or clean (perhaps too clean and neat)?
  - Are there indications in view of the children's activities (e.g., paintings, crafts, writing)?
  - Are the infants all in swings or cribs or on the floor with toys and gyms?
  - Cleanliness—Are the diaper-changing areas clean? Does the staff wash their hands after changing diapers or wiping up messes? Are the eating areas clean? Is all food in the kitchen covered?
  - Safety—Are all the outlets covered? Are stairs protected with carpet? Are gates in place where necessary? Is the facility well lit?
  - Food—Is it nutritious? Is the amount appropriate? Do the meals include age-appropriate foods?
  - Observe how the "teacher" interacts with the children. Question them about the children. Are they truly familiar with the child, knowing each child's likes and dislikes and personality? How do they handle discipline? Do they interact with the children on their level—eye to eye?
- Request at least two references from parents with a similar-age child.
- How does the center communicate with the parents regarding activities, the child's progress, and any problems?
- Are unannounced visits okay?

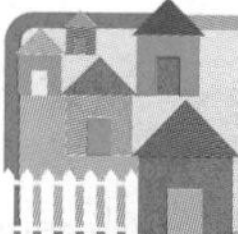

Chart 5–9
Community Care

What Parents Should Tell Baby Sitters

- Always leave number of where you can be reached.
- Have emergency numbers posted near the phone, including
  - Police
  - Fire department
  - Poison control
  - Pediatrician
  - Dentist
  - Nearest relative or neighbor
- Have your address and phone number posted near the phone as well.
- Let the sitter know how long you will be gone and return when stated.
- If there is a delay, be sure to call the sitter and let him or her know.
- Instruct sitter in child's routine with any tips that work for you (e.g., special story, music, comforting toy).
- If the child is breast-fed, introduce the bottle before going out for the first time.
- Possibly leave an article of clothing with similar scent on it for sitter to have to adjust infant to new caregiver.
- Instruct sitter as to when the child will need to be fed and what the child should be fed and be sure that supplies are available.
- Set clear guidelines in regard to handling emergency situations and disciplinary methods.
- Ask sitter to write down any questions or comments he or she may have while caring for the child.

Care is provided at the level the parent can give at home. The care is not comparable to an in-patient health care setting (Briggs, 1987).

Alert: *In any daycare environment, concerns as to the potential for neglect and/or abuse of the child must be addressed. If a child's personality suddenly changes, and there are no other outside apparent causes (e.g., recent move, divorce, death of a family member), a look at the child care provision may be indicated. Clinging behavior, excessive crying when dropping a child off with the care provider, or more subtle signs such as a child not looking at an adult in the face, weight loss, refusing to eat, a sad worried look, withdrawal, and being unable to be comforted are potential signs of neglect or abuse.*

Injury and Illness Prevention

During the first year, parents of healthy infants are likely to visit their health care provider more often than at any other time in the child's life, unless an acute condition arises. The frequency of contacts with the infant and the family provides ample opportunity for the nurse to complete developmental surveillance. As discussed in Chapter 4, developmental surveillance encompasses all activities related to the detection of developmental problems and the promotion of healthy development (Curry & Duby, 1994). The nurse uses techniques such as direct observation of the child, eliciting parental concerns, and completing developmental screening to identify infants who may be "at risk" for developmental delay. Each encounter with the family is an opportunity to provide guidance and education regarding the needs of the infant. Chart 5–4 summarizes important topics to discuss and activities to engage in with the family who has an infant.

Injury Prevention

One of the first priorities of the new parents is to babyproof the home. Although most parents think of babyproofing once the infant is crawling, it is never too early to start thinking of safety—in cribs, car seats, and the newborn's immediate environment (Chart 5–10).

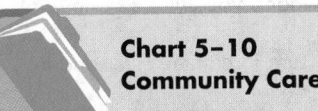

Chart 5–10
Community Care

Injury Prevention Guidelines for the Family with an Infant

Home Safety

- Ensure that the crib is safe. The slats should be no more than 2⅜ inches apart, and the mattress should be firm and fit snugly. The side rails should be all the way up when the child is sleeping. As the child learns to sit and stand the mattress should be lowered.
- Put the infant to sleep on his or her back or side.
- Do not drink hot liquids or smoke while holding the infant.
- Keep all poisonous substances, cleaning agents, health and beauty supplies, medicines, and home improvement materials in a locked safe place out of sight and reach of the infant.
- Use safety locks on cabinets.
- Keep sharp objects (e.g., scissors, knives) out of reach.
- Get down on the floor and check for hazards at the infant's eye level.
- Place plastic plugs in electrical sockets.
- Do not leave heavy objects or containers of hot liquids on tables with tablecloths that the infant may pull down.
- Install gates at the top and bottom of stairs.
- Place safety devices on windows and make sure screens are secure.
- Avoid dangling electrical and drapery cords.

Play Safety

- Keep toys with small parts or other small objects out of infant's reach.
- Do not use an infant walker at any age.
- Do not give the infant plastic bags, latex balloons, or small objects such as marbles.
- Teach siblings which of their toys are unsafe for the infant to play with.

Water Safety

- Set hot water thermostat at less than 120°F.
- Test the temperature of the bath water with your wrist to make sure it is not too hot for the infant.
- Never leave the infant alone in a tub of water or on high places.
- Empty buckets, tubs, or small pools immediately after use.
- Ensure that swimming pools are enclosed by a four-sided fence with a self-closing, self-latching gate.

Crib Safety

Safety should be addressed even before the infant is born, when the parents-to-be are beginning to purchase the equipment an infant will use. Cribs are usually the first item that is either purchased or obtained through a friend or family. All cribs manufactured since 1973 in the United States are required to meet stringent federal regulations for safety. If a crib is borrowed or obtained used, the following checklist should be used: the side slats should be no less than 2⅜ inches apart, decorative cutouts should be avoided, mattress must fit snugly on all sides, and drop sides must have safety latches and lower only part of the way. The mattress should be firm, not soft, and no pillow is needed for an infant. Bumper pads should fit around the entire interior of the crib and be secured in at least six places; and if ties are used, these should be trimmed after they are secured, so the infant will not be caught on them or choke on them. If an older crib is obtained that has been painted, the paint should be stripped off (not sanded) and the crib should be repainted with a high-quality enamel paint. Some new parents are opting for cribs with mesh sides rather than the old wooden ones. In this situation, the sides must be kept raised because the mesh causes pockets that can trap an infant and be hazardous when they are lowered.

Car Seat Safety

The next major purchase is the car seat. Most hospitals will not discharge an infant home unless there is a car seat available to transport the child. Many acute care facilities have a car seat loan program or other means to provide car seats to those unable to purchase their own. Car seats that were manufactured before January 1981 should not be used because of newer more stringent

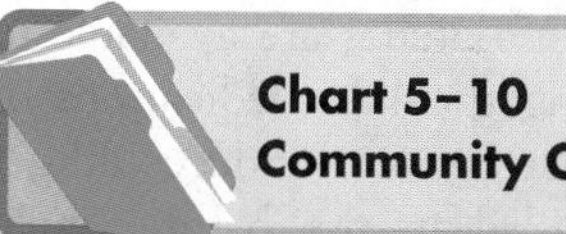

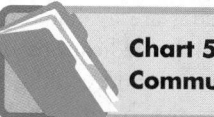

Chart 5–10
Community Care

Injury Prevention Guidelines for the Family with an Infant *Continued*

Car Safety

- Use an infant seat that is properly secured at all times.
- Place the car seat in the back seat of the car, facing backward toward the backrest of the car.

Safety with Others

- Never leave the infant alone or with a young sibling or pet.
- Keep the infant away from cigarette smoke. Do not allow people to smoke around the infant.
- Use baby sitters who have received CPR training.
- Provide the baby sitter with a list of emergency phone numbers, the home address and phone number, your location, and how you can be reached.
- Keep food for animals out of child's reach. Do not let the child approach an animal that is eating.

Outdoor Safety

- Avoid overexposure to the sun.
- Use straps in strollers to contain the child.
- Do not allow the child to be outdoors unattended.

Emergency Preparation

- Keep own address and phone number posted near the phone.
- Keep list of emergency numbers (doctor, hospital, nearest neighbor, poison control center) near the phone.
- Keep a 1-oz bottle of syrup of ipecac in the home and use as directed by the poison control center or health care provider.
- Learn first aid and infant CPR.

Adapted from Green, M. (Ed.). (1994). *Bright futures: Guidelines for health supervision of infants, children, and adolescents.* Arlington, VA: National Center of Education in Maternal and Child Health. *Bright Futures* was supported by the Maternal and Child Health Bureau and the Medicaid Bureau.

safety standards that were implemented at that time (see Resources).

There are three basic types of car safety seats: infant seats that are installed in a rear-facing position only and used until the infant is about 20 lb, convertible seats that can be used in both rear-facing and front-facing positions, and booster seats that are only forward facing and have a removable shield (this one is for older children). Parents should look at all types and decide on one that fits their usage style and size of their car. If the infant is a newborn up to 20 lb, an infant seat should be used. Some convertible seats are also manufactured with infant specifications and can be used as well. Many parents find purchasing two or more car seats to be cost prohibitive and want to spend more on one type that will take the child through more ages. A convertible seat should be used forward facing from the time the infant weighs 20 lb until about 40 lb. At that time, the convertible seat needs to be converted to a booster seat, or a booster seat needs to be obtained. Once the child is over 60 lb, he or she should use the regular automobile seat with a lap belt, adding a shoulder harness when he or she is more than 48 inches tall. When using car seats, it is important to always follow the manufacturer's directions regarding installation and proper use to protect the child.

caREminder: *Car seats should be placed in the back seat of the automobile because it is much safer than in the front seat, owing to the potential of rapid inflation of airbags on impact.*

Home Safety

To prepare the home environment, start with general home-safety issues. Ideally all parents should know cardiopulmonary resuscitation (CPR) and first aid and make emergency plans for accidents and fires including escape route planning. Emergency numbers should be posted near the telephone along with the address and phone number of the residence. This information is helpful to the parent who in times of emergency may temporarily be unable to state his or her own address and phone number.

Smoke alarms should be installed on every level of the home, and carbon monoxide detectors are recommended to be installed near the sleeping quarters or according to the manufacturer's directions. Every home should be equipped with a working flashlight and fire extinguisher (kept near the kitchen).

Hot water heaters should be turned down to 120°F to prevent scalding of the child's skin. Lamps and appliances should have the cords shortened and covered or hidden out of view of the child. Electrical outlets should be covered. Windows should have locks and screens that are securely attached, and the window cords should be rolled up or placed out of reach with the use of rubber bands or twist ties. As the infant begins to crawl, safety gates need to be installed to prevent entrance up or down stairwells and in rooms with computer or office equipment.

Two areas that are always thought of as hazardous are the kitchen and the bathroom. Children have more potential to injure themselves in these two locations owing to the types of activities and equipment that are available. To babyproof the kitchen, babyproof locks should be installed on all the cabinets. One or two cabinets may be left open if they contain items for the child to play with such as plastic bowls, spoons, and pan lids. All sharp scissors and knives should be kept in drawers or cupboards with child-resistant latches. When cooking, pot handles should be turned away from the front of the range. All cleaning supplies should be placed up high out of reach and/or kept in a childproof cupboard.

In the bathroom, the toilet lid should be kept lowered to prevent drowning. Safety latches are available to prevent the child from opening the lid. Medications or toiletries should not be kept out where a child could get to them. Nonskid strips installed in the bathtub help prevent falls. A cushioned cover placed over the faucet will prevent the child from becoming injured by the faucet. When bathing the infant or child, caregivers are instructed to never leave the child unattended in the water.

The infant spends a lot of time unsupervised in his or her bedroom, so the "nursery" must be inspected carefully for any hazards. The parents should be encouraged to get down on their hands and knees and see the environment from the perspective of the child. All potential hazards are removed from this level. Next, other areas of the child's environment need to be evaluated for safety. Crib mobiles and monitors should be out of reach. The infant should never be left unattended on a changing table even if strapped in place.

Outdoor Safety

Outside areas must be policed with the same rigorous attention with which the interior of the home is assessed. Playgrounds can be a tremendous opportunity for a child to explore and expand his or her physical capability. Risks can be minimized if the equipment is kept in good condition and the area is appropriately designed. The area needs to be arranged to allow enough room between equipment to prevent collision with other equipment or interference with other play areas. The equipment should be placed far enough away from off-limit areas such as trafficked streets, railroad tracks, and so on, and it should be in good condition (e.g., no broken pieces, rusted or exposed bolts, splinters). A soft, shock-absorbing material under the equipment (at least 6 inches of sand, mulch, or bark or rubberized matting) is required by many building codes. The area must be well maintained, with no overgrown bushes interfering with the equipment. Overgrown grass or an abundance of leaves can cause slippery areas. Cleanliness must be maintained, with no broken glass or trash accessible to the child, who is prone to put foreign objects in his or her mouth. These are guidelines that can be applied to both public and home playgrounds. Home playgrounds may have additional issues to be assessed, such as whether they are fenced, what kind of vegetation is being grown around the yard (poisonous or not), whether pesticides or herbicides have been used in proximity to the play environment, and whether there are animals in the neighborhood that might present a hazard to children playing in the yard.

Toys

The first gift a newborn will probably receive is a toy of some type. All children need toys to learn from and to assist in meeting developmental milestones. Toys are the tools of play for children. But, as with any tool, they must be appropriate for the job and safe. Toys must match the child's age and development. Manufacturer's guidelines may help, but the parents know whether their child is mature and skilled enough for a particular toy. Rattles should be at least 1⅝ inches in diameter to prevent them from becoming lodged in the child's throat. All toys should be well constructed with no loose pieces that can be removed and potentially swallowed. This is of particular importance with stuffed animals or dolls, because some toys have eyes or noses that may be loosened and possibly swallowed. Small toys should be avoided until the child is at least 3 years old. A small device has been developed to assist parents and health care professionals in determining what toy or toy part is too small. This device is a small cylinder designed to be the approximate size of a child's throat. If the object can fit into the cylinder, do not allow the child to play with the object (see Resources).

Balloons, although they are fun to look at and part of many birthday parties, should not be allowed to be blown up or played with by children younger than 5 years old. If a balloon pops, be sure all the pieces are collected, because a crawling infant can pick up a loose piece. Toys need to be inspected periodically to be sure they remain in good condition; if they become broken or overly worn, they should be repaired or discarded. Projectile toys should be avoided as well as toys that produce loud noises. It has been documented that noise levels at or about 100 dB (the sound of a typical cap gun at close range) can damage an infant's hearing. A quick clue to a safe toy is to look for the letters ASTM. This indicates the product meets the national safety standards for the American Society for Testing and Materials.

Health Supervision

The American Academy of Pediatrics recommends that the infant be seen by a health care provider within the first week after birth and at 1, 2, 4, 6, 9, and 12 months of age. Table 5–4 summarizes the aspects of the health supervision that will be covered at each visit. In addition, Chapter 6 provides a more detailed description of the aspects of the physical examination that should be completed at each visit. Chapter 6 also discusses the particular immunizations and routine diagnostic tests that are completed throughout the childhood years.

A primary focus of illness prevention is centered on encouraging parents to pay attention to the schedule of health care visits with their infant. Regular and periodic assessment by the same health care provider can assist in the early detection of developmental problems. In addition, frequent visits with a primary health care provider assists in establishing a trusting relationship between the family and the health care team. Therefore, when problems do arise the family is likely to feel more comfortable seeking advice and support from the health care team as opposed to relying on home remedies and advice of friends. Common maladies that can affect the infant include fever, colds, diarrhea, otitis media, rashes, and communicable diseases.

Developmental Surveillance

Chart 5–11 is a summary of the developmental milestones that are accomplished in the first year. This information is useful to provide the nurse with direction for specific trigger questions that can be asked of the parent to determine the infant's developmental progress. It is not effective to simply ask an open-ended question such as "Is your child developing well?" Most parents would respond positively despite the fact that they may lack the information about what developmental milestones their child should be reaching at any given point in time. The information presented in Chart 5–11 can also be used to summarize for the family the developmental achievements that they should be expecting to see and promoting as the infant matures.

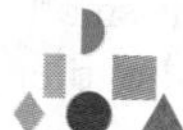

Toddlers

Toddlerhood is the period from 1 to 3 years of age. During this time, the child's rate of growth slows com-

Table 5–4
Health Supervision Interventions: Infancy

	Newborn	1 Mo	2 Mo	4 Mo	6 Mo	9 Mo	1 Yr
Physical Examination	X	X	X	X	X	X	X
Growth Parameters (height, weight, head circumference)	X	X	X	X	X	X	X
Immunizations	X	X*	X	X	X	X	X
Metabolic and Hemoglobinopathy Screening as Required by State	X						
Hearing Screening	X†	X†	X†				
Assessment of High-Dose Lead Exposure		X			X	X	X
Anemia Screening					X‡		
Lead Screening					X§		X§
Hematocrit or Hemoglobin Screening						X‖	X‡‖
Tuberculin Test						X¶	X**

* If not administered previously.
† Completed before 3 months of age.
‡ If certification needed for WIC (Special Supplemental Food Program for Women, Infants and Children).
§ At 6 months if infant is high risk or 12 months if low risk.
‖ At 9–12 months for certification for WIC or if certain risk factors are present.
¶ If certain risk factors are present.
** At 12 or 15 months before administration of measles, mumps, rubella (MMR) vaccine.
From Green, M. (Ed.). (1994). *Bright futures: Guidelines for health supervision of infants, children, and adolescents.* Arlington, VA: National Center for Education in Maternal and Child Health. *Bright Futures* was supported by the Maternal and Child Health Bureau and the Medicaid Bureau.

pared with the growth that occurred in infancy; however, many changes physically and developmentally can still be expected. The child starts to walk and talk and begins to test boundaries and assert some independence.

Nutrition

Once the child reaches the first birthday he or she should have already been started on table food. As his or her rapid growth rate has decreased, the child needs less calories per day than needed in infancy (Table 5–5). After gaining 3 to 4 lb every 2 to 3 months during the first year, the toddler now gains only 3 to 5 lb per year.

The toddler should be introduced to a schedule revolving around 3 meals per day with a mid-morning and a mid-afternoon snack. The stomach of a toddler is small, and frequent small meals are more desirable. The diet should consist of the four basic food groups, with a variety of foods with different textures and tastes offered (see Table 5–5). The toddler should be able to have the same foods that the rest of the family is eating. The portion size for the toddler should be about one fourth of the amount a normal adult would be served. Heavily spiced or salted foods should be avoided because these may not be palatable for the toddler. Foods should be mashed or cut into small pieces to prevent choking.

caREminder: *To prevent a toddler from choking, never give small hard foods such as peanuts or hard candies. Even soft small foods such as grapes could be a hazard. Carrots and hot dogs should be cut lengthwise and then in quartered pieces to prevent choking.*

The young toddler has not mastered use of the spoon or fork; therefore, finger foods are highly recommended. A plastic mat placed underneath a highchair and use of bibs help contain some of the mess the toddler will make as he or she uses the hands to experiment with food and as attempts are made to use the spoon. By 18 months, the toddler has enough control over the movements of the hands and fingers to navigate food to the mouth pretty consistently using a spoon.

At 1 year of age, the child can begin drinking whole cow's milk instead of formula or breast milk. Some mothers may continue to offer breast-feeding at bedtime. The toddler should be receiving 24 to 32 oz of milk per day, taking this fluid primarily from a cup. If the toddler is

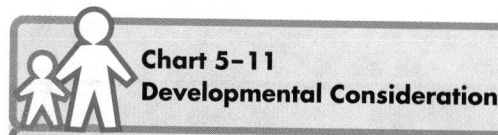

Chart 5-11
Developmental Considerations

Milestones of the Infant (Newborn to 12 Months)

Physical Development

Newborn

10% loss of birth weight in first 3–4 days of life
73% of body weight is fluid
Head circumference is 70% of adult size
Needs to consume 120 cal/kg of weight per day
Sleeps 20–22 hr/day, with brief waking periods of 2–3 hr
Grows about 1 inch/mo
Gains 5–7 oz/wk
Feeds every 2½–5 hr

2–5 Mo

Posterior fontanelle closes
Obligate (preferential) nose breathers until about 5 mo
Drooling begins

5–6 Mo

Doubles birth weight
Teeth may begin to erupt
Moves food to back of mouth and swallows during spoon feedings
Sleeps through the night for up to 8 hr
Goes 4–5 hr between feedings
Has 2–4 naps/day

7–9 Mo

Begins teething with lower central incisors, followed by two upper incisors
Mashes food with jaws
Sleeps 14–16 hr/day including naps

10–12 Mo

Sleeps 14–16 hr/day and still naps
Drooling stops
Grows about ½ inch/mo

Sexual

All infants

Oral stage: oral gratification and sucking needs

10 Mo

Begins sexual identity

Language

Newborn

Alerting
Social smile

2–3 Mo

Laughs and squeals
Cooing
Utters single vowel sounds such as "ah" and "eh"

4 Mo

Utters two-syllable vowel sounds
Includes consonant sounds such as "m" and "b"
Produces belly laughs
Orients to voice

5 Mo

Razzing
Intersperses vowel and consonant sounds

6 Mo

Babbling
Uses about 12 speech sounds

7 Mo

Makes "talking sounds" in response to caregiver or while others are talking
Coos and squeals
Vocalizes up to four different syllables

8–10 Mo

Uses "dada" and "mama" in nonspecific way
Responds to own name (receptive language skills develop first)
Babbles to produce consonant sounds
Vocalizes to toys

9–12 Mo

Imitates speech sounds
Understands name and "no"
Understands "bye" and "pat-a-cake"
Imitates facial expressions
Imitates definite speech sounds
Uses jargon
Communicates by pointing to objects and by using gestures
Responds to simple verbal requests

12 Mo

Has one word (or a few) in vocabulary
Comprehends "give" and stops when told "no"
Has receptive vocabulary of several dozen words
Deaf infants lose ability to vocalize by age 1
Jabbers expressively
Experiments with "pseudowords"

Chart continued on following page

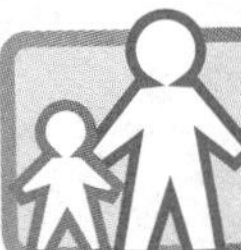

Chart 5–11
Developmental Considerations

Milestones of the Infant (Newborn to 12 Months) *Continued*

Vision

Newborn
Fixates on human face and demonstrates preference
Blink reflex present

2 Mo
Follows to midline
Produces tears
Visual acuity is hyperoptic

4 Mo
Follows objects to 180 degrees

5 Mo
Visual acuity 20/200
Recognizes feeding bottle

6 Mo
Inspects hands
Can fixate on object 3 feet away
Strabismus no longer within normal limits
Develops hand–eye coordination

8 Mo
Has permanent eye color
Depth perception developing

10 Mo
Tilts head backward to see up

12 Mo
Shows smooth visual pursuit of objects with 20/100 vision
Can follow rapidly moving objects

Hearing

Newborn
Startles to loud noises
Prefers high-pitched voices
Low-pitched noises have quieting effect
Responds to human voice over other noises
Auditory behavior is reflexive; generalized body movement (blinking or crying)
Recognizes certain sounds, ignores others; attends to quiet sounds more than loud ones—these are learned rather than reflexive behaviors
Turns to voice (quiet listening)

5 Mo
Orients to bell (looks to side)
Stops crying in response to music

7 Mo
Orients to bell (looks to side, then up)

10 Mo
Localizes sound from above or below
Orients to bell (turns directly to bell)

Gross Motor

Newborn
Turns head when prone but cannot support head
Adjusts posture when held at shoulder
May squirm to corner or edge of crib when prone
Arm and leg movements are reflexive

6 Wk–2 Mo
Holds head up 45–90 degrees when prone
May hold head steady when in supported sitting position

3 Mo
Rolls over from back to side
Holds head erect and steady

4 Mo
When supported, sits with rounded back and flexed knees
May bear weight on legs when assisted to stand
Head lag disappears when pulled to sitting position

5 Mo
Pulls to sitting position
Rolls from back to stomach
Sits alone momentarily
Shows unilateral reaching

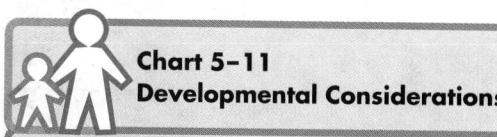

Chart 5–11
Developmental Considerations

Milestones of the Infant (Newborn to 12 Months) *Continued*

Gross Motor *Continued*

6 Mo
Sits without support
May creep an inch forward or backward
Moves from place to place by rolling
Begins drinking from a cup

7 Mo
Stands while holding on
Early stepping movements
Begins to crawl or hitch
Raises head spontaneously when supine

8 Mo
Pulls to standing position
Raises self to sitting position
Palmar grasp disappears

9 Mo
Walks with help
Crawls, creeps, or hitches when permitted
Sits down
Holds own bottle
Drinks from cup or glass

10 Mo
Continues walking skill development with help
Stands alone
May climb up and down stairs
Sits without support
Recovers balance
Changes from prone to sitting position

11 Mo
May walk alone
Begins to stoop and recover
Pushes toys
"Cruises"

12 Mo
Continues walking skills
Climbs onto sofas and chairs

Fine Motor

Newborn
Follows to, and slightly past, midline

2–3 Mo
Keeps hands open predominately
Reflex grasp replaced by voluntary grasping
Grasps objects such as rattle in open hand
May bring hands together at midline

3–4 Mo
Uses ulnar-palmar prehension with a cube
Reaches for objects
Hands predominantly open

5 Mo
Attempts to "catch" dangling objects with two hands
Begins use of forefinger and thumb in pincer grasp (opposible thumb-prehension)
Retains two cubes
Recovers rattle
Reaches for and grasps objects

6–7 Mo
Can grasp at will
Holds and manipulates objects
Scoops pellet
Transfers from hand to hand
Demonstrates inferior pincer
Bangs objects together
Can release objects

8–9 Mo
Combines spoons or cubes at midline
Retains two of three cubes offered
Achieves neat pincer grasp of pellet
Feeds self finger foods using only one hand
Releases objects at will
Rings bell
Holds bottle and places nipple in mouth when wants it

10–11 Mo
Plays "pat-a-cake" (a midline skill)
Puts several objects in a container
Holds crayon adaptively
Bangs two cubes together
Looks for hidden object (object permanency)
Achieves neat pincer grasp

Chart continued on following page

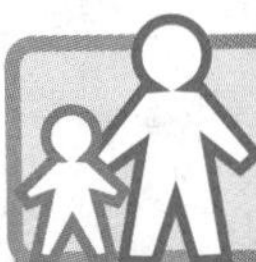

Chart 5-11
Developmental Considerations

Milestones of the Infant (Newborn to 12 Months) *Continued*

Play

All Infants
Solitary play
May be imitative
Explorative and manipulative

5–7 Mo
Resists toy pull
Picks up tiny objects
Plays "peek-a-boo"
Works for toy out of reach

8–9 Mo
Plays "pat-a-cake"
Recognizes self in mirror

10–12 Mo
Plays ball with examiner
Achieves object permanence (searches for dropped objects)

Cognitive

Newborn
Substage I
Practice of reflexes and reflex-like actions

1–4 Mo
Substage II: Purposeful
Reproduction of reflex actions

4–8 Mo
Substage III: Objects
Oriented and imitative actions
Accidental actions are repeated
Develops habits
Responds negatively to removal of a toy

8–12 Mo
Substage IV
Coordination, intentional goal direction, and achievement
Experimentation of object permanence
Imitates and models behavior
No concept of death
Enjoys "peek-a-boo" game
Attempts to flee from unpleasant events
Recognizes anticipatory signs
Repeats actions that elicit response from others
Dislikes restrictions
Shakes head for "no"
Appears interested in picture book

Social

Newborn
Regards face and establishes eye contact

1–2 Mo
Smiles responsively
Enjoys cuddling and motion

2–3 Mo
Smiles spontaneously

3–5 Mo
Smiles at mirror image
Shows interest in siblings
Invites social interactions by smiling

6 Mo
Exhibits stranger anxiety
Extends arms to be held

7–9 Mo
Waves hands

12 Mo
Demonstrates emotions of fear, anger, affection
Can indicate desires without crying
Offers object to a familiar adult
Talks to mirror

drinking more than 32 oz of milk per day, this will interfere with the amount of solid food that the child will want to eat. Unless the toddler has an underlying medical condition (e.g., diabetes), low-fat or skim milk should not be introduced until the child is older than 2 years of age.

Food strikes are not uncommon at this age. If a toddler refuses to eat a meal, he or she should not be

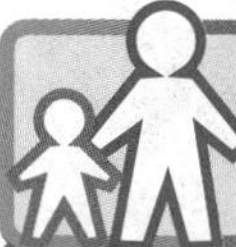

Chart 5-11
Developmental Considerations

Milestones of the Infant (Newborn to 12 Months) *Continued*

Interpersonal

0–3 Mo
Normal autism; self-absorbed, egocentric

4–18 Mo
Symbiotic phase—mother seen as an extension of child's body and needs, and vice versa

6–10 Mo
Stranger anxiety
Waves arms and legs when frustrated

8–24 Mo
Separation anxiety
Trust vs. mistrust

Emotional

Newborn–3 Mo
Feeling regulated and interested in the world
Sensitive to parent's joyful interest in him or her

3–7 Mo
Forming attachments
Highly specialized interest in the human world

4–10 Mo
Purposive communication
Can connect small units of feelings into simple patterns
Purposeful expression of wants and needs
Fluctuates easily between laughing and crying

10–18 Mo
Complex sense of self
Communication is truly interactive, enabling toddler to tune into parent and to appropriately build on parent's response

Moral/Spiritual

All Infants

Moral
Stage I: Preconventional Level
Beginning of punishment (by deprivation or injury, but makes no cognitive connection)
No moral concepts or rules exist

Spiritual
Stage 0: Undifferentiated
Not capable of formulating or communicating any conceptual ideas about self or environment
Trust vs. mistrust: sets foundation for subsequent development of faith

forced to do so, because this can lead to eating disorders later in life. As the toddler's taste buds mature, physiologic anorexia is experienced. The toddler goes through periods in which he or she is very particular about which foods are eaten. The toddler also begins to be attracted by the color, smell, and shape of food. Foods that seem familiar, that is, that look like or smell like other foods he or she enjoys, are most likely to be eaten. Food should not be used as a reward or a punishment (Smith, 1991). Mealtimes should be nonstressful but not "play" times. Plates should be attractive and not overfilled with food.

Table 5–5
Food Guide for Children

	1–3 Yr	4–6 Yr	7–10 Yr	11–14 Yr	15–21 Yr
Calorie Requirement					
Range	1100–1550	1400–1800	1900–2400	2200–2700	2558
Calories/kg/day	102	90	70	Male, 55 Female, 47	Male, 45 Female 40
Components					
Protein (g)	33–37	45–60	55–60	90–115	92
Fat (g)	50–75	70–90	90–110	90–115	90–115
Carbohydrate (g)	130–165	155–200	220–285	280–335	345
Menu Guidelines					
Breads/cereals	2–4 servings (2–3 slices bread, ¼ c potatoes)	3–5 servings	4–7 servings	4–7 servings	6–11 servings
Vegetables	½ c cooked or tender raw vegetables	½ c cooked or raw vegeta-bles	2 servings	2–3 servings	3–5 servings
Fruits (may include 100% fruit juice)	1 citrus and 2 others	1 citrus and 2–3 others	1 citrus and 3–4 others	1 citrus and 3–4 others	2–4 servings
Dairy products (including yo-gurt, cheese products)	2–3 c serving	2–3 c servings	2–3 c servings	2–3 c servings	2–3 c servings
Meats/poultry/ beans/nuts	2 servings = 1 oz chopped meat, poultry, or fish; 1 egg; 1 oz cheese	2 servings = 1½ oz meat, poultry, or fish; 3 oz cottage cheese; or 1½ oz cheese; 1–2 eggs	2 servings = 2 oz meat, poultry, or fish; 2 oz cheese; 4 oz cottage cheese; or 2 eggs	2 servings = 2 oz meat, poultry, or fish; 2 oz cheese; 4 oz cottage cheese; or 2 eggs	2 servings = 2 oz meat, poultry, or fish; 2 oz cheese; 4 oz cottage cheese; or 2 eggs
Fats	30% of calo-ries should be from fat	Moderately re-duced fat diet	Low-fat diet	Low-fat diet	Low-fat diet

Adapted from *FDA food pyramid* and *ARA nutrition care manual* (12th ed.). (1992). Philadelphia: ARAMARK Corp.

Oral Health

Over the toddlerhood period, the child gains a full set of 20 primary teeth. As the teeth continue to erupt, the toddler may experience some of the same discomfort as was experienced during infancy when the teeth started to come in. The act of chewing food brings comfort to the toddler's gums, just as biting on a teething ring did for the infant. An increase in the amount of drooling may occur when teeth are erupting.

If the child has not had a visit to the dentist, the ideal time is when the child has a full set of 20 teeth. The dentist will check the child's mouth for the placement of the teeth, note any problems with the initial eruption of the teeth, assess the size of the jaw for future molars, and give recommendations for follow-up visits and fluoride treatments. The first trip to the dentist should be a non-threatening experience for the child. Children's books that have stories about trips to both the doctor and dentist are good tools to help the child prepare for the visit. In addition, after the visit the books can be read again to compare the child's experience with that discussed in the story and allow the child to verbalize his or her feelings about the visit. Pediatric dentists are very sensitive to the needs and fears of children and usually go very slowly, allowing the child to become familiar with the equipment and procedures.

Parents need to help toddlers brush their teeth. Toddlers do not possess the manual dexterity needed to effectively brush their own teeth. Encouraging toddlers to participate in the routine develops good dental hygiene habits; although at this time, the parent must assume complete responsibility. Brushing in front of a mirror or allowing the toddler to sit with his or her head in the parent's lap and having the parent brush the toddler's teeth and then having the toddler "brush" the parent's teeth is a good starting point. The easiest technique to teach at this time is the horizontal brushing technique. As the child matures, a more sophisticated up-and-down technique can be taught. Any single approach to preventive care is not good enough. The child's teeth should be brushed at least twice daily. After the child has had the opportunity to brush the teeth, the parent should finish brushing the teeth to ensure that all areas of the mouth are cleansed. Flossing may be introduced at this time, although the child does not have the manual dexterity to accomplish flossing and needs a parent's assistance.

A small, child-size, soft toothbrush should be used with only plain warm water on the brush to begin. The foaming and flavor of the toothpaste may deter the young child from getting used to brushing. Only a tiny, pea-sized amount of fluoridated toothpaste should be used. There are many toothpastes developed just for children that are made with appealing flavors. A potential problem with these toothpastes is that the flavors are so good that the child wants to eat the paste off the brush rather than use the brush to make the up-and-down movements against the teeth. The toothpaste should be kept out of reach of the child so that he or she does not try to eat the paste directly from the tube.

Even though water in the community may be fluoridated, the dentist may recommend fluoride treatments or fluoride supplements based on the level of fluoride in the drinking water and on the child's daily ingestion of water. The use of fluoride supplements should be monitored because excessive ingestion of fluoride can cause fluorosis, which is characterized by staining of the teeth. The child should be monitored to prevent excessive swallowing of fluoridated toothpaste, and the use of fluoride dentifrice should be delayed until the child is older than 2 years of age.

The dentist may recommend coating the child's teeth with a plastic occlusal sealant as a preventive measure against tooth decay. If the enamel of a child's tooth is impaired, this procedure is usually recommended. Although the procedure is entirely painless, it does require the cooperation of the child; thus, attempting to coat the teeth of the young toddler may not be successful.

A continuing concern at this age is baby bottle tooth decay (BBTD), caused by the child's being put to bed with either milk or juice in a bottle. The child does not rinse the teeth, and the sugars in the milk or juice settle on the teeth for the night and promote caries development. Parents should be reminded to never put the toddler to bed with a bottle of juice or milk.

Many parents also find that this is the time to encourage the weaning of pacifiers to coincide with weaning from the bottle. Methods to wean from the pacifier were presented in the infancy section.

Hygiene and Personal Care

Bathing

The toddler's increased activity level necessitates bathing on a daily or every-other-day basis. Hair should be washed two to three times per week. Most toddlers enjoy taking a bath, although they may not like having their hair washed. A good time to bathe the child is after eating, either in the evening or after breakfast. During the meal, the toddler is likely to have spread food in the hair as well as all over clothing. By the evening, the toddler is fairly dirty from a full day of play. Evening bath time provides an opportunity for cleansing and a method to relax the child in preparation for bedtime.

Bath time is usually viewed as another opportunity for play by the child. Plastic bath toys should be provided, with caution used in regard to the size of the toy and the presence of removable parts. Bubble baths should be avoided to prevent any urethral irritation and possible development of cystitis. Mild shampoos can be used to wash the hair. During rinsing, a washcloth placed over the child's eyes can prevent the shampoo from irritating the eyes. The toddler should never be left alone or be monitored by young siblings while bathing. Placing a young sibling in the bathtub with the toddler while the parent leaves the room does not guarantee the safety of either child.

The toddler is becoming more self-aware of body parts and spends time in the bath exploring his or her naked body and enjoying the unencumbered feeling without clothing. He or she will have discovered his or her genitalia and may touch them frequently when the diaper is removed. The toddler should not be punished for exploring the body in this fashion.

During bath time, the parents should observe the condition of the child's skin and for symmetry of body parts. Any unusual findings should be reported to a health care provider. Bruises or other unusual marks

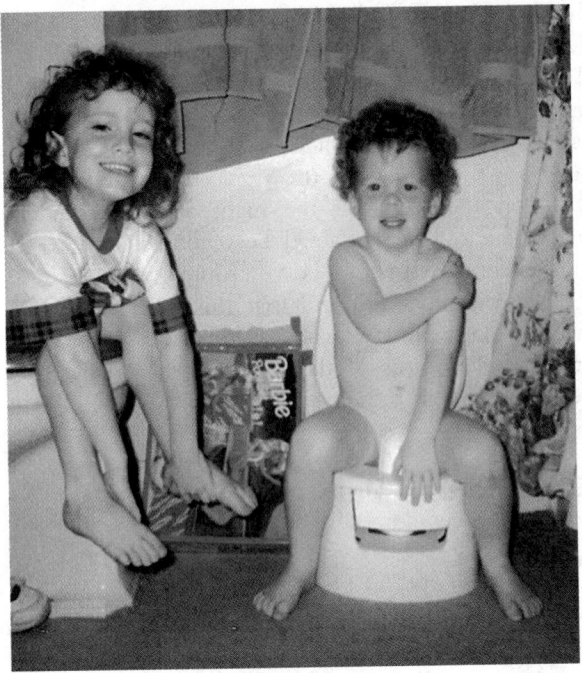

Figure 5–4
The toddler may be encouraged to use the toilet by watching and following the lead of an older sibling.

around the genitalia and buttocks area should especially be noted because these may be signs of physical abuse.

Dressing

During the toddler years, the child begins to participate in dressing and undressing. This may begin with the toddler simply lifting a foot to have a shoe put on or learning to slip an arm in a sleeve hole. By age 3, the toddler is able to undress without assistance (except for removal of shoes) and may be able to put on most simple pieces of clothing. Clothes should be purchased that are easy for the toddler to learn to put on. For instance, shirts with large neck openings and pants made of stretchy fabrics are easy for the toddler to don. Velcro used on shoes as well as for closures on clothes is easier for the toddler than buttons, zippers, snaps, and shoelaces. The toddler is generally not very particular about selecting the clothes he or she is wearing. If the parent wishes to offer a choice, only two items should be presented because the child will not fare well with too many choices.

Toilet Training

As the toddler approaches the second birthday, parents may start thinking about toilet training (Fig. 5–4). There are many books available that indicate toilet training can be done quickly. The key is the readiness of the child. Parents usually find that the older child is the more successful. Some of the signals that indicate a child is ready for toilet training are a predictable bowel movement schedule, diapers remaining dry for longer periods, the ability to follow instructions, the child showing an interest in imitating family members in the bathroom, and an indication either by a facial expression or some other change in activity that the bladder is full or the bowel needs to be evacuated. These readiness signals may occur at the age of 2 but more commonly are seen at 2½ to 3 years of age (Frauman & Brandon, 1996; Shelov, 1993) (Chart 5–12).

Sleep

During the toddler years, the active and exuberant child continues to require 12 or more hours of sleep each day. The 1-year-old spends approximately 13¾ hours a day sleeping. This time is slowly tapered to 13 hours a day by age 2 and 12 hours a day by age 3. There is no magic hour in which the toddler should be placed in bed for

Chart 5–12

Strategies for Successful Toilet Training

- Be sure toddler is ready for toilet training (usually between 18 and 36 months)
  - Understands meanings of words used for toileting
  - Has been able to remain dry for periods of time
  - Has some regularity to bowel and bladder episodes
  - Indicates that there is an awareness of when to evacuate the bowel or bladder
  - Understands what the "potty" is used for
  - Is able to follow simple instructions
  - Shows interest in the "potty" and becoming more independent
- Use child-size "potty" that sits firmly on the floor.
- Use any number of videos or books to introduce the concepts.
- Use adult words for urine and bowel movements ("pee" and "poop" are acceptable).
- Start by increasing the child's awareness of bodily functions.
- Praise the child for attempts even if they are not totally successful.
- Avoid scolding the child for "accidents"; make a matter of fact comment about how the child will be more successful the next time.

the night. Eight o'clock in the evening is a reasonable time, allowing parents to have some moments to themselves before they retire for the evening. Most parents gauge bedtime based on their own routines; that is, those who like to retire very late often enjoy having their children stay awake until 10 or 11 P.M. This is quite acceptable as long as the child is able to sleep for a 10-hour stretch. In the home in which the caregivers must rise early and take the children to daycare, managing a late night/early morning schedule deprives the child of some much needed hours of sleep.

Naps

Naps continue to be an essential component of the child's daily routine. Until about the 16th month, the toddler takes two naps a day, one in the morning and one in the evening, each lasting 2 hours. Between the 16th and 20th month, the morning nap will be dropped, leaving one afternoon nap lasting 2 to 2½ hours. Although some parents assert that their 3-year-old will not take a nap, the need for a mid-afternoon period of rest is warranted in most children. Many children resist "shutting down" and ceasing all play activities to engage in quiet time. Once quiet time has been imposed, these same children are often the first to fall asleep. For the child who will not sleep, an extended period of quiet activity, such as looking at books, can be beneficial as a structured period of rest before the busy activities of the evening when all the family members gather at home. Toddlers who are consistently cranky in the early evening hours are usually those who have not napped but would benefit greatly from this activity as part of their daily routine.

Promotion of Social Competence

Personality Development

This is the age that is known as the "terrible twos" because this is the time that the child is starting to assert his or her independence. This is the time that he or she acquires a sense of autonomy and independence through the mastery of various specialized tasks, such as the control of bodily functions, refinement of motor and language skills, and acquisition of socially acceptable behaviors. Temper tantrums are common during this age, and discipline must be consistent.

Building self-esteem in a toddler is quite challenging because there is quite a lot of negativism occurring during this age. The child acts on the impulse of the moment and is not able to completely understand what the parent wants. At this time, it is important to have the positives outweigh the criticisms (Shelov, 1993). Keep the rules to a minimum if possible. Toddlerproofing the house will assist by not having tempting things around that the child can get into unexpectedly. This keeps the environment explorable and gives the child the ability to expand on the skills that need mastering (e.g., fine motor and gross motor skills).

Temperament

The temperament that the child displayed as an infant may well continue into toddlerhood. If the infant was a fussy, difficult infant, the child may or may not be the same way as a toddler. During this period of time, the toddler becomes frustrated easily and wants to do as much as possible for himself or herself (part of asserting independence). Temper tantrums are a common way of dealing with this frustration.

When dealing with temper tantrums, it is important to remain calm. If dealt with in a controlled manner, the tantrums may actually diminish over time. It is sometimes effective to use humor to redirect the tantrum. A funny face or a joke may distract the child. When disciplining, positive redirection and firm tones with eye contact are usually very effective, but often short "time-outs" (timed to equal 1 minute per age) or a reward system may be helpful. It is important for the parent to be consistent in the communication of the infraction to prevent the child from receiving confusing messages.

Parents should pick their battles; if the issue is not life endangering, or unsafe, or amoral, let it go (e.g., allow the toddler to wear one red shoe and one blue shoe). The toddler should not be allowed to become overtired. This often causes many more arguments than necessary. The child is too young to say, "Hey, I've had a really busy day and need to relax for a while." The toddler also needs to learn how to pace himself or herself and slow down. The child should be allowed a period of time when he or she can learn how to occupy himself or herself for short periods of quiet time. Alerting the toddler to transition times is very important. Many daycare settings use songs to let the toddler know that it is now time for cleanup and to start to get ready for a change in routine. The parent can use a similar technique by giving the child at least 5-minute notices that something else is going to happen. It is also helpful to give options that are attractive to the child to assist with transition. A choice between just leaving and going home to something the toddler likes to do (e.g., a bath, play with the pet) is much easier to negotiate. A parent should not overnegotiate: pleading and expecting the child to understand and agree are unrealistic. There will come the time that even when the parent has negotiated, not allowed the child to become overly tired, and offered appealing options, the child will still be uncooperative and will need to be gently but physically moved to the next task or place. A parent can learn to anticipate the child's limit, such as discussing the toys that will be shared at an upcoming visit with another child (Chart 5–13).

Parents want their children to have a very healthy sense of self-esteem. Building self-esteem starts when the child is an infant with the parent showing unconditional love and focused attention to the child. As the child becomes a toddler, the child develops new needs for self-expression and power. As a child tests the limits of independence, parents find that rules and limits will be tested. Two areas that are usually the first that the toddler tests are feeding and dressing. The child should be given as many opportunities to succeed as possible by supplying him or her with the tools to succeed, such as child-sized utensils for eating and clothing that is easy for the child to select, put on, and fasten. As the child develops language skills, the parent should listen to the child talk, even if it is for just a few minutes a day to have eye contact and really become engaged in what is being "discussed." Unsuccessful attempts should be applauded as much as the successful attempts at learning new skills. If possible, the parent can discuss in very simple terms what happened and what other choices could have been made to possibly make this a successful attempt. The goal is to create a positive nurturing environment in which the toddler can explore and cultivate experiences to build self-esteem (Chart 5–14).

Chart 5–13

Avoiding Temper Tantrums

- "Childproof" the home to reduce the number of times the parent must say "no" to the child's actions and activities.
- Allow the young children to make frequent small choices, providing clearly defined, acceptable parameters.
- Evaluate the child's temperament and changes that occur in temperament over the course of the day. Plan activities accordingly.
- Make sure "no" really means "no" and not "well, maybe." Even if the child protests vehemently, the parent should not back down from his or her stand; otherwise, the child learns that "if I protest enough, Mom or Dad will give in."
- Once a tantrum has started, ignore the child's behavior. The parents should stand about 5 feet away from the child and keep doing the activity they were previously engaged in. The parent should not speak to the child and should avoid eye contact until the child has calmed. Move objects out of the way or move the child, if necessary, to prevent injury. Do not let the child hurt him- or herself or others. The tantrums may increase for a while as the child tries harder to gain parental attention; however, this method is effective in heading off tantrums and not reinforcing them.
- After the tantrum, discuss the child's behavior with him or her in a calm neutral tone. Discuss ways the child can get "in control." Do not talk excessively about the tantrum because this can negatively impact the child's self-esteem.

Adapted from Needlman, R. (1995). Temper tantrums. In S. Parker & B. Zuckerman (Eds.), *Behavioral and developmental pediatrics* (pp. 306–309). Boston: Little, Brown & Company.

Chart 5–14

Strategies for Enhancing Self-Esteem

- Help the child build a healthy relationship with peers because children are sensitive to evaluation of peers.
- Treat the child with respect—ask their view and opinions and respond seriously.
- Use physical contact to communicate feelings of love and acceptance.
- Talk to the child (even as an infant or toddler) using the child's name frequently; give hugs, smile, and use eye contact.
- Applaud unsuccessful attempts as well as successes.
- Develop a positive, nurturing environment.
- Do not belittle the child.
- Use positive reinforcement whenever possible and avoid negative criticism.
- Include the child in activities that interest the adult.

Fears

The most common fears for toddlers are the fear of separation from the parent and loud noises. Fears are common in children of all ages, changing as the child matures and obtains a more concrete level of cognitive ability (Fig. 5–5). Usually there is a triggering event for some fears, such as the fear of dogs or falling. Because of the limited cognitive understanding of the toddler, some fears that are irrational surface as the toddler does not have enough information to self-reassure and allay the fear (Table 5–6).

Play

The play interaction for an infant occurs primarily between the parent and the infant. As the infant matures and becomes more social, the play interaction with peers evolves into several different types of play styles. On-

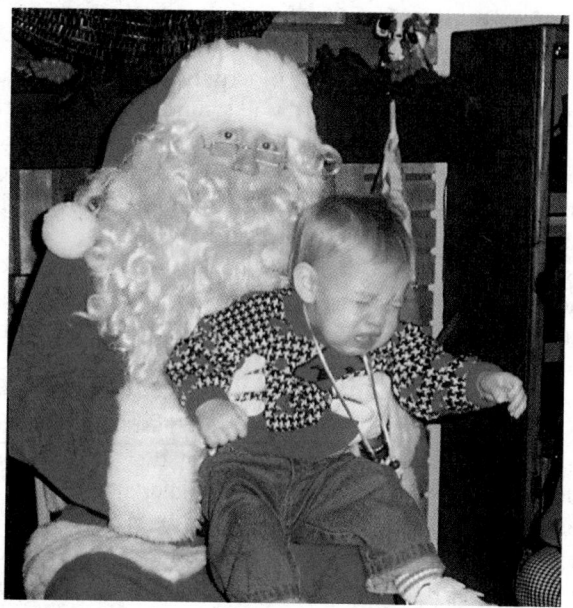

Figure 5–5
Santa Claus and other costumed characters can be very frightening to a toddler.

looker play is when the child is an observer of the actions of other children and does not attempt to interact with them. Solitary play is when a child is playing by himself or herself, absorbed in an activity and uninterested in the play of other children. Parallel play occurs when children play with similar toys, beside other children, but are not influenced by other children's play activities (Fig. 5–6). The child may have an identical toy but play with it in a different manner. Play is considered *associative* when children are playing together in a group but there is no organization or leadership; however, there may be sharing of materials or following of one another (Fig. 5–7). An example would be two children drawing pictures, sharing paper and crayons, and discussing what they are drawing, but neither is suggesting they draw the same thing. Once the play is organized, with a leader/follower type of relationship established, the play is considered to be *cooperative*.

The major accomplishment of the second year of life is learning to walk. By the time the toddler is 2 years old, he or she is able to walk, run, carry several large objects while walking, and go up and down stairs. This

Table 5–6
Common Childhood Fears

Type of Fear	Age Ranges								
	5–8 Mo	8 Mo–1 Yr	2 Yr	3 Yr	4–5 Yr	6–8 Yr	9–10 Yr	11–13 Yr	13+ Yr
Abandonment	X	X							
Separation	X	X	X						
Noises		X	X						
Strangers		X	X	X					
Falling		X				X			
Animals		X		X	X				
Bath/toilet		X	X						
Dark		X							
Nightmares (monsters)				X	X				
Becoming lost				X	X				
Divorce/death of parent				X	X				
New situations					X	X			
Hospitals/doctors/needles						X			
Ghosts/supernatural						X	X		
School failure						X	X	X	
Peer rejection							X		
Burglars							X	X	X
Accidents/death								X	
Peer pressure								X	X
Sexual experiences								X	X

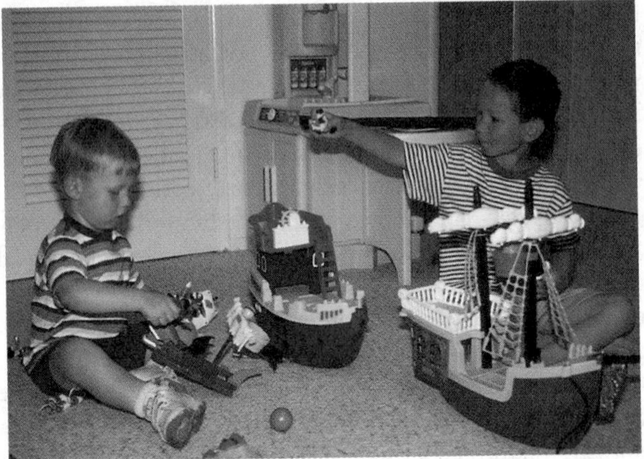

Figure 5–6
During parallel play, children may play side by side but do not influence each other's play activities.

occurs over several months, starting out with the toddler having a wide base of support with the feet and using the hands and arms for balance. It is not uncommon for the toddler to "cruise" furniture—using tables, sofas, and chairs as crutches to assist with the balancing act. This is a time when falls are frequent, and the parents must be aware of sharp table edges and small wrinkles in carpets or rugs that may mean disaster to the toddler.

Fine motor skills are also being perfected. At 1 year of age, it is still very difficult for the toddler to use a pincer grasp to pick up small items (between thumb and forefinger). As the toddler matures during the second year, these skills become easier.

Figure 5–7
During associative play, children play together, although there is no specific organization to, nor leader guiding, their activities.

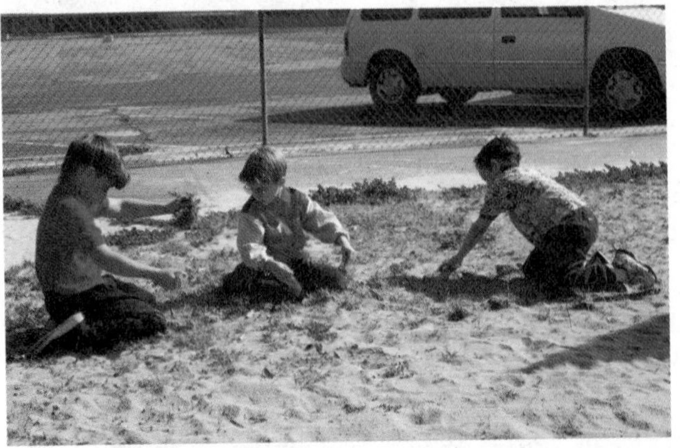

Age-Appropriate Activities

At 1 year of age, gross motor activities take precedence. The toddler is learning to walk, run, and explore the environment from a new level. The child prefers objects that make noise in response to this effort, and because attention spans are still short, the toddler needs a wide variety of objects to play with and touch. Filling containers with objects and dumping them out, stacking blocks and knocking them over, scribbling, and painting are activities that are good for this age. Playing games that also teach spatial concepts such as "under," "in," "over," and so on, helps the child develop skills. Another developmental milestone is the child's understanding of language. Now the parents may find that they need to spell out words they would rather the toddler not hear (e.g., "Should we buy some C-A-N-D-Y?"). The toddler is more responsive to conversations and pays more attention, so songs and music are good games as well as nursery rhymes. By the end of this first year, the toddler has a vocabulary of about 50 words and is using pronouns; by the time the toddler is 3 years old, he or she is using sentences of two and three words and understands most of what is said to him or her. The toddler enjoys examining pictures in books and having stories read to him or her (Fig. 5–8).

Mechanical toys give 2-year-olds a sense of accomplishment because they have a cause-and-effect mechanism—something happens because the toddler caused it to happen. Memory games, matching games, hide and

Figure 5–8
The toddler enjoys examining pictures in books and listening as stories are read.

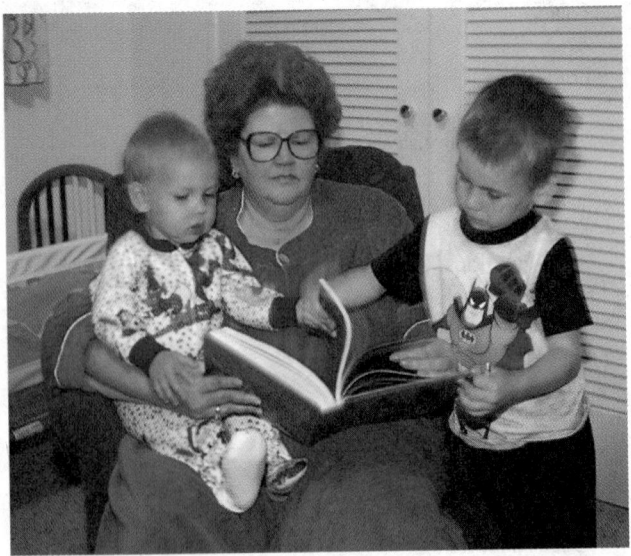

seek, pretend games, and "Simon Says" are great fun to the toddler because the child is the center of attention.

As the toddler becomes 2, and his or her gross motor skills are more developed, the child will be interested in a tricycle, kicking balls, and running games. The child's fine motor skills are developed enough to color with crayons, turn pages in books, and operate small mechanical-type toys that produce action or sounds. All toys still need to meet the appropriate safety standards.

Styles of Play

During the second year of life, the toddler is very self-centered. The child is primarily interested in how people and things react in relation to him or her. At this time, the toddler plays alongside children without truly interacting with them. The child watches other children, even imitates some things they are doing. The child may compete for an adult's attention or a toy but is unable to play cooperatively. Sharing is not a concept that the child understands at all. Imitation is a game that he or she finds impossible to resist—it is not uncommon to hear a child use exactly the same tone and verbiage that the parent uses in similar circumstances.

Exposing the toddler to a wide variety of types of interactions (playing alone, in peer groups, or with older children or adults), locations for play (home, friend's home, parks, libraries), and types of activities (structured, group, quiet, spontaneous) is beneficial. Because toddlers are very active, the parent must be sure to provide enough physical space for the child to play in. Tactile exploration is important to the child. Water tables, sand, soap bubbles, and clay provide excellent opportunities for the toddler to explore different textures and develop creativity. Safety must always be considered, and toys must be appropriate with no sharp edges. Adult supervision is necessary with many of the opportunities the toddler will use for exploration.

Daycare and Baby Sitters

The parent should already have a regular baby sitter, and the child may have already experienced some time in daycare. Many of the daycare programs "graduate" their charges into preschool programs within the same building. If the child has only experienced a home-based sitter, au pair, or relative or has been in a home daycare setting, this may be the age that the parent wishes to start looking for a preschool.

Preschool refers to an organized program of early childhood education. Preschools can be extremely important to the child's overall development because the child receives stimulation in areas that are not normally addressed in the home environment. They are also valuable as a resource for discovering potential learning disabilities at a very early phase (Franck & Brownstone, 1991).

How to Choose a Preschool

Many of the same questions that are asked when a daycare center is chosen are the same questions that need to be asked when a preschool is chosen. Besides location, hours the center is open, numbers and ages of the other children, and cost, the "instructional" capacities of the preschool need to be evaluated. The parent should be cautious of preschools that promise "speed-up" learning techniques.

If the child has never attended a daycare setting, the initial strategy is to allow the child to adjust to the separation from parent to center. The preschool is not designed to begin meeting the child's academic needs but just to offer the building blocks to prepare for the more "academic environment" of kindergarten (the "official" start of school) (Shelov, 1993). The goals should allow the child to be comfortable with a few hours of separation and familiarize him or her with group activities and the learning process.

A good preschool will encourage the children to gain independence and self-confidence and to develop interpersonal skills. The preschool should have the resources to identify any learning disorders; or if the child has already been identified with a special need, the preschool should have the appropriate resources in place to comprehend what is needed (most general preschools are not equipped to do this, and the parents should speak with the director).

The program should have relatively small class sizes, about 10 or fewer, and the "teacher" or aides should have early childhood development or education experience. In many states, this is mandated by the daycare or preschool regulations. The health care professional should advise parents to be sure to investigate the disciplinary methods used and be sure they are in line with the home discipline techniques. The entire center and grounds should be childproofed and under adult supervision at all times. A parent should be encouraged to visit the center whenever he or she would like. One should be suspicious of centers that have very strict visiting procedures.

Health issues should be addressed, such as what happens when a child becomes ill at the center and what are the policies regarding accepting children with apparent illness. There should be strict policies regarding infectious diseases. Hand washing by both staff and children should be encouraged. Child-size sinks should be available, and the toilet-trained children should be expected to wash their hands after having used the facilities. If there are children who are still in diapers, there should be a separate diaper station that is cleaned after each use with the appropriate disinfectant.

It is extremely important that the parent agree with the overall theory of the program. Although some children thrive in a structured environment, many need to have an opportunity to socialize and learn to control emotions and explore their own ideas (Ryval, 1994). There are many different types of methods used today in preschool. Montessori is one of the more popular types of daycare settings at this time, but parents should be encouraged to investigate all available programs to find the type that may be the most suitable for the child. The health care professional should become familiar with all types of preschools and options in the area.

Injury and Illness Prevention

Injury Prevention

Although the home has been babyproofed, it is now time to toddlerproof the home (Chart 5–15). Cribs, playpens, and highchairs will no longer contain a curious active toddler. All cupboards at the toddler's level should have

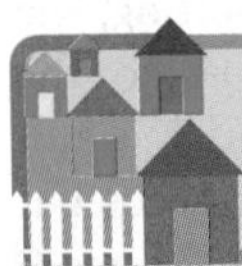

Chart 5–15
Community Care

Injury Prevention Guidelines for the Family with a Toddler

Home Safety

- Get down on the floor and check for new hazards now that the toddler is walking.
- Test smoke detectors to ensure that they work properly. Change batteries yearly.
- Do not leave heavy objects or containers of hot liquids on tables with tablecloths that the child may pull down.
- Turn pan handles toward the back of the stove.
- Keep the toddler away from hot stoves, fireplaces, irons, curling irons, and space heaters.
- Ensure that all electric wires, outlets, and appliances are inaccessible or protected.
- Keep all poisonous substances, cleaning agents, health and beauty supplies, medicines, and home improvement materials in a locked safe place out of sight and reach. Never store poisonous substances in empty jars or soda bottles.
- Keep cigarettes, lighters, matches, and alcohol out of the toddler's sight and reach.
- Use safety gates at the top and bottom of stairs. Supervise the toddler closely when he or she is on stairs.
- Place safety devices on windows and make sure screens are secure.
- Ensure that guns, if in the home, are locked up and that ammunition is stored separately. A trigger lock is an additional important precaution.

Play Safety

- Do not give the toddler plastic bags, latex balloons, or small objects such as marbles.
- Teach siblings which of their toys are unsafe for the toddler to play with.
- Confine the toddler's outdoor play to areas with fences and gates, especially at a child care facility, unless he or she is under close supervision.
- Ensure that playgrounds are safe. Check for impact- or energy-absorbing surfaces under playground equipment. Make sure playground equipment is not over 3 ft tall and not made of pressure-treated wood.

Water Safety

- Ensure that the hot water heater is set at less than 120°F.
- Test the bath water temperature with your wrist to make sure it is not hot before bathing your toddler.
- Supervise the toddler constantly whenever he or she is around water, buckets, the toilet, or the bathtub.
- Empty buckets, tubs, or small pools immediately after use.
- Ensure that swimming pools are enclosed by a four-sided fence with a self-closing, self-latching gate.
- Ensure that the toddler wears a life vest if boating.
- Use flotation devices on the toddler when he or she is in the pool or jacuzzi. Note that inflatable flotation devices or "knowing how to swim" do not make a toddler safe in the water.

safety locks or have nothing in them that could ever be injurious to a child. Small sharp objects, such as jewelry or pins, should be kept out of reach. All filmy type of plastic bags (e.g., dry cleaning bags) should be discarded as soon as possible. Toys should be checked and discarded if any have broken pieces and sharp edges. Selected toys should be appropriate for the child's age group per the manufacturer's recommendations.

Electrical outlets should be covered and electrical cords kept out of reach by hiding them behind furniture and using a minimum of extension cords. Guards on sharp coffee table edges can be used to prevent injuries. Valuable or heavy objects should be placed out of the toddler's curious reach. If there are stairs in the house, a gate should be used to block the upper and lower areas to prevent falls.

In the kitchen, pot handles should be turned inward on the stove. All cleansers and chemicals are stored in high places and out of reach. Knives, skewers, and other sharp objects should be kept toward the back of the cabinets or drawers. One should never leave a child alone in a kitchen. Parents should be aware that they should never walk with a child while holding a hot beverage.

In the bathroom, a child should never be left unattended for even a moment in a bathtub. Also, the top of

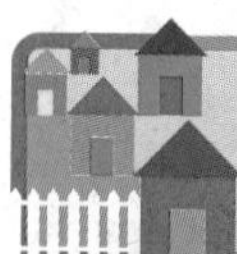

Chart 5–15
Community Care

Injury Prevention Guidelines for the Family with a Toddler *Continued*

Car Safety

- Change to a toddler care seat. Make sure it is properly secured at all times. The car seat should face toward the front of the car but remain in the back seat.
- Never leave the toddler alone in the car or in the house.

Safety with Others

- Do not leave young siblings alone to supervise the toddler (e.g., in the bathtub or in the house).
- Keep the infant away from cigarette smoke. Do not allow people to smoke around the toddler.
- Choose caregivers carefully. Discuss with them their attitudes about behavior in relation to discipline. Prohibit corporal punishment.
- Teach the child to use caution when approaching animals, especially if the animals are unknown or eating.
- Teach the child not to talk to strangers.

Outdoor Safety

- Put sunscreen on the toddler before he or she goes out to play.
- Keep the toddler away from moving machinery, lawn mowers, overhead garage doors, driveways, and streets.
- Ensure that a toddler riding in a seat on an adult's bicycle is wearing a helmet. Wear a helmet yourself.
- Supervise the child whenever he or she is outside. Know where your child is at all times. A toddler is too young to be roaming the neighborhood alone.
- Teach the toddler pedestrian safety skills.

Emergency Preparation

- Keep your address and phone number posted near the phone.
- Keep a list of emergency numbers (doctor, hospital, nearest neighbor, poison control center) near the phone.
- Keep a 1-oz bottle of syrup of ipecac in the home and use as directed by the poison control center or health care provider.
- Enroll in a child CPR course.
- Discuss with the health care professional what to do for falls, cuts, puncture wounds, bites, bumps on the head, bleeding, and broken bones.

Adapted from Green, M. (Ed.). (1994). *Bright futures: Guidelines for health supervision of infants, children, and adolescents.* Arlington, VA: National Center of Education in Maternal and Child Health. *Bright Futures* was supported by the Maternal and Child Health Bureau and the Medicaid Bureau.

the toilet should be put down after each use. The medicine cabinet should be cleaned out and old or not used medicines discarded by flushing them down the toilet. The temperature of the hot water heater should be lowered to 120°F. After running the bath, the hot water is turned off first and the cold water last to prevent scalding. Soft protectors should be used on the tub spouts to prevent bumps on the head. Floors should be wiped frequently to be kept dry and not slippery.

Developmental Surveillance

Chart 5–16 is a summary of the developmental milestones that are accomplished in the toddler years. This information is useful to provide the nurse with direction for specific trigger questions that can be asked of the parent to determine the toddler's developmental progress. Questions regarding how the child attempts to communicate, what the child understands, and how the child maneuvers to get from one place to another should be formulated as open ended as possible to elicit more information. By the time the child is a toddler, the child should have a vocabulary of three to six words, understand simple commands, be able to walk, feed himself or herself with fingers, and drink from a cup. By age 2 years, the child should have increased his or her vocabulary to at least 20 words, use two-word phrases, go up and down stairs one step at a time, and be able to kick a ball (Green, 1994). Health supervision interventions are presented in Table 5–7.

Preschoolers

Preschoolers are children who range in age from 3 to 6 years old. Although a child may have already attended daycare and started in "preschool" while 2 years of age, most children begin preschool at the age of 3 or older.

Nutrition

By the age of 3, a preschooler should be eating only table food and no longer drinking formula but rather low-fat milk. The child should be feeding himself or herself most of the food, with occasional help from the parent in regard to cutting larger pieces, and so on. Food should be varied, and the child should be offered a variety of different textures and types of food. One should not assume that an initial turndown of a new food is a permanent dislike and label the child as a "picky eater." The food

Table 5–7
Health Supervision Interventions: Toddler

	1 Yr	15 Mo	18 Mo	2 Yr	3 Yr
Physical Examination	X	X	X	X	X
Growth Parameters (height, weight, head circumference)	X	X	X	X	X
Immunizations	X	X	X‡		
Assessment of High-Dose Lead Exposure	X	X	X	X	X
Lead Screening	X			X	
Hematocrit or Hemoglobin Screening	X*				
Tuberculin Test	X†	X†		X§	X§
Assessment of Risk for Hyperlipidemia				X	X
Vision Screening					X‖
Hearing Screening					X
Blood Pressure Screening					X

* At 9–12 months if needed for certification for WIC (Special Supplemental Food Program for Women, Infants and Children) or if certain risk factors are present.
† At 12 or 15 months before administration of measles, mumps, rubella (MMR) vaccine.
‡ If not previously administered.
§ Annual test if certain risk factors are present.
‖ Rescreen vision in 6 months if child is uncooperative.
From Green, M. (Ed.). (1994). *Bright futures: Guidelines for health supervision of infants, children, and adolescents.* Arlington, VA: National Center for Education in Maternal and Child Health. *Bright Futures* was supported by the Maternal and Child Health Bureau and the Medicaid Bureau.

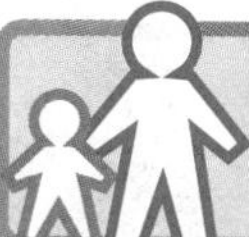

Chart 5–16
Developmental Considerations

Milestones of the Toddler (12–36 Months)

Physical

12 Mo
Head circumference equals chest circumference
Triples birth weight to 20 lb
Half of adult height
Height increases 3 in/yr for next 7 years
Weight increases 4–6 lb/yr

18–24 Mo
10–14 temporary teeth
Anterior fontanelle closes
Cuspids and first and second molars appear
Toilet training may be initiated
Chest circumference exceeds head circumference

24 Mo
16 temporary teeth
Average weight is 30 lb
Toilet training may begin; voluntary control of anal and urethral sphincters occurs
Average 10–14 hr of sleep, including afternoon naps

36 Mo
Nighttime control of bowel and bladder may be achieved
Weight increases 4 to 6 lb/yr
Height increases 3 in/yr

Sexual

All Toddlers
Anal stage
Sensual pleasure shifts to anal and urethral areas
Identification with male/female sex roles

36 Mo
Knows own sex

Language

12–18 Mo
Beginning of spoken language; may occur at same time as walking, although concentration on one or the other may occur
Recognizes nouns that stand for objects
Uses gestures to make needs known
Develops from 3 to 20 words
Use of telegraphic speech; use of noun and verb to convey meaning
Use of words may be quite inconsistent

18–24 Mo
Follows directions
Points to nose, hair, eye, etc. on demand
Comprehends "give me that" when accompanied by a gesture

24 Mo
300-word vocabulary
Gives first and last name
Progressive comprehension of speech
Talks without trying to convey ideas

36 Mo
900-word vocabulary
Uses complete sentences of 3 to 4 words
Talks incessantly
Asks many questions

Vision

18 Mo
Displays interest in pictures

24 Mo
Identifies forms
Snellen testing
20/40 Vision

36 Mo
20/30 vision

Chart continued on following page

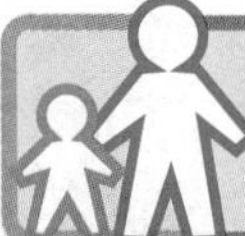

Chart 5–16
Developmental Considerations

Milestones of the Toddler (12–36 Months) *Continued*

Gross Motor

12–18 Mo
Walks well
Throws ball
Stoops and recovers
Walks up stairs with help
Begins to run
Walks sideways and backward for 10 ft
Stands on one foot with help
Sits down from standing by self
Falls frequently, often used as a way of sitting down
Rolls large ball on floor

18–24 Mo
Kicks ball forward
Throws overhand
Walks down stairs with help—one at a time
Climbs
Sits self in a small chair

24–36 Mo
Jumps and runs well
Jumps from bottom step
Jumps in place
Balances on one foot for 1 second
Pedals tricycle
Walks on a straight line
Tiptoes
Broad jumps 4–14 in
Can pick up objects on floor without losing balance

Fine Motor

12–18 Mo
Scribbles spontaneously
Builds tower of two blocks, then four blocks
Dumps raisins from container after demonstration, then spontaneously
May untie shoes
Uses opposable thumb well (prehension)
Shows preference for handedness
Turns pages in a book
Uses spoon with frequent spills when getting food to mouth

18–24 Mo
May remove articles of clothing
Holds pencil well enough for scribbling
Builds tower of four cubes
Imitates vertical line within 30 degrees
Turns doorknobs within reach

24–36 Mo
Unbuttons large buttons
Builds tower of 6–8 cubes
Can use paintbrush
Imitates scribble
Copies a circle
Begins to wash and dry hands
Drinks from cup
Can begin brushing teeth 1–2 times a day
Can take off socks and other easy to manipulate clothing
Snaps large snaps
Zips large zippers with help
Twists caps off bottles
Places simple shapes in correct holes
Will disassemble objects

Play

12–24 Mo
Parallel play
Imitates adult roles
Imitates housework
Will do simple household tasks

24–36 Mo
Parallel and associative play
Uses colors
Begins to play interactive games, such as tag
Plays with sand, clay, puzzles
Fantasy and make-believe play
Action games/ritualistic, such as tag or "hide and seek"

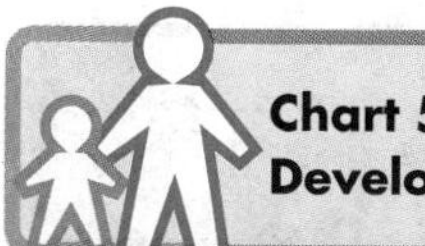

Chart 5-16
Developmental Considerations

Milestones of the Toddler (12–36 Months) *Continued*

Cognitive

2–7 Yr—preoperational and preconceptual

12–18 Mo

Substage V

Uses imitation to discover new ways of acting
Experiments to discover how objects behave and how they can be manipulated

18–24 Mo

Substage VI

Concept of object permanency fully achieved
Symbolic plane
Limited concept of time (no "tomorrow")
Very egocentric
Animist (talks to stuffed animals)
Imaginary playmates
Premature sense of cause/effect
Goal-directed behavior
Death is reversible; a temporary restriction, departure or sleep
Bedtime very ritualistic

Social

12–18 Mo

Responds to limit setting
Anal stage

18–36 Mo

Attempts to please parents and conform to their expectations
Aware of family relationships and roles

Interpersonal

12–24 Mo

Differentiation between "good mother/bad mother" to "good me/bad me" or "not me"
Swings from love to hate

36 Mo

Self-concept begins
Egocentric in thought and behavior

Emotional

30–48 Mo

Uses symbolic communication to convey ideas in terms of complex intentions
Explores different emotions in pretend play
Can communicate and comprehend emotions of self and others

Chart continued on following page

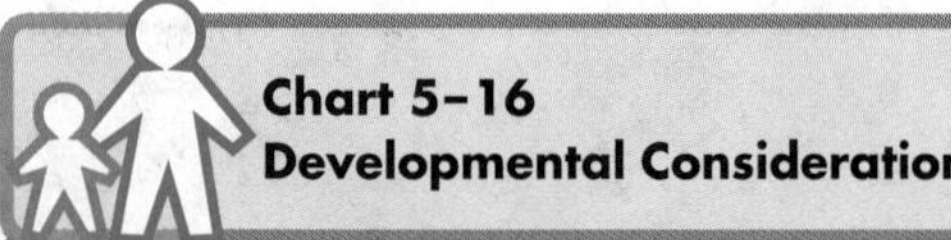

Chart 5–16
Developmental Considerations

Milestones of the Toddler (12–36 Months) *Continued*

Moral/Spiritual

All Toddlers

Moral

Stage 2: Preconventional Level

Detects concepts of fairness and sharing
"Instrumental-relationistic" orientation
Satisfaction of own needs
Conventional level; beginning "good girl/nice boy"
Approval-seeking behavior coupled with desire to please

Spiritual

Stage I: Intuitive/Projective

Learns to imitate the religious affect and behavior of parents
Mimics religious gestures although does not comprehend meaning
Formulates own conceptions and explanations of faith and belief
Cannot separate feelings from intellect
Formulates imagined descriptions of God (angel, friend child can communicate with)

should be offered again; if the child is not forced to eat it, often it will be accepted. As with toddlers, attempts should be made to keep mealtimes free of tension and stress and to serve appropriate-sized portions. Loading a child's plate can be overwhelming for the child and present an unrealistic amount of food for the child to consume. Between meals, nutritious snacks should be encouraged and junk food discouraged. Enough time should be allowed at mealtime for the child to feed himself or herself, but mealtimes should not continue past 20 to 30 minutes. If the child has not finished by then, he or she should be allowed to leave the table. A child should never be kept at the table after the other family members have left because this may appear to be a punishment. Food should never be used as a reward or a punishment. This can cause mixed messages and confuse the child.

Foods are offered that are age appropriate for the preschooler to perfect newly developed skills. Finger foods such as diced fruit, steamed diced vegetables, shredded cheese, or cereals are ideal for the child to utilize the pincer grasp. Child-size utensils are offered for use, such as chunky handled spoons and forks that fit his or her hands, and the child is allowed to feed himself or herself. When introducing a new food, the parents can be encouraged to offer a taste or combine a new food with an old favorite. If it is refused, it can be tried again in a few days but not forced. The child will have personal likes and dislikes as all individuals do. If the child consistently refuses a particular food or food group, one can become creative. For instance, if the child refuses to eat raw apples, try steaming or baking them or grating them onto a plate with a dip. Desserts may be part of the meal and should not be held as a reward for a clean plate. Many parents will seek advice from the health care professional regarding feeding and food strikes.

The diet should be developed around the food pyramid, and amounts should be limited to approximately 1 tablespoon per year of age for each food served (see Table 5–5). At this age, a child may be switched to low-fat milk or skim milk from whole milk to reduce the fat in the child's diet. The latest recommendations are a total fat intake of no more than 30% for anyone age 2 years or older. The usual source for most of the fat in preschoolers' diets appears to come from dairy products. It is believed that by utilizing lower-fat alternatives to these dairy products, the total fat intake can be easily reduced to the recommended amounts.

Occasionally a preschooler will develop a "feeding

strike." This is a very normal situation encountered by many parents. As long as there is no underlying physical problem, and the child is at an adequate weight for his or her height, the preschooler will eat when he or she becomes hungry. It is important for the nurse to determine whether the family dynamics are allowing food to be used as a power source. One should determine whether the child is being offered a variety of foods and an opportunity to make choices regarding those foods (offer an either/or situation, such as eggs or cereal for breakfast). Often a preschooler is offered too much food on a plate, and it is overwhelming. The child will not eat or simply picks at the food. Occasionally, a preschooler only wants a few items of food (possibly all white foods) or a very limited variety of foods. The parent can continue to offer a wide variety of foods but should not force the child to eat them. The parent can encourage the child to taste the food when serving it to the rest of the family. The pediatrician can be consulted to prescribe a vitamin supplement (Parker & Zuckerman, 1995).

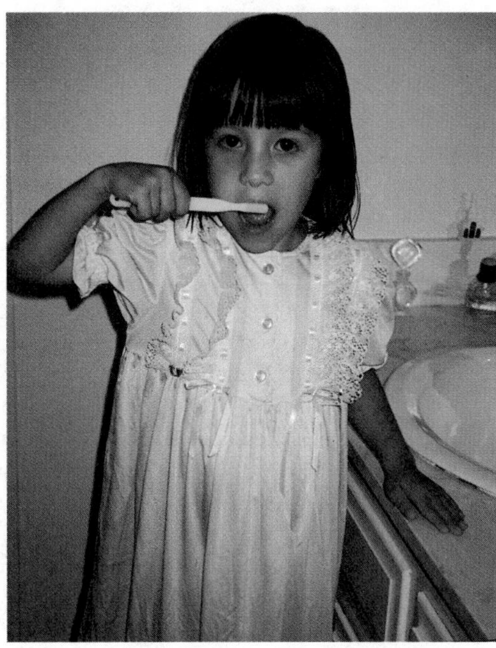

Figure 5–9
To promote good oral hygiene, the preschooler should brush her or his teeth once in the morning and once in the evening.

Oral Health

If the preschooler has not been seen by a dentist during the toddler years, now is the time for the first dental appointment. By the time the child is 5, some of the permanent teeth may start to erupt, and preventive care at an early age will forestall any problems. The number one dental problem among preschoolers is tooth decay. There is a fallacy that because the cavities are in the baby teeth, which will be lost, it is nothing to worry about. However, the premature loss of baby teeth may cause a shift in other baby teeth and not allow the permanent teeth room to come in at a much later date.

The best method of preventive care is for the child to develop good dental hygiene habits at an early age (Fig. 5–9). As a toddler, the child should be having the teeth brushed at least once or twice a day. Although the child may now be an active participant in this endeavor, owing to limited manual dexterity, the preschooler still needs close supervision and assistance by the parent.

The use of a soft bristled toothbrush in a child size and a dab of fluoride toothpaste is recommended. It is cautioned not to overuse a fluoride toothpaste because the child may swallow the toothpaste in amounts that may cause dental fluorosis, which produces staining on the permanent teeth. For many years, dentists recommended only brushing up and down. It is now thought that any direction of brushing is fine as long as each tooth is thoroughly brushed from gum line to the crown and the plaque that forms on a daily basis is removed. Children usually concentrate on the teeth that are in the front because they can easily see these teeth and "forget" about the teeth in the back. This is when parental assistance is needed to be sure those "forgotten teeth" are brushed as carefully.

It is important to monitor the amount of sweets that the child eats. Fresh fruits and vegetables are good for healthy teeth, and candy is a real culprit of tooth decay. If a child does eat sweets, he or she should brush the teeth immediately afterward to remove the sugars and not allow them to remain in the mouth. If this is not feasible, he or she can at least rinse the mouth with plain water.

Using many of the same techniques as with a toddler, preparing a preschooler for the first visit to the dentist should not be difficult. The parent may want to talk to the dentist before the first visit to find out exactly what the dentist will be doing and then in simple terms describe to the child what will occur. Using words such as "tickle" helps describe the feeling of the vibration of the tooth cleaning equipment without making it scary. If the first visit is for something that is likely to be painful, such as an extraction, the child should not be told that it will be painless, because then the child will feel that his or her trust has been violated.

The dentist will check the teeth for cavities, placement, and potential problems and may recommend a fluoride treatment. Occasionally, the dentist will also suggest that a sealant be applied to weak areas of the teeth to prevent tooth decay. Once the preschooler starts seeing the dentist, the visits should be scheduled about every 6 months.

Hygiene and Personal Care

Sleep

It is not uncommon for the preschooler to maintain similar sleep patterns to those that were held in the toddler years. A 3-year-old still requires approximately 12 hours of sleep a day. By 6 years of age, 10 to 11 hours of sleep a day will suffice. Around the age of 4, many children discontinue the afternoon nap. In many daycare centers and preschools, the afternoon nap period is continued because a great number of children can still benefit from a scheduled period of rest in the middle of the day. During this time, many preschoolers do not "sleep" but are encouraged to remain on a mat or blanket quietly playing to develop the ability to relax or unwind from the tension of the day's activities.

A bedtime routine should be developed. A winding-down routine possibly consisting of a bath, story, and lights out should be established. Rowdy play should be avoided close to the bedtime because this tends to excite the preschooler and make it more difficult to get the child to bed, let alone to sleep. At this age, the preschooler may dispute going to bed, particularly if there are older siblings who have later bedtimes. A calm, firm attitude should be used to put the child to bed.

Sleep problems encountered around the age of 3 may occur in a child who has a bad dream, awakes, and is unable to return to sleep. By the age of 5, the child understands that dreams are not real and is able to return to sleep easier. When the 3-year-old awakes, he or she needs to be reassured that the images he or she saw were not real nor harmful. The parent can comfort the child and allow him or her to remain in bed and return to sleep. Several books are available about dreams that can be read to the preschooler to assist with this transition (see Resources). If this becomes an overwhelming problem, the parents should consult with a health care provider.

Self-Care

Preschoolers are in an independent stage and have lost their "baby look." At 3 years old, the child understands some colors and matching; by the time the child is 5, he or she will be deciding what to wear and dressing himself or herself completely. Outfits that are easy to don with stretchy waistbands and easy-to-pull-on shirts should be continued. If there are buttons, large ones with large buttonholes work best, and Velcro closures can be used. Items that close in the back should be avoided. A way to avoid arguments about outfits is to try to keep everything as color coordinated as possible. Many clothing manufacturers develop clothing lines that are interchangeable. The order in which clothing is put on is very confusing to preschoolers, and if the parent places the clothes out in the order in which they are to be put on, this helps the child. Shoes need to be fitted correctly and checked periodically for fit. At this age, the child may grow out of shoes faster than any other clothing item.

Promotion of Social Competence

Personality Development

Self-Esteem

Self-esteem involves the development of a sense of self-worth and identity. This is a lifelong task that begins at birth but is truly fostered in the toddler and preschool years (see Chart 5–14). Preschoolers love to pretend they are adults and do appear very grown up at times. Their self-esteem is significantly tied to their learning new skills. They are developing an awareness of their own skills and interests. As these children become more competent and more self aware, and more aware of peers, parents may hear them express a lot of dissatisfaction with their achievements. They may want their drawing to look like "Peter's drawing" or to look like a "real" flower. Parents as well as nurses who work with children need to nourish these feelings of self-esteem by showing respect and support to the child, allowing the child to make decisions, listening to the child, and spending time with the child. The parent needs to be a "coach" to the child rather than just a "cheerleader." A "cheerleader" just stands at the sidelines and praises the accomplishments of the child; a "coach" uses the praise to instill self-worth and teach the child the skills he or she needs by reinforcing specific actions that the child performed ("You did such a good job setting the table by putting the napkins and forks in exactly the right place!").

Some other ways to foster good self-esteem are to provide opportunities for the child to make choices and decisions (this allows the child some control over his or her life). To offer encouragement and positive feedback, the child should not constantly be berated and "put down." The child should be allowed to establish self-discipline so he or she understands logical consequences and can make appropriate choices, and the parent should help the child learn how to deal with mistakes and failures so the child will not avoid attempting new things (Parker & Zuckerman, 1995). Spending just a few minutes each day talking with the child about the events of the day, or praising the child for his or her accomplishments (with specific examples), or providing an environment where the child can play without being restrained by "no," "don't touch," and so on will do much to foster a healthy self-esteem.

Temperament

How the preschooler adapts to the new challenges of his or her life and meets developmental milestones may be determined by the child's temperament. An "easy" child with high adaptability will accept new activities and experiences easily. A "difficult" child is the exact opposite, will not make these transitions easily, and may be very loud and vocal regarding these changes. The "slow to warm up" child will react with some negativity and produce more positive responses with repeated exposures (Zuckerman, 1995).

Tantrums may not have totally disappeared by the time the child is 3; but by the time the child is 5, tantrums should be at a minimum. The best method to deal with tantrums is to first remain calm; second, to exit the scene if at all possible; third, to call a time-out to allow the child time to regain control; and, fourth, to attempt to verbalize empathy to the child. Using these techniques should help a parent or a nurse survive a tantrum.

If at all possible, the very best technique is to avert the tantrum altogether. This is easier to do now that the child has language skills, although not sufficient language skills to verbalize frustration. Preschoolers become easily overwrought when they are overly tired, hungry, and feeling helpless. Sometimes parents find keeping a log of their child's "meltdowns" (when they occurred and what caused them) helps discern a pattern and give the parents an opportunity to avert the tantrums by interceding before the child reaches a level of extreme frustration or helplessness.

Discipline and Limit Setting

At age 3, there are still signs of the "terrible twos," but by the time the child is 5 these signs are almost gone. During this transitional stage, many of the same tactics that were used when the child was a toddler are still very effective. Limits are needed to define acceptable behaviors. These limits will be tested in many ways. At the age of 3, the child is unable to verbalize many feelings and becomes frustrated. Frustration is exhibited by the child's acting out or perhaps by hitting. A child welcomes limit setting because this defines the boundaries that are expected. When boundaries are crossed, then disciplinary actions need to be taken. Positive redirection, guiding the child toward the accepted behavior verbally may be effective. If this is not effective, often health care professionals have recommended the use of time-outs (Chart 5–17).

Chart 5–17

Discipline Measures

- Set realistic limits.
- Be consistent with consequences.
- Do not be overly negative.
- Use positive redirection whenever possible—distracting the child toward a more positive action.
- Selectively ignore situations if the behavior is not a major issue; ignore it, but compliment and reward the more positive behavior.
- Use time-outs when appropriate (when the child is 18 to 24 months old)—1 minute of time out for each year of age. Time-outs should be used to allow both the adult and the child cooling off time.
- The use of corporal punishment (spanking, hitting) only reinforces violent behavior and may confuse the child.
- Childproof the home so there are less opportunities for the child to be in a situation where he or she could get into trouble.
- Provide the child with a good role model.

Time-outs can be an extremely effective tool for the parent to use for discipline. It is important the parent use it appropriately for it to be effective. A child should not stay in a time-out situation until he or she does what the parent wants done. A time-out is a method of teaching the child how to regain self-control and calm down (Fig. 5–10). Therefore, it is appropriate to use a time-out when a preschooler is hitting or screaming but not appropriate to use it when he or she will not pick up his or her toys. A time-out should be timed appropriately. It is more effective to have a short time-out than a very long one because a long time-out allows the child to redirect his or her attention from calming down to being resentful. The maximum time-out should be 1 minute for each year of age, but it may be necessary to start with much shorter time-outs (Christophersen, 1990). A time-out should end as soon as the child is calm.

Time-outs do not have to occur in the child's room; any location where the child is removed from activity and has an opportunity to become calm will do. The nurse or parent must explain to the child why the child is receiving the time-out.

Establishing a consistent routine for the child is very helpful in preventing a child from developing frustration when he or she is unprepared to move to a new activity. Preschoolers love to imitate their parents and other adults. Consistently setting a good example helps the preschooler understand the expectations. Using natural or logical consequences helps the child understand the association between an action and the result. Redirection of the child's behavior when the child is doing some-

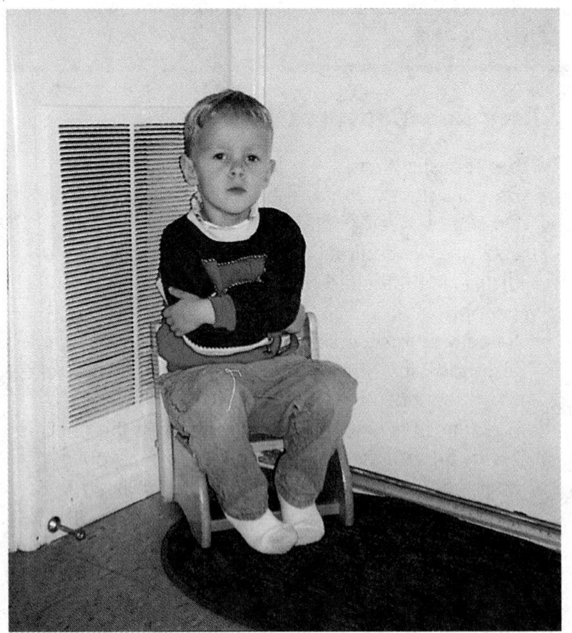

Figure 5–10
Time-outs are a disciplinary measure used to remove the child from an activity and allow him or her to calm down and consider what was wrong in his or her actions.

thing that is not appropriate is always one of the best ideas.

Sexuality

No parent should be surprised by the emerging awareness the child has of his or her body at the ages of 3 to 5. Parents may find preschoolers examining each other's genitalia and laughing about a "bathroom" joke. Any effort to reprimand the child or forbid these actions could lead to unwanted consequences at a later time because this will increase his or her guilt and remorse. It may be difficult for an adult not to act shocked at a 3-year-old masturbating, but a 3-year-old already has built-in guilt regarding this sexual exploration, and if it is handled in a punitive manner, it could lead to permanent consequences at a later time. Therefore, a more casual response on the part of the parent is recommended.

Children at this age have normal curiosity about their bodies. Questions that they ask should be answered simply and honestly. Preschoolers have active imaginations, and if they are told not to ask such questions, they will come up with their own answers, which may not be totally accurate. The parents should investigate the actual intention behind the "question." Most have heard the old joke about the child asking where he or she came from and the parents going into a long detailed explanation of childbirth only to discover the child wanted to know the town where he or she was born. It is important for the parents not to let their own bias or prejudice influence their answers. A 3-year-old girl is very curious about the "thing" that the 3-year-old boy has that she does not. And the 3-year-old boy is just as mystified that the girl can urinate without having a penis. When children ask about sexual issues, parents should use the correct terms for all the body parts, including genitalia. This is also a good time to introduce to the child the idea that certain body parts are private and should not be touched by "strangers" (Green, 1994).

Relationships

By the age of 3, the child is less egocentric and can actually interact with other children. These children start to play together rather than side by side. During this time, these children may also start to develop friends, and by the age of 4 they will have a very active social life and possibly even "best" friends. The child is also learning to use words instead of actions to work out situations, particularly disagreements.

At age 3, the child is still quite involved with fantasy and will drift from reality to fantasy often. Once the child is 4, there is more reality in his or her life. The child can distinguish that he or she is not a "superhero" or "storybook princess." He or she will want to please friends and show off to them.

During this age, the child initially identifies more with one parent than another as if to learn all he or she can about his or her parents one at a time. It is important that the parents understand that this "bonding" is a normal part of development, and the parents should not display disappointment or jealousy when it occurs (Fig. 5–11).

It is common for a child to have siblings at this age. It is important that the new older brother or sister be given the support needed during the time when much of the parental attention is going to the new sibling. When the preschooler does something to cause the newborn to cry, many parents discipline the preschooler and comfort the infant. This may lead to further jealousy on the part of the preschooler. It is better to investigate the reasoning behind the action and talk to the preschooler about alternatives. If it is jealousy, the parents need to look at the type of time they are spending with each child. One parent could spend quality time with the older child while the other parent cares for the newborn. Once the children are old enough to play together, it is best to allow them to work out differences themselves. It has been found that parents who do not take sides but assist the children in working out their differences can turn sibling rivalry into a positive advantage (Franck & Brownstone, 1991).

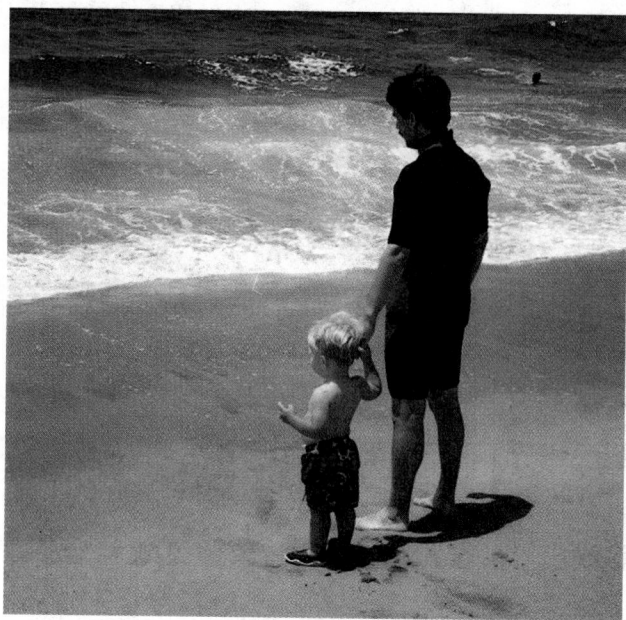

Figure 5–11
Bonding is promoted by allowing the preschooler to spend special time with each parent.

Fears

A preschooler is still learning to differentiate between reality and fantasy. With a very vivid imagination, a 3- to 5-year-old can have some very definite fears. These fears may be of real objects (e.g., dogs) as well as imaginary things (e.g., monsters in the dark). Ten of the most common fears found among preschoolers are dogs, insects, monsters, the dark, thunder, water, the moon, strangers, unfamiliar places, and clowns (Ryval, 1994).

When a child experiences a fear, it is important that the parent takes it seriously and comforts the child and then discusses the fear with the child. The parent should not belittle the fear and never use it as a threat, because this could exacerbate the fear. Sometimes the parent may need to use concrete actions to remove an imaginary fear, such as "monsterproofing" the bedroom (Green, 1994).

Most of these fears are a perfectly normal part of development and will disappear as the child matures. There are some situations that may exacerbate the fears, such as a move to a new house, divorce, death in the family, or a serious accident or illness. The child may ask a lot of repetitious questions. If the parent or the nurse is caught off guard and cannot think of an answer, one should be honest and state, "I need to think about that one." But one must be sure to get back to the child with a simple and concrete answer as soon as possible (Ucci, 1995). Sometimes reading books about the scary situations helps a child regain control and understand the situation is not to be feared. Another common technique is desensitization, when a fear is conquered by approaching it little by little. For example, a fear of water can be conquered by playing with water in a basin, then in a sink, then from the side of the tub (always with adult supervision) until enough confidence is obtained to get into the tub. If a fear becomes a phobia, then the health care team needs to be consulted.

Play

From ages 3 to 5, the preschooler develops much more control over gross and fine motor skills, allowing the child to play more actively. The preschooler is able to run, jump, hop, and possibly skip without as much concentration. Although he or she still may demonstrate some "stiffness" in certain areas, he or she can catch bounced balls, go up and down stairs, throw a ball overhand, swing, and climb. Manual dexterity is developing, and the child should be able to hold a crayon as an adult does and not in a fist position. The preschooler is full of energy and often "all over the place." Therefore, constant supervision is needed to prevent injuries.

Age-Appropriate Activities

By age 3, the child has developed the gross motor skills to jump, kick a ball, ride a tricycle, and walk upstairs with alternating steps, although he or she may still use the same feet to come down stairs. The child has understandable speech and a vocabulary of about 900 words and has some self-control and a beginning concept of time. Play needs to expand on these skills. The child should have a tricycle, large sturdy toys such as big blocks, active toys like a pounding bench, and musical toys that encourage rhythmic movement. The preschooler also likes show and tell, guessing games (because his or her memory is improving), and big-pieced jigsaw puzzles. At age 3, play is still egocentric, but the child is becoming more tolerant of play companions.

At the age of 4, the child is now able to jump on one foot, skip, walk down the stairs with alternating feet, and throw a ball overhand. His or her vocabulary has expanded to 1500 words, and he or she is using full sentences and can understand simple analogies. The preschooler is able to use scissors well, and his or her fine manual dexterity is improving. Construction toys, jigsaw puzzles, memory games, and fantasy play are favorites for this age (Fig. 5–12). The child will tell family secrets and exaggerate stories. He or she loves to listen to books and music. During ages 3 to 4 years, the child has an insatiable curiosity and will constantly ask "why" questions. These children are developing a sense of their world around them. The play is now becoming interac-

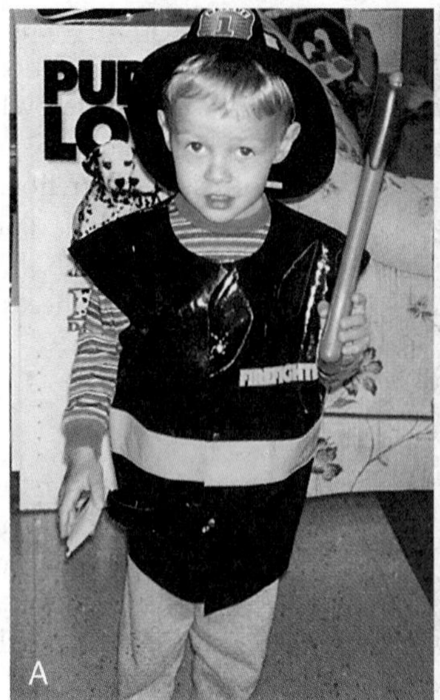

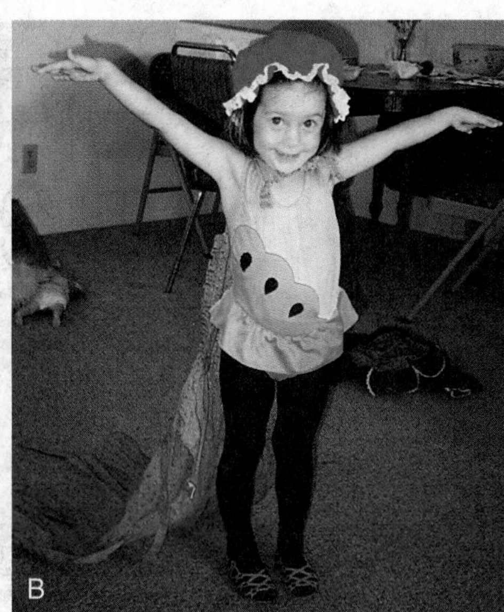

Figure 5–12
The preschooler enjoys dressing up and pretending to be different real and make-believe characters.

tive, and the child can obey limits but still does not have a sense of true right or wrong. Imaginary friends are a very common occurrence around this age.

When the child reaches 5, he or she has developed very good balance and coordination. This child can hop and skip on alternate feet, throw and catch a ball, dress himself or herself, and complete total self-care. Pretend play, playing with puppets, and dressing up in clothes are favorite games to be added to the list. The child has a speech capacity of about 2100 words and is almost 100% understood, even by strangers. This is the age when the child starts to mimic his or her parents and behave in a gender-specific fashion. The preschooler has developed some impulse control and is able to play in groups well and may be introduced to sports activities.

Generally, toys for the 3- to 5-year-olds need to be sturdy with no sharp edges or small pieces. Preschoolers learn many things by doing. It is an age when they will pretend to be a mother or father, doctor or nurse, which is why pretend play and dress up are so important. They have a lot of energy, and as their manual dexterity is improving they need large balls to bounce and tricycles to ride. Electrical toys should be avoided unless they are battery operated and used under adult supervision only. Toys should always be chosen according to the child's age and size and should be checked often to be sure that they have not become broken or developed a dangerous sharp edge.

Early Introduction of Organized Sport Activities

Most experts believe that children should be 7 to 8 years old before they engage in team sports. At the age of 5, the child has enough skills to start the rudimentary learning of certain sports skills, such as throwing a baseball or kicking a soccer ball. Generally, the 5-year-old has enough skill to actually participate in low-level sports such as T-ball, soccer, gymnastics, karate, bicycling, or dance.

An emphasis on physical fitness for children has emerged recently, even to the point that some experts believe exercise improves a child's performance in school. It is important for children to develop a healthy exercise habit in early years to improve their general well-being throughout their life. An introduction to sports may assist in this endeavor, because it is thought that sedentary children become sedentary adults.

Children will not benefit from sports unless they are suited for the sport in both age and temperament. The parent needs to work hard to find the right sport for the child and make the experience a positive one. A parent should not be as concerned with who won the game as with how the game was played—did everyone have a good time and play their best? Praising the child's efforts and not giving tips on how the child could have done something better or differently is more positive.

The child should be allowed to quit a sport he or she does not care for or finds too hard. Many parents believe that this allows the child to become a "quitter," but if the child has a very bad experience with a coach or someone on the team, there can be permanent repercussions and the child may never again participate in a sport. Remember that the main reason for sports is to have fun, get exercise, and enjoy the sport—all the other benefits come second.

Television

Today many parents and child care providers are realizing that television can be used in a constructive and positive manner. In recent years, television has received a bad reputation as being the "electronic baby sitter" and used as a substitute for education or playing. The child of today often views his or her first television program as an infant and by 3 years of age will have several regular favorite programs. Some of these programs can be very helpful by introducing colors or the alphabet in a creative stimulating way. Many of the programs that are on the television today are not appropriate for younger viewing (Shelov, 1993).

Young children believe that everything they see on television is real. They develop a distorted view of how to deal with problems because their favorite cartoon character is successful at using violence as a method to cope with anger and frustration. Cartoons contain much more violence than adult programming; therefore, the young child assumes that violence is then an acceptable option for them. Television can contribute to many psychological and physical problems because it lessens the creative ability of the child and can undermine the child's capacity for individual thinking.

It is almost impossible to ban television from a child's life, but parents should monitor carefully what a child is watching and how much a child watches. There are devices that can be used to limit a child's television watching such as "TV allowance" and "TV lockout," which are electronic devices that are installed between the television set and the cable input or the antenna to prevent unauthorized television watching (see Resources). It has been documented that children who watch a great deal of television are more likely to become obese (Shelov, 1993). As a general rule, 1 to 2 hours of quality television per day should be the limit. The parent should watch with the child to explain about the programs and commercials (not a part of the program, but an advertisement) and talk with the child about the program and what actually was the message. This helps develop critical viewing skills for the child and allows the child to make better choices about television programming when he or she is older (Chart 5–18).

Chart 5–18

Guidelines for Television and Video Viewing

- Limit children's television viewing time to no more than 1 to 2 hours per day.
- Parents should control which shows their children watch.
- Parents should watch television with their children, especially if the child is viewing a new show or a new videotape.
- If the child is allowed to watch television while the parent cooks dinner, showers, or engages in other activities in which the play activities cannot be adequately supervised, encourage parents to select videotapes for the child to view.
- Parents and daycare providers should familiarize themselves with high-quality low-cost videotapes that are available from the library or for purchase.
- Parents should not assume that videotapes produced by a major "family" entertainment company are appropriate for children of all age levels. Fighting scenes or death of a mother or father may be very disturbing for the young child.
- Parents should be encouraged to provide feedback to the networks regarding the quality of programming for children.

Daycare and Baby Sitters

If the child has not as yet attended daycare, now is the time many parents wish to enroll the child in preschool to prepare him or her for kindergarten. Perhaps the family has had a change in status and now the "at-home" parent must return to work. The same guidelines that were used for infants or toddlers should be used to choose a daycare center for a preschooler.

Usually by this age, the child has been left with a sitter or family member to allow the parents some time alone. When the parents are looking for a "permanent" sitter for when the parents need to go out or to work, care must be taken to select the appropriate individual to provide care for the child at home. An interview should take place and appropriate questions asked regarding the caregiver's approach to discipline, general child-rearing beliefs, providing appropriate activities for the child, and so on. The ideal candidate will have local references and be a person with whom the parents feel they can develop an open relationship.

Preparation for School

Preschools

If the child has not been enrolled in a group daycare center before, many parents choose at this age to enroll the child in either nursery school or preschool to prepare the child for kindergarten. Although these programs usually do not start academic learning, they do provide stimulation for the child in areas that are often neglected at home. They also provide the child an opportunity to get used to leaving home for a period of time and be exposed to group activities (Shelov, 1993) (Fig. 5–13). It is important to monitor the child's behavior when starting preschool because some children may be too young to adapt to a very structured environment and may actually show signs of stress. The program should fit the child's

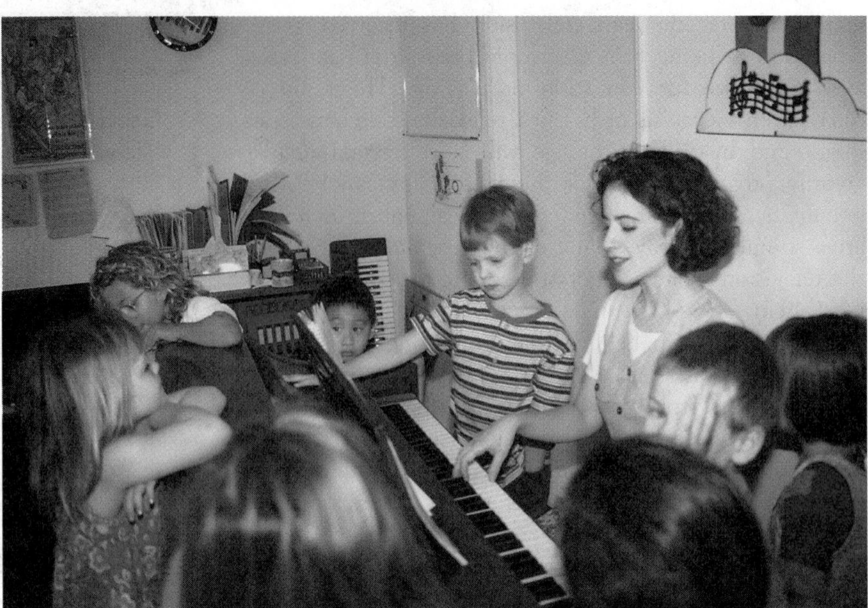

Figure 5-13
In the preschool setting, children are exposed to a variety of activities to enhance development of multiple intelligences.

temperament; for example, a child who is very active may need more play time (Ryval, 1994). One of the most important aspects of preschool is *not* to pressure the child to develop reading and writing skills. Usually the kind of learning that the children did to learn to read at age 3 or do math was not of help once the child was in school. The child had not developed the independent thinking skills that are needed to continue learning and therefore did not continue to excel. What also had been missed were the socialization skills that are needed to relate to other children.

To make good-byes easier, the parent should develop a morning routine, prepare as much as possible the night before, and do not rush in the morning. The rushing tends to cause stress for the parents, and the child feels the tension and may become upset when the parent leaves, thinking that he or she did something wrong. When the parent and child arrive at the center, the parent can spend a few minutes to settle the child in, perhaps read a book, start a group activity, and so on. The ultimate good-bye should be short—the parent should not linger as if unsure whether he or she should leave or not. If it is the first time the child and parent have been separated, it may take a few days of adjustment, such as spending more time the first day and decreasing it each day. Once the day is over, the parent should not be surprised if the child appears preoccupied and ignores him or her, or the child might burst into tears because he or she really missed the parent.

Preparing the Child for Kindergarten

Kindergarten is the child's first "real" school experience. Kindergarten is usually half or full day, and the child must be 5 years old by the "cutoff" date for the school district. The kindergarten is usually centered in the elementary school and focuses on social skills of the child and elementary academics. Before entrance into the kindergarten many school districts require testing to assess the child's readiness or to see if the child has the necessary skills to succeed (Franck & Brownstone, 1991).

The parents can prepare the child by talking to him or her about kindergarten. They can explain how it will be different from the preschool experience, with new children to meet and different things to "play" with. The school may expect the child to have more control, particularly if the child has already attended preschool. He or she will have more independence and more responsibilities (Shelov, 1993).

Injury and Illness Prevention

The preschooler is now old enough to be asked to wash his or her hands after toileting and when they are dirty from play. It is a good time to reenforce the concept of cleanliness. This is one of the most important ways to prevent illness. Another preventive area is to be sure the preschooler's immunizations are up to date. In many states, it is a requirement that certain immunizations be completed.

Injury Prevention

The home of the preschooler should be "babyproofed and toddlerproofed" and all of the considerations for infants and toddlers should still be in place. Preschoolers are slightly taller now and just as curious but more inventive and may stack furniture to get to items. Medications should be locked away, and the Poison Center number should always be near the telephone (Chart 5–19).

Appropriately fitting car seats and seat belts should always be used when the child is in the car or truck. The parent should not start the car unless everybody (including the parent) is buckled up. The preschooler will follow the parent's lead; if the parent buckles up, the preschooler will imitate this behavior. If the preschooler should unbuckle during the car ride, the parent should pull over and stop the car until the child is re-restrained.

The preschooler is now able to ride a tricycle and may be able to ride a bicycle by the time he or she is 5. Although many communities do not require the use of a helmet, it can reduce the risk of head injury by 85%. A proper-fitting helmet should be one of the first items purchased when purchasing a bicycle for a preschooler. The helmet should be approved by either SNELL (Snell Memorial Foundation) or American National Standards Institute (ANSI) because these are the two most rigorous testing agencies for bicycle helmets. The child needs to start learning the laws of the road. Preschoolers who ride bikes should understand that it is necessary to follow the same type of traffic laws cars do and go with the flow of traffic, signal when stopping or turning, and obey stop signs and stop lights. Light or reflective clothing is recommended when riding at dusk. Bikers should be encouraged to ride on paths as much as possible and avoid the streets, because they are eight times more likely to have an injury on a street than on a bike path.

Drowning is the most common injury among children younger than 4 years of age (Ellis, 1995). Although teaching preschoolers to swim helps, children should never be around water without adult supervision (Fig. 5–14). Swimming in partially covered pools should be avoided because the child may become trapped underneath the cover. When a pool is not in use, the stairs should be removed and at least a 5-foot-high fence around the pool with a latched and locked gate is usually required by local codes. When boating, every person in the craft is required to have a flotation device and be wearing it.

Young children have thinner and much more sensitive skin than adults. When they are to be out in the sun for a prolonged period of time, sunscreen of at least a sun-protective factor of 15 to 30 should be applied frequently and liberally. If it is hot, children should be sure to drink plenty of fluids because they tend to become dehydrated easily.

Preschoolers now have the memory capability to learn their own telephone numbers and addresses. If they are ever lost, they can assist the police in locating the parents.

Choking is another hazard that faces these independent little people. They are now eating table food but still have tiny windpipes that can easily be occluded. It is best to avoid hard candy, hot dogs (unless cut up), popcorn, and peanuts until the child is older.

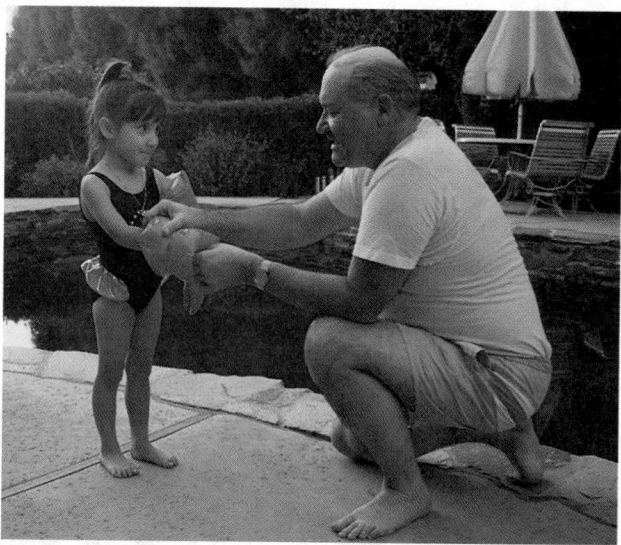

Figure 5–14
The preschooler should wear safety equipment while swimming and be accompanied by an adult.

Developmental Surveillance

Chart 5–20 is a summary of the developmental milestones that are accomplished in the preschool years. This information is useful to provide the nurse with direction for specific trigger questions that can be asked of the parent to determine the preschooler's developmental progress. Trigger questions should include concerns the parent may have regarding the child's overall development, how the child communicates and comprehends instructions, how the child walks, and whether the child is toilet trained. By the age of 3, the child should be able to ride a tricycle, kick a ball, balance on one foot, and feed and dress himself or herself (Green, 1994) (Table 5–8).

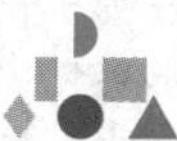

School-Age Children

Nutrition

By the age of 5 to 12 years, the child's diet should be a healthy combination of the foods made up from the food pyramid recommended by the Food and Drug Administration. Because this is the age when most food preferences are determined, it is important that the parents

Text continued on page 308

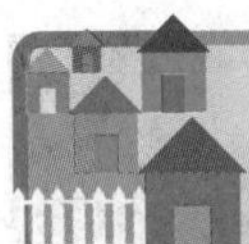

Chart 5–19
Community Care

Injury Prevention Guidelines for the Family with a Preschooler

Home Safety

- Establish and enforce consistent, explicit, and firm rules for safe behavior.
- Test smoke detectors to ensure that they work properly. Change batteries yearly.
- Keep all poisonous substances, cleaning agents, health and beauty supplies, medicines, and home improvement materials in a locked safe place. Have safety caps on all medications.
- Keep cigarettes, lighters, matches, and alcohol out of the child's sight and reach.
- Ensure that guns, if in the home, are locked up and that ammunition is stored separately. A trigger lock is an additional important precaution.
- Teach the child safety rules for the home. Conduct fire drills at home.

Play Safety

- Ensure that playgrounds are safe. Check for impact- or energy-absorbing surfaces under playground equipment.
- Teach the child about playground safety.
- Teach the child about sports safety, including the need to wear protective sports gear.

Water Safety

- Ensure that home and neighborhood swimming pools are enclosed by a four-sided fence with a self-closing, self-latching gate. Children should be supervised by an adult whenever they are in or around water.
- Ensure that the child wears a life vest if boating.
- Teach the child how to swim.
- Teach the child safety rules for swimming pools.

Car Safety

- Continue to use a car seat or a properly secured booster seat until the child weighs 60 lb or his or her head is higher than the back of the seat. The child weighing more than 60 lb should wear a seat belt at all times.
- Never leave the child alone in the car or in the house.

Safety with Others

- Keep the child away from cigarette smoke. Do not allow smoking in the home.
- Choose caregivers carefully. Discuss with them their attitudes about behavior in relation to discipline. Prohibit corporal punishment.
- Teach the child safety rules regarding interacting with strangers.
- Ensure that the child is supervised before and after school in a safe environment.

Outdoor Safety

- Put sunscreen on the child or teach the child how to put sunscreen on before he or she goes out to play.
- Supervise all play near streets or driveways.
- Teach the child pedestrian and neighborhood safety skills.
- Teach the child about safety rules for getting to and from school.
- Teach the child about safety rules for bicycles. Teach the correct signals for traffic safety.
- Ensure that the child wears a bicycle helmet when riding a tricycle or a bicycle with or without training wheels.

Emergency Preparation

- Keep your address and phone number posted near the phone.
- Keep list of emergency numbers (doctor, hospital, nearest neighbor, poison control center) near the phone.
- Keep a 1-oz bottle of syrup of Ipecac in the home and use as directed by the poison control center or health care provider.

Adapted from Green, M. (Ed.). (1994). *Bright futures: Guidelines for health supervision of infants, children, and adolescents.* Arlington, VA: National Center of Education in Maternal and Child Health. *Bright Futures* was supported by the Maternal and Child Health Bureau and the Medicaid Bureau.

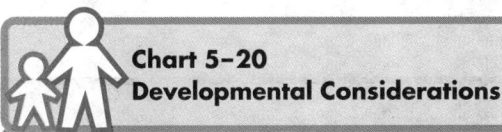

Chart 5–20
Developmental Considerations

Milestones of the Preschooler (3–6 Years)

Physical

All Preschoolers
Walks erect, swings arms
Rapid skeletal development taking place
Nutritional needs: 1400–1800 cal/day
Loses baby fat and tummy
Needs 12 hours of sleep a night

5 Yr
Three teeth decayed
Is one half of adult height

6 Yr
First permanent tooth erupts; begins loss of deciduous teeth
Brain is 90% adult weight
Needs 2000 cal/day

Sexual

All Preschoolers
Phallic Stage
Much genital manipulation and exploration (particularly with other children)
Shows intense attraction and love for parent of opposite sex (Oedipus conflict in males/Electra conflict in females)
Rivalry with parent of opposite sex
Castration anxiety; mutilation fears
Intrusive procedures threaten body integrity
Masturbation

Language

3–4 Yr
Uses four to five words in sentences with adult sense of syntax
Names body parts; recognizes some colors
Talks fluently and listens
Comprehends "cold, tired, hungry" or at least two of these three words
900-word vocabulary
Repeats sentences of three to four words

4–5 Yr
Knows opposites analogies
Recognizes most colors
1500-word vocabulary
Knows simple songs
Tells exaggerated stories
Questioning at a peak
Asks permission
Relates experiences and tells about activities in sequential order
Counts to 30

5–6 Yr
Can identify all coins
Defines words
Knows composition of objects
2100-word vocabulary
Can repeat sentence of 10 syllables or more
Knows names of days, weeks, months
Can follow commands in succession
Recognizes shapes

Vision

3 Yr
20/30 vision
Copies a circle
Color vision fully intact

4 Yr
Cooperates with Snellen testing
Copies crosses
Maximum potential for developing amblyopia

5 Yr
Recognizes colors
Copies a square

6 Yr
Full visual maturity achieved

Chart continued on following page

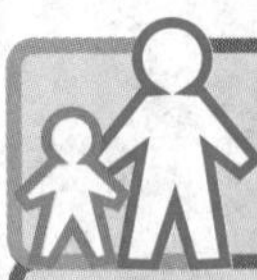

Chart 5–20
Developmental Considerations

Milestones of the Preschooler (3–6 Years) *Continued*

Hearing

All Preschoolers
Cooperates on systematic audiometric tests
Clues to hearing deficit include volume of television program, whether child responds to you, audiometric test results, intelligible speech continuing at age 5

Gross Motor

3 Yr
Hops on one foot
Rides tricycle
Can undress self in most situations
Catches soft object with both hands
Jumps from low step

4 Yr
Skips
Balances on one foot for 5 seconds (two of three tries)
Catches bounced ball (two of three tries)
Dresses without supervision
Walks downstairs using alternating feet
Twists upper body while holding feet in one place

5–6 Yr
Walks backward heel to toe (two of three tries)
Balances on one foot for 10 seconds (two of three tries)
Skips and hops on alternating feet
Throws and catches ball well
Jumps rope
Jumps from height of 12 inches and lands on toes
Enjoys participating in sports activities
Rides a bike

Fine Motor

3–4 Yr
Picks longer line (three of three tries)
Begins to use blunt scissors
Strings large beads on shoe lace

4–5 Yr
Ties shoe laces
Draws a man with three to six parts
Copies a square
Uses scissors

5–6 Yr
Draws a man with six parts
Copies a triangle
Dresses without supervision
Can print letters or numbers

Play

All Preschoolers
Parallel/associative play
Defines own rules
Cooperative play
Joins in play with others
Plays interactive games
Imitative play
Dramatic play
Solitary play
Play with parents
Onlooker play
Imaginary playmates

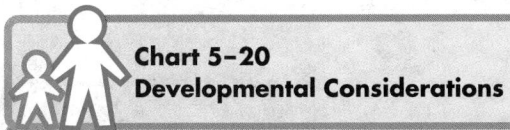

Chart 5–20
Developmental Considerations

Milestones of the Preschooler (3–6 Years) *Continued*

Cognitive

All Preschoolers

Preoperational

Egocentrism

Omnipotence (inability to distinguish between one's own perception and that of someone else)

Thinking is concrete and tangible; becomes more intuitive toward end of this stage

"Transductive reasoning" from a particular event to another event

Animism

Magical thinking

Artificialism (all things are "made for a purpose")

Irreversibility (cannot backtrack steps in a thinking pattern)

Centration (inability to consider several aspects of the situation simultaneously)

Trial vs. error

Primitive concepts of space, time, and causality

Uses memory

Death is reversible, a temporary restriction, departure, or sleep

Juxtaposition—no relationship between stated ideas

Social

All Preschoolers

Separates easily from mother

Magical thinking

When permitted freedom, creativity is enhanced

Many fears that are very real and logical to the child

Interpersonal

All Preschoolers

Primitive sense of body image begins

Initiative vs. guilt

Emotional

All Preschoolers

Emotional thinking

Can understand that feelings are connected ("mad because")

Added logic to expression of ideas dealing with complex intentions, wishes, and feelings

Moral/Spiritual

All Preschoolers

Moral

Stage 3: Conventional Level

Desires to please others

Seeks approval or attention-getting through behaviors

Social concern

Spiritual

Stage I: Intuitive/Projective

Learns to imitate the religious affect and behavior of parents

Mimics religious gestures although does not comprehend meaning

Cannot separate feelings from intellect

Formulates imagined descriptions of God (angel, friend child can communicate with)

Table 5–8
Health Supervision Interventions: Preschooler

	3 Yr	4 Yr	5 Yr	6 Yr
Physical Examination	X	X	X	X
Growth Parameters (height, weight)	X	X	X	X
Immunizations		X‡	X‡	X‡
Assessment of High-Dose Lead Exposure	X	X	X	X
Tuberculin Test	X*	X*§	X*§	X*§
Assessment of Risk for Hyperlipidemia	X	X	X	X
Vision Screening	X†	X	X	X
Hearing Screening	X	X	X	X
Blood Pressure Screening	X	X	X	X

* Annual test if certain risk factors are present.
† Rescreen in 6 months if child is uncooperative.
‡ Administer between ages 4 and 6 before school entry to bring immunization status up to date.
§ Perform once between age 4 and 6 before school entry.
From Green, M. (Ed.). (1994). *Bright futures: Guidelines for health supervision of infants, children, and adolescents.* Arlington, VA: National Center for Education in Maternal and Child Health. *Bright Futures* was supported by the Maternal and Child Health Bureau and the Medicaid Bureau.

offer the child a wide variety of foods. Family food habits influence children the most during this period of time.

The amount of food that the child eats is still not in the equivalent amounts to an adult portion (see Table 5–5). Monitoring the child's weight occasionally assists in determining whether the child is getting an appropriate amount of food. Overestimating the amount of food a child needs is detrimental because the child could be encouraged to overeat. Obesity is a common nutritional problem in children, with prevalence estimated to range between 25% and 30% of prepubertal children and between 18% and 25% of adolescents (Keller & Stevens, 1996). The health care professional can guide the parent in assisting the child to make correct choices of healthy foods and to stay away from an overabundance of salt or sugar consumption. With growth spurts and extra activity between the ages of 7 and 10, both boys and girls consume between 1600 and 2400 calories per day. Because of the difference in body size, boys may require more calories than girls (Shelov, 1993).

If a child is eating a well-balanced diet, the American Academy of Pediatrics does not recommend the use of vitamin supplements. All the nutrients a child needs should be coming from the food eaten. The most recent recommendation is to introduce a low-fat diet consisting of less than 30% fat at this age. This also helps the child start a lifelong habit of healthy eating.

As the child enters school and begins eating lunch at school, it is difficult to monitor what the child is eating away from home. Many children participate in a school lunch program or may "brown bag" their lunch from home. If the child is bringing a lunch from home, it should be varied, with interesting tasty foods that the child likes.

School cafeteria lunches have been a focus in the media because it is believed they do not have enough healthy choices for children. The National School Lunch Act has stated that the lunches provided by schools contain one third of the daily recommended amounts of key nutrients and include a meat (or meat substitute), vegetable, fruit, bread, and milk. The law does not address issues of freshness of food, cooking methods, or fat content. One of the disadvantages with school lunch programs is that the children may pass up the school lunch altogether if it is not appealing and buy a "vending machine" lunch or trade with friends for non-nutritious choices. One of the successful strategies offered by schools today is teaching children about healthy food at an early grade level and eliciting their help in making appropriate decisions.

This is also an ideal age to encourage children to assist with the preparation of meals (Fig. 5–15). Adult supervision is needed when the child is 5 to 8 years old; but by the time the child is 12, the child should be able to prepare a simple meal without assistance. Allowing children to prepare their own school lunches encourages them to make choices of foods that they will eat and not discard or trade.

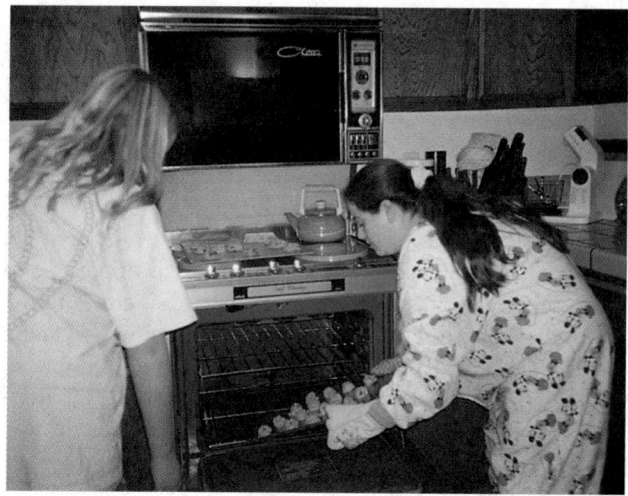

Figure 5–15
Learning to cook can be an enjoyable activity for the school-age child.

Oral Health

Until the child is 7 to 10 years old, the child may need assistance with the actual brushing of teeth. If the child is developing good oral hygiene habits, he or she does not run the risk of developing dental caries and problems that cause premature tooth loss. If the child has lost a tooth prematurely, space retainers may be used to maintain the appropriate alignment of the teeth while waiting for the eruption of the permanent tooth.

At the twice-a-year dental checkups, the dentist will monitor the child for the placement of teeth and may recommend an appointment with an orthodontist if the dentist discovers some abnormalities. Earlier orthodontic treatment is becoming the trend, because it has been proven that if the problem is treated earlier, the child may need less treatment because the teeth are easier to move. It is also believed that early treatment reduces the risk of relapse. If the child does need orthodontic intervention, there are several issues that the health care professional can help the parent determine. The child must be compliant with the care that is needed for the braces (e.g., cleanliness) and also have a good rapport with the orthodontist and staff because they will be seeing each other at least every month for about 2 years. In some cases, there is no problem with waiting to have the orthodonture work done, and it is not uncommon to have more than one opinion.

At the age of 5½ to 6, the 6-year molars appear. These are the first of the permanent teeth to appear and usually do not cause the same problems as teething does in an infant. Many parents are not even aware that they are erupting. At the age of 6 to 7, the first of the primary teeth begin to be replaced by permanent teeth, starting with the central incisors. At 7 to 8 years old, the lateral incisors develop. The primary bicuspids are lost at 10 to 11 years, and by 12 years old the permanent bicuspids erupt. With the eruption of these teeth, there is not the same amount of fussiness or discomfort as the infant appeared to experience. It is important that if the primary tooth is lost before the eruption of the permanent tooth that the dentist be consulted for the possibility of the placement of a spacer to allow the teeth to remain in their optimal position.

Hygiene and Personal Care

Sleep

During the school-age years, sleep disturbances are a relatively uncommon occurrence. The child should be averaging 8 to 10 hours of sleep per night, although this can vary considerably and still be considered a normal range.

The most common sleep disturbances at this age can be traced to several origins: a general behavioral problem, separation anxiety, wanting to have special time with a parent without sibling interruptions, having an altered sleep cycle that may need some adjustment, or attention deficit hyperactivity disorder, in which children have great difficulty settling down at bedtime and tend to sleep less than their counterparts of the same age. Some other causes of sleep disturbances can be nightmares, fears of the dark, night terrors, or sleepwalking. Although the child may not wake fully with some of the these problems, the child may be less alert in the morning. Most of these sleep disturbances are usually limited as to length and resolve without intervention (Shelov, 1993). If a child should continue to have sleep disturbances, a pediatrician should be consulted in regard to interventions.

Physical Fitness

Physical fitness helps start healthy behavioral habits that will allow a child to be a healthy and fit adult. What starts out as fun play can set up a lifetime of healthy activities for an adult to pursue to remain fit and healthy. From 5 to 8 years old, children want to have fun and be with peers. An introduction of team sports that are loosely structured and not too aggressive toward winning are good options. From years 8 to 10, a variety of sports, both team and individual, are a good way for a child to find something that he or she enjoys (Fig. 5–16). After age 10, with the advancement of puberty and fragile egos, it is necessary to match sports to the physical and emotional development of the child.

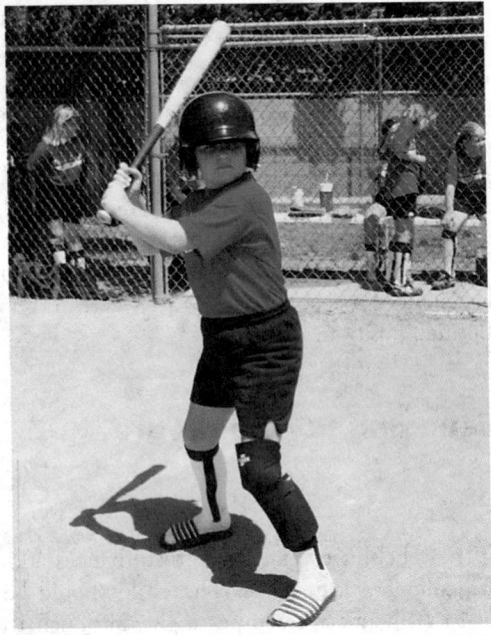

Figure 5–16
Girls and boys enjoy participating in team sports and can benefit from the physical activity.

Promotion of Social Competence

Personality and Temperament

As discussed earlier, the temperament of the child, whether "easy," "difficult," or "slow to warm up," assists in determining how a child adjusts to the environment and will influence his or her personality. The "difficult" child is usually the child that is most challenging to live with. The nurse may need to assist the parents in determining good strategies to use when dealing with a "difficult child." The nurse can coach the parents to remain neutral or objective in emotional situations and not take the behavior that is being exhibited personally. Are their expectations realistic? Parents need to learn to attempt to anticipate high-risk situations and strategize how to effectively deal with them to avoid potential disasters. Parents may need to take into consideration their own temperaments when dealing with "difficult" children. Health care professionals may find it necessary to counsel the parent to adjust his or her behavior as well (Shelov, 1993).

This is also the period of childhood when individuality is being experienced at much higher levels. By the time the child is 7, there is less of a sense of globalness and the child is more earthbound and becomes more introverted. By the time the child is 9, he or she is much more aware of the reality of the world and also the faults of parents. At this age, the child is independent and critical and may actually feel alienated by parents. The common statement of the day may be "you are not my boss" or "you can't make me" as the child tests the limits and boundaries. Setting fair, firm limits with consistency is the most successful strategy to utilize. This is a critical stage for the child who needs mature, compassionate adults to be role models because these adults can be a positive influence on the child's future life.

As the child reaches the age between 7 and 14, emotions run rampant. The child has vivid, intense, and overstated emotions that almost run the child rather than the opposite. At this stage, adults must be careful not to feed into the child's feelings of self-criticism, because the child is very vulnerable. A stimulating environment where a child can invent, create, experiment, and "grow" builds self-confidence in the child.

Relationships

During the school-age years, making friends is one of the most important accomplishments. The school-age child is able to form complex relationships, and communication has developed to a point that the child can share feelings and understand spatial concepts of time. During this period, peers become very important to the child (Fig. 5–17). A child may develop a "best" friend that usually complements himself or herself and provides a person with whom he or she can feel completely comfortable (Shelov, 1993). Parents may feel left out of their child's life, but health care professionals can assist the parents to understand that it is necessary for the child to differentiate himself or herself from parents and siblings. The nurse can help a parent develop a good relationship with the child by encouraging the parent to be a "sounding

Figure 5–17
In the early school-age years, same-sex activities are customary.

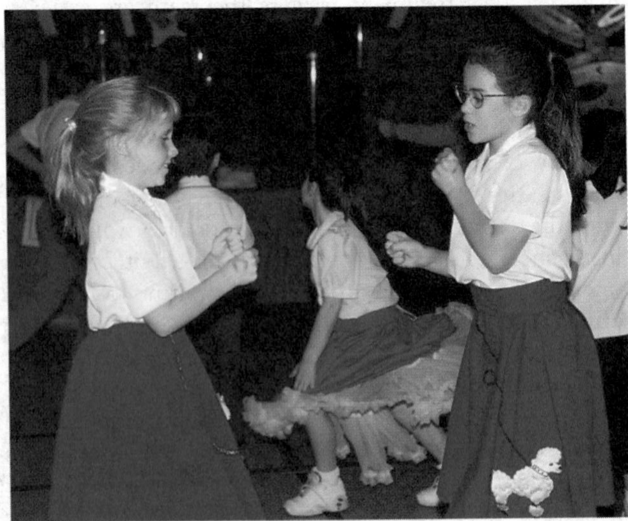

board," by building in extra time to talk, for instance before bed, or by having the child accompany the parent while he or she is running errands in the car.

Sexuality

The child actually starts the process of learning about sex as a toddler. By the time the child is 7 to 12 years old, the child has a great curiosity about sex. This is a critical time for the discussion to start about sex and should include the social implications as well as the biological factors. It is important that the parent be involved in delivering the information about sexuality to the child so that the parental values can be communicated. Parents may be uncomfortable discussing different aspects of sex education with the child and may seek the health care professional's advice in regard to how to answer the questions presented to them. If a parent has established open lines of communication about sex from an early age, it is easier for the child to approach the parent with questions and not utilize peers for this information. Parents should be encouraged to use correct terminology of the sexual organs and simple but honest explanations of the functions of the body parts and the actions that cause pregnancy, for example. Many parents believe that open, frequent discussions about sex cause a teenager to become promiscuous, whereas actually the opposite is true. Usually teenagers have intercourse as a result of social and peer pressure and with appropriate information may actually delay having sex.

The onset of puberty takes place during this period of childhood, occurring in boys at about age 13 to 15 years and in girls as early as age 9 to 16 years. As the children become more aware of their changing bodies and as they experience hormonal changes (see Chart 5–26), many questions arise.

Menarche usually occurs at about 12 years of age, with a range of 9 to 16 years of age not being abnormal. This is a symbolic achievement of womanhood in a young girl's life, yet very often it is not discussed openly nor is the girl given accurate information. Nurses are traditionally perceived as the group to be the resource for this information because male physicians may not be comfortable discussing these issues with a young "woman" nor are they perceived as having the time to spend answering questions. Girls will have questions about exercise, hygiene, sanitary protection, and pain. Single male parents may feel the need to find a female to discuss these issues with their daughters, but many male parents are fully capable of giving the information and having a unique bond with their daughters.

Another area of concern for girls is the formation of their breasts. A girl may feel very self-conscious about the development of her breasts. She may also be concerned if they are asymmetrical or "lumpy." The girl needs to be reassured that this is normal during this stage. Young girls may also feel the need to camouflage their appearance by wearing large, loose-fitting clothing to mask the development. Parents should be encouraged to be supportive and understanding with the changes that are occurring, both physically and emotionally.

As boys enter puberty, they usually lag slightly behind girls. The girls may for a short period of time be taller and show more traits of puberty than boys (see Chapter 4 and the section on Tanner staging). Boys experience voice changes (cracking of the voice), growth spurts, and possibly "wet dreams" or spontaneous erections. Neither the spontaneous erection nor the wet dreams (nocturnal seminal emissions) means that the child is sexually active or having overactive sexual thoughts. Parents may need to be instructed that these occurrences are spontaneous and the child is not doing anything to cause these ejaculations or erections.

During this period of time, the child may become very modest and self-conscious. Adults need to avoid even good-natured teasing because this may cause embarrassment as the child becomes extremely sensitive about his or her body image.

Activities (Play)

Up to now most of the play activities that the child has engaged in have been fantasy play that has very few structured rules. Now the child is becoming very aware of the need for rules and structure. This need for rituals and rules translates well into team sports and other activities that have rules and structure. The group the child participates with may actually develop very rigid and outlandish rules for some group games.

Team play is a more complex version of group play and an ideal time for the child to learn the importance of being a team player and achieving goals set for the team, not just the individual. They also learn how to work cooperatively in a group to achieve a goal, which can later be transferred to other situations. They learn about competition and the importance of attaining the goal. Through these accomplishments they develop self-esteem, physical skills, and improved manual dexterity. Another focus of the ritualistic behavior is collecting. The school-age child may develop the desire to collect all sorts of matching and nonmatching items. School-age children have a greater ability to concentrate and participate in self-initiated quiet activities that challenge their cognitive skills, such as reading and playing computer and board games (Fig. 5–18).

Sports

Because physical fitness is an important element of a healthy lifestyle, parents should be encouraged to have

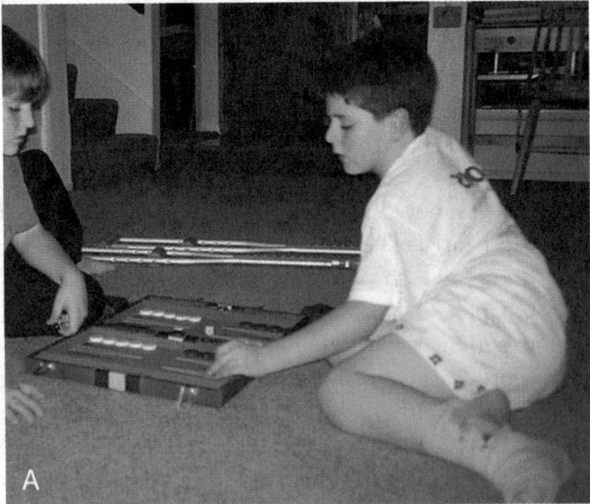

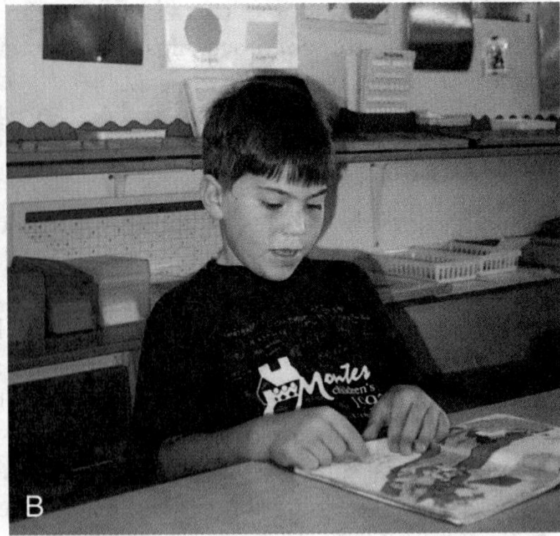

Figure 5–18
A, Board games can be used to sharpen the child's cognitive skills. *B*, Reading should be encouraged in both school and home settings.

the child participate in sports activities. The American College of Sports Medicine recommends that health care professionals actively promote physical fitness in children. School-age children should be encouraged to participate in 20 to 30 minutes of vigorous physical activity at least three times per week. These should be activities that can be easily incorporated into the child's routine, that the child enjoys, and that could be continued into adulthood. These activities can include bicycling, walking, running, or swimming. Also team sports such as baseball, basketball, soccer, or football allow the child to develop group play skills. These can be introduced as early as at 6 to 8 years old and be continued through adolescence into adulthood.

This is an ideal age to introduce musical instrument instruction. The child has the manual dexterity, attention span, and the rule rigidity to allow this experience to be a positive one.

School

Even if the child has attended preschool, kindergarten is a big step in any child's life. Parents may approach the physician or the nurse to determine whether the child is "ready" for kindergarten.

To be ready for school, a child should be able to play well with others, be toilet trained, have fine manual dexterity to use a crayon or fasten buttons, be able to sit quietly and listen to a story, and have enough memory skills to memorize his or her name and address and phone number (Shelov, 1993). School personnel may conduct other readiness testing that determines academic readiness, but they will also be looking at fine and gross motor skills and attention span. None of these "tests" is infallible, and the child who may not do well when tested still may be very successful in the kindergarten environment, particularly with the right teacher.

One of the best teachers that a child can have is his or her parent. There are many things that a parent can do at home to enhance a child's learning skills for school, such as allowing the child to assist in the kitchen to learn fractions (e.g., using ¼ cup, ½ cup), giving the child the opportunity to add and subtract the money in a wallet or coin purse, and allowing the child to read an article from a child's magazine, a recipe, or a billboard to enhance reading skills.

Although parents may be aware their child is unusually early in some of the developmental milestones or possesses extraordinary capabilities (e.g., early advanced language development, unusually retentive memories), it is usually the school system that identifies a child as being potentially gifted. The definition of giftedness varies with each source. Initially it was thought that simply a high IQ (top 1%) defined a child as gifted. More recently, the definition has been expanded to include three areas: an above-average intelligence, a high level of creativity, and a high level of task commitment (Schechter, 1994). Occasionally, children's academic or behavioral problems may be attributed to the boredom the child experiences with the school curriculum. Many children who have been identified as gifted often have difficulties relating with peers owing to the contrast between their chronological age and their intelligence. Also siblings who are not gifted often feel inferior to their gifted brother or sister. School often provides testing for the child and offers special programs to enhance learning capabilities and expand areas of potential. Parents and teachers often find it challenging dealing with gifted children because they often have the ability to question traditional facts and conclusions and have an insatiable curiosity that can be irritating to authority figures. Although gifted children need to be challenged in their areas of excellence, they should be offered the basic instruction that all children receive, although possibly to an accelerated degree (Chart 5–21).

Once the child has started school and is attending on a regular basis, each new year should be approached with a positive feeling (see Fig. 5–18*B*). The parents should not allow any negative experiences from a previous school year or from their own personal background to influence the child's expectations of the new year.

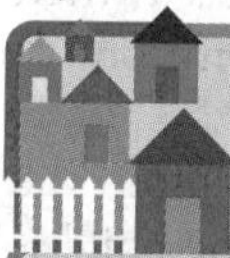

Chart 5–21
Community Care

Responsibilities of the Health Care Team to Gifted Children and Their Families

Identification

- Awareness of margins of normal development and appreciation of markers of developmental precocity
- Identifying resources within the community to help evaluate gifted children
- Helping children and families understand the concept of giftedness

Management

Home

- Helping parents prevent creating excessive vulnerability or privilege in the identified child
- Helping family deal with siblings of identified child
- Helping family avoid overstimulation of child
- Awareness of enrichment and supportive resources in the community

School

- Advocacy of appropriate educational resources in the school system
- Awareness that gifted children may have behavioral and learning problems that require intervention
- Fostering communication between the school and the family

Source: Schechter, N. (1994). The gifted child. In S. Parker & B. Zuckerman (Eds.), *Behavioral and developmental pediatrics* (pp. 165–167). Boston: Little, Brown & Company.

Homework

Homework is a natural consequence of school. Homework usually starts at the third-grade level at about 15 to 30 minutes several times per week, increasing to up to 2 hours each night by the time the child is in high school. Homework should not be a power struggle between the parent and the child. Parents need to allow the child to complete the homework, with assistance and support. Good homework habits should be developed at an early age, and the child should have a specific time, place, and tools to complete the assignments. The decision as to where and when a child does homework needs to be determined by the family dynamics. Some children do best by doing the homework immediately after school, whereas others have too many distractions and do better when they do it after dinner. Both are acceptable, as long as the child develops the habit of completing the homework.

Parents may seek advice from the health care professional if there are school problems particularly involving the lack of completed homework. The health care professional should encourage the parent to allow the child to suffer the natural consequences of not doing homework. This need not be a power struggle at home. The parent can be supportive and open and show interest but not insist the homework be completed perfectly or argue with the child about homework. The professional can encourage the parents to meet with the school personnel regarding the problems of homework, working with the school and coordinating with the teacher to develop delineation of responsibilities for the school and the child. Parents need to be encouraged not to do their child's homework and to avoid criticizing the child about homework.

After-School Care

A parent is usually somewhat relieved when a child starts school on a full-day schedule. If the parent has not been working, now is an opportunity to return to work, but usually school is 5 to 6 hours long and not the 8 to 10 hours that a parent needs for work and to travel to and from work. Until a child is 12 or 13 years old, a child should continue to have some after-school care. Latchkey kids (children who are unsupervised at home after school at an early age) are becoming a more common occurrence in today's society. Children younger than the age of 13 usually do not have the maturity to make decisions in an emergency situation. Some children may have the skills needed to make these decisions as young as 8, but legal authorities usually do not allow a parent to leave the child in an unstructured environment until the age of at least 12 or 13. Many children who are allowed to be home after school by themselves may develop fears or anxieties because they feel isolated and lonely. Nurses should be aware of the resources in the community to assist families in locating programs to care for children after school. The nurse may also be helpful in assisting the family to develop rules for when the child must stay at home alone, such as locking doors, never opening the door to strangers, and having a neighbor or close friend available by phone if there is a question or problem (Chart 5–22). The child should be taught how to use the telephone, and a list of emergency phone numbers should be posted next to the telephone, including the home address and telephone number, because it is easy for a child to forget his or her own address and phone number in an emergency.

Fears

During the school-age years, the most common fears are still some of the same fears experienced to a lesser degree as a preschooler, such as a fear of darkness, separation, and injury. Some newer fears that are now experienced have to do with failure at school and peer relationships (see Table 5–6). These fears intensify and diminish during the period of middle childhood. This is a normal part of childhood, and most fears will subside on their own. Yet, some fears may become so persistent as to become phobias. Many parents may seek professional assistance to determine whether a fear has become a phobia (when a fear reaches abnormal proportions and becomes irrational).

Nurses can assist parents in dealing with the fears of the child by understanding which fears are normal at each age and encouraging the parent to use sympathy, empathy, and open communication to allow the child to express the fears. The child should never be ridiculed or forced to "be brave," because these techniques could backfire and cause the fear to increase rather than diminish and ultimately become a true phobia.

Injury and Illness Prevention

During the middle childhood years, as the child increases his or her independence, the potential for accidents is also increased. The child does not have the maturity to accurately judge speeds or distances and may also be compelled to play unsafe "games" with matches or loaded firearms on a "dare." Most of these accidents are preventable, and with a little forethought the child will not be at risk for lifelong injuries or death.

By implementing simple routines and enforcing rules, children can be kept reasonably safe. The parent should insist on the use of seat belts when the child is in the car and/or the use of the appropriate type of car seat. As the child grows and weighs more than 60 lb (some jurisdictions may have lower weight requirements) or head is higher than the back of the seat, the child should be using a regular adult seat belt without a booster seat. Doors should be locked at all times, and a child should never be allowed to be alone in the car.

Crossing the street may also be a challenge for the 6- to 10-year-old who is still unable to judge the speed of an oncoming car or the distance it is from the intersection. Adult supervision should be used until the child is older than 10.

The bicycle is one of the most popular "toys" of children aged 6 to 12. Mastering the skill of riding a two-wheeled bicycle means independence, a mode of independent transportation, and freedom. Because bicycles can pose serious risks to safety, a child must learn the rules of the road and abide by them. Most of the accidents between bicycles and automobiles are caused when a child does not obey the rules and darts out in front of a car or rides against traffic.

A properly fitted bicycle helmet that can absorb the impact of a crash should be worn at all times the child is on the bicycle. Many communities are enacting laws that require all bicyclists to wear helmets.

Helmets are one of the safety elements that should also be used when a child is using a skateboard or skates. In addition, the child should have protective knee and elbow pads as well as wrist guards to prevent serious injury during falls off the skateboard or skates or during collision with another object.

Although the number one cause of death in middle childhood is accidental injuries, the second most common cause of death is drowning. As parents see the child mature, they may have more confidence in allowing the child more independence as they overestimate the child's survival skills. The child must have adult supervision whenever he or she is around water. Swimming instruction from a qualified instructor is of primary importance but should not be done in lieu of adult supervision. There should be very specific rules enforced whenever a child is to be around water such as never swimming alone, no diving unless the depth of the water is determined, and/or wearing a personal flotation device when riding in a boat.

School-age children are often captivated by guns. In television and movies, handgun violence does not appear as devastating as it actually is. Children should never be allowed access to firearms. Even with instruction, they are not mature enough to handle a potentially lethal weapon. A loaded gun should never be kept in a car or a home. The gun should be kept unloaded and the ammunition in another location under lock and key.

Even with all these precautions, many children are allowed access to firearms through friends or family members. The parents must have discussions with their children in regard to tactics to use if they are approached by a friend with a gun or encounter a gun in another home or at school. They should be encouraged to stay away

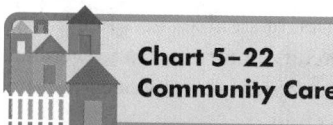

Chart 5–22
Community Care

Injury Prevention Guidelines for the Family with a School-Age Child

General Safety

- Reinforce important safety considerations. Anticipate that the child may make errors in judgment because he or she is trying to imitate peers.
- Anticipate providing less supervision.

Home Safety

- Establish and enforce consistent, explicit, and firm rules for safe behavior.
- Test smoke detectors to ensure that they work properly. Change batteries yearly.
- Lock up poisons, matches, and electrical tools.
- Ensure that guns, if in the home, are locked up and that ammunition is stored separately. A trigger lock is an additional important precaution.
- Reinforce the child safety rules for the home, including what to do when home alone. Discuss visitors, not tying up the telephone for long periods of time, and what to do in case of fire or other emergencies. Conduct fire drills at home.

Activity Safety

- Reinforce sports safety with the child, including the need to wear protective sports gear.
- Teach the child to avoid high noise levels, especially when using music headsets.

Water Safety

- Ensure that home and neighborhood swimming pools are enclosed by a four-sided fence with a self-closing, self-latching gate. Children should be supervised by an adult whenever they are in or around water.
- Teach the child how to swim.
- Reinforce safety rules for swimming pools.

Car Safety

- The child should wear a seat belt in the car at all times.

Safety with Others

- Keep the child away from cigarette smoke. Do not allow smoking in the home.
- Teach the child safety rules regarding interacting with strangers. Ensure that the child's school curriculum has information on how to deal with strangers.
- Ensure that the child is supervised before and after school in a safe environment.

Outdoor Safety

- Ensure that the child puts on sunscreen before he or she goes outside for long periods of time.
- Reinforce the child's knowledge of neighborhood safety skills.
- Reinforce child safety rules for bicycles, including use of proper traffic signals.
- Ensure that the child wears a bicycle helmet when riding a bicycle.
- Do not allow the child to operate a power lawn mower or motorized farm equipment.

Emergency Preparation

- Keep your address and phone number posted near the phone.
- Keep list of emergency numbers (doctor, hospital, nearest neighbor, poison control center) near the phone.

Adapted from Green, M. (Ed.). (1994). *Bright futures: Guidelines for health supervision of infants, children, and adolescents.* Arlington, VA: National Center of Education in Maternal and Child Health. *Bright Futures* was supported by the Maternal and Child Health Bureau and the Medicaid Bureau.

from it, not to touch it, and to report it to their parent. Frequent discussions with children about what is being observed on television in comparison to reality of life will help them understand that guns are not toys and need to remain with adults (see Chart 5–22).

Developmental Surveillance

Chart 5–23 presents a summary of the developmental milestones that are accomplished in the school-age years. This information is useful to provide the nurse with direction for specific trigger questions that can be asked of the parent to determine the child's developmental progress. Trigger questions should also include school performance as well as the usual concerns regarding general developmental issues. Health supervision interventions for this age group are listed in Table 5–9.

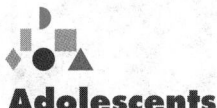

Adolescents

Nutrition

Within the next 7 years, the adolescent will have a growth rate that is second only to that of an infant. Typically, the adolescent's weight doubles and height increases by about 25%. Heredity, nutrition, and general health must be taken into account as influences on the predominant stature for the child.

Obesity (body weight more than 20% above the ideal weight) is of some concern at this age. Preserving self-esteem is crucial at this age, and obesity carries with it a stigma in today's society. Families should be encouraged not to use food as a power struggle and to be flexible about the personal choices of the teenager. The teenager should be receiving a balanced diet based on the food pyramid with a caloric intake of 1500 to 2400 calories, although some athletes may need substantially more. Dietary counseling is recommended to prevent the obese teenager from becoming an obese adult because this is associated with increased mortality and morbidity from heart disease and other disorders.

Teenagers are growing quickly and using enormous amounts of energy. This keeps them hungry most of the time, and as they test their independence, food may be one of the issues discussed. It is important that the child be allowed to make some choices and that food not be a battleground. Most teenagers today do not eat a good breakfast. They skip breakfast because they tend to be in a hurry in the morning or believe that it is not important. A good breakfast gives the teenager the energy for a good day at school or to accomplish athletics before school.

Table 5–9
Health Supervision Interventions: School-Age

	6 Yr	8 Yr	10 Yr
Physical Examination	X	X	X
Growth Parameters (height, weight)	X	X	X
Tanner Stage or Sexual Maturity Rating			X
Immunizations	X*		
Assessment of High-Dose Lead Exposure	X		
Tuberculin Test	X†‡	X†	X†
Assessment of Risk of Hyperlipidemia	X	X	X
Vision Screening	X	X	X
Hearing Screening	X	X	X
Blood Pressure Screening	X	X	X
Scoliosis Screening		X	X

* Administer at 4 to 6 years of age, before school entry to bring immunization status up to date.
† Annual test if certain risk factors are present.
‡ Performance between ages 4 and 6 before school entry.
From Green, M. (Ed.). (1994). *Bright futures: Guidelines for health supervision of infants, children, and adolescents.* Arlington, VA: National Center for Education in Maternal and Child Health. *Bright Futures* was supported by the Maternal and Child Health Bureau and the Medicaid Bureau.

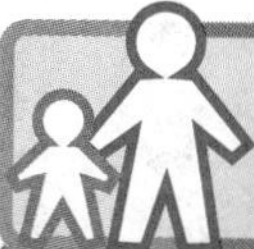

Chart 5-23
Developmental Considerations

Milestones of the School-Age Child (7–11 Years)

Physical

All School-Age
- Females by age 11 have achieved 90% adult height and 50% adult weight
- Males at 12 have achieved 80% of adult height and 50% of adult weight
- Striking changes in growth of long bones
- Begins Tanner stages of prepubertal development
- By age 12 have all permanent teeth except second and third molars

6–9 Yr
- Sleep 11–12 hr/day
- Gains 3–5 lb/yr
- 10–11 permanent teeth
- Arms grow longer in proportion to body

10–11 Yr
- Sleep 10 hr/day
- 12-year molars erupt
- Posture similar to adults
- Prepubescent changes may begin in girls

Sexual

All School-Age
- Some females capable of menarche at 11–12 yr
- Normal homosexual interest

Vision

7 Yr
- 20/20 vision

Gross Motor

6 Yr
- Walks a straight line
- Has mastered all skills on Denver Developmental Screening Test

8 Yr
- Crouches on tiptoes
- Puts right or left foot forward on command

9–11 Yr
- Balances on one leg with eyes closed
- Catches tennis ball with one hand

Fine Motor

All School-Age
- Continually refines and improves previously learned skills
- Movements are more graceful
- Bathes self unassisted
- Uses tools

Play

All School-Age
- Cooperative "team" play
- Skill play (jump rope, skating)
- Testing, model building, exploration
- Collects things and classifies them
- Hobbies
- Board games
- Reads for pleasure
- Easily engrossed in long hours of television watching

Chart continued on following page

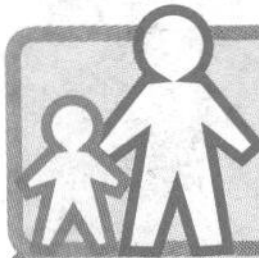

Chart 5-23
Developmental Considerations

Milestones of the School-Age Child (7–11 Years) *Continued*

Cognitive

All School-Age
Concrete Operations
Ability to reason
Concept of reversibility
Classifies objects according to their characteristics
Concept of conservation
Concept of relativism
Can place self in another's situation
Serialization—masters the ordinal number line; can group and sort/place in logical order
Fundamental skills of reading, writing, and grammar develop
Concept of reciprocity
Concept of identity
Combination skills
Tells time
Decentration—ability to focus on many aspects of experience

11 Yr
Capable of abstract and deductive reasoning
Death is irreversible but capricious
Uses external/internal physiologic explanations
Knows coin exchange

Social

All School-Age
Social participation in school, neighborhood, scouting groups
Begins to manage cooperative and competitive relationships
Demonstrates affection to others
Enjoys friendship with same-sex peers
Respects parents

Interpersonal

All School-Age
Independence within family
Self-regulation of behavior
Industry vs. inferiority

Anorexia Nervosa and Bulimia

These two conditions are related, although they have different etiologies. Usually seen in female adolescents, both have the possibility of life-long complications. Anorexia nervosa is characterized by the child having a distorted image of herself—feeling she is too fat, when she may actually be 20% or more underweight. The anorexic limits food intake severely, drinks large amounts of water, and may exercise strenuously. These adolescents usually need to be hospitalized and may need intravenous or nasogastric feedings along with psychotherapy to return them to a desired weight and normal lifestyle.

Whereas the anorexic patient invariably appears emaciated, the bulimic teenager is usually either slightly overweight or slightly underweight and rarely near death. Bulimia is characterized by frequent repeated episodes of binge eating followed by induced vomiting or overuse of laxatives to eliminate the foods from the body. Bulimic teenagers do develop other complications (e.g., electrolyte imbalances, tears in the esophagus) from the induced vomiting or overuse of laxatives.

Both of these conditions are psychological illnesses that present as physical symptoms. Many of these adolescents attempt to hide the symptoms from their parents or health care professionals. Bulimics rarely admit to forcing

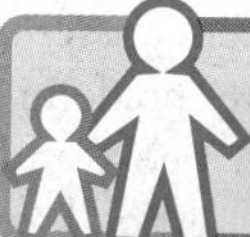

Chart 5–23
Developmental Considerations

Milestones of the School-Age Child (7–11 Years) *Continued*

Emotional

All School-Age

Uses coping behaviors (strategies): avoidant coping, active coping, avoidant-active coping

Moral/Spiritual

All School-Age

Moral

Stage 4: Conventional

Concern with authority figures, fixed rules in moral decisions
Concern with obligation to duty
A "bad" act breaks a rule or does harm
Accidents or misfortunes may be interpreted as punishment
Develops a conscience and sense of values

Spiritual

Stage II: Mythical/Literal

Distinguishes religious fact from fantasy
Respects and relies on authoritative figures such as parents, priest, rabbi
Attitude of peers toward faith is influential
Monomythic attitude; uses fantasies to explain events or facts he or she doesn't understand
Learns to differentiate between natural and supernatural
God is perceived in anthropomorphic imagery (has human qualities)
Description of God implies a formation of a reciprocal relationship

themselves to vomit after binging. Anorexics may take to wearing loose-fitting clothes and lie about eating elsewhere so they do not have to eat with the family. These conditions are discussed further in Chapter 29.

Treatment is not simple with either disorder. The diagnosis of an eating disorder should be contemplated when a teenager presents to the health care professional who appears to be underweight, not of appropriate height, or of normal sexual maturation for gender but following unhealthful dietary habits (Rees, 1996). Teenagers with either anorexia nervosa or bulimia may need to be hospitalized. Patients with either disorder definitely need psychotherapy and possibly family counseling, because often dysfunctional family dynamics may be a contributing factor. Medications and behavior modification programs are used to treat both of these disorders.

Oral Health

By the time the child has reached adolescence, twice-a-year dental checkups should have been established, as well as good oral hygiene habits. The adolescent should have been evaluated for and possibly have orthodonture work initiated. The teenager needs to be instructed in the care of the teeth with the orthodontic appliances in place because there is an increased opportunity for dental caries with poor dental hygiene. The incidence of dental caries usually declines as the child matures, so it is not as much of a concern as it was when the child was a toddler; however, the risk of gingivitis does increase. This is also the age of experimentation and possible initiation of tobacco use, in the form of either cigarettes or smokeless tobacco. Adolescents who use smokeless tobacco are at a greater risk of developing gingivitis, gum recession, stained teeth, or halitosis and should be counseled not to start smoking or use smokeless tobacco products (American Academy of Family Physicians, 1993).

Hygiene and Personal Care

Changes Related to Puberty

As the teenager reaches puberty, there are many changes that occur physically (Fig. 5–19). In females, the earliest sign is usually thelarche, or the development of breast tissue, followed by the development of pubic hair and then the ultimate hallmark of late puberty—menarche, or the first menstruation. In males, the earliest sign of puberty is testicular enlargement, followed by some penile growth and the development of pubic hair. Boys also experience a "cracking of the voice" as the larynx and vocal cords grow to their full size and the male voice becomes deeper and more resonant. Both boys and girls usually experience a growth spurt of 3 to 4 inches over the next 2 years (see Tanner staging in Chapter 4).

During the time teenagers are developing pubic hair, the males are also developing some chest hair, and both sexes are developing axillary hair. This is a time to discuss the use of deodorants and regular bathing schedules. Boys will need to be taught how to shave because they will start to develop a light mustache on their upper lip.

A common occurrence in both boys and girls in the teenage years is the appearance of acne vulgaris or common acne. Acne vulgaris is an inflammation of the sebaceous glands and hair follicles of the skin characterized by comedones, papules, and pustules. Cysts and nodules may develop, and scarring is a common occurrence. Acne appears in both males and females but more predominantly in males. It usually occurs on the face, neck, and upper chest; and although it may last into adulthood, it is usually most severe during adolescence.

Figure 5–19
The adolescent is very concerned about personal appearance.

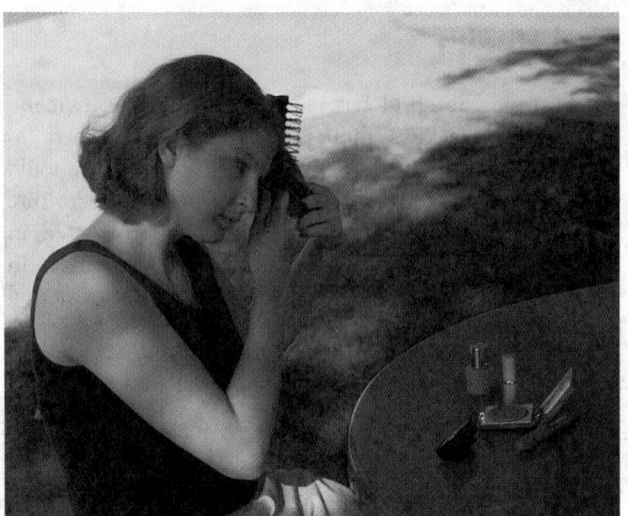

The cause of acne vulgaris is not known, although it is believed that heredity does play a predisposing factor. There have been many statements about certain foods causing acne breakouts, but as yet there has been no scientific evidence linking foods to acne, with the exception of some very specific allergic reactions.

The real cause of acne vulgaris appears to be the increased production of sebum by the sebaceous follicles of the skin in response to increased hormone levels during puberty. Treatment is individualized depending on the severity of the symptoms. Although acne is not caused by dirt or excessive oil on the skin, gentle cleansing of the skin should occur at least twice a day. The use of skin cleansers or antibacterial cleansers may be too drying and actually cause more problems. There is a wide variety of topical medications for use with acne that may alleviate scarring and reduce the severity of a flare-up. A physician should be consulted if the acne is so severe as to need the use of prescription medications. The physician may also prescribe a systemic antibiotic for the teenager with severe acne. These antibiotics decrease the colonization of the bacteria and decrease inflammation. The use of the tetracycline collection of drugs has been proven safe over long periods of time. Occasionally, oral contraceptives have been prescribed for use with teenage females with good results.

Sleep

The teenager needs 8 to 8½ hours per night of sleep. During this age, with an increase in social activities, school commitments, and possibly work activities, it is important that the adolescent receive enough sleep at night.

Parents and health care professionals need to be alert to abnormal sleep patterns because these could indicate some other underlying problem, such as drug abuse or depression. Teenagers should be sleeping uninterrupted through the night without nightmares or sleepwalking. If any of these aberrations is present, then the child should be seen by a physician to determine whether there is an underlying cause.

Physical Fitness

If physical fitness has been introduced at an early age, most likely the adolescent is exercising regularly through competitive or individual sports. Many adolescents are still not as physically active as they should be, and they should be encouraged to develop some healthy lifestyle

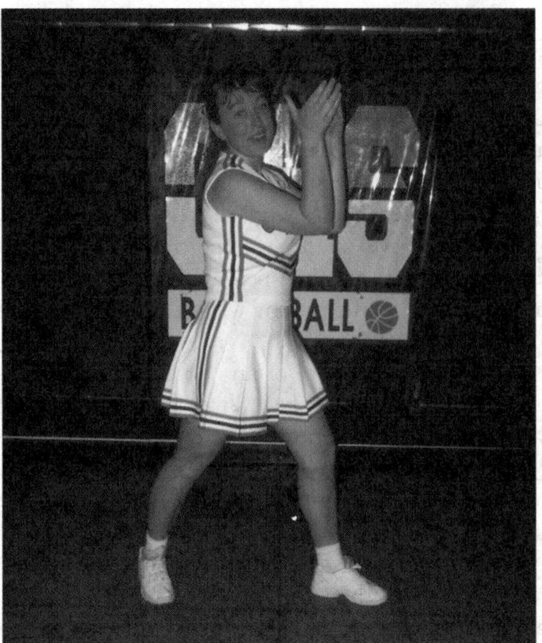

Figure 5–20
Cheerleading is an example of an activity that promotes physical fitness and helps the adolescent learn to work with others in a small group.

habits. Enjoyment of the particular activity appears to enhance the motivation to participate in that activity (Fig. 5–20).

Teenagers still need to develop their coordination and are still gaining muscle strength. Female adolescents stop increasing muscle strength at the time of their first menses, but males continue to increase their strength until they reach adulthood.

If the teenager is an active participant in sports, either individual or competitive, he or she may need to adjust his or her caloric intake accordingly. Some athletes may need to ingest as much as 4000 to 6000 cal/day to maintain a constant weight. The health care professional should be alert to the nutritional needs of the teenage athlete.

Promotion of Social Competence

Temperament

During this period, adolescents are leaving childhood behind and entering maturity. As teenagers gain independence, they begin to challenge values that have been established. They may become critical about household rules and challenge the adult authority from time to time. It is still necessary for the adult to set appropriate, constant limits. During middle adolescence, the teenager may spend more time ignoring adult authority and become much more reliant on peer relationships. Mood swings are not an uncommon occurrence during the early adolescent period and tend to smooth out during the middle adolescent period when the teen will be more introspective and have a tendency to feel inadequate. By late adolescence, the emotions will have smoothed out and become more consistent.

Relationships

This is the time that adolescents must establish an identity for themselves outside the family. They will use their friends to elicit a response to their ideas and actions as they evolve into adults. During the early part of adolescence, teenagers usually are preoccupied with what is happening to themselves physically. They use peer groups to stabilize themselves while entering puberty. Young adolescents usually have one very "best" friend of the same sex. Parents are still important to them, even though they are trying to separate from the family.

As the adolescent enters middle years, making friends will be easier and the teenager will again use peers for the validation they were seeking from the parents in earlier years. Peer relationships are extremely important, as the group forms the criterion the teen uses to measure himself or herself (Fig. 5–21). This is usually the low point in the parental relationship as the adolescent pushes for independence and separation. There may be major conflicts as the child detaches himself or herself from the parental bond.

Figure 5–21
When not with friends, the teenager will often spend many hours monopolizing the family phone to talk with friends.

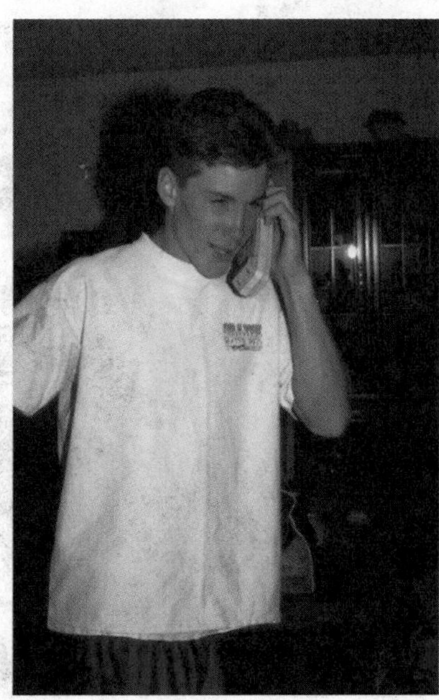

By late adolescence, the teenager is less dependent on peer groups and develops more individual relationships, including heterosexual relationships. The emancipation from the parental bond is complete, and the teenager has far less conflict with the family.

Sexuality

During middle adolescence, the teenager also starts forming attachments with the opposite sex and wants to start dating. Heterosexual relationships are important for the teenager to develop emotional and behavioral autonomy (Fig. 5–22). Around the age of 13 or 14, adolescents may question their sexual identity as they find a friend or mentor of the same sex attractive. Statistics show 5% to 10% of adolescents are homosexual (Greydanus, 1991). What stimulus causes a child to choose homosexuality as a lifestyle is still unclear. Usually by middle adolescence, most teenagers will firmly establish heterosexual relationships; by late adolescence or early adulthood, there may be the teenager who has determined he or she is homosexual.

In early adolescence, there is still some self-exploration, and many questions may be asked in regard to what is happening to the individual physically. As the teenager enters puberty, it is important that the correct information be shared. Through either the parent or the health care professional, accurate information regarding the physical changes that will occur and what is normal should be provided. Because of the influence of television and movies, many teenagers have an idealized body image and/or misinformation about sex. Some of the correct information may be provided by a school sex education course, but there still may be issues the teenager needs answers about that he or she may be reluctant to discuss in a classroom setting. Family values also need to be communicated and defined for the teenager. Parents as a whole seem to shy away from discussing anything about sex with the teenager, owing to discomfort or lack of information. Above all, it is important for the lines of communication to remain open with the parent so the teenager can go to the parent with a problem or a question.

Figure 5–22
The adolescent develops strong intimate relationships that provide a source of support and companionship.

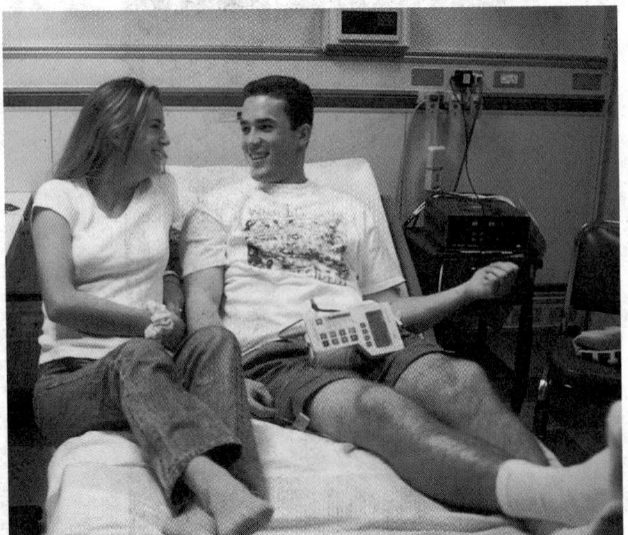

As the sexual identity of an adolescent emerges, sexual motivation may change. With appropriate information regarding prevention of sexually transmitted diseases, or pregnancy, a teen may choose to delay sexual activity, although many times this is not the case (Hockenberry-Eaton, Richman, DiIorio, Rivero, & Maibach, 1996). Often peer pressure and self-esteem influence adolescents in their actions more than the influence of education. Physicians have not been an active participant in the delivery of information because they often do not have the access to the teenagers nor the incentive to do preventive care (Igra & Millstein, 1993). Therefore, it may fall to the nurse interacting with the adolescent, either in the physician's office or in the school, to be the individual to impart the responsibilities regarding sexual intercourse.

By middle adolescence, pairing off in couples is common. The type and depth of the relationships vary, but as the teenager experiences his or her first "love" the potential for sexual activity becomes more prevalent. Many teenagers find it hard to believe that love can exist without sexual activity. By the late adolescence, a consolidated sexual identity has appeared and the teenager is more comfortable.

School

School for the adolescent is very important. It is a center for socialization as well as learning. High school is sometimes intimidating for the student coming from an elementary type of education, and many schools are preparing the students before admission with orientation days and visits. The high school is responsible for counseling the student for higher learning and/or vocational training (Elkind, 1993), and high school today is usually not the end of formal education. Most students are at least encouraged to apply to colleges. Sometimes teenagers feel a great deal of pressure to achieve high academic or athletic accomplishments, which can produce bouts of depression (see Chapter 29).

Homework may also be an issue for the teenager because at a high school level it is usually more intense. At this time, the parents should not be as involved with homework as they were when the child was a school-ager. The basics should have been developed at an early age and may just need to be reinforced. Arrangements for homework should be worked out at the beginning of the school year—when it will be done and where, along with the consequences that will occur if it is not completed. Nagging, threats, and bribery do not appear to be effective with teenagers, but occasional monitoring and negotiations with the student usually produce better results (Elkind, 1993).

Illness and Injury Prevention

Prevention of Substance Use and Abuse

One of the foremost concerns of parents of adolescents is the prevention of the use of drugs and alcohol. Education about drugs and alcohol does have a significant effect on the attitudes of the adolescent. The best time to start this education is when the child is still a school-ager, and if it is reinforced during adolescence, it is even more effective. One of the best ways for a teenager to learn about drugs and alcohol is through parental modeling. If the parent abstains from using drugs, tobacco, or alcohol, usually the teenager will adopt a similar value (Chart 5–24).

Tobacco and alcohol symbolize adult status to the adolescent, and parental warnings can be perceived as a mechanism to block them from achieving independence. Although the Food and Drug Administration has restricted the advertising of tobacco products and banned the sale of tobacco products to teenagers younger than the age of 18, it is still a very prevalent trend. Cigarette smoking has declined overall in the past decade, but the current rate of use among teenagers has hardly declined at all (Satcher & Ericksen, 1994). The number of 8th graders smoking increased 30% from 1991 to 1994, and 10th graders who smoke increased 20%. The percentage of high school seniors who smoke is greater than the percentage of adults ("Fighting a losing battle," 1995). Even though the long-term consequences of smoking are known, adolescents appear to have little concern with the outcomes that may occur 20 or 30 years from now. Peer pressure and the belief that tobacco use is enjoyable were the most influential factors (Fig. 5–23). A better focal point for teaching teens that smoking is not beneficial is the immediate adverse side effects on health: wheezing, phlegm production, aggravation of asthma, and diminished athletic ability. Because adolescents are also very concerned about personal appearance and social acceptability, the detractions of yellowing teeth and bad breath may also be used as a convincing argument. Of great concern is that Columbia University's Center on Addiction and Substance Abuse found that 12- to 17-year-olds who smoked were much more likely to use harder drugs (Henderson, 1994).

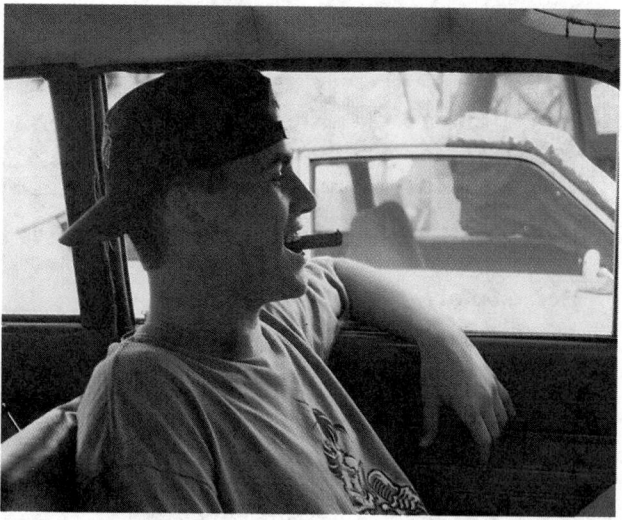

Figure 5–23
Peer pressure heavily influences an adolescent's decision to try tobacco, alcohol, and drugs.

Alcohol abuse is extremely prevalent in the teenage population. The average age at which adolescents begin to drink alcohol is about 12 years old. By the time a teenager becomes a high school senior, 92% will have tried alcohol and 4% of high school seniors will be using it regularly (Elkind, 1993).

Again, parental modeling appears to be one of the most effective methods for the teenager establishing appropriate standards regarding drinking. Many teenagers actually obtain their alcohol from their parents, either directly or indirectly.

According to the Alcohol, Drug Abuse, and Mental Health Administration, an adolescent can become addicted to alcohol within 6 months because he or she usually drinks in large quantities, whereas it may take several years for an adult to become addicted. There are four stages of becoming addicted:

1. Experimental stage: when the teenager tries out alcohol and likes its effect
2. Seeking-out stage: when the teen seeks out opportunities to drink
3. Dependency stage: when the alcohol-induced high becomes top priority for the teen
4. Addiction stage: when the teenager needs alcohol just to feel "normal"

Many teenagers will try alcohol but will never be addicted. Thirty percent of boys and 20% of girls before the 10th grade will have experimented with drinking. Many parents do not take drinking as seriously as drug abuse because they perceive it as the "lesser of two evils" because alcohol is a legal substance (Greydanus, 1991).

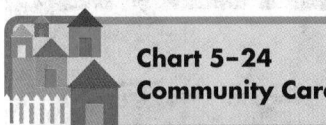

Chart 5–24
Community Care

Injury and Violence Prevention Guidelines for the Adolescent

Home Safety

- Ask your parents to check smoke detectors to ensure that they are working properly and to change batteries yearly.
- Discuss with your parents safety rules for the home, including those about visitors, use of the telephone, and what to do in case of fire or other emergencies. Conduct fire drills at home.

Activity Safety

- Wear protective sports gear.
- Wear appropriate protective gear at work and follow job safety procedures.
- Avoid high noise levels, especially when using music headsets.
- Always wear a helmet when on a motorcycle, in an all-terrain vehicle, or when riding a bicycle. Even with a helmet, motorcycles and ATVs are very dangerous.

Water Safety

- Learn how to swim. Do not swim alone.
- Do not drink alcohol especially while boating or swimming.

Car Safety

- Wear a seat belt in the car at all times.
- If you are driving, insist that your passengers wear seat belts.
- Follow the speed limit and traffic rules.
- Do not drink alcohol and drive. Plan to have a designated driver if drinking.

Outdoor Safety

- Protect yourself from skin cancer by putting sunscreen on before you go outside for long periods of time. Avoid tanning salons.

Emergency Preparation

- Make sure your address and phone number are posted near a phone at your house.
- Know where the list of emergency numbers (doctor, hospital, nearest neighbor, poison control center) is kept in your home.
- Know how to contact your parents in case of an emergency. Keep their work phone numbers in your purse, wallet, or school notebook.
- Keep some loose change with you at all times so that you can make an emergency call if needed.

Violence Prevention

- Do not carry or use a weapon of any kind.
- Develop skills in conflict resolution, negotiation, and dealing with anger constructively.
- Learn techniques to protect yourself from physical, emotional, and sexual abuse, including rape by either strangers or acquaintances.
- Seek help if you are physically or sexually abused or fear that you are in danger.

Adapted from Green, M. (Ed.). (1994). *Bright futures: Guidelines for health supervision of infants, children, and adolescents.* Arlington, VA: National Center of Education in Maternal and Child Health. *Bright Futures* was supported by the Maternal and Child Health Bureau and the Medicaid Bureau.

The negative effects of alcohol can be devastating when teens mix drinking and driving. The leading cause of adolescent death is driving while under the influence of alcohol (American Academy of Family Physicians, 1994).

Alcoholism is difficult to treat but must not be ignored. Professional intervention and programs developed to treat alcoholic adolescents can be of assistance. The health care professional should always be observing adolescents for potential drug or alcohol abuse. The most common signs a clinician should be alert for are physiologic dependence or withdrawal, such as craving, compulsive alcohol-seeking behavior, tremulousness, agitation, weight loss, headaches, and changes in mental status. The American Academy of Pediatrics recommends counseling regarding abuse of alcohol as part of routine well-child care by the primary care clinician (American Academy of Family Physicians, 1994).

Although most adolescents limit their experimentation to alcohol, tobacco, and marijuana, the Substance Abuse and Mental Health Services Administration reports that 23 million people over the age of 12 have used illegal drugs (Monroe, 1996).

The chief groups of drugs that are abused are cannabis, barbiturates and tranquilizers, stimulants, hallucinogens, and narcotics (see Chapter 29 for more descriptions of psychoactive substances). Although there appears to be a decline in the use of illegal drugs by teenagers, 1 in every 6 high school seniors has experimented with cocaine and 1 in every 18 has tried crack (Elkind, 1993).

Cannabis or marijuana is not the "safe" drug it was once thought to be. There is now evidence indicating that, particularly with overuse, it can have significant health consequences. It alters perception and emotions, affects short-term memory, reduces concentration and coordination, and may cause violent mood swings. It increases the appetite, which may cause weight gain (Monroe, 1996). Smoking marijuana also has all the detrimental effects on the lungs as smoking cigarettes. Marijuana actually contains more carcinogenic chemicals than an equal amount of tobacco smoke; and because many marijuana users hold the smoke in their lungs for a period of time, the potential for damage may be greater (Greydanus, 1991). Marijuana also contains a mood-altering chemical, tetrahydrocannabinol (THC), that attaches to organs and can cause hallucinations, disrupt menstrual cycles, and be a threat to genetic fragmentation of chromosomes, affecting the formation of DNA.

Barbiturates and tranquilizers are types of depressants that depress the central nervous system activity, causing the teenager to feel calm and perhaps inducing sleep. Besides alcohol, which is a depressant, other drugs that produce similar effects are phenobarbital, amobarbital (Amytal), pentobarbital (Nembutal) (also known on the street as "yellow jackets" and "nembies"), and secobarbital (Seconal) ("red devils" or "reds"). There are also nonbarbiturate drugs that cause similar effects, such as methaqualone (Quaaludes) and benzodiazepines (Valium, Librium). All these drugs cause the user to develop a tolerance level, and the teenager must take more and more to obtain the same feeling. Many teens combine these drugs with alcohol, which potentiates the effects of the drugs and can perhaps be fatal (Monroe, 1996). These drugs do produce physical dependence and will produce withdrawal symptoms if discontinued abruptly.

Stimulants include crack, cocaine ("coke," "snow," "blow," "toot," "nose candy," or "flake"), amphetamines ("uppers"), and methamphetamine ("speed" and "ice"). Cocaine and crack are highly addictive and produce a decreased appetite, abnormal sleep patterns, erratic behavior, sweating, anxiety, and tremors. Crack is cocaine that has been chemically altered to form a substance that can be smoked. Cocaine is usually taken through the mucous membranes of the nares by insufflation and produces a telltale side effect of a "runny nose." These drugs produce a euphoria and an energizing effect. Once the high is achieved, there is a swift backlash effect, causing depression, anxiety, irritability, and fatigue. This causes the person to take more cocaine to alleviate these feelings, potentially inducing an overdose and risking heart attack, stroke, seizure, or respiratory arrest (Monroe, 1996). These side effects are potential even with a first-time user. Withdrawal from cocaine does not cause the same physical effects as withdrawal from other substances, but there is a psychological dependence on the drug that makes withdrawal very difficult.

Hallucinogens such as LSD ("acid") or PCP ("angel dust" or "crystal") are mind-altering drugs that affect a teenager's perception, emotions, and thinking. LSD causes panic, confusion, anxiety, and terror by hallucinations. PCP can elicit bizarre behavior that can cause the teenager to be combative with wide mood swings. Both increase the heart rate and blood pressure and can cause muscle tremors, seizures, and coma. Because these drugs do not produce physical dependence, the withdrawal can be done swiftly, but studies have shown some long-term recurring effects of mind-altering drugs (Monroe 1996).

Narcotics are opium based and usually derived from the juice of poppy seeds, but today some narcotics are produced synthetically. Narcotics include opium (Dover's powder) and heroin ("junk," "smack," "brown sugar"), and all are extremely addictive. Because users develop a tolerance, larger and larger doses must be taken to obtain the same effect (Monroe, 1996). Synthetic narcotics as well as opium-based narcotics relieve pain and induce sleep, thus causing a euphoric feeling. These drugs are usually introduced by needles and not ingested or smoked, and telltale needle puncture wounds or "tracks" may indicate usage. Because narcotics are physically as well as psychologically addicting, withdrawal can be very disagreeable, causing such symptoms as vomiting, severe diarrhea, cramping, and watery eyes and nose. Because these symptoms begin within 4 to 8 hours after the last dose, teenagers demonstrate a drug-seeking posture to secure more of the drug. Because heroin is injected, often in "social" situations where needles are shared or are not sterile, the risk of infection with the human immunodeficiency virus is very high (Monroe, 1996).

Inhalants and solvents such as glue, typewriter correction fluid, paint, aerosols, and gasoline are more of the substances adolescents will use for euphoric purposes. These products are easy to carry and conceal. Inhalants are frequently used in the classroom without other students and teachers knowing (Espeland, 1997). Most often the substance is either placed on a rag and sniffed or put in a plastic or brown bag and inhaled ("huffing"). In addition to the side effects of the substances causing irregular heartbeats and liver and kidney damage, many adolescents may become asphyxiated when they lose consciousness before removing the plastic bag from their face.

When interacting with a teenager, the clinician needs to be alert for signs of use and abuse, such as reddened eyes; constant runny nose or sniffles; rapid mood swings; history of bizarre behavior; withdrawal from friends, former activities, and family; and a dropping of grades. Other signs would be the smell of smoke, alcohol, or burnt marijuana on the adolescent's person, signs of needle tracks, unusual sleep patterns, loss of coordination, weight loss or gain, or pinpoint pupils (Chart 5–25).

Chart 5–25

Signs of Substance Abuse

- Red eyes
- Runny or stuffy nose (constant)
- Rapid mood swings
- History of bizarre behavior
- Withdrawal from friends, activities, and family
- Smell of smoke
- Signs of needle tracks
- Unusual sleep patterns
- Loss of coordination
- Pinpoint pupils
- Weight loss or gain—change in eating habits
- Gastrointestinal upset (diarrhea)
- Tremors
- Depression or agitation
- Hallucinations or disorientation

If the adolescent is suspected of using some type of drug, the nurse may be the first to identify the problem by putting together the pieces of history, activity, and physical signs and symptoms. If there is an overdose potential, the adolescent must seek medical treatment as soon as possible because to delay may be fatal. Long-term management is more complex, requiring physical and psychological support systems for both the adolescent and the family. It is essential to keep communication open with the teenager to build self-esteem and find a "high" without drugs.

Gang Activity

Youth gangs exist all over the country, in cities large and small. Gangs are not new to the United States; they have been around since the 18th century. As of 1991, gang members number about 130,000 (Oliver, 1995). Easy access to guns makes gangs of today especially dangerous.

Gangs come in all size groups: very large with subdivisions and very small with just a few members. If a group or clique meets the three following criteria, according to experts, it can be defined as a "gang":

1. There must be distinct group recognition by the members (e.g., use of signs, colors).
2. The gang must be identified by the community as a gang group.
3. The gang must be involved in some illegal activities to get a reputation within the community that is not positive (Oliver, 1995).

Gangs are usually classified in three types:

1. Territorial gangs: This group controls a specific geographic area.
2. Organized gangs: There is more of a military type of organization with a definite structure with a leader, "warlord," treasurer, enforcer, and foot soldiers. This group usually is involved in illegal activities that involve large amounts of money.
3. Scavenger gangs: This group has common behaviors, is usually smaller, and may not have other gang characteristics. Members are usually attracted for a sense of belonging (Oliver, 1995).

Usually gangs develop from a group of "troublemaking" adolescents who share a common neighborhood, school, or interest. Traditionally, gang members were exclusively male, but now it is not uncommon for a gang to recruit female members. The most common recruits are from the inner city, the poor, and adolescents with low self-esteem, gathering together for mutual support and understanding. Usually these adolescents have little family support. The feelings of poor self-esteem are negated by being accepted by a group that has "power" (and money). Ninety-six percent of gang members are younger than the age of 25, and 90% are between the ages of 12 and 21 (Goldentyer, 1994). Gangs group together adolescents of similar cultural backgrounds and usually exclude anyone who is not the same.

Getting out of gangs is very difficult. Many ex–gang members state that the easiest way is to just "fade" away, by not attending the activities as often and not being part of the crowd. After a while, the gang member is "forgotten." Unfortunately, physicians and nurses usually see the gang members in the emergency department after a confrontation. Education is one of the best tools to prevent adolescents from joining gangs. The health care professional can talk to the teenager about alternatives to a gang lifestyle and can assist the teen in finding non-gang role models. Group counseling with the parents may assist in the development of a stronger family relationship. Programs can be offered to keep the teenagers busy after school, perhaps allowing them to develop other peer relationships outside of gangs, within sports, art, music, and so on. Teenagers can be encouraged to plan their future. The professional should not sugarcoat the possibilities of what will occur if the adolescent joins a gang or remains in a gang. Arrest, prison, injury, and possibly death all are very real outcomes of gang membership.

Prevention of Pregnancy and Sexually Transmitted Diseases

Studies indicate that between 36.9% and 66.4% of high school students are sexually active. One in every 10 adolescent girls between the ages of 15 and 19 becomes pregnant. Annually, 2.5 million teenagers in the United States contract a sexually transmitted disease (Harbin, 1995; Moriarty, 1997).

Sexual education courses alone have had little impact on reducing adolescent pregnancies because it was

Table 5–10
Contraception Methods

Method	Effectiveness for Contraception	Effectiveness Against Sexually Transmitted Diseases	Side Effects
Abstinence	Excellent	Excellent	None
Birth control pills	Most effective	None	Potential stroke, blood clots, heart attacks, and cancer
Condoms (both male and female)	Very effective with proper use	Very effective	None
Spermicides	Most effective when used with condom	None unless used with condom	Occasional irritation due to allergic reaction to spermicide
Norplant	Highly effective	None	Potential for bleeding, irregular menses, amenorrhea, dermatitis, acne, infection at implant site; occasionally removal is difficult
Depo-Provera	Highly effective	None	Migraine, lethargy, depression, weight gain, irregular menses, or amenorrhea, pulmonary embolism, breast tenderness or enlargement
Rhythm method	Not very effective	None	None
Withdrawal	Not effective	None	None
"Morning after" pill (combination of estrogen and progestin with ethinyl estradiol)	Effective if given within appropriate time frame	None	Occasionally nausea; may experience breakthrough bleeding, rashes, breast tenderness or enlargement

assumed the pregnancies were unintentional. However, adolescent decision-making as to intercourse with or without protection is a complex fabric of many factors, including socioeconomic conditions, psychological factors, race, peer relationships, and family values (Gordon, 1996).

The form of contraception most commonly used among adolescents is low-dose contraceptive pills (OCPs), with condoms being the second most favored and the one used most often at the initial coitus opportunity (Table 5–10). Condoms also play the critical role in reducing sexually transmitted diseases. Condoms used solely as the method of contraception have a typical failure rate of about 20%. Sexual education programs with an abstinence theme that encourage role playing using concrete techniques to enable an adolescent to say "no" help create alternatives (Moriarty, 1997; Nelson, 1996a).

Other methods of birth control such as Norplant, Depo-Provera, and intrauterine devices are convenient and well tolerated by teens and have very low failure rates (Nelson, 1996b). Coitus interruptus (withdrawal before ejaculation) or "rhythm" methods (determining "safe" days according to menstrual cycle), spermicides, and the vaginal sponge are other alternatives. These may not be as effective as the other contraceptives but are available without prescription or the involvement of a health care professional.

The most effective prevention of sexually transmitted diseases such as gonorrhea, chlamydia, herpes, syphilis, and the acquired immunodeficiency syndrome is, of course, abstinence. The second most effective method of protection is the use of condoms. Many teenagers are not aware of the modes of transmission of these diseases and with misinformation do not effectively protect themselves against exposure because they believe that any form of

Table 5–11
Health Supervision Interventions: Adolescent

	11–14 Yr	15–17 Yr	18–21 Yr
Physical Examination	X	X	X
Growth Parameters (height, weight)	X	X	X
Immunizations	X*	X*	X*
Tanner Stage or Sexual Maturity Rating	X	X	X
Scoliosis Screening	X	X	X
Females (breast exam, pelvic exam, Papanicolaou smear)	X†	X	X
Males (evaluate for gynecomastia, hernias, testicular cancer)	X	X	X
Vision Screening	X	X	X
Hearing Screening	X	X	X
Tuberculin Test	X‡§	X‡§	X‡
Blood Pressure Screening	X	X	X
Hematocrit or Hemoglobin Screening for Females	X∥	X∥	X∥
Hyperlipidemia Screening	X∥	X∥	X∥††
Annual Screening for Gonorrhea and Chlamydia	X¶	X¶	X
Syphilis Screening (VDRL/RPR)	X**	X**	X**
HIV Screening	X**	X**	X**
Screening for Behavioral or Emotional Concerns	X	X	X
Nonfasting Blood Cholesterol Level			X

* Administered if immunization status is not up to date.
† Perform pelvic examination and Papanicolaou smear annually if teenager is sexually active.
‡ Once at 14 to 16 years of age.
§ Annual if certain risk factors present.
∥ If certain risk factors are present.
¶ For sexually active adolescents.
** If adolescent asks to be tested or if certain risk factors are present.
†† Annual screening for adolescents older than age 19.
From Green, M. (Ed.). (1994). *Bright futures: Guidelines for health supervision of infants, children, and adolescents.* Arlington, VA: National Center for Education in Maternal and Child Health. *Bright Futures* was supported by the Maternal and Child Health Bureau and the Medicaid Bureau.

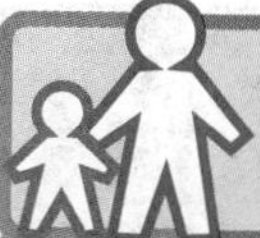

Chart 5–26
Developmental Considerations

Milestones of the Adolescent

Physical

Full height not attained until ages 20 to 24 yr when epiphyseal plates close
Marked increase in muscle mass in males related to androgen
By age 17, muscle mass is 2 times greater in males than females, resulting in strength two to four times greater in males
Adult cardiovascular rhythms by age 16

Great nutritional needs:
Males: 3600 cal/day
Females: 2600 cal/day
At end of adolescence, male basal metabolic rate is about 10% greater than female
Nutrition needs: pregrowth spurt—1500–2400 cal/day; pubertal girls—2000–2500 cal/day; pubertal boys—2500–3000 cal/day

Sexual

Genital Stage
Learning appropriate outlets for sexual drives
Menarche 10–15 yr in girls
Usually cannot reproduce for 1–2 yr after menarche because of anovulation
Early use of oral contraceptives will limit potential height
Male attains puberty between 12–16 yr
Tanner steps I–V usually attained between early and late adolescence

Approximate sequence of appearance of sexual characteristics in adolescence:

Females

8–9 Yr
Hormones begin to release, sometimes causing moodiness and skin sensitivity

9–10 Yr
Hips start rounding out
Breast nipples start to grow

10–11 Yr
Breast tissues around and under nipples begin to grow
Downy hair near labia
Growth spurt may begin

11–12 Yr
Internal and external organs continue growing (vagina, uterus, breasts, ovaries)
Pubic hair becomes darker, coarser, and curlier

12–13 Yr
Underarm hair growth
Onset of menstruation (average age 12.8 years and approximately 2 years after breasts start growing)
Pregnancy is now possible

13–14 Yr
There may be times when underpants are wet with a clear mucus; this is often heavier in teen years and will continue naturally during adulthood, especially with ovulation and sexual arousal

14–15 Yr
Earliest normal pregnancy possible
Majority of growth spurt complete (height)

15–16 Yr
Acne
Deepening of voice, though not as much as males

16–17 Yr
Full height achieved

Males

9–10 Yr
Hormones begin to release, sometimes causing moodiness and skin sensitivity

10–11 Yr
Testes become larger
Scrotal skin becomes redder and coarser

11–12 Yr
Prostate begins functioning
Penis begins to lengthen

12–13 Yr
Pubic hair growth
May experience wet dreams, spontaneous erections, ejaculations (about 1 year after testes begin to grow)
Growth spurt may begin

Chart continued on following page

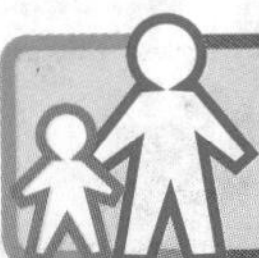

Chart 5-26
Developmental Considerations

Milestones of the Adolescent *Continued*

Sexual *(Continued)*

13–14 Yr
Rapid growth of the penis—especially enlargement occurring about 1 year after testes begin to grow
Testes color deepens
Two thirds of boys may experience slight growth of their breast tissue, which generally subsides within 1 year but may last 3 years

14–15 Yr
Underarm hair
Mustache begins as fine hair starting at outside lip edges about 2 years after pubic hair
Voice change begins

15–16 Yr
Average age that sperm matures and can cause pregnancy; average age 14.6 years; 50% of boys reach this stage within the past 2 years
Majority of growth spurt complete (height)

16–17 Yr
Chest and shoulders fill out
Facial and body hair becomes heavier
Acne

21 Yr
Full height achieved

Play

Group/peer activities such as sports, academic teams
Seeks parental-adult "limit setting"
Thrill-seeking behaviors

Cognitive

Pseudo-stupidity: asks "dumb" questions
Difficulty reconciling concrete and formal operations
Imaginary audience: super self-consciousness; believes everybody is watching and evaluating
Personal fable: belief of being special and not subject to rational laws
Apparent hypocrisy: act of expressing an idea tantamount to working for and attaining it

Formal Operations
Abstraction and hypothetical/deductive reasoning
Adaptability and flexibility
Thinking in abstract terms
Uses abstract symbols
Makes conclusions drawn from set of observations
Develops hypotheses and tests them
Considers abstract, theoretical, and philosophical matters
Problem solving
Ability to comprehend purely abstract or symbolic content exists
Ability to solve math and logic problems
Comprehends value and belief systems in the philosophical, moral, and political realms
Reality vs. possibility—views only one arrangement of the possible
Combinational reasoning
Propositional thinking
Hypothetical-deductive reasoning
Death is irreversible, universal, personal, but distant
Uses natural, physiologic, and theological explanations of death

Social

Capable of sharing self with others to foster intimate relationship
Inability to form intimate relationships may lead to sense of isolation

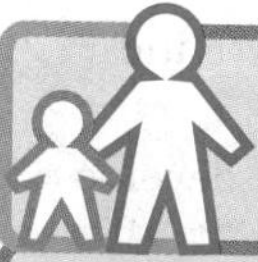

Chart 5–26
Developmental Considerations

Milestones of the Adolescent *Continued*

Interpersonal

Identity vs. role confusion

Moral/Spiritual

Moral

Stage 4: Conventional (12–16 Yr)
Fixed rules in moral decisions
Obligation to do no harm and to do duty

Stage 5: Postconventional (16 Yr)
Social contracts understood and formulated
Laws recognized as changeable
Correct actions depend on standards and individual rights

Stage 6: Adulthood
Abstract moral principles govern behavior
Morality is easily separated from legality
Orientation is based on universal, ethical orientation
Can apply situational ethics

Spiritual

Stage III: Synthetic/Invention (Preadolescent)
Reflects and questions religious beliefs as gains more contact with people whose values and beliefs are different
Seeks to resolve moral conflicts by appealing to outside authority figures rather than using own inner resources
Learns to distinguish more clearly between supernatural vs. natural
Perceives God as a spirit
Begins to understand spiritual component of individuals

Stage IV: Individuating/Reflexive (Adolescent)
Seeks to establish and maintain balance regarding religious/spiritual questions and beliefs; may adapt "devil may care" attitude or go to other extreme and join zealous religious group or may suspend effort to resolve conflict

contraception is a preventive measure. The health care professional plays a key role in the education and allaying of myths regarding the transmission of these diseases.

Developmental Surveillance

Chart 5–26 presents a summary of the developmental milestones that are accomplished in the adolescent years. This information is useful to provide the nurse with direction for specific trigger questions that can be asked of the parents or child to determine the adolescent's developmental progress. Trigger questions should also include social and sexual activity and school and vocational performance, as well as the health activities for this age (Table 5–11). A primary goal of developmental surveillance is to promote adolescent self-advocacy, that is, to assist the adolescent in seeking out, evaluating, and using information to promote his or her own health. Nurses can prepare adolescents for self-advocacy by teaching the adolescent to ask for information and make decisions about his or her own care, by encouraging health promotion activities, and by providing the adolescent with age-appropriate and correct health care information (Vessey & Miola, 1997).

Summary of Key Concepts

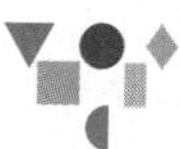

- Infants develop at an accelerated rate during the first year of life. Learning to sit, crawl, stand, and develop fine motor abilities during this period of time is an extraordinary accomplishment.
- Toddlers with the need to explore and test boundaries need definite limits set and boundaries prepared so the child can grow within safe limitations.

- Introducing the preschooler to the school environment and activities should be addressed during this period.
- Parents will focus on adapting to the school environment and development of interpersonal relationships.
- The most important issues to assess during the adolescent period are alcohol usage, potential drug abuse, and sexual relationships potentially leading to intercourse.

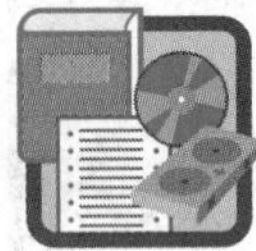

Resources

Organizations

American Academy of Pediatrics
Division of Public Education
141 Northwest Point Boulevard
P.O. Box 927
Elk Grove Village, IL 60009-0927

Children with Attention-Deficit Disorder (CHADD)
499 Northwest Seventieth Avenue
Suite 308
Plantation, FL 33317
(305) 587-3700

Council for Exceptional Children
1920 Association Drive
Reston, VA 22091
(703) 620-3660

International Lactation Consultants Association (ILCA)
201 Brown Avenue
Evanston, IL 60202-3601
(847) 260-8874

La Leche League International Headquarters
1400 North Meacham Road
Schaumburg, IL 60173-4840
(800) LA-LECHE

Medela, Inc.
P.O. Box 660
McHenry, IL 60051
(800) TELL-YOU
Resource on breast-feeding and breast pumps

Mothers Against Drunk Driving
511 East John Carpenter Freeway, Suite 700 Irving, TX 75062
(800) 438-6233

National Association for Gifted Children
1155 15th Street NW
Suite 1002
Washington, DC 20005
(202) 785-4268

National Highway Traffic Safety Administration
400 7th Street SW, Room 5319
Washington, DC 20005
(800) 424-9393

National Runaway Switchboard
3080 North Lincoln
Chicago, IL 60657
(800) 621-4000

National Safety Council
1121 Spring Lake Drive
Itasca, IL 60613-0429
(800) 621-7619

Runaway Hotline
P.O. Box 12428
Austin, TX 78711
(800) 231-6946
(800) 392-3552 (within Texas)

Safe Sitter
1500 North Ritter Avenue
Indianapolis, IN 46219
(800) 255-4089
Information regarding developing classes for prospective teen sitters

Hotlines

The American Baby Helpline
(900) 860-4888 (cost $ .95 per minute)
24-hour, 7-day-a-week helpline

National Highway Traffic Safety Administration Hotline
(800) 424-9393

Books and Printed Materials

American Baby Magazine
Cahners Publishing Company
475 Park Avenue South
New York, NY 10016

Bright Futures: Guidelines for Health Supervision of Infants, Children, and Adolescents
National Maternal and Child Health Clearinghouse/Circle Solutions Inc.
Greensboro Drive
Suite 600
McLean, VA 22102
(703) 821-8955 ext. 254 or 265
FAX: (703) 821-2098

DeFrancis, B. (1994). *The Parents' Resource Almanac*. Holbrook, MA: Bob Adams, Inc.

The Exceptional Parent Magazine
Psy-Ed Corporation
209 Harvard Street, Suite 303
Brookline, MA 02146-5005

Ezzo, G., & Buckham, R. (1995). *Baby Wise*. Sisters, OR: Questar Publishers, Inc.
Written for parents, the book suggests ways to introduce order and stability into the routine care of the infant.

Franck, I., & Brownstone, D. (1991). *The Parent's Desk Reference*. New York: Prentice-Hall.

Gifted Child Today
P.O. Box 6448
Mobile, AL 36660-0448

✏ *A Very Special Critter* by Mercer Mayer
Story about a child who is handicapped

✏ *Bedtime for Frances* by Russell Hoban

✏ *In the Night Kitchen* by Maurice Sendak

✏ *Just Me and My Brother* by Mercer Mayer

✏ *Just Me and My Little Sister* by Mercer Mayer

✏ *The New Baby* by Mercer Mayer

✏ *The New Baby* by Stanley and Janice Berenstain

✏ *There's a Nightmare in My Closet* by Mercer Mayer

Public Playground Handbook for Safety
U.S. Consumer Product Safety Commission
Washington, DC 20207
(800) 638-CPSC

Children's Videos

✏ *A New Baby at My House*—Sesame Street

Computer Resources

Consumer Product Information Safety Commission
(800) 638-2772
Web: http://www.cpsc.gov

Nutrition
Web: http://www.fsci.umn.edu/tools.htp
By typing a specific food into the search form, you can discover the amount of nutrient contained in the food.

Safety Equipment

No-Choke Test Tube
Toys to Grow On
P.O. Box 17
Long Beach, CA 90801

✏ Resources specifically for children.

References

American Academy of Family Physicians. (1993). Oral health in children and adolescents. *American Family Physician, 47*(5), 1285–1286.

American Academy of Family Physicians. (1994). Alcohol and other drug abuse in adolescents. *American Family Physician, 50*(8), 1737–1740.

Brazelton, T. B. (1992). *Touchpoints*. Reading, MA: Addison-Wesley Publishing Company.

Briggs, N. (1987). Day care for medically fragile children. *Pediatric Nursing, 13*(2), 120–121.

Christophersen, E. (1990). *Beyond discipline*. Kansas City, MO: Westport Publishers.

Corbett-Dick, P., & Bezek, S. (1997). Breastfeeding promotion for the employed mother. *Journal of Pediatric Health Care, 11*(1), 12–19.

Curry, D., & Duby, J. (1994). Developmental surveillance by pediatric nurses. *Pediatric Nursing, 20*(1), 40–44.

Dennison, B. E., Rockwell, H., & Baker, S. (1997). Excess fruit juice consumption by preschool-aged children is associated with short stature and obesity. *Pediatrics*, 99(1), 15–22.

Elkind, D. (1993). *Parenting your teenager in the 1990s*. Rosemont, NJ: Modern Learning Press.

Ellis, A. (1997). Swimming pool drownings and near-drownings among California preschoolers. *Public Health Reports, 112*(1), 73–78.

Espeland, K. (1997). Inhalants: The instant, but deadly high. *Pediatric Nursing, 23*(1), 82–86.

Fighting a losing battle. (1995). *Pediatrics for Parents. 16*(4), 7–8.

Franck, I., & Brownstone, D. (1991). *The parent's desk reference*. New York, NY: Prentice-Hall.

Frauman, A., & Brandon, D. (1996). Toilet training for the child with chronic illness. *Pediatric Nursing, 22*(6), 469–472.

Froese-Fretz, A., & Keefe, M. (1997). The irritable infant. *Advance for Nurse Practitioners, 5*(2), 63–66.

Goldentyer, D. (1994). *Gangs*. Austin, TX: Raintree Steck-Vaughn Publishers.

Gordon, C. P. (1996). Adolescent decision making: A broadly based theory and its application to the prevention of early pregnancy. *Adolescence, 31*(123), 561–585.

Green, M. (Ed.). (1994). *Bright futures: Guidelines for health supervision of infants, children, and adolescents*. Arlington, VA: National Center for Education in Maternal and Child Health.

Greydanus, D. (1991). *The American Academy of Pediatrics: Caring for your adolescent ages 12 to 21*. New York, NY: Bantam Books.

Harbin, R. E. (1995). Female adolescent contraception. *Pediatric Nursing, 21*(3), 221–226.

Henderson, C. (1994). Study links teenage smoking to harder drugs. *Cancer Researcher Weekly*, April 11, 19–20.

Hockenberry-Eaton, M., Richman, M. J., Dilorio, C., Rivero, T., & Maibach, E. (1996). Mother and adolescent knowledge of sexual development: The effects of gender, age, and sexual experience. *Adolescence, 31*(121), 35–48.

Igra, V., & Millstein, S. G. (1993). Current status and approaches to improving preventative services for adolescents. *JAMA, 269*(11), 1408–1413.

Keefe, M., Froese-Fretz, A., & Kotzer, A. (1996). The REST regimen: An individualized nursing intervention for infant irritability. *MCN, 22*, 16–20.

Keller, C., & Stevens, K. (1996). Childhood obesity: Measurement and risk assessment. *Pediatric Nursing, 22*(6), 494–499.

Lerner, H. (1993). Sleep position of infants: Applying research to practice. *MCN, 18*, 275–277.

Lombardi, J. (1995). Involving working parents. *Children Today, 23*(4), 2–10.

Monroe, J. (1996). Recognizing signs of drug abuse. *Current Health 2, 23*(1), 16–20.

Moriarty, A. (1997). Contraceptive use options for adolescents. *Journal of Pediatric Health Care, 11*(3), 144–146.

Munson, M. (1996). Breast-feeding basics: Position yourself for success. *Prevention*, 48(2), 44–46.

Nelson, A. (1996a). Adolescent contraception. *The Western Journal of Medicine, 165*(6), 374–377.

Nelson, A. (1996b). Counseling issues and management of side effects for women using depot medroxyprogesterone acetate contraception. *The Journal of Reproductive Medicine, 41*, 391–400.

Oliver, M. T. (1995). *Gangs: Trouble in the streets*. Springfield, NJ: Enslow Publishers.

Parker, S., & Zuckerman, B. (1995). *Behavioral and developmental pediatrics*. Boston: Little, Brown & Company.

Peters, S. (1997). The mystery of insufficient milk syndrome. *Advance for Nurse Practitioners*, *5*(2), 57–58.

Rees, J. (1996). Eating disorders in adolescents: A model for broadening our perspective. *Journal of the American Dietetic Association*, *96*(1), 22–24.

Ryval, M. (1994). Starting preschool: How to ensure it's right for your child. *Chatelaine*, *67*(9), 40 –41.

Satcher, D., & Ericksen, M. (1994). The paradox of tobacco control. JAMA, *271*(8), 627–629.

Schechter, N. (1994). The gifted child. In S. Parker & B. Zuckerman (Eds.), *Behavioral and developmental pediatrics* (pp. 165–167). Boston: Little, Brown & Company.

Shelov, S. (1993). *The American Academy of Pediatrics: Caring for your baby and young child, birth to age 5*. New York: Bantam Books.

Smith, D. (1991). *Comprehensive child and family nursing skills*. St. Louis: Mosby–Year Book.

Snow, L., & Fry, M. (1990). Formula feeding in the first year of life. *Pediatric Nursing*, *16*(5), 442–446.

Turecki, S. (1995). Temperamentally difficult children. In S. Parker & B. Zuckerman (Eds.), *Behavioral and developmental pediatrics* (pp. 310–314). Boston: Little, Brown & Company.

Ucci, M. (1995). Coping with children's fears. *Child Health Alert*, *13*, 3.

Vessey, J., & Miola, E. (1997). Teaching adolescents self-advocacy skills. *Pediatric Nursing*, *23*(1), 53–56.

Victora, C., Tomasi, E., Olinto, M., & Barros, F. (1993). Use of pacifiers and breastfeeding duration. *Lancet*, *341*, 404–407.

Von Burg, M., Sanders, B., & Weddell, J. (1995). Baby bottle tooth decay: A concern for all mothers. *Pediatric Nursing*, *21*(6), 515–519.

Wong, D. (1986). Helping parents select day-care centers. *Pediatric Nursing*, *12*(3), 181–187.

Zuckerman, B. (1995). Healthy parenting choices: Children's temperament styles and parent's expectations. *Pediatric Basics*, *74*, 2–8.

Bibliography

Balsmeyer, B. (1990). Sleep disturbances of the infant and toddler. *Pediatric Nursing*, *16*(5), 447–452.

Beauchesne, M. (1997). Violence prevention: A community approach. *Journal of Pediatric Health Care*, *11*(4), 155–164.

Chandler, L. (1996). Changing children in a changing society. *Childhood Education*, *72*(5), 294–296.

DeFrancis, B. (1994). *The parents' resource almanac*. Holbrook, MA: Bob Adams, Inc.

Furman, L. (1995). A developmental approach to weaning. MCN, *20*(6), 322–325.

Hendricks, C., & Reichert, A. (1996). Parents' self-reported behaviors related to health and safety of very young children. *Journal of School Health*, 66(7), 247–251.

Honig, J. (1986). Preparing preschool-aged children to be siblings. MCN, *11*(1), 37–43.

Kaste, L., & Gift, H. (1996). Inappropriate infant bottle feeding. *Journal of the American Medical Association*, *275*(2), 88T.

Levine, E. (1995). *The Good Housekeeping illustrated book of childcare from birth to preteen*. New York, NY: Hearst Corporation.

McEvoy, M., Montana, B., & Panettieri, M. (1996). A nursing intervention to ensure a safe playground environment. *Journal of Pediatric Health Care*, *10*, 209–216.

McKimmey, M. (1994). Child's play is serious business. *Children Today*, *22*(2), 14–17.

Myerhoff, M. (1995). Babies, daycare, and social skills. *Pediatrics for Parents*, *16*(3), 8.

Needlman, R. (1995). Sibling rivalry. In S. Parker & B. Zuckerman (Eds.), *Behavioral and developmental pediatrics* (pp. 384–386). Boston: Little, Brown & Company.

NCAST. (1990). *Keys to caregiving*. Seattle, WA: NCAST Publications.

Oberklaid, F., Sanson, A., Pedlow, R., & Prior, M. (1993). Predicting preschool behavior problems from temperament and other variables in infants. *Pediatrics*, *91*(1), 113–120.

Poulton, S., & Sexton, D. (1995). Feeding young children: Developmentally appropriate considerations for supplementing family care. *Childhood Education*, *72*(2), 66–72.

Rollins, J. (1991). Focus on summertime. *Pediatric Nursing*, *17*(3), 317–319.

Roberts, P., & Moseley, B. (1996). Father's time: Importance of fathers in child rearing. *Psychology Today*, *29*(3), 48–57.

Sears, W. (1991). *Keys to calming the fussy baby*. New York: Barron's Educational Series.

Schor, E. (1995). *The American Academy of Pediatrics: Caring for your school age child ages 5 to 12*. New York: Bantam Books.

Schmitt, B. (1992). *Instructions for pediatric patients*. Philadelphia: W. B. Saunders.

Swingle, M. (1984). How to prepare the family for sibling rivalry. *Children's Nurse*, *2*(2), 1–3.

Trippe, H. (1996). Children and sport: Encouraging a healthy attitude to exercise should start in primary school. *British Medical Journal*, *312*, 199–201.

Troy, P., Wilkinson-Faulk, D., Smith, A., & Alexander, D. (1988, January). Sibling visiting in the NICU. *AJN*, 70H–70J.

Vaughan, V. (1995). Critical life events: Sibling births, separations, and deaths in the family. In M. Levine, W. Caret, & A. Crocker (Eds.), *Developmental-behavioral pediatrics* (pp. 128–134). Philadelphia: W. B. Saunders.

Weigley, E. (1990). Changing patterns in offering solids to infants. *Pediatric Nursing*, *16*(5), 439–446.

Health Assessment and Well-Child Care

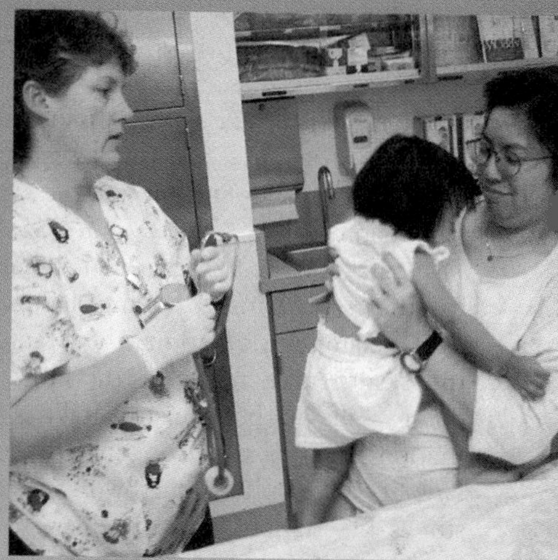

CHAPTER

6

OUTLINE

Levels of Prevention

Immunization

- Historical Perspectives
- Recommended Childhood Immunization Schedule
- Contraindications and Precautions for Immunization
- Routine Childhood Immunizations: Individual Vaccines
- Strategies for Improving Immunization Status

Health Assessment from Infancy Through Adolescence

- Communication Skills
- Health History
- Physical Examination
- Database and Interpretation

Health Surveillance Visits

Anticipatory Guidance

- Symptom Management and Teaching Principles

OBJECTIVES

- Describe the levels of prevention that are used as primary approaches to pediatric health assessment and teaching.
- List the childhood immunizations and their schedule of administration for those routine vaccines and identify the side effects associated with each of the vaccines.
- Discuss key points in the health assessment of children from infancy through adolescence.
- Elicit a pediatric health history pertinent to either the health supervision needs or illness-related problems of children from birth through adolescence.
- Discuss key approaches to interviewing the child and the family based on developmental considerations, psychosocial/emotional considerations, and level of acuity of illness.
- Perform a basic physical examination on a child that reflects knowledge of the developmental differences in the various body systems from birth through adolescence.
- Identify how the physical examination process may need to be altered based on developmental considerations.
- Differentiate normal from abnormal findings obtained while either taking historical information or performing the physical examination.
- Discuss the health care areas that are covered during health surveillance visits of children of each age group.
- Select age-appropriate teaching techniques to relay anticipatory guidance and disease prevention information.

KEY TERMS

acquired immunity
antibody
antigen
herd control/herd immunity
immunity
immunization
natural immunity
passive immunity
toxoid
vaccination
vaccine

This chapter focuses on the steps in complete health assessment of children from the neonatal period through adolescence. The various components of health supervision are identified, including childhood immunizations and anticipatory guidance issues. An in-depth discussion of the various components of the pediatric health history is presented, as is an overview of the comprehensive pediatric physical examination. Tips about examination techniques to use with children and how to communicate with parents, children, and teenagers are also provided. Subsequent chapters of the text contain information on the focused health history and physical assessment specific to each body system and expand on the information found in this chapter.

Data obtained from a comprehensive health history, together with clinical findings based on a complete physical examination, form the framework for assessing the health care needs of the child and family. Developing skills in both history taking and physical examination requires that the nurse have a solid knowledge base to assess physical growth and developmental milestones of children and a framework from which to address anticipatory guidance needs. In addition, the nurse must be an astute listener, an inquisitive interviewer, and an observant clinician with the necessary skills to perform a physical assessment and the knowledge to enable differentiation of normal from abnormal findings.

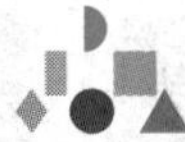

Levels of Prevention

Health is more than the absence of disease. Being healthy is being whole in mind, body, and spirit. Many of the conditions that affect health—food, shelter, education, income, sustainable resources, peace, social justice, and equity—are not readily amenable to intervention through the health care system.

Worldview: *In developing countries, overpopulation, poor sanitation, contaminated water, malnutrition, and inadequate housing present major threats to health. In developed countries such as the United States, major health problems are more likely to be lifestyle related and the result of accidents, alcohol and substance abuse, tobacco use, violence, or environmental pollution. Poverty is a linking factor and threatens health in all societies.*

Since the beginning of the 20th century, child health has improved remarkably in the United States. This progress resulted from a combination of social and economic changes, advances in therapeutic medicine and surgery, and implementation of public health measures such as immunization programs aimed at prevention of specific childhood diseases. Today, health care is more prevention focused than ever. The objectives set forth in the *Healthy People 2000* report (U.S. Department of Health and Human Services, 1990) clearly establish a health care agenda in which solutions to medical and social problems lie in preventive strategies rather than in emphasizing only the treatment of a disease or an injury.

Preventive health care is viewed as part of a continuum of intervention that includes a primary, secondary, and tertiary level of prevention. **Primary prevention** is directed at recognizing susceptibility to disease and employing strategies to prevent it from occurring. Primary prevention efforts often target those individuals at increased risk of developing a disease or condition. The use of immunizations is an excellent example of primary prevention. Other examples of primary prevention include chlorination and fluoridation of water and anticipatory guidance given to parents of toddlers about the need to keep poisons and medications out of their child's reach.

Secondary prevention is directed at early identification of risk factors for specific diseases or disabilities and initiation of early intervention to prevent the development of such diseases or their sequelae. Because of the increased awareness of specific social, occupational, environmental, and behavioral factors known to be antecedents of childhood illnesses and disabilities, the care of children is becoming more focused on illness and injury prevention. Many secondary prevention efforts are the result of governmental or social agency initiatives. Examples of secondary prevention strategies include state-mandated neonatal screening for inherited metabolic disorders such as phenylketonuria, hearing and vision screening in schools, and special screening programs for genetic diseases such as sickle-cell anemia or Tay-Sachs disease in at-risk populations.

For those children with known diseases, disabilities, or medical conditions (special needs children), a major emphasis in their health care is the avoidance of complications and additional disability. Therefore, **tertiary prevention** is an important educational strategy because it focuses on eliminating or halting the progression of disability associated with existing disease states. An example of tertiary prevention is the provision of chest physiotherapy to a child with cystic fibrosis.

Prevention efforts can be targeted at the individual child, the family, or the community. Preventive strategies can decrease the probability that low- or medium-risk children will develop particular diseases or conditions and subsequently enter high-risk categories of disease states or impaired health status. Therefore, this group of children benefits the most from participation in prevention programs.

Nurses play important roles in protecting children's health at all three levels of prevention. As health care continues to move from acute care settings to the community, home, short-stay centers, day-care centers, and school-based clinics, nurses have opportunities to provide direct clinical prevention services such as immunizations, to coordinate services, to provide leadership in the development and implementation of community-based prevention strategies, and to continue to advocate for children's health.

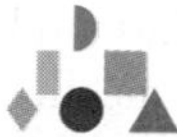

Immunization

Routine childhood immunization is an integral part of health maintenance for children. In the United States, the Advisory Committee on Immunization Practices (ACIP) of the Centers for Disease Control and Prevention (CDC) and the American Academy of Pediatrics (AAP) Committee on Infectious Disease share the responsibility for establishing recommendations for the administration of vaccines in the public and private sector. To ensure that all children are adequately protected from disease, health care providers are encouraged to follow the recommended immunization schedules and administration guidelines from the ACIP and the AAP (Chart 6–1). The World Health Organization (WHO) provides guidelines for immunization practices for the rest of the world because many developing countries do not have their own infrastructure to generate national guidelines.

The pediatric nurse needs to be familiar with issues

Chart 6–1
Nursing Interventions Classification (NIC)

Immunization/Vaccination Administration

Definition

Provision of immunizations for prevention of communicable disease

Activities

Teach parent(s) recommended immunization schedule (diphtheria, tetanus, pertussis, polio, measles, mumps, and rubella*) necessary for children, their route of medication administration, reasons and benefits of use, adverse reactions, and side effects.
Teach individual/families about vaccinations available in the event of special incidence and/or exposure (e.g., cholera, influenza, plague, rabies, Rocky Mountain spotted fever, smallpox, typhoid fever, typhus, yellow fever, and tuberculosis).
Provide immunization information in written form.
Provide diary for recording date and type of immunizations.
Identify proper administration techniques.
Identify latest recommendations about use of immunizations.
Administer injections to infant in the anterolateral thigh, as appropriate.
Inform patient/families which immunizations are required by law for entering school.
Follow the American Academy of Pediatrics and U.S. Public Health Service guidelines for immunization administration.
Inform travelers of vaccinations appropriate for travel to foreign countries.
Identify contraindications for administering immunizations, such as fever, another infectious disease, or skin lesions at site of immunization.
Recognize that a delay in series administration does not indicate restarting the schedule.
Secure informed consent to administer vaccine.
Help family with financial planning to pay for immunizations (e.g., insurance coverage and health department clinics).
Inform parent(s) of comfort measures helpful after medication administration to child.
Observe patient for a specified period after medication administration.
Restrain child during immunization, as needed.
Schedule immunizations at appropriate time intervals.

* Hepatitis B and varicella vaccines are also recommended.
From McCloskey, J., & Bulechek, G. (1996). *Nursing interventions classification (NIC)* (2nd ed.). St. Louis: Mosby–Year Book. Reprinted with permission.

regarding childhood immunizations. Vaccine research is ongoing, and new vaccines continue to be developed. Additional information about specific vaccines is continually being discovered, and recommendations for their use often change. Excellent resources for current information regarding immunization practices in the United States include the following:

- *The Red Book: Report of the Committee on Infectious Disease*, published every 2 years by the AAP
- Recommendations of the Advisory Committee on Immunization Practices (ACIP) of the CDC
- *Morbidity and Mortality Weekly Report* (MMWR), a newsletter issued weekly by the CDC
- The National Immunization Program (NIP) of the CDC
- *Physicians' Desk Reference*
- Package inserts accompanying the vaccines

Historical Perspectives

The widespread use of immunization against disease remains one of the most dramatic advances in pediatrics, altering the morbidity and mortality associated with once common and feared childhood diseases. However, the history of immunization in the United States is a mixture of success and failures. The elimination of smallpox in 1980, the near-elimination of meningitis caused by *Haemophilus influenzae* type b with the development of a vaccine administered in infancy, the establishment of universal hepatitis B immunization guidelines in 1991, and the approval of the varicella-zoster (chickenpox) and hepatitis A vaccines in 1995 can be counted among the successes resulting from immunization programs. The use of vaccines has clearly and repeatedly been demonstrated to be the most cost-effective way of eliminating vaccine-preventable diseases against which children are now routinely immunized.

Unfortunately, success has been accompanied by failures, as evidenced by unacceptably low rates of immunization due to complacency and unwarranted fears. Although completion of the recommended childhood immunization schedule is a requirement for entrance into school, children younger than age 2 years—the group at greatest risk for developing vaccine-preventable disease—have the worst rates (between 40% and 70%) of vaccine completion in the United States (Arbiter et al., 1993; Zell, 1994). These rates should be at a minimum level of 80% to provide protection to the general population, a concept known as *herd immunity*. The recent resurgence of measles and pertussis was particularly devastating to children younger than age 6 months. Reasons for low immunization rates include failure of health care providers to use every encounter as a chance to vaccinate; failure to administer vaccines to vulnerable children on time; unnecessary delays in vaccine administration based on misinformation about contraindications; and the erroneous beliefs held by parents and caretakers that the diseases are no longer a health threat.

Vaccine failures and waning vaccine immunity also contribute to the inability to eradicate infectious and highly communicable diseases. The resurgence of measles in college-age students in the 1980s led to further study of the vaccine's immunogenic properties and identification of the need for a booster vaccination when the levels of protection begin to fall around the age 12 years. Tetanus is another example of a vaccine given in infancy that needs to be boosted around age 12, every 10 years thereafter, and at times of injury to provide adequate levels of protection.

Recommended Childhood Immunization Schedule

The recommended age for beginning primary immunization of infants is at birth (Table 6–1; see Appendix 8). In the first year of life, three doses each of diphtheria and tetanus toxoids and pertussis vaccine (DTP or DTaP [Tripedia]), *Haemophilus influenzae* type b (Hib) vaccine, and oral polio vaccine (OPV) are recommended at age 2, 4, and 6 months. The third dose of OPV may be administered any time at age 6 to 18 months. In late 1996 the ACIP recommended a change in the routine polio vaccination schedule with a switch to a two-dose schedule of inactivated polio vaccine (IPV) at age 2 and 4 months, followed by two doses of OPV (the first OPV at 12 to 18 months and the second dose at 4 to 6 years). Either polio vaccination option (OPV only or combination IPV and OPV) is acceptable.

Four types of Hib vaccine are available for use in infants. Infants given PedvaxHIB (PRP-OMP) at age 2 and 4 months do not require a third dose at age 6 months. The AAP and the CDC recommend administration of hepatitis B vaccine to all infants at birth. The recommended three-dose schedule of hepatitis B vaccination for infants born to hepatitis B surface antigen (HBsAg)-negative mothers is dose one at birth, dose two 1 month after dose one, and dose three at age 6 to 18 months. Routine testing of infants to determine the presence of anti-HBsAg is not recommended, except in infants whose mothers tested positive for HBsAg during pregnancy.

A child born prematurely should receive the full dose of each vaccine at the appropriate chronologic age.

Table 6–1
Recommended Childhood Immunization Schedule—United States, February–December 1997*

Vaccines[1] are listed under the routinely recommended ages. Bars indicate range of acceptable ages for vaccination. Shaded bars indicate catch-up vaccination: at 11 to 12 years of age, hepatitis B vaccine should be administered to children not previously vaccinated, and varicella vaccine should be administered to children not previously vaccinated who lack a reliable history of chickenpox.

Age ▶ Vaccine ▼	Birth	1 mo	2 mo	4 mo	6 mo	12 mo	15 mo	18 mo	4–6 yr	11–12 yr	14–16 yr
Hepatitis B[2,3]	Hep B-1										
		Hep B-2			Hep B-3					Hep B[3]	
Diphtheria, Tetanus, Pertussis[4]			DTaP or DTP	DTaP or DTP	DTaP or DTP		DTaP or DTP[4]		DTaP or DTP	Td	
H. influenzae type b[5]			Hib	Hib	Hib[5]	Hib[5]					
Polio[6]			Polio[6]	Polio		Polio[6]			Polio		
Measles, Mumps, Rubella[7]						MMR			MMR[7] or	MMR[7]	
Varicella[8]						Var				Var[8]	

* Approved by the Advisory Committee on Immunization Practices (ACIP), the American Academy of Pediatrics (AAP), and the American Academy of Family Physicians (AAFP).

[1] This schedule indicates the recommended age for routine administration of currently licensed childhood vaccines. Some combination vaccines are available and may be used whenever administration of all components of the vaccine is indicated. Providers should consult manufacturer package inserts for detailed recommendations.

[2] Infants born to HBsAg-negative mothers should receive 2.5 μg of Merck vaccine (Recombivax HB) or 10 μg of SmithKline Beecham (SB) vaccine (Engerix-B). The second dose should be administered ≥1 month after the first dose.

Infants born to HBsAg-positive mothers should receive 0.5 mL hepatitis B immune globulin (HBIG) within 12 hours of birth, and either 5 μg of Merck vaccine or 10 μg of SB vaccine at a separate site. The second dose is recommended at 1–2 months of age and the third dose at 6 months of age.

Infants born to mothers whose HBsAg status is unknown should receive either 5 μg of Merck vaccine or 10 μg of SB vaccine within 12 hours of birth. The second dose of vacine is recommended at 1 month of age and the third dose at 6 months age. Blood should be drawn at the time of delivery to determine the mother's HBsAg status; if it is positive, the infant should receive HBIG as soon as possible (no later than 1 week of age). The dosage and timing of subsequent vaccine dosses should not be based on the mother's HBsAg status.

[3] Children and adolescents who have not been vaccinated against hepatitis B in infancy may begin the series during any childhood visit. Those who have not previously received three doses of hepatitis B vaccine should initiate or complete the series during the 11- to 12-year-old visit. The second dose should be administered at least 1 month after the first dose, and the third dose should be administered at least 4 months after the first dose and at least 2 months after the second dose.

[4] DTaP (diptheria and tetanus toxoids and acellular pertussis vaccine) is the preferred vaccine for all doses in the vaccination series, including completion of the series in children who have received ≥1 dose of whole-cell DTP vaccine. Whole-cell DTP is an acceptable alternative to DTaP. The fourth dose of DTaP may be administered as early as 12 months of age, provided 6 months have elapsed since the third dose, and if the child is considered unlikely to return at 15- to 18-months of age. Td (tetanus and diphtheria toxoids, absorbed for adult use) is recommended at 11- to 12-years of age if at least 5 years have elapsed since the last dose of DTP, DTaP, or DT. Subsequent routine Td boosters are recommended every 10 years.

[5] Three *H. influenzae* type b (Hib) conjugate vaccines are licensed for infant use. If PRP-OMP (PedvaxHIB) is administered at 2 and 4 months of age, a dose at 6 months is not required. After completing the primary series, any Hib conjugate vaccine may be used as a booster.

[6] Two poliovirus vaccines are currently licensed in the US: inactivated poliovirus vaccine (IPV) and oral poliovirus vaccine (OPV). The following schedules are all acceptable by the ACIP, the AAP and the AAFP, and parents and providers may choose among them:

1. IPV at 2 and 4 months; OPV at 12 to 18 months and 4 to 6 years;
2. IPV at 2, 4, 12 to 18 months and 4 to 6 years;
3. OPV at 2, 4, 6 to 18 months and 4 to 6 years.

The ACIP routinely recommends schedule 1. IPV is the only poliovirus vaccine recommended for immunocompromised persons and their household contacts.

[7] The second dose of MMR is routinely recommended at 4 to 6 years of age or at 11 to 12 years of age, but may be administered during any visit, provided at least 1 month has elapsed since receipt of the first dose and that both doses are administered at or after 12 months of age.

[8] Susceptible children may receive varicella vaccine (Var) at any visit after the first birthday, and those who lack a reliable history of chickenpox should be immunized during the 11–12 year-old visit. Children ≥13 years of age should receive 2 doses, at least 1 month apart.

From Peters, S. (1997). The state of pediatric immunizations today. *Advance for Nurse Practitioners, 5*(2), 44. Reprinted with permission.

OPV is not given to an infant who is hospitalized to prevent transmission of the live virus, which is shed in stool for days to weeks following receipt of the vaccine. Table 6–1 presents a recommended schedule for children not immunized during infancy.

Children who began primary immunization at the recommended age but did not complete the immunization series according to the recommended schedule should receive only the missed doses, rather than beginning the series again. HBV, DTP or DTaP, IPV or OPV, measles, mumps, and rubella (MMR), and Hib vaccines can be administered simultaneously to children younger than age 7 years who start the series late or who are more than 1 month behind in the immunization schedule and in whom compliance with the optimum schedule is doubtful.

Worldview: *Many children adopted from abroad have not been properly immunized before their arrival in the United States. Immunizations should begin immediately, according to the recommendations of the AAP. Immunization status of refugee or immigrant children should also be reviewed on arrival in the United States and deficiencies addressed.*

Immunizations recommended at age 12 to 15 months include a DTP and a single dose of MMR. The booster dose of DTaP is recommended at age 15 to 20 months. DTaP contains only parts of the pertussis bacterium, not the whole bacterium as does DTP. Data suggest that DTaP is effective in decreasing the incidence of adverse reactions while maintaining a high immunogenicity against contracting pertussis.

The second dose of the MMR vaccine may be given at entry to kindergarten (age 4 to 6 years) or during middle school (age 11 to 12 years). Varicella vaccine (Varivax) is recommended for administration as a single dose in children age 12 to 18 months and in children age 18 months to 12 years with no history of chickenpox.

Due to recent changes in the immunization recommendations, the 1997 immunization schedule recommends the following immunizations for all 11- to 12-year-old children: Hepatitis B vaccine series; a booster with combined diphtheria and tetanus toxoids (Td); and a second dose of MMR vaccine. The Td booster may be given through age 14 to 16 years. When the Td vaccine is given at age 11 to 12 years, health care providers should also ensure that the child has received the second dose of MMR (CDC, 1995). For adolescents aged 13 years and adults who have not had chickenpox, Varivax administration is recommended to be followed by a second dose of Varivax 4 to 8 weeks later.

Contraindications and Precautions for Immunization

Unfounded fears and lack of knowledge regarding contraindications to immunization can needlessly interfere with a child receiving protection against life-threatening, but vaccine-preventable, disease. Awareness of the reasons for withholding immunizations, both for the child's safety in minimizing adverse reactions and in achieving maximum benefit, is important for the pediatric nurse.

The only true contraindications to immunization are a history of severe anaphylactic reaction to a vaccine or vaccine component or encephalopathy within 7 days after a dose of DTP/DTaP. MMR vaccines contain minute amounts of neomycin, and measles and mumps vaccines are derived from chick embryo tissue cultures, which may contain substances allergenic to egg-sensitive individuals. Although a history of anaphylactoid reaction to neomycin or to egg is considered a contraindication to the MMR vaccine, one study demonstrated safe administration of a single-dose MMR vaccine to children with allergy to eggs, even to those with severe hypersensitivity (James, Burks, Roberson, & Sampson, 1995). The ACIP advises careful weighing of risks and benefits before making this decision.

Alert: *As with any medication, rare severe systemic reactions such as anaphylaxis or generalized urticaria are possible. Because of the potential for anaphylaxis with the administration of a vaccine, any patient receiving a vaccine should be observed for several minutes after the vaccine is given for signs of immediate allergic/anaphylactic reaction.*

Local reactions at the injection site, such as redness or swelling, are not uncommon and are self-resolving. Systemic reactions may occur up to 7 days after administration of DTP (most reactions occur within 72 hours), 5 to 15 days after MMR, and between 30 days to 6 months after OPV.

Evidence regarding the exact cause of adverse events associated with the pertussis vaccine is not conclusive. At best, a temporal relationship exists bewteen DTP administration and acute encephalopathy (primarily within 3 days of vaccination but possibly up to 7 days) with associated chronic nervous system dysfunction (CDC, 1996d). However, the estimated risk is none to 10.5 incidents per million DTP vaccinations. The issue of pertussis vaccine safety should finally be put to rest now that the 1997 vaccine schedule recommends DTaP for all childhood doses.

There are no documented cases of central nervous system injury or death temporally associated with DTaP administration. Generally, immunizations should not be given to a child with high fever and serious illness. Exercising this precaution avoids adding the risk of adverse side effects from the vaccine to a child who is already ill or confusing symptoms of the illness with a side effect of the vaccine.

caREminder: *High fevers and severe illness are reasons to delay immunization, but only until the child has recovered from the acute stage of the illness. Minor illnesses such as a cold, otitis media, or mild diarrhea without fever are not contraindications to immunization.*

A guide discussing contraindications to childhood vaccinations is available at no charge from the CDC.

Vaccines derived from live viruses are generally not administered to any child with an altered immune system, because severe vaccine-induced illness may result. Because the polio vaccine is derived from live virus, OPV should not be given to an immunosuppressed child or to a child with either symptomatic or asymptomatic human immunodeficiency virus (HIV) infection. OPV is also contraindicated for a child who has close personal contact with an HIV-infected or severely immunosuppressed person. Because poliovirus is shed in the stool for several days to weeks after receipt of the oral polio vaccine, immunosuppressed contacts would be placed at unnecessary risk for contracting vaccine-related polio. Inactivated polio vaccine (IPV) should be administered in children whose contact with immunocompromised individuals precludes use of OPV.

MMR is recommended for all asymptomatic HIV-infected persons and should be considered for all symptomatic HIV-infected persons because of the severity of the illness if an HIV-positive individual were to contract measles. However, because of a case of pneumonitis associated with MMR vaccination in a person with advanced acquired immunodeficiency syndrome (AIDS), the CDC is rethinking its recommendations and currently believes it may be prudent to withhold MMR for HIV-infected individuals with evidence of severe immunosuppression (CDC, 1996d). Immunization with MMR is generally deferred during pregnancy.

Routine Childhood Immunizations: Individual Vaccines

Diphtheria-Tetanus-Pertussis

DTP or DTaP is a combination of three killed vaccines given as a series of five injections. Four are administered over the first 15 months of age, with a booster at primary school entry. The vaccine is injected intramuscularly in either the vastus lateralis or the deltoid muscle, depending on the child's muscle mass. Occasionally, there may be tenderness, redness, or swelling at the site of the injection. This can be relieved with ice packs for the first 24 hours, followed by warm compresses if the inflammation persists. Fever has been reported in approximately 1 in 100 to 1000 children after administration of DTP. Acetaminophen should be given prophylactically before the vaccine is administered and continued every 4 hours for 24 hours.

Rarely, a child may spike a temperature of 104°F or higher after DTP immunization. The increased temperature has been attributed to the pertussis component of the vaccine.

caREminder: *Precautions to subsequent vaccination with DTP include convulsions with or without fever occurring within 3 days after vaccination and the following events occurring within 48 hours of vaccination: fever to 105°F or higher that is not attributed to another cause, collapse or shock-like state, and persistent and inconsolable crying lasting 3 hours or more.*

Diphtheria and tetanus are rare diseases in the United States. Those infected are usually elderly people who had not received Td boosters in the previous 10 years. Serologic tests indicate that naturally acquired immunity to tetanus and diphtheria toxin does not occur in the United States. Universal vaccination with appropriately spaced boosters at 10-year intervals is necessary to provide continued protection (CDC, 1995).

Worldwide, 350,000 people contract pertussis (whooping cough) each year and 50,000 die of it. The great majority of deaths are children younger than 6 months of age. The pertussis vaccine is a whole cell killed bacterium, rather than a toxoid like the other vaccines with which it is combined for administration. Because the vaccine is made from the whole *Bordetella pertussis* bacterium and contains multiple antigens, it has been implicated as the cause of a higher rate of local and systemic reactions. As mentioned previously, there is a causal relationship between DTP and acute encephalopathy; however, studies have demonstrated no causal relationship between DTP and sudden infant death syndrome, infantile spasms, hyperactivity, learning disorders, or infantile autism (CDC, 1996d).

In 1979, an acellular pertussis vaccine, containing one or more immunogens derived from the *B. pertussis* organism, was developed in Japan. In 1991 an acellular vaccine (DTaP [ACEL-IMUNE]) was developed and first licensed in the United States for use only as the fourth and fifth doses for children previously immunized with at least three doses of the DTP vaccine. After careful analysis of clinical trials involving children given DTaP as their primary series of vaccination, the ACIP and the AAP recommended the use of acellular pertussis vaccine (Immunization Action News, 1996).

Multiple doses of DTP/DTaP vaccine are necessary to provide adequate and lasting immunity. Antibody titers fall over time; therefore, immunity is boosted with recommended administration of Td (tetanus and a much lower dose of diphtheria toxoid) every 10 years. Currently, pertussis vaccine is not administered to anyone older than age 7 years because the risk of receiving the vaccine increases as the incidence, severity, and fatality of the disease decrease. Studies are now underway to determine if booster shots including the pertussis component should be given to the adult and adolescent community to decrease the incidence of carriers of *B. pertussis* in the general population (Mokotoff et al., 1994).

Haemophilus influenzae Type b

Hib vaccine is administered intramuscularly in either the vastus lateralis or the deltoid muscle depending on the muscle mass. The vaccines against *H. influenzae* type b are major weapons in the prevention of childhood bacterial meningitis. The vaccine era began in 1985, with the licensure of a polyribosylribitol phosphate (PRP) vaccine for routine use in children age 24 months and older. Further research led to the development of vaccines with improved immunogenicity in younger infants, a development accompanied by a dramatic decline in the incidence of invasive infections due to *H. influenzae* type b.

Four conjugate vaccines (PRP-D [Prohibit], Connaught Laboratories; HbOC [HIBTITER], Lederle-Praxis; PRP-OMP [Pedvax HIB], Merck, Sharp, & Dohme; PRP-T [ActHIB/Omni Hib], Pasteur-Merleux Vaccines) and two combination vaccines that combine the DTP vaccine with HIB (HbOC/DTP [Tetramune], Lederle-Praxis; PRP-DTP [ActHIB/DTP]) are licensed for use in the United States. PRP-D is recommended only for infants age 12 months and older; HbOC, PRP-OMP, and PRP-T are recommended for infants beginning at age 2 months. Aside from a slight fever and soreness at the injection site, no other side effects are commonly associated with this vaccine. In the combination product with DTP, the risk of local and systemic effects is similar to those following concurrent administration of its individual component vaccines.

Hepatitis B

Hepatitis B virus (HBV) is a potentially fatal viral infection, frequently culminating in cirrhosis or liver cancer during adulthood. Because HBV infection can occur perinatally or any other time during childhood, HBV is an important pediatric disease. Hepatitis B vaccine is given in a series of three intramuscular doses. Approximately 95% of infants and 90% of adults who receive three injections develop immunity to the virus. Universal vaccination of all infants is recommended, and adolescents who have not previously received three doses of HBV vaccine should initiate or complete the series by 11 to 12 years of age (CDC, 1995). No follow-up antibody testing is needed for infants born to HBsAg-negative mothers (see Chapter 24).

Infants born to HBsAg-positive mothers should receive hepatitis B immunoglobulin (HBIG) within 12 hours of birth in addition to completing the series of three vaccines. Those infants who do not receive HBIG have a 90% risk of developing chronic hepatitis B and subsequently developing liver cancer or cirrhosis in their mid 30s to early 40s. Within 6 months of the last dose of vaccine, these infants should be tested to determine if they are immune. If they are not immune, anti-HBs and HBSAg-negative additional vaccinations are given along with repeated testing for the presence of protective antibodies. Five percent of these children do not seroconvert.

Two hepatitis B vaccines are available in the United States. One is plasma derived for people with an allergy to yeast. The other is a recombinant product grown in common baker's yeast. The most common side effect observed after vaccination with each of the available vaccines has been soreness at the injection site.

Measles-Mumps-Rubella

Measles-mumps-rubella (MMR) should be administered between age 12 and 15 months and a second dose at age 4 to 6 or 11 to 12 years. Because of continued outbreaks of measles among unvaccinated preschool-age children and among vaccinated school-age children and college students in the 1980s, a second dose of MMR was added to the schedule to provide lasting immunity. The mumps virus vaccine is combined with measles and rubella; it should not be administered to infants younger than age 12 months because persisting maternal antibodies can interfere with the immune response. Rubella, while a relatively mild infection in children, presents a serious risk to the developing fetus in a pregnant woman. The goal of rubella immunization is protection of future unborn children rather than the recipient of the immunization. Vaccination of pregnant women with MMR is contraindicated.

MMR is administered by subcutaneous injection. Because of the risk of a diminished immune response or tissue damage, intramuscular injection is not recommended (AAP, 1994). Occasional soreness, redness, or swelling at the site of the injection can result after administration of the vaccine. Ice packs for the first 24 hours and warm compresses thereafter can relieve local symptoms. In occasional cases, 1 to 2 weeks after the first dose there may be a rash; fever; swelling of the lymph nodes in the cheeks, neck, or under the jaw; or a seizure related to a high fever. One to 3 weeks after the first dose there may be pain, stiffness, or swelling in one or more joints lasting up to 3 days. In rare cases this stiffness may last up to a month but is self-resolving (CDC, 1994).

Polio

There are two types of trivalent polio vaccine: liquid oral polio vaccine (OPV) administered by mouth and an enhanced, injectable inactivated polio vaccine (eIPV) for subcutaneous administration. The inactivated vaccine is highly immunogenic; after three doses it induces immunity equal to or greater than that of the OPV. The oral vaccine gives gut immunity (IgA) that provides resistance to reinfection with wild polioviruses, is easy to distribute, is well accepted by the community, and has worked successfully. In addition, the live poliovirus can be shed to contacts, who become immunized through this exposure.

In rare instances (1 in approximately 1.5 million first doses and 1 in 30 million later doses), OPV has been associated with paralytic disease in vaccine recipients or their close contacts (Strebel et al., 1994). As of December 1993, all cases of polio in the United States (an average of nine cases per year) have been associated with the oral vaccine. It is theorized that the attenuated vaccine, derived from three wild polioviruses, mutates after ingestion and reverts to the wild virus, causing paralysis. The remaining cases of polio have been demonstrated to have been imported from other areas of the world.

There have been no documented cases of vaccine-associated polio paralysis (VAPP) with the use of the inactive vaccine. Because of the risk of vaccine associated polio, the ACIP now recommends a sequential childhood schedule of two doses of IPV followed by two doses of OPV. This transition recommendation is expected to reduce the frequency of VAPP by 50% to 75% or more and could facilitate the final transition to an all IPV schedule in the United States.

Varicella-Zoster

Chickenpox, the primary infection caused by the varicella-zoster virus, is an extremely contagious type of herpesvirus. It is generally considered a benign, self-limited infection in the usually healthy child. However, chickenpox is a costly disease, in terms of its financial impact and the harm it inflicts in certain populations, in particular neonates and immunocompromised children. About 5% of individuals become adults without having had chickenpox. Varivax (manufactured by Merck, Sharp & Dohme) is a live, attenuated varicella-zoster virus vaccine that was approved for use in the United States in May 1995.

The Varivax vaccine is well tolerated. Five to 10 percent of children receiving the vaccine develop localized reactions with mild fever and/or rash development in the month after immunization. Lesions, usually located on the face, chest, and back, usually resemble mosquito bites and can last up to a few days. Other adverse reactions include pain at the site of injection and fever, similar to the reactions associated with other vaccines.

The vaccine is given subcutaneously in the outer part of the upper arm or anterolateral thigh.

Alert: *It is contraindicated in individuals with a history of hypersensitivity to any component of the vaccine, including gelatin, and in individuals with a history of anaphylactoid reaction to neomycin (CDC, 1996b).*

Vaccines for Children with Special Needs

Four vaccines are recommended only for children with special needs: influenza, pneumovax, hepatitis A, and bacille Calmette-Guérin (BCG). Influenza vaccine is strongly recommended for children younger than age 6 months who have underlying medical conditions that place them at risk for complications of influenza. Included in this list are children with cardiovascular or pulmonary problems (including asthma), chronic metabolic disorders (including diabetes mellitus), renal disease, hemoglobinopathies, immunosuppression (including immunosuppression by medications), and children on long-term aspirin therapy. Only split virus vaccine should be used in children younger than age 12 years because of its lower potential for causing febrile reactions. A two-dose schedule is recommended for children younger than 9 years of age who are receiving the vaccine for the first time. The route of administration is intramuscular, and dosage is age dependent (CDC, 1996a). The preferred injection site is the anterolateral aspect of the thigh for infants and young children and the deltoid for older children.

BCG vaccination, derived from a strain of *Mycobacterium bovis*, is rarely indicated but is recommended only for infants or children who are tuberculin skin test negative and fall into two select groups:

- Those who are exposed continually to untreated or ineffectively treated individuals with infectious pulmonary tuberculosis and cannot be separated from the infected person or given long-term primary preventive therapy
- Those who are exposed continually to an individual with infectious pulmonary tuberculosis caused by *M. tuberculosis* strains resistant to isoniazid and rifampin and cannot be separated from the infected person

The BCG vaccination is given percutaneously by means of a multiple-puncture disk in the lower deltoid area (CDC, 1996c).

Hepatitis A vaccine is recommended for children older than age 2 years who have chronic liver disease or clotting factor disorders, male adolescents who have sex with other males, and illicit drug users. Two vaccines—Havrix and Vaqta—are approved for intramuscular administration in a series of two doses. The second dose of Havrix is given 6 to 12 months after the first dose. The second dose of Vaqta is administered 6 months after the first dose.

The prevention of *Streptococcus pneumoniae* disease or its complications is important in children with chronic illnesses associated with an increased risk of pneumococcal disease. Vaccination with a 23-valent pneumococcal polysaccharide vaccine (Pneumovax 23 or Pnu Immune

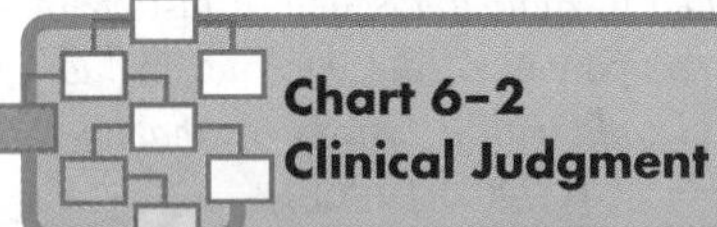

Chart 6–2
Clinical Judgment

An Unimmunized Toddler

Manuel is a 15-month-old brought into the clinic by his mother because he has a cold and has been very fussy and has been pulling at his ears. He has not been to your clinic before.

Questions

1. What other information should the nurse obtain?
2. What are the major issues that must be addressed at this visit?
3. Is Manuel too sick to receive immunizations today?
4. Which immunizations should Manuel receive today?
5. What should Manuel's mother be taught about potential reactions to the vaccines?

Answers

1. The history of present illness:
    How long has Manuel been sick? (3 days)
    Has he had a fever? (he has felt pretty warm but not hot)
    What, if anything, has been done to treat him? Has it helped? (no treatment)
    Is anyone else sick at home? (brothers have colds)
   Review of systems
   Past medical history
    Birth history
    Previous illnesses (colds, diarrhea, no injuries, serious or chronic illnesses)
    Current medications (none)
    Allergies (none known)
    Immunization status (received hepatitis B vaccine in hospital at birth, none since)
    Growth and development
   Family and social history
   Physical examination: normal except bilateral mucoid discharge from nares and bulging, erythematous tympanic membranes; rectal temperature of 100°F
2. A) Upper respiratory tract infection and bilateral otitis media
   B) Deficient immunization status.
3. No—he does not have a high fever or serious illness.
4. HBV (second dose), DTP, IPV, MMR, Hib
5. Acetaminophen should be given prophylactically before the injection and every 4 hours for 24 hours.
   Apply ice at injection site, if needed, for 24 hours, and then warm compresses.
   Immunization-specific reactions (e.g., soreness at site, rash)
   Notify health care provider of:
    Fever >105°F
    Seizure
    Persistent and inconsolable crying lasting ≥3 hours
    Collapse or shock-like state
   Importance of continuing immunization series

23) is recommended for children 2 years or older in the following categories: splenic absence or dysfunction; sickle cell disease; nephrotic syndrome; immunosuppression including HIV; and cerebrospinal fluid leaks. The vaccine is given either intramuscularly or subcutaneously. Revaccination is recommended in children with a high risk for severe pneumococcal infection, including those likely to have a rapid decline in their serum antibody concentration (e.g., nephrotic syndrome, anatomic asplenia, or sickle cell disease) 3 to 5 years after initial vaccination who will be 10 years old or younger at revaccination. For children older than 10, the interval for revaccination is 6 years or more. Local reactions are most common; fever and myalgias occur in less than 1% of vaccinations, and severe adverse events are rare (Peter & Klein, 1996).

Strategies for Improving Immunization Status

Education remains the most important tool in increasing immunization rates in this country and the world. Nurses should not assume that the general public understands and accepts the premises for routine childhood immunizations. It is important to first assess the parent's or caretaker's level of knowledge about immunization and the disease it prevents. A 1995 study conducted by the American Nurses Association revealed that 47% of respondents had no idea that polio was contagious and 59% did not know that children should receive their first immunizations against pertussis by age 2 months (Burgraf, 1995). Keane and colleagues (1993) found that caretakers who knew that the schedule printed on their child's immunization record was to be completed by age 24 months were compliant and their children had a positive vaccination status at 19 months. More than 40% of caretakers interviewed did not know that the immunization schedule should be completed by age 24 months, whereas 27% did not know their children's immunization status or incorrectly stated the child's status. Work by Arbiter and colleagues (1993) suggests that if a mother is informed of the importance of immunizations before leaving the birthing hospital, her child would begin immunizations on time and have a much higher probability of continuing to be current with immunization.

Without a doubt the risk from disease is always greater than the risk from vaccine for all individuals for whom vaccines are not contraindicated. Vaccination decreases the probability that a person will contract a disease and spread that disease to the greater population. Informed consent needs to be obtained before vaccinations are given. The health care provider needs to explain the risks and benefits of immunization; it is the caretaker's responsibility to decide whether the child should be immunized (Chart 6–2). Laws in most states require a minimum number of immunizations before school entry. Parents may decline immunizations on religious or, in some states, ideologic grounds. However, in the event of an epidemic, the health of the greater community takes precedence over the rights of the unimmunized individual.

The general public in the United States has no first-hand experience with most vaccine-preventable illnesses that are now part of routine childhood immunizations. The phenomenon of "out of sight, out of mind" is operational; the longer it has been since a disease was prevalent, the harder it is to convince people that there is still a threat. The potential health risk for spread of disease is there if children, especially those younger than age 2 years, are not immunized. Pediatric nurses must educate parents and caretakers about the need to vaccinate to ensure a healthy start and a healthy tomorrow for children.

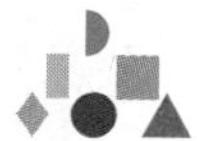

Health Assessment from Infancy Through Adolescence

Communication Skills

Developing communication skills that are essential for both obtaining a health history and performing a physical examination requires a conscientious and concerted effort. The nurse must be able to receive and send information while concentrating on both verbal and nonverbal messages that are being exchanged. Internal factors that relate to one's ability to successfully communicate include the ability to be empathetic (i.e., understanding how the person perceives or feels), to be an active listener (i.e., listening to what is said, or not mentioned, and how it is said), and to convey respect.

External considerations that affect communication include privacy, interruptions, comfort in the physical environment, and note taking. The need to ensure privacy involves arranging a setting so that conversations are not overheard by others or, if interviewing must be done at the bedside, pulling bedside curtains to partition the area and asking visitors (non-parents) to step out of the room. Interruptions break the flow of communication and are distracting; therefore, unnecessary interruptions should be discouraged and the nurse should ask not to be disturbed except for an emergency. Considerations in the physical environment include a comfortable room temperature, adequate lighting, a quiet setting, and a place for the child or parent and examiner to sit and see each

Chart 6–3
Nursing Interventions

Communication Techniques for Conducting a Health History

- Introduce yourself, your title, and the purpose of the interview.
- Ask the parent/caregiver and child how they wish to be addressed.
- Use open-ended questions as much as possible but follow with closed or direct questions when specific information is needed.
- Ask one question at a time and use language that the adult and child understand.
- Ask for clarification, if confused by the person's choice of words or explanation.
- Summarize to ensure that you correctly understand what was said.
- Close the interviewing by giving the parent/caregiver and child an opportunity to reflect to determine whether any additional information should be shared.

other. If the nurse stands during the interview, the message conveyed is that of the need for haste. Note taking should be kept to a minimum, so the nurse can focus attention on who is speaking and what is being said (Jarvis, 1996).

The nurse must be aware of the previously mentioned communication skills and techniques when conducting an interval or episodic history interview related to a specific health problem (Chart 6–3). Familiarity with a child and family can sometimes result in failure to actively listen or communicate as effectively by taking issues for granted.

Health History

The complete health history is divided into component parts that are addressed in a systematic fashion (Chart 6–4). This information can be obtained through either a direct interview alone or through a combination of direct interview and a health questionnaire. If a questionnaire is used, the nurse needs to verify that the informant can both read and write and that the questionnaire is at an appropriate level of understanding.

Worldview: *The services of an interpreter who is fluent in the language of the informant and preferably trained to perform interpreter duties should be sought whenever the historian and interviewer are not fluent in the same language. Asking a sibling to interpret for the parent may be perceived by the parent as a sign of disrespect. Parents also may be reluctant to disclose information about a genetic problem or sexual issue if their child is interpreting for them.*

Accurate data collection is of paramount importance, and cultural dynamics are essential to consider (see Chapter 4 for cultural and spiritual assessment). Specific items related to the adolescent health history are discussed at the end of this chapter under developmental considerations related to the adolescent history and physical examination.

Identifying or Biographic Data

The interviewer starts by obtaining certain identifying data that include the child's name, nickname, birth date, gender, and the identity of the person providing the information (i.e., how is the historian related to the child). If an interpreter is used, the name of this individual is also included. In the written notes about the health history, a statement about the reliability of the informant is made.

caREminder: *Even if the informant is a parent, he or she may not be knowledgeable regarding the child or current condition (e.g., the child is in daycare, or the parent only sees the child occasionally).*

Chart 6–4

Components of a Complete Pediatric History

Identifying or biographical data
Reason for seeking care (chief complaint)
History of the present illness
Past medical history
- Obstetric and perinatal history
- Hospitalizations, accidents, surgical procedures, ingestions, and injuries
- Previous illnesses (serious or chronic)
- Current medications
- Allergies
- Immunizations
- Nutrition
- Growth and development
- Habits and behaviors

Family history
Social and environmental history
Review of systems

Reason for Seeking Care (Chief Complaint)

This section of the health history was once called the "chief complaint" but is now more appropriately designated as the "reason for seeking care." The term *chief complaint* is restrictive and is not inclusive of the need for preventive care. The reason for seeking health care is stated in the parent's, caretaker's, or child's own words. This statement is put in quotation marks and represents the historian's spontaneous response to a simple, open-ended question such as "What brings you here today?" or "What seems to be the matter?"

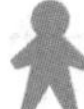

Tip: *Ask the child "Why did you come to see me today?" The child's perception of the reason for the visit may differ from the caretaker's.*

If the interviewer identifies a symptom or problem, the duration of this concern is included in the statement (e.g., "My baby's been throwing up for 2 days.").

History of the Present Illness

This section provides much of the key data that will direct the physical examination and determine the final health assessments. It includes information about the onset of each symptom, duration and nature of the symptoms, any precipitating or related factors, and relief measures or remedies taken. Eight factors should be investigated for each symptom identified (Chart 6–5).

Location. For symptoms such as pain, rash, lesions, or paresthesia, inquiry is made as to the specific body location or locations, whether the symptom is localized or generalized, and, for pain, whether it is deep or superficial.

Quality or Character. The character or quality of the symptom is assessed by asking the historian to describe the symptom. For example, is the pain dull, sharp, aching, or throbbing? Is the rash a bright red or pink? Does the child's cough sound like a bark or a whooping noise? Is the symptom getting better, worsening, or staying about the same?

Chart 6–5

Symptom Assessment

Location
Quality or character
Quantity or severity
Timing
Setting
Aggravating or alleviating factors
Perceptions of the child and parent
Associated factors

Quantity or Severity. Questions must be asked about the amount and/or severity of the symptom. When the infant vomits, how much formula or breast milk is vomited—a tablespoonful or 2 to 3 ounces? With heavy menstrual bleeding, does the teen completely saturate a pad? How often must the pad be changed?

Timing. Timing of a symptom relates to its onset, duration, and frequency. If possible, the nurse should try to determine the exact date or time that the symptom appeared and how long it lasted. Were there any periods when the symptom abated (i.e., was it intermittent or steady)?

Setting. The setting in which the symptom appeared is often relevant. For example, is the child's stomachache present only during math class at school?

Aggravating or Relieving Factors. The patient should be asked about any factors that may seem to make the symptom better or worse. Does the pain subside if the child does not put weight on the leg? What medications or alternate therapies has the adolescent tried for menstrual cramps and have they helped relieve the cramping?

Perceptions of the Child and Parent. How the parent/caregiver and child perceive the symptom alerts the nurse to areas of potential anxiety. For instance, parents of a child who has frequent epistaxis may be concerned about leukemia.

Associated Factors. The patient should be queried about associated factors or symptoms that might be present and not mentioned by the historian. A review of systems related to the symptom is done at this point in the health history. Many health care professionals do the total review of systems here rather than after the family health history.

Past Medical History

This section of the history is a profile of the child's past illnesses, health care, health promotion activities, growth and development, injuries, and hospitalizations. The information obtained provides additional clues as to the child's overall health status and helps determine whether past events might have influenced the current problem or situation.

Obstetric and Perinatal History. The examiner should obtain information about the duration of gestation and whether the pregnancy, labor, and delivery were normal. When did the mother obtain prenatal care? The mother should be asked about the infant's birth weight, length, and Apgar score, if known, whether the child was born prematurely, and whether the infant went home with the mother after birth or if any complications, such as ABO incompatibility or hyperbilirubinemia, occurred.

Hospitalizations, Accidents, Surgeries, Ingestions, and Injuries. The parent is asked about any hospitalizations, emergency department visits, ingestion of poisonous substances, surgeries/special procedures, accidents, or injuries that required sutures, x-rays, or medical intervention. The date of the event or approximate age of the child should be included.

Tip: *Ask the child what it was like when he or she was in the hospital.*

Previous Illnesses (Serious or Chronic). This category includes serious or chronic health problems, a prior life-threatening illness, and any significant communicable diseases.

Current Medications. The historian needs to list all prescription medications, creams, and over-the-counter preparations that the child is currently taking or recently completed. The name and dosage are listed as well as the route, frequency, and duration of administration. Also important is inquiry into the use of folk remedies (e.g., herbal teas).

Allergies. Any allergies to drugs, foods, contact agents, or other substances (e.g., ragweed, dust, mold, pollen) are noted. Does the child have any history of asthma, allergic rhinitis or conjunctivitis, or atopic skin disease? The nurse should ask the parent to describe the type and severity of symptoms associated with any allergic response and how the child was treated.

Immunizations. The nurse should review the child's immunization record and list all immunizations given and their dates. The parent is asked whether any untoward reactions occurred related to an immunization. If a reaction did occur, he or she is asked to describe what happened. The date of the last tuberculin skin test should be listed as well.

Nutrition. For an infant, the parent is asked about the frequency of breast feeding or the type and amount of formula given over the past 24 hours to calculate caloric intake. As solids are introduced, the examiner should determine from the parent what is being offered, how much, and how frequently. Is the younger child still feeding from a bottle or has he or she switched to a cup? For the older child, the examiner should ask about milk intake over a 24-hour period and the number and type of meals and snacks eaten each day (i.e., description of typical breakfast, lunch, dinner, and snacks). Questioning about the number and types of servings using food groups or the food pyramid as guidelines is another approach. Special cultural practices or ethnic foods should be listed. A 3-day or 1-week food diary is useful if a nutritional disorder is suspected. See Chapter 5 for additional discussion about nutritional assessment.

Growth and Development. The examiner should seek validation about the attainment of developmental milestones by performing an appraisal of key developmental areas—fine and gross motor, language, personal social, psychosocial, and cognitive (see Chapter 4). Growth parameters are best assessed by measuring height, weight, and head circumference; sequential measurements on a growth chart provide useful data (see the section on Physical Assessment in this chapter).

For the school-aged child and adolescent, inquiry is made into school performance (grades) and the child's socialization with peers (e.g., "What do you do after school?", "What hobbies or recreational activities interest you?", or "Are you involved in sports or organized club activities?"). The nurse can ask how the child is doing in spelling, reading, or math and whether the child is in an age-appropriate grade or in any special education classes or programs in school.

The nurse may want to develop a quick personal checklist for this assessment or use a printed form that lists developmental milestones for the various age groups. *Bright Futures: Guidelines for Health Supervision of Infants, Children and Adolescents* (Green, 1994) is an easy-to-use resource for developmental milestones. Refer to Chapter 5 for summary tables.

Habits and Behaviors. Does the child have any unusual habits, activities, or behaviors? Sleep patterns are frequently mentioned as problematic. The older child or teenager should be asked about gang involvement, tobacco (cigarettes and chewing tobacco) and drug use, and alcohol consumption.

Family History

In the family history section, the interviewer obtains information about the age and health or the age and cause of death of the child's family members—biologic siblings, parents, and grandparents. The use of a genogram to diagram relationships and to identify health problems in specific family members readily provides data in a visual fashion (see Chapter 8). The nurse should inquire about any family history of heart disease, high blood pressure, kidney disease, diabetes, allergies, or asthma; any genetically inherited diseases, mental retardation, or illnesses; seizures; learning disability; and alcoholism. In addition, the nurse may ask about whether there is anyone else in the family with symptoms similar to the child's presenting problems (e.g., headaches in a child whose mother has a history of migraine headaches).

Social and Environmental History

The family unit and support system are important factors in health promotion and disease prevention. Family cohesiveness and interpersonal relationships can be determined by seeking information about who lives with the child, who is the primary caregiver, and whether the family has a support system to help them with child care or in times of need. If the biological parents are separated or divorced, the nurse should inquire about involvement of the out-of-home parent. Family living arrangements, home environment, and economic status or hardships have implications for health care planning and management strategies. Information should be sought about the safety of the home setting and community (e.g., If a child lives in a house or apartment with iron bars on the windows, can the bars be released in case of fire? If the home or apartment has a swimming pool, do the parents know cardiopulmonary resuscitation?). For older children, peer relationships should be discussed. Health promotion practices or behaviors (e.g., use of car seat restraints and bicycle helmets, exposure to passive smoke, poison control measures, smoke detection devices, and removal of firearms from the home) can be identified (see Chapter 5).

Review of Systems

The review of systems serves to evaluate the past and present health state of each body system, is a double check to determine whether significant data were omitted, and also functions as a means to inquire about health promotion needs. The historian is questioned about the presence or absence of specific signs and symptoms for each body system and also queried about health promotion activities related to a particular body system.

Each Health Challenge chapter in this text (Chapters 14 through 30) discusses alterations in a body system or systems and includes a section called Focused Health History. The focused health history section discusses pertinent information that should be obtained for a review of that particular body system.

Physical Examination

The usual approach to the physical examination of infants and young children is to start with the chest and work downward and then finish with the head and neck. The traditional sequence in preschool and older children starts with inspection of the head and works downward ("head to toe"). The usual sequence may need to be altered in certain children, however, based on such factors as the child's developmental age and presenting symptoms. The important point is to eventually cover all aspects of the examination.

caREminder: *Wait until the end of the examination to perform the more intrusive procedures that are likely to distress the child, such as inspection of the mouth and otoscopic examination of the ears.*

Modesty is an issue that surfaces with some preschool children but takes on heightened importance beginning with school-age children. Every effort should be made to provide appropriate covering and to expose only the area to be examined. The examiner should wash his or her hands before beginning and put on gloves to examine the genital and rectal areas. Hands should be warmed with water or by rubbing them before palpation. A cold stethoscope should also be warmed by rubbing it in the hands. All needed equipment should be readily available, and safety measures should be followed when examining infants and young children. Chart 6–6 identifies age-appropriate approaches to the physical examination from infancy through the school-age period. Additional developmental considerations related to the physical examination of the adolescent are discussed at the end of this chapter.

Vital Signs

The examination begins by measuring the child's vital signs: temperature, pulse, blood pressure, and respiration. Pulse, blood pressure, and respiratory findings are compared to normal ranges for the child's age.

Tip: *Choose your words carefully when explaining vital sign measurements to a young child. Avoid saying, for example, "I'm going to take your pulse now." The child may think that you are going to actually remove something from his or her body. A better phrase would be "I'm going to count how fast your heart beats."*

Temperature. Normal body temperature is roughly 37°C (98.6°F) measured orally. Body temperature can be influenced by many non–illness-related factors. Active exercise, stress, crying, environmental heat, and excessive clothing can increase body temperature. In contrast, lack of clothing and exposure to environmental cold air can lower body temperature.

Diurnal variations in body temperature also occur. Body temperature is generally lowest between 1 and 4 A.M. and highest between 4 and 6 P.M. (Engel, 1993). Chart 6–7 outlines some important considerations to keep in mind when measuring temperature in children.

Pulse. In infants and young children (younger than 2 years), the apical pulse is more reliable for recording rates than other sites. The apical pulse rate is assessed for 1 full minute preferably when the child is quiet; if the child is crying or fussy, this should be noted. The child's activity during pulse assessment should be documented. Variations in heart rate generally are much more dramatic in children than in adults. Factors known to affect heart rate include medication, activity, hyperthermia or hypothermia, hypoxia, apprehension, pain, and hemor-

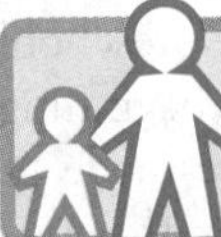

Chart 6–6
Developmental Considerations

Physical Examination from Infancy Through the School-Age Years

Infants

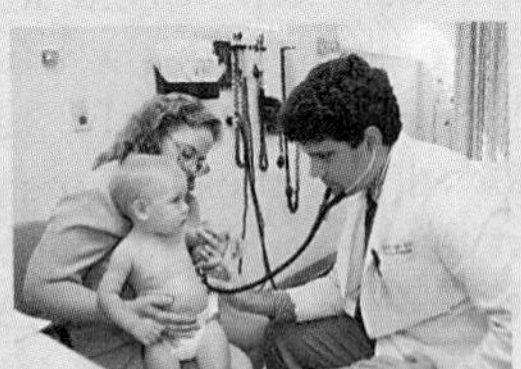

Examine an infant in a parent's lap or on the examination table if the infant is quiet. Leave diaper on and wrap young infant in a blanket to maintain warmth and security. Use comfort measures such as pacifier or a bottle if the infant becomes fussy. Talk softly and establish eye contact. Avoid sudden, startling movements. Parents can help with the ear examination by having the older infant rest head against their shoulders.

Toddler

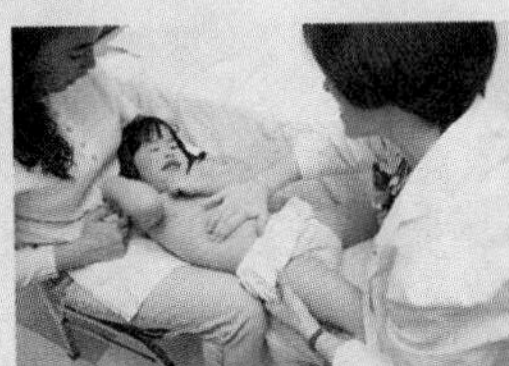

It is best to examine a toddler while he or she is sitting in a parent's lap. Examiner and parent sit opposite each other with knees touching to use knees as an examination surface. Use play techniques to gain attention and distract child with stories. Let toddler handle equipment but be mindful of safety issues. If toddler is uncooperative, quickly perform what has to be done. Call child by name and praise frequently.

Preschool Child

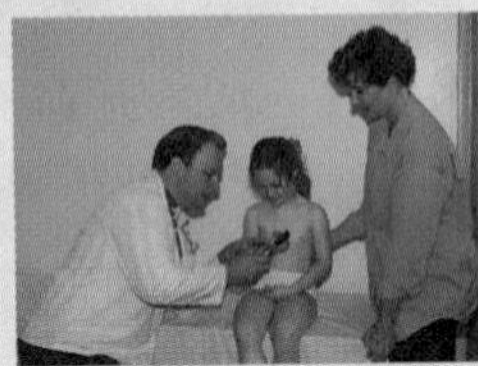

Give child the choice of either sitting on a parent's lap or sitting on the examination table. Tell parent to stay close to and within eye contact of the child. Explain procedures and what is being done in simple terms that the child understands. Interact with the child, allow to handle equipment, and encourage child to talk about self. Modesty concerns start to emerge.

School-Age Child

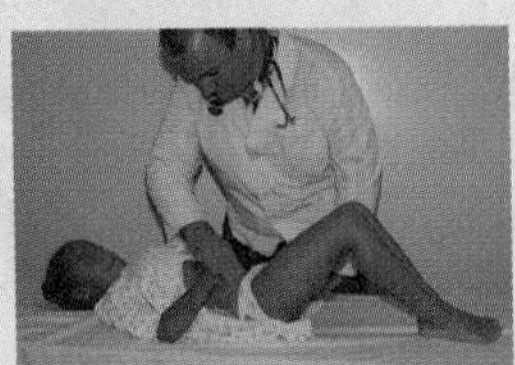

Be cognizant of need for privacy and modesty concerns. Explain procedures and equipment (e.g., allow child to listen to own heart). Teach about body function while examining. Focus on dialoguing and interacting with the child. Common issues are ticklishness when palpating and hesitancy to allow genitalia to be checked. To reduce ticklishness when palpating the abdomen place the child's hand under your hand, have the child bend at the knees, or use a stethoscope to apply pressure to palpate. These are also useful techniques to use if the child is complaining of abdominal pain and is fearful of having his/her abdomen palpated. Provide for covering of genitalia and be matter of fact with the child about examining the genitalia (i.e., explain that you look at all children's private parts to be sure that everything is fine). This is also an opportunity to teach about approaching sexual development. Allow the older school-age child the choice of whether to have a parent present.

rhage. Chart 6–8 presents some nursing considerations to keep in mind while assessing pulse rate, along with normal ranges by age.

Blood Pressure. Measurement of blood pressure is a routine part of physical assessment in children older than age 3 years and in younger children and infants who have symptoms that warrant investigation (e.g., those suggestive of cardiac pathology and pulse strength difference between upper and lower extremities). Various devices can be used to measure blood pressure, including mercury-gravity or aneroid sphygmomanometers and electronic devices that use oscillometric or Doppler tech-

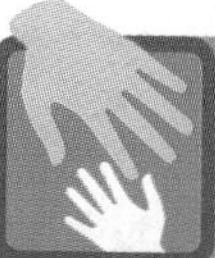

Chart 6–7
Nursing Interventions

Temperature Assessment

- Recording the route of temperature measurement (i.e., oral, rectal or axillary) is always an important consideration.
- The use of tympanic membrane measurements remains controversial. Tempa-DOT is an accurate and reliable method especially for temperatures below 38°C. Electronic thermometers are commonly used for children.
- The recommended duration of measurement for oral, rectal, and axillary temperatures using a mercury thermometer vary from institution to institution but generally average around 7, 4, and 5 minutes, respectively.
- Oral temperatures are the preferred site in children older than 5 to 6 years of age. Place under tongue in right or left posterior sublingual pocket. Oral temperatures are influenced by such factors as crying, eating, drinking, and the location of the thermometer in the mouth.
- Oral temperatures may be contraindicated if a child is on oxygen, had oral surgery, is comatose, has a seizure disorder, is a mouth breather, or is dehydrated.
- Axillary temperatures can be taken in all age groups; this is the preferred route for routine temperatures in preschoolers. Place under arm with tip in center of the axilla next to skin and forearm held firmly against the child's side.
- The axillary route may not be sensitive to early changes in body temperatures.
- Rectal temperatures can be taken in all age groups, but caution is required in children younger than age 2 years, because of potential for breakage (mercury thermometers) or perforation. Insert lubricated-tip not more than 2.5 cm (1 inch) into the rectum and hold securely in place.
- Rectal temperatures are contraindicated if the child has had anal surgery, diarrhea, or rectal irritation.
- The traditional gold standard of estimating rectal temperature by adding 1°F to the oral temperature reading and 2°F to axillary temperature does not always hold up (Haddock, Merrow, & Swanson, 1996).

niques. Using the proper-size cuff is vital for accurate blood pressure readings. Chart 6–9 presents some nursing considerations to keep in mind while assessing blood pressure, along with normal ranges by age.

Respiration. Respiratory rate is assessed by counting the number of breaths the child takes for 1 full minute. In infants, abdominal movement should be observed rather than chest movement, because the respiratory effort is primarily diaphragmatic. Chart 6–10 provides nursing considerations and age-related norms for respiratory rate.

Anthropometric Measurements

Accurate measurement and recording of height (length), weight, and head circumference offer valuable information about how a child is growing. Plotting this information on a growth chart is important for comparison with other children of the same age and to ascertain the child's own pattern of growth (see Appendix 1). Height and weight are also discussed in Chapter 4.

Height. For infants and toddlers up to age 24 months, height measurement is best done by using a flat board placed across and perpendicular to an examining table in contact with the vertex of the infant's head and soles of the feet (Fig. 6–1). Care must be taken to extend the hips and knees fully for accurate measurement.

For children older than age 2 years, a wall-mounted apparatus known as a stadiometer provides the most ac-

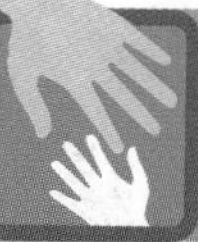

Chart 6–8
Nursing Interventions

Assessing Pulse Rate

- Count the pulse rate for 1 full minute as a baseline; if frequent readings are required, use shorter times (15 to 30 seconds).
- Consider the following age-related norms when assessing pulse rate (Jarvis, 1996):

Age	Normal range (beats per minute)	Average
Neonate	70–190	120
1 year	80–160	120
2 years	80–130	110
4 years	80–120	100
6 years	75–115	100
10 years	70–110	90
14 years		
Female	65–105	85
Male	60–100	80
18 years		
Female	55–95	75
Male	50–90	70

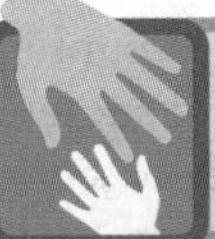

Chart 6–9
Nursing Interventions

Blood Pressure Measurement

- Cuff size is an important determinant for accurate readings in children; the width of the rubber bladder should cover two thirds of the circumference of the arm, and the length should encircle 100% of the arm without overlap.
- Crying can cause electronic blood pressure devices to read blood pressure inaccurately; take readings when the child is calm. Document the child's activity.
- An alternative method to auscultation of blood pressure is palpation. To palpate the blood pressure, place one finger over the artery (brachial or radial in the arm, tibialis dorsalis in the leg), inflate the cuff until the pulse is obliterated, slowly deflate the cuff until the pulse is felt. This point is documented (e.g., 70/p). No diastolic pressure is obtained using this method.
- Consider norms for age when evaluating blood pressure.

The following are systolic blood pressures based on 50th percentile of height and 90th percentile of blood pressure. Height percentile should be based on standard growth curves.

Age in Years	Boys	Girls
1	98/53	100/54
2	102/57	102/58
3	105/61	103/62
4	107/64	104/65
5	108/67	106/67
6	110/70	107/69
7	111/72	109/70
8	112/73	111/71
9	113/74	113/73
10	115/75	115/74
11	117/76	117/75
12	119/77	119/76
13	122/77	121/78
14	125/78	122/79
15	127/79	124/79
16	130/81	125/80
17	133/83	125/80

Data from National High Blood Pressure Education Program Working Group on Hypertension Control in Children and Adolescents. (1996). Update on the 1987 Task Force Report on High Blood Pressure in Children and Adolescents: A working group report from the National High Blood Pressure Education Program. *Pediatrics, 98,* 649–658.

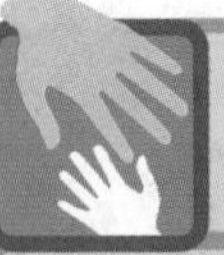

Chart 6–10
Nursing Interventions

Assessing Respiratory Rate

- Count the respiratory rate for 1 full minute.
- In infants, observe abdominal movement, as the respiratory effort is primarily diaphragmatic.
- Consider age-related norms when assessing respiratory rate, as follows (Behrman & Kliegman, 1994):

Age	Rate (breaths per minute)
Preterm	40–60
Term	30–40
5 years	25
10 years	20
15 years	16

curate standing height measurement. The child is measured while standing in stocking or bare feet with the heels back and shoulders just touching the wall. The child is instructed to look straight ahead without tilting the head.

Weight. First, the scale is checked to ensure that it is calibrated correctly. An infant is weighed on an infant scale in the nude (Fig. 6–2). The same scale should be used to weigh an infant returning for assessment of weight gain or loss.

A child old enough to stand should be weighed on a stand-up scale, wearing underpants. A very young child may be scared to stand on the scale alone. If this is the case, both the parent and the child are weighed together, and the parent's weight is subtracted.

Head Circumference. Head circumference (occipitofrontal circumference) should be measured at every well-child visit up to age 2 years. To measure head circumference, a paper tape measure is wrapped around the maximum occipitofrontal circumference (Fig. 6–3). Three separate readings are taken, and the largest value is recorded.

Body Fat Percentage

Fat is a constituent of all body tissues. It serves several important functions, including energy storage, insulation, and a cushion for internal organs. In term neonates, fat accounts for about 4% of total body weight (compared with 10% to 30% or more in adults).

Body fat content varies with age and sex. The ado-

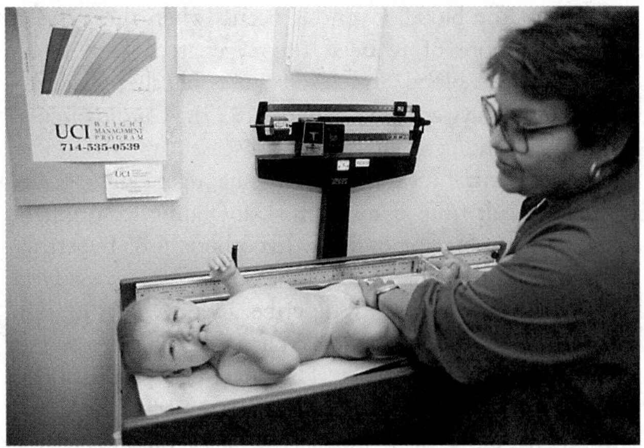

Figure 6–1
To ensure accurate height measurement, the examiner makes sure that the infant's head is against the end point and his or her hips and legs are fully extended on the measuring board. The measurement scale is calibrated from the head end point (e.g., in this example, the scale starts at 1 inch).

lescent growth spurt in lean body mass is considerably greater in boys than in girls, and girls generally have higher percentages of body fat than boys. Those who subscribe to evolutionary explanations of gender differences attribute the higher percentages of body fat in females to women's traditional role in feeding infants, making it a survival mechanism. Regardless of the veracity of this view, adequate fat stores are known to play a role in the onset of menarche in adolescent females.

Baseline and follow-up measurement of body fat percentage is one of the best indicators of progress in health-related fitness. An appraisal of body composition is a significantly more accurate reflection of fitness than height and weight percentile comparisons. Body cavities are not considered in growth charts' percentile comparisons of height and weight. A muscular or larger-framed child or adolescent, for example, may have a low percentile of body fat but have a weight percentile greater than height percentile when plotted on a growth chart. This is because muscle is more dense and thus weighs more than fat.

Several methods are available for measuring body composition. The use of skin calipers is the most convenient method. When using skin calipers, the more sites that are measured, the more accurate the determination of body fat percentage. The triceps and calves are the most common sites of measurement. Hydrostatic (or underwater) weighing is considered the most accurate method of determining body fat percentage; however, it is often impractical. Electrical impedance techniques are becoming more readily available and may one day become the method of choice for measuring body composition.

General Appearance

The child's general appearance is an important indicator of wellness or the severity of an illness. In a complete physical examination, a section called the "general appearance" is included as an introductory statement to the physical assessment of the individual body systems. It represents the examiner's subjective impression of the child's overall state of health based on observations made during the time spent interviewing the child, parent, or both and performing the physical examination. The nurse should note whether the child appears sick or well, functions at a developmentally appropriate level for age, and appears well nourished and hydrated.

In addition, other indicators that have relevance to an overall impression and deserve mention are the child's state of hygiene in terms of body odor, general grooming and cleanliness, and condition of clothing, as well as the child's behavior, specifically remarking on interactions with others, the overall personality, and activity level. For infants and young children who are ill, the type of cry or voice (e.g., hoarse, husky, weak, or high-pitched) is an important clinical assessment. Likewise, altered state of consciousness, coma, apathy, restlessness, delirium, and irritability are descriptors that, if present, should be reported as part of the initial impression. Any unusual postures, positions, or body movements should be noted as well as facial expressions (e.g., frozen watchfulness [hypervigilant and fearful], grimacing from pain, or no eye-to-eye contact), because these often are important assessment clues.

Figure 6–2
Older infants are usually more cooperative with being weighed when allowed to sit on the scale. Note the close proximity of the nurse's hands for safety.

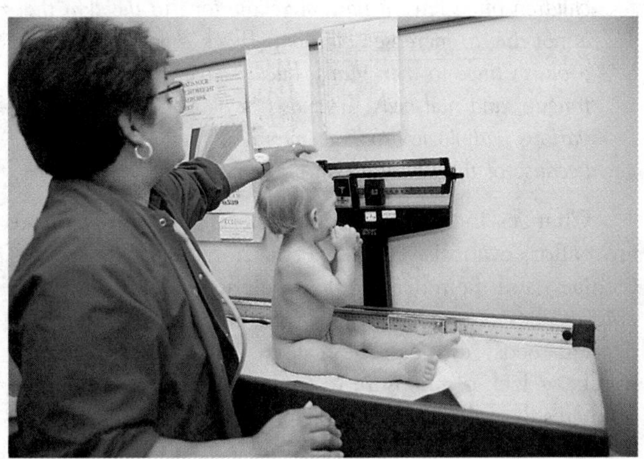

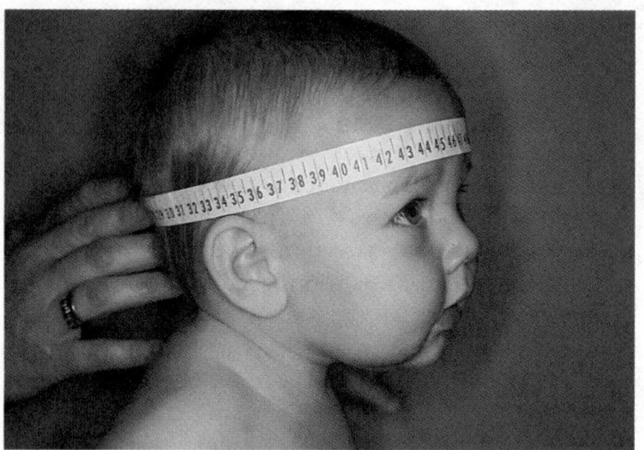

Figure 6–3
Head circumference is measured by wrapping the paper tape over the eyebrows and around the occipital prominence.

Integument

Physical assessment of the integumentary system (the skin, hair, and nails) involves careful observation and, at times, palpation. A well-illuminated room or natural daylight is essential for accurate assessment. Room temperature is another important consideration, because cold-induced cyanosis or flushing with heat can alter physical findings, especially in the newborn and young infant. In an adolescent female, removal of nail coloring and cosmetics may be needed. The entire body surface must be observed; otherwise, lesions or rashes under clothing can be missed. Maintaining modesty is always an important consideration.

Skin. The skin is assessed for odor, color and pigmentation, texture, temperature, moisture, and turgor. Usual and distinctive odors can be due to metabolic disease, poor hygiene, or infection.

Worldview: *A child's skin color and pigmentation are influenced by racial characteristics. For example, Asian children often have a natural yellow tone to the skin that is not due to increased bilirubin. Black children may have a bluish tinge to their gums, buccal cavity, borders of the tongue, and nail beds. Cyanosis in black children due to various pathologic processes may be difficult to detect because of their darker skin pigmentation.*

Changes in skin coloring that are important to note are pallor, cyanosis, erythema, plethora, ecchymoses, petechiae, and jaundice. Pallor, paleness, or an ash-gray color is best observed in the face, mouth, conjunctivae, or nail beds and can be caused by anemia, syncope, shock, or lack of exposure to sunlight. Peripheral cyanosis often results from cold or anxiety and is due to temporary vasoconstriction; central cyanosis involves the lips, mouth, and trunk and indicates reduced oxygen-carrying capacity of the blood. Cyanosis occurs when there is 4 to 5 g/dL or more of reduced (deoxygenated) hemoglobin present in the blood and results in a bluish tone (Hay, Groothuis, Hayward, & Levin, 1995). Cardiovascular, respiratory and/or hematologic disease are the major causes of central cyanosis. Erythema or redness of the skin can result from many factors, including local inflammation, infection, exposure to hypothermia or hyperthermia, alcohol, blushing, allergy, or other dermatoses. *Plethora* is the term used to describe redness of the skin, especially the cheeks and lips, that is due to an increased number of red blood cells. The increased production of red blood cells is a compensatory mechanism from chronic hypoxia. Ecchymoses are large, diffuse areas of black and blue color due to bleeding into the skin and commonly result from injury. In contrast, petechiae are small ($\leq$ 2 mm), distinct pinpoint hemorrhages into the skin or mucous membranes often seen with blood disorders or systemic infection. Jaundice is a yellowish pigmentation resulting from depositions of bile pigment in the skin, sclerae, and mucous membranes. Jaundice is indicative of hepatic disease and severe infections in infants. In contrast, carotenemia is a yellowish discoloration of the skin from deposits of carotene caused by excess ingestion of yellow and orange vegetables. In carotenemia, the sclerae and mucous membranes are not involved.

Pressing the skin or nail bed causes blanching or a whitening appearance that is useful to contrast color changes. Pressing the skin with a glass slide to produce a blanching effect helps in the assessment of jaundice (yellow remains), pallor (the color change in the skin is slight), and petechiae (lesions remain).

Assessing skin texture and moisture involves inspection and palpation. Children's skin is normally smooth, soft, and slightly dry to the touch. Any variations such as scars, keloids, excessive dryness, or dermatitis should be noted. Temperature is assessed by palpating the skin with the back of the hand comparing both symmetrical parts and the lower and upper extremities of the body for degree of warmth or coolness. Skin turgor, or tissue elasticity, is assessed by grasping a fold of skin on the upper arm or abdomen between the fingers and quickly releasing the tissue (Fig. 6–4). State of hydration and nutrition affects tissue turgor. Skin that immediately returns to place without residual marks has good turgor or adequate hydration. Skin that only slowly returns to place (tents) or retains marks indicates decreased turgor and poor hydration. The presence of edema is determined by pressing the thumb into any area that looks swollen or puffy (see Chapter 17).

All skin lesions or rashes should be carefully inspected. Gloves should be worn when palpating lesions and areas of rash. The location, size, distribution of the lesions over the body, and distinguishing features of the

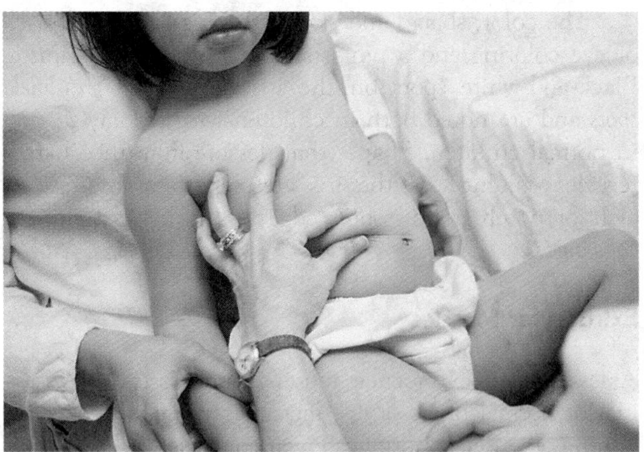

Figure 6–4
To assess skin turgor, the examiner grasps a fold of skin on the child's abdomen and quickly releases it.

primary or secondary lesion, including color, shape, raised, crater-like or flat and exudate, should be noted. (Common primary and secondary skin lesions in children and adolescents are described in Chapter 25.) In addition, the presence of warmth or scratch marks are noteworthy. Using a body diagram to sketch lesions or indicate their distribution is helpful in recording physical findings.

Nails. Assessment of the nails involves inspection for color, shape, and texture. The nails are normally pink, convex, smooth, and hard but flexible. Two significant deviations in nail shape to note are clubbing, in which the base of the nail becomes enlarged and swollen, and spoon nails (koilonychia), in which the nail assumes a concave curve. Clubbing is associated with chronic hypoxia; spoon nails are sometimes noted in a patient with iron-deficiency anemia. The dermatoglyphics, or skin patterns, of the hands and feet become important in the infant or child with a suspected genetic defect or condition (e.g., presence of simian crease with trisomy 21).

Assessment of nails and hair is also discussed in Chapter 25.

Hair. The hair is inspected for distribution, color, texture, amount, and quality. In children, scalp hair is normally shiny, silky, and strong. Genetics influences the appearance and texture of hair. However, unusual hairiness anywhere in the body, hairlines that extend to mid forehead, or tufts of hair on the skin over the spine or sacrum represent deviations from normal. Similarly, white locks of hair, loss of hair (alopecia), and dry, brittle hair are important clinical findings. In newborns, lanugo is normal and is the soft, downy hair that covers the infant. The presence of pubic and axillary hair in the adolescent is one of the secondary sex characteristics. White ova (nits) attached to the hair shafts indicate pediculosis.

Head and Neck

The head is observed for shape and symmetry from different angles and palpated for signs of fractures or swelling. The shape of a newborn or infant's head can be influenced by unusual positioning in utero, oligohydramnios (deficiency of amniotic fluid), length of pushing during labor, positioning after birth, genetic disorders, or congenital anomalies. The suture lines and fontanelles of the infant are palpated to check for overriding sutures and flat, depressed, or bulging fontanelles. The anterior fontanelle measures 1 to 5 cm in length and width until it normally closes at around age 9 to 18 months; the posterior fontanelle closes around age 2 months. Head posture and control in the infant, which is a sign of developmental maturation, should be noted. Head measurements from the most prominent point of the occiput around the head just above the eyebrows and pinna are serially measured in children until age 24 months (Green, 1994).

The head and neck is assessed for full range of motion to determine any limitation of movement. The face is inspected for symmetrical appearance proportions and movement of its structures. The sinuses of children are palpated and, if warranted, percussed, depending on the stage of sinus development, which is age dependent.

The major structures of the neck are the trachea, which is normally midline, and the thyroid, located at the base of the neck. The neck is inspected for any swelling, webbing, or venous distention. The trachea is palpated with the thumb and index finger on opposite sides to detect any deviations. The thyroid gland is not normally palpable in children. To palpate for an enlarged thyroid, the examiner should stand behind the child and place the fingers over the gland at the base of the neck and then ask the child to swallow. Infants and young child have short necks, making thyroid palpation difficult. Lying the infant or young child supine across the parent's lap may facilitate palpation for an enlarged thyroid.

Eyes

External Structures

Assessment of the external eye involves inspection for position, placement, size, symmetry, color, and movement. The distance between the inner canthi of the eyes determines whether the eyes are wide set (hypertelorism) or close set (hypotelorism), with 2.5 cm being the average distance between canthi (Engel, 1993); wide- or close-set spacing of the eyes can be a normal variant or associated with a genetic condition.

caREminder: *Vertical folds of excess skin (epicanthal folds) that partially or completely cover the inner canthi* *and an upward slanting of the eyes are normal findings in Asian children but may be markers of various chromosomal conditions (e.g., trisomy 21) in other children.*

(See Chapter 28 for illustrations of eye structure, eye placement, and epicanthal folds.)

When the eyelids are open, their placement should be somewhere between the upper border of the iris and the upper border of the pupil. Deviations from normal placement of the eyelids is referred to as ptosis when the lids droop and cover the pupil and sunset eyes when the sclera is apparent between the upper lid and the iris. Eyelids that roll abnormally inward or outward are termed *entropion* and *ectropion*, respectively. Discoloration of the eyelids (e.g., erythema or bluish coloration from a hematoma), change in size such as seen with edema, discharge, lesions (e.g., blocked sebaceous glands), and movement problems should be noted. Excessive tearing or discharge from the eyes should be noted. In young infants, the eyes should be inspected for any swelling of the nasolacrimal sac area and, if present, the area should be palpated for tenderness. The eyebrows are normally symmetrical in both shape and movement and do not meet in the midline. The eyelashes curve outward and are inspected for any debris or nits.

The edges and lining of the eyelids are also inspected for signs of inflammation (blepharitis or conjunctivitis) or lesions (stye or chalazion). The palpebral conjunctivae are normally pink and glossy and can be inspected easily by gently pulling the lower lid downward while the child looks up. To inspect the lining of the upper lid, the nurse should either hold the lashes and pull downward and forward while the child looks down or roll the upper eyelid over a cotton-tipped applicator. The bulbar conjunctiva is transparent; however, dilatation of its blood vessels results in redness. The sclera is the white, opaque covering of the eye and is inspected for any changes in coloring. Examples of color changes include a yellow tinge due to jaundice, a bluish tint that may be associated with osteogenesis imperfecta, or black marks that are frequently a normal finding in dark-skinned people or may be associated with an imbedded foreign body.

The pupils are inspected for size, equality, and response to light by darkening the room and separately shining light directly into the pupil of each eye. The pupils are normally equal and should respond with brisk constriction. The opposite eye should also show a consensual reflex movement (constriction) to the light. To test for accommodation, the child should look at a penlight that is held at a distance and then quickly brought toward the midline of the child's nose. The normal response is pupillary constriction and convergence of the axes of the eyes. The pupils should constrict as the object comes near. The normal pupillary response is PERRLA: pupils equal, round, react to light and accommodation.

The color, shape, and size of the iris are noted. Lack of eye coloring and a pinkish glow are seen in albinism. Black-and-white spots on the iris are termed *Brushfield spots* and are noted both in children with trisomy 21 and in normal children. Shapes that deviate from the characteristic roundness of the iris are important findings. A cleft or notch of the outer edge of the iris is termed a *coloboma.*

Extraocular Muscles

Assessment of extraocular muscle function involves testing for normal range of eye muscle movement and determining whether abnormal movements, such as strabismus and nystagmus, are present. The corneal light reflect test and the cover tests are the two key means to assess extraocular function and binocular vision (using both eyes for vision). A penlight is shone into the eye from a distance of about 16 inches. Normally the light shines symmetrically in the middle of both pupils. This is termed the *corneal light reflex,* and the test is called the corneal light reflex test or Hirschberg test (see Chapter 28).

Any malalignment should be investigated for muscle imbalance. A tendency to have strabismus or intermittent crossing of eyes either inward or outward is normal during the first 6 months of life. The cover test can detect either a phoria (tendency to deviate from alignment) or trophia (overt malalignment). The cover test is performed at both near and far gaze. While the child is gazing at a near object (13 inches) and then again at a far object (20 inches), one eye is covered with a hand, eye patch, or nontransparent piece of paper and then uncovered. Movement of the uncovered eye indicates malalignment. The examiner should uncover the occluded eye and observe whether the occluded eye moves; normally the eyes remain fixated. In the alternating cover/uncover test, the patch is moved from one eye to another while the child is fixating on an object. Movement noted in the eyes during the covering or uncovering is an attempt to reestablish fixation and indicates muscle malalignment (Hay et al., 1995). Nystagmus, or rapid, oscillating, jerky eye movements, is elicited by instructing the child to follow either a light, finger, or tiny object, held about 12 inches away, through the six cardinal fields of gaze (i.e., lateral, medial, superior, and inferior). A few beats of nystagmus are normal only if present in the far lateral gaze.

Ophthalmoscopic Examination

The ophthalmoscopic examination is a specialized skill that involves practice and a cooperative child. The intent of this section is to give an overview of the examination of the interior eye and to describe its normal structures. To see the various eye structures, it is best to

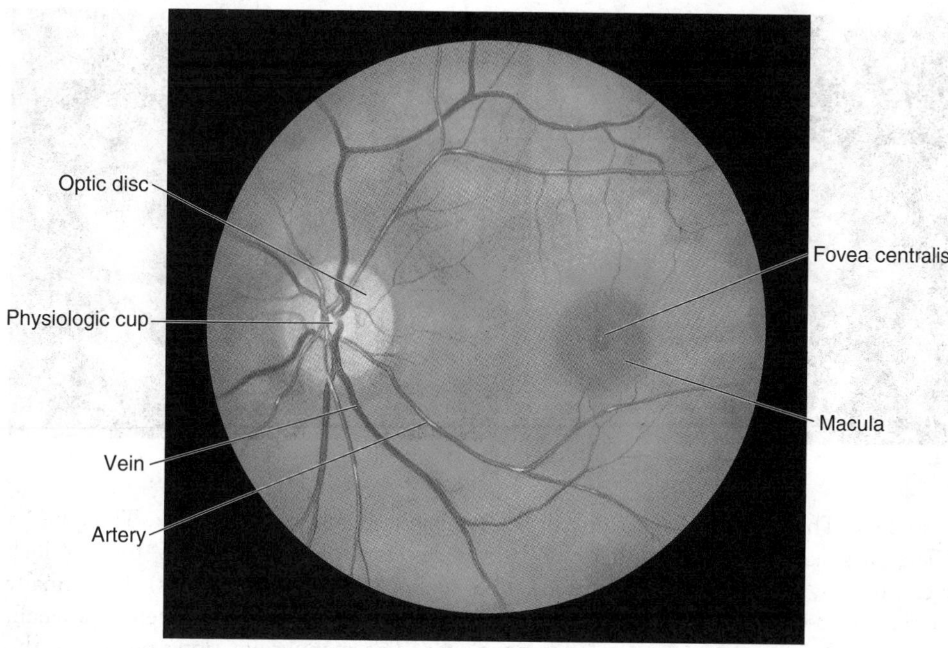

Figure 6–5
Structures seen on funduscopic examination. The pupil appears to have a red glow if the lens and cornea are transparent and the retina is normal. (From Jarvis, C. [1996]. *Physical examination and health assessment* [2nd ed., p. 304]. Philadelphia: W. B. Saunders. Reprinted with permission.)

perform this examination in a darkened room. The child's right eye is examined with the examiner's right eye and the child's left eye with the examiner's left eye. The diopter reading is set at +8 to +2 and the eye is examined from a distance of 10 to 12 inches, moving inward at an angle until the child's face is reached. The pupil reveals a red reflex or glow if the lens and cornea are transparent and the retina is normal (Fig. 6–5). In newborns and young infants, the red reflex appears lighter; in darker-skinned individuals the red reflex often appears darker. While slowly moving inward, the examiner should adjust the diopter setting to see the fundus clearly. If the examiner and the child have normal vision, a reading of 0 diopter results in a sharp focus of the fundus (Jarvis, 1996). Moving the diopters compensates for nearsighted or farsighted eyes. If the examiner with normal vision must use red diopter lenses to focus the fundus, the child is nearsighted. If the examiner needs black diopter lenses to focus the fundus, the child is farsighted.

The optic disk appears creamy white, yellow-orange, to pinkish; is round or oval; and normally has clear margins. Arteries are smaller and brighter than veins and have a thin stripe of light down the middle. The macula is similar in size to the optic disk and located to the temporal side of the disk. The macula is somewhat darker than the rest of the fundus. The fovea centralis, the area of almost perfect vision, appears as a tiny white glistening dot in the center of the macula (see Fig. 6–5).

Visual Acuity

Testing for visual acuity in young infants is generally done by testing certain reflexes and attending behaviors. Normal visual milestones are presented in Chapter 4. Light perception is tested by observing whether the infant blinks in response to a bright light and has pupillary constriction. An examiner should be able to elicit certain attending behaviors in a newborn or infant when an object is placed in the line of vision. These responses are age dependent. At age 3 months, an infant should be able to fixate and attempt to follow an object such as a toy, penlight, or face; by 5 months, the infant can follow these objects or fixation targets through all fields of gaze (Zitelli & Davis, 1992). There are various letter or symbol vision tests. Commonly used tests include the Allen picture cards, for children aged 2 to 3 years; the Snellen E chart, for children aged 3 to 6 years; and the standard Snellen chart, used as soon as the child knows the alphabet. Color deficiency (or colorblindness) is a result of an X-linked disorder. It is primarily seen in males. In the Ishihara and Hardy-Rand-Ritter tests, the child is asked to look at pseudoisochromatic cards and identify the numbers or the symbols hidden by certain confusion colors. Failure to recognize the number or symbol against the color field is diagnostic.

Ears

External Structures

The external ear is inspected first for placement and position. The top of the ear should meet or cross an imaginary horizontal line drawn from the inner eye to the occiput, and the pinna should angle no more than 10 degrees from a line drawn perpendicular from the imaginary horizontal line. Low-set or obliquely set ears are

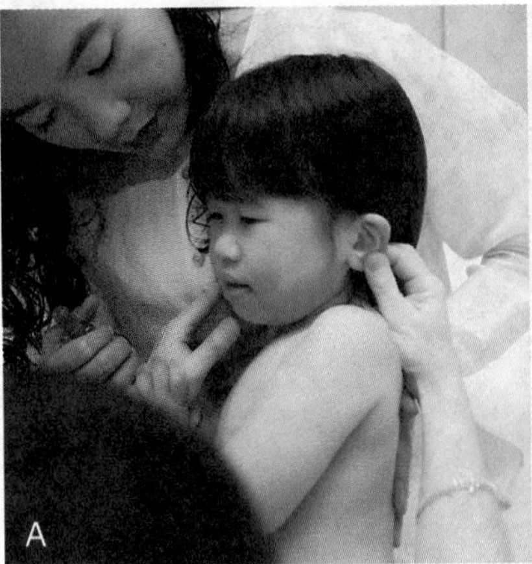

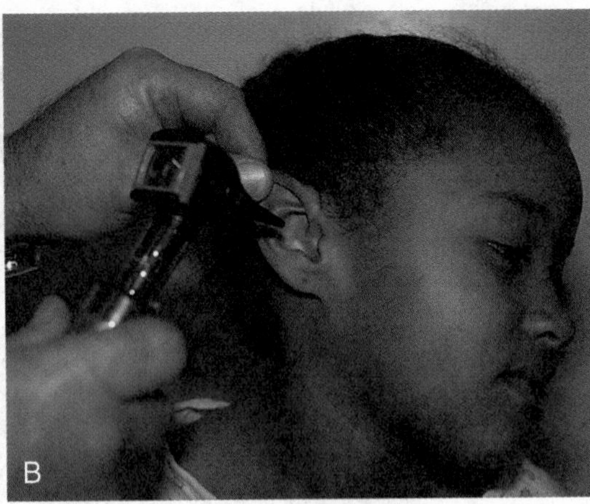

Figure 6–6
Ear examination. A, In children younger than age 3 years, the pinna is pulled down and back to straighten the ear canal and visualize the tympanic membrane. B, In children older than age 3 years, the pinna is pulled up and back.

associated with chromosomal disorders. The newborn's ears are flat against the head. The mastoid area is inspected and palpated behind the ear; redness and swelling of this area and a protruding pinna are associated with mastoiditis.

The structures of the external ear including the helix, tragus, concha, and lobule are inspected for abnormalities in shape or structure; tenderness on movement is abnormal. Any skin tags, nodules, sinus tracts, or pits in the skin found around the pinna should be noted. Discharge from the external canal can be cerumen (soft, yellow-brown) or a finding of external otitis (yellow or greenish discharge).

Otoscopic Examination

The otoscope is used to visualize the canal and structures of the middle ear and is held like a pencil so that the examiner's little finger rests on the child's head and the otoscope moves with the child. To maximize the visual area, the examiner should use the largest speculum that can fit into the ear canal. To straighten the ear canal, the pinna is pulled down and back or out in infants and children younger than age 3 years (Fig. 6–6A). For children older than age 3 years, the pinna is pulled up and back to the 10 o'clock position (Fig. 6–6B). Individual variations may require manipulating the earlobe in a slightly different direction than what is the usual practice. The speculum is inserted into the auditory meatus slowly and carefully, and the canal is inspected. Normally, the canal is pink with small hairs. Any lesions, discharge, or foreign bodies in the canal are noted.

The tympanic membrane is inspected for color and landmarks. The color is normally translucent, light pearly pink, or gray. Erythema can be a normal finding if the infant or child is crying or has a fever; however, marked erythema is associated with infection (otitis media). Serous otitis media can present as a dull yellow, yellow-amber, or gray color. Perforations leave scarring and an ashen-gray color. In assessing landmarks, one should think of the tympanic membrane as a clock. The cone of light or light reflex is seen around the 5 to 7 o'clock position. The umbo (tip of the malleus) is normally found at the center of the clock and is seen as a small, round opaque spot. The manubrium (long process of the malleus) is the white line extending from the umbo upward to a knob-like protuberance (the short process of the malleus) around the 1 o'clock position.

caREminder: *Fluid behind the tympanic membrane causes bulging that distorts or obliterates the appearance of the landmarks. Negative pressure in the middle ear causes retraction of the tympanic membrane with abnormally prominent landmarks.*

Compliance or mobility of the tympanic membrane can be evaluated by tympanometry testing or pneumatic otoscopy. In this procedure, the examiner exerts pressure against the tympanic membrane by creating a seal with the speculum and using a bulb attachment to puff air into the canal (Fig. 6–7).

Figure 6–7
A pneumatic otoscope is used to evaluate mobility of the tympanic membrane. Note the mother helping to restrain and position the infant.

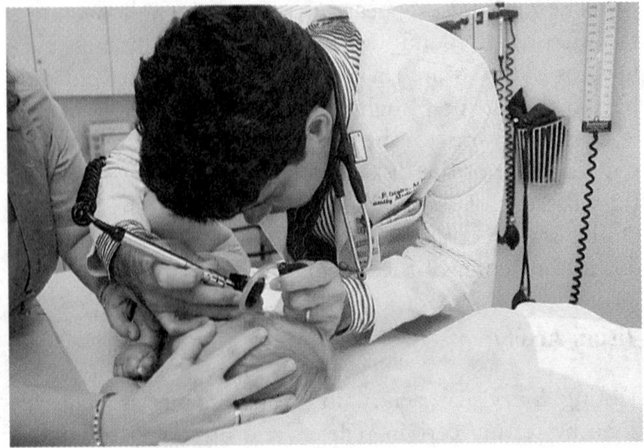

Hearing Acuity

An assessment of hearing acuity can be performed by play audiometry in specialized settings or by audiometry using earphones in children age 4 years and older. Other, more sophisticated tests, such as evoked otoacoustic emissions and brain stem auditory evoked response, may be performed for an infant or a child at risk for hearing loss (see Chapter 25).

Face, Nose, and Oral Cavity

Face and Nose

Having completed the eye and ear examination, the examiner next observes the face for symmetry, spacing, and sizing of its structures and for facial expression. The nose should be symmetrical and midline to an imaginary line drawn from between the eyes to the center of the notch in the upper lip. Genetic differences can be observed in the shape of the bridge of the nose with a characteristic flattened appearance in Asian and some black children. The external nares are inspected for patency, discharge, flaring, and any lesions. To check for patency in newborns, the nurse should block one nostril and at the same time close the infant's mouth and see if the infant continues to breathe smoothly. A penlight or an otoscope is used to visualize the internal nasal cavity by pushing the tip of the child's nose upward while the neck is tilted backward.

For a closer inspection of the mucous lining of the inferior and middle turbinates, a nasal speculum is inserted gently into each nostril. The color, consistency, and integrity of the nasal membranes and septum as well as the septal alignment should be noted. The mucosa is normally pink, and the septum should be midline. Mucosal membranes that are pale, grayish, boggy (spongy texture), bright red, or excoriated are noteworthy.

The amount, color, and texture of any nasal discharge is noted. Watery discharge associated with crying is normal. In contrast, a thin, clear discharge is seen with allergies and sinusitis (either clear or mucopurulent rhinorrhea). Purulent discharge indicates either a viral or a bacterial infectious process. The finding of unilateral nasal discharge is significant.

Oral Cavity

Assessment of the mouth and throat begins at the lips. They should be pink, firm, symmetrical, and moist and with no lesions or excoriations. The buccal mucosa, gingivae, tongue, and palate are observed. These structures are normally pink, firm, smooth, glistening, and moist. The examiner should note the presence of texture changes, increased size, furrows in or limited movement of the tongue, as well as notches, clefts, or unusual arches in the hard palate or any unusual odor (halitosis). Any lesions, swelling, excoriations, or bleeding in these structures is abnormal. While observing the teeth, one can assess for number, hygiene, and the presence of malocclusion, caries, or staining (see Chapter 4). The uvula should be midline and move upward when a gag reflex is elicited.

The tonsils, which are part of the lymphatic system, normally undergo hypertrophy during early childhood, followed by gradual shrinkage beginning around age 10 years (Zitelli & Davis, 1992). The tonsils are normally the same color as the surrounding buccal mucosa and often have crypts on their surface (see Chapter 16). Increased redness or exudate indicates infection. Table 6–2 provides a guide for assessing tonsil size.

Table 6–2
Guide to Tonsillar Size

Scale	Tonsillar Position
1+	Just visible
2+	Halfway between the tonsillar pillars and uvula
3+	Touching the uvula
4+	Touching each other

The use of a tongue blade to view the oral cavity is helpful but can also frighten the young child or cause respiratory arrest if the epiglottis is inflamed. If a clear view of the buccal mucosa is not obtained, the tongue blade can be slipped between the inner cheeks and the gum line. Often an examiner can obtain a clear view of the back of the mouth without the use of a tongue blade in several ways. For the infant or toddler, the mouth can be inspected when the child cries. By tilting the young child's head backward and asking the child to say "ahhh," the examiner is often able to get a clear view of the tonsils, uvula, and oropharynx. If these techniques do not work, the tongue blade can be lightly inserted along the side of the tongue.

▽ **Alert:** *A tongue blade should never be inserted in the mouth of a child who exhibits signs or symptoms of epiglottitis.*

Thorax and Lungs

Chest Configuration and Movement

Assessment of the thorax and lungs begins with inspection of chest configuration, movement, and symmetry. Any abnormalities should be recorded, such as unusual roundness (barrel shape), protuberant or depressed ster-

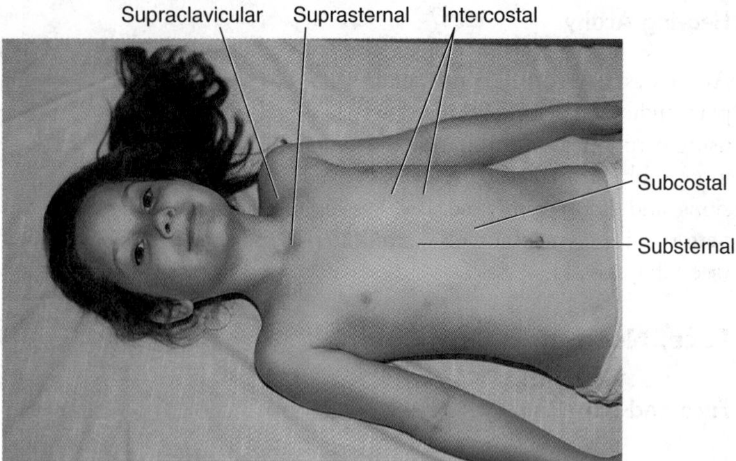

Figure 6–8
Possible sites of retractions.

num, unusual knobbing of the rib cage, or asymmetrical movement—including retractions and their locations—above the clavicles, suprasternal, substernal, and/or intercostal area (Fig. 6–8). Chest movement associated with breathing varies with age. Abdominal or diaphragmatic breathing is characteristic of children younger than age 6 to 7 years. In older children, particularly females, thoracic respirations are predominant. However, the abdomen and chest should always move together in a synchronous fashion.

The rate, depth, quality, and regularity of respiration should be noted as well as the ratio of the inspiratory to expiratory phase of breathing. Respiratory rate is influenced by age and other factors, such as fever and disease status.

Breath Sounds

The examiner listens for audible sounds that may be associated with impaired respiratory efforts, such as stridor, barky or staccato cough, or grunting. Palpating the chest for tactile fremitus (a vibratory sensation) and percussion to determine dullness, resonance, or tympany can sometimes give the examiner additional information about the lungs. However, auscultation of the lungs provides essential information for evaluating the child's respiratory status. Both the open-bell and closed diaphragm should be used for assessment. The lung fields (front, back, and axillary areas) should be auscultated by systematically and symmetrically (comparing one side to another) listening for breath sounds as the child

Table 6–3
Characteristics of Normal Breath Sounds

Sound	Quality	Relationship of Inspiration (I) to Expiration (E)	Normal Location
Vesicular	Soft, swishing	I is longer, louder, and higher pitched than E (I > E)	Throughout lung field
Bronchovesicular	Louder and higher pitch than vesicular; Mixed	I and E are equal (I = E)	Over manubrium and upper intrascapular region where trachea and bronchi bifurcate
Bronchial	Tubular, harsh, hollow	I is short, E is long (I < E)	Over trachea

Table 6–4
Characteristics of Adventitious (Abnormal) Breath Sounds

Sound	Description	Pathology and Examples
Crackles		
Fine	Intermittent, high-pitched, soft popping sounds. Hear late in inspiration. Sound similar to hair rolling between fingers. Not cleared by coughing.	Fluid in alveoli (pneumonia)
Medium	Intermittent and medium-pitched sounds that are loud and noncrackling. Heard early or mid-inspiration.	Fluid in bronchioles and bronchi (pulmonary edema)
Coarse	Loud, bubbling, low-pitched sounds. Heard on expiration. Clear with coughing.	Fluid in bronchioles and bronchi that is resolving (bronchitis)
Friction Rub		
	Superficial, coarse, low-pitched, grating sound. Sounds similar to two pieces of leather rubbing together. Heard in inspiration and expiration.	Pleural inflammation due to loss of normal lubricating fluid (pleuritis)
Rhonchi (Wheezes)		
Sonorous	Continuous, snoring, low-pitched, moaning, vibrating sound that clears with coughing. Heard throughout respiratory cycle.	Air flow obstruction (mucus) in large bronchi and trachea (bronchitis, upper respiratory tract infection)
Sibilant	Continuous, high-pitched, musical, hissing sound. Heard predominately in mid to late expiration.	Air flow through narrowed passageway because of inflammation, collapsing, secretions, or tumors (asthma)
Wheezes (Audible)		
Inspiratory	Sonorous, musical sounds heard on inspiration	High obstruction (croup)
Expiratory	Whistling, sighing sounds heard on expiration	Low obstruction (bronchial foreign body)

takes a deep breath in and blows out. Pretending to blow out the light of an otoscope or penlight is one of many useful games that can be played to encourage deep breathing.

Breath sounds are classified as vesicular, bronchovesicular, or bronchial depending on the sound's loudness and duration during inspiration versus expiration (Engel, 1993; Jarvis, 1996). These various types of breath sounds are normally heard in a distinct area of the chest but become abnormal findings when absent or heard in noncharacteristic locations (Table 6–3). Adventitious sounds that are not normally heard include crackles (discontinuous, interrupted explosive sounds), which can be course, medium, or fine; rhonchi (continuous low-pitched sound); friction rubs; or wheezing (continuous high-pitch sound) (Table 6–4). Absent or diminished breath sounds in any area are also pathologic.

caREminder: *In infants and young children, lack of subcutaneous fat and smaller distances between structures may make breath sounds readily transmitted across lung fields. This must be kept in mind when assessing the presence, location, and nature of breath sounds in infants and young children.*

Cardiovascular System

The child is observed for signs of cyanosis, edema (peripheral, sacral, or periorbital), mottling of the skin (in young infants), clubbing of the nail bed, distended neck veins, or squatting posture. Inspection of the chest in infants and young children with thin chest walls often reveals a cardiac pulsation, the apical impulse (AI) or point of maximal impulse (PMI), which is a normal finding. In contrast, any visible pulsation of the chest caused by a heave or lift of the ventricle, a sustained forceful thrusting of the ventricles during systole, is an abnormal finding. The fingers are used to determine the AI, the apex beat, or the PMI (area of most intense pulsation, which may or may not be the AI). These two terms are not interchangeable.

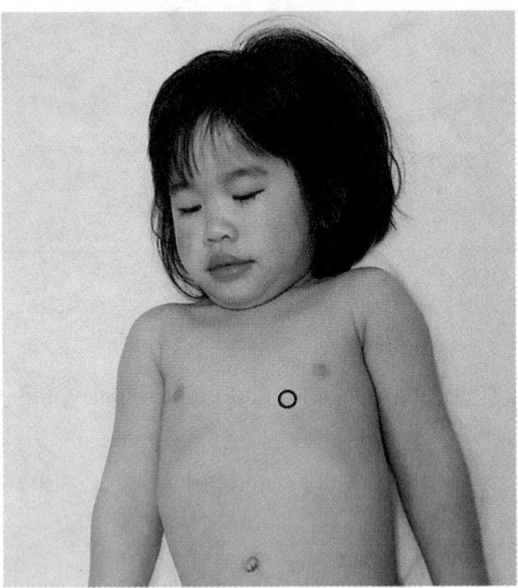

Figure 6–9
Location of the apical impulse in a child younger than age 7 years.

caREminder: *The location of the AI varies with age. In children younger than age 7 years, it is found just left of the midclavicular line and fourth intercostal space; in children older than 7 years, it is located at the left midclavicular line and fifth intercostal space (Fig. 6–9).*

The ball of the hand is used to palpate for the presence of a thrill, a vibratory sensation that feels like the belly of a purring cat. Thrills are pathologic findings. Percussion of the heart has limited usefulness in the cardiac examination of children.

Heart Sounds

Auscultation of heart sounds is an essential assessment skill. Practice and experience enable the examiner to identify the various hearts sounds and murmurs. Heart sounds are produced by the opening and closing of the valves and by vibrations of blood against the walls of the heart and its vessels. Table 6–5 lists the sites of cardiac auscultation and provides descriptions of the various heart sounds that may be heard. The stethoscope's bell is used to detect low-pitched heart sounds; the diaphragm is used to detect high-pitched heart sounds.

The examiner begins at the second right intercostal area, where the closure of the aortic valve is best heard, and then moves to the second left intercostal space to best hear the sound of the pulmonic valve closing. Because the second heart sound (S2) represents closure of both the aortic and pulmonic valves together, the aortic and pulmonic areas are the sites where the S2 is heard loudest. The sound made by the closing of these two valves can sometimes be heard as a split sound. A normal physiologic split sound of S2 can often be heard in the pulmonic area and is a factor of hearing the aortic valve close slightly before the pulmonic valve. Inspiration affects the timing of the closure of these two valves. Therefore, a normal physiologic split varies with inspiration and fades out with expiration. A fixed split S2 that does not vary with respiration is abnormal.

Next, while carefully listening, the examiner then inches down the left sternum to Erb's point at the second and third left intercostal space close to the sternum (Fig. 6–10). Here S1 and S2 are of equal intensity. S1 is heard loudest at the tricuspid and mitral or apical areas. The tricuspid area is at the fifth right and left intercostal space close to the sternum and represents the area where closure of the tricuspid valve is best heard. The mitral area is located at the third to fourth intercostal space and lateral to the left midclavicular line in infants and at the fifth intercostal space, left midclavicular in children around age 7 years. Mitral valve closure is heard best here.

Two additional hearts sounds—S3 and S4—warrant consideration. S3 is a normal sound, produced by vibrations during ventricular filling. It is often a difficult sound for unskilled examiners to detect. S4 can be a normal finding in some children and young adults but is an abnormal sound in older adults.

When listening to the heart, the examiner is evaluating the quality and the intensity of the heart sounds,

Table 6–5
Differentiation of Heart Sounds by Site, Location, and Characteristics

Cardiac Auscultatory Site	Location	Characteristics
Aortic area	2nd right IC space	S2 heard louder than S1; S2 is "dub" sound
Pulmonic area	2nd left IC space	S2 split heard best
Erb's point	2nd and 3rd IC space	S1 and S2 equal loudness; common site of innocent murmurs
Tricuspid area	5th right and left IC space	S1 heard as louder sound than S2; S1 is "lub" sound
Mitral or apical area	3rd to 4th IC space and lateral	S1 heard loudest; S1 is synchronous with carotid pulse

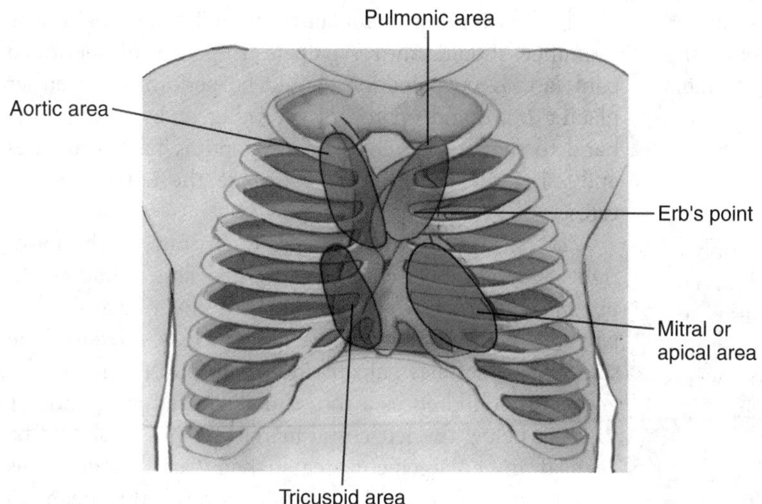

Figure 6–10
Normal location of heart sounds.

its rate, and its rhythm. S1 and S2 should be clear and distinct sounds. In addition, their intensity should be consistent with what would be expected normally at a particular auscultatory site. The rate should be synchronous with the radial pulse and consistent with the norms for cardiac rate by age of the infant or child.

caREminder: *Many young children have periods of sinus arrhythmia, in which the heart rate increases with inspiration and decreases with expiration. This common finding is considered a variant of normal if the arrhythmia disappears during breath holding.*

Fever and anemia also increase cardiac rate and the S1 intensity.

Murmurs

Murmurs are blowing or swooshing sounds caused by turbulent blood flow in the chambers of the heart or its vessel. Infants and children often have innocent or functional murmurs that must be differentiated from the serious organic murmurs. Innocent murmurs are frequently heard in young children and have no pathologic process associated with them. They are thought to be a factor of a child's thin chest wall that makes it easy for these sounds to be transmitted. Functional murmurs are due to certain physiologic conditions such as fever and anemia that cause increase blood turbulence; when these conditions are corrected the murmur disappears. Organic murmurs are associated with pathology of the chambers, valves, or vessels.

When a murmur is detected, the following information is noted:

- *Location:* where it is heard the best and whether it is heard in other auscultatory areas (i.e., where, if anywhere, does it radiate?)
- *Timing:* Does the murmur occur during S1, which represents ventricular systole; during S2, which represents diastole; or throughout the entire cardiac cycle?
- *Intensity:* see Table 6–6
- *Pitch:* low, medium, or high
- *Variation with position:* heard when sitting, standing, supine, or squatting
- *Quality:* describe the sound using terms such as musical, blowing, harsh, or rumbling (Hay et al., 1995).

Characteristics of innocent murmurs of childhood that differentiate them from pathologic murmurs include the following: soft sounding, relatively short in duration, occurring during systole, vibratory and of medium pitch, heard best at the left lower sternal or midsternal border, not associated with physical findings of cardiac pathology, and does not radiate (Behrman, Kliegman, Arvin, & Nelson, 1996; Jarvis, 1996). One must remember to auscul-

Table 6–6
Grading Scale for Classification of Heart Murmurs by Intensity

Grade	Characteristics
Grade I	Soft and difficult to hear
Grade II	Soft but easily heard
Grade III	Loud but no associated thrill
Grade IV	Loud with an associated thrill
Grade V	Loud and audible with edge of the stethoscope; thrill present
Grade VI	Very loud and heard with stethoscope off the chest; thrill present

tate with the child in at least two positions—supine, sitting, or lying on the left side—and to use both the bell and diaphragm of the stethoscope. Innocent murmurs often disappear with a change of position.

Vasculature

Assessment of the vascular system involves palpation of the peripheral arteries for equality, rate, and rhythm. The radial, femoral, popliteal, and dorsalis pedis pulses are palpated to determine blood flow for vascular integrity. To assess these pulses in infants, light palpation works best using one or two fingers for the femoral pulses.

Abdomen

Inspection of its contour and the skin covering the abdomen is the first step in the assessment process. Any unusual shapes or tenseness that denote pathology should be sought, such as organomegaly, ascites, inguinal or femoral bulging, malnutrition, or tumor. The pot-bellied or prominent abdomen is a normal characteristic of infants and children until puberty. Skin markings such as distended veins or striae should be noted. Detection of unusual movements (e.g., peristaltic waves or abdominal respirations in children younger than age 7 years) can indicate gastrointestinal or pulmonary problems. In newborns and young children, the umbilicus should be inspected for discharge, fistulas, or signs of inflammation and palpated for herniation.

Next, auscultation of the abdomen for bowel sounds or bruits (murmurs) should be performed in a systematic fashion by firmly pressing the stethoscope and listening to all four (right and left upper and lower) quadrants of the abdomen. Normally, bowel sounds are heard every 10 to 30 seconds. Always listen for bowel sounds before palpation. Gently stroking the abdomen with one's fingers can help elicit bowel sounds; the examiner should listen for at least 5 minutes before determining that bowel sounds are absent (Engel, 1993). Percussion to determine areas of dullness, flatness or tympany has limited clinical usefulness in pediatrics but can assist the examiner in assessing for liver enlargement.

The examiner's hand and fingers should be warm when palpating the abdomen. Both superficial and deep palpation are useful in assessing pain and organomegaly or determining the presence of a mass. A useful technique to use with a crying infant is to put one hand behind the infant's legs and bend them at the knees while at the same time gently palpating the abdomen with the index finger of the other hand when the infant exhales with each cry.

Tip: *To help with young children who are ticklish, ask them to bend their knees and distract them by having them tell a story.*

If a child has complaints of abdominal pain, the examiner should always palpate the area of identified pain last. Deep palpation should be performed by either placing one hand on top of the other or by placing one hand to support the child's corresponding back structures and using the other hand to palpate the anterior structures.

To palpate the liver, the examiner starts in the lower right quadrant by using two to three fingers and works up. In infants and young children, the liver edge is often palpable 1 to 2 cm below the right costal margin. The spleen is sometimes palpable during inspiration in infants and young children as a soft, thumb-shaped mass about 1 to 2 cm below the left costal margin. Palpation should be deep. If any enlargement greater than 2 cm is found, this is abnormal and needs referral. Beyond the neonatal period, kidneys are normally difficult to palpate unless enlarged. Sometimes the tip of the right kidney can be felt in the neonate as a normal finding. Palpation for a femoral hernia is done by placing the index finger on the femoral pulse and the middle and ring fingers just medially on the skin just over the area where a femoral hernia occurs. To check for an inguinal hernia in a young male child, the examiner's baby finger should be gently slid into the external inguinal canal at the base of each scrotum to determine whether bowel is present.

Lymphatic System

Assessment of the lymphatic system involves palpation to detect lymph node enlargement (Fig. 6–11). If lymph nodes are felt, the examiner notes their size, color of the overlying skin, location, temperature, consistency, and whether tenderness is present. Nodes in the areas anterior and posterior to the sternocleidomastoid muscle are sought by sliding one's fingers against this muscle. The preauricular, mastoid, submandibular, and supraclavicular areas are palpated. To assess for the presence of axillary nodes, the child's arm is held in a slightly abducted position at the sides while palpating this area. For the inguinal area, the child should be in a supine position while the examiner is palpating. The assessment of the spleen was discussed in the section on the abdomen.

External Genitalia and Breasts

Assessment of the external genitalia should be done in a matter-of-fact manner that takes into consideration issues of privacy and modesty. These are particularly important points to remember when examining an adolescent. Assessment of sexual maturation should be noted using Tanner's stages of sexual development for males and females as outlined in Chapter 4.

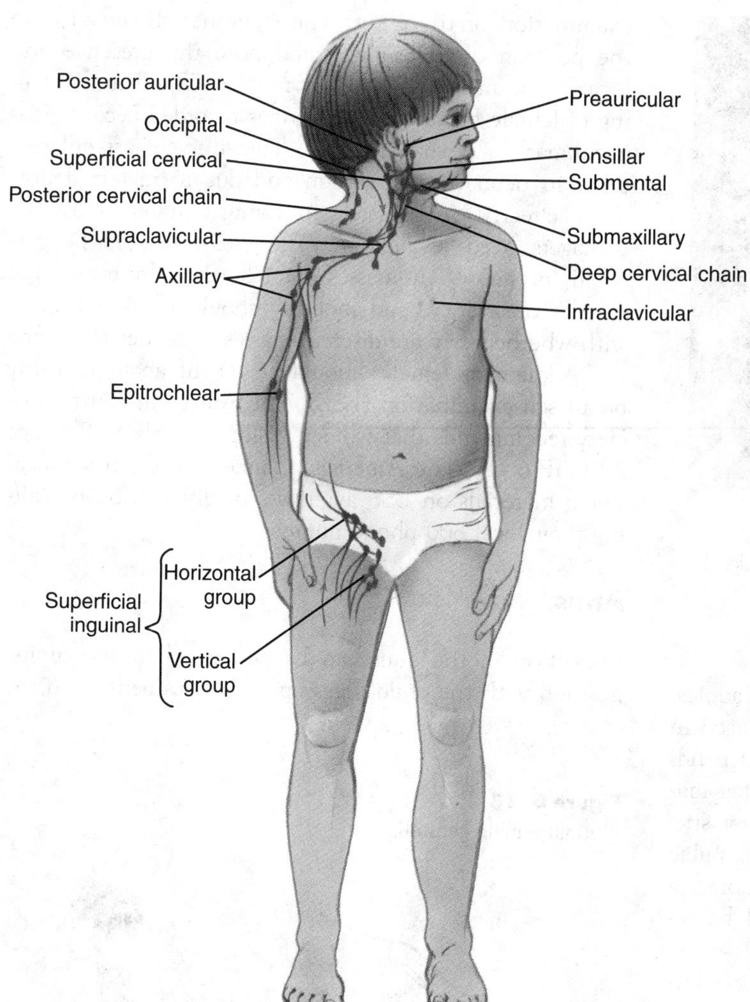

Figure 6–11
Superficial lymph nodes and lymph drainage.

Male Genitalia

In assessment of the male genitalia, the examiner first inspects the penis for size, color, and the presence of any skin lesions or discharge. Notation is made as to whether the male is circumcised and, if not, whether the foreskin retracts easily.

Alert: *Never forcefully retract the foreskin.*

The foreskin is normally adherent in infants and young males until approximately age 3 years. The meatus is inspected for shape (slit-like), placement, and whether ulceration or discharge is present. If pubic hair is present, its distribution, quantity, and quality is described using Tanner's staging. Pubic lice or nits are a significant finding.

The scrotal sac is then inspected for color, size, symmetry, presence of rugae, masses, and lesions. The left scrotum commonly hangs lower than the right. To palpate the testes in an infant or young male, the thumb and index finger of one hand are held over the inguinal canal area to prevent the testes from retracting (the cremasteric reflex) while at the same time palpation is done with the other hand (Fig. 6–12). If the testes cannot be felt, the examiner should have the child sit in an Indian fashion or stand and see if the testes can be palpated. If they still cannot be felt, the examiner should feel the inguinal canal and, if the testes are present there, try to milk them down the canal and into the sac. Cold, excitement, touch, and stimulation are factors that can stimulate the cremasteric reflex, causing the testes to temporarily ascend. Normally, the testes are equal in size and oval; the size of the testes depends on the stage of sexual development. The epididymis is the ridge of soft tissue behind the testes. Note any masses, swelling, tenderness, or asymmetry of the testes and refer to the physician or advanced nurse practitioner.

Female Genitalia

Inspection of the external female genitalia requires that the examiner be able to visualize the external genitalia and the vestibule (the area between the labia minora). Gloves should be worn and the child's legs placed in a

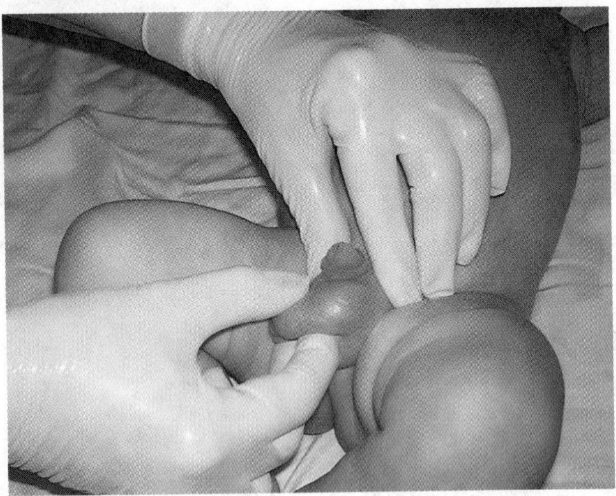

Figure 6–12
To palpate the testes in a young male the examiner blocks the inguinal canal to prevent the testes from retracting into it.

frog-leg (soles of the feet touching) position. The adolescent female is more comfortable if her legs are placed in stirrups. The appearance of the external genitalia depends on the child's stage of sexual maturation. The labia majora, labia minora, and the clitoris are observed for size, color, skin lesions, and masses. The presence of pubic hair and the appropriate Tanner stage should be noted; a child with pubic hair before age 8 years should be referred for an endocrinologic evaluation.

Gentle traction of the labia majora allows a thorough inspection of the vestibule area, including the urethral meatus, vaginal opening, and hymen as well as the fossa and posterior fourchette (Fig. 6–13). Any unusual redness, discharge, edema, scarring, or lesions should be noted. The female genitalia is responsive to estrogen. Maternal estrogen is responsible for the redundant hymen and prominent labia seen in the young infant. Likewise, the effect of endogenous estrogen during puberty again changes the appearance of the labia and the hymenal tissue (which becomes flowery and pale pink).

Ambiguous genitalia and fused labia in infants are abnormal findings and indicate significant pathology. Minor labial adhesions are a common problem seen in young children and are treated only if there is interference with urinary or vaginal drainage. Treatment consists of application of estrogen-containing cream and good hygiene until separation occurs, followed by long-term use of petrolatum to the area.

Breasts

Inspection and examination of the breasts is usually done immediately before or after the respiratory and cardiac examinations. Breast assessment logically is part of the examination of the chest. The examiner should observe the position of the nipples and note the presence and location of any supernumerary nipples. The Tanner staging of female breast development is recorded because it is a hallmark of sexual maturity. Transitory breast enlargement in neonates is common and due to maternal hormone effect. Gynecomastia in young children and male teenagers needs evaluation. The breasts should be palpated for masses. If masses are felt, their location, size, shape, consistency, and mobility should be noted along with whether they are discrete masses or tender to touch.

Adolescent females should be taught about monthly breast self-examination (BSE). The American Cancer Society recommends that women begin monthly BSE at age 20 (TIP 6–1). The American Cancer Society has educational materials on BSE available for distribution by calling their local 800 phone number.

Anus

Inspection of the anus can be performed in the supine position with the child's legs up and knees bent or in the

Figure 6–13
Normal female genitalia.

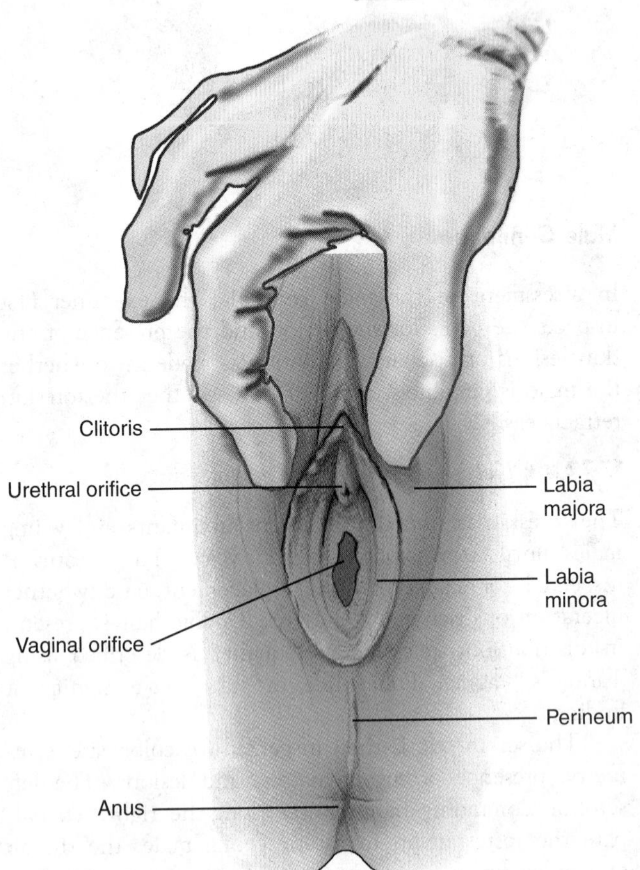

TIP 6–1 A Teaching Intervention Plan for Breast Self-Examination

Nursing Diagnosis and Outcomes

- Knowledge deficit: breast self-examination techniques

Outcome: The adolescent will demonstrate correct breast self-examination techniques.

- Health seeking behaviors: breast self-examination

Outcome: The adolescent will routinely perform breast self-examination.

Interventions

Teach the adolescent:

Steps of Breast Self-Examination

- Perform visual inspection in the following positions: standing with arms raised above the head, hands on hips, bending forward, arms relaxed at side.
- Lie down and put a pillow under the right shoulder. Place the right arm behind the head. Adolescents with large breasts should also examine their breasts in the side-lying position.
- Use the finger pads of the three middle fingers on the left hand to feel for lumps. The finger pads are the top third of each finger. Move the fingers in circles about the size of a dime.
- Press firmly enough to know how one's breasts feel.
- Examine by starting at the armpit moving downward and proceeding in a vertical fashion. The perimeters are bounded by the line that extends down from the middle of the armpit to just beneath the breast, continues across the underside of the breast to the middle of the breast bone, and then moves up to and along the collar bone and back to the middle of the armpit.
- Squeeze the nipples to check for discharge and examine the breast tissue that extends into the armpit with one's arm relaxed at one's side.
- Repeat the examination on your left breast, using the right hand finger pads.

Contact Health Care Provider if

Any changes from normal are detected.

knee chest, prone, or side-lying recumbent position depending on the age of the child. The anus is observed for tone by scratching the anal area and noticing the "wink" response (anal reflex). Any unusual laxity that is not associated with the presence of stool in the ampulla is noted. Gentle traction allows for a closer view of the anal folds or rugae, which should have a wrinkled rather than a smooth appearance. The location of anal tags, scars, fissures, hemorrhoids, or lesions is recorded. Perianal rashes or hyperpigmentation should also be noted.

Musculoskeletal System

The musculoskeletal system is subject to tremendous changes from infancy through adolescence. For example, joint range of motion (ROM) changes with age. In infancy, the normal arc of motion is greatest and declines as the child matures. Therefore, the examiner must be familiar with normal physiologic findings seen in the musculoskeletal system as the child matures. The physical examination should include two components: an age-specific screening evaluation to give the examiner an overview of the musculoskeletal system and a more thorough examination to assess specific musculoskeletal problems.

Screening of the infant involves observing the infant for general body configuration and spontaneous and symmetrical movements of the extremities. The back and the neck are inspected for full range of motion. The examiner should look for obvious deformities or any unusual findings such as a sacral dimple, extra digit, metatarsus adductus, or congenital torticollis. The clavicles, limbs, back, and neck are palpated for signs of tenderness, swelling, masses, or deformities; and range of motion is assessed in all joints. Muscle strength is assessed by picking up the infant with the examiner's hands under the infant's axillae. Normal infants wedge their body against the examiner's hands. The hips should be evaluated for developmental dysplasia of the hip by performing a care-

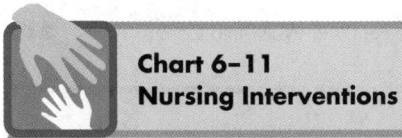

Chart 6–11
Nursing Interventions

Assessment for Development Dysplasia of the Hip (DDH)

The technique of manual examination of an infant hip should only be performed by a trained examiner. The child should be lying supine and as relaxed as possible. Allowing the infant to suck on a pacifier or bottle may help to keep the child calm. Stand at the foot of the infant. First, place your thumbs on the inside of the infant's thighs. Place the forefinger along the top of the thigh and the middle finger down the outside of the infant's thigh, feeling for the head of the femur with the fingers. The hip and knee should be flexed. Both hips are grasped simultaneously to provide stability for the examination, but each should be examined independently. When in doubt about what is felt, stabilize the infant's pelvis with the thumb of one hand over the pelvis and the fingers under the sacrum. To examine an infant's left hip, use one's left hand to stabilize the pelvis; use the other hand to manipulate the hip.

Technique	Positive Findings in the Neonatal Period
Ortolani maneuver	To perform this maneuver, which attempts to reduce a hip that has been dislocated, abduct the hip and lift the head of the femur anteriorly into the acetabulum. If the hip is reducible, it may be felt or heard moving into the acetabulum. The examiner feels a palpable "clunk."

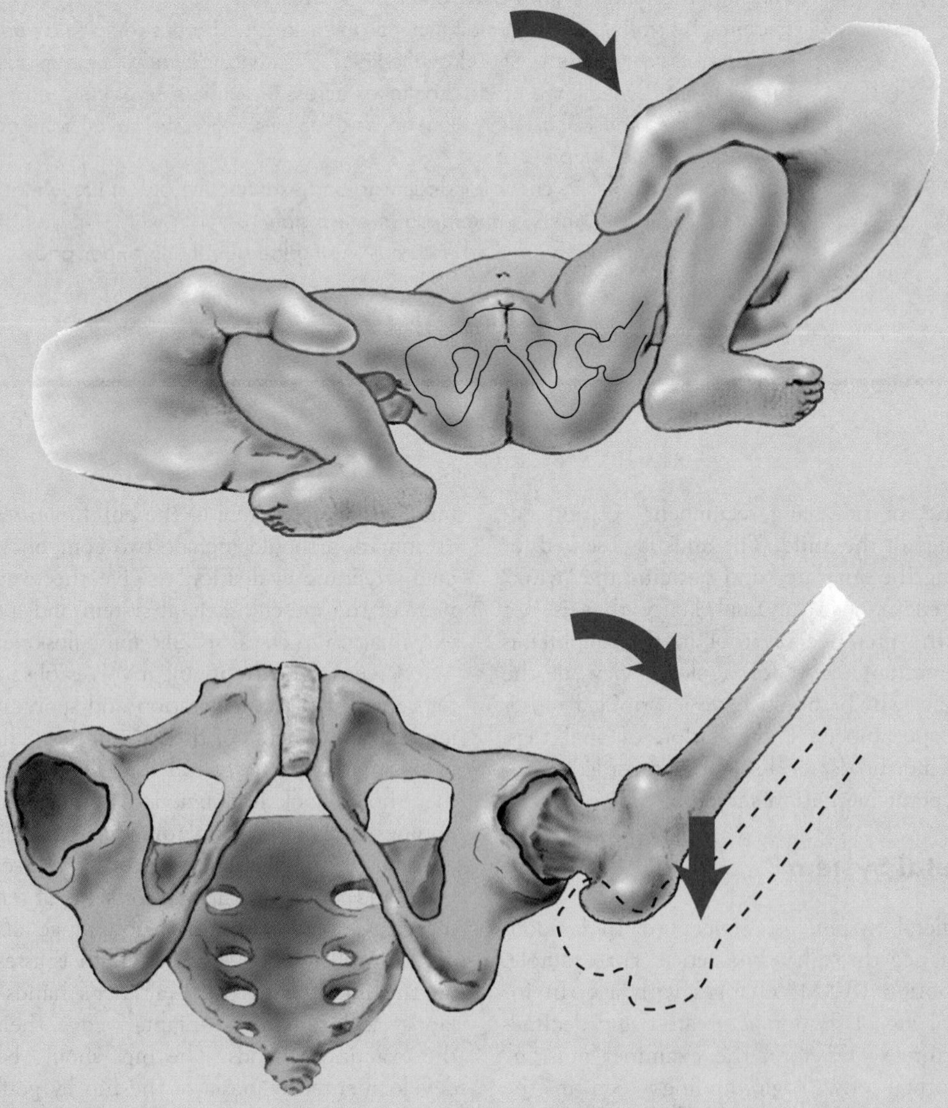

Chart 6–11
Nursing Interventions *Continued*

Assessment for Development Dysplasia of the Hip (DDH)

Technique	Positive Findings in the Neonatal Period
Barlow maneuver	To perform this maneuver, which attempts to dislocate an unstable hip, adduct the hip (bring 10 to 20 degrees past midline) and apply a gentle posterior force with the palm to the knee. If the hip is dislocatable, it can usually be felt slipping out of the acetabulum.

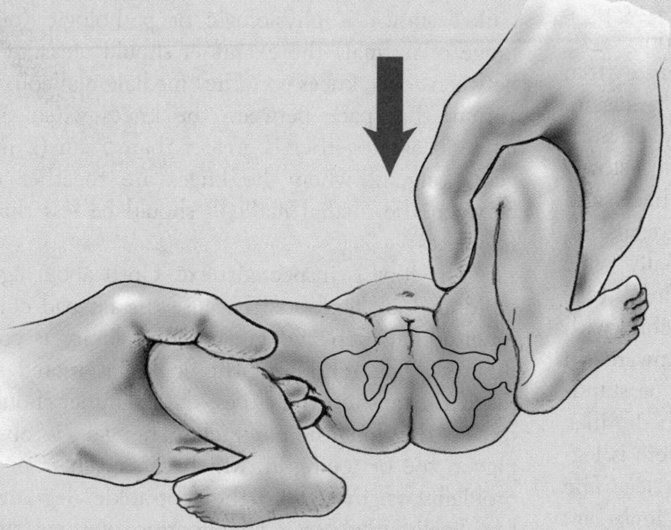

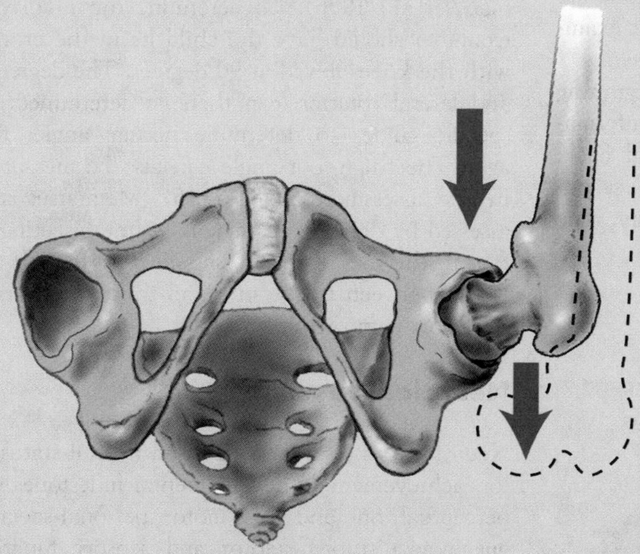

Technique	Positive Findings in Older Infants and Children
Abduction	Limited abduction of the hips
Allis sign	Compare leg lengths by placing the infant in the supine position; flex them at the knees, and compare their heights.
Trendelenburg gait	When the child bears weight on the dislocated side, the unaffected side of the pelvis drops.

ful evaluation of the hip joint and determining the presence of key positive signs as identified in Chart 6–11 (see also Fig. 6–14).

Alert: *Never repeatedly manipulate a hip that is reducible or dislocatable. Doing so may cause vascular compromise.*

An important point to remember in the screening examination of the child and adolescent is to ensure that clothing is not obstructing the examiner's view and shoes are not worn, which can interfere with gait analysis. It is best to have the child dressed in only underwear or a swimsuit at this point in the physical examination.

The child stands, and the examiner observes from front, back, and side views to assess body configuration, symmetry, and proportions and to detect any physical deformities. The examiner has the child walk slowly without shoes and then walk on his or her heels and toes, looking for evidence of gait asymmetry, irregularity, or weakness. The gait of a toddler is normally wide spaced but is symmetrical. In contrast, a painful (antalgic) gait has a shortened stance phase and a child with in-toeing walks with one foot or both turned inward. In assessing the pelvis and back, the child should be standing and the examiner places his or her hands on the iliac crests to observe whether they are level or if there is leg-length discrepancy. The child then raises each leg. The neck and the joints of the upper and lower limbs are tested for range of motion; muscle strength and tone are determined by having the child push against the examiner's hand.

Children should be screened for scoliosis beginning at age 8 to 9 years (see Chapter 20 for more information). The child is observed from the front and back; there should be no differences in shoulder height, scapular prominence, flank crease, and pelvis symmetry. The child should be told to slowly bend forward holding the hands together in a prayer-like fashion while the examiner sits level with and facing the child. Each level of the spine is observed. A "rib hump" is an abnormal finding and suggestive of scoliosis (Staheli, 1992).

Figure 6–14
Assessment for developmental dislocation of the hip.

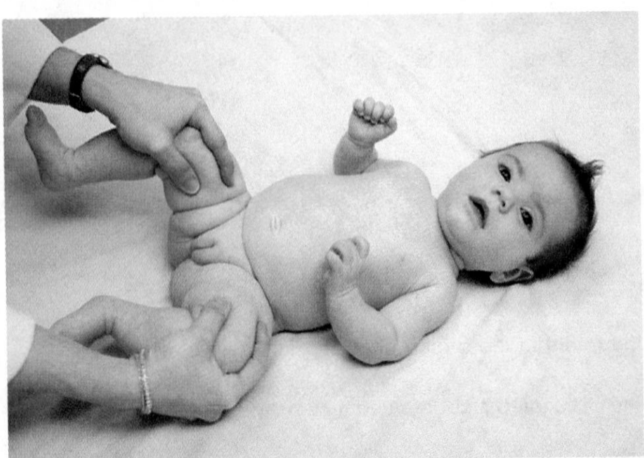

There is a normal range of findings of the lower extremities based on developmental considerations. A "bowlegged" (genu varum) appearance is due to lateral bowing of the tibia and is normal in the toddler years until 1 year after the child started walking. A "knock knee" (genu valgum) appearance is a common finding between 3 and 4 years. To help determine whether the child's stance is physiologic or pathologic (outside the range of normal) the examiner should measure the space between the knees or the medial malleoli. In genu varum, the space between the knees when the medial malleoli are together is greater than 5 cm (2 inches). In genu valgum, when the knees are together the space between the medial malleoli should be less than 7.5 cm (3 inches).

The foot is inspected next. Until about age 3 years, children look flatfooted because the fat pad conceals the longitudinal arch and greater joint laxity is common in infants. Older children who look flat footed should be asked to stand on their toes; the examiner should be able to see the longitudinal arch. The gait is observed for pigeon toe or toeing-in, which can result from rotational problems originating at the foot-ankle, leg-knee, femur-hip, acetabulum, or a combination of these sites (Behrman, et al., 1996). To determine hip involvement, the examiner should have the child lie in the prone position with the knees flexed at 90 degrees, The degree of medial and lateral rotation can then be determined. There are specific guides to determine normal angles for specific ages. The thigh-foot angle can also be measured to help in the assessment (Fig. 6–15). Metatarsus adductus is assessed by drawing an imaginary line bisecting the hindfoot to the toes. The line should pass through the second toe or between the second and third toe (Burns, Barber, Brady, & Dunn, 1996).

Neurologic System

Neurologic assessment focuses on mental status or behavior, achievement of developmental milestones (cognitive-perceptual, fine and gross motor, personal-social, and language acquisition), motor and sensory functions, deep tendon and infant reflexes, and cranial nerve function. Although the findings from assessment of the nervous system are reported under the name of the neurologic system, the actual neurologic assessment is integrated throughout the physical examination. For example, the cranial nerves are assessed when examining the head and the deep tendon reflexes are tested when examining the extremities.

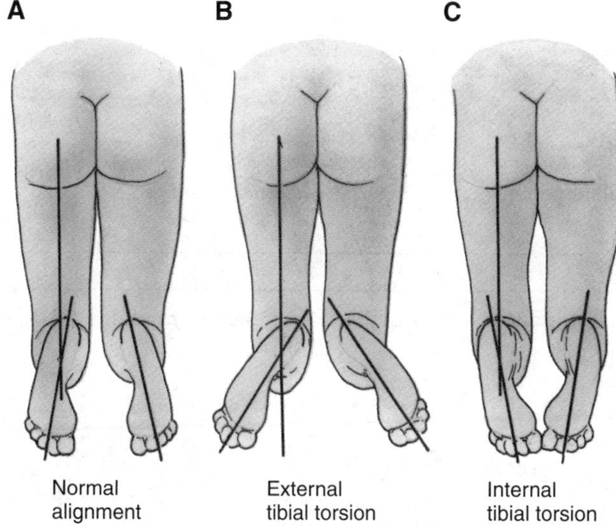

Figure 6–15
Thigh–foot angle. With the child in the prone position and the knees flexed and approximated, the long axis of the foot can be compared with the long axis of the thigh (femur). The long axis of the foot bisects the heel and the second toe or lies between the second and third toes. Normal alignment *(A)* is characterized by slight external rotation. External tibial torsion *(B)* produces excessive outward rotation. Internal tibial torsion produces inward rotation of the foot and is a negative angle *(C)*. (Adapted from Thompson, G. H. [1996]. Gait disturbances. In R. M. Kliegman, M. L. Nieder, & D. M. Super [Eds.], *Practical strategies in pediatric diagnosis and therapy* [p. 761]. Philadelphia: W. B. Saunders. Used with permission.)

Behavioral and Developmental Assessment

In infants and children a behavioral assessment is important and was discussed previously in the history section of this chapter. While taking a history and performing the physical examination, the examiner assesses the child's state of consciousness and looks for clues of neurologic problems, such as hyperirritability, restlessness, hyporeactivity, tics, or unusual repetitive behaviors, as well as indicators of alterations in level of consciousness.

The assessment of developmental milestones in infants and children is best done by determining whether the child has mastered certain tasks (see Chapter 5). Standardized tests such as the Brazelton Neonatal Behavioral Assessment Scale (NBAS), Denver Developmental Screening Test (DDST) II, the Early Language Milestone (ELM), or the Clinical (Capute) Linguistic and Auditory Milestone Scale are useful screening tests, especially if questions arise about the child's development. (Chapter 4 summarizes these tools.) The child is then referred for other more sophisticated testing if problems are found at the screening level.

Motor and Sensory Function

Motor functioning usually is assessed as part of the musculoskeletal examination. The development of motor skills is age related, and there is a cephalocaudal progression of development. In infancy, the examiner looks for the presence or absence of specific infant reflexes (Table 6–7). In the older child, muscle strength and symmetry are tested by the examiner telling the child to "squeeze against my fingers, press the soles of your feet against my hands, and push your arms and legs against my hands."

Several tests of cerebellar functioning can be performed with an older child. Having the child hop, skip, jump, and walk heel-to-toe tests cerebellar functioning. The child is asked to extend an arm and then touch a finger to the nose with eyes open and then shut. Similarly, the child then stands and rubs the heel of one foot down the shin of the other leg with eyes open and closed. While the child is standing with heels together, the examiner should have the child close his or her eyes and note whether the child leans or falls to one side; this is an abnormal finding known as Romberg's sign.

Additional tests may elicit "soft" neurologic signs—performance on selected motor or sensory tests that is abnormal for a child of that age. Minimal choreoathetoid (involuntary purposeless and uncontrollable) movements in the fingers of an extended arm in a child younger than age 4 years is one example of a "soft" neurologic sign. Another example is mirror movement of the fingers of the child's opposite hand when he or she is asked to perform a finger to thumb movement with one hand. These findings may or may not indicate an abnormality, and their significance as an indication of a neurologic disorder should be interpreted cautiously, because these signs may disappear as the child gets older. Children with hyperactivity or attention-deficit disorder may exhibit these signs. However, once again, the significance of "soft" neurologic signs is controversial.

Sensory functioning includes vision, hearing, and peripheral sensation. Vision and hearing are assessed as part of the evaluation of cranial nerves and also through separate auditory and visual testing (see Chapter 28 for more information). Peripheral discrimination can be assessed in children old enough to cooperate by having the child close his or her eyes and touching different parts of the body with either a pin or cotton or a warm or cold object. The child is asked to identify which object is being used. Again with the child's eyes closed, the examiner touches different parts of the body at the same time and asks the child to tell what body part is being touched.

Assessment of cranial nerve function is outlined in Table 6–8. Some of the techniques used to assess individual cranial nerves are age dependent (e.g., an infant will not follow commands). If a neurologic problem or

Table 6–7
Assessment of Infant Reflexes

Reflex	How to Test	Usual Response	Abnormal Findings
Newborn Reflexes			
Babinski's sign	Stroke sole of foot along lateral edge from heel upward.	Toes fan, dorsiflexion of big toe.	Persistence beyond age 24 months
Crawling	Place infant on abdomen.	Crawling movements with arms and legs.	Asymmetrical movements
Dance or stepping	Hold infant with feet lightly touching firm surface.	Feet move up and down.	Persistence beyond age 4–8 weeks
Extrusion	Touch tip of infant's tongue.	Tongue extends out.	Persistence beyond age 4 months
Galant's 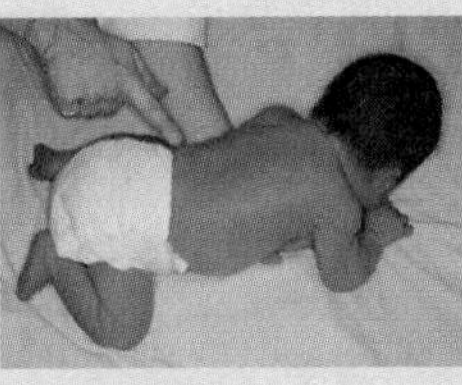	Stroke lateral side of spine from shoulder to buttocks.	Back moves to side being stroked.	Persistence beyond age 4–8 weeks
Moro's	Place infant semi-upright position; let head fall backward with immediate resupport with the examiner's hands.	Symmetrical abduction and extension of arms, flexion of thumb, followed by flexion and adduction of upper limbs.	Persistence beyond age 4 months; asymmetrical or absent response
Palmar grasp 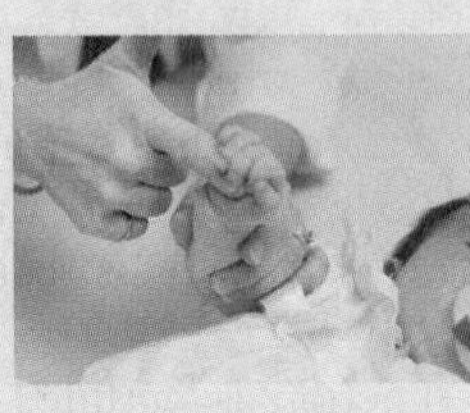	Place finger or object in infant's open palm.	Infant's fingers curve around finger or object and resist its removal.	Absence or persistence beyond age 10 months

Table 6–7
Assessment of Infant Reflexes *Continued*

Reflex	How to Test	Usual Response	Abnormal Findings
Newborn Reflexes			
Rooting 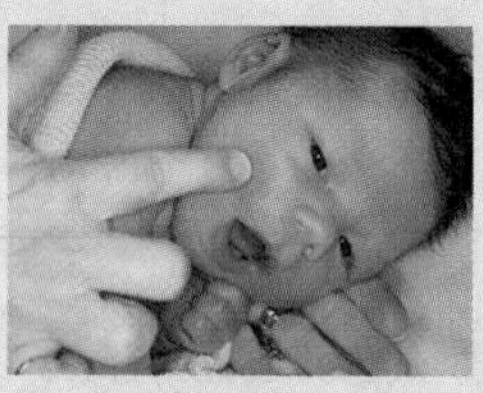	Stroke corner of infant's mouth.	Infant opens mouth and turns head to side being stroked.	Absence or depressed; disappears by age 3–4 months when awake
Startle 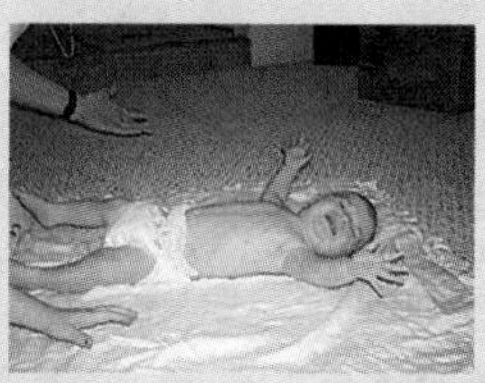	Clap hands loudly.	Infant extends and flexes arms quickly.	Absence or persistence beyond age 4 months
Sucking	Place nipple 3–4 cm into the infant's mouth.	Infant begins sucking.	Absence or depressed; disappears at age 3–4 months when awake
Later Reflexes			
Neck righting 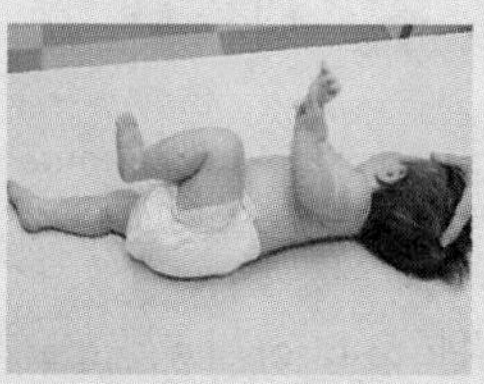	Place infant supine and turn the head to one side.	Infant's trunk and pelvis turn in the direction that the head is rotated.	Absence after age 6 months or persistence beyond age 2 years
Parachute 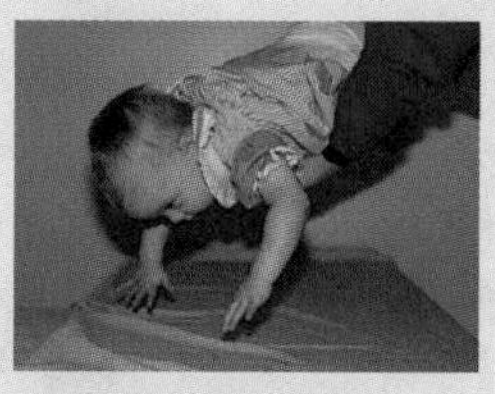	Suspend the infant by the trunk and suddenly flex body forward.	Infant spontaneously extends arms, hands, and fingers.	Should appear by age 6–8 months
Tonic neck 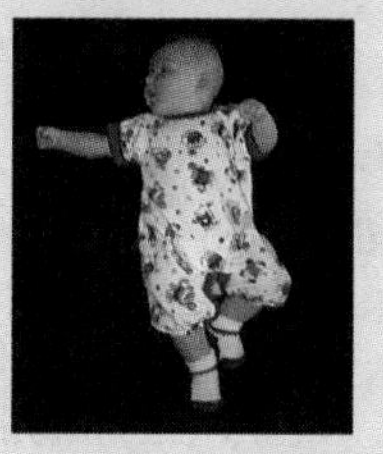	Turn infant's head quickly to one side when supine.	Extension of arm and leg on side that head turned with flexion in opposite limbs	If locked in the "fencer's position"; normal from age 2–6 months

Table 6–8
Assessment of Cranial Nerve Function

Cranial Nerve	Assessment of Function
I, Olfactory	Not routinely tested. Have child close one eye, occlude one nostril at a time, and ask him or her to identify various common aromatic scents (e.g., vanilla, orange, peanut butter, peppermint).
II, Optic	Test for visual fields and visual acuity; fundoscopic examination.
III, Oculomotor	Check pupil size and reactivity. Have child follow the light in the six cardinal positions of gaze and raise eyebrows.
IV, Trochlear	Have child move eyes downward and inward.
V, Trigeminal	Palpate jaw and temple muscles for symmetry and strength as child bites down (motor function). Test for corneal reflex by lightly touching the cornea with a wisp of cotton; have the child close both eyes and see if the child can tell when the forehead, cheeks, and chin are touched with a cotton wisp (sensory function).
VI, Abducens	Check for ability to move the eyes side laterally.
VII, Facial	Have the child smile, lift eyebrows, or show his or her teeth (motor function). For an infant, observe for facial symmetry when crying. Ask child to identify various tastes of substances (e.g., sugar, salt, or lemon juice) placed on the anterior two thirds of the tongue with an applicator. This evaluates sensory function and is a test not routinely done.
VIII, Acoustic	Test hearing. Clap hands from behind (not next to ear so air movement is felt) to see if infant responds; whisper to child from behind so they do not see your lips moving. (See Chapter 28 for more information on audiometry and other selected hearing tests.)
IX, Glossopharyngeal	Test the child's ability to identify the taste of various substances (see CN VII) placed on the posterior of the tongue. This test is not routinely done. Phonation and swallowing are tests of motor function.
X, Vagus	Elicit gag reflex by placing a tongue blade to the posterior palate; check ability to swallow; and note hoarseness. Check that uvula and soft palate rises when child says "ahhh."
XI, Accessory	Have child shrug shoulders while pressure is applied by the examiner's hands to determine strength. Similarly, tell the child try to turn his or her head to the side while the examiner places a hand against the face to resist this movement.
XII, Hypoglossal	Ask child to stick out his or her tongue and move it in all directions. Place a tongue blade against the side of the child's tongue and ask the child to move it away.

symptom is present, a complete neurologic examination is needed. Otherwise, a screening examination is usually done.

Reflexes

Testing reflexes is a routine part of the neurologic examination. Testing can be done with a reflex hammer, the flat of the fingers, the edge of the stethoscope diaphragm, or the side of the hand. The usual deep tendon reflexes that are tested include the biceps, triceps, brachioradialis, quadriceps (patellar), and the Achilles. The area over the tendon is tapped, and the examiner looks for either extension or flexion (Fig. 6–16). To test for the plantar response, the examiner lightly strokes the lateral side of the sole of the foot and across the ball of the foot with an upward motion. The normal response is plantarflexion of the toes and sometimes the whole foot. Table 6–9 describes how to test for deep tendon reflexes and normal findings.

The superficial reflexes that are commonly tested are the abdominal, cremasteric, and anal reflexes. The abdominal reflex is tested by stroking the abdominal skin with the handle of a reflex hammer or with a wooden applicator tip, moving from the side toward the midline in all four quadrants. The umbilicus moves toward the

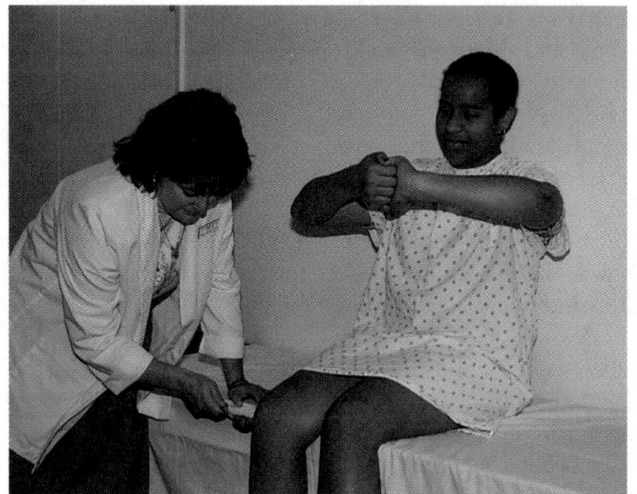

Figure 6–16
To facilitate evaluation of deep tendon reflexes in a child's lower extremities, the child may be distracted by having him or her lock the fingers together and then try to pull his or her hands apart.

stroking. This reflex may not be present in infants younger than age 6 months. The cremasteric reflex is elicited by gently stroking the inner aspect of the thigh of the male. Elevation of the testis on that side is the normal response. The anal reflex is tested by stroking the perianal skin and observing a brisk contracture of the anal sphincter (the "anal wink").

The neurologic system undergoes dramatic growth and maturation during the infancy period. The presence and disappearance of primitive infant reflexes occurs in a sequence during specific periods of development (see Table 6–7). Therefore, the absence or persistence of these reflexes is cause for alarm; these reflexes are important considerations in the assessment of a child during the first year of development. The Moro, grasp, tonic neck, and parachute are the most important primitive reflexes. Their presence or absence during specific periods of development or an abnormal reflex response can signal a central nervous system disorder (Behrman et al., 1996).

Developmental Considerations: Adolescents

Issues related to sexual development, the establishment of sexual identity, and preparation for adulthood emerge as major areas in the adolescent health assessment. In addition to the traditional areas covered in the comprehensive pediatric health history, a comprehensive adolescent sexual history is obtained (Burns et al., 1996). The content areas discussed for females include the following:

Table 6–9
Assessment of Deep Tendon Reflexes

Deep Tendon Reflex	Method of Testing	Normal Finding
Biceps	Flex the forearm, place your thumb over antecubital space, and tap with reflex hammer.	Slight flexion of forearm
Triceps	Abduct arm and support forearm with your hand, child's forearm hangs free; or, hold child's wrist over his chest to flex arm at elbow. Tap directly above elbow.	Partial extension of forearm
Brachioradialis	Place child's arm and hand in relaxed position with arm flexed and palm down. Tap the radius about 1 inch (2.5 cm) above wrist.	Flexion of forearm and palm turns upward
Quadriceps	Have child's legs flexed at the knees and dangling. Tap midline just below the patella. Distract an older child by asking him or her to lock the fingers of their hands tightly together and try to pull them apart. Tap while the child is busy doing this task.	Partial extension of the lower leg
Achilles	Use same position as for quadriceps testing or, in supine position, flex knee and support that leg on the other leg. Lightly support foot in your hand in dorsiflexion and tap Achilles tendon.	Foot plantarflexes (downward)

Note: A four-point scale is typically used to grade the level of response: 4+, hyperactive, very brisk; 3+, brisker than average; 2+, average; 1+, diminished; and 0, no response. If the child tenses the muscle and tendon group to be tested, the deep tendon reflex is difficult to elicit.

- *Menarche/menses:* age at onset; duration, quantity of flow, and frequency of menses; last menstrual period; and any problems with dysmenorrhea
- *Sexual activity:* sexual behaviors and practices (include questions from kissing, necking, petting, to intercourse); if applicable, frequency of sexual coitus and age of debut; sexual orientation (males, females, bisexual), number of sexual partners; issues of date rape, prior sexual molestation, or prostitution
- *Contraceptive history:* understanding of various types of contraceptives for females and males; current and past use of contraceptives
- *Obstetric and gynecologic history:* number of pregnancies, past gynecologic procedures or illnesses (pelvic inflammatory disease)
- *History of sexually transmitted diseases:* type, dates, and treatment; sexually transmitted disease history in partner; any current signs or symptoms
- *Body image:* perceptions about her body and sexual identity
- *Anticipatory guidance:* preparation for her emerging sexual development
- *Partner:* involvement and commitment to family planning

Important content areas for males include the following:

- *Spermarche:* age of first ejaculation
- *Sexual activity:* sexual behaviors and practices (include questions from self-masturbation, kissing, necking, petting, to intercourse); if applicable, frequency of sexual coitus and age at debut; sexual orientation (females, males, bisexual), number of sexual partners
- *Contraceptive history:* knowledge about condoms to prevent pregnancy and sexually transmitted diseases; consistency of condom use or other methods of birth control; whether he and his female partner discuss using a method of birth control; and male responsibility if he fathers a child
- *History of sexually transmitted diseases:* type, dates, and treatment; sexually transmitted disease history in partner; any current signs or symptoms
- *Body image:* perceptions of his body and sexual identity
- *Anticipatory guidance:* preparation for his emerging sexual development
- *Partner:* involvement and commitment to family planning

General issues to be discussed that pertain to all adolescents include a tobacco, alcohol, and drug history (the onset, duration, frequency, and type), risk-taking behaviors (e.g., driving under the influence, drag racing cars, and hitch hiking), exposure to violence in the home or community, emotional stability (suicide and depression), school performance and vocational development, family life and involvement, future plans, and the presence of a support system (profile of parents, friends, and others).

The young adolescent (age 12 to 14 years) should be given the choice of whether the parent is present during the interview and examination, but time should always be allowed to talk alone with the adolescent. The older adolescent should be interviewed alone. Issues of confidentiality need to be addressed with both the adolescent and parent. Both the child and parent should be told that what each one says in confidence will not be discussed with the other unless the information is something that the individual agrees to share (Hahn, 1996). Issues of confidentiality generally center around sexual activity, birth control, and feelings about oneself or the parent–child relationship. The adolescent should be told from the start of the interview that thoughts about harming himself or herself or others cannot be kept confidential.

Tip: *Allow the adolescent to undress in private before the physical examination. Explain what is being done and why in terms easy for the adolescent to understand. Actively talk with the adolescent during the examination and frequently emphasize normal findings (e.g., your ears are fine, your eyes are great). Ask the adolescent questions about sexual changes to let the teen know that these changes are normal and expected. When examining the genitalia of an adolescent of the opposite sex or if a male examines the breasts of a female, it is common and standard practice to always have someone present who is of the same sex as the adolescent being examined.*

Many adolescents are afraid to ask questions and are grateful when the topic is approached by the nurse. The examination is ended only after time is allowed for the adolescent to ask questions and to clarify what, if any, physical findings are found. In addition, the examiner should establish with the adolescent what information will be discussed with the parent, either by the examiner alone or by the adolescent and examiner together. Positive communication between parent and adolescent should be encouraged and promoted.

Database and Interpretation

Having conducted a health history and performed a physical examination, the nurse has a database from which to derive a plan of action. As additional data are received, such as laboratory and other radiographic information, modifications in the assessment and plan can be made. Knowledge and skills of pediatric health assessment develop over time and with practice. Often health care professionals think that the biggest challenge they face is to learn physical examination techniques and skills. However, it is the astute nurse who realizes more often than not the real challenge lies in becoming a skilled interviewer.

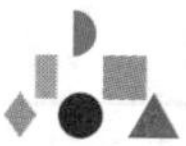

Health Surveillance Visits

At the beginning of the 20th century, infectious diseases caused most of the morbidity and mortality in children and health supervision consisted primarily of cursory examination to detect contagious diseases. The childhood mortality rate was reduced dramatically by the first public health revolution that brought with it immunization against infectious and potentially life-threatening diseases, pasteurization, and improved nutrition and sanitation.

Children of today face new issues as major economic, social, and demographic changes have significantly affected American families. Today, 25% of infants and toddlers and 20% of older children live in poverty. More than 25% of the nation's children now live in single-parent households, usually with their mothers, a percentage that continues to increase. Today's children are growing up in step, blended, sequential, homeless, or foster families. Over 1 million children each year are affected by divorce, and another million infants are born each year to unmarried mothers. Task overload and role strain are experienced by single parents as well as families with two working parents. Almost 11 million mothers of preschool children are employed outside the home.

These societal changes are accompanied by new morbidities and mortalities among children and adolescents that must be addressed by health supervision guidelines. Injuries are the leading cause of death in children older than 1 year. Conservative estimates suggest that 12% to 15% of American children have mental and emotional disorders. Among 15-year-olds, one in seven smokes, one in three has consumed alcohol excessively, one in five smokes marijuana daily, and one in four girls and one in three boys are sexually active.

In providing health supervision for today's children, the health care professional must recognize that physical well-being, mental health, cognitive development, the new morbidities, and social efficacy are influenced by socioeconomic variables, behavior factors, family and cultural considerations, environment, education, access to health care, and the availability and quality of community resources.

Guidelines developed for health surveillance of infants, children, and adolescents are based on the beliefs that health supervision is as follows (Green, *Bright Futures*, 1994, p. xv):

- A longitudinal process that promotes a partnership and shared agenda between the health care professional, the child, and the family
- Personalized to fit the individual
- Contextual (i.e., views the child in the context of the family and the community)
- Supportive of the child's self-esteem, sense of competence, and mastery
- Based on a health diagnosis
- Focused on the strengths as well as the problems and issue of the family and community
- Part of a seamless system that includes community-based health, education, and human services
- Complementary to health promotion and disease prevention efforts in the family, the school, the community, and the media

The need for definitive health supervision research is critical to provide scientific support for disease prevention and health promotion strategies and interventions. Effective health promotion and prevention has far greater implications for infants, children, adolescents, and their parents or caretakers than with any other population group.

Pediatric health supervision involves promoting health, preventing mortality and morbidity, and enhancing development and maturation. Prevention requires both an orderly and routine schedule of activities based on knowledge of predictable physical and psychosocial development (attainment of developmental milestones), as well as recognition of prevention as a constant, ongoing process rather than an episodic one. Table 6–10 presents guidelines for preventive health supervision visits based on recommendations by the AAP and Bright Futures and developed by Behrman, Kliegman, and Arvin (1996). Health promotion visits for children acknowledge the first aspect of prevention: predictable physical and psychosocial development. This model of prevention recommends activities at each visit that include screening procedures and health promotion and disease prevention strategies, primarily the use of immunization and the physical examination. Should a scheduled well-child care visit be used to address an identified health problem, then the well-child care visit should be rescheduled.

Table 6-10
Guidelines for Preventive Health Supervision Visits*

Activity	1st week	1 mo	2 mo	4 mo	6 mo	9 mo	12 mo	15 mo	18 mo	2 yr	3 yr	4 yr	5 yr	6 yr	8 yr	10 yr	11–14 yr	15–17 yr	18–21 yr
Interview (for special attention)	✓	✓	✓	✓	✓	✓	✓	✓		✓	✓	✓	✓	✓	✓	✓	✓	✓	✓
Family history	✓	✓	✓											✓				✓	
Pregnancy and delivery	✓																		
Neonatal course	✓	✓																	
Developmental evaluation	✓	✓	✓	✓	✓	✓	✓	✓	✓	✓	✓	✓	✓	✓	✓	✓	✓	✓	✓
Anticipatory guidance	✓	✓	✓	✓	✓	✓	✓	✓	✓	✓	✓	✓	✓	✓	✓	✓	✓	✓	✓
Body systems (for special attention)																			
Hearing/vision	✓	✓	✓	✓	✓	✓	✓		✓	✓	✓	✓	✓		✓	✓	✓	✓	
CNS (including sleep)	✓	✓	✓	✓	✓	✓	✓		✓	✓	✓	✓							
Gastrointestinal/feeding	✓	✓	✓	✓	✓	✓	✓		✓	✓	✓	✓	✓		✓	✓	✓	✓	
Urinary	✓									✓									
Dental care							✓	✓	✓	✓	✓	✓	✓	✓	✓	✓	✓	✓	
Drugs, alcohol, tobacco															✓	✓	✓	✓	✓
Pica							✓	✓	✓	✓	✓	✓							
Sexual behavior															✓	✓	✓	✓	✓
Physical Examination (complete) (for special attention)	✓	✓	✓	✓	✓	✓	✓	✓	✓	✓	✓	✓	✓	✓	✓	✓	✓	✓	✓
Parent–child interaction	✓	✓	✓	✓	✓	✓	✓	✓	✓	✓	✓	✓	✓	✓	✓	✓			
Height and weight	✓	✓	✓	✓	✓	✓	✓	✓	✓	✓	✓	✓	✓	✓	✓	✓	✓	✓	✓
Head circumference	✓	✓	✓	✓	✓	✓	✓	✓											
Blood pressure											✓	✓	✓	✓	✓	✓	✓	✓	✓
Acne																	✓	✓	✓
Vision																			
Tear ducts	✓	✓																	
Fixed eyes	✓	✓																	
Red reflex	✓	✓	✓	✓	✓	✓	✓												
Fundus	✓				✓														
Strabismus	✓	✓	✓	✓	✓	✓				✓									
Hearing	✓	✓	✓			✓	✓	✓	✓	✓	✓	✓	✓	✓					
Speech			✓	✓	✓	✓	✓	✓	✓	✓	✓	✓	✓	✓					

Neurologic problems			√	√	√	√	√												
Cardiac murmurs	√	√	√	√		√	√												
Abdominal masses	√	√	√																
Hip dysplasia	√	√	√	√	√	√	√		√	√									
Gait							√	√	√		√								
Metatarsus adductus		√																	
Sexual development															√	√	√	√	
Scoliosis															√	√	√	√	√
Evidence of neglect/abuse		√	√	√	√	√	√	√	√	√	√	√	√	√	√	√	√	√	
Counseling (for special attention)																			
Diet	√	√	√	√	√	√	√	√	√	√	√					√	√	√	√
Sleep	√	√	√	√	√		√		√	√	√			√		√	√	√	√
Toilet training								√	√	√	√								
Accidents										√	√	√	√	√	√	√	√	√	√
Child care		√	√	√	√	√	√	√	√	√	√		√						
School problems													√	√	√	√	√	√	√
Puberty and sexuality															√	√	√	√	√
Substance abuse															√	√	√	√	√
Laboratory																			
Hgb/Hct					√ or	√ or	√			√					√		√	√	
Urinalysis					√					√					√				
Urine culture (girls)							√						√			√	√		
Tuberculin						√ or	√			√				√	√	√	√	√	√
Screening																			
Lipids										√	or	√		√		√	√	√	√
Metabolic	√																		
Lead			√		√ or	√ or	√ or	√		√	√		√						
Audiometer	√ (Prior to 3 mo)												√	√					
Snellen chart											√		√	√		√			
Sexually transmitted diseases																	√	√	√
Immunizations	√	√	√	√	√	√	√	√	√			√ or	√				√		

* These suggestions or guidelines represent an analysis of recommendations by the American Academy of Pediatrics and Bright Futures. They are not intended to be all-inclusive but rather to serve as reminders for some of the important preventive and health promotion activities that should be considered at various ages when physician–patient encounters may occur. The content and timing of visits will need to be altered according to special needs and the presence or absence of risk factors for the child and his or her family.

From Behrman, R. E., Kliegman, R. M., & Arvin, A. M. (Eds.). (1996). *Nelson textbook of pediatrics* (15th ed., pp. 20–21). Philadelphia: W. B. Saunders. Reprinted with permission.

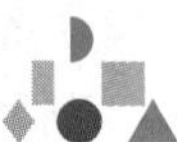

Anticipatory Guidance

The components of anticipatory guidance for children of all ages and their parents or caretakers include discussions about healthy habits, social competence including family relationships and parent/child interactions, and community interactions (Green, 1994). These discussions should focus on age-appropriate topics in each of these areas (see Chapter 5 for more information). Issues about healthy habits center on lifestyle choices, injury and violence prevention (Chart 6–12), nutrition and healthy eating choices (Chart 6–13), oral health (Chart 6–14), mental health (issues of self esteem, depression, anger, and suicide), and sexuality education.

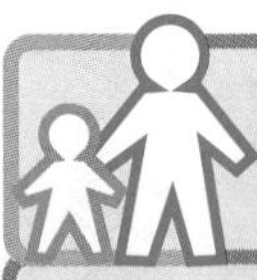

Chart 6–12
Developmental Considerations

Healthy Habits—Lifestyles and Preventable Injury

Health Lifestyles Discussion Issues

- Physical activities (avoidance of sedentary activities—limit television viewing)
- Avoidance of drugs, alcohol, and tobacco
- Exposure to second-hand smoke
- Personal hygiene
- Need for adequate sleep
- Sunscreen protection
- Violence prevention, including firearms removed from home or locked and out of reach
- Smoke and carbon monoxide detector in home

Injury Prevention by Age Group

Infant, Toddler, and Preschool Children

- Child-proof home (hot liquids, water temperature <120°F, poisons, medicines, irons, sharp objects, plastic bags, stairs, window guards, matches, outlets, cords, small and sharp objects)
- Car seat installation, use, and position in car
- No baby walker
- Water safety (pools, bodies of water, buckets, toilets)
- Supervision around animals, driveways, streets, equipment
- Playground and stranger safety starting at preschool age

School-Age Children

- Firm rules for behavior—neighborhood, sports, school, home
- Seat belt use
- Helmets—bike, roller blade or skating—and other safety equipment for sport activities
- Safe after school environment plus home alone rules
- Good touch versus bad touch education
- Pedestrian and playground safety
- Water safety

Adolescence

- Firm rules for behavior
- Job and sport safety issues—protective equipment and rules for safe participation
- Seat belt use
- Substance abuse—alcohol, tobacco, or drugs
- No carrying or use of weapons
- Safe driving rules both as a responsible driver and passenger
- Learn to protect self from abuse (e.g., physical and emotionally abusive relationships, sexual abuse, and date rape)
- Dealing with anger and conflict resolution in a nonviolent manner

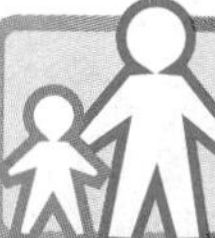

Chart 6–13
Developmental Considerations

Healthy Habits—Nutrition and Healthy Eating Choices

Infants and Preschool Children

- Breast feeding (correct positioning, normal infant patterns of feeding, frequency, nipple care, and maternal issues)
- Formula feeding (formula preparation, iron fortified, techniques, no heating in microwave, positioning)
- Introduction of solids (age, cues, types of foods and amounts)
- No solid foods mixed with bottles
- No honey
- Iron-deficiency anemia due to excessive milk intake
- Foods associated with choking (e.g., peanuts, popcorn, carrot sticks, raisins, whole beans, hard candy, touch meats, grapes, hot dogs)
- Introduction of cup around age 6 months; feeding self around age 15 months
- Introduction of table and finger food; provide healthy choices
- Do not force eating

Preschool Children

- Limit sweets
- Provide healthy choices of three meals a day and nutritious snacks
- Do not get into battle about eating
- Picky eater but will over time eat a variety of food

School-Age Children and Adolescents

- Provide healthy choices for meals
- Teach how to choose healthy foods
- Limit high-fat and high-sugar foods
- Manage weight through appropriate eating and regular exercise
- Eat food rich in calcium and iron (adolescent)

Social competence discussions emphasize the need for the following: teaching family and societal rules about resolving conflict; age-appropriate discipline; developmentally appropriate behaviors; praise and encouraging expression of feelings; the ability to show respect for and communicate in a positive manner with siblings, peers, parents, and individuals in authority positions; showing affection; positive role modeling by parents; inquiring about school-related progress and career choices for teenagers; and allowing opportunities for socialization and to achieve developmental milestones. Community interaction discussions acquaint parents and caregivers with available community resources that are family and child focused, such as parent and community support groups, early intervention programs for at-risk children, community and after-school activities for children and teenagers, and child care resources and guidelines. The need for financial assistance, Medicaid, food, housing, and transportation are also items that are addressed under this heading.

The nurse needs to assume a proactive role in discussing anticipatory guidance issues with children and their families. Emphasizing and teaching about the value of a healthy lifestyle and behaviors is the responsibility of all members of the health care team. Every health care encounter is an opportunity for health teaching that should not be overlooked. A pediatric or adolescent health assessment is never complete if anticipatory guidance issues are not identified and addressed whether through discussion, providing written literature, or stressing the need for a follow-up health surveillance visit (Chart 6–15).

Symptom Management and Teaching Principles

Well-child care encompasses health assessment and management of symptoms commonly seen in minor illnesses.

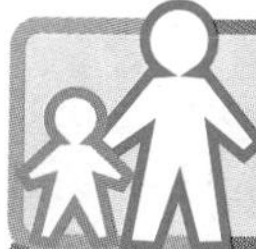

Chart 6–14
Developmental Considerations

Healthy Habits—Oral Health

Infants and Toddlers

- No bottle in bed or carrying around bottle of milk or juice
- Fluoride (begin at age 6 months)
- Brush teeth (begin about age 9 months)
- Dental visit (at age 1 year)

Preschool and School-Age Children and Adolescents

- Discourage sucking habits at around age 4 years
- Routine dental visits
- Brush teeth
- Learn dental emergency care
- Fluoride
- Discuss dental sealants

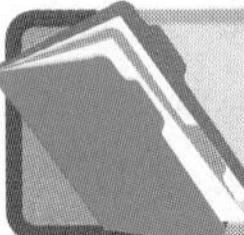

Chart 6–15
Nursing Interventions Classification (NIC)

Anticipatory Guidance

Definition

Preparation of patient for an anticipated developmental and/or situational crisis

Activities

- Assist the patient to identify possible upcoming, developmental, and/or situational crisis, and the effects the crisis may have on personal and family life.
- Instruct about normal development and behavior, as appropriate.
- Provide information on realistic expectations related to the patient's behavior.
- Determine the patient's usual methods of problem solving.
- Assist the patient to decide how the problem will be solved.
- Assist the patient to decide who will solve the problem.
- Use case examples to enhance the patient's problem-solving skills, as appropriate.
- Assist the patient to identify available resources and options for course of action, as appropriate.
- Rehearse techniques needed to cope with upcoming developmental milestone or situation crisis with the patient, as appropriate.
- Assist the patient to adapt to anticipated role changes.
- Provide a ready reference for the patient (e.g., educational materials/pamphlets), as appropriate.
- Suggest books/literature for the patient to read, as appropriate.
- Refer the patient to community agencies, as appropriate.
- Schedule visits at strategic developmental/situational points.
- Schedule extra visits for patient with concerns or difficulties.
- Schedule follow-up phone calls to evaluate success or reinforcement needs.
- Provide the patient with a phone number to call for assistance, if necessary.
- Include the family/significant others, as appropriate.

From McCloskey, J., & Bulechek, G. (1996). *Nursing interventions classification (NIC)* (2nd ed.). St. Louis: Mosby–Year Book. Reprinted with permission.

It also involves effective health teaching of children and their families (Chart 6–16).

The nurse's role in managing common pediatric illnesses involves planning and delivering treatments and medications, evaluating the effectiveness of therapies, teaching patients and their families, assessing the urgency of a situation (see Chapter 30 for information about telephone triage), and giving feedback to physicians and other health care professionals. Specific disease management is covered throughout this text (Table 6–11).

When instructing family on home management, the nurse must be cognizant of certain factors that will impact teaching effectiveness. The following factors should be considered:

- The family's financial resources (e.g., pre-packed oatmeal bath for a rash is fairly expensive. For families with limited resources, corn starch may be suggested as an alternative)
- Literacy level—ability to read, write, and follow written instructions
- Home environment—safety factors, sanitation, physical surroundings
- Lifestyles—work commitments of parents and schooling considerations
- Previous skill levels and available equipment (e.g., Do they have a thermometer? Do they know how to use it?)
- Social network to assist with other children or provide needed relief for parents
- Willingness to perform the required treatment (i.e., emotional readiness and stability)
- Access to home health care resources such as a visiting nurse or respiratory therapist

The nurse should take time to practice procedures or administration of medications with the parent or child and plan for return demonstrations to assess competency

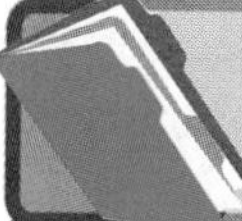

Chart 6–16
Nursing Interventions Classification (NIC)

Learning Facilitation

Definition

Promoting the ability to process and comprehend information

Activities

- Begin the instruction only after the patient demonstrates readiness to learn.
- Set mutual, realistic learning goals with the patient.
- Identify learning objectives clearly and in measureable/observable terms.
- Adjust the instruction to the patient's level of knowledge and understanding.
- Tailor the content to the patient's cognitive, psychomotor, and/or affective abilities/disabilities.
- Provide information appropriate to developmental level.
- Provide an environment conducive to learning.
- Arrange the information in a logical sequence.
- Arrange the information from simple to complex, known to unknown, or concrete to abstract, as appropriate.
- Differentiate "critical" content from "desirable" content.
- Adapt the information to comply with the patient's life-style/routines.
- Relate the information to the patient's personal desires/needs.
- Provide information that is consistent with the patient's values/beliefs.
- Provide information that is compatible with the patient's locus of control.
- Ensure that the material is current and up-to-date.
- Provide educational materials to illustrate important and/or complex information.
- Use multiple teaching modalities, as appropriate.
- Use familiar language.
- Define unfamiliar terminology.
- Relate new content to previous knowledge, as appropriate.
- Present the information in a stimulating manner.
- Introduce the patient to persons who have undergone similar experiences.
- Encourage the patient's active participation.
- Use self-paced instruction, when possible.
- Avoid setting time limits.
- Provide adequate time for mastery of content, as appropriate.
- Keep teaching sessions short, as appropriate.
- Simplify instructions, as appropriate.
- Repeat important information.
- Provide verbal prompts/reminders, as appropriate.
- Provide memory aids, as appropriate.
- Avoid demands for abstract thinking, if patient can think only in concrete terms.
- Ensure that consistent information is being provided by various members of the health care team.
- Use demonstration and return demonstration, as appropriate.
- Provide opportunities for practice, as appropriate.
- Provide frequent feedback about learning progress.
- Correct information misinterpretations, as appropriate.
- Reinforce behavior, as appropriate.
- Provide time for the patient to ask questions and discuss concerns.
- Answer questions in a clear, concise manner.

From McCloskey, J., & Bulechek, G. (1996). *Nursing interventions classification (NIC)* (2nd ed.). St. Louis: Mosby–Year Book. Reprinted with permission.

Table 6–11
Common Childhood Symptoms of Illness

Symptom	Information Covered in Chapter
Runny nose/cough/sore throat/wheezing	16, Health Challenge: Alterations in Respiratory Status
Earache	28, Health Challenge: Alterations in Vision, Hearing, and Communication
Rash/itching	25, Health Challenge: Alterations in Skin Integrity 24, Health Challenge: Pediatric Infections
Abdominal pain/nausea/vomiting/diarrhea	18, Health Challenge: Alterations in Gastrointestinal Status 24, Health Challenge: Pediatric Infections 17, Health Challenge: Alterations in Fluid and Electrolyte Status
Headache/seizure	21, Health Challenge: Alterations in Neurologic Status
Limp/fractures	20, Health Challenge: Alterations in Musculoskeletal Status
Fever	30, Health Challenge: Pediatric Emergencies
Anemia	23, Health Challenge: Alterations in Hematologic Status
Dysuria/frequency	19, Health Challenge: Alterations in Genitourinary Status

level (TIP 6–2). The parent or child, depending on his or her age, needs specific information about signs and symptoms that indicate a worsening or an improvement in the child's condition. Finally, access to a telephone and an emergency plan of action if the child's condition suddenly worsens are important considerations for planning home management care.

The nurse plays a key role in promoting health maintenance behaviors in children and their families. Careful listening and observation during the history and physical examination and effective teaching techniques optimizes the nurse's effectiveness in fulfilling this role.

TIP 6–2 A Teaching Intervention Plan for Administration of Oral Medications at Home

Nursing Diagnosis and Outcome

- Knowledge deficit: correct techniques for medication management

Outcome: The child and family will appropriately store, administer, and monitor for side effects of medications.

Interventions

Teach the child and family the following about medications:

Storage

- Store all medications out of children's reach, in a locked cupboard, if possible.
- Never remove medication labels.
- When medication is no longer needed, flush it down the toilet.
- Check all medications once a year and discard all leftover, outdated, or unlabeled medications.

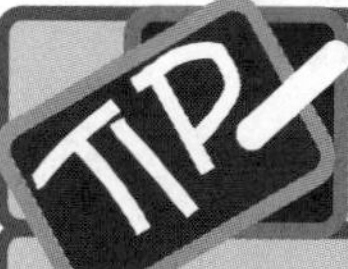

TIP 6–2 A Teaching Intervention Plan for Administration of Oral Medications at Home *Continued*

Administration

- Follow label instructions or administer as indicated by your health care practitioner or pharmacist.
- Refrigerate medication if label indicates; do not freeze.
- Give most medications on an empty stomach for better absorption; for exceptions (e.g., erythromycin) read and follow label instructions.
- Use oral syringes or medication measuring spoons to measure doses; household teaspoons are not accurate for medication measurement.
- Do not tell a child that medication is "candy."
- If needed, mix in small amounts of nonessential foods (e.g., applesauce, jelly), not in favorite or staple foods (see Chapter 9 for more oral medication administration techniques).
- If child immediately vomits the entire dose, readminister recommended dose.
- If child vomits more than 1 hour after a dose was administered, wait and give the next scheduled dose.
- Give the entire course of antibiotics, even if the child's condition improves, unless otherwise instructed.
- Never give medications prescribed for someone else, even if the illnesses seem similar.

Cancel Health Care Provider if

- The child vomits more than one dose of the medication.
- The symptoms of illness that the medication is to treat do not improve.
- The child's condition appears worse or changes occur, such as a rash or trouble breathing.

Summary of Key Concepts

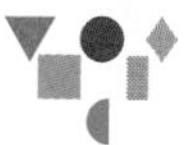

- In children, primary, secondary, and tertiary prevention focuses on preventing illness and injury.
- Routine immunization of children has significantly reduced morbidity and mortality associated with previously common childhood illnesses.
- High fever and severe illness are reasons to delay immunization until the child has recovered. Minor illnesses are not contraindications for immunization.
- To obtain an accurate and complete health history and physical assessment, the nurse must incorporate developmentally appropriate techniques and evaluate findings based on the child's age and developmental norms.
- Age-focused health surveillance improves wellness by screening for physical issues (problems or changes) commonly found at that age and promoting discussion of developmentally appropriate psychosocial issues.
- Anticipatory guidance regarding home management of symptoms associated with common childhood illnesses can help the family manage these symptoms more effectively.

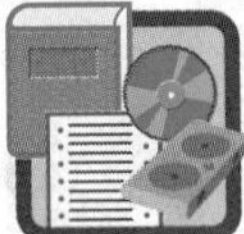

Resources

Organizations

National Association of Pediatric Nurse Associates and Practitioners
1101 Kings Highway North, Suite 206
Cherry Hill, NJ 08034-1912
(609) 667-1773

Printed Materials

American Academy of Pediatrics. (1997). *Guidelines for Health Supervision III*. Elk Grove Village, IL: AAP.

Tappero, E. P., & Honeyfield, M. E. (1996). *Physical assessment of the newborn* (2nd ed.). Petaluma, CA: NICU Inc. (888) 642-8465.

Audiovisuals

Charsha, D. (1996). *Neonatal physical assessment*. St. Louis: C. V. Mosby. (3 videotapes: Gestational Age and Size Evaluation; Respiratory and Cardiovascular Assessment; Neurologic, Gastrointestinal, Genitourinary, Musculoskeletal and Skin Assessment).

Lehrer, S. (1992). *Understanding pediatric heart sounds*. Philadelphia: W. B. Saunders (book and cassette tape).

National Association of Pediatric Nurse Associates and Practitioners. (1996). *Pediatric assessment*. Baltimore, MD: Williams & Wilkins (3 videotapes: Infants and Toddlers; Preschool and School-Age Children; and the Adolescent).

Hotlines

Vaccine Adverse Event Reporting System
(800) 822-7967

Computer Resources

American Nurses Association and Association of Teachers of Preventive Medicine. Immunization: You Call the Shots.
Healthsoft, Inc.
P. O. Box 3069
Orlando, FL 32802
(800) 235-0882
(Interactive software on two disks including a tutorial on immunizations and decision-making simulation)

Pediatric Points of Interest, established by the Department of Pediatrics at Johns Hopkins University, Baltimore, MD, and Marshall University School of Medicine, Huntington, WV (Provides links to children's hospitals, health organizations, parenting resources and links for children)
http://www.med.jhu.edu/peds.neonatology/poi.html

Digital Anatomist (interactive anatomy atlas)
http://www1.biostr.washington.edu/DigitalAnatomist.html

Healthnet Connection by Blue Cross & Blue Shield United of Wisconsin (Provides links specific to children and families, as well as adults)
http://www.healthnetconnect.net/linx.html

The Nemours Foundation from the duPont Hospital for Children (Provides health topics for children)
http://www.kidshealth.org

References

American Academy of Pediatrics. (1994). *1994 Red Book: Report of the Committee on Infectious Diseases* (23rd ed.). Elk Grove Village, IL: Author.

Arbiter, A., Ross, R., Levenson, R., Eikner, D., Dillon, C., Thompson, T., & Divack, M. (1993, April). *A study to increase immunization coverage of inner city children in Philadelphia.* Presented at a symposium conducted by the National Immunization Conference, Washington, DC.

Behrman, R. E., & Kliegman, R. M. (Eds.) (1994). *Nelson essentials of pediatrics* (2nd ed.). Philadelphia: W. B. Saunders.

Behrman, R. E., Kliegman, R. M., Arvin, A. M., & Nelson, W. E. (Eds.) (1996). *Nelson textbook of pediatrics* (15th ed.). Philadelphia: W. B. Saunders.

Burgraff, V. B. (1995). The vaccine report: Parents speak out on immunization. *Immunization Action News*, 2(4), 4.

Burns, C. E., Barber, N., Brady, M. A., & Dunn, A. M. (Eds.) (1996). *Pediatric primary care: A handbook for nurse practitioners*. Philadelphia: W. B. Saunders.

Centers for Disease Control and Prevention (CDC). (1994). General recommendations on immunization. *Morbidity and Mortality Weekly Reports*, 43(1), 1–21.

Centers for Disease Control and Prevention (CDC). (1995). Recommended childhood immunization schedule. US, 1995. *Morbidity and Mortality Weekly Reports*, 44(RR-5), 1–9.

Centers for Disease Control and Prevention (CDC). (1996a). Recommendations of the Advisory Committee on Immunization Practices (ACIP). Prevention and control of influenza. *Morbidity and Mortality Weekly Reports*, 45(RR-5), 1–24.

Centers for Disease Control and Prevention (CDC). (1996b). Recommendations of the Advisory Committee on Immunization Practices (ACIP). Prevention and control of varicella. *Morbidity and Mortality Weekly Reports*, 45(RR-11), 1–36.

Centers for Disease Control and Prevention (CDC). (1996c). Recommendations of the Advisory Committee on Immunization Practices (ACIP). The role of BCG vaccine in the prevention and control of tuberculosis in the United States. *Morbidity and Mortality Weekly Reports*, 45(RR-4), 1–18.

Centers for Disease Control and Prevention (CDC). (1996d). Recommendations of the Advisory Committee on Immunization Practices (ACIP). Update: Vaccine side effects, adverse reactions, contraindications, and precaution. *Morbidity and Mortality Weekly Reports*, 45(RR-12), 1–35.

Engel, J. (1993). *Pocket guide: Pediatric assessment* (2nd ed.). St. Louis: Mosby–Year Book.

Green, M. (Ed.). 1994. *Bright futures: Guidelines for health supervision of infants, children and adolescents*. Arlington, VA: National Center for Education in Maternal and Child Health.

Haddock, B. J., Merrow, D. I., & Swanson, M. S. (1996). The falling grace of axillary temperatures. *Pediatric Nursing*. *22*(2), 121–125.

Hahn, M. S. (1996). Talking to teens: What clinicians need to know. *Advance for Nurse Practitioners*, *4*(2), 49–51.

Hay, W. W., Groothuis, J. R., Hayward, A. R., & Levin, M. J. (1995). *Current Pediatric Diagnosis and Treatment* (12th ed.). East Norwalk, CT: Appleton & Lange.

Immunization Action News. (1996). FDA Approves DTaP Vaccine for Use in Infants. Department of Health and Human Services: Centers for Disease Control and Prevention. Vol. 3, No. 5 August 1996, pp. 1–4.

James, J., Burks, W., Roberson, P. K., & Sampson, H. A. (1995). Safe administration of the measles vaccine to children allergic to eggs. *New England Journal of Medicine*, *332*, 1262–1266.

Jarvis, C. (1996). *Physical examination and health assessment* (2nd ed.). Philadelphia: W. B. Saunders.

Keane, V., Stanton, B., Horton, L., Aronson, R., Galbraith, J., & Hughart, N. (1993). Perceptions of vaccine efficacy, illness, and health among inner city parents. *Journal of Clinical Pediatrics*, *1*, 2–7.

Mokotoff, E. D., Dunn, R. A., Johnson, D., Wilcox, K., Burgher, L, & Lett, S. (1994). Pertussis transmission from adult to infant—Michigan, 1993. *Journal of the American Medical Association*, *273*, 768–769.

Peter, G. & Klein, J. O. (1996). Pneumococcal vaccine. *Pediatrics in Review*, *17*, 335–341.

Staheli, L. T. (1992). *Fundamentals of Pediatric Orthopedics*. New York: Raven Press.

Strebel, P. M., Aubertlon-Cambiescu, A., Nedelcu, N. I., Biberi-Moroeanu, S., Suttyer, R. W., Kew, O. M., Pallansch, M. A., Patriarca, P. A., & Cochi, S. L. (1994). Paralytic poliomyelitis in Romania, 1984–1992. *American Journal of Epidemiology*, *140*, 1111–1124.

U.S. Department of Health and Human Services. (1990). *Healthy people 2000: National health promotion and disease prevention objectives for the year 2000*. (PHS) 91-50212. Washington, DC: U.S. Government Printing Office.

Zell, E. R. (1994). An analysis of doctor certified medical records of children entering school in 19 urban and one rural area in Arkansas. *Journal of the American Medical Association*. *16*, 331–403.

Zitelli, B. J., & Davis, H. W.(Eds.) (1992). *Atlas of pediatric physical diagnosis* (2nd ed.). New York, NY: Gower Medical Publishing.

Bibliography

American Academy of Pediatrics, Committee on Practice and Ambulatory Medicine. (1996). The use of chaperones during the physical examination of the pediatric patient. *Pediatrics*, *98*, 1202.

American Academy of Pediatrics, Committee on School Health. (1993). *School health: Policy and practice* (5th ed.). Elk Grove Village, IL, American Academy of Pediatrics.

Axton, S. E., & Hall, B. (1994). An innovative method of administering IV medications to children. *Pediatric Nursing*, *20*, 341–344.

Bass, J. L., Christoffel, K. K., Widome, M., Boyle, W., Scheidt, P., Stanwick, R., & Roberts, K. (1993). Childhood injury prevention counseling in primary care settings: A critical review of the literature. *Pediatrics*, *92*, 544–550.

Beckstrand, R. L., Moran, S., Wilshaw, R., & Schaalje, G. B. (1996). Supralingual temperatures compared to tympanic and rectal temperatures. *Pediatric Nursing*, *22*, 436–438.

Berkowitz, C. D. (1996). *Pediatrics: A primary care approach*. Philadelphia: W. B. Saunders.

Boekeloo, B. O., Schamus, L. A., Cheng, T. L., & Simmens, S. J. (1996). Young adolescents' comfort with discussion about sexual problems with their physician. *Archives of Pediatric and Adolescent Medicine*, *150*, 1146–1152.

Brynes, K. (1996). Conducting the pediatric health history: A guide. *Pediatric Nursing*, *22*, 135–137.

Curry, D. M., & Duby, J. C. (1994). Developmental surveillance by pediatric nurses. *Pediatric Nursing*, *20*, 40–44.

Elster, A. R., & Kuznets, N. J. (1994). *American Medical Association Guidelines for Adolescent Preventive Services (GAPS): Recommendations and rationale*. Baltimore, MD: Williams & Wilkins.

Engel, J. K. (1996). *Pocket guide to pediatric assessment* (3rd ed.). St. Louis: C. V. Mosby.

Evans, G. (1996). National childhood vaccine injury act: Revision of the vaccine injury table. *Pediatrics*, *98*, 1179–1181.

Ford, C. A., Millstein, S. G., Eyre, S. L., & Irwin, C. E. (1996). Anticipatory guidance regarding sex: Views of virginal female adolecents. *Journal of Adolescent Health*, *19*, 179–183.

Green, M. (1992). 20 interview questions that work. *Contemporary Pediatrics*, 9(11), 47–71.

Jarvis, C. (1996). *Physical examination and health assessment* (2nd ed.). Philadelphia: W. B. Saunders.

Kelly, L., Morin, K., & Young, D. (1996). Improving caretakers' knowledge of fever management in preschool children: Is it possible? *Journal of Pediatric Health Care*, *10*, 167–173.

Laing, I. A., & McIntosh, N. (1994). *Paediatric history and examination*. Philadelphia: Balliere Tindall/W. B. Saunders.

Miller, N. P. (1993). Guidelines for primary care follow-up of premature infants. *Nurse Practitioner*, 8(10), 45–48.

Mitchell, M. A. S., & Jenista, J. A. (1997). Health care of the internationally adopted child. Part 1: Before and at arrival into the adoptive home. *Journal of Pediatric Health Care*, *11*, 51–60.

Mitchell, M. A. S., & Jenista, J. A. (1997). Health care of the internationally adopted child. Part 2: Chronic care and long-term medical issues. *Journal of Pediatric Health Care*, *11*, 117–126.

Neifert, M. (1996). Early assessment of the breastfeeding infant. *Contemporary Pediatrics, 13,* 142–166.

Royce, C. F. (1995). Breaking through to the adolescent patient. *American Journal of Nursing, 95*(12), 19–23.

Schmitt, B. D. (1992). *Instructions for pediatric patients.* Philadelphia: W. B. Saunders.

Schubiner, H., & Eggly, S. (1995). Strategies for health education for adolescent patients: A preliminary investigation. *Journal of Adolescent Health, 17*(1), 37–41.

Selekman, J. (1996). Revision in pediatric immunization schedules and policy updates. *Pediatric Nursing, 22,* 424–426.

Sharp, L., Pantell, R. H., Murphy, L. O., & Lewis, C. C. (1992). Psychosocial problems during child health supervision visits: Eliciting, then what? *Pediatrics, 89,* 619–623.

Tappero, E. P, & Honeyfield, M. E. (1996). *Physical assessment of the newborn: A comprehensive approach to the art of physical examination.* Petaluma, CA: NICU, Inc.

Thomas, K. A., Savage, M. V., & Brengelmann, G. L. (1997). Effect of facial cooling on tympanic temperature. *American Journal of Critical Care,* 6(1), 46–51.

Unti, S. M. (1994). The critical first year: History, physical examination, and general developmental assessment. *Pediatric Clinics of North America, 41,* 859–873.

U.S. Public Health Service. (1996). Put prevention into practice: Dental and oral health. *Journal of the American Academy of Nurse Practitioners, 8,* 293–297.

U.S. Public Health Service (1997). Put prevention into practice: Blood pressure. *Journal of the American Academy of Nurse Practitioners, 9,* 27–32.

Vessey, J. A. (1995). Developmental approaches to examining young children. *Pediatric Nursing, 21,* 53–56.

Vessey, J. A., & Stueve, D. L. (1996). A comparison of two techniques for weighing young children. Pediatric Nursing, *22,* 327–329, 341.

Wells, N. King, J., Hedstrom, C., & Youngkins, J. (1995). Does tympanic temperature measure up? *American Journal of Maternal Child Nursing, 20,* 95–100.

Zimmerman, R. K., Ahwesh, E. R., Mieczkowski, T. A., Block, B., Janosky, J. E., & Barker, D. W. (1996). Influence of family functioning and income on vaccination in inner-city health centers. *Archives of Pediatric and Adolescent Medicine, 150,* 1054–1061.

Health Promotion Through Community Care

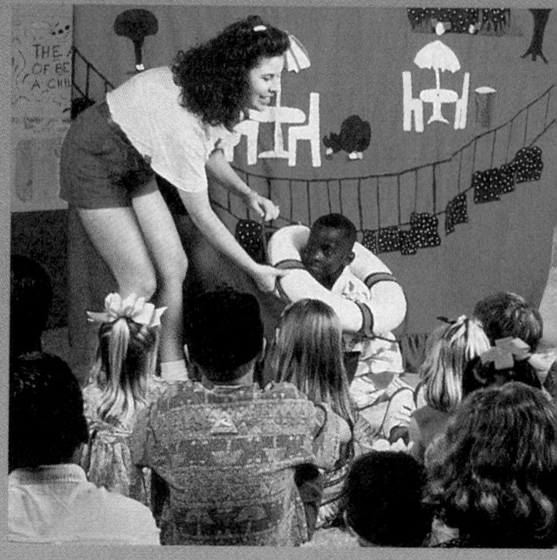

OUTLINE

Standards and Guidelines

Community Resources

Public Health Programs for Children and Their Families

- Medicaid
- Early and Periodic Screening, Diagnosis and Treatment Program (EPSDT)
- Special Supplemental Food Program for Women, Infants and Children (WIC)
- Supplemental Security Income for the Aged, Blind and Disabled (SSI)
- Maternal and Child Health Services Block Grant
- National Health Service Corps
- Community and Migrant Health Centers

Community Education Programs for Children with Special Health Care Needs

- Education for All Handicapped Children Act
- Education of the Handicapped Act, Amendment of 1986
- Individuals with Disabilities Education Act (IDEA)
- Head Start

Private Programs for Community Care Services

Scope of Child Health Care Services in the Community

- Parents'/Caregivers' Role
- Community's Role
- Employer's Role
- Nurse's Role

OBJECTIVES

- Describe public health programs designed to meet the needs of children and their families.
- Describe public education programs available for children with special health care needs.
- State the role of private organizations in meeting the health needs of children and their families.
- Select strategies to be used by parents/caregivers, the community, employers, and nurses to promote health maintenance in children.

KEY TERMS

Community and Migrant Health Centers (C/MHCs)

Early and Periodic Screening, Diagnosis and Treatment Program (EPSDT)

entitlement program

Head Start

Maternal and Child Health Services Block Grant

Medicaid

National Health Service Corps (NHSC)

Special Supplemental Food Program for Women, Infants and Children (WIC)

Supplemental Security Income for the Aged, Blind and Disabled (SSI)

CHAPTER

7

Nurses have a long history of working in communities and using or obtaining public health resources for children and adults. From Lillian Wald's 1893 district nursing service in New York to current public health programs and visiting nurse services, nurses have long been concerned with meeting families' health care needs in homes, in schools, and in communities (Swanson & Albrecht, 1993).

As medical economics and technology change, more children are being cared for in community settings. Many clients receive health care in managed care organizations, which discourage expensive inpatient treatment and promote outpatient, community-based care. Medical technologies have changed such that early discharge, home care, and outpatient options are safer and more available. As a result, nurses are providing more care in the community and will continue to do so in the future.

Nurses have an increasing number of roles to play in community settings, including primary care practitioner, care coordinator, client advocate, and health program planner (Fig. 7–1). Whether the nurse works in a hospital, an outpatient setting, or a clinic, most of the nurse's clients will return to their communities. Hence, no matter where children and their families come into initial contact with the health care team, community services and public health are almost always a component of care.

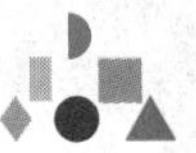

Standards and Guidelines

The American Nurses' Association (ANA) has defined Standards of Community Health Nursing Practice to characterize, measure, and provide guidance in achieving excellence in care (Council of Community Health Nurses, American Nurses' Association, 1986). These standards should be used to guide the practice of all nurses working in the community (Chart 7–1).

In 1991, the American Public Health Association (APHA) published the third edition of *Health Communities 2000: Model Standards* (Model Standards Work Group, American Public Health Association, 1991). This volume describes in detail guidelines for community attainment of the Year 2000 National Health Objectives. Of particular interest are the specific guidelines for infants, children, and adolescents (Chart 7–2). A community can use these to set health goals and devise ways to meet these goals.

Whereas the ANA standards define the process of providing care in community settings, the APHA model standards define the goals of public health in communities. To work successfully in this setting, the nurse must be aware of the needs and the strengths of communities and their members, including public health and community resources, to link children and families with available resources and advocate for the establishment of those resources that are unavailable.

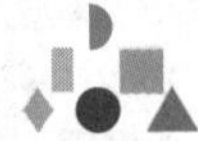

Community Resources

Nurses who care for children and families must be aware of the community resources available to their clients for several reasons. First, a working knowledge of these programs lets the nurse make appropriate referrals for services to meet specific client needs. Second, by knowing

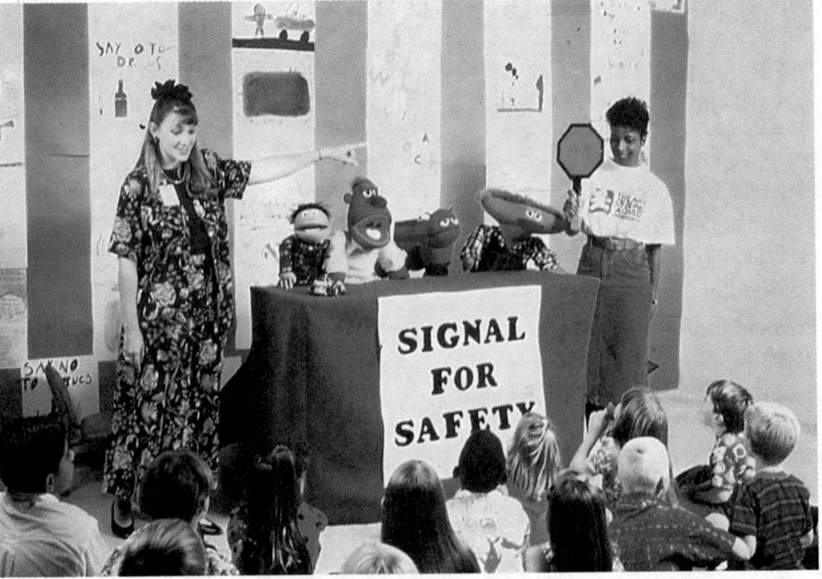

Figure 7–1
A health fair, one of many settings in which nurses provide community health care services.

Chart 7–1

Standards of Community Health Nursing Practice

Standard I. Theory
The nurse applies theoretical concepts as a basis for decisions in practice.

Standard II. Data Collection
The nurse systematically collects data that are comprehensive and accurate.

Standard III. Diagnosis
The nurse analyzes data collected about the community, family, and individual to determine diagnoses.

Standard IV. Planning
At each level of prevention, the nurse develops plans that specify nursing actions unique to client needs.

Standard V. Intervention
The nurse, guided by the plan, intervenes to promote, maintain, or restore health; to prevent illness; and to effect rehabilitation.

Standard VI. Evaluation
The nurse evaluates responses of the community, family, and individual to interventions in order to determine progress toward goal achievement and to revise the database diagnoses and plan.

Standard VII. Quality Assurance and Professional Development
The nurse participates in peer review and other means of evaluation to assure quality of nursing practice. The nurse assumes responsibility for professional development and contributes to the professional growth of others.

Standard VIII. Interdisciplinary Collaboration
The nurse collaborates with other health care providers, professionals, and community representatives in assessing, planning, implementing, and evaluating programs for community health.

Standard IX. Research
The nurse contributes to theory and practice in community health nursing through research.

From Council of Community Health Nurses, American Nurses' Association. (1986). *Standards of community health practice.* Washington, DC: Author. Reprinted with permission.

Chart 7–2

Healthy Communities 2000: Model Standards and Goals for Children

- All infants, children, and youth will participate in a comprehensive health program that emphasizes preventive care.
- Child abuse and neglect will be eliminated.
- The incidence of preventable injuries and deaths occurring among children will be reduced.
- All children, including those with chronic handicaps, will function at their optimal level.
- Indicators for the health of any financial, ethnic, socioeconomic, or geographic subgroup will not be significantly more adverse that those for the entire community.
- Children and adolescents will develop and mature in good health, secure in the prospects for a productive and happy future.

From Model Standards Work Group, American Public Health Association. (1991). *Healthy communities 2000: Model standards: Guidelines for community attainment of the year 2000 national health objectives.* Washington, DC: Author.

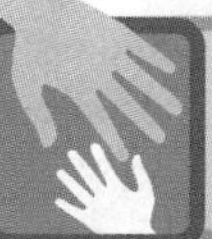

Chart 7–3
Nursing Intervention

Helping Families Stay Organized

Many families, especially those with children with special health care needs, interact with a number of different programs. The nurse can suggest ways in which families can keep track of paperwork—the various plans, copies of forms, applications, correspondence, and the like—that they may receive. One simple method is to ask the family to purchase, or provide for them, a three-ring binder and dividers so that all paperwork can be filed by agency/program name. Likewise, medical reports, special school papers, and other material can be filed in this notebook as well. Some families like to include a zippered pencil case that fits into the notebook to keep immunization records, parking tokens, clinic registration cards, and pens within easy reach. Simple strategies for reducing confusion and anxiety can help families deal more effectively with the multiple service systems with which they must interact.

how to access the programs and what services are offered, the nurse can educate families to apply for appropriate services efficiently. Applying for public services can be a difficult task, because not all service systems are client-friendly. If families know what to expect, what paperwork to bring to appointments, and which services are available, they may be more likely to access and use these services. Third, by being aware of the individual programs and the service systems offered, the nurse can help coordinate resources and provide referrals in a way that avoids gaps, duplication, and confusion. Finally, by knowing about these programs, the nurse can help redirect the family if they receive inaccurate or confusing information or cannot access services for other reasons (Chart 7–3).

When working within a particular community, the nurse should establish relationships with professionals from other agencies who may also serve the same clients. The school nurse, for instance, should develop relationships with professionals from the local health department clinics, the office of the Special Supplemental Food Program for Women, Infants and Children (WIC), the Head Start program, and others. In this way, the school nurse can serve clients more effectively through enhanced collaboration and coordination.

TIP 7–1 A Teaching Intervention Plan for the Family Accessing Needed Services

Nursing Diagnosis and Family Outcomes

- Family coping: potential for growth related to self-actualization of needs
  Outcomes:
  Family will successfully receive services to meet client and/or family needs.
  Family members will verbalize feelings of personal growth.

Guidance for Families

- Through careful assessment, assist the family in identifying strengths and needs.
- Identify resources in the community that may be available to meet client/family needs. If none appear to be available, call closely related programs and agencies to ask for referrals or information about needed services.
- Contact prospective agencies to determine services available, eligibility criteria, application procedures (including what the client should bring to apply), location, transportation routes, and any other information specific to the program.
- Present the information to the family, including your rationale for selecting the program. Identify benefits to be gained as a result of program participation. In addition to sharing the information verbally, write down key points and give this information to the family. If anything additional is known about the agency that will help promote follow-up, share this with the family as well (e.g., if waits are long and food is unavailable or expensive, advise parents to bring a lunch or snacks; if there is a long walk between the bus stop and the office, inform the parents so they may choose to bring a stroller, an umbrella in case of inclement weather, etc.).
- Ask the family to help identify impediments to follow-up or use of services so that these can be minimized whenever possible (e.g., "Is there anything you can think of that will keep you from applying for WIC services?").
- Some agencies/programs allow person-to-person referrals. If this is the case and families request or require this kind of assistance, seek parent consent and then contact a key individual at the referral agency. Briefly describe family needs and inform the individual of the referral. Define a follow-up date with both agency staff and families to keep everyone focused on obtaining services.
- Relay any additional information to family members and assist them as necessary if obstacles arise.
- Advise families to maintain a file of all correspondence, appointment notices, and so on and to request the name of the individual whenever contact with the agency is made.
- Some parents with poor reading skills or who are unable to speak, read, or write English may need additional assistance to obtain information, gather materials, or read or complete necessary paperwork.

The nurse should also obtain in-depth information about commonly used programs. If the nurse routinely refers clients to the WIC program, for instance, these clients will be better served if the nurse has a working knowledge of services provided, eligibility requirements, application procedures, waiting periods, any costs, and the local office's address and telephone number. Simply giving a family an agency name and telephone number is not enough to promote access to the services. Through appropriate referrals to community health programs, the nurse can help ensure the health of the child as well as the entire family (TIP 7–1).

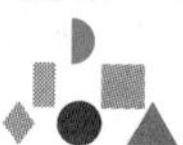

Public Health Programs for Children and Their Families

Many publicly funded health programs serve children and families. Some programs serve selected clients, such as those who meet certain income eligibility criteria; others are available to all who apply.

Medicaid

Medicaid is a form of health insurance for low-income and disabled individuals. Established in 1965 as Title XIX of the Social Security Act, Medicaid is a federal entitlement program (an open-ended program serving all eligible individuals entitled to the service without regard to a budgetary cap). It is financed by federal and state funds and administered by the states (Hill, 1992). The federal government pays from 50% to 80% of each state's medical assistance payments (Parette, 1993). Medicaid is not a direct provider of service, but rather provides compensation for health care services. Federal guidelines define the scope of basic services, the extent of coverage, and certain administrative requirements. The states administer the program and determine income eligibility criteria, specific services to be covered, and payment levels and methods. States may offer additional services beyond those required by federal statute (Saunders, 1994; Schwartz, 1990).

Table 7–1 describes services covered by Medicaid. Of particular relevance to community-based nurses is the ability to use Medicaid as a source of payment for home or extended care. Because long-term hospitalization can negatively affect a child's growth and development and the entire family's well-being, the option of home care for a seriously ill or disabled child is very important. Through home and community-based waivers, authorized under the Omnibus Reconciliation Act of 1981 (OBRA 81) and the Tax Equity and Fiscal Responsibility Act of 1982 (TEFRA), states can coordinate medical and support services to children living at home, thus avoiding costly institutional care (Hall, 1990). Eligibility criteria for these programs are broader than standard Medicaid eligibility. Thus, more children and families may be served. In addition, individual states may offer expanded medical services and respite care.

Chart 7–4 describes individuals eligible for Medicaid. Because Medicaid is a state-based program, clients must be residents of the state in which they apply for services.

Worldview: *To be eligible to receive Medicaid, an individual must be a citizen or lawfully admitted to the United States. Income-eligible children can qualify if they were born in this country, even if their parents are not citizens or reside in this country without appropriate legal documentation. There are provisions for undocumented clients to receive Medicaid for medical emergencies and prenatal care and delivery (Orloff, Rivera, & Rosenbaum, 1992).*

Families may apply for Medicaid at their local welfare office or at "outstationed" sites in federally qualified health centers and disproportionate-share hospitals (hospitals that receive extra federal funding to care for large numbers of clients receiving Medicaid.) Waits in welfare offices can be long, and the application process itself can be difficult. This may discourage some families from seeking out much-needed assistance.

The current trend in Medicaid is to encourage recipients to enroll in managed care programs to help contain

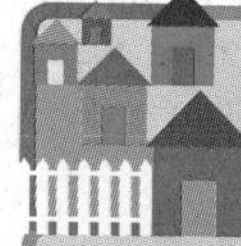

Chart 7–4
Community Care

Individuals Eligible for Medicaid

- Recipients of Aid to Families with Dependent Children (AFDC)
- All pregnant women, infants, and children younger than 6 years of age with family income up to 133% of the federal poverty level, whose resources do not exceed state-set limits
- All children born after September 30, 1993, with family incomes up to 100% of the federal poverty level
- All infants born to Medicaid-enrolled women without separate application, for up to 1 year
- Supplemental Security Income (SSI) recipients
- May cover "medically indigent" clients who fall below a certain income level
- Certain additional low-income pregnant women and children as determined by individual states
- Children in federally assisted foster care and adoption placements

Table 7-1
Services Covered by Medicaid

Mandatory	Optional*
Inpatient hospital services	Services in an intermediate care facility
Outpatient hospital services	Services in an intermediate care facility for the mentally retarded
Laboratory and x-ray services	Dental care
Physician services	Clinic services
Nurse midwife services	Private duty nursing
Rural health clinic services	Pediatric services
Ambulatory services provided by federally qualified health care centers	Optometrist services
Nursing facility services for individuals 21 or older	Chiropractic services
Early and periodic screening, diagnostic, and treatment services for individuals younger than age 21	Physical therapy
Home health care for adults entitled to nursing facility services	Speech, hearing, and language disorder services
Family planning services for individuals of childbearing age	Prescription drugs
Services of certified pediatric or family nurse practitioners practicing within the scope of state law, regardless of whether they are under the supervision of or associated with a physician	Dentures
A 60-day continuation of Medicaid services for pregnant women who were eligible for and received Medicaid coverage during their pregnancy for pregnancy-related and postpartum services (coverage extends until the last day of the month in which the 60-day period beginning from birth ends)	Prosthetic devices
	Eyeglasses
	Diagnostic, screening, preventive and rehabilitative services
	Hospice services
	Case management services
	Respiratory care services
	Inpatient hospital and nursing facility
	Services for individuals 65 or older in an institution for mental diseases
	Home and community-based care for functionally disabled elderly individuals
	Community-supported living arrangement services
	Any other appropriate medical care and other remedial care recognized under state law, specified by the Secretary of Health and Human Services

* Optional services determined by individual states.

program costs. As of 1995, 7.8 million recipients, or 23%, were enrolled in managed care plans. This number is expected to continue to rise in the future (Kaiser Commission on the Future of Medicaid, 1995). In a managed care system, a defined package of services is offered for a preset monthly fee (a premium) paid by Medicaid (Rivera, Regan, & Rosenbaum, 1995). Some states have obtained a federal waiver to require this of all Medicaid recipients; others encourage enrollment in managed care plans, most often health maintenance organizations (HMOs). (See Chapter 1 for more discussion of managed care.)

Each Medicaid recipient enrolled in a managed care program chooses a primary care provider who coordinates and oversees the delivery of health care services to that client. This approach should result in increased access to preventive and primary care and decreased fragmentation of care, especially for low-income individuals who previously had poor access to providers. This is also expected to decrease the use of inappropriate sources of health care, such as emergency departments used for primary care. However, because the managed care plan is receiving one preset monthly amount to provide all care to a client, the provider may be reluctant to make referrals to expensive specialists or use high-cost diagnostic tests.

At times, Medicaid has been the target of political criticism and threatened budget cuts, because it is designed to serve the poor—those least likely to have political clout. Despite this, during the 15 years after Medicaid's inception, physician visits by the poor have increased by 40%, and first-trimester prenatal care for blacks has increased by 18% (Saunders, 1994). Such statistics demonstrate that Medicaid has indeed improved access to health care for low-income individuals.

OBRA 89 and 90 expanded enrollment in Medicaid for pregnant women and children, made enrollment simpler, broadened and strengthened the benefits for children, and improved payments to providers (Orloff et al., 1992). By 1990, Medicaid paid for 30% to 50% of all births in the United States. By 1991, it had become the primary source of health insurance for 20.3% of all children (Orloff et al., 1992). In 1995, 35 million individuals were covered by this program (Kaiser Commission, 1995).

Although Medicaid provides tremendous benefits to eligible recipients, it has several shortcomings. Because of eligibility requirements, the program serves only a portion of those who need it. Eligible individuals may see their benefits cut with minor income increases. This is a particular problem for children with special health care needs, for whom ongoing care is vital. Additionally, the near poor or working poor who are uninsured may not qualify, but still have no health care insurance. There is a shortage of providers willing to accept Medicaid because of low reimbursement rates, especially in certain areas, which may result in lack of care and inappropriate use of emergency departments (Orloff et al., 1992).

Early and Periodic Screening, Diagnosis and Treatment Program

A very important component of Medicaid for children is the Early and Periodic Screening, Diagnosis and Treatment (EPSDT) Program. This separately mandated program serves Medicaid-eligible individuals younger than age 21. As with the basic Medicaid program, providers are reimbursed for services; EPSDT is not a direct service program.

The EPSDT program was enacted in a 1967 amendment to the Social Security Act as a mandatory service under Medicaid (Smith, 1994). It was established as a federally financed, state-administered program whose goal is to ensure that children enrolled in Medicaid receive a basic set of comprehensive services to promote health and identify and treat health problems at early stages.

The mission of EPSDT is to prevent unnecessary childhood illness, disability, and death by offering prevention services and identifying problems before they become serious. Under the EPSDT program, children are screened for health deficiencies and diagnosed and treated with services covered under Medicaid (Schwartz, 1990). The program combines screening for health problems with outreach, follow-up care, and case management (Rivera et al., 1995). States must assist children to receive these services by

- informing eligible clients about the program
- helping families make appointments
- arranging transportation
- providing services in a timely fashion
- ensuring an adequate supply of providers (Johnson & Moore, 1990)

EPSDT services may be provided by physicians, nurse practitioners, and physician assistants in clinics, schools, hospitals, health departments, and Head Start programs.

The EPSDT program has had three principal effects:

- It has eliminated the differences that previously existed between the amount of care received by poor and nonpoor children.
- It has dramatically improved access to preventive, primary, and specialty care for poor children.
- It has resulted in improved use of prenatal care, improved rates of childhood immunization, and overall improvement in child health outcomes (Rivera et al., 1995).

Although the EPSDT program has provided comprehensive primary care to scores of children, it has had some problems. For the first 22 years of the program, well-child examinations were scheduled too far apart, interperiodic examinations were not covered, gaps existed between specialty visits (e.g., dental), access to the program was limited if a single provider could not provide the full range of EPSDT services, and some federally reimbursable treatment services (particularly for mental health services) were not provided (Smith, 1994). OBRA 89 aimed to correct these deficiencies by increasing access to the program and expanding treatment services (Chart 7–5). OBRA-mandated changes to the EPSDT program included screening requirements, a periodicity schedule for examinations, and the mandate for services to be performed between specified intervals if they are medically necessary to identify and treat a suspected illness or condition, even if the service is an optional one that the state does not cover in its Medicaid program (Schwartz, 1990).

Chart 7–5

EPSDT Required Services

- Comprehensive health and developmental history (including physical and mental health and nutritional status)
- Comprehensive unclothed physical examination with appropriate follow-up care
- Vision and hearing service with appropriate follow-up care
- Immunizations
- Appropriate laboratory tests including lead level and x-ray services
- Comprehensive preventive, restorative, and emergency dental care
- Health education
- Anticipatory guidance
- Any medically necessary treatment for identified conditions

caREminder: *Although they are too often overlooked, adolescents are eligible to receive EPSDT benefits and should be encouraged to do so. Developmentally appropriate examinations and anticipatory guidance for the prevention of sexually transmitted diseases, pregnancy, and drug and alcohol use are components of the program. The examinations may be used as a camp or sports physical to allow teenagers the opportunity to participate in these activities.*

EPSDT also allows for pregnancy testing. A pregnant teen may be offered extensive medical and emotional support services including health, psychosocial, and nutritional assessments; counseling on hazards of tobacco, drug, and alcohol use; vitamins; childbirth education; and parent training (Fig. 7–2). Family planning services may also be included (Healthy Mothers, Healthy Babies Coalition, 1986).

As more Medicaid recipients are being forced or encouraged to enroll in managed care plans, concern is growing that these plans may not be providing the legally mandated services under EPSDT. A 1994 study found that states often failed to detail service obligations related to EPSDT standards in their managed care contracts. Therefore, it concluded that children may not be receiving the level of service to which they are entitled (Children's Defense Fund, 1995).

Nurses are an integral part of the EPSDT program. Many nurses perform outreach services to identify eligible clients and encourage participation. Nurses also may serve as program administrators, overseeing their operations, ensuring the quality of care offered by various providers, and training providers and their staff in program specifics. Some nurses serve clients directly by providing primary care as nurse practitioners or work in supportive and facilitative roles providing immunizations, teaching patients and families, and coordinating services through case management. To date, only about 35% of eligible children receive EPSDT services (Smith, 1994). Through their numerous contacts with families, nurses are in a position to work toward increasing this number.

Special Supplemental Food Program for Women, Infants and Children

The Special Supplemental Food Program for Women, Infants and Children (WIC) provides nutritious food, health education, and links to health care resources to pregnant and lactating women, infants younger than age 1 year, and children up to age 5 years who are at risk for nutritional problems. The WIC program was enacted in 1972 as an amendment to the Child Nutrition Act of 1966. It was designed to make supplemental foods available to pregnant or lactating women and to infants who are determined by a health professional to be at nutritional risk because of inadequate nutrition or income (Hynes & Schwartz, 1991). Since its inception, the WIC program has expanded to serve more clients and provide other activities such as outreach. The program is funded by the Food and Nutrition Service of the United States Department of Agriculture and is administered via grants to states and then to local health and human services organizations. Some states offer additional financial support. Approximately 7900 WIC clinics exist nationwide (Food Research and Action Center, 1991).

Eligibility for the program is based on financial need and a demonstrated risk for the development or presence of a nutrition-related health problem, such as iron defi-

Figure 7–2
EPSDT benefits include education and counseling to teen mothers and fathers.

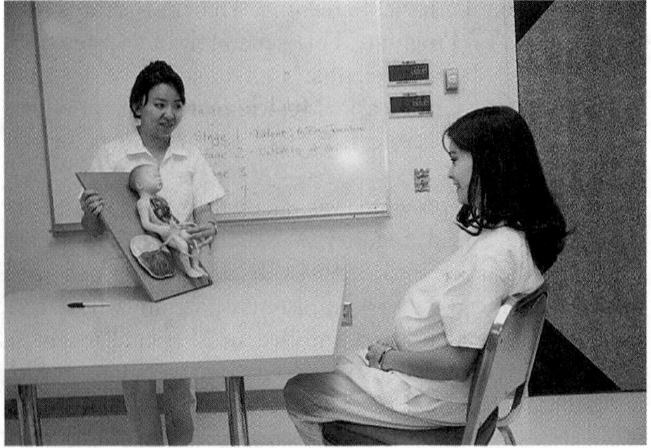

ciency anemia. The program is not an entitlement; thus, it operates within a fixed budget determined each year by Congress. As a result, not all eligible clients can be served. Pregnant and lactating women and infants up to age 1 receive priority, followed by children up to age 5. In 1991, 4.7 million women and children, or approximately 55% of the eligible population, received WIC benefits (Hynes & Schwartz, 1991). Almost all pregnant women with a family income at or below 185% of the federal poverty level qualify for WIC (Avruch & Cackley, 1995).

WIC provides coupons that clients use to purchase specific foods meant to provide certain key nutrients, such as protein, iron, calcium, and vitamins A, C, and D. Typically, such foods include formula, cheese, eggs, iron-fortified baby and regular cereals, fruit juice, beans, and peanut butter. The coupons can be used at most grocery stores, although some agencies distribute food directly (Fig. 7–3).

caREminder: *Some mothers may feel self-conscious using coupons, feeling that others view them in a negative light. Frequent reminders and support by the nurse about the importance of good nutrition during pregnancy and infancy may help mothers refocus on the importance and necessity of this program.*

WIC includes an educational component. Each client meets with a nutritionist for an assessment and discussion of specific needs. In addition, classes are held periodically on nutrition-related topics as well as such topics as breast-feeding, car seat use, and immunizations.

WIC provides important links to health care providers, social services, and other public programs (such as Medicaid) to ensure that all clients receive appropriate care. Some WIC offices are free standing. Many are located in health department clinics so that clients can access many services in one location. The program also includes outreach and, in certain areas, transportation to WIC offices.

Figure 7–3
WIC provides coupons so eligible recipients can purchase healthy food items for their families.

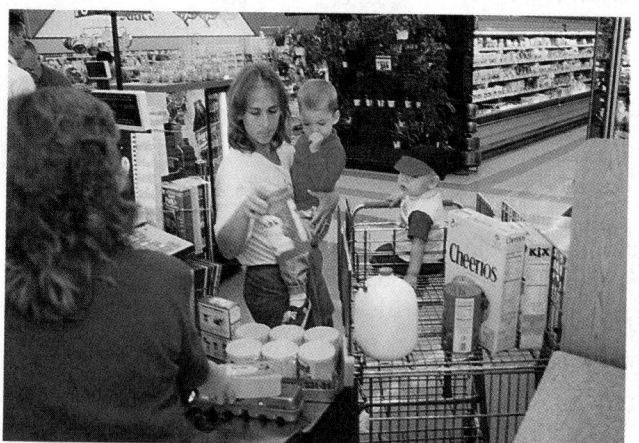

Evaluations of WIC have shown that women receiving prenatal benefits have lower rates of low-birth-weight infants. In addition, studies have shown lower hospitalization costs for mothers receiving Medicaid and for their infants when WIC services have been received (Avruch & Cackley, 1995). Nurses can positively affect the health of mothers and children by informing clients about and referring them to this important program.

Supplemental Security Income for the Aged, Blind and Disabled

Supplemental Security Income for the Aged, Blind and Disabled (SSI) is a program that provides monthly payments to income-eligible individuals who are older than age 65, blind, or disabled. Payments vary based on income, living arrangements, and other factors (U.S. Department of Health and Human Services, Social Security Administration [SSA], 1992). The money can be used as income or to purchase services not otherwise available, including caregiving assistance. For parents of a disabled child, the money also can pay for incidental expenses related to health care, such as parking or child care, or can help compensate for the loss of income resulting from the need to care for the child.

The program was enacted as part of the Social Security Amendments of 1972. The federal government provides matched funds to the states, who determine income eligibility guidelines and payment levels (Schwartz & Hynes, 1991). In most states, clients receiving SSI also receive Medicaid and may receive food stamps (SSA, 1992).

In order to be eligible for SSI benefits, a child must be a citizen or a lawful permanent resident of the United States, even if the parents are neither. Also, a child must meet certain income eligibility criteria based on his or her family's income and resources. Finally, the child must be medically eligible for the program.

Children may be determined to be disabled by physical, mental, or developmental disorders. There is an appeals process for children found to be ineligible for SSI benefits. Parents may initiate this process if they feel an erroneous determination has been made. If an appeal is filed, the child may be required to see a medical provider with whom the family is unfamiliar, one chosen by the SSA to offer an additional opinion about the child's eligibility. This examination is provided at no cost to the family.

Nurses play an important role in ensuring that all potentially eligible clients are referred to the SSI program. Because supportive documentation is needed to establish eligibility, nurses may help families gather and submit appropriate records.

caREminder: *Families should be instructed to save all correspondence from the SSA as well as copies of any documentation sent to the agency, in the event that additional or duplicate information is needed.*

Maternal and Child Health Services Block Grant

The Maternal and Child Health Services Block Grant (Title V of the Social Security Act), originally enacted in 1935, provides federal funds to the states for preventive, primary, and specialty care for pregnant women, mothers, infants, children, and adolescents. In this federal–state partnership, the states contribute $3 for each $4 of federal money received.

The states must use the block grant funds to develop a maternal and child health (MCH) system that ensures comprehensive, coordinated services to improve the health of all mothers and children. They must direct these services to low-income clients and those with poor access to services (Aliza, 1993; Johnson, 1994; Saunders, 1994; United States Department of Health and Human Services, Public Health Service [U.S. DHHS/PHS], 1992). Chart 7–6 defines states' goals for the MCH block grant funds. They may carry out this mandate by providing services directly or by promoting access to services through program development, coordination, or oversight. Individual states may establish their own priorities and use the money to provide MCH services within the state according to local, regional, and statewide needs.

At the state level, MCH services are managed through the state health agency. Services are usually delivered by local health departments. Private physicians, hospital-based clinics, community health centers, and school-based clinics may also be involved in MCH service delivery through grants, contracts, or reimbursement to independent community agencies and providers. The organizational structure, staff responsibilities, and specific programs and services vary from state to state (Chart 7–7) (Hess, 1994). The states must coordinate and integrate services with other programs, including health (such as EPSDT), social services, child nutrition (such as WIC), and education at the state and local levels to avoid duplication and ensure effectiveness (National Governors' Association, 1995).

Before 1981, Title V included two programs: the MCH program and the Crippled Children's Services (CCS) program. In 1981, OBRA 81 combined these programs to create the currently titled Maternal and Child Health Services Block Grant. This consolidated the MCH

Chart 7–6

States' Goals for the Use of MCH Block Grant Funds

- To provide and ensure mothers and children access to quality maternal and child health services.
- To reduce infant mortality and the incidence of preventable disease and handicapping conditions in children.
- To provide rehabilitation services for blind and disabled individuals younger than age 16 years receiving benefits under Title XVI (Supplemental Security Income [SSI]) when services are not provided by Medicaid.
- To provide family-centered, community-based coordinated care to children with special health care needs and their families.

Chart 7–7

Examples of Maternal and Child Health Services

Preventive health care
- Newborn screening
- Immunizations
- Injury prevention

Primary health care

Specialized health care
- Services for children with special health care needs
- Purchase of specialized equipment (e.g., wheelchairs, adaptive equipment)

Regionalized systems of care

Family support services
- Case management
- Transportation
- Home visiting

Health education
- State and community needs assessments
- Guidelines/standards development and monitoring for preventive, primary, and specialty care
- Technical assistance and training for specific programs
- Infrastructure development
- Service integration
- Planning, coordinating, and ensuring the quality of MCH services

and CCS programs and added five other programs previously funded separately: the SSI Disabled Children's program and programs for genetic disease testing and counseling for hemophilia, lead prevention, sudden infant death syndrome (SIDS), and adolescent pregnancy prevention (Aliza, 1993; National Governors' Association, 1995). Grants were given to states, who in turn determined how funds would be used for these programs.

OBRA 89 further amended Title V to include new data and reporting requirements. It also required that a specific percentage of the funds be set aside to provide services for children with special health care needs (30%) and preventive and primary care for children and youth (30%). Further, it required each state to submit an application for the block grant. The application demands a statewide needs assessment for all mothers and children and children with special health care needs, a definition of health status measures and measurable objectives for programs, a description of the use of federal funds and state matching funds, and documentation verifying the ongoing activities of all existing programs (U.S. DHHS/PHS, 1992).

Currently, Title V includes three components: the MCH program, the Children with Special Health Care Needs (CSHCN) program (formerly the Crippled Children Services program), and two discretionary grant programs—Special Projects of Regional and National Significance (SPRANS) and Community Integrated Service Systems (CISS). Eighty-five percent of the federal allocation goes to state health agencies on the basis of a predetermined formula, and 15% is allocated to SPRANS and CISS projects. SPRANS programs provide grants through a competitive process to health departments, universities, and other community agencies for research, training, genetic disease education, testing, counseling, referral and follow-up, regionalized hemophilia care, and innovative demonstration projects (U.S. DHHS/PHS, 1992). CISS grants for home visiting programs, projects to integrate service delivery systems, and development of community-based services are also provided for in this legislation. There is no matching requirement for these grants.

There is often confusion between Title V and Medicaid. Title V provides money to states, which determine how it will be used to improve the health of *all* women and children. It requires the states to develop systems that ensure access to high-quality care. It is not an entitlement program; rather, it provides a set level of funding to each state as determined by Congress. As discussed earlier, Medicaid is a form of health insurance for low-income, disabled, and elderly persons. It focuses on primary and acute care. Medicaid only *reimburses* for services; in contrast, Title V programs may provide services directly—for instance, in a community prenatal clinic (Johnson, 1994; National Governors' Association, 1995). In fact, a client may visit a prenatal clinic established with Title V funds but pay for the clinic's services with Medicaid.

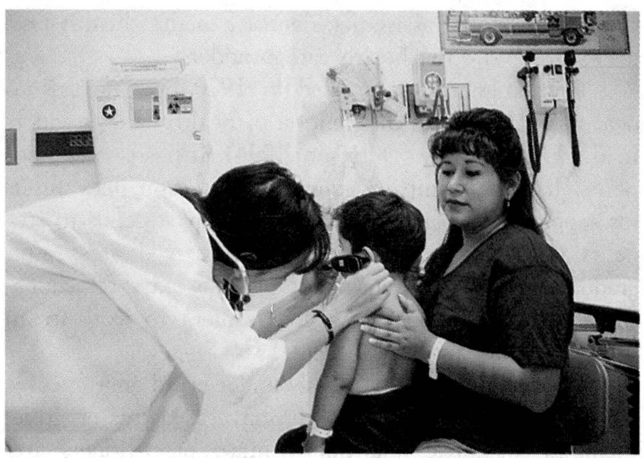

Figure 7–4
Utilizing Title V funds, nurse practitioners can provide child health care to eligible families.

Nurses play various important roles in MCH programs. For instance, in a maternity care program utilizing Title V funds, nurses may serve as nurse midwives or nurse practitioners delivering primary care (Fig. 7–4). They may also be involved in the delivery of clinic, patient education, case management, or care coordination services. Within a CSHCN program, nurses may be responsible for a range of services from case finding to determining client eligibility, developing plans of care, making referrals, coordinating services, and providing patient care. In a number of states, the director of the CSHCN program is a nurse.

Besides working directly with clients, nurses often administer programs. They may be responsible for program development as well as for planning, budgeting, and performing quality assurance activities. As for other public health programs, all nurses should understand which clients can receive which services, in order to refer clients appropriately, coordinate services among and between agencies, and educate families properly.

National Health Service Corps

The National Health Service Corps (NHSC) is a federally funded program designed to encourage primary care practitioners to practice in medically underserved areas, including inner city neighborhoods, rural communities, and Indian reservations. The program's mission is to deliver primary care health services to areas with severe shortages of health care providers and reduce the numbers of these areas by providing health care professionals and resources (Harmon, 1992). Primary care professionals include physicians, certified nurse midwives, nurse practitioners, physician assistants, dentists, mental health professionals, and other health care providers.

The program was created in 1970 by Congress to deal with an uneven distribution of health care providers in the United States (Johnson, 1994). It has two components. Its scholarship program awards tuition, fees, funds for supplies and equipment, and monthly stipends to students in return for services in underserved areas after graduation. Its loan repayment program pays off educational loans in return for a commitment to work in an underserved area (Harmon, 1992).

Many children in medically underserved areas receive primary care from providers who have used this program, including pediatric and family nurse practitioners and certified nurse midwives. NHSC not only benefits clients who previously had no access to primary care, but it also assists health care professionals who need financial aid for education and an opportunity to practice.

Community and Migrant Health Centers

Authorized by Title II of the Public Health Service Act, Community and Migrant Health Centers (C/MHCs) are federally funded comprehensive primary care clinics located most often in medically underserved areas. The program was established in 1965 and is administered by the Bureau of Primary Care, United States Public Health Service. Nationwide, approximately 600 clinics serve more than 5 million clients, three quarters of whom are women of childbearing age and children. Approximately 60% of C/MHC community health centers and almost all of its migrant health centers are located in rural areas (Johnson, 1994). Clinics are supported through federal grants, Medicare and Medicaid reimbursements, the National Health Service Corps, the Rural Health Clinic Program, WIC, and Title X Family Planning grants. In addition, they may receive Title V (MCH services block grant) funds directly or through SPRANS grants (Lecks, Mitchem, & Weiss, 1992).

C/MHCs must serve areas designated as medically underserved and provide basic primary care and supportive and facilitative services on a sliding scale basis. They are each governed by a board, of which the majority of members are users of the clinic services (Hill, 1992). They provide comprehensive medical care and support services through an interdisciplinary approach directly or by arrangement with community-based facilities. A major component of these clinics is maternal and child health services, which are designed to decrease infant mortality and improve the health of mothers and children, especially those from low-income families (Chart 7–8).

Nurses perform a variety of roles in these clinics. They may provide direct services, such as primary care, core public health functions, traditional clinic support, patient and family teaching, and case management. They may be involved in clinic administration. Because a center may offer a wide range of services, from prenatal to pediatric to adult care, the nurse has an opportunity to draw on expertise from a variety of areas. Also, because the center may provide preventive and primary care to all members of a particular family, the nurse may get to know the entire family and to have a positive effect on the family's overall health and well-being.

To refer clients and coordinate care properly, nurses who work outside C/MHC clinics should have knowledge of the system, the services it offers, and methods of accessing its services.

Chart 7–8

Services Provided by C/MHC

- Primary and preventive health services including pediatric care
- Comprehensive prenatal services
- Diagnostic laboratory tests
- Diagnostic x-ray examinations
- Preventive dental services
- Emergency care
- Pharmacy services
- Transportation
- Translation
- Environmental health services
- Outreach
- Case management
- Home health services*
- Rehabilitation services*

* Optional.

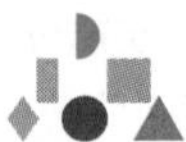

Community Education Programs for Children with Special Health Care Needs

Many nurses play a critical role in providing health services in schools and early intervention programs for children with special health care needs and their families. Nurses who do not work in these areas must understand the types of services offered and which children may be eligible to receive them (Chart 7–9). This section describes the most pertinent education and early intervention legislation aimed at children with special needs. It also discusses how the nurse may assist in the provision of services.

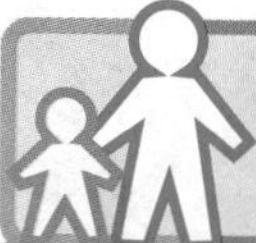

Chart 7–9
Developmental Considerations

Children with Special Needs

Children with special health care needs are those who have, or are at increased risk for, chronic physical, developmental, behavioral, or emotional conditions and who also require health and related services of a type or amount beyond that required by children generally (Division of Children with Special Health Care Needs, 1996).

Education for All Handicapped Children Act

Public Law 94-142, the Education for All Handicapped Children Act, was enacted in 1975 and became effective in 1977. This law represented an educational bill of rights for handicapped children. It required free, appropriate, and individualized education in the least restrictive environment for individuals 6 to 21 years of age (Fig. 7–5) (Aliza, 1993; Jenkins, Covington, & Plotnick, 1994). Services for children ages 3 to 5 (Part B) were optional, to be provided at each state's discretion, but were encouraged. Preschool services could be provided in conjunction with other government programs (e.g., Head Start), in private programs, or in regular public schools.

One component of the law requires an Individual Education Program (IEP) for all children receiving services. The plan is to be child centered and address the long-term developmental needs of the child. Parents should be encouraged to be actively involved in the IEP process, which includes assessments, plan development, referrals, and periodic reevaluation.

caREminder: *Parents must be notified of IEP meetings. They may bring additional support persons of their choosing, such as child advocates, lawyers, psychologists, and other relatives. Parents must sign a form indicating they have been informed about the program. They do not have to agree with the program and may request or appeal for changes.*

Individual states have guidelines indicating time frames in which the steps of the IEP must take place. In addition, an appeals process exists to allow parents an avenue for resolving conflicts with school or other professionals about the plan.

Nurses may be involved in the IEP process in a variety of ways. They may inform team members about the child's health care needs, they may help interpret complicated medical reports, they may be involved in making referrals or recommendations, and they may also provide support to families through appropriate advocacy (Fig. 7–6). Although these tasks are most likely carried out by the school nurse, they may also be performed by a child's home health care, hospital, or clinic-based nurse or one involved in providing transition for the child from another program.

Education of the Handicapped Act, Amendment of 1986

In 1986, the Education of the Handicapped Act, Amendment of 1986 (PL 99-457) was passed. This mandated early intervention services for 3- to 5-year-olds (previously an optional service to be provided at states' discretion) through the development of comprehensive, coordinated, and interdisciplinary statewide programs utilizing family-centered principles (Jenkins et al., 1994). In addition, it required each state to develop a plan to serve children from birth to 2 years old at risk for developmental disabilities (Part H). The law provided financial assistance to states to develop and implement the plan, facilitate coordination of payments for early intervention services, and provide for quality services (Hansen, Holaday, & Miles, 1990). The law included interagency and interdisciplinary collaboration, a child identification system, a family designated case manager, and a definition of developmental delay (Burns & Thornam, 1993). Agencies to be involved included those dealing with education, health, human services, developmental disabilities, mental health, public welfare, and children and youth through an interagency coordinating council. Each state would determine who was eligible to receive ser-

Figure 7–5
Federal legislation has ensured that children with disabilities have equal access to school programs and activities.

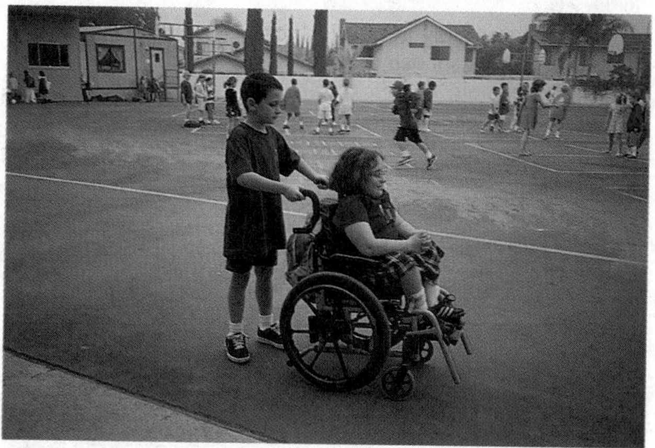

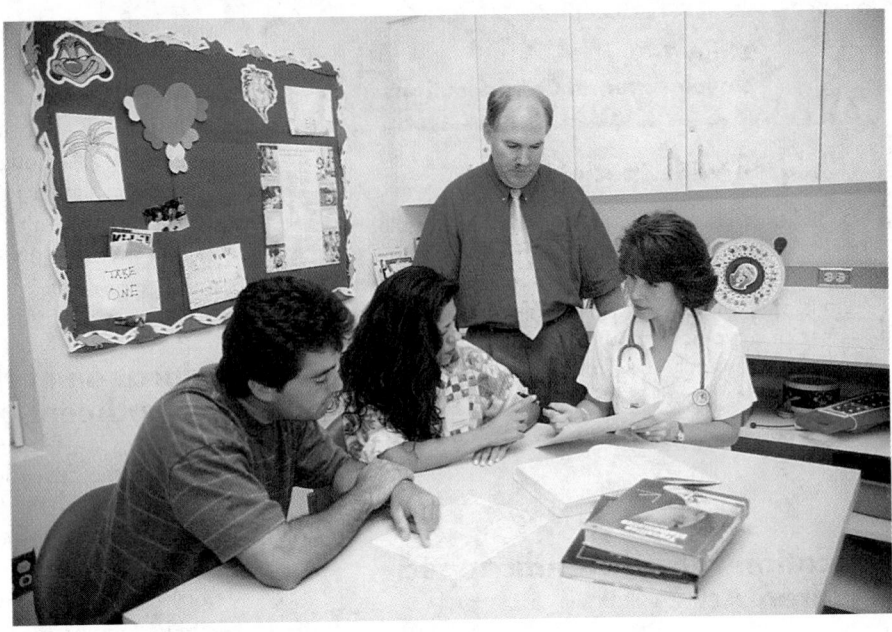

Figure 7–6
The nurse plays an active role in initiating and implementing Individual Education Programs (IEPs) in the school.

vices. Early intervention services were described as those that meet the developmental need of infants and toddlers in one or more of the following areas: physical, cognitive, communication, socio-emotional, and adaptive (Jenkins et al., 1994). Table 7–2 describes which children must be served, professionals who may be involved, and which services may be provided.

The law also requires that care be provided in a family-centered manner, with active participation of family members in developing the plan, choosing providers, and designating a service coordinator. (See Chapter 1 for a discussion of family-centered care.) It requires the development of an Individualized Family Service Plan (IFSP) for each child served. The plan follows assessments done by professionals from a variety of different disciplines to identify child and family strengths and needs. Specific components of the plan are described in Chart 7–10. The plan is similar to the IEP described earlier but is family focused rather than child focused.

Early intervention programs are the payers of last resort. Private health insurance, Medicaid, or special grant funded or charity programs may pay for direct services, or in the event that these are unavailable, the early intervention program provides funding. The role of

Table 7–2
Public Law 99-457 Education of the Handicapped Act, Amendment of 1986

Who Will Be Served	Who May Provide Services	Services That May Be Provided
Child with a delay in physical, cognitive, language and speech, psychosocial, and/or self-help skills Child with a known physical or mental condition resulting in developmental delay (e.g., Down syndrome) Child who is at risk for developmental delay (this may be a biological or environmental risk, e.g., perinatal substance abuse)	Nurses Physicians Special educators Speech-language professionals (pathologists and audiologists) Occupational and physical therapists Psychologists Social workers Nutritionists	Assessments Speech therapy Physical therapy Occupational therapy Infant stimulation Counseling Home visits Case management Psychological services Health services Special education Family training

Chart 7–10

Components of the Individualized Family Service Plan (IFSP)

Statement of family's concerns
Assessment of family strength and needs
Present level of development (physical, cognitive, communicative, socio-emotional, and adaptive)
Major outcomes for the child and family
Specific services to meet needs, including frequency, intensity, and method of delivery
Dates for initiating and completing the services
Any modifications of outcomes or services needed
Identification of a case manager
Transition plan (to other services providers)

the early intervention program is to coordinate services first and secondarily to provide a means to pay for services if no other funding exists.

Individuals with Disabilities Education Act

In 1993, Public Law 102-119, the Individuals with Disabilities Education Act (IDEA), reauthorized the Education of the Handicapped Act of 1986. Focus shifted from planning to implementing systems to serve children from birth to age 3 years.

Nurses help identify appropriate infants, toddlers, and their families and assist them in accessing the early intervention system through appropriate referrals, education about potential services, and follow-up. Prospective early intervention clients may be identified in neonatal or pediatric intensive care units, general pediatric units or newborn nurseries, outpatient clinics, physicians' offices, or anywhere else the nurse has contact with children and families. In a truly family-centered approach to delivering care, the nurse may even identify siblings or children of clients who may benefit from early intervention services.

Within the early intervention service system, nurses play a variety of important roles while working in schools, agencies for children with special health care needs, regional centers for the developmentally disabled, home health agencies, private case management companies, or outpatient clinics. Nurses may be involved in interdisciplinary assessments, serve as case managers, provide education and support to families as they work their way through the system, or provide direct service as defined in the IFSP. Whatever the role of the nurse in referrals to or work within the early intervention system, principles of family centeredness remain an important focus.

Head Start

Another program serving preschoolers with special health care needs is the Head Start program. Head Start, begun in 1965 by the United States Office of Economic Opportunity, is funded by the federal Department of Health and Human Services, Administration for Children, Youth and Families. It is a child development program aimed at preparing low-income preschoolers for entry into school by providing opportunities for learning, social development, and health care (Kassebaum, 1994; Schmidt & Wallace, 1994). The program is locally administered by community-based, nonprofit organizations and school systems (U.S. DHHS/PHS, 1986).

There are four major components to the Head Start program, including health (which includes medical, dental, mental health, and nutrition services), education, parent involvement, and social services (Mangu, 1991) (Fig. 7–7). The health component includes examinations, immunizations, health education for children, families, and staff and meals and snacks that meet at least one third of the daily nutritional needs of the children.

The education component is designed to meet a preschooler's individual learning needs, such as an introduction to the concepts of numbers. Additionally, it meets the ethnic and cultural needs of the communities it serves, for instance, providing bilingual teachers. Parents are encouraged to be actively involved in the program by helping in the classroom, serving on advisory committees, and attending parent education programs. The social ser-

Figure 7–7
Head Start programs provide health services, nutritional services, and education to help low-income preschoolers gain developmental advantages in preparation for entry into school.

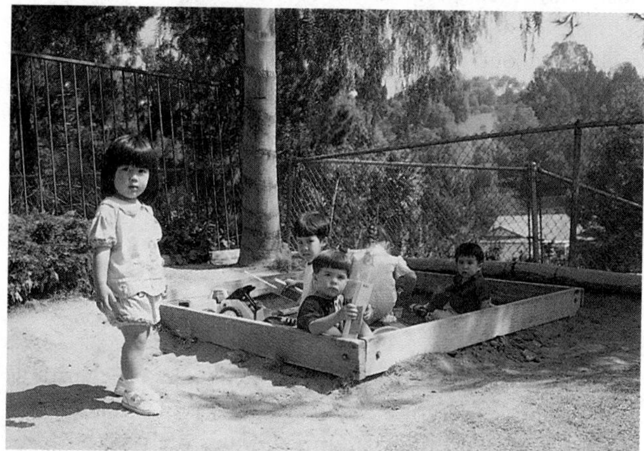

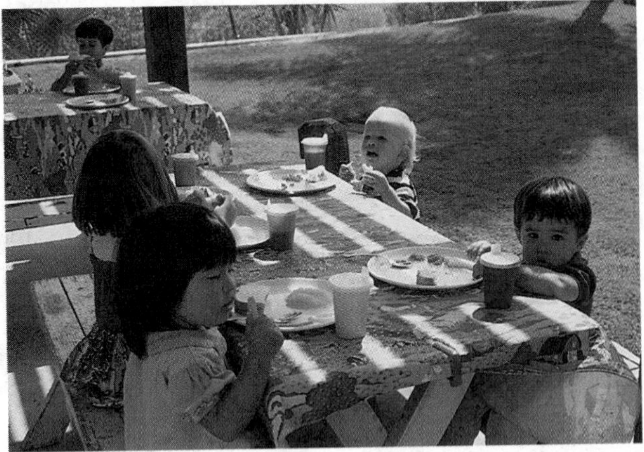

Figure 7–8
Nutritious meals are provided to these children in daycare courtesy of a state-sponsored health program for young children.

vices component offers families referrals to other programs and resources.

Head Start is mandated to provide services to children with special health care needs. Ten percent of its enrollment must be available to these children. Head Start programs may coordinate with other programs, such as public school special education, to meet the special needs of individual students. Because of funding constraints, only about one third of eligible children are able to receive Head Start services (Johnson, Sum, & Weill, 1992). Nurses are often involved in Head Start programs by serving on advisory boards and providing direct services to children.

Through all this legislation, children with special health care needs from birth to 21 years have access to appropriate developmental and educational services. Nurses play a vital role in helping to ensure these services.

In addition to the federal programs described here, there are numerous state and local programs serving children and families (Fig. 7–8). And many of the previously described programs have a different name at the state or local level. The nurse should make every effort to learn about these local resources and utilize them to meet client needs.

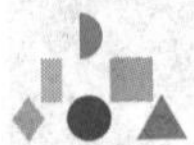

Private Programs for Community Care Services

Besides publicly funded programs, a number of charitable and nonprofit organizations exist to serve children with special needs and their families. Groups such as the Muscular Dystrophy Association, the American Cancer Society, Easter Seals, and others may provide direct assistance to families in the form of transportation, equipment, or special camps for children. They may also aid families by providing educational materials geared toward children and adults. Often services are offered free or at a minimal cost. Many of these organizations also provide written resource materials or courses and conferences for professionals and fund research activities (Thomas, 1994).

Nurses should identify resources such as these within their clients' communities and become familiar with the eligibility requirements and services offered. In addition, nurses can support the work of these groups by sitting on advisory committees, volunteering within the organization, or supporting fundraising efforts. See the resource section at the end of each chapter in this text for lists of directories containing information about these programs as well as other disease-specific groups providing concrete, educational, and supportive services to children and families.

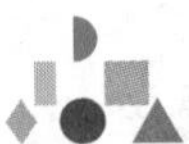

Scope of Child Health Care Services in the Community

A wide range of community-based services, from preventive, primary, and specialty care to respite and long-term care, is available to children and families in a variety of different settings. Children may receive health and related services in schools, clinics, daycare programs, Head Start programs, camps, homeless shelters, and other locations. Nurses are often key to service delivery in these settings. Table 7–3 describes the health care settings and services in which nurses can work to meet the needs of children and families.

As discussed earlier, many programs have a legal mandate to provide services to eligible clients and families, often within a specific time frame. An awareness by the nurse of legal requirements for service provision can help ensure that clients receive services to which they are entitled in a timely manner.

Because community-based service delivery often involves more than one agency, the nurse must be especially sensitive to issues of confidentiality. Conversations, forms, and medical records may not be shared with another agency without specific consent by the family. When consent is given, it is important to share only relevant information to protect client and family privacy. Agencies that routinely share and receive information often have release of information forms for this purpose.

Table 7–3
Community Health Care Services for Children and Their Families

Location	Services Provided by the Nurse or APN
Schools	
Health office School-based clinics	Preventive care Primary care Coordination of services (case management) Client/family advocacy Client/family teaching Consultation to teachers and administrators Program development
Homes	
Home health care Hospice Public health	Direct patient care Environmental assessments Care planning Coordination of services (case management) Client/family teaching Consultation with other health professionals Program development
Community Based Facilities	
Skilled nursing facilities Community nursing centers Extended care facilities Shelters Daycare/respite facilities Community clinics	Direct patient care Environmental assessments Care planning Coordination of services (case management) Client/family teaching Consultation with other health professionals Program development
Specialty Camps	
	Preventive care Primary care Direct patient care Client/family teaching Consultation with camp staff Program development Environmental assessment First aid/injury education Outdoor safety education

Parents'/Caregivers' Role

A variety of strategies exist to improve child health, from additional funding for key programs to serve greater numbers of children, to creating healthier and more supportive communities, to helping families learn to ask for needed services and advocate for themselves. The potential roles for nurses are limitless. In caring for children and families, nurses should look for any and all opportunities to achieve this goal of improved health for all children. Because parents and caregivers have primary responsibility for meeting the health needs of their children, most strategies to improve child health should be appropriately adapted to meet the cultural, language, and learning needs of this particular group. Although a few strategies are solely the responsibility of parents and caregivers, most rely on a service system that is easily accessible, community-based, family-centered, coordinated, and culturally relevant (Koop, 1987). It is up to nurses and other health professionals to ensure that service systems possess these characteristics.

Parents can, however, be encouraged to take responsibility for learning about resources for their family members and following up when referrals have been offered to them. Likewise, parents should be encouraged to ask questions and challenge information that appears to be incorrect or otherwise limits access to needed services. Nurses can be very helpful in this arena, teaching parents to effectively advocate for themselves (Chart 7–11).

Community's Role

Communities can help improve the health of children and families by ensuring the presence of appropriate resources and access to resources by those who need them. For families of children with special health care needs, communities should also ensure access to community activities and resources and nurture the children's participation in them (Hobbs et al., 1985).

In order to ensure the most comprehensive set of resources to its community members, communities should undertake periodic needs assessments to determine what service demands are not being met. Nurses are well positioned to take part in these needs assessments because they are often involved in multiple facets of community life and have contact with many diverse members of the community in schools, public health clinics, private offices, hospitals, home health agencies, and other local programs, where they become aware of their client's unmet needs.

Once a needs assessment is completed and strengths and deficiencies identified, communities can develop multiagency collaborations to meet the needs of community members. Nurses can be involved in this effort to ensure seamless transitions from one program to another as well as identify gaps and areas of duplication in the service

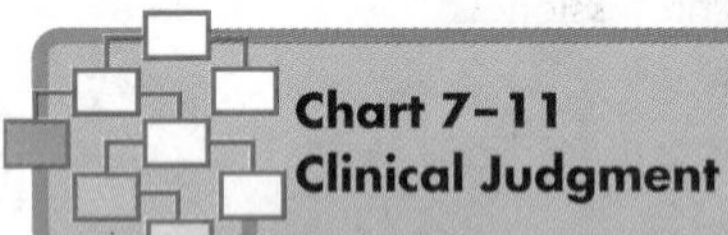

Chart 7–11
Clinical Judgment

The Child with Multiple Special Needs

Mrs. Thompson has recently moved to the area and is beginning prenatal care in a family practice clinic for low-income families. With her for today's visit is her 2-year-old daughter. Her daughter is not yet walking, appears small for her age, and has visible dental caries. At the end of Mrs. Thompson's prenatal visit, you ask to speak with her regarding her daughter.

Questions

1. What information do you want to illicit from Mrs. Thompson about her daughter?
2. When Mrs. Thompson answers your questions, which information may be particularly relevant to you?
3. What are the current possible problems for this child?
4. What interventions or referrals are appropriate for the child and family?
5. What factors would indicate that this child is receiving appropriate services to meet her needs?

Answers

1. What are Mrs. Thompson's perceptions about her daughter? Does she have any concerns about her health or development? Does she have a regular provider of health care? Has she received services from any agency or program in the past? What is her daughter's general health/developmental history?
2. A history of health problems or developmental delays, her mother's affirmation or denial of the existence of potential health or developmental problems, her history of past service utilization.
3. Dental caries, possible developmental delay, possible poor nutritional status.
4. Depending on need and current service utilization, referrals to a primary health care provider, the local early intervention program, the Special Supplemental Food Program for Women, Infants and Children (WIC), a pediatric dentist, and the local social services agency to apply for food stamps, Medicaid, and Aid to Families with Dependent Children (AFDC) as needed.
5. The child has an ongoing source of preventive and primary health care; she is enrolled in an early intervention program for assessment, monitoring, and intervention as needed; she receives WIC food coupons to meet her nutritional needs; she receives regular dental care and her mother has received information about preventing dental caries. She and her family are receiving AFDC, Medicaid, and food stamps if determined to be eligible. Additionally, her mother receives WIC coupons as well to promote good nutrition during pregnancy.

delivery system. Nurses may also participate in community planning meetings to develop strategies for providing services. This may also involve opportunities to seek funding for proposals, such as grant writing or making presentations to community groups. Chart 7–12 summarizes the nursing diagnoses pertinent to the nurse's work within a community.

Communities should develop strategies to enhance

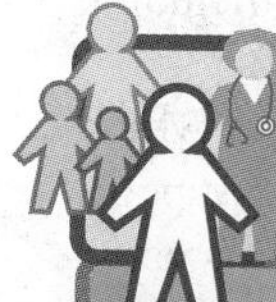

Chart 7–12
Nursing Diagnoses and Outcomes

Provision of Community Care

Ineffective community coping related to increased levels of gang violence, drug use, teen pregnancy, sexually transmitted diseases

Outcomes: Community members express awareness of the specific problems.
Community members state need for development and implementation of plan for addressing specific problems.
Community members evaluate program and revise as needed.

Potential for enhanced community coping related to child safety (drowning prevention, poison prevention), child health, cardiovascular fitness, nutrition, immunizations

Outcomes: Community members express understanding of problems associated with failure to implement prevention programs.
Community members develop plan to increase child health and safety awareness.
Community members evaluate established plans (e.g., have increased immunization rates), revise plans as needed.

Ineffective management of therapeutic regimen, community, related to gang violence, drug abuse, teen pregnancy

Outcomes: Community members express awareness of the specific problems.
Community members state need for development and implementation of plan for addressing specific problems.
Community members evaluate program and revise as needed.

Family coping: Potential for growth related to self-actualization of needs

Outcomes: Family members discuss impact of and feelings about child's illness.
Participate in development and management of plan that coordinates with lifestyle.
Provide care to maintain/promote child's health.
Use available community support systems.

Ineffective management of therapeutic regimen, family, related to socioeconomic deprivation, complex health care needs, lack of understanding of or unwillingness to manage health care needs

Outcomes: Family members express desire to effectively manage child's health care needs.
Family members state knowledge of community resources/support.
Family members demonstrate effective care behaviors.

Impaired home maintenance management related to inadequate support, lack of knowledge

Outcomes: Family members express need to modify home to more effectively manage child's health care needs.
Family members develop and discuss resources available to provide support to effectively manage care at home.

Altered parenting/risk for altered parenting related to lack of knowledge; ineffective role models, ill child

Outcomes: Parents demonstrate appropriate bonding behaviors (good eye contact, comfortable physical contact, talk lovingly to child).
Demonstrate correct care techniques.
State knowledge of age-appropriate growth and development and provide appropriate play opportunities.

access to services that already exist. This may involve such ideas as providing free or low-cost local transportation, providing low-cost child care at service delivery sites or local parks and schools, or co-locating services, with one or more programs at the same site. Improving access may also involve working with individual programs to increase "client friendliness" with extended hours, bilingual/bicultural workers, printed materials in easy-to-read formats, and a clear and simplified application process. Input from the community can be very powerful in promoting these changes.

Finally, communities should offer support to all its members, well and ill, able-bodied and disabled. Support often comes by providing tangible services such as self-help groups, counseling, food banks, and homeless shelters (Fig. 7–9). In addition, support is achieved by a spirit of inclusion of all members through regular dialogue, community forums, and an awareness of the needs of others.

Employer's Role

Employers can also use strategies to improve the health of their employees' children and the community in which they are located. To ease the burden on families of providing health care, employers can provide health insurance, family leave to care for ill family members, or other flexible benefit arrangements to meet individual family's needs. In addition, employers can establish information and referral services for their employees and the community at large to encourage the effective utilization of existing services.

Employers can provide a healthy work environment for their own employees and promote healthful living through on-site educational programs, for instance, smoking cessation, weight loss, or prenatal education programs. Employers may also offer an employee assistance program with counseling and other supportive services to help employees and their families in crisis, including health-related crises.

Employers can also serve the communities in which they are located by providing funding or in-kind support such as advertising and meeting space for locally based services. In addition, employers can contribute to the health of the community through responsible use of environmental resources.

Figure 7–9
Communities can sponsor health care activities to enrich and benefit all members of the society, such as this homeless shelter.

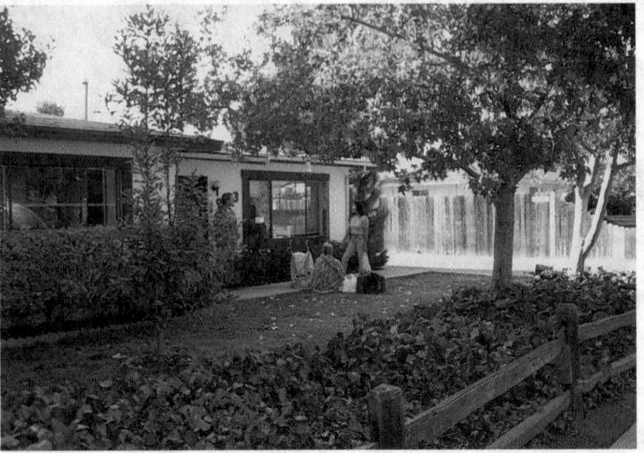

Nurse's Role

Nurses serve in a myriad of ways to improve child health. Although nurses work in a variety of different practice settings, most work directly with clients in hospitals, public health clinics, physicians' offices, home health agencies, and community programs. Promoting child health is an obvious function in all of these sites through teaching, direct service, client advocacy, and coordination of care.

Effectively teaching clients about resources, self-care, and other health promotion activities is a key role for nurses. Chart 7–13 describes health education interventions that can be used during these opportunities. Because an adult, a child, or both may be the intended audience, teaching strategies must effectively meet the needs of both learners.

An important role for nurses in relation to public health programs and third-party payers is that of client advocate. Not all service systems are client friendly, easy to access, or understandable to those outside the program. Eligibility criteria can be confusing, the application process complicated, or the services offered inadequate (Chart 7–14).

Advocacy can take a number of forms, from calling an agency on behalf of a client to working to change agency policy to better meet the needs of the families it serves. In addition, families can be taught to advocate for themselves by teaching them about programs and providing support while they speak out on behalf of their children. If parents need assistance beyond that which can be offered by the nurse, a referral can be made to a local protection and advocacy agency. (See Chapter 1 for additional discussion regarding a nurse's advocacy role.)

Another key role for nurses is that of care coordinator or case manager. In this capacity, the nurse attempts to improve access to needed care and reduce gaps or duplication in services through the development and implementation of an appropriate plan of care. An additional goal of care coordination may be cost containment.

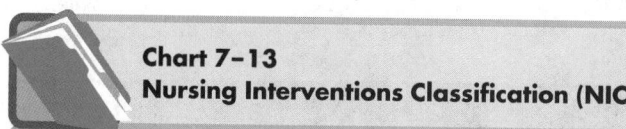

Chart 7–13
Nursing Interventions Classification (NIC)

Health Education

Definition

Developing and providing instruction and learning experiences to facilitate voluntary adaptation of behavior conducive to health in individuals, families, groups, or communities

Activities

Target high-risk groups and age ranges that would benefit most from health education.
Target needs identified in Healthy People 2000: National Health Promotion and Disease Prevention Objectives or other local, state, and national needs.
Identify internal or external factors that may enhance or reduce motivation for healthful behavior.
Determine personal context and sociocultural history of individual, family, or target group.
Assist individuals, families, and communities in clarifying health beliefs and values.
Identify characteristics of target population that affect selection of learning strategies.
Prioritize identified learner needs based on client preference, skills of nurse, resources available, and likelihood of successful goal attainment.
Formulate objectives for health education program.
Identify resources (e.g., personnel, space, equipment, and money) needed to conduct program.
Consider accessibility, consumer preference, and cost in program planning.
Strategically place attractive advertising to capture attention of target audience.
Avoid use of fear or scare techniques as strategy to motivate people to change health or lifestyle behaviors.
Emphasize immediate or short-term positive health benefits to be received by positive lifestyle behaviors, rather than long-term benefits or negative effects of noncompliance.
Incorporate strategies to enhance the self-esteem of target audience.
Develop educational materials written at a readability level appropriate to target audience.
Teach strategies that can be used to resist unhealthful behavior or risk taking, rather than give advice to avoid or change behavior.
Keep presentation focused, short, and beginning and ending on main point.
Use group presentations to provide support and lessen threat to learners experiencing similar problems or concerns, as appropriate.
Use peer leaders, teachers, and support groups in implementing programs to groups less likely to listen to health professionals or adults (i.e., adolescents), as appropriate.
Use lectures to convey the maximal amount of information when appropriate.
Use group discussions and role playing to influence health beliefs, attitudes, and values.
Use demonstrations/return demonstrations, learner participation, and manipulation of materials when teaching psychomotor skills.
Use computer-assisted instruction, television, interactive video, and other technologies to convey information.
Use teleconferencing, telecommunications, and computer technologies for distance learning.
Involve individuals, families, and groups in planning and implementing plans for lifestyle or health behavior modification.
Determine family, peer, and community support for behavior conducive to health.
Use social and family support systems to enhance effectiveness of lifestyle or health behavior modification.
Emphasize the importance of healthful patterns of eating, sleeping, exercising, and so on to individuals, families, and groups who model these values and behaviors to others, particularly children.
Use a variety of strategies and intervention points in educational programs.
Plan long-term follow-up to reinforce health behaviors or lifestyle adaptations.
Design and implement strategies to measure client outcomes at regular intervals during and after completion of the program.
Design and implement strategies to measure the program and the cost-effectiveness of education, using these data to improve the effectiveness of subsequent programs.
Influence development of policy that guarantees health education as an employee benefit.
Encourage policy whereby insurance companies give consideration for premium reductions or benefits for healthful lifestyle practices.

From McCloskey, J., & Bulechek, G. (1996). *Nursing interventions classification (NIC)* (2nd ed.). St. Louis: Mosby–Year Book. Reprinted with permission.

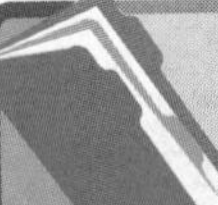

Chart 7–14
Nursing Interventions Classification (NIC)

Insurance Authorization

Definition

Assisting the patient and provider to secure payment for health services or equipment from a third party

Activities

Explain reasons for obtaining preapproval for health services or equipment.
Explain consent for release of information.
Obtain signature of patient or responsible adult on release of information form.
Obtain information and signature of patient or responsible adult on assignment of benefits form, as needed.
Obtain information for third-party payer about the necessity of the health service or equipment.
Obtain or write a prescription for equipment, as appropriate.
Submit a prescription for equipment to the third-party payer.
Record evidence of preapproval (e.g., validation number) on the patient's chart, as necessary.
Inform the patient or responsible adult of the status of the preapproval request.
Discuss financial responsibilities of client (e.g., out-of-pocket expenses), as appropriate.
Notify appropriate health professional if approval is refused by the third-party payer.
Negotiate alternative modalities of care, as appropriate, if approval is refused (e.g., outpatient status or change in care/acuity level).
Provide preapproval information to other departments, as necessary.
Document care provided, as required.
Assist with the completion of claim forms, as needed.
Facilitate communication with third-party payers, as needed.
Collaborate with other health professionals about continued need for health services, as appropriate.
Document continued need for health services, as required.
Provide necessary information (e.g., name, Social Security number, and provider) to third-party payer for billing, as needed.
Assist the client in accessing needed health services or equipment.

From McCloskey, J., & Bulechek, G. (1996). *Nursing interventions classification (NIC)* (2nd ed.). St. Louis: Mosby–Year Book. Reprinted with permission.

In the care coordination process, the nurse assesses the client and family to determine strengths and needs. In collaboration with the family, the nurse establishes goals and a plan of care is developed. The plan is explicit as to who will do what and when, specifying, in particular, who will assume accountability for each component. The child and family are periodically reevaluated to determine the appropriateness of the plan and the need for any revision. Case closure occurs when the client has been transferred to another agency or is no longer in need of services. Case closure is a key element of care coordination, not merely the end. Clients and families should be told how and under what circumstances they may reenter the service system. If they are no longer receiving services because they are ineligible, every effort should be made to refer them to a program that may be able to serve them.

In addition to working directly with clients, nurses may work toward improving child health through the development of needed programs or policies that better meet the needs of children and families. Chart 7–15 summarizes the many interventions the nurse can use to support community health needs. Opportunities to work in the community are available in public health agencies, hospitals, and community-based programs. Nurses can also promote child health by being aware of relevant legislative issues and responding to them when necessary.

Systems serving children and families, including those with special needs, are constantly in flux. Legislation changes the eligibility, services, and funding for these programs, often from year to year. The programs described in this chapter are, for the most part, susceptible to legislative change and may look different in the future. To be effective in planning, providing, and directing care for children and families, nurses must be aware of these changes and their impact. This self-education

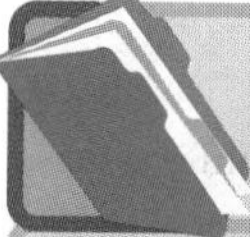

Chart 7–15
Nursing Interventions Classification (NIC)

Environmental Management: Community

Definition

Monitoring and influencing of the physical, social, cultural, economic, and political conditions that affect the health of groups and communities

Activities

Initiate screening for health risks from the environment.
Participate in interdisciplinary teams to identify threats to safety in the community.
Monitor status of known health risks.
Participate in community programs to deal with known risks.
Collaborate in the development of community action programs.
Promote governmental policy to reduce specified risks.
Encourage neighborhoods to become active participants in community safety.
Coordinate services to at-risk groups and communities.
Conduct educational programs for targeted risk groups.
Work with environmental groups to secure appropriate governmental regulations.

From McCloskey, J., & Bulechek, G. (1996). *Nursing interventions classification (NIC)* (2nd ed.). St. Louis: Mosby–Year Book. Reprinted with permission.

can be achieved in a number of ways, including membership in professional organizations; attendance at conferences; regular review of newsletters, journals, and newspapers; participation in advisory boards; and contact with legislators. Because nurses have a knowledge of the needs of the populations they serve, they must keep themselves apprised of the issues and speak out on their clients' behalf when necessary.

Summary of Key Concepts

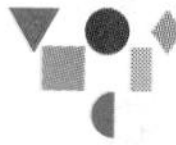

- As medical economics and technology change, more clients are being cared for in community settings.
- A number of public health programs exist to serve children and families. Knowledge of these programs aids the nurse in appropriately referring clients to needed services.
- Medicaid is a form of health insurance for low-income individuals. A specific component of this, the Early and Periodic Screening, Diagnosis and Treatment (EPSDT) Program, mandates a basic set of comprehensive services to promote health and identify and treat health problems in infants, children, and adolescents.
- The Special Supplemental Food Program for Women, Infants and Children (WIC) provides nutritious food, health education, and links to health care resources to low-income pregnant and lactating women, infants to 1 year of age, and children to age 5 at risk for nutritional problems.
- Supplemental Security Income for the Aged, Blind and Disabled (SSI) provides financial support to low-income elderly, blind, or disabled individuals, including children. In most states, clients also receive Medicaid.
- The Maternal and Child Health Services Block Grant provides for funds from the federal government to the states for preventive, primary, and specialty care for women and children. Examples of programs funded by

this grant include services for children with special health care needs, prenatal care, and genetic disease testing and counseling.

- The National Health Service Corps (NHSC) is a federal program awarding scholarships and loans to students within the health professions who in turn agree to work in medically underserved areas. This program thus increases the number of health care providers in areas where services are lacking but the need is great.
- Community and Migrant Health Centers (C/MHCs) provide comprehensive, primary care to families, primarily in medically underserved areas. There are approximately 600 clinics nationally serving more than 5 million clients, three quarters of whom are women of childbearing age and children.
- Public education programs exist that provide services for children with special needs. The Education for All Handicapped Children Act of 1975 requires free, appropriate, and individualized education in the least restrictive environment for handicapped individuals 6 to 21 years of age. The 1986 Education of the Handicapped Act mandates services for 3- to 5-year-olds and requires states to develop a plan for children birth through age 2 at risk for developmental disabilities. The 1993 Individuals with Disabilities Education Act requires implementation of systems to serve children from birth to 3 years.
- The Head Start program prepares low-income preschoolers for entry into school by providing opportunities for learning, social development, and health care. This program is mandated to provided services to children with special needs as well.
- Private, nonprofit organizations are also a source of care for children. These may be disease-specific or serve broad categories of children. Additionally, they may offer supportive services such as transportation or respite care to needy families.
- Children and families may receive health care in a variety of settings, including schools, clinics, daycare programs, Head Start programs, camps, and homeless shelters.
- Parents and caregivers can improve and enhance child health by learning about available resources, asking questions, and challenging information that limits access to services.
- Communities can work toward improvement of child and family health by ensuring that appropriate resources are locally available. Additionally, providing a healthful living environment should be a goal for communities as well as employers.
- Nurses are obviously well positioned to improve child and family health in a number of ways, including direct service, client advocacy, teaching, and coordination of care. In addition, nurses may be involved in the development of new programs geared to meet the emerging needs of clients.

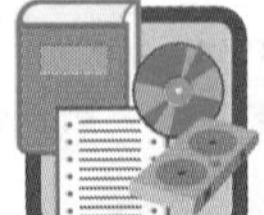

Resources

Organizations

American School Health Association
7263 State Route 43
Kent, OH 44240
(216) 678-1601

Child Welfare League of America
440 First Street, NW, Suite 310
Washington, DC 20001-2085
(202) 638-2952
Web: http://www.cwla.org

Children's Defense Fund (CDF)
25 E Street, NW
Washington, DC 20001
(202) 628-8787
Web: http://www.childrensdefense.org

Department of Health and Human Services
200 Independence Avenue, SW
Washington, DC 20201
(202) 619-0257
E-mail: hhsmail@os.dhs.gov
Web: http://www.os.dhs.gov

Family Resource Coalition
200 South Michigan Avenue, Suite 1520
Chicago, IL 60604
(312) 341-0900

National Association of Community Health Centers
1330 New Hampshire Avenue, NW, Suite 122
Washington, DC 20036
(202) 659-8008

National Association of School Nurses
P.O. Box 1300
Scarborough, ME 04070
(207) 883-2117
E-mail: nasn@aol.com

National Center for Networking Community-Based Services
Georgetown University Child Development Center
3800 Reservoir Road, NW
Washington, DC 20007
(202) 687-8837

Parent Action
2 N. Charles Street, Suite 960
Baltimore, MD 21201
(410) 727-3687

Social Security Administration
6401 Security Boulevard
Baltimore, MD 21235
(800) 772-1213

Visiting Nurse Association of America
3801 E. Florida Avenue, Suite 900
Denver, CO 80216
(303) 753-0218

Hotlines

Health Insurance Association of America
(800) 635-1271

Maternal and Child Health Services
An 800 number is available in each state.

Books and Other Printed Materials

Maternal and Child Health Publications Catalog

United States Department of Health and Human Services, Public Health Service

Health Resources and Services Administration

Maternal and Child Health Bureau

These four publications can be obtained from:

National Maternal and Child Health Clearinghouse
2070 Chain Bridge Road, Suite 450
Vienna, VA 22182-2536
(703) 821-8955
FAX: (703) 821-2098

Exceptional Parent
Annual Resource Guide
January 1997 (and annually)
(800) 562-1973

Pickett, O. K., Clark, E. M. & Kavanaugh, L. D. (Eds.). (1994). *Reaching out: A directory of national organizations related to maternal and child health.* Arlington, VA: National Center for Education in Maternal and Child Health
(703) 524-7802
FAX: (703) 524-9335

Directory of Federally Funded Resource Centers. (1993). National Center for Service Integration. Child and Family Policy Center.
(515) 280-9027

National Directory of Children, Youth and Family Services (1995–96)
(800) 343-6681
FAX: (800) 845-6452

Aron, L. Y., Loprest, P. J., & Steverle, C. E. (1996). *Serving children with disabilities: A systematic look at the programs.* Washington, DC: Urban Institute Press.

References

Aliza, B. (1993). *Building systems: A report on Title V programs' collaboration with the part H early intervention initiative.* Washington, DC: Association of Maternal and Child Health Programs.

Avruch, S., & Cackley, A. P. (1995). Savings achieved by giving WIC benefits to women prenatally. *Public Health Reports, 110*(1), 27–34.

Burns, M., & Thornam, C. B. (1993). Broadening the scope of nursing practice: Federal programs for children. *Pediatric Nursing, 19*(6), 546–552.

Children's Defense Fund. (1995). *The state of America's children yearbook.* Washington, DC: Author.

Council of Community Health Nurses, American Nurses' Association. (1986). *Standards of community health practice.* Washington, DC: Author.

Division of Children with Special Health Care Needs. (1996). Washington, DC: Division of Children with Special Health Care Needs, Maternal Child Health Bureau, Health Resources and Service Administration, U.S. Department of Health and Human Services.

Food Research and Action Center. (1991). *WIC: A success story* (3rd ed.). Washington, DC: Author.

Hall, L. (1990). *Medicaid home care options for disabled children.* Washington, DC: National Governors' Association.

Hansen, S., Holaday, B., & Miles, M. S. (1990). The role of pediatric nurses in a federal program for infants and young children with handicaps. *Journal of Pediatric Nursing, 5*(4), 246–251.

Harmon, R. G. (1992). The national health service corps: Bridging the gap in health care. *Academic Medicine, 67*(11), 758–759.

Healthy Mothers, Healthy Babies Coalition. (1986). *Healthy mothers, healthy babies: A compendium of program ideas for serving low-income women* (DHHS Publication No. PHS 86-50209). Washington, DC: U.S. Public Health Service, Division of Maternal and Child Health.

Hess, C. A. (1994). The organization of maternal and child health services. In H. M. Wallace, R. P. Nelson, & P. J. Sweeney (Eds.), *Maternal and child health practices* (4th ed., pp. 131–140). Oakland, CA: Third Party.

Hill, I. T. (1992). The role of Medicaid and other government programs in providing medical care for children and pregnant women. *The Future of Children, 2*(2), 134–153.

Hobbs, N., Perrin, J. M., & Ireys, H. T. (1985). *Chronically ill children and their families.* San Francisco: Jossey-Bass.

Hynes, M., & Schwartz, R. E. (1991). *MCH related federal programs: Legal handbooks for program planners: The Special Supplemental Food Program for Women, Infants and Children (WIC).* Washington, DC: Association of Maternal and Child Health Programs.

Jenkins, J. R., Covington, C., & Plotnick, J. (1994). Early childhood intervention: The law. *MCN, 19*(3), 135–142.

Johnson, C. M., Sum, A. M., & Weill, A. D. (1992). *Vanishing dreams: The economic plight of America's young families.* Washington, DC: Children's Defense Fund.

Johnson, K. A. (1994). Rural maternal and child health services. In H. M. Wallace, R. P. Nelson, & P. J. Sweeney (Eds.), *Maternal and child health practices* (4th ed., pp. 166–173). Oakland, CA: Third Party.

Johnson, K., & Moore, A. Y. (1990). *Improving health programs for low-income youths*. Washington, DC: Children's Defense Fund.

Kaiser Commission on the Future of Medicaid. (1995). *Medicaid and managed care*. Washington, DC: The Henry J. Kaiser Family Foundation.

Kassebaum, N. (1994). Head Start. *American Psychologist, 49*(2), 123–126.

Koop, C. E. (1987). *Surgeon General's report: Children with special health care needs: Campaign '87: Commitment to family centered coordinated care for children with special health needs* (DHHS Publication No. HRS/D/MC 87-2). Washington, DC: U.S. Department of Health and Human Services, Public Health Service.

Lecks, M., Mitchem, F., & Weiss, S. (1992). *A report on coordination between community and migrant health centers and Title V maternal and child health services programs*. Washington, DC: National Association of Community Health Centers.

Mangu, P. B. (Ed.). (1991). *1990 Head Start Health Institute Proceedings*. Washington, DC: National Center for Education in Maternal and Child Health.

McCloskey, J., & Bulechek, G. (1996). *Nursing Interventions Classification (NIC)* (2nd ed.). St. Louis: Mosby–Year Book.

Model Standards Work Group, American Public Health Association. (1991). *Healthy communities 2000: Model standards: Guidelines for community attainment of the year 2000 national health objectives*. Washington, DC: Author.

National Governors' Association, Health Policy Studies Division. (1995). *Promoting the health of all women and children through Title V*. Washington, DC: Author.

Orloff, T. M., Rivera, L. A., & Rosenbaum, S. (1992). *Medicaid reforms for children: An EPSDT chartbook*. Washington, DC: Children's Defense Fund.

Parette, H. P., Jr. (1993). High-risk infant case management and assistive technology: Funding and family enabling perspectives. *Maternal-Child Nursing Journal, 21*(2), 53–64.

Rivera, L., Regan, C., & Rosenbaum, S. (1995). *Managed care and children's health: An analysis of early and periodic screening, diagnosis, and treatment services under state Medicaid managed care contracts*. Washington, DC: Children's Defense Fund.

Saunders, S. E. (1994). Medicaid, maternal and child health, and programs for children with special needs. In H. M. Wallace, R. P. Nelson, & P. J. Sweeney (Eds.), *Maternal and child health practices* (4th ed., pp. 166–173). Oakland, CA: Third Party.

Schmidt, W. M., & Wallace, H. M. (1994). The development of health services for mothers and children in the United States. In H. M. Wallace, R. P. Nelson, & P. J. Sweeney (Eds.), *Maternal and child health practices* (4th ed., pp. 166–173). Oakland, CA: Third Party.

Schulzinger, R. (1993). Infants, toddlers, and SSI: Changing the rules, reaching the children. *Zero to Three, 13*(3), 27–30.

Schwartz, R. E. (1990). *MCH related federal programs: Legal handbooks for program planners: Medicaid*. Washington, DC: Association of Maternal and Child Health Programs.

Schwartz, R. E., & Hynes, M. (1991). *MCH related federal programs: Legal handbooks for program planners: Supplemental security income (SSI) for disabled children*. Washington, DC: Association of Maternal and Child Health Programs.

Smith, K. (1994). EPSDT and health care reform. *Pediatric Nursing, 20*(1), 66–67.

Swanson, J. M., & Albrecht, M. (1993). *Community health nursing: Promoting the health of aggregates*. Philadelphia: W. B. Saunders.

Thomas, H. (1994). Conceptual underpinnings of the family support movement. *Journal of Pediatric Health Care, 8*, 57–62.

United States Department of Health and Human Services, Public Health Service. (1992). *Understanding the Title V of the Social Security Act: A guide to the provisions of federal maternal and child health services legislation after the enactment of the Omnibus Reconciliation Act (OBRA) of 1989* (PL Publication No. 101–239). Washington, DC: Author.

United States Department of Health and Human Services, Social Security Administration. (1992). *Understanding SSI* (SSA Publication No. 17-008). Washington, DC: Author.

Bibliography

American Academy of Pediatrics. (1995). The pediatrician's role in family support programs. *Pediatrics, 95*, 781–783.

Aron, L. Y., Loprest, P. J., & Steuerle, C. E. (1996). *Serving children with disabilities: A systematic look at the programs*. Washington, DC: The Urban Institute Press.

Center for the Future of Children, The David and Lucile Packard Foundation. (1996). *The future of children: Special education for students with disabilities*. 6(1), Spring: Author.

Ferretti, C., Verhey, M. & Isham, M. (1996). Development of a nurse-managed, school-based health center. *Nurse Educator, 21*(5), 35–42.

Swanson, J. M., & Albrecht, M. (1993). *Community health nursing: Promoting the health of aggregates*. Philadelphia: W. B. Saunders.

U.S. Department of Health and Human Services. (1991). *Health people 2000: National health promotion and disease prevention objectives*. Washington, DC: U.S. Government Printing Office.

Wallace, H. M., Nelson, R. P., & Sweeney, P. J. (1994). *Maternal and child health practices* (4th ed.). Oakland, CA: Third Party.

Wallace, H. M., Biehl, R. F., MacQueen, J. C., & Blackman, J. A. (1997). *Mosby's resource guide to children with disabilities and chronic illness*. St. Louis: Mosby–Year Book.

Maintaining Health Across the Continuum of Care

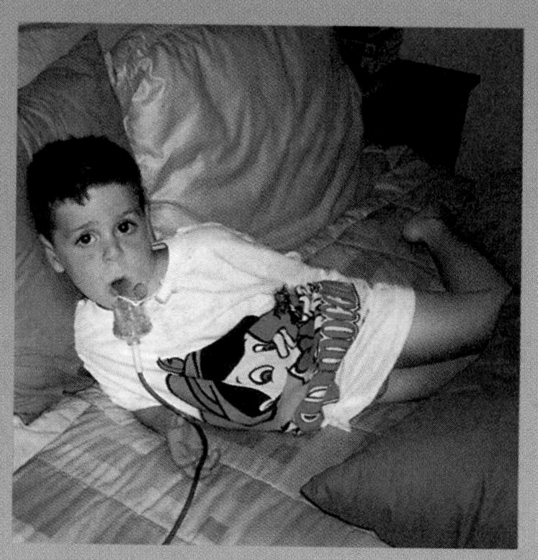

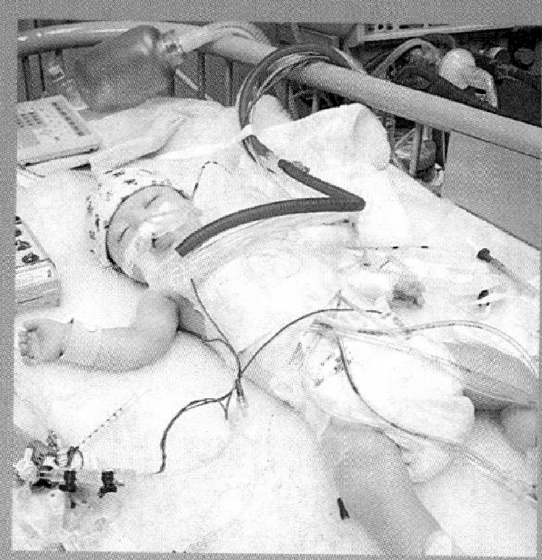

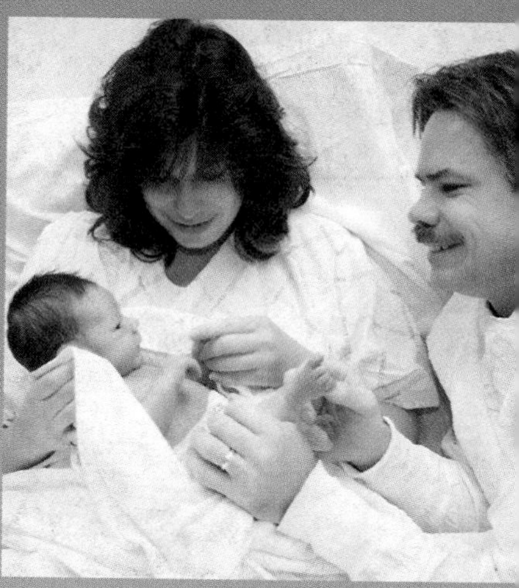

UNIT

3

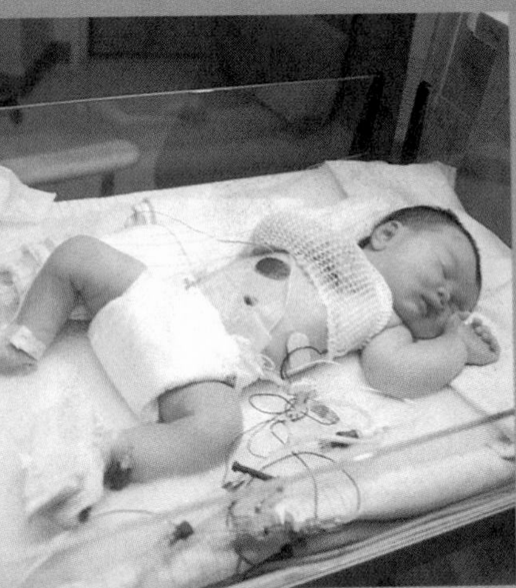
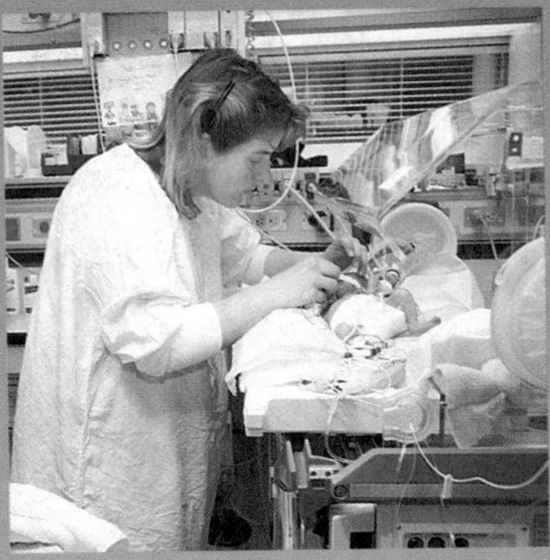
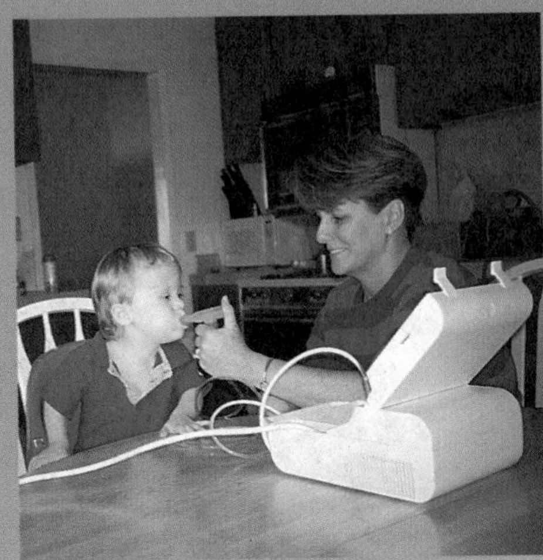

In this unit, the focus shifts from the well child to the child facing a serious acute or chronic health condition. Nurses are in a key position to assess family needs and work collaboratively to select a course of action that will help the child and family adapt and adjust to changes in the child's health status. Most families are unprepared for the challenges brought by a serious illness in a child. The chapters in this unit discuss the current research, theories, and practice interventions that can be used to help the child and family manage their needs over the entire continuum of care.

Many children with an acute or a chronic condition may require some form of rehabilitation or home care. These care services are discussed, with emphasis given to the nurse's role in these settings. An entire chapter is devoted to managing pain in children. Monitoring and managing this aspect of the child's care is a critical component of the interdisciplinary approach needed to help the child maintain comfort and have the physical and psychological resources necessary to achieve optimal health outcomes.

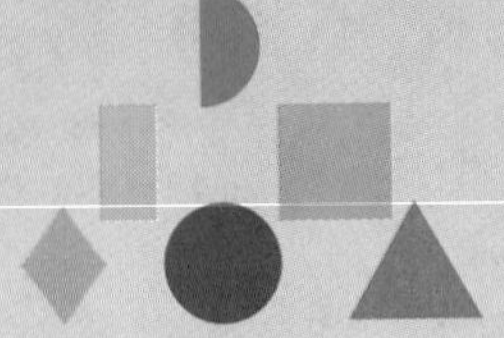

Unexpected Outcomes of Childbearing

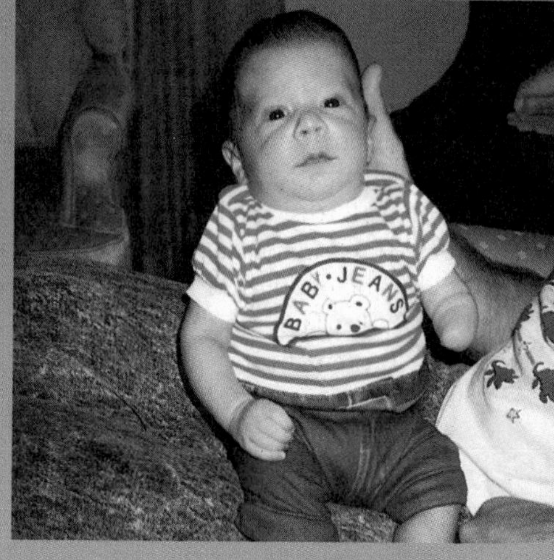

OUTLINE

Providing Support to the Family
- Presentation of Bad News
- Perinatal Infant Death

Genetic Counseling
- Genograms

Genetic Screening and Fetal Diagnostic Tests
- Maternal Serum Alpha-Fetoprotein
- Triple Marker Screening
- Chorionic Villus Sampling
- Fetal Ultrasonography
- Amniocentesis

Genetic and Multifactorial Disorders
- Overview of Genetic Theory
- Patterns of Inheritance in Genetic Disorders
  - Monogenic Conditions at the Single Gene Locus
  - Chromosomal Aberrations
- Congenital Anomalies
- Teratogens and Environmental Exposures
  - Chemicals
  - Infectious Agents
  - Ionizing Radiation
  - Other Teratogens

Long-Term Implications

OBJECTIVES

- Define unexpected outcomes of childbearing and discuss their impact on individual and family development.
- Examine issues surrounding perinatal loss as an unexpected outcome of pregnancy.
- Examine aspects of genetic counseling, including the use of genograms.
- Discuss information a parent needs to bring to a genetic counseling session.
- Explain the rationales for genetic screening tests.
- Review conditions related to genetic inheritance.
- Describe the principles of teratogenesis and the impact of teratogens on the affected child.
- Present the concept of the high-risk newborn as an unexpected outcome of pregnancy.

KEY TERMS

allele
aneuploidy
autosome
consanguinity
deletion
folate deficiency
genome
genotype
heterozygote
homozygote
inborn error
karyotype
mutation
phenotype
polygenic
sex-linked genes
teratogen
X chromosome
Y chromosome

CHAPTER

8

Many perinatal conditions contribute to morbidity and mortality in children. Some are readily apparent at birth; others manifest themselves over time at the molecular and microscopic levels. Unexpected outcomes of childbearing and pregnancy can take many forms, including maternal feelings of loss of control during the labor process; expectation of a delivery without analgesia or anesthesia, replaced by the need for an emergency cesarean section; postpartum depression; an unsuccessful breast-feeding experience; a fussy, colicky infant; hyperbilirubinemia; a normal infant coupled with inappropriate developmental expectations on the part of the parents; birth of a male child when a female child was expected (or vice versa); multiple births; visible or invisible anomalies; complications of perinatal infections; perinatal morbidity to the mother or child; and neonatal and possibly even maternal death. The most common type of unexpected outcome is prematurity.

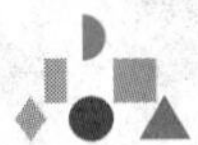

Providing Support to the Family

All of the previously described conditions may influence the way in which parents handle and feel about their new child. Mothers of all infants must master the maternal thinking and problem-solving process of learning the baby (Sullivan, 1997). Mothers of preterm infants experience significant levels of stress and depression during the early postpartum period (Younger, Kendell, & Pickler, 1997). Early delivery results in lost time to emotionally prepare for the delivery and motherhood, creating an added major stressor in family life (Fig. 8–1).

Mothers and fathers may react differently to their perinatal status (Chart 8–1). Often, people expect them to have identical thoughts, feelings, and reactions to their perinatal status because they are "a couple." In a situation in which the pregnancy has resulted in an unexpected outcome, it may be useful to intervene with parents separately, so each may express private feelings safely, rather than editing them for the benefit of the partner.

The nurse is in a unique position to help family members express and resolve some unhappy reactions to the addition of a child who has increased care requirements or characteristics that they did not envision in their fantasy of the perfect child (Fig. 8–2). This will eventually benefit all members of the infant's family. Even if an infant falls well within normal parameters in every assessment category, the astute nurse will notice family members' remarks and attempt to explore further emotional reactions or make appropriate referrals. For example, a new father may come to a newborn nursery to visit his infant and make a remark such as, "Yes, I wanted to have children . . . but not with this woman." There is significant emotional content in such a remark. Perhaps all that can be said is a therapeutic response, such as, "I'm sorry that this has happened this way for you." The nurse should try to avoid attempting to control another person's emotional response to an unexpected situation. Extreme sensitivity is required to handle unexpected outcomes, and the nurse is often the only person with such close access to the patient. The nurse's empathetic words may provide welcome emotional relief or may cause internalization and damaging negative emotions for a long time (Fig. 8–3).

Dysfunctional grieving may result from unexpected

Figure 8–1
A, Unexpected outcomes of childbearing often require many hands and much sophisticated equipment to ensure optimal neonatal health. B, Most parents expect their newborn to look healthy and adapt well to life outside the womb.

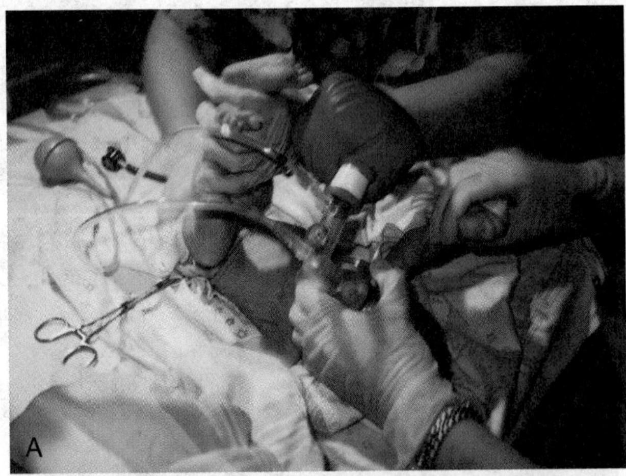

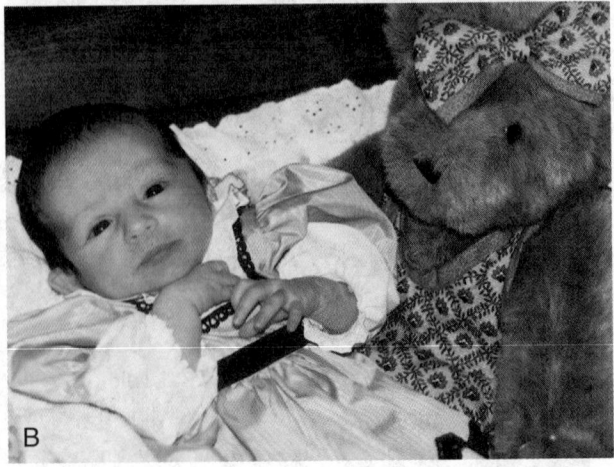

Chart 8–1

First Visit to the Neonatal Intensive Care Unit

Brandon Gregory lay on his back asleep. Beneath him, on a sheet printed with little girls in sunbonnets, was a standard diaper that could have served him as a hammock. Over him, to minimize heat loss while permitting close observation, was a square blanket of Saran Wrap bordered in adhesive tape. His legs were splayed and drawn up sharply at the knees. His arms lay bent at the elbows, the tiny hands palm up, the tiny fingers curled into calyxes beneath the tiny ears. Brandon's elbows were two pale brown lines. His incipient hair was pale brown. His temples and much of the rest of his body were dusted with fine fetal down that would eventually disappear. Blood vessels showed in and under the translucent marbled skin of his abdomen as reddish-purple traces.

A green tube in the baby's mouth connected him to the respirator. The tube had been anchored with tape to his upper lip and cheeks from ear to ear. A clear tube had been taped into his umbilicus for painless blood sampling. Two more clear tubes had been inserted into his foot and right wrist for medications and fluids in the form of intravenous feedings. Both those tubes were taped in place over foam blocks and rolled gauze that protected the baby's skin from direct contact with the adhesive.

In the anteroom, Tom Gregory showed his wife how to scrub at the sink. Each tied a clean yellow gown on the other. They approached the closed glass door. Somewhat tentatively, Tom knocked.

Robin began to feel shaky. Through the glass she caught sight of a baby who looked terrible, and suddenly she became afraid.

Someone let them in. Ordinarily, the nursing staff prepares a parent visiting for the first time. Apparently, no one realized that Robin had not been in before. The Gregorys proceeded on their own. Once they got past the baby she'd seen first, Robin breathed a sigh of relief. The other babies seemed bigger and not so badly off.

Ahead of Robin, her husband turned a corner and stopped. Still in his sunglasses, he faced her. "Here he is."

Rounding the corner herself, she glanced down, stopped short, took a step back, and felt her heart break.

She burst into tears. Tom led her out of the unit and into the small waiting room. There, a few minutes later, Brandon's nurse, a man, stocky and curly-headed, and about their age, found them. Robin thought he was an aide.

The nurse apologized. He felt so bad not to have been there when the parents came in. He'd been to lunch, he explained. If he'd been in the unit, he could have prepared Mrs. Gregory.

Robin shook her head. Nothing could have prepared her.

The nurse begged them to go back in with him. As if dreaming, Robin followed the young man and her husband back to Brandon's bedside. Speaking slowly and in everyday language, the nurse explained about all the equipment. Robin could not begin to keep up with all the information he was giving her. She could not imagine how a baby who looked as Brandon did could possibly survive.

The nurse urged Robin to touch the baby.

She could not bring herself to do so.

From Anderson, P. (1985). *Children's hospital* (pp. 194, 198). New York: Harper & Row. Used with permission.

outcomes with the pregnancy or the infant. Few people, regardless of their profession, are well equipped to recognize and assist the grieving process after the immediate period following the loss (James & Cherry, 1988). The loss may not be a death but the loss of the expectation of the fantasy of a normal child. Chronic sorrow may ensue if the defects are significantly life altering (Olshansky, 1962). Chapter 12 provides more information about the experiences of loss and grieving in a family.

Many individuals have been separated from the customs of their cultures of origin that helped their predecessors deal with significant losses. The nurse should study the customs of other cultures and subcultures to learn how loss and death are handled within them. This is especially important when working with members of a particular culture different from one's own. The nurse should never assume that his or her culture is the same as a patient's or parent's, even if both are part of the same larger culture. The family's particular needs need to be explored with a member of that family. In addition, extended family members may be apart from one another or be separated by financial concerns (such as long-distance telephone bills). Perhaps people are isolated in their own areas by living alone or by having financial distress or underlying psychiatric conditions. Attempts to place the parents in some form of contact with the

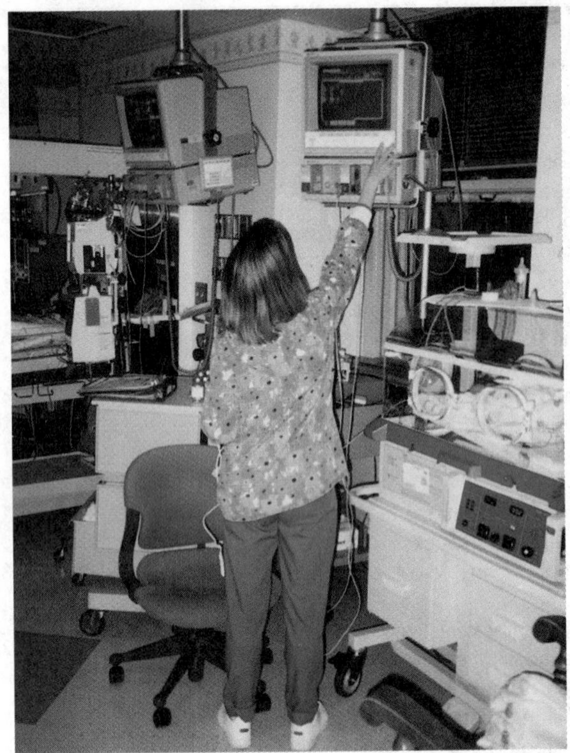

Figure 8–2
The neonatal intensive care unit is full of complicated equipment, which parents may find confusing and overwhelming.

child's caregivers and their significant others, by telephone, may be useful.

Presentation of Bad News

The way in which parents are presented with bad news about their infant significantly affects how they will handle the child in the future. Separation anxiety is very high, especially when parents have fantasized about having a perfect child during the pregnancy. There is a disruption of family boundaries, particularly when the infant is transferred to another institution for tertiary care or surgery.

caREminder: *Prompt, honest, and complete notification* ***to parents only*** *of the infant's condition is imperative. The infant's parents can decide what information to disclose to others of their choice.*

Telephone calls should be screened carefully to identify the caller. The parents may use a "password" so that staff members can identify them as individuals appropriate to receive information. Parents can be offered the opportunity to see and hold their infant, even for the most severely ill or deceased child.

Presentation of harsh realities may be painful but may help parents deal realistically with the situation, especially if they are using denial as a defense mechanism. Parents who are usually very competent in their own worlds may exhibit denial by asking questions that seem odd to the nurse, such as whether mechanically ventilated children may go home with them. The nurse helps such parents by presenting basic reality in a supportive and nonjudgmental manner.

The nurse must consider parents' fears when discussing problems with them. Parents may ask, Are we the cause? Is our infant going to die? By exploring such fears, the nurse can help prevent them from becoming an obstacle to attachment. Persistent fear that the infant may not be normal can interfere with attachment.

To avoid misunderstanding, the nurse must choose his or her words carefully. For example, family members may misconstrue the words "blood type incompatibilities" as an antagonism between the mother's and infant's personalities. Parents may have difficulty accepting that their beloved infant is "allergic" to the mother's blood type. They may suffer guilt, self-blame, or spiritual distress surrounding these physiologic outcomes. Lack of successful treatment for physical conditions creates psychological problems.

Before telling families that the infant is "doing well," the nurse must consider what "well" means. If the infant is stabilized on a ventilator in a critical care unit, this does not seem "well" to most parents and families.

Parents deal with continuing anxiety through a vari-

Figure 8–3
Preterm infants are often born intact and healthy.

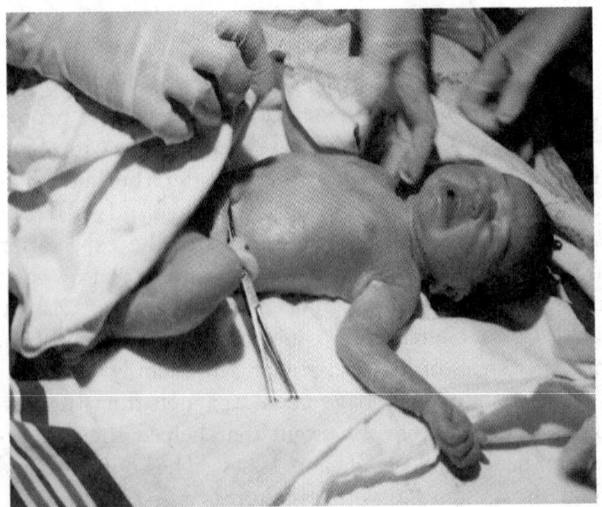

ety of maladaptive and/or adaptive responses (Fig. 8–4). Stress further alienates them from their children. Their needs and readiness to take in information must be assessed. If they ask many or too simple questions, they may be seeking emotional support. Parents who have been given unreasonably grim predictions build walls of pessimism to protect themselves. This has important implications for attachment and anticipatory grieving. In addition, providers should be careful about giving information selectively. This includes withholding information (to a point of negligent nondisclosure) and distortion of truth. The provider/patient power differential is rarely more exaggerated when information is being delivered about one's child. Frequently, a parent's desire is an unfulfillable wish to switch places with one's child so that the child need not undergo painful procedures and other consequences of the condition.

Discussing prognosis is the physician's domain. When parents are told what an illness means, it may be just as important for them to hear what it does not mean. They may ask questions about this later. It is helpful to ask directly if parents are concerned about whether their child will be normal or whether they fear his or her death.

The world of sick infants, oxygen requirements, and monitors is alien to families. Sometimes they may distract themselves from the pain and dealing with the infant as a person, for example, by calling to discuss laboratory values with the nurse. A strategy for intervention is to refocus them on the unique qualities of the infant as an

Figure 8–4

Adaptive and maladaptive parental responses to serious deviations in a child's health. (Adapted from Grant, P. [1978]. Psychosocial needs of families of high-risk infants. *Family and Community Health*, 1[3], 93. Used with permission.)

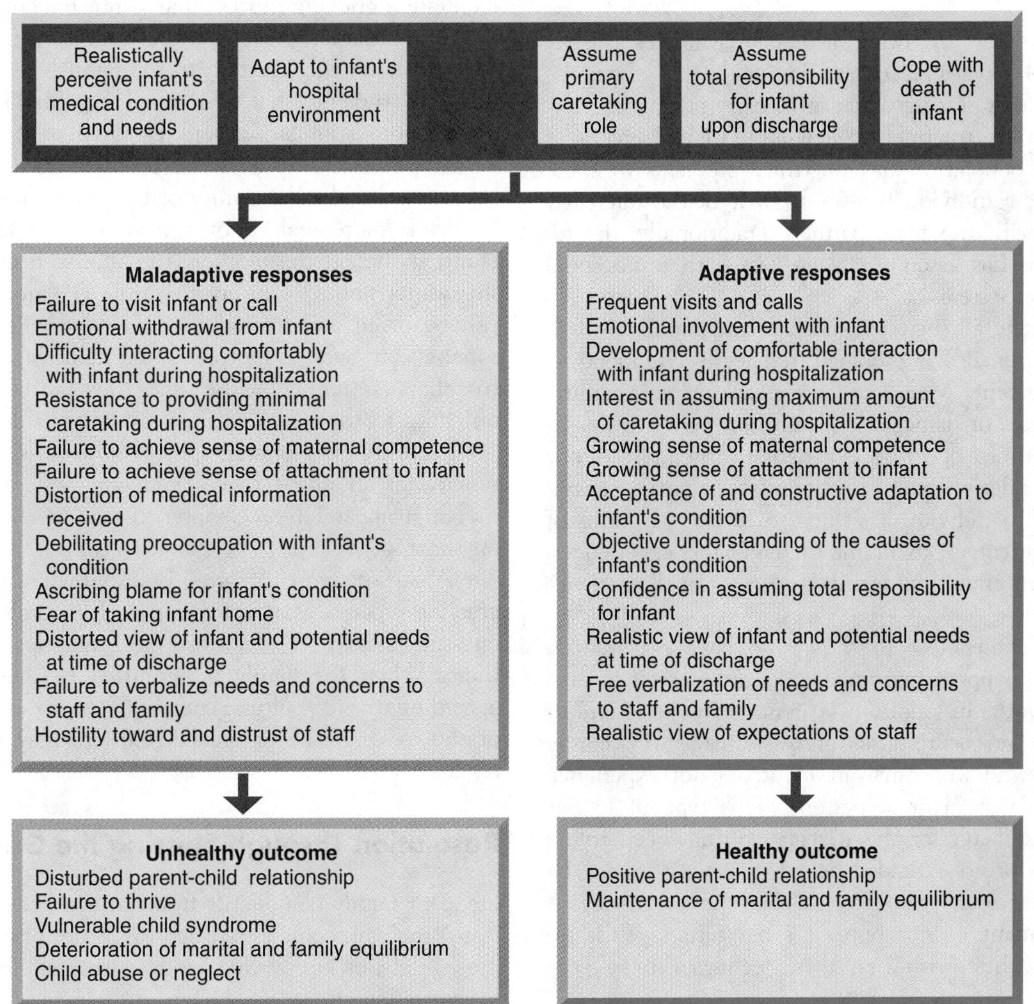

individual, including positive characteristics. The importance of parental involvement is stressed throughout this text. Close physical contact and caregiving behaviors help parents feel closer and more confident in their abilities as parents.

Perinatal Infant Death

Spontaneous Abortion

Even if spontaneous abortion occurs as early as the first trimester, it is an unexpected death experience. At best, there is meaning that the pregnancy was in some way defective. Acute grief responses may be experienced. There may be feelings of relief, as well. Even if the woman had considered therapeutic termination of the pregnancy, a spontaneous loss will trigger feelings of loss of control. Some women may brush off an unexpected early pregnancy loss as if it were just another menstrual period. In other situations, a complex set of emotions may characterize individuals and families when there is such a loss.

Some women are aware of their pregnancies as early as 10 to 14 days after conception with the advent of home pregnancy testing or sensitive early pregnancy testing in infertility treatment follow-up. Twenty percent of the general population has infertility problems in some form. Of these individuals, 40% to 50% of the infertility causes rest with the male partner. Traditionally, the female partner has assumed "blame" in both professional and lay belief systems.

In virtually all societies, much of the population (especially the female) is groomed from early childhood to become a parent. Memories of experiences surrounding perinatal losses or damaged children may persist throughout the lifetimes of those experiencing them. It is not unusual for elderly women to recount their entire perinatal histories to individuals willing to listen! All forms of pregnancy outcomes, including the enjoyable experiences, are significant emotional events to the persons experiencing them.

Many people close to those who have experienced losses make inappropriate remarks in the interest of providing comfort. In addition, parents may be attempting to bear an acute grief process unaided by family and friends who were unaware of or did not experience the pregnancy as a "real person." This type of loss is particularly difficult for the woman who has been trying to conceive for an extended period of time. She may be the only individual who experienced the pregnancy as the embodiment of her hopes for her future. With no one to empathize with her, these feelings can be very alienating.

Fetal Loss

If a pregnancy has progressed far enough to get to the fetal period (after the first 8 weeks of a gestation), there may be significant parental, and especially maternal, investment. This is particularly true if the couple has experienced difficulty conceiving. Parents should be offered the option of touching, fondling, or holding the deceased fetus/infant, even if it is grossly malformed. This is not unduly upsetting to most mothers. Fathers should not be permitted to decide if the mother is to see her deformed or deceased child. This decision should always be offered to the infant's mother independently of family input. If the woman is incapable of doing so at the time of the infant's death, an option to visit at the morgue may be provided in some settings. Parental fantasies are often much worse than the reality of any anomalies or the visual condition of the deceased fetus.

In the past, parents were not permitted contact with the dead or dying infant because it was believed to be "too upsetting" for them. It probably was more difficult for providers to deal with openly emoting families. To facilitate a grieving process that is not fraught with regret and recriminations, every effort should be made by the nurse to tailor the situation to the family's requests.

It is thought that affectional bonding is enhanced with tactile stimulation and caregiving for all infants. This type of activity does not result in pathologic grieving. It may make the reality of this particular infant and its death more real. Photographs may be taken if the family wishes. If the mother is unable to decide whether she wants photographs at the time, Polaroid snapshots can be taken and offered to her, along with other personal effects, such as footprints and name bracelets. If the snapshots are refused at the time, they can be kept in the unit files for over a year after the infant's death. In the 19th century after photography was invented, it was customary for an infant to be "laid out" and photographed in burial apparel (see Chapter 12 for more information on this topic).

A strong sense of grief is a normal aspect of the grieving process. Many providers feel uncomfortable with outward display of emotions and attempt to squelch them. When the family is permitted to show emotions according to its cultural norms, a sense of resolution of the loss may be enhanced. Closure may occur more readily.

Resolution Through Sharing the Grief

Frequent family complaints from mishandled death situations include comments such as "the physicians and nurses did not know what to do with me." Families may be treated with a "conspiracy of silence" as if nothing happened to them. Nurses should express sorrow or sympathy to the family. Although this may elicit outward expression of emotion, such as crying, this is a form of therapeutic communication, because it facilitates resolution through sharing. Talking about this family's tragedy should be permitted.

caREminder: *Avoid platitudes such as "Please don't feel so bad . . . you have other children at home" or "You can always have another baby."*

This type of remark usually inflicts a lot of emotional damage by negating the reality and individuality of the particular lost infant. It may seem especially callous if a couple has made many unsuccessful attempts to conceive over a long period of time.

There are many options with respect to a fetal/neonatal death experience. It is the family's role, particularly the mother's, to choose. Some options include autopsy (possibly required by law), donation of the body to science, having the institution dispose of the body, and planning a funeral. Funerals for infants are much less expensive than those of adults. Many families do not know what they want to do, especially right away. Sufficient time should be provided without pressure so that family decisions may be made.

If an autopsy is required by law or circumstances may require reporting the loss to the medical examiner's office, the nurse should check the policy in his or her institution or call the local medical examiner's office. It is the physician's responsibility to obtain consent for autopsy when it is optional. In cases determined to have circumstances that may require reporting the death to the medical examiner's office, autopsy is not optional. Nurses should avoid witnessing consent for autopsies because they may be construed to be in legal collusion with the physician, should it be called to question. It is best to ask a "noninterested third party" such as an admissions clerk or unit secretary to witness signatures for such consents.

Multicultural Considerations Regarding Death

The hospital chaplain, parish priest, rabbi, or other family-requested member of the clergy should be consulted if the patient's religious/spiritual needs are beyond the nurse's ability to help.

Worldview: *Christian baptism is within the province of the nurse or other laypersons when death is imminent or has already occurred. The nurse may want to notify the member of the clergy designated by the family if there is time. This requires their permission. The parents should be notified as quickly as possible about changes in the infant's status. A baptismal certificate is completed and presented to the parents as official documentation of the ritual. Baptism may be performed by anyone when a member of the clergy cannot be summoned quickly enough. The act is accomplished by touching water to the child's scalp and saying, "I baptize you Baby Jane (or John) Doe in the name of the Father, the Son and of the Holy Spirit. Amen." The baptism is recorded on the child's chart and bed.*

The nurse should support the family religion or belief systems in all dealings with young patients and be aware of the parents' desires. Bias concerning the religious practices of patients or families should not be displayed, and the nurse should avoid inflicting his or her own values and beliefs on those not interested. Some of the most overwhelming emotions occur at times of serious illness in both the families of an ill child and the health care providers. Among them are intense anxiety, fear, and feelings of powerlessness. If the infant's mother and other immediate family members are unable to speak the language of the attending health care providers, a translator can be called to make sure their wishes are considered fully. If it is not feasible to do so at the time of the infant's death, a social service consultation and referral to a bereavement counselor may be in order.

Genetic Counseling

The nurse's role in genetic counseling includes answering the spontaneous questions of families in health care settings. To fufill this responsibility, the nurse must keep up to date with advances in science. This is very difficult in the field of genetics, because new information is presented all the time. The International Society of Nurses in Genetics, Inc. (ISONG) (see Resources at the end of this chapter) is actively involved in promoting education and support for nurses who provide genetic health care. Members act formally and informally with other national genetics groups, such as the American College of Medical Genetics, the American Society of Human Genetics, and the National Society of Genetics Counselors (Anderson, 1996). See Chapter 27 for Nursing Interventions Classification (NIC) guidelines on genetic counseling.

A good example of knowledge increasing is the explosion of information known about a heritable disorder called *cystic fibrosis of the pancreas*. This condition was thought to have been transmitted by autosomal recessive inheritance at a single gene locus. In 1987, the gene locus was identified. Now, several hundred alleles and sites are known to contribute to the genetic code for cystic fibrosis, with more information being refined day to day. If the nurse is uncertain of the accuracy and timeliness of the information requested, appropriate referrals should be made to the patient's physician or a genetic counselor.

The *genome* is defined as the totality of genes of an organism making up its hereditary constitution. In humans, an estimated 3 billion pairs of amino acids are arranged in the double helix of DNA molecules that make up the 23 pairs of human chromosomes. Approximately 100,000 genes constitute the human genome (Jonsen, 1996). The Human Genome Project is an international endeavor in progress with hundreds of geneticists at work to unravel the secrets of how humans are "put together" genetically (Bishop & Waldholz, 1990; Jonsen, 1996; Williams & Lessick, 1996). The central idea for this work in progress is that the tens of thousands of genes that make up each human chromosome are arranged in an orderly fashion. The order of these genes is to be mapped or sequenced so that *phenotypic* (the individual's structure and physiologic functioning) characteristics can be located and potentially engineered or managed in a way that they are no longer problematic to an individual (Jonsen, 1996). It is beyond the scope of this text to explain the basics of DNA replication, and the reader is referred to a basic text on genetics to enhance or reinforce previous learning.

Old genetic and scientific paradigms are replaced as new information becomes available. A prime example of this is the heritable nature of schizophrenia. Although currently theories suggest a strong genetic influence on this condition, a former theory of its origins was the "schizophrenogenic mother." Health care professionals who subscribed to the older theory may have contributed to emotional damage to the families of individuals with schizophrenia by applying an unproven theory.

Genetic study, manipulation, engineering, and discovery have profound implications for appropriate ethical use of the information. The implications of genetic research and testing for children are controversial when there is no available benefit (curative or preventive treatment) (Williams & Lessick, 1996). The United States government is concerned with such implications and has published the *ELSI Bibliography: Ethical, Legal and Social Implications of the Human Genome Project* (Yesley, 1993). This is an evolving computer database that can be rapidly searched and sorted on a variety of parameters and their combinations.

Families may assume that the terms *genetic engineering* or *genetically engineered* apply to permanent changes in the genome rather than to somatic cell therapy to improve the medical outcomes of a chronic condition, such as cystic fibrosis.

The outcomes of the Human Genome Project have profound implications for most areas of human concern—science, ethics, the professions, biology, and religion, to name a few.

For children identified prenatally or at birth with inborn errors of metabolism, such as phenylketonuria, such information is invaluable, because it allows for early dietary treatment, which decreases the degree and probability of mental retardation for that condition. This is also true for their families and society for the prevention of severe retardation in an individual who cannot provide self-care throughout life. For others identified with genetic diseases such as Huntington's disease, there is reason to fear the development of a "biological underclass" in which individuals are discriminated against by employers, insurance companies, and others (Bishop & Waldholz, 1990, p. 21).

Professionals with graduate preparation in genetic counseling devote a life's work to keeping abreast of sensitive approaches and new knowledge in the field (Bartels, LeRoy, & Caplan, 1993). This field is well established and carries its own value system, ethic for professional training, workplace ideology, and approaches to patients that minimize physical and emotional damage, no matter what genetic heritage the family brings to the counseling situation (Bosk, 1993; Marks, 1993; Sorenson, 1993).

Genograms

The use of genograms has been adapted to many professional settings as an instrument for screening genetic or heritable conditions and as an avenue into other forms of inquiry, such as a family's psychological dynamics. Family-of-origin work helps to reveal behavioral patterns and cultural styles transmitted over generations. However, this chapter focuses on genograms of individuals with inherited conditions and genetic diseases that create alterations in the family. The genogram is the first tool used to unravel the genetic "story" of a family and a unique, inherited trait (Fig. 8–5).

Genograms are the primary tool of the genetic counselor and other professionals interested in inherited characteristics. Genograms create a family systems perspective that might otherwise be unappreciated by the health care provider (Jackson, 1996; McGoldrick & Gerson, 1985). Genograms are an excellent way to demonstrate critical family events, such as birth dates, death dates, marital and other childbearing relationships, and interfamily relationships. Frequently, when an unusual genetic manifestation occurs in an individual, a careful interviewer might find a common ancestor among spouses who did not perceive that they had married a relative. In most societies, the incest taboo holds among parents and their

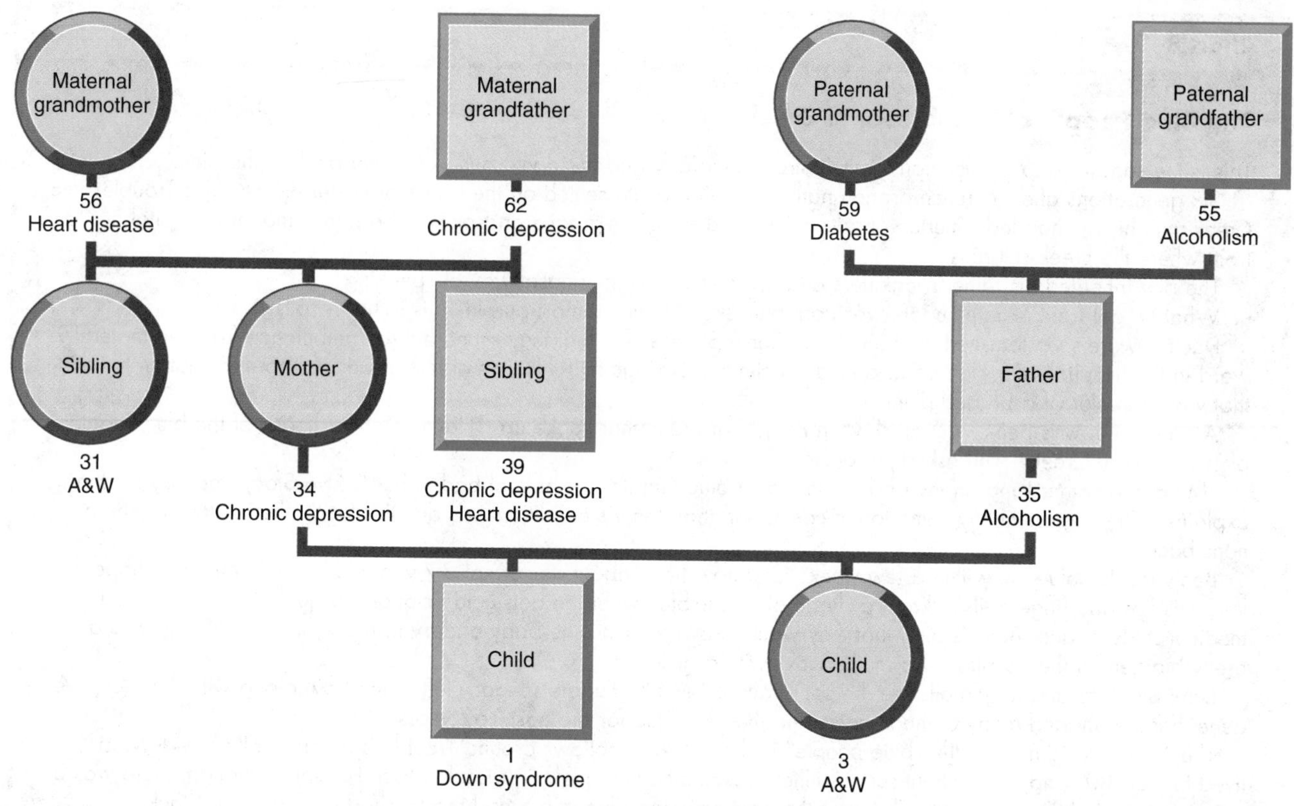

Figure 8–5
Family genogram of disease patterns. Circles represent females; squares, males. A & W indicates alive and well, in good health. (Adapted from Betz, C. L., Hunsberger, M. M., & Wright, S. [Eds.] [1994]. *Family-centered nursing care of children* [2nd ed., p. 46]. Philadelphia: W. B. Saunders. Used with permission.)

offspring, siblings, grandparents, aunts, and uncles. However, it is not uncommon or illegal to marry one's cousins, second cousins, and so on. This is known as *consanguinity* when offspring are concerned. Completing a genogram becomes complex when an incestuous relationship results in offspring with genetic diseases, especially when not all family members are aware of the nature of the child's conception.

The construction of a genogram and eliciting of relevant information from a family during the assessment require precision and careful listening skills (McGoldrick & Gerson, 1985). A family member might call a genetic disease by a colloquial term that an untrained ear might miss. Chart 8–2 describes how a mutation for methemoglobinemia was traced by many descendants to a common ancestor. This anecdote includes examples of genogram construction and demonstrates how a number of descendants of the first person exhibiting the mutation grew apart in the family tree. Generations later, the gene was expressed through a number of consanguineous marriages.

Genetic Screening and Fetal Diagnostic Tests

Families make many choices with their prenatal care providers during a pregnancy about undergoing genetic screening tests. Sometimes these tests are perceived to be routine, not a matter of choice. When a woman chooses to use prenatal diagnostic testing, her experience of the pregnancy and her relationship with the fetus may change. She may feel unwilling to commit fully to the pregnancy until after receiving negative test results. The nurse's role in this situation is to provide supportive and nonjudgmental care by actively listening. Other women approach pregnancy in different ways. For example, they may have a name and collection of personal articles for their fantasy infant even before conception, because they believe such a child is an eventuality in their lives.

The goal of prenatal testing is to evaluate the status

Chart 8–2

The Blue People of Troublesome Creek

This is the saga of an Appalachian family's strange malady and the doctor who put them back in the pink.

Six generations after a French orphan named Martin Fugate settled on the banks of Eastern Kentucky's Troublesome Creek with his red-headed American bride, his great-great-great-great-grandson was born in a modern hospital not far from where the creek still runs.

The boy inherited his father's lankiness and his mother's slightly nasal way of speaking.

What he got from Martin Fugate was dark blue skin. "It was almost purple," his father recalls.

Doctors were so astonished by the color of Benjy Stacy's skin that they raced him by ambulance from the maternity ward in the hospital near Hazard to a medical clinic in Lexington. Two days of tests produced no explanation for skin that was the color of a bruised plum.

A transfusion was being prepared when Benjy's grandmother spoke up. "Have you ever heard of the blue Fugates of Troublesome Creek?" she asked the doctors.

"My grandmother Luna on my dad's side was a blue Fugate. It was real bad in her," Alva Stacy, the boy's father, explains. "The doctors finally came to the conclusion that Benjy's condition was due to blood inherited from generations back."

Benjy lost his blue tint within a few weeks, and now he is about as normal a 7-year-old boy as you could hope to find. His lips and fingernails still turn a shade of purple-blue when he gets cold or angry, a quirk that so intrigued medical students after Benjy's birth that they would crowd around the baby and try to make him cry. "Benjy was a pretty big item in the hospital," his mother says with a grin.

Dark blue lips and fingernails are the only traces of Martin Fugate's legacy left in the boy, along with the recessive gene that has shaded many of the Fugates and their kin blue for the past 162 years.

They're known simply as the "blue people" in the hills and hollows around Troublesome and Ball Creeks. Most lived to their 80s and 90s without serious illness associated with the skin discoloration. For some, though, there was a pain not seen in laboratory tests. That was the pain of being blue in a world mostly shades of white to black.

There was always speculation in the hollows about what made the blue people blue—heart disease, a lung disorder, the possibility proposed by one old-timer that "their blood is just a little closer to their skin." But no one knew for sure, and doctors rarely paid visits to the remote creekside settlements where most of the "blue Fugates" lived until well into the 1950s. By the time a young hematologist from the University of Kentucky came down to Troublesome Creek in the 1960s to cure the blue people, Martin Fugate's descendants had multiplied their recessive genes all over the Cumberland Plateau.

Madison Cawein began hearing rumors about the blue people when he went to work at the University of Kentucky's Lexington medical clinic in 1960. "I'm a hematologist, so something like that perks up my ears," Cawein says, sipping a whiskey sour and letting his mind slip back to the summer he spent "tromping around the hills looking for blue people."

of the fetus. Its main advantage is the attainment of knowledge; the chief disadvantage is the potential moral and ethical dilemma faced by the parents should they be faced with a decision of what to do about a fetus with a now known defect. Such decisions may include whether to terminate or maintain the pregnancy. The screening tests described below include the most current guidelines (National Institutes of Health, 1995).

Maternal Serum Alpha-Fetoprotein

Maternal serum alpha-fetoprotein (MSAFP) measurement is recommended for all pregnant women between 16 to 18 weeks' gestation in centers with counseling and follow-up services, skilled ultrasound and amniocentesis capabilities, and reliable, standardized laboratories. MSAFP screens for neural tube defects (NTDs) and Down syndrome. This test is performed to measure the amount of fetal glycoprotein in the amniotic fluid or in maternal blood. The accuracy of this test requires knowing the exact gestational age of the fetus at the time the maternal blood sample is drawn, because there are false-positive and false-negative results associated with inaccurate dating of the fetus.

The MSAFP test detects approximately 80% of open NTDs (lesions not covered by skin) and 20% of infants with Down syndrome. The MSAFP level is *elevated* in the case of NTDs and *low* in Down syndrome (Moore &

Chart 8–2 *Continued*

The Blue People of Troublesome Creek

Cawein is no stranger to eccentricities of the body. He helped isolate an antidote for cholera, and he did some of the early work on levodopa, the drug for Parkinson's disease. But his first love, which he developed as an Army medical technician in World War II, was hematology. "Blood cells always looked so beautiful to me," he says.

Cawein would drive back and forth between Lexington and Hazard—an 8-hour ordeal before the tollway was built—and scour the hills looking for the blue people he'd heard rumors about. The American Heart Association had a clinic in Hazard, and it was there that Cawein met "a great big nurse" who offered to help him.

Her name was Ruth Pendergrass, and she had been trying to stir up medical interest in the blue people ever since a dark blue woman walked into the county health department one bitterly cold afternoon and asked for a blood test.

"She had been out in the cold and she was just *blue*!" recalls Pendergrass, who is now 69 and retired from nursing. "Her face and fingernails were almost indigo blue. It like to scared me to death! She looked like she was having a heart attack. I just knew that patient was going to die right there in the health department, but she wasn't a'tall alarmed. She told me that her family was the blue Combses who lived up on Ball Creek. She was a sister to one of the Fugate women."

About this same time, another of the blue Combses, named Luke, had taken his sick wife up to the clinic at Lexington. One look at Luke was enough to "get those doctors down here in a hurry," says Pendergrass, who joined Cawein to look for more blue people.

Trudging up and down the hollows, fending off "the two mean dogs that everyone had in their front yard," the doctor and nurse would spot someone at the top of a hill who looked blue and take off in wild pursuit. By the time they'd get to the top, the person would be gone. Finally, one day when the frustrated doctor was idling inside the Hazard clinic, Patrick and Rachel Ritchie walked in.

"They were bluer'n hell," Cawein says. "Well, as you can imagine, I really examined them. After concluding that there was no evidence of heart disease, I said 'Aha!' I started asking them questions: 'Do you have any relatives who are blue?' Then I sat down and we began to chart the family."

Cawein remembers the pain that showed on the faces of the Ritchie brother and sister. "They were really embarrassed about being blue," he says. "Patrick was all hunched down in the hall. Rachel was leaning against the wall. They wouldn't come into the waiting room. You could tell how much it bothered them to be blue."

After ruling out heart and lung diseases, the doctor suspected methemoglobinemia, a rare hereditary blood disorder that results from excess levels of methemoglobin in the blood. Methemoglobin, which is blue, is a nonfunctional form of the red hemoglobin that carries oxygen. It is the color of oxygen-depleted blood seen in the blue veins just beneath the skin.

Adapted from Trost, C. (1982). The blue people of Troublesome Creek. *Science '82*. Used with permission.

Persaud, 1993). About 90% of cases with elevated MSAFPs are not caused by NTDs but by multiple gestations, fetal death, other congenital anomalies, and erroneous calculation of the pregnancy's dates. A positive (elevated) MSAFP value must be followed by a repeat measurement; however, up to one third of repeated measurements are false positive. To discern the cause of elevated MSAFP, a level II ultrasound examination is often done. If the results are not clear, an amniocentesis may then be performed to measure amniotic alpha-fetoprotein (AFP) level. In fetuses with open NTDs and ventral wall defects (e.g., gastroschisis and omphalocele), AFP escapes into the amniotic fluid and the AFP level is quite high (National Institutes of Health, 1995).

Triple Marker Screening

Triple marker screening is a cluster of three maternal blood tests that has supplanted the use of MSAFP testing alone. These are MSAFP, human chorionic gonadotropin (hCG), and unconjugated estriol (UE). The screening is completed about week 16 of the pregnancy and beyond, at the same time the MSAFP test is done. Taken together, these three values provide a better basis for prediction for the presence of certain genetic conditions, including Down syndrome, trisomy 18, open NTDs, and other birth defects. The triple marker screening, like other screening tests, estimates the risk of the fetus having specific birth defects. The individual patient's results are compared in the computer with a large database of women her age, and the risk for a range of birth defects is calculated by comparison to this large sample size.

Chorionic Villus Sampling

Chorionic villus sampling (CVS) obtains trophoblastic tissue to detect chromosomal aberrations (National Institutes of Health, 1995). The physician obtains biopsy specimens by inserting either a needle through the mother's abdominal wall or a cannula through the vagina and cervical canal, guided by ultrasonography. The advantages of CVS are that it permits *karyotyping* (analysis of the fetal chromosomes) at 10 to 12 weeks' gestation and yields more rapid results than an amniocentesis, which cannot be done until week 14 or 15 at the very earliest. Its disadvantages include discrepancies between the karyotype of the villi and the fetus owing to contamination of the sample by nonfetal cells or placental mosaicism (nonfetal cells with different genetic material), miscarriage, chorioamnionitis (infection), and membrane damage; foreshortened limbs in some newborns; and a slightly higher complication rate than amniocentesis (National Institutes of Health, 1995).

Fetal Ultrasonography

The fetal ultrasound examination (sonogram) is a screening procedure that uses sonar (high-frequency sound waves) that is directed at the fetus to provide a detailed image of organs and skeletal structures. This can be done transvaginally, by the insertion of a probe into the mother's vagina, or transabdominally, by passing a transducer over the mother's skin where the uterus is palpated. The sonogram provides information about the placenta, umbilical cord, amniotic fluid volume, and fetal organs and skeletal structure. The procedure is performed early in pregnancy to determine presence of a heartbeat (as early as week 3 or 4 of postconception age), activity level, intrauterine gestational age, and structural defects such as NTDs and congenital heart disease. The procedure is noninvasive and readily available.

If problems are detected on the first, or level I, sonogram, subsequent and more detailed, level II (targeted) sonograms may be performed. Level II sonograms provide information such as

- Limb length
- Presence of a nuchal fold
- Bladder filling and voiding
- Condition of spinal column
- Outflow tracts and number of chambers in the heart
- Placental location and structure

Limb length and presence of a nuchal fold, among other characteristics, may indicate the possibility of chromosomal aberrations known as the trisomies, discussed later in this chapter. For accurate screening, the age of the pregnancy must be determined accurately. Level II sonograms are done at 17 weeks' gestation and beyond, with most of them being done before 20 weeks when used as a screening device for chromosomal aberrations. When hydrocephalus, NTDs, kidney problems, diaphragmatic hernias, or heart defects are suggested, level II ultrasonography and fetal echocardiography yield much information later in the pregnancy.

Amniocentesis

Actual diagnosis of chromosomal aberrations of some diseases transmitted at the single gene locus, and of the fetal gender can be made. The primary vehicle for this is amniocentesis. The most common prenatal test for detecting genetic disorders, amniocentesis should be offered routinely to pregnant women who will be 35 years old and older at the time of delivery because of their increased risk of chromosomal aberrations. The following list includes other candidates for amniocentesis (Hall, 1996):

- Women who have already given birth to a child with a chromosomal anomaly such as Down syndrome
- Couples who are known heterozygous carriers for an autosomal recessive disorder, such as Tay-Sachs disease
- Suspected or known carriers of a sex-linked recessive disorder
- Women who have had a child with an NTD and have an abnormal MSAFP in the current pregnancy

Pre-procedure counseling should include possible risks to the fetus (e.g., approximate 1% risk of miscarriage as a result of the procedure), the probability of a chromosomal aberration (given the patient's age), and any other information related to potential risks identified during genetic history-taking.

Amniocentesis is performed by inserting a fine needle through the wall of the uterus and into the amniotic sac of fluid containing the fetus. Amniotic fluid is withdrawn for DNA and biochemical analysis.

Ultrasonography is used to help guide the physician in inserting the needle properly. Assessment for NTDs and chromosomal disorders is routinely done with an amniocentesis. The procedure is performed at 14 to 16 weeks' gestation and beyond; before this time, there is very little amniotic fluid. Results usually take 10 days to 4 weeks to process. The advantages of amniocentesis are only a small risk of miscarriage, detection of approximately 90% of open NTDs, and very good resolution of chromosome structure. The disadvantages are that it must be done relatively late in the pregnancy and that the turnaround time for results is long.

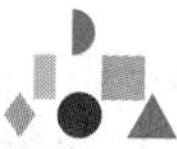

Genetic and Multifactorial Disorders

Perinatal and pediatric nurses must understand the principles of heredity and the sequence of organogenesis. They must be able to identify infants and children who vary from developmental norms. From 2% to 5% of genetic coding results in errors that become dysfunctional structures or physiologic functions. Some are deadly. Most errors in coding are not lethal but may cause some structural or physiologic alteration. Lethal errors are eventually selected out of the gene pool by evolution, because many of the affected do not survive to reproduce. For example, females with Turner's syndrome (46XO chromosome complement) cannot reproduce. Many females and most males with cystic fibrosis lack the ability to reproduce. This is changing with advances in science, and an increased number of females with cystic fibrosis are able to conceive and bear infants. Thus, individuals with formerly "lethal" genetic diseases are now "surviving to reproduce." Phenylketonuria is another example; a generation of phenylketonuric females who have been treated with exclusion diets are now of age to reproduce. Potential return to elevated levels of serum phenylalanine in the mother also has implications for the fetus. The scientific knowledge base regarding outcomes is incomplete.

A newborn nursery nurse might be the first individual to notice the appearance of an infant that sets it apart from others. The infant may have no obvious malformations, but other variations from normal may add up to a genetic syndrome. Some of the most common physical findings for infants at risk for a genetic disorder include polydactyly (extra fingers or toes); low-set ears; "rocker-bottom" feet (abnormally shaped like the rockers on a rocking chair); distinctive weak cries; "fright wig" pattern of hair distribution; and evidence of cardiac disease (difficulty eating and breathing).

When one defect is present, the nurse must suspect internal anomalies, such as heart or kidney malformations. An infant or child should never be labeled as abnormal or a "funny-looking kid." This label may be overheard by family members and be emotionally upsetting.

Heredity is the process by which all living things produce offspring like themselves. This capacity for self-reproduction involves the transmission from parent to offspring of information that specifies a certain pattern of growth and organization. *Genetics* is the study of heredity, examining the physical and chemical properties of hereditary material, how the material is transmitted in successive generations, and how the information is expressed in the development of an individual.

No one is immune to genetic anomalies. Each individual carries anywhere from 6 to 20 potentially fatal recessive genes, which are only expressed if two people who have the same gene have children. Genetic disorders are not always inherited; mutations or chromosomal aberrations can occur at any time.

Overview of Genetic Theory

This section presents fundamental concepts of genetics and selected, common genetic disorders. For more in-depth information, see the reference list, bibliography, and resources.

DNA (deoxyribonucleic acid) is the molecule that carries hereditary information and forms the chromosomes. *Chromosomes* are rod-shaped structures that contain genes or genetic information. Present in every cell, chromosomes are made up of protein and DNA. DNA stores genetic material. The *gene* is the basic unit of heredity; each gene has a specific location (locus) on a specific chromosome. There are thousands of genes in each cell controlling a specific function or trait. Genes function by controlling the function of other genes, specifying the structure of proteins, and specifying the structure of RNA (ribonucleic acid), which is necessary in the assembly of proteins (Raff, 1994).

DNA is a large molecule built from four different nucleotides (guanine, adenine, thymine, and cytosine) that are grouped in specific sequences to encode information. The order of the nucleotides determines the information that is carried. This information is transcribed into messenger RNA (mRNA), which provides a working copy of the genetic information from which proteins are made (Pickler & Munro, 1995).

Humans have 22 pairs of *autosomes* (chromosomes that transmit most traits and characteristics) and 1 pair of (two) *sex chromosomes* (that determine the gender of offspring) in each somatic cell of their bodies. Females have the genotype 46XX; males carry the 46XY genotype. All somatic cells of the body divide by *mitosis*, giving rise to two daughter cells. Each daughter cell contains the same number and type of chromosomes as the parent cell.

The sex cells in the parents' reproductive organs divide by *meiosis*, resulting in cell nuclei that contain half the chromosomal material. This condition is known as the *haploid complement* of genetic material. Until the ova (egg) and sperm from each parent unite to form a *zygote* (new individual), the chromosomal complement of the gamete cells remains haploid.

Cell division does not always occur perfectly. Chromosomal anomalies may result from a *disruption in the control of chromosome movement* during cell division or an *alteration in chromosome structure* that leads to abnormal chromosome behavior or a change in the number of genes (Raff, 1994).

Patterns of Inheritance in Genetic Disorders

Monogenic Conditions at the Single Gene Locus

When a gene cannot carry out the specific function, it is called *recessive*, and a lower-case letter is used to represent it. Two recessive genes are not always necessary for expression of a recessive characteristic. One alone will be expressed if there is no dominant allele present.

Not all traits coded at the single gene locus form genetic disorders. The clinical expression of a mutant allele results in a phenotype that is described in terms of inheritance patterns. Some traits form ordinary characteristics and features of an individual, such as eye color and familial baldness. Blue eye coloring is an autosomal recessive trait. Familial baldness in some males follows an X-linked inheritance pattern, passed on from mother to son. Because females have two X chromosomes, familial baldness is not expressed in the female offspring. The woman passes the trait to her male offspring with her X chromosome.

X-Linked Inheritance

The genes on the X chromosome are inherited and expressed differently from the genes on the autosomes. For instance, a man expresses a recessive gene on his X chromosome but it is not expressed in any of his children. Subsequently, some of the sons of his daughters exhibit the trait, but it does not appear in any of his son's children. This is called *skip-generation inheritance* (Nora & Fraser, 1989).

Most genes on the X chromosome do not have alleles (corresponding sites) on the Y chromosome. Allelic genes pair such that all the autosomes pair for their entire lengths; however, the X and Y pair only at a small region at their ends (allelic genes are present only at this small region). A male, therefore, will express almost all the genes on his single X (remember, male = XY), including those that are recessive. Females (XX) express only those recessive genes that are homozygous (carry the same trait). The genes on the X chromosome that have no allele on the Y chromosome are referred to as *X-linked*, or *sex-linked, genes*. Two well-known examples of X-linked recessive inheritance are color blindness and hemophilia (Leroy, 1992).

Autosomal Dominant Disorders

Autosomal dominant disorders (Table 8–1) include those associated with learning disabilities, behavioral abnormalities, or mental retardation, such as neurofibromatosis, tuberous sclerosis, and Huntington's disease (Leroy, 1992). Hereditary blindness and deafness are also inherited as autosomal dominant traits, but they do not adversely affect intellectual capabilities. Other examples of autosomal dominant disorders include Waardenburg's syndrome and achondroplasia. It is beyond the scope of this chapter to define each of these conditions. The reader is referred to the references, bibliography, and resources for further information.

Autosomal Recessive Disorders

Inherited metabolic diseases, or *inborn errors of metabolism*, result in an *enzyme deficiency* blocking a specific metabolic pathway (Table 8–2). When a genetic defect alters protein production, the body's metabolic processes are affected because the enzyme's function is altered. Enzyme deficiencies result in accumulation of harmful mate-

Table 8–1
Selected Autosomal Dominant Disorders

Disorder	Characteristic Features
Huntington's disease	Adult onset, progressive mental and motor deterioration
Neurofibromatosis (von Recklinghausen's disease)	Café au lait spots, internal and external tumor formation, growth abnormalities, highly variable expressivity; incidence, 1 in 3000 to 1 in 4000
Holt/Oram syndrome	Cardiac anomaly (atrial or ventricular septal defect), hypoplastic or absent thumb, occasionally anal atresia
Marfan syndrome	Long, thin extremities, joint laxity, pectus excavatum or carinatum, frequent femoral and inguinal hernias; variable expressivity, 1 in 60,000
Tuberous sclerosis	Intellectual impairment, seizures, adenoma sebaceum in "butterfly" distribution on face, bone cysts especially in hands; incidence, 1 in 100,000

Table 8–2
Selected Recessive Disorders

	Characteristic Features
X-Linked Recessive Disorders	
Hemophilia	Excessive bleeding from minor injuries; incidence, 1 in 10,000
Ichthyosis (also autosomal dominant and autosomal recessive forms)	"Fish-skin" appearance, especially on head, abdomen, and flexures
Menkes' syndrome	Progressive brain deterioration, tortuous cerebral and other arteries, bone changes, kinky hair
Lesch–Nyhan syndrome	Self-mutilation, spastic cerebral palsy, mental retardation
Duchenne muscular dystrophy	Progressive skeletal/cardiac muscle deterioration; one third are mentally retarded
Autosomal Recessive Disorders	
Sickle cell anemia	Chronic anemia, vaso-occlusive crises (due to intravascular sickling), poor growth, and development
Cystic fibrosis	Extremely thick mucus clogs passageways in lungs, liver, and pancreas; 1 in 1000 to 1 in 37,000 whites
Albinism	Decrease or absence of pigmentation of skin, hair, and eyes; seven types, different frequencies
Cooley anemia (true beta-thalassemia)	Severe anemia, frequent infections, hepatosplenomegaly, poor growth, hemochromatosis

rial or creation of abnormal metabolites. These metabolites build up to create biochemical abnormalities, many of which ultimately are incompatible with life. In an affected infant who appears normal at birth, developmental delays may be picked up at well-baby visits or the infant may die unexpectedly.

Most inborn errors of metabolism are rare. The more common ones are covered in detail in Chapter 27. Inborn errors of metabolism include disorders of amino acid metabolism, organic acid metabolism, lysosomal storage, carbohydrate metabolism, and lipid metabolism.

Disorders of amino acid metabolism include maple syrup urine disease and phenylketonuria. Amino acids are the primary components of proteins, and some also function as neurotransmitters or act as intermediates in metabolic cycles. Because their functions are essential to life, defects in their metabolism can have significant effects. (For details, see Chapter 27.)

Disorders of organic acid metabolism (or organic acidemias) are due to catabolic defects of amino acid(s) or pyruvate. Symptoms occur at any time between the neonatal period and early childhood. The striking presentation of these diseases is *unexplained severe ketoacidosis*. Other laboratory findings include hypoglycemia (from the interference of gluconeogenesis by metabolites) and hyperammonemia (from suppressed urea cycle enzyme function).

Lysosomal storage diseases are largely inherited in an autosomal recessive manner. They result from the deficiency of one or more lysosomal enzymes, which causes an accumulation of mucopolysaccharides (mucus forming), glycoproteins, or sphingolipids (phospholipids found in the brain and other nerve tissue), or a combination of these substances. Lysosomal storage diseases involve the skeleton, central nervous system, and viscera (Pennock, 1994).

Galactosemia is the classic carbohydrate disorder. Most galactose in the diet comes from the breakdown of lactose, the major disaccharide found in milk. Normal metabolism of large amounts of galactose is typically not a problem. However, in classic galactosemia, an inborn error in galactose metabolism is inherited as an autosomal recessive disorder and causes serious problems if lactose is consumed. The frequency is approximately 1 in 50,000 (Dunger & Holton, 1994). Although lipid disorders of metabolism are rare, the two most common ones are Tay-Sachs disease and Gaucher's disease type I. Both are especially prevalent among those with Ashkenazi Jewish genetic heritage.

Chromosomal Aberrations

When a genetic disorder is the result of an entire chromosome being repeated more than once (nondisjunction) or of a large piece of one chromosome erroneously attaching to another (translocation) during meiosis, the result is a chromosomal aberration. Chromosomal aberrations may be present with either the autosomes or the sex chromosomes. Down syndrome, for example, can occur either through a trisomy of autosome 21 (there are three chromosomes 21 instead of two) or through a translocation of chromosome 21 that attaches to another one of the autosomes. Chromosomal aberrations occur during the process of meiosis of the parental gametes, usually oogenesis in the mother, resulting in aneuploidy.

Trisomies are the result of an extra, or third, chromosome (nondisjunction) going to one of the gamete cells during meiosis (haploid reproduction) or a large additional piece of genetic material (translocation) to a chromosome that subsequently causes congenital malformations. Persons with trisomies 13, 18, and 21 present with remarkable, consistent features. Other trisomies, such as trisomy 8 and trisomy 22, may occur but are rare.

Trisomy 13: Patau's Syndrome

The infant with trisomy 13 is distinguishable at birth, presenting with a small cranium, broad nose, hypotelorism (eyes set closely together), and, frequently, cleft lip and palate. These midline abnormalities of the face predict the abnormalities of the brain, together known as holoprosencephaly. Cardiac defects may include ventral and atrial septal defects, dextrocardia, and anomalous valves. Approximately 50% of these infants also present with myelomeningocele. Severe mental retardation is associated with this disorder. Most infants do not survive past age 1. The frequency is approximately 1 in 15,000 live births (Moore & Persaud, 1993).

Trisomy 18: Edwards' Syndrome

Infants born with trisomy 18 also have specific characteristics. These include low-set ears, hypotonia, short palpebral fissures (eye slits), micrognathia (small chin), small mouth (pinched-face appearance), and epicanthal folds. They also have clenched fists, with the index and pinky finger characteristically overlapping the third and fourth fingers; rocker-bottom feet; mottled skin; cardiac and renal abnormalities; skeletal deformities; and a feeble cry. These infants are smaller than normal. Severe mental retardation occurs with this syndrome, and survival is about 10 weeks of age, although some children do survive into childhood.

Trisomy 21: Down Syndrome

Down syndrome produces specific physical characteristics, including a broad, flat face; round cheeks; eyes obliquely placed; narrow palpebral fissures; a small nose; a long, thick tongue; broad hands; and stubby fingers (Pueschel, 1992). Down syndrome causes limited intellectual ability, owing to the presence of three chromosomes 21 rather than two for most people. Most children with Down syndrome (92% to 95%) have trisomy 21. Translocation accounts for approximately 5% of Down syndrome, and mosaicism occurs in 3%. Advanced maternal age is an established factor in the occurrence of Down syndrome. No paternal age is associated with an increase in new autosomal gene mutations.

Down syndrome is the most common autosomal chromosomal aberration in live-born infants, with an incidence of 1 in 1000 (Pueschel, 1992). At present, less than 20% of children with Down syndrome are born to women older than 35 years of age at the time of delivery, whereas 30 years ago, approximately 50% were offspring of mothers older than 35 (Pueschel, 1992). The decline is attributed to prenatal testing such as amniocentesis or chorionic villus sampling. Down syndrome is not race specific.

Theories about the causes of Down syndrome include a genetic predisposition to nondisjunction, maternal ovarian or other radiation exposure, infectious diseases, autoimmune disorders, and hormonal alterations in women of advanced maternal age. Evidence supports multiple causality (Pueschel, 1992).

Phenotypic expression of Down syndrome can vary dramatically. Some characteristics change over time; for example, palpebral fissures and abundant neck tissue become less prominent with increasing age, but a fissured tongue becomes more apparent as the child grows (Pueschel, 1992). Some characteristics commonly occur and are considered to be typical of the person with Down syndrome. However, all physical features do not appear in every child with the syndrome (Chart 8–3). Many of these features do not inhibit the child's abilities. For example, slanted palpebral fissures, heavy epicanthal

Chart 8–3

Common Clinical Features in Infants with Down Syndrome

Separated sagittal suture
Oblique palpebral fissure
Wide space between first and second toes
False fontanelle
Plantar crease between first and second toes
Hyperflexibility
Increased neck tissue
Abnormally shaped palate
Hypoplastic nose
Muscle weakness
Hypotonia
Brushfield spots
Mouth kept open
Protruding tongue
Epicanthal folds
Single palmar crease
Brachyclinodactyly
Short, stubby hands
Flattened occiput
Abnormal size of ears
Short, stubby feet
Abnormal structure of ears

From Pueschel, S.M. (1992). The child with Down syndrome. In M. D. Levine, W. B. Carey, & A. C. Crocker (Eds.), *Developmental-Behavioral Pediatrics* (2nd ed., p. 221). Philadelphia: W. B. Saunders. Reprinted with permission.

folds, and Brushfield spots (in the iris of each eye) do not interfere with the child's vision. Other defects, such as congenital heart disease and duodenal atresia, are life threatening and require prompt medical attention.

Developmental Expectations. In children with Down syndrome, mental abilities range from severe retardation to near-average intelligence. Most of them function in the mild to moderate range of mental retardation. Some have been found to have intelligence in the borderline to low-average range of intelligence, and only a few are severely retarded. Behavior and emotional disposition also vary from the placid, inactive child to one who is aggressive and hyperactive, with most falling in between. Stereotyped expectations are problematic for families where there is a person with Down syndrome.

Classic research revealed that the responses of infants with Down syndrome in strange situations are qualitatively similar to those of nonretarded children (Berry, Gunn, & Andrews, 1980). It appears that children with Down syndrome were more sensitive in unfamiliar situations, when separated from their mother, and in the presence of a new person, indicating that early social awareness of infants with Down syndrome seems to be quite developed. Other studies (Pueschel, 1992) noted the same range of behavior in children with Down syndrome as children of 46XX or 46XY karyotypes: there were remarkable similarities in terms of social behavior and interaction patterns.

The growth rate of children with Down syndrome is slower than normal. Children with Down syndrome may also have significant gastrointestinal problems, such as Hirschsprung's disease, or severe cardiac conditions.

caREminder: *Advise parents to promote good eating habits in the very young child, when slow growth is most commonly a problem.*

Parents often ask about the child's motor development and want to know if the child will achieve developmental milestones within the "normal" range (Table 8–3). Children with Down syndrome display varying degrees of developmental delay.

caREminder: *Point out to parents that their child will make steady progress in overall development. Also note that there is no reason for them not to become productive, self-assured members of society, from whom nonaffected individuals can learn a great deal.*

Children whose parents provide a nurturing and stimulating environment and who are enrolled in an early intervention program should exhibit relatively advanced development. Children with severe cardiac disease cannot be expected to develop as well because much of their energy is going into the exchange of oxygen and nutrients.

Table 8–3
Developmental Milestones and Skills in Children with Down Syndrome

	Average (months)	Range (months)
Milestone		
Smiling	2	1.5–3
Rolling over	6	2–12
Sitting	9	6–18
Crawling	11	7–21
Creeping	13	8–25
Standing	10	10–32
Walking	20	12–45
Talking, words	14	9–30
Talking, sentences	24	18–46
Skill		
Eating		
Finger feeding	12	8–28
Using spoon/fork	20	12–40
Toilet training		
Bladder	48	20–95
Bowel	42	28–90
Dressing		
Undressing	40	29–72
Putting clothes on	58	38–98

From Pueschel, S. M. The child with Down syndrome. (1992). In Levine, M. D., Carey, W. B., & Crocker, A. C. (Eds.), *Developmental-behavioral pediatrics* (2nd ed., p. 225). Philadelphia: W. B. Saunders. Reprinted with permission.

Well-Child Care. Children with Down syndrome need the same kind of well-child care as any other children, including immunizations, attention to medical emergencies, and family support. They also require some special health care attention (Chart 8–4).

Educational Intervention. Reports suggest that early learning interventions and experiences may result in progress that would normally not be observed in infants with Down syndrome who did not have such learning opportunities. Children in early intervention programs can benefit from sensory stimulation, exercises involving fine and gross motor activities, and instruction in language acquisition (Pueschel, 1992).

Self-help skills, such as feeding, toilet training, and dressing foster independence and should be taught. Parents can be guided in continuing to provide a rich environment that will promote the child's development and

Chart 8–4

Special Health Care Needs of Children with Down Syndrome

- Audiometric assessment should be done early. Hearing deficits occur in 70% to 80%. If significant impairment or chronic otitis media is present, refer patient to audiologist.
- Congenital heart disease occurs in 40% to 45% of population. Best evaluation and follow-up is done by a pediatric cardiologist.
- Errors of visual refraction and cataracts are common ocular disturbances. Best initial evaluation and necessary treatment is done by an ophthalmologist.
- Appropriate anticipatory nutritional guidance is indicated, with best results measured by outcomes (e.g., growth parameter comparisons). In infancy, failure to thrive is common and related to congenital conditions such as cardiac disease or duodenal atresia. In adolescence, obesity may become problematic for some.
- Uncompensated or compensated hypothyroidism occurs in 20% of population. This can further contribute to brain function; therefore, testing of thyroid function studies (TSH, T_3 and T_4) is recommended at regular intervals. Initiate thyroid hormone replacement on diagnosis, so that normal learning processes may be optimized.
- Skeletal, immunologic, metabolic, biochemical, and oncologic issues may require the attention of respective specialists.

enhance family life. Each child, as an individual, has the basic right to quality of life.

Turner's Syndrome

The cause of Turner's (45XO) syndrome is a chromosomal aberration in the number of sex chromosomes present (Hagerman, 1992). One of the two X chromosomes normally found in females is missing (Nora & Fraser, 1989). It produces short stature, webbed neck, gonadal dysgenesis (lack of sexual development), low hairline in the back, and cubitus valgus (arms that turn out at the elbow). Turner's syndrome is a relatively common genetic disorder (1 in 2000) that affects only females. It occurs as result of nondisjunction (Nora & Fraser, 1989).

All females do not exhibit all features of the Turner syndrome constellation. In an infant, the astute nurse may notice lymphedema (puffy hands and feet). In a prepubescent girl, other common features may include micrognathia (small jaw), fingernails that turn up at the end, short metacarpals (especially the fourth and fifth), and pigmented nevi (small moles on the skin). Cardiovascular malformations occur in 25% of these individuals (Rieser & Underwood, 1989).

The most common feature of Turner's syndrome is short stature. Infants with this syndrome are often less than 18½ inches long at birth. Until age 3 years, growth may proceed at a normal pace, then it slows down. The female with this syndrome notices that she is relatively shorter than her friends of the same age. If the individual is untreated, the pubertal growth spurt does not occur, and many females grow at a slow rate into their 20s. The adult woman with Turner's syndrome reaches an average height of 142 cm (4′8″). The cause of short stature in females with Turner's syndrome is not fully understood, but one important factor is the impaired ability of their bones to grow. Lack of growth hormone has been implicated by some researchers, but further research is needed to find effective treatment (Rieser & Underwood, 1989).

The other hallmark of Turner's syndrome is lack of sexual maturation, that is, lack of breast development, menses, and feminine body contours. This occurs because the ovaries, which produce female hormones (estrogen and progesterone) and ova, are not completely developed. If estrogen and progesterone are not produced, sexual development occurs only by replacing hormones with medication. With incomplete ovarian development, few or no ova are stored. Therefore, most females with Turner's syndrome cannot conceive a child, even though their fallopian tubes, uterus, and vagina function normally. Some females (5%–10%) exhibit signs of breast development between age 10 and 12 years, but rarely does it continue through puberty (Hagerman, 1992).

In the mosaic form of this syndrome, some of the individual's somatic cells contain a normal complement of chromosomes whereas others do not (46XX, 45X). There are more likely to be signs of sexual development without treatment, although it is unlikely that menstruation or full development will occur. In untreated girls from age 10 to 12 years, sparse pubic and axillary hair may be present owing to the normal amounts of androgens produced by the adrenal glands.

Individuals with Turner's syndrome typically have normal IQs. However, they may have a visuospatial deficit, which may lead to problems with drawing, handwriting, map reading, and related tasks (Nora & Fraser, 1989). If school performance is a concern, psychological testing should be performed so that appropriate teaching strategies can be implemented before the child falls behind. Parents and teachers should have the same academic expectations for the child with Turner's syndrome as for other children but should remain alert for clues to potential problems.

Androgen therapy is frequently used to stimulate growth in females with Turner's syndrome. Low doses achieve the desired results without causing adverse effects. Unfortunately, androgens may expedite bone maturation by premature closure of epiphyseal plates, hastening the end of growth. See Chapter 26 for further details of hormonal treatment of the child with Turner's syndrome. It is important to bear in mind that women with Turner's syndrome may expect to have a healthy and satisfying sexual life, just as any other woman.

Growing up is challenging for any child. Growing up with an obvious difference in height or appearance may create challenges that may impede abilities to develop a strong sense of self. Parents are instrumental in their child's development and adjustment. The nurse should give appropriate information to the parents, while reiterating that the learning process will continue over the months and years as issues arise. Parents need support in raising their child in a world that can be unkind to anyone who is different. However, they are not encouraged to overprotect the child. The nurse can offer ways for the parents to make life easier for a short child (Chart 8–5). At some point, the young woman with Turner's syndrome may seek professional counseling or a support group, such as a local chapter of the Turner's Syndrome Society of America (see Resources).

Women with Turner's syndrome should be offered the same options for having children as other women with fertility problems. Anticipatory guidance is an important aspect of nursing care for patients with Turner's syndrome and their families. The knowledgeable nurse can help parents of toddlers and preschoolers with Turner's syndrome develop a plan to explain how women can become mothers. A developmentally simple approach is used depending on the girl's age. Introducing adolescents and young adults to the possibility of in-vitro fertilization with donor ova, including potential benefits and limitations, can bring a sense of hopefulness to the young woman with Turner's syndrome (Vockrodt & Williams, 1994).

Chart 8–5
Community Care

Facilitating Adjustment to Short Stature

- Lower mirrors and closet rods, and have steady footstools throughout the house.
- Give the child the same responsibilities at home (no excuses from household chores just because of his or her size).
- Dress the child according to his or her age, not size, realizing that this may involve having clothes altered.
- Encourage activities that allow for competition and the chance to learn to work and play with others (e.g., drama, dance, sports, 4H clubs).
- Refer to support groups, such as a chapter of the Turner's Syndrome Society of America.

Klinefelter's Syndrome

Klinefelter's syndrome is considered to be the most common sex chromosomal aneuploidy, a result of nondisjunction during meiosis of the mother's ovum. These individuals have one or more extra X chromosomes (Hagerman, 1992). The basic abnormality is when a male has 47 chromosomes with a sex chromosome complement of XXY, rather than 46XY. The incidence is approximately 1 in 800 live births (Cohen & Durham, 1985).

There are no distinguishing characteristics at birth, although up to 25% of infants may exhibit anomalies such as malformed ears, clinodactyly, genitourinary anomalies, and various skeletal deformities (Cohen & Durham, 1985). During childhood, these males appear to be normal. Many individuals are detected during adolescence because of delayed development of secondary sex characteristics or learning/behavioral difficulties or in adult life because of infertility.

During puberty, the testes do not fully develop, remaining only about half the size of those of normal males. Penile growth and size is normal. Owing to the low testosterone level and the high follicle-stimulating hormone level, these boys develop fatty deposits on their hips and may develop gynecomastia (breast enlargement). Individuals with Klinefelter's syndrome can have sexual intercourse, but they are sterile because of abnormal spermatogenesis.

The male with Klinefelter's syndrome is often tall with disproportionately long lower limbs. He may experience gross motor incoordination that causes feelings of awkwardness (Collins, 1995). Boys with this syndrome have exhibited difficulties with school performance, possibly owing to reduction in auditory processing, storage, retrieval ability, and language development (Cohen & Durham, 1985). Intelligence testing reveals normal performance IQ but reduced verbal IQ (Cohen & Durham, 1985).

The individual with Klinefelter's syndrome is also at risk for psychosocial problems because of an altered body image (Connaughty, 1992). Puberty is stressful enough for normal adolescents; those with Klinefelter's syndrome experience even more stress, with gender confusion due to breast enlargement, sparse facial hair, fatty deposits on the hips, and alienation as peer comparisons are made. Delay in language development and inadequate verbal skills contributes to the difficulties such boys have in

Chart 8–6

Nursing Considerations for Patients with Klinefelter's Syndrome

- Recognize each family member's need for time to process feelings about this diagnosis.
- Assess the client/family's need for education.
- Assess the need for counseling related to sexuality, gender identification, and infertility.
- Address the question to whom the family wants to disclose this information.
- Provide information about increased health and educational risks.

dealing with their peers. Any problems not resolved during adolescence may lead to inferiority feelings that persist throughout life.

Medical treatment of Klinefelter's syndrome involves administering testosterone injections to induce a more masculine appearance and to improve emotional maturity. If these injections are continued during adulthood, careful monitoring is advised (Collins, 1995).

Nursing can be of great assistance to the patient and family with Klinefelter's syndrome through case finding, counseling, referral, and education (Chart 8–6). The nurse must first be comfortable with and knowledgeable about this disorder and key issues.

Fragile X Syndrome

In 1991, the gene coding for fragile X syndrome was isolated and was designated *FMR1* (fragile X mental retardation). Fragile X syndrome is the most common human chromosomal anomaly associated with heritable mental retardation in males (Tarleton & Saul, 1993). Males and females may be affected, thus, fragile X syndrome is considered to be a dominant X-linked disorder with reduced penetrance in females (approximately one third will express clinical findings).

The characteristic long, narrow face with prominent ears is common in adults. However, prepubertal males more typically exhibit puffiness around the eyes, strabismus (crossed-eyes), elongated and narrow palpebral fissures, large head (greater than 50th percentile) relative to body size, and prominent ears (long, wide, or protruding). Other findings, such as epicanthal folds and low-set ears, are much less common. Macro-orchidism (large testes) is the next physical finding most commonly seen in fragile X syndrome (Goldson & Hagerman, 1992).

Orthopedic problems in children with the fragile X syndrome are pes planus (flatfoot), scoliosis, and joint laxity. Joint laxity occurs in approximately 73% of children younger than 11 years of age, and the incidence decreases with age. Musculoskeletal hypotonia is also a common finding.

Behavioral characteristics are striking in fragile X syndrome and have been significant in leading clinicians to the diagnosis. Hyperactivity, autism, tics, and aggressive outbursts are the presenting complaints of many males with this condition (Goldson & Hagerman, 1992). Autistic-like behaviors occur in some fragile X syndrome boys, with the most severely retarded carrying the diagnosis of autism. However, most children with fragile X syndrome are interested in relating socially but are anxious and easily overstimulated. They also exhibit hand biting, hand flapping, hyperactivity, and poor eye contact. Aggressive outbursts may be triggered by environmental stress, causing the child to lose control. In addition, they may misinterpret social approaches as threatening, which may lead to aggressive responses.

Cognitive patterns are confusing. Fragile X syndrome males may exhibit strength in areas of memory, vocabulary, and visual-perceptual tasks, such that reading and spelling are surprisingly better than their IQ would predict. However, they are weak in abstract reasoning (noticeable in the school-age child), sequential processing, and mathematics. These children are typically impulsive, making it difficult for them to focus on a cognitive task for more than a few minutes. As a result, tasks that require sequential processing are difficult for them. Enormous advances in cytogenetics led to the recognition and description of the fragile X syndrome, so named because of its association with a rare folate-sensitive fragile site in chromosomal band Xq27.3. The cytogenetic test for this syndrome has been available for a number of years, but there are some problems (Tarleton & Saul, 1993). Not all cells in affected males show the fragile site. Also, transmitting males do not demonstrate a cytogenetic abnormality, and many carrier females appear cytogenetically normal. Recent advances include the sequencing of the *FMR1* gene and the identification of an unstable repetitive sequence within the FMR1 region. When the number of repetitions becomes excessive, silencing of the *FMR1* gene occurs, and the FMR1 protein is not produced. Fragile X syndrome is caused by the lack of this protein, although the function of the protein is not known.

DNA testing has identified many more carriers who were previously cytogenetically negative. This testing has shown that all mothers of fragile X syndrome–positive males are carriers. It has also been suggested that the carrier rate may be as high as 1 in 500 in the general population. However, large-scale screening has not been done. Therefore, all individuals with mental retardation or autism of unknown etiology should be screened with

DNA testing to detect the fragile X chromosome or any other chromosomal abnormality causing developmental delays (Tarleton & Saul, 1993).

No cure exists for fragile X syndrome, but the child's development and behavior can be improved through the combined efforts of professionals in education, language and motor therapy, counseling, and medicine. Infants and toddlers are hypotonic and have temper tantrums and sleeping difficulties. Infant stimulation and early intervention programs in a developmental preschool should include occupational, physical, and language therapy. All members of the interdisciplinary team should work closely with the parents to help them understand their child's strengths and weaknesses and to help them deal with behavior problems. Infants and toddlers do not usually receive medications, except for folic acid, and its use is controversial.

School-age children present with attention deficits, language difficulties, and impulsivity. These are significant problems for approximately 80% of fragile X syndrome males and 30% of the females. Speech and language therapy is essential and should focus on auditory processing and abstract reasoning skills. Occupational therapy is helpful in improving fine and gross motor coordination. Sensory integration therapy helps with attention deficits and tantrums related to overstimulation. Stimulant medications may be used in some children but can cause such adverse effects as mood lability and irritability.

Congenital Anomalies

Congenital anomalies (birth defects or congenital malformations) are defects that are present at birth. They may be caused by genetic factors, environmental factors, or both (multifactorial inheritance). Congenital anomalies are a leading cause of infant mortality in the United States. Anomalies may exist as a single or multiple occurrence, and they may be of minor or major clinical significance. An example of the gravity of one form of these anomalies serves to illustrate possible outcomes for the child and family. When a child is born, the first news the parents and other family members want to hear is whether it is a boy or girl. When an infant is delivered with ambiguous-appearing genitalia, it is imperative that a delay phase be built in before announcing the infant's gender to extended family and friends. Extreme emotional damage can ensue in a family when the gender of an infant has been announced to family and friends and then changed.

There are many other situations in which there may be an extreme emotional impact on the family without the correct psychosocial interventions.

Approximately 90% of infants born with three or more minor anomalies also have one or more major anomalies (Moore & Persaud, 1993). Major defects are more common in early embryos, but, when affected, most result in spontaneous abortions. Chromosome abnormalities account for 50% to 60% of spontaneous abortions. Most of the major anomalies are fully covered in Unit 4, Managing Health Challenges. Table 8–4 lists selected congenital anomalies.

Teratogens and Environmental Exposures

Embryonic or fetal growth may be disturbed so that a structural or functional defect is produced. An agent ca-

Text continued on page 443

Table 8–4
Summary of Selected Congenital Anomalies

System	Specific Anomaly	Clinical Manifestations	Interventions
Nervous System			
Neural tube defects		Most CNS anomalies occur during weeks 3–8 of embryonic development.	
Spinal column	Spina bifida cystica	Many variations; nonfusion anomalies of vertebral arches; spinal cord spills out into meningeal sac.	Surgical repair of open sac; shunting if hydrocephalus is present
	Spina bifida occulta	Small, pilonidal dimple, often with tuft of hair in L5 or S1 vertebrae; incidence: 1 in 10 people.	No treatment or cosmetic repair in later life

Table continued on following page

Table 8–4
Summary of Selected Congenital Anomalies *Continued*

System	Specific Anomaly	Clinical Manifestations	Interventions
Nervous System *Continued*			
Brain	Congenital hydrocephalus	Increased intracranial pressure and all of its symptoms: decreasing level of consciousness; widening pulse pressure; rising and elevated systolic blood pressure; sunset sign (top of sclera over iris becomes visible when eyes are open); bulging anterior fontanelle; lethargy; somnolence.	Surgical placement of shunts
	Anencephaly	Congenital absence of all major structures of the brain; death usually precedes birth or occurs shortly afterward.	None; referral to transplant program as appropriate
Eye		In general, eye anomalies are uncommon. Most result from defects in closure of the optic fissure during week 4 of embryonic development.	Symptomatic as per degree of impaired vision
	Coloboma of eyelid	Uncommon; small or large notch in upper eyelid	None or cosmetic
	Coloboma of iris	"Keyhole" appearance in pupil; possible involvement of ciliary body and retina	Visual correction as indicated
	Congenital cataract	Lens opaque; grayish white; possibly related to galactosemia or teratogens (such as rubella)	Surgical correction
	Congenital ptosis of the eyelid	Drooping of one or both upper eyelids.	Visual correction
Ear	Many minor, clinically insignificant abnormalities of the auricle. Severe malformations are often associated with chromosomal aberrations.	Low-set pinna top is observable below eye–occiput line.	Cosmetic; presence alerts observer to look for more serious, associated anomalies (cardiac and renal).
Integumentary System			
Ichthyoses	Develop during weeks 3–8 of embryonic development and beyond; genetic.		
	Harlequin fetus	Skin is extremely thick, rigid, and cracked. Death usually occurs within first week of life.	None
	Collodion baby	Covered by thick, taut membrane that cracks with initiation of respirations; membrane sheds after several weeks.	None
	Lamellar ichthyosis	Autosomal recessive; appears similar to collodion baby, except scaling persists; development of sweat glands hampered; hair growth impaired.	Keep in cool environment, especially in hot weather.
	Congenital ectodermal dysplasia	Hereditary: rare; partial failure of the epidermis to develop; dental abnormalities; absence of body hair.	Supportive; prosthetic

Table 8–4
Summary of Selected Congenital Anomalies *Continued*

System	Specific Anomaly	Clinical Manifestations	Interventions
Integumentary System *Continued*			
Angiomas	Nevus flammeus	Flat, pink or red flamelike blotch usually seen on back of neck.	No specific treatment
	Port wine stain (hemangioma)	Larger and darker than nevus flammeus; usually on anterolateral face or neck. When found in distribution of trigeminal nerve, it is sometimes associated with Sturge-Weber syndrome (angioma of meninges and brain).	No specific treatment
	"Strawberry" marks	Very common in neonates; regress with growth	No specific treatment
Hair anomalies	Albinism	Hypopigmentation due to lack of melanin in the skin	No specific treatment
	Alopecia	Absence or loss of hair due to failure of follicles to develop or those that produce poor quality hairs	No specific treatment
	Hypertrichosis	Excessive hair due to supernumerary follicles or persistence of hairs that normally disappear after birth	No specific treatment
	Pili torti	Familial disorder in which hairs are twisted and bent; associated with other ectodermal defects.	No specific treatment
Nail anomalies	Anonychia	Rare; absence of nails; permanent and associated with poor development of hair and dental anomalies	Cosmetic
Respiratory System			
Pharyngeal apparatus anomalies	Arise from gill arch mesodermal layer during weeks 3–8 of embryonic development; there are cysts or possible sinus tracts to the outer layer of the skin; may affect tongue, thyroid gland, and palate.		
	Tongue surface	Unusual to see abnormalities; most fissures common in Down syndrome.	Surgical reduction for cosmetic effect in extreme cases of enlargement
	Papillae of tongue	Hypertrophy	
	Congenital cysts and fistulas	Derived from remnants of the thyroglossal duct; pharyngeal discomfort and dysplagia (difficulty swallowing)	Surgery as necessary; speech therapy and other supportive care as necessary.
	Ankyloglossia (tongue-tied)	Frenulum (normally connects inferior surface of tongue to floor of mouth). Free protrusion impaired; speech difficulties with letters and sounds that require tongue thrust (T, D, L, N, S, Z, R, Th); poor sucking in neonates; poor chewing and swallowing; incidence, 0.2–6.8 in 1000	Frenulum may split naturally or require surgical release.

Table continued on following page

Table 8-4
Summary of Selected Congenital Anomalies *Continued*

System	Specific Anomaly	Clinical Manifestations	Interventions
Respiratory System *Continued*			
	Macroglossia	Excessively large tongue; uncommon; most often seen in Down syndrome and other chromosomal aberrations; generalized hypertrophy, usually due to a lymphangioma (benign lymph tumor)	Surgical reduction (elective)
	Microglossia	Extremely rare; abnormally small tongue often associated with micrognathia (small mandible, recessed chin) and limb defects (Hanhart syndrome)	No treatments or cosmetic surgery in conjunction with other anomalies
	Thyroid-ectopic gland	Incomplete descent of the thyroid so that gland remains high in the neck; possible erroneous excision, creating permanent dependence on thyroid medication	Endocrinologist follow-up
	Accessory thyroid tissue	Can be found in tongue or in neck above the gland; an accessory gland may develop in the neck, but usually there is not enough tissue to sustain function.	Endocrinologist follow-up
	Thyroglossal duct cysts and sinuses	Persistence of embryonic thyroglossal duct; results in cysts in tongue or neck structures inferior to hyoid bone; swelling develops as a progressively enlarging, movable mass; asymptomatic if uninfected; sinus tracts to the skin sometimes follow infection and skin is perforated.	Surgical excision when symptomatic
	Cleft palate and lip	Weeks 6–9 of embryonic development; split or fissure often occur together; can occur separately; classified according to developmental criteria; atypical facial appearance, feeding problems and speech impediments; related to many causes: multifactorial, single mutant genes, pharmaceutical teratogens, chromosomal aberrations (especially trisomy 13); incidence of cleft lip, 1 in 1000; incidence of cleft palate, 1 in 2500	Surgical repair in stages
	Chest anomalies		
	Diaphragm	Possibly life threatening, especially in transition to extrauterine environment; includes eventration and congenital diaphragmatic hernia (CDH); protrusion of abdominal contents into chest cavity in CDH; 97% of CDHs are unilateral; both conditions are life threatening	Surgical palliation and long-term ventilatory support as indicated; fetal surgery for CDH.

Table 8–4
Summary of Selected Congenital Anomalies *Continued*

System	Specific Anomaly	Clinical Manifestations	Interventions
Respiratory System *Continued*			
	Tracheoesophageal fistulas (four major types)	Incomplete partitioning by tracheoesophageal septum; abnormal communication between trachea and esophagus; incidence, 1 in 2500; more males affected; 85% associated with esophageal atresia (blind pouch); saliva accumulates in the mouth and upper respiratory tract; chemical pneumonitis (burns of lungs by gastric contents) as a result of stomach contents reflux	Surgical repair
	Hypoplastic lung(s)	Poor lung development in utero	Death usually ensues shortly after birth.
Cardiovascular System			
	Congenital heart defects	Many; common, affecting about 6 in 1000 live births; causes mostly unknown; occur between weeks 3–8 of embryonic development.	Surgical repair or palliation now possible for most anomalies.
Digestive System Anomalies			
	General defects	Foregut, midgut, and hindgut anomalies form in week 4 of embryonic development.	
	Esophageal atresia	Blockage of esophagus resulting in polyhydramnios	Surgical correction
	Esophageal stenosis	Narrowed esophageal lumen—usually in distal third	Surgical correction
	Pyloric stenosis	Thickened pyloric sphincter leading to narrowed canal and projectile vomiting	Surgical correction
	Duodenal atresia	Partial occlusion of lumen; bile-stained vomitus	Surgical correction
	Extrahepatic biliary atresia	Obstruction at porta hepatis; jaundice	Surgical palliation; possible liver transplantation
	Annular pancreas	Ringlike band of pancreas obstructs duodenum; pancreatitis.	Supportive care
	Most are related to changes on the genome; may accompany other anomalies or occur by themselves		
Musculoskeletal System			
	Accessory ribs	May be either primitive and vestigial or well developed; lumbar most common—no problems; cervical less common, genetic; may be unilateral or bilateral; symptoms related to pressure on brachial plexus or subclavian artery	Symptomatic
	Hemivertebra	Failure of half of the vertebra to form embryonically creating scoliosis (lateral curvature)	Surgery as indicated

Table continued on following page

Table 8–4
Summary of Selected Congenital Anomalies *Continued*

System	Specific Anomaly	Clinical Manifestations	Interventions
Musculoskeletal System *Continued*			
	Rachischisis (cleft vertebral column)	Complex group of vertebral abnormalities that affect axial structures; vertebral and neural defects may be extensive or restricted to a small area.	Symptomatic
	Craniosynostosis	Premature closure of skull sutures; probably genetic in origin. The particular suture that closes determines the shape of the deformity; more common in males.	Surgical release
	Achondroplasia (dwarfism)	Specific constellation of abnormalities including short stature and other differently formed bones; associated with sperm in older fathers; incidence, 1 in 10,000 live births; trunk is normal, limbs short, head large and nose appears "scooped out"; autosomal dominant; 80% new mutations; 20% inherited from parents.	No treatment
	Cleft hand/cleft foot	"Lobster claw" deformities; hand or foot is divided into two opposing parts; rare.	Surgical release
	Absent radius	Partial or complete absence of radius; hand deviates laterally; genetic.	No treatment
	Polydactyly	Extra digits of hand(s) or feet; often poor muscle development; often attached by a narrow stalk; common, dominant trait.	Surgical removal or tie-off
	Syndactyly	"Webbing" of digits is most common with complete fusion in some cases; most often seen in third and fourth fingers and between second and third toes; trait may be dominant or recessive.	Surgical release
	Congenital clubfoot	Talipes equinovarus is the most common of several possibilities. Sole of foot is inverted; may be unilateral or bilateral; incidence, 1 in 1000; male:female ratio is 2:1.	Serial casting shortly after birth
	Congenital hip dislocation	Relaxed hip joint capsule; abnormal development of acetabulum; incidence, 1 in 1500; more common in females.	Triple diapering at birth; Frejka splinting and surgery may be necessary.
Urologic System Anomalies			
	Renal agenesis	Unilateral—refers to absence of kidney on one side; incidence, 1 in 1000; more males; left kidney is usually the absent one; contralateral kidney usually compensates; two vessel umbilical cord is primary finding; bilateral renal agenesis (no kidneys) occurs in 1 in 3000 and death ensues.	No treatment

Table 8–4
Summary of Selected Congenital Anomalies *Continued*

System	Specific Anomaly	Clinical Manifestations	Interventions
Urologic System Anomalies *Continued*			
	Horseshoe kidney	Inferior poles of both kidneys (usually lower) are fused; this U shape is from failure of ascent during embryonic development; incidence, 1 in 500; asymptomatic because collecting system develops normally; in Turner syndrome, 7% have horseshoe kidney.	No treatment
	Congenital polycystic kidneys	Small to large cysts in both kidneys create severe renal insufficiency. Some individuals are less severely affected and may have normal renal function.	Dialysis and renal transplantation
	Exstrophy of the bladder	An outpouching (beyond the skin) of the posterior wall of the bladder appears as a bright red, everted bulging mass inferior to the umbilicus. Urine dribbles from the bladder.	Surgical repair
Reproductive System Anomalies			
	Some conditions that appear to be congenital malformations are really endocrine disorders.		When an infant is born with ambiguous genitalia, sexual reassignment may be necessary. Most born with condition are reared as females.
	True hermaphroditism	Both testicular and ovarian tissue are present; usually not functional; very enlarged clitoris appears to be a penis	
	Hypospadias	External urethral opening is either on the ventral surface of the glans penis or the shaft of the penis; incidence, 1 in 300 live males	Surgical correction
	Cryptorchidism (undescended testes)	Common in premature males (about 30%); may be unilateral or bilateral; descent usually occurs naturally by the end of the first year.	Surgery when failure to descend occurs spontaneously
	Absence of the vagina and uterus	Failure of sinovaginal bulbs to develop and form vaginal plate; uterus is also absent; incidence, 1 in 4000 female births	Cosmetic surgery

Data from Fonkalsrud, Smith, Shaw, Borick, & Shaw, 1993; Graham, 1992; Moore & Persaud, 1993; Rosenberg et al., 1993; Rosenberg et al., 1983; Werler, Louik, Shapiro, & Mitchell, 1994; Werler, Mitchell, & Shapiro, 1989; Werler, Mitchell, & Shapiro, 1992a, 1992b; Mitchell, Rosenberg, Shapiro, & Slone, 1981; Mitchell, Schwingl, Rosenberg, Louik, & Shapiro, 1983.

pable of producing such an effect is called a *teratogen*. The science of teratology includes the study of how birth defects occur on the biochemical, morphologic, or behavioral levels. Many teratogenic defects are not detectable at birth, but some become evident later in life. All events happen through some alteration in genetic material to some of the developing embryonic or fetal cells. Some may be in the form of behavioral disorders, whereas others are visible (extra fingers, missing parts). In the case of biochemical defects, an enzymatic path may be missing that is essential to life-sustaining biochemistry.

Environmental influences that adversely affect the developing embryo and fetus usually occur after conception. However, a preconception teratogenic event can occur, such as significant doses of radiation to an individual's gametes. (See Chapter 4 for more information regarding teratogens that can affect the fetus and growing child.) Most teratogenic effects occur within a set of circumstances that adhere to basic principles (Chart 8–7). Large, multi-institutional and demographically diverse studies of birth defects in the United States are under way (Mitchell, 1988; Werler, Mitchell, & Shapiro, 1992c). Such studies permit methods other than speculation to account for teratogenic events surrounding the birth process.

The susceptibility of an embryo or fetus to environmental damage is determined by its stage of development. Figure 8–6 depicts the most susceptible areas to teratogenic events at different times during organogenesis. The timing of toxicity is the idea that the damaging event occurs during a critical period of development (Moore & Persaud, 1993), such as week 4 of embryonic development. The three germ layers (endoderm, ectoderm, and mesoderm) and their derivatives (e.g., neuroectoderm and gill arch mesoderm) are forming at this time. All major organ systems are derived from these tissues. Many important events, such as formation of the neural tube, transpire during this and the other weeks of the embryonic period (weeks 3 through 8 of postconception development) (Moore & Persaud, 1993).

A teratogen's effect depends on the genetic predisposition (possible susceptibility) of the developing organism, including before conception. The toxic agent may affect an embryo even before conception (such as radiation damage to ovaries or testes). Some genetic changes may not be manifested for several generations if they are autosomal recessive. Women in industrial jobs have a much higher rate of children with anomalies than the general population. Men are not tested enough, although certain exfoliants, pesticides, and agents of chemical warfare have been considered as causes of birth defects in children (Miller, 1995).

Chart 8–7

The Principles of Teratogenesis

- The susceptibility of the embryo or fetus is determined by its stage of development. Timing of toxicity has greater implications for damage during critical periods, such as the embryonic period (weeks 3 through 8) when the germ layers are developing.
- The effect of a teratogen depends on the genetic predisposition (possible susceptibility) of the developing organism, including prior to conception.
- A single agent may produce a variety of anomalies at different levels of biological organization (biochemical, physiological, and behavioral).
- Viruses, chemicals, or radiation may produce similar-looking defects, which may be mistaken for inherited malformations.
- Many teratogens have no adverse effect on the mother and may even be beneficial to her well-being.

A single agent may produce various anomalies at different levels of biological organization (biochemical, physiological, and behavioral). For example, congenital rubella (German measles) may produce anomalies such as cataracts, heart defects, deafness, and mental retardation.

Many teratogens have no adverse effect on the mother and may even be beneficial to her well-being. The classic example of teratogenesis is when thalidomide was widely used as a sedative and antinauseant from 1957 to 1962 (Moore & Persaud, 1993). Although the effect on the mother was a sense of well-being, exposure of the embryo to maternal ingestion of thalidomide before day 33 of gestation created severe limb foreshortening (meromelia) or amelia (complete absence of limbs) (Moore & Persaud, 1993).

Pregnancy can be determined biochemically as early as 12 days after fertilization with a sensitive early pregnancy test known as a quantitative beta–human chorionic gonadotropin serum level. Home urine testing kits purchased commercially may take 1 or 2 weeks longer for positive results revealing pregnancy. However, because approximately 50% of the pregnancies in the United States are unplanned, it is neither practical nor reasonable to expect that a woman knows this early of her own positive pregnancy status (USDHHS, 1990, 1992).

caREminder: *During weeks 3 through 8 after conception inclusively (the embryonic period) the embryo is most sensitive to teratogens.*

At this time, all major organ systems are developing, including the central nervous system and cardiovascular system. The woman who is unaware of the pregnancy may ingest or expose herself to agents that endanger embryonic development.

Chemicals

Many inhaled or ingested substances are teratogenic. Exposure to pesticides is of great danger to developing embryos, fetuses, infants, and small children especially. Pesticides, created to reduce insect and rodent populations work similarly on fetuses when they cross the acid mantle of their mother's skin or are inhaled. The exfoliant Agent Orange, used widely in the Vietnam War, was thought to have altered spermatogenesis in exposed males. Maternal exposure to spermicides has been implicated in relation to certain birth defects (Louik, Mitchell, Werler, Hanson, & Shapiro, 1987).

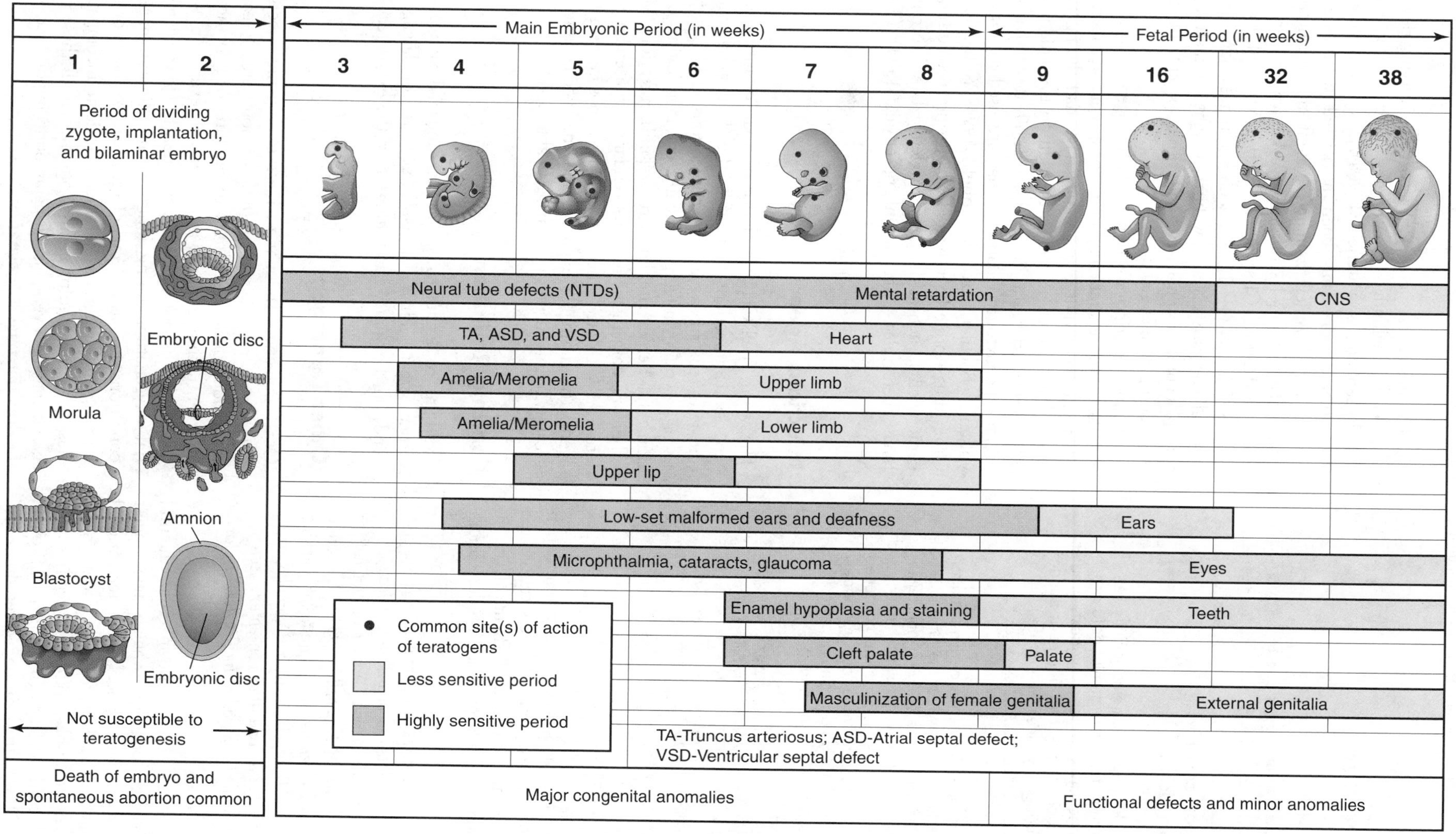

Main Embryonic Period (in weeks)
Fetal Period (in weeks)
1
2
3
4
5
6
7
8
9
16
32
38
Period of dividing zygote, implantation, and bilaminar embryo
Morula
Embryonic disc
Blastocyst
Amnion
Embryonic disc
Not susceptible to teratogenesis
Death of embryo and spontaneous abortion common
Neural tube defects (NTDs)
Mental retardation
CNS
TA, ASD, and VSD
Heart
Amelia/Meromelia
Upper limb
Amelia/Meromelia
Lower limb
Upper lip
Low-set malformed ears and deafness
Ears
Microphthalmia, cataracts, glaucoma
Eyes
Enamel hypoplasia and staining
Teeth
Cleft palate
Palate
Masculinization of female genitalia
External genitalia
● Common site(s) of action of teratogens
Less sensitive period
Highly sensitive period
TA-Truncus arteriosus; ASD-Atrial septal defect; VSD-Ventricular septal defect
Major congenital anomalies
Functional defects and minor anomalies

Figure 8–6
Fetal development and relative sensitivity to teratogenesis. (From Moore, K. L., & Persaud, T. V. N. [1998]. *The developing human* [6th ed., p. 182]. Philadelphia: W. B. Saunders. Reprinted with permission.)

Table 8–5
Environmental Teratogens

Type of Exposure	Possible Teratogenic Effects
Chemicals	
Pesticides	Death of embryo
Industrial wastes	Birth defects
Degradation products of pesticides and industrial wastes	Mutagenicity, carcinogenicity (Although the experimental data are inconclusive, evidence suggests greater toxicity in prenatal age period than during any other time of life.)
Radiation	
	The peak incidence of gross malformation occurs when the fetus is irradiated during the early organogenetic period. However, cellular, tissue, and organ hypoplasia can be produced by radiation throughout organogenetic, fetal, and neonatal periods if the dose is high enough.

Data from Hunon, O., Slone, D., & Shapiro, S. (1977). *Birth defects and drugs in pregnancy*. Littleton, MA: Publishing Sciences Group. From Wieczorek, R. R., & Natapoff, J. R. (1981). *A conceptual approach to the nursing of children: Health care from birth through adolescence* (p. 102). Philadelphia: J.B. Lippincott. Reprinted with permission.

Disease states in the mother, such as insulin-dependent diabetes mellitus or gestational diabetes (either recognized or unknown), may produce biochemicals in the mother's body that cross the placenta and produce anomalies in the infant.

Alert: *Nutritional deficiencies in the mother, such as a folate deficiency, are related to neural tube defects (NTDs) in the embryonic period (Werler & Mitchell, 1993; Werler, Shapiro, & Mitchell, 1993). This condition is easily changed when women planning pregnancies ingest folate (folic acid) supplements, a B-complex vitamin, in the months before and after conception occurs. The U.S. recommended daily allowance is 400 μg for pregnant women.*

Table 8–5 lists a number of known environmental teratogens. The average pregnant woman may ingest many over-the-counter, prescription, and recreational drugs during pregnancy, usually before she knows she is pregnant. Caffeine in soft drinks, coffee, and tea has been related to selected birth defects (Rosenberg, Mitchell, Shapiro, & Slone, 1982). In addition, street drugs and popular substances such as tobacco cause varying degrees of damage (Haglund & Cnattingius, 1990; Werler, Lammer, Rosenberg, & Mitchell, 1990a). Too much vitamin A supplementation has been associated with assorted birth defects (Werler, Lammer, Rosenberg, & Mitchell, 1990b). Fetal alcohol syndrome is a known problem discussed in depth in Chapter 14 (Werler, Mitchell, Rosenberg, & Lammer, 1991). All such substances have direct prenatal effects, such as low birth weight, premature labor, placental insufficiency, and other potentially life-threatening problems.

Many prescription drugs pose teratogenic threats. It is difficult to separate exposure to specific agents from other exposures that women may have had during their pregnancies (Mitchell, 1994). In addition to thalidomide, other suspected agents include hydantoin derivatives, especially phenytoin (Dilantin), that are used as anticonvulsants (Buehler, Rao, & Finnell, 1994; Yerby, 1994). Other drugs formerly suspected of creating specific teratogenic events, such as diazepam in cleft palate deformities, have been ruled out (Rosenberg et al., 1983) (Table 8–6).

Infectious Agents

The word "TORCH" stands for a group of intrauterine, teratogenic infections that affect the developing embryo and fetus: toxoplasmosis, other infections such as hepatitis or parvovirus infection, rubella, cytomegalovirus infection, and herpes simplex virus type II infection. Many other microorganisms may also endanger the embryo and fetus. As with any other intrauterine exposure to a toxic agent, the timing of exposure and the specific infection create varying degrees of damage (Table 8–7).

Ionizing Radiation

Exposure to gamma rays, x-rays, and radioactive substances creates birth defects. The degree of damage depends on the amount and duration of the exposure.

Other Teratogens

Other influences thought to have teratogenic effects include high altitude (as in mountainous areas), carbon monoxide poisoning (related to smoking or poor heating and ventilation during winter), anoxic events in which the mother is not affected permanently (lowered maternal oxygenation during long airplane flights), maternal conditions such as toxemia of pregnancy or heart or renal disease, and maternal-fetal blood antigen incompatibilities. Protecting the pregnant woman from all these possible damaging events is of paramount importance for a healthy outcome of pregnancy.

Table 8–6
Pharmaceutical Teratogens

Drug	Time of Ingestion	Teratogenic Effect
Drugs with Definite Teratogenic Implications		
Thalidomide	20th to 35th day of gestation	Musculoskeletal deformities
Androgenic hormones	Before 12th gestational week	Pseudohermaphroditism
Folic acid antagonists	Embryonic period	Various skeletal and systemic disorders
Nicotine (smoking)	Continuous during pregnancy	Low birth weight, prematurity
Drugs Suspected of Teratogenic Effects		
Anticonvulsants	Embryonic period	Cleft lip or cleft palate, congenital heart disease
Neurotropic-anorexigenic	Embryonic period	Biliary tract atresia and various other multiple deformities
Oral hypoglycemics	Embryonic period	Malformed infants
Alkylating agents	Embryonic period	Multiple musculoskeletal defects, intrauterine death
Alcohol	Large amounts ingested during pregnancy	Microcephaly, fetal growth retardation, mental retardation
Drugs with Potential Teratogenic Properties*		
Aspirin	Malformations, growth retardation	
Antibiotics (streptomycin, tetracycline, penicillin, streptomycin mixtures, dactinomycin, mitomycin C, puromycin, lincomycin)	Pregnancy wastage	
Antituberculotic drugs (streptomycin, isoniazid, *p*-aminosalicylic acid)	Inconclusive	
Imipramine	Reduction deformities of upper limb	
Insulin	Malformed fetus, mentally defective children	
Female sex hormones	May be one of multifactorial causes of congenital heart disease; diethylstilbestrol given to pregnant women has resulted in vaginal or cervical adenocarcinoma in the female offspring when they are between 8 and 24 years of age.	

* Teratogenic effects were found in laboratory animals but rarely implicated in humans.
From Wieczorek, R. R., & Natapoff, J. R. (1981). *A conceptual approach to the nursing of children: Health care from birth through adolescence* (p. 102). Philadelphia: J. B. Lippincott. Reprinted with permission.

Table 8–7
Infectious Teratogens

Type of Infection	Time After Conception	Teratogenic Effect
Rubella virus	First and second trimesters	Deafness, congenital heart disease, microcephaly, hepatosplenomegaly, mental retardation, fetal death; elevated IgM levels in newborn (virus may be systemic or local in fetus).
Cytomegalovirus (Most common cause of congenital infections)	Increased incidence late in pregnancy	Mental-motor retardation, microcephaly; elevated IgM levels in newborn (isolate virus from nasopharynx and urine).
Herpes simplex virus (Type I—oral area causes common cold sore or fever blister. Type II—cervicitis and vaginitis, venereally transmitted.)	Transplacental or transamnionic near delivery	1. Vesicular skin lesions 2. Central nervous system 3. Systemic disease, hepatitis, jaundice, pulmonary effects, hepatomegaly, and thrombocytopenia
Venezuelan equine (encephalomyelitis virus)	100 days after conception	Hydrocephalus, cataracts
Varicella-zoster virus (chickenpox, shingles)	Throughout pregnancy	Prematurity, stillbirth, abortion, reduction and deformity of limbs, skin scars, low birth weight, chorioretinitis, dysphagia, meningoencephalitis
Coxsackievirus	Throughout pregnancy	Myocarditis, urogenital anomalies, digestive system defects, low birth weight
Mumps	First trimester	Fetal mortality, endocardial fibroelastosis
Rubeola	First trimester	Newborns develop measles.
Echoviruses	Any time during pregnancy	Generalized infection, with massive terminal hemorrhage involving most organs of the body
Western equine encephalomyelitis	Any time during pregnancy	Congenital encephalitis
Vaccinia virus	Primary maternal vaccination in the first or second trimester	Fetal infection, stillbirth, abortion, prematurity, and death
Variola virus (smallpox)	Any time during pregnancy	Death, abortion, skin lesions, smallpox, pneumonia
Hepatitis Type A—infectious hepatitis, short incubation Type B—infectious hepatitis, long incubation	Can be transmitted any time during pregnancy or in the neonatal period	Stillbirth, abortion, jaundice, hepatosplenomegaly, hemolytic anemia with a liver function test indicating an obstructive type of jaundice
Type C—influenza bacteria and protozoa	Any time during pregnancy	Data inconclusive: potential fetal malformations, disease, and death
Group B streptococci	At birth: found in positive vaginal and anal cultures of mother. Fathers have positive prostatic and urethral secretions	Respiratory failure, pneumonia
Listeria monocytogenes	Any time during pregnancy	Circulatory collapse, meningitis, fetal wastage
Syphilis	Any time during pregnancy	Fetal damage and severe disease, stillbirths; symptoms may appear after the newborn period, such as failure to thrive, fever, anemia, rashes, rhinitis, moist lesions
Parvoviruses	First trimester	Embryonic/fetal death
Sepsis neonatorum	Results from premature rupture of membranes	Systemic infection of blood stream and meninges

Table 8–7
Infectious Teratogens *Continued*

Type of Infection	Time After Conception	Teratogenic Effect
Congenital pneumonia	Within first 12 hours of extrauterine life	Meningitis, splenitis, sepsis, necrotizing enterocolitis
Chlamydia	Third trimester	Transmitted through vaginal flora; chlamydial pneumonia
Ophthalmia neonatorum	Immediately after birth	May progress to panophthalmitis
Toxoplasmosis	Any time during pregnancy; can be transmitted by the ingestion of infected raw meat	Microcephaly, hydrocephaly, chorioretinitis, anemia
Mycoplasma infections	Transmitted through vaginal flora	Fetal wastage
Human immunodeficiency virus	All trimesters	Life-threatening viral load

Adapted from Wieczorek, R. R., & Natapoff, J. R. (1981). *A conceptual approach to the nursing of children: Health care from birth through adolescence* (pp. 103–104). Philadelphia: J. B. Lippincott. Used with permission.

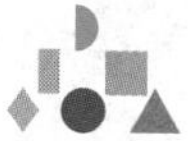

Long-Term Implications

The newborn may be classified as high risk for any condition mentioned in this chapter. High risk refers to a range of actual or potential disabilities resulting from genetic, teratogenic, or iatrogenic abnormalities. Such disabilities may be life threatening. Others may be health threatening but not of immediate danger to the child and family. Other conditions may simply shorten the life expectancy. Some conditions may permit a normal life expectancy but significantly alter or hinder the child's ability to function fully in society. The reader is encouraged to explore other chapters in this text for specific conditions and the ways in which they explicitly affect the child and family (Fig. 8–7).

Specific outcomes of prematurity are explored in depth in Chapter 14. However, the impact of the birth

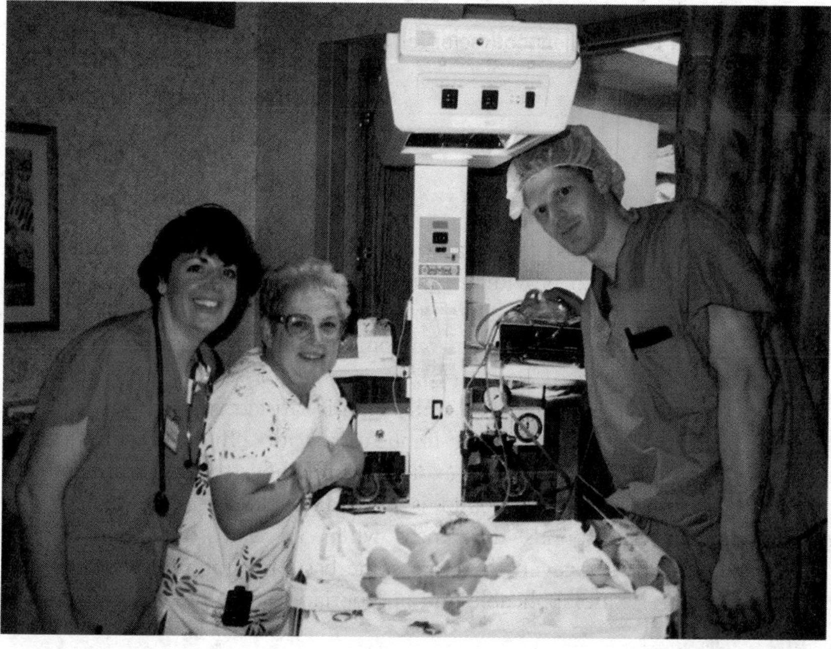

Figure 8–7
The competent obstetric team works very hard to ensure that the best possible outcomes are realized for the neonate.

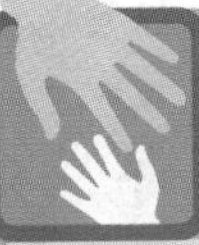

Chart 8–8
Nursing Interventions

Acute Unexpected Outcomes of Childbearing

- Intervene with parents separately, so each may express private feelings in a safe environment, rather than editing for the benefit of the other partner.
- Avoid attempting to control another person's emotional response to an unexpected situation.
- Recognize your own discomfort with a situation.
- Avoid letting personal value judgments become obvious.
- Study the customs of other cultures and subcultures, even though on an informal basis, so that you know how loss and death are handled within them.
- Do not make assumptions that your culture of origin is the same as another's, even if you grew up in the same larger culture.
- Provide prompt, honest, and complete notification *to parents only* of the infant's condition.
- Consider parental fears when discussing problems.
- Be careful with your choice of words.
- Before telling families that the infant is "doing well," consider what "well" means.
- When parents are told what an illness means, it may be just as important for them to hear what it does not mean.
- Recognize that repeated or "dumb" questions may be a support-seeking behavior.
- Recognize that lack of success with physical conditions creates psychological problems.
- Ask directly if parents are concerned about whether their child will be normal or whether they fear its death.
- Refocus them on the unique qualities of the infant as an individual, including positive characteristics.
- Avoid taking over aspects of the parental role that parents can become invested in with your encouragement.
- Let parents know that someone will be available to help them.
- Give them the phone number of the infant's unit and invite them to call at any time.
- Assure them that information regarding the specifics of the child's condition will be given only to them.
- Politely discourage other callers from seeking information other than a general condition report.
- Determine who is placing the call before disclosing information.
- Make regular calls to families who do not initiate contact themselves.
- Keep detailed records of staff interactions with families.
- Avoid platitudes such as "Please don't feel so bad . . . you have other children at home" or "You can always have another baby."
- Consult the hospital chaplain, parish priest, rabbi, or other family-requested member of the clergy if the patient's religious/spiritual needs are beyond the nurse's ability to help.
- Perform baptism on appropriate infants when a member of the clergy cannot be summoned quickly enough.
- Call a translator, when needed, to make sure a family's wishes are considered fully.
- Suggest a social service consultation and referral to a bereavement counselor for high-risk individuals.

of a child with significant problems has a fairly predictable set of emotional responses among parents and other family members. Most premature infants gain health in a predictable pattern and grow up to be fine (Fig. 8–8). The emotional impact of prematurity on the family may not be appreciated by individuals close to them. Premature infants generate a lot of anxiety and changes in plans. Preparations are incomplete for the infant's homecoming. Work situations and commitments may have to be postponed or abandoned by the parents. The premature ending of a pregnancy may have a significant emotional and physical impact on the mother and the involved father as well as the infant. Parental competence with providing physical care to a premature infant in the home may have little to do with the emotional impact of this unexpected outcome or the coping skills of the parents (Chart 8–8). It is a major stressor even if everybody's physical well-being is satisfactory.

Long-term implications for children with specific conditions are explored throughout this book as appropriate. Every child is an individual, and each child/family responds differently when a health deviation occurs. However, there are some basic nursing interventions that are applicable and appropriate to families with a develop-

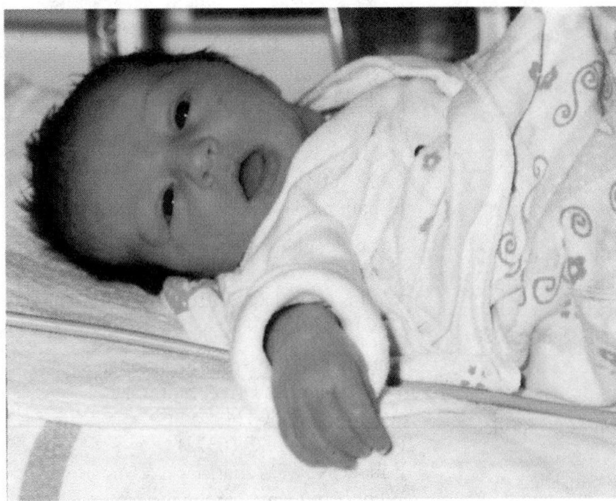

Figure 8–8
Most preterm infants gain health in a predictable pattern and grow up to be healthy children and adults.

mentally delayed child. The nurse is in the optimal position to discern, based on close observation and interaction with the child and family, how the family may best be served by the available resources. It is also his or her responsibility to provide follow-up care, ensuring that services are continued.

Public Law 99.457 mandates early intervention for children 3 years and younger who are developmentally delayed, or at risk for delay. This legislation not only provides standard therapies but also incorporates provisions for parent support groups, respite programs, innovative financial programs, networking, and discharge planning. *Each state manages its early intervention program (EIP) differently.*

When an infant or child is identified as a candidate for receiving these services, the nurse works in collaboration with the family to develop a plan of care. Referral to an EIP is indicated if the infant or child would benefit from occupational, physical, and language therapy and the input of an interdisciplinary team.

Specific nursing interventions include, but are not restricted to, the following:

- Referring the child for early intervention services.
- Alleviating the family's fears by providing information.
- Acting as a family advocate by helping them find the best care, technological advice, and treatment available.
- Forming parent support groups that provide opportunities for sharing of information.

Summary of Key Concepts

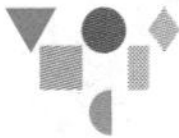

- Many aspects of childbearing can have unexpected outcomes for parents and family members.
- Prematurity is the most common unexpected outcome of childbearing.
- Presentation of bad news by nurses and other providers is part of one's professional responsibility. Specific ways to do this are discussed with specific conditions.
- Perinatal infant deaths can affect the rest of the family's life; how the nurse handles such situations may alleviate suffering.
- Nurses will be called on more and more to provide genetic information about specific conditions to children and their families.
- Genograms are useful tools for understanding heritable disorders. The nurse must understand them.
- Genetic screening and fetal diagnostic tests reveal important prenatal information that the nurse uses in providing support to families.
- Genetic and multifactorial disorders sometimes mimic one another. An understanding of the basics clears up confusion for children and their families.
- Congenital anomalies account for the leading causes of infant mortality in the United States. There are thousands of possibilities ranging from minor defects to fatal defects.
- Teratogens and other environmental exposures may result in congenital anomalies. The principles of teratogenesis are explored with an emphasis on prevention of future problems.

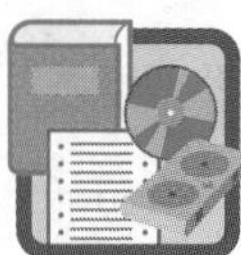

Resources

Organizations

The Access Group
1776 Peachtree Road NW
Atlanta, GA 30309
(800) 821-8580
Children with disabilities born to Vietnam veterans

Alcohol, Drug and Pregnancy Helpline
National Center for Perinatal Addiction, Research and Education (NAPARE)
200 North Michigan Avenue, Suite 1000
Chicago, IL 60611-1676
(800) 638-2229

California Teratogen Information Service and Clinical Research Program
University of California at San Diego
Department of Pediatrics
225 Dickinson Street
San Diego, CA 92103
(800) 532-3749 (within California)

CDC National AIDS Clearinghouse
P.O. Box 6003
Rockville, MD 20850
(800) 458-5231
(800) 243-7010 (hearing impaired)

Cornelia de Lange Syndrome Foundation
60 Dyer Avenue
Collinsville, CT 06022
(800) 223-8355
(800) 735-2357 (Connecticut and Canada only)
Birth defects information

Devereux Foundation
19 South Waterloo Road
Devon, PA 19333
(800) 345-1292
Treatment of emotionally, developmentally, and mentally handicapped

Good Samaritan Project Teen
Teaching AIDS Prevention Program
3030 Walnut Street
Kansas City, MO 64108
(800) 234-8336 (4–8 PM central time)

Grief Recovery Helpline
8306 Wilshire Boulevard, Suite 21A
Beverly Hills, CA 90211
(800) 445-4808

Human Growth Foundation
7777 Leesburg Pike, Suite 202S
Falls Church, VA 22043
(800) 451-6434
Child growth abnormalities

Institute of Logopedics
2400 Jardine Drive
Wichita, KS 67219
(800) 835-1043
Programs for multiply handicapped children

International Society of Nurses in Genetics, Inc.
Eileen Rawnsley, Executive Director
7 Haskins Road
Hanover, NH 03755
(603) 643-5706
FAX: (603) 643-3169
E-mail: erawn@valley.net

Little People of America
P.O. Box 9897
Washington, DC 20016
(800) 243-9273

National Down Syndrome Congress
1605 Chantilly Drive, Suite 250
Atlanta, GA 30324
(800) 232-NDSC (6372)
E-mail: NDSC@charities usa.com
Web: http://www.carol.net/ndsc

National Down Syndrome Society
666 Broadway
New York, NY 10012
(800) 221-4602
Web: http://www.pcsltd.com/ndss/

National Easter Seal Society
70 East Lake Street
Chicago, IL 60601
(800) 221-6827

National Fragile X Foundation
1441 York Street, Suite 215
Denver, CO 80206
(800) 688-8765

National Information Center for Children and Youth with Handicaps
P.O. Box 1492
Washington, DC 20013
(800) 695-0285
Web: http://www.aed.org/nichy/

National Information Clearinghouse for Infants with Disabilities and Life-Threatening Conditions
P.O. Box 8057
Gaithersburg, MD 20898-8057
(800) 854-7013

National Organization for Rare Disorders
P.O. Box 8923
New Fairfield, CT 06812
(800) 999-6673

National Organization on Disability (NOD)
910 16th Street, NW, Suite 600
Washington, DC 20006
(800) 248-ABLE (2253)

National Pesticide Telecommunications Network
Texas Tech University
Thompson Hall, Room S129
Lubbock, TX 79430
(800) 858-7378

Shriners Hospital Referral Line
2900 Rocky Point Drive
Tampa, FL 33607
(800) 237-5055
Free orthopedic, burn, or other care for children

Sudden Infant Death Syndrome Alliance
10500 Little Patuxent Parkway, Suite 420
Columbia, MD 21044
(800) 221-SIDS (7437)

Turner's Syndrome Society of the United States
811 Twelve Oaks Center
15500 Wayzata Boulevard
Wayzata, MN 55391
(800) 365-9944
FAX: (612) 475-9949
E-mail: tesc0016@maroon.tc.umn.edu

Hotlines

CDC National HIV/AIDS Hotline
Centers for Disease Control and Prevention
Atlanta, GA 30333
(800) 342-AIDS (2437)
(800) 344-SIDA (Spanish)
(800) AIDS-TTY (hearing impaired)

Center for Substance Abuse Treatment Hotline
11426-28 Rockville Pike, Suite 410
Rockville, MD 20852
(800) 662-4357

Emergency Planning and Community Right-to-Know/Superfund Hotline
Environmental Protection Agency
401 M Street SW
Washington, DC 20460
(800) 535-0202
(800) 553-7672 (hearing impaired)

National Cocaine Hotline
P.O. Box 100
Summit, NJ 07902-0100
(800) 262-2463

National STD Hotline
(sexually transmitted diseases)
Centers for Disease Control and Prevention
Atlanta, GA 30333
(800) 227-8922

Safe Drinking Water Hotline
EPA, Mail Stop 4604
401 M Street, SW
Washington, DC 20460
(800) 426-4791

Computer Resources

Down Syndrome WWW Page
http://www.nas.com/downsyn/index.html

Sibling Support (Down Syndrome) Project's web site
http://www.chmc.org/departmt/sibsupp

Parents Helping Parents
http://www.portal.com/~cbntmkr/php.html

Books and Printed Materials

The Best Toys, Books & Videos for Kids
Exceptional Parent Library
(800) 535-1910

Down Syndrome Quarterly
Denison University
Granville, OH 43023
Subscriptions $24/year (4 issues)
http://www.denison.edu/dsq/

Your Baby Has Down Syndrome (video)
http://www.nb.net.mall/d/MSNCT_order.html
The Mackenzie Sara Noca Charitable Trust
1510 Greendale Drive
Pittsburgh, PA 15239
(412) 798-0794

Medical and Surgical Care for Children with Down Syndrome, A Guide for Parents (1995). D. C. Van Dyke & P. Mattheis (Eds.) ISBN 0-933149-54-9
Woodbine House
6510 Bells Mill Road
Bethesda, MD 20817
(800) 843-7323

Medical Care in Down Syndrome: A Preventive Medicine Approach
P. T. Rogers & M. Coleman
ISBN 0-8247-8648-X
Marcel Dekker, Inc.
New York, NY

Advances in Down Syndrome
V. Dmitriev & P. Oelwein (Eds.)
Special Child Publications
ISBN 0-87562-092-2

The Language of Toys: Teaching Communication Skills to Special-Needs Children: A Guide for Parents and Teachers (1988)
S. Schwartz & J. E. Heller Miller
Woodbine House
6510 Bells Mill Road
Bethesda, MD 20817
(800) 843-7323

Teaching Strategies for Children with Down Syndrome: A Resource Guide (K-6)
B. Tien & C. Hall, (Eds.)
Jointly prepared by the PREP Program and the Ups & Downs Association of Calgary, Alberta
Ups & Downs
Calgary Down Syndrome Association
1001-17 Street NW
Calgary, Alberta, Canada T2N 2E5
(403) 289-4394

Toys and Product Catalog Listing for Children with Special Needs

ABLEDATA
8455 Colesville Road, Suite 935
Silver Spring, MD 20910-3319
(800) 227-0216

Achievement Products, Inc.
P.O. Box 9033
Canton, OH 44711
(216) 453-2122

References

Anderson, G. W. (1996). The evolution and status of genetics education in nursing in the United States 1983–1995. *Image, 28*(2), 101–106.

Bartels, D. M., LeRoy, B. S., & Caplan, A. L. (1993). *Prescribing our future—ethical challenges in genetic counseling.* New York: Aldine de Gruyter.

Berry, P., Gunn, P., & Andrews, R. (1980). Behavior of Down syndrome infants in a strange situation. *American Journal of Mental Deficiency, 85,* 212.

Bishop, J. E., & Waldholz, M. (1990). *The story of our astonishing attempt to map all the genes in the human body—genome.* New York: Simon & Schuster.

Bosk, C. L. (1993). The workplace ideology of genetic counselors. In D. M. Bartels, B. S. LeRoy, & A. L. Caplan (Eds.), *Prescribing our future—ethical challenges in genetic counseling* (pp. 25–37). New York: Aldine de Gruyter.

Buehler, B. A., Rao, V., & Finnell, R. H. (1994). Biochemical and molecular teratology of fetal hydantoin syndrome. *Neurologic Clinics, 12,* 741–748.

Cohen, F. L., & Durham, J. D. (1985). Klinefelter syndrome. *Journal of Psychosocial Nursing, 23*(1), 19–25.

Collins, C. (1995). Klinefelter's syndrome. *Nursing Times, 91*(12), 48–53.

Connaughty, M. S. (1992). Accelerated growth in children. *Journal of Pediatric Health Care,* 6, 316–324.

Dunger, D. B., & Holton, J. B. (1994). Disorders of carbohydrate metabolism. In J. B. Holton (Ed.), *The inherited metabolic diseases* (2nd ed., pp. 21–41). New York: Churchill Livingstone.

Fonkalsrud, E. W., Smith, M. D., Shaw, K. S., Borick, J. M., & Shaw, A. (1993). Selective management of gastroschisis according to the degree of visceroabdominal disproportion. *Annals of Surgery, 218,* 722–747.

Goldson, E., & Hagerman, R. J. (1992). The fragile X syndrome. *Developmental Medicine and Child Neurology, 34,* 822–832.

Graham, J. M. (1992). Congenital anomalies. In M. D. Levine, W. B. Carey, & A. C. Crocker (Eds.), *Developmental-behavioral pediatrics* (2nd ed., pp. 229–243). Philadelphia: W. B. Saunders.

Hagerman, R. J. (1992). Chromosomal disorders. In M. D. Levine, W. B. Carey, & A. C. Crocker (Eds.), *Developmental-behavioral pediatrics* (2nd ed., pp. 213–220). Philadelphia: W. B. Saunders.

Haglund, B., & Cnattingius, S. (1990). Cigarette smoking as a risk factor for sudden infant death syndrome: A population based study. *American Journal of Public Health, 80*(1), 29–32.

Hall, J. G. (1996). Genetic counseling. In R. E. Behrman, R. M. Kliegman, & A. M. Arvin (Eds.), *Nelson textbook of pediatrics* (15th ed., pp. 327–328). Philadelphia: W. B. Saunders.

Jackson, J. F. (1996). *Genetics and you.* Totowa, NJ: Humana Press.

James, J. W., & Cherry, F. (1988). *The grief recovery handbook: A step-by-step program for moving beyond loss.* New York: Harper & Row.

Jonsen, A. R. (1996). The impact of mapping the human genome on the patient–physician relationship. In T. H. Murray, M. A. Rothstein, & R. F. Murray (Eds.), *The human genome project and the future of health care* (pp. 1–20). Bloomington, IN: Indiana University Press.

Leroy, J. G. (1992). Heredity, development, and behavior. In M. D. Levine, W. B. Carey, & A. C. Crocker (Eds.), *Developmental-behavioral pediatrics* (2nd ed., pp. 195–212). Philadelphia: W. B. Saunders.

Louik, C., Mitchell, A. A., Werler, M. M., Hanson, J. W., & Shapiro, S. (1987). Maternal exposure to spermicides in relation to certain birth defects. *New England Journal of Medicine, 317,* 474–478.

Marks, J. H. (1993). The workplace ideology of genetic counselors. In D. M. Bartels, B. S. LeRoy, & A. L. Caplan (Eds.), *Prescribing our future—ethical challenges in genetic counseling* (pp. 15–24). New York: Aldine de Gruyter.

McGoldrick, M., & Gerson, R. (1985). *Genograms in family assessment.* New York: W. W. Norton.

Miller, K. (1995, November). The tiny victims of Desert Storm. *Life,* 46–62.

Mitchell, A. A. (1988). Slone Epidemiology Unit Birth Defects Study. Massachusetts Department of Public Health. *Genetic Resource, 4*(3), 1–2.

Mitchell, A. A. (1994). Special considerations in studies of drug-induced birth defects. In B. L. Storm (Ed.), *Pharmacoepidemiology* (2nd ed., pp. 595–608). New York: Wiley.

Mitchell, A. A., Rosenberg, L., Shapiro, S., Slone, D. (1981). Birth defects related to bendectin use in pregnancy. *Journal of the American Medical Association, 245*(22), 2311–2314.

Moore, K. L., & Persaud, T. V. N. (1993). *The developing human* (5th ed.). Philadelphia: W. B. Saunders.

National Institutes of Health (1995). *Clinical preventive services* [Electronic data transfer via Internet World Wide Web]. Washington, DC: National Library of Medicine, NIH [producer and distributor].

Nora, J. J., & Fraser, F. C. (1989). *Medical genetics* (3rd ed.). Philadelphia: Lea & Febiger.

Olshansky, S. (1962). Chronic sorrow: A response to having a mentally defective child. *Social Casework, 43,* 190–193.

Pennock, C. A. (1994). Lysosomal storage disorders. In J. B. Holton (Ed.), *The inherited metabolic diseases* (2nd ed., pp. 205–228). New York: Churchill Livingstone.

Pickler, R. H., & Munro, C. L. (1995). Gene therapy for inherited disorders. *Journal of Pediatric Nursing, 10*(1), 40–47.

Pueschel, S. M. (1992). The child with Down syndrome. In M. D. Levine, W. B. Carey, & A. C. Crocker (Eds.), *Developmental-behavioral pediatrics* (2nd ed., pp. 221–228). Philadelphia: W. B. Saunders.

Raff, B. S. (1994). Nursing and genetics for the 21st century. *Journal of Obstetric, Gynecologic, & Neonatal Nursing, 23*(6), 477–480.

Rieser, P. A., & Underwood, L. E. (1989). *Turner syndrome: A guide for families.* Wayzata, MN: The Turner Syndrome Society.

Rosenberg, L., Mitchell, A. A., Shapiro, S., & Slone, D. (1982). Selected birth defects in relation to caffeine-containing beverages. *Journal of the American Medical Association, 247*(10), 1429–1432.

Rosenberg, L., Mitchell, A. A., Parsells, J. L., Pashayan, H., Louik, C., & Shapiro, S. (1983). Lack of relation of oral clefts to diazepam use during pregnancy. *New England Journal of Medicine, 309,* 1282–1285.

Sorenson, J. R. (1993). The workplace ideology of genetic counselors. In D. M. Bartels, B. S. LeRoy, & A. L. Caplan (Eds.), *Prescribing our future—ethical challenges in genetic counseling* (pp. 3–14). New York: Aldine de Gruyter.

Sullivan, J. M. (1997). Learning the baby: A maternal thinking and problem-solving process. *Journal of the Society of Pediatric Nurses, 2*(1), 21–28.

Tarleton, J. C., & Saul, R. A. (1993). Molecular genetic advances in fragile X syndrome. *Journal of Pediatrics, 12,* 169–184.

U.S. Department of Health and Human Services (1990). *Healthy people 2000.* Boston: Jones & Bartlett.

U.S. Department of Health and Human Services (1992). *Healthy children 2000.* Boston: Jones & Bartlett.

Vockrodt, L., & Williams, J. K. (1994). A reproductive option for women with Turner's syndrome. *Journal of Pediatric Nursing,* 9(5), 321–325.

Werler, M. M., Lammer, E. J., Rosenberg, L., & Mitchell, A. A. (1990a). Maternal cigarette smoking during pregnancy in relation to oral clefts. *American Journal of Epidemiology, 132,* 926–932.

Werler, M. M., Lammer, E. J., Rosenberg, L., & Mitchell, A. A. (1990b). Maternal vitamin A supplementation in relation to selected birth defects. *Teratology, 42,* 497–503.

Werler, M. M., Louik, C., Shapiro, S., & Mitchell, A. A. (1994). Ovulation induction and risk of neural tube defects. *Lancet, 344,* 445–446.

Werler, M. M., Mitchell, A. A., Rosenberg, L., & Lammer, E. J. (1991). Maternal alcohol use in relation to selected birth defects. *American Journal of Epidemiology, 134,* 691–698.

Werler, M. M., Mitchell, A. A., & Shapiro, S. (1989). The relation of aspirin use during the first trimester of pregnancy to congenital cardiac defects. *New England Journal of Medicine, 321,* 1639–1642.

Werler, M. M., Mitchell, A. A., & Shapiro, S. (1992a). First trimester maternal medication use in relation to gastroschisis. *Teratology, 45,* 361–367.

Werler, M. M., Mitchell, A. A., & Shapiro, S. (1992b). Demographic, reproductive, medical and environmental factors in relation to gastroschisis. *Teratology, 45*, 353–360.

Werler, M. M., Mitchell, A. A., & Shapiro, S. (1992c). Commentary: Analyses and reanalyses of epidemiologic data: Learning lessons and maintaining perspective. *Teratology, 46*, 209–211.

Werler, M. M., & Mitchell, A. A. (1993). Case-control study of vitamin supplementation and neural tube defects: Consideration of potential confounding by lifestyle factors. *Annals of the New York Academy of Sciences, 678*, 276–283.

Werler, M. M., Shapiro, S., & Mitchell, A. A. (1993). Periconceptual folic acid exposure and risk of occurrent neural tube defects. *Journal of the American Medical Association, 269*, 1257–1261.

Williams, J. K., & Lessick, M. (1996). Genome research: Implications for children. *Pediatric Nursing, 22*(1), 40–46.

Yerby, M. S. (1994). Pregnancy, teratogenesis and epilepsy. *Neurologic Clinics, 12*, 749–772.

Yesley, M. S. (1993). *ELSI Bibliography: Ethical, Legal & Social Implications of the Human Genome Project*. Washington, DC: U.S. Department of Energy—Office of Energy Research.

Younger, J. B., Kendell, M. J., & Pickler, R. H. (1997). Mastery of stress in mothers of preterm infants. *Journal of the Society of Pediatric Nursing, 2*(1), 29–35.

Bibliography

Carpenter, N. J. (1994). Genetic anticipation: Expanding tandem repeats. *Neurologic Clinics, 12*, 683–698.

Naidu, S., & Moser, H. W. (1994). Peroxisomal disorders. *Neurologic Clinics, 12*, 727–740.

Miller, R. G., & Hoffman, E. P. (1994). Molecular diagnosis and modern management of Duchenne muscular dystrophy. *Neurologic Clinics, 12*, 699–726.

Murray, T. H., Rothstein, M. A., & Murray, R. F. (1996). *The Human Genome Project and the Future of Health Care*. Bloomington, IN: Indiana University Press.

Scanlon, C., & Fibison, W. (1995). *Managing genetic information: Implications for nursing practice*. Washington, DC: American Nurses Publishing.

Schaffer, G. B., & Bodensteiner, J. B. (Eds.) (1994). Pediatric neurogenetics [special issue]. *Neurologic Clinics, 12*(4).

Wang, P. P., & Jernigan, T. L. (1994). Morphometric studies using neuroimaging. *Neurologic Clinics, 12*, 789–802.

Weaver, D. D. (1989). *Catalog of prenatally diagnosed conditions*. Baltimore: Johns Hopkins University Press.

Wilson, G. N. (1994). Atypical inheritance: New horizons for neurology. *Neurologic Clinics, 12*, 663–682.

Yesley, M. S. (May, 1993). *ELSI bibliography: Ethical, legal & social implications of the Human Genome Project*. Washington, DC: U.S. Department of Energy—Office of Energy Research. Searches conducted via Internet on request at roth_michael_r@ofvax.lanl.gov or at msy@lanl.gov

Acute Illness as a Challenge to Health Maintenance

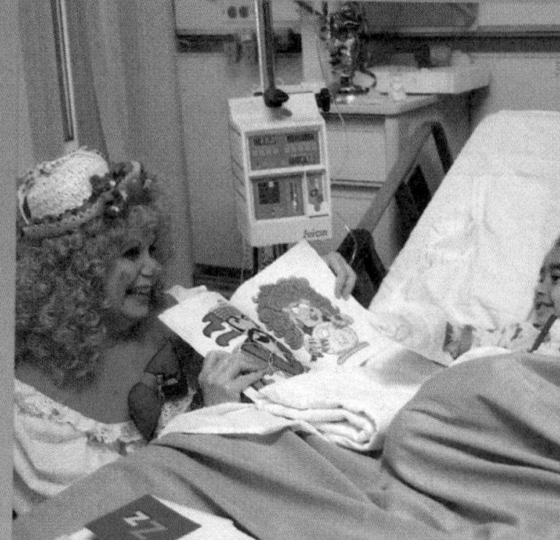

OUTLINE

The Acute Care Experience
- Care Management Systems
- Admission Process
- Intensive Care Unit
- Adolescent Unit
- Ambulatory Care Settings in the Hospital

Responses to a Child's Acute Illness
- Child's Response to Hospitalization
- Family's Response to Hospitalization
- Prolonged Hospitalization
- Hospitalization as a Threat to Family Cohesion

Support for the Child and Family During Acute Illness
- Education to Support the Child and Family
- Programs to Support the Child and Family

Care of the Child in the Acute Care Setting
- Activities of Daily Living
- Safety
- Latex Allergy
- Routine Procedures
- Medication Administration
- Infection Control
- Visitation Policies

Care of the Child Going to Surgery
- Preoperative Care
- Surgical Suite
- Postanesthesia Care
- Same-Day Surgery

Preparation for Discharge from Acute Care

OBJECTIVES

- Facilitate care during acute illness to minimize stress for the child and family.
- Discuss the impact of hospitalization on the child's and family's coping and adaptation responses.
- Select nursing interventions to provide basic care needs for the child during an episode of acute illness.
- Examine interventions that provide psychosocial support to the family during hospitalization.
- Describe nursing care of the child having surgery.
- Identify factors that prepare the child and family for a smooth transition from the acute care environment to a community setting.

KEY TERMS

adaptation
atraumatic care
child life programs
coping
support groups
therapeutic play

CHAPTER

9

An acute illness is a threat to the child and his or her family characterized by suddenness, severity, and disruption of the normal patterns of everyday life. The critical nature of the illness and the uncertainty regarding its outcomes challenge the child's emotional well-being and integrity of the family system. An acute illness is generally unexpected. Prior to accessing the acute care setting, some children may have had an illness that was treated unsuccessfully in the home. The caregiver's inability to recognize the severity of the illness or to prevent it from worsening may impair the child's overall health status.

This chapter views acute illnesses as those in which changes occur relatively rapidly, reach a certain level of acuity, then subside. Chronic illness, in contrast, is present for a prolonged period, potentially never resolving. For some children the acute illness may be an exacerbation of a chronic illness or the terminal stages of a life-threatening condition. Although the child's current acute status may be an "expected" part of the disease process, the child's debilitated state is likely to distress the child and family. Traumatic events such as drowning, motor vehicle accidents, poisonings, and injuries are also sources of acute or life-threatening illness in children that will lead them to the acute care setting.

Acute illness encompasses the minor illnesses that are frequent in childhood and those of a more serious nature. This chapter focuses on care delivery in the hospital as providing the greatest threat to child well-being and family cohesion. Principles of atraumatic care should be implemented regardless of the setting in which care is delivered.

The acute care setting is a busy and noisy environment, full of unexpected and often unpleasant events for the child. Anxiety, fear, pain, discomfort, surprise, separation, loss, fatigue, frustration, mistrust, and anger are common experiences for the child and the family. It is the responsibility of all members of the health care team to be aware of and sensitive to this general problem and also to be well trained in making assessments and designing interventions that enhance family function and reduce the trauma associated with interaction with the acute care setting—be it clinic, outpatient unit, or hospital. In acute care, skilled interventions are critical to successfully guiding the child and family away from harm and toward benefit. These interventions include the following:

- Integrating age-appropriate principles of growth and development in all care
- Responding to the unique psychosocial needs of the child and family
- Facilitating entry into the acute care setting
- Maintaining appropriate hygiene and safety
- Supervising or implementing routine care and procedures in a non-threatening way
- Monitoring visitation
- Implementing effective discharge

The Acute Care Experience

Proponents of family-centered care have long been concerned with aspects of the acute care experience that are problematic for the child and family. The Association for the Care of Children's Health (ACCH) has been a leader in promoting family-centered care strategies (see Chapter 1). ACCH provides excellent resource materials and guidelines for tailoring acute care in a way that minimizes the stressful impact of the event on the child and family (Johnson, Jeppson, & Redburn, 1992). For years, research has documented that illness and subsequent hospitalization are stressful events for families (Youngblut & Shiao, 1993). The family-centered care approach has developed hand in hand with this knowledge and has become the philosophical underpinning for the care of children and their families. Treating the whole family as the patient and involving all family members in decision-making and care delivery become important approaches in child health care.

Family-centered care necessitates liberal 24-hour visitation policies, sibling involvement in hospitalization, pet visitation policies, family conferences about decision-making, promotion of family use of support systems, and family education and training with regard to the care of the child. Unfortunately, some hospitals have been slow to embrace all aspects of family-centered care, especially changes in visitation policies (Johnson et al., 1992).

Care Management Systems

Care delivery in the acute care setting is currently approached in a variety of ways, which include primary care, team nursing or functional nursing, and case management systems (Manthey, 1991). During the admission process, families need explanations of how care in that environment is organized. In any system in which responsibility for care is divided among various personnel, families must be oriented to the roles and expectations of health team members to prevent confusion about the delivery of care. With this knowledge, families can work better with the health care team as partners to meet the needs of the child.

The nurse is often responsible for delegating tasks to unlicensed assistive personnel (UAP).

caREminder: *When delegating acts of nursing, the nurse still remains accountable, and legally liable, for the completion and outcome. Appropriate delegation to UAP includes an assessment of the UAP's qualifications and job description, how these match with the task, and clear communication of what is expected (see Chart 1–13).*

In **primary care** systems of delivery, the primary nurse is responsible for clinical decision-making on a 24-hour basis. The primary nurse develops the plan of care, coordinating with other team members (e.g., pharmacist, dietitian, child life specialist, etc.) to provide a comprehensive plan that meets the needs of the individual child and family. The primary nurse may provide the daily total care for the patient or may delegate some daily care to other providers (Manthey, 1991). For example, if the primary nurse is not working that shift, others provide care to the child following the plan of care developed by the primary nurse. The nurse delivering care makes clinical decisions based on changes in the child's needs and responses to treatment but follows the plan whenever possible. If primary nursing is used with case management, the primary nurse is the case manager. Primary nursing care systems are not to be confused with total care systems. In the latter, the key difference is that work allocation is delivery of total patient care for that shift and clinical decision-making by the registered nurse is shift based. Clearly in such a system, the coordination of care is not addressed by the bedside role of providing nursing care, making case management a desirable component of care coordination.

Similarly, **team nursing** and **functional nursing** are systems in which clinical decision-making is shift based; the registered nurse is responsible for ensuring that care tasks are completed for a large group of patients, but work is allocated to other personnel with mixed skill levels. Work may be divided by function or by groups of patients based on geography within the health care setting or diagnosis. Interdisciplinary team members provide individual input. Again, these systems of care delivery clearly do not incorporate comprehensive care coordination in bedside nursing roles; consequently, care coordination must be addressed through other mechanisms, case management being one that is widely used.

Case management refers to the manner in which care is coordinated. Care coordination involves planning and oversight of care by the case manager to ensure that proper care is delivered and services are not duplicated over the continuum from preadmission to post-discharge. Case management is a popular form of care coordination that may be used with any system of nursing care delivery. If the patient falls into a diagnostic category that is case managed in the particular setting, this needs to be explained to the patient/family. Case management may be explained by the case manager during the preadmission visit or at the time of admission by the case manager or admitting nurse. Case management is a process for coordinating the care of patients that have diagnoses frequently seen in the setting (e.g., gastroenteritis with dehydration) or those with complex needs so as to ensure quality and control cost. Case management may also include a risk assessment component to optimize outcomes (e.g., the case manager calls the patient when an appointment is missed). The case manager communicates with the interdisciplinary team members to facilitate timely care delivery. The goal of case management is to provide the patient/family with the best service possible without problems of redundancy, inefficiency, or missed care (Bower, 1992). Research shows that patient satisfaction improves and that hospitals cut costs with case management (Wesp & Hartman, 1996).

The case management process is often guided by a tool called a critical pathway, care pathway, or interdisciplinary action plan that specifies that events and intervention will happen to a patient with a particular diagnosis on each day (or time period) of the treatment plan (see Chapter 1). The patient and family should be introduced to the case manager before or at the time of admission. The case manager can then inform the family about what to expect during the acute care experience and how to contact the case manager by phone if needed. In complex, acute, and chronic illness situations, the family must be able to reach the case manger or designee at "off" hours. Ideally this introduction should relieve some of the patient's and family's concerns about their treatment plan and the care they are receiving.

Admission Process

The admission process is the beginning of the relationship between the child, family, and the health care staff. It assumes great importance because if hospitalization begins problematically, the negative first impression tends to color the entire acute care episode. If a positive first impression is made by all the parties, this serves as the basis for establishing a trusting and supportive relationship between the health care team, the child, and the family, leading to improved outcomes.

Accessing the acute care setting includes both an unanticipated visit to the family health care provider that is relatively low stress and an unanticipated, abrupt, and distressing trip to the hospital. The admission process may be as simple as signing in on the clipboard at the doctor's office or medical clinic. On the other hand, the process may be more complex, as in hospital admission. The process of obtaining insurance information and often

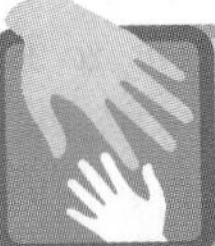

Chart 9–1
Nursing Interventions

Guidelines for the Preadmission Experience

- Ensure that the child knows why he or she is going to the hospital.
- Incorporate parents'/caregivers' feedback regarding methods or tools that have helped the child adjust to past experiences.
- Encourage use of familiar, comforting toys and belongings during the admission.
- Explain in age-appropriate terms the steps to the admission process (admission, laboratory work, patient unit, etc.).
- Use multisensory mechanisms for preparation, such as play materials, books, and videos that illustrate aspects of hospitalization.
- Determine whether a preadmission tour would benefit or frighten the child.

preapproval for admission can be time-consuming. Most hospital admissions of children younger than the age of 6 years are unplanned (Melnyk, 1994).

One survey of hospitals in the United States and Canada found that, in 1988, only 20% of pediatric patients were recipients of a preadmission experience (Maieron & Roberts, 1993). In an effort to counter this problem, pediatric hospitals have implemented programs for visiting schools and parent and community groups that are geared to educating prospective clients about the hospital experience. These programs allow the family and the child to come to the hospital in advance of admission and receive information that explains what will happen while the child is in the hospital and, if appropriate, receive a facility tour. This is particularly useful for preschool-age children who may be especially frightened by hospitalization but are old enough to benefit from the desensitization effects of a preadmission program (Chart 9–1).

Communicating with the Child and Family

Communication is a dynamic two-way process that involves a sender and receiver. All behavior is communication; to help avoid faulty communication, engage in interpersonally effective communication with the child and family. Some basic strategies for effective communication involve

- Clearly stating one's case
- Clarifying and qualifying statements
- Asking for feedback regarding what the listener heard
- Being receptive to feedback received

In the acute care experience, assessing the individual's readiness for communication becomes a key component of effective communication. Parents and children are involved in a stressful situation, so determining the level at which they can participate in communication is a vital skill (e.g., if they are anxious, only simple, basic concepts should be discussed or they may need to discuss what is distressing them before progressing to other topics). Your receptivity to feedback from the child or family is key in this determination. Some families use maladaptive coping mechanisms to deal with the stress of a child's hospitalization. The nurse needs to recognize the maladaptive behavior, interpret it as such, and respond therapeutically (Baker, 1994). For example, when a parent criticizes the care the nurse delivers, the parent may be angry or frustrated. Defending oneself may lead to further confrontation. Conversely, acknowledging the emotion ("You sound like you are angry. Tell me about it") may address the parent's issues and lead to effective problem-solving.

Communication or sharing of information is the cornerstone of building a trusting, supportive relationship with a family (Chart 9–2). Important facts must be learned from the family and child regarding why they have come to the acute care setting and what their expectations are of the health care team. In addition, information about what the family may expect during their visit must be shared. If this exchange does not occur in a timely fashion, the family's trust of the hospital staff can be undermined. Unfortunately, cost containment issues have led to decreased staff-to-patient ratios, making timely communication a greater challenge. Nonetheless, priorities need to be set that support this initial in-depth exchange of information. The best context in which this exchange can occur is during the admission assessment.

Admission Assessment

Admission assessments need to include physiologic and psychosocial data. Ideally, the assessment occurs when the child's primary caregiver is present. Psychosocial assessments of younger children, especially infants, toddlers, and preschoolers, cannot be completed without the assistance of a parent or caregiver. The exception to this is the adolescent whose privacy and confidentiality needs may preclude the presence of a parent. Ultimately, the admission assessment cannot be completed without the information of the caregiver, who is able to give historical information about the child's health status, such as childhood illnesses and immunizations.

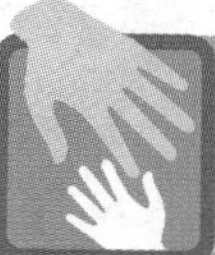

Chart 9–2
Nursing Interventions

Facilitating Communication with Parents of Acutely Ill Children

- Use active listening techniques:
  - Convey a non-hurried demeanor, and minimize interruptions.
  - Position self at same level when communicating (e.g., sit down).
  - Be aware of nonverbal messages conveyed in body stance and voice inflection.
  - Consider cultural background of parents when using some techniques (e.g., maintaining eye contact is considered disrespectful in many Asian cultures).
  - Clarify what you think you heard (e.g., "You are angry because the doctors did not talk with you this morning.").
  - Encourage and accept expression of feelings (use statements such as "This is a difficult time for you.").
  - Reflect parents' statements (e.g., "You feel guilty because you didn't call the doctor sooner.").
  - Ask the parents specific questions about their needs (e.g., "Do you need to go get something to eat? I will sit with Sandy while you are gone.").
  - Do not take anger personally.
- Provide information:
  - Give honest, accurate information.
  - Use short, simple explanations.
  - Be tactful in stating information, but do not try to minimize the seriousness of a situation.
  - Avoid letting long periods of time pass without giving information—especially in critical situations—even if it is only to tell the parents that the child's condition has not changed and what is being done to support the child.
  - Volunteer information freely to promote trust.
  - Teach and reinforce knowledge of disease process, treatments, and how parents can support their child.
- Be consistent:
  - Give same information over time and by different health team members.
  - Minimize the number of health team members interacting with the parents.
- Reinforce importance of the parent's role:
  - Acknowledge parents' expertise in knowing their child.
  - Encourage and provide opportunities for parents to provide physical care for the child; parents may need to be shown how they can do this (e.g., demonstrate how to bathe a child with an IV).
  - Ensure parent involvement in care conferences.

Communication with the caregiver must be in a context of respect for their role as the person most knowledgeable about the child, whether this individual is the parent, grandparent, or other legal guardian.

caREminder: *The objective of the assessment is to learn what information is needed to provide the best possible care for the child.*

If the caregiver understands this point, he or she will be more willing to cooperate with the assessment. The setting should provide as much privacy as possible, with minimal noise and stimulation. Learning from the caregiver how the child copes with new situations and what the child has been told about the current situation is important in planning how to approach the child. In addition, approaching the child with a communication style that matches developmental age is a key ingredient in completing an assessment that is most productive for the nurse and least frightening for the child (Chart 9–3).

Most acute care settings have standardized forms for the admission assessment (Fig. 9–1). These forms can cue the nurse to elicit all the important information in the most efficient manner possible. Such approaches to assessment may or may not be based on a nursing model. The tool's design helps the staff better understand the child's physiologic and developmental needs as well as the social, religious, and cultural practices that might be affected by hospitalization. The tool must be comprehensive and useful in order to serve as a sufficient mechanism for determining the child's condition on admission. It should cover key assessment areas of the child's history, including the following:

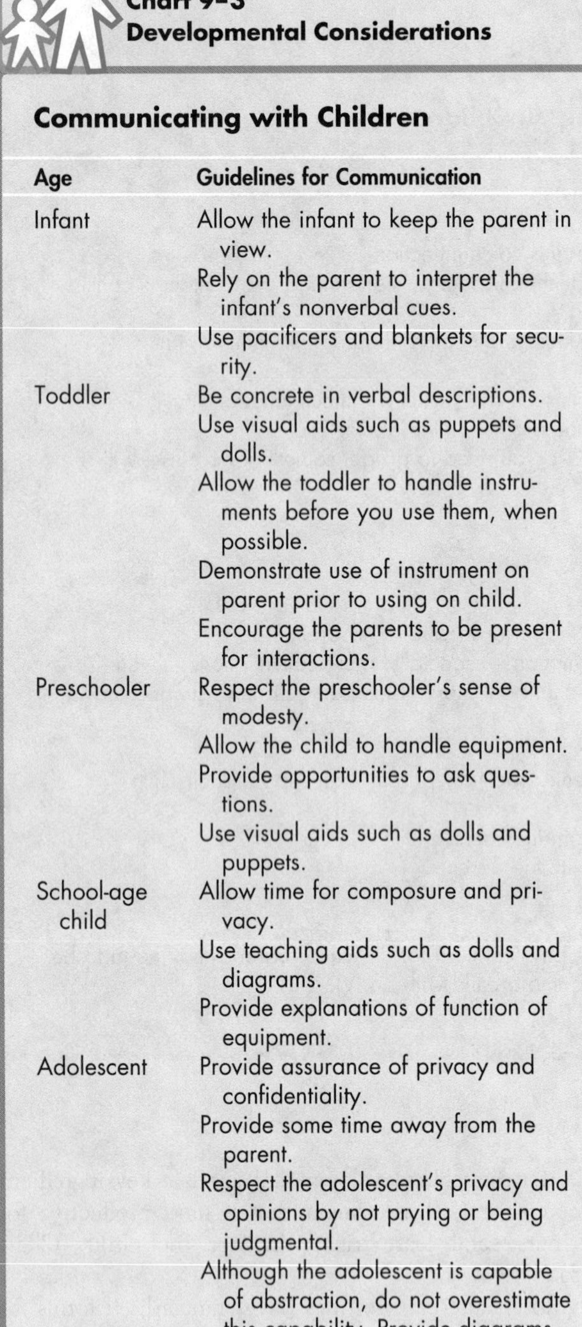

Chart 9–3
Developmental Considerations

Communicating with Children

Age	Guidelines for Communication
Infant	Allow the infant to keep the parent in view. Rely on the parent to interpret the infant's nonverbal cues. Use pacificers and blankets for security.
Toddler	Be concrete in verbal descriptions. Use visual aids such as puppets and dolls. Allow the toddler to handle instruments before you use them, when possible. Demonstrate use of instrument on parent prior to using on child. Encourage the parents to be present for interactions.
Preschooler	Respect the preschooler's sense of modesty. Allow the child to handle equipment. Provide opportunities to ask questions. Use visual aids such as dolls and puppets.
School-age child	Allow time for composure and privacy. Use teaching aids such as dolls and diagrams. Provide explanations of function of equipment.
Adolescent	Provide assurance of privacy and confidentiality. Provide some time away from the parent. Respect the adolescent's privacy and opinions by not prying or being judgmental. Although the adolescent is capable of abstraction, do not overestimate this capability. Provide diagrams and models to ensure comprehension.

- Present illness or reason for seeking health care
- Birth history
- Previous health challenges
- Childhood illnesses
- Immunizations
- Allergies
- Current medications
- Nutritional assessment
- Family medical history
- Environmental history
- Social history
- Growth and developmental history

At minimum, it should also guide a general head-to-toe assessment that examines

- Skin, head, eyes, ears, nose, and throat
- Cardiovascular and respiratory systems
- Gastrointestinal system
- Genitourinary/reproductive system
- Musculoskeletal system
- Neurologic system

Based on this general examination, priorities are established for more in-depth assessment in a particular area. For example, if an infant has no bowel sounds, the need for further immediate assessment and intervention becomes the priority of the examination. The documentation of findings, reporting of variances from the norm to appropriate personnel, and the development of a plan of care are also key ingredients of admission care (Chart 9–4).

Intensive Care Unit

The intensive care experience occurs in an environment that is truly a world unto itself, apart and different from the rest. If the hospitalization experience threatens family coping and health maintenance, the intensive care experience intensifies this threat. In terms of stress reduction, the needs of the child in the intensive care unit (ICU)

Figure 9–1
Documenting admission assessment findings in a computerized database organizes the information and makes it accessible to all health care providers.

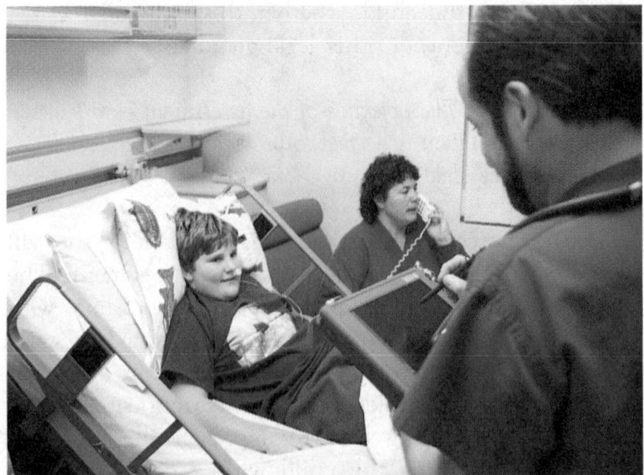

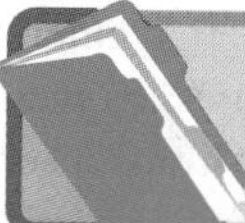

Chart 9–4
Nursing Interventions Classification (NIC)

Admission Care

Definition

Facilitating entry of a patient into a health care facility

Activities

- Introduce yourself.
- Provide appropriate privacy for the patient/family/significant others.
- Orient patient/family/significant others to immediate environment.
- Orient patient/family/significant others to agency facilities.
- Perform admission history.
- Perform admission physical assessment, as appropriate.
- Perform admission financial assessment, as appropriate.
- Perform admission psychosocial assessment, as appropriate.
- Perform admission religious assessment, as appropriate.
- Provide patient with "Patient's Bill of Rights."
- Document pertinent information.
- Maintain confidentiality of patient data.
- Identify patient at risk for readmission.
- Establish nursing diagnoses.
- Begin discharge planning.
- Implement safety precautions, as appropriate.
- Label patient's chart, room door, and/or head of bed, as indicated.
- Notify physician of admission and patient status.
- Obtain physician's orders for patient care.

From McCloskey, J., & Bulechek, G. (1996). *Nursing interventions classification (NIC)* (2nd ed.). St. Louis: Mosby–Year Book. Reprinted with permission.

and the needs of the family are separate. However, their effects on each other are highly interdependent in terms of outcome and cannot be addressed without that perspective. Certain factors that affect the child and family are the environment, routines, and family support and visitation policies.

The environment is one of noise and light. It has been demonstrated that noises in ICUs are often equal to that of rush-hour traffic (65 to 100 dB) and that sounds of 50 dB and above raise the perception of pain (Johnson et al., 1992). The sources of noise include alarms on monitors, pumps, machines, telephones, and staff communication. Overhead lighting is bright; in addition, phototherapy and heat lamps add additional light and heat to the environment. It is important to implement strategies to reduce such noxious stimuli (Chart 9–5).

The routines and procedures of the critical care unit make it confusing, frightening, and threatening for children. Protecting children from this milieu as much as possible is desirable (Johnson et al., 1992), including preventing children from seeing what is happening to other children, especially when other children are bleeding profusely or there are frightening aspects of care occurring. Family visitation and support is key in ameliorating this threat. Child life personnel who can interact with the children in the ICU also promote their adjustment to the process. An important nursing intervention is communication with the child to the extent possible, explaining what is happening in a manner that is developmentally appropriate for the child. For the child with impaired communication due to intubation or other reasons, communication supports may be used. These supports may include alphabet boards, picture boards, or word cards. In addition, the use of hand and eye signals can be very useful. Allowing the child to indicate his or her choice whenever possible may enhance a sense of control and increase the feeling of security and competence.

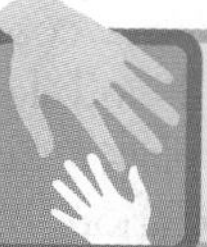

Chart 9–5
Nursing Interventions

Eliminating Noxious Stimuli

- Coordinate care to decrease noise.
- Place noisy equipment away from the head of the bed.
- Keep alarms turned low and promptly respond to them.
- Guard against loud talking, laughing, music.
- Decrease volume on overhead paging system.
- Provide acoustic design measures in the building (e.g., carpet, padded trash can lids, acoustical ceiling tile).
- Cycle light to maintain day and night differentiation.
- Control bright light through dimmed lighting.
- Replace white light with soft yellow lighting.
- Turn off overhead lighting when possible; use direct light at individual bedside as needed; use flashlights to check on children.
- Drape isolettes/cribs to prevent bright light.
- Shield infant's/child's eyes and ears.
- Evaluate benefit of providing soft music with a low pitch, slow tempo to promote relaxation.

Policies need to reflect a philosophy of family-centered care (see Chapter 1). The relationships between parents and children should be preserved to the extent possible through liberal visitation policies and other strategies (Committee on Hospital Care, American Academy of Pediatrics, 1993; Johnson et al., 1992). A 1988 ACCH survey concluded that significant progress had been made in establishing open 24-hour visitation for parents in critical care units; of the hospitals surveyed, 83% allowed 24-hour visitation for pediatric ICUs, and 93% allowed it for neonatal intensive care units (NICUs) (Johnson et al., 1992). However, these policies are often limited to parents, eliminating other important family supports, such as grandparents and siblings.

The rationales for these limitations have been that visits are upsetting for children and other family members, that visitation leads to cross-infection for the patient, and that it is physiologically damaging to the patient and disrupts the unit (Tughan, 1992). Staff attitudes and misconceptions of parental needs are the primary barriers that prevent implementation of open visitation (Page & Boeing, 1994). ACCH is a proponent of more open visiting, voicing the belief that the child and family can cope better with the stress of the situation through extended family support.

Another important policy consideration is the provision of information to parents. Successful coping is greatly dependent on timely information delivered in a coordinated, knowledgeable manner. Designating a coordinator for communication leads to improved and less confusing communication. Such persons can play a key role in building a supportive and trusting relation between family and staff. Interventions for facilitating communication between parents and staff are presented in Chart 9–2.

Inevitably one cannot discuss intervention in the intensive care setting without discussing grief and loss. As parents face the realities of losing their child, they greatly need supportive interventions that facilitate grief. These interventions include

- Listening while parents express their feelings
- Allowing them to acknowledge their loss
- Being available to the family no matter how uncomfortable the experience
- Helping parents realize that grieving occurs differently in each individual

See Chapter 12 for an in-depth discussion of grief and bereavement.

No less important in achieving family-centered care in the intensive care setting is the issue of staff competency. The staff should be prepared with knowledge and skills regarding disease and equipment management that is pertinent to pediatric critical care, communication theory, skills, and techniques that include crisis intervention, promotion of child and family coping, bereavement counseling, ethical decision-making with families, as well as providing developmentally supportive care (Johnson et al., 1992). This is a national standard of care and should be met in all pediatric critical care delivery settings.

Adolescent Unit

Another specialty unit is the adolescent unit. Characteristics of adolescent development dictate the need for special requirements in unit design. Adolescents have the need for establishment of a separate identity, peer interaction, and privacy. The environment should reflect that the unit is a place for teens. Desks should be available for schoolwork; each bed should have a telephone; bathrooms should afford privacy; and a lounge for recreation should be established (Johnson et al., 1992).

Unit operations should reflect the adolescent's autonomy by including them as partners in the health care team. This may be done by

- Teaching the adolescents about their illness
- Encouraging them to participate in decision-making about their condition
- Supporting the adolescents in managing their health (in such areas as medications, diet, and pain management)

Finally, promoting the continuance of their education through in-hospital school and school reintegration and providing supportive services such as teen rap groups, support groups, and peer and role-model visitation are components of designing an adolescent unit that is conceptually and developmentally well founded (Johnson et al., 1992).

Ambulatory Care Settings in the Hospital

As cost containment pressures increase, much of the care that had been delivered in hospitals is being moved to outpatient settings, such as primary and specialty care clinics, ambulatory surgery centers, and day hospitals. A special subset of ambulatory care is the emergency department. Although each setting delivers different types of care, they share some common design objectives. Waiting room design should address comfort, education and information needs, facilitation of social interaction, as well as privacy needs (Johnson et al., 1992). Play area design should be appropriate to the ages and physical conditions of the children served. Privacy and noise reduction are important factors in designing treatment rooms so that children are not frightened by what they see and hear. The latter guideline holds especially true for emergency departments, which can be chaotic, and consequently terrifying for children (Fig. 9–2).

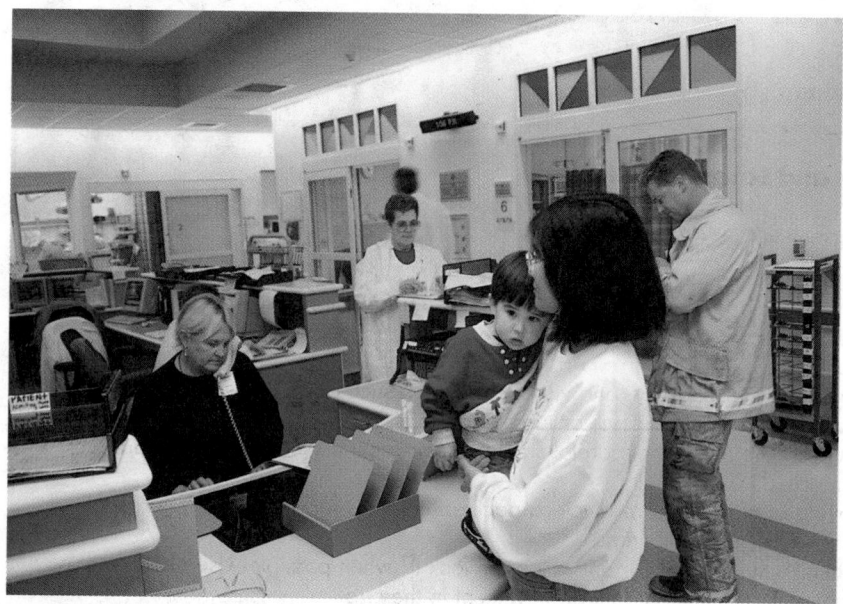

Figure 9–2
A child may be overwhelmed by the sights, sounds, and bustle of the emergency room. A parent's presence can help the child cope with this unfamiliar, sometimes frightening environment.

Day hospitals are a developing trend in care delivery and have been used for renal dialysis, hematology-oncology care, rehabilitation, and acquired immunodeficiency syndrome (AIDS)–related care (Johnson et al., 1992). Day hospitals usually have fixed hours of operation, most commonly during daylight hours. These units provide a setting to deliver time-limited, technically oriented procedures that for whatever reasons (i.e., environment, equipment, personnel, need for high technology support) cannot be done at home. They are less threatening to the health maintenance of the patient and family than inpatient settings. However, they are arenas in which painful and unpleasant experiences for the child occur. Time spent in the day hospital often means an absence from school or a missed opportunity doing some preferred activity. If the child's emotional, cognitive, social, and educational needs are not addressed, professional standards of care delivery will not be achieved, and positive patient outcomes will not be maximized (Johnson et al., 1992).

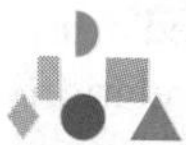

Responses to a Child's Acute Illness

Family coping skills are important factors to consider during a child's acute illness because families who face serious illness in a child (or family member) are at risk for psychosocial maladjustment (Tomlinson, Kirschbaum, Harbaugh, & Anderson, 1996; Youngblut & Shiao, 1993). However, not all families have difficulty coping with such a situation (LaMontagne, Johnson, & Hepworth, 1995). Those with effective coping skills fare much better. Therefore, the nurse must assess the family's coping skills, promote the use of effective ones, and teach additional skills if needed. Because pediatric care is family-centered, the nurse must understand the effects of hospitalization on the patient and family and must intervene to promote effective coping by all family members.

Child's Response to Hospitalization

Children tend to respond to hospitalization with emotional upset. Seminal work by Prugh, Staub, Sands, Kirschbaum, and Lenihan (1953) revealed how children react negatively to the stress of hospitalization with separation anxiety, loss of control, and unrealistic fears. These responses are often manifest in aggressive behaviors including crying, screaming, withdrawing, kicking, biting, hitting, physically resisting procedures, or ignoring requests. Hospitals have become more family-focused, but acute illness and hospitalization remain a threat to child development and family cohesion.

Separation Anxiety. Hospitalized children between the ages of 6 months and 4 years are at the greatest risk for separation anxiety (Bonn, 1994). Older children are still at risk, but increasing cognitive abilities and concept of time help them cope. Classic work by Robertson (1958) described the phases through which young children progress when separated from their parents:

- **Protest**—The child searches for the lost parent, angrily protests, cries frequently, and rejects hospital staff. When the parent returns, the child readily goes to him or her.

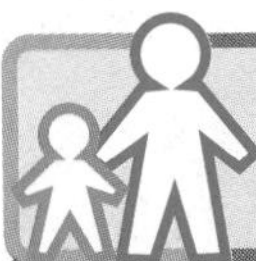

Chart 9–6
Developmental Considerations

Minimizing Separation Anxiety and Loss of Control

Age	Stressor	Intervention
Infant	Separation	Promote rooming-in of parents. Play peek-a-boo to promote mastery of the separation experience. Seek volunteer support for holding and stimulating the infant in the parent's absence. Provide tactile, auditory, and visual stimulation such as mobiles over the crib, cuddly toys, musical toys, or tape recordings. Minimize the number of caretakers; have consistent nurse assigned to care for the child. Provide comfort measures such as pacifier, holding, rocking, talking in a soothing voice, and cuddling.
	Loss of Control	Minimize the use of restraints. Heparin lock IV when possible. Use a crib with a canopy to allow freedom of movement in the crib. Alter the environment by using infant seat, buggy, or stroller and bringing the infant to playroom or nursing station when possible. Provide toys, such as stuffed animals, mirrors, and mobiles.
Toddler	Separation	Encourage rooming-in of parents. Teach parents to assess symptoms of stress, such as protest and withdrawal. Encourage parents to provide comfort measures. Play hide-and-seek with the child to promote mastery of the separation experience. Use doll-play to demonstrate that parents will return. Give the child time frames when parent will return: "After Sesame Street is over." Have parents bring in "transitional objects" from home to promote familiarity with the environment (e.g., favorite toys, clothes, tapes of family members' voices, photographs of family members, and pets).
	Loss of Control	Promote home rituals, such as feeding and bedtime rituals. Promote dietary practices similar to those at home. Encourage autonomy by giving choices when possible, such as with toys or games. Take the child to the playroom. Provide an opportunity for medical play. Teach the parents that regression is a typical response to hospitalization and will usually resolve when the child returns home.

- **Despair**—The child becomes more sad and apathetic, mourning the lost parent, crying less, and searching the environment less. When the parent returns, the child may not readily approach him or her or may cling to the parent.
- **Denial or Detachment**—The child becomes cheerful, interested in the environment and new persons, seemingly unaware of the lost parent, friendly with staff, and developing superficial relationships.

caREminder: *Because the child becomes increasingly "easier" to work with, it may be mistakenly interpreted that the child is coping effectively.*

However, children who progress to denial suffer long-term impaired parental relationships and impaired trust, which can lead to problems in establishing close relationships, attention deficits, self-centeredness, and decreased intellectual functioning. Therefore, the pediatric nurse must develop interventions that reduce separation anxiety (Chart 9–6).

Separation anxiety is not unique to younger children. Preschoolers exhibit fewer symptoms of restlessness, hyperactivity, and irritability but more somatic symptoms (such as vomiting, urinary frequency, diarrhea, and dizziness) (Chart 9–7).

School-age children manifest anxiety but exhibit

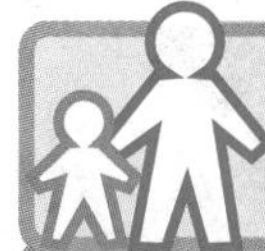

Chart 9–6
Developmental Considerations *Continued*

Minimizing Separation Anxiety and Loss of Control

Age	Stressor	Intervention
Preschooler	Separation Loss of Control	Use interventions for toddlers. Encourage autonomy by offering choices and participation in self-care. Take the child to the playroom. Urge the child to participate in medical and therapeutic play. Be truthful with the child.
School-age child	Separation	Promote communication with siblings and friends. Maintain normalcy by encouraging the child to do homework from school. Be available to talk to the child. Be supportive when the child expresses feelings of loneliness. Take the child to the playroom. Explain to the parents the importance of frequent visits. Rooming-in is not necessary.
	Loss of Control	Provide opportunities to discuss the medical situation. Encourage the child to discuss his or her understanding. Provide explanations of the medical situation, using diagrams, equipment, and concrete explanations. Allow opportunities for the child to achieve the developmental goal of "industry" by helping with tasks. Promote choices in care, if possible.
Adolescent	Separation	Promote peer interactions. Promote parent visitation. Teach parents the importance of the adolescent's need for control. Provide activities, such as "rap sessions," dances, and make-up sessions.
	Loss of Control	Develop the plan of care with the adolescent. Respect the adolescent's need for independence. Offer choices in routines, if possible. Allow for privacy. Be open and forthright about the medical situation. Allow time to discuss this with the adolescent.

fewer panic reactions than younger children. Children of this age have a concept of time and understand that parents need to leave and that parents will return. Their anxiety is related to fear of the unknown or unexplained, and their coping mechanisms are denial and rationalization.

The adolescent suffers separation anxiety when separated from peers rather than parents, but it is still crucial that they are confident in their parents' commitment to them (Armsden & Lewis, 1993). The adolescent's efforts to maintain peer contact may break hospital rules. For example, the adolescent may leave the hospital without permission, leave the unit after hours to meet peers in the lobby, use the telephone excessively (to the exclusion of participating in the hospital regimen), or refuse hospital treatments that are viewed as disfiguring or displeasing to peers.

Loss of Control. Hospitalized children commonly experience loss of control. Unlike separation anxiety, which decreases as the child ages, control issues persist because the child is removed from the normal environment. Minimizing separation anxiety and loss of control is crucial to promoting effective coping for the hospitalized child.

Fears. General fears by developmental age (see Chapter 5) are important to keep in mind when children are hospitalized:

- Infants fear loud noises, sudden movements, and loss of physical and emotional support.
- Older infants fear separation, strangers, and heights.

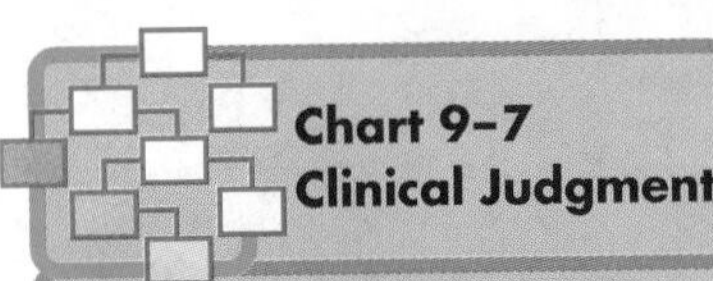

Chart 9–7
Clinical Judgment

Separation Anxiety

Darlene, age 4, was admitted to the hospital for intravenous antibiotic therapy for severe periorbital cellulitis. She cried in response to any interventions, but stopped quickly when her mother was present. However, when her mother, Mrs. G., tried to leave, Darlene clung to her and screamed. Soon, Mrs. G. began to leave without telling Darlene. The first time this occurred, Darlene cried most of the night. The nurse asked Mrs. G. to tell Darlene when she planned to leave and when she would return, to allay the child's anxiety. However, Mrs. G. felt bad when she told Darlene because Darlene started to "act up." After the first two nights, Darlene stopped crying, but began bed-wetting and waking frequently during the night, calling for her mother. During the day, she was listless and had decreased appetite. Mrs. G. became concerned about her daughter's regressive behaviors and asked the nurse for help.

Questions

1. How well is Darlene adapting to hospitalization? How is her mother responding?
2. What factors did you consider in making your assessment?
3. Which nursing diagnosis is applicable in this situation?
4. What should the nurse do to help Darlene and Mrs. G. cope more effectively?
5. What behaviors will indicate that Darlene is coping more effectively?

Answers

1. Darlene is not adapting well. Mrs. G. is responding by avoiding the situation.
2. Initially, Darlene showed normal behaviors expected in response to the acute stressor of hospitalization: crying with treatments and clinging to her mother when she tried to leave. When Mrs. G. started leaving without telling Darlene, Darlene cried even without the stimulation of treatments. Darlene then stopped crying but was listless and had decreased appetite. She also wet the bed and woke frequently.
3. Ineffective family coping: disabling.
4. Listen to Mrs. G.'s concerns, eliciting reasons for why she leaves without telling Darlene. If Mrs. G. thinks that she upsets Darlene more by telling her, because Darlene then clings to her and screams, explain that this is an expected, healthy reaction to separation. Have Mrs. G. agree that she will always let Darlene know when Mrs. G. is leaving and when she will return. The nurse can be present at this time and comfort Darlene when her mother leaves. Ask Mrs. G. if any other family or friends can stay in Mrs. G.'s absence. Encourage Mrs. G. to bring in photographs, personal objects (favored objects of Darlene's, a piece of Mrs. G.'s clothing), and tapes of Mrs. G. or her husband reading stories. Arrange for child life specialist to implement doll-play with Darlene depicting mother leaving and returning. Reinforce with Darlene that "Mommy will come back ________" (after your nap, when Sesame Street is over).
5. Darlene is more animated, involved in playing, and responding to her environment; her appetite and sleep patterns improve; there is a decreased frequency of bed-wetting. It would be expected that Darlene will continue to protest when Mrs. G. leaves.

- Toddlers fear the dark, being alone, animals, some machines, and draining tubs.
- Preschoolers fear mutilation, the unknown, the supernatural, and separation.
- School-age children fear bodily injury, death, unsafe situations, loss of control, having a parent die, and school-related concerns.
- Adolescents fear loss of peer relationships, body disfigurement, loss of physical abilities, and death in the family.

Fears more specific to children who are ill or hospitalized are of intrusive procedures, body distortion, or mutilation (Brennan, 1994). Needles and shots are often cited as what children fear most (Rice, 1993). When asked which things they were fearful of, hospitalized school-age children ranked highest separation from family, having shots and fingersticks, having to stay in the hospital a long time, and being told something was wrong with them (Hart & Bossert, 1994). Children with higher trait anxiety and from lower income families reported higher amounts of fear (Hart & Bossert, 1994).

Fears of the child need to be considered during all interventions. Many of a child's fears are actualized in the hospital: separation, loss of control, body mutilation, and painful events. The nurse must provide developmentally appropriate explanations to counter unrealistic fears and intervene to minimize trauma caused by those fears that are real (e.g., encourage parental presence during procedures or in the postanesthesia care unit [PACU], have child make decisions/allow choices whenever possible, use topical anesthetics and/or oral medications to reduce pain from needle sticks).

Promoting Coping in Hospitalized Children

The nurse needs to support the child in developing effective coping behaviors. The predominant patterns of coping by preschoolers and school-age children were found to be taking direct action and information-seeking (Corbo-Richert, Caty, & Barnes, 1993). However, other children cope by information limiting or avoiding (Thompson, 1994). This reinforces the need for individualized intervention. It is often thought that a well-prepared child will cope better. When teaching, the nurse needs to be alert to the child's cues indicating how much information is desired and prepare the child based on this.

Teach the child strategies that can reduce stress and promote coping, such as relaxation, imagery, distraction, and positive self-talk (see Chapter 13 for further discussion). Parental involvement also helps the child cope. A positive relationship between the number of activities a parent participates in and the child's behavior during hospitalization has been demonstrated (Jones, 1994). Simple hand-holding has also been shown to promote coping. Adolescents preferred to hold their mother's hand. If she was unavailable, then they preferred a specific nurse's hand (Weekes, Kagan, James, & Seboni, 1993).

Therapeutic play can also be used to promote coping by helping children work through hospital experiences. This may be effective for a number of reasons: It provides the child with information; the child feels a sense of control and mastery when able to manipulate the equipment and play situation; and the nurse or child life specialist can use the session to model effective coping behaviors.

Children often reveal their fears and concerns through drawing. Based on knowledge of growth and development, the nurse can use drawings as an effective method of assessment and vehicle for communication with the child. In identifying the child's concerns and perceptions, the nurse can correct misconceptions and support coping skills. A nurse should use drawings for psychotherapy only if trained for such. Drawing materials are familiar to the child and non-threatening and may support coping through distraction. Most children draw without prompting; some ask for guidance about what to draw. A broad, non-directive response may help elicit issues of concern to the child (e.g., "what it will be like after surgery" or "what you are thinking of right now"). What children draw and how they draw it may be significant. For example, very large things may imply aggressive tendencies (often the health care team or equipment such as needles are large), tiny things (the child in bed) may imply feelings of insignificance or inferiority (O'Malley & McNamara, 1993). Remember that not every drawing has therapeutic significance—a picture may just be a picture.

Music can also be used to promote coping. The child can select the music, giving him or her control over the situation and providing a familiar milieu and distraction. The child's preference should be honored, although music that has a slow tempo (60 to 80 beats per minute) with low pitch at low volume is best for promoting relaxation and reducing tension (Kaminski & Hall, 1996; Klein & Winkelstein, 1996) (Fig. 9–3).

Assisting the family in obtaining a temporary pager may enhance coping and satisfaction for children and families (Ashenberg, Maier, Lambert, & McAliley, 1996). Treatment of acute illness frequently involves waiting, which exacerbates anxiety and frustration. Having a pager may enable the child and family to leave the clinic or child's room to go to the cafeteria or playroom and return when paged. Having a pager also lets the parents run errands, eat, or just get out of the room while the child sleeps, knowing they can be paged when the child awakens. These options allow the family choices that increase their control and promote coping.

Family's Response to Hospitalization

Family members are affected by hospitalization based on their relationship to the child and their role in the family. The parents' coping abilities may be reduced by fi-

Figure 9–3
This adolescent listens to soothing music to promote relaxation and coping during stressful procedures.

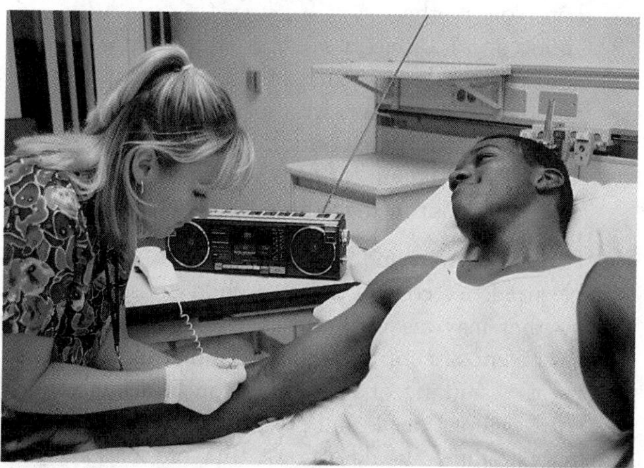

nancial, emotional, or work-related stressors, as well as the need to care for their other children as well as the hospitalized child. Siblings' coping skills can be affected by misperceptions about the sick child's condition and feelings of loss, parental neglect, isolation, or loneliness. The nurse needs to know how parents and siblings may be affected by the child's hospitalization.

Coping by Parents

In acute care, parental coping is just as important as the child's coping. Hospitalization of a seriously ill child can precipitate a crisis for the family. Parents may become anxious and confused and may develop psychosomatic symptoms, guilt, and denial (Kruger, 1992). They may respond with defensiveness and projection of anger onto staff members.

The nurse needs to know how to support parents during this time (see Chart 10–3). By providing appropriate information to parents about hospitalization, the nurse can reduce their anxiety during the child's hospital stay. By enhancing the parents' understanding of the child's illness, the nurse can promote their ability to cope with it (Melnyk, 1995; Tomlinson et al., 1996).

The child's hospitalization may make the parents feel a loss of control, which can become a barrier to family-centered care in that parents lose their normal parenting roles. Loss of control over the care of one's child may cause humiliation or anger. A different perspective from the traditional view of health care providers is that the parent should always be viewed as the "expert in charge," because parents have the right to make most decisions about care, not the medical staff. Parents have identified the need to have information (e.g., the prognosis, why things are done to the child, knowing the child is being treated for pain) as very important (Fisher, 1994). In their role as "protector" of their child, having information may help them maintain control. Schepp (1992) identified four factors that affect the need for control:

- Mother's age: Younger mothers needed more control than older mothers.
- Child's age: Mothers of younger children needed more control than mothers of older children.
- Hospital time: Mothers who spent more time in the hospital needed more control.
- Number of children: Mothers with fewer children need more control than those with more children.

These research findings suggest that parents have variable needs for control during a child's hospitalization. One mother may regard a nurse's action as an excellent relinquishment of control. Another mother may see these actions as a shirking of duty. Therefore, the nurse must assess the parents' needs and preferences for participation in care. The nurse should also use this information when planning interventions in order to promote parent coping and satisfaction with care. Similarly, the nurse's expectations regarding parental participation in their child's care must be individualized and clearly discussed with the parent at the onset of the hospital stay.

Coping by Siblings

Family-centered care also addresses the needs of siblings. Therefore, the nurse should assess each sibling for risk factors that affect coping and signs of stress and ineffective coping (Chart 9–8). Children who perceived more changes in their parents' behavior were found to experience more stress (Simon, 1993).

Tip: *Ask the siblings how they think things are different since the child has been sick or in the hospital.*

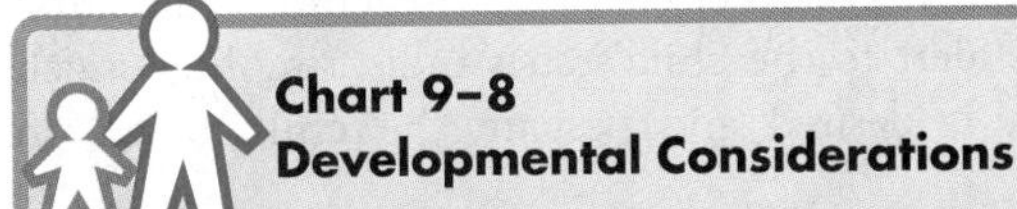

Chart 9–8
Developmental Considerations

Sibling Coping with Hospitalization

Risk Factors in the Sibling

- Sibling is undergoing stress in other areas, such as school or peer relationships.
- Sibling has a poor relationship with the parents or the ill child before the illness began.
- Sibling has not developed effective coping skills as part of general life strategies.
- Sibling is cared for outside of own home.
- Increased change in parents' behavior.

Risk Factors in the Ill Child

- Ill child is developmentally delayed.
- Ill child has multiple handicaps.
- Ill child has chronic or genetically transmitted disorder.
- Ill child has an altered body image, such as that caused by amputation, burns, disfigurement, or scars.
- Ill child has a terminal condition.
- Ill child is in an intensive care unit.
- Ill child is undergoing prolonged or repeated hospitalizations.

Signs of Stress

- Somatic symptoms—vomiting, diarrhea, or abdominal pain.
- Change in appetite.
- Change in academic performance.
- Change in temperament—irritability, nervousness, sorrow, difficulty concentrating.

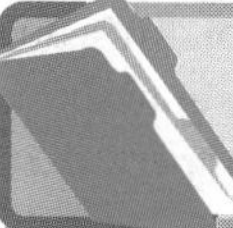

Chart 9–9
Nursing Interventions Classification (NIC)

Sibling Support

Definition

Assisting a sibling to cope with a brother's or sister's illness

Activities

- Explore what sibling knows about ill brother or sister.
- Appraise stress in sibling related to condition of ill brother or sister.
- Appraise sibling's coping with illness of brother or sister.
- Facilitate family members' awareness of sibling's feelings.
- Provide information about common sibling response and what other family members can do to help.
- Perform sibling advocacy role (e.g., in case of life-threatening situations when anxiety is high and parents or other family members are unable to perform that role).
- Recognize that each sibling responds differently.
- Encourage parents or other family members to provide honest information to sibling.
- Encourage parents to arrange for care of young siblings in their own home, if possible.
- Assist sibling to maintain and/or modify usual routines and activities of daily living, as necessary.
- Promote communication between well sibling and ill brother or sister.
- Encourage sibling to visit ill brother or sister.
- Explain to visiting sibling what is being done in care of ill brother or sister.
- Encourage well sibling to participate in care of the ill brother or sister, as appropriate.
- Recognize and respect sibling who may not be emotionally ready to visit an ill brother or sister.
- Encourage maintenance of parental or family interactional patterns.
- Assist sibling to clarify and explore concerns.
- Use drawings, puppetry, and dramatic play to see how younger sibling perceives events.
- Clarify sibling concern for contracting the illness of the affected child, and develop strategies for coping with concern.
- Teach pathology of disease to sibling, according to developmental stage and learning style.
- Use concrete substitutes for sibling who is unable to visit ill brother or sister (e.g., pictures and videos).
- Explain to young siblings that they are not the cause of illness.
- Teach siblings strategies for meeting own emotional and developmental needs.
- Provide referral to peer sibling group, as appropriate.
- Provide community resource referrals to sibling, as necessary.
- Communicate situation to the school nurse to promote support for young sibling, in accord with parental wishes.

From McCloskey, J., & Bulechek, G. (1996). *Nursing interventions classification (NIC)* (2nd ed.). St. Louis: Mosby–Year Book. Reprinted with permission.

Parental perceptions of effects of illness on the siblings have not been found to correlate with siblings' self-report, therefore it is more accurate to obtain information directly from the sibling (Craft, 1993). On the basis of assessment findings, the nurse should intervene to promote sibling coping (Chart 9–9).

Prolonged Hospitalization

Advances in technology have made it possible for many children who would have died years ago to survive critical illness. Some of these children are acutely ill for a period of time, and although their health status stabilizes, they continue to have care needs that necessitate hospitalization. These children may remain in the hospital for many months, or even years. To a child and their family, the hospital environment can be confusing and overstimulating. Periods of rest are often broken by painful events and procedures. It is not an environment that is conducive to normal parenting or achievement of tasks that promote growth and development in the child. Incorporation of the family's cultural mores is hampered during prolonged hospitalization because exposure to the foods, language, and traditions of the culture is usually limited.

Parenting. Prolonged hospitalization imposes different parenting demands than those in the home. Initially, parents need to deal with the child's illness and uncertainty regarding the outcome (see Chapter 10 for discussion of chronic conditions). Parents may feel that their role is less important because the health care team has the technological expertise to care for the child's physical needs.

The health care team can do a number of things to strengthen the parent–child bond. Identify a few key staff members for the family to communicate with. This enables these staff members to become familiar with the family's needs and strengths and how to best support these. If parents are unable to stay with the child, minimize interruptions when they do visit. Encourage parents to perform normal parenting tasks (e.g., providing physical care, promoting acquisition of developmental tasks, setting limits) and reinforce how important they are to their child. Offer information freely to make parents feel they are an integral part of the child's care. There will be times when parents cope better than at other times; negotiate with them about how involved they want to be in the child's care (e.g., some days they are ready to learn new skills, others they may only have the emotional energy to rock their child) (Wells, DeBoard-Burns, Cook, & Mitchell, 1994b). When hospitalization is prolonged, families often become close to each other, sharing information about themselves and their child.

caREminder: *It is important to keep information confidential. If families want to share information with the families of other patients, it is the parents' prerogative. The health team should not make those decisions for them.*

Financial concerns often become more of an issue with prolonged hospitalization. Initially parents may have been given a paid leave from work. After a period of time, parents may need to return to work in order to maintain insurance benefits. They may feel powerless and guilty because they must work and thus cannot be with the child as much as they would like. Parents may feel stuck in a position, unable to change jobs because of preexisting condition exclusions on much-needed insurance. All of these factors may make the parent less able to support their child during their hospitalization.

Effect on the Child. Growing up in the hospital may lead to delayed development of psychosocial skills (Wells, DeBoard-Burns, Cook, & Mitchell, 1994a). Prolonged hospitalization may interfere with the development of trust and attachment. This is of particular concern in infants, who may not form a primary attachment with parents as a result of multiple caretakers meeting the child's needs in often inconsistent ways. It is important to have consistent caretakers, who all follow a consistent plan, maintain the child's routine, and set consistent limits on behavior. The plan should be developed jointly with the parents, health team, and child if he or she is old enough to participate in the discussion.

Early developmental intervention to prevent the negative effects of prolonged hospitalization is preferable (Fig. 9–4). Nurses are often task-oriented and less developmentally focused and must strive to encourage developmentally appropriate tasks, even though they may take longer to perform. For example, a toddler needs to learn to feed himself, a preschooler needs to dress herself. Doing it themselves fosters a sense of control, difficult to achieve in the hospital. This bolsters self-esteem and socialization skills. Create personal space for the child,

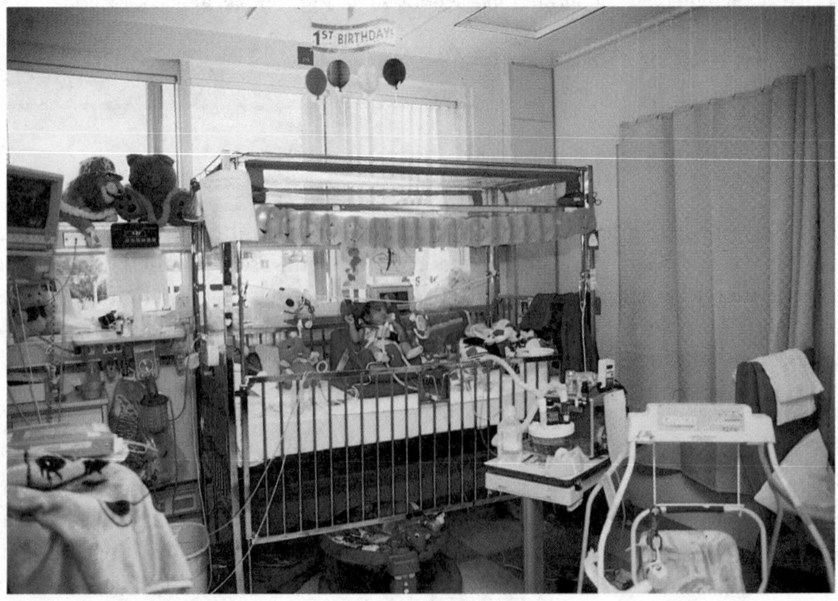

Figure 9–4
Celebration of special events and developmental milestones is important in normalizing a child's life when hospitalization is prolonged. "Lucky" celebrates his first birthday in the hospital. He was hospitalized for 10½ of his first 12 months of life.

even if it is only a small area, which also helps develop a sense of control. Help the child identify acceptable outlets for expressing negative feelings such as gross motor activity, pounding toys, or words to use. Take infants to the playroom; provide school for older children (Standiford, Ahlrichs, Carmicle, & Wells, 1993). Children of any age benefit from trips outside. Remember to treat the child as a child, not as a disease.

Discharge. After a prolonged hospitalization, discharge presents a greater challenge than normal. The child must adjust, or readjust, to the home environment, with resultant changes in lifestyle. Parents often need to change their schedule and demands of care. Family routines and dynamics will change with the introduction or reintroduction of the child who has been hospitalized. Siblings may need to adjust to changing behavioral expectations, household chores, and routines.

The child and family benefit from a period of transition prior to the actual discharge (Wells et al., 1994b). Assess what will be needed in the setting the child will be going to; not all children may be able to be discharged home. Determine what equipment, schooling, therapy, respite care, home care, and transportation will need to be arranged. (See Chapter 11 for more information.)

Tip: *Remember to talk to the child about the planned discharge. Home passes may help the child and family adjust to the change. When the child returns to the hospital, talk concretely about how it was: what they did, ate, saw, where they slept, etc. This will make the impending discharge more real to the child and help ease the transition.*

Have the parents assume total care of the child in the hospital for 24 hours in order to gain familiarity and comfort with the process while still having medical support close at hand.

Hospitalization as a Threat to Family Cohesion

Hospitalization can threaten family cohesiveness by affecting the patient, the parents, and the siblings. Each person suffers a different kind of trauma from hospitalization. Consequently, the nurse must meet their needs with different interventions. The nurse must also determine how the family as a system is affected. Previous family routines, roles, and structures may need to be changed or abolished to meet the needs of the sick child. This can involve giving up pets (as with an asthmatic child), changing sleeping arrangements (as for a child with cystic fibrosis who needs nighttime therapy), and changing foods (as for a child with diabetes). Hospitalization may place extra stress on an already strained family, pushing the family into crisis and possible loss of cohesiveness.

Research suggests that families who can maintain cooperation, social support, and understanding of the medical situation, have open communication with the health care team, are self-directed, and use problem-focused coping strategies are better able to adapt to the ill child (LaMontagne et al., 1995). These factors also may help them maintain cohesiveness and support each other. See Chapter 3 for additional information regarding family assessment and interventions to maintain integrity during maturational and situational crises.

Financial Considerations. Parents of ill children face increased financial demands. They may have such expenses as surgeries, medications, equipment, supplies, travel, and baby-sitting for siblings. If both parents must work to pay for these expenses, they may find it difficult to visit the hospital to support the child. For such parents, the nurse's encouragement to visit and promote child coping may become another stressor, producing guilt and anger. That is why the nurse should include financial concerns in all family assessments. Also, the health care team should be sensitive to the family's financial situation and help them find other means of support for the child, such as visits by grandparents or friends.

A family's socioeconomic class can affect its financial concerns. For example, families from lower socioeconomic classes face greater financial burdens and practical difficulties from a child's hospitalization. Transport may be a barrier to visitation if families depend on public transportation. Lack of money for the care of other siblings may also affect the family's visitation.

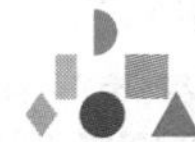

Support for the Child and Family During Acute Illness

During a child's acute illness, the crux of family-centered care is consistent support of the family and child. This support requires interdisciplinary teamwork directed and monitored by a case management process, child life programs, referrals to support groups or other resources such as social work, and child life or psychiatric counseling.

caREminder: *Support is provided by an underlying philosophy of atraumatic care. Most diagnostic procedures and interventions to restore health are psychologically distressing, if not invasive and painful. The goal when implementing interventions using principles of atraumatic care is to minimize the emotional and physical trauma associated with procedures and the health care environment (Chart 9–10).*

Chart 9–10
Nursing Interventions

Delivering Atraumatic Care

Aspect of Care	Interventions
Psychological	Always explain what is happening to the child—in their terms, not in adult and medical terms. Do not go into a lot of detail; keep it simple, direct, and honest. Do not tell the child it is not going to hurt if it is, but do not dwell on the pain factor. The use of topical anesthesia and medications assists in obtaining the cooperation of the child in the procedure. Ask the child to draw a picture of what is going to happen—you may find many misconceptions as well as open opportunities for discussion. Keep the parents involved as much as possible nurturing and supporting the child; do not isolate the child from parent. The parent's absence may be more traumatic to the child than the procedure.
Environment	Keep the child's environment as non-threatening as possible. Interpret the surroundings from the child's point of view. What does that large machine look like—possibly a monster? Are there all types of implements out that cause pain or look scary? Is the room very sterile with no friendly items around? The machines can be draped with sheets or put in other areas; the implements can be put away. To soften the area and to distract the child from any potential procedures, add pictures (even handdrawn) of rainbows, butterfly, or flowers, or a stuffed animal.
Restraints	Use restraints as minimally as possible and use the least restrictive one that provides safety (e.g., start with mittens first before a full arm restraint). Attempt at first to distract the child with games or toys, sing songs, read stories, or tell silly jokes. If the IV is in the child's right hand and the child is right-handed, both the nurse and the child should draw left-handed, make designs, "silly" pictures, or play board games only require that one hand, etc. If it is absolutely necessary to restrain a child, allow periods of freedom while supervised, e.g., during bath or meals.
Pain	Medicate freely. Do not withhold medication after surgery because the infant or child is not crying. Look for other signs of distress: pallor, furrowed brow, grimaces, shallow and rapid breathing, withdrawal of limb or area in pain, or thrashing around. Obtain the child's subjective rating of pain if possible.
Surgery	Prepare child prior to hospitalization if possible with a visit to see the environment and play with the items to be used to gain familiarity (blood pressure cuff, masks [both surgical and anesthesia], IV equipment, etc.) and to have the schedule explained. Have the child draw pictures and tell a story about the experience to get a better idea of the child's true impressions.
Suturing	Use topical anesthesia prior to injecting the area with an intradermal anesthetic. Use as fine a needle as possible (30 gauge if possible). Cover the wounds with as small a dressing as possible, and decrease size of dressings as the wound improves. A child will correlate the size of the dressing with the severity of the wound.
Blood drawing	Draw blood as infrequently as possible. Attempt to draw as few specimens as possible for the maximum amount of tests. When doing heelsticks on infants, first use a topical anesthetic, such as EMLA cream, and use a non-traumatic lancet such as a Tenderfoot rather than a regular lancet or a scalpel blade. When doing venous draws, the use of EMLA cream at least 1 hour prior to the draw allows for sufficient anesthesia.
IVs	Prior to the insertion, use EMLA cream. Attempt to place the IV in a location where the child or infant will not need a lot of restraints or arm boards. If not possible, use padded or air-filled arm boards of the appropriate size, with a non-threatening look (e.g., colorful covers with pediatric designs) to provide extra cushioning. Allow the older child to become familiar with the IV equipment by using tubing for play or creative endeavors. Soften the impact of IV poles and pumps by attaching pictures of animals, butterflies, or rainbows or stuffed animals to them.
Injections	Use the appropriate length and bore needle. Administer medication in the largest muscle mass possible, as deep as possible. Use a topical anesthetic such as EMLA cream 1 to 2 hours prior to injection to increase local anesthesia. If medication is very irritating, mix with a small amount of lidocaine, unless it is contraindicated.

With the increasing emphasis on family-centered care, there has been a reorientation from regarding the health professional as the expert to viewing the parents as expert in care of their child, therefore encouraging continued parental involvement in care of their child during hospitalization (Johnson & Lindschau, 1996) (see Chapter 1). Most parents actively participate in caring for their child, believing that it is beneficial for the child. Ongoing assessment and a positive attitude toward parent participation help guide the nurse in developing interventions that are individualized to best support the family. Parent's readiness to care is fostered by familiarity and experience with care, a supportive family network, and support from other parents (Coyne, 1995). The nurse and family need to negotiate to develop mutual understanding of what will be done by whom (Evans, 1994). Recognize that parents' ability to provide care varies depending on the parents' psychological and physiologic status, the situation, the child's status, and other stressors. At times, parents are ready to learn new skills. At other times, parents can provide previously mastered care or only routine hygiene and nutrition or simply provide psychological support with no physical care. Occasionally parents may need to withdraw and regroup before being able to actively participate in their child's care again. Supporting parental involvement is usually beneficial for both child and family.

Acute illness affects children and families in variable ways depending on the child's age, developmental needs, and diagnosis. The family's coping skills and resources also influence reaction to the illness and interventions needed to support the child and family.

Assessment identifies nursing diagnoses pertinent to the individual child and family. Nursing diagnoses usually applicable to the hospitalized child and family are identified in Chart 9–11. To identify nursing diagnoses most

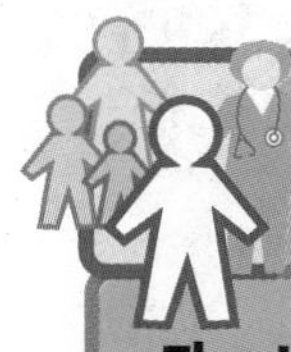

Chart 9–11
Nursing Diagnoses and Outcomes

The Hospitalized Child and Family

Ineffective family coping related to hospitalization of child

Outcomes:
Family will exhibit adequate internal levels of cooperation to organize daily family activities during hospitalization.
Family will accept need for hospitalization and adopt strategies for maintaining relationship with hospitalized child during hospitalization.
Family will articulate an optimistic, but realistic, definition of the situation by discharge.
Family will recognize and utilize resources by discharge.

Knowledge deficit: child's diagnosis and treatment, hospital routine

Outcomes:
Child/Family will be knowledgeable regarding disease process and necessary medical intervention during hospitalization and after discharge.
Child/Family will be knowledgeable about and understand rationale for hospital routines.

Ineffective individual coping related to effects of hospitalization

Outcomes:
Child will utilize age-appropriate developmentally effective coping strategies to deal with the process of hospitalization:
- Engage in play or discussion to decrease fear of procedures
- Feel a sense of trust and security in relation to continued family integrity
- Obtain sleep and rest necessary for achieving wellness

Anxiety and fear related to procedures/unknown processes

Outcomes:
Child will engage in play to decrease fear of procedures.
Child/Family will practice developmentally appropriate coping strategies.

Powerlessness related to reaction to new environment

Outcomes:
Child will gain age-appropriate mastery of environment through play and establishment of routines that mimic home environment to the extent possible.
Child/Family will perform activities of daily living in new environment through support of caregivers.

likely to apply to the specific physiologic problem, refer to the chapter dealing with that pathology.

Education to Support the Child and Family

Before providing information, the nurse must determine the learning needs of the child and family. Throughout the initial interview, the nurse collects data about their physical and psychosocial needs. Then the nurse analyzes the data to determine whether the child and family understand the situation. By identifying knowledge deficits on admission, the nurse can plan effective teaching strategies that address parents' and family's deficits and promote coping.

Learning needs are affected by many factors, including prior experience with illness, cultural background, language skills, the patient's and family's educational levels, and the patient's developmental level (Rakel, 1992). An educational plan must address factors to meet the patient's and family's information needs.

Patient teaching may be classified in several ways. The nurse may teach individuals or groups. The acute care nurse commonly teaches about diseases, preoperative care, procedures or treatments, prescribed medications, prescribed diet, prescribed activity, and psychomotor skills. Sometimes a teaching plan incorporates several of these topics.

The process of patient teaching resembles the nursing process. Teaching begins with assessment of the problem and of readiness to learn. Then it progresses to de-

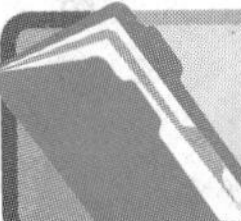

Chart 9–12
Nursing Interventions Classification (NIC)

Play Therapy

Definition

Purposeful use of toys or other equipment to assist a patient in communicating his/her perception of the world and to help in mastering the environment

Activities

- Provide developmentally appropriate play equipment.
- Provide safe play equipment.
- Provide equipment that stimulates creative, expressive play.
- Provide equipment that stimulates role playing.
- Provide equipment that stimulates aggressive or regressive play, as appropriate.
- Provide real or simulated hospital equipment to encourage expression of knowledge and feelings about hospitalization, treatments, or illness.
- Provide a quiet environment that is free from interruptions.
- Communicate acceptance of feelings, both positive and negative, expressed through play.
- Set limits for therapeutic play session.
- Communicate purpose of play session.
- Supervise play therapy sessions.
- Discuss play activities with family.
- Encourage patient to share feelings, knowledge, and perceptions.
- Observe the patient's use of play equipment.
- Record observations made during play session.
- Structure play session to facilitate desired outcome.
- Allow patient to manipulate play equipment.
- Validate patient feelings expressed during the play session.
- Compare data gathered from observations of behavior during play session with data obtained from history.
- Continue play sessions on a regular basis to establish trust and reduce fear of unfamiliar equipment or treatments.
- Determine patient's misconceptions through comments made during hospital role-playing sessions.
- Determine family interaction patterns through doll role play, as appropriate.

Note: Similar activities are used for play therapy and therapeutic play. The nurse or child life specialist may use these activities for therapeutic play. One does not perform play therapy unless specially trained to do so.
From McCloskey, J., & Bulechek, G. (1996). *Nursing interventions classification (NIC)* (2nd ed.). St. Louis: Mosby–Year Book. Reprinted with permission.

velopment of a plan, implementation of the plan, and evaluation of its effectiveness (Rakel, 1992). During the assessment step, the nurse should determine the learner's cultural background and establish a rapport, especially when the nurse and learner come from different cultures.

To promote positive patient outcomes, the nurse must adopt education strategies that enhance learning readiness and facilitate effective learning. Providing effective patient and family education has long been a professional practice standard. Because failure to teach essential information regarding health care and maintenance has recently became grounds for lawsuits, effective education now is also a legal requirement for nurses.

Programs to Support the Child and Family

Therapeutic Play

For sick children, play is the mechanism through which they cope, learn, test new ideas, and test newly acquired psychomotor skills. In other words, play is the medium through which children grow and develop. Play also provides the child with a sense of control (Chambers, 1993). Normative play is different from therapeutic play. Normative play is activity in which children spontaneously engage and from which they derive pleasure. Therapeutic play is activity directed by the health care team to promote emotional and physical well-being. Unlike normative play, therapeutic play is goal-directed. Nevertheless, both types of play should be provided in the hospital.

Although often used interchangeably, therapeutic play is different from play therapy. Play therapy is play that helps a child express and work through emotional or psychological issues. It is usually considered a form of psychotherapy that is supervised by a professional educated in play therapy methods. Play therapy may be directed by the therapist or by the child with the therapist guiding the session. Nurses and child life specialists most commonly guide children during therapeutic play sessions (Chart 9–12).

Therapeutic play sessions should be conducted in a non-threatening environment. This time is protected. No treatments, doctors, or other distressing interruptions are allowed. The health professional guiding the session should be accepting of the child's play behaviors and avoid expressing approval or disapproval.

Therapeutic play includes instructional play, emotional outlet play, and physiologically enhancing play (Vessey & Mahon, 1990). These types of play are always geared to the child's physical, emotional, and cognitive abilities (Chart 9–13). The nurse must incorporate play into the plan of care and value this time as essential to

Chart 9–13

Materials/Methods for Use in Therapeutic Play

Instructional Play

- Dolls dressed as doctors, nurses, children, and family members
- Hospital gowns and pajamas
- Identification bracelets
- Surgical hats, masks, and booties
- Stethoscopes
- Blood pressure cuff, thermometers, and tape
- Large syringes without needles
- Bandages and dressing materials
- Equipment such as an IV pole, stretcher, and bed
- Oxygen masks
- Wash basin and towels
- Laboratory coats
- "Good Patient" stickers

Dramatic Play

- Punching bags
- Paints and crayons
- Inflatable bopper clowns
- Pegboard and hammers
- Dress-up clothes
- Puppets
- Blank books for writing stories or poetry
- Interactive video games
- Opportunities to play "doctor and nurse"
- Games such as peek-a-boo, hide-and-seek
- Sessions for telling "hospital stories"
- "Rap" groups
- Skits
- Song-writing sessions
- Water play
- Aggression play toys, such as blocks, clay, Play-Doh, punch pillows, squirt guns, and tin cans

Physiology Enhancing Play

- Lung expansion—straw blowing, tuned bottle blowing, blowing bubbles, blowing up and popping paper bags, pinwheel spinning, kazoo or woodwind instrument playing
- Pain management—reading stories, pop-up books, telling jokes, playing musical tapes, playing video games
- Improve range of motion/muscle strength—leave toys just out of reach, take a doll on an airplane ride, arm wrestle, reach to hang up decorations, throw bean bags

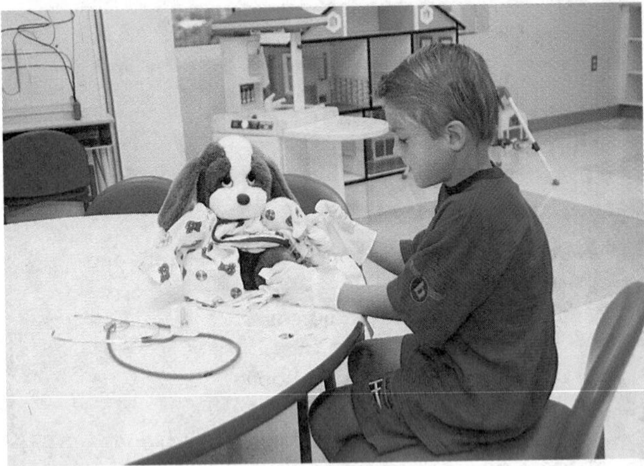

Figure 9–5
Instructional play can help prepare a child for surgery.

the child's development and emotional well-being (LeVieux-Anglin & Sawyer, 1993).

Instructional Play. This type of play may be used to prepare the child for a procedure or to help the child learn about his or her disease (Fig. 9–5). For instance, permitting the child to play with a urinary catheter, squirt water through it, and see a diagram of it in the bladder helps the child understand urinary catheterization. Instructional play can enhance teaching about a disease by permitting the child to draw pictures of affected body parts.

Worldview: *For children who do not understand the language spoken by the health team, medical play on dolls or puppets can help the child understand experiences (Loranger, 1992).*

Emotional Outlet Play. Also called *dramatic play,* this type of play gives the child an opportunity to express anxiety through play. This is useful because children are not always able to articulate their fears. This type of play is useful if the timing is right. The child should not be forced into it if he or she is not emotionally or physically ready. That is why the assessment skills of the pediatric nurse and child life specialist are so important to this activity (Hart, Mather, Slack, & Powell, 1992).

Physiology-Enhancing Play. This type of therapeutic play enables children to improve their physical health. For a child with asthma, for example, physiology-enhancing play may include breathing games to promote lung expansion (Fig. 9–6). To manage pain, play may include relaxation techniques or distraction games. A child who needs to increase range of motion or strengthen muscle groups can also benefit from directed play activities.

Child Life Programs

Child life programs became popular in the United States in the 1960s as a way to enhance family-centered care. These programs are designed to minimize stress for children and families during hospitalization and to promote the hospitalized child's continued growth and development. The American Academy of Pediatrics mandates that acute care pediatric services provide child life programs (Committee on Hospital Care, 1993).

To help the child cope successfully with hospitalization, child life programs organize interventions in the following categories:

- Play
- Preparation for hospitalization, procedures, and surgery
- Emotional support for parents and siblings
- Patient advocacy with hospital staff
- Promotion of family-centered environment

The child life specialist is responsible for designing and implementing interventions in each category that meet the needs of the patients and their families. To do this, child life specialists must be trained in child development and in techniques to address anxieties and fears regarding children's condition, impending procedures, and hospitalization. They also must be able to work in an interdisciplinary setting so that therapeutic activities incorporate all aspects of care.

Figure 9–6
Physiology-enhancing play at asthma camp includes blowing bubbles.

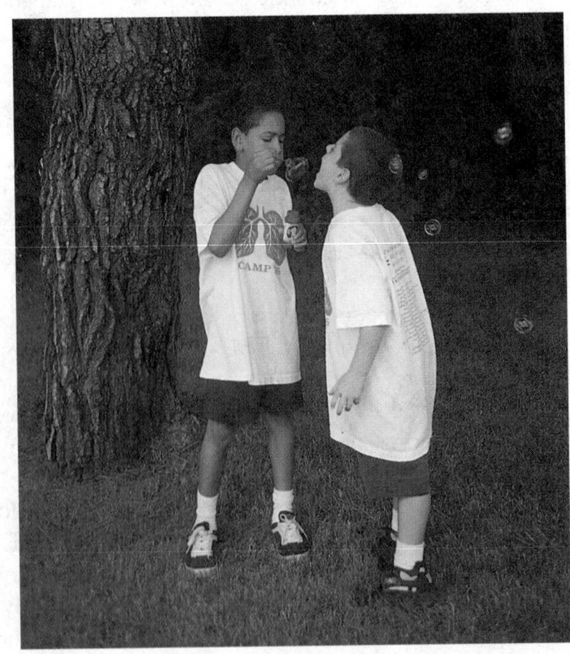

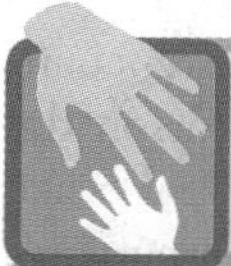

Chart 9–14
Nursing Interventions

Infection Control in the Playroom

All personnel and visitors must wash hands with antimicrobial soap:

- Upon entering and leaving the unit
- When serving food to patients
- After assisting patients with toileting or diapering
- After blowing or wiping a patient's or own nose
- After removing gloves used for handling body fluids
- When leaving an isolation area or handling articles from that area
- When leaving the toilet

Prevent toys and equipment from becoming vectors for infectious agents by

- Not allowing stuffed or unwashable toys in the playroom
- Scrubbing all toys handled by infectious or drooling patients in warm soapy water and rinsing for at least 30 seconds with manual friction; spray with disinfectant, leave on surface for amount of time specified by manufacturer, rinse with water
- Wiping all non-submersible toys with cloth saturated with disinfectant, leave on surface for amount of time specified by manufacturer, wipe with water-moistened cloth

Because child life specialists are one of the few health care professionals who do not cause the child pain or discomfort, this specialist is often the one with whom the hospitalized child feels comfortable. The child life specialist may become the primary health care professional to whom the child expresses feelings of anxiety, fears, and anger.

For hospitalizations more than a few days, a teacher may be provided through the local school district or the child life program. Teachers provide programmed instruction and assist children in keeping current in the homework they would be completing if they were in school with other children.

Playroom

This distinctive area should be equipped to meet the unique, cultural, age-appropriate developmental needs of the population being served. Children and families should be encouraged to engage in activities there and always feel welcome to enter.

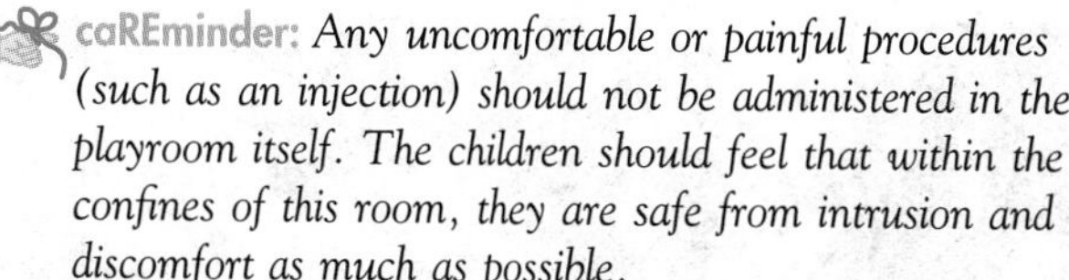

caREminder: *Any uncomfortable or painful procedures (such as an injection) should not be administered in the playroom itself. The children should feel that within the confines of this room, they are safe from intrusion and discomfort as much as possible.*

To prevent the spread of infection in the playroom, follow standard precautions. Ensure that body fluids are not spread in the playroom. If a child's infectious secretions cannot be safely contained, do not permit that child in the playroom. To help minimize spread of infection, wash toys with soap and water or a 10% hypochlorite (chlorine bleach) solution after use. Also, follow the facility's guidelines for infection control in the playroom (Chart 9–14). Effective control is enhanced by consistent adherence to the policy.

Hospital Tours

Whenever possible, patients and families (or prospective patients and their families) should have an opportunity to tour the acute care setting (Chart 9–15). It is espe-

Chart 9–15

Guidelines for Conducting a Hospital Tour

- Keep groups small—about 10 children per group.
- Conduct the tour for 20 to 30 minutes depending on the children's attention span. The nurse or child life specialist conducting the tour should have time dedicated for the tour with no interruptions.
- Encourage parents to join the tour.
- Present the tour in a non-threatening environment, such as the hospital playroom, school classroom, or child's home.
- When unable to actually tour the site (e.g., emergency on unit, presenting at a school), use an indirect method of presenting the hospital tour, such as a puppet, film, or slide show.
- Present the tour and explanations at the child's developmental level.
- Avoid dwelling on unpleasant or threatening events or intrusive procedures.
- Give the child and parents an opportunity to ask questions.
- Give the children an opportunity for therapeutic play, using dolls and hospital equipment.
- Give the children something to take home to remind them of the hospital tour, such as a coloring book, mask, or head cover.
- Encourage parents to discuss the tour afterward with the child and clarify any concerns they may have.

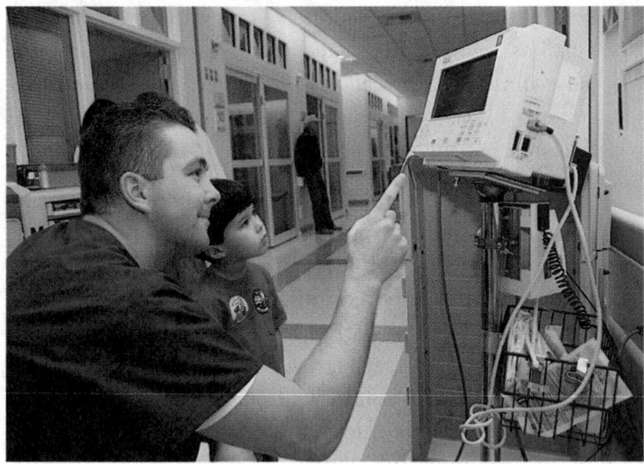

Figure 9–7
A hospital tour familiarizes the child with the new environment.

cially useful before hospital admission or surgery. A successful perioperative tour can create a positive impression of the surgical experience and defuse a potentially threatening event for the child and family. It lets the child and family meet the care providers and other staff members and begin getting accustomed to the environment (Avigne & Phillips, 1991). A successful tour shows the enthusiasm, dedication, and commitment of an interdisciplinary team of nurses, recovery room personnel, physicians, and other personnel who may work with the child.

If an older child is especially anxious about surgery, the facility may arrange for a tour through an operating room that is not in use, a preoperative area, and a PACU. The perioperative nurse can make the tour more child-friendly by using a large doll or stuffed animal to help demonstrate machinery that the child will encounter. A child may be delighted to see a teddy bear on the operating table "take a nap for surgery" and then "wake up" to be hugged. The nurse should explain the purposes of hospital pajamas, masks, caps, shoe covers, and gloves and let the child try them on. The nurse may let the child hear the beeps of an electrocardiograph (EKG) machine and feel the stickiness of the EKG pads (Fig. 9–7), or the nurse may place a pulse oximeter probe on the child's fingers or toes, put a blood pressure cuff on the child, or let the child listen to his or her own heartbeat through a stethoscope.

If the facility cannot provide tours of the operating room, it may substitute a photograph album, slide show, or a videotape presentation of a tour. No matter what form the tour takes, the nurse may present a certificate to each child upon completion of the tour.

Some facilities have taken the hospital tour to the local community. In this outreach program, health care personnel use a videotape and discussion to present the hospital tour to schools and other community organizations. These presentations also act as marketing tools, enhancing the image of the hospital or surgery center to potential patients (Fig. 9–8).

Support Groups

Parents usually find it helpful to discuss concerns about their ill child with other parents who have similar experiences (Amico & Davidhizar, 1994). To facilitate this, the nurse can introduce parents to each other or refer them to a specific support group. Many types of support groups exist, ranging from disease-specific support groups to support groups for siblings, grandparents, or others.

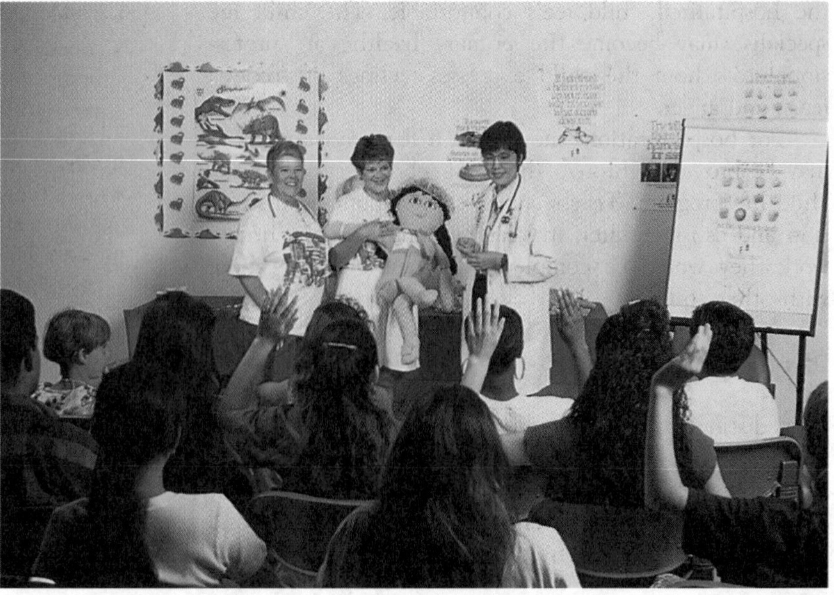

Figure 9–8
Presentations at school familiarize children with the environment and routines, which may reduce distress during later interactions with the acute care setting.

However, available groups vary from region to region. To find out what groups are available in a particular region, the nurse can ask a social worker or contact ACCH for referrals. ACCH has promoted the establishment of family resource libraries in hospitals. If the facility has one of these libraries, the nurse can easily check for services at the regional and national levels (Johnson et al., 1992). Computer support groups are rapidly evolving and have the potential to be a powerful support tool as more families become computer literate.

The unit-based support group is a particular type of support group. It is especially useful during hospitalization because it can provide a brief escape from the stress of the hospital environment. In this support group, parents can discuss their immediate concerns about hospitalization. The presence of other parents makes it easier for parents to discuss issues that they may have difficulty addressing individually with a staff member. These support groups usually are led by a professional such as a pediatric nurse, child life specialist, or social worker (Ladebauche, 1992). The group leader must have an understanding of group theory and excellent communication skills.

Having a hospital staff member lead the group helps parents solve problems that they identify in the group such as displeasure with routines or concern over a child's behavior. In a support group for an infant special care unit, for example, the support group may be led by the unit-based social worker and a Spanish translator to provide a means for families to better understand hospitalization and vent their frustrations with it. Each week, a member of a different discipline attends the support group so parents can discuss specific questions with that representative. This type of group helps parents feel like part of the team.

Another type of support group is an organization that provides services for children, such as the Make-A-Wish Foundation, which grants the wishes of terminally ill children. Through such organizations, athletes, celebrities, and entertainers have visited ill children, talked with them, and given them hope and encouragement during their illness. (See Resources section for a list of some available support groups.)

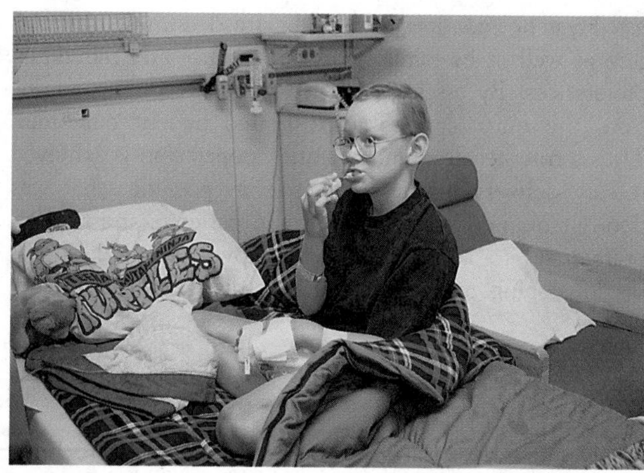

Figure 9–9
Familiar objects and maintaining home routines normalize the environment and help the child cope with hospitalization.

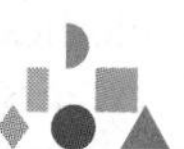

Care of the Child in the Acute Care Setting

Soon after admission, the child and family encounter experiences related to the routines of the acute care setting. These routines include procedures that are part of the child's diagnostic evaluation and treatment as well as care that affects activities of daily living (ADLs). The most common of these routines are hygiene, safety, routine procedures, medication administration, infection control issues, and visitation policies. Each of these categories provides in its own way an intrusion into the child's and family's privacy, for it represents and mandates a departure from their way of life at home. Continuity between home life and hospital life is often difficult to achieve; nonetheless, an admission assessment that reveals as much as possible about home routines, likes, dislikes, coping mechanisms, favorite toys, and activities can help the nursing staff assist the child and family in bridging the gap between home and hospital (Fig. 9–9). Many routines from the home environment can be transferred, or adapted with minor changes, to the hospital environment.

caREminder: *Every contact with the child and family is a teaching opportunity. After evaluating readiness to learn, present content at this level (e.g., if anxious, present simple, focused information; if asking appropriate questions, proceed to more complex topics). Issues taught may range from specific care of the child to anticipatory guidance regarding well-child care.*

Activities of Daily Living

Perhaps the hospital routines that are most disruptive to home patterns are those regarding hygiene and ADLs. Bathing, oral care, dressing, toileting, and sleeping are such basic functions that the ways in which one performs them are taken for granted. Acute illness changes the way in which these functions are performed as a result of the child's physical condition and restrictions caused by treatment devices.

Hygiene practices and ADLs are determined by culture as well as by family practices, rituals, and individual preferences. By assessing them thoroughly during admission, the nurse can enhance desired patient outcomes. This is true because much greater cooperation is achieved if care delivery mimics as closely as possible what was done at home. Communicating the patient's and family's preferences to all involved care providers is a key part of developing an interdisciplinary plan of care for the child.

Bathing

Safety and privacy are the greatest concerns in bathing. Infants through preschoolers should never be left alone when bathing. Infants who can sit alone may be allowed to sit in a tub but need to be bathed. Toddlers also need to be bathed, but they can help. Preschoolers can be more independent with bathing but still need assistance. Children of these ages are more comfortable if a parent or grandparent helps them with their bath, especially after they reach the stage of stranger anxiety, which begins around age 6 to 8 months. School-age children can bathe themselves, especially after age 8, barring developmental or physical handicaps, but may not be as thorough as they should. School-age children who have the physical strength to bathe alone are not at risk for accidents while bathing, as are infants toddlers, and even preschoolers. However, developmental capacities must be assessed before making this professional judgment. Developmentally delayed children of school age and older may require constant supervision during the bath. Adolescents are often preoccupied with hygiene and the primary concern becomes having the "space" and time to carry out the desired hygiene rituals in the most private, autonomous way possible. For patients who are too ill to get into a tub or shower, the bed bath becomes a necessity. For children hospitalized for longer than a few days, periodic hair washing is necessary. An infant's hair should be washed daily or every other day to prevent cradle cap. Infants younger than the age of 1 month do not require soap. Older children typically need one or two shampoos per week.

Frequency and timing of bathing are often culturally determined and should be respected within the confines of standards acceptable for infection control and scheduling. Some children are accustomed to bathing in the morning, while others prefer to do this before bed. If the child is fairly independent, arranging for a shower or bath before bedtime may greatly increase their personal satisfaction. A bath every day is not necessary, providing that the patient is clean enough for infection control. Cultural practices also determine the nature of hair care, and the family and patient preferences should be respected.

Worldview: *The hair care needs of African-American children can be met by providing wide combs and pomades (oil-based pastes used to facilitate hair combing and styling). Do not use petroleum jelly.*

Checking with the parents for assistance and asking them to bring in supplies is helpful. Hair care may be left to willing family members as long as it does not jeopardize patient safety.

Oral Care

Providing oral care for children is a necessary and challenging aspect of hygiene. Young children often do not like to have their teeth brushed and resist it. Children younger than the age of 6 need assistance with mouth care. Although it is important to permit preschool-age children to begin brushing their own teeth, they need one thorough brushing per day with the assistance of an adult. Several ineffective brushings a day cannot replace one thorough brushing. Infants whose teeth have not erupted need mouth care; this can be provided by using a washcloth or sponge-tipped applicators to rub the gums and oral cavity. Once the teeth have erupted, a soft toothbrush and fluoride toothpaste can be used in combination with dental floss to remove plaque. Preschoolers often like to use a familiar brush, although supervision is required to ensure that the child does not ingest large quantities of fluoridated toothpaste. School-age children can brush their teeth but need reminders to be thorough. Adolescents are sensitive about "bad breath" and are usually compliant with oral care.

Children who have been treated with certain types of immunosuppressive or chemotherapeutic agents may experience stomatitis. Oral care for these children is key in minimizing the occurrence of infection and/or severity of the condition (see Chapter 22).

Clothing

Some hospitalized children are too sick to dress in anything other than a gown or pajamas. Parents may wish to select outfits for the infant or toddler to wear that are more attractive and warmer than the hospital gown. Older children may feel like donning play clothes from home. The child should be allowed to choose the clothes to wear. This may be especially important to adolescents whose chief developmental concerns are body image and personal appearance.

Toileting

It has long been recognized that many children regress developmentally during hospitalization. Toddlers who have just begun to master toilet training may revert to diapers. No interventions usually are needed. Once the child returns home, they usually resume their former developmental level. If a child has recently been toilet trained, the nurse should make a concerted effort to assist the child in maintaining continence. The key guideline in toileting is to ensure the patient's privacy and dignity, no matter what the age. Adolescents may be particularly embarrassed by the use of a bedpan, especially in a shared room. Male patients of school-age and older may be embarrassed by assisted toileting from female nurses, particularly in the use of urinals. Being direct and matter-of-fact and allowing as much privacy as possible are the preferred interventions in these situations. Keeping toileting implements, such as urinals and bedpans, out of sight when not in use and keeping bedside commodes emptied, clean, and stored as covertly as possible are also commonsense interventions related to toiling. Promptly answering the call light promotes trust that assistance is available when needed. This decreases a sense of humiliation and anxiety.

Sleep

Sleep is necessary to maintaining and promoting health. It is theorized to be essential in curing or effectively adapting to disease (Parker, 1995). Sleep deprivation has deleterious effects on the immune system and can impair healing. The hospital environment is notorious for promoting sleep pattern disturbances. Because deep sleep is thought to be necessary to growth hormone secretion (Parker, 1995), sleep pattern disturbances are a serious concern for care providers in pediatric hospitals.

In the hospital, sleep pattern disturbances can result from three basic types of sources: physiologic, psychological, and environmental. Physiologic factors can include diseases that cause pain, such as juvenile rheumatoid arthritis, and medications that decrease rapid eye movement (REM) sleep, such as barbiturates, opiate derivatives, and benzodiazepines. Separation anxiety may be the most prevalent cause of sleep disturbance. Another psychological factor may be a preexisting stressor, such as a dysfunctional family. The hospital environment has many factors that can precipitate sleep pattern disturbance; these include noise (such as monitors and alarms), too much light, and treatments and assessments that frequently wake the child.

Assessment of home preferences and routines for sleeping is a step toward eliminating sleep pattern disturbance in the hospital. Determining the child's bedtime, sleep duration, bedtime rituals, and nap pattern helps the nurse develop a plan of care that prevents sleep pattern disturbance (Chart 9–16). Minimizing noise and light in

Chart 9–16
Developmental Considerations

Sleep Promotion in Hospitalized Children

Developmental Age	Developmental Guideline
All ages	Post daily schedule at child's bedside, include nap times and bedtime. Establish light-dark cycle if room has no window. Eliminate noxious stimuli. Synchronize hospital routines with child's normal routines. Treat the child's pain.
Infant	Provide a sense of security for the infant by rocking and holding during the evening. Swaddle a younger infant. Adhere to home bedtime rituals, such as taking a bottle while rocking. Place cuddly toys in the crib. Play a familiar lullaby using a musical toy.
Toddler or preschooler	Adhere to home bedtime rituals, such as reading a story, having a snack, and brushing teeth. Use transitional objects from home such as toys, blankets, and clothes. If the parents cannot be present, encourage them to leave pictures of themselves and the family or tape-recorded stories. Permit telephone calls to parents at bedtime.
School-age child	Allow the child to express fears of separation through imaginary play with puppets, dolls, or drawings. Adhere to bedtime rituals. Permit telephone calls to family at bedtime.
Adolescent	Enforce mutually agreed upon bedtime. Encourage quiet activity in the hour before bedtime: relaxing music, reading, television. Give back rub. Maintain home bedtime rituals.

the environment can also promote healthy nighttime sleep patterns.

caREminder: *The nurse is key in ensuring that medication schedules, whenever possible, do not interrupt sleep. Also, schedules for weighing and vital signs should be planned to coincide with sleep patterns.*

Nutrition

Nutrition can become a major challenge in the care of the hospitalized child. Interruption of personal preferences, habits, or family and cultural practices along with malaise from illness can decrease the child's appetite. Therefore, assessment must take into account all these factors. Working with the dietitian, to determine the optimal diet within the bounds of diet orders, can improve a sick child's nutritional intake. Developmentally appropriate foods should be selected, with input from children who are old enough. Foods may also be brought in by family members. Provision should be made for appropriate storage and refrigeration of this food.

Worldview: *The child may be accustomed to having certain staple foods at every meal (e.g., rice for Asian children, beans and tortillas for Hispanic children). Accommodating these preferences may improve the child's intake as well as satisfaction with care.*

Safety

Injuries are the leading cause of death in children and adolescents and often require treatment in the hospital setting (Behrman, Kleigman, & Arvin, 1996). To prevent future injuries, the nurse should identify the family's learning needs and provide safety education, because

Chart 9–17
Developmental Considerations

Ensuring Child Safety in the Acute Care Setting

Developmental Age	Age-Specific Activities and Risks	Guidelines During Hospitalization
Infant	*Activities:* Rolls over Creeps Crawls Pulls to stand Walks *Risks:* Suffocation Falls Choking Drowning	Keep the side rails up on the crib at all times. Always leave the infant in a secure environment, such as a crib with side rails up or strapped in a stroller with wheels locked. Do not leave in prone position or propped with pillows. Do not use pillows or soft bedding. Do not allow parents to sleep while holding or rocking infant. Do not leave infant with bottle propped. Put a net or Plexiglas dome over crib after age 6 months. Never leave the infant unattended near water. Avoid wearing removable jewelry when caring for an infant.
Toddler	*Activities:* Walks Explores environment Put objects in mouth Feeds self *Risks:* Falls Burns Suffocation Poisoning Electrical shock from uncovered outlets Drowning	Keep sharp objects out of reach. Keep out of reach any small hard objects, such as buttons or coins, or balloons that could be aspirated. Keep medication and poisons out of reach. Ensure that the crib is covered and side rails are up. Do not leave the child unattended near water. Do not leave the child unattended when not secured, such as with a stroller or wheelchair strap. Supervise feeding. Avoid foods that present a choking hazard, such as whole grapes, hot dogs, peanuts. If the parents request a large bed because the child sleeps in one at home, evaluate toddler's motor skills for safety of this and obtain consent for release of side rails.

most injuries occur under fairly predictable circumstances. Efforts should not be focused on only those who have been injured, but should include all hospitalized children, because all children are at high risk for injuries.

The nurse should provide a safe environment for children in the hospital. This is a particular challenge when caring for children for the following reasons:

- Children are statistically at greater risk for accidents.
- Staffing levels do not permit one-to-one monitoring for children.
- The environment is potentially harmful (equipment, toxic substances).

The challenge is to maintain a developmentally appropriate approach. As the child matures, the safety risks and safety precautions change (Chart 9–17). Some general safety principles include security measures, proper identification of the child, and safety mechanisms.

Infant and Child Security

Crime and violence against children have drawn much attention at the national level in recent years. Missing children hotlines have been established at national and state levels. Several cases of kidnapping of children from hospitals and nurseries have occurred. Gang violence has become a concern in the pediatric setting as younger and younger children are victims of gang crimes in urban settings and are hospitalized with injuries. Security measures to protect these victims from further retaliation have become necessary. This general climate has led acute care settings to become increasingly concerned with the protection and safety of their patients and others.

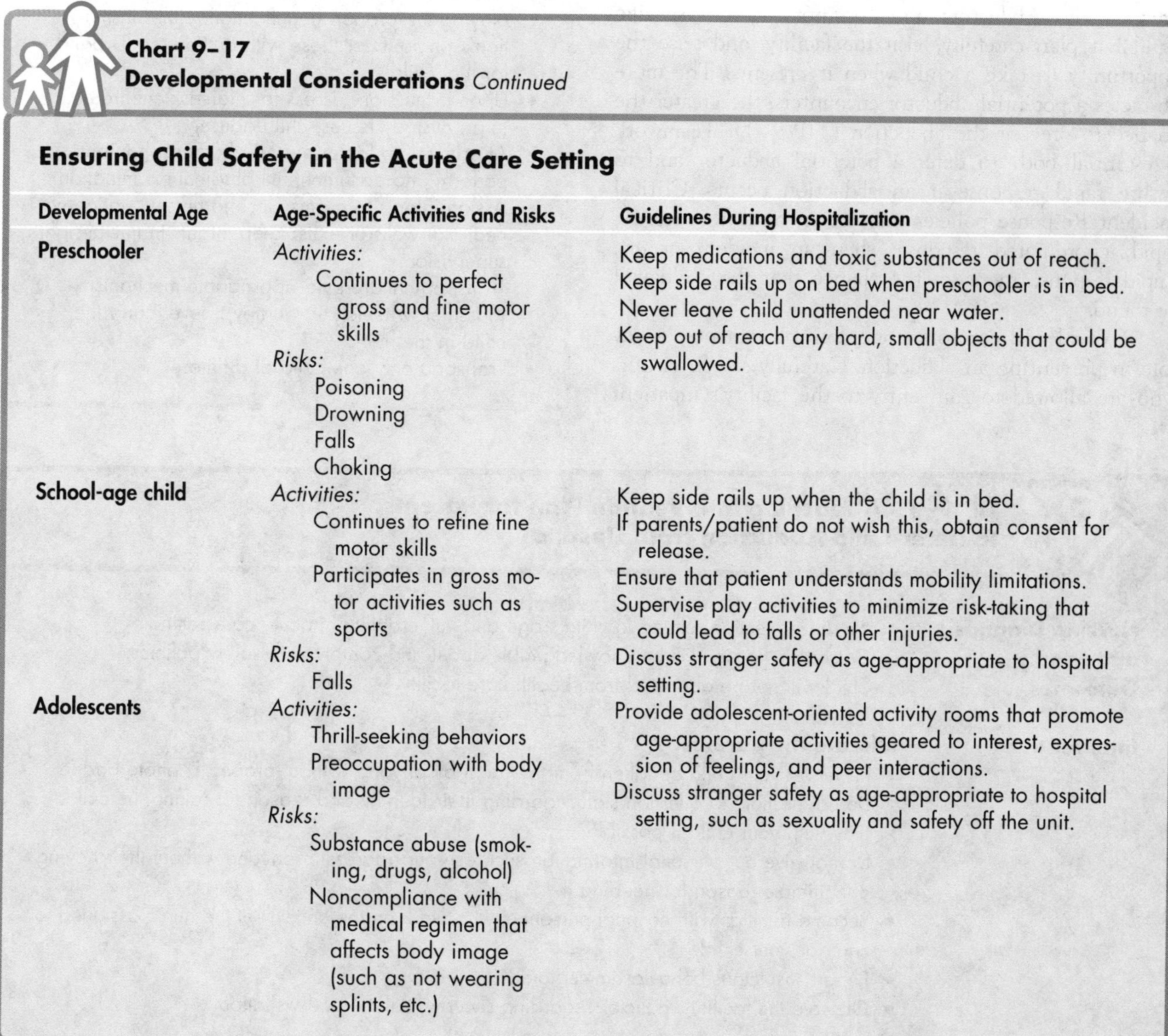

Chart 9–17
Developmental Considerations *Continued*

Ensuring Child Safety in the Acute Care Setting

Developmental Age	Age-Specific Activities and Risks	Guidelines During Hospitalization
Preschooler	*Activities:* Continues to perfect gross and fine motor skills *Risks:* Poisoning Drowning Falls Choking	Keep medications and toxic substances out of reach. Keep side rails up on bed when preschooler is in bed. Never leave child unattended near water. Keep out of reach any hard, small objects that could be swallowed.
School-age child	*Activities:* Continues to refine fine motor skills Participates in gross motor activities such as sports *Risks:* Falls	Keep side rails up when the child is in bed. If parents/patient do not wish this, obtain consent for release. Ensure that patient understands mobility limitations. Supervise play activities to minimize risk-taking that could lead to falls or other injuries. Discuss stranger safety as age-appropriate to hospital setting.
Adolescents	*Activities:* Thrill-seeking behaviors Preoccupation with body image *Risks:* Substance abuse (smoking, drugs, alcohol) Noncompliance with medical regimen that affects body image (such as not wearing splints, etc.)	Provide adolescent-oriented activity rooms that promote age-appropriate activities geared to interest, expression of feelings, and peer interactions. Discuss stranger safety as age-appropriate to hospital setting, such as sexuality and safety off the unit.

A good security program combines several approaches. The institution must develop and adhere to policies that safeguard children; educate and promote teamwork by all staff, parents, and visitors; and provide physical and electronic security measures (Rabun, 1996).

Security policies vary according to setting. Most units that deal with newborns have strict policies regarding infant, mother, and father identification (ID) banding; saving cord blood; obtaining footprints and photographs of the infant shortly after birth; and identifying the person to whom the infant is discharged. Pediatric units must have similar policies in place (Chart 9–18). The institution should post and enforce the policy that parents are not allowed to leave children unattended in waiting rooms.

All staff (e.g., nurses, physicians, therapists, security and support personnel), parents, and visitors must be familiar with security policies and adhere to them. Everyone must be alert for suspicious behavior and report it immediately. Abductors often do not target a specific child but plan carefully, visit the facility, and seize the opportunity to take a child when it presents. The more obstacles a potential abductor encounters, the greater the chance to prevent the abduction (TIP 9–1). Teamwork is essential both to deter a potential abductor and to ensure rapid response if an abduction occurs. Critical Incident Response policies must be in place to ensure a rapid, coordinated response when an incident occurs. Rapid response increases the chance that the child will be found.

Physical and environmental controls can play a key role in preventing an abduction. Carefully screen visitors who are allowed to gain entry to the facility's inpatient

Chart 9–18

Sample Security Policies for Pediatric Unit

- All staff must wear institution's photo ID above the waist; consider adding some other identification to indicate those who are allowed to transport child.
- All staff are to monitor and report any suspicious behavior by visitors (e.g., visiting "just to see" infants, questioning the facility's procedures or physical layout, carrying large package off unit, taking hospital lab coats or scrubs).
- Keep staff locker rooms locked; do not let visitors borrow scrubs or lab coats.
- All visitors must enter and exit through access controlled corridor.
- Parents or visitors must wear ID wristband or show photo ID.
- Question anyone transporting a child without displaying the proper identification, either institution's photo ID or those with authorized ID band for that child.
- Upon admission, assess for high-risk children (e.g., custody issues, child abuse).
- At admission, footprint and photograph infants, perform and document full physical examination.
- Assign infants to rooms close to nurses' station not near stairwells or exits; keep infants in line-of-sight supervision.
- Transport children via appropriate mechanism (bassinet, wheelchair, gurney); *never* carry the child in the halls.
- Transport only one child at a time.

TIP 9–1 A Teaching Intervention Plan for Parents to Deter Child Abduction from Hospital

Nursing Diagnosis and Family Outcomes

- Altered protection related to child's age and vulnerability in acute care setting
  Outcomes: Family will be knowledgeable about and comply with safety policies.
  Child will not be abducted from health care facility.

Interventions

Educate the parents:

- Never let your child be taken from the room by anyone without proper ID photo badge.
- Do not hesitate to question staff regarding their identity and reason for taking the child.
- Stay with your child if possible.
- Do not give out personal information such as your address to anyone without their having a legitimate reason for needing it.
- Become familiar with hospital personnel who work on the unit; meet the nurse assigned to care for your child.
- Report suspicious behavior immediately.
- Observe the facility's policies regarding security, safety, and visitation.

area. In cases of individual need for increased protection, use visitor restrictions that designate who may and may not visit the child. This helps prevent harm to the child and others. In newborn nurseries, arrange visitation hours that permit viewing without physical access to the infants. Ensure that identifying data, such as mother's full name, is not displayed on the crib card or where visitors could view it. The abductor may attempt to take the child from the home. Measures such as surveillance cameras and door alarms increase environmental security.

Alert: *Specific photo IDs should be mandatory for personnel allowed to transport children.*

Health care facilities are also increasing their security staff, so these armed personnel have high visibility. Emergency rooms are improving security by having armed personnel on guard at all times and limiting access through the use of locked doors that, with the exception of employees, can be entered only with permission. These constraints may seem excessive and annoying to the patients and families if they do not understand the reasons for them. The nurse should review the rationale for implementing security precautions, and all staff should reinforce and comply with these precautions.

Identification

Accurate identification of the child in the acute care setting is aided by placement of an ID band on the child's wrist or ankle upon admission. If the child has any known allergies, these should be identified in a similar manner. This is often done with a separate, brightly colored band placed on the same extremity as the ID band. If the bands are removed (e.g., for IV placement in that extremity), they should be replaced immediately.

Figure 9–10
Safety is always a priority. The nurse must keep at least one hand on the infant at all times when not properly secured.

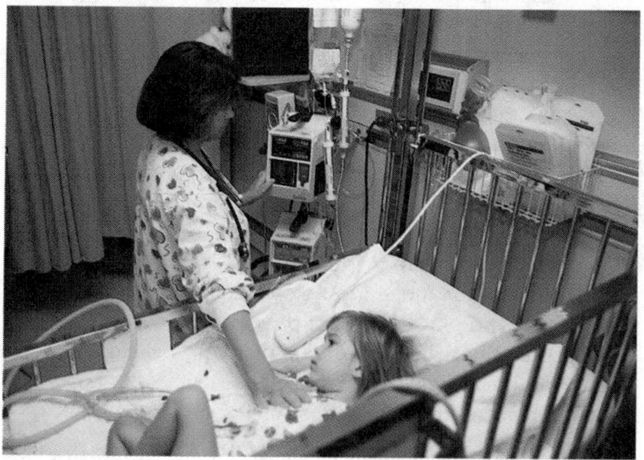

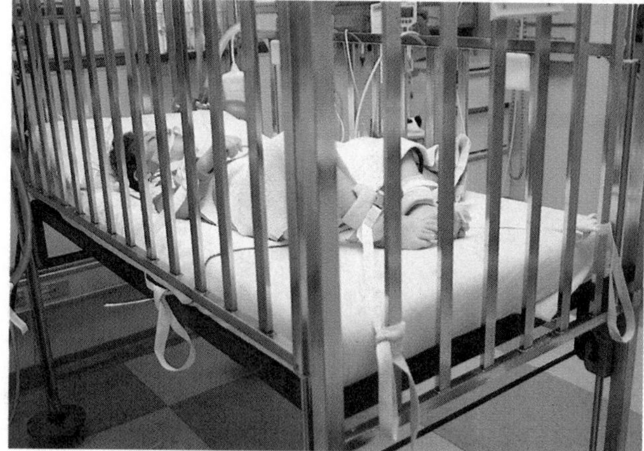

Figure 9–11
To promote safety, restraints should be attached to the bed frame *under* the side rails, not to the side rails.

Alert: *To ensure that the appropriate child receives the correct treatment, ID bands should be checked prior to administration of medications or performing treatments. It is not permissible to only verbally verify the child's name (e.g., "Are you Johnny?") before implementing medical procedures.*

Safety Mechanisms

In the acute care setting, several mechanisms exist for ensuring child safety. These include side rails, cribs, safe modes of transport, and restraints. General engineering controls that enhance environmental (electrical and mechanical) safety contribute to the patient's overall safety. Close monitoring can prevent the child from getting into dangerous situations. When providing care to an infant or toddler with the side rails down, stand next to the child to prevent him or her from rolling off the crib. If you must turn your back or reach for something, always keep one hand on the child's trunk to prevent him or her from rolling (Fig. 9–10).

Side rails are commonly used in the hospital to prevent the patient from falling out of bed. Because side rails vary in design, learn how to operate them in that particular setting. One needs to ensure that they are locked in place when leaving the bedside and know how to lower them quickly in an emergency. Also, never tie restraints to side rails because raising and lowering of the rail could injure the restrained limb (Fig. 9–11).

Covers for cribs are also commonly used in the pediatric setting. These typically are Plexiglas domes, plastic, or netting and should be used when the child is old enough to pull to stand and could thus conceivably fall out of the crib (Fig. 9–12).

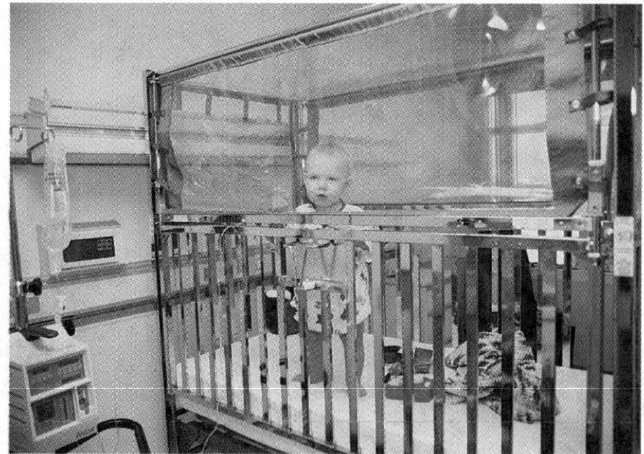

Figure 9–12
A crib cover can be used to restrain a child who is old enough to stand up.

In *transport or transfer* of the child, several actions can increase safety (Murphy, 1992). First, never leave the pediatric patient alone when being transported, whether by gurney, wheelchair, or other means. Also, have ready, easy access to the child's head at all times, should vomiting or respiratory distress occur. When the child is being transferred in or out of a gurney or wheelchair, lock the wheels in place to prevent falls. Always secure the safety straps or "seatbelts" on wheelchairs, strollers, and wagons.

It is unsafe to carry a child for a long distance because of the risk of tripping, slipping, falling, or fatiguing. Walking for a distance is not an appropriate option for sick children. Transport devices, such as wheelchairs and gurneys, should be used to transport children from the pediatric unit to other areas of the hospital, such as radiology or the laboratory. A crib-type stretcher with side rails covering the entire length should be used for infants and toddlers requiring gurney transport.

Nurses report using *physical restraint* to promote inactivity or immobility, prevent interference with tubes or dressings, prevent touching or scratching healing tissue, facilitate administration of medications or treatments, prevent children from getting out of bed or into dangerous place, or to protect staff from combativeness (Selekman & Snyder, 1995). Reasons for restraint use varied depending on child's age and type of unit.

caREminder: *Because use of restraint can result in complications such as falls, incontinence, and pressure sore formation, it is prudent to minimize use of restraints while still providing a safe environment and preventing disruption of medical treatments (Chart 9–19).*

The Joint Commission on Accreditation of Healthcare Organizations (JCAHO) plays a leadership role in ensuring that hospitals are protecting consumer rights through the appropriate use of restraints. The JCAHO requires that patients with arm, leg, or jacket restraints be checked periodically for neurovascular integrity and general safety and that this assessment information is documented in the patient's chart. Hospital policy dictates the frequency of assessment, but assessment must be performed at least every 15 minutes in behavioral health care settings. The nurse must release restraints and document assessment of the child's overall status, including hygiene, elimination, and nutrition at least every 2 hours. A physician's order stating the reason for the restraints, type of restraint, and duration of restraint is required and must be rewritten every 24 hours. This standard does not apply to the use of restraint for procedures (e.g., holding the arm down to start an intravenous [IV] line, putting the child in a mummy restraint to suture a laceration). Treatment restraints need to be removed as soon as the procedure is completed.

A serious infringement of patients' rights is the use of restraints for punishment. A restraint should never be used to place a child in "time-out." Time-outs are used to help the child regain self-control of behavior. The use of

Chart 9–19
Nursing Interventions

Alternatives to Use of Physical Restraint

- Increase supervision of child by parents, family, friends, volunteers, or nurses.
- Have windows to increase ability to observe the child when not physically in the same room.
- Actively listen to the child.
- Ask the parent the most effective methods of obtaining compliance and distracting the child.
- Take child to nurses' station or playroom, unless contraindicated by child's condition.
- Provide activities to distract the child and to promote expression of feelings such as anger or aggression.
- Prepare the child for procedures as developmentally appropriate, because a prepared child may maintain better control and need less restraint.
- Hold the child's hand or foot, simple touch may comfort the child and "help remind them to hold still."
- Protect and cover the site (e.g., tape IVs well, cover with a cup or gauze); put clothes on the child, which make it physically more difficult to pull out a tube or disrupt a wound.
- Ensure that child's hygiene, nutrition, toileting, and comfort needs are met.
- Minimize environmental stimuli if they trigger the child's loss of control.

restraints imposes an external control, rather than allowing the child to develop internal control.

Limb restraints are used when children could harm themselves if not restrained, such as when ensuring the integrity of IV sites, catheter, endotracheal tubes, feeding tubes, and surgical sites and dressings. Many commercial restraints are available; most include a soft sponge to protect circulation. Use caution that the restraint cannot tighten around the extremity and impair circulation.

caREminder: *When restraining limbs, use padding to protect circulation and fasten restraints in a way that prevents impaired circulation.*

Elbow restraints are sometimes used to prevent the child from reaching the face to do harm. These prevent elbow flexion but leave the hands free for play and exploration. Elbow restraints may be needed after cleft lip and palate repair or to prevent oral or nasal feeding tubes from being pulled out. There are commercial sleeves into which tongue blades can be inserted to prevent elbow flexion. These can also be fabricated at the bedside using rolled gauze and gauze dressing pads to pad the tongue blades to prevent skin abrasion (Fig. 9–13A).

Jacket restraints are useful when the child needs to remain supine and is too young to do this by himself or herself.

Alert: *The jacket restraint needs to be applied properly and the child monitored closely. The child may potentially shift position enough to be improperly restrained, causing airway or circulatory problems (Fig. 9–13B).*

Mummy restraints are useful when performing procedures for which the infant or toddler will not hold still. With appropriate teaching, they may be used by a parent who must perform procedures with the child at home, such as changing tracheostomy tubes or performing wound care. The child is placed on the diagonal of a blanket with the feet and head at opposite corners. The sides are wrapped over the child's chest and the feet are secured by tucking the lower corner over them. Tape can be used to hold the folds in place (Fig. 9–13C).

Belt restraints should always be used when young children are placed in infant seats, swings, or high chairs. A strap should be secured to the chair running between the child's legs up to the belt, to prevent the child from sliding down and injuring himself or herself.

Figure 9–13
Three types of restraints: *(A)* elbow restraint; *(B)* jacket restraint; *(C)* mummy restraint.

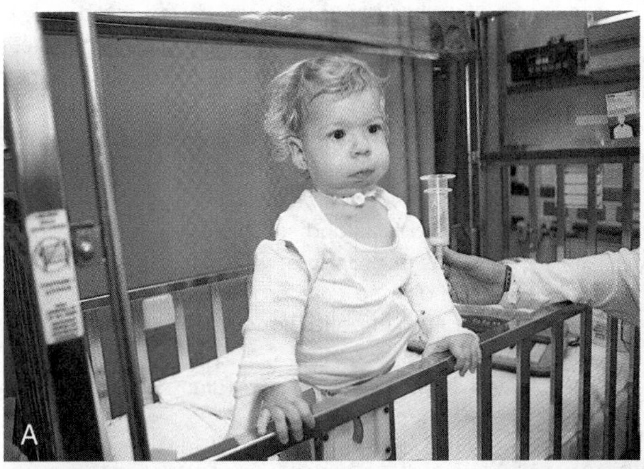

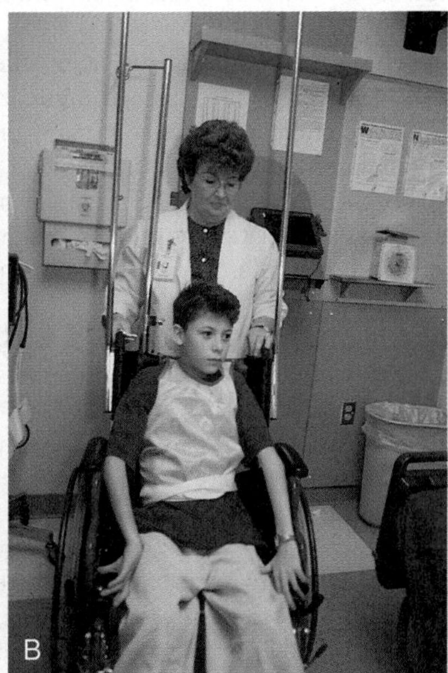

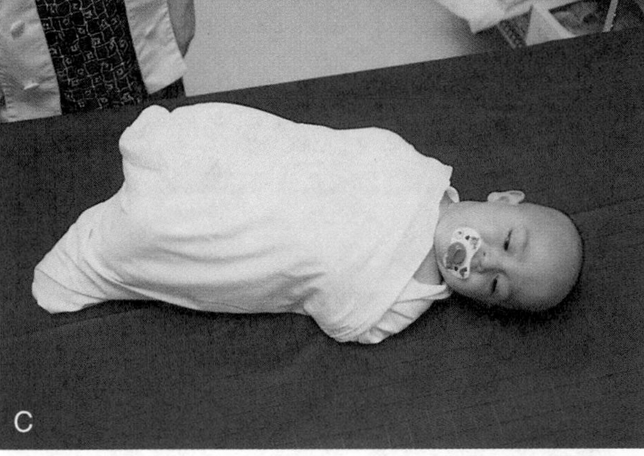

Latex Allergy

Although measures are taken to provide a safe environment for children, families, and health care workers, the acute care setting may pose an additional hazard for those who are allergic to latex. This is because the health care environment contains many products that contain latex as well as airborne latex allergens (particularly from powdered latex gloves). Those with increased exposure to latex are at highest risk of developing latex allergy. Early reports of latex sensitivity were from patients with myelomeningocele (Slater, 1989). The use of latex gloves by health care workers has increased dramatically with the initiation of universal precautions in the late 1980s, which is the probable cause for the increase in latex allergies seen in this population. It is now recognized that patients who have undergone multiple surgeries (Kinnaird, McClure, & Wilham, 1995) and those with a history of atopy (Young & Meyers, 1997) are also at high risk for developing latex allergy.

The most common allergic reaction to latex is a delayed hypersensitivity presenting as contact dermatitis (Sussman & Beezhold, 1995). A less common, but more serious, reaction is an immediate response that presents as urticaria, rhinoconjunctivitis, bronchospasm, and anaphylaxis (Heinzerling & Johnson, 1996). A high index of suspicion regarding latex allergy must be maintained because its symptoms are difficult to distinguish from other allergic reactions or causes.

Treatment. The best treatment for latex allergy is identification of high-risk populations and minimizing latex exposure in these children. Latex is in many products found in the home and those used in health care (Table 9–1); latex-free substitutions should be made when possible. The Spina Bifida Association of America maintains a current list of latex-safe alternatives (see Resources at end of chapter).

Children at high risk for, or identified with, latex allergy should have their medical and dental charts flagged with this information. The school or daycare center should be notified, have non-latex gloves and an Epi-Pen available, and notify health care providers in an emergency.

In the acute care setting, latex avoidance is particularly important because many products contain latex. Latex precautions need to be initiated and family teaching done (Chart 9–20). In addition to using latex-free products, medications must be carefully administered to prevent latex exposure. Do not puncture latex rubber stoppers on vials to withdraw medications because this may introduce latex into the medication. Use latex-free IV tubing and injection ports. It is questionable whether syringes with rubber stoppers on the plunger may leach latex into the medication (Young & Meyers, 1997). Therefore, medications should be drawn up immediately before administration.

The high-risk child going to surgery should be scheduled as the first case of the day to minimize exposure to

Chart 9–20
Nursing Interventions Classification (NIC)

Latex Precautions

Definition

Reducing the risk of a systemic reaction to latex

Activities

- Question patient or appropriate other about history of neural tube defect (e.g., spina bifida) or congenital urological condition (e.g., exstrophy of the bladder).
- Question patient or appropriate other about history of systemic reactions to natural rubber latex (e.g., facial or scleral edema, tearing eyes, urticaria, rhinitis, and wheezing).
- Refer patient to allergist for allergy testing, as appropriate.
- Record allergy or risk in patient's medical record.
- Place allergy band on patient.
- Post sign indicating latex precautions.
- Survey environment and remove latex products.
- Monitor latex-free environment.
- Monitor patient for signs and symptoms of a systemic reaction.
- Report information to physician, pharmacist, and other care providers, as indicated.
- Administer medications, as appropriate.
- Instruct patient and family about risk factors for developing a latex allergy.
- Instruct patient and family about potential for reaction.
- Instruct patient and family about latex content in products and substitution with nonlatex products, as appropriate; wearing a medical alert tag; and notifying care providers.
- Instruct patient and family about signs of a reaction.
- Instruct patient and family about emergency treatment.
- Instruct patient and family about administration of epinephrine, as appropriate.
- Instruct visitors about latex-free environment.

From McCloskey, J., & Bulechek, G. (1996). *Nursing Interventions classification (NIC)* (2nd ed.). St. Louis: Mosby–Year Book. Reprinted with permission.

Table 9–1
Examples of Latex Items in the Hospital and Community Environment

Hospital	Community
Ace wraps	art supplies
Ambu bags	balloons
Band-Aids	balls
blood pressure cuff tubing	cleaning gloves
catheters	condoms/diaphragms
diapers	diapers
drains	elastic (hair accessories)
elastic bandages	elastic (in clothing)
gloves (surgical and examination)	feeding nipples
intravenous tubing injection ports	food handled with latex gloves
medication vial rubber stoppers	handles on racquets, some tools
molded surgical masks with elastic band	infant toothbrush massager
moleskin adhesive	pacifiers
Pleurovac, chest drain, tubing	tires
pulse oximeter probes	toys (check per manufacturer)
rubber dams	water toys
shoe covers (elastic portion)	wheelchair cushions, tires
sleeves (sterile, elastic portion)	
socks (patient hospital supply socks)	
specimen trap	
syringes (rubber plunger)	
tape	
test tube rubber stopper	
tubing (multiple sources)	
arthroscopy	
irrigation	
blood pressure cuff	
cystocatheter	
Pleurovac	
stethoscope	
tourniquet	
Urimeter (drainage port)	

Some, not all, of these items may contain latex. Many manufacturers currently produce nonlatex items. Latex content depends on the specific manufacturing brand name and product number.
From Young, M. A., & Meyers, M. (1997). Latex allergy considerations for the care of pediatric patients and employee safety. *Nursing Clinics of North America, 32,* 169–182. Reprinted with permission.

airborne latex. The anesthesia care practitioner must be notified of the latex allergy. Histamine blockers such as diphenhydramine, methylprednisolone, and cimetidine may be given preoperatively (Kinnaird et al., 1995). With early identification of children at risk for developing latex allergy and meticulous attention to latex avoidance, latex allergy and the resultant deleterious effects may be minimized.

Routine Procedures

Performing procedures, including specimen collection, on children can be time-consuming at best. At worst, it can be frustrating or even impossible without taking extreme measures, such as using restraints. Small children are afraid of procedures and often are very unwilling to cooperate. Knowing how to minimize trauma to the child and the parent but also perform the task requires skill. It begins with clear communication with the child and parent, explaining the purpose of, steps to, and outcomes expected from the procedure. This requires knowing the major fears of the child's age group, understanding the best time to give information as determined by the child's developmental level, providing preparation at that time, and addressing fears by using language or props that the child can understand.

Use honest, understandable language when talking to children about pain and procedures. Ambiguity or unfamiliarity with language is especially a problem for preschoolers, but toddlers and school-age children are also subject to misunderstanding, especially if ambiguous or unfamiliar terms are used (Table 9–2). Include explanations about what will happen and why, what the effects will be, and how the child can help during the procedure. Choose vivid language and sensory information for preparations, such as color, sound, size, or shape. Avoid jargon, fantasy, and ambiguity when asked if a procedure is going to hurt. Do not be dishonest about the outcome or the pain involved; try to describe it as well as possible.

Table 9–2
Language Considerations for Pediatric Patients

Potentially Ambiguous	Clearer
The doctor will give you some "dye." *To make me die.*	"The doctor will put some medicine in the tube that will help her be able to see your ______ more clearly."
Dressing, dressing change *Why are they going to undress me? Do I have to change my clothes? Will I be naked?*	"Bandages; clean new bandages."
Stool collection *Why do they want to collect little chairs?*	Use child's familiar term, such as "poop," "BM," or "doody."
Urine *You're in?*	Use child's familiar term, such as "pee."
Shot *Are they mad at me? When people get shot, they're really badly hurt. Are they trying to hurt me?*	"Medicine through a (small, tiny) needle."
CAT scan *Will there be cats? Or something that scratches?*	Describe in simple terms, and explain what the letters of the common name stand for (if child is old enough).
PICU *Pick you?*	Describe in simple terms, and explain what the letters of the common name stand for (if child is old enough).
ICU *I see you?*	Describe in simple terms, and explain what the letters of the common name stand for (if child is old enough).
IV *Ivy?*	Describe in simple terms, and explain what the letters of the common name stand for (if child is old enough).
Stretcher *Stretch her? Stretch who? Why?*	"Bed on wheels."
Special; funny *It doesn't look/feel special to me.*	"Odd; different; unusual; strange."
Gas; sleeping gas *Is someone going to pour gasoline into the mask?*	"Medicine, called anesthesia. It is a kind of air you will breathe through a mask like this to help you sleep during your operation so you won't feel anything. It is a different kind of sleep." Explain differences.
Put you to sleep *Like my cat was put to sleep? It never came back.*	"Medicine, called anesthesia. It is a kind of air you will breathe through a mask like this to help you sleep during your operation so you won't feel anything. It is a different kind of sleep." Explain differences.
Move you to the floor *Why are they going to put me on the ground?*	"Unit; ward." Explain why the child is being transferred, and where.

Table 9–2
Language Considerations for Pediatric Patients *Continued*

Potentially Ambiguous	**Clearer**
OR (or treatment room) table *People aren't supposed to get up on tables.*	"A narrow bed."
Take a picture (x-rays, CT, and MRI machines are far larger than a familiar camera, move differently, and don't yield a familiar end product.)	"A picture of the inside of you." Describe appearance, sounds, and movement of the equipment.
Flush your IV *Flush it down the toilet?*	Explain in simple terms, "Put some water in your IV tube."
Potentially Unfamiliar	**Concrete Explanation**
Take your vitals	"Measure your temperature; see how warm your body is; see how fast and strongly your heart is working." Nothing is "taken" from the child.
Electrode, leads	"Sticky like a Band-Aid, with a small wet spot in the center, and small strings that attach to the snap" (monitor electrodes) "Paste like wet sand, with strings with tiny metal cups that stick to the paste" (EEG electrodes) "The paste washes off easily afterwards; the strings go into a box that will make a picture of how your heart (or brain) is working." Show child electrodes and leads before using. Let child handle them and apply them to a doll or to self.
Intravenous, IV	"Medicine that works best when it goes right into a vein" (intravenous). "It's the quickest way to help you get better." First ask the child if he or she knows what a vein is, and why some medicine is OK to take by mouth and others work best in a vein. Explain concept of initials if child is old enough.
Hang your (IV) medication	"Bring in new medicine in a bag, and attach it to the little tube already in your arm. The needle goes into the tube, not into your arm, so you won't feel it."
NPO	"Nothing to eat. Your stomach needs to be empty." Explain why. "You can eat and drink again as soon as . . ." Explain with concrete descriptions.
Anesthesia	"The doctor will give you medicine; you may hear it called 'anesthesia.' It will help you go into a very deep sleep. You will not feel anything at all. The doctors know just the right amount of medicine to give you so you will stay asleep through your whole operation. When the operation is over, the doctor stops giving you that medicine and helps you wake up."
Incision	"Small opening." Follow with discussion of how cuts and scrapes received while playing have healed in the past.
Hard Impact	**Softer Impact**
This part will hurt.	"It (Your ________) may feel (or feel very) sore, achy, scratchy, tight, snug, full, or . . . [other descriptive term]."

Table continued on following page

Table 9–2
Language Considerations for Pediatric Patients *Continued*

Hard Impact	Softer Impact
The medicine will burn.	"Some children say they feel a very warm feeling."
The room will be very cold.	"Some children say they feel very cool."
The medicine will taste (or smell) bad.	"The medicine may taste (or smell) different than anything you have tasted before. After you take it, will you tell me how it was for you?"
Cut, open you up, slice, make a hole	"The doctor will make a small opening." Use concrete comparisons, such as "your little finger" or "a paper clip" if the opening will indeed be small.
As big as . . . (e.g., size of an incision or of a catheter)	"Smaller than."
As long as . . . (e.g., for duration of a procedure)	"For less time than it takes you to . . ."
As much as . . .	"Less than . . ."
You will have to say good-bye to your parents.	"That will be the time when you say 'See you later' to your parents."
Lots of children feel sick to their stomachs and throw up when they wake up.	"Your stomach has also been asleep and resting. It may need time to wake up. As your stomach wakes up, you will slowly be able to drink and then eat food again. Some children say they feel sick while their stomachs wake up; other children say they feel fine."
You will have a sore throat when you wake up.	"Your throat may feel very dry when you wake up."
You are angry/scared/sad. That was very hard for you.	"How was that for you? Was it the way you thought it would be? or harder or easier? Is there something else we should tell people about this?"

Adapted with permission of the Association for the Care of Children's Health, 7910 Woodmont Avenue, Suite 300, Bethesda, MD 20814, from Gaynard, L., Wolfer, J., Goldberger, J., Thompson, R., Redburn, L., & Laidley, L. (1990). *Psychosocial care of children in hospitals: A clinical practice manual from the ACCH Child Life Research Project* (pp. 62–65). Bethesda, MD: ACCH.

Research suggests that parental participation can play a major role in reducing a child's experience of pain during invasive procedures (George & Hancock, 1993). However, successful parental involvement depends on both parents' and staff's attitudes and willingness to work together (Palmer, 1993). If parents cannot or do not wish to be present, support them in this.

Children's fears of body intrusion and pain are developmentally based. Therefore, the caregiver must perform a careful developmental assessment of the child and use appropriate intervention to promote coping (see Chapter 13). For example, preschoolers believe that all their blood can be lost from a cut, so Band-Aids are important. They also fear body mutilation, so they need reassurance that taking specimens will not mutilate them.

In addition to preparing the child and family, successful procedure performance also depends on knowledge of age-dependent variances and proper equipment selection and use (Chart 9–21).

Medication Administration

Medication administration reflects one of the finer points of the art of pediatric nursing. The resistance of the infant, toddler, or preschooler to swallowing foul-tasting or -smelling medications can be dramatic in its display and time-consuming for the nurse. Soliciting the aid of the parents can be especially useful, because they may have already developed a form of medication administration that is acceptable to the child. Successful medication administration must focus on safety and development.

caREminder: *Safety is the predominant consideration in medication administration, because an error in this area can be lethal. Pediatric drug dosing requires specialized knowledge because children physiologically process medications differently from adults.*

Neonates have less plasma albumin available for drug binding than adults. Infants have prolonged gastric emp-

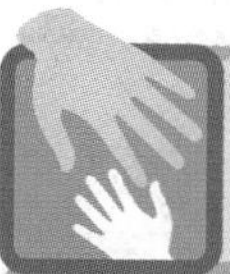

Chart 9–21
Nursing Interventions

Procedures

Procedure	Variances	Rationale	Nursing Considerations
All	Children understand and react to situations based on cognitive maturity. Teaching and support must be geared to cognitive level.	Developmentally appropriate support helps child maintain control.	Prepare for procedure as developmentally appropriate. Give choices as appropriate. Offer coping strategies (e.g., pacifier for infant, distraction for toddler). Teach parents techniques to support child during procedure. Have another staff member available to hold/assist as needed. After procedure, provide comfort measures, positive reinforcement. See Chapter 13 for considerations for painful procedures.
Blood Specimen Collection	Small total blood volume in young children. Iodine is easily absorbed through infant's skin.	Need to monitor for anemia and/or fluid volume deficit. Most laboratories can analyze values based on a small amount of blood.	Use a topical anesthetic (EMLA) on site prior to non-urgent blood draws (not in neonates). Use a Band-Aid to prevent bleeding after specimen is obtained, especially in preschoolers. In neonates and children requiring frequent blood sampling, maintain an ongoing tally of the amount of blood extracted (in cubic centimeters [cc]) Collect minimal amount of blood required to perform laboratory analysis. Do not put child in bed to obtain the specimen; keep the bed a safe area. When povidine-iodine is used, be certain it is cleansed from skin afterward.
Venipuncture	Common sites are veins on dorsum of hand, antecubital flexor surface of foot, wrist (very sensitive area).		Help child maintain control of situation; if appropriate, offer choice of sites, have child help cleanse site. If unable to obtain venous access after two or three attempts, find another practitioner to do the puncture. After procedure, apply pressure to site until bleeding stops, then cover as appropriate (e.g., no tape for premature infant, Band-Aid for preschooler).

Chart continued on following page

Chart 9–21
Nursing Interventions *Continued*

Procedures

Procedure	Variances	Rationale	Nursing Considerations
Capillary puncture 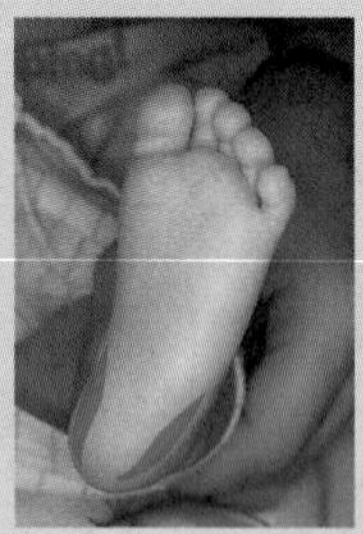	Can use lateral aspect of the heel up to about 1 year of age; do not use side of finger until 5 or 6 years of age.	To avoid striking the medial plantar artery or the periosteum of the bone, because these are relatively superficial in young children To reduce discomfort afterward	Choose site carefully (check landmarks). Warm the extremity prior to drawing blood; wet a disposable diaper with warm water and wrap around the foot or hand. Do not squeeze extremity excessively when drawing blood (causes cells to hemolyze; so may obtain false high K^+ level from heelstick or fingerstick).
Urine Specimen Collection	Child may have difficulty understanding request. Adolescent may be reluctant to have test completed or may be unable to void on request. Urine may be aspirated from cotton balls for small-volume tests such as specific gravity, pH, or glucose.	Language used by the nurse may be misunderstood by the child. Concerns over body image, body functions, and privacy; perhaps suspicious that urine specimen is requested for drug testing Disposable diapers with absorbent gel are difficult to aspirate from and yield inaccurate results.	Use child's words such as "pee pee" to make request. Provide privacy for older child, adolescent. Clean area or teach child/parent correct cleaning method for clean-catch specimen. Provide potty chair or urine collector in toilet for preschool or school-age child. Explain to adolescent why test is needed. Offer child something to drink; most infants void shortly after feeding. Too much fluid may dilute the specific gravity of the urine. Cotton balls may be placed near the urethra inside the diaper to squeeze out urine for small volume testing; do not aspirate urine from diaper. Run water in sink to trigger urge to void.
Urine Bag 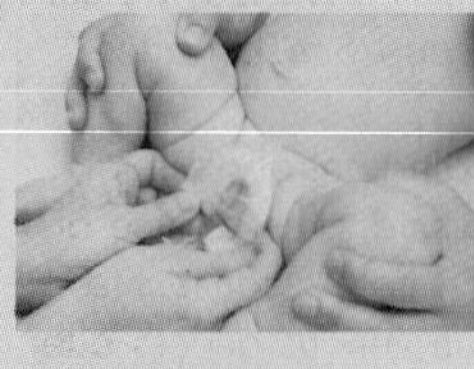 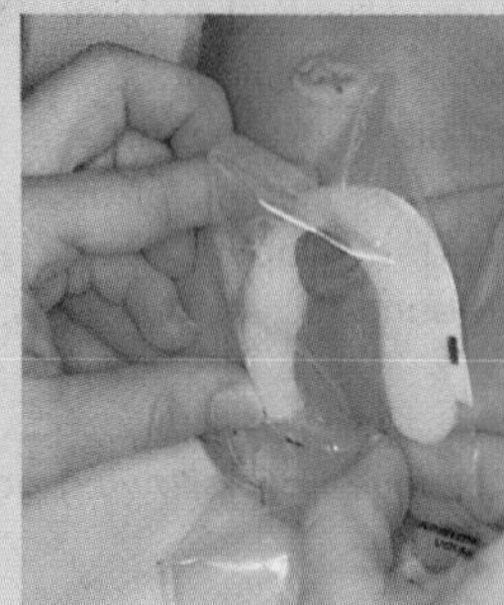	Urine bags must be used to collect urine from infants/toddlers for larger amounts, e.g., routine urinalysis.	Lack of bowel/bladder control does not allow young children to voluntarily cooperate with specimen collection.	Clean and dry perineal skin. Apply chemical adhesive (e.g., tincture of benzoin) to help maintain seal (do not use on premature infants, neonates). To place on female: position lower half of adhesive on bag on perineum first, then press on adhesive up toward symphysis. To place on male: insert penis and scrotum into bag opening, adhesive adheres to perineum and symphysis. Make sure bag does not cover anus, to reduce contamination. Cut a hole in the diaper, pulling the urine bag through the opening; thus, when the child voids, it is easily visible and the urine bag can be removed immediately.

Chart 9–21
Nursing Interventions *Continued*

Procedures

Procedure	Variances	Rationale	Nursing Considerations
Urine catheterization	Difficult to find urethral opening in female infants; may have excess tissue overlying opening. Choose urinary catheter size depending on child's age: Neonate: 5–6 French Infant: 5–8 French Toddler/preschooler: 8 French School-age: 8, 10, 12, 14 French Adolescent: 10, 12, 14 French	Swelling of the labia in neonates, due to maternal hormones, makes it difficult to visualize urethral opening. Smaller catheter size promotes comfort and is adequate for specimen collection. Feeding tubes are usually less expensive than catheters but are more prone to knotting in the bladder (Carlson & Mowery, 1997). Use of shorter length urinary catheters, and basing length of insertion on sex and age, can reduce incidence of knotting (e.g., for toddler and younger females insert 2 inches, for male infants insert 3 inches, male toddlers 3–4 inches) (Carlson & Mowery, 1997).	Have second person maintain child in frog-leg position. Use thumb and forefinger to spread labia. Exert slight pressure up and out to reveal urethral opening in female. Insert sterile lubricant, using specific adapter containing 2% Xylocaine into urethra; 5 mL for girls and young boys, 10 mL for adolescent boys (Gray, 1996). Have extra catheter ready; if the first is contaminated or inadvertently placed in vagina, leave it in place, and put the second catheter in other opening (urethra). Insert indwelling catheters to the hub of the catheter, and do not inflate balloon until urine is seen; after balloon inflation, pull catheter back to seat at bladder base (Carlson & Mowrey, 1997). If indwelling catheter or urine bag with drainage tubing is used, ensure collection tubing is out of young child's reach, out of view.
Suprapubic aspiration	Procedure used to collect urine from infants who cannot void. Needle is inserted through abdominal wall into bladder.	Theoretically, the risk of bladder infection from needle insertion is less than that from catheter insertion.	Performed by physician or nurse practitioner
Stool Collection	May be particularly embarrassing for school-age child and adolescent.		Know the words the child uses for stool. If the child is not toilet trained, scrape stool from a diaper using tongue blade and place in stool collection cup. Children who are toilet trained should be asked to use a potty seat or have a collection container placed in the toilet. Provide privacy.

Chart continued on following page

Chart 9–21
Nursing Interventions *Continued*

Procedures

Procedure	Variances	Rationale	Nursing Considerations
Sputum Specimen Collection	Must use suctioning to obtain specimen from infants and toddlers.	Infants/toddlers will not cough productively on command.	Do not exceed 80–100 mmHg suction pressure. Limit suctioning time to 10 seconds.
Nasogastric/ Orogastric Tube Placement	Placement of nasogastric tube in infants/toddlers should be completed as quickly as possible.	The young child cannot cooperate by swallowing during tube insertion.	Measure tip of tube from child's nose to earlobe to xiphoid process. Mark level on tube with tape, lubricate tip with water or soluble lubricant, and quickly insert. In young child, may need to angle tube toward occiput rather than up. Do not exert pressure on nares when taping tube to cheek.

tying and immature renal function (Sagraves, 1995). Some children metabolize drugs rapidly; periods of rapid growth may lead to subtherapeutic drug levels; and some drugs may have paradoxical effects in children. Also, preverbal children cannot describe symptoms associated with side effects. Therefore, the nurse must ensure that the correct medication in the correct dose is being administered to the correct patient.

The physician, nurse practitioner, or pharmacist may prescribe medications. All health professionals are responsible for administering safe dosages and monitoring for toxic effects and side effects of drugs. The nurse must know how to calculate therapeutic dosages to determine whether they are safe to administer and what toxic effects and side effects are associated with the drugs being administered.

In children, the therapeutic dose of medication is determined using body weight or body surface area (BSA). When using body weight, verify the correct dose from a reference source and calculate it for that child. For example, if the dose is 10 mg/kg/24 hours divided every 6 hours, then for a 10-kg child, the dose would be 100 mg/24 hours or 25 mg given every 6 hours. BSA is computed as a relationship between height and weight using a nomogram (Fig. 9–14). Infants have more BSA than would be expected from their weight because the ratio of BSA to weight varies inversely with length. To predict dose based on BSA, determine the safe dose from a reference source and calculate. For example, if a child's BSA is 0.5 m^2 and the recommended dose is 100 mg/m^2/24 hours in 2 divided doses, then 0.5 $m^2 \times 100$ mg = 50 mg/24 hours or 25 mg every 12 hours.

Besides addressing safety concerns, the nurse must administer medications to children in a developmentally appropriate manner (Chart 9–22).

Oral Medications

The gastrointestinal tract provides a vast absorptive area for medications. Administration by that route is also less invasive, thus less traumatic, than intramuscular or intravenous injection. Therefore, the oral route should be used to administer medications whenever possible. Children have a natural aversion to foul-tasting and smelly substances. They may cry and refuse to take medication or may try to spit out the dose.

Alert: *For liquid medications, an oral syringe or medication cup should be used to ensure accurate dosage measurement. Use of a household teaspoon or tablespoon may result in dosage error because they are inaccurate.*

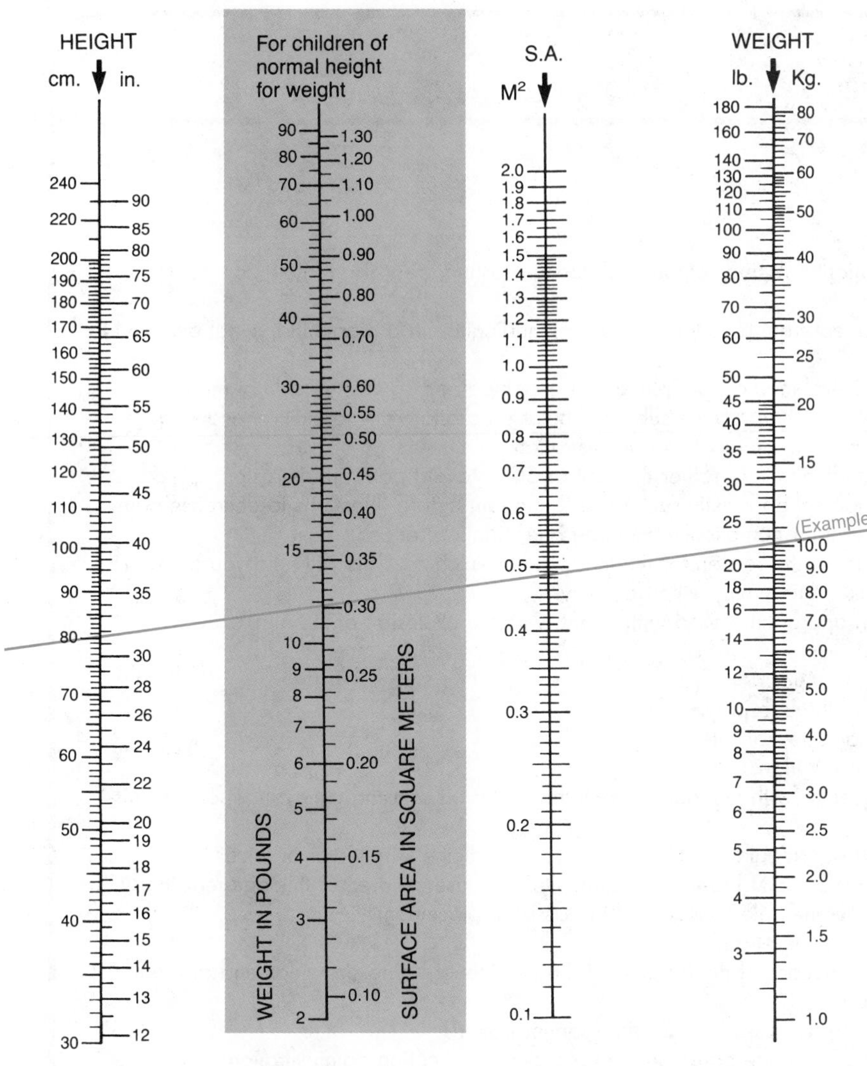

Figure 9–14
Nomogram for estimation of body surface area. The surface area is indicated where a straight line that intersects the height and weight levels intersects the surface area column; or, if the patient is roughly of average size, from the weight alone (shaded area). (Nomogram modified from data of E. Boyd by C. D. West.) (From Betz, C. L., Hunsberger, M. M., & Wright, S. [1994]. *Family-centered nursing care of children* [2nd ed., p. 864]. Philadelphia: W. B. Saunders.)

When administering oral medication, NEVER

- Mix it with the infant's formula or necessary food source (e.g., cereal).
- Mix it with the child's favorite food.
- Deceive the child about the fact that you are administering medication (e.g., by pretending that you are giving the child something good to eat).
- Use the medication as a reward or punishment.

Mixing medications with formula or preferred foods may lead to the dislike of that food, as well as to a distrust of the caregiver or a generalized distrust of the hospital staff. Similarly, such distrust may be created with the pretense that what is being given to the child is good or desirable. The overall objective is to administer the entire dose of medication while creating the least aversion to medication possible for the child (Fig. 9–15).

Tip: *Tell the child to drink juice or milk after distasteful medications. Older children can suck the medication from a syringe, pinch their nose, or drink through a straw to decrease the input of smell, which adds to the unpleasantness of oral medications.*

Intramuscular Medications

When delivering care using principles of atraumatic care, administration of medications via the intramuscular (IM) route should be rare. Children fear invasive procedures, needles, and shots. Using an IM injection to deliver pain medication in itself causes pain—and frequently psychological distress in the child. Most drugs, including pain medications and antibiotics, can be given orally or intravenously (IV). The rectal route may be psychologically traumatic but should not be physically painful.

If a medication is ordered IM, the nurse needs to advocate for the child. Consider whether the medication can be given via another, less traumatic, route, such as orally or rectally. If the child has an IV line, can that route be used to administer the drug? If the drug is to be given routinely, it is probably less traumatic to insert an

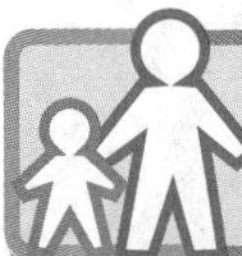

Chart 9–22
Developmental Considerations

Medication Administration

Developmental Age	Guidelines
Infant	Place oral medication in a *small* amount of pleasant-tasting food, if an infant can eat from spoon. If the infant cannot eat from a spoon, place oral medication in a nipple that is not attached to a bottle. If the infant refuses oral medication, place it in a syringe and squirt it in side of mouth, toward back of jaw. Then rub the submandibular area bilaterally to elicit swallowing. Ask the parent to assist in medication administration. If possible, give medications IV rather than IM or SQ to avoid pain and intrusion. If possible, use a topical anesthetic such as EMLA cream before injections to decrease pain. Praise an older infant for compliance. Comfort after administration.
Toddler	Explain in simple terms the reason for the medications, such as "This will help you get well" or "This will make your tummy-ache go away." Use administration approaches used with infant, with the exclusion of the nipple. Provide distraction. Permit expression of anger. Provide preparation through play. Place a Band-Aid on injection site. Comfort after administration.
Preschooler	Use same techniques as with the toddler, with the exclusion of using the syringe for administration. Offer choices such as "Would you like to take your medicine with water or juice?" Immediately place a Band-Aid on the injection site, because children of this age fear their blood will "run out the hole." Allow child to assist in placement. Praise the child for cooperation.
School-age child	Give concrete explanations of the purpose of the medication using drawings and diagrams of targeted body parts. Give as much choice as possible regarding administration. Allow independence from the parent in the process of medication administration.
Adolescent	Use approaches suggested for school-age child. Depending on maturity of the adolescent, use more abstract rationales for medication.

IV line and give the medication IV than to give repeated injections. Check with the pharmacist and/or physician to change the route of administration.

caREminder: *If the medication must be administered IM, use a topical anesthetic (EMLA) prior to giving the injection.*

Complications associated with giving IM injections in children include intra-arterial or intravenous injection, nerve injury, muscle fibrosis or contracture, and infection at the injection site. Again, IM injections should be avoided when possible. If necessary to use this route, meticulous attention must be given to proper technique and landmark location to avoid complications.

Prior to administering an IM injection, the nurse must evaluate the child's size, muscle development, motor capabilities, and diagnosis. These factors help determine the most appropriate site for injection (Fig. 9–16). For example, a child must have been walking at least a year before the dorsogluteal site is used. Even then, the muscle is small, poorly developed, and close to the sciatic nerve, which is relatively large in young children. Therefore, the ventrogluteal or vastus lateralis site is a safer choice in an infant. If multiple injections are necessary, injection sites must be rotated.

Tip: *Tell the child it is all right to make noise or cry out during the injection. His or her job is to try not to move the extremity.*

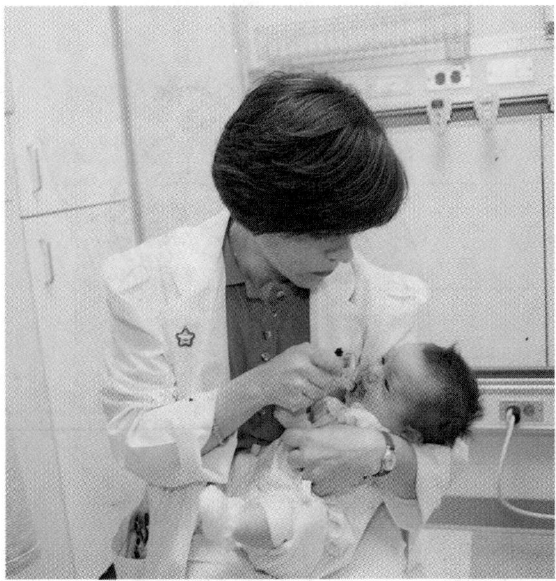

Figure 9–15
Administering oral medication to an infant. Note how the nurse can control the infant's movements by holding the infant's left arm (the infant's right arm is tucked under the nurse's left arm) and tucking the infant's head in the crook of her arm.

Volume of fluid to be injected and needle size must also be considered when administering IM injections. The maximum volume that the muscle will accommodate depends on muscle size, thus it varies with age of the child and the site used. Needle gauge and length also vary depending on the muscle mass. Generally, a 25-gauge needle is used for neonates, a 23-gauge for infants, and 22- to 20-gauge needles for older children.

Intravenous Medications

The IV route provides direct access into the vascular system. For this reason, it is ideal to use when drugs must be delivered rapidly, high serum concentrations of a drug must be maintained, or reliable absorption is necessary. For the child with established IV access, administration of medications via this route can be done in a manner that is relatively non-threatening to the child. (See Chapter 17 for an in-depth discussion of venous access and IV therapy.)

Adverse effects of IV medication administration include extravasation of the drug into surrounding tissue, resulting in temporary or permanent damage, and reaction to the drug, including side effects and anaphylaxis. The nurse must intervene to minimize these hazards (Chart 9–23). Before administering an IV medication, check the site to ascertain that the IV fluid has not infiltrated the tissue. Medications given IV enter the vascular system quickly. Anaphylaxis or toxic side effects (e.g., respiratory or cardiac depression) may manifest immediately or after a period of time. The nurse must know the medication's potential side effects and adverse reactions, monitor the child for these, and teach the child and family to notify the health professional if these or any other unusual signs or symptoms appear. Check your institution's policy on which drugs must be administered by a physician and which must be verified for accuracy by another nurse.

Many medications are incompatible with other drugs, diluents, and IV solutions. Check a reference source for compatibilities, flush well between administration of incompatible drugs, or give via different IV access. Do not mix medications or give medications in the same line when administering blood products.

To minimize adverse effects associated with high serum drug levels (e.g., nephrotoxicity, ototoxicity) and to avoid venous irritation from concentrated solutions, IV medications are usually diluted. Young children may develop fluid overload from the extra 50 mL of fluid commonly given to administer medication "piggybacks" to adults. Most institutions have specific policies on diluting drugs and administering diluted drugs. IV medications can be delivered in various ways, depending on the drug (e.g., pain medications or diuretics may be given IV push, whereas antibiotics are often given over 30 to 60 minutes) and the child's fluid status (e.g., infants cannot handle large fluid volumes; children with renal, cardiac, or other problems may require fluid restriction).

▽ **Alert:** *The extra fluid given to administer IV medications and flush the tubing must be included in the calculation of the child's total fluid intake, particularly in young children or those with unstable fluid balance.*

Some medications are very irritating to the veins. Giving them over a longer period or in more fluid can help minimize this irritation.

IV medications can be given directly into the IV tubing (IV push), retrograde, or via buretrol or syringe pump. Medications given **IV push** immediately enter the vascular system with almost instantaneous effects (Fig. 9–17). IV push medications are usually administered over a few minutes and necessitate small amounts of extra fluid intake. Medications given **retrograde** are administered in a tubing port with the flow to the child blocked, so the medication is injected back up the tubing. Thus, the fluid in the tubing is displaced by the amount of medication fluid administered. Most systems are set up so this displaced fluid backs up into the drip chamber (which can accommodate about 3 mL) or

Ventrogluteal: Use the hand opposite the side for injection to locate landmarks (e.g., to give in child's left hip, use your right hand to locate landmarks). Locate by placing your palm on the greater trochanter, index finger on the anterior superior iliac spine, and middle finger on the posterior edge of the iliac spine. Inject into center of the V formed by the index and middle fingers.

caREminder: Insert needle at 90 degrees but directed slightly upward toward iliac crest. Use in any age. Use 5/8–1-inch needle. Limit injectate volume to 0.5 mL in infant, 1.5 mL in preschooler, 2 mL in older child. Free from major nerves and blood vessels.

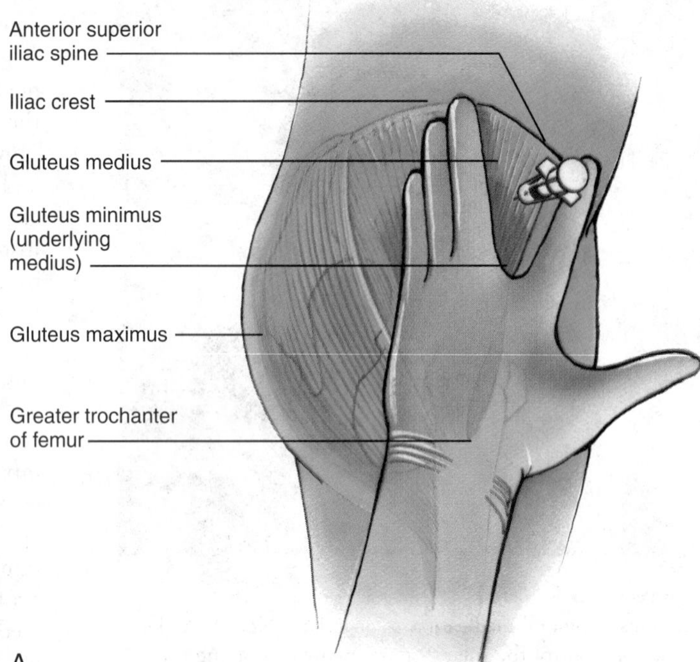

Vastus Lateralis: Palpate greater trochanter and knee. Divide into thirds; site is in middle third. Draw two imaginary lines from greater trochanter to knee—one mid-anteriorly, one mid-laterally. Injection site is located between these lines in mid-lateral, anterior thigh.

caREminder: Insert needle at 90 degrees. Largest muscle available in infants and young children. Use 5/8–1-inch needle. Limit injectate volume to 0.5 mL in infant, 1 mL in toddler, 2 mL in school-ager. Site can be used in older children but is more painful than other sites. Relatively free from major nerves and blood vessels.

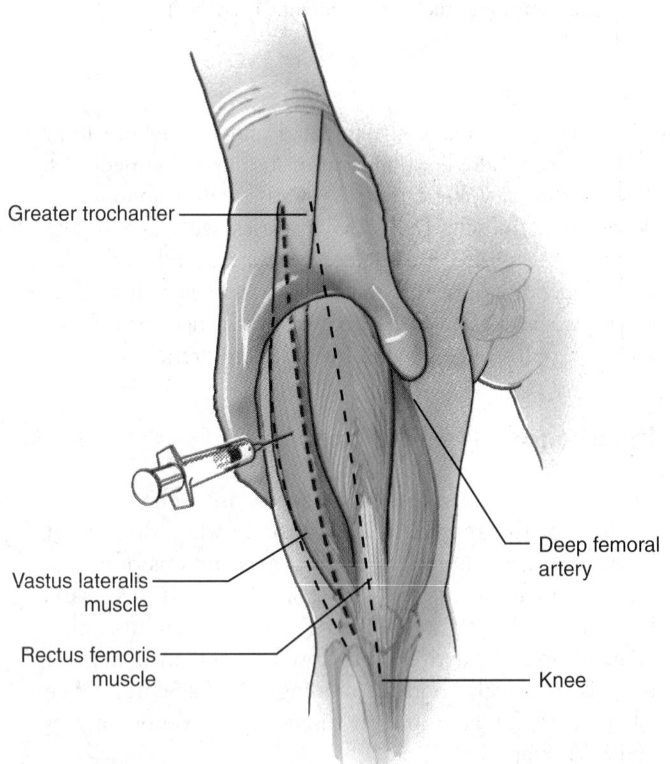

Figure 9–16
See legend on opposite page

into a syringe placed in the tubing for this purpose. The IV flow rate remains unchanged. If the fluid backs up into the syringe and is discarded, the child does not receive any extra fluid. Retrograde administration is being used less frequently as **syringe pumps** are becoming more readily available (Fig. 9–18). Low-volume tubing can be used to minimize the amount of drug wasted in the tubing. The pump is set to administer the drug over

Deltoid: Identify lower edge of acromium process and point on arm in line with axilla. Site is 1–3 fingerbreadths (depending on size of child) below acromium process and just above axilla. Inject into mid-deltoid region.

caREminder: Insert needle into muscle at 90 degrees, pointed slightly toward acromium process. Use ½–1-inch needle. Muscle mass limited, use small injection volumes (0.5–1 mL) and avoid irritating solutions and repeated injections. Provides more rapid medication absorption than gluteal regions. Radial nerve lies under deltoid muscle.

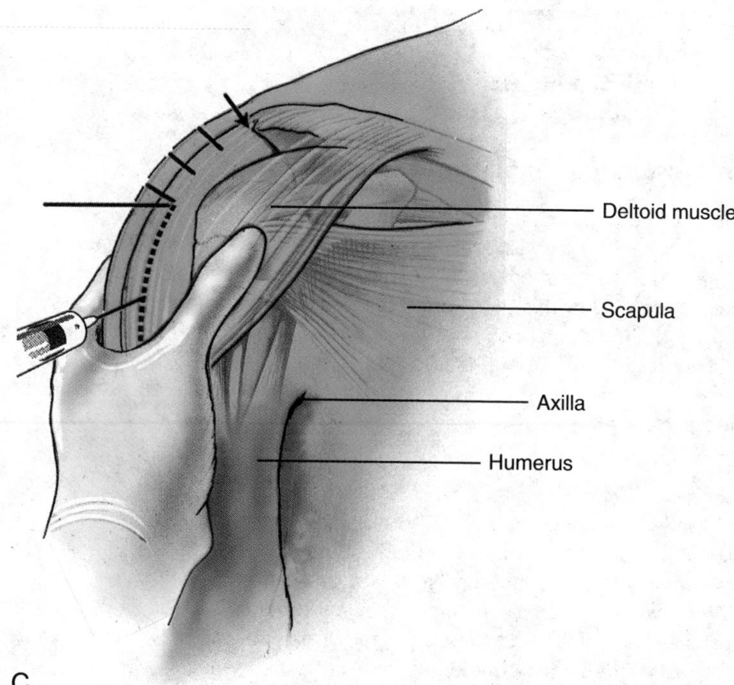

Dorsogluteal: Locate posterior superior iliac spine and the greater trochanter; imagine a line between the two. Inject in the upper outer region above this line into the gluteus medius muscle.

caREminder: Have child lie prone and toe-in to relax muscle. Insert needle at 90 degrees to surface on which child is lying. Should not be used in children younger than 5 years of age; site is not well developed, thus the margin of error is very small. Use ½–1½-inch needle depending on child's size. Can accommodate larger injectate volumes (1.5 mL in school-age, 2 mL in adolescent). Close to sciatic nerve and superior gluteal artery.

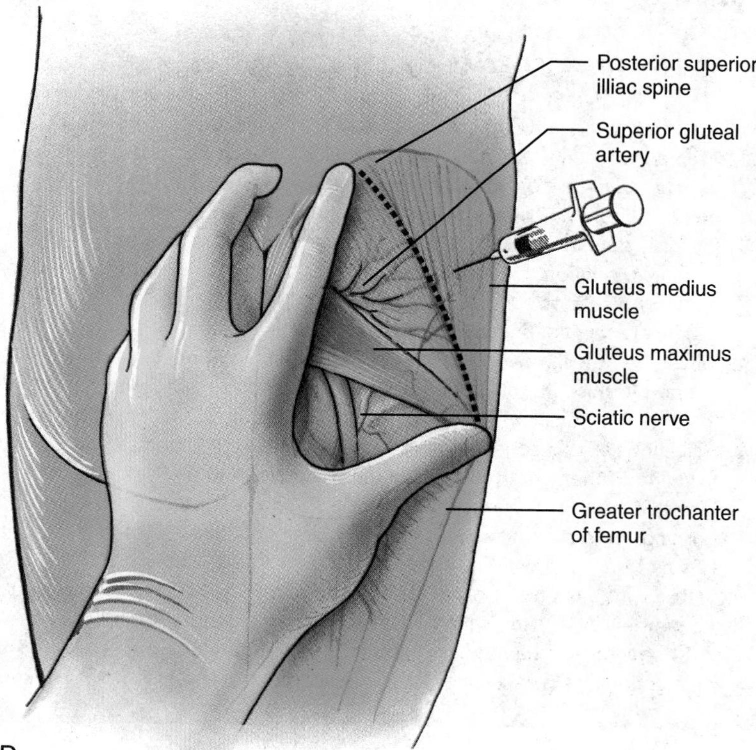

Figure 9–16
Intramuscular injection sites in children: *(A)* ventrogluteal; *(B)* vastus lateralis; *(C)* deltoid; *(D)* dorsogluteal.

the predetermined period. Minimal amounts of extra fluid are needed to administer the medications. For children who can tolerate extra fluid volume, IV medications can be administered via **buretrol**. The drug is diluted in a specific amount of fluid in the buretrol, taking into account how much fluid the drug must be diluted in, the child's IV flow rate, and the fluid volume in the tubing. After the buretrol is empty, the drug remains in the tubing. Therefore, it is necessary to know how much fluid the tubing holds (commonly

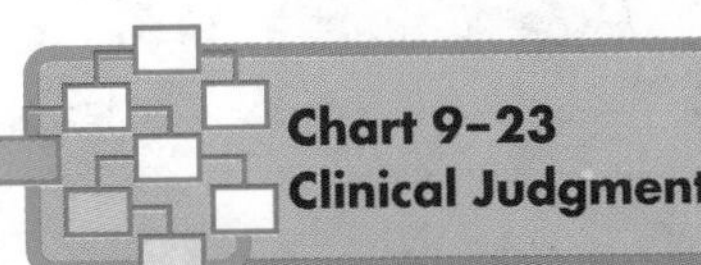

Chart 9–23
Clinical Judgment

Intravenous Medication Administration

Ari is a 14-year-old, hospitalized for the past 4 days with staphylococcal pneumonia. His current weight is 40 kg. As part of his treatment he is receiving intravenous (IV) fluid at 125 mL/hr and nafcillin 1300 mg every 4 hours via peripheral IV. The reference source says that nafcillin must be diluted 10 to 20 mg/mL and given over 30 to 60 minutes. Ari has had his IV restarted four times since admission and complains bitterly that the IV site burns during nafcillin administration. You review his chart and find that the nafcillin has been given in 65 mL of fluid followed by 15 mL to flush the IV tubing, then 45 mL to maintain his 125 mL/hr IV rate.

Questions

1. The recommended dose of nafcillin is 100 to 200 mg/kg/24 hours given every 4 to 6 hours. Is Ari's dose within suggested range?
2. What factors concerning Ari's IV may indicate a problem?
3. Is the nafcillin being diluted in the best way to manage this situation?
4. How will you dilute the nafcillin based on Ari's current IV rate?
5. What will indicate that the more prolonged administration of a less concentrated solution has addressed the problem? If nafcillin administration remains problematic, what are alternatives for you to consider or address with the rest of the health care team?

Answers

1. Yes:
   40 kg × 100 mg = 4000 mg/24 hours = 666.6 mg every 4 hours
   40 kg × 200 mg = 8000 mg/24 hours = 1333.3 mg every 4 hours
   Ari is receiving 1300 mg every 4 hours, almost 200 mg/kg/24 hours.
2. Ari's IV has been restarted on an average of once every 24 hours, which is too frequent. In this situation it may indicate that the nafcillin is injuring the veins. Nafcillin is very irritating to the veins, but when well managed, the patient should not be very uncomfortable during administration.
3. No, it is diluted in the maximum concentration recommended (1300 mg ÷ 65 mL = 20 mg/mL, which is the maximum dilution concentration), and the nafcillin is administered over 40 minutes (65 mL + 15 mL flush = 80 mL given at a rate of 125 mL/hr = 2 mL/min = 40 minutes for 80 mL), a period of time slightly longer than the shortest recommended administration time of 30 minutes.
4. Infuse the nafcillin over a longer period of time (60 minutes), diluted in more fluid. Subtract the 15 mL of fluid needed to flush the medication through the tubing in order to find out the amount of fluid left for that hour in which to dilute the nafcillin. 125 − 15 = 110 mL to dilute the 1300 mg of Nafcillin. 1300 mg ÷ 100 mL = 11.8 mg of nafcillin/mL. This concentration is closer to the recommended minimal dilution of 10 mg/mL and should be less irritating to the vein than the previously administered 20 mg/mL.
5. Effective management may be indicated by maintenance of one peripheral IV site for 72 hours and the nafcillin not burning upon administration. If the problem continues, dilute the nafcillin in even more fluid, either manipulating the IV rate to end up with the same fluid balance (e.g., giving 150 mL the hour the nafcillin is administered and then 100 mL the next hour) or, if Ari can tolerate the extra fluid, increasing the fluid amount for the hour the nafcillin is administered. Consult with the clinical pharmacist. The length of time over which the nafcillin is administered should not be increased beyond 60 minutes because this may affect serum drug levels and administration of other medications he is receiving. It may be appropriate to insert a PICC line (peripherally inserted central catheter).

15 mL) so at least that amount can be given to flush the medication through the tubing into the vein. The buretrol is tagged with tape or a designated sticker, so that everyone is aware that a medication or flush is infusing (Fig. 9–19).

Infection Control

Infection control is an increasingly important focus in health care settings. Although much of the public concern is with HIV, the risk of acquiring hepatitis B in

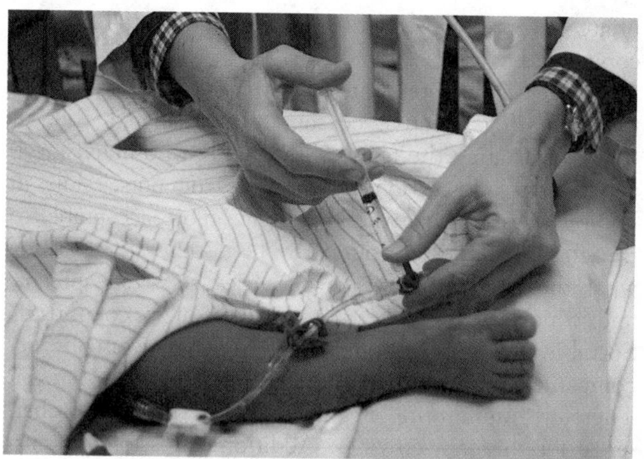

Figure 9–17
Medications administered IV push enter the vascular system immediately.

unvaccinated health care workers is even greater than the risk of HIV (Valenti, 1993). Recently the spread of non-resistant tuberculosis has increased the need for hospitals to provide exposure-control plans that protect patients, visitors, and health care workers. Federal and state regulatory agencies (such as the Occupational Safety and Health Administration) monitor facilities for exposure-control plans and workplace and engineering controls that minimize the threat of infection. However, the most important way to minimize exposure to and transmission of pathogens is by following standard precautions (see Chapter 24 for discussion).

caREminder: *All body fluid must be handled using standard precautions, whether or not it has been tested and identified as containing contagions. This includes wearing gloves to change diapers.*

The control of potential infections is of critical importance in pediatric care because nosocomial infections are primary contributors to mortality and morbidity in young hospitalized patients (Peters, Lepow, McCracken, & Phillips, 1991). In response to this high level of risk, all hospitals have implemented routine guidelines and policies designed to prevent or reduce the spread of infection. Many of these policies, such as isolation practices, have proved their value to such an extent that they are found in some form in every acute care setting.

The overriding goal of infection control programs is the protection of all patients and staff at all times from infectious disease. Although health care providers can be infected by contact with patients, patients are more susceptible to infection. This is due to the fact that hospitalization is more likely to occur when the general state of health is impaired, and the ability of the immune system to ward off infection is likely compromised. Furthermore, many patients experience invasive procedures, which allow a port of entry for exogenous bacteria to enter the body. To reduce the spread of microorganisms by direct contact with patients, hands must be washed before *and* after contact with each child.

Appropriate disinfection of patient care materials between children, or single-use, disposal equipment can reduce the spread of microorganisms by indirect contact. Airborne contamination can be addressed by having children and employees cover their nose and mouth when sneezing and coughing, using disposable tissues if possible, and then washing their hands.

When following standard precautions, health care personnel should wear gloves and other personal protective equipment as needed for protection from contact with blood and other body fluids. Hands should be washed after gloves are removed. Gloves need to be changed between patients and taken off before contact with inanimate objects such as the telephone or pens.

Strict adherence to standard precautions can become another stressor for the child and family in the acute care setting. Children and families may be approached by personnel wearing protective devices, such as gowns, masks, and goggles. Parents may be required to wear this personal protective equipment when caring for their children. Children in isolation may be sequestered from others in the environment. Such measures can be frightening for the child and annoying and cumbersome for parents.

Figure 9–18
Syringe pump used to administer IV medication.

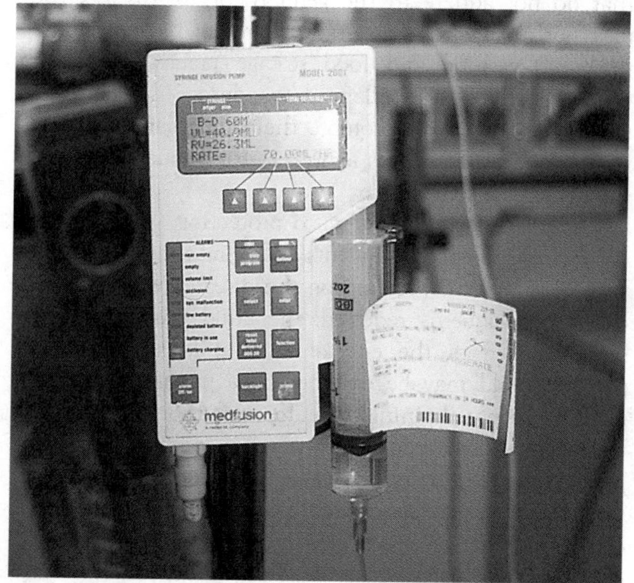

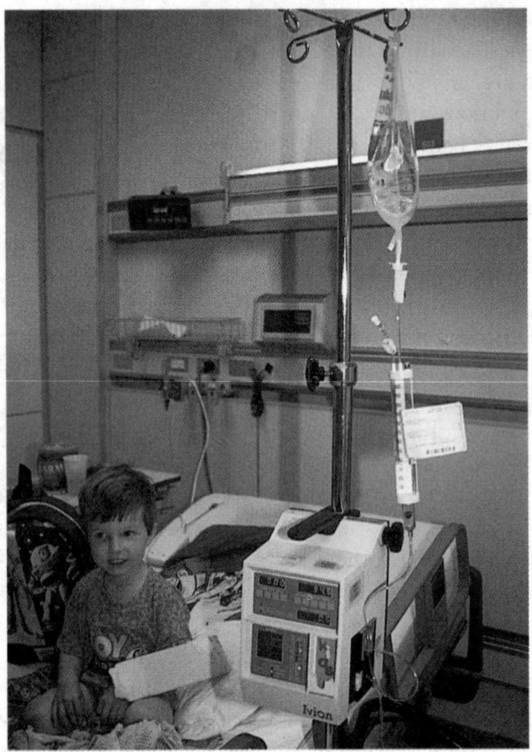

Figure 9–19
IV medication being administered via buretrol. Note the sticker on the buretrol to alert all staff that medication is infusing.

Further, infection control measures may impede family and cultural practices. Some families may want to store food in the room. Others may want to keep plants, flowers, or small pets there. All these items can harbor bacteria or act as vectors for insect infestations. To compound the problem, some families may belong to cultures that do not adhere to the germ theory of disease; they may not adhere to Western standards of hygiene related to hand washing and food storage practices. In such cases, the nurse is challenged to educate the family in such a manner as to promote their compliance with infection control standards as well as their satisfaction with the acute care experience.

Isolation. Isolation refers to protecting the child and others from infectious agents. This may be done in a variety of ways, depending on the disease. Whatever isolation technique is required, the child usually must be sequestered from the environment at large. For example, the child may be confined to a private room, may need to keep a draining wound covered, or may need to wear a mask when leaving the room. Sequestration can impair the child emotionally and socially. Toddlers and preschoolers cannot fully understand these processes and, hence, have greater difficulty coping during periods of required isolation. Thus, the pediatric nurse must intervene by providing developmentally appropriate diversional activities for the child to enhance coping.

Perhaps the intervention of the greatest importance for promoting effective coping of the isolated child is that of educating the family. The family who understands the reason for isolation can become the nurse's ally in finding ways to make the experience more acceptable to the child. Families are often the best source for learning what the child fears, which activities he or she prefers, and which measures he or she finds most comforting. Social isolation is an unpleasant experience usually accompanied by depression, fatigue, frustration, and anger. Therefore, minimizing its impact is an important challenge for the care provider. Additional tips for minimizing social isolation for an isolated child include the following:

- Discuss with the parents and significant others the importance of their visiting the child.
- Include parents in the process of explaining the isolation to the child when developmentally appropriate.
- Encourage picture videos of family, friends, and pets.
- Provide access to telephone or "video-tel" where available.
- Arrange for the child life specialist to visit the child for therapeutic play.

Visitation Policies

Separation of hospitalized children from their parents adds to the difficulty of adjusting to hospitalization. Yet, the development of visitation policies that give parents full visitation rights has been an uphill struggle with hospital administrations. In a study that supports visitation, Tughan (1992) examined parent, patient, and staff perceptions of visitation in the pediatric ICU with regard to the facilitation of family-centered care. Some recommendations for change based on this study were that

- Visitation should be open to grandparents and siblings with parents' permission.
- The number of visitors may need to be limited because of space and patient access considerations.
- The parents should have 24-hour access, but daily rest is important.
- The nursing staff should be able to ask visitors to leave for organizational purposes.
- In cases of a grave prognosis, any person so designated by the parents should be allowed to visit.
- Exceptions to the guidelines should be determined collaboratively by the patient, parents, and interdisciplinary team.

True family-centered care views parents as partners in care, not as visitors. Some myths commonly cited by opponents of liberalized visitation policies are as follows (Johnson et al., 1992):

- Myth 1: Children are upset by their parents' visitation. This is often substantiated by nothing more than the fact that the child cried in the presence of the parent, a rather simplistic view of what might be upsetting a hospitalized child. Often the child may feel more comfortable expressing emotion in front of the parents.
- Myth 2: Visitation leads to increased infection. Although increased exposure may increase risk of infection (Stover & Burgess, 1996), this remains controversial. Screening visitors may limit the risk while providing psychological benefit to child and family (Hamrick & Reilly, 1992; "ICP's Develop Policies for Pet and Sibling Visitation," 1994).
- Myth 3: Rooming-in has special room design requirements. This is an uncreative approach, whereas adaptation to rooming-in is relatively easy for motivated staff and parents (e.g., cots at the bedside are often sufficient).
- Myth 4: Liberalized visitation policies will lead to chaos. This may be a valid concern but can be addressed through quotas of visitors at any one time for any one patient.

Fortunately, the proponents of liberalized family visitation policies have had some influence. Today, most facilities that care for children have 24-hour open visiting for parents and grandparents. This policy encourages them to participate in their child's care and to room-in when possible. The Pediatric Bill of Rights (Association for the Care of Children's Health, 1991) pledges to the family the right to feel welcome in the hospital and to have a place for at least one family member to spend the night. If parents cannot be present to support the child in person, it should not be assumed they do not care or are "bad" parents. Encourage participation in the child's care to the extent they are able, and encourage the participation of significant others.

If parents are reluctant to visit because the child cries and protests when they leave, explain that this is a normal response to separation. If parents are absent as a result of work, sibling care, or other responsibilities, reinforce that the child will be attended to. Provide the family with the name and telephone number of a contact person knowledgeable about the child; the nurse can also initiate regular telephone contact with the family. When appropriate, assist the child in calling home. Assisting the family with logistics (e.g., handouts regarding hospital, visitation policies, support services; transportation, meal and lodging assistance; etc.) may increase visitation (Stepanek & Ahmann, 1995).

Siblings

Another aspect of family visitation is sibling visits. Sibling visitation is an important aspect of meeting the developmental needs of the hospitalized child (Whitis, 1994). Unfortunately, Whitis (1994) found that 64% of hospitals restricted visiting to children older than the ages of 12 to 14. This study supported earlier findings.

The benefits from sibling visitation are multiple, but probably the most important is that seeing one's brothers and sisters helps normalize hospitalization for the patient, especially a child with a condition that requires a prolonged stay, such as cancer or certain traumatic injuries. For prolonged hospitalizations, videophones can play a key role in supplementing sibling visitation to promote increased contact between siblings on an ongoing basis. Sibling visitation promotes adaptation of the sibling to the situation. It easily dispels misconceptions the sibling may have about the hospitalized child, such as things are "worse" than reported or the child is dead. It helps reduce separation anxiety that affects siblings when parents spend time at the hospital. Sibling visitation also promotes effective coping for the siblings at home because it provides opportunities for nurses to intervene directly, educate, allay fears, and promote a realistic understanding of the situation (Craft, 1993). Finally, it eases the strain on parents who often face conflict between being in the hospital and supervising the children at home.

ACCH supports visitation for siblings of all ages. Opponents' concerns must be addressed through policy changes. Chaos can be reduced by controlling the hours for visitation and limiting the number of persons who visit a patient at any one time. Sibling visitation may lead to greater cross-infection (Stover & Burgess, 1996). Screening siblings for infectious symptoms or exposures may protect vulnerable patients and their visitors. This type of screening can limit potential exposures to varicella (chickenpox), measles, and respiratory syncytial virus (RSV).

Having a policy on sibling visitation helps provide a consistent approach that the staff can follow and present to families (Chart 9–24). Patients and families come from diverse cultural and socioeconomic backgrounds and have varying expectations of their hospital experience. Guidelines that define how the hospital can meet the family's visitation needs can serve as a useful communication tool. Guidelines can also maintain infection control and safety standards and enhance the family's satisfaction with the facility.

Pets

A recent trend in acute care is pet visitation or animal-assisted therapy (Fig. 9–20). The touching, holding, or cuddling of animals is therapeutic. Pet visits distract chil-

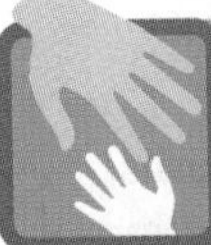

Chart 9–24
Nursing Interventions

Sibling Visitation

- Establish specific times for sibling visitation, preferably times when siblings will be out of school and when many procedures are not being carried out.
- Screen siblings to identify symptoms of communicable disease, such as rash, runny nose, cough; many institutions have a standard form:
  - Teach the family about sibling screening policy.
  - Identify key personnel who will perform sibling screenings.
  - Perform screenings every 24 hours.
  - Once screening is completed, indicate clearance of sibling for visitation on the unit, for example, by providing a visitor sticker.
- Find out if a brother or sister would like to visit. Respect the child's feelings.
- Explore the visiting child's understanding and provide age-appropriate information before the child comes to the unit. Visual aids such as picture books, photographs, or drawings can familiarize children with what they will see.
- If visiting children must wear isolation clothing, allow them to dress in gowns, gloves, and masks and role play before the visit.
- Ask parents if they want help responding to sibling's questions, concerns, anger, frustrations, or fears during the visit.
- Control the environment to make it as familiar and non-threatening to the visiting sibling as possible.
- Use drapes or dividers to provide privacy and shield the visiting sibling from confusing or disturbing sights.
- Avoid interrupting the visit for intrusive procedures or examinations.
- Be sure the sibling is always accompanied by a family member.
- Ensure that the sibling performs hand washing upon entering and leaving room.

Adapted with permission of the Association for the Care of Children's Health, 7910 Woodmont Ave., Suite 300, Bethesda, MD, 20814, from Johnson, B., Jeppson, E., & Redburn, L. (1992). *Caring for children and families: Guidelines for hospitals* (pp. 411–412). Bethesda, MD: ACCH.

dren from the confines of their illness. Children can openly display affection and joy toward the pet. Pet visits also give children an opportunity to learn about animals. Organizations exist that provide trained animals expressly for this purpose. Or with the proper screening, the child's own animal may visit ("ICP's Develop Policies for Pet and Sibling Visitation," 1994; Yamauchi & Olmsted, 1996). Reuniting a child with a beloved pet is an inter-

Figure 9–20
Pet visits can help reduce the stress of hospitalization for a child.

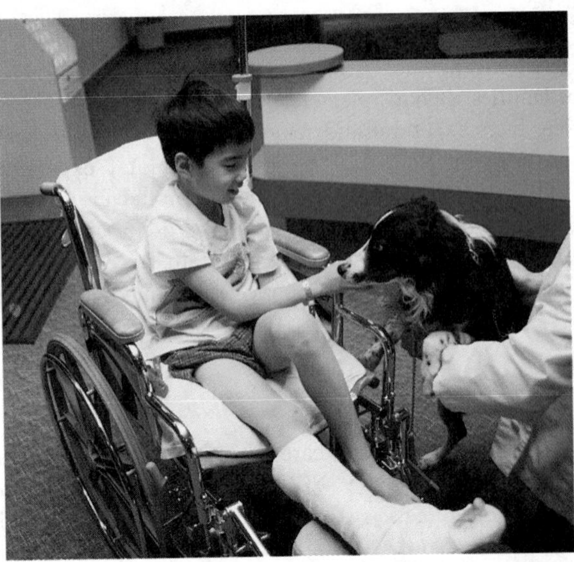

Chart 9–25

Guidelines for Pet and Animal Visitation

- Establish a mechanism for screening and approval of animals.
- Obtain parent's consent for the child to participate in the pet program.
- Ensure that the choice of animals complies with state and local health department regulations.
- Identify designated areas for animal visitation.
- Identify key personnel who will manage animals on location in the facility.
- Consult with the infectious disease or immunology department to determine patient restrictions regarding pet visitation.

vention that supports the philosophy of holism. When developing such a program, some key points must be addressed (Chart 9–25). If pet visitation is not possible, the videophone or use of videotapes may provide some comfort to the child during the parent–child separation.

Care of the Child Going to Surgery

Preoperative Care

Preparation of the child and family for surgery can be a highly specific process, tailored to the child's needs and developmental status and to the procedure required. In many facilities, the nurse is a primary source of information for the patient and family. It is not unusual for families under stress to ask the nurse for the same information that the physicians provided about the potential risks and benefits of surgery. The family may be unsure that they heard the information clearly, feel that they may have forgotten part of it, or want a verification of what they have been told. The nurse may need to clarify information and misconceptions or counsel the patient and families as the emotional impact of the need for surgery is understood. The family may be reluctant to ask the nurse to clarify information because they may feel that it would appear they were not paying attention.

caREminder: *The nurse should clarify family understanding by routinely reviewing discussions with the surgeon, anesthesiologist, and other members of the health team.*

Details of information sometimes differ between health care personnel. For instance, the parents may ask the nurse how long their child's operation will take. When told that a particular procedures usually takes 3 hours, the family may say, "The doctor told us it will take 2 hours." Then the nurse must explain that it takes time to attach monitors and electrodes, and administer anesthesia; furthermore, when the surgery is over, waking the patient also typically takes some time. Thus, although the surgery may last only 2 hours, the child may be in the operating room closer to 3 hours. If the parents expect their child to emerge from surgery in 2 hours, yet the child does not come out for another hour, the parents may spend the extra hour in worry or near-panic as they wonder if something has gone wrong.

Teaching. Preoperative anxiety has been identified as a universal phenomenon and can be expected to affect young children as well as older patients (Maligalig, 1994). A goal of preparing children and families for surgery is to minimize the impact of the unexpected and endeavor to make the unknown known in a non-threatening manner, understandable to the child. By doing so, the anxiety of facing the unfamiliar can be reduced. Adequate preparation may also bolster feelings of control. Preparation for procedures by providing adequate information has been demonstrated to influence children's coping and the outcome of the child's hospitalization (Corbo-Richert et al., 1993; LaMontagne, 1993; Ziegler & Prior, 1994).

Preoperative teaching strategies should be individualized based on the child and family's developmental level, anxiety level, and previous experiences and whether the surgery is done emergently or is a planned event. Keeping in mind that children usually regress when stressed and that high anxiety levels interfere with information processing, present information in simple terms, providing sensory descriptions (e.g., what the child will feel, see, taste, smell, or hear) (Chart 9–26). Explain the expected sequence of events and help identify appropriate coping strategies. Demonstrate relaxation methods, distraction, and/or deep breathing techniques so that the child can practice them in advance and they may be sufficiently useful for the child to maintain control. (See Chapter 13 for a discussion of these techniques.)

caREminder: *Build on the previous experiences of the child when presenting new information. In addition, the use of videos, tours, pictures, written material, hands-on manipulation of medical equipment, and role playing increases the effectiveness of the information and can help allay fears and correct misconceptions (Ziegler & Prior, 1994).*

Provide opportunities for the child and family to express emotions, fears, and anxieties and to ask questions. Evaluate understanding and clarify misperceptions. When surgery is planned, preparation should be done a few days to weeks prior—the timing depends on developmental level and individual characteristics (e.g., toddlers may be taken on a tour a day or two prior to surgery; an anxious adolescent may cope with 1 to 3 weeks preparation, thus having time to incorporate the information and practice coping techniques). When surgery is done on an emergent basis, teaching may need to be condensed and essential information presented, perhaps just as events are occurring.

Consents. During admission, the family is generally required to sign a bewildering array of forms, most of which contain a large amount of material in relatively small type. One of these forms requiring signature is a general or "blanket" consent from, which is required before any patient is admitted. The amount of information provided to the family at this time varies greatly depending on the facility or the person who asks the family to sign.

Informed consent is the standard for all patients who are admitted to the hospital or undergo medical procedures. When the patient is a child, it is particularly important to keep the parents informed, so that they can

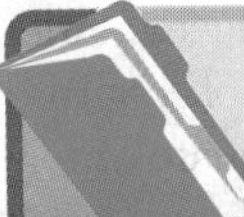

Chart 9–26
Nursing Interventions Classification (NIC)

Teaching: Preoperative

Definition

Assisting a patient to understand and mentally prepare for surgery and the postoperative recovery period

Activities

- Inform the patient and significant other(s) of the scheduled date, time, and location of surgery.
- Inform the patient/significant other(s) how long the surgery is expected to last.
- Determine the patient's previous surgical experiences and level of knowledge related to surgery.
- Appraise the patient's/significant other's anxiety relating to surgery.
- Provide time for the patient to ask questions and discuss concerns.
- Describe the preoperative routines (e.g., anesthesia, diet, bowel preparation, tests/labs, voiding, skin preparation, IV therapy, clothing, family waiting area, and transportation to operating room), as appropriate.
- Describe any preoperative medications, the effects these will have on the patient, and the rationale for using them.
- Inform the significant other(s) of the location to wait for the results of the surgery, as appropriate.
- Conduct a tour of the postsurgical unit(s) and waiting area(s), as appropriate.
- Introduce the patient to the staff who will be involved in the surgery/postoperative care, as appropriate.
- Reinforce the patient's confidence in the staff involved, as appropriate.
- Provide information on what will be heard, smelled, seen, tasted, or felt during the event.
- Discuss possible pain control measures.
- Explain the purpose of frequent postoperative assessments.
- Describe the postoperative routines/equipment (e.g., medications, respiratory treatments, tubes, machines, support hose, surgical dressings, ambulation, diet, and family visitation), and explain their purpose.
- Instruct the patient on the technique of getting out of bed, as appropriate.
- Evaluate the patient's ability to return demonstrate getting out of bed, as appropriate.
- Instruct the patient on the technique of splinting incision, coughing, and deep breathing.
- Evaluate the patient's ability to return demonstrate splinting incision, coughing, and deep breathing.
- Instruct the patient on how to use the incentive spirometer.
- Evaluate the patient's ability to return demonstrate proper use of the incentive spirometer.
- Instruct the patient on the technique of leg exercises.
- Evaluate the patient's ability to return demonstrate leg exercises.
- Stress the importance of early ambulation and pulmonary care.
- Inform patient about how they can aid in recuperation.
- Reinforce information provided by other health care team members, as appropriate.
- Determine the patient's expectations of the surgery.
- Correct unrealistic expectations of the surgery, as appropriate.
- Provide time for the patient to rehearse events that will happen, as appropriate.
- Instruct the patient to use coping techniques directed at controlling specific aspects of the experience (e.g., relaxation and imagery), as appropriate.
- Include the family/significant others, as appropriate.

From McCloskey, J., & Bulechek, G. (1996). *Nursing interventions classification (NIC)* (2nd ed.). St. Louis: Mosby–Year Book. Reprinted with permission.

make treatment decisions for their child based on the most complete information available. The explanations should be comprehensive and should describe the potential benefits and risks of each procedure or regimen (see Chapter 2 for more information on consent and assent).

The parent or guardian is asked to sign a consent form(s) for any specific procedure to be performed, whenever possible. In an emergency, when a delay in obtaining consent is likely to lead to loss of the patient's life or significant functioning, the physician can authorize an emergency procedure. The institution should have a clear written policy for these cases.

Generally, the procedural or surgical consent form is more detailed than the general consent form required for hospital admission. These specific authorizations are used in obtaining informed consent. Informed consent is based on the concept that the child, parent, or guardian has the right to receive details and information about the child's health, as well as the expected risks and benefits of the specific procedures and alternative methods of treatment. It gives the child and family clear explanations, in language that they can comprehend. Based on this information, the family can weigh the implications, analyze expected outcomes, consider alternatives, and then decide to approve or refuse the procedure based on the child's best interests. Informed consent requires the physician and family to collaborate with respect to health care.

Presurgical Assessment. One of the nurse's principal responsibilities when caring for a child before surgery is the preoperative assessment of the child and family. By using a methodical, comprehensive assessment, the nurse can anticipate the patient's specific needs and prepare to meet them. By doing so, the nurse can ensure continuity of care as the pediatric surgical patient progresses through the various areas before surgery (LaRosa Nash & O'Malley, 1997).

One of the primary goals of presurgical assessment is to identify factors that may affect the child's recovery from surgery. These factors include the child's age and developmental level, surgical procedure to be performed, concomitant illnesses and treatments, presurgical preparation, and the psychological status of the child and family (Planchock & Wiggins, 1994). After identifying the factors that may influence a child's surgery and recovery, the nurse should develop and implement strategies to facilitate the most positive outcome.

In many acute care settings, preoperative assessments are also done by other health care professionals, including the surgeon, anesthesiologist, pediatrician, and specialists from other disciplines. These evaluations do not negate the value of the nursing assessment; instead, multiple appraisals serve to complement and augment patient care. Not only does this give the health care team members a greater sense of the child's history and psychosocial needs, but it also provides the child and family with more opportunities to interact with the professionals who will provide the care. In addition, face-to-face interviews during assessment serve to foster greater opportunity for the patient and family to consider the child's condition, discuss concerns, and attain a more thorough understanding of instructions and explanations.

Because innocent heart murmurs are common in children, the nurse or other health care professional may detect a heart murmur during the presurgical assessment (see Chapter 6 for discussion of innocent murmurs). It is important to identify children with cardiac anomalies prior to anesthesia because of the changes in vascular resistance that occur, potentially altering intracardiac shunts. If the child has signs of a potentially pathologic murmur detected, then further follow-up with EKG and evaluation by a pediatric cardiologist are suggested preoperatively (Maxwell, Deshpande, & Wetzel, 1994).

In the child with a known cardiac anomaly, details of the type of defect, previous surgeries, and current status should be obtained and the anesthesia care provider notified prior to surgery. Antibiotic prophylaxis to prevent bacterial endocarditis may be ordered.

Laboratory tests that are not indicated by history in healthy children very rarely show any abnormalities of consequence (LaRosa Nash & O'Malley, 1997). Therefore, routine laboratory tests for elective surgery are usually not done. Laboratory tests, if deemed necessary by the presence of signs of infection, other illness, abnormality, or chronic disease, are usually completed 24 to 48 hours prior to surgery.

caREminder: *The nurse should review the laboratory test results during the presurgical assessment and notify the surgeon of abnormal findings. A decision will be made whether to cancel the surgery or not.*

The child coming for surgery may have a cold, fever, or other infection. During admission, the nurse must determine whether the child's illness requires that surgery be canceled. If the child has allergic rhinitis, the surgery does not need to be postponed. If the child has an infection, elective surgery should be postponed. The surgeon should be notified to make that decision.

Preoperative Fasting. Pediatric surgical patients must remain on NPO (nothing by mouth) status for a minimum time before scheduled surgery. This practice is based on the need for the patient to have a relatively empty stomach, which reduces the risk of aspiration if vomiting occurs after anesthesia administration. Although the requirement to maintain a preoperative NPO status is universal, the amount of time required is under debate. Historically, long periods of preoperative fasting, such as 8 to 12 hours, were the norm. As a result, many facilities used automatic orders, such as "NPO after midnight," regardless of whether the operation was scheduled at 7 o'clock in the morning or 7 o'clock that night.

Research has found that liquids, especially clear fluids, are generally emptied from the stomach in less than 2 hours, and that solid foods take several hours longer (Schreiner, 1994). Allowing the child to drink *clear* fluids until 2 hours prior to the operation does not result in any increased postsurgical problems (Schreiner, 1994). In light of this finding, the standardized order of "NPO after midnight" is increasingly being replaced with shorter, more individualized time frames. For example, some facilities use NPO requirements for healthy infants and young children of 4 hours before a scheduled surgery; others may allow clear oral fluids to be taken up to 2 to 3 hours before the procedure. This reduced NPO time has en-

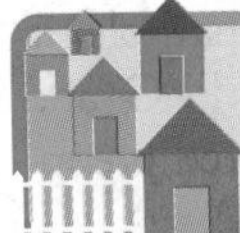

Chart 9–27
Community Care

Preoperative Fasting Instructions

- Normal meals and snacks may be eaten until bedtime on the evening before the day of surgery.
- After bedtime, no foods or fluids should be ingested, except for **clear** fluids such as water, apple juice, cranberry juice, Jell-o, ginger ale, etc. These clear fluids may be ingested until 2 hours before you arrive at the hospital. Fluids that should NOT be ingested include milk, orange juice, and other fluids that contain particulate matter and are not "clear."
- Infants who receive formula should finish their last feeding 6 hours before the start of surgery. Like older children, they may drink **clear** fluids up to 2 hours before coming to the hospital.
- Infants who are breast-fed may nurse until 3 hours before scheduled to arrive at the hospital.
- Exceptions to the above rules may be made by the anesthesiologist, taking into account the health status and special considerations of the individual child.
- If the child must take any oral mediation, generally it may be taken with a small sip of water. Medications that are important to continue include antibiotics, anticonvulsants, bronchodilators, as well as other drugs ordered by the surgeon or anesthesiologist. The health care team should be informed of these and any other medications that your child is currently taking.

This is an example of information the nurse may provide to the patient and family before surgery. Specific instructions may vary. Check your facility's protocol.

hanced child and family satisfaction, because the distress of hunger and thirst in children waiting for surgery had been a source of anxiety and apprehension for the young patient and family members.

caREminder: *To avoid misunderstanding and potential delay or cancellation of surgery, specific, written instructions must be given to the family (Chart 9–27).*

These guidelines apply to healthy children. The anesthesiologist orders the specific time period the child is to remain NPO. Patients who are at higher risk of aspiration include those with delayed gastric emptying, esophageal reflux, obesity, pregnancy, a tenuous airway, systemic disease, previous vomiting during induction, and emergency surgery. Except when surgery is unanticipated, high-risk patients have food withheld for 12 hours and clear fluids for 8 hours. An IV line may be started to avoid dehydration.

Skin Preparation. Because everyone's skin ordinarily sustains a wide variety of potentially infectious bacteria and other microorganisms, many hospitals sanction skin cleansing prior to surgery. Bacterial counts can be significantly reduced by mechanical scrubbing with an antimicrobial soap solution. The rationale behind this type of skin preparation stems from the observation that such a regimen removes not only the microbes, but flakes of dead skin cells, oils, and other debris that foster the growth of the bacteria. Even with the most thorough skin cleansing, live human skin can never be completely "sterilized" of all microorganisms.

Some facilities aspire to achieve such a progressive reduction of bacteria that children are instructed to begin antimicrobial skin preparation before admission to the hospital for elective procedures. Although the particular techniques, time frames, and endorsed products vary among different hospitals, all share the same goal of reducing the risk of postoperative wound infection (AORN, 1995).

Hair removal is rarely deemed necessary in prepubescent children because they have scant amounts of body hair. If hair removal is necessary, it is completed with the goal of preserving skin integrity. Therefore, clippers are usually used. Razors, although able to remove hair closer to the root than clippers, are more apt to produce microscopic abrasions and nicks in the skin that serve as a port of entry and thus potential source of infection. Because many individual are sensitive to depilatories, their use requires testing on a patch of skin 24 hours prior to use. Children, in particular, because of their skin structure, develop adverse reactions to depilatories, therefore their use is rarely indicated. Hair removal is performed as close to the time of operation as possible, again with the goal of reducing opportunity for bacterial colonization. This is preferably completed in the induction room, not the operating room (OR), to avoid releasing loose hairs into the environment. Advantages of hair removal after the child is anesthetized, although prolonging anesthesia time, are reduction of anxiety in the child and minimizing scratches and nicks because the risk for the child making sudden movements is eliminated.

Surgical Suite

Just prior to transporting the child to the OR, one last assessment is performed. Most facilities have a form that must be completed that covers standard assessment parameters (Table 9–3).

Some facilities may allow parents to be present during the initial administration of anesthesia, in a designated "anesthesia induction area" or preoperative holding

Table 9–3
Pediatric Presurgical Check

Aspect of Care	Nursing Action	Rationale
Identification verification	Verify that identification band corroborates with patient/family statement and chart documentation.	The identification band functions as a safety measure so that the proper patient receives the correct surgery.
Preoperative work-up within hospital parameters (often 72 hours)	Check that laboratory values are in the chart. Assess laboratory values for relationship to normalcy, and identify any values that lie outside normal ranges.	Special attention should be paid to potentially significant outliers that may indicate change in patient status or electrolyte imbalance.
Consents completed: General consent Surgical consent	Confirm that all required consent forms are fully filled out, with dates, proper procedure identified, and witness.	Lack of properly signed consents can result in litigation and refusal of reimbursement to the institution.
Surgical attire	Dress child per facility's policy regarding perioperative attire.	Some facilities allow children to wear underwear to the OR in order to reduce anxiety.
Family notification	Verify that the family/guardian is informed regarding location of surgical waiting room, anticipated length of surgery, and areas to obtain amenities such as coffee and refreshments.	Concerned family members generally want to remain nearby when possible, in order to be notified as to the ongoing status or outcome of surgery as soon as possible.
Allergy status	Prominently note known or suspected allergies in the chart.	Patient or family members should be asked about any allergies, including episodes of hives and food or medication allergy.
Familial history of problems with anesthesia	Elicit family history of reaction to anesthesia.	Intolerance or adverse reactions to anesthesia can be life-threatening and may be hereditary.
Familial history of problems with anesthesia	Elicit family history of reaction to anesthesia.	Intolerance or adverse reactions to anesthesia can be life-threatening and may be hereditary.
Vital signs	Chart current vital signs; identify any unusual trends or values outside the norm.	Unusual patterns or change in vital signs may indicate change in patient status.
Body weight and height	Document current height and weight.	Height and weight are the primary parameters used to determine drug dosages, blood volume, and fluid requirements.
Urine	Encourage child to void prior to surgery, and document; note any changes or unusual appearance in urine.	The opportunity to void in the OR may be limited, and the child will receive generous amounts of IV fluids intraoperatively.
NPO status	Keep the child NPO as ordered; inform family of underlying rationale.	Stomach contents may be aspirated during intubation. Anesthesia may reduce gastric motility, as well as cause nausea and vomiting.
Removal of foreign objects or personal belongings	Check for and ask the child about the possible presence of hair pins, jewelry, etc. Remove these prior to transport to the OR. If items (such as a ring) are not removable, the OR nurse should be notified of their presence, so that any hazard that these may produce can be minimized.	Metal or other materials may be a risk factor for burns from the cautery used in surgery or form pressure sores during prolonged surgery. Check even infants for earrings; older children may have other body areas pierced, such as umbilicus.
Removal of prostheses	Remove contact lenses, eyeglasses, and orthodontic appliances prior to transport to the OR. Note any exceptions.	Items such as contact lenses and orthodontic appliances are commonly encountered in the preadolescent and adolescent population.

Table continued on following page

Table 9–3
Pediatric Presurgical Check *Continued*

Aspect of Care	Nursing Action	Rationale
Nail bed assessment	Remove any nail polish from fingers and toes prior to transportation to the OR.	Nail polish can obscure the ability to accurately assess for oxygenation and capillary refill.
Dentition	Examine the mouth, and inquire about potentially loose teeth. If identified, note and report to the OR nurse or anesthetist.	Children intermittently loosen their "baby teeth," which can pose a hazard should the patient be intubated.
Preoperative medication	Administer any prescribed medications prior to transport to OR. If IM medications are ordered, check with anesthesia care practitioner to give via different route.	Light sedation is often desirable to allay anxiety associated with surgery. Medication should be administered with enough time to achieve desired effect, and the patient monitored or observed for any adverse reactions.
Operative site preparation	Comply with facility standards for skin preparation for cleansing or shaving of operative skin.	The skin at the operative site should be as free of oil and debris as possible, to reduce risk of infection.

area (Fig. 9–21). A few facilities allow parents to be present when the initial anesthesia takes place in the sterile environment of an operating room. These practices attempt to address the child's fear and separation anxiety and cultivate a smoother induction, particularly when the child has not received prior sedation. Another benefit to eliminating preoperative sedation in selected procedures is that recovery time after anesthesia is shortened (LaRosa Nash & Murphy, 1997).

Parents can help calm an anxious child in the seemingly bizarre perioperative setting (Henderson, Baines, & Overton, 1993). Some legal and other concerns may argue against such practices. For one, parents may not fully comprehend the OR routine and interpret an unremarkable event or comment as malevolent circumstance. Another concern is about the reaction of an unprepared "civilian" in the OR and the possibility that an unpredictable reaction (such as fainting) may occur. These concerns may have some basis, but they may be addressed with proper screening of child, parent, and situation and with adequate preparation.

In order to determine appropriateness of parental presence during induction, several factors need to be assessed. These include predictors of problematic behavior with separation from parent and not taking a preoperative tour, history of previous surgery, and preoperative displays of overt parental dependence or withdrawn affect (Vetter, 1993). Additionally, developmental level, age, willingness to cooperate, previous hospital experiences, and level of anxiety need to be considered (LaRosa Nash & Murphy, 1997). The parent who wishes to be present needs to be prepared for how the OR will look, the sequence of events, how the child may react (e.g., eyes rolling back, drooling, involuntary movements), and specific actions they can do to support the child (sitting next to him or her, maintaining physical contact, talking to the child). This can be an emotional experience for the parent, and support should be provided before and after the induction.

When the facility does not permit parents into the OR, the anesthesiologist may administer an anesthetic either nasally or orally to the child in the preoperative

Figure 9–21
A parent's presence in the preoperative area can help reduce the child's separation anxiety. The child must be prepared for the parent's appearance in operating room garb.

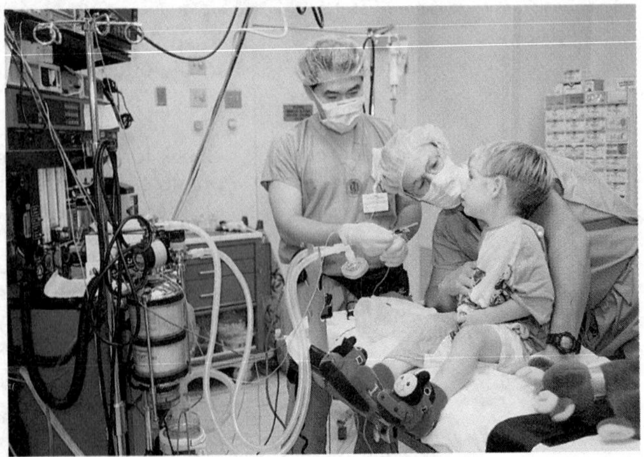

holding area. This is usually a combination of drugs, such as ketamine, atropine, and midazolam (Douglas, 1995). These agents relax the child and create an amnesiac effect, so that the child accepts separation from the parent and remembers little about it.

Postanesthesia Care

After surgery, most patients are taken to the postanesthesia care unit (PACU) (which is also called the postanesthesia room or recovery room) or the ICU. This unit provides resources and skilled nursing personnel for closely monitoring the patient who is emerging or recovering from the effects of the anesthesia. The need for intensive surveillance and immediate effective intervention is essential because the pediatric surgical patient is physiologically unstable as a result of the anesthesia.

Children differ from adults in their response to surgery in several ways (Chart 9–28). For example, they are at greater risk of surgical hypothermia, unlike adults who are better able to maintain standard body warmth. The child's inability to sustain optimal body temperature stems from four reasons. First, the mechanism responsible for thermoregulation is immature and developing, as are most of the child's physical systems. Second, a child is prone to increased heat loss from the body because there is relatively little subcutaneous tissue. Third, a child has relatively large proportion of body surface area to body weight, which further facilitates heat loss. Finally, a pediatric patient loses more heat through respiration than the adult. The ability to achieve and maintain optimal body temperature is inversely proportional to the patient's age; that is, the younger the child, the more likely he or she is to have difficulty maintaining body temperature.

The nurse can perform several postoperative interventions to help prevent hypothermia. Exposed body areas can be covered; including the extremities and top of the head, to reduce heat loss to the environment. The room temperature can usually be adjusted to a warmer level. If necessary, a radiant warmer or mechanical warming blanket can be used to help the child maintain warmth. Postoperative fluids can be warmed. Whenever measures are used to alter the patient's temperature, the nurse should check the patient's temperature frequently to evaluate their effectiveness.

Postoperatively, children can suffer many of the same sequelae as adults. They may suffer headache, especially after receiving an inhalational agent. Nausea and vomiting are common, particularly in children who have undergone strabismus or orchiopexy surgery (Parnass, 1993).

Chart 9–28
Nursing Interventions

Post-Anesthesia Concerns for the Pediatric Patient

Aspect of Care	Reasons for Concerns	Interventions
Airway Management	Laryngospasm after extubation	Position the child to maintain airway; head midline, may need to displace mandible anteriorly, open mouth. Administer 100% oxygen via positive pressure ventilation if laryngospasm occurs. Anesthesia care practitioner may administer a dose of succinylcholine. Assist with reintubation, if needed.
	Post-intubation croup	Provide humidified mist to child. Give racemic epinephrine treatment via aerosol nebulizer as ordered. Give corticosteroids before extubation, if ordered. If croup persists longer than 2 to 4 hours, expect to hospitalize the child overnight for observation.
	Apnea	Use a cardiac monitor, apnea monitor, and pulse oximeter to monitor the child's status. Provide assisted ventilation as necessary. Keep appropriate pediatric resuscitative equipment available at the bedside.

Chart continued on following page

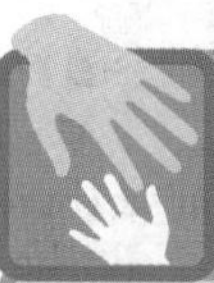

Chart 9–28
Nursing Interventions *Continued*

Post-Anesthesia Concerns for the Pediatric Patient

Aspect of Care	Reasons for Concerns	Interventions
Airway Management	Airway complications caused by bleeding after nasopharyngeal surgery	Assess the oral and nasal cavities for bright red blood. Observe for excessive swallowing. Monitor for changes in vital signs. Provide fluid resuscitation. Elevate the head of the bed. Apply an ice pack to neck or nose. Keep the child as quiet as possible. Do not remove clots. Administer pain medications as needed.
	Aspiration	Suction the mouth, pharynx, and trachea if vomiting or excessive accumulation of secretions occurs. Administer oxygen. Position the patient prone or on the side.
	Delayed return to consciousness	Before extubation, assess child's muscular strength, respiratory effort, airway protection, and eye opening. Identify any residual effects of drugs.
Fluid Maintenance	Preexisting volume depletion due to illness NPO status before surgery	Closely monitor intake and output. Urine output should average 1 mg/kg/hr. Establish and protect venous access.
	Child's body surface area is greater than adult's; during illness, trauma, or stress, the child's extracellular fluid is easily depleted.	Administer maintenance fluids that are hypotonic and contain glucose.
	Although child has relatively greater fluid demands than adult, actual amount of fluids required is small.	Prevent fluid overload by administering all fluids, blood, and blood products with a volumetric infusion pump.
	Accelerated hypoglycemic reactions due to fluid loss and stress of illness and surgery	Monitor for symptoms of hypoglycemia; check blood glucose if symptoms present.
	External loss of fluid from vomiting, diarrhea, and nasogastric suctioning	Administer isotonic replacement fluids.
	Postoperative hemorrhage due to bleeding of an open vessel, continuous third-spacing fluid shift, or coagulopathy	Monitor circulatory status by assessing vital signs, urine output, central venous pressure, and pulmonary artery pressure. Give blood or blood products as needed.
Seizures	Risk factors, such as previous history of seizures; intracranial injury, hemorrhage, or tumor; increased intracranial pressure; or metabolic or nutritional disorders that may result in electrolyte imbalances, such as hypoglycemia, hypocalcemia, and hyponatremia	Assess the child for predisposing factors that increase risk for seizures. Treat seizures promptly with diazepam or lorazepam as ordered. Ensure that the child's airway is maintained. Provide additional respiratory support after any drug therapy begins. Keep resuscitative equipment immediately available. Prepare the child for a complete diagnostic work-up as needed to determine the cause of the seizure.

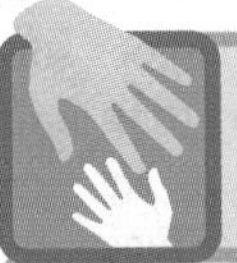

Chart 9–28
Nursing Interventions *Continued*

Post-Anesthesia Concerns for the Pediatric Patient

Aspect of Care	Reasons for Concerns	Interventions
Thermoregulation	High ratio of body surface area to body mass and large heads in relation to body size, thus lose heat readily Hypothermia with increased risk of apnea, hypoventilation, hypotension, hypoglycemia, and metabolic acidosis (in neonates) Cool operating room Postoperative shivering, which can increase oxygen requirements by 400–500% Hypothermia causes slowed recovery from anesthetic agents and may delay elimination of muscle relaxants. Heat loss via vasodilation, lack of muscle tone, and inhibition of temperature regulation caused by general anesthesia and neuromuscular block	Use warming lights and heating blankets to keep the child warm. Wrap the child's head to preserve body heat. Give the child supplemental oxygen. Use pulse oximetry to monitor the adequacy of oxygen therapy. Treat shivering with small dose of IV meperidine, or place heat on the child's skin.
Emergence Delirium	Increased prevalence in children and young adults. May be exacerbated by hypoxia, nausea, dizziness, inability to move, pain, fear, anxiety, full bladder, hypotension, gastric distention, and pharmacologic agents or postoperative medications	Involve the parent or guardian in recovery by having them hold, reassure, and comfort the child. Immediately rule out hypoxia as the cause. Give narcotics to treat pain. Catheterize the bladder if warranted. Use a soft, soothing voice and light touch to calm the child. Protect the child from self-injury by padding the bed or crib rails. Relax physical restraints if they cause the child to fight harder. Secure all venous access devices, tubes, drains, and dressings.
Emergency Resuscitation	Equipment too large for the child Immediate need for pediatric dosages of resuscitation medications	Always use equipment specifically designed for pediatric patients. Organize resuscitation equipment for pediatric patients on a cart, including defibrillator paddles, intraosseous and IV needles, and oxygen equipment. Ensure that the staff is competent in using pediatric equipment. Keep essential resuscitation medications immediately available in pediatric dosages. Ensure that the child's age and weight are easily retrieved from the chart. Keep pediatric emergency drug dosage calculation cards handy.

Information from Meyer-Pahoulis, E., Williams, S. L., Davidson, S. I., McVey, J. R., & Mazurek, A. (1993). The pediatric patient in the post anesthesia care unit. *Nursing Clinics of North America, 28,* 519–530.

Sore throat also is common, even after surgery that did not involve endotracheal intubation. Postoperative bleeding, dizziness, vertigo, loss of appetite, and muscle soreness and pain are also prevalent.

The nurse must also monitor for signs of malignant hyperthermia (MH): tachypnea, tachycardia, and chaotic dysrhythmias. Later signs are increased temperature, muscle rigidity, hyperkalemia, hypercalcemia, and myoglobinuria (Meyer-Pahoulis, Williams, Davidson, McVey, & Mazurek, 1993). MH is an inherited syndrome in which succinylcholine and inhalation agents trigger a fulminant hypermetabolic state. The incidence of MH is greater in children than adults, perhaps as a result of differences in anesthetic techniques (Meyer-Pahoulis et al., 1993).

Visitation in the Postanesthesia Unit. The presence of a parent or other trusted family member provides invaluable support and reduces the hospitalized child's sense of isolation and separation anxiety (Bru, Carmody, Donohue-Sword, & Bookbinder, 1993). Children's crying decreased by 54% when parents were present in the PACU (Fiorentini, 1993). For these reasons, many PACUs allow or actively encourage one parent to visit at the bedside, when the child is physiologically stable.

At times, hospitals may restrict a parent's visitation rights, especially when the child is not fully recovered from the effects of anesthesia or when recovery takes place in an adult PACU where the patient's acuity level requires a high level of technical nursing interventions. However, many facilities recognize the strong bond between parents and children and relax their visitation rules for parents. Many facilities now welcome parents in the immediate postanesthesia area, when the child is awake enough to ask for or want them there.

Safety and Restraints. At times during the postoperative period, the child's normal movements may need to be restricted to ensure safety or keep IV lines or nasogastric tubes in place. One or more of the child's limbs may be restrained, for example, when the child is disoriented, combative, or receiving an IV infusion.

Application of an IV protective restraint should limit limb movement but allow some range of motion. The nurse must perform neurovascular assessments frequently to ensure that distal areas retain normal pulses, color, and sensation. The nurse should perform skin care, such as gentle massage with a moisturizer, if the nearby area shows signs of irritation. Generally, the nurse should remove any restraints and change the patient's position at least once every 2 hours.

Same-Day Surgery

Since the early 1980s, a trend has developed toward using less expensive forms of patient management. In surgical care, this trend has led to same-day surgery. In this type of surgery, the patient comes to the surgical setting in the morning or early afternoon, undergoes surgery and, upon recovery, returns home later that day. Some facilities call this day surgery or outpatient surgery. No matter what it is called, same-day surgery reduces the number of labor-intensive hospital days and the cost of surgery.

Generally, the child must meet several criteria to be eligible for same-day surgery. The pediatric patient must be healthy and meet the standards for the American Society of Anesthesiology (ASA) Classification I (have no active infection, symptoms of a cold, or history of sleep apnea or bleeding disorders). Also, a history of prematurity may preclude same-day surgery, as well as being under the facility's minimum age, although infants younger than age 1 month can successfully undergo same-day surgery if they have compliant parents.

One day before the surgery, the child is assessed, at which time required laboratory studies, if indicated, are performed. If assessment reveals cold symptoms, such as excessive mucus production, that could interfere with anesthesia and physically stress the child further, elective same-day surgery may be postponed.

For many types of surgeries and patients, outpatient procedures can be performed safely and efficiently. However, same-day surgery has one major disadvantage: ab-

Chart 9–29

Discharge Criteria for Same-Day Surgery Patients

Child must:

- Have vital signs stable, similar to preoperative baseline vital signs, with no signs of respiratory distress.
- Have no signs of complications as related to anesthesia or specific to type of operation, e.g., no excessive bleeding from wound, minimal nausea, vomiting, dizziness.
- Have pain well controlled.
- Regain preoperative cognitive functioning; may still be very sleepy and need assistance with motor functions.
- Have ingested fluid and retained. Some facilities are eliminating this requirement, because letting the child choose whether to drink or not reduces the incidence of vomiting immediately postoperatively (Schreiner, 1994).
- Have voided.
- Have caregivers state understanding of postoperative care and signs of complications and when to call health care provider, and be given written instructions and prescriptions as indicated.

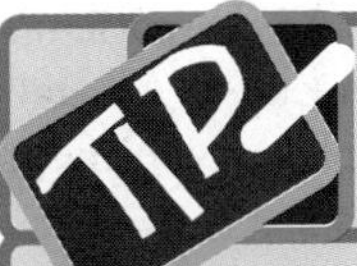

TIP 9–2 A Teaching Intervention Plan for the Child After Same-Day Surgery

Nursing Diagnoses and Family Outcomes

- Knowledge deficit: postoperative care, expected postoperative course, signs of complications
  Outcome: Child/family will verbalize and demonstrate appropriate postoperative care and state signs of complications.
- Pain related to effects of surgery
  Outcome: Child will have pain adequately managed and verbalize or display minimal pain behaviors.
- Risk for infection related to effects of invasive procedures, break in skin integrity
  Outcome: Child will not develop infection.

Interventions

Educate the parents:

- *Activity restrictions*—Usually restrict to quiet activities for 24 hours because of effects of anesthesia; no unsupervised activities for 24 hours that require coordination, e.g., stair climbing, sports; then as appropriate to the procedure, e.g., when myringotomy tubes placed, child must wear earplugs when in water (baths, swimming)
- *Intake*—Clear liquids, then increase as tolerated or as specific to procedure (e.g., posttonsillectomy soft foods); how to tell if drinking enough, if voiding once every 8 hours probably has sufficient intake; tips to promote fluid intake: popsicles, serve fluid in small cups, encourage a few sips with every television commercial
- *Incision/wound care*—If appropriate, whether to change dressing or not; amount and type of drainage expected; any special site care: elevation, ice, cleansing
- *Pain management*—How to assess as age and child appropriate; pharmacologic and nonpharmacologic management strategies with potential side effects of drugs and actions to minimize these (e.g., drink plenty of fluids with codeine to counter constipating effects)
- *Proper use of any equipment*—e.g., crutch walking
- *Number, name of contact person, and when to notify health care provider*—Signs of complications pertinent to procedure: excessive bleeding; acute onset, excessive or poorly controlled pain; unable to tolerate oral fluids; insufficient urine output; altered motor or cognitive functioning, lethargic, unable to arouse

breviated contact with health care personnel. As a result, the child and family have less time to learn about the child's preparation and follow-up. Yet, the family is expected to learn all information to provide postoperative care for the child at home. To compensate for the shortened time for patient and family interactions, the nurse must provide thorough postoperative assessment and interventions (Chart 9–29, TIP 9–2).

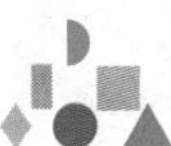

Preparation for Discharge from Acute Care

For years, it has been said "discharge planning begins on the day of admission." Although this statement remains true today, the scope of discharge planning has expanded. Aside from motivational and educational level and cultural considerations, other components must be included in discharge planning for children. These components include the child's diagnosis or condition, how care will be provided (by parent, other family members, nurse, or daycare provider; the child usually needs to be school-age or older to perform self-care), community medical resources, educational interventions (early intervention or special education programs, issues related to home tutoring or returning to school, therapy), and financial resources (Hamilton & Vessey, 1992). Because patients are now discharged earlier and often require home care, discharge may be complex and require more family preparation, including education, skill development, and supply acquisition. Although who is responsible for aspects of discharge planning varies in different facilities, it is a standard of practice that the registered nurse is responsible for family education. The faster the nurse identifies the family's needs and begins the teaching, the more time the family has to master the information and make the necessary adaptations to the home.

In addition to meeting educational needs, the nurse prepares the child and family for discharge by addressing financial issues. In this era of skyrocketing medical costs, ensuring reimbursement has become important. During discharge preparation, the nurse should also discuss follow-up. Because hospital stays are shorter than ever, follow-up appointments or arrangements are crucial to the patient's health and safety. Follow-up appointments are used to periodically assess the patient's progress toward wellness or adaptation. Special arrangements may be made for schooling, outpatient therapies, home health referrals, and in-home equipment, supplies, services, and medications (Chart 9–30). (See Chapter 11 for more in-depth discussion.)

A documentation system that shows the patient's progress helps the team continue its efforts toward preparing the patient and family for discharge. Another useful tool is a discharge planning checklist. As the patient's needs are met, they are marked on the checklist. All staff members can refer to the checklist and plan teaching or supply ordering as needed.

Follow-up after discharge helps parents obtain more information regarding care of their child and provides support to parents in reassuming (or assuming) their role as caregiver (Snowdon & Kane, 1995). Support after discharge may be more effective because parents may be less anxious, more able to assimilate information, and have had an opportunity to identify specific questions and issues. Postdischarge follow-up can be performed easily through a telephone call or a home visit if needed.

Acute illness and hospitalization of a child are stressors that jeopardize the emotional and physical well-being of the child and threaten family cohesiveness. Using developmentally and culturally appropriate approaches to provide information and emotional support while addressing the child's physiologic needs in the most atraumatic manner possible, the interdisciplinary team can minimize the negative consequences of acute illness and hospitalization.

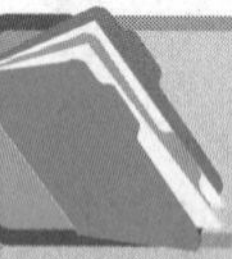

Chart 9–30
Nursing Interventions Classification (NIC)

Discharge Planning

Definition

Preparation for moving a patient from one level of care to another within or outside the current health care agency

Activities

- Assist patient/family/significant others to prepare for discharge.
- Collaborate with the physician, patient/family/significant others, and other health team members in planning for continuity of health care.
- Coordinate efforts of different health care providers to ensure a timely discharge.
- Identify patient's and primary caregiver's understanding of knowledge or skills required after discharge.
- Identify patient teaching needed for post-discharge care.
- Monitor readiness for discharge.
- Communicate patient's discharge plans, as appropriate.
- Document patient's discharge plans on chart.
- Formulate a maintenance plan for post-discharge follow-up.
- Assist patient/family/significant others in planning for the supportive environment necessary to provide the patient's post-hospital care.
- Develop a plan that considers the health care, social, and financial needs of patient.
- Arrange for post-discharge evaluation, as appropriate.
- Encourage self-care, as appropriate.
- Arrange discharge to next level of care.
- Arrange for caregiver support, as appropriate.
- Discuss financial resources, if arrangements for health care are needed after discharge.
- Coordinate referrals relevant to linkages among health care providers.

From McCloskey, J., & Bulechek, G. (1996). *Nursing interventions classification (NIC)* (2nd ed.). St. Louis: Mosby–Year Book. Reprinted with permission.

Summary of Key Concepts

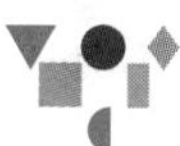

- A child's acute illness is a major stressor for the entire family. With appropriate interventions, nurses and other health care professional can promote effective family coping.
- The role of the family cannot be overemphasized in pediatric health care. The expert practitioner incorporates the view of the parent/caregiver as the "expert in charge" into the plan of care.
- The potential for ineffective coping develops during admission, which often requires in-depth questions about family life. The nurse can reduce this potential problem by using culturally and developmentally appropriate communication techniques with the child and establishing a trusting relationship with the parents.
- Intensive care can be exhausting for the patients and shattering for parents and siblings. By minimizing noise and overstimulation, communicating honestly with families, and promoting 24-hour visiting policies, the nurse can help offset the hardship of the intensive care experience.
- Family cohesiveness and coping can be promoted through child life programs, therapeutic play for the patient and siblings, and support groups and resources for the parents.
- Hospital routines can be very constricting for patients and families. Routine activities, such as performing procedures, collecting specimens, administering medications, providing hygiene, and adjusting ADLs, may cause upset and disruption for the patient. By taking age-appropriate and atraumatic approaches to these routines, the nurse lessens their seeming invasiveness.
- Safety, visitation, and infection-control policies may be frustrating to parents and children because these policies can limit their movement and control. By taking an enlightened approach to these policies, the nurse and facility can limit such frustration.
- The stress of surgery may be reduced by the presence of appropriately prepared parents during induction of anesthesia and in the PACU.
- Preparation for discharging the child from the acute care setting begins upon admission. Discharge planning includes evaluation of the child's care needs and teaching the child and caregiver how to meet these needs.

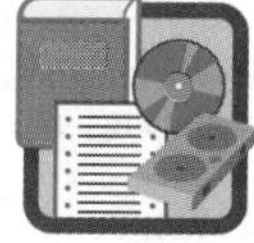

Resources

Organizations

Association for the Care of Children's Health
7910 Woodmont Avenue, Suite 300
Bethesda, MD 20814
(301) 654-6549
(800) 808-ACCH

Federation for Children with Special Needs
95 Berkeley Street, Suite 104
Boston, MA 02116
(617) 482-2915

Institute for Family Centered Care
7900 Wisconsin Avenue, Suite 405
Bethesda, MD 20814
(301) 652-0281

The National Association of Children's Hospitals and Related Institutions (NACHRI)
401 Wythe Street
Alexandria, VA 22314
(703) 684-1355

National Center for Parent Directed Family Resource Centers
535 Race Street, Suite 140
San Jose, CA 95126
(408) 288-5010

Videotapes

Communicating with children: Supportive interactions in hospitals. (1991).
Available from ACCH, #7777.

Family-centered care. (1991).
Available from ACCH, #7505.

Protecting against latex allergy. (1996).
Available from:
Spina Bifida Association of America
4590 MacArthur Blvd., NW, Suite 250
Washington, DC 20007-4226

Safeguard their tomorrows. (1991).
Available from Mead Johnson Nutritionals (contact your local representative).

Pamphlets

A guide for teachers: Children and hospitals (2nd ed.). (1990).
Available from ACCH, #8007.

A pediatric bill of rights. (1991).
Available from ACCH, #1000 (English), #3100 (Spanish).

Changes in behavior when your child returns home from the hospital. (1992).
Available from:
MaxiShare
P.O. Box 2041
Milwaukee, WI 53201

Preparing your child for the hospital: A checklist (2nd ed.).
Available from ACCH, #8247.

Your child goes to the hospital (2nd ed.). (1991).
Available from AACH, #8006.

Latex Allergy Resources

ALERT (Allergy to Latex Education and Resource Team)
P.O. Box 23722
Milwaukee, WI 53223
(414) 677-9707

Canadian Latex Allergy Association
(905) 885-9708

ELASTIC (Education Latex Allergy Support Team and Information Coalition)
196 Pheasant Run Road
West Chester, PA 19380
(610) 436-4801

FDA Latex Allergy Hotline
(301) 594-3060

Latex Allergy News
176 Roosevelt Ave.
Torrington, CT 06790
(860) 482-6869

NO Latex Industries
(800) 296-9185

Spina Bifida Association of America
4590 MacArthur Boulevard, NW, Suite 250
Washington, DC 20007-4226
(800) 621-3141

References

Amico, J., & Davidhizar, R. (1994). Supporting families of critically ill children. *Journal of Clinical Nursing, 3*, 213–213.

AORN. (1995). *Standards and recommended practices*. Denver, CO: Author.

Armsden, G. C., & Lewis, F. M. (1993). The child's adaptation to parental medical illness: Theory and clinical implications. *Patient Education and Counseling, 22*, 153–165.

Ashenberg, M. D., Maier, N. P., Lambert, S. A., & McAliley, L. G. (1996). Easing the wait: Development of a pager program for families. *Pediatric Nursing, 22*, 103–107.

Association for the Care of Children's Health. (1991). *A pediatric bill of rights*. Bethesda, MD: Author.

Avigne, G., & Phillips, T. L. (1991). Pediatric preoperative tours: Successful hospital program expands to community. *AORN Journal, 53*(6), 1458–1465.

Baker, N. A. (1994). Avoiding collisions with challenging families. *American Journal of Maternal Child Nursing, 19*, 97–101.

Behrman, R. E., Kliegman, R. M., & Arvin, A. M. (1996). *Nelson textbook of pediatrics* (15th ed.). Philadelphia: W. B. Saunders.

Bonn, M. (1994). The effects of hospitalisation on children: A review. *Curationis: South African Journal of Nursing, 17*(2), 20–24.

Bower, K. (1992). *Case management by nurses*. Kansas City, MO: American Nurses Publishing.

Brennan, A. (1994). Caring for children during procedures: A review of the literature. *Pediatric Nursing, 20*, 451–458.

Bru, G., Carmody, S., Donohue-Sword, B., & Bookbinder, M. (1993). Parental visitation in the post-anesthesia care unit: A means to lessen anxiety. *Children's Health Care, 22*, 217–226.

Carlson, D., & Mowrey, B. D. (1997). Standards to prevent complications of urinary catheterization in children: Should and should-knots. *Journal of the Society of Pediatric Nurses, 2*, 37–41.

Chambers, M. A. (1993). Play as therapy for the hospitalized child. *Journal of Clinical Nursing, 2*(6), 349–354.

Committee on Hospital Care, American Academy of Pediatrics. (1993). Child life programs. *Pediatrics, 91*, 671–673.

Corbo-Richert, B., Caty, S., & Barnes, C. M. (1993). Coping behaviors of children hospitalized for cardiac surgery: A secondary analysis. *Maternal-Child Nursing Journal, 21*, 27–36.

Coyne, I. T. (1995). Partnership in care: Parent's views of participation in their hospitalized child's care. *Journal of Clinical Nursing, 4*, 71–79.

Craft, M. J. (1993). Siblings of hospitalized children: Assessment and intervention. *Journal of Pediatric Nursing, 8*, 289–297.

Douglas, E. (1995). Cocktail of oral midazolam and ketamine hailed as effective form of premedication. *Anesthesiology News, 21*(9), 29.

Evans, M. A. (1994). An investigation into the feasibility of parental participation in the nursing care of their children. *Journal of Advanced Nursing, 20*, 477–482.

Fiorentini, S. E. (1993). Evaluation of a new program: Pediatric parental visitation in the post anesthesia care unit. *Journal of Post Anesthesia Nursing, 8*, 249–256.

Fisher, M. D. (1994). Identified needs of parents in a pediatric intensive care unit. *Critical Care Nursing, 14*(6), 82–90.

George, A., & Hancock, J. (1993). Reducing pediatric burn pain with parent participation. *Journal of Burn Care and Rehabilitation, 14*, 104–107.

Gray, M. (1996). Atraumatic urethral catheterization of children. *Pediatric Nursing, 22*, 306–310.

Hamilton, B., & Vessey, J. (1992). Pediatric discharge planning. *Pediatric Nursing, 18*, 475–478.

Hamrick, N. B., & Reilly, L. (1992). A comparison of infection rates in a newborn intensive care unit before and after adoption of open visitation. *Neonatal Network, 11*, 15–18.

Hart, D., & Bossert, E. (1994). Self-reported fears of hospitalized school-age children. *Journal of Pediatric Nursing, 9*, 83–90.

Hart, R., Mather, P. L., Slack, J. F., & Powell, M. A. (1992). *Therapeutic play activities for hospitalized children*. St. Louis: Mosby.

Heinzerling, S., & Johnson, M. F. (1996). Latex allergy: One emergency department's response. *Journal of Emergency Nursing, 22,* 67–69.

Henderson, M. A., Baines, D. B., & Overton, J. H. (1993). Parental attitudes to presence at induction of paediatric anaesthesia. *Anaesthesia and Intensive Care, 21,* 324–327.

ICP's develop policies for pet and sibling visitation. (1994). *Hospital Infection Control, 21,* 108–112.

Johnson, A., & Lindschau, A. (1996). Staff attitudes toward parent participation in the care of children who are hospitalized. *Pediatric Nursing, 22,* 99–102, 120.

Johnson, B., Jeppson, E., & Redburn, L. (1992). *Caring for children and families: Guidelines for hospitals.* Bethesda, MD: Association for the Care of Children's Health.

Jones, D. C. (1994). Effect of parental participation on hospitalized child behavior. *Issues in Comprehensive Pediatric Nursing, 17,* 81–92.

Kaminski, J., & Hall, W. (1996). The effect of soothing music on neonatal behavioral studies in the hospital newborn nursery. *Neonatal Network, 15,* 45–53.

Kinnaird, S. W., McClure, N., & Wilham, S. (1995). Latex allergy: An emerging problem in healthcare. *Neonatal Network, 14,* 33–38.

Klein, S. A., & Winkelstein, M. L. (1996). Enhancing pediatric health care with music. *Journal of Pediatric Health Care, 10,* 74–81.

Kruger, S. (1992). Parents in crisis: Helping them cope with a seriously ill child. *Journal of Pediatric Nursing, 7,* 133–140.

Ladebauche, P. (1992). Unit-based family-support groups: A reminder. *American Journal of Maternal Child Nursing, 17,* 18–21.

LaMontagne, L. L. (1993). Bolstering personal control in child patients through coping interventions. *Pediatric Nursing, 19,* 235–237.

LaMontagne, L. L., Johnson, B. D., & Hepworth, J. T. (1995). Evolution of parental stress and coping processes: A framework for critical care practice. *Journal of Pediatric Nursing, 10,* 212–218.

LaRosa Nash, P. A., & Murphy, J. M. (1997). An approach to pediatric perioperative care: Parent-present induction. *Nursing Clinics of North America, 32,* 183–199.

LaRosa Nash, P., & O'Malley, M. (1997). Streamlining the perioperative process. *Nursing Clinics of North America, 32,* 141–151.

LeVieux-Anglin, L., & Sawyer, E. H. (1993). Incorporating play interventions into nursing care. *Pediatric Nursing, 19,* 459–463.

Loranger, N. (1992). Play intervention strategies for the Hispanic toddler with separation anxiety. *Pediatric Nursing, 18,* 571–575.

Maieron, M., & Roberts, M. (1993). Psychosocial policies in hospitals serving children: Comparative characteristics. *Children's Health Care, 22*(2), 143–167.

Maligalig, R. M. (1994). Parents' perceptions of the stressors of pediatric ambulatory surgery. *Journal of Post Anesthesia Nursing,* 9(5), 278–282.

Manthey, M. (1991). Delivery systems and practice models: A dynamic balance. *Nursing Management, 22*(1), 28–30.

Maxwell, L. G., Deshpande, J. K., & Wetzel, R. C. (1994). Preoperative evaluation of children. *Pediatric Clinics of North America, 41,* 93–110.

Melnyk, B. M. (1994). Coping with unplanned childhood hospitalization: Effects of informational interventions on mothers and children. *Nursing Research, 43,* 50–55.

Melnyk, B. M. (1995). Parental coping with childhood hospitalization: A theoretical framework to guide research and clinical intervention. *Maternal-Child Nursing Journal, 23,* 123–131.

Meyer-Pahoulis, E., Williams, S. L., Davidson, S. I., McVey, J. R., & Mazurek, A. (1993). The pediatric patient in the post anesthesia care unit. *Nursing Clinics of North America, 28,* 519–530.

Murphy, L. (1992). Safety measures are important in the operating room. *Plastic Surgical Nursing, 12*(4), 162.

O'Malley, M. E., & McNamara, S. T. (1993). Children's drawings: A preoperative assessment tool. *AORN Journal, 57,* 1074–1089.

Page, N. E., & Boeing, N. M. (1994). Visitation in the pediatric intensive care unit: Controversy and compromise. *AACN Clinical Issues in Critical Care Nursing, 5,* 289–295.

Palmer, S. (1993). Care of sick children by parents: A meaningful role. *Journal of Advanced Nursing, 18,* 185–191.

Parker, K. P. (1995). Promoting sleep and rest in critical ill patients. *Critical Care Nursing Clinics of North America, 2,* 337–349.

Parnass, S. M. (1993). Ambulatory surgical patient priorities. *Nursing Clinics of North America, 28,* 531–545.

Peters, G., Lepow, M. L., McCracken, G. H., & Phillips, C. F. (Eds.). (1991). *Report of the Committee on Infectious Diseases.* Elk Grove, IL: American Academy of Pediatrics.

Planchock, N. Y., & Wiggins, M. V. (1994). Preoperative assessment and teaching: Physiologic and psychological preparation. *Seminars in Perioperative Nursing,* 3(2), 161–169.

Prugh, D., Staub, E., Sands, H., Kirschbaum, R., & Lenihan, E. (1953). A study of the emotional reactions of children and families to hospitalization and illness. *American Journal of Orthopsychiatry, 23*(1), 80–106.

Rabun, J. B. (1996). *For healthcare professionals: Guidelines on prevention of and response to infant abductions* (4th ed). Available from the National Center for Missing and Exploited Children, 2101 Wilson Blvd., Suite 550, Arlington, VA, 22201-3052.

Rakel, B. A. (1992). Interventions related to patient teaching. *Nursing Clinics of North America, 27*(2), 397–423.

Rice, L. J. (1993). Needle phobia: An anesthesiologist's perspective. *The Journal of Pediatrics, 122,* 59–513.

Robertson, J. (1958). *Young children in hospitals.* London: Tavistock.

Sagraves, R. (1995). Pediatric dosing information for health care providers. *Journal of Pediatric Health Care,* 9, 272–277.

Schepp, K. (1992). Correlates of mothers who prefer control over their hospitalized children's care. *Journal of Pediatric Nursing, 7,* 83–89.

Schreiner, M. S. (1994). Preoperative and postoperative fasting in children. *Pediatric Clinics of North America, 41,* 111–120.

Selekman, J., & Snyder, B. (1995). Nursing perceptions of using physical restraints on hospitalized children. *Pediatric Nursing, 21,* 460–464.

Simon, K. (1993). Perceived stress of nonhospitalized children during the hospitalization of a sibling. *Journal of Pediatric Nursing,* 8, 298–304.

Slater, J. E. (1989). Rubber anaphylaxis. *New England Journal of Medicine, 29,* 1126–1130.

Snowdon, A. W., & Kane, D. J. (1995). Parental needs following the discharge of a hospitalized child. *Pediatric Nursing, 21,* 425–428.

Standiford, D. A., Ahlrichs, J., Carmicle, C., & Wells, P. W. (1993). Extended day program: Bringing preschool to the hospital. *Pediatric Nursing, 19,* 238–241.

Stepanek, J. S., & Ahmann, E. (1995). Parent-professional collaboration when hospital visits are infrequent. *Pediatric Nursing, 21,* 466–468.

Stover, B. H., & Burgess, C. O. (1996). Pediatrics. In R. N. Olmsted (Ed.), *Infection control and applied epidemiology* (pp. 96-1–96-31). St. Louis: Mosby–Year Book.

Sussman, G., & Beezhold, D. (1995). Allergy to latex rubber. *Annals of Internal Medicine, 122,* 143–146.

Thompson, M. L. (1994). Information-seeking, coping and anxiety in school-age children anticipating surgery. *Children's Health Care, 23*(2), 87–97.

Tomlinson, P. S., Kirschbaum, M., Harbaugh, B., & Anderson, K. H. (1996). The influence of illness severity and family resources on maternal uncertainty during critical pediatric hospitalization. *American Journal of Critical Care, 5*, 140–146.

Tughan, L. (1992). Visiting in the PICU: A study of the perceptions of patients, parents, and staff members. *Critical Care Nursing Quarterly, 15*(1), 57–68.

Valenti, W. M. (1993). Infection control and the pregnant health care worker. *Nursing Clinics of North America, 28*, 673–686.

Vessey, J. A., & Mahon, M. M. (1990). Therapeutic play and the hospitalized child. *Journal of Pediatric Nursing, 5*(5), 328–333.

Vetter, T. R. (1993). The epidemiology and selective identification of children at risk for preoperative anxiety reactions. *Anesthesia and Analgesia, 77*, 96–99.

Weekes, D. P., Kagan, S. H., James, K., & Seboni, N. (1993). The phenomenon of hand holding as a coping strategy in adolescents experiencing treatment-related pain. *Journal of Pediatric Oncology Nursing, 10*, 19–25.

Wells, P. W., DeBoard-Burns, M. B., Cook, R. C., & Mitchell, J. (1994a). Growing up in the hospital: Part I, Let's focus on the child. *Journal of Pediatric Nursing, 9*, 66–73.

Wells, P. W., DeBoard-Burns, M. B., Cook, R. C., & Mitchell, J. (1994b). Growing up in the hospital: Part II, Nurturing the philosophy of family-centered care. *Journal of Pediatric Nursing, 9*, 141–149.

Wesp, C. E., Jr., & Hartman, D. E. (Eds.). (1996). *Clinical maps for acute care: Managing care through collaborative practice*. Gaithersburg, MD: Aspen.

Whitis, G. (1994). Visiting hospitalized patients. *Journal of Advanced Nursing, 19*, 85–88.

Yamauchi, T., & Olmsted, R. N. (1996). Animal-assisted therapy. In R. N. Olmsted (Ed.), *Infection control and applied epidemiology* (pp. 97-1–97-5). St. Louis: Mosby–Year Book.

Young, M. A., & Meyers, M. (1997). Latex allergy considerations for the care of pediatric patients and employee safety. *Nursing Clinics of North America, 32*, 169–182.

Youngblut, J. M., & Shiao, S. Y. P. (1993). Child and family reactions during and after pediatric ICU hospitalization: A pilot study. *Heart & Lung, 22*, 46–54.

Ziegler, D. B., & Prior, M. M. (1994). Preparation for surgery and adjustment to hospitalization. *Nursing Clinics of North America, 29*, 655–669.

Bibliography

Axton, S. E., & Hall, B. (1994). An innovative method of administering IV medications to children. *Pediatric Nursing, 20*, 341–344.

Azarnoff, P. (1985). Preparing well children for possible hospitalization. *Pediatric Nursing, 11*(1), 53–56.

Beachy, P., & Deacon, J. (1992). Preventing neonatal kidnapping. *Journal of Obstetric, Gynecologic & Neonatal Nursing, 21*, 12–16.

Bent, K. N., Keeling, A., & Routson, J. (1996). Home from the PICU: Are parents ready? *American Journal of Maternal/Child Nursing, 21*, 80–84.

Carmichael, K. D. (1993). Play therapy and children with disabilities. *Issues in Comprehensive Pediatric Nursing, 16*, 165–173.

Carmichael, K. D. (1994). Play therapy for children with physical disability. *Journal of Rehabilitation, 60*, 51–53.

Case management opportunities expand in pediatric care delivery. (1993). *Case Management Advisor, 4*, 101–102, 105.

Caty, S., Ellerton, M. L., & Ritchie, J. A. (1984). Coping in hospitalized children: An analysis of published case studies. *Nursing Research, 33*, 277–282.

Chesla, C. A., & Stannard, D. (1997). Breakdown in the nursing care of families in the ICU. *American Journal of Critical Care, 6*(1), 64–71.

Coffman, S., Edwards, J. A., & Piskosz, Z. (1994). Support groups: Working side by side with parents. MCN, *19*, 281–284.

Committee on Hospital Care. (1996). Physician's role in coordinating care of hospitalized children. *Pediatrics, 98*, 509–510.

Coyne, I. T. (1996). Parent participation: A concept analysis. *Journal of Advanced Nursing, 23*, 733–740.

Cureton-Lane, R. A., & Fontaine, D. K. (1997). Sleep in the pediatric ICU: An empirical investigation. *American Journal of Critical Care, 6*(1), 56–63.

Darbyshire, P. (1993). Parents, nurses and pediatric nursing: A critical review. *Journal of Advanced Nursing, 18*, 1670–1680.

Greenberg, J. A., & Davis, P. J. (1996). Premedication and induction of anesthesia in pediatric surgical patients. *Anesthesiology Clinics of North America, 14*, 781–802.

Jay, S. S., & Youngblut, J. M. (1991). Parent stress associated with pediatric critical care nursing: Linking research and practice. *AACN Clinical Issues in Critical Care Nursing, 2*(2), 276–284.

Kain, Z. N., Mayes, L. C., O'Connor, T. Z., & Cicchetti, D. V. (1996). Preoperative anxiety in children: Predictors and outcomes. *Archives of Pediatric and Adolescent Medicine, 150*, 1238–1245.

Kennedy, C. M., Gyr, P. M., & Garst, K. F. (1991). A nursing tool to assess children upon hospital admission. *American Journal of Maternal-Child Nursing, 16*, 79–82.

Knafl, K. A., Cavallari, K. A., & Dixon, D. M. (1988). *Pediatric hospitalization: Family and nurse perspectives*. Glenview, IL: Scott, Foresman.

Leff, P. T., Chan, J. M., & Walizer, E. M. (1991). Self-understanding and reaching out to sick children and their families: An ongoing professional challenge. *Children's Health Care, 20*(4), 230–239.

Lewis, C. C., Alford-Winston, A., Billy-Kornas, M., McCaustland, M. D., & Tachman, C. P. (1992). Care management for children who are medically fragile/technology-dependent. *Issues in Comprehensive Pediatric Nursing, 15*(2), 73–91.

Meyer, E. C., Kennally, K. F., Zike-Beres, E., Cashore, W. J., & Oh, W. (1996). Attitudes about sibling visitation in the neonatal intensive care unit. *Archives of Pediatric and Adolescent Medicine, 150*, 1021–1026.

Paarette, H. P. (1993). High-risk infant case management and assistive technology: Funding and family enabling perspectives. *Maternal-Child Nursing Journal, 23*(2), 53–64.

Petrillo, M., & Sanger, S. (1980). *Emotional care of hospitalized children* (2nd ed.). Philadelphia: J. B. Lippincott.

Rapp, S. E. (1996). Recovery and discharge. *Anesthesiology Clinics of North America, 14*, 817–834.

Rennick, J. E. (1995). The changing profile of acute childhood illness: A need for the development of family nursing knowledge. *Journal of Advanced Nursing, 22*, 258–266.

Rubin, S. (1992). What's in a name? Child life and the play lady legacy. *Children's Health Care, 22*(1), 4–13.

Sheldon, L. M. (1996). An analysis of the concept of humor and its application to one aspect of children's nursing. *Journal of Advanced Nursing, 24,* 1175–1183.

Shelton, T. L., Jeppson, E. S., & Johnson, B. H. (1992). *Family-centered care for children with special health care needs* (2nd ed.). Bethesda, MD: Association for the Care of Children's Health.

Slusher, I. L., & McClure, M. J. (1992). Infant stimulation during hospitalization. *Journal of Pediatric Nursing, 7*(4), 276–279.

Thompson, R. H. (1995). Documenting the value of play for hospitalized children: The challenge in playing the game. *The ACCH Advocate, 2*(1), 11–14.

Topf, M., Bookman, M., & Arand, D. (1996). Effects of critical care unit noise on the subjective quality of sleep. *Journal of Advanced Nursing, 24,* 545–551.

Vessey, J. A., Holland, C. V., McVay, C. J., Williams, S. D., & McNatt, S. (1993). Latex allergy: A threat to you and your patients? *Pediatric Nursing, 19,* 517–520.

Wilson, K., Kendrick, P., & Ryan, V. (1992). *Play therapy: A non-directive approach for children and adolescents.* London: Bailliere Tindall.

Chronic Conditions as a Challenge to Health Maintenance

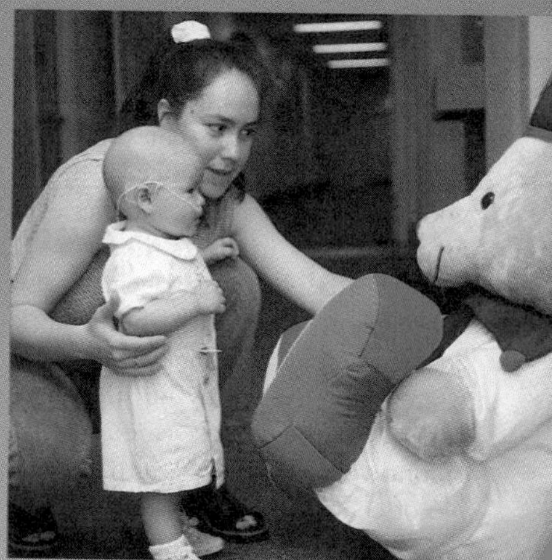

OUTLINE

OBJECTIVES

- Define "chronic condition."
- Analyze the impact of a chronic condition on the child, family, and individual family members.
- Discuss methods to assess family functioning in a family that has a child with a chronic condition.
- Identify critical points that may cause disequilibrium in the family of a child with a chronic condition and discuss appropriate nursing interventions.
- Implement interventions to promote health and normalization for the child with a chronic condition.
- Describe measures to provide well-child care to the chronically ill child.
- Relate the names and functions of support resources for the child with a chronic condition.

KEY TERMS

chronic condition
chronic sorrow
critical period
family equilibrium
normalization

CHAPTER

10

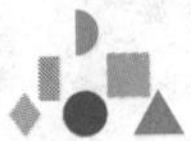

Chronic Conditions in Childhood

Nurses working with chronically ill children need a keen understanding of family dynamics as well as knowledge of the pathologic processes involved in the chronic conditions of childhood. Expert assessment skills and a knowledge of normal growth and development help the nurse determine the specific impact of the condition and its treatment on the child. This information helps the nurse design interventions that promote growth and development despite the presence of the chronic condition. An understanding of the economics of health care reimbursement policy as it affects the individual child and family is also essential. Case management and teaching skills allow the nurse to work with the child and the family as they adapt to change. Nursing research has clearly demonstrated that the family has the ability to become the true experts in the child's care. Families learn to work collaboratively with the health care provider and are capable of coordinating the child's care (Perkins, 1993).

The diagnosis of the chronic condition, the ongoing care requirements, and the changes in family structure and function that it causes have a long-term impact on the child and family. From the time of the actual diagnosis, most families move from a period of disorganization to one of recovery and reorganization. At the point of reorganization, many families find themselves stronger, with a whole new repertoire of coping mechanisms, child care skills, and family interactions that help them effectively face the challenges and changes to come (Austin, 1991; Hymovich, 1976; Lindsey, 1996).

However, not all families react to the diagnosis or care of the child's chronic condition positively. An increase in stress has been documented in families of children with chronic conditions (Eiser, 1993). This can cause some families to become weaker and develop (or continue use of) coping patterns that negatively affect one or more family members (Austin, 1991). Although the divorce rate is no higher in families of chronically ill children, some families dissolve through separation or divorce or after the death of the child. The chronic condition can be a major contributing factor to these changes.

Because each family is structured differently, the nurse must determine a family's unique response to the child's chronic condition (Fig. 10–1). Core nursing strategies include assessment, support and provision of direct physical care, and education. The desired nursing outcome is that the family deals effectively with the challenges the chronic condition presents. The health care team assists the family in moving toward normalization, a situation in which they see their lives more like the lives they planned before the chronic disorder. Normalization activities are also undertaken to try to make their lives as close to that of other families as possible, despite the restrictions of the chronic condition.

The knowledge needed to effectively care for a child with a chronic condition—for example, normal growth and development and theories about family structure and function—is provided throughout this text. This knowledge forms the basis for recognizing and analyzing the impact of the chronic condition on the child and family. The goal is to develop and implement family-centered, community-based plans of care, in collaboration with the

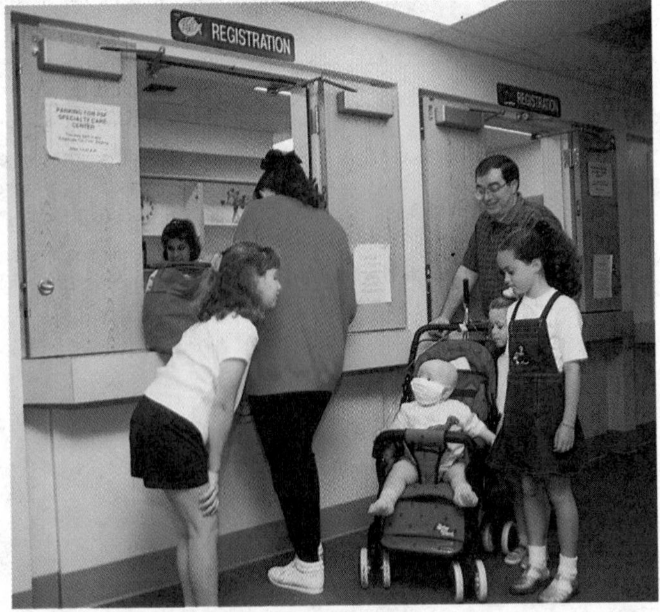

Figure 10–1
When the child has a chronic condition, participation by the entire family may promote family cohesiveness.

child, family, and a interdisciplinary team of care providers.

What Is a Chronic Condition?

A chronic condition interferes with daily functioning for more than 3 months in a year, causes hospitalization longer than 1 month in a year, or is likely to do either of these (Lawrence, 1990). Chronic conditions take many forms in childhood. Some children have a congenital anomaly (e.g., clubfoot) or genetic defect (e.g., cystic fibrosis) that caused structural or functional damage to a body sysem to be present at birth. Others have an acquired disease or injury (e.g., brain damage secondary to closed head injury) that causes repeated, intermittent, long-term, or permanent impairments or deviations from normal physiologic function. Many chronic conditions can have minimal effects on the child's ability to engage in usual childhood activities, do regular school work, and achieve independent mobility. Some conditions have a profound effect on the child's activities and life expectancy. The exact effect of a chronic condition on any child is not always related to the severity of the disease. Some children with very complex problems adapt quite well, whereas others with less serious conditions have great difficulty (Eiser, 1993).

When identifying applicable nursing diagnoses for these children, the assessment data must be examined carefully to ensure that the data have been grouped properly so that patterns are viewed as a whole and not as isolated events. In addition, the cause of each diagnosis must be written carefully because the plan of care directly addresses the cause of the identified problem or strength for that family. For example, a sleep pattern disturbance could be caused by a need to take medications during the night, excessive daytime sleeping, or pain. A selection of common nursing diagnoses for the child, parents, and other family members is presented in Charts 10–1 and 10–2.

Chronic conditions can involve one organ system (e.g., sensory in the case of blindness) or multiple organ systems (e.g., respiratory, exocrine, gastrointestinal in the case of cystic fibrosis). It is not unusual for a particular chronic condition to directly affect one aspect of the child's physical, psychological, or social functioning (e.g., muscular control in cerebral palsy), which then affects other areas, such as the ability to socialize or to eat.

Chronic conditions can also have varying effects on the child's cognitive functioning. In some cases, decreased cognitive ability is the primary problem. Cognitive impairment can also be the result of a physiologic injury (anoxia at birth) that also caused a physical impairment (cerebral palsy). However, in some cases, cognitive impairment may appear to be present when it is not because the child has not received the needed level of environmental stimulation at home, play, or school, resulting in learning deficits. It may not be possible for members of the health care team to assess cognitive ability in a child with a particular physical condition.

Examples of chronic conditions in childhood include asthma, diabetes, renal or liver anomalies, the sequelae of spina bifida, congenital heart defects, epilepsy, deafness, gastroesophageal reflux, hydrocephalus (congenital or acquired), cancer, and even chronic otitis media. A need for enteral feedings, ventilatory support, continuous apnea monitoring, or parenteral nutrition are also examples of situations in which a child could be siad to have a chronic condition (Office of Technology Assessment, 1978). In 1995, 9.3% of children in the United States were classified as having a disability (Centers for Disease Control and Prevention, 1995).

Chronic conditions can vary in course, intensity, and severity over the life of the child. Most children and their families come to view the chronic condition simply as a characteristic of the child and not as an illness (Fig. 10–2). Having a urinary tract infection or diabetic ketoacidosis is being ill, having spina bifida or being a diabetic is not. The chronic condition may require substantial modifications in the family's lifestyle from that originally expected, but the family reaches equilibrium and often finds purpose in the challenges the condition has brought them (Donnelly, 1994; Simon & Smith, 1992; Teague et al., 1993).

Figure 10–2
Not all children with chronic conditions have clear physical signs of the presence of their condition, such as these boys playing at asthma camp.

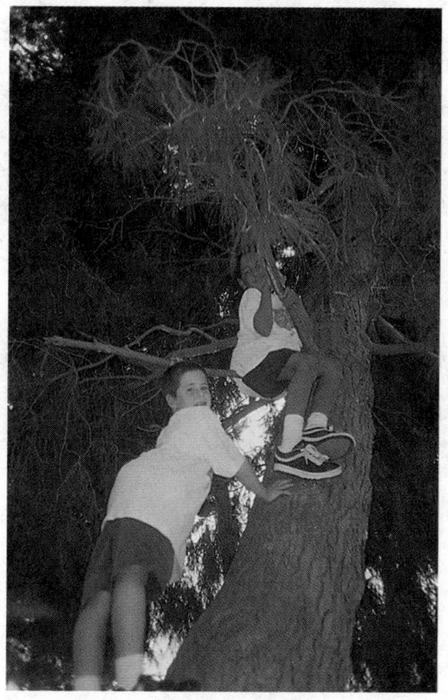

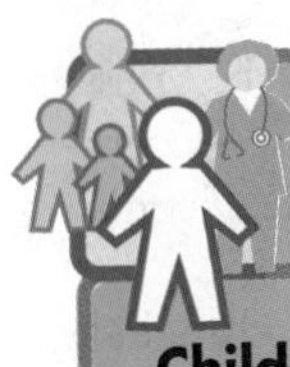

Chart 10–1
Nursing Diagnoses and Outcomes

Child

Altered growth and development related to physical effects of the chronic condition or its treatment; decreased access to usual socialization experiences

Outcomes: The child will have growth along own growth curve optimized within the restrictions imposed by the chronic condition.
The child will participate in developmentally appropriate socialization experiences.

Anxiety related to uncertain prognosis; actual or perceived loss of body integrity; threat to self-concept

Outcomes: The child will verbalize feelings of anxiety.
The child will identify and use methods to reduce feelings of anxiety.

Body image disturbance related to being different than peers, perceiving self as sick

Outcome: The child will verbalize a positive body image.

Grieving, dysfunctional related to inability to accept the chronic condition; failure to restructure life after diagnosis of chronic condition

Outcome: The child will successfully work through the grieving process and create a new definition of self and life goals.

Hopelessness related to failing physiologic condition; prolonged pain; prolonged activity restriction; loss of something valued (ability to socialize, perform in school, belief in God)

Outcomes: The child will have interventions implemented to promote comfort (manage pain, help with activities of daily living).
The child will verbalize a sense of control and a positive outlook on life.

Self-care deficit related to pathophysiologic change (specific to condition); decreased motivation; anxiety; fatigue

Outcome: The child will perform self-care as developmentally and physically able.

Sexual dysfunction related to specific effect of condition or its treatment on libido or sexual maturation; nonavailability of partners

Outcome: The adolescent will verbalize acceptance of, satisfaction with sexual functioning.

Sleep pattern disturbance related to frequent awakening secondary to condition or treatment of condition; excessive daytime sleeping; pain

Outcome: The child will develop regular sleep patterns that provide energy to carry out activities of daily living and play.

Social isolation related to lack of social skills; embarrassment, limited mobility or energy secondary to specific condition; communication barrier

Outcome: The child will participate in developmentally appropriate social activities.

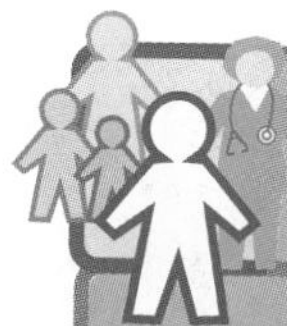

Chart 10–2
Nursing Diagnoses and Outcomes

Family Members and Caregivers

Altered family processes related to disruption of family routines due to demands of treatment of condition; physical changes of child; hospitalization of child

Outcomes: The family will discuss methods to minimize alterations in family functioning.
The family will demonstrate adaptive coping and family functioning.

Altered parenting due to interruption in the bonding process; separation of child from parents; unrealistic expectations of child by parents; knowledge of how to adapt parenting skills to accommodate child's condition; interruption of family life secondary to the treatment of the chronic condition

Outcome: The parents will demonstrate parenting skills that support the physical, developmental, and psychosocial needs and capabilities of the child with a chronic condition and of the siblings.

Anxiety related to uncertain prognosis; actual or perceived loss of child; concerns about ability to provide child's care needs

Outcomes: The parents will verbalize feelings of anxiety.
The parents will identify and use methods to reduce anxiety.

Caregiver role strain, risk for related to multiple care needs of child; no other caregivers

Outcomes: Parents will identify and use other caregivers for child.
Parents will take time away from child to meet own needs.

Family coping: potential for growth related to need for family to work together to accomplish tasks and develop new ways to meet needs of individual members

Outcome: The family will cope with demands imposed by child's chronic condition, develop new coping strategies to manage demands and promote family functioning, and feel a sense of achievement that they were able to do so.

Grieving, anticipatory related to anticipated shortened life expectancy of child due to chronic condition; change in family life plan as was envisioned prior to child's diagnosis

Outcome: The parents will progress through grieving process in an adaptive manner, still able to effectively communicate and support self and family functioning.

Grieving, dysfunctional related to inability to accept the presence of the child's chronic condition; failure to restructure personal and family life after diagnosis of chronic condition

Outcome: The parents will successfully work through the grieving process and create a new family life plan that incorporates changes necessitated by the child's chronic condition.

Hopelessness related to failing physiologic condition of child; loss of something valued (wished for child; belief in God)

Outcome: The parents will identify positive aspects of the situation and a feeling of hope.

Ineffective family management of therapeutic regimen related to lack of education, support, or physical ability to carry out plan of care; complexity, cost, side effects; knowledge deficit about how to implement regimen; failure to accept seriousness of problem or benefits of regimen; fear of being different

Outcome: Family will successfully manage child's care needs and will identify sources of support to help in managing the child's condition.

Chart continued on following page

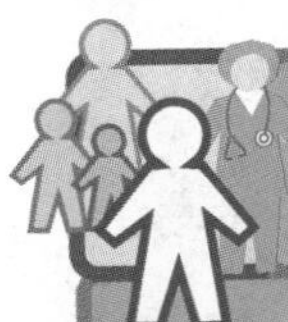

Chart 10–2
Nursing Diagnoses and Outcomes *Continued*

Family Members and Caregivers

Powerlessness related to lack of ability to control progression of condition; inability to communicate with health care provider

Outcomes:	Family will verbalize feelings of powerlessness and impact it has on the family. Family will identify positive coping strategies to deal with child's chronic condition. Family will be involved in decisions made regarding the child and treatment plan.

Sexual dysfunction related to fatigue secondary to care of child; lack of privacy secondary to presence of other caregivers in home

Outcome:	Parents will identify factors that might interfere with meeting own need for intimacy and deal with these in order to meet sexual needs.

Sleep pattern disturbance related to physical care needs of child

Outcome:	Caregivers will identify own sleep needs and develop strategies to meet these.

Social isolation related to care requirements of child

Outcomes:	Caregivers will verbalize need to maintain social relationships outside of those that focus on the child with a chronic condition. Caregivers will take time to get away from caregiving situations, with and without the child with a chronic condition, and enjoy social activities.

How Do the Family and the Child Maintain Equilibrium?

Equilibrium is the state of balance in which needs of individual family members are met and the family is able to carry out desired activities. To achieve equilibrium, different family members take on specific roles and the family constructs an effective support structure, often with the help of extended family, friends, health care providers, and the community.

For some families, roles are clear, the work is evenly distributed, and the support structure is broad, strong, and resilient. In other families, one or more members take little or no part in maintaining equilibrium, whereas the others take on much of the illness care and home maintenance. Family members may be unwilling to participate, or a family member may not allow participation by other members. These families may be in equilibrium, but if the support structure is limited or weak, the family may be at greater risk for problems if there is any additional stress.

When interactions within the family unit are mapped out, the patterns of interaction that produce equilibrium can be seen. In two-parent households there can be a *parent-shared pattern*, wih both parents helping with the care and sustenance of the child and family unit. A parent-shared pattern can be present even if only one parent is seen by health care providers (Clements, Copeland, & Loftus, 1990). For example, the mother may be the person who brings the child to the hospital, whereas the father handles the clinic visits. Or the mother and father may both work, and the family may negotiate with other family members or friends to assist with the day-to-day care of their child.

Figure 10–3
To manage the many health care needs of a child with a chronic condition, single-parent families often draw on the support of family or friends to maintain equilibrium in their family.

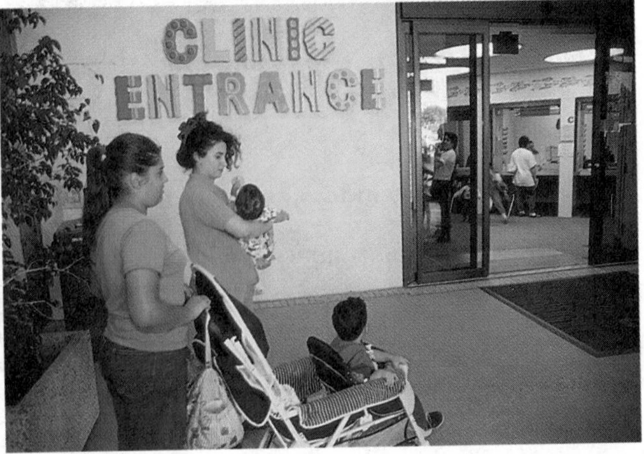

With a *mother-* or *father-centered pattern*, one parent takes on most of the caretaking and household maintenance roles. He or she provides all support to the child and must take on more and more responsibilities when the needs of the child, family, or either parent change. As with a single-parent family, a strong support structure with a great deal of assistance from friends and extended family is usually needed to maintain equilibrium (Fig. 10–3).

When there is a change in the needs of any one family member (as may happen with the diagnosis or exacerbation of a chronic condition), or the nature of the support structure changes (as may happen if a trusted friend moves away), there will be a period of disequilib-

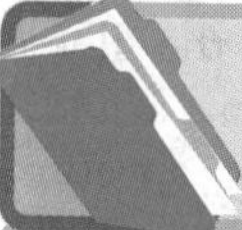

Chart 10–3
Nursing Interventions Classification (NIC)

Family Support

Definition

Promotion of family values, interests, and goals

Activities

Assure family that best care possible is being given to patient.
Appraise family's emotional reaction to patient's condition.
Determine the psychological burden of prognosis for family.
Foster realistic hope.
Listen to family concerns, feelings, and questions.
Facilitate communication of concerns/feelings between patient and family, or between family members.
Promote trusting relationship with family.
Accept the family's values in a nonjudgmental manner.
Answer all questions of family members or assist them to get answers.
Orient family to the health care setting, such as hospital unit or clinic.
Provide assistance in meeting basic needs for family, such as shelter, food, and clothing.
Identify nature of spiritual support for family.
Identify congruence between patient, family, and health professional expectations.
Reduce discrepancies in patient, family, and health professional expectations through use of communication skills.
Assist family members in identifying and resolving a conflict in values.
Respect and support adaptive coping mechanisms used by family.
Provide feedback for family regarding their coping.
Counsel family members on additional effective coping skills for their own use.
Provide spiritual resources for family, as appropriate.
Provide family with information about patient's progress frequently, according to patient preference.
Teach the medical and nursing plans of care to the family.
Provide necessary knowledge of options to family that will assist them to make decisions about patient care.
Include family members with patient in decision-making about care, when appropriate.
Encourage family decision-making in planning long-term patient care affecting family structure and finances.
Acknowledge understanding of family decision about postdischarge care.
Assist family to acquire necessary knowledge, skills, and equipment to sustain their decision about patient care.
Advocate for family, as appropriate.
Foster family assertiveness in information seeking, as appropriate.
Provide opportunities for visitation by extended family members, as appropriate.
Introduce family to other families undergoing similar experiences, as appropriate.
Give care to patient in lieu of family to relieve them and/or when family is unable to give care.
Arrange for ongoing respite care, when indicated and desired.
Provide opportunities for peer group support.
Refer for family therapy, as appropriate.
Tell family members how to reach the nurse.
Assist family members through the death and grief processes, as appropriate.

From McCloskey, J., & Bulechek, G. (1996). *Nursing interventions classification (NIC)* (2nd ed.). St. Louis: Mosby–Year Book. Reprinted with permission.

rium until new patterns of interaction are established (Clements et al., 1990). A major role of the nurse is to implement nursing interventions that promote family equilibrium and a strong support structure to maintain that equilibrium (Chart 10–3).

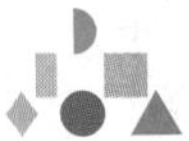

Responses to a Child's Chronic Condition

Parents of a child with a chronic condition are challenged to learn more than the normal repertoire of parenting skills. These parents must develop the additional skills needed, meet the demands of the child's chronic condition, and help the child cope with his or her condition. Optimally, parents reach the point at which they are fully committed and actively involved in their child's care (Perkins, 1993).

Perkins (1993) has studied how parents change their involvement in their child's care after the diagnosis of a chronic condition. Soon after the diagnosis, parents are usually onlookers who assist the health care provider only when requested. They may take in and use all information offered in a fairly indiscriminate way, expressing uncertainty about their ability to care for their child. As their knowledge and confidence increase, parents participate more actively with the care of the child and begin to work to normalize the family and the child's lives. New parents begin to filter information provided and check out answers. Perkins found that parents can become the primary performer of care, with the health care providers taking the assistant role. Parents can become expert investigators of new information and approaches to their child's care who take on the role of coordinator of the child's care.

As the child matures, the parents must relinquish control to accommodate the child's needs to become independent. Parents who have been highly participative in their child's care may need assistance in this transfer of control to their child. This occurs even when the child's condition does not permit him or her to actually provide self-care. These children also need to take a more active role in planning their care and making decisions about that care as they mature.

Initial Impact

The reaction of the family to the discovery or diagnosis of a chronic condition in the child has been called initial impact. This usually occurs at the time of diagnosis, when a name is placed on the condition. However, the initial impact may occur over time when the recognition of the condition or the assignment of a diagnosis takes longer (Clements et al., 1990; Copeland, 1993). For the child with asthma, the initial impact may be on the afternoon when the child is admitted to the emergency department with his or her first acute attack. In the case of a child with cerebral palsy, the initial impact may occur over the first year of life as the full scope of the motor deficiencies is determined.

Cohen (1995a) has studied parents in the time following the diagnosis of a chronic condition (her example was cancer). She found that when the signs of the illness first appear, the parent often views the symptoms as ordinary day-to-day occurrences. Fatigue, lack of appetite, and a big bruise are a part of childhood. The initial actions taken to address these illness cues are usually standard interventions drawn from the parent's repertoire of parenting skills, such as an extra nap, favorite foods, or using more protective gear during sports activities.

When these actions do not work, the parent may try another strategy until he or she accepts that the actions are not working because the child does not have a common childhood problem. Many parents carefully consider how they will present the problem to the health care provider, because they want to be sure their complaint is seen as legitimate, while, at the same time, they want to be sure they are not embarrassed if there is nothing wrong. One strategy is to wait until the next routine visit. This is often detrimental or impossible if the problem, such as new onset diabetes or acute asthma, is progressing rapidly. Another strategy is to seek help on a different issue that they known will get attention. The parent then asks the health care provider to check out the symptoms that have been actually causing them concern (Cohen, 1995a).

Once the child has entered the health care system, health care providers seek to identify the problem, prescribe an appropriate treatment strategy, and determine its effectiveness. The most obvious or common explanations are often considered first, delaying the definitive diagnosis. This period of uncertainty is very difficult for the parent (Cohen, 1993a, 1995a, 1995b; Knafl, Ayres, Gallo, Zoeller, & Breitmayer, 1995).

During the initial diagnostic period, parental responses and actions should be evaluated with an understanding that the parent may be basing his or her interpretation of the child's symptoms on prior knowledge and experiences (Fig. 10–4). This limited viewpoint can make it difficult for parents to comprehend or accept information presented by health care providers. It can also cause them to take actions or ask questions that appear inappropriate when viewed with hindsight or with more diagnostic knowledge. For example, the father of an infant who was severely impaired secondary to prolonged anoxia at birth interpreted the posturing and rigidity of his daughter Karin as a sign she was a fussy baby. Another example is the mother of a 5-week-old boy who is

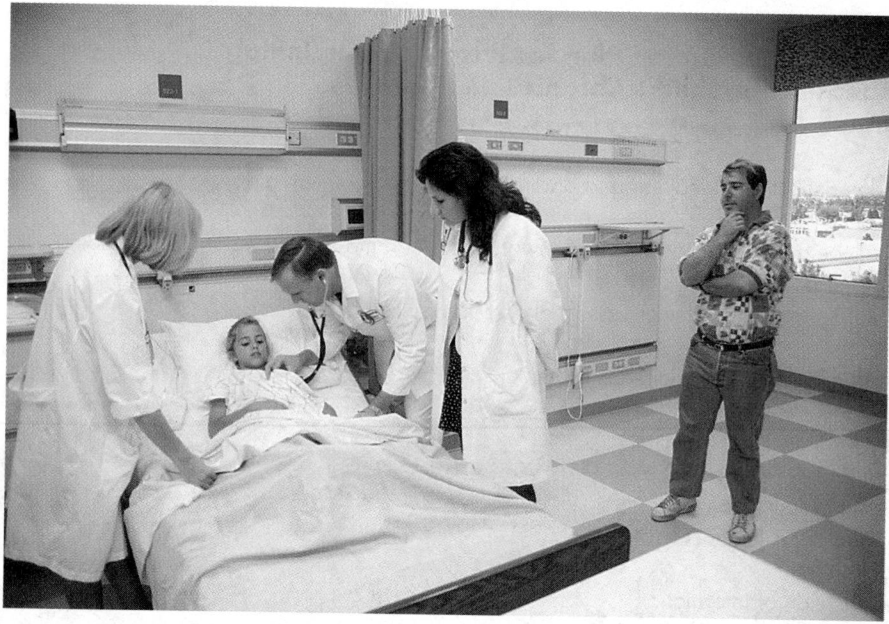

Figure 10–4
Early after the diagnosis, the parents are often not comfortable participating in assessment and care planning discussions, especially if the health care provider makes no effort to include them.

going home with a tracheotomy and gastrostomy tube. Although no one in his family has shown a readiness or willingness to learn to care for his special needs at home, she is asking many questions about the type of preschools her son can attend.

Family Needs at the Time of Diagnosis

At the time of diagnosis, families express a need for education a well as for psychosocial, physical, financial, and spiritual support. Because they draw on existing coping mechanisms to deal with the crisis of diagnosis, coping mechanisms are often found to be inadequate and they must develop or expand them. The health care team can work together to ensure that family members are provided with the information needed to adjust and adapt to the child's condition. TIP 10–1 provides a summary of the teaching interventions needed with these families.

Understanding the Child's Condition

The family may have inadequate understanding of the child's condition. Psychological support, spiritual support, and care of basic needs must be addressed. To deal effectively with the condition, the family must learn new skills to manage the day-to-day demands of the child's illness. Parents, children, and other family members often have trouble absorbing the large volume of information presented at the time of diagnosis. For some conditions, the parent must make only minor adjustments in parenting skills to meet the child's new needs. For other conditions, families must learn a whole new repertoire of skills.

Parents must learn about the condition itself and the specific steps they must take to safely care for their child. The family must also become familiar with aspects of the health care system with which they have never interacted. Parents report a need and desire for control (Cohen, 1995a). To take control they need the knowledge base necessary for making decisions.

Unfamiliarity with medical terms and techniques can make learning even more difficult. The teaching atmosphere must be kept open and accepting. Nursing research indicates that parents may be afraid to ask questions because they fear they will be evaluated negatively by a health care provider (Simon & Smith, 1992).

Even young children not ready for formal teaching sessions need education. This could be as simple as feeding 2-day-old Sara, scheduled for a cleft lip repair, with a syringe on the day before her surgery to allow her to become familiar with this method of receiving her formula. One-year-old Jose can hold and play with oxygen administration devices and do practice blood pressure measurements the week before he has his second-stage repair for a congenital heart defect. Teaching the child in this way, helps him or her gain some personal control over experiences that are an ongoing part of life with a chronic illness. It also provides the foundation for the child to assume self-care activities. Child life staff are excellent resources for the development and implementation of programs to prepare children for procedures and to educate them about their conditions. Videos and computer-assisted instruction can be engaging ways for a child to learn about his or her illness and its care (Peterson, 1996).

caREminder: *The child's knowledge needs change as the child moves on to new developmental stages (e.g., begins school and travels on the school bus), the condition takes*

TIP 10–1 A Teaching Intervention Plan for Parents in the Initial Period After Diagnosis of a Child's Chronic Condition

Nursing Diagnosis and Family Outcomes

- Knowledge deficit: the condition and parents' role in the treatment plan

  Outcomes:

  Family will be given instruction geared toward their learning style, level of understanding, and knowledge deficits.

  Family will be able to implement essential care for the child.

Instructional Interventions

Verify cause of knowledge deficit. For example:

- Excessive anxiety
- Fear of condition
- Illiteracy
- Impaired communication
- Lack of prior teaching
- Language different
- Misinterpretation of information
- Unwillingness to learn

Assess baseline knowledge or experience with the chronic condition.

- What has the parent already been taught?
- Does the parent know anyone else with this condition?
- What have they heard about children with this condition?
- Is there any aspect of the child's care that is of particular concern to them?

Assess family structure, function, and usual patterns as they impact care.

- Who will be providing care to the child?
- Who will be backup for care?
- Where is the child when not with the family?
- What does the parent need to know to care for child safely at home?
- Will any family routines be affected by the presence of the chronic condition?
- What will be the child's involvement in his or her care, based on age and cognitive development?
- What will be the siblings' involvement in the child's care, based on age and cognitive development?
- How are siblings and friends affected by the presence of the child's chronic condition?
- What does the parent want to learn first?

Design teaching plan based on family assessment.

- Involve all caregivers and significant family members.
- Adapt teaching plan to accommodate the usual patterns of family or help the parents change these patterns.
- Begin with essential skills needed for the child's safe care and move on to those needed for long-term care and in-depth understanding of the child's condition and needs.

Present content using standard teaching principles.

- Use language best comprehended by the parent (e.g., English, Spanish, Creole).
- Use vocabulary understood by parent while teaching them to understand medical language that they may hear in future.
- Use a variety of teaching techniques to meet unique learning styles.

  Discussion
  Direct demonstration
  Video/audio tape
  Books
  Practice equipment
  Computer programs
  Meetings with other parents, children with the condition

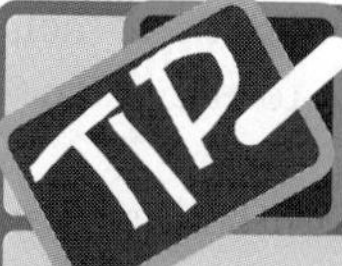

TIP 10–1 A Teaching Intervention Plan for Parents in the Initial Period After Diagnosis of a Child's Chronic Condition *Continued*

- Encourage questions.
- Explore questions for possible concerns not evident in questions.
- Be alert for information overload.
- Allow practice and return demonstration of skills.
- Provide source of backup for later questions.
  - Home nursing
  - Phone calls from care provider
  - Support group
  - Written material

Educate for future.

- Expand natural parenting skills to promote development despite presence of chronic condition.
- Learn how the child can continue prior activities or activities can be adapted to accommodate limitations of condition.
- Learn to find new knowledge on own.
  - Support groups
  - Reading
  - Electronic support groups
- Learn to question and collaborate with health care providers.
- Learn to evaluate accuracy of information provided.
- Learn to educate staff and other caregivers about child's unique needs.
- Prepare for changes in care brought on by progression or improvement of condition, developmental changes of child/caregivers, need for child to increase self-care.

on a new dimension (e.g., more labile diabetes as the child moves through puberty), or the family changes (e.g., divorce, remarriage, birth of a child, departure of a sibling for college). As the child develops cognitively and emotionally, the need and ability to learn about his or her condition also evolve.

The ongoing assessment of learning needs of the parent and child, even when they appear quite knowledgeable, should be a part of each health care encounter. The depth and scope of the education of the parent, child, and family support persons should be gradually increased with every encounter with the family. Begin with information needed to safely care for the child and make immediate decisions, and progress to information that helps the parent and child make informed decisions about future care options and increases their knowledge of the condition.

Even when in-home care will be provided after discharge, the parents need education to help them progress to the point where they can be the coordinator of care and their child's advocate. Parents need to be in a position of knowledgeable strength to direct the care provided, evaluate the health care providers, and maintain control. Parents must be prepared to provide care if a health care provider fails to arrive or is unable to provide the needed care. Many parents who initially think they need and want continuous help in the home find that, despite the value of the health care providers, there are times they simply want their homes to themselves (Leonard, Brust, & Nelson, 1993; Nuttall, 1988; Patterson, Jernell, Leonard, & Titus, 1994; Teague et al., 1993).

Other family members must be taught to care for the child. This will allow them to assist with the child's physical care and decrease their fear of interacting with the child. This fear can make them afraid to engage in the normal interactions so essential to the child's development (Fig. 10–5).

Parents report that one of the most difficult things they face is having an individual they expect to accept and support the child, such as the grandparents, display fear about being left with the child (Nuttall, 1988). In addition to losing the emotional support, the parent may be losing a source of respite care if the child's physical care needs are ongoing.

Psychosocial Support

The family's response to the crisis of the diagnosis of a chronic condition often resembles the grief reaction. The

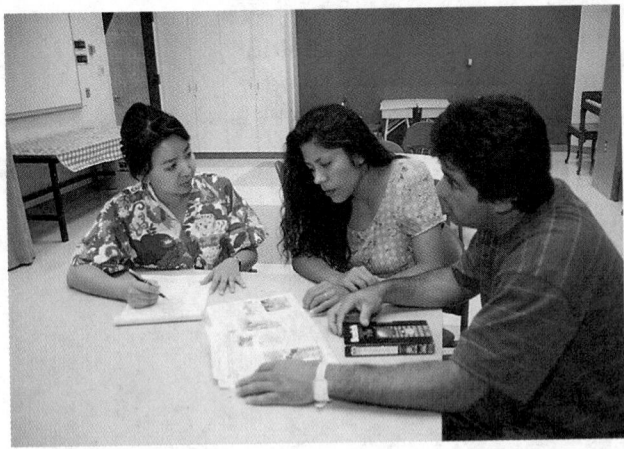

Figure 10–5
A variety of educational tools should be used to prepare the family and child for care.

family mourns the loss of the dreamed of child and their life as they planned it would be. Although some of these responses may appear abnormal, they can also be evidence of a healthy response to the problem (Austin, 1991; Johnston & Marder, 1994).

Worldview: *Each family's response is influenced by their cultural background. Some may be very verbal about feelings, whereas others may not be willing to discuss feelings with those outside their family. For instance, in some families the father may assume the dominant role as breadwinner and decision maker of the family. If only the mother is seen in the health care setting, there may be a need to verify that essential information is communicated to the father so that decisions can be made supported by the existing family structure. Be certain to ask specific questions in order to determine how each family is responding to the diagnosis, how health care decisions will be made, and how they expect to care for the child (Geissler, 1993).*

A common response to the diagnosis of a chronic condition is *denial*. This response must be carefully assessed, because what looks like denial can actually be evidence that the parents are still viewing the illness as a normal childhood problem that they can treat using their usual repertoire of interventions. As they realize this is not correct, they will begin to accept the information the health care providers are offering more readily.

True denial occurs when the individual continues to not accept the diagnosis. This can be a problem if the denial causes family members to distrust the health care provider or to interfere with treatment. Disbelief may cause the family members to bring the child to other care providers so they can find one who will not make the same "erroneous" diagnosis, which can delay initiation of care. Chart 10–4 presents nursing interventions to help parents displaying this and other reactions to the diagnosis of a chronic condition.

Another reaction at the time of the initial diagnosis can be *guilt*. Parents often examine their behavior to find what they did or did not do to cause the condition (Johnson & Marder, 1994; Simon & Smith, 1992). This makes the wording of interview questions crucial.

caREminder: *Asking "When did you first notice she was going to the bathroom more than usual?" allows the parent of a child newly diagnosed with type I diabetes to report his or her observations. Asking "How long was she going to the bathroom more than usual before you brought her to the doctor?" reinforces guilt.*

Anger is another common response. Anger can be manifested as aggression, hostility, and demanding behavior directed against themselves, health care providers, family, friends, or their God. Including the parent and child in treatment planning may reduce anger and the displacement of feelings of rage and helplessness against others. Health care providers must remain non-defensive and avoid personalizing the anger that may be inappropriately directed against a caregiver. The health care worker should consider how he or she would feel in the same situation, as this helps establish empathy.

caREminder: *Teach family members that the anger of the parents, child, or siblings may be inappropriately directed against them. If they are prepared for this, it is less likely they will terminate their relationship with the family at a time when the family needs them most.*

Loneliness is another emotion experienced by families of a child with a chronic condition (Johnson & Marder, 1994). Changes in relationships with family and friends, some of which may occur as a part of a very constructive attempt to deal with the challenges they face, can isolate family members (Donnelly, 1994; Teague et al., 1993; Williams, Lorenzo, & Borja, 1993). An assessment finding might be a parent who does not discuss any activities except those revolving around care of the child. Another parent may state there is no one who can understand their needs.

Loneliness can result in marital difficulties if one parent withdraws from the relationship or begins to increase socialization outside the home without including the spouse. Home care by professional nurses, hospice care, and participation in parent support groups are three interventions that have been shown to reduce stress and allow the parents to expand the scope of usual social activities (Patterson et al., 1994; Sherman, 1995; Smith, Gabard, Dale, & Drucker, 1994).

Fear is another common emotional reaction to the diagnosis of a chronic condition in a child (Donnelly, 1994; Johnston & Marder, 1994; Teague et al., 1993).

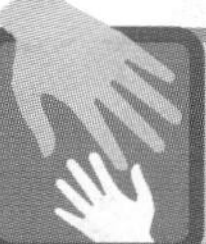

Chart 10–4
Nursing Interventions

Supporting the Emotional Responses of Parents

Emotion	Examples	Problematic Examples	Nursing Interventions	Outcomes
Grief	Despair, remorse	Withdrawal; unrelenting sadness	Validate feelings Offer support Help parents reestablish structure in life	Parents begin to integrate fact that child has chronic condition into how they view the child in a positive way
Denial	Forgetting Overcompensation Disbelief	Interference with treatment Distrust	Reflect back statements Clarify feelings Offer feedback Help parents recognize that responses are normal	Parents begin to make appropriate plans for future Parents ask questions that show understanding of condition
Guilt	Self-blame	Spousal blame Continual self-recrimination	Give information Explore ideas about why child has condition	Self-blame comments subside Projection of blame onto others decreases Coping with realistic guilt
Anger	Aggression Hostility	Acts helpless Interferes with treatment plan	Include parents when developing treatment plan Remain non-defensive	Parents begin to actively participate in planning care Parents accurately and constructively directs anger
Fear	Anxiety Self-doubt Disoriented	Hypochondriacal Panic attacks Avoidance	Have parents participate in development and implementation of treatment plan Point out parental competence Repeat instructions, if needed	Parent initiates discussion of new treatment approaches Parent carries out needed treatments
Loneliness	Quiet Isolated	Marital discord Job difficulties	Assist in establishing contact with potential support persons/groups Help family reestablish or develop social connections	Family contacts support group and goes to meetings Family reports social activities that give them enjoyment

Adapted from Johnston, C., & Marder, L. (1994). Parenting the child with a chronic condition: An emotional experience. *Pediatric Nursing, 20,* 611–614. Used with permission.

Parents fear they will not be able to care for their child, and they find it difficult to be unable to foresee the future clearly. Accurate information given at the appropriate level and paced for the individual family empowers the family to become as active in their child's care as they desire and helps reduce these problems but may not alleviate them. For some of the chronic conditions experienced by children, there is a great deal of uncertainty about the future and fear is a natural response.

Many families come to a point where they find purpose in the presence of the chronic condition. Research with these families indicated that they develop a personal philosophy about the family, living, and sharing. They see the child and the child's condition as a source of strength, which promotes development of all members (Donnelly, 1994; LoBiondo-Wood, Bernier-Henn, & Williams, 1992; Simon & Smith, 1992; Teague et al., 1993).

Physical Needs

Fatigue and physical demands usually compound family problems. At the time of diagnosis, there is often an exhausting series of visits to health care providers and hospitalization. Fatigue from lack of sleep is aggravated by the stress of the diagnostic process (Cohen, 1993a; Ray & Ritchie, 1993; Teague et al., 1993).

Interdisciplinary clinics can decrease the fatigue of the parents of children with a complex problem by decreasing the number of times they must bring their child for evaluation and follow-up. At these clinics, members from different health care disciplines all are present on the same day and in the same location. A program serving the child with spina bifida should have nursing, social work, orthopedics, orthotics, and renal specialists ready to evaluate the child at each clinic (Fig. 10–6). An oncology program for children with brain tumors should be staffed with neurosurgeons, neurologists, and endocrinologists in addition to nurses and social workers.

Fatigue can impair otherwise effective coping abilities. If the condition is one that requires around-the-clock care, parents will have their sleep disrupted over a long period of time. This is aggravated by the decrease in socialization and the loss of a major source of relaxation (Donnelly, 1994; Teague et al., 1993; Williams et al., 1993).

Fatigue can also result from the physical demands of the child's care. For the child with a mobility impairment, lifting and positioning the child becomes more difficult as the child's height and weight increase. Transporting equipment such as oxygen or a wheelchair takes strength and physical dexterity. Parents and caregivers must learn all the basic principles of body mechanics to provide safe care to the child and to protect themselves from injury. Caregivers often neglect their own physical needs in their love and dedication to the child. Nurses should help families recognize their physical needs and find realistic ways to have those needs met (Chart 10–5).

Chart 10–5
Nursing Interventions

Helping Parents Meet Their Own Physical Needs

- Encourage accepting offers of help from friends or family members to:
  - Watch siblings
  - Bring meals
  - Learn to provide care to child
- Suggest use of a babysitter who is comfortable with child's needs.
- Suggest that parent naps when child does.
- Adapt environment to make provision of care easier:
  - Elevate bed.
  - Position tables to make equipment accessible during care.
  - Modify daily care to better accommodate family's activities (e.g., bath in evening).
- Teach proper body mechanics for lifting, turning, positioning, and transporting child (e.g., from bed to chair to car).
- Have child begin self-care activities as soon as developmentally appropriate.
- Work with family to limit number of health care visits.
- Use community resources for respite care.
- Work with interdisciplinary team to ensure that all services available are accessed when needed.
- Provide sleeping facilities for parent during hospitalizations.

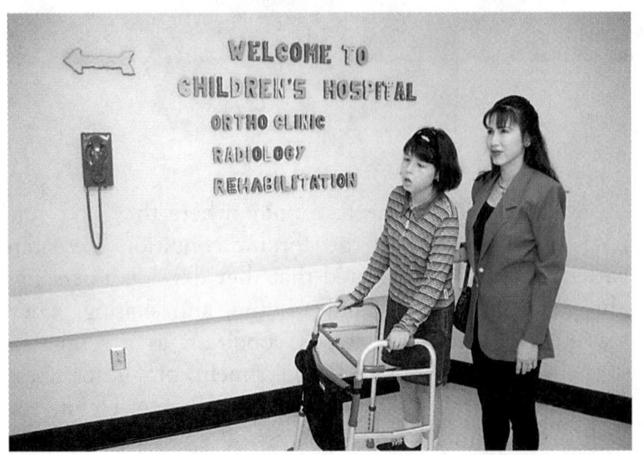

Figure 10–6
Interdisciplinary clinics allow full evaluation of the child without requiring the parents and child to make multiple visits to health care providers.

Knowledge Regarding Care Needs of the Child

Parents need to enhance their existing parenting skills to incorporate caregiving skills needed to meet the care needs of their child. Each physical symptom—difficulty breathing because of asthma, frequent loose stools due to celiac disease, ineffective swallowing because of cerebral palsy, hair loss as the result of chemotherapy—causes a unique response in the child, parents, siblings, other family members, friends, and all those around them (Cohen, 1993a; Horner, 1992; Perkins, 1993).

Worldview: *To facilitate family adaptation, the treatment plan should be developed with a consideration of family lifestyle, cultural, and ethnic preferences: for example, dietary considerations if the family follows strict vegetarian dietary restrictions or the need to avoid blood products if the family are Jehovah's Witnesses.*

A particularly difficult physical symptom for parents to cope with is the child's pain (Rao & Kramer, 1993; Simon & Smith, 1992). Pain can result from the illness, as with sickle cell anemia, or from the treatment of the illness, as with surgery to correct an orthopedic anomaly. Parents need to be able to act as advocates for their child at times when the assessment or treatment of the condition causes the child pain or discomfort and health care providers do not provide needed interventions. For example, a parent may need to ensure that his or her child, admitted to the hospital because of a seizure that morning, is fed to decrease hunger pains. Another parent may work with the nurse anesthetist to plan the optimal type of sedation for the child during an endoscopy procedure.

Spiritual Support

The spiritual needs of the child and family should be determined. The family can then be helped to access needed spiritual support. Many families draw great strength from their faith, although this is not always expressed by their involvement with a particular church and religion (Chart 10–6). Concepts such as hope and faith are directly tied to the spiritual domain and are often great sources of support to the family (Fish & Shelly, 1978; Highfield & Cason, 1983).

To assess the family's spiritual beliefs, the nurse can look for evidence of involvement with a church, such as religious symbols, medals, statues, books, or music. These may be used to initiate discussion of spiritual strengths or needs. Parents should be encouraged to include their minister, priest, rabbi, or member of their church in these discussions if desired. The plan of care should be modified to accommodate religious practices (Fulton & Moore, 1995) (see Chart 3–20, Worldview: Questions for Spiritual Assessment).

Assessment should explore other aspects of spirituality, such as the presence of hope and a sense of purpose and meaning in life. A need to both give and receive love has also been identified as a component of spirituality (Highfield & Cason, 1983) (see Chart 3–18, Nursing Interventions Classification (NIC): Spiritual Support).

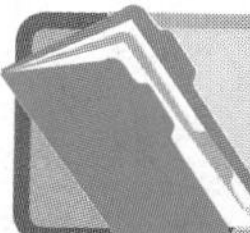

Chart 10–6
Nursing Interventions Classification (NIC)

Hope Instillation

Definition

Facilitation of the development of a positive outlook in a given situation

Activities

- Assist patient/family in identifying areas of hope in life.
- Inform the patient about whether the current situation is a temporary state.
- Demonstrate hope by recognizing the patient's intrinsic worth and viewing the patient's illness as only one facet of the individual.
- Expand the patient's repertoire of coping mechanisms.
- Teach reality recognition by surveying the situation and making contingency plans.
- Assist the patient to devise and revise goals related to the hope object.
- Help the patient expand spiritual self.
- Avoid masking the truth.
- Facilitate the patient's incorporating a personal loss into his or her body image.
- Facilitate the patient's/family's reliving and savoring past achievements and experiences.
- Emphasize sustaining relationships, such as mentioning the names of loved ones to the unresponsive patient.
- Employ guided life review and reminiscence, as appropriate.
- Involve the patient actively in own care.
- Develop a plan of care that involves degree of goal attainment, moving from simple to more complex goals.
- Encourage therapeutic relationships with significant others.
- Teach family about the positive aspects of hope (e.g., develop meaningful conversational themes that reflect love and need for patient).
- Provide patient/family opportunity to be involved with support groups.
- Create an environment that facilitates the patient's practicing religion, as appropriate.

From McCloskey, J., & Bulechek, G. (1996). *Nursing interventions classification (NIC)* (2nd ed.). St. Louis: Mosby–Year Book. Reprinted with permission.

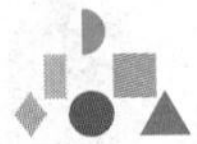

Assessment of the Family

Families of children with a chronic condition have common, but not universal, experiences. Often the response to the condition is based on a *perception* of the severity of the problem, not its actual severity. Nursing strategies that help parents and children have a more positive perception of the condition have the potential of benefiting the family.

Common issues faced by the child include decreased participation in normal childhood activities, pain and discomfort, and experience with hospitalizations. Some children experience loneliness, loss of control, concerns that they are different from their peers, and fears of dependence on parents and caregivers. For families, common issues include the burden of care, finances, and a need to interact with complex medical systems and many care providers. Difficulties with child care and worries about long-term care can complicate feelings of loneliness, guilt, and anger already discussed (Perin, 1995).

The nurse must accept the family at the stage and with the reactions and coping mechanisms (both effective and ineffective) they bring to the situation. A coping mechanism should not be judged as good or bad based on a personal value system. The nurse cannot presume that a family will be at a particular point in their response to the identification of a chronic condition simply because the child's problem was just diagnosed or has been present for years. Verifying assessment findings with the family must be done before the nurse can interpret their reaction to the situation (Johnston & Marder, 1994).

Each family responds to the presence of a chronic condition in one of their children in a unique manner. One nursing objective is to determine what that response is. Before labeling a family's behavior (such as not rooming in) as dysfunctional, verify that the response is, in fact, dysfunctional for that family. Forcing the family to change to a more "functional" pattern may actually be damaging (Johnston & Marder, 1994).

For example, a mother who continues to go to work every day despite her child's hospitalization for newly diagnosed diabetes, may be doing so to maintain some control in at least one aspect of her life. Having this small degree of control may help her deal more effectively with the very "out of control" situation she feels when facing the newly diagnosed illness of her child.

Verifying who lives with the child and which family members provide support can also be helpful. Family assessment tools such as the Family APGAR (Smilkstein, Ashworth, & Montano, 1982) and HOME Inventory (Caldwell & Bradley, 1984) provide data on individual family members' perceptions of their support from the family and the family's interaction with the children at home. (See Chapter 3 for detailed information on these assessment tools.) The family Apgar appraises each member's perception of support. Their responses are charted on a grid similar to that for the infant Apgar to give a total score. The HOME Inventory is designed for focused assessment in the home environment. In addition to summarizing data about members of the household, the tool has a list of assessments that focus on family interaction both in and out of the home. Both total and subscores are generated, and these can help the caregiver focus on specific areas of family function that may warrant attention (see Table 3–4, Family Assessment Tools).

Tools such as the CICI: PQ (Chronicity Impact and Coping Instrument: Parent Questionnaire) (Hymovich, 1983) and the CHIP (Coping Health Inventory for Parents) (McCubbin, McCubbin, Cauble, & Nevin, 1979) provide further data on indivdual parental responses. These tools focus on the response of the family to the chronic condition in their child.

Other useful assessment tools are kinetic family drawings (Rollins, 1990) and conjoint family drawings. In kinetic family drawings, the child is asked to draw a picture of the family "doing something." In a conjoint family drawing, the family works together to produce a picture. These drawings provide insight into relationships within the family and can reflect the feelings of both children and adults.

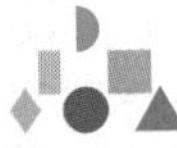

Critical Points in the Trajectory of the Chronic Condition

Families of children with chronic conditions face numerous critical points caused by increases in the needs of individual members or changes in the family support as previously assigned roles and responsibilities are renegotiated (Clements et al., 1990; Copeland, 1993). Nurses must be alert for the occurrence of one of these critical points and intervene appropriately (Chart 10–7).

Increase in Physical Symptoms

One critical point for the family is any time the child's physical symptoms increase. The family and child must learn to cope with new physical demands and alter patterns that are no longer effective (Cohen, 1993a; Clements et al., 1990). The stress from the increase in the symptoms is compounded by guilt over why the treat-

Chart 10–7

Critical Points in the Trajectory of the Chronic Condition

Change in physical symptoms
Relocation
Parental absence
Developmental advance
Birth of a subsequent child

Data from Clements, D., Copeland, L., & Loftus, M. (1990). Critical times for families with a chronically ill child. *Pediatric Nursing, 16*, 157–161.

ment provided was not successful and fear that the illness is getting worse or is out of control.

Relocation

Relocation of the child from home to a hospital or long-term care facility or from such a facility to home is another critical point (Clements et al., 1990). When the child is rehospitalized, the family and child must renegotiate roles with health care providers. This can be very stressful because the parents often feel their position as expert is neither recognized nor respected by the health care providers with whom they must now work (Burkhart, 1993; Copeland, 1993; Nuttall, 1988; Perkins, 1993; Simon & Smith, 1992).

When the child moves from the hospital to home, care needs depend on the reasons the child was hospitalized. If the child was admitted for a procedure that is "routine" for him or her, such as a dose of chemotherapy, the parents and child may be very aware of how to meet care needs at home. However, all short admissions are not for procedures for which the family is so well educated. For example, the child with a long-term feeding tube may have a new type of tube implanted. Education and support to care for this new tube are essential.

The most complex transition is from hospital to home when the child has been hospitalized for a long time (see Chapter 9 for further discussion). Even if the parents have been fully participative in their child's care, they need time to prepare to take on the home care roles independently. This may necessitate establishing a transitional care-by-parent unit or perhaps setting aside a room where parents can room in and take on all responsibilities, asking for support only as needed (Fig. 10–7).

This transition also requires that the home be prepared for the child's arrival (see Chapter 11). The case manager can work with the family to obtain needed equipment, and the home care nurse can do a predischarge visit to assist with any needed modifications in the home environment. If the child is dependent on electricity or phone contact, the utility companies need to be notified. The family also needs to ensure that they are prepared to transport the child. They need to practice placing the car seat and any needed equipment in the automobile before the day of the discharge.

These transitions can be difficult for the parents; they also can be difficult for the staff. If the child has been on the unit for a long period—in some cases, from birth—staff members will also experience a sense of loss when the child leaves the unit. Staff may also fear for the child's safety and need to examine their feelings that the parents are not as capable as they are.

By working with the families and establishing partnerships throughout hospitalizations, even if parent visits are infrequent, the staff can better prepare the parents for home care and increase their own ability to let the child go to his or her home and family (Barnsteiner & Gillis-Donnovan, 1990; Stepanek & Ahmann, 1995; Wells, DeBoard-Burns, Cook, & Mitchell, 1994a, 1994b).

Relocation can also occur as the result of positive events such as the child's going to camp, a school trip, or moving out to live independently. Such events can cause the parents to fear for the well-being of the child. Will the substitute caregivers see and act on potential conditions quickly and effectively? Will the child be safe traveling in vehicles the parents cannot control? Will the child comply with treatment regimens that have been taught but can no longer be tightly monitored?

When the relocation is from home to another site, parents and families may have dramatic changes in their day-to-day responsibilities once they no longer need to

Figure 10–7
Encouraging parents to stay in the room with their child allows them to gradually take on full responsibility for the care needs of a child requiring complex physical care.

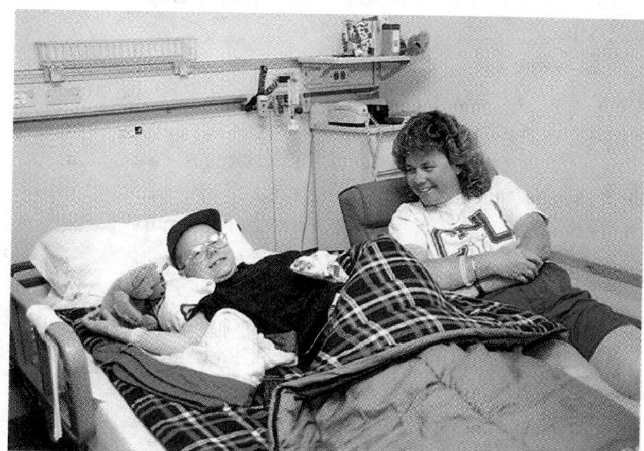

provide direct care for the child. Suddenly, hours that were absorbed with the planning or implementation of care of the child are unfilled, and a sense of emptiness ensues (Clements et al., 1990).

When the relocation of the child is to a long-term care facility, families report a mix of feelings, which can range from guilt, to loneliness, to relief. Often, after the child is relocated, the family members realize that the problems they hoped such a move would solve are problems that could not be solved simply by the relocation of the child.

Relocation of the child can also be seen positively by the family. For both the child and family, the need to hospitalize the child may be a sudden and welcome relief from the day-to-day responsibilities for monitoring and implementation of care to the child. Someone else does the glucose monitoring, offers to carry out the intermittent catheterization, provides the round-the-clock antibiotic at the right time, or brings in the nutritional supplements with each meal.

The nursing staff should clarify with the family what they want the staff to help them with or take responsibility for during a hospitalization or clinic visit. Some families want to maintain full control and provide all care, whereas others want to be there as parents only, with staff providing all physical care. There are also parents who desire a middle ground. They may want to coordinate and direct care but not carry out all care.

caREminder: *Specific roles and activities for the family members and health care providers should be clearly identified and communicated to avoid increasing parental stress.*

Parental Absence

Another critical point is parental absence (Clements et al., 1990). Absences can be caused by parental illness, vacations, divorce, or the psychological withdrawal of a parent from caretaking responsibilities. Routine reassessment of the family structure and support helps illuminate such changes.

In some cases, the sudden absence of a primary caregiver can so negatively affect the child's care that an emergent health situation arises, resulting in hospitalization of the child. Absences, for whatever cause, can influence the quality of care provided to the affected child. In the absence of a parent or other primary caregiver, children may have to "fend for themselves."

In other cases, another caregiver may take over the parenting responsibilities yet not have a full understanding of the child's needs. To prevent such lapses in quality care, the parents or primary caregivers should always have a backup plan as to who can assist the child in his or her care. Written instructions should be kept updated and should be left in an easily located place. The child's health care records and other important documents (insurance forms, addresses for supplies) should be included. Should an unexpected absence of the parent occur, others would have easy access to important health care information.

When parental absences are planned, the substitute caregiver needs written permission from the parents to make health care decisions should an emergency situation arise. The temporary caregiver should be given ample opportunity to demonstrate care skills. Extra supplies should be available in case the parents planned time of leave is extended. The child should feel as comfortable as possible with the substitute caregiver and should be reassured that the parents will return.

Developmental Advances

The movement of the child from one developmental stage to the next is another critical point (Clements et al., 1990; Cohen, 1993a, 1995b). The usual fears of parents as their child experiences normal developmental changes are aggravated when there is the very real possibility that the developmental change will increase the chance of acute illness or other negative outcome. Examples of normal developmental changes that impact the care of a child with a chronic condition are provided in Chart 10–8.

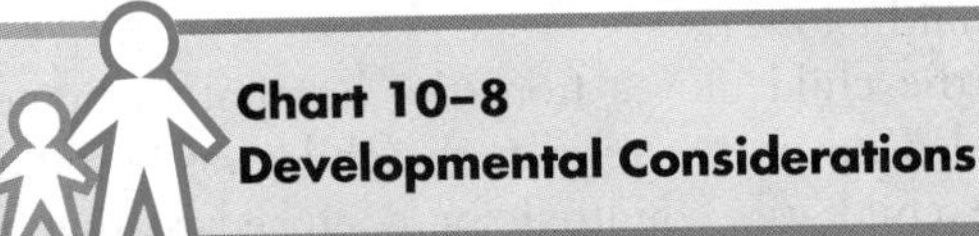

Chart 10–8
Developmental Considerations

Examples of Changes That Affect Chronic Conditions

- Newborn with a gastrostomy tube becomes an active infant, crawling across the rug, dragging his tube behind him
- Toddler with cerebral palsy shows readiness for toilet training but cannot pull her pants down over braces
- Preschooler with hemophilia is ready to start kindergarten, where a teacher will need to recognize and begin care for a bleeding joint
- School-age child with spina bifida wants to take on greater responsibility for her own urinary and bowel management and does not want Mommy's help at all
- Adolescent with sickle cell anemia begins to develop sexually and expresses hopes for marriage and children

caREminder: *Help parents learn to differentiate between behaviors resulting from developmental changes and those resulting from the chronic condition. For instance, a 2-year-old with hydrocephalus may be irritable and cranky because that is common for 2-year-old children. However, these same behaviors can be the result of increased intracranial pressure from shunt failure.*

Birth of a Subsequent Child

The birth of a subsequent child can be another critical point. Parents report they are often anxious about the new baby, as they fear the development of the symptoms that indicated the sibling's chronic condition. They may seek additional reassurance that the subsequent child is healthy or request assessment of the child even if there is no evidence that the child has any problem.

If the earlier child's problems resulted in developmental delays, the parents are often astonished, and sometimes frightened, by the rapidity of developmental change in a child without the condition. They may find the high level of activity of the unaffected child surprising. The achievements of this child can illuminate areas in which the child with the chronic condition was not able to achieve fully.

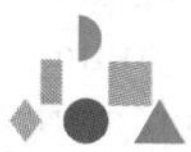

Family Responses Over the Trajectory of the Chronic Condition

Each family member responds to a chronic condition in an individual manner. Because the family is a system, these distinctive individual reactions combine to create a unique response in the family. This response is influenced by factors such as the steps the family usually takes to maintain equilibrium, the roles assumed by each family member, the family's support structures, and their prior experience with the chronic condition.

Chronic Sorrow and Sustained Uncertainty

Chronic sorrow is described by Olshansky (1962) as a natural response to a tragic event. Parents who experience chronic sorrow have recurrent and intermittent feelings of sadness, anger, guilt, or failure caused by recognition or reinforcement of the fact that their child is different. There is never full acceptance and closure. These families do not report that they are always sad. Rather they report sadness at specific times, often when the child would have achieved some developmental or social milestone but does not, or does so only with great difficulty because of the chronic condition. (See chapter 12 for further discussion of this concept.)

Sustained uncertainty is another common emotional reaction (Cohen, 1993a, 1993b, 1995b; Donnelly, 1994; Horner, 1992). Parents fear they will not be able to care for their child and find it difficult to foresee the future clearly. Parents report that these feelings are worse at the times previously described as critical points. Many report increased uncertainty when words like "high risk" are used by health care providers, when there is any change in the treatment, when symptoms increase, and at night when they find themselves alone (Cohen, 1995b; Horner, 1992). Nursing interventions to address these problems include giving accurate, clear information as soon as it is known. Test results should be reported to the parent as soon as possible after they become available. The nurse should assist the parents in their search for answers and be sure the family is fully included in the development of the plan of care (Cohen, 1995b). The nurse must be careful to review the language used to discuss the child's condition and to reassess the family continually to determine whether any words or phrases are particularly upsetting. It is part of the nurse's role to anticipate and encourage questions and expressions of concern whenever the treatment or symptoms change. When parents report fear and uncertainty associated with certain times, such as night, the health care team should work with them to identify ways they can increase support at those points.

All members of the family do not experience chronic sorrow or sustained uncertainty in the same way (Clubb, 1991; Cohen 1993b, 1995b; Shepard & Mahon, 1996). Such differences in response can be a source of additional stress between family members. They can also necessitate different approaches and nursing strategies for each family member.

The Affected Child

The response of a child to a chronic condition varies with the child's age, his or her emotional and cogniitve development, the specific condition, and the response of the individual family. The core principle is that the child is first and foremost a child. These children have been described as normal children in abnormal situations (Teague et al., 1993). Children respond with resilience and survival, not trauma and maladjustment (Eiser, 1993).

caREminder: *To keep the focus on the child as an individual, a helpful question to ask is, "What would this child be doing if he did not have this chronic condition?" Would he be playing on the rug in the living room, out in the woods with his brother, learning to use the slide at the neighborhood playground, auditioning for the school play, or quietly sleeping in his crib in a back bedroom?*

The answer to this question often gives excellent focus to a plan to promote the child's development.

Many factors influence the individual child's reaction to the presence of a chronic condition (Chart 10–9). The nurse should determine the impact of each factor on that child, because they do not affect all children the same or as may be expected (Ryan-Wenger, 1996). For example, a condition that prevents the child's attendance at school would be expected to have a negative impact on the child's learning. But if the child has access to home schooling and computer networks, or enjoys reading on many topics, the impact may be minimal.

Most children with chronic conditions progress through the usual stages of growth and development. Even those children with cognitive, developmental, or physical impairments and those whose illness makes it difficult for the child to engage in activities normal for their age group will grow and develop over time, although they may set their own pattern and pace. Each unique pattern must be recognized, assessed, and monitored if the child is to achieve optimal development (Chart 10–10).

Chart 10–9

Factors Affecting the Child's Experience of a Chronic Health Condition

Characteristics of the Child

Age of onset
Personality/temperament
Intelligence
Self-concept
Gender
Ethnic background
Developmental level
Understanding of illness
Locus-of-control beliefs

Characteristics of the Illness

Age of onset
Stable or unpredictable
Prognosis
Interference with mobility
Interference with normal activities
Visibility
Academic effects
Medications and other treatments
Intensity of care requirements
Discomfort
Nervous system involvement

Characteristics of the Family

Marital status
Number and ages of children
Parents' education
Parents' occupations
Financial situation
Strength of parents' relationship
Parents' self-esteem
Extended family support
Social support network
Ethnic background

From Perin, E. (1995). Chronic conditions. In S. Parker & B. Zuckerman (Eds.), *Behavioral and developmental pediatrics. A handbook of primary care* (pp. 95–100). Boston: Little, Brown. Reprinted with permission.

Infants

For the infant, the major psychosocial developmental milestone is the achievement of a sense of trust. Cognitively, infants progress through sensorimotor development and continue the rapid physical growth and development begun before birth.

An infant does not know that he or she has what adults call a "chronic condition." Infants do not know that their body structure, abilities, or health is any different from that of anyone else. And, when they begin to perceive themselves as different, it is simply that—different. Just as boys and girls are different, children with different body structures and abilities are different. Their major concern is anything that affects their comfort (Vessey & Swanson, 1996). The infant's major need is care that will promote his or her complex, multifaceted growth and development needs with a consideration for the unique effect of the condition on this process.

The infant with a chronic condition needs the same consistent care from consistent caregivers, preferably his or her parents, as any other infant. This care should be responsive to his or her cues and give the infant an opportunity to respond to the cues of those around him or her. The infant needs to be exposed to the same wide array of tactile, olfactory, gustatory, auditory, and sensory stimulation as infants without the condition (Lipsi, Clements-Shafer, & Rushton, 1991; Nugent, 1989; Verzemnieks, 1984) (Fig. 10–8).

Parents must refine or, in the case of a new parent, develop parenting skills that help their child achieve normal developmental milestones. This allows them to design daily activities that allow the chld to have usual experiences for infants his or her age despite restrictions caused by the condition. Research with parents has documented a strong desire in the parent to normalize the child's experience and the home environment. This can drive them to take steps to actively involve themselves and their child in all usual day-to-day events after mak-

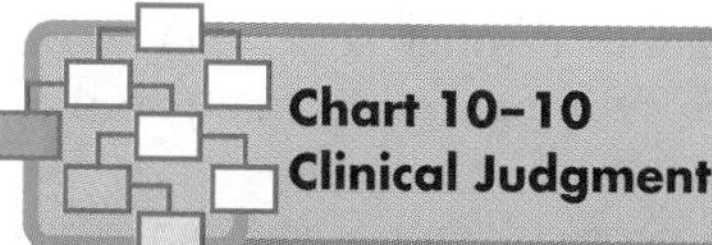

Chart 10–10
Clinical Judgment

An Adolescent with Newly Diagnosed Diabetes

David A. was 16 when he developed type I diabetes. His initial hospitalization was only 5 days long. Seven days after diagnosis, he returned to school, where he worked with his teachers and guidance counselor to modify his school day. David asked that he be moved to a different English class so that he could have lunch earlier than the 1 P.M. sixth period slot he was assigned to and for permission to leave the classroom to check his blood glucose if he felt unusual during the class day.

He continued to play soccer and socialize with his friends. This included a late night pizza party 2 nights after his discharge from the hospital. His glucose level the next morning was 385 mg/dL.

David's friends were intensely curious about his shots and diet and nicknamed his diabetes his "diabolical" condition. He was pleasantly surprised as he realized that he could do almost anything with a little preplanning. He began recording serum glucose levels between 60 and 70 mg/dL and was slow to increase his food intake after repeated counseling by the clinical nurse specialist. Six months after his diagnosis, David compared his problem with that of his friends with vision conditions. They needed glasses or contacts. He needed insulin, exercise, and a good diet.

Questions

1. What other data about David's family, friends, and health status would help you better appraise David at the time of diagnosis?
2. What assessment findings indicate that David was attempting to normalize his life after the diagnosis of type I diabetes?
3. Are there are indications that David is denying the seriousness of the diabetes?
4. You are planning to review David's self-care with him. What would you want to include in this session?
5. What outcome criteria would indicate that David has successfully adapted to the presence of his condition?

Answers

1. Which members of his family provide his greatest support? Who does he live with? Does David have any other chronic condition? What are the activities he enjoys participating in with his friends?
2. Meeting with guidance counselor, continuing prediagnosis sports activities, going out for pizza with friends and eating pizza, comparing his condition with his friends' vision problems, preplanning as needed to participate in usual activities.
3. Failing to eat enough to keep his glucose level in a normal range. Not following the prescribed diet.
4. Reassess his baseline knowledge. Discuss what is working well and what areas he is finding to be a problem. Review information about type I diabetes based on his response or the educational plan developed with David. Reinforce content on maintaining a high enough glucose level. Discuss level of participation of family in his care. (The vignette gives no indication of their knowledge level or level of participation.)
5. David is able to fully participate in prediagnostic activities with modifications needed to maintain normal glucose level, good nutrition. There are no episodes of hypo- or hyperglycemia. David is able to identify and discuss areas of concern and participate in planning actions to address these concerns. Family members are knowledgable about David's condition and how they can help him manage the condition. Family members are aware of signs of serious problem and knowledgable about actions to protect David.

ing the adaptations needed to accommodate the chronic problem. Chart 10–11 illustrates some of the ways parents can modify one aspect of infant care—feeding—to meet the normal newborn needs of a child with a chronic condition.

Many parents need to learn how to interpret the responses and behaviors of their infant. For example, the parent of a blind child needs to learn that if their child does not look at them when they talk to him or her, this does not mean the child has not heard them. Instead, this unexpected response occurs because the infant is not getting the visual reinforcement for looking back at the parent that would occur if he or she could see (Holaday, 1987).

Other parents have difficulty organizing the environment around their infant. In an attempt to be sure they

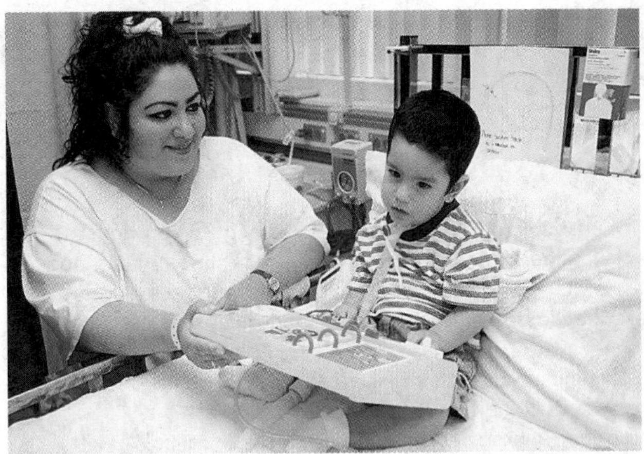

Figure 10–8
The presence of a chronic condition does not necessarily prevent the child from engaging in age-appropriate activities.

are providing enough stimulation, they offer it when the infant has not displayed any readiness cues. Later, when the child does express readiness for interaction, they fail to provide it (Phillips & Hartley, 1988).

Toddlers

Toddlers need to develop autonomy and self-control. They refine communication, fine and gross motor, social, and psychological skills through the use of language and interactions with those around them. Play is an active part of this learning, as is the chance to freely explore the environment.

An apparent need to set limits on the child's activities owing to demands of the condition, such as the use of a wheelchair or a hookup to oxygen therapy, can greatly limit the child's ability to have the learning experiences needed for development. The nurse should continually reassess whether the chronic condition is preventing the child from engaging in activities usual for his or her age and work with the family to design modifications in the environment and equipment to eliminate barriers. Constructing wide doors to allow movement from room to room, providing long oxygen tubing, or placing the non-ambulatory child on the kitchen floor so he or she can play with the pots in the cabinets support normalization activities. The child is able to do what other children his or her age can do.

Preschoolers

Preschoolers are developing a sense of initiative and need a chance to explore their environment freely. They have an initial understanding of their internal body and can comprehend simple explanations of their condition. Because the chronic condition is often one they have known all their lives, the condition itself is rarely seen as an illness, although complications can be.

Preschoolers are still very egocentric and can see a direct causal relationship between their actions and any problem that may develop. For example, the child with hemophilia who gets angry at a parent and throws all his books on the floor may see this misbehavior as the cause of his visit to the clinic the next day for administration of his routine dose of factor VIII. Preschoolers must be listened to carefully to ensure that such incorrect associations are recognized and corrected.

Preschoolers need to be around other children and adults to develop social skills. The child whose condition has limited such activities must be helped to expand his cadre of friends. Daycare centers for children with chronic illness can be instrumental in getting these children into social environments. In addition, such children are eligible for the school services discussed later in this chapter. Referral to school resources is essential.

The child must be continually reassessed to verify that special services are necessary for the child to begin school. The use of a wheelchair or adaptive device is not an absolute reason for exclusion from a regular school

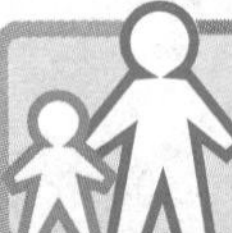

Chart 10–11
Developmental Considerations

Example of Modifications on Usual Care Activities

Situation: Infant with unrepaired esophageal stenosis has gastrostomy tube for all feedings because he cannot coordinate his ability to suck and swallow.

- Learn to identify hunger cues (crying and fussiness 2 to 3 hours after his last feeding, sucking vigorously on his pacifier, turning to items placed near his mouth with an attempt to suck), and feed him on demand.
- Pick up and hold infant while feeding is given; hold him snugly as if he was being fed orally.
- Provide a pacifier for sucking during feeding.
- Place a small amount of formula in his mouth or on his pacifier to stimulate olfactory and gustatory senses.
- Administer the feeding over the usual 10 to 15 minutes he would be expected to take the feeding orally.
- Talk and sing to him as the feeding progresses.
- Stop feeding if he stops actively sucking on the pacifier, falls asleep, or otherwise indicates that he is full.

setting. Assumptions about reasons for exclusion must be challenged frequently because we have come to realize that in the past these children were kept much too isolated and were presented with challenges much below their abilities.

School-Age Children

The major developmental task of the school-age child is the achievement of a sense of industry and accomplishment from achievement. This is most clearly seen in school but involves other aspects of the child's life, such as sports or hobbies.

Most school-age children with chronic conditions can meet these developmental achievements without difficulty. However, some conditions do make it difficult for the child to accomplish normal developmental tasks. There may be fewer opportunities for the child to have a sense of achievement. In some cases, the child does not have the physical stamina to fully participate in school activities (Vessey & Swanson, 1996). The child may have difficulty attending school regularly and, when there, may not do well because of frequent absences. Even with accomplishments in school activities, the child may find it difficult to participate in the many other activities such as sports and clubs that allow them to develop social skills and have a sense of accomplishment and pride in their work (Chart 10–12).

Parents of the school-age child may see their child as vulnerable (Ahmann & Bond, 1992), making it very difficult for them to allow the child to move on to activities outside of their direct control. The family cohe-

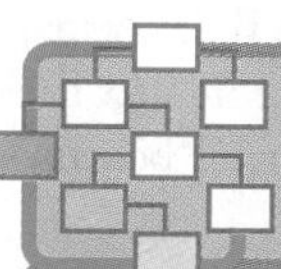

Chart 10–12
Clinical Judgment

A Child's Adaptation to Restrictions of Condition

Six-year-old Jenny G. was on bedrest at home because of recurrent congestive heart failure caused by myocarditis. Despite the fact that anything more than quiet activity made her short of breath and often worsened her failure to the degree where she would be too tired to even eat the next day, she was always sneaking out of her room and playing actively in the hall. She talked about being bored and missing all her friends and activities at school.

Jenny's teacher worked with her mother to develop a special project to be completed in conjunction with her classmates. She was put in charge of updating the classroom's dinosaur display. A giant dinosaur had been placed on a bulletin board near the front of the room. Using a collection of dinosaur cut-out books, Jenny was to get pictures of all the types of dinosaurs they discussed each day. She was also asked to practice her writing skills by putting her classmates' names on the cut-out dinosaurs that were put on the big one. To practice her arithmetic, she kept track of the number of dinosaurs she made each day and how many she sent in to her classmates by way of her friend who stopped by two or three times a week. Jenny had a great sense of pride in her accomplishment, along with quiet activity. Now that her friends have a reason to visit, they are more likely to stay to play a game after school, although they still want to play outdoors and the visits are still fairly brief. Jenny also got a 92 on her last math quiz.

Questions

1. Are these activities addressing the identified reason Jenny is not staying quiet?
2. What data from the vignette support your conclusion?
3. What other data would help confirm this conclusion?
4. What strategies would you use to promote Jenny's continued good health?
5. What outcomes would indicate that Jenny is doing well?

Answers

1. She reported feeling restless and bored and that she missed her friends from school. These activities gave her something focused to accomplish each day and allowed her to do the same activities as her classmates.
2. She is making the dinosaurs for the class, sending them in as requested, learning her math, and seeing her friends. She is also spending more quiet time at home as desired.
3. Her episodes of fatigue could be tracked. In addition, other physiologic parameters such as heart rate or blood pressure should indicate improvement.
4. Work with Jenny and her family to identify additional interventions such as this that can meet both her physiologic and psychosocial needs. Encourage Jenny to discuss her illness with her friends and to answer their questions.
5. Jenny is able to move back into the classroom easily with minimal loss of achievement as a result of her absence.

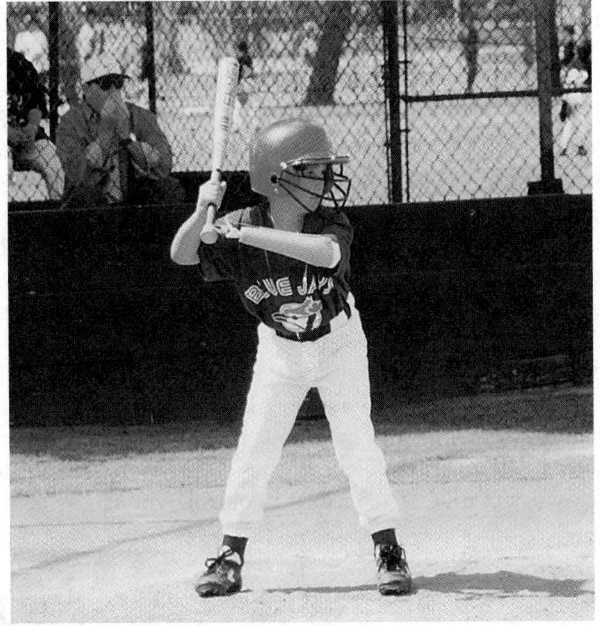

Figure 10–9
The child should be allowed to set his or her own limits and to participate in the usual wide range of activities.

sion, so beneficial earlier in the child's life, may have a negative effect on the child's development of autonomy (Dashiff, 1993).

School-age children are able to learn about their condition. With adult supervision, they can often provide for their own care needs. Parents of all school-age children need to gradually give up control of their child's day-to-day activities. This is no less true when the child has a chronic condition. However, when one of the parent's coping mechanisms has been to maintain tight control over the child's care, these normal developmental changes can be more stressful. Parents may need help identifying things the child can do on his or her own and areas where the parent needs to decrease existing levels of participation and supervision.

School-age children may also be so strongly drawn to achievement of developmental tasks of the school-age period that they find it difficult to tolerate the essential restrictions of the condition. Where the restrictions are unnecessary, they can be eliminated; where they are needed for the health of the child, they should be enforced in a way that allows to child to continue to meet developmental needs (Fig. 10–9).

Adolescents

The major task of the adolescent is the development of identity. The teen undergoes the physiologic changes of puberty and needs to integrate beliefs learned and taken in over their childhood with those they will retain as they move into adulthood. The adolescent with a chronic health condition must also face the actual and potential impact of the chronic health condition on their future and take on the responsibility for the management of the condition so they can move on to the independence of adulthood. The usual rebellion of the teenager, their strong desire to be like their peers, and difficulty in believing anything bad can happen to them are common impediments to successful completion of this stage of life (Fig. 10–10). The nurse can help the child and the family explore ways for the teen to become an active participant in their own health care, family, and community.

The adolescent must temper future plans according to the limitations of their health conditions while not overemphasizing barriers to goals or rejecting realistic possibilities (Vessey & Swanson, 1996). Often they must fight the fears and prejudices of those around them, especially adults who are ready to assign a "sick role" to the adolescent or to discourage specific activities because "they are just not realistic."

The adolescent with a chronic health condition goes through the usual developmental stages of adolescence. Changes in physical size and strength, puberty, behavioral changes, and a need to explore the world beyond that which they have known occur for them, just as they do for "normal" adolescents. Fear of rejection because they are different, as well as risk taking and rebellion directed toward treatment, is common (Ahmann & Bond, 1992). This can cause a child who has been successfully managing a condition to show a high degreee of noncompliance.

Adolescent development is more complicated in situations in which the child is not able to achieve full, or even any, independence. Such children must participate

Figure 10–10
The presence of a chronic condition does not make an adolescent immune to the usual mood swings of adolescence.

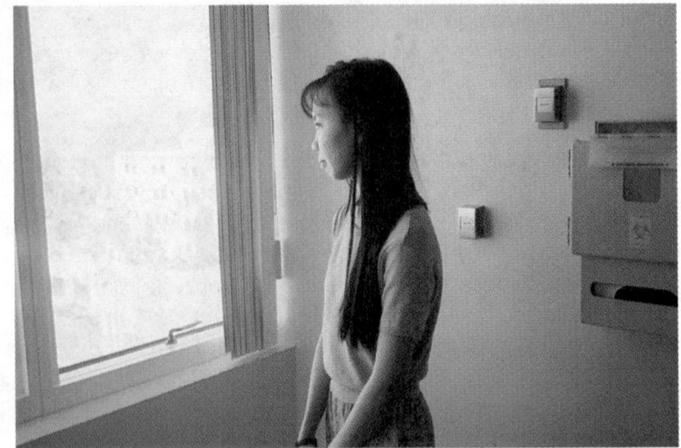

in planning for their future and be given the opportunity to achieve as many of the normal developmental tasks as possible. Even the most profoundly affected child should have responsibilities like preparing menus for the week, scheduling their own appointments, or tutoring siblings and others (Ahmann & Bond, 1992).

Opportunities for the adolescent with a chronic condition to interact with peers may be decreased. This can be caused by peer rejection, withdrawal, embarrassment, or conflict between the adolescent's perceptions of the desired self and the real self. Many of the specific challenges facing the adolescent with a chronic condition revolve around self-image and relationships with peers. This includes the development of sexuality (Selekman & McIlvain-Simon, 1991). Adolescents must deal with any direct physical effects of their condition which interfere with the development of close relationships with friends. These can include pain, fatigue, motor instability and offensive odors. The condition can alter body image, and the treatment of the condition can have detrimental effects on the adolescent's appearance, activity level, and sexual development (Selekman & McIlvain-Simon, 1991).

Nursing strategies are modifications of those used with all adolescents. The nurse must remain sensitive to the child's cultural beliefs and practices. It should be made clear to the adolescent with a chronic illness that the health team members do not expect him or her to know everything, and the nurse should try to anticipate the child's questions, and allow the adolescent to take an active part in any planning (Selekman & McIlvain-Simon, 1991).

Adolescents interviewed about activities that they found supportive identified six such activities. One was additional material support, for example, receiving more gifts or clothes than their siblings or peers. Others identified what has been called situational humanistic support. This is voluntary support offered by persons such as teachers or neighbors when they help the adolescent engage in activities or access information and advice from individuals outside the family. Professional support was that received from the health care professionals with whom they interacted. Affiliative support was that shared with children of the same age and with those who had had similar life experiences. Emotional support had multiple dimensions. Advisory support was that which helped them learn how to handle bothersome situations. Safety support was that which helped them remain safe, whether they were in the neighborhood or in the hospital. Self-ideal emotional support was the support in the assurance that you are loved for yourself (Brydolf & Segesten, 1996). Nurses can help children with chronic conditions access each of these types of support and help their parents understand their potential value to the adolescent.

An additional concern of the adolescent is the need to move from pediatric service providers to those who work primarily with adults (Telfair, Myers, & Drezner, 1994). Many adult care practitioners have little experience in the treatment of these problems previously limited to childhood only. Both the adolescent and health care providers need help in the transition of care (Chart 10–13).

Response of Parents

Parental response to the presence of a chronic condition in one of their children is highly individualized. Although the presence of a chronic condition in a child can be a source of stress and family dysfunction, there is no significant difference in divorce rates between these parents and parents with unaffected children (Eiser, 1993). However, with the overall high divorce rate, many chronically ill children live with a divorced parent and often with a step-parent.

Assessment of the parents should include exploration of the parents' perception of how well the child is able to participate in normal age-appropriate activities (Ahmann & Bond, 1992). Interviews should be adapted to the developmental stage of the child and his or her chronic condition and should include discussion of how the condition affects the child, family, and the child's and the family's friends (Chart 10–14).

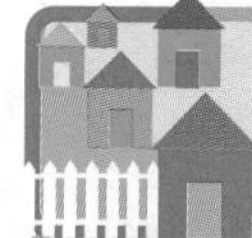

Chart 10–13
Community Care

Information Needs of Adolescents with a Chronic Condition

- How to solve their own health care problems and care for their own health needs
- How to locate and access adult health care programs and providers who can meet their needs
- How to educate others about their chronic condition
- How to deal with health care providers who are not familiar with their condition
- How to help adult health care providers learn what works for them as individuals

Adapted by permission of Elsevier Science, Inc., from Telfair, J., Myers, J., & Drezner, S. (1994). Transfer as a component of the transition of adolescents with sickle cell disease to adult care: Adolescent, adult, and parent perspectives. *Journal of Adolescent Health, 15*, 558–565. Copyright 1994 by the Society for Adolescent Medicine.

Chart 10–14

Parental Interview Questions on Impact of Condition on Child and Family

- Tell me how you think your child's condition has affected him/her and your family.
- Tell me about your child and school.
  Explore:
  Transportation concerns
  Academic achievement
  Reactions of classmates and teacher
  Participation in field trips and other special activities
- Tell me about your child's ability to dress and toilet himself/herself.
  Explore:
  Concerns about appearance
  Detail regarding self-care abilities
- Tell me about your child's participation in chores around the house. How does this compare with that of your other children?
- Tell me about disciplining your child. How does this compare with discipline for your other children?
- Tell me about your child's friendships.
  Explore:
  Rejections by previous friends
  Having friends over
- Tell me about what your child does for fun.
  Explore:
  Previous favorite pastimes
  Group activities
- Tell me about what you do together as a family.
- What are some things you would like to be able to do?

Adapted from Ahmann, E., & Bond, N. J. (1992). Promoting normal development in school-age children and adolescents who are technology dependent: A family centered model. *Pediatric Nursing, 18,* 399–405. Used with permission.

The parents' responses would guide the remainder of the interview and the subsequent teaching and support interventions. If the parent reported few family activities or a list of things they wish they could do but feel are forbidden to them now, an in-depth discussion of perceived barriers and an exploration of ways they can be eliminated or overcome can follow. If the parent discusses only the child with the chronic illness or seems to treat him or her unnecessarily differently from siblings, discussion of the needs of the other children can be pursued. If a rich variety of friends and activities are reported, the positive nature of these interactions can be reinforced and the parent encouraged to share his or her and the children's plans for the future.

Parents express a need for information, interpersonal interactions, and support (Edwards-Beckett & Cedargren, 1995). They focus on actions that help them maintain family stability (Hayes, 1992). Parents constantly work to resolve the uncertainty of the chronic condition and to normalize the experience of both the child with the chronic condition and the family as a whole (Cohen, 1995b). Many parents work to maintain their relationship to the child as a parent not simply as a paraprofessional, even when they are able to provide much of the care and do the case management themselves. This enables them to step back and allow health professionals to provide care in many situations while they meet the child's needs through their parental role.

Parents also engage in normalization activities. Parents work to engage in behaviors that demonstrate to others that this is a family just like any other. The child with the chronic condition is often teated as just another member of the family with a full share of responsibilities (Shepard & Mahon, 1996). This can be very positive because the child has all the usual childhood needs and generally benefits from being challenged just like his or her siblings.

Much of the research on parenting a child with a chronic condition has focused on mothers because they are often the primary caregivers for the child. Mothers tend to focus their efforts on managing the child's symptoms. Some choose not to work and others are not able to work because of the care demands of the child. Mothers must be carefully assessed and supported; studies evaluating the functional status of the chronically ill child indicate that the child's adjustment related more to the mother's stress level than to the intensity of the child's symptoms (Shepard & Mahon, 1996).

Studies of the fathers of children with chronic conditions indicate that many are actively involved, although their concerns may differ from those of mothers (Fig. 10–11). For example, some fathers are less concerned with physical symptoms because they are less involved with dealing with those symptoms. Other fathers are concerned with the financial aspects of the care and take on full responsibility for one or more areas of the child's care (Boyd, Vollmer, & Valanis, 1993; May, 1991).

Another concern of some fathers is continued involvement in the child's treatment decisions if the parents are divorced and the child lives with the mother. This is an issue even when the parents have joint custody (May, 1991).

Not all children with chronic conditions are cared for by their biological parents. Many live with foster families, making it essential that issues related to custody and consent by clarified. Foster parents need education

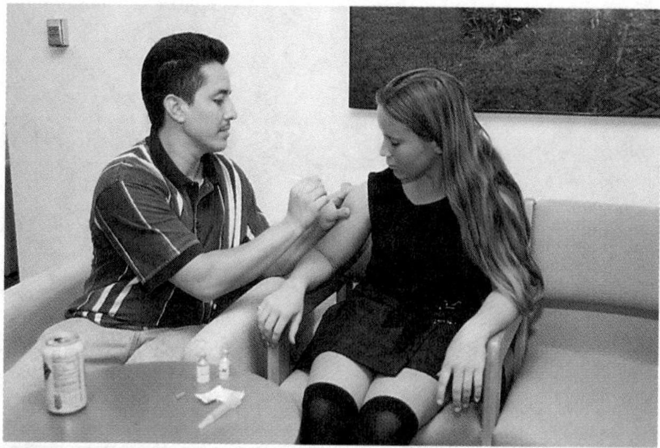

Figure 10–11
Fathers should be encouraged to participate in the care of their child.

and support just as do natural parents. A unique characteristic of these families that they often have several special needs children in the home, making interactions with the health care system difficult.

Another group of children with chronic conditions live in their adopted families. Adoptive parents report less guilt than biological parents, because they know they are not the cause of the condition if it was congenital. However, they still face the other challenges of the parent of a child with a chronic condition, and they need the same level of education and support (Smith & Sherwen, 1984).

Response of Siblings

Although it is widely believed that siblings of children with chronic conditions have additional problems when compared with siblings of children without chronic conditions, this does not occur universally (Thompson, Curtner, & O'Rear, 1944). In fact, on measures of social competence or behavior maladjustment, siblings of chronically ill children do not consistently demonstrate any deficits (Eiser, 1993; Gallo, Breitmayer, Knafl, & Zoeller, 1992; Stewart et al., 1993). When there are problems, they often relate more to family structure, their inability to control the illness, and personal characteristics of the child or parents (Gallo, Breitmayer, Knafl, & Zoeller, 1993; Thompson et al., 1994). Siblings were found to have more household responsibilities and child care responsibilities (Faux, 1993; Williams et al., 1993).

Even though the research studies on siblings of children with chronic conditions did not demonstrate a higher rate of difficulties, this does not mean that individual children do not have problems (Stewart et al., 1993). Each family, and the siblings within each family, must be evaluated as a unique unit, just as it would be done in any other aspect of nursing practice (Chart 10–15).

In many cases, the distress of the siblings is related to higher degrees of parental, particularly maternal, stress. Thus steps that help to decrease this stress may be beneficial to the children as well as the parents. Siblings often find support groups to be helpful (Faux, 1993).

Often the response of the nonaffected child is one of jealousy of the attention given to the affected child. This

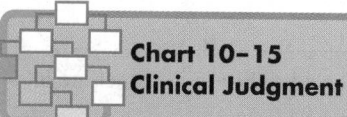

Chart 10–15
Clinical Judgment

Sibling of a Child with a Chronic Condition

Lili and Nica are 3½-year-old twins. Lili has spastic diplegia cerebral palsy (CP), which has necessitated her wearing braces, using a walker, and receiving assistance getting on and off the toilet. Nica has no health problems. Their parents report that sometimes Lili says she wishes that she "had legs like Nica's," but more often Nica says, "I wish I had cerebral palsy." Their parents report the following story during a routine health assessment for Lili and ask for your guidance in handling the situation.

One day, a piano tuner came over to check the family piano. Lili and Nica were sitting on the couch and were introduced. Lili piped up, "I have cerebral palsy, my legs aren't strong like Nica's, and I can't run to the potty myself. I wear braces because I have cerebral palsy, but I'm getting stronger, and I can walk in my walker." The piano tuner said to her, "Well, I'm sure there are lots of people to help you to the potty and to walk." To which Lili replied, seriously "Yes, that's right." Nica looked sad that she didn't have something special to tell the piano tuner. She put down the picture she had been enthusiastically working on for the last half hour and went out of the room.

Chart continued on following page

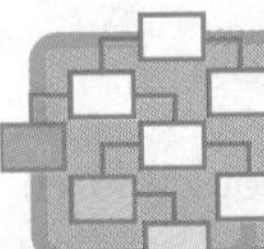

Chart 10–15
Clinical Judgment *Continued*

Sibling of a Child with a Chronic Condition

Questions

1. What additional information would you try to elicit from the twins' parents before addressing their concerns? What would you look for in the twins' interactions if they were both present?
2. What are the signs that Nica may be having difficulty adapting to having a sibling with a chronic condition?
3. Do you think Nica is having a problem because her sister has a chronic condition?
4. What steps could the family take to assist and support Nica?
5. What outcomes would indicate that the twins are developing as expected?

Answers

1. Is this common behavior or does it occur only occasionally? Are there times when Nica is the one who is boasting rather than Lili? What other indications of expected sibling rivalry are present? Are there any times when it seems to occur more or less often? If Lili and Nica are both present, how do they interact with each other? Does Lili dominate the interaction, or does Nica appear to be on an even par with her sister?
2. Her comments about her sister and her failure to engage in the common sibling exchange in which each tries to best the other in achievements and for attention. The fact that she did not show off her drawing.
3. Without repeated observations it is impossible to answer this question. Although the behaviors indicated that she is having difficulties and may be depressed, the practitioner would need to verify this as part of a pattern.
4. Fully inform both girls of all events in the family, including facts about Lili's condition. Reassess their interactions to see whether they are focusing more than is needed on Lili and her accomplishments and problems to the exclusion of Nica. Work with family to develop a plan to have times at which Nica is the center of attention to balance the time Lili must be. If Nica's behavior remains negative or if she begins to actively withdraw or stop engaging in activities, refer to a family counselor.
5. Both girls continue to develop a relationship as sisters; each has opportunities to develop personal interests. Each sister may still want something that the other sister has, while still being happy for who she is.

normal sibling reaction is aggravated by the presence of real situations in which the brother or sister does in fact get more attention as a result of his or her health condition. The parents face the conflict of wanting and needing to support and encourage the child with the chronic condition without ignoring, abandoning, or failing to meet the needs of the child without the condition.

As siblings of a child with a chronic condition get older, it is not uncommon for them to take an active role in the care of the affected sibling. This is more noticeable in female siblings of the affected child, who commonly take a greater role in the caretaking activities (Faux, 1993). Parents need to remain sensitive to the fact that the sibling should not be made to feel that they must provide the care.

Siblings should be assessed at the time of diagnosis and periodically thereafter to determine their support needs, comprehension of the illness, and learning needs

Figure 10–12
Siblings need to be fully informed about their sibling's care needs and condition and should be allowed to participate in care activities as much as they wish to.

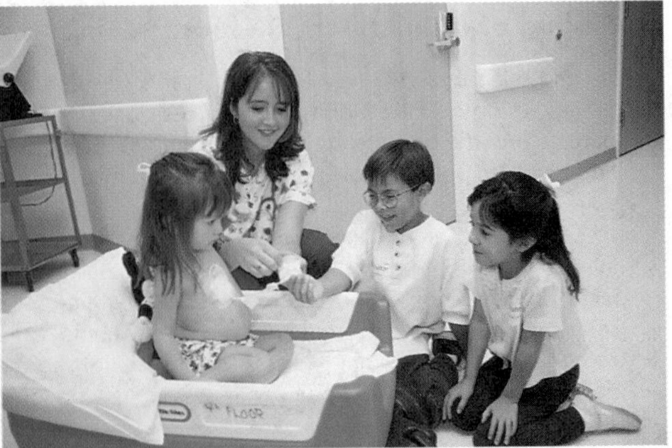

(Faux, 1993). (TIP 10–2). Because siblings are also at risk of stress during hospitalization and surgery of their brother or sister, they should be included in preparation activities. Infants and toddlers should be well supported at home if they cannot accompany the family to the hospital. Sibling visitation for older children should be allowed if desired by the sibling and family (Faux, 1993) (see Chapter 9).

Researchers have found that healthy siblings are often poorly informed about their sibling's illness (Eiser, 1993). Assessing what parents have discussed with them and what parents have avoided discussing illuminates areas in which the family needs assistance (Fig. 10–12). Communication techniques such as active listening should be taught as needed. Parents may need help initiating discussions of the implications of marriage and childbearing with the siblings as well as the child with the chronic condition. This area can be especially difficult if the chronic condition in the sibling has a potential impact on childbearing in all of the children, as often occurs in genetic diseases (Faux, 1993).

Anticipatory guidance about developmental issues can help parents understand normal sibling responses. This will help the parent gear communication to the

TIP 10–2 A Teaching Intervention Plan for the Sibling of a Child with a Chronic Condition

Nursing Diagnosis and Family Outcomes

- Knowledge deficit: condition and the effect it will have on the affected sibling, their family, and themselves

Outcomes:

Sibling will understand the reason actions related to the chronic condition are being taken.
Sibling will identify how he or she can participate in the child's care.

Instructional Interventions

Verify baseline knowledge.

- What have they been told by their sibling, their parents, friends, or health care providers?
- What questions do they have about the condition, how it affects their sibling, and how it affects themselves?
- Do they know anyone else with this condition?
- What do they most want to learn now?

Assess sibling's involvement with child with chronic condition.

- Do they ever need to help with care?
- What do they wish they could do? What do they wish they did not have to do?
- Are there any activities they would like to participate in which are not allowed because of their sibling's needs?
- How are their friendships affected by the presence of the sibling's chronic condition?

Design teaching plan based on sibling assessment.

- Be specific and increase detail as cognitive ability, age, and interest increase. Do not hide facts of the condition.
- Begin teaching items they are most curious and concerned about.

Present content using standard teaching principles.

- Use vocabulary understood by the child while teaching medical language that he or she may hear in the future.
- Adapt teaching approach to accommodate the sibling's cognitive and physical development (more pictures with preschoolers; pamphlets, books, and computer programs for school-age siblings).
- Encourage questions.
- Explore questions for possible concerns not evident in questions.
- Provide source of backup for later questions.

Sibling support group

- Provide sibling support group.

child's personality and development while not supressing normal sibling responses like jealousy and envy (Faux, 1993).

Response of Other Family Members

Parents consistently report that support from family members and friends is valuable. The social support they receive from these individuals helps them establish and maintain equilibrium within their lives.

Determination of who these other family members are should be a part of the initial and ongoing assessment. The genogram can illuminate such relationships. Family members who are supportive of the parents should be included in teaching sessions when possible, to increase their ability to provide specialized care such as use of an apnea monitor or application of braces. The nurse should assess the family members for fears of caring for the child or doing what they would like to do with the child because of the condition. Because these fears are usually unfounded, gentle encouragement may help them go beyond them.

In cases in which the care is very complex, not all family members will be able to learn to participate in the child's care. In these cases, they can be encouraged to continue to do the non–care-related activities they would do if the child did not have the condition. Grandparents can hold, snuggle, read to, and play with children even if there is some aspect of their condition they cannot care for.

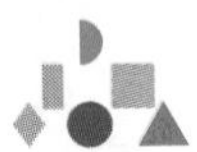

Interventions to Promote Health and Normalization

Regardless of the impact of the chronic condition on the child's day-to-day life, interventions aimed at promoting the child's optimal health and well-being are needed. The goals of these interventions are both to maximize health despite the presence of the condition and to address the health maintenance issues faced by all children discussed in Chapter 6. The outcome will be that the child establishes a normal state for himself or herself that meets his or her needs.

Management by the Interdisciplinary Team

Children with chronic conditions often need the help of many individuals; including nurses, nurse practitioners, clinical nurse specialists, physicians of many types, social workers, dietitians, other family members, and friends. This makes an interdisciplinary approach to care with high-level case management essential (Davis & Steel, 1991; Urbano, von Windeguth, Siderits, & Studenic-Lewis, 1989).

Parents report that they often go from agency to agency where individual aspects of the chronic condition are addressed. This necessitates repeated visits to agencies and clinics, which can be stressful, expensive, and exhausting for all involved. Despite all the visits and all the specialists they see, often no one asks about or monitors normal developmental issues or helps them pull it all together.

Consistent care by professional nurses, both nurse practitioners and general practice pediatric nurses, improves the ability of the child and family to adjust to the chronic condition. Children whose care was managed by nurses have been found to have significantly less anxiety, better scholastic competence, and better scores on behavioral and self-worth measures (Pless et al., 1994). Families report that they prefer care provided in the home by professional nurses (Patterson et al., 1994; Ray & Ritchie, 1993; Scannell, Gilles, Biordi, & Child, 1993).

The services parents want from a case manager include help in finding community resources and understanding individual educational plans (Davis & Steele, 1991). Parents also want information about the condition itself, treatment options, parent suport groups, and ways to contact other families with similar needs. Assistance with completing applications for services and help with obtaining family counseling, adaptive equipment, and respite services are expected of case managers. Calls and home visits as well as direct care activities are also desired by some parents. The need for parents to remain central and in control of child care is evidenced by the fact that in one study 32 of 58 parents stated that they preferred to be the case manager themselves or to comanage the child's care with a health care provider (Davis & Steele, 1991).

Well-Child Care in the Presence of a Chronic Condition

The interventions needed to promote well-child care can be overlooked because of the intensity of actions required to manage the chronic condition. Careful assessment and a focus on the developmental needs of the child can ensure that such interventions are not omitted. Developmental surveillance, an active and continuous assessment process of the child, should be instituted to identify and to intervene with children at risk for developmental problems. (See Chapter 4 for more discussion of this concept.)

Although care paths are typically used to guide care

during episodes of acute exacerbations (e.g., sepsis, pneumonia), interdisciplinary plans can also be useful to direct care that promotes and maintains wellness. A care path for the child with a chronic condition has specific outcomes that address the condition itself (e.g., when anticonvulsant dosages should be reevaluated as the child gains weight) and more general outcomes with plans for the child's need for education, health promotion, and changes in self-care activities. The specific items that are monitored for each child are based on his or her individual needs (Care Path 10–1). The health care team can utilize the care path to ensure that all aspects of care are being monitored and reevaluated as necessary over the course of time.

Promoting Growth and Development

Recurrent hospitalizations, limited mobility, decreased opportunities to interact with family and peers, altered nutrition, the condition itself, and the side effects of needed medications are but a few of the reasons individual children with chronic health conditions are at risk for al-

Text continued on page 561

Care Path 10–1 An Interdisciplinary Plan of Care for the Child with a Chronic Condition

Nursing Diagnosis	Patient/Family Intermediate Outcomes			
	Time of diagnosis	Discharge from agency to home	Six months	One year and yearly
Altered growth and development due to presence of a chronic condition	Family will have knowledge of child's current developmental capabilities.	Family will have knowledge of developmental milestones the child should achieve in next year.	Child will progress developmentally according to his or her own ability.	Family will have clear picture of child's current developmental capabilities and what milestones child should achieve in next year.
Self-care deficit related to impairments associated with chronic condition	All family members will acquire knowledge about chronic condition.	Family members will be able to carry out needed skills to manage child's chronic condition. Child will receive needed care in safe, supportive home environment.	Family members incorporate new repertoire of skills as necessitated by child's condition. ⟶	Child will increase participation in care as appropriate to physical, cognitive, and social development.
Alteration in family processes secondary to diagnosis, and adjustments to child's chronic condition	Family will acknowledge potential impact of child's condition in family life.	⟶	Family will exhibit positive adjustment to child's condition and related changes in family lifestyle. Siblings will have own developmental needs met.	⟶ ⟶
Grieving (potentially dysfunctional) secondary to diagnosis of chronic condition	Family will verbalize feelings regarding child's condition.	⟶	Family will develop repertoire of coping mechanisms to successfully deal with child's condition.	Family will successfully complete the grieving process.

Care Path continued on following page

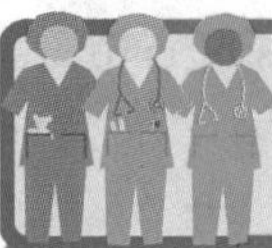

Care Path 10-1 An Interdisciplinary Plan of Care for the Child with a Chronic Condition *Continued*

Nursing Diagnosis	Patient/Family Intermediate Outcomes			
	Time of diagnosis	Discharge from agency to home	Six months	One year and yearly
Risk for caregiver role strain secondary to demands of child's care and other personal responsibilities	Caregiver will identify role and responsibilities in relation to self, other family members, and affected child.	⟶	Caregiver will participate in activities to relieve role strain. Caregiver will have positive balance between demands of illness and other personal needs.	⟶ ⟶
Risk for impaired social interaction secondary to limitations and stigma associated with chronic condition	Child will gain support from familiar social interactions during initial stages of condition.	⟶	Child will have maximum possible participation in peer and school activities and learning.	⟶
Care Intervention Categories				
Consults	Needed medical and nursing specialists for diagnosis and treatment of condition. Social worker for assistance to condition-specific programs and services. Home care agency/nursing for continued care of complex problems. School health to facilitate continued education or return to school.	Assign/identify case managers. Verify that initial consultations/referrals have been accomplished. Provide names of parent/community support persons. Make initial contact, if needed.	Reassess adequacy of initial referrals. Work with family to make additional referrals, modify contacts. Verify that family is using support services. If not, or if not effective, modify plan.	Modify referrals as needed by changes in child's condition or child/family's continued development.
Developmental Assessment	Complete baseline developmental assessment appropriate to child's physical and cognitive abilities. Compare with prior assessments, if available.	Parents/caretakers will describe how to adapt usual activities to continue to promote growth and development.	Assess growth and development and implement interventions to correct any areas with deficits. Work with family to adapt care to promote usual developmental activities.	Reassess growth and development. Assist family/child to take steps necessary to ensure exposure to usual experiences that promote development. As child matures, increase child's involvement in care.

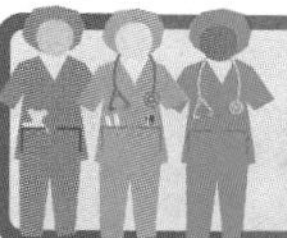

Care Path 10-1 An Interdisciplinary Plan of Care for the Child with a Chronic Condition *Continued*

Care Intervention Categories	Time of diagnosis	Discharge from agency to home	Six months	One year and yearly
Family Support	Support family's initial reaction: grief response, shock, fear, anxiety. Educate family and members of their support systems regarding normalcy of reaction. Help family modify reactions that are not helping them cope effectively.	Verify family has begun to make needed changes to adapt to presence of chronic condition. Confirm referral to support programs in community (parent support group, home care, social worker).	Determine whether new patterns are conducive to function of family, adaptive to presence of chronic condition. Family taking active role in making needed changes in structure, function, and relationships. Help family modify interactions as needed.	Evaluate patterns to verify they are changing as child and family continue to develop and mature. Make additional referrals as warranted, based on reassessment of family.
Immunizations	Assess current immunization status. Identify needed immunization. Clarify valid contraindications to immunizations.	Administer immunizations identified as needed or past due. Add special immunization as needed because of condition to immunization schedule.	Review immunization history. Administer immunizations identified as needed or past due. Initiate steps to eliminate/bypass barriers to immunization.	Verify that immunizations are up to date. Administer immunizations needed at this time.
Medications	Provide family with information regarding medications child is receiving. Discuss which of these may be continued upon discharge.	Evaluate family knowledge regarding medications. Discuss methods of home administration of the medications. Determine whether family has necessary equipment and supply of medication to administer at home. Discuss side effects of medications and administration when the child is ill.	Evaluate medication dosage, compliance, and need based on child's current health status, weight, age, and any side effects noted by family.	⟶

Care Path continued on following page

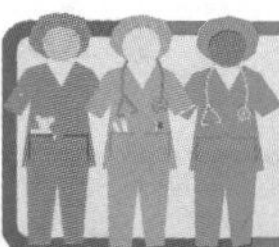

Care Path 10–1 An Interdisciplinary Plan of Care for the Child with a Chronic Condition *Continued*

Care Intervention Categories	Time of diagnosis	Discharge from agency to home	Six months	One year and yearly
Nutrition	Complete nutritional assessment. Develop plan to modify family diet if needed to meet child's current health needs.	Implement changes in child and family's diet as needed. Evaluate child's ability to have nutritional plan followed at daycare or school settings.	Evaluate child's growth and nutritional status. Based on this evaluation, implement retraining of family and/or dietary changes if needed.	⟶
Pain Management	Assess need for pain management. Develop consistent method to evaluate child's level of pain. Implement pain management measures.	Evaluate continuing need for pain management measures. Teach parents how to assess child's pain and intervene. Teach child nonpharmacologic and pharmacologic measures to manage pain.	⟶ ⟶	⟶ ⟶
Play/School	Determine impact of chronic condition on child's ability to participate in school activities.	Contact school nurse/teacher to discuss any needed modifications in child's activities.	Verify that needed modifications have been implemented and that unneeded restrictions are not in place.	Assess for needed changes based on child's physical and cognitive development and progression through school. Implement new teaching support as needed.
Psychosocial	Assess for signs of grief reaction: denial, anger, bargaining, acceptance.	Acknowledge grief reaction. Support family. Educate family and support persons of normal grief reaction.	Evaluate ongoing grief reaction and signs of resolution. Refer for continued support, as needed.	Assess for ongoing grief or for events that cause new grief reaction.
Rehabilitation and Habilitation	Assess home for barriers to care of child and his or her condition. Initial home care referral.	Help parents/caregivers learn new care activities. Verify that modifications in home environment have been made. Confirm home care referral complete: equipment delivered to home, family knows how to use it, and it is appropriate to that home.	Reassess home care needs. Further modify environment to meet child/family's social, safety, and developmental needs. Initiate additional interventions to meet needs.	⟶ ⟶

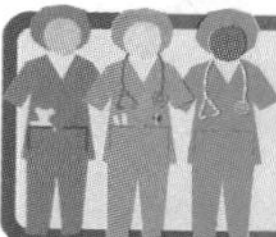

Care Path 10–1 An Interdisciplinary Plan of Care for the Child with a Chronic Condition *Continued*

Care Intervention Categories	Time of diagnosis	Discharge from agency to home	Six months	One year and yearly
Self-Care	Determine child's ability to participate in own care. Educate child regarding self-care. Determine baseline knowledge, skills, experiences of family, existing parenting skills, learning style.	Assess parents for fear of allowing child to do self-care. Verify that child's self-care activities are appropriate for condition and age. Provide education regarding care essential to safety of child. Give additional learning materials in format appropriate to family. Refer to visiting nurse/home care/other source of support to assist with complex care.	Determine effectiveness of self-care activities. Assess child to determine whether there are additional areas where he or she can or should care for self. Reevaluate self-care skills of child. Initiate teaching in style appropriate to child/family to supplement skills, correct problems. Determine future needs based on changes in condition of child/family.	Reevaluate self-care and increased responsibilities as child matures. Help parents release responsibilities to child. Assess whether child has decreasing ability to care for self (e.g., with muscular dystrophy) and work with him or her to allow others to help. Reevaluate and modify as needed.
Sibling Support	Determine number, age, sex of all siblings and their usual level of interaction with child/family. Explore siblings' knowledge of condition and family's expectations of siblings.	Discuss sibling needs with family. Include siblings in education settings, health care visits. Help family understand that even young children (3–5 yr) feel changes because of chronic illness diagnosis.	Analyze impact of chronic condition of child on sibling. Initiate needed education and support for child and family.	Reassess sibling needs as they change as a result of their development or changes in child's condition. Work with family to implement support care for sibling.

tered growth and development (Chart 10–16). Nursing's role is to recognize the barriers to achieving developmental milestones faced by each child and then to collaborate with the family and child to design interventions to overcome or ameliorate the barriers (Chart 10–17) (Revell & Liptak, 1991).

Chapter 4 provides a summary of the numerous developmental assessment tools available to evaluate children of all ages and physical capabilities. When selecting an assessment tool, consider the child's specific condition and whether or not that condition, in and of itself, would make it impossible for the child to demonstrate the skills or competencies reflected on that test (Vessey & Swanson, 1996). For example, many of the tests of cognitive ability designed for infants assume that the child has normal motor development; such tests may not be appropriate for a child with spastic cerebral palsy or spina bifida.

Assessment of development has multiple components, and each of these must be evaluated in the child with a chronic condition. These include physical, behavioral, psychodynamic, sociologic, family and child interac-

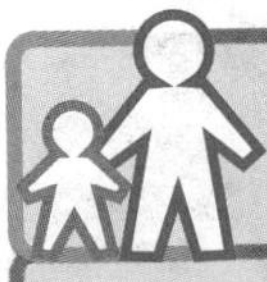

Chart 10–16
Developmental Considerations

Potential Effects of Chronic Conditions on Development

Stage	Expected Developmental Achievements	Potential Barriers to Developmental Achievements	Strategies to Promote Development
Infant	Sense of trust and security Sensorimotor skills Gross motor control	Parental grief Altered feeding experiences Restriction of movement Hospitalization(s) Painful procedures Chronic discomfort Multiple caregivers Inconsistent routines Lack of consistent response to infant cues	Provide consistent care from a limited number of caregivers Establish reciprocity—caregiver responds to infant's cues and infant is given opportunity to respond to caregiver's cues Expose infant to normal range of environmental stimuli while ensuring periods without stimuli Assist parents in the development of attachment and caregiving/parenting roles Enroll in early intervention program if appropriate
Toddler	Autonomy and self-control Increasing gross and fine motor skills Independent activity Development of speech Cognitive and social growth Initial development of egocentric thought Normal negativism; confrontations over everyday activities, especially feeding and discipline	Negative responses to anything that is restrictive Parents desire to control all activities Limited interaction with other children and adults beyond family Parental conflict between need to discipline and need to complete life-sustaining care Decreased quality and quantity of play opportunities	Teach and support development of usual parenting skills Encourage active interactions with environment and people in the environment (e.g., mobility devices as needed; playing on floor; going out in neighborhood, to mall, to see family and friends) Encourage full range of play activities to develop social, fine and gross motor ability, and cognitive skills Set limits as usual Support parents as child becomes more active and less under their complete control
Preschool	Initiative Egocentrism increases Beginning to understand internal body, but thought processes still pre-operational Still understands events only through his or her own experience with them Varying understanding of body function and illness	Medication requirements Dietary restriction Mobility restriction or inability to be mobile without assistance Need for adult supervision but need to be with peers Repeated separations from famiily Caregiver difficulty with limit setting	Promote active involvement with environment Enroll in activities (preschool, daycare) that allow interaction with other children Identify and correct incorrect associations between events and causes Begin education about condition Allow and encourage participation in self-care activities

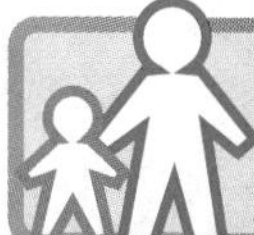

Chart 10–16
Developmental Considerations *Continued*

Potential Effects of Chronic Conditions on Development

Stage	Expected Developmental Achievements	Potential Barriers to Developmental Achievements	Strategies to Promote Development
School-Age	Industry Sense of accomplishment/mastery from activities undertaken Begin development of independence from family Develop relationships with peers, school, play groups Refine gross and fine motor, cognitive, and social skills	Differences from peers Dependence on medical care Restriction on independence Requirements for adult monitoring Medication, dietary, activity requirements/restriction School absences Inability to fully participate in desired activities	Promote full participation in school Explore ways to increase stamina and decrease exhaustion Help parents deal with fears related to vulnerability of child Identify barriers to achievement and develop plan to overcome or bypass them Educate about normal changes caused by conditions Encourage increasing self-care Encourage child to develop strategies to deal with negative aspects of condition
Adolescence	Sense of identity Increased independence from family Develop problem-solving skills, abstract thought Fuller understanding of body function and condition Accept changes in body image: rapid physical growth, sexual maturation Prepare for life as an adult; choice of vocation Reluctance to accept own vulnerability, leading to increased risk-taking activities	Altered body image Decreased growth Visible deformity Need for adult supervision and/or assistance with daily activities Medication and dietary requirements Possible vocational limitation Development of sexuality Need to explain condition to others	Educate about normal changes of adolescence Explore questions related to sexuality Prepare for transition to adult caregivers Explore sources of social problems Continue education about condition, care of condition Encourage active participation in decisions about own care Reevaluate level of participation in own care and increase if appropriate Integrate care requirements into daily activities

tion, and cognitive development (Revell & Liptak, 1991).

Physical development includes the progressive attainment of abilities such as gross and fine motor skills, vision, speech, and language. Behavioral development addresses the social learning, bonding, and attachment that occurs over childhood as well as the achievement of coping and self-help skills. Psychodynamic development describes the psychosocial development of the child throughout childhood. Sociologic development examines the nature and types of unique relationships the child has with adults and other children. Family systems describe the relationship (fit) between the child's personality (temperament, ability to interact) and that of each parent and the family unit (Revell & Liptak, 1991).

The last of the development areas that must be evaluated is cognitive. Children with certain conditions, such as Down syndrome, often have cognitive deficits that are part of the the pathology of the condition. But other children, such as those with cerebral palsy, may appear to have cognitive deficits because of a lack of exposure to significant learning activities or a failure of the instru-

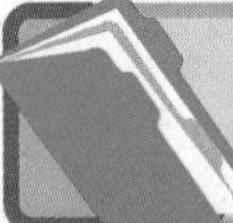

Chart 10–17
Nursing Interventions Classification (NIC)

Normalization Promotion

Definition

Assisting parents and other family members of children with chronic illnesses or disabilities in providing normal life experiences for their children and families

Activities

Promote development of membership of child into family system without letting child become central focus of family.
Assist family to view affected child as a child first, rather than a chronically ill or disabled individual.
Provide opportunities for child to have normal childhood experiences.
Encourage interaction with normal peers.
Deemphasize uniqueness of child's condition.
Encourage parents to make child appear as normal as possible.
Assist family in avoiding potentially embarrassing situations with child.
Assist family in making changes in home environment that decrease reminders of child's special needs.
Determine accessibility of activity and child's ability to participate in activity.
Identify adaptations needed to accommodate child's limitations, so child can participate in normal activites.
Communicate information about child's condition to those who need this information to provide safe supervision or appropriate educational opportunities for child.
Assist family in altering prescribed therapeutic regimen to fit normal schedule, when appropriate.
Assist family in advocating for child in school system to ensure access to appropriate education programs.
Encourage child to participate in school and community activities appropriate for developmental and ability level.
Encourage parents to have same parenting expectations and techniques for affected child as with other children in family, as appropriate.
Encourage parents to spend time with all children in family.
Involve siblings in care and activities of child, as appropriate.
Determine need for respite care for parents or other care providers.
Identify resources for respite care in community.
Encourage parents to take time to care for their personal needs.
Provide information to family about child's condition, treatment, and associated support groups for families.
Encourage parents to balance involvement in special programs for child's special needs and normal family and community activities.
Encourage family to maintain usual social network and support system.
Encourage family to maintain usual family habits, rituals, and routines.

From McCloskey, J., & Bulechek, G. (1996). *Nursing interventions classification (NIC)* (2nd ed.). St. Louis: Mosby–Year Book. Reprinted with permission.

ment to accurately evaluate children who do not have the motor skills needed to demonstrate intelligence on that instrument (Revell & Liptak, 1991).

Nutrition

Many chronic conditions make it difficult for the child to remain well nourished. Nutrition should be evaluated in two ways. The first way is to verify that the child is taking in an appropriate mix of nutrients. The second step is to evaluate the effect of that nutrition on the child's physical growth. The first assessment ascertains whether the needed nutrients are available, and the second verifies that desired outcomes are being achieved.

Nutrient intake may be determined by a careful history that obtains information about the child's typical dietary intake. Elicit the route (oral/enteral/parenteral), types, and amounts of nutrients. To evaluate the effect of nutrition on physical growth, the nurse should determine whether the child has achieved normal parameters for physical growth. Is the child on target for height, weight, head circumference, and other relevant measures of growth? In young children, because brain growth is a priority, nutritional deficiency is first reflected in decreased height and weight growth along the child's growth curve. Growth of head circumference eventually decreases if inadequate nutrition continues. For some children, the reason for nutritional deficit is that the child's actual condition (e.g., celiac disease) has made it impossible for the child to absorb nutrients, and this is reflected in his or her height and weight. The intervention plan would be to educate the family and child on the diet modifications needed and to work with the family to identify and overcome barriers to maintaining the diet.

For other children, such as those with esophageal anomalies, growth parameters may not be achieved because the child cannot take in a sufficient quantity or quality of nutrients orally to meet nutritional needs. The nurse should verify that the alternate enteral route (e.g., gastrostomy tube) is being used properly. In other cases, such as with chronic congestive heart failure due to a congenital cardiac anomaly, the child's energy needs may far exceed his or her ability to take in nutrients. In this case, the child may need carefully timed feedings of a nutrient-enhanced formula (e.g., with additional fats and carbohydrates), with supplemental formula given via orogastric tube passed at the time of the feeding.

caREminder: *Not all children who are below targeted growth parameters have impaired growth. It is important to evaluate whether a child is following his or her own growth curve. A child at the 10th percentile at birth who remains between the 10th and 15th percentiles throughout the first year of life may be doing well, although he or she is clearly smaller than most children of the same age. Other children have conditions that make use of the growth charts inappropriate. In a child with idiopathic scoliosis or scoliosis secondary to meningomyelocele, height may indicate very little about the child's actual development, although it can be used as part of the evaluation of the progression of the vertebral defect.*

School

School is a significant experience for all children (Fig. 10–13). Not only does the child develop much of the cognitive and analytic knowledge and skill needed for life in school, school is also a major setting for social development. Some chronic conditions have minimal or no impact on the child's ability to go to school. Attendance and school progress should be monitored to be sure that exacerbations of the condition or a prolonged hospitalization does not interfere with the child's performance in school (Chart 10–18).

Children with chronic illness should be monitored for evidence that they are using their illness to avoid school. If this problem is identified, the child should return to school as soon as possible. After a comprehensive evaluation to determine why the child does not want to attend school, a plan to address any problems identified should be implemented.

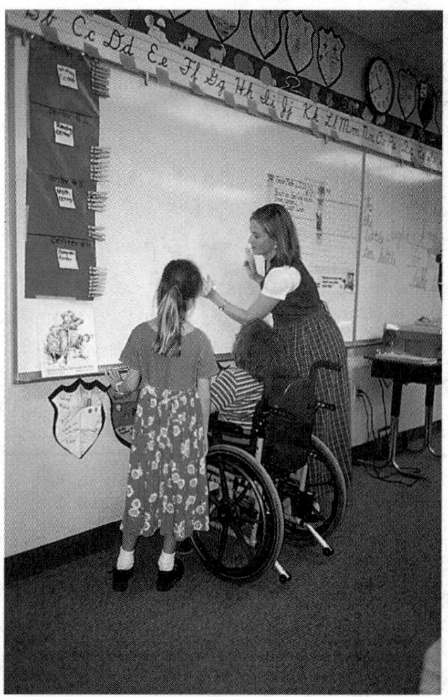

Figure 10–13
School attendance allows the child with a chronic condition to develop both socially and cognitively.

For other children, particularly those with mobility impairments, developmental delays, and technologic intervention that requires ongoing care (e.g., oxygen therapy or continuous total parenteral nutrition), school attendance can be difficult. The Education of All Handicapped Children Act (PL 94-142) and the 1986 amendments to this law to include infants and toddlers (PL 911-457) have greatly expanded the scope of services to children in schools. (See Chapter 7 for a detailed explanation of these federal laws.) These laws mandate early intervention programs, family training, counseling, home visits, diagnostic evaluation, and special education and related services. The law addresses children with physical and emotional disturbances, cognitive impairment, and any problem serious enough to impede success in regular education programs (Vessey, Jackson, Rabin, & McFadden, 1996; Walker, 1991).

Individualized Education Plan

A key part of such programs is the development of both short- and long-term goals for each child and a plan for how services will be provided. This is summarized in the individualized education plan (IEP) (see Chapter 7 for more detailed discussion). An IEP includes a current statement of the child's educational performance, short-

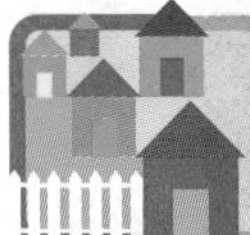

Chart 10–18
Community Care

Interdisciplinary School-Based Care for the Child with a Chronic Condition

Actions for the School Nurse

- Maintain individualized health care plan (IHP) for every student who may need treatment at school. Include information on medications, dosages, triggers, and emergency procedures.
- Alert staff members about students with a history of conditions likely to manifest themselves in the classroom.
- Assist with the administration of medication in accordance with school policy.
- Monitor response to treatment using criteria appropriate to condition.
- Communicate with parents about problems at school and the student's general progress in controlling his or her condition at school.
- Conduct inservice training on chronic conditions as needed.
- Consult with staff to help develop appropriate school activities for students with specific conditions.
- Collaborate with the Parent Teacher Association to offer family education programs in school if numerous children have similar conditions or children with multiple chronic conditions have common needs.
- Collaborate with community-based treatment and support groups.

Actions for the Guidance Counselor

- Recognize that learning to cope with any chronic illness can be difficult. Teachers may notice low self-esteem, withdrawal from activities, discouragement over the steps needed to control the condition, or difficulty making up schoolwork.
- Offer special counseling with the faculty, student, and/or parents to help the student handle problems more effectively.

Actions for the Principal

- Involve staff in the IHP, which should be a cooperative effort involving the student, parents, teachers, school staff, and physicians.
- Develop a clear policy on taking medication during school hours.
- Designate one person on the school staff to be responsible for maintaining each student's IHP.
- Provide opportunities for staff to learn about the chronic conditions.
- Establish a resource file for the staff to get additional information about the chronic conditions. Make general information available to students as well.
- Support and encourage communication with parents to improve school health services.

term objectives, long-term goals, and a description of services to be provided. Although health care providers are not required to participate in the development of the IEP, the school nurse can play a major role in its development and monitoring.

These federal laws also address transportation needs of the child and the implementation of support services. Even with these major federal initiatives, parents often have difficulty accessing needed educational services for their children. Common barriers are inability of the school system to provide the needed services and disputes about the setting in which those services should be provided. The school nurse is often in the best position to be case manager, both because she or he often identifies deficits that must be addressed and because she or he has repeated contact with the rest of the interdisciplinary team (American Academy of Pediatrics, 1990; Joachim, 1989; Pesata, 1994; Vessey et al., 1996; Walker, 1991).

A special focus of the plan of care for children with chronic conditions should be the continuation of school activities when it is impossible for the child to attend school regularly (Rabin, 1994). For some children, it is necessary to modify the school environment to allow the child to participate without barriers, both environmental and physical (McCarthy, Williams, & Eidahl, 1996). For example, the child on chemotherapy may need an opportunity to take a nap while his or her peers are at gym, and the child with spina bifida may need a private place to do self-catheterization. The child who needs to miss school frequently may need a source of ongoing educa-

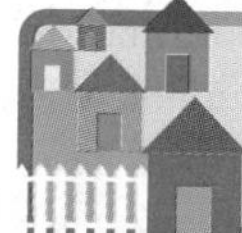

Chart 10–18
Community Care *Continued*

Interdisciplinary School-Based Care for the Child with a Chronic Condition

Actions for the Physical Education Instructor and Coach

- Encourage exercise and participation in sports for students with chronic conditions that impact their ability to engage in usual physical education programs.
- Support the student's IHP if it requires premedication before exercise.
- Understand what to do if an acute episode occurs during exercise. Have the child's IHP available.
- Encourage students with chronic conditions to participate actively in sports, but also recognize and respect their limits. Permit less strenuous activities if a recent illness precludes full participation.
- Refer your questions about a student's ability to fully participate in physical education to the parents and school nurse.

Actions for the Classroom Teacher

- Know the early warning signs of problems for specific chronic conditions (e.g., wheezing with asthma, irritability with hypoglycemia).
- Have a copy of the child's IHP in the classroom. Review it with the student and parents. Know what steps to take in case of a problem.
- Develop a clear procedure with the student and parent for handling schoolwork missed.
- Understand that students with some chronic conditions may feel drowsy or tired, different from the other kids, anxious about access to medication, embarrassed about the disruption to school activities that their condition causes, and/or withdrawn.
- Help the student feel more comfortable by recognizing these feelings. Try to maintain confidentiality. Work with the student and plan education of classmates about the child's condition.
- Know the possible side effects of the child's medications and how they may impact the student's performance in the classroom. Refer any problem to the school nurse and parent(s).
- Encourage the student with a chronic condition to participate fully in physical activities.
- Allow a student to engage in quiet activity if recovery from an acute episode precludes full participation.

Adapted from *Managing asthma: A guide for schools.* National Heart, Lung, and Blood Institute (NHLBI), National Institutes of Health, U.S. Department of Health and Human Services, and the Fund for the Improvement and Reform of Schools and Teaching, Office of Educational Research and Improvement (OERI), U.S. Department of Education. September 1991. (NIH Publication No. 91-2650).

tion on those days he or she is not at school or a preplanned intervention to help him or her make up deficits upon return to school.

Individualized Health Care Plan

School nurses should develop individualized health care plans (IHPs) for children with chronic conditions. Although not mandated by the special education laws, IHPs are valuable because they integrate assessment data from health care providers, teachers, parents, the child, and anyone else involved in the child's care. IHPs should be developed for all children with physical or emotional chronic conditions, not only those covered by the federal laws. They are also useful for children with short-term health care needs (Hass, 1993).

A typical IHP includes assessment data, nursing diagnoses, and specific goals and outcome statements for that child. The IHP's nursing interventions reflect the unique needs of the child and family and include interventions that support the child's ability to perform in the school setting. Supplemental materials such as treatment authorization forms, assessment worksheets specific to the condition, checklist to help parents decide whether the child should attend school, emergency treatment plans, transportation plans, referral checklists, medication administration records, guides for self-medication, and health care education plans for the child, teachers, and other children are often a part of the IHP (Hass, 1993) (Fig. 10–14).

Immunization

Full immunization is a goal for children with chronic conditions, as it is for their unaffected peers. (See Chap-

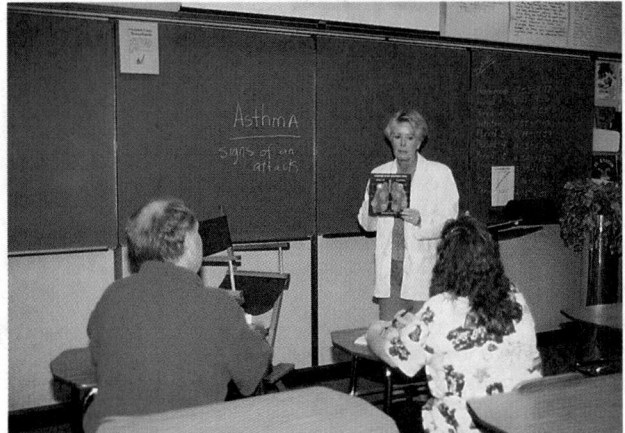

Figure 10–14
Teachers can benefit from education about the health care needs of a chronically ill child in their class.

ter 6 for a full discussion of childhood immunizations.) True contraindications should be the only reason why immunizations are delayed or omitted. It is rare that even a child with a chronic condition has one of these contraindications. The nurse can educate parents about immunization patterns as well as risks and benefits of specific immunizations. Non-mandated vaccines such as those for influenza, chickenpox, and pneumococcus are often of value to the child with a chronic condition, and each child should be evaluated to see if these would be beneficial.

The nurse must monitor the immunization status of the child carefully, because children with chronic illnesses are often underimmunized despite frequent contacts with health care professionals (Havens & Bodenham, 1992). Immunization visits may be scheduled with other visits when possible. Preferably, the parents should view each visit with a health care provider as an immunization opportunity. The nurse can evaluate the child's immunization status and administer all immunizations due. This facilitates full immunization with the smallest number of additional health care visits for the child and family. If many children in a practice setting are not fully immunized, the health care workers must examine their practice patterns to eliminate actual or perceived barriers (as seen by the parents or care providers). This step requires good communication between the child's multiple health care providers and can be an activity of the case manager.

Immunizations should be free or low cost (Havens & Bodenham, 1992). Often this is possible through federal or state immunization programs, and the steps to promote access to such services should be integrated into the child's plan of care.

Accurate and complete recording and tracking of immunizations is needed. This is facilitated by coordination and communication between health care providers who the child may visit for care for their conditions (e.g, orthopedist or endocrinologist) and their primary care provider and is monitored best by the case manager.

Because staff in specialty health settings are not usually familiar with immunization products, one person should be responsible for monitoring their storage and the development and implementation of immunization protocols such as mandatory record keeping. These specially identified staff should stay updated about current immunization standards and could be responsible for reporting adverse events to the Vaccine Adverse Event Reporting System (VAERS; 1-800-822-7967).

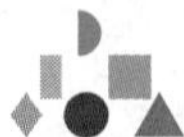

Support for the Child and Family Facing Chronic Conditions

Support for the child and family takes many forms. Most families need assistance in gaining and maintaining the financial resources needed to pay for treatment of the condition. They also need emotional support to help them cope with the challenges faced on a daily basis.

Financial Support

A major impediment to the achievement of full abilities for the child with a chronic condition is the difficulty of accessing all the needed services. One of the reasons for this difficulty is the expense of such services. Although the current thrust of private and government efforts is toward universal health insurance, this does not guarantee that there will be access to all needed services. For example, a family may be at risk of losing coverage if the parent carrying the health policy changes jobs. Another potential problem is that the lifetime maximum payout of the plan may be reached early in the child's life.

There are multiple ways to finance health care for chronic conditions, and most families use more than one. (See Chapter 7 for a comprehensive discussion of federal assistance programs for children.) One major source is commercial insurance. Such plans offer the advantage of access to a wide variety of health care providers and agencies but may be limited by high co-payments and deductibles and limits on treatment of preexisting conditions. A variation is the inclusion of a preferred provider limitation on the commercial plan. Such options offer lower co-payments if preferred providers are used and put limits on the ability of the family to choose providers and agencies. Another variation is the health maintenance organization (HMO). Such groups offer managed care and coordination of all health care services between providers and agencies. Many HMOs have little or no restrictions on the treatment of preexisting condition. The major limitation is that the family can use only providers and agencies with which the HMO has contracts unless they are willing to pay for the services themselves (Kaufman, 1991a, 1991b; O'Grady, 1996). For example, the HMO may provide ear, nose, and throat (ENT) services through a general ENT physician but not by a pediatric ENT subspecialist.

Another source of financial support is the Civilian Health and Medical Program of the Uniformed Services (CHAMPUS), the health insurance program for those in the military. In addition to providing routine health and illness care, CHAMPUS provides special programs for children with chronic health conditions, and this may include home care. Some branches of the armed services attempt to assign parents to bases located near the services that their child needs (Kaufman, 1991a, 1991b). The Indian Health Service provides a similar scope of services to the Native Americans they serve (O'Grady, 1996).

Eligibility of individuals with chronic conditions for the Medicaid program, administered by each state, is based on income. Most Medicaid programs offer a full range of preventive and illness-related services, including Early and Periodic Screening, Diagnosis and Treatment Program (EPSDT). EPSDT is designed to identify children needing services.

A major modification in Medicaid took place in 1981 when a program known as the Katie Beckett Waiver was implemented. Through this program, children who would have been eligible for services only in a hospital were able to receive care at home. Katie Beckett Waivers are currently available in most, but not all, states (Kaufman, 1991a).

Title V of the Social Security Act, through the MCH Service block Grants, funds programs to serve children with a wide variety of cognitive and physical disabilities. Programs for Children with Special Health Care Needs (CSHCN) were formerly called Crippled Children's Services and are now called Children's Medical Services (CMS) in most states. Specific eligibility criteria and decisions related to the scope of services for CSHCN agencies are formulated and implemented by each state (Kaufman, 1991a; O'Grady, 1996). Nurses working with children with chronic conditions must become familiar with CSHCN programs in their state and work with them to help eligible children access services. Nurses working from within CSHCN must work to coordinate the care the child receives from outside of the CSHCN system.

Another major, but underused, source of funding for children with chronic conditions is the Supplemental Security Income (SSI) program. SSI provides cash and Medicaid coverage for selected blind and disabled children younger than the age of 16 so they may obtain rehabilitation services. The eligibility requirements for children allow an individualized functional assessment based on children their own age (Farel, McCarraher, Cotten, & McLaurin 1995; Kaufman, 1991b). Children with cognitive delays may be served through the state's developmental disabilities system.

Emotional and Educational Support

Given the inherent, ongoing nature of a chronic condition, emotional and educational support can play a key role in optimizing family functioning. Direct teaching by health care professionals, modeling of practices needed for the care of the child, and the use of books and videotapes and computer assisted instructions are some of the interventions that work.

Support Groups

Support groups, where families and children can share experiences with others in similar situations, can be valuable resources. Most support organizations have national and regional offices. Many have local chapters. In addition to providing emotional support, these organizations distribute educational materials and offer assistance in finding and evaluating treatment.

A list of support groups for children with chronic conditions and their families is provided at the end of this chapter and other chapters in this text.

Some groups, such as the Special Olympics, do not focus on the chronic condition at all. Instead, they provide opportunities for the child to engage in social and athletic activities that promote the development of the whole child. Although there are constant efforts to promote the child's access to all experiences they would have if they did not have the chronic condition, activities like Special Olympics offer a place to achieve for the child who does not have the ability to participate in such integrated activities. Both parents and professionals find the Special Olympics highly beneficial, particularly in terms of social adjustment and life satisfaction. Some experts expressed concerns about the potentially segregative aspects of the program, whereas parents focused on administrative issues of the program (Klein, Gilman, & Zigler, 1993).

Bibliotherapy

Bibliotherapy allows children and families to explore their own feelings by reading about other families in similar situations. As opposed to the books and pamphlets designed to help the child and family learn how to provide care needed because of the disease, bibliotherapy

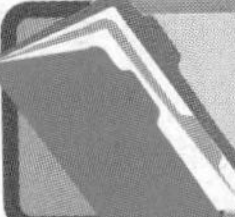

Chart 10–19
Nursing Interventions Classification (NIC)

Bibliotherapy

Definition

Use of literature to enhance the expression of feelings and the gaining of insight

Activities

Determine the particular needs of the situation.
Set therapy goals.
Select books that reflect the situation or the feelings the patient is experiencing.
Consult with a librarian who is skilled in book finding.
Consult guides to recommended books from self-help groups.
Make selections appropriate for reading level.
Read aloud, as needed or feasible.
Use pictures and illustrations.
Encourage reading and rereading.
Talk about the feelings expressed by the characters.
Follow up reading sessions with play sessions or role modeling work, either individually or in therapy groups.
Evaluate goal attainment.

From McCloskey, J., & Bulechek, G. (1996). *Nursing interventions classification (NIC)* (2nd ed.). St. Louis: Mosby–Year Book. Reprinted with permission.

addresses the emotional reactions they commonly experience.

Readers can gain insight into their own feelings as they learn about the experiences of other families in both fictional and true life accounts. Children and families can read how other children successfully dealt with the challenges they are facing. Bibliotherapy provides examples of positive and negative coping behaviors and responses in a non-threatening way. Such books can also be the genesis for questions and a starting point for discussion about issues that must be addressed. The nurse can utilize bibliotherapy as a strategy to assist families in the process of adapting to the child's changing condition (Chart 10–19). The Resources section of this chapter lists a wide variety of books available for the child and family.

Electronic Networks

Another source of family education and support are electronic networks. Parents and children familiar with access to the Internet can reach all the research and scientific data available over this vast electronic network (Chart 10–20). Families often need help interpreting what they find on electronic networks and discerning what applies to them or their child. Also, they may need help discriminating between formal, well-reviewed materials, such as the information posted on a cancer association web site, and a posting that is no more than the personal opinion of someone who sounds knowledgeable but is not.

Electronic networks are the source of a new type of support group—electronic discussion groups. Some take place on the commercial networks (such as CompuServe or America Online), but most are open to everyone on the Internet. These discussion groups focus on specific conditions (such as spina bifida), the general challenges of raising (or being) a child with a chronic condition, or day-to-day parenting issues (Wink, 1995, 1996; Yerks, 1996).

Electronic discussion groups offer parents the constant and willing ear of other persons facing similar problems. The discussions are often about the care of the child's chronic condition. For example, parents may share opinions about the effectiveness of a specific anticonvulsant or the ketogenic diet as treatments for epilepsy. There are frequent discussions about accessing services, such as dental care for a child with spastic cerebral palsy or full education for a child with autism. There are tips for dealing with the health care system and health care professionals. Parents also express their needs to be respected for their knowledge and to stay in control of their child's health care, as well as their frustration when health care providers do not recognize these needs. How to simply be a good parent is another common thread, with discussion about how to handle discipline problems, sibling conflict, and the school system and how to plan

Figure 10–15
Caregivers can access electronic networks to learn more about their child's condition and communicate with other families who are sharing similar experiences.

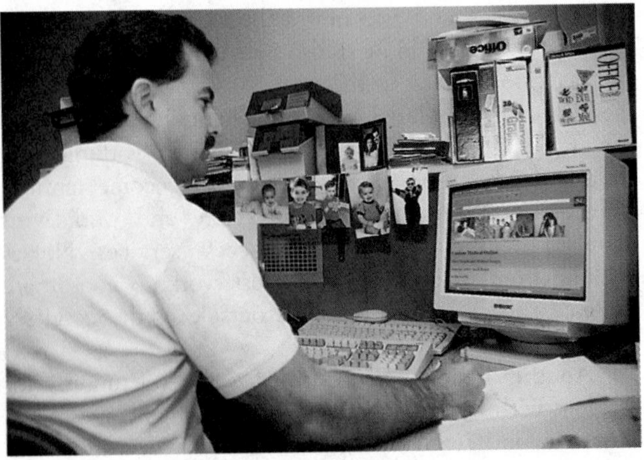

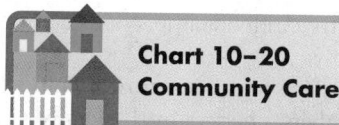

Chart 10–20
Community Care

Using Electronic Networks

A computer, modem, communication software, and an account with an Internet service provider (ISP) allow access to the international computer network known as the Internet. Internet users can send and receive electronic mail (e-mail), participate in discussion groups, and access and use resources stored on computers around the world.

Electronic discussion groups (also called listservers and mailing lists) allow participants to share experiences and both give and receive support from others with similar concerns. Participants receive all messages sent to the group and can send messages to the entire group. The universality of the concerns of parents and children is evident in the messages posted to the lists.

To subscribe to a discussion group, send a message to the electronic address of the computer on which the group is based. The "Subject" field is usually left blank. In the message field, enter the phrase "sub" followed by the name of the list and then your name. For example, to subscribe to our-kids, the subscription message would be sent to

majordomo@tbag.osc.edu

The message field would contain the phrase

Sub our kids ⟨your name⟩ *(do not include the brackets!)*

Occasionally, the computer through which the discussion group is processed requires a different subscription message in which case an error message is sent that often states the correct information.

Confirmation messages are then sent by the computer. These include important computer commands such as how to digest the list (so you get all messages once a day instead of as they come in—helpful with very active groups like our-kids) and unsubscribe (essential if you go on vacation).

To send messages to the group, use the discussion list address, not the computer's address. To send messages to an individual who has posted a message to the group, use their individual e-mail address.

The Internet has thousands of files that benefit nurses, families, and children. Each file must be evaluated to be sure the source is reliable and the information is valid. For example, a posting from the National Cancer Institute on the treatment of a particular cancer is both reliable and valid; a posting by someone with that cancer probably reflects only the experiences of that one person.

The best way to access Internet resources is through a WWW browser. After entering the Universal Resource Locator (URL) of a site, you are electronically transported to that site. The WWW has search programs that allow users to search for the desired information. The Resources section lists some of the major electronic discussion groups and WWW sites for children, families, and nurses.

and have a good family vacation (Wink, 1995, 1996; Yerks, 1996).

Most important, electronic discussion groups offer a constant source of support. Even though most parents of children with chronic conditions report a decreased ability to socialize, electronic support groups are always there. At the end of a long, trying day, the computer and modem allow access to other caring parents who can encourage and boost the spirits of parents who doubt their ability to continue to care for their child and even to continue to face life (Wink, 1995, 1996; Yerks, 1996) (Fig. 10–15). The Resource section of this chapter contains a list of World Wide Web sites focusing on nursing or on children with chronic conditions.

Summary of Key Concepts

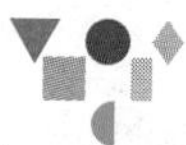

- The initial impact of the diagnosis of a chronic condition usually occurs at diagnosis, but can occur over time when the diagnostic period is prolonged.
- Emotional reactions to the diagnosis of a chronic condition include grief, denial, guilt, anger, loneliness, and fear.
- Each member of the family responds to the presence of a chronic condi-

tion in an individual manner. These distinctive individual reactions combine to create a unique response in the family.

- Families of children with chronic conditions face numerous critical points caused by increased needs of individual members, changes in the family support, relocation of the child or a family member, parental absence, developmental advances of the child, or the birth of a subsequent child.
- Siblings of children with chronic conditions do not always have additional problems when compared with siblings of children without chronic conditions.
- Emotional and educational support play a key role in optimizing family functioning.
- Families need ongoing assessment of learning needs as the child's condition changes and the child and family develop.
- Interventions aimed at promoting optimal health and well-being maximize health despite the presence of the condition.
- Nurses working with children with chronic conditions should understand the economics of health care reimbursement and possess case management skills.
- Educational and electronic resources can be used by children and their parents to learn more about the child's condition and to network with families facing similar circumstances.

Resources

Organizations

American Bar Association
Child Advocacy Center
1800 M Street, NW, Suite 200
Washington, DC 20036

Association for the Care of Children's Health (ACCH)
7910 Woodmont Avenue, Suite 300
Bethesda, MD 20814
(800) 808-ACCH

Canadian Rehabilitation Council for the Disabled
One Yonge Street, Suite 2110
Toronto, Ontario, Canada M5S 1ES

Challenge International
6710 Lowell Avenue
McLean, VA

Children's Defense Fund
122 C Street, NW, Suite 400
Washington, DC 20001

Hospice Association of America
228 Seventh Street, SE
Washington, DC 20003
(202) 547-7424

Hospice Nurses Association
Medical Center E, Suite 375
211 N. Whitfield
Pittsburgh, PA 15206
(412) 687-3231
E-mail: hnsfan@usa.pipeline

National Hospice Organization
1901 N. Moore Street, Suite 901
Arlington, VA 22209
(703) 243-5900
Web site: http://www.nho.org

National Information Center for Children and Youth with Disabilities
P.O. Box 1492
Washington, DC 20013

National Maternal and Child Health Clearinghouse
8201 Greensboro Drive, Suite 600
McLean, VA 22102-3810
(703) 821-8955, ext. 254

Hotlines

American Association of Disabled Persons
(800) 642-8775

Center for Rehabilitation Technology
(800) 726-9119

Center for Special Education Technology
(800) 873-8255

Cleft Palate Foundation
(800) 242-5338

National Association for the Dually Diagnosed
(800) 331-5362

National Autism Hotline
(304) 525-8014

National Center for Research in Vocational Education
(800) 762-4093

National Center for Youth with Disability
(800) 333-6293

National Easter Seal Society
(800) 221-6827

National Hospice Organization
(800) 658-8898

National Information Center for Children and Youth with Disabilities
(800) 695-0285

National Information Center for Orphan Drug and Rare Diseases
(800) 456-3505

National Information Clearinghouse for Infants with Disabilities and Life-threatening Conditions
(800) 922-1107

Social Security Administration
(800) 234-5772

United Cerebral Palsy Association, Inc.
(800) 872-5827

Books and Printed Materials

ACCH has many publications available that pertain to the family of a child with a chronic condition. The following are some examples. Contact ACCH for a catalog or to obtain resources.

Children with Special Needs (2nd ed.)
L. Bradway, L. A. Block, 1990
Designed as a quick reference for teachers.

Circles of Care and Understanding: Support Groups for Fathers of Children with Special Needs
J. May, 1992

Counseling Parents of Children with Chronic Illness or Disability
H. Davis, 1993

Deciphering the System: A Guide for Families of Young Children with Disabilities
P. Beckman, G. Beckman Boyes, 1993

A Difference in the Family: Life with a Disabled Child
H. Featherstone, 1990

Family-Centered Care for Children Needing Specialized Health and Developmental Services
T. Shelton, J. Stepanek, 1994

Family/Professional Collaboration for Children with Special Health Needs and Their Families
K. Bishop, J. Woll, P. Arango, 1993

✏ *It Isn't Fair! Siblings of Children with Disabilities*
S. D. Klein, M. J. Scheifer (Eds.), 1993

Organizing and Maintaining Support Groups for Parents of Children with Chronic Illness and Handicapping Conditions
M. Nathanson, 1986

Raising a Child Who Has a Physical Disability
D. G. Albrecht, 1995

Sibshops: Workshops for Siblings of Children with Special Needs
D. J. Meyer, P. F. Vadasy, 1994

✏ Resources specifically for children.

Your Child and Health Care: A "Dollars and Sense" Guide for Families with Special Needs
L. R. Rosenfield, 1994

After the Tears: Parents Talk About Raising a Child with a Disability
by Robin Simons
Harcourt Brace & Company, 1987

Bibliography on Self-Management for People with Chronic Disease
Center for the Advancement of Health and Center for Health Studies of Group Health Cooperative of Paget Sound
(202) 387-2829
An indexed bibliography of research, meta-analysis, and review articles for 18 chronic conditions.

Breaking New Ground Resource Center
Purdue University
1146 Agricultural Engineering Building
West Lafayette, IN 47907-1145
(317) 494-5088
FAX: (317) 496-1115
Breaking New Ground *is a newsletter for farmers with disabilities.*

Directory of College Facilities and Services for the Disabled
by Carol Thomas, James Thomas
Oryx Press
2214 N. Central at Encanto
Phoenix, AZ 85004

Exceptional Parent
P.O. Box 3000
Department EP
Denville, NJ 07834

Financial Aid for the Disabled and Their Families
by Gail Ann Schlachter, David Weber
Reference Service Press
1100 Industrial Road #9
San Carlos, CA 94070

✏ *Harry and Willy and Carrothead*
by Judith Caseley
Book about a child with no left hand and how he deals with kindergarten.

✏ *How it Feels to Fight for Your Life,*
by Jill Krementz
Little, Brown and Company, 1989
Essays by children who have chronic illnesses.

✏ *How it Feels to Live with a Physical Disability*
by Jill Krementz
Simon & Schuster, 1992
Essays by kids ages 6 through 16. Focuses on "positive attributes and unique abilities." Photographs show daily life, including school, sports, and therapy sessions.

Job Opportunities for the Blind
National Federation of the Blind
1800 Johnson Street
Baltimore, MD 21230

✏ *Kids Explore the Gifts of Children with Special Needs*
Westridge Young Writers Workshop
Santa Fe, NM: John Muir Publications, 1994
Each section is written by the classmates of special needs kids. Includes black and white photographs and drawings.

Peterson's Guide to Colleges with Programs for Learning Disabled Students
Peterson's Guides
P.O. Box 2123
Princeton, NJ 08543

Superkids
60 Clyde Street
Newton, MA 02160
A newsletter for families and friends of children with limb differences.

Uncommon Fathers: Reflections on Raising a Child with a Disability
Edited by Donald J. Meyer
Bethesda, MD: Woodbine House, 1995

Unlocking Potential
by Barbara Scheiber, Jeanne Talpers
Adler & Adler Publishers
4550 Montgomery Avenue
Bethesda, MD 20814

✏ *A Very Special Critter*
by Gina and Mercer Mayer
Racine, WI: Western Publishing, 1992
Preschool story told by a little critter who learns that a critter who uses a wheelchair is going to be in his class.

Computer Resources

CaringKids
Internet discussion forum for children age 18 and younger who have family members or friends with serious illness.
E-mail: CaringKids
Request@sjuvm.stjohns.edu

SickKids
Internet discussion forum for sick children age 18 and younger.
E-mail: SickKids
Request@sjuvm.stjohns.edu

Worldwide Web Sites

American Academy of Pediatrics
http://www.aap.org/dogl/dogl.html

Amputee Home Page
http://www.portal.ca/~igregson/amputee.html

Cerebral Palsy
http://www.iinet.com.au/~scarffam/cpa.html

Down Syndrome
http://www.nas.com/downsyn/

Hospital Web
http://neuro.www.mgh.harvard.edu/hospitalweb.nclk

HyperDOC: The National Library of Medicine (NLM)
http://www.nlm.nih.gov/

MCHNet Gopher
gopher://mchnet.ichp.ufl.edu/1

Morbidity and Mortality Weekly Report
http://www.cdc.gov/epo/mmwr/mmwr.html

National Institute of Health
http://www.nih.gov/

Nemours Foundation
http://kidshealth.org/ai

Our-Kids
http://wonder.mit.edu/our-kids.html

ParentsPlace
http://www.parentsplace.com

PEDINFO
http://www.lhl.uab.edu/pedinfo

Sudden Infant Death Syndrome
http://q.continuum.net/~sidsnet/

References

Ahmann, E., & Bond, N. J. (1992). Promoting normal development in school-age children and adolescents who are technology dependent: A family centered model. *Pediatric Nursing, 18*, 391–405.

American Academy of Pediatrics (AAP), Committee on Children with Disabilities, Committee on School Health. (1990). Children with health impairments in schools. *Pediatrics*, 86, 636–638.

Austin, J. (1991). Family adaptation to a child's chronic illness. In J. Fitzpatrick, R. Taunton, & A. Jacox (Eds.), *Annual review of nursing research*. New York: Springer.

Barnsteiner, J. H., & Gillis-Donovan, J. (1990). Being related and separate: A standard for therapeutic relationships. *MCN, The Journal of Maternal and Child Nursing; 15*, 223–228.

Boyd, S. T., Vollmer, W., & Valanis, B. (1993). Parental roles in a family with an asthmatic child. *Sigma Theta Tau Electronic Databases*.

Brydolf, M., & Segesten, K. (1996). "They feel your needs in the air": Experiences of supportive activities among adolescents with ulcerative colitis. *Journal of Pediatric Nursing, 11*, 71–78.

Burkhart, P. V. (1993). Health perceptions of mothers of children with chronic conditions. *Maternal-Child Nursing Journal, 21*, 122–129.

Caldwell, B., & Bradley, R. (1984). *Home observation for measurement of the environment* (rev. ed.). Little Rock, AR: University of Arkansas.

Centers for Disease Control and Prevention. (1995). Disabilities among children aged ≤17 years—United States, 1991–1992. *Morbidity and Mortality Weekly Report*, 44(33), 611–612.

Clements, D., Copeland, L., & Loftus, M. (1990). Critical times for families with a chronically ill child. *Pediatric Nursing, 16*, 157–161.

Clubb, R. L. (1991). Chronic sorrow: Adaptation patterns of parents with chronically ill children. *Pediatric Nursing, 17*, 461–466.

Cohen, M. H. (1993a). The unknown and the unknowable: Managing sustained uncertainty. *Western Journal of Nursing Research, 15*, 77–96.

Cohen, M. H. (1993b). Diagnostic closure and the spread of uncertainty. *Pediatric Nursing, 16*, 135–146.

Cohen, M. H. (1995a). The stages of the pre-diagnostic period in chronic, life threatening childhood illness: A process analysis. *Research in Nursing & Health, 18*, 311–348.

Cohen, M. H. (1995b). The triggers of heightened parental uncertainty in chronic, life threatening childhood illness. *Qualitative Health Research, 5*, 63–77.

Copeland, L. G. (1993). Caring for children with chronic conditions: Model of critical times. *Holistic Nursing Practice, 8*, (1), 45–55.

Dashiff, C. J. (1993). Parents' perceptions of diabetes in adolescent daughters and its impact on the family. *Journal of Pediatric Nursing*, 361–369.

Davis, B. D., & Steele, S. (1991). Case management for young children with special health care needs. *Pediatric Nursing, 17*, 15–19.

Donnelly, E. (1994). Parents of children with asthma: An examination of family hardiness, family stressors, and family functioning. *Journal of Pediatric Nursing*, 9, 398–408.

Edwards-Beckett, J., & Cedargren, D. (1995). The family management style of families with a child with myelomeningocele. *Sigma Theta Tau Electronic Databases*.

Eiser, C. (1993). *Growing up with a chronic disease. The impact on children and their families*. Philadelphia: Jessica Kingsley Publishers.

Farel, A. M., McCarraher, D. R., Cotten, N., & McLaurin, J. A. (1995). Opportunities for older children and adolescents with disabilities through the supplemental security income program. *Children's Health Care, 24*, 21–32.

Faux, S. A. (1993). Siblings of children with chronic physical and cognitive disabilities. *Journal of Pediatric Nursing, 8*, 305–317.

Fish, S., & Shelly, J. (1978). *Spiritual care: The nurse's role*. Downers Grove, IL: InterVarsity.

Fulton, R. A., & Moore, C. M. (1995). Spiritual care of the school-age child with a chronic condition. *Journal of Pediatric Nursing, 10*, 224–231.

Gallo, A., Breitmayer, B., Knafl, K., & Zoeller, L. (1992). Well siblings of children with chronic illness: Parents' reports of their psychologic adjustment. *Pediatric Nursing, 18*, 23–27.

Gallo, A., Breitmayer, B. J., Knafl, K. A., & Zoeller, L. H. (1993). Mothers' perceptions of sibling adjustment and family life in childhood chronic illness. *Journal of Pediatric Nursing, 8*, 318–324.

Geissler, E. M. (1993). *Pocket guide to cultural assessment*. St. Louis: Mosby–Year Book.

Hass, J. (Ed.). (1993). *The school nurse's source book of individualized healthcare plans*. North Branch, MN: Sunrise River Press.

Havens, D. M., & Bodenham, K. (1992). Standards for pediatric immunization practices. *Journal of Pediatric Health Care*, 6, 275–278.

Hayes, V. E. (1992). The impact of a child's chronic illness on the family system. *Sigma Theta Tau Electronic Databases*.

Highfield, M., & Cason, C. (1983). Spiritual needs of patients: Are they recognized? *Cancer Nursing*, 6, 187–192.

Holaday, B. (1987). Patterns of interaction between mothers and their chronically ill infants. *Maternal-Child Nursing Journal, 16*, 29–45.

Horner, S. D. (1992). Groping in the dark: Uncertainty in family caring. *Sigma Theta Tau Electronic Databases*.

Hymovich, D. (1976). Parents of sick children. Their needs and tasks. *Pediatric Nursing*, 3(5), 9–13.

Hymovich, D. (1983). The chronicity impact and coping instrument: Parent questionnaire. *Nursing Research, 32,* 275–281.

Joachim, G. (1989). The school nurse as a case manager for chronically ill children. *The Journal of School Health, 59,* 406–407.

Johnston, C. E., & Marder, L. R. (1994). Parenting the child with a chronic condition: An emotional experience. *Pediatric Nursing, 20,* 611–614.

Kaufman, J. (1991a). An overview of public sector financing for pediatric home care: Part 1. *Pediatric Nursing, 17,* 280–281.

Kaufman, J. (1991b). An overview of public sector financing for pediatric home care: Part 2. *Pediatric Nursing, 17,* 380–381, 422.

Klein, T., Gilman, E., & Zigler, E. (1993). Special Olympics: An evaluation by professionals and parents. *Mental Retardation, 31*(1), 15–23.

Knafl, K., Ayres, L., Gallo, A., Zoeller, L., & Breitmayer, B. (1995). Learning from stories: Parents' accounts of the pathway to diagnosis. *Pediatric Nursing, 21,* 411–415.

Lawrence, K. S. (1990). *Guidelines for reporting and writing about people with disabilities* (3rd ed.). Research and Training Center on Independent Living.

Leonard, B. J., Brust, J. D., & Nelson, R. P. (1993). Parental distress: Caring for medically fragile children at home. *Journal of Pediatric Nursing, 8,* 22–30.

Lindsey, E. (1996). Health within illness: Experiences of chronically ill/disabled people. *Journal of Advanced Nursing, 24,* 465–472.

Lipsi, K., Clements-Shafer, K., & Rushton, G. H. (1991). Developmental rounds: An intervention strategy for hospitalized infants. *Pediatric Nursing, 17,* 433–437, 468.

LoBiondo-Wood, G., Bernier-Henn, M., & Williams, L. (1992). Impact of the child's liver transplant on the family: Maternal perspective. *Pediatric Nursing, 18,* 461–465.

May, J. (1991). *Fathers of children with special needs: New horizons.* Bethesda, MD: Association for the Care of Children's Health.

McCarthy, A., Williams, J., & Eidahl, L. (1996). Children with chronic conditions: Educators' views. *Journal of Pediatric Health Care, 10,* 272–279.

McCloskey, J., & Bulechek, G. (1996). *Nursing interventions classification (NIC)* (2nd ed.). St. Louis: Mosby–Year Book.

McCubbin, H., McCubbin M., Cauble A., & Nevin, R. (1979). *Coping health inventory for parents* (CHIP). St. Paul, MN: Family Social Services, University of Minnesota.

Nugent, K. E. (1989). Routine care: Promoting development in hospitalized infants. *MCN, The Journal of Maternal and Child Nursing, 14,* 318–323.

Nuttall, P. (1988). Maternal responses to home apnea monitoring of infants. *Nursing Research, 37,* 354–357.

Office of Technology Assessment. (1978). *Technology-dependent children: Hospital vs. home care. A technical memorandum* (OTA-TM-H-38). Washington, DC: U.S. Congress.

O'Grady, R. S. (1996). Financing health care for children with chronic conditions. In P. Jackson, & J. Vessey (Eds.), *Primary care of the child with a chronic condition* (2nd ed., pp. 100–117). St. Louis: Mosby–Year Book.

Olshansky, S. (1962). Chronic sorrow: A response to having a mentally defective child. *Social Casework, 43,* 190–193.

Patterson, J. M., Jernell, J., Leonard, B. J., & Titus, J. C. (1994). Caring for medically fragile children at home: The parent-professional relationship. *Journal of Pediatric Nursing, 9,* 98–106.

Perin, E. (1995). Chronic conditions. In S. Parker & B. Zuckerman (Eds.), *Behavioral and developmental pediatrics. A handbook of primary care.* Boston: Little, Brown & Co.

Perkins, M. T. (1993). Parent-nurse collaboration: Using the caregiver identity emergence phase to assist parents of hospitalized children with disabilities. *Journal of Pediatric Nursing, 8,* 2–9.

Pesata, V. L. (1994). Applying Benner's model to school nursing of multiple handicapped children. *Clinical Nurse Specialist, 8,* 230–233.

Peterson, M. (1996). What are blood counts? A computer-assisted program for pediatric patients. *Pediatric Nursing, 22,* 16–20.

Phillips, S., & Hartley, J. T. (1988). Developmental differences and interventions for blind children. *Pediatric Nursing, 14,* 201–204.

Pless, I. B., Freeley, N., Gottlieb, L., Rowat, K., Dougherty, G., & Willard, B. (1994). A randomized trial of a nursing intervention to promote the adjustment of children with chronic physical disorders. *Pediatrics, 94,* 70–75.

Rabin, N. B. (1994). School reentry and the child with a chronic illness: The role of the pediatric nurse practitioner. *Journal of Pediatric Health Care, 8,* 227–232.

Rao, R. P., & Kramer, L. (1993). Stress and coping among mothers of infants with a sickle cell condition. *Children's Health Care, 22,* 161–188.

Ray, L. D., & Ritchie, J. A. (1993). Caring for chronically ill children at home: Factors that influence parents' coping. *Journal of Pediatric Nursing, 8,* 217–225.

Revell, G. M., & Liptak, G. S. (1991). Understanding the child with special health care needs: A developmental perspective. *Journal of Pediatric Nursing, 6,* 258–267.

Rollins, J. A. (1990). Childhood cancer: Siblings draw and tell. *Pediatric Nursing, 16,* 21–26.

Ryan-Wenger, N. (1996). Children, coping and the stress of illness: A synthesis of the research. *Journal of the Society of Pediatric Nurses,* 1(3), 126–138.

Scannell, S. S., Gilles, D. A., Biordi, D., & Child, D. A. (1993). Negotiating nurse-patient authority in pediatric home health care. *Journal of Pediatric Nursing, 8,* 70–78.

Selekman, J., & McIlvain-Simon, G. (1991). Sex and sexuality of the adolescent with a chronic condition. *Pediatric Nursing, 17,* 535–538.

Shepard, M., & Mahon, M. (1996). Chronic conditions and the family. In P. Jackson & J. Vessey (Eds.), *Primary care of the child with a chronic condition,* (2nd ed., pp. 41–57). St. Louis: Mosby–Year Book.

Sherman, B. R. (1995). Impact of home-based respite care on families of children with chronic illness. *Children's Health Care, 24,* 33–45.

Simon, N. B., & Smith, D. (1992). Living with chronic pediatric liver disease: The parents' experience. *Pediatric Nursing, 18,* 453–458.

Smilkstein, G., Ashworth, C., & Montano, D. (1982). Validity and reliability of the family APGAR as a test of family function. *Journal of Family Practice, 15,* 303–311.

Smith, D., & Sherwen, L. (1984). The bonding process of mothers and adopted parents. *Topics in Clinical Nursing, 6,* 38–48.

Smith, K., Gabard, G., Dale, D., & Drucker, A. (1994). Parental opinions about attending parent support groups. *Children's Health Care, 23,* 127–136.

Stepanek, J. S., & Ahmann, E. (1995). Parent-professional collaboration when hospital visits are infrequent. *Pediatric Nursing, 21,* 466–468.

Stewart, S. M., Kennard, B. D., DeBolt, A., Petrik, K., Waller, D. A., & Andrews, W. S. (1993). Adaptation of siblings of children awaiting liver transplantation. *Children's Health Care, 22,* 205–215.

Teague, B. R., Fleming, J. W., Castle, A., Kiernan, B. S., Lobo, M. L., Riggs, S., & Wolfe, J. G. (1993). "High tech" home care for children with chronic health conditions: A pilot study. *Journal of Pediatric Nursing, 8,* 226–232.

Telfair, J., Myers, J., & Drezner, S. (1994). Transfer as a component of the transition of adolescents with sickle cell disease to adult care: Adolescent, adult and parent perspectives. *Journal of Adolescent Health, 15,* 558–565.

Thompson, A. B., Curtner, M. E., & O'Rear, M. R. (1994). The psychosocial adjustment of well siblings of chronically ill children. *Children's Health Care, 23,* 211–226.

Urbano, M. T., von Windeguth, B. V., Siderits, P., & Studenic-Lewis, C. (1989). Developing case managers for chronically ill children: Florida's registered nurse specialist program. *The Journal of Continuing Education in Nursing, 22,* 62–66.

Verzemnieks, I. O. (1984). Developmental stimulation for infants and toddlers. *American Journal of Nursing, 85,* 741–752.

Vessey, J., Jackson, P., Rabin, N., & McFadden, E. (1996). School and the child with a chronic condition. In P. Jackson & J. Vessey (Eds.), *Primary care of the child with a chronic condition* (2nd ed., pp. 86–99). St. Louis: Mosby–Year Book.

Vessey, J., & Swanson, M. (1996). Chronic conditions and child development. In P. Jackson & J. Vessey (Eds.), *Primary care of the child with a chronic condition* (2nd ed., pp. 16–40). St. Louis: Mosby–Year Book.

Walker, O. (1991). Where there is a way, there is not always a will: Technology, public policy, and the school integration of children who are technology-assisted. *Children's Health Care, 20,* 68–73.

Wells, P. W., DeBoard-Burns, M. B., Cook, R. C., & Mitchell, J. (1994a). Growing up in the hospital: Part I, Let's focus on the child. *Journal of Pediatric Nursing, 9,* 66–73.

Wells, P. W., DeBoard-Burns, M. B., Cook, R. C., & Mitchell, J. (1994b). Growing up in the hospital: Part II, Nurturing the philosophy of family-centered care. *Journal of Pediatric Nursing, 9,* 141–149.

Williams, P., Lorenzo, F., & Borja, M. (1993). Pediatric chronic illness: Effects on siblings and mothers. *Maternal-Child Nursing Journal, 21,* 111–121.

Wink, D. M. (1995). An introduction to nursing on the Internet: Part 1. *Nurse Educator, 20,* 9–13.

Wink, D. M. (1996). An introduction to nursing on the Internet: Part 2. *Nurse Educator, 21,* 8–12.

Yerks, A. M. (1996). The Internet and pediatric nursing: Guide to the information superhighway. *Pediatric Nursing, 22,* 11–15.

Bibliography

Armstrong, F. D., Lemanek, K. L., Pegelow, C. H., Gonzalez, J. C., & Martinez, A. (1993). Impact of lifestyle disruption on parent and child coping, knowledge, and parental discipline in children with sickle cell anemia. *Children's Health Care, 22,* 181–203.

Carpenito, L., (1995). *Nursing diagnosis. Application to clinical practice* (6th ed.). Philadelphia: J. B. Lippincott.

Clawson, J. (1996). A child with chronic illness and the process of family adaptation. *Journal of Pediatric Nursing, 11,* 52–61.

Erikson, E. H. (1963). *Childhood and society* (2nd ed.). New York: W. W. Norton.

Failla, S., & Jones, L. C. (1991). Families of children with developmental disabilities: An examination of family hardiness. *Research in Nursing and Health, 14,* 41–50.

Fosdal, M. O. (1992). Living with spina bifida. *Journal of Neuroscience Nursing, 24,* 286–289.

Futcher, J. A. (1988). Chronic illness and family dynamics. *Pediatric Nursing, 14,* 381–385.

Havighurst, R. J. (1979). *Developmental tasks and education* (4th ed.). New York: McKay.

Ho, H. H., Miller, A., & Armstrong, R. W. (1994). Parent-professional agreement on diagnosis and recommendations for children with developmental disorders. *Children's Health Care, 23,* 137–148.

Holman, A., Hochstadt, J., & Yost, D. (1991). A nationwide director of resources for medically complex children. In J. Hochstadt & D. Yost (Eds.), *The medically complex child. The transition to home care.* New York: Harwood Academic Publishers.

Jackson, P., & Vessey, J. (Eds.) (1996). *Primary care of the child with a chronic condition* (2nd ed.). St. Louis: Mosby–Year Book.

Jessop, D. J., & Stein, R. E. K. (1994). Providing comprehensive health care to children with chronic illness. *Pediatrics, 93,* 602–607.

Kelly, M. (1993). Safe transport of technology-dependent children. *MCN, The Journal of Maternal Child Nursing, 18,* 211–232.

Leonard, B. J., Johnson, A. L., & Brust, J. D. (1993). Caregivers of children with disabilities: A comparison of those managing "OK" and those needing more help. *Children's Health Care, 22,* 93–105.

Lewandowski, L. (1996). A parent has cancer: Needs and responses of children. *Pediatric Nursing, 22,* 518–521.

Lipman, T. H., DiFazio, D. A., Meers, R. A., & Thompson, R. L. (1989). A developmental approach to diabetes in children: Birth through preschool. *MCN, The Journal of Maternal and Child Nursing, 14,* 255–259.

Lipman, T. H., DiFazio, D. A., Meers, R. A., & Thompson, R. L. (1989). A developmental approach to diabetes in children: School age–adolescence. *MCN, The Journal of Maternal and Child Nursing, 14,* 330–332.

Piles, C. (1990). Providing spiritual care. *Nurse Educator, 15*(1), 36–41.

Romaniuk, D. K., & Kristjanson, L. J. (1995). The parent-nurse relationship from the perspective of parents of children with cancer. *Journal of Pediatric Oncology Nursing, 12,* 80–89.

Sabbeth, B. (1984). Understanding the impact of chronic childhood illness on families. *Pediatric Clinics of North America, 31,* 47–57.

Schilling, L. S., & DeJesus, E. (1993). Developmental issues in deaf children. *Journal of Pediatric Health Care, 7,* 161–166.

Strauss, S., & Munton, M. (1985). Common concerns of parents with disabled children. *Pediatric Nursing, 11,* 371–375.

Tetrick, A. P. (1989). *Guidelines for families with a chronic disease. Division of Maternal and Child Health*. Washington, DC: U.S. Department of Health and Human Services.

Visscher, E. M., & Clore, E. R. (1992). The genogram: A strategy for assessment. *Journal of Pediatric Health Care, 6*, 361–367.

Wilson, D. & Ralekin, C. (1990). An introduction to using children's drawings as assessment tools. *The Nurse Practitioner, 15*(3), 23–35.

Wuest, J., & Stern P. N. (1990). Childhood otitis media: The family's quest for relief. *Issues in Comprehensive Pediatric Nursing, 19*, 25–39.

Rehabilitation, Habilitation, and Home Care: Supporting Health Maintenance

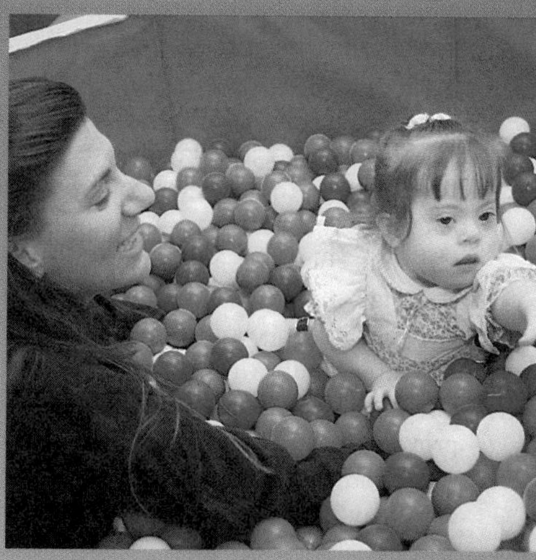

OUTLINE

OBJECTIVES

- Describe the differences between adult and pediatric rehabilitation.
- Examine the philosophy and goals of pediatric rehabilitation and habilitation.
- Recognize the levels of rehabilitative care and the team models used to provide care.
- Identify measurement tools that can be used to assess the child with habilitative needs.
- Delineate health care interventions involved in the management of functional health patterns for the child with rehabilitative and habilitative needs.
- Discuss issues related to the child's return to the community and ongoing health care needs.
- State the types of home care available to families.
- Discuss assessment and preparation of the home that are necessary to enable the family to care for the child in this environment.
- Identify the reasons why a family may select not to care for their child at home.

KEY TERMS

adaptive device
advocacy
assistive device
chronic illness
disability
habilitation
handicap
impairment
rehabilitation
technology-dependent child
transdisciplinary approach

CHAPTER

11

Like adults, children can acquire an injury or illness causing an impairment that results in a long-term disability. Brain injury, spinal cord injury, and burns are examples of such injuries. Children can also sustain a long-term disability as a result of an injury, an illness, or a condition occurring in utero or during delivery. Examples include cerebral palsy, spina bifida, and Down syndrome. These children have rehabilitative, habilitative, and home care needs as they pursue the lifelong task of developing to their highest level of ability. Through rehabilitation, the child is assisted to restore functions lost through an injury or illness. The child and family are provided support to help them adjust to an altered level of functional capacity. Habilitation focuses on helping the child develop new skills and abilities, although developmentally these abilities may not have been previously attained. Home care provides an opportunity for the child to be in the home with the family while undergoing medical therapy. Rehabilitation, habilitation, and home care are disciplines that provide services to support the health maintenance of the child who has a chronic condition or disability or who may be recuperating from an acute illness.

Rehabilitation and home care services for children have dramatically expanded over the past decade. As a result of ongoing advances in technology and medical science, the percentage of Americans with chronic conditions continues to grow. This trend includes large numbers of children. In the United States an estimated 7.5 million children have chronic conditions such as developmental disabilities, chronic diseases, and mental health problems (Vessey, 1994). More than 68,000 children who are not in acute care require some form of medical technology support as a result of conditions that have led to the loss of normal body functions or are otherwise severe enough to affect activities of daily living (Ahmann & Lierman, 1992: Office of Technology Assessment, 1987; Strutts, 1994). Technology support ranges from simple, non-invasive equipment such as an apnea monitor to complicated systems such as a ventilator (Britton & Johnston, 1993). Health care services to provide for the needs of these children range from care provided in the home by trained caregivers to around-the-clock monitored care in a long-term care facility.

The expansion of rehabilitation and home care services for children has also been influenced by the changing nature of hospital reimbursement, decreased lengths of hospital stays, the belief that outpatient and home care services reduce costs, patient preferences, and legislation that has supported the rights of handicapped individuals (McClowry, 1993; McClung, 1995). Although a child may not know life without a disability, the handicapping nature of these conditions, that is, the child's social barriers to independence, depends greatly on society accepting and making adaptations for these children in the schools, social settings, and the workplace. The Education for All Handicapped Act (Public Law 94-142) mandates that states provide free and appropriate education in the least restrictive setting for children with disabilities. In 1986, the amendment to this act, Public Law 99-457, required states to provide early assessment and intervention programs for high-risk children and mandated involvement by the family (Kaufman, 1991; Selekman, 1991). Chapter 7 provides an in-depth discussion of the legislation that has affected care of the child requiring special community services.

The increased growth in rehabilitation and home care services has created a need for nurses with the professional skills and knowledge to provide care to this expanding population. The nurse serving in these arenas must be independent in providing care and acting as a case manager in a variety of settings. Conversely, she or he must also be able to function as a team member, coordinating a broad range of services and resources for children and their families. Also required are knowledge of the developmental capabilities of children and the skills needed to work collaboratively with the families. The child requiring rehabilitative care or ongoing support by medical technology faces many challenges to normal development. Long-term hospital stays, frequent visits to rehabilitation centers, and medical treatments provided in the home can interfere with parent-child attachment and with the development of peer relationships. Cumbersome equipment can make it difficult for the toddler to move about and to explore his or her world. Visible tubes and catheters may influence the school-age child's emerging self-esteem. Required daily treatments may meet with noncompliance by the adolescent who is asserting his or her independence. Knowledge of child development and family theory is essential to promote the well-being of all family members as they face issues associated with care of the physically and developmentally challenged child.

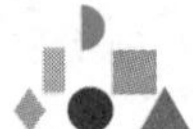

Pediatric Rehabilitation and Habilitation

Rehabilitation of children differs from that of adults in several ways (Chart 11–1). The difference that forms the basis for understanding all other variation is that adults have reached a level of physical and mental maturity and children have not. Children are in the midst of their growth and development, learning new skills and tasks. Children heal faster, generally have a higher metabolic rate, and have greater nutritional needs than adults. The

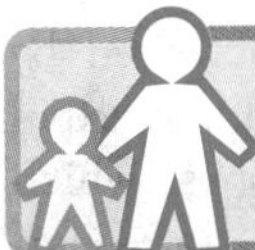

Chart 11–1
Developmental Considerations

Differences Between Rehabilitation of the Adult and of the Child

In Adult Rehabilitation . . .	In Pediatric Rehabilitation . . .
The focus is on reintegrating or compensating for what is lost.	The focus is on helping the child to attain skills and abilities at a level that may have been previously unknown to the child.
The needs for rehabilitation involve suddenly acquired conditions such as trauma, stroke, and heart disease or debilitating conditions such as diabetes, arthritis, and pulmonary disease.	The needs for habilitation involve some form of chronic illness, congenital anomaly, or disabling condition acquired as a result of medical interventions that have sustained the child's life.
Physical development is complete for the most part. Emotional development and cognitive development have also reached a plateau, with growth continuing but with less variance than in the pediatric population.	The child continues to experience a tremendous amount of physical, emotional, sexual, social, and cognitive development.
The family is important as a source of support and as an adjunct to treatment.	The family must simultaneously learn to care for the child and foster the child's development as well as learn to manage their own individual and family needs.
The goal is to teach the adult to care for himself or herself.	The goal is to teach the child to care for himself or herself as appropriate for age and capabilities.
The focus is on vocational rehabilitation, teaching skills and knowledge so that the adult can perform or resume an occupation.	The focus is on educational rehabilitation, reaching the highest academic level possible, while teaching the child life skills that would be accomplished by any child, such as ordering food in a restaurant, receiving change from a purchase, and using public transportation. Therapeutic support services also assist in developing skills such as walking, building a block tower, combing hair, and learning to color.
The necessity for rehabilitation is a new concept. Before the condition that brought him or her to the point of requiring rehabilitation, the adult was able to care for himself or herself and to complete daily activities.	The child's disability is the norm. The child has a known dependence and, depending on the age at onset, is likely not to have known a life without his or her chronic condition.
Experiencing chronic pain, discomfort, or the need for treatment as a result of the condition and undergoing rehabilitation may be relatively new experiences.	The experience of chronic pain or discomfort or the need for treatment may not be new to the child. The child with a disability or a chronic condition may already have spent many years with these experiences as a result of the condition.

Information adapted from Selekman, J. (1991). Pediatric rehabilitation: From concepts to practice. *Pediatric Nursing, 17,* 11–14, 33.

child's cognitive level continues to change, as do his or her emotional, psychosocial, and sexual areas of development (Strutts, 1994).

The child's learning process is affected by cognitive and developmental factors that may not have an influence on the adult's ability to learn. For example, toddlers and preschoolers learn through exploration, by discovering their world. If a child's environment is limited to the length of an oxygen or ventilator tube, or if experiences are limited by physical immobility, the focus of habilitative care would be on assisting the child to compensate for this limitation. For instance, the family would be instructed to use extra lengths of oxygen tubing and/or a small oxygen tank that could be easily moved from room to room to broaden the world of the oxygen-dependent child. Or perhaps the young child with limited physical mobility would be encouraged to explore his or her environment and experience independent exploration on a scooter board or while seated in a small wheeled cart. Unlike an adult, the child may not be aware that there is a world full of exciting adventures and experiences beyond the scope of what can be immediately seen and touched. The goal of pediatric rehabilitation and habilitation is to help the child and family adapt their environment so as to allow the child to achieve his or her highest possible developmental level despite physical and environmental limitations.

The adult in rehabilitation often has a repertoire of past experiences from which to build new adaptive tasks and to learn to reintegrate and to compensate for what he or she has lost because of illness or injury (Burkett, 1989). However, the child may not have such a strong experiential basis on which to build (Fig. 11–1). For example, a kindergartner who experiences disfiguring burns on the arms and upper chest must learn all over again how to hold a spoon and a drinking cup, as well as how to acquire the new ability of writing.

caREminder: *The child must be habilitated to his or her new developmental age, not the level at which the injury occurred (Selekman, 1991).*

Although experts may dispute the correct terminology for describing this process, in these instances "habilitation" and "rehabilitation" are used interchangeably.

Adults most often require rehabilitation because of a sudden disability resulting from a stroke or an injury. In contrast, children most commonly need rehabilitation because of a chronic illness or congenital defect (Selekman, 1991). These conditions are generally characterized by periods of exacerbation during which the child may experience loss of certain developmental milestones, which must be reattained once the child's health status improves. Unlike most adult situations, the family may not have a diagnosis or "label" for the underlying cause of the disability. This is particularly true for rare diseases and conditions, in which it might be years before a diagnosis is determined and the family has a true idea of what the future may hold for their child (Selekman & Synder, 1996). Without clear guidelines, parents may be at a loss as to which developmental and physical goals are attainable for their child. The future is not guaranteed for anyone, but most children have a reasonable expectation of being able to walk, to talk, to go to school and interact with others, and to achieve a certain level of independence. If a child is blind, therapy includes ways of helping the child to succeed without sight. When the sequelae of an impairment are unknown, it becomes difficult to plan the best way to help the child deal with an unknown outcome. Lack of information is one of the most unsettling aspects of caring for or being a child with an undiagnosed disability (Seltzer & Krauss, 1994).

Figure 11–1
Prolonged hospitalization and dependence on respiratory support make achievement of normal developmental milestones difficult. A therapist can come to the child's bedside to facilitate rehabilitative goals.

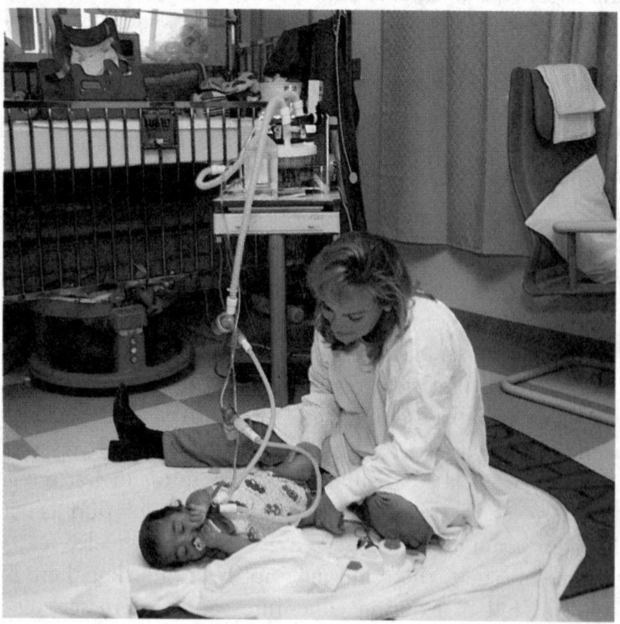

Philosophy and Goals of Pediatric Rehabilitation

The late 19th and early 20th centuries brought improved hygiene and nutrition, the development of immunization programs, and the introduction of new medications, all of which significantly contributed to the decrease in mortality and the improvement in health status of modern societies (McKeown, 1979). The beginning of the 20th century saw a shift in the focus of society toward individuals with specific disabilities. The first pediatric rehabilitation facility in the United States was established in 1872. Many of the early facilities focused on the care of children with nutritional and vitamin deficiencies, debilitating infectious diseases such as tuberculosis and poliomyelitis, and neurologic and orthopedic conditions.

Over the years, the specialty care area of pediatric rehabilitation and habilitation has continued to evolve. Current areas of care are not limited to neurologic or orthopedic conditions. Nutritional and respiratory conditions continue to be a primary focus, although with advances in technology and medical science, the care needs of children are quite different. Instead of the vitamin deficiencies commonly seen in the past, metabolic disturbances and feeding disorders are a focus of care. Tuberculosis was once a primary cause of respiratory distress; now children are receiving ventilator assistance while their lungs continue to develop after premature birth. Many of the children successfully treated in rehabilitation and habilitation today would not have survived their illness or condition 20 years ago.

Pediatric rehabilitation programs continue to focus on a continuum of care within a developmental, educational, and family systems framework (McCourt, 1993). Advances in technology, lifesaving measures throughout the early developmental stages, and more successful treatment of disease have led to a new focus on restorative and preventive care.

The philosophy of rehabilitation rests on the following principles:

- Rehabilitation recognizes the uniqueness and wholeness of each individual and views each person and his or her own environment as interdependent systems (Sayles, 1981).
- Despite the severity of an injury or illness, each individual has the potential to maintain or to regain self-esteem and dignity and to transcend disability. Individuals can obtain optimal independence within the limits of disability when they participate fully in making decisions about their rehabilitation (Dittmar, 1989).
- Through rehabilitation, persons with disabilities are enabled to mobilize their own resources, to decide what they wish to do and what they are able to be, and to achieve goals through their own efforts and in their own way (Wright, 1983).
- Each individual is a social organism motivated to work and to contribute as a member of society; this contribution begins with self-support and extends to a commitment to family, community, nation, and the world (Wright, 1983).

Using these tenets as a foundation, the developing specialty of pediatric rehabilitation builds on them to encompass the unique influence of the growth and developmental process. As previously stated, rather than assisting a child to a level of ability and independence previously known, the focus of care of the pediatric client is on achieving a level of development and ability not yet attained (Fig. 11–2). A young child who sustains a traumatic injury does not have his or her previous level of function as the rehabilitation goal because the developmental process continues while the healing occurs. The goal is to achieve age-appropriate ability and to enable continued growth and development.

Terminology

Frequently, terminology used in rehabilitation leads to incorrect meaning and stimulates confusion and inconsistency between and among professionals and their clients. A primary example of such an error can be seen when the term *impairment*, *disability*, or *handicap* is selected to describe or to explain a condition. Many persons interpret these terms as having a hierarchic relationship, with impairment connoting the least significant disability and handicap the most. Others view the same terms as being related to specific conditions, with impairment or disability referring to mental or cognitive deficiency and handicap referring to physical inability. Still others may see little difference in meaning and use these terms interchangeably, perhaps selecting the one that seems "nicer" or more "politically correct."

The World Health Organization makes the following

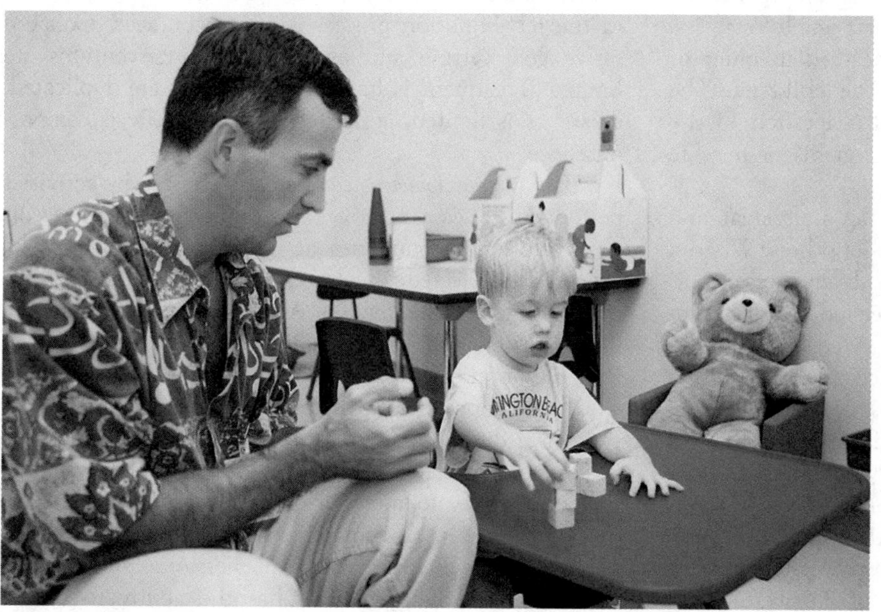

Figure 11–2
Pediatric rehabilitation and habilitation services help the child attain skills that are new to the child, yet appropriate to his or her developmental age.

distinctions among an impairment, a disability, and a handicap (Storck & Thompson-Hoffman, 1991):

- An *impairment* is defined as "a loss or abnormality of a psychological, physiological, or anatomical structure and function" (p. 6).
- A *disability* occurs when there is a "restriction or lack (resulting from an impairment) of ability to perform an activity in the manner or within the range considered normal for a human being" (p. 6).
- A *handicap* occurs when there is "a disadvantage for a given individual resulting from impairment or disability that limits or prevents fulfillment of a role that is normal for that individual" (p. 7).

Using these definitions as a framework, an impairment is related specifically to an injury or a body part that is altered. For instance, a visual impairment indicates an anatomic condition contributing to altered visual acuity. A neurologic impairment indicates that an aspect of the neurologic system (i.e., the brain, spinal cord, nerve cell, or neurotransmission) has sustained damage or is not functioning as it should. Rehabilitative care centers on the continued healing of an injury or recovery from an illness that causes an impairment. Another primary focus of rehabilitation is the prevention of complications of a condition or illness that would cause, or further, an impairment.

A *disability*, or *functional limitation*, is specifically related to what an individual is not able to do as a result of an impairment. A function cannot be performed, or does not develop, as it would have had there been no impairment. This is a central focus in rehabilitation. When a child cannot perform a function as he or she could once before or as others can, steps can be taken to assist the child in a return to this level of function. If the impairment is such that return is not possible, assistive devices or adaptive techniques can be used in order to achieve a higher degree of ability. The child must be supported in his or her psychological adaptation to the altered function and the effect it has on his or her life style.

A *handicap* has less to do with an individual and much more to do with the perceptions of others. When a child with a disability is placed at a disadvantage compared with others, because of his or her functional limitation, a handicapping situation exists. A person is handicapped only by the lack of acceptance or adaptation in society. A handicap, in many ways, is *imposed* on an individual rather than being an intrinsic characteristic of the individual. In a model of disability published in 1991 by the Committee on a National Agenda for the Prevention of Disabilities, Division of Health Promotion, Institute of Medicine, the term handicap was deleted and the concepts of risk factors and quality of life were added (Pope & Tarlov, 1991).

The Rehabilitation Team

Rehabilitative and habilitative care are team efforts. The child and the family are linked to many people who are working toward helping the child attain his or her highest potential (Chart 11–2). To achieve this, the family must become knowledgeable about the specific disability and must practice care procedures under the supervision of health care professionals until they can perform them independently.

Various team models can be used in the rehabilitation process, both in facilities and in the community. The models can be described as multidisciplinary, interdisciplinary, or transdisciplinary. The types of team models used may vary according to the practice setting; benefits and limitations can be identified for each model.

Core functions of the rehabilitative team include:

- Assessment of the patient's needs and functional ability
- Development and documentation of an interdisciplinary treatment plan based on the client's and the team's goals
- Implementation of the treatment plan in an interdisciplinary manner
- Evaluation of the treatment plan by the extent to which goals are achieved by the patient
- Planning for patient discharge (CARF, 1996; JCAHO, 1996)

The *multidisciplinary team* is characterized by the activities of individuals from various disciplines who are required to know only the skills of their own discipline. The benefits of this model include minimal coordination efforts and less time spent in team meetings. This model poses limitations in that patient and family participation in the rehabilitation process is not encouraged. Collaborative goal setting and evaluation of interventions are limited. Treatment is fragmented, services are duplicated, creativity is limited, and effectiveness of care is compromised.

The *interdisciplinary team* is characterized by activities performed by team members from different disciplines directed toward a common goal. This model is required by agencies that accredit health care and rehabilitation facilities (Joint Commission on Accreditation of Healthcare Organizations and the Commission on Accreditation of Rehabilitation Facilities). This model involves members who have knowledge of therapeutic interventions beyond their own discipline and who can collaboratively achieve goals far greater than their own. Benefits of this model include the development of a team with a holistic view of clients' needs. A comprehensive, consistent, nonfragmented approach fosters optimal client outcome. An effective interdisciplinary team has the ability to reduce health care costs and to improve client outcomes

Chart 11–2

The Rehabilitation Team

Title	Responsibilities
Rehabilitation or home care nurse	Provides direct and indirect nursing care to prevent further disability, maintain present ability, and restore lost ability. Teaches the child to use remaining abilities in adapting to or altering lifestyle. Monitors all aspects of the child's physical and developmental well-being and coordinates services for the family.
Physical therapist	Evaluates, prevents, and manages disorders of human motion. Assists clients in regaining function and in preventing pain and disability after disease, injury, or loss of a body part. Evaluates muscle strength, range of joint motion, posture and gait, limb length and condition, activities of daily living, sensory and motor function, orthotic and prosthetic fit and function, reflexes and muscle tone, and sensorimotor performance. Treatments include hydrotherapy, diathermy, ultrasonography and ultraviolet radiation, and electrical stimulation. Performs massage and assists clients in performing therapeutic exercises. Works to reeducate muscles, improve coordination, and teach relaxation techniques. Uses biofeedback, orthotics or prosthetics, and other assistive devices such as crutches, canes, walkers, and wheelchairs.
Occupational therapist	Assists child to maintain and restore physical and psychological ability to function in preparation for return to work, family, school, or community. Assesses muscles that need strengthening and coordination and recommends practical activities to improve strength. Assesses age-appropriate tasks and roles in family and community, including activities of daily living, work activities, play activities, and driving capabilities. Teaches homemaking skills, energy conservation, and work simplification methods to improve work tolerance. Works with the client to improve communication skills such as reading, writing, and using the telephone. Designs assistive and adaptive devices to help the client in activities of daily living, as well as splints for the prevention and control of potential deformities of the hand and upper extremity.
Speech/language pathologist	Evaluates and treats communication disorders that result from physical and developmental disorders or from illness or surgical procedures. Speech therapy is concerned with resolving speech, language, and hearing problems that may affect expression, reception, or both. Treatment techniques are designed to facilitate communication with staff and family members, and speech and language recovery. Receives specialized training in oromotor function and feeding and works with the client toward improved motor function and coordination, facilitating safe oral feeding.
Nutritionist	Attends to the nutritional needs of clients, assessing nutritional history and determining ideal body weight. With the speech therapist, identifies foods that facilitate swallowing. Plans and modifies special and therapeutic diets, educates team members in basic and therapeutic nutrition, and counsels clients and family members about dietary modifications and preparation related to the client's needs.
Psychologist	Performs psychometric assessments to analyze the intellectual, cognitive, and emotional status of the client and evaluates the stimulus situations and reinforcers that influence behavior. Counsels clients and families in institutions and communities, acts as primary therapist, and conducts research. Instructs clients, families, and staff about expectations of cognitively impaired individuals, emotional adaptation to disability, and behavioral management techniques.
Social worker	Assesses family structure and support systems and assists clients and families in problem-solving efforts related to work, finance, living situations, social life, marriage, child care, and emotional well-being. Assists the family and the rehabilitation team in the discharge planning process, identifying ways to obtain coverage for care, equipment, home modifications, and transportation. Facilitates the referral to other care facilities, if necessary.

Chart continued on following page

Chart 11–2 *Continued*

The Rehabilitation Team

Title	Responsibilities
Physician	Responsible for the medical management of clients and evaluation of the comprehensive treatment plan. Prescribes therapeutic aids and prosthetic and orthotic devices.
Educator	Evaluates and implements adaptations required for the child to optimize his or her school experience and facilitate learning.
Vocational rehabilitation counselor	Works with the educator and the child as the child nears the end of the high school years. Assesses the child's limitations, strengths, and interests to identify potential employment opportunities. Develops the training program for the child to become employable.
Child life specialist	Minimizes or prevents the developmental and psychological disruptions associated with hospitalization, illness, injury, and disability in childhood and adolescence. Uses directed and expressive play, recreation, creative arts, education, and social and family activities to promote growth and maturation, help children cope with the psychosocial stressors of treatment and rehabilitation, and teach modifications that allow children to participate with their peers in recreation and leisure activities with a focus on inclusion rather than on disability.

(O'Toole, 1992). The limitations of the interdisciplinary team model include its complexity and the amount of time required to maintain communication and collaborative efforts.

The *transdisciplinary team* is characterized by the utilization of professionals who have had instruction and experience across all disciplines. It is similar to the interdisciplinary team model; however, in this model, one or two individuals are responsible for implementing the treatment plan. Members of individual disciplines are available for consultation. A high degree of communication, interaction, staff development, and open thinking is involved (Hoeman, 1992). The benefits of this model include less stress on the client, who works with only a limited number of professionals. Staff resources are also conserved. The primary care provider may not demonstrate expertise in all areas of the treatment plan, however. The clear cost savings and effectiveness of this model have not yet been demonstrated.

Levels of Rehabilitative Care

Rehabilitative services are provided in three primary settings. The choice of setting for an individual child is dependent on the child's level of medical acuity and the availability of such services in the community. It is important to remember that rehabilitation as a process depends more on the team members and treatment implemented than on the setting where the care is provided.

Acute rehabilitation refers to the phase of rehabilitative services provided immediately after an injury or illness. Once medically stable, the patient receives therapeutic services in an acute care unit or is transferred to a rehabilitation unit or facility that is in close proximity to emergency care facilities, should complications occur.

Subacute rehabilitation refers to the phase of care that extends for up to 6 months after an injury or illness. Therapeutic services are typically provided in a freestanding rehabilitation facility where ongoing recovery and prevention of complications continue. Patient and family teaching is emphasized with a goal of return to the home and to the community.

Postacute rehabilitation refers to the phase of care extending up to 12 months or longer after an injury or illness. Care may be delivered in a residential setting or in the home and the school with supportive services. The goal of care at this level includes educational or vocational interventions, along with the reinforcement of adaptive techniques to optimize functional ability and independence.

Assessment of the Child with Rehabilitative and Habilitative Needs

Assessment of the child with a long-term disability requires the use of standardized measurement tools and ongoing assessment information gathered by members of the rehabilitation team. Measurement tools in rehabilitative care provide an objective measure of the child's functional abilities. They also provide information regarding needs of the child and the family, the effectiveness of

Table 11–1
Measurement Tools Used in Pediatric Rehabilitation

Measurement Tool	Age	Focus, Design	Administration
BDI (Battelle Developmental Inventory, DLM Teaching Resources)	Birth to 8 yr	Incorporates a number of developmental and adaptive activities in the personal-social, adaptive activities of daily living, motor, communication, and cognitive performance areas. Many of the motor and adaptive items are developmental in nature, with only a subset of items relevant for functional assessment of the child with severe disabilities.	Administered using structured interviews, observation, and direct testing. A brief screening version is available.
VABS (Vineland Adaptive Behavior Scale, American Guidance Service)	Birth to 19 yr	Assesses ability to perform necessary activities of daily living. Covers a wide range of areas, including communication, daily living skills, and motor ability. This test is useful for overall descriptions of function in school-age children and adolescents but does not provide sufficient analysis of dependence in functional items for extremely young children or those with severe physical or cognitive delays.	Available in three forms: a survey, an expanded version, and a classroom edition.
GMFM (Gross Motor Function Measures) (Russell et al., 1989)	Young children with cerebral palsy	The test identifies developmental performance and mobility in the following positions and activities: supine, prone, quadruped, sitting, kneeling, standing, walking, and the use of stairs. The focus is exclusively on gross motor function; however, important items such as wheelchair mobility and transfer are not addressed. The child is evaluated on a four-point rating scale measuring the level of the activity completed: cannot initiate, initiates independently, partially completes, and completes independently.	Direct assessment of gross motor function.
Wee FIM (Functional Independence Measure for Children, Research Foundation, State University of New York)	6 mo to 7 yr and older	Captures measurements of levels of dependence or independence in the following areas: eating, grooming, bathing, dressing upper body, dressing lower body, toileting, bladder management, bowel management, transfers to chair or wheelchair, transfers to toilet, transfers to tub or shower, locomotion, stairs, comprehension, expression, social interaction, problem solving, and memory. It is constructed to mimic the FIM used for adults and is intended to help facilitate growth of the disabled child into an independent adult. It serves as a basic indicator of severity of disability and does not identify an impairment.	For use by a trained clinician in any discipline.
PEDI (Pediatric Evaluation of Disability Inventory, Department of Rehabilitation Medicine, New England Medical Center Hospitals)	6 mo to 7 yr	Provides a descriptive measure of the child's current functional performance. Measures both capability and performance of functional activities in three content domains: self-care, mobility, and social function. Designed primarily for the functional evaluation of young children; however, it can also be used for the evaluation of older children if their functional abilities fall below that expected of 7-yr-old children without disabilities.	Can be administered by a clinician or educator who is familiar with the child or via a structured interview with the parent.
FRESNO (Fresno Rehabilitation Evaluation of Sensori-Neurologic Outcomes, Valley Children's Hospital, Fresno, CA)	Birth to 3 yr	This tool targets the skills of infants and young children in three main self-help areas, feeding or eating, dressing, and toileting, providing a descriptive measure of the child's functional ability.	Can be administered by a clinician in any discipline who is familiar with the child and the areas that the tool addresses or may be administered by a team of professionals.
SIB (Scale of Independent Behavior, DLM Teaching Resources)	Infant to adult; best used between 6 yr and adolescence	Addresses four adaptive skill clusters: motor, social interaction and communication, personal living, and community living. Part of the Woodcock-Johnson Psychoeducational Battery. Identifies functional skills needed at home and in social and community settings.	Individually administered by structured interview. Short form available for rapid screening.

Table 11–2
Focus of Treatment in Pediatric Rehabilitation

Type of Disorder	Examples	Focus of Treatment
Neurodevelopmental conditions	Cerebral palsy Down syndrome Spina bifida Learning disabilities Mental retardation Autism or pervasive developmental disabilities Dual diagnoses Fetal alcohol syndrome Fragile X syndrome Rett's syndrome	Education or vocational training · Program early intervention before preschool age, stimulation of developmental skills and milestones. · Support development of cognitive skills. · Support development of social skills. · Provide training in life skills (e.g., money management, transportation, shopping). Physical therapy · Maximize gross motor balance, strength, and endurance. · Maintain range of motion, muscle tone, and reflexes. · Improve perceptual-motor ability. · Develop and use splints or braces for support or to maintain or improve function. · Promote independence and safety in mobility. · Train in ambulation with or without assistive devices or use of a wheelchair. · Transfers, gait training, ability to ascend and descend stairs. · Treatment modalities including hydrotherapy, hippotherapy, transcutaneous electrical stimulation, biofeedback, weight training, hot and cold applications. Occupational therapy · Maximize fine motor strength and ability to support gross motor function. · Hand-eye coordination. · Sensory integration. · Development and use of splints for support or to maintain or improve function. · Safety in judgment (recognition of hot and cold, sharp and dull). · Ability to manipulate objects and perform tasks of daily living (toileting, hygiene, grooming, dressing, feeding). · Training in activities of daily living with or without adaptive devices. · Support in ability to perform life skills (manipulate coins, prepare meals, sew or mend garments, perform cleaning and household activities). · Support fine motor skills to permit activities of leisure and recreation (sewing, crafts, art, music). · Support in ability to perform skills related to education or vocational training (coloring, writing, copying, typing). · Treatment modalities including vestibular stimulation. Speech therapy · Ability to perform oromotor function for safe feeding and airway protection. · Improve skill in eating or feeding. · Improve skills in perception of language. · Improve skills in expressive language. · Treatment modalities including oromotor desensitization and stimulation, exercises for language perception and articulation, methods of augmentative communication. Child life and recreation therapy · Support participation in activities of leisure or recreation (art, crafts, music, athletics). Sensory treatment · Evaluation of hearing ability and use of assistive device. · Evaluation of vision ability and use of assistive device.

Physical conditions	Fracture Legg-Calvé-Perthes Avascular necrosis Developmental dysplastic hip Juvenile rheumatoid arthritis Arthrogryposis multiplex congenita Amputation Spinal cord injury Brain injury Burns Muscular dystrophy Epidermolysis bullosa	Surgical intervention · Reduction, osteotomy, tendon release, prosthetic implantation, bone grafting, external fixation. Physical therapy · Maximize gross motor balance, strength, and endurance. · Maintain range of motion, muscle tone, and reflexes. · Development and use of splints or braces for support or to maintain or improve function, independence, and safety in mobility. · Training in ambulation with or without assistive devices or use of a wheelchair. · Transfers, gait training, ability to ascend and descend stairs. · Treatment modalities including hydrotherapy, hippotherapy, transcutaneous electrical stimulation, biofeedback, weight training, hot and cold applications. Orthotics or prosthetics · Construction of support devices or braces or artificial limbs.
Chronic conditions	Asthma Diabetes mellitus Encopresis Acute lymphocytic leukemia Bronchopulmonary dysplasia Psychiatric disorders Systemic lupus erythematosus	Medical management · Monitor health status and response to treatments. · Ensure that medical regimen is achievable and can be maintained considering individual resources and home environment. Individual and family knowledge · Support development of knowledge about condition. · Support development of skill in procedures necessary for self-care. · Support understanding of effect of condition on growth and development and effect of developmental tasks on medical management of condition. Individual and group counseling · Support self-concept, self-esteem, and body image. · Monitor risk for complications for further illness (including infection). Pharmacology
Complex medical conditions	Reflex sympathetic dystrophy Organ transplantation Acquired autoimmune deficiency Blount's disease Pain Behavioral disorders Ventilator assistance	Medical management · Monitor health status and response to treatments. · Ensure that medical regimen is achievable and can be maintained considering individual resources and home environment. Technological support · Ventilator. · Infusion pump. · Feeding tube. Behavior management · Positive, negative, and differential reinforcement. · Punishment, time out, response cost, overcorrection. Individual and group counseling Transcutaneous electrical neuronal stimulation Biofeedback Individual and family teaching · Support development of knowledge about condition. · Support development of skill in procedures necessary for self-care. · Support understanding of effect of condition on growth and development and effect of developmental tasks on medical management of condition.

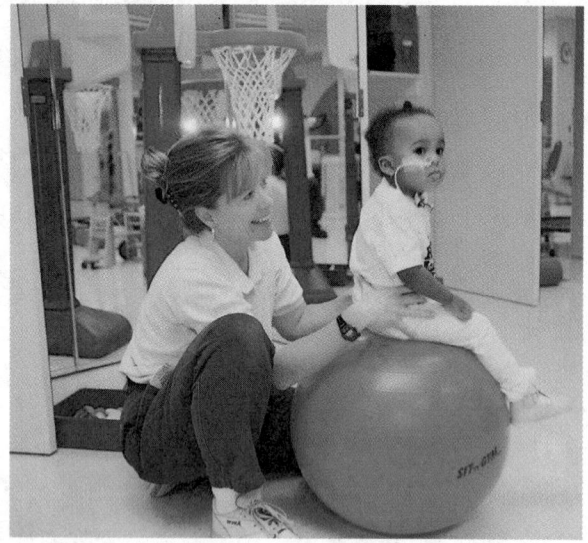

Figure 11–3
Rehabilitation provides purposeful stimulation to facilitate development of physical, cognitive, and psychosocial skills.

interventions, and the success of a specific rehabilitative program. Few tests are available that address the special needs of children and their families. The measurement tools should not be used in isolation, as no single tool provides a complete picture of a child's needs. Rehabilitation teams generally find it useful to adopt two or more pediatric measurement tools, tailoring aspects of each to capture the specific needs of a specific patient population. Table 11–1 provides a summary of seven tools that can be used by the pediatric rehabilitation team.

Health Challenges of the Child Receiving Rehabilitative and Habilitative Services

The conditions of children requiring rehabilitation and habilitation vary widely but share many commonalities in the functional limitations that can affect the child (Table 11–2). The general types of conditions that can benefit from rehabilitative services are discussed in the following. More complete discussions of specific disease processes can be found in Chapters 14 through 30 of this text, in which alterations in specific body systems are presented.

Neurodevelopmental Conditions

Neurodevelopmental conditions are characterized by an impairment of the neurologic system that causes a delay in one or more areas of development. These conditions can be genetic, perinatal, or congenital. Examples include cerebral palsy, spina bifida, and Down syndrome.

Cerebral palsy is a nonprogressive condition in which an abnormality occurs in the brain before it reaches maturity, resulting in disorders of movement and posture. Spina bifida is a congenital malformation of the neural tube such that the child is born with a portion of the spinal cord in a sac presenting outside the body. The spinal cord does not develop below the level at which the sac appears on the spinal column. Down syndrome, or trisomy 21, results from a chromosomal abnormality. Children with these conditions may have a degree of mental retardation, as well as physical disability.

In caring for the child with a neurodevelopmental condition, it is important to accurately identify developmental levels in the areas of physical, cognitive, and social or emotional development (Fig. 11–3). The child's abilities may be widely disparate from his or her chronologic age in these areas of development.

Physical Conditions

Rehabilitation is frequently characterized by conditions requiring attention to the physical aspects of disability, often acquired as the result of illness or injury (Strutts, 1994). Such conditions often have intensive or critical care periods at their onset. Once medical stability is achieved, the focus of care turns toward restoration of function and ability while maintaining health status and preventing complications, or rehabilitation (Fig. 11–4).

Figure 11–4
Therapeutic interventions include using technology to promote recovery and restore function and ability.

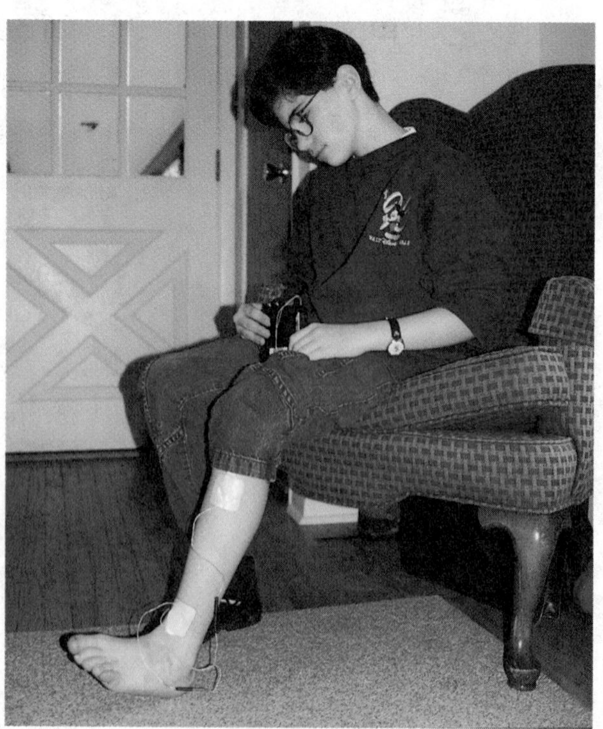

Conditions that require this approach include brain injury, spinal cord injury, burn, and musculoskeletal disorders.

A child may incur a brain injury as the result of trauma, the growth of a tumor, or an infection. The scope of the injury can be local, limited to a specific area, or diffuse, involving several areas of the brain. A spinal cord injury, although most often caused by trauma, can also result from a tumor or an infection. The degree to which a child is impaired is directly related to the area(s) of the central nervous system that is injured or not functioning properly and the part(s) of the body that is controlled by the nonfunctioning area of the nervous system. Musculoskeletal disorders may be congenital (e.g., arthrogryposis multiplex congenita), diagnosed at a young age (e.g., juvenile rheumatoid arthritis), or result from trauma or infection. When the structure of the body is disrupted, the child's ability to function is significantly altered. Burns result from injury or trauma, although some congenital conditions require a similar type of treatment (e.g., epidermolysis bullosa). The function of the area of the body that is burned is directly affected.

Chronic Conditions

Childhood chronic illness often results in frequent hospitalization, lost school days, and greatly increased family stress (Martinez, Schreiber, & Hartman, 1991). Extended periods of bed rest, inactivity related to fatigue, and immobility related to confining treatment modalities cause a child to need rehabilitative services. Care is often directed toward helping the child regain physical strength and abilities (Fig. 11–5). In addition, if the child's health status has been compromised for a long period, habilitation services are provided to advance the child's abilities to a new, more appropriate level. For instance, the toddler who has had a bone marrow transplant may be hospitalized for 3 to 6 months or longer. Over a 3-month period, a healthy toddler can advance from walking with an unsteady gait to running with confidence. The same child may also advance from self-feeding finger foods to competent use of a spoon. Because of extensive medical interventions and the critical nature of the child's condition, the toddler having a transplant may have had limited opportunity to walk and no opportunity

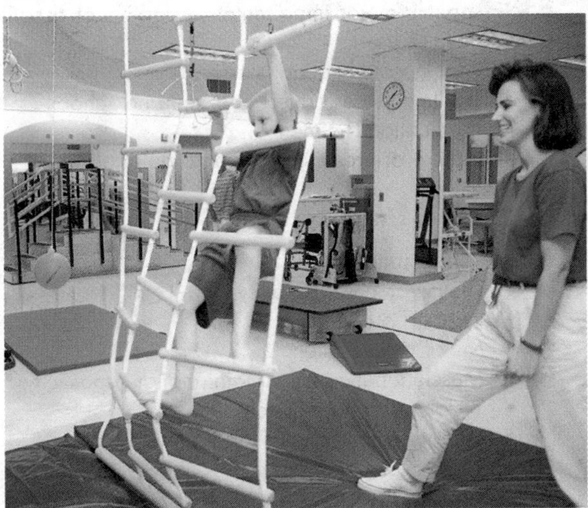

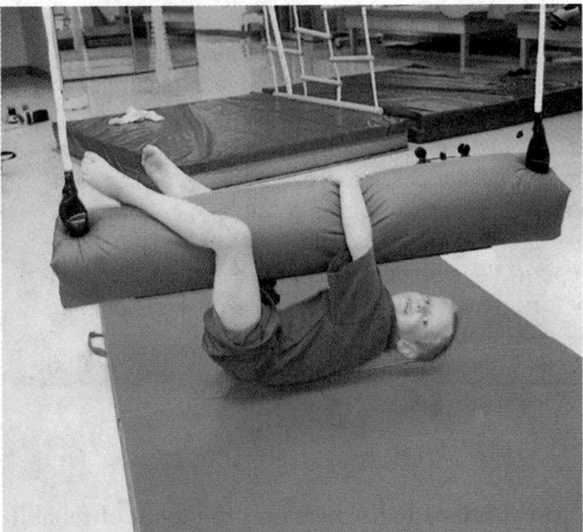

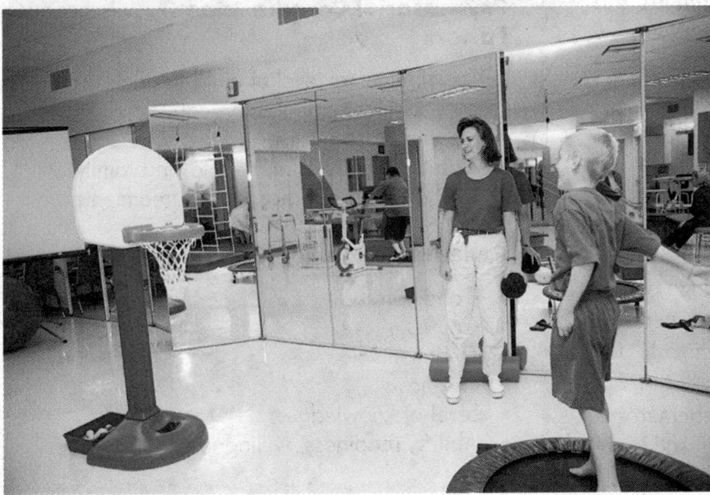

Figure 11–5
During physical rehabilitation, a therapist uses specially designed equipment to encourage activities that strengthen certain muscle groups and promote coordination.

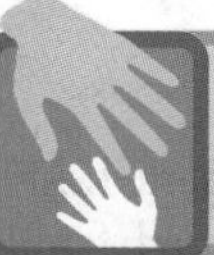

Chart 11–3
Nursing Interventions

Strategies for Normalizing Care of the Child

- Use a transdisciplinary approach to health care to minimize the number of professionals the family has to deal with, while still maintaining access to the expertise and professional services the child requires.
- Provide consistent caregivers.
- Establish daily routines.
- Maintain a schedule for the child to monitor health maintenance issues such as immunizations, vision and hearing examinations, and dental screening.
- Select medical equipment that meets the child's developmental needs (e.g., standing frame to foster participation in activities, lightweight infusion pumps for the child attending school).
- Develop all goals and a plan of care for the child in collaboration with the family.
- Establish guidelines for discipline and limitations that parents and other caregivers consistently follow.
- Optimize opportunities for experiences that enhance the child's growth and development. For instance, encourage play, weekly outings, and participation in special events with other children.
- Encourage the child to provide for his or her own personal care as much as possible (e.g., brushing teeth, hair care, dressing).
- Support development of the child's role in the family (assigning chores for which he or she is able to be responsible).

to learn to eat unassisted. Therefore, the focus of rehabilitative and habilitative care is on increasing strength and endurance and on helping the child to attain the new developmental skill of self-feeding.

Another characteristic of chronic conditions is their episodic nature. A child may go for long periods with good health and suddenly have an exacerbation or worsening of his or her condition. Conditions in which this occurs include diabetes, asthma, and systemic lupus erythematosus. Children with these conditions are not generally recognized as having a disability, although when their disease "flares," they may be unable to perform many functions that previously were not difficult for them.

An adolescent with systemic lupus erythematosus may have a flare of the condition and may suddenly become quite ill, weak, and fatigued. Rehabilitation efforts focus on promoting strength and endurance while managing the medical condition. Continued education for children and their families about the condition and the steps toward disease management is essential. Support services help them to cope with having a chronic illness.

Complex Medical Conditions

Rehabilitation interventions are frequently needed to support the health care needs of children with complex medical conditions. Examples include children who have

Chart 11–4

Focused Health Assessment of the Child with Rehabilitation/Habilitation Needs

Pertinent History

- Birth history, complications
- Complications associated with disability: seizures; cognitive status; problems with vision, hearing, speech; motor impairments; adaptive or assistive devices used
- Prior hospitalization, surgery
- Treatments performed at home and school
- Medication regimen
- Nature of present condition requiring treatment

Physical Findings

- Reflex patterns
- Temperament, irritability
- Feeding problems
- Motor development
- Muscle tone, range of joint motion, spasticity
- Vision, hearing, speech
- Weight, vital signs, level of consciousness
- Functional limitations

Psychosocial Concerns and Developmental Factors

- Developmental level of child in each area (cognitive, socioemotional, physical)
- Coping mechanisms
- Habits, daily routine of child and family
- Likely response to hospital or treatment

Patient and Family Knowledge

- Condition
- Causes
- Treatments
- Prognosis
- Level of knowledge
- Ability, readiness, willingness to learn

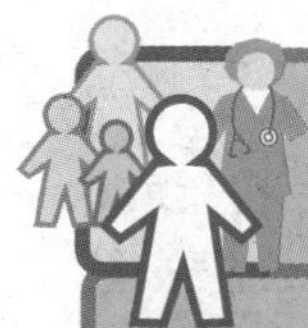

Chart 11–5
Nursing Diagnoses and Outcomes

The Child with a Disability

Self-care deficit: feeding, bathing and hygiene, dressing and grooming, toileting related to physical/mental deficit

Outcomes: Child will achieve/maintain functional abilities to be as independent as possible.
Child will achieve/maintain adequate weight and level of hydration.
Child will maintain adequate personal hygiene.

Altered growth and development related to mental/emotional/cognitive deficit

Outcomes: Child will maintain/improve level of development.
Child will participate in activities with family, siblings, peers.

Impaired verbal communication related to inability to articulate/hear spoken words

Outcome: Child will achieve/maintain communication skills, utilizing augmentative devices as necessary.

Impaired physical mobility related to muscle weakness, spasticity, or paralysis

Outcomes: Child will maintain/improve range of joint motion and mobility.
Child will remain free from accidents or injury.
Child will use adaptive/assistive devices correctly.

Family coping: potential for growth related to adjustment in lifestyle in caring for a child with a disability

Outcomes: Family will develop collaborative relationships with caregivers.
Family will participate in decision making about the child's care.

Knowledge deficit regarding treatment, and skills necessary to care for the child at home and measures to promote independent function and prevent complications and exacerbations of condition

Outcomes: Child and family will describe the care needs accurately.
Child and family will demonstrate skills and procedures to be performed after discharge.
Child and family will schedule follow-up appointments.
Child and family will identify community services available.
Child and family will demonstrate home management skills and use of medical or adaptive equipment.
Child and family will describe potential complications and actions to be taken for each.

Alteration in health maintenance related to a chronic condition that may have periodic exacerbations and need for intensified treatment

Outcomes: Child and family will be maintained at home as well as possible, without hospitalization.
Child and family will participate in illness management tasks as able.
Child and family will establish an efficient daily routine for ongoing home treatment.

Disturbance in self-concept: body image, self-esteem, role performance, and personal identity related to the impact of a chronic condition and its effects (i.e., visibility, prognosis, treatment requirements, functional capabilities)

Outcomes: Child will perform self-care activities as developmentally able.
Child will participate in social activities with peers.

Social isolation related to family withdrawal from friends and community because of demands of a child with a chronic condition

Outcome: Family will participate in social activities.

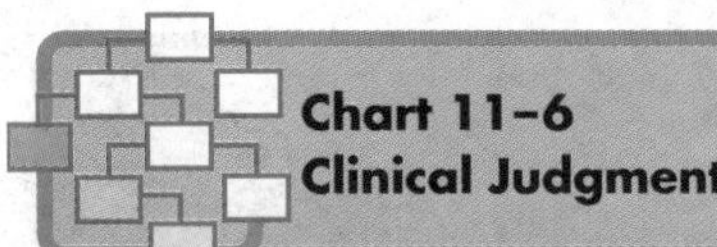

Chart 11–6
Clinical Judgment

Developmentally Appropriate Interventions for the Child with Down Syndrome

Sara is a 4-year-old girl with trisomy 21 (Down syndrome). She is admitted to the hospital in order to have her tonsils and adenoids removed. This has been determined to be necessary by her doctor because periods of sleep apnea have been noted. Sara is happy and playful in her room. Her mother describes this as her usual behavior.

Questions

1. During your assessment, what information should you ask Sara's mother about the child's development?
2. While you are talking with the mother, what observations about Sara's behavior might be useful in planning her care?
3. Sara's mother states that her daughter does not have intelligible speech but has learned several sign language terms. Her daughter can walk and run with ease. She cannot feed herself well with a spoon. Do you think these milestones are age appropriate?
4. On the morning of surgery, how would you prepare Sara for the events that will occur?
5. After surgery, Sara refuses to drink and continually cries for her mother, indicating that she wants to be picked up and held.

Answers

1. Assess her speech, hearing, and visual skills. Children with Down syndrome often have speech delays and hearing or vision problems. Determine how Sara communicates her desires and how she can be best approached to follow instructions. Assess whether she has had prior experiences with surgery or hospitalization.
2. Does she readily make contact with strangers? Does she readily explore her surroundings? How does she respond to hospitalization?
3. Sara exhibits speech delays and delays with hand-eye coordination. A 4-year-old should be able to feed herself or himself easily using a fork and spoon and should have speech that is essentially completely intelligible.
4. Have Sara sit with her mother. Provide an additional opportunity to review the process of preparing for surgery and what occurs afterward, using actual pieces of equipment (e.g., mask and IV tubing, cup for drink). Allow Sara to practice using these things on a favorite doll or bear. Have Sara teach the nurse how she says "hurt."
5. Allow Sara to sit on her mother's lap in a well-supported chair. Encourage Sara to drink fluids or eat popsicles in flavors that she likes (not citrus). Encourage saliva production with a lollipop (if permitted by the physician) or lemon glycerin swab. Administer pain medication as ordered.

had organ transplantation, acquired autoimmune deficiency, or conditions resulting in obesity (i.e., Blount's disease, Pierre Robin syndrome) and those who are dependent on ventilator assistance. The physiologic nature of these conditions requires careful medical management, but factors in the environment equally influence the child's well-being. Support of the child's nutritional status and control of exposure to infection are of primary concern, and continued stimulation and activity are essential to foster development and to maintain overall physical strength and ability.

Management of Functional Limitations

The focus of care for the child dealing with the effects of a sudden illness or injury or a chronic condition is to enable the child to lead a life as "normal" as possible. Achieving that goal requires that all aspects of the child's growth and development needs be considered and addressed by the health care team (Chart 11–3). Therefore, when caring for the child with a disability, it is important to have a firm sense of the child's developmental level in all areas and the impact of the disability on his or her physical ability. Many times, important areas of care are overlooked when the caregiver is unfamiliar with the child's condition and the best way to meet his or her needs. A focused health assessment identifies areas requiring special attention (Chart 11–4). Only through a careful assessment of the child, the child's condition, and the family's ability to care for the child can appropriate nursing diagnoses and patient outcomes be identified to direct the plan of care (Chart 11–5).

As with all children, the approach to care should be guided by the child's understanding of and ability to cope with a given situation. For example, an 8-year-old with a developmental disability undergoing orthopedic surgery may not benefit from a coloring book depicting the operating room and recovery room. If his or her cognitive ability is at a 4-year-old level, it may be more beneficial to have the child handle equipment such as the face mask used by the anesthetist, trying it on a doll's face and then on his or her own face. Likewise, placing a bandage "cast" on a doll's leg helps prepare the child for what he or she will find after surgery. The child with physical impairments, regardless of his or her level of intelligence, should be afforded every opportunity to participate in self-care activities that will foster independence (Chart 11–6).

Regardless of the reason for the child needing rehabilitative and habilitative services, the basic components of the treatment program identify and address the child's functional limitations. These functional limitations include ambulation and mobility issues, dressing skills, personal hygiene, grooming activities, language and communication skills, eating skills, and acquiring vocational skills.

Ambulation depends on an ability to perceive one's position in space (proprioception), to maintain a sense of balance, and to support the body while shifting weight to move the feet in sequence. Children with hemiplegia or diplegia may learn to walk if spasticity and impaired control are not too severe. These children may require a cane, crutches, and/or long- or short-leg braces for support. Children with quadriplegia, depending on the severity and type, more rarely walk except in sheltered conditions. Children with lower extremity weakness or paralysis may learn to walk with the support of long-leg braces and crutches or with a walker (Fig. 11–6). This means of ambulation is frequently limited to sheltered conditions and short distances.

Wheelchair mobility requires the ability to sit with fair stability in a chair and the strength either in the upper extremities to be able to reach the wheels and move them with the hands or in the lower extremity to be able to touch the floor and move the wheelchair with the feet. Proper seating is essential and is a particular challenge with growing children. An ill-fitting wheelchair exaggerates abnormal movement. A power wheelchair can be considered if strength and endurance are a problem, although the controls may require adaptation. Individuals with perceptual deficits have difficulty steering properly. Safety factors to be considered include the child's level of development and judgment.

Transfers are essential in many activities of daily living. Although ambulation may be independent, the child may not be able to get in and out of the bathtub. Balance depends on specific muscle groups; poor muscle control or contracture may interfere with the child's ability to maneuver. If there are visual problems or difficulties orienting, supports are available as an aid. Generally, children with spastic diplegia with upper extremity function can use a slide board independently or assist with a pivot transfer. Moderately affected children who are able to support their weight on their lower extremities and maintain balance can also pivot transfer. When an impairment to the spinal cord is involved, the transferring situations are usually from one seated surface to another (e.g., bed to wheelchair, wheelchair to toilet or shower chair). Children who are more disabled may require a two-person lift transfer or the use of assistive equipment.

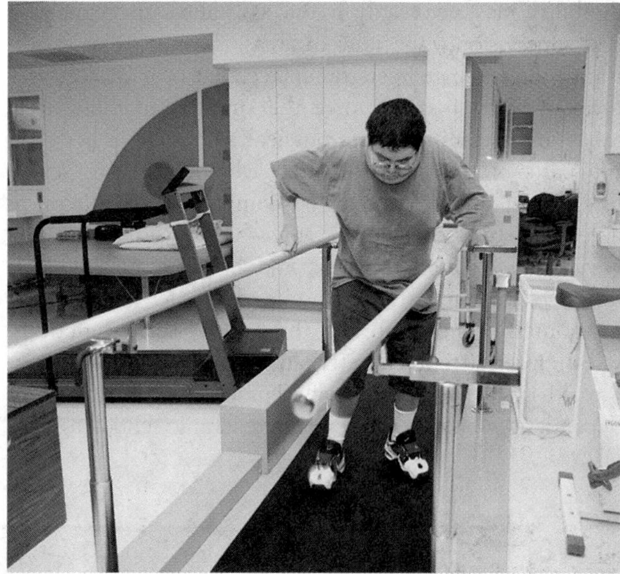

Figure 11–6
In the rehabilitation center, assistive devices can be used to support the return of strength and skill in ambulation, while also serving to build the child's confidence in his or her returning ability.

Dressing is a developmental milestone and is a basic activity of daily living. When a child has physical limitations, the caretaker frequently fosters dependence without intending to do so. The functional abilities necessary for independence in dressing include cognitive recognition of the garments that are appropriate for the weather conditions, the planned activities, and in relationship to overall outfitting; the ability to access clothing from storage areas; the strength in shifting weight and in maintaining balance in a sitting position while negotiating limbs into the garment; the flexibility to reach parts of the body; eye–hand coordination; and the manual dexterity to maneuver the garments and/or assistive devices.

Personal hygiene, like dressing, is an activity of daily living that in our culture generally commands respectful privacy. Personal hygiene includes activities related to bathing, washing, and toileting. These activities require accessibility of bathroom fixtures. Safety in performing these activities is also a concern. Children with a mild disability may need only initial assistance in preparation and supervision, especially in areas of safety (e.g., monitoring the water temperature, placement of bath mat, and level of water in the tub or the sink). Children with a moderate disability require physical assistance in performing parts of the care. Children who have more severe functional limitations may be completely dependent or able to assist the caretaker only partially in these areas. For example, a child with spina bifida faces the challenges of implementing a bowel and bladder management program to compensate for the loss of these functions. Clean intermittent catheterization may need to be performed by a caregiver initially but can be performed independently by the child upon reaching school age. A bowel program may continue to be administered by the caregiver for a longer period (Chart 11–7).

Grooming activities include hair brushing and oral hygiene, as well as shaving or makeup application in adolescence and adulthood. Although perhaps not considered as critical as dressing and personal hygiene, these activities of daily living are vitally important to the child's self-esteem. Generally, these activities require upper extremity strength, manual dexterity, and visual acuity with eye–hand coordination.

Language and communication are essential functional components. Language development involves the ability to hear, to interpret, and to understand situations encountered in the environment. It also involves the ability

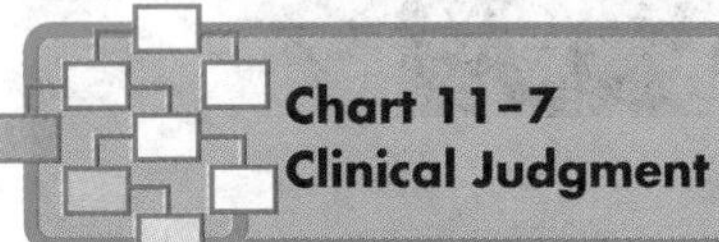

Chart 11–7
Clinical Judgment

The Child with Spina Bifida Admitted for a Self-Catheterization Program

Five-year-old Michelle was born with myelomeningocele at the L-1 level. She is admitted to the rehabilitation facility for an instructional program in self-clean intermittent catheterization (CIC). Until now, Michelle has been incontinent and has continued to wear diapers. This has not presented a problem in the past, but she is now preparing to enter the public school.

Questions

1. What information will you need regarding Michelle's elimination patterns?
2. What self-care techniques should be introduced to Michelle?
3. How would you determine that Michelle is ready to participate in this program?
4. What steps would be followed in introducing self-clean intermittent catheterization to Michelle?
5. How would you determine that Michelle is ready for discharge?

Answers

1. How much fluid does Michelle usually drink per day, especially in the evening? How frequently is her diaper changed? When changed, is the diaper damp, wet, or fully saturated? How soon is Michelle again wet?
2. Perineal care, recognition of relationship of volume of intake and types of fluids to output of urine.
3. Michelle shows interest in "keeping dry" and wearing underwear. Michelle is able to understand that she will be able to "go to the bathroom" using the catheter and will not be wet in between times.
4. A clean intermittent catheterization program should be initiated by the nurse, explaining the purpose and technique to Michelle step by step.
   An anatomically correct doll can be used to introduce the topic and explain how the body works. This can also be used to have Michelle "try" the techniques.
   Michelle should assist in gathering supplies and in setting up for the procedure, and watch the catheterization, using a mirror.
   Michelle should initiate steps of the procedure (cleansing with soap and water, identifying urethral opening with mirror).
   Michelle should try to insert the catheter after she has been cleansed and prepared by the nurse.
   Michelle should try the procedure independently while in bed.
   Michelle should try the procedure while sitting on the toilet.
5. Michelle is able to perform each step of the procedure independently with only occasional reminders or verbal cues. Michelle's parent(s) demonstrate independence in performing the procedure. Michelle's parents support their daughter in completing each task and understand the steps that Michelle must practice to gain complete independence.

to formulate thoughts and to interact with the environment and with other persons in it. Communication skills are essential to interacting with others. Making one's needs known in a manner that is understood by others is a basic function of all humans. Compromise of this process can be related to several conditions: cognitive deficits, sensory impairment (e.g., vision, hearing), motor impairment (e.g., dysarthria, or difficulty forming words with the structures of the mouth), or an alteration in physical structures (e.g., tracheostomy).

Eating problems may include poor control of the lips, the tongue, and the airway protective mechanisms; slow eating; and poor chewing and swallowing ability. Visuomotor problems interfere with the coordination of motions for scooping and carrying the food to the mouth. Feeding problems may also be related to a variety of other clinical problems, such as hypotonia, a weak suck, poor coordination of swallow, tonic bite reflex, hyperactive gag reflex, exaggerated tongue thrust, drooling, risk of aspiration, gastroesophageal reflux, and the child's inability to communicate hunger. Constipation can also affect the child's appetite.

Vocation and employment options are a key aspect of function and development. Cognitive deficits and mobility limitations are the greatest factors in determining the vocational possibilities for an individual with a disability. The young adult may achieve development of skills and enter the work force in competitive employment, supported employment, or a sheltered workshop.

In determining life skill and adaptation, it is also important to consider the child's ability to socialize with peers and to experience success. Recreational activities for children with disabilities may be as therapeutic in facilitating physical function as they are in teaching them alternative ways to participate in activities (Fig. 11–7). Each experience brings an opportunity for the child to achieve and obtain mastery of age-appropriate developmental skills and abilities.

Adaptive and Assistive Devices

To maximize the child's functional abilities, the nurse needs to know what adaptive and assistive devices the child uses and to become familiar with their use. The nurse must pay extremely close attention to this to support the child's recovery from an injury or illness, to maintain the child's functional ability, and to prevent further complications. The use of positioning devices to maintain alignment at all times is essential. In addition, positioning the child in relation to his or her external environment can positively foster the child's function. For example, speaking to a child from above his or her line of sight fosters poor muscular alignment; speaking at eye level promotes positive alignment. Positioning in bed a child who favors his or her right side with all toys and other items of interest on the right side of the bed fosters continued preference and possible contracture development. Contractures may develop when muscles consistently have increased tone and remain in shortened positions for prolonged periods. Positioning the child with

Figure 11–7
Therapeutic riding and adapted sports are rehabilitative activities that provide socialization and an opportunity to achieve.

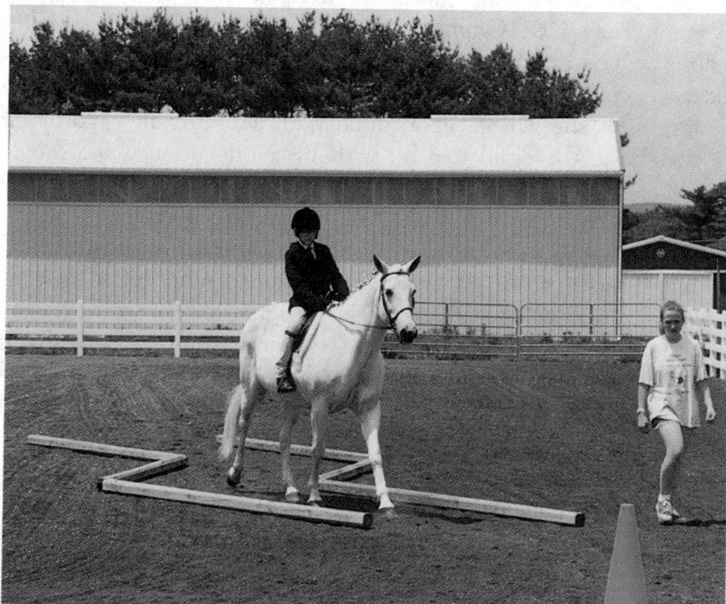

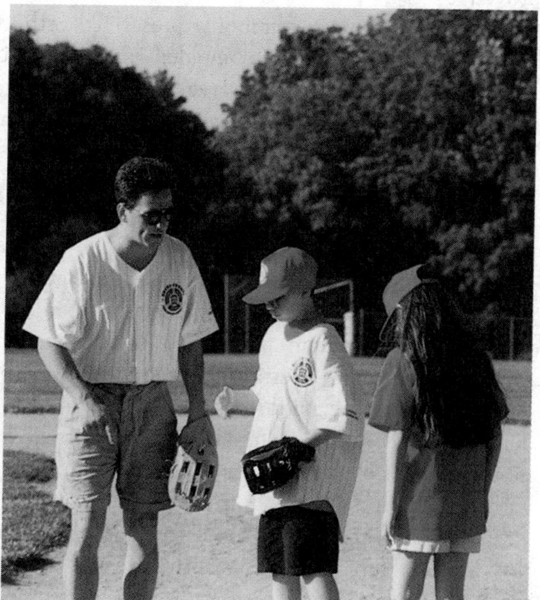

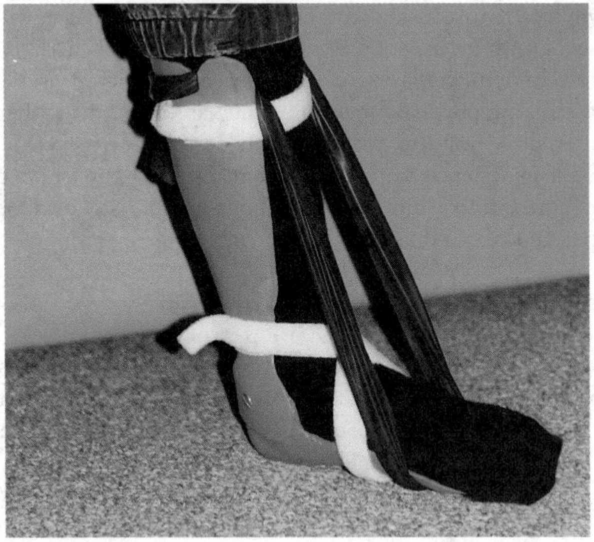

Figure 11–8
Splints can be fabricated by a bioengineering company or by the therapist using temperature-sensitive moldable plastic. Worn while the child sleeps, this foot splint includes a hinge at the ankle. With the use of an elastic band, the splint maintains correct foot position while stretching the heel cord.

items of interest to the left side enhances the child's desire to turn in this direction.

The use of sidelyers and corner seats for infants and young children promotes flexion and appropriate positioning for play and functional activities. Supportive orthotics also act to reduce spasticity, maintain range of motion, prevent contractures, and promote function. Orthoses may be used to maintain a group of muscles in a lengthened state so that function of the joint is improved.

One of the most commonly prescribed orthotics is a short leg brace called a molded ankle-foot orthosis (MAFO) (Fig. 11–8). This serves to decrease foot extension and may further decrease muscle tone in the hips, providing a more stable sitting position. Correcting the child's abnormal foot position may alter the position of the hips and knees when the child stands, thereby improving gait.

A variety of splints may be used to improve hand function. A common one is the resting hand splint. In this splint, the thumb is held in an abducted position with the wrist in a neutral or slightly extended position. This maintains the hand in an open position to prevent deformity and maintain function. Even with loss of fine motor control of the hand and fingers, a functional grasp with fingers and opposing thumb is a tremendously advantageous ability for the child to maintain. The loss of this level of function significantly affects the child's degree of independence.

Other devices include the prone stander, which promotes skeletal alignment, preserves bone mineralization, and allows the child to participate in activities. Scooters, tricycles, and wheelchairs provide a means of moving independently within the environment to increase opportunities to explore and gain social interactions.

Community Reentry and Ongoing Health Care Needs

Preparing the child for discharge from the inpatient rehabilitation stay to home begins even before admission. When goals are set during the preadmission process, discharge to home is the primary outcome identified. Every member of the team maintains this focus during their assessment of the child and integrates it into the development of the patient's plan of care. In addition to identifying the child's health status and functional ability, key assessments include the level of coping and adaptation, skill in performing the care required, and compatibility with the home environment and lifestyle. Of immediate concern in addressing the goal of discharge to the home is whether the physical environment can accommodate the needs of the child. These issues are explored in the initial interviews at the time of admission. Parents are asked to describe their home environment: type of community, transportation available, type of dwelling, number of stairs or rails, location and description of principal rooms in the house, and specifics regarding the supply of utility services as necessary.

Services in the community are explored throughout the admission. Depending on the needs of the child, a home visit by key rehabilitation team members may be conducted before discharge. In this manner, potential obstacles to the success of a home care program can be identified. Often, children are permitted to have a therapeutic home pass (THP). This allows a planned overnight stay in the child's home (or the home to which he or she will go upon discharge), affording an opportunity for the child to visit with his or her friends and family while implementing the care skills learned during the hospitalization. In this way, unforeseen problems or obstacles can be identified and discussed with the team upon return to the rehabilitation center. These new issues can then be more closely addressed before discharge.

Referral to community services is initiated as early as possible in the admission but requires having a firm sense of the child's continued needs. Home care agencies and community providers are notified and provided with essential information. At times, members of the home care and equipment companies meet with the child and the family during the inpatient stay. In cases in which care is complex, home care nurses are invited to the rehabilitation facility to participate in teaching regarding the

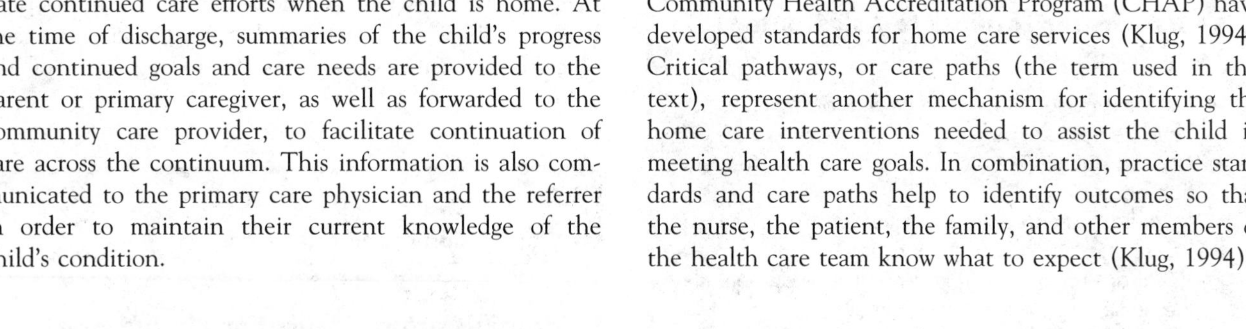

child's care needs. The parent or primary caregiver is an important participant in this process. Efforts are focused on assisting the parents or caregivers to know the child's ongoing care needs so that they will be able to coordinate continued care efforts when the child is home. At the time of discharge, summaries of the child's progress and continued goals and care needs are provided to the parent or primary caregiver, as well as forwarded to the community care provider, to facilitate continuation of care across the continuum. This information is also communicated to the primary care physician and the referrer in order to maintain their current knowledge of the child's condition.

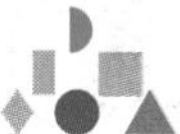

Pediatric Home Care

As recently as the mid-1970s, the options open to families of a child with long-term rehabilitative and health care needs were limited to either placing the child in a group home equipped to meet his or her basic needs or bringing the child home and hoping for the best with extremely limited professional help in the community. Families whose children had more short-term but nonetheless life-altering needs, such as intravenous (IV) therapy for treatment of osteoporosis or phototherapy for treatment of hyperbilirubinemia, had only one option: hospitalization (Schuman & Karush, 1992). In all of these cases, the family's need to remain together and the child's developmental needs were not addressed.

With the recognition that even the most compromised child has a right to live as full and normal a life as possible, support for bringing children home has become the norm rather than the exception (Ahmann & Lipsi, 1992). One study concluded that parents, with support of home care nurses, were able to give care that equaled or surpassed that provided in hospitals (Schreiner, Donar, & Kettrick, 1987). Children in home care also acquire fewer infections and achieve optimal socialization and gross motor skills (Futcher, 1988). Early intervention programs, teachers, therapy centers, rehabilitation nurses, pediatric home care nurses, and families all work together to ensure that on the way to becoming medically stable and physically independent, "a kid can be a kid" (Gorski, 1991). For the child who is technology dependent or medically fragile, home care provides a major alternative to long-term hospitalization if the caregiver is willing and able to provide for the child's care needs.

Standards of care have been developed that identify the home health nurse's responsibilities. The *Scope of Home Health Practice* and the *Standards of Community Health Nursing Practice* developed by the American Nurses' Association (1992, 1986) are examples of professional performance standards that can guide home care practices. In addition, the Joint Commission on Accreditation of Healthcare Organizations (JCAHO) and the Community Health Accreditation Program (CHAP) have developed standards for home care services (Klug, 1994). Critical pathways, or care paths (the term used in this text), represent another mechanism for identifying the home care interventions needed to assist the child in meeting health care goals. In combination, practice standards and care paths help to identify outcomes so that the nurse, the patient, the family, and other members of the health care team know what to expect (Klug, 1994).

Selecting Appropriate Home Care Services

When the child's condition has stabilized, the family and health care team can focus on making the arrangements for discharge from the acute care or acute rehabilitation setting to the home. When health care interventions must continue in the home, the inpatient facility and/or the insurance agency can provide the family with a choice of two or three different home care agencies to provide services. A social worker or case manager can work with the family to determine what home care services, supplies, and activities will be funded under a medical insurance plan or other funding source. Unfortunately, many insurance plans can be quite restrictive in the home care services that are considered to be a benefit or covered expense. Families may incur many out-of-pocket expenses, such as transportation to the hospital or clinic for periodic evaluations, parking fees, and lost income from work (Ladden, 1990). The health care team should encourage the family to interview prospective home care agencies to select the one that best meets their needs, is compatible with their other commitments, and is covered by their insurance (Chart 11–8).

When a home care company has been selected, representatives from the company are expected to participate in the discharge planning activities, including arrangement for home equipment (Klug, 1992). The home care company also helps to determine the level of nursing that is most appropriate to meet the needs of the child. There are two primary types of home care services: private duty and skilled intermittent visits. With private duty care, there is a nurse at the child's side up to 24 hours a day. Private duty nursing is similar to the care received in the hospital, in that the nurse provides most of the child's care needs. The nurse teaches the parents how to provide the care with a goal of enabling the family to independently provide care at least 8 hours of the day or night.

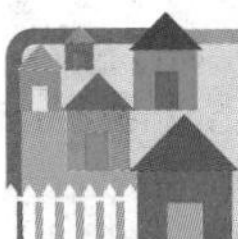

Chart 11–8
Community Care

Questions for Families to Ask Home Care Agency

- Does the nurse who will be caring for my child have pediatric experience?
- Has the agency handled children with this condition before?
- If we have any problems or questions, will there be a nurse on call 24 hours a day?
- What are my options if I do not like or agree with the nurse who comes to my home?
- How often will the nurse talk with my child's doctor?
- Does your agency provide other services such as case management and therapy?
- (Private duty) How often does your agency not have enough nurses to cover the number of cases? What can we do if a nurse is not available to care for our child?
- Will the nurse call and make an appointment with us for her visits or just show up?
- How will the billing be handled? Do you work directly with the insurance company?
- Will your agency arrange for the equipment that we need?
- Who do we call if there is a problem with the equipment and/or it needs to be repaired or replaced?
- Will your agency arrange for the medical supplies that we may need? Who reorders them?

With intermittent care, a nurse may visit the home from two or three times a day to two or three times a week. A typical intermittent home care visit lasts about 1½ hours. Before discharge to the home, the health care team teaches the parents or primary caregivers to perform the majority of tasks to meet the child's care needs. During the home visit, the nurse completes a head-to-toe assessment of the child and evaluates the child's progress. The caregiver's knowledge and proficiency are assessed. Family teaching about the diagnosis, monitoring of equipment, and treatment is provided as indicated by the individual situation and the caregiver's questions (Martinez et al., 1991). Even such traditionally high-technology tasks as intravenous infusion can be performed by the family. Nurses need to be prepared to provide extensive education to parents or caregivers to enable them to safely deliver care that was formerly in the domain of licensed professionals (Chart 11–9).

Preparing for the Transition to Home Care

It may seem fairly simple to arrange for a child's care to be given in his or her own home instead of the hospital; however, there are processes that must occur to ensure successful transition and ongoing management of the

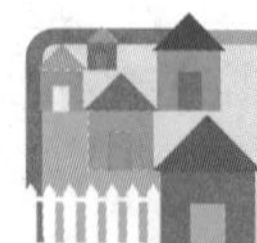

Chart 11–9
Community Care

Administering Medications in the Home

If the child is to receive IV medications through a peripheral line:

- Before the first visit, request that a new IV access be obtained before discharge from the hospital.
  Not having to deal with starting a new line during the initial visit increases the amount of time for education and return demonstration, enabling the family to become independent in their care of the child.
- Have a backup plan already worked out in case the IV line needs to be restarted and you are unsuccessful in restarting it.
  The doctor may give you orders to give oral medication until a line can be placed. If you are unable to start the IV line, another nurse can come to the home to attempt to obtain access, or the child can be taken to an outpatient center or emergency room for the IV insertion.
- Always carry extra IV supplies in your nursing bag.
  There are usually no supplies in the home should equipment be defective or become contaminated.

If the child is receiving multiple oral medications:

- Make a color-coded chart with the times and doses of the medications all listed. Show the family how to notate on the chart that a dosage has been given.
- Have the family post the chart in a prominent place, such as the refrigerator door.
- Make a calendar indicating when refills will be needed. To avoid running out of medication, mark the medication bottles with colored tape that matches the color-coded chart.
- Be sure that administration of medications does not conflict with mealtimes and with the schedule the family usually maintains. This helps to ensure that the family and the child will adhere to the medication schedule.

child's care in the home. Although every situation is unique, there are common threads that apply to all children being evaluated for home care (Klein-Berndt, 1991).

Assess the Child's Needs

The goals of home care are to normalize the life of the child in a family and a community and to foster the child's maximal growth and development (Fleming et al., 1994). Therefore, to begin the transition process the nurse and the family must have a good understanding of the child's medical condition. Understanding the complexities of the child's condition helps in recognizing the child's limits and stress signals, which indicate the child's tolerance for certain activities (Ahmann & Lipsi, 1992). This information also assists the family in selecting opportunities that can maximize the child's developmental skills and abilities. The family must be included as central members of the assessment and planning team (Sterling, Jones, Johnson, & Bowen, 1996). This team should begin to come together when it is first evident that the child's health care needs may exceed those that can be offered in the doctor's office, in the emergency department, or during a short hospital stay. The team evaluates the type of support or care the child requires to be cared for in the home and to minimize the child's need for frequent, unscheduled acute care services.

Assessment tools may be used by the nurse to record observed behaviors and functional skills of the child. Table 11–1 identifies pediatric tools that are used by the rehabilitative team and are equally applicable to the home care team. In addition, Chapter 4 presents a summary of several tools that can be used to assess the child's development and the home environment. Chapter 3 contains a summary of measurement tools to assess family functioning.

Identify the Caregivers

A major task of the team is to determine who the actual caregivers in the home will be. When the child is in the hospital, it is important to note individuals who come to visit and to assist with the child's care. Regardless of the level of family involvement, the responsibility of care for the child continues to be held by the nursing staff. When planning for home care, the focal point changes. Most typically, it is the parents or other family members who will be responsible for providing the care and bringing the child to the follow-up visits. In some cases, the parents may not be available to provide the child's care at home. Changes in family and economic demographics have shown an estimated 75% of all mothers work outside the home (Zigler & Gilman, 1993). In most cases, parents are able to take time off from work when their child is first involved in an accident or becomes ill. However, by the time their child is sent home, many parents have to return to work (Strutts, 1994). Therefore, the first question that should be asked is, "Who will actually be in your home or available nearby to help you with your child's care?" The people identified need to be included as much as possible in all of the discharge teaching and planning. Ideally, the parents and the other selected home caregivers are introduced to information about the child's medical condition, treatment, and potential complications as quickly as possible (Mitchell, 1996). If home care nurses, aides, or therapists are to be involved, they should also be identified as early as possible and included in all aspects of this transition process.

Determine the Level of Support Services

When it has been determined who will be providing the care in the home, the level of nursing expertise and home care support services needed to augment family efforts is ascertained (Chart 11–10). The medical equipment and supplies to be used, the availability of family resources, and family living arrangements also need to be investigated before the child's return home. Other questions that should be addressed include the following: will the child be able to attend school or require home instruction (the decision may depend on whether the school is accessible as defined by the child's needs or by the child's abilities)? How will the child be transported to and from school? What school will the child attend? Will respite care be available for the family? How will the family obtain supplies for their child's care and where will they store them? How will the child's care needs affect needs of other children in the home? How will caring for other family members affect the parents' or caregivers' ability to care for the child (Phillips & Brostoff, 1989)?

Develop the Home Care Path

With this assessment completed, a home care path is developed. The home care path is another mechanism that should be used to clearly define standards of care. This plan of care begins with the determination of goals for the child and the family. For example, if a child's apneic spells are the concern and the focus of home care services, then teaching the family to respond to, record, and treat apneic events is a primary goal elaborated on the home care path. The resources needed to achieve the goals are also indicated on the care path. The creativity of the parent–home care nurse team effort knows no bounds when it comes to determining how to implement the required care and at the same time allow for developmental and family considerations. For example, a trip to the zoo can easily be planned around a total parenteral nutrition (TPN) infusion or a physical therapy session

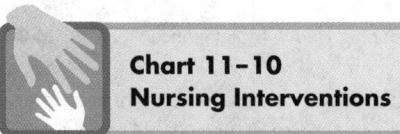

Chart 11-10
Nursing Interventions

Family and Home Assessment

Expected Outcome	Intervention
Family caregivers will have adequate training and preparation to care for the child at home.	Before discharge or at the first visit, identify the family members who will actually be providing the care. Review all written instructions with the caregivers. Observe the caregivers' demonstrations of any medically related task they will be completing independently. Leave booklets with pictures and/or videos that can be used as references with the caregivers in the home. Review the care path with the caregivers and make changes as needed to meet the child's and the family's needs.
Family caregivers will respond appropriately to situations that indicate potential medical problems.	Provide the family with written lists of signs and symptoms that signal potential variances from what is considered the baseline for the child. Review steps to be taken should a medical problem arise. Alert emergency services in the community to the presence of a child in the home who may need their assistance. Post important phone numbers in a prominent location in the home.
Telephone service will be available to the family.	Identify a local business or neighbor who will allow the family to use their phone in an emergency. If no phone is in the home, cell phones can be rented through many home care companies or through local fire departments.
Basic utilities will be available to the family.	Assist the family to secure the basic utilities needed to provide for the child's needs. • Bottled water can be used if there is no running water. • Electrical generators can be rented from local utility companies. If equipment required for the child's care and electricity are not available, battery-powered equipment should be used. • Many local governments assist with heating costs in an emergency. Many churches stock blankets and warm clothing for families in need. • If electricity is available to the family, the local utility company should be alerted and the family placed on a priority service list. • If refrigeration is required and there is none, dry ice can be obtained from any food market at little or no cost. If dry ice is used, care must be taken not to touch it directly and not to store the medication directly on it.
The home will be a safe environment.	Assess the home for safety. • If electrical equipment is used, a three-pronged grounded plug should be used. Extension cord use should be avoided. • To avoid overheating and the risk of fire, plywood or other wood should be placed under the electrical equipment, rather than having it rest directly on carpet. • Knobs and buttons on all equipment should be covered with clear tape. This enables them to be checked while lessening the risk of accidentally changing the setting. • Medications, needles, syringes, sharps, and sharps container should be stored in a locked container. • A list of all medications and their dosages should be attached to a list of emergency phone numbers. • All medications should be properly stored. • All equipment should be unplugged when not in use. • Throw rugs should be avoided to lessen the possibility of tripping on them.

scheduled so that it does not interrupt the family dinnertime (Chart 11–11).

The plan of care is determined in collaboration and cooperation with the family. The family provides valuable insight into the strengths and needs of the child and home situation, allowing the care path to be tailored and individualized (Ahmann & Lierman, 1992; Nissim & Sten, 1991). Both the nurse and the family caregiver should sign the care path document when they agree that the instructions are understood and that they have been safely demonstrated (Care Path 11–1).

As care of the child in the home continues, so do the needs of family members. Changes in the child's condition (both positive and negative) require the family and the health care team to reframe their understanding of the child's capabilities and their perception of the future. Changes in family structure may alter the previous arrangement of who has been defined as the primary

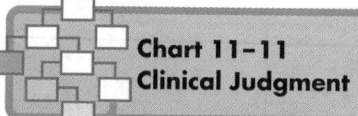

Chart 11–11
Clinical Judgment

Home Care of the Child with Pneumonia

Six-year-old Sarah has been hospitalized for 3 days for treatment of acute respiratory distress related to pneumonia. She is discharged to home to recover and to complete her 10-day course of intravenous antibiotics. She is being cared for by her grandmother while her mother returns to work. The grandmother speaks limited English and was not included in any of the discharge teaching in the hospital. As a home care nurse, you have been contracted to make two home visits, 8 hours apart, and then visit three times a week for the duration of the IV treatment. The family is expected to be independent in the administration of the IV antibiotic after the first two visits from the home care nurse.

Questions

1. During the first home visit, what is your assessment of the nursing needs of this family?
2. What would you include in an "absolutely must teach" list for the first visit?
3. What two problems would you consider to be of the highest priority?
4. With a known language barrier situation, how would you carry out the teaching with this family?
5. If the family is not able to care for Sarah's health needs independently by the end of your second visit, what should you do?

Answers

1. Sarah needs to be monitored for changes in her respiratory status. The mother and the grandmother must be taught how to assess when Sarah's condition has worsened. They must also be taught how to administer the IV antibiotics and to assess for problems with the infusion site. The fact that one of the two caregivers in the family speaks a different language from the nurse must be addressed. Fears of the family may play a major role in the success or failure of this home care situation.
2. Assessment of Sarah's respiratory status, when to get help, and whom to call should be included. The antibiotic teaching must include storage, dosage, side effects, and times given. The IV information must include site verification, hookup and administration, and an understanding of how the IV delivery system works.
3. The highest concern is appropriate monitoring and response to changes in Sarah's respiratory status. Responsibility for the administration of the IV antibiotic is the second concern.
4. The mother must be in the home during your opening visit to sign the consent-for-treatment documents. Take advantage of this fact to have her translate communications with the grandmother. Have the mother write the instructions that you are giving in both languages. Sarah is old enough to help with some of the translation. Include Sarah in all of the teaching. Ask the mother if there is a relative or a neighbor who speaks both languages who is willing to serve as a backup translator. Use color charts to teach about dosage and times. Arrange for the simplest IV system to be used. Use pictures of symptoms, such as a child gasping for air, to demonstrate complications. Set up a relay system from the grandmother to the mother to the health care professionals in case an emergency arises.
5. If a situation is not safe for any reason, extra visits must be arranged. Rarely does an insurance company or state agency deny a home care nurse extra visits when safety is an issue. It is important to document the exact, extenuating circumstances that necessitate the added support. Included in this document should be a plan to remedy the situation. If extra visits are denied, arrange for the child to be taken to an outpatient clinic for assessment and for IV administration.

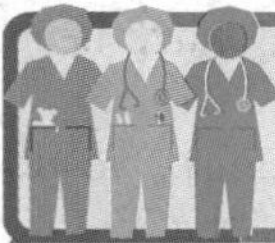

Care Path 11-1 An Interdisciplinary Plan of Care for the Child Receiving Home Care

Nursing Diagnosis	Patient/Family Intermediate Outcomes			
	Before discharge	**First day at home**	**Second day at home**	**Third day at home**
Knowledge deficit: management of IV therapy	Child and family will meet the home care nurse. Family will be introduced to home care equipment.	Family will participate in administration of IV medication to the child.	⟶	Family will demonstrate setup and infusion of IV medication.
Potential for impaired skin integrity related to presence of IV access device	Child will have patent IV access and will be free from signs and symptoms of infection.	⟶	⟶	⟶ Family will be competent in completing head-to-toe assessment of the child.
Potential for ineffective family management of therapeutic regimen	Family members will openly express feelings and concerns regarding their caring for the child.	⟶	⟶	Family members will express confidence in caring for the child.
Care Intervention Categories				
Medications and IVs	New IV started or percutaneous intravenous central catheter (PICC) or medial intravenous device (MID) inserted.	Nurse and caregiver assess the IV site for patency and signs or symptoms of infection at the insertion site.	Nurse and caregiver assess the IV.	If peripheral IV used, nurse will change site.
Psychosocial	Family assessed as to any religious and/or cultural beliefs that may affect child's home therapy. Social service's or nurse's assessment of family dynamics and actual caregiver identified.	Nurse discusses with family any information that in-hospital staff have given her or him about the family's religious and/or cultural beliefs. Works with family to incorporate their wishes into the plan. Nurse assesses family and environment for safety and understanding of all that is involved in administration of IV therapy.	Discuss with the family whether they feel that their needs are being met. Family is encouraged to discuss any problems that they are having coping with home treatment. Compliance assessment made.	⟶ ⟶ ⟶

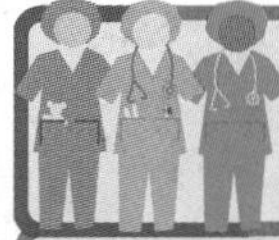

Care Path 11-1 An Interdisciplinary Plan of Care for the Child Receiving Home Care *Continued*

Care Intervention Categories	Before discharge	First day at home	Second day at home	Third day at home
Teaching	Home care nurse to visit family or caregivers. Introduce IV equipment that will be used in the home.	Demonstrate infusion device. Initial guided return demonstration by caregiver of IV infusion. Discuss medical necessity for IV therapy. Setup, storage, schedule, and dosage discussed. Discuss side effects. Discuss complications with IV site.	Caregiver return demonstrates setup and infusion of IV. Review medical necessity for IV therapy. All aspects of IV therapy reviewed.	Caregiver demonstrates setup and infusion of IV. Review all aspects that are still questioned by family.
Vital signs and baseline parameters	Expected vital sign limits determined. Determine physician's guidelines about when to be notified of changes.	Head-to-toe assessment by nurse made. Family aware of all of nurse's findings. Physician notified of status.	Family and nurse do head-to-toe assessment. Findings discussed with physician.	⟶

caregiver. Changes occur as the child develops, acquiring more self-care skills and a more complete understanding of his or her condition (Fig. 11–9). The health care team must manage all of these changes by being flexible and adaptive to the family. The child's plan of care must be continually reevaluated to determine its applicability to present conditions and to be centered around the family's needs and abilities.

Address Family Concerns

This time of planning and preparation for home care can be one of extreme stress for the family. They are torn between looking forward to having their child out of the hospital and at home and fear of what having the child at home may mean for them. Parents have both a desire to verbalize their concerns and have them openly addressed and a desire to hide their fears so that no one will misinterpret them as indicating lack of competence in caring for their child at home (Faulkner, 1996). Families can be best supported by listening to them tell the story of the child's illness and their experiences and feelings at the time of diagnosis and throughout the hospitalization. Having a compassionate understanding of how this situation has affected the family helps in determining how best to help them. The family may be afraid of giving the impression to the nurse that they do not understand the instructions and therefore are not able to take care of the child. The nurse should never assume that the family members understand what has been explained. A nod from the family members may be just a reflex to hide a fear of being less than capable. The nurse should be certain to repeat information over the course of several teaching sessions with the family. Written instructions are essential to provide the family with further reference material to reinforce the verbal message. Ample time must be allowed for the family to participate in return demonstration of any psychomotor skills (Snowdon & Kane, 1995). Optimally, the home caregivers are given the opportunity to provide for the child's care needs while the child is still in the inpatient setting and can be monitored several times by the nursing staff.

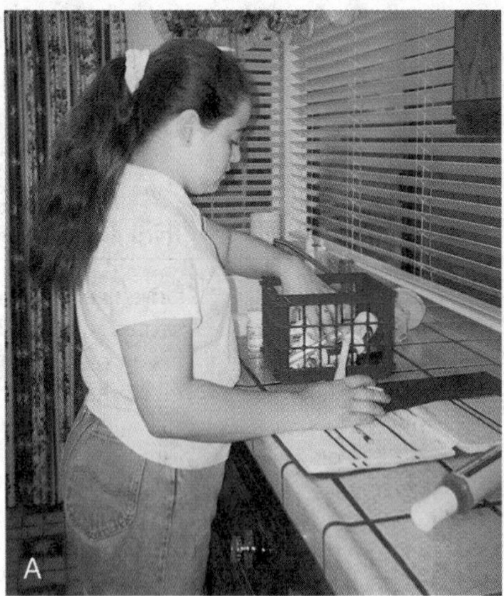

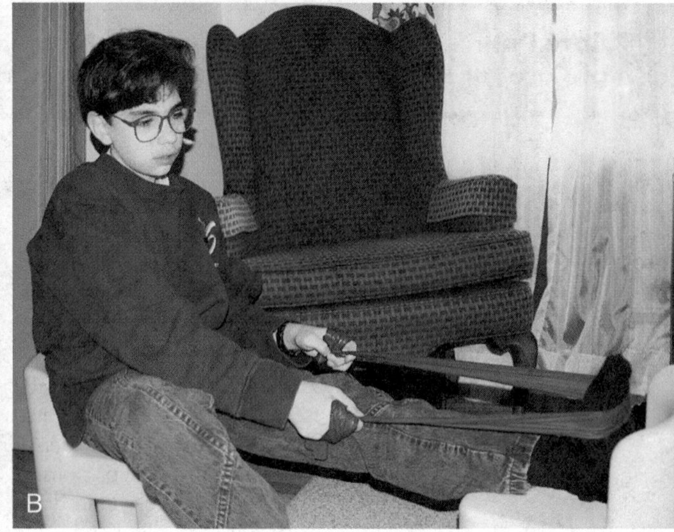

Figure 11–9
The child with a chronic condition should be encouraged to become more and more responsible for managing his or her own treatments and medications.

Home Care Equipment and Supplies

During preparations for discharge, the health care team should take into consideration the fact that there may well be great differences between the equipment used in the home and the equipment used in the hospital (Richardson, Student, O'Boyle, Smyth, & Wheeler, 1992). In the inpatient setting, nursing energies should not be spent teaching parents how to use equipment and supplies that are not to be used in the home. Before the child's discharge, the durable medical equipment company and/or infusion therapy company that will be providing equipment to the family should be notified. Representatives come to the inpatient setting or arrange to meet the parents at their home to demonstrate equipment use. It is most beneficial for the family if the home equipment can be used with the child in the inpatient setting before discharge. This allows the family to have easy access to professionals who can demonstrate proper use of the equipment and who can troubleshoot any anticipated problems and ensures that equipment is available at discharge. In addition, all equipment and supplies should be delivered to the home at least the day before the discharge date.

caREminder: *Planning for the proper equipment must include an assessment of the home.*

Every home care nurse's nightmare is to go into the home of a newly discharged child to find a major problem such as no electricity for the fiberoptic blanket or no refrigerator to store the IV medication. The home care nurse must make a complete home assessment as part of the first visit (see Chart 11–10). As a foundation for the assessment, the nurse should use information obtained from a consultation with the discharge team. Household safety must be evaluated, including the presence of smoke detectors, electrical outlets for medical equipment, adequate lighting, and heating or cooling. A list of emergency telephone numbers should be posted near the telephone. If the family does not have a telephone, the location of one within easy access must be determined. The home assessment should also include an evaluation of infection control and environmental factors that may be hazardous to the child's health. For instance, the number of visitors to the home may need to be reduced. Effective hand washing should be reviewed. Cigarette smoke should be eliminated in the home of a child with respiratory difficulties. The ability to dispose of medical supplies properly should be reviewed. Space to accommodate the child and his or her equipment may pose a problem. Siblings may have to change bedroom and storage spaces to provide space for the medical supplies.

Durable Medical Equipment

An astounding array of highly technological and simplified medical supplies are commonly used in the home that are rarely used in the hospital. For example, in the course of providing IV therapy, the hospital nurse probably uses standard delivery tubing, extension tubing, an infusion pump, an IV pole, and a large amount of adhesive tape to secure this equipment in place. In the home, IV therapy can be given by simply attaching a premixed ball or bag of medication with attached and preprimed

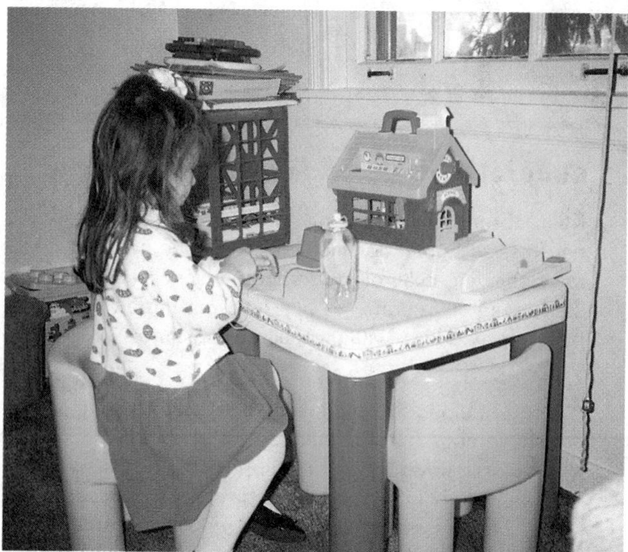

Figure 11–10
The bottle on the table is an intravenous medication administration device. The use of portable equipment permits the child to play and move about freely.

tubing to the IV site, a device known as a "snap" (Fig. 11–10). The child wears the medication bag in a belt, back pack, or shoulder pack. No pump is used, because the timing is preset within the medication delivery system. This piece of home equipment allows the child freedom to move about easily, to receive medications at school, and to continue all of his or her normal activities during a treatment.

Home phototherapy is another example of high technology made simple. In the typical hospital treatment, a baby with hyperbilirubinemia is kept in an enclosed isolette or warm bed, unclothed except for a diaper, and eyes covered to prevent ocular injury from the lights. The phototherapy light must be monitored for strength and the isolette must be monitored for proper warmth. The baby is not held by the staff except during feedings, when the child may be taken out of the bed and the phototherapy lights turned off. In the home, a fiberoptic blanket or pad is widely used (Fig. 11–11). A study completed in 1991 demonstrated that fiberoptics and conventional bilirubin lights were equally effective (Schuman & Karush, 1992). The advantages of fiberoptics are that the baby may sleep in his or her own crib and the eyes do not have to be covered. The infant may be held as much as the parents desire, may be breast-fed or bottle-fed, and may be dressed normally. During the treatment, the baby wears a fiberoptic blanket or pad next to his or her skin. The blanket or pad is attached by a long cord to a light source. There is no transmission of heat, only light. Once again, the equipment for the home provides more freedom of movement and allows the child's developmental needs to be met.

Adaptive or Assistive Devices

In addition to an array of medical equipment used in the home, other adaptive devices are used to enhance the mobility and function of children with physical impairments. For instance, the use of positioning devices to maintain proper body alignment at all times is essential. The positioning of the child in relation to his or her external environment positively fosters the child's function. Adaptations to the home environment may be needed to help the child to rise from a sitting position or to go up and down a step. Floor coverings may have to be altered. For instance, the home of the child with a walker or crutches should not have loose rugs on the floor that could cause the child to stumble and fall. The child in a wheelchair may have difficulty maneuvering over thick carpeted areas. Ramps may have to be added to enable the child to enter the home or move from room to room if there are steps in entryways that hinder the child's mobility.

Working Effectively with Families

Family Needs

The child with either short-term or long-term rehabilitative and home care needs places a tremendous amount of stress on the family. Having a technology-dependent or disabled child at home can have both a positive and a negative effect on the family. Health care literature notes that depression among family members is greater because of intrafamily and marital strains. Families have stated that they felt as though they had given up many things because of the ill child. For instance, the family income became more restricted, they saw friends less, and plans to go out were often changed at the last minute. Parents

Figure 11–11
Using home phototherapy, the family with a newborn can be together while the child receives therapy for hyperbilirubinemia.

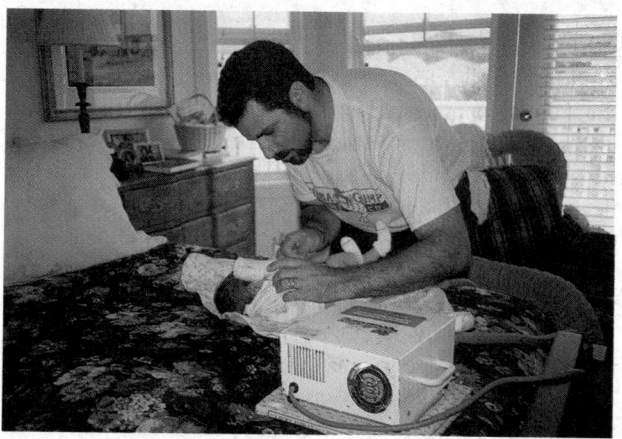

reported that personal privacy, family rituals, and control over their child were compromised. Caregiver fatigue was a major problem, as was finding reliable people to care for the child. Siblings resented the time, money, and attention their brother or sister was receiving. Marital roles had to be renegotiated, and career plans had to be altered or put on hold (Aqazio, 1997; Snowdon & Kane, 1995; Sterling et al., 1996; Teague et al., 1993; Worthington, 1995).

Chapter 10 provides an in-depth discussion of the impact of a child's long-term illness on the child and on the family system. Chapter 3 discusses some of the theoretical models that explain how families may interpret stressful situations and may use various coping strategies to manage crisis events. The reader is encouraged to review both of these chapters to understand further the needs of children and their families who participate in rehabilitation and home care activities.

The nurse can play a vital role in helping the family to cope with and to adjust to their life circumstances. This process begins by focusing on the parents' actual needs, not only on the "perceived needs" as seen by health care professionals. Each family is unique. The experiences, coping styles, and pattern of family interactions differ from family to family. These differences must be respected and must form the basis of individualized family care. The objective of nursing care is to support family unity, to promote optimal adjustment, and to help integrate the child into the family and community (Phillips & Brostoff, 1989). The family looks to the nurse as a professional with whom they can share their concerns, frustrations, and goals for the future. The nurse is in an optimal position to build up the family and to bolster family optimism and cohesion. The nurse can assist the family in identifying and evaluating available resources. The nurse who enables and empowers the family helps them to see their strengths and facilitate their actions to reach their maximum potential (Nissim & Sten, 1991; Sterling et al., 1996).

Chart 11–12
Worldview

Cultural Considerations in the Home

Keen observation, sensitivity to culturally based mannerisms, and open communication are the best tools for identifying cultural factors that influence care in the home (Grossman, 1996). There are three rules of thumb for working within a cultural structure:

- Preservation: keeping the practices or beliefs that are of help to the child, such as acupressure to relieve pain in Asian cultures
- Adaptation: adapting or adjusting the practices or beliefs that neither help nor harm, such as spreading of cornmeal around the bed in Native American cultures
- Repatterning: avoiding the practices or beliefs that may cause harm, such as holding a baby upside down over water in Hispanic culture (Leininger, 1994)

The nurse should look around the home and see if there are any clues as to possible cultural influences for the family, such as statues, special candles, or sprinkled spices. The nurse should ask the family whether there is a special religious practice that will be followed to help the child heal. The nurse can assess the interaction and the communication style of the family to see if there are any cultural taboos that should be avoided (Grossman, 1966).

Boundaries

When a child is being cared for in a clinic or hospital, there are fairly clear boundaries between the nurses and the family members. Even if the parents and the child have a rooming-in situation before discharge, the parents generally follow the dictates of the institution and the health care providers if there is any question about the child's care (Lantos & Kohrman, 1992). In the home, the parents set the pace of the care and have the final say about the treatment of the child. The nurse is an invited guest providing a service in the home. Before discharge, the parents may have been instructed in a certain way of doing a given task. For example, the parents and the home care nurse may have different methods of verifying the placement of a nasogastric (NG) tube. Not uncommonly, parents are led to believe that there is only one way of doing a task or procedure. Parents typically are most concerned about doing everything just right. They were taught one way, and that is the way they believe it must be done. The home care nurse has three options: adopt the parents' method, show the parents a new method, or create a new method based on both the parents' and the nurse's intervention style. As in all venues of nursing care, an awareness of and respect for the family's cultural beliefs and practices must be integrated into the home care interventions (Yoos, Kitzman, Olds, & Overracker, 1995) (Chart 11–12). If the nurse has succeeded in gaining their trust and respect, the parents are much more open to alternative ways of carrying out procedures and the nurse is more cognizant of the issues that affect family caregiving practices (Klug, 1993). Families want recognition for their contributions to their child's care and for their level of expertise regarding the child's condition and needs. By working in collaboration with the family, as a member of *their* team, the nurse acknowledges the family's opinion, skills, and abilities.

To promote a therapeutic environment in the home, the nurse must form a strong, mutually respectful relationship with the family. This mutual respect forms the basis of the decisions about the child's care (Ahmann, 1994). To set the stage for this trusting relationship, the nurse and the family should establish clear house rules (Chart 11–13). These rules define the nurse's role and reinforce the family's primary control over the child and the environment (Klug, 1993). The house rules include negotiating aspects of the physical environment, such as where to park, areas of privacy in the home, responsibilities of the nurse toward the child, interactions with other family members, and lines of authority and decision-making.

caREminder: *While providing care services to the family, the nurse must always be cognizant of monitoring and maintaining his or her own personal safety (Chart 11–14).*

In long-term home care, the question of boundaries may reach into such areas as discipline of the child. Ahmann and Bond (1992) suggest that in general the nurse should respect the wishes of the parents in regard to the type of discipline used unless there is risk or harm to the child. In home care, the needs of the child and family must take precedence over scheduled interventions (Mitchell, 1996).

Termination

The nurse-family home care relationship may be terminated because the child's condition no longer warrants professional home care, the child is in need of more acute care services, or the child has died. Although professional boundaries and interactions have been maintained, over any lengthy period of time the nurse is likely to have become an integral part of the family system. The family may be fearful of managing the child without the visible presence of the home care nurse. The family may be anxious about finding a safe and competent nonprofessional caregiver or baby sitter. Marital and sibling relationships may change because of the realignment of household and childcare responsibilities (Aqazio, 1997).

Whatever circumstances surround the termination of service, the family and the nurse should express their feelings to one another. Feelings of sadness should be acknowledged as appropriate to the situation. The family may also express anxiety regarding the new responsibilities they must now shoulder. When a therapeutic relationship exists, the nurse has a responsibility to help the family understand and accept the necessity for changes in service and look with optimism on the future.

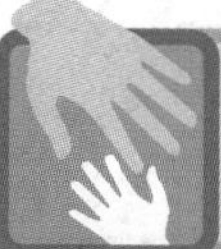

Chart 11–13
Nursing Interventions

House Rules for the Home Care Nurse

Determine with the family:

- Where should you park?
  Check local ordinances about on-street parking and/or overnight parking.
- Should you knock or ring the doorbell?
- What bathroom may you use?
  You may want to bring your own liquid soap to avoid use of the family's bar soap.
- Where should you store your meal?
  Bringing a frozen coolant with your meal avoids use of the family refrigerator.
- Where can you safely place your nursing bag and personal equipment?
  Bring clean newspaper or piece of plastic to place under your bag to reduce contamination from home to home.
- Where should medical supplies and/or equipment be stored?
  This should be a locked area. When ordering supplies, remember that once the supplies are in the home, they cannot be returned, even if they are in sealed bags or boxes. Families are charged for all supplies in the home, whether they are used or not.
- In case of an emergency, who should be called if the parents are not home?
- Who may visit the child while your care is being given?
- In what rooms will the nursing care be given?
  Limiting your care space to the child's immediate environment increases the amount of privacy for the family.
- Clearly define what you will and will not be doing in the home. What is the family's understanding of your scope of responsibilities?
  Care of siblings, transportation of the child to doctor's appointments, and household tasks not related to the nursing support of the child are areas in which nurses are commonly asked to participate. A home care nurse may not do any of these.
- If the child misbehaves, what disciplinary measures can you institute?
  Discipline parameters should be clearly established. This not only relates to who should discipline the child and what form this discipline should take but also reflects safety issues from a nursing standpoint.

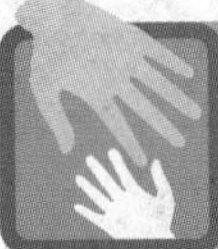

Chart 11–14
Nursing Interventions

Safety Precautions for the Home Health Nurse

A home care nurse may be in situations that require a little more caution than is needed when working with others in a hospital or clinic. The following are suggestions for enhancing the nurse's safety when working in the community:

- Do not carry a purse into a patient's home. Lock all personal items in the trunk of your car.
- Do not wear expensive jewelry or an expensive watch.
- Wear comfortable, flat shoes in which you can easily run.
- If your home care agency does not require uniforms, wear slacks and top in muted colors.
- Inform at least one other person of where you are going and when you expect to return.
- If you do not need to carry a nursing bag, don't. Put needed equipment in the pockets of a fishing jacket, for instance.
- Phone ahead to the patient's home and inform the family when they can expect you. Verify the patient's address and directions.
- Have a cellular phone in your car.
- If you are traveling to a known or suspected unsafe area, arrange with the local police for an escort.

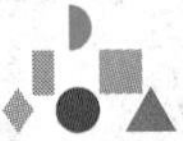

Alternatives to Home Discharge

Discharging the child to the home may not always be feasible or in the best interest of the child or the family. Home care requires parental dedication, commitment, and courage. Some families may be ambivalent about caring for their child at home. In other cases, the family may want to take the child home but be anxious about providing the necessary level of care. These families may benefit from a gradual transition to the home. It may prove beneficial in the long run to discharge the child to a subacute care or to a postacute rehabilitation facility for a temporary period. This allows further opportunity for the family to learn about the child's care, to slowly assume more ongoing responsibility, and to make the adjustments to their home to accommodate the child (Ladden, 1990; Nissim & Sten, 1991). In some instances, it is best to pursue a medical foster home placement. This kind of placement offers the child a homelike environment until his or her medical needs either resolve or at least become more manageable, allowing a return to home. In other cases, home care may be attempted if the parents wish, then discontinued at a later date owing to the child's debilitating condition or to the family's inability to provide for the child's care. The parents may have felt obligated to care for the child at home but may now feel overwhelmed by the responsibility. Other parents are enthusiastic at the onset but reconsider their decision as the full impact of the child's care is realized.

In response to these situations, should the family elect not to care for the child or provide medical therapies at home, alternative plans should be made. Alternatives to home care include specialized foster care, chronic or long-term care pediatric facilities, pediatric nursing homes, and residential and hospice facilities. With the development of these alternative care environments, long-term hospitalization in acute care and pediatric rehabilitation facilities is no longer necessary. The health care team works with the family to ensure that professional goals, family needs, and the child's welfare are congruent. Decisions by the family are respected and a collaborative approach is maintained, regardless of the setting in which care is provided to the child.

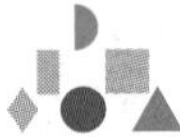

The Future of Pediatric Rehabilitation and Home Care

Children with conditions requiring rehabilitation and/or home care present many challenges in ensuring that their needs are met and in providing opportunities to achieve their optimal level of development. These challenges include overcoming the actions, attitudes, and barriers that are a result of discrimination directed toward those who are chronically ill or disabled. Turner-Henson, Holaday, Corser, Ogletree, and Swan (1994) examined mothers' perceptions of discrimination experienced by chronically ill school-age children. Thirty-five percent of the sample perceived that their child experienced problems with discrimination. These problems were perceived as human-made barriers that made it difficult to care for the child, to allow the child to participate in age-appropriate activities, and to take the child out in public places.

Other barriers that must be addressed are those created by health care personnel and the health care system. The health needs of the child can involve an array of personnel, services, and treatments. Services may be inadvertently duplicated or omitted, and information given to the family may be contradictory and confusing. The family has the added burden of coordinating their lives around multiple visits to multiple care providers. A transdisciplinary approach to the child's care could ease the burden and sense of confusion that families often experience. Having one or two professionals from key disciplines address the child's primary needs would provide more consistent care to the child and his or her family (Ahmann & Lierman, 1992). This approach requires professionals to cross-train in areas that involve specific aspects of the child's care. For instance, the physical therapist would instruct the nurse in specific techniques to encourage musculoskeletal development. These specialists would remain a vital part of the health care team and would be used as needed for consultation and for periodic evaluation of the child's progress.

The limited health care dollars available for rehabilitation and home care services also represent a problem that needs to be addressed. As more and more children have a need to receive these services, insurance and reimbursement agencies must recognize the need to provide more comprehensive coverage to support the child and the family. More home care services and innovative supportive programs need to be developed.

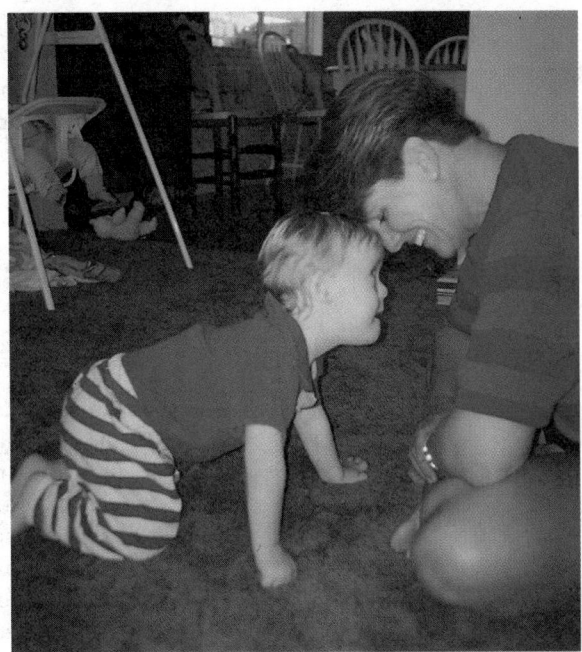

Figure 11-12
Rehabilitation, habilitation, and home care services aim to help the child and family reach their optimum potential.

Chart 11-15

Measures to Improve Health Care Services for Rehabilitation and Home Care

- Expand financing mechanisms and insurance plans to be more comprehensive of children's care needs.
- Develop policies to extend public and private insurance benefits to cover such expenses as transportation to and from the hospital or medical facility; lost income from work; and parking, meal, and motel expenses associated with extended hospitalizations.
- Provide low-cost parking permits at hospitals and rehabilitative facilities for families whose children require services for longer than 1 or 2 months.
- Decrease the number and frequency of clinic and physician encounters for the family by consolidating clinic services and incorporating transdisciplinary care.
- Provide education to assist inpatient health care providers in better managing the preparation and transition of the family to home care services.
- Change inpatient care interventions to be consistent with the manner in which these interventions are being carried out in the home.

Nurses can take an active role in changing public policy and health care delivery standards for rehabilitation and home care (Wegener & Aday, 1989). Nurses can also participate in research that articulates the needs of children requiring long-term rehabilitation and home care. More literature is needed that discusses the interventions that the rehabilitation and home care teams have found to be effective. Measurement tools need to be developed that accurately assess family needs, the developmental and educational needs of the child, and the child's progress in meeting identified needs (Chart 11–15).

These are the things that make rehabilitation and home nursing so wonderfully special: watching a 5-year-old with cerebral palsy take his or her first steps, helping the father of an infant with a cardiac defect bottle-feed his child instead of tube feeding, watching a 12-year-old finally take a breath on his or her own after being on a ventilator for an extended period. Touching the lives of these children helps bring them a brighter future (Fig. 11–12).

Summary of Key Concepts

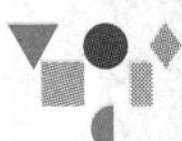

- Rehabilitation is a dynamic, goal-oriented process that facilitates the child's progression toward health and assists in restoring functions lost through injury or illness.
- Habilitation is the process in which the child develops new skills and abilities to achieve a maximum level of functioning that is appropriate for the child's developmental age.
- Rehabilitation and habilitation services can be provided by a transdisciplinary team approach in which one or two providers directly implement the plan of care of multiple disciplines.
- The focus of care for the child dealing with the effects of a sudden illness or injury or a chronic condition is to enable the child to lead as "normal" a life as possible.
- The two primary types of home care services available are private duty and skilled intermittent visits. With private duty care the nurse is at the bedside for up to 24 hours a day. With intermittent care, the nurse may visit the home several times a day or several times a week.
- To prepare for the transition to home care, the nurse and family must have a thorough understanding of the child's condition and health care needs. The health care team must identify the home caregivers and determine the level of support services that are needed in the home.
- A home care path should be developed in collaboration with the family and altered as needed to reflect changes in the child's condition and the family's abilities.
- There may be great differences between the equipment used in the home and the equipment used in the hospital. In the inpatient setting, the nurse should not teach the parents to use equipment and supplies that will not be used at home. It would be more beneficial to the family to obtain the home care supplies and have an opportunity to practice using them in the inpatient setting before discharge.
- To work effectively with a family, the home care nurse must respect the family's privacy and strive to develop a trusting relationship in which roles and expectations are clearly defined.
- A family may decide that they are unable or unwilling to care for their child in the home. In these cases, medical foster home placement, a pediatric nursing home, a hospice facility, a pediatric long-term care facility, or a residential facility may be selected as an alternative to home care of the child.
- Nurses can take an active role in changing public policy and health care delivery standards to improve the services available for children needing rehabilitation and home care.

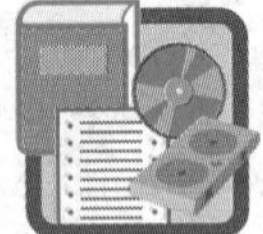

Resources

Organizations

American Academy of Ambulatory Care Nursing
East Holly Avenue, Box 56
Pitman, NJ 01071
(609) 256-2350
E-mail: aaacn@mail.ajj.com

American Association of Spinal Cord Injury Nurses
75-20 Astoria Boulevard
Jackson Heights, NY 11370
(718) 803-3782

American Association on Mental Retardation
1719 Kalorama Road NW
Washington, DC 20009
(800) 424-3688

American Congress of Rehabilitation Medicine
4700 West Lake Avenue
Glenview, IL 60025
(847) 375-4725
Web: http://www.amctec.com/amc

American Rehabilitation Association
1910 Association Drive, Suite 200
Reston, VA 22090

American Subacute Care Association
1440 Kennedy Causeway, Suite 421
North Bay Village, FL 33141
(305) 864-0396
E-mail: ascamail@aol.com
Web: http://www.subacute.org/ascamail

Association of Rehabilitation Nurses
4700 West Lake Avenue
Glenview, IL 60025-1485
(800) 229-7530
E-mail: info@rehabnurse.org

Children's Hospice International
700 Princess Street
Alexandria, VA 22314
(800) 346-2742

Developmental Disabilities Nurses Association
1720 Willow Creek Circle, Suite 515
Eugene, OR 97402
(800) 888-6733

Hospice Association of America
228 7th Street SE
Washington, DC 20003
(202) 547-7424

Hospice Nurses Association
5512 Northumberland
Pittsburgh, PA 15217
(412) 687-3231

Information Center for Individuals with Disabilities
Fort Point Place, 27-43 Wormwood Street
Boston, MA 02210-1606

National Association for Home Care
228 7th Street SE
Washington, DC 20003
(202) 547-7424

National Information Center for Children and Youth with Disabilities (NICHCY)
PO Box 1492
Washington, DC 20013-1492
(800) 999-5599

National Rehabilitation Association
633 South Washington Street
Alexandra, VA 22314
(703) 836-0850

National Rehabilitation Information Center (NARIC)
8455 Colesville Road, Suite 1540
Arlington, VA 22209
(703) 524-6686
(800) 346-2742
Web: http://www.naric.com/naric

Nurses of the Developmentally Disabled
PO Box 134
Convent Station, NJ 07961
(201) 887-6145

Visiting Nurse Association of America
3801 East Florida Avenue, Suite 900
Denver, CO 80210
(303) 753-2018

Rehabilitation Products and Assistive Devices

Ablsdata, National Rehabilitation Information Center (NARIC)
8455 Colesville Road, Suite 935
Silver Spring, MD 20910-3319
(310) 588-9284

Accent on Information
PO Box 700
Bloomington, IL 61702
(309) 378-2961

Independent Living Aids
27 East Mall Street
Plainfield, NY 11803
(516) 752-3135

Computer Resources

The American Physical Therapy Association
http://www.apta.org

Occupational Therapy Talk Back
http://home.erathlink.net/-whitson/talkback.htm/

Nursing Net
http://www.communique.net/-nursgnt/

Respiratory Care Home Page
http:www.theshop.net/kuhlman/resp.htm

Virtual Nursing Center
http://www-sci.lib.uci.edu/HSG/Nursing.htm/

References

Ahmann, E. (1994). Family centered care: The time has come. *Pediatric Nursing, 20,* 52–53.

Ahmann, E., & Bond, N. (1992). Promoting normal growth in school-age children and adolescents who are technology dependent: A family centered model. *Pediatric Nursing, 18,* 399–405.

Ahmann, E., & Lierman, C. (1992). Promoting normal development in technology-dependent children: An introduction to the issues. *Pediatric Nursing, 18,* 143–148.

Ahmann, E., & Lipsi, K. (1992). Developmental assessment of the technology-dependent infant and young child. *Pediatric Nursing, 18,* 299–305.

American Nurses' Association. (1986). *Standards of community health nursing practice*. Kansas City, MO: Author.

American Nurses' Association. (1992). *A statement on the scope of home health nursing practice*. Washington, DC: Author.

Aqazio, J. (1997). Family transition through the termination of private duty home care nursing. *Journal of Pediatric Nursing, 12*(2), 74–84.

Britton, L., & Johnston, J. (1993). Dependent on technology: A child grows up hospitalized. *Pediatric Nursing, 19,* 579–584.

Burkett, K. W. (1989). Trends in pediatric rehabilitation. *Nursing Clinics of North America, 24,* 239–255.

Commission on Accreditation of Rehabilitation Facilities (CARF). (1996). *Standards manual for facilities serving people with disabilities*. Tucson: Author.

Dittmar, S. (Ed.). (1989). *Rehabilitation nursing: Process and application*. St. Louis: C. V. Mosby.

Faulkner, M. (1996). Family responses to children with diabetes and their influences on self care. *Journal of Pediatric Nursing, 11,* 82–93.

Fleming, J., Challela, M., Eland, J., Hornick, R., Johnson, P., Martinson, I., Nativio, D., Nokes, K., Riddle, I., Steele, N., Sudela, K., Thomas, R., Turner, Q., Wheeler, B., & Young, A. (1994). Impact on the family of children who are technology dependent and cared for in the home. *Pediatric Nursing, 20,* 379–388.

Futcher, J. (1988). Chronic illness in family dynamics. *Pediatric Nursing, 14,* 381–385

Gorski, P. (1991). Promoting infant development during neonatal hospitalization. *Children's Health Care, 20*(4), 205–257.

Grossman, D. (1996). Cultural dimensions in home health nursing. *American Journal of Nursing, 7*(96), 33–34.

Hoeman, S. P. (1992). Community-based rehabilitation. *Holistic Nursing Practice, 6*(2), 32–41.

Joint Commission on Accreditation of Healthcare Organizations (JCAHO). (1996). *Rehabilitation services: Accreditation manual for hospitals*. Oakbrook Terrace, IL: Author.

Kaufman, J. (1991). An overview of public sector financing for pediatric home care: Part one. *Pediatric Nursing, 17*, 280–281.

Klein-Berndt, S. (1991). Bronchopulmonary dysplasia in the family: A longitudinal case study. *Pediatric Nursing, 17*, 607–611.

Klug, R. (1992). Selecting a home care agency. *Pediatric Nursing, 18*, 504–506.

Klug, R. (1993). Clarifying roles and expectations in home care. *Pediatric Nursing, 19*, 374–376.

Klug, R. (1994). Setting home care standards. *Pediatric Nursing, 20*, 404–406.

Ladden, M. (1990). The impact of preterm birth on the family and society. Part 2: Transition to home. *Pediatric Nursing, 16*, 620–622, 626.

Lantos, J., & Kohrman, A. (1992). Ethical aspects of pediatric home care. *Pediatrics, 89*, 920–924.

Leininger, M. (1994). *Transcultural nursing concepts, theories, and practice*. Columbus, OH: Greyden Press.

Martinez, N., Schreiber, M., & Hartman, E. (1991). Pediatric nurse practitioners: Primary care providers and case managers for chronically ill children at home. *Journal of Pediatric Health Care, 5*, 291–296.

McClowry, S. (1993). Pediatric nursing psychosocial care: A vision beyond hospitalization. *Pediatric Nursing, 19*, 146–148.

McClung, R. (1995). Considerations for the use of a conceptual model in home health nursing. *Pediatric Nursing, 21*, 68–70.

McCourt, A. (Ed.). (1993). *The speciality practice of rehabilitation nursing: A core curriculum* (3rd ed.). Skokie, IL: Rehabilitation Nursing Foundation of the Association of Rehabilitation Nurses.

McKeown, T. (1979). *The role of medicine: Dream, mirage or nemesis*. Princeton, NJ: Princeton University Press.

Mitchell, S. (1996). Infants with bronchopulmonary dysplasia: A developmental perspective. *Journal of Pediatric Nursing, 11*(3), 145–151.

Nissim, L., & Sten, M. (1991). The ventilator-assisted child: A case for empowerment. *Pediatric Nursing, 17*, 507–511.

Office of Technology Assessment. (1987). *Technology-dependent children: Home care vs. Home care. A technical memorandum*. Washington, DC: Congress of the United States.

O'Toole, M. T. (1992). The interdisciplinary team: Research and education. *Holistic Nursing Practice, 6*(2), 76–83.

Phillips, M., & Brostoff, M. (1989). Working collaboratively with parents of disabled children. *Pediatric Nursing, 15*, 180–185.

Pope, A. M., & Tarlov, A. R. (Eds.). (1991). *Disability in America: Toward a national agenda for prevention*. Washington, DC: National Academy Press.

Richardson, M., Student, E., O'Boyle, D., Smyth, M., & Wheeler, T. (1992). Establishment of a state-supported, specialized home care program for children with complex health-care needs. *Comprehensive Pediatric Nursing, 15*, 93–122.

Russell, D., Rosenbaum, P., Cadman, D., Gowland, C., Hardy, S., & Jarvis, S. (1989). The gross motor function measure: A means to evaluate the effects of physical therapy. *Developmental Medicine and Child Neurology, 31*, 341–352.

Sayles, S. M. (Ed.). (1981). *Rehabilitation nursing: Concepts and practice—A core curriculum*. Evanston, IL: Rehabilitation Nursing Institute.

Schreiner, M., Donar, M., & Kettrick, R. (1987). Pediatric home ventilation. *Pediatric Clinics of North America, 34*(1), 47–60.

Schuman, A., & Karush, G. (1992). Fiberoptic vs. conventional home phototherapy for neonatal hyperbilirubinemia. *Clinical Pediatrics, 31*, 345–352.

Selekman, J. (1991). Pediatric rehabilitation: From concepts to practice. *Pediatric Nursing, 17*, 11–14, 33.

Selekman, J., & Synder, M. (1996). *Primary care of the child with a chronic condition*. St. Louis: Mosby–Year Book.

Seltzer, W., & Krauss, M. (1994). Binding ties: Roles of adults with siblings of persons with mental retardation. *Journal of Mental Retardation, 34*, 83–93.

Snowdon, A., & Kane, D. (1995). Parental needs following the discharge of a hospitalized child. *Pediatric Nursing, 21*, 425–428.

Sterling, Y., Jones, L., Johnson, D., & Bowen, M. (1996). Parents' resources and home management of the care of chronically ill infants. *Journal of the Society of Pediatric Nurses, 1*(3), 103–109.

Storck, I. F., & Thompson-Hoffman, S. (1991). Demographic characteristics of the disabled population. In S. Thompson-Hoffman & I. F. Storck (Eds.), *Disability in the United States: A portrait from national data* (pp. 1–12). New York: Springer Publishing Company.

Strutts, A. (1994). Selecting outcomes of technology dependent children receiving home care and prescribed child care services. *Pediatric Home Care, 20*, 501–505.

Teague, B., Fleming, J., Wolfe, J., Castle, G., Kiernan, B., Lobo, M., & Riggs, I. (1993). "High-tech" home care for children with chronic health conditions: A pilot study. *Journal of Pediatric Nursing: Nursing Care of Children and Families, 8*, 226–231.

Turner-Henson, A., Holaday, B., Corser, N., Ogletree, G., & Swan, J. (1994). The experiences of discrimination: Challenges for chronically ill children. *Pediatric Nursing, 20*, 571–577.

Vessey, J. (1994). Improving the primary care pediatric nurses provide to children and their families. *Pediatric Nursing, 20*, 64–65.

Wegener, D., & Aday, L. (1989). Home care for ventilator-assisted children: Predicting family stress. *Pediatric Nursing, 15*, 371–376.

Worthington, R. (1995). Effective transitions for families: Life beyond the hospital. *Pediatric Nursing, 21*, 86–87.

Wright. B. (1983). *Physical disability: A psychological approach*. New York: Harper & Row.

Yoos, L., Kitzman, H., Olds, D., & Overracker, I. (1995). Child rearing beliefs in the African-American community: Implications for culturally competent pediatric care. *Journal of Pediatric Nursing, 10*, 343–352.

Zigler, E., & Gilman, E. (1993). Day care in America: What is needed. *Pediatrics, 91*, 175–178.

Bibliography

Batshaw, M. L., & Perret, Y. M. (1992). *Children with disabilities: A medical primer* (3rd ed.). Baltimore: Paul H. Brooks.

Cady, C., & Yoshioka, R. (1991). Using a learning contract to successfully discharge an infant on home total parenteral nutrition. *Pediatric Nursing, 17,* 67–72.

Clements, D. B., Copeland, L. G., & Loftus, M. (1990). Critical times for families with a chronically ill child. *Pediatric Nursing, 16,* 157–161.

Davis, B. D., & Steele, S. (1991). Case management for young children with special health care needs. *Pediatric Nursing, 17,* 15–19.

Edwards, P. A. (1992). The evolution of rehabilitation facilities for children. *Rehabilitation Nursing, 17,* 191–192, 195.

Griebel, M., Pakes, W., & Worley, G. (1991). The Chariari malformation associated with myelomeningocele. In H. L. Rekate (Ed.), *Comprehensive management of spina bifida* (pp. 69–92). Boca Raton, FL: CRC Press.

Haley, S. M., Baryza, M. J., & Webster, H. C. (1992). Pediatric rehabilitation and recovery of children with traumatic injuries. *Pediatric Physical Therapy,* 4(1), 24–30.

Heery, K. (1992). Restoring childhood through rehabilitation. *Rehabilitation Nursing, 17,* 193–195.

Kalscheur, J. A. (1992). Benefits of the Americans with Disabilities Act of 1990 for children and adolescents with disabilities. *American Journal of Occupational Therapy,* 46, 419–433.

Koop, C. (1987). *Children with special health care needs: Campaign '87.* U.S. Department of Health and Human Services, Washington, DC: U.S. Government Printing Office.

Lynch, E., & Hanson, M. (1995). *Developing cross cultural competence: A guide for working with young children and their families.* Baltimore: Paul H. Brooks.

Mariano, C. (1989). The case for interdisciplinary collaboration. *Nursing Outlook, 37,* 285–288.

Martinson, I. (1995). Pediatric hospice nursing. *Annual Review of Nursing Research, 13,* 195–214.

Molnar, G. E. (1988). A developmental perspective for the rehabilitation of children with physical disability. *Pediatric Annals, 17,* 766–776.

Nehring, W. (1994). The nurse whose specialty is developmental disabilities. *Pediatric Nursing, 20*(1), 78–81.

Newacheck, P., & McManus, M. (1988). Financing health care for disabled children. *Pediatrics, 81,* 385–394.

NICHCY. (1991). The education of children and youth with special needs: What do the laws say? *NICHCY News Digest, 1*(1), 1–16.

Perrin, J., Guyer, B., & Lawrence, J. (1992). Health care services for children and adolescents. *The Future of Children, 2,* 58–77.

Sterling, Y. (1991). Resource needs of mothers managing chronically ill infants at home. *Neonatal Network,* 9(1), 55–58.

Trachtenberg, S. (1990). Rights of children with developmental disabilities. In M. W. Schwartz (Ed.), *Pediatric primary care: A problem-oriented approach* (2nd ed.). Chicago: Year Book Medical Publishers.

Trueman, M. S. (1989). Collaboration: A right and responsibility of professional practice. *Critical Care Nurse, 11*(1), 70–71.

Yoos, L. (1987). Chronic childhood illness: Developmental issues. *Pediatric Nursing, 13,* 25–28.

The Grieving Family

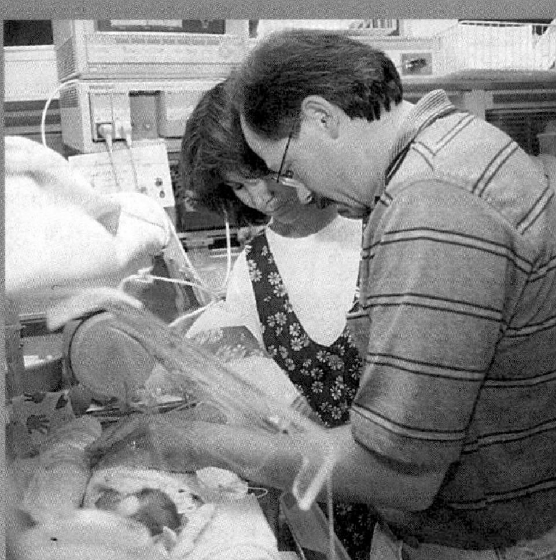

OUTLINE

OBJECTIVES

- Examine the process of grief and bereavement in the family coping with the death of a child.
- Analyze the effect of cultural and religious practices and influences on the family coping with grief.
- Differentiate between the child's understanding of and the ability to cope with death and grief as he or she matures.
- Describe the unique responses of the family coping with a child's death.
- Describe the needs of the family facing the death of a child in the hospital and at home.
- Discuss the unique needs of the family who has lost a child during the perinatal period.
- Relate the names and functions of organizations that assist families in coping with the loss of a child.

KEY TERMS

bereavement
grief
life transition

CHAPTER

12

The death of a child at any age is difficult for the parents and family. The loss can be equally difficult for the siblings, friends, nurses, and other health care professionals who care for the child and the child's family.

The care of the child and family facing death is not simple. Adults helping children must deal with their own grief and need to mourn while helping the child do the same. The child may be the one who is dying, or the child may be a sibling or friend of a child who has died. The loved one whom the child loses through death can be a parent, a sibling, a family member, or a friend. For the child, resolution of the experience of the loss of a loved one involves both progression through the bereavement process and achievement of normal developmental milestones.

An important part of the nursing care of the dying child is the care of the physical illness. This chapter focuses on the child's understanding of death and interventions to help the child successfully cope with the loss of a loved one. The unique physical care needs of the dying child in the months, weeks, and hours before death and the psychosocial aspects of the care of the child and family when they experience a death are also presented.

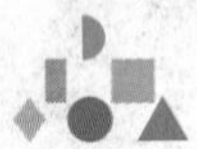

Grief and Bereavement

Grief is the painful, sad, and anguished feeling accompanying loss. Grief is usually thought of as a reaction to the death of a loved one. Other losses, however, such as the loss of an object (e.g., a special ring or long-term home), of a relationship (e.g., a best friend moves away), or the loss of anything, tangible or intangible, that is highly valued, can result in a grief reaction. The family who has eagerly anticipated the arrival of their healthy newborn experiences grief and bereavement if the child is born with a congenital abnormality. The unanticipated diagnosis of leukemia or diabetes in a previously healthy teenager elicits grief within the family and for the afflicted child. When grief from any type of loss is unresolved, it can reappear during an attempt to resolve the grief associated with a later loss. Bereavement, often called mourning, is the mental work following the loss, which allows adaptation to that loss (Hughes, 1995).

Reaction to Grief

Grief caused by the potential or actual loss of a loved one or by an anticipated outcome results in both physiologic and emotional responses. Physiologic symptoms include waves of physical distress including shortness of breath, an empty feeling in the stomach or heart, physical weakness, and a loss of appetite. An inability to concentrate or sleep, a general sense of unreality, and a need to withdraw from others is also common (Hughes, 1995).

Kubler-Ross (1969) described five common reactions to death or approaching death: denial and isolation, anger, bargaining, depression, and acceptance. These stages of death, or reactions to mourning, explain the coping mechanisms people use to deal with losses. Even though Kubler-Ross presented these mechanisms as sequential reactions, they actually occur more randomly, with individuals moving from one reaction to another before achieving full resolution. Not all persons experience all the reactions.

Denial and Isolation

The first reaction is denial and isolation. Denial can be overt, such as when a parent says, "The doctor told us Sammy has a very bad head injury, but with all these new machines he will be back at school in no time." Signs of denial can be more subtle, such as when the family attempts to go on with life as usual with no adaptation for essential disease care. At times, the denial is in the form of psychological isolation. In this case, the child or parent is able to talk about the illness, or the potential or actual death with no emotion or acknowledgment of what the death will mean.

Denial can be therapeutic if it allows individuals to distance themselves from the trauma of the diagnosis or death itself in order to activate coping mechanisms or reach out for help. Prolonged denial, however, can cause missed opportunities for needed emotional care or for actual disease treatment or amelioration of negative symptoms.

Anger

The second reaction is anger, which can be quite pronounced. Often, the trigger is the loss of the person who is dying or has died, but anger can also be triggered by the loss of the expected future. It is not unusual for displaced anger to be directed at persons who have no role or culpability in the death or loss. These persons can be health care workers, family members, friends, or anyone with whom the person interacts. The anger can also be self directed because of actual or perceived personal failure in preventing the loss from occurring. Anger can be directed at family members whose children are alive and thriving, at health care providers, or at a higher power.

caREminder: *The anger of a grieving person should not be taken personally. Specific issues should be addressed and corrected if possible, and the angry person should be allowed the time needed to overcome this reaction and move on in his or her grieving process.*

By not overreacting to the angry person, the nurse allows continued development of the therapeutic relationship that the person needs to complete the grieving and bereavement process. To help prevent disruption of family relationships, family members should be taught that anger is a normal part of the grief reaction.

Bargaining

In bargaining, the grieving person offers some action, perhaps to a higher being, in exchange for a cure or the return of the loved one. Promising good behavior, returning to active participation in religious activities, and offering to support a special cause are all examples of bargaining. A major component of bargaining is the maintenance of hope.

Bargaining can be therapeutic and may actually help the person look to the future, even when that future is not clear. On the other hand, bargaining can cause individuals to seek out alternative but ineffective treatments "just in case" they might work. These can be physically, emotionally, and financially draining on the family and may delay use of traditional, but not so promising, approaches to care.

Depression

Depression can be based on both current and prior losses. Expressing underlying fears and concerns helps the person move beyond the depression. The depressed person prepares for the altered future, which may encompass dealing with a chronic or acute illness in the family, coping with the person's own death and the loss of all that is associated with life, or preparing for the loss of a loved one who is dying. This behavior should be accepted and supported. Attempts to cheer up the person ignore the real concerns and issues that the depressed person is trying to deal with.

Acceptance

Acceptance or resolution of the fact that the loss will occur or has occurred is necessary for the grieving person to move on with life. Acceptance helps the dying person peacefully move on to death. For the family of a child with an unexpected illness, acceptance helps them incorporate the diagnosis and all associated health care needs into their lifestyle and routine.

Chart 12–1

Bereavement Tasks

- Recognizing the loss
- Reacting to the separation
- Recollecting and reexperiencing the deceased and the relationship
- Relinquishing old attachments to the deceased and to the shared world
- Readjusting to allow movement into a new world without the loved one, but without forgetting the old world
- Reinvesting in the new world

From Rando, T. (1993). *Treatment of complicated mourning.* Champaign, IL: Research Press. Reprinted with permission.

Bereavement Tasks

A person must complete six bereavement tasks (Chart 12–1). Working through these tasks facilitates adjustment to the loss.

Recognizing the Loss

In recognizing the loss, a person accepts the reality of the loss. Parents of a child with a chronic illness, congenital defect, or disfigurement must accept the reality that their child will not be like other children. For the parents of a dying child, they must accept that their child will not recover or return and that the child will not be a part of their lives again (Rando, 1993).

During this task, ill, disabled, or disfigured children recognize that they are different from their peers. The child's level of cognitive understanding impacts this perception of the loss. The dying child needs to understand what it means to be dead and what causes a person to die. The child should be asked about his or her observations so that misconceptions can be corrected. These discussions should occur as soon as possible after the diagnosis, death, or loss to avoid missed opportunities to talk and to avoid sending the message that the loss is not to be discussed. Often, the challenge is not to get the child to talk, but to be sure that, when the child wants to talk, someone is there to listen. This person should be willing to answer questions and to talk about what the child is feeling (Walker, 1993).

caREminder: *Children should not be given more information than they request or can comprehend.*

Reacting to the Separation

Reaction to the separation has been described as experiencing the pain. The grieving person must feel, identify, accept, and express the psychological reactions to the loss (Rando, 1993). This can bring out intense and painful feelings.

There is also a need to identify and mourn secondary losses that occurred with the primary loss (Rando, 1993). For the parents whose child has died, this can mean loss of the socialization they enjoyed when they served as class parents in their child's school. For the boy whose father died, this might mean there is no one to take him on the father–son camping trip. An illness can separate a child from peers and family, with frequent exacerbations of the illness and hospitalizations curtailing previously enjoyed activities.

Often, a child displays aggression (McCown & Davies, 1995), sadness (Mahon & Page, 1995), anger, or other strong emotional reactions. These reactions should be addressed when they occur, and appropriate methods to express the emotions should be discussed. Most important, the source of the emotional reaction should be determined. Strong emotional responses frequently result from unexpressed fears and concerns or from a misunderstanding of the relationship between events (Whittam, 1993) (Chart 12–2).

Recollecting and Reexperiencing the Deceased and the Relationship

The next task is to review and remember realistically the relationship with the person who died or to remember how relationships were before the onset of illness or other loss. This often involves reviving and reexperiencing the feelings that come with these memories. This process allows the grieving person to acknowledge both the good memories and the unpleasant events and prevents memorializing the person as a saint when it is not warranted (Rando, 1993). For the parents of a child who dies, this can mean realizing that the child made them angry, too, and that the surviving sibling is not their only child who could be difficult. For the child, it may mean acknowledging that not everything an older sibling did was good and that not all of the older child's behaviors should be emulated.

In cases of loss in which severe dysfunction or death of a child occurs, the sibling child may take on roles and attributes of the affected child (Whittam, 1993). These roles can be positive, such as taking on the love of a sport, or negative, such as taking on the physical symptoms of the child's illness or a love of the reckless driving that led to the accident or subsequent death. The sibling may want to keep possessions and pictures of the affected child (when healthy). The sibling should be given the opportunity to choose these items. The sibling

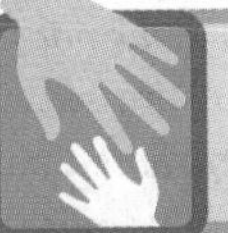

Chart 12–2
Nursing Interventions

Responding to Children's Feelings Associated with Loss

Confusion

Situation: A bereaved 3-year-old announces that her brother called to say that he will be coming home for dinner that night.
Response: "I think that you wish he could have dinner with us. I do, too, but he can't."
Rationale: Avoidance of facts adds to confusion and hinders the child's ability to cope with the loss.

Guilt

Situation: A 5-year-old fears that he caused his sister's death by wishing that she would go away.
Response: "We all have bad feelings about people—even those we love the most. But even the worst feelings can't kill someone."
Rationale: Consistent reassurance that the child is not responsible for the death aids the young child in relieving guilt.

Anxiety

Situation: A 7-year-old asks whether he will die of the same disease that resulted in his sibling's death.
Response: "Your sister was sick for a very long time. You are well. You cannot catch what she had."
Rationale: Facts help the child to gain emotional distance from the situation and to resolve anxiety.

Anger

Situation: A 10-year-old becomes enraged when her sibling is killed in an accident and says that life is not fair.
Response: "I'm very angry too. It isn't fair. We may never understand why this happened."
Rationale: Acknowledgment of feelings facilitates self-expression, which may diffuse anger.

Sorrow

Situation: A 12-year-old finds that she cannot escape the sadness she feels after her brother's death.
Response: "I know because I hurt too. It happens when you lose someone you love."
Rationale: Acceptance of feelings permits the child to experience feelings such as sorrow and to learn to tolerate them.

Adapted from Gibbons, M. (1992). A child dies, a child survives. The impact of sibling loss. *Journal of Pediatric Health Care, 6,* 65–72. Used with permission.

may also reenact rituals or events that were a part of the previous life with the loved one. The child should be allowed to do so, but the feelings behind these activities should be addressed to help the child acknowledge and deal with them.

Relinquishing Old Attachments to the Child and the Shared World

To go on with life without the deceased child or with the child in an altered state and appearance, the grieving individuals must give up their ties to the world they shared. This does not mean that they must dramatically change their lives, but it does mean that they must acknowledge that the child is no longer a part of their life or that the future will be different from the one they *would* have shared (Rando, 1993). For the parents, it can mean recognizing that life no longer revolves around the activities shared with the child. For a child, it might mean accepting that the loved one will not be the person who will provide help and support as the child moves into adulthood and begins to raise a family.

Moving into a New World Without the Loved One, but Without Forgetting the Old World

Bereaved persons must begin to move into a new reality in which the deceased person does not have an active part (Rando, 1993). Parents of a child who died may plan a vacation in the middle of the school year. A child whose best friend died of complications of cystic fibrosis may join the soccer team, even though they made a pact not to do things that they could not both participate in.

Reinvesting in the New World

An active reinvestment in the new world without the loved one, or with the loved one's new limitations, is the final step. It is not enough to simply move on; the person must become involved in the world again (Rando, 1993). Parents may begin planning for other children who are wanted for themselves, not as replacements for the child who has died or who is severely ill. Siblings must continue normal physical and emotional development. A toddler needs to develop autonomy and increased physical abilities, such as bladder and bowel control. The school-age child needs to increase participation in activities in school and with peers. Continued achievement in school and other activities is also important. The adolescent needs to begin to differentiate from the family, even if the death of a family member has drawn the adolescent into new and closer attachments to family members.

The time for the completion of the bereavement process is much longer than was once thought. For most individuals, the time period is 18 months. When a child has died, the time can be much longer. It is not unusual for a parent to have a resurgence of the grief reaction at certain trigger points long after the date of a death, such as when the child would have been starting high school or a first job. Grieving persons must be prepared for the occurrence of these feelings and must be helped to understand that the feelings are normal. Healing takes time and cannot be rushed.

Cultural and Religious Influences

When dealing with the grieving child and family, cultural and religious concerns should be recognized and addressed. Grieving and bereavement are treated differently in different cultures, and this influences the response of the child and family. When assessing the family, it is important for the nurse to seek out such factors and to take steps to accommodate the family's wishes, even if their requests are unfamiliar. If the nurse is unsure of the family's cultural beliefs or needs, the family should be asked to share them.

It is important to be cognizant of differing cultural practices and beliefs and to understand behavior based on these ideas. It is equally important not to expect certain behaviors based on cultural influence. The following are examples of how care might need to be modified in different situations.

In Japanese culture, there is emphasis on the importance of the family over the individual. Siblings are expected to be patient with the sick or dying child. Research by Saiki, Martinson, and Inano (1994) found that siblings usually did not complain when attention was focused on the dying child, but that, in some siblings, physical or emotional problems did develop. Japanese mothers are the primary caregivers, and families are not comfortable receiving support from outside the family. Therefore, Japanese families, especially mothers, struggle to provide care on their own at the expense of their own health and the needs of siblings (Saiki et al., 1994). An appropriate intervention would be to remind parents to pay attention to the needs of siblings.

Nurses often offer support with a pat on the hand or the back. For Native Americans, touching is reserved for family or very close friends (Nishimoto, 1996); therefore, touching is not an appropriate method of providing support for Native Americans.

The subculture of gender may influence patterns of Native Americans' grieving. Females often openly and emotionally express their grief, whereas males may show little emotion and seek no support. These patterns are not exclusively related to gender (Nishimoto, 1996), and interventions should be tailored to the individual response.

Many families draw great strength from their faith, although spiritual beliefs are not always expressed by in-

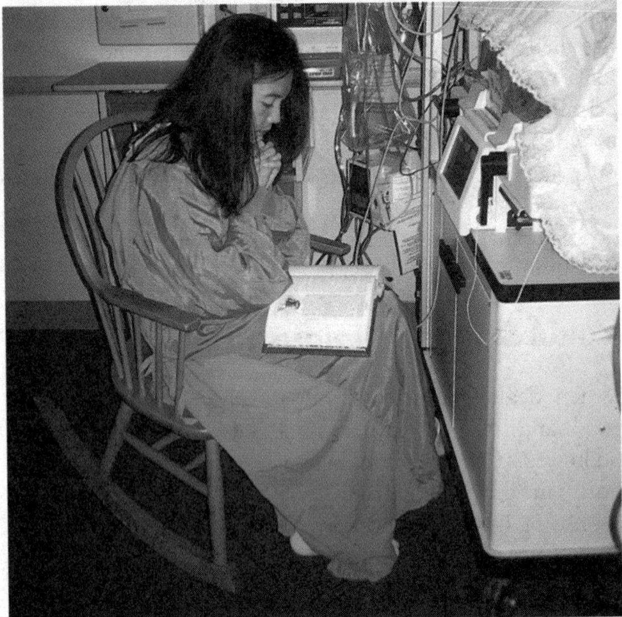

Figure 12–1
A family's religious practices, a source of spiritual support, should be incorporated into care.

volvement with a particular church or religion. Concepts such as hope, faith, and a sense of meaning and purpose in life are directly tied to the spiritual domain. Spirituality or religion may or may not be a source of support for the family (Dowden, 1995; Whittam, 1993). Some families hope for religious miracles at the time of their child's diagnosis or death. If desired, parents should be encouraged to seek their minister, priest, rabbi, or members of their church for support, and the plan of care should be modified to accommodate religious practices (Fig. 12–1).

To assess the family's spiritual beliefs, the nurse should look for evidence of involvement with a religion such as religious symbols, medals, statues, books, or music. (See Chapter 3 for a discussion of spiritual assessment.) These may be used to initiate discussion of spiritual strengths or needs. Many religions have specific death services or rituals, and every effort should be made to allow for these (Chart 12–3). If death occurs, the family may wish to complete special prayers or services and death rites to prepare the body for burial.

Promoting Successful Bereavement When Death Has Occurred

Each death is different and these differences affect the child's reaction to the death (Chart 12–4). After a death, some changes in the child's life are inevitable. Behavior of adults around the child changes as they

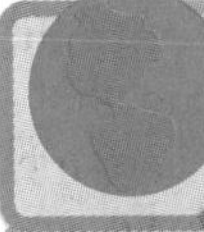

Chart 12–3
Worldview

Death Rituals of Different Religions

Muslim

Organ donation or transplants may be opposed. The dead must be buried intact so autopsy is uncommon and cremation not permitted. Grief is not shown in the dying person's presence, and impending death is hidden from the person. After the death, loud expressive mourning occurs. The body is wrapped in special cloth and buried in ground.

Hindu

Hindus believe in reincarnation. Death may be seen as God's will, and believers need time for prayer readings from holy Sanskrit books. Strings (to signify a blessing) may be tied around the wrist or neck of the child. Families may want to wash the body after death, and they may not want the body to be touched by non-Hindus. Transfusions, transplants, and autopsies are permissible; cremation is preferred.

Jewish

Burial usually takes place within 24 hours of death. The body must not be mutilated so autopsies, embalming (which removes blood that is considered a body part), and cremation are forbidden. The body must return to the earth. The body of the deceased is never left unattended until buried.

Christian Scientists

Believers may oppose the use of drugs, blood transfusions, or other treatments. Healing is seen as spiritual renewal, so Christian Scientists may want treatment or support from another Christian Scientist. Autopsy is permitted only in cases of sudden death.

Episcopal or Catholic

Infant baptism is not mandatory, but can be done if the parents desire. If a priest is unavailable, nurses can baptize by pouring a small amount of water over the child's head and saying "I baptize you in the name of the Father, the Son, and the Holy Spirit." Sacrament of the sick is offered to all seriously ill patients. It is often given to those who are dying and is no longer given only if death is imminent. Donation and transplantation of organs is permitted, and believers do not think that extraordinary artificial means of sustaining life must be used.

Chart 12–4

Factors That Affect the Child's Reaction to a Death

- Age of the child
- Developmental level of the child
- Relationship of the child to the person who died
- Suddenness of the death
- Child's knowledge about death before the death occurred
- Cause of the death: accident, sudden illness, prolonged illness, suicide, violence
- Amount and nature of discussion about the death with the child before the death occurred
- Coping abilities of the parents and family members
- Support resources of the child and family

Adapted from Castiglia, P. T. (1988). Death of a parent. *Journal of Pediatric Health Care, 2,* 157–159. Used with permission.

grieve. The child's daily routine may change during the acute phase surrounding the death and the funeral, and because of the absence of the loved one.

The health care team should help parents understand how important it is to have as few additional changes around the time of the death as possible. A safe, familiar environment and routine are essential for the child during the bereavement period. Unnecessary changes in the child's daily life (e.g., changing sleeping arrangements, place of residence, degree of contact with remaining family members, school, or daycare center) should be avoided. For example, a parent may need to choose between seeking a full-time job with full financial security but which leads to many changes in the child's environment and a part-time job with less financial security but which allows a fairly stable home environment. The part-time job may be the better choice. See Chart 12–5 for specific nursing interventions that can help the child during the bereavement process.

Successful bereavement is facilitated when family members are helped to recognize that they will each mourn differently. Individual parents and siblings of similar age or experience may progress through grieving differently. Members of the extended family vary in both degree and display of response and speed with which they achieve resolution. Individual reactions change over time. Each person comes to the end of the acute grief reaction at a different point during the ensuing 1 to 2 years.

Even the most skillful and sensitive care does not guarantee that each child will have a smooth progression through the bereavement process. But, when the child's needs and reactions are recognized and addressed, the child has the opportunity to successfully navigate the painful time following the death.

Dysfunctional Bereavement

Anyone who experiences a loss or the death of a loved one is at risk for dysfunctional or complicated bereavement. Complicated bereavement is present if, based on the time since the loss or death, there is some compromise, distortion, or failure of one or more of the six processes of bereavement. Such individuals are unable to accept the loss, experience the pain, or move on to a life that is different. Such mourners often try to deny, repress, or avoid aspects of the loss, including the step of relinquishing the relationship with the deceased child or other loved ones (Rando, 1993).

Parents are at high risk for complicated bereavement. Individuals are also at risk if the loss was sudden or unexpected, or if the relationship with the child or other family members was characterized by anger, ambivalence, or dependency. Other risk factors for complicated bereavement occur when losses are perceived as preventable, there are unaddressed loss issues from the past, there are mental health problems, and the mourner perceives a lack of support. Although research verifies that support groups may be of assistance to such individuals (Heiney, Ruffin, & Goon-Johnson, 1995), referral for mental health counseling may be needed for persons experiencing dysfunctional bereavement.

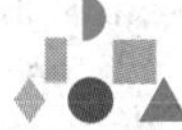

Care of the Caregiver

Before discussing how health care providers can help others, it is important to look at how caregivers can help themselves and their peers. The death of a child can be a traumatic event for the care provider. This occurs whether interactions with the child and family were brief or long-standing and whether the child's death was unexpected or the anticipated outcome of an illness or injury.

Even the most emotionally balanced nurse can experience an acute response to the death of a child. This may not happen with each child's death, but it does happen and it is normal. Nurses must learn to care for and support themselves and their peers when faced with the strong emotions and responses that accompany death. The concepts and intervention strategies presented in this section should be examined as they apply to individual nurses and the families for whom they provide nurs-

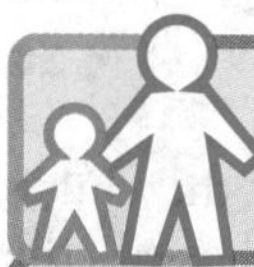

Chart 12–5
Developmental Considerations

A Child's Understanding of and Reaction to Fatal Illness and Death

Nursing Concern	Infant to Young Toddler (to age 2)	Older Toddler to Preschooler (ages 2 to 6)	School-Age Child (ages 6 to11)	Preadolescent to Adolescent (ages 11 to 18)
Developmental task	Achievement of awareness of being separate from significant other; development of trust and autonomy	Development of autonomy and initiative	Development of a sense of industry	Achievement of a sense of identity
Cognitive age/ stage	Sensorimotor	Preoperational thought: egocentric, magical, little concept of body integrity. Tendency to use and repeat words they do not understand, providing own explanations and definitions. Literal translation of words. No abstract thought.	Concrete operational thought (ages 7 to at least 10); beginning of logical thought but tendency to be literal	Formal operational thought; beginning of ability to think abstractly. Continued existence of some magical thinking (e.g., feeling guilty for illness) and egocentrism.
Major fears	Separation, strangers	Separation, loss of control, bodily injury, mutilation, the unknown, the dark, being left alone	Loss of control; bodily injury and mutilation; failure to live up to expectations of important others; monsters in their room, ghosts, and bogeyman coming to get them (or their parents)	Loss of control; altered body image; separation from peer group
Understanding of death	Perceives death as separation or abandonment; feels a sense of loss; realizes something is different	Feels it is reversible; may ascribe blame for the death to self because of magical thinking and egocentricity; may think dead person is somewhere else; perceives external, unrelated, concrete phenomena as cause of death (e.g., dying because you go to the hospital); perceives cause of death as proximity between two events (e.g., dying because you are near someone who died); early understanding of universality of death; may think that biological functions continue; may fear loving anyone else because that may cause them to die.	Time and place of death is better understood; developing understanding of irreversibility, cessation of bodily function, and multiple causes of death	Full comprehension of subconcepts of death possible; understands reality of own death but may deny own vulnerability and display risk-taking behavior

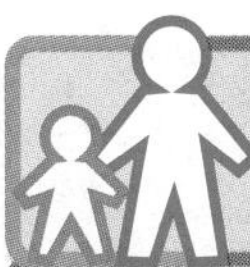

Chart 12–5
Developmental Considerations *Continued*

A Child's Understanding of and Reaction to Fatal Illness and Death

Nursing Concern	Infant to Young Toddler (to age 2)	Older Toddler to Preschooler (ages 2 to 6)	School-Age Child (ages 6 to11)	Preadolescent to Adolescent (ages 11 to 18)
Impact of illness/death of significant person	Potential distortion of differentiation of self from parent or significant others; fear of new caretakers or acceptance of all caretakers with no preference for prime caretakers; may change eating and sleeping patterns; may increase self-comforting behaviors such as thumb sucking and rocking. Long-term negative effects include failure to develop or maintain attachments and a sense of trust and autonomy.	Interference with/loss of developing sense of control and independence; interference with/loss of accomplishments such as walking, talking, toileting; strong fears of separation, abandonment, rejection, and threat to own security; clinging, fearful to be away from parents or to try new activities; repetition of questions that reflect an attempt to understand what "dead" means: "When will Johnny be back? Will God make Johnny better and send him back? Can we go to see Johnny now?"	Potential feelings of inadequacy or inferiority if autonomy and independence are compromised; may have extremes of behavior: withdrawal, acting out; may ask for guidance about how to act and what to say; may be judgmental about their own behavior and that of others, getting upset with "gross" displays of emotion; may act silly or laugh or suddenly become very quiet when death is discussed because of a lack of knowledge of how to respond. Surviving children's playmates in particular may show increased interest in staying at home or in their parents' health and well-being because of fear that they, too, will die. Play may involve violence, such as having cars crash and burn. May display self-consciousness about expressing their feelings and about their behavior not seeming different from their peers; may take on role of protector of parents, siblings, or other family members.	Potential alteration/relinquishment of newly acquired roles and responsibilities; may show extremes of behavior, hysterically crying one minute followed by embarrassed laughter the next; embarrassed to show their emotions in front of their friends, they may isolate themselves or go to great lengths to give the impression that "everything is fine"; may take on role of protector of parents, siblings, or other family members

Chart continued on following page

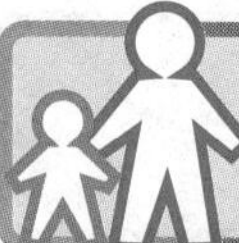

Chart 12–5
Developmental Considerations *Continued*

A Child's Understanding of and Reaction to Fatal Illness and Death

Nursing Concern	Infant to Young Toddler (to age 2)	Older Toddler to Preschooler (ages 2 to 6)	School-Age Child (ages 6 to11)	Preadolescent to Adolescent (ages 11 to 18)
Nursing interventions	Provide consistent care with the same caretakers in a familiar environment; minimize separation from parents or significant others; decrease parental anxiety, which is projected to infant.	Minimize separation from parents or significant others; keep security objects at hand; provide simple, correct, brief explanations; explain and maintain consistent limits; provide opportunities for play or play therapy; encourage questions; provide honest, simple, direct explanations and answers; use pictures, models, actual equipment, medical play; reassure child that he or she is not responsible for the death; reassure and demonstrate that the child will be cared for; assess for actions or words that show fear that something the child did caused the death or that behavior, such as being very good, might bring the person back; allow and encourage play showing a reenactment of events such as the funeral; read stories about dead pets and other animals to help the child express feelings; encourage drawings to allow the child to express feelings without using words.	Provide choices whenever possible to increase the child's sense of control; stress and facilitate contact with peer group; use diagrams, pictures, and models for explanations; emphasize the "normal" things the child can do; reassure the child that he or she has done nothing wrong and that hospitalization is not "punishment"; use physiologic reasons for death; encourage group activities to deal with grief; answer questions and discuss death-related concerns.	Allow adolescent to be an integral part of decision-making regarding care; give information sensitively; allow as many choices and as much control as possible; be honest about treatment and consequences; stress what the adolescent can do for himself or herself; assist in maintaining contact with peer group; use physiologic reasons for death; answer questions and discuss death-related concerns; discuss values; encourage group activities to deal with grief.

Data from Davis, B. (1993). Helping the siblings. In A. Armstrong-Dailey & S. Goltzer (Eds.). *Hospice care for children.* New York: Oxford University Press; Faulkner, K. (1993). Children's understanding of death. In A. Armstrong-Dailey & S. Goltzer (Eds.). *Hospice care for children.* New York: Oxford University Press; Furman, E. (1985). Children's patterns in mourning the death of a loved one. *Issues in Comprehensive Pediatric Nursing, 8,* 185–203; Gibbons, M. (1993). Psychosocial aspects of seious illness in childhood and adolescence. In A. Armstrong-Dailey & S. Goltzer (Eds.). *Hospice care for children.* New York: Oxford University Press.

ing care. Nurses with clear beliefs are better able to respond to the needs of each client without interference from their unexamined values, beliefs, fears, or personal grief.

When the child dies at home or on a general inpatient unit after a period of illness, the focus of care is helping the child and family experience a peaceful death. Even though there is sadness when the child dies, there has been time to prepare for the death and the desired outcomes are often achieved. The death of a child in a critical care setting can be exceptionally difficult for the staff, however, because the goal in such settings is the saving of life, and death can be seen as a sign of failure (Miles & Warner, 1992).

The death of a favorite patient can be stressful and painful for nurses working with dying children. Yet, nurses often report personal renewal from the experience of helping the child and family. They simultaneously grieve for the loss of the child while renewing their personal and professional commitment to the larger mission of achieving a cure for most of the children in their care (Hinds et al., 1994). Unit-based interventions and activities (Chart 12–6) give all hospital personnel involved with the care of the child a chance to remember the child and express their grief (Lunny, 1994). They also reinforce the fact that not all children die and that some children treated for serious or terminal illness survive and flourish. Such programs are found to be helpful by staff members, even if the programs do not decrease their stress or physical responses experienced following a significant death (Hinds et al., 1994). The programs legitimize the staff's grief experience (Heiney, Wells, & Ruffin, 1996).

Chart 12–6

Care for the Staff Members Who Work with Dying Children

- Plan unit-based memorial services to be held throughout the year.
- Provide support sessions for staff members from all services (nursing, social work, medicine, housekeeping).
- Keep a memorial book on the unit with pictures, letters, and poems about the children.
- Provide critical stress debriefings after particularly difficult deaths.
- Identify specific nurses who will care for the dying child and who can offer support to each other as well as to the family and the child.
- Plan a yearly party with survivors.
- Rotate staff members to settings where they see children who are doing well.

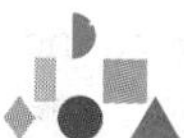

The Child's Understanding of Death

Children do not understand death all at once. Instead, they gradually increase their comprehension of the various subconcepts of death: universality, irrevocability, cessation of biological function, and causality (see Chart 12–5). Children usually master the subconcepts of death between 5 and 7 years of age (Schonfeld, 1993), with almost all children having an accurate concept by 9 years of age (Mahon, 1993). Individual children do not develop an understanding of all four subconcepts at the same rate or at the same age. Increased comprehension of the meaning of death is more dependent on the child's cognitive functioning than chronologic age (Mahon, 1993). In all cases, the child can explain death only within his or her understanding, based on personal experience.

Universality, or inevitability, another subconcept of death, develops as children realize that everyone will die. An understanding of the *irreversibility*, or irrevocability, of death is developed as the child comprehends that life will not return to the body. Full comprehension of *finality* comes with the realization that there is complete cessation of biological functions after death. Understanding of multiple *causality*, the true causes of death, incorporates the concepts of death by internal forces (old age, illness), external forces (trauma, accident, intentional harm), or suicide. Children who have experienced the death of a loved one do not have an accelerated progression in the comprehension of these subconcepts (Mahon, 1993).

Developmental Considerations

Children must be assessed individually to determine their unique understanding of each subconcept to allow the individualization of care. Simple stories about the death of a person or animal can open the door for such an assessment discussion. After the story is read, the child can be asked the following questions: "How did this person die?" "Will this person ever come back to life?" "Will everyone die?" The child should be asked to support his or her answers because the child's reasoning may reveal a lack of understanding of a subconcept. Hypothetical situations can be discussed with adolescents.

Infants and Young Toddlers

Infants and young toddlers (birth to age 2 years) have no comprehension of death and they react to death as abandonment. Infants and young toddlers are aware of changes in their patterns of care although they cannot directly express this awareness. They react when they sense that their needs are not met.

When a sibling or other non-parental family member dies, the reaction of the infant or young toddler depends on the reactions of the adult caretakers, primarily the mother. If she is upset or distracted and not as responsive to the child's cues, then the child reacts.

Older Toddlers and Preschoolers

Older toddlers and preschoolers (age 2 to 6 years) still have little understanding of death (see Chart 12–5). Most see death as reversible. They may compare it to sleep. This undeveloped conceptualization of death is reinforced by popular media in which cartoon figures and real characters die freely, then reappear later, often with no evidence of wounds or injuries. Older toddlers and preschool children do not understand that all people die. They believe biological processes continue after death. Because their cognitive development is preoperational, their thinking is also characterized by egocentricity and the belief that what they wish for can happen. This includes a belief that they can wish for the disappearance or death of another person (Gibbons, 1992, 1993).

Older toddlers and preschoolers can benefit from hearing stories with themes that relate to death. This allows the permanency of death to be presented gently and opens the door to questions. Stories give the child a chance to talk about what they are feeling and learn the normalcy of the feelings of sadness, anger, and abandonment that accompany the death of a person they love.

Older toddlers and preschoolers often have limited experience with death and they often draw incorrect conclusions from what they do see. This makes it especially important to answer their questions simply but honestly. Nurses should be alert for any behavior, question, or comment that indicates the child has misunderstood some aspect of the death process. Natural opportunities to talk about death, for example, when a pet dies or a dead animal is seen on the roadside, should be taken. In talking about death, explanations should be kept accurate and simple. Children's comments should be listened to carefully to be sure their concerns and questions are really being addressed (Gibbons, 1992, 1993).

The absence of full comprehension of death subconcepts in the preschooler helps explain their many misconceptions. For example, 4-year-old Mary is very concerned that her grandpa will be hungry if he cannot get food after he is buried. Three-year-old Jose is sure that his pet dog Ruff will come back to life, and he wants to keep Ruff's toys and bed. Five-year-old Manuel has become withdrawn and fearful after his infant brother, whom he had wished would just go away, dies of sudden infant death syndrome.

School-Age Children

School-age children (ages 6 to 11 years) are often fascinated with the details of death and commonly ask about what happens to the body in the coffin or about the spiritual aspects of death. There can still be major areas of misunderstanding, depending on the child's exposure to death and on how the information was presented (or not presented) in the past. It is during the school-age period that most children develop their understanding of the four death subconcepts.

School-age children still have concerns about isolation and abandonment. Their need to be with both family and friends can be strong. They need to be treated with respect. School-age children can use written and verbal communication to express their feelings and concerns. They also enjoy drawing and expressing themselves creatively. These activities provide a window into the child's understanding of death, feelings about their own death, and their reaction to the death of a loved one (Faulkner, 1993; Gibbons, 1992, 1993).

Preadolescents and Adolescents

Preadolescents and adolescents (ages 11 to 18 years) have a full cognitive understanding of death, although they still may have some misconceptions based on either inaccurate information or lack of personal experience with death. They are not only able to comprehend all the subconcepts of death but they are also able to understand the effect that death has on other people and on society. Despite this cognitive maturity, few adolescents see themselves as vulnerable or likely to die and a sense of omnipotence is common.

When adolescents must acknowledge their own vulnerability and face their own death, their feelings can be displayed indirectly through their behavior. Some adolescents express anger by being non-compliant; others express their feelings by isolating themselves. Sorrow about the loss of a future can be shown by wanting to marry in order to make the potential future a reality in the present. To deal with these powerful feelings, adolescents need privacy without abandonment. They also need continued opportunities to interact with peers and to make a contribution to the world around them (Faulkner, 1993).

Helping the Child Learn to Cope with Grief or Loss

The more children know, the more knowledge and coping strategies they have to draw on when they need to cope with personal grief or the death of a loved one. Development of a realistic concept of grief and death, of their causes and consequences, and of what happens to the body when death occurs is important. Children also need to learn how to cope with the strong negative emotions that they experience.

Learning About Grief and Loss

Children do not need to have a loved one die or to experience a great loss themselves to learn to cope with grief. As children see grief and loss around them, it should be discussed. This prevents development of the belief that discussion of grief and death is taboo. The loss of a pet can be a powerful learning experience. If a pet runs away, the child can be encouraged to discuss feelings about the missing animal. If the pet dies, this is a chance for the child to talk about how the pet died, why it died, and how that death makes both the adult and child feel. The child can also be introduced to the rituals that the family's culture uses to say good-bye to a dead loved one and to express grief and sadness.

Causes of loss should be discussed honestly with both internal and external causes acknowledged. When the cause of a death is unknown, this uncertainty can be stated. Flowery analogies or stories may only confuse the child.

Tip: *When a child has lost a sibling, it is better to say "Your brother has died and he is not going to be with us any more" rather than "The angels came and took your brother to heaven." Children may interpret such statements literally and become fearful that angels will come for them, too.*

In the case of suicide, saying that the person was sick in the mind, causing the person to take his or her life, is a better explanation than saying that the person was unhappy or disappointed with life. For the child who was a significant part of the suicide victim's life, this explanation helps alleviate misconceptions if the child thinks he or she was a cause of the person's unhappiness.

Even young children benefit from discussions of what happens to the body after death. If the child asks or indicates a desire to go to the funeral, this request should be granted. The child should be prepared before attending the funeral. Explanations can be given regarding the events that will occur during the funeral service, how people may respond during the service, and how witnessing these events may make the child feel.

Tip: *The child should be told specifics about what will happen and what will be seen. The child should be prepared for how the coffin looks and that the dead person will look asleep. The child should be told that people may cry and be upset because they are sad that the person has died. If the child goes to the cemetery, the child should be told that the coffin will be placed in the ground. The child should be told that it is all right if he or she wants to leave at any time during the ceremony.*

Throughout the service, the child should be accompanied by a trusted adult who can maintain enough control to serve as a resource and support for the child (Schonfeld, 1993).

Learning to Cope with Strong Negative Feelings

To be able to deal with the powerful reactions experienced after the death of a loved one or the grief associated with an unexpected personal loss, children must learn to deal with strong feelings such as longing, anger, sadness, and confusion. When children display behaviors that indicate they are having these feelings, regardless of the reason, the feelings should be addressed and the names of the feelings used. Parents should be taught to not ignore strong or negative feelings or to do things to take the child's mind off the feelings. This approach does not make the feelings, or the events that caused them, go away. When well-meaning adults seek to protect the child in this way, they deny the child the opportunity to acknowledge and then learn to cope with feelings and fears. Acknowledging strong and unpleasant feelings and helping the child work through those feelings lets the child know, via both verbal and non-verbal messages, that the feelings are normal. The child will also develop the cadre of skills needed to deal with such emotions throughout life.

Even very young children are aware when someone around them has died. The child senses and observes the changes, without being told. All children need an opportunity to discuss the emotions that accompany their grief and to learn about the ramifications of a particular death on themselves and their family.

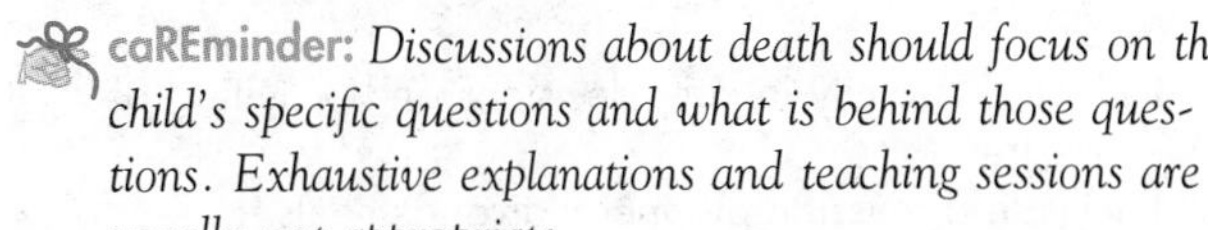

caREminder: *Discussions about death should focus on the child's specific questions and what is behind those questions. Exhaustive explanations and teaching sessions are usually not appropriate.*

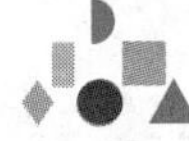

Interdisciplinary Care of the Dying Child

A team of professionals, lay persons, family members, and friends provide care for the dying child. The role of each member of this team changes over time, especially as the focus of the care becomes the support of a peaceful death rather than the promotion of continued life. For the

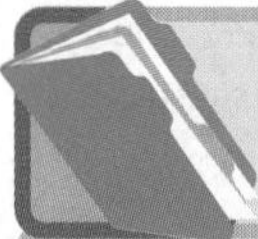

Chart 12–7
Nursing Interventions Classification (NIC)

Dying Care

Definition

Promotion of physical comfort and psychological peace in the final phase of life

Activities

Reduce demand for cognitive functioning when patient is ill or fatigued.
Monitor patient for anxiety.
Monitor mood changes.
Communicate willingness to discuss death.
Encourage patient and family to share feelings about death.
Support patient and family through stages of grief.
Monitor pain.
Minimize discomfort, when possible.
Medicate by alternate route when swallowing problems develop.
Postpone feeding when patient is fatigued.
Offer fluids and soft foods frequently.
Offer culturally appropriate foods.
Monitor deterioration of physical and/or mental capabilities.
Provide frequent rest periods.
Assist with basic care, as needed.
Stay physically close to frightened patient.
Respect the need for privacy.
Modify the environment, based on patient's needs and desires.
Identify the patient's care priorities.
Facilitate obtaining spiritual support for patient and family.
Respect the patient's and family's specific care requests.
Support the family's efforts to remain at the bedside.
Include the family in care decisions and activities, as desired.
Facilitate discussion of funeral arrangements.

From McCloskey, J., & Bulechek, G. (1996). *Nursing interventions classification (NIC)* (2nd ed.). St. Louis: Mosby–Year Book. Reprinted with permission.

dying child, the maintenance of relationships with family members, friends, and trusted health care providers and the maintenance of personal dignity can be of utmost importance. The care of the dying child should focus on emotional and physical needs. Care for only one of these two major areas is never adequate (Chart 12–7).

Assessment

To plan interventions appropriate for the child and family, a baseline assessment should be completed (Chart 12–8). The health care provider's attitudes, strengths, and limitations in working with children and families who have experienced loss influence the relationship with the grieving family. A structured assessment should be completed in a private area, conveying an unhurried, non-judgmental attitude. All interaction with the child and family provide opportunity for informal data collection regarding the family's grief and loss. The nurse

Chart 12–8

Factors to Evaluate During Grief Assessment

- Type of loss (death—relationship to deceased; chronic or terminal illness; disfigurement; material possession)
- Circumstances surrounding the loss
- Stage of acute grief or bereavement; period of time since loss
- History of other significant losses (persons, pets, objects) and response to them
- Understanding of the grieving process
- Child's cognitive level and accuracy of understanding of the four subconcepts of death. The following are suggested questions to use in this evaluation:
  - *Universality*—Does everyone die eventually?
  - *Irreversibility*—Can someone come back to life again after he dies?
  - *Cessation of bodily function*—What happens after a living thing dies? Can it hear or feel? Does it still need to eat?
  - *Causality*—What causes someone to die?
- Perceived value of what may be, or was, lost
- Usual patterns of coping—what comforts the child?
- Sense of control in the present situation and how this impacts the ability to deal with the loss
- How the child or family is responding to this loss:
  - *Behavioral manifestations of grieving* (aggressiveness, anger, anxiety, sadness, depression, withdrawal, attention-seeking behavior)
  - *Somatic problems associated with grieving* (change in eating patterns, sleep pattern disturbance, change in activity level)
- Usual support systems (family, spiritual, community) and the availability of these support systems in the present situation

should *listen astutely to the family and answer their questions honestly*.

Emotional Care

Assessment focuses care so that it meets the needs of the individual child and family (Chart 12–9). Dying children are usually aware of their illness and the fact that they are dying (Walker, 1993). The nurse should remain alert to the child's desire to talk about death and the child's condition. This may be expressed by behavioral changes or questions about other topics because it is rarely expressed directly.

If their impending death is not discussed, children do not always initiate the discussion because they sense that such discussions make their parents sad. Children can feel guilty that they caused their parents' sadness and then they may try to protect their parents by not talking about the things that concern them most. Parents and other family members must be helped to understand that the child knows that he or she is very sick and dying. Not talking about these issues actually adds to

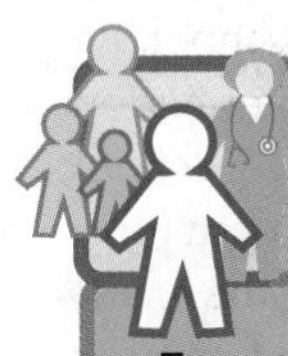

Chart 12–9
Nursing Diagnoses and Outcomes

Emotional Care of the Dying Child and the Family

Anticipatory grieving related to loss of function resulting from terminal illness; recognition of own terminal illness

Outcome: The child verbalizes feelings and positively progresses through the stages of grief.

Altered growth and development related to inability to engage in usual age-appropriate activities

Outcome: Alternative activities appropriate to age, energy level, and functional ability are made available to the child.

Anxiety related to concerns about own death or death of child; changes in family

Outcome: The child or family verbalize feelings and practice techniques to reduce anxiety (e.g., deep breathing); identify how to cope with family changes.

Caregiver role strain related to demands of care of dying child; changed needs of family members; insufficient support

Outcome: Family caregivers have respite from providing care (alternate care among family members or health team); identify ways to meet family needs; identify sources of support.

Body image disturbance related to physical effects of terminal illness or treatment of the illness

Outcome: The child verbalizes feelings regarding change in appearance; identify methods to offset these changes.

Powerlessness related to loss of control, inability to perform roles and responsibilities secondary to terminal illness, and lifestyle restriction

Outcome: The child is offered as many choices as possible; identify methods to overcome restrictions.

Situational low self-esteem related to inability to engage in usual activities or activities at same level of involvement or performance

Outcome: The child verbalizes feelings and engages in or masters other activities.

Sleep pattern disturbance related to fear, anxiety, need to be with dying child

Outcome: The child or family obtain adequate amounts of sleep, in blocks of time.

Spiritual distress related to crisis of the illness, suffering, death of self or child

Outcome: The child or family verbalize feelings and identify and use spiritual or religious supports.

the child's burdens because he or she must then expend energy to leave this very important topic out of conversations.

caREminder: *Parents know their child best and, if they feel strongly that their child should not be told of his or her impending death, the nurse should elicit their reasons. Parents' wishes should be respected, but it is not appropriate to lie to or deceive the child.*

Even if the facts of the illness are discussed openly, the child may need help expressing feelings such as fear of the unknown about dying or sadness about not being able to play with friends. Art, play therapy, music, books, and writing can all help the child express and explore those feelings. By examining these creative efforts and discussing them with the child, the parent and nurse can help the child understand what is happening and develop needed and effective coping techniques. As children deal with their impending death, they may designate who they want their treasured belongings to be given to after they die. This is a method of coping and should not be discouraged.

School-age children and adolescents need to be involved in purposeful activity and spend time with peers. Adolescents, with their more comprehensive understanding of death and dying, often express concerns about their individuality and body image as well as concerns about the future. They expect and need honesty from adults.

Care of the siblings and parents is also a part of the psychosocial care of the dying child. Family members must be encouraged to assist the child, but they must also be given support to care for themselves and each other, so that they may eventually move on to life without the dying child.

Continuing in School

As the illness of the terminally ill child progresses, a frequent question is whether the child should continue to go to school. The answer is usually yes. School plays a very important part in a child's life. In addition to helping the child acquire knowledge, school activities promote self-esteem and allow the child to be identified as an important member of society. At school, the child can continue to gain independence and maintain some degree of control over the environment.

School provides opportunities for socialization. The child should be encouraged to maintain contact with peers, and peers should be helped to maintain contact with the child. Attendance at school also minimizes exclusion from school activities that are important to the child.

Whether or not the child goes to classes regularly, the school-age child needs to maintain academic success. Both the child and teacher must set attainable goals without the child being relieved of responsibility for learning and completing assignments. Making no academic demands can lead the child to believe that he or she has no value in life or is close to death.

Some parents may be concerned about the child attending school because they see it as a potential site of physical and emotional danger. Other parents want to spend more time with their child and see school attendance as an impediment. These issues should be identified and discussed so that the child may still attend school.

Teachers and school staff members need information and support for themselves (Chart 12–10). The school nurse should work with the child and parents to establish the nature of the material to be discussed and the manner of its presentation. Accurate information and answers help prevent incorrect conclusions. Some children want to present this information to their peers themselves. Others want the teacher or school nurse to tell their fellow students about their loss of hair or need for a wheelchair or other assistive device.

Regardless of what the classmates and the school staff are told, the child should be prepared for the questions and changes in relationships that arise after returning to school. By practicing responses and role playing possible situations, the child learns how to answer questions and to understand peer reactions.

When working with students, faculty, and staff, the nurse should stress the need for openness and free communication. Fears should be acknowledged and addressed. Few adults and older children are comfortable discussing or facing death, which can make them avoid the affected child. They need to learn that the child knows that he or she is sick and that avoiding opportunities to discuss the illness robs the terminally ill child of needed opportunities to share the experience (Kalb, 1993). The child also wants to participate in life. Full and open discussion of day to day events should be continued.

Physical Care

The dying child often has many physical needs that must be addressed (Chart 12–11). The goal is to optimize quality of life and promote comfort.

Environment

The physical environment of the dying child includes the actual bed or chair where the child spends time. Both should be comfortable and able to support the child physically. The child's environment should be amenable to the child's activities, such as sleeping, reading,

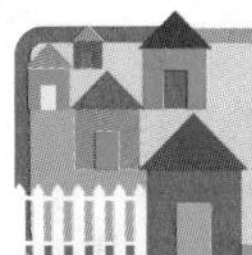

Chart 12–10
Community Care

Focus on Terminally Ill Children in the School

Address the staff's personal concerns and attitudes toward terminal illness, death, and dying:
- Evaluate prior personal experiences with death.
- Discuss fears of working with a child who is dying.
- Discuss concerns about other students and how they are coping with having a terminally ill peer.
- Evaluate uneasiness about teacher–pupil ratio.

Educate the staff about the needs of the terminally ill student:
- Encourage meaningful communication.
- Respect the need to live with dignity.
- Listen without anger and with acceptance.
- Encourage hope.
- Tell the student that he or she is a valuable person and will not be forgotten.
- Promote self-esteem.

Discuss ways to individualize instruction:
- Work with the child and family to modify the child's instructional program in light of fatigue, absences, and effects of medications.
- Allow rest periods while at school.
- Send work home on the weekend before it is assigned so work can be done at the student's own pace.
- Hold the student to whatever academic and behavioral standards he or she is able to meet.
- Do not isolate the student from activities or peers.

Teach ways to protect the child from injury or illness:
- Have the student sit in the front row.
- Teach the child not to share utensils.
- Wash hands after blowing nose, toileting.
- Ask parents to keep children who are sick at home.

Address fears that a medical emergency will occur in the classroom:
- Teach about disease.
- Contact health personnel, parents, and the child to determine the best ways to meet the child's needs.
- Develop written instructions for emergency care of the specific child.

Develop a plan for after the death of a child:*
- Share reactions within the class through discussions and writing.
- Listen to what students have to say.
- Correct misunderstandings about the illness and death or the student's responsibility for it.
- Encourage creative expressions of grief such as letters and memorials.
- Present information about death rituals and funerals.
- Listen to and empathize with the children, hear what they say.
- Respond with real feelings, express own grief.
- Allow crying and other expressions of grief.
- Expect unusual behavior, inability to concentrate, increased daydreaming, withdrawal, physiologic reactions such as insomnia, headaches, increased appetite.
- Refer students for additional help when needed.
- Recognize that grief may last 6 months or more.

* This section can be modified to meet the needs of children who have had any significant loss (parent, sibling, public figure).
Adapted from Davis, K. (1989). Educational needs of the terminally ill student. *Issues in Comprehensive Pediatric Nursing, 12,* 235–245. Taylor & Francis. Used with permission.

playing games, or visiting with friends (Miser & Miser, 1993).

The child needs to be able to move within the environment—to spend time with people, to spend time alone, to spend time sleeping. This may require placing a commode in a private place near the family room or a cot in the corner of the dining room. The environment should be repeatedly evaluated to ensure that it remains

Chart 12–11
Nursing Interventions

Physical Problems of the Dying Child

Diagnoses and Assessment Findings	Possible Causes	Nursing and Collaborative Care
Pain **Chronic pain** Restlessness Expressions of discomfort Refusal to participate in activities	Tissue damage Pressure Ischemia	Use nonpharmacologic pain relief (guided imagery, music, distractions, TENS, heat/cold application). Administer pharmacologic intervention (NSAID, narcotics, adjuctive drugs). Position for comfort.
Sleep pattern disturbance Daytime sleeping Intermittent dozing Inability to sleep at night	Lack of consistent daily routine	Establish pattern of activities during day and sleep at night with consistent bedtime routine. Use sleeping area only for sleep or change area between use for sleep and wake activities (e.g., open curtains, have child lie on quilt during day, dim lights, sleep under quilt and sheets at night).
	Frequent procedures that interrupt sleep	Eliminate all unnecessary procedures during sleep time (e.g., vital signs, administration of non-essential medications). Explore ways to do essential activities without waking child.
	Anxiety or other emotional problems disturbing sleep	Assess child for emotional issues that may be increasing anxiety and disturbing sleep.
	Drowsiness from drugs given for pain, inability to sleep at night	Adjust narcotic dose or timing of analgesics if possible. Administer sedatives or sleeping medications cautiously (may interact with narcotics).
Impaired gas exchange Deleterious changes in pulse, blood pressure, respiratory rate, respiratory effort Hypoxia	Anemia Progressive cardiac failure Upper airway obstruction Pneumonia Prolonged immobility	Administer oxygen to correct hypoxia. Treat pneumonia if appropriate. Administer diuretics, sedatives. Position for optimal ventilation.
Risk for infection Fever Increased fatigue or lassitude (expected inflammatory reaction may be absent if neutrophil count is low)	Immunocompromised state	Assess continuously for sign of infection. Avoid contact with individuals with active infections, flu, chickenpox. Avoid contamination of intravenous lines. Do not administer live virus vaccines.
Signs of urinary tract infection Fever Lower abdominal pain Back pain Dysuria Frequency Foul-smelling urine	Poor fluid intake Intermittent or continuous bladder catheterization	Increase fluid intake orally or parenterally. Assess daily for signs of infection. Use clean/sterile technique for all catheterizations. Prevent urine reflux from indwelling catheter, hold below level of bladder. Treat active urinary tract infection with antibiotics.

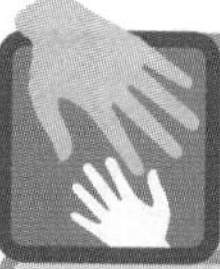

Chart 12–11
Nursing Interventions *Continued*

Physical Problems of the Dying Child

Diagnoses and Assessment Findings	Possible Causes	Nursing and Collaborative Care
Signs of respiratory system infection Fever Tachypnea Shortness of breath Abnormal breath sounds	Immobility Aspiration	Position to prevent aspiration. Administer supportive treatments (oxygen and sedation). Suction if needed for comfort.
Signs of fungal infection White patches on tongue Perineal itching	Prolonged antibiotic or steroid therapy Immunocompromised state Neutropenia	Assess comfort level and whether oral lesions interfere with intake. Administer clotrimazole troches or mycostatin (after feeding if oral infection is present).
Impaired tissue integrity Skin breakdown Erythema Pain Blisters Decubitus	Prolonged bed rest	Assist child out of bed several times per day. Turn every 2 to 3 hours if not asleep. Active or passive range of motion four times a day. Gently massage areas at risk for pressure. Use air mattress, elbow pads, other protective devices to relieve pressure. Avoid pressure on areas at risk for breakdown, such as ankles, heels, elbows, ears, back of head, lower back.
	Urinary or bowel incontinence	Promote urinary and bowel continence, and respect child's privacy during toileting. Remind child to use bathroom or bedpan at regular intervals. Keep child clean and dry at all times. Use barrier ointments to protect skin.
	Poor nutrition Denervation of skin resulting from tumor	Increase hydration and improve nutrition. Assess potential problem areas for breakdowns not felt by child.
Risk for disuse syndrome Contractures Muscle weakness	Inappropriate alignment of extremities and joints	Use pillows and other positioning aids to align extremities and joints.
Constipation Change in frequency, consistency of bowel movement	Inactivity	Help child to get out of bed several times per day.
	Embarrassment about bowel function	Provide privacy for bowel movement.
	Changes in diet Decreased oral intake Narcotic analgesics	Offer favorite foods that promote bowel function. Encourage at least small amounts of fluids and foods. Adjust narcotic dosages, use NSAIDs to lower narcotic requirements, if possible.
	Neurologic impairment resulting from tumor	Administer stool softeners/other drugs; may require combination of interventions such as Colace, mineral oil, Senokot, Dulcolax, enemas given multiple times per day. Assist with treatment to reduce tumor size if appropriate (irradiation, steroids).

Chart continued on following page

Chart 12–11
Nursing Interventions *Continued*

Physical Problems of the Dying Child

Diagnoses and Assessment Findings	Possible Causes	Nursing and Collaborative Care
Fluid volume deficit Signs of dehydration	Bowel dysfunction (diarrhea)	Prevent/treat diarrhea.
	Poor intake	Increase intake orally or via central line.
	Poor oral hygiene	Provide oral care two to three times per day with non-irritating/non-drying fluids (no alcohol or glycerin).
	Oral pain/mucositis	Apply topical analgesics (lidocaine, dyclonine) or administer systemic narcotics for pain.
	Fungal infection causing oral discomfort	Treat fungal infection with mycostatin.
	Fatigue	Organize care. Ensure adequate rest.
	No fluids available	Offer fluids frequently.
Altered nutrition: less than body requirements Weight loss Does not maintain growth curve Vomiting with and without nausea	Catabolism Anorexia Malaise Fever	Offer small, frequent feedings of favorite foods. Increase caloric load of foods. Administer hyperalimentation as appropriate.
	Narcotic analgesics	Administer antiemetics: phenothiazines (Thorazine), lorazepam (Ativan). Change to narcotic with a decreased emetic effect.
	Chemotherapy	Administer drugs to prevent chemotherapy-induced vomiting: sondansetron.
	Increased intracranial pressure	Reduce intracranial pressure: assist with administration of steroids, cranial radiation.
	Gastritis	Reduce gastric secretions: avoid offending foods; administer H_2 antagonist.
	Bowel obstruction	Assist with treatment of bowel obstruction: gastric decompression, reduction of tumor, surgical resection, increased activity.

TENS, transcutaneous electrical nerve stimulation; NSAID, non-steroidal anti-inflammatory drug.
Data from Miser J., & Miser, A. (1993). Pain and symptom control. In A. Armstrong-Dailey & S. Goltzer (Eds.). *Hospice care for children* (pp. 140–153). New York: Oxford University Press.

appropriate for the child and the family (Fig. 12–2). What works well early in the terminal phase may not work as the disease progresses and the child's physical condition deteriorates.

Pain Control

One of the most important aspects of the physical care of the dying child is pain control (see Chapter 13). Physiologic tolerance to the narcotics, dealing with side effects, and determining the best route of administration must all be considered when the pain control program is developed and continually reevaluated.

caREminder: *Children who require long-term pain control often need to have narcotic dosages increased periodically, possibly by 30% to 50% at a time, to maintain comfort. Meperidine (Demerol) should never be used for such long-term pain control because of the resultant accumulation of a toxic metabolite (normeperidine) after as few as 3 days of treatment.*

Parents are often concerned about narcotic addiction. The difference between physiologic dependence and drug addiction with drug seeking activity should be explained and reinforced (see Chart 13–19). Some parents may fear specific drugs and may prefer alternative narcot-

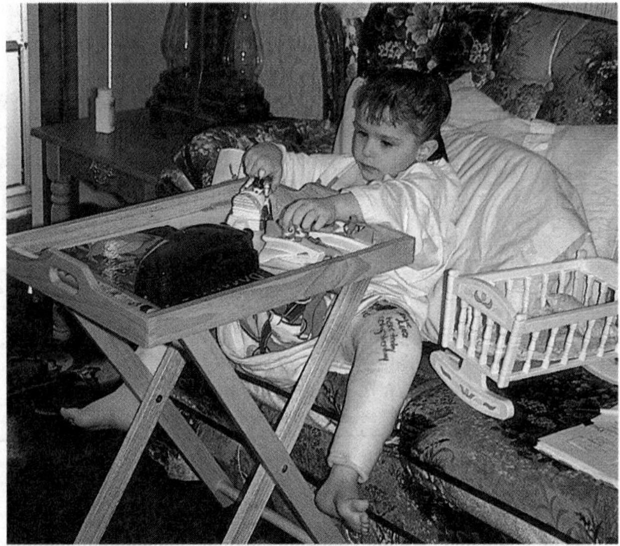

Figure 12–2
To optimize comfort, the environment must be equipped and organized to meet the child's physical needs. (Courtesy of Judy Gross and Children's Hospital, Orthopediatric Unit, Medical University of South Carolina, Charleston, South Carolina.)

ics. In almost all cases, the goal is to maximize the child's comfort and quality of life.

Symptom Management

In addition to pain, other physical problems include nausea and vomiting, sleep disturbances, skin breakdown, contractures, constipation, infections, dehydration, inadequate nutrition, neurologic abnormalities, and cardiovascular dysfunction (Miser & Miser, 1993).

Individual children need help dealing with symptoms of their particular terminal illness. The cause of each symptom must be determined so that correct treatment can be given. Many problems (e.g., the child does not eat) require intervention by members of the health care team.

Treatment of specific physical problems in the dying child should be considered as part of the child's long-term care. For example, constipation, which may be caused by high-dose narcotic administration, continues until the child dies. Thus, laxatives, normally given on an as-needed basis, must be administered daily. The presence of a daily bowel movement is an indication that the medication is working, not that it is time to stop giving the laxative.

The child should be kept clean, dry, well hydrated, and physically comfortable. Excretions and secretions must be removed to prevent skin breakdown. Loss of urinary and bowel control may occur and steps to prevent this or to clean the child immediately should be taken. A child who can drink should be encouraged to drink fluids. If the child is receiving parenteral or enteral fluids, a volume sufficient to maintain full hydration should be given to help make the child comfortable. Oral care is especially important when the child is not drinking or cannot brush his or her teeth.

Tip: *Even if the child does not appear to be conscious, the nurse should talk to the child during care and explain what is happening and why. The nurse can talk about the weather, television programs, and other interests of the child. Pictures from home or school should be posted if the family desires.*

Discontinuing Treatment

A difficult aspect of the care of the terminally ill child is deciding what care to carry out and what to omit.

caREminder: *When making choices about care, the context of the decision must be carefully examined. The choice that initially seems to be right is not always in the best interest of the child.*

New treatments are usually not initiated if there is no chance of cure. This is often a requirement for participation in hospice programs. However, some treatments are given for palliative as well as curative reasons.

Radiation therapy, usually given to "cure" the tumor, can also reduce its size and reduce pain. Giving antibiotics to cure the constant colonization of an indwelling urinary catheter is probably a futile effort. But, treatment of a urinary tract infection that is causing dysuria, frequency, and pain can improve the child's quality of life. A child may receive oxygen or be suctioned to promote comfort. Increased parenteral fluids can be appropriate to maintain hydration when the child ceases to drink.

A decision about continuing treatment for the dying child may be necessary when the care being given is causing discomfort with no benefit to the child. Hemodynamic monitoring, insertion of central lines to administer total parenteral nutrition to meet *long-term* nutrition needs, even doing daily weights or laboratory studies are examples. The parents and health care team must work together to determine when these interventions should be stopped (Miser & Miser, 1993).

Another important decision is determining what, if any, resuscitation measures will be implemented. When it is apparent that the child is close to death, no interventions are usually appropriate. The resuscitation status of the child should be communicated to all those involved in the child's care, including ancillary staff.

Care at the Time of Death

Each child's death is a special, albeit sad, moment. The fact that the child will die soon is often known when the child is terminally ill. Parents, siblings, and other support persons who the child or parents wish to have present should be allowed to be with the child if possible.

caREminder: *As death nears for the child, direct care activities, except for comfort measures, should be omitted to allow the environment to be peaceful.*

Emotional Support

Direct, clear communication is essential. Religious rituals are often important to families at the time of death. Families should be encouraged to invite their clergy member, priest, or rabbi to join them. The child's ability to hear and communicate is not always clear to caregivers, but this should not stop efforts to talk to and communicate with the child.

Many parents wish to hold their child, and every effort should be made to accommodate this desire. The presence of multiple intravenous lines, tubes, and even ventilatory support, are not reasons to deny this request (Fig. 12–3).

caREminder: *The parents should be offered the opportunity to be with their child after the death and before the child receives postmortem care. Parents should be asked if they want someone to be with them or if they want to be alone with their child. Some parents welcome the option of giving care such as the final bath. The nurse should stay with the parents if they request.*

Figure 12–3
Parents' wishes to hold their dying child should be respected and facilitated.

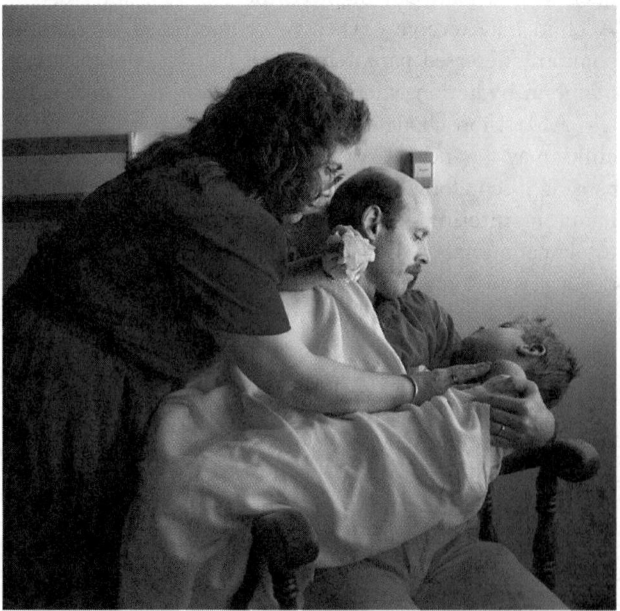

Personal items of the child should be returned to the parents. If a parent does not want these items, they should be carefully stored and the parents should be told they can return for them whenever they wish. This may be many years after the child's death.

Parents are often in a state of shock. Their decision-making ability should be assessed carefully. Assistance with driving home or caring for other children may be needed.

Time of Death Decisions

In approaching parents about decisions that must be made at the time of death, the nurse must be sensitive to the family's cultural and ethnic background (see Chart 12–3). Some interventions, such as organ donation, are not permitted in certain cultures. The subject of **organ donation** should be discussed only after the parents have been told that their child is dying and the feasibility of organ donation is confirmed. It is important for the nurse to be familiar with the state and agency's protocol for identification of potential organ donors (Chart 12–12).

When discussing organ donation with the parents, the nurse should be alert for comments that indicate that the parents do not understand the process. The concept of brain death is often poorly understood by the general public. Parents may not comprehend that the child has been pronounced dead and that equipment, such as a ventilator, is being used to maintain circulation to organs that will be donated, not to preserve the child's life (Miles & Warner, 1992).

caREminder: *Do not let preparation for the donor process interfere with the parents' wishes to be with their child before ventilatory support is removed (Miles & Warner, 1992). Throughout the process, the child's body should be treated with respect.*

The decision about an **autopsy** is often made by the medical examiner's office but may be left up to the parents. Facts about the autopsy (TIP 12–1) should be sensitively presented and the parents given enough time to make the decision.

Funeral arrangements need to be made by the parents. This is something few parents are prepared to do. If local mortuaries offer free or low-cost funerals for infants and children, such information should be made available to the parents. For the parent whose child has just died, talk about a funeral may be very disturbing.

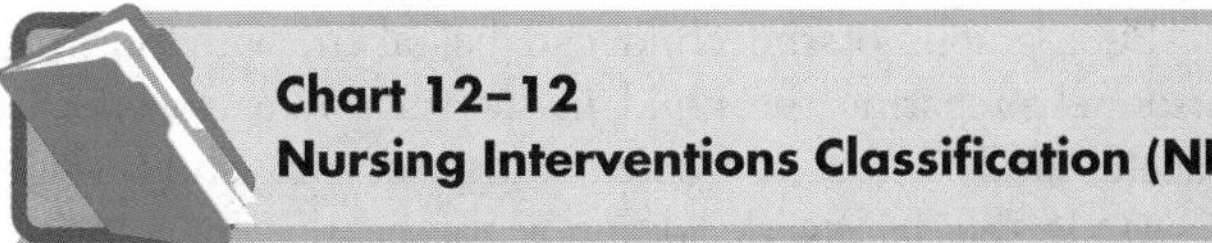

Chart 12–12
Nursing Interventions Classification (NIC)

Organ Procurement

Definition

Guiding families through the donation process to ensure timely retrieval of vital organs and tissue for transplant

Activities

Review institutional policy and procedures for organ donation.
Review potential donor medical history for contraindications to donation.
Anticipate organ suitability for donation, depending on criteria of death.
Determine whether patient has an organ donation card.
Provide emotional support for families when donation is desired but contraindicated.
Alert organ procurement team of potential donor.
Participate in obtaining specimens to verify donor suitability.
Prepare to articulate current criteria for brain death in terms that family members can understand.
Obtain consent for organ donation from family, as appropriate.
Collaborate with the family to complete separate consent forms that specifically name the organs and tissues authorized for removal.
Allow family time for grieving.
Provide emotional support for family.
Answer commonly asked questions about financial responsibility for procurement, criteria for transplant, and length of procedure.
Take actions to preserve viability of organ (e.g., supplying intravenous fluids and ventilation).
Participate in organ procurement procedures, as appropriate.
Provide postmortem care.
Offer the family postmortem viewing of the body, when possible.
Participate in postprocedure conference.

From McCloskey, J., & Bulechek, G. (1996). *Nursing interventions classification (NIC)* (2nd ed.). St. Louis: Mosby–Year Book. Reprinted with permission.

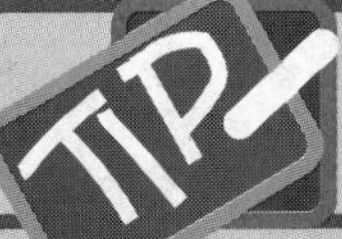

TIP 12–1 A Teaching Intervention Plan for the Family Considering an Autopsy

Nursing Diagnosis and Outcome

- Knowledge deficit: autopsy
  Outcome: The family makes an informed decision regarding performance of an autopsy.

Interventions

- If the autopsy is not mandated, advise the parents that they have a choice as to whether or not it is done.
- Advise that health insurance companies may not cover the cost of an autopsy.
- Instruct that the autopsy may help to clarify the cause of death.
- Educate that the autopsy can help the medical team to understand the disease or the impact of the injury and thus help other children.
- Clarify that the child will feel no pain.
- Advise that the child's body will be respected and there will be no obvious indication of an autopsy.
- Indicate that the family will get feedback about the autopsy from their family doctor.

The Type and Place of Death: Special Considerations

The type of death (expected, unexpected, or traumatic) and place where the death occurs impact the choice of health care provider interventions and the family's response to the loss. The type and place of death must be considered to meet the needs of the family when delivering care.

Perinatal Loss

In perinatal loss, a parent can experience a significant grief reaction, even when a pregnancy has been brief. As the pregnancy becomes real to the parents, particularly to the mother, there can be significant investment and bonding, even before the signs of pregnancy are clear to others.

Nurses in many settings care for families experiencing perinatal loss—miscarriage, stillbirth, and neonatal death. This could be in the emergency department (ED), labor and delivery unit, neonatal care unit, mother–baby and women's units, or primary care settings in the community. The goals of care are to meet the family's medical needs, validate the loss, and teach about usual responses to the loss. It is thought that, to facilitate grief resolution, parents must first attach to, then detach from, their deceased infant (Schlomann & Fister, 1995).

Regardless of the setting of a perinatal death, the parents should be offered the option of touching, fondling, or holding the deceased fetus or infant, even if it is grossly malformed. This gives parents a chance to attach to their infant.

Parental fantasies about the infant's appearance are often worse than the reality of the anomalies or condition of the deceased infant. Seeing and holding the infant validates the existence of the infant and makes the reality of the death more clear. The infant should be cleaned and wrapped as appropriate for the gestational age in preparation for this visit, and the appearance of the baby should be described to the family before the visit. The nurse should stay with the family at the beginning of the visit and then offer them time alone with the infant. Decisions about the length of this visit and the individuals who will be present should be left up to the family.

caREminder: *Fathers or other family members should not be permitted to decide whether the mother is to see her deceased child. This opportunity should always be offered to the infant's mother independently of family input. If the woman is incapable of seeing the child or making the decision at the time of the infant's death, an option to visit at the morgue should be provided if the baby cannot be taken from the morgue.*

Photographs of the child can be taken, with nursing personnel preparing the child in such a way as to offer a peaceful and attractive remembrance of the child (Fig. 12–4). If the family decides not to see the infant, the body should be kept on the unit as long as possible, for at least 2 hours, to allow them time to change their minds.

Immediately after the death, activate the perinatal bereavement protocol. Bereavement team support persons, who may be nurses, social workers, physicians, or other parents who have experienced perinatal losses, should be notified immediately so they can visit as soon as possible after the death. *Resolve Through Sharing* is an example of a program that is used internationally to support families experiencing a perinatal loss. This program trains health care providers to serve as counselors who can intervene with families to facilitate coping with their loss.

Figure 12–4
Identical twins Kyle Allen (*A*) and Brian James (*B*) Messner were born on March 14, 1995. Kyle was stillborn; Brian lived for 9 days. The twins died as a result of twin-to-twin transfusion syndrome. Presenting the deceased child to the family in an esthetically pleasing manner and taking keepsake photographs of the child are two interventions to support the family in the grieving process.

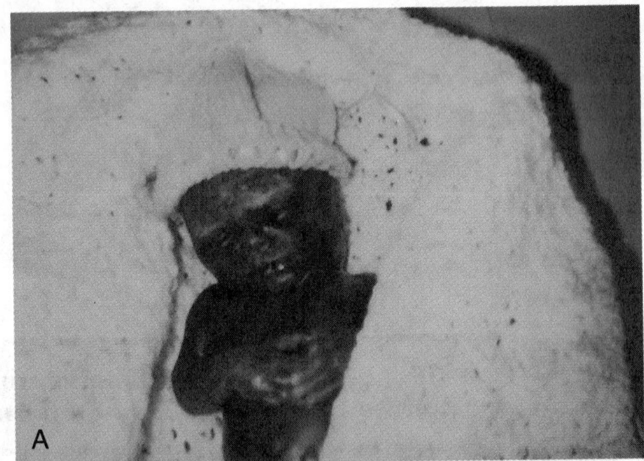

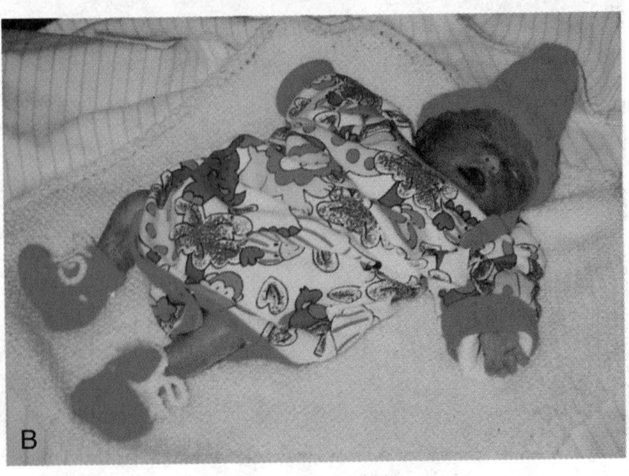

A strong sense of grief is a normal aspect of the bereavement process and one that the parents may have great difficulty with, especially if the death was unexpected. Nurses should facilitate expression of these emotions according to cultural norms to increase the opportunity for resolution of the grief. The nurse should consult the hospital chaplain, family priest, rabbi, or other family-requested clergy member to support the family's spiritual beliefs, without promoting his or her own personal beliefs.

Nurses should express their sympathy to the family. Families should not be treated with a "conspiracy of silence," as if nothing happened to them. Nurses should encourage and remain open to talking about the family's tragedy. Remarks such as "Please don't feel so bad, you have other children at home" or "You can always have another baby" negate the reality and individuality of the lost infant. Such comments can be especially distressing if a couple has had unsuccessful attempts to conceive or deliver a healthy baby. Furthermore, medical jargon and comments can increase the parents' sense of guilt that they caused the death.

The bereavement team members can help parents make the many decisions needed in the immediate postdelivery period (Chart 12–13). Each time parents make a decision, they are able to take control in a very difficult situation. An autopsy may be desired by the parents or required by law. For some infants, the option to donate organs may be viable.

The parents must determine how and where the infant will be buried. Requirements for burial vary from state to state, but it is usually required for all births after 20 weeks' gestation. Parents may choose to have the institution dispose of the body. If the infant is to be buried, the parents can be asked whether there is a special outfit, blanket, or other object they would like to have buried with the infant. Sufficient time should be provided without pressure so that a family decision may be made.

When an infant's death occurs on the perinatal unit, a decision must be made about where the mother will be placed in the immediate postdelivery period. Parents should be involved in this choice because it is an action that can increase their sense of control. Many agencies attempt to place a woman whose infant has died on a non-obstetric unit. Regardless of the unit where she stays, all staff members should be alerted to her loss. The *Resolve Through Sharing* program recommends placing a simple card with a photo of a flower on the door to the woman's room (Fig. 12–5). The photo is a visual reminder to all personnel that a loss has occurred. This prevents inadvertent comments about the infant who has died and reminds caregivers that this woman and her family need more than the usual postpartum care.

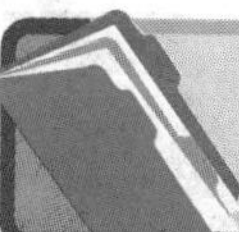

Chart 12–13
Nursing Interventions Classification (NIC)

Grief Work Facilitation: Perinatal Death

Definition

Assistance with the resolution of a perinatal loss

Activities

Encourage participation in decisions about discontinuing life support.
Assist in keeping infant alive until parents arrive.
Baptize the infant, as appropriate.
Encourage parents in holding infant while it dies, as appropriate.
Determine how and when the fetal or infant death was diagnosed.
Discuss plans that have been made (e.g., burial, funeral, and infant name).
Discuss decisions that need to be made about funeral arrangements, autopsy, genetic counseling, and family participation.
Describe mementos that will be obtained, including footprints, handprints, pictures, caps, gowns, blankets, diapers, and blood pressure cuffs, as appropriate.
Discuss available support groups, as appropriate.
Discuss differences between male and female patterns of grieving, as appropriate.
Obtain infant footprints, handprints, length and weight, as needed.
Prepare infant for viewing by bathing and dressing, including parents in activities as appropriate.
Encourage family members to view and hold infant for as long as desired.
Discuss appearance of infant based on gestational age and length of demise.
Focus on the normal features of infant, while sensitively discussing anomalies.
Encourage family time alone with infant, as desired.
Provide referrals to the chaplain, social service, grief counselor, and genetic counselor, as appropriate.
Create keepsakes and present them to the family before discharge, as appropriate.
Discuss characteristics of normal and abnormal grieving, including triggers that precipitate feelings of sadness.
Notify the laboratory or funeral home, as appropriate, for disposition of body.
Transfer infant to the morgue or prepare the body to be transported to a funeral home.

From McCloskey, J., & Bulechek, G. (1996). *Nursing interventions classification (NIC)* (2nd ed.). St. Louis: Mosby–Year Book. Reprinted with permission.

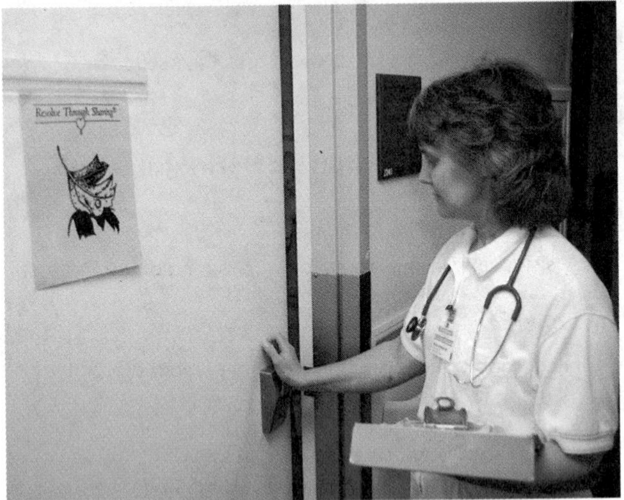

Figure 12–5
The Resolve Through Sharing purple rose on the door alerts all staff to the family's loss.

When the perinatal death occurs in the ED, the nurse should take special care to protect the family and to provide them with an opportunity to see and hold the infant. Terms such as "spontaneous abortion" should be avoided because the term "abortion" is more closely associated with voluntary termination of pregnancy. The nurse should be especially careful of where the fetus is placed. Putting the fetus in a cold metal tray can be very disturbing to the parents. A remembrance packet should be offered to the parents. This packet may include a photograph of the child and a lock of the child's hair.

Referral to a support group and teaching about the normal reactions that follow perinatal death are essential components of the care provided to these families, even if the interactions with the health care system are brief. Parents should be prepared for the intensity of their reactions and for the fact that they will each react differently. If the loss was early in the pregnancy, other family members may act as if they are ignoring the loss because they are afraid to hurt the couple by talking about it. Pamphlets with suggestions for the family and friends should be offered to the parents to share with their support persons (Chart 12–14). If the death is in a later stage of pregnancy when many people know about the expected birth, the parents should be helped to plan how to respond to questions about their new baby. One such response is "Thank you for asking. I am doing well, but, my baby died just after he was born."

Much of the grief work of parents who have experienced a perinatal loss occurs after discharge from the acute care institution. Use of detailed perinatal loss follow-up tools assists primary care providers in community settings to thoroughly address the parents' physical and emotional status, autopsy results, and the parents' support network and ability to communicate with significant others and to give anticipatory guidance regarding grief reactions and future pregnancies (Ewton, 1993). If symptoms of unresolved grief are present 12 to 18 months after the loss, referral for in-depth counseling should be made.

Death in the Hospital

Children who die in the hospital may be in the general pediatric unit, ED, critical care unit, or an operating room (OR). The principles of care are the same in all locations but the site of death and the circumstances that bring the child to the unit can have a significant bearing on the needs of the family.

General Pediatric Unit

When a child dies on a general pediatric unit, the child is often at the terminal stage of long-term disease. Care is similar to that described for the emotional and physical care of the dying child. Open visiting should be encouraged. Families who spend a lot of time at the hospital during the child's illness may need health care provider support and encouragement to leave the room and the unit to meet their own needs and the needs of their other children. After the child's death, the staff working with the child may also need support. Children on the unit who knew the child may also need help to address their grief.

Emergency Department or Critical Care Unit

Children who die in an ED or a critical care unit are often the victims of accidental or intentional trauma. Others die because of sudden illness such as respiratory failure, sudden infant death syndrome (SIDS), or fulminating meningitis. In addition, children who have been in treatment for a chronic condition and who are admitted to an ED or critical care unit may die because of an acute crisis that does not resolve.

When the death is from trauma, other family members or friends may have been injured or killed. The relationship of the victims should be determined and support appropriate to the situation offered. When one or both parents are injured or dead, the emotional support of surviving children is essential. Issues of authority for consent must be clarified. When the affected family members are in different facilities, lines of communication between family members and the health care team must be established.

When the child's death is the result of violence, steps to document the injuries, preserve evidence, and notify law enforcement authorities, if they are not already

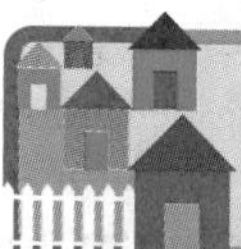

Chart 12–14
Community Care

Suggestions for Family and Friends After the Death of a Child

Be yourself. Show your concern and sorrow in your own way. You will not be effective without natural and total sincerity.

Be there. Brief telephone calls and visits say "I care and I want to help."

Say "I'm sorry." Once you have expressed your sorrow, allow the parents or family to respond. Don't be afraid of silence. Often, your caring presence is enough.

Touch. A hug or a hand to hold can sometimes say more than words.

Find helpful activities. Don't wait to be asked to do something. Look around for what is needed. Provide a meal, do errands, or babysit the other children.

Don't protect. There are many helpful things to do, but shielding the family from the reality of the situation is not one of them. They need to make their own decisions and work through their grief.

Talk about the child. Don't be afraid that mentioning the child will remind them of their grief. They haven't forgotten. They need to talk about their child. When you avoid the subject, it seems that you are saying that the child didn't exist.

Cry with them. Family members and friends often feel that they must "hold up" to be supportive. This is not necessarily true. Your tears show that you care. However, if your own grief is so overwhelming that you cannot function, it is probably best to wait to interact with the parents or family until you can function.

Laugh with them. It is important to recall humorous incidents and endearing qualities about the child. These memories may bring mutual smiles and laughter. Remember, though, that jokes and trivial discussions are not appropriate at this time.

Don't look for something positive. There is nothing positive in the situation, and anything you try to point out as positive may be perceived by the parents or family as a lack of understanding for their pain.

Avoid stock responses. Don't use such cliché phrases as "I know how you feel." "Be thankful that. . . " "Don't cry." "It's better this way." "You have other children." "You can have other children." "It's God's will."

Listen with understanding.

Acknowledge the family's feelings and questions. You cannot answer these questions, so don't try. Just acknowledge their right to be angry.

Reassure. It is common for those who are grieving to feel guilt and to engage in an "if only" type of exercise. Although this is normal, repeated reassurance is necessary.

Be patient. Every person grieves differently and on his or her own timetable. You cannot rush the process.

Modified from the Bereavement Packet from the Arnold Palmer Hospital for Children & Women, Orlando, FL. Used with permission.

involved, are needed. Nurses must also work with social service, pastoral care, and other support personnel to initiate crisis support care for the parents and other children.

When the death is suspected to be the result of family violence, the nurse must report suspected abuse. Social workers and law enforcement authorities then have a major role in initiating child protection activities for other children and initiating action against the perpetrator. The nursing role is one of assessment, documentation, and parent and family support. The facts of the case are rarely clear when the child is first brought to the ED.

caREminder: *A non-judgmental approach to all family members should be taken to avoid the damage that can be caused by the false accusation of an innocent parent.*

In other cases, the child's fatal injury may occur because the parent or another person did not use safety precautions to protect the child. For example, a mother did not clean out the drawers in the bathroom cabinet when she had her first baby. As a result, she did not discard the half-full bottle of antimalarial pills, which poisoned her 2-year-old when she ate them thinking they were candy. Or, an aunt decided to hold her infant nephew in the front seat rather than getting the car seat from her brother's car. They were just going down the block and she never thought they would be hit from behind. The baby died the next day from a ruptured spleen and liver. Such parents and family members need supportive care and may need referral to a mental health professional to resolve their guilt about their accidental role in the child's death.

When the child is admitted to the ED or critical care unit, the family assessment process must be accelerated. The nurse must determine what the family knows and expects, and then reinforce and clarify that information. Comments should be focused on what parents want and need to know. The critically ill or injured child is often fully alert and aware of the surrounding activities despite serious injuries.

caREminder: *The nurse should answer the child's questions. The child should be given opportunities to express concerns and, if age appropriate, participate in care decisions (Miles & Warner, 1992).*

The family must be helped to comprehend a rapidly evolving series of events concerning their child's condition and the multiple decisions they need to make. Parents need rapid preparation for what they will see, feel, and experience. The possibility of the child's death should be discussed as soon as such an outcome seems likely (Miles & Warner, 1992). Questions should be encouraged, even when they are repeated.

caREminder: *Caregivers should use specific language when speaking to parents. Saying "Your child's heart has stopped and we are giving him medicines to try to get it restarted" is better than saying "Your child has arrested and is being resuscitated." Saying "We have tried three treatments to stop the bleeding but they did not work" is better than saying "He was non-responsive to any of the anticoagulants and just bled out."*

Parents should be asked whether a clergy member, either the hospital chaplain or someone from their place of worship, should be called. Their need to carry out specific religious rituals for the time of death should be respected.

Give parents frequent updates on the child's condition. Parents unfamiliar with ED and critical care environments may need permission to approach or touch their child. They may also welcome being asked to help with simple care (Nelson, 1995). This allows them to have a sense that they are caring for and comforting their child even at the time of death. When answering questions, caregivers should be as direct and complete as possible, and they should try to not rush the parents as they work to absorb the reality of the impending or actual death of their child (Miles & Warner, 1992; Nelson, 1995).

Parents should be encouraged to participate in decision-making about subsequent treatment to the extent that they desire to do so. Decisions may include whether to initiate more aggressive treatment when the possibility of a positive outcome still exists or whether to discontinue or not begin treatment when the child's survival is unlikely. Parents may need to decide whether to have the child's organs donated and whether an autopsy will be performed (see Chart 12–12 and TIP 12–1). Some parents feel ill-equipped to make many of these decisions and freely defer to the judgment of the health care professionals (Miles & Warner, 1992). Although contrary to the policies of most hospitals, consideration may be given to allowing the parents to remain in the room during resuscitation efforts. Parents, when given clear instructions, feel more satisfied with the care their child received because they perceive the frenzy of a code situation as meaning that everything possible is being done for their child (Yoder, 1994).

When death is clearly inevitable, the parents should be given the option of being with their child. If possible, the parents should be queried separately because their decisions may otherwise be made simply to meet the perceived needs of the other parent (Miles & Warner, 1992).

Parents should determine who will attend the final visit with the child—family, siblings of the child, clergy, or friends. In cases of severe injuries, the parents should be prepared for how the child looks (Miles & Warner, 1992). The child and room should be prepared for the parents' visit, but it may be beneficial to leave much of the resuscitation equipment in the room to reinforce the fact that efforts were taken to save the child.

Parents who do not want to see their child after the death can be gently encouraged to do so. Even when the death was the result of severe trauma, parents who see their child have fewer fantasies about the event. The parents should be offered the opportunity to hold their child, and the length of the final visit should be determined by the needs of the individual family (Nelson, 1995; Wells, 1996). Mementos should be given to the parents, and the rest of the agency's bereavement protocol should be initiated. Caregivers should give written information about support available for the family over the difficult months ahead.

The nurse can act as the gatekeeper who helps the parents find needed privacy and facilitates communication among family members. The nurse should suggest ways for parents to discuss the events with their other children. Nurses should be prepared for the family to express grief in a variety of ways, including anger and rage, and should not take negative responses personally.

Siblings of dead children need care also. If they are present in the hospital, they should be informed about what is happening and given an opportunity to express their questions and fears. If children want to see their brother or sister, it is generally preferable to honor this request. This issue should be discussed with parents.

If the siblings are not present, parents should be advised on ways to talk to them about their brother or sister's death. Fantasies and misunderstandings are common, and some children see themselves as responsible for the death. These ideas must be identified and dispelled. If the sibling is responsible, however, for example, after a firearm injury or fatal accident, emergency emotional support for the sibling must be initiated immediately (Chart 12–15).

Operating Room

Another possible place of death for the hospitalized child is the OR. Parents may express a need to be with their child when it becomes clear that the child will die in the OR. Individual units should have procedures regarding such eventualities because the decision to grant a parental request to enter the OR or to ask parents whether they want to enter the OR often must be made quickly (Fina, 1994).

One member of the OR team should be designated as the person who confirms that death is likely. The parents should then be offered the chance to be with their child in the OR. Other persons who can be with parents, such as the child's siblings, clergy, extended family, or friends, should be identified. Caregivers should be careful not to give parents the message (verbally or nonverbally) that they must go into the OR.

If the parents choose to go to the OR suite, they should be prepared for what they will see and how the child will look. The OR environment and staff should be prepared for the parents' visit. Visible blood on the child, the bed, or on surgical instruments should be cleaned or covered up. One staff member, preferably a nurse, should support the parents during the visit. If possible, the parents should be offered a place to sit during the visit. Parents should be helped to approach and touch their child because they may need to receive permission from the health care team to do this. Parents should be given the opportunity to be present when life support is discontinued (Fina, 1994).

After the child's death, the parents should be offered additional time to be with their child before, during, or after postmortem care is completed. At this point, movement of the child to the recovery area should be considered.

Hospice Programs

Another option for children who are approaching death is enrollment in a pediatric hospice program. Hospice programs all subscribe to similar standards and practices. The child must be in the terminal phase of illness, usually with death expected in the ensuing 4 to 6 months. The child and family must have decided to forgo any further treatments or diagnostic efforts to sustain life.

Support and education for family and friends is an essential part of hospice care. The initial visit of the hospice worker is usually made within 24 hours of the

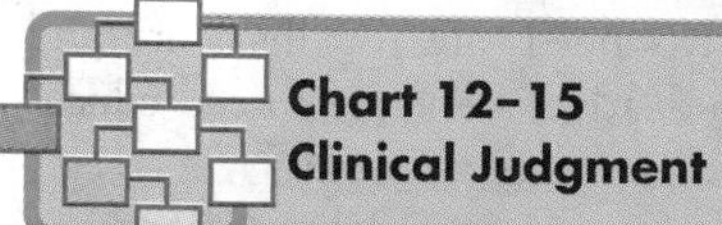

Chart 12–15
Clinical Judgment

A Child Experiencing the Traumatic Death of a Sibling

Nine-year-old Eric G. and his 4-year-old sister Sara were playing at home while their parents worked in the garden. Eric and Sara had been carefully instructed to never play with the gun that Mr. G. kept in a cabinet over the refrigerator. Around 4 P.M., Eric and Sara were searching for snacks to eat before dinner. Eric pulled a chair up to the kitchen counter and began searching the cabinets. He finally found a full bag of chips hidden in the cabinet over the refrigerator, just behind the gun. When he moved the gun, he was fascinated by how it felt and looked and brought it down "just for a minute." The gun discharged, hitting Sara in the chest. The emergency response team transported Sara to the hospital. After briefly interviewing Eric and his parents, the police helped them get to the hospital. There, Eric tells you that the policeman said he killed his sister.

Questions

1. What other data about Eric and his family should be obtained at the time of their admission?
2. What assessment finding indicates that Eric was misinterpreting comments made to him?
3. What simple tools can be used to help Eric express his feelings?
4. What immediate referrals would you make for Eric's care?
5. What types of concerns would you have about Eric's reaction to his sister's injury and possible death?

Answers

1. Who do the children live with? Which members of Eric's family provide his greatest support? Has Eric had any prior experience with such an event?
2. Eric says that the policeman said that he killed his sister, but the police officers only remember asking Eric what happened to his sister.
3. Drawing, storytelling, and reading stories that contain the themes that Eric expresses in his comments to staff and family.
4. A child life worker, social worker, psychologist, or psychiatrist should see Eric within an hour of his sister's admission.
5. Eric is likely to react strongly to any comments made in the hours and days after the accident. Even supportive comments of caring adults may be misinterpreted by him. He will feel responsible for her death.

referral because the family's needs are usually acute and the child may be close to death. Parents also need education about the physiologic processes of death.

The site where hospice services are delivered and the scope of services provided differ from hospice to hospice and even from family to family. Most children enrolled in hospice are cared for at home. The hospice staff helps the child and family deal with pain, manage symptoms, and maintain nutrition; they do anything needed to promote the comfort of the child. Respite care to allow the parents and family to leave the child and the assistance of a home health aide or hospice volunteer to allow the parents to return to work can also be a part of the hospice program (Chart 12–16). Emotional support for the entire family is an essential component of hospice care both before and after the child's death.

The main need of the child and family is for help with pain and symptom control. Parents provide most of the care and, with respite care, can continue to work and participate in activities that the dying child cannot attend. Parents report that the illness is less disruptive to family life when the child is at home. Even though they are better able to maintain control, the parents still experience stress as a result of the illness, the child's care, and their own fatigue (Martinson, 1993).

Parents and other relatives are more likely to be with the child at the time of death if the death takes place at home. Although nurses are often in the home at the time of the death, many parents choose not to call the nurse until after the death so that the family can be alone with the child (Martinson, 1993). Most hospice programs continue to support the family after the child's death because the acute stage of grief can extend for 2 years after the child's death (Martinson, 1993).

In some cases, the child needs to be admitted to an **inpatient hospice**. Inpatient hospice units meet the needs of families who cannot provide care in the home when the child is not a candidate for admission to an acute care or rehabilitative setting. The inpatient hospice can address the psychological and physical needs of children and their families while providing the excellent nursing and medical care needed (Lombardi, 1993).

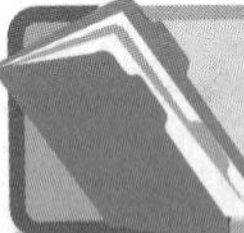

Chart 12–16
Nursing Interventions Classification (NIC)

Respite Care

Definition

Provision of short-term care to provide relief for the family caregiver

Activities

Establish a therapeutic relationship with patient/family.
Monitor endurance of caregiver.
Inform patient/family of available state funding for respite care.
Coordinate volunteers for in-home services, as appropriate.
Arrange for a substitute caregiver.
Follow the usual routine of care.
Provide care, such as exercises, ambulation, and hygiene, as appropriate.
Obtain emergency telephone numbers.
Determine how to contact usual caregiver.
Provide emergency care, as necessary.
Maintain normal home environment.
Provide a report to usual caregiver on return.

From McCloskey, J., & Bulechek, G. (1996). *Nursing interventions classification (NIC)* (2nd ed.). St. Louis: Mosby–Year Book. Reprinted with permission.

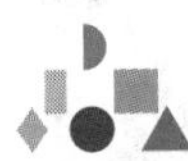

Care of the Family After the Death of a Loved One

When a person significant to a family has died, each member of the family is in need of immediate help and assistance. If family members have the needed knowledge and coping mechanisms, that immediate help assists them until their resources can be mobilized. For family members without needed resources, the nurse's role is one of educator and support person as the family is helped to move through the bereavement process to life without the loved one. Many nursing diagnoses might be applicable to the grieving family (Chart 12–17). Family assessment identifies pertinent issues that need to be addressed when working with individual families (see Chart 12–8).

Parents

The death of a child is one of the most difficult experiences that a parent can face. The child whose parent has died loses a part of himself or herself. So, too, the parent whose child has died loses a part of himself or herself, as well as losing the child.

Grief Reactions in Parents

For some parents, the death of a child is a time of great personal growth accompanied by great pain. For others, it is a time of overwhelming sadness that does not remit for

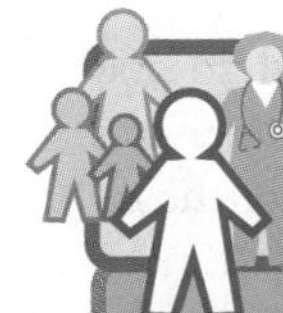

Chart 12–17
Nursing Diagnoses and Outcomes

Emotional Care of the Grieving Family

Altered family processes related to changes in relationships and roles in the family secondary to death of a family member

Outcome: The family will remain supportive of all members.

Anxiety related to concerns about death of a child or changes in the family

Outcome: The family will verbalize feelings of anxiety and identify methods of dealing with them.

Caregiver role strain related to necessity of meeting needs of family members in ways not done before, insufficient support

Outcomes: The caregivers will develop new methods of accomplishing necessary tasks.
Caregivers will identify support networks.

Grieving related to death of a loved one

Outcome: The family will verbalize feelings and will work through bereavement tasks.

Dysfunctional grieving related to death of a loved one

Outcome: The family will have dysfunctional responses recognized early and will be offered psychosocial counseling.

Spiritual distress related to crisis of the illness, suffering, or death of a child

Outcome: The family will verbalize distress and will have spiritual counselors available for support.

Sleep pattern disturbance related to need to be with dying child, fear, or anxiety

Outcome: The family will resume previous sleep patterns and state they feel rested.

Powerlessness related to inability to perform roles and responsibilities secondary to terminal illness or death of a child secondary to terminal illness

Outcome: The family will verbalize feelings of powerlessness; will be given opportunities to make decisions regarding care.

years, if ever. The time and pattern of the bereavement process for the grieving parent is much longer than for bereavement from other losses and often there is never full resolution of the grief. With skilled care by the entire health care team, however, the parent can be helped to successfully complete the bereavement process and move on to a life without the child (Kachoyeanos & Selder, 1993; Worder & Monahan, 1993).

Even though each parent reacts to the death of the child in a unique way, several patterns are seen. Parents who had ambivalent relationships with their child or were unable to help their child in the time before death report more problems with bereavement than those who had a good relationship and were able to support the child at the time of death. Parents whose child dies after a chronic illness have less acute responses than those whose child dies after an accident or brief illness. The ability to clearly identify the cause of death also helps parents in their time of grief. Parents who are with their child at the time of death or who see their child soon after the death are better able to realize that the child is dead. Such a visit also reduces concerns about the nature and extent of the damage to the child's body and decreases fantasies about the child's death and hope that the child is not in fact dead and will someday reappear (Kachoyeanos & Selder, 1993).

Parental responses to the death of their child continue long after the classic 1- or 2-year grieving period common with the death of friends, grandparents, or parents when the child is an adult. Parents must undergo a life transition as they move from the old reality to a new reality—from life with their child to life after their child's death. This transition process is characterized by a sense of uncertainty and a variety of trigger events (Kachoyeanos & Selder, 1993).

The sense of uncertainty pervades the total experience. Parents report that they do not know how to act or communicate their needs. This includes having a sense that they have no language to express themselves. Because information helps decrease uncertainty, having questions answered is helpful to bereaved parents; however, the new information can also raise more questions (Kachoyeanos & Selder, 1993).

Trigger events reinforce the fact that the parent's reality has changed. The first trigger event is the actual death of the child. At this time, the parents must accept the irrevocability of the death.

caREminder: *Clear, gentle discussions of the child's death, in which the child is called by name and the word "death" is used, helps dissipate the uncertainty inherent at this time. This initial transition is facilitated if the nurse keeps the focus on the child's death and the parent's needs.*

If procedural items (e.g., gathering information for the death certificate or making funeral arrangements) must be processed, they should be presented in such a way that recognition of the value and dignity of the child is demonstrated. Parents often find it difficult to make decisions at this time, and encouragement to see their child and to involve the siblings is appropriate (Kachoyeanos & Selder, 1993).

Trigger events continue long after the child's death. Doing something that was previously done with the child, passing the site of the accident where the child died, or hearing music that the child liked are examples of events that can reactivate memories of the child and feelings about the child's death. The reality of the child's death is reinforced when special dates such as birthdays or family holidays occur (Fig. 12–6). These dates can be used as special occasions to remember the child. The dates may also have been times when developmental achievements (e.g., beginning to walk, joining the Girl Scouts, graduation, marriage, or birth of a grandchild) would have taken place. Triggers are experienced by parents regardless of how old the child was at death or how much time has elapsed since the child's death (Kachoyeanos & Selder, 1993).

Parents need to structure a new reality after the child's death. This effort is apparent in many of their actions. Parents often compare themselves to others to judge how well they are doing. Talking with other parents who have lost a child and participating in support groups help the parents learn that their reactions are normal. These activities help parents learn strategies for coping with their pain and the challenges they face. They learn that they will emerge from the period of deep and painful grief (Kachoyeanos & Selder, 1993).

Parents also need to know that they were good parents. They may overtly ask whether they provided good care to the child or brought the child for treatment at the right time. Others seek affirmation of their parenting skills indirectly by listening to comments of those who cared for their child. Thus, a random remark while looking at pictures of the child such as "Aren't those pajamas pretty" can provide positive feedback whereas a simple statement such as "Look at how messy that bib was" can be interpreted as a negative evaluation of the parents' ability to meet even the most basic hygienic need of their child.

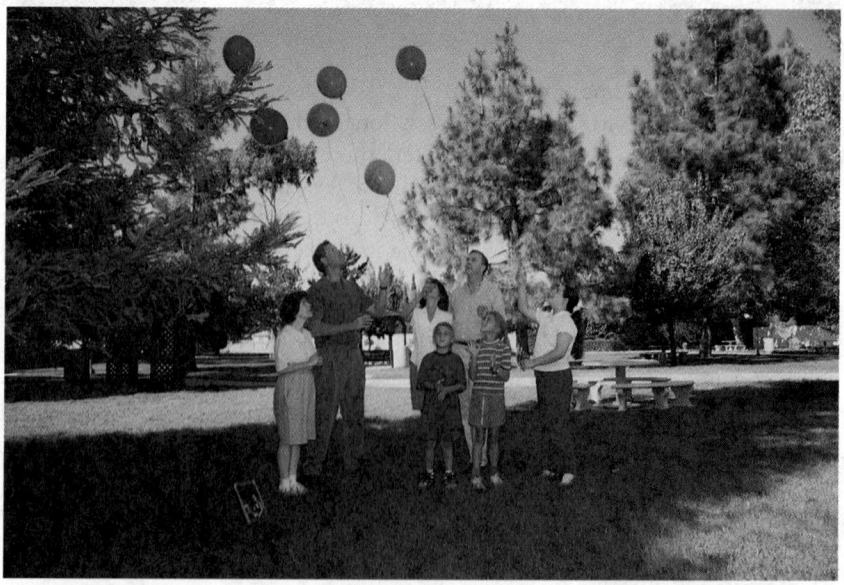

Figure 12–6
On the anniversary of a child's death, family members and friends meet to send balloons (non-Mylar) with messages inside up to heaven for the deceased child.

Parents have a strong desire to return to the "normal" world they knew before the child's death (Kachoyeanos & Selder, 1993). This desire may lead the parent to engage in an activity, such as suddenly taking a family vacation to a theme park with the other children, which appears inappropriate in light of the recent death. Often, such activities are undertaken with the hope that they will make the negative and painful emotions dissipate. This rarely happens.

Parents may also be afraid that they will forget the child. As a result, they engage in "presencing" by looking at pictures or videotapes in which the child appears and keeping the child's possessions for months, sometimes years. When the possessions are given away, they are given away to someone meaningful. Although keeping the possessions intact permanently may be a sign of dysfunctional grief, it is generally better for the parents to delay dismantling the child's room and disposing of the child's possessions for several months (Kachoyeanos & Selder, 1993). This allows them time to thoughtfully decide what they want to keep and what they want to give away.

Helping Grieving Parents

A bereavement program can be very helpful to the parents and siblings of a deceased child. The foundation of such a program is an educated staff that knows how to work effectively with grieving families and that helps each other with their own grief reactions. Knowledge of the characteristics of parental grief, children's grief, and staff grief is essential (Heiney, Hasan, & Price, 1993).

The staff can help the family by establishing a relationship, by being present both physically and emotionally, and by continuing to focus on the family as a system (Chart 12–18). The family should be educated about normal grieving and should be encouraged to talk about the death, their reaction to it, and their feelings. Siblings also should receive education, attention, and support. When necessary, the family should be referred for counseling (Stewart, 1995).

Often, the staff nurse caring for the dying child is in an excellent position to initiate the bereavement support process. Follow-up efforts can then be made by the staff or a bereavement coordinator.

caREminder: *Immediate follow-up efforts should include communication of information to the staff about funeral arrangements and specific needs of the family. Parents should be given mementos of the child such as a lock of hair or a final picture. A sympathy card and any personal message from the staff can be sent to the family (Heiney et al., 1993).*

Follow-up efforts can include sending a personal letter from the nursing staff to the family followed by a call within 2 weeks of the child's death, at which time additional support can be offered and referral to counseling can be made if needed. The family can be contacted at times likely to trigger resurgence of the grief response, such as the child's birthday, major holidays, or the anniversary of the child's death, so that additional support can be provided. A tracking card and check sheet can be used to identify dates for follow-up interventions (Heiney et al., 1993).

The bereavement program for parents of older children who died resembles that for the family who has had a perinatal loss. A bereavement packet with information about sources of support, the grieving process, helpful books and videotapes, and poems and stories written by parents whose children died should be developed. Discus-

Chart 12–18
Nursing Interventions

Helping Parents Face the Death of Their Child

Communication

- Listen attentively.
- Find out what the family knows and what they want to know.
- Use language that family members can understand.
- Call the child by name.
- Use silence as an ally but watch for signs that parents need to talk.
- Encourage questions.
- Do not offer platitudes.
- Do not automatically offer tissues.

Facilitate Family Grieving

- Offer a private place for the family to retreat.
- If death occurs, allow the family time with the child after the death.
- Encourage involvement of siblings.
- Preserve memories of the child: last height, weight, lock of hair, hospital name band, plaster of Paris hand- or footprint, picture of the child, child's blanket and clothes in a plastic bag (to preserve scent).
- Help establish links with a social worker, spiritual support person (chaplain, priest, rabbi, healer), funeral director.
- Provide specific information about how the needs of siblings can be met.
- Provide pamphlets for family members and friends to give them tips about how to help the parents.

sions about the care of siblings and having additional children are an important part of a bereavement follow-up program.

Siblings

Siblings of the deceased child need care based on their age, developmental stage, and relationship with their sibling. They should not be protected from information about the child's illness or given evasive answers to their questions about the death.

There has been a dramatic improvement in the emotional health of siblings of children who have died. Studies of bereaved siblings indicate that they are often more mature than their peers. They have similar, or higher, scores on measures of adjustment and self-concept than their peers who did not lose a sibling. This is a very different finding from that of 10 to 15 years ago when as many as 50% of siblings of children who died had behavioral or emotional problems (Walker, 1993).

These positive changes have been attributed to alterations in how death is dealt with in American society. Death is spoken of more openly than it once was, and care for the siblings is integrated into plans of care. Because nurses and other health care providers are more attuned to the child's psychological needs, they are more responsive to those needs.

caREminder: *Siblings of a child who has died should be involved to the degree that they wish to be involved. Their questions and concerns should be addressed freely and openly.*

Siblings of deceased children experience stress as the result of the death. If the child was ill before the death, this stress is compounded by the changes in family structure and environment as a result of the illness. But, this stress passes if the siblings are given the help and support they need during and after the acute phase of grief. Siblings need to grieve, to say good-bye.

Outdoor activities, yelling (Lehna, 1995), play therapy, support groups, and art therapy have been found to help the grieving child. A multidimensional home care program that addresses physical, emotional, and other needs of the family during the terminal phase of an illness is also beneficial. Parents should be taught about the needs of the siblings and ways to help them progress through the bereavement process (Chart 12–19).

Parents should be taught that the child who died was unique and their remaining children cannot, and should not, take over the life of that child. Neither current nor future children should be made into "replacement" children to compensate for the lost child. Replacement children are given the burden of assuming their own identity as well as that of the dead child (Gibbons, 1992).

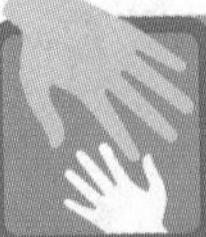

Chart 12–19
Nursing Interventions

Helping Siblings Grieve

Educate the sibling about death:
- Assess what the sibling knows and wants to know and provide necessary teaching.
- Involve siblings in family discussions about the dying child and after the child's death.
- Spend time with the sibling, explaining what happened and answering questions.
- Look for opportunities to give information.
- Do not be evasive.

Teach the sibling about the normal emotions that accompany grief and bereavement:
- Share your own memories and feelings with the sibling.
- Let the sibling know that feeling sad, angry, or scared is okay for adults and for the children, and that crying is okay (even for boys).
- Allow laughter and fun times, which can occur even in the midst of great sadness.

Meet the sibling's need for support and comfort:
- Decrease the sense of abandonment by being with the sibling both physically and emotionally.
- Consider whether the sibling relationship was positive or negative and how that has impacted grieving.
- Use physical touch as a way of reassuring and comforting the sibling.
- Help the sibling identify and express feelings about the child who has died.
- Reassure the sibling that it is not likely that anyone else (particularly the parents) will also die within the near future.
- Encourage siblings to express their feelings and thoughts in their own way through discussion, writing letters, poetry, art.
- Look for evidence that the sibling is protecting the parents (e.g., by not telling them his or her fears and concerns or trying to lessen the parents' grief).

Promote normalcy in the sibling's life and routines:
- Continue to expect the sibling to have responsibilities at home and at school.
- Give simple directions or use reminder lists for things that need to be done if the sibling has trouble remembering.
- Encourage the sibling's involvement with friends and peers.

Adapted from Davis, B. (1993). After a child dies: Helping the siblings. In A. Armstrong-Dailey & S. Goltzer (Eds.), *Hospice care for children* (p. 150). New York: Oxford University Press. Used with permission.

TIP 12–2 A Teaching Intervention Plan for Helping Parents Promote Self-Esteem of a Sibling After a Child's Death

Nursing Diagnosis and Outcomes

- Self-esteem disturbance related to not feeling as worthwhile as the child who died
  Outcome: The parents will promote feelings of realistic self-appraisal, positive self-concept, and high self-esteem in the siblings of the child who died.

Interventions

Instruct parents to

- Speak with pride about the child for what he or she is.
- Describe the child as different (in a positive way) from his or her peers as a result of the experience of the sibling's death.
- Be aware that, if other children are added to the family (e.g., by adoption or birth), the sibling of the child who died may feel displaced by the new addition.

Educate parents not to

- Give any indication that the surviving child is not "as good" as the deceased sibling.
- Indicate that the surviving child is in any way responsible for the sibling's death.
- Express a preference for or wish to have a child who in some way (e.g., gender, ability) is like the child who died.
- Display a preference for the deceased child by comments or comparisons.

Adapted from Martinson, I., Davies, E., & McClowry, G. (1987). The long-term effects of sibling death on self-concept. *Journal of Pediatric Nursing, 2,* 227–235. Used with permission.

Parents need help to understand how their actions and the home environment can positively or negatively affect the future self-concept and emotional health of surviving siblings (TIP 12–2). Children who demonstrate a positive self-concept have been made to feel special and are reported as being highly competent. Children who experience low self-concept report that they feel that they do not compare favorably with the deceased child or that they have been displaced by another child.

Personal Response of the Nurse

Often, an individual nurse wants to attend the funeral or reach out to the family. This may be an essential step to help the nurse resolve his or her own grief. Families can find such expressions of caring and grief both helpful and comforting. To be most therapeutic with the family, the nurse should keep the focus on the family (Chart 12–20).

caREminder: *When visiting the family, nurses should avoid platitudes. The nurse should call the child by name and use direct language. For example, the nurse should say "I'm so sorry that Mary died" rather than "Your child has expired." This lets the parent know that the nurse sees the child as a unique special person, and it helps the parents internalize the reality of the death (Miles, 1990).*

When a nurse does attend the funeral or visit the family at home, the visit should not be so brief that the family feels further abandonment and isolation. However, the nurse should be sensitive to whether the family welcomes the visit. If a personal telephone call is made, the family should be given the opportunity to decline to talk. The nurse can tell the family member that he or she was thinking of them and then ask whether it is a good time to talk (Miles, 1990).

Special Situations

Death of a Parent

A child whose parent has died needs special attention. Because of the unique bond between the child and parent, particularly the infant and mother, death of a parent results in both loss of self (the part that was bound to the parent) and loss of other (the parent who died). The remaining parent and other family members are also grieving, making it hard for them to meet the child's

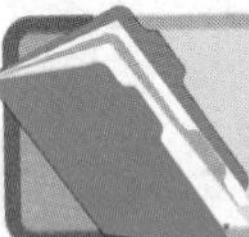

Chart 12–20
Nursing Interventions Classification (NIC)

Presence

Definition

Being with another during times of need

Activities

Demonstrate accepting attitude.
Verbally communicate empathy or understanding of the patient's experience.
Be sensitive to the patient's traditions and beliefs.
Establish trust and a positive regard.
Listen to the patient's concerns.
Use silence, as appropriate.
Touch patient to express concern, as appropriate.
Be physically available as a helper.
Remain physically present without expecting interactional responses.
Provide distance for the patient and family, as needed.
Offer to remain with patient during initial interactions with others on the unit.
Help patient to realize that you are available, but do not reinforce dependent behaviors.
Stay with patient to promote safety and reduce fear.
Reassure and assist parents in their supportive role with their child.
Stay with the patient and provide assurance of safety and security, during periods of anxiety.
Offer to contact other support persons (e.g., priest/rabbi), as appropriate.

From McCloskey, J., & Bulechek, G. (1996). *Nursing interventions classification (NIC)* (2nd ed.). St. Louis: Mosby–Year Book. Reprinted with permission.

needs for consistent support and attachment. The child may worry that the surviving parent will die too. The loss of a parent is difficult for the child. Adults often have several significant persons in their life with whom they form attachments; however, a child usually has only two significant attachments—those to each parent. The parent meets the child's physiologic and emotional needs and gradually helps the child meet those needs independently. When a parent dies, someone else must take over the missing parent's role, be it the other parent or someone else. Infants and young toddlers need immediate and consistent replacement of this primary caretaker role.

Activities shared with the dead parent may no longer be enjoyed. For the infant or toddler, this can be eating or the development of new abilities like smiling, rolling over, or toilet training. For the older child, this could be going to the movies or special school events.

The child often regresses for a short time. Young children who cannot express themselves verbally may display emotions through play or other behaviors. In some cases, problems may not be evident initially; they may occur at the beginning of the next developmental phase such as the progression from school age to adolescence.

Death of a Friend

Children may face death in the ranks of their peers, school staff, family, or community. The cause is often acute or chronic illness, but increasing numbers of children are exposed to death as a result of violence. Schools need to include content about death and dying in the school curriculum and have a crisis plan that can be activated quickly after a death in the school community. The school nurse plays a significant role in the development and implementation of death education curriculum and crisis plans.

Educational programs about the facts of death, recognizing depression, understanding grief, and effective communication between child and teacher, child and child, and child and family should be implemented. Discussion should include how to interact with a bereaved student who is returning to school, how to accept and address their grief, and the importance of resuming a normal relationship. Staff and students should be taught how to recognize students who are grieving or who are at risk for suicide. Detailed information on ways to help those individuals obtain assistance should be provided.

▽ **Alert:** *Emphasize with students that, when a friend talks about taking his or her own life, it is essential to share this information with a counselor, teacher, or some other trusted adult. In this case, getting the friend help is more important than keeping their secret.*

The school crisis plan should detail all needed steps from the notification of student, faculty, and staff about the death to the implementation of long-term support services. The crisis plan should be flexible enough to be used if the person who died is a student, faculty or staff member, or significant person in the community, and whether death is from illness, suicide, or violence.

The crisis management team might include the school nurse, counselors, teachers, and administrators as well as community-based personnel (e.g., health care, fire, police, and emergency professionals) (Oates, 1993). One person should be designated as spokesperson and someone should be identified to notify the family if the death occurred at the school. A plan to notify staff, students, and parents should include prepared scripts and memos that can be modified based on the specific situation (Oates, 1993).

Policies about holding memorial services on campus and student attendance at funeral services on school days should be developed. The plan should also include a detailed plan about how the students' and staff's emotional needs will be met on both an acute and long-term basis. A training program for staff and teachers for both the acute event and the residual problems is needed. A plan to evaluate the outcome each time the plan is implemented is essential.

The suicide of a student, staff member, or community member requires special attention. Students may want to follow the example of the student who committed suicide because they desire the same attention or because it appears to be a particularly attractive way to deal with the concerns of adolescence. The death must be acknowledged and the usual grief activities completed. Memorializing the child who committed suicide, even if he or she was popular, however, is not recommended because such activities indirectly condone suicide as an acceptable action.

A recurrence of grief reactions can occur on anniversary dates, for example, 1 year after a bus crash that killed members of the junior class on the way to school. Faculty should be reminded to look for signs of an increased grief response on significant occasions, such as the day the star football player would have received the district trophy if he had not died after a car accident.

Grief support groups have been found to be very helpful for school-age and adolescent children (Chart 12–21). Sessions held at school have the advantage of being easy to attend and occurring in a setting familiar to the child. Support groups can also be based at sites where the loved one of a child was treated.

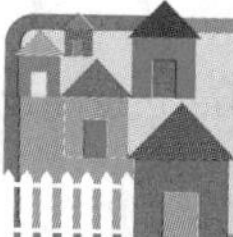

Chart 12–21
Community Care

Suggested Content of a Grief Support Program

Education

- Discuss normal grief, emotional pain, healthy and unhealthy reactions, depression.
- Read and discuss stories related to death and loss.
- Put comments, poems, questions in a jar, and discuss some each day to help participants share what they are feeling.

Creative Activities

- Draw pictures of activities that participants liked doing with the person who died.
- Create a memorial tribute to the person who died (photograph album, scrapbook, poems, play).
- Develop loss graphs to identify personal significant losses over time.

Simple Writing Assignments

When ________ died, I lost ________________.

Complex Writing Assignments

In a letter to the person who died:

- Tell what you remember about his or her death.
- Ask any questions you have about the death or anything else that is puzzling to you.
- Say what you wish you had said before he or she died or that you wish you had said more often.
- List any regrets you have about your relationship.
- Make any apologies you think are necessary.
- Tell him what you really liked or appreciated and how you wish he or she had been different.
- State specifically what you lost when he or she died.
- Discuss the feelings you have had since his or her death and how your life is now.
- Discuss how you think your life would be different if he or she had not died.

Adapted from Oates, M. A. (1993). *Death in the school community: A handbook for counselors, teachers, and administrators.* Alexandria, VA: American Counseling Association. Used with permission. No further reproduction authorized without written permission of the American Counseling Association.

Care of Extended Family and Friends

Extended family members and friends should be included in the bereavement programs as previously described based on their degree of involvement with the person who has died. Persons such as out-of-state grandparents, spouses of the non-custodial parent, daycare providers, and parents of the child's friends are often not seen, thus overlooked, by the health care providers who are caring for the child and family.

When these individuals are seen in other settings for reasons unrelated to the death of the child, skillful assessment often identifies concerns of these individuals and enables the nurse to implement needed bereavement care. A collection of pamphlets and books on bereavement should be available to clients, regardless of the focus of the setting. Lists of local support groups and counselors can often be helpful.

Extended family and friends are often unsure of how they can help the grieving family. They fear they will do something wrong when they call or visit so they do neither. This contributes to the isolation of the grieving family in a time of great need.

caREminder: *Friends and family should be reassured that, if they act genuinely and with sincerity when they are with the grieving family, what they do will rarely be wrong. Suggestions of helpful activities should be provided to them (see Chart 12–14).*

Continued Family Care After Death

The family needs ongoing care after the death of a child. This is provided through multiple support networks and special bereavement services of the agencies where their child received care.

Support Networks

There are several major national support networks for families whose children have died and for children who have had significant losses through death. These groups, such as Compassionate Friends, offer many materials useful to the grieving family. Local chapters are located across the country. The national office can help families find such groups.

Other support networks help families whose children have died from specific causes. Examples are groups for victims of SIDS, murder, and suicide. Again, referral to such groups can be through national chapters and local chapters. Many agencies that serve dying children offer support services for the families of the children in their care. Such groups help the family contact groups whose members are facing similar problems.

Bibliotherapy

Another major way that family members can be helped in the time after the death of a child is through bibliotherapy (Bowden, 1993; Corr, 1993). Bibliotherapy usually takes one of three forms. The first is through books that present facts about the child's illness and death. The second is through books written by parents or children who have had similar experiences. The third is through books that deal with the general themes of grief and loss.

Bibliotherapy can also be used effectively with children. Everything from simple stories to full-length novels help the child learn about death and the feelings that accompany death.

Summary of Key Concepts

- Nurses caring for the grieving family must clarify their own beliefs if they are to respond therapeutically to the needs of the family.
- Children gradually increase their comprehension of the various subconcepts of death.
- Children learn to cope with grief by development of a realistic concept of death and learning how to cope with strong negative emotions.
- Grief caused by the potential or actual loss of a loved one results in both physiologic and emotional responses.
- The time for the completion of the bereavement process is at least 18 months.
- After a death, major changes in the surviving child's daily life should be avoided.
- Successful bereavement is facilitated if the family members are helped to understand that they will each mourn differently.
- After the death of their child, parents must undergo a life transition as they move from life with their child to life after their child's death.
- Children whose loved ones have died should not be protected from information or given evasive answers to questions about the death.
- Play therapy techniques, support groups, and art therapy have been found to help the grieving child.
- When choices about care of the dying child are made, the context of the decision must be carefully examined.
- Parents should be encouraged to be with their child after the child's death and before the child receives postmortem care.
- The family needs continued care after the death of the child.

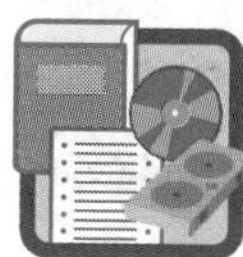

Resources

Support Groups

Bereaved Survivors of Homicide Group

Candlelighters Childhood Cancer Foundation *for parents and families of children with cancer*
7910 Woodmont Ave.
Bethesda, MD 20814
(301) 657-8401
(800) 366-2223

Children's Hospice International
2202 Mt. Vernon Ave.
Suite 3C
Alexandria, VA 22301
(800) 24-CHILD

The Compassionate Friends *for bereaved parents and siblings*
P. O. Box 3696
Oak Brook, IL 60522-3696
(630) 990-0010

H. E. A. L. (Helping Endure Infant Loss) *for parents who have experienced miscarriage, stillbirth, or newborn death*

MADD, Inc. *assists victimized families of drunk driving*
511 East John Carpenter Freeway
Suite 700
Irving, TX 75062
(800) GET MADD

Make A Wish Foundation fulfills favorite wish of a child with life-threatening or terminal illness
100 W. Clarendon
Suite 2200
Phoenix, AZ 85013
(602) 279-9474

Resolve Through Sharing *for parents experiencing a perinatal loss*
Lutheran Hospital–LaCrosse
1910 South Ave.
LaCrosse, WI 54601
(608) 791-4747

SHARE for families experiencing pregnancy and infant loss
St. Joseph's Health Center
Attn: National SHARE Office
300 First Capitol Dr.
St. Charles, MO 63301
(800) 821-6819

SIDS Alliance *provides assistance and information to anyone dealing with sudden infant death syndrome*
1314 Bedford
Suite 210
Baltimore, MD 21208
(800) 221-7437

✏ Resources specifically for children

Bibliotherapy

For Adults

Grollman, E. (1977). *Living when a loved one died.* Boston: Beacon Press.

Grollman, E. (1977). *Talking about death: A dialogue between parent and child.* Boston: Beacon Press.

Grollman, E. (1981). *What helped me when my loved one died.* Boston: Beacon Press.

Horchler, J. N., & Morris, R. R. (1994). *The SIDS survival guide.* Cheverly, MD: SIDS Educational Services Inc. (301) 322-2620.

Ilse, S. (1990). *Empty arms: Coping with miscarriage, stillbirth, & infant death.* Maple Plain, MN: Wintergreen Press, 3630 Eileen St., Maple Plain, MN 55359 (612) 476-1303.

Kubler-Ross, E. (1969). *On death and dying.* New York: Macmillan Publishing Co.

Kubler-Ross, E. (1975). *Death: The final stage of growth.* Englewood Cliffs, NJ: Prentice-Hall.

Kubler-Ross, E. (1978). *To live until we say goodbye.* Englewood Cliffs, NJ: Prentice-Hall.

Kubler-Ross, E. (1983). *On children and death.* New York: Macmillan.

Kushner, H. (1982). *When bad things happen to good people.* New York: Avon Books.

Rank, M. (1985). *Free to grieve: Miscarriage and stillbirth.* Minneapolis, MN: Bethany House Publishers.

Schiff, H. (1977). *The bereaved parent.* New York: Crown Publishers, Inc.

✏ Books for Children

Alderman, L. (1989). *Why did Daddy die?* New York: Pocket Books.

Buscaglia, L. (1982). *The fall of Freddie, the leaf.* Thorofare, NJ: Charles B. Slack, Inc.

Hazen, B. (1985). *Why did Grandpa die? A book about death.* Racine, WI: Western Publishing Company.

Johnson, J., & Johnson, M. (1978). *Tell me, Papa.* Omaha, NE: Centering Corporation.

Krementz, J. (1988). *How it feels when a parent dies.* New York: Alfred A. Knopf.

Krementz, J. (1989). *How it feels to fight for your life.* Boston: Little Brown & Company.

Kubler-Ross, E. (1982). *Remember the Secret.* Berkeley, CA: Celestial Arts.

Mellonie, B., & Ingpen, R. (1983). *Lifetimes: A beautiful way to explain death to children.* New York: Bantam Press.

Sesame Street (1984). *I'll Miss you, Mr. Hooper.* New York: Random House.

Viorst, J. (1971). *The tenth good thing about Barney.* New York: Aladdin Books.

Grief Periodicals for Adults and Children

Bereavement: A Magazine of Hope and Healing
Andrea Gambell, editor
350 Gradle Dr.
Carmel, IN 46032

Fernside Inside
Newsletter of the Fernside Center for Grieving Children
2303 Indian Mound Ave.
Cincinnati, OH 45212
(513) 841-1012
✏ *Just for Us: A bereavement newsletter for children and teens*

St. Mary's Hospital for Children
29-01 216th St.
Bayside, NY 11360
(718) 281-8800

Resource Distributors

Centering Corporation
1531 N Saddle Creek Rd.
Omaha, NE 68104-5064
(402) 553-1200

The Good Grief Program
Judge Baker Children's Center
295 Longwood Ave.
Boston, MA 02115
(617) 534-4005

Medic Publishing Company
P. O. Box 89
Redmond, WA 98073-0089
(206) 881-2883

The Rainbow Connection
477 Hannah Branch Rd.
Burnsville, NC 28714
(704) 675-5909

Professional Associations

Association for Death Education and Counseling
Association Resources
638 Prospect Ave.
Hartford, CT 06105

The Center for Death Education and Research
1167 Social Science Bldg.
University of Minnesota
Minneapolis, MN 55455

The Foundation of Thanatology
630 W 168th St.
New York, NY 10032

American Association of Suicidology
4201 Connecticut Ave. NW
Suite 310
Washington, DC 20008
(202) 237-2280

References

Bowden, V. (1993). Children's literature: The death experience. *Pediatric Nursing, 19*, 17–21.

Corr, C. (1993). Children's literature on death. In A. Armstrong-Dailey & S. Goltzer (Eds.), *Hospice care for children* (pp. 266–286). New York: Oxford University Press.

Dowden, S. (1995). Young children's experiences of sibling death. *Journal of Pediatric Nursing, 10*, 72–79.

Ewton, D. (1993). A perinatal loss follow-up guide for primary care. *The Nurse Practitioner, 18*(12), 30–36.

Faulkner, K. (1993). Children's understanding of death. In A. Armstrong-Dailey & S. Goltzer (Eds.), *Hospice care for children* (pp. 9–21). New York: Oxford University Press.

Fina, D. (1994). A chance to say goodbye. *American Journal of Nursing, 94*(5), 42–45.

Gibbons, M. (1992). A child dies, a child survives. The impact of sibling loss. *Journal of Pediatric Health Care, 6*, 65–72.

Gibbons, M. (1993). Psychosocial aspects of serious illness in childhood and adolescence. In A. Armstrong-Dailey & S. Goltzer (Eds.), *Hospice care for children* (pp. 60–74). New York: Oxford University Press.

Heiney, S., Hasan, L., & Price, K. (1993). Developing and implementing a bereavement program for a child's hospital. *Journal of Pediatric Nursing, 8*, 385–391.

Heiney, S. P., Ruffin, J., & Goon-Johnson, K. (1995). The effects of a support group on selected psychosocial outcomes of bereaved parents whose child died from cancer. *Journal of Pediatric Oncology Nursing, 12*(2), 51–61.

Heiney, S. P., Wells, L., & Ruffin, J. (1996). A memorial service for families of children who died from cancer and blood disorders. *Journal of Pediatric Oncology Nursing, 13*, 72–80.

Hinds, P., Puckett, P., Donohoe, M., Milligan, M., Payne, K., Phipps, S., Davis, S., & Martin, G. (1994). The impact of a grief workshop for pediatric oncology nurses on their grief and perceived stress. *Journal of Pediatric Nursing, 9*, 388–397.

Hughes, M. (1995). *Bereavement and support. Healing in a group environment.* Washington, DC: Taylor & Francis.

Kachoyeanos, M., & Selder, F. (1993). Life transitions of parents at the unexpected death of a school-age and older child. *Journal of Pediatric Nursing, 8*, 41–49.

Kalb, K. (1993). IHP: Grief–loss–divorce. In M. Hass (Ed.), *The school nurse's source book of individualized healthcare plans* (pp. 275–282). North Branch, MI: Sunrise River Press.

Kubler-Ross, E. (1969). *On death and dying.* New York: Macmillan.

Lehna, C. R. (1995). Children's descriptions of their feelings and what they found helpful during bereavement. *American Journal of Hospice & Palliative Care, 12*(5), 24–30.

Lombardi, N. (1993). Palliative care in an inpatient hospital setting. In A. Armstrong-Dailey & S. Goltzer (Eds.), *Hospice care for children* (pp. 248–265). New York: Oxford University Press.

Lunny, M. (1994). Giving caregivers permission to grieve. *Journal of Pediatric Oncology Nursing, 11*(Suppl. 1), 57–58.

Mahon, M. (1993). Children's concept of death and sibling death from trauma. *Journal of Pediatric Nursing, 8*, 335–344.

Mahon, M. M., & Page, M. L. (1995). Childhood bereavement after the death of a sibling. *Holistic Nursing Practice*, 9(3), 15–26.

Martinson, I. (1993). A home care program. In A. Armstrong-Dailey & S. Goltzer (Eds.), *Hospice care for children* (pp. 231–247). New York: Oxford University Press.

McCown, D. E., & Davies, B. (1995). Patterns of grief in young children following the death of a sibling. *Death Studies, 19*(1), 41–53.

Miles, A. (1990). Caring for families when a child dies. *Pediatric Nursing, 16*, 346–347.

Miles, M., & Warner, J. (1992). The dying child in the intensive care unit. In M. F. Hazinski (Ed.), *Nursing care of the critically ill child* (2nd ed.). St. Louis: Mosby–Year Book.

Miser, J., & Miser, A. (1993). Pain and Symptom Control. In A. Armstrong-Dailey & S. Goltzer (Eds.), *Hospice care for children* (pp. 140–153). New York: Oxford University Press.

Nelson, L. (1995). When a child dies. *American Journal of Nursing, 95*(3), 61–64.

Nishimoto, P. (1996). Venturing into the unknown: Cultural beliefs about death and dying. *Oncology Nursing Forum, 23*, 889–894.

Oates, M. A. (1993). *Death in the school community: A handbook for counselors, teachers, and administrators*. Alexandria, VA: American Counseling Association.

Rando, T. (1993). *Treatment of complicated mourning*. Champaign, IL: Research Press.

Saiki, S. C., Martinson, I. M., & Inano, M. (1994). Japanese families who have lost children to cancer: A primary study. *Journal of Pediatric Nursing, 9*, 239–250.

Schlomann, P., & Fister, S. (1995). Parental perspectives related to decision-making and neonatal death. *Pediatric Nursing, 21*, 243–247, 254.

Schonfeld, D. J. (1993). Talking with children about death. *Journal of Pediatric Health Care, 7*, 269–274.

Stewart, E. S. (1995). Family-centered care for the bereaved. *Pediatric Nursing, 21*, 181–184, 187.

Walker, C. L. (1993). Sibling bereavement and grief responses. *Journal of Pediatric Nursing, 8*, 325–334.

Wells, E. J. (1996). Assisting parents when a child dies in the ICU. *Critical Care Nurse, 16*, 58–62.

Whittam, E. H. (1993). Terminal care of the dying child. *Cancer, 71*(Suppl. 10), 3450–3462.

Worder, W., & Monahan, J. (1993). Caring for bereaved parents. In A. Armstrong-Dailey, & S. Goltzer (Eds.), *Hospice care for children* (pp. 122–139). New York: Oxford University Press.

Yoder, L. (1994). Comfort and consolation: A nursing perspective on parental bereavement. *Pediatric Nursing, 20*, 473–477.

Bibliography

Armstrong-Dailey, A., & Goltzer, S. (Eds). (1993). *Hospice care for children*. New York: Oxford University Press.

Arnold, J. H., & Gemma, P. B. (1983). *A child dies. A portrait of family grief*. Rockville, MD: Aspen Systems Corporation.

Attig, T. (1996). Beyond pain: The existential suffering of children. *Journal of Palliative Care, 12*(3), 20–23.

Blake, M. (1992). A lullaby for Bobby. *American Journal of Nursing, 92*(10), 112.

Bourne, V., & Meier J. (1988). What happens now? A book to be read to children who have lost a loved one. *Oncology Nursing Forum, 15*(1), 81–85.

Bowlby, J. (1960). Grief and mourning in infancy and early childhood. *Psychoanalytic Study of the Child, 15*, 9–52.

Bowlby, J. (1961). Childhood mourning and its implication for psychiatry. *American Journal of Psychiatry, 118*, 481–498.

Brown, C. E., & Kozick, P. (1994). Impressioning: A way to preserve memories. MCN, *19*, 285–287.

Cayse, L. (1994). Fathers of children with cancer: A descriptive study of their stressors and coping strategies. *Journal of Pediatric Oncology Nursing, 11*, 102–108.

Davies, B., Clarke, D., Connaughty, S., Cook, K., MacKenzie, B., McCormick, J., O'Loane, M., & Stutzer, C. (1996). Caring for dying children: Nurse's experiences. *Pediatric Nursing, 22*, 500–507.

Fulton, R. A., & Moore, C. M. (1995). Spiritual care of the school-age child with a chronic condition. *Journal of Pediatric Nursing, 10*, 224–231.

Glazer, H., & Landreth, G. (1993). A developmental concept of dying in a child's life. *Journal of Humanistic Education and Development, 31*, 98–105.

Kleiber, C., Montgomery, L. A., & Craft-Rosenberg, M. (1995). Information needs of the siblings of critically ill children. *Children's Health Care, 24*, 47–60.

Mahon, M. M. (1994). Death of a sibling: Primary care interventions. *Pediatric Nursing, 20*, 293–295, 328.

Murray, J. (1995). Social support for siblings of children with cancer. *Journal of Oncology Nursing, 12, 62–70*.

Opie, N. D. (1992). Childhood and adolescent bereavement. *Annual Review of Nursing Research, 10*, 127–141.

Prong, L. L. (1995). Childhood bereavement among Cambodians: Cultural considerations. *Hospice Journal—Physical, Psychosocial & Pastoral Care of the Dying, 10*(2), 51–64.

Richmond, T., & Craig, M. (1995). Timeout: Facing death in the ICU. *Dimensions of Critical Care Nursing, 4*(1), 41–45.

Schlomann, P., & Fister, S. (1995). Parental perspectives related to decision-making and neonatal death. *Pediatric Nursing, 21*, 243–247, 254.

Soutter, J. (1994). A strategy for caring for families in bereavement. *Nursing Times*, 90(30), 37–39.

Stewart, E. (1995). Family-centered care for the bereaved. *Pediatric Nursing, 21*, 181–184.

Pain Management in Children

OUTLINE

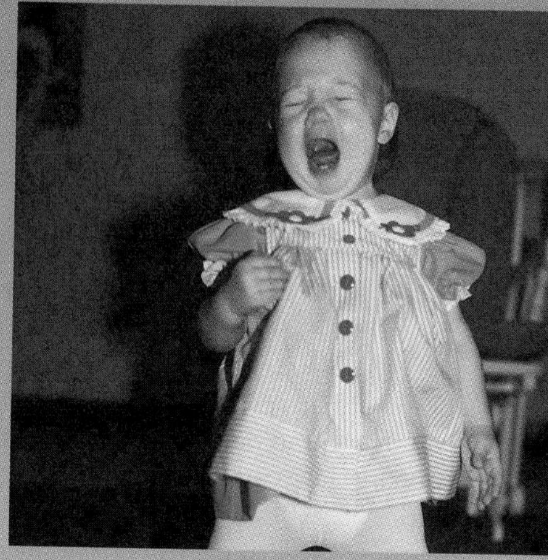

OBJECTIVES

- Explain the physiologic mechanisms that lead to the sensation of pain in a child.
- Identify various factors that may intensify or modify the pain experience.
- Discuss the assessment techniques and tools utilized to evaluate pain in children.
- Describe nonpharmacologic nursing interventions to decrease pain in children.
- Describe pharmacologic interventions used to manage pain in the pediatric patient.
- Contrast manifestations of chronic pain with acute pain and how management strategies for children in special pain situations may differ.
- Discuss the role of the nurse on the interdisciplinary pain team.
- Identify topics regarding pain in children that require further research.

KEY TERMS

Acute pain
Chronic pain
Conscious sedation
Nociception
Patient-controlled analgesia (PCA)
Recurrent pain

CHAPTER

13

Pain has historically been ignored or undertreated in children, particularly infants. Research supports the fact that children are indeed capable of experiencing pain, possibly to an even greater degree than adults.

Some of the most common misperceptions about pain in children include the following:

- Infants are neurologically immature and therefore cannot conduct pain impulses.
- Even if infants experience pain, they do not remember it, because of cortical immaturity.
- Children do not report pain while sleeping or playing, so they must get over it quickly or not be experiencing it.

All of these statements are inaccurate. The health care provider must be cognizant of information that negates these statements and prepare arguments to counter the inaccurate perceptions of children's pain experiences. Pain has deleterious effects. It must be recognized and treated. The position of the American Academy of Pediatrics (AAP) is that infants should be evaluated for anesthesia risk using the same medical criteria as for older patients. They do not recommend that treatment decisions be made solely on the basis of age (AAP, 1987).

Assessment findings and management are different for each child. These are dependent on existing pathology and individual characteristics such as age, physiology, previous experiences, and temperament. Knowledge of developmentally appropriate pain physiology, assessment, and management techniques is necessary for the nurse to care and advocate for this vulnerable population.

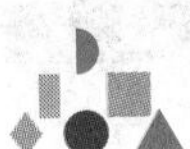

Neurophysiology of Pain

Historically, pain impulse transmission was viewed as a predictable response pattern. A certain stimulus produced a certain response; the impulse went from point A to point B along specified tracts that did not vary. However, research indicates that the nociceptive system is "plastic"—changeable and variable between and within individuals, even to the same stimuli at different points in time (Anand & Carr, 1989). Many factors influence how the stimulus is transmitted, the path it takes, how it changes (or is modulated) along the way, and how the person perceives it.

Pain is a highly complex, dynamic, subjective process that is generally useful to the growing child. It warns the child of danger and serves to limit further injury. The rare child with congenital insensitivity to pain often suffers severe injury or infection because the child's early warning system does not function normally. Acute pain elicits a reflexive withdrawal, with physiologic, metabolic, and behavioral responses. In contrast, an individual tends to adapt to pain that is chronic in nature. Thus, the response to pain may be attenuated, but chronic pain is just as valid and debilitating to the child as acute pain.

Pain Impulse Transmission

The basic mechanisms of pain impulse transmission in children are similar to those of adults. A brief review is presented here, emphasizing the developmental and maturational changes that occur as they influence pain transmission and perception. For a more in-depth study of the pathophysiology of pain, the reader is referred to the numerous reviews that exist (Bonica, 1990; Wall & Melzack, 1989; Wallace, 1992).

Peripheral Transmission

Nerves, referred to as primary afferent fibers, transmit information about noxious stimuli from the periphery to the dorsal horn of the spinal cord (Fig. 13–1). The two types most involved in pain transmission are A delta and C fibers. A delta fibers are larger and myelinated; C fibers are smaller and unmyelinated and thus conduct more slowly. When these afferent fibers are excited by mechanical, thermal, or chemical stimuli to a sufficient degree, they depolarize and transmit the impulse to the dorsal horn of the spinal cord.

The "first pain" that occurs with injury is transmitted by the A delta fibers. It is sharp, localized, and stinging. The dull, aching "second pain" that occurs next is transmitted by the C fibers. A different group of afferent fibers, A beta, transmit low-intensity, mechanical information (e.g., touch, pressure) from the periphery. A beta fibers help regulate how the body responds to pain because the stimuli they carry compete with the incoming noxious stimuli and serve to decrease the number of noxious signals that get through. For example, ice applied to a bump on the head helps decrease the amount of pain the child feels. This is the basis of the gate control theory of pain (Melzack & Wall, 1965), which proposes that incoming benign stimuli (sensation of cold) reach the dorsal horn first and "close the gate" to the painful stimuli (head bump) trying to get through.

Depolarization of the fibers by the incoming messages activates the release of neurotransmitters. Neurotransmit-

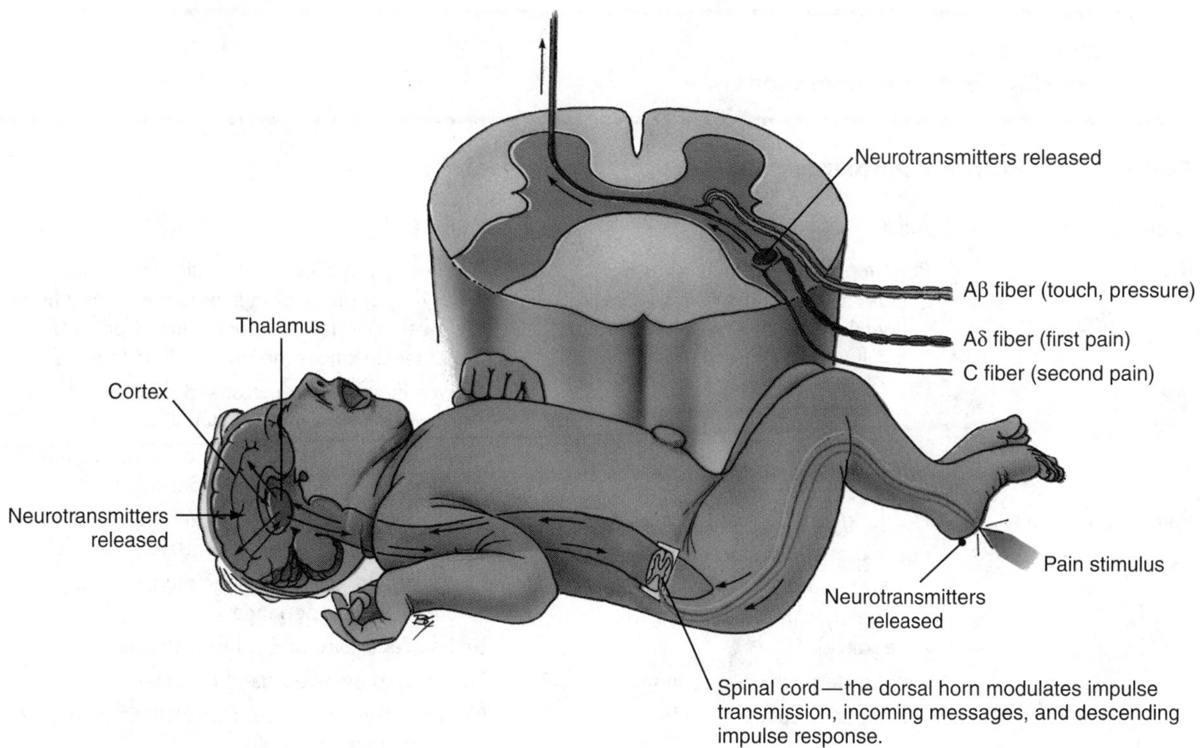

Figure 13–1
Transmission of pain impulse in an infant.

ters are chemical substances that mediate transmission of the pain impulse. They may be either excitatory or inhibitory. Some excitatory neurotransmitters are substance P, somatostatin, cholecystokinin, and neurotensin. Inhibitory substances are enkephalin, endorphins, and norepinephrine.

Central Transmission

All incoming information related to pain crosses the dorsal horn of the spinal cord on its entry into the central nervous system (CNS). This information excites secondary neurons in the spinal cord via neurotransmitters that carry the signals to the higher centers in the CNS. The CNS rapidly sends descending messages back through the dorsal horn. On the basis of the incoming and descending messages traveling through it, the dorsal horn modulates the organism's resulting response to the stimuli.

Developmental Patterns

Even premature infants have the physiologic structures in place to transmit pain impulses. The argument that lack of myelination makes pain impulse transmission difficult in children is invalid because it is known that adults transmit impulses over poorly myelinated or unmyelinated fibers (Chart 13–1). Any slower conduction rate related to lack of myelination is offset by the shorter interneuronal and neuromuscular distances that the impulse needs to travel (Anand & Carr, 1989).

The neonate transmits the pain impulse quite slowly and does not have the ability to inhibit the transmission (Fitzgerald & Anand, 1993). There are a number of reasons for this. C fibers transmit pain impulses from the periphery to spinal cord neurons, but these neurons do not transmit the signal well to higher brain centers. Thus, the signal stays in the system. Mechanisms that inhibit pain impulse transmission, neurotransmitters and receptors, are not mature in the neonate. There is a lack of precision in signal transmission, a lack of inhibition, and an increased chance of the stimulus persisting in the system. Therefore, it is likely that the neonate feels even more pain with the same stimulus than an adult would. Younger infants may also perceive pain more intensely than older children or adults because their descending control mechanisms are immature, limiting their ability to modulate the experience (McGrath & Craig, 1989).

It has been argued that infants cannot feel or remember pain because of cortical immaturity. There are several reasons to discount this argument. Functional ma-

Chart 13–1
Developmental Considerations

Contrasts in Pain Mechanisms

Characteristic	Adult	Young Child
Conduction	Pain impulses transmitted via nerves that have myelin sheaths (A delta fibers) and via nerves that are not myelinated (C fibers)	Myelination in process; A delta nerves have varying degrees of myelin present, may have slower conduction velocity that is offset by shorter distances the impulse has to travel Nerves in skin have increased density at birth, increasing sensitivity to stimuli Newborns may be deficient in neurotransmitters that inhibit pain impulse transmission
Perception of pain	Has language to express pain Past experience affects present situation Coping style in place (positive or negative) Able to deal with abstractions Understands cause and effect	Dependent on age, may be unable to verbalize pain in terms that adults understand Lack of control or unfamiliar situations may intensify pain experience Limited repertoire of coping methods Pain may be viewed as punishment Cannot understand cause and effect (medicine makes pain go away)

turity of the fetal cerebral cortex has been demonstrated by (1) electroencephalogram (EEG) patterns and cortical evoked potentials; (2) measurement of cerebral glucose utilization showing maximal metabolic rates in sensory areas of the brain, including the cortex; and (3) well-defined periods of sleep and wakefulness, regulated by cortical functioning, from 28 weeks' gestation (Anand & Carr, 1989). Therefore, the infant demonstrates functional cortical maturity, a component of pain perception and memory. Memory for pain may be inferred in infants who show changes in behavior after undergoing unanesthetized circumcision (Emde, Harmon, Metcalf, Koenig, & Wagonfeld, 1971; Richards, Bernal, & Brackbill, 1976). By 6 months of age infants start to show fear of painful situations (McGrath & Craig, 1989), thus demonstrating memory of painful events. It is probable that newborns also have the ability to remember painful events and react defensively (Dalla Barba et al., 1991).

The nervous system of a young child is still developing and malleable. It is important to remember that subjecting infants and young children to painful stimuli may permanently alter the way they transmit and process stimuli for the rest of their lives (Anand & Carr, 1989).

Effects of Acute Pain on Children

Although pain can be beneficial in warning the child of injury, the effects of pain are generally deleterious. Pain, in children of any age, evokes negative physiologic, metabolic, and behavioral responses. These include increased heart rate, respiratory rate, and blood pressure and increased secretion of catecholamines, glucagon, and corticosteroids (for more detailed discussion, see the section on assessing pain). Pain leads to anorexia, causing poor nutritional intake and delayed wound healing; impaired mobility; sleep disturbances; withdrawal; irritability; and developmental regression. Consequent to these responses, untreated pain affects length of convalescence and hospitalization. The body adapts to pain that is chronic; thus vital sign changes are usually not significant.

Pain has a significant impact on morbidity and mortality. Premature infants undergoing cardiac surgery who received less anesthesia had more postoperative complications and deaths than infants given deeper anesthesia (Anand & Hickey, 1992). Critically ill adults who reported greater pain intensity had an increased incidence of atelectasis as a postoperative complication (Puntillo & Weiss, 1994).

Pain is a major source of iatrogenic stress in prematurely born infants. To stabilize and deliver lifesaving care to premature infants, they are frequently subjected to stressful, invasive, and painful procedures. Unstable vital signs, particularly blood pressure, as a result of pain may result in additional complications such as intraventricular hemorrhage in the premature infant. The physiologic effects of pain result in a catabolic state that has the potential to be more damaging to infants and young children, who have higher metabolic rates and less nutritional reserves than adults. Medical and developmental outcomes can be improved by care delivery that recognizes early signs of stress and attempts to minimize stressful episodes (Als et al., 1986).

caREminder: *The nurse is in a key position to assess for cues indicating stress (e.g., gaze aversion, hiccups, yawning, flaccid posture) and physiologic instability (vital sign changes) resulting from pain. Interventions need to be implemented as appropriate for the situation, for example, allowing rest periods for the infant to regroup or stopping the procedure, giving pain medication, and providing physical boundaries and support.*

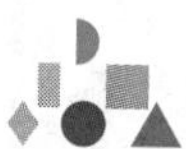

Factors That Influence the Pain Experience

Perception of pain may be positively or negatively influenced by the factors listed in Chart 13–2. These factors do not operate in isolation. They are listed separately for ease of discussion; all contribute in varying degrees to the totality of the pain experience. It is important to consider them when providing care and to remember that children react individually given their unique characteristics and situation.

Chart 13–2

Pain Perception in the Child—Influencing Factors

- Developmental level
  - Influences cognitive processing
- Type of injury or pain experience
  - Time (acute, chronic, recurrent)
  - Degree (extensive, minor injury)
  - Cause (traumatic, surgical, diagnostic test or treatment)
  - Meaning of or attitude toward pain
- Genetic characteristics
  - Varying levels of neurotransmitters
  - Varying response to medications
- Gender
  - Males may have higher pain tolerance, or it may be that it is more socially acceptable for females to express pain
- Temperament
  - Regular versus irregular patterns
  - Negative versus positive in mood and reactions
  - Ability to adapt to situations
  - Level of perseverance
- Social and cultural influence
  - Transmits accepted standards of behavior, how to react to and communicate pain (e.g., good to express pain, let it out, share with others; or do not express pain, accept it stoically, be brave, do not shame self and family by succumbing to pain)
- Individual coping style
  - Coping style (attender versus distracter)
  - Previous coping techniques learned (successful or not)
- Perception of control
  - Lack of control tends to intensify perceived pain.
- Achievement of secondary gains
  - Does the child gain anything from experiencing pain?
- Parents
  - Parental reaction to the child's situation influences the child's perception of and reaction to pain.

One cannot differentiate between these factors; all contribute to the totality of the child's unique response to the situation. Care must be taken to assess and treat pain on the basis of the individual child's response, not on possibly inaccurate stereotypical expectations.

Type of Pain Experience

Obviously, the severity of a physical injury plays a role in the pain experience. The more extensive the tissue damage, the greater the number of signals being transmitted through the nociceptive system. Exceptions to this occur with injuries in which nerve tissue has been destroyed, for example, severe burns or injuries resulting in paralysis.

The child experiencing pain may be able to cope for a time. The persistence of pain leading to sleep disturbances, depletion of inhibitory neurotransmitters, and activity limitation may reach a point at which the child feels as if the pain is in control, a feeling that exacerbates the pain. Conversely, children who learn techniques to control the pain may be able to minimize their perception of pain and thus feel a sense of mastery of the situation.

Pain that occurs interspersed between pain-free intervals is called recurrent pain; examples are colic, abdominal pain, limb pain, and headaches. Children with recurrent pain may also feel controlled by the pain. Their complaints are often labeled "psychosomatic." They differ from those with chronic persistent pain whose pain can often be traced back to surgical or physical injury. Recurrent pain may go untreated if adults discount the complaints from the child.

Psychological Factors

The meaning that the pain has for the child may affect the perception of it. For example, surgical pain after correction of a disfiguring birthmark might be better tolerated than surgical pain after removal of a cancerous tumor. The former may be considered positive and the latter more frightening and threatening.

The child's level of cognitive development affects the pain experience (Chart 13–3). How the pain is perceived influences both reaction to it and treatment options. In one study, older patients with juvenile rheumatoid arthritis reported higher levels of pain than younger ones (Beales, Keen, & Lennox Holt, 1983). The authors concluded that because of their greater insights into concepts of illness and disease, the older children were more

Chart 13–3
Developmental Considerations

Cognitive Level—Impact on the Pain Experience

It is important to remember that developmental gains build on each other and that children often regress when stressed. The behaviors that were achieved most recently are the first lost.

Infant

No words for pain
Has memory for painful events by 6 months, probably much earlier
Responds to parent's temperament (anxiety).

Toddler

Uses words for pain (e.g., owie, boo-boo, hurt)
Has developed object permanence
Egocentric; needs autonomy, sense of control

Preschooler

Has language to express pain but differs from an adult in how he or she understands the world, so words often misinterpreted
Often thinks he or she did something to incur pain as punishment
Mixes fact and fiction; has magical thinking
No cause-and-effect thinking
Beginning concept of time (medicine will start working when the television show is over)
Fears bodily injury or mutilation
Thinks the more blood there is, the worse the injury must be
Uses delays to put off treatments
Does better if can handle equipment and see how it works
Needs some control over situation

School-Age Child

Fears body mutilation
Has logical reasoning but needs to be related to concrete things
Beginning cause-and-effect understanding
Can delay gratification
Understands time
Relies less on parent and more on self-initiated coping resources

Adolescent

Understands abstractions
Needs to maintain self-esteem, control
Benefits from practice of nonpharmacologic techniques beforehand to maintain control
Feels omnipotent—nothing can harm him or her, so may not comply with treatment or medication regimens
Thinks that the nurse knows when pain medication is needed, so may not request this

able to consider the meaning and long-term consequences of this pain and thus reacted more, reporting higher pain levels.

The term "behavioral distress" has been used to refer to both children's pain and their anxiety because of the difficulty in distinguishing between the two by observation (Jay, Ozolins, Elliott, & Caldwell, 1983). The subjective feeling of pain may be intensified by anxiety and vice versa. Caution must be used when interpreting observations of pain, because behaviors may also reflect underlying emotions rather than directly reflecting the strength of the pain experienced.

Even if the child's cause of distress cannot be directly attributed to pain, interventions should be implemented. Psychological pain is just as important as physical pain. Children's overt signs of distress may be attenuated by distraction or having a calm parent to support the child.

Temperament has been described as the innate personality of the child that predisposes him or her to a certain behavioral style (Chess & Thomas, 1985). This is a relatively stable trait that correlates with the child's response to pain. "Difficult" children (intense, more negative in mood, poorly adaptable, irregular) were more prone to display distress behaviors (Schechter, Bernstein, Beck, Hart, & Scherzer, 1991) than "easy" children (adaptable, positive, regular patterns). More intense children also tended to receive more postoperative pain medications (Wallace, 1989). It has not been shown that temperament influences the actual intensity of the pain experience, but it does seem to influence the demonstration of pain behaviors.

Coping style, the strategies a child uses to cope with stressors, is another individual characteristic influencing pain. Examples of different coping styles are information seeking or avoiding and focusing attention toward or away from the painful stimuli (Fanurik, Zeltzer, Roberts, & Blount, 1993).

caREminder: *Coping style assumes particular importance when considering the type of pain reduction or coping intervention to use with a specific child. If there is a mismatch between coping style and intervention, the intervention may have reduced efficacy.*

Past experience with pain has an impact on present behavior. When previous situations have resulted in successful coping behaviors, the child is more likely to feel in control and respond in an adaptive manner. Fear and/or anxiety may intensify the perception of the pain, especially if previous experiences have been negative. Pain perception may also be intensified if the child has not had the experience before and has no coping skills to call upon. Noxious thermal stimuli have been shown to activate parts of the cortex of the brain and the area of the limbic system that is thought to control emotion, particularly anxiety (Talbot et al., 1991). This helps to explain the effectiveness of cognitive and behavioral strategies in helping children to cope with pain.

Biological Factors

Different ethnic groups may possess varying levels of neurotransmitters or respond to medications differently. These would influence how the person transmits, inhibits, and feels pain. Chinese children were reported to need less analgesia after burns than is common in children from Western countries (Hu, Zhang, & Chen, 1991). The authors hypothesized that this was due to different pain tolerance levels.

Gender may also influence pain manifestation (Faucett, Gordon, & Levine, 1994; Vallerand, 1995). Subtle sex differences have been found, such as girls requiring more time to calm after immunization than boys (Schechter et al., 1991). This may be due to biological differences or influenced by societal expectations. Many societies discourage boys from crying or demonstrating pain, whereas this behavior may be more tolerated in girls.

Cultural and Societal Factors

The majority of the research on how culture influences pain responses has been done with adults. Although it is logical that similarities exist in children's responses because of acculturation, research is needed to substantiate this. It should be noted that differences within a cultural group are often greater than those found between groups—reinforcing the point that beliefs about pain and responses to it are unique to the child.

Children are socialized in the social and cultural mores of their family system. As with other behaviors, parents teach a child how to express and respond to pain and methods that are helpful in pain relief (Villarruel & de Montellano, 1992) (Chart 13–4).

It has been suggested that different pain response patterns exist among various cultural groups. Italian and Jewish patients were more emotional and dramatic about their pain and usually uninhibited about communicating their distress. "Old Americans" (white Anglo-Saxons who had been in the United States for generations) and Irish patients were less expressive and emotional and wanted to hide their pain. The Irish also tended to deny pain (Zborowski, 1952). These differences may be due to physiologic differences or to socialization.

Few cross-cultural differences were found in pain descriptors of Asian American, Latin American, Arab American, and Dutch children (Abu-Saad, 1984a, 1984b, 1990). Children in the first three groups were all born in the United States and the interviews were done in English. Therefore, it might be assumed that the children

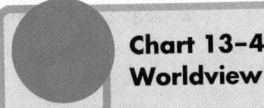

Chart 13-4
Worldview

A Sampling of Folk Beliefs About Causes and Remedies for Pain*

Chinese	*Belief:* Yin and yang. *Remedy:* Acupuncture.
Filipino	*Remedy:* Gather roots and herbs from the hinterland, mix with oil, and gently rub on painful area.
Indian	*Remedy:* Collect the dew from split pea plants and give a teaspoon for abdominal cramps.
Mexican American	*Belief:* Pain is a consequence of immoral behavior; in order to maintain equilibrium in body, want to maintain a balance between hot and cold; it is courageous and pious to endure pain stoically. *Remedy:* Sulfur and steam baths; bleeding (removes excess blood that causes headaches); herbs, tobacco, coconut, wormwood.
Native American	*Remedy:* Brewed tea with the bark of a willow tree to decrease the pain of headache.
Vietnamese	*Belief:* Sickness, evil spirits, or imbalances in life's elements cause pain; children older than 8 years should accept pain stoically and not be physically comforted, younger children may cry or complain but should not show any hurtful physical behavior (biting, kicking). *Remedy:* Balms, cupping, coining.
Zimbabwean	*Belief:* Pain (or, more generally, disease) is caused by displeasing ancestral spirits—"Vidzimu." *Remedy:* Traditional ceremonies to appease ancestral spirits; scarification ("Kutema nyora"), similar to acupuncture, around the painful area.
Remedies That Have Widespread Acceptance	Chicken soup, herb teas, tea with lemon and/or honey.

* See Chapter 3 for further explanation of some of these beliefs.

References: Fritz, K.I., Schechter, N., & Bernstein, B. (1991). Cultural components of pain behavior in Vietnamese refugee children. *Journal of Pain and Symptom Management, 6,* 205; Sonqishe, M., & Levy, L. (1990). Pain control in a patient with myeloma in Zimbabwe. *Cancer Nursing, 13,* 198–200; Villarruel, A., & Ortiz de Montellano, B. (1992). Culture and pain: A Mesoamerican perspective. *Advances in Nursing Science, 15,* 21–32.

were acculturated to the American lifestyle, which may have diluted any cultural differences.

A child (or parent) may be embarrassed when pain involves certain body systems such as the genitourinary (GU) system. Social and cultural taboos exist concerning this "private" area. Individuals of some cultures discuss GU problems only with health care providers of the same sex and/or if no one of the opposite sex, including a spouse, is in the room.

Tip: *Find out what words the child uses for genitalia, voiding, and stooling and use these words in questioning or discussion. Provide privacy and expose the area only as much as needed for assessment or treatments.*

It is unclear how culture or ethnicity influences responses to pain but care should be delivered in a culturally sensitive manner. Avoid stereotypes but be aware that cultural and individual factors influence a child's behavioral response to pain. Country of origin, often related to culture, may affect reaction to pain (Chart 13–5). Pain assessment should take all factors into account and the treatment plan should accommodate cultural beliefs as much as possible.

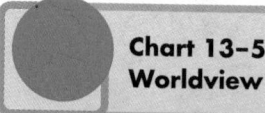

Chart 13–5
Worldview

Pain Reactions in Various Cultures

Algeria, Bahrain, Egypt, Iraq, Kuwait, Morocco, Saudi Arabia, Tunisia
Request or expect immediate pain relief; express pain only to relatives, close friends.

Cambodia, Laos, Vietnam
May not request relief until pain is severe.

China
Pain may not be demonstrated because showing emotion is considered a weakness; may need to offer interventions more than once because it is not polite to accept something the first time.

India
Acceptance of pain, may allow some pain interventions.

Ireland
Stoic, do not express pain.

Korea
Stoic, may display no facial expression.

Mexico
Stoic, may express pain in order to relieve it, may refuse pain interventions as a method of atonement.

Philippines
Stoic, may believe pain is God's will and God will help them endure.

Turkey
Pain is a part of life to be tolerated.

Reaction to pain and expression of it vary between countries; this is a sampling based on information from Geissler, E. M. (1994). *Pocket guide to cultural assessment.* St. Louis: Mosby–Year Book. Refer to this for more complete discussion.

Sense of Control

Feelings of lack of control may intensify the pain experience. When something is being done to (versus done with) a child, the child has no power. This exacerbates fear and anxiety, thus amplifying the pain experience. Many of the cognitive-behavioral techniques for pain reduction (relaxation, deep breathing, distraction) work because they reduce anxiety and fear and increase the child's sense of control or mastery over the situation. Children who have a perception of control over a situation and are involved in it respond with more adaptive behaviors (Ellis & Spanos, 1994). For example, the child who helps remove bandages often tolerates a painful dressing change better than one who is restrained and has the procedure done to his or her body.

Secondary Gains

Another psychological factor to consider when evaluating the pain experience is that of secondary gains. Does the child gain anything from reporting pain? Does she or he get to miss school or other activities, get more attention, or have other such secondary benefits? If so, this may influence the perceived intensity of the pain.

Parental Influence

Separation from parents is a stressor for children and may intensify the pain experience. Separating a child from a parent results in the well-known "separation anxiety" manifested by often dramatic behavioral demonstrations. Separation anxiety generally occurs between 9 and 12 months of age and often extends to 5 years of age in a stressful situation such as one involving pain. Older children state that what helps them cope in painful situations is parental presence (Watt-Watson, Evernden, & Lawson, 1990). Whenever possible, the parent should be present to support the child.

The parents' perception and handling of the situation strongly influence the child's perception of the pain and reaction to it. There is a relationship between parental anxiety and increased distress in the child (Jay et al., 1983). Parents should be carefully prepared for what will happen to the child so that they can help the child to cope (TIP 13–1). When prepared, parents often choose to stay with the child because they feel that they may be helpful, not in the way (Watt-Watson et al., 1990). The child may display more distress behaviors with the parent present. This behavior should not be taken as a negative sign. The child may feel more comfortable in displaying these signals of distress to the parent (Shaw & Routh, 1982). Expression of feelings is known to be a positive coping strategy.

Factors That Influence Health Care Team Decisions

Assessment and treatment decisions made by the health care team affect the adequacy of pain management. Children are often undermedicated and pain management is suboptimal (Altimier, Norwood, Dick, Holditch-Davis, & Lawless, 1994).

TIP 13–1 A Teaching Intervention Plan for Parents of a Child Undergoing a Painful Procedure

Nursing Diagnosis and Family Outcomes

- Knowledge deficit: supporting the child undergoing a painful procedure

  Outcomes:

  Child will be supported by family during painful procedure.

  Parents/family members will discuss interventions they can implement to support the child during a painful procedure.

Interventions

Include the parents when teaching the child about the procedure.

Speak with the parents after teaching, not in the child's presence:

- Clarify interpretations of what was taught.
- Correct misconceptions.
- Discuss how the child may respond before, during, and after the procedure.

Discuss how parents can help the child cope; give concrete, specific, and developmentally appropriate suggestions for how they can assist their child:

- Hold the child's hand.
- Speak in a low soothing tone, maintain eye contact with the child.
- Touch other parts of the child's body depending on the child's preference (firm touch, pressure, stroking).
- Keep the child informed of the procedure's progress (e.g., "It's half over now").
- Assist the child with previously practiced relaxation techniques (e.g., deep breathing, counting).
- Use distraction (e.g., blow bubbles, read stories).
- Use positive reinforcement of desired behaviors (e.g., "You are breathing so deep"; "You are holding your hand so still").
- Avoid threats, such as painful procedures (e.g., injections), in an attempt to get the child to behave.

Give the parents the option to stay with their child during the procedure:

- Reinforce that parental presence is for support of their child, not for restraint.
- If the parents opt not to stay, reassure them that someone will be there to provide support for the child.

Nursing and medicine both contribute to the problem of suboptimal pain management. Physicians tend to order inadequate amounts and occasionally inaccurate doses of pain medications to be given on an as-needed basis (Schechter, Allen, & Hanson, 1986). Nurses tend to undermedicate by not administering dosages (Hester, Foster, Kristensen, & Bergstrom, 1989) or administer at the longest dosing interval. Nurses often choose the lowest opioid dose or administer non-narcotic analgesics (Gadish, Gonzales, & Hayes, 1988). Many health care providers do not recognize subtle pain behaviors in children such as lying quietly, poor appetite, clinging to parents, or disturbed sleep patterns. Thus, these children are not treated for pain.

Increased education and research regarding children's pain within the past two decades may be heightening awareness of this issue, but inappropriate utilization of pain medication continues to be a problem (Tesler, Wilkie, Holzemer, & Savedra, 1994). One survey found that 87% of 150 hospitalized children, 4 to 14 years old, reported pain during the previous 24 hours (Johnston, Abbott, Gray-Donald, & Jeans, 1992). Analgesics were administered to only 38% of these children. Another study of 24 school-age children's experience with postoperative pain showed a more positive trend. All children received some analgesia, usually narcotics, given postoperatively (Alex & Ritchie, 1992). This demonstrates a more liberal use of medications than previous research had found. Children in the study still reported a high prevalence of moderate to severe pain, indicating further need for improving pain management.

There remain inconsistencies between nurses' attitudes toward pain management and actual clinical practice. Several factors such as demographic variables, nursing education, patient age, and years of nursing experience have been investigated as influencing pain management decisions, often with conflicting results.

Burokas (1985) found that demographics such as age, educational preparation, and personal pain experience did not significantly influence nurses' decisions when medicating children. There were differences in medication practices related to the practice setting (neonatal intensive care unit [ICU], pediatric ICU, or surgical unit). Treatment decisions were influenced by having offspring who had experienced pain and by the nurses' goal of pain relief (Burokas, 1985). Conversely, other researchers found that personal pain experience did influence their assessment of patients experiencing pain (Holm, Cohen, Dudas, Medema, & Allen, 1989). Bradshaw and Zeanah (1986) found few differences in nurses' pain assessment related to years of experience or type of practice setting. Nurses with higher levels of education demonstrated the most insight concerning pain management (Margolius, Hudson, & Michel, 1995). Nurses' answers to questionnaires about their beliefs and nursing practice regarding pain did not coincide with actual assessment and treatment behaviors (Burokas, 1985; Gadish et al., 1988).

Nurses need to identify their own feelings and preparation when assuming responsibility for appropriate pain assessment and management in children and to recognize how these factors may affect their clinical practice in effectively addressing and alleviating pain. The priority the nurse places on pain relief influences how well the patient's pain relief needs are met.

caREminder: *Pain management is a major facet of nursing care. This needs to be recognized as a priority and time allotted for appropriate assessment and management of pain.*

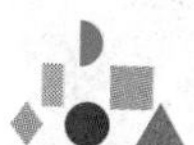

Assessing Pain in Children

At present, there is no easily administered, widely accepted, uniform technique for assessing pain in children, particularly infants, although it is an area of active research. Assessment techniques can be classified as subjective reports, physiologic monitoring, and behavioral observations. Assessments that use a combination of the three usually result in the most accurate appraisal of pain. Factors that influence the pain experience must be considered, a pain history obtained, and expectations for pain relief discussed with both the child and parents or caregivers.

It is optimal if the child and family can be introduced to the selected method of pain assessment before they are experiencing pain (e.g., preoperatively). This gives them a chance to incorporate the concept and practice under conditions of reduced stress. It also provides information regarding the child's baseline pain level. If the assessment method does not seem to be appropriate, another can be introduced. Once an acceptable method is chosen, this method should be the one that is consistently used. It is confusing to the child, family, and health team if, for example, at different times a 6-point scale (0 being no pain, 5 the most pain you could have) is used and at other times an 11-point scale or different method is used. Lack of consistency makes it difficult to assess effectiveness of management or patient improvement.

Subjective Reports of Pain

Pain is a subjective experience. Thus, self-report of pain is a critical component in pain assessment. Subjective reports of pain may include verbalizations or nonverbal reports such as coloring the parts that hurt on a body outline tool. Children in pain have consistently reported that needles and shots are what they fear the most (Broome, 1985; Eland, 1985). They may deny having pain to avoid an injection. This fear may influence the data gathered during assessment.

Tip: *To increase the accuracy of assessment data, the nurse should implement anticipatory interventions such as telling the child that medicine to make the pain go away is given through an intravenous (IV) tube.*

If this is not the case, and intramuscular (IM) injections are ordered, the nurse should consult the health care provider ordering the IM injection to discuss changing to another route, according to current practice guidelines (Acute Pain Management Guideline Panel, 1992).

A low correlation was found between mothers' (Stein, 1995) and nurses' judgments of children's pain and the children's self-reports of pain (Rømsing, Møller-Sonnergaard, Hertel, & Rasmussen, 1996; Teske, Daut, & Cleeland, 1983). Assessment of the child's pain by the mother correlated more with the child's self-report than did the nurse's assessment (Miller, 1996). Correlation of nurses' and children's pain ratings was even lower when there was a discrepancy between the patient's report and nonverbal behavior, such as often occurs in chronic pain. Nurses rated pain as less intense when no signs of pathology were present and when it was of long-term duration (Taylor, Skelton, & Butcher, 1984), thus not identifying this pain as readily as acute pain or viewing it as being as significant as acute pain. Although assessing chronic pain requires different techniques than assessing acute pain, this difference may not be reflected in actual practice.

Infants

Infants are preverbal and thus cannot communicate their pain in words. Therefore, reliance on physiologic monitoring and behavioral observations and maintenance of a high index of suspicion about the presence of pain are necessary. The parent may be able to aid the nurse in obtaining a subjective report of the infant's pain.

Toddlers and Preschoolers

A common myth is that if a child does not report pain or request pain relief, the child does not have pain. Pain is an abstract concept. Toddlers, preschool children, and younger school-age children are limited by their cognitive abilities in localizing and expressing pain intensity, understanding reasons for the pain, and effectively using internal and external cues to cope (Broome, 1985). Toddlers and preschoolers may not understand the word pain but can report "hurt," "owie" (Eland, 1985), "boo-boo," or "ouch." It is important to find out what words the child uses to describe pain and to use these terms during interactions with the child.

Because toddlers and preschoolers do not comprehend abstractions, they may be able to indicate where their pain is but not be able to describe its intensity. If they are having difficulty localizing the pain, it may be helpful to tell them to point to their pain (using the child's term for it) with just one finger or have them show you where they would need a bandage placed.

Preschoolers, depending on developmental maturity, may be able to localize their pain using a body outline tool, originally developed by Eland (1981) (Table 13–1). This tool consists of a line drawing of a child showing both front and back (Fig. 13–2). Often, hair and genitals are not included and the facial features are drawn so as not to represent a specific gender or ethnicity. The body outline may be used by having the child either make an X where the pain is or color the body. Colors may be used to indicate pain intensity. The child can be given six to eight crayons and instructed to arrange them in order by color representing the most hurt to no hurt. Although there is individual variation in pain color choices, children often pick red, black, or purple to indicate severe pain (Abu-Saad, 1981). The child then colors the body outline using the selected colors to indicate

Table 13–1
Self-Report Methods for Pain Assessment

Method	Description	Comments
Direct questioning *Measures pain location, intensity, qualities* Age: children as young as 2–3 yr	Ask the child, using his or her word for pain, if he or she has pain, how the pain feels, where it is, when it occurs, and what helps relieve it; children who understand numeric value can rate pain on a 0–10 scale (0 being no pain, 10 the worst pain you could have)	Verbalizations by the child are the best marker of the subjective experience of pain; in nonverbal children, parents should be questioned; advantages to using a 0–10 rating scale are that it requires no equipment and is quick to administer
Adolescent Pediatric Pain Tool (APPT) *Measures pain location, intensity, and quality* Age: 8–17 yr	Consists of a front and back body outline, a 100-mm word-graphic rating scale, and a pain descriptor list	Evaluates three components of pain, so should provide a more precise description than a method that evaluates only one component
Body outline tool (originally developed by Eland) *Measures pain location and intensity (if colors are ranked)* Age: 4 yr and older	Line drawing of child's body, unclothed, non–gender specific, front and back; child marks an X or colors the painful area; colors can be ranked in order of increasing pain intensity before coloring	Young children may reverse right and left sides, front and back of body; validate responses and color choices with the child

Table 13–1
Self-Report Methods for Pain Assessment *Continued*

Method	Description	Comments
Faces *Measures amount of pain* Age: children as young as 3 yr	Cartoon drawings or pictures ranging from no pain to crying (intense pain); the child chooses the picture that is most like how he or she is feeling at that time	Quick to administer and does not require verbal responses
Oucher (original Caucasian version developed by Beyer) *Measures amount of pain* Age: photographs as young as 3 yr, generally school-age and older children can use numeric scale	Six photographs depict a young child's facial expression of no hurt to the biggest hurt you could ever have; children point to the picture that most closely approximates their own level of discomfort; also has numerical 0–100 scale	Three versions have been developed to accommodate for cultural bias—Caucasian, African American, and Hispanic versions; to use the numeric scale must be able to understand sequencing and numeric value (able to count to 100 by ones)
Pain diary *Evaluates various aspects of the pain experience* Age: children who can write and record events	Child records events preceding pain onset, precipitating factors, rates the severity, activity level, events out of the ordinary that occurred; may also record medications or psychological techniques used	Inexpensive to use; information is recorded shortly after it happens so should not be subjected to recollection distortion; child is actively involved in managing pain, which contributes to a sense of control; information obtained is not as structured as in other methods, may obtain superfluous data; subject to the child's biases
Poker Chip Tool (developed by Hester) *Measures amount of pain* Age: 4½–13 yr (probably older)	Four red poker chips represent "pieces of hurt"; child chooses chips from 0 (no hurt) up to 4 (most hurt you could have)	Good for preschool children—concrete, simple to use, and resembles a toy, so is nonthreatening; easy to carry and disinfect; nonverbal response (intubated patients, language barrier)
Varni-Thompson Pediatric Pain Questionnaire *Measures pain intensity, quality, location and sensory, affective, and evaluative aspects of pain perception* Age: 8 yr and older	Has child, adolescent, and parent forms that use a selection of (1) VAS, (2) color-coded scale and body outline, (3) pain descriptors to circle, (4) questions about family history and socioenvironmental influences	Designed to assess chronic, recurrent pain; applicability to other pain syndromes is being investigated (e.g., sickle cell disease); does provide detailed history but is somewhat lengthy for routine clinical use
Visual Analogue Scale (VAS) *Measures amount of pain* Age: children as young as 4½ yr	A single horizontal or vertical line, typically 10 cm long, anchored by descriptors of pain at each end, such as "absent" to "severe"; child marks the line at any point on the continuum to indicate pain intensity	Sometimes constructed with hash marks at equal intervals (a true VAS contains no markings between the anchors), which adds a numeric dimension to the tool; 10-cm line shows smaller measurement error than length of 5 or 20 cm (Seymour, Simpson, Charlton, & Phillips, 1985); can be a vertical or horizontal scale

All responses require careful validation with the child.
Recommended ages are for cognitive age of the individual (developmentally delayed, mentally retarded).
It has been suggested that, of these methods, only the Poker Chip Tool, Oucher, and the Adolescent Pediatric Pain Tool have undergone enough testing to demonstrate reliability and validity (Hester, 1993).

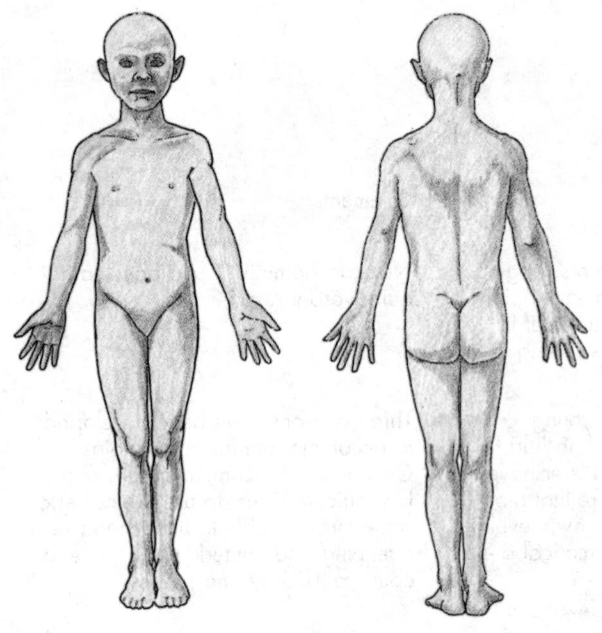

Figure 13–2
Body outline pain assessment tool.

areas of hurt. One may discover unanticipated information, such as that a nasogastric (NG) tube hurts more than an abdominal incision. Thus, the drawing has the potential to provide a depth of information about the child's pain and pain perception. Coloring on serial outlines may help track the trajectory of the pain, which is particularly useful with children dealing with chronic pain.

The Poker Chip Tool helps children 4½ to 13 years old describe the intensity of their pain. Children are given four poker chips and told that one chip is a little bit of hurt and four is the most hurt they could have (Hester, 1979). They are then instructed to pick the number of pieces of hurt that they have. A few different self-report scales have been developed that use cartoon drawings or pictorial representations of faces depicting varying degrees of discomfort or pain (Beyer, Denyes, & Villarruel, 1992; Kuttner & LePage, 1989; Wong & Baker, 1988) (Fig. 13–3). The Oucher (Fig. 13–4) combines pictures with a vertical visual analogue scale so it can be used with both preschool and school-age children, 3 to 12 years of age (Knott et al., 1994). Examples of visual analogue scales are shown in Figure 13–5.

Worldview: *Tools used to assess pain should be appropriate for race as well as age. African American and Hispanic versions of the Oucher have been developed and tested for reliability and validity. Chinese characters are read vertically downward and from right to left. Thus, horizontally oriented scales are probably less appropriate for this population. Vertically oriented visual analogue scales give more reliable results (Aun, Lam, & Collett, 1986).*

School-Age Children

School-age children begin to have the ability to communicate pain in the more abstract terms that adults use. They are able to communicate effectively concerning their pain and generate excellent descriptors of pain such as squeezing, stabbing, and burning (Ross & Ross, 1984). School-age children can describe the pain they have and can list things that help alleviate their pain (Savedra, Gibbons, Tesler, Ward, & Wegner, 1982).

School-age children usually respond to direct questioning regarding their pain. Use of projective techniques such as the body outline tool, face scales, Poker Chip Tool, visual analogue scale, and Oucher is also effective (see Table 13–1). Often, older children use the pictures of the Oucher as a cue and then refer to the corresponding numerical value to report intensity, but the two scales are not interchangeable (Knott et al., 1994).

Children with chronic pain present their own unique assessment challenges. The Varni-Thompson Pediatric Pain Questionnaire was first used to assess chronic pain in children with juvenile rheumatoid arthritis (Varni, Thompson, & Hanson, 1987). It uses a variety of methods to provide a comprehensive pain assessment (see Table 13–1). Pain symptom diaries may provide useful information, particularly in assessment of chronic pain. The reason for collecting information should be identified so that the child can focus the narrative. For example, if the aim is to identify the etiology of recurrent pain, the child should record events preceding pain onset, precipitating factors, and so forth. If the goal is to evaluate effectiveness of ongoing management, the child may record medications or psychological techniques used, record activity level, and rate the intensity at specified intervals during the day.

Adolescents

The expanding cognitive abilities of adolescents should enable them to understand abstractions and describe pain

Figure 13–3
Faces pain rating scale. (Redrawn from Whaley, L., & Wong, D. [1987]. *Nursing care of infants and children* [3rd ed., p. 1070]. St. Louis: Mosby. Used with permission.)

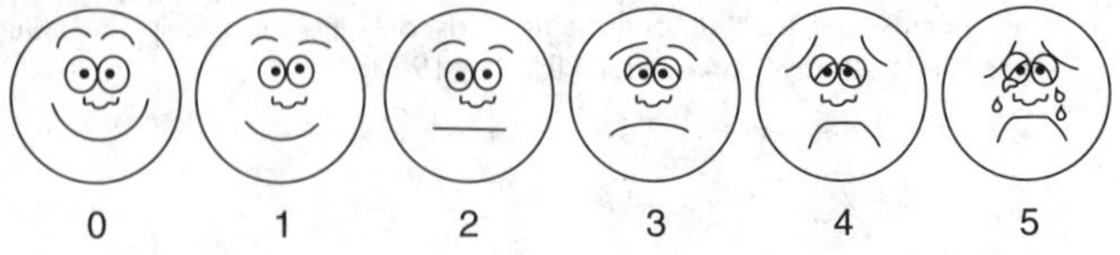

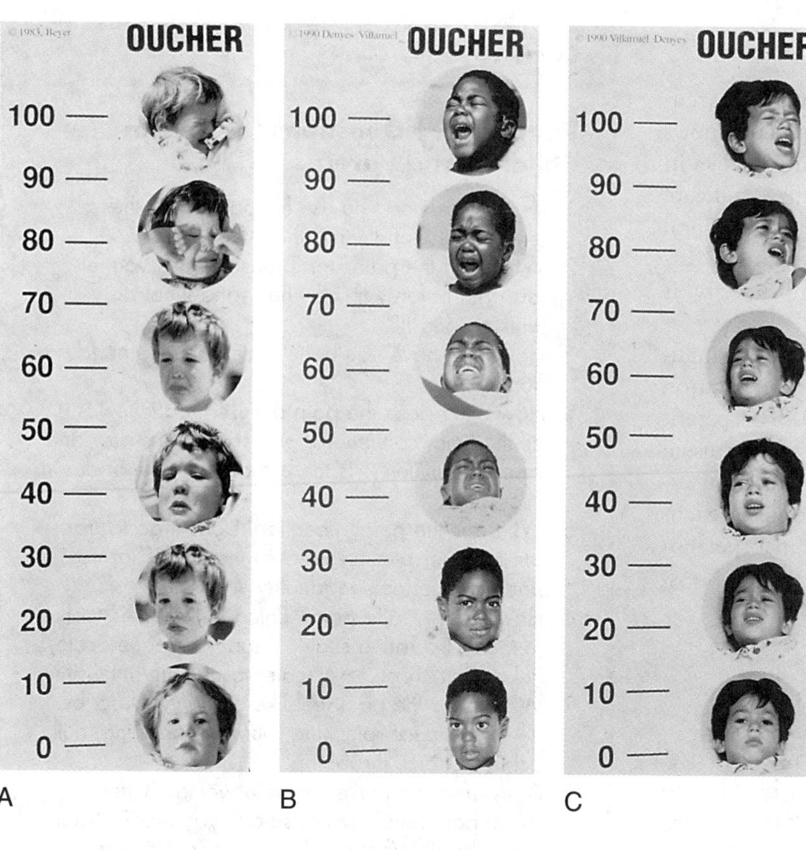

Figure 13–4
The Oucher pain assessment tool: (A) Caucasian version; (*B*) black version; (C) Hispanic version. (*A*, Developed and copyrighted by Judith E. Beyer, R.N., Ph.D., 1983; *B*, developed and copyrighted by Mary J. Denyes, Ph.D., R.N., and Antonia M. Villarruel, Ph.D., R.N., 1990; C, developed and copyrighted by Antonia M. Villarruel, Ph.D., R.N., and Mary J. Denyes, Ph.D., R.N., 1990. Used with permission.)

in adult terms. Adolescents may not verbalize that pain is being experienced. This may happen because they think the nurse knows they are in pain (Favaloro & Touzel, 1990) and will do something if and when it can be done (e.g., giving medications), so nothing is said. Adolescents may also be afraid to say they are in pain because their peers and/or parents may consider them to be "babies." Fear of addiction is another factor that may play a role in children, adolescents, and parents not verbalizing or denying offers of medications.

Tip: *The nurse should explain that narcotic use for moderate to severe pain will not lead to addiction (Schechter, 1989), the psychological craving for the drug. Physical dependence can be managed by tapering the drug. The difference between "good drugs" and "bad drugs" can be discussed and that "say no to drugs" does not apply to analgesics given for pain and monitored by the health care team.*

Many of the self-report tools employed with school-age children may be suitable for use with adolescents. These include face scales, the Poker Chip Tool, 0 to 10 rating scales, and visual analogue scales. A body outline tool may not only provide valuable information about the adolescent's pain but also give an outlet for expression of fears regarding body image. The Adolescent Pediatric Pain Tool has been developed especially for this age group (see Table 13–1). Older adolescents may be able to use the McGill Pain Questionnaire developed for use with adults (Melzack, 1983).

One should remember that pain, when combined with the other stressors of rapid physical and psychological change that an adolescent undergoes, may cause regression. This impairs coping abilities, and the adolescent (younger child and even adult) may not function at the level at which she or he did previously. The potential for regression should be recognized when selecting assessment methods for any age. If the individual is functioning at a less sophisticated developmental level, assessment methods should be chosen as appropriate for this lower level.

Figure 13–5
Visual analogue scales: true VAS *(top)*; numeric VAS *(bottom)*.

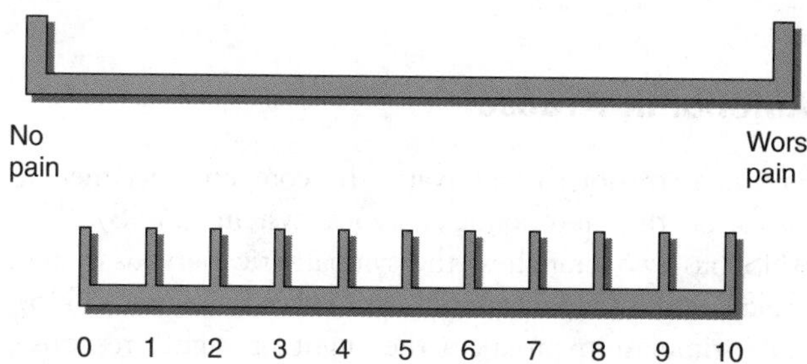

Parents

It is important to solicit parental input to increase accuracy of the assessment (Chart 13–6). The parent knows the child's normal behaviors and can be invaluable in detecting and interpreting changes that may indicate pain. These assessments might be classified as behavioral observations, but they are susceptible to the parent's interpretations and biases, so a degree of subjectivity is inevitable.

Parental appraisal of the child's pain may be influenced by the parents' perception of their own preparation for a procedure (Watt-Watson et al., 1990). The parent is also a good resource when assessing the child's usual coping style, which has a later impact on planning decisions regarding nonpharmacologic interventions. Teaching parents about children's pain cues and management strategies can further add to the precision of the assessment process.

Chart 13–6

Pain History Questions for Verbal Children and Parents

1. What words do you use for pain? (Use these terms when conducting the interview.)
2. When did the pain start? *(onset)* Have you felt this pain before? If so, when, and what do you think caused it?
3. How long have you been feeling this pain? *(duration)*
4. How often does the pain occur? *(frequency)* Is it all the time *(continuous)* or just happens now and then *(intermittent)*? Is there a certain time of day it occurs?
5. Where is the pain? *(location)* Does it go to *(radiate to)* other places? Point to the area(s) or use body outline tools to identify site.
6. How severe is the pain? *(intensity)* Use this tool (e.g., 0–10 rating scale, Visual Analogue Scale, Poker Chip Tool, face scale) to quantify intensity.
7. What does the pain feel like? *(quality)* Describe it—for instance, pinching, burning, stabbing, dull, aching, sharp, throbbing.
8. Does anything make the pain worse? Better? What pain relief methods have you tried? What works best? What would you do/not do again?
9. How does the pain affect you? Can you put the pain out of your mind and carry on normal activities of daily living? Or does the pain keep you from doing things you want to do?

Physiologic Monitoring

Several physiologic parameters have been investigated as pain indices. These include heart rate (HR), blood pressure (BP), transcutaneous oxygen levels, palmar sweating, and hormone levels. Most are thought to reflect a global response to stress, crying, or handling or positioning for procedures and, although giving an indication of physiologic status, are not necessarily specific to pain. Changes in these parameters most likely include components of anxiety, fear, or anger. Because of this, it may be that these indices are more valid pain indicators in young infants (whose pain may not be influenced by fear, anger, or anxiety). As the child matures, with increasing cognition, language skills, and control over behavioral manifestations, these other parameters may assume primary importance while physiologic indices become secondary.

caREminder: *Assessment of pain is most accurate if it is multidimensional.*

Persistent pain results in the body adapting to it, with a gradual stabilization of autonomic responses. Therefore, depending primarily on physiologic indices (which have since stabilized) may result in lack of recognition of many instances of pain.

Autonomic Arousal

Pain is a stressor that activates the compensatory mechanisms of the autonomic nervous system (ANS). The ANS has two branches: the sympathetic nervous system (SNS) and the parasympathetic nervous system (PNS). SNS stimulation produces the "fight or flight" response, which results in tachycardia, peripheral vasoconstriction, diaphoresis, pupil dilation, and increased secretion of catecholamines as well as adrenocortical, thyroid, and pancreatic hormones.

Other signs of autonomic arousal are found in response to painful stimuli (Fig. 13–6). Respiratory rate, systolic blood pressure, transcutaneous oxygen ($TcPO_2$) levels (Brown, 1987), heart rate, and intracranial pressure (Stevens & Johnston, 1994) have been found to increase with painful stimuli. Conversely, decreased respiratory rate, oxygen saturation, and $TcPO_2$ levels have also been noted in response to pain (Craig, Whitfield, Grunau, Linton, & Hadjistavropoulos, 1993). When assessing changes in vital signs, it is important to consider how they are related and how other factors such as the child's position, fear, and anxiety and medications given may affect the parameters being evaluated.

Research yields conflicting results, possibly because of differences in measurement, populations, and pain situations. Vital sign changes may be seen as a general reaction to physiologic stress rather than as specific to pain. Vital sign changes should be used as an indicator of

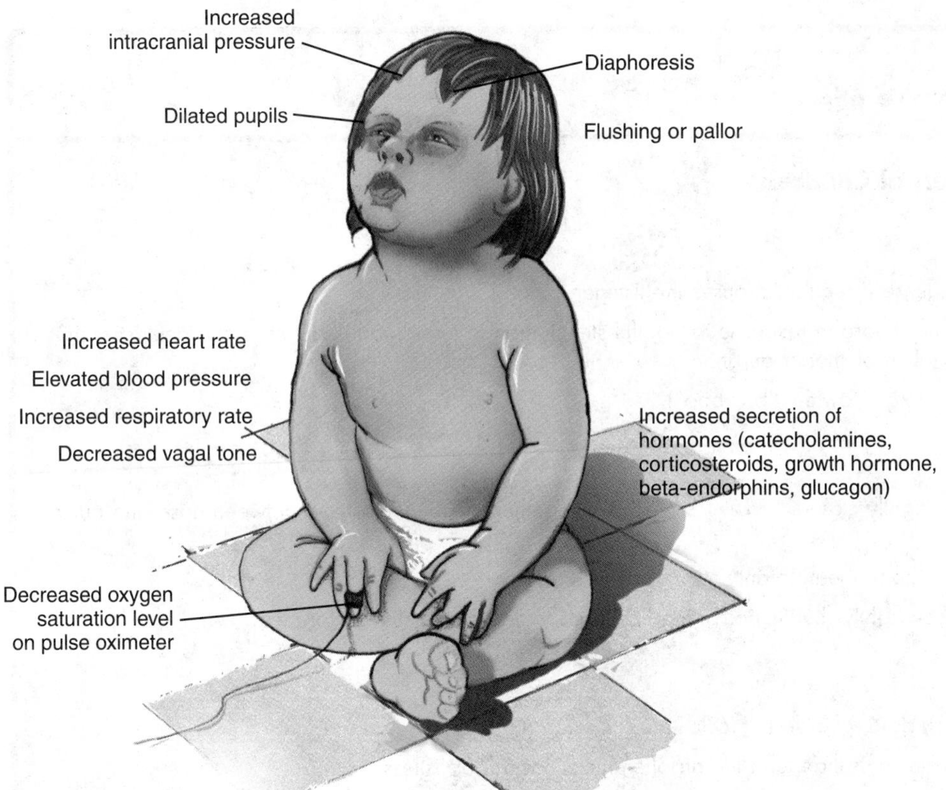

Figure 13–6
Physiologic responses to acute pain.

response with consideration given to the child's situation, behavior, and subjective reports.

Dilated pupils, another sign of autonomic arousal, may also be found in response to pain. Pupil size can be used as a component of pain assessment and as a barometer for adequacy of treatment (e.g., small or decreased pupil size may indicate that the interventions were effective, and dilated pupils may signal untreated pain).

The PNS reaction to a painful stimulus is mediated through the vagus nerve and is thought to be reflected in vagal tone. Computer analysis of the electrocardiogram generates a value for vagal tone by measuring the amplitude of respiratory sinus arrhythmia. Respiratory sinus arrhythmia is defined as the slowing of the heart rate during expiration and increasing of the rate during inspiration. Vagal tone is a physiologic measure that may be a reliable index of pain.

Vagal tone decreases with increasing invasiveness of a painful procedure (Porter, Porges, & Marshall, 1988). Resting vagal tone may be predictive for magnitude of response. Infants with higher resting values showed a greater magnitude of change from baseline during circumcision than infants with lower resting vagal tones (Porter et al., 1988). The infants who seemed to react more may be at greater risk for adverse outcomes in response to painful procedures. These adverse outcomes may include fluctuation in vital signs, crying, and hypoxic episodes that potentially contribute to the occurrence of intraventricular hemorrhage. This has implications for preemptive pain management, that is, treating pain before it causes detrimental effects. If children who will have a more detrimental response are identified, more aggressive treatment can be implemented to avert negative outcomes. The technique for measuring vagal tone is used in pain research but is currently too cumbersome to be used clinically.

Hormonal or Metabolic Responses

Hormonal and metabolic changes have been demonstrated in premature and term infants undergoing the stress of lightly anesthetized surgery. There is increased secretion of catecholamines, growth hormones, beta-endorphins, glucagon, cortisol, and other corticosteroids (Anand, Hansen, & Hickey, 1990; Anand & Hickey, 1987). This results in the breakdown of carbohydrate and fat stores, leading to marked hyperglycemia and lactic acidosis. Hormonal and metabolic responses were decreased in infants given more potent anesthetic agents. The lightly anesthetized infants also had significantly increased postoperative mortality and morbidity.

Neuroendocrine hormone response is closely correlated with the immune system response. Psychological and physical stress has been shown to depress immune responsiveness, which can be associated with an increased incidence of infections (Cohen, Tyrrell, & Smith, 1991; Hauser, Chan, Casey, Midgley, & Holbrook, 1991).

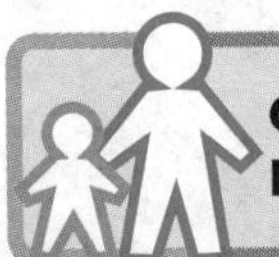

Chart 13–7
Developmental Considerations

Pain Indicators in Preverbal Children*

Verbalizations

Term Infant. Cry: high pitched, tense, irregular, arouses the listener

Preterm Infant. Cry: less frequently heard in response to painful stimuli than in term infant; has more characteristics that arouse listener, higher pitched, often of shorter duration

Toddler. Cry, pet terms for pain (e.g., "owie," "boo-boo")

Facial Expression

Term Infant. Pain grimace (eyes tightly closed, brows lowered and together, deepened furrow between nose and outer corner of lip)

Preterm Infant. Weaker grimace than in term infant

Toddler. Grimace, clenched teeth, tightly shut lips or biting lips, eyes wide open, wrinkled forehead

Body Movement

Term Infant. Withdrawal of limb, rigid, guarded, flaccid

Preterm Infant. Less vigorous movements than term infant; often limp, flaccid, or listless

Toddler. Self-limited movement, flexed or rigid extremities, guarding of painful area, restless (flailing, kicking, rolling head side to side, frequent position changes), touching or pointing to painful area, aggressive actions (biting, hitting, pushing caregiver)

Physiologic Changes

In an unstable child, you may just see greater instability:

↑ HR, RR, shallow respirations

↑ ICP

↓ oxygen saturation

↑ or ↓ BP

Dilated pupils

Diaphoresis

Behavior

Infants. Change in sleep patterns, may see more or less sleep; irritable, unable to comfort; avoidance of eye contact

Toddlers. Same behaviors as in infants, plus changes in activity level, anger, self-consolation (e.g., "rub my tummy," rubbing own tummy)

Parental Input

How do the parents perceive their child's level of comfort? Is this typical behavior? What are the changes? Does anything help alleviate the pain?

* Keep in mind that the context in which the painful event is experienced affects the response; for example, if the infant is in a deep sleep state, often see less vigorous response to stimuli; severely ill children often show less vigorous movements and a greater variability (greater changes, wider ranges) in physiologic parameters.

Hormonal and metabolic responses are quite variable and none has been shown to be a definitive measure of pain. In the current state of technological development, measurement of hormonal response is invasive and expensive and results are not immediately available, so assessment of these is not appropriate for clinical decisions regarding pain management.

Behavioral Observations

Infants

In the absence of precise physiologic measures and a self-report of pain in the infant, other indices of pain such as behavioral observations must be used. Cry patterns, facial expressions, and body movements have been investigated as behavioral measures of infant pain (Chart 13–7).

Crying is a behavior that is one of the most widely accepted indicators of pain in infants (Porter, 1993). The cry of an infant generally evokes a response in its caretaker. This may be evolutionary in that a cry signal from an infant elicits a response from the caretaker that ensures survival of the species. A pain cry is high pitched, tense, and irregular and arouses the listener. Cry has been experimentally analyzed for frequency, pitch, oscillation, and other characteristics using a spectrograph. Researchers have been able to distinguish cries associated with pain from other cries such as those associated with stress and discomfort (Levine & Gordon, 1982). Unfortunately, spectrographic analysis of cry requires training and the equipment is not readily available in the clinical area and is costly; therefore it is not practical for clinical use at present. It is difficult to distinguish between a pain cry and cries related to hunger or stimulated by startle (Porter, Miller, & Marshall, 1986). Therefore, the listener must rely on contextual cues to judge the eliciting stimulus.

Crying is one way that an infant communicates to others. Although it is a subjective method of assessing the distress of an infant, it still has face validity and needs to be recognized and responded to. Situational aspects must be considered (has it been a while since the last feeding? is the diaper wet? has the infant experienced a painful procedure recently? how long has the baby been crying?) when assessing the infant's behavior to arrive at appropriate interpretations and actions.

Facial expression has been studied to identify the expressions unique to different emotions and to investigate developmental changes. A fairly consistent facial expression in infants in response to painful stimuli has been described. Specifically, this consists of eyes forcefully closed, brows lowered and together, nasal roots broadened and bulged, deepened nasolabial furrow, and a square mouth and taut, cupped tongue (Grunau & Craig, 1987; Izard, Hembree, & Huebner, 1987) (Fig. 13–7). Grunau and Craig (1987), in a study of newborns reacting to the stimulus of a heel lance, noted a state-dependent difference in that alert infants responded with significantly more facial movement than sleeping infants.

Historical studies that included body movements as indicators of infant response to noxious stimuli concluded that reflex withdrawal was the most common response (Lipsitt & Levy, 1959; Sherman & Sherman, 1925). The fact that neonates subjected to heelsticks make swiping movements by the unaffected leg at the lanced leg (Franck, 1986) calls into question whether withdrawal is merely reflexive. The velocity of withdrawal may also be related to the intensity of the stimulus.

More complex behavioral changes that are unique to the individual child may also occur in response to pain. Some infants respond to the pain of circumcision by becoming more withdrawn and quiet, whereas others become more active and agitated (Marshall, Stratton, Moore, & Boxerman, 1980). Sleep disturbances have also been noted (Emde et al., 1971). Infant state influences the behavioral response to pain—infants in deeper sleep states are less likely to demonstrate as robust a response to pain as active awake infants. The

Figure 13–7
Facial expression of pain in an infant, with forcefully closed eyes, lowered brows, deepened furrow between nose and outer corner of lip, and square mouth with cupped tongue.

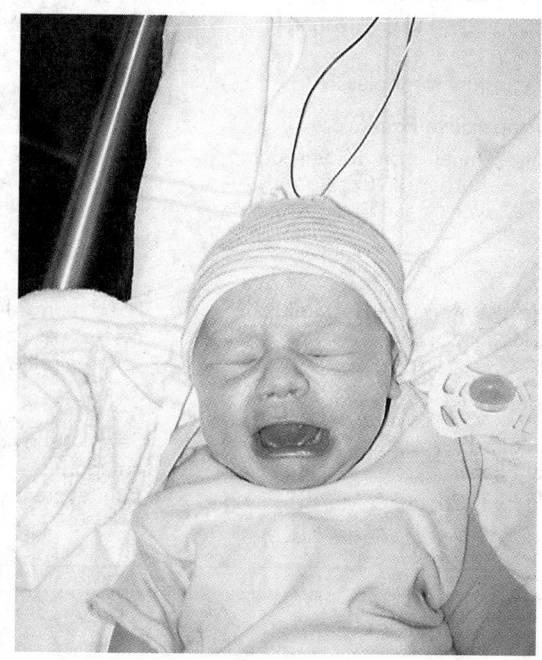

nurse should take this into consideration when assessing for pain.

caREminder: *If an infant is not responding vigorously, it should not be assumed that the infant is not in pain. It may be that the infant is in a sound sleep state or is too weak to respond.*

Observing multiple behaviors instead of only one indicator gives the potential to obtain a more objective, accurate assessment of an infant's pain. Because of the inherent difficulties, there are few published pain assessment tools for use with preverbal infants that have demonstrated acceptable reliability and validity (Table 13–2).

Table 13–2
Behavioral Tools for Pain Assessment

Tool	Behaviors	Comments
Children's Hospital of Eastern Ontario Pain Scale (CHEOPS) (McGrath et al., 1985) Age: 1–7 yr	Six categories: crying, facial expression, verbalizations, torso activity, if/how child touches wound, leg position	Tested in acute postoperative pain, insensitive to pain of longer duration; easy to learn; time considerations in that many behaviors are evaluated across the six categories
Gustave-Roussy Child Pain Scale (Gauvain-Piquard, Rodary, Rezvani, & Lemerle, 1987; Gauvain-Piquard et al., 1991) Age: 2–6 yr	Three categories: pain items, psychomotor atonia, anxiety items	Evaluates cancer pain intensity of longer duration, thus rates behaviors at times other than during procedures; depression closely associated with pain; variability in scores suggests scale discriminates between pain levels
Neonatal Facial Coding System (Grunau & Craig, 1987) Age: preterm to 4 mo (Johnston, Stevens, Graig, & Grunau, 1993)	Facial muscle group movement: brow bulge, eye squeeze, nasolabial furrow, open lips, stretch mouth (horizontal and vertical), lip purse, taut tongue, chin quiver	Focuses on only one aspect of pain behaviors; clinical use limited by time involved in training to score and analysis of videotape; measures response to acute pain stimuli
Neonatal Infant Pain Scale (Lawrence et al., 1993). Age: preterm to 6 wk	Six behaviors: facial expression, cry, breathing patterns, arms, legs, state of arousal	Easy to use clinically for acute pain, needs further testing for more ongoing pain (e.g., postoperative)
Pain/Discomfort Scale (Broadman, Rice, & Hannallah, 1988) Age: infant to adolescent	Six criteria: blood pressure, cry, movement, agitation, posture, pain complaints	Assesses postoperative pain (Hannallah, Broadman, Belman, Abramowitz, & Epstein, 1987); easy to use
Postoperative Pain Score (Attia, Amiel-Tison, Mayer, Shnider, & Barrier, 1987; Barrier, Attia, Mayer, Amiel-Tison, & Shnider, 1989) Age: 1–7 mo	Ten behaviors: sleep, facial expression, cry, motor activity, excitability, digit flexion, sucking, tone, consolability, sociability	May assess distress behaviors, not pain specific; may not provide valid indicators of pain beyond immediate postoperative period; easy to use
Princess Margaret Hospital Pain Assessment Tool (Robertson, 1993) Age: 7–14 yr	Five criteria: facial expression, nurse's assessment, position in bed, sounds, self-assessment	Not suitable for assessment of spasmodic pain; quick and easy to use
Toddler-Preschooler Postoperative Pain Scale (Tarbell, Cohen, & Marsh, 1992) Age: 1–5 yr	Seven behaviors divided into three categories: vocal, facial, and bodily pain expression	Developed for postoperative pain; limited number of items and easy to score

Not an all-inclusive listing. Responses should be evaluated in a situational context (stimuli, pain event) and validated with self-report or physiologic parameters as appropriate.

Preterm Infants

Nurses' judgments of pain in newborns are influenced by the vigor of the baby's response (Shapiro, 1993). Because the preterm infant's response to pain is less robust than that of a term infant, the health care team needs to be cognizant of subtle pain cues in premature infants (Fig. 13–8). Preterm infants often become limp, flaccid, or listless. Caretakers should take preventive measures to help support the infant during painful and stressful procedures (Fig. 13–9). The cry of a premature or medically compromised infant is higher pitched than that of a healthy term infant (Porter et al., 1988) and has more characteristics that arouse a caregiver. This finding may be related to the inability of preterm infants to demonstrate the strong grimace (because of neurologic immaturity or just weakness) and vigorous body movements that term infants display.

It is important to distinguish between agitation and pain, particularly in preterm infants, who may show more physiologic instability in response to these stressors. Behaviors of agitation and pain are related and may resemble each other but interventions, although having some overlap, are different. Agitation generally refers to excessive gross motor activity with whining, crying, irritable, restless behavior (Broome & Tanzillo, 1990). The infant is usually difficult to console. To distinguish between pain and agitation, one must assess the infant in terms of the nature of the painful stimuli, the environment, and behaviors (Table 13–3).

Figure 13–8
Lack of physical boundaries adds to the disorganization of this baby showing stress cues of crying, finger extension and splaying, and some leg extension.

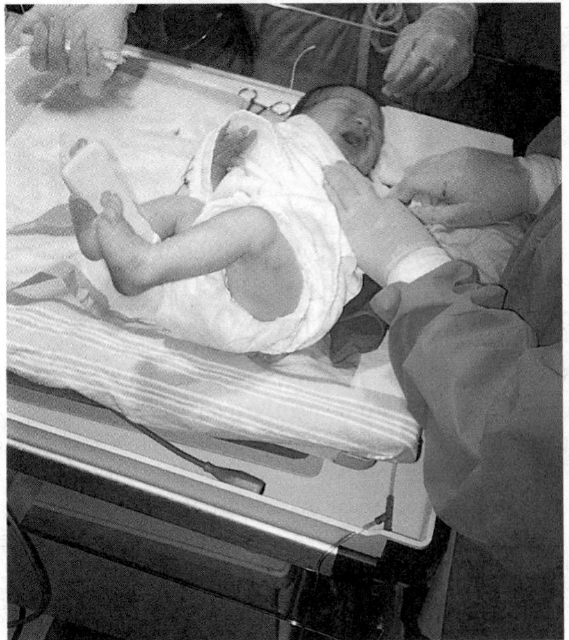

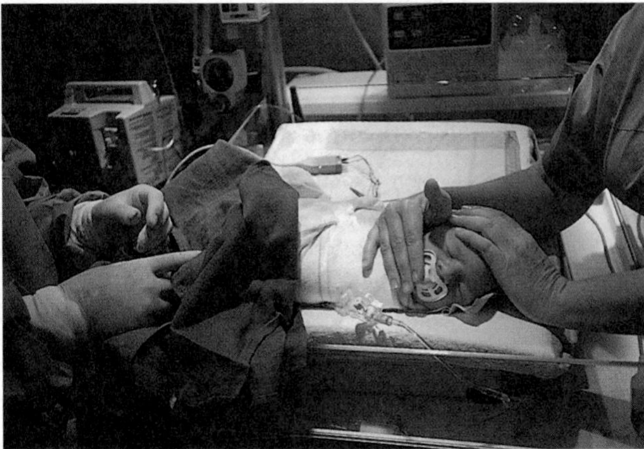

Figure 13–9
Appropriate management of a baby undergoing a painful procedure includes physical support and containment.

Toddlers and Preschoolers

Behaviors in the toddler and preschooler that are thought to be attributable to pain reflect developing cognition and motor skills (Mills, 1989; Taylor, 1983) (see Chart 13–7). A common myth is that an active child who is playing or one who is sleeping or can be distracted from pain does not have pain. Young children often use physical activity as a coping strategy (McCaffery & Beebe, 1989). From their perspective, if they stay in bed they become "sitting ducks" for painful procedures that are common to hospitals (McCaffery & Beebe, 1989). The young child may sleep as a coping mechanism or may fake sleep in an attempt to avoid painful procedures (McCaffery & Beebe, 1989). Children may sleep for other reasons. They may have been experiencing pain, obtained relief, and are finally able to sleep. They may also be sleeping because of exhaustion but are still in pain. They may have been medicated with opioids and sedated yet still not provided with sufficient pain relief. Further assessment should determine whether pain management is adequate in a sleeping child.

caREminder: *Do not assume adequate pain relief in a sleeping child.*

School-Age Children and Adolescents

School-age children and adolescents may show fewer overt behaviors in response to pain than younger children. This may be due to the fact that children older than 7 years are starting to recognize the psychological

Table 13–3
Is the Infant in Pain or Is It Agitation?

Environmental Issues

May exacerbate perceived pain intensity or precipitate agitation

- *Recent occurrence or presence of any presumed painful stimulus:* overt and covert such as incision pain, fracture, otitis media, postextubation edema.
- *Routine care* is a stressor for sick and compromised infants who have a greater degree of autonomic instability; care should be planned to allow for undisturbed time and delivered in a developmentally supportive manner; assessment should include consideration of basic infant care issues (e.g., time since last feeding, dry diaper).
- *Noise and light levels:* low levels contribute to an atmosphere of calm; high levels may have no effect on an infant in pain or may exacerbate the intensity of the pain; high levels further disorganize an agitated infant and escalate the situation.
- *Caretaker* who does not routinely care for the child will not be as sensitive to the infant's subtle cues, particularly of agitation, and may not as readily calm the child or know what is most effective in doing so.
- *Lack of physical boundaries:* well-defined boundaries (blankets, nests, buntings, something to push against to feel contained and keep extremities from flailing) assist an infant to stay organized; this is particularly important with preterm infants, who do better with looser wrapping, whereas a term infant may need to be tightly swaddled.

Behaviors

	Pain	Agitation
Cry	Greater intensity, high pitched, tense, sudden, loud	Whining, tends to be more annoying than alerting to the caretaker
Facial expression	Pain facies, grimace, preterm show weaker response	Frowning, may look more "wild eyed," out of control
Activity	Tensed muscles, flexed extremities, may swipe at painful area; preterm may be limp, listless	Random movements of head and flailing extremities, hypertonic, arched posture
Sleep	Altered patterns	More regular patterns, agitated during awake state
Arousal	Greater intensity, wider fluctuations in vital signs, shallow breathing	Vital signs more stable, see decompensation as agitation is prolonged

These are generalizations; each infant is unique in response to situations and behaviors and must be evaluated individually.

components of pain, that it causes either physical or mental suffering (Gaffney & Dunne, 1986). Older children can use behavioral and cognitive coping strategies when dealing with pain (McGrath & Craig, 1989). They are also beginning to understand the need for aversive procedures. School-age children are at a developmental stage in which approval is sought.

School-age children and adolescents may try to rest quietly when in pain. Observed body movements might be lying still, rigid, or curled in a fetal position; guarding or touching the painful area; and clenching fists. Facial expression may be the same as described for the toddler or preschooler. Children of these age groups may also have a change in demeanor and be irritable, angry, sad, or depressed (Alex & Ritchie, 1992). They may also show restlessness, withdrawal, and aggressiveness and/or have a change in sleep patterns.

Depending on individual coping style, school-age children or adolescents may want to look at what is causing the pain (attend to the pain) or may look away and try to distract themselves from it. Remaining in control is particularly important to an adolescent, which may be reflected in decreased manifestation of overt behaviors indicating pain. This does not mean that the adolescent is experiencing less pain.

If pain is of longer duration, the child may forget how it feels to be pain-free and think such a degree of pain is the norm. When children are questioned later

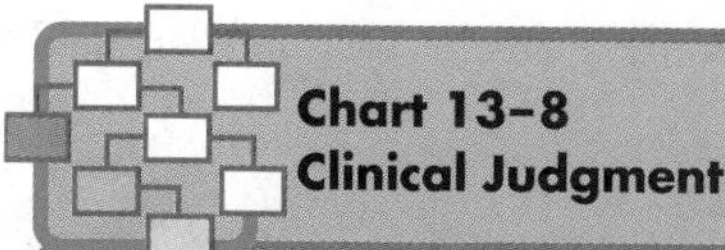

Chart 13–8
Clinical Judgment

A School-Age Child in Pain

Carmen is a 7-year-old weighing 23 kg, who was hit by a car while riding her bike yesterday. She has a left femur fracture and is in traction with an IV line. Her mother is staying with her. Both Carmen and mother were taught how to use the Poker Chip Tool to rate pain when she was admitted. Carmen has orders for acetaminophen with codeine elixir (5 mL of elixir = 12 mg codeine, 120 mg acetaminophen), 10 mL q 3–4 hr PO PRN; ibuprofen, 230–460 mg q 4–6 hr PO PRN; morphine sulfate, 2–4 mg q 3–4 hr IM or IV PRN. Carmen received acetaminophen with codeine elixir 2 hours ago. When you go in to take her vital signs she rates her leg pain as "one chip of hurt." HR = 100 beats per minute, RR = 28 breaths per minute, BP = 120/80, she cries or moans frequently and is lying rigid in bed.

Questions

1. Do you think Carmen is in pain?
2. What behaviors indicate that she is or is not in pain?
3. What would you do to reevaluate Carmen's pain?
4. When Carmen's pain is reassessed, she picks four chips of hurt. What would you do at this time?
5. When you evaluate Carmen 3 hours later, she has two chips of hurt, vital signs are at baseline values, and she cries with movement but is engrossed in the television show she is watching. What should you do?

Answers

1. Yes.
2. Her subjective rating of her pain is one chip of hurt, which would indicate a small amount of pain. Nonverbal cues that indicate that she is having pain are elevated HR, RR, and BP; crying; and unwillingness to move.
3. Carmen's subjective rating of pain is incongruent with objective findings; therefore, review how to use the Poker Chip Tool.
4. Give morphine at 2 mg IV and ibuprofen at 300 mg PO (comes as 100 mg per 5 mL; it is easy to dispense this lower dose and evaluate response in conjunction with morphine). Consult physician regarding giving ibuprofen around the clock because it is particularly effective for musculoskeletal pain.
5. She seems more comfortable but is still rating mild to moderate pain. Because she fractured her femur yesterday, it is anticipated that it would still be quite painful. Give the morphine IV and evaluate response. In 24 to 48 hours try acetaminophen with codeine for pain management.

about why pain was not complained of, they frequently reply they did not realize they were in pain.

Because self-report is considered the most reliable gauge of pain and most children in this age group are able to do this, asking the child about the pain experience should provide the most accurate method of assessment. This avoids the problem that arises when there is a discrepancy between the amount of pain the patient says he or she is experiencing and the overt behavioral demonstration (Chart 13–8). When self-report is not possible, as with an intubated, comatose, or developmentally delayed child, assessment tools developed for younger children may provide information regarding the pain.

Tools That Assess Distress

Emotions such as anxiety may be manifest as distress, reflected as an upset child. Tools that assess distress may not evaluate behaviors that are pain specific, but it needs to be recognized that distress may intensify the pain experience and should be addressed. Often, psychological interventions (e.g., preparation, distraction, imagery) are effective in reducing distress.

The COMFORT scale was designed to measure children's distress in a pediatric intensive care unit. It looks at eight dimensions in assessing distress: alertness, calmness, respiratory response, movement, mean arterial pressure, heart rate, muscle tone, and facial expression (Ambuel, Hamlett, Marx, & Blumer, 1992). The COMFORT scale shows preliminary evidence of reliability and validity and promise as a measure of distress in children of all ages.

Several tools have been developed to assess behavioral distress (pain plus anxiety) in children with cancer. The Procedure Behavior Rating Scale (Katz, Kellerman, & Siegel, 1980) and the Observation Scale of Behavioral Distress (Jay et al., 1983) were designed to measure distress related to procedural pain. Both tools showed similar developmental trends in that younger children tended to demonstrate more intense overt distress (crying, screaming) and children older than 7 years demonstrated less intense overt distress. These tools were tested in children with cancer and cannot be generalized to other populations.

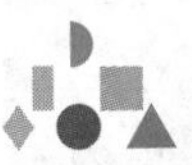

Nursing Diagnoses and Outcomes

Identification of nursing diagnoses applicable to the child in pain is based on assessment findings. This process may seem simple, but psychological aspects of the pain must also be considered (Chart 13–9). Appropriate management techniques are determined on the basis of identified diagnoses.

Chart 13–9
Nursing Diagnoses and Outcomes

The Child in Pain

Pain related to effects of disease, treatment, injury	
Outcome:	Pain will be alleviated or reduced to an acceptable level as defined by the child.
Pain, chronic related to effects of disease state; altered pain processing	
Outcome:	Pain will be alleviated or reduced to an acceptable level as defined by the child.
Fear related to inadequate preparation; anticipation of pain; lack of adequate pain control	
Outcome:	Child will not be fearful, will be prepared for pain situations, will have pain controlled at acceptable levels.
Anxiety related to effects of pain, lack of control over pain	
Outcome:	Child will not show behaviors of or verbalize anxiety, will be prepared for pain situations to increase feelings of control, will have pain controlled at acceptable levels.
Knowledge deficit: pain causes and interventions	
Outcome:	Child and family members will have age and culturally appropriate explanations given and understanding of pain and what they can do to relieve pain.

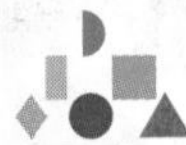

Managing Pain in Children

The role of the health team in pain management is to listen to the child and family, provide relevant education, maintain continuity of care, strive for the best pain assessment, and intervene appropriately. Inadequate pain management results in needless physical and psychological suffering of the patient and family system. These adverse outcomes can be avoided with appropriate pain management (Chart 13–10).

Alert: *Severe, unrelenting pain should be considered a medical emergency.*

The Agency for Health Care Policy and Research (AHCPR) has produced two Clinical Practice Guidelines specifically on pain: *Acute Pain Management: Operative or Medical Procedures and Trauma* and *Management of Cancer Pain*. The guidelines address overall pain control and strategies for pain management in specific groups, including infants, children, and adolescents. The guidelines also mandate that institutions take responsibility for ensuring adequacy of pain management via interdisciplinary collaboration and ongoing quality monitoring.

The expectations of the child and family regarding pain relief should be discussed. Is it expected that there will be complete pain relief? Is this realistic in the specific situation? Is it expected that pain will be relieved enough so that the child can participate in certain activities? Realistic goals should be mutually decided upon by the child, family, and health care team to avoid misunderstanding and mismanagement of the pain.

Suspicion of pain may arise from observations of behavior or knowledge that similar conditions in an adult (surgery, procedures, disease state) would cause subjective reporting of pain and a subsequent request for intervention. Assessments should be conducted at routine intervals and at an appropriate interval after interventions are implemented (e.g., 15 minutes after IV administration of medications, 30 minutes after oral medications are given, 30 minutes after changing position). One must develop a trusting relationship with the child and family—believe that the pain exists if verbalizations or behaviors indicate that it does. Remember that chronic pain behaviors differ from those of acute pain.

caREminder: *Maintain a high index of suspicion regarding the presence of pain, and actively advocate for pain relief on behalf of the child. Children of all ages have the ability to experience pain and interventions must be implemented when the presence of pain is suspected.*

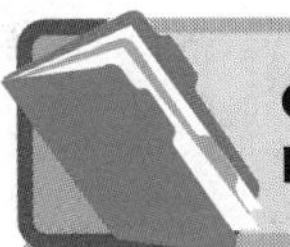

Chart 13–10
Nursing Interventions Classification (NIC)

Pain Management

Definition

Alleviation of pain or a reduction in pain to a level of comfort that is acceptable to the patient

Activities

Perform a comprehensive assessment of pain to include location, characteristics, onset/duration, frequency, quality, intensity or severity of pain, and precipitating factors.

Observe for nonverbal cues of discomfort, especially in those unable to communicate effectively.

Ensure that the patient receives appropriate analgesic care.

Use therapeutic communication strategies to acknowledge the pain experience and convey acceptance of the patient's response to pain.

Consider cultural influences on pain response.

Determine the impact of the pain experience on quality of life (e.g., sleep, appetite, activity, cognition, mood, relationships, performance of job, and role responsibilities).

Evaluate past experiences with pain to include individual or family history of chronic pain or resulting disability as appropriate.

Evaluate, with the patient and the health care team, the effectiveness of past pain control measures that have been used.

Assist patient and family to seek and provide support.

Utilize a developmentally appropriate assessment method which allows for monitoring of change in pain and that will assist in identifying actual and potential precipitating factors (e.g., flow sheet, daily diary).

Determine the needed frequency of making an assessment of patient comfort, and implement monitoring plan.

Provide information about the pain, such as causes of the pain, how long it will last, and anticipated discomforts from procedures.

Control environmental factors that may influence the patient's response to discomfort (e.g., room temperature, lighting, and noise).

Reduce or eliminate factors that precipitate or increase the pain experience (e.g., fear, fatigue, monotony, and lack of knowledge).

Consider the patient's willingness to participate, ability to participate, preference, support of significant others for method, and contraindications when selecting a pain relief strategy.

Select and implement a variety of measures (e.g., pharmacologic, nonpharmacologic, and interpersonal) to facilitate pain relief as appropriate.

Consider type and source of pain when selecting pain relief strategy.

Encourage patient to monitor own pain and to intervene appropriately.

Teach the use of nonpharmacologic techniques (e.g., biofeedback, TENS, hypnosis, relaxation, guided imagery, music therapy, distraction, play therapy, activity therapy, acupressure, hot/cold application, and massage) before, after, and, if possible, during painful activities; before pain occurs or increases; and along with other pain relief measures.

Collaborate with the patient, significant other, and other health professionals to select and implement nonpharmacologic pain relief measures as appropriate.

Provide the person optimal pain relief with prescribed analgesics.

Implement the use of patient-controlled analgesia (PCA) if appropriate.

Use pain control measures before pain becomes severe.

Medicate before an activity to increase participation, but evaluate the hazard of sedation.

Ensure pretreatment analgesia and/or nonpharmacologic strategies before painful procedures.

Verify level of discomfort with patient, note changes in the medical record, and inform other health professionals working with the patient.

Evaluate the effectiveness of the pain control measures used through ongoing assessment of the pain experience.

Institute and modify pain control measures on the basis of the patient's response.

Promote adequate rest/sleep to facilitate pain relief.

Encourage patient to discuss the pain experience, as appropriate.

Chart continued on following page

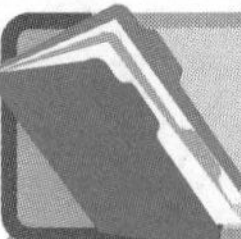

Chart 13–10
Nursing Interventions Classification (NIC) *Continued*

Pain Management

Activities

Notify physician if measures are unsuccessful or if current complaint is a significant change from patient's past experience of pain.
Inform other health care professionals/family members of nonpharmacologic strategies being used by the patient to encourage preventive approaches to pain management.
Utilize a multidisciplinary approach to pain management, when appropriate.
Consider referrals for patient, family, and significant others to support groups and other resources, as appropriate.
Provide accurate information to promote family's knowledge of and response to the pain experience.
Incorporate the family in the pain relief modality if possible.
Monitor patient satisfaction with pain management at specified intervals.

From McCloskey, J., & Bulechek, G. (1996). *Nursing interventions classification (NIC)* (2nd ed.). St. Louis: Mosby–Year Book. Reprinted with permission.

To make appropriate diagnostic and management decisions, the specific situation (age, coping style, environment) and type and intensity of pain should be considered. The most successful pain management strategy is a dynamic, proactive approach (Chart 13–11). This involves maintaining control of the pain with around-the-clock management. Interventions can be classified as nonpharmacologic or pharmacologic. These methods can be used alone or in conjunction with each other to augment their effects.

Nonpharmacologic Pain Management

Nonpharmacologic interventions usually fall under nursing's domain. Although they do not have the potency of narcotics, particularly for severe pain, nonpharmacologic interventions provide coping strategies that may help to reduce pain perception and increase comfort. For example, cognitive-behavioral interventions may alter perception of the pain being experienced. Nonpharmacologic interventions should not be used as a substitute for analgesics, rather as adjuvants (Chart 13–12). When nonpharmacologic methods are used in addition to analgesics, particularly during conscious sedation, the child must be monitored closely. Occasionally, the techniques seem to have an additive effect and vital signs (HR, BP, respiratory rate, oxygen saturation) may drop to a point where the sedative drugs must be reduced.

Depending on the individual child and situation, the following interventions, used alone or in various combinations, may prove effective. Consideration of developmental level of the child, individual patient needs, and pain situation is important when selecting these techniques. Attention must also be directed toward needs of the parents.

Chart 13–11

ABCDEs of Pain Management

Assessment is multidimensional.
Believe that the child has pain if the history supports it or the child reports it (either by behavior or words).
Communication is clear, concise, and patient focused.
Do something/intervene—interventions implemented with consideration of developmental age, type and intensity of pain.
Evaluate effectiveness of interventions; go back to assessment.

Parental Involvement

Parents who are knowledgeable about what is going to happen and about specific things they can do to facilitate pain management generally feel less helpless, are less anxious, and are better able to support their child. A parent's sensitive response to the child's reaction can promote the child's coping skills (Carpenter, 1992).

Assessment methods and management plan should be discussed, agreed upon, and used consistently by the family and health team. The extent to which the parents wish to be involved should also be discussed. In addition, parents should be allowed time away from the child to ask questions privately of the health care team.

Parents should be encouraged to maintain an active

Chart 13–12

Nonpharmacologic Pain Relief Methods—Advantages and Disadvantages

Advantages

- Potential for avoiding the side effects associated with medications
- Efficacy in alleviating pain and other uncomfortable sensations such as nausea, fear, and anxiety
- Ability to help the child maintain control

Disadvantages

- Limited effectiveness with severe pain
- Variable effectiveness in individual children
- Amount of time required to implement some techniques
- May not have good role model or coach available to implement some of these (imagery, relaxation)

role in assessment and management of pain and in being an advocate for their child. They might do this by evaluating the effectiveness of medications and requesting a change in dosing if the desired response is not obtained or by decreasing external stimuli (visitors, noise, light). Parents should also be given the option of requesting a break if procedures are prolonged and their child is not coping well. The health team should ensure that events or procedures are explained before implementation. If the health team overlooks this preparation, the parent should make sure that explanations are given to the child. Parents can also ensure that the child is told before anything is done (e.g., "the doctor is going to wash your back now" or "what are you going to do now, doctor?").

Parents should be allowed and encouraged to stay with their child, even during procedures (see TIP 13–1). Aspects of support such as not using threats and giving positive reinforcement ("I know you tried to hold still" or "you are standing straighter when you walk now") can be presented. Some parents feel that it is not proper for the child to cry. They should be told that this is acceptable behavior that may even help the child cope. A parent can model desired behaviors such as deep breathing and muscle relaxation and help the child practice these skills. Parents can also provide distraction by such means as blowing bubbles, reading books, telling stories, and helping the child go on imaginary trips.

Parents are often concerned about their child being given narcotics and the potential for addiction. The role of prescription medications, particularly opioids, in pain management and the parent's feelings regarding this issue should be discussed. Education may be needed for the parent to sanction use of these drugs and provide appropriate guidance for the child.

Cognitive-Behavioral Interventions

Cognitive-behavioral interventions usually have three main objectives:

- To provide information to prepare the child and family for what will happen
- To focus the child's attention on something so that the child does not attend to or perceive pain at the usual intensity
- To provide the child with coping skills or emotional support to modify behaviors that may initiate or exacerbate the pain

Advantages of using cognitive-behavioral interventions are that they are generally independent nursing actions that are noninvasive, are inexpensive, can be used in many situations, and provide the child and family with some control over the pain. General principles of psychological care should not be overlooked (Chart 13–13).

For these interventions to be effective, the child must have the energy and be willing to participate (Kachoyeanos & Friedhoff, 1993). The person supporting the child should not be performing the procedure and the child must trust this person. Use of these techniques may require time and practice and may not achieve the desired results when first used.

Preparation

Both the child and parents must be given explanations about their situation. These may be general explanations about hospitalization and the health care environment or more specific to preparation for a procedure.

Some parents and health team members feel that preparation takes too much time and that the procedure could be finished in less time. Children who have been prepared for a procedure demonstrate less distress during the procedure (Manne et al., 1990), although cognitive preparation may not have the same effect in preoperational children (Gedaly-Duff, 1987). If there is no intervention, children who are distressed during painful procedures have increased distress behaviors over time (Katz et al., 1980).

It is important to reinforce that pain is not a punishment for misdeeds. Because of their cognitive abilities, preschool and younger school-age children frequently assume that their wrongdoing caused the pain. Inform the child that the pain will go away, if that is the case as with postoperative or procedural pain. Young children

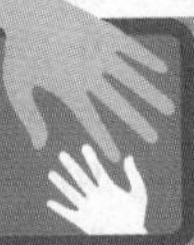

Chart 13–13
Nursing Interventions

Providing Psychological Support for the Child in Pain

- Encourage use of previously learned coping skills; remember that children regress when stressed.
- Painful procedures should be performed in designated areas, *not* in the child's room or playroom.
- Do not talk over the child—talk to the child or leave the vicinity.
- Reinforce that pain is not a punishment for misdeeds.
- Be honest; clarify communication.
- Ask the child "what do you think will help you in this situation?" and "what can I do to help?"
- Give the child control whenever possible—let the child remove a dressing, help set up for a fingerstick, prepare a site by wiping with alcohol, choose an IV site.
- Suggest what the child *can* do ("hold your leg still"), not what the child cannot do ("do not move your leg").
- Have the child and parents practice appropriate coping actions before they will be needed; give positive reinforcement for desired behaviors.
- Use the power of suggestion to help increase the efficacy of any strategy (e.g., "when you go on an imaginary trip the LP seems to be over faster" or "this cold massage can make your leg feel better").

may think it will go on forever, which adds to their anxiety and distress.

Be honest if pain is anticipated. If the child is not told honestly what to expect, trust will not develop.

Tip: *Tell the child it may hurt but that there are things that can be done to help make it not so bad.*

Specific details regarding procedural and sensory information should be given as developmentally appropriate (Chart 13–14).

The child and family should be taught that they need to tell the health team when pain is present. They should be introduced to a developmentally and culturally appropriate assessment tool and practice using it. If it does not seem to be effective, another tool should be selected. The goal is to find a tool or method that elicits the desired information regarding pain presence and then to use this consistently in evaluating pain.

The infant probably does not need psychological preparation in the typical manner, although even infants should be talked to and told what is being done. As mentioned previously, attention to preparing parents for what will occur may lower their anxiety, enabling them to better support their child.

Toddlers and preschoolers may be told about upcoming hospitalization a day or two beforehand. In anticipation of this, they may be introduced to the hospital and routines via a tour of the facility, videos, coloring books, or having age-appropriate books read to them (see Resources at the end of the chapter).

Children younger than 7 should be prepared about an hour before a procedure (Patterson & Ware, 1988). Children of this age usually do not remember much information given far in advance of a procedure. A toddler does not understand the rationale for a painful procedure; preschoolers are unable to reason beyond the immediate event and do not understand cause and effect. Explain the procedure sequentially using simple explanations or drawings and allow the child to see and manipulate equipment. Other methods of preparation include books, puppet shows, or videotapes. Use of videotapes may serve two purposes. One is to demonstrate what will happen. The other is to model, or demonstrate, coping behaviors that may be adaptive in the specific situation. It may be beneficial to older children for preparation to be done several days in advance (Broome, 1990). A prolonged time period gives older children time to think about what methods they can use to cope in the situation. In addition to the methods discussed for younger children, an increasing amount of detail regarding the procedure should be added with rationales for actions given. Questions should be elicited and answered. Discuss what they think will happen, how they usually respond to similar situations, and things they might do to cope with this.

Ideally, preparation is done before the child is in pain. When a painful event happens under emergency conditions, preparation occurs almost concurrently with the procedure. As with any situation, tell the child what you are doing.

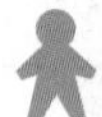

Tip: *Give sensory information such as "this may feel like it is pinching, stinging, poking, cold" or "you might not feel much of anything; tell me what it feels like for you."*

All children should have basic comfort measures addressed such as hunger and thermal regulation and should be allowed to void prior to a procedure. These may help decrease anxiety and increase comfort. EMLA cream, discussed under pharmacologic management, should be applied when needles are to be used (e.g., IV insertion, lumbar puncture, bone marrow aspiration).

Desensitization

Desensitization is a method of dealing with stress-inducing situations in which the child is helped to learn differ-

Chart 13–14
Nursing Interventions

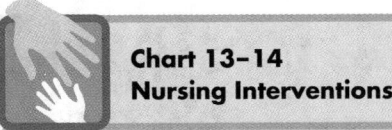

Helping the Child Cope with Planned Painful Events

Before the Procedure

- Be honest and specific about what will happen.
- Give information as appropriate to the child's developmental level and previous experiences—the older the child, the more details should be included and the further in advance of the event they should be told:
  - Infant: as the procedure is carried out
  - Toddler: immediately before the procedure
  - Child younger than age 7: about an hour before the procedure
  - Older child: several days in advance
- Give procedural information:
  - What is to be done and why
  - Where the procedure will occur (treatment room, operating room)
  - How the child will get to where the procedure will be performed
  - What equipment will be used
  - Who will be in the room
  - Who will do the procedure
  - How long it will take
  - Show the child the room and let him or her manipulate equipment when possible.
- Give sensory information:
  - What the room will look like
  - Sounds the child may hear (e.g., beeping from the pulse oximeter, buzzing alarms, machinery moving)
  - Smells to expect
  - How it will feel (e.g., hard table, cold antiseptic, pressure, pinch)
- Prepare room and equipment before bringing child to room; seeing things being set up or delays in performing procedure heighten anxiety.

During the Procedure

- Implement nonpharmacologic interventions:
  - Ensure the presence of favorite objects (blanket, stuffed animal).
  - Minimize extraneous noise: move noisy machines, mute alarms; speak quietly in a low tone.
  - Avoid sudden, jarring movements.
  - Position the child for comfort within restrictions for the procedure.
  - Have adequate light, direct light to procedure site, away from child's eyes or shield eyes if child will tolerate.

After the Procedure

- Give a clear signal when procedure is finished (pick up, sit up, "it's done now").
- Review the experience with child and family (play therapy).
- Clarify perceptions.
- Reinforce or reward positive coping behaviors.
- Discuss alternatives for future success.

ent responses to use in the specific situation. Positive self-talk is one method of doing this. The child is taught to say out loud or think statements that reframe the situation into one that is manageable. Examples are "I can do this, it's not that bad," "I've handled this before, I can do it again," "Stay calm, it will be over soon." Positive self-talk tends to be more effective with older school-age children and adolescents.

Play therapy can also be used to change the child's response to a situation (see Chapter 9). The child is encouraged to manipulate the actual equipment used and act out a situation using a doll, which gives the child

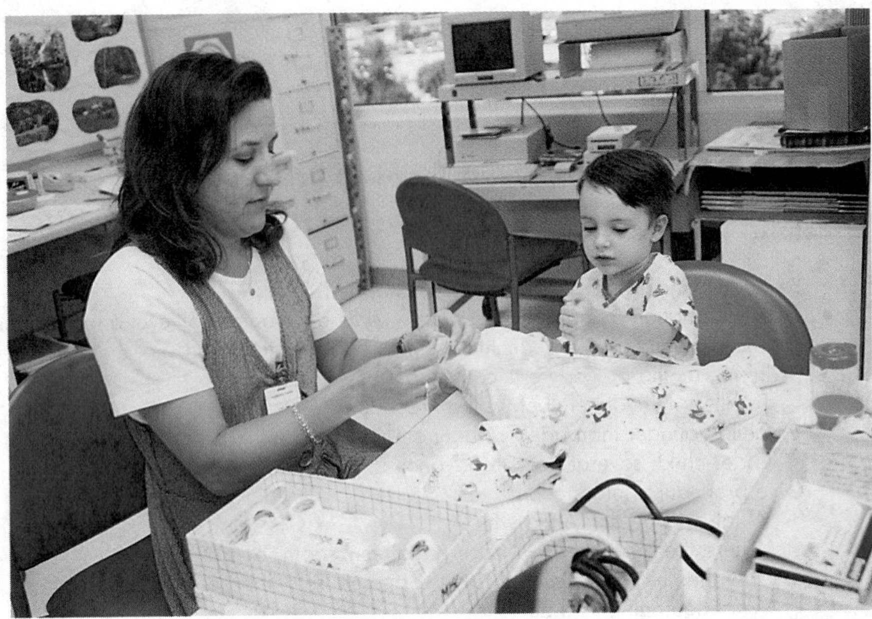

Figure 13–10
Play therapy after a painful event can be used to reinforce positive coping strategies.

control over the situation. The child's response gives the nurse insight into how the child is interpreting the experience. This is a good time to demonstrate adaptive coping skills. If the child is fearful, do not force him or her to become involved. Rather, the nurse might play with the equipment and act out the scenario as if the child were not present. The child may pay attention from afar and later feel more comfortable playing. Therapeutic play should continue after the event so that the child has the opportunity to express feelings in a safe environment (Fig. 13–10).

Distraction

A goal of cognitive interventions is to divert the child's attention away from the pain via controlled, purposeful behaviors. The focus needs to be on what will draw the individual child's attention from the pain. It is not realistic to expect to eradicate the pain; it is realistic to expect a reduction in perceived intensity. Simple distraction, as discussed in this section, is a practical method of diversion to use because little training or preparation is needed. Imagery and hypnosis are diversionary methods but require more practice and training and are not appropriate with infants and toddlers.

Passive means of accomplishing distraction may be watching television or a mobile hung from the ceiling, playing video games, or listening to music. Music therapy has been used to treat pain in adults (Bailey, 1986) and may be therapeutic in children (Collins & Kuck, 1991; Ryan, 1989). Music listened to through headphones may be most effective because it can help filter out some of the external noises in the environment. Playing tapes of uterine sounds (sounds heard in the womb—whooshing of maternal heartbeat) is appropriate for infants. Playing soothing instrumental music or carrying or talking to an infant may provide distraction and possibly encourage relaxation.

More active methods of distraction involve children doing something. They might be instructed to squeeze a parent's hand so tightly that it hurts, hug a stuffed animal, yell, or help blow bubbles. Use of a kaleidoscope was found to reduce pain perception and behavioral distress during an acute pain experience (Vessey, Carlson, & McGill, 1994). Reading stories can be an effective diversionary technique; especially effective are pop-up books or ones with parts the child can manipulate to become more involved in the story.

Imagery

Imagery is another method of distraction and can also enhance relaxation. Children are actively involved in visualizing a situation that decreases the amount of pain perceived either by picturing themselves engrossed in a different scenario or visualizing something done to their body to decrease pain messages traveling through.

Talk with the child before deciding on the scenario to be imagined. Ask what the child's favorite place or activity is and try to base an active, sensory scene on this experience (Chart 13–15). Try to ascertain whether the child would be more open to a male or female voice. It is also necessary to be aware of fears the child has, such as of water, animals, or activities, so that they are not brought into the imagery and make it a negative experience.

Chart 13–15

Favorite Imaginary Trips

The Beach. Where you can walk and feel the sand between your toes; sun warming your body; cool water on your feet, knees, thighs; hear the waves crashing on the beach and birds squawking

A Field. See all the colorful flowers, smell the flowers, feel the breeze and warm sun

Lying in a Hammock. Very relaxed, your arms and legs sink into the hammock, see the blue sky and the clouds moving overhead, feel the sun and breeze as the hammock gently rocks

An Amusement Park. Smell the popcorn, hear the people, see the lights, ride the roller coaster

Imagery can also be used effectively to create a situation that blocks the travel of pain messages. Imagining a pain switch or magic glove has been found to be effective (Kuttner, 1986). The pain switch controls the area of pain (leg, arm, abdomen) and the child visualizes turning the pain switch off to that area so that messages cannot travel, much as a light switch controls electricity. Color can also be incorporated into the imagery, having the child picture a color, for example, red when pain can travel or is present, with the area turning black when the switch is turned off. A magic glove can be put on the hand, finger by finger, suggested to diminish the pain associated with venipuncture or fingerstick. It might also be useful in other situations; children are susceptible to the power of suggestion. A magic blanket might be used in areas where a glove would not work, such as the back or abdomen. The hands are extremely sensitive parts of the body. One can take the magic glove and hold it over other parts of the body (e.g., over the cheek before dental work) to induce numbness or decrease pain.

Relaxation

Anxiety and feelings of helplessness may be reduced by use of relaxation techniques, indirectly reducing intensity of perceived pain. These techniques may also be effective alone in bringing the child to a different level of consciousness, thus altering pain perception. To learn and practice relaxation techniques successfully, children need to be with someone with whom they feel safe such as a parent, nurse, or social worker. Relaxation techniques need to be practiced with a support person before use. Under stressful conditions, children often cannot implement these alone and need the support person to guide them.

If psychological factors such as anxiety seem to exacerbate the child's reaction, encourage the child to take an active role in managing the situation. Feeling in control of a situation may reduce anxiety. The child might help remove a dressing; pick the site in which to insert an IV line, prepare tape and cleanse the insertion site, and then help tape the line once it is placed; or the child might arrange a schedule for the day given that certain events must occur. Use of transcutaneous electrical nerve stimulation (TENS) or cutaneous stimulation gives other opportunities for the child to exert control.

When teaching relaxation techniques to the child and family, keep the environment quiet. It may help to hang a "do not disturb" sign on the door to limit interruptions. The child may sit or lie in a supportive chair or bed. To enhance relaxation, children may be told to feel their body sinking into the furniture. They may also be told to make their brain like a blackboard that has been wiped clean, thinking of nothing but the words that you are telling them. Speak in a calm, low, measured tone.

Muscle relaxation can be taught in a variety of ways. A descriptive way to help children learn what tenseness and relaxation may feel like is to tell them to "hold your arms (legs) out very straight, tense or squeeze your muscles until the count of 10, 1 . . . 10, now let go" or to "breathe in and hold it, feel the tightness in your chest, breathe out all at once, feel the tension leaving your body completely." Another method of muscle relaxation is to work from the feet up the body (e.g., "feel your feet relaxing, sinking into the mattress, they are very heavy. Now feel your calves sinking further down, very relaxed.").

Various **breathing methods** may effectively induce relaxation. Monitor for hyperventilation as you implement these. One method is to have the child slowly take five deep breaths in through the nose and slowly exhale through pursed lips. Another method is to have the child count with the support person from 1 to 10, saying the number with each exhalation (McDonnell & Bowden, 1989), and gently inhale through a slightly open mouth. These can be repeated until a calm is experienced, remembering that this may take practice. "Blowing the pain away" can be particularly effective with younger children. At the first sign of pain, the children are taught to take a breath and blow out as hard as they can. This helps them to maintain control by taking the aversive stimulus and acting upon it rather than letting it overwhelm them.

Meditation is another method for aiding relaxation (Smith & Womack, 1987). This might be achieved by concentrating on a visual, mental, or auditory focal point. Children are told to sit quietly with their eyes shut, to empty their mind of other things, and to be aware of their breathing. With each exhalation they repeat a simple phrase to themselves ("relax") or might focus on a chant ("ohmmmm"), brushing aside distracting thoughts. This should be performed for at least 20 minutes.

Biofeedback training involves giving information to the child about a physiologic function such as heart rate, skin temperature, or muscle tension. The information is given in the form of an analogue signal, usually a visual display via digital readout or line graph or by using a variably pitched tone (children tend to prefer visual feedback). The child is instructed to use mental imagery to increase or decrease reactivity in the system being monitored. Reinforcement occurs when the child is able to effect change in the desired direction, thus strengthening self-control over the physiologic function. Use of biofeedback requires specialized training and equipment and may be more appropriate for pain of longer duration.

Hypnosis

Hypnosis is considered as an altered state of consciousness characterized by focused attention and profound relaxation. Hypnotic state induction needs to be done under the supervision of an experienced practitioner. Variability exists between individuals in receptivity and ability to be hypnotized. Children can often use hypnosis more readily than adults because of their capacity for imagination.

Hypnotic induction in children younger than 6 is usually most successful via guided imagery (Morgan & Hilgard, 1979) or using favorite stories (Kuttner, 1988). For school-age children guided imagery or eye fixation (watching a coin or other image) is suggested. Adolescents might use imagery or progressive relaxation.

Humor

The use of humor can be successful in reducing perceived pain intensity. It may work by inhibiting impulse transmission via the gate theory or by release of endorphins (Smith, 1986). This intervention is obviously more appropriate for mild to moderate pain. This can be implemented by spontaneous use of situations (someone wearing two differently colored socks), telling jokes, funny stories, or movies. Humor that induces laughter may not be effective after abdominal surgery, when it might increase pain. It must always be used judiciously, considering the patient and situation. For example, it may not help an extremely anxious child or in a serious situation.

Biophysical Interventions

Biophysical management techniques attempt to affect physiologic responses directly during painful experiences. It is thought that these techniques work by sending benign messages that compete with the painful messages to the dorsal horn of the spinal cord and brain. The benign messages get to the dorsal horn first or in greater numbers and block the transmission of painful messages. Biophysical techniques, particularly cutaneous stimulation, may be detrimental in preterm infants. Touch in conjunction with painful stimuli results in greater changes of HR, BP, and transcutaneous arterial oxygen tension from baseline (Beaver, 1987). Because of the intense physiologic response that is evoked, these strategies are not appropriate for use in preterm infants. Fluctuations in vital signs may cause intraventricular hemorrhage. The nurse should provide supportive care, monitor the infant's cues for signs of stress, and intervene as indicated (Chart 13–16).

Sucking during painful stimuli attenuates pain distress behaviors and has a pacifying effect (Campos, 1989; Miller & Anderson, 1993). Non-nutritive sucking helps an infant to organize behaviors and adapt to stimuli (Kimble, 1992) and may increase the release of pain-alleviating neurotransmitters, thus aiding in stress reduction (Field, 1993). Therefore, non-nutritive sucking may augment other interventions aimed at pain alleviation and provide the benefit of stress reduction. This can be achieved by giving a pacifier or having an infant breastfeed immediately after the procedure.

Use of a **sucrose-coated pacifier** during a painful procedure has been investigated as a potential method of pain relief. This intervention is based on studies demonstrating raised pain thresholds with use of sucrose in rats (Blass, Fitzgerald, & Kehoe, 1987). The pain threshold elevation was shown to be reversible by use of an opioid antagonist. Thus, it was hypothesized that sucrose may have analgesic properties that are mediated through the opioid pathways. Human infants undergoing painful procedures cried most when given no intervention, less when offered a water-moistened pacifier, and least when offered a sucrose-coated pacifier (Blass & Hoffmeyer, 1991). Use of 25% or 50% sucrose before a pain stimulus reduced crying and heart rate more effectively than 12.5% sucrose or water (Haouari, Wood, Griffiths, & Levene, 1995). Sucrose may be a relatively benign, yet effective, easy-to-use method of pain relief for infants.

Swaddling soothes infants subjected to painful stimuli (Campos, 1989). **Holding** is comforting for children of all ages and often helps them achieve a more relaxed state. Both methods serve to limit excessive, uncontrolled movements that may exacerbate pain. They also provide physical boundaries that may assist infants in organizing themselves. Infants older than 3 to 6 months often fight against swaddling, which may intensify anxiety and pain. The amount of comfort derived from being held is a function of the individual child's personality and situation. Holding a child on the chest of an adult, on the

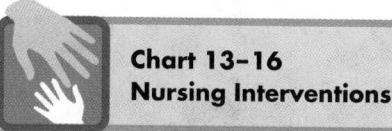

Chart 13–16
Nursing Interventions

Nonpharmacologic Pain Management for Infants

Soothing may be enhanced by use of multiple modalities. Infants should be monitored for cues indicating stress—for example, gaze aversion, hiccups, finger splaying (rigid extension and separation of fingers), yawning, fussing, becoming limp, going into a sleep state or "shutting down," bradycardia—and interventions implemented or withdrawn on the basis of infant's response. Ability to comfort is a function of the child's unique response, the pain situation, the interventions implemented, and the caretaker's sensitivity in reading the baby's cues.

- Provide supportive boundaries—blankets, bunting, adult hands surrounding infant containing the child but not moving.
- Encourage hand-to-mouth behaviors.
- Sucking—pacifier or thumb or fingers.
- Sucrose—give oral sucrose solution or coat a pacifier with sucrose and let the infant suck on it 2 minutes prior to and during painful procedures (may decrease pain perception); remove the pacifier when the procedure is completed and infant is calm.
- Auditory stimuli—uterine sounds, instrumental music, humming, parent's voice (more effective with older infant); make sure not to overstimulate the child.
- Swaddling—tightly wrapping in blanket with extremities flexed and hands uncovered to facilitate hand-to-mouth behavior; tight wrapping provides too much stimuli for preterm infants, who should be loosely wrapped with boundaries to push against, which gives a feeling of containment and security.
- Positioning—decrease muscle tension and pull on painful area, limit movement; for example, support legs in a flexed position if there is an abdominal incision, elevate extremity.
- Holding—support caregiver with proper armrests, footrests, pillows so the caregiver is comfortable.
- Rocking—rhythmic, continuous, horizontal (the person holding stands and gently turns trunk side to side, with feet stationary, so that the child moves in the horizontal plane).
- Touch—firm pressure or stroking; preterm infants do better with firm touch on their head or heels, not the trunk.
- Visual stimuli—more effective with older infant; use parent's face, pictures, mobiles.
- Allow recovery periods—if infant is showing signs of stress, stop procedures when possible and allow infant to reorganize; implement other comfort measures to augment those already in use.

left side over the heart, works particularly well in calming. **Rocking** soothes children as measured by quieting behaviors. Continuous, horizontal rocking appears to be the best way to induce drowsiness in infants (Byrne & Horowitz, 1981), relaxing them and decreasing tension that may worsen perceived pain intensity.

Proper **positioning** provides support for and decreases muscle tension over painful areas; for example, if the child has an abdominal incision, place pillow under legs when lying on back and bend knees up when lying on side (Fig. 13–11). The patient's situation dictates appropriate actions: pressure on an incision may exacerbate pain but might be helpful when a child with an abdominal incision has to cough and deep breathe; pressure may reduce abdominal pain caused by gas; elevation of a swollen extremity may decrease swelling and thus pain.

Cutaneous Stimulation

The mechanism by which cutaneous stimulation provides an analgesic effect is not clear. It may provide additional sensory input to "close the gate" to nociceptive stimuli. The nurse must watch for cues indicating stress in children of all ages.

Alert: *These strategies are not for use in preterm infants.*

Cutaneous stimulation is often applied over the painful area. This may not be possible, as with an extremely painful area, altered skin integrity, and cast or dressing placement. When direct cutaneous stimulation is not feasible, alternative sites may be used (Chart 13–17).

Massage may be done on the total body or localized to the back, extremities, or painful area (use alternative sites if this is not tolerated). This may interrupt pain signals and also enhances relaxation. Massage with a firm movement, particularly with ticklish children.

Thermal application may involve cold, ice, or heat. It is not suggested for use in infants, who are more prone to thermal injury because of their skin structure. Cold is often more effective in relieving pain than heat, but heat is usually better accepted. Alternating between heat and cold may prove more effective than using either alone.

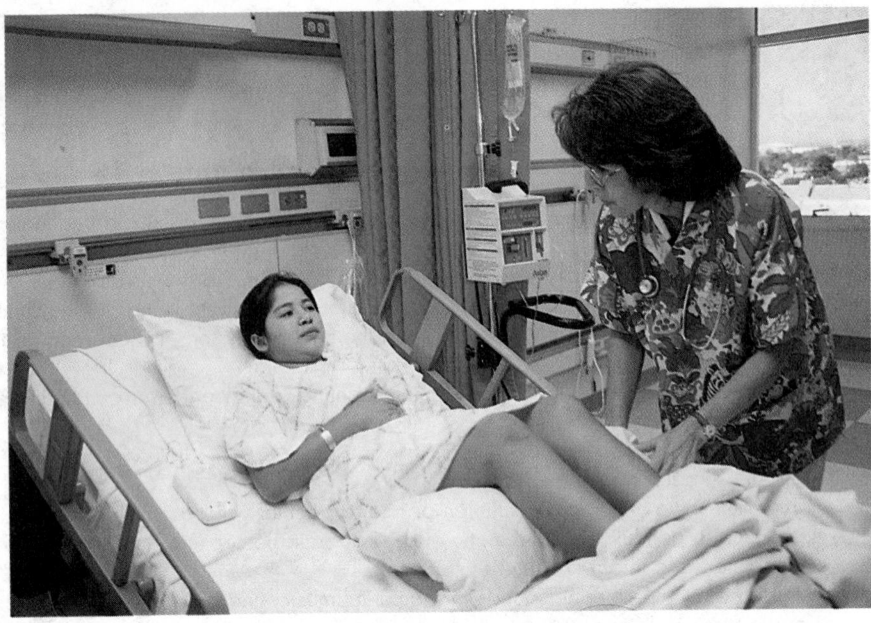

Figure 13–11
Proper positioning may help alleviate pain.

Application of cold is thought to slow noxious impulse conduction and cause vasoconstriction (Ernst & Fialka, 1994), which may reduce release of irritating substances at the site. In pain associated with trauma, cold may reduce swelling and muscle spasms. A cold pack should be wrapped well enough so that it feels cool but is not uncomfortable. Ice massage is effective for injection and musculoskeletal pain, headaches, toothaches, or brief,

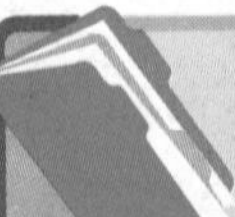

Chart 13–17
Nursing Interventions Classification (NIC)

Cutaneous Stimulation

Definition

Stimulation of the skin and underlying tissues for the purpose of decreasing undesirable signs and symptoms such as pain, muscle spasm, or inflammation

Activities

Discuss various methods of skin stimulation, their effects on sensation, and expectations of patient during activity.
Select a specific cutaneous stimulation strategy, based upon the individual's willingness to participate, ability to participate, preference, support of significant others, and contraindications.
Select the most appropriate type of cutaneous stimulation for the patient and the condition (e.g., massage, cold, ice, heat, menthol, vibration, TENS).
Instruct on indications for, frequency of, and procedure for application.
Apply stimulation directly on or around the affected site as appropriate.
Select stimulation site, considering alternate sites when direct application is not possible (e.g., adjacent to, distal to, between affected areas and the brain, contralateral to).
Consider acupressure points as sites of stimulation as appropriate.
Determine the duration and frequency of stimulation based on method chosen.
Encourage the use of an intermittent method of stimulation as appropriate.
Allow the family to participate as much as possible.
Select alternate method or site of stimulation if altered sensation is not achieved.
Discontinue stimulation if increased pain or skin irritation occurs.
Evaluate and document response to stimulation.

painful procedures. Ice massage may be done using an ice cube. Another convenient method is to fill a paper cup with water and freeze it; the water expands over the cup edges and the cup is held at the bottom to massage. Use circular or back-and-forth motions. Have the patient lie on a plastic-backed pad to absorb melting water.

Alert: *Do not use ice massage on one site for longer than 7 to 10 minutes or in infants younger than 3 months of age (McCaffery & Beebe, 1989). Stop if the child complains or blanching occurs.*

Use of heat promotes circulation to the area, which may promote removal of pain-causing substances. A hot pack should be wrapped well enough to be comfortably warm.

Alert: *Caution should be taken to prevent burns—do not use longer than 20 to 30 minutes; do not use with sleeping patients; monitor skin integrity.*

Transcutaneous Electrical Nerve Stimulation

TENS is a method by which a small electrical current is applied to the skin via conductive pads attached to a battery-operated generator. Parameters such as amplitude (amount of energy applied to skin), rate (number of times the nerve is stimulated per second), and pulse width (depth of stimulation) (Eland, 1989) can be variably set depending on the effect desired. The TENS electrode needs to be placed so that the stimulus generated is directed at the central nervous system, for example, at points where peripheral nerves are superficial, acupuncture and trigger points (Eland, 1993). The mechanism of action is thought to be inhibition of afferent nociceptive impulse transmission via stimulation of large myelinated fibers (Chart 13–18).

When used at conventional settings, TENS causes a tingling, buzzing sensation. This sensation, coupled with being unfamiliar with the machine, may produce fear in the child. Demonstrate use of the equipment on a parent, and then suggest the child try it on a nonpainful area. When the child appears comfortable with this, suggest using TENS for a painful area (Eland, 1993). Advantages of using TENS are that it is safe, efficacious (Lander & Fowler-Kerry, 1993), and simple to use with training and gives the child a sense of control.

Acupressure

Although acupuncture is available for pain management, needles often frighten children, a fear that begins in older infancy. Acupressure is a noninvasive derivative of acupuncture in which manual pressure is applied to the skin at appropriate acupuncture or trigger points by experienced practitioners. Acupressure is more readily acceptable to children and may be quite effective in pain management.

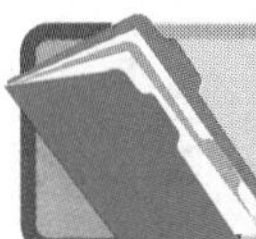

Chart 13–18
Nursing Interventions Classification (NIC)

Transcutaneous Electrical Nerve Stimulation (TENS)

Definition

Stimulation of skin and underlying tissues with controlled, low-voltage electrical vibration via electrodes

Activities

Discuss the rationale for and limits and potential problems of TENS with the patient, family, and/or significant others.
Determine whether a recommendation for TENS is appropriate.
Discuss therapy with physician and obtain prescription for TENS if appropriate.
Select stimulation site, considering alternate sites when direct application is not possible (e.g., adjacent to, distal to, between affected areas and the brain, and contralateral).
Determine therapeutic amplitude, rate, and pulse width.
Give thorough verbal and written instruction on the use of TENS and its operation.
Apply electrodes to the site of stimulation.
Adjust the amplitude, rate, and/or pulse width to predetermined settings indicated.
Maintain stimulation for predetermined interval (continuous or intermittent).
Instruct the patient to adjust the site and settings to achieve the desired response based on individual tolerance if appropriate.
Observe patient application of TENS and inspection of skin surfaces.
Inspect or instruct patient to inspect sites of electrodes for possible skin irritation at every application or at least every 12 hours as appropriate.
Use TENS alone or in conjunction with other measures as appropriate.
Evaluate and document the effectiveness of TENS in altering pain sensation periodically.

From McCloskey, J., & Bulechek, G. (1996). *Nursing interventions classification (NIC)* (2nd ed.). St. Louis: Mosby–Year Book. Reprinted with permission.

Pharmacologic Pain Management

Drug therapy is an important component of managing both acute and chronic pain. Nurses play a key role in monitoring for efficacy and side effects of medications. A thorough knowledge of drug pharmacokinetics, accurate assessment of type and intensity of pain, and education

Chart 13–19
Nursing Interventions Classification (NIC)

Analgesic Administration

Definition

Use of pharmacologic agents to reduce or eliminate pain

Activities

Determine pain location, characteristics, quality, and severity before medicating patient.
Check medical order for drug, dose, and frequency of analgesic prescribed.
Check history for drug allergies.
Evaluate the patient's ability to participate in selection of analgesic, route, and dose, and involve the patient as appropriate.
Choose the appropriate analgesic, or combination of analgesics when more than one is prescribed.
Determine analgesic selections (narcotic, non-narcotic, NSAID) based on type and severity of pain.
Determine the preferred analgesic, route of administration, and dosage to achieve optimal analgesia.
Choose the IV route, rather than IM, for frequent pain medication injections when possible.
Sign out narcotics and other restricted drugs, according to agency protocol.
Monitor vital signs before and after administering narcotic analgesics with first time dose or if unusual signs are noted.
Attend to comfort needs and other activities that assist relaxation to facilitate response to analgesia.
Administer analgesics around-the-clock to prevent peaks and troughs of analgesia, especially with severe pain.
Set positive expectations regarding the effectiveness of analgesics to optimize patient response.
Administer adjuvant analgesics and/or medications when needed to potentiate analgesia.
Consider use of continuous infusion, either alone or in conjunction with bolus opioids, to maintain serum levels.
Institute safety precautions for those receiving narcotic analgesics as appropriate.
Instruct to request p.r.n. pain medication before the pain is severe.
Inform the individual that with narcotic administration drowsiness sometimes occurs the first 2 to 3 days and then subsides.
Correct misconceptions/myths patient or family members may hold regarding analgesics, particularly opioids (e.g., addiction, risks of overdose).
Evaluate the effectiveness of analgesic at regular frequent intervals after each administration, but especially after the initial doses, also observing for any signs and symptoms of untoward effects (e.g., respiratory depression, nausea and vomiting, dry mouth, constipation).
Document response to analgesic and any untoward effects.
Evaluate and document level of sedation for patients receiving opioids.
Implement actions to decrease untoward effects of analgesics (e.g., constipation, gastric irritation).
Collaborate with the physician if drug, dose, route of administration or interval changes are indicated, making specific recommendations based on equianalgesic principles.
Teach about the use of analgesics, strategies to decrease side effects, and expectations for involvement in decisions about pain relief.

From McCloskey, J., & Bulechek, G. (1996). *Nursing interventions classification (NIC)* (2nd ed.). St. Louis: Mosby–Year Book. Reprinted with permission.

of patients, families, and other health team members are essential (Chart 13–19).

Drug Administration Considerations

Scheduling

Pain is best managed by a proactive, preemptive approach. It is much more effective and humane to anticipate and treat pain than to try to manage pain once it is present. See Chart 13–20 for definition of terms important in discussion of analgesics.

If pain is present for the majority of the day, medications need to be scheduled and administered around the clock (ATC), not PRN (pro re nata, as necessary). If pain is present during a limited portion of the day, PRN administration may be adequate. PRN administration of pain medication tends to propagate a pain cycle with the peaks (sedation) and troughs (pain) of drug action. In addition, the child must recognize the pain and commu-

Chart 13–20

Concepts Related to Analgesia Administration

Ceiling Effect. There is a maximum dose beyond which added analgesia does not occur; doses higher than recommended dose do not produce greater pain relief; for example, giving ibuprofen at 10 mg/kg q 6 hr may give pain relief to a pain rating of 4 out of 10, administration of 25 mg/kg does not result in more pain relief or change the pain rating from 4 out of 10.

Tolerance. A larger dose of the medication is required to maintain the same effect. For example, Maria, an 8-year-old with cancer, has been receiving morphine at 0.2 mg/kg IV q 2 hr for bone pain that has been rated 3 out of 10, vital signs are stable, and oxygen saturation is in the 90s. Today, Maria has been complaining of increased pain, ratings are 6 out of 10, heart rate is increased more than 20% over baseline, respiratory rate is increased, oxygen saturations are 75 to the 80s, BP is labile, and morphine is increased to 0.3 mg/kg IV q 2 hr; 30 minutes later Maria reports pain as 3 out of 10, and vital signs are back to baseline values.

Physical Dependence. The physiologic requirement for the drug and presence of withdrawal symptoms with sudden termination of the drug. For example, a neonate has been receiving fentanyl as a continuous IV infusion for 4 days and has the drip suddenly discontinued; the infant starts demonstrating signs of withdrawal—irritability, tremors, and increased crying.

Psychological Dependence (Addiction). Characterized by a compulsive craving for the drug and its use for effects other than pain relief. For example, a 17-year-old with no pain history has been using IV narcotics because he "likes how they make him feel and has to get them every day."

nicate it to the nurse. The nurse must receive the request, get the drug, and administer it, which delays the time between pain stimulus and relief.

Scheduling takes into account the duration of action and half-life of the specific drug. When sustained-release or long-acting drugs are given, it may be necessary to use quick-acting preparations for a rescue dose during breakthrough pain episodes.

Route of Administration

If the patient is able to take medications **orally** and pain can be controlled, this is optimal. This may be more feasible with chronic pain. For more acute (e.g., postoperative) or severe (e.g., cancer) pain, injectable administration may be needed.

Intramuscular injections, although common, are not recommended. There is wide variability in drug absorption and this route is painful. Children are fearful of needles and often deny the existence of pain and suffer rather than have an injection.

Intravenous administration of opioids (some drugs, particularly adjuvants, cannot be given intravenously) provides a rapid onset of action and is most effective when treating severe pain. Opioids can be given as an IV bolus, subcutaneously (SQ), and/or as a continuous infusion.

Patient-controlled analgesia (PCA) is a technique in which patients administer their own opioid medication via a computer-controlled infusion pump connected to the infusion tubing (Fig. 13–12). When an IV line is present, PCA provides a much more palatable alternative to IM injections. Children with cancer pain, in particular, may obtain pain relief via a PCA opioid infusion administered through a small needle inserted into the abdominal SQ tissue.

The PCA pump is programmed for dosage and "lockout" intervals to ensure safety, and the patient pushes the button to administer a bolus of the drug. Medication can be administered as a patient-demanded bolus, or the bolus mode can be superimposed on a continuous infusion. The goal of PCA is to maintain an even level of drug in the blood stream. PCA saves nursing time compared with IM administration. It also saves the child from the pain

Figure 13–12
PCA is an effective method of opioid administration.

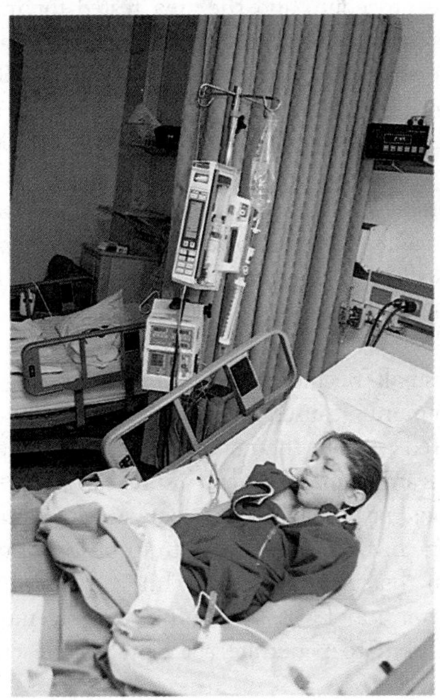

of an injection and gives the child control, which may be the important factor in decreasing the amount of pain perceived.

PCA has been used successfully in children as young as 3 (Gureno & Reisinger, 1991), but questions remain about the age at which they become cognitively capable of using it. The push-button device is easy to use and concrete, something the child can touch and hold. It takes a few minutes for the child to experience pain relief; there is not immediate feedback when the button is pushed, so the child may stop using it, not believing it works. The family and visitors need to be taught how to facilitate the child's use of PCA and not to push the button for the child. Although the total amount of opioid that can be administered is preset, someone else pushing the button bypasses one of the built-in safety features of the system, that an oversedated patient cannot self-administer medication.

Parent-controlled analgesia has also been used effectively. The concept is similar to that of PCA but parents control the opioid administration. Targeted populations are children too young to self-administer medication, those unable cognitively to understand the concept (e.g., developmentally delayed children), and those physically unable to manipulate the button (e.g., children with cerebral palsy). Parents should be taught the basic concept of PCA, side effects associated with opioids, and simple methods of pain assessment covering both indicators of pain and oversedation. For this to be effective, parents must be present the majority of the time.

Local anesthetics (lidocaine, procaine) can alleviate procedural pain (lumbar puncture [LP], venipuncture, wound repair). Local anesthetics are injected subcutaneously with a small needle into the skin around the area to be manipulated. This should be done 5 to 10 minutes before the procedure and the area tested for insensitivity before beginning the procedure. Arguments against using locals are that the "caine" stings for about 30 seconds after injection and the child is subjected to an additional injection.

caREminder: *The stinging sensation can be reduced by buffering the lidocaine solution (9 parts lidocaine to 1 part sodium bicarbonate), which raises the pH of the solution.*

The small needle used for infiltration of the tissue most commonly causes less pain than if the area was manipulated without the benefit of the local anesthetic.

The **transdermal (topical)** route can be used to give medications painlessly or to reduce the pain of local infiltration. *EMLA* (eutectic mixture of local anesthetics) is a cream that can be used in children over 1 month of age. Do not rub EMLA into the skin; it must thickly cover the skin to penetrate adequately. The cream must be applied to intact skin an hour before a procedure and covered with an occlusive dressing (Fig. 13–13).

caREminder: *If inserting an IV line, cover two potential sites in case the first stick is unsuccessful.*

Organizing nursing care to take the time required into account or having the child or family apply EMLA on an outpatient basis may eliminate this as a detrimental issue.

TAC (tetracaine, epinephrine, cocaine) is an anesthetic used for lacerations requiring suturing. It is not effective through intact skin. A gauze soaked with TAC is placed in the wound for about 15 minutes until anesthesia is achieved.

Alert: *TAC can be rapidly absorbed through mucosal surfaces, leading to toxic reactions (Berde, 1993). Use caution around the nose, mouth, and genitals; do not let infants inadvertently suck on the gauze.*

LET (lidocaine, epinephrine, tetracaine) is another mixture of local anesthetics used for suturing lacerations. It should not be used on mucous membranes. LET is thought to involve fewer adverse reactions than TAC, is less expensive, and does not entail the controlled substance monitoring issues involved with TAC. LET is prepared by the pharmacy as a liquid or gel. The gel form contains the medication at the application site and prevents it from running into the mucous membranes. LET should be placed on the wound for 10 to 30 minutes, no longer.

Figure 13–13
EMLA cream reduces the pain of IV catheter insertion and reduces the child's distress.

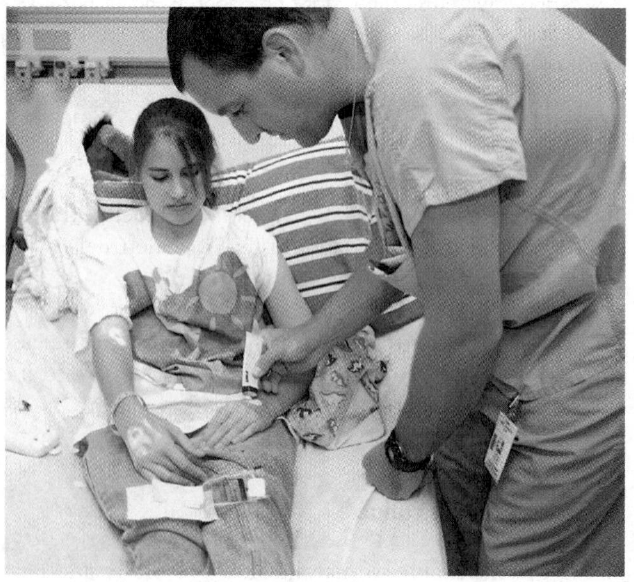

Tip: *Older children may want to help with the application of LET; younger children may tolerate the procedure better if parents assist.*

Skin refrigerants such as *dichlorotetrafluoroethane* (Frigiderm) (Maikler, 1991) and *ethyl chloride* (Zappa & Nabors, 1992) have been shown to be effective in reducing procedural pain such as that resulting from injections and LPs. The latter is flammable and must be used with adequate ventilation. Refrigerants cool the skin, which may decrease the number of pain impulses being transmitted. The refrigerant is sprayed for a few seconds onto the cleansed and prepared site immediately before needle insertion.

Fentanyl and *clonidine* can be administered via patch, usually for pain of a more chronic nature. Fentanyl is a potent opioid. The mechanism of action of clonidine in alleviating pain is not known. Clonidine is a noradrenergic agonist, and it is possible that it mimics the pain-inhibiting effects of similar substances that are naturally released by the body.

When patches are used there is a long onset and offset of action, so it is necessary to have already titrated the child's dose to effect and know the dose that works. To convert the child receiving other opioids to the fentanyl patch, the equianalgesic dose must be calculated. This is done by determining the amount of opioid required in the past 24 hours and converting this to its equianalgesic morphine dose. The corresponding fentanyl dose is then derived from this.

Depending on the type of patch, other analgesics need to be given for the first 24 to 48 hours after the patch is applied. The patch should be placed on intact skin on a flat area of the upper torso. A child who has an adverse reaction to fentanyl needs to be monitored for 12 to 24 hours after patch removal until the serum drug levels begin to drop.

Rectal administration of many medications is effective, particularly in infants and toddlers. This route is not well accepted by children older than 2 years.

Regional analgesia encompasses a variety of techniques including epidural infusion and peripheral nerve blocks. *Epidural* administration of opioids (morphine, fentanyl) and/or local anesthetics (bupivacaine, lidocaine) provides excellent pain relief for postoperative (Grass, 1992) and cancer pain. The child can usually cough, deep breathe, and ambulate comfortably (Schryer, 1989).

caREminder: *No systemic opioids should be given, because this increases the risk of respiratory depression. The nurse must routinely assess for level of sensation, especially if local anesthetics are given, and for catheter integrity.*

Peripheral nerve blocks, administered by the anesthesiologist, can be quite effective in managing pain. They can be used for procedures or injuries (femoral nerve block for fractured femur), for surgery without anesthesia (dorsal penile nerve block for circumcision), during surgery (which may lighten general anesthesia requirements), or to manage postoperative pain (ilioinguinal block for herniorrhaphy).

Conscious sedation is a depressed state of consciousness induced via the use of medications. It is generally used for painful procedures such as bone marrow aspiration, lumbar puncture, laceration repair, and fractures, but may be used for nonpainful procedures such as magnetic resonance imaging (MRI) or computed tomography (CT). When conscious sedation is planned, diet is restricted to clear liquids for 4 to 8 hours as age appropriate and nothing is given by mouth for 2 hours before the procedure.

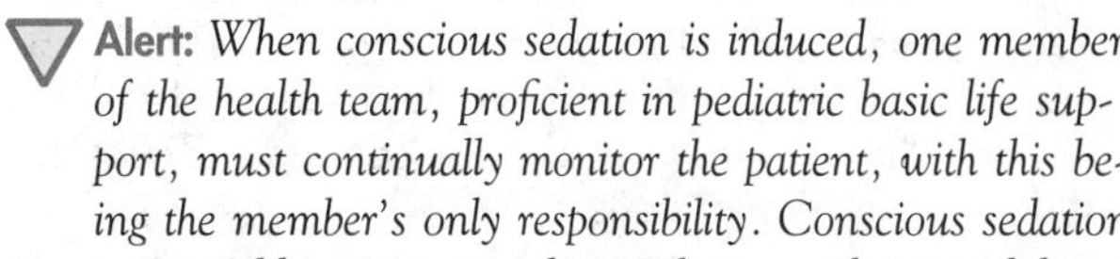

Alert: *When conscious sedation is induced, one member of the health team, proficient in pediatric basic life support, must continually monitor the patient, with this being the member's only responsibility. Conscious sedation may readily progress to deep sedation with an inability to maintain protective reflexes and a patent airway.*

Personnel competent to perform pediatric advanced life support, particularly airway management and intubation, and equipment for resuscitation must be readily available. The patient must be continuously monitored with at least pulse oximetry (American Academy of Pediatrics, 1992). Vital signs such as heart rate, respiratory rate, BP, oxygen saturation, and level of consciousness must be documented at least every 5 minutes (Chart 13–21).

Documentation should also include all medications and fluids administered (dose, route, time), monitoring devices used (continuous pulse oximetry), untoward or significant reactions and actions taken, and discharge instructions given.

The child must be sufficiently recovered from the effects of medications and return to a baseline level of functioning to be safely discharged. Discharge criteria include requirements that the child has stable cardiovascular function and airway patency, is arousable and can talk and follow directions as age appropriate, has age-appropriate motor skills (infant can sit, older child can walk), and has an adequate state of hydration. Handicapped children should be evaluated for return to baseline status. Families should be given written discharge instructions.

Medications

Medications used for pain management are classified into three categories, depending on their mechanism of action:

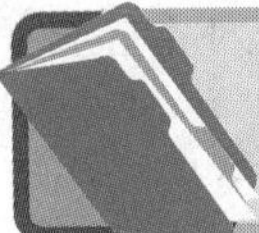

Chart 13–21
Nursing Interventions Classification (NIC)

Conscious Sedation

Definition

Administration of sedatives, monitoring of the patient's response, and provision of necessary physiological support during a diagnostic or therapeutic procedure

Activities

Review patient's health history and results of diagnostic tests to determine whether patient meets agency criteria for conscious sedation by a registered nurse.
Ask patient or family about any previous experiences with conscious sedation.
Check for drug allergies.
Verify that patient has complied with dietary restrictions, as determined by agency criteria.
Review other medications patient is taking and verify absence of contraindications for conscious sedation.
Instruct the patient and/or family about effects of sedation.
Evaluate the patient's level of consciousness and protective reflexes before conscious sedation.
Obtain baseline vital signs.
Obtain baseline oxygen saturation and EKG rhythm, as appropriate.
Initiate an IV line, as appropriate.
Administer medication as per physician's order or protocol, titrating carefully according to patient's response.
Monitor the patient's level of consciousness and vital signs, as per agency protocol.
Monitor oxygen saturation, as appropriate.
Monitor the patient's EKG, as appropriate.
Monitor the patient for adverse effects of medication, including agitation, respiratory depression, undue somnolence, hypoxemia, arrhythmias, apnea, or exacerbation of a preexisting condition.
Restrain the patient, as appropriate.
Ensure availability of and administer benzodiazepine receptor antagonist (flumazenil), as appropriate per physician's order or protocol.
Ensure availability of and administer narcotic antagonists, as appropriate per physician's order or protocol.
Determine whether the patient meets discharge or unit transfer criteria.
Discharge or transfer patient, as per agency protocol.
Document actions and patient response, as per agency policy.

From McCloskey, J., & Bulechek, G. (1996). *Nursing interventions classification (NIC)* (2nd ed.). St. Louis: Mosby–Year Book. Reprinted with permission.

- Nonopioid analgesics
- Opioid analgesics
- Adjunctive medications

Nonopioid Analgesics

Nonopioid analgesics are most effective for mild to moderate pain. They differ from opioids in that they are antipyretic, have a ceiling effect, and do not produce tolerance or physical or psychological dependence. Nonopioid analgesics (except acetaminophen) reduce nociceptor stimulation by inhibition of prostaglandin synthesis and are considered integral to any analgesic regimen (American Pain Society, 1992). Nonopioids can be used alone or in conjunction with an opioid for severe pain to achieve peripheral and central mechanisms of action. They are useful when pain involves an inflammatory process (Table 13–4).

Opioid Analgesics

This category includes centrally and peripherally acting opioids such as codeine, hydrocodone, morphine, meperidine, hydromorphone, methadone, oxycodone, and fentanyl (Table 13–5). Opioid effects are mediated by different receptors in the central nervous system. The different opioid drugs are classified, according to their receptor binding properties, as agonists, antagonists, or agonists-antagonists.

Agonists (e.g., morphine, hydromorphone) produce analgesia; agonists may have different effects on different receptors so different side effects may be seen.

Table 13-4
Dosing Nonsteroidal Anti-inflammatory Drugs (NSAIDs)

	Dose*			
Drug	Adult or adolescent	Child less than 50 kg	Infant younger than 6 mo	**Comments**
				Useful for mild to moderate pain or to augment and decrease narcotic requirements with severe pain; good for musculoskeletal pain. They differ in chemical structure, so if one drug is not effective, another should be tried. All except acetaminophen have anti-inflammatory properties. Side effects: gastritis, platelet dysfunction (except acetaminophen and choline magnesium trisalicylate), and renal insufficiency; monitor for bleeding and oliguria.
Acetaminophen	650–975 mg q 4 hr PO	10–15 mg/kg q 4 hr PO 15–20 mg/kg PR	10–15 mg/kg q 4–6 hr PO	No anti-inflammatory properties. Prolonged half-life in neonates, so see peak serum concentration at ~60 min (30 min in older children), may need longer dosing intervals; good for premature infants because it does not interfere with platelet function, so does not increase chance of bleeding and intraventricular hemorrhage.
Aspirin	650–975 mg q 4 hr PO	10–15 mg/kg q 4 hr PO 15–20 mg/kg PR		The standard against which other NSAIDs are compared. Possible association with Reye's syndrome—not recommended for children under 12 yr, do *not* give in the presence of fever, varicella, known or suspected viral illness.
Choline magnesium trisalicylate (Trilisate)	1000–1500 mg b.i.d. PO	25 mg/kg b.i.d. PO		Contains salicylate—do not use with known or suspected viral infection.
Ibuprofen (Motrin, Advil)	400 mg q 4–6 hr PO	10–20 mg/kg q 6–8 hr PO		
Naproxen (Naprosyn)	500 mg PO initial dose, then 250 mg q 6–8 hr PO	5 mg/kg q 8–12 hr PO		
Ketorolac (Toradol) (parenteral NSAID)	30 or 60 mg IM/IV initial dose, then 15 or 30 mg q 6 hr	1 mg/kg IM/IV loading dose, then 0.5 mg/kg q 6 hr		Not yet approved for use in children; use not to exceed 5 days.

PO, oral; PR, per rectum; IM, intramuscular; IV, intravenous; b.i.d., twice daily.

References: Acute Pain Management Guideline Panel. (1992). *Acute pain management: Operative or medical procedures and trauma. Clinical practice guideline* (AHCPR Publication, No. 92-0032). Rockville, MD: Agency for Health Care Policy and Research, Public Health Service, U.S. Department of Health and Human Services; American Pain Society. (1992). *Principles of analgesic use in the treatment of acute pain and cancer pain* (3rd ed.). Skokie, IL: American Pain Society; Lau, N. (1992). Pediatric pain management—part I. *Journal of Pediatric Health Care, 6,* 87–92; Management of Cancer Pain Guideline Panel (1994). *Management of cancer pain. Clinical practice guideline* (AHCPR Publication No. 94-0592). Rockville, MD: Agency for Health Care Policy and Research, Public Health Service, U.S. Department of Health and Human Services.

Table 13-5
Dosing Opioids

Drug	Dose: Adult or adolescent	Dose: Child less than 50 kg	Dose: Infant younger than 6 mo	Comments
				Opioids—useful for moderate to severe pain. Most effective to anticipate pain and treat before onset. Physical dependence may occur rapidly (3 days or less). Side effects: respiratory depression (most common in first days of treatment in children who have not been receiving opioids), pruritus, nausea, diarrhea, constipation, orthostatic hypotension, sedation, agitation.
Agonists				
Morphine	30 mg q 3–4 hr PO 10 mg q 3–4 hr IV	0.3 mg/kg q 3–4 hr PO 0.1–0.2 mg/kg q 3–4 hr IV PCA load 0.03–0.05 mg/kg PCA 0.02–0.03 mg/kg basal 0.01–0.02 mg/kg/hr	0.05–0.2 mg/kg q 3–4 hr IV IV gtt—50 μg/kg load, then 10–15 μg/kg/hr	Agonists do not have a ceiling; that is, they can be administered in increasingly large doses, limited only by the occurrence of side effects. Morphine—↑ ICP (caution with premature infants, children with head injuries), may cause bronchospasm.
Fentanyl		2–3 μg/kg q 1–2 hr IV IV gtt—0.5–1.0 μg/kg/hr	1–2 μg/kg q 1–2 hr IV IV gtt—1–2 μg/kg load, then 1–5 μg/kg/hr	Rapid onset of action, short duration. Side effects: chest wall rigidity if given rapidly, bradycardia, does not ↑ ICP.
Meperidine (Demerol)	100 mg q 3 hr IV	0.75 mg/kg q 2–3 hr	1.0 mg/kg q 3 hr	*Not* recommended, particularly for multiple doses, because the end product of metabolism, normeperidine, may accumulate and cause CNS irritability (tremors, muscle twitching, seizures); use only if intolerant to all other drugs. Causes less respiratory depression than morphine.
Hydromorphone (Dilaudid)	6 mg q 3–4 hr PO 1.5 mg q 3–4 hr IV	0.06 mg/kg q 3–4 hr PO 0.015 mg/kg q 3–4 hr IV		Less histamine release than morphine, better initial opioid for patients with reactive airways.
Codeine	60 mg q 3–4 hr PO 60 mg q 2 hr IM/SQ	0.5–1 mg/kg q 3–4 hr PO, not recommended IM		Generally combined with a nonopioid (e.g., acetaminophen—dose must not exceed acetaminophen safe dose of 90 mg/kg/day)
Methadone	20 mg q 6–8 hr PO 10 mg q 6–8 hr IV	0.2 mg/kg q 6–8 hr PO 0.1–0.2 mg/kg load IV, then 0.05–0.1 mg/kg q 4–12 hr IV	0.4–0.7 mg/kg per 24 hr IV divided into four doses	Prolonged duration of action; useful in weaning from opioids

Table 13-5
Dosing Opioids *Continued*

Drug	Dose			Comments
	Adult or adolescent	Child less than 50 kg	Infant younger than 6 mo	
Agonist-Antagonists and Partial Agonists				
Buprenorphine (Buprenex)	0.4 mg q 6–8 IV	0.004 mg/kg q 6–8 hr IV		Have an analgesic ceiling: increasing analgesia is produced with increasing the dose up to a certain point, where increasing the dose does not produce additional analgesia; these drugs can cause dysphoria and hallucinations, so are less useful for pain relief in children.
Nalbuphine (Nubain)	10 mg q 3–4 hr IV	0.1 mg/kg q 3–4 hr IV		Useful when side effects of agonists prevent giving enough drug to obtain adequate analgesia. Need to give high doses initially when switching from agonist in order to overcome antagonistic effects.

PO, oral; IV, intravenous; IV gtt, continuous intravenous drip; IM, intramuscular; SQ, subcutaneous; ICP, intracranial pressure.
These are recommended starting doses in children who are not tolerant to opioids; optimum doses are determined by titrating to effect. Starting doses do not apply to children with renal/hepatic insufficiency or other conditions affecting drug metabolism. IM/SQ not recommended (except parenteral codeine in adults). Antagonist (naloxone) and appropriate resuscitation equipment should be readily available when IV narcotics are administered.
References: Acute Pain Management Guideline Panel. (1992). *Acute pain management: Operative or medical procedures and trauma. Clinical practice guideline* (AHCPR Publication No. 92-0032). Rockville, MD: Agency for Health Care Policy and Research, Public Health Service, U.S. Department of Health and Human Services; American Pain Society. (1992). *Principles of analgesic use in the treatment of acute pain and cancer pain* (3rd ed.). Skokie, IL: American Pain Society; Truog, R., & Anand, K. J. S. (1989). Management of pain in the postoperative neonate. *Clinics in Perinatology, 16,* 61–78; Yaster, M., & Maxwell, L. G. (1993). Opioid agonists and antagonists. In N. L. Schechter, C. B. Berde, & M. Yaster, (Eds.), *Pain in infants, children, and adolescents* (pp. 145–171). Baltimore: Williams & Wilkins.

Antagonists (e.g., naloxone) bind to opioid receptors. They have no intrinsic activity of their own and do not initiate a pharmacologic effect. Thus, they do not produce analgesia but they block the site from use by agonists to produce analgesia. Administration of small amounts of naloxone may reverse some of the side effects of opioids without affecting their analgesic properties. Larger doses cause sudden reversal of the analgesic properties and result in sudden and severe pain in a child being treated for pain; they also precipitate acute withdrawal in a child who has become physically dependent on opioids.

Agonists-antagonists (e.g., nalbuphine, buprenorphine) can provide analgesia but also reverse the effect of other opioids.

A common misconception is that it is too dangerous to administer narcotics to young children. Close monitoring for side effects, most notably respiratory depression, is indicated in all children, especially after IV or epidural administration (Chart 13–22). Opioid clearance is slow in infants younger than 3 months compared with older children (Tyler, 1994). This does not mean that infants should not receive opioids. It means that the dose needs to be titrated to effect and that intensive monitoring of infants up to 6 to 12 months of age is warranted (Acute Pain Management Guideline Panel, 1992) (Chart 13–23).

A closely related myth is that children may become addicted to opioids. This is propagated by those who do not understand the difference between physical and psychological dependence (see Chart 13–20) and the role opioids play in pain management. Development of tolerance may be delayed by combining opioids and nonopioids or changing to another opioid (American Pain Society, 1992). When switching to another opioid or to a different route of administration (e.g., IV to oral), an equianalgesic conversion must be calculated and the patient monitored for response (American Pain Society, 1992; McCaffery & Beebe, 1989).

caREminder: *Equianalgesic tables can be obtained from various sources (e.g., Acute Pain Management Guideline*

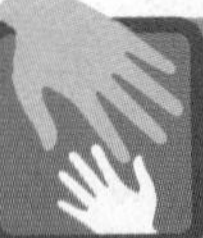

Chart 13–22
Nursing Interventions

Opioid Side Effects

Common Opioid Side Effects	Interventions*
Respiratory depression (especially with IV, epidural, high doses)	Assess respiratory rate and depth, have resuscitation equipment and naloxone available.
Sedation	Assess level of consciousness, for chronic therapy add stimulant as ordered (e.g., caffeine, dextroamphetamine, methylphenidate).
Constipation	Assess bowel sounds, encourage ambulation, increase fluid and fiber intake, administer a stool softener and a laxative, as ordered.
Nausea	Administer hydroxyzine or a phenothiazine antiemetic as ordered.
Pruritus	Administer an antihistamine as ordered, apply cool compresses to the site.
Urinary retention	Monitor intake and output, apply a warm compress over the bladder, have the patient ambulate if possible.

* American Pain Society. (1992). *Principles of analgesic use in the treatment of acute pain and cancer pain* (3rd ed.). Skokie, IL: Author.
Treatment of side effects is also dependent on the specific situation and how they interfere with activities of daily living. For example, sedation may be desired in the immediate postoperative period but not desired for the patient with cancer.

Panel, 1992, p. 112) These tables generally compare the analgesic effect of a drug with that of morphine, 10 mg IM (e.g., the equianalgesic dose of oral morphine would be 30 mg every 3 to 4 hours with around-the-clock dosing). Equianalgesic tables provide an approximate point to dose from. The child's clinical response to analgesic dose must be evaluated and the dose titrated to provide effective pain relief.

Physical dependence on opioids may develop if used for more than 3 to 4 days, even fewer days when administered via continuous infusion. To decrease the risk of withdrawal or the occurrence of side effects, the dose should be gradually decreased (10% to 20% per day) or the time between doses gradually increased; do not simply eliminate doses. Use caution with children who may have developed physical dependence; use of antagonists (naloxone) to reverse side effects may precipitate sudden withdrawal. Withdrawal symptoms include irritability, abdominal cramps, vomiting, diaphoresis, and insomnia. Infants may also demonstrate increased crying, poor feeding (but show ravenous sucking), and increased muscle tone, tremors, and jitteriness. If withdrawal symptoms are present, ensure a quiet, darkened environment; handle an infant as little as possible, and ask older children what their needs are; and provide comfort measures (offer pacifier, swaddle infants, apply cool cloth to forehead for older children). Sedatives may be used to manage symptoms. Use of a scoring method similar to one developed for neonatal abstinence syndrome (NAS) (for infants born to opioid-addicted mothers) helps in consistent monitoring and tracking of opioid weaning (Franck & Vilardi, 1995). Children should be monitored for at least 48 hours after discontinuing continuous opioid infusions (French & Nocera, 1994).

Adjuncts

These drugs play a role in pain management by their effects on potentiating analgesic actions of other drugs, reducing anxiety, and/or exerting an analgesic effect of their own. **Tricyclic antidepressants** (e.g., imipramine, amitriptyline) are given in small doses that are subtherapeutic for treatment of depression. They are thought to work by blocking reabsorption of some neurotransmitters (norepinephrine, serotonin). Side effects are somnolence, dry mouth, and occasionally blurred vision. To ensure better patient compliance, teach that these side effects are common in the first few days and then usually diminish. Encourage the child to put up with the side effects and give the drug adequate time to have an impact on the pain. These drugs are more frequently used for chronic pain, so the side effect of somnolence may be a benefit for patients who have had altered sleep patterns.

Benzodiazepines (e.g., diazepam, lorazepam, midazolam) are used to reduce anxiety and produce amnesia.

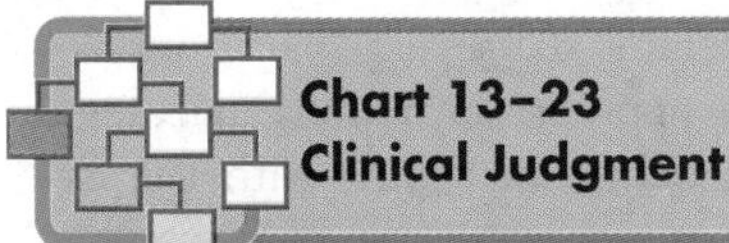

Chart 13–23
Clinical Judgment

An Infant in Pain

Diep is a 3-kg, 1-week-old patient 20 hours post major abdominal surgery. Vital signs are HR 166 beats per minute, RR 50 breaths per minute and shallow, oxygen saturation 90%. She has slept for brief periods since surgery and has a high-pitched cry that is more intense after repositioning. She keeps her eyes closed most of the time and is not interested in her environment. She has had 0.1 mg of morphine IV every 4 hours since surgery.

Questions

1. Is Diep's pain being relieved by the doses of IV morphine?
2. What behaviors indicate that Diep is in pain?
3. Is Diep receiving adequate analgesia for her level of pain?
4. What should you do to better manage Diep's pain?
5. When should you reevaluate Diep's pain level, and what will indicate that your interventions have been effective?

Answers

1. No.
2. Increased HR, RR and shallow respirations, decreased oxygen saturation, intense high-pitched cry, sleep pattern disturbance, lack of socialization.
3. Pain behaviors indicate severe pain. She is not receiving adequate analgesia as indicated by demonstrated pain behaviors and on morphine dose administered (recommended morphine dose for an infant is 0.05 to 0.2 mg/kg q 3 to 4 hr = 0.15 to 0.6 mg per dose). Both dose and frequency could be increased.
4. Increase both dosage and frequency of administration of morphine, might give 0.2 to 0.4 mg and reevaluate pain status, consider starting IV morphine with continuous drip at 30 to 45 μg/hr (dose is 10 to 15 μg/kg/hr). Implement nonpharmacologic interventions: position with knees bent to avoid tension on abdominal incision; place firm boundaries around her, blanket rolls or parent's (nurse's) hands, to help her feel more secure; swaddle; offer pacifier. Monitor for respiratory depression, as with anyone receiving IV morphine.
5. Evaluate about 20 minutes after morphine dose. Effectiveness of interventions would be demonstrated by vital signs returning to baseline values and decreased amount and intensity of cry. Possibly may see increased interest in environment but, given the stress of recent surgery and altered sleep patterns for the past 20 hours, would anticipate catch-up sleep to occur with longer periods of deep sleep.

These drugs have few analgesic properties themselves but are used to enhance the analgesic effects of other drugs and to counteract the side effects.

caREminder: *Painful procedures should not be performed without the addition of analgesic drugs.*

Benzodiazepines block rapid eye movement (REM) sleep; thus, caution should be used if these drugs are administered to young children for longer than 1 day. No research has been done on the impact these drugs may have on long-term memory and cognition, especially when used in young infants with rapidly developing nervous systems.

Phenothiazines (e.g., chlorpromazine, promethazine) are antiemetic and decrease anxiety but may actually increase pain perception. For this reason the use of a "cocktail" of meperidine (Demerol), promethazine (Phenergan), and chlorpromazine (Thorazine) for pain relief and sedation during painful procedures is *not* recommended (Acute Pain Management Guideline Panel, 1992).

Alert: *When phenothiazines are used in conjunction with opioids there is an increased risk of excessive sedation and respiratory depression.*

Sedatives cause drowsiness, which, when combined with fear and anxiety, may heighten the child's feelings of loss of control.

Anticonvulsants (e.g., carbamazepine, phenytoin) and both Ca^{2+} and Na^{+} channel blockers (verapamil, mexiletine) can be useful in treatment of neuropathic pain. They are thought to work by suppressing peripheral nerve excitability (Zeltzer, Anderson, & Schechter, 1990).

Chart 13–24

Checklist for Assessing Adequacy of Pain Management in Children

Pharmacologic Strategies

- ☐ Have the child and parent(s) been asked about their previous experiences with pain and their preferences for use of analgesics?
- ☐ Does the child or parent(s) have reservations about the use of opioids for pain treatment?
- ☐ Is the child being adequately assessed at appropriate intervals?
- ☐ Are analgesics ordered for prevention and relief of pain?
- ☐ Is the analgesic strong enough for the pain expected or the pain being experienced?
- ☐ Is the timing of drug administration appropriate for the pain expected or experienced?
- ☐ Is the route of administration appropriate for the child?
- ☐ Is the child adequately monitored for the occurrence of side effects?
- ☐ Are side effects appropriately managed?
- ☐ Has the analgesic regimen provided adequate comfort and satisfaction from the perspective of the child or parent(s)?

Nonpharmacologic Strategies

- ☐ Have the child and parent(s) been asked about their experience with and preferences for a given strategy?
- ☐ Is the strategy appropriate for the child's developmental level, condition, and type of pain?
- ☐ Is the timing of the strategy sufficient to optimize its effects?
- ☐ Is the strategy adequately effective in preventing or alleviating the child's pain?
- ☐ Are the child and parent(s) satisfied with the strategy for prevention or relief of pain?
- ☐ Are the treatable sources of emotional distress for the child being addressed?

From *Management of cancer pain* (AHCPR Publication No. 94-0592) (p. 128). (1994). Rockville, MD: Agency for Health Care Policy and Research, Public Health Service, U.S. Department of Health and Human Services.

Ensuring Effective Outcomes of Pain Management

For the child experiencing mild to moderate pain, nonpharmacologic interventions alone may adequately manage the pain. For moderate to severe pain, use of medications coupled with appropriate nonpharmacologic strategies best supports the child in coping with the experience. Pharmacologic management of pain can be achieved using a single drug or combinations of the drugs discussed earlier. Dose, schedule, route, and combinations must be titrated so that an optimal effect is obtained. Side effects must be anticipated and managed. The adequacy of pain management must be evaluated on a routine basis (Chart 13–24).

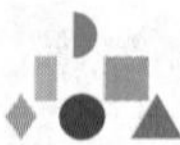

Special Pain Situations

Chronic Pain

Pain that persists a month beyond the usual expected disease or injury course is considered chronic (Bonica, 1990). In contrast to acute pain, chronic pain does not have a biologically protective function. Some causes of chronic pain in children are cancer, sickle cell disease, juvenile rheumatoid arthritis, and recurrent pains (headache, abdominal and limb pain). The importance of distinguishing between acute and chronic pain lies in the differences of assessment and management.

Impact on the Child

The effects of chronic pain on the child may include sleep disturbances, exhaustion, irritability, mood disturbances, and depression. These effects are probably related to depletion of serotonin and endorphins. Many children respond to chronic pain by regression to earlier developmental stages. Another reaction may be an increased response to minor injuries. For example, an exaggerated response would occur when a child bumps his or her knee and then reports that it hurts horribly and cries for 20 minutes.

The primary task of childhood is achievement of developmental milestones, socialization, and self-differentiation. Chronic pain may delay acquisition of normal skills (Chart 13–25). The extent of the impact is dependent on the interplay between the child's physical limitations caused by the pain and the degree to which physical and emotional factors interfere with activities of daily living. Children may restrict themselves to activities that are easy for them, not trying new activities that promote a sense of success and accomplishment, in addition to acquisition of new skills. Achievement of milestones may also be delayed because parents are overprotective and limit the child's experiences for fear they may exacerbate the pain.

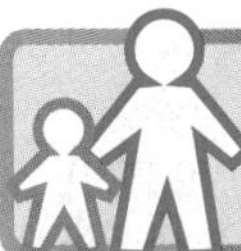

Chart 13–25
Developmental Considerations

Impact of Chronic Pain, Potential Reactions

Children of all ages respond to ongoing pain by regression to earlier stages of development.

Infant

- Withdrawal or difficulties in social interactions
- Feeding problems
- Sleep pattern disturbances
- Motor development delays related to limitation of movement

Toddler and Preschooler

- Withdrawal, aggression
- Motor lags
- Loss of recently achieved developmental milestones (e.g., toileting, motor skills)

School-Age Child

- Withdrawal, aggression, out-of-control behaviors, depression
- Delay in achieving self-care skills
- Delay in achieving socialization skills (school and peer involvement)

Adolescent

- Alteration in body image and peer relationships
- Withdrawal, oppositional behavior, depression
- May affect achievement of independent self-care skills

Impact on the Family

Negative repercussions are usually seen in the family system when a member suffers from chronic pain. In addition to the patient, the needs of the parents and siblings must be recognized and addressed. The ongoing nature of the child's suffering may result in exhaustion and ensuing irritability. Parental employment may be jeopardized by the time and energy demands imposed by the situation. Other financial problems may occur because of expenditures related to the pain problem.

Siblings of the child in pain may feel neglected because of the increased attention focused on the child experiencing pain. Marital difficulties may be caused by the prolonged stress on the family system. The parents may feel inadequate that they are unable to help their child or prevent the child's suffering. This feeling of inadequacy can manifest itself as anger, directed inward as depression, directed at each other, or, not uncommonly, directed at health care providers. Inadequacy may also be manifest in controlling behaviors by the parents such as stating that only a certain nurse can take care of the child. The nurse needs to remember that the parent is generally acting out of concern for the child and may use control as a coping strategy. The nurse needs to be sensitive to the parent's needs, recognizing that the parent knows the child better than other members of the health care team.

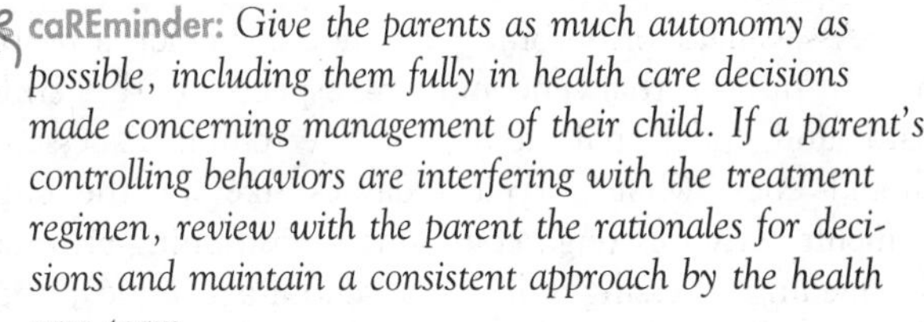

caREminder: *Give the parents as much autonomy as possible, including them fully in health care decisions made concerning management of their child. If a parent's controlling behaviors are interfering with the treatment regimen, review with the parent the rationales for decisions and maintain a consistent approach by the health care team.*

Children experiencing chronic pain may find that others discredit their complaints or label them as psychosomatic. Assessment and management of these children require astute perception and a holistic approach, embracing the philosophy that the health team is working *with* the family in achieving the desired outcomes.

Assessing Chronic Pain

When pain is chronic in nature, the methods and tools used for acute pain may assist in the assessment process. Often, because chronic pain results in adaptation, one does not see the more dramatic response behaviors as seen with acute pain (Chart 13–26). Vital sign changes

Chart 13–26

Signs and Symptoms of Chronic Pain in Children

- Vital signs stable
- Altered muscular movement → misused, tense muscles → ↓ movement → altered sensory input
- Disrupted sleep → tires readily, ↑ irritability, ↓ ability to concentrate
- Developmental regression
- Change in eating patterns
- Behavior or school problems
- Withdrawal from peer group activity
- Depression
- Aggression

seen with acute pain have stabilized, so one cannot rely on these. The initial response to chronic pain can result in behavior and school problems before a diagnosis is even made. A frequent marker of the degree of disability or dysfunction caused by the pain is school avoidance (not attending school regularly) by the patient.

caREminder: *Family, teachers, and health team members need to remember that the body adapts to pain that is ongoing and the child may not demonstrate behaviors that are typical of acute pain.*

This should help avoid a common assumption that the child is not experiencing pain and is exaggerating the pain ratings.

Assessment of chronic pain should include a routine health history that encompasses aspects of the child's pain and functional ability of the child. Assessment should elicit what a typical day is like for the child. Difficult activities (e.g., comfortably positioning an infant for feeding, dressing self for a school-age child), those that exacerbate pain (no nap for a toddler, participation in sports for an adolescent), and activities that reduce the pain (position, distraction, medications) should be identified. Keeping a symptom diary may help identify proactive steps to avoid exacerbation of pain. A diet history should also be obtained, because chronic pain may cause loss of appetite. Aspects of family functioning should be evaluated, such as parental mental health, stressors in the family, other siblings with the same disease, pain that started after a grandparent died of cancer, and perceptions such as that relatives have migraines and they "are genetic, so nothing can be done."

A thorough physical examination should be completed. This serves a dual purpose. The first is to evaluate the child's baseline status. The second is to assure the child and family that the child's pain is being taken seriously and they are believed. When the child is followed for a period of time, health care providers may feel comfortable that they know the situation and become biased in their assessments and conclusions.

Alert: *A new disease or advancing pathology may have occurred since the last visit; this should not be overlooked as a potential cause of pain. Increased or different pain complaints need to be investigated.*

The family is helped to establish realistic goals and set priorities. The goals should not be too basic or easy, as the child needs to be challenged, but, conversely, should not be so difficult that they cause frustration.

Managing Chronic Pain

Many of the techniques previously discussed are applicable to the management of chronic pain in children. Obviously, strategies are influenced by the origin and type of pain. Pathology should be addressed and treated. The focus in acute pain is on rest, symptomatic treatment, and avoiding stress. The focus shifts with chronic pain to helping the child regain or achieve appropriate developmental tasks, decreasing attention to pain behaviors (while making sure that pain control is as good as possible), and emphasizing a productive role.

Children with chronic pain benefit from an interdisciplinary approach that combines behavioral, biophysical, and pharmacologic strategies. Interventions are planned on the basis of assessment findings, goals, and priorities of the family (Chart 13–27). Parents should reward positive behavior; that is, praise the child for performing activities of daily living even when having pain. Less attention should be paid to complaining, after it is determined that this is not caused by new or different pain. The child should resume self-care and activity to the fullest extent possible. School attendance should be strongly encouraged as this is a normalizing activity for children. If the child has missed school for a period of time, school reintegration needs to be addressed (Rabin, 1994).

Reassessment of pain and reevaluation of the treatment program need to be done on a routine basis. The benefit of an interdisciplinary approach can be realized by utilizing the strengths of different team members: the nurse should be a contact person for the family and coordinate team member activities. This may involve coordinating with the physician and pharmacist for medication schedule, dose, or drug changes; psychologist for behavioral and coping strategies; physical therapist for functional activity and strength training; nutritionist for diet modifications; or social worker for family support issues (Chart 13–28).

Pain in the Emergency Department

The child presenting to the emergency department (ED) should have the ABCs (airway, breathing, circulation) addressed first. Severe pain is considered an emergency in itself and requires immediate attention after evaluation and stabilization of the ABCs. The child in the ED may experience pain resulting from pathology and/or from diagnostic or therapeutic procedures. If painful procedures are necessary, prepare the child before the procedure when possible. When interventions need to be done on an emergent basis, explain what is being done as it is happening. Position the child securely for procedures. Restrain as needed so that the child's movement does not prolong the procedure or increase pain.

Tip: *Tell the child "I am helping you to hold still," which gives the child more of a perception of control, versus "I have to hold you so you won't move." Tell children what they can do to make it easier for themselves "Squeeze*

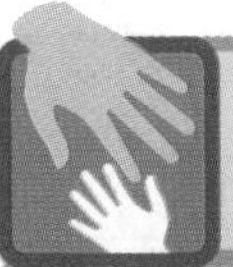

Chart 13-27
Nursing Interventions

Chronic Pain

- Believe that the child has pain.
- Help the child and family establish realistic goals—steadily work toward these with small steps; reinforce the fact that overexertion is usually counterproductive.
- Provide environmental manipulation:
  - Coordinate with physical therapy to evaluate need for and providing adaptive aids such as a cane, slip-on shoes; adding a railing to the stairway.
  - Evaluate the effect of different positions to promote comfort and functional activity.
  - Rearrange the daily schedule to provide more time for difficult activities or to allow the child to perform them in the morning when fatigue may be less of an issue.
  - Schedule rest periods, promote uninterrupted sleep.
- Optimize nutritional intake.
- Teach stress reduction techniques: biofeedback, exercise, relaxation.
- Implement biophysical interventions: TENS, cutaneous stimulation, nerve blocks.
- Provide pharmacologic interventions:
  - The oral route is preferable for nonmalignant pain, transdermal patches convenient to use.
  - Medicate to provide pain relief or at least so child can participate in normal activities.
  - Single-drug therapy may be tried but complex pain problems often require combinations of drugs (acetaminophen, NSAIDs, antidepressants, anticonvulsants, benzodiazepines, opioids).
  - Individualize schedule, around-the-clock dosing with additional dosing available for breakthrough pain.
  - If opioids are used, tolerance may develop; if so, dosages need to be adjusted.
  - Watch for signs of withdrawal when discontinuing medications; reduce dosage slowly to avoid withdrawal and acute exacerbation of pain; wean from sedatives first.

your mommy's hand as hard as this hurts" or "count to 10." Tell them what they can do ("hold your leg still") versus what they cannot do ("don't move your leg").

Whenever time permits, use EMLA cream for venipunctures, lumbar punctures, and so forth or TAC for lacerations. IV opioids or conscious sedation should be used for more painful procedures. Children undergoing conscious sedation in the ED should be assumed to have a full stomach.

Pain management should be addressed early to avoid escalating the pain and the child's and family's distress. Psychological support should always be given and nonpharmacologic techniques used when possible. In the ED drugs are usually given to control pain because of the amount of pain experienced and time constraints.

Children in shock should not be given opioids until hemodynamic stability is achieved. If severe pain is present in a child with potential hemodynamic compromise, small doses of short-acting opioids may be given repeatedly (e.g., morphine or fentanyl every 5 minutes). Headache associated with head injuries can often be managed with nonopioid analgesics. This is preferable because opioids may mask signs of changing neurologic status. If opioids are required, small amounts that do not affect level of consciousness should be used. Aggressive pain management is required for children with burns. Opioids combined with nonopioids should be given as soon as possible. Dressing the wounds and cold compresses aid in pain relief. Fractures can be extremely painful; short-acting IV opioids should be given. If pain is less severe, ibuprofen or acetaminophen with codeine and application of cold may be effective. Pain resulting from minor injuries may be managed with acetaminophen, ibuprofen, or another nonsteroidal anti-inflammatory drug (NSAID) as age appropriate or a weak opioid such as codeine. Reevaluation of pain intensity and efficacy of interventions should be done frequently, at least every time vital signs are taken.

A Handicapped Child Experiencing Pain

The child who is handicapped still has the capability to experience both acute and chronic pain, although the child may be lacking in ability to communicate this effectively. The handicapped child should have pain managed as any other child does. If the child has cognitive deficits, use tools for pain assessment that are appropriate for developmental level. Do not use chronologic age as a basis for pain assessment.

When the child is unable cognitively to communicate pain, assessment methods used for infants may be employed (e.g., vital sign changes, crying, moaning, refusal to move, decreased appetite, irritability, sleep disturbance). The child's typical behaviors when pain free should be used as a baseline to evaluate for pain and response to treatment. The method the child usually uses to communicate should be used (e.g., letter board, shaking head, blinking eyes, specific words for pain).

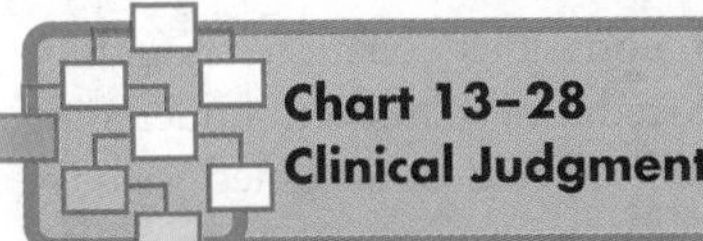

Chart 13–28
Clinical Judgment

An Adolescent in Pain

Charles is a 14-year-old with hemophilia who weighs 50 kg. He is well known to your clinic because he has a history of multiple bleeding episodes. He is not receiving routine medication, only factor XIII for acute bleeding episodes. He comes in today limping and complaining of joint pain at 8 on a 10-point scale. Charles greets all the nurses with a hug and smile but seems much less cheerful than normal. Vital signs are normal for age.

Questions

1. What more would you ask Charles about his current complaints?
2. Charles indicates that this pain is primarily in his left knee and ankle, although all lower extremity joints are painful intermittently. This has been present for about 7 months, becoming increasingly painful until reaching its present level about 2 weeks ago. He has lost 2 kg since last weighed 6 months ago and is not sleeping well ("I can't get comfortable"). He misses at least 1 day of school a week, and his grades are dropping. He still swims and ropes but can't ride his bike to school anymore. On the basis of this history, what are your concerns?
3. What is his current problem?
4. How should this be managed?
5. When and how will you reevaluate Charles?

Answers

1. History of current pain complaint—did he hurt himself recently? Does he think it is an acute bleed? Where is the pain? What does it feel like? How long has it been present? Is it always at this level or is it intermittent? Is pain interfering with activities of daily living, including eating and sleeping, school attendance and performance, and with activities that he enjoys (swimming, bike riding, and roping)? If pain is interfering, to what extent? Does anything help relieve the pain?
2. The pain is affecting Charles' quality of life—sleeping and eating disturbances, interfering with school, socialization, and potentially his ability to achieve independence and self-care skills.
3. Chronic arthritic pain from previous bleeding episodes.
4. Start oral nonsteroidal anti-inflammatory drug and weak opioid around the clock. Physical therapy consultation. Discuss nonpharmacologic methods of pain relief—cutaneous stimulation (cold, massage) and cognitive-behavioral methods (progressive muscle relaxation, meditation, guided imagery, self-hypnosis). Have Charles select one to learn and use until next appointment. Have Charles keep symptom diary.
5. Reevaluate in 1 month (takes about this time for NSAID effects to occur). Charles should call clinic sooner if the pain worsens or is not below 4 out of 10 in 2 days (Charles' goal). At this time, review symptom diary. Ask if Charles is satisfied with management plan. Develop plan to wean from opioid if he has not already reduced his dosage (this pain will be chronic; it is optimal to manage without opioids, although they should be used when the situation dictates). Is the behavioral technique working, does he like it, does he want to learn another?

Community Care: Focus on the Child in Pain at Home

The majority of children who experience pain are not seen in the health care setting. Well-child care can include anticipatory guidance regarding management of minor pain at home. Ice, massage, Band-Aids, rest, distraction, or other nonpharmacologic interventions may be quite effective. Acetaminophen or ibuprofen, particularly effective for musculoskeletal pain, may be given.

Alert: *Aspirin use is thought to be associated with an increased incidence of Reye's syndrome and should not be given, particularly when a viral infection is present, unless instructed by a health care provider.*

Aspirin may be used to manage chronic inflammatory disease such as juvenile rheumatoid arthritis. When pain is associated with signs of systemic disease, the health care provider should be consulted.

The child and parents being discharged from a health care setting should always be sent home with written instructions. Instructions should include intensity of pain to expect with the condition or procedure and how long it might last; how to use a developmentally appropriate assessment tool, preferably a method that was used in the health care setting; and how to assess pain level. Interventions appropriate for pain management in this situation should be given, ranked in order of what to try first or what to do for certain pain levels (e.g., if pain is severe give the opioid, if mild give acetaminophen). Activity restrictions, if any, should also be included (e.g., after conscious sedation child requires close supervision for at least 8 hours and should participate in no potentially dangerous activities such as bathing, use of tools, bike riding, skating, or using playground equipment). Parents should be taught to evaluate the effectiveness of interventions. If medications are used, reinforce that regular dosing is most effective; include side effects of medications and how to prevent them or what to do if they occur (e.g., if receiving opioids increase fluid and fiber intake to decrease constipation). The number of the person to call if pain management is inadequate also needs to be given.

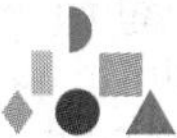

The Interdisciplinary Pain Team

Effective management of pain in the pediatric population requires the efforts of many individuals, sharing their expertise. These include, but are not limited to, nurses, pediatricians, anesthesiologists, pharmacists, psychologists, physical therapists, social workers, and child life workers. Some centers are large enough to support a specific pediatric pain program. This is optimal, because pain management is an expanding field of research and practice patterns change with new knowledge. Some centers incorporate the pediatric population into the general pain program. Others rely on individuals with knowledge in the field.

Nursing's Role in Pain Management

Nursing makes significant contributions to and should take a lead role in the management of pain in children. Assessment of pain must be performed during initial patient contact and routinely when assessing vital signs. Realistic goals and a plan for action must be agreed upon with the family ("Ashley will walk to the end of the hall. She will take her pain medication 30 minutes before this and use cold packs.") The interventions and goals must be reevaluated at appropriate intervals.

The nurse is pivotal in ensuring the effectiveness of medications and has a role in educating the other health team members who write the orders (Chart 13–29). Discuss the rationale for why using the IM route for pain medications or giving Demerol-Phenergan-Thorazine combinations for procedural pain is not appropriate. Question less than optimal medication choices, both dose and drug (e.g., using acetaminophen when a narcotic is indicated). Encourage use of opioids and nonopioids in combination. To ensure optimal efficacy of medications, be familiar with mechanism of action, peak and duration of action, and side effects. Plan care on the basis of this information. This plan should include preventing pain when possible, observing for effectiveness of and tolerance of medications, and scheduling to keep pain intensity at a minimal level. Around-the-clock management is imperative. If PRN medications are ordered the nurse must make sure they are administered properly. Do not interpret PRN to mean as little as possible or as infrequently as possible. Combine pharmacologic and nonpharmacologic methods as appropriate to age and situation.

Chart 13–29

Do's and Don'ts of Pain Management

Do

- Treat pain as a medical emergency.
- Use age-appropriate assessment methods.
- Use the same assessment method over time to compare adequacy of management.
- Consider individual child, pain history, and situation when determining treatment.
- Combine opioids and nonopioids (e.g., nonsteroidal anti-inflammatory drugs), as prescribed.
- Adhere to an around-the-clock administration schedule.
- Use nonpharmacologic interventions as appropriate, for example, positioning properly, promoting adequate rest, providing distraction, helping the patient use imagery, playing soothing music, applying ice to relieve musculoskeletal pain.
- Evaluate the effectiveness of treatments.
- Remain alert for causes of pain other than the primary diagnosis or complaint.

Don't

- Forget that signs and symptoms are different in chronic pain and acute pain.
- Withhold opioids for a child in pain because of fear of addiction or respiratory depression.
- Give IM injections.
- Administer meperidine, particularly for long-term use.
- Switch analgesics without first consulting with the physician; first, make sure that adequate to maximal doses are being given; it is appropriate to switch drugs if child is experiencing side effects.
- Forget that breakthrough pain may occur even with around-the-clock drug administration.

The nurse needs to advocate for the patient. This may involve convincing a parent that opioids are appropriate for the situation or consulting with the physician regarding an ineffective medication regimen. Health team members need to collaborate to promote effective communication and decrease the amount of frustration that may be involved in this process (Chart 13–30).

Chart 13–30
Nursing Interventions

Optimizing Pain Management

- Make sure that the currently ordered regimen has been followed and utilized to the fullest (highest doses, most frequent intervals).
- Keep the focus on the patient (not "what you ordered is not working" or "I cannot stand his crying anymore").
- Believe that everyone is trying to provide excellent patient care.
- Offer objective physiologic and behavioral evidence of pain, not vague statements ("HR is 140s, up from baseline of 100, RR is in the 50s, baseline is in the 20s, oxygen saturation is in the low 90s, down from 98%, during the past 4 hours he has slept fitfully for no longer than 20 minutes at a time, he lies stiffly in bed, grimaces and cries when moved, he is consolable with a pacifier but this is not sustained longer than 2 minutes" versus "he appears to be in pain"). Knowing the physician's criterion for pain indicators is a benefit; the patient report can address these (e.g., if the physician believes that all toddlers are irritable and cry after surgery because they are in a strange environment but takes vital sign changes as valid, emphasize vital sign changes).
- State current management regimen, both pharmacologic and nonpharmacologic (morphine at 1 mg IV is ordered every 3 hours, it was last given 90 minutes ago, his mother is holding him and his favorite video is on).
- Ask the physician or pharmacist for management suggestions. If the physician has no suggestions or is reluctant to change regimen, reiterate your assessment that the child is experiencing pain and your suggestion for management ("what about increasing the morphine to 1.5 mg or giving it every 2 hours?"); encourage a 24-hour trial period of revised pharmacologic management, which may convince the physician of its effectiveness.
- Be persistent in advocating for the child, do not get angry, remember everyone is working toward the same goal.

Documentation

However pain is managed, the plan must be clear, consistent, and well documented so that all team members can work efficiently together. An effective way to achieve these goals is to utilize interdisciplinary protocols for pain management. Standards for pain management have been developed by various organizations such as the Acute Pain Management Guideline Panel (AHCPR), American Pain Society, American Academy of Pediatrics, Oncology Nursing Society, and the World Health Organization. Protocols should include institution- or unit-specific guidelines for pain assessment for children of various ages. These guidelines should outline the specific behaviors to be included, tools to be utilized, frequency of assessments, interventions, and documentation requirements. Inclusion of psychosocial and developmental issues is particularly critical if the team cares for adults as well as children and the physician members are not pediatricians. Child life workers can be particularly valuable in this situation, providing nonpharmacologic pain management such as relaxation, distraction, and procedural preparedness. Assessment of pain by nurses is most consistently performed when pain is viewed as the fifth vital sign. To facilitate consistent documentation of pain assessments, there should be a designated area next to the vital sign recordings on the child's flow sheet. Management of more complex pain problems, rapidly changing regimens, or weaning from opioids may best be documented on a separate pain flow sheet. Other issues that should be addressed by the pain team or person responsible for pain management in the institution are quality improvement and outcome monitoring; home care needs, community resources, and school integration; and research utilization or implementation of clinical research.

Children in Pain: What Still Needs to Be Done?

Much still needs to be done to improve management of pain in children. There has been a tremendous increase of interest in and research on the topic in the past two decades but issues still remain. Children of all ages would benefit from increased research. There has been a particular paucity of research on older infants; many infant studies have investigated newborns and infants younger than 6 months.

Neurophysiology

Questions still remain regarding the neurophysiology of pain. What are the differences in how the pain impulse is transmitted and responded to in relation to the child's level of maturation? What impact does anatomy (thin skin structure in infant making terminal nerve fibers more superficial, increased number of cutaneous nerve fibers, size of child and distance the impulse has to travel) have on impulse transmission and response? How do changing levels of myelin, excitatory and inhibitory neurotransmitters, and drug kinetics and metabolism affect pain perception and response? What are the long-term effects of painful experiences for children?

Assessment

Clinically applicable, multidimensional, quick and easy to use, noninvasive pain assessment tools have been developed. Research needs to confirm their reliability and validity and determine whether any of the existing tools are superior. Ideally, tools would detect the presence or absence of pain and differentiate between pain intensity levels. The inability of infants to self-report pain makes identification of valid tools particularly important for this population. Because of the inherent response differences in children of various ages and abilities (preterm infant, neonate, older infant, toddler, ventilated, developmentally delayed, paralyzed), behavioral assessment tools may need to be population specific.

Vagal tone, a physiologic index, may provide a precise assessment of pain that can be used across age groups. Further investigation of what this value indicates and how it can be evaluated at the bedside is required. How can the interrelatedness of changes in vital signs with pain and other factors such as position, fear, anxiety, and anger be evaluated? If the child was in a curled position for a lumbar puncture, could decreased tidal volume resulting from pressure on the diaphragm be responsible for the decreased oxygen saturation levels noted? If oxygen saturation was decreased, would not one expect to see a resultant increase in heart rate? What is the contribution of pain and of positioning to the change from baseline?

Are there cultural or ethnic variances in response to pain and, if so, how can assessment be done? Will management of the pain change?

Nonpharmacologic Pain Management

A number of nonpharmacologic pain management interventions are implemented on the basis of anecdotal evidence of efficacy. Research into degree of efficacy and most effective method of implementation is needed. For example, does the rate of rocking affect pain? Does sucking really reduce perceived pain or does it just decrease the amount of crying? What new and different nonpharmacologic methods can be used? Folk remedies may provide valuable lessons in nonpharmacologic (and possibly pharmacologic if herbs and roots are included) pain management.

Pharmacologic Pain Management

Many avenues remain to be explored to improve pharmacologic management of children's pain. What are the most appropriate dosing guidelines for younger children, particularly infants? Is there a "best" age to start use of PCA? Are there cognitive (versus chronologic) issues that identify who can use PCA? Do other versions of PCA (nurse or parent controlled) improve management or save nursing time? Are they safe?

Children still report experiencing moderate to severe pain postoperatively. Why? Is the reason physician ordering practices (no drug or wrong drug ordered, inadequate dose, inappropriate route or schedule)? Is the problem with nursing assessment or administration practices? Is more education needed? Will increased use of protocols help improve management and decrease pain? Existing drugs may prove beneficial in treatment of acute and chronic pain. What are these and what are appropriate doses?

These are but a sampling of topics that need to be addressed. Assessment and management of pain in children are challenging. We must continue to meet this challenge; the comfort and well-being of children depend on it.

Summary of Key Concepts

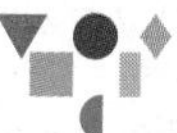

- Infants and children have the physiologic structures and capability to feel pain, possibly to an even greater extent than adults.
- The experience of pain is unique to each individual; many factors influence the experience.
- Pain is what the experiencing person says it is; self-report is the most accurate method of pain assessment. When self-report cannot be obtained (preverbal infants, developmentally delayed or critically ill children), physiologic and behavioral cues may provide data regarding pain. Assessments that are multidimensional provide the most accurate information.

- Undermedicating is the biggest nursing or medical problem.
- Pharmacologic and nonpharmacologic methods of managing pain augment each other; one does not replace the other.
- Management decisions are made on the basis of influencing factors (age, coping style, pain situation).
- Analgesics need to be administered on an around-the-clock basis. It is safe to administer opioids to infants, although monitoring for respiratory depression, as with any patient, is indicated.
- Signs and symptoms of acute pain differ from those of chronic pain. The body adapts to chronic pain, so vital sign changes are not readily apparent. Different behavioral cues may be seen (depression with chronic pain versus lying rigid in bed when in acute pain).
- A cohesive, interdisciplinary approach to pain management, including child and parents, produces the best outcomes.
- Knowledge of pain neurophysiology and pain assessment and management techniques is increasing, but more research is needed.

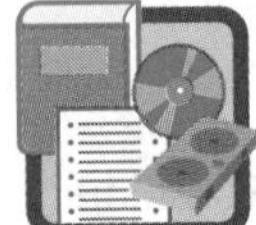

Resources

Organizations

American Academy of Pain Management
13947 Mono Way, Suite A
Sonora, CA 95370
(209) 533-9744
web: http://www.aapainmanage.org

American Chronic Pain Association
PO Box 850
Rocklin, CA 95677
(916) 632-0922

American Pain Society
4700 West Lake Avenue
Glenview, IL 60025
(847) 375-4715

American Society of Pain Management Nurses
2755 Bristol Street, Suite 110
Costa Mesa, CA 92626
(714) 545-1305

International Association for the Study of Pain
909 NE 43rd Street, Suite 306
Seattle, WA 98105-6020
(206) 547-6409

Books for Children

✏ Berenstain, S., & Berenstain, J. (1981). *The Berenstain Bears go to the doctor.* New York: Random House.

✏ Berger, K., Tidwell, R. A., & Haseltine, M. (1977). *A visit to the doctor.* New York: Grossett & Dunlap.

✏ Ciliotta, C., & Livingstone, C. (1980). *Why am I going to the hospital?* New York: Lyle Stuart.

✏ Hautzig, D. (1985). *A visit to the Sesame Street hospital.* New York: Random House.

✏ Howe, J. (1981). *The hospital book.* New York: Crown Publications.

✏ Reit, S. (1978). *Bugs Bunny goes to the dentist.* New York: Western Publishing.

✏ Reit, S. (1984). *Jenny's in the hospital.* New York: Western Publishing.

✏ Rey, M., & Rey, H. A. (1966). *Curious George goes to the hospital.* Boston: Houghton-Mifflin.

✏ Scarry, R. (1972). *Nicky goes to the doctor.* New York: Golden Press.

Books for Parents

McGrath, P. J., Finley, A., & Ritchie, J. (1994). *Pain, pain go away: Helping children cope with pain.* Bethesda, MD: Association for the Care of Children's Health. Available from ACCH, 7910 Woodmont Avenue, Suite 300, Bethesda, MD, 20814.

Videotapes

Children in pain. L. Kuttner. Available from Suncoast Media, 2938 West Bay Drive, Suite B, Largo, FL 34640, (800) 899-1008.

No fears—No tears: Children with cancer coping with pain. L. Kuttner. Available from Canadian Cancer Society, 955 West Broadway, Vancouver, BC VSZ 3X8, Canada, or to borrow free of charge from local branches of the American Cancer Society.

The nursing management of pediatric epidural (530 series). Texas Scottish Rite Hospital for Children. Available from TSMedia, 18 Halley Court, Fairfield, CT, 06430, (800) 876-6334.

✏ Resources specifically for children.

Pain management in children. Available from Maxishare, P.O. Box 2041, Milwaukee, WI 53201.

Pain in infants and children. B. Stevens & M. Broome. Available from Williams & Wilkins Electronic Media, 428 E. Preston Street, Baltimore, MD 21202, (800) 527-5597.

Pediatric conscious sedation [Book and video series]. T. J. Abramo. Available from Mosby–Year Book, 11830 Westline Industrial Drive, P.O. Box 46908, St. Louis, MO 63146-9934.

Taming the hurting things. Available from Association for the Care of Children's Health, 7910 Woodmont Avenue, Suite 300, Bethesda, MD 20814, (301) 654-6549, extension 327.

Audiotapes

Most are appropriate for pain and stress in general.

Instrumental Music

Good for any age, particularly infants, to create a soothing atmosphere of sound.

When You Wish Upon A Star, Somewhere Over the Rainbow, and others by D. Kobialka.

Lullabies & Sweet Dreams, Spectrum Suite, and others by S. Halpern, Ph.D.

Recordings from both artists available from Willow Tree/Sound Rx, P.O. Box 11439, San Rafael, CA 94915, (800)726-3924.

Transitions, for infants—sounds of the womb.

Guided Imagery with Music

Ages 4–12

The Star Within, The Healing Heart, by R. Daleo, Ph.D. Available from Mindworks for Children, P.O. Box 2494, Cambridge, MA 02238-2493.

Ages 12 and Up

Healing Journey, Rainbow Butterfly, Letting Go of Stress, and others by E. Miller, M.D. Available from Source Cassette Learning Systems, P.O. Box W, Stanford, CA 94309, (800) 52-TAPES.

Health Journeys for General Wellness, Health Journeys for People Preparing for Surgery, and others by B. Naparstek. Available from Image Paths, P.O. Box 5714, Cleveland, OH 44101-0714, (800) 800-8661.

Most of these audiotapes are also available from Nightingale Knowledge, 11053 Bel Aire Court, Cupertino, CA 95014, (408) 253-2770.

Guidelines /Position Statements

Acute Pain Management Guideline Panel. (1992). *Acute pain management: Operative or medical procedures and trauma. Clinical practice guideline* (AHCPR Publication No. 92-0032). Rockville, MD: Agency for Health Care Policy and Research, Public Health Service, U.S. Department of Health and Human Services.

To order call (800) 358-9295 or write Center for Research Dissemination & Liaison, AHCPR Clearinghouse, P.O. Box 8547, Silver Spring, MD 20907.

American Academy of Pediatrics. (1992). Guidelines for monitoring and management of pediatric patients during and after sedation for diagnostic and therapeutic procedures. *Pediatrics, 89,* 29–34.

American Nurses' Association. (1991). Position statement on the registered nurses' (RN) role in the management of patients receiving IV conscious sedation for short-term therapeutic, diagnostic, or surgical procedure. Kansas City: Author.

American Pain Society. (1992). *Principles of analgesic use in the treatment of acute and chronic pain.* Skokie, IL: Author.

Management of cancer pain (AHCPR Publication No. 94-0592). (1994). Rockville, MD: Agency for Health Care Policy and Research, Public Health Service, U.S. Department of Health and Human Services.

To order call the National Cancer Institute at (800) 4-CANCER or write AHCPR Clearinghouse, Cancer Pain Guideline, P.O. Box 8547, Silver Spring, MD 20907.

Oncology Nursing Society position paper on cancer pain. (1991). Oncology Nursing Society. Dept. 1889, Pittsburgh, PA, 15278-1889.

References

Abu-Saad, H. (1981). The assessment of pain in children. *Issues in Comprehensive Pediatric Nursing, 5,* 327–335.

Abu-Saad, H. (1984a). Cultural components of pain: The Asian-American child. *Children's Health Care, 13,* 11–14.

Abu-Saad, H. (1984b). Cultural group indicators of pain in children. *Maternal Child Nursing Journal, 13,* 187–196.

Abu-Saad, H. (1990). Toward the development of an instrument to assess pain in children: Dutch study. In D. Tyler & E. Krane (Eds.), *Advances in pain research and therapy: Pediatric pain* (vol. 15, pp. 101–106). New York: Raven Press.

Acute Pain Management Guideline Panel. (1992). *Acute pain management: Operative or medical procedures and trauma. Clinical practice guideline* (AHCPR Publication No. 92-0032). Rockville, MD: Agency for Health Care Policy and Research, Public Health Service, U.S. Department of Health and Human Services.

Alex, M. R., & Ritchie, J. A. (1992). School-aged children's interpretation of their experience with acute surgical pain. *Journal of Pediatric Nursing, 7,* 171–180.

Als, H., Lawhon, G., Brown, E., Gibes, R., Duffy, F., McAnulty, G., & Blickman, J. G. (1986). Individualized behavioral and environmental care for the very low birth weight preterm infant at high risk for bronchopulmonary dysplasia: Neonatal intensive care unit and developmental outcomes. *Pediatrics, 78,* 1123–1132.

Altimier, L., Norwood, S., Dick, M. J., Holditch-Davis, D., & Lawless, S. (1994). Postoperative pain management in preverbal children: The prescription and administration of analgesics with and without caudal analgesia. *Journal of Pediatric Nursing, 9,* 226–232.

Ambuel, B., Hamlett, K., Marx, C., & Blumer, J. (1992). Assessing distress in pediatric intensive care environments: The COMFORT Scale. *Journal of Pediatric Psychology, 17,* 95–109.

American Academy of Pediatrics. (1987). Neonatal anesthesia. *Pediatrics,* 80, 446.

American Academy of Pediatrics. (1992). Guidelines for monitoring and management of pediatric patients during and after sedation for diagnostic and therapeutic procedures. *Pediatrics,* 89, 29–34.

American Pain Society. (1992). *Principles of analgesic use in the treatment of acute pain and cancer pain* (3rd ed.). Skokie, IL: American Pain Society.

Anand, K. J. S., & Carr, D. B. (1989). The neuroanatomy, neurophysiology, and neurochemistry of pain, stress, and analgesia in newborns and children. *Pediatric Clinics of North America,* 36, 795–822.

Anand, K. J. S., & Hickey, P. (1987). Pain and its effects on the human neonate and fetus. *New England Journal of Medicine, 317,* 1321–1329.

Anand, K. J. S., & Hickey, P. (1992). Halothane-morphine compared with high-dose sufentanil for anesthesia and postoperative anesthesia in neonatal cardiac surgery. *New England Journal of Medicine, 326,* 1–9.

Anand, K. J. S., Hansen, D. D., & Hickey, P. (1990). Hormonal-metabolic stress responses in neonates undergoing cardiac surgery. *Anesthesiology, 73,* 661–670.

Attia, J., Amiel-Tison, C., Mayer, M.-N., Shnider, S., & Barrier, G. (1987). Measurement of postoperative pain and narcotic administration in infants using a new clinical scoring system. *Anesthesiology,* 67(3A), A532.

Aun, C., Lam, Y. M., & Collett, B. (1986). Evaluation of the use of visual analogue scale in Chinese patients. *Pain, 25,* 215–221.

Bailey, L. (1986). Music therapy in pain management. *Journal of Pain and Symptom Management, 1,* 25–28.

Barrier, G., Attia, J., Mayer, M. N., Amiel-Tison, C., & Shnider, S. M. (1989). Measurement of post-operative pain and narcotic administration in infants using a new clinical scoring system. *Intensive Care Medicine, 15,* S37–39.

Beales, J. G., Keen, J. H., Lennox Holt, P. J. (1983). The child's perception of the disease and experience of pain in juvenile chronic arthritis. *Journal of Rheumatology, 10,* 61–65.

Beaver, P. K. (1987). Premature infants' response to touch and pain: Can nurses make a difference? *Neonatal Network,* 6(3), 13–17.

Berde, C. (1993). Toxicity of local anesthetics in infants and children. *Journal of Pediatrics, 122,* S14–S20.

Beyer, J., Denyes, M., & Villarruel, A. (1992). The creation, validation, and continuing development of the Oucher: A measure of pain intensity in children. *Journal of Pediatric Nursing, 7,* 335–346.

Bildner, J., & Krechel, S. W. (1996). Increasing staff nurse awareness of postoperative pain management in the NICU. *Neonatal Network, 15,* 11–16.

Blass, E., & Hoffmeyer, L. (1991). Sucrose as an analgesic for newborn infants. *Pediatrics,* 87, 215–218.

Blass, E., Fitzgerald, E., & Kehoe, P. (1987). Interactions between sucrose, pain and isolation distress. *Pharmacology Biochemistry and Behavior,* 26, 483–489.

Bonica, J. J. (1990). *The management of pain* (2nd ed.) Philadelphia: Lea & Febiger.

Bradshaw, C., & Zeanah, P. (1986). Pediatric nurses' assessments of pain in children. *Journal of Pediatric Nursing, 1,* 314–322.

Broadman, L., Rice, L. J., & Hannallah, R. (1988). Testing the validity of an objective pain scale for infants and children. *Anesthesiology,* 69(3A), A770.

Broome, M. (1985). The child in pain: A model for assessment and intervention. *Critical Care Quarterly,* 8, 47–55.

Broome, M. (1990). Preparation of children for painful procedures. *Pediatric Nursing, 16,* 537–541.

Broome, M., & Tanzillo, H. (1990). Differentiating between pain and agitation in premature neonates. *Journal of Perinatal and Neonatal Nursing, 4,* 53–62.

Brown, L. (1987). Physiologic responses to cutaneous pain in neonates. *Neonatal Network,* 6(3), 18–22.

Burokas, L. (1985). Factors affecting nurses' decisions to medicate pediatric patients after surgery. *Heart and Lung, 14,* 373–378.

Byrne, J., & Horowitz, F. D. (1981). Rocking as a soothing intervention: The influence of direction and type of movement. *Infant Behavior and Development,* 4, 207–218.

Campos, R. G. (1989). Soothing pain-elicited distress in infants with swaddling and pacifiers. *Child Development,* 60, 781–792.

Carpenter, P. J. (1992). Perceived control as a predictor of distress in children undergoing invasive medical procedures. *Journal of Pediatric Psychology, 17,* 757–777.

Chess, S., & Thomas, A. (1985). Temperamental differences: A critical concept in child health care. *Pediatric Nursing, 11,* 167–171.

Cohen, S., Tyrrell, D. A. J., & Smith, A. P. (1991). Psychological stress and susceptibility to the common cold. *New England Journal of Medicine, 325,* 654–656.

Collins, S. K., & Kuck, K. (1991). Music therapy in the neonatal intensive care unit. *Neonatal Network,* 9, 23–26.

Craig, K. D., Whitfield, M. F., Grunau, R. V., Linton, J., & Hadjistavropoulos, H. D. (1993). Pain in the preterm neonate: Behavioural and physiological indices. *Pain, 52,* 287–299.

Dalla Barba, B., Gatto, C., Valenza, E., Calabro, L., Cavedagni, M., Prandoni, S., & Benini, F. (1991). Pain memory in full-term newborns. *Journal of Pain and Symptom Management,* 6, 206.

Eland, J. (1981). Minimizing pain associated with prekindergarten intramuscular injection. *Issues in Comprehensive Pediatric Nursing,* 5, 361–372.

Eland, J. (1985). The child who is hurting. *Seminars in Oncology Nursing, 1,* 116–122.

Eland, J. (1989). The effectiveness of transcutaneous electrical nerve stimulation (TENS) with children experiencing cancer pain. In S. Funk, E. Tornquist, M. Champagne, L. A. Copp, & R. Wiese (Eds.), *Key aspects of comfort: Management of pain, fatigue, and nausea* (pp. 87–100). New York: Springer.

Eland, J. (1993). The use of TENS with children. In N. L. Schechter, C. B. Berde, & M. Yaster (Eds.), *Pain in infants, children, and adolescents* (pp. 331–339). Baltimore: Williams & Wilkins.

Ellis, J. A., & Spanos, N. P. (1994). Cognitive-behavioral interventions for children's distress during bone marrow aspirations and lumbar punctures: A critical review. *Journal of Pain and Symptom Management,* 9, 96–108.

Emde, R., Harmon, R., Metcalf, D., Koenig, K., & Wagonfeld, S. (1971). Stress and neonatal sleep. *Psychosomatic Medicine, 33,* 491–497.

Ernst, E., & Fialka, V. (1994). Ice freezes pain? A review of the clinical effectiveness of analgesic cold therapy. *Journal of Pain and Symptom Management,* 9, 56–59.

Fanurik, D., Zeltzer, L., Roberts, M., & Blount, R. (1993). The relationship between children's coping styles and psychological interventions for cold pressor pain. *Pain, 53,* 213–222.

Faucett, J., Gordon, N., & Levine, J. (1994). Differences in postoperative pain severity among four ethnic groups. *Journal of Pain and Symptom Management,* 9, 383–389.

Favaloro, R., & Touzel, B. (1990). A comparison of adolescents' and nurses' postoperative pain ratings and perceptions. *Pediatric Nursing, 16,* 414–424.

Field, T. (1993, Spring). Sucking for stress reduction, growth and development during infancy. *Pediatric Basics, 64,* 13–16. (Available from Gerber Products, Fremont, MI.)

Fitzgerald, M., & Anand, K. J. S. (1993). Developmental neuroanatomy and neurophysiology of pain. In N. L. Schechter, C. B. Berde, & M. Yaster (Eds.), *Pain in infants, children, and adolescents* (pp. 11–31). Baltimore: Williams & Wilkins.

Franck, L. (1986). A new method to quantitatively describe pain behavior in infants. *Nursing Research, 35,* 28–31.

Franck, L., & Vilardi, J. (1995). Assessment and management of opioid withdrawal in ill neonates. *Neonatal Network, 14,* 39–48.

French, J., & Nocera, M. (1994). Drug withdrawal symptoms in children after continuous infusions of fentanyl. *Journal of Pediatric Nursing, 9,* 107–113.

Gadish, H., Gonzalez, J., & Hayes, J. (1988). Factors affecting nurses' decisions to administer pediatric pain medication postoperatively. *Journal of Pediatric Nursing, 3,* 383–390.

Gaffney, A., & Dunne, E. (1986). Developmental aspects of children's definitions of pain. *Pain, 26,* 105–117.

Gauvain-Piquard, A., Rodary, C., Francois, P., Rezvani, A., Kalifa, C., Lecuyer, N., Cosse, M., & Lesbros, F. (1991). Validity assessment of DEGR[R] Scale for observational rating of 2–6-year-old child pain. *Journal of Pain and Symptom Management, 6,* 171.

Gauvain-Piquard, A., Rodary, C., Rezvani, A., & Lemerle, J. (1987). Pain in children aged 2–6 years: A new observational rating scale elaborated in a pediatric oncology unit—preliminary report. *Pain, 31,* 177–188.

Gedaly-Duff, V. (1987). Preparing young children for painful procedures. *Journal of Pediatric Nursing, 3,* 169–179.

Grass, J. (1992). Fentanyl: Clinical use as postoperative analgesic—epidural/intrathecal route. *Journal of Pain and Symptom Management, 7,* 419–430.

Grunau, R., & Craig, K. (1987). Pain expression in neonates: Facial action and cry. *Pain, 28,* 395–410.

Gureno, M. A., & Reisinger, C. (1991). Patient controlled analgesia for the young pediatric patient. *Pediatric Nursing, 17,* 251–254.

Hannallah, R., Broadman, L., Belman, B., Abramowitz, M., & Epstein, B. (1987). Comparison of caudal and ilioinguinal/iliohypogastric nerve blocks for control of post-orchiopexy pain in pediatric ambulatory surgery. *Anesthesiology, 66,* 832–834.

Haouari, N., Wood, C. Griffiths, G., & Levene, J. (1995). The analgesic effect of sucrose in full term infants: A randomised controlled trial. *British Medical Journal, 310,* 1498–1500.

Hauser, G., Chan, M., Casey, W., Midgley, F., & Holbrook, P. (1991). Immune dysfunction in children after corrective surgery for congenital heart disease. *Critical Care Medicine, 19,* 874–881.

Hester, N. O. (1979). The preoperational child's reaction to immunization. *Nursing Research, 28,* 250–255.

Hester, N. O. (1993). Pain in children. *Annual Review of Nursing Research, 11,* 105–142.

Hester, N. O., Foster, R., Kristensen, K., & Bergstrom, L. (1989). *Measurement of children's pain by children, parents, and nurses: Psychometric and clinical issues related to the Poker Chip Tool and the Pain Ladder* [Abstract](Grant No. R23 1382). National Institutes of Health, National Center for Nursing Research.

Holm, K., Cohen, F., Dudas, S., Medema, P. G., & Allen, B. L. (1989). Effect of personal pain experience on pain assessment. *Image, 21,* 72–75.

Hu, Yh., Zhang, Gq., & Chen, Zh. (1991). Pain after burn injuries among Chinese children: A further study on transcultural and ethnic differences of pain [Abstract]. *Journal of Pain and Symptom Management, 6,* 155.

Izard, C., Hembree, E., & Huebner, R. (1987). Infant's emotion expressions to acute pain: Developmental change and stability of individual differences. *Developmental Psychology, 23,* 105–113.

Jay, S., Ozolins, M., Elliott, C., & Caldwell, S. (1983). Assessment of children's distress during painful medical procedures. *Health Psychology, 2,* 133–147.

Johnston, C. C., Abbott, F. V., Gray-Donald, K., & Jeans, M. E. (1992). A survey of pain in hospitalized patients aged 4–14 years. *Clinical Journal of Pain, 8,* 154–163.

Johnston, C. C., Stevens, B., Craig, K., & Grunau, R. (1993). Developmental changes in pain expression in premature, full-term, two- and four-month-old infants. *Pain, 52,* 201–208.

Kachoyeanos, M. K., & Friedhoff, M. (1993). Cognitive and behavioral strategies to reduce children's pain. *American Journal of Maternal Child Nursing, 18,* 14–19.

Katz, E., Kellerman, J., & Siegel, S. (1980). Behavioral distress in children with cancer undergoing medical procedures: Developmental considerations. *Journal of Consulting and Clinical Psychology, 48,* 356–365.

Kimble, C. (1992). Nonnutritive sucking: Adaptation and health for the neonate. *Neonatal Network, 11*(2), 29–33.

Knott, C., Beyer, J., Villarruel, A., Denyes, M., Erickson, V., & Willard, G. (1994). Using the Oucher—Developmental approach to pain assessment. *American Journal of Maternal Child Nursing, 19,* 314–320.

Kuttner, L. (1986). *No fears—No tears: Children with cancer coping with pain* [Videotape]. Vancouver, Canada: Canadian Cancer Society.

Kuttner, L. (1988). Favorite stories: A hypnotic pain-reduction technique for children in acute pain. *American Journal of Clinical Hypnosis, 30,* 289–295.

Kuttner, L., & LePage, T. (1989). Face scales for the assessment of pediatric pain: A critical review. *Canadian Journal of Behavioural Science, 21,* 198–209.

Lander, J., & Fowler-Kerry, S. (1993). TENS for children's procedural pain. *Pain, 52,* 209–216.

Lawrence, J., Alcock, D., McGrath, P., Kay, J., MacMurray, S. B., & Dulberg, C. (1993). The development of a tool to assess neonatal pain. *Neonatal Network, 12,* 59–66.

Levine, D., & Gordon, N. G. (1982). Pain in prelingual children and its evaluation by pain-induced vocalization. *Pain, 14,* 85–93.

Lipsitt, L., & Levy, L. (1959). Electrotactual threshold in the neonate. *Child Development, 30,* 547–554.

Maikler, V. E. (1991). Effects of a skin refrigerant/anesthetic and age on the pain responses of infants receiving immunizations. *Research in Nursing & Health, 14,* 397–403.

Manne, S. L., Redd, W. H., Jacobsen, P. B., Gorfinkle, K., Schorr, O., & Rapkin, B. (1990). Behavioral intervention to reduce child and parent distress during venipuncture. *Journal of Consulting and Clinical Psychology, 58,* 565–572.

Margolius, F. R., Hudson, K. A., & Michel, Y. (1995). Beliefs and perceptions about children in pain: A survey. *Pediatric Nursing, 21,* 111–115.

Marshall, R., Stratton, W., Moore, J. A., & Boxerman, S. (1980). Circumcision. I: Effects upon newborn behavior. *Infant Behavior and Development, 3,* 1–14.

McCaffery, M., & Beebe, A. (1989). *Pain: Clinical manual for nursing practice.* St Louis: Mosby.

McDonnell, L., & Bowden, M. L. (1989). Breathing management: A simple stress and pain reduction strategy for use on a pediatric service. *Issues in Comprehensive Pediatric Nursing, 12,* 339–344.

McGrath, P. J., & Craig, K. (1989). Developmental and psychological factors in children's pain. *Pediatric Clinics of North America, 36,* 823–836.

McGrath, P. J., Johnson, G., Goodman, J., Schillinger, J., Dunn, J., & Chapman, J. A. (1985). CHEOPS: A behavioral scale for rating postoperative pain in children. In H. L. Fields, R. Dubner, & F. Cervero (Eds.), *Advances in pain research and therapy* (pp. 395–402). New York: Raven Press.

Melzack, R. (1983). The McGill Pain Questionnaire. In R. Melzack (Ed.), *Pain measurement and assessment* (pp. 41–47). New York: Raven Press.

Melzack, R., & Wall, P. (1965). Pain mechanisms: A new theory. *Science, 150,* 971–979.

Miller, D. (1996). Comparisons of pain ratings from postoperative children, their mothers, and their nurses. *Pediatric Nursing, 22,* 145–149.

Miller, H. C., & Anderson, G. C. (1993). Nonnutritive sucking: Effects on crying and heart rate in intubated infants requiring assisted mechanical ventilation. *Nursing Research, 42,* 305–307.

Mills, N. (1989). Pain behaviors in infants and toddlers. *Journal of Pain and Symptom Management, 4,* 184–190.

Morgan, A. E., & Hilgard, E. (1979). The Stanford hypnotic clinical scale for children. *American Journal of Clinical Hypnosis, 21,* 148–169.

Patterson, K., & Ware, L. (1988). Coping skills for children undergoing painful medical procedures. *Issues in Comprehensive Pediatric Nursing, 11,* 113–143.

Porter, F. (1993). Pain assessment in children: Infants. In N. L. Schechter, C. B. Berde, & M. Yaster (Eds.), *Pain in infants, children, and adolescents* (pp. 87–96). Baltimore: Williams & Wilkins.

Porter, F., Miller, R., & Marshall, R. E. (1986). Neonatal pain cries: Effect of circumcision on acoustical features and perceived urgency. *Child Development, 57,* 790–802.

Porter, F., Porges, S., & Marshall, R. (1988). Newborn pain cries and vagal tone: Parallel changes in response to circumcision. *Child Development, 59,* 495–505.

Puntillo, K., & Weiss, S. J. (1994). Pain: Its mediators and associated morbidity in critically ill cardiovascular surgical patients. *Nursing Research, 43,* 31–36.

Rabin, N. B. (1994) School reentry and the child with a chronic illness: The role of the pediatric nurse practitioner. *Journal of Pediatric Health Care, 8,* 227–232.

Richards, M. P. M., Bernal, J. F., & Brackbill, Y. (1976). Early behavioral differences: Gender or circumcision? *Developmental Psychobiology,* 9(1), 89–95.

Robertson, J. (1993). Pediatric pain assessment: Validation of a multidimensional tool. *Pediatric Nursing, 19,* 209–213.

Rømsing, J., Møller-Sonnergaard, J., Hertel, S., & Rasmussen, M. (1996). Postoperative pain in children: Comparison between ratings of children and nurses. *Journal of Pain and Symptom Management, 11,* 42–46.

Ross, D., & Ross, S. (1984). Childhood pain: The school-age child's viewpoint. *Pain, 20,* 179–191.

Ryan, E. (1989). The effect of musical distraction on pain in hospitalized school-aged children. In S. Funk, E. Tornquist, M. Champagne, L. A. Copp, & R. Wiese (Eds.), *Key aspects of comfort: Management of pain, fatigue, and nausea* (pp. 101–104). New York: Springer.

Savedra, M., Gibbons, P., Tesler, M., Ward, J., & Wegner, C. (1982). How do children describe pain? A tentative assessment. *Pain, 14,* 95–104.

Schechter, N. (1989). The undertreatment of pain in children: An overview. *Pediatric Clinics of North America, 36,* 781–794.

Schechter, N., Allen, D., & Hanson, K. (1986). Status of pediatric pain control: A comparison of hospital analgesic usage in children and adults. *Pediatrics, 77,* 11–15.

Schechter, N., Bernstein, B., Beck, A., Hart, L., & Scherzer, L. (1991). Individual differences in children's response to pain: Role of temperament and parental characteristics. *Pediatrics, 87,* 171–177.

Schryer, N. M. (1989). Epidural catheters: Pain management in the child. *Dimensions of Critical Care Nursing, 8,* 347–355.

Seymour, R. A., Simpson, J. M., Charlton, J. E., & Phillips, M. E. (1985). An evaluation of length and end-phrase of visual analogue scales in dental pain. *Pain, 21,* 177–185.

Shapiro, C. (1993). Nurses judgments of pain in term and preterm newborns. *Journal of Obstetric, Gynecologic, and Neonatal Nursing, 22,* 41–47.

Shaw, E. G., & Routh, D. K. (1982). Effect of mother presence on children's reaction to aversive procedures. *Journal of Pediatric Psychology, 7,* 33–42.

Sherman, M., & Sherman, I. (1925). Sensori-motor responses in infants. *Journal of Comparative Psychology, 5,* 53–68.

Smith, D. P. (1986). Using humor to help children with pain. *Children's Health Care, 14,* 187–188.

Smith, M., & Womack, W. (1987). Stress management techniques in childhood and adolescence. *Clinical Pediatrics, 26,* 581–585.

Stein, P. R. (1995). Indices of pain intensity: Construct validity among preschoolers. *Pediatric Nursing, 21,* 119–123.

Stevens, B., & Johnston, C. C. (1994). Physiological reposes of premature infants to a painful stimulus. *Nursing Research, 43,* 226–231.

Talbot, J., Marrett, S., Evans, A., Meyer, E., Bushnell, M. C., & Duncan, G. (1991). Multiple representations of pain in human cerebral cortex. *Science, 251,* 1355–1358.

Tarbell, S., Cohen, T., & Marsh, J. (1992). The Toddler-Preschooler Postoperative Pain Scale: An observational scale for measuring postoperative pain in children aged 1–5. Preliminary report. *Pain, 50,* 273–280.

Taylor, A., Skelton, J., & Butcher, J. (1984). Duration of pain condition and physical pathology as determinants of nurses' assessments of patients in pain. *Nursing Research, 33,* 4–8.

Taylor, P. (1983). Post-operative pain in toddler and pre-school age children. *Maternal Child Nursing Journal, 12,* 35–50.

Teske, K., Daut, R, & Cleeland, C. (1983). Relationships between nurses' observations and patients' self-reports of pain. *Pain, 16,* 289–296.

Tesler, M., Wilkie, D., Holzemer, W., & Savedra, M. (1994). Postoperative analgesics for children and adolescents: Prescription and administration. *Journal of Pain and Symptom Management, 9,* 85–95.

Tyler, D. (1994). Pharmacology of pain management. *Pediatric Clinics of North America, 41,* 59–71.

Vallerand, A. H. (1995). Gender differences in pain. *Image, 27,* 235–237.

Varni, J., Thompson, K., & Hanson, V. (1987). The Varni/Thompson pediatric pain questionnaire. I. Chronic musculoskeletal pain in juvenile rheumatoid arthritis. *Pain, 28,* 27–38.

Vessey, J. A., Carlson, K. L., & McGill, J. (1994). Use of distraction with children during an acute pain experience. *Nursing Research, 43,* 369–372.

Villarruel, A., & de Montellano, B. O. (1992). Culture and pain: A Mesoamerican perspective. *Advances in Nursing Science, 15,* 21–32.

Wall, P. D., & Melzack, R. (1989). *Textbook of pain* (2nd ed.). New York: Churchill Livingstone.

Wallace, K. (1992). The pathophysiology of pain. *Critical Care Nursing Quarterly,* 15(2), 1–13.

Wallace, M. (1989). Temperament: A variable in children's pain management. *Pediatric Nursing, 15,* 118–121.

Watt-Watson, J., Evernden, C., & Lawson, C. (1990). Parents' perceptions of their child's acute pain experience. *Journal of Pediatric Nursing, 5*, 344–349.

Wong, D., & Baker, C. (1988). Pain in children: Comparison of assessment scales. *Pediatric Nursing, 14*, 9–17.

Zappa, S., & Nabors, S. (1992). Use of ethyl chloride topical anesthetic to reduce procedural pain in pediatric oncology patients. *Cancer Nursing, 15*, 130–136.

Zborowski, M. (1952). Cultural components in response to pain. *Journal of Social Issues, 8*, 16–30.

Zeltzer, L., Anderson, C., & Schechter, N. (1990). Pediatric pain: Current status and new directions. *Current Problems in Pediatrics, 20*, 411–486.

Bibliography

Adrian, E. R. (1994). Intranasal Versed: The future of pediatric conscious sedation. *Pediatric Nursing, 20*, 287–292.

Alfieri, D. R., & Cagan, D. (1995). Transdermal fentanyl. *Pediatric Nursing, 21*, 72–74.

Anand, K. J. S., & McGrath, P. J. (1993). *Pain in neonates*. Amsterdam: Elsevier.

Bhatt-Mehta, V., & Rosen, D. (1991). Management of acute pain in children. *Clinical Pharmacy, 10*, 667–684.

Carlson, K. L. (1996). Pediatric nonpharmacologic pain management: A review of intervention research. *Capsules and Comments in Pediatric Nursing, 2*, 269–277.

Cote, C. J. (1994). Sedation for the pediatric patient: A review. *Pediatric Clinics of North America, 41*, 31–58.

Dick, M. J. (1993). Preterm infants in pain: Nurse's and physician's perceptions. *Clinical Nursing Research, 2*, 176–187.

Fuller, B. F., & Conner, D. A. (1995). The effect of pain on infant behaviors. *Clinical Nursing Research, 4*, 253–273.

Johnston, C. C., & Stevens, B. (1990). Pain assessment in newborns. *Journal of Perinatal and Neonatal Nursing, 4*, 41–52.

Levine, M. (Ed.). (1984). Recurrent pain in children. *Pediatric Clinics of North America, 31*, 947–1152.

McGrath, P. A. (1987). An assessment of children's pain: A review of behavioral, physiological and direct scaling techniques. *Pain, 31*, 147–176.

McGrath, P. A. (1990). *Pain in children: Nature, assessment, and treatment*. New York: Guilford Press.

National Institute of Nursing Research. (1994). *Symptom management: Acute pain* (NIH Publication No. 94-2421). Bethesda, MD: U.S. Department of Health and Human Services.

Nelson, M. S., Walters, V. E., & Watkins, L. M. (1996). Competency verification for conscious sedation. *Journal of Emergency Nursing, 22*, 116–119.

Schechter, N. (1989). Acute pain in children. *Pediatric Clinics of North America, 36*, 781–964.

Schechter, N., Altman, A., & Weisman, S. (Eds.). (1990). Report of the consensus conference on the management of pain in childhood cancer. *Pediatrics*, 86(Suppl. 5), 813–834.

Schechter, N., Berde, C., & Yaster, M. (1993). *Pain in infants, children, and adolescents*. Baltimore: Williams & Wilkins.

Wetzel, R. C. (Ed.). (1994). Pediatric anesthesia. *Pediatric Clinics of North America, 41*, 1–256.

Managing Health Challenges

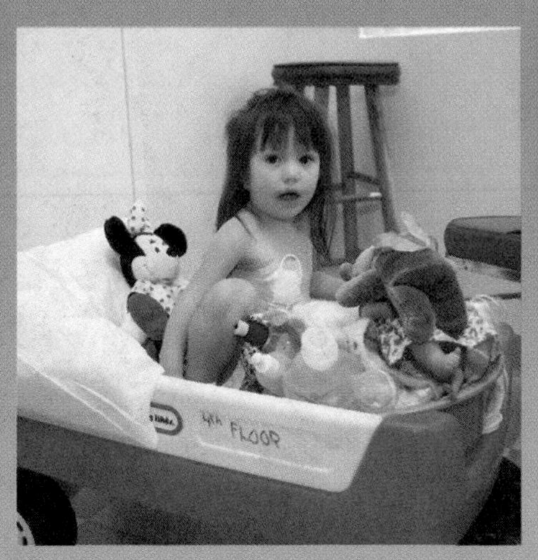

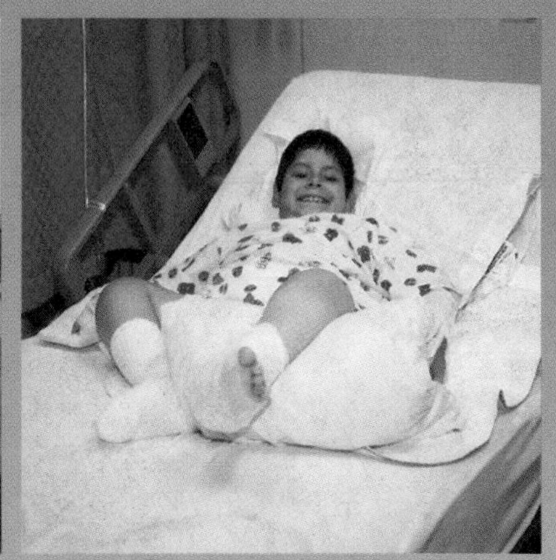
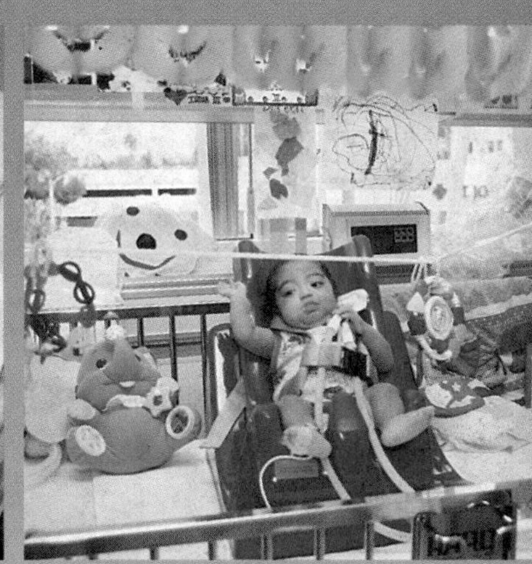

UNIT

4

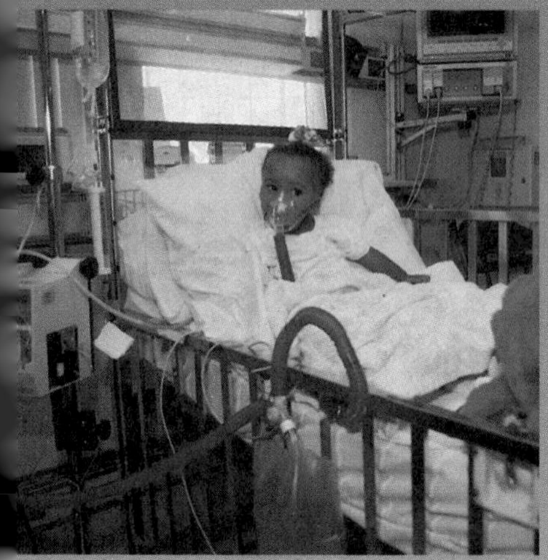
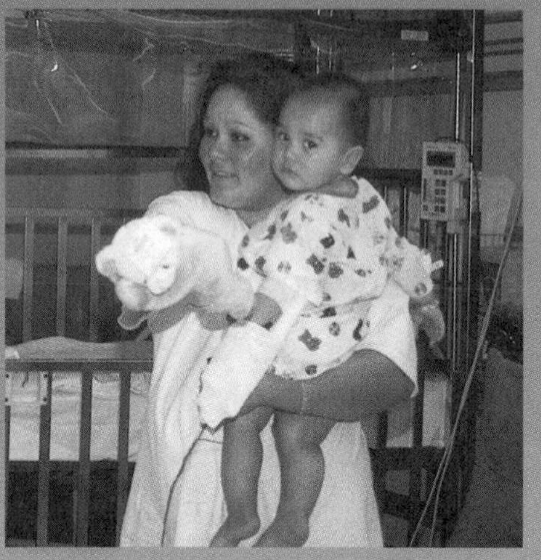
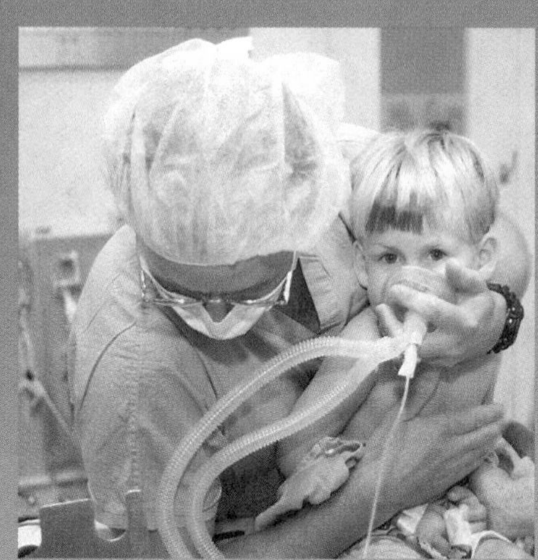

The chapters in this unit cover acute and chronic conditions that can affect infants, children, and adolescents. Disease conditions are grouped with like conditions that primarily affect a specific body system. Each chapter begins with several features to assist the nurse in summarizing the assessment data specific to that system. These features include charts on focused health history, focused physical assessment, and nursing diagnoses and outcomes. Also, developmental and biological variances are highlighted; these summarize system changes that occur with age throughout life. The diagnostic criteria section discusses laboratory tests and diagnostic procedures used to diagnose specific conditions. The treatment modalities section summarizes the methods used by the interdisciplinary team to manage health challenges in a child afflicted with a disorder affecting the subject body system. In the discussion of a particular condition, interventions, teaching intervention plans (TIPs), care paths, community care highlights, and other features are integrated into the discussion to emphasize the care of the child and family across the continuum of the family life cycle and the unique life circumstances of each child.

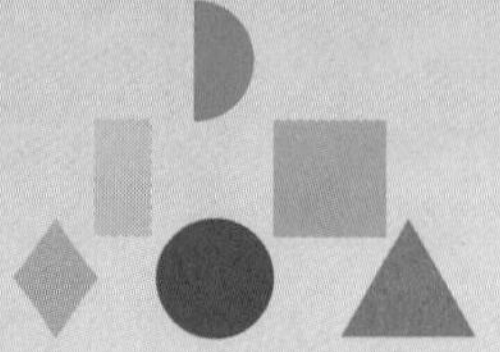

HEALTH CHALLENGE:

The Neonate

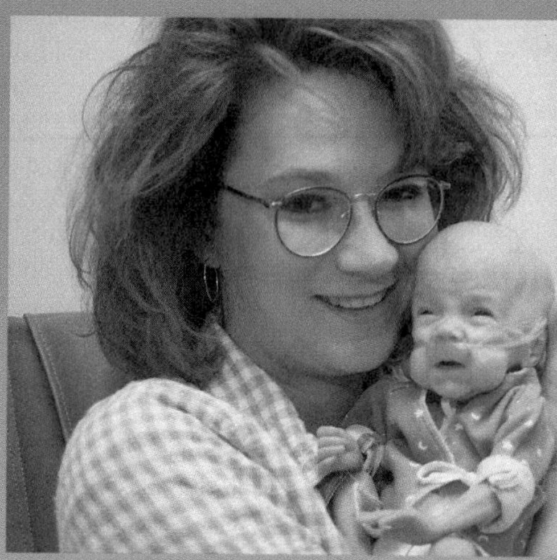

OUTLINE

Assessment of the Neonate with a Health Challenge
- Focused Health History
- Focused Physical Assessment
- Nursing Diagnoses and Outcomes
- Developmental and Biological Variances

Diagnostic Criteria for Evaluating the Neonate with a Health Challenge
- Ballard Scale
- Neonatal Behavioral Assessment Scale
- Assessment of Preterm Newborn Behavior Scale

Treatment Modalities
- Skin-to-Skin Care
- Developmental Care

Health Challenges in the Neonate
- Disorders of Prematurity and Low Birth Weight
    - Thermoregulatory Problems
    - Surfactant Deficiency
    - Patent Ductus Arteriosus
    - Neonatal Sepsis
    - Intraventricular Hemorrhage
    - Apnea of Prematurity
    - Feeding and Nutrition Problems
    - Necrotizing Enterocolitis
    - Retinopathy of Prematurity
- Birth Injuries
    - Soft Tissue Injuries
    - Extracranial Hemorrhage
    - Skull Fracture
    - Clavicular Fracture
    - Peripheral Nerve Injuries
- Perinatal Asphyxia
- Infants of Diabetic Mothers
- Fetal Alcohol Syndrome
- Intrauterine Exposure to Cocaine or Narcotics
- Infants of Tobacco Smokers
- Prenatal and Neonatal Exposure to Varicella
- Neonatal Hyperbilirubinemia
- Neonatal Hypoglycemia
- Meconium Aspiration

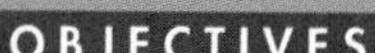

OBJECTIVES

- Describe the nursing assessment measures that would assist in identifying developmental disorders and common problems associated with the high-risk neonate.
- Identify the appropriate use of the Ballard scale, the neonatal behavioral assessment scale, and the assessment of the preterm newborn behavioral scale that assist the health care team in the identification of developmental disorders and health care problems of high-risk neonates.
- Explain the etiology, prognosis, and patient outcomes of common disorders affecting the preterm neonate.
- Describe significant pathophysiologic principles and their impact on developmental alterations in the neonate.
- Discuss nursing care for a neonate with a health challenge.
- Identify interdisciplinary interventions commonly used for each health challenge in neonates.

KEY TERMS

apnea
appropriate for gestational age (AGA)
caput succedaneum
cephalhematoma
extremely low birth weight (ELBW)
hyperbilirubinemia
intrauterine growth retardation (IUGR)
jaundice
kernicterus
large for gestational age (LGA)
low birth weight (LBW)
neonatal abstinence syndrome (NAS)
orogastric tube
periodic breathing
postconceptual age
small for gestational age (SGA)
very low birth weight (VLBW)

CHAPTER

14

The neonatal period is one of the most vulnerable times in the human life cycle. Normal neonates are challenged to adapt to the extrauterine environment and use newly functioning independent biological systems. It is a time when mothers seek help to ensure the neonate's well-being. This care is initiated in a social context (Pridham, 1997). The premature or ill term neonate faces additional challenges as a result of prematurity or intrauterine exposures that increase the likelihood of morbidity or death. Neonatal mortality is largely dependent on birth weight and gestational age. Lowest mortality is associated with birth weights of 3000 to 4000 g and a gestational age of 38 to 42 weeks (Behrman, Kliegman, & Arvin, 1996).

Nurses caring for neonates during this vulnerable period use acute assessment skills and definitive interventions to assist and support the transition to extrauterine life. Neonates demonstrate illness through insidious signs and symptoms. Therefore, astute assessment skills are needed to identify early signs of impending problems. For example, subtle changes in the neonate's breathing or feeding patterns and behavior may be the first signs of neonatal sepsis (systemic infection). Early recognition of these signs is vital to provide prompt interventions.

Neonatal intensive care units (NICUs), introduced in the 1960s, have lessened neonatal morbidity and mortality. Along with the recent advances in technology, NICUs have improved the success of intensive care for neonates. As technology advances, there has been an increase in the survival of neonates with low birth weight along with an improvement in the morbidity associated with premature birth. This technology is expensive and is in part contributing to the current high cost of health care in the United States.

The special challenges that face the high-risk neonate, including prematurity, birth trauma, and intrauterine exposures, are explored in this chapter. The focus is on nursing assessment and interdisciplinary interventions used to assist and support the high-risk neonate's transition to extrauterine life and continued growth and development.

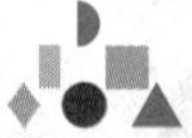

Assessment of the Neonate with a Health Challenge

Historically, physicians and nurses working in the NICU have focused on developing new technology and therapies to better understand and treat problems in the ill neonate. Not until recently has there been a focus on the neurobehavioral development of the neonate. Both the disease process and the NICU environment present challenges to optimizing the neurobehavioral development of the ill term and preterm neonate. Surgery, premature body systems, and withdrawal from intrauterine drug exposure are examples of factors that may inhibit the natural progression of neurobehavioral development. Additionally, results of studies on the NICU environment have shown that the bright lights and noise as well as the common and frequent procedures, such as suctioning the endotracheal tube, changing the infant's position, or assessing vital signs, can cause severe hypoxemia (Harrison, 1997). Although techniques to assess and manage pain in the hospitalized infant have progressed greatly over the past 20 years (Hudson, 1997), they still may impede the neurobehavioral development of the neonate.

Assessing for developmental problems in the neonate involves evaluating neurologic and behavioral functioning. The neurologic examination focuses on the presence of reflexes such as the grasp and Moro reflexes and the quality of muscle tone. The behavioral examination complements the neurologic examination and seeks to describe the quality of behavioral performance. The combination of these two assessments is the neurobehavioral assessment that determines the neonate's behavioral capabilities, interactive qualities, and adaptations to the extrauterine environment. Information obtained from this assessment can be used to plan interventions that support and optimize the neonate's development.

Focused Health History

The purpose of the health history is to collect data regarding the quality of the progression of development of the high-risk neonate. Whether the nurse is caring for the neonate in the normal newborn nursery, the NICU, or the family's home, specific health patterns are important to assess for all newborns. After delivery, a healthy term neonate is generally cared for in a normal neonatal nursery where the nurse focuses on the establishment of feedings and normally functioning body systems. The nurse caring for the neonate reviews the labor and delivery records to determine the presence or absence of prenatal care, general health of the mother, length of labor, and any difficulties encountered during labor, such as maternal fever or fetal distress. Delivery difficulties are also important, such as the need to use forceps or vacuum extraction at the time of delivery. Knowing this information assists the nurse to be alert to any potential problems in the neonate and education of the caregivers.

In the delivery room or within the NICU, the nurse reviews the labor and delivery records and begins neonatal records, to help identify potential problems. The focus is on the primary problem of the neonate that prompted an admission to the NICU.

In the home or at a clinic visit, the primary caretaker is the best source for information related to the neonate's current health and developmental status. This interview process also lets the nurse assess the quality of the caretaker's attachment and responsiveness to the neonate's needs. Assessment of feeding, stooling, and activity patterns also is essential to determine the neonate's well-being (Chart 14–1). The nurse obtains information related to the health of the mother during pregnancy, quality of the labor and delivery, and the initial newborn course. This information assists the nurse to focus on specific health patterns and physical characteristics that may be altered if the pregnancy or neonatal course was difficult. Specific at-risk neonates include those who were admitted to the NICU, born prematurely, or experienced a difficult transition, as evidenced by a low Apgar score (less than 6) at 5 minutes. Responses to the nurse's health history questions can suggest developmental delays and can guide the physical examination.

Focused Physical Assessment

Physical assessment of the neonate involves inspection, observation, smell, palpation, percussion, and auscultation. The key parameters are assessed during the examination of all newborns (Chart 14–2). The purpose of the neonatal examination is to identify existing abnormalities and provide baseline data for comparison as the newborn adapts to the extrauterine environment. The neonate should be assessed at delivery, immediately on admission to the nursery, and then frequently thereafter.

Apgar scoring (Fig. 14–1) was developed in 1952 by Dr. Virginia Apgar, an anesthesiologist, as a quick delivery suite evaluation for newborns' immediate adjustment to extrauterine life. The Apgar score is recorded at 1 and 5 minutes after birth and repeated until the infant's condition stabilizes. The infant is rated on a scale of 0 to 2

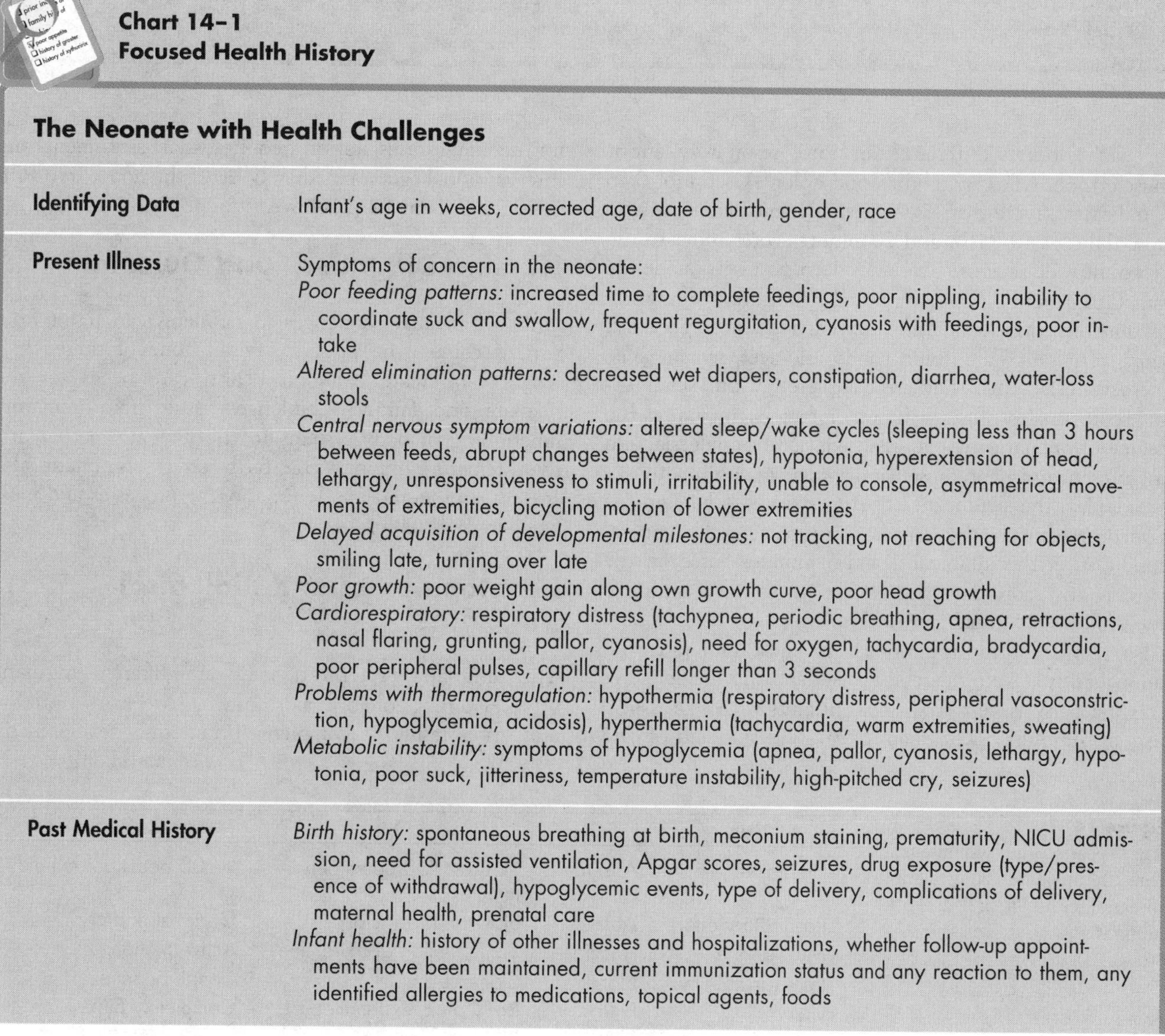

Chart 14–1
Focused Health History

The Neonate with Health Challenges

Identifying Data	Infant's age in weeks, corrected age, date of birth, gender, race
Present Illness	Symptoms of concern in the neonate: *Poor feeding patterns:* increased time to complete feedings, poor nippling, inability to coordinate suck and swallow, frequent regurgitation, cyanosis with feedings, poor intake *Altered elimination patterns:* decreased wet diapers, constipation, diarrhea, water-loss stools *Central nervous symptom variations:* altered sleep/wake cycles (sleeping less than 3 hours between feeds, abrupt changes between states), hypotonia, hyperextension of head, lethargy, unresponsiveness to stimuli, irritability, unable to console, asymmetrical movements of extremities, bicycling motion of lower extremities *Delayed acquisition of developmental milestones:* not tracking, not reaching for objects, smiling late, turning over late *Poor growth:* poor weight gain along own growth curve, poor head growth *Cardiorespiratory:* respiratory distress (tachypnea, periodic breathing, apnea, retractions, nasal flaring, grunting, pallor, cyanosis), need for oxygen, tachycardia, bradycardia, poor peripheral pulses, capillary refill longer than 3 seconds *Problems with thermoregulation:* hypothermia (respiratory distress, peripheral vasoconstriction, hypoglycemia, acidosis), hyperthermia (tachycardia, warm extremities, sweating) *Metabolic instability:* symptoms of hypoglycemia (apnea, pallor, cyanosis, lethargy, hypotonia, poor suck, jitteriness, temperature instability, high-pitched cry, seizures)
Past Medical History	*Birth history:* spontaneous breathing at birth, meconium staining, prematurity, NICU admission, need for assisted ventilation, Apgar scores, seizures, drug exposure (type/presence of withdrawal), hypoglycemic events, type of delivery, complications of delivery, maternal health, prenatal care *Infant health:* history of other illnesses and hospitalizations, whether follow-up appointments have been maintained, current immunization status and any reaction to them, any identified allergies to medications, topical agents, foods

Chart continued on following page

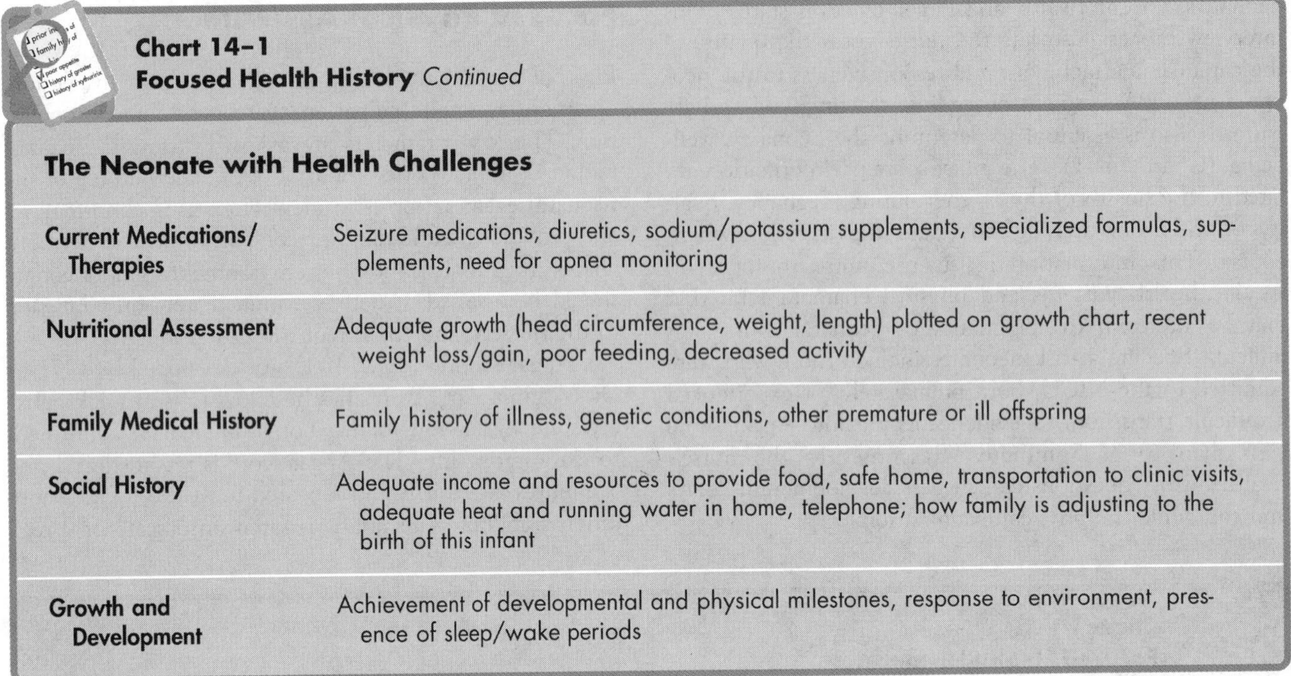

Chart 14–1
Focused Health History *Continued*

The Neonate with Health Challenges	
Current Medications/ Therapies	Seizure medications, diuretics, sodium/potassium supplements, specialized formulas, supplements, need for apnea monitoring
Nutritional Assessment	Adequate growth (head circumference, weight, length) plotted on growth chart, recent weight loss/gain, poor feeding, decreased activity
Family Medical History	Family history of illness, genetic conditions, other premature or ill offspring
Social History	Adequate income and resources to provide food, safe home, transportation to clinic visits, adequate heat and running water in home, telephone; how family is adjusting to the birth of this infant
Growth and Development	Achievement of developmental and physical milestones, response to environment, presence of sleep/wake periods

for each of five criteria: heart rate, respiratory effort, muscle tone, reflex irritability, and color. A score of 0 to 3 indicates severe distress, requiring immediate resuscitation. The 5-, 10-, 15-, and 20-minute scores indicate the probability of success. Scores of 4 to 6 signify moderate difficulty, whereas scores of 7 to 10 indicate the absence of difficulty. Many healthy newborns do not receive a score of 10 because their hands and feet remain blue (acrocyanosis) until they are completely warm. The Apgar score is also affected by other factors, including the degree of prematurity, maternal sedation or analgesia, and the presence of neuromuscular disorders in the infant.

Today, the significance of Apgar scores is being questioned. Although the Apgar score reflects the general condition of the infant at 1 and 5 minutes based on the criteria, the score does not predict neonatal mortality or the infant's eventual physical or neurologic outcomes. Also, Apgar scores are normal in most children who subsequently develop cerebral palsy, and the incidence of cerebral palsy is very low among infants with scores of 0 to 3 at 5 minutes (Kliegman, 1996). The standard of care for neonatal resuscitation requires that assessment and intervention begin immediately at birth, not a full minute later (Bloom & Cropley, 1995).

Nursing Diagnoses and Outcomes

Although health challenges in neonates can result from various causes, the presence of any one of these challenges can create common health care needs for the neonate and family. Challenges result from immature functioning of body systems in the neonate, particularly the premature infant. The birth of a sick infant also stresses coping and family functioning processes and must be addressed (Chart 14–3).

Developmental and Biological Variances

The term and preterm neonate are different in many ways. A term neonate is born after 37 weeks of gestation and, as a result of complete intrauterine development,

Text continued on page 729

Figure 14–1
The Apgar scoring system evaluates the neonate's adjustment to extrauterine life at 1 and 5 minutes.

Sign	0	1	2
Heart rate	Absent	Slow, <100 beats per minute	>100 beats per minute
Respiratory effort	Absent	Slow and irregular	Good, strong cry
Muscle tone	Flaccid	Some flexion of extremities	Active motion
Reflex irritability	None	Grimace	Cough or sneeze
Color	Pale, blue	Body pink, extremities blue	Completely pink

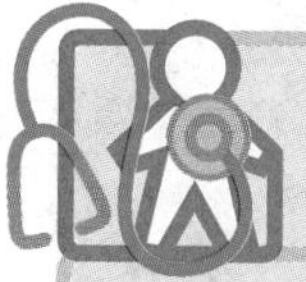

Chart 14–2
Focused Physical Assessment

The Neonate with Health Challenges

Parameter	Normal	Abnormal	Cause
Birth history	Apgar score >7 at 5 min	Apgar score <7 at 5 min	Asphyxia, traumatic delivery, hemorrhage, nuchal cord
Color	Pink Acrocyanosis during first 24 hours of life	Cyanosis (central)	Congenital heart disease
		White/pale	Respiratory distress, hypothermia, hypovolemia, anemia, sepsis
		Mottled	Acidosis, hypotension, hypothermia, shock
		Jaundice in first 24 hours of life	Hemolysis, sepsis, biliary atresia
		Jaundice after first 24 hours of life	Immature liver
		Plethoric, ruddy	Polycythemia, hyperthermia
Skin	Mature, intact, presence of subcutaneous fat, vernix, scant lanugo, milia, erythema toxicum	Thin, transluscent blood vessels; lack of vernix, abundant lanugo	Prematurity
		Lack of subcutaneous fat	Prematurity, IUGR
		Petechiae	Trauma, sepsis
		Edema	Trauma
		Peeling, long fingernails and toenails	Post-term
		Meconium staining	Meconium aspiration, fetal distress
		Forceps marks	Trauma, asphyxia
	Capillary refill <3 sec	Prolonged capillary refill	Hypovolemia, acidosis, hypothermia
Position/activity	Spontaneous movements	Frog position of legs, decreased tone, weak grasp	Prematurity
	Flexed position, palmar grasp, lusty cry, normal tone	Decreased movement	Birth asphyxia, neurologic damage
		Weak palmar grasp	Prematurity
		High-pitched cry	Neurologic abnormality, drug withdrawal
		Increased tone	Drug exposure/birth asphyxia
		Hypotonia	Neurologic damage
Head	Normocephalic/minimal head lag	Microcephalic	TORCH syndrome/transplacental infections, congenital anomalies
		Hydrocephalic	Congenital anomalies, IVH, meningomyelocele
		Encephalocele	Herniated brain
		Anencephaly	Absent cerebral tissue/neural tube defect
		Molding	Difficult delivery, prolonged labor

Chart continued on following page

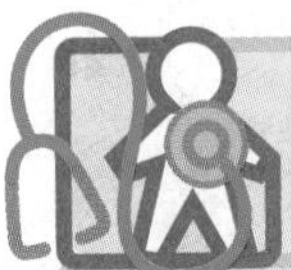

Chart 14–2
Focused Physical Assessment *Continued*

The Neonate with Health Challenges

Parameter	Normal	Abnormal	Cause
Head *continued*		Cephalhematoma	Difficult delivery, use of vacuum extraction
		Caput succedaneum	Pressure on presenting part, prolonged labor
		Full anterior fontanelle	Increased ICP, IVH
		Sunken anterior fontanelle	Dehydration
		Increased head lag	Hypotonia/prematurity
Eyes	Clean/white sclera	Yellow sclera	Jaundice
		Hemorrhages	Birth trauma
	Blink reflexes present	Absent reflex	Neurologic damage
			Facial nerve paralysis
	Presence of red reflexes	Absent red reflex	Congenital cataracts
	Eyes on line with ears	Low-set ears	Down syndrome
Ears	Adequate cartilage formation	Cartilage flattened/folded	Prematurity
Nose	Midline	Off midline	Congenital malformation
	Nares patent	Not patent	Choanal atresia
Mouth	Intact hard/soft palate	Not intact	Cleft lip/palate
	Present gag reflex	Not present	Neurologic abnormalities
	Present sucking reflex	Not present	Prematurity, neurologic difficulties
	Present rooting reflex	Not present	Prematurity, neurologic abnormality
Neck	Normal tonic neck reflex	Asymmetrical	Prematurity/neurologic dysfunction
	Full ROM	Decreased ROM	Fetal position
	Clavicles intact	Fractured	Birth trauma
Respiratory	Equal expansion	Asymmetrical	Pneumothorax, phrenic nerve damage
	No distress	Grunting, flaring, retractions	Surfactant deficiency/pneumonic sepsis, retained lung fluid
	Respiratory rate: 40–60 breaths per minute	Tachypnea	Congenital heart disease/respiratory distress
	Clear breath sounds	Rales/rhonchi/wheezing	Fluid in alveoli, decreased ventilation, PDA
		Decreased breath sounds	Pneumothorax, diaphragmatic hernia
	Normal peripheral pulses	Decreased	Congenital heart disease
		Increased	PDA
Cardiac	Regular rate and rhythm	Irregular	Supraventricular tachycardia, congenital heart block
	Heart rate: 80–150 beats per minute (term)	Bradycardia	Hypothermia, sepsis, apnea

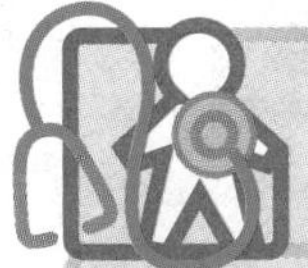

Chart 14–2
Focused Physical Assessment *Continued*

The Neonate with Health Challenges

Parameter	Normal	Abnormal	Cause
Cardiac *continued*	Heart rate: 120–160 beats per minute (preterm)	Tachycardia	Hypovolemia, hyperthermia, anemia, acidosis, congestive heart failure
	Murmur first 24 hours of life	Murmur prolonged	Congenital heart disease, PDA, acidosis, anemia
	Quiet precordium	Active precordium	PDA of prematurity
Abdomen	Rounded, symmetrical bowel sounds present	Distention	Obstruction, NEC, renal abnormality, fetal hydrops
		Scaphoid	Diaphragmatic hernia
		Decreased bowel sounds	Obstruction, NEC
		Hyperactive bowel sounds	Hypermotility, colitis
	Soft/non-tender	Tense/tender	NEC, abdominal mass
	Liver: sharp edge 1–2 cm below costal margin	Enlarged	Hepatosplenomegaly, hemolysis, sepsis
	Umbilical cord: three vessels	Two-vessel cord	Congenital anomalies, renal anomalies
	Smooth	Bowel loops	Obstruction, feeding intolerance
	Meconium passage within 24 hours after birth	No stool within first 24 hours	Obstruction, imperforate anus Hirschsprung's disease
	Normal stooling pattern/type	Water-loss stools	Diarrhea, colitis, rotavirus, feeding intolerance
		OB+ stools	Anal fissure, NEC, colitis
		Reducing substance positive	Carbohydrate intolerance
		Bright red streaks	Anal fissure, colitis
		Meconium plugging	Hirschsprung's disease, cystic fibrosis
Genitourinary tract	Vagina patent with white discharge	Blood-tinged discharge	Maternal hormones
		Ambiguous genitalia	Congenital anomalies, adrenal hyperplasia
	Anus patent	Nonpatent	Imperforate anus
	Urinary meatus midline	Meatus displaced to ventral surface	Hypospadias
		Meatus displaced to dorsal surface	Epispadias
	Urination within first 24 hours	Failure to void within first 24 hours	Renal obstruction, polycystic kidneys
	Testes descended	Undescended	Prematurity
		Fluid-filled scrotal sac	Hydrocele
Extremities	Full ROM in all four extremities	Limited ROM in all four extremities	Clavicle injury, brachial plexus injury
	Ten fingers, toes	More/less than 10 digits/webbing	Congenital syndromes
	Buttock creases symmetrical	Asymmetrical	Congenital hip dysplasia

Chart continued on following page

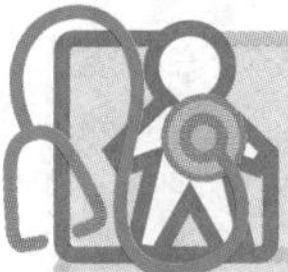

Chart 14–2
Focused Physical Assessment *Continued*

The Neonate with Health Challenges

Parameter	Normal	Abnormal	Cause
Torso	Spine intact	Spine not intact	Meningomyelocele
Growth	AGA	SGA/IUGR	Smoking during pregnancy, poor maternal nutrition, transplacental infection, drug exposure
		LGA	Diabetic mothers/post term

AGA, appropriate for gestational age; ICP, intracranial pressure; IUGR, intrauterine growth retardation; IVH, intraventricular hemorrhage; LGA, large for gestational age; NEC, necrotizing enterocolitis; OB+, occult blood–positive; PDA, patent ductus arteriosus; ROM, range of motion; SGA, small for gestational age.

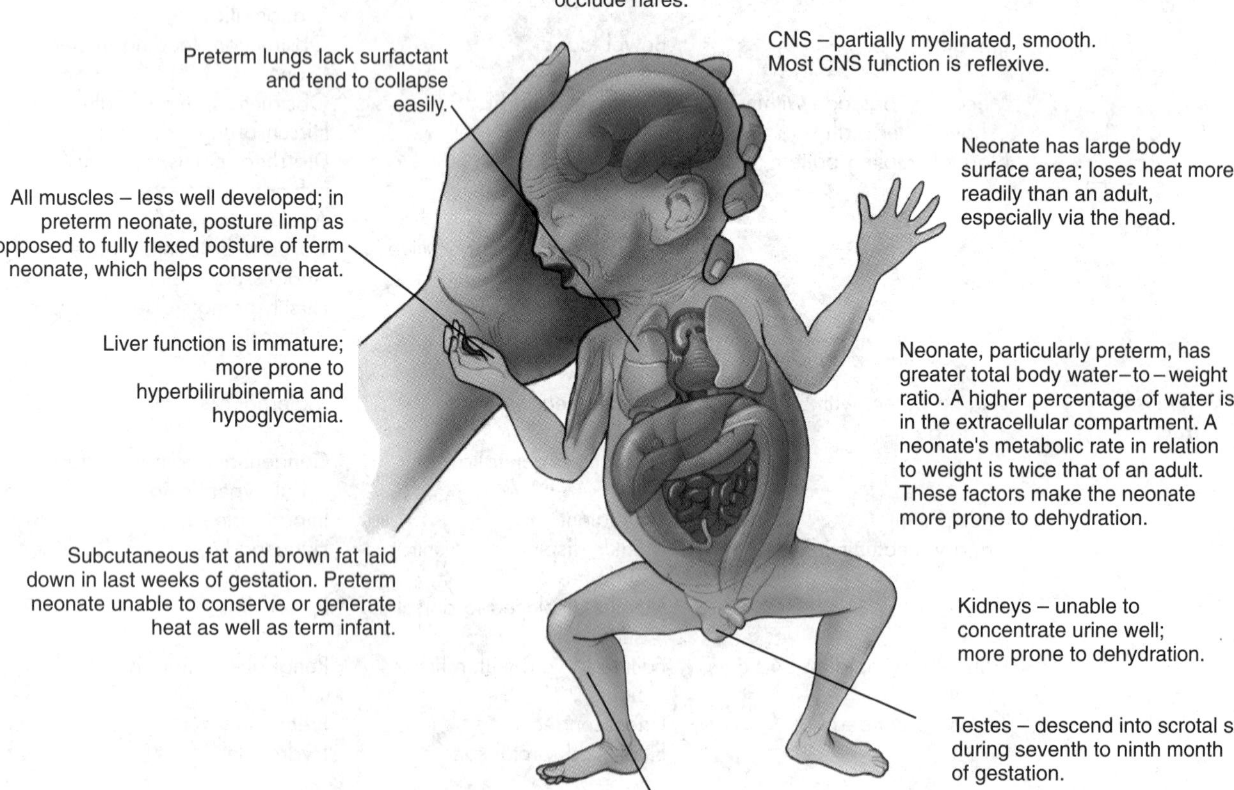

Neonates are obligate nose breathers for approximately the first 5 months; do not occlude nares.
Preterm lungs lack surfactant and tend to collapse easily.
CNS – partially myelinated, smooth. Most CNS function is reflexive.
Neonate has large body surface area; loses heat more readily than an adult, especially via the head.
All muscles – less well developed; in preterm neonate, posture limp as opposed to fully flexed posture of term neonate, which helps conserve heat.
Liver function is immature; more prone to hyperbilirubinemia and hypoglycemia.
Neonate, particularly preterm, has greater total body water–to–weight ratio. A higher percentage of water is in the extracellular compartment. A neonate's metabolic rate in relation to weight is twice that of an adult. These factors make the neonate more prone to dehydration.
Subcutaneous fat and brown fat laid down in last weeks of gestation. Preterm neonate unable to conserve or generate heat as well as term infant.
Kidneys – unable to concentrate urine well; more prone to dehydration.
Testes – descend into scrotal sac during seventh to ninth month of gestation.
Skin less well connected between dermis and epidermis; slight friction causes blistering.
Neonates, particularly preterm, have an increased susceptibility to infection. Ability to produce an inflammatory response, which helps localize the infection, is immature. Signs of infection are usually subtle and generalized.

Figure 14–2
Developmental and biological variances: the neonate.

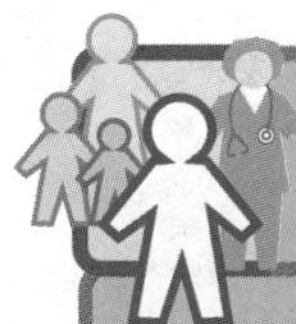

Chart 14–3
Nursing Diagnoses and Outcomes

Neonates with a Health Challenge

Ineffective thermoregulation related to immature skin structure and decreased amount of subcutaneous tissue

Outcomes: Neonate will be maintained within a neutral thermal environment.
Neonate will have a stable temperature between 36.4° and 37.0°C

Risk for infection related to effects of immature immune system

Outcome: Neonate will remain infection free.

Risk for impaired skin integrity related to thin skin from immaturity

Outcome: Neonate will have intact skin.

Altered growth and development related to poor feeding and weight gain

Outcome: Neonate will demonstrate adequate growth and feeding patterns.

Risk for altered parent/infant attachment related to effects of hospitalization, sick infant's ability to interact with parents

Outcome: Parents will participate in the neonate's care, as appropriate, and begin to verbalize positive statements regarding the neonate.

Altered family processes related to reaction to an acutely ill neonate

Outcome: Family will visit the neonate frequently, maintain mutual support, and seek external resources as needed.

Knowledge deficit: well-child care or complicated home care

Outcome: Parents will be able to provide competent care of the neonate after discharge.

possesses the necessary physical attributes to successfully adapt to the extrauterine environment. A healthy term neonate at birth exhibits strong muscle tone and reflexes, vigorous cry and respiratory effort, normal respiratory rate, and a normal cardiac rate and rhythm.

The preterm neonate is defined as one born before 37 weeks' gestation and is extremely vulnerable to developmental problems because the central nervous system (CNS) is immature and still developing. The premature neonate in the NICU is subjected to loud and sudden noises, constant bright light, painful procedures, irregular patterns of handling, and rapid temperature changes, all of which may have detrimental effects on the developing immature systems of the premature neonate. The uterus provided a warm, slightly oscillating, fluid-filled, quiet environment in which all physiologic and developmental needs were met. The NICU environment may precipitate hypoxia as a result of needed medical and nursing procedures, leading to damage of the developing CNS. Reducing light, noise, and temperature changes and providing periods of "hands off" care have been shown to improve weight gain and behavioral assessment scores (Als et al., 1994).

The sick term neonate is less vulnerable to developmental problems owing to the more mature and organized CNS and in most cases, a higher proportion of subcutaneous fat. However, because of the disease process the term neonate may experience difficulty in interacting with the environment in ways that a healthy term neonate would (Fig. 14–2).

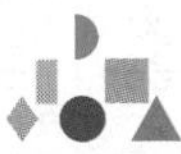

Diagnostic Criteria for Evaluating the Neonate with a Health Challenge

The specific diagnostic tests and procedures used to assess a neonate depend on the suspected disorder (Table 14–1). Prenatal tests commonly performed are fetal ultrasonography and determination of alpha-fetoprotein levels. These and other prenatal diagnostic measures are discussed in Chapter 8.

Several assessment scales are available to assist in evaluating the progression of development in the neonate. The most common are the Ballard scale, the Brazelton neonatal behavioral assessment scale (NBAS), and the assessment of preterm newborn behavior (APIB) scale.

Ballard Scale

Ballard and colleagues (1991) presented a tool used to assess specific neuromuscular and physical characteristics of the neonate (Fig. 14–3). Posture, square window (wrist flexion), arm recoil, popliteal angle, scarf sign, and heel to ear are the neuromuscular indicators that are scored. Physical indicators include skin, presence or ab-

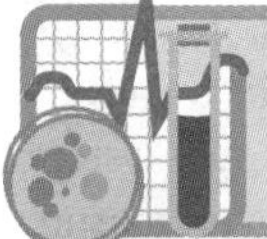

Table 14–1
Diagnostic Tests and Procedures for Evaluating the Neonate with a Health Challenge

Diagnostic Test or Procedure	Purpose	Findings and Indications	Health Care Provider Responsibilities
Chest radiography (also abdominal)	To examine soft tissue and bony structure. Abdominal: to diagnose free air in abdomen and evaluate bowel and other organs	Evaluate lung aeration, lung expansion, lung disease, heart size; bony structures density; intramural air = necrotizing enterocolitis	Shield newborn with gonad shield; protect self with lead apron; keep others 10 feet away from area. Hold newborn during procedure to ensure adequate positioning and avoid rotation.
Pulse oximetry	To measure oxygen saturation of blood; noninvasive; measures amount of light absorbed by hemoglobin in the blood	Saturations <80 may indicate poor blood oxygen content. Saturations >100 may indicate hyperoxia.	Protect probe from phototherapy light. Ensure correlation with heart rate. Change site every 12 hours to avoid skin breakdown due to pressure. Test may be inaccurate in anemic patients.
Ultrasound (head, abdominal, fetal)	Evaluates internal anatomic structures through emission of sound waves to evaluate tissue density, movement of tissue, and flow of blood	Heart defects and pulmonary artery pressures; presence of blood in ventricles, brain masses, and in fetal structures	Assist to position newborn. Sedate as needed.
Pneumogram	Twelve- to 24-hour sleep study to measure the presence of apnea, bradycardia, and desaturations	Results read by physician; presence of apnea/bradycardia indicates need for apnea monitor at home.	Ensure monitor is on and apnea/bradycardia episodes are documented on test strip.
Transcutaneous monitoring (TCM)	Measurement of CO_2 and O_2 transcutaneously that correlates with blood CO_2 and O_2. Skin is heated to measure values.	Transcutaneous CO_2 values more accurate than O_2 values. High CO_2 readings may indicate hypoventilation.	Change probe site every 2–4 hours. Monitor for skin burns. Obtain blood gas sample to correlate findings.
Arterial blood gas	Analysis of arterial oxygenation, CO_2 retention, and loss or gain of buffer system acid versus base by the blood system	Normal findings: pH: 7.35–7.45 $Pa{CO_2}$: 35–45 mmHg $Pa{O_2}$: 50–80 mmHg HCO_3: 22–26 mEq/L BE: 5 to +5 Elevated $Pa{CO_2}$ indicates hypoventilation. Decreased $Pa{O_2}$ indicates hypoxemia.	Avoid allowing air into sample. If sample obtained from heel as capillary blood gas: warm heel 5 minutes before draw; use appropriate site on heel; avoid excessive squeezing of heel which will cause erroneous results. Extremity must have good perfusion to obtain accurate results. Capillary blood values for pH and CO_2 usually correlate with arterial values; O_2 values do not correlate well and should not be relied on.
Hemoglobin/hematocrit	To determine the amount of circulating red blood cells (hematocrit) and oxygen-carrying capacity of the blood (hemoglobin)	Range for hemoglobin values is 17–19 g/dL; for hematocrit value is 50-63 mL/dL.	Heelstick samples may have higher values, owing to sludging of red blood cells.
Serum glucose	To detect the presence of hyperglycemia or hypoglycemia.	Normal values: Term newborn: 40–120 mg/dL Preterm newborn: 30–160 mg/dL	Do not draw sample from a central line with glucose infusing because erroneous values may result. Capillary samples may be lower if heel site is not warmed before sample is drawn

MATURATIONAL ASSESSMENT OF GESTATIONAL AGE (New Ballard Score)

NAME ____________ DATE/TIME OF BIRTH ____________ SEX ____________

HOSPITAL NO. ____________ DATE/TIME OF EXAM ____________ BIRTH WEIGHT ____________

RACE ____________ AGE WHEN EXAMINED ____________ LENGTH ____________

APGAR SCORE: 1 MINUTE ________ 5 MINUTES ________ 10 MINUTES ________ HEAD CIRC. ____________

EXAMINER ____________

NEUROMUSCULAR MATURITY

NEUROMUSCULAR MATURITY SIGN	SCORE							RECORD SCORE HERE
	-1	0	1	2	3	4	5	
POSTURE								
SQUARE WINDOW (Wrist)	>90°	90°	60°	45°	30°	0°		
ARM RECOIL		180°	140°-180°	110°-140°	90°-110°	<90°		
POPLITEAL ANGLE	180°	160°	140°	120°	100°	90°	<90°	
SCARF SIGN								
HEEL TO EAR								
							TOTAL NEUROMUSCULAR MATURITY SCORE	

PHYSICAL MATURITY

PHYSICAL MATURITY SIGN	SCORE							RECORD SCORE HERE
	-1	0	1	2	3	4	5	
SKIN	sticky friable transparent	gelatinous red translucent	smooth pink visible veins	superficial peeling &/or rash, few veins	cracking pale areas rare veins	parchment deep cracking no vessels	leathery cracked wrinkled	
LANUGO	none	sparse	abundant	thinning	bald areas	mostly bald		
PLANTAR SURFACE	heel-toe 40-50 mm:-1 <40 mm:-2	>50 mm no crease	faint red marks	anterior transverse crease only	creases ant. 2/3	creases over entire sole		
BREAST	imperceptible	barely perceptible	flat areola no bud	stippled areola 1-2 mm bud	raised areola 3-4 mm bud	full areola 5-10 mm bud		
EYE/EAR	lids fused loosely: -1 tightly: -2	lids open pinna flat stays folded	sl. curved pinna; soft; slow recoil	well-curved pinna; soft but ready recoil	formed & firm instant recoil	thick cartilage ear stiff		
GENITALS (Male)	scrotum flat, smooth	scrotum empty faint rugae	testes in upper canal rare rugae	testes descending few rugae	testes down good rugae	testes pendulous deep rugae		
GENITALS (Female)	clitoris prominent & labia flat	prominent clitoris & small labia minora	prominent clitoris & enlarging minora	majora & minora equally prominent	majora large minora small	majora cover clitoris & minora		
							TOTAL PHYSICAL MATURITY SCORE	

SCORE

Neuromuscular ________

Physical ________

Total ________

MATURITY RATING

score	weeks
-10	20
-5	22
0	24
5	26
10	28
15	30
20	32
25	34
30	36
35	38
40	40
45	42
50	44

GESTATIONAL AGE (weeks)

By dates ________

By ultrasound ________

By exam ________

Reference
Ballard JL, Khoury JC, Wedig K, et al: New Ballard Score, expanded to include extremely premature infants. *J Pediatr* 1991; 119:417-423. Reprinted by permission of Dr Ballard and Mosby-Year Book, Inc.

Figure 14–3
The new Ballard scale estimates gestational age based on the neonate's neuromuscular and physical maturity.

sence of lanugo, presence or absence of creases on the plantar surfaces, breast development, and eye and ear formation. Genitalia are scored as to gender-specific characteristics. The Ballard tool may be used from birth for the extremely premature and term neonate through day 5 of life. After completing the gestational age assessment, the weight, length, and head circumference are plotted to identify appropriate for gestational age (AGA), large for gestational age (LGA), or small for gestational age (SGA) neonates because each have specific clinical and risk factors. Based on the intrauterine growth chart, babies are classified as AGA if they weigh between the 10th and 90th percentiles, LGA if they weigh more than the 90th percentile, and SGA if they weigh less than the 10th percentile (Dodd, 1996). Although easy to administer, the Ballard score may give erroneous results in cases of prematurity, neurologic disorders, and asphyxiated neonates.

Neonatal Behavioral Assessment Scale

The NBAS is a comprehensive tool used to assess the healthy full-term neonate's behavior (see Table 4–15). This tool combines evaluation of the reflexes (Pressler & Hepworth, 1997), motor capacity, state regulation, and interactive abilities (Brazelton, 1984). To use the tool the examiner observes the neonate through various states of sleep, arousal, and wakefulness and the interactions between the neonate and the environment. The results obtained demonstrate the neonate's ability to organize states, habituate to the external environment and stimuli, regulate motor activity, respond to reflex testing, orient to visual and auditory stimuli, interact with the caregiver, and self-console (Brazelton, 1984). The tool is also useful to demonstrate to parents how their neonate responds to caregiving.

The preterm neonate may also be assessed utilizing a modified NBAS that includes both the original full-term scale and additional subscales specifically focused on the preterm neonate's behavior. The preterm neonate behaves differently from the full-term healthy or ill neonate. The preterm neonate may be better served if tested using the APIB, which is more discrete in its assessment of preterm neonatal functioning.

Assessment of Preterm Newborn Behavior Scale

The APIB is useful for preterm and high-risk full-term newborns from birth to 44 weeks' postconceptual age. Administration of the APIB requires specialized training and an experienced clinician. The focus of this assessment is to determine how neonates cope with the intense environment of the NICU and the degree of organization of the CNS (Als, Duffy, & McAnulty, 1988). The information gained from this tool assists the NICU staff and the family in assessing the degree of fragility and tolerance the neonate has to interactions.

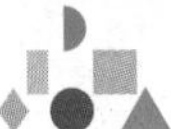

Treatment Modalities

Care for the neonate focuses on assisting the infant in transitioning to extrauterine life and then maintaining physiologic stability, particularly thermoregulation and prevention of hypoglycemia and infection.

Neonates are more likely to require resuscitation than any other age group, and how the infant is cared for at birth may have lifelong effects (Bloom & Cropley, 1995). In order to train health care professionals to skillfully perform neonatal resuscitation in a standardized, methodical manner, the Neonatal Resuscitation Program (NRP) was developed. NRP, according to American Academy of Pediatrics and American Heart Association guidelines, teaches steps in evaluating the infant, decision-making, and actions based on the evaluation. A goal is that at least one person skilled in neonatal resuscitation is present at every delivery.

Most infants respond to warming, drying, positioning, suctioning, and stimulation. Some infants require more vigorous steps such as ventilation, chest compression, endotracheal intubation, and administration of medications.

Figure 14–4
Kangaroo care involves skin-to-skin contact between parent (the mother in this photograph) and newborn.

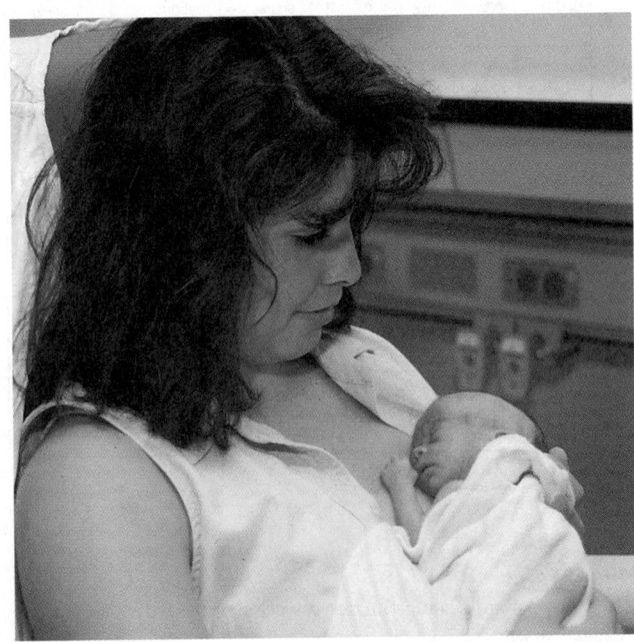

Decisions for care must be based on the infant's response to previous actions.

After immediate stabilization at birth, the infant must be monitored, and interventions implemented as indicated, to ensure adequate cardiorespiratory adaptation, thermoregulation, normoglycemia, initiation of feedings, and bonding with parents. Specific treatments for the unique health challenges that neonates face are discussed in the individual sections. An overriding dictate of neonatal care, especially important for premature infants with a more immature CNS, is that care is delivered in a developmentally appropriate manner. Two treatment modalities that meet this mandate are kangaroo care and developmental care.

Skin-to-Skin Care

Skin-to-skin holding, or kangaroo care (Fig. 14–4), is the practice of holding an infant, clothed only in a diaper, skin-to-skin against the bare chest of the father or between the breasts of the mother (Chart 14–4).

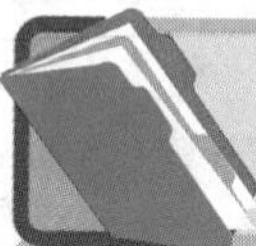

Chart 14–4
Nursing Interventions Classification (NIC)

Kangaroo Care

Definition

Promoting closeness between parent and physiologically stable preterm infant by preparing the parent and providing the environment for skin-to-skin contact

Activities

Discuss parent reaction to premature birth of infant.
Determine image parent has of premature infant.
Determine and monitor parent's level of confidence in caring for infant.
Encourage parent to initiate infant care.
Explain kangaroo care and its benefits to parent.
Determine whether infant's physiological status meets guidelines for participation in kangaroo care.
Prepare a quiet, private, draft-free environment.
Provide parent with a reclining or rocking chair.
Have parent wear comfortable, open front clothing.
Instruct parent how to transfer infant from incubator, warmer bed, or bassinet and how to manage equipment and tubing, as appropriate.
Position diaper-clad infant in prone upright position on parent's chest.
Wrap parent's clothing around or place blanket over infant to maintain infant's position and temperature.
Encourage parent to focus on infant, rather than high technological setting and equipment.
Encourage parent to gently stroke infant in prone upright position, as appropriate.
Encourage parent to gently rock infant in prone upright position, as appropriate.
Encourage auditory stimulation of infant, as appropriate.
Reinforce eye contact with infant, as appropriate.
Support parent in nurturing and providing hands-on care for infant.
Encourage parent to hold infant with full, encompassing hands.
Encourage parent to identify infant's behavioral cues.
Point out infant state changes to parent.
Instruct parent to decrease activity when infant shows signs of overstimulation, distress, or avoidance.
Encourage breast-feeding during kangaroo care, as appropriate.
Encourage parent to provide kangaroo care from 20 min to 3 hr at a time on a consistent basis, as appropriate.
Encourage postpartum mothers to change position and get up every 90 min to prevent thrombolytic disease.
Monitor parent's emotional reaction to kangaroo care.
Monitor infant's physiological status (e.g., color, temperature, heart rate, and apnea), and discontinue kangaroo care if infant becomes physiologically compromised or agitated.

From McCloskey, J. C., & Bulechek, G. M. (1996). *Nursing interventions classification (NIC)* (2nd ed.). St. Louis: Mosby–Year Book. Reprinted with permission.

Worldview: *In European and Scandinavian nurseries, skin-to-skin holding began in the early 1980s. Modern-day skin-to-skin holding was first described in 1983 in Bogota, Colombia, where mothers held their premature neonates skin-to-skin on their bare chest to provide warmth. In the nursery at Bogota, there were not enough isolettes for every premature neonate and neonates frequently shared isolettes. As a result, sepsis and mortality rates were high among these premature neonates. After instituting skin-to-skin holding, mortality and infection rates were significantly decreased (Rey & Martinez, 1983).*

Chart 14–5
Nursing Interventions

Providing Developmentally Appropriate Care

Element	Intervention
Environment	Provide calm and soothing ambiance. Avoid loud, sudden noises: pad trashcan lids, close isolette portholes gently, carefully place items on top of isolettes, decrease decibel level of telephones, intercoms, and overhead music. Lighting should be modifiable to provide adequate lighting for examinations and procedures but be able to dim for rest and to facilitate eye opening in the infant to interact with parents or the environment.
Positioning	Support the infant in a flexed, tucked position either with a positioning aid (bumper, nest, blankets) for rest or with the caregiver's hands during procedures. Side-lying or prone positioning is best. Change position gently while supporting the infant in a tucked position; avoid extreme limb extension.
Handling	Avoid giving too much stimulation at one time. Approach the child slowly (e.g., place your hands on the infant gently for a few seconds then gently turn infant over instead of abruptly opening isolette and flipping infant on his or her back). Observe the infant's cues for tolerance of handling and indications to reduce or stop stimulation. Procedures may need to be implemented in stages, allowing the infant to recover before proceeding (e.g., pause and provide containment or a pacifier to suck on).
Self-regulation	Observe the infant for behaviors used to self-soothe (e.g., hand to mouth movements). Support self-soothing behaviors or positions of the infant. Post a list of the infant's stress cues, cues that indicate relaxation, and self-soothing methods of the infant.
State regulation	Observe infant for differentiated sleep–wake cycles. Provide a calm, stable environment. Time activities to coincide with the infant's patterns (e.g., offer feedings when the infant is in a quiet awake state).
Caregiving event	Incorporate all the above into care delivery: Provide care when the infant is in a quiet awake state, if medically feasible. Observe the infant's cues and modify care based on these. Have two caregivers perform noxious procedures: one to perform the procedure and one to support the infant with containment and promotion of self-soothing behaviors. Plan procedures prior to implementation; consider necessity of procedure versus physiologic cost to the infant; have all equipment readily available.

Research has demonstrated the benefits of kangaroo care for both infants and parents. During kangaroo care, preterm infants had a significant increase in sleep time and a reduction in activity, demonstrated less agitation, apnea, and bradycardia, and maintained stable oxygen saturation (Ludington-Hoe, Hadeed, & Anderson, 1991; Ludington-Hoe, Thompson, Swinth, Hadeed, & Anderson, 1994; Messmer et al., 1997). Mothers report improved lactation with kangaroo care (Wallace & Ridpath-Parker, 1993). Parents who participate in kangaroo care increase their comfort level in providing care and report increased fulfillment and ability to know their infants, thus promoting parental attachment (Gale, Franck, & Lund, 1993; Legault & Goulet, 1995; Messmer et al., 1997). Kangaroo care is well tolerated by infants and their families and should be incorporated as a standard of nursing practice (Messmer et al., 1997).

Developmental Care

Developmental care is a philosophical approach to caring for the neonate that is based on the individual relationship between the caregiver and infant (VandenBerg, 1997). The focus of developmental care is on supporting the sick infant's neurobehavioral and physiologic organization. Health care providers must understand and interpret the meaning of infant behaviors. The caregiver must watch each infant for behavioral and physiologic cues and vary care based on the infant's response. Sick premature infants respond differently than healthy term infants.

caREminder: *Behaviors that indicate stress in the premature infant include facial grimace, yawning, tongue protrusion, hiccoughing, finger splaying, gaze aversion, fussing, crying, and vomiting. Physiologic stress cues include changes in heart or respiratory rates (tachycardia, bradycardia, tachypnea, apnea), grunting, gasping, cyanosis, and decreased blood oxygen levels (reflected in decreased oxygen saturation or* $TcPCO_2$ *levels). The infant exhibits these signs when the environment is stressful, such as in the presence of bright lights and loud noises or when handled excessively.*

To effectively deliver developmentally appropriate care, specific elements must be considered. These include the environment, positioning and handling of the infant, promoting self-regulation and state regulation in the infant, and implementation of all caregiving events (VandenBerg, 1997) (Chart 14–5).

Implementing developmental care has shown to decrease the time the premature neonate is on the ventilator and on supplemental oxygen, improve weight gain, and shorten hospital stays (Als et al., 1994). Individualizing care by offering nipple feedings when infants are in quiet awake states results in more successful feeding, an important discharge criterion for the premature infant (McCain, 1997). Additionally, premature neonates provided with developmental care have improved neurodevelopmental outcomes at 2 weeks and at 9 months (Als et al., 1994). Developmental care is a family centered concept that improves both medical and developmental outcomes for premature neonates.

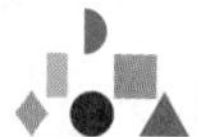

Health Challenges in the Neonate

Several disorders place the neonate at risk for ongoing health problems. Such disorders as prematurity, low birth weight, perinatal asphyxia, and birth trauma are examples of conditions that require skilled nursing assessment and interventions to promote healing and optimal development. In addition, there are specific diseases of the newborn that follow predictable trajectories. The most common are discussed in this section.

Disorders of Prematurity and Low Birth Weight

Low birth weight (LBW) is defined as a birth weight less than 2500 g (5.5 pounds), and *very low birth weight* (VLBW) is a birth weight less than 1500 g (3.5 pounds). *Extremely low birth weight* (ELBW) is a birth weight less than 1000 g (2.2 pounds).

The causes of premature delivery remain unknown. Maternal or fetal sepsis and high-risk pregnancies, such as those with multiple gestation, abruptio placentae, and pregnancy-induced hypertension, can all contribute to premature delivery. In many cases no specific causal factor can be identified, and in some cases there are multiple causal factors.

Premature delivery occurs in approximately 1% of all pregnancies and is defined as any neonate born before 37 weeks' gestation regardless of birth weight (Harlow et al., 1996). Approximately 3.6% of infants born in the United States are premature and have LBW (McCormick, 1991).

Currently, more than 270,000 neonates are born with LBW and 48,000 with VLBW (McCormick, 1991). Approximately 13% of all black neonates were born with LBW in 1988, and the likelihood of having LBW was almost 2½ times greater for black neonates than for whites (McCormick, 1991). Prematurity and LBW are the major contributors to the newborn mortality rate, because neonates born at these weights are 40 times more likely to die in the first year of life (McCormick, 1991).

LBW without prematurity (i.e., a birth weight that is low despite carrying the pregnancy to term) is considered intrauterine growth retardation (IUGR) and is associated with poor placental circulation such as maternal hypertension, smoking during pregnancy, substance abuse, and cardiac or pulmonary problems. Often, no cause can be identified in the newborn with IUGR. Neonates may be symmetrically growth retarded, in which all growth parameters are compromised, or asymmetrically growth retarded, in which head circumference is AGA but birth weight and other growth parameters are compromised.

Prevention of prematurity and LBW is clearly related to adequate and early prenatal care. The rate of LBW may be reduced significantly if all women began prenatal care in the first trimester and continued it throughout the pregnancy (Leveno, Cunningham, Roark, Nelson, & Williams, 1985). Nonwhites (i.e., blacks, Hispanics, Native Americans), women with less than a high school education, and adolescents are less likely to receive early prenatal care (Leveno et al., 1985).

Pathophysiology

Neonates born prematurely have a higher incidence of morbidity and mortality than term neonates. This is likely due to LBW. Prematurity and LBW are the major contributors to the newborn mortality rate, because neonates born at these weights are 40 times more likely to die in the first year of life (McCormick, 1991). Premature birth before 23 weeks' gestation is generally not compatible with life, owing to the lack of alveoli and other lung tissue necessary for respiration. Neonates born at 23 to 25 weeks' gestation are at the edge of viability, weigh 500 to 700 g, and have a 34% to 50% chance for survival (Hack et al., 1991).

Although they have the necessary anatomic structures, many problems occur due to the extreme immaturity of all body systems. This can lead to problems with thermoregulation, surfactant deficiency, patent ductus arteriosus (PDA), sepsis, intraventricular hemorrhage (IVH), apnea of prematurity, feeding and nutrition problems, necrotizing enterocolitis (NEC), and retinopathy of prematurity (ROP). Because each of these disorders requires different care, they are covered in detail after a general discussion of assessment and care of premature and LBW neonates.

Assessment

The premature neonate has physical characteristics different from term neonates. Observation reveals that the premature neonate's posture is lacking flexion and that muscle tone is decreased. This is obvious when the very premature neonate is supine, because the arms and legs remain extended. Also, the arm recoil is slow. As the neonate grows and matures, so does the ability for flexion.

The skin is thin and may be transparent. Blood vessels are easily discernible. The skin can be very moist and even gelatinous, depending on gestational age. The more premature the neonate, the thinner and more gelatinous the skin. The thin skin is very absorptive, and exposure to caustic agents may not only impede skin integrity but also may lead to systemic effects. Alcohol burning and toxicity in the extremely premature neonate have been reported (Watkins & Keogh, 1992). The skin of the premature neonate consists of only four layers, compared with the nine layers of the term neonate (Malloy & Perez-Woods, 1991).

If the neonate is extremely premature (between 20 and 22 weeks' gestational age), lanugo is not present. Lanugo is very fine, downy body hair that is shed during the seventh to eighth month of gestation (Fig. 14–5). However, as the fetus grows, lanugo is abundant and then decreases again near term.

Color is an important indicator of well-being in any neonate. The mucous membranes, including the lips and tongue, are inspected for central cyanosis. Other color abnormalities, including jaundice and ruddiness, must be evaluated, especially if they occur within the first 24 hours.

The nurse should assess the quality and quantity of respirations. Signs of respiratory distress are noted, including sternal, intercostal, and substernal retractions, nasal flaring, grunting, and tachypnea. Periodic breathing is common in the premature neonate, and apnea may indicate sepsis, especially in the first 12 hours of life. Lung sounds may be diminished if the premature neonate has surfactant deficiency or pneumonia. Lung sounds are auscultated in the premature neonate's axillae.

The chest is observed to assess movement and symmetry, as well as the presence or absence of an active precordium. An active precordium is easily seen on the thin chest of a premature neonate and may indicate a

Figure 14–5
Lanugo in a premature neonate.

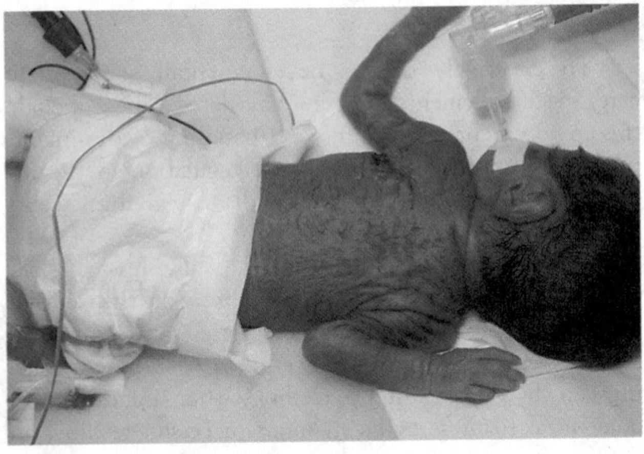

PDA. All heart borders are auscultated. Murmurs are common to the premature neonate and should be noted for quality and location.

The head of the premature neonate is larger in proportion to the rest of the body. This reflects the cephalocaudal progression of growth. The anterior fontanelle is gently palpated to assess for fullness or depression. Normally, the anterior fontanelle is soft and flat. Often, the sutures of the premature head are overriding, especially after the first 4 to 5 days of life.

The abdomen of a premature neonate is soft and slightly rounded but not generally distended unless resuscitation at birth included bag and mask ventilation by which air may be forced into the stomach. The abdomen is auscultated for bowel sounds in all four quadrants. Abnormal abdominal examination findings are distention, discoloration, observable bowel loops, and absence of bowel sounds. If the premature neonate is receiving enteral intake, the abdominal examination should be performed before every feeding and include measuring the abdominal girth for baseline and comparison data. Feeding residuals (food that is present in the stomach 3 hours after feeding) should also be noted, including amount and color. Stools are tested for presence of occult blood and reducing substance. Stools containing microscopic amounts of blood will test positively for occult blood, which may be an early sign of NEC or another feeding disorder. Stools that contain more than 0.5% sugar will test positive for reducing substance and is an abnormal finding that may indicate feeding malabsorption.

Interdisciplinary Interventions

The sick neonate or premature infant must have basic care needs met, such as thermoregulation, prevention of infection, providing caloric and nutritional needs, in addition to addressing existing pathology as discussed under the specific disorder. Meeting the needs of the family is also an integral component of care.

The birth of a sick or premature infant is a stressor for the family (see Chapter 8). Sources of parental stress include the setting and timing of first interaction with the infant; appearance, behavior, and pain responses of the infant; perceived morbidity of the infant; and preparation for the NICU and appearance of the infant (Shields-Poë & Pinelli, 1997; Wereszczak, Miles, & Holditch-Davis, 1997). Parents vividly remember positive and negative staff behaviors and view support from nurses as very helpful in coping with the birth and hospitalization of a high-risk infant (Miles, Carlson, & Funk, 1996). Support from nurses in establishing caring relationships with parents, treating parents as partners in the care of their infant, providing technically competent care to the infant and clear explanations to the parents, and giving parents an opportunity to see and touch their infant in the delivery room or prior to transport may reduce parental stress.

Community Care

In general, as immaturity increases and birth weight decreases, the likelihood of intellectual and neurologic deficits (e.g., cerebral palsy, hearing and vision defects, learning difficulties) increases (Behrman et al., 1996; Schraeder, Heverly, O'Brien, & Goodman, 1997). Long-term follow-up, surveillance for neurodevelopmental delays or problems, and provision of early intervention and special education resources are necessary.

Thermoregulatory Problems

Thermoregulation is a common problem for premature neonates, owing to their lack of subcutaneous and brown fat stores, thin skin, immature CNS, limited ability to assume a flexed posture, and increased surface area/body mass ratio (Thomas, 1994). The maintenance of a normal temperature is vital to the premature neonate because hypothermia leads to an increased metabolic rate and oxygen demand, apnea, respiratory distress, and cyanosis.

Term neonates respond more efficiently to hypothermia than preterm neonates. In response to hypothermia, the term neonate is able to increase muscle activity, initiate nonshivering or chemical thermogenesis, and utilize brown fat stores to generate heat. The preterm neonate is unable to increase muscle activity or to assume a flexed position due to poor motor tone and has limited brown fat stores. Additionally, premature neonates may be unable to initiate thermogenesis, owing to limited stores of fat and insufficient amounts of other chemicals such as glucose, liver enzymes, and hormones. In summary, limited methods to produce heat coupled with many mechanisms of heat loss make the premature neonate very susceptible to hypothermia.

Nonshivering thermogenesis involves the release of norepinephrine to mobilize brown fat to increase metabolic rate and generate heat (Thomas, 1994). The quantity of brown fat increases with increasing gestational age. In the term newborn, brown fat is located in the axillae, between the scapulae, in the mediastinum, around the liver, and down the spine (Fig. 14–6). Utilization of brown fat increases the metabolic rate significantly and is initiated when the newborn is in an environment below the neutral thermal range. A neutral thermal environment is one at which the neonate maintains a normal core temperature with minimal oxygen consumption and calorie expenditure (Thomas, 1994). Heat loss is generated through radiation, convection, conduction, and

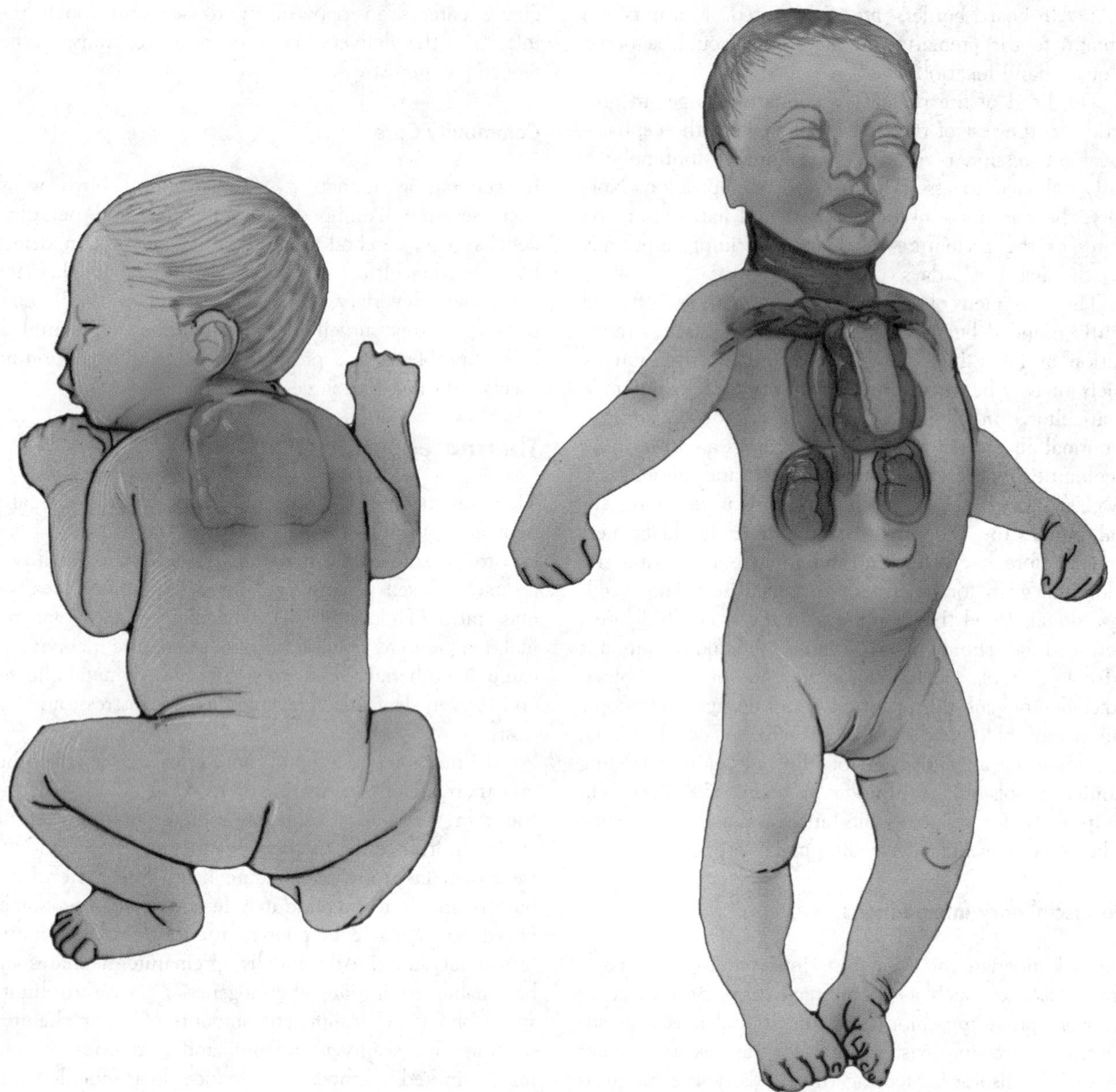

Figure 14–6
Location of brown fat in term neonates.

evaporation (Table 14–2). The nurse caring for premature neonates must understand the concepts of thermoregulation and mechanisms of heat loss to prevent hypothermia.

Assessment

Neonates who are hypothermic may appear pale with acrocyanosis or central cyanosis, mottling, and signs of respiratory distress. Consistently cold-stressed neonates exhibit poor weight gain, metabolic acidosis, and apnea and bradycardia.

Interdisciplinary Interventions

Preventing cold stress and promoting a neutral thermal environment and monitoring for hypothermia are cornerstones to caring for all neonates, especially premature

Table 14–2
Mechanisms of Heat Loss and Prevention Techniques

Heat Loss Mechanism	Example	Prevention Techniques
Convection: Heat loss occurring when heat is exchanged between two objects within the same environment	Loss of heat from the neonate's skin to the cooler, surrounding air. For example, cold drafts in the delivery room or nursery will lead to heat loss through convection. The premature neonate is especially vulnerable to this type of heat loss, because the amount of body surface exposed is increased owing to lack of a flexed posture from poor muscle tone.	Warm the delivery room or nursery. Avoid drafts. Prewarm the isolette. Transport the neonate in an isolette. Use plastic sleeves on the isolette portals. Swaddle the neonate with warmed blankets.
Conduction: Loss of heat through direct contact with an object that is cooler	Placing a neonate on a cold scale or next to cool blankets	Pad the scale with a warm blanket before weighing. Use warm blankets to dry the neonate.
Evaporation: Loss of heat through conversion of water to its gaseous state	A newly delivered neonate who is wet with amniotic fluid and a neonate receiving a bath. Extremely premature neonates are very vulnerable to evaporative heat loss due to thin and extremely permeable skin.	Dry the neonate quickly after delivery or bathing. Warm all solutions before applying to the neonate. Administer warmed oxygen.
Radiation: Loss of heat between two objects in the environment across a gradient that are not in direct contact with each other	Loss of neonate's body heat to the surrounding, cooler incubator walls	Avoid placing the bassinette/isolette near cold walls or windows. Use a double-walled isolette. Prewarm the isolette.

infants (Chart 14–6). If hypothermia occurs, intervening during apnea and bradycardic spells also becomes critical. Nursing interventions to decrease heat loss begin at delivery by warming the delivery room and quickly drying the neonate to prevent evaporative heat loss. Warming scales, stethoscopes, and blankets are other effective interventions to prevent heat loss. Finally, placing a cap on the head is an easy and effective manner to prevent heat loss in the premature neonate. Other devices that may be used in the NICU to promote a neutral thermal environment include radiant warmers, isolettes, heat shields, plastic wraps, and warming pads (Fig. 14–7).

The neonate's skin and core temperatures and the isolette or ambient temperature are closely monitored. All premature neonates under a radiant warmer or in an isolette must have a skin probe in place to continuously monitor skin temperature. The skin temperature is the first to fall in cold stress (Thomas, 1994). Skin probes must be in appropriate places on the neonate to obtain the most accurate readings. Areas over brown fat and bone, such as over the liver and the spine, are avoided. The lower left abdomen is the ideal place for a skin probe. The skin probe must be secured in place, because accidental dislodgment may lead to overheating. Troubleshooting thermoregulation problems includes monitoring the location of the probe and not allowing the neonate to lie on it, which may increase the temperature readings artificially. Also, ensuring that the probe is on and not accidentally removed is important to obtain accurate measurements. If the probe is dislodged, it may sense cooler room air, generate heat in response, and overheat the infant.

The neonate's core temperature is monitored by the axillary route every hour until stable and then every 2 to 3 hours.

caREminder: *Routine rectal temperatures are avoided because they may cause tissue damage and are stressful to the neonate.*

The isolette ambient temperature is compared with previous measurements of ambient temperature to detect temperature instability, which is an early sign of sepsis. As the neonate's skin temperature drops, the ambient temperature will increase accordingly. Any changes in ambient temperature should be investigated further.

caREminder: *Instruct others to avoid opening the isolette unnecessarily.*

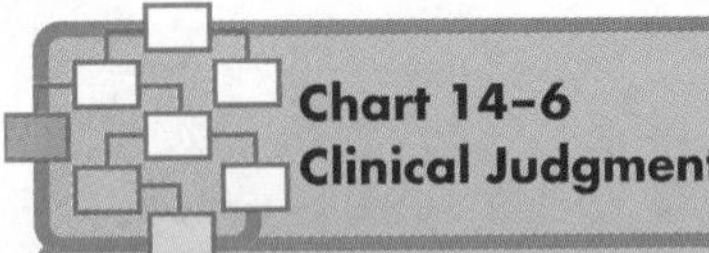

Chart 14–6
Clinical Judgment

Preterm Infant with Hypothermia

Yolanda is an infant, 32 weeks' gestation, just admitted to the NICU after a precipitous delivery in the Emergency Department. She was placed under the radiant warmer on admission. Vital signs: HR, 160; RR, 80, T, 96.4°F axillary; weight, 2330 g. Yolanda has nasal flaring with grunting; pulse oximeter readings are dropping into the 80's. She is pale with acrocyanosis, has a weak cry, is floppy, and shows minimal response to stimulation. Laboratory values: pH, 7.31; blood bicarbonate, 18 mEq/dL; serum glucose, 25 mg/dL.

Questions

1. What data from the assessment are indicative of a clinical problem?
2. What are pertinent nursing diagnoses that must be considered at this time?
3. Considering Yolanda's history, which nursing diagnosis must be addressed immediately and why?
4. What nursing actions must be implemented to prevent further deterioration in Yolanda's status?
5. What parameters must be monitored carefully until Yolanda is normothermic, and routinely after that?

Answers

1. Low temperature, symptoms of respiratory distress (grunting, nasal flaring, tachypnea), oxygen saturation in the 80's, pale, floppiness with minimal response to the environment. Acrocyanosis would be normal in the first hours after birth; central cyanosis would indicate a problem. An infant of 32 weeks' gestation would be hypotonic but demonstrate limb recoil with stimulation and would respond to the environment. Abnormal laboratory values: pH and bicarbonate levels reflect acidosis; serum glucose of 25 mg/dL indicates hypoglycemia.
2. Hypothermia
   Altered tissue perfusion: cardiopulmonary, cerebral, gastrointestinal, peripheral, renal
   Impaired gas exchange
   Risk for infection
   Risk for disorganized infant behavior
   Risk for altered infant/parent attachment
3. Hypothermia must be addressed immediately because it will create or exacerbate other clinical problems such as respiratory distress, acidosis, and hypoglycemia. Tachypnea is caused by the increased oxygen demand from the increased metabolic rate to keep warm. Hypothermia leads to peripheral vasoconstriction, resulting in decreased tissue perfusion and subsequent hypoxia and metabolic acidosis. These lead to pulmonary vasoconstriction, which results in increased pulmonary artery pressure and right-to-left shunting of blood, worsening the hypoxia. Hypoxia may impair surfactant release, further worsening the respiratory distress and acidosis. Increased metabolism also consumes glucose, leading to hypoglycemia. Breakdown of glycogen to glucose while hypoxic generates extra lactic acid, worsening the acidosis.
4. Ensure that the temperature probe for the radiant warmer is positioned on a solid mass surface or the trunk or lower extremities, not air-filled cavities such as stomach or lungs. Position the probe on the surface of the infant that faces the heat source; the infant must not lie on the probe. Ensure that the warmer is on servocontrol (controlled by the infant's temperature, not manually). Position the warmer away from drafts and opening doors. Make sure that Yolanda is dry and on dry linen. If these are in place, Yolanda may require an additional heat source such as a heat lamp, warmed blankets, or artificial heat blankets. Prewarm equipment such as stethoscopes and scales.
5. Temperature 97.2° to 99.1°F axillary (36.2° to 37.3°C), cardiorespiratory status, arterial blood gases (pH, bicarbonate, oxygen), blood glucose.

Neonatal care can be clustered, with many tasks performed at the same time. This limits the amount of temperature fluctuations. Collaborating with other members of the health care team in timing of procedures and examinations serves to limit heat losses and provide extended sleep periods. Neonates who exhibit apnea and bradycardia require prompt interventions, as detailed in the section on apnea of prematurity.

Radiant Warmers. Radiant warmers provide heat quickly and efficiently and allow access to the neonate for stabilization and resuscitation measures. However, they allow for convective heat loss and an increased

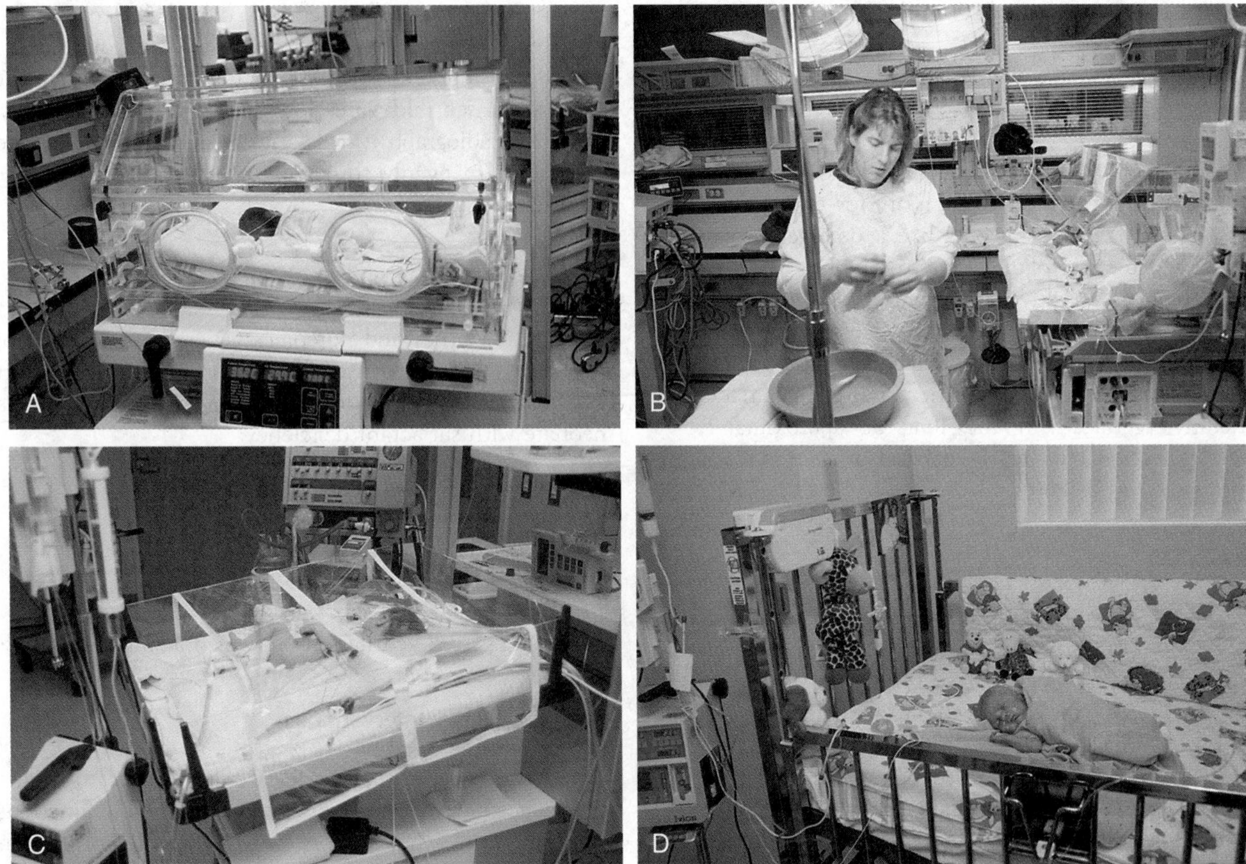

Figure 14–7
Various methods help neonates maintain thermoregulation: *A*, Isolette. *B*, Radiant warmer. *C*, Plastic wrap. *D*, Swaddling with blankets.

insensible water loss from the skin, especially in the extremely LBW neonate. Therefore, radiant warmers should be utilized for initial stabilization only and the neonate should be moved to an isolette as soon as possible.

Isolettes. An isolette provides minimal radiant and convective heat losses and allows for constant visual observation of the neonate. Portholes allow for minimal heat loss during nursing care and should be used at all times. Double-walled isolettes buffer radiant heat loss because the inside wall is warmed by the ambient air temperature of the isolette. Double-walled isolettes are often reserved for the neonate who weighs 1200 g or less or if the neonate demonstrates difficulty in maintaining a stable temperature.

Heat Shields. Heat shields are effective in decreasing convection and radiant heat loss. Made of Plexiglas or plastic, heat shields are an additional tool to assist with temperature instability. However, because these devices may also block the warming equipment from providing heat to the neonate they may be inappropriate for use in the cold-stressed neonate.

Plastic Wraps. Plastic wraps have been used to reduce evaporative heat losses. These devices are often reserved for the neonate with extreme LBW who may have excessive insensible losses from thin, gelatinous skin.

Warming Pads. Warming pads including heated water pads have been effective in decreasing heat loss and improving thermal stability. Some manufacturers have produced temporary warming pads that can be activated at the time of delivery or during transport of the neonate that produce heat for up to 6 hours. This warming device must be padded with a blanket to avoid thermal burns to the skin.

Surfactant Deficiency

Respiratory distress is common in premature neonates and may be due to such problems as sepsis, hypoglycemia, hypothermia, or lung immaturity. In utero, the placenta performs respiratory functions because the fetus' lungs are filled with fluid and do not participate in air exchange. At delivery, the lungs normally become air filled, are perfused by blood, and participate in oxygen and carbon dioxide exchange. To perform this function, the lungs must inflate properly.

Pathophysiology

The lungs of a premature neonate lack a phospholipid called surfactant, which is necessary for effective respiratory function. Surfactant acts like a detergent to reduce the surface tension of the lungs, promoting their expansion (Stevens, Wright, & Clements, 1989). Without surfactant, the lung collapses after every expiration and reinflates with great difficulty, requiring the neonate to generate intense pressures with every breath. Surfactant is generally produced in the lung at approximately 35 weeks' gestation but may be delayed by maternal complications such as diabetes.

Assessment

The diagnosis of surfactant deficiency is based on maternal history, neonatal physical examination, and laboratory and radiographic findings (Table 14–3). The typical maternal history includes preterm labor, fetal gestational age of less than 37 weeks, lecithin/sphingomyelin ratio less than 2:1, and absence of phosphatidylglycerol.

The neonate with surfactant deficiency displays signs of moderate to severe respiratory distress, including sternal, substernal, and intercostal retractions, grunting, and nasal flaring. Central cyanosis is common, and hypotension may be present if the neonate is severely distressed and acidotic.

Diagnostic Tests. Laboratory studies include a lung profile that may reveal an immature lecithin/sphingomyelin ratio. The lung profile may be done on the amniotic fluid at the time of rupture of the membranes, or a tracheal aspirate may be obtained from the neonate. Analysis of arterial or capillary blood gases may reveal respiratory acidosis from carbon dioxide retention and hypoxemia. Electrolyte levels may show dehydration, especially in the extremely premature neonate from the increased insensible water loss due to thin skin. Finally, the chest radiograph reveals a reticulogranular or "ground glass" pattern evenly throughout the lungs from massive atelectasis.

Nursing Diagnoses and Outcomes

Nursing diagnoses and outcomes generally applicable for neonates with a health challenge are presented in Chart 14–3. In addition, the following may be applicable for a neonate with surfactant deficiency:

- **Impaired gas exchange related to effects of poor lung compliance and atelectasis**
  Outcomes: The neonate will display blood gas levels within normal limits.
  The neonate will show no signs of adverse effects from assisted ventilation or oxygen administration.

Interdisciplinary Interventions

Care of the neonate in respiratory distress due to surfactant deficiency involves monitoring of all body functions and supporting the neonate with supplemental oxygen and assisted ventilation if needed. However, the mainstay of treatment for surfactant deficiency is the administration of exogenous surfactant, either artificial (Exosurf) or bovine-extracted (Survanta). Both types require intratracheal administration. They coat the lungs to improve ventilation and oxygenation and protein leakage that commonly accompanies surfactant deficiency (Jobe, Ikegami, & Jacobs, 1983). Protein leakage occurs in damaged lungs, causing pulmonary edema. Overall, the most commonly reported response after administration of sur-

Table 14–3
Indicators of Surfactant Deficiency

Maternal History/Factors	Physical Examination of Newborn	Lab/Radiology Findings
Premature labor Lack of treatment with corticosteroids Lecithin/sphingomyelin ratio <2:1 on amniotic fluid Absent phosphatidylglycerol	Cyanosis Labored breathing Retractions Tachypnea Grunting Nasal flaring Poor tissue perfusion Skin mottling Hypotension	Lecithin/sphingomyelin ratio <2:1 on tracheal aspirate Respiratory/metabolic acidosis Reticulogranular pattern on chest radiograph Massive atelectasis on air bronchogram

factant is rapidly improved oxygenation and decreased need for respiratory support.

The use of exogenous surfactant for surfactant deficiency has changed the outcomes for neonates with surfactant deficiency. However, the incidence of chronic lung disease, a morbidity associated with surfactant deficiency, has not changed over many years.

Surfactant administration may have adverse effects on the neonate. Surfactant instillation into the trachea may cause acute reduction in oxygenation by blocking large and small airways. Careful ventilation is needed to minimize this effect. Other side effects are pneumothorax and pulmonary hemorrhage. Because of the rapid changes in lung compliance, pneumothorax may occur if ventilation requirements are not monitored carefully and decreased according to the neonate's response. When surfactant is administered, there may be a sudden increase in the lung compliance. Subsequently, the ventilator pressures must be decreased to avoid overdistention of the lungs and pneumothorax. Pulmonary hemorrhage occurs as a result of pulmonary edema and the fragile capillary bed of the premature lung.

The nurse, in collaboration with respiratory therapists and the medical team, must be vigilant in monitoring chest wall expansion, improved breath sounds, and a decreased need for oxygen. The nurse can decrease the amount of supplemental oxygen according to the neonate's overall skin color and the pulse oximeter readings. The nurse has an important role in monitoring the neonate before, during, and after administration of surfactant (Chart 14–7).

Chart 14–7
Nursing Interventions

A Neonate Receiving Surfactant Administration

Before Surfactant Administration

- Obtain and record baseline vital signs.
- Note ventilator settings, oxygen settings, pulse oximeter readings, and transcutaneous monitor readings.

During Surfactant Administration

- Note amount instilled and neonate's response.
- Monitor vital signs continuously.
- Watch for cyanosis and improved chest wall movement.
- Increase oxygen and ventilation as needed.

After Surfactant Administration

- Avoid suctioning for at least 4 hours if possible.
- Monitor vital signs frequently.
- Carefully observe for signs of improvement, including increased oxygenation, decreased need for respiratory support, and improved chest movement.
- Wean ventilator settings as needed.

Patent Ductus Arteriosus

The ductus arteriosus is a fetal shunt located between the pulmonary artery and the aorta. In fetal circulation, the ductus arteriosus allows oxygenated blood from the placenta to flow directly to the systemic circulation, bypassing the lungs. After birth, the ductus arteriosus functionally closes, owing to the increased oxygen content of the blood. PDA is a persistence of that fetal shunt after delivery and is common in preterm newborns because of decreased pulmonary vascular resistance and decreased responsiveness of the PDA to close in the presence of high oxygen levels (Park, 1988). The presence of a PDA leads to pulmonary overcirculation and pulmonary edema. Diagnosis includes the presence of congestive heart failure, unstable blood pressures and widened pulse pressures, metabolic acidosis, and increasing oxygen support. PDA is diagnosed from a bedside echocardiogram, a chest radiograph, and the presence of clinical symptoms (see Chapter 15).

Initially, treatment of PDA in the neonatal period includes fluid restriction, diuretics, and ventilator support. If the PDA remains problematic and the neonate symptomatic, indomethacin is administered intravenously. Indomethacin is a prostaglandin inhibitor that promotes ductal closure. This drug is most effective in preterm neonates if given before age 4 weeks. Side effects include elevated blood urea nitrogen and creatinine, decreased urine output, and decreased platelets and platelet function (Park, 1988). These values are evaluated before administration of each dose.

If the administration of indomethacin is ineffective, the premature neonate may need to have the PDA surgically corrected. This procedure maintains a mortality rate of approximately 2%. Its potential complications include phrenic nerve paralysis, lung contusions, sepsis, and ligation of the pulmonary artery (Park, 1988). Mortality and morbidity is highest in the very sick, unstable neonate. Details of surgery and complications are discussed in Chapter 15.

Neonatal Sepsis

Sepsis is a common complication in premature neonates owing to their inability to adequately respond to sepsis, their exposure to bacteria from invasive devices, their thin skin, and their poor nutritional state. Additionally, infection may result from direct contact with the vaginal canal during birth, transplacentally before birth, and from prolonged rupture of membranes. Maternal or fetal sepsis may be a cause of premature delivery, and this often complicates the neonate's hospital course, resulting in increased mortality (Gerdes, 1991). The premature neonate's immune system responds poorly to infection because the inflammatory response is weakened by limited neutrophil storage and altered neutrophil function (McCourt, 1994).

Assessment

Signs of sepsis in premature neonates are often vague, subtle, and nonspecific, making diagnosis difficult. Apnea, lethargy, temperature instability, poor feeding, respiratory distress, increasing oxygen requirements, and hyperbilirubinemia are all signs of sepsis in the neonate. Cardinal signs of sepsis include poor feeding, increased apneic spells, jaundice, temperature instability, increased oxygen requirement, and lethargy (see Chapter 24 for further discussion of sepsis).

Diagnostic Tests. When infection is a potential problem, the physician will initiate a specific (septic) work-up that commonly includes the following:

- Complete blood cell count showing an elevated or decreased white blood cell count, an increased number of immature white cells, and decreased platelets
- Blood cultures testing positive for specific organisms
- Tracheal aspirate for culture
- Urine culture
- Chest radiograph
- Lumbar puncture, to determine if meningitis is present

Additional tests may be done on the cerebrospinal fluid (CSF) to determine the presence of infection and include glucose levels, white blood cell count, and protein level.

Interdisciplinary Interventions

Sepsis can kill a neonate within hours because of the infant's inability to wall off and localize infections as older people with better developed immune responses can. The nurse must constantly be vigilant to any signs of sepsis and must articulate these to the other members of the health care team. Early identification and treatment of infection can prevent serious complications.

Because of the neonate's decreased ability to respond to infection, broad-spectrum antibiotics are initiated immediately; waiting for any of the laboratory test results would delay treatment. The nurse's role is to assist with the diagnostic work-up, including obtaining many of the blood samples. Additionally, the nurse's ongoing assessment of the neonate is documented and communicated with the team. Sepsis in the neonate can escalate quickly, necessitating vigorous interventions such as intubation, volume resuscitation, initiation of dopamine and dobutamine drips, and other resuscitative efforts. Each of these interventions has specific indications. For example, intubation is required when the neonate is apneic or in respiratory failure. Volume resuscitation, or the administration of normal saline or albumin, is performed to restore intravascular volume that may be depleted owing to capillary leak of fluid into the subcutaneous tissue. Finally, dopamine and dobutamine are medications that are used to maintain blood pressure and improve cardiac contractility.

caREminder: *Every member of the family and health care team has a role in the prevention of infection. Hand washing is the number one way to prevent the transmission of nosocomial infections. Hand washing must be performed by all individuals before and after handling of any neonate.*

Additionally, sterile technique must be used for all invasive procedures such as suctioning the endotracheal tube and initiating intravenous lines. Central lines must also be handled with sterile technique because these lines are an easy portal of entry for sepsis.

Intraventricular Hemorrhage

Intraventricular hemorrhage, bleeding within the ventricles in the brain, is almost exclusively a problem related to prematurity, specifically in infants of less than 32 weeks' gestation.

The incidence of IVH varies from 25% to 40% in premature neonates (Hill & Volpe, 1994). Neonates weighing less than 1000 g are at highest risk. The incidence is likely to escalate as the survival rate of extremely premature neonates continues to improve.

The causes are not completely understood but may involve the dynamic interaction between the hemodynamic status of the neonate and the fragility of the capillary bed. Clearly, preterm neonates with respiratory distress are at an increased risk for IVH.

Pathophysiology

Normally, the blood vessels of the brain are protected from fluctuations in blood flow through autoregulation. Autoregulation allows the arterioles to constrict and dilate despite fluctuations in systemic pressure to ensure constant blood flow to the brain. The premature neonate is unable to autoregulate due to immaturity of the CNS, resulting in the brain receiving variable blood flow. This directly affects the flow to the germinal matrix that houses thin-walled blood vessels that are easily ruptured. The germinal matrix is a temporary structure in the brain of premature neonates that is highly vascularized. The purpose of the germinal matrix is to produce precursor cells that will later develop into neurons and glial cells for eventual migration into the cerebral cortex.

Positive-pressure ventilation, hypoxia, hypotension, and rapid volume expansion can contribute to IVH (Volpe, 1989). A very sick premature neonate may have hypotension from a persistent PDA and require assisted ventilation, which increases the risk for the development of an IVH. An IVH is due to rupture of the blood vessels in the subependymal space and bleeding into the lateral ventricle. If the hemorrhage is large, a blood clot may form within the ventricle or blood may spread throughout the ventricular system and into brain tissue. IVH is categorized as grades I through IV (Chart 14–8), based on results of cranial ultrasonography.

Prognosis. Prognosis for a neonate with IVH depends on the severity of the hemorrhage and presence of associated problems, such as asphyxia and sepsis. Overall mortality for neonates with IVH is 25% to 50% (Volpe, 1989). Neonates with grade I or II hemorrhages generally have a low incidence of long-term neurologic sequelae (Van De Bor et al., 1993). Neonates with more severe hemorrhages have a mortality of 50% to 60% that increases if ventricular dilatation and posthemorrhagic hydrocephalus develops. The chance for long-term deficits and neurologic sequelae in these neonates is 40% to 90% (Van De Bor et al., 1993).

Common complications of IVH are ventricular dilatation, posthemorrhagic hydrocephalus, and periventricular leukomalacia. Ventricular dilatation occurs in approximately 50% of neonates with IVH and is due to a clot that blocks the flow of CSF. Posthemorrhagic hydrocephalus results from progressive ventricular dilation and occurs in 15% of all IVHs. Moderate to severe IVH has the highest incidence of developing hydrocephalus. Signs and symptoms of hydrocephalus include increasing head circumference, apnea and bradycardia spells, and increasing need for respiratory support.

Periventricular leukomalacia is an ischemic injury to the white matter in the brain. This is commonly noted in neonates who die of IVH (Takashima, Mito, & Houdou, 1989). The true incidence of periventricular leukomalacia is unknown because it cannot be accurately detected with bedside cranial ultrasound testing.

Chart 14–8

Classification of Intraventricular Hemorrhage

Grade I: Germinal matrix hemorrhage only
Grade II: Germinal matrix hemorrhage with extension into the ventricles
Grade III: Germinal matrix hemorrhage with dilated ventricles
Grade IV: Intraventricular hemorrhage with extension into brain tissue

Assessment

Common symptoms of IVH include a sudden decrease in hematocrit, severe and sudden unexplained deterioration of vital signs, bulging fontanelles, changes in activity level, and sudden lethargy (Dietch, 1993). The diagnosis is confirmed by cranial ultrasonography. More than 90% of neonates with IVH bleed within the first 4 days of life, and 50% bleed within 24 hours of birth (Hill & Volpe, 1994).

Nursing Diagnoses and Outcomes

Nursing diagnoses and outcomes generally applicable for neonates with a health challenge are presented in Chart 14–3. In addition, the following may be applicable for a neonate with IVH:

- **Altered cerebral tissue perfusion related to effects of blood within the ventricle**
  Outcome: The neonate will maintain cerebral perfusion pressure adequate to provide oxygen and nutrients to the brain.

Interdisciplinary Interventions

Prevention of IVH is the most important goal, and nurses are instrumental in this (Chart 14–9). Nursing procedures such as endotracheal tube suctioning and rapid infusions of fluid can cause IVH. Acute management of IVH includes support of all vital functions, including increasing ventilation pressures and supplemental oxygen to maintain normal ventilation and oxygenation, providing packed red blood cells to correct anemia due to bleeding, and infusing volume replacement to maintain tissue perfusion. During the acute event of an IVH, the nurse should be monitoring all vital signs carefully and frequently, as often as every 15 minutes, because the neonate's condition may be extremely unstable.

Apnea of Prematurity

Apnea is defined as a cessation of respiratory air flow for 20 seconds or longer in the preterm neonate and 15 seconds or longer in the term neonate (see Chapter 16). *Apnea of prematurity* refers to apnea in neonates of less than 37 weeks' gestation. As the premature neonate develops and matures, the incidence of apnea decreases. All neonates are periodic (irregular) breathers. However, the

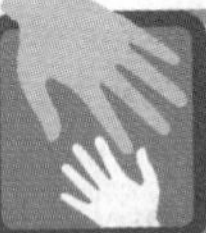

Chart 14–9
Nursing Interventions

Reducing the Risk of Intraventricular Hemorrhage

- Minimize stressors: Reduce environmental noise, light, and noxious stimuli; support infant in a flexed, tucked position; avoid unnecessary procedures.
- Monitor infant for stress cues, and alter interventions based on these.
- Promote self-comforting behaviors in infant.
- Avoid tight Bili masks.
- Maintain the head in midline position.
- Avoid overhydration.
- Perform vigilant monitoring of hemodynamic and respiratory status to avoid rapid changes in these vital functions that may lead to IVH.

cessation of breathing for longer than 20 seconds is abnormal and requires intervention.

Apnea in the neonate can result from many disorders, such as sepsis, seizures, metabolic disturbances, gastroesophageal reflux, and intrauterine drug exposure (Chasnoff, Hunt, & Kletter, 1989; Walsh, Farrel, & Keeman, 1978).

Pathophysiology

Apnea of prematurity is a result of the immaturity of the CNS, which fails to initiate breathing. The medulla oblongata, the most inferior part of the brain stem, controls respiratory drive. Owing to prematurity, the patterned firing of the neurons in this section of the brain is altered. Additionally, premature neonates have a diminished response to hypoxemia and hypercarbia, leading to apnea. Often after the neonate becomes apneic, bradycardia ensues.

Assessment

Apnea occurring in premature neonates with no underlying disease such as sepsis, anemia, or gastroesophageal reflux is generally categorized as apnea of prematurity. The physical examination reveals a vigorous premature neonate with no signs of sepsis or metabolic disturbances. It is important to investigate all potential causes of apnea to initiate the appropriate treatment.

One diagnostic study specific to determining the cause of apnea is the pneumocardiogram. This study continuously measures heart rate, respiratory rate, and pulse oximetry values during a specified time period. This information is plotted on a graph and can clearly demonstrate the occurrence of apneic spells and subsequent bradycardia and desaturation. Results from this study are used to determine the type of apnea and to rule out any possible treatable cause.

Nursing Diagnoses and Outcomes

Nursing diagnoses and outcomes generally applicable for neonates with a health challenge are presented in Chart 14–3. In addition, the following may be applicable for a neonate with apnea of prematurity:

▶ **Ineffective breathing pattern related to an immature CNS**

Outcomes: The infant will have apnea and bradycardia spells recognized immediately and stimulation initiated.

The infant will experience no adverse sequelae resulting from ineffective breathing pattern.

Interdisciplinary Interventions

Nursing interventions include close monitoring for apnea and subsequent bradycardia and appropriate documentation. During a spell, the neonate can be lightly stimulated by rubbing his or her back or foot to initiate breathing. If this is not effective, more vigorous stimulation should be provided, progressing to bag-and-mask ventilation as necessary (Fig. 14–8).

Documentation is extremely important and should include the following:

- Duration of apneic episode
- Lowest heart rate during the episode
- Time of last feeding, to determine whether reflux is associated with the apnea spell (If the spell is due to reflux, often it occurs shortly after a feeding.)
- Interventions performed

Nurses may be instrumental in minimizing the number of apneic episodes by positioning the neonate in the prone position. The prone position improves oxygenation and decreases the work of breathing. Additionally, the prone position is associated with fewer apnea spells (Heimler, Langlois, Hodel, Nelin, & Sasidharan, 1992).

The medical team initiates pharmacotherapy if the spells are severe or frequent. Severe or frequent spells cause the body to shunt blood from nonvital organs such as the bowel to vital organs such as the heart and brain. Treatment must be initiated to control the spells and avoid ischemic damage to the bowel and prevent the development of NEC.

Treatment includes respiratory stimulants such as the methylxanthines (aminophylline, theophylline, and caffeine) and, when needed, doxapram to decrease the occurrence of apnea. These drugs act by stimulating the CNS and increasing alveolar ventilation (Gerhardt &

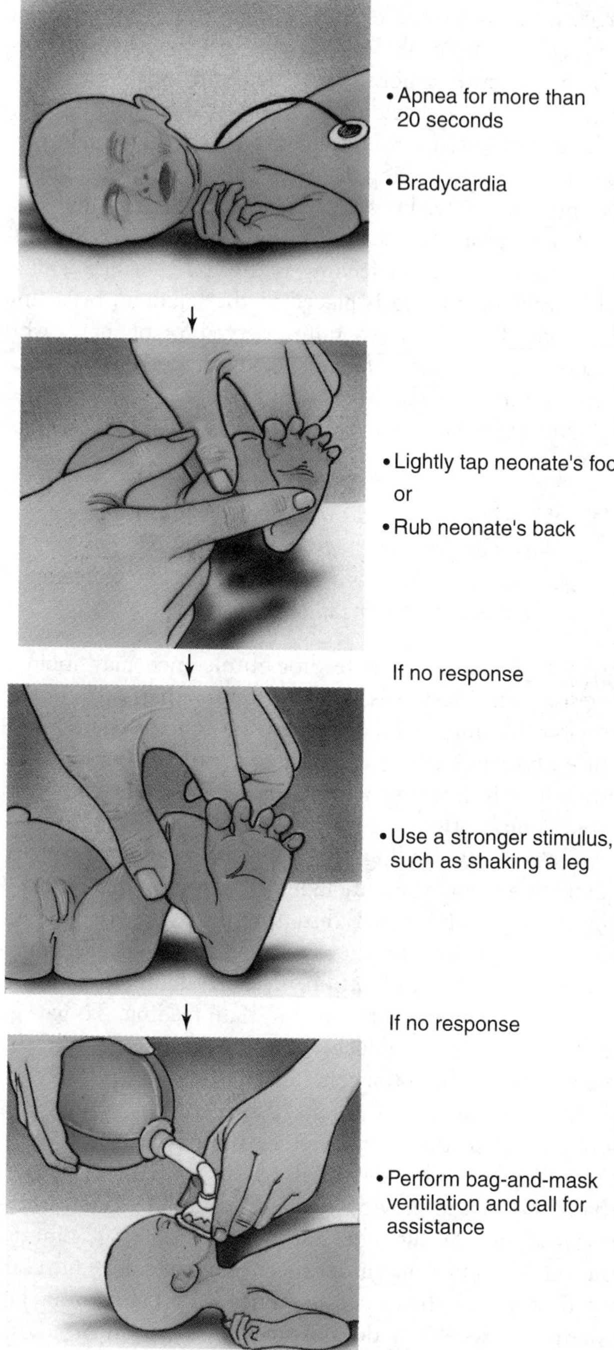
Nursing Interventions in Apnea
• Apnea for more than 20 seconds
• Bradycardia
• Lightly tap neonate's foot
or
• Rub neonate's back
If no response
• Use a stronger stimulus, such as shaking a leg
If no response
• Perform bag-and-mask ventilation and call for assistance

Figure 14–8
Nursing interventions progressively increase in invasiveness for apnea of prematurity.

McCarthy, 1983). Common side effects of caffeine and theophylline are tachycardia and irritability. Additionally, oral medications may be irritating to the gut and lead to feeding intolerance. These medications should not be given if the heart rate is more than 180 beats per minute. If medications are not successful, continuous positive airway pressure may be initiated through an endotracheal tube or nasal device to help decrease the work of breathing and improve lung compliance.

Most neonates outgrow apnea of prematurity and can be successfully weaned from medications and continuous positive airway pressure. However, some symptomatic neonates, those with cyanotic color changes and bradycardia, require medications at discharge and home apnea monitoring. The nurse's role is critical in teaching parents how to correctly administer medications and monitor for side effects. The nurse also provides teaching related to the apnea monitor and newborn cardiopulmonary resuscitation (see TIP 16–4).

Community Care

Neonates discharged with home apnea monitors and medications to treat apnea need close follow-up. There are follow-up visits provided in the home by nurses and respiratory therapists to ensure that the family is comfortable with the home apnea monitor and techniques for handling emergencies. Ongoing reinforcement of teaching is done at this time.

Typically, the neonate is seen in the clinic 1 to 2 weeks after discharge, depending on his or her stability. At this first clinic visit, the physician reviews with the primary caretaker the number and severity of apneic spells and interventions required, if any. Adjustments are made to the home apnea monitor alarms as needed, and the medications are reviewed for appropriate dosing. Weaning of medications is done according to the neonate's progress and number of apnea spells.

Feeding and Nutrition Problems

Premature neonates have immature gastrointestinal systems and require additional specialized support to obtain nutrition and maintain growth. Effective suck-swallow reflexes are not present until 33 to 34 weeks' gestation. Suck reflexes are present before this age. However, sucking and swallowing does not become coordinated until this time. Therefore, providing enteral nutrition to the premature newborn is a challenge.

Assessment

The premature neonate requires calories for growth and the repair of injured tissue. The premature newborn should grow along the natural progression of intrauterine growth had the pregnancy carried to term. To determine if adequate growth is occurring, the nurse plots the weight, length, and head circumference of the neonate on the appropriate intrauterine growth curve. Neonates falling below the curve are not growing appropriately, and treatment must be initiated.

Nursing Diagnoses and Outcomes

Nursing diagnoses and outcomes generally applicable for neonates with a health challenge are presented in Chart 14–3. In addition, the following may be applicable for a neonate with feeding and nutrition problems:

- **Altered nutrition: less than body requirements, related to inability to take enteral feedings and acute illness**
  Outcome: The neonate will have caloric and nutritional needs met via enteral or parenteral routes.
- **Ineffective breast-feeding related to inability or decreased ability to breast-feed and acute illness**
  Outcomes: The neonate will demonstrate normal growth as measured on the intrauterine growth curve. The neonate will gain weight at a rate of 15 to 30 g/day.

Interdisciplinary Interventions

Premature neonates require a high caloric intake for growth, tissue repair, and laying down of subcutaneous fat. Parenteral nutrition is used initially until the neonate has become stable and ready to handle enteral feeding. Parenteral nutrition includes the administration of total parental nutrition (TPN) and lipids through a peripheral or central venous catheter. Common central lines include peripherally inserted lines that are threaded to the entry of the right atrium or the inferior vena cava. A Broviac catheter may also be placed into the upper chest with the tip located at the entry of the heart. Weaning from TPN is begun slowly as enteral feedings are introduced.

Initially, enteral feedings are offered slowly and are termed *stimulation* or *"stim" feeds* because they are used to prime the gut for absorption. Premature neonates are fed slowly and gradually, taking up to 3 weeks to achieve complete enteral feeds (Neu, Valentine, & Meetze, 1990). This is due to the common initial problems premature newborns experience and the instability of other body systems that make enteral feeding undesirable.

caREminder: *Breast milk is the enteral feeding of choice owing to the presence of easily digested proteins, antibodies and immunoglobulins, and high protein content (Lawrence, 1994).*

Breast milk from the premature newborn's mother has both a higher protein and fat content than breast milk from a term infant's mother. If breast milk is unavailable, specially designed premature formulas are utilized because they contain additional minerals, different types of fat, and protein to support the growth of premature neonates. Initially, formulas are introduced at half strength and slowly increased in both volume and strength as the neonate demonstrates tolerance.

Because of their inability to suck and swallow efficiently, premature neonates are fed through intermittent or continuous gavage feedings. Intermittent bolus gavage feedings are more physiologic and may improve production of the enteric hormones required for successful feeding (Romero & Kleinman, 1993). Continuous gavage feedings are often better tolerated by the extremely premature neonates owing to their small gastric volumes. During gavage feedings the infant should be offered a pacifier to promote the association of sucking with feeding. Another route of feeding is the use of a nasojejunal tube in which the tip is placed in the jejunum, bypassing the stomach. This is generally reserved for neonates who do not tolerate gastric feedings and is used only for continuous drip feedings.

Nutrition is one of the most important assessment areas for nurses caring for premature neonates.

caREminder: *Often, the quality of feeding tolerance and behavior are the first clues to other problems. For example, one of the first signs of an infection in a premature neonate may be feeding intolerance.*

Signs and symptoms of feeding intolerance may include emesis, gastric residuals that are greater than 30% of the previous feeding, or bilious emesis or aspirates. The astute nurse observes these subtle changes and collaborates with other health care team members to intervene early and avoid complications.

Before any feeding the nurse must perform an abdominal examination, including measuring the girth. If bowel loops, abdominal distention, or decreased bowel sounds are present, the nurse notifies the medical team to determine a course of action. If the abdominal examination is normal, the nurse may initiate feeding. To gavage feed, the nurse introduces a feeding tube through the mouth into the stomach. Then the nurse aspirates slightly to measure a residual, that is, the amount of formula left in the stomach since the previous feeding. If the residual is not abnormal (green, bilious, or greater than 30% of the previous feeding), the nurse administers the feeding. During tube insertion and feeding administration, the nurse monitors the neonate's color and ability to tolerate the process. Apnea and bradycardia are potential side effects during tube insertion, and cyanosis may occur during the feeding. If these complications occur, the nurse should immediately discontinue the feeding, clear the airway if needed, and administer supplemental oxygen.

Necrotizing Enterocolitis

Necrotizing enterocolitis is an acquired disease characterized by necrosis of the mucosal and submucosal layers of the gastrointestinal tract. It commonly occurs in premature neonates weighing less than 1500 g and accounts for 3% to 15% of all admissions to NICUs (Kliegman, 1990). In the United States, NEC develops in 2000 to 4000 neonates each year (Rushton, 1990a). The overall mortality is 4% to 40% depending on the severity of the disease and associated problems (Kliegman, 1990).

Pathophysiology

Prematurity and LBW are highly associated with the development of NEC, although there are reports of it developing in term neonates (Wiswell, Robertson, & Jones, 1986). The premature neonate around 30 to 32 weeks' gestation is the most commonly affected (Rushton, 1990a). The causes of NEC are not completely understood. It appears to be initiated when the body shunts blood away from vital organs (such as the bowel) during hypoxemia. This leads to decreased blood flow to the bowel, causing bowel wall ischemia. Then bacteria colonize in the bowel and form a substrate (formula) that allows bacterial invasion of the bowel wall.

Timing and method of feeding premature neonates and the incidence of NEC continue to be controversial. Some authorities state that premature neonates should not be enterally fed at all until complete stability of body functions has been established (Goldman, 1980). Others state that avoiding enteral feedings until the neonate is stable leads to long-term TPN, placing the neonate at risk for poor nutrition, neonatal rickets, and chronic lung disease (Ostertag, LaGamma, Reisen, & Ferrentino, 1986). Additionally, enteral feedings appear to assist with maturation and growth of the intestine in the premature neonate.

Assessment

Necrotizing enterocolitis produces gastrointestinal and systemic signs and symptoms that must be immediately reported to the medical team and include abdominal distention, visible bowel loops, and a shiny, possibly discolored abdomen. Additionally, bilious or large feeding residuals, grossly bloody or occult positive stools, lethargy, decreased bowel sounds, and sepsis-like symptoms occur with NEC. Sepsis-like symptoms are further described as temperature instability, poor perfusion, metabolic acidosis, and hypotension.

Radiography of the abdomen reveals dilated bowel loops, ileus, or the classic sign of NEC—pneumatosis intestinalis, which is air in the bowel wall. Perforation may ensue with late NEC, requiring immediate surgery.

Nursing Diagnoses and Outcomes

Nursing diagnoses and outcomes generally applicable for neonates with a health challenge are presented in Chart 14–3. In addition, the following may be applicable for a neonate with NEC:

- **Altered gastrointestinal tissue perfusion, related to effects of hypoxic insult**
  Outcome: The neonate will demonstrate adequate circulation to intestines, as evidenced by tolerance to feedings or no signs of NEC.

Interdisciplinary Interventions

Nursing interventions revolve around immediate recognition of early signs of NEC, including increasing gastric residuals and abdominal distention. An abdominal examination includes the inspection of the abdomen for the presence of loops or distention, auscultating for bowels sounds, palpating for distention, and presence or absence of blood in the stools. Additionally, the nurse must evaluate gastric residuals for amount and color. If the residuals are greater than 30% of the previous feeding or bilious, the nurse holds the feeding and notifies the medical team.

Once NEC is diagnosed, the nurse assesses the condition of the neonate and is alert to signs of a worsening condition, including unstable vital signs, increasing blueness of the abdomen, increasing abdominal girth, hypotension, and metabolic acidosis. Restarting of enteral feeds may not begin until 7 to 10 days after the initial event and then is done with great caution.

Surgical intervention is initiated if bowel perforation occurs. NEC is a dynamic disease in which segments of bowel wall worsen while others recover. The timing of surgery will dictate what is seen when the abdomen is entered. The goal is to remove the necrotic areas of the bowel and save as much of the bowel as possible. One complication of surgery for NEC is short-bowel syndrome, in which a large portion of the gut is removed owing to necrosis and the newborn is left with minimal amounts of intestine for absorption. These neonates have long-term feeding and nutrition difficulties and may be frequently hospitalized throughout infancy and childhood.

Retinopathy of Prematurity

Retinopathy of prematurity is a common disorder in extremely premature neonates who survive. It is a pathologic fibrous process that results from injury to the developing premature retinal vasculature. ROP occurs in premature neonates; neonates born at 38 weeks' gestation or later are unlikely to develop ROP. The incidence ranges from 16% to 56% in neonates weighing less than 1500 g or less than 30 weeks' gestation (Greven & Tasman, 1990). Incidence is 90% in neonates weighing less than 750 g, 78% in those weighing 750 to 999 g, and 47% in those weighing 1000 to 1250 g (Phelps, 1992). More information on ROP is presented in Chapter 28.

Birth Injuries

Traumatic injury can occur to the neonate during the perinatal period. It is estimated that birth injury occurs in 2% to 7% of every 1000 live births (Mimouni, Midovnik, Rosenn, Khoury, & Siddiqi, 1992). Perinatal events and conditions associated with birth injuries include the following (Levine et al., 1984):

- Use of forceps
- Shoulder dystocia
- LGA
- Second stage of labor exceeding 60 minutes

Birth injuries such as lacerations and bruising may also occur during cesarean sections or during resuscitation.

Injuries that occur intrapartally are often related to an abnormal fetal presentation, such as breech or abnormal fetal position leading to compression fractures. Additionally, oligohydramnios (decreased amniotic fluid) may be associated with epidermal shearing of the skin due to excessive rubbing against the uterine wall without the amniotic fluid as a cushion. The risk of nerve injury is increased with breech positions, prolonged or precipitate labor, prematurity, multiple gestation, and shoulder dystocia (Levine et al., 1984).

Common birth injuries are soft tissue injury, extracranial hemorrhage, fracture, and peripheral nerve injury. Soft tissue injuries include bruising, abrasions, and petechiae over the presenting part. Edema may also be present. Because each of these injuries requires different care, they are covered in detail after a general discussion of assessment and care of neonates with birth injuries.

Assessment

A complete and thorough physical examination is imperative to quickly identify birth traumas. Any history of a difficult or prolonged labor, LGA status, or birth to a diabetic mother is noted. Birth injury may cause reduced range of motion in the extremities. The skull may have edema, petechiae, or soft tissue swelling. Skin tears and bruising suggest soft tissue injuries. Radiographs reveal any bone fractures.

Nursing Diagnoses and Outcomes

In addition to the nursing diagnoses listed in Chart 14–3, the following may be applicable to the neonate with a birth injury:

- **Pain related to fracture, skin breakdown, or edema**
  Outcome: The neonate will show no signs of pain such as increased crying, heart rate, and respiratory rate or poor feeding.
- **Risk for injury related to improper positioning of paralyzed extremity**
  Outcome: The neonate will have affected extremity positioned properly and will display normal joint range of motion.
- **Impaired skin integrity related to disruption of skin surface from trauma**
  Outcome: The neonate will show adequate wound healing.

Interdisciplinary Interventions

The nurse is in an ideal position to identify birth injuries early and provide interventions. Most injuries need supportive care only, such as a fractured clavicle or caput succedaneum. Other injuries need splinting and immobilization. The nurse collaborates with other health care team members including the physician and occupational therapist to provide needed interventions.

Soft Tissue Injuries

These injuries are generally self-limiting and require only supportive care and reassurance to parents. Scleral hemorrhages may be noted soon after birth and are a result of increased pressure on the fetal head during delivery. Edema, petechiae, and bruising also result from increased pressure on the presenting part of the fetus. Petechiae must be followed closely because they also may be a symptom of a bleeding disorder or sepsis.

Extracranial Hemorrhage

Caput succedaneum and cephalhematoma are the most common birth injuries (Fig. 14–9). Caput succedaneum is edema that occurs over the presenting part in a vertex delivery. The edema is often marked with bruising, petechiae, and broken skin. The edema is above the periosteum and crosses the suture lines of the skull. This benign injury resolves within 2 to 3 days after birth.

Cephalhematoma is subperiosteal bleeding over the cranial bone. This type of hemorrhage commonly occurs after traumatic deliveries in which forceps were used, prolonged and difficult labors, and primiparous births.

The descent through the birth canal can be stressful to the fetus. For successful vaginal delivery to occur, the fetal skull bones override one another to accommodate the small space of the pelvic inlet and vaginal tract. As a result, molding of the head may be seen. Additionally, the delivery of the fetal head may be facilitated by the obstetrician by applying forceps or vacuum extraction. Forceps are metal tongs applied to the sides of the fetal head to assist with its delivery. Vacuum extraction is an

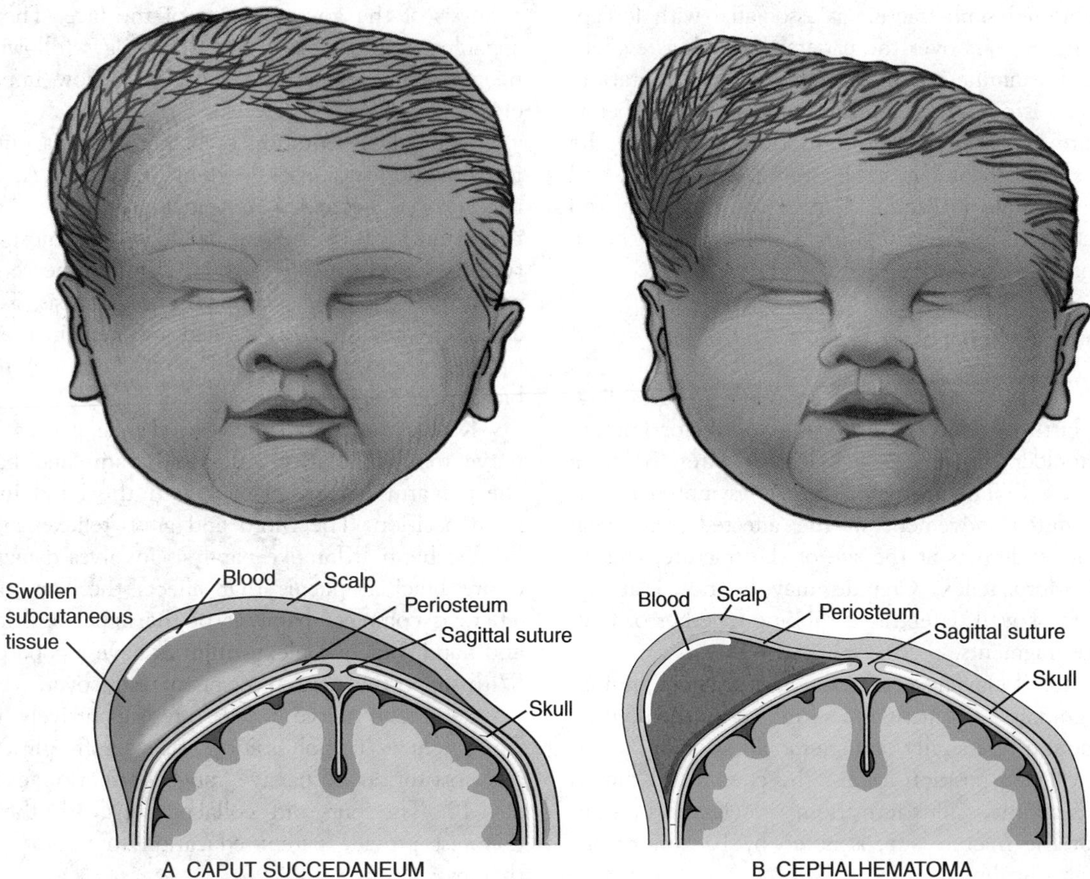

Figure 14–9
Caput succedaneum *(A)* and cephalhematoma *(B)* are common birth injuries.

application of a suction device to the fetal presenting part to assist delivery. Both forceps and vacuum extraction devices may potentially cause trauma to the fetal head, leading to edema and bleeding.

The nurse assesses for skull and scalp abnormalities, the location of edema, petechiae, and bruising. Edema that crosses the suture line suggests caput succedaneum; edema that does not cross these lines indicates a cephalhematoma. Skull indentation is significant, possibly indicating an underlying fracture, and requires further investigation such as a radiograph. Signs of increased intracranial pressure may occur, including a full or tense anterior fontanelle, irritability, poor feeding, and apnea.

Compared with a caput succedaneum, a cephalhematoma does not cross suture lines, has little or no ecchymosis, and takes longer to resolve—up to 2 months (Brann & Schwartz, 1987). Also, a cephalhematoma can continue to bleed, leading to anemia. Hyperbilirubinemia may also be a prolonged problem owing to lysis of the blood underneath the periosteum. If this is the case, close monitoring of the serum bilirubin level is necessary to provide prompt interventions for hyperbilirubinemia, including phototherapy. On occasion, an underlying skull fracture is present.

Skull Fracture

Skull fractures may result from fetal skull passage through the maternal ischial spines, sacral promontory, or symphysis pubis or from the use of forceps. Normally, the fetal skull tolerates the pressure generated by birth because of its flexibility from poorly ossified bone. However, application of forceps or a traumatic delivery may result in a skull fracture.

Skull fractures may be linear or depressed. Linear skull fractures are most often present over the frontal or parietal bones and rarely over the occipital bone. The neonate is often asymptomatic and with only a cephalhematoma noted on physical examination. Diagnosis is made by skull radiography. Healing takes place without intervention and only monitoring for increased intracranial pressure is needed. This includes measuring the head circumference, monitoring for a bulging or tense anterior fontanelle, and noting irritable or lethargic behavior.

A depressed skull fracture is associated with forceps delivery and appears over the parietal bone. It is evident on physical examination as a visible skull indentation. The neonate is often asymptomatic unless the dura below the fracture has been lacerated. In this severe case the neonate is very ill and unstable, may need surgery, and may suffer neurologic deficits. With good follow-up and early treatment the neonate with a skull fracture has a good prognosis.

Clavicular Fracture

Clavicular fractures are the most common fractures diagnosed as birth trauma. Clavicles are at risk for fracture during shoulder dystocia or with arms extended in a breech delivery. The neonate is often asymptomatic or exhibits limited movement in the affected arm, local swelling or tenderness at the site of the fracture, and an abnormal Moro reflex. Crepitus may be noted at the fracture site as well. Crepitus is rubbing together of fractured bone fragments.

A fractured clavicle is diagnosed by physical findings and radiography. Treatment is determined by the severity of the fracture. Generally, arm immobilization by a soft splint in a flexed position against the chest is all that is needed. Generally, callus formation, as detected by radiography at the fracture site, is noted by 10 days of age and indicates healing.

Nursing interventions include periodically checking for skin breakdown, removing the splint for bathing, and teaching the parent. Parent education includes the correct application of the splint, frequency of skin checks, and follow-up appointments.

Peripheral Nerve Injuries

Peripheral nerve injuries result from stretching or hyperextension of nerve tissue. They generally occur during birth or traumatic or difficult delivery. Nerve damage ranges from very limited edema that resolves quickly to complete paralysis. The most common peripheral nerve injuries are facial nerve palsy and brachial plexus palsy (Fig. 14–10).

Facial nerve palsy is a common type of peripheral nerve palsy, occurring in 1% to 7% of 1000 live births (Levine et al., 1984). Facial nerve damage results from prolonged pressure on the facial nerve from the maternal pelvis or forceps.

Brachial plexus palsy results when the cervical and thoracic nerve roots are damaged as a result of excessive lateral flexion and traction on the neck. The injury is usually unilateral and occurs most frequently on the left side.

Presentation of facial nerve palsy varies and ranges from inability to close the eye or open the mouth to paralysis of the lower portion of the face. The injury is apparent at birth or within a few days following. Most neonates recover spontaneously with slow improvement of movement within 3 weeks.

Clinical presentation of brachial plexus injuries varies with the location and extent of damage. At birth, the neonate has decreased movement from the shoulder to the hand. Erb-Duchenne paralysis, the most common type, is due to damage to the C5 and C6 nerve roots and presents as shoulder and upper arm paralysis. The arm is adducted and internally rotated and kept in the "waiter's tip" position with decreased or absent Moro reflex and biceps and radial reflexes.

Klumpke's paralysis involves damage to the C8 to T1 nerve roots that affects the lower arm and hand. The affected arm remains flaccid with the hand in a claw-hand position. The Moro and grasp reflexes are absent. Erb-Duchenne-Klumpke paralysis involves damage to the entire brachial plexus that affects the hand and arm. There is complete paralysis of the upper and lower arm and hand. Brachial plexus injuries have a good prognosis. With supportive care, most neonates recover.

Peripheral nerve palsies are supportively managed. This includes immobilization with a soft splint or brace and institution of passive range of motion exercises at day 10. The nurse in collaboration with the physical therapist provide parent education to reinforce ongoing therapy.

Perinatal Asphyxia

Causes of perinatal asphyxia include interrupted umbilical blood flow, abruptio placentae, and inadequate placental perfusion. A common cause of fetal hypoxia is cord compression during birth (Jacobs & Phibbs, 1989). The easily compressed vein in the umbilical cord interrupts blood flow to the fetus, and the less distensible arteries continue to pump blood into the placenta, causing fetal hypotension.

Placental insufficiency is another cause of perinatal asphyxia and is most likely to result in long-term sequelae (Jacobs & Phibbs, 1989). Common causes are maternal anesthesia, pregnancy-induced hypertension, and oxytocin (Pitocin) hyperstimulation that does not allow for adequate placental perfusion. The fetus responds to placental insufficiency with bradycardia and decreased variability as noted on the fetal monitor.

Trauma during delivery is another potential cause of fetal asphyxia. Cephalopelvic disproportion may lead to the fetus becoming "stuck" in the birth canal or cord compression while moving through the canal. In some cases the clavicle is purposefully fractured to deliver the neonate quickly. The use of high forceps also denotes a difficult delivery and failure of the fetus to easily fit through the birth canal. These situations may lead to

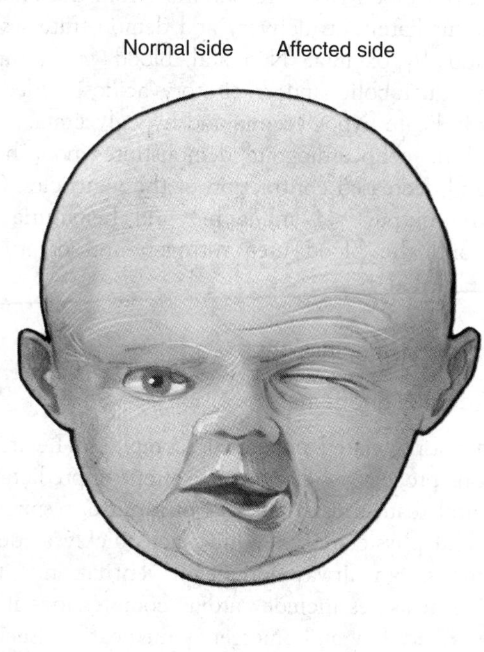

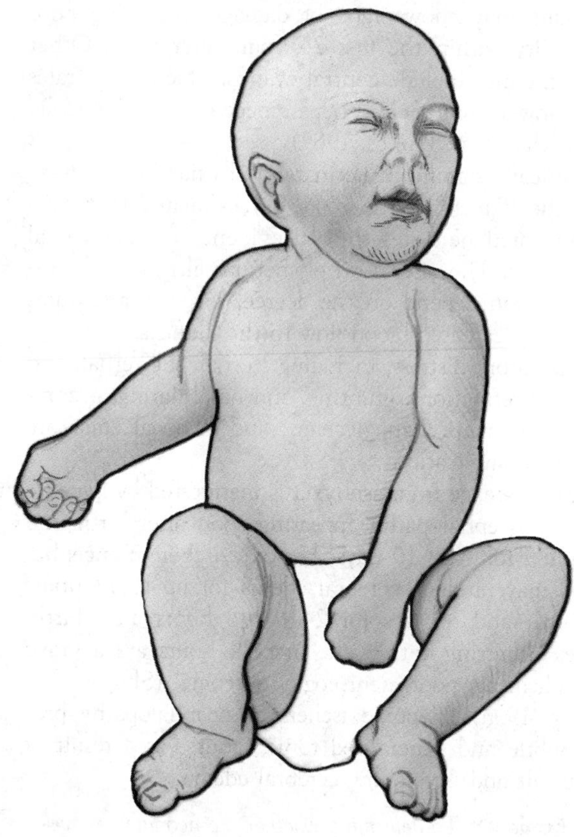

Figure 14–10
Facial nerve palsy *(A)* and brachial plexus palsy *(B)* are common peripheral nerve injuries in neonates.

fetal asphyxia. Neonates with these risk factors and history must be evaluated carefully.

Pathophysiology

The fetus initially responds to hypoxia with bradycardia. This increases cardiac output by shunting blood away from the kidneys and gut to the heart and brain. With worsening fetal hypoxia and acidosis, hypotension results from cardiac and respiratory failure. The heart rate may increase slightly but eventually decreases, and bradycardia ensues. These events are often recorded on the fetal monitor during labor. The fetal monitor reveals a loss of beat-to-beat variability, fetal tachycardia then bradycardia, and poor short-term variability and late decelerations (Eden & Boehm, 1990).

Prognosis. The prognosis for perinatal asphyxia and resultant hypoxic ischemic encephalopathy is variable and ranges from death immediately after birth to severe neurologic deficits to no sequelae. Hypoxic ischemic encephalopathy is a clinical syndrome present in neonates with brain injury caused by perinatal asphyxia. Apgar scores alone are poor predictors of the adverse neurologic sequelae of perinatal asphyxia (Clark & Hakanson, 1988). Therefore, combining the Apgar score with the entire clinical picture, including timing of onset and severity of seizures and neurologic examination findings, gives a better estimation of outcome.

Assessment

The initial signs of perinatal asphyxia appear immediately after birth. The neonate is limp, cyanotic, bradycardic, and apneic. Muscle tone, reflexes, and spontaneous movement are extremely depressed in the asphyxiated neonate and are often the last parameters to return during recovery. The intrapartum history may reveal significant fetal distress, including prolonged bradycardia, late decelerations, and poor fetal heart rate variability.

All body systems may be affected, including the

heart, kidneys, lungs, metabolic system, and the brain. The heart may show signs of damage, including poor contractility within the first 24 hours after birth. Other clinical findings include central cyanosis, tachypnea, rales in the lower lung fields, hepatomegaly, and a systolic murmur (Jacobs & Phibbs, 1989).

Clinically significant perinatal asphyxia almost always affects the kidneys. Perlman (1989) estimated that 50% of asphyxiated neonates showed evidence of acute renal involvement. The effects on glomerular filtration and tubular function depend on the degree, severity, and duration of the decreased blood flow to the kidneys.

Respiratory distress, including sternal, substernal, and intercostal retractions, grunting, and nasal flaring, is common. Also, acute hypoglycemia and hypocalcemia are metabolic complications.

Brain damage from asphyxia is manifested by hypoxic ischemic encephalopathy appearing soon after birth and continuing for 7 to 10 days. Hypoxic ischemic encephalopathy may produce cerebral edema for up to 72 hours after birth and seizures for 24 to 48 hours after birth. Seizures occurring within the first 24 hours are a grave sign indicating poor neurologic outcome (Shaywitz & Fletcher, 1993). Hypoxic ischemic encephalopathy produces subtle and generalized tonic seizures as a result of CNS insult and developing cerebral edema.

caREminder: *To determine whether the neonate's movements are tremors or seizure activity, check for subtle signs of seizures, such as lip smacking, rapid eye movements, and tongue thrusting (Table 14–4).*

Nursing Diagnoses and Outcomes

Nursing diagnoses and outcomes generally applicable for neonates with a health challenge are listed in Chart 14–3. In addition, the following may be applicable to a neonate with perinatal asphyxia:

- **Sensory-perceptual alterations (all forms), related to effects of anoxia**
  Outcome: The neonate will show no signs of neurologic deterioration and will respond appropriately to the environment.

Table 14–4
Differentiating Seizures from Jitteriness

Assessment Findings	Seizures	Jitteriness
Ceases with passive flexion	No	Yes
Activity induced	No	Yes
Associated with cyanosis or bradycardia	Yes	No
Eye deviations	Yes	No

Assessment

Many blood tests are used to determine the presence of asphyxia. Cord blood gases are obtained from the umbilical cord immediately on delivery and demonstrate severe acidosis and hypoxemia. Neonatal blood gas samples demonstrate metabolic and respiratory acidosis. Electrolyte levels indicate hypoglycemia and hypoglycemia.

A bedside echocardiogram demonstrates poor heart function and decreased contraction of the ventricles. Oliguria (urine output <1 mL/kg/hr) and hematuria are common, and the blood urea nitrogen and creatinine levels are elevated.

Interdisciplinary Interventions

Delivery Team Management

Care of the asphyxiated neonate is complex. The initial stabilization process is labile and often unpredictable. The neonatal team usually consists of a nurse, respiratory therapist, and physician. They must act quickly at delivery to establish an airway and begin ventilation. Other resuscitative measures include cardiac compressions if the heart rate is very low and emergency medications such as epinephrine administered through the endotracheal tube or through an umbilical venous catheter inserted by the physician. The nurse's role in the resuscitation of an asphyxiated neonate involves assessing heart rate and initiating compressions. Also, the nurse may assist the respiratory therapist in establishing and maintaining an adequate airway by stabilizing the endotracheal tube, applying positive-pressure ventilation, and assessing for breath sounds. The team must work together, because these neonates are critically ill. Quick and efficient stabilization is imperative to the neonate's survival.

Apgar scoring, while helpful in objectively determining the neonate's response to resuscitation, should not be used to determine when resuscitation is initiated. The initiation and further decisions related to resuscitation are based on the neonate's responses to early resuscitative efforts. Respiratory effort, heart rate, color, presence of reflexes, and muscle tone are ongoing evaluation assessments during resuscitation.

NICU Team Management

On the neonate's arrival to the NICU, the nurse quickly ensures the presence of a patent airway, establishes baseline vital signs, and promotes thermoregulation. A complete physical examination is performed to detect any congenital anomalies or other complications. Focusing on the neonate's muscle tone, response to care, and reflexes, the nurse begins to establish a baseline neurologic status that will be helpful for later comparison.

The nurse assists with placement of invasive lines to better monitor blood pressure and obtains specimens for laboratory tests. Close monitoring is done for aberrations in all laboratory values, and bedside glucose, hemoglobin, and hematocrit testing is done.

The nurse monitors the neonate's response to treatments and assists to determine the extent of organ involvement. For example, meticulous monitoring of urine output aids in assessing renal damage. Documenting neurologic symptoms helps to determine CNS damage.

The medical team aggressively treats the neonate by promoting oxygenation, by providing ventilation, and with medications. The physician evaluates chest radiographs, serial blood gas levels, and other laboratory studies to guide treatments. The goals of treatment are to avoid hypercarbia, control seizures, and restrict intravenous fluids to prevent cerebral edema.

Other nursing interventions include monitoring for signs of cerebral edema and increasing intracranial pressure. Signs of increasing intracranial pressure in the neonate include the following:

- Increasing lethargy
- Increasing head circumference
- Tense anterior fontanelle
- Widening sutures
- Apnea
- Deteriorating vital signs

Phenobarbital is the medication of choice to control seizures. If seizures continue after intravenous administration of phenobarbital, phenytoin (Dilantin) may be initiated. Other supportive therapies with seizures include correcting any metabolic abnormalities, ensuring an adequate airway, and promoting oxygenation and ventilation.

The nurse monitors the neonate's response to the seizure medications by noting the time that the seizures stopped and monitoring for side effects. The most common side effect of phenobarbital is respiratory depression.

The family is often distressed by the unexpected events of the birth and will need reassurance and frequent updating of the neonate's condition. The nurse explains the current treatments and the neonate's responses to the family and facilitates communication with the physician. Involving the social worker as soon as possible will provide additional support to the family.

Infants of Diabetic Mothers

The infant of a diabetic mother is at risk for many problems. To decrease the risk to the neonate, the mother's blood glucose level must be assessed and properly controlled during pregnancy to minimize hypoglycemia and hyperglycemia. Diabetes screening should begin at week 26 to 28 of gestation. Common problems in infants of diabetic mothers include macrosomia (increased adipose tissue) and subsequent traumatic delivery, hypoglycemia within a short time after delivery, respiratory distress from surfactant deficiency, electrolyte disturbances, polycythemia, and congenital anomalies (Suevo, 1997).

Pathophysiology

Insulin does not cross the placenta. The fetus increases its own production of insulin in response to the high glucose levels from the mother. This state of hyperinsulinism leads to macrosomia, increased fat accumulation, and LGA. The hyperinsulinemia continues after delivery, reaching a level 10 times higher than that in normal neonates (Knip, Lautala, Leppaluoto, Akerblom, & Kouivalainen, 1983).

Because of the hyperinsulinemia, hypoglycemia occurs rapidly after delivery when the supply of glucose is abruptly ceased. The hyperinsulinemia may last for several days and require intravenous therapy to maintain normal glucose values.

Infants of diabetic mothers have a higher incidence of respiratory distress and surfactant deficiency when compared with normal neonates. Poorly controlled maternal diabetes and the effects on the neonate appear to impair the development of surfactant (Landon & Gabbe, 1992). This has led many obstetricians to deliver these infants at 37 to 38 weeks to ensure adequate lung maturity.

Hypocalcemia and hypomagnesemia are also common problems of infants of diabetic mothers owing to decreased hypoparathyroid functioning. The frequency and severity of abnormal maternal blood glucose levels can contribute significantly to the occurrence of congenital abnormalities such as congenital heart disease and central nervous system defects such as caudal regression syndrome (Suevo, 1997).

Assessment

A maternal history of diabetes mellitus or gestational diabetes is usually present, but many mothers exhibit no history or have not obtained appropriate prenatal care. Infants of diabetic mothers have a characteristic appearance owing to the increased subcutaneous fat, full face, smaller head circumference to weight ratio, and a larger weight to length ratio. The placenta and umbilical cord are often very large.

A complete assessment is vital to detect congenital anomalies, specifically congenital heart defects. Close observation is necessary to detect hypoglycemia. Hypoglycemia may be asymptomatic or may be marked by lethargy, a high-pitched cry, jitteriness, and seizures. The nurse monitors for respiratory distress and auscultates for cardiac murmurs. A hemoglobin and hematocrit is sent to the laboratory to monitor for polycythemia. A polycythemic newborn appears ruddy. Electrolytes are also monitored for the presence of hypocalcemia, and supplemental calcium may be necessary.

Because of the infant's large size, traumatic deliveries and subsequent birth traumas are common. If there is decreased movement or crying with movement of an extremity, further investigation for birth trauma is necessary. Not all diabetic mothers are identified before delivery. Therefore, LGA neonates are at risk for blood glucose problems and should have serial blood glucose determinations after birth.

Interdisciplinary Interventions

The nurse closely monitors for the signs and symptoms of hypoglycemia, obtains blood glucose values every 30 to 60 minutes after birth until stable, then every 2 to 4 hours for 24 hours until stable, and initiates early feedings, as appropriate (Care Path 14–1). Feedings are contraindicated if respiratory distress is present, because there is a risk of aspiration. Intravenous fluids are initiated if feedings are withheld.

Fetal Alcohol Syndrome

Ethyl alcohol ingestion by pregnant women can lead to the largest identified cause of teratogenesis (chemically induced physical or mental anomalies) in a fetus: fetal alcohol syndrome (FAS). FAS is a syndrome of growth deficiency in length and weight, microcephaly, low-set ears, and short palpebral fissures at birth (Fig. 14–11) (Chasnoff, Landress, & Barnett, 1990). Additionally, mild to moderate retardation and delayed motor and language development is recognized early in infancy. Neonates with FAS have lower levels of arousal and are more restless and irritable when compared with normal neonates. A milder form of FAS presents with only partial expression and is known as fetal alcohol effects (FAE). FAE is not immediately apparent at birth. The neonate develops poorly and may fail to thrive and make poor progress in school, manifesting learning disabilities and behavioral problems associated with hyperactivity and problems of impulse control.

The incidence of FAS in the United States is estimated at 1 in 1000 (Abel, 1995). Research has not been able to demonstrate a dose-response relationship between alcohol exposure and the development of neurologic problems, but any amount of alcohol taken by a pregnant woman constitutes a risk to the fetus.

Pathophysiology

The active ingredient of alcohol is ethanol. Ethanol's metabolites are readily transferred across the placenta and to the fetus (Lipson, 1988). Ethanol is a CNS depressant and migrates into the fetal brain as well as the liver, kidneys, and pancreas. Fetal ethanol metabolism is half that of the adult, and the fetus relies on the placenta for ethanol clearance. Consequently, this produces amniotic fluid with high ethanol levels and a neonate who may appear intoxicated at birth.

Ethanol and its metabolites are teratogens depending on the time of exposure. Weeks 3 through 8 of gestation are the most vulnerable times for toxicity because cells are dividing and organs are developing (Ernhart, Sokol,

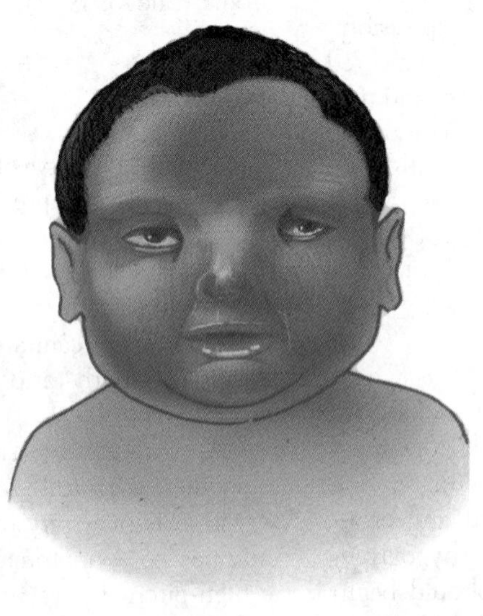

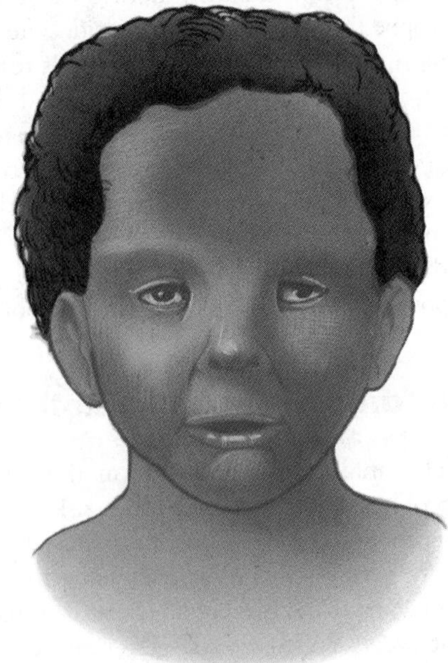

Figure 14–11
Typical facial characteristics of fetal alcohol syndrome in infant at age 1 week *(A)* and 1 year *(B)*.

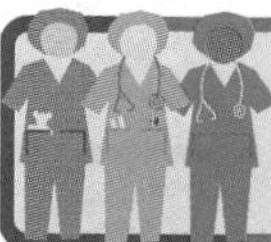

Care Path 14–1 An Interdisciplinary Plan of Care for the Infant of a Diabetic Mother

Nursing Diagnosis	Patient/Family Intermediate Outcomes			
	Admission	**Day 1**	**Day 2**	**Days 3–4**
Altered nutrition less than body requirements related to increased glucose utilization	Infant will have adequate nutrition as evidenced by intake at 60–80 kcal/kg.	⟶	⟶	⟶
Risk for injury related to effects of hyperinsulinism secondary to maternal diabetes	Infant will maintain blood glucose value between 45–100 mg/dL.	⟶		Patient will experience normal glucose value with enteral intake only.
	Infant will have normal electrolyte balance.		Infant will have normal electrolyte balance on full enteral feeding or need only calcium supplements.	
	Infant will have symptoms of hypoglycemia recognized immediately and treatment initiated.	⟶	⟶	⟶
Risk for impaired gas exchange related to effects of surfactant deficiency	Infant will have signs and symptoms of RDS recognized immediately and treatment initiated.	Infant will experience adequate gas exchange.	⟶	⟶
Care Intervention Categories				
Consults	Genetics if other abnormalities are present. Cardiology, if CHD.			
Labs	Electrolytes Blood gases Septic work-up if indicators present Bedside blood glucose q 1–3 hr	Blood glucose q 2–4 hr	Bedside blood glucose before every feeding	Discontinue bedside blood glucose monitoring
Medications and IVs	$D_{10}W$ continuous IV as needed for hypoglycemia, may require up to $D_{20}W$	⟶	Wean IVs as glucose levels stabilize.	⟶
	Supplemental electrolytes, p.r.n.	⟶	Begin electrolyte supplements as needed.	⟶
	Corticosteroids if needed to control hypoglycemia	⟶		

Care Path continued on following page

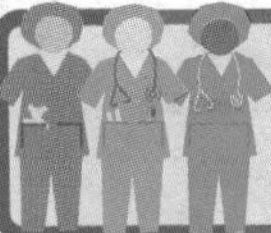

Care Path 14–1 An Interdisciplinary Plan of Care for the Infant of a Diabetic Mother *Continued*

Care Intervention Categories	Admission	Day 1	Day 2	Days 3–4
Nutrition	Initiate early feedings, if tolerated, with formula or follow breastfeeding with formula. NPO if RDS or RR > 80 Strict intake and output	→ → →	Frequent feeds to control hypoglycemia	→ →
Procedures	Echocardiogram to rule out CHD, if indicated Chest radiograph to rule out lung and cardiac disease			
Psychosocial	Clinical social work on admission	Provide support and reassurance if guilt displayed related to poor maternal glucose control	→	Ongoing support as needed
Teaching	Orient to NICU, breast pumping and storage, environment, equipment	Begin disease process teaching.	Begin medication teaching, if applicable (e.g., calcium supplements)	Formula preparation, home care Follow-up care needed When to notify health care provider
Vital signs/ baseline parameters	VS q 1–2 hr Daily weights Cardiorespiratory Pulse oximeter Transcutaneous monitor, if RDS	VS q 2–3 hr → →	VS with feedings. → Discontinue monitors when stable.	→

CHD, congenital heart disease; ECG, electrocardiogram; NICU, neonatal intensive care unit; NPO, nothing by mouth; RDS, respiratory distress syndrome; RR, respiratory rate; TPN, total parenteral nutrition; VS, vital signs.

Martier, Moron, & Nadler, 1987). The exact amount of maternal alcohol ingestion that causes FAS is not clear, but there appears to be a "threshold level" at which a disruption of the organogenesis occurs. This threshold is unknown.

Prognosis. The prognosis for these neonates is poor in that the damage done to the CNS is irreversible. As these children grow and develop, educational programs can help these individuals realize their potential but cannot offer a cure. Early diagnosis and interventions are important to help these neonates develop into self-sufficient adults. Some will require constant supervision, whereas others may live independent lives. One study noted that the craniofacial malformations of FAS diminished over time but the inadequate weight gain and microcephaly persist (Spohr, Willms, & Steinhausen, 1993).

Assessment

Physical manifestations of FAS range from mild to severe. Common signs of FAS include SGA, microcephaly, poor growth, microphthalmia (small eyes), short palpebral fissures, and micrognathia (small chin) (Appelbaum, 1995). Additionally, congenital heart disease such as ventricular septal defect, atrial septal defect, and tetralogy of Fallot are associated with alcohol exposure prenatally. Renal anomalies may also occur in 10% to 20% of affected neonates. The diagnosis is made by reported maternal alcohol consumption during pregnancy and the presence of a cluster of anomalies.

The CNS is affected in over 80% of neonates with FAS in the form of microcephaly. Alcohol withdrawal often presents within 24 hours after birth with tremors, irritability, and abdominal distention. Neonates with FAS are less able to habituate to aversive stimuli as measured by the NBAS (Richardson, Day, & Taylor, 1989). The most profound effect of FAS is CNS dysfunction and poor academic performance during the school years. Approximately 3% are severely to profoundly retarded (Spohr, Willms, & Steinhausen, 1993).

FAS neonates are smaller at birth and fail to grow normally or demonstrate appropriate catch-up growth. Head growth is often below the tenth percentile. Facial anomalies are common and affect the midface. Other complications of FAS include irritability, poor feeding due to ineffective coordination of suck and swallow, and hypersensitivity to external stimuli (Appelbaum, 1995).

Nursing Diagnoses and Outcomes

Nursing diagnoses and outcomes generally applicable for neonates with a health challenge are presented in Chart 14–3. In addition, the following may be applicable for a neonate with FAS:

- **Altered nutrition: less than body requirements, related to poor nippling**
  Outcomes: The neonate will ingest adequate calories and nutrients. The neonate will display adequate growth.

Interdisciplinary Interventions

Nursing interventions are mainly supportive during the neonatal period. To minimize CNS irritability and hypersensitivity to the environment, nursing interventions are geared at maintaining a quiet environment that promotes normal wake and sleep patterns. Additionally, clustering care and minimizing unnecessary handling are vital in the nursing care of these neonates.

Nutritional management is critically important for the neonate with FAS, because poor feeding is common. Optimizing calories and promoting normal suck-swallow patterns are important nursing interventions.

Intrauterine Exposure to Cocaine or Narcotics

The incidence of substance abuse among pregnant women has been reported to be approximately 10% (Farkas & Parran, 1993). Cocaine has been reported to be the most common illicit drug used by women of childbearing age, with estimates of up to 30% in some communities (Baxter, Butler, Brinker, Frazier, & Wedgeworth, 1995). This degree of prenatal drug exposure has far-reaching implications for the health professional caring for these mothers and neonates.

Methamphetamine, cocaine, and heroin are the common drugs abused prenatally. Polydrug use, or use of more than one drug, is most common (Chasnoff, 1988). The fetus exposed to intrauterine drugs may exhibit withdrawal symptoms after birth (neonatal abstinence syndrome [NAS]). These classifications of drugs are considered together despite their major pharmacologic differences, because many substance-using mothers are polydrug users. In addition, withdrawal symptoms may be similar.

Cocaine

Cocaine is a stimulant that increases the dopamine release and decreases uptake of norepinephrine (Dixon, 1989). When used while pregnant, stimulants cause massive vasoconstriction throughout the body, including the vessels in the uterus and placenta. This often leads to preterm labor, placental insufficiency, or abruptio placentae. Additionally, studies have demonstrated that cocaine can cause significant vasoconstriction, subsequently leading to short-term hypoxic episodes to the fetus (Collins, 1989).

Cocaine use during pregnancy increases the risk of birth anomalies because it has teratogenic effects, especially in the first 3 months of gestation. Cocaine crosses the placenta quickly, and metabolites can be detected in the fetus for up to 4 days after exposure. Common birth defects associated with cocaine use include genitourinary malformations, prune belly syndrome, limb defects, cardiovascular defects, brain lesions, and cerebral infarcts (Chasnoff, Chisum, & Kaplan, 1988; Norris & Hill, 1992). Additionally, maternal cocaine abuse contributes to the development of NEC in the neonate (Czyrko, Del Pin, O'Neil, Peckham, & Ross, 1991).

Maternal cocaine use is associated with IUGR, including reduced head circumference. Other malformations associated with cocaine use include congenital heart disease, encephalocele, and microcephaly. Withdrawal symptoms are uncommon and usually mild when present. Perhaps the most serious complications of cocaine use during pregnancy are the increased risks of preterm delivery and abruptio placentae.

Narcotics

Narcotics are CNS depressants that produce feelings of peace and relaxation. Codeine, heroin, methadone, and morphine are the most common narcotics. Heroin is six times as potent as morphine and highly addictive. These drugs readily cross the placenta; and at birth, when the supply is ceased, the neonate may show signs of withdrawal at 24 to 72 hours (Levy & Spino, 1993).

Heroin reduces uteroplacental blood flow and inhibits fetal growth. Combined with inadequate maternal calorie and protein intake, it produces IUGR, including poor brain growth. During pregnancy, maternal heroin use creates fetal addiction. If the mother attempts to stop using heroin or if her intake is erratic, fetal withdrawal and possible death may occur. Often, the mother is placed on methadone maintenance during her pregnancy to avoid fetal death. Methadone is a synthetic opioid drug that works as a substitute for heroin. The benefit of methadone maintenance is that the level of drug can be maintained as a constant at an exact dose and does not exert the mood-altering effects of heroin.

The heroin or methadone exposed newborn is often SGA, has LBW, and has a smaller head circumference (Chasnoff, Hatcher, & Burns, 1986). LBW neonates have a higher morbidity and mortality than AGA neonates (Boobis & Sullivan, 1986). Mothers abusing narcotics such as heroin are often living in substandard conditions and may be homeless. This leads to poor nutrition because food is scarce and to a lack of prenatal care. Additionally, some addicts resort to prostitution to continue their habit, which increases their risk of sexually transmitted diseases such as syphilis, gonorrhea, and human immunodeficiency virus infection. These diseases, along with poor nutrition, lead to a high-risk pregnancy and an increased risk for delivery of a neonate with LBW.

Neonates exposed to intrauterine narcotics generally recover with little to no long-term effects. Several studies have shown that when environmental factors are controlled, there is not a significant drug-imposed effect on later growth and development (Carta et al., 1994). However, these neonates have been shown to be at high risk for child abuse owing to their withdrawal behaviors, such as irritability and decreased sleep (Kelley, 1992). These behaviors are difficult to manage especially when combined with a drug-abusing mother who has limited coping skills or resources. Withdrawal behaviors may last for up to 6 months.

Assessment

The neonatal abstinence scoring system is a tool used to assess the severity of drug withdrawal behaviors. Finnegan (1985) published this scoring system in an attempt to rate withdrawal behaviors on an objective scale. This tool lists 21 symptoms commonly seen in neonates during withdrawal. The neonate is scored at 2 hours after birth and then every 4 hours for the first 5 days of life. If the symptoms are increasing in severity, then the neonate is scored every 2 hours.

Neonates whose mothers are suspected drug users are scored every 2 hours for the first 48 hours of life, regardless of the score (Finnegan, 1985). Thereafter, if the scores are 7 or less, the scoring is completed every 4 hours for 48 hours. A score of 7 or less is categorized as mild withdrawal. Nursing judgment is used to avoid waking the neonate unnecessarily.

If the score is 8 or greater, medication is initiated and the scoring continues for 5 days. Each scoring interval rates the newborn's behavior during the entire 2- or 4-hour interval, not just the behavior present at the time of scoring. The newborn should be awakened to elicit reflexes and specified behavior.

Cocaine-exposed neonates demonstrate increased muscle tone, tremors, and prolonged retention of primitive reflexes (Chasnoff, 1988). The cocaine-exposed neonate does not present with specific withdrawal behaviors and may only demonstrate irritability several weeks after birth. Premature delivery and associated problems are the primary challenges for the cocaine-exposed neonate (see earlier discussion of prematurity and LBW). One study demonstrated significant impairment in motor control and state regulation in full-term neonates exposed prenatally to cocaine (Delaney-Black et al., 1996).

For narcotic-exposed neonates, the prenatal and labor and delivery history may show high-risk maternal factors such as the lack of prenatal care or an admitted history of drug use. Drug-addicted pregnant mothers commonly do not obtain prenatal care or obtain it sporadically. The labor and delivery events are also significant, including the presence of meconium or fetal distress. Heroin-addicted neonates have a greater incidence of meconium aspiration (Philips, 1986).

The physical examination findings and mental state of the mother are also helpful. Often, the mother admits to heroin use or of having taken illicit drugs in the past. Needle tracks from illicit drug injections are also high-risk findings. The mental status examination findings may be helpful if the mother was able to answer questions coherently.

At birth, gestational age assessment determines whether the newborn has appropriately grown in utero. Many drug-exposed neonates are SGA and have a head circumference that is normally larger than the rest of the body. This is described as head-sparing SGA.

On admission to the nursery, the neonate is assessed further. Neonates exposed to narcotics display withdrawal symptoms within 2 to 6 days after delivery, when the drug level becomes critically low. The symptoms that appear gradually and progress in severity and frequency include the following (Chasnoff et al., 1986; Oro & Dixon, 1988):

- Tremors
- High-pitched cry
- Sneezing
- Irritability
- Increased muscle tone
- Poor feeding
- Diarrhea
- Weight loss and inadequate weight gain
- Decreased sleep
- Poor state control
- Increased sensitivity to environmental stimuli
- Increased activity

The CNS symptoms appear first, followed by gastrointestinal disturbances. Finnegan (1985) determined that the most common symptom of NAS is tremors.

The increased activity, poor feeding, irritability, increased metabolic rate, and decreased sleep leads to inadequate weight gain and growth (Oro & Dixon, 1988). Weinberger and Kendall (1986) found the neonates suffering from moderate to severe NAS demonstrated abnormal weight change patterns: the most severe NAS resulted in almost twice the number of days to regain birth weight.

Each withdrawal symptom should be investigated as it appears to help rule out other causes, such as hypoglycemia or hypocalcemia. Tremors are not uncommon with other abnormalities, such as hypoglycemia, hypocalcemia, or hypomagnesemia; and these conditions must be ruled out before treating for drug exposure.

Diagnostic Tests. At the time of admission, maternal blood work and urine samples may be sent based on the mother's history and presentation. Legal issues regarding such testing are determined on a state-by-state basis.

Generally, if the maternal history poses a risk, the neonate's urine sample is sent to the laboratory for drug testing immediately after birth. Urine collected after 36 hours is more likely to be negative for qualitative toxicologic assessment. If available, meconium or hair samples can be sent for toxicology because these samples show long-term drug exposure.

Nursing Diagnoses and Outcomes

Nursing diagnoses and outcomes generally applicable for neonates with a health challenge are presented in Chart 14–3. In addition, the following may be applicable for a neonate with intrauterine drug exposure:

- ▶ **Risk for impaired skin integrity, related to frequent diarrheal stools**
  Outcome: The neonate's skin will remain intact.
- ▶ **Ineffective breathing pattern, related to impaired CNS function, as evidenced by a respiratory rate above 60 breaths per minute and respiratory alkalosis**
  Outcomes: The neonate's respiratory rate will remain below 60 breaths per minute.
  The neonate will show no signs of alkalosis.

Interdisciplinary Interventions

Quieting and darkening the environment is a vital nursing function to assist the neonate to calm and sleep.

caREminder: *Advise other health care workers not to disturb the newborn and to talk quietly while near the bedside. The nurse must provide periods of undisturbed sleep, limiting examinations and procedures.*

Providing boundaries in the crib with blankets, offering the pacifier, and swaddling are all interventions the nurse can do to help calm the irritable neonate. The nurse clusters care activities to promote longer periods of sleep and to avoid unnecessary handling.

Skin care can be a challenge in these neonates owing to frequent watery stools. Also, it is common to have skin breakdown at the knees and nose from rubbing against the blankets during irritability spells. Nurses prevent skin breakdown by applying barrier creams to the diaper area. Knees may be protected by use of sheepskin, or occlusive dressings can be used for added protection.

Teaching the parents about the withdrawal symptoms and treatment is another important nursing intervention (TIP 14–1). The nurse provides this teaching objectively and clearly, avoiding causal and accusatory statements. It is vital that the family understand the withdrawal course, treatment, and expected behaviors. The mother learns coping and calming skills for her newborn by observing the nurse. The nurse also teaches the mother about medication administration.

Based on the Neonatal Abstinence Score, the physician may start medications such as phenobarbital or pare-

TIP 14–1 A Teaching Intervention Plan for the Child with Neonatal Abstinence Syndrome

Nursing Diagnoses and Family Outcomes

- Impaired skin integrity related to frequent, loose stools
  Outcomes: Family will state reason for skin breakdown.
  Family will demonstrate appropriate cleansing and application of diaper cream.
- Sleep pattern disturbance related to irritability
  Outcomes: Family will state importance of sleep to overall health.
  Family will demonstrate swaddling and calming techniques, darkening environment.
  Family will safely and accurately administer medications.
- Altered nutrition less than body requirements related to increased activity and poor sleep cycles
  Outcomes: Family will feed newborn safely and efficiently.
  Family will state need for increased calories.
  Family prepares specialized formula accurately and stores safely.
- Altered parenting related to drug abuse and decreased resources/support
  Outcome: Family will complete needed referrals and seek resources.

Interventions

Teach parent/caregivers about:

Medications

Measure medication carefully and give at designated times.
Administer medications as prescribed, and give phenobarbital in small amount of formula.
Monitor for lethargy or increased irritability; give only what is prescribed to avoid overdose.
Keep medications out of reach of children.

Nutrition

Promote small, frequent feedings; use high calorie (24 cal/oz) formula.

Special Considerations

Promote adequate sleep by providing quiet environment, swaddling, offering pacifier; allow prolonged periods of sleep.

Skin

Protect diaper area with barrier creams.

Psychosocial

Provide referrals to community resources (public health department, mental health services, addiction treatment center, food subsidy programs).
If caregiver feels "out of control" and unable to cope, call a friend to watch newborn, call health care provider, close door and allow newborn to cry.

Contact Health Care Provider if

The neonate develops water-loss stools; increase in irritability; vomiting; fever >38°C; lethargy; poor feeding; accidental overdose

goric to control the withdrawal symptoms. Finnegan (1985) recommends initiating pharmacotherapy only after other common metabolic conditions have been ruled out. The need for pharmacologic interventions is indicated if the score is more than 8 for three consecutive scores or if the average of three consecutive scores is 8 or greater (Finnegan, 1985). Additionally, if the total score is 12 or greater for two consecutive intervals, therapy should also be initiated before the 4-hour interval has elapsed.

Phenobarbital is used to suppress the major CNS

aberrations. Effective in controlling irritability and improving sleep patterns, phenobarbital is often used in polydrug exposure. In contrast, paregoric is most effective in pure narcotic withdrawal because it actually replaces what is missing in the body. Paregoric contains opium alkaloids that are antispasmodics and phenanthrene derivatives that are analgesics and narcotics. Therefore, this drug decreases diarrhea. However, paregoric contains alcohol (44% to 46%), is difficult to titrate, and may require a longer course of therapy than other drugs (Finnegan, 1985).

A nutritional consultation may be helpful to optimize caloric intake. A formula with 24 calories per ounce may be needed to meet the metabolic needs of these neonates. Nipple feeding may be ineffective, and an experienced occupational therapist may assist with nippling evaluation and interventions. Breast-feeding is not recommended for neonates of mothers with a drug history. Some drugs, especially cocaine, are passed to the infant through breast milk. Often the neonate will need intravenous fluid and nutrition to maintain proper growth. This requires a longer hospitalization.

Community Care

A clinical social worker assists with the placement of the neonate if the mother is unable or unwilling to care for her newborn. Working closely with the clinical social worker is vital to provide the best home care situation for the mother and newborn. Additionally, the clinical social worker assists the mother to obtain necessary social services, parenting classes, and referrals (Chart 14–10.).

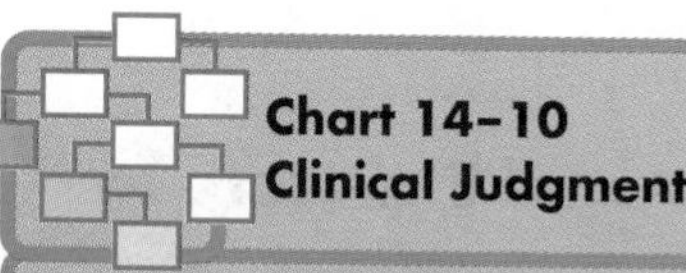

Chart 14–10
Clinical Judgment

Infant of a Substance-Abusing Mother

Hannah is a 3-day-old term newborn who is small for gestational age (SGA), delivered to a mother who is taking methadone and abusing heroin. Hannah is irritable and has increased muscle tone, diarrhea, frantic sucking, and vomiting. Vital signs: HR, 180; RR, 70; no other signs of respiratory distress; T, 100.5°F axillary; weight, 1800 g.

Questions

1. What other assessment data should the nurse collect?
2. Which assessment findings are abnormal?
3. What is the cause for Hannah's symptoms?
4. What nursing interventions should initially be implemented?
5. How will the nurse know that Hannah is improving?

Answers

1. Quality of Moro's reflex, presence of skin breakdown (knees, chin), number of hours spent sleeping between feedings, comparison of birth weight to current weight to determine presence of significant weight loss (>10% of birth weight), presence of tremoring (while disturbed or undisturbed), nasal congestion or rhinorrhea, sweating, and mottled skin.
2. Irritability, increased muscle tone, diarrhea, frantic sucking, vomiting, rapid respiratory rate, elevated temperature, weight indicates SGA.
3. Hannah is experiencing neonatal abstinence syndrome. After delivery, when the supply of heroin and methadone is gone, the infant responds with active withdrawal symptoms. These may occur any time after delivery but are most common within 48–72 hours. The most common symptoms include central nervous system irritability and gastrointestinal hypermotility. Weight loss is due to the hypermetabolic state in which there is increased oxygen consumption at the cellular level.
4. Initiate the Neonatal Abstinence Score Sheet to provide ongoing documentation of behaviors in an objective format. Provide a quiet and darkened environment. Swaddle with blankets and provide rhythmic rocking. Provide small, frequent, and calorie-dense feedings. Offer a pacifier. Collaborate with the medical team to initiate medications to alleviate the withdrawal symptoms. Include the parents by demonstrating appropriate interventions that assist in calming the infant.
5. Neonatal Abstinence Score Sheet scores of 8 or less. Daily weight gain. Sleeping at least 3 hours between feedings. Coordinated suck-swallow patterns with minimal spillage of formula; no vomiting or regurgitation. Infant is able to have awake/alert states and responds to caregiver interactions appropriately.

Infants of Tobacco Smokers

Tobacco smoke reduces maternal oxygen levels, and nicotine readily crosses the placenta, appearing in fetal blood at levels higher than those seen in maternal serum (Mactutus, 1989).

Approximately 30% of women in the United States smoke cigarettes (Bendich, 1993); approximately 29% of pregnant women smoke during their pregnancy (Khalsa & Gfroerer, 1991). Maternal smoking doubles the risk for spontaneous abortion and increases the risk of preterm delivery by about 36% (Meyer, Jonas, & Tonascia, 1976). Smoking is associated with dose-related IUGR. Heavier smoking is correlated with lower birth weight. Neonates born of smokers have a higher mortality rate than neonates born of nonsmokers.

Pathophysiology

The components of cigarette smoke, including nicotine and carbon monoxide, inhibit cell uptake of amino acids in the placenta. These amino acids are the building blocks of proteins that are essential for adequate fetal growth. Without these proteins, LBW may occur. Additionally, nicotine produces vasoconstriction and may lead to reduced placental blood flow. This reduces blood flow to the fetus and limits the availability of nutrition and oxygen.

In response to this vasoconstriction and limited blood flow, the fetus increases its production of fetal red blood cells, inducing polycythemia. Although compensatory, polycythemia has inherent problems because the blood can begin to sludge, owing to its increased viscosity, which leads to further hypoxia from blockage of blood vessels.

The risk to the neonate born to a mother who smokes is ongoing. Research has indicated that neonates exposed to cigarette smoke have an increased incidence of sudden infant death syndrome (Cutz, Perrin, Hackman, & Czegledy-Nagy, 1996).

Assessment

Obtaining a complete maternal history regarding all drug use—legal, illegal, over-the-counter, and prescription—is important to identify neonates at risk.

Interdisciplinary Interventions

Nursing interventions are geared at the prevention of smoking and the support of smoking cessation programs and techniques. Recognition of smoking as an addiction is an important concept to truly assist the individual with cessation. Nurses should encourage the cessation of smoking during pregnancy and at least the reduction of the number of cigarettes smoked. Additionally, neonates exposed postnatally to tobacco smoke are more likely to be hospitalized, to suffer from respiratory illnesses, and to be irritable (Minchin, 1991). Cessation of smoking will improve not only the health of the fetus but also that of the neonate.

Cigarette smoking and breast-feeding are controversial because nicotine can be found in the breast milk in dose-dependent amounts. However, mothers are encouraged to breast-feed because qualities of breast milk are still beneficial to the neonate (Minchin, 1991). The nursing care of neonates exposed to nicotine in utero is identical to care of the LBW neonate discussed earlier in this chapter.

If parents are unwilling to stop smoking, encourage them to refrain from smoking inside the home. At the very least, do not smoke in the same room with the infant.

Prenatal and Neonatal Exposure to Varicella

Fetal infection due to maternal varicella in the first or early second trimester of pregnancy may result in varicella embryopathy. This condition is characterized by limb atrophy, scarring of the skin, and CNS and eye manifestations. Fetal exposure to maternal varicella infection during the late second trimester and third trimester results in a one in four chance of being affected. However, there is minimal risk of developing congenital varicella syndrome, owing to exposure late in pregnancy, after the critical developmental period.

Etiology and Incidence

Varicella is a member of the herpesvirus family that causes chickenpox as well as varicella zoster. Most women in the United States have been exposed to varicella; the incidence of the virus in pregnant women is estimated at 0.5 in 10,000 pregnancies (Gershon, 1990).

Pathophysiology

Varicella is a teratogen to the fetus and affects the musculoskeletal, neurologic, and ocular systems. It may cause limb defects, cicatricial skin lesions (zigzag scarring, often in a dermatomal pattern), microcephaly, cortical atrophy, cataracts, and chorioretinitis (Gracey, 1997). Mothers who contract varicella infection early in pregnancy are often counseled to abort the fetus because of varicella's deleterious affects on the developing fetus.

The severity of neonatal varicella infection depends on the timing of the exposure. Infections in the neonate are severe if contracted within 4 days before and 2 days after delivery, possibly owing to the lack of passive immunity to the neonate from the mother. Infections are milder when maternal varicella occurs between 5 and 21 days before delivery. The mortality associated with varicella in neonates is approximately 20% and poses a significant risk to premature neonates, owing to their immunocompromised states.

Assessment

Physical findings include a generalized vesicular rash and a known history of exposure. Diagnosis is confirmed by isolation of the virus from a vesicle or by a rise in antibody titer. Symptoms in the neonate range from mild (e.g., fever and cutaneous lesions) to severe (hemorrhagic rash, cyanosis, respiratory distress, and pneumonia).

Interdisciplinary Interventions

The American Academy of Pediatrics (1994) recommends the administration of varicella-zoster immunoglobulin (VZIG) as soon as possible to neonates born to women with the onset of a varicella rash within 5 days before delivery or within 2 days after delivery. Approximately one half of these neonates are expected to develop varicella even if VZIG is given, but the disease severity is lessened.

VZIG is not indicated for healthy term neonates exposed postnatally to varicella or those born to mothers whose rash developed more than 48 hours after delivery. Premature neonates exposed postnatally should receive VZIG because of their immunocompromised state and lack of maternal antibody transfer during the third trimester.

The newborn who develops vesicles should be treated with acyclovir. Neonates exposed or infected and in the hospital are isolated for 21 days or 28 days if VZIG was given or until all vesicles have crusted over. The mother and newborn are isolated together, if possible.

Neonatal Hyperbilirubinemia

In utero, the placenta serves as the primary organ to clear bilirubin from the fetus's system. After birth, the neonate is challenged to excrete bilirubin in the presence of an increased production of bilirubin from excessive breakdown of red blood cells.

Jaundice or *physiologic jaundice* is a term used to describe a yellowing of the skin and is one of the most common physical findings during the initial neonate period. Jaundice appears when bilirubin is deposited into the subcutaneous tissue and becomes visible when the serum bilirubin levels exceed 7.0 mg/dL (Wilkerson, 1988). Jaundice due to normal physiologic processes occurs in 45% to 60% of all healthy term neonates and in up to 80% of preterm neonates within the first week of life, most often by 2 days of age (Blackburn, 1995).

Alert: *Jaundice occurring within the first 24 hours of life or after 2 weeks of life signifies an abnormal physiologic process and should be followed up immediately.*

Hyperbilirubinemia describes excessive levels of bilirubin in the blood that are often due to a pathologic process. Common causes of hyperbilirubinemia in the neonate are increased bilirubin production, decreased excretion of bilirubin, or both (Table 14–5).

Hemolytic disease of the newborn (Rh or ABO incompatibility) is discussed in Chapter 23.

Bacteremia—specifically that caused by gram-negative organisms—is known to increase the breakdown of red blood cells, leading to hyperbilirubinemia. Also, the liver may be affected in sepsis, leading to decreased excretion. Other common causes of increased breakdown of red blood cells leading to an increased production of bilirubin include drug reactions, extravascular blood in

Table 14–5
Common Causes of Hyperbilirubinemia

Increased Bilirubin Production	Decreased Bilirubin Excretion	Increased Production and Decreased Excretion
Hemolytic disease	Prematurity	Prematurity
Bacteremia	Bowel obstruction	Bacterial infections
Cephalhematoma	Hypothyroidism	Congenital infections
Excessive bruising	Hypoxia	
Polycythemia	Breast milk jaundice	

cephalhematomas, and excessive bruising. Decreased excretion of bilirubin leads to an increased amount of circulating bilirubin. Common causes include prematurity, bowel obstruction, breast milk jaundice, hypothyroidism, hypoxia, and asphyxia.

Premature neonates are at risk for hyperbilirubinemia owing to immaturity of the liver, relatively limited albumin binding sites, and severe illness. Premature neonates often present with elevated bilirubin levels that peak at about 1 week of life versus the term newborn, in whom levels peak around day 4 of life.

Bowel obstruction leads to hyperbilirubinemia as stool is obstructed, causing an increased absorption of bilirubin through the intestinal tract. Also, any damage to the liver may hinder its ability to metabolize and excrete bilirubin.

Breast milk jaundice has received increased attention as a cause for unconjugated hyperbilirubinemia. The theory suggests that substances in breast milk appear to interfere with bilirubin conjugation or increased resorption of bilirubin from the intestine (Wilkerson, 1989). Another facet of breast milk jaundice is related to the quality of suckling at the breast. Neonates having difficulty breast-feeding may develop jaundice from dehydration and caloric deprivation. If the newborn is healthy with no signs of other causes of jaundice, it is recommended to continue breast-feeding the newborn frequently.

Hypoxia and subsequent asphyxia drops the pH of the blood, impairing the ability of albumin to bind bilirubin, leading to elevated bilirubin levels. Asphyxia also causes damage to other organs, such as the liver, which may impair its ability to metabolize and excrete bilirubin.

Hypothyroidism leads to increased bilirubin levels, possibly owing to a delay in the development of necessary enzymes that convert bilirubin to its excretable form. Additionally, the plasma membrane of the liver may be altered in hypothyroidism, leading to an impaired ability of the bilirubin to be carried into the hepatic cell.

Prognosis. If the hyperbilirubinemia has been controlled and the level of unconjugated bilirubin has been kept to a minimum, the prognosis for a full recovery with no sequelae is good for the term newborn (Wilkerson, 1989). Conversely, if the unconjugated bilirubin is high and the neonate is very ill, kernicterus may develop. Kernicterus is a neurologic syndrome resulting from the deposition of unconjugated bilirubin into the brain cells. Neonates with this condition have obvious yellowing of the brain tissue on autopsy. Kernicterus and its subsequent neurologic sequelae are directly related to the high serum levels of bilirubin.

The development of kernicterus leads to severe motor and sensory deficits, mental deficits, and death (Wilkerson, 1989). Any newborn with a bilirubin level that meets the requirements for an exchange transfusion is at risk for hearing deficits and must be screened for this before discharge.

Pathophysiology

Bilirubin is the end product of the breakdown of heme, a substrate of hemoglobin. It is released into the blood stream as red blood cells are broken down. Neonates produce bilirubin at more than twice the rate of the adult, about 8 mg/kg/day (Tan, 1991). This large bilirubin production is due to a short red blood cell life span and higher circulating red blood cell volume. Neonates have a higher number of circulating red blood cells, owing in part to the naturally occurring hypoxic intrauterine environment.

In utero, bilirubin produced by the fetus crosses the placenta to maternal circulation and is excreted by the maternal liver. After delivery, the neonate begins to build up levels that exceed the capacity of the neonatal liver to excrete the bilirubin (the neonate's liver has the ability to excrete approximately two thirds of the circulating bilirubin). After the red blood cell has been broken down and the bilirubin is released into the blood stream, it is bound to albumin in the plasma. Once all the albumin-binding sites are saturated, bilirubin circulates freely in the plasma. This freely circulating bilirubin has a high affinity for fatty tissue such as brain tissue and can cause serious neurologic sequelae if allowed to remain at high levels.

After the bilirubin reaches the liver, it is transferred from the albumin to the liver cell. In the liver, the bilirubin is transformed in the presence of the enzyme glucuronyl transferase and conjugated for excretion into bile. The majority of the bilirubin, approximately 95%, is excreted into bile. The bile is secreted into the intestine, and the bilirubin is expelled through the stool. Neonates may have delayed intestinal motility coupled with poor fluid intake that leads to decreased urine and stool output and delayed bilirubin excretion. In this situation, the bilirubin in the stool is reabsorbed through the intestine, causing higher levels of circulating bilirubin.

There are two types of bilirubin: conjugated and unconjugated. Unconjugated bilirubin has not been converted in the liver and is fat soluble. Fat-soluble bilirubin has a high affinity for extravascular tissue, including fatty tissue and brain. Conjugated bilirubin has been conjugated in the liver and is water soluble and easily excreted in the biliary tree.

The neonate's liver is immature, and the large amount of bilirubin that is produced and cannot be excreted is deposited in the skin, producing jaundice. This accounts for the jaundice occurring in healthy term neonates after 24 hours of life and is a common identified problem during the neonatal nursery stay or in the postnatal home visit.

Assessment

As described earlier, jaundice is the first clinical manifestation seen in neonates with elevated bilirubin levels. Noting the onset of clinical jaundice is important because the appearance of jaundice before the first 24 hours of life is abnormal and may indicate a hemolytic process, sepsis, or other abnormal condition requiring prompt intervention.

The blood types of the mother and neonate are assessed to determine if risk factors for the development of jaundice are present. Additionally, the obstetric history is helpful to determine if the delivery was complicated or traumatic.

Inspection of the neonate is the most effective determination of jaundice, along with blood studies including total and direct bilirubin, Coombs' tests, and blood grouping. Visible jaundice tends to progress from the face downward. Guidelines to use when estimating the extent of involvement of jaundice are as follows:

- Light jaundice: appears on the face
- Slightly higher jaundice: appears on face, trunk, abdomen
- Hyperbilirubinemia: visible orange color extending to the thighs or the entire abdomen. Once visible jaundice appears, a blood sample is sent to the laboratory for serum bilirubin determination and further follow-up is indicated.

caREminder: *The accepted upper limit of physiologic jaundice in the healthy term neonate with no high-risk factors is 15 mg/dL on the third day of life (Wilkerson, 1989).*

The term newborn's serum bilirubin levels peak at the fifth postnatal day. Neonates who have elevated levels that increase greater than 5 mg/dL/day are at high risk for treatment of hyperbilirubinemia.

The nurse assesses the neonate's liver size, presence of bruises or petechiae, and level of activity. Neonates with a hemolytic process often have hepatosplenomegaly. Neonates with hyperbilirubinemia may have excessive extravascular blood or bruising. High levels of bilirubin may lead to lethargy and decreased tone.

Close observation of the neonate's intake and amount of weight loss is also an important assessment component. A neonate who feeds poorly at the breast or is disinterested in feeding after 24 hours is at risk for developing hyperbilirubinemia. Neonates often lose weight during the first week of life, but excessive weight loss (more than 10%) may indicate dehydration, which hemoconcentrates the blood, leading to an elevated serum bilirubin level.

Anemia is rare in neonates with physiologic jaundice but may occur in hemolytic jaundice. Neonates who appear pale should have screening hemoglobin assessment. Other clinical signs of anemia include tachycardia and hypotension.

Neonates with a high unconjugated or indirect bilirubin level often have a hemolytic or physiologic process. In contrast, those neonates with an elevated conjugated or direct bilirubin have an obstructive jaundice, such as with biliary atresia. Neonates with direct hyperbilirubinemia have a dark yellow color rather than the lighter yellow color of physiologic jaundice.

Neonates born severely affected by Rh incompatibility may present with erythroblastosis fetalis, which is so named chiefly owing to the presence of immature circulating red blood cells (erythroblasts) in the blood of the fetus (see Chapter 23). Erythroblasts appear owing to the rapid occurrence of anemia and the body's attempt to increase production of red blood cells, producing more immature red blood cells. These neonates are severely ill, with hepatosplenomegaly, congestive heart failure, and severe generalized edema (hydrops fetalis), including pleural effusions and ascites.

Nursing Diagnoses and Outcomes

Nursing diagnoses and outcomes generally applicable for neonates with a health challenge are listed in Chart 14–3. In addition to these and those discussed with hemolytic disease of the newborn in Chapter 23, the following may be applicable to a neonate with jaundice or hyperbilirubinemia:

- ▶ **Risk for impaired skin integrity related to dryness of skin and phototherapy rash**
  Outcome: The neonate will maintain intact skin.
- ▶ **Fluid volume deficit related to increased insensible water loss from phototherapy, poor feeding, and lethargy**
  Outcomes: The neonate will ingest fluid to meet needs. The neonate will remain normovolemic during phototherapy.

Interdisciplinary Interventions

Acute assessment skills are vital to initiate early treatment for jaundice. As discussed earlier, jaundice appearing after the first 24 hours of life in a healthy term newborn is physiologic jaundice and often requires no treatment. The nurse must monitor feeding behavior and number of wet diapers to ensure adequate intake. Daily total and direct bilirubin levels may be ordered by the physician if jaundice continues to increase. Increasing lethargy, poor feeding, and decreasing output are all signs of worsening jaundice and require evaluation by a physician or nurse practitioner (Care Path 14–2). Hyperbiliru-

Care Path 14–2 An Interdisciplinary Plan of Care for the Child with Hyperbilirubinemia

Nursing Diagnosis	Patient/Family Intermediate Outcomes			
	Admission	Day 1	Day 2	Days 3–4
Risk for impaired skin integrity related to phototherapy	Infant will have little/minimal skin breakdown	→	→	→
Fluid volume deficit related to increased insensible water loss and lethargy water-loss stools	Infant will have normovolemic state and/or limited s/s of dehydration.	Infant will have normal electrolytes and results of a physical examination consistent with normovolemia.	→	→
Impaired thermoregulation related to phototherapy	Infant will experience a temperature within normal limits in an isolette	→	Infant will maintain normal temperature in room air	→
Altered nutrition less than body requirements related to lethargy	Infant will be supported with gavage feedings and/or IV feedings until nippling.	→	Infant will nipple all feedings and receive 80–120 kcal/kg/day.	→
Care Intervention Categories				
Consults	Clinical social work as indicated	Consider hematology if hemoglobin falls <7.		
Discharge planning			Consider home phototherapy if adequate feeding is established and there are no other illnesses.	Begin teaching of medications, signs and symptoms of dehydration and jaundice, and use of home medical equipment
Labs (septic work-up if risk factors present)	Monitor bilirubin levels q 12hrs. Obtain mother and newborn blood type to determine set-up. Obtain baseline electrolyte levels if dehydrated.	Follow bilirubin levels. Determine rate of water-loss stools; strict intake and output.	Continue daily bilirubin testing.	→

binemia is treated with sunlight when levels are mildly elevated, phototherapy, exchange transfusions, or medications.

Phototherapy. Phototherapy is indicated in healthy term neonates if the indirect bilirubin levels are ≥18 to 20 mg/dL by the second day of life (Behrman et al., 1996) (Chart 14–11). Using a range of bilirubin levels rather than an absolute number allows the clinician to

Care Path 14–2 An Interdisciplinary Plan of Care for the Child with Hyperbilirubinemia *Continued*

Care Intervention Categories	Admission	Day 1	Day 2	Days 3–4
Medications and IVs	IV fluids if unable to nipple or take enough to meet fluid requirements.	Wean IV and increase PO feeding.	→ Full PO feeds.	→
Nutrition	Encourage feeding if no other problems and no RDS.	Increase calories and volume as tolerated.	→	→
Safety and activity	No oils/lotion on skin	→	→	→
	Cover eyes while under lights.	→	→	→
		Maintain under light as much as possible; take out for feedings	→	→
	Check bilimeter q 12 hr.	→	→	→
	Check eyes with each feeding.	→	→	→
Special considerations	Watch skin for breakdown from bilistools; no oils/lotions to skin	Complete physical assessment		
Teaching	Encourage visitation. Orient to environment and equipment in use. Teach breast milk pumping and storage.	Begin disease process education.	Begin jaundice teaching and treatment. Educate when to call physician. Begin pushing feedings.	Begin home medical equipment teaching if home on phototherapy.
Visitors	Open visitation for parents	→	→	→
Vital signs/ baseline parameters	VS every feeding (q 3–4 hr) Daily weights Baseline parameters with VS Cardiorespiratory monitor if indicated			

RDS, respiratory distress syndrome; VS, vital signs.

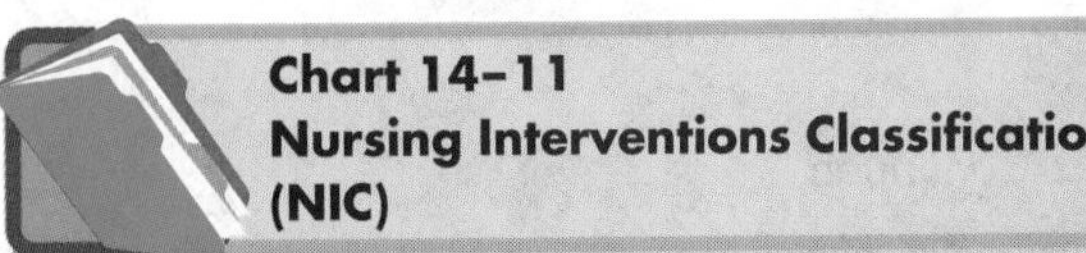

Chart 14–11
Nursing Interventions Classification (NIC)

Phototherapy

Definition

Use of light therapy to reduce bilirubin levels in newborn infants

Activities

Review maternal and infant history for risk factors for hyperbilirubinemia (e.g., Rh or ABO incompatibility, polycythemia, sepsis, prematurity, and malpresentation).
Observe for signs of jaundice.
Order serum bilirubin levels, as appropriate, per protocol or primary practitioner request.
Report lab values to primary practitioner.
Place infant in isolette.
Instruct family on phototherapy procedures and care.
Apply patches to cover both eyes, avoiding excessive pressure.
Remove eye patches every 4 hr or when lights are off for parental contact and feeding.
Place phototherapy lights above infant at appropriate height.
Check intensity of lights daily.
Monitor vital signs, per protocol or as needed.
Change infant position every 4 hr or per protocol.
Monitor serum bilirubin levels, per protocol or practitioner request.
Evaluate neurological status every 4 hr or per protocol.
Observe for signs of dehydration (e.g., depressed fontanels, poor skin turgor, and loss of weight).
Weigh daily.
Encourage eight feedings per day.
Encourage family to participate in light therapy.
Instruct family on home phototherapy, as appropriate.

From McCloskey, J. C., & Bulechek, G. M. (1996). *Nursing interventions classification (NIC)* (2nd ed.). St. Louis: Mosby–Year Book. Reprinted with permission.

assess many clinical variables of each neonate. For example, a neonate with severe bruising from a traumatic delivery who is not breast-feeding well may need phototherapy initiated at the lower range. In contrast, a healthy vigorous breast-feeding newborn may not need phototherapy for hyperbilirubinemia until the higher levels are achieved. This approach has evolved from the research findings, indicating that healthy term neonates have a low risk of developing kernicterus at bilirubin levels less than 20 mg/dL (Tan, 1991).

Phototherapy works by converting bilirubin in the skin to a water-soluble form that can be excreted by the liver without conjugation (Wilkerson, 1989). It is initiated for any form of unconjugated hyperbilirubinemia and can be used in conjunction with other treatments such as exchange transfusion. Phototherapy is most effective in treating slowly developing hyperbilirubinemia and is an adjunct treatment for the more rapidly rising forms of hyperbilirubinemia, such as those caused from hemolytic processes (Tan, 1991).

White, blue, and green lights can be used to deliver phototherapy. Only light of certain wavelengths can be absorbed by bilirubin. The differences between the colored lights is the spectral band each one emits. The blue lights have been shown to be more effective in photodegradation, owing to the narrow spectral band emitted (Tan, 1989). Although more effective, the special blue lights may cause headaches in health care workers. Additionally, they may hinder observing the neonate's color because the blue hue emitted is deceiving. There have been no known hazards or complaints noted with the other colored lights.

Phototherapy is delivered by placing the neonate unclothed underneath the phototherapy lights to allow exposure of skin to the light. To improve efficiency of the treatment, as much of the skin should be exposed to the light as possible. Additionally, the neonate must be exposed to the light as much as possible. Diapering the neonate may be needed to contain urine and stool. This diapering serves also to protect the reproductive organs because the side effects of phototherapy on these organs is unknown.

Phototherapy lights can be used in the home setting with select neonates and their parents. Also available is the BiliBlanket (Ohmeda), which is easier to manage both in the hospital and home setting. The BiliBlanket is a bank of phototherapy lights that is flexible and is wrapped around the neonate much like a blanket. Studies have demonstrated that a fiberoptic device such as the phototherapy blanket is as effective and safe as conventional phototherapy (Gale, Dranitzki, Dollbery, & Stevenson, 1991; Rosenfeld, Tuest, & Concepcion, 1991).

The advantage to the fiberoptic blanket is that the overall body is exposed to the phototherapy during normal caregiving activities such as feeding, holding, and sleeping. There is no need to protect the eyes unless the face is directly next to the light. Additionally, the fiberoptic blanket is easily managed in the home or in the mother's hospital room (Fig. 14–12; see Figs. 23–13 and 23–14).

Before initiating home phototherapy, whether the fiberoptic blanket or the traditional bank of lights is used, the neonate and the parents must be assessed as to the appropriateness of home treatment. The ideal candidate is a healthy and full-term neonate with no other underly-

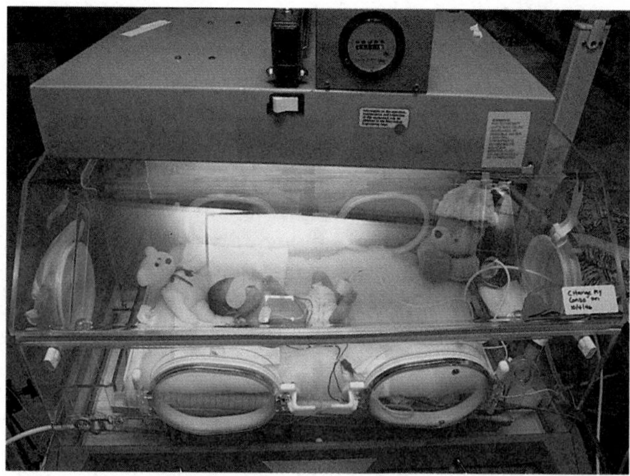

Figure 14–12
It is important to protect the infant's eyes and maintain a normal temperature in an infant undergoing phototherapy.

ing disease or problems who has a well-established feeding pattern. The parents must be willing and able to provide the phototherapy treatment and to carefully monitor the color of the neonate's skin, feeding vigor, and activity. Detailed parent training and education is a must for home phototherapy to be successful (see Chart 23–24).

During phototherapy, the neonate's eyes must be covered to prevent microscopic injury to retinal cells. Eye patches or phototherapy masks are applied and secured at the initiation of phototherapy and kept in place at all times while the neonate is under phototherapy to protect the eyes from damage. When properly applied, the mask covers the eyes and does not occlude the nares.

Alert: *Check the position of the phototherapy mask frequently to ensure it has not shifted and obstructs the nares. Also ensure that excess pressure is not applied across the nose in positioning the mask.*

During feedings, the lights are turned off and the eye patches removed to provide stimulation and to allow the caregiver to inspect the eyes for drainage or edema.

Metabolic rate and insensible water loss are both increased during phototherapy (Tan, 1991). Metabolic rate changes may be due to hyperthermia, which is a common problem for neonates because the phototherapy lights emit heat. Neonates require increased calories to balance this metabolic rate and to assist with the elimination of bilirubin through the intestinal tract.

Frequent feedings are also essential to prevent dehydration. Dehydration is common in neonates who have poorly established feeding patterns and lethargy. High bilirubin levels tend to make the neonate listless and lethargic, leading to poor feeding. Also, water loss stools, commonly referred to as "bili stools," may occur as a result of photodegradation of bilirubin. Breast-feeding or bottle-feeding should be increased during treatment to offset both calorie loss and dehydration.

Skin care is essential for the neonate undergoing phototherapy because the frequent water loss stools in combination with dry skin can lead to skin breakdown. Frequent diaper changes and position changes may prevent breakdown of the skin. It is also common for the neonate to develop a rash while under phototherapy similar to a heat rash. It requires no treatment and often resolves with discontinuation of the phototherapy treatment.

Avoiding application of lotions or baby oils to the skin during phototherapy treatment is an important nursing intervention. Applying lotion to the skin leads to excessive skin redness and burns. Reinforcement of this to the parents is also important.

It is the nurse's responsibility to ensure that the phototherapy light is not too close or too far away from the neonate. The light must be no closer to the newborn than 18 cm and not more than 30 to 40 cm away. The nurse measures the distance at least once per shift and at every home visit. The luminosity intensity of the light must also be measured at least once per shift. This is done by using a phototherapy meter placed at the level of the neonate while he or she is undergoing phototherapy. The purpose of measuring the intensity is to ensure a minimum level of microwatts emitted from the lights. If the level is too low, the lights must be replaced or a new phototherapy unit obtained to ensure maximum therapy. Usually, a measurement of 10 to 12 $\mu W/cm^2$ exposed to the skin surface is effective.

The neonate's temperature must also be monitored closely, because hyperthermia is not uncommon. Hypothermia may also be a problem if the room has drafts, leading to convective heat loss. Axillary temperatures are performed regularly on neonates under phototherapy.

Neonates with a high direct bilirubin level (exceeding 2.0 mg/dL) should not receive phototherapy. A high direct hyperbilirubinemia is associated with liver disease, such as neonatal hepatitis or congenital obstructive jaundice. Although conjugated bilirubin is generally not toxic to the neonate's CNS, it must be evaluated carefully. "Bronze baby" syndrome occurs when direct bilirubin is exposed to phototherapy, producing a gray-brown discoloration of the skin and darkening of both serum and urine.

Exchange Transfusion and Medications. If phototherapy is ineffective in resolving the hyperbilirubinemia and the level continues to rise approaching levels at which kernicterus may occur, more drastic interventions, such as exchange transfusion or medications, may be required (see Chapter 23). Exchange transfusion involves the removal of the neonate's blood and replacement with new blood. This procedure is rarely done for neonates with physiologic jaundice and is most commonly used for severe hemolytic processes involving intractable anemia.

Administration of phenobarbital assists to increase the hepatocyte microsomal enzyme glucuronyl transferase. This will stimulate the rate of bilirubin excretion.

Community Care

With mothers and neonates discharged from the hospital within 12 hours of delivery, it is imperative that parents know how to assess jaundice. Nurses are the primary educators of parents with neonates and are in a pivotal role to provide vital information related to general neonatal care. Discharge teaching related to jaundice includes an explanation of (1) jaundice and its common signs and symptoms, (2) how to evaluate feeding and output quantities, (3) how to monitor for changes in activity level and skin color, and (4) when to call the physician.

The parents are taught how to assess the jaundice in their neonate's skin by focusing on the progression of jaundice, which begins in the face and moves to the abdomen and lower extremities. They are taught to monitor the number of wet diapers per day to assist in evaluating adequate intake. Also, the nurse stresses the importance of noting the neonate's activity, because increasing jaundice leads to lethargy and poor feeding. Finally, the use of indirect sunlight through a window assists to decrease jaundice because it works to photodegrade bilirubin from the skin much like phototherapy.

Neonatal Hypoglycemia

The brain is glucose dependent and must have a continual supply of glucose to function properly. Newborns who use up energy supplies for temperature regulation are at higher risk than older people who have physiologic pathways for gluconeogenesis firmly established for hypoglycemic events.

Hypoglycemia in the neonatal period is a significant problem, occurring in approximately 4 per 1000 live births (Denne & Kalhan, 1986). Hypoglycemia is defined as a blood glucose value less than 40 mg/dL in the term and preterm newborn (Brooks, 1997).

Alert: *Serious consequences of hypoglycemia include brain damage resulting in developmental delay and learning disabilities (Sann, 1990). Prompt assessment of neonates with risk factors can prevent such complications.*

Neonates with symptomatic and recurrent hypoglycemia are more likely to have long-term sequelae than those neonates who are asymptomatic (Sann, 1990). However, transient hypoglycemia is the most common type in the neonatal period. This type is of short duration and rarely recurs (Baird, 1996).

The fetus receives a continuous supply of glucose from the placenta. During the third trimester, the fetus begins to store energy in preparation for delivery and the first few hours after birth. At delivery, the maternal supply of glucose ceases and the neonate initiates glycolysis, glycogenolysis, and gluconeogenesis. These processes mobilize liver glycogen to maintain normal serum glucose levels. Glucose values decrease rapidly after birth and stabilize by 3 to 4 hours of life. At this time, enteral feedings (breast-feeding or formula) must be initiated to maintain normal glucose values.

Neonates at risk for hypoglycemia include those with decreased substrate, endocrine disorders, and increased utilization of glucose. Other causes of hypoglycemia include sepsis and congenital heart disease. Finally, specific procedures may induce hypoglycemia such as exchange transfusion. Hypoglycemia is common in the SGA and premature neonate owing to the decreased amounts of available substrate, rapid utilization of glucose, and the instability of glucose metabolism (Holtrop, 1993). It is estimated that transient hypoglycemia develops in 40% to 50% of all SGA neonates (Haymond, 1989). Endocrine disorders that induce hypoglycemia through a hyperinsulinemia process include those affecting neonates of diabetic mothers, Beckwith-Wiedemann syndrome, and nesidioblastosis. Increased utilization of glucose occurs in neonates with sepsis, perinatal asphyxia, and hypothermia.

Assessment

Most normal neonatal nurseries and NICUs have specific protocols for screening high-risk neonates for hypoglycemia. SGA and LGA neonates and those of diabetic mothers should all receive a screening bedside glucose evaluation shortly after birth and then at regular intervals. Signs and symptoms of hypoglycemia are nonspecific and variable. The most common and classic symptoms are as follows:

- High-pitched cry
- Apnea
- Cyanosis
- Irritability
- Lethargy
- Respiratory distress
- Hypotonia
- Pallor
- Seizures
- Tremulousness

Many of the signs and symptoms mimic other diseases, such as sepsis. Because of the lack of obvious symptoms in some infants, the nurse must maintain a high index of suspicion of hypoglycemia based on history or presence of subtle signs.

The prognosis is related to the duration and severity

of the hypoglycemia as well as to the underlying cause. Major long-term sequelae of severe, prolonged hypoglycemia are neurologic, including mental retardation and cerebral atrophy.

Interdisciplinary Interventions

Nursing interventions include prevention of hypoglycemia and early identification of neonates at risk. Neonates at risk may be fed early either at the breast or with formula. If the newborn is unable to feed well or is in respiratory distress, intravenous therapy is initiated to maintain normal glucose levels. In severe cases of refractory hypoglycemia, corticosteroids may be administered either intravenously or intramuscularly. Corticosteroids such as hydrocortisone are used to decrease peripheral glucose utilization and increase gluconeogenesis.

Neonates treated for hypoglycemia should have bedside glucose measurements taken every 30 minutes until stable values are achieved and then every hour for 3 hours to ensure stability. The nurse should assess for the presence of symptoms of hypoglycemia, as mentioned earlier.

Meconium Aspiration

Meconium aspiration is a condition in which the infant, either before or during the birth process, passes its first meconium stool and sucks the material into the respiratory tract with some of its first breaths. Meconium is a very viscous, sticky forest-green liquid that consists of gastrointestinal secretions, bile acids, salts, mucus, pancreatic juice, cellular debris, amniotic fluid and swallowed vernix caseosa, lanugo, and blood. The substance can first be found in the fetal gastrointestinal tract as early as the 16th week of gestation.

Meconium staining of the amniotic fluid (indicating that the substance was passed before birth) is seen in 10% to 15% of all deliveries (Co & Vidyasagar, 1990). About 5% of these neonates will develop meconium aspiration syndrome (MAS). The clinical picture includes radiographic findings and respiratory distress in the infant whose symptoms cannot otherwise be explained (Wiswell & Bent, 1993). The most widely accepted theory regarding the reason for the passage of meconium into the amniotic fluid is related to relaxation of the anal sphincter during an episode of fetal hypoxia. In response to intrauterine asphyxia, insufficient oxygen transported to the fetal intestine is followed by relaxation of anal sphincter tone and evacuation of meconium. Passage of meconium may, however, also represent a maturational event in that it is rare before 37 weeks' gestation but may occur in 35% or more of pregnancies lasting longer than 42 weeks (Eden, Seifert, & Winegar, 1987).

Pathophysiology

Regardless of the cause, when meconium is passed into the amniotic fluid it then can be aspirated into the lungs, creating many mechanical and physiologic changes. The degree of severity of the condition at times is related to the viscosity of the meconium, which is usually described as thick, moderate, or thin. A large amount of thick meconium could rapidly cause complete obstruction of the upper airways with associated hypoxia, hypercapnia, and acidosis. More commonly, diffuse particles of meconium migrate to smaller peripheral airways. Partial or complete mechanical obstruction results in air trapping, atelectasis, overdistended or hyperexpanded regions, and possible pneumothoraces. This is due to a ball/valve effect in which air is allowed into the lung but obstructed from exiting.

Chemical inflammation and/or infection in the lower airways is also seen in this syndrome. Ventilation-perfusion mismatches ensue, creating hypoxia and acidosis. These factors produce pulmonary vasoconstriction, resulting in persistent pulmonary hypertension of the newborn.

Historically, the diagnosis of meconium aspiration held connotations of high morbidity and mortality, especially related to poor neurologic outcomes. The majority of infants with meconium-stained amniotic fluid suffer little or no pulmonary sequelae. Of the infants who develop MAS, approximately 30% require mechanical ventilation and 4% die (Wiswell & Bent, 1993). Cerebral palsy has been implicated in some cases of as a possible sequela of meconium staining and aspiration. Insufficient data exist to prove or refute this contention. Anoxic encephalopathy is an uncommon but tragic outcome in some instances of meconium aspiration.

Prognosis. Several reports have documented abnormal long-term pulmonary function among children who had MAS as newborns (MacFarlane & Heaf, 1988; Swaminathan, Quinn, & Stabile, 1989). The most common abnormalities noted were spontaneous wheezing and exercise-induced bronchospasm, suggesting small airway injury and disease. Bronchopulmonary dysplasia may occur when a prolonged period of mechanical ventilation is required. When severe MAS is accompanied by persistent pulmonary hypertension of the newborn, it is usually associated with a higher mortality rate.

Assessment

Neonates with MAS are often term, post mature, or SGA (Co & Vidyasagar, 1990). Symptoms range from mild respiratory distress to severe hypoxemia and respiratory failure. Infants with minimal meconium aspiration characteristically present with tachypnea and mild cyanosis. Those with more severe MAS have marked respiratory distress with cyanosis, irregular or gasping respirations, grunting, and intercostal and substernal retractions. The chest is typically hyperinflated, with increased anteroposterior diameter of the thoracic cage (Co & Vidyasagar, 1990). Arterial blood gas values show evidence of severe hypoxemia, hypercapnia, and combined respiratory and metabolic acidosis. Lung sounds may be diminished.

As in other diagnoses involving illness in the newborn, the psychosocial/emotional manifestations in parents and family members include shock, fear, anxiety, and grief over the loss of the expected "perfect" or "normal" infant. Mothers especially require sensitivity and honest, supportive communication regarding the infant's prognosis because they are undergoing fatigue, pain, and hormonal fluctuations immediately after childbirth.

Nursing Diagnoses and Outcomes

In addition to the nursing diagnoses discussed in Chart 14–3, the following are applicable to the neonate with MAS:

- **Ineffective airway clearance related to effects of meconium in lungs**
  Outcome: Neonate will maintain patent airway.
- **Impaired gas exchange related to effects of altered ventilation and perfusion of lungs**
  Outcome: Neonate will maintain oxygen saturation of at least 92%.

Interdisciplinary Interventions

The infant with meconium-stained amniotic fluid or MAS should be provided with the optimal ventilatory support, based on accurate respiratory assessment. Milder cases often require endotracheal suctioning at birth, supplemental oxygen, possible antibiotic therapy, and supportive care. Aggressive postpartum suctioning and airway management have decreased the incidence and severity of MAS (Wiswell & Bent, 1993).

The nurse monitors for development of pneumothorax and deterioration. Signs and symptoms include bradycardia, hypotension, carbon dioxide retention, and hypoxemia. When this happens, the air source is immediately removed.

Infants with severe MAS who develop respiratory distress in the delivery room are intubated, suctioned, ventilated with a resuscitation bag and 100% oxygen, and admitted immediately to an NICU where they are placed on mechanically assisted ventilation. The reader should refer to a neonatal critical care or maternity text for techniques of neonatal resuscitation at the delivery of an infant. Nutritional support and pharmacologic therapy are provided, as well as aggressive chest physiotherapy (with evaluation for low platelet counts to prevent ecchymosis) if breath sounds are coarse or a chest radiograph reveals patchy, irregular infiltrates suggestive of MAS (Co & Vidyasagar, 1990). The high-frequency oscillatory ventilator is useful in treating severe MAS.

If there is no medical response to the high-frequency oscillatory ventilator, surfactant therapy, and/or vasodilators, the infant is referred to a center where extracorporeal membrane oxygenation (ECMO) is available. ECMO is a highly invasive therapy involving temporary cardiopulmonary bypass (Fig. 14–13). It is generally used when infants have not responded to more conservative management and are at high risk of death. The goal of ECMO therapy is to allow the lung disease to improve over a period of days by giving the lungs a "rest." ECMO therapy carries many potential complications, such as alterations in cerebral blood flow. The survival rate of ECMO therapy is approximately 85% (Wiswell & Bent, 1993).

ECMO therapy for MAS is very expensive, both financially and emotionally. Intensive nursing care (sometimes with a 2:1 or greater ratio of specialized pump technicians and nursing staff to one infant) is needed as well as specific technological requirements. Care of the infant on ECMO therapy is similar to care of the infant undergoing cardiopulmonary bypass surgery for congenital heart defects. It is beyond the scope of this chapter to discuss such care in depth; the reader is referred to texts concerning pediatric critical care for further information.

Social service and other counseling interventions are imperative for family support. Because tertiary centers are often located many miles away from homes and the usual support systems, assistance with securing food, transportation, lodging, and resources for sibling care is required.

Figure 14–13
Extracorporeal membrane oxygenation (ECMO) is a highly invasive therapy involving temporary cardiopulmonary bypass.

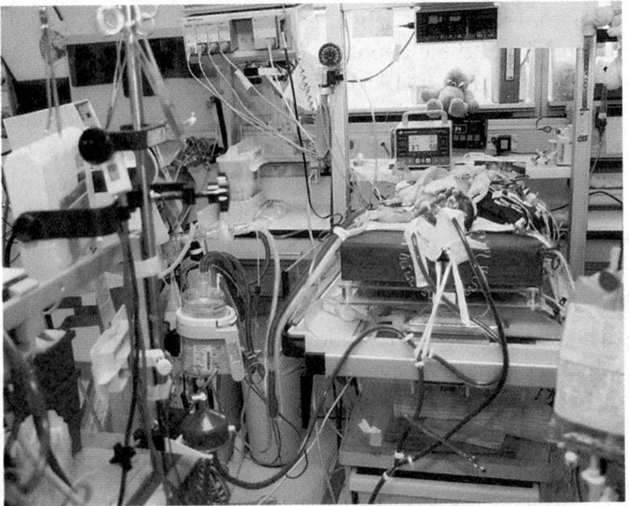

Summary of Key Concepts

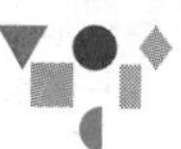

- The neonatal period is a vulnerable time in the life cycle in which the body systems are adapting to the extrauterine environment. The high-risk neonate faces many challenges during this adaptive phase.
- The premature neonate faces many challenges as the various body systems mature in the extrauterine environment. All body systems of the premature neonate are immature, and supportive interventions are applied to promote optimal growth and development.
- Intrauterine drug exposure may lead to premature labor and birth, undergrown neonates, and congenital anomalies. Specialized nursing interventions are needed to assist these neonates in developing and growing normally and to support the family.
- Birth injuries include soft tissue injury, extracranial hemorrhages, fractures, and peripheral nerve injury. They add additional challenges to the neonate's transition efforts. Many injuries resolve without complications but may cause long-term neurologic sequelae.
- Perinatal asphyxia can be a devastating condition leading to long-term neurologic deficits. Effective neonatal resuscitation and other treatments are initiated to correct the acidosis and hypoxemia.
- Infants of diabetic mothers face challenges including congenital anomalies, birth trauma, and postnatal hypoglycemia. Close monitoring of the neonate during the postnatal period is vital to identify birth trauma and hypoglycemia and provide early interventions.
- Jaundice is a common finding in the first few days after birth. Hyperbilirubinemia is a condition in which the bilirubin levels become elevated and treatment is necessary. Education of the family to monitor for increasing jaundice at home is an important nursing intervention.
- Hypoglycemia may occur during the neonatal period as a result of many physiologic processes. Additionally, specific high-risk conditions increase the chance of the occurrence of hypoglycemia. Monitoring for signs and symptoms of hypoglycemia is an important nursing intervention to ensure prompt treatment is initiated.
- Aspiration of meconium-stained amniotic fluid at the delivery process may result in a severe and life-threatening chemical pneumonia if left untreated. Treatment consists of intubation and visualization of the vocal cords as soon as possible after birth. Vigorous removal by suctioning is done to prevent meconium from being sucked farther into the tracheobronchial tree.

Resources

Organizations

Association of Women's Health, Obstetric and Neonatal Nurses (AWHONN)
700 14th Street NW, Suite 600
Washington, DC 20005-2019
(202) 662-1600

Be Healthy, Inc.
Positive Pregnancy and Parenting Fitness
51 Saltrock Road
Baltic, CT 06330
(800) 433-5523

La Leche League International
P.O. Box 1209
Franklin Park, IL 60131-8209
(800) 525-3243

National Association of Neonatal Nurses
1304 Southpoint Boulevard, Suite 280
Petaluma, CA 94954-6859
(800) 451-3795

National Cocaine Hotline
P.O. Box 100
Summit, NJ 07902-0100
(800) 262-2463

National Council on Alcoholism and Drug Dependence Hopeline
12 West 21st Street, Suite 700
New York, NY 10010
(800) NCA-CALL (622-2255)

National Information Clearinghouse for Infants with Disabilities and Life-Threatening Conditions

NICU Ink Book Publishers

The Annual Review of Research for Neonatal Nurses
1304 Southpoint Boulevard, Suite 280
Petaluma, CA 94954-6861
(707) 762-2646

Sudden Infant Death Syndrome Alliance
10500 Little Patuxent Parkway, Suite 420
Columbia, MD 21044
(800) 221-SIDS (7437)

Books and Printed Materials

Shelov, S. P., & Hannemann, R. E. (1993). *The American Academy of Pediatrics—Caring for Your Baby and Young Child Birth to Age Five—the Authoritative Guide*. New York: Bantam.

Guidelines/Position Statements

Early Discharge of the High Risk Neonate Position Statement. (1997). National Association of Neonatal Nurses.

Infant Developmental Care Guidelines. (1993). National Association of Neonatal Nurses.

Neonatal Follow-up Care of the High Risk Neonate: Position Statement. (1997). National Association of Neonatal Nurses.

Newborn Discharge and Follow-up Care: Position Statement. (1997). National Association of Pediatric Nurse Associates and Practitioners.

Video

American Academy of Pediatrics (1988). *Baby Alive—Emergency Treatment—Accident Prevention*. Action Films and Video, Ltd.

References

Abel, E. (1995). An update on incidence of FAS: FAS is not an equal opportunity birth defect. *Neurotoxicology and Teratology, 17*(4), 437–443.

Als, H., Duffy, F., & McAnulty, G. (1988). Behavioral differences between preterm and full term neonates as measured on the APIB system scores. *Newborn Behavior and Development, 11*, 305–318.

Als, H., Lawhon, G., Duffy, F., McAnulty, G., Gibes-Grossman, R., & Blickman, J. (1994). Individualized developmental care for the very low birth weight preterm infant: Medical and neurofunctional effects. JAMA, *272*(11), 853–858.

American Academy of Pediatrics. (1994). *Report of the Committee on Infectious Diseases: The red book*. Elk Grove Village, IL: Author.

Appelbaum, M. (1995). Fetal alcohol syndrome: Diagnosis, management, and prevention. *Nurse Practitioner, 20*(10), 27–31.

Baird, P. B. (1996). Neonatal glucose screening. *Neonatal Network, 15*(7), 63–66.

Ballard, J. L., Khourg, J. C., Wedig, K., Way, L., Eilers-Watsman, B., & Lipp, R. (1991). New Ballard score expanded to include extremely premature neonates. *Journal of Pediatrics, 119*, 417–423.

Baxter, A., Butler, L. S., Brinker, R. P., Frazier, W. A., & Wedgeworth, D. M. (1995). Effective early intervention for children prenatally exposed to cocaine in an inner-city context. In M. Lewis & M. Bendersky (Eds.), *Mothers, babies, and cocaine*. Hillsdale, NJ: Lawrence Erlbaum Associations.

Behrman, R. E., Kliegman, R. M., & Arvin, A. M. (Eds.). (1996). *Nelson textbook of pediatrics* (15th ed.). Philadelphia: W. B. Saunders.

Bendich, A. (1993). Lifestyle and environmental factors that can adversely affect maternal nutritional status and pregnancy outcomes. *Annals of New York Academy of Sciences, 678*, 255–263.

Blackburn, S. (1995). Hyperbilirubinemia and neonatal jaundice. *Neonatal Network, 14*(7), 15–25.

Bloom, R. S., & Cropley, C. (1995). *Textbook of neonatal resuscitation*. Elk Grove Village, IL: American Academy of Pediatrics/American Heart Association.

Boobis, S., & Sullivan, F. (1986). Effects of life-style on reproduction. In S. Fabro & A. Scialli (Eds.), *Drug and chemical action in pregnancy: Pharmacologic and toxicologic principles* (pp. 373–425). New York: Marcel Dekker.

Brazelton, T. (1984). *Neonatal behavioral assessment scale* (2nd ed.). Philadelphia: J. B. Lippincott.

Brooks, C. (1997). Neonatal hypoglycemia. *Neonatal Network, 16*(2), 15–21.

Carta, J. J., Sideridis, G., Rinkel, P., Guimaraes, S., Greenwood, C., Baggett, K., Peterson, P., & Atwater, J. (1994). Behavioral outcomes of young children prenatally exposed to illicit drugs: Review and analysis of experimental literature. *Topics in Early Childhood Special Education, 14*, 184–216.

Chasnoff, I. (1988). Drug use in pregnancy: Parameters of risk. *Pediatric Clinics of North America, 35*(6), 1403–1411.

Chasnoff, I., Chisum, G., & Kaplan, W. (1988). Maternal cocaine use and genitourinary tract malformations. *Teratology, 37*, 201–204.

Chasnoff, I., Hatcher, R., & Burns, W. (1986). Prenatal drug exposure: Effects on neonatal growth and development. *Neurobehavioral Toxicology and Teratology, 8*, 351–362.

Chasnoff, I., Hunt, C., & Kletter, R. (1989). Prenatal cocaine exposure is associated with respiratory pattern abnormalities. *American Journal of Diseases in Children, 143*, 583–587.

Chasnoff, I., Landress, H., & Barnett, M. (1990). The prevalence of illicit drug or alcohol use during pregnancy. *New England Journal of Medicine, 322*, 1202–1206.

Clark, D., & Hakanson, D. (1988). The inaccuracy of Apgar scoring. *Journal of Perinatology, 8*, 203–208.

Co, E., & Vidyasagar, D. (1990). Meconium aspiration syndrome. *Comprehensive Therapy, 16*(10), 34–49.

Collins, E. (1989). Perinatal cocaine intoxication. *Medical Journal of Australia, 150*, 331–333.

Cutz, E., Perrin, D., Hackman, R., & Czegledy-Nagy, E. (1996). Maternal smoking and pulmonary neuroendocrine cells in sudden infant death syndrome. *Pediatrics*, 98(4), 668–672.

Czyrko, C., Del Pin, C., O'Neil, J., Peckham, G., & Ross, A. (1991). Maternal cocaine abuse and necrotizing enterocolitis: Outcome and survival. *Journal of Pediatric Surgery, 26*(4), 414–421.

Delaney-Black, V., Covington, C., Ostrea, E., Romero, A., Baker, D., Tagle, M., Nordstrom-Klee, B., Silvestre, M., Angelilli, M., Hack, C., & Long, J. (1996). Prenatal cocaine and neonatal outcome: Evaluation of dose-response relationship. *Pediatrics*, 98(4), 735–740.

Denne, S., & Kalhan, S. (1986). Glucose carbon recycling and oxidation in human neonates. *American Journal of Physiology, 252,* 71–75.

Dietch, J. (1993). Periventricular-intraventricular hemorrhage in the very low birth weight neonate. *Neonatal Network, 12*(1), 7–16.

Dixon, S. (1989). Effects of transplacental exposure to cocaine and methamphetamine on the neonate. *Western Journal of Medicine, 150,* 436–442.

Dodd, V. (1996). Gestational age assessment. *Neonatal Network, 15*(1), 27–36.

Eden, R., & Boehm, F. (1990). *Assessment and care of the fetus.* Norwalk, CT: Appleton & Lange.

Eden, R. D., Seifert, L. S., & Winegar, A. (1987). Perinatal characteristics of uncomplicated postdate pregnancies. *Obstetrics and Gynecology,* 69(3), 296–299.

Ernhart, C., Sokol, R., Martier, S., Moron, P., & Nadler, D. (1987). Alcohol teratogenicity in the human: A detailed assessment of specificity, critical period, and threshold. *American Journal of Obstetrics and Gynecology, 156,* 33–39.

Farkas, K. J., & Parran, T. V. (1993). Treatment of cocaine addiction during pregnancy. *Clinics in Perinatology, 20,* 29–45.

Finnegan, L. (1985). Neonatal abstinence. *Current Therapy in Neonatal-Perinatal Medicine, 21,* 236–240.

Gale, G., Franck, L., & Lund, C. (1993). Skin-to-skin (Kangaroo) holding of the intubated premature infant. *Neonatal Network, 12*(6), 49–56.

Gale, R., Dranitzki, Z., Dollbery, S., & Stevenson, D. (1991). A randomized, controlled application of the Wallaby Phototherapy System compared with standard phototherapy. *Journal of Perinatology, 10*(3), 239–242.

Gerdes, J. (1991). Clinicopathologic approach to the diagnosis of neonatal sepsis. *Clinics in Perinatology, 18*(2), 362–365.

Gerhardt, T., & McCarthy, J. (1983). Effects of aminophylline on the respiratory center and reflex activity in the premature newborn with apnea. *Pediatric Research, 17,* 188–191.

Gershon, A. (1990). Chickenpox, measles, and mumps. In J. S. Remington & J. O. Klein (Eds.), *Infectious diseases of the fetus and neonate newborn* (3rd ed., pp. 345–445). Philadelphia: W. B. Saunders.

Goldman, H. (1980). Feeding and NEC. *American Journal of Diseases in Children, 134,* 553–555.

Gracey, K. (1997). Maternal varicella infection: Risks to the mother and baby? *Neonatal Network, 16*(7), 43–45.

Greven, C., & Tasman, W. (1990). Scleral buckling in stages 4b and 5 ROP. *Ophthalmology, 97,* 817–820.

Hack, M., Horbar, J., Malloy, M., Tyson, J., Wright, E., & Wright, L. (1991). Very low birth weight outcomes of the National Institute of Child Health and Human Development Neonatal Network. *Pediatrics, 87,* 587–597.

Harlow, B., Frigoletto, F., Cramer, D., Evans, J., LeFevre, M., Bain, R., & McNellis, D. (1996). Determinants of preterm delivery in the low-risk pregnancies. *Journal of Clinical Epidemiology,* 49(4), 441–8.

Harrison, L. (1997). Research utilization: Handling preterm infants in the NICU. *Neonatal Network 16*(3), 65–69.

Haymond, M. W. (1989). Hypoglycemia in infants and children. *Endocrinology Clinics of North America, 18,* 211–252.

Heimler, R., Langlois, J., Hodel, D., Nelin, D., & Sasidharan, P. (1992). Effect of positioning on the breathing pattern of preterm infants. *Archives of Diseases in Childhood, 67,* 312–314.

Hill, A., & Volpe, J. J. (1994). Neurologic disorders. In G. B. Avery, M. A. Fletcher, & M. G. MacDonald (Eds.). Neonatology: *Pathophysiology and management of the newborn* (4th ed., pp. 1117–1138). Philadelphia: J. B. Lippincott.

Holtrop, P. (1993). The frequency of hypoglycemia in full-term large and small for gestational age neonates. *American Journal of Perinatology, 10*(2), 150–154.

Hudson, D. C. (1997). Pain management in the hospitalized infant. *Journal of the Society of Pediatric Nursing, 2*(2), 93–96.

Jacobs, M., & Phibbs, R. (1989). Prevention, recognition and treatment of perinatal asphyxia. *Clinics in Perinatology, 16*(4), 785–807.

Jobe, A., Ikegami, M., & Jacobs, H. (1983). Permeability of premature lamb lungs to protein and the effect of surfactant on that permeability. *Journal of Applied Physiology,* 55, 169–176.

Kelley, S. (1992). Parenting stress and child maltreatment in drug exposed children. *Child Abuse and Neglect, 16,* 317–328.

Khalsa, J., & Gfroerer, J. (1991). Epidemiology and health consequences of drug abuse among pregnant women. *Seminars in Perinatology, 15,* 265–270.

Kliegman, R. (1990). Neonatal necrotizing enterocolitis: Bridging the basic science with the clinical disease. *Journal of Pediatrics, 117,* 5, 833–835.

Kliegman, R. M. (1996). The fetus and the neonatal infant. In R. E. Behrman, R. M. Kliegman, & A. M. Arvin (Eds.), *Nelson textbook of pediatrics* (15th ed.). Philadelphia: W. B. Saunders.

Knip, M., Lautala, P., Leppaluoto, J., Akerblom, H., & Kouivalainen, K. (1983). Relation of enteroinsular hormones at birth to macrosomia and neonatal hypoglycemia in neonates of diabetic mothers. *Journal of Pediatrics, 103,* 603–611.

Landon, M. B., & Gabbe, S. G. (1992). Diabetes mellitus and pregnancy. *Obstetrics and Gynecology Clinics of North America, 19,* 633–651.

Lawrence, R. (1994). *Breast-feeding: A guide for the medical professional* (4th ed.). St. Louis: C. V. Mosby.

Legault, M., & Goulet, C. (1995). Comparison of kangaroo and traditional methods of removing preterm infants from incubators. *Journal of Obstetric, Gynecologic, and Neonatal Nursing, 24,* 501–505.

Leveno, K. J., Cunningham, F. G., Roark, M. L., Nelson, S. D., & Williams, M. L. (1985). Prenatal care and the low birth weight newborn. *Obstetrics and Gynecology,* 66, 599–605.

Levine, M. G., Holroyde, J., Woods, J. R., Siddiqi, T. A., Scott, M., & Miodovnik, M. (1984). Birth trauma: Incidence and predisposing factors. *Obstetrics and Gynecology, 63,* 792–794.

Levy, M., & Spino, M. (1993). Neonatal withdrawal syndrome: Associated drugs and pharmacologic management. *Pharmacotherapy, 13*(3), 202–210.

Lipson, T. (1988). Fetal alcohol syndrome. *Australian Family Physician, 17,* 385–386.

Ludington-Hoe, S., Hadeed, A., & Anderson, G. (1991). Physiologic responses to skin-to-skin holding contact in hospitalized premature infants. *Journal of Perinatology, 11*(1), 19–24.

Ludington-Hoe, S., Thompson, C., Swinth, J., Hadeed, A., & Anderson, G. (1994). Kangaroo care: Research results, and practice implications and guidelines. *Neonatal Network, 13*(1), 19–27.

MacFarlane, P. I., & Heaf, D. P. (1988). Pulmonary function in children after neonatal meconium aspiration syndrome. *Archives of Diseases in Children, 63,* 368.

Mactutus, C. (1989). Developmental neurotoxicity of nicotine, carbon monoxide, and other tobacco smoke constituents. *Annals of New York Academy of Science, 562,* 105–120.

Malloy, M., & Perez-Woods, R. (1991). Neonatal skin care: Prevention of skin breakdown. *Pediatric Nursing, 17*(1), 41–48.

McCain, G. C. (1997). Behavioral state activity during nipple feedings for preterm infants. *Neonatal Network, 16*(5), 43–47.

McCormick, M. (1991). Trend in rates of low birth weight in the United States. In H. L. Berendes, S. Kessel, & S. Yafee (Eds.), *Advances in the prevention of low birth weight: An international symposium* (pp. 3–17). Washington, DC: National Center for Education in Maternal and Child Health.

McCourt, M. (1994). At risk for infection: The very low birth weight newborn. *Journal of Perinatal Nursing, 7*(4), 52–64.

Messmer, P. R., Rodriguez, S., Adams, J., Wells-Gentry, J., Washburn, K., Zabaleta, I., & Abreu, S. (1997). Effect of kangaroo care on sleep time for neonates. *Pediatric Nursing, 23,* 408–414.

Meyer, M., Jonas, B., & Tonascia, J. (1976). Perinatal events associated with maternal smoking during pregnancy. *American Journal of Epidemiology, 103,* 464–476.

Miles, M. S., Carlson, J., & Funk, S. (1996). Sources of support reported by mothers and fathers of infants hospitalized in a neonatal intensive care unit. *Neonatal Network, 15*(3), 45–52.

Mimouni, F., Miodovnik, M., Rosenn, B., Khoury, J., & Siddiqi, T. A. (1992). Birth trauma in insulin-dependent diabetic pregnancies. *American Journal of Perinatology, 9,* 205–208.

Minchin, M. (1991). Smoking and breastfeeding: An overview. *Journal of Human Lactation, 7,* 183–188.

Neu, J., Valentine, C., & Meetze, W. (1990). Scientifically-based strategies for nutrition of the high-risk low birth weight infant. *European Journal of Pediatrics, 150,* 2–13.

Norris, M., & Hill, C. (1992). Assessing congenital heart defects in the cocaine-exposed neonate. *Dimensions of Critical Care Nursing, 11*(1), 6–12.

Oro, A., & Dixon, S. (1988). Waterbed care of narcotic-exposed neonates. *American Journal of Diseases in Children, 142,* 106–108.

Ostertag, S., LaGamna, L., Reisen, C., & Ferrentino, F. (1986). Early enteral feeding does not affect the incidence of NEC. *Pediatrics, 77,* 275–280.

Park, M. K. (1988). *Pediatric cardiology for practitioners.* Chicago: Mosby–Year Book.

Perlman, J. (1989). Systemic abnormalities in term neonates following perinatal asphyxia: Relevance to long-term neurologic outcome. *Clinics in Perinatology, 16,* 475–484.

Phelps, D. (1992). Retinopathy of prematurity. *Current Problems in Pediatrics, 22*(8):349–371.

Philips, K. (1986). Neonatal drug addicts. *Nursing Times, 82*(12):36–38.

Pressler, J. L., & Hepworth, J. T. (1997). Newborn neurologic screening using NBAS reflexes. *Neonatal Network, 16*(6), 33–46.

Pridham, K. (1997). Mothers' help seeking as care initiated in a social context. *Image, 29*(1), 65–70.

Rey, E., & Martinez, H. (1983). Rational management of the premature newborn. Paper presented at the First Course Fetal and Neonatal Medicine, Bogota, Colombia, March 17–19, 137–151.

Richardson, G., Day, N., & Taylor, P. (1989). The effect of prenatal alcohol, marijuana, and tobacco exposure on neonatal behavior. *Newborn Behavior and Development, 12,* 199–209.

Romero, R., & Kleinman, R. (1993). Feeding the very low birth weight infant. *Pediatrics in Review, 14*(4), 123–132.

Rosenfeld, W., Tuest, R., & Concepcion, L. (1991). A new device for phototherapy treatment of jaundiced neonates. *Journal of Perinatology, 10*(3), 243–248.

Rushton, C. (1990a). NEC part I: Pathogenesis and diagnosis. *Maternal Child Nursing, 15,* 296–300.

Sann, L. (1990). Neonatal hypoglycemia. *Biology of the neonate, 58,* 16–21.

Schraeder, B. D., Heverly, M. A., O'Brien, C., & Goodman, R. (1997). Academic achievement and educational resource use of very low birth weight (VLBW) survivors. *Pediatric Nursing, 23,* 21–25, 44.

Shaywitz, B., & Fletcher, J. (1993). Neurological, cognitive, and behavioral sequelae of hypoxic-ischemic encephalopathy. *Seminars in Perinatology, 17*(5), 357–366.

Shields-Poë, D., & Pinelli, J. (1997). Variables associated with parental stress in neonatal intensive care units. *Neonatal Network, 16*(1), 29–37.

Spohr, H., Willms, J., & Steinhausen, H. (1993). Prenatal alcohol exposure and long-term developmental consequences. *Lancet, 341,* 907–910.

Stevens, P. A., Wright, J. R., & Clements, J. A. (1989). Surfactant secretion and clearance in the neonate. *Journal of Applied Physiology, 67,* 1597–1605.

Suevo, D. M. (1997). The infant of the diabetic mother. *Neonatal Network, 16*(5), 25–33.

Swaminathan, S., Quinn, J., & Stabile, M. W. (1989). Long term pulmonary sequelae of meconium aspiration syndrome. *Journal of Pediatrics, 114,* 356.

Takashima, S., Mito, T., & Houdou, S. (1989). Relationship between periventricular hemorrhage, leukomalacia and brain stem lesions in prematurely born neonates. *Brain Development, 11,* 121–124.

Tan, K. (1989). Efficacy of fluorescent daylight, blue and green lamps in the management of non-hemolytic hyperbilirubinemia. *Journal of Pediatrics, 114,* 132–135.

Tan, K. (1991). Phototherapy for neonatal jaundice. *Clinics in Perinatology, 18,* 423–439.

Thomas, K. (1994). Thermoregulation in neonates. *Neonatal Network, 13*(2), 15–20.

Van De Bor, M., Ens-Dokkum, M., Schreuder, M., Veen, S., Brand, D., & Verloove-Vanhoreck, P. (1993). Outcome of periventricular-intraventricular hemorrhage at 5 years of age. *Developmental Medicine and Child Neurology, 35,* 33–41.

VandenBerg, K. A. (1997). Basic principles of developmental caregiving. *Neonatal Network, 16*(7), 69–71.

Volpe, J. J. (1989). Intraventricular hemorrhage and brain injury in the premature newborn. *Clinics in Perinatology, 16*(2), 361–387.

Wallace, J., & Ridpath-Parker, J. (1993). Kangaroo care. *Quality Management in Health Care, 2,* 1–5.

Walsh, J., Farrel, M., & Keeman, W. (1978). GER in neonates: Relationship to apnea. *Journal of Pediatrics, 92,* 73–75.

Watkins, A., & Keogh, E. (1992). Alcohol burns in the neonate. *Journal of Paediatrics and Child Health, 28,* 306–308.

Weinberger, S., & Kendall, S. (1986). Early weight change patterns in neonatal abstinence. *American Journal of Diseases in Children, 140,* 829–832.

Wereszczak, J., Miles, M. S., & Holditch-Davis, D. (1997). Maternal recall of the neonatal intensive care unit. *Neonatal Network, 16*(4), 33–39.

Wilkerson, N. (1988). A comprehensive look at hyperbilirubinemia. *Maternal-Child Nursing, 13,* 360–364.

Wilkerson, N. (1989). Treating hyperbilirubinemia. *Maternal-Child Nursing,* 14, 32–36.

Wiswell, T. E., & Bent, R. C. (1993). Meconium staining and meconium aspiration syndrome. *Update on Neonatology, 40*(5), 955–981.

Wiswell, T. E., Robertson, C. F., & Jones, T. A. (1986). NEC in full term neonates. *American Journal of Diseases in Children, 142,* 532–535.

Bibliography

Barras, F. C. (1992). Comparison of the causes and consequences of prematurity and intrauterine growth retardation: A longitudinal study in southern Brazil. *Pediatrics, 90,* 238–244.

Bell, E. H., Geyer, J., & Jones, L. (1995). A structured intervention improves breast-feeding success for ill or preterm infants. *MCN, 20,* 309–314.

Goldman, D. J., & Goldman, S. L. (1992). Prematurity. In P. L. Jackson & J. A. Vessey (Eds.), *Primary care of the child with a chronic condition* (pp. 446–464). St. Louis: Mosby–Year Book.

Kenner, C., Brueggemeyer, A., & Gunderson, L. (1993). *Comprehensive neonatal nursing: A physiologic perspective.* Philadelphia: W. B. Saunders.

Loughead, M. K., Loughead, J. L., & Reinhart, M. J. (1997). Incidence and physiologic characteristics of hypothermia in the very low birth weight infant. *Pediatric Nursing, 23,* 11–15.

Meisels, S. J., & Fenichel, E. (1996). *New visions for the developmental assessment of infants and young children.* Washington, DC: National Center for Infants, Toddlers and Families.

Mitchell, A., Steffenson, N., Hogan, H., & Brooks, S. (1997). Neonatal group B streptococcal disease. *MCN, 22,* 249–253.

Philbin, M. K. (1997). Some implications of early auditory development for the environment of hospitalized preterm infants. *Neonatal Network, 15*(8), 71–73.

Pickler, R. H., Higgins, K. E., & Crummette, B. D. (1993). The effect of nonnutritive sucking on bottle-feeding stress in preterm infants. *Journal of Obstetric, Gynecologic, and Neonatal Nursing, 22,* 230–234.

Pickler, R. H., & Terrell, B. V. (1994). Nonnutritive sucking and necrotizing enterocolitis. *Neonatal Network, 13*(8), 15–18.

Pokorni, J. L., & Stanga, J. (1997). Serving infants and families affected by maternal cocaine abuse: Part I. *Pediatric Nursing, 22,* 439–442.

Polin, R., & Fox, W. (1992). *Fetal and neonatal physiology* (vols. 1 & 2). Philadelphia: W. B. Saunders.

Pomerance, J., & Richardson, C. (1993). *Neonatology for the clinician.* Norwalk, CT: Appleton & Lange.

Sastry, B., Mouton, V., & Kambam, J. (1993). Tobacco smoking by pregnant women: Disturbances in metabolism of branched chain amino acids and fetal growth. *Annals of New York Academy of Sciences, 678,* 361–363.

Smitherman, C. (1994). The lasting impact of fetal alcohol syndrome and fetal alcohol: Effect on children and adolescents. *Journal of Pediatric Health Care, 8,* 121–125.

HEALTH CHALLENGE:

Alterations in Cardiovascular Status

OUTLINE

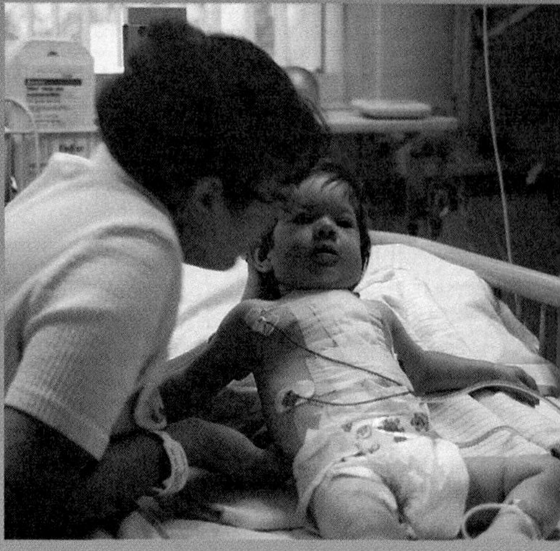

OBJECTIVES

- Describe specific assessment skills that assist in the identification and care of the child with an alteration in the cardiovascular status.
- Identify invasive and non-invasive diagnostic tools that help in evaluating children with the suspected diagnosis of heart disease.
- Describe information to be taught to the pediatric cardiac patient preparing for a procedure.
- List nursing interventions and potential complications during the acute and the convalescent phases of the postoperative cardiac patient.
- Recognize multifactorial, genetic, and environmental influences on congenital heart disease.
- Explain the pathophysiology, presentation, and clinical management of the child with congestive heart failure, cyanosis, and acquired heart disease.
- Recognize the anatomic variations associated with the more common congenital defects, and give the hemodynamic consequences of these defects.
- Relate the various congenital defects to appropriate medical and surgical treatments, and differentiate uses of palliative procedures.

KEY TERMS

acquired heart disease
atelectasis
cardiomegaly
cyanosis
diastole
diuretic
gradient
inotropic
palliative procedure
shunt
systole
pulmonary collaterals
pulmonary hypertension

CHAPTER

15

There are two primary types of heart disease that occur in children: congenital and acquired. Congenital heart disease (CHD) refers to a functional or structural disease of the heart that is present at birth, even though the illness may not manifest itself clinically until later in life. Cardiac conditions that develop after birth are known as acquired heart disease. Heart disease in children occurs in all cultures and in all ethnic populations. The incidence of CHD, or the number of children born with congenital heart disease annually as compared with all children born, is approximately 8 of 1000 live births (Hoffman, 1990; Zita & Roberts, 1995). There are factors that cause an underestimation of the occurrence of CHD. Efforts to record all the cases of children who actually have CHD are limited. Researchers may have difficulty ascertaining statistics on children with CHD in rural areas, in areas with a high population of indigent families, and in underdeveloped nations. Another reason for faulty statistics may be the failure to record children with mild versions of a defect, such as mild pulmonary stenosis or mild coarctation of the aorta.

caREminder: *Nurses need to realize that the presence of CHD is diagnosed by 1 month after birth in only 50% to 60% of all cases. The nurse should not assume that the presence of a cardiac condition would already have been ruled out in the older child who presents with questionable symptomatology (Hoffman, 1990).*

Stillborn fetuses have an incidence of CHD that is up to 10 times higher than that of a liveborn infant, and miscarried fetuses are also thought to have a much greater incidence of CHD (Hoffman, 1990).

There are a variety of factors that are related to the incidence of CHD. Parents of a child with CHD may express concerns about the risk of recurrence of the condition if they have a *family history* of CHD or if one of their other children was afflicted with a congenital heart defect. The likelihood of recurrence of CHD depends on specific lesions, chromosomal issues, gender, race, and environmental factors. It is known that risks are much higher for more serious versions of a lesion; and the closer lineage the relative has to the afflicted child, the higher the risk. Recurrent risk to subsequent siblings in a family is approximately 2% to 6%. The risk of parents with CHD passing on heart abnormalities to their own children increases to 5% to 10%. The risk increases by three to four times if more than one child in a family has a heart defect (Hoffman, 1990).

Environmental or teratogenic insults, such as the ingestion of drugs (recreational or prescribed) or alcohol during pregnancy, can increase the risk of heart defects in the fetus. *Toxic exposure* of the mother to some drugs such as lithium carbonate, especially early in the pregnancy, is known to be associated with heart disease in the child. Aspirin products have long been implicated as teratogens in CHD, but evidence in the scientific knowledge base is inconclusive (Werler, Mitchell, & Shapiro, 1989). *Maternal conditions* such as diabetes or lupus have caused offspring with cardiac problems. Most of the cases of congenital heart disease fall into the *multifactorial*, or random accidents of nature, category. In these cases, the mother has no known environmental exposures or illnesses that are documented as leading to CHD and there is no known family history of congenital heart disease. When discussing the reasons for heart disease with family members, the nurse should explain that the death of an elderly family member from atherosclerotic heart disease is different from the incidence, if any, of childhood heart disease that may have affected the family.

Syndromes that affect other body systems can be associated with congenital heart defects. For example, Down syndrome, trisomies 13 and 18, asplenia syndrome, and DiGeorge syndrome all are associated with congenital heart defects. Approximately 5% to 8% of children with CHD have a concurring chromosomal defect (Hoffman, 1990).

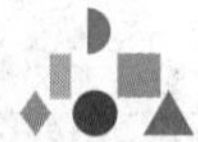

Assessment of the Child with Alterations in Cardiovascular Status

Focused Health History

A comprehensive pediatric evaluation must include a recording of the child's chief complaint, the maternal/fetal history, the postnatal history, and the family history (Chart 15–1).

The chief complaint is the reason that the child and family are seeking an evaluation. For example, if the child is being seen for a history of chest pain, the nurse needs to note whether the pain was related to activity, the duration of the chest pain, whether the pain occurs while taking a breath, and whether the child has episodes of syncope or palpitation. For complaints of tachycardia or palpitation, the nurse should also note whether these episodes coincide with the ingestion of cold medications or anti-asthmatic drugs.

Any potential maternal/fetal teratogenic event that could have influenced cardiac development is noted. A severe infection such as measles or influenza, especially when accompanied by high temperatures during the first trimester, has the potential to alter fetal cardiac development. The nurse should make certain to note whether the mother ingested medications before realizing that she was pregnant.

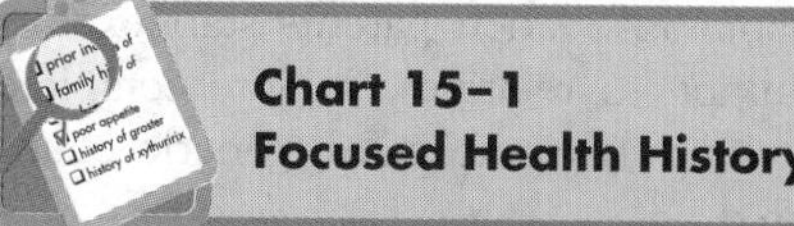

Chart 15–1
Focused Health History

Cardiovascular System

Identifying Data	Age, gender, place of birth (e.g., metropolitan area, foreign country), religious affiliation, number of other siblings in family
Present Illness	Identify who is giving history, in their own words. Chest pain—sporadic and short, with exertion Parents deny any symptoms, and a pediatrician or RN heard a murmur. Complaint of heart palpitations, tachycardia, syncope, or parents feel baby's heart races Tires while feeding; sucks vigorously, then fatigues Gains weight inadequately but may have normal height for age Vomits frequently Sweats while eating Cyanotic, which worsens with feeding or activity Becomes irritable easily or cries weakly Has limited activity level, has trouble keeping up with siblings Most comfortable in preferred position; more calm with head of bed elevated; squats when playing
Past Medical History	*Maternal fetal history:* maternal exposure to teratogens, infections, prescription and over-the-counter medications; illicit drug or alcohol use during pregnancy; mother's history of chronic illness *Previous health challenge:* previous illness and/or injuries and child's response to illness; history of heart palpitations, tachycardia, or syncope, or baby's heart races. *Childhood illnesses:* history of common communicable diseases and ability to recover; children with heart disease frequently have repeat upper respiratory tract illnesses *Immunization:* status of current immunizations
Allergies	Medications, animals, foods, and others. What are the symptoms? Does the child receive any treatment?
Current Medications	Over-the-counter and prescription and others (home remedies, herbs)
Family Medical History	Any family history of childhood cardiac diagnosis, miscarriages, stillbirths for mother or on either grandparent's side. Family history of cardiac disease occurring before age 55, any deaths related to cardiac disease. Other siblings with similar cardiac diagnosis.

caREminder: *In order not to inflict guilt feelings on the mother for actions she may have taken during her pregnancy that may have affected the child, the nurse must be sensitive about the wording of questions during the interview.*

The fetal environment of a mother with a chronic illness such as diabetes or lupus can also cause negative outcomes on fetal development. Any history of drug or alcohol use and the severity of abuse, if any, must be documented, because drugs and alcohol are known to have adverse effects on fetal development. The information is limited by what the mother can, or is willing to, reveal. See Chapters 4 and 8 for an in-depth discussion of teratogenesis.

A postnatal history includes growth and development patterns, symptoms, and illness patterns. Data collection should include the parents' description of their child's feeding and weight gain patterns. Questions should be asked to ascertain whether the child has met major developmental milestones. The nurse should note whether the child has dysmorphic features or a diagnosis of a chromosomal defect, such as Down syndrome, that is associated with heart disease. Some chromosomal defects can lead the diagnostician to suspect a cardiac lesion. A history of puffy eyelids, tachypnea, and dyspnea can be indicative of congestive heart failure (CHF). Frequent respiratory infections are a common problem of some children with congenital heart disease.

A family history relevant to cardiac problems and to other medical events should also be completed. Family histories are sometimes obtuse or vague. A typical vague historical account from a worried parent might be: "My mother said she had a baby that died and it was blue," or "My husband says his mother lost a child as an infant but she won't talk about it." When parents start exploring their past and talking to relatives, a more complete family history may evolve. In some cases, genetic counseling may be warranted.

Focused Physical Assessment

Physical assessment of the cardiovascular system uses the techniques of inspection, palpation, and auscultation (Chart 15–2). Cardiac inspection of a child can be completed without waking a sleeping child or disturbing an

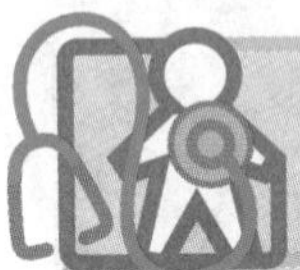

Chart 15–2
Focused Physical Assessment

Cardiac

Inspection	Normal Findings	Alterations
General appearance Nutritional state	Happy, interacting Well nourished Height and weight within normal limits for age	Cranky, in distress, weak Undernourished Underweight, height below average or normal
Size, shape, and symmetry of chest	Infant's thorax is rounded, transverse diameter increases until chest assumes elliptic shape of the adult by age 6	Presence of chest retractions Presence of heaves or lifts Enlargement over heart Asymmetrical movement of chest
Skin	Warm, dry, pink skin	Pallor Cyanosis Note mucous membranes, sclera, palms, and soles of feet for cyanosis or mottling Jaundiced
	Skin color stays the same, even with activity	Clammy sweating with activity or feeding
	No edema	Periorbital or peripheral edema
	No scars	Scars from previous heart surgeries
Nail beds	Pink, flat nail	Clubbed (widened terminal phalanges) Cyanotic nail beds
Respiratory	Rate normal for age Effortless and silent	Increased, even with rest With CHF, can be labored and more comfortable with head elevated
Pulses Blood pressure	No difference between femoral and brachial pulses No difference in BP in arms and legs	Bounding pulses Differentiation in BP and pulses can be an indicator of coarctation of the aorta
Heart auscultation	Apical pulse may be visible Is louder than in adults because chest wall is thinner Regular rate and rhythm	Murmur (turbulence of blood flow) may or may not be present with a heart lesion and murmurs vary with lesion If murmur present, note intensity, location, quality, and timing and whether systolic or diastolic Irregular rhythm

awake child. During the inspection, the nurse observes the child's overall appearance and activity level. Children with cardiac conditions are often small for their age and may appear to be malnourished. The child may appear lethargic, fretful, or agitated. Skin color is assessed for cyanosis or pallor, or both. Mottling of the skin may be noted. Diaphoresis may occur in children with left-to-right shunts. The presence or absence of edema should be noted. Inspection of the chest may reveal bulging or prominence on the chest wall, especially on the left side where the apex of the breast is most commonly situated. The point of maximum impulse (PMI) is visually apparent as a pulsation in children with thin chest walls or with enlarged hearts. If possible, the nurse should observe the infant while the child is being fed. This provides the opportunity to determine whether the child is becoming easily tired when feeding or whether skin color changes are noted when the child is feeding.

Palpation should include feeling the quality of peripheral pulses and noting any irregularities in rate and volume between right and left arms and legs. Palpation also includes taking the child's blood pressure. When taking blood pressures, it is imperative that the child be in a relaxed state. If the child is stressed or fidgety, there is a high risk of artificially high or low pressures.

Alert: *If weak pulses or low blood pressure is identified in the lower extremities as compared with the upper extremities, this can be an indication of coarctation of the aorta. Bounding pulses can be an indication of a patent ductus arteriosus or aortic insufficiency.*

The cardiac assessment should include palpation of the liver borders to document evidence of hepatomegaly from right-sided heart failure. In smaller, thinner children, the liver is more easily palpable. When assessing a child, palpate the distended liver borders, and chart how many centimeters below the rib cage the borders of the liver are palpable.

Cardiac auscultation is another aspect of the physical examination. Auscultation of heart sounds requires more skill than other portions of the child's physical assessment. The nurse should not expect to hear a murmur from all children with known cardiac lesions, because some malformations seldomly produce abnormal heart sounds. It is important that the nurse listen carefully and describe exactly what is heard (see Chapter 6 for more information regarding physical assessment of the cardiovascular system). When listening to the child's chest, the nurse should auscultate the anterior chest, as well as the lateral and the posterior chest area. On assessment, the nurse should note the rate and the regularity of the heartbeat and the intensity and quality of the heart sound. Any abnormality of the first and second heart sounds should be documented, such as a split heart sound. Any extra heart sounds such as murmurs, gallops, or rubs are also documented. The location on the thorax where the extra heart sound is heard most distinctly can assist in giving information about the anatomic origin of a murmur. A murmur is also graded for its intensity, to identify the loudness of the murmur. Further evaluation may be required to distinguish an innocent, or asymptomatic, murmur from one that indicates the presence of a pathologic condition. The term *innocent* indicates that the murmur represents a normal finding with no implication of the presence of a pathologic condition or process (Gessner, 1997; Smith, 1997). Innocent murmurs can be exacerbated by conditions such as fever, anemia, anxiety, and exercise. These situations can accentuate an innocent murmur that would not normally be audible.

Nursing Diagnoses and Outcomes

The impact of heart disease on the child and the family is both acute and long term. When heart disease is suspected, the health care team acts rapidly to ensure that the child's physiologic status is stabilized. Nursing diagnoses during the early critical stages focus on the oxygenation, cardiac output, and fluid volume concerns related to the child's specific condition (Chart 15–3).

Because the heart is viewed as vital to human existence, the presence of a cardiac condition is likely to cause significant fear for the parents and the family. The plan of care for the child with a cardiac condition must help the parents cope with their feelings so that they are able to deal with the facts related to their child's illness. A significant role of the nurse is to assist the family in understanding the child's condition and the treatment plan.

The majority of children affected with CHD or an acquired heart condition are able to lead normal lives. Nursing diagnoses that address alterations in development, body image, and self-esteem concerns may be applicable in cases in which it is assessed that the child's condition is perceived as severely limiting or disabling.

Developmental and Biological Variances

Embryologic Development

The heart starts to form early in the first 3 weeks of embryologic development. Fetal cardiac circulation is essentially developed before the eighth week. In this fragile stage of fetal development, congenital heart lesions can occur (Zita & Roberts, 1995). The heart in the fetus begins as a simple tube that, over a short period of time, is transformed into a functional, complex organ (Fig. 15–1). One end of the primitive linear tube eventually gives rise to the arterial system, and the opposite end

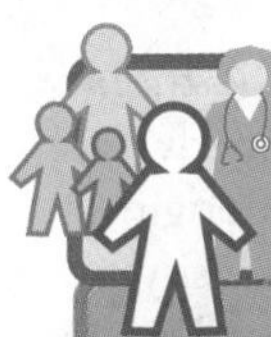

Chart 15–3
Nursing Diagnoses and Outcomes

Alterations in Cardiovascular Status

Thermoregulation, ineffective (post-surgically) related to cardiopulmonary bypass, immaturity of the thermoregulation centers, low cardiac output state, cool surgical suite

Outcome: Child will maintain normothermia.

Alteration in cardiac output related to decreased preload/hypovolemia, postoperative bleeding, increased afterload, altered myocardial contractility, arrhythmias

Outcome: Child will maintain a cardiac output adequate to maintain perfusion of body as evidenced by stable vital signs, level of consciousness within normal limits, hemodynamic stability, adequate tissue perfusion, and no signs of venous congestion.

Alteration in fluid and electrolytes related to cardiopulmonary bypass, fluid overload/dehydration, diuretics, poor nutritional status, anesthesia, bleeding

Outcomes: Child will have clear breath sounds and no signs of edema and return to preoperative body weight.
Laboratory values will be within normal limits.

Impaired gas exchange related to effects of cardiac surgery/anesthesia, fluid shifts, hypoventilation, atelectasis, effusions, pulmonary congestion, pain, immobility, underlying congenital disease

Outcome: Child will demonstrate adequate ventilation and gas exchange by adequate arterial blood gas results, minimal pulmonary secretions, and normal breath sounds.

Potential for injury (neurologic) related to cardiopulmonary bypass, intracardiac mixing (emboli), low cardiac output, hypotension, hypoxia, electrolyte imbalances/fluid shifts, narcotics, anesthesia

Outcome: Child will sustain no neurologic deficits. Seizures will be controlled with appropriate anticonvulsant therapy.

Potential for infection related to pulmonary status, congenital defect/mixing or poor pump, prolonged operative time, excessive postoperative bleeding, prosthetic devices, compromised nutritional status, indwelling catheters, CHF, poor cardiac output

Outcomes: Incision will be free of infection.
Child will be afebrile, with a white blood cell count (WBC) within normal limits.

Pain related to surgical incision, invasive lines, and restraints

Outcomes: Child will demonstrate pain relief by absence of crying, restlessness, agitation, irritability, facial grimacing, splinting, or rigid body posture.
Child will progress to ambulation and playing in age-appropriate manner.

Anxiety related to unfamiliar environment and people, and overstimulation

Outcomes: Child will be comforted by parental presence and holding (when stable).
Child will experience adequate periods of rest.

Alteration in parenting related to symbolic meaning of the heart, separation, lack of control and fear of the unknown, alterations in routine, financial as well as social constraints

Outcomes: Parents will demonstrate appropriate bonding and attachment behaviors.
Parents will verbalize feelings regarding their child's illness.
Parents will demonstrate knowledge and understanding of discharge instructions.

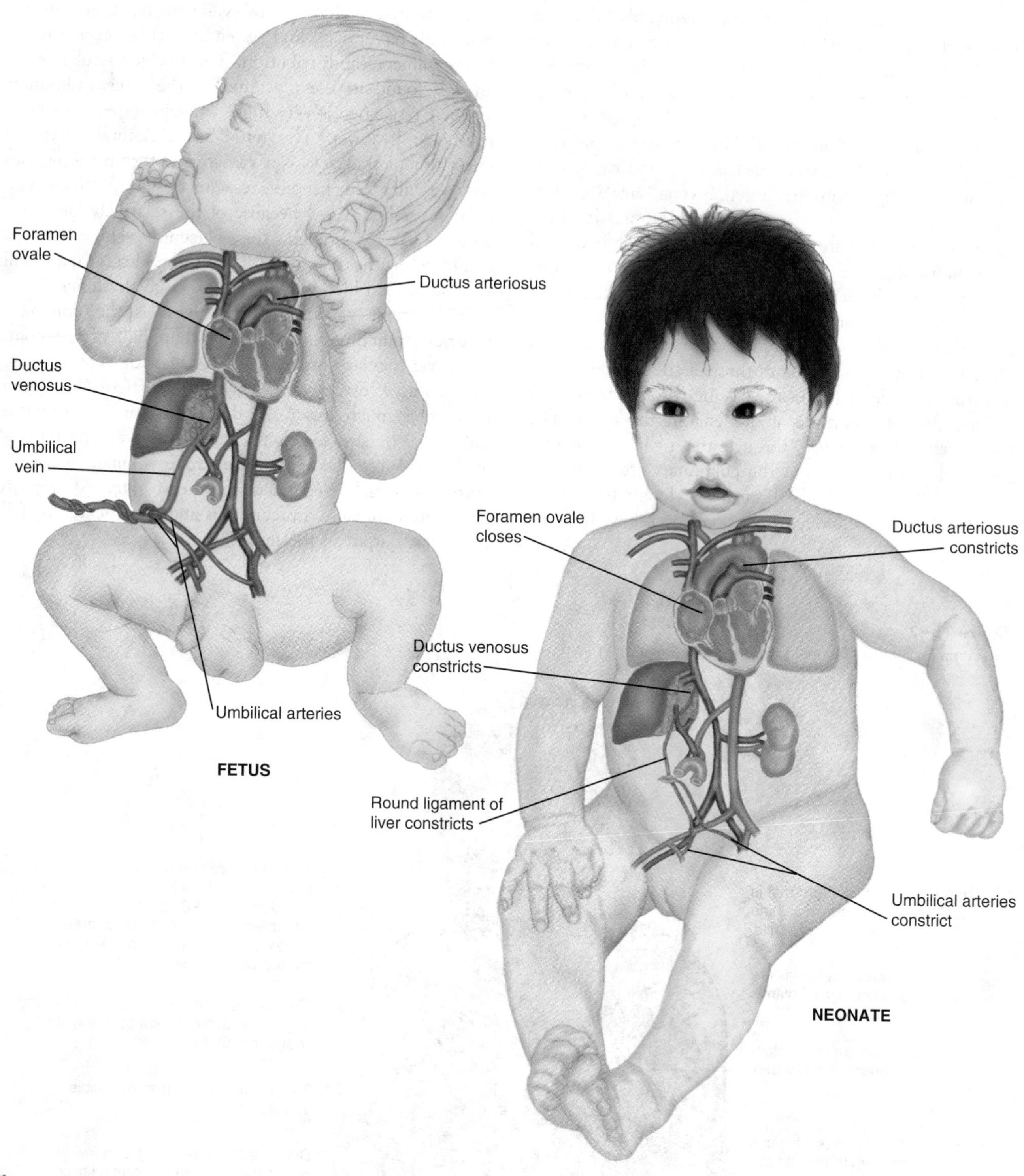

Figure 15–1
Fetal circulation and changes at birth. (From Ashwill, J. W., & Droske, S. C. [Eds.] [1997]. *Nursing care of children: Principles and practice* [p. 910]. Philadelphia: W. B. Saunders. Reprinted with permission.)

becomes the venous system. As the tube widens, it folds and bulges, evolving into four separate chambers. By the end of the third week of gestation, the heart is beating; and by the fourth week, the atrium and the ventricles, are visible heart structures (Alyn & Baker, 1992; Witt, 1997).

In fetal circulation, blood flows from the placenta through the umbilical vein, to the liver and the ductus venosus, and then into the inferior vena cava (see Fig. 15–1). At the vena cava, fetal blood from the liver mixes with blood from the lower portion of the body and then drains into the right atrium. Blood from the upper portion of the body, the head, the arms, and the brain returns to the right atrium through the superior vena cava. Once in the right atrium, a division occurs wherein some blood bypasses the lungs through the foramen ovale into the left side of the heart, passing through to the left atrium, the left ventricle, and then out the aorta. The rest of the blood travels through the right atrium into the right ventricle and out the pulmonary artery. A portion of this blood travels through the lungs; the rest of the blood crosses the ductus arteriosus and flows into the descending aorta.

Fetal blood flow through the heart has more than one potential pathway. The vascular resistance in the placental, pulmonary, and systemic circulation is a major factor influencing distribution. The lowest vascular resistance is found in the placenta. In the fetus, pulmonary vascular resistance is very high, whereas systemic vascular resistance is lower. The fetus has a naturally hypoxic environment that acts as a vasoconstrictor on the pulmonary vascular bed, keeping resistance high. Systemic vascular resistance is low because of the relatively large volume of flow through the placenta. These factors, combined with the areas of shunting, lead to a small volume of fetal blood circulating through the lungs.

The right ventricle in the fetus is the dominant ventricle, pumping slightly more than half of the combined ventricular output. Pressures in both ventricles are equal, unlike in the adult, where normal right ventricular pressure is much lower. In the adult, cardiac output is influenced by stroke volume and heart rate. The fetus is unable to substantially increase stroke volume, so cardiac output is largely dependent on heart rate. A drop in heart rate can cause a precipitous and life-threatening fall in cardiac output in the fetus.

Figure 15–2
Developmental and biological variances: cardiovascular system.

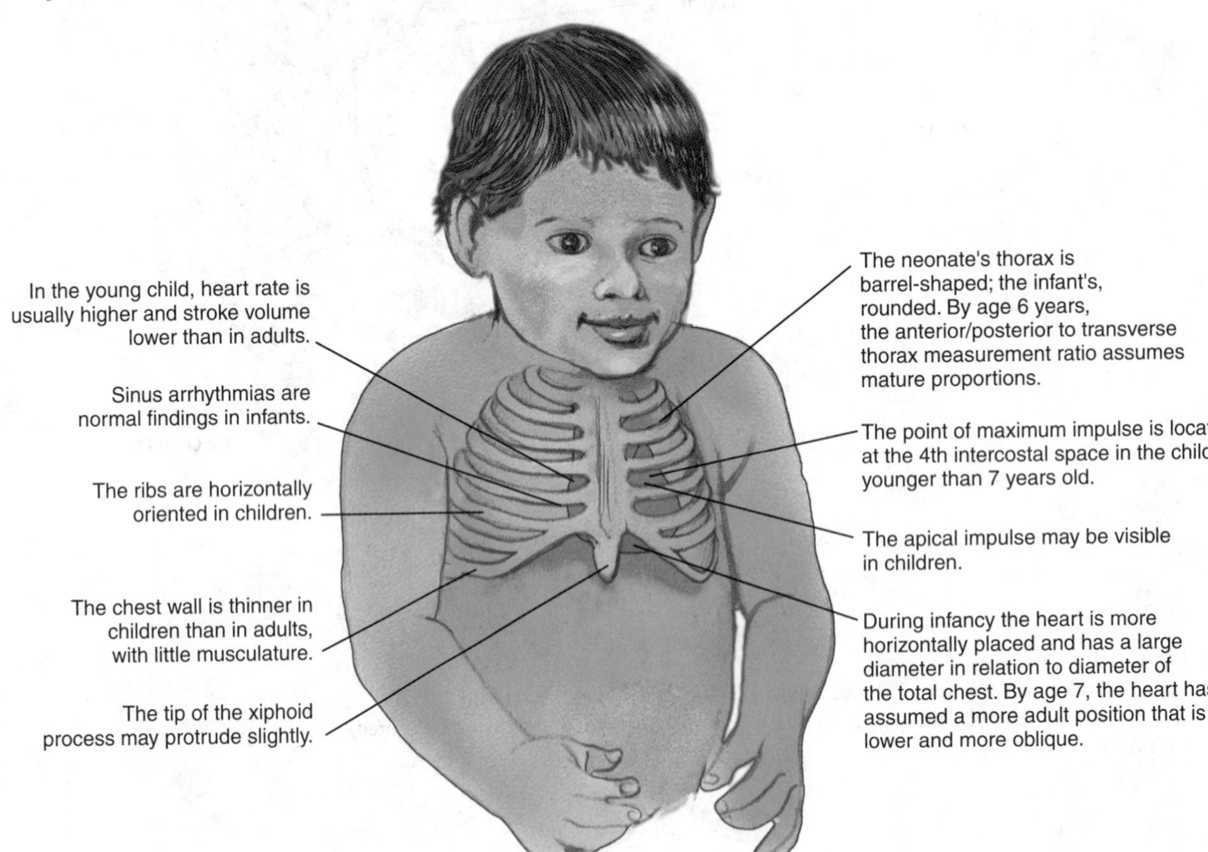

In the young child, heart rate is usually higher and stroke volume lower than in adults.
Sinus arrhythmias are normal findings in infants.
The ribs are horizontally oriented in children.
The chest wall is thinner in children than in adults, with little musculature.
The tip of the xiphoid process may protrude slightly.
The neonate's thorax is barrel-shaped; the infant's, rounded. By age 6 years, the anterior/posterior to transverse thorax measurement ratio assumes mature proportions.
The point of maximum impulse is located at the 4th intercostal space in the child younger than 7 years old.
The apical impulse may be visible in children.
During infancy the heart is more horizontally placed and has a large diameter in relation to diameter of the total chest. By age 7, the heart has assumed a more adult position that is lower and more oblique.

Cardiovascular Changes at Birth

At birth, the organ responsible for oxygenation changes from the placenta to the lungs. Circulatory apparatus that are unique to the fetus—the placenta, the foramen ovale, and the ductus arteriosus—undergo abrupt changes at birth. In the fetus, the collapsed lungs have a high pulmonary vascular resistance (PVR), which makes the pressure on the right side of the heart high and limits blood flow to the lungs. At birth, there is an increase in alveolar oxygen tension, and a large volume of circulating blood shifts from placental flow to the pulmonary arteries. Together, these conditions cause vasodilatation in the pulmonary vascular bed, thereby creating a lower PVR and lower right-sided heart pressure. This change in blood flow causes a rise in left atrial pressure forcing the closure of the flap-like foramen ovale and creating higher pressures on the left side of the heart. Elevated arterial oxygenation and other factors stimulate the cessation of shunting across the ductus arteriosus. Constriction of the ductus arteriosus is generally achieved within the first 3 days of life. With closure of the ductus arteriosus and the foramen ovale, the two levels of circulatory shunting in the heart cease (Sansoucie & Cavaliere, 1997). When these anatomic shunts are no longer present, the transition to extrauterine circulation is complete (see Fig. 15–1).

At birth, the ventricular muscles are of equal wall thickness. Eventually, the left ventricle becomes thicker from the work of pumping blood to the systemic circulation. This explains why neonatal systemic blood pressure is low in the early days after birth: the ventricular strengthening and pressure changes are still occurring.

Cardiovascular Changes Throughout Childhood

When compared with the cardiac assessment of an adult, there are normal biological and developmental variations of the cardiovascular status of infants and children. Cardiac assessment variations are related to the natural progression of growth and development in children (Fig. 15–2).

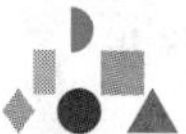

Diagnostic Criteria for Evaluating Cardiovascular Disorders

There are several diagnostic procedures that augment information obtained from the history and physical examination of the cardiovascular system and give direction to the diagnosing and management of these children. Commonly employed tests and the rationales for their use are described in this section (Table 15–1).

Cardiac Enzymes

The presence of elevated cardiac enzymes may assist in the diagnosis of myocardial stress and injury. Serum creatine kinase (CK) and lactate dehydrogenase isoenzyme (LDH) have been used to evaluate myocardial stress in adults; more recently these tests are being used to evaluate myocardial compromise in infants. Myocardial insult can occur in infants as a result of asphyxia, tricuspid insufficiency, and papillary muscle infarcts. Increases in CK can also be produced by central nervous system damage such as cerebral infarct and periventricular hemorrhage. Evaluation of cardiac enzymes should be completed on the stressed neonate to evaluate the possibility of cardiac compromise (Verklan, 1997).

Chest Roentgenography

A chest roentgenogram (x-ray) is an essential tool in the diagnosis and evaluation of the heart and provides information about the heart size and shape, enlargement of the chambers, and the status of pulmonary blood flow. Cardiomegaly (enlarged heart) visualized on a chest x-ray is commonly the first piece of evidence that causes medical personnel to consider the presence of a heart defect. Chest roentgenography is also traditionally performed before cardiac surgery to provide a baseline chest film to compare with cardiac changes postoperatively. The status of the lungs and other noncardiac tissues (e.g., size of thymus, rib notching) that may be affected by compromised cardiac function can be assessed with chest radiographs.

Pulse Oximetry

Transcutaneous pulse oximetry is a noninvasive method of assessing arterial oxygen saturation. Pulse oximetry is accomplished by beaming a light through tissue and measuring the amount of light absorbed by oxygen-saturated hemoglobin with a light-receiving sensor. Data shown on the monitor readout generally include heart rate and oxygen saturation. Normal readings for children with congenital heart disease vary depending on the actual lesion; but for most children without congenital heart disease, normal oxygen saturation is 94% to 100%.

Oxygen saturation values should measure close to arterial blood gas saturations. Use of oximetry can reduce the need for arterial blood gas testing and can assist in titrating oxygen administration. When reading a pulse oximeter monitor, a good arterial wave form should be present and should correlate to the heart rate indicated with the child's auscultated heart rate to ensure a more

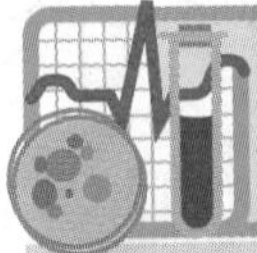

Table 15-1
Diagnostic Tests and Procedures for Evaluating Cardiovascular Status

Diagnostic Test or Procedure	Purpose	Findings	Health Care Provider Responsibilities
Chest roentgenography (x-ray)	Define and silhouette heart, show pulmonary markings (use posterior and lateral views)	Heart size Shape of heart Pulmonary vascular markings Cardiothoracic ratio	Advise parents that variations from normal can help in the differential diagnosis of heart disease and allow for documentation of trends such as increasing heart size.
Pulse oximetry	Identify patient's oxygen saturation Can reduce the need for arterial blood gases in the postoperative period Helps the practitioner know when to wean a child off oxygen Quick and easy non-invasive test	Normal 94–100% Pulse oximetry values below "normal" can be acceptable and expected in a cyanotic child.	Alarm parameters need to be set and checked at beginning of each shift. If readings fall below parameters, assess child immediately for respiratory distress.
Electrocardiogram	Graphic display of the electrical activity of the heart Non-invasive, inexpensive test 12-lead ECG done as preoperative baseline Continuous monitor used in immediate postoperative period Holter monitor used to determine arrhythmias during day-to-day activity	Diagnostic of conduction disturbances Detects hypertrophy of ventricles and atria Helps in the diagnosis of heart defects	Small children are required to be very still for about 1 minute and tolerate leads stuck to skin.
Cardiac enzymes (serum creatine kinase [CK] and lactate dehydrogenase isoenzyme)	These enzymes are released when myocardial stress and cardiovascular injury have occured. Also seen with central nervous system injury, pulmonary infarct, necrosis of the kidney, liver damage, and ischemic rhabdomyolysis.	Normal total CK = 70–380 IU/L Normal total lactate dehydrogenase = 327–874 IU/L	In children, myocardial damage causes elevations for about 7–10 days after the insult. Therefore, analyses for cardiac enzymes in infarcts need not occur immediately.
Echocardiogram	Uses ultrasound to show anatomic visualization of heart structure and functional information. Noninvasive.	Shows image of heart in motion Can provide specific diagnosis of heart abnormalities, trends, and function	Requires patient to be still approximately 45 minutes. Toddlers may require sedation.
Transesophageal pacing/echocardiography	Esophageal probe placed to provide ultrasonic pictures or to pace heart	Assessment of cardiovascular structures and function Through esophageal placement of probe, practitioner can better view atrial activity and control tachyarrhythmias. Helps in diagnosis of complex arrhythmias	Patient must be cooperative or sedated. Can be done at the bedside in a monitored situation

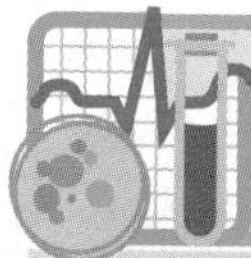

Table 15–1
Diagnostic Tests and Procedures for Evaluating Cardiovascular Status *Continued*

Diagnostic Test or Procedure	Purpose	Findings	Health Care Provider Responsibilities
Cardiac catheterization	Invasive diagnostic procedure Catheters are placed in various locations in heart, dye is injected, and pictures are taken. Helps in making diagnosis and planning surgery Some patients' cardiac defect can be treated through catheters.	Visualization of heart and great vessels Also can be used as interventional procedure to treat heart defects	Provide pre-catheterization teaching Performed in specialized suite for heart catheterization Post-catheterization: monitor insertion site for bleeding. Monitor affected extremity circulation.
Angiography	X-ray visualization of the anatomy of the heart chambers or blood vessels during or after the introduction of a radiopaque contrast medium into either an umbilical or percutaneous femoral site (i.e., completed during cardiac catheterization procedure)	Procedure is completed if further anatomic clarification after non-invasive imaging is needed, if child's history and assessment is not consistent with non-invasive imaging findings, or child has very complex lesion.	Complications can include catheter-related problems such as vascular/arterial occlusion, venous thrombosis, air embolism, coronary arterial injection, myocardial stain (injection of contrast medium into the myocardium), and myocardial perforation. Child must be monitored for these complications.

accurate reading. The probe can be clipped onto fingers, toes, earlobes, or the spongy tissue between the thumb and the index finger. Inaccurate values are more likely to exist if the child is peripherally vasoconstricted, cold, or in shock, or if the child has low cardiac output. Also, if the child is moving, the values are likely to be inaccurate.

Electrocardiogram

Electrocardiographic techniques utilize the electrical impulse each heart beat generates to provide a graphic tracing of the electrical activity produced by the heart from different sides and different planes of the body. Electrodes are applied to the body surface with special adhesive pads and conductive gel to detect the magnitude and the duration of electrical currents produced in the heart (Fig. 15–3). An electrocardiogram (ECG or EKG) assists in determining the anatomy of a defect and in diagnosing disturbances in conduction and produces data about the size and workload on the heart.

Continuous bedside electrocardiographic monitoring is usually a three-lead system used to provide a constant monitor of the child's heart rhythm at the bedside. It is used to track heart rate, changes in rhythm, and frequency of arrhythmias, but it is a limited diagnostic tool. Because some children may have skin that is sensitive to the tape and gel of commercial pads, the sites should be inspected daily and changed frequently. The nurse is responsible for setting minimum and maximum limits and seeing that alarms are functioning and activated.

Multilead electrocardiography is used for diagnostic purposes when there is a cardiac defect or arrhythmia that is auscultated or suspected. The traditional 12-lead ECG is performed by simultaneously recording six limb leads and six precordial leads that are placed in specific locations. Variations are noted that might indicate cardiac lesions and normal deviations. For example, the electrocardiogram of a newborn is characterized by right ventricular dominance that is normal at that age. Nurses assist in obtaining the most accurate reading by encouraging the child to keep very still while the strip is running.

caREminder: *Although most modern multilead ECG machines print out a diagnosis at the top of the ECG strip, the information given must be verified by a cardiac specialist, as this information may be inaccurate for the pediatric patient.*

A **Holter monitor** is an ambulatory 8- to 24-hour electrocardiogram. Electrocardiographic electrodes are placed on the chest wall and are connected to a small recorder carried by the child that continuously tapes the ECG rhythm. The family is given a diary in which they record the timing of the day's activities and any symptoms. The tape is then fed into a computer that scans the types, number, and duration of arrhythmias. Holter monitors can be obtained to document the presence of arrhythmias, to determine precipitous or detrimental

Figure 15–3
A normal ECG waveform. (From Black, J. M., & Matassarin-Jacobs, E. [Eds.] [1997]. *Medical-surgical nursing: Clinical management for continuity of care* [5th ed., p. 1222]. Philadelphia: W. B. Saunders. Reprinted with permission.)

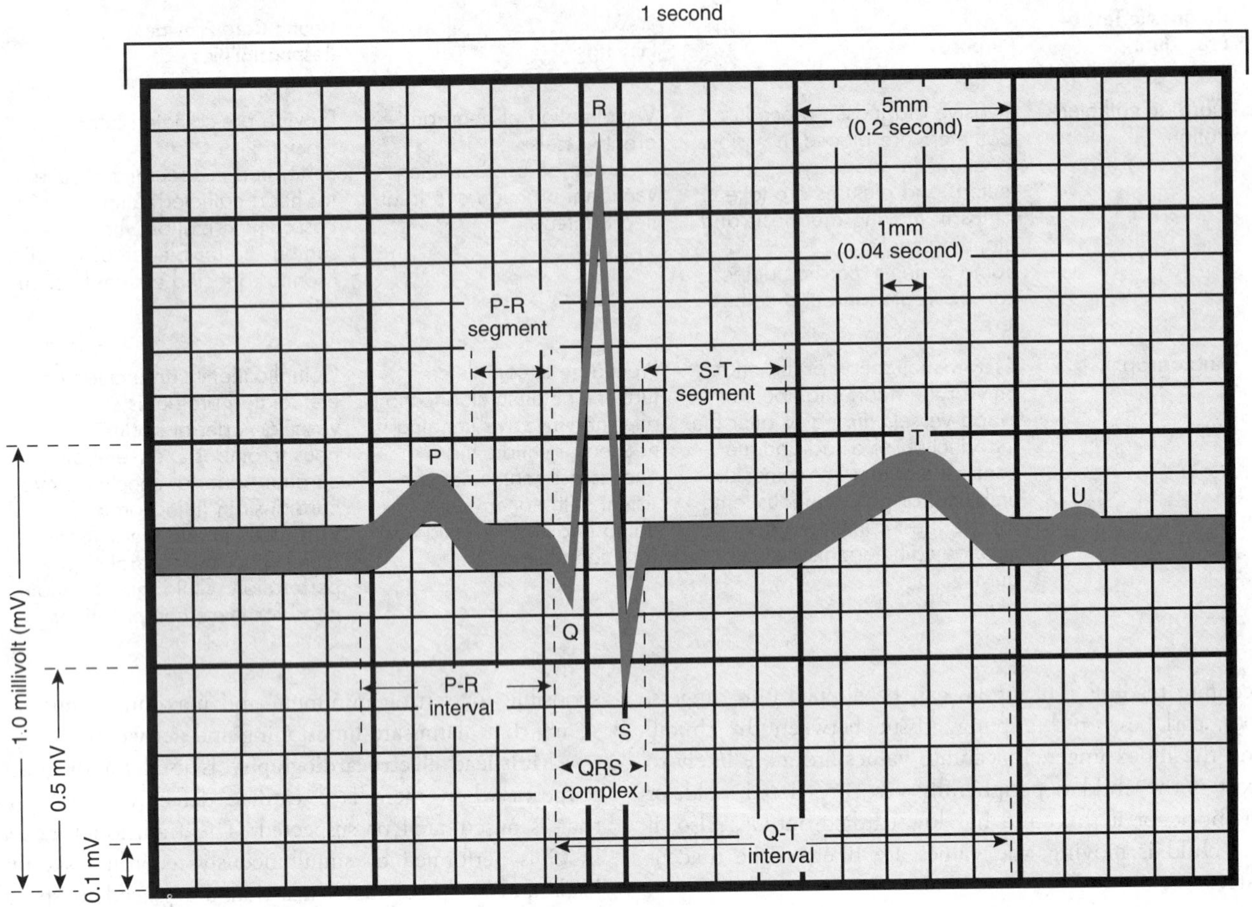

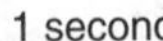

ECG Wave Forms

The letters, P, QRS, and T are used to label the ECG waveforms produced.

The **P wave** is the first wave of the ECG complex and represents atrial depolarization and contraction or the spreading of the impulses from the sinus node through the atria. The P wave is normally upright, smooth, and rounded.

The **P-R interval** represents the time it takes an impulse to trace from the AV node to the bundle of His, which is timed from beginning of the atrial depolarization to the beginning of ventricular depolarization. Normal P-R interval is 0.12 to 0.20 second.

The **QRS complex** reflects ventricular depolarization and contraction. This complex consists of three separate waves. The first negative deflection is the Q wave; the R wave is the positive or upright stroke; and the S wave is the negative deflection that follows. Not all rhythm strips show all three waves.

The **T wave** signifies the repolarization of the ventricles. Normally it has a smooth, rounded shape and points in the same direction as the QRS complex. Variations of T waves can indicate electrolyte imbalances and myocardial injury.

The **Q-T interval** is measured from the beginning of the Q wave to the end of the T wave. It reflects the total time of ventricular depolarization and repolarization or electrical systole. Normal length varies with age, gender, and heart rate.

The **S-T segment** is an isoelectric line that reflects the time that ventricles are in an absolute refractory period between ventricular repolarization and depolarization. It runs from the end of the QRS complex to the beginning of the T wave.

events, and to evaluate the efficiency of antiarrhythmic drugs.

Echocardiogram

The echocardiogram is a non-invasive diagnostic tool that permits the visualization of valves, ventricles, septa, the atria, and vessels. Echocardiography can measure chamber enlargement, wall thickening, stroke volume, and blood shunting and is sensitive enough to measure small amounts of fluid between the pericardial membranes. Without increasing the risk of operative morbidity and mortality, some children can have an echocardiogram and thereby avoid catheterization (Krabill et al., 1987; Verklan, 1997).

Echocardiography uses ultrasound (high frequency sound waves) to produce an image of the heart in motion. A transducer is placed on the chest wall, and, through ultrasonic gel, the ultrasonic pulses are bounced off the structures of the heart. The returned echoes, or signals, are then processed into a visual image. The test is painless, yet it requires a child to lie still for up to an hour. Obesity, a thick chest, or motion by the child can obstruct the visualization of structures. Frequently, infants and toddlers are sedated for this procedure, because it is unlikely that the young child will hold still for the duration of the study. In many cases, an accurate diagnosis via echocardiography can circumvent the need for cardiac catheterization for diagnostic purposes.

The advent of real-time imaging and cross-sectional imaging and the development of the expertise of fetal echocardiographers have resulted in the ability to diagnose CHD prenatally. In as early as 16 to 18 weeks' gestation, fetal cardiac ultrasound may diagnose problems. However, this can occur only if the obstetrician recommends a level II sonogram, by which such problems are initially detected. Routine level I sonograms do not detect CHD (Allen, 1990; Ardinger, 1997; Derek & Kline, 1990). Expectant mothers selected for a fetal echocardiogram are those who are considered to be at high risk for problems. This group includes mothers with a history of CHD in the family, maternal diabetes, maternal drug abuse, and other factors. When a prenatal diagnosis determines the presence of congenital heart disease, it may alter the plan for a routine delivery. Options in these cases include delivery of the infant in a high-risk unit and the provision of life-sustaining measures if required for the neonate.

Transesophageal Pacing/ Echocardiography

Transesophageal echocardiography (TEE) is an invasive diagnostic procedure that assesses cardiac vascular structures and function. TEE utilizes high-frequency ultrasound waves transmitted from a probe in the esophagus. The ultrasonic transducer is advanced orally into the esophagus, allowing tomographic imaging of the heart and thoracic areas. Images obtained supplement information gathered from a standard transthoracic echocardiogram. It can be performed as an outpatient procedure or in the critical care unit. This procedure is becoming more common in the intraoperative setting to assess surgical repairs once the child is disconnected from cardiopulmonary bypass and before the child's chest is sutured closed.

Esophageal electrocardiography is helpful in developing the differential diagnosis of complex arrhythmias. These procedures consist primarily of esophageal placement of nasogastric tubes containing the ECG electrodes. Activity recorded in the esophagus amplifies atrial depolarization and identifies otherwise easily obscured arrhythmias. The probe can also pace and capture the rhythm of the heart for treatment of tachyarrhythmias and perform stress testing of children who are unable to exercise. The role of the nurse is to coordinate the procedures, administer the medications, provide teaching, and assess and monitor the child.

Cardiac Catheterization

Cardiac catheterization is an invasive diagnostic procedure that provides visualization of the heart and the great vessels and also provides information about cardiac function.

Specific information obtained during this procedure includes

- Size and morphology of the heart to identify anatomic abnormalities
- Blood gas values with oxygen saturation in different chambers and vessels
- Direction and amount of shunting
- Intracardiac pressure gradient
- Evaluation of cardiac muscle and pumping function

The procedure is used to diagnose CHD, to complete electrophysiologic studies of the heart, and as an interventional technique to assist in the treatment of the child's condition. The procedure involves passing a thin, flexible radiopaque catheter into the chambers of the heart via a peripheral vessel, usually the femoral vein or artery. In the neonate, the umbilical vein or artery may be used. A percutaneous needle puncture is all that is needed to introduce the catheter into the femoral vessel. In some children with very small vessels that are difficult to reach, a cutdown may be necessary.

Catheterization of the right side of the heart is completed by passing the catheter into the femoral vein and advancing it through the inferior vena cava and into the right atrium, the right ventricle, and the pulmonary artery. If the foramen ovale is patent or if an atrial septal defect is present, the catheter may be advanced into the left atrium through these openings to evaluate the left side of the heart. If there is no atrial or ventricular communication, then evaluation of the left side of the heart is completed by passing the catheter into the femoral artery and into the descending aorta to the left.

Angiography is performed when a contrast medium is injected into a chamber or vessel of the heart during catheterization. A video recording of the x-ray film is made to allow the health care team to replay the tape at a later time and to further analyze the structure of the heart. Many, if not most, diagnostic pediatric cardiac catheterizations are performed as outpatient procedures, as are some interventional catheterizations. A cardiac catheterization suite is a specially equipped area in the hospital with an operating table, fluoroscopy cameras, hemodynamic monitoring equipment, and specialized personnel.

Pre-Catheterization Care

When preparing a child for cardiac catheterization, baseline assessment includes an evaluation of the child's physiologic status, with an emphasis on the cardiac state and on the peripheral extremities. Lower extremity pulses are palpated and marked with a pen for easy location. Documentation of accurate height and weight is essential for drug dose and other calculations performed for catheterization. If a child has signs of systemic infection, such as a runny nose, fever, or skin rash, the catheterization may be delayed. The nurse should verify that the child has had nothing to eat or to drink prior to the procedure, noting when the last fluids or food was ingested. A careful history for allergies is ascertained, because contrast dyes are used during angiography. Information about any adverse reactions from a previous catheterization, such as vomiting, should also be elicited.

When children are sent to the catheterization laboratory, they are confronted with technical equipment and a room full of strangers where they may feel defenseless. Preparation for this procedure should be provided before the day of the procedure to both guardians and patients in an honest, open way and in a relaxed setting. The nurse should consider the age and maturity of the child when preparing an explanation of the environment and of the catheterization routine, utilizing a chronological description from admission to discharge (Fig. 15–4). Teaching can include a tour of the catheterization laboratory and recovery area. Children can also be shown the areas where their families and friends will be waiting. It is helpful if the child is able to meet a staff member and recognize that person on the day of the study. Discussions should be oriented toward de-escalating anxiety in the child. The nurse should explain the rationale for restraints, and, if the child has a clear concept of time, tell the child how long the procedure will last. The nurse should also include a description of how the staff will be dressed and the importance of being on bed rest and of keeping the affected leg immobilized.

Tip: *During pre-catheterization teaching, assure the older child that the procedure will be done in the fold of the leg and that his or her genitalia will be covered. The child will probably not know where the "groin" is located, or what it is. Using the word "fold" or "bend" of the leg is much clearer to the child.*

Assure the child that there is little pain or discomfort, but that the procedure does require cooperation by lying still for a period of time. A relaxed, informed child can develop a sense of personal control, anticipate events, and overcome misconceptions. At the beginning of the teaching and tour, the nurse should ascertain whether the child has undergone a catheterization before and what he or she remembers about the other experiences. It is not unusual for a child with complex CHD to have had multiple catheterizations. Preparing the children and the caregivers helps decrease anxiety and allows them to be better informed and prepared.

Tip: *Encourage the child to pick out a favorite toy, doll, or blanket to keep throughout the procedure and in the recovery area.*

A peripheral intravenous line is started before catheterization for medication access and to prevent dehydration in cyanotic children. During the catheterization, the child's feet are not easily accessible for inspection or to assess for infiltrations; therefore, intravenous lines in the feet are avoided whenever possible.

Before the catheterization, the child is sedated. The choice of medication varies depending on the institution, the age of the child, and the type of catheterization planned. Conscious sedation is provided for routine catheterizations. General anesthesia may be used for procedures that place the child at greater risk or for more complex interventional catheterization. Before sedation, the nurse should have the toilet-trained child void, preferably before he or she is transported to the catheterization laboratory. Once the child has been sedated, he or she should be kept flat in bed to avoid the risk of injury due to the altered mental state and due to potential complications from the catheterization process.

Catheterization

During the procedure, the child is monitored with automatic blood pressure cuffs, pulse oximetry, and cardiac rhythm monitors. Emergency drug dosages are calculated before the procedure. The catheterization laboratory can

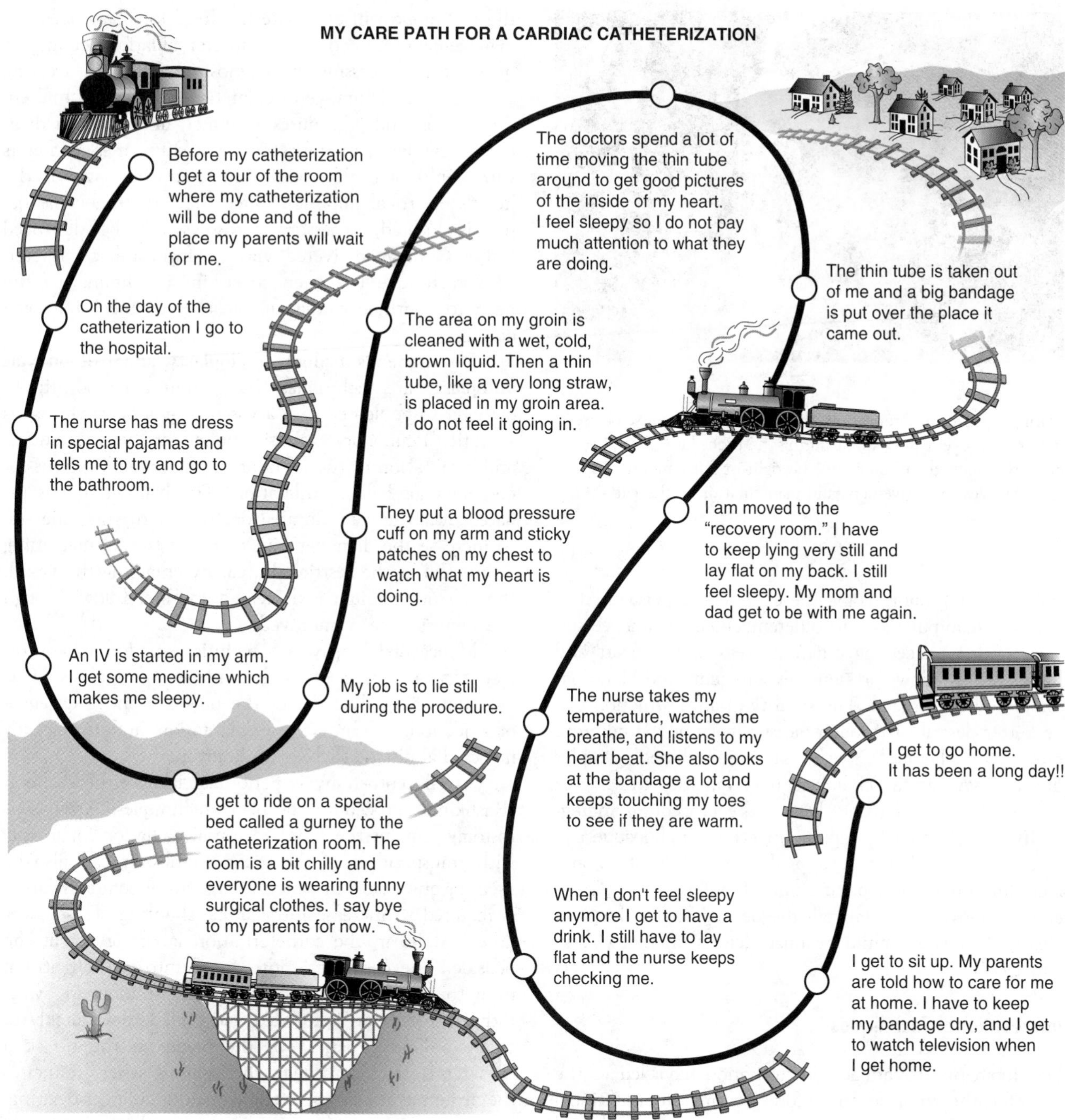

MY CARE PATH FOR A CARDIAC CATHETERIZATION
Before my catheterization I get a tour of the room where my catheterization will be done and of the place my parents will wait for me.
On the day of the catheterization I go to the hospital.
The nurse has me dress in special pajamas and tells me to try and go to the bathroom.
An IV is started in my arm. I get some medicine which makes me sleepy.
I get to ride on a special bed called a gurney to the catheterization room. The room is a bit chilly and everyone is wearing funny surgical clothes. I say bye to my parents for now.
My job is to lie still during the procedure.
They put a blood pressure cuff on my arm and sticky patches on my chest to watch what my heart is doing.
The area on my groin is cleaned with a wet, cold, brown liquid. Then a thin tube, like a very long straw, is placed in my groin area. I do not feel it going in.
The doctors spend a lot of time moving the thin tube around to get good pictures of the inside of my heart. I feel sleepy so I do not pay much attention to what they are doing.
The thin tube is taken out of me and a big bandage is put over the place it came out.
I am moved to the "recovery room." I have to keep lying very still and lay flat on my back. I still feel sleepy. My mom and dad get to be with me again.
The nurse takes my temperature, watches me breathe, and listens to my heart beat. She also looks at the bandage a lot and keeps touching my toes to see if they are warm.
When I don't feel sleepy anymore I get to have a drink. I still have to lay flat and the nurse keeps checking me.
I get to sit up. My parents are told how to care for me at home. I have to keep my bandage dry, and I get to watch television when I get home.
I get to go home. It has been a long day!!

Figure 15-4
A care path for a child undergoing cardiac catheterization.

be quite cool. Wrap the head and extremities of small children and infants in blankets or use a mechanical warming blanket. An infant's temperature should be monitored continuously by a rectal probe. After the child is positioned and restrained, the site for catheter insertion is prepared. This usually involves cleansing the side with iodine solution and injecting topical lidocaine over the site where the skin is to be punctured.

Catheters are introduced into the cardiovascular system through the central venous system (or right side of the heart) to the right atrium, or the left side of the heart (that is retrograde up the abdominal aorta) through the arterial system. A percutaneous sheath is placed, usually using the groin's femoral artery and/or vein. This allows various catheters to be taken in and out without creating any new insertion sites and minimizes vessel

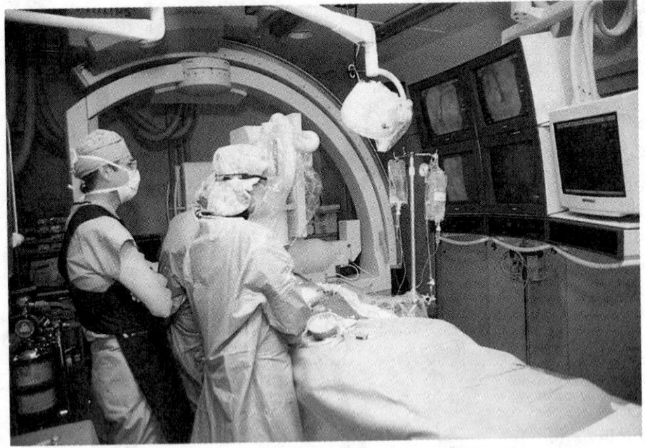

Figure 15–5
During cardiac catheterization, the child is under conscious sedation to prevent movement during the procedure. The physician introduces a catheter into the right or left femoral vein and observes the movement and manipulation of the catheter on a monitor.

trauma. Using fluoroscopy, the catheters are visualized as they are manipulated into different chambers and vessels (Fig. 15–5). Accessing different areas of the heart and blood vessels allows pressure measurements and blood gas sampling in each area. The severity of an obstruction can be better described through measurement of the different pressure gradients. Oxygen saturation blood samples drawn from various chambers help quantify the degree and location of shunting. During the procedure, **angiography** is performed by rapidly injecting a radiopaque dye through the catheter at a predetermined location and recording on motion picture film. The fluoroscopic cameras are moved to obtain all the desired angles that will clearly delineate a child's cardiac defects on film (Verklan, 1997).

Interventional Techniques

Developments in cardiac catheterization have led to the use of catheterization to perform routine interventional procedures. Some interventional procedures are performed urgently to save a life, whereas others may eliminate or delay surgery for some children with cardiovascular diseases. Interventional catheterization can provide the child with a procedure that has less physical and emotional trauma, faster recovery, and a shorter, less expensive hospital stay than surgery.

Standard interventional procedures include electrophysiology studies with ablation, percutaneous balloon angioplasty, myocardial biopsy, atrial septostomy, vascular occlusion devices, and stents. **Electrophysiology studies (EPS)** are used for dysrhythmias that do not respond to pharmaceutical management or when it is believed that the technique will eliminate the need for pharmaceutical management. Closed chest catheter ablation techniques have been successful in diagnosing and then treating ventricular and supraventricular tachycardias in children. Preparation and procedures are much like those for diagnostic cardiac catheterization, but EPS uses catheters with multipolar electrodes that map the path of the heart's electrical impulses. Once the arrhythmogenic tissue is located, accessory pathways can be destroyed through energy delivered via the intracardiac catheter. This technique has been successful in eliminating the need to continue cardiac medication regimens for some children.

Percutaneous balloon angioplasty and balloon valvuloplasty are techniques that permit a balloon-tipped catheter to be floated into a vascular area or valve that is stenotic. Pulmonary stenosis, pulmonary valve stenosis, and coarctation of the aorta are common applications for percutaneous balloon dilatation. The balloon that is inflated over the stenotic area deforms or ruptures the site to increase the diameter by expanding the intimal lining of a vessel at the restricted area. By enlarging the vessel, the pressure gradient is decreased and blood flow through the stenotic area is improved.

Myocardial biopsy is a technique performed to collect a small piece of cardiac tissue for analysis. This procedure is used to detect the presence and the degree of rejection in cardiac transplantation and to identify myocardial disease such as cardiomyopathy.

Atrial septostomy is performed using either balloon (Rashkind's procedure) or blade techniques. Atrial septostomy remains the standard initial palliation for infants with transposition of the great arteries. It can also be used for any lesion in which a large atrial communication is required to increase intracardiac shunting. This procedure is done in the catheterization laboratory or at the bedside. The catheter is introduced into the left atrium from the right atrium through a patent foramen ovale. Either the balloon is inflated and pulled back quickly to create a larger opening or the blade on the tip of a catheter is crossed through the opening where it incises the atrium as it crosses, thereby creating a larger opening. These techniques may sound crude, but they can provide an effective tool in saving and improving the lives of infants.

There are various techniques developed to perform transcatheter vascular occlusion. A device can be implanted to embolize vessels such as the patent ductus arteriosus or systemic to pulmonary collaterals. **Coil embolization** is one device used to occlude a vessel. A coil wire is delivered through an end-hole catheter that is extruded out the end of the catheter at a predetermined location. On extrusion, the piece of steel coils back on itself, and this promotes clot formation and acts to embolize the vessel. Soon after coil placement, fibrous tissue grows around the device, ensuring its immobility. Successful closure using such devices can allow for selected children to avoid surgical intervention. Of the occlusion devices in use, coil embolization is a commonly seen technique. Coil embolization in the patent ductus arteriosus, or collateral vessel to occlude systemic to pulmonary collaterals, can allow some children to bypass the need for surgery, resulting in lower risks and trauma.

Stainless steel **stents** can be placed in areas of the branch pulmonary artery system that are stenotic. They are made of a stainless steel mesh compressed into a small diameter tube that is etched with multiple rows of staged rectangles that expand when extruded into placement. Once expanded, the slots assume a diamond shape, appearing much like a very small version of "chicken wire," and can be further expanded with a balloon. Through expansion, the stent effectively increases the diameter of the vessel and endothelializes into the vessel wall over time.

Post-Catheterization Care

The child's cardiovascular status is continuously assessed after undergoing a cardiac catheterization. Nursing measures are directed toward prevention and/or monitoring of complications that may occur (Chart 15–4). Assessment of the child's cardiovascular status includes recording of vital signs, checking the insertion site, monitoring and comparing catheterized extremities, and assessing the child's level of consciousness. Post–cardiac catheterization vital signs are performed much like for a postoperative surgical recovery patient. Generally, these observations are taken every 15 minutes until the child is awake and stable, then every half hour for 3 hours, then hourly up to 6 hours or more, if needed. When checking the child, assessment for signs of hypotension, such as cold clammy skin, increased heart rate, or dizziness, is done. Cardiac monitoring and pulse oximetry are used to aid in assessment of the child's status until the child is stabilized. During the recovery period, the child remains on bed rest with the head of the bed flat or elevated only slightly (Care Path 15–1).

Nurses participate in the facilitation of recovery by encouraging the child to remain flat in bed, keeping the punctured leg straight for the prescribed time. Toddlers may be more cooperative if placed in the prone position in a parent's lap. The need for immobilization and frequent monitoring should be explained to family members. The nurse should caution the child to avoid sitting, raising the head, straining the abdomen, or coughing during the post-catheterization recovery period.

When vital signs are taken, the dressing on the groin is inspected for evidence of bleeding or hematoma. If a hematoma is observed, the nurse should mark the margins with a felt-tipped pin and monitor for changes.

Chart 15–4

Potential Complications After Cardiac Catheterization

Complication	Description
Hemorrhage	Vessel bleeding at insertion site, decreased hematocrit
Hematoma	False aneurysm, subacute hematoma
Vomiting	Caused by anxiety, NPO status, sedative drugs
Hypovolemia	Status, blood loss, diuretic action of dyes
Hypotension	Caused by medications, bleeding, contrast media
Arrhythmia	Transient bradycardia, premature ventricular contractions
Venous occlusion	Usually transient, from a clot, intimal tear, or herniation
Loss of pulses	Loss of pulse in catheterized extremity, usually transient, caused by vessel vasospasm, usage of larger catheters; smaller child at greater risk
Arterial thrombus	Aggregation of blood factors causing arterial occlusion
Renal damage	Clearance of contrast media, hematuria, oliguria, anuria
Fever/infection	Low-grade, 4–8 hours, catheter-induced (rare)
Pulmonary embolus	Risks greater in patient with intracardiac mixing and polycythemia from venous stasis pressure at puncture site
Allergic reaction	From sedatives, contrast media (rare)
Perforation	Tamponade, cardiac perforation by angiographic catheter (rare)
Arteriovenous fistula	When both the artery and vein are punctured, a communication between them shunting blood from the distal extremity
CNS insult	Strokes, seizures from air embolus (rare)
Death	Highest occurrence in infants (rare)

Alert: *Even though clot formation has occurred at the catheter insertion site, hemorrhaging could occur during the recovery period. The groin dressing should remain on the child, and the site should not be covered with blankets to allow any blood drainage to be noted immediately by health care personnel.*

With each set of vital signs, there should be an assessment of both lower extremities, with bilateral palpation for the presence of dorsalis pedis and posterior tibial pulses and inspection for color, temperature, and capillary refill and for continued immobilization of the affected leg. The affected foot may be cyanotic or cooler temporarily, especially if there is vasospasm of the vessel or if the child's core temperature is also low.

Level of consciousness is assessed, and clear liquids are initiated once the child is fully awake. Fluids are encouraged to help the kidneys filter out contrast dyes. Children and their guardians are given written and verbal discharge instructions before returning home of signs and symptoms to assess for (TIP 15–1).

Care Path 15–1 An Interdisciplinary Plan of Care for the Child with Diagnostic Cardiac Catheterization

Nursing Diagnosis	Patient/Family Intermediate Outcomes		
	Day: Preoperative Teaching	Day: Pre-catheterization	Day: Post-catheterization
Anxiety related to fear of physical harm, knowledge deficit, separation of child from parents, home care	Child and family will schedule preoperative tour and teaching. Child and family will express understanding and will ask pertinent questions, expressing feelings and concerns. Patient will receive an age-appropriate explanation of sensations to expect, in an honest, simple way.	Family will provide comfort and encouragement to child. Child will be interested, at ease, and playful. Reinforce teaching. Child will receive preoperative medications in a timely manner and will take a comfort toy to procedure. Family will be encouraged to stay with child right up until procedure.	Family/child will verbalize discharge instructions and will express understanding of them. Child will remain calm and cooperative.
Alteration in cardiac output related to underlying cardiac defect, fluid imbalance, dehydration, from NPO preoperatively, contrast media, narcotics, blood loss, alteration in temperature and mechanical forces		Child will maintain cardiac output within precatheterization parameters. Child's vital signs will remain stable.	Child will take adequate PO; urine output will be adequate. → →
Potential alteration in tissue perfusion related to presence of catheters in vein and artery, bleeding, embolus, hematoma		Child will maintain adequate nutrition and oxygenation at the cellular level. Child's extremities will remain warm, well perfused, and with normal movement and sensation. Child's pulses remain strong and palpable.	→ → → Child experiences no bleeding or hematoma at insertion site.

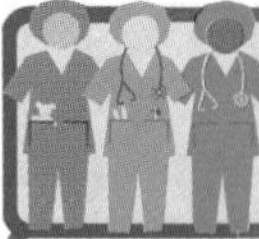

Care Path 15-1 An Interdisciplinary Plan of Care for the Child with Diagnostic Cardiac Catheterization *Continued*

Care Intervention Categories	Day: Preoperative Teaching	Day: Pre-catheterization	Day: Postcatheterization
Consults	Catheterization laboratory personnel Clinical nurse specialist (CNS)	Catheterization staff	Recovery staff Clinical nurse specialist (CNS) Pediatric cardiologist
Discharge planning	Predict special needs of individual patients.		Test results reviewed with family. Family given written and oral instructions with signs and symptoms to call for.
Labs	CBC, ECG, chest x-ray, electrolytes, and typing and crossmatching of blood		CBC if blood loss was substantial.
Medications and IVs		Maintenance IV; NPO—hold routine medications.	IV until taking PO fluids well; resume precatheterization medication.
Monitors		Baseline vital signs and oxygen saturation	ECG until stable, pulse oximetry, and vital signs
Nutrition	Routine	NPO	Once alert, clear liquids; advance as child tolerates.
Pain management		Pre-catheterization sedation	Avoid sedatives—child needs to wake up so he or she can be discharged. Encourage comfort measures and parent contact.
Play therapy/school	Therapeutic play, tour of the catheterization laboratory, playroom visit.	Review teaching; remind child that he or she can end the day in the playroom.	To playroom before discharge
Psychosocial	Reinforce teaching; encourage parents to ventilate anxieties and to ask questions.	Reinforce teaching; encourage parents to ventilate anxieties and to ask questions.	Reinforce teaching, encourage parents to ventilate anxieties and to ask questions. Encourage a parent to stay with patient.
Radiology	Pre-catheterization x-ray		

Care Path continued on following page

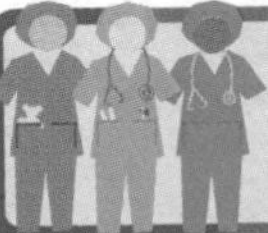

Care Path 15–1 An Interdisciplinary Plan of Care for the Child with Diagnostic Cardiac Catheterization *Continued*

Care Intervention Categories	Day: Preoperative Teaching	Day: Pre-catheterization	Day: Post-catheterization
Safety and activity		Once sedated, keep child in bed.	Leg immobilized, rails up, bed flat
Self-care	Normal ADLs	May help with care	Once child is discharged, limit rough play; no baths—short shower only for 2 days.
Teaching	Explain procedures to child and family. Give them a tour of catheterization laboratory. Describe the procedure in chronological order.	Reinforce teaching.	Discharge instructions both written and oral.
Visitors	Include all significant others and siblings as family wishes.	Limit to immediate family.	Minimize visitors to keep child quiet and calm. Encourage parents to stay at bedside.
Vital signs/baseline parameters		Baseline height and weight with vital signs. Vital signs monitored frequently during procedure	Every 15 minutes until stable, then every half hour for 2 hours, then every hour for a total of 6 hours.

ADLs, activities of daily living; CBC, complete blood count; ECG, electrocardiogram; IM, intramuscular; NPO, nothing by mouth; PO, by mouth.

TIP 15–1 A Teaching Intervention Plan for the Child Going Home After Cardiac Catheterization

Nursing Diagnosis and Family Outcomes

- Knowledge deficit: Management of the child at home after a cardiac catheterization.

  Outcomes:

  Child and family will express concerns and will remain calm and supportive of the child.

  Child and family will follow written discharge instructions for care of the child and the puncture site.

  Family will contact physician to make follow-up appointments and if any complications occur.

Treatment of the Child

Activity

- A child may resume normal activities, but no running, bike riding, skating, jumping, swimming, or other vigorous "roughhousing" or sports for the next 3 days.
- Children may return to school 2 days after discharge.

TIP 15-1 A Teaching Intervention Plan for the Child Going Home After Cardiac Catheterization *Continued*

Catheterization Site

- Inspect the catheterization site daily for a week. Some bruising at the catheterization site is common. If there is drainage from the catheterization site, call your doctor.
- A small amount of blood on the bandage is normal. If bleeding that soaks through the bandage has occurred, hold pressure on the catheterization site until the bleeding stops and call the doctor.

Bathing

After a catheterization, a child should avoid prolonged bathing for 2 days. A sponge bath or brief shower is permitted.

Diet

Resume previous diet at home.

Pain

Most children do not need any medicine for pain once home, although a child may have some slight groin discomfort.

Behavior

- Even after a short stay in the hospital, it is possible to see temporary changes in the child's behavior (i.e., irritability, irregular sleep pattern, bad dreams, an increase in "childish ways"). It is important to be understanding but at the same time keep basic discipline rules.
- Because illness and hospitalization affect the whole family, parents may see changes in the child's behavior at home or in school *and* in the behavior of siblings.

Follow-up

You should schedule a follow-up appointment within a week. After reviewing the catheterization procedure, the doctor will discuss the results and the plan of care with you.

Contact Health Care Provider if

- Your child has a fever higher than 101°F during the next week after the heart catheterization.
- The leg in which the catheterization was done becomes cooler, paler, or more numb than the other leg.

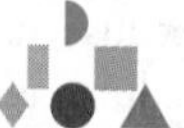

Treatment Modalities

The Interdisciplinary Cardiac Health Care Team

The cardiac team is composed of an interdisciplinary group of health care professionals who together create goals and a treatment plan in collaboration with the child and the family. The cardiac team includes nurses, surgeons, cardiologists, social workers, anesthesiologists, and other ancillary personnel (Chart 15–5). In pediatric cardiac programs, health care team members meet on a regular basis to discuss the children with a cardiovascular diagnosis and determine appropriate plans of care. Selected potential surgical and catheterization cases are reviewed for input from team members to determine the most effective regimen of care. This promotes an interdisciplinary approach to care and encourages open dialogue regarding all children in a specific cardiac care program. The treatment options available for children with cardiac disease include interventional catheterization, cardiac surgery, pacemakers, and medical management using pharmaceutical, dietary, and activity interventions.

Chart 15–5

Interdisciplinary Members of the Pediatric Cardiac Care Team

Cardiovascular Surgeon. Preoperative examination and screening; recommends and performs surgery; postoperative management

Cardiologist. Referring physician; performs diagnostic evaluation, including cardiac catheterization, and medical management of patient

Anesthesiologist. Committed anesthesiologist to care specifically for cardiac patients; facilitate continuity of care for this patient population

Clinical Nurse Specialist/Nurse Practitioner. Provides continuity and emotional support for patients and families throughout hospital stay; family teaching and support pre- and postoperatively; daily rounds and assessment; collaborates with physicians in direction of care; program coordination and administration

Nursing Staff. Cardiovascular nursing is a subspecialty of critical care nursing. It is a selective group of staff trained in specific protocols and adept in caring for this patient population. Once a patient is convalescing, he or she is generally placed on the regular pediatric ward.

Social Worker. Provides counseling and guidance for families coping with emotional and economic stresses of illness or hospitalization; supplies crisis intervention, assesses home and social environment, and makes referrals to appropriate community resources

Play Therapist/Child Life Specialist. Provides play-related growth and development interventions; assists with emotional support and recreational diversional activities for pediatric patients

Financial Screen/Clerical Support. Provides financial clearance for procedures and hospitalization; arranges accommodations for out-of-town families and scheduling of events

Volunteers/Community Networking. Varies in communities; some hospitals have specific heart family volunteers, others have scheduled support groups

Cardiac Surgery

Pediatric cardiovascular surgical advances over recent decades have been instrumental in reducing mortality and allowing for definitive repairs at an earlier age. The focus of care has moved beyond survivability in short-term years to a greater number of children with complex congenital heart disease living to become adults.

Palliative Procedures

Surgeries that are not curative, but rather are performed for heart defects as a surgical bridge, are called palliative procedures. These types of surgical interventions can allow the child's condition to become more stable and to provide time for the child to grow until a more definitive surgical correction is viable. Sometimes palliative procedures are performed because there are no curative surgical options for a particular heart defect.

Pulmonary Artery Banding

Pulmonary artery banding is provided to children who have conditions in which there is excess pulmonary blood flow to the lungs. These children cannot tolerate or are not ready for total surgical repair, yet the failure of medical interventions to manage the child's CHF necessitates the performance of this procedure. The banding causes a narrowing of the pulmonary artery, which minimizes pulmonary blood flow. Banding is performed with a lateral thoracotomy incision and placement of a Teflon tape band around the main pulmonary artery. If the band is too tight, it can result in reversal of the shunt and cyanosis. If the band is too loose, excess blood flow to the lungs will continue.

Shunts

Shunts are placed to increase pulmonary blood flow for cyanotic infants by creating an extra pathway for blood to reach the lungs. Some common lesions for which a shunt may be placed in the neonate are pulmonary atresia, tricuspid atresia, tetralogy of Fallot, or severe pulmonary stenosis. Any infant less than 6 months of age with medically unmanageable hypoxic spells or cyanosis may require shunt placement.

Infants with severe cyanosis from restricted blood flow to the lungs may benefit from a systemic to pulmonary artery shunt. A **Blalock-Taussig** shunt is a procedure in which the subclavian artery is turned down and anastomosed to the pulmonary artery. Access to the vessels is through a lateral thoracotomy incision. Because it is not an open heart surgery, the shunt procedure is completed without putting the child on cardiopulmonary bypass. Even children who are very small or quite ill can usually tolerate this procedure without major complications. Common problems of a Blalock-Taussig (BT shunt) procedure are a thrombus or closure of the shunt, congestive heart failure from excessive pulmonary blood flow if the shunt is too large, and hypoperfusion of the affected arm. A modification of this procedure is more frequently used in which there is placement of a Gore-Tex tube graft from the subclavian artery to the pulmonary artery. The shunt's size is selected to be large enough to maximize pulmonary flow while avoiding excessive flow and CHF.

Slightly older children who have obstructive flow to the lungs may require a **Glenn's procedure**. The Glenn's procedure is a palliative surgery that optimizes the child's cardiovascular status and is frequently used as a staging procedure as part of the Fontan surgery (discussed later in this chapter). Glenn's procedure is an anastomosis of the superior vena cava to the pulmonary artery, which allows some blood to flow to the pulmonary system by bypassing the right side of the heart. This surgery also can be done through a thoracotomy incision.

Corrective Procedures

The surgical trend in recent years has been toward surgical intervention early in life, often in infancy. The timing of surgeries depends on the anatomy of the lesion, the child's growth and development, any concurrent illnesses, and family needs. Parents are encouraged to schedule the surgery when other family events and sources of stress are minimized. Issues that can hasten the time frame for completion of the surgeries include risks of pulmonary hypertension, prevention of aorta pulmonary collateral vessel development, and avoidance of deterioration of ventricular function. Children who develop irreversible pulmonary hypertension can become inoperable. Delay of surgeries may be required because of the presence of other medical conditions that make the child a poor surgical candidate. Surgery may also be delayed to allow the child to grow. For example, if the child needs a valve replacement, it is to the child's advantage that surgery be delayed to allow the heart to grow larger. This allows for placement of a larger valve that will not be quickly outgrown by the child.

Preoperative Teaching

As with any patient scheduled for surgery, the information given by the health care provider to the child and the family should include an explanation of the intended surgery and of complications that may occur and a description of the medical equipment that will be used to support the child during the recovery period. It is especially helpful to give the child and the family a chronological explanation of the events that will occur during the period from admission to discharge (Chart 15–6). (See Chapter 9 for preparing a child for surgery.) All questions should be answered honestly and kept in simple terms so families can comprehend them. The nurse should allow the parents to absorb information and to ask questions at their own pace. The preoperative teaching period is a good time for the nurse to assess family needs and family patterns of coping and interaction. This information should be incorporated into the plan of care for the child in order to ensure that the unique needs of the family are being met (Chart 15–7).

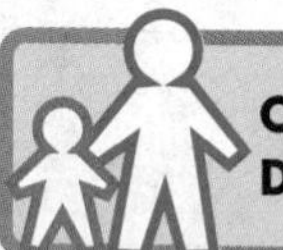

Chart 15–6
Developmental Considerations

Preparation of the Child for Cardiac Surgery

Infants

Avoid making changes in an infant's routine prior to surgery (e.g., starting to introduce solids or changing sleeping schedules).
Infants who are used to being around a variety of people will be less cranky in the unfamiliar environment of the acute care setting.
Place familiar items in bed with child, such as a music box or stuffed animal.

Toddler/Preschooler

Provide detailed information to parents; give simple and brief information to child.
Allow time to play, and space for exploration.
Encourage contact with security object.
Utilize imitation.
Dispel misconceptions.
Reinforce that there will be parental presence.

School-Age

Give more detailed explanation.
Reinforce peer involvement.
Introduce to hospital units and equipment.
Dispel myths.
Respect privacy; reduce exposure of body.
Provide simple reading materials.

Adolescent

Encourage peer interaction, and telephone access when possible.
Emphasize positive attributes; consider body image changes.
Use reading materials/videos.
Explain all activities; include patient in all decisions.
Respect need for privacy and allow for private teaching.

All Age Groups

Provide diversional activities when stable (VCRs, TV, books, toys).

A preoperative tour of the intensive care unit (ICU) helps alleviate stress for the older child and for parents and family members who have had no prior experience of the conditions in an ICU. It can be overwhelming for

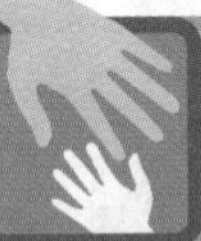

Chart 15-7
Nursing Interventions

Cardiac Preoperative Teaching Topics

Chronological Course of Events

Family blood donation
Preoperative day: intensive care unit (ICU) tour
Surgical procedure
ICU stay
Convalescence
Discharge planning
Follow-up

Child's General Appearance

Monitors
Sedation/pain management
Ventilator support
Chest tubes
Arterial and intravenous lines
Pacemaker

Postoperative Respiratory Needs

Ventilation: tube, suctioning
Turn, cough, deep breathing, incentive spirometry
Nasotracheal suctioning
Nasal cannula, oxygen mask or tent

Activity Progression

How to pick up child after surgery
ICU: bedrest, chair
Ambulation/playroom

Nutrition

NPO (nothing by mouth): preoperatively, ICU
IVs
How eating is advanced

Wound

Care and dressing

Sensory Stimuli

Noises, personnel
Child interactions/coping
Restraints
Pain management

parents to see ventilators, monitors, and a large variety of tubes and lines entering and exiting any small child, much less one's own. During preoperative teaching, parents should be allowed to visit another parent and child in the ICU. This may alleviate some of their fears.

The type of chest incision that the child will have should be explained to the parents. The surgeon makes this decision based on the type of surgery that is scheduled. All **cardiopulmonary bypass (pump) cases** require separation of the sternum. Either a midsternal or a lateral thoracotomy incision is used. Some surgeons use a mammary incision for female patients. This allows a V-neck shirt or swimsuit to be worn without showing a scar.

Parents should be told that there is no way to predict exactly how long the presence of various tubes and lines will be required or how long a child will be in the hospital after surgery. General guidelines can be given with an explanation that parents will be updated daily on how their child progresses. For many routine surgeries, a child spends most of the hospital stay in the ICU. Typically, a child who was once quite ill achieves a particular level of stability and may progress so quickly toward being able to return home that it is a surprise to the parents (Fig. 15–6).

Many hospitals have designated blood donor systems to encourage the family to have members donate blood for the child's surgery. Once the blood has been drawn, it is screened for suitability and then is designated for use during the child's surgery.

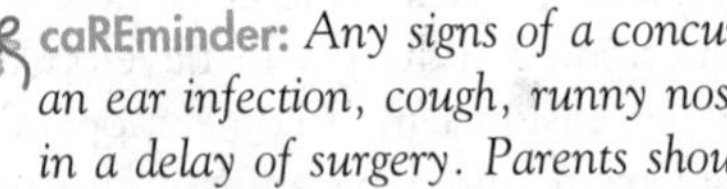

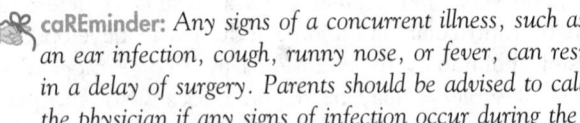

caREminder: *Any signs of a concurrent illness, such as an ear infection, cough, runny nose, or fever, can result in a delay of surgery. Parents should be advised to call the physician if any signs of infection occur during the immediate preoperative period.*

Intraoperative Care

In the surgical suite, the child is intubated and most of the monitoring and intravenous lines are placed before the chest incisions are made. Monitoring and invasive lines include ECG leads, nasogastric tube, pulse oximetry, Foley catheter, peripheral intravenous lines, intra-arterial line, and triple lumen central line with **central venous pressure (CVP)** monitoring.

Cardiopulmonary Bypass

Cardiopulmonary bypass incisions are placed midsternally by separating the skin and then splitting the sternum. The heart and lungs are connected to a cardiopulmonary bypass pump to oxygenate and perfuse the rest of the body while the heart is stopped to be repaired. The right side of the heart is cannulated, capturing venous blood before it returns to the heart. Venous blood is shunted to the pump, where it is oxygenated and circulated and the temperature is regulated. The oxygenated blood is returned to the body through the cannulas in the ascending aorta. During the time that it is on the pump, the heart is stabilized with an electrolyte solution called cardioplegia that helps immobilize and protect the heart

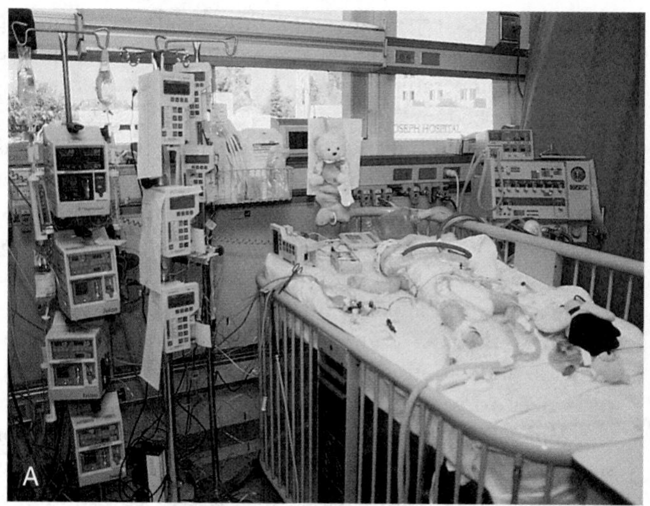

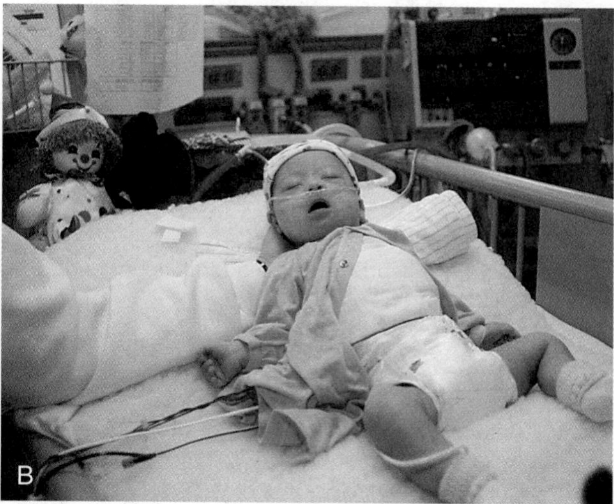

Figure 15–6
A, A child immediately after cardiac surgery. *B*, The same child 1 week later.

during the surgery. The cardiopulmonary bypass pump also reduces the body's metabolic rate and decreases oxygen demand during surgery by creating a hypothermic state.

Once the cardiac surgical repairs are done, the child is rewarmed and the heart is restarted by the surgeon. Before closing the chest, temporary pacing wires may be placed on the outside of the heart and passed through the chest wall. Chest tubes are placed to evacuate any bleeding from around the heart. Depending on the nature of the surgery and the monitoring needs, transthoracic central lines may be placed in the right or left atrium and/or the pulmonary artery. These allow for more detailed hemodynamic monitoring than can be provided by a CVP line alone. The sternum is closed and secured with wire. Finally, the skin is sutured shut.

Non-Pump Cases

Non-pump cases are those cases that do not require entering the heart and thus can be done without the technique of cardiopulmonary bypass. Examples are repairs of coarctation of the aorta or patent ductus arteriosus. These surgeries are usually completed using a lateral thoracotomy approach. In this approach, the pleural space is entered, therefore chest tube placement is required before the chest is closed. Generally, non-pump cases do not require placing of pacing wires or transthoracic lines in the child at the end of the surgery.

Postoperative Care

In caring for open heart surgical patients, small or abrupt changes in the status of a patient must be efficiently noted and acted on in the critical postoperative period. During the acute phase of care assessment, interventions are aimed at stabilizing the child, minimizing complications, and facilitating progression through the recovery process.

Vital sign parameters are defined by the surgical team and may vary from those of a normal heart, depending on the specific needs of an individual patient. If the patient still has intracardiac mixing after surgery, a liberalized range of oxygen saturation is considered acceptable. Continuous blood pressure monitoring is provided in the critical care unit through intra-arterial catheters connected to a transducer and monitor (Chart 15–8). These are located in the femoral artery or the radial artery. For neonates, a catheter is usually threaded through the umbilical artery for hemodynamic monitoring. Vital signs are routinely taken, and deviations from expectations are recorded, quickly responded to, and reported. A head-to-toe assessment, concentrating on the cardiopulmonary status of the child, is performed and recorded by the nurse every shift and done as needed for changes in the child's status.

Interdisciplinary Interventions

Managing Changes in Body Temperature. Hypothermia occurs in the immediate postoperative period, resulting from core temperature cooling associated with cardiopulmonary bypass. Warming measures are initiated on arrival to the ICU. Temperature can be monitored continuously by a rectal probe. The child is assessed for any signs of cold stress such as shivering, low core/skin temperature, cold or cyanotic extremities, pallor, and/or metabolic acidosis. A neutral thermal environment is maintained. Techniques for warming include using warming lights and

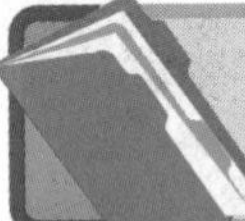

Chart 15–8
Nursing Interventions Classification (NIC)

Hemodynamic Regulation

Definition

Optimization of heart rate, preload, afterload, and contractility

Activities

Recognize presence of blood pressure alterations.
Auscultate lung sounds for crackles or other adventitious sounds.
Auscultate heart sounds.
Monitor and document heart rate, rhythm, and pulses.
Monitor electrolyte levels.
Monitor systemic and pulmonary vascular resistance, as appropriate.
Monitor cardiac output and/or cardiac index and left-ventricular stroke work index, as appropriate.
Administer positive inotropic/contractility medications.
Evaluate side effects of negative inotropic medications.
Monitor peripheral pulses, capillary refill, and temperature and color of extremities.
Elevate the head of the bed, as appropriate.
Place in Trendelenburg position, if appropriate.
Monitor for peripheral edema, jugular vein distention, and S3 and S4 heart sounds.
Monitor pulmonary capillary/artery wedge pressure and central venous/right-atrial pressure, if appropriate.
Maintain fluid balance by administering IV fluids or diuretics, as appropriate.
Administer vasodilator and/or vasoconstrictor medication, as appropriate.
Monitor intake/output, urine output, and patient weight, as appropriate.
Insert urinary catheter, if appropriate.
Minimize/eliminate environmental stressors.
Administer antiarrhythmic medications, as appropriate.
Monitor effects of medications.
Monitor pacemaker functioning, if appropriate.
Evaluate effects of fluid therapy.

From McCloskey, J., & Bulechek, G. (1996). *Nursing interventions classification (NIC)* (2nd ed.). St. Louis: Mosby–Year Book. Reprinted with permission.

warm blankets (especially around the head) and changing the temperature setting on the ventilator. Neonates are kept in a temperature-regulated warmer isolette or a radiant warmer bed.

As the child recovers, an elevated temperature is frequently associated with the need for pulmonary toilet or the evacuation of accumulated mucus from the lungs. Cooling measures are initiated for elevated temperatures. These include a cool bath, ice bags to the groin and axillae, cooling blanket, and administration of antipyretics. After the first postoperative day, spikes in temperature are indications that blood, sputum, and urine cultures need to be drawn.

Maintaining Cardiac Output. The child is assessed for signs and symptoms of decreased cardiac output such as hypotension, edema, increased liver size by palpation, low toe temperature (cool extremities), delayed capillary refill, weak peripheral pulses, mottled extremities, abnormal filling pressures, low urine output, and mental status changes.

Evaluation of hemodynamic lines, vital signs, peripheral pulses, and the warmth and color of extremities can provide valuable information about the child's preload status. Problems with preload can be related to excessive chest tube drainage causing hypovolemia or fluid leaking into the interstitial spaces from the vascular bed. Volume replacement is administered as required. A 5% albumin solution is a commonly used intravascular volume expander, unless the child is bleeding.

The child's afterload is continuously evaluated by assessing systemic pressure, systemic vascular resistance, and pulmonary vascular resistance. Afterload may be increased in the vasoconstricted patient as a result of hypothermia or poor cardiac output. Vasodilators, such as nitroprusside or nitroglycerin, infused intravenously can reduce afterload. In the presence of poor cardiac function, vasoactive and inotropic agents are administered intravenously and titrated to maintain adequate cardiac output. Commonly infused inotropic medications are dopamine, dobutamine, and amrinone.

If diminished cardiac output is refractory to large dosages of multiple inotropic infusions, cardiac assist devices may be used. Ventricular assist devices (VADs) are pumps used to provide critical support to a patient in severe refractory heart failure or as a bridge to transplantation. Extracorporeal membrane oxygenation (ECMO) is prolonged external cardiopulmonary bypass that allows the cardiopulmonary system to rest while permitting resolution of reversible pathology. Left ventricular assist devices (LVADs) support heart function, but the heart must maintain circulation. Blood is diverted from the left heart and returned back to the aorta via a pump. Intraaortic balloon pumps (IABPs) are useful for larger children to augment the existing circulation. All support devices are invasive and have a variety of complications associated with them. Once the patient's cardiac strength returns, he or she is weaned from support devices.

caREminder: *Peripheral vasoconstriction, assessed as cold feet and poor capillary refilling time, can be an early sign of diminished cardiac output. A thermometer probe placed on the toes can be used to monitor subtle changes in peripheral temperatures.*

Cardiac Tamponade. Cardiac tamponade occurs when a volume of fluid large enough to interfere with ventricular filling and pumping collects in the pericardial sac and causes a critical suppression of cardiac output. It is most likely to occur in the immediate postoperative period but can also occur during later stages of recovery. Signs and symptoms of cardiac tamponade include hypotension, muffled heart sounds, decreased systemic perfusion, sudden cessation of chest drainage, narrowing pulse pressures, widening mediastinum on chest x-ray film, and increased right and left atrial pressures. Cardiac tamponade can cause a child to go into cardiac arrest and can necessitate surgical re-exploration of the chest cavity. If this condition is not picked up by early assessment, death may ensue.

Arrhythmias. Arrhythmias may occur from surgical injury to the heart or fluid and electrolyte imbalances, primarily hypokalemia. The ECG, which runs continuously, is monitored and evaluated by the nurse, who documents the rhythm and notes changes. If temporary pacing wires are present, they are connected to a temporary pacemaker as per the hospital protocols. Antiarrhythmic agents are administered as ordered while the child is monitored for signs of side effects.

Temporary Pacing Wire Management. Temporary pacing wires are placed in the heart muscle and brought out through the chest at the close of an open heart surgical case. The wires may be connected to an external temporary pacemaker and placed next to the patient. The wires are left connected to a temporary pacemaker as an emergency backup pacer and used only if needed. The wires are usually left connected to the temporary pacemaker for 48 hours or until the patient is out of danger of dysrhythmia. In some cardiac programs, the wires are just taped to the anterior chest wall. Nursing interventions related to care of the child with pacing wires are discussed in Chart 15–9.

Maintaining Fluid and Electrolyte Balance. As a response to surgery and cardiopulmonary bypass, aldosterone and antidiuretic hormone are secreted. They cause an increase in sodium and water retention and excretion of potassium. Over the postoperative period, excess fluid, which had settled into the interstitial spaces, diffuses back into the systemic system. Because of excessive total body fluids, patients are frequently placed on diuretics and fluid restrictions.

Postoperative hydration assessment includes palpating fontanelles in infants, checking mucous membranes, checking skin turgor, and assessing for signs of edema. Edema is most evident in the hands, feet, sacrum, and periorbital areas. Fluid restrictions are calculated, and intake is adjusted to meet limitations. Patients are weighed daily, and intake and output is monitored closely and documented. Hypotensive episodes can be treated with small intravenous fluid volume boluses given as ordered. Once a patient is tolerating oral intake, fluid limits are advanced slowly.

Urine output is an indicator of fluid volume status as well as end-organ perfusion and is monitored hourly while Foley catheters are in place. Renal failure is more likely to occur in children with cyanotic heart disease and in those with periods of hypotension. The child's electrolytes, as well as other laboratory values, are monitored. Acid-base deficits can be related to poor pulmonary function, but acidosis is also an indicator of poor

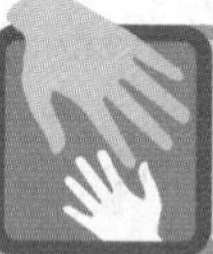

Chart 15–9
Nursing Interventions

Caring for the Child with Temporary Pacing Wires

- Wires should be secured to the child's chest, avoiding tension on the wires and preventing them from dangling so they cannot be pulled out by accident.
- In general, the wires on the right side of the chest are atrial wires and the wires on the left side of the chest are ventricular wires. (This may vary; for example, in patients with dextrocardia [congenital growth of heart inside the right side of the chest], wires will be reversed.)
- The wires should be marked either positive or ground and negative.
- Attach pacemaker control boxes to the bed with a safety pin. That way, when a child is held or is up in the chair, it minimizes the risk that the pacemaker could fall on the floor.
- If wires are disconnected from the pacemaker, place them in a finger cot or part of a disposable glove and tape wires to chest.
- Protect pacer wires from microshock. Avoid placing any electrical equipment on bed, such as infusion pumps or tape recorders. Remove all liquids from near electrical equipment or pacing wires.
- Temporary wires are pulled out before discharge by the surgeon, and this can be done at the bedside.
- After discontinuation of pacing wires, the child is monitored for signs and symptoms of cardiac decompensation.

cardiac output. Hypokalemia is treated with intravenous potassium boluses while the child is in the ICU.

Respiratory Function. The patency of chest tubes is maintained, drainage is monitored and evaluated, and its consistency and color are noted (Fig. 15–7). Surgeons discontinue mediastinal chest tubes once drainage subsides, which is usually by the second postoperative day. Although the procedure is quick, removing tape from dressings and skin is painful, and removal of the chest tubes is uncomfortable. The child should be medicated for pain in advance of pulling chest tubes.

Alert: *More than 1 cc/kg/hr of chest tube drainage in the immediate postoperative period is considered excessive. If a coagulopathy is ruled out, too much bleeding can necessitate the child's return to the surgical suite for the surgeon to explore the chest and search for potential bleeding vessels.*

Signs of acute bleeding can be increased heart rate, narrowing pulse pressures, decreased perfusion, and decreased blood pressure. Bleeding can occur from the numerous suture lines in the heart and great vessels. Cardiopulmonary bypass also traumatizes blood from the mechanical actions of the blood passing through the pump and tubing. While on bypass, the patient is fully heparinized to keep blood from clotting in the pump tubing. This is reversed once the surgical repairs are complete but can lead to clotting abnormalities postoperatively. Blood in the blood bank and an active blood clot for crossmatching blood are kept available. Patient clotting factors, complete blood count, and platelets are routinely monitored. Blood is replaced as necessary, but judiciously. Cardiac nursing units have an emergency sternotomy tray available and a protocol for reopening a chest incision in the ICU in the event of an emergency. For example, sudden and/or excessive bleeding may necessitate emergency reopening of the chest.

Figure 15–7
The child returning from cardiac surgery often has a chest tube in place to drain blood and fluids that collect in the mediastinal and pleural spaces.

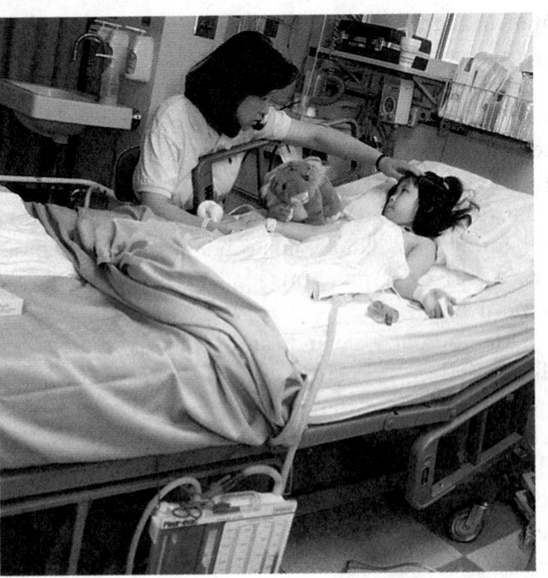

While on the pump, the lungs are deflated, causing atelectasis. Also, cardiopulmonary bypass causes water and sodium retention and potassium depletion, so fluid settles in the interstitial spaces of the pleura, which increases body weight temporarily. Changes occur in the alveoli, and small pulmonary vessels become more permeable, resulting in interstitial pulmonary edema. This causes leukocyte aggregation and sequestration in the lung, creating a mild decrease in lung compliance. Sternal pain can deter a patient from coughing and taking deep breaths to re-expand the lungs.

Pulmonary assessment is performed, and changes are documented as they occur. Assessment includes the child's general appearance and color. Mild tachypnea and decreased tidal volume usually occur postoperatively. Signs and symptoms of impaired pulmonary function include dyspnea, tachycardia, tachypnea, pallor, diaphoresis, adventitious breath sounds, poor cough, and use of accessory muscles. Irritability, exhaustion, and an alarmed look can also be signs of respiratory distress. Cyanosis, abnormal arterial blood gas values, and low oxygen saturations can be normal in children with intracardiac mixing.

Extubation may occur in the surgical suite for older children and for those children who are predictably stable patients. Most children are extubated within 24 hours of surgery. Critically ill postoperative patients can require ventilation for cardiopulmonary support over many days. Endotracheal suctioning is done as needed, noting the character, amount, and consistency of pulmonary secretions.

Once the child has been extubated, the patency of the airway must be ensured and monitored for stridor or wheezing. Infants are put in the "sniffing position," with the head cocked back and nose pointing up. Supplemental oxygen is administered and weaned as tolerated. Chest wall rise and expansion and respiratory rate and quality are assessed. The head of the bed is elevated to encourage lung expansion and ease the work of breathing. Pulmonary hygiene includes coughing, deep breathing, breathing treatments, incentive spirometry, and nasotracheal suctioning. Chest physiotherapy is used to mobilize secretions and reinflate regions of atelectasis. Nursing care is scheduled and tasks are clustered to prevent exhaustion and hypoxia. As the child tolerates it, activity is encouraged. Pain medication is administered on a regular basis. Here, the nurse must balance minimizing pain and maximizing alertness so that the patient can still elicit a strong cough.

Postoperative cardiac surgical patients are at risk for

the development of pleural effusions. These can develop from an imbalance between filtration and reabsorption of pleural fluids. A chylothorax is the drainage of chyle into the chest. A chylothorax can develop when a thoracic duct is injured and occurs most commonly after thoracotomy incisions.

Monitoring Neurologic Functioning. Potential causes of neurologic insults could be hypotensive states, hypoxia, or an embolic event. The causes of postoperative neurologic deficits are not always clear. Some children have marginal cerebral blood flow during surgery, just above the threshold for infarction. A neurologic examination includes level of consciousness, pupillary response, movement of extremities, and responses to stimuli. Other changes that may indicate alterations in neurologic status are irritability, a high-pitched cry, poor feeding, or rigidity. Subtle neurologic changes, such as poor eye focusing or confusion, are usually normal and transient. More severe changes include seizures, coma, and one-sided weakness.

Seizures that are related to neurologic dysfunction or electrolyte imbalances can occur. Seizures may be difficult to distinguish from normal jitteriness. Subtle signs of focal seizure activity might include chewing, eye deviation, or hypotonia. Anticonvulsant medications are administered to suppress seizure activity.

Preventing Infection. Children who are more debilitated pre- or postoperatively, who require prolonged ventilation, or who are malnourished are especially at risk for infection. Prophylactic antibiotics are usually administered for 48 hours or until invasive lines are removed.

All dressings are assessed frequently and changed based on unit standards. The nurse should document the absence or presence of redness, exudate, or granulation of the chest incision and any invasive line insertion sites. Pacing wires are dressed and secured to the chest and labeled for easy access in case of an emergency. White blood count values are monitored daily.

Sedation and Pain Management. While a child is critically ill, sedation can be a part of hemodynamic management. Because sedation reduces systemic vascular resistance and pulmonary vascular resistance, it improves cardiac performance. When a child is heavily sedated or paralyzed, the eyelids may not completely shut, thus the eyes should be lubricated and taped shut with paper tape to prevent corneal damage.

Pain and anxiety are major issues for patients and families once a child is hemodynamically stable. After patients are assessed for possible causes of pain and adequacy of pain control interventions, they are medicated appropriately. It is important for children to be comfortable enough to take deep breaths, cough, and be involved in activities between resting. Signs and symptoms of pain are crying, restlessness, irritability, grimacing, splinting, rigid posture, increased heart rate, and/or increased respiration or increased blood pressure. The nurse should position the child for comfort. This may include bundling of infants, placing the child in a particular position, or providing a pacifier. Other non-invasive procedures that can augment the effectiveness of narcotic pain medications are cartoons, music, favorite or new toys, and a soothing voice or music. Supplement narcotic analgesia with acetaminophen. Administered on a regular basis, it alleviates the general soreness of surgery, does not suppress respirations, and allows a child to be alert and interact.

Nutritional Management After Cardiac Surgery. If a child is extubated, has active bowel sounds, is passing flatus, and has a soft, non-distended abdomen, he or she may be ready to resume oral feeding.

Infants are started on a 5% dextrose solution or pediatric electrolyte solution. The older child is given ice chips and sips of water. When ingesting fluid, the child's head should be propped up 30° to 40°, or the child should be held in the parent's lap. The nurse should observe whether or not the suck-swallowing reflex is normal. After the feeding, the child's head should remain elevated for half an hour to prevent vomiting and spitting up. As the child demonstrates tolerance of fluids by mouth, the maintenance intravenous fluids are decreased. Twenty-four-hour fluid totals are calculated based on ordered fluid limit and subtracting out the ordered intravenous therapy fluids to determine the amount of remainder of the fluid limit for oral intake per hour. Fluid limits are ordered by the surgeon and are based on the child's "dry weight." Once the child is allowed to eat, daily nutritional intake is documented. A dietary consult is provided if the child has the diagnosis of failure to thrive or demonstrates poor nutritional intake.

Psychosocial Support. Once a child is extubated and is hemodynamically stable, he or she can increase activity and can sit up in a chair, even before most invasive lines are discontinued. When lines are removed, children can ambulate and can begin to participate in activities in the playroom. Part of a nurse's postoperative interaction is confidence boosting. Children may be afraid to move and to walk out of fear and pain. Positive reinforcement and prodding a child to increase activity can help smooth recovery from surgery.

An important nursing intervention is to lessen the negative impact on the child's physical, emotional, and social well-being. Negative behavioral changes are normal and are to be expected. Changes may include clinging behavior, fear of uniforms, depression, or regression in behaviors. Uncooperative behaviors are self-protective and are an expression of anger. A combination of medications for pain, distraction techniques, and comfort measures, prodding the child to advance activities, and accepting negative behaviors can help a child cope with the pain and stresses of hospitalization.

Tip: *When a child is overwhelmed by multiple lines and tubes, he or she may choose one item to constantly complain about. This item may even be an insignificant issue like some tape on an arm. The child may need to focus on something because of the lack of the ability to fight all the current stresses. Reassure parents that this is a normal coping mechanism.*

Parents suffer greatly at the sight of ill children and their inability to protect them from pain. Parents usually protect and comfort their child continually in their day-to-day life. Normally, a parent controls every aspect of a child's life and meets all physical and emotional needs. At home, parents decide when to feed, bathe, change diapers, put down for naps, and plan activities. Suddenly they are compelled to give their child up to strangers whom they allow to perform strange, painful, and unusual procedures on their child in hopes of an improved future. This can be overwhelming and can cause parents to feel guilty, saddened, and stressed.

The nurse can help by encouraging parents to express fears and concerns regarding their child's condition. Families should be encouraged to participate in a child's care as often as they can and to do as much as they feel comfortable with. Nurses can promote parents' touching and comforting of their child and allow them to hold the child as much as is practical. All procedures should be explained to parents, while encouraging questions and allowing them to verbalize concerns. Parents benefit from continual updates of the child's status and progression. Also, nurses are instrumental in making referrals to support systems when needed.

Community Care. Discharge planning needs are assessed in advance and follow-up referrals provided, if necessary. Discharge teaching includes postoperative expectations and written discharge instructions (TIP 15–2). Parents need to be comfortable with activity restrictions for discharge and not over- or underprotect their child during the recovery process.

Discharge instructions should include discussion of a

TIP 15–2 A Teaching Intervention Plan for the Child After Cardiac Surgery: Discharge Instructions

Nursing Diagnosis and Family Outcomes

- Risk for ineffective individual and family (child and family) coping related to knowledge deficit about postoperative home care.

Outcomes:

Family will provide child with support, assistance, and encouragement to manage or master tasks related to the postoperative care.

Family will follow written discharge instructions and seek health care assistance as needed to ensure safety and promote well-being of the child.

Treatment of the Child

Medications

- Carry a list of your child's medications with you at all times (the name of each medication, the dosage, and how often it is taken).
- Always get your prescriptions filled before you run out.
- Never stop giving any medicine. Your cardiologist will determine when the medication is to be changed or stopped.
- Bring the medications and the list when you come in for your first follow-up visit.

Wound Care

- Only sponge bathe your child the first week. Do not apply lotions or powders to the incision site during the first 2 weeks after surgery.
- Keep the incision area clean and dry. If the incision area should get dirty or soiled, cleanse the area with mild soap and water.
- Steri-Strips over the incision site should be left in place until your child's first office visit. Occasionally these strips become loose and fall off. Do not worry if this should occur.
- Observe the incision site daily for redness, swelling, or drainage.
- Tingling, itching, and numbness are normal sensations from the wound and will eventually go away.
- Areas of the incision that are constantly irritated by clothing or the chin rubbing can be covered with a Band-Aid to prevent irritation and promote faster healing.

TIP 15-2 A Teaching Intervention Plan for the Child After Cardiac Surgery: Discharge Instructions *Continued*

- Keep a shirt over the incision when your child is outside. This will lessen the scar by protecting it from the sunlight.

Activity

- When children go home after cardiac surgery, they generally recover quickly and are able to participate in most of their normal activities. We encourage patients to gradually increase activity each day. They may rest more and take it easy and even may not enjoy or try to do some of the things they did before coming to the hospital. This will improve as a child recovers.
- Infants and children tend to pace themselves and will rest if they feel tired. A sensible balance of rest and exercise is recommended.
- Avoid lifting your child under the arms, as this may cause discomfort by placing stress on the surgical site. Instead, slide your hands under your child's buttocks and support his or her chest as you lift.
- The breast bone (sternum) needs approximately 6 weeks to heal. During that time, the child should not be involved in rough play or activities such as bicycling, climbing, skateboarding, or contact sports. Avoid activities that would put pressure on the child's chest, such as heavy lifting, or any activity that might cause a blow to the chest.
- Try to avoid large crowds and/or people with active infections for at least 2 weeks (e.g., birthday parties, church, school, shopping malls).
- Initially, children may experience clinging behavior and/or sleep disturbances after discharge. Usually positive reassurance and returning to a normal routine will encourage getting back to regular behavior.

Diet

Children can return to their normal diet with no restrictions.

Immunizations

Immunizations are normally delayed for 6–8 weeks after surgery.

Dental Care

Whenever possible, routine dental care should be delayed 4–5 months after your child's surgery. Remember, some children with cardiac problems are required to take antibiotics for dental work or other procedures. This is done to prevent an infection in the child's heart.

Discomfort

Your child may continue to experience some incisional or chest discomfort after discharge from the hospital. Tylenol may be given unless otherwise ordered by your physician.

Contact Health Care Provider if

You think there is a change in your child's behavior; it could be a sign of illness. This may or may not be important, but it is prudent to check. Signs of illnesses may include

- A change in feeding pattern
- Breathing harder or faster
- Puffiness of the hands, feet, or face, especially around the eyes
- Excessive sweating, especially evident on the forehead
- Weakness, irritability, weak cry in infant
- Cool, pale, mottled hands or feet
- Few wet diapers or poor urine output
- Temperature higher than 101°F

child's need for immunizations. Immunizations are avoided around the time of surgery. Otherwise, despite illnesses and hospitalizations, families should be instructed to try to maintain immunizations at scheduled times. Small, cachectic (extremely thin and poorly nourished) infants often receive half doses of immunizations.

Medic Alert bracelets are recommended for children with pacemakers, heart transplants, or automatic implantable cardioverter defibrillators (AICDs) and for those on anticoagulant therapy. It is not considered necessary for all children with cardiac conditions to wear Medic Alert bracelets. Children who had a history of seizure activity after the surgery may wear bracelets as recommended by the physician until they are seizure-free for a period of time.

Pacemakers

Pacemakers can be used in children who have impaired impulse formation or conduction problems and who are symptomatic. Bradycardia requiring pacemaker insertion are of primarily two types. One type, **sick sinus syndrome or sinus node dysfunction**, occurs when the heart's pacemaker functions normally but not fast enough to provide an adequate cardiac output. **Atrioventricular (AV) block,** the second category of bradycardia, occurs when the normal pacemaker functions appropriately but the signal is not transmitted through to the AV node and to the ventricles. The second type may be caused by a congenital heart block, medications, an infection of the heart, or as a post-surgical complication.

The components of a pacemaker are the generator and pacing leads. Pacing leads attach from the heart to the pulse generator. Modern pacemakers can sense the atrial and ventricular heart rhythms and can respond to them based on set limits and with a set spacing of the paced beats. Pacemakers also have the capability to inhibit their response at each chamber based on parameters set on the pacemaker. Some pacemakers have the ability to sense the patient's activity level and give the patient an appropriate heart rate. The energy amount provided with each beat is also controlled. Lithium pacemaker batteries have lives of 4 to 10 years depending on the frequency of impulse usage and amplitude (Yerby & Hubbard, 1985).

Leads are placed on the atrium and the ventricles and screwed into the heart muscle. The location of lead placement depends on the type of heart problem and the size of the patient. In children, the wires are placed on the external heart and the generator is inserted in the abdominal space. Surgical placement involves a thoracotomy and an abdominal incision. In the past, permanent pacemakers were too large to be placed in small children, but modern pacemakers are small and lightweight and have been placed in infants.

Community Care. Children have their pacemakers checked as outpatients on a regular basis. A specialized computer and magnet that communicates through radiofrequency signals is placed over the pacemaker generator and is used to change settings and to evaluate the pacemaker. It is a non-invasive way to check the activities of the pacemaker and the battery usage.

As part of the pacemaker package, children are given a transtelephonic system to take home. This allows them to periodically transmit electrocardiograms to the clinic over their home telephone. The placement of a pacemaker requires long-term follow-up and future surgeries. Periodically, a minor surgery is required to replace the battery in the pacemaker. Lead wires can be fractured, and replacing them involves a surgery that is more extensive than just battery replacement.

Psychosocial responses to pacemaker insertion depends on the personal responses of individual families. The child may have body image disturbance or self-concept changes caused by scars, activity restrictions, and continual follow-up. If parents change a job, it can create insurance problems, and this preexisting condition may affect their insurability. In the future, limitations on employability of the child can impose an extra burden on the patient and family.

Parents of children with pacemakers are instructed to have them avoid contact sports such as gymnastics and football. High magnetic areas such as MRI machines should be avoided. High-voltage areas such as high-tension wires can also interfere with the function of a pacemaker. Modern microwave ovens do not affect pacemakers.

Cardiac Transplantation

In recent years, cardiac transplantation has become a viable option for extending the length and quality of life of children who have exhausted available medical treatment and palliative surgeries and are no longer surviving well as demonstrated by disabling cardiac symptoms or limited life expectancy. The diagnosis that most often leads to cardiac transplantation in older children is cardiomyopathy. Some of the congenital cardiac defects associated with cardiac transplantation are hypoplastic left heart syndrome and other complex single ventricle hearts.

Before 1980, fewer than five children per year received a heart transplant. Transplant survival improved with the discovery of cyclosporine, an immunosuppressive drug, and the population receiving transplantations expanded to younger and older patients. One study that evaluated the survival of 111 neonate transplant recipients showed an 81% survival rate at 5 years (Chiavarelli, Gundry, Razzouk, & Bailey, 1993).

Pediatric Donors

Although the list of infants and children waiting for transplantation is shorter than for adults, there is an extremely limited supply of donor pediatric hearts. Those children waiting on the list currently outnumber donor heart supplies. Most pediatric donors die from sudden infant death syndrome, trauma, or birth asphyxia.

It is difficult to determine when to time the listing of a patient to wait for an available heart. Decisions depend on the expected natural history of the particular underlying heart problem. Decisions as to when the heart failure is terminal and shortages of available donors severely limit the timing of transplantation surgeries.

In order for a child to be included on the waiting list, the presence of any other systemic diseases that might rule out the viability of transplantation must be evaluated. Also, a psychosocial profile of the family is developed. This profile considers resources and commitment to the program. The depth of ethical decisions, the financial burden, the need for patient compliance with medications, and constant follow-up make the care of these children complex.

Once listed with the United Network for Organ Sharing (UNOS) on the national computer, patients and donors are matched based on blood type, body weight, length of time on the waiting list, and the child's medical stability. Orthoptic heart transplantation, replacing a recipient's heart with one from a human organ donor, is the commonly accepted mode of cardiac transplantation today.

Maintaining Immunosuppression

After a heart transplant, the major challenge in caring for children is maintaining the balance between immunosuppression and factors such as adverse medication side effects, infection, and rejection of the donor organ. For the health care practitioner, the balance between infection and rejection may be viewed as the largest issue. For the child, side effects from immunosuppressive medications, expenses, and constant follow-up care are generally the areas of most concern. Rejection of the foreign heart is attempted by all recipients' immune systems. The recipient's body never learns to accept the foreign tissue. Rejection occurs because of an incompatibility of cell surface antigen, which invokes a humoral and cellular immune response.

Management of rejection traditionally has included triple medication therapy of cyclosporine, azathioprine (Imuran), and prednisone. This triple therapy is ordered so that the practitioner can prescribe lower dosages of each, thus decreasing overall side effects. Susceptibility to infections is a complication of all the immunosuppressive medications used today. Cyclosporine inhibits T-cell function, but exactly how it works is unclear. Cyclosporine is the number one immunosuppressive drug taht has led to an increase in the survival of transplant recipients. Side effects include tremors, gum hyperplasia, hirsutism, flushing, nephrotoxicity, seizures, and hypertension. Imuran (azathioprine) is another immunosuppressive drug given to transplant recipients. It is a bone marrow suppressor that inhibits purine synthesis and metabolism. The white blood cell count of children receiving this drug is followed closely to monitor for the side effect of bone marrow depression.

Prednisone, a corticosteroid, influences the immune system through its strong anti-inflammatory action and immunologic effect. Because of the severity of side effects of prednisone, transplant recipients with minimal rejection episodes may be weaned off prednisone therapy. Side effects of corticosteroids include poor wound healing, ulcers, growth impairment, delayed sexual maturation, glucose intolerance, increased appetite, hyperlipidemia, cushingoid appearance, acne, and sun sensitivity. When a school-age child is overweight, excessively hairy, and has a moon-shaped face, this appearance can be a great source of stress for him or her. Adolescents need to be monitored closely for issues of noncompliance. Usually, most of the symptoms subside in those children able to tolerate lower dosages of the immunosuppressive medications.

Serial myocardial biopsies are the most reliable predictor of rejection. They are performed in toddlers and children but are technically more difficult in infants. Children are also followed up closely through non-invasive clinical evaluation including echocardiography, chest x-ray films, and patient signs and symptoms. Episodes of rejection may be managed by pulse courses of intravenous steroid therapy or other strong immunosuppressive medications.

Over a life span, the long-term effects from suppression therapy on small children are unknown. Chronic usage of drugs for immunosuppression has led to renal dysfunction, malignancies, and hypertension. One important limiting factor for long-term survival of heart transplant recipients is cardiac allograft vasculopathy, which is an accelerated form of coronary artery disease. It occurs in 40% of patients at 5 years after transplant, and the only treatment is re-transplantation (Yeatman, Smith, Dunning, Large, & Wallwork, 1995).

Routine immunizations are still given to transplant recipients, but no live viruses are used. Normal childhood infections are well tolerated in these children. Although transplantation has allowed many children to survive otherwise terminal diseases, it is not a panacea and is still an evolving field of care.

Supportive Care

When parents learn that their child has the diagnosis of CHD or another cardiac condition, there are significant psychological and social impacts for the family. Parents usually need time to come to grips with the realities of having a child with a cardiac condition. There is an emotional symbolism associated with the heart. Many cultures place the heart as an organ of great importance. Parents may view their child as having a "broken heart," a term associated with sadness in Western civilization.

Parents of children with a correctable cardiac lesion may be just as anxious, if not more anxious, than those of a child with a very complex congenital lesion. Many children with cardiac lesions have no outward signs of cardiac disease. There may be no specific symptoms that would cause the parents to feel that their child has a problem. These parents may also have fear and guilt about putting their otherwise "perfect child" through medical interventions. It can seem almost easier to accept for parents whose children are cyanotic, with tetralogy of Fallot for instance, than for parents of an asymptomatic child with an atrial septal defect (ASD). The parents with the cyanotic child are immediately emotionally rewarded by a child who has turned pink after the surgery. The parents of the "healthy child" with an ASD, who never even realized there was a problem, take home a sore, cranky child with a large scar on his or her chest. It seems to help the parents accept the child's condition if the practitioner can point out some measurable feature the parents can relate to in order to convince and reassure them that corrective interventions must be completed. The practitioner can show parents the echocardiogram results and the location of the lesion. Visualizing the chest roentgenogram of an enlarged heart with CHF, or comparing a poor growth curve with that for other children, can help parents realize the existence of the heart defect.

Parental support groups or parent meetings with other families of children with CHD can be a source of support for these parents, helping them to sort out the emotions and stresses of having a child diagnosed with CHD.

Parents of symptomatic children are often emotionally drained and have infrequent breaks from child care responsibilities. Baby sitters are often fearful to take on the management of medication administration and the emotional burden of an ill child. Parents of these children may be frightened and fearful of creating situations in which their child becomes symptomatic. The simple activities one normally does with an infant, such as feeding, can become tedious and painstaking events.

Options for "fixing" a child with heart disease are not always clear and usually include expensive and invasive procedures. At times, families of children with complex heart disease are forced to make choices for their child that will markedly alter the course of a child's life. Financial and religious factors may influence the decisions that parents make in regard to the care of their child with CHD. Many parents have continued a job they may have otherwise quit to maintain their health insurance benefits, whereas other parents may refuse a job transfer to another city, so they can stay located near a medical center where they are comfortable with the staff and the facility. The needs of families in a world that can provide high technology care are multifaceted, involving ethical, religious, financial, and emotional components.

Community Care

Most school-age children with CHD are able to attend normal schools. If a child is being kept out of school, contact should be made with a social worker or with the child's cardiologist to confirm that there is a medical need for the child to be denied access to school. Some parents may have inappropriate fears over the vulnerability of their child and may overprotect a child by keeping him or her out of the school system. Most children can be encouraged to participate in school playground activities at their level of tolerance but should not be pressured to exercise beyond their personal limits.

Children with severe cardiac lesions that need a more sedentary lifestyle require a modification of school programs on an individual basis. This allows the child to participate at an appropriate level of toleration. For instance, a nap time could be substituted for a recess time period for a child who has a cardiac condition. Transportation to and from school could be arranged instead of having the child walk. If there is a period of missed school time, it is often associated with a procedure such as surgery or cardiac catheterization (Chart 15–10). Classmates should be encouraged to keep in contact with the ill child, perhaps visiting the child's home and sending cards to the hospital.

Children with minor cardiac issues or those whose lesions are repaired can generally travel without limitations. Extreme heat and a sudden climate change can stress ill children and can cause venous pooling from vasodilation. Aggressive travel itineraries may overtax the endurance level of a child with limited reserve. Children with unrepaired lesions, CHF, cyanosis, or the propensity for sudden illness or complications need to have ready access to appropriate emergency care. After cardiac transplantation, children are not allowed to travel with families who go to underdeveloped countries because there is a greater risk of illness from water sources and limited medical care.

If traveling to large metropolitan areas, it is usually possible for the child's cardiologist to have a contact

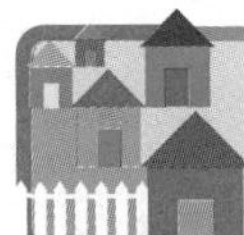

Chart 15–10
Community Care

Activity Recommendations for the Child with Cardiac Disease

Post–Cardiac Catheterization Routine

- Keep the child out of school for 2 or 3 days or over a weekend.
- No gym class or playground activities for 1 week.
- After 1 week, the child can return to normal activities.

Post–Cardiac Surgical Care

- Keep the child out of school 1 week after discharge from hospital.
- Encourage fellow students to send cards and drawings to post on the wall in the ICU.
- School nurse may be involved in administering midday dosages of required medications.
- Child will refrain from gym classes or playground activities for 6 weeks to allow time for the sternum to heal.
- Any situation that could induce a blunt chest trauma should be avoided.

physician in the vacation area to call if necessary. At all times, parents should carry a list of emergency contact medical personnel, a list of medications, and a short written synopsis of the child's history.

Airplane travel or travel to areas of high altitude are restricted in children with cyanotic heart disease, pulmonary hypertension, and severe CHF. Higher elevations have a lower partial pressure of oxygen, which may further compromise the child's oxygen-carrying capacity. Supplemental oxygen is used if altitude travel is necessary. Commercial airlines will not allow families to bring their own oxygen tank. If oxygen support is necessary, arrangements need to be made in advance with the airlines and with a medical supply company at the family's destination.

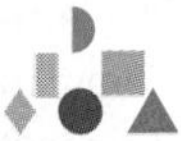

Alterations in Cardiac Status

Cardiac Hemodynamics

Cardiac output is the volume of blood ejected by the heart in 1 minute. It can be calculated by taking the number of times the child's heart beats in a minute and multiplying that number by the stroke volume. Stroke volume is the volume of blood ejected by the ventricles per beat, in milliliters.

$$\text{Cardiac output} = \text{Heart rate} \times \text{Stroke volume}$$

Heart rate is influenced by the autonomic nervous system. An increase in heart rate will shift the formula to cause an increase in cardiac output, and a decrease in heart rate causes an decrease in cardiac output unless stroke volume is increased. For a child with perfusion problems, an increase in the heart rate could improve cardiac output. However, a heart rate that is too high can diminish cardiac output. An extremely fast heart rate shortens diastolic filling time and limits coronary artery perfusion. Because neonates do not have the ability to increase their stroke volume in order to increase cardiac output, an increase in cardiac output in the neonate depends on heart rate. Factors that affect stroke volume are preload, contractility, and afterload. Preload can be described as the amount of volume in the heart at the end of diastole, causing the stretching or tension of cardiac muscle fibers. This volume of blood returned to the heart, or preload, is also referred to as the left ventricular end-diastolic volume. Starling's law of the heart states that the larger the volume of blood flow, the greater the stretch on the cardiac muscle fibers and, therefore, the greater the force of contraction. This law also tells us that there is a point of diminishing returns: if the cardiac muscle is stretched maximally, the heart fails.

Shunting. Normally, oxygen-depleted blood drains into the right heart from the venous system via the inferior and superior vena cava. From there, blood is pumped to the lungs to pick up oxygen. The oxygen saturation of blood returning to the right heart and the pressures in the right chambers are normally low. The blood that enters the left atrium from the lungs is normally fully saturated and is pumped under high pressure to the systemic circulation via the left ventricle (Fig. 15–8).

In cyanotic heart disease, blood pumped to the systemic circulation is mixed with unoxygenated blood. In acyanotic heart disease, blood pumped to the systemic circulation is not mixed with unoxygenated blood.

Shunting occurs when blood abnormally crosses from one chamber, artery, or vein to another. When shunting occurs in a cardiac lesion, this causes the mixing of oxygenated and deoxygenated blood. Fluid naturally flows along the path of least resistance. In the presence of an abnormal communication between the left and right side of the heart, blood will flow from the left to the right side of the heart because the pressures are so much greater on the left side of the heart. This is referred to as a left-to-right shunt. This occurs as long as the pressures on the left side of the heart remain greater than those on

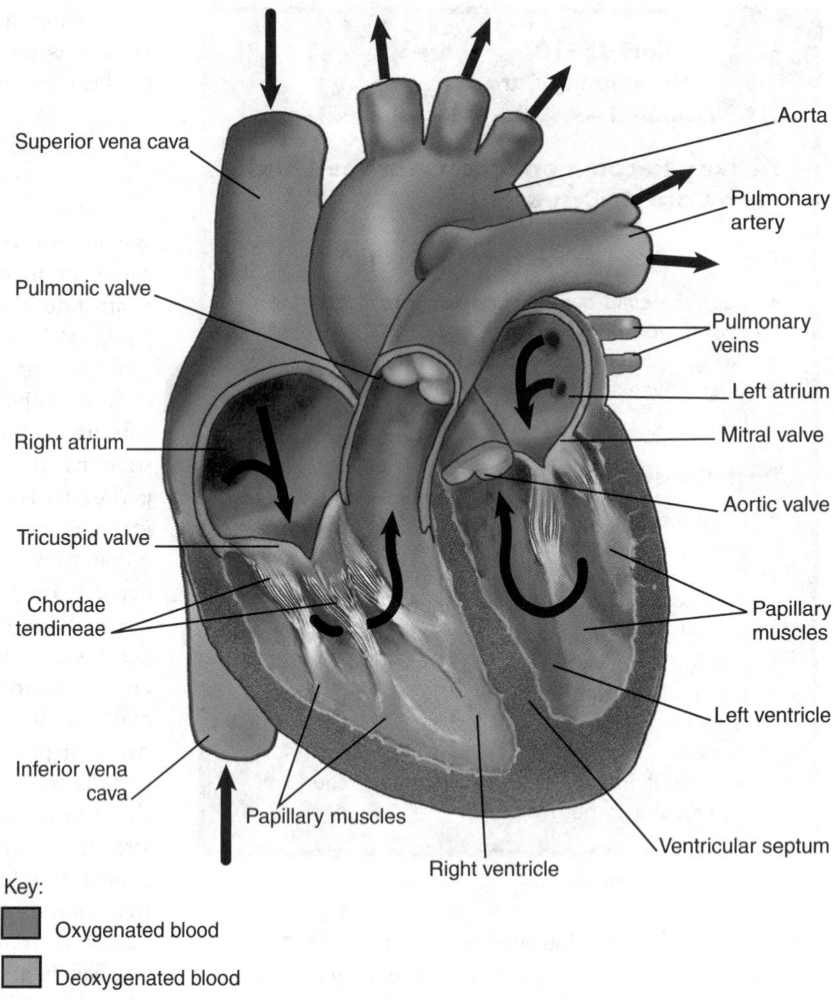

Figure 15–8
Normal heart structure.

the right. The lesions where this phenomenon occurs are called acyanotic lesions and can cause overcirculation of the lungs, which may result in a child's having congestive heart failure.

Right-to-left shunting occurs when pressures on the right side of the heart exceed the normally higher pressures on the left, causing some of the unoxygenated blood to shunt through an abnormal opening into the left heart before flowing to the lungs, resulting in cyanosis. Generally this condition exists with an obstructive lesion on the right side of the heart.

Contractility is the ability of the cardiac muscle fibers to shorten and therefore to pump the blood efficiently. Reduced contractility, or snap of the heart muscle, can diminish cardiac output. Excessive increase in contractility, such as for a child receiving high doses of inotropic medications, can overwork the heart muscle. Fluids flow from an area of high pressure to an area of lower pressure, taking the pathway of least resistance. Pressures that cause fluids to flow are influenced by resistance. Resistance to flow is dependent on the friction of flow against the blood vessel and the size of the vessel. Changes in pressure or resistance influence flow. Afterload is a label given to the peripheral resistance in vessels against which the left ventricle has to eject a volume of blood. An increase in afterload can cause the heart to work harder, pumping against the increased resistance. Prolonged or extensive resistance to pumping can lead to ventricular hypertrophy, an increase in the size of the ventricular muscle mass. This can occur in any age group.

Congestive Heart Failure

Congestive heart failure (CHF) is one of the major manifestations of cardiac disease. It is a clinical syndrome in which the heart's pumping ability is inadequate to meet the metabolic demands of the body (Kohr & O'Brien, 1995). Congestive heart failure is usually seen in infants, because most cardiac lesions are repaired or palliated in the first year of life of children living in the United States. If a well child presents with CHF beyond the first year of life, it may be due to an acquired cardiac disease such as rheumatic fever, bacterial endocarditis, or viral cardiomyopathy. Older children may present with CHF later in life because of the presence of a previously undiscovered lesion.

Pathophysiology

In congenital heart disease, CHF can be a result of overcirculated lungs, volume and/or pressure overloading, or poor myocardial function. It can be a right- or a left-sided heart problem, although children usually present in biventricular failure. Right ventricular dysfunction causes right ventricular end-diastolic pressure (RVEDP) to increase, leading to pulmonary venous engorgement. Left ventricular dysfunction causes left ventricular end-diastolic pressure (LVEDP) to increase, causing systemic engorgement. The ventricles dilate in response to elevated pressures.

The presence of a congenital heart defect is the most common reason for children to have CHF (Kohr & O'Brien, 1995). Lesions that cause volume overloading are those that have left or right shunts, such as an AV canal or ventricular septal defect. For example, a child with a large ventricular septal defect has shunting from the left side of the heart to the right. Because blood travels the path of least resistance, some blood crosses from the left ventricle to the right side without exiting the aorta and circulates to the lungs repeatedly, causing an extra load on the lungs.

Pressure overloads can be caused by an obstructive lesion on the left side of the heart. For example, in the case of aortic stenosis, the left ventricle is constantly pumping against a restricted valve. Depending on stressors and the severity of the stenosis, this could lead to failure of the left side of the heart. Neonates with a severe left-sided obstruction may be without symptoms initially because their patent ductus is open; therefore pressures may be relieved by shunting across the patent ductus. Symptoms appear as the ductus closes.

A child who presents in CHF usually has an underlying anatomic disorder but could have a non-structural condition such as a chronic heart rhythm disturbance or cardiomyopathy, causing poor myocardial function. Arrhythmias that can cause CHF are chronic supraventricular tachycardia, atrial fibrillation/flutter, and congenital heart block. Occasionally, the presentation of these arrhythmias is in utero, and the fetus is treated via medications given to the mother. In dilated cardiomyopathy, there is a dilation of cardiac chambers and a weakening of myocardial contraction, leading to CHF.

Assessment

The diagnosis of CHF is based on the judgment of the practitioner; there is not a single diagnostic test that can confirm the diagnosis of CHF. A diagnosis can be based on findings from the child's history, physical assessment, and a chest radiograph. A positive radiograph shows cardiomegaly and increased pulmonary vascular markings from excessive pulmonary blood flow. The clinical manifestations seen in CHF are elicited because of pulmonary congestion, systemic venous backup, and poor myocardial pumping (Chart 15–11). Symptoms occur when the heart's compensatory mechanisms have exceeded the point of efficiency and cardiac output is diminished.

As the heart fails, the body utilizes available compensatory mechanisms in an attempt to meet the circulatory needs. Tachycardia occurs as a compensatory response to decreased cardiac output. When auscultation of the heart is performed, a gallop rhythm may be heard, and on palpation, the pulse may be weak and thready. Tachycardia is a result of increased catecholamine (epinephrine and norepinephrine) release, which causes rapid filling of stiff ventricles in an attempt to increase the force and rate of myocardial contraction. Tachycardia also increases oxygen consumption of the heart. Tachycardia that is too rapid decreases the heart's filling time and coronary perfusion. Although it has a compensatory advantage, excessive tachycardia can become destructive, ultimately impeding cardiac output.

Chart 15–11

Clinical Manifestations of Congestive Heart Failure

Systemic Venous Congestion

Weight gain
Hepatomegaly
Edema
Jugular venous distention (children)

Pulmonary Venous Congestion

Tachypnea
Dyspnea
Cough (children)
Wheezes
Rales
Retractions (infants)
Nasal flaring (infants)

Compensatory Response

Tachycardia
Cardiomegaly
Gallop murmur
Diaphoretic
Fatigue
Failure to thrive

Cardiomegaly occurs as a muscular response to the need to increase cardiac output. When viewing the child's chest, a hyperactive precordium may be caused by cardiac enlargement. The heart dilates to increase the stretch on fibers in order to improve the force of contraction. Stretching and dilation are advantageous to increasing cardiac output within limits. After a certain point, the heart stretches beyond efficiency and fails. An extra heart sound, an S_3 gallop murmur, may be audible. It occurs from excessive preload and ventricular dilation.

Systemic Venous Congestion (Right-Sided Failure). When there are elevated right atrial filling pressures, the emptying of the vena cava into the right atrium is restricted. Blood pooling in the venous circulation raises systemic venous pressures; this in turn leads to fluid settling in the interstitial spaces. With diminished blood flow to the kidneys, the renin-angiotensin system is stimulated to vasoconstrict, causing aldosterone secretion that causes salt and water retention, which further compounds fluid retention and decreases urine output. Weight gain can be caused by swelling of soft tissue in dependent or sensitive areas, such as sacrum, scrotum, or eyelids. Distended neck veins (despite sitting up) and ankle edema are other areas less commonly used to assess fluid retention in children. In the presence of right-sided heart failure, hepatomegaly occurs from distended vessels that back up in the liver. When there is systemic venous distention, blood pools in the venous portal circulation, engorging the liver.

Pulmonary Venous Congestion (Left-Sided Failure). Imbalances between filtration and reabsorption of fluid in the pulmonary capillary bed caused by increased pulmonary capillary pressures can lead to respiratory symptoms. Pulmonary congestion can cause tachypnea (shallow and rapid breathing) that worsens with feeding or activity. Dyspnea or increased effort of breathing is exhibited by grunting, nasal flaring, and/or retractions that worsen in recumbent positions.

Irritation from bronchial edema can cause a chronic, dry, hacking cough. Pulmonary obstruction, which causes edema of the bronchial mucosa from a distended airway, can cause wheezes. One of the late signs of heart failure is when rales are heard on auscultation. Rales occur from fluid settling into the alveolar spaces, causing pulmonary edema.

Diaphoresis, Fatigue, and Exercise Intolerance. During an infant feeding or during physical activity, the child with CHF may be diaphoretic. This is usually seen as a cool sweat on the forehead. Diaphoresis occurs because of an increased sympathetic change stimulated by increasing cardiac output that stimulates the stretch receptors and baroreceptor in the blood vessels.

Children in CHF may fatigue easily and may exhibit poor exercise tolerance. Infants may tire with feedings and may appear anxious, irritable, and difficult to console. A typical diagnosis given to these children may be failure to thrive, growth retardation, or poor weight gain. Failure to thrive is related to poor nutritional intake, nausea, and increased metabolic needs. Infants in CHF tend to fall in the bottom percentiles of their growth charts for weight and may have normal height development. The decision to time a surgical intervention may be made from following a child's physical development and recognizing indications of a flattened growth curve. Children with CHF frequently do not meet their developmental milestones at a normal pace. They may have delays in gross motor skills. Learning to sit up and to walk and other gross motor activities require extra energy that a child with limited cardiac reserve may not have to spare. As the child's condition allows, age-appropriate play should be encouraged to enhance cognitive and motor development. After surgical repair, and once a child is no longer in CHF, children tend to catch up developmentally with their peers.

Nursing Diagnoses and Outcomes

In addition to the nursing diagnoses prescribed in Chart 15–3, the following are applicable to the child with CHF.

- **Alteration in cardiac output related to altered myocardial contractility**
  Outcome: The child will maintain adequate cardiac output as measured by adequate tissue perfusion, hemodynamic stability, and no signs of systemic venous congestion.
- **Ineffective breathing pattern related to excessive fluid in lung spaces, also breathing difficulties from poor cardiac output and increased respiratory rate required to compensate**
  Outcomes: The child will maintain normal respiratory rate and will perform normal work of breathing.
  Breath sounds will be clear, and oxygen saturations will be within normal limits for child.
- **Alteration in fluid volume: increase related to volume overloading from myocardial dysfunction; altered ratio of electrolytes from diuretic therapy; and risks of dehydration from poor oral intake and usage of diuretics**
  Outcomes: Fluid balance will be monitored continuously as evidenced by documentation in the intake and output sheet and daily weight.
  The child will have an adequate or negative fluid balance.
- **Alteration in nutrition less than body requirements related to increased work of feeding and increased calorie requirements**
  Outcomes: Parents will verbalize understanding of nutritional needs of child and feeding techniques. The child will maintain growth curve appropriate for age.

Interdisciplinary Interventions

When caring for a child with CHF, interventions are directed at conserving energy and decreasing metabolic demands on the weakened myocardium. Interventions are also directed toward removing excess accumulated fluids so that the pump has less preload of circulating blood volume. Nursing interventions to maximize cardiac function are an augmentation to pharmacologic agents. If there is an exacerbation of symptoms from an underlying problem, such as a viral infection, they should be treated.

Promote Rest. In the presence of impaired circulation and pulmonary congestion, the child's caretakers should limit his or her energy expenditures by promoting rest. This will lower metabolic requirements and oxygen needs on an already strained pump. Hematocrit levels and blood values are maintained at or above normal to maximize oxygen-carrying capacity. Nursing care should be timed so that activities are clustered together and are followed by long periods of undisturbed rest. Sedation can be provided for an acutely ill child with CHF who is restless and irritable. For toddlers and older children, television and video games allow for an emotional distraction and encourage inactivity. Breathing and eating are strenuous activities for infants in CHF, leaving no extra energy for the work of play or motion. They tend to limit their own activity by falling asleep.

Positioning. Along with the overcirculated lungs of a child in CHF, there is also decreased lung compliance causing more utilization of energy resources. A child can be positioned in a semi-Fowler's position to facilitate lung expansion, provide less restrictive movement of the diaphragm, and relieve pressure from abdominal organs. Small children can be propped up in an infant seat. An upright position also decreases pulmonary congestion by encouraging pooling of blood in dependent areas, which minimizes the work of breathing.

Nutrition and Feedings. Feeding issues can be perplexing. Both the increased metabolic needs of the child's overworked heart and the extra work of breathing demand extra energy. The logical deduction is to encourage an infant to eat as much as possible. The drawback is that feeding takes energy, too. Also, feeding distends the abdomen in infants, which pushes up on the diaphragm and decreases lung expansion. Feeding also increases fluids in the circulatory system. Fluid restriction may be employed for older children, but an infant's nutritional requirement is dependent on fluid needs.

Because infants with CHF fatigue easily, feedings may take longer than with healthy children. Smaller and more frequent feedings are better tolerated and decrease the likelihood of vomiting. Formulas with increased calories and nutritional supplements are given to meet the greater caloric requirements from the overworked heart and labored breathing.

Children are weighed daily to follow trends in nutritional stability and diuresis. It is imperative to monitor the child's condition through daily weights and accurate intake and output documentation. Because of variations between different scales, the child should be weighed on the same scale daily, at the same time period, and before feeding. Most children are not fluid and sodium restricted, although some older children may be. This form of management is individualized to the specific child. For instance, a child from an Asian cultural background may overuse salt-laden soy sauces and retain extra fluids, requiring diet modification limiting sodium.

Oxygen. Oxygen is administered judiciously. Oxygen decreases the work of breathing by allowing blood to be fully saturated and by increasing the arterial oxygen levels, which relieves respiratory distress. Detrimentally, oxygen is also a pulmonary bed dilator and can further exacerbate CHF in cases in which the lungs are overloaded. Oxygen is generally administered at low levels through humidification (Palmisano, Martin, Krauzowicz, Truman, & Meliones, 1990).

Pharmacologic Management. Diuretics are medications given to lessen the workload on the heart by removing extra fluids the heart has to pump, ultimately decreasing reload. In CHF, the renal tubular system tries to increase reload by retaining salt and water to therefore increase circulating volume. Diuretics are given to counteract this compensatory mechanism. Furosemide (Lasix) is the most commonly used diuretic, which inhibits electrolyte reabsorption at the loop of Henle. Spironolactone (Aldactone) is a potassium-sparing diuretic used in conjunction with furosemide to prevent excessive potassium loss.

Alert: *Diminished cardiac output compromises perfusion to the kidneys, requiring close monitoring of renal function. Diuretics improve urine output but do not specifically help renal perfusion.*

In order to relieve symptoms and to improve the heart's pumping ability, current methods of treatment include preload and afterload reduction. Positive inotropic agents are administered to improve myocardial contractility by providing enhanced contractility. Digoxin (Lanoxin) is a commonly used cardiac glycoside administered orally or intravenously as a positive inotrope. It decreases workload of the heart and improves myocardial function. Dosages are given based on the child's size (weight). Blood levels of digoxin can be checked by drawing blood periodically and when symptoms occur to ensure the levels are within normal limits.

caREminder: *Digoxin toxicity is a serious complication of therapy in any age group. Signs and symptoms of digoxin toxicity in infants and children include nausea, vomiting and anorexia, and an irregular, low apically auscultated heart rate.*

The telephone number of a poison control center should be at hand in any household. In case of accidental ingestion or overdose of digoxin, an immediate call should be made to poison control to avoid fatality. Digoxin should be kept out of the reach of children at all times, and only those family members who have been carefully trained should administer this medication because it has a very narrow safety margin between therapeutic value and toxicity.

Sympathomimetic agents, the rapidly acting catecholamines dopamine and dobutamine, are positive inotropic drugs that are administered as an intravenous drip, most often in an intensive care unit. Common side effects are tachycardia and arrhythmias that are more likely to occur as dosages are increased.

Vasodilators enhance cardiac output by decreasing afterload through a decreased left ventricular end-diastolic volume and pulmonary capillary wedge pressure. Venous dilators such as nitroglycerin dilate the systemic veins, leading to lowered blood pressure, and reduce venous congestion, which in turn decrease preload. They also dilate the coronary arteries, improving myocardial blood flow. See a critical care pediatric text for elaboration of these concepts.

Captopril (Capoten) and enalapril (Vasotec) are angiotensin-converting enzyme (ACE) inhibitors. They are used to block the conversion of angiotensin I to II in the kidneys, which cause vasoconstriction from aldosterone. Decreased formation of angiotensin II and aldosterone causes vasodilatation and increased sodium excretion. Another arterial vasodilator is hydralazine (Apresoline), which also reduces vascular resistance by manipulation of afterload. The amount of medication given is titrated by slowly increasing dosages based on the child's weight, symptoms, and level of tolerance.

Improving cardiac output from manipulation of preload and afterload can have a potent hemodynamic effect, so children must be monitored closely for tolerance and for negative side effects. Parents are taught the signs and symptoms of CHF and parameters for which they should notify medical personnel. The term "heart failure" conjures up the image in the parents' mind of a terminal state. This frightens families. Parents associate the terminal idea of the heart stopping suddenly. For many children, heart failure is a condition that can be medically managed and stopped with surgical repair. Teaching should include an explanation of the warning signs that indicate that a child's condition is deteriorating and that medical interventions are necessary. Parents are given specific guidelines on how to administer medications, the rationale for each medication, and potential adverse reactions.

Cyanotic Heart Disease

Cyanosis is caused by circulating deoxygenated hemoglobin and is reflected in a bluish hue to skin, nail beds, and mucous membranes. When there is a reduced saturated hemoglobin, but a normal ability to carry oxygen, the circulation compensates by increasing the extraction of oxygen by peripheral tissues.

There are reasons, other than cardiac issues, for a child to appear cyanotic. Structural changes in the lungs, such as bronchopulmonary dysplasia (BPD), pulmonary edema, pulmonary-arterial venous fistulas, and some neurologic abnormalities can cause cyanosis in a child. The health care provider cannot assume that the child who is assessed and who appears dusky or cyanotic has a primary cardiac problem.

Pathophysiology

Cyanosis in CHD results mainly from two anatomic situations. The first is that pulmonary venous blood is not being delivered to the systemic circulation, as occurs in transposition of the great arteries and total anomalous pulmonary venous return. The second is restricted pulmonary blood flow, as occurs in pulmonary atresia and tetralogy of Fallot (TOF). The severity of cyanosis depends on the volume of pulmonary blood flow or the degree of intracardiac mixing (shunting) (Nouri, 1997).

Hematologic problems associated with cyanotic heart disease include polycythemia, dehydration, bleeding, clubbing of nail beds, hypoxic spells, central nervous system (CNS) injury, and negative developmental outcomes. Polycythemia is caused by low arterial oxygen levels that trigger erythropoietin production in the kidneys, which stimulates the bone marrow to increase red blood cell (RBC) production. Polycythemia is a compensatory mechanism in which the body attempts to have more hemoglobin available to increase oxygen-carrying capacity and thereby improve oxygenation to tissues. Once the hematocrit reaches a level of 65% or higher, there is such an increase in blood viscosity that there is a risk of complications such as cerebrovascular accidents or strokes (Park, 1996). Children can also be anemic if there is not enough iron present for the creation of the excess hemoglobin.

Chronic tissue hypoxia stimulates an increase in production of red blood cells, creating a condition of polycythemia. This compensation causes increased available hemoglobin to carry oxygen to tissue. When a child who is polycythemic from cyanosis contracts a virus, especially in the presence of vomiting and/or diarrhea, he or she must be monitored closely for dehydration. When the vascular space is crowded with extra hemoglobin, this minimizes the space available for fluids and the children are at greater risk for hemoconcentration.

Excessively increased hemoglobin limits space in the vascular bed for platelet and other coagulation factors. Therefore, children with chronic polycythemia tend to have abnormalities of hemostasis. These children may tend to bleed postoperatively, bruise easily, or be prone to epistaxis (nosebleeds).

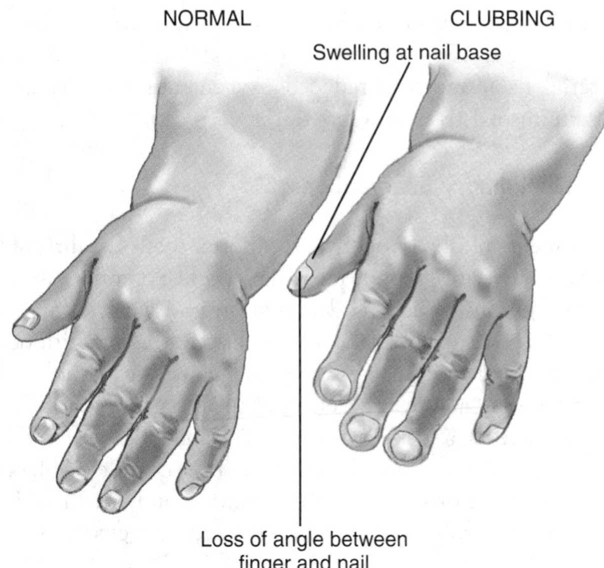

Figure 15–9
Clubbing of the nails.

Clubbing is a thickening, widening, and flattening of the toes and fingernails (Fig. 15–9). For unknown reasons, it slowly develops from chronic arterial denaturation and polycythemia. Clubbing is not seen solely in children with cyanotic heart disease but may be associated with other diseases, such as cirrhosis of the liver, chronic respiratory conditions, or hereditary nonspecific clubbing.

Children with tetralogy of Fallot (TOF) and with some other cyanotic defects *may* have hypercyanotic spells, commonly referred to as TET spells. These spells commonly occur when a child's heart has not yet been repaired and when systemic vascular resistance is at its lowest (Pinsky & Arciniegas, 1990; Harris & Valmorida, 1997; Nouri, 1997). The actual mechanism of action of these spells is not completely understood. Characteristics of a spell are worsening cyanosis, uncontrollable crying, and hyperpnea (increased rate and depth of respiration). These symptoms can be short-lived and subtle or can last for hours (Chart 15–12). A child may become limp or faint. Convulsions or death may even occur.

▽ **Alert:** *TET spells may arise without warning or after a predictable precipitating event. To decide whether a child is having a TET spell, the nurse should auscultate the heart. There is a decreased intensity of murmur during a spell.*

Significant neurologic complications are a risk of chronic cyanosis. Chronic hypoxia and underperfusion put these children at greater risk of stroke, increased incidence of meningitis, and brain abscesses. Hyperviscosity of blood from polycythemia increases the chances of thromboembolic events such as thrombus, brain abscesses, and abnormal neurologic development. Neurologic growth and development are impaired from chronic hypoxia. This is indicated by factors such as lower intelligence quotients and poorly developed gross motor functions (Walsh, Morrow, & Jonas, 1995). With modern management techniques, a larger group of the cyanotic cardiac population are candidates for earlier surgical repair. Earlier intervention can lead to fewer neurologic complications from chronic cyanosis.

Assessment

The ability to visibly assess for cyanosis depends on the degree of denaturation and the skin hue of the individual. The more hemoglobin not bound to oxygen that is circulated in the body, the more likely the child is to appear cyanotic. Cyanosis is more easily seen in lighter-skinned individuals and in natural light. In children with darker complexions, cyanosis appears dark purplish-black, an aubergine or eggplant color. When assessing a child with dark pigmentation, it is best to look at the nail beds, mucous membranes, the palms of hands, and the soles of feet. In the newborn, it is more difficult to determine whether the child actually has clinically significant cyanosis, because acrocyanosis (peripheral cyanosis) is normally present. Other data must be collected, such as the presence of poor feeding and tachypnea, to gain a more complete clinical picture of the child.

Diagnostic Tests. One of the compensatory mechanisms for low arterial oxygenation is increased red blood cell (RBC) production in an attempt to improve oxygen-carrying capacity. Clinical inspection for cyanosis is made by measuring the child's hemoglobin level. A child who is severely anemic and has a large left-to-right shunt may not appear cyanotic because the hemoglobin level may be too low for the child to appear blue. Further assessment, including a complete blood count, arterial blood gases, chest roentgenogram, and electrocardiogram, assists in developing an accurate diagnosis.

Administering oxygen is a tool used in the diagnosis

Chart 15–12

Characteristic Signs and Symptoms of Hypercyanotic Spells

Worsening cyanosis
Disappearance or decrease in intensity of heart murmur
Hyperpnea
Irritability or prolonged crying
Limpness, fainting
Convulsing

of CHD. If 100% oxygen is administered to an infant with intracardiac shunting from CHD or central cyanosis, there may be only inconsequential improvements of partial pressure of serum oxygen concentration (PaO_2) on arterial blood gases. It can actually destabilize some children with severe forms of CHD. Yet, an infant with an underlying pulmonary problem may significantly improve with supplemental oxygen. Also, children with intracardiac mixing may worsen their cyanosis with crying and activities, whereas the child who is cyanotic for other reasons, such as BPD, may improve with supplemental oxygen or crying.

Normal oxygen saturation of RBCs is 95% to 100%. Depending on the cyanotic heart defect, a child might have an expected saturation level ranging from 85% to 89% or less. A PaO_2 of 87 millimeters of mercury (mm of Hg) would be considered normal in an arterial blood gas (ABG), but a cyanotic child may be expected to show a PaO_2 around 45 mm Hg. Hypoxia is defined as a reduced arterial PaO_2 and as a reduced oxygen saturation leading to diminished tissue oxygenation.

Interdisciplinary Interventions

Treatment of TET or hypercyanotic spells is directed toward preventing conditions that would potentiate a cyanotic response, such as dehydration or crying. When a child has a known cyanotic condition, the practitioner must respond more aggressively and quickly to childhood illnesses that may cause dehydration (Chart 15–13). Because there is a risk of the child's blood becoming too viscous from a high hematocrit, the complete blood count is monitored closely in cyanotic children. In addition, these children must be assessed for evidence of

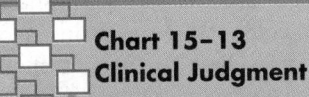

Chart 15–13
Clinical Judgment

Dehydration in the Child with Congenital Heart Disease

Eleven-month-old Rochelle presents at the clinic with what is described as 24 hours of vomiting and diarrhea. She is cyanotic, listless, and tachypneic (abnormally rapid respiratory rate) and has a temperature of 38.6°C. The mother states that her child has a heart problem.

Questions

1. What historical data would be helpful to clarify the diagnosis?
2. What are potential complications of dehydration and diarrhea particular to this child that the nurse needs to consider in her nursing care?
3. Does the child need to be admitted to the hospital?
4. What would be appropriate interventions?
5. What factors would indicate that the child has recovered with no ill side effect from this dehydration episode?

Answers

1. What is the actual cardiac diagnosis of the child? Is there a history of any cardiac surgery? Is the child normally cyanotic, and how do past episodes compare with the present one? What is the child's normal oxygen saturation? What medications, if any, is the child taking? How many dosages of the medications were missed? Has she been exposed to anyone with a history of vomiting and diarrhea? How many, and how large, were the stools the child had? When did she last urinate?
2. Children with cyanotic heart disease may be at risk for hypercyanotic spells, and dehydration can be a triggering response. The complete blood count may be too high as a result of hemoconcentration. Also, cyanotic children are at increased risk for stroke and brain abscess.
3. Yes. Because the child is listless and tachypneic, she is exhibiting clinical signs of deterioration from dehydration. Also, reasons for the vomiting and diarrhea, other than a virus, need to be ruled out.
4. Administer intravenous fluids, low-flow oxygen supplementation, antipyretics, and antiemetics and begin pulse oximetry monitor. If the patient was taking digoxin, a blood level should be obtained, because one symptom of an elevated or toxic digoxin level is vomiting. The patient's pediatric cardiologist should be notified of the admission. Send stool cultures for evaluation. Routine laboratory values should include a blood culture with routine blood work (complete blood count [CBC] and an electrolyte panel). Anemia and electrolyte imbalances need to be ruled out.
5. The child has no vomiting or diarrhea. She is interacting playfully and tolerating oral intake, and her oxygen saturation levels on room air are at baseline.

bruising, petechiae of the skin, or epistaxis. In treating a cyanotic spell, interventions are aimed at raising the systemic vascular resistance (SVR). Calming and comforting measures are provided to decrease oxygen demand and hyperventilation. Oxygen is administered as well as morphine sulfate in an attempt to relax the right ventricular infundibulum, which increases pulmonary blood flow and therefore decreases the right-to-left shunt. During a cyanotic spell, the child is placed in the knee-chest position, which blocks flow to the legs and decreases venous return from the legs. This raises SVR. A cyanotic toddler may occasionally squat while playing, eliciting the same effect as does the knee-chest position. Decreasing venous return from the legs reduces left-to-right shunts, resulting in improved blood flow to the lungs. Oral propranolol (Inderal) is useful in controlling spells by stabilizing the reactivity of peripheral vasculature. In severe cyanotic spells, as the child becomes more hypoxic and pulmonary blood flow decreases, the child can develop metabolic acidosis. Acidosis necessitates immediate correction with sodium bicarbonate intravenously.

Collateral vessels develop in patients with cyanotic lesions such as pulmonary atresia. These vessels are the body's attempt to improve oxygenation. They usually arise from the thoracic aorta and supply parts of the pulmonary system. These vessels tend to be fragile and tortuous. When a surgon is correcting lesions to improve a child's oxygenation, these vessels are a nuisance, as they can be numerous and difficult to reach surgically. Many collaterals can be occluded in the catheterization laboratory with occlusion devices such as coils or ligated in surgery if they can be reached. Taking out collaterals can be laborious and may require repeat procedures.

Palliative surgeries to improve cardiac mixing or increase blood flow to the lungs can be performed to allow for growth and development. Definitively, a permanent cardiac repair, which can remove areas of shunting and/or allow normal blood flow to the lungs, can fix cyanosis so that the previous compensatory responses diminish. Cardiac transplantation may become the only option for a child with worsening symptoms who has received maximum medical management and for whom there are no surgical options.

Parents of cyanotic children must be taught how to differentiate between worsening blueness and cyanotic spells. It is not surprising to see a cyanotic infant who is obese. Parents fear his or her crying and turning blue, so they may continually pacify the infant with a bottle. Teaching should include a discussion of aggressively preventing dehydration to avoid an overly viscous blood volume. Another fear for parents is having their child turn more cyanotic with increased activity. Most cyanotic children limit their own activity levels. They may be as active as their peers but do tend to fatigue sooner (Koster, 1994).

Chart 15–14

Common Abbreviations in Congenital Heart Disease

AS	Aortic stenosis
ASD	Atrial septal defect
CO	Cardiac output
CATH	Heart catheterization
CHD	Congenital heart disease
CHF	Congestive heart failure
COA	Coarctation of the aorta
ECHO	Echocardiography
IHSS	Idiopathic hypertrophic subaortic stenosis
IVC	Inferior vena cava
LA	Left atrium
LPA	Left pulmonary artery
LV	Left ventricle
LVOT	Left ventricular outflow tract
MPA	Main pulmonary artery
MPA	Mean pulmonary artery
MR	Mitral regurgitation
MS	Mitral stenosis
PA	Pulmonary atresia *or* pulmonary artery
PAP	Pulmonary artery pressure
PDA	Patent ductus arteriosus
PS	Pulmonary stenosis
PVR	Pulmonary vascular resistance
RA	Right atrium
RPA	Right pulmonary artery
RV	Right ventricle
RVOT	Right ventricular outflow tract
SVC	Superior vena cava
SVR	Systemic vascular resistance
TA	Truncus arteriosus
TAPVR	Total anomalous pulmonary venous return
TGA	Transposition of the great arteries
TOF	Tetralogy of Fallot
TR	Tricuspid regurgitation
TS	Tricuspid stenosis
VSD	Ventricular septal defect

Congenital Heart Defects

It is important to have an understanding of a given child's precise cardiac defect because management and health outcomes depend on the specific pattern that a defect follows. Each lesion has its own natural history of adverse effects on pulmonary vascular resistance and on both ventricles, valves, or other structures. Survival and/or prevention of complications can require prompt diagnosis and treatment in early infancy, whereas with other conditions, children may grow into adulthood before becoming symptomatic. Hospitalized children with a cardiac diagnosis may be in various stages of repair, may have surgical trauma, or may have a possible inadequate or disrupted surgical repair. Chart 15–14 provides a list of common terms that are used to discuss CHD.

When categorizing CHD, lesions are commonly listed as cyanotic or acyanotic based on the individual heart anomaly (Table 15–2). These guidelines cannot be *strictly* applied, because many defects can present with different degrees of severity, with variations on the lesion, and with more than one defect of the same heart (multiple complex lesions). When a child has a multiple complex lesion, the plan of care is not always clearcut and there may be much debate among practitioners as to what action to take.

Acyanotic Defects with Increased Pulmonary Blood Flow

Patent Ductus Arteriosus

Pathophysiology

Patent ductus arteriosus (PDA) is the persistence of the fetal vessel that connects the aorta and the pulmonary artery (PA). It is generally at the lesser curvature of the aortic arch distal to the subclavian artery and connected to the left or main PA. This vessel normally closes completely by 6 weeks of age (it is believed it constricts in response to oxygen). At birth, the newborn's lungs ex-

Table 15–2
Classification of Congenital Heart Defects

Defect	Incidence
Acyanotic Defects with Increased Pulmonary Blood Flow	
Patent ductus arteriosus (PDA)	10% of all congenital defects; female to male, 3 : 1
Atrial septal defect (ASD)	10% of all congenital defects; more frequent in females than males
Ventricular septal defect (VSD)	25% of all congenital defects; more common in males than females
Atrioventricular canal defect (AV canal)	5% of all congenital defects
Acyanotic Defects That Obstruct Flow from the Ventricles	
Coarctation of the aorta (COA)	4–10% of all congenital defects; more frequent in males than females
Aortic stenosis (AS)	5% of all congenital defects; more frequent in males than females
Pulmonary stenosis (PS)	8% of all congenital defects; sibling reoccurrence is 2.9%
Cyanotic Defects with Decreased Pulmonary Blood Flow	
Tricuspid Atresia	1–3% of all congenital defects
Tetralogy of Fallot (TOF)	10% of all congenital defects; more common in males than females
Pulmonary atresia	1% or less of all congenital defects
Cyanotic Defects with Increased Pulmonary Blood Flow	
Total anomalous pulmonary venous return (TAPVR)	1% or less of all congenital defects; more common in males than females
Truncus arteriosus	1% of all congenital defects
Hypoplastic left heart syndrome (HLHS)	1–2% of all congenital heart disease; more common in males than females
Cyanotic Defects with Variable Pulmonary Blood Flow	
Transposition of the great arteries (TGA, TGV)	5% of all congenital defects; more common in males than females
Single ventricle	Less than 1% of all congenital defects; occurs equally in males and females.

pand, and the right side of the heart and pulmonary artery pressures decrease. When the umbilical cord is cut, systemic pressures increase, causing arterial blood to shunt from the aorta to the PA. Oxygenated blood normally causes the ductus to constrict; failure to close leaves the patient with a PDA. If it remains open, blood flows from the high pressure in the aorta to the path of least resistance through the ductus, thus causing excessive blood flow to the lungs (Fig. 15–10) (Hoffman, 1990; Park, 1996; Wood, 1997).

A PDA in the premature infant is not considered a congenital lesion but a situational defect, as it occurs functionally as a result of the premature delivery. Congestive heart failure commonly occurs in premature infants with a PDA.

Assessment

Symptoms that occur in the presence of a PDA vary depending on the age of the child and the size of the shunt. In general, the larger the shunt, the greater the likelihood that the child will have symptoms of CHF. Slight flow from a small PDA may not clinically overstress a heart, but the child is still at a greater risk than other children of air embolus, bacterial endocarditis, or clots. Also, if a PDA is left untreated, over time it puts the patient at risk for developing pulmonary hypertension.

On assessment, the murmur of a PDA is continuous, machinery-like, and best heard at the second and third intercostal spaces (McNamara, 1990). Peripheral pulses are bounding from the runoff of blood from the aorta to the PA. These children also have a widened pulse pressure. The diagnosis of PDA can be confirmed and treated through data obtained by x-ray two-dimensional echocardiography, Doppler and color-flow studies (Wood, 1997).

Children who have their initial diagnosis made past the toddler years may often be described by parents as frequently having pulmonary infections. They may be thinner than other children and show an enlarged heart on the chest roentgenogram.

Figure 15–10
Patent ductus arteriosus.

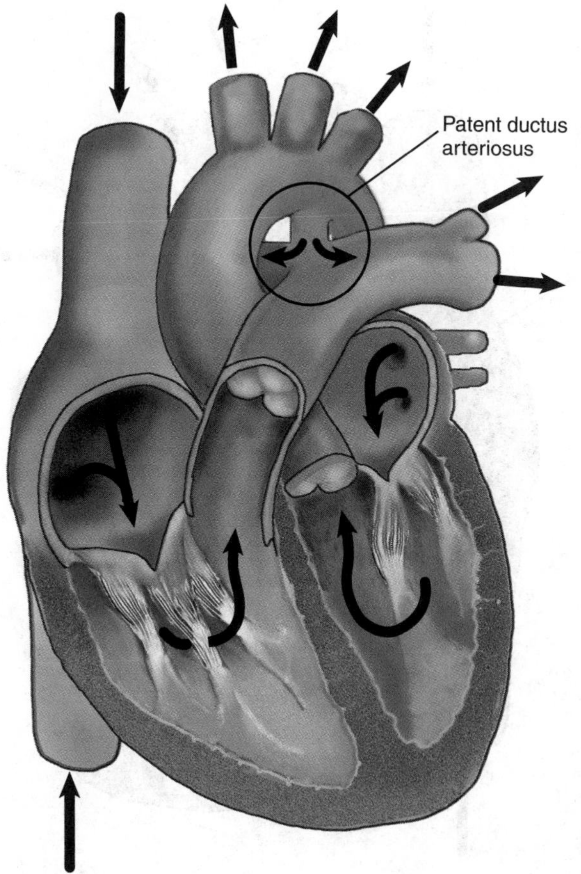

Interdisciplinary Interventions

Preterm infants without bleeding tendencies who have good renal function may receive an oral administration of indomethacin, a prostaglandin inhibitor, to encourage ductal closure. Success in closure of PDAs with indomethacin is variable (Kirsten, 1996). Interventions, both surgically and in the catheterization laboratory, are low risk. In recent years, PDAs have been successfully occluded using devices in the catheterization laboratory. If the child is not a good candidate for PDA closure in the laboratory, surgical ligation is usually done in early childhood. The procedure is a "non-pump" case and is accomplished through a left thoracotomy incision. A non-pump case means that the heart continues to beat during surgery and no cardiopulmonary bypass pump is required. Although uncommon, potential complications include phrenic nerve damage, diaphragmatic paralysis, laryngeal nerve damage, chylothorax, transient hypertension, and atrial flutter. A chylothorax is the leaking of lymphatic fluid into the thoracic space caused by surgical trauma that results in a leaking thoracic duct. There is an increased risk of a chylothorax with any thoracotomy incision. Nursing care postoperatively should include aggressive chest physiotherapy and pulmonary toilet. Adequate pain medication needs to be provided to discourage chest splinting and encourage deep breathing.

A PDA can be protective in an infant with a cardiac lesion where adequate circulation is dependent on an open ductus arteriosus. The PDA acts as a natural shunt, allowing blood flow to mix and bypass an obstructed area. These infants receive prostaglandin E_1 infusion to ensure patency of the PDA. This substance is widely found throughout the body and is involved in the regulation of virtually all organ systems. Intravenously, it is a potent dilator of the ductus arteriosus and is used for left-sided obstructive lesions to improve systemic perfusion, acid-base balance, and urine output.

Atrial Septal Defect

Pathophysiology

An atrial septal defect (ASD) is a communication between right and left atria through the septum that persists beyond the newborn period. Blood shunts from the left atrium to the right atrium because pressures are greater on the left side of the heart. This left-to-right shunt can cause the mean pressure in the right atrium and left atrium to be similar. The amount of blood that shunts across the septum is relative to the size of the hole. If the ASD is large enough, there is a burden on the right side of the heart. This occurs from excess circulating blood volume in the right heart circulation and the pulmonary bed (Fig. 15–11) (Hoffman, 1990; Park, 1996; Samanek et al., 1989; Wood, 1997).

There are three classifications of ASD, which are based on the actual location of the hole in the atrial septum. If the hole in the atrial septum is high in the septum, it is called a sinus venosus defect. Sinus venosus ASDs are the second most common ASD and are located near the junction of the superior vena cava (SVC) and the right atrium. These are often associated with anomalous pulmonary venous return, which will be discussed later. These require a patch closure of the hole, and the surgeon must avoid damage to the sinoatrial node to prevent arrhythmias.

The most common ASD, an ostium secundum defect, is located midseptum. It is located in the fossa ovalis center of the septum and can be surgically closed with a suture or patch. Ostium primum defects, the third classification of ASD, are located low in the septum. These lie inferiorly to the foramen ovale in the lowest portion of the septum. Ostium primum ASDs can also be associated with a cleft in the mitral valve and mitral insufficiency.

Assessment

Because in the fetus the foramen ovale is naturally open, a diagnosis of ASD cannot be made in utero. Children with an ASD may be on the slender side with slight growth retardation. They may tire more easily than their peers during athletic activities. They also have a greater likelihood of having a history of repeat pulmonary infections. Because they generally lack any obvious symptoms, they are frequently identified during a physical examination only as having a murmur. If the ASD is not detected in early childhood, they can remain asymptotic until adulthood. ASDs are usually clearly delineated through the use of echocardiography, and if surgical re-

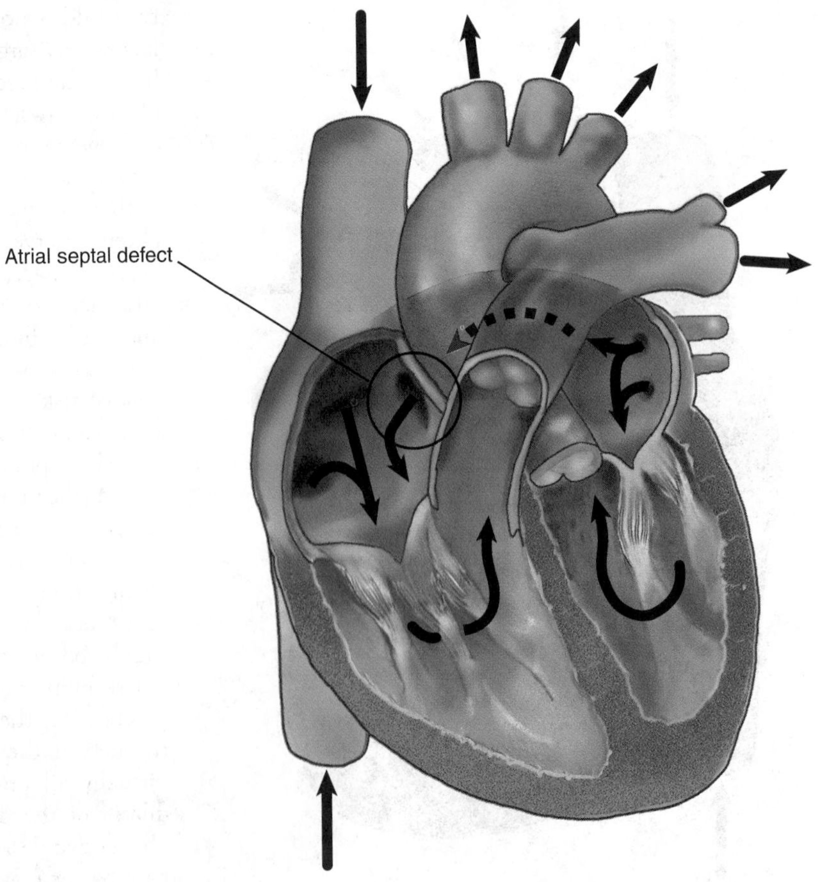

Figure 15–11
Atrial septal defect.

pair is planned, they rarely require a cardiac catheterization preoperatively.

Children are usually asymptomatic, but in severe cases they can have CHF. If the child is symptomatic, a chest roentgenogram may show cardiomegaly with an enlarged right atrium and right ventricle and increased pulmonary blood flow. If left unrepaired, as time passes, there is an increased likelihood of right and left cardiac hypertrophy, and as the atrium enlarges and stretches, the patient may have atrial arrhythmias. With chronic excessive pulmonary blood flow, there is a risk of increased pulmonary vascular resistance leading to pulmonary hypertension and the risk of pulmonary emboli.

Interdisciplinary Interventions

Treatment is provided in infancy if the child has CHF. If asymptomatic, the ASD is generally closed in early childhood. Spontaneous closure of the defect has been reported, as well as decrease in size of the ASD in infancy and early childhood. Surgical repair is completed on cardiopulmonary bypass and through a median sternotomy incision. A rare surgical complication of repairing an ASD is complete heart block from suture damage causing edema at the AV node and bundle of His. If a partial anomalous venous return exists, the patch closure is placed so that it directs venous return to the left atrium with a baffle. Instead of the septum being repaired straight up and down, it angles over to envelope the oxygenated blood returning to the right atrium and direct it to the left atrium.

Although the technique is still considered experimental, ASDs can be closed in the catheterization laboratory with an implantable umbrella. A device is placed through the atrial septum and is opened in the left atrium and pulled against the opening to occlude the ASD.

Ventricular Septal Defect

Pathophysiology

A ventricular septal defect (VSD) is an opening or communication in the septum, usually the membranous portion, between the right and left ventricles. A VSD can be located in multiple and various places in the septum. Physiology of a VSD depends on the size and location of the defect and the effects on pulmonary vascular resistance (Fig. 15–12) (Hoffman, 1990; Park, 1996; Samanek et al., 1989; Wood, 1997).

The types of VSDs are membranous, muscular, and

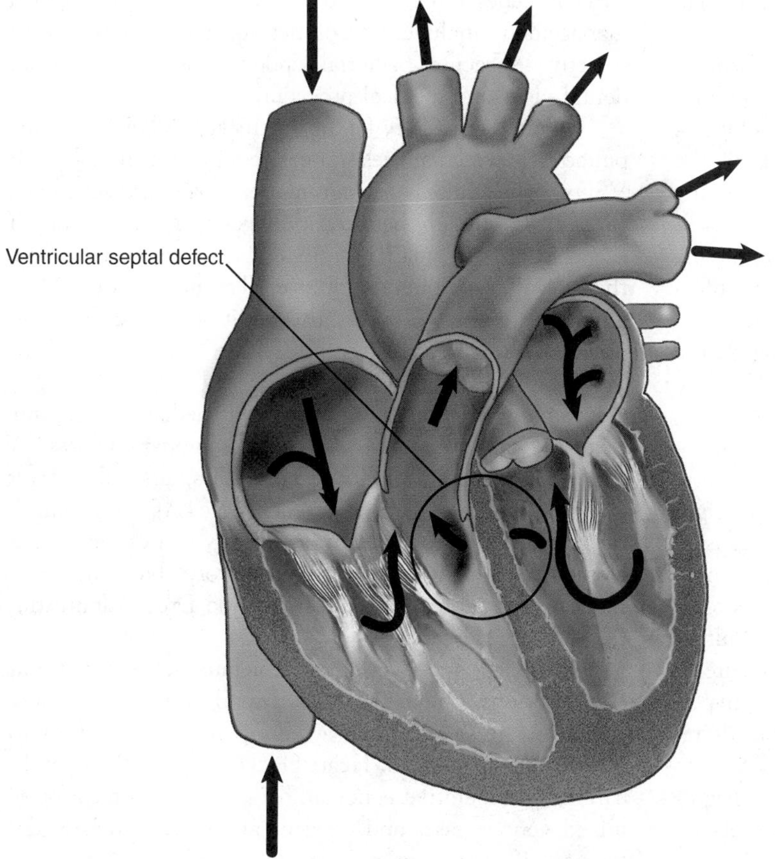

Figure 15–12
Ventricular septal defect.

supracristal. The most common VSD, occurring in 70% to 80% of cases, is the membranous VSD, which exists in the outflow tract of the left ventricle below the aortic valve. The muscular VSD occurs 25% of the time and is located entirely within the muscular septum. Muscular VSDs, found in around 5% of the population, commonly exist in multiple locations, giving a Swiss cheese effect. The overlapping holes can limit the surgeon's ability to find the VSDs. Supracristal VSDs exist in the infundibular septum and can result in prolapsing aortic valve cusps (Park, 1996).

The larger the VSD, the larger the shunt, which will rob the systemic circulation of a considerable portion of blood flow. Excessive flow through the right ventricle can overwork it and overcirculate the pulmonary bed as well.

Assessment

In the presence of a small VSD, there is normal growth and development without symptoms. To be classified as small, a VSD must be smaller than the orifice of the aortic valve and restrictive to flow across it, therefore shunting a limited volume of blood. Depending on the situation, the practitioner may elect for surgical repair to alleviate the risk of infective endocarditis. A decrease in the size or spontaneous closure of defects has been reported. Also, large defects tend to become smaller over time. If a defect closes, it is most likely to occur in the first year or not at all (Kidd, 1992). Children with small VSDs have a very good prognosis.

An infant born with a VSD may not have an audible murmur until 6 to 8 weeks after birth, when pulmonary vascular resistance falls and CHF can develop. A larger VSD is one that is larger than the orifice of the aortic valve and is unobstructive in nature; thus, pressure can equalize between the left and right ventricles. Children with moderate to large VSDs are prone to having decreased exercise tolerance, repeated pulmonary infections, slowed to impaired growth and development, and CHF. Chest roentgenogram results vary depending on the amount of the shunting but can exhibit increased pulmonary vascular markings and cardiomegaly.

If moderate to large VSDs are left untreated, pulmonary vascular resistance will eventually increase from constant excess flow. Over time, pressures in the right ventricle and the left ventricle may change, causing higher pressures in the right rather than the left ventricle. When this occurs, the shunt reverses and becomes right to left, then cyanosis and clubbing develop. Pulmonary vascular resistance exceeding systemic pressure is called Eisenmenger's complex. Severe pulmonary hypertension can cause the condition to be inoperable. If repaired, the sudden alteration of the excess blood flow to the lungs by patching the VSD may prove fatal. Right-sided heart failure occurs because pulmonary vessels remain constricted postoperatively. The high pressure in the lungs overburdens the right ventricle, which no longer has the pop-off valve of the VSD. Because of advances in postoperative management of pulmonary hypertension, a greater number of patients considered to be high risk have successfully had their pulmonary hypertension managed. Management in the intensive care unit includes sedation, hyperventilation, inotropes for right ventricular failure, and prostaglandin E_1 to decrease pulmonary vascular resistance. New inhalation therapies, such as nitric oxide, that decrease pulmonary blood flow assist in the management of pulmonary hypertension. Other defects putting the patients at risk for pulmonary hypertension are atrioventricular canal and truncus arteriosus (Rykerson, Thompson, & Wessel, 1995). To prevent lung disease and CHF, it is beneficial to repair a VSD early in life.

VSDs are the most common lesion to coexist with other cardiac anomalies. A VSD in combination with other lesions can have different effects on the heart. Depending on the specifics of the individual's lesion combinations, a VSD could be an asset that counters problems caused by another defect.

Interdisciplinary Interventions

Children with a VSD are monitored for signs and symptoms of CHF, poor growth and development, and poor feeding. In the presence of CHF, standard treatment for VSD includes diuretics and digoxin (Lanoxin). Medical management includes antibiotics for prophylaxis against infective subacute bacterial endocarditis (SBE) for all dental visits and medical procedures.

Infants with CHF, failure to thrive, and/or increasing pulmonary vascular resistance require repair of their VSD. If the child is asymptomatic, repairs are scheduled early in life, usually between the ages of 1 and 4 years. If the child is too small or too ill, but is in heart failure, then a palliative pulmonary artery banding is done. Most children are able to bypass this additional procedure and undergo one surgery to complete the repair (Care Path 15–2).

Surgery is completed through a median sternotomy incision with the heart on cardiopulmonary bypass. A stitch closure is done for small VSDs, and, for larger defects, a patch is sewn over each hole. At some pediatric cardiac centers, VSDs from selective cases have been closed in the catheterization laboratory, but this technique is not approved by the Food and Drug Administration for general care yet.

Although most children tolerate surgery without complications, they do occur. Septal sutures can cause edema in the surgical area, which is in close proximity to the conduction system. Heart block is a potential complication. Postoperative echocardiography and monitoring of mixed venous gases and oxygen saturations can help determine if there are any residual VSDs left after the

Care Path 15–2 An Interdisciplinary Plan of Care for the Child with Surgical Repair of a VSD

Nursing Diagnosis	Patient/Family Intermediate Outcomes						
	Preoperative Day	OR-ICU	Postoperative Day 1	Postoperative Day 2	Postoperative Day 3	Postoperative Day 4	Postoperative Day 5
Alteration in cardiac output related to cardiopulmonary bypass, surgical heart incisions, manipulation, preoperative CHF		Child will remain hemodynamically stable. Child will have good urine output ≥ 1 cc/kg/hr.	Child remains hemodynamically stable. Child has minimal drainage from chest tubes.	→ →	→	→	→
Impaired gas exchange related to sternal wound, anesthesia, fluid retention, atelectasis	Child will receive preoperative incentive spirometry teaching age-appropriate.	Child's respiratory parameters maintained within expected limits.	Child will increase activity and have adequate cough. →	→ →	→ →	→ →	→ →
Pain related to surgical wound, multiple tubes	Child will be playing on ward and in playroom. Preoperative age-related pain teaching given.	Child will remain free from pain.	→ Child will tolerate progressive increase in activities and will receive regular pain medication.	→ →	→ →	→ →	→ →
Anxiety related to altered family process, strange environment, activities restricted.	Family will receive preoperative teaching and tour. Parents and child will express concerns and will ask questions. Child will be playful.	Family and child asking appropriate questions and expressing concerns. Child will interact well and will remain calm. Orientation to ICU reinforced.	→ →	→ →	→ →	→ →	→ →
Care Intervention Categories							
Consults	Clinical nurse specialist Cardiologist Surgeon Social worker Anesthesiologist	→ → → → →					
Discharge planning	Discuss length of stay with parents and time away from school.					Initiate discharge instructions, both written and verbal.	Review discharge instructions. Schedule follow-up.
Labs	CBC and differential, typing and crossmatching 4 units of blood, Chem 6, PT, PTT	CBC, Chem 10, ABG on admission, K every 6 hours	CBC, Chem 6, ABG, in addition K and ABG p.r.n. ABG with extubation prn	am Hct, K	am CBC, K	am K	

Care Path continued on following page

Care Path 15–2 An Interdisciplinary Plan of Care for the Child with Surgical Repair of a VSD *Continued*

Care Intervention Categories	Preoperative Day	OR-ICU	Postoperative Day 1	Postoperative Day 2	Postoperative Day 3	Postoperative Day 4	Postoperative Day 5
Medications and IVs	Routine medications	Antibiotic, IV, dopamine or dobutamine as needed	Antibiotic, diuretic, dopamine p.r.n., IV	Antibiotic, diuretic, dc dopamine, IV	Diuretic, dc antibiotics	Diuretic as needed	Diuretic as needed
Monitors		ECG monitor, CVP, transthoracic left atrial pressure line, arterial line, O_2 saturation, Foley, pacing wire	ECG, CVP, arterial line, O_2 saturation, Foley	ECG, CVP, vital signs every 1–2 hours, O_2 saturation, dc arterial line, dc Foley, dc pacing wire	ECG, dc CVP, vital signs every 2–4 hours	Vital signs every 4 hours	⟶
Nutrition	Regular diet NPO after midnight	NPO Nasogastric tube	Clear liquids after extubation	Liquid; advance as tolerated	Regular diet for age	⟶	⟶
Pain management		Anesthesia, IV pain medication prn	IV pain medication prn	Oral pain medication prn		Oral Tylenol with codeine or plain Tylenol	Tylenol p.r.n.
Procedures (diagnostics)	12-lead ECG Echocardiogram if not done recently	Admit to ICU 12-lead ECG				12-lead ECG	
Psychosocial	Arrange for parents to stay close to child. Encourage visiting.	Encourage parents at bedside.	⟶	⟶	⟶	Encourage parents to plan with child for going home. Encourage visitors, with break times for rest.	⟶

Respiratory	Chest x-ray	Ventilator Postoperative chest x-ray Chest tubes	Extubate, O_2 by nasal cannula am chest x-ray ⟶ Cough and deep breathe	Discontinue O_2 ⟶ Chest x-ray after chest tubes discontinued ⟶	⟶ ⟶		am chest x-ray
Safety and activity	Up ad lib on unit to playroom	Surgery Bed rest in ICU	Up with assistance in ICU	Up ad lib in ICU or stepdown unit	Up ad lib in stepdown unit	Up ad lib in pediatric ward to playroom	Up ad lib Discharge
Special considerations	Betadine bath	Turn quarter-turn I&O, dressing clean and intact, maintain 24-hour fluid restriction	⟶	I&O, wound clean and dry Dressing discontinued Maintain 24-hour fluid restriction	⟶ ⟶ ⟶	⟶	⟶
Teaching	Preoperative teaching and tour of ICU	Orient parents to ICU routine and child's status.	Teach parent how to assist in eliciting cooperation and motivating child.	⟶ Explain expected day's events.	⟶ ⟶	⟶	⟶
Vital signs/baseline parameters	Preoperative weight Routine vital signs	Vital signs every 15 minutes until stable, then every hour	Weigh daily, vital signs every 1–2 hours Strict I&O	Weigh daily, vital signs every 2 hours ⟶	Weigh daily, vital signs every 4 hours ⟶	⟶ ⟶	⟶ ⟶

ABG, arterial blood gases; ad lib, as desired; am, morning; Chem 6, potassium, sodium chloride, glucose, CO_2; Chem 10, potassium, sodium chloride, glucose, CO_2, creatine, blood urea nitrogen, calcium; CVP, central venous pressure; dc, discontinue; Hct, hematocrit; ICU, intensive care unit; I&O, intake and output; K, potassium; NPO, nothing by mouth; OR, operating room; p.r.n., as required; PT, prothrombin time; PTT, partial thromboplastin time.

repair is done. Inotropic medications are generally administered to support cardiac output in the immediate postoperative period.

Atrioventricular Canal Defect, Atrioventricular Septal Defect, or Endocardial Cushion Defect

Pathophysiology

Normally, in utero, the endocardial cushions grow and separate into two openings that develop into the tricuspid and mitral valves. The cushions also contribute to the development of both the atrial and ventricular septa (Hoffman, 1990; Park, 1996; Wood, 1997).

An AV canal consists of a large central hole, where the cushion did not develop properly, that allows blood to flow among all four chambers. Levels of shunting occur where the lower portion of the atrial septum and the upper portion of the ventricular septum do not meet in the middle. Along with the left-to-right shunting, at the atrial and ventricular levels, there exist varying degrees of valve insufficiency. This is present as a result of inadequate fusion of the centrally located endocardial cushion tissue. During development, both the septum and the mitral and tricuspid valve leaflets are underdeveloped (Fig. 15–13).

Directions and pathways of flow between chambers depend on pulmonary and systemic resistance, pressure in chambers, and compliance of chambers. Because of the free flow of blood among the chambers, children are at risk for pulmonary hypertension and CHF.

For an incomplete or partial AV canal, there are varying degrees of partial fusion of the endocardial cushion that result in variable atrial and ventricular valve abnormalities. If this is mild, it can be treated much like an ASD.

Assessment

Diagnosis of AV canal can be made in utero by a level II ultrasound examination. If the defect is undiagnosed at birth, these children tend to present early in life with failure to thrive, repeated pulmonary infections, and congestive heart failure. They may be underweight, tachypneic, and tachycardic. Varying degrees of cyanosis are present that worsen with activity. The presence of this defect is frequently associated with Down syndrome and asplenia (absent spleen) or with polysplenia (multiple splenic tissue). These children generally die early in life without surgical intervention. Their longevity depends on the size of the communication between chambers and the degree of AV valve incompetence. Early surgical correction can help avoid the development of pulmonary hypertension from excessive pulmonary blood flow.

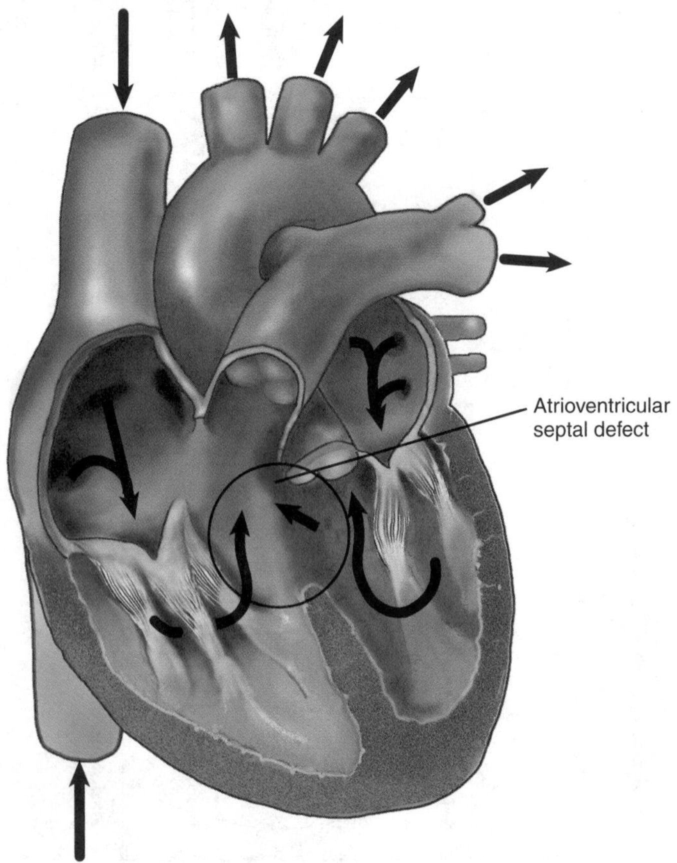

Figure 15–13
Atrioventricular canal defect.

Interdisciplinary Interventions

Medical management includes controlling congestive heart failure by using diuretics and digoxin (Lanoxin). Caloric supplements are provided to support the increased metabolic demand and so that each feeding provides more calories to the infant and allows the infant to expend less energy.

If the child is asymptomatic, repairs are scheduled early in life, usually toward the end of the first year. If the child is too small or too ill for surgery but is in heart failure, a palliative pulmonary artery band is done. Most children are able to bypass this additional procedure and have a complete surgical repair.

Surgical repair is through a median sternotomy incision, and deep hypothermia is used. A Dacron patch is used to surgically close the septal defects. The mitral and tricuspid valves are reconstructed or replaced when necessary.

Complete heart block can occur after AV valve repair. Postoperatively, echocardiography is done to monitor for valvular dysfunction in the reconstructed valves. If pulmonary hypertension is present preoperatively, then postoperatively one can expect instability if the patient has to do the work of breathing. These patients must be weaned from the ventilator slowly over days.

Acyanotic Defects That Obstruct Flow from the Ventricles

Coarctation of the Aorta

Pathophysiology

Coarctation of the aorta (COA) is a deformity that is created by localized constriction or narrowing of the aortic wall. This lesion is typically located at the junction of the aortic arch and descending aorta distal to the origin of the left subclavian artery. The COA location is the area directly opposite of where the ductus arteriosus existed. Coarctation can be preductal, where the area of narrowing is proximal to the ductus, or postductal, where the obstruction is distal to the ductus. Any length of the aorta can have an obstruction, but it usually occurs in the upper thoracic arch (Fig. 15–14).

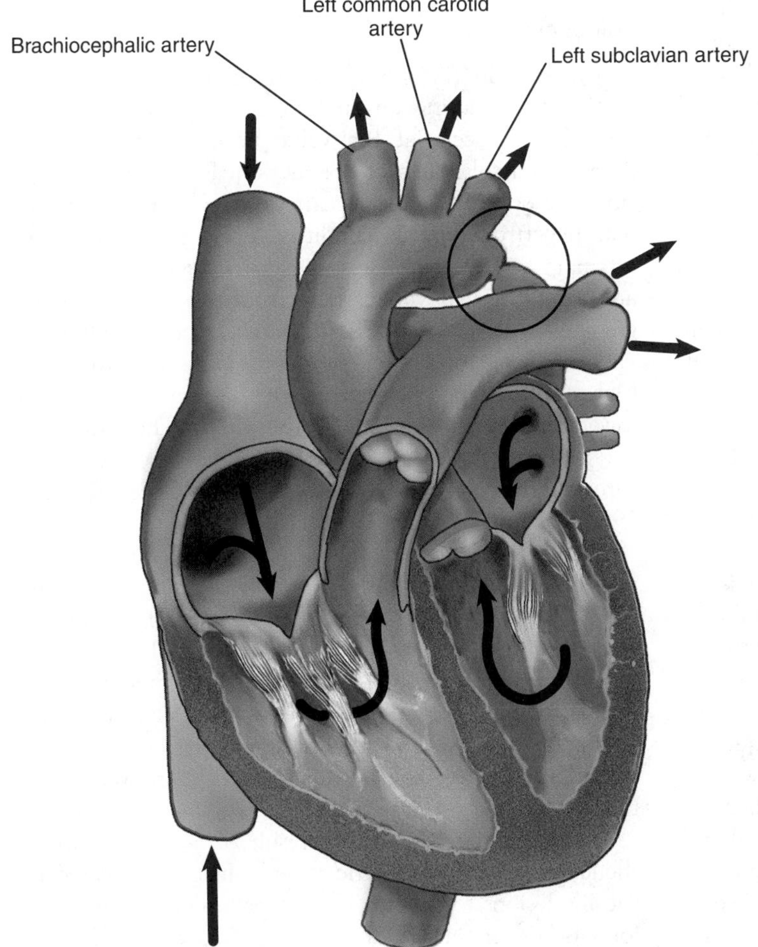

Figure 15–14
Coarctation of the aorta.

Narrowing of the aorta mechanically obstructs the pumping of the left ventricle, therefore putting a strain on the left ventricle. When there is an obstruction or narrowing of the aorta, there is still normal pulmonary blood flow and no areas of intracardiac mixing unless the patient has a coexisting lesion. As blood is pumped out of the left ventricle to the aorta, some blood flows to the head and upper extremities at a high pressure. The rest of the blood meets the obstruction and jets through the constricted area, traveling on down the descending aorta. Therefore, pressures are greater in the upper extremities and as compared with the lower extremities.

Assessment

As in other defects, manifestations depend on the severity of the narrowing of the aorta. On assessment, these children can have decreased or absent pulses in the lower extremities.

caREminder: *The nurse should measure four extremity blood pressures to document hypertension and the blood pressure gradient between the upper and lower extremities. A finding of a pressure gradient in an infant should be reported promptly.*

The actual mechanism for hypertension in children with coarctation is unclear. Normal heart function produces a pulsatile flow to the organs. When an aortic coarctation is present, organs receive a non-pulsatile flow caused by the obstructed area. It is thought that the renin-angiotensin cycle is stimulated via non-pulsatile renal blood flow and causes arterial vasoconstriction to maintain what it thinks is adequate blood flow to the body.

Infants with moderate to severe narrowing can have failure to thrive and CHF. Adolescents have upper extremity hypertension. Infants with severe coarctation can have renal shutdown and early death from CHF if not treated. Approximately 6% of the patients with COA also have other defects. Thirty percent of patients with Turner's syndrome have COA (Hoffman, 1990; Park, 1996).

Interdisciplinary Interventions

Balloon angioplasty in the catheterization laboratory is an option for some types of COA lesions. These children can have excellent results while avoiding the more invasive, traumatic surgical repair. Balloon angioplasty patients run the risk of not being provided with adequate relief of the pressure gradient and subsequently requiring surgical repair.

If surgically repaired, the aorta is cross-clamped through a posterior lateral thoracotomy incision, and the aorta can be repaired without the patient being put on cardiopulmonary bypass. There are several ways to repair a COA depending on the specifics of the lesion. A primary end-to-end anastomosis is done for a discrete localized constriction. A patch angioplasty using a Dacron patch to widen the area of flow around the COA is a commonly used technique. For more elongated coarctations, a Dacron conduit used as a bypass tube graft is inserted to act as a bridge over the space. In infants, the subclavian artery may be sacrificed and used as a flap aortoplasty to patch the constriction of the aorta.

In the immediate postoperative period, the child's blood pressure is tightly managed and is kept low. This is done so there is no excessive pressure on the fresh suture lines of the aortic repair site. A child can have residual hypertension even after successful surgical repair. Complications are not common but include infection, hemorrhage, renal dysfunction, paralytic ileus, or spinal cord ischemia producing paraplegia. These may occur from cross-clamping the aorta during the repair, which causes lack of blood flow below the aorta.

In children with complicated multiple lesions as well as a COA, the coarctation is surgically repaired. This relieves obstruction to the heart's pumping action. Subsequently, other surgical cardiac repairs may be scheduled.

Aortic Stenosis

Pathophysiology

Aortic stenosis (AS) is a narrowing in the area of the aortic valve causing obstruction to left ventricular outflow. It can occur at the valve itself, or it may be a discrete muscular area of obstruction. Resistance to ejection of blood through the heart can result in left ventricular hypertrophy. This condition develops as the heart attempts to overcome resistance through the stenotic area. In a normal valve, there would be no measurable gradient when pressures are measured before and after the valve orifice. In a stenotic valve, pressures would be higher before blood passes through the stenotic valve and lower after it passes through the valve. The ascending aorta dilates from the turbulent jet of blood shooting through the constricted area (Fig. 15–15) (Hoffman, 1990; Park, 1996; Samanek et al., 1989).

As with pulmonary stenosis, there are three categories of AS. In valvular AS, the most common lesion, the valve leaflets are abnormal, such as a small annulus or thickened cusps. The second most common lesion is subvalvular, where there is a fibromuscular membrane below the valve that is localized or long and tubular. The least common lesion is supravalvular, consisting of an annular constriction where the aortic lumen is narrowed above the valve.

Aortic stenosis can be a result of a birth defect or rheumatic fever. Rheumatic fever damages the valve by causing lesions to develop on the leaflets and causing scar formation over time (Ohler, Fleagle, & Lee, 1989).

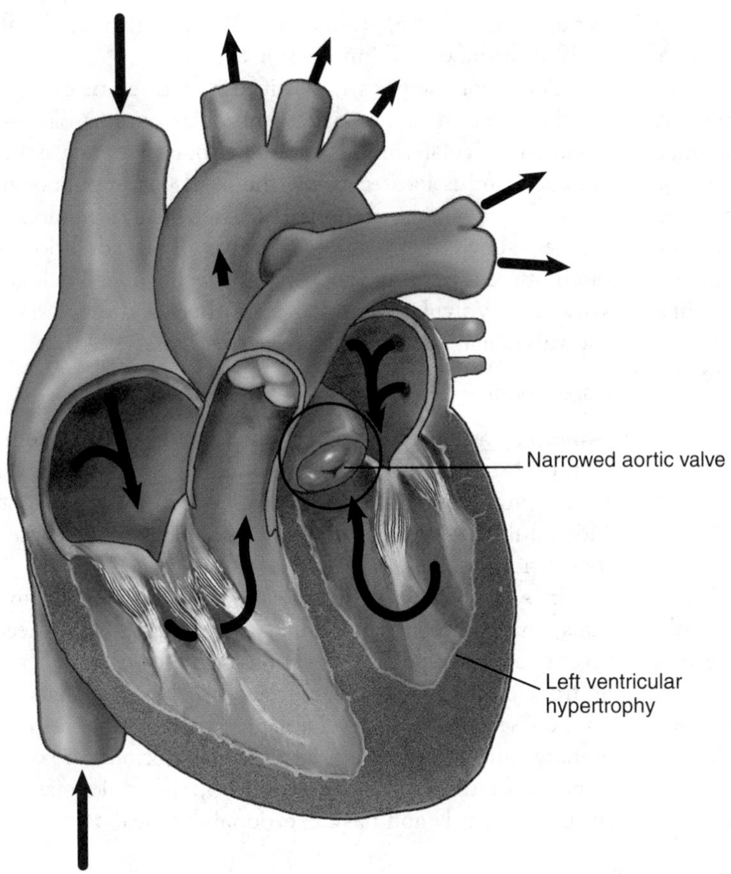

Figure 15–15
Aortic stenosis.

Assessment

The severity of signs and symptoms associated with AS depends on the amount of valvular deformity and blockage. Children with mild to moderate AS are usually asymptomatic but may have exercise intolerance. Stenotic aortic valves may go undetected for many years or present early in life with severe hemodynamic changes. Stenosis and calcification of valves tend to progressively worsen with age. Older children with AS are at risk for arrhythmias and for sudden death (Davis & Small, 1995).

In severe cases, there is a decreased cardiac output from a poor left ventricular ejection fraction. Infants with critical AS have CHF. Symptoms in older children with severe AS may include angina, syncope, left ventricular heart failure, dyspnea, fatigue, and palpitations (Ohler et al., 1989). Chest x-ray films can show left ventricular enlargement with dilation of the ascending aorta.

Interdisciplinary Interventions

Children with moderate to severe AS are instructed to restrict exercise by avoiding sustained strenuous activity. Critically ill newborns may require management in the neonatal intensive care unit with oxygen and prostaglandin E_1 (PGE_1). PGE_1 infusion maintains the patency of the ductus arteriosus. This allows for improved systemic blood flow, avoiding both decreased extremity and organ perfusion and acidosis.

Balloon valvuloplasty in the cardiac catheterization laboratory can be performed. This procedure includes the risk of inducing aortic regurgitation and has not been as successful as valvuloplasty of the pulmonic valve.

If the child is symptomatic and if there is significant left ventricular dilation and dysfunction, surgical repair is done through a sternal incision. The surgical procedure varies depending on the type and severity of the lesion. Valvular repair may involve an aortic valve commissurotomy (dilating the valve and incising the commissures of the valve). Potential postoperative complications include residual stenosis and aortic insufficiency.

If the risk of aortic valve insufficiency is too great, the child may require an aortic valve replacement. It is advantageous, if possible, to delay valve replacement until the child is large enough to receive an adult size valve, with the goal being to limit the total number of valve replacement surgeries required throughout a lifetime. If the valve is replaced with a metal valve, it requires the child to be on long-term anticoagulant therapy.

Recently the trend in valve replacement surgery is to use a pulmonary autograft, which allows some adolescents to avoid anticoagulant therapy. The stenotic aortic valve is removed and the patient's own pulmonary valve is transplanted in its place. The root where the patient's own pulmonary valve was located is replaced with a homograft valve. It is thought that the patient's own valve will last longer and function better than a homograft valve in the aortic position. Because the left side of the heart has high pressures, it is thought that the patient's own valve should last longer. This of course involves a more complicated surgery, because two valves are replaced (Davis & Small, 1995).

Pulmonary Stenosis

Pathophysiology

Pulmonary stenosis (PS) is a narrowing at some location along the right ventricular outflow tract. Pulmonary valvular stenosis is the most common lesion producing obstruction to flow of the right ventricular systolic ejection. Therefore, there are increased right ventricular pressure and increased right ventricular stroke volume workload. The cusps of the three-leafleted pulmonary valve may be thickened and fused, and the diameter of the opening varies (Fig. 15–16) (Hoffman, 1990; Samanek et al., 1989; Warshaw & Winn, 1988).

Pulmonary stenosis is classified into three types based on the location of the right ventricular outflow obstruction. Subvalvular stenosis or infundibular stenosis is uncommon and is located below the level of the pulmonary valve. Supravalvular stenosis is located in the pulmonary arteries above the pulmonary valve. This condition is often associated with congenital rubella and Williams' syndrome. Valvular stenosis, where there is a dysplasia of the valve, makes up 90% of the cases (Park, 1996).

Assessment

Symptoms associated with PS are related to the severity of the obstruction. A child with mild stenosis may have no symptoms and may not require invasive interventions. Most children with PS are acyanotic and have no activity restrictions.

In severe cases, an infant may be cyanotic and have signs and symptoms of CHF. These infants may need urgent surgical repair or palliation. Some cases may benefit from dilatation in the cardiac catheterization laboratory. In severe cases, development of the peripheral pulmonary arteries may be affected by various areas of stenosis. In the case of moderate PS, the child may fatigue more easily and have exertional dyspnea.

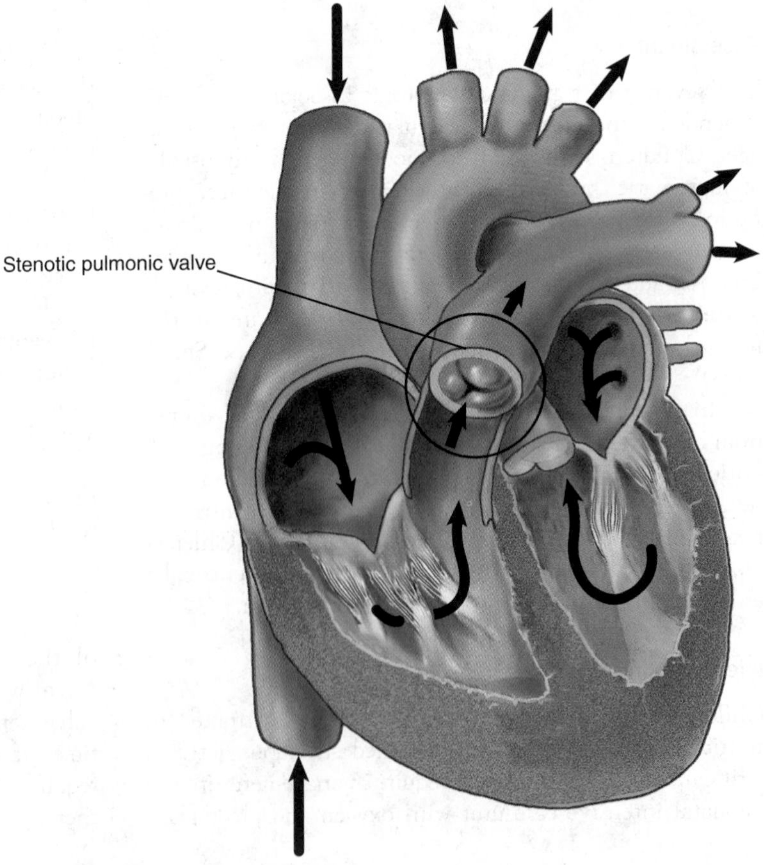

Figure 15–16
Pulmonic stenosis.

Interdisciplinary Interventions

A balloon valvuloplasty in the cardiac catheterization laboratory may be performed to dilate and rupture the deformed valve through circumferential stress. Intervention in the catheterization laboratory is the procedure of choice because it is less invasive than surgery, has low risks, and produces good outcomes.

Surgical repair involves a pulmonary valvulotomy with resection of any muscle mass and patch widening of the pulmonary arteries as required. The surgery is completed through a sternal incision and sometimes requires the use of cardiopulmonary bypass. If the pulmonary arteries are stenotic, they may require a patch widening or a stent placement in the catheterization laboratory. After repair, the pulmonary valve is regurgitant, yet most patients are asymptomatic and merely require follow-up the rest of their lives.

Cyanotic Defects with Decreased Pulmonary Blood Flow

Tricuspid Atresia

Pathophysiology

Tricuspid atresia is a cardiac lesion in which the tricuspid valve is missing, so there is no connection between the right atrium and the right ventricle (Fig. 15–17). Generally, the right ventricle is hypoplastic, and the inflow portion of the right ventricle is missing. In infants, survival depends on the presence of an associated defect that allows some cardiac mixing, such as an ASD, VSD, or PDA. Coexisting lesions associated with tricuspid atresia might include pulmonary stenosis, transposition of the great arteries, coarctation of the aorta, and hypoplastic pulmonary arteries (Hoffman, 1990; Park, 1996; Sade & Fyfe, 1990).

Assessment

These infants are cyanotic from restricted pulmonary blood flow and can have hypoxic spells. These infants may require a shunt in early infancy to increase pulmonary blood flow. Clinical manifestations include poor feeding and tachypnea. Cardiac roentgenography shows a normal or slightly increased heart size with decreased pulmonary vascular markings. Without interventions, children die early in infancy.

Interdisciplinary Interventions

Palliation to increase pulmonary blood flow to the lungs can be provided from placement of a Blalock-Taussig shunt. If the neonate has inadequate intracardiac mixing, a balloon atrial septostomy can be done to increase right-to-left shunting. Depending on the specifics of the partic-

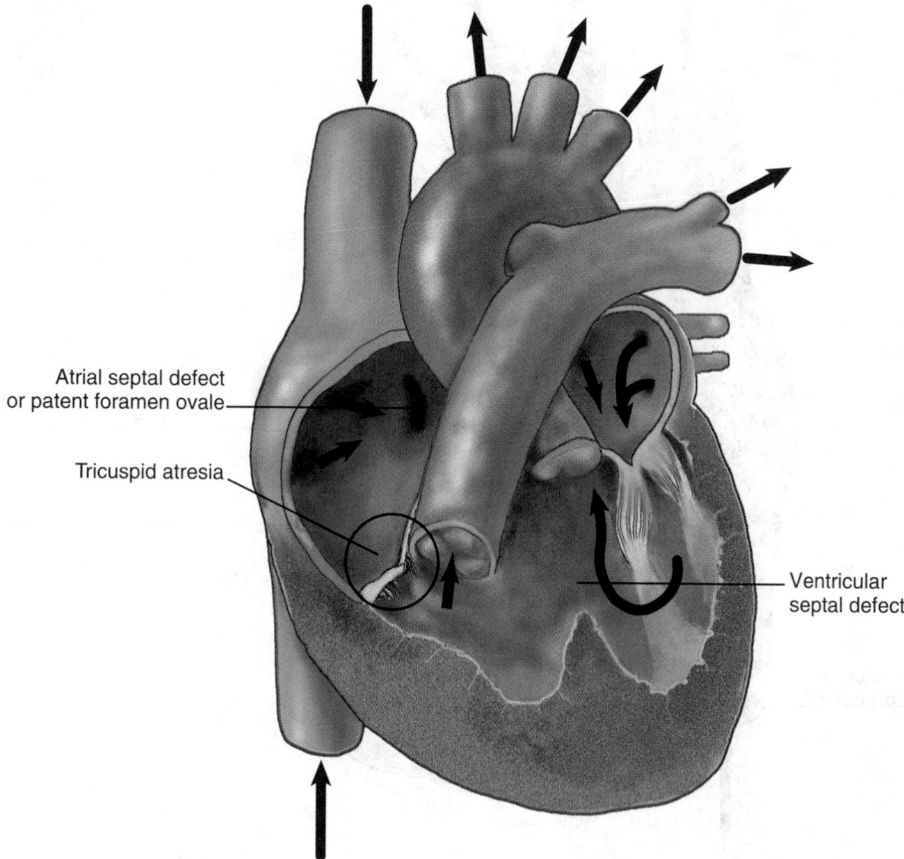

Figure 15–17
Tricuspid atresia.

ular lesion, some children have excessive pulmonary blood flow. In these cases, a pulmonary artery banding procedure is desirable to control CHF, limiting the excessive pulmonary blood flow.

A hemi-Fontan or bidirectional Glenn shunt is the preparatory surgery performed before the Fontan procedure. This is essentially an anastomosis (connection) of the superior vena cava to the pulmonary artery. It redirects partial venous return straight to the lungs.

The final repair is the Fontan procedure, which allows the single usable ventricle to act as the systemic pump. All the systemic venous return is directed to the lungs and bypasses the ventricle. This is accomplished through a surgical connection completed between the right atrium and the pulmonary artery. Some surgeons choose to leave a small fenestration, or opening, between the atrial baffle that acts like an ASD. This allows a small amount of intracardiac mixing and acts as pressure relief in the right atrium.

Tetralogy of Fallot

Pathophysiology

Tetralogy of Fallot (TOF or TET) is a name given to a commonly occurring combination of four problems whose manifestations and course are somewhat predictable. The child with TOF has

- A large ventricular septal defect.
- Some degree of right ventricular outflow tract obstruction or pulmonary stenosis.
- An aorta that is positioned such that it overrides the ventricular septum.

Because of these three defects, the right ventricle becomes hypertrophic from continually pumping against an obstruction to flow from the ventricle (Fig. 15–18). The amount of shunting through the VSD varies depending on the amount of right ventricular outflow obstruction and the size of the VSD. These children have diminished blood flow to the lungs and excessive blood flow to the body of poorly oxygenated blood (Hoffman, 1990; Park, 1996).

Assessment

Congestive heart failure is rarely a problem with TOF. Children with TOF have varying degrees of pulmonary stenosis, with correlating proportions of cyanosis. As discussed in the section on cyanosis, these children are mildly cyanotic at rest and have increasing cyanosis with crying, activity, or straining such as with a bowel move-

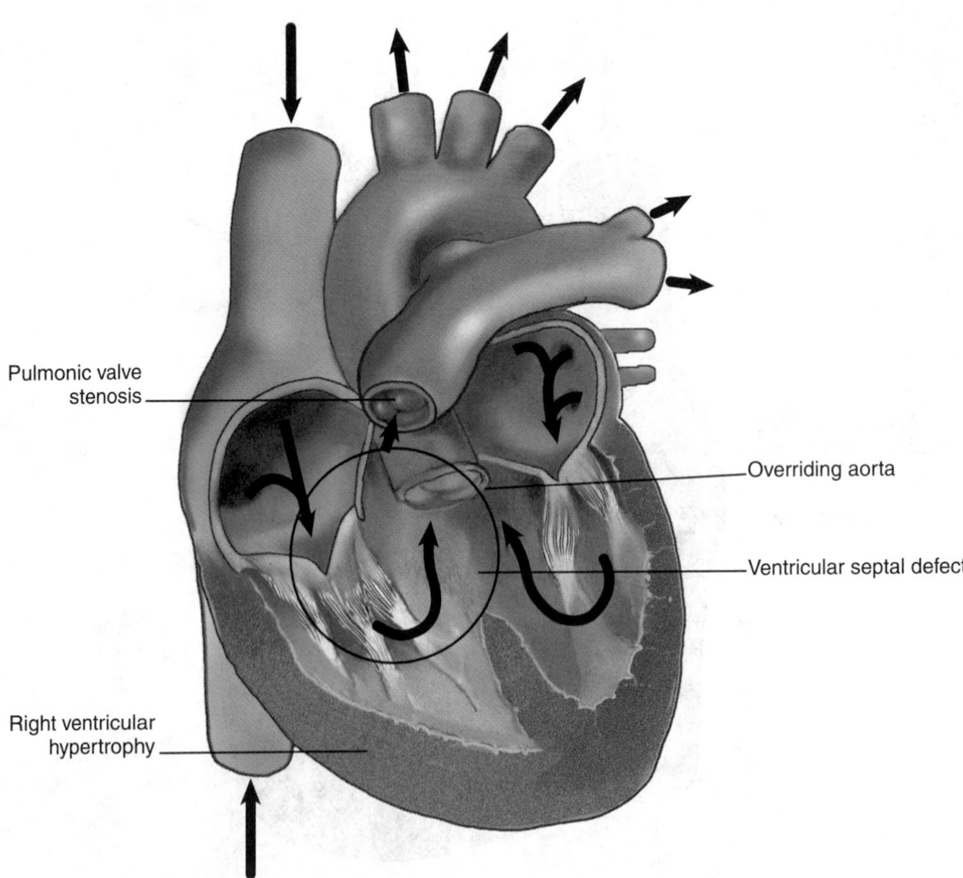

Figure 15–18
Tetralogy of Fallot.

ment. Cyanosis may not be obvious in the neonate, but as early months pass there is an increase in infundibular pulmonary stenosis, which also increases the right-to-left shunting through the VSD.

Children with TOF have normal growth and development, but they tend to limit their own activity levels relative to their level of hypoxic tolerance. If left untreated, they eventually suffer worsening cyanosis, clubbing, polycythemia, and exercise intolerance.

Some children with TOF can be acyanotic. If, along with a large VSD, there is mild or moderate pulmonary stenosis such that the amount of intracardiac mixing is limited, they may not be blue. When the secondary lesion of pulmonary stenosis is present, with the right balance, it can act as a left ventricular outflow obstruction to decrease pulmonary blood flow from excessive shunting across the VSD. This may help prevent congestive heart failure but further complicates surgical repair of the heart. These children are often referred to as "pink TETs."

Chest roentgenogram of the child with TOF shows decreased pulmonary blood flow and a normal heart size. The heart shows a boot-shape silhouette from right ventricular hypertrophy pushing the heart apex upward (Park, 1996). Echocardiography can provide information that clearly defines the defect. If the coronary anatomy cannot be clearly delineated by echocardiography, a diagnostic heart catheterization is performed. Catheterization provides specific preoperative information about the direction and the amount of shunting, about the coronary anatomy, and about each portion of this heart defect.

Interdisciplinary Interventions

Medical management includes monitoring children via their oxygen saturation for the degree of hypoxia, optimization of oxygenation, and recognition and treatment of hypoxic spells (see description and management of cyanosis earlier in this chapter).

Some children require a palliative procedure to increase pulmonary blood flow. A Blalock-Taussig shunt can decrease cyanosis and eliminate TET spells. Children who may benefit from a shunt placement before total corrective surgery are those who are too ill or small for complete repair. Also, if the coronary artery crosses the right ventricular outflow tract, standard surgical repair is ruled out. If a shunt is placed, it is removed at the time of the definitive surgical repair. At some cardiac centers, selected patients have undergone balloon dilatation of the outflow tract in the cardiac catheterization laboratory in an effort to widen the pulmonary artery and increase pulmonary blood flow before surgical repair.

Surgical repair is done through a median sternotomy incision with the heart on cardiopulmonary bypass. The VSD is patched in such a way as to direct blood flow to include the overriding aorta toward the left ventricle. The right ventricular outflow tract is widened by resecting the infundibular tissue and placement of a patch.

Most children survive surgery without long-term problems. Possible surgical complications include bleeding, heart conduction problems, pulmonary valve regurgitation, residual VSD, and persistent right ventricular failure.

Pulmonary Atresia

Pathophysiology

Pulmonary atresia is a severe version of pulmonary stenosis in which there is failure of the pulmonary valve to develop and the valve is imperforated. Generally, but not always, the right ventricle is also poorly developed. Pulmonary atresia can occur with or without an intact ventricular septum (Fig. 15–19) (Park, 1996).

Assessment

These children present in severe cyanosis and with tachypnea. Without medical intervention, these children have a very poor prognosis.

Interdisciplinary Interventions

As with most heart lesions, antibiotics are provided as prophylaxis against infective endocarditis for dental care and medical interventions. Goals of care are oriented toward minimizing cyanosis. In infancy, these children undergo heart catheterization to define anatomic and physiologic features. A balloon atrial septostomy may be done to improve shunting across the atria. In infancy, a systemic to pulmonary artery shunt surgery is performed to increase pulmonary artery blood flow by creating a right-to-left shunt.

Once the child is a little larger and if there is an adequate sized right ventricle, a valved conduit is placed using a homograph to provide circulation from the right ventricle to the pulmonary arteries. Homograft tissue is tissue donated from a cadaver and preserved for later surgical insertion. This surgery allows biventricular function and separation of the pulmonary and systemic circulations.

Depending on the specific dynamic of the child's pulmonary arteries and if the right ventricle is of adequate size, some children benefit from a surgery that includes placement of a patch on the right ventricular outflow tract and a pulmonary valvulotomy. This procedure opens communication between the right ventricle and the pulmonary arteries. Blood passes through the right ventricle and the pulmonary arteries and can stimulate growth of those areas.

Children with pulmonary atresia and poor distal pulmonary artery development can require multiple heart catheterizations and surgeries and still may have a limited quality of life. When the right ventricle is hypoplastic, a

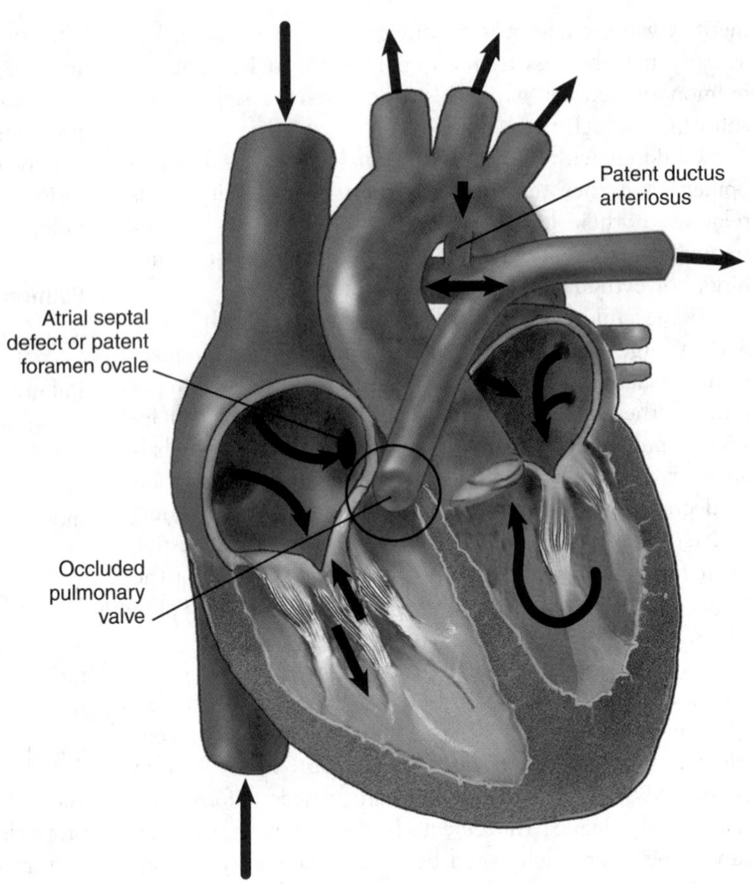

Figure 15–19
Pulmonary atresia.

modified Fontan procedure is used to provide separate pulmonary and systemic circulations.

Cyanotic Defects with Increased Pulmonary Blood Flow

Total Anomalous Pulmonary Venous Return

Pathophysiology

In newborns with total anomalous pulmonary venous return (TAPVR), the pulmonary veins do not return to the left atrium, instead they abnormally return to the right side of the heart. This blood returning back to the right side of the heart can go to the systemic venous circulation first and then to the right atrium or just directly to the right atrium (Fig. 15–20) (Hoffman, 1990; Park, 1996).

Because the systemic and pulmonary circulations are mixed, these infants are cyanotic. The presence of an ASD is necessary for cardiac mixing and survival. In these children, the left atrium is relatively small from lack of blood flow, and the right atrium may be distended from excessive blood flow.

There are different ways that the pulmonary veins are abnormally routed. The most common type is called supracardiac, where the pulmonary veins drain directly into the superior vena cava. Another type of TAPVR is called cardiac, where the pulmonary veins drain into the coronary sinuses or directly flow into the right atrium. The supracardiac and cardiac types of TAPVR are generally non-obstructive. With infracardiac TAPVR, the common pulmonary vein runs below the diaphragm into the portal system. A fourth type of TAPVR is a mixed combination of the other types.

Assessment

A newborn's degree of cyanosis depends on the adequacy of mixing through the foramen ovale and the amount of obstruction of flow via the misdirected pulmonary veins themselves. These children have CHF, poor feeding, and failure to thrive. Chest roentgenography shows cardiomegaly of the right atrium and right ventricle with increased pulmonary vascular markings. These children are also prone to repeat pulmonary infections.

Interdisciplinary Interventions

Newborns with TAPVR can deteriorate quickly if left untreated. Anticongestive medications that include digitalis and diuretics are administered. Some infants can benefit from a balloon atrial septostomy for inade-

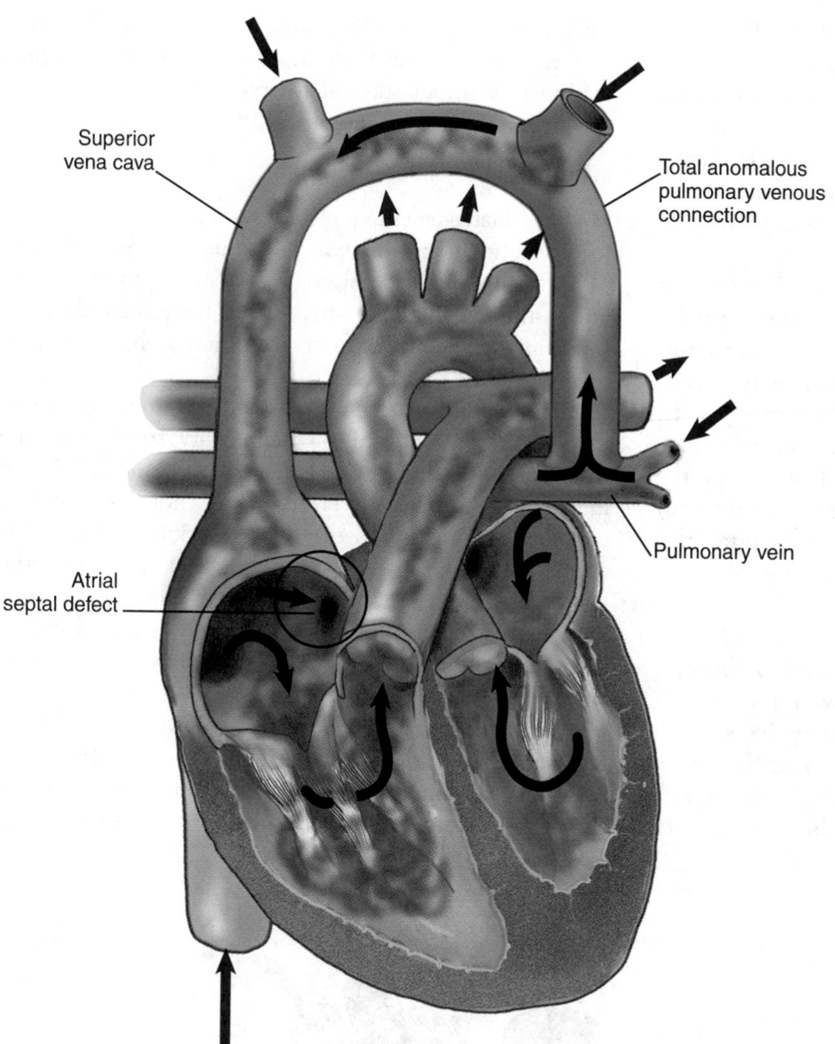

Figure 15–20
Total anomalous pulmonary venous return.

quate intracardiac mixing to encourage right-to-left shunting.

Surgical repair is done in infancy; mortality is high, and those surviving have a prolonged postoperative recovery. Surgical correction varies depending on the location of the veins. It is done via a median sternotomy incision and on cardiopulmonary bypass. In supracardiac lesions, the pulmonary veins are anastomosed to the left atrium and the ASD is patched. For the cardiac type of TAPVR, a communication is created from the coronary sinus and the left atrium and the ASD is patched. For an infracardiac lesion, an anastomosis is created from the pulmonary veins and patched to the left atrium, and the pulmonary vein that extends below the diaphragm is ligated.

These children are sensitive to fluid volume loading because of the small left atrium. They may require a high right atrial pressure to ensure left atrial filling. Postoperative complications include atrial arrhythmias, pulmonary hypertension, and pulmonary vein obstruction. Mortality for this operation is high, but when there is also pulmonary vein obstruction, long-term outcomes are much worse.

Partial anomalous pulmonary venous return (PAPVR) is when one or more but not all of the pulmonary veins drain into the venous system. If the partial vein drains into the right atrium, many of these defects can be repaired by simply widening the ASD patch to direct flow of the anomalous pulmonary veins toward the left atrium.

Truncus Arteriosus

Pathophysiology

In the lesion known as truncus arteriosus, the embryonic division of the primitive fetal truncus into the aorta and pulmonary artery did not occur. At birth, a single large vessel, the common trunk, arises from both ventricles astride a large VSD. The orifice of the common trunk has one valve that has three to four leaflets. The common trunk leaves the heart and gives rise to the systemic and pulmonary circulations. Systemic and pulmonary blood mix completely (Fig. 15–21) (Hoffman, 1990).

There are four categories of truncus arteriosus. Type I is the most commonly occurring version of truncus, defined by a partial separation of the aorta and pulmonary artery. A short pulmonary trunk arises from the posterior aspect of the large truncus or aorta. Type II truncus is when two pulmonary arteries arise from the posterior aspect of the truncus. Each one is connected separately to the truncus instead of a main pulmonary artery. Therefore, there is no main pulmonary artery. Type III truncus is much like type II, except the two pulmonary arteries arise separately from the lateral aspect of the truncus. In type IV, there are no pulmonary arteries, just bronchial arteries arising from the descending aorta. This fourth type is not considered a true truncus.

Assessment

Diagnosis of truncus arteriosus can be made in utero by a fetal cardiologist using echocardiography. Physical findings depend on the amount of pulmonary blood flow. These children generally present with varying degrees of cyanosis and signs and symptoms of CHF. They are susceptible to frequent pulmonary infections, failure to thrive, and dyspnea with feeding. Chest x-ray films show marked cardiomegaly with increased pulmonary vascular markings. Without surgical intervention, within 6 to 12 months most children die of CHF (Park, 1996).

Interdisciplinary Interventions

Medical management includes anticongestive measures for CHF, including digoxin and diuretics. Severely cyanotic infants may be helped by a systemic to pulmonary artery shunt. Pulmonary artery bands have been placed in some infants, but this form of palliation has met with high mortality.

The definitive surgical repair, the Rastelli operation, involves detachment of the pulmonary trunk from the truncus so the truncus can pump the systemic circulation independently. Then a prosthetic or homograft valved conduit is connected to the right ventricle to direct flow to the pulmonary arteries. The VSD is closed so that the left ventricle pumps exclusively to the aorta. Even though this surgery is complicated and associated with a high mortality, surgery is done in infancy because most children do not survive past that age without repair.

Repeat surgeries are done through the child's life to replace conduits that have been outgrown or that malfunction. Potential postoperative complications are arrhythmias, pulmonary problems, and persistent CHF. The

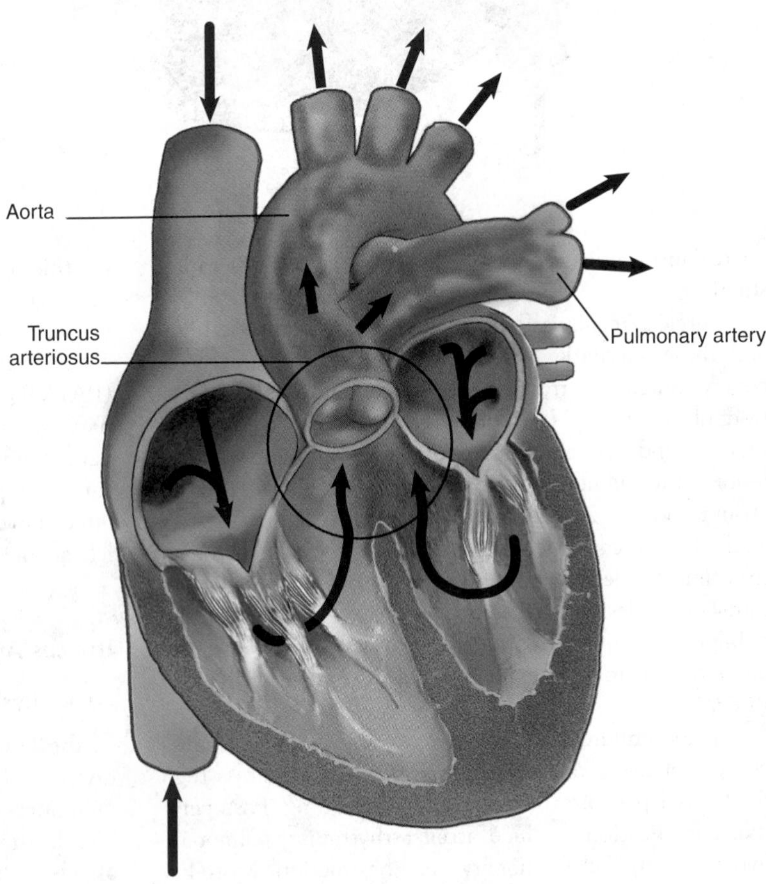

Figure 15–21
Truncus arteriosus.

imperfect truncal valve may have worsening regurgitation over time.

Hypoplastic Left Heart Syndrome

Pathophysiology

Hypoplastic left heart syndrome (HLHS) is the lesion that is the most common cause of death during the first month of life (Bailey & Gundry, 1990; Hoffman, 1990). HLHS is a diagnostic label given to a syndrome that includes a group of related anomalies characterized by hypoplasia of the left ventricle, mitral atresia, aortic atresia, and hypoplasia of the ascending aorta and aortic arch. The left ventricle and mitral valve may be entirely absent or poorly developed; therefore, systemic circulation is provided by the right ventricle through the ductus arteriosus (Fig. 15–22).

Assessment

Without intervention, these infants are critically ill at birth or within the first couple of days of life and develop progressive hypoxia, acidosis, and shock as the ductus arteriosus closes and systemic perfusion diminishes. Death generally occurs within the first few days of life without intervention. Not all children present prior to early discharge despite the severity of this condition. Chest x-ray films show cardiomegaly, and generally these children do not have an audible murmur. If adequate information is received from the echocardiogram, a cardiac catheterization may not be necessary. Hypoplastic left heart syndrome can be detected prenatally with a level II ultrasound examination.

Interdisciplinary Interventions

Historically, infants with HLHS died because there were no viable treatment interventions available. Currently, there are three treatment options: palliative surgery, cardiac transplantation, or no intervention (therefore death would occur). Religious backgrounds and family interactions can affect the family's decision. It is imperative that the health care team be as realistic and honest as possible in allowing parents to express their feelings and to comprehend the potential implications of each choice. Each option has its own medical, emotional, and economic burdens.

If parents choose not to provide any surgical intervention, they may leave the newborn in the hospital and visit with the baby at the bedside. Others have taken a relatively stable newborn home after medical interventions have been withdrawn and have allowed him or her to die with family support at home. The choice of allowing the child to die is an extraordinary situation for

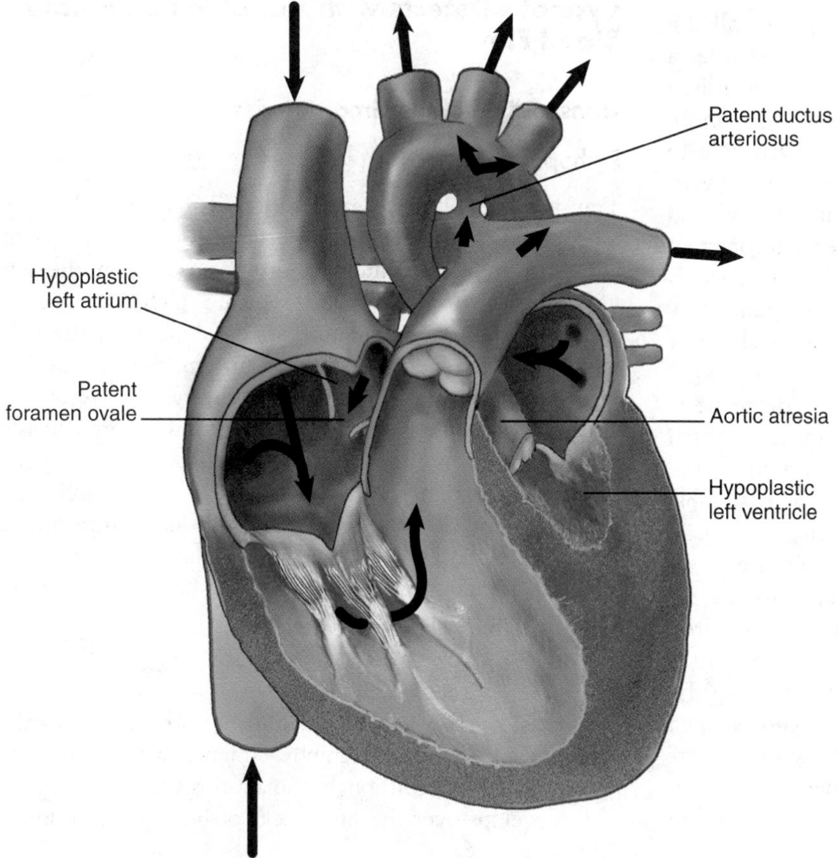

Figure 15–22
Hypoplastic left heart syndrome.

nurses. They must provide emotional support to a family in the grieving process as well as help them resolve any guilt or anger over their child's cardiac defect.

If the parents choose to stabilize the newborn for surgery, interventions are made to maintain adequate systemic perfusion and a balanced pulmonary circulation. Interventions include keeping the ductus open with an intravenous infusion of prostaglandin E_1 and low-dose dopamine. Usually newborns are maintained on mechanical ventilation until stabilized. Acidosis is treated aggressively, and digoxin and diuretics are administered to manage CHF. It is recommended that infants be maintained on 21% oxygen to keep the PaO_2 in the high 30s. This helps balance pulmonary and systemic vascular resistance.

A newborn waiting for cardiac transplantation remains hospitalized. A percentage of this population dies waiting for a heart to become available for transplantation. One study looked at 111 HLHS infants whose parents chose to wait for a transplant. Twenty-four percent did not survive the waiting period (Chiavarelli et al., 1993). If the diagnosis of HLHS is known in the fetal state and parents choose transplantation, there remains a level of unpredictability related to when a donor heart could become available. Some cardiac centers place a fetus on the transplantation computer waiting list before it is born.

For those parents who select surgical palliation, their child receives a multi-stage surgical intervention called a Norwood procedure, followed by a Fontan procedure at a later point in time. Stage I, the Norwood or the initial palliative surgery, has the goal of creating an unobstructed and permanent flow from the right ventricle to the aorta. The right ventricle becomes the systemic ventricle by using the proximal pulmonary artery and patches of pericardial or homograph tissue to reconstruct the aorta. Usually an atrial septostomy is done to encourage adequate mixing. Also, the distal main pulmonary artery is attached to a systemic-pulmonary artery shunt or a modified Blalock-Taussig shunt.

This first stage creates pulmonary blood flow at near-normal levels and adequate systemic perfusion, which helps preserve ventricular function. The goal is to set the child up for survival and create anatomy that is suitable for a Fontan repair, or stage II. After the stage I surgical repair, blood enters the right atrium and exits the single ventricle from the pulmonary artery stump into the repaired aorta. From there, most of the blood travels out the aorta into the systemic system. Some of the blood passes through the shunt to the lungs and returns to the heart oxygenated. This portion of blood is again pumped by the right ventricle out the aorta to the systemic system. Problems can arise in the management of flow to the lungs. A shunt that is too small can lead to severe hypoxia, but a shunt that is too large will steal from the systemic circulation, leading to poor systemic perfusion and acidosis.

When the child outgrows the Norwood shunt he or she received in surgery as a newborn, he or she is scheduled for the next surgery. Stage II consists of the hemi-Fontan procedure or a variation of the Glenn shunt done to decrease the volume load on the right ventricle. This procedure is basically an anastomosis of the superior vena cava to the pulmonary artery and removal of the newborn shunt that was placed in the first surgery.

The final surgery involves the completion of the Fontan procedure, which allows separation of the pulmonary and systemic circulations. This surgery entails the direct connection of venous return through the right atrium to the pulmonary artery. This leaves the systemic blood flow to be pumped via the single ventricle. Therefore, systemic flow is separated from the returning venous blood that goes directly to the lungs. The original Fontan procedure has evolved into different variations that are generally referred to as a modified Fontan.

Historically, limited numbers of children with HLHS survived through the final surgery. However, with recent increased experience in postoperative management by large centers, there has been much improvement in survival rates (Norwood, 1991).

Cyanotic Defects with Variable Pulmonary Blood Flow

Transposition of the Great Arteries

Pathophysiology

Transposition of the great arteries (TGA or TGV) is a malformation in which the aorta arises from the right ventricle and the pulmonary artery arises from the left ventricle. Two parallel and separate circulations exist (Fig. 15–23). One circulation system consists of the pulmonary veins traveling to the left atrium, then to the left ventricle, then to the pulmonary artery, and returning again to the pulmonary veins. The second system consists of blood flowing from the venae cavae, to the right atrium, to the right ventricle, then to the aorta and back again. Patient survival depends on adequate intracardiac mixing of blood between the two circulations via a PDA, a patent foramen ovale, or a VSD (Hoffman, 1990; Park, 1996; Samanek et al., 1989).

Assessment

Diagnosis of TGA can be made in utero by a fetal cardiologist using echocardiography. Infants with TGA are cyanotic at birth, although the cyanosis may be subtle. CHF develops over the first weeks of life. These children

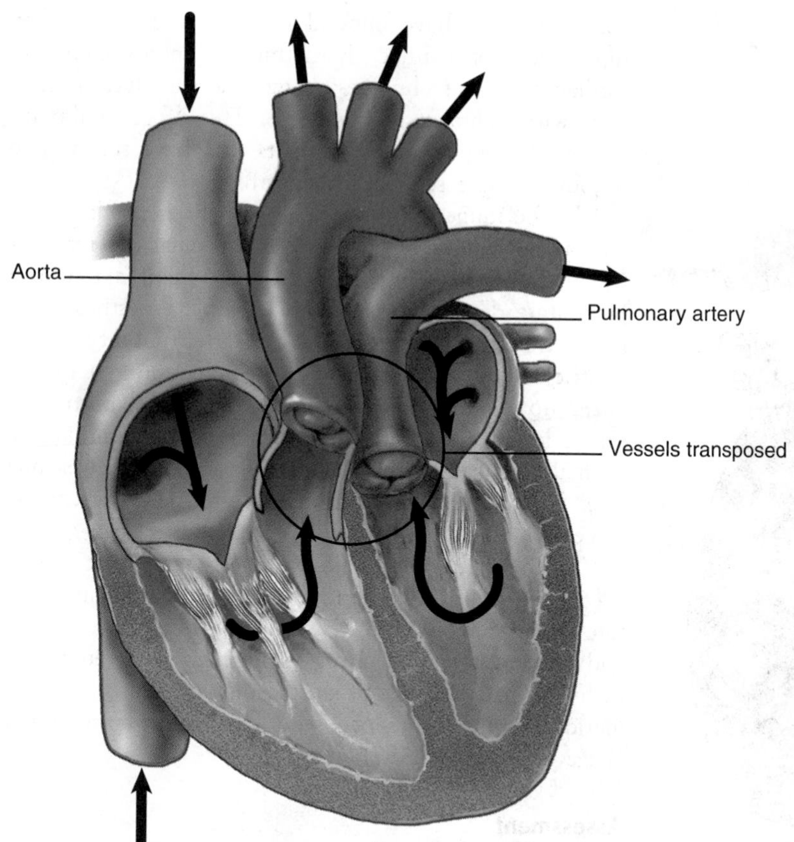

Figure 15–23
Transposition of the great arteries.

present with hepatomegaly, are poor feeders, and develop dyspnea. In infancy, progressive acidosis and hypoxemia occur unless adequate intracardiac mixing is established.

Diagnosticians need an accurate preoperative view of the coronary artery anatomy before surgical repair. In some cases this can be defined with echocardiography alone; otherwise, catheterization is required. Chest x-ray films show cardiomegaly with increased pulmonary vascular markings on cardiac silhouette.

Interdisciplinary Interventions

Preoperatively, intravenous prostaglandin E_1 might be used to maintain patency of the PDA and to improve systemic arterial flow in children with inadequate intracardiac mixing. A palliative balloon atrial septostomy may be urgently performed in those children without a coexisting lesion. A coexisting lesion allows for stabilization without a prostaglandin E_1 infusion. Heart failure is treated with digoxin and diuretics.

The Jantene operation, or the arterial switch surgery, is the surgical repair of choice for TGA and corrects the parallel circulations. In the arterial switch surgery, the trunks of the aorta and the pulmonary artery are dissected and reversed onto their appropriate ventricular outflow tracts. Also, the coronary arteries are reimplanted into the stump of new aorta. This surgical repair is frequently done during the first weeks of life. Long-term survival for these children is excellent (Pinsky & Arciniegas, 1990). Complications include coronary artery occlusion and pulmonary artery stenosis.

Single Ventricle

Pathophysiology

When the diagnosis of single ventricle is made, it denotes a condition in which both the right atrium and the left atrium empty into one ventricular chamber. The second ventricle may be a tiny chamber or be a remnant of the one larger chamber. Both great vessels usually come off the single ventricle, so oxygenated and unoxygenated blood are completely mixed in the chamber (Fig. 15–24). These children also have a high incidence of asplenia and polysplenia syndrome (Hoffman, 1990; Park, 1996).

Assessment

Clinical manifestations vary depending on the specific combination of problems. Cyanosis, failure to thrive. and difficulty fighting pulmonary infections are common manifestations.

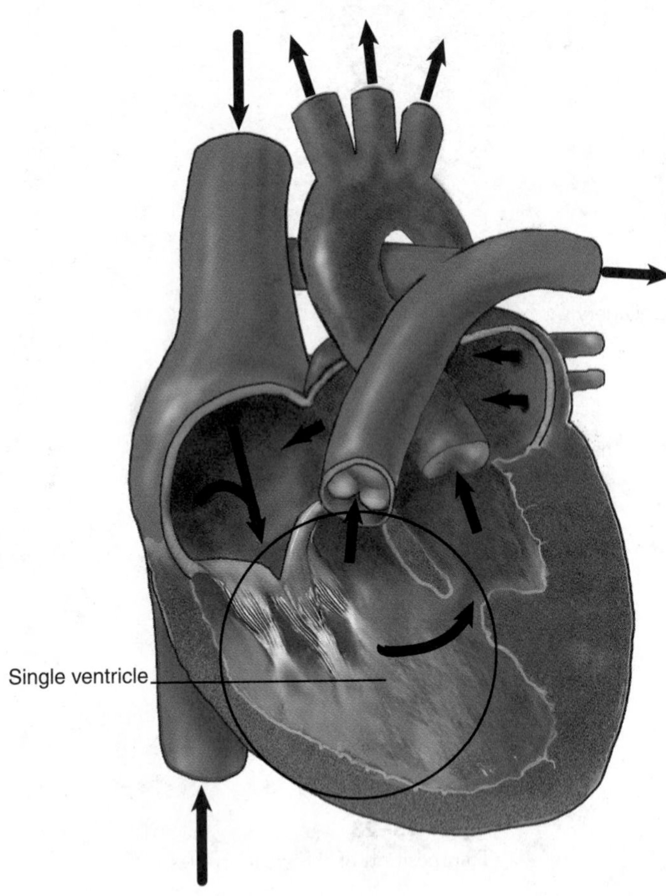

Figure 15–24
Single ventricle.

Interdisciplinary Interventions

Palliative surgical interventions include a Blalock-Taussig shunt if there is restricted pulmonary blood flow. When medical management of CHF is not adequate, a pulmonary artery band may be placed to restrict pulmonary blood flow. If the dynamics of a particular child's heart allows for it, many of these children may benefit from a modified Fontan procedure.

Acquired Heart Disease

Acquired heart disease refers to those disorders of the heart that are not present at birth. This includes cardiac disorders other than anatomic defects, although some illnesses such as dysrhythmias and cardiomyopathy can also have a congenital origin. Some acquired problems such as dysrhythmias can develop as sequelae of congenital heart disease and/or surgery.

Dysrhythmias

Dysrhythmias and arrhythmias are generic terms for a variety of classifications of abnormal heart rhythms. Advances in care have allowed for improved control and suppression of cardiac dysrhythmias. Improvements in cardiac surgical techniques promote longer lives in children with complex heart disease. This progress also increases the population of patients that have survived to become at increased risk for arrhythmias.

In the immediate postoperative period, children who are cardiac surgical patients are at particular risk for electrolyte imbalances and hemodynamic changes that can precipitate dysrhythmias (Chart 15–15). Anesthesia and medications can cause depression and irritability of the ventricles. Direct damage to the conduction system can occur from suture lines, dissection, and mechanical manipulation of the heart chambers. Sinus tachycardia is a normally configured rhythm that has a faster than normal rate. Sinus tachycardia is common after pediatric cardiac surgery.

In the first week of life, it is estimated that 1% to 5% of newborns experience some disturbance in heart rate or rhythm. Most of these disturbances are transient and benign, rarely requiring treatment. Supraventricular tachycardia (SVT) is the most common form of symptomatic rhythm disturbance seen in the newborn period (Page & Hosking, 1997).

Assessment

When caring for children with the potential for cardiac dysrhythmias, the nurse must first identify children at risk. Once a rhythm disturbance occurs, there is a need to identify the dysrhythmia and evaluate the clinical significance of the dysrhythmia. When evaluating the clini-

Chart 15–15

Underlying Causes of Dysrhythmias

Hypovolemia
Hypoxia
Fever
Hypothermia
Gastric dilatation
Metabolic and electrolyte disturbances: acidosis, K, Mg, Ca
Intracardiac monitoring lines
Chest trauma
Sympathetic catecholamine discharge from pain, anxiety, fear
Central nervous system diseases
Drug toxicity
Primary congenital cardiac arrhythmia
Newborn maternal disease (diabetes, toxemia)
Arrhythmogenic medications (including antiarrhythmic medications with pro-arrhythmic effects)

cal significance of a dysrhythmia, the nurse should assess the blood pressure, urine output, peripheral pulses, toe temperature, skin color, capillary refill, and level of consciousness. Dysrhythmias require prompt treatment if they affect cardiac output. The nurse should continuously assess and monitor the child's response to the dysrhythmia and treatments. Nursing care includes ruling out potential precipitating events and considering underlying causes before intervening (Chart 15–16).

Diagnostic Tests. Irregularities in cardiac rhythms can be documented and diagnosed through continuous ECG monitors, 12-lead ECG, Holter monitors, transesophageal probes, and electrophysiology studies (EPS), described earlier in this chapter. Despite all these diagnostic tools and treatments, it remains important for the nurse to integrate the needs of the child at the appropriate developmental level.

Interdisciplinary Interventions

The therapies available for children with recurring arrhythmias include pharmacologic management and suppression, ablative therapy, implantable antiarrhythmia devices, cardioversion, and pacemakers. Utilization of specific tools depends on the needs of each patient. Ablation therapy and pacemakers are discussed in the Treatment Modalities section of this chapter.

Pharmacologic management and suppression make up the simplest approach to controlling arrhythmias. Drawbacks include noncompliance with the medication

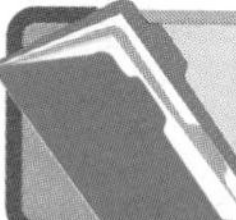

Chart 15–16
Nursing Interventions Classification (NIC)

Dysrhythmia Management

Definition

Preventing, recognizing, and facilitating treatment of abnormal cardiac rhythms

Activities

Ascertain patient and family history of heart disease and dysrhythmias.
Monitor for and correct oxygen deficits, acid-base imbalances, and electrolyte imbalances, which may precipitate dysrhythmias.
Apply EKG electrodes and connect to a cardiac monitor.
Set alarm parameters on the EKG monitor.
Ensure ongoing monitoring of bedside EKG by qualified individuals.
Monitor EKG changes that increase risk of dysrhythmia development: prolonged QT interval, frequent premature ventricular contractions, and ectopy close to the T wave.
Facilitate acquisition of a 12-lead EKG, as appropriate.
Note activities associated with the onset of dysrhythmias.
Note frequency and duration of dysrhythmia.
Monitor hemodynamic response to the dysrhythmia.
Determine whether patient has chest pain or syncope associated with the dysrhythmia.
Ensure ready access of emergency dysrhythmia medications.
Initiate and maintain IV access, as appropriate.
Administer Advanced Cardiac Life Support, as indicated.
Administer prescribed IV fluids and vasoconstrictor agents, as indicated, to facilitate tissue perfusion.
Assist with insertion of temporary transvenous or external pacemaker, as appropriate.
Teach patient and family the risks associated with the dysrhythmia(s).
Prepare patient and family for diagnostic studies (e.g., cardiac catheterization or electrical physiological studies).
Assist patient and family in understanding treatment options.
Teach patient and family about actions and side effects of prescribed medications.
Teach patient and family self-care behaviors associated with use of permanent pacemakers and AICD devices, as indicated.
Teach patient and family measures to decrease the risk of recurrence of the dysrhythmias.
Teach patient and family how to access the emergency medical system.
Teach a family member CPR, as appropriate.

From McCloskey, J., & Bulechek, G. (1996). *Nursing interventions classification (NIC)* (2nd ed.). St. Louis: Mosby–Year Book. Reprinted with permission.

regimen, especially in the adolescent population, adverse side effects, and failure of the medications to control the arrhythmia. The availability of a variety of drugs and advancements in pharmacotherapeutics are overshadowed by the lack of information about long-term efficacy of using toxic antiarrhythmia medications in the growing child.

Arrhythmias have been managed through the implantation of devices such as an **automatic implantable cardiac defibrillator** (AICD) and pacemakers. AICDs are used in a select group of patients for whom ablation and medical management have not controlled the arrhythmia. These devices are expensive, implantation requires surgery, and follow-up is extensive. AICD is a system that senses the heart's rhythm and can provide defibrillation for ventricular tachycardia and ventricular fibrillation. The system consists of epicardial sensing leads attached to the heart to sense the rhythm, wire mesh patches on the epicardium for defibrillation, and a pulse generator placed in the abdominal cavity. AICD devices have limited usage in the pediatric population. Unmanageable ventricular tachyarrhythmias are not common in children, and the relative size of the device creates a space limitation for placement in small children. Even though current usage is low, there is a growing population of children surviving complex surgeries, so there may be a growing population of older children benefitting from the use of an AICD device (TIP 15–3).

Sinus Tachycardia. Sinus tachycardia is a rhythm disturbance that is normal in configuration but with a rate that is faster than the acceptable parameters for the age of the child. It is not regarded as abnormal depending on the age and situation the child is in. A fussy or crying infant's heart rate may be situationally faster than normal

TIP 15–3 A Teaching Intervention Plan for the Child with an Automatic Implantable Cardiac Defibrillator: Discharge Instructions

Nursing Diagnosis and Family Outcomes

- Knowledge deficit: management of the child with an AICD at home

Outcomes:

Family/child will describe the activity restrictions for the child.

Family/child will participate in activities to promote safety and prevent harm to the child.

Family will identify symptoms of dysrhythmia and state actions to take if symptoms occur.

Treatment of the Child

Activity

- Avoid heavy lifting and "roughhousing" until the wound is completely healed (6 weeks).
- Always avoid any contact sport that may injure the pulse generator (e.g., karate, wrestling).
- Children may return to school after their first follow-up appointment, limiting gym and recess for 6 weeks.

Wound Care

Monitor the incision site for blood, drainage, redness or swelling at the incision.

Avoid strong magnetic fields

- Contact with strong magnets may inadvertently deactivate the device. Avoid strong magnetic fields (e.g., arc welders, large transformers, electrocautery, lithotripsy, radiation therapy, computed tomography scan, magnetic resonance imaging, airport security wands). In general, avoid construction sites and some hospital equipment. Also, avoid direct contact with an alternator of a large running motor, such as a car or boat.
- If you hear beeping sounds coming from your pulse generator, move away from the area. Also, do not place magnets close to your pulse generator.

Clothing

Wear loose, comfortable clothing around the waist to avoid irritating the pulse generator incision site.

Chart 15–17

Causes of Sinus Tachycardia

Congestive heart failure
Fever
Pain
Anxiety
Hypotension
Dehydration
Sepsis
Acidosis
Catecholamines
Drugs
Anemia

for the child's age but requires no medical intervention. Sinus tachycardia is commonly seen in children after cardiac surgery, in febrile children, and in dehydrated children (Chart 15–17). Medical treatment for sinus tachycardia is rarely necessary. Interventions are focused toward treatment of the underlying causes, because a fast heart rate is frequently a compensatory mechanism for some underlying problem.

Sinus Bradycardia. The conduction system in newborns is not completely matured, predisposing neonates to dysrhythmias. Sinus bradycardia is a rhythm that is normal in configuration but too slow for the age of the child. These episodes are most common in premature newborns. Bradycardia is more likely to occur during suctioning, feeding, or passing of a nasogastric tube because newborns are more susceptible to stimulation of the va-

TIP 15–3 A Teaching Intervention Plan for the Child with an Automatic Implantable Cardiac Defibrillator: Discharge Instructions *Continued*

Carrying Proper Identification

A Medic Alert bracelet should be considered in addition to the permanent ID card the child will receive from the AICD manufacturer. This ID can be used to explain that the AICD is an implanted device that may set off airport security systems.

Cardiopulmonary Resuscitation (CPR) Instruction

Family members should learn CPR and the importance of beginning CPR immediately. This can be beneficial for the patient as well as for any outside public emergency. Persons administering CPR may feel a slight buzz or tingling of the child's skin.

Shock Initiation

A child who receives a shock or has symptoms should record the event in a diary and report it to the physician. Information should include the number of shocks, symptoms before and after time of each shock, activity at time of shock, and action taken. Keep a record of audible beeping tones and report them.

Actions for Symptoms

Procedures to follow if symptoms of dysrhythmia occur (feel faint, dizzy, weak, black out, or have a rapid heart rate):

- Lie down or sit with back supported.
- Take a pulse to identify rhythm.
- Call for help if symptomatic.

Contact Health Care Provider if

- Child complains of dizziness or weakness.
- Child has rapid heart rate.
- Child has fainting spells.
- Child has fever.
- Incision site is red, swollen, or has drainage.

gus nerve (cranial nerve X). In the postoperative cardiac child, damage to the sinoatrial node can also induce sinus bradycardia. In children without cardiac disease, bradycardia may be a late sign of hemodynamic compromise and requires an immediate intervention. If left untreated, it may lead to death within a short period.

Supraventricular Tachycardia. A common significant irregularity of the heart that occurs in children is SVT. This rhythm occurs as a sudden burst of heart rate exceeding 200 without variations in the pulse rate. It may subside spontaneously. Cardiac output may be compromised by this rhythm. Once SVT is identified and documented with a 12-lead ECG and rhythm strip, the rhythm may be disrupted through nursing interventions called vagal maneuvers. Having the child gag, cough, or create the motion of holding one's breath as if to strain when having a bowel movement can sometimes disrupt the SVT rhythm. Also, mimicking the diving reflex by pressing an ice bag to the forehead may elicit this reflex, which slows the heart rate (Page & Hosking, 1997). If the child has a pacemaker, the rate can be increased to a rate much higher than the child's and overdrive pace the abnormal rhythm while decreasing the heart rate to normal. Another tool used to interrupt an SVT rhythm is cardioversion. **Cardioversion** is a controlled bolus of energy directed transthoracically to depolarize the cardiac cells and allow the heart to return to a normal sinus rhythm.

Medications used to control SVT include digitalis, propranolol (Inderal), verapamil, and amiodarone. Intravenous esmolol is a rapid and short-acting beta-blocker used to break SVT and has minimal side effects. SVT can occur in the postoperative cardiac surgery patient and is also one of the most common dysrhythmias that occurs in infants. Wolff-Parkinson-White syndrome (WPW) is one cause of SVT. In this syndrome, the heart has an accessory pathway providing a reentry mechanism for impulses. This creates atrial tachycardia. Most infants with WPW have a structurally normal heart; however, there are some associations with Ebstein's anomaly, tricuspid atresia, corrected transposition of the great vessels, and hypertrophic cardiomyopathy (Page & Hosking, 1997).

Nursing Responsibilities. The nurse provides teaching and emotional support to families, prepares children for procedures or testing, and monitors children during diagnostic testing and procedures. Parents have fears and anxiety when caring for a child with a dysrhythmia. These issues include concerns over the long-term requirements of drug therapy and their side effects. The nurse needs to routinely protect the child from injury during procedures, while also maintaining readiness for any necessary emergency support in case the child becomes hemodynamically compromised (Chart 15–18).

Cardiomyopathy

Cardiomyopathy is a myocardial disease in which the muscular pump is no longer effective, resulting in heart failure. The name *cardiomyopathy* is given to a disease that has multiple causes but that basically leads to the same clinical picture.

Etiology

For the vast majority of cases, the underlying impetus for development of cardiomyopathy is unknown. Because the causes of cardiomyopathy are not fully understood, preventive education cannot be provided. Such types of cardiomyopathy are referred to as **primary** or idiopathic, because there is no known insult such as a virus or a metabolic disorder that caused the heart muscle to fail.

The origin of **secondary** cardiomyopathy, or cardiomyopathy from a known cause, can vary. A history of exposure to toxins, including cancer therapy with chemotherapeutic agents like doxorubicin (Adriamycin), has been known to induce cardiomyopathy. Some children present after an infection, in acute heart failure. Acquired immunodeficiency syndrome (AIDS) has also been associated with cardiomyopathy. Coronary artery diseases such as Kawasaki disease can lead to heart failure. Other possible causes include nutritional diseases, glycogen storage diseases, systemic connective tissue diseases, tumors of the heart, and chronic supraventricular tachycardia (SVT) (McCance & Huether, 1994).

The functional classifications of cardiomyopathy in children are dilated, hypertrophic, and restrictive. These classifications are based not on the causes of failure, but on the mechanism of heart failure, which can be systolic impairment or compliance abnormalities.

Dilated cardiomyopathy is also called congestive cardiomyopathy. It is characterized by cardiac dilation and enlargement of all four chambers with progressive deterioration of cardiac output and CHF. The decreased stroke volume and decreased cardiac output lead to systemic and pulmonary congestion, which are compensated for by increased heart rate, increased sympathetic stimulation, and dilated chambers.

Medical management includes diuretics such as furosemide (Lasix) to help decrease preload and digoxin to treat CHF. Therapies to decrease afterload, such as captopril or hydralazine, are also used.

Hypertrophic cardiomyopathy is a form of cardiomyopathy that causes impairment of ventricular filling from gross ventricular hypertrophy. This thickening of the ventricular wall narrows the ventricular cavity, restricting its ability to fill and causing abnormal stiffness of the left ventricle.

This form of cardiomyopathy can occur but is rarely seen in infants. It is usually noted in adolescence and

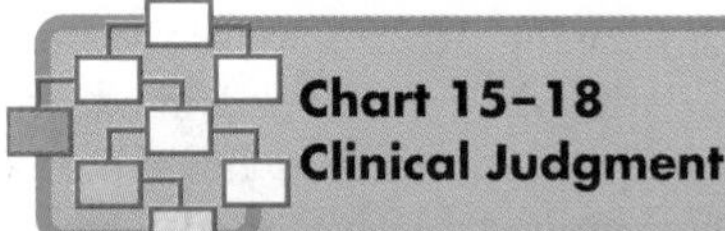

Chart 15–18
Clinical Judgment

A Child with Alterations in Cardiovascular Status

Rick is a 14-year-old male admitted to the emergency room after passing out while playing basketball with his brother in their backyard. He has a permanent cardiac pacemaker that was inserted 5 years ago. Now Rick is awake and complaining about having to go to the hospital. His mother states he has been easily fatigued lately.

Questions

1. During your assessment, what other information would you elicit about Rick's present illness?
2. What are reasons for syncope in a child with a permanent pacemaker?
3. What would be your initial intervention?
4. What information might be gained by placing the patient on the cardiac monitor?
5. If he is currently hemodynamically stable and his rhythm on the monitor is normal, what further action is required?

Answers

1. What is his underlying cardiac problem? When was his last cardiac follow-up appointment? Does he take any antiarrhythmic medications? Did he miss any dosages? What are his previous cardiac surgeries? Is this his first episode of syncope? What are his pacemaker settings? What are his heart rate and blood pressure?
2. It is important to make sure Rick has been seen recently for a checkup, because the pacemaker battery is 5 years old and it may have reached its limits. He could be having an arrhythmia that is abnormal and faster than the pacemaker settings. He could have a cracked pacing lead causing the pacemaker to malfunction. If he is taking antiarrhythmic medications to suppress a tachyarrhythmia and has been noncompliant in taking the medications, he could have a breakthrough arrhythmia.
3. Place Rick on the cardiac monitor to see what his current heart rhythm is.
4. This will depend on the reason for his syncope. Information gained from a basic ECG will simply let you know if he is currently using his pacemaker and if his rhythm is normal at this time. It is also possible that his syncope was caused by a rhythm disturbance that occurred on exertion when playing basketball.
5. His cardiologist should be notified of his admission to the emergency room. The patient should be referred to his pacemaker clinic and placed on a 24-hour Holter monitor to see what his heart rhythm is over this period of time. Also, if there was a lapse in taking his medications, teaching and behavior modification efforts should be used.

early adulthood after symptoms begin to express themselves. It is believed that hypertrophic cardiomyopathy is often genetically transmitted.

Beta-blockers, such as propranolol (Inderal), are administered to decrease outflow tract obstruction and minimize arrhythmias. Calcium channel blockers, such as verapamil or nifedipine, may be used to improve diastolic filling. Surgical removal of excessive obstructive heart tissue is done in severely obstructed cases.

Restrictive cardiomyopathy is the least common form of cardiomyopathy and involves impaired diastolic ventricular filling related to excessive stiffness of the ventricular walls. Despite poor filling, contractile function is normal in these patients. Secondary factors that can cause restrictive cardiomyopathy include glycogen deposits, neoplastic infiltrates, and iron deposits. Interventions include diuretics, but not digoxin, because systolic function is adequate. Steroids are administered to patients with known inflammatory disease.

Prognosis. In general, the prognosis is poor. The clinical course of patients varies. Death can be sudden (presumably from a lethal arrhythmia) or progressive with slow deterioration of heart function and worsening symptoms of CHF. Yet, other children with the diagnosis of cardiomyopathy can have cardiac function that remains stationary for many years and can live a relatively active life (Friedman, Moak, & Garson, 1991).

Assessment

Children present with a murmur or signs and symptoms of CHF such as hepatomegaly (enlarged liver), tachycardia, jugular venous distention, fatigue, dyspnea on exertion, and orthopnea (difficulty breathing while lying down).

The chest roentgenography shows four-chamber enlargement and pulmonary congestion. This pulmonary congestion can lead to pulmonary hypertension and possible pleural effusions. As heart function worsens, the likelihood of arrhythmias increases. Common initial symptoms include shortness of breath, dyspnea on exertion, paroxysmal nocturnal dyspnea, peripheral edema, and history of syncope or palpitation. An echocardiogram is the main diagnostic tool, which diagnoses as well as monitors changes in the size of the heart walls and cardiac output.

Interdisciplinary Interventions

If a specific reason for the child to have cardiomyopathy can be found (such as a carotene deficiency), some of these children can benefit from interventions directed specifically to treat the origin of the illness. Otherwise, management is aimed at extending the length and improving quality of life for the child by minimizing symptoms and complications. Medications given vary somewhat depending on the type of cardiomyopathy.

These children are at risk for clot formation and benefit from anticoagulant medications such as aspirin or warfarin (Coumadin). Myocardial biopsy is done when cardiomyopathy is suspected. It can be useful to rule out some of the causes of cardiomyopathy but generally does not add to the treatment plan.

Activity restriction or bed rest is recommended to reduce the workload on the heart. As children become ill, fatigue is the limiting factor on activities. As heart functions worsen, children are subjected to increasing frequency of hospital admissions for inotropic support such as intravenous dobutamine.

One of the more complicated features of caring for a child with cardiomyopathy is determining the proper timing for a heart transplant. It is a tragedy for a child to die prematurely when survival with transplantation was a wanted and viable option. Yet the practitioner does not want to prematurely recommend transplantation for a child who could have maintained a relatively decent quality of life with cardiomyopathy.

Caretakers should provide emotional support and strategic management of activities that are enjoyable to a child yet do not overtax the heart. When increasing activity is a drain on energy reserves, appetites tend to decrease as well. Nutritional consultation and encouraging families to bring in favorite foods that are nutritionally balanced can be beneficial.

Dyslipidemia

Dyslipidemia, formally known as hyperlipidemia, is an abnormal level of blood lipids and lipoproteins. There is an apparent association between high-fat diets, elevated serum cholesterol levels, and adult atherosclerosis. Individuals with abnormal lipid profiles in childhood have a much greater chance of developing atherosclerotic vessel disease in adulthood. Educational promotions aimed at reducing serum cholesterol levels in children have been made in the hopes of establishing good childhood health habits that will extend into adulthood and reduce adult atherosclerotic disease.

Pathophysiology

Cells require cholesterol in order to survive. Cholesterol allows the synthesis of cellular membranes and steroid production to occur. Because the body has the ability to produce cholesterol, it is impossible to completely remove cholesterol through diet restriction.

Lipoproteins are protein-coated packages that carry cholesterol and fat in the blood. When obtaining a fasting lipid profile, results include total cholesterol, total triglycerides, high-density lipoprotein (HDL) cholesterol, and low-density lipoprotein (LDL) cholesterol. LDL levels are not drawn but can be calculated based on the three other components drawn. Plasma lipids are separated via a centrifuge and are grouped based on size and density.

For **LDL cholesterol**, a value of less than 130 mg/dL is a desirable level. LDL cholesterol is the main transporter in the plasma of cholesterol to cells and is synthesized in the liver. Because LDL deposits cholesterol on the artery walls, promoting atherosclerosis, it is considered an undesirable cholesterol. Individuals with high levels of LDL cholesterol are at higher risk for the development of coronary heart disease.

For **HDL cholesterol**, a value of more than 45 mg/dL is desirable. HDL cholesterol transports cholesterol from the blood stream to the liver for secretion in the bile. It is the most dense lipoprotein because it contains the least amount of fat and the greatest amount of protein. Higher levels of HDL are considered to shield against vessel disease.

Triglycerides are compounds of fatty acids synthesized from carbohydrates and are the main storage fuel for energy. Triglycerides are carried on **very-low-density lipoprotein** (VLDL) molecules.

Desirable total cholesterol levels are less than 200 mg/dL (Schell, 1990). More important than the total cholesterol levels is the ratio of HDL to LDL cholesterol. The total cholesterol to HDL ratios in children should be less than 3.5 (Baker, Roberts, & Gothing, 1995).

There are three forms of lipoprotein abnormalities: genetic, disease related, and environmental. Genetic causes of elevated lipoproteins are the primary form of the disease. Children from families in which there is a known family history of dyslipidemia or premature death from atherosclerotic heart disease should be tested early with a lipid screen. Parents with a background of familial lipid diseases have a 50% chance of passing it on to their children (Baker et al., 1995).

There are several genetic disorders in children that lead to dyslipidemia. In familial **hypercholesterolemia,** there is faulty gene coding of LDL receptors causing ineffective LDL clearance and resulting in elevated plasma levels. It is a rare genetic disease that does not respond well to treatment and causes young children to develop coronary artery disease. In children, **hypertriglyceridemia** causes elevated triglyceride levels and, frequently, low HDL values. Another genetic disorder of lipids is familial **hypoalphalipoproteinemia,** which causes low HDL values. These children are at risk for developing early heart disease, especially if early interventions are not taken.

In childhood, some of the secondary disease-related causes of dyslipidemia are diabetes mellitus, hypertension, hypothyroidism, liver disease, and nephrotic syndrome. In infancy, dyslipidemia is usually related to glycogen storage diseases or congenital biliary atresia (Baker, et al., 1995; Gerchufsky, 1996). Secondary environmental causes of dyslipidemia include obesity, inactivity, smoking, steroids, oral contraceptives, and, especially, a diet high in cholesterol and fats.

Assessment

In the majority of individuals, atherosclerosis, or hardening of the arteries, is not diagnosed until adulthood when they are already symptomatic and have substantial disease present. It can be assumed that this disease develops slowly throughout life, starting in childhood, and may be well under way by adolescence. Screening is recommended for children and adolescents whose parents or grandparents, at age 55 or younger, had coronary atherosclerosis, a myocardial infarction, angina pectoris, peripheral vascular disease, cerebrovascular disease, or sudden cardiac death. In addition, a child whose parent has high blood cholesterol (240 mg/dL or higher) should be screened (Gerchufsky, 1996).

Interdisciplinary Interventions

Modification of risk factors is the goal for all children with dyslipidemia. Because there have been no lifelong studies showing the results of childhood preventive measures to lower cholesterol levels, it can only be assumed that early treatment can minimize the risk of developing coronary artery disease as an adult. Cholesterol testing for children should be done if there is a family history of dyslipidemia or if any risk factors such as obesity or secondary diseases known to be associated with increased lipids are present.

Community Care

Children at risk for, or with, dyslipidemia can benefit from counseling by a registered dietitian. A dietary plan can be outlined and follow-up care can be provided over many months. Adult studies show that controlling dietary intake to reduce saturated fats and cholesterol can reduce total cholesterol levels (Baker et al., 1995). Nutritional education includes teaching about a diet low in total fat, cholesterol, and saturated fat. It is also imperative to educate mothers of children younger than age 2 years that they should not restrict their child's dietary intake of fat because it is essential for normal development, especially myelination of the nervous system.

Obesity education focuses on achieving a proper weight ratio for height, age, and body structure. Obese children tend to come from obese families. In those cases, behavior modification and education have to meet the needs of the family as a whole. If an obese child is living in a family of normal weight individuals, there may be an emotional component to overeating habits, and those problems as well as dietary adjustments should be addressed. Nutritional education has to stress the permanency of changing habits for a lifetime.

The current culture of our society popularizes sedentary activities such as television and computers or video games. Maintenance of cardiovascular fitness requires regular physical activity. It may be helpful for a family to document hours participating in sedentary activities as compared with physical activities to increase awareness.

Smoking habits generally begin in the adolescent years. If a teenager is diagnosed with dyslipidemia and the parents deny the child's usage of oral contraceptives or cigarettes, the child should be counseled separately. The nurse should expect some parents to be naive as to their child's activities. Preemptive education of children can help alleviate the potential problem of smoking.

If diet therapy and exercise alone are not successful in controlling resistant cholesterol levels, drug therapies are administered judiciously. Two bile acid–binding resins, cholestyramine resin and colestipol, are the recommended drugs for pediatric patients. They work by binding bile acids in the intestines; they are excreted in the feces and therefore are not absorbed systematically. Occasionally, niacin is taken alone or as adjunct therapy with resin binders. High doses of niacin suppress production of LDL cholesterol by the liver. Liver function tests should be ordered routinely while taking niacin because it can cause hepatic inflammation.

Through behavior modification, most individuals are able to regulate their blood cholesterol levels. Nurses must develop a thorough understanding of dyslipidemia, risk factors, and preventive care. Cholesterol awareness and education is an important teaching tool in all aspects of nursing care.

Bacterial/Infective Endocarditis

Some children with heart defects may develop a serious infection of the endocardial surface of the heart called endocarditis. It is theorized that bacteremia induced in the blood stream is more likely to lodge as a complication of having CHD or, in the rare case of a child with Kawasaki disease or rheumatic heart disease, with valve dysfunction. This occurs because these children have areas in their heart with abnormal flow, turbulence, or artificial materials. Bacterial endocarditis can also occur in a child without any heart disease. Children at greatest risk for endocarditis are those with prosthetic valves (Freed, 1992). Other children at risk include any with a previous history of bacterial endocarditis, most cardiac defects, or cardiomyopathy (Dajani et al., 1991).

Pathophysiology

Infectious organisms that are most likely to be found in a positive blood culture, in the presence of endocarditis, are *Candida*, *Staphylococcus aureus*, and *Streptococcus* (Freed, 1992; Zales & Wright, 1997). Bacteria causing endocarditis are introduced into the blood stream by procedures that cause damage to mucosal surfaces or contaminated tissue. Germs may enter the blood stream from the mouth after dental office procedures or after an infection in the throat, ears, or chest. Intestinal, urinary tract, and vaginal procedures or surgeries also are events that put the patient at increased risk for bacterial endocarditis. The wave of improvement in cardiac surgical repair techniques, having pediatric conditions repaired at an earlier age, and giving prophylactic antibiotics have improved outcomes for patients at risk for bacterial endocarditis.

Assessment

Signs and symptoms of endocarditis can be elusive. The practitioner relies on a high index of suspicion in diagnosing infective endocarditis. Symptoms might include fever, decreased activity level, new or changes in a murmur, and neurologic symptoms such as seizures. Laboratory values showing a decrease in hemoglobin, increased sedimentation rate, and hematuria can help in making the diagnosis. Skin changes such as petechiae (minute hemorrhages from fragile capillaries) are rare in children and are probably caused by microemboli.

Diagnostic Tests. When endocarditis is suspected, a definitive diagnosis is achieved through blood cultures drawn from two separate places. A negative blood culture does not rule out the existence of endocarditis, it just indicates a lesser likelihood of its existence.

Routine chest x-rays, echocardiography, and transesophageal echocardiography are tools used to aid in the diagnosis of endocarditis by locating vegetation within the heart. This is an area where growth of infection on tissue may be seen. If no vegetation is found, this does not rule out endocarditis (Bisno et al., 1989; Zales & Wright, 1997).

Interdisciplinary Interventions

If the diagnosis of bacterial endocarditis is suspected, antibiotics are administered after blood cultures are drawn. Antibiotic selection is based on culture and sensitivity results. Antibiotics are administered continually over a 4- to 6-week period. The most effective and economically sound treatment of endocarditis is preventive therapy with antibiotics. The American Heart Association recommendations include oral amoxicillin for prophylaxis with routine dental office work and upper respiratory tract procedures. Clindamycin or erythromycin is taken if the patient is unable to take amoxicillin. These antibiotics are recommended to be taken 1 hour before a procedure, with a follow-up dose given 6 hours after (Blake, 1995; Zales & Wright, 1997).

Prevention of endocarditis is important. Parents should be taught the importance of notifying any physician or dentist caring for their child that he or she should be treated with prophylactic antibiotics for any procedures. The American Heart Association produces several patient education pamphlets with complete guidelines that can be useful to give to patients who are at risk for endocarditis. Nurses should be proactive in counseling those parents whose children could benefit from prophylactic antibiotics and teach parents the signs and symptoms of bacterial endocarditis.

Kawasaki Disease

This disease was first described by Kawasaki in 1967 as mucocutaneous lymph node syndrome (Fujita et al., 1989). Kawasaki disease is an acute, usually self-limiting multiple organ system disease of childhood that occurs both epidemically and endemically worldwide. The etiology of the disease is unknown but may involve an infectious agent. Kawasaki disease occurs most frequently in Japan and in children of Japanese heritage. Black children are at intermediate risk, and Caucasian children are at lowest risk (Shreve, 1993). Kawasaki disease most commonly occurs in winter and spring and most often affects children younger than 5 years of age, with the peak incidence occurring between 6 months and 2 years. Kawasaki disease is more common in males than females, with a ratio of 1.6:1 (Wartmann, 1992).

The importance of Kawasaki disease relates to the fact that approximately 20% of children develop coronary artery abnormalities, which in some children lead to ischemia, myocardial infarction, and death. Kawasaki disease has become a leading cause of acquired heart disease in children. Therefore, follow-up care in community settings is an important piece in the continuum of pediatric care for this disease.

Assessment

The diagnosis of Kawasaki disease is established on clinical grounds because no specific laboratory test exists (Pahl, 1997). The diagnosis of Kawasaki disease is confirmed if the child has been febrile for at least 5 days and demonstrates four of the remaining diagnostic features (Chart 15–19). Laboratory features associated with Kawasaki disease, but not diagnostic of it, may include a leukocyte count of more than 20,000 with left shift, an erythrocyte sedimentation rate (ESR) of 770, a platelet count of more than 800,000, the presence of circulating immune complexes, and pyuria with sterile urine (Fujita et al., 1989).

Kawasaki disease is generally regarded as a triphasic disease comprising acute, subacute, and convalescent stages. The acute phase (1 to 11 days) is characterized by progressive inflammation of the small vessels, and complications may include early arthritis, uveitis, meningitis, perivasculitis, myocarditis, pericarditis, mitral insufficiency, and congestive heart failure. During the subacute phase (11 to 21 days), inflammation of the medium sized muscular arteries leaves the patient at risk for coronary artery aneurysm and at greatest risk for serious cardiovascular complications, as well as late-onset arthritis, gallbladder hydrops, fingertip and toe desquamation, thrombocytosis, mitral insufficiency, and coronary artery thrombosis. The convalescent phase (21 to 60 days) is signaled as the walls of the vessels begin to heal inward. Complications of this phase may include the persistence of arthritis, aneurysms may persist, and long-term scarring may form in affected vessels. The children at greatest risk are infants and children with prolonged fever (Fujita et al., 1989).

Chart 15–19

Clinical Criteria for Kawasaki Disease

Fever that persists for more than 5 days
Bilateral conjunctivitis (without exudate)
Changes in the mucosa of the oral cavity, such as dry, cracked lips and tongue, a strawberry tongue, and diffuse reddening of the oral and pharyngeal mucosa
Changes in the extremities, such as edema of the hands and feet, reddening of the palms and soles, and membranous desquamation of the fingertips and toes
Erythematous rash (often in the perineal area)
Non-purulent swelling of cervical lymph nodes larger than 1.5 cm in diameter

Interdisciplinary Interventions

Children with Kawasaki disease may need hospitalization for diagnostic purposes, for medical indications, or for initiation of therapy. Joint pain may limit a child's mobility and may require comfort measures. Frequent oral care and a clear liquid diet is provided to minimize mucous membrane pain. Intravenous gamma globulin is administered during the acute phase to reduce the risk of coronary artery abnormalities. This therapy may be continued for 6 to 8 weeks. Initial treatment includes high-dose aspirin as an anti-inflammatory, and it is subsequently stopped if no coronary artery involvement develops (Wartmann, 1992). Aspirin may be continued indefinitely if there are coronary arterial abnormalities (Belkengren & Sapala, 1997). An echocardiogram is obtained at baseline and throughout the disease course and convalescence, at regular intervals, to monitor myocardial and coronary artery status.

Nursing care initially centers around observing for signs of congestive heart failure (increased respiratory rate, increased heart rate, dyspnea, rales, abdominal distention). Monitoring of children receiving IVIG is similar to that of any patient receiving a blood product, including frequent observation for signs of allergic reaction. Particularly while high-dose aspirin therapy is delivered, the nurse should be alert to signs and symptoms of bleeding caused by the anticoagulant effect of aspirin, such as tarry stools, excessive bruising, altered mental status, or excessive bleeding from the gums. Mobility should be assessed, and passive range of motion and elevation of affected limbs may be used if arthralgia develops.

Child life and volunteer services should be used to provide age-appropriate bed rest activities to minimize the child's activity and irritability. Efforts should be made to modify the environment to also reduce irritability; these modifications may include dim lighting and noise control.

Community Care

Discharge teaching focuses on follow-up, cardiopulmonary resuscitation (CPR) instruction if cardiac damage has occurred, and signs of congestive heart failure. Home care includes teaching of potential cardiac sequelae and compliance with therapy. The child should follow a low-cholesterol diet, and his or her temperature should be monitored for several days after the return home. The family should understand that the disease is not spread from person to person.

caREminder: *Live virus vaccine should not be administered for at least 5 months after gamma globulin therapy (Belkengren & Sapala, 1997).*

Other immunizations can be given at their scheduled times. To reduce the risk of Reye's syndrome (associated with the aspirin therapy), it is recommended the child have an influenza vaccine.

Families should be encouraged to obtain school work for the child to do at home and should facilitate the return to school when the child is cleared by the physician. The school nurse should be alerted to any limitation or follow-up necessary. All discharge instructions should be written down, so that they are available for future reference.

Follow-up visits during the first two months post-hospitalization will occur frequently. The child is assessed for cardiac dysrhythmias, heart failure, valvular problems, and myocarditis. Serial ECGs and echocardiograms will be used to assess for these conditions. All other symptoms of Kawasaki disease are self-limiting and will resolve within 6 to 8 weeks (Belkengren & Sapala, 1997).

Acute Rheumatic Fever

Acute rheumatic fever (ARF) is a sequela of group A beta-hemolytic streptococcal respiratory infections. It is a multi-system disorder that may involve the heart, joints, central nervous system, and the skin. A latency period of about 20 days intervenes between a reported incidence of pharyngitis and the onset of symptoms of ARF. During the latency period, patients are asymptomatic.

The incidence of rheumatic fever in the United States has dramatically decreased over the past 50 years. Improved socioeconomic conditions in the United States have played a major factor in reducing the incidence of this disease. Additionally, the aggressive treatment of streptococcal pharyngitis with antibiotics and the initiation of long-term prophylactic therapy for those children who have had a prior episode of rheumatic fever have contributed to the reduction in incidence and severity.

Worldview: *ARF remains prevalent in socially and economically deprived population groups in which widespread poverty and overcrowding exist. Children should be considered at risk if their living situation is characterized by poor sanitation practices and crowding. When the child presents with a cold or any of the clinical manifestations noted in the Jones criteria (discussed later), the current or past presence of a streptococcal infection should be determined.*

The increased incidence of streptococcal infections in fall, winter, and early spring is associated with an increased incidence of ARF at these same time periods. Children age 5 to 15 years are more susceptible to group A streptococcal infections and therefore are also more susceptible to ARF. However, the condition has also been noted in older age groups where close personal quarters are maintained (i.e., the military services) (Todd, 1996). The disease is slightly more common in girls than in boys and is now more common in blacks than in other ethnic groups.

Recent outbreaks of rheumatic fever have not led to an overall increase in the incidence rate. In contrast to previous outbreaks in which overcrowding and poor sanitation were important predisposing conditions, the new outbreaks have occurred in middle-income and rural populations in which adverse social economic conditions could not be implicated. Investigators have speculated that virulence factors associated with group A beta-hemolytic streptococcus may have played a greater role in these incidents.

Pathophysiology

Group A beta-hemolytic streptococcal infection of the respiratory tract is the essential environmental trigger that acts on predisposed individuals. Host susceptibility implicates immune response (IR) genes, which are present in approximately 15% of the population. The immune response triggered by colonization of the pharynx with group A streptococci consists of

- Sensitization of B lymphocytes by streptococci antigens
- Formation of immune complexes that cross-react with cardiac sarcolemma antigens
- Myocardial and valvular inflammatory response

Prognosis. Acute rheumatic fever is rarely fatal. Arthritic symptomatology and chorea subside over several months. Mortality and permanent effects are primarily due to cardiac involvement.

Assessment

The diagnosis of ARF is made by clinical diagnosis, lacking a single laboratory test. The Jones criteria remain the guideline in establishing the diagnosis of ARF (Chart 15–20). Traditionally, two major, or one major and two minor, criteria (plus supporting evidence of streptococcal infection) justified the diagnosis of rheumatic fever. However, physical findings may be so subtle and transient that the child's symptoms are marginal with respect to the standards of the criteria. If rheumatic fever appears likely on the basis of appropriate evaluation but does not fully meet the revised Jones criteria, a diagnosis of sus-

Chart 15–20

Jones Criteria (Revised)

Major Manifestations

- Carditis
- Polyarthritis (two or more joints with heat, pain, redness, and tenderness and swelling)
- Sydenham's chorea
- Erythema marginatum (macular erythematous rash with a circinate border on trunk and extremities)
- Subcutaneous nodules (non-tender, movable on scalp, over joints, and spinal column)

Minor Manifestations

- Polyarthralgia (pain in two or more joints without heat, swelling, and tenderness)
- Fever (low-grade)
- Previous rheumatic or heart disease

Acute Phase

- Elevated erythrocyte sedimentation rate (ESR)
- C-reactive protein
- Leukocytosis
- Prolonged P-R interval on ECG

pected ARF is appropriate, owing to the serious consequences of missing the diagnosis.

The most serious manifestation of ARF is carditis. It is the only manifestation that can cause mortality during the acute stage of the illness or that may result in long-term sequelae. Rheumatic carditis affects the endocardium and the pericardium. Overall, endocarditis is the most significant manifestation, because it is the only finding that results in residual chronic cardiac disease. There are four main clinical signs of acute rheumatic carditis:

- Regurgitant murmur
- Cardiomegaly
- Congestive heart failure
- Pericardial friction rubs

The absence of a murmur makes the diagnosis of rheumatic carditis unlikely. Patients should be carefully and frequently examined for the presence of a new murmur. The most common murmur is one of mitral regurgitation and generally occurs early in the acute attack. The murmur is holosystolic, is heard best at apex, and radiates to the left axilla. The murmur also has a high-pitched, blowing quality, is unchanged by position, and has an intensity of two or greater on a scale of six.

The chorea of ARF (Sydenham's chorea, chorea minor, St. Vitus' dance) indicates involvement of the central nervous system by the rheumatic process. The latency period for chorea is from 1 to 6 months after an upper respiratory infection. Chorea is characterized by purposeless, involuntary movements, emotional lability, and muscular incoordination. The onset of the disease is usually insidious. Initially, the child is more clumsy than usual and may have a shortened attention span, which may lead to school-related problems.

Interdisciplinary Interventions

Treatment of ARF should match the manifestations and severity of the attack. A definitive diagnosis is essential before aspirin or corticosteroids are administered, as these anti-inflammatory agents can mask other diagnoses, such as septic arthritis. Supportive management of carditis includes inotropic agents, diuretics, vasodilators, and, occasionally, corticosteroids. Chorea is treated in a quiet environment with sedatives and minor tranquilizers, as required.

Community Care

Prevention must be a priority for all health care professionals working with pediatric patients. All children older than 3 years of age with the symptoms of fever and sore throat should be cultured for streptococcus, and those with positive cultures should be treated with penicillin. The nurse can include this preventive teaching in anticipatory guidance discussions starting with preschool, stressing the importance of contacting the physician for sore throat and/or fever lasting for 24 hours, or rash. Also, the nurse can mention the importance of notifying the physician of contact when another child with strep throat is in school. Most schools send notification of contact with such illnesses home to the parents.

Asplenia

Asplenia is a congenital absence of the spleen and occurs in conjunction with complex uncorrectable congenital heart disease. It is an immunodeficiency syndrome that is also called Ivemark's syndrome. These children are at high risk for severe infections. Clinical examination shows an abdominal roentgenogram with the liver lying midline and a blood smear with the presence of Howell-Jolly bodies. This blood test identifies remnants of RNA, which tells the practitioner that there is no spleen activity. Children with asplenia take daily doses of amoxicillin throughout their lives as prophylaxis against systemic bacterial infection. Children with complicated cardiac anomalies can also have polysplenia. This occurs when multiple splenic tissue exists (Phoon & Neill, 1994).

Summary of Key Concepts

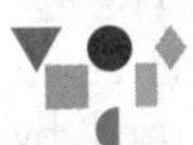

- Prenatal factors that predispose a newborn to heart disease can be genetic, environmental, maternal, or multifactorial.
- Symptoms that may indicate a cardiovascular dysfunction are poor weight gain, feeding difficulties, sweating with feeding, frequent respiratory infections, activity intolerance, tachycardia, and cyanosis.
- A variety of tests are used to assess cardiac function, including electrocardiography, radiography, echocardiography, and cardiac catheterization techniques.
- Nursing care responsibilities for the child after cardiac catheterization include monitoring the insertion site for bleeding and assessing perfusion of the extremity that is distal to the puncture site.
- Clinical manifestation of CHF includes cardiomegaly, tachycardia, tachypnea, gallop rhythm, decreased urine output and edema, decreased peripheral pulses and mottling of the extremities, sweating, hepatomegaly, failure to thrive, feeding difficulties, and decreased exercise intolerance.
- Digoxin (Lanoxin) is administered to children with CHF to improve myocardial efficiency. In the acute care setting, the dose of digoxin should be checked by two nurses prior to administration to prevent dosing errors.
- Congenital heart defects can be divided into five main categories: acyanotic defects with increased pulmonary blood flow (PBF), acyanotic defects that obstruct flow from the ventricles, cyanotic defects with decreased PBF, cyanotic defects with increased PBF, and cyanotic defects with variable PBF.
- Cyanotic children should be kept well hydrated to avoid further increasing their blood viscosity.
- Although dysrhythmias are relatively uncommon in children, those more likely to occur include supraventricular tachycardia, tachycardia, and bradycardia.
- Heart transplantation may be the only option for children with cardiomyopathy or CHD with deteriorating cardiac function.
- A low-fat and low-cholesterol diet should be promoted in all children older than the age of 2 years.
- Prophylactic antibiotics are administered with dental or medical procedures to prevent bacterial endocarditis in many children with heart disease.
- Kawasaki disease is acute mucocutaneous lymph node syndrome, which can affect multiple organ systems. The most serious complication is cardiac involvement. Intravenous gamma globulin is administered in the acute phase to reduce the risk of coronary artery abnormalities.
- Rheumatic heart disease is thought to be caused by an autoimmune response from an episode of group A hemolytic streptococcal upper respiratory infections. Rheumatic fever can cause damage to heart valves and carditis.
- Asplenia is a congenital absence of the spleen that occurs in conjunction with complex, uncorrectable congenital heart disease.

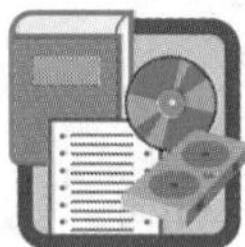

Resources

Organizations

American Association of Critical Care Nurses
101 Columbia
Aliso Viejo, CA 92656
(800) 899-2226
FAX: (714) 362-2020
Web: http://www.aacn.org

American Heart Association
7272 Greenville Avenue
Dallas, TX 75231-4586
(800) 242-8721
Web: http://www.amhrt.org

Association for Children with Down Syndrome
2616 Martin Avenue
Bellmore, NY 11710
(516) 221-4700

Congenital Heart Anomalies—Support, Education, Resources
2112 North Wilkins Road
Swanton, OH 43558

The Heartline Group, Inc.
229 Loving Court
Sewell, NJ 08080-3005

Mended Hearts Association
National Office
7320 Greenville Avenue
Dallas, TX 75231

National Cholesterol Education Program
NHLBI Information Center
P.O. Box 30105
Bethesda, MD 20824-0105

National Down Syndrome Society
666 Broadway
New York, NY 10012
(800) 221-4602

National Heart, Lung and Blood Institute Information Center
P.O. Box 30105
Bethesda, MD 20824-0105
(800) 757-9355

U.N.O.S. The United Network for Organ Sharing
1100 Boulder Parkway, Suite 500
P.O. Box 13770
Richmond, VA 23225

Books and Printed Materials

The Heart of a Child by Catherine Neill
Baltimore: Johns Hopkins Press
For families of children with heart defects and is available in book stores.

National Cholesterol Education Program
U.S. Department of Health & Human Services
Public Health Service—National Institutes of Health
National Heart, Lung and Blood Institute

Parent's Guide:
Cholesterol in Children—Healthy Eating is a Family Affair (NIH Publication No. 92-3099, Nov. 1992)

✏ *7- to 10-Year-Olds:*
Eating With Your Heart in Mind (NIH Publication No. 92-3099, Sept. 1995)

✏ *11- to 14-Year-Olds:*
Heart Health ... Your Choice (NIH Publication No. 92-3101, Nov. 1992)

✏ *15- to 18-Year-Olds:*
Hearty Habits—Don't Eat Your Heart Out (NIH Publication No. 92-3102, Sept. 1993)

What is a Pediatric Cardiologist? (pamphlet)
American College of Cardiology
Old Georgetown Road
Bethesda, MD 20814-1699

American Heart Association National Center (or local chapter)
7272 Greenville Avenue
Dallas, TX 75231-4596
Feeding Infants with Congenital Heart Disease

If Your Child Has a Congenital Heart Defect: A Guide for Parents

Abnormalities of Heart Rhythm: A Guide for Parents

You, Your Child and Rheumatic Fever

Dental Care for Children with Heart Disease

✏ Children's Help Your Heart Cookbook

Kawasaki Disease—An Explanation

Caring For A Child With A Heart Condition: A Guide for Parents
American Heart Association, San Francisco Chapter
120 Montgomery, Suite 1650
San Francisco, CA 94104

Henrietta Egleston Hospital for Children
Cardiology Department
Atlanta, GA

✏ Your Heart Test

✏ So You are Going to Have a Heart Cath (coloring books)

Association for the Care of Children's Health
3615 Wisconsin Avenue, N.W.
Washington, DC 20016

✏ A Child Goes to the Hospital

✏ About Your Heart Test (coloring book)

✏ About the ICU (coloring book)

Preparing Your Child for Extended or Repeated Hospitalizations

Kushner, H. (1981). *When Bad Things Happen to Good People*. New York: Avon Books.
Religious and ethical view on life's losses.

✏ Resources specifically for children.

References

Allen, L. (1990). Echocardiographic detection of congenital heart disease in the fetus: Present and future. *British Heart Journal, 74*(2), 103–106.

Alyn, I., & Baker, L. (1992). Cardiovascular anatomy and physiology of the fetus, neonate, infant, child, and adolescent. *Journal of Cardiovascular Nursing,* 6(3), 1–11.

Ardinger, R. (1997). Genetic counseling in congenital heart disease. *Pediatric Annals,* 26(2), 99–104.

Bailey, L., & Gundry, S. (1990). Hypolpastic left heart syndrome. *Pediatric Clinics of North America, 37*(1), 137–149.

Baker, A., Roberts, C., & Gothing, C. (1995). Dyslipidemias in childhood. *Nursing Clinics of North America,* 30(2), 243–259.

Belkengren, R., Sapala, S. (1997). Pediatric management problems: Kawasaki disease. *Pediatric Nursing, 23*(4), 404–405.

Bisno, A., Dismukes, W., Duraxck, D., Kaplan, D., Karchmar, A., Kaye, D., Rahimtoola, S., Sande, M., Sanford, J., Watanakunakorn, C., & Wilson, W. (1989). Antimicrobial treatment of infective endocarditis due to viridans streptococci, enterococci, and staphylococci. *JAMA, 261*(10), 1471–1477.

Blake, G. (1995). Combating infection: Managing antibiotic prophylaxis for dental and upper respiratory tract procedures. *Nursing 95, 25*(1), 18, 21.

Chiavarelli, M., Gundry, S. R., Razzouk, A., & Bailey, L. (1993). Cardiac transplantation for infants with hypoplastic left-heart syndrome. *JAMA, 270*(24), 2944–2947.

Dajani, A., Bisno, A., Kyung, C., Durack, D., Gerber, M., Kaplan, E., Millard, D., Randolph, M., Shulman, S., & Watanakunakorn, C. (1991). Prevention of bacterial endocarditis. *Circulation, 83,* 1174–1178.

Davis, J., & Small, B. (1995). Advances in the treatment of aortic stenosis across the lifespan. *Nursing Clinics of North America,* 30(2), 317–331.

Derek, F., & Kline, C. (1990). Fetal echocardiographic diagnosis of congenital heart disease. *Pediatric Clinics of North America, 37*(1), 45–67.

Freed, M. (1992). Infectious endocarditis in children. *Current Opinion in Pediatrics, 4,* 821–827.

Friedman, R., Moak, J., & Garson, A. (1991). Clinical course of idiopathic dilated cardiomyopathy in children. *Journal of American College of Cardiology, 18*(1), 152–155.

Fujita, Y., Nakamura, Y., Sakata, K., Hara, N., Kobayashi, M., Naga M., Yanagawa, H., & Kawasaki, T. (1989). Kawasaki disease in families. *Pediatrics, 84,* 666–669.

Gerchufsky, M. (1996). Lipid dilemmas in pediatrics. *Advance for Nurse Practitioners,* 4(12), 14–18, 21, 50.

Gessner, I. (1997). What makes a heart murmur innocent. *Pediatric Annals,* 26(2), 83–91.

Harris, M., & Valmorida, J. (1997). Neonates with congenital heart disease, Part III: Congenital cardiac defects with decreased pulmonary blood flow. *Neonatal Network, 16*(2), 59–63.

Hoffman, J. (1990). Congenital heart disease: Incidence and inheritance. *Pediatric Clinics of North America, 37*(1), 33–43.

Kidd, L. (1992). The history of the common forms of congenital heart disease including ventricular septal defect, pulmonary stenosis, and aortic stenosis. *Current Opinion in Pediatrics, 4,* 842–847.

Kirsten, D. (1996). Patent ductus arteriosus in the preterm infant. *Neonatal Network, 15*(2), 19–25.

Kohr, L., & O'Brien, P. (1995). Current management of congestive heart failure in infants and children. *Nursing Clinics of North America,* 30(2), 261–290.

Koster, N. (1994). Physical activity and congenital heart disease. *Nursing Clinics of North America,* 29(2), 345–56.

Krabill, K., Ring, S., Foker, J., Braunlin, E., Einzig, S., Berry, J., & Bass, J. (1987). Echocardiographic versus cardiac catheterization diagnosis of infants with congenital heart disease requiring cardiac surgery. *American Journal of Cardiology,* 60, 351–354.

McCance, K., & Huether, S. (1994). *Pathophysiology: The biologic basis for disease in adults and children* (2nd ed.). St. Louis: Mosby–Year Book.

McNamara, D. (1990). Value and limitations of auscultation in the management of congenital heart disease. *Pediatric Clinics of North America, 37*(1), 93–113.

Norwood, W. (1991). Hypoplastic heart syndrome. *Annals of Thoracic Surgery, 52,* 688–695.

Nouri, S. (1997). Congenital heart defects: Cyanotic and acyanotic. *Pediatric Annals,* 26(2), 92, 95–98.

Ohler, L., Fleagle, D., & Lee, B. (1989). Aortic valvuloplasty: Medical and critical care nursing perspectives. *Focus On Critical Care, 16*(4), 275–287.

Page, J., & Hosking, M. (1997). An approach to the neonate with sudden dysrhythmia: Diagnosis, mechanisms and management. *Neonatal Network, 16*(6), 7–18.

Pahl, E. (1997). Kawasaki disease: Cardiac sequelae and management. *Pediatric Annals,* 26(2), 112–115.

Palmisano, J., Martin, J., Krauzowicz, B., Truman, K., & Meliones, J. (1990). Effects of supplemental oxygen administration in an infant with pulmonary artery hypertension. *Heart and Lung, 19*(6), 627–630.

Park, M. (1996). *Pediatric cardiology handbook* (3rd ed.). St. Louis: Mosby–Year Book.

Phoon, C., & Neill, C. (1994). Asplenia syndrome—risk factors for early unfavorable outcome. *American Journal of Cardiology, 73,* 1235–1237.

Pinsky, W., & Arciniegas, E. (1990). Tetralogy of Fallot. *Pediatric Clinics of North America, 37*(1), 179–191.

Rykerson, S., Thompson, R., & Wessel, D. (1995). Inhalation of nitric oxide. *Nursing Clinics of North America,* 30(2), 381–389.

Sade, R., & Fyfe, D. (1990). Tricuspid atresia: Current concepts in diagnosis and treatment. *Pediatrics Clinics of North America, 37*(1), 151–166.

Samanek, M., Slavik, Z., Zborilova, B., Hrobonova, V., Vorisov, M., & Skovranek, J. (1989). Prevalence, treatment, and outcome of heart disease in live-born children: A prospective analysis of 91,823 live-born children. *Pediatric Cardiology, 10*(4), 205–211.

Sansoucie, D., & Cavaliere, T. (1997). Transition from fetal to extrauterine circulation. *Neonatal Network, 16*(2), 5–12.

Schell, M. (1990). Cholesterol, lipoproteins, lipid profiles: A challenge in patient education. *Focus on Critical Care, 17*(3), 203–211.

Shreve, B. (1993). Kawasaki disease: Early treatment/positive results—One family's story. *Pediatric Nursing, 19*(6), 607–610.

Smith, K. (1997). The innocent heart murmur in children. *Neonatal Network, 11*(5), 207–214.

Todd, J. (1996). Rheumatic fever. In R. Behrman, R. Kliegman, & A. Arvin (eds.), *Nelson textbook of pediatrics* (pp. 754–760). Philadelphia: WB Saunders.

Verklan, M. (1997). Diagnostic techniques in cardiac disorders: Part II. *Neonatal Network, 16*(5), 7–13.

Walsh, A., Morrow, D., & Jonas, R. (1995). Neurologic and developmental outcomes following pediatric cardiac surgery. *Nursing Clinics of North America, 30*(2), 347–363.

Warshaw, M., & Winn, C. (1988). Pulmonary valvuloplasty as an alternative to surgery in the pediatric patient: Implications for nursing. *Heart and Lung, 17*(5), 521–526.

Wartmann, D. D. (1992). Kawasaki syndrome. *Seminars in Dermatology, 116,* 37–47.

Werler, M. M., Mitchell, A. A., & Shapiro, S. (1989). The relation of aspirin use during the first trimester of pregnancy to congenital cardiac defects. *New England Journal of Medicine, 321,* 1639–1642.

Wolf, C. (1997). Cardiac embryology. *Neonatal Network, 16*(1), 43–49.

Wood, M. (1997). Acyanotic lesions with increased pulmonary blood flow. *Neonatal Network, 16*(3), 17–25.

Yeatman, S., Smith, J., Dunning, J., Large, S., & Wallwork, J. (1995). Cardiac transplantation: A review. *Cardiovascular Surgery, 3*(1), 1–14.

Yerby, A., & Hubbard, J. (1985). Cardiac pacemakers in children. *Critical Care Quarterly, 8*(3), 19–28.

Zales, V., & Wright, K. (1997). Endocarditis, pericarditis and myocarditis. *Pediatric Annals, 26*(2), 116–121.

Zita, J., & Roberts, P. (1995). Patient care for interventional cardiac catheterization. *Nursing Clinics of North America, 30*(2), 333–345.

Bibliography

Bando, K., Turrentine, M. W., Sun, K., Sharp, T. G., Ensing, G. J., Miller, A. P., Kesler, K. A., Binford, R. S., Carlos, G. N., Hurwitz, R. A., et al. (1995). Surgical management of complete atrioventricular septal defects. *Journal of Thoracic and Cardiovascular Surgery, 110*(5), 1543–1552.

Bell, P., & Diffee, G. (1991). Cardiopulmonary bypass. *AORN Journal, 33*(6), 1480–1496.

Brannon, P., & Johnson, R. (1992). The internal cardioverter defibrillator: Patient-family teaching. *Focus on Critical Care, 19*(1), 41–46.

Callow, L. (1989). A new beginning: Nursing care of the infant undergoing the arterial switch operation for transposition of the great arteries. *Heart and Lung, 18*(3), 238–255.

Callow, L. (1994). Nursing implications of interventional device placement in pediatric cardiology and pediatric cardiac surgery. *Critical Care Nursing Clinics of North America, 6*(1), 133–151.

Carpenter, K. (1993). A comprehensive review of cyanosis. *Critical Care Nurse, 13*(4), 66–72.

Castiglia, P. (1996). Kawasaki disease. *Journal of Pediatric Health Care, 10,* 124–126.

Cetta, F., Bell, T. J., Podlecki, D. D., & Ros, S. P. (1993). Parental knowledge of bacterial endocarditis prophylaxis. *Pediatric Cardiology, 14,* 220–222.

DiLucente, L., & Gorcsan, J. (1991). Transesophageal echocardiography, application to the postoperative cardiac surgery patient. *Dimensions of Critical Care Nursing, 12*(2), 74–80.

Douville, C., Sade, R., & Fyfe, D. (1991). Hemi-Fontan operation in surgery for single ventricle: A preliminary report. *Annals of Thoracic Surgery, 51,* 893–900.

Driscoll, D. (1990). Evaluation of the cyanotic newborn. *Pediatric Clinics of North America, 37*(1), 1–23.

Evans-Berro, E. (1991). How to defeat a "TET spell." *American Journal of Nursing, 91*(7), 46–48.

Finkelmeier, B. (1994). Ablative therapy in the treatment of tachyarrhythmias. *Critical Care Nursing Clinics of North America, 6*(1), 103–110.

Fyfe, D., & Kline, C. (1990). Fetal echocardiographic diagnosis of congenital heart disease. *Pediatric Clinics of North America, 37*(1), 45–67.

Garasen, A., Briden, T., & McNamara, D. (1990). *The science and practice of pediatric cardiology.* Philadelphia: Lea & Febiger.

Gersony, M. (1991). The child with dilated cardiomyopathy: Prognostic considerations and management decisions. *Journal of the American College of Cardiology, 18*(1), 152–154.

Human, D., McIntyre, L., Gniewek, A., & Hanna, B. D. (1995). Technology assessment of surgical closure of patent ductus arteriosus: An evaluation of the clinical effectiveness and costs of a new medical device. *Pediatrics,* 96(4), 703–706.

Jacobs, M., Rychik, J., Murphy, J., Nicolson, S., Steven, J., & Norwood, W. (1995). Results of Norwood's operation for lesions other than hypoplastic left heart syndrome. *Journal of Thoracic and Cardiovascular Surgery, 110*(5), 1555–1561.

Jensen, C. (1992). Nursing care of a child following an arterial switch procedure for transposition of the great arteries. *Critical Care Nurse, 12*(8), 51–57.

Johnston, J. (1991). A new beginning: Current trends in pediatric heart transplantation. *Focus on Critical Care, 18*(1), 23–28.

Kirklin, J., Colvin, E., McConnel, M., & Bargeron, L. (1990). Complete transposition of the great arteries: Transposition in the current era. *Pediatric Clinics of North America, 37*(1), 171–177.

Kothari, S. (1992). Mechanisms of cyanotic spells in tetralogy of Fallot—the missing link? *International Journal of Cardiology, 337,* 1–5.

Kulick, D., & Rahimtolla, S. (1991). Current role of digitalis therapy in patients with congestive heart failure. *JAMA, 265*(22), 2995–2997.

Moser, S., Crawford, D., & Thomas, A. (1993). Updated care guidelines for patients with automatic implantable cardioverter defibrillators. *Critical Care Nurse, 13*(2), 62–74.

Noonan, D., Koster, N., & White-Traut, R. (1991). Nursing considerations for the neonate awaiting heart transplantation for the hypoplastic left heart syndrome. *Journal of Pediatric Nursing, 6*(5), 322–330.

Norwood, W. (1992). Fontan procedure for hypoplastic left heart syndrome. *Annals of Thoracic Surgery, 54,* 1025–1030.

O'Brien, P., & Smith, P. (1994). Chronic hypoxemia in children with cyanotic heart defects. *Critical Care Nursing, 6*(1), 215–226.

Pennington, D., & Swartz, M. (1993). Circulatory support in infants and children. *Annals of Thoracic Surgery, 55*(1), 233–237.

Ritchie, J., Phillips, K., & Luft, H. (1993). Coronary angioplasty. Statewide experience in California. *Circulation,* 88(6), 2735–2743.

Starnes, V., Griffin, M., Pitlick, P., Bernstein, D., Baum, D., Ivens, K., & Shumway, N. (1992). Current approach to hypoplastic left heart syndrome. *Journal of Thoracic and Cardiovascular Surgery, 104*(1), 189–195.

Sullivan, M. (1995). Facilitating continuity of care. *Nursing Clinics of North America, 30*(2), 221–229.

Thurlow, T. (1995). The role of the cardiovascular social worker. *Nursing Clinics of North America, 30*(2), 211–219.

Wiles, H. (1990). Imaging congenital heart disease. *Pediatric Clinics of North America, 37*(1), 115–136.

Wolfgang, R., & Lock, J. (1990). Balloon dilation. *Pediatric Clinics of North America, 37*(1), 193–209.

Zahka, K., Spector, M., & Hanisch, D. (1993). Hypoplastic left-heart syndrome Norwood operation, transplantation, or compassionate care. *Clinics in Perinatology, 20*(1), 145–154.

HEALTH CHALLENGE:

Alterations in Respiratory Status

OUTLINE

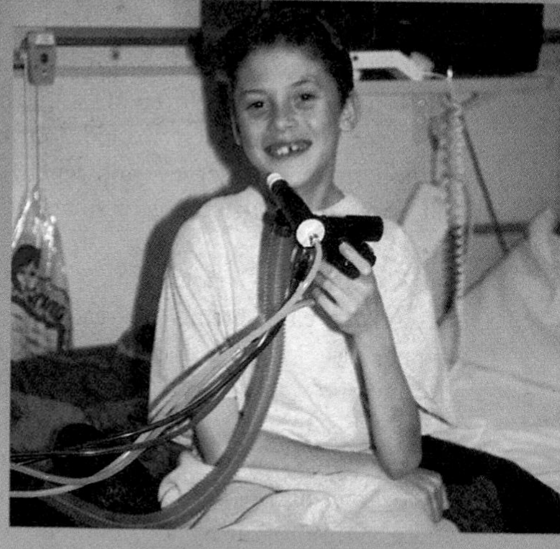

OBJECTIVES

- Describe the nursing assessment of the child experiencing compromises in respiratory function.
- Describe the developmental and biological variances in the child's respiratory system that predispose them to respiratory problems.
- Explain the nursing responsibilities associated with the diagnostic phase of children experiencing respiratory difficulties.
- Describe the common alterations in health patterns within the respiratory system in children in terms of etiology, pathophysiology, clinical manifestations, and interdisciplinary interventions.
- Select the treatment modality that is the most effective intervention for a selected respiratory condition.
- Select nursing care interventions to support the child with an acute or chronic respiratory illness.

KEY TERMS

apnea
atelectasis
atopy
bradycardia
cor pulmonale
cyanosis
dyspnea
hemoptysis
hypercarbia
hypoxemia
hypoxia
pallor
respiratory distress
respiratory failure
retractions
tachypnea
ventilation-perfusion mismatch

CHAPTER

16

Respiratory illnesses are the most common conditions encountered by the nurse caring for infants and children. These disorders can be acute, life-threatening, or chronic in nature and can present as either the primary clinical problem or a secondary complication from other conditions (Zander & Hazinski, 1992). The physiologic processes of respiratory control and gas exchange in children, although immature, are determined by respiratory mechanisms similar to those of adults. However; structural variations in the respiratory tract of infants and young children result in significant differences in the manifestation of respiratory disturbances. In addition, children have fewer cardiopulmonary reserves, and when challenged with insult or injury to these systems, decompensate more quickly.

Key functions of the nurse in the acute or ambulatory health care setting are readily identifying respiratory compromise in the child and quickly instituting corrective measures. The development and refinement of assessment skills in order to meet this challenge comfortably and accurately is a formidable accomplishment for the practitioner and is one of the hallmarks of the age-appropriate nature of caring for children. Therefore, the skilled nurse must have an excellent working knowledge and a keen understanding of the clinically significant and unique anatomic and physiologic features of the respiratory tract in children. Additionally, an awareness of how infections occur in children, especially as they affect the respiratory system, is important because of the relatively common and often debilitating nature of these problems. Knowledge of both acute and chronic respiratory conditions helps the nurse provide appropriate care, which sometimes continues throughout the life span of the child.

Assessment of the Respiratory System

Collecting the health history and performing the physical assessment of the child with a respiratory disturbance is the first step in the nursing process. Important information is shared and observations are made that will assist the health care team in planning interventions and monitoring the progress of treatment. At the time of the history and physical examination, the child and/or family have an opportunity to tell their story about the illness that prompted them to seek care from the health care team. The assessment can be made a more positive experience when the nurse is able to allay the child's fears and discomfort and establish a relationship of trust and communication between the child, parent, and nurse.

Focused Health History

A wealth of data is obtained when the nurse listens carefully and can translate the information directly into improving care for the child and the family. An exploration of the structure, function, and characteristic environment and routines of the family may yield important information about the child's respiratory status. Noting which family members are present and listening to the interaction and remarks made between family members are also valuable.

The history begins with the reason for the visit or hospitalization. All descriptions of the child's symptoms or condition should be documented in the child's or parents' own words when possible (Chart 16–1). The problem should be followed chronologically from the first symptoms to the present. Questions to ask include the following: Have the symptoms been getting worse, and over what length of time? Are symptoms continuous, or do they come and go? What factors make symptoms better or worse? What therapies or remedies have been tried, and what was the child's response? Clear and detailed information about the present illness helps the nurse initially formulate a plan of care and directs further questioning to confirm or refute any hypothesis regarding diagnosis.

The child's past medical history, including birth history, previous health challenges, childhood illnesses, immunizations, and allergies, helps put the present illness into perspective. For example, a child presenting with paroxysmal coughing episodes may cause the nurse to consider bronchitis, pneumonia, or foreign body aspiration, depending on the presence of other accompanying symptoms. However, if the child was never immunized against pertussis or screened for tuberculosis, additional possibilities for the symptoms must be considered.

Family medical history, especially the presence of infectious or genetic disorders, and an environmental history are also essential elements of a respiratory assessment. Irritants in the home such as smoke from tobacco or wood-burning stoves, excessive dust, pet dander, and paint fumes all can exacerbate wheezing.

caREminder: *If the child spends large amounts of time out of the house—at the baby sitter's, school, grandparents' or friends' homes—these environments should also be explored for possible contributing factors and irritants.*

Lastly, the respiratory health history should include assessment of nutrition and general growth and development factors. Growth impairment due to chronic hypoxia and poor nutritional intake is sometimes the first sign of

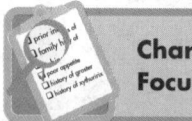

Chart 16–1
Focused Health History

Respiratory

Identifying Data	Specifically note the child's age and race
Present Illness	Chest pain with breathing Shortness of breath (with activity) Difficulty eating Cough (duration, onset, intermittent or continuous, paroxysmal, worse at night, production of sputum) Nasal congestion Runny nose (color of mucus) Sore throat Airway noise (barking cough, dry cough, stridor or wheeze) Easy fatigability Anyone else in the household ill
Past Medical History	
Birth History	Spontaneous breathing at birth Meconium-stained amniotic fluid Prematurity Required mechanical ventilation Prenatal maternal infections (i.e., chlamydia or herpes simplex) Maternal smoking history, marijuana, heroin, cocaine
Previous Health Challenges	History of respiratory illness such as strep throat, tonsillitis Number of colds per year including "typical course" Do colds include coughing, wheezing, or other noisy breathing History of otitis media
Childhood Illnesses	History of tuberculosis History of pertussis
Immunizations	Status of current immunizations (especially pertussis) Recent tuberculosis test and results
Allergies	Animals Plants Other irritants Foods Medicines
Current Medications	Medications related to current treatment of any chronic respiratory problems Medications (including over-the-counter medications) related to home remedies for current respiratory problems
Nutritional Assessment	Weight loss Failure to gain weight between office visits Decrease in physical activity Decreased appetite
Family Medical History	Family history of allergies, asthma, tuberculosis, pertussis, cystic fibrosis Focus on sibling history of respiratory illness
Environmental History	Environmental exposures that may affect breathing, such as smog, allergens, animals, powders, aerosols, household irritants Smoking behaviors of other household members
Social History	Psychosocial Cultural (any customs that may affect treatment) How many persons living in the household and whom Who is the child's primary caretaker?
Growth and Development	Physical milestones Developmental milestones Habits: play, sleep School attendance and performance

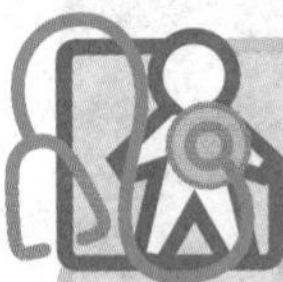

Chart 16–2
Focused Physical Assessment

Respiratory System

Assessment	Normal Findings	Alterations/Clinical Significance
Shape, size, and symmetry of the thoracic cavity	The infant's thorax is rounded, with anterior/posterior diameter equal to transverse diameter. The transverse diameter gradually increases, reaching adult radios at about 6 years of age.	Pectus excavatum (deep collapse of the tissue around and below the sternum) and pectus carinatum (a protuberant sternum) are asymmetric deformities of the chest. Either may compromise lung expansion. A round chest in an older child is usually indicative of chronic lung disease.
Type of breathing	In the child younger than 7 years, respirations are diaphragmatic. The abdomen rises with inspiration. Later, the breathing becomes thoracic.	Abdominal breathing in an older child may indicate a respiratory disorder or a fractured rib.
Depth/regularity of respirations (duration of inspiration relative to expiration)	Inspiratory phase of respiration is slightly longer than, or equal to, the expiratory phase.	Prolonged expiratory phase may indicate an obstructive respiratory disorder, such as asthma. Prolonged inspiratory phase may indicate an upper airway obstruction, such as croup.
Color of face, trunk, nail beds Shape of nail beds	Skin and mucous membranes are pink. Nail beds are pale or pink. Nails are flat with the angle between nail and nail base at approximately 160 degrees.	Cyanosis is indicative of inadequate oxygenation. Mottling of the trunk may indicate severe hypoxemia. Mottling and cyanosis may also be related to vasoconstriction or polycythemia. Digital clubbing (tissue proliferation on terminal phalanx) is indicative of chronic hypoxemia.
Quality of breathing	Quiet, non-labored breathing at a respiratory rate normal for age	Presence of tachypnea, dyspnea, or orthopnea indicates respiratory difficulty. Retractions are associated with both obstructive and restrictive lung diseases. Nasal flaring—bilateral widening on respiration—is associated with the child's attempt to improve oxygenation.
Quality of breath sounds	*Vesicular* are low-pitched, soft sounds (insp > exp) heard throughout lung field. *Bronchovesicular* are moderately pitched, harsh sounds (insp = exp) heard over the manubrium. *Bronchotubular* are high pitched, hollow sounds (insp < exp) heard over the trachea.	Absent or diminished breath sounds are associated with obstruction or pneumothorax. Adventitious breath sounds, including rales, rhonchi, and wheezes, are associated with fluid, secretions, pulmonary edema, inflammation, exudate, tumors, and foreign bodies.

insp, inspiration; exp, expiration.

decompensation in the child with chronic respiratory problems.

Focused Physical Assessment

When performing a physical assessment of the respiratory system in infants and children, the nurse uses the techniques of inspection, palpation, and auscultation. Advanced clinicians sometimes use percussion to locate areas of fluid accumulation and/or a mass in the lungs. Chart 16–2 summarizes possible physical assessment findings and highlights abnormalities and their implications.

Tip: *The following suggestions can help facilitate the physical assessment of the child:*

- *Allow the younger child to play with the stethoscope before starting your examination, or have the child listen to his or her own chest or that of the parent.*
- *Remove the infant or young child's shirt as early as possible in the assessment so that you can visualize the chest during rest (while you are conducting the health history). This may not be appropriate for the older child, who can be modest.*
- *Infants and toddlers are best assessed while held on their parent's lap.*
- *Try to count respirations first before touching the child, and then auscultate heart and lung sounds while the child is quiet and not crying.*
- *To allay the child's fear, warm the stethoscope with your hand and place it first on the child's hand before placing it on his or her chest.*

Observations to make during inspection include the rate, rhythm, and depth of respirations. Respiratory effort and appearance of retractions, nasal flaring, and use of accessory muscles should also be noted. The best indicator of pulmonary function in young children and infants is the respiratory rate (Cloutier, 1994). The respiratory rate should be counted for one full minute, ideally when the child is asleep or quiet (Chart 16–3). Tachypnea may also be expected to be observed in the presence of fever, anxiety, or stress. The child's general appearance, skin color, mental status, and nutritional status are also important to observe and note.

Chart 16–3

Normal Respiratory Rates in Children

Age	Average Respiratory Rate (breaths per minute)
Infant	30–60
1–2 years	24–40
3–4 years	20–30
5–8 years	20–24
9–12 years	18–22
13–18 years	12–16

Palpation of the chest involves assessing for chest expansion, tenderness, pulsations, and/or masses in the thoracic region. Subcutaneous emphysema or crepitus is a manifestation of free air that has leaked from the respiratory system into the subcutaneous tissue, most commonly resulting from a pneumomediastinum or pneumothorax. It can usually be palpated over the neck, shoulders, and upper chest. Symmetry of chest wall excursions should be assessed and palpated, especially in a child in whom trauma is suspected. Trauma to the rib cage can cause fractures and flail chest, which may manifest as paradoxical movement of the chest and decreased movement of the affected side. Position of the trachea may deviate from the midline in the presence of atelectasis and with pneumothorax, therefore palpation of this structure is important.

During auscultation, the quality and intensity of the breath sounds should be assessed as well as noting the area of the chest where they are heard. Familiarity with normal breath sounds are (including vesicular, bronchotubular, and bronchovesicular) and where they are best heard is important in differentiating abnormal from normal findings. Adventitious breath sounds that can be auscultated include wheezes, crackles (rales), and rhonchi (Table 16–1).

Audible abnormal noises to observe and listen for include stridor and grunting. Stridor is a harsh, grating, whistling sound heard on inspiration and produced by turbulent airflow through laryngeal or tracheal obstruction. It is usually more pronounced when the child is crying or agitated. Grunting is a noise the infant may make as he or she attempts to provide a self-induced positive end-expiratory pressure (PEEP). By grunting, the infant closes the glottis and applies positive pressure to the airway to increase the resting volume of the lung (Cloutier, 1994).

Alert: *Grunting is usually an ominous sign and may indicate impending respiratory failure in the infant or young child. Other clinical signs of impending respiratory failure that require immediate attention include increased work of breathing (severe retractions and grunting), diminished or absent breath sounds, development of hypoventilation (apnea or gasping respirations), altered level of consciousness (lethargy or inability to be consoled by parents), poor systemic perfusion (capillary refill of more than 2 seconds and/or mottling), tachycardia, and bradycardia (late sign) (Fig. 16–1).*

Table 16–1
Adventitious Breath Sounds

Breath Sound	Characteristics	Cause
Rales/crackles (fine or coarse)	Intermittent, medium- to high-pitched crackling or popping sounds, often heard on inspiration. Coarser rales occasionally clear with coughing or suctioning.	Associated with diseases of the smaller airways, including cystic fibrosis, pneumonia, and pulmonary edema.
Rhonchi (bubbly rales)	Continuous snoring, low-pitched sounds, often heard on expiration; occasionally on inspiration. Usually clear with cough or suctioning.	Associated with involvement of the upper airways, such as in bronchitis.
Wheeze	Continuous, whistling, musical, high-pitched sounds heard during expiration. Associated with a prolonged expiratory phase. May be audible without a stethoscope.	Associated with obstruction in the lower airways, such as in asthma or bronchiolitis.
Stridor	A sonorous, musical sound heard on inspiration. Associated with a prolonged inspiratory phase. Usually audible without stethoscope.	Associated with obstruction of the upper airways, such as in foreign body aspiration, laryngotracheomalacia, or croup.

Nursing Diagnoses and Outcomes

After a thorough assessment of the child, the nurse uses the data to identify patient needs and related nursing diagnoses. There are several nursing diagnoses that address alterations in respiratory function (Chart 16–4). In addition, respiratory distress in children may lead to correlating problems in other body systems (e.g., cardiac, immune). The nurse's plan of care should encompass all primary and secondary effects of the child's respiratory illness.

Similarly, promoting growth and development and ensuring adequate home management of a child's condition are of specific interest. Care directed in these areas can reduce exacerbations of the child's condition and/or prevent recurrence of respiratory illnesses.

Figure 16–1
An infant in respiratory distress. (© 1988, American Heart Association. Used with permission.)

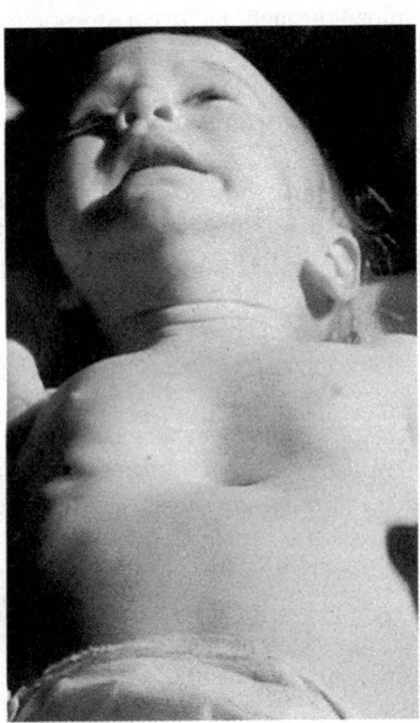

Developmental and Biological Variances

The child's respiratory system differs in many ways from that of the mature adult, and children are more vulnerable to respiratory illnesses or complications of respiratory diseases than adults (Chart 16–5). The child is physically smaller and functionally immature, thus the pediatric respiratory system has much less reserve capacity. Children develop respiratory distress and/or respiratory failure much more readily than adults as a result of specific anatomic and physiologic variations that exist in the pediatric respiratory system. Differences in the size, structure, and function of the respiratory system in children, as compared with adults, account for the majority of the variances in respiratory symptomatology seen in the child (Fig. 16–2). The five major anatomic components of the respiratory system include the central nervous system, the airways, the chest wall, the respiratory muscles, and the lung tissue. These structures function respectively to

Chart 16–4
Nursing Diagnoses and Outcomes

Alterations in Respiratory Status

Altered growth and development related to underlying chronic lung disease

Outcome: Infant/child/adolescent demonstrates maintenance of or improvement toward ideal body weight, developmental milestones, or level- and age-appropriate skills.

Alterations in health maintenance related to home management of respiratory illness

Outcome: Parent/caretaker attains/maintains safe home management skills, identify and access appropriate resources, and exhibit increased confidence with home care management.

Non-compliance related to extensive treatment plan and self-care management

Outcome: Child/parent attains/maintains behaviors consistent with the goals of therapy, willingness to follow therapy, and communicates consequences.

Risk for infection related to respiratory disorder

Outcome: Child is free from infection, and the parent/caretaker shall demonstrate adequate knowledge of risk for infection and the signs/symptoms of infection and practice precautionary measures.

Alterations in nutrition: less than body requirements related to underlying chronic lung disease and increased work of breathing

Outcome: Child demonstrates adequate nutritional intake for age, and the parent/caretaker shall identify steps to achieve/maintain ideal body weight.

Ineffective airway clearance related to excess thick secretions, obstruction, or infection

Outcome: Child or parent/caretaker demonstrates ability to effectively clear the child's airways.

Ineffective breathing pattern related to respiratory disease process

Outcome: Child demonstrates an effective respiratory rate, rhythm, and effort and experience improved gas exchange in the lungs.

Impaired gas exchange related to underlying respiratory disease process

Outcome: Child demonstrates adequate oxygenation and ventilation.

Decreased cardiac output related to respiratory distress and failure

Outcome: Child demonstrates adequate cardiac output.

Knowledge deficit related to new and complex treatment regimen and/or home care needs

Outcome: Parent/caretaker identifies and demonstrates all home care needs of the child.

Alterations in family processes related to chronic health care needs of child with a respiratory disease

Outcome: Parents and/or family maintain communication, participate in care of the child, assist in identifying resources, and identify/delegate role functions.

Ineffective family/individual coping related to chronic nature of underlying respiratory disease

Outcome: Family and/or individual child demonstrates effective coping by seeking assistance, providing supportive nurturing behaviors, and actively participating in care.

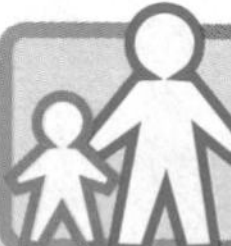

Chart 16–5
Developmental Considerations

Anatomic and Physiologic Differences Between Adults and Children

Infants and children are more susceptible to respiratory distress and compromise because of the following factors:

- The chest wall is primarily cartilage, therefore, more compliant.
- Children use diaphragmatic breathing, or abdominal versus costal breathing, up to about age 7.
- The intercostal muscles are underdeveloped and less able to help with breathing.
- Children have lower tidal volumes (amount of air inspired and expired with each breath) and therefore have less pulmonary reserves.
- Infants are obligate nose breathers up to 4 to 6 weeks of age and have irregular respirations with short apnea spells up to 15 seconds.
- Up to about age 8, the child's trachea is shorter, and the narrowest portion of the larynx occupies a more superior anterior position at the cricoid area.
- Airway diameters are smaller, therefore relatively small amounts of secretions or edema can significantly reduce the diameter, resulting in significant increased resistance to airflow and work of breathing.
- The alveoli are smaller in number and are more immature.

(1) control the rate and depth of respiration; (2) conduct gases to and from the lungs; (3) provide a structural enclosure and protection for the lungs and contribute to expansion of the lungs, stabilization of skeletal structures, and patency of airways; and (4) provide a surface for gas diffusion/exchange (Hazinski, 1996). Variances in these structures are summarized in this section, with suggestions provided regarding modification of assessment skills and intervention techniques that can assist the nurse in providing optimal care to the child.

Central Nervous System Control of Breathing

Respiratory rate and depth are controlled by central and peripheral chemoreceptors located in the circulatory system. These receptors are present at birth, but fewer numbers exist in the infant and young child than in an adult. Term infants and young children respond to hypoxemia and hypercarbia normally, by increasing the rate and depth of respiration in an attempt to normalize blood gas concentrations of oxygen and carbon dioxide. The premature infant, however, may respond to low blood oxygen levels initially by increasing the rate of respiration, followed by a slowing of respiratory rate and/or apnea. The astute pediatric nurse monitors infants with bronchopulmonary dysplasia, pneumonia, or bronchiolitis very closely for hypoxia and possible apneic episodes.

Airways

There is perhaps no more striking or clinically significant anatomic variation related to respiratory function in children than the airways. Although the full array of conducting airways is present at birth, the airways continue to grow in length and diameter throughout childhood. The diameter of the airways in the infant and young child is very small. A small amount of edema or mucus in the airway produces a critical decrease in the airway diameter and increases the resistance to air flow dramatically (Fig. 16–3). Conditions that involve increased production and accumulation of mucus, such as asthma and cystic fibrosis, or even a severe upper respiratory infection, may result in significant respiratory distress because of this phenomenon. The tongue in children is larger in relation to the mouth and can also cause airway obstruction.

The position and shape of the larynx in children up until approximately age 8 is different from that of the adult (it is higher and more anterior). The narrowest portion of the larynx is at the level of the cricoid ring (Fig. 16–4).

caREminder: *The child younger than age 8 requiring intubation usually does not need a cuffed endotracheal tube (ET tube). The cricoid provides a "natural physiologic cuff" around the uncuffed or straight tube.*

In adults, the narrowest portion of the larynx is at the vocal cords. The cartilage surrounding the entire larynx is quite soft and can easily be compressed when the neck is flexed or hyperextended. Maintaining an optimal neck position (sometimes called the "sniffing position") by placing a towel under the occiput of the head is an important nursing consideration and may be needed for a child in acute respiratory distress.

The pediatric trachea is also shorter than in the adult. In newborns, the trachea is 4 cm long, and in 18-month-old infants, it is 7 cm. In adults, it is 12 cm long (Seidel, 1996). The cartilaginous rings surrounding the trachea in some infants are weak and are not able to provide adequate support for the airway during inspiration. Collapse of the airway results, causing the characteristic stridor heard in patients with tracheomalacia. The right mainstem bronchus arises from the trachea at a

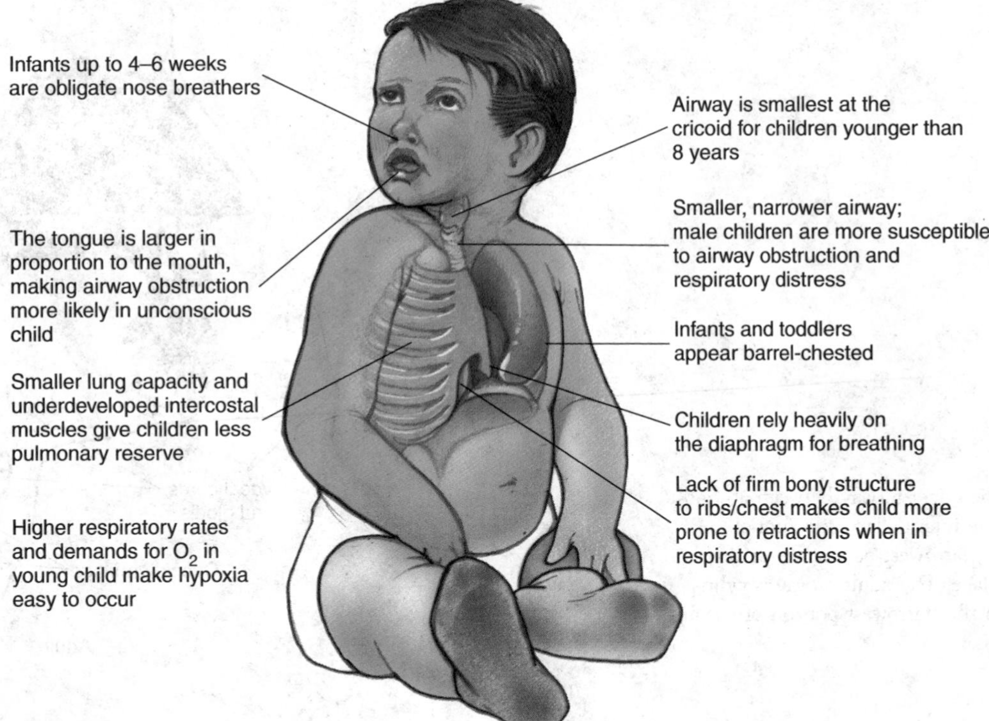
Infants up to 4–6 weeks are obligate nose breathers
The tongue is larger in proportion to the mouth, making airway obstruction more likely in unconscious child
Smaller lung capacity and underdeveloped intercostal muscles give children less pulmonary reserve
Higher respiratory rates and demands for O_2 in young child make hypoxia easy to occur
Airway is smallest at the cricoid for children younger than 8 years
Smaller, narrower airway; male children are more susceptible to airway obstruction and respiratory distress
Infants and toddlers appear barrel-chested
Children rely heavily on the diaphragm for breathing
Lack of firm bony structure to ribs/chest makes child more prone to retractions when in respiratory distress

Figure 16-2
Developmental and biological variances: respiratory.

wide angle (versus the much sharper angle of the left mainstem bronchus). Therefore, the pediatric nurse must assess carefully for symmetry of breath sounds in the pediatric patient, as the right mainstem bronchus is a common location for aspirated foreign bodies.

Chest Wall

Chest retractions are a clinical phenomenon unique to pediatric patients because their cartilaginous chest wall is twice as compliant or flexible as the bony chest wall of

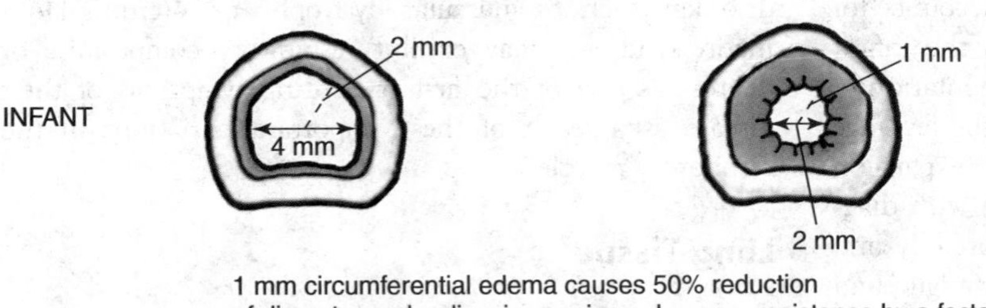
INFANT
2 mm
4 mm
1 mm
2 mm
1 mm circumferential edema causes 50% reduction of diameter and radius, increasing pulmonary resistance by a factor of 16.

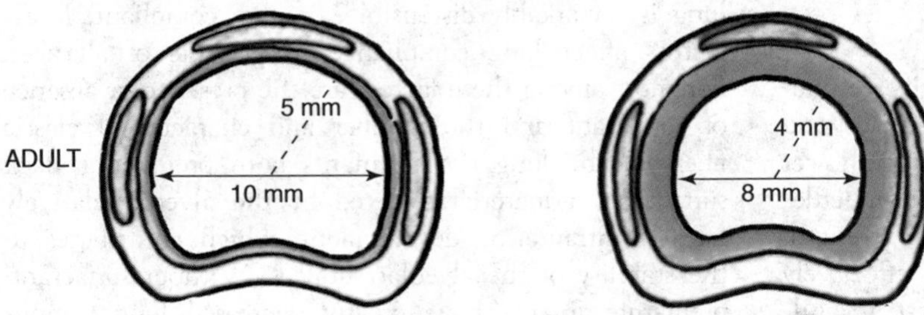
ADULT
5 mm
10 mm
4 mm
8 mm
1 mm circumferential edema causes 20% reduction of diameter and radius, increasing pulmonary resistance by a factor of 2.4.

Figure 16-3
A small amount of mucus can produce significant obstruction of the pediatric airway. (Modified from Coté, C. J., Ryan, J. F., Todres, I. D., & Goudsouzian, N. G. [1993]. A *practice of anesthesia for infants and children* [2nd ed., p. 62]. Philadelphia: W. B. Saunders.)

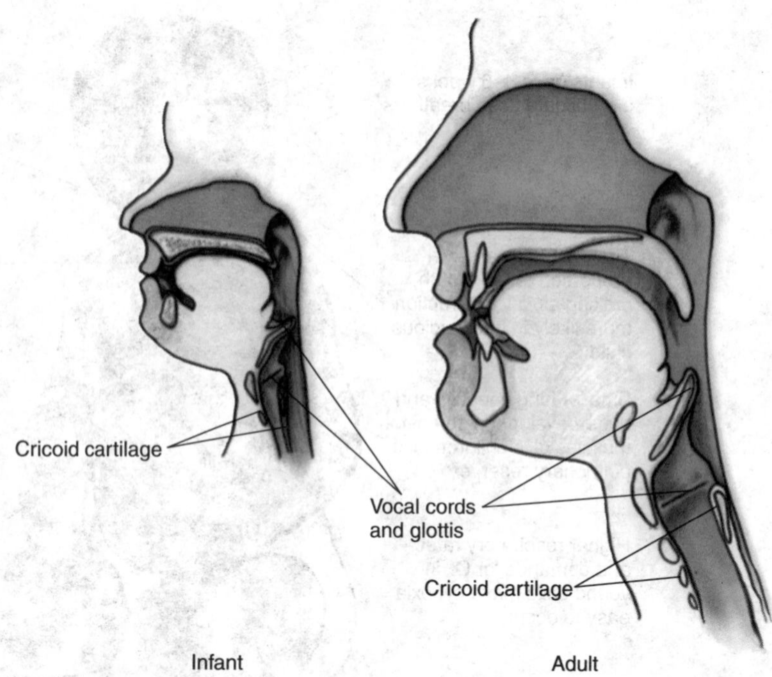

Figure 16–4
Differences in the upper airway between a child and an adult. The infant's larynx is funnel-shaped, with the narrowest part of the airway at the cricoid cartilage. The adult airway is cylinder-shaped, with the narrowest portion of the airway at the glottis.

the adult (Hazinski, 1996). Chest retractions increase the work of breathing and reduce the efficiency of ventilation during periods of respiratory distress. Other anatomic variations of the chest wall that adversely affect the mechanical efficiency of breathing in the infant and young child are the shape of the chest and the angle of rib articulation relative to the sternum and vertebrae. Until the child reaches 7 or 8 years of age, the ribs are horizontal in orientation, in contrast to a 45-degree angle present in the older child and adult. This accounts for the barrel-shaped appearance of the chest in the infant and young child. Because of this horizontal orientation of the ribs, the intercostal muscles do not have the leverage necessary to lift the ribs and aid in chest expansion during respiration. Young infants and children with diagnoses such as pneumonia must be assessed carefully and frequently for the development of respiratory fatigue and subsequent respiratory failure as a result of these variations.

Respiratory Muscles

The muscles important for efficient and effective respirations include the diaphragm, the intercostal muscles, and the muscles supporting the head and the upper and lower airways. In general, these muscles are relatively underdeveloped in pediatric patients—lacking the tone, strength, and coordination necessary to prevent and/or effectively manage episodes of respiratory distress. The head in children is proportionally larger and also has less muscular support.

The diaphragm, which is the main muscle of respiration in patients of all ages, is located higher in the thorax in the infant and young child and is inserted horizontally—versus obliquely, as in the adult. Any condition that impedes diaphragmatic movement, such as abdominal distention as a result of the accumulation of air or fluid, can significantly compromise the child's respiratory status. In addition, the intercostal muscles are underdeveloped and function only to stabilize rather than actually lift the chest wall (Hazinski, 1996). Children with neuromuscular weakness or paralysis secondary to disorders such as muscular dystrophy or Werdnig-Hoffmann syndrome may exhibit respiratory compromise or distress as one of the first presenting symptoms of their disease as a result of these important variations in the respiratory muscles.

Lung Tissue

Lung compliance is the volume of air moved per unit pressure change. Compliance refers to the relative "ease" of inflation and deflation of the lungs. The normal adult lung is remarkably distensible, or very compliant. Many factors affect lung compliance in patients of all ages. Foremost among these factors are the presence or absence of surfactant and the number and character of elastic fibers in the lung tissue. Infants born prematurely lack surfactant, a material secreted by the alveoli relatively late in intrauterine development, which contributes to the stability of the alveolar surfaces. Without surfactant, premature infants have greatly decreased lung compliance, leading to severe respiratory distress and even death. Lung compliance gradually increases throughout childhood, as lung tissue grows and the existing tissue matures.

Another variation in the lung tissue of the pediatric patient is a decreased amount of elastic tissue in the septa of the alveoli. This causes an increased tendency for loss of patency of the alveoli, leading to a higher incidence of pulmonary edema, pneumomediastinum, and pneumothorax. Low elastic recoil properties cause a higher incidence of atelectasis in pediatric patients as compared with adults. In addition, poorly developed pathways of collateral ventilation can lead to rapid small airway obstruction and significant respiratory distress. Because of all these variations, neonates are especially susceptible to the development of pulmonary edema. Therefore, in addition to careful assessment of respiratory status, fluid and electrolyte balance is also a very important consideration. Patients with bronchiolitis or bronchopulmonary dysplasia may need to have their oral fluid intake limited to prevent pulmonary edema.

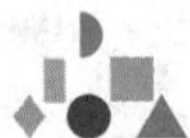

Diagnostic Criteria for Evaluating Alterations in Respiratory Status

There are four major groups of diagnostic tests and procedures used in the evaluation of the respiratory system and respiratory disorders in children:

- Measurement of lung volumes and flow rates
- Direct or indirect blood and body fluid analysis
- Imaging techniques
- Direct visualization of the respiratory tree

These diagnostic tests, used alone or in combination with others, yield information necessary in the diagnosis and treatment of acute and chronic lung disease. Table 16–2 describes the purpose, findings, and indications of

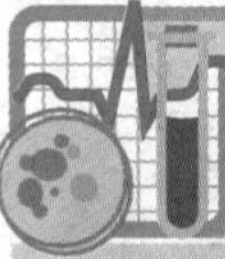

Table 16–2
Diagnostic Tests and Procedures for Evaluating Respiratory Status

Diagnostic Test or Procedure	Purpose	Findings and Indications	Health Care Provider Responsibilities
Pulmonary function tests (spirometry, gas dilution, and body plethysmography)	Measures airway function, lung volumes, and gas exchange. Used to determine the presence, nature, and extent of pulmonary disease. Does not indicate the cause of the dysfunction.	Abnormalities of particular measurements may occur in different diseases. Restrictive diseases have a decreased vital capacity (VC) and total lung capacity (TLC). Obstructive diseases may show an increase in TLC and residual volume (RV), decreased VC, and decrease in forced expiratory volume in 1 sec (FEV_1) and forced expiratory flow between 25% and 75% VC ($FEF_{25\%-75\%}$).	Most results are effort dependent. Emphasize the need for maximum cooperation during the test to achieve valid results. Some tests require that the child's nose be clamped. Child should not have eaten immediately prior to exam—coughing required during the test may stimulate vomiting. Test may be performed before and after bronchodilator therapy.
Peak flow measurement	Used to measure the greatest flow velocity during a forced expiration. Child exhales forcefully and quickly into the meter while taking maximal deep inhalation (total lung capacity).	Peak flow rate decreases as airway obstruction increases. Values should be compared with the individual child's baseline or "personal best" vs. average predicted normal values.	Must be developmentally able to follow instructions, generally >age 4–5. May not be appropriate if child is in severe respiratory distress. Accurate peak flow measurement is effort dependent.
Arterial blood sample	Used to measure and analyze arterial oxygen levels, CO_2 retention, and alterations in the pH.	The arterial PCO_2 is an indicator of adequacy of ventilation. Arterial PO_2 is an indication of altered gas exchange, and pH indicates whether hypo- or hyperventilation is chronic or acute.	Avoid getting air in syringe with the sample; this can alter the findings. Firm pressure should be applied to the puncture site for 5 min after draw to prevent hematoma or bleeding. Most reliable when obtained from an indwelling arterial catheter. Arterial puncture is painful and may be associated with altered findings.

Table continued on following page

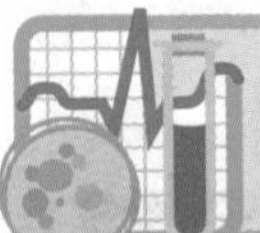

Table 16–2
Diagnostic Tests and Procedures for Evaluating Respiratory Status *Continued*

Diagnostic Test or Procedure	Purpose	Findings and Indications	Health Care Provider Responsibilities
Sputum culture/ tracheal aspiration	Used to examine and identify presence of bacterial, viral, fungal, or other respiratory pathogens.	Presence of pathogens usually indicates infection. Observe sputum for color, consistency, and odor. Yellow or green sputum that is thick indicates infection. Infection with *Pseudomonas aeruginosa* causes the sputum to have a distinct "sweet" odor.	Specimen should be collected within 3–7 days after onset of signs and symptoms and before antimicrobial therapy is initiated, unless the culture is being completed to examine the effectiveness of therapy. The specimen should be placed in a sterile container for culture or a tube with appropriate medium. Specimen must be from bronchial tree, not just saliva from mouth. Specimens should not be frozen, and should be transported as soon as possible.
Throat culture (throat swab)	Used to determine viral or bacterial cause in pharyngitis. Reliable method to differentiate infection with group A beta-hemolytic *Streptococcus pyogens* from viral organisms.	Positive throat culture for *S. pyogens* indicates "strep throat."	Specimens should be obtained from the posterior pharynx and each tonsillar area. Any white patch on inflamed area should be cultured. Results take 24–48 hr to obtain. Special test kits for strep throat are available that should yield results in 7 min.
Nasal and nasopharyngeal culture or washing	Preferred method used to detect bacterial, viral, and other respiratory pathogens, because large number of ciliated epithelial cells are essential for optimal recovery of the pathogens.	Able to detect *Bordetella pertussis, Candida albicans, Corynebacterium diphtheriae, Neisseria* meningitis, *Haemophilus influenzae,* and others. Coagulase-positive staphylococcus may be present in 50% of people who have nasopharyngeal cultures done.	For a culture, the flexible swab should be inserted into the nose and rotated against the anterior hairs for a good specimen. For a washing, normal saline should be instilled into the nostril and then immediately suctioned with a catheter into a specimen container.
Sweat chloride test	Used in diagnosis of cystic fibrosis. Measures amount of sodium and chloride content in the sweat.	Sweat chloride of $\geq$ 60 mEq/L indicates positive test for cystic fibrosis. Levels of 40–60 mEq/L are highly suggested to be positive.	Test takes about an hour for enough sweat to be collected.
Lung biopsy and/or thoracentesis	A needle is inserted through an intercostal space into lung tissue to obtain a lung aspirate specimen for histology and culture.	Purulent fluid is indicative of infection (empyema). Presence of lymphocytes with chyle indicates chylothorax. Presence of lymphocytes may indicate malignancy, and bloody fluid may indicate hemothorax.	Bleeding and pneumothorax are potential complications.
Chest x-ray	The best initial imaging technique to detect abnormalities of the pulmonary, mediastinal, and musculoskeletal structures of the thorax.	Air or fluid in the pleural space indicates a pleural effusion or pneumothorax. Hyperinflation often implies air trapping seen in bronchiolitis or asthma, and atelectasis and/or infiltrates may indicate pneumonia.	Determine whether adolescent female patients may be pregnant. Anteriposterior (AP) view more appropriate for the younger child (younger than 2 years).

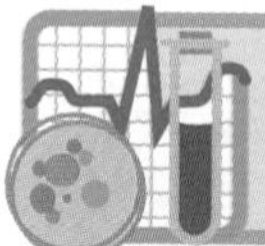

Table 16–2
Diagnostic Tests and Procedures for Evaluating Respiratory Status *Continued*

Diagnostic Test or Procedure	Purpose	Findings and Indications	Health Care Provider Responsibilities
Fluoroscopy	Related to chest x-ray films, but image is continuous on a television monitor to allow for continuous observation of chest movements during inspiration and expiration.	Useful in the assessment of diaphragmatic movement; air trapping and presence of pulsation in intrathoracic masses.	Child should be immobilized. Determine whether adolescent female patients may be pregnant. Personnel should protect radiosensitive areas such as gonads and thyroid gland with lead shields.
Bronchography	Uses a contrast medium instilled directly into the tracheobronchial tree to visualize the bronchi for narrowing obstruction or dilation or malformation of the bronchial tree.	Provides information about the most peripheral bronchioles. Chronic distal bronchial obstruction and dilation are indicative of bronchiectasis.	Signed consent required. Child NPO 6–12 hr before test and after test until gag reflex returns. Check whether child has any loose teeth prior to test. Usually performed with child under general anesthesia.
Computed Tomography (CT) scan	A sequence of x-ray films that show a cross-sectional view of the thorax. Used to detect masses or locate lesions.	Presence of mediastinal mass may indicate tumor; hilar adenopathy may indicate infection with tuberculosis.	Sedation or immobilization of child usually required. NPO 3–4 h prior to examination because IV contrast media may be used to further visualize cardiac chambers and vessels.
Radionuclide scintigraphy Lung scan (V/Q Scan) Radionuclide scintigraphy	A nuclear medicine scan performed to detect alterations or defects in perfusion (Q) and/or inequalities in ventilation (V).	Scintigraphy is able to detect non-infectious inflammatory diseases, presence of pulmonary emboli, pulmonary complications of HIV infection, and evaluations of tumors.	Signed consent required for injection of radionuclides IV. Child may not be NPO. Young child or uncooperative child may be sedated and thus should be NPO 4 hr before procedure.
Magnetic resonance imaging (MRI)	Uses magnetic waves to provide two- and three-dimensional views on the transaxial, coronal, and sagittal planes.	Easily detects abnormalities of soft tissues, presence of solid masses, chest wall deformities, and vascular abnormalities.	Child must be able to cooperate and lie still; the younger child may need to be sedated. Any clothing with metal snaps or metal items, such as barrettes, should be removed.
Laryngoscopy/bronchoscopy rigid (can remove foreign bodies from major airways) or flexible fiberoptic (more detailed visualization of mucosa)	Procedure similar to insertion of an endotracheal tube used to provide direct visualization of the airways using a lighted laryngoscope.	Aids in diagnosing cause of upper airway obstructions (including foreign bodies), abnormalities in major airways, aspiration of thick mucous plugs; obtaining secretions for bronchial lavage and cultures, aspiration of thick mucous; and obtaining secretions for cultures.	Requires signed consent. Suction equipment and oxygen should be ready and available at bedside. Conscious sedation required for flexible bronchoscopy; general anesthesia required for rigid bronchoscopy.

individual diagnostic tests, as well as the specific responsibilities and considerations for the health care provider. It is important to remember that the degree of sensitivity and specificity associated with each test varies with the disease (Voter & McBride, 1996). Sensitivity refers to the accuracy with which the test yields desired information, and specificity is the degree to which the test confirms or rules out a particular abnormality. For example, the chest x-ray examination is a sensitive but nonspecific imaging technique in that it is used to evaluate many different pulmonary conditions. It can be very accurate in the evaluation of conditions such as atelectasis and pulmonary edema. It indicates the presence and exact location of abnormalities. However, a chest x-ray examina-

Table 16-3
Pediatric Arterial Blood Gases

	pH	$PaCO_2$	PaO_2	HCO_3	BE	Causes of Imbalance
Normal Values						
Preterm Infant	7.11–7.36	27–40 mmHg	55–85 mmHg	21–28 mEq/L	±2	
Term Infant	7.35–7.45	27–41 mmHg	54–95 mmHg	21–28 mEq/L	±2	
Child	7.35–7.45	35–45 mmHg	80–100 mmHg	21–28 mEq/L	±2	
Abnormal Values						
Respiratory acidosis (acute alveolar hypoventilation)	<7.30	>50 mmHg	WNL or <80 mmHg	WNL	WNL	Chronic lung disease (chronic bronchitis, asthma), respiratory depression from drugs or anesthesia pneumonia, respiratory distress
Respiratory alkalosis (acute alveolar hyperventilation)	>7.50	<30 mmHg	WNL	WNL	WNL	Anxiety, fear, pain, improperly adjusted ventilator (overventilation), salicylate toxicity, fever, hyperventilation, hypoxia, tetany, head trauma, gram-negative septicemia
Metabolic acidosis	<7.30	WNL	WNL	<21 mEq/L		Severe diarrhea, kidney failure, diabetic ketoacidosis, shock, burns, malnutrition, ingestion of salicylates
Metabolic alkalosis	>7.50	WNL	WNL	>28 mEq/L		Loss of bicarbonate by intestines, severe vomiting, cystic fibrosis, gastric suctioning, severe diarrhea, renal failure, diuretics
Respiratory acidosis with compensation (chronic alveolar hypoventilation)	WNL	>50 mmHg	WNL or <80 mmHg			Kidneys try to retain more HCO_3 by increasing retention.
Respiratory alkalosis with compensation (chronic alveolar hyperventilation)	WNL	<30 mmHg	WNL			Kidneys try to reduce HCO_3 by increasing excretion.
Metabolic acidosis with compensation	WNL	<30 mmHg	WNL			Lungs try to reduce PCO_2 by increasing ventilation.
Metabolic alkalosis with compensation	WNL	>50 mmHg	WNL			Lungs try to increase PCO_2 slightly by hypoventilation.

WNL, within normal limits.

tion is less useful in the evaluation of possible foreign body aspiration, as the absence of abnormalities on the x-ray film does not rule out the diagnosis. In contrast, a sweat chloride measurement is sensitive *and* specific for the diagnosis of cystic fibrosis (in most age groups). It confirms this particular diagnosis but has little value in the evaluation of other lung diseases.

Blood Gases

Measurement of blood gases is considered one of the most useful diagnostic tests when a child is in respiratory distress and/or impending cardiopulmonary failure, therefore knowledge of normal arterial blood gas values for children is important for assessing and evaluating the child (Table 16–3). The values of importance for evaluation of lung function, gas exchange, and tissue perfusion include the pH, $PaCO_2$, and PaO_2. Determination of blood gases is useful in the management of the child in acute respiratory distress because the information helps the health care team make decisions regarding interventions such as necessity for intensive care, administration of oxygen, and mechanical ventilation management.

Pulse Oximetry

Pulse oximetry is a relatively accurate, portable, and noninvasive method for monitoring arterial hemoglobin saturation (SaO_2). It has been used in a variety of clinical situations in evaluating respiratory function and the presence of hypoxemia and is now a widely used and available technology. Important to note is that pulse oximetry measures the arterial hemoglobin saturation, not arterial PaO_2 as obtained in an arterial blood gas specimen. However, it allows for continuous monitoring and evaluation of hemoglobin saturation, which can be used to estimate the child's PaO_2 using the oxyhemoglobin dissociation curve. Monitoring pulse oximetry allows the advantage of being able to detect cases of clinically unsuspected hypoxemia in a variety of clinical settings, such as in the operating or emergency room and even in an ambulatory setting (Hanna, 1995; Murray & Loughlin, 1995).

Pulse oximetry works by using a photodetector and light-emitting diodes that are aligned across from one another on a pulsatile tissue bed such as the ear or a distal extremity (Fig. 16–5). The diodes emit infrared light through the tissue bed while the photodetector determines the amount of light that is absorbed within the tissue. Oxygenated hemoglobin absorbs infrared light, and it is the differential light absorbance of saturated (oxygenated) and unsaturated hemoglobin that is used to calculate the hemoglobin oxygen saturation. Additionally, the monitor is able to detect a pulse signal, and it provides a digital display of the pulse rate (Chart 16–6).

Figure 16–5
Child with a pulse oximeter. The finger probe has a red sensor light that fascinates some children.

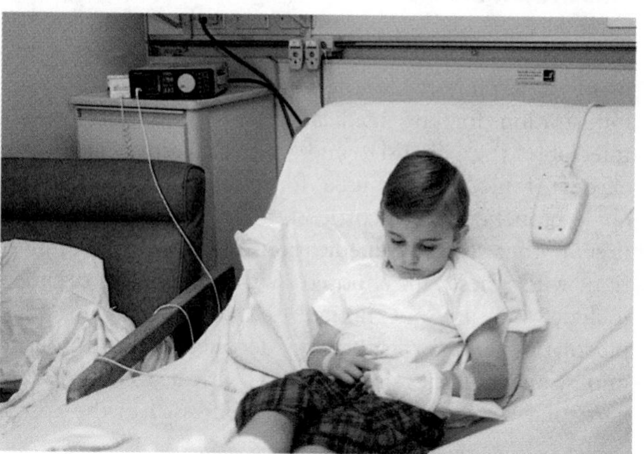

Chart 16–6
Nursing Interventions

Pulse Oximetry

Nursing implications for pulse oximetry use and monitoring include clinical judgment to interpret the readings, identification of factors that may cause potential errors in readings, and sensor application. The nurse should evaluate the readings in the context of trends documented over time, the clinical symptoms of the child, and influential factors such as patient motion (Hanna, 1995). Choosing the appropriate sensor size for the child according to the weight is essential to limit inaccurate readings. The sensor package indicates which size is appropriate for the child's weight. The sensor is placed with the light source directly opposite the photodetector. Other sources of potential errors in the oximeter readings are abnormal hemoglobin, poor peripheral perfusion, motion artifact, and ambient light interference (Carroll, 1993). Hemoglobin saturated with carbon monoxide causes the oximetry readings to remain in the 90s despite hypoxemia; therefore it should not be used on patients with carbon monoxide poisoning. Readings may be inaccurate in patients with poor perfusion to the extremities or those who are hypotensive. The sensor has difficulty picking up the signal when there is a lot of movement or if bright light is shining directly on the sensor, and this may affect the readings because the photodetector measures light. To avoid this, simply place a sock over the child's foot or place the hand or foot under the sheet or blanket to protect it from light. Any nail polish, especially blue, black, or green, should be removed, as this may affect readings as well.

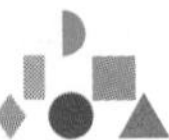

Treatment Modalities

Respiratory illnesses in children, both acute and chronic conditions, require aggressive and immediate intervention by members of the health care team. Respiratory failure is the leading cause of cardiopulmonary arrest in children. A thorough assessment of the child's status, followed by quick actions that support the child's oxygenation and ventilation, can serve to avert an impending arrest situation. In the case of acute respiratory problems, children generally respond well and promptly to the simple administration of oxygen and medications. For the child with a chronic respiratory condition, oxygen, medications, airway clearance techniques, and nutritional support are treatment modalities that can assist the child through exacerbations of the illness as well as provide them with the strength to maintain a high level of wellness despite their chronic condition.

Administration of Oxygen

Oxygen is indicated for the treatment of hypoxemia and is considered the most dramatic, life-saving intervention and/or drug administered by the health care provider for the treatment of hypoxemia. Oxygen is indicated for the presence of or risk of low PaO_2 and is also indicated to improve oxygenation when cardiac output is low, to decrease pulmonary vascular resistance, to enhance elimination of CO_2, or to accelerate removal of nitrogen from air-containing spaces such as in a pneumothorax.

Oxygen can be administered or delivered via mask (Fig. 16–6), nasal cannula, oxygen hood, oxygen tent, or mechanical ventilation. The mode of oxygen delivery used is based on the concentration or percentage of oxygen (FiO_2) desired for the child as well as the ability of the child to cooperate with therapy. To ensure patient safety, the concentration of inspired oxygen should be measured and monitored carefully, and the child's response during oxygen therapy should be documented. To help reduce the risk of oxygen toxicity, use the least amount of oxygen required to normalize PaO_2 (more than 60 to 80 mmHg) and SaO_2 (more than 93%), use an FiO_2 of 50% or less whenever possible, and decrease the percentage of oxygen as soon as the child's condition permits. Table 16–4 describes the different modes of oxygen delivery.

Figure 16–6
Child receiving oxygen via a face mask.

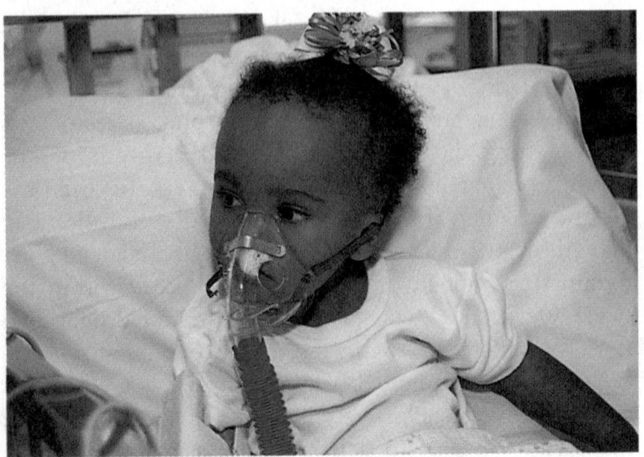

A function of the upper respiratory tract is to warm and humidify inspired air. Inspired air is normally warmed to body temperature and fully saturated with water (100% relative humidity). When these two processes are bypassed, as in the case of providing oxygen via an artificial airway such as an endotracheal tube or a tracheostomy tube, it is necessary that the child receive heated, humidified inspired gases. Medical gases such as oxygen that flow from a central source or a cylinder and are at room temperature with 0% humidity also necessitate humidification and heating of the inspired gas before administration to the child.

caREminder: *To decrease the risk of mucociliary dysfunction, injury to the respiratory epithelium, and thickening of secretions, children receiving oxygen therapy through an artificial airway for more than 1 to 2 hours should receive warmed, humidified inspired oxygen.*

The use of oxygen therapy in the home is becoming more prevalent. Possible respiratory complications requiring children to have home oxygen therapy include irreversible damage to the lung tissue and alveoli from bronchopulmonary dysplasia, the presence of severe infection, or the presence of airway obstruction. TIP 16–1 describes care of the child receiving home oxygen therapy and the educational needs of the family and/or caretakers.

Medications

Medications are an important component in the treatment of respiratory disorders in children. Routes of administration for the medications are oral, intravenous, injectable (SQ or IM), and via inhalation. The main classes of medications used for respiratory disorders include bronchodilators, corticosteroids, and mast cell stabilizers. Other groups of medications often used in conjunction with these in children with respiratory disorders include, but are not limited to, antibiotics, antivirals, mucolytics and expectorants, decongestants, antihistamines, and diuretics. The pharmaceutical agents used for particular respiratory disorders are addressed in the appro-

Table 16–4
Modes of Oxygen Delivery

Method of Delivery	Percentage of O_2 Delivered	Liter Flow	Comments
Nasal cannula	21% O_2 plus 3% per liter	0.5–6 L/min	Dries mucosa, give with humidification Provides limited O_2 delivery Easy to use and well tolerated
Nasal catheter	—	—	Not recommended No advantage over nasal cannula Can cause trauma or gastric distention
O_2 hood	Can deliver FiO_2 up to 100%	10–15 L/min	Difficult to assess baby Need to remove baby for feeding and care Need oxygen analyzer to gauge percentage of oxygen delivered
O_2 tent (mist tent)	Up to 40–50% FiO_2	10–15 L/min	Infant or child can get cold If $FiO_2 > 30\%$, tent is not satisfactory
Venturi mask	24–50% FiO_2	3–15 L/min	Adjustable to control percentage of oxygen delivered
Simple face mask	<40% FiO_2	4–8 L/min	Not a stable delivery system of $FiO_2 > 40\%$
Partial re-breathing mask	50–60% FiO_2	6–10 L/min	Allows greater concentration of O_2 to be delivered
Non-rebreathing mask	90–95% FiO_2	6–10 L/min	
Bag-valve mask	65–95% FiO_2	10–15 L/min	Excellent method for assisted ventilation Mask is selected to fit over the child's mouth and nose
O_2-powered device	—	—	Never use in children

priate sections. Principles of inhalation therapy and aerosolized medications are addressed here.

Aerosol Therapy

Bronchodilators, corticosteroids, and mast cell stabilizer medications are prescribed as inhalers or for nebulization. However, bronchodilators and corticosteroids are also available in oral and intravenous forms. Administering medications via inhalation is effective because the medication reaches the small airways and works directly on the lungs. Nebulization or aerosolization of medications is done by using compressed air or oxygen. There are a variety of machines (compressors) for use with a hand-held nebulizer that are often available for use in the home. Most children younger than 5 years of age or older children who may have difficulty coordinating a metered dose inhaler should use a nebulizer with either a mask or mouthpiece. The hand-held nebulizer has the advantages of being able to aerosolize almost any drug available in liquid form, allowing modification of dose volume and concentration, and requiring minimal patient coordination (Rau, 1991). The child or infant usually uses a mask attached to the nebulizer cup, which is held over the nose and mouth. The medication is dispersed as a mist. Older children can use the mouthpiece and should be instructed to take slow, deep breaths through the mouth during the treatment (Fig. 16–7).

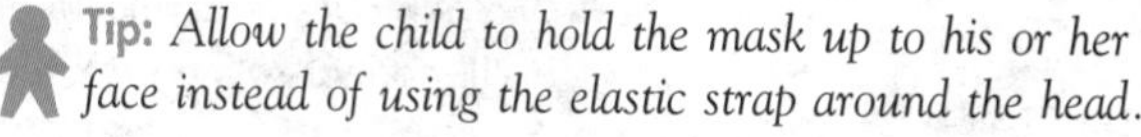

Tip: *Allow the child to hold the mask up to his or her face instead of using the elastic strap around the head.*

Figure 16–7
Child receiving treatment with a nebulizer.

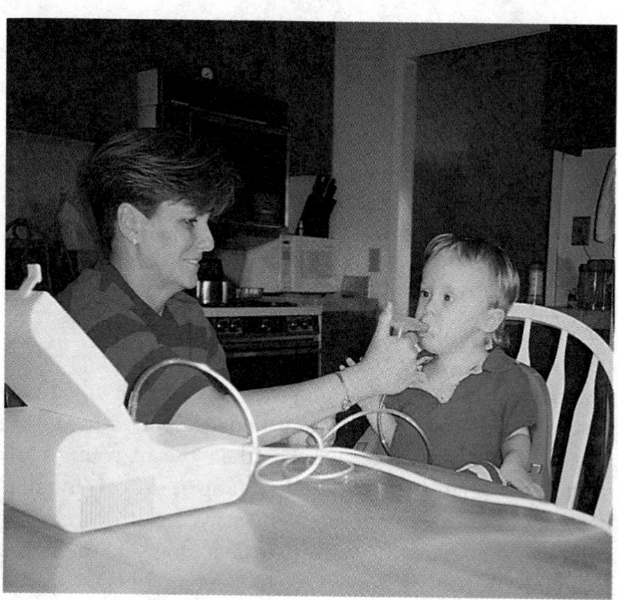

TIP 16–1 A Teaching Intervention Plan for the Child on Home Oxygen Therapy

Nursing Diagnoses and Outcomes

- Knowledge deficit related to care of the infant/child and home management with oxygen therapy
  Outcome: Parents/caregivers shall verbalize the need for oxygen, care of the infant/child while on oxygen therapy, and safety precautions and demonstrate care of the child and use of the oxygen.
- Risk for injury related to use of oxygen in the home and fire hazards
  Outcome: Family shall remain free of injury, and the potential for fire or explosion shall be minimized.
- Impaired gas exchange related to underlying respiratory disease process
  Outcome: Infant/child will have adequate oxygenation and ventilation as evidenced by normal (for age and child) respiratory rate and effort and color of child.

Instructional Interventions

Physiology and Need for Oxygen

- Discuss with parents/caregivers how oxygen enters the body and how it is used by the body. Explain the need/rationale for oxygen for their child.

Use of Oxygen

- Explain and demonstrate how to place/change the nasal cannula under the nose and over the ears with the portion with the holes positioned under the nose, and how to attach the cannula to the flowmeter on the tank.
- Show parents/caregivers how to open the oxygen device and how to regulate the flow (depends on device being used in the home).

Physical Care

- Provide appropriate skin care on the face. Use hypoallergenic tape or skin protectant on the areas where the cannula is secured on the face.
- Oxygen can be drying to the nares; provide humidity with oxygen if flow >1 L/min, or instill normal saline drops to nares, p.r.n.

When the child is getting the treatment, he or she may like to have "teddy" or "dolly" wear a mask and "get a treatment" too.

The metered-dose inhaler (MDI) is a simple and portable self-contained hand-held canister that is able to deliver a predetermined amount of the specified medication to the patient. Most bronchodilators, corticosteroids, and mast cell inhibitors are available as an MDI. Although MDIs have the advantage of being very portable and are able to provide efficient drug delivery with rapid preparation and administration time, they do have the disadvantage of being difficult to coordinate and use correctly (Chart 16–7). This disadvantage makes their use in young children questionable. Additionally, proper use of inhalers has been found to be deficient in many health care practitioners, complicating effective teaching of their use (Hanania, Wittman, Kesten, & Chapman, 1994).

For the child younger than 6 to 8 years of age, a spacer device that is attached to the MDI should always be used (Fig. 16–8). Use of a spacer allows time for the propellant to remain suspended and achieve smaller particle size and also provides ease of coordination. Some of these devices use a whistle to cue the child who is inhaling too fast (Dettenmeier, 1992). Another device for inhalation that is available is the drug-powder inhaler (DPI), which consists of a suspension of microfine solid particles of drug contained in a small MDI-sized device with a mouthpiece. These devices are marketed more in Europe and Canada, but Ventolin Rotacaps with Rotahaler (Glaxo Wellcome) are available in this formulation in the United States (Rau, 1991).

When the infant or child is receiving aerosol or inhalation therapy, it is necessary to assess the child's response to treatment. Assess the child's breath sounds and respiratory effort before and after the treatment for

TIP 16–1 A Teaching Intervention Plan for the Child on Home Oxygen Therapy *Continued*

- Provide nasopharyngeal suctioning to nares with bulb syringe as needed to keep nares patent and to allow adequate flow of oxygen to child.
- Do not use petroleum-based creams or ointments or oil-based products on the child (they are combustible).

Health Maintenance

- Describe and have parents/caregivers identify "normal" color and respiratory status for their infant.
- Teach parents/caregivers how to detect changes in color (blueness of lips/nail beds, pale, or dusky) and respiratory status (retractions, nasal flaring, accessory muscle use, and increased respiratory rate). Instruct caregivers on need to notify physician if these changes are present.
- Stress importance of regular follow-up visits with health care provider.

Home Safety and Modifications

- Family should have the following available in the home:
  - Notification sticker (OXYGEN IN HOME) for fire department. Place on front window where easily visible.
  - Fire extinguisher and label for area where kept
  - Smoke detector
  - Battery-operated flashlight on hand in child's room in event of power failure
  - List of emergency numbers posted by all phones
- Do not allow smoking in the home. Post "No Smoking" signs. Do not burn incense, candles, or fires in the home. Keep the oxygen tank more than 5 feet away from the heater.
- Reduce static electricity of clothes by using fabric softener.
- Keep oxygen source upright and secured in holder at all times!
- If traveling, keep portable oxygen source in upright position and secure at all times. Keep window open slightly in car to allow ventilation. Avoid places that allow smoking.

effectiveness. For the child receiving bronchodilators (beta-adrenergic agents), it is also important to assess the heart rate, as tachycardia is a common side effect of these medications.

caREminder: *Be sure to have the child rinse out the mouth after use of an MDI, especially if using a corticosteroid. This is done to decrease the chance of systemic absorption and side effects related to the medications.*

Airway Clearance Techniques

Traditionally, chest physiotherapy—postural drainage and percussion—has been the primary intervention for pulmonary conditions with hypersecretion or retained bronchial secretions. For example, children with conditions such as cystic fibrosis, bronchiectasis, or dysfunctional motility of cilia or those receiving mechanical

Figure 16–8
Commercial spacer device.

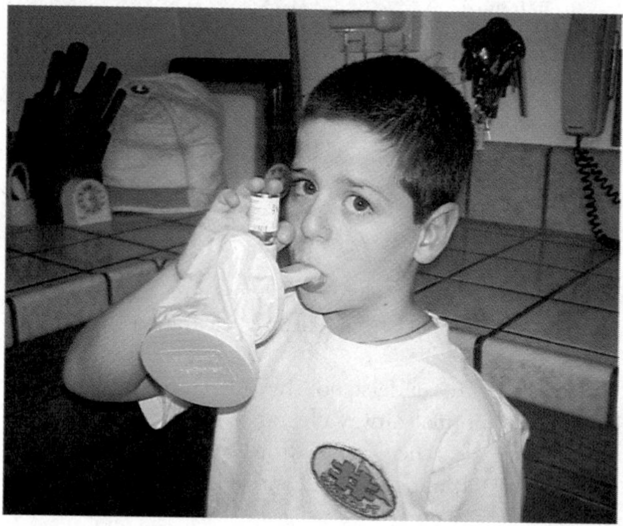

Chart 16–7

Use of a Metered-Dose Inhaler

Steps:

1. Remove cap from metered-dose inhaler (MDI), and hold canister upright.
2. Shake the inhaler 3 or 4 times.
3. Tilt the head back slightly and exhale normally.
4. Position the inhaler in one of the following ways:
   Close lips around the mouthpiece of the inhaler.
   Open mouth and hold mouthpiece 2 fingerbreadths from the mouth.
   Use a spacer (best for young children).

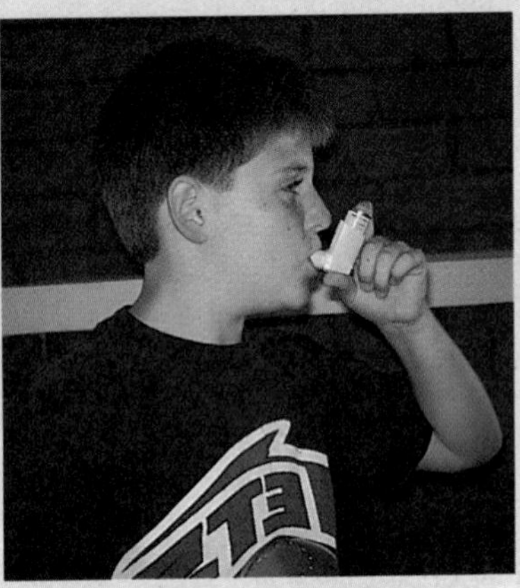

5. Start to breathe in slowly and press down on the inhaler to release the medication as you are inhaling.
6. Continue inhaling slowly and deeply (3 to 5 seconds).
7. Hold breath for a count of 10 (5 to 10 seconds) to allow the medicine to reach the lungs, then exhale.
8. Wait 1 to 2 minutes, and repeat puffs as directed (steps 2 through 7).
9. Rinse out mouth with water and spit out after using an inhaled corticosteroid.

ventilation or with acute problems after general anesthesia can benefit from airway clearance techniques (ACTs).

In order to understand the ACTs, it is helpful to first review normal airway clearance. The process of normal airway clearance results from several functions: (1) mucociliary clearance, (2) characteristics of mucus, and (3) an effective cough. The cilia that line the airways beat in constant rhythmic fashion to sweep the mucus and particulate matter from the more distal airways to the larger airways. When the mucus is mobilized to the larger airways, an effective cough causes an air–liquid interaction, which is essential for effective airway clearance. An effective cough consists of three phases: (1) an inspiratory gasp that facilitates an increase of lung volume to total lung capacity; (2) compression phase, during which the epiglottis closes along with the vocal cords, increasing intrathoracic pressure; and (3) the expulsive phase, during which the epiglottis relaxes and suddenly opens so that air under pressure in the lungs explodes outward, producing a cough (Guyton, 1981). This increased velocity of air flow increases the gas–liquid interaction along the central airways, creating detachment of mucus from the airway wall.

In abnormal situations, any portion of the airway clearance process may be dysfunctional, leading to retained secretions, or there may be hypersecretion of mucus in the airways. Accumulation of secretions in the airways leads to partial or total obstruction. Ventilation and gas exchange are altered, and a favorable environment for infection is produced.

Recently, newer methods for airway clearance have been described in the literature. Although these techniques offer independence and, it is hoped, greater compliance, they have raised concerns and controversies regarding effectiveness of therapy and "best therapy." These techniques are gaining greater acceptance and have been implemented for routine care of cystic fibrosis in several areas around the world. They are now gaining interest in the United States, especially for older children and adolescents, because they allow for more independence and compliance. There are now more therapy options for airway clearance than were available in the recent past. Ongoing research to continue to support findings to match the most effective therapy with the individual will contribute to quality of life issues in this rapidly expanding area. Table 16–5 summarizes information on these techniques as well as traditional ACTs. Advantages and disadvantages of the new techniques are also addressed, along with age indicators. For further reading, Hardy (1994) provides a comprehensive review of the newer ACTs.

The patient approach for these newer interventions must include assessment of the following: severity and type of lung disease, physical ability to perform the technique, effectiveness of the particular technique, and age of the child. Other psychosocial factors to be considered are motivation to learn, compliance, cost, and payer or reimbursement. The skill level of the "educator" is another factor to consider. The educator or health care provider must carefully evaluate the child's response to

Table 16–5
Airway Clearance Techniques (ACTs)

Airway Clearance Technique (ACT)	Description	Benefits/Advantages	Disadvantages/Problems
Postural Drainage and Percussion (PD&P)	Mobilizes secretions by using dependent positioning, gravity, and percussion Vibration with expiration can be used Mechanical percussor can be used (vs. cupped hands)	Gold standard Localize therapy to involved segment Can be assisted with mechanical percussor Used by all ages; especially infants, toddlers, and preschool children	Time-consuming Usually needs another person to do all lobes Difficult to apply in any setting Difficult to tolerate with O_2 dependency, gastroesophageal reflux, and implanted venous access devices Does not foster independence Adherence problems Carpal tunnel syndrome reported by some caregivers
Autogenic Drainage (AD) (Self-Drainage)	Controlled method of breathing using three different lung volumes	Effective Needs no external devices Allows for independence	Labor- and time-intensive to teach and learn Must be able to take directions >12 yr of age
Active Cycle of Breathing Technique (ACBT)	Combines three methods: 1. Thoracic expansion exercises 2. Breathing control 3. Forced expiratory techniques in a set cycle	Allows for independence Absence of desaturation or compromise during therapy No costly equipment	Not useful for infants and young children
Positive Expiratory Pressure (PEP)	Breathes out 10–20 times through a flow resister, creating positive pressure in airway to about 15–20 cm H_2O during exhalation, followed by 2–3 "huff" coughs Cycle repeated up to 20 min	Allows for independence Not reported to cause compromise with desaturation Can be done by children >3 yr of age	Potential complication of pneumothorax
High-Frequency Chest Compression (HFCC)	High-frequency oscillation to chest wall delivered by a vest	Allows for independence for older children Possible future application for younger children	Trial time to determine effectiveness prior to rental/purchase Patients may not tolerate the feeling from the compression Equipment must be rented or purchased Requires storage space Requires concentration May be uncomfortable if child has venous access device that is being used during the respiratory treatment
Exercise	Many choices of activities An activity that requires physical exertion, endurance, and upper body strengthening Consult CF team physical therapist for individual program	May not cost anything May apply in many situations Socially acceptable May also improve cardiovascular fitness, self-esteem, and general health	May cost for membership to clubs or gyms; depends on climate Limited to physical ability
Flutter Valve	Small pipe-like device with a metal ball rotating freely within pipe Patients inhale and actively exhale through pipe, which generates positive pressure to about 15–25 cm H_2O. Oscillations are transmitted to airways. This is done for 5–15 breaths, followed by 2–3 huffs through flutter until lungs are clear, or for 20 min.	Allows independence Requires cooperation	Requires purchase of the device

Personal communication, Tom Newton, RCP Memorial Miller Children's Hospital, 1995.

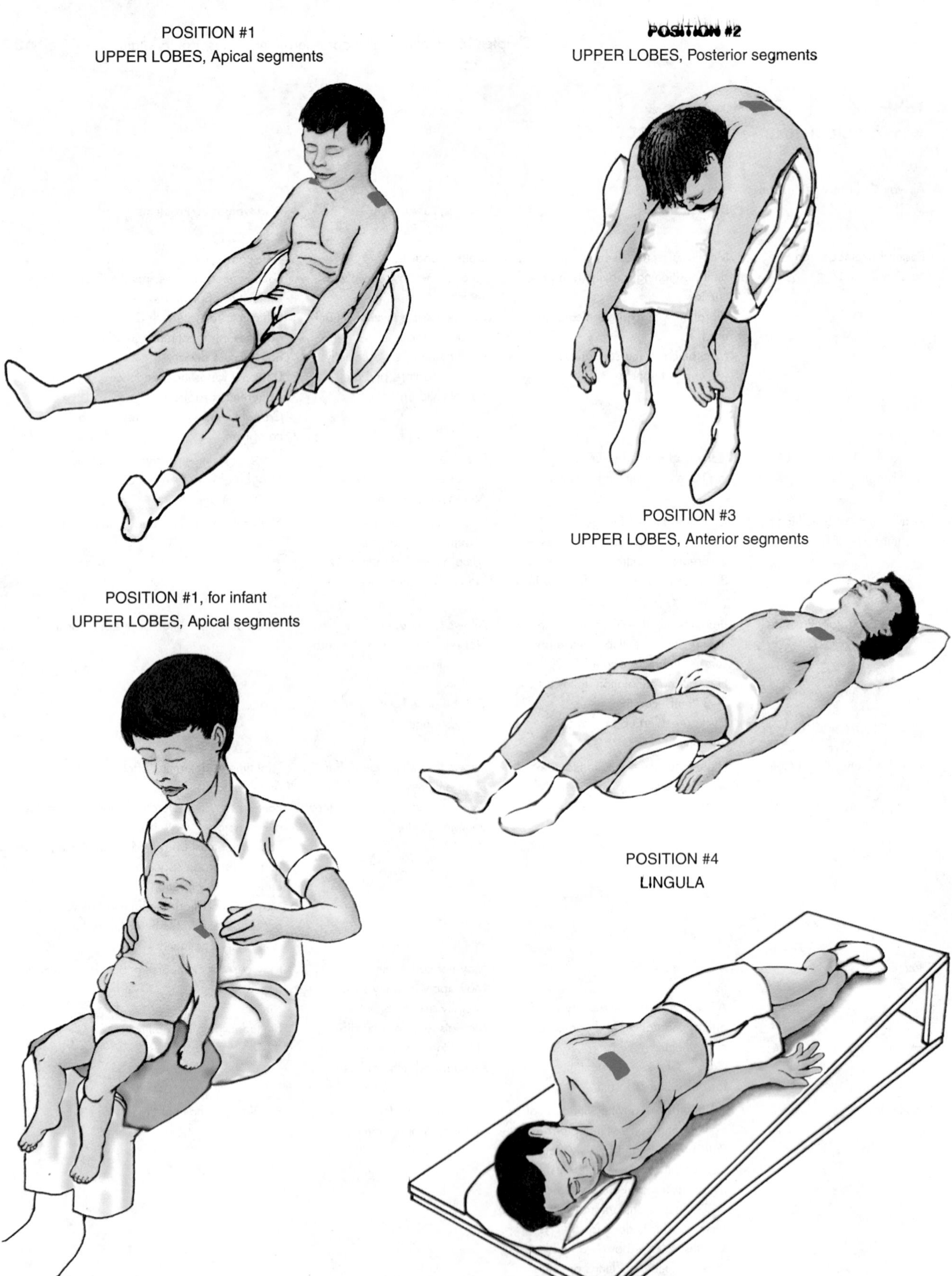

Figure 16–9
Postural drainage in children. (© Cystic Fibrosis Foundation, 1992. Used with permission.)

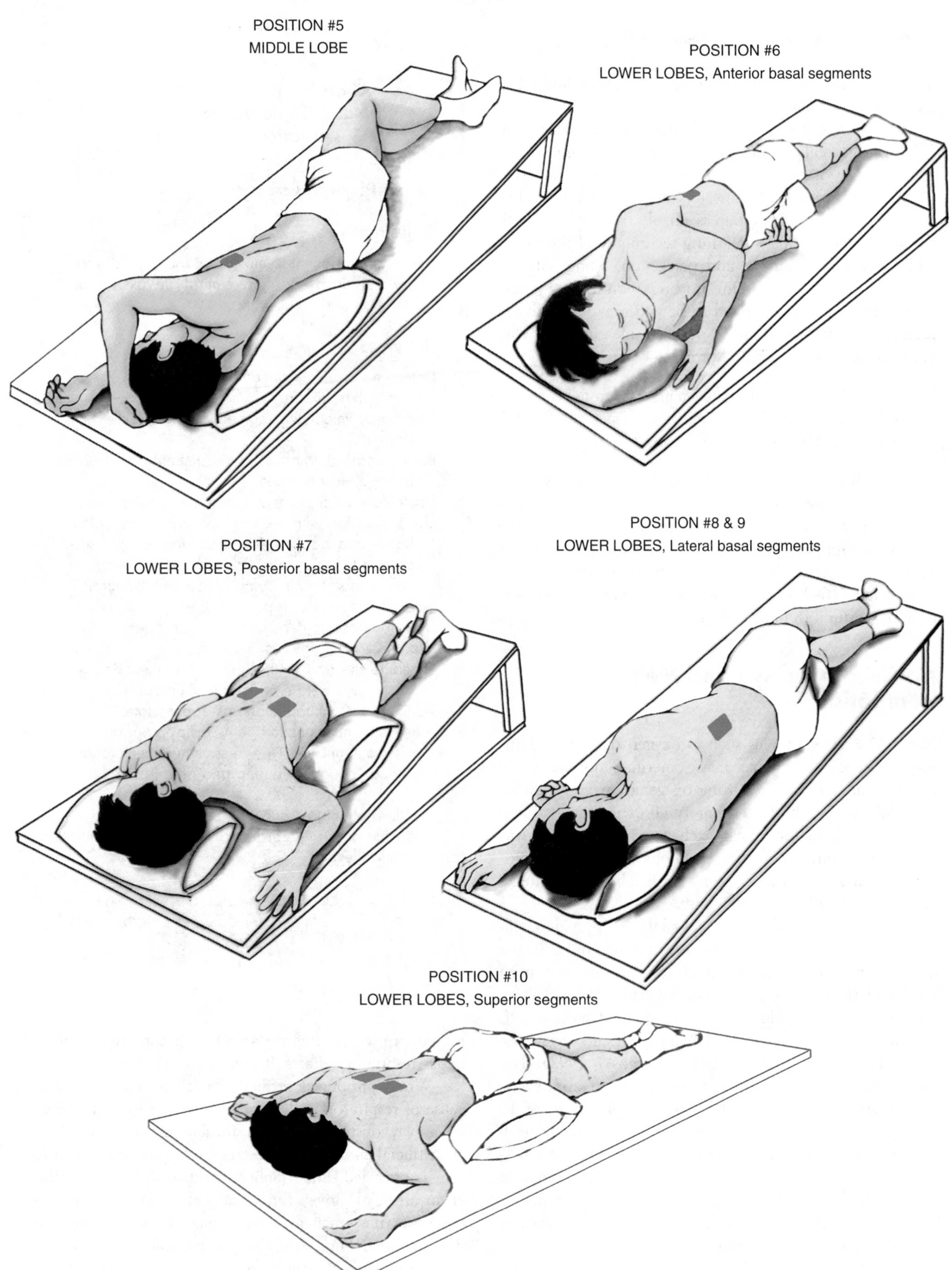
POSITION #5
MIDDLE LOBE
POSITION #6
LOWER LOBES, Anterior basal segments
POSITION #7
LOWER LOBES, Posterior basal segments
POSITION #8 & 9
LOWER LOBES, Lateral basal segments
POSITION #10
LOWER LOBES, Superior segments

Figure 16–9 *Continued*

any airway clearance technique so that appropriate effectiveness can be determined.

In practice today, postural drainage and percussion (PD&P), also called chest physiotherapy, continues to be the mainstay of therapy in the United States (Fig. 16–9). It is the primary therapy for infants and young children, because this age group is unable to cooperate with the required controlled breathing techniques of the newer ACTs. Postural drainage and percussion, along with all the ACTs, requires careful nursing monitoring. These techniques are recommended to be performed 30 minutes prior to mealtimes. This is a safety measure to avoid vomiting and aspiration and promote comfort.

caREminder: *Supplemental continuous gastrostomy tube or nasogastric tube feedings must be discontinued for at least 30 minutes prior to the therapy.*

The health care provider must exercise caution for individuals with gastroesophageal reflux. Oxygen saturations are monitored during therapy, particularly when the Trendelenburg position is used, because this position may be poorly tolerated by patients with respiratory compromise. Chart 16–8 outlines nursing interventions for performing postural drainage and percussion.

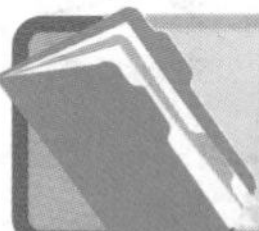

Chart 16–8
Nursing Interventions Classification (NIC)

Chest Physiotherapy

Definition

Assisting the patient to move airway secretions from peripheral airways to more central airways for expectoration and/or suctioning

Activities

Determine presence of contraindications for use of chest physiotherapy.
Determine which lung segment(s) needs to be drained.
Position patient with the lung segment to be drained in uppermost position.
Use pillows to support patient in designated position.
Use percussion with postural drainage by cupping hands and clapping the chest wall in rapid succession to produce a series of hollow sounds.
Use chest vibration in combination with postural drainage, as appropriate.
Use an ultrasonic nebulizer, as appropriate.
Use aerosol therapy, as appropriate.
Schedule chest physiotherapy around meal times—30 minutes before or 1 hour after meals.
Administer bronchodilators, as appropriate.
Administer mucokinetic agents, as appropriate.
Monitor amount and type of sputum expectoration.
Encourage coughing during and after postural drainage.
Monitor patient tolerance via SaO_2, respiratory rhythm and rate, cardiac rhythm and rate, and comfort levels.

Adapted from McCloskey, J., & Bulechek, G. (1996). *Nursing interventions classifications (NIC)* (2nd ed.). St. Louis: Mosby–Year Book. Used with permission.

Artificial Airways and Mechanical Ventilation

Non-invasive techniques such as oxygen therapy and airway clearance techniques may sometimes not meet the needs of all children requiring oxygenation and ventilation. When the child's respiratory effort is increased and inadequate to maintain gas exchange because of airway obstruction, intrapulmonary pathophysiology, neuromuscular disease, or other factors, artificial or mechanical ventilation may become necessary.

There are several methods available to provide artificial ventilation. A bag-valve-mask unit or Ambu bag is used to manually ventilate a child who has not been intubated (placement of an endotracheal tube). Effective bag-valve-mask ventilation is best provided with a self-inflating bag and a mask that properly fits over the child's nose and mouth (Zander & Hazinski, 1992). The nurse ensures that the bag is connected to an oxygen source with oxygen being delivered at a flow rate of 10 to 15 L/min. To provide an open airway, the child's neck is slightly extended in the sniffing position and the jaw is lifted (Fig. 16–10). Caution is taken in the pediatric trauma victim with possible spinal injury or in infants for whom overextending the neck can occlude the airway. A seal is created with the mask, held with the non-dominant hand, placed over the nose and mouth of the child. The dominant hand compresses the bag rhythmically and in synchrony (or slightly faster) with the child's spontaneous respiratory efforts, if present.

When prolonged artificial ventilation is needed because of respiratory failure or anesthesia, or when there is an airway obstruction, then intubation or placement of an artificial airway is necessary and mechanical ventilation is provided. Endotracheal intubation is the insertion of an artificial airway (endotracheal tube) through either the nose (nasotracheal) or the mouth (orotracheal) into the trachea (Fig. 16–11). Mechanical ventilation replaces the work of breathing and involves inflation of the lungs with compressed gas applied by either positive or

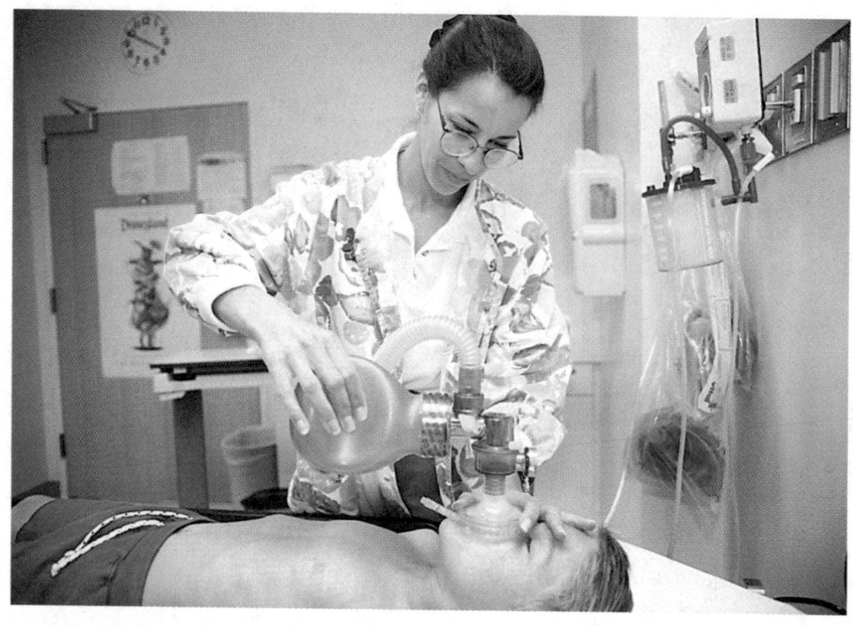

Figure 16–10
Child being ventilated using the bag-valve-mask technique.

negative pressure. Positive pressure ventilators are more commonly used than negative pressure machines. They work by creating pressure at the airway opening that is greater than the intra-alveolar pressure, thus forcing pressurized gas into the lungs. This flow of compressed gas improves gas exchange and inflation of poorly ventilated portions of the lungs. Negative pressure machines are more cumbersome and are primarily used for long-term ventilation in persons with respiratory failure caused by neuromuscular diseases. The machines consist of a body shell or tank (iron lung) that works by creating intermittent negative pressure around the thorax, causing the chest to be drawn outward and inspiration to occur. Negative pressure machines do not require an artificial airway. A newer mode of providing mechanical ventilation is called high-frequency ventilation. This machine works by delivering oxygen under high pressures at a rapidly cycling rate. Chart 16–9 outlines nursing interventions in caring for the intubated child receiving mechanical ventilation.

Figure 16–11
An intubated child. The tube has not yet been secured in place.

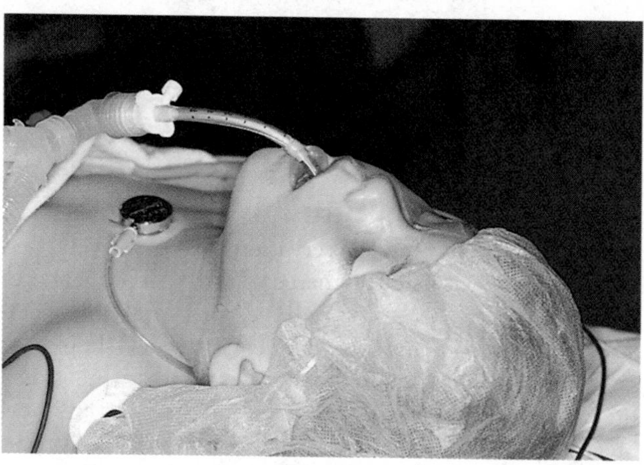

Tracheostomy

A tracheostomy consists of the surgical placement of an artificial airway directly into the trachea below the larynx. Many conditions in children that can cause upper airway obstruction, respiratory failure, or prolonged intubation may need to be managed with placement of a tracheostomy tube. In some clinical conditions such as laryngotracheomalacia, subglottic stenosis, or vocal cord paralysis, the tracheostomy may be long-term, until the condition is outgrown or corrected. Emergencies such as epiglottitis or foreign body aspiration may require a tracheostomy for more short-term management. In some cases, such as in chronic respiratory failure with long-term mechanical ventilation, the tracheostomy may be permanent.

Tracheostomy tubes are made of Silastic, silicone, or metal and are available in various sizes and lengths. The appropriate size is determined based on the child's age and size. Single cannula tracheostomy tubes are most commonly used in pediatric patients because they have a smaller inner diameter and are usually made of Silastic, which better conforms to the shape of the trachea. For older children, a tracheostomy tube with an inner cannula may be used. The inner cannula is removed for cleaning while the outer cannula is left in place. Additionally, some tracheostomy tubes have external cuffs.

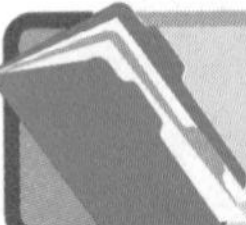

Chart 16–9
Nursing Interventions Classification (NIC)

Mechanical Ventilation

Definition

Use of an artificial device to assist a patient to breathe

Activities

Monitor for respiratory muscle fatigue.
Monitor for impending respiratory failure.
Consult with other health care personnel in selection of a ventilator mode.
Initiate setup and application of the ventilator.
Instruct the patient and family about the rationale and expected sensations associated with use of mechanical ventilators.
Routinely monitor ventilator settings.
Monitor for decrease in exhale volume and increase in inspiratory pressure.
Ensure that ventilator alarms are on.
Administer muscle-paralyzing agents, sedatives, and narcotic analgesics, as appropriate.
Monitor the effectiveness of mechanical ventilation on patient's physiologic and psychological status.
Initiate calming techniques, as appropriate.
Provide patient with a means for communication (e.g., paper and pencil or alphabet board).
Check all ventilator connections regularly.
Empty condensed water from water traps, as appropriate.
Ensure change of ventilator circuits every 24 hours, as appropriate.
Use aseptic technique, as appropriate.
Monitor ventilator pressure readings and breath sounds.
Stop nasogastric feedings during suctioning and 30 to 60 minutes before chest physiotherapy.
Silence ventilator alarms during suctioning to decrease frequency of false alarms.
Monitor patient's progress on current ventilator settings and make appropriate changes as ordered.
Monitor for adverse effects of mechanical ventilation; infection, barotrauma, and reduced cardiac output.
Position to facilitate ventilation/perfusion matching ("good lung down"), as appropriate.
Collaborate with physician to use CPAP or PEEP to minimize alveolar hypoventilation, as appropriate.
Perform chest physical therapy, as appropriate.
Perform suctioning, based on presence of adventitious sounds and/or increased ventilatory pressures.
Promote adequate fluid and nutritional intake.
Provide routine oral care.
Monitor effects of ventilator changes on oxygenation: ABG, SaO_2, SvO_2, end-tidal CO_2, Q_{sp}/Q_1, and A-aDO_2 levels and patient's subjective response.
Monitor degree of shunt, vital capacity, V_d/V_1, MVV, inspiratory force, and FEV_1 for readiness to wean from mechanical ventilation, based on agency protocol.

CPAP, continuous positive airway pressure; PEEP, positive end-expiratory pressure; ABG, arterial blood gases; MVV, maximal voluntary ventilation.
From McCloskey, J., & Bulechek, G. (1996). *Nursing interventions classification (NIC)* (2nd ed.). St. Louis, MO: Mosby–Year Book. Reprinted with permission.

Most pediatric tubes do not have an external cuff because of the small airway diameter and increased risk of trauma to the airway caused by the cuff. Because cuffless single cannula tracheostomy tubes are used in the majority of children, explanation of the nursing care focuses on these.

While the child is hospitalized, nursing care involves preparing the child and family preoperatively, providing skilled nursing care and observation postoperatively, and facilitating a successful discharge plan for home management if the tracheostomy will be long-term. Preoperatively, the child and the family/caregivers should be given an explanation of the need for the tracheostomy tube, basic anatomy and physiology of the airway, how breathing will be different, what to expect postoperatively, and how the child will look when he or she returns from surgery. If possible, allow the family to see a tracheostomy tube and supplies to help decrease anxiety about what to expect.

Postoperative nursing care should focus on close observation to maintain a patent airway and monitoring of possible complications such as hemorrhage, edema, subcutaneous emphysema, pneumothorax, and accidental decannulation. Because infants and children are at greater risk for tracheostomy obstruction related to the relatively smaller airway, they should be initially managed in an intensive care or close observation unit postoperatively (Fitton, 1994).

▽ **Alert:** *All children with a tracheostomy should have an extra tracheostomy tube of the same size available at the bedside in case the tube in place becomes obstructed and unable to clear or is dislodged.*

Respiratory assessments include vital signs and examination of the child's color, respiratory rate and effort, breath sounds, and type and amount of secretions and should be performed every 15 minutes until the patient is stable and then every 1 to 2 hours for the first 24 hours postoperatively. For the first 5 to 6 days, until the tracheocutaneous tract is well formed, long sutures (stay sutures) attached to the trachea are taped to the chest. The sutures can be used to keep the stoma open in the event of an accidental decannulation. The surgeon removes the sutures when the tract in the trachea is formed.

It is important that the airway remain patent to prevent obstruction and possible complications. The child may require frequent suctioning for several hours immediately after the procedure because there are often excessive and sometimes bloody secretions. Frequency of suctioning should then be provided on an as-needed basis to prevent occlusion of the tracheostomy tube from secretions and mucous plugs. Complications of suctioning can include hypoxemia, hypotension, bradycardia (vasovagal responses), laryngospasm, bronchospasm, atelectasis, and trauma to the airway. Precautions the nurse should take when suctioning the child with an artificial airway include gauging the suction pressure (should be between 80 and 100 mmHg), limiting the time for suctioning (no longer than 4 to 5 seconds) and the number of suction passes, monitoring the depth of the suction catheter (¼ to ½ inch beyond the tip of the length of the airway), and providing manual ventilations with oxygen and/or rest time between suction passes (Fitton, 1994; Runton, 1992). Sterile isotonic saline without preservatives may be instilled (0.5 to 3 mL, depending on the child's size) to help loosen secretions and mucous plugs for easier removal.

The functions of warming, filtering, and humidification of inspired air that the upper respiratory tract normally performs are bypassed in a child with a tracheostomy. Therefore, humidification and warming of the inspired air are necessary to maintain loose secretions, prevent occlusion of the tube from secretions, and prevent drying of the tracheal mucosa. Nursing care is directed toward maintaining appropriate humidification via a mist collar. In addition, promoting adequate fluid intake to keep the child well hydrated is important. To prevent infection and irritation of the skin around the tracheostomy tube, stoma care should be provided to keep the skin clean and dry. The secretions around the stoma can be gently removed by using half-strength hydrogen peroxide and either gauze or cotton-tipped swabs. Tracheostomy ties should also be kept clean and dry and should be changed daily and as needed when soiled. The schedule of tracheostomy tube changes varies depending on the institution or physician preference, but they are generally performed once a week in the child with a well-healed tracheostomy stoma (Chart 16–10).

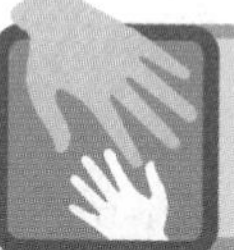

Chart 16–10
Nursing Interventions

Tracheostomy Tube Changes

The first tracheostomy tube change usually is done by the surgeon approximately 5 days after the tracheotomy is performed. Subsequent tracheostomy tube changes are performed by the nurse or respiratory therapist, depending on the institution. There is no standard schedule of when tracheostomy tubes should be changed; although it is recommended that the tube be changed before a feeding or meal to avoid stimulation that could cause emesis. Once the tract and stoma are well healed, tube changes can be done once a week. Smaller-diameter tubes may need to be changed more frequently because of risk of occlusion from mucous plugs. Changing of the tracheostomy tube should be done using sterile technique while the child is hospitalized to reduce risk of infection; however, "clean" technique is taught to parents once the child is home because tracheostomy tubes are often cleaned and reused for a period of time at home. Prepare the new tube with the tracheostomy ties attached and the obturator in place. It is helpful to have a second person help hold and position the child during the procedure. Suction the child to minimize secretions. While holding the old tracheostomy tube in place, cut the old tracheostomy ties and remove the tube from the stoma. Gently insert the new tube into the stoma using a forward and downward motion following the natural curve of the trachea. Immediately remove the obturator and assess for adequacy of ventilation by listening for air movement from the tracheostomy tube and auscultating breath sounds.

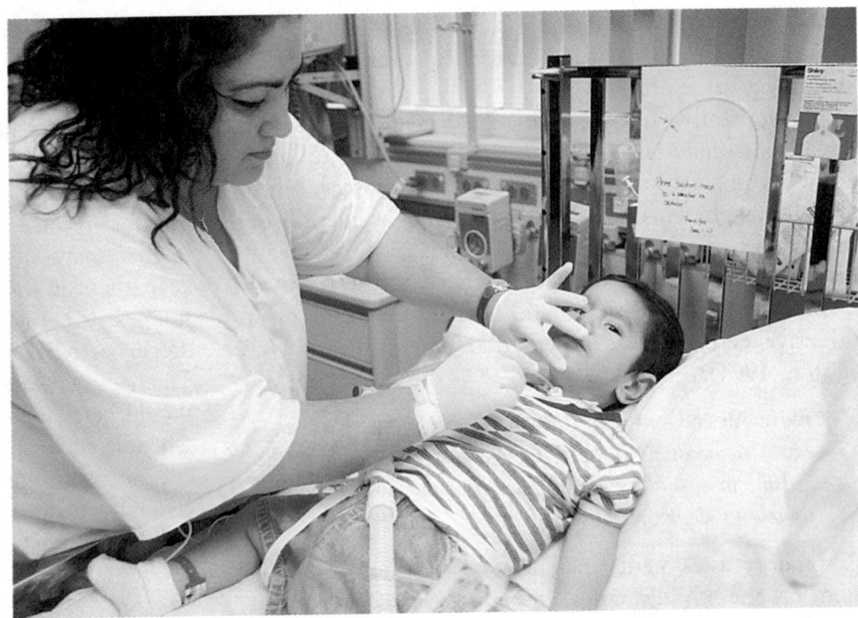

Figure 16–12
Caregivers should be given ample opportunity to take care of the child's tracheostomy before the child is discharged.

Because many children are going home with tracheostomy tubes, it has become necessary to teach parents and/or other significant caretakers how to care for the child at home (Fig. 16–12). TIP 16–2 outlines a teaching instructional plan for the child who has had a tracheostomy tube placed. It is also helpful to ensure that visiting nursing is provided following discharge to assist the family with the routine care of the child.

TIP 16–2 A Teaching Intervention Plan for the Child Receiving Home Tracheostomy Care

Nursing Diagnoses and Family Outcomes

- Risk for injury related to management of tracheostomy
  Outcome: Family will verbalize and identify factors in handling an airway emergency with a tracheostomy.
- Knowledge deficit related to home maintenance management of tracheostomy
  Outcome: Family will identify and demonstrate all aspects of home care of the child prior to discharge.

Instructional Interventions

Suctioning

- Identify need for suctioning: sound of mucus in the tracheostomy tube; breathing sounds "rattled"; child is restless or appears anxious; child's color is pale or dusky; there is difficulty feeding.
- Connect suction catheter to suction tubing and be careful not to touch tip of catheter. Instill a few drops of sterile saline (0.5 to 2 cc, depending on size) into the tracheostomy tube, and allow child to take a few breaths.
- Insert the suction catheter to the predetermined depth (depending on tracheostomy tube size) and place thumb over port to apply suction. Pull back catheter while twirling catheter between thumb and index finger.
- Rinse mucus from catheter with sterile saline, and repeat as necessary.

TIP 16–2 A Teaching Intervention Plan for the Child Receiving Home Tracheostomy Care *Continued*

Stoma Care

- Tracheostomy site requires daily care and observation for signs of infection or complications.
- Keep skin and stoma site clean and dry. Gently clean skin and stoma with a clean wet washcloth. Use half-strength hydrogen peroxide to remove thicker, crusted secretions if necessary.
- Inspect stoma site for signs of infection or breakdown of the skin around the stoma.
- Change tracheostomy ties daily and as needed when soiled or wet. Ties should be kept clean and dry and should be made of durable non-fraying material. Inspect skin around neck for redness, irritation, and/or breakdown from the ties.

Tracheostomy Tube Change

- Routine tracheostomy tube changes are usually done once a week or more often as needed or ordered by the physician.
- Gather all supplies, wash hands thoroughly, and prepare child for procedure. A second person is needed to assist with positioning of the child. Position child with neck slightly extended; may use a towel roll placed under the shoulders.
- Suction child to minimize secretions. Cut old ties while holding tracheostomy tube in place. Remove old tube from stoma and gently insert new tracheostomy tube with obturator into the stoma using a downward and forward motion following the curve of the trachea.
- Quickly remove the obturator, assess for adequacy of ventilation, and secure the tracheostomy ties.

Daily Care and Home Environment

- Caution should be taken when feeding the infant or child so that food or formula does not get into the tracheostomy. If this should occur, suction the tracheostomy immediately. Never prop a bottle or leave the infant or child unattended while feeding.
- Child may be bathed in a tub, being sure to keep the water shallow and not allowing water to get into the tracheostomy tube. Never leave the child unattended in the tub, and do not put the child in a shower. Avoid use of talcum and baby powders on the infant or child.
- Encourage normal play both indoors and outdoors as much as possible. Avoid toys that are fuzzy or have small removable parts. On cold and windy days outside, the tracheostomy may be loosely covered with a mask or 100% cotton scarf. Children should avoid play in sandboxes, in or around pools/lakes/ocean, and participation in contact sports.
- When buying clothes, avoid those with high, tight necklines that may cover the tracheostomy opening.
- Do not allow smoking in the child's home or around the child.

Safety and Emergency Care

- The tracheostomy tube should be changed or replaced immediately if accidental dislodgement or occlusion of the tube should occur.
- Keep all emergency telephone numbers by the telephone and a copy with the family at all times.
- Be sure to have all necessary equipment (extra tracheostomy tube with ties, suction machine and catheters, Ambu bag, etc.) with child when traveling or going on "outings" outside the home.
- Keep flashlight handy in case of power failure, and notify electric and telephone companies that there is a child with special health care life-sustaining needs in the home.

TIP continued on following page

TIP 16–2 A Teaching Intervention Plan for the Child Receiving Home Tracheostomy Care *Continued*

- Keep all immunizations up to date.
- Tension on tracheostomy ties should be checked daily. Tracheostomy ties should be tight enough to allow the smallest finger to be slipped underneath. Twill tape tracheostomy ties can stretch after being initially secured, so recheck in 1 to 2 hours for appropriate tightness.
- Tracheostomy ties should be tied on the side of the neck to prevent skin breakdown on the back of the neck.

Contact Health Care Provider if

- There is a fever higher than 101°F.
- The child is having difficulty breathing or the breathing pattern changes.
- The child's lips or nail beds become bluish or dusky.
- There is an increase in secretions or change in color, odor, or consistency of the secretions.
- There is blood (greater than a teaspoon) coming from the tracheostomy.
- There is difficulty inserting the tube with a routine tracheostomy tube change.
- There is a rash, drainage, or unusual odor around the tracheostomy stoma.
- Food or formula is coming through the tracheostomy tube.

Alterations in Respiratory Status

Congenital Abnormalities of the Respiratory System

Congenital abnormalities or malformations of the respiratory systems are fortunately rare. These disorders result in respiratory dysfunction primarily caused by airway obstructions or collapse. The specific conditions discussed in this section are choanal atresia, Pierre Robin syndrome, laryngomalacia, and tracheomalacia.

The diagnosis of these abnormalities is generally made at birth or shortly thereafter, when the child exhibits varying degrees of respiratory distress. The treatment is largely supportive. Surgical interventions to relieve the obstruction or structurally support the airway are uncommon. Adequate nutritional support to promote optimal weight gain is a key intervention. These conditions improve with growth, and in the absence of other congenital anomalies, the prognosis for normal respiratory function is good.

Choanal Atresia and Pierre Robin Syndrome

Severe acute airway obstruction in the newborn is rare and is usually the result of congenital anomalies and malformations or sequences of combined anomalies. Choanal atresia and Pierre Robin syndrome are two of the relatively common examples of congenital anomalies that can cause acute and/or chronic upper airway obstruction and lead to respiratory distress, feeding problems, or even death.

Pathophysiology

Choanal atresia, the most common congenital anomaly of the nose, consists of a unilateral or bilateral bony or membranous septum between the nose and the pharynx. In some cases, only stenosis is present. When only one side is affected, the infant does not usually have severe symptoms at birth, and the diagnosis may be suggested only at the time of the first respiratory infection, when there is unilateral nasal discharge or disproportionately severe upper airway obstruction (Arnold, 1996).

Pierre Robin syndrome was first reported in 1923 by a French physician, for whom the condition was later named. He described the association of newborn micrognathia (abnormally small jaw, especially the lower portion) with upper airway obstruction caused by glossoptosis (a prolapse of the tongue into the pharyngeal airway) and cleft palate (Robin, 1923) (Fig. 16–13). Like choanal atresia, this syndrome is a congenital disorder. It occurs approximately once in every 30,000 live births. It is thought to be initiated by hypoplasia of the mandible before 9 weeks' gestation. This malformation of the mandible restricts the tongue to a posterior position, which

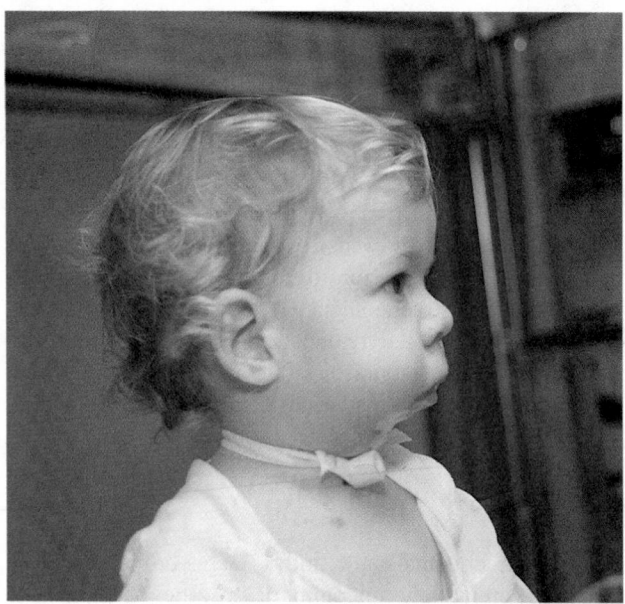

Figure 16–13
In the child with Pierre Robin syndrome, malformation of the mandible makes the chin appear recessed and restricts the tongue to a posterior position, causing easy occlusion of the airway. A tracheostomy is necessary to maintain an open airway.

then interferes with fusion of the growing palatal shelves and results in a wide, U-shaped palatal cleft. Thus, the cleft palate and glossoptosis occur sequentially from the initial effect of the mandibular anomaly (Shprintzen, 1988).

Assessment

Because most newborns are obligate nose breathers, bilateral choanal atresia is usually associated with immediate apnea and cyanosis requiring endotracheal intubation and resuscitation. Infants who must be able to mouth breathe immediately experience difficulty with sucking and swallowing and become cyanotic with feeding. These infants require intubation for maintaining the mouth in an open position by taping of a large oral airway in place and require nutritional supplementation by using gavage feedings.

Intermittent upper airway obstruction is the hallmark manifestation of Pierre Robin syndrome. Obstruction and sudden death are more common in the supine position, during feeding, and in active sleep cycles when pharyngeal muscle tone is weak or absent. Obstruction is generally relieved by crying, which causes pharyngeal muscles to become taut and stimulated. The child with Pierre Robin syndrome is often cyanotic during feedings and is subject to frequent severe respiratory tract infections or pneumonia. Normal feeding is difficult because the pharyngeal obstruction predisposes the infant to aspiration. Failure to gain weight is common, and gavage or gastrostomy feedings may be necessary. Chronic obstruction may result in pulmonary edema, pulmonary hypertension, and cor pulmonale. Pierre Robin syndrome, like choanal atresia, may occur in sequence with other congenital anomalies, yet may also occur in otherwise normal infants.

Interdisciplinary Interventions

Respiratory assessment of the infant with choanal atresia or Pierre Robin syndrome should focus on adequacy of oxygenation. Respiratory rate, presence of tachypnea, skin color and temperature, retractions, transcutaneous oxygen, carbon dioxide level, and oxygen saturation all are important parameters to monitor. The presence of cyanosis during feeding is, especially, a key assessment finding. Polysomnographic recordings, which provide data regarding heart and respiratory rate, oxygen saturation, breathing effort, and airflow during sleep, are helpful assessments in determining the severity of airway obstruction. Observing and assessing for signs of chronic obstruction (cor pulmonale) is also important.

Surgical excision of the obstruction is most often a successful treatment for choanal atresia. Some surgeons advise immediate correction, whereas others feel that if the infant's respiratory status is not significantly compromised, surgery can be scheduled electively after the infant's condition stabilizes. Postoperatively, both nares are intubated to prevent recurrence of the obstruction by swelling. Although the prognosis for an infant having a surgically corrected choanal atresia is good related solely to respiratory function, the presence and severity of other multiple birth defects that often occur simultaneously with choanal atresia affect long-term general prognosis.

Methods of treatment for Pierre Robin syndrome include (1) positional therapy only, (2) placement of an oral or nasopharyngeal airway (a clear plastic tube positioned in the oral cavity or nasopharynx to maintain a patent airway), (3) surgical creation of a tongue-lip adhesion to hold the tongue forward, and (4) tracheostomy. With adequate nutrition and growth of the mandible, the problems may resolve by 6 to 12 months of age (Corbett, 1990).

Proper positioning of the infant with Pierre Robin syndrome is a key nursing intervention.

Alert: *The infant must be maintained in the prone position as much as possible to prevent the tongue from obstructing the pharynx and causing respiratory distress. Improper positioning can quickly result in complete obstruction and death.*

A tracheostomy is necessary for infants unresponsive to conservative airway management. Maintaining adequate pulmonary toilet by tracheal suctioning then becomes an important intervention, as does parental education regarding care of the tracheostomy and safety considerations (see TIP 16–2).

Community Care

Feeding and nutritional assessments of the child with choanal atresia or Pierre Robin syndrome are crucial. Oral feeding patterns should be carefully evaluated for signs of cyanosis and/or aspiration, with safe airway management and careful observation for airway obstruction being the primary objective. For children with gavage or gastrostomy tube feedings, the possibility of vomiting and/or gastroesophageal reflux also mandates diligent airway assessment during and after feedings. These children's growth should be plotted against norms for age on a regular basis and close attention paid to the potential for failure to thrive. Feeding problems caused by a cleft palate and/or small mandible and prolapsed tongue can sometimes be effectively managed with modified nipples. If gavage or gastrostomy feedings are necessary, parental education on feeding techniques is a key intervention provided by nurses, occupational therapists, or feeding therapists. Nutritionists provide information on preparing special high-calorie formulas, if needed. Providing adequate nutritional support promotes optimal growth of the mandible and possible resolution of the airway obstruction.

As described here, early and ongoing support and education of parents of a child with choanal atresia and/or Pierre Robin syndrome and any other associated congenital anomalies is of utmost importance. A diagnosis of a congenital defect in a child creates a crisis for the family. Parents of the infant with a congenital anomaly exhibit a myriad of emotions and behaviors as they grieve for the "lost" perfect child. They may express concerns and feelings of fear of the unknown, guilt, anger, grief, and inadequacy. Guilt is a common reaction when parents are told their infant has a congenital anomaly. It is important to reinforce the concept that in most cases the cause of the defect is unknown and not the fault of the parents. One of the first tasks of the nurse is to provide the necessary education to help clarify information related to the diagnosis. Education and support must then focus on facilitating the parent's understanding of the infant's needs. Most commonly this includes appropriate positioning and feeding techniques, possible home apnea/bradycardia monitoring, and instruction on tracheostomy or gastrostomy feedings. Teaching appropriate skills for meeting those needs and aiding the parents in acquiring confidence in their capacity to care for their child facilitates discharge from the hospital. An interdisciplinary approach, including occupational therapists/feeding specialists, nutritionists, and social workers, in collaboration with physicians and nurses, will have the highest degree of success in supporting and educating families in their transition to independent care of their child with choanal atresia or Pierre Robin syndrome.

Laryngomalacia and Tracheomalacia

Laryngomalacia and tracheomalacia are defects of the airways characterized by weakness and poor tone in a particular area of the respiratory tree. A child can have laryngomalacia, tracheomalacia, tracheobronchomalacia, or a combination. Laryngomalacia is the congenital abnormality of the larynx. Tracheomalacia and tracheobronchomalacia are classified as either primary (congenital) or secondary (acquired) conditions.

Pathophysiology

Primary tracheomalacia and tracheobronchomalacia, which are relatively uncommon, are the result of the congenital immaturity of the airway cartilages. Secondary conditions, which are more common, are due to a degeneration of the previously normal cartilaginous support. This occurs most often in premature infants as a result of prolonged intubation and mechanical ventilation, oxygen toxicity, or recurrent infections. In infants, the lumen of the airway remains intact largely because of the support of the tracheal cartilage. If the cartilaginous rings are congenitally absent, small, malformed, or too pliable, essential support of the trachea is lacking. This lack of support is the most common cause of tracheomalacia. Fortunately, these conditions are generally a benign form of mild respiratory distress and rarely require intervention. The condition improves as the airway enlarges, and the infant generally outgrows the condition by 6 months to 1 year of age.

Assessment

As tracheal expansion and contraction occur normally with respiration, slight variations in the size of the airway are seen. These variations are minimal—for example, during sleep, when respirations are shallow, and during forceful breathing or crying, when they are more pronounced.

In the child with laryngomalacia or tracheomalacia, the affected portion of the infant's airway collapses during inspiration. This collapse creates a narrowing and is accompanied by a loud stridor. The stridor is worse when the infant is crying, positioned with neck flexed, or has a respiratory infection. Other symptoms often include cough, wheezing, and tachypnea. Retractions and labored breathing are also common symptoms. Severe respiratory distress and cyanosis can occur, but are rare. Secondary tracheobronchomalacia may also be produced by compression of blood vessels or a tumor or by aspiration of a foreign body and can cause wheezing, hyperinflation, atelectasis, and possible cyanotic spells. The diagnosis of tracheobronchomalacia is confirmed by flexible bronchoscopy under local anesthesia. This allows a view of the respiratory tree during normal spontaneous respirations.

The infant's noisy, labored breathing can be very distressing to the parents. Advice from family or friends to "do something about it" may also be upsetting. With support from health care personnel, parents gradually become very accustomed to the child's baseline respiratory status and become skilled at detecting a deviation from the baseline. In general, this condition does not affect the infant's ability to sleep, feed, or interact with the environment. Infants with laryngomalacia and/or tracheomalacia generally grow and develop normally.

Interdisciplinary Interventions

The infant will outgrow this condition as the supporting cartilage matures and enlarges. Medical management involves the control of bacterial infection and secretions with antibiotics and humidification therapy. Most cases of laryngomalacia and tracheomalacia/tracheobronchomalacia resolve completely with few residual symptoms. Rarely, a tracheostomy is indicated if the infant's respiratory distress affects the ability to ingest feedings and gain weight. Severe tracheomalacia may require stenting—a surgical reconstructive procedure to the trachea that provides additional support for the airway as it matures.

Nursing interventions include observation of the degree of respiratory distress, assessment of the infant's ability to feed, and plotting serial growth parameters (including height, weight, height-for-weight, and head circumference) on standardized growth charts with each outpatient visit. Reassure parents that the infant will outgrow the condition, usually by the end of the first year. During that time, teach parents about their child's baseline respiratory status and how to recognize variations from this. Occasionally home apnea/bradycardia monitoring is indicated, especially if the child has a history of cyanotic episodes.

Chart 16–11

How Parents Can Respond to Unsolicited Advice

- Gently remind the individual that the child's condition is being well monitored.
- Thank them for their concern, but assure them that you are following advice from health care professionals.
- Discuss baseline respiratory status and potential deviations from baseline.
- Change the subject.
- Limit contact with an especially persistent or upsetting individual.

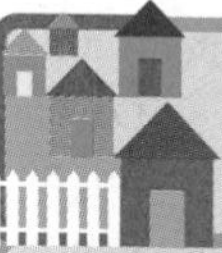

Chart 16–12
Community Care

Respiratory Distress: When to Seek Help from the Health Care Provider

- Infant/child's respiratory rate (at rest or during sleep) is more than 60 breaths per minute.
- Child seems to be "working hard" to breathe. This may include moving his or her head and moving shoulders up and down with each breath, grunting, or gasping.
- There is bluish coloration of lips, nail beds, and/or oral mucosa.
- There is "pulling" or "caved in" appearance of skin and musculature between ribs, below sternum, or under ribcage with each inspiration.
- Child demonstrates extreme irritability or restlessness and is not interested in feeding (infants) or meals (older children).
- Child has no interest in usual activities or is unable to play as a result of breathing difficulties.

Community Care

The role of the nurse is also to assist the family to ensure adequate intake of formula or breast milk (either by actual breast-feeding or breast milk expressed into a bottle) and solid foods as the infant reaches the appropriate age for their introduction. Routine infant health care is administered. Teach parents appropriate responses to unsolicited advice (Chart 16–11). Role playing may be useful. Parents need to be informed that the infant's symptoms may worsen during respiratory illnesses. If they have any concern about worsening respiratory distress, instruct them when to seek assistance from their health care professional (Chart 16–12). Parents should also be instructed in cardiopulmonary resuscitation technique.

Upper Respiratory Infections and Obstructions

Upper respiratory tract infections are extremely common in infants and young children. The upper respiratory tract, or upper airway, consists primarily of the nose, mouth, and oral pharynx. For purposes of this discussion, infections of the epiglottis, larynx, and trachea are considered in the upper respiratory tract as well. Infections of this area of the respiratory system are usually viral and self-limiting. Although the respiratory tract is equipped with several natural defense mechanisms, invading organisms frequently gain access to these structures, resulting in mild to life-threatening respiratory problems. Once infection has occurred, organisms travel freely among the structures of the upper airway, including through the eustachian tubes to the inner and middle ears. The severity of resulting illness depends on the age of the child, the nature of the organism, and the integrity of the child's immune response. Some infections can lead to inflammation and/or obstructions of the airway, or obstruction can result from noninfectious causes. Most upper respiratory conditions are treated in the home or in ambulatory care settings.

Allergic Rhinitis

Allergic rhinitis is a condition characterized by sneezing; nasal itching; thin, watery rhinorrhea; and nasal congestion. The conjunctivae and posterior pharynx may also be involved. Allergic rhinitis may be seasonal, with symptoms that correspond to specific pollen peaks in the spring or fall, or may be perennial (year-round symptoms). Some children have perennial symptoms with additional flares during pollen seasons. Allergic rhinitis is the most common of all allergic disorders, affecting 10% to 20% of the population. Allergic rhinitis accounts for 2 million days lost from school, 28 million days of restricted activity, and a cost of more than $1 billion for physician visits annually (Milgrom, 1993).

Pathophysiology

Airborne allergens come into contact with mast cells and basophils at mucosal surfaces. Mast cells have immunoglobulin E (IgE) receptors on their membrane surfaces that bind in serum. Exposure to the appropriate airborne allergens cross-links the mast cell IgE receptors and triggers the release of chemical mediators such as histamine, tryptase, leukotrienes, and prostaglandins. This mediator release causes an immediate reaction, which includes sneezing, itching, nasal congestion, and mucus secretion accompanied by nasal mucosa edema. Four to 12 hours later, there is a late-phase reaction involving cellular infiltration with basophils and eosinophils. This late-phase response causes a second, more prolonged period of nasal congestion.

Assessment

Diagnosis of allergic rhinitis is based on clinical history, family history, physical findings, and laboratory (skin test) evaluation. The child generally presents with nasal congestion, pruritus, clear rhinorrhea, and paroxysms of sneezing. The nasal congestion may be bilateral, unilateral, or variable and is often worse at night. Parents may tell you that their children sniff, snort, and frequently clear their throats. They may also twitch, pick or rub their nose, and have episodes of repetitive sneezing. There may also be itching and watering of the eyes in conjunction with nasal symptoms. Bronchospasm with coughing, shortness of breath, or chest tightness may occur in children who also have asthma. Other symptoms may include fatigue, irritability, headache, depression, and anorexia.

Allergic rhinitis is often inherited, therefore it should be determined if other family members (parents, siblings, grandparents) have a history of hay fever or allergies. Determining the presence of familial tendencies assists in making the diagnosis for the child under observation (Cornell, 1997).

On physical examination, the nurse should look for the presence of certain characteristic features that distinguish allergic rhinitis from the common cold (rhinitis) (Table 16–6). The child may have "ocular shiners," which is a bluish discoloration of the infraorbital area caused by increased venous flow related to the local allergic vigor. There may be a transverse crease across the lower third of the nose caused by the child's rubbing the nose (referred to as the "allergic salute"). Examination of the nasal cavity using a nasal speculum may reveal edematous mucosa, with swollen, boggy, and pale pink to blue-gray turbinates. Nasal secretions are generally clear, watery, or white. Microscopic examination of the nasal secretions reveals abundant eosinophils. Skin testing for sensitivity to allergens believed to contribute to the nasal symptoms may help establish specific triggers for the allergy symptoms (e.g., dust mite, cat, dog, trees, grass, or ragweed).

Interdisciplinary Interventions

The mainstay of treatment for allergic rhinitis is avoidance of the offending allergen(s). Regardless of other

Table 16–6
Differences Between Allergic Rhinitis and the Common Cold

Symptoms	Allergic Rhinitis	Common Cold
Family history of atopy	Yes	No (±)
Conjunctival pruritus	Yes	No
Fever	No	Yes (±)
Pharyngitis/laryngitis	No	Yes
Purulent secretions	No	Yes
Sinus pain	Yes	(±)

treatments used, patients must minimize contact with the offending allergen. Environmental control measures that can help relieve symptoms by limiting exposure to common indoor allergens are shown in Chart 16–13. Parents of children with seasonal (pollen-induced) allergic rhinitis must be cautioned that pollen counts are highest in the mornings between 5 and 10 A.M. Bedroom windows should be kept closed at night to limit pollen exposure. One may be able to further limit exposure by washing the child's hair each night, by drying linens indoors, and by keeping household pets either completely indoors or outdoors during pollen seasons.

Medical management involves the use of antihistamines and decongestants. Antihistamines are use to antagonize histamine at its H_1 receptor site, thereby blocking the vasodilatation, sneezing, and hypersecretion it causes. Decongestants may be helpful in reducing nasal obstruction through vasoconstriction. However, there is no evidence that has demonstrated the effectiveness of over-the-counter cold and allergy relief preparations in infants and preschool children. In addition, there are no proven recommended dosages for the young child.

Cromolyn sodium acts by stabilizing mast cell membranes; this decreases mediator release in hypersensitivity reactions. Therefore, cromolyn sodium is most helpful when used prophylactically before a pollen season begins. Cromolyn sodium is available as a topical nasal spray. Severe nasal symptoms require the addition of topical nasal steroids, which act on several levels to block local inflammation. Immunotherapy involves the subcutaneous injection of increasing amounts of an allergen to which the patient is sensitive in an attempt to decrease sensitivity and reduce the severity of clinical symptoms; it is an effective option that must be considered for those individuals who have not responded well to medications.

The nurse must educate the parents and child regarding the uses of and side effects of the medication (antihistamines, decongestants, and mast cell stabilizers). Many of the medications have not been shown to be effective, and the potential side effects and recommended dosing have not been adequately examined in infants and young children. Parents should be informed that current antihistamines can be divided into two basic types: sedating and non-sedating. Terfenadine, astemizole, and loratadine are examples of non-sedating antihistamines. These medications are not recommended for children younger than 12 years of age and have potential drug interactions that parents and health care professionals must be alerted to. The less expensive and usually shorter-acting diphenhydramine, chlorpheniramine, brompheniramine, and clemastine are a few examples of sedating antihistamines. These medications are more commonly available in cold and allergy preparations for younger children (Table 16–7).

Table 16–7
Cold and Allergy Preparations

First Generation	Side Effect	Second Generation	Side Effect
Non-selective; cross the blood-brain barrier		Selective; non-sedating; do not cross the blood-brain barrier	Not approved for children younger than the age of 12
Chlorpheniramine	Drowsiness, insomnia, nervousness, irritability, disturbed coordination, dryness of mucous membranes, urinary hesitancy, gastrointestinal upset, constipation. Potentiates central nervous system depression with alcohol.	Terfenadine	Dizziness, hypotension, insomnia, visual disturbances, dry mouth, anaphylaxis, bronchospasm, and angioedema. May not be given with antibiotics such as erythromycin or antifungals such as ketoconazole because of increased risk of hepatic dysfunction, electrolyte abnormalities, and arrhythmias.
Brompheniramine		Astemizole	Long half-life, may suppress a positive skin test for up to 6 weeks. May stimulate appetite.
Diphenhydramine	Can be sedative; can also cause mouth dryness, blurred vision, and urinary retention.		
Hydroxyzine	Can cause drowsiness and mouth dryness.		

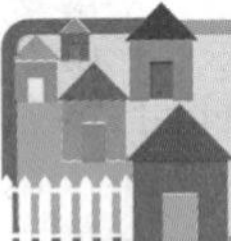

Chart 16–13
Community Care

Home and School Environmental Control of Allergies

Management of allergies and asthma consists of not only medications and family/patient education but also focuses on reducing allergen and irritant exposure in the home. Factors in the home and school, particularly smoke, dust mites, and cockroaches, may be contributing to allergy and asthma exacerbations. Identification of triggers and irritants can be explored with the child and family. Suggestions for eliminating or reducing triggers can be provided to families.

Possible suggestions include the following:

Home

- At minimum, smoking should not be allowed in the child's bedroom, in the car, and other rooms in which the child is in contact with the smoker. Have the smoker smoke outside. Ideally, smoking should be eliminated altogether.
- Encase mattresses, box springs, and pillows with airtight hypoallergenic covers. The child should avoid sleeping or lying on rugs or upholstered furniture. Use synthetic materials for all bedding, and wash bed linens and stuffed toys weekly in hot water (130°F).
- Eliminate clutter (dust collectors) including knickknacks, pictures, wall hangings, trophies, and stuffed toys from the child's bedroom. Clean and dust the child's bedroom twice a week.
- Use washable shades, vertical blinds, or curtains that are washable in hot water (130°F). Curtains should be washed every 1 to 2 weeks.
- Hardwood floors are preferred to carpeting. If able, remove carpeting from the child's room. If unable, vacuum twice a week. The child should be out of the room or house during vacuuming.
- Pets, particularly dogs and cats, should not be allowed in the child's bedroom. Wash the pet weekly; ideally, the pet should be kept outdoors.
- Avoid painting or using cleaning products around the child. The child should not be in the house when itis being cleaned. Avoid perfumes, powders, and hair sprays around child.
- Clean and dust the kitchen floor and cabinets 1 to 2 times a week to remove cockroach allergen present in house dust (especially in apartment buildings). Keep brown paper grocery bags, cardboard boxes, and newspapers outside.
- Avoid using humidifiers in the house as they promote the growth of dust mites and can harbor fungi and molds if not cleaned properly. Ideal humidity level in the house should be kept at 25% to 40%.

School

- Chalkboards should be cleaned when students are not in the classroom. Erasers should be cleaned outside.
- Paints and markers often have strong fumes; replace tops when they are not in use.
- Stuffed animals and toys should be made of synthetic washable material, stored in plastic bags, or washed several times a year.
- Teachers should use non-furbearing pets such as fish or snakes. The allergen particle from furbearing pets is smaller than the dust particle and remains in the air for a longer period of time.
- Bookshelves trap dust easily and should be dusted weekly.
- Lamps should have plain shades rather than pleated shades that can trap more dust.
- Furniture should be made of vinyl, leather, or wood. Avoid upholstered furniture.
- If possible, remove rugs and keep floors clean. Bare wood or tile floors are best.
- Carpet squares trap dust and should be cleaned weekly.
- Pollen count should be checked before opening windows for "a little fresh air."
- Clean fan blades and front grate monthly.
- Clean or change window air conditioner filters every 2 weeks.
- Use air conditioners or a dehumidifier to keep relative humidity in the classroom low, between 35% and 45%.
- Teachers and staff should avoid perfumes, scented talcum powder, and hair sprays.
- Many children cannot read. If you have cleaning materials (chemical) in the classroom, be sure there is a danger sticker on it. Some cleaning products have strong fumes; replace caps quickly. Use natural cleaning agents:
- White or apple cider vinegar can be used to remove mold, mineral deposits, and crayon marks.
- Baking soda is a good general cleaner that can also be used as a room rug deodorizer or refrigerator deodorizer.
- Club soda is a good spot remover.
- Use liquid rather than bar soap (mild or unscented) for hand washing.
- Treat carpets and soft furniture with 3% tannic acid or benzoate (Acarosan).

Sinusitis

Infection of the paranasal sinuses in children is a frequent occurrence. The exact incidence and prevalence of this disorder are unknown because of the difficulty in definitive diagnosis, especially in younger children. Sinusitis characteristically responds well to antibiotic therapy, although prolonged courses are generally required. Complications can occur as a result of local extension of the disease. Orbital cellulitis is the most common serious complication. Intracranial infection with associated neurologic symptomatology is also a potential sequela of sinusitis. Prompt appropriate antibiotic therapy usually prevents the onset of these potentially life-threatening neurologic and ophthalmologic complications.

Pathophysiology

The paranasal sinuses are hollow areas in the skull beneath the turbinates in the nasopharynx. The various functions of the sinuses include warming and humidifying inspired air, trapping inspired particles, secreting mucus, and reducing the weight of the skull. The sinuses are prone to infection most frequently after a viral upper respiratory tract infection because the sinus cavities in children are smaller in area than in the adult (Fig. 16–14). Inflammation and edema of the mucous membranes during an upper respiratory tract infection can lead quickly to obstruction of the opening to the nasopharynx. The normally sterile sinus cavity is then invaded by bacteria. Bacterial pathogens in acute sinusitis are the same as those found in acute otitis media, with *Streptococcus pneumoniae* and *Haemophilus influenzae* predominating. *Moraxella (Branhamella) catarrhalis* is also a common cause of acute sinusitis in children (Wilder, 1996).

Assessment

Children with sinusitis have various clinical manifestations and histories. Fever and irritability following a viral upper respiratory tract infection may be the only manifestation in the infant or young child. Other possible clinical symptoms in the older child may be purulent rhinorrhea, malodorous breath, headache, anorexia, sore throat, a feeling of fullness or pain in the face, cough, and a disturbed sense of smell.

Diagnostic Tests. The diagnosis of sinusitis can be made only with certainty by obtaining a positive culture from sinus aspiration. Nasopharyngeal culture results have shown poor correlation with sinus culture results. Plain radiography and/or a computed tomography (CT) scan may be helpful in the diagnosis of acute sinusitis. Areas of varying degrees of mucosal thickening, frank opacification, or air-fluid levels have been accepted as criteria for diagnosis (Smith, 1994).

Interdisciplinary Interventions

Antimicrobial therapy, symptomatic relief measures, and drainage are the main types of interventions for sinusitis.

Figure 16–14
Development of the frontal, ethmoid, and maxillary sinuses.

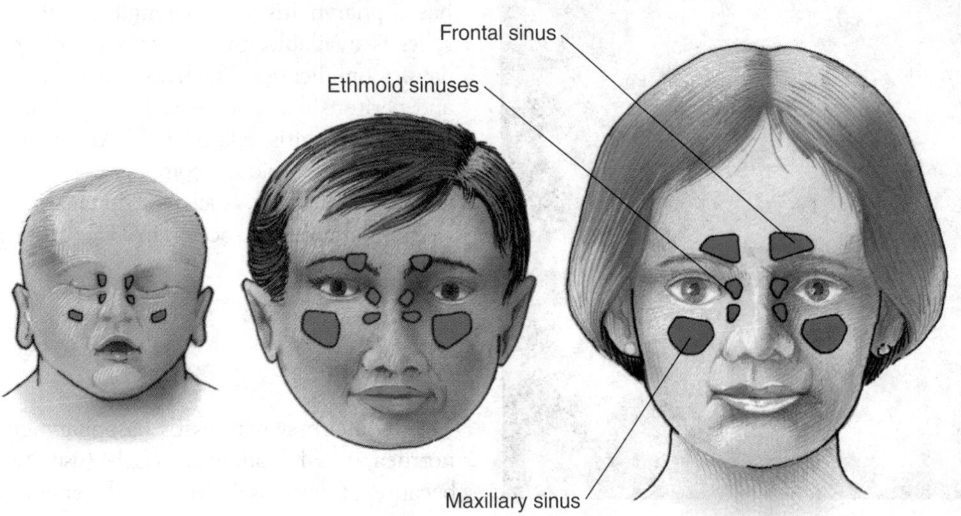

Antibiotics are given orally, are usually the same as those used for otitis media, and may be required for up to 6 weeks. Rarely, hospitalization is required for an advanced infection or complication requiring more intense neurologic monitoring and/or parenteral antibiotic therapy. Decongestants and antihistamines have been used to promote drainage from the sinuses. No documentation of the efficacy of these agents in children exists, and use should be discouraged, especially in infants and very young children, because of lack of information about the potential side effects.

Nasopharyngitis and Pharyngitis

Nasopharyngitis (common cold) and pharyngitis (throat infections) are among the most frequently encountered complaints in the pediatric ambulatory care setting. One group of researchers reported that in the first 3 years of life, children cared for at home averaged about four respiratory infections per year, whereas those in group daycare with two to six children averaged about five or six infections, and those in group daycare with seven or more children averaged about six or seven infections per year (Wald, Guerra, & Byers, 1991). These inflammatory syndromes of the nasopharynx and oropharynx are attributed predominantly to infectious agents, or less commonly, to secondary involvement in systemic or noninfectious illnesses (Fig. 16–15).

Figure 16–15
Common signs and symptoms of a cold include runny nose, red eyes, and fatigue.

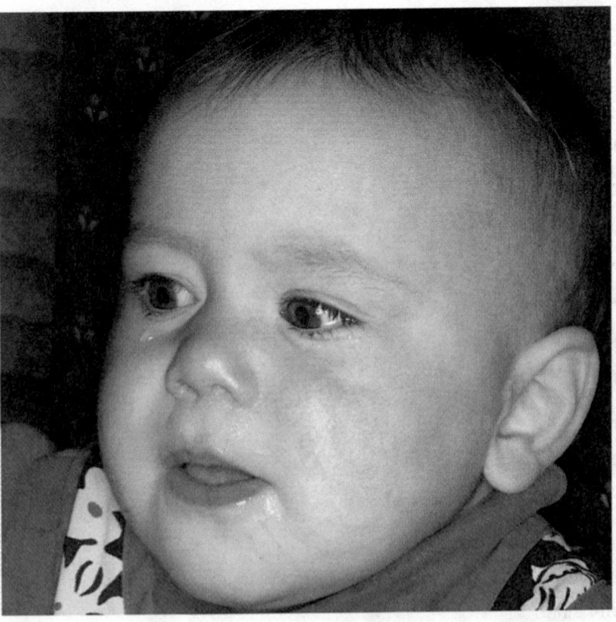

Etiology

Viral upper respiratory infections constitute the vast majority of cases of pharyngitis and nasopharyngitis. Rhinovirus, respiratory syncytial virus, coronavirus, and adenovirus are the most common pathogens in children younger than 3 years of age. Influenza, parainfluenza, Epstein-Barr virus, and coxsackievirus A are among the more prevalent causative agents in older children and adolescents. Pharyngitis is most commonly attributed to group A beta-hemolytic streptococcus (GABHS). Other etiologic agents include *Corynebacterium diphtheriae*. Infection with diphtheria was common at the turn of the century; however, nonimmunized and/or immigrant populations in the United States remain at risk for contracting this organism today. *Mycoplasma pneumoniae* can also cause pharyngitis that is clinically indistinguishable from GABHS, most commonly in the adolescent population. Gonococcal pharyngitis may be seen in sexually active or sexually abused children. Table 16–8 compares pharyngitis caused by viral versus bacterial agents.

Pathophysiology

The nasopharynx and oropharynx consist of mucous membrane layers composed of stratified squamous epithelium and are where the inflammatory process is initiated. The lymphatic drainage system is involved in a secondary capacity. Excessive drying of the mucous membranes during the winter months and passive or active smoking are other potential contributing factors (Feldman, 1993). The virulence of viral or bacterial pathogens depends on mucosal cell wall antigens. Viral particles are transmitted in an airborne manner, by direct contact, and rarely by food-borne transmission (Vukmir, 1992).

Prognosis. There is no specific treatment for viral nasal pharyngitis or pharyngitis, although symptomatic relief is available. Symptoms generally resolve in 5 to 7 days. Complications such as otitis media, lymphadenitis, and peritonsillar abscess may occur. If left untreated, bacterial pharyngitis related to GABHS resolves in 5 to 7 days. More serious complications resulting from a GABHS infection, such as rheumatic fever and acute glomerulonephritis, occur in 3% of untreated patients (Knudtson, 1994).

Assessment

The hallmark symptoms of nasopharyngitis are clear rhinorrhea, nasal stuffiness, cough (usually worse at night because of postnasal drip), and generalized malaise and

Table 16–8
Comparison of Viral and Bacterial Pharyngitis

	Viral Pharyngitis	Streptococcal Pharyngitis
Symptomatology	WBC usually normal	WBC count elevated (15,000–20,000/mm^3)
	Gradual onset	Abrupt onset
	Headache, low-grade fever	Headache, fever up to 104°F
	Rhinitis, cough, and hoarseness common	Rhinitis, cough, and hoarseness uncommon
	Abdominal discomfort uncommon	Often complaints of abdominal discomfort and trouble swallowing
	Slightly red pharynx with moderately enlarged tonsils	Erythema and enlargement of tonsils with white exudate on posterior pharynx and tonsils
	Marked cervical lymphadenopathy usually not present	Firm, tender cervical lymph nodes present
Treatment	Symptomatic treatment only: · Provide rest · Reduce fever · Prevent spread of infection · Facilitate breathing · Promote comfort · Prevent dehydration	Antibiotics to eradicate organisms, either penicillin or erythromycin for 10 days, plus symptomatic treatment listed under viral pharyngitis
Complications	Few complications	Complications include otitis media, sinusitis, peritonsillar abscesses, acute cervical adenitis, rheumatic fever, meningitis, and acute glomerulonephritis
Duration	Usually self-limiting, lasting 1–5 days	Without antibiotics, child may be acutely ill for 2 weeks

irritability. Extreme throat discomfort is the chief complaint in most cases of pharyngitis. White exudate and/or petechiae may be visible on the posterior palate and/or tonsils with both GABHS and C. *diphtheriae* infections. High fever, scarlatiniform rash, and tender cervical lymphadenopathy may also be present in bacterial pharyngitis. Dysphasia, hoarseness, and/or laryngitis may accompany either pharyngitis or nasal pharyngitis.

Community Care

Pharyngitis and nasal pharyngitis are treated in the home by the parents, often in collaboration with the pediatrician or pediatric nurse practitioner. Bacterial pathogens can be identified by throat culture and treated with the appropriate antibiotics. Teaching parents careful monitoring for signs of complications or disease progression and prompt seeking of medical attention is an important health care provider intervention. Parents may also be advised to position the infant in an infant seat or with the head of the bed elevated for comfort and to facilitate drainage of nasal secretions. A bulb syringe may also be used to clear nasal passages before feedings, especially for infants, to promote feeding/nippling. Supportive care, including rest, nutritious foods, and cool fluids, is the primary intervention. Acetaminophen should be given for fever higher than 101°F axillary, and cool mist air via vaporizer or humidifier helps to thin secretions. Comfort measures such as cool fluids and ice pops may be given to the child, and warm saline throat irrigations (salt water gargle) may be comforting for the older, cooperative child.

Although the sight of a young child struggling with the symptoms of a bacterial or viral upper respiratory

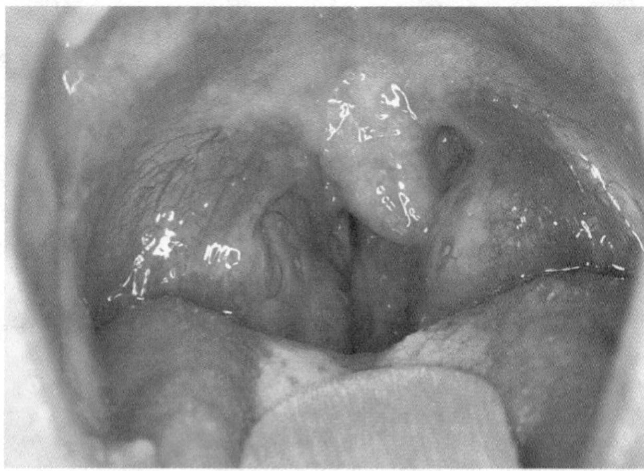

Figure 16–16
"Kissing tonsils" occur when the tonsils are so enlarged that they touch the uvula and/or each other, greatly narrowing the airway.

infection is distressing, however common, parents should be discouraged from using remedies such as heated vapor and over-the-counter antihistamines and decongestants. Some over-the-counter preparations may moderately reduce symptoms in older children and adolescents (Macknin, 1992).

Tonsillitis

The tonsils are located on either side of the pharyngeal cavity and are part of the lymphatic system. There are four pair of tonsils located in the nasal and oral pharynx; however, it is the palatine, or faucial, tonsils that enlarge and are readily seen behind the faucial pillars at the sides of the oropharynx. Adenoids are the nasopharyngeal tonsils and are located adjacent to the palatine tonsils on the posterior wall of the nasopharynx (Fig. 16–16). Tonsils and adenoids are important to the normal development of the body's immune system, because they serve as part of the body's defense against infection; but they may become a site of acute or chronic infections (tonsillitis). Tonsillar tissue increases in size during childhood as a result of acute nasopharyngeal infections that commonly occur in the school-age child. Tonsils reach their maximum size between 8 and 12 years of age, then begin to involute, or shrink, during adolescence.

Etiology

Acute infection of the palatine tonsils is thought to result largely from group A beta-hemolytic streptococcus (GABHS) infection, although other causative organisms include *Haemophilus influenzae*, pneumococcal infection, and viral agents. The GABHS agent is particularly problematic because it cannot be identified except by throat culture, which may be difficult to obtain and is at times inconclusive. Children generally recover from tonsillitis, but if caused by GABHS that is not completely eradicated, sequelae such as rheumatic fever or acute glomerulonephritis may occur.

Pathophysiology

Acute infection of the tonsils and/or adenoids is considered to be acute pharyngitis and is discussed in that section of the chapter. Chronic tonsillitis is a common affliction of childhood; exact incidence, however, is largely unknown. Repeated acute infections centered in lymphoid tissue such as the tonsils draw the body's defenses to that location, causing swelling of the tissue. It most often affects school-age children. Enlarged tonsils and adenoids impinge on the pharyngeal opening of the eustachian tube, preventing it from ventilating and draining the middle ear, thus contributing to incidence of otitis media as a sequela to tonsillitis.

Assessment

Children with acute and/or chronic tonsillitis present with clinical signs and symptoms similar to pharyngitis. Inflammation of the tonsils and surrounding tissues is accompanied by varying degrees of soreness of the mucosa. This soreness may cause the child to refuse to eat or drink because of discomfort on swallowing. Additional clinical manifestations may include exudate on the tonsillar surface, significant erythema, recurrent and/or persistent sore throats, and possible obstruction to swallowing or breathing by hypertrophied tonsils and/or adenoids. Occasionally there may be dryness and irritation in the throat and offensive breath. Rarely, hypertrophied tonsils and adenoids obstructing the upper airway can cause respiratory distress, with chronic hypoxia and the development of pulmonary hypertension. Children with tonsils or adenoids that are significantly enlarged so as to partially obstruct the upper airway often present as being "mouth-breathers" and often snore during sleep.

Hypertrophy of the tonsils and/or acute infection must be carefully evaluated by the health care professional. Many enlarged tonsils are in fact normal in size. The misinterpretation results from failure to appreciate that tonsils are normally larger during early childhood years as a result of frequent infections of the nasopharynx. Tonsils may virtually meet in the midline in some normal, asymptomatic children, especially when the child is gagged. It must also be ascertained whether hypertrophy is chronic or the result of a recent acute infection. Tonsils can increase in size tremendously with an acute infection and recede after the infection subsides.

Inspection of tonsils is usually easily accomplished in the older child by asking the child to say "aaah." If the child is unable to hold the tongue down, use of a tongue blade lightly on the tongue may be helpful. Younger children consider the examination of the mouth and throat intrusive and may be uncooperative. Infants and young children whose cooperation cannot be gained will usually open their mouths during crying to allow a good view of the oropharynx. If a tongue blade is needed, it should be used with caution and quickly.

Tip: *Demonstration of examining the throat through play with a doll or with the parent may be helpful. Drawing a happy face or cartoon character on the end of the tongue blade that you will hold or drawing on a tongue blade for the child to take home may be sufficient to gain the young child's cooperation.*

Interdisciplinary Interventions

When tonsillitis is present, it is necessary to screen for GABHS by culturing the tonsillar surface that may contain the exudate. A throat culture can be best obtained using the same techniques as when inspecting the throat. Identification of the causative organism is helpful in determining the antibiotic course that will be used. Oral antibiotics are ordered for administration at home. The recommended treatment for acute tonsillitis secondary to GABHS is penicillin administered orally or intramuscularly and should be given for 10 days (the oral dose). It is important to educate the parent/caretaker of the importance of administering the complete course of penicillin because, although symptoms may subside in 24 to 72 hours, it is necessary to prevent complications such as rheumatic fever and glomerulonephritis (see Pharyngitis). Erythromycin (30 to 50 mg/kg/day) is an effective, inexpensive alternative antibiotic for the child who is allergic to penicillin.

Community Care

The symptoms of a sore throat may be treated in the home with acetaminophen, throat lozenges or hard candies, cool fluids, ice chips or ice pops, and salt water gargles to keep the throat moist. The use of topical anesthetics such as the aqueous solution of lidocaine should be discouraged because their efficacy in young children is unproven and because of the risk of systemic absorption and allergic sensitization. The nurse should stress the importance of hydration through use of frequent small sips of cold liquid beverages.

The child with uncomplicated acute tonsillitis is usually managed on an ambulatory basis. Rarely, the swelling of the throat is severe or symptoms seem to indicate that the child has epiglottitis, or the child may become severely dehydrated and therefore require hospitalization for treatment with intravenous fluids, parenteral antibiotics, and emergency equipment available in case of airway obstruction.

Tonsillectomy and Adenoidectomy

Tonsillectomy and adenoidectomy (T&A) are controversial surgical interventions for chronic tonsillitis. Although these procedures have been widely practiced for over a century, no definite criteria have been established as absolute indications for surgery. Recurrent throat infections (documented with positive throat cultures) remain one of the leading indications for surgery. Tonsillectomy has been documented to decrease the number of infections in these children in the subsequent 2 years; however, many children who have not had tonsillectomies also have a decline in the number of throat infections (Arnold, 1996). Chronic upper airway obstruction is also a major indication for surgery. Symptoms of upper airway obstruction are more prominent during sleep and include mouth breathing, loud snoring, and, in extreme cases, apnea. The child with upper airway obstruction significant enough to warrant tonsillectomy may also exhibit sleep disturbances and enuresis. Patients with severe obstruction improve after surgery; patients with mild to moderate symptoms improve with no treatment. Health care professionals, in collaboration with parents, should carefully document that sore throats caused by GABHS are frequent (more than five per year), symptomatic (fever, exudate, erythema, adenitis), and costly (missed school/work days and medical expenses) before considering tonsillectomy (Arnold, 1996).

Tonsillectomy and adenoidectomy, if performed, are done ideally 2 to 3 weeks after an acute infection. This procedure can be done safely and cost effectively on an outpatient basis. The nurse prepares the child and family for the surgery and orients both child and family to the postoperative care protocol. Prior to the surgery, baseline vital signs should be obtained along with a history of any bleeding disorders because of the risk of hemorrhage. The child will receive general anesthesia for the surgery and continuous nursing care and monitoring during the immediate postoperative period for bleeding, pain control, and encouragement of oral intake when stable, as necessary (TIP 16–3).

The child should be observed for the possibility of hemorrhage during the postoperative period. An ice collar is applied externally around the neck, and as soon as the child is awake he or she may take ice chips. The most comfortable and safe position for the child is prone (on the abdomen) with the head turned to the side so that mouth drainage can be observed. Small amounts of bright red blood may be present soon after the surgery. It is normal for the child to have one emesis of old blood

TIP 16–3 A Teaching Interventional Plan for the Child After Tonsillectomy or Adenoidectomy

Nursing Diagnoses and Outcomes

- Pain related to surgical procedure
  Outcome: Child will be comfortable and will receive adequate periods of rest.
- Fluid volume deficit related to decreased intake of fluids and loss of fluids (vomiting, secretions)
  Outcome: Child will have adequate fluid intake with minimal fluid losses.
- Knowledge deficit regarding signs of postoperative complications
  Outcome: Family/caretaker verbalizes and describe home treatment and early signs of postoperative complications.

Home Management of the Child

- The child should engage in quiet activity for the first week following surgery. The child may return to school in 1–2 weeks or after the follow-up appointment.
- Administer analgesics for pain every 4–6 hours as needed. Use acetaminophen for pain relief; avoid aspirin and ibuprofen because these may increase bleeding tendencies.
- An ice collar on the child's neck may help in pain management.
- Halitosis is common for 1–2 weeks following surgery. Provide mouth care by providing mouth rinses, instructing the child not to gargle.
- Encourage plenty of fluids (1–1½ quarts) daily.
- Offer tepid fluids or slow-melting fluids such as ice pops or Italian ices and offer a soft diet, avoiding spicy, rough, or coarse foods, for the first 7–10 days.
- Use caution with straws, utensils, and sharp, pointed toys that may be put in the mouth and injure the surgical site.
- Avoid crowds and protect child from contact with persons who are ill.
- Emphasize importance of surgical follow-up appointment, usually 1–2 weeks after surgery.

Contact Health Care Provider if

- There is persistent bleeding, frequent swallowing, coughing, or blood in vomitus.
- The child complains of an earache.
- The child has a fever higher than 101°F.

after the surgery and small amounts of blood-streaked mucus within the first few hours after the surgery.

caREminder: *Any needed suctioning should be done with caution to avoid trauma to the oropharynx and surgical site. The child is instructed to avoid too much coughing, talking, clearing of the throat, or blowing of the nose after surgery so as not to disturb the surgical site.*

If the child spits up bright red blood frequently or has repeated emesis of old blood from the stomach, or if he or she becomes tachycardic (heart rate >120 beats per minute), pale, and restless, the surgeon should be notified immediately. Occasionally it may be necessary for the child to return to surgery to ligate a bleeding vessel.

If no bleeding occurs, ice chips and water may be given soon after surgery after the child is fully alert. The diet should be advanced from clear liquids to full liquids as tolerated. The child should be given pain medication, often in the form of a liquid or syrup, within the first 2 hours after surgery. The child should receive pain medication every 4 hours during the first 24 to 48 hours to control pain and make swallowing fluids more comfortable.

The child may be discharged on the day of surgery or the following day, but should convalesce at home for several days. Instructions are given to the parent or caretaker that the child should get plenty of rest, drink plenty of fluids, and eat soft foods in several small meals throughout the day. Popsicles, puddings, cream soups (not hot), fully cooked vegetables, and mashed potatoes are recommended soft foods. Any bleeding should be reported immediately to the physician. Delayed hemorrhage is possible up to 7 to 10 days after surgery.

Croup

Croup is a general term that refers to the clinical syndrome of hoarseness, inspiratory stridor, a "croupy" or barking cough, and varying degrees of respiratory distress. It is commonly referred to as laryngotracheobronchitis (LTB) because it involves inflammation of one or more of the following structures:

- the vocal cords and larynx
- subglottic tissue
- trachea
- bronchi
- bronchioles

This syndrome may be infectious or noninfectious in nature. The peak incidence of this illness is in the 1- to 2-year-old age group but can commonly be seen in children age 6 months to 4 years (Cressman & Myer, 1994). Before age 6, males are affected more commonly than females. In older children, males and females are affected equally (Grad & Taussig, 1990). Croup usually occurs during the fall and winter months.

Infectious agents associated with croup may be bacterial or viral; the vast majority of cases being viral in origin and affecting the subglottic region. Viruses, predominantly parainfluenza 1, 2, and 3, influenza A and B, adenovirus, and respiratory syncytial virus (RSV), are common etiologic agents. Enterovirus and measles have also been identified. Noninfectious croup may be caused by asthma or allergic reactions, or it may follow endotracheal extubation or foreign body aspiration.

Pathophysiology

Subsequent to a viral infection or other type of irritant to the epithelial tissue of the airway, an inflammatory response results. Vascular congestion and edema then develop. This inflammation accounts for the narrowing of the subglottic region, the smallest portion of the upper airway in children, thus producing the classic symptoms of upper airway obstruction found in children with croup (Cressman & Myer, 1994). In addition to edema, laryngeal muscle spasm and accumulation of secretions also contribute to airway obstruction. As this process progresses, surface mucosal ulcerations may also occur.

Prognosis. Croup is generally a self-limiting illness in which children's symptoms subside in 3 to 5 days, and full recovery without complications is the norm. Respiratory arrest and the need for a tracheostomy are rare.

Assessment

Onset of croup is usually gradual. The child with croup may have a history of a mild upper respiratory infection for several days, with or without fever. The onset of croup is then marked by the development of the characteristic "barking" cough, hoarse phonation, and inspiratory stridor. The child rarely looks ill or toxic but presents with an increased respiratory rate. Additional clinical signs, depending on the severity of airway obstruction, may include suprasternal, substernal, and intercostal retractions; intermittent cyanosis during coughing; and altered mental status related to hypoxia and carbon dioxide retention. A thorough respiratory assessment is important because the child with upper airway obstruction with mild hypoxia develops muscle fatigue and hypoventilation that can result in severe hypoxemia and hypercapnia (Schidlow & Smith, 1994). Occasionally endotracheal intubation is necessary because of complete airway obstruction or respiratory distress.

Parental anxiety is also a characteristic assessment finding, the degree of which depends on many factors, including parental experience with previous croup episodes, lack of sleep from child's "barking," and the severity of the child's respiratory distress and degree of anxiety and irritability. Sometimes parents lack understanding of bacterial versus viral illnesses and are distressed when antibiotics are not prescribed.

Acute spasmodic laryngitis, or "midnight croup," refers to a distinct entity in which the child goes to bed without a cough, but often with other mild symptoms of an upper respiratory infection, and suddenly awakens several hours later with a croupy cough and marked inspiratory stridor (Schidlow & Smith, 1994). These children are usually asymptomatic the following morning, and recurrence on the following night is not uncommon. Spontaneous recovery is expected.

Interdisciplinary Interventions

Management of croup includes identification of the severity of respiratory distress and collaboration with the parents and health care team to determine the need for hospitalization and/or intubation. Children who present with cyanosis and who are severely hypoxic, fatigued, in respiratory distress, or unable to drink sufficient fluids are hospitalized in order to receive intravenous fluid, oxygen, and airway support. The child with croup should be observed for any deteriorating respiratory status, and monitoring of vital signs must include rate, rhythm, and depth of respirations and cardiac rate and rhythm. Tachycardia and/or cardiac arrhythmias may be seen with hypoxia. Equipment for intubation and/or tracheostomy should be readily available. Body temperature should be evaluated and antipyretics administered for fever higher than 38.5°C (101°F).

It is controversial whether providing an environment rich in humidity via continuous fine mist ("croup tents") has any therapeutic benefit. Parents may find that their child will improve after being taken out in the cool night air or into the bathroom with a warm, running shower. Mist may be helpful to moisten and decrease the viscosity of airway secretions, making it easier for the child to remove them by coughing. Dry, warm air may cause exudates to adhere to the airway wall. Studies have failed to demonstrate, however, any beneficial effect of humidified air as compared with room air on subglottic edema (Bourchier, Dawson, & Fergusson, 1984; Henry, 1983).

Although mist was widely used in the past, current therapy relies more on aerosol inhalation therapy with medications such as racemic epinephrine. Racemic epinephrine is believed to work via topical alpha-adrenergic stimulation, which causes mucosal vasoconstriction leading to decreased edema in the subglottic region. Mist tents may be used to deliver oxygen therapy to children unable to tolerate a mask or nasal cannula. Nurses should facilitate the administration of respiratory inhalation treatments at the prescribed frequency, disrupting the child's regular feeding and sleep patterns as little as possible.

Community Care

Nutritional supports for children with croup are generally short term. Clear oral fluids should be encouraged, unless respiratory distress is severe, in which case the child should have nothing by mouth and should be hydrated intravenously. Fluids should be encouraged, choosing those the child prefers. When solid food is resumed, frequent small nutritious snacks are usually more appealing than an entire meal.

Two of the most important nursing interventions for the child with croup are minimization of anxiety and maximization of opportunities for rest. Providing a comfortable environment free from noxious stimuli lessens respiratory distress. Children should be encouraged to engage in quiet play that provides diversion and reduces anxiety. Coloring books, watching favorite videotapes, listening to music, reading stories, and doing puzzles are some examples.

Teaching parents and other caretakers about medications and respiratory inhalation treatments and how to assess their child's respiratory status is also important. Although most children recover without complications, caretakers must be able to verbalize and describe signs of impending respiratory failure and know how to access emergency services. A home health referral may be indicated if the parent's assessment ability is in question and the child's condition does not warrant hospitalization. The child should be afebrile and free from cough before returning to school or daycare environment. In the acute phase of the illness, parental anxiety may be very high. Health care professionals should provide information and support, emphasizing the short-lived nature of the illness. Provide the opportunity for parents to get adequate rest. For the child who remains at home, assist the parents in mobilizing their resources in extended family and community to relieve them of some of the responsibility for care. Facilitating sibling care is also a helpful intervention.

Epiglottitis

Epiglottitis is an acute inflammation of the supraglottic structures, the epiglottis and aryepiglottic folds. It characteristically does not involve the subglottic and tracheal regions. Epiglottitis is significant because it constitutes one of the true pediatric emergencies. If treatment is delayed, it may rapidly progress to complete airway obstruction, cardiopulmonary arrest, and a potentially fatal outcome. When prompt diagnosis and coordinated, well-organized management occur, the prognosis for full and uncomplicated recovery is excellent.

Epiglottitis is a rare disease. Its incidence nationwide is unknown, but it is thought to constitute fewer than 10 per 10,000 pediatric hospital admissions (Hoekelman, 1994). It affects persons in all age groups, including infants, but occurs most often in children 2 to 7 years of age, with 80% of the cases occurring before 5 years of age. It occurs year round, but more frequently during winter and early spring.

Etiology

Epiglottitis most commonly results from infection of the supraglottic structures by *Haemophilus influenzae* type B (HIB). Group A beta-hemolytic streptococci, *Streptococcus pneumoniae*, and, rarely, other bacteria and some viruses have also been reported. The infecting organism can be isolated from the upper airway as well as from the blood. Direct invasion by HIB causes inflammation of the supraglottic structures with subsequent edematous swelling of these structures and bacteremia. Since 1985, with the licensing of the HIB vaccines, there have been reports of dramatic declines (up to 73%) in the incidence of diseases caused by HIB nationwide (Adams et al., 1993). This does not mean pediatric health professionals should dismiss the risks of epiglottitis and its consequences, however, because organisms other than HIB are possible infectious agents in epiglottitis. All patients having the clinical picture of this disease must be managed with the same cautious approach used prior to the introduction of the HIB vaccine.

Assessment

Epiglottitis is characterized by the sudden onset of respiratory distress (including stridor) over a few hours, with a high fever (>39°C). The child has a sore throat, hoarseness, dysphagia, and drooling (Fig. 16–17). Often these symptoms were preceded by symptoms of an upper respiratory infection. Rarely is the disorder accompanied by the characteristic "barking" cough of croup. Agitation, characterized by irritability and restlessness, is almost always present, as is the child's refusal to lie down, preferring to sit upright and lean forward, mouth open, to attain the best airway possible, and to allow secretions to run out of the mouth. This is known as the "tripod" position and is the hallmark of epiglottitis. As the obstruction increases, retractions of the supraclavicular and substernal area and cyanosis may be present. Parents are very fearful and anxious as they witness and describe the child's rapid onset of symptoms.

Direct visualization of the upper airway is discouraged and should be attempted only by a person skilled in intubation and with all necessary equipment present at the bedside. This direct visualization procedure may be dangerous because it may precipitate complete airway obstruction and respiratory arrest. The epiglottis is visualized as cherry red; it and surrounding structures are extremely swollen, with severe narrowing of the laryngeal orifice. There is often pooling of mucous secretions.

caREminder: *The use of tongue blades or other instrumentation to visualize the epiglottis should be avoided. Such actions can cause the epiglottis to spasm and totally occlude the airway.*

The diagnosis is more safely made primarily on clinical signs and should be considered in every child with acute upper airway obstruction who has a high fever, sore throat, and looks "toxic," especially if these signs have developed over only a few hours. A lateral neck radiograph is also a diagnostic technique. It shows the epiglottis as a large, rounded soft mass below the base of the tongue.

Figure 16–17
Child with epiglottitis in distress. (© 1988, American Heart Association. Used with permission.)

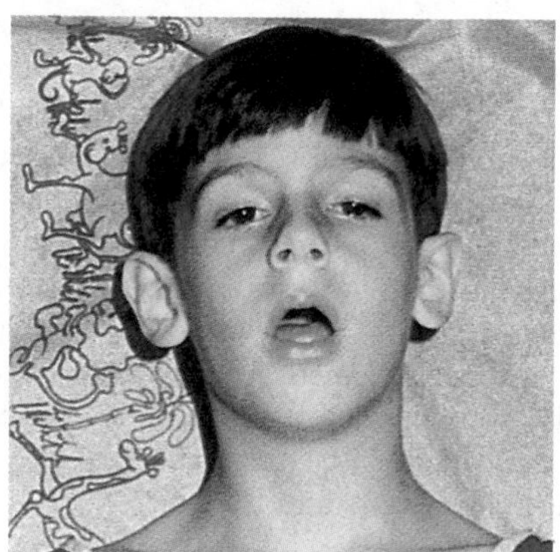

Interdisciplinary Interventions

Children for whom the diagnosis of epiglottitis is suspected should be carefully monitored by skilled personnel at all times. The nurse should expect that the child and parents will be extremely anxious. The most important interdisciplinary intervention is keeping the child quiet and undisturbed until endotracheal intubation is performed. The nurse should minimize episodes of crying by allowing the child, if possible, to sit upright in the parent's arms. The child should never be forced into the supine position because this may cause the inflamed epiglottis to obstruct the airway, compromise diaphragmatic excursion and air movement, or create choking on swallowed secretions.

Respiratory status, including rate and depth of respirations and the presence of retractions, nasal flaring, and stridor, must be carefully monitored. The child should be given humidified oxygen by face mask, with the head of the bed elevated at all times. Continuous pulse oximetry should be instituted to obtain information on arterial oxygen saturation. Intravenous antibiotics (usually ampicillin or cefuroxime) must be given as soon as possible. Upon strong suspicion or confirmation of the diagnosis, intubation should be performed, ideally in the operating room under general anesthesia. Rarely intubation is not possible secondary to laryngospasm and/or severe swelling, and placement of a tracheostomy is required (see Treatment Modalities).

Other important nursing interventions include administration and monitoring of sedative medication, as there can be a high risk of accidental extubation. Mild sedation, combined with the use of restraints, prevents this complication and allows the child to breathe spontaneously, making mechanical ventilation unnecessary. Assessment for possible respiratory complications, monitoring of body temperature, and provision of adequate fluid and calorie intake are also crucial to the care of the child with epiglottitis. The child must have nothing by mouth during the acute phase of the illness, and oral fluids and soft foods should not be provided until the child has demonstrated tolerance of extubation (Chart 16–14).

As in any hospitalization, parental anxiety is high. This is especially true if the child is admitted in acute respiratory distress. Calm, factual, step-by-step information should be provided during this period, with full realization that this information may need to be repeated as the family's stress level decreases and they are able to formulate questions. Initial information should include

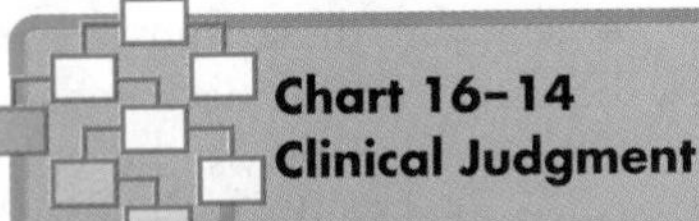

Chart 16–14
Clinical Judgment

The Drooling Child

Jimmy, a 5-year-old child, presents in the emergency room with respiratory stridor upon inspiration and a temperature of 102.5°F. He is drooling and prefers to sit forward with his chin slightly protruded. His mother states that he developed the difficulty breathing "so suddenly," and both mother and child appear anxious.

Questions

1. What additional data would you collect during your initial assessment?
2. Is this an upper or lower respiratory problem?
3. What actions would your initial interventions include?
4. Is obtaining a throat culture indicated at this time? Why or why not?
5. What interventions should be implemented to maintain a patent airway in this child?

Answers

1. Heart rate. Duration of fever and other signs of respiratory illness. Is the child voiding, and when did he last eat or drink (to assess for dehydration and shock)? If the child opens his mouth wide, can you visualize the epiglottis or tonsils? Are they enlarged? Is there any history of tonsillitis?
2. An upper respiratory problem, as distinguished by inspiratory stridor due to an obstruction. In this case, the obstruction is a swollen cherry-red epiglottis.
3. Interventions include establishing and maintaining an airway. Keep the child with his mother to help reduce anxiousness and allow him to remain in "tripod position," as this helps maintain an open airway. Provide oxygen via mask or blow-by oxygen. If respiratory distress becomes severe, ventilate with a bag-valve mask.
4. A throat culture should not be obtained, because manipulation of the oropharynx for visualization or when obtaining a culture may precipitate airway (trachea) spasm and obstruction from the swollen epiglottis.
5. The primary therapy is to maintain the airway; therefore, provide oxygen support via face mask or bag-valve mask ventilation as needed until the physician is ready to intubate the child.

the course of events in the immediate future, for example, when and where the child will be intubated; where the family may wait; when they may first visit the child after airway management is accomplished; how the child will be given nutrition, hydration, and medication; and how long they should expect he or she will need to remain intubated and sedated.

Recovery from epiglottitis is usually rapid, with endotracheal extubation occurring in 2 to 3 days as the fever dissipates, the child can handle secretions, and airway narrowing is resolved. Parental reassurance and support are key during this recovery phase because the rapid progression and critical nature of this disorder render it extremely frightening. Nurses and social workers can assist families by providing frequent accurate education and update on the child's condition and allowing parental visitation or "rooming-in" as much as possible. Parents should be informed as to when they should expect the child to resume normal dietary habits and when discharge from the hospital is expected. Teaching regarding the administration of oral antibiotics at home (to complete a 7-day course) should begin at the time the child's intravenous line is discontinued.

Community Care

If not already done, immunization with the HIB capsular polysaccharide vaccine should be urged for the patient and all siblings of appropriate age (see Chapter 6). Prophylaxis with rifampin (20 mg/kg/day, maximum 600 mg/day) by mouth is recommended to all household contacts, if at least one contact is younger than 4 years, regardless of the immunization status of the child (American Academy of Pediatrics, 1984). The management of daycare and nursery school contact groups should be individualized. A definitive recommendation regarding rifampin prophylaxis in daycare centers has not been made, rather, prompt medical evaluation of febrile episodes in attendees is urged (American Academy of Pediatrics, 1984). The HIB vaccine and rifampin prophylaxis can both be obtained free of charge from the county public health agency in many states.

Bacterial Tracheitis

Bacterial tracheitis is a relatively uncommon, but potentially life-threatening, infection of the upper trachea. It is also referred to as membranous laryngotracheitis or membranous croup. It is commonly seen in children between 1 and 6 years of age. The cause of bacterial tracheitis is believed to be a complication of viral croup and superinfection with *Staphylococcus aureus*, although other organisms have also been implicated.

Assessment

Typically, the child presents with a more toxic appearance than if the child had viral croup. There is a history of a prior upper respiratory tract infection and/or viral croup, and then the child develops a high fever, cough, increasing inspiratory stridor unaffected by position, and a toxic appearance. The trachea is inflamed and appears erythematous and edematous with thick, tenacious, purulent secretions. Early recognition of bacterial tracheitis and prompt attention to the child's airway are necessary to prevent obstruction secondary to the thick secretions.

Interdisciplinary Interventions

The treatment and management of bacterial tracheitis should be approached promptly and vigorously. The child should be hospitalized, and appropriate emergency airway management equipment should be available. Frequent tracheal suctioning is necessary to keep the airway patent, and often the child has an artificial airway (endotracheal tube) in place. This management is especially true in the younger child who is at risk for abrupt airway obstruction. Additionally, the child requires humidified oxygen, parenteral antibiotics, and antipyretics for fever and discomfort.

Apnea

Apnea is defined as the cessation of airflow into and out of the lungs. Apneic episodes lasting longer than 20 seconds and/or shorter respiratory pauses associated with cyanosis, bradycardia, pallor, or limpness are considered pathologic. This definition is simply a description of a characteristic clinical syndrome, not a specific disease process. There are two general types of apnea:

- *Central apnea* is an impairment of control of breathing mechanisms resulting in absence of nasal airflow and ventilatory effort.
- *Obstructive apnea* is usually caused by anatomic abnormalities and occurs when there is an absence of nasal air flow despite normal or exaggerated respiratory effort.

Central and obstructive apnea can occur together and is referred to as mixed apnea. Periodic breathing (PB) is a pattern of breathing characterized by short apneas occurring at regular intervals and is frequently seen in premature infants. PB is defined as three episodes of apnea lasting longer than 3 seconds, interrupted by respiration lasting 20 seconds or less (Gaultier, 1994). This section focuses on central apnea as manifested in apnea of prematurity, apnea of infancy, and apparent life-threatening events.

Incidence

Although apnea can occur at any age, the premature infant is at a greater risk. Normal respiratory system development is such that the lungs and respiratory center of the brain are designed to breathe and control respiration at term, although they are capable of breathing air by 23 weeks' gestation. Therefore, the lungs and respiratory center have not fully matured in the premature infant, leading to disruptions in the regularity of respiration. *Apnea of prematurity* (AOP) is the occurrence of pathologic apnea and periodic breathing in a premature infant. AOP is a common, natural consequence of immaturity and need not be viewed as a disease entity. It is estimated that at least 50% of premature infants with PB develop AOP (Carroll, Marcus, & Loughlin, 1993). AOP has been documented to occur in up to 25% of premature infants less than 37 weeks' gestation or less than 2500 g in weight and in 84% of those weighing less than 1000 g (Morriss, 1984). It is expected that premature infants will outgrow AOP, usually by 40 weeks postconceptual age. Studies of sudden infant death syndrome (SIDS) have indicated that apnea of prematurity in and of itself was not a precursor or predictor of subsequent SIDS death. It had been previously speculated that PB is a precursor to longer, more serious episodes of AOP, but studies have demonstrated that although most preterm infants exhibit PB, this pattern of breathing decreases by 40 weeks postconceptual age, and that there does not appear to be a relationship between prolonged apnea and the incidence of PB (Barrington & Finer, 1990; Glotzbach, Baldwin, Lederer, Tansey, & Ariagno, 1989).

Apnea of infancy (AOI) describes episodes of cessation of breathing or respiratory pauses in a previously healthy infant at least 40 to 42 weeks postconceptual age. The healthy infants who present with a history of AOI or an apparent life-threatening event for whom the obvious treatable causes have been ruled out present a greater challenge in evaluation and management. The

Chart 16–15

Causes of Apnea in Previously Healthy Infants

- Laryngeal chemoreceptor apnea
- Seizure disorder
- Infection (sepsis, meningitis, respiratory syncytial virus, *Bordetella pertussis*)
- Upper airway obstruction (croup, epiglottitis)
- Breathholding spells
- Congenital heart disease
- Cardiac dysrhythmia
- Hyponatremia, hypoglycemia, hypocalcemia, hypoxemia, hypocarbia
- Failure of automatic ventilation (congenital central hypoventilation syndrome)
- Central nervous system tumor (brain stem compression)
- Anemia
- Alcohol, sedatives, narcotics

current term for these more significant disturbances, *apparent life-threatening events* (ALTEs) describes their frighteningly serious nature. These episodes have been formerly termed a "near-miss SIDS episode"; however, it is believed the term ALTE more accurately describes the occurrence. An ALTE is defined as an event in which an infant has a convincing history of an episode of apnea that is sudden in onset, considered frightening to the observer, and is characterized by color change (cyanosis or pallor), marked change in muscular tone (limpness, rarely stiffness), choking and/or gagging, and requires significant intervention (vigorous shaking, mouth-to-mouth breathing, or full cardiopulmonary resuscitation) to revive the infant and restore normal breathing (National Institutes of Health, 1987).

Acute apneic episodes with cyanosis in the post-term infant can have a variety of treatable causes (Chart 16–15). ALTE can also be the result of a profound central nervous system insult or depression involving structural damage to the brain stem, as in trauma, infection, or edema, or interference with cerebral metabolic function (e.g., drug overdose, hypotension, severe hypoxia). The prognosis for these infants depends on the etiology and treatment of the underlying cause.

Assessment

Apnea may present simply as a parental report of prolonged asymptomatic respiratory pauses during sleep or as dramatically as a complete witnessed cessation of breathing and absence of a heart rate. Because apneic episodes, regardless of their severity, typically occur away from the view of the medical team, the significance of the event is based largely on the caregiver's recollection of the event. A single mild episode that required little or no intervention does not necessitate an extensive diagnostic evaluation or aggressive therapy and has little prognostic significance. Infants usually appear entirely normal by the time they reach medical attention following an ALTE. The most important assessment is obtaining a careful history from the person witnessing the event. Medical and nursing personnel should collaborate to gain as much detail as possible about the event itself, the physical condition of the infant before and after the event, and circumstances surrounding its occurrence (Chart 16–16). Reliability of the historian and signs of child abuse or neglect should be assessed, as well as the evaluation of sepsis.

Diagnostic Tests. Further assessments include, but are not limited to, the following:

- Arterial blood gases (persistent acidosis indicates a severe event or a chronic metabolic disorder)
- Complete blood counts (anemia may precipitate apnea; polycythemia reflects chronic hypoxia; elevated white blood cell count indicates infection)
- Serum electrolyte, glucose, and blood urea nitrogen levels (numerous abnormalities, such as hypocalcemia and hypoglycemia, may contribute to the development of apnea)

Chart 16–16

Acute Life-Threatening Episode: History and Physical Findings

- Change in body color to very pale or blue/cyanotic
- Loss of normal body tone (limp)
- Apneic
- Usually discovered while asleep, but can occur when awake
- May be evidence of vomiting
- Vigorous stimulation and/or cardiopulmonary resuscitation needed to revive the infant and restore normal breathing
- May take several minutes for the infant to regain improved color and tone after respiration is restored

Interdisciplinary Interventions

Optimal care of infants who have had an episode of apnea accompanied by color change or who present with a serious ALTE includes hospitalization for observation, monitoring by health care personnel, a thorough evaluation for possible causes, and parent training (Care Path 16–1). Continuous cardiorespiratory monitoring and frequent assessment of color, breathing patterns and effort, and tone are appropriate health care interventions for the hospitalized infant with apnea or history of an ALTE. Methods of continuous cardiorespiratory monitoring by which to record and save information (such as pneumograms, documented or "memory" monitoring with automatic event recorders, and polysomnography) yield useful assessment data during the initial evaluation, as well as later in the home setting.

Alert: *In cases in which no treatable cause for an ALTE is found, numerous studies have demonstrated that these infants have a risk that is 15 times greater for subsequent death from SIDS than that of the general population (Kelly, Shannon, & O'Connell, 1978; Oren, Kelly, & Shannon, 1986; Ward et al., 1986).*

As a group, these infants also have a high incidence of subsequent episodes of apnea (Keens et al., 1982). The preterm infant who continues to exhibit symptomatic apnea during the hospital stay should also be evaluated carefully for hypoxia or anemia, which can cause apnea in the premature infant. In the absence of hypoxia or anemia, preterm infants who are still having clinical episodes of apnea can be discharged with home apnea/bradycardia monitoring equipment.

Respiratory stimulants such as theophylline or caffeine are sometimes useful in decreasing the severity and/or frequency of apneic episodes. Theophylline and caffeine are central nervous system stimulants that act on the respiratory center of the brain and therefore are sometimes effective in treating central apnea only. Besides stimulating the respiratory center, these drugs also act on the kidney, heart, and skeletal and smooth muscles. Side effects include tachycardia and increased diuresis. Parents and caregivers must be taught to draw up and administer the medications and observe for toxic side effects (tachycardia, vomiting, excessive irritability). Therapeutic drug levels should be monitored, and toxic levels should be reported.

Community Care

Because there is currently no specific treatment for infants with AOI or ALTE of unknown etiology, home apnea/bradycardia monitoring is the primary therapy. Ongoing therapy can be equally anxiety-producing as the initial ALTE for parents and families. Home monitors serve only to alert the caregiver that an apneic episode is occurring (Fig. 16–18). The parent or caregiver must then respond and act to evaluate and terminate the apneic episode. Most parents feel the need to use the monitor at all times when the infant is not being directly observed. Home apnea monitoring often adversely affects parents' ability to work, socialize, nurture their other children, and generally maintain their former life functions because of their obsessive focus on the monitor and its every nuance (Nuttall, 1988).

Before initiation of home apnea monitoring, the nursing assessments for this population should begin while the infant is hospitalized. Before discharge, the nurse should conduct a thorough review of the family's living arrangements and verification of the presence of appropriate resources to successfully support a home apnea monitoring program. Minimum environmental requirements include electricity, a telephone in the home, and availability of caregivers trained to respond to the apnea alarm. The inpatient evaluation of the family system prior to discharge is crucial in determining the teaching plan and coordinating follow-up. It may be necessary to contact community resources when appropriate according to the family's needs (Spinner, Gibson, Wrobel, & Spitzer, 1995).

Parental education for home apnea/bradycardia monitoring includes information on when to use the monitor,

Figure 16–18
Child with a home apnea monitor.

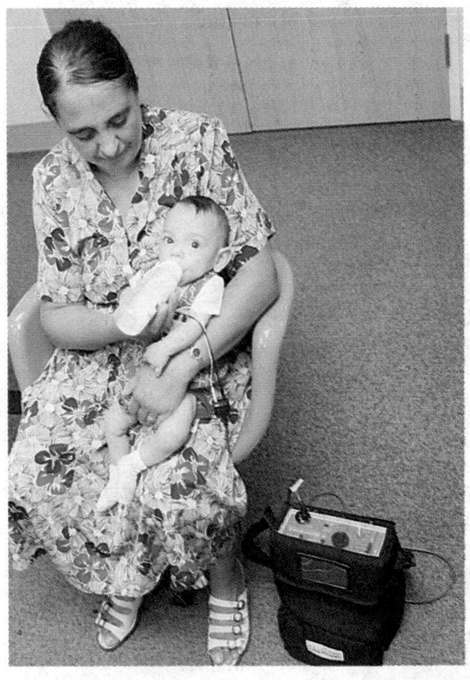

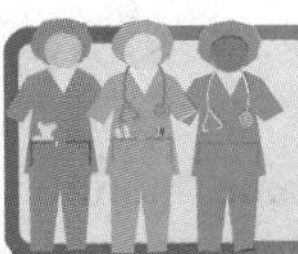

Care Path 16-1 An Interdisciplinary Plan of Care for the Child with Apnea

Nursing Diagnosis	Patient/Family Intermediate Outcomes			
	Day: Admission	Day 1	Day 2	Day 3: Discharge
Ineffective breathing pattern related to apneic episodes	Child will have effective breathing pattern without apneic spells throughout hospitalization.	⟶	⟶	⟶
Impaired home management maintenance related to change in home care regimen	Parents will verbalize understanding of necessary diagnostic tests and consultations.	⟶	Parents will verbalize and demonstrate understanding of CPR and home apnea monitor prior to discharge.	⟶
Altered family processes related to anxiety associated with threat of infant death	Parents will develop open communication with health care team and receive patient information in a timely manner.	⟶	⟶	Parents will verbalize understanding of need to develop support system to provide respite care.
Care Intervention Categories				
Consults	Social service Gastroenterology	Basic life support instructor		
Discharge planning	Notify discharge planner of need for home nursing referral at time of discharge. Find out whether family has telephone.	Advise family of home nursing referral. Complete home health care referral. Contact home health agency.	Discharge conference with parents to review teaching needs, follow-up clinic visits, equipment needs, and financial resources. Provide parents with information on support group or name of other family with child on apnea monitoring at home.	Home visit by home care agency is scheduled.
Labs	Possible tests include CBC, capillary blood gases, calcium, electrolytes, glucose, septic work-up	If theophylline is given, theophylline level after third dose.		
Medications and IVs	If needed, theophylline or caffeine.	⟶	⟶	Gastroesophageal reflux medications, if indicated
Monitors	Cardiorespiratory monitor Pulse oximetry	⟶ ⟶	Place home monitoring device on child	⟶

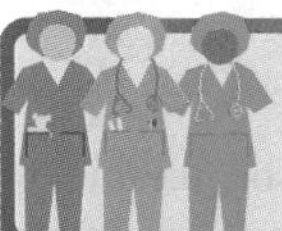

Care Path 16–1 An Interdisciplinary Plan of Care for the Child with Apnea *Continued*

Care Intervention Categories	Day: Admission	Day 1	Day 2	Day 3: Discharge
Nutrition	Diet for age as tolerated	→	→	→
		Reflux precautions if diagnosed with reflux	→	→
	Accurate intake and output	→	→	→
Procedures (diagnostics)	Pneumogram (pneumocardiogram) ECG, EEG Chest x-ray	If history indicates, upper GI series, reflux scan, Ph probe, polysomnography		
Safety and activity	Head of bed elevated.	→	→	→
	Position on abdomen between feedings.	→	→	→
	Avoid hyperflexion of neck.	→	→	→
Teaching	Orient family to hospital and primary caregivers. Have family verbalize understanding of monitors and diagnostic studies.	Have family verbalize understanding of infant's cardiopulmonary system. Have family demonstrate reflux precautions, medication administration, monitor application, steps to answer monitor alarms. Begin CPR teaching.	Have family demonstrate use of home monitor. Have family demonstrate CPR. Review guidelines for using home monitoring with parents.	Suggest to parents that other child care providers (grandparents, babysitters) learn monitor use and CPR
Vital signs/ baseline parameters	Check vital signs every 4 hr	→	→	→
	Daily weights	→	→	→
	Height on admission	→	→	→
	Complete assessment with emphasis on respiratory system.	Assess response to reflux precautions.	→	→
	Assess and document respiratory responses to care.	→	→	→

CBC, complete blood count; CPR, cardiopulmonary resuscitation; EEG, electroencephalogram; ECG, electrocardiogram; GI, gastrointestinal.

how to respond to alarms (including appropriate assessments and interventions), when and from whom to seek help, and infant cardiopulmonary resuscitation. Parents and caregivers are also taught to keep a log or diary of all apnea and bradycardia alarms, especially those requiring any intervention. If both parents work outside the home, alternative caregivers (extended family members, daycare providers, etc.) must also receive this education (TIP 16–4).

The National Institutes of Health Consensus Development Conference on Infantile Apnea and Home Monitoring (National Institutes of Health [NIH], 1987) suggested that an adequate monitoring support system include medical, technical, psychosocial, and community support services. As in the case of AOP, the nurse or social service professional conducts an assessment of the family's strengths, weaknesses, and support resources and provides families with anticipatory guidance to help prepare for the demands of home monitoring. Ideally, there should be monitor program support staff available to parents on a 24-hour basis after discharge from the hospital, as well as access to other psychosocial support mechanisms (Ahmann, 1992). Most infants with ALTE require 4 to 6 months of home monitoring. The decision to discontinue the apnea monitor should be made jointly between the family and the health care professionals. If the decision to end monitoring is made, parents should receive a clear statement of the status of the problem, that it appears to have resolved, and that the infant can be expected to grow and progress normally (National Association of Apnea Professionals, 1996). Discontinuation of monitoring is accomplished using a similar protocol as in persistent AOP, in that the monitor may be safely discontinued after 2 to 3 months of no apnea or bradycardia spells that require intervention (NIH, 1987). Because of the diligence required for successful home monitoring, many parents find it difficult to stop home monitoring when it is no longer required for their infant. The caregiver has learned to rely on the monitor to provide a comforting reassurance that the child is well. Nurses in home apnea monitoring programs should provide anticipatory guidance and psychological preparation regarding this issue. Some infants have died as a result of noncompliance or errors in home monitoring techniques (Ward et al., 1986). This highlights the extreme importance of parental teaching and assessment/reassessment of home monitoring skills.

Parental anxiety is characteristically the foremost psychosocial issue challenging nurses and other members of the health care team in working with the infant and family after admission to the hospital with an apneic episode or after an ALTE. The parents of these infants, especially if one or both were the observers of the initial episode, may believe that the infant was in the process of dying. They are often terrified that a similar event will occur in the future from which they will be unable to revive their infant. Much guidance and reassurance is needed in conjunction with education to increase parental confidence and problem-solving skills.

Foreign Body Aspiration

Foreign body aspiration (FBA) remains a persistent problem and an important cause of morbidity and mortality in the pediatric age group. Foreign bodies retained in the airway can be potentially life-threatening and/or can produce severe lung damage. Commonly aspirated objects include foods such as hot dogs, peanuts, other nuts and seeds, grapes, popcorn, and carrots as well as items such as small plastic toys, marbles, buttons, earrings, and latex balloons. Factors related to a young child's physical and developmental status predispose him or her to the risk of foreign body aspiration. Young children explore the environment by putting objects in their mouths. In addition, seeking relief from the teething process by chewing on hard objects is also a contributing factor to the occurrence of foreign body aspiration. Exposure to certain foods may be inappropriate for a young child's cognitive and dental stage of development, leading to incidence of choking and aspiration.

Incidence

It is difficult to quantify overall incidence of this phenomenon because the vast majority of foreign bodies aspirated into the respiratory tract are probably expelled immediately by spontaneous coughing, never requiring medical intervention. The Consumer Product Safety Commission monitors emergency room encounters for 119 hospitals representing all geographic regions of the United States. They reported a 2-year analysis (1988–1989) of more than 1100 emergency room encounters for foreign body aspirations in children aged 0 to 3 years. Seventy-seven percent of these children were between 1 and 3 years old, with the average age of 23 months. Overall, more than half (52%) were boys, and 87% of the children older than 3 years were boys. The increased incidence of foreign body aspiration in boys is attributed to their increased activity level. The home was the most common site of injury (Reilly, 1992).

Pathophysiology

The pathophysiology of foreign body aspiration is variable depending on the substance or object aspirated, the size of the foreign body, the location of the object in the respiratory tract, and the acute or chronic nature of the condition. If an object is too large or of a shape that does not allow it to be expelled by coughing, respiratory

TIP 16-4 A Teaching Instructional Plan for the Infant on Home Apnea Monitoring

Nursing Diagnoses and Family Outcomes

- Ineffective breathing pattern related to apneic episodes
  Outcome: Infant demonstrates an effective respiratory rate, rhythm, and effort and will not experience any apneic episodes.
- Knowledge deficit related to management of therapeutic regimen including home apnea monitor use and infant cardiopulmonary rescucitation.
  Outcome: Parents/caregivers verbalize understanding of rationale for home apnea monitoring, demonstrate proper technique in home monitor use, and demonstrate appropriate infant CPR technique.
- Altered family processes related to having infant with apnea
  Outcome: Family shall maintain open communication, participate in care of the infant, assist in identifying resources, and identify role functions.

Instructional Interventions

Monitor Use

- Instruct parents or caregivers on use of the home apnea monitor:
  - Rationale for use
  - When to use the monitor
  - How to respond to alarms
  - Documentation of alarms
  - What to do in the event of an emergency
- Instruct parents/caregivers on proper technique of monitor use:
  - Application of electrodes
  - Cleaning equipment
  - Trouble-shooting false alarms

Medications

- Instruct parents/caregivers about the rationale for any medications prescribed, including theophylline or caffeine and medications for gastroesophageal reflux if present.
  - Dosage and times of administration
  - Drug/food interactions
  - Potential side effects and/or toxic effects

Infant Cardiopulmonary Resuscitation

- Instruct parents/caregivers on proper CPR and airway obstruction techniques for the infant.

Follow-up Care

- Discuss with family the importance for follow-up care with physician and other health care providers involved with the infant's care. Physician is to be available 24 hours a day for consultation.
- Equipment vendors should be available by telephone 24 hours a day in the event of monitor problems.
- Refer family for appropriate psychosocial support if family is experiencing concerns and increased stress related to infant's being monitored.

Community Care

- Refer parents/caregivers to community resources for additional CPR training if requested: American Heart Association or American Red Cross.
- Help identify support groups or parent-to-parent telephone contact.

symptoms result. Foreign bodies in the upper airway often cause a mechanical obstruction or partial obstruction that results in non-specific respiratory signs and symptoms such as cough, wheeze, stridor, dyspnea, voice changes, cyanosis, retractions, and/or hemoptysis. These symptoms are usually exhibited at the time of the aspiration, although in 10% to 20% of patients, symptoms subside or are not present at all until days or weeks following the event (Wagner, 1994). At times, a carefully assessed history reveals an episode of coughing, choking, or breathing difficulty that can be traced back to an aspiration event, but on many occasions, the discovery of a foreign body aspiration is made without ever obtaining such a history from the child or caregivers (Wagner, 1994).

Prognosis. The prognosis for a child returning to his or her previous respiratory status following aspiration of a foreign body is good if evaluation is made quickly and the object is extracted by bronchoscopy as soon as possible. Complications that arise related to foreign body aspiration events are most often linked to a delay in proper diagnosis and treatment (Wagner, 1994). In extreme cases, the child may require a tracheostomy, depending on where the obstruction is, if there is persistent airway obstruction due to tissue damage and edema. Asphyxiation and death can occur following complete laryngeal or tracheal obstruction.

Assessment

The location of the foreign body is a key factor in determining the sign, symptoms, and physical assessment findings (Table 16–9). Although nearly all children who have aspirated a foreign body exhibit a chronic cough and/or a history of an acute coughing episode, other symptoms vary according to where in the respiratory tract the object is lodged.

The child with a foreign body that lodges in the upper airway, such as the larynx or trachea, usually presents with an acute and rather fierce onset of stridor and respiratory distress necessitating immediate intervention to dislodge the foreign body. A foreign body lodged in the bronchus may act as a ball valve, obstructing the airway perhaps partially on inspiration and completely on expiration. Wheezing localized to one side of the chest on inspiration and diminished breath sounds on expiration result. In children with an esophageal foreign body, the trachea is impinged upon by compression from a nearby distended esophagus, causing respiratory distress. Physical assessment findings may reveal asymmetry of chest wall movement and/or wheezing or diminished breath sounds in a localized area of the lungs. If the obstruction is located in the upper airway, stridor is common.

Diagnostic Tests. Chest x-ray findings are varied. X-ray films may be normal, may allow clear visualization of the presence of a foreign body, or may show changes related to the foreign body directly or caused by secondary inflammatory changes. Abnormalities are less likely to be noted on the chest x-ray films for foreign bodies located above the bifurcation of the mainstem bronchus (Mu, Sun, & He, 1990). Lateral neck films are obtained when this is suspected. If a delay in diagnosis has occurred, radiographic abnormalities are more likely (Blazer, Naveh, & Friedman, 1980).

"Chronically" retained foreign bodies can lead to a marked inflammatory response in the respiratory tract and, possibly, death. The right mainstem bronchus is a

Table 16–9
Locations of Foreign Body Aspirates

Location of Foreign Body	Clinical Findings
Supraglottic	Cough, dyspnea, drooling, gagging, changes in phonation
Larynx	Cough, stridor, changes in phonation, at time severe respiratory distress
Trachea—intrathoracic	Expiratory wheeze, inspiratory noise
Trachea—extrathoracic	Inspiratory stridor, expiratory noise
Bronchi	Cough, asymmetric breath sounds or wheeze, hyperresonance
Esophageal	Drooling, dysphagia, stridor, respiratory distress

common site for foreign body lodgment because of its angle. Airway inflammation and narrowing secondary to edema often occurs. Materials such as nuts, which contain fats, cause an especially intense inflammatory response. Recurrent infections such as lipoid pneumonia or a lung abscess may ensue. Chronic obstruction of air exchange to the alveoli could result in a picture of obstructive emphysema on chest x-ray films. Foreign bodies that have been dislodged by coughing can lead to involvement as described here in different lung segments.

Psychosocial Assessment

The psychosocial manifestations of a foreign body aspiration incident vary in intensity, depending on the severity of the event. The most dramatic scenario involves the infant or child with a complete airway obstruction who is experiencing respiratory arrest and requires immediate resuscitation. This is an extremely terrifying experience for both the child and the caregivers. Asphyxiation with subsequent brain damage and/or death may occur. The grief and guilt that parents and caregivers experience in this situation are tremendous and often incapacitating. The availability of extensive support and counseling services is crucial for these families. Families with less severe episodes of foreign body aspiration may also express feelings of guilt or embarrassment at inadequate supervision of their young child or at unrecognized symptoms resulting in a delay in seeking medical attention. Education on the prevention of foreign body aspiration is an effective nursing intervention for such situations (Chart 16–17).

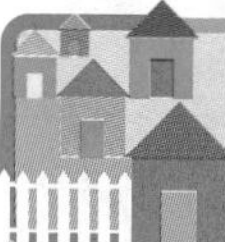

Chart 16–17
Community Care

Preventing Foreign Body Aspiration

- No small, hard candies, raisins, popcorn, or nuts should be given to children younger than 3 to 4 years of age.
- Cut hot dogs, Vienna sausages, and grapes into small pieces.
- Supervise children well during snacks and meals, and minimize distractions (such as watching television).
- Insist that children be seated while eating.
- Caution children about running, jumping, or talking with food in their mouth.
- Inspect toys for small, removable parts.
- Keep coins, latex balloons, and earrings out of young children's reach.

Interdisciplinary Interventions

Emergency treatment for the choking child includes the use of abdominal thrusts (the Heimlich maneuver) in the child older than 1 year of age and use of back blows and chest thrusts in the infant younger than 1 year. (See Chapter 30 for a discussion of these techniques.) These methods should be used in situations in which the aspiration was witnessed or strongly suspected and the child has an ineffective cough with increasing stridor and respiratory distress or has become unconscious and apneic.

In many cases, the object is not coughed up spontaneously and is lodged further down in the respiratory tree; therefore, the foreign body has to be removed as soon as possible to prevent further airway damage. Rigid bronchoscopy to remove the foreign body after aspiration is the most common medical intervention. This procedure is very safe and effective when carried out by an experienced physician. Rigid bronchoscopy allows removal of the object and any associated inflammatory material, as well as providing an assessment of the condition of the airway. Flexible fiberoptic bronchoscopy is considered for the infant or child without a conclusive history of foreign body aspiration but with persistent unexplained respiratory symptoms.

Nursing care responsibilities for the infant or child undergoing rigid bronchoscopy should focus on preoperative preparation and postoperative monitoring. Provide an explanation to the family regarding the reason for the procedure. Intravenous hydration, emptying of stomach contents, and preoperative assessment of respiratory status are fundamental interventions. A respiratory therapist should be available to assist the physician during the procedure and to assess the patient. Postoperative assessment of respiratory status is imperative. Frequent assessment of the quality and symmetry of breath sounds is essential, along with the careful documentation of vital signs, color, and respiratory effort. Atelectasis, bronchospasm, and pneumothorax all are possible postbronchoscopy complications.

Community Care

The most effective "therapy" for foreign body aspiration is prevention. Anyone who works with children should be certified in cardiopulmonary resuscitation, including airway obstruction management. Health care providers should encourage parents and others involved in caring for young children to be taught and certified in these procedures to be able to deal effectively in the event of a foreign body aspiration. Providing education for parents and other caregivers of infants and young children regarding aspiration risk factors is an essential role for all pediatric health care providers. Information on common items aspirated, especially risky age groups, and developmental and environmental considerations can help parents be more aware of potential dangers and take proper precautions. Children in the age range of 6 months to 2 years commonly place objects in their mouth as a way of exploring their environment and are at highest risk for aspiration events. They also have insufficient size and number of teeth to thoroughly chew foods.

Objects most commonly aspirated are small and have a smooth surface and a round or cylindrical shape. The most common offenders are foods such as hot dogs and Vienna sausages, small candies, peanuts, and grapes. An additional risk factor for foods are items that are hard or tough (peanuts, carrots) and difficult to chew. The most commonly ingested nonfood items are coins, balloons, small balls, marbles, and earrings. In April 1990, the Consumer Product Safety Commission recommended that warning labels be placed on all packages of the toys named here, as these objects were associated with the highest aspiration mortality rates (Reilly, 1992).

Environmental factors such as a high degree of distraction during play and meal times and insufficient adult supervision may also contribute to foreign body aspiration. Parents must be reminded that watching television during meals can be a dangerous distraction to toddlers and young children and should be avoided. Caregivers of children at play must be cautioned about being vigilant with small children, to keep them from putting objects in their mouths. Visitors to the home should place their purse and other personal items out of reach of the small child. Lastly, products containing any small, cylindrical components should contain labels discouraging use around young children and detail the age groups particularly affected.

Lower Respiratory Infections and Obstructions

The lower respiratory system consists of the conducting airways beneath the trachea and the organ of respiration, the lungs. The structures of the lower respiratory system constitute the reactive portion of the airway because of their smooth muscle content and ability to constrict. Infection and inflammation of these structures can quickly result in increased mucus production, edema, altered gas exchange, and air trapping.

Lower respiratory tract infections can be a serious threat to the health of any child but are especially dangerous to the child with underlying conditions such as congenital heart disease or chronic lung disease. Lower respiratory tract disorders are treated with supportive care as well as oral or parenteral antibiotics, oxygen, respiratory therapy measures, nutritional support, and aerosolized medication.

Influenza

Influenza illnesses have been described and defined epidemiologically for centuries. Influenza viral agents were the first proved to be respiratory tract pathogens. Consequently, the terms "flu" and "influenza" are perhaps the most overused diagnostic labels for nondescript infectious conditions in both medical and lay circles. This confusion is probably due to an extremely broad range of clinical manifestations of influenza infection and its wide prevalence in the community.

Etiology

There are three influenza virus types, specific in their protein and antigen composition: influenza A, B, and C. There are literally hundred of subtypes of these categories that "shift" their complement of antigens on a regular basis. These mutations largely account for the ability of influenza to produce serious epidemics in populations of people who have been previously immunized or have experienced influenza infection. This makes the preparation and distribution of influenza vaccines necessary on an annual basis.

Influenza infection often occurs in epidemics that sweep throughout a community in a matter of 6 to 8 weeks. Thousands of individuals die from influenza infections in the United States each year. Morbidity is highest in susceptible populations such as infants and persons older than 65 years of age. The incidence of infection is highest, however, in children of school age. Infection with influenza A virus is approximately four times more common than infection with influenza B virus.

Pathophysiology

The influenza viruses are large, single-stranded RNA viruses. One of the predominant pathogenic characteristics of influenza viruses is its affinity for epithelial cells of the respiratory tract mucosa. The virus causes a lytic infection of the respiratory epithelium with a loss of ciliary function, decreased mucus production, and desquamation of the epithelial layer. The incubation period for influenza virus can be as short as 2 to 3 days, and viral replication usually continues for 10 to 14 days after primary infection (Wright, 1996).

Prognosis. In most children, influenza is a self-limiting, febrile, respiratory illness. Subglottic croup is a common manifestation, especially in infants. Some children experience complications including sepsis, laryngotracheobronchitis, pneumonia, myocarditis, acute myositis, and Reye's syndrome in children who may have received salicylates. Children with compromised respiratory status, such as those with cystic fibrosis, bronchopulmonary dysplasia, severe asthma, and cardiac disease, may develop acute respiratory failure. Fatality in previously healthy children is rare and is generally the result of viral pneumonia or a secondary bacterial infection.

Assessment

Infections with influenza viruses may be manifested by mild, moderate, or severe clinical symptoms. Generally a child with influenza infection has a more sudden onset of these symptoms than do children with parainfluenza, respiratory syncytial virus, or adenovirus infections. Children with influenza present with a fever of sudden onset accompanied by a flushed face, dry throat and nasal mucous membranes with dry cough, sore throat, muscle pain, headache, and malaise. During the acute phase of the illness, the child may be quite ill and require hospitalization if dehydrated or if a secondary infection develops. Fever, sore throat, and headache normally subside in 3 to 5 days, whereas other symptoms such as fatigue and malaise may persist for several weeks. Supportive interaction with parents is necessary because anxiety often exists regarding progression of the illness and complications. Children are often disappointed at missing important events and activities, yet they do not have the strength to participate.

Interdisciplinary Interventions

Interventions for the child with influenza include supportive care to alleviate or minimize symptoms. Administration of acetaminophen every 4 to 6 hours for fever and muscle aches is beneficial.

Alert: *It is never appropriate to treat children 18 years of age or younger with aspirin or other salicylate derivatives because of the relationship between viral syndromes, aspirin, and Reye's syndrome.*

Other antipyretic therapies include undressing the child with a persistent fever to permit radiant heat loss and giving tepid sponge baths.

caREminder: *Do not bathe a shivering child, as it is likely the child will shiver more and remain febrile.*

Parents should be taught the signs and symptoms of respiratory deterioration, the signs of dehydration as well as its prevention and treatment, and the contraindication of aspirin administration in children.

Clear liquids for children and oral rehydration formulas for infants replace losses from fever, tachypnea, and vomiting. Oral fluids should be offered in small amounts (30–60 mL) on a frequent basis. If the child becomes dehydrated and requires hospitalization, he or she should receive parenteral fluids. Rest and bed rest is important to the child and should be encouraged for the first 3 to 5 days. The hospitalized child should be assessed for hydration status (i.e., skin turgor, presence of tears, last void), and respiratory status should be monitored for signs of increasing respiratory distress related to complications. If the child is home, the nurse should instruct the parents or caretaker what to watch for, such as increased lethargy, excessive vomiting, or respiratory distress that may indicate that the child needs to be seen by a health care professional.

Alert: *Supplemental oxygen may be needed for chronically ill children with an influenza infection because of their poor respiratory reserves and increased propensity to develop hypoxemia.*

Community Care

In the community, use of inactivated influenza vaccine is recommended to prevent influenza for the following categories of individuals:

- Infants and children 6 months of age or older who would be at high risk if they contracted influenza.
- Medical care providers or household contacts of infants and children listed in Chart 16–18.
- Children and adolescents who are receiving long-term aspirin therapy and thus might have an increased risk of acquiring Reye's syndrome as a result of influenza virus infection.
- Other children whose families wish to reduce their chances of acquiring influenza.

The American Academy of Pediatrics has further defined specific recommendations for targeted at-risk children (Chart 16–18). The only specific contraindication for the use of this inactivated vaccine is anaphylactic hypersensitivity to eggs.

Bronchiolitis

Bronchiolitis is an acute inflammation and obstruction of the bronchioles, the smallest, most distal sections of the respiratory airway network. It generally occurs during the first 2 years of life, with a peak incidence between 2 and 6 months of age. Infant susceptibility may be due to the lack of full maternal antibody protection that is universally present at birth and for the first few months of life (Schwartz, 1995). In some areas, it is the most frequent cause for hospitalization of infants younger than the age of 1 year. The incidence is highest during winter and

Chart 16–18

Recommendations for Administering the Influenza Vaccine to Children Who Are at High Risk of Infection

- Chronic pulmonary disease (cystic fibrosis, asthma, bronchopulmonary dysplasia)
- Congenital heart diseases and hemodynamically significant diseases
- Those receiving immunosuppressive therapy
- Sickle cell disease and other hemoglobinopathies
- Diabetes and other chronic metabolic diseases
- Chronic renal disease
- Symptomatic human immunodeficiency virus (HIV) infection

From American Academy of Pediatrics. (1988). Immunization practices committee: Prevention and control of influenza. *Morbidity and Mortality Weekly Report, 37*, 361.

early spring. Many infants can be managed at home; a few may require hospitalization.

Etiology

Acute bronchiolitis most often has a viral cause. In more than one half of the cases (up to 85%), respiratory syncytial virus (RSV) is the cause (McIntosh, 1991) (Chart 16–19). Infections with other viruses, primarily adenovirus, parainfluenza, and influenza, have been associated with bronchiolitis in smaller numbers of cases. In a small percentage of infants with bronchiolitis, suprainfection with a bacterial pathogen can occur. RSV is transmitted by direct contact with infected secretions. Adults as well as children are infected with RSV disease, thus the source of viral infection in an infant is usually a family member with a mild respiratory illness. Infants who are at particular risk for developing respiratory failure and complications related to bronchiolitis include infants with chronic lung disease such as bronchopulmonary dysplasia, congenital heart disease, or immunodeficiency.

Pathophysiology

In bronchiolitis, the bronchioles become narrowed, and some even become totally occluded as a result of the inflammatory process, edema of the airway wall, accumulation of mucus and cellular debris, and smooth muscle spasm. There may also be thickening of the muscular wall and destruction of ciliated cells. This narrowing of the airway lumen can cause a profound decrease in air flow. Impaired clearance of secretions and decreased air flow lead to bronchiolar obstruction, atelectasis, and hyperinflation, causing impaired gas exchange that results in hypoxemia. Carbon dioxide retention occurs in the severely affected infant. It is not uncommon for respiratory rates to be more than 60 breaths per minute and as high as the low 100's per minute.

Prognosis. Infants with moderate to severe respiratory distress due to bronchiolitis are usually hospitalized. Although they may appear extremely ill on admission to the hospital, these infants, given proper supportive care, show clinical improvement within 3 to 4 days. However, the clinical course may be prolonged. Some infants have a protracted course, with persistent wheezing and abnormalities in gas exchange that may take months to resolve.

Assessment

The infant with bronchiolitis has typically had an upper respiratory infection for 2 to 3 days. Parents report sneezing and nasal discharge initially, and then the infant develops a harsh dry cough and low-grade fever. Wheezing is often heard on auscultation, and the infant may develop increasingly distressed breathing and tachypnea. These infants have feeding difficulties with loss of appetite because of nasal congestion and increased work of breathing. Respiratory distress with feeding difficulties is usually the reason for admission to the hospital.

Hospitalized infants with RSV bronchiolitis are at high risk for respiratory failure and may require a course of mechanical ventilation during the acute phase of the illness. Generally the most critical phase of the disease is

Chart 16–19

What Is RSV?

- It is a highly contagious respiratory virus that is extremely prevalent in communities in the winter and early spring months.
- RSV has a high affinity for respiratory tract mucosa.
- Most children develop infection within the first 3 years of life.
- Most children tolerate infection without problems.
- RSV can cause severe lower respiratory tract infections (and sometimes death) in some children with underlying chronic conditions.
- RSV is commonly spread through direct contact with infectious secretions via hands, droplets, and fomites.

the first 24 to 72 hours. At highest risk are those infants with underlying cardiac or pulmonary conditions. Clinical indications for mechanical ventilation include worsening respiratory distress with increased work of breathing, heart rates of more than 200 beats per minute, poor peripheral perfusion, apnea and/or bradycardia, and hypercarbia.

Because a major consequence of airway obstruction is impaired gas exchange, the child with bronchiolitis has many of the signs and symptoms of hypoxia and respiratory distress. The respiratory rate is increased, often to rates of more than 60 breaths per minute. Chest retractions are visible; rhonchi and wheezes or crackles are generally heard in all lung fields. Respiratory distress often prevents adequate oral fluid intake; thus, the child with bronchiolitis may be significantly dehydrated. In addition, there is insensible fluid loss due to elevated respiratory rate. When the infant becomes ill during winter months, dry air may further exacerbate the condition. Hypoxia and hypercarbia result in restlessness and irritability, making the child difficult to console, even by parents.

Interdisciplinary Interventions

The care of a child with bronchiolitis involves respiratory, pharmacologic, and nutritional support (Care Path 16–2). The child's caretakers play an active role in the health management of the child, because most children are not hospitalized and do not require 24-hour care by the health care team.

Because RSV and other causative agents are shed in high titers for days after the onset of the illness, contact isolation of other patients and family members is strongly recommended. Transmission of infection to staff and other patients in the hospital is not uncommon, as RSV is also easily transmitted on hands, clothing, equipment, cribs, etc. Limitation of child-to-child contact, washing toys between children's use of them, and careful hand washing are the most effective methods of preventing nosocomial infections.

Respiratory Support

Oxygen should be administered to infants with all but the mildest cases of bronchiolitis. The oxygen is optimally humidified and of a concentration sufficient to maintain arterial oxygen saturations greater than or equal to 92%. Continuous pulse oximetry is recommended for infants in acute distress (see Diagnostic Criteria). Care should be taken to document oxygen saturations when the child is awake during quiet time, asleep, and with crying. Desaturations less than 90% with crying would be expected, therefore close monitoring until saturations return to baseline (more than 92%) is essential.

Pharmacologic Support

Bronchodilators, aminophylline, and corticosteroids have not been documented to be effective in viral bronchiolitis and are not recommended for use (Rakshi & Couriel, 1994). They are, however, sometimes used in infants with more severe respiratory distress.

Ribavirin (Virazole) is an antiviral agent that has been demonstrated to reduce significantly the severity of bronchiolitis caused by RSV when administered early in the course of the illness. In mechanically ventilated infants, most of whom were previously healthy and had no underlying conditions, ribavirin treatment has been demonstrated to be safe and was associated with a reduced need for mechanical ventilation and supplemental oxygen, shorter duration of hospitalization, and cost-effectiveness (American Academy of Pediatrics, 1993). Other candidates for ribavirin therapy include infants at increased risk for respiratory complications and respiratory failure because they have an underlying cardiac, lung (bronchopulmonary dysplasia or cystic fibrosis), or immunodeficiency disease.

The drug can be used on the intubated mechanically ventilated patient as well as the nonintubated patient. It is administered as an aerosolized particle mist, typically over 12 to 18 hours daily, for 3 to 5 days. Adverse reactions to ribavirin therapy include anemia, conjunctivitis, and rash. Nurses and respiratory therapists administering ribavirin should wear a specially designed mask to prevent exposure to ribavirin particles released into the air and seek further information if additional concerns about personal safety exist (Chart 16–20).

Chart 16–20

Hazards of Ribavirin Therapy

- Precipitation of ribavirin in the ventilator apparatus can result in obstruction or malfunction of the expiratory valve, resulting in high positive end-expiratory pressure (PEEP).
- Although ribavirin has shown no embryo toxicity in primates, it has been shown to be reabsorbed in fetuses of pregnant rabbits and to cause malformation of offspring in rodents. Even though there have been no validated detrimental effects to human fetuses after several years of clinical use, it is not recommended that pregnant health care professionals care for a patient receiving ribavirin therapy.
- Precipitation of the drug on contact lenses has been associated with conjunctivitis and damage to contact lenses.

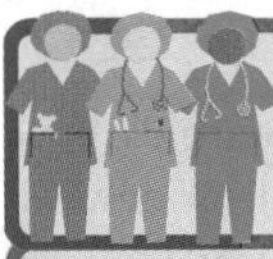

Care Path 16–2 An Interdisciplinary Plan of Care for the Child with Bronchiolitis

	Patient/Family Intermediate Outcomes		
Nursing Diagnosis	**Day 1**	**Day 2**	**Day 3**
Ineffective breathing pattern related to inflammatory process of mucous membranes in bronchioles	Child will demonstrate and maintain an improved breathing pattern throughout hospitalization as evidenced by decrease or absence of tachypnea, retractions, nasal flaring, grunting, wheezing, cyanosis, and/or cough.	Child will demonstrate an improved breathing pattern throughout therapy with ribavirin (if ordered).	⟶
Impaired gas exchange related to bronchiolar obstruction, atelectasis, and hyperinflation	Infant demonstrates adequate oxygenation and ventilation as evidenced by oxygen saturations >92% and decreased work of breathing.	⟶	⟶
Alteration in nutrition: less than body requirements related to decreased oral intake and increased metabolic rate from fever and tachypnea	Infant demonstrates adequate nutritional and fluid intake for age as evidenced by tolerating feeds and weight maintenance.	⟶	⟶
Parental knowledge deficit related to home management of bronchiolitis	Family verbalizes and demonstrates an understanding of home medication administration.	⟶	⟶
Care Intervention Categories			
Consults	Infectious disease physician Pediatric pulmonologist prior to initiation of ribavirin, if needed		
Discharge planning		Possible discharge if ribavirin therapy not needed. Return to clinic if signs/symptoms of respiratory distress recur.	If ribavirin therapy is given, consider discharge after 3 days of therapy if clinically stable. For persistent moderate wheezing, arrange for home nebulizer.

Day 4	Day of Discharge
⟶	⟶
⟶	⟶
⟶	⟶
⟶	Family will demonstrate home medication administration.

Care Path continued on following page

RespiGam (respiratory syncytial virus immune globulin intravenous [Human]) has been approved by the United States Food and Drug Administration (FDA) for prevention of serious lower tract respiration infection caused by RSV. The medication is indicated for children younger than 24 months of age with bronchopulmonary dysplasia or a history of premature birth (≤35 weeks' gestation). The first dose should be given prior to RSV season, with subsequent doses given monthly throughout the season for protection ("First RSV Prevention Drug," 1996; Oertel, 1996).

Nutrition and Rest

Nutritional care for the infant with bronchiolitis includes supportive fluid and electrolyte replacement. In the case of severe respiratory distress and/or a respiratory rate of 60 breaths per minute or more, the infant should have nothing by mouth and fluid should be given intravenously. If the patient was malnourished prior to the onset of the illness and/or requires longer term mechanical ventilation, nutritional support with hyperalimentation and intralipids is required. Close monitoring of fluid and electrolyte status, including accurate measurement of intake and output with urine specific gravities, is essential to assess for dehydration.

Respiratory distress or air hunger creates anxiety in both infant and parents. The irritable, crying, inconsolable infant is unable to drink fluids and is exhausting to care for. Parents are often suffering from frustration and worry about the child's condition, as well as being completely exhausted at the time of admission to the hospital. Parents of a child with a chronic condition such as bronchopulmonary dysplasia may experience guilt for not having prevented exposure to infection in their already fragile child. Seeking medical attention may also have been delayed because of knowledge deficit or a variety of reasons. These parents need the opportunity to express their feelings and receive support. Nurses or social service personnel are the ideal members of the health care team to provide these interventions to the family of an ill infant.

Infants hospitalized with acute bronchiolitis are using all their energy to breathe. These infants are too uncomfortable to respond to the social stimuli they are accustomed to, such as television or interaction with siblings. As the child's condition improves, quiet play activities may be gradually reintroduced. Minimizing energy expenditure and oxygen consumption should remain a primary goal of therapy until the child's oxygen saturation levels are continuously within normal limits. Soothing activities, such as musical toys and holding and rocking by parents, will help the infant relax.

Family Education

Education of the parent or caregiver of an infant with bronchiolitis is essential, especially if the child is not

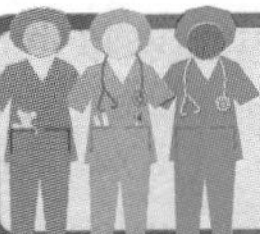

Care Path 16–2 An Interdisciplinary Plan of Care for the Child with Bronchiolitis *Continued*

Care Intervention Categories	Day 1	Day 2	Day 3
Labs	CBC with differential Blood culture (if patient appears toxic or temperature > 102°F). Consider blood gas measurements. Nasal washing for RSV panel.		Repeat laboratory tests that have shown abnormal results.
Medications and IVs (consider if wheezing)	IV fluids at maintenance if clinically dehydrated or not taking PO feeds. IV antibiotics if suspicion or evidence of bacterial infection. Acetaminophen p.r.n. for fever. Neo-Synephrine ⅛% 2–3 drops each nostril every 6 hr p.r.n. for nasal congestion.	IV fluids if clinically dehydrated. Consider ribavirin for premature infants, RSV, or children with underlying chronic condition. ⟶	Maintain IV fluids if not taking PO feeds well or Hep-Lock. ⟶ ⟶
Monitors	Cardiorespiratory monitor Continuous pulse oximetry	⟶ ⟶	⟶ ⟶
Nutrition	NPO if in respiratory distress. PO feedings if RR < 60.	Diet appropriate for age. Encourage PO feeds.	⟶ ⟶
Psychosocial	Parental support for anxiety. Rest for parents if sleep-deprived.		
Radiology	Chest x-ray		
Respiratory	Suction p.r.n. Oxygen to keep O_2 saturation >92%. Raise head of bed.	⟶ Oxygen to keep O_2 saturation >92%. ⟶	⟶ Begin weaning oxygen to keep O_2 saturation >92%. ⟶

Day 4	Day of Discharge
→ → →	Discontinue IV. Discontinue ribavirin.
→ Pulse oximetry check every 4 hr.	Discontinue cardiorespiratory monitor. Discontinue pulse oximeter.
→ →	→ →
→ Continue to wean O_2. →	Discontinue O_2.

Care Path continued on following page

hospitalized and is cared for at home. The parent must be taught to recognize the signs of increasing respiratory distress, such as grunting, retractions, pallor, and/or cyanosis. Teach parents how to count the respiratory rate for a full minute, during both sleep and awake times. Teach parents to encourage fluids and to measure and record the infant's oral intake during the illness and observe for signs of dehydration. Other issues relevant to the care of the infant with bronchiolitis in the home could include use of cool mist to replace insensible fluid loss, positioning the child with the head of the bed elevated for comfort and to facilitate removal of secretions, and quiet play activities as the child's energy level permits. Encourage parents to call their health care provider if they have any doubts about their infant's respiratory status.

The parents caring for their ill child at home may need some respite. Explore with the family their resources, such as extended family, friends, or neighbors who may relieve them, and encourage them to ask for assistance. Parents who have been awake for several nights with an ill, irritable infant need time free of child care responsibilities to sleep. Nurses can assist also by providing support and positive feedback as the infant's condition improves.

Bronchitis

Bronchitis is defined as a transient inflammatory process involving the distal trachea and major bronchi. The pharynx and nasopharynx may also be involved; the laryngeal and subglottic regions are not. Bronchitis can exist in acute, chronic, and recurrent forms. In the child with a competent immune system, bronchitis usually has a viral cause. Most episodes of acute bronchitis caused by bacteria occur as secondary infections while airways are vulnerable following a prior viral attack or other insult. Although exposure to irritants such as gastric acid or passive smoke and environmental pollutants can produce acute symptoms, these insults are more significant in their contribution to symptoms in children with reactive airways (see Asthma). As with most viral respiratory infections, the peak incidence is in winter and early spring. The disease appears to be more common in younger children and in males.

Pathophysiology

The pathologic characteristics of bronchitis include similarities to other respiratory conditions, including bronchiolitis and asthma (Table 16–10). Viral or bacterial agents attack the airway mucosa, causing inflammation and edema. The ciliated epithelium becomes damaged, and there is increased mucous gland activity and infiltration by neutrophils into the airway wall and lumen. This

Care Path 16–2 An Interdisciplinary Plan of Care for the Child with Bronchiolitis *Continued*

Care Intervention Categories	Day 1	Day 2	Day 3
Safety and activity	Activity as tolerated Crib rails up at all times.	⟶ ⟶ Bed rest during ribavirin therapy	⟶ ⟶ ⟶
Special considerations	Contact isolation.	⟶ Visitors must wear mask. No pregnant women if infant receiving ribavirin.	⟶ ⟶
Teaching	Rationale for admission and what to expect during hospitalization	Ribavirin precautions. Use of normal saline drops and bulb syringe.	Home medication administration. Home nebulizer if indicated. Avoid exposure to passive smoke. Appropriateness of over-the-counter medications.
Vital signs/baseline parameters	Check vital signs every 2 hr. Strict intake and output.	Check vital signs every 2–4 hr. ⟶	Check vital signs every 4 hr. ⟶

CBC, complete blood count; NPO, nothing by mouth; PO, by mouth; RR, respiratory rate; RSV, respiratory syncytial virus.

accounts for what sometimes appears to be purulent sputum, in the absence of a bacterial infection. Mucociliary transport is disrupted, and this contributes to secondary bacterial infection. Acute bronchitis is most often a mild and self-limiting condition. Cough is the primary symptom, and it usually resolves within 2 weeks without therapy. There is an extremely low mortality associated with acute bronchitis. Chronic and recurrent bronchitis in children are conditions that are not clearly understood. Pathologic changes commonly seen in chronic bronchitis in childhood include thickened bronchial walls, mucous gland hypertrophy, and chronic inflammation. As these characteristics are commonly seen in asthmatic patients as well, a pathologic link between the two conditions is suspected (Daigle & Cloutier, 1994). Chronic bronchitis in children, however, is a symptom of an underlying pulmonary disorder and may be a significant factor in predisposing the child to chronic respiratory symptoms and lung dysfunction even into the adult years (Burrows & Taussig, 1980).

Assessment

The onset of viral bronchitis is generally gradual, beginning with upper respiratory symptoms such as rhinitis and a minimal cough. Three to 4 days later the cough becomes more pronounced. Cough begins as dry and non-productive and progresses to a looser and more productive nature. Low-grade fever (less than 101°F) is common. Young children generally swallow the mucus, often resulting in vomiting and paroxysmal coughing. Auscultation of the chest may be unremarkable in the early stages; rhonchi and wheezing may be heard as the cough progresses. During the recovery phase of the last 7 to 10

Day 4	Day of Discharge
→	→
→	→
→	
→	→
→	→
→	→

days, the cough subsides and the fever resolves. If the cough or fever persist beyond 2 weeks, a secondary bacterial infection should be suspected, and the child should be referred for appropriate medical treatment.

Interdisciplinary Interventions

Treatment for acute bronchitis is largely supportive. Adequate rest and humidification of room air improve the child's comfort. Exposure to irritants such as cigarette smoke should be strictly avoided. A productive cough is common, so the use of cough suppressants should be discouraged so as to allow the child to cough and expectorate if able. Antibiotics should be reserved for conditions in which a bacterial infection has been confirmed by culture. Acetaminophen may be administered to help reduce the fever. Bronchodilators, such as albuterol, and/or oral steroids may be considered for the child with known or suspected asthma or who is clinically wheezing.

The child with acute bronchitis should be comforted and monitored for respiratory distress. Nutritional support should be focused on maintaining adequate hydration. The child should be encouraged to drink plenty of fluids and eat foods such as ice pops, fruit ices, broth, and Jell-O to prevent dehydration. The child's appetite for foods is usually diminished and post-tussive emesis is common. Small frequent feedings (or clear liquids if vomiting is frequent) are appropriate for the acute phase of the illness. As cough diminishes, regular diet may be gradually resumed.

Community Care

Quiet activities such as watching television, playing with puzzles, and reading books are recommended for the toddler or school-age child while recovering from bronchitis. Allowing for adequate rest is an important consideration, as frequent coughing may disrupt sleep. After the first 3 to 5 days, when the child is feeling better, school homework should be resumed. The child may return to school when he or she receives adequate rest at night, is not coughing, and is afebrile. Normal energy level may not be restored for several days to weeks. Parents should consider half-day school attendance during the recovery period. Teach parents and caregivers that it is important for the child to avoid passive smoke and other environmental pollutants, especially in the case of recurrent bronchitis. Dust- and allergy-proofing the home environment, especially the child's sleeping quarters, helps prevent subsequent recurrences.

Pneumonia

Pneumonia accounts for only 10% to 15% of all respiratory tract infections, but represents a significant cause of morbidity and mortality in children worldwide. Although most deaths occur in third world countries, pneumonia remains a major factor in morbidity in developed countries, especially among the chronically ill pediatric population.

The term pneumonia describes any inflammatory condition of the lung, resulting most frequently from infection, in which the alveoli are filled with fluid and/or blood cells, causing an impairment of oxygen exchange. Pneumonia can be either a primary illness or become a complication of another respiratory infection or underlying illness. It is distinguished from the more common upper respiratory tract infections by the presence of lower respiratory tract signs and symptoms such as tachypnea and rales and associated areas of infiltration on chest x-ray films.

Table 16–10
Characteristics of Acute Bronchitis, Bronchiolitis, and Asthma

	Acute Bronchitis	Bronchiolitis	Asthma
Pathology	Transient inflammation of lower airways from trachea to bronchi Sloughing of respiratory mucosa and mucosal congestion No decrease in air flow or gas exchange	Infectious inflammation of small bronchioles Sloughing of respiratory epithelium into airway Tissue edema and mucus production Leads to decreased air flow and decreased gas exchange	Recurrent airway inflammation on response to allergens or irritants Bronchoconstriction decreases air flow and leads to decreased gas exchange Mucous plugging occurs in the airways
Clinical symptoms	Primary symptom is cough, which may be loose and productive Low-grade fever lasts 3–5 days Rhinitis Some wheezing possible on expiration Severe hypoxia uncommon	Starts with upper airway infection of 1–3 days' duration Progresses to tachypnea (>60 breaths/min), retractions, rales and cough over the next 3–5 days Fever Wheezing variable Severe hypoxia can occur	Episodic expiratory wheezing (sometimes inspiratory wheeze if severe)—can be brief or prolonged Non-productive cough Severe hypoxemia common
Treatment	Bronchodilators if wheezing Antibiotics for documented bacterial infection Avoidance of irritants	Oxygen therapy Fluid support Respiratory support with bronchodilator therapy may be used Corticosteroids rarely helpful Antiviral agents	Brochodilators and corticosteroids Respiratory support if respiratory failure imminent Preventive and environmental control measures Education stressing prevention and/or early detection and treatment
Etiology	Viral or bacterial infection	Usually viral infection	Bronchial hyperreactivity Hereditary component Allergic component Exacerbated by infections

Etiology

The causes of pneumonia in children vary depending on the season and the age and the health status of the child (Chart 16–21). In the newborn infant, pathogens that can cause pneumonia are acquired by several means. Transplacental infection, aspiration of organisms during passage through the birth canal, and contact with humans or contaminated equipment immediately after birth are the most common mechanisms. Organisms contracted during the birth process, such as *Chlamydia pneumoniae* and *Streptococcus pneumoniae*, may cause illness immediately or later in infancy. Newborn infants are also very susceptible to viral organisms in the community, especially during the winter months. Common viruses transmitted by siblings or other family members include respiratory syncytial virus (RSV), enterovirus, rhinovirus, and parainfluenza virus.

After 1 month of age, viruses become the most common cause of pneumonia. RSV is the major cause, occurring mostly in winter and early spring. The parainfluenza viruses occur primarily in spring and fall. Influenza viruses are most prevalent in winter; adenovirus infections occur year round. Bacterial pneumonias occur year round but are most common in the winter months.

Once children reach school age, *Mycoplasma pneumoniae* becomes the most common etiologic agent. Infections occur year round, with sporadic peaks in incidence in the fall or early winter. In this older age group, as in younger children, the influenza and parainfluenza viruses, as well as adenovirus, are common pathogens for pneumonia.

Not all inflammation of the lung is infectious in origin; thus, pneumonia can be caused by aspiration of foreign substances into the lungs. Gastroesophageal reflux with aspiration, smoke inhalation, hydrocarbon ingestion, aspiration of baby talcum powder, near-drowning, and some autoimmune processes (such as pulmonary hemosi-

Chart 16–21

Viral Causes of Pneumonia

Virus	Age	Season
Respiratory syncytial virus (RSV)	Infants, young preschool	Winter
Parainfluenza viruses 1 and 2	Preschool	Fall
Parainfluenza virus 3	Infants and preschool	Spring
Influenza viruses A and B	Preschool, school-age	Winter
Adenoviruses	All ages	Year round

derosis) all can result in a pneumonia-like syndrome. When gastric contents, secretions, blood, or volatile chemical compounds enter the lung, the presence of one or more of these irritants initiates the characteristic inflammatory response. Gastroesophageal reflux, the retrograde movement of gastric contents into the esophagus, is common in normal individuals following meals. It is associated with pneumonia when the acidic contents enter the pharynx, where, if protective mechanisms fail, it is aspirated. Use of baby talcum powder or any other fine-particle material should be avoided, as it can be inhaled into the pharynx and lower airways and precipitate inflammation of tissue (see "Hazards of Baby Powder" in Chapter 25).

Hydrocarbons are organic solvents found in many settings as components of gasoline, furniture polish, cleaning compounds, lighter fluid, paint thinner, and kerosene. The viscosity and chemical composition of these compounds render them readily aspirated and result in damaging sequelae to the respiratory system. Upon entering the alveolar space, they dissolve surfactant lipids and impair surface tension, thereby reducing activity of surfactant. Atelectasis, alveolar cell damage, edema, granulocyte infiltration, hemorrhage, and/or necrosis result.

Smoke inhalation, too, results in similar pathology due to chemical irritation. The irritants involved depend on the source of the smoke. Hydrochloric acid, acrolein and aldehydes are common findings in victims of smoke inhalation from household fires.

Pathophysiology

Although the term pneumonia refers to a multitude of disorders that differ widely depending on causative agent, a common feature is that each involves an inflammatory response. The respiratory tract is normally equipped with a variety of natural mechanisms to guard the lungs against infection. The nose filters air; the cough reflex serves to expel objects or organisms in the laryngeal airway; cilia in the walls of the trachea and bronchi trap small particles and remove them via mucus. When any of these defenses is impaired, viral or bacterial pathogens invade and initiate the inflammatory response.

Viral agents enter the upper respiratory tract and spread via the airways. The severity of the inflammatory response and the associated pathophysiology vary. Characteristic features include loss of alveolar cell wall integrity, resulting in accumulation and stasis of fluid and mucus, and smooth muscle contraction. These changes result in obstruction of airflow and diminished alveolar-capillary gas exchange. Hypoxia ensues as a result of ventilation-perfusion mismatch.

Bacteria are introduced into the lungs through the inhalation of infectious droplets or through the blood stream. The alveolar involvement is characteristically more intense in bacterial pneumonia than that seen in viral infections. The alveoli can fill rapidly with proteinaceous fluid, causing the similar picture of ventilation-perfusion mismatch, or bacterial agents can cause necrosis of intra-alveolar septa, causing abscesses and destruction of lung architecture.

Prognosis. Significant sequelae or long-term alteration of pulmonary function as a result of pneumonia is rare. In developed countries, death is limited almost exclusively to children with underlying conditions such as chronic lung or cardiac diseases. There is an accumulating body of evidence that recurrent viral pulmonary infections in childhood associated with environmental irritants (e.g., secondhand smoke, smog) can lead to chronic lung disease in adults.

Assessment

The signs and symptoms of a respiratory infection also vary depending on the pathogen, the age of the child, and the child's ability to fight infection. Generally, younger children, especially those younger than 3 years of age, exhibit more severe symptoms than older children. Pneumonia, regardless of etiology, is generally distinguished from less severe respiratory tract infections by the cough, tachypnea, crackles, and cyanosis. Although it is not usually possible to distinguish viral versus bacterial pneumonia by clinical manifestations alone, it is important to understand the characteristic presentation of each.

Viral pneumonia typically has a gradual onset, beginning with an upper respiratory tract infection of 3 to 4 days' duration. This initial illness may include low-grade fever and rhinorrhea, with a gradual development of cough and increasing respiratory distress. The child in respiratory distress may manifest cyanosis, grunting respirations, retractions, coarse crackles, and/or wheezing.

In contrast to pneumonia of viral etiology, a more acute pattern of onset is suggestive of bacterial pneumonia. In addition to the previously mentioned symptomatology, a more ill or toxic appearance with cough productive of thick green, yellow, or blood-tinged sputum and chest pain may also be present. Common bacterial pathogens include *Streptococcus pneumoniae*, *Haemophilus influenzae*, *Staphylococcus aureus*, group B streptococcus, *Chlamydia pneumoniae*, and *Mycoplasma pneumoniae*. Fever and increased respiratory rate are hallmark manifestations of most cases of bacterial pneumonia. Poor oral intake and increased insensible losses from fever and tachypnea may lead to symptoms of dehydration. The child with sepsis and early shock will have tachycardia, hypotension, and poor perfusion.

The young child or infant with fever, retractions, tachypnea, and/or grunting will be irritable and difficult to console. Hypoxia and hypercarbia result in decreased level of consciousness in a child of any age. Parental anxiety is common because of the often severe acute onset of respiratory symptoms in the child.

Children with chronic illnesses, such as asthma, bronchopulmonary dysplasia, or cystic fibrosis, often develop recurrent and/or persistent pneumonias because of respiratory compromise. Immunodeficiencies, congenital heart disease, neuromuscular diseases, and various hematologic and oncologic diseases all are conditions that can render the child compromised in the ability to fight pneumonias and other infections. Varicella zoster and measles virus, for example, are common childhood viral infections with generally mild respiratory symptoms that can be life-threatening to an immunocompromised child. Families of chronically ill children live with the constant fear of exposure to a potentially fatal infection and may exhibit feelings and behaviors of guilt and anger upon diagnosis of yet another pneumonia. Counseling and support for these families during acute illness episodes is imperative.

Interdisciplinary Interventions

Interventions for the child with pneumonia involve careful assessment of respiratory status and general supportive care (Care Path 16–3). Whether or not a child with pneumonia requires hospitalization depends on the child's age, general health status, and the suspected organism. Because infants readily develop respiratory distress with accompanying hypoxia, apnea, poor feeding, and dehydration, hospitalization is common. Home health support regarding respiratory assessment and medication administration is an option for the older child being treated at home.

For the hospitalized child, close and frequent respiratory assessment, including evaluation of respiratory rate and effort, color, presence and location of retractions, breath sounds, and oxygen saturation levels, is done for the infant or child with pneumonia. Changes in the respiratory status are to be immediately reported for further medical evaluation. Supplemental oxygen may be needed to keep saturation levels greater than or equal to 92%. For some children, continuous pulse oximetry is indicated. Chest physiotherapy (percussion, vibration, and postural drainage) should be implemented to facilitate clearing of secretions, with special attention paid to any identified areas of involvement or infiltration on the chest x-ray film (see Treatment Modalities).

In the majority of viral pneumonia cases, especially in infants, antibiotics are given because secondary bacterial involvement cannot be ruled out. Many experts consider this the safest and most practical approach, although it may not alter the course of the illness. Infants are generally treated with broad-spectrum antibiotics such as ampicillin and an aminoglycoside. Specific antiviral therapy for respiratory syncytial virus (ribavirin) is considered for infants and children with chronic illnesses (see Bronchiolitis). After age 3 months, and up to 5 years in a child with severe illness, cefuroxime, vancomycin, or ampicillin and gentamicin intravenously are recommended and usually administered while the child is hospitalized. In older children with less severe illness, oral antibiotic therapy is indicated.

caREminder: *Children in severe respiratory distress should receive nothing by mouth (NPO) because of the increased work of breathing and the risk of aspiration.*

Fluids and medications are administered via the intravenous route. Fever and tachypnea result in insensible fluid loss; thus, the child with pneumonia is at risk for dehydration. Accurate intake and urine output and urine specific gravity are measured frequently, and assessment of skin turgor is done to monitor hydration status. Body temperature is monitored and fevers are treated with acetaminophen, because a high body temperature can increase oxygen requirements and exacerbate insensible fluid loss. As the child's respiratory status improves, the diet can be advanced from clear liquids to regular diet as tolerated. For the child with recurrent aspiration pneumonias, suck and swallow coordination and gastroesophageal reflux evaluations may be done to identify risk for aspiration before full oral feedings are resumed. If oral intake is allowed, they should be given with caution to avoid aspiration.

Constant information and support for the child and/or family from all health professionals during an acute pneumonia episode is essential. Social services may provide counseling services or referrals in the event of life-threatening and/or chronic illness. Once the child's con-

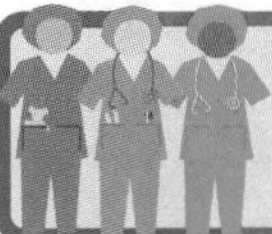

Care Path 16–3 An Interdisciplinary Plan of Care for the Child with Pneumonia

Nursing Diagnosis	Patient/Family Intermediate Outcomes			
	Day 1	Day 2	Day 3	Day 4
Ineffective breathing pattern related to an inflammatory infection of the lower airway	Child demonstrates and maintains an improved breathing pattern throughout hospitalization as evidenced by decrease in or absence of tachypnea, retractions, nasal flaring, grunting, wheezing, cyanosis, and/or cough.	⟶	⟶	⟶
Knowledge deficit related to disease process and home management of child upon discharge	Family verbalizes understanding of illness and rationale for treatment plan.	By discharge, family will verbalize/demonstrate an understanding of home medication administration, how to perform PD&P, how to use a bulb syringe and a metered dose inhaler (MDI) as appropriate, and when to notify physician of changes in respiratory status.	⟶	⟶
Care Intervention Categories				
Discharge planning			Discharge to home if on room air, respiratory treatment not needed more than every 4–6 hr, and tolerating PO feeds. For bacterial pneumonia, discharge on PO antibiotics to complete a 10-day course.	Instruct parent to call physician if respiratory distress is noted. Ensure that parent makes a follow-up appointment within 1 week of discharge.
Diagnostic tests	CBC with differential Consider blood culture and cold agglutinins. Chest x-ray			

Care Path continued on following page

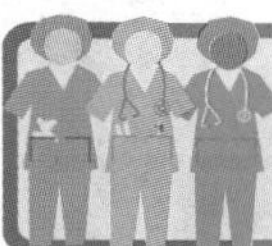

Care Path 16–3 An Interdisciplinary Plan of Care for the Child with Pneumonia *Continued*

Care Intervention Categories	Day 1	Day 2	Day 3	Day 4
Medications and IVs	Cefuroxime 75–150 mg/kg/day IV q 8 hr for bacterial pneumonia (maximum dose, 6 g/day). Heparin lock or consider IV fluids if unable to take PO feeds. Neo-Synephrine ⅛% 2–3 drops each nostril every 6 hr, p.r.n. for nasal congestion.	⟶	⟶	Discontinue Neo-Synephrine. Change to oral antibiotics.
Monitors	Consider apnea monitor for infants <6 mo with moderate to severe respiratory distress. Saturation check once, and then check p.r.n. for respiratory distress.	⟶	⟶	Discontinue apnea monitor
Nutrition	NPO	Diet for age as tolerated	⟶	⟶
Respiratory treatment	Oxygen to keep saturations ≥93%	Consider weaning oxygen	Wean oxygen	Discontinue oxygen
	Bulb or wall suction p.r.n.	⟶	⟶	
	PD&P with nebulized treatments, if clinically indicated (atelectasis or lobar pneumonia by chest x-ray)	⟶	⟶	
	Albuterol 0.15 mg/kg in 2 cc normal saline via nebulizer every 2–4 hr and p.r.n. (minimum diluted dose 0.25 cc)	Consider alternating nebulized treatments with MDI treatment	⟶	Discontinue nebulized treatments and use albuterol MDI 2–4 puffs via aerochamber every 4–6 hr, if clinically indicated.
		Or		
		Discontinue nebulized treatments and use albuterol MDI 2–4 puffs every 4–6 hr, if clinically indicated.	⟶	

Care Path 16–3 An Interdisciplinary Plan of Care for the Child with Pneumonia *Continued*

Care Intervention Categories	Day 1	Day 2	Day 3	Day 4
Safety and activity	Activity as tolerated	⟶	⟶	⟶
Special considerations	Contact isolation	⟶	⟶	Discontinue isolation
Teaching	Use of a bulb syringe Signs and symptoms of respiratory distress	How to do respiratory treatments	Home medication administration, including discontinuation and follow-up instructions	Review all teaching content.
Vital signs/ baseline parameters	Check vital signs every 4 hr Strict intake and output	⟶	⟶	⟶

MDI, metered-dose inhaler; NPO, nothing by mouth; PD&P, postural drainage and percussion; PO, by mouth.

dition becomes more stable, parents, nurses, and child life specialists should collaborate in planning quiet diversionary activities appropriate for the child's age.

Children with pneumonia are evaluated in an ambulatory care setting 2 to 3 weeks after completion of treatment. Repeat chest radiographs are necessary to evaluate persistent symptoms or confirm complete recovery.

Chronic Conditions of the Respiratory System

Chronic conditions of the respiratory system affect children in all age groups and account for significant alterations in their quality of life and physical and social development and, at times, early death. Asthma, bronchopulmonary dysplasia, and cystic fibrosis can be debilitating diseases in which the child's respiratory status affects all other aspects of the child's and family's physical and emotional health. There are no "cures" for these chronic disorders. They are best managed through extensive patient and family education related to prevention and minimization of symptoms, early and ongoing medical treatments, and optimization of self-care and home care strategies. These conditions are characterized by periods of relative wellness interspersed with periods of acute exacerbation, often necessitating hospitalization.

Asthma

Asthma is the most common chronic condition in childhood, affecting approximately 4 million children in the United States (Taylor & Newacheck, 1992). Among children, acute exacerbations of asthma account for a loss of more than 10 million school days and are responsible for more hospitalizations, restricted activity, and significant health care costs than any other pediatric chronic illness (Weiss, Gergen, & Hodgson, 1992). Some sources cite both the presence and severity of asthma to be increasing around the world, the cause of which is unclear. A greater understanding of the pathophysiology of asthma in recent years has led to dramatic changes in the child's care. Comprehensive treatment programs that address important issues such as accurate diagnosis, patient/family education, and environmental control have been shown to significantly improve the overall health of children with asthma. (National Heart, Lung and Blood Institute [NHLBI], 1991; Scott, 1997).

Worldview: *Increasing prevalence of asthma has become a world concern. Many countries, not just the United States, are seeing growing numbers of children and adults affected by asthma. It is estimated that more than 100 million people worldwide have asthma. Asthma has had a significant impact on mortality and morbidity in countries* *such as Australia, New Zealand, France, England, Japan, and Singapore and is the most common and important chronic airway disease in most African nations. Together with the World Health Organization (WHO), the National Heart, Lung and Blood Institute (NHLBI) convened two workshops on Global Strategy for Asthma Management and Prevention with participants from every region of the world. The purpose was to develop information, recommendations, and tools to assist health care professionals and public health officials in designing and delivering effective asthma management and prevention programs (National Institutes of Health, 1995).*

Incidence

Asthma is a chronic illness characterized by frequent acute exacerbations sometimes necessitating emergency room treatment and hospitalization, but rarely death. The mortality rate, however, has increased in the 1980s and 1990s. Statistics show that asthma prevalence rates among children are increasing 6.9% (4.8 million children) in the United States (Centers for Disease Control and Prevention, 1996). Some epidemiologic work has suggested that asthma is strongly associated with a Western lifestyle, in that the prevalence among children in developing countries is less than 1%, as compared with more than 20% in some industrialized countries (Sears, 1990). In the United States, asthma is more common in males, in certain geographic regions (e.g., the South and West), in urban areas, and in blacks. Poor and minority populations, particularly blacks living in urban areas, have had a disproportionate prevalence rate of asthma and increase in morbidity and mortality as compared with whites (CDC, 1996; Taylor & Newacheck, 1992; Wing, 1993). The racial discrepancy in the prevalence of childhood asthma in the United States appears to be due largely to social and environmental factors rather than to genetic differences (Schwartz, Gold, Dockery, Weiss, & Speizer, 1990; Weitzman, Gortmaker, & Sobol, 1990).

Studies have revealed risk factors for asthma mortality. Foremost among these is a lack of appreciation of the severity of the child's asthma by the parents and medical personnel. Over-reliance on bronchodilators in lieu of other medications, specifically anti-inflammatory drugs, and delay in seeking treatment during an asthma attack are also significant factors (Birkhead, Attaway, Strunk, Townsend, & Teutsch, 1989; Lanier, 1989). Erratic compliance with medications and medical follow-up and nonwhite and low socioeconomic status were also identified. The unfortunate fact is that deaths from asthma are usually preventable. Children at risk require more intense treatment, education, monitoring, and family support to prevent negative outcomes.

Pathophysiology

Because the pathology of childhood asthma is incompletely understood, the disease is best defined as a condition characterized by reversible (in most cases) airway obstruction, airway inflammation, and increased airway responsiveness to a variety of stimuli (NHLBI, 1991). Although the precise pathogenesis of asthma is yet to be discovered, the airways are hyperresponsive to a number of precipitants or triggers (e.g., inhaled antigen, respiratory infections, exercise, irritants, emotional stress) (Chart 16–22), and the condition is manifested by exaggerated bronchoconstriction of the airways. Mast cells in the airways release inflammatory and chemotactic mediators, such as histamine, that cause smooth muscle contraction and bronchoconstriction. Goblet cells hypersecrete mucus, and there is epithelial damage that leads to increased permeability and sensitivity to inhaled allergens, irritants, and inflammatory mediators. The result is airway edema, mucous plugging, and significant airway narrowing, leading to rapid airway obstruction (Fig. 16–19). This acute reaction is called the *early asthmatic re-*

Chart 16–22

Common Asthma Triggers

Housedust Mites and Dust. Collected in rugs, bedding, upholstered furniture, draperies, stuffed animals

Pollens. From flowers, trees, grasses, hay, ragweed, and other plants

Mold. Spores outdoors or mold found in bathrooms, damp areas

Smoke. From cigarettes, cigars, wood-burning stoves, kerosene heaters

Animals. Cats, dogs, rabbits, gerbils, chickens, hamsters, horses, birds, goose down (feathers), insect parts from dead cockroaches

Inhalants/Chemicals. Vapors and sprays from cleaning products, paint, paint thinner, furniture polish, air fresheners, perfumes, hair spray, talcum powder, incense, etc.

Foods/Medications. Nuts, chocolate, eggs, milk, orange juice, peanut butter, fish, sulfites in shrimp, dried fruits and food dyes, salicylates

Weather. Excessively cold air, wet or humid, changes in weather and seasons, air pollution

Infections. Colds, other viruses, sore throat

Exercise. After overexertion, or in cold weather

Emotions. Fear, anger, crying, laughing

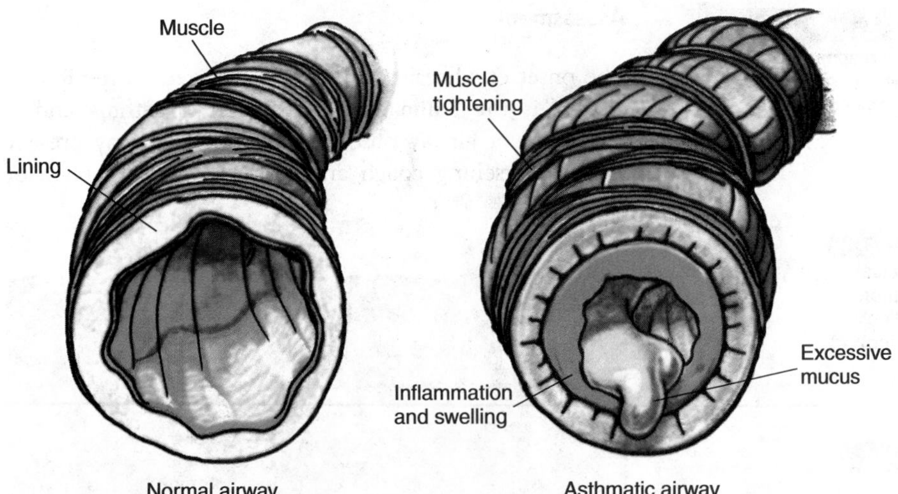

Figure 16–19
Asthmatic airway compared with a normal airway.

sponse (EAR) and generally resolves with treatment with bronchodilators within 1 to 3 hours.

A key development in the study of asthma has been recognition of the *late asthmatic response* (LAR). Mediator release from the mast cells causes direct migration and activation of inflammatory infiltrates, predominantly eosinophils and neutrophils, and mast cell degranulation causes the release of leukotrienes and prostaglandins, which further lead to inflammation. In the LAR, airway obstruction persists or reappears. It occurs 4 to 6 hours later and can last 24 hours or more. The LAR has a number of features characteristic of chronic asthma: less responsiveness to bronchodilators, increased mucus secretion, heightened airway responsiveness, and the development of airway inflammation. With the onset of the LAR, a vicious self-perpetuating cycle of asthma symptoms ensues.

In addition to bronchoconstriction, the other contributors to the process of airway obstruction, including airway inflammation and mucus secretion, have recently become recognized as essential features of asthma. *Airway inflammation*, in particular, long identified as a pathologic finding in severe fatal asthma, has been noted in patients with relatively mild asthma. Inflammation is probably a crucial component in the chronicity of asthma and the intensity of airway hyperreactivity. Although the degree of airway reactivity is thought to be related to the extent of inflammation, the clinical manifestations of this reactivity are determined by complex interactions between genetic, allergic, and environmental factors (Fig. 16–20).

The physiologic changes that occur during an acute episode contribute to the clinical findings characteristic of asthma exacerbation. Air becomes trapped behind the narrowed airways and the functional residual capacity rises, causing hyperinflation of the lungs, which can be seen on a chest x-ray film. This hyperinflation helps keep the airways open that are already narrowed from bronchoconstriction, mucosal edema, and mucus. Accessory muscles of respiration are used to help maintain the lungs in a hyperinflated state, therefore the child has retractions. Hypoxemia results from ventilation-perfusion mismatch, as areas of the lung are not being well ventilated.

There is evidence that asthma is partly hereditary in nature. Studies have shown that the risk of having an asthmatic child is significantly greater when one or both parents have asthma than if neither parent is affected (Horwood, Fergusson, & Shannon, 1985). Atopy (an increased predisposition to form antibodies on exposure to common environmental antigens) is present in the majority of patients with asthma. Atopy is at least partially hereditary, although it is possible that exposure to certain allergens early in life (e.g., pollens, animal danders) may influence the development of asthma in a child who is genetically predisposed. Food allergens, however, are rarely responsible for airway reactions in children. Although the link between asthma and atopy is not completely clear, it is possible that exposure to allergens produces airway inflammation, thus leading to increased airway responsiveness. This in turn is responsible for the development of asthma.

Other factors felt to be involved in the development of airway reactivity and asthma include respiratory infections and environmental factors. RSV bronchiolitis, for example, has been linked in a causal fashion to enhanced airway reactivity, especially in children with a family history of atopy. In children with asthma, parental (particularly maternal) smoking has been associated with increases in the severity of symptoms and hospitalizations. The relationship of passive smoking and the development

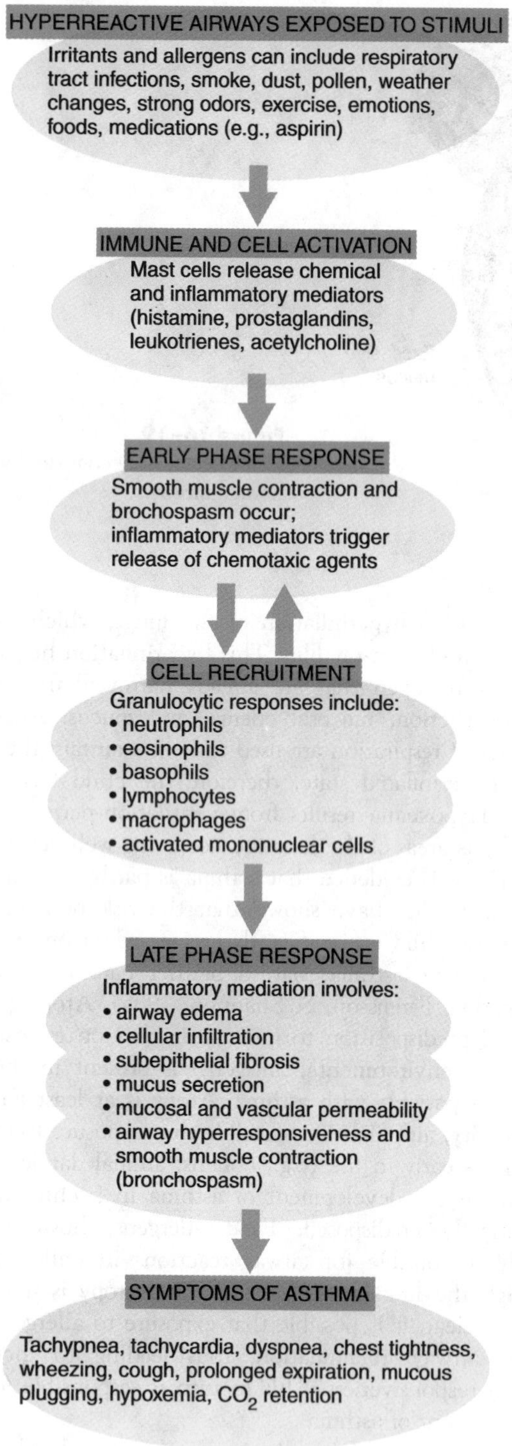

HYPERREACTIVE AIRWAYS EXPOSED TO STIMULI

Irritants and allergens can include respiratory tract infections, smoke, dust, pollen, weather changes, strong odors, exercise, emotions, foods, medications (e.g., aspirin)

IMMUNE AND CELL ACTIVATION

Mast cells release chemical and inflammatory mediators (histamine, prostaglandins, leukotrienes, acetylcholine)

EARLY PHASE RESPONSE

Smooth muscle contraction and brochospasm occur; inflammatory mediators trigger release of chemotaxic agents

CELL RECRUITMENT

Granulocytic responses include:
- neutrophils
- eosinophils
- basophils
- lymphocytes
- macrophages
- activated mononuclear cells

LATE PHASE RESPONSE

Inflammatory mediation involves:
- airway edema
- cellular infiltration
- subepithelial fibrosis
- mucus secretion
- mucosal and vascular permeability
- airway hyperresponsiveness and smooth muscle contraction (bronchospasm)

SYMPTOMS OF ASTHMA

Tachypnea, tachycardia, dyspnea, chest tightness, wheezing, cough, prolonged expiration, mucous plugging, hypoxemia, CO_2 retention

Figure 16–20
Sequence of events in an asthma attack.

of asthma is less well defined; however, some research has preliminarily suggested that maternal smoking may cause alteration in the developing lung before birth. The role of air pollution in the development of asthma remains controversial.

Assessment

The onset of wheezing with varying degrees of respiratory distress is the hallmark manifestation of asthma and is the result of airway obstruction. The child may present with a worsening cough and wheezing and complain of

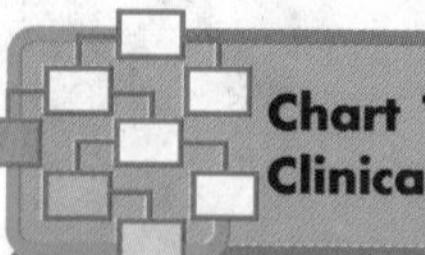

Chart 16–23
Clinical Judgment

The Child in Respiratory Distress

Six-year-old Danielle comes to the community health clinic with her mother. The child presents with a history of onset of wheezing, shortness of breath, chest tightness, and cough that developed the previous night. Danielle is lethargic and pale and her skin is cool and clammy. She is sitting in a tripod position; her eyes are open wide with a fearful countenance.

Questions

1. What historical data would help to clarify the diagnosis?
2. Is this an upper or lower respiratory problem?
3. Is the child in respiratory distress?
4. What would be your initial intervention?
5. How would you determine whether oxygen therapy and bronchodilators are effective in relieving the child's respiratory problems?

Answers

1. Number of similar occurrences of these respiratory signs the child has had in the past year. Family history of asthma. Introduction of new animals, products, or other environmental factors at home or school. Occurrence of respiratory illness in other family or friends at this time.
2. Lower respiratory, as distinguished by wheezing and chest tightness due to bronchial constriction.
3. Yes. Respiratory distress occurs when there is an inadequate ability to meet the oxygenation needs of the body. Signs of respiratory distress include nasal flaring, retractions, poor chest expansion, cool extremities, poor peripheral pulses, and changes in level of consciousness.
4. Provide oxygenation to the child 100% O_2 at 6 liters, given via face mask or nasal cannula. Do not have her lie down; let her assume a position of comfort.
5. The signs and symptoms of respiratory distress would be alleviated. The child would become more alert and pink and appear calm and able to verbalize that the tightness in her chest has diminished or that she is able to breathe easier.

chest tightness. Because of bronchospasm, airway inflammation, and mucous plugging, expiration becomes increasingly difficult for the child and there is air trapping (Bechler-Karsch, 1994). Other assessment findings that may be present in the child with a moderate to severe asthma exacerbation are the inability or unwillingness to lie flat and a prolonged expiratory phase (Chart 16–23). Status asthmaticus is an acute state of *severe* asthma that fails to respond readily to usual methods of therapy, resulting in the need for hospitalization. Clinical evaluation of the asthma patient should be assessed and classified according to severity (Table 16–11). Accurate recognition of severity and initiation of immediate appropriate therapy are proven factors in avoiding deaths.

▽ **Alert:** *Special attention must be paid to children at high risk of asthma-related death. Children with a history of the following are at an increased risk for asthma-related death:*

- *Prior admission to an intensive care unit for asthma (with or without intubation)*
- *Two or more hospitalizations for asthma and/or three or more emergency room visits for asthma in the past year*
- *A recent hospitalization or emergency room visit for asthma in the past month*
- *Current use of, or recent withdrawal from, systemic corticosteroids*
- *History of psychiatric disease or psychosocial issues*
- *History of noncompliance with asthma treatment plan (NHLBI, 1991)*

Hypoxemia is universal in the child with moderate to severe symptoms. Carbon dioxide retention is also a common finding. Hypoxemia and hypercarbia result from air trapping in the alveoli and ventilation-perfusion mismatch. $PaCO_2$ higher than 50 mmHg is indicative of ventilatory failure unless the child has a preexisting chronic lung disease. Typical x-ray findings in the child with significant asthma symptoms are hyperexpansion, atelectasis, and a flattened diaphragm. Younger children are particularly prone to the development of atelectasis because of small airways and underdeveloped collateral ventilation. Infiltrates and/or pneumothoraces are uncommon findings.

Table 16–11
Clinical Assessment According to Severity

	Mild	Moderate	Severe
Appearance			
Alertness	Normal	Normal/may be irritable	May be decreased
Color	Good	Pale	Possibly cyanotic
Dyspnea	Absent to mild	Moderate	Severe
Speaks:			
Sentences	Complete	Partial	(−)
Phrases	(+)	(+)	Short
Words	(+)	(+)	Single
Accessory muscle use and retractions			
Intercostal	Absent to mild	Moderate	Marked
Sternocleidomastoid	Absent	(+)	(+)
Tracheosternal	Absent	(+)	(+)
Nasal flaring	Absent	Absent	(+)
Auscultation of wheeze	End expiratory	Expiratory and inspiratory	Breath sounds becoming inaudible, poor air exchange
Laboratory values			
$PaCO_2$	<35 mmHg	<40 mmHg	>40 mmHg
SaO_2	>95%	90–95%	<90%
PEFR	70–90% of predicted or personal best	50–70% of predicted or personal best	<50% of predicted or personal best

PEFR, peak expiratory flow rate.
Modified from NHLBI Guidelines.

The presence of pulsus paradoxus (a fall in systemic blood pressure with inspiration) occurs because the negative pleural pressures become more negative as a result of lung hyperinflation. A fall of 12 mmHg or more in systolic blood pressure with inspiration versus expiration indicates moderate distress. A fall of 20 mmHg or more occurs in severe status asthmaticus. Pulsus paradoxus may be difficult to assess in the young child because of rapid heart and respiratory rates. In the preverbal child, quality of cry (weak versus lusty) should also be evaluated.

Children in the midst of an acute asthma exacerbation, or status asthmaticus, are frightened as well as short of breath. Parents are equally frightened and anxious and may or may not be able to adequately comfort the child. Unless the child is in impending respiratory failure, allow the child to remain in the parent's lap if this is the most comforting position for him or her. Even in the most acute situations, it is reassuring to provide care in a calm, organized, and confident manner. Most children can be cared for quickly, efficiently, and with a minimum of painful or distressing procedures. Factual information relayed to parents and family members in a calm and timely manner also helps allay fears. Because obtaining an accurate history is essential to the care of the child with status asthmaticus, it is important for parents to remain calm and able to coherently answer vital questions.

Some children may have early or prodromal signs and symptoms hours to days before an asthma exacerbation. Early warning symptoms include throat tightness, itchy or scratchy throat, headache, earache, lethargy, and puffy face, and the child is just not his or her usual self. It is important to help the family identify early warning signs that their child may exhibit to help with treatment and identification of when the asthma may become worse.

A careful history is one of most important elements in the evaluation of the patient with mild, moderate, or severe asthma. Historical data provide information in identifying possible high-risk patients and planning for the appropriate interventions they require. The key information to compile in the history is listed in Table 16–12. It is important that other conditions that may present with wheezing and shortness of breath are ruled

Table 16–12
History Data for Assessing Asthma

Nature of symptoms	Shortness of breath, wheeze, cough, chest tightness, rhinorrhea, conditions such as sinusitis, eczema
Pattern of symptoms	Continuous vs. episodic, onset and duration, severity, frequency, seasonal, perennial, diurnal variation
Aggravating factors or triggers	Upper respiratory infections, environmental allergens and irritants, smoke, emotions, exercise, weather changes, pets, air pollution
Typical exacerbation	Prodromal signs and symptoms, temporal progress, and usual management and response to treatment
Previous and current drug therapy	Dosage, mode of delivery, response, side effects
Development of disease	Age at onset, age at diagnosis, progress of disease, previous evaluations, treatments, and response to present management
Impact of disease	Number of emergency room visits, hospitalizations and intensive care unit admissions in past year, school attendance and performance, activity limitations and exercise tolerance, sleep disturbances, child's growth and development, child's behavior, effect on siblings, economic impact
Living situation/environment	Presence of smokers in home, pets, housing conditions, home age, heating/air conditioning, carpeting, humidifier, cockroaches
Family and patient perception of asthma	Knowledge of and belief in chronicity of asthma, coping styles, family support systems, capacity to recognize exacerbation, economic resources
General medical history	Presence of or history of allergic disorders (allergic rhinitis, atopic dermatitis), recurrent respiratory tract infections, birth history (early injury to lung tissue), symptoms of gastroesophageal reflux, detailed review of systems
History of allergies	History of adverse reactions to medications, food, or allergens (pollen, mold, pets)
Family medical history	History of IgE-mediated allergy in close relatives, asthma in close relatives

out. Additionally, if the child presents with recurring episodes, it is helpful to identify possible precipitating factors and what has been effective in terms of treatment in the past. The physical examination should focus on the child's general health condition, including growth and development, as well as hydration status and any signs of drug-related side effects.

Diagnostic Tests. Diagnostic studies helpful in the evaluation of the child with acute asthma symptoms include peak expiratory flow rate (PEFR), arterial blood gases, pulse oximetry, and chest x-rays. PEFR is a valuable measurement in the assessment of asthma severity, as well as the response to therapy. PEFR is the greatest velocity of flow that can be generated in forced expiration, starting with fully inflated lungs. PEFR should be evaluated in a serial manner and compared with the baseline or "personal best" for the individual rather than with normal values (NHLBI, National Asthma Education Program Expert Panel Report, 1991). PEFR decreases as airway obstruction and inflammation worsen. Children younger than 4 years of age are generally not able to perform PEFR tests, and they may be too stressful for the child in severe distress, potentially worsening his or her status.

Interdisciplinary Interventions

Until recently, asthma was viewed as a disease of acute airway obstruction. Consequently, therapy consisted largely of bronchodilators to relieve bronchospasm. Currently, it is felt that asthma is not primarily an acute bronchospastic disease, but rather a condition of airway hyperreactivity and inflammation. Treatment for asthma now aggressively focuses on anti-inflammatory medications and prevention of exacerbations (Table 16–13). It is believed that by reducing the airway inflammation, airway hyperreactivity will be reduced. In addition to pharmacotherapy, other areas of focus in the management of asthma include patient and family education and preventive and environmental control measures (Care Path 16–4).

Acute Asthma Attack

For children presenting in severe respiratory distress with an acute asthma attack unresponsive to home medical management, nursing assessments and interventions in the first hour are critical to achieving a favorable outcome. Heart rate, respiratory rate, breath sounds, pulse oximetry, PEFR (if patient is able), and use of accessory

Table 16–13
Pharmaceutical Agents Used in the Care of the Child with Asthma

Generic Name (Brand)	Route Given	Action	Side Effects
Beta$_2$-agonists			
Albuterol (Proventil, Ventolin)	PO/Inhaled	Rapid-acting bronchodilator—opens the airways by relaxing smooth muscle contraction, enhances mucociliary clearance, reduces bronchospasm.	Nervousness, skeletal muscle tremors, tachycardia, insomnia, irritability, headache. Inhaled drugs have less side effects than those taken orally.
Terbutaline (Brethine/Brethaire)	PO/Inhaled	Rapid-acting bronchodilator—opens the airways by relaxing smooth muscle contraction, enhances mucociliary clearance, reduces bronchospasm.	Nervousness, skeletal muscle tremors, tachycardia, insomnia, irritability, headache. Inhaled drugs have less side effects than those taken orally.
Metaproterenol (Alupent)	PO/Inhaled	Rapid-acting bronchodilator—opens the airways by relaxing smooth muscle contraction, enhances mucociliary clearance, reduces bronchospasm.	
Salmeterol (Serevent)	Inhaled	Long-acting bronchodilator—opens airways by relaxing smooth muscle contraction, reducing bronchospasm; enhances mucociliary clearance and decreases vascular permeability. **Not to be used for an acute exacerbation.**	Anxiety, nervousness, tachycardia, pyosis, skeletal muscle tremor, headache or hypokalemia.

Table continued on following page

Table 16–13
Pharmaceutical Agents Used in the Care of the Child with Asthma *Continued*

Generic Name (Brand)	Route Given	Action	Side Effects
Beta$_2$-agonists			
Epinephrine (Adrenalin)	Injectable	Rapid-acting bronchodilator—opens airways by relaxing smooth muscle contraction. Also used to treat anaphylaxis, angioedema, and cardiac arrest.	Skeletal muscle tremor, tachycardia, irritability, palpitation.
Anticholinergics			
Ipratropium bromide (Atrovent)	Inhaled	Bronchodilator effect by reducing vagal tone to the airways; less potent activity than beta-agonists.	Tachycardia, dry mouth, blurred vision, headache.
Methylxanthines			
Theophylline Aminophylline	PO/Injectable	Bronchodilator effect—exact mechanism not clear, may enhance mucociliary clearance, increase diaphragmatic contractility and have some anti-inflammatory effects.	Normal serum levels (10–20 mg/L): jitteriness, nausea, vomiting, headache, relaxes lower esophageal sphincter and increases acid secretion. Toxic effects: seizures, tachycardia, arrhythmias.
Corticosteroids			
Methylprednisolone (Medrol or Solu-Medrol) Prednisone, Prednisolone (Deltasone)	PO or IV PO	Anti-inflammatory—affects by decreasing airway hyperreactivity, prevents and suppresses activation and migration of inflammatory cells in the airways. Short bursts can interrupt acute asthma episodes.	Increased appetite, fluid retention, mood changes. Long-term use may lead to adrenal suppression, osteoporosis, muscle weakness, cataracts, hypertension, and glucose intolerance.
Beclomethasone (Beclovent, Vanceril) Flunisolide (AeroBid) Triamcinolone (Azmacort)	Inhaled	Anti-inflammatory—affects by decreasing airway hyperreactivity, prevents and suppresses activation and migration of inflammatory cells in the airways. Short bursts can interrupt acute asthma episodes. Reduces airway inflammation, maintains airway stability, prevents hyperreactibility and enhances effects of beta-agonists.	Rarely systemic side effects compared with the oral medications. Oral candidiasis, hoarseness.
Mast Cell Inhibitors			
Cromolyn sodium (Intal)	Inhaled	Anti-inflammatory—affects by inhibiting activation and release of mediators from mast cells. Maintains airway stability. Takes 3–4 weeks for therapeutic effects to be demonstrated.	Minimal side effects. Rarely: irritation of throat, or cough.
Nedocromil sodium (Tilade)	Inhaled	Anti-inflammatory—affects by inhibiting activation and release of mediators from mast cells. Maintains airway stability. Takes 3–4 weeks for therapeutic effects to be demonstrated.	Minimal side effects. Rarely: irritation of throat, or cough.

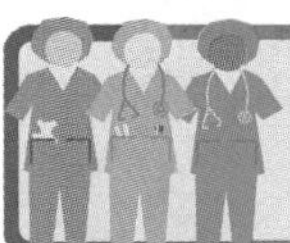

Care Path 16–4 An Interdisciplinary Plan of Care for the Child with Status Asthmaticus

Nursing Diagnosis	Patient/Family Intermediate Outcomes			
	Day: Admission	**Day 1**	**Day 2**	**Day 3**
Ineffective breathing pattern related to an ineffective gas exchange and acute respiratory distress	Child will have decreased signs and symptoms of acute respiratory distress as evidence by decreased retractions, accessory muscle use, and respiratory rate.	Child demonstrates improved oxygenation and ventilation as evidenced by decreasing demands for O_2 and respiratory treatments and oxygen saturations >95%.	Child demonstrates continued improvement in breath sounds and gas exchange and will tolerate less frequent nebulizer use.	Child will have normal respiratory rate for age and good gas exchange.
Activity intolerance related to ineffective O_2 consumption and O_2 demand	Child activities and environment will foster a calm and restful atmosphere.	Child will increase level of activity and will be given developmentally appropriate diversional activities.	Child will increase level of activity and will be given developmentally appropriate diversional activities.	⟶
Altered family processes related to having child with chronic condition (asthma)	Family members verbalize understanding of need to hospitalize child and expected course of hospitalization.	Family members participate in child's care and help identify appropriate community resources for asthma care.	⟶	⟶
Alterations in health maintenance related to home management plan for asthma		Family members verbalize understanding of disease definition, symptomatology, and triggers of asthma episodes.	Family members demonstrate competency in use of home nebulizer and administration of home medications. Child will demonstrate appropriate use of a peak flow meter and MDI with spacer if ordered.	Family verbalizes knowledge of signs and symptoms of respiratory distress, asthma triggers, and emergency plan. Family verbalizes approaches to environmental control of triggers.
Care Intervention Categories				
Discharge planning		Assess need for home compressor/nebulizer machine.	Assess home environment. Modify home environment accordingly.	Assess need for visiting nurse.
Labs	If on theophylline at home, obtain blood levels. Electrolytes, ABG (p.r.n.).	Theophylline levels if on IV theophylline. Electrolytes, ABG, as needed.		

Care Path continued on following page

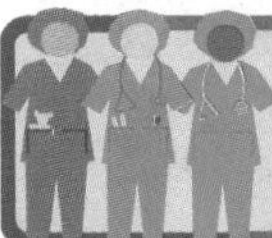

Care Path 16–4 An Interdisciplinary Plan of Care for the Child with Status Asthmaticus *Continued*

Care Intervention Categories	Day: Admission	Day 1	Day 2	Day 3
Medications and IVs (consider if wheezing)	Aerosolized bronchodilators q 1–2 hr Corticosteroids, oral, or IV Theophylline preparation, oral or IV p.r.n. IV fluids at maintenance if not taking PO feeds or dehydrated Acetaminophen p.r.n. for fever Continued use of any inhaled corticosteroids or cromolyn sodium if used at home Sodium bicarbonate if pH <7.25	Continue aerosolized bronchodilators q 2–3 hr and adjust to home schedule (TID) IV fluids if not taking PO feeds or heparin lock. Change to oral corticosteroids and oral theophylline Inhaled anti-inflammatories if needed	If IV discontinued, continue oral medications. Continue aerosolized bronchodilators q 4 hr.	Aerosolized bronchodilators q 4 hr (to be discharged on 3–4 times/day). Continue oral medications.
Monitors	Pulse oximetry Cardiorespiratory monitor if respiratory rate >60, if HR, or there are signs of respiratory distress	⟶ Discontinue cardiorespiratory monitor if stable	Pulse oximetry spot checks	Discontinue pulse oximetry
Nutrition	NPO if dyspneic Diet appropriate for age Accurate intake and output if on IV, then discontinue	⟶ ⟶	⟶	⟶
Radiology	Chest x-ray if first wheeze or if temperature >102°F			
Respiratory	Oxygen to maintain saturations >95% Measure peak expiratory flow rate before and after treatments	Oxygen to maintain saturations >95% Peak expiratory flow rate before and after treatments	Wean oxygen to maintain saturations >95% ⟶	Discontinue oxygen if saturations >95% ⟶

Care Path 16-4 An Interdisciplinary Plan of Care for the Child with Status Asthmaticus *Continued*

Care Intervention Categories	Day: Admission	Day 1	Day 2	Day 3
Safety and activity	Encourage quiet activities	Quiet activities; television, puzzles, books if no respiratory distress	Activity ad lib	⟶
	Side rails up	⟶		
	Position for comfort	⟶		
Teaching		Begin generalized asthma education with child and family members. Begin teaching child breathing exercises.	Instruct child and family on use of home nebulizer and/or MDI with spacer and peak flow meter.	Discuss home management plan and emergency treatment plan.
Vital signs/ baseline parameters	Strict I&O	⟶	⟶	⟶
	Admission height/ weight			
	Check vital signs every 2 hr	Vital signs and respiratory assessments every 2–4 hr	Vital signs and respiratory assessment every 4 hr	⟶
	Respiratory assessment every 2 hr			

ABG, arterial blood gases; ad lib, as desired; I&O, intake and output; MDI, metered-dose inhaler; NPO, nothing by mouth; PO, by mouth.

muscles should be continuously monitored. The child should receive supplemental humidified oxygen via mask or nasal cannula (2 to 6 L/min) to maintain oxygen saturation of 95% or more. Pharmacotherapy includes epinephrine 1 : 1000 aqueous 0.01 mL/kg/dose SQ (maximum single dose 0.3 mL) immediately if the patient is unable to generate sufficient flow for PEFR or if he or she is exhibiting a depressed level of consciousness. Nebulized albuterol 0.15 mg/kg (maximum 5 mg/dose) should be administered with high-flow oxygen every 20 minutes up to 1 hour. Corticosteroids (methylprednisolone, prednisone) are given either intravenously or orally and should be started if the child had a poor response to the initial treatment or if the child is steroid dependent (Roncolli, 1996).

After the first hour, the child's response to therapy should be comprehensively reassessed. For the child with an acute exacerbation who has exhibited a poor response to initial interventions, hospitalization is indicated. Hospitalization may also be necessary for other individual considerations, such as the family with a history of poor compliance and/or a child with a history of multiple admissions. The child is generally admitted to an age-appropriate medical unit. The child will prefer a high Fowler's position or sitting up and leaning slightly forward. Nebulized albuterol treatments should continue for these children every 1 to 2 hours, with a measurement of PEFR before and after treatments if possible. PEFR should be maintained at more than 40% of baseline.

For some children experiencing an acute episode, continuous nebulization of albuterol over several hours versus intermittent treatments has been shown to be an effective treatment modality and is considered safe in combination with accurate ongoing clinical assessments and effective interdisciplinary communication (Ferrante & Painter, 1995). Blood gas analysis and pulse oximetry should be monitored. PCO_2 should remain less than 40 mmHg, with O_2 saturation (while receiving supplemental O_2) higher than 90%. Methylprednisolone is given orally or intravenously 1 to 2 mg/kg/dose every 6 hours. Pulsus paradoxus should be assessed, with acceptable findings being less than or equal to 15 mmHg. If intravenous theophylline is started, the nurse monitors the infusion for side effects and toxicity as well as effectiveness of therapy in relieving respiratory distress. Strict avoidance in the hospital setting of all environmental irritants such as smoke, paint, glue, or perfume is imperative; therefore encourage activities that do not involve the use of paint, glue, or pens with strong odors.

As the child's condition improves, the albuterol treatments are extended to be given every 3 to 4 hours, and corticosteroids are given orally if they were given intravenously on admission. If the patient's clinical assessment does not improve (i.e., PEFR is less than 40% of baseline, PCO_2 is more than 40 mmHg, O_2 saturation is less than 90% on high-flow supplemental oxygen, continued severe wheezing and use of accessory respiratory muscles despite albuterol therapy, pulsus paradoxus is more than 15 mmHg), transfer to an intensive care setting is warranted. Endotracheal intubation and assisted ventilation must be considered if there is a steady clinical deterioration despite continued intensive therapy.

Combined with management of the child's clinical symptoms, nursing care must be focused on allaying the anxiety of the child and parents. Social service professionals may also intervene in this area by encouraging parents to be at the bedside as much as possible, perhaps assisting with resources for child care and/or transportation to make prolonged visitation possible. After the acute phase of illness, social workers may be instrumental in reintegrating the child into their daycare or school setting and collaborating with nurses to provide the necessary education for safe management in the community. Play therapists also provide education through the use of techniques such as puppet shows, games, and arts and crafts to help children learn about the management of their disease. Supervised medical play—handling and directly manipulating intravenous equipment, nebulizers, and syringes in a nonthreatening environment—encourages the child to express fears and anxieties.

Community Care

Although hospitalization for treatment of acute asthma exacerbation is a common occurrence, the management of children with asthma should primarily and ideally take place in outpatient settings and the community. The child who presents in the doctor's office with an acute exacerbation has the same symptoms but possibly to a lesser degree. It is important to assess the respiratory status, including rate, effort, presence of wheezing, color, PEFR, and alertness. The child should be given albuterol via nebulization or metered-dose inhaler every 20 minutes up to an hour and then reassessed. If there is a poor response, the child may need to be hospitalized. The child who responds to the albuterol should continue on albuterol treatments every 4 hours at home. The parents should be instructed on signs and symptoms of respiratory distress that may necessitate emergency treatment. If the child is going to receive a short course of corticosteroids, instruct the family on the importance of this medication to reduce the airway inflammation. The child may be prescribed inhaled anti-inflammatory drugs, therefore it is important to instruct the child and family in the reason for taking the medicine on a daily basis to prevent exacerbations.

The goals of asthma therapy are to minimize symptoms, maximize lung function, and allow children to lead normal lives with minimal interference from their illness. The primary goal is the promotion of optimal physical growth and function through minimizing airway obstruction, maximizing physical function despite airway obstruction, and preventing and treating exacerbations and complications of asthma and its therapy. Secondly, the child should achieve and maintain normal psychosocial growth and function through maintenance of optimal psychosocial development and maximal participation in his or her own health care. Lastly, normal family functioning should be maintained by promoting optimal family functioning and integrating the child's care needs into the daily lifestyle of the family.

In order to achieve these objectives, patient and family education must be an integral part of asthma care. Parents and children with asthma often have a poor or incomplete understanding of the disease and its management, and this may lead to increased need for hospitalization and increased health care costs. In 1991, the National Asthma Education Project (NAEP) and the Executive Summary Board's National Guidelines for the Diagnosis and Management of Asthma were implemented to increase public and professional awareness about asthma and to improve effective control of asthma with updated treatment information (NHLBI, National Asthma Education Program Expert Panel Report, 1991). The guidelines emphasize patient and family education. A number of asthma self-management programs have been developed in recent years to address the issue of adherence to treatment plan and lack of patient and family knowledge and awareness. Several of these programs are available through the American Lung Association (AirWise, AirPower, Open Airways) or the Asthma and Allergy Foundation of America (Asthma Care Training for Kids). Research has been conducted to look at the effectiveness of asthma management programs on children's self-management behaviors and health-related outcomes (Clark et al., 1981; Deaves, 1993; Evans et al., 1987; Lewis, Rachelefsky, Lewis, de la Sota, & Kaplan, 1984; McNabb, Wilson-Pessano, Hughes, & Scamagas, 1985; Yoos et al., 1997). Educational programs that focus on self-management skills help shift the often crisis-ori-

Chart 16–24
Community Care

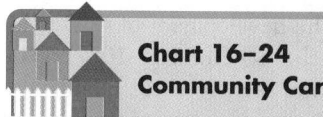

Components of an Asthma Education Program

Topic	Content
Definition of Asthma	Emphasize chronic nature of asthma, prognosis, and goals of therapy
Signs and Symptoms	Discuss main symptoms of an acute episode, variability of symptoms, recognition of mild/prodromal symptoms
Pathophysiology	Characteristic changes that occur in the airways (inflammation, bronchospasm, mucus) and role of medications
Asthma Triggers and Avoidance of Triggers	Help family/patient identify possible aggravating factors that may exacerbate asthma. Offer suggestions for home environment modification (see Chart 16–13)
Treatment of Asthma	Discuss medications (dose, frequency, actions, and side effects), need for individualized continuing care, need for preventive treatment, importance of early treatment of asthma episodes
Written Guidelines	Plan for what to do during an acute exacerbation, medication plan for maintenance, use of diaries to monitor symptoms and peak flow meter readings
Correct Use of Inhalation Devices	Demonstrate correct use of metered dose inhalers, nebulizer treatments, spacing devices, and care of these devices
Peak Expiratory Flow Meter	For children >5 years of age, teach use of peak flow meter and instruct to keep record of readings to identify "personal best," instruct when to initiate or change treatment based on peak flow readings
Fears and Misconceptions/Feelings about Asthma	Respond to patient and family concerns regarding medications, clear up any misconceptions (asthma not caused by psychological factors, deaths usually related to undertreatment of asthma, children should maintain active lives), acknowledge negative feelings of having asthma, refer to appropriate self-management programs/community resources
Communication with Child's School, Daycare, Camp, etc.	Importance of notifying school of child's condition, need for medication in school, participation in sports and physical education

ented nature of asthma care to one of proactive intervention and prevention.

The essential components of a parent/patient education program are outlined in Chart 16–24. Chart 16–13 provides information to help the family reduce exposure to environmental allergens within the home that may exacerbate asthma. The nurse, when working with the family, must be sensitive to the social, educational, environmental, and cultural issues many families face, and after careful assessment of the family and the environment, the nurse can make recommendations that are the most economical and feasible (Kuster, 1996).

Any education and/or materials given to the child and family should be geared toward the child's cognitive, affective, and developmental levels (Ladebauche, 1997). Several appropriate educational booklets are available through community resources such as the American Lung Association or the National Asthma Education Program (see Resources at the end of this chapter). The information given to parents and families should also be provided to the child's school teachers, school nurse, coaches, camp counselors, and other community personnel to ensure awareness of asthma, ensure continuity of treatment, and facilitate problem-solving if the child should have an acute episode. The importance of regular follow-up with a *consistent* heath care provider cannot be overemphasized. The child's progress must be closely monitored in relation to responses to therapy, compliance, and history of acute exacerbations.

Bronchopulmonary Dysplasia

Bronchopulmonary dysplasia (BPD) is a chronic lung disease of children that begins in infancy. It occurs in newborns who are born prematurely and/or have a variety of pulmonary disorders and who require ventilatory support with high positive airway pressures and oxygen in the first 2 weeks of life. The effects of BPD may last several months to years. BPD was first described by Northway, Rosan, and Porter (1967) as the radiographic and clinical syndrome seen in infants who had been treated with mechanical ventilation and high levels of inspired oxygen and who survived respiratory distress syndrome. Although timing of diagnosis varies, the clinical diagnosis is generally made at approximately 1 month of age in infants who required mechanical ventilation for at least 1 week, have symptoms of persistent respiratory distress, are dependent on supplemental oxygen, and have chest x-ray films that show hyperinflation, atelectasis, increased density, and fibrotic areas.

Incidence

Because the diagnostic criteria for BPD are not precise and universally distinct, the incidence of this disease is difficult to ascertain. Some retrospective studies of neonates suggest that BPD occurs in 12% to 70% of premature births, the incidence being inversely related to birth weight (Parker, Lindstrom, & Cotton, 1992; Tooley, 1979). The impact of therapies such as high-frequency oscillatory ventilation (HFOV) and surfactant replacement on the overall incidence of BPD remains to be fully demonstrated. HFOV delivers gas at extremely high frequencies (>200 "breaths"/min) and considerably lower pressures, thus reducing barotrauma to the alveoli. Studies have shown surfactant therapy to reduce the severity of respiratory distress syndrome and decrease the amount of time on mechanical ventilation. Many clinicians speculate, however, that there will be little decrease in the actual incidence of BPD, because surfactant therapy may allow smaller, sicker infants to survive who otherwise would have died during their early neonatal course (Ackerman, 1994).

Pathophysiology

The pathophysiology of BPD is complex and of multietiologic and multisystem origins. It starts with an acute insult to the neonate's lungs, such as respiratory distress syndrome, pneumonia, or meconium aspiration, that requires positive pressure ventilation and high concentrations of oxygen over extended time. These therapies result in tissue and cellular injury to the immature lung. The epithelium of the conducting airways develops lesions from injury thought to be related to hyperoxia and positive pressure. Excessive pulmonary fluid and collection of cellular debris in the alveoli, and recurrent bacterial and viral infections, are additional factors contributing to the alveolar tissue damage. Genetic factors, especially family history of airway hyperreactivity, may predispose some infants to the development of BPD (Motoyama, Fort, Klesh, Mutich, & Guthrie, 1987). The state of chronic undernutrition seen in these infants also affects the ability of the lung to resist injury and repair damaged tissue (Frank & Sosenko, 1988).

The most significant underlying pathologic process in BPD is the profound alteration of lung compliance. Pulmonary compliance is reduced as a result of a combination of factors:

- Fibrosis of the airways and marked hyperplasia of the bronchial epithelium, which occur secondary to alveolar damage
- Increased fluid in the lung, as a result of disruption of the alveolar-capillary membrane
- Overdistention due to damage to alveolar supporting structures, resulting in air trapping (Ackerman, 1994)
- Fibrosis, airway edema, and bronchoconstriction, increasing airway resistance

Decreased compliance and increased airway resistance increase the work of breathing, resulting in tachypnea and wheezing.

Pulmonary gas exchange is impaired by several factors in the infant with BPD. Hypoxia occurs secondary to ventilation-perfusion mismatch in the areas of alveolar collapse. Increased pulmonary vascular resistance causes intrapulmonic shunting, thus also contributing to hypoxia. Hypercarbia is common and is also caused by ventilation-perfusion mismatch, as well as by hypoventilation.

Large airway pathology (i.e., in the trachea and bronchi) was not originally described as a component of BPD but has since been recognized to be a frequent finding as the disease progresses (Ackerman, 1994). Both tracheomalacia and bronchomalacia are commonly found in this population and are postulated to be the cause of acute severe cyanotic episodes in the older BPD infant (McCubbin, Frey, Wagener, Tribby, & Smith, 1989).

Growth failure in infants with BPD is almost universal, resulting from increased caloric needs, caused by creased work of breathing, and high resting oxygen nsumption. Growth and lung disease may also be complicated by gastroesophageal reflux with frequent emesis, poor oral feeding skills, and recurrent respiratory infections (Kurzner et al., 1988).

Pulmonary hypertension is a sometimes terminal complication of BPD resulting from fibrosis and chronic hypoxia. The pulmonary vasculature of these infants develops increased reactivity to hypoxia, resulting in pulmonary hypertension and right ventricular hypertrophy with congestive heart failure. Pulmonary hypertension responds at least in part to oxygen, a potent pulmonary vasodilator (Abman et al., 1985). Low-flow supplemental oxygen is administered in these infants, at times on a long-term basis, in an attempt to prevent chronic hypoxia and subsequent pulmonary hypertension.

Prognosis. Approximately 25% of patients with severe BPD die (Ackerman, 1994). Early deaths are generally from untreatable respiratory failure, with later deaths being associated with infection or pulmonary hypertension/cor pulmonale, or an acute severe cyanotic episode, unresponsive to rapid institution of cardiopulmonary resustation (Abman et al., 1985). Although it is well documented that BPD infants have a prolonged and complicated neonatal course, the long-term pulmonary prognosis for survivors of BPD is relatively good. Young adults with BPD born in the 1960s and 1970s have pulmonary function and airway abnormalities, but only a small percentage have persistent symptoms of respiratory difficulty (Northway, Moss, & Carlisle, 1990). Chest x-ray films have also continued to show abnormalities years after the initial lung injuries (Griscom, Wheeler, & Sweezey, 1989; Northway et al., 1990), but the impact of these insults on health and quality of life is largely unknown. As the earliest survivors of BPD are now just in their early 20s, more research is needed regarding the long-term implications of their early lung disease.

The prognosis for the survivors of BPD from a nonpulmonary perspective is also quite promising. Unless there was a perinatal central nervous system insult or injury, neurodevelopmental outcome was found to be normal by 10 to 12 years of age in 60% of patients (Vohr et al., 1991). The majority of infants grow well beyond 2 years of age, but approximately 35% remain below the 10th percentile for weight and 25% are below the 10th percentile for length (Robertson, Etches, Goldson, & Kyle, 1992).

Assessment

The clinical manifestations of BPD are a direct reflection of the pathophysiology of this disorder. Tachypnea, dyspnea, and wheezing are intermittently or chronically present secondary to airway obstruction and increased airway resistance. Increased work of breathing, as evidenced by intercostal and/or substernal retractions, and use of accessory muscles are common in the infant with BPD. Infants who have been intubated for long periods of time may develop subglottic stenosis, which results in inspiratory stridor. Furthermore, hypoxemia and hypercapnia are chronic states that contribute to the problem. The child might turn cyanotic when crying or after a few moments of missing his or her supplemental oxygen. Infants with moderate to severe BPD are frequently described as irritable and difficult to comfort. This behavior may result from hypoxia or underlying neurologic dysfunction. They may develop irregular sleep patterns as a result of frequent medical treatments, medications, and therapies. Inguinal hernias are often present, which may be a result of the continuous increase in abdominal pressure caused by high airway resistance and use of accessory respiratory muscles. These infants also have extraordinarily insensible fluid losses because of tachypnea and excessive perspiration related to hypercarbia.

Pallor, digital clubbing, and severe growth failure are found in the most severe cases of BPD. These manifestations are due to chronic hypoxia (despite oxygen therapy) and myocardial dysfunction secondary to cor pulmonale. Infants with severe BPD often experience serious episodic cyanotic "spells" that are very difficult to treat. These episodes may be precipitated by agitation and are thought to be caused by the sudden development of partial or complete airway obstruction secondary to tracheomalacia and/or bronchospasms. These episodes are frightening, potentially life-threatening spells in which manual ventilation is often required. Other therapy depends on etiology, but prevention of agitation through the use of sedation and comfort measures is an important intervention.

The incidence of neurologic abnormalities and developmental delay in infants with bronchopulmonary dysplasia is variable, but they are known to occur in children with BPD. Infants who are born prematurely likely experience some degree of developmental delay with or without neurologic insult. Even if there is no evident damage to the neurologic system during hospitalization in the neonatal intensive care unit, these children with BPD may show signs of problems when school-age. These problems can range from vision and hearing losses to speech delays, learning disabilities, and poor attention span (Abham & Groothius, 1994). Developmental delays result from long-term ventilatory support, poor nutritional status, inadequate sensory stimulation, neurologic sequelae, and decreased energy and respiratory reserves (Mitchell, 1996).

Psychosocial Assessment

The emotional impact on parents and family of having a child with BPD is a topic of critical importance for nurses and other health professionals involved in the care of these children. The illness of a child is clearly a crisis for the family unit. The development of a chronic condition with life-threatening implications in a premature infant, followed by the complex home care of that child, is a situation so laden with stress and anxiety that it is often described by families as an "emotional roller coaster" from which there is no opportunity to "get off." The specific psychosocial assessment areas that are discussed in this section include grief/sorrow, social isolation, and financial demands.

The birth of an infant is generally a happy time for parents. However, when the child is delivered prematurely and/or has severe respiratory distress, which may lead to BPD, the parents experience grief and fear instead of happiness. Their vision of a "perfect" infant is shattered, and they must deal with a new reality that has been presented. They may grieve over losing the concept of an "ideal" child, the child they never had. The health care professional must be aware that this chronic sorrow is part of the natural process of coping with the loss of a healthy child and is not a maladaptive response (Lemons & Weaver, 1986).

Social isolation is also a prevalent psychosocial manifestation of families with an infant with BPD. The care of a frequently hospitalized infant with a chronic illness can absorb virtually all the time and energy of parents. They must attempt to balance time with the ill child and time for their other children and for themselves. This balancing of time is often a difficult task, and family sacrifices have to be made. Parents and older siblings may be required to adjust work and school schedules and adjust or eliminate recreational activities so that the needs of the child with BPD can be met. Social interactions are often drastically reduced because of lack of time, energy, transportation, and/or financial resources. In addition, clear-cut social guidelines for approaching families with chronically ill children are limited. At a time when support is most important, individuals in social networks may feel awkward and tend to withdraw. As a result, the family becomes socially isolated at times when resources and support are greatly needed. Assessment of social support and interactions is crucial in planning the care of a family with an infant or child with BPD.

Financial issues are a major concern. Hospital costs are extremely high for these children. Care of ventilator-dependent children can exceed thousands of dollars per day (McAleese, Knapp, & Rhodes, 1993). Although home care represents a significant savings, costs for these children may surpass $10,000 per month for therapies, equipment, drugs, supplies, and nursing services. The availability of third-party payer or Medicaid monies for home care services varies widely from state to state. Regardless of payer status, families often incur large financial costs. Loss of parental wages as a result of direct caregiving or frequent follow-up appointments; insurance co-payments and deductibles; increased home heating, air conditioning, and electricity bills; and the need for items not covered by payers (such as special formulas, corrective lenses, and rehabilitative equipment) all place significant financial demands on families (McAleese et al., 1993). A thorough financial assessment of a family's resources and assets is an important tool in planning for safe and cost-effective care for infants and families with BPD. These avenues should be explored jointly by a social services professional and the family's self-selected financial planner.

Interdisciplinary Interventions

Just as the pathophysiology of BPD is multifactorial, its treatment is multifaceted. Medical management of BPD is centered on

- Prevention and minimization of hypoxia and hypercarbia
- Treatment of bronchoconstriction and airway hyperreactivity and inflammation
- Treatment of pulmonary edema
- Promotion of repair of chronic lung injury

These desired ends are achieved in varying degrees by medical therapies such as supplemental oxygen, diuretics, bronchodilators, anti-inflammatory agents, and various modes of assisted mechanical ventilation. Tracheostomy is considered for those who require assisted ventilation for more than 3 months as a neonate or who have chronic hypercarbia and increased work of breathing (Ackerman, 1994; Doyle, 1996).

Prevention and Minimization of Hypoxia

The primary and most important aspect of therapy in infants with BPD is the management of hypoxia. Maintaining adequate tissue oxygenation is imperative in preventing significant morbidity and potential mortality. Supplemental oxygen therapy is prescribed to promote growth and neurodevelopment and prevent or control pulmonary hypertension. The administration and monitoring of oxygen therapy is a major nursing responsibility in the care of an infant with BPD. Pulse oximetry or transcutaneous oxygen monitors are used to continuously or intermittently display oxygen saturation. Oxygen saturations of 92% to 95%, depending on severity of illness, are necessary to facilitate an improved rate of weight gain (Hudak, Allen, & Hudak, 1989) and control pulmonary hypertension (Goodman et al., 1988). The nurse must respond to the infant's changing oxygen needs, titrating oxygen flow to keep saturations within the prescribed parameters. Feedings, periods of increased activity, and periods of sleep are occasions when desaturations are most likely (Ackerman, 1994).

The mode of oxygen delivery should be tailored to the specific needs of the infant. Most infants with mild to moderate BPD can tolerate a nasal oxygen cannula. Children with tracheostomies may use a tracheostomy mist collar (Fig. 16–21). Humidification is necessary for liter flow equal to or greater than 1 L/min to prevent airway irritation and mucous plugging. The nurse should make an ongoing assessment of increased demand for

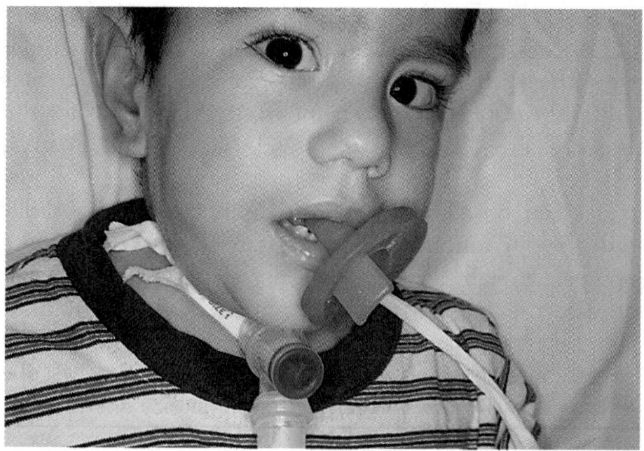

Figure 16–21
Humidified oxygen is provided to the child using a mist delivery device.

oxygen by the infant, especially during acute illnesses, fever, stress, and/or increased periods of activity. Reassessment should include child's color, presence and degree of respiratory distress (possibly including retractions, nasal flaring, and use of accessory respiratory muscles), breath sounds, vital signs, and level of consciousness.

Other nursing interventions for the infant with BPD include administering multiple oral and inhaled pharmacologic agents, monitoring of their effectiveness, and identifying possible adverse side effects (Table 16–14).

Respiratory Care

Because excessive airway secretions are difficult problems for the infant or child with BPD, diligent airway clearance is needed to prevent mucous plugging and airway obstruction. Cough is often ineffective in these children because of generalized debilitation and tracheomalacia. Nasal-pharyngeal or tracheal suctioning is needed frequently to maintain patent airways, especially during illnesses or respiratory tract infections. Chest physiotherapy may also help improve secretion clearance and lessen atelectasis. Always collaborate with respiratory therapists and/or parents to schedule chest physiotherapy to occur 30 minutes before feedings and before rest periods if possible. Suctioning should immediately follow chest physiotherapy, and other times as needed.

For the infant with severe long-term BPD, home assisted ventilation can be a safe and cost-effective alternative to chronic hospitalization (DeWitt, Jansen, Ward, & Keens, 1993). Home ventilation allows a degree of normalization for the family and provides opportunities for the enhancement of the social development of the infant. Because of the excessive care demands, there is the potential for parent or family burn-out. As with all complex home care situations, support with staffing of

Table 16–14
BPD Medications and Side Effects

Type of Medication	Action	Possible Side Effects
Bronchodilators		
Theophylline Metaproterenol sulfate Albuterol (Ventolin) Terbutaline	Bronchodilators open the airways of the lungs. They work by relaxing the muscles around the airways. These medicines can be used alone or in groups.	Increased heart rate Shakiness or tremors Hyperactivity Possibly nausea and vomiting (theophylline)
Diuretics		
Furosemide (Lasix) Spironolactone (Aldactone) Hydrochlorothiazide (Aldactazide) Chlorothiazide (Diuril)	Diuretics cause an increased amount of water and salt to be excreted in the urine. They also decrease the amount of fluid in the lungs.	Decreased serum potassium (hypokalemia) and calcium (hypocalcemia). Muscle cramps and irregular heart rhythm are signs. Serum electrolytes must be closely monitored.
Anti-inflammatory Drugs		
Pediapred (oral liquid) Cromolyn sodium (Intal) (inhaled)	Anti-inflammatory drugs are used in children whose wheezing is not controlled with bronchodilators. These medicines do not reverse or stop existing wheezing. They are used on a long-term basis to prevent wheezing and respiratory distress. They work well only if taken continuously.	Short-term use causes little or no side effects. Longer-term effects include impaired growth and decreased ability to fight infections.

nurses in the home is crucial to the success of a home ventilation program.

Positioning and comforting interventions are of extreme importance in caring for the infant with BPD. Ill or premature infants who are chronically air-hungry are extremely irritable and may be difficult to console. With the collaboration of physical and occupational therapies, nurses should develop individualized plans for the handling and activity level of these infants that takes into consideration the developmental level and ability to tolerate stimulation. Frequent and prolonged rest periods are necessary because of increased energy demand and sleep deprivation. Signs of overstimulation in the neurologically immature child include cyanosis, avoidance of eye contact, vomiting, diaphoresis, and/or falling asleep.

Nutritional Support

Because growth failure is common in the infant with BPD, providing nutritional support is one of the most crucial, although difficult, aspects of caring for these children. Management of feedings in infants and young children with BPD has direct implications for long-term outcome, because an adequate caloric intake is necessary for growth of healthy lung tissue and resolution of the disease. Yet these infants suffer from a myriad of conditions that impair their ability to feed: gastroesophageal reflux, often with aspiration; emesis; chronic fatigue; behavioral oral aversion; and swallowing dysfunction due to poor oral-motor development. Feeding is generally viewed for the normal infant as a pleasant and positive experience; however, for the BPD child it is often perceived as a battle. It can seem the more that nurses and parents are concerned and anxious about nutrition and place pressure on the infant or child to eat, the less the child eats. Feeding issues with the BPD infant or child can be a frustrating and challenging experience, but coordinated interdisciplinary effort is the key to successfully approaching these problems.

Nutritional assessment of the child with BPD is the initial step. This includes documentation of anthropometric (precise measurement of the body includes weight, height, and head circumference) and biochemical data, dietary intake, and clinical status. Strategies in nutritional support then focus on optimizing the caloric intake to meet the individual needs of the child. Concentrating formula to provide more calories per ounce, medication to control gastroesophageal reflux, and small frequent feedings all are appropriate for the child with mild to moderate growth failure.

Infants with severe growth failure, or for whom the previously listed strategies are unsuccessful, should be considered for surgical placement of a gastrostomy tube or percutaneous endoscopically placed gastrostomy (PEG) tube. This may or may not be performed in conjunction with a Nissen fundoplication, depending on the severity of gastroesophageal reflux. Although parents sometimes view the need for a gastrostomy tube as a sign of their "failure" to orally feed their infant, it is important for the entire health care team to provide support and to stress the benefits of this mode of therapy. Calorie-dense formulas can be administered with minimal risk of aspiration, in a continuous infusion if necessary, to promote optimal growth. Feeding specialists and caregivers can provide therapy to develop and refine suck and swallow coordination skills concurrently, so that as the infant's growth, strength, and ability to orally feed improve. Tube feedings can be slowly weaned and frequency and amount of oral feedings increased (Chart 16–25). This strategy temporarily relaxes the intense focus on eating and can transform parental anxiety into energy devoted to interventions such as positive oral stimulation and non-nutritive sucking during tube feedings.

Family Education and Support

Other nursing and social service interventions with the child and family with BPD should focus on providing education and support. Parents must be taught about all aspects of their child's disease, especially topics relating to home care. If the child is to receive oxygen, arrangements must be made for administering the oxygen (Chart 16–26). Medication administration, feeding and nutrition, developmental interventions, chest physiotherapy, and suctioning are among the most important topics of education for the parents and family of a child with BPD. Family members are taught cardiopulmonary resuscitation. Instruction is given regarding the symptoms indicating that the child's respiratory condition is worsening and when to seek medical attention.

Parent support groups facilitated by nursing or social service professionals are often successful in addressing parental anxiety and promoting positive coping. Sibling reactions and coping, financial stress, profound chronic fatigue, and uncertainty about their child's physical and intellectual future all are topics many parents find comforting to discuss with others who have had similar experiences and concerns. Some families too are referred by social services for private counseling to address and facilitate stress management.

Prevention of BPD remains the ultimate goal. Ensuring that all pregnant women receive adequate prenatal care (even before conception) eliminates or alleviates many poor birth outcomes, especially low birth weight (Institute of Medicine, 1985). Decreasing the incidence of premature birth by socioeconomic and political action is the avenue that has been least explored and holds much promise for future success. Nurses and other health professionals can be instrumental in this movement by becoming informed and communicating with public pol-

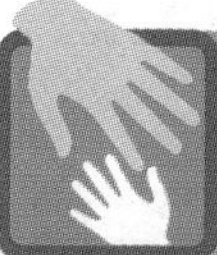

Chart 16–25
Nursing Interventions

How to Improve Feeding Capabilities in an Infant with BPD

1. Have baby in *calm,* alert state before beginning to feed.
2. *Gently* normalize total body posture. Position baby in caregiver's lap with neck in neutral position, hips and knees 90 degree flexion, both upper extremities with elbows flexed 90 degrees and swaddled across chest. *Note:* If baby becomes excessively hot or sweaty with swaddling of entire body, then fold a thin pillowcase or light towel in a long rectangle and swaddle *only* around the arms and partial trunk to prevent excessive scapular retraction, arching, and flailing of the upper extremities.
3. Careful monitoring of physiologic parameters, especially respiratory rate, is necessary. Feedings may need to be limited or postponed if the infant remains tachypneic.
4. Choose a nipple that allows moderate resistance to flow without excessive energy expenditure. Standard-shaped nipples are preferred for several reasons.
5. Present nipple slowly and calmly, with minimal intraoral stimulation.
6. Head and neck posture can alter oral-motor patterns during sucking. Normalization of total body posture should be emphasized during feeding. Ideally, marked neck extension should be reduced to aid oral-motor control. The goal of improved head and neck positioning may need to be addressed slowly, to minimize stress to the infant.
7. Allow baby to set the nippling pace, with rests as needed.
8. Stop nippling if baby begins to sweat or cries inconsolably for 1 minute; if excessive increased respiratory rate or heart rate as determined by physician; if takes longer than 20 minutes.
9. Oral-tactile hypersensitivity is not uncommon in the infant with BPD. This is evidenced by pulling back as the nipple is placed on the lips, and becoming agitated or gagging as the nipple is placed in the mouth. Treatment strategies include

   Maximize pleasurable oral-tactile input such as non-nutritive sucking and stroking of the head, face, and lips.

   Minimize aversive oral input by early utilization of nasal intubation if possible, and by care practices that support the infant's neurobehavioral organization.

BPD Nippling Evaluation

	Absent 0	1	2	Normal 3	4	Excessive 5
Gag						
Rhythmic suck on pacifier						
General irritability:						
• Before nippling						
• During nippling						

icy makers individually or through involvement in professional organizations. Experts in the care of these infants and families are clearly in a prime position to facilitate change.

Cystic Fibrosis

Cystic fibrosis (CF) is now described as the most common life-shortening condition affecting those with a European Caucasian background. This description is a departure from the recent past, when CF was described as the most lethal genetic disease of childhood. The primary reason for the changes in life expectancy is earlier diagnosis, allowing for initiation of therapy with more effective medicines. CF is an autosomal recessive genetic condition. This means that both parents carry the gene and with each pregnancy there is a 25% chance the baby will have CF, a 50% chance the baby will be a carrier, and a

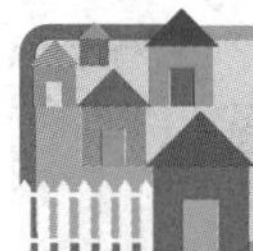

Chart 16–26
Community Care

Methods of Home Oxygen Delivery

Method	Advantages	Disadvantages	Special Considerations
Compressed gas in tank	Usually the least expensive system Can be used with any flow rate; continuously or intermittently (with proper flow meter)	Large tanks take much storage space Under very high pressure. If valve were broken or jarred loose, tank would behave like a high-powered rocket. Heavy, cumbersome	Tanks vary in size from very large, to portable (with a cart) All tanks must be stored with a stable base and secured against falling over When traveling, the system should be secured in the vehicle to prevent rolling or other movement.
Liquid oxygen	Twice as much oxygen can be stored in the same amount of space as tanks Very light and portable; the most convenient system May be more cost effective than tanks if high flow is required	Usually the most expensive system Evaporates when not being used continuously Not practical with low flow rates	Portable system is filled from a larger reservoir When traveling, the system should be secured in the vehicle to prevent rolling or other movement.
Oxygen concentrator	Machine separates oxygen from nitrogen in the room air. Never needs to be "refilled." Practical for rural areas or areas not routinely serviced by oxygen companies	Runs by electricity. Backup system needed for power outages Noisy Increases electric bills Difficult to transport in a two-story home or outside the home	Must have grounded electrical outlet When traveling, the system should be secured in the vehicle to prevent rolling or other movement. A portable system of compressed gas should be dispersed for emergency use and transport to clinic for illnesses.

All oxygen systems should be kept away from any open flame, combustible materials, or sources of sparks.

25% chance the baby will neither be a carrier nor have CF (Fig. 16–22).

The frequency of CF carriers in Caucasians is 1 in 25 (Aitken & Fiel, 1993), and the estimated incidence in live Caucasian births in 1990 was 1 in 3500. The incidence of live births is less frequent in other ethnic and racial groups. FitzSimmons (1993) reports the following data from an epidemiologic study in 1990: 1 in 11,500 in Hispanic live births, 1 in 14,000 African American live births, 1 in 25,500 in Asian live births, and 1 in 10,500 American Indian, Eskimo, and Aleut live births. Since the early 1980s, advances in the care of CF have led to an increased life expectancy and have contributed to a positive impact on the quality of life.

Pathophysiology

The CF gene, identified in 1989, is located on chromosome 7. The protein product of this gene, referred to as cystic fibrosis transmembrane regulator (CFTR), is defective. This defect leads to abnormal electrolyte and fluid transport across epithelial cell membranes by mechanisms

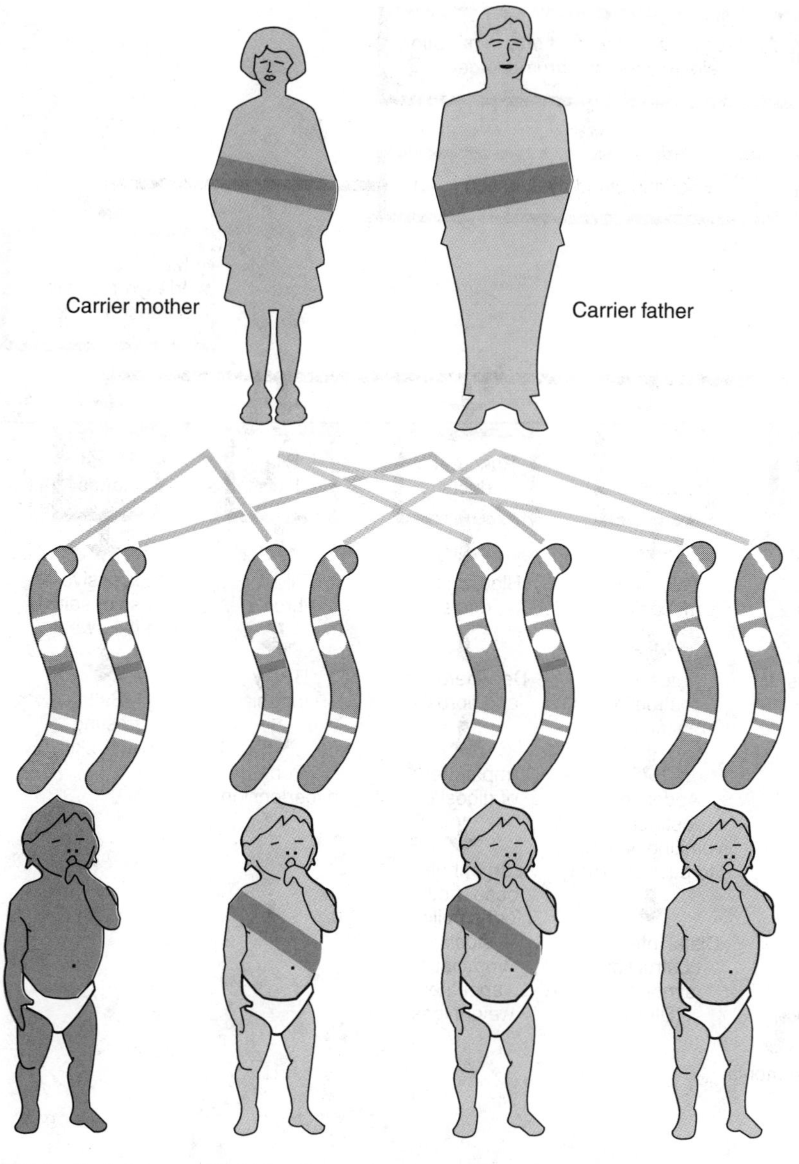

Figure 16–22
Genetic transmission of cystic fibrosis: autosomal recessive inheritance.

still not well understood. This alteration explains the thickened mucus and secretions of the pulmonary, gastrointestinal, and reproductive systems. It also explains the abnormality in the sweat glands accounting for an elevated sodium and chloride concentration from blocked or abnormal transport (Wilmott & Fiedler, 1994) (Fig. 16–23).

There are more than 500 gene mutations of CF (Marelich & Cross, 1996). Approximately 70% of these mutations are identified to be the ΔF508. A small number of these mutations occur with reasonable frequency, whereas the majority are rare. This finding helps explain the wide variation of the clinical manifestations of the phenotypic expression of CF. For example, 99% of those who are homozygous for the ΔF508 allele have pancreatic insufficiency, whereas only 36% of CF people with other mutations are pancreatic insufficient (Orenstein, 1993). Carrier testing for the general population is still not widely available but can be done. Prenatal diagnosis is available on request for those couples with known or suspected family histories. Prenatal testing is also done when obstructed fetal bowel is detected by ultrasound, because of its association with meconium ileus. Carrier diagnosis for individuals with confirmed or suspected fam-

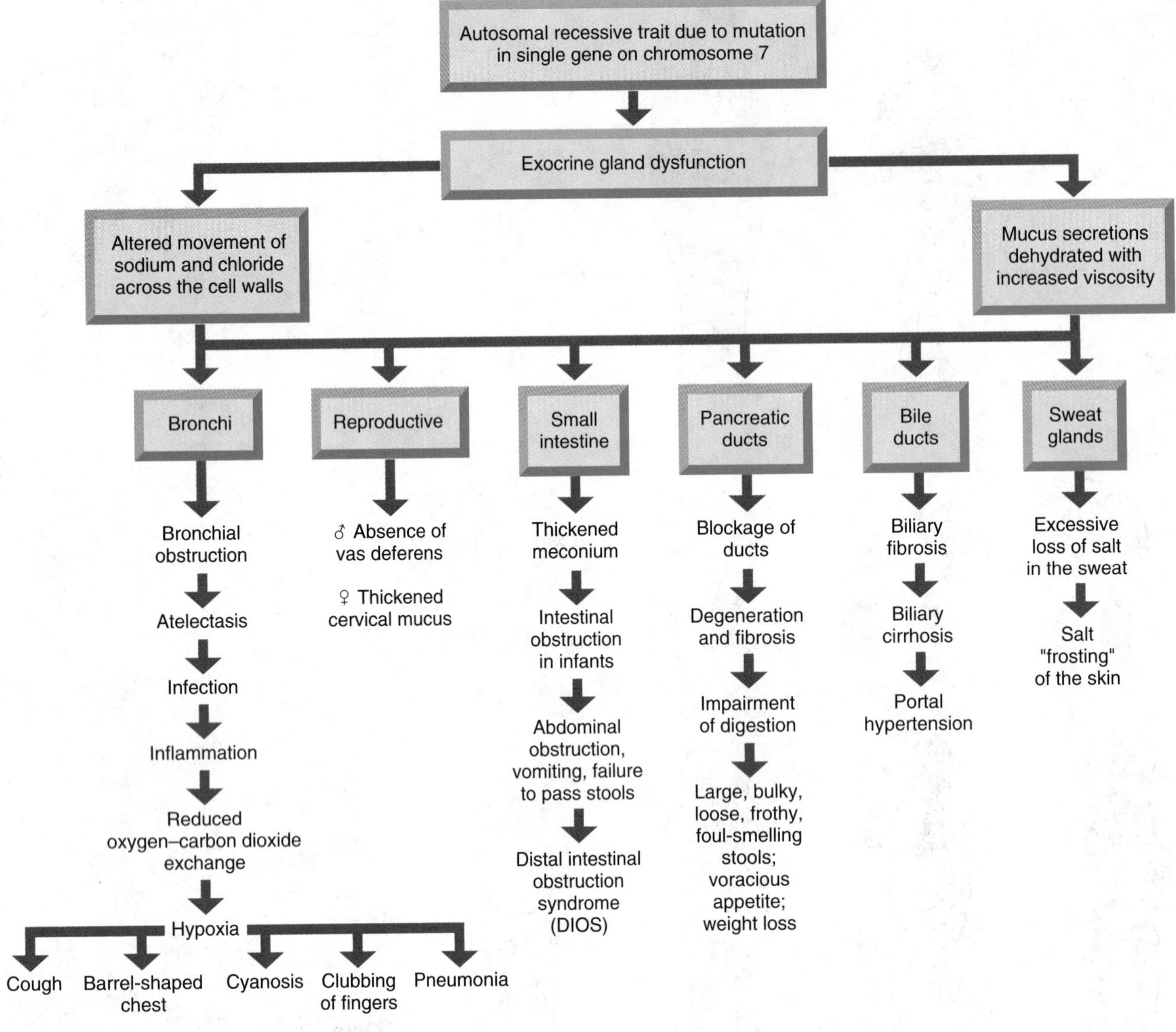

Figure 16–23
Manifestations of cystic fibrosis. (Modified from Orenstein, D. M. [1991]. Cystic fibrosis. *Respiratory Care*, 36(7), 748.)

ily histories can also be done. A buccal smear for DNA analysis may be obtained when neonates present with a clinically suspicious picture, allowing for diagnosis at an earlier age.

Prognosis. Today when an infant has been diagnosed with CF, the family is informed that his or her average life span is 30.1 years (Cystic Fibrosis Registry, 1996). However, more and more people are living with CF into their 30s and 40s. Pediatric health care teams must be prepared to foster a "wellness" focus for these individuals. Planning for a productive life is the norm in the clinical care delivered from a skilled interdisciplinary team.

Assessment

Cystic fibrosis is a multisystem condition. The main systems affected are related to the sweat glands and the exocrine glands in the pulmonary and digestive systems. Exocrine glands secrete substances to the body's surface or organ lumen. CF is characterized by cycles of relatively symptom-free periods interspersed with periods of illness. It should be noted, however, that each child with CF has very individual clinical manifestations. For example, some children may never be hospitalized until adolescence or older, yet there are many children who require hospitalization multiple times during infancy and throughout childhood.

There is no cure for CF. It follows a pattern of progressive lung damage over time. The course of the disease generally begins with increased secretions leading to airway obstruction, inflammation, infection, scarring, bronchiectasis, and cor pulmonale with eventual respiratory failure. Early in life the sputum and throat cultures are positive for *Staphylococcus aureus* and *Haemophilus influenzae*. At some stage the cultures become positive for *Pseudomonas aeruginosa* and the patient remains colonized with this organism, which is never eradicated from the lungs.

Alert: *More recently an organism Pseudomonas (Burkholderia) cepacia has been cultured from the sputum (Kotloff & Zuckerman, 1996). This organism has been associated with a relatively rapid deterioration of the child's condition.*

The presence of this organism, *Burkholderia cepacia,* has also been responsible for altering the activities and lifestyles for those with CF because of its communicability among the CF population. During hospitalization, these patients have been restricted from the recreation room, one of the few places that helps create a more tolerable hospital stay. Individuals with CF are no longer cohorted in the same room when hospitalized, unless their sputum cultures are known to be negative for *B. cepacia.* The Cystic Fibrosis Foundation has recommended terminating CF camps to avoid cross-colonization of this potentially devastating organism (Pegues et al., 1993). A concern for antibiotic-resistant organisms is gaining similar attention.

The need for more aggressive therapy and hospitalization is referred to as a pulmonary exacerbation. This occurs when the following symptoms exist: fatigue, decreased appetite, weight loss, increased sputum production; increased cough, hemoptysis, decreased spirometry values, and poor response to outpatient therapeutic measures such as oral antibiotics and increased pulmonary treatments at home.

The respiratory assessment findings for an infant or child may reveal increased anterior-posterior diameter, or "barrel"-shaped, chest due to hyperaeration and increased work of breathing. The nail beds may show mild to severe clubbing, the mechanism of which is unclear. There is a characteristic cough that may increase during pulmonary exacerbations. The cough can be paroxysmal in nature and frequently ends with post-tussive emesis. Breath sounds are assessed for equal aeration and the presence or absence of rales, crackles, and wheezing throughout all lung fields, particularly in the upper lobes and the right middle lobe. Respiratory rate has been found to be a sensitive indicator of respiratory dysfunction, when counted accurately and for one full minute (Browning, D'Alonzo, & Tobin, 1990). Oxygenation is assessed by inspection of color changes of mucous membranes, nail beds, and general skin color. Pulse oximetry is used to monitor oxygen saturation. Breathing is assessed for rate, depth, effort, and use of accessory muscles. A history is obtained on sputum characteristics, including the color changes, volume, viscosity, and presence or absence of blood. Cough pattern, changes in breathing during activities of a typical day, and history of headaches and pain are also elicited. Current chest radiographs are compared with baseline films, and spirometry values are compared with prior results.

The newborn may present with meconium ileus and bowel obstruction and perforation requiring surgical intervention. Young infants may be irritable and present with failure to thrive despite a history of a good appetite. The infant or child with CF may appear physically small for his or her age in both linear growth and weight. Approximately 80% to 85% of children are pancreatic insufficient, resulting in malabsorption of important nutrients, fats, and proteins. Thus, the stool is described as foul smelling, greasy, and bulky.

The overall size of the child is noted on physical examination. The general condition, muscle tone, and muscle mass are noted. Some children with CF may demonstrate a protuberant abdomen. The skin is assessed for bruising, old surgical scars, and indicators of adequate, excessive, or inadequate fluid balance. The oral mucous membranes, especially of infants, need to be assessed. Oral lesions may result from enzymes or from thrush, a monilial superinfection that may be caused by oral antibiotics. Thrush may also manifest as candidal vaginitis in the female adolescent or monilial diaper rash in the infant. The rectal area of infants should be examined for perirectal irritation from unabsorbed enzymes. Inspection of the condition of the skin in the diaper area is also needed. A history from the caregiver of a prolapsed rectum should be elicited. Other history and symptoms that require assessment are irritability and any associated behaviors; emesis; stool pattern with frequency and characteristics; and verbal reports of abdominal pain, discomfort, and/or "heartburn," which may indicate gastroesophageal reflux (GER). A careful history and assessment is done when children are in the high-risk group for a more recently described gastrointestinal problem termed fibrosing colonopathy (Borowitz, Grand, Durie, & the Consensus Committee, 1995). This condition includes the presence of true colonic strictures and the prestricture state (Borowitz et al., 1995). The factors identified that place individuals at greater risk were patients taking more than 6000 lipase units/kg/meal for longer than 6 months, those who are younger than 12 years of age and have had a history of meconium ileus or distal intestinal obstruction syndrome, and intestinal surgery (Smyth et al., 1995).

Adolescents may have delayed secondary sexual development from the chronicity of CF and from difficulty meeting nutritional needs throughout their life. This type of delay may cause the teen to look younger than his or her peers. There is then a mismatch between their normal cognitive development and their immature or underdeveloped appearance. These children may be labeled as "precocious" and be sensitive about their young physical appearance.

> **Tip:** *The parent may assist the child in developing a prerehearsed script to respond to common and potentially uncomfortable situations regarding their maturity. This may help reduce the feelings of uneasiness and increase his or her confidence.*

It is during the adolescent years that the patient may learn about the reproductive associations of CF. Approximately 98% of males are sterile because of the blockage of the vas deferens from thick secretions or from abnormal development resulting in absent passage of sperm. Females may become pregnant, but the thick cervical mucus may act as a natural barrier to sperm. Infertility, however, must not be assumed for either gender. Appropriate referrals for informed family planning and life decisions are recommended and supported.

General nursing assessment must also include a history of changes in activity tolerance, exercise program, sleep and rest disturbance, and sleep position. Overall health maintenance such as immunizations, annual flu vaccine (McMullen, 1992), and compliance history is important to document.

Delays in the diagnosis of CF may result from the patient's expressing minimal symptoms. For example, there have been reports of adults diagnosed with CF after identification of nasal polyps or from an infertility evaluation. As people live longer with CF, other symptoms and/or complications may manifest themselves (Chart 16–27). Infections such as respiratory syncytial virus (RSV) may result in severe pulmonary complications, particularly in infants (Abman, Ogle, Butler-Simon, Rumack, & Accurso, 1988).

Diagnostic Tests. The sweat test is the diagnostic test for CF. An elevated sweat sodium chloride (NaCl) level of ≥60 mEq/L is a positive diagnostic result that is confirmed by a second test. The sweat sample is usually obtained by stimulating a small patch of sweat glands on the inner aspect of the forearm. An adequate quantity of sweat, between 50 mg and preferably 100 mg, must be collected to ensure reliability (Rosenstein, 1990). A diagnosis is made with two positive sweat chloride study results and the presence of clinical symptoms or a family history. The siblings are also tested when a diagnosis is confirmed (McMullen, 1992).

Psychosocial Assessment

The presence of a chronic condition in an infant or child may have an impact on his or her development. However, the acquisition and progression of these milestones may not be adversely affected, depending on the severity and frequency of illness. Many children report living a daily life "just like their friends." Self reports such as these are validated when talking to young adults about growing up. Infants and children who require frequent hospitalizations and who have repeat cycles of illness may demonstrate developmental lags. Many children who experience long-term hospitalization may lag in their gross motor skills because they have not had the opportunities and/or energy for this aspect of development. Their confinement in the hospital has not allowed them the chance to jump and climb for gross motor development, and the work of breathing expends so much energy, there is little left for other areas of day-to-day living. Similarly, these same children demonstrate age-appropriate fine motor, language, and social skills. The adjustment of the child and family living with CF depends on how much the child is affected by the condition. Therefore, health care providers may observe a range of coping styles and behaviors. More recent research studies have reported that the majority of families do cope successfully (Patterson, McCubbin, & Warwick, 1990). Earlier studies reported somewhat mixed findings, attributed, in part, to not taking the severity of illness into account (Gibson, 1988; Lask, 1992; Sawyer, 1992; Stullenbarger, Norris, Edgil, & Prosser, 1987).

The general approach for children with CF is to "normalize" their daily living within the child's specific limitations. For example, because a cold can create significant effects for a child with CF, a parent may need to request friends and neighbors to cooperate in keeping the children separated when illnesses or colds develop. Parents and children may benefit from assistance to sort out appropriate measures for daily living.

"Out of home" daycare for the working parent is a frequent and practical concern of many families. This type of daycare is not contraindicated. These choices and decisions are explored with each family on an individual basis. Advantages and disadvantages are evaluated with consideration given to the individual infant or child's health status. It is helpful to plan for a reevaluation of health status 3 to 6 months after such a change is initiated to determine the frequency of acute illnesses.

School attendance is another major concern for children. Children are encouraged to attend school. The school-age child may have many new hurdles to confront about CF. Parents are encouraged to educate teachers about their child's condition in hopes of facilitating an understanding about the specialized needs of their child.

Chart 16–27

Complications of Cystic Fibrosis

Complications	Causes
Pulmonary:	
Minor Hemoptysis	Common after age of 10 years. Blood streaking is from mucosal irritation in the airway. (1,2)
Major Hemoptysis	Occurs more frequently with age; in less than 10% of adults. Bleeding caused from high systemic pressure of bronchial circulation when infection erodes a blood vessel. (1,2)
Pneumothorax	Incidence increases with age (approximately 16–20% patients older than 18 years experience this complication). Rupture of subpleural blebs through visceral pleura. High rate of recurrence. (1,2)
Nasal Polyps	Occurs in 10–25% of CF patients; most common in older children and adolescents; etiology unknown. (1)
Chronic Sinusitis	Occurs in >90% of CF patients. Etiology is thought to be from abnormal occlusion of the ducts and prevention of mucus drainage; maxillary and ethmoid sinuses most commonly involved. (1)
Cor Pulmonale	Occurs in advanced disease. Right ventricular hypertrophy, chronic hypoxemia and pulmonary hypertension, and right-sided heart failure.
Pulmonary Hypertrophic Osteoarthropathy	Occurs in approximately 4% of older pateints; etiology is unclear.
Gastrointestinal:	
Cystic Fibrosis Diabetes	Occurs in up to 8–15% of patients with onset in adolescence. Etiology is unknown. It is postulated that deficiency is secondary to fibrosis of the pancreas, destroying the islet's architecture; usually non-ketotic. (1,3)
Distal Intestinal Obstruction Syndrome Equivalent (DIOS) (formally called meconium ileus equivalent)	Incidence is up to 10–20% of adult CF patients. Usually occurs during adolescence or later. May be partial or complete obstruction; etiology is multifaceted; intestinal mucoproteins may be more viscous, enteroglucagon release results from increased undigested fats that slow transit time; a fecal mass forms at the ileocecal region and extends distally. (1,4)
Cholelithiasis	Occurs in up to 12% of patients, rarely represents symptomatically prior to teenage years. Stones are usually cholesterol. Etiology from alterations in bile lipid composition. (1)
Liver Disease	Occurs in about 4% of patients, peaking in adolescence and decreasing after 20 years.
Multilobar Cirrhosis	Results from thickened secretions in bile ductules causing plugging, ductular proliferation, inflammation, and cirrhosis. (1)
Gastroesophageal Reflux (GER)	Occurrence of symptoms varies. There is a transient inappropriate relaxation of the lower esophageal sphincter. Contributing factors include positioning, cough, and increased intra-abdominal pressures vs. thoracic pressure gradient. (1,4)
Pancreatitis	Acute pancreatitis occurs in approximately 10% of patients. It can occur with pancreatic sufficiency. It is an inflammatory response. Exact causative mechanism is unclear.
Fibrosing Colonopathy	Occurs in a small percentage of patients. Risk factors include children younger than the age of 12 years. Strong association with oral pancreatic high-dose enzyme intake for >6 months.

1. Aitken & Fiel (1993)
2. Schidlow, Taussig, & Knowles (1993)
3. Cystic Fibrosis Foundation Consensus Conference (1990)
4. Shalon & Adelson (1996)

Booklets are available for teachers through local CF centers. The decision to tell classmates and peers about CF is a very personal one. Families are encouraged to discuss these issues with their CF team to obtain direction and support for these decisions. Parent–teacher conferences at the beginning of each school year are an effective way to provide the needed information and establish a communication channel to successfully reduce the sense of difference the child may feel at school.

Children must be prepared to take their medicines at school, take rest time when they are unable to keep up with their peers, use the bathroom facilities more often, and adjust their school schedule to minimize stresses when trying to get to classes on time. Assisting the child with a rehearsed script to respond to frequently asked questions about CF symptoms and management may help to strengthen the child's confidence and coping ability. Maintaining school attendance is encouraged so that the child has the opportunity to socialize and diversify his or her strengths to prepare for future goals. Social isolation because of sporadic school attendance can lead to other psychosocial issues such as depression. The child's condition must be addressed individually for appropriate modifications.

The family may request assistance from the CF center nurse or social worker to intervene with school issues. The physical therapist can also provide valuable input for guidelines in physical education activities related to exercise tolerance and endurance.

During adolescence, planning for the future and choosing a career are central tasks to accomplish. Attention must be also directed to a career that will fulfill the ability to work in spite of changing conditions. Career and vocational counselors are resources that may assist in this planning process.

For the parents of a newly diagnosed infant or child, the process of adjustment may be compared with the grief process. Parents often report feeling that they cannot get on with their lives and that they have difficulty regaining stability for 6 months to 1 year after diagnosis. Patients and their families may function adequately for a while and then need some additional support during high crisis times. Some examples are the first hospitalization after diagnosis, the death of another child at the same CF center, making the transition to adult care, taking on new home therapies such as oxygen or intravenous antibiotics, or attending the first day of school. Lask's (1992) review of the psychosocial literature indicates that the psychosocial research must include the severity of illness to make the findings more meaningful. More research is needed on affected individuals and their functioning within the family unit as well as the father's role. Research on issues such as the transition for the older adolescent or young adult with CF from a pediatric care team to an adult counterpart team and identified outcomes for care will enable CF care teams to better address developmentally sensitive issues within more appropriate time frames.

Interdisciplinary Interventions

The care and treatment of CF uses an interdisciplinary model. In addition, the care of CF is carried out at an accredited CF center. These centers meet the criteria set forth by the Cystic Fibrosis Foundation to deliver the quality of care and maintain the standard of practice. Most CF centers are directed by a pediatric pulmonologist. Additional pediatric specialists function as part of the team or are consulted on an as-needed basis. They include pediatric specialists of gastroenterology, infectious diseases, genetics, and endocrinology. Other integral team members include the following: clinical social worker, advanced practice nurse (pediatric nurse practitioner [PNP] or clinical nurse specialist [CNS]), respiratory care practitioner, registered dietitian, physical therapist, child

Chart 16–28
Worldview

Cystic Fibrosis

Because CF is primarily a condition that affects people of European-Caucasian genetic backgrounds, the CF care team must be sensitive to the cultural issues for minority individuals and families. Families may experience a sense of isolation within their cultural environment. There may be lifestyle practices that are not part of the norm and may have an impact on the care of an infant or child. For example, some cultures may support breast-feeding for a longer duration than current practices in the American culture. The CF team members must work to understand these cultural differences and support choices that will not jeopardize the condition of the patient. For this example, this may mean more frequent monitoring of growth parameters to ensure that the child's nutritional needs are being met while supporting cultural practices. Additionally, the CF care team must facilitate availability of educational materials in the family's native language as well as linking parents and families with culturally matched support. The team must also ensure that these families have a clear understanding of the genetics so that they may respond to questions and concerns among family and extended family to avoid further feelings and experiences of isolation. The cultural differences and practices related to CF are a ripe area for nursing research so that the family's needs may be addressed in a more sensitive environment.

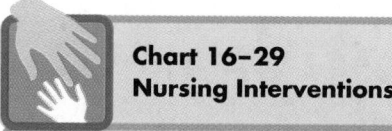

Chart 16–29
Nursing Interventions

Administering Pancreatic Enzymes

Greater attention in the recent past has focused on the dosing of pancreatic enzymes. There have been reports in the past several years identifying a new clinical complication with cystic fibrosis, *fibrosing colonopathy* (Borowitz, Grand, Durie, & the Consensus Committee, 1995). These reports speculate the correlation of this gastrointestinal complication with the introduction of high-dose pancreatic enzymes containing 25,000 to 32,000 lipase units/capsule. These products were voluntarily removed from the market in response to the reported observations. Health care providers became more aware and cautious about the potential problems that may result from pancreatic enzyme. The CF Foundation organized a Consensus Conference in conjunction with the Food and Drug Administration with the following recommendations:

- Recommended *starting* dose of lipase is
  - For infants: 2000 to 4000 lipase units/120 mL of formula or per breast-feeding
  - For children younger than 4 years of age: 1000 lipase units/kg/meal
  - For children older than 4 years of age: 500 lipase units/kg/meal (older patients ingest less fat per kilogram of body weight)
- Usually half the standard pancreatic lipase dose is given with snacks.
- Nursing considerations include the following:
  - Encourage three meals and two to three snacks per day.
  - Discourage eating throughout the entire day.
  - Administer enzymes before or with meals (and with vitamins); with snacks; with milk and oral or bolused nutritional supplements; and before nocturnal feeds begin (and occasionally after completion, as prescribed).
- Capsules may be opened and contents mixed with small amount of applesauce or other non-alkaline food.
- Microcapsules should not be crushed.
- Avoid allowing microcapsules to sit in food that disrupts the enteric coating.
- Do not give enzymes with clear liquids, popsicles, or frozen juice bars.
- Assess the oral mucosa and perirectal area for irritation from contact with unswallowed or unabsorbed enzymes.
- Monitor stool pattern and characteristics.
- Be alert to complaints such as bloating, flatus, abdominal pain, loose and frequent stools *with* steatorrhea, *and/or* poor growth.
- Instruct parent/patient not to adjust the dose.
- Instruct parent/patient to check expiration dates and store in cool place.

life specialist, genetic counselor, the parents/caregivers, and the child, when developmentally appropriate. These health team members work together to treat the complex needs of the children and their families (Care Path 16–5). Although each discipline has a specialized knowledge base and clearly defined roles, overlap in role functions may occur depending on individual family needs and their identification of team members with whom a preferred rapport has developed. The goal of the team is to "normalize" the lives of the families and to maintain and/or prevent further pulmonary damage so the child may benefit as newer treatment options become available (Chart 16–28).

Medical Management

The medical management of the child with CF is multifaceted. A child may have early symptoms of a pulmonary exacerbation and be managed at home with oral antibiotics, aggressive pulmonary therapy, and close follow-up at the CF center or with the pediatrician. If a poor response to oral therapy is determined, then a "tune-up" is required. "Tune-ups" have traditionally necessitated hospitalization. During a 10- to 14-day hospital stay, aggressive pulmonary and nutritional therapy is instituted, along with intravenous antibiotics and an exercise program. Today, with a shift toward ambulatory services, many individuals with CF may initiate their "tune-up" in the hospital for the first several days and complete it at home. During this first phase of the "tune-up," appropriate antibiotics are administered based on findings from the sputum culture and sensitivities. This home care approach depends on factors such as severity of illness, venous access, ability and resources of the family, and payer source.

Medical management includes aggressive therapeutic interventions and evaluation of the response to these

Table 16–15
Pharmaceutical Agents Used in the Care of the Child with Cystic Fibrosis

Category	Purpose	Example
Aerosols		
Bronchodilators (aerosols and metered-dose inhalers)	Open up airways	Albuterol (Proventil) Terbutaline
Antibiotics	Antimicrobial for *P. aeruginosa* locally	Tobramycin; colistin
Enzyme	Thins mucus	DNase
Pancreatic Enzymes	Increase food/nutrient absorption	Cotazym Creon Pancrease Ultrase
Vitamins/Minerals	Fat-soluble vitamin supplement in water miscible form; supplement overall diet	Vitamins A, D, E, and K; Aquasol A Multivitamin
H_2 Blocker	Alters GI acidic environment; GER therapy	Ranitidine (Zantac) Cimetidine (Tagamet)
Prokinetic Agents	Enhances GI motility; GER therapy	Cisapride (Propulsid)
Antibiotics	Antimicrobial for:	
Oral	*S. aureus*	Cloxacillin, dicloxacillin, cephalexin, clindamycin
	H. influenzae	Amoxicillin, cefaclor, cefprozil, trimethoprim sulfamethoxazole, amoxicillin and clavulanic acid
	P. aeruginosa	Ciprofloxacin, ofloxacin
Intravenous	*S. aureus*	Oxacillin, nafcillin, methicillin
	P. aeruginosa	Gentamicin or tobramycin, Amikacin Ticarcillin Carbenicillin Piperacillin Mazlocillin Timentin Imipenem/cilastatin Aztreonam Timentin (ticarcillin/potassium clavulanate) Piperacillin/tazobactam (Zosyn)

Personal communication, Jane Hodding, Pharm. D., Memorial Miller Children's Hospital, 1995.

therapies. Therapies for the pulmonary system include identification of organisms from sputum cultures and sensitivities. Intravenous antibiotics and monitoring of drug levels, increased frequency of aerosol treatments, and airway clearance therapies are prescribed. Assessment of exercise and activity endurance is completed. A daily program to increase the client's endurance or to prevent its loss during hospitalization is part of the plan of care. The gastrointestinal therapies include nutritional assessment and evaluation of blood chemistries for nutritional deficits, including measurement of hematocrit, hemoglobin, albumin, prealbumin, and vitamins A and E levels. The dietitian assesses the actual and ideal body weight and develops and monitors a plan for a calorically dense diet to provide nutritional and caloric needs. Enzyme use and tolerance are evaluated and adjusted as indicated (Chart 16–29). Identifying new symptoms that may contribute to the diagnosis of complications is an ongoing process. The management of CF with early interventions for new symptoms contributes to improved outcomes. Monitoring the therapies with laboratory tests, pulmonary function tests (PFTs), and radiologic studies and coordinating the team consults are both a part of the medical management of CF. The daily medication lists required to maintain the baseline health include a long list of pharmaceutical agents (Table 16–15).

Another medication has been released specifically for CF. It is an enzyme, DNase, which thins the viscous secretions by acting on the DNA in the sputum. DNA exists in the sputum as a result of the destruction of neutrophils and bacteria, and leads to the production of thick, sticky mucus. Thinner secretions enable better mucociliary action and airway clearance. The medication is administered via nebulizer at a dose of 2.5 mg once or twice a day in conjunction with standard therapies. It has reduced the use of parenteral antibiotics for pulmonary infections by approximately 30% and has improved pulmonary functions in one of the clinical trials (Wilmott & Fiedler, 1994). The medication is currently recommended for children older than 5 years of age. Pulmonary function test values assist in determining those individuals who may benefit from this therapy. An added benefit of this therapy is self-reports from individuals with CF stating it not only improved airway clearance but also improved a sense of well-being. The main side effect is voice alteration. The American Hospital Formulary Service (1995) lists sore throat, chest pain, rash, and conjunctivitis as other side effects that occur with greater frequency with patients receiving DNase than in those receiving placebo. Otherwise the medication has been well tolerated. The health care provider should have knowledge that this medication must be stored properly in the refrigerator. The overall cost-benefit analysis is carefully considered. More long-term studies are needed to direct long-term use and the benefits of this therapy (Fuchs et al., 1994).

All team members provide age-appropriate education about the care of CF to the patients and families as a primary role function. The following discussion outlines team functions and specific interventions from each discipline. All ancillary team members function in collaboration with the primary CF team physician.

Nutritional Support

The registered dietitian assesses physical growth and conducts a nutritional assessment at each admission. Serum laboratory results such as albumin, prealbumin, glucose, electrolytes, and complete blood count (CBC) are assessed. Levels of vitamins A and E are assessed annually, and skinfold measurements are obtained as indicated. Physical growth is plotted on the growth chart to monitor progress and response to therapeutic interventions. The dietitian identifies dietary requirements and goals and initiates an overall plan to meet the high caloric nutritional needs. Guidelines for administration of pancreatic enzymes are provided. Effectiveness of replacement enzymes is also monitored through fecal fat studies. Infants are usually placed on an elemental formula to optimize absorption. Elemental formulas are composed of simple and easily absorbed forms of carbohydrates (glucose polymers or monosaccharides), proteins (amino acids or casein hydrolysates), and fat as medium-chain triglycerides (MCT). The most common elemental formula is Pregestimil (Brady, Rickard, Fitzgerald, & Lemons, 1986). This is a relatively expensive preparation and costs may vary across individual pharmacies. There are special state-funded programs that may provide assistance in obtaining this formula. Infants may receive breast milk or standard infant formula and thrive adequately without gastrointestinal complications as long as enzymes are adjusted appropriately. The older child is managed with a high-calorie, high-protein diet, including snacks and nutritional oral supplements, as indicated, to boost calories and nutrition. Pancreatic enzymes are administered at each feeding, meal, and snack to optimize absorption of the nutrients consumed.

Children with CF tend to have increased duodenal acidity (Kuhn & Horn, 1994), which may counteract the effects of pancreatic enzymes. H_2 blockers are often added to treatment to enhance pancreatic enzyme activity while remaining within the recommended range of ≤ 2500 lipase units/kg/meal (Borowitz et al., 1995; Duffield, 1996). If weight gain and progress toward nutritional goals are not demonstrated, then alternate feeding routes are considered. Gastrostomy tubes, (such as percutaneous endoscopic gastrostomy [PEG] tubes), low-profile gastrostomies such as the Button, or jejunostomy tubes (J-tubes) are possible options. A program of nocturnal drip feedings through the gastrostomy tube is recommended to assist the individual in supplementing oral intake.

Placement of feeding tubes is generally well tolerated using conscious sedation. However, the parent and child must have preparation for the procedure by the CNS/PNP and/or the child life specialist. They must also know that the postprocedure discomfort will be managed so that secretion clearance is not altered. The factors that are considered when recommending gastrostomy tube feedings include the nutritional assessment, the overall health status of the child, adherence to prescribed care, and the timing of the procedure. A child may have this procedure done at the completion of a tune-up so that his or her health status is optimal.

Salt supplementation is recommended for CF patients to prevent dehydration. The infant's formula is supplemented with ⅛ teaspoon of table salt in a 24-hour supply of formula. Older children are generally recommended to eat salty foods and snacks. Salt supplements, which are usually implemented during the warmer months, are also considered with active sports participation. These practices may vary by geographic regions because of climate differences. Adequate fluid consumption is also important.

Respiratory Support

A respiratory care practitioner (RCP) works under the supervision of the physician, as do all team members. The RCP instructs the families on the most effective airway clearance technique that is individualized to the patient. The gold standard for airway clearance consists of postural drainage and percussion (PD&P) done after

Text continued on page 968

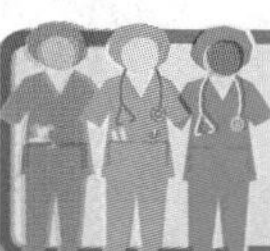

Care Path 16–5 An Interdisciplinary Plan of Care for the Child with Cystic Fibrosis (CF): Pulmonary Exacerbations

Nursing Diagnoses	Day 1: Admission	Day 2	Day 3
Alteration in gas exchange related to decreased airway clearance and sputum production		Child demonstrates improved gas exchange with improved airway clearance measured by: · Increased O_2 saturations · Decreased respiratory rate · Decreased use of accessory muscles	⟶
Alteration in nutrition secondary to decreased appetite and increased metabolic requirements due to work of breathing, infection, and malabsorption		Child demonstrates progress toward nutritional goals evidenced by: · Increased appetite · Increased weight · Tolerance to nocturnal feedings/supplements	⟶
Potential for nonadherence to self-care related to chronic nature of condition and developmental level	Child and family will attain and maintain behaviors consistent with goals of therapy evidenced by: · Willingness to follow treatment plan · Communicating consequences of nonadherence	⟶	⟶
Potential for alteration of effective coping related to initial or repeated hospitalizations	Child/family confirm receipt of information about support group.	Child participates in recreational and therapeutic play/activities.	⟶
Care Intervention Categories			
Consults	CF team and specialists as needed (e.g., endocrine, ENT).	Psychosocial assessment: medical social worker/psychologist, with interventions as appropriate	

Days 4–11	Day 12	Day 13	Discharge
⟶	Child demonstrates continued improvement evidenced by: · Decreased secretions · Increased airway clearance · Improved or back to baseline PFTs · Increased O_2 saturation/baseline · Decreased cough · Increased exercise tolerance	⟶	⟶
⟶	Child continues to demonstrate movement toward nutritional goals	⟶	⟶
⟶	Child will verbalize a plan of self-care skills/behaviors related to CF care.	⟶	⟶
⟶	⟶	⟶	⟶
Consider patient/family care conference.			

Care Path continued on following page

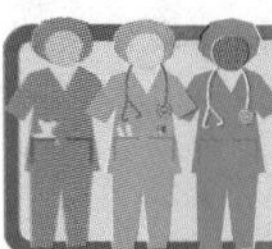

Care Path 16–5 An Interdisciplinary Plan of Care for the Child with Cystic Fibrosis (CF): Pulmonary Exacerbations *Continued*

Care Intervention Categories	Day 1: Admission	Day 2	Day 3
Discharge planning		Resource assessment	Coordinate home care plan.
Labs	CBC with differential Sputum culture and sensitivity labeled for CF Basic biochemical panel to include renal and liver functions and glucose Other laboratory tests p.r.n.: UA, AFB, sputum for fungal cultures, IgE, HbA_{1c}	Assess aminoglycoside therapy. Levels with third to fourth dose; repeat if dose adjusted. Follow up on abnormal laboratory values.	Assess culture results and sensitivities.
Medications and IVs	Determine venous access option: initiate IV, PICC, or access implanted venous access device.	IV care maintenance	⟶
	Standard IV solution for pediatric patients, unless patient has glucose intolerance. Normal saline or heparin lock may be used.	⟶	⟶
	Pulmonary medications/aerosolized/antibiotics/DNase	⟶	⟶
	Pancreatic enzymes	⟶	⟶
	Vitamins	⟶	⟶
	H_2 blockers	⟶	⟶
	Prokinetic agents	⟶	⟶
	Antibiotics	⟶	⟶
	NSAIDs/analgesics	⟶	⟶

Days 4–11	Day 12	Day 13	Discharge
Identify home care needs and initiate referrals: · Nutritional/enteral supplements · Respiratory durable medical equipment for airway clearance, O_2; etc. · Home IV antibiotics and labs Track progress of education for new home care skills. Consider home health referral.	Verify discharge plan.	Obtain prescriptions for discharge needs.	Confirm understanding of discharge: · Follow-up plan/medical appointment · Return to school/work
Prealbumin p.r.n. Consider work-up for allergic bronchopulmonary aspergillosis (ABPA).			
→ → → → → → → → →	→ → → → → → → → →	→ → → → → → → → →	→ → → → → → → → →

Care Path continued on following page

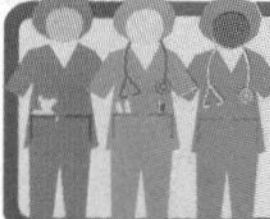

Care Path 16–5 An Interdisciplinary Plan of Care for the Child with Cystic Fibrosis (CF): Pulmonary Exacerbations *Continued*

Care Intervention Categories	Day 1: Admission	Day 2	Day 3
Monitors	Spot pulse oximetry for O_2 saturations ≥92% Continuous pulse oximetry for O_2 saturations ≤92%	⟶ ⟶	⟶ ⟶
Nutrition	Regular diet (high calories) Snacks t.i.d. Night supplemental feeds for 10–12 hours as indicated Monitor stool pattern. Calorie count p.r.n.	⟶ ⟶ ⟶ ⟶ ⟶	⟶ ⟶ ⟶ ⟶ ⟶
Pain management	Assess comfort level Assess for pain using age-appropriate systematic method and intervene p.r.n.	⟶ Assess response to pain interventions.	⟶ ⟶
Play therapy/school/activity	Initiate therapeutic play/recreational activities as appropriate. Incorporate schoolwork into daily schedule Ad lib activities of daily living (ADLs)	Activities as appropriate	Consult child life specialist to prepare for procedures p.r.n. Physical therapist (PT) to assess exercise tolerance
Procedures/diagnostics	Chest x-ray posteroanterior and lateral views Spirometry PFTs for ≥5 years ABG as indicated		

Days 4–11	Day 12	Day 13	Discharge
→ →	→ →	→ →	→ →
→ → →	→ → →	→ → →	→ → →
→ Nutrition follow-up Assess need for home enteral program and placement of gastrostomy tube (GI)	→	→	→
→ →	→ →	→ →	→ →
Activities as appropriate Daily exercise program with PT	→	→	→
Consider work-up for cor pulmonale, ECG, O_2 desaturation study, or other tests as indicated by clinical status.			

Care Path continued on following page

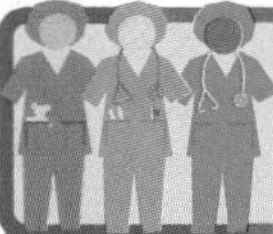

Care Path 16–5 An Interdisciplinary Plan of Care for the Child with Cystic Fibrosis (CF): Pulmonary Exacerbations *Continued*

Care Intervention Categories	Day 1: Admission	Day 2	Day 3
Special considerations	Infection control measures for multiple resistant organisms Assess need for implanted venous access device.	Diversional activities for child on barrier precautions	
Teaching	Assess self-care behaviors and provide age-appropriate education.	Assess changes from baseline and provide education p.r.n. Assess/instruct airway clearance techniques.	Assess/instruct in nutritional care.
Treatment and interventions	PD&P and airway clearance techniques (ACTs) while awake O_2 as indicated	⟶ ⟶	⟶ ⟶
Vital signs/baseline parameters	Admittance weight; height; and head circumference (≤3 yr) Vital signs every 4 hours Respiratory assessment	Weight every morning ⟶	⟶ Vital signs every 4 hours while awake if stable

ABG, arterial glood gases; AFB, acid-fast bacilli; CBC, complete blood count; ECG, electrocardiogram; GI, gastrointestinal; HbA_{1c}, hemoglobin A_{1c}; IgE, immunoglobulin E; NSAID, nonsteroidal anti-inflammatory drug; PD&P, postural drainage and percussion; PFT, pulmonary function test; PICC, peripherally inserted central catheter; p.r.n., as needed; UA, urinalysis.

aerosolized treatments BID to QID (see Chart 16–8). More recently, alternate airway clearance techniques (ACTs) have been found to be effective when individualized to patient response. Most of these techniques require that a patient can follow instructions and be cooperative. These newer techniques have been readily accepted by families, patients, and the CF team because they allow for greater independence. There are many factors to assess for appropriate matching of the ACT to the patient, including history of adherence, age, effectiveness measured by PFTs, motivation, and cost (Hardy, 1994) (see Table 16–5).

Nursing Interventions

The role of the clinical nurse is primarily to provide direct care. This role is central to the hospitalized child because the nurse is the person most consistently at the bedside. Coordinating care and monitoring the overall response to therapies (i.e., breathing treatments, self-care participation, activity level, elimination pattern, and appetite) are essential information to determine progression toward clinical outcomes. The clinical nurse also initiates and maintains intravenous lines for antibiotic therapy and other intravenous medications as needed. Measure-

Days 4–11	Day 12	Day 13	Discharge
Assess/instruct in adherence to treatments/medications. Symptom management Promote age-appropriate CF self-care.	Assess/instruct in exercise program. Home care and follow-up plan		
→ →	→ →	→ →	→ →
→ →	→ →	→ →	→ →

ment of accurate height and weight on admission is essential, along with daily weight measurement to monitor nutritional progress. Additionally, the nurse is able to provide feedback from observations of the interactions between the child, parent, and caregiver and their responses to each other.

The CF team nurse, usually an advanced practice nurse, assists in coordinating the overall care, ensuring that all team members have provided consultation during hospitalization. Assessing for the need for team and family conferences and education regarding treatment, medicines, options related to venous access, and alternate routes for nutritional supplementation are also important functions of the CF team nurse. Assessment for home intravenous antibiotic therapy and discharge readiness are also conducted by the CF team nurse. In many CF centers, it is the CF team nurse who performs the follow-up telephone calls to the caregivers and to the schools, when indicated. In addition, the CF team nurse participates in the continuum of care by providing care at office or clinic visits. This puts the nurse in a unique position to follow up the child and provide interventions from an ambulatory and an inpatient perspective. The nurse, in some centers, may be able to perform school visits and assist with school reintegration, if indicated. Early identification and preparation for procedures, including preparation for changes in level of care, are also central to the CF team nurse's role. An additional role function is the education and coordination of team involvement when a new diagnosis is made.

In the past, when an infant or child was newly diagnosed, he or she was admitted to the hospital. The hospital admission was justified for a "tune-up" and also used for comprehensive education of home care management of CF from the interdisciplinary team. In the managed care environment of today's practice, hospitalization is not justified for education for a new diagnosis, unless the infant or child is acutely ill. The CF team nurse often functions as the overall coordinator of the CF center to ensure smooth functioning of the center, understanding of role functions within the team, and coordination of the clinical care.

Social Service

The clinical social worker assists the caregivers and the children with coping and integrating CF into their life. The families are helped to obtain linkage with the appropriate state and federal programs for medical care, such as Children's Medical Services, state Medicaid, Aid to Families with Dependent Children (AFDC), and Supplemental Security Income for the Aged, Blind and Disabled (SSI). The social worker also is a source of emotional support and provides appropriate referrals as needed. The social worker acknowledges that each family is unique, with individual needs and stresses. Many social workers facilitate support groups and provide parent-to-parent networking.

Physical Therapy

The physical therapist evaluates the muscles used for breathing, posture, and the child's ability to carry out daily activities. The physical therapist also prescribes individualized exercise programs and monitors endurance. The roles of the physical therapist and respiratory care practitioner may overlap in certain regions of the country. The child with CF is assessed on a regular basis and provided a home exercise program.

Child Life Services

The child life specialist's focus of practice is on therapeutic play along with recreational and diversional activities. They assist the child in coping with hospitalization, medical visits, and procedures through play. The child life specialist can provide input into developmentally based motivational and behavioral programs to encourage the children to do their treatments, drink their nutritional supplements, cooperate with therapy, and take medicines. Child Life Departments usually have scheduled tours to prepare children for hospitalization or procedures prior to the event. This is particularly helpful for children being admitted for the first time or when a child has progressed to the next developmental level between hospitalizations. Some Child Life Departments may offer school programs or assist with arrangements for homebound teachers.

New Treatment Approaches

The approach to treatment of CF today is one with greater optimism. Promising new therapies and interventions, such as medications (i.e., antibiotics and enzymes for pancreatic replacement and for thinning secretions [DNase]), transplantation, and identification of the basic genetic defect, have provided hope for improved quality of care and longer life. Lung transplantation is now an established treatment option for CF.

It is beyond the scope of this section to discuss in detail the many issues of lung transplantation, such as surgical technique, indications, and complications. Kotloff and Zuckerman (1996) present a comprehensive discussion of CF and its special considerations for transplantation for further reading. Heart-lung transplantation (HLT) was the first type of transplant done in 1984 in a CF patient (Kotloff & Zuckerman, 1996). Since these initial attempts, transplantation techniques have undergone numerous modifications to improve outcomes. Now, the procedure of choice is the bilateral sequential lung transplantation (BSLT). As of 1996, more than 150 CF patients worldwide have undergone HLT and more than 500 have undergone double BSLT. Because of the limited and suitable organ supply for lung transplant use, and because CF patients waiting for transplant have such a high mortality rate, living donor bilateral lobar transplantation is also an option. This procedure involves the donation of a lobe from a compatible living related donor. The actuarial survival rate from data compiled from major worldwide CF transplant centers is, collectively, approximately a 70% survival rate at 1 year post transplant (Kotloff & Zuckerman, 1996). Complete normalization of pulmonary function values usually occurs approximately 6 months after transplant. Unfortunately, the complication of bronchiolitis obliterans occurs in up to 40% to 50% of long-term survivors.

There continue to exist many difficult issues surrounding lung transplantation. One is the initiation of the referral for transplantation. CF centers approach this issue by describing a "window of opportunity" for transplant referral. Because of the waiting period between listing the patient as a transplant candidate and the actual transplant, the patient and family must understand that there may be up to a 2-year wait. The patient must be ill enough to qualify as a transplant candidate yet well enough to endure and survive the surgery. The patient and family are usually given information about the transplant, with the understanding that the procedure does not treat all of the affected organ systems. The CF patient's lungs are free of CF after the transplant. The patient may have other affected organ systems from CF that will continue to necessitate treatment. The family and patient are also approached to help them understand that transplantation is not a cure for CF. It is a treatment option, exchanging one medical problem for another. With increased experience in CF lung transplantation, more data will contribute to the increasing knowledge toward better outcomes and quality-of-life issues for individuals with CF.

Much of the current research surrounding CF involves the pulmonary system because it is the severity of lung disease that determines the quality and length of life. Immunotherapy is directed toward reducing the lung inflammation from the organisms that colonize the lungs and cause repeated infections. When taken consistently, ibuprofen, a nonsteroidal anti-inflammatory drug (NSAID), has been found to retard the progression of CF lung disease in patients with mild disease (Konstan, Byard, Hoppel, & Davis, 1995). The study was aimed at individuals between 5 and 39 years with a FEV of <60%. However, the study had the most pronounced effect in those 13 years old and younger. The dosing is 20 to 30 mg/kg twice a day, with monitoring of blood levels to achieve a level between 50 and 100 μg/mL, which ensures the antineutrophil effects. The side effects reported of gastrointestinal complaints were infrequent. One of 85 patients reported exacerbation of conjunctivitis, and one reported exacerbation of epistaxis.

Prednisone has been studied extensively with application to CF individuals. A multicenter trial study in 1986 compared two dosing schedules and a placebo (Thompson, Smits, & Fick, 1992). The study was discontinued when an increase in cataracts, growth retardation, and glucose intolerance in the high-dose group was observed.

Gene therapy, defined as the introduction of genetic material into cells for therapeutic purposes (Rosenfeld & Collins, 1996; Shalon & Adelson, 1996), is another therapy currently receiving much attention and research worldwide. The normal gene is attached to a virus and administered by way of aerosol to replace the abnormal CF gene. Research in this area is progressive and is building excitement for a "cure" for CF. There are many questions and concerns surrounding this mode of therapy. For example, one important question involves identification of target cells in the lungs for directing this therapy; another concern is about the duration of the therapeutic effects and frequency of administration. Gene therapy is still in an infancy stage, yet it does hold future promise to further the quality of life and decrease the mortality and morbidity from complications of CF. This is a most challenging and stimulating time in the history of CF. The scientific breakthroughs have created more realism about transforming dreams into realities for the patients and families as well as for those who deliver their care.

Education regarding self-care and integrating the CF care into daily schedules is necessary to assist the family fostering independence and age-appropriate skills of daily living. All too often the health care team may be so focused on the disease process that there may be lags in educating families to integrate developmentally appropriate strategies as a part of the care. For example, instruction on time management skills for a first-time parent may be helpful (Sawyer, 1992). Each developmental stage merits review with the family and the patient, when age appropriate, to facilitate strategies that will allow this specialized care to be provided daily. Parents and caregivers need to have guidance about home care strategies based on developmental frameworks. They must understand concepts such as offering the toddler a choice of juice to take with medicines; thus, there is no unacceptable choice and the toddler maintains the "control" for mastery of that stage (Chart 16–30).

Parents, caregivers, and patients must also be kept informed regarding changes in condition and updates on the expanding and newer therapies. They must be educated when new therapies are introduced for maintenance care, such as oxygen, enteral home nutrition programs, home intravenous antibiotic administration, home maintenance of venous access devices, administration of aerosolized antibiotics, or the use of DNase.

Community Care

The CF team members work in concert with each other, the families, and the children to support a common goal. Because of the complexities and variations of CF, many of the team's functions overlap or may be carried out differently across different centers. For example, referrals for transplantation and issues on making the transition to adult care may be coordinated by the clinical social worker or the CF team nurse. Supporting a family through the decision-making process of end-stage care is generally a shared process by all team members but may be the primary responsibility of the clinical social worker. It is also critical for the CF team members to acknowledge the support systems of the family and consult other professionals, such as pastoral care services or psychologists.

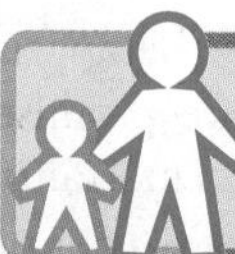

Chart 16–30
Developmental Considerations

Self-Care Strategies for the Child with Cystic Fibrosis

Nursing Strategies for Self-Care Skills					
Infant (0–12 mo)	**Toddler (1–3 yr)**	**Preschool (3–5 yr)**	**Childhood (6–12 yr)**	**Adolescence (12–18 yr)**	**Adolescence (continued)**
Institute measures to promote age-appropriate behaviors Provide information of "self-care skills": • Discuss age-appropriate behaviors • Response to crying promptly (0–3 mo) • Response to cues as indicated (>3 mo) • Establishment of regular routines • Incorporation of special care into routines • Provide reinforcement about PD&P and comfort r/t "sensorimotor stimulation" Monitor all developmental progress Provide recommendations for home schedule/time management Provide health care teaching: • Disease management • Normal acquisition of developmental skills, especially for first-time, new parent	Discuss normal developmental behaviors Assess and monitor feeding behaviors: provide information regarding age-appropriate behavioral management Provide information for self-care skills: • Incorporate distraction techniques for resistant behaviors • Use games to gain cooperation • Allow for simple choices that are all acceptable • Encourage sharing of care between primary caregivers at home • Assist with scheduling therapies into rituals • Provide opportunities for therapeutic play • Offer medications in a medicine cup • Allow to help gather supplies "Blowing" activities, such as bubbles, horns, pinwheels Provide information on disease management	Institute measures to promote age-appropriate behaviors Discuss normal developmental behaviors Support choices for beginning of "day-care"/out-of-home care: • Discuss home care and small daycare program advantages • Discuss information needed for alternate caregiver Provide information for self-care skills: • Assistance with pill swallowing • Allow choices with food/snack selection • Begin PEP therapy (~4 yr) • Coughing secretions "up" and in tissue • Provide information to identify basic symptoms indicating need for health care team/doctor visit Support for exercise as part of ADLs: • Running • Tricycle • "Blowing" activities Provide information on disease management	Institute measures to promote age-appropriate behaviors Assess understanding of the following: • Medications • Nutrition/snacks • Respiratory treatments Provide information for self-care skills: • Give responsibilities for simple tasks regarding therapies: • Set up nebulizer • Prepare medications • Clean nebulizer • Remind to initiate ACT time • Have child answer health team's questions • Include in decision-making Incorporate exercise as part of ADLs: • Group or solo sports • Encourage use of wind instruments (horns) • Coach during PEP/ACT therapy by caregiver Discuss school performance/attendance and ways to ensure self-care at school Provide information on disease management	Institute measures to promote age-appropriate behaviors Discuss/assess/monitor normal developmental concerns/issues Provide information to facilitate increased self-care skills: • Self-administration of medications, aerosol treatments, snack/meals, ACT • Take inventory of medications • Arrange for refills for medications • Schedule clinic appointments • Set up nocturnal/daily O_2 with checking flow rate Assess and monitor the following: • Understanding of disease process • Medication • Problem-solving skills • Current self-care behaviors Provide information on disease management	Encourage and facilitate the following with individual and caregiver: • Monitoring of self-care by caregiver from afar • Decision for when parental presence is desired at clinic • Involvement in decision-making • Negotiation of schedule with special events Support exercise as part of ADLs: • Aerobic and anaerobic • Upper body strengthening • Stretching • Energy conservation techniques Provide information on education and career planning Facilitate discussion on peer relationships/dating Discuss transitioning plans and process Initiate referrals to support choices: • Genetic counseling • Sexuality issues Provide information on insurance and health care systems

ACT, airway clearance time; ADLs, activities of daily living; PD&P, postural drainage and percussion; PEP, positive expiratory pressure.
Developed by Linda Tirabassi Davidson. Used with permission of Long Beach Memorial Medical Center, Long Beach, CA.

Summary of Key Concepts

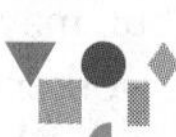

- Certain anatomic and structural features of the respiratory tract in infants and young children predispose them to develop respiratory distress more readily than older children or adults.
- Respiratory illnesses are the most common reason for pediatric hospital admissions and ambulatory center visits, especially during winter and early spring.

- Viral and bacterial infections of the respiratory system are common and relatively unavoidable in childhood.
- Children with chronic conditions, especially those involving the respiratory or cardiac systems, are at highest risk for serious morbidity or mortality associated with common childhood respiratory infections.
- Worsening respiratory distress can be identified by frequent and thorough respiratory assessments. The ideal respiratory care in pediatric patients involves recognizing signs and symptoms of respiratory distress and instituting appropriate interventions before respiratory failure develops.
- In childhood respiratory conditions, parents must be educated on how to recognize signs and symptoms of respiratory compromise and to notify their health care provider immediately. They must be taught when and how to access emergency medical personnel if needed.
- Many pediatric respiratory conditions, especially those of a chronic nature, are best managed by regular follow-up visits with health care providers and by taking proactive and/or preventive measures.

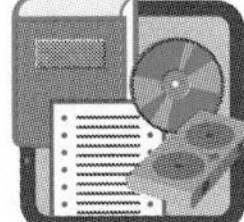

Resources

Organizations

American Association for Respiratory Care (AARC)
11030 Ables Lane
Dallas, TX 75229-2750

American Cleft Palate-Craniofacial Association
1218 Grandview Avenue
Pittsburgh, PA 15211
(800) 24-cleft
(412) 481-1376

American Lung Association
1740 Broadway
New York, NY 10019-4374
(contact your local chapter listed in the phone book)

Asthma and Allergy Foundation of America (AAFA)
1125 Fifteenth Street, NW, Suite 502
Washington, DC 20005
(800) 7-ASTHMA or
(202) 466-7643

Cystic Fibrosis Foundation
6931 Arlington Road
Bethesda, MD 20814
(301) 951-4422 or (800) FIGHT CF

International Cystic Fibrosis Association
3567 East 49th Street
Cleveland, OH 44105

National Allergy & Asthma Network/Mothers of Asthmatics
3554 Chain Bridge Road, Suite 200
Fairfax, VA 22030
(800) 878-4403

National Asthma Education Program
NHLBI Information Center
P.O. Box 30105
Bethesda, MD 20824-0105
(301) 951-3260

National Foundation for Asthma, Inc.
P.O. Box 50304
Tucson, AZ 85703
(602) 624-7481

National Heart, Lung and Blood Institute
National Institutes of Health
9000 Rockville Pike
Building 31, Room 4A21
Bethesda, MD 20892
(301) 496-4236

National Jewish Center for Immunology & Respiratory Medicine
1400 Jackson Street
Denver, CO 80206
(800) 222-5846

Respiratory Nursing Society
5700 Old Orchard Road, First Floor
Skokie, IL 60077
(708) 966-8673

Books and Printed Materials

Asthma management in minority children: Practical insights for clinicians, researchers and public health planners.
Available from National Heart, Lung and Blood Institute.

✏ CF Family Education Project at Baylor College of Medicine and Texas Children's Hospital. (1995). *Cystic Fibrosis Family Education Program*. Genentech, Inc., 460 Point San Bruno Blvd. South San Francisco, CA 94080-4990.

✏ Resources specifically for children.

This is a developmentally based program (from early an childhood level through adolescents) with 4 topics about living with CF: Respiratory, Nutrition and malabsorption, Communication and Coping. There is a companion workbook for the parent to assist the child. The books are intended to facilitate developmentally appropriate self-care behaviors. There is also a booklet in this program series for the newly diagnosed patient and family. This booklet is directed to parents of children under three years of age.

✏ Croal, D. A. (1994). *CF and your tomorrow: A guide to surviving and thriving with cystic fibrosis*. Solvay Pharmaceuticals, 901 Sawyer Road, Marietta, GA 30062.
This presents a comprehensive and sensitive discussion, authored by an adult with CF. It is directed for an adolescent or young adult.

✏ Cunningham, J. C., and Taussig, L. M. (1989). *A guide to cystic fibrosis for parents and children*. McNeil Pharmaceuticals.
This book provides basic information on CF is a easy to read format. It is also available in Spanish. There is a companion video available in English only.

✏ Greibel, K. W. (1987). *This is Paul*. McNeil Pharmaceutical. McNEILab, Inc., Springhouse, PA 19477.
This booklet is written for the child 5 years of age or older.

✏ Mondolfo, A. (1988). *Cystic fibrosis*. Reid-Rowell Pharmaceuticals, Marietta, GA.
This booklet is written for children between 6 to 12 years of age.

✏ Mulligan, C., & Simpson, V. S. (1985). *Asthma and you*. Glaxo Pharmaceuticals, Research Triangle, Park, NC, and St. Joseph's Hospital and Medical Center, Phoenix, AZ.
This is a coloring booklet for children 7 years of age and older.

✏ Orenstein, D. M. (1997). *Cystic fibrosis: a guide for patient and family*. Philadelphia: Lippincott-Raven.
This is a comprehensive book covering the many aspects of CF.

Plaut, T. F. (1988). *Children with asthma: A manual for parents* (2nd ed.). Pedipress, Inc.
This is a comprehensive book written for parents, discussing all components of asthma care.

✏ Plaut, T. F. (1992). *One-minute asthma*. Pedipress, Inc.
This is a booklet written for parents of children, or adults, who have asthma.

✏ Publications from the Cystic Fibrosis Foundation:

Cystic fibrosis and exercise: a beginners guide
A teacher's guide to cystic fibrosis
The genetics of cystic fibrosis
Living with cystic fibrosis: A guide for adolescents

Ryan, L. (1996). *Cystic fibrosis: A handbook for teachers*. Solvay Pharmaceuticals, 901 Sawyer Road, Marietta, GA 30062.

✏ Sander, N. (1993). *So you have asthma, too*. Allen & Hanbury's Respiratory Institute, A division of Glaxo, Inc., Research Triangle Park, NC.
This is a booklet written for children 5 and older that discusses asthma. It is also available in Spanish. It has a companion video, as well.

✏ Sander, N. (1994). *I'm a meter reader*. Allen & Hanbury's Respiratory Institute, A division of Glaxo, Inc., Research Triangle Part, NC.
This booklet is written for children 5 and older who are using a peak flow meter to monitor their asthma. IT is also available in Spanish, and has a companion video.

Sindel, S., & Hartman, L. (1989). *A way of life: cystic fibrosis nutrition handbook and cookbook*. University of Wisconsin Hospital and Clinics, Madison, WI 53792.
This is a recipe book as well as a book on nutrition as it relates to CF.

✏ Stanzione, A., & Goodwin, S. L. *Let's look at me*. Marietta, GA: Reid-Rowell.
This is a workbook for ages 6 years through 12 years and has a facilitator's guide for directing the child.

Young, A. (1994). *Cystic fibrosis in the classroom*. Scandipharm.
This booklet is written for teachers and provides information about supportive strategies in the classroom.

Audiovisuals

Managing Childhood Asthma (1994)
Medcom, Inc.
Garden Grove, CA
A video for parents on childhood asthma.

✏ *Winning Against Asthma* (1994)
Medcom, Inc.
Garden Grove, CA
A video on asthma for children 7 and older.

References

Abham, S. H., & Groothius, J. R. (1994). Pathophysiology and treatment of bronchopulmonary dysplasia. *Pediatric Clinics of North America, 41*, 277–315.

Abman, S. H., Ogle, J. W., Butler-Simon, N., Rumack, C. M., & Accurso, F. J. (1988). Role of respiratory syncytial virus in early hospitalizations for respiratory distress of young infants with cystic fibrosis. *Journal of Pediatrics, 113*, 826–830.

Abman, S. H., Wolfe, R. R., Accurso, F. J., Koops, B. L., Bowman, C. M., & Wiggins, J. W., Jr. (1985). Pulmonary vascular response to oxygen in infants with severe bronchopulmonary dysplasia. *Pediatrics, 75*, 80–84.

Ackerman, V. L. (1994). Bronchopulmonary dysplasia. In G. M. Loughlin & H. Eigen (Eds.), *Respiratory diseases in children: Diagnosis and management* (pp. 383–392). Baltimore: Williams & Wilkins.

Adams, W. G., Deaver, K. A., Cochi, S. L., Phikaytis, B. D., Zell, E. R., Broome, C. V., & Wegner, J. D. (1993). Decline in childhood Haemophilus influenzae type b (HIB) disease in the Hib vaccine era. *Journal of the American Medical Association, 209*, 221–226.

Ahmann, E. (1992). Family impact of home apnea monitoring: An overview of research and its clinical implications. *Pediatric Nursing, 18*, 611–616.

Aitken, M., & Fiel, S. B. (1993). Cystic fibrosis. *Disease-a-Month, 39*(1), 1–52.

American Academy of Pediatrics, Committee on Infectious Diseases. (1984). Revision of recommendations for use of rifampin prophylaxis of contacts of patients with Haemophilus influenzae infection. *Pediatrics, 74*, 301.

American Academy of Pediatrics, Committee on Infectious Diseases. (1993). Use of ribavirin in the treatment of respiratory syncytial virus infection. *Pediatrics, 92*, 501–504.

American Hospital Formulary Service. (1995). *Drug information* (pp. 1836–1838). Bethesda, MD: American Society of Health Systems Pharmacists.

Arnold, J. (1996). Upper respiratory tract. In R. Behrman, R. Kliegman, & A. Arvin (Eds.), *Nelson textbook of pediatrics* (pp. 1185–1195). Philadelphia: W. B. Saunders.

Barrington, K. J., & Finer, N. N. (1990). Periodic breathing and apnea in preterm infants. *Pediatric Research, 27*(2), 118–121.

Bechler-Karsch, A. (1994). Assessment and management of status asthmaticus. *Pediatric Nursing, 20*, 217–223.

Birkhead, G., Attaway, N. J., Strunk, R. C., Townsend, M. C., & Teutsch, S. (1989). Investigation of a cluster of deaths of adolescents from asthma: Evidence implicating inadequate treatment and poor patient adherence with medications. *Journal of Allergy and Clinical Immunology, 84*(4), 484–491.

Blazer, S., Naveh, Y., & Friedman, A. (1980). Foreign body in the airway: A review of 200 cases. *American Journal of Diseases in Children, 134*, 68–71.

Borowitz, D. S., Grand, R. J., Durie, P. R., & the Consensus Committee. (1995). Use of pancreatic enzyme supplements for patients with cystic fibrosis in the context of fibrosing colonopathy. *Journal of Pediatrics, 127*, 681–684.

Bourchier, D., Dawson, K. P., & Fergusson, D. M. (1984). Humidification in viral croup: A controlled trial. *Australian Pediatric Journal, 20*(4), 289–291.

Brady, M. S., Rickard, K. A., Fitzgerald, J. F., & Lemons, J. A. (1986). Specialized formulas and feedings for infants with malabsorption or formula intolerance. *Journal of the American Dietetic Association, 86*, 191–200.

Browning, I. B., D'Alonzo, G. E., & Tobin, M. J. (1990). Importance of respiratory rate as an indicator of respiratory dysfunction in patients with cystic fibrosis. *Chest, 97*, 1317–1321.

Burrows, B., & Taussig, L. M. (1980). As the twig is bent, the tree inclines (perhaps). *American Review of Respiratory Diseases, 122*, 813.

Carroll, J. L., Marcus, C. L., & Loughlin, G. M. (1993). Disordered control of breathing in infants and children. *Pediatrics in Review, 14*(2), 51–66.

Centers for Disease Control and Prevention. (1996). Asthma mortality and hospitalization among children and young adults—United States, 1980–1993. *Morbidity and Mortality Weekly, 45*, 350–353.

Clark, N. M., Feldman, C. H., Evans, D., Millman, E. J., Wailewski, Y., & Valle, I. (1981). The effectiveness of education for family management of asthma in children: A preliminary report. *Health Education Quarterly*, 8, 166–174.

Cloutier, M. M. (1994). History and physical examination. In D. V. Schidlow & D. S. Smith (Eds.), *A practical guide to pediatric respiratory diseases* (pp. 1–8). Philadelphia: Hanley-Belfus.

Corbett, A. (1990). Respiratory disorders of the newborn. In V. Chernick (Ed.), *Disorders of the respiratory tract in children* (pp. 265–296). Philadelphia: W. B. Saunders.

Cornell, S. (1997). Allergic rhinitis in children. *Advances for Nurse Practitioners, 5*(2), 30–34.

Cressman, W. R., & Myer, C. M. (1994). Diagnosis and management of croup and epiglottitis. *Pediatric Clinics of North America, 41*, 265–276.

Cystic Fibrosis Foundation Consensus Conference. (1990). The consensus conference on CF-related diabetes mellitus. *Consensus Conferences: Concepts in Care, 1*, Section IV, January 11–12.

Cystic Fibrosis Registry. (1996, August). *Cystic fibrosis foundation patient registry annual data report 1995*. Bethesda, MD.

Daigle, K. L., & Cloutier, M. M. (1994). Bronchitis. In G. M. Loughlin & J. Eigen (Eds.), *Respiratory disease in children* (pp. 301–305). Baltimore: Williams & Wilkins.

Deaves, D. M. (1993). An assessment of the value of health education in the prevention of childhood asthma. *Journal of Advanced Nursing, 18*, 354–363.

Dettenmeier, P. A. (1992). *Pulmonary nursing care*. St. Louis: Mosby–Year Book.

DeWitt, P. K., Jansen, M. T., Ward, S. L., & Keens, T. G. (1993). Obstacles to discharge of ventilator-assisted children from the hospital to home. *Chest, 103*(5), 1560–1565.

Doyle, P. (1996). Bronchopulmonary dysplasia and corticosteroid therapy: A case review. *Neonatal Network, 15*(6), 35–39.

Duffield, R. (1996). Cystic fibrosis and the gastrointestinal tract. *Journal of Pediatric Health Care, 10*(2), 51–62.

Evans, D., Clark, N. M., Feldman, C. H., Rips, J., Kaplan, D., Levison, M. J., Wailewski, Y., Levin, B., & Mellins, R. (1987). A school health education program for children with asthma aged 8–11 years. *Health Education Quarterly, 14*, 267–279.

Feldman, W. E. (1993). Pharyngitis in children. *Post Graduate Medicine, 93*(3), 141–144.

Ferrante, S., & Painter, E. (1995). Continuous nebulization: A treatment modality for pediatric asthma patients. *Pediatric Nursing, 21*, 327–331.

First RSV prevention drug. Advance for nurse practitioners. (1996). *Drug News, 4*(5), 61.

Fitton, C. M. (1994). Nursing management of the child with a tracheostomy. *Pediatric Clinics of North America, 41*, 513–524.

FitzSimmons, S. C. (1993). The changing epidemiology of cystic fibrosis. *Journal of Pediatrics, 122*, 1–9.

Frank, L., & Sosenko, I. R. (1988). Undernutrition as a major contributing factor in the pathogenesis of bronchopulmonary dysplasia. *American Review of Respiratory Diseases, 138*, 725–729.

Fuchs, H. J., Borowitz, D. S., Christiansen, D. H., Morris, E. M., Nash, M. L., Ramsey, B. W., Rosenstein, B. J., Smith, A. L., & Wohl, M. E., for the Pulmozyme Study Group. (1994). Effect of aerosolized recombinant human DNase on exacerbations of respiratory symptoms and on pulmonary function in patients with cystic fibrosis. *New England Journal of Medicine, 331*, 637–642.

Gaultier, C. (1994). Maturation of respiratory control. In G. M. Loughlin & H. Eigen (Eds.), *Respiratory disease in children* (p. 14). Baltimore: Williams & Wilkins.

Gibson, C. (1988). Perspective in parental coping with a chronically ill child: The case of cystic fibrosis. *Issues in Comprehensive Pediatric Nursing, 11*, 33–41.

Glotzbach, S. F., Baldwin, R. B., Lederer, N. E., Tansey, P. A., & Ariagno, R. L. (1989). Periodic breathing in preterm infants: Incidence and characteristics. *American Journal of Diseases in Childhood, 144*, 785–792.

Goodman, G., Perkin, R. M., Anas, N. G., Sperling, D. R., Hicks, D. A., & Rowen, M. (1988). Pulmonary hypertension in infants with bronchopulmonary dysplasia. *Journal of Pediatrics, 112*, 67–72.

Grad, R., & Taussig, L. (1990). Acute infections producing upper airway obstruction. In V. Chernick (Ed.), *Disorders of the respiratory tract in children* (pp. 336–348). Philadelphia: W. B. Saunders.

Griscom, N. T., Wheeler, W. B., & Sweezey, N. B. (1989). Bronchopulmonary dysplasia: Radiographic appearances in middle childhood. *Radiology, 171*, 811–814.

Guyton, A. C. (1981). *Textbook of medical physiology*. Philadelphia: W. B. Saunders.

Hanania, N. A., Wittman, R., Kesten, S., & Chapman, K. R. (1994). Medical personnel's knowledge of and ability to use inhaling devices. *Chest, 105*, 111–116.

Hanna, D. (1995). Guidelines for pulse oximetry use in pediatrics. *Journal of Pediatric Nursing, 10*, 124–126.

Hardy, K. A. (1994). A review of airway clearance techniques: New techniques, indications, recommendations. *Respiratory Care, 39*, 440–454.

Hazinski, M. F. (Ed.). (1996). *Nursing care of the critically ill child*. St. Louis: Mosby–Year Book.

Henry, R. (1983). Moist air in the treatment of laryngotracheitis. *Archives of Diseases in Childhood, 58*(8), 577.

Hoekelman, R. A. (1994). Epiglottitis: Another dying disease? *Pediatric Annals, 23*(5), 229–230.

Horwood, L. J., Fergusson, D. M., & Shannon, F. T. (1985). Social and familial factors in the development of early childhood asthma. *Pediatrics, 75*(5), 859–868.

Hudak, B. B., Allen, M. C., & Hudak, M. L. (1989). Home oxygen therapy for chronic lung disease in extremely low birth weight infants. *American Journal of Diseases in Childhood, 143*, 357–360.

Institute of Medicine, Committee to Study the Prevention of Low Birth Weight. (1985). *Preventing low birth weight.* Washington, DC: National Academy Press.

Keens, T. G., Sargent, C. W., Denies, P. C., Bookout, S. M., Gates, E. P., & Platzker, A. G. (1982). Pneumograms do not predict subsequent apnea in near-miss sudden infant death syndrome infants [Abstract]. *American Review of Respiratory Diseases, 125*, 192.

Kelly, D. H., Shannon, D. C., & O'Connell, K. (1978). Care of infants with near-miss sudden infant death syndrome. *Pediatrics, 61*, 571–514.

Knudtson, M. D. (1994). Differential diagnosis of pharyngitis in children. *Journal of Pediatric Health Care, 8*(1), 33–35.

Konstan, M. W., Byard, P. J., Hoppel, C. L., & Davis, P. B. (1995). Effect of high-dose ibuprofen in patients with cystic fibrosis. *New England Journal of Medicine, 332*, 848–854.

Kotloff, R. M., & Zuckerman, J. B. (1996). Lung transplantation for cystic fibrosis. *Chest, 109*, 787–798.

Kuhn, R. J., & Horn, L. (1994). Pancreatic enzyme therapy in patients with cystic fibrosis: The high dose lipase issue. *Pediatric Nursing, 20*, 623–624.

Kurzner, S. I., Garg, M., Bautista, D. B., Bader, D., Merritt, R. J., Warburton, D., & Keens, T. J. (1988). Growth failure in infants with bronchopulmonary dysplasia: Nutrition and elevated resting metabolic expenditure. *Pediatrics, 81*, 379–384.

Kuster, P. A. (1996). Reducing risk of house dust mite and cockroach allergen exposure in inner-city children with asthma. *Pediatric Nursing, 22*(4), 297–303.

Ladebauche, P. (1997). Managing asthma: A growth and development approach. *Pediatric Nursing 23*(1), 37–44.

Lanier, B. (1989). Who is dying of asthma and why. *Journal of Pediatrics, 115*, 838–840.

Lask, B. (1992). The need for psychosocial interventions: How to convince the skeptic [Summary]. *Pediatric Pulmonology*, 8, 232–234.

Lemons, P. M., & Weaver, D. D. (1986). Beyond the birth of a defective child. *Neonatal Network, 5*, 13–20.

Lewis, C. E., Rachelefsky, G., Lewis, M. A., de la Sota, A., & Kaplan, M. (1984). A randomized trial of A.C.T. (Asthma Care Training for Kids). *Pediatrics, 74*, 478–486.

Macknin, M. (1992). Respiratory infections in children: What helps and what doesn't. *Post Graduate Medicine, 92*, 235–250.

Marelich, G. P., & Cross, C. E. (1996). Cystic fibrosis in adults. *Western Journal of Medicine, 164*, 321–334.

McAleese, K. A., Knapp, M. A., & Rhodes, T. T. (1993). Financial and emotional cost of bronchopulmonary dysplasia. *Clinical Pediatrics, 12*, 393–400.

McCubbin, M., Frey, E. E., Wagener, J. S., Tribby, R., & Smith, W. L. (1989). Large airway collapse in bronchopulmonary dysplasia. *Journal of Pediatrics, 114*, 304–307.

McIntosh, K. (1991). Pathogenesis of severe acute respiratory infections in the developing world: RSV and parainfluenza viruses. *Reviews of Infectious Diseases, 13*(Suppl. 6), S492–S500.

McMullen, A. H. (1992) Cystic fibrosis. In P. Ludder-Jackson & J. A. Vessey (Eds.), *Primary care of the child with a chronic condition*. St. Louis: Mosby.

McNabb, W. L., Wilson-Pessano, S. R., Hughes, G. W., & Scamagas, P. (1985). Self-management education of children with asthma: AIR WISE. *American Journal of Public Health, 75*, 1219–1220.

Milgrom, E. C. (1993). Practical approach to diagnosing and treating sinusitis. *Western Journal of Medicine, 158*(5), 517–518.

Mitchell, S. H. (1996). Infants with bronchopulmonary dysplasia: A developmental perspective. *Journal of Pediatric Nursing, 11*(3), 145–151.

Morriss, F. C. (1984). Apnea. In D. L. Levin, F. C. Morriss, & G. C. Moore (Eds.), *A practice guide to pediatric intensive care*. St. Louis: Mosby.

Motoyama, E. K., Fort, M. D., Klesh, K. W., Mutich R. L., & Guthrie, R. D. (1987). Early onset of airway reactivity in premature infants with bronchopulmonary dysplasia. *American Review of Respiratory Disease, 136*, 50–57.

Mu, L., Sun, D., & He, P., (1990). Radiologic diagnosis of foreign body aspiration in children: Review of 343 cases. *Journal of Laryngeal Otology, 104*, 778–782.

Murray, C. B., & Loughlin, G. M. (1995). Making the most of pulse oximetry. *Contemporary Pediatrics, 12*(7), 45–52, 55–57, 61–62.

National Association of Apnea Professionals. (1996). Guidelines for the provision of services to families using infant apnea monitors. *Neonatal Intensive Care, 9*(3), 10–15.

National Heart, Lung and Blood Institute. (1991). *Guidelines for the diagnosis and management of asthma* (DHHS NIH Publication No. 91-3042). Washington, DC: U.S. Government Printing Office.

National Heart, Lung and Blood Institute, National Asthma Education Program Expert Panel Report. (1991). Guidelines for the diagnosis and management of asthma. *Pediatric Asthma Allergy and Immunology, 5*, 57–188.

National Institutes of Health Consensus Development Conference on Infantile Apnea and Home Monitoring. (1987). *Pediatrics, 79*, 292–299.

National Institutes of Health. (1995). *Global initiative for asthma: Global strategy for asthma management and prevention. NHLBI/WHO Workshop Report* (NHLBI Publication No. 95-3659). Washington, DC: U.S. Government Printing Office.

Northway, W. H., Moss, R. B., & Carlisle, K. B. (1990). Late pulmonary sequelae of bronchopulmonary dysplasia. *New England Journal of Medicine, 323*, 1793–1799.

Northway, W. H., Rosan, R. C., & Porter, D. Y. (1967). Pulmonary disease following respiratory therapy of hyaline membrane disease. *New England Journal of Medicine, 276*, 357–368.

Nuttall, P. (1988). Maternal responses to home apnea monitoring of infants. *Nursing Research, 37*, 354–357.

Oertel, M. (1996). Respigam: An RSU immune globulin. *Pediatric Nursing, 22*(6), 525–528.

Oren, J., Kelly, D., & Shannon, D. C. (1986). Identification of a high risk group for sudden infant death syndrome among infants who were resuscitated for sleep apnea. *Pediatrics, 77*, 495–499.

Orenstein, D. M. (1993). Cystic fibrosis. *Current Problems in Pediatrics, 23*(1), 4–15.

Parker, R. A., Lindstrom, D. P., & Cotton, R. B. (1992). Improved survival accounts for most but not all of the increase in BPD. *Pediatrics*, 90, 663–668.

Patterson, J. M., McCubbin, H. I., & Warwick, W. J. (1990). The impact of family functioning on health changes in children with cystic fibrosis. *Social Science Medicine, 31*(2), 159–164.

Pegues, D. A., Carson, L. A., Tablan, O. C., FitzSimmons, S. C., Roman, S. B., Miller, J. M., Jarvis, W. R., & Summer Camp Study Group. (1993). Acquisition of pseudomonas cepacia at summer camps for patients with cystic fibrosis, part I. *Journal of Pediatrics, 124*, 694–792.

Rakshi, K., & Couriel, J. M. (1994). Management of acute bronchiolitis. *Archives of Disease in Childhood, 71*, 463–469.

Rau, J. L. (1991). Delivery of aerosolized drugs to neonates and pediatric patients. *Respiratory Care, 36*, 514–545.

Reilly, J. S. (1992). Airway foreign bodies: Update and analysis. *International Anesthesiology Clinics, 30*(4), 49–55.

Robertson, C. M. T., Etches, P. C., Goldson, E., & Kyle, J. M. (1992). Eight-year school performance, neurodevelopmental, and growth outcome of neonates with bronchopulmonary dysplasia: A comparative study. *Pediatrics, 89*, 365–372.

Robin, P. (1923). La chute de la base de la langue considérée comme une nouvelle cause de gene dans la respiration nasopharyngienne. *Bulletin de l'Academie Nationale de Medecine (Paris), 89*, 37–41.

Roncolli, M. (1996). Asthma medications for children: Guidelines for the primary care practitioner. *Journal of the American Academy of Nurse Practitioners, 8*(5), 243–252.

Rosenfeld, M. A., & Collins, F. S. (1996). Gene therapy for cystic fibrosis. *Chest, 109*, 241–252.

Rosenstein, B. (1990). Interpreting sweat tests in the diagnosis of cystic fibrosis. *Journal of Respiratory Diseases, 11*, 519–528.

Runton, N. (1992). Suctioning artificial airways in children: Appropriate technique. *Pediatric Nursing, 18*, 115–118.

Sawyer, E. H. (1992). Family functioning when children have cystic fibrosis. *Journal of Pediatric Nursing, 7*(5), 304–311.

Schidlow, D. V., & Smith, D. S. (1994). Stridor and upper airway obstruction. In D. V. Schidlow & D. S. Smith (Eds.), *A practical guide to pediatric respiratory diseases* (pp. 31–38). Philadelphia: Hanley-Belfus.

Schidlow, D. V., Taussig, L. M., & Knowles, M. R. (1993). Cystic Fibrosis Foundation consensus conference report on pulmonary complications of cystic fibrosis. *Pediatric Pulmonology, 15*, 187–198.

Schwartz, J., Gold, D., Dockery, D. W., Weiss, S. T., & Speizer, F. E. (1990). Predictors of asthma and persistent wheeze in a national sample of children in the United States. Association with social class, perinatal events, and race. *America Review of Respiratory Diseases, 142*, 555–562.

Schwartz, R. (1995). Respiratory syncytial virus in infants and children. *Nurse Practitioner, 20*(9), 24–29.

Scott, S. (1997). Partnership in asthma care. *Advances for Nurse Practitioners, 5*(5), 50–86.

Sears, M. R. (1990). Epidemiology of asthma. In P. M. O'Byrne (Ed.), *Asthma as an inflammatory disease*. New York: Marcel Dekker.

Seidel, J. S. (1996). Respiratory distress. In C. D. Berkowitz (Ed.), *Pediatrics—A primary care approach* (pp. 135–138). Philadelphia: W. B. Saunders.

Shalon, L. B., & Adelson, J. W. (1996). Cystic fibrosis: Gastrointestinal complications and gene therapy. *Pediatric Clinics of North America, 43*, 157–191.

Shprintzen, R. J. (1988). Pierre Robin, micrognathia, and airway obstruction: The dependency of treatment on accurate diagnosis. *International Anesthesiology Clinics, 1*, 64–71.

Smith, D. S. (1994). Sinusitis. In D. V. Schidlow & D. S. Smith (Eds.), *A practical guide to pediatric respiratory diseases* (pp. 15–18). Philadelphia: Hanley-Belfus.

Smyth, R. L., Ashby, D., O'Hea, U., Burrows, E., Lewis, P., van Velzen, D., & Dodge, J. A. (1995). Fibrosing colonopathy in cystic fibrosis: Results of a case-control study. *Lancet, 346*, 1247–1251.

Spinner, S., Gibson, E., Wrobel, H., & Spitzer, A. R. (1995). Recent advances in home infant apnea monitoring. *Neonatal Network, 14*(8), 39–46.

Stullenbarger, B., Norris, J., Edgil, A. E., & Prosser, M. J. (1987). Family adaptation to cystic fibrosis. *Pediatric Nursing, 13*, 29–31.

Taylor, W. R., & Newacheck, P. W. (1992). Impact of childhood asthma on health. *Pediatrics, 90*, 657–662.

Thompson, A. B., Smits, W. L., & Fick, R. B. (1992). Immunomodulatory therapies for cystic fibrosis. *Seminars in Respiratory Infections, 7*(3), 218–226.

Tooley, W. H. (1979). Epidemiology of bronchopulmonary dysplasia. *Journal of Pediatrics, 95*, 851–858.

Vohr, B. R., Coll, C. G., Lobato, D., Yunis, K. A., O'Dea, C. & Oh, W. (1991). Neurodevelopmental and medical status of low birthweight survivors of bronchopulmonary dysplasia at 10 to 12 years of age, *Developmental Medicine and Child Neurology, 33*(8), 690–697.

Voter, K. Z., & McBride, J. T. (1996). Diagnostic tests of lung function. *Pediatrics in Review, 17*(2), 53–63.

Vukmir, R. B. (1992). Adult and pediatric pharyngitis: A review. *Journal of Emergency Medicine, 10*, 607–616.

Wagner, M. H. (1994). Foreign body aspiration. In J. Eigen & G. M. Loughlin (Eds.), *Respiratory disease in children*. Baltimore: William & Wilkins.

Wald, E. R., Guerra, N., & Byers, C. (1991). Frequency and severity of infections in day care: Three-year follow-up. *Journal of Pediatrics, 118*, 509–514.

Ward, S. L., Keens, T. G, Chan, L. S., Chipps, B. E., Carson, S. H., Deming, D. D., Krishna, V., MacDonald, H. M., Martin, G. I., Meredith, K. S., et al. (1986). Sudden infant death syndrome in infants evaluated by apnea programs in California. *Pediatrics, 77*, 451–455.

Weiss, K. B., Gergen, P. J., & Hodgson, T. A. (1992). An economic evaluation of asthma in the United States. *New England Journal of Medicine, 326*, 862–866.

Weitzman, M., Gortmaker, S., & Sobol, A. (1990). Racial, social and environmental risks for childhood asthma. *American Journal of Diseases in Children, 144*, 1189–1194.

Wilder, B. (1996). Management of sinusitis. *Journal of the American Academy of Nurse Practitioners, 8*(11), 525–529.

Wilmott, R. W., & Fiedler, M. A. (1994). Recent advances in the treatment of cystic fibrosis. *Pediatric Clinics of North America, 41*, 431–451.

Wing, J. S. (1993). Asthma in the inner city—A growing public health concern in the United States. *Journal of Asthma, 30*, 427–430.

Wright, P. (1996). Influenza viral infections. In R. E. Behrman, R. M. Kliegman, & A. M. Arvin (Eds.), *Nelson textbook of pediatrics* (15th ed.). Philadelphia: W. B. Saunders.

Yoos, H., McMullen, A., Bezek, S., Hondorf, C., Berry, S., Herendeen, N., MacMaster, K., & Schwartzberg, M. (1997). An asthma management program for urban minority children. *Journal of Pediatric Health Care, 11*, 66–74.

Zander, J., & Hazinski, M. F. (1992). Pulmonary disorders. In M. F. Hazinski (Ed.), *Nursing care of the critically ill child* (2nd ed.). St. Louis: Mosby–Year Book.

Bibliography

Aitken, M., Burke, W., McDonald, G., Shak, S., Montgomery, A. B., & Smith, A. (1992). Recombinant human DNase inhalation in normal subjects and patients with cystic fibrosis. *Journal of the American Medical Association, 267*(14), 1947–1951.

American Academy of Pediatrics. (1996). Reassessment of the indications for ribavirin therapy in respiratory syncytial virus infections. *Pediatrics*, 97(1), January, 137–140.

Balfour-Lynn, I., Girdhar, D., & Aitken, C. (1995). Diagnosing respiratory syncytial virus by nasal lavage. *Archives of Disease in Childhood, 72*(1), 58–59.

Capen, C., Dedlow, E., Robillard, R., Fuller, B., & Fuller, C. (1994). The team approach to pediatric asthma education. *Pediatric Nursing, 20*(3), 231–237.

Carey, B. (1996). Bronchopulmonary dysplasia. *Neonatal Network, 15*(4), 73–77.

Carroll, P. (1993). Clinical applications of pulse oximetry. *Pediatric Nursing, 19*, 150–151.

Castiglia, P. (1996). Adjusting to childhood asthma. *Journal of Pediatric Health Care, 10*(2), 82–84.

Colin, A. A., & Wohl, M. E. B. (1994). Cystic fibrosis. *Pediatrics in Review, 15*(5), 192–200.

Cystic Fibrosis Foundation. (1993). *Cystic Fibrosis Foundation patient registry annual data report 1992*. Bethesda, MD: Author.

Denny, F. W., & Clyde, W. A., Jr. (1986). Acute lower respiratory tract infections in non-hospitalized children. *Journal of Pediatrics, 108*, 635–646.

Dickson, S. (1995). Understanding the oxyhemoglobin dissociation curve. *Critical Care Nurse, 15*(5), 54–58.

Dougherty, J. (1990). Negative pressure devices in pediatric practice. *Pediatric Nursing, 16*, 135–138.

Eagan, T. M. (1992). Lung transplantation in cystic fibrosis. *Seminars in Respiratory Infections, 7*(3), 227–239.

Fackelmann, K. (1996). 100-day cough. *Science News, 150*, 46–47.

Fackelmann, K. (1996). A link between pertussis and crib death. *Science News, 150*, 47.

Fields, A. I., Rosenblatt, A., & Pollack, N. M. (1991). Home care cost-effectiveness for respiratory technology-dependent children. *American Journal of Diseases of Children, 145*, 729–733.

Fink, R. B., & Lynch, J. P. (Eds.). (1992). Cystic fibrosis [Special issue]. *Seminars in Respiratory Infections, 7*(3).

FitzSimmons, S. C. (1994). The changing epidemiology of cystic fibrosis. *Current Problems in Pediatrics, 24*(5), 171–179.

Geller, G. (1995). Cystic fibrosis and the pediatric care giver: Benefits and burdens of genetic technology. *Pediatric Nursing, 21*(1), 57–61.

Gibbons, M. (1996). Rx for asthma. *Advance for Nurse Practitioners*, 4(7), 45–47.

Gregg, R. G., Wilfond, B. S., Farrell, P. M., Laxova, A., Hassemer, D., & Mischler, E. (1993). Application of DNA analysis in population-screening program for neonatal diagnosis of cystic fibrosis (CF): Comparison and screening protocols. *American Journal of Human Genetics, 52*, 616–626.

Groothuis, J. (1994). Role of antibody and use of respiratory syncytial virus (RSV) immune globulin to prevent severe RSV disease in high-risk children. *The Journal of Pediatrics, 124*(5), s28–s32.

Groothuis, J., Simoes, E., & Hemming, V. (1995). Respiratory syncytial virus (RSV) infection in preterm infants and the protective effects of RSV immune globulin (RSVIG). *Pediatrics*, 95(4), 463–467.

Groothuis, J., Simoes, E., Levin, M., et al. (1993). Prophylactic administration of respiratory syncytial virus immune globulin to high-risk infants and children. *The New England Journal of Medicine, 329*(21), 1524–1530.

Hagemann, T. (1996). Cystic fibrosis—Drug therapy. *Journal of Pediatric Health Care, 10*(3), 127–134.

Hanson, M. (1996). Bronchiolitis in children. *The Nursing Spectrum*, February 26, 12–13.

Hardy, K. A. (1993). Advances in our understanding and care of patients with cystic fibrosis. *Respiratory Care, 38*(3), 282–289.

Kamada, A. K. (1994). Therapeutic controversies in the treatment of asthma. *The Annals of Pharmacotherapy*, 28, 904–914.

Keens, T., Jansen, M. T., DeWitt, P. K., & Ward, S. L. D. (1990). Home care for children with chronic respiratory failure. *Seminars in Respiratory Medicine, 11*, 269–281.

Keller, K., et al. (1994). Acute asthma management in children: Factors identifying patients at risk for ICU treatment. *Journal of Asthma, 31*(5), 393–400.

Lowe, D. (1994). Practical aspects of oxygen therapy. In D. V. Schidlow & D. S. Smith (Eds.), *A practical guide to pediatric respiratory diseases* (pp. 289–300). Philadelphia: Hanley-Belfus.

Meng, A., & Martorell, N. (1997). The hospitalized child with asthma. *MCN, 22*(3), 128–134.

Middleton, A. (1997). Managing asthma: It takes teamwork. *American Journal of Nursing*, 97(1), 39–43.

Moler, F., Khan, A., Meliones, J., Custer, J., Palmisano, J., & Shope, T. (1992). Respiratory syncytial virus morbidity and mortality estimates in congenital heart disease patients: A recent experience. *Critical Care Medicine, 20*(10), October, 1406–1413.

Orenstein, D. M. (1991). Cystic fibrosis. *Respiratory Care, 36*(7), 746–756.

Padur, J., Raposs, M., Houston, B., Barnard, M., Danovsky, M., Olson, N., Moore, W., Vats, T., & Lieberman, B. (1995). Psychosocial adjustment and the role of functional status for children with asthma. *Journal of Asthma, 32*(5), 345–353.

Phillips, O. P., Elias, S., Woods, D., Hanissian, A. S., Schumacher, R. A., & Bishop, C. (1993). Cystic fibrosis mutations in white and black Americans: An approach to identification of unknown mutations with implications for cystic fibrosis screening. *American Journal of Obstetrics and Gynecology, 168*(4), 1076–1082.

Ryan, L., & Williams, J. (1996). A cystic fibrosis handbook for teachers. *Journal of Pediatric Health Care, 10*(4), 174–179.

Ryan-Winger, N., & Walsh, M. (1994). Children's perspectives on coping with asthma. *Pediatric Nursing, 20*(3), 224–228.

Sherman, L., & Rosen, C. (1990). Development of a preschool program for tracheostomy dependent children. *Pediatric Nursing, 16*, 357–361.

Smith, M. B., & Feldman, W. E. (1993). Over-the-counter cold medications. *Journal of the American Medical Association, 269*, 2258–2263.

Spahis, J. (1994). Sleepless nights: Obstructive sleep apnea in the pediatric patient. *Pediatric Nursing, 20*, 469–472.

Swartz, M. (1996). Environmental control of allergens and irritants. *Journal of Pediatric Health Care, 10*(3), 145–146.

Thompson, R. J., Gustafson, K. E., Hamlett, K. W., & Spock, A. (1992). Stress, coping, and family functioning in the psychological adjustment of mothers of children and adolescents with cystic fibrosis. *Journal of Pediatric Psychology, 17*(5), 573–585.

White, K. R., Munro, C. L., & Pickler, R. H. (1995). Therapeutic implications of recent advances in cystic fibrosis. *MCN*, 20, November-December, 304–308.

Wilson, J., Arnold, C., Connor, R., & Cusson, R. (1996). Evaluation of oxygen delivery with the use of nasopharyngeal catheters and nasal cannulas. *Neonatal Network, 15*(4), 15–22.

HEALTH CHALLENGE:

Alterations in Fluid and Electrolyte Status

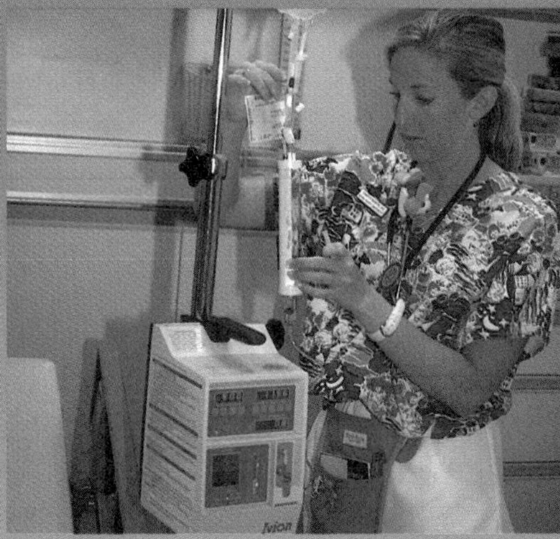

OUTLINE

OBJECTIVES

- Discuss the physiologic principles that regulate fluid and electrolyte balance.
- Compare total water distribution, intracellular fluid, and extracellular fluid in infants, children, and adults.
- Review assessment parameters for a child at risk for fluid or electrolyte imbalance.
- Identify laboratory tests used to assess fluid and electrolyte balance.
- Calculate maintenance fluid therapy requirements and identify nursing care priorities for a child receiving intravenous fluid therapy.
- Discuss nursing care measures for the child receiving total parenteral nutrition.
- Describe the assessment and treatment of hypertonic and hypotonic dehydration.
- Explain the principles of acid-base balance.
- Discuss the causes and treatment of specific electrolyte imbalances.

KEY TERMS

acidosis
alkalosis
dehydration
edema
electrolyte
extracellular fluid
extravasation
hypertonic fluid
interstitial fluid
intracellular fluid
ion
isotonic fluid
oncotic pressure
osmolality
osmotic pressure
osmosis
pH
vesicant

CHAPTER

17

Water is critical to human survival. Not only is it the primary fluid within the body, it also provides a medium in which body solutes (electrolytes) are dissolved and metabolic reactions occur. Alterations in fluid and electrolyte balances can occur as a result of a disease, injury, or therapeutic intervention that hinders the body's normal physiologic mechanisms that regulate fluid intake and output.

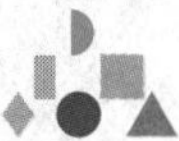

Principles of Fluid and Electrolyte Balance

In the human body, water is distributed in two main compartments: intracellular fluid (ICF) and extracellular fluid (ECF). ECF is further divided into intravascular fluid and interstitial fluid. The cell membrane provides a barrier between the ECF and ICF; fluid moves through this barrier by osmosis. Fluid movement between the two ECF compartments occurs through filtration.

Electrolyte concentrations are not uniform and differ between the ECF and the ICF. Fluid and electrolytes continuously move from one compartment to another. This movement is influenced and controlled by various regulatory mechanisms (Chart 17–1).

To help illustrate the concept of movement and transportation of fluids between compartments, consider this example. Sodium is the principal cation in ECF, and potassium is the principal cation in ICF. To maintain an equilibrium between sodium and potassium concentrations, water moves from ICF to ECF through passive transport mechanisms, whereas sodium and potassium move between cells through active transport mechanisms. Maintaining this equilibrium is a continuous, ongoing process.

Chart 17–1

Physical Factors That Affect Fluid Balance

Pressure Gradients

Hydrostatic Pressure

- Pressure exerted by fluid in a closed system (e.g., blood in capillaries)
- The force that pushes water out of the blood vessels into the interstitium
- Provided by contractions of the heart
- Highest pressures are within the capillary beds

Osmotic Pressure

- Moves water from a low solute concentration to a high solute concentration
- Equalizes the concentration of solvents on both sides of a semipermeable membrane
- Intracellular and extracellular fluid solutes (e.g., Na^+, proteins) participate in this process

Oncotic Pressure

- Generated by colloids in solution (e.g., plasma proteins, albumin)
- The force that draws water into the blood vessels
- Balances capillary hydrostatic pressure
- Allows kidneys to regulate filtration and reabsorption

Transport Mechanisms

Passive Transport

- Movement of solutes across membrane from area of greater concentration to area of lesser concentration
- Occurs automatically
- Requires no energy output

Active Transport

- Movement of solutes against a pressure gradient
- Facilitated by energy released through the Na^+-K^+ ATP pump

Several physiologic mechanisms regulate fluid and electrolyte homeostasis in the body. The *kidneys* regulate fluid balance through their ability to concentrate and dilute urine. Antidiuretic hormone (ADH), a hormone produced by the hypothalamus and stored in the pituitary gland, stimulates renal reabsorption of water. When serum sodium levels are high, ADH secretion increases the permeability of the kidneys' distal tubules and collecting ducts to water. This enables the kidneys to retain more water.

The angiotensin-renin system, along with aldosterone, also assists the kidneys in regulating fluid and electrolyte homeostasis. When reduced blood flow is detected by the kidney, renin is produced, which in turn stimulates angiotensin within the blood vessels. The release of aldosterone is then stimulated by angiotensin. As a result, sodium and water reabsorption is increased in the renal tubules. This mechanism produces (1) increased blood flow to the kidney, (2) increased intravascular volume, and (3) increased blood pressure.

In the *gastrointestinal tract*, changes occur in the electrolyte levels of gastrointestinal secretions. Water and sodium are reabsorbed, and potassium is excreted. Normally, fluid is replaced through oral fluid intake. Because of the large absorptive surface area of the gastrointestinal tract, changes in fluid and electrolytes can occur rapidly. Imbalances must be treated quickly and appropriately to prevent decompensation in the child's health status.

Insensible water loss refers to invisible, continuous, and passive water loss from the skin and lungs resulting from heat expenditure (Finberg, Kravath, & Hellerstein, 1993). No electrolytes are lost or excreted in insensible water loss. This process is one method that the body utilizes to regulate temperature.

The *integumentary system*, as a thermoregulatory mechanism, impacts fluid and electrolyte balance. Losses of fluid, sodium, potassium, and chloride occur in sweat. In contrast to insensible water loss, this process is intermittent and is more dependent on environmental temperature.

Most regulatory mechanisms involve the excretion of fluid and electrolytes. The exception is thirst, the impetus to ingest water. The thirst center is located in the hypothalamus. As a major regulatory mechanism, thirst is unreliable. It is stimulated by a decrease in the intravascular volume and/or an increase in the osmolality of ECF. The infant and young child can experience thirst but have a limited ability to take action to meet this need. They depend on others to provide oral fluids and to appropriately regulate the type and amount of fluid intake.

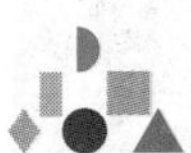

Assessment of the Child with an Alteration in Fluid and Electrolyte Status

Disease, age, environment, and activity level all affect fluid and electrolyte status. Imbalances in fluids and electrolytes are reflected in many body systems. Thus, assessment of a child with a known or suspected fluid or electrolyte imbalance requires a multisystem evaluation.

Focused Health History

A health history pertinent to fluid and electrolyte status includes present and previous illnesses, health habits, and fluid intake and output (Chart 17–2).

Intake and output profoundly affect fluid and electrolyte balance. The health history should include questions about the amount as well as the type of fluids ingested. The nurse needs to investigate fluid intake carefully to uncover possible causes of imbalance. For instance, feeding an infant formula prepared with too much water, either as a cost-saving measure or through error, may lead to water intoxication. Conversely, feeding formula prepared with too little water (which results in a formula with high osmolality that pulls water into the gut) can lead to dehydration and electrolyte imbalance. An older child or an adolescent with an eating disorder (i.e., anorexia or bulimia) may also have insufficient fluid intake and thus be at risk for severe, possibly life-threatening electrolyte imbalances.

Major routes of fluid output are urine, stool, and vomiting. To assess voiding patterns, ask the parent how many wet diapers the infant or young child has each day, and ask an older child how often he or she voids.

Tip: *When asking a child about output patterns, clarify the type of output using age- and culturally appropriate terms for urine and stool.*

Vomiting usually occurs early if high bowel obstruction is present. In appendicitis and bowel obstruction beyond the small intestine, vomiting is usually delayed several hours after onset of pain. In children, vomiting is

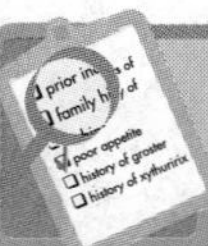

Chart 17–2
Focused Health History

Fluid and Electrolyte Status

Demographic Data

- Child's age, height, weight
- Source of data (historian)

Reason for Seeking Care

- In child's, or historian's, own words, why he or she has accessed the health care system (present illness)
- When symptoms started and duration and nature of symptoms, precipitating factors, and home management of current illness

Chart continued on following page

Chart 17–2
Focused Health History *Continued*

Fluid and Electrolyte Status

Reason for Seeking Care *Continued*

- Note, in particular, presence of the following:
  Recent weight change
  Fever, diaphoresis
  Edema
  Change in level of consciousness or behavior (e.g., lethargy, irritability, weakness), headaches
  Change in sleep patterns (describe)
  Number of voidings in past 24 hours; time of last void/wet diaper, urine amount, color, odor
  Stool appearance, consistency, amount
  Nausea, vomiting, or abdominal pain
  Relation of symptoms to food ingestion
  Presence of sore throat or oral lesions that interfere with intake

Past Medical History

- Birth history—presence of congenital defects, especially those involving gastrointestinal/genitourinary system
- Previous health challenges—recurrent, chronic, or episodic illness or surgery, how managed; child's response to previous illnesses, hospitalizations
- Childhood illnesses—recent contact with someone who is sick; describe symptoms
- Immunizations received, when, reaction to them
- Allergies to drugs, food, or other sensitizing agents (describe reaction)

Current Medications

- List all medications (e.g., diuretics, digitalis, potassium supplements), home remedies (e.g., teas, herbs), vitamins or food supplements the child is currently receiving

Nutritional Assessment

- Time the child last ate; type of food or fluid and amount ingested
- Is the child retaining food and fluid?
- Describe typical intake of food and fluid—type, how prepared, frequency and quantity; for infants or toddlers include if intake is via bottle, breast, or cup; if breast fed, note any change in mother's diet; if a commercial formula is used, note formulation (e.g., ready-to-feed, powder) and how formula is prepared (dilution amounts)
- Any change in the child's appetite or oral intake; is the child complaining of thirst?

Family Medical History

- History of same illness in other family members (describe symptoms and any treatments)

Environmental History

- Known or possible ingestion of poisons
- Exposure to high environmental temperatures

Social History

- Psychosocial: financial status, issues regarding obtaining adequate food supply, sanitation for food storage and preparation
- Child care issues: who cares for child and where (e.g., child care center, home)
- Cultural: practices that may overheat infants (e.g., wrapping in blankets even in hot temperatures); administration of home remedies that may cause fluid or electrolyte imbalance

Growth and Development

- Physical and developmental milestones; age-appropriate achievement
- Daily routines and habits: sleeping, feeding, toileting

associated with many common disorders, including otitis media, sinusitis, pharyngitis, and pneumonia.

Fever, which increases metabolic rate, increases the rate of fluid loss. Various toxins can interfere with cellular function and metabolism, leading to fluid and electrolyte imbalances.

Focused Physical Assessment

Physical assessment for a child with altered fluid and electrolyte status includes a general survey and a system-specific examination focusing on level of hydration (Chart 17–3). The general survey evaluates the child's appearance and level of distress. It always includes weighing the child and comparing the result to previous weights. Any significant fluid loss or gain will be reflected in weight changes.

Fluid deficit may compromise peripheral perfusion, as reflected in changes in vital signs and level of consciousness. The child may report dizziness when standing up after lying down. Electrolyte imbalance may also cause altered vital signs and level of consciousness, as well as more system-specific findings (e.g., impaired muscle function).

Specific vital sign changes point to the type and degree of imbalance. For example, temperature elevation typically occurs in hypernatremia (sodium excess), because hypernatremia causes excessive fluid loss, making less water available for heat loss through sweating. Conversely, temperature may be subnormal in fluid volume deficit. Pulses may be rapid and weak in fluid deficit and bounding in fluid overload. Cardiac dysrhythmias may occur in various imbalances, notably hyperkalemia (potassium excess) and hypokalemia (potassium deficit). Blood pressure may be elevated in fluid volume excess and decreased in fluid volume deficit. (Because a child's young, healthy blood vessels normally compensate well in response to decreased fluid volume, blood pressure is a late sign of volume deficit, however.)

Other physical assessment findings suggest specific fluid and electrolyte imbalances. Delayed capillary refill, a sign of inadequate peripheral perfusion, points to fluid volume deficit. Altered level of consciousness may indicate insufficient blood flow to the brain owing to lack

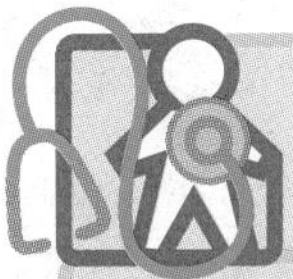

Chart 17–3
Focused Physical Assessment

Fluid and Electrolyte Imbalances

Parameter	Factors to Note
General appearance	Level of distress
Skin	Decreased or increased skin temperature Dry skin and mucous membranes; diaphoresis; flushing Poor turgor, tenting, dough-like feel to skin; edema Sunken eyeballs; absence of tears Pale, ashen, or cyanotic nailbeds or mucous membranes Delayed capillary refill (>3 sec)
Neuromuscular	Change in level of consciousness: unresponsiveness, irritability, lethargy, confusion Weak, high-pitched cry Sunken or bulging fontanelle in infant Change in muscle tone: hyperreflexia or hyporeflexia; positive Chvostek's sign (i.e., facial twitching as the facial nerve is tapped); weakness or flaccidity; tetany Seizures
Cardiovascular	Change in pulse rate or quality: rapid, weak, thready, bounding, arrhythmias Increased or decreased blood pressure Neck vein distention
Respiratory	Change in respiratory rate and quality: tachypnea, apnea, deep, shallow Moist breath sounds Cough
Gastrointestinal	Abdominal distention Abnormal peristaltic waves

of blood volume. Other signs of fluid deficit include dry mucous membranes, sunken eyeballs, lack of tears when crying, sunken fontanelle in infants, and poor skin turgor.

caREminder: *To evaluate skin turgor, gently lift the child's abdominal skin between the thumb and forefinger, then release. Skin that does not return to its original shape but stays raised or "tented" indicates poor turgor.*

Fluid overload may produce moist breath sounds, edema, and a bulging fontanelle in infants.

Electrolytes play a vital role in cellular metabolism and neuromuscular function. Electrolyte imbalances may produce neurologic symptoms, muscle cramps, increased or decreased muscle tone, and hypoactive or hyperactive reflexes. For example, a positive Chvostek's sign (facial twitching when the facial nerve is tapped) may indicate hypocalcemia or hypomagnesemia.

Nursing Diagnoses and Outcomes

Nursing diagnoses that may be appropriate for the child with altered fluid and electrolyte status, along with desired patient outcomes, are listed in Chart 17–4. Because fluid and electrolyte imbalances produce widely varying effects, additional diagnoses not listed may be appropriate for children with specific alterations.

Developmental and Biological Variances

Infants and children are more susceptible than adults to fluid and electrolyte imbalances (Fig. 17–1). In an infant, for example, a high basal metabolic rate makes the normal turnover rate of water and electrolytes two to three faster than in an adult. Approximately 50% of ECF in the infant is exchanged each day (Hazinski, 1988). This makes an infant more susceptible to significant physical changes from fluid deficit.

The amount of total body water and the proportional sizes of the ICF and ECF compartments change from infancy to adolescence (Fig. 17–2). Infants and young children have a higher proportion of total body water, stemming from a higher proportion of ECF and

Figure 17–1
Developmental and biological variances: fluid and electrolyte balance.

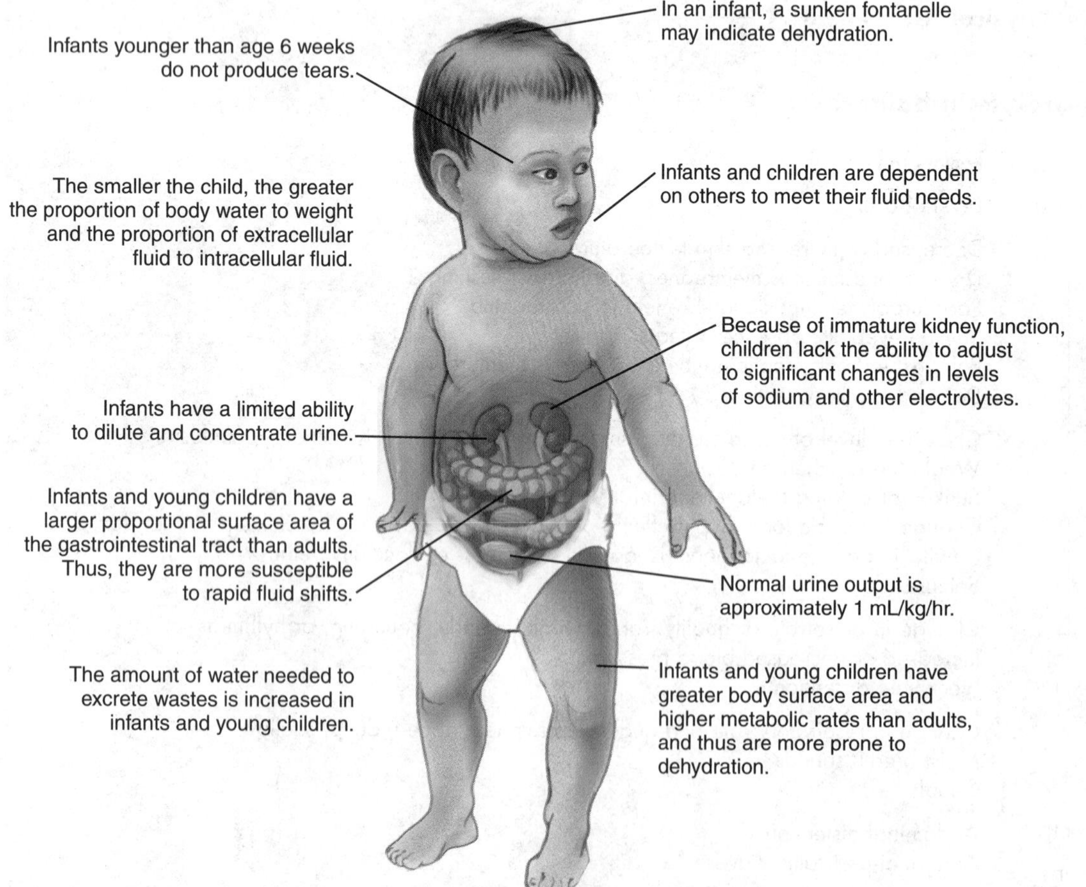

In an infant, a sunken fontanelle may indicate dehydration.
Infants younger than age 6 weeks do not produce tears.
The smaller the child, the greater the proportion of body water to weight and the proportion of extracellular fluid to intracellular fluid.
Infants and children are dependent on others to meet their fluid needs.
Because of immature kidney function, children lack the ability to adjust to significant changes in levels of sodium and other electrolytes.
Infants have a limited ability to dilute and concentrate urine.
Infants and young children have a larger proportional surface area of the gastrointestinal tract than adults. Thus, they are more susceptible to rapid fluid shifts.
Normal urine output is approximately 1 mL/kg/hr.
The amount of water needed to excrete wastes is increased in infants and young children.
Infants and young children have greater body surface area and higher metabolic rates than adults, and thus are more prone to dehydration.

Chart 17–4
Nursing Diagnoses and Outcomes

The Child with a Disturbance in Fluid and Electrolyte Balance

Nursing Diagnosis	Desired Outcome
Altered tissue perfusion (specify type: renal, cerebral, cardiopulmonary, gastrointestinal, peripheral) related to effects of fluid deficit, electrolyte imbalance	The child will have signs of altered tissue perfusion recognized promptly and interventions instituted to maintain adequate perfusion.
Altered nutrition: less than body requirements related to effects of disease process	The child will take in (PO, enteral, IV) sufficient fluid and nutrients based on age and medical needs. The child will gain weight at a rate appropriate for his or her age.
Activity intolerance related to weakness from disease process	The child will be able to perform activities normal and appropriate for his or her developmental level.
Knowledge deficit: recognition and management of fluid and electrolyte imbalance	The child and parents will demonstrate understanding of the tests and procedures performed. The child, if old enough, and parents will recognize early symptoms of fluid and electrolyte imbalance and implement appropriate interventions.

Figure 17–2
Total body water distribution by age. Note the changes in intracellular and extracellular fluid volume.

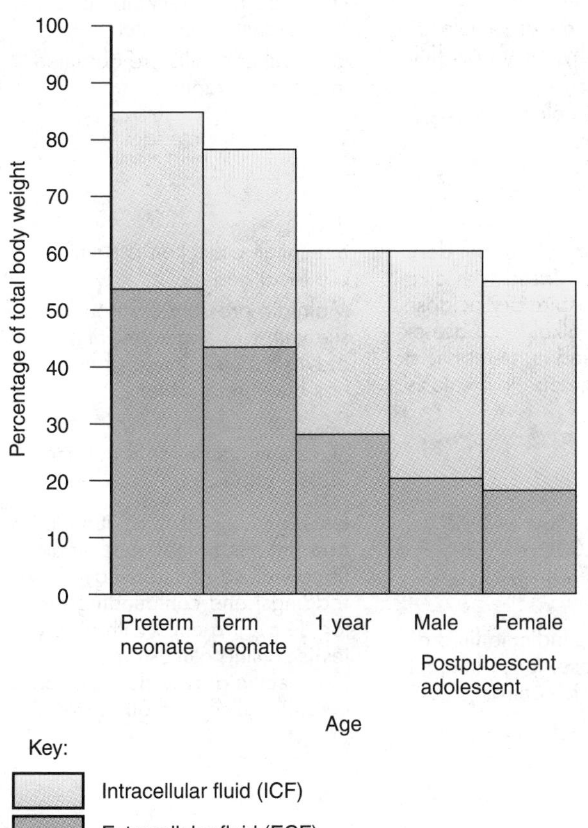

lower total body fat. Total body fat increases dramatically in the first year of life, with a concurrent decrease in the amount of total body water. Total body water content is 85% to 90% of weight in a preterm infant and 78% in a full-term infant. This proportion remains fairly constant until adolescence, when characteristic sex differences occur. Normally, males have greater muscle mass and less body fat than females. Therefore, the sexually mature male has about 60% total body water; the female, about 55%.

Children are more prone than adults to diseases that affect fluid and electrolyte status. They can rapidly lose large amounts of fluid and electrolytes through diarrhea, vomiting, and high fever. Moreover, infants and young children are dependent on others to meet their fluid needs; and when these needs are not met, imbalances can develop rapidly.

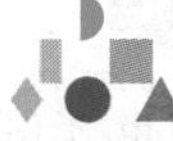

Diagnostic Criteria for Evaluating Alterations in Fluid and Electrolyte Status

Diagnostic tests performed to evaluate fluid and electrolyte imbalances include blood chemistry and serum electrolyte analyses, hemoglobin and hematocrit levels, arterial blood gas values, urine studies (specific gravity, osmolality, pH), and stool analysis (Table 17–1). Nurs-

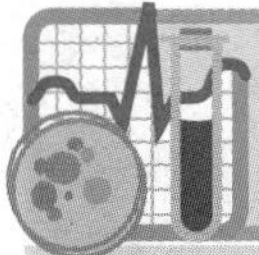

Table 17–1
Diagnostic Tests and Procedures for Evaluating Fluid and Electrolyte Imbalance

Diagnostic Test or Procedure	Purpose	Findings/Indications	Health Care Provider Responsibilities
Blood chemistry/electrolyte analysis (Na^+, K^+, Ca^{2+}, Cl^-, Mg^{2+}, PO_4^-, albumin, blood urea nitrogen [BUN], creatinine)	Analyzes various chemical components of blood	Few disorders produce a single abnormality; several components are usually analyzed to detect a pattern of abnormal results that may point to a disorder. Na^+, K^+, and Cl^- help maintain osmotic pressure and acid-base balance; decreased Na^+ associated with severe diarrhea, vomiting, edema; increased Na^+, with dehydration; decreased K^+, with diarrhea, severe vomiting; increased K^+, with renal disease, massive cell damage, acidosis. Decreased protein levels result in decreased Ca^{2+} levels, because half of blood Ca^{2+} is protein bound; Ca^{2+} and PO_4^- have an inverse relationship; hypoalbuminemia often results in edema (albumin helps maintain normal body water distribution). Increased BUN may occur in kidney disease, shock, dehydration; decreased BUN may occur in negative nitrogen balance and overhydration.	Obtain specimens correctly (e.g., get free flow of blood because when hemolyzed, cells break, releasing potassium, resulting in elevated K^+ levels and an inaccurate analysis of actual serum K^+ values). Do not draw blood from same extremity an intravenous line is infusing in. Provide psychologic and physical support when specimen is obtained; use topical anesthetic when possible. Evaluate results based on patterns of findings, including child's symptoms.
Blood hemoglobin (Hgb) and hematocrit (Hct)	Measures Hgb, the main component of erythrocytes, which is the vehicle for transporting O_2 and CO_2, and Hct, the concentration of erythrocytes in plasma	Increased Hgb and Hct in extracellular fluid volume decrease (decreased in blood loss) and hyperosmolar fluid imbalance Decreased Hgb and Hct in extracellular fluid volume excess and hypo-osmolar fluid imbalance Hgb is important buffer in blood; helps maintain acid-base balance	Support child when obtaining specimen. Put blood in correct tube and label specimen accurately. Ensure that results are obtained in a timely manner.
Arterial blood gases (ABGs)	Assesses acid-base status	Based on uncompensated values: pH decreased with acidosis, increased with alkalosis; PCO_2 elevated in respiratory acidosis, decreased in respiratory alkalosis; base excess and HCO_3^- decreased in metabolic acidosis and increased in metabolic alkalosis	Specimen collection is painful; use local anesthetic. Maintain pressure over puncture site with two fingers for minimum of two minutes, longer if child has bleeding problems. Expel air bubbles in syringe. Place sample on ice if not immediately analyzed.
Urine specific gravity	Measures kidney's ability to dilute and concentrate urine	Normal values: neonate, 1.001–1.020; over 1 month, 1.001–1.030 Low specific gravity may indicate fluid excess or kidney disease High specific gravity may indicate fluid deficit, the presence of glucose, large amounts of protein, or radiographic contrast media elevates results.	Evaluate findings in relation to age (infants do not concentrate urine well so normally have low readings) and confounding factors (e.g., if a child with diabetes is spilling glucose in urine, the specific gravity does not accurately reflect hydration status).

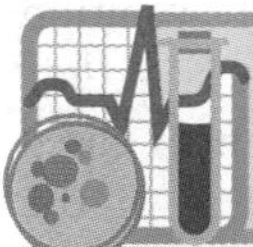

Table 17–1
Diagnostic Tests and Procedures for Evaluating Fluid and Electrolyte Imbalance *Continued*

Diagnostic Test of Procedure	Purpose	Findings/Indications	Health Care Provider Responsibilities
Urine osmolality	More exact measure of urine concentration than specific gravity	Normal value: 50–1400 mOsm/kg H_2O, depending on fluid intake Value after 12-hour fluid restriction: >850 mOsm/kg H_2O is normal	Evaluate findings in relation to age and confounding factors.
Urine pH	Measures acidity/alkalinity of urine; reflects ability of renal tubules to maintain normal hydrogen ion concentration in plasma and extracellular fluid	Varies widely with kidney function, averages 6 Acid urine (pH <7) found with high-protein diet or acidosis (e.g., diarrhea, dehydration, respiratory disease, uncontrolled diabetes) Alkaline urine (pH >7) found with vegetarian diets and those high in citrus fruits and dairy products and with diseases associated with hyperventilation, urinary tract infection, or chronic renal failure	Obtain freshly voided specimen for most accurate results; otherwise, refrigerate specimen.
Stool analysis	Evaluates stool for consistency, color, odor, absence or presence of blood, mucus, food residue, tissue fragments, bacteria, and parasites	Diet influences color; normal brown color is due to breakdown of bile; if passage is rapid (e.g., diarrhea), stool may be yellow or green (this is normal in breast-fed infant). Evaluation of consistency may indicate amount of water loss. Characteristics may help diagnose disease: for example, diarrhea with mucus and blood (typhus, cholera, amebiasis) and diarrhea with mucus and pus (ulcerative colitis, shigellosis, salmonellosis).	Fresh stools provide the most accurate results; warm stools are best for ova and parasite detection. Avoid testing stool contaminated with urine or toilet bowl water.

ing responsibilities related to diagnostic studies include obtaining specimens, accurately labeling and sending specimens to the laboratory, and following up on results. Follow-up involves evaluating results and notifying the physician or advanced nurse clinician of values outside normal age-appropriate ranges.

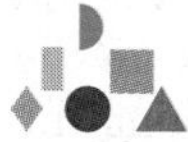

Treatment Modalities

Alterations in fluid and electrolyte balance are managed by correcting the specific imbalance (e.g., giving fluid when the child is dehydrated) and treating the underlying cause (e.g., controlling diarrhea). Whenever possible, fluid and electrolyte imbalances are treated with oral fluid ingestion. When oral fluids cannot be given, intravenous fluids or total parenteral nutrition (TPN) must be administered to meet the child's fluid, electrolyte, and/or nutrition needs.

Intravenous Therapy

Intravenous (IV) therapy is used in clinical situations requiring administration of fluids (and sometimes medications) to a child who cannot maintain a normal fluid balance by oral ingestion. The route, volume, and type of fluid administration are key factors in managing the child receiving IV therapy.

Route of Administration

IV fluids can be given by peripheral vein, central vein, or intraosseous access. The route of fluid administration depends on the child's clinical situation, the type of fluids and medications administered, and the duration of IV fluid therapy.

Peripheral Venous Access

Peripheral IV lines are used for short-term administration of fluids and medications. Potential sites of peripheral IV catheter placement include the scalp, the back of the hand, the arm (including the antecubital fossa), the foot, and the leg. Factors considered in determining placement site include the child's age and condition, comfort, safety, positioning or securing needed, and condition of the vein. In infants, for instance, the scalp veins generally are easier to cannulate than extremity veins, and so the scalp is a common placement site. Many parents find a scalp IV line in their infant quite distressing. The nurse should discuss the scalp placement procedure, including the rationale, with the parents before placing the IV line and offer to save any hair that is shaved from the infant for them.

Worldview: *Touching of a child's head by strangers may be offensive to some Asians. Explain the need to touch the child's head to the parents before starting a scalp IV line.*

When placing IV lines in extremities, the most distal sites should be accessed first. The antecubital fossa should not be used until other sites have been exhausted. A catheter in the antecubital region, or any joint, is easily disturbed by joint flexion, and the immobilization required may cause joint stiffness and pain. An older child should be allowed a choice of catheter placement sites, as appropriate. If the arm is used, it should be the nondominant one; and in an ambulatory child, one should avoid using the feet or legs, if possible.

Tip: *When securing an IV line with an armboard, tell the child that the armboard is there to help him or her remember not to move that arm too much.*

When a peripheral IV line is needed for intermittent administration of medication but is not required for continuous IV fluid administration, an IV lock may be used. Catheter gauge, the child's diagnosis, the medication administered, the flush solution used, and the length of time between flushes are all variables that impact longevity of the IV site. Whether to use heparin or saline solution to flush the IV lock is controversial (Bossert & Beecroft, 1994). Some studies found that saline flush was sufficient to maintain the IV line (Hanrahan, Kleiber, & Fagan, 1994); others found saline sufficient except for smaller 24-gauge catheters (Danek & Noris, 1992). Still other studies found that heparin flushes contribute to IV line patency and decreased phlebitis (Gyr et al., 1995). Definitive recommendations for type of flush solution cannot be made at this time. The nurse must follow facility-specific protocols for IV lock maintenance, based on patient population and standards of practice in the community.

Central Venous Access

Central venous catheters (CVCs) are larger-bore catheters that are inserted either percutaneously or by cutdown and advanced into the superior or inferior vena cava (Fig. 17–3). The umbilical vein may be used in an infant during the first few days after birth.

CVCs are used in situations that require long-term venous access. They are particularly good for administering fluids with high glucose concentrations, blood and blood components, medications that are irritating to peripheral vessels, and chemotherapy agents and for obtaining blood samples. CVCs can be multilumen, designed to deliver multiple therapies concomitantly. When a small-gauge CVC is in place, as is common in infants, administration of blood may clot the catheter. The manufacturer's recommendations for appropriate usage should be checked. When a CVC does not have an infusion running, it must be flushed with heparin to maintain patency. Again, facility protocol and manufacturer's recommendations should be checked. If a peripherally inserted central catheter (PICC) or tunneled catheter is damaged, it usually can be repaired.

Generally, CVCs are classified as nontunneled, tunneled, implanted ports, or peripherally inserted central catheters (Keegan-Wells & Stewart, 1992). *Nontunneled* catheters are generally used for short-term central access in the acute care setting. They are placed percutaneously, usually into the subclavian or jugular vein, using local or general anesthesia. Because of the insertion method (direct puncture into a large vein, not tunneled under the skin), nontunneled catheters carry an increased risk of dislodgement and infection compared with tunneled catheters.

Broviac, Hickman, and Groshong catheters are *tunneled* beneath the skin for several inches (may be shorter in infants and young children) from the skin exit site to the vein insertion point. These catheters have a Dacron cuff 1 to 2 inches proximal to the exit site to secure the catheter and reduce the risk of infection by blocking the migration of pathogens from the skin along the catheter tunnel to the central circulation. General anesthesia is usually required to place tunneled catheters in children. Broviac and Hickman catheters require a heparin flush when not used for infusion. Facility and manufacturer's recommendations should be checked. A Groshong catheter requires a saline flush.

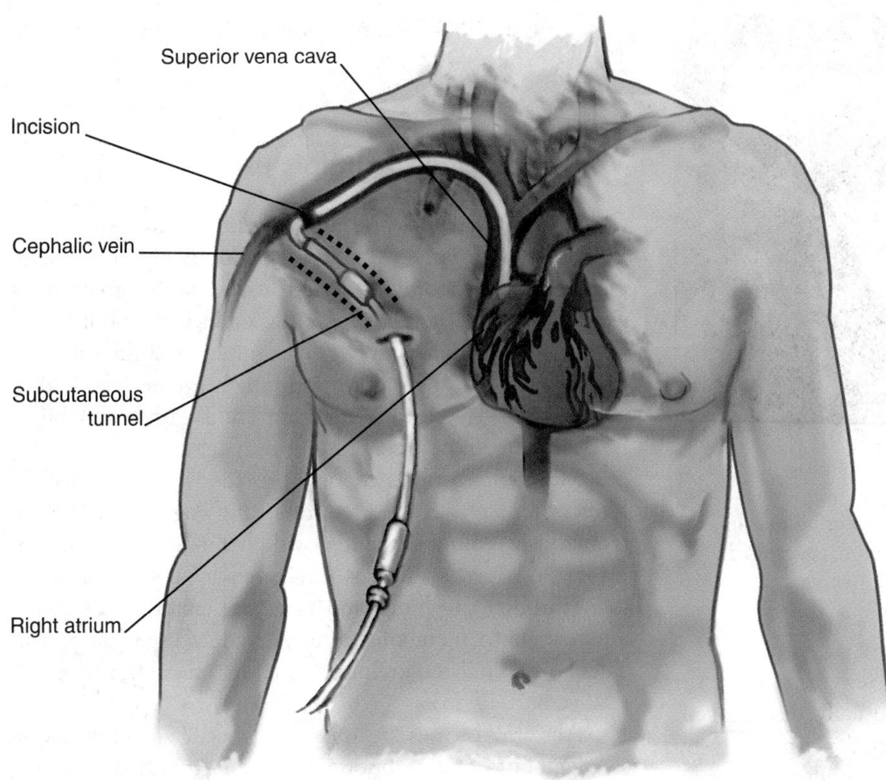

Figure 17–3
Position of a tunneled central venous catheter in the superior vena cava. Note that the skin insertion site is a distance from the vein entry site, with the catheter being tunneled under the skin for this distance.

A tunneled catheter exits the skin and is visible, although it can be hidden under clothing (Fig. 17–4). Because of its visibility, it may have a negative impact on the child's body image. Participation in contact sports may be limited in a child with a tunneled catheter.

Implantable ports (e.g., Port-A-Cath, Infuse-A-Port, Omega) are surgically placed under the skin and sutured to the chest wall with the child under general anesthesia. No part of the port is external. Implantable ports have a self-sealing silicon septum (which can be palpated under the skin) enclosed in a metallic chamber. This provides a reservoir that connects to a large central vein by means of a Silastic catheter.

The port is accessed with deflected-tip, noncoring needles to prevent leakage. Patients generally report that accessing the port with a needle is less traumatic than venipuncture, although some children still react negatively to the needlestick associated with port access (Keegan-Wells & Stewart, 1992). To make port access more tolerable, topical anesthetic (e.g., EMLA cream) can be used. To insert the needle, the skin over the port is palpated to identify the septum (Fig. 17–5). Needles can be left in place for a maximum of 7 days (Hughes, 1996). The port should be flushed with heparin to maintain patency.

Because an implanted port is placed under the skin, it is less visible than other catheters and may have less negative impact on body image, although alteration in body image may still be present. Once the site has healed

Figure 17–4
A tunneled central venous catheter should have an occlusive dressing in place. Although it can be hidden under clothing, it often has a negative impact on body image.

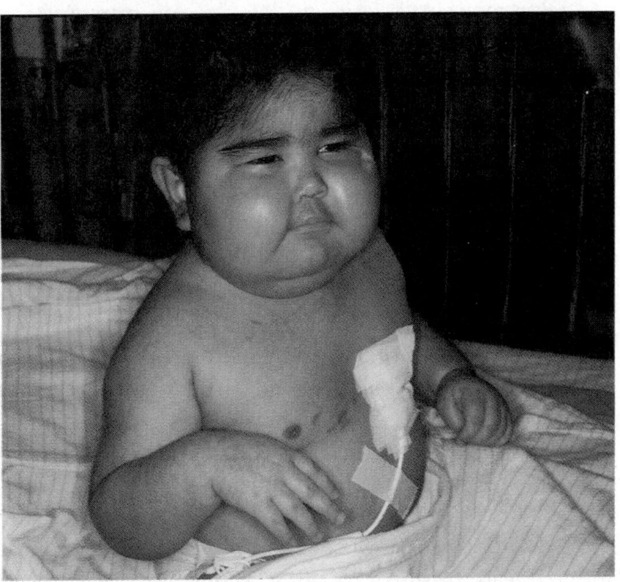

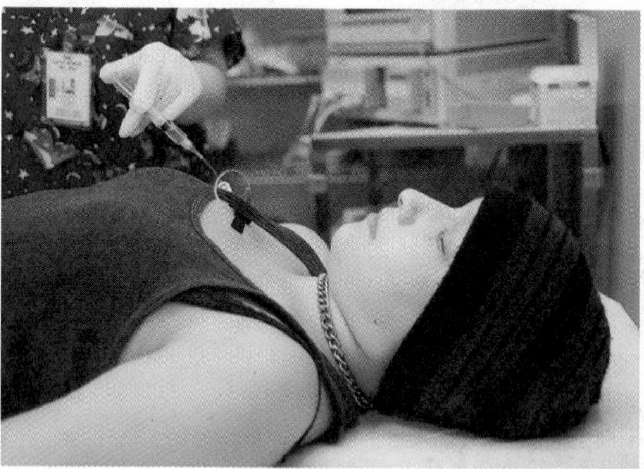

Figure 17–5
Implanted ports are accessed with special noncoring needles, and an occlusive dressing is used when the port is accessed.

after placement, the child usually has few restrictions on activity, although contact sports are usually discouraged.

A PICC line (Fig. 17–6) is inserted peripherally by means of a percutaneous puncture. It is generally inserted at the antecubital fossa into the basilic or cephalic vein and threaded into the subclavian or superior vena cava. In infants, other sites may be used. A PICC line is a good choice for the child requiring long-term antibiotic therapy. Insertion is usually done under local anesthesia only. However, in infants, local anesthesia often causes the vessels to constrict; thus, IV sedation may be given before PICC insertion.

caREminder: *PICC lines are usually not sutured in place. During dressing changes, extreme care must be taken to avoid displacing the catheter. Any extra length of tubing must be coiled under the dressing.*

Intraosseous Access

The intraosseous (IO) route provides temporary vascular access in children age 6 years and younger in emergency situations until venous access can be obtained. A large-bore needle is placed into the bone marrow cavity, optimally in the proximal tibia (Fig. 17–7). Fluids, blood, and most medications (cytotoxic drugs should be avoided) are rapidly absorbed into the systemic circulation from this site. The marrow space can be rapidly accessed, even in hypotensive children or when cardiopulmonary resuscitation is in progress. After initial fluid resuscitation, vascular access may be more readily achieved. Bone marrow obtained when the IO needle is inserted can be used to assess hemoglobin, electrolyte levels, blood chemistry values, and blood gases (Orlowski, 1994).

Volume of Fluid Administered

Calculation of fluid and electrolyte requirements takes into consideration the child's maintenance needs, replacement of ongoing abnormal losses, and correction of existing fluid deficits. The child's clinical condition is also a determining factor. For example, a child with impaired renal or cardiac function may be given less fluid to prevent fluid overload, whereas a child with major burns likely will require increased fluid intake.

Maintenance fluid therapy provides fluid and electrolytes in amounts equal to normal ongoing losses. Normal metabolism produces solutes, which must be excreted in urine, and heat, which is dissipated by insensible water loss (through the lungs and skin). Therefore, fluid needs are related to metabolic rate. A widely used method of calculating fluid requirements is based on caloric expenditure (Chart 17–5).

Abnormal losses are those that occur either in excessive amounts or by abnormal routes. Abnormal ongoing losses are calculated based on measurement of vomitus, gastrointestinal suction losses, diarrhea, and excessive urine output and on increased insensible water loss: increased ambient temperature, use of radiant warmers, fever, hyperventilation, burns, or excessive sweating. Abnormal losses are corrected on an ongoing basis to prevent further fluid and electrolyte deficits.

Figure 17–6
Peripherally inserted central catheter (PICC) line in place; caution must be used not to displace the catheter.

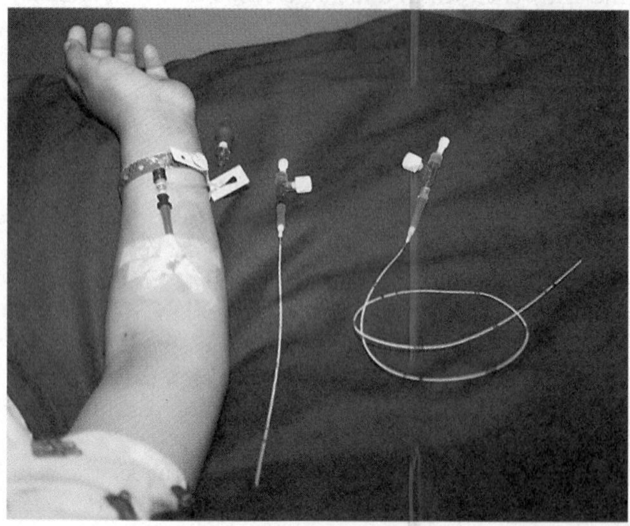

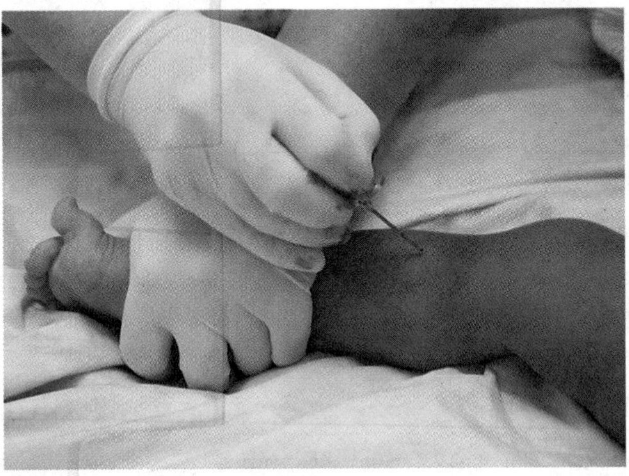

Figure 17–7
Intraosseous needle in place for emergency vascular access.

Correction of fluid deficits replenishes fluids lost before initiation of treatment. This is calculated based on measured weight loss or on estimated percentage of fluid lost based on clinical signs of dehydration.

Type of Fluid Administered

Both glucose and electrolytes should be included in maintenance IV solutions administered to children. In short-term IV therapy, 5% dextrose solutions help minimize protein catabolism, ketosis, and negative nitrogen balance, although they do not provide total caloric needs. A 10% dextrose solution is usually administered to neonates.

Glucose is metabolized rapidly, which decreases the osmolality of the solution. This allows the "free water" to rapidly move to a more hypertonic space—often the brain in young children, causing cerebral edema. Electrolytes in solutions help prevent fluid from shifting out of the vascular space. A hypotonic solution (e.g., D_5 0.2 NS) is usually given, because children need more free water than adults owing to their higher daily fluid turnover. The optimum concentration of these components depends primarily on the child's serum electrolyte values and also on the underlying disease process.

Two basic types of IV fluid preparations are used: crystalloid and colloid (Table 17–2). The type used for volume replacement depends on the nature of the loss, as well as on ongoing maintenance needs. Crystalloids are solutions that equilibrate rapidly between the vascular and interstitial space. Because crystalloids do not stay in the vascular space, two to four times more crystalloid volume than colloid volume must be given to correct deficits (Kuhn, 1991).

Colloids help maintain plasma oncotic (osmotic) pressure. Because of their large size, colloids remain in the vascular space and exert osmotic force to pull fluid into the circulatory space, thus maintaining intravascular volume. Albumin is the most abundant plasma protein. It is compatible with any blood type, because it does not contain any blood antibodies.

Interdisciplinary Interventions

Preparation of the child and the family is essential in easing the anxiety and fear related to IV fluid therapy. The nurse should clearly describe the equipment, supplies, and the procedure itself to the child and family. An older child should be allowed to make certain choices about the therapy whenever it is medically safe to do so. Permitting the child to choose the extremity to

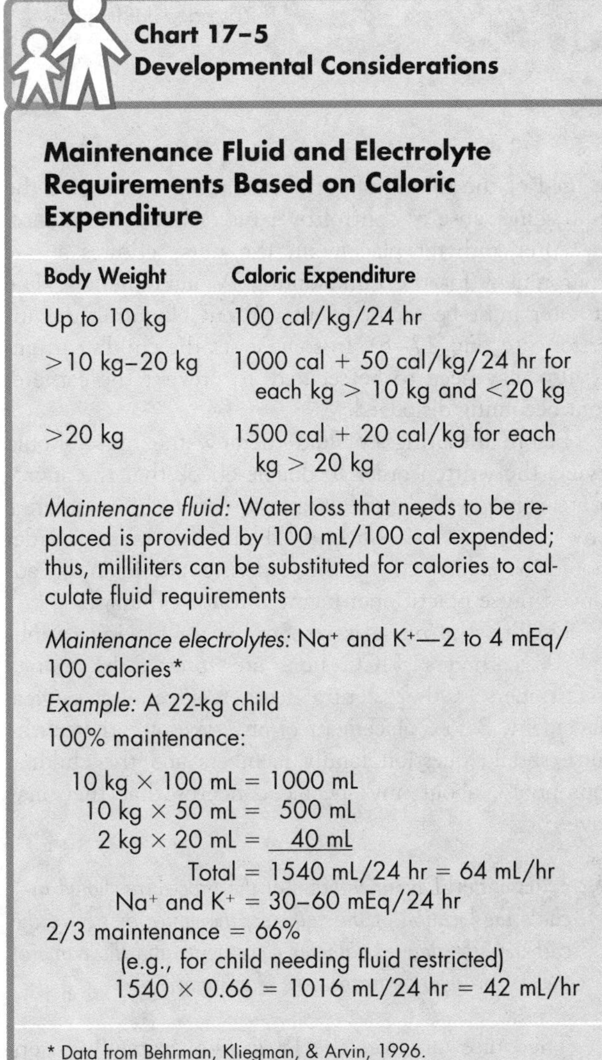

Chart 17–5
Developmental Considerations

Maintenance Fluid and Electrolyte Requirements Based on Caloric Expenditure

Body Weight	Caloric Expenditure
Up to 10 kg	100 cal/kg/24 hr
>10 kg–20 kg	1000 cal + 50 cal/kg/24 hr for each kg > 10 kg and <20 kg
>20 kg	1500 cal + 20 cal/kg for each kg > 20 kg

Maintenance fluid: Water loss that needs to be replaced is provided by 100 mL/100 cal expended; thus, milliliters can be substituted for calories to calculate fluid requirements

Maintenance electrolytes: Na^+ and K^+—2 to 4 mEq/100 calories*

Example: A 22-kg child

100% maintenance:

10 kg × 100 mL = 1000 mL
10 kg × 50 mL = 500 mL
2 kg × 20 mL = 40 mL
Total = 1540 mL/24 hr = 64 mL/hr
Na^+ and K^+ = 30–60 mEq/24 hr

2/3 maintenance = 66%
(e.g., for child needing fluid restricted)
1540 × 0.66 = 1016 mL/24 hr = 42 mL/hr

* Data from Behrman, Kliegman, & Arvin, 1996.

Table 17–2
Crystalloids versus Colloids

Fluid	Indications	Advantages	Disadvantages
Crystalloid			
Normal saline (0.9% NS) Ringer's lactate (RL) (contains NaCl, K, Ca, Na lactate)	Ongoing maintenance Replacement of gastrointestinal losses Acute volume expansion in shock	Less expensive than colloid Readily available	Does not stay within the vascular system as long as colloid solutions
Colloid			
Albumin Synthetic plasma substitutes: hetastarch, dextran Blood products: whole blood, packed cells, fresh frozen plasma	Shock Adult respiratory distress syndrome Renal failure Burns Liver failure Hypoproteinemia Third-space fluid shifts	Remain within the vascular compartment Smaller amounts of fluid More effective in achieving hemodynamic stability	Expensive Blood products less readily available Greater potential for fluid overload

be used or the timing of catheter placement can give the child some sense of control over his or her environment.

After catheter placement, the nurse ensures a safe environment for the child during IV fluid therapy. The catheter must be secured, but without obscuring the insertion site (Fig. 17–8). In some cases the child's extremity also may need to be secured, to prevent the catheter from becoming dislodged.

Before initiating IV fluid therapy, the nurse should review the written order to double-check that the appropriate solution and rate of infusion have been ordered. Any questions or concerns about the written order should be addressed to the ordering physician or advanced nurse practitioner before initiating therapy.

Usually, the nurse is responsible for placing peripheral IV catheters. PICC lines are inserted by trained practitioners. Other central catheters require surgical placement. Before placement of any type of catheter, the nurse should question family members and the child, if appropriate, about any specific concerns that they may have.

caREminder: *Documentation of the procedure should include the location of the catheter, the gauge or size of the catheter, the date of catheter placement, and the name of the person who performed the placement.*

The nurse monitors the IV infusion carefully to ensure that the child receives the correct volume of fluid at the correct rate of infusion. Infusion pumps are usually used for IV therapy in infants and young children. One aspect of this monitoring includes verifying that the pump is set correctly and is delivering the ordered infusion rate. If an infusion pump is not used or if it malfunctions, the nurse can deliver the IV fluid through a microdrip-type tubing that delivers fluid at a slow rate.

The nurse observes the child and site of IV infusion

Figure 17–8
Peripheral intravenous catheter in place. The insertion site and surrounding area must be easy to visualize, to enable prompt detection of signs of complications.

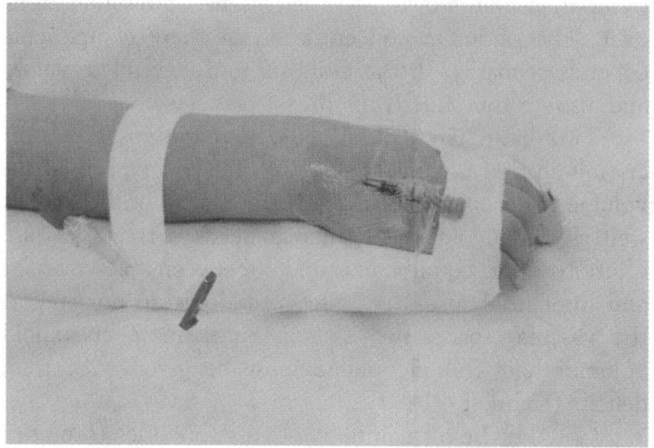

for signs of complications every 1 to 2 hours. Potential complications include infiltration of fluid into the surrounding tissue, air emboli, venous phlebitis, and infection (Chart 17–6). Vascular overload or electrolyte imbalance may also occur. The nurse should teach the older child, the parents, and other caretakers to observe for and report any signs of complications, particularly infiltration (Chart 17–7).

Because of the CVC's central access and long-term use, infection is a particular concern when these catheters are used. Children are at increased risk for catheter-related infection and skin irritation (which can lead to infection) because they tend to play with the dressing or tubing, which can introduce contamination from soiled hands, vomit, or stool (Freiberger, 1994). One study identified several factors associated with increased incidence of bacteremia in infants and toddlers with CVCs, including parenteral alimentation infusions, use of the line for medication administration and blood withdrawal, increased accidental line disconnections, and tunneled Silastic catheters infusing into the subclavian vein (Long, Byrnes, Leclair, Stashinko, & Molchan, 1996).

Pneumothorax, hemothorax, and perforation of the central vessel are possible complications directly related to the CVC placement procedure. Single-lumen CVCs have a lower rate of complications, including infection and sepsis, than multilumen CVCs (Ford, 1996).

Protocols for CVC insertion site and line care must be meticulously followed by all health care team members. These should include how often to clean the site and the proper cleansing technique, how often to flush the catheter and the appropriate flushing solution, how often to change tubing, and how to properly maintain an occlusive dressing. (Implanted ports need an occlusive dressing only when accessed.)

Playing with or pulling at the catheter or tubing increases the risk of line breakage, with the resulting complications of exsanguination and air embolism. Regardless of the type of venous access device used, it must be protected as developmentally appropriate (Chart 17–8). If the child attends school or daycare, teachers and care providers must be given guidelines for catheter care (see Chart 22–10).

Nursing responsibilities also include assessment of the child's overall status and careful monitoring of intake and output. This includes both IV and oral intake as well as all output. Daily weights should be recorded to assess the adequacy of fluid volume management.

Alert: *During IV fluid therapy, monitor for and promptly report signs of overhydration, such as increased respiratory rate, respiratory distress, and rales on lung auscultation. Support the child's respiratory effort, elevate the head of the bed, and check the infusion set-up for errors (e.g., inaccurate programming of the pump infusion rate).*

Parenteral Nutrition

The parenteral method of delivering fluids, electrolytes, and calories into the central venous system bypasses the gastrointestinal tract, the central thirst mechanism, and the hunger regulatory mechanism. Children have enormous metabolic needs and require high amounts of energy and protein to support their continued growth (Ford, 1996).

The basic purpose of IV nutritional support is to restore or maintain optimum nutritional status. IV nutrition also provides fluid to aid excretion of waste and to replace insensible fluid losses (Ford, 1996). The gut should be used whenever possible to provide nutrition (see Chapter 18 for further discussion). Enteral (oral or tube) feedings, even in small amounts of 5 to 10 mL/hr, are beneficial in helping maintain gut structure, integrity, and function. Use of the gut maintains intestinal villi (which atrophy if not stimulated) and enzyme activity and prevents breaks in the mucosal wall through which bacteria can enter the system and cause sepsis. Use of the gut also helps avoid the hypermetabolic state that occurs after major stress or critical illness.

TPN provides complete nutrition for children who cannot consume sufficient nutrients through the gastrointestinal tract to meet and sustain metabolic requirements (Skaer, 1993). TPN solutions provide protein, carbohydrates, electrolytes, vitamins, minerals, trace elements, and fats.

Good candidates for TPN include children with short gut syndrome, cancer, or increased metabolic needs due to injury. Contraindications to the use of TPN include an anticipated course of less than 5 days; after surgery, in the immediate postoperative period; when the risk exceeds the perceived benefit; and when aggressive nutritional support is not desired. A child rarely receives TPN exclusively, with no oral intake, for prolonged periods. Partial therapy, in which enteral intake is supplemented with TPN, provides the benefits of gut stimulation while still providing adequate calories, nutrition, and fluids.

TPN can be provided by peripheral or central venous access. Peripheral delivery of IV nutrition should be restricted to a maximum of 10% glucose (Ford, 1996; Hughes, 1996). Concentrations higher than this frequently produce a chemical phlebitis. Peripheral TPN is most appropriate for short-term support of older children.

caREminder: *Peripheral IVs used for TPN should be changed every 2 to 3 days to decrease the risk of phlebitis and local wound infection (Ford, 1996).*

Chart 17–6
Nursing Interventions

Complications of Intravenous Therapy

Complication	Signs and Symptoms	Nursing Interventions*
Infiltration (extravasation): *fluid leaks into subcutaneous tissues*	Fluid leakage around the catheter site Swelling when compared with the opposite extremity Site cool to the touch Decreased rate of infusion Tenderness, pain	Site, especially distal to catheter insertion, should be readily observable. Monitor the area distal to catheter insertion site and dependent area for signs of complications at least every hour. If complications occur, discontinue IV, elevate extremity, apply warm moist compress (ice may be applied instead of heat if certain medications have extravasated). Notify advanced nurse practitioner or physician if medications have extravasated. As ordered, administer drugs (e.g., hyaluronidase) to neutralize or help diffuse extravasated vesicants (medications that cause tissue damage on extravasation). Usually, no neutralizing drugs are given when fluid or nonvesicant medications have infiltrated.
Catheter occlusion: *blockage of catheter usually by clotted blood, or precipitates such as incompatible solutions, TPN, antibiotics*	Fluid will not infuse or unable to flush Frequent infusion pump alarms	Maintain fluid infusion rate. If catheter appears occluded, *gently* flush line (avoid exerting too much force, which may push clot into vascular system or cause rupture of the vein or catheter); use a 3- to 5-mL syringe to flush line (smaller syringes create greater pressures, which increase the chance of vein or catheter rupture); use normal saline initially to flush. If saline is unsuccessful, then use lytic agents for central lines per facility protocol: Urokinase for blood clot or thrombus HCl for mineral precipitant $NaHCO_3^-$ for medication incompatibility precipitant Ethyl alcohol for lipid precipitant
Air embolism: *air enters the circulation and travels to the right side of the heart*	Respiratory distress Cyanosis Tachypnea Hypotension	Secure all tubing connections. Use air-eliminating filters on tubing. Use IV pumps that alarm when air in tubing is detected. When air is detected, clamp IV catheter or tubing or remove air to prevent further air entry. Place the child in left lateral Trendelenburg position to try to prevent air entering left side of heart and circulating to system. Promptly aspirate air from catheter with syringe. If symptoms occur, notify advanced nurse practitioner or physician immediately; may be a medical emergency. Support cardiorespiratory function; administer oxygen as ordered.

Chart 17-6
Nursing Interventions *Continued*

Complications of Intravenous Therapy

Complication	Signs and Symptoms	Nursing Interventions*
Phlebitis: *injury to the vein without clot*	Red streak along the vein Warmth along the vein Possible edema	Dilute antibiotics in adequate amount of fluid, infuse over longest period recommended to provide better hemodilution of drug. Change insertion site routinely per facility protocol. Apply moist heat to site for 20 minutes several times a day.
Thrombophlebitis: *injury to the vein with a clot*	Tenderness Edema Area warm to touch Additionally, with a central venous catheter: Signs and symptoms related to impeded venous return—edema of the neck, chest, or affected extremity, leading to facial swelling and neck vein distention with complete vein occlusion Moderate pain in neck that may radiate down arm or to the back	Monitor for signs and symptoms; notify advanced nurse practitioner/physician if any develop. Elevate the affected extremity.
Infection: *introduction of pathologic organisms locally or systemically*	Redness at the catheter insertion site Exudate from the catheter insertion site Fever Elevated white blood cell	Wash hands before and after contact with child. Maintain sterile or clean technique for IV insertion and dressing and tubing change. Minimize manipulation of, or trauma to, the insertion site. Change IV solution per protocol, usually within 24 hours. Change tubing per protocol, usually within 24 to 72 hours.
Metabolic derangement: *imbalance in electrolytes, minerals, glucose, and proteins*	Signs vary depending on the specific imbalance: Hyponatremia: muscle cramps, nausea, diarrhea, lethargy, seizures Hypokalemia: diarrhea, muscle weakness, nausea, abdominal distention, tachycardia, irritability, confusion Zinc deficiency: poor wound healing, impaired protein synthesis and cellular immunity, skin hyperpigmentation (especially around lips) Copper deficiency: skin depigmentation, skeletal demineralization, microcytic hypochromic anemia, leukopenia, neutropenia Hypoglycemia: hungry, shaky, weak, dizzy, headache, diaphoresis, blurred vision, slurred speech, seizures, coma Hyperglycemia: increased thirst and urination	Consult with dietitian, pharmacist, and physician/advanced nurse practitioner, to ensure appropriate intake (oral and/or IV) for needs. Monitor for signs of imbalance. Intervene as needed for specific imbalance (e.g., for hypoglycemia, PO or IV glucose, depending on severity and child's status).

* Documentation of assessments and interventions is required.

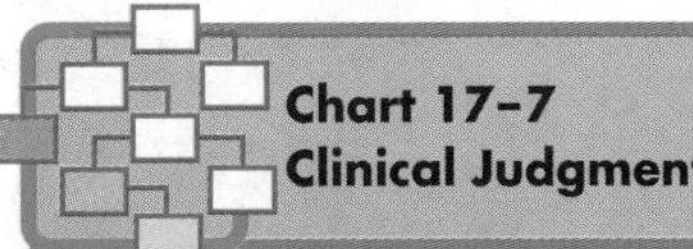

Chart 17–7
Clinical Judgment

Child with Phlebitis

Tran is a 3-year-old who has a peripheral IV for antibiotic therapy. His present IV has been in place 2 days. Shortly after the nurse started this antibiotic dose, Tran started crying and picking at the IV site in his left hand.

Questions

1. What assessment data regarding the IV site should the nurse collect?
2. Are any of the IV site assessment findings abnormal? If so, which ones?
3. Should the IV be taken out?
4. After discontinuing the IV in the left hand, what should be done to care for the site?
5. What is the usual course of symptom resolution with phlebitis?

Answers

1. Color of the site—redness, streaking, pallor (there is a faint red line proximal to the IV site); temperature of the surrounding skin (left wrist is warmer than right); presence of edema (left hand and wrist appear slightly more swollen than right); palpate the site (unremarkable—no fibrosis or hardened line felt)
2. Yes; a faint red line proximal to site, site warmer than opposite limb with slight edema. Tran is also complaining of pain at the site.
3. Yes
4. Apply warm compresses; elevate the extremity if swelling is present; monitor site for symptom resolution; teach parents, and child if old enough, these interventions.
5. Swelling, redness, and pain will decrease over the next 1 to 3 days.

Sufficient nutritional support in older children may be provided peripherally to allow protein sparing, but this is limited by nutrient concentrations and fluid volume (Ford, 1996). In younger children, the high amounts of protein and calories needed for growth necessitate prohibitively high fluid volumes for peripheral delivery. Even with calorie supplementation with fat emulsions, the full caloric needs of smaller children usually cannot be met by peripheral TPN (Ford, 1996). For these children, TPN infusion through a CVC is usually required.

Daily caloric requirements are calculated along with disease-specific needs when administering TPN. Caloric intake must be above the child's maintenance requirements (which are based on body weight) to allow for growth and any necessary healing. Caloric requirements are increased in many clinical situations, including burns,

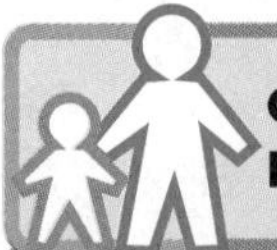

Chart 17–8
Developmental Considerations

Securing Venous Access Devices

Infants

After applying transparent dressing:

Coil catheter on top of or beside occlusive dressing and secure well with paper or clear tape.

Use only Luer-Lok equipment; tape all connections for additional security.

For child receiving home IV therapy; if infant is old enough to chew IV tubing, tunnel IV tubing under child's clothing and have it exit out the back of the child's garment.

Infants may require extra length of tubing to allow the IV pump to be out of reach of the crib/playpen and allow for crawling around.

Toddlers

The same considerations for infants applies to toddlers with one addition: If the toddler makes attempts at handling the catheter, the child may need to wear a tight fitting shirt with a catheter tape tab placed on the catheter and then pinned to the shirt. Another layer of clothing on top will prevent easy access to the catheter by the child.

School-Age Children

This age group can usually understand explanations regarding their catheter. It may be necessary to keep infusion pumps out of reach to prevent them from adjusting their IV rate. They may also need extra length tubing to allow them to engage in play activities without putting tension on the catheter. If developmental delays exist, consider the age at which the child is functioning for guidelines for securing their catheter.

Adolescents

There are no specific age-appropriate considerations, unless developmental delay is present. Consider age at which the adolescent is functioning for guidelines about securing the catheter.

Keegan-Wells, D., & Stewart, J.L. (1992). The use of venous access devices in pediatric oncology nursing practice. *Journal of Pediatric Oncology Nursing, 9*(4), 159–169. Reprinted with permission.

sepsis, major surgery or injury, cardiac dysfunction, fever, and chronic illness.

To balance nutrition during prolonged therapy and prevent fatty acid deficiency, IV fat solutions (lipids) are required. The younger the child, the more quickly fatty acid deficiency can occur. Sick newborns maintained on IV alimentation with no fat supplements develop changes indicative of fatty acid deficiency within the first week of life; changes occur in premature infants in 2 to 3 days (Ford, 1996).

Fat emulsions have a low osmolarity; therefore, they may help decrease the incidence of phlebitis associated with peripheral administration of solutions with high glucose concentrations. Administration of fat emulsions has been associated with detrimental effects, such as decreased pulmonary diffusion and peripheral oxygenation, bilirubin displacement from albumin, alteration in leukocyte function, hyperphospholipidemia, hypercholesterolemia, and changes in prostaglandin metabolism (Ford, 1996). Serum triglyceride levels must be monitored periodically in the child receiving IV fat emulsions.

Complications of Parenteral Nutrition

Possible complications of parenteral nutrition include all of those commonly seen in any form of IV therapy (see Chart 17–6). Sepsis is a constant danger. In addition, metabolic complications such as hyperglycemia and hypoglycemia, acidosis, calcium and phosphorus abnormalities, and trace metal deficiencies may occur (Hughes, 1996). Electrolyte and mineral levels, blood urea nitrogen (BUN), creatinine, liver enzymes, bilirubin, total protein, albumin, and a complete blood cell count are some of the values that should be monitored on a routine basis during prolonged therapy. Liver dysfunction is rare but does occur. The cause of this complication is not known.

Other complications are associated with too-rapid infusion of the TPN solution. These can include respiratory distress, nausea, and electrolyte imbalances.

Interdisciplinary Interventions

Care responsibilities for a child receiving parenteral nutrition include those for any child receiving IV therapy: site, catheter, and tubing care and close monitoring for signs of complications from the catheter (infiltration, occlusion, infection, phlebitis) and from the IV infusion (fluid and electrolyte imbalances, metabolic complications). Clean technique should be vigilantly maintained for catheter site and tubing care. TPN solutions provide an excellent medium for bacterial growth; thus, sterile technique must be maintained when preparing and administering these solutions.

The child's rate of growth is monitored by recording daily weights and evaluating growth on a standardized growth chart. Careful intake and output records are kept.

caREminder: *The TPN infusion rate should remain fairly constant to avoid glucose overload. The infusion rate should never be abruptly increased or decreased in an attempt to "even out" the infusion, unless otherwise ordered.*

Laboratory values are monitored according to institutional protocol, and abnormal results are noted and investigated. Monitoring serum glucose level is particularly important, because the child receiving TPN is adapting to a high glucose solution. Glucose monitoring can be done by serum laboratory values or by the Chemstrip method at the bedside.

The health care team promotes developmentally appropriate tasks that might be limited by restrictions imposed by long-term TPN infusions. For example, for a child learning to walk, tubing length may be increased (taking care that the child does not play with the tubing or become entangled in it) or a portable infusion pump can be used. Depending on the child's needs, parents, the nurse, a child life specialist, and a physical or occupational therapist may all be involved in promoting the child's physical and emotional development.

Consideration of the child and family's psychological needs is important in both hospital and home care situations. Lack of, or restrictions on, oral intake can be very frustrating for the child and family. Many social situations have eating as a focal point; to many parents, being able to feed their child is a central facet of being a "good" nuturing parent. All health team members should use principles of therapeutic communication when dealing with the child and family.

Children receiving TPN who have other medical needs may associate oral intake (stimulation) with uncomfortable procedures such as suctioning, nasogastric or orogastric tube insertion, or endotracheal intubation. This underscores the importance of providing positive oral experiences such as sucking on a pacifier for younger children or hard candy, if allowed, for older children. A proactive approach should be taken to prevent adverse psychosocial and developmental effects of prolonged restriction of oral intake during TPN therapy. The child should receive a program of oral stimulation, coordinated by the occupational therapist, as well as positive tactile and social stimulation during TPN infusion. The *oral stimulation program* promotes dealing with textures, tastes, and movement of food in the mouth and decreases aversive responses to the introduction of food. The program may include complete oral motor and feeding evaluation and may involve gum massage and oral motor exercises to promote muscle strengthening for specific muscle groups noted to have increased or decreased tone during assessment.

TIP 17–1 A Teaching Intervention Plan for the Family with a Child Requiring Home TPN

Nursing Diagnoses and Family Outcomes

- Risk for injury related to ongoing TPN infusion
  Outcome: Child will suffer no injury associated with TPN infusion
- Knowledge deficit: management of TPN therapy
  Outcome: Parents, caregivers, and the child, if old enough, will be knowledgeable about and appropriately manage home TPN

Interventions

Teach the parents, caregivers, and child as appropriate:

Safety Issues Regarding Child Health

- How to assess fluid balance
- Assessment for signs of electrolyte imbalance and infection

Safety Issues Regarding Child Development

- Use techniques to promote achievement of age-appropriate developmental milestones (e.g., place infant who is learning to crawl, or toddler learning to walk, on the floor with enough tubing to be mobile; monitor to prevent child chewing on, pulling on, or getting entangled in tubing; ensure close monitoring of a preschooler who is using scissors so the catheter or tubing is not inadvertently cut; involve school-agers and adolescents in their own care to promote independence).
- Stabilize infusion pumps and poles so they will not fall on child.
- Have plastic cover over pump controls so the child cannot change the infusion settings; turn pump face away from child so the lighted numbers are not tempting to play with (check pump settings frequently).
- Use developmentally appropriate methods to secure venous access device (see Chart 17–8).
- Often home TPN is cyclically delivered, usually during sleep time; encourage gross motor activity during infusion-free periods; if awake during infusion, limit activities to circumscribed areas and arrange quiet activities (e.g., doing homework at the kitchen table, watching television in the family room).
- Promote mealtimes as pleasant social events; encourage the entire family to eat together.

Other challenges associated with resumption of oral intake are also best addressed by anticipating them and taking a proactive approach. Because TPN provides all needed calories and nutrients, the child may not be hungry and may not want to eat. Parenteral nutritional support should be decreased as oral intake is increased. Intake should be monitored, but the focus should not be centered on how much is eaten, nor should the child be forced to eat. Mealtimes should be promoted as pleasant social situations. Ill children often have little control over situations; one situation in which they often can exert control is refusing to eat when allowed oral intake. Not focusing on the issue, offering as many choices as possible (e.g., type of food, where to eat, when to eat), and emphasizing control in other areas (which games to play, when to have rest periods) may help defuse the situation.

The dietitian should be involved in ensuring that TPN infusions are nutritionally complete and, along with the occupational therapist, should facilitate the transition to oral intake. If the child is experiencing discomfort related to an underlying disease process, adequate pain relief should be provided, to facilitate positive interactions during mealtime.

Home TPN Therapy

Teamwork is essential to ensure the successful administration of TPN therapy at home. Child, parent, and caregiver education is a major component of discharge planning. Social, financial, and medical issues need to be addressed. Parent and caregiver limitations must also be considered. If the child requires a continuing program of oral motor stimulation, parents may be taught what to do under the direction of a trained therapist in the area of

TIP 17–1 A Teaching Intervention Plan for the Family with a Child Requiring Home TPN *Continued*

Basic Emergency Measures

- General problem-solving techniques
- How to clamp the catheter if it breaks or becomes disconnected
- What to do if the infusion infuses too rapidly (slow infusion rate, monitor child, test blood glucose level, notify health care provider as listed below)
- Keep a list of emergency phone numbers posted by every phone in the house.
- Notify local electric and utility companies of the child's medical situation in case of a power outage.
- Pumps need to be plugged into a three-pronged outlet for grounding; an adaptor can be obtained from a hardware store if needed.

Safety Issues for Night TPN Infusion

- Adapt sleeping arrangements so the parents can hear and respond to pump alarms.
- Keep the path clear to the child's room to avoid parental injury from tripping over obstacles.

Management of TPN Therapy

- Review and observe return-demonstration on central line site and catheter care.
- Properly store supplies (clean, dry place away from high traffic areas; e.g., the kitchen counter is not a good place for storage) and parenteral solutions (keep in small cardboard box in top shelf of refrigerator to avoid anything spilling on them).
- Take a small bag of supplies (syringe heparin, tape, clamp, extra cap) when going away from home.
- Know procedure for initiating and maintaining the TPN infusion (visual inspection of solution, expiration date, clean technique, managing infusion device).

Contact Health Care Provider if

- Child develops signs of fluid or electrolyte imbalance or infection
- Catheter problems occur

oral-motor dysfunction (e.g., occupational or speech therapist).

Caregiver and child education should begin in the hospital as soon as the need is identified. Coordination between the hospital, the home care agency, and all caregivers is a priority when planning for discharge. Financial support is a major concern for many families. Social services personnel, the case manager, and others involved in discharge planning should help the family assess their financial and social support resources and provide assistance before the decision to discharge the child on parenteral nutrition. Care needs of the child with a chronic condition are discussed in Chapter 10. Home care needs are addressed in Chapter 11.

Children discharged on home TPN therapy and their parents have multiple teaching needs (TIP 17–1). Ongoing follow-up care is essential to assess knowledge and safe practice, as well as the effectiveness of the therapy.

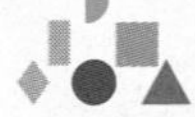

Alterations in Fluid and Electrolyte Balance

Fluid Imbalances

Dehydration

Dehydration occurs when fluid loss exceeds fluid intake. The primary cause can be an overall increase in fluids lost or a decreased intake. Dehydration can also result when fluid shifts occur and the fluid accumulates in a space outside ICF and ECF spaces, such as the abdominal cavity (a phenomenon sometimes called third spacing). Because fluid moves from the intravascular space, this shift results in intravascular fluid deficit and dehydration.

The body maintains equal osmolality between ICF and ECF compartments. Osmolality changes in one compartment lead to compensatory water shifts as the body attempts to restore equality of osmolality between compartments.

In adults, the greatest proportion of water is stored in the intracellular space. Therefore, water must shift out of the intracellular space into the extracellular space to be lost from the vascular volume. Children have a greater proportion of body water in the extracellular space (see Fig. 17–2), which makes it easier for water to be lost from the intravascular space. This is one of the reasons why children are more prone to dehydration than adults.

Gastrointestinal output, in the form of diarrhea and emesis, is the most common cause of dehydration in children. Worldwide, diarrheal disease is one of the leading causes of morbidity and mortality in children, causing 3 to 5 million deaths yearly (Pickering & Snyder, 1996). Each year in the United States, 20 to 35 million episodes of diarrhea occur in children younger than age 5, resulting in 400 to 500 deaths (Pickering & Snyder, 1996). Fever, increased respiratory rate, diuretics, hemorrhage, burns, and adrenal insufficiency can also lead to dehydration.

Assessment

Dehydration is classified as mild, moderate, or severe. Clinical manifestations depend on the type of dehydration, its cause, and the severity of fluid loss (Table 17–3). Infants and children are more susceptible to dehydration and may have more severe manifestations.

Types of dehydration include isotonic, hyponatremic (hypotonic), and hypernatremic (hypertonic). Classification is made based on the child's sodium level: 130 to 150 mEq/L in isotonic dehydration, below 130 mEq/L in hyponatremic dehydration, and above 150 mEq/L in hypernatremic dehydration (Behrman, Kliegman, & Arvin, 1996).

Isotonic dehydration occurs when sodium and water are lost in proportional amounts. The net result is a reduction in the circulating blood volume. The major fluid loss is from the ECF compartment, which in children is proportionally larger than the ICF compartment. Signs and symptoms may be similar to those of hypovolemic shock.

Hyponatremic dehydration, also commonly referred to as hypotonic dehydration, can result from either water retention or sodium loss. Defects in renal water excretion are almost always the cause of water retention, resulting in hyponatremia. Hypotonic dehydration can occur when sodium is lost with water but the net loss of fluid is replaced by hypotonic solutions, either orally or intravenously. This may occur with the use of formula diluted with water beyond manufacturer's recommendations or fluid replacement with electrolyte-free water. Because sodium is more abundant in the extracellular space, fluid in the intracellular space is normally hypotonic in relation to the extracellular space. In hypotonic dehydration, the

Table 17–3
Clinical Signs of Dehydration

	Severity		
Sign	Mild	Moderate	Severe
Loss of body weight	5%	5%–9%	>10%
Level of consciousness	Alert to restless, irritable	Restless to lethargic	Lethargic to comatose
Blood pressure	Normal	Normal; may be low when upright	Low
Heart rate	Normal	Increased	Increased
Pulse	Normal	Faint, thready	Unpalpable
Mucous membranes	May be dry	Dry	Dry, parched
Eyeballs, fontanelle	Normal	May be normal or sunken	Sunken
Skin turgor	May be normal	Poor	Poor; tenting
Skin temperature	Normal	Cool	Cool, mottled, cyanotic
Urine output	May be low (normal is 1–2 mL/kg/hr)	Low, concentrated, oliguric	Low, anuric

ICF becomes relatively more concentrated because the sodium in the extracellular compartment is diluted. Because water follows sodium, water shifts from the ECF to the ICF compartment.

The risk of hypotonic dehydration is increased in infants with immature renal function and those whose oral intake after diarrhea is treated with hypotonic or electrolyte-free solutions. The most common solutions erroneously used in these situations are water or sugar water. Clinical signs include those of poor skin turgor and vascular collapse: increased heart and respiratory rates, decreased blood pressure, and delayed capillary refill. Neurologic manifestations may occur as brain cells swell.

Hypernatremic dehydration is marked by elevated sodium levels in the ECF compartment. Thus, water shifts from the ICF to the ECF compartment in an effort to restore equality of osmolality. This significantly decreases intracellular volume, but clinical signs of fluid loss are not as apparent as in other types of dehydration, even in the presence of similar fluid loss, because the shifting of fluid into the extracellular space helps maintain vascular volume. Clinical manifestations of hypertonic dehydration include a dough-like feel to the skin, lethargy, irritability, and seizures. Neurologic signs are related to the decreased intracellular volume of brain cells.

Interdisciplinary Interventions

Dehydration with clinical manifestations calls for prompt fluid replacement. The priority intervention is to restore and maintain intravascular volume. Once this is accomplished, any remaining fluid and electrolyte deficit can be corrected by administering an appropriate solution at an appropriate rate. This solution is in addition to any normal maintenance fluids that the child needs.

Mild to moderate dehydration can be corrected with oral intake of fluids (Holliday, 1996). Moderate and severe dehydration may require intravenous (IV) fluid replacement therapy (Care Path 17–1). Indications for IV therapy to correct a fluid deficit include shock and impaired circulation, severe dehydration, uncontrollable vomiting, or inability to ingest oral fluids, as in lethargy, coma, or severe gastric distention (Behrman et al., 1996).

Isotonic solutions (never hypotonic solutions) should be used for initial rehydration therapy. (Hypotonic fluid shifts out of the extracellular space and so does not help restore vascular volume.)

Alert: *Using isotonic fluids is even more critical in children with hypernatremia, because hypotonic solutions cause water to move intracellularly into brain cells, causing cerebral edema, seizures, and profound neurologic sequelae. The rate of fluid replacement should also be*

Care Path 17–1 An Interdisciplinary Plan of Care for the Child with Moderately Severe Isotonic Dehydration

Nursing Diagnosis	Patient/Family Intermediate Outcomes		
	0–8 hr	**8–24 hr**	**Days 2–3**
Fluid volume deficit related to excessive gastrointestinal output	Child will regain adequate intravascular volume, will not demonstrate signs of shock (capillary refill >3 seconds, ↑ HR), will have urine output of at least 0.5–1 mL/kg/hr	Child will have fluid deficits replaced and maintenance fluid and electrolyte needs met.	Child will have maintenance fluid needs met and potassium deficits being corrected.
Altered nutrition: less than body requirements related to inability to ingest or retain nutrients	Child will have decrease in number of diarrhea/vomiting episodes. Child will tolerate small amounts of oral electrolyte solution.	Child will tolerate small amounts of oral electrolyte solution. Child will have nutritional status evaluated.	Child will tolerate oral feedings.
Alteration in skin integrity related to frequent diarrheal stools	Child will have perineal area cleaned immediately after stooling.	Child will not experience impaired perineal skin integrity or will show improvement if present.	⟶

Care Path continued on following page

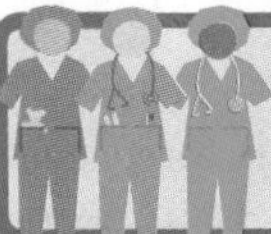

Care Path 17–1 An Interdisciplinary Plan of Care for the Child with Moderately Severe Isotonic Dehydration *Continued*

Nursing Diagnosis	Patient/Family Intermediate Outcomes		
	0–8 hr	**8–24 hr**	**Days 2–3**
Knowledge deficit: treatment regimen, signs of complications.	Child/family will be prepared for and state rationale for treatments, including IV or oral rehydrating regimen.	⟶	Child/parents will list signs of complications and when to notify health care provider.
Care Intervention Categories			
Consults	Social Services p.r.n. for family with great psychosocial support needs or who need help in identifying or accessing resources		
Labs	CBC, serum electrolytes, creatinine, BUN, urine specific gravity, stool C&S, O&P if diarrhea present		Serum electrolytes, creatinine, BUN p.r.n.
Medications and IVs	IV: start hourly maintenance fluid (add K^+ *after* child has voided); if signs of shock present, give 20 mL/kg fluid boluses until stable; *plus* replace one half of calculated fluid deficit *plus* replace ongoing fluid losses, if not tolerating oral rehydration. Give antimicrobial agents as indicated for infectious process.	IV: continue hourly maintenance fluid *plus* replace second half of calculated fluid deficit *plus* replace ongoing fluid losses, if not tolerating oral rehydration.	IV: maintenance fluid; discontinue when oral intake exceeds output
Monitors	Cardiorespiratory monitor if signs of shock present; discontinue when no signs of shock		
Nutrition	Oral maintenance electrolyte solution (Infalyte, Pedialyte) Continue breast-feeding if tolerated	⟶	Infants: continue breastfeeding or reintroduce formula. If diarrhea increases, dilute the formula or switch to a nonlactose formula. Older children: milk products if tolerated, starchy foods (avoid foods high in sugar or fat) Resume normal diet as tolerated.

Care Path 17–1 An Interdisciplinary Plan of Care for the Child with Moderately Severe Isotonic Dehydration *Continued*

Care Intervention Categories	0–8 hr	8–24 hr	Days 2–3
Play therapy/school	Age-appropriate diversional activities as child's activity level dictates	⟶	⟶
Safety and activity	Side rails up IV well-secured, monitor every hr Out of bed ad lib, as tolerated		
Vital signs/baseline parameters	HR, RR, BP, temperature on admission, hourly if signs of shock present; if no signs of shock, every 4 hr and p.r.n. Baseline weight Intake and output Assessment of hydration status	Vital signs q 4 hr Weight q 24 hr Intake and output	⟶
Tests	Urine specific gravity q 8 hr	⟶	⟶
Discharge planning/ teaching	Teach child/family about acute care regimen, procedures, and treatments. Evaluate for home care needs.	⟶ Review importance of good hand washing, especially if child has diarrhea.	Teach child/family about dietary restrictions and how long to continue; how to evaluate hydration status; signs of complications and when to notify health care provider; about how to avoid repeat episodes by early recognition of symptoms and prompt intervention to reduce severity of dehydration; when to follow up with health care provider. *Discharge when:* · Child has stable cardiovascular status and intake exceeds output · Parents state understanding of importance of maintaining oral intake and how to do so, of signs of complications and when to notify health care provider

ad lib, as desired; BP, blood pressure; BUN, blood urea nitrogen; CBC, complete blood count; C&S, culture and sensitivity; HR, heart rate; O&P, ova and parasites; p.r.n., as needed; RR, respiratory rate.

more gradual, over 48 hours rather than 24 hours, in the case of hypertonic dehydration (Finberg et al., 1993). When the sodium level falls too quickly, similar fluid shifts occur in the brain.

IV fluids should contain sodium when the serum sodium level is below normal limits. Common solutions include lactated Ringer's (LR), normal saline (NS), ½ NS, and ¼ NS. If the child is hemodynamically unstable, 20-mL/kg boluses of isotonic solutions should be given until vital signs indicate stability.

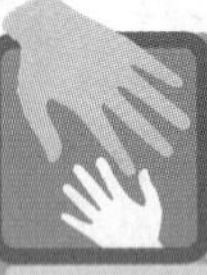

caREminder: *To avoid serious cardiac sequelae associated with hyperkalemia, potassium should not be added to IV fluids until the child has voided, demonstrating adequate renal function.*

Therapy, whether oral or IV, should continue until

- Vital signs are stable.
- Weight gain is steady.
- Adequate urine volume is present.
- Serum electrolytes are within normal limits.
- Acidosis, if present, has been corrected.

Nursing responsibilities when caring for a child with dehydration include initial assessment and ongoing monitoring (Chart 17–9). The underlying cause of the dehydration also should be investigated (Chart 17–10). The nurse assesses cardiac output by measuring blood pressure with the child in both the upright and supine positions. Lower blood pressure in the upright position may indicate a decrease in ECF volume. The nurse can expect the child to exhibit tachycardia as a compensatory measure to maintain cardiac output in the presence of decreased vascular volume. Assessing temperature is also important. Increased body temperatures can lead to increased respiratory rate and a resulting increase in metabolic needs. This can cause increased insensible fluid loss through skin and lungs.

Chart 17–9
Nursing Interventions Classification (NIC)

Fluid/Electrolyte Management

Definition

Regulation and prevention of complications from altered fluid and/or electrolyte levels

Activities

Monitor for abnormal serum electrolyte levels, as available.
Obtain laboratory specimens for monitoring of altered fluid or electrolyte levels (e.g., hematocrit, BUN, protein, sodium, and potassium levels), as appropriate.
Weigh daily and monitor trends.
Restrict free water intake in the presence of dilutional hyponatremia with serum Na level below 130 mEq per liter.
Give fluids, as appropriate.
Promote oral intake (e.g., provide oral fluids that are the patient's preference, place in easy reach, provide a straw, and provide fresh water), as appropriate.
Administer prescribed nasogastric replacement based on output, as appropriate.
Administer fiber as prescribed for the tube-fed patient to reduce fluid and electrolyte loss through diarrhea.
Minimize the number of ice chips consumed or amount of oral intake by patients with gastric tubes connected to suction.
Irrigate nasogastric tubes with normal saline.
Provide free water with tube feedings, as appropriate.
Set an appropriate intravenous infusion (or blood transfusion) flow rate.
Monitor laboratory results relevant to fluid balance (e.g., hematocrit, BUN, albumin, total protein, serum osmolality, and urine specific gravity levels).
Monitor laboratory results relevant to fluid retention (e.g., increased specific gravity, increased BUN, decreased hematocrit, and increased urine osmolality levels).
Monitor hemodynamic status, including CVP, MAP, PAP, and PCWP levels, if available.
Keep an accurate record of intake and output.
Monitor for signs and symptoms of fluid retention.
Institute fluid restriction, as appropriate.

Community Care

Oral fluid replacement therapy is commonly provided in the home care setting. Commercial oral solutions (e.g., WHO oral rehydration salts, Rehydralyte) contain water, electrolytes, bicarbonate or citrate, and glucose. Glucose is necessary to facilitate transport of sodium and water across the bowel wall (Acra & Ghishan, 1996).

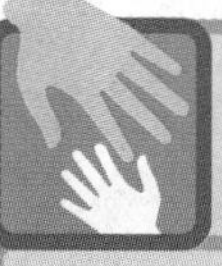

Worldview: *Oral rehydration therapy (ORT) is commonly used, particularly in developing countries, to treat diarrheal dehydration. ORT is simpler to implement than IV rehydration and effectively treats dehydration (Holliday, 1996). In developed countries, IV therapy is still commonly used to treat dehydration, probably because of the ease of access and established care patterns.*

Oral rehydration should be given frequently and in small amounts (TIP 17–2). When educating parents and other caregivers, the nurse needs to provide detailed, specific information on the type of fluids to give, how much to give, and how long to continue rehydration therapy.

Edema

Fluid movement between the vascular and interstitial compartment is regulated by hydrostatic pressure and osmotic pressure (see Chart 17–1). Edema, abnormal accumulation of fluid in the interstitial tissues, results from an imbalance in the physiologic forces that regulate fluid movement. This imbalance either causes excess fluid to enter the interstitial fluid compartment or causes excess fluid to remain in this compartment. Filtration, the movement of fluid across a semipermeable membrane that occurs across capillary beds, also influences the movement of fluid into the interstitium. Hypoproteinemia (low serum protein level), for instance, results in decreased oncotic pressure in the capillaries; thus, due to osmotic pressure, fluid shifts out of the vascular bed into the interstitial space, resulting in edema. In another example,

Chart 17–9
Nursing Interventions Classification (NIC) *Continued*

Fluid/Electrolyte Management

Activities

Monitor vital signs, as appropriate.
Correct preoperative dehydration, as appropriate.
Maintain intravenous solution containing electrolyte(s) at constant flow rate, as appropriate.
Monitor patient's response to prescribed electrolyte therapy.
Monitor for manifestations of electrolyte imbalance.
Provide prescribed diet appropriate for specific fluid or electrolyte imbalance (e.g., low sodium, fluid restricted, renal, and no added salt).
Monitor for side effects of prescribed supplemental electrolytes (e.g., GI irritation).
Assess patient's buccal membranes, sclera, and skin for indications of altered fluid and electrolyte balance (e.g., dryness, cyanosis, and jaundice).
Consult physician if signs and symptoms of fluid and/or electrolyte imbalance persist or worsen.
Administer prescribed supplemental electrolytes, as appropriate.
Administer prescribed electrolyte binding/excreting resins, as appropriate.
Institute measures to control excessive electrolyte loss (e.g., by resting the gut, changing type of diuretic, or administering antipyretics), as appropriate.
Institute measures to rest the bowel (e.g., restrict food or fluid intake and decrease intake of milk products), if appropriate.
Follow quick-acting glucose with long-acting carbohydrates and proteins for management of acute hypoglycemia, as appropriate.
Prepare patient for dialysis (e.g., assist with catheter placement for dialysis), as appropriate.
Monitor for fluid loss (e.g., bleeding, vomiting, diarrhea, perspiration, and tachypnea).
Promote a positive body image and self-esteem, if concerns are expressed as a result of excessive fluid retention, if appropriate.

From McCloskey, J., & Bulechek, G. (Eds.). (1996). *Nursing interventions classification (NIC)* (2nd ed.). St. Louis: Mosby–Year Book. Reprinted with permission.

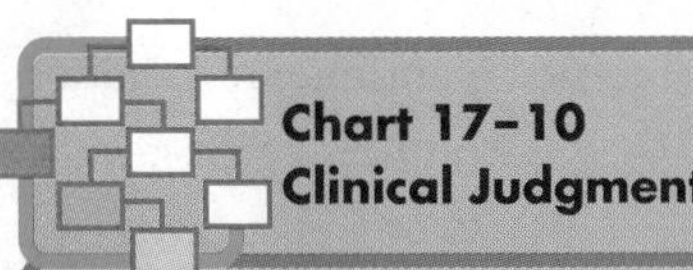

Chart 17–10
Clinical Judgment

A Dehydrated Infant

Ten-day-old Dan is brought to the clinic by his mother. She states that he is sleeping a lot, feeding poorly, and very fussy when awake. The nurse's physical assessment findings include

- Heart rate: 160 beats per minute
- Respiratory rate: 60 breaths per minute
- Capillary refill: 2 seconds
- Skin and mucous membranes: dry
- Abdominal skin remains raised for 2 seconds after being pinched
- Fontanelle: sunken
- Weight: 3.5 kg

Questions

1. What questions should the nurse ask the mother?
2. What signs and symptoms indicate dehydration?
3. What is the problem? How severe is it?
4. What interventions should be implemented?
5. What follow-up is appropriate?

Answers

1. How many wet diapers has the baby had in the past 24 hours? (three)
   How much stool? (no change in stooling patterns—about 3/24 hours)
   Any fever? (no)
   Is the baby breast or bottle fed? If bottle fed what type and how is formula prepared? For any feeding method: How often does the baby eat? How much? (Dan is breast fed three to four times in 24 hours, 10 minutes each side is attempted; he latches intermittently during feeding; mother complains of sore, cracked, bleeding nipples)
   What did the baby weigh at birth? (3.8 kg)
2. Three wet diapers in past 24 hours; normal is six to eight. Increased heart rate, respiratory rate, delayed capillary refill, dry skin and mucous membranes, poor skin turgor, sunken fontanelle, behavior changes. Only three to four feedings per 24 hours; normally should nurse 10 to12 times in 24 hours.
3. Dehydration secondary to poor feeding. Dan has lost 0.3 kg since birth. He is moderately dehydrated.

   $$\frac{3.5}{3.8} = 0.92 = 92\% \text{ of birth weight} = 8\% \text{ weight (fluid) loss}$$

4. The dehydration needs to be addressed while supporting continued breast-feeding, if possible. Have mother breast-feed Dan and observe latch, suck, and swallow for problems. Supplement with formula as needed. Review breast-feeding techniques with mother. Instruct mother to breast-feed every 2 to 3 hours around the clock; call health care provider if Dan does not have six to eight wet diapers in 24 hours, if increasing lethargy, or if he does not eat well (if poor breast-feeding and then refuses supplemental formula).
5. Return to clinic tomorrow to ensure Dan has sufficient intake, as evidenced by weight gain, voiding six to eight times in 24 hours, normal vital signs and capillary refill, good skin turgor, moist mucous membranes, decreased fussiness, and sleepiness. Observe feeding technique, refer to lactation consultant if problems continue with breast-feeding.

increased fluid in the blood vessels causes vascular congestion. As a result, fluid leaks from the vessels, across the capillary membrane, and into the interstitial space, causing edema.

Edema can be local or generalized throughout the body. Severe edema in all body tissues is known as anasarca.

Various physiologic conditions influence the formation of edema. A primary cause is renal dysfunction that influences sodium reabsorption and retention. Administration of corticosteroids also can cause sodium retention and subsequent edema formation. Liver dysfunction (which often causes hypoproteinemia) and cerebral edema caused by infection, trauma, or a vascular condi-

TIP 17–2 A Teaching Intervention Plan for Home Management of the Dehydrated Child

Nursing Diagnoses and Family Outcomes

- Fluid volume deficit related to effects of increased fluid losses or needs or of decreased intake
  Outcomes: The child will maintain vascular volume as evidenced by normal heart rate and blood pressure.
  The child will have urine output of at least 1 mL/kg/hr.
- Knowledge deficit: management of dehydration
  Outcome: The child's parents will verbalize understanding of the treatment of episodes of vomiting and diarrhea and state methods to manage fluid loss at home.

Interventions

Teach the child and parents:

- Signs of dehydration (decreased urine output, dry mucous membranes, lack of tears, sunken eyeballs or fontanelle, change in level of consciousness)
- *Not* to use boiled skim milk or other concentrated solutions because they contain too much salt
- *Not* to use home remedies (decarbonated soda, Jell-O, fruit juice, tea) because they usually have low sodium concentrations, which can cause hyponatremia, and have inappropriately high osmolality from excessive carbohydrates, which can exacerbate diarrhea
- Proper methods of diluting infant formula; not to overdilute to make more formula
- The importance of good hand washing, particularly in the presence of infectious diseases
- Components of
  1. *Oral rehydration therapy (ORT)* to replace existing losses
  2. *Maintenance therapy* to replace continuing losses after ORT is completed combined with adequate dietary intake

Type of Solution to Use:

- *ORT:* rehydrating solutions are available commercially in the United States (e.g., Rehydralyte); worldwide the World Health Organization provides an oral rehydration solution (ORS); lower sodium solutions, as used in the maintenance phase, should *not* be used as rehydrating solutions
- *Maintenance:* solutions with lower sodium concentrations (e.g., Infalyte, Pedialyte) are used to prevent hypernatremia associated with lower fluid volume intake during this phase.

Amount of Solution to Give:

- ORT for mild dehydration 50 mL/kg over 4 hours; for moderate dehydration 100 mL/kg over 6 hours
- For children younger than age 2, give 4 oz; if older than age 2, give 4 to 8 oz, slowly every hour, divided into small amounts every 15 to 20 minutes.
- If vomiting occurs, give 1 to 2 teaspoons every few minutes until vomiting stops, then give 4 to 8 oz of ORT as above; continue to repeat unless emesis consistently occurs in an amount that exceeds the intake
- Increase the amount of solution if diarrhea continues or symptoms of dehydration continue
- Decrease the amount of solution if the child appears well hydrated or periorbital edema develops
- Breast-feeding or oral feedings should be resumed as soon as possible
- Stop giving ORT when hydration is normal
- Maintenance therapy of 150 mL/kg/24 hours plus 10 mL/kg for each stool and 2 mL/kg with each emesis

TIP continued on following page

TIP 17–2 A Teaching Intervention Plan for Home Management of the Dehydrated Child *Continued*

Contact Health Care Provider if

- The amount or frequency of vomiting or diarrhea is increasing
- Diarrhea or vomiting does not improve after 24 hours of treatment
- The child appears worse (decreased level of consciousness, decreasing urine output, becomes dizzy when upright, increased fever, seizures)
- The child's fluid status does not improve (no urine output within 8 hours, tongue and cheeks do not become moist, no tears with crying)
- The child refuses to eat or is unable to ingest more solution than is vomited

Data from Behrman, Kliegman, & Arvin, 1996; Straughn & English, 1996.

tion are a challenge to manage in the presence of any coexisting cardiovascular compromise.

Assessment

Excess fluid in the ECF compartment can be detected through a rapid gain in body weight. As discussed earlier, daily weighing is a vital part of the focused physical assessment for a child with altered fluid and electrolyte status. Parents may be the first to note a child's unusual weight gain by observing that his or her clothes suddenly do not fit.

caREminder: *One kilogram of body weight equals the weight of 1 L of water; thus, the amount of fluid gain or loss can be calculated from weight gain or loss.*

Edema in a child usually occurs first in dependent areas (the sacrum, ankles, and feet) or in the periorbital area. Pitting edema is observed when finger pressure exerted on an area leaves an indentation once that pressure is removed. This commonly occurs in significant generalized edema.

Other physical signs of edema include a bounding pulse and hepatomegaly (enlarged liver). In the presence of respiratory distress, crackles can be heard on auscultation of the lungs. Distended neck veins may be visible in an older child assessed in a supine or semi-Fowler position.

Nursing Diagnoses and Outcomes

In addition to the nursing diagnoses listed in Chart 17–4, the following may be applicable to the child with edema:

- **Fluid volume excess related to effects of disease process or treatment, inability to excrete fluid, osmolality imbalance**
  Outcomes: The child will have symptoms of respiratory distress, as evidenced by increased respiratory rate, retractions, nasal flaring, and cyanosis of nail beds and mucous membranes recognized promptly and treatment initiated.
  The child will maintain baseline weight, without rapid gain from fluid excess, and will demonstrate slow long-term weight gain along his or her growth curve.
- **Risk for impaired skin integrity related to easily friable skin**
  Outcomes: The child will have intact skin, without any evidence of breakdown.
  Interventions will be implemented to prevent tissue breakdown at pressure sites and dependent areas.
- **Impaired physical mobility related to restriction of normal range of motion**
  Outcomes: The child will maintain maximum range of motion while edema is present.
  The child will remain as independent as possible within the limits set by the edema.
- **Body image disturbance is related to perception of the edema**
  Outcomes: The child will verbalize acceptance of his or her physical appearance.
  The child will continue to have social interactions with peers, consistent with his or her age and developmental milestones.
- **Knowledge deficit: care of the child with edema**
  Outcomes: The child and parents will demonstrate an

understanding of cause of edema and of all tests and procedures.

The parents will provide care to their child, including providing appropriate nutritional intake and preventing the sequelae of edema such as skin breakdown.

The child will provide self-care, as appropriate.

Interdisciplinary Interventions

Interventions for the child with edema focus on determining and treating the underlying cause. Diuretic administration may be ordered to promote renal excretion of water and sodium and help remove excess fluid. Diuretics are indicated in children with pulmonary edema, increased cerebral edema, generalized edema, hypertension, or renal dysfunction. Serum potassium levels must be carefully monitored if a potassium-wasting diuretic is administered.

Nursing care of the child with severe edema requires strict and accurate monitoring of intake and output. Discrepancies between intake and output must be noted and discussed with the health care team. The child should be weighed each day. Weighing should be done at the same time of day, on the same scale, and with the child wearing the same amount of clothing.

caREminder: *Daily weight is compared with previous measurements, and trends are noted. If a significant weight gain occurs, the child should be assessed for other signs of fluid retention, such as rales or periorbital or dependent edema.*

Edematous tissue is easily injured and must be protected. A child with limited mobility needs regular position changes. Low-pressure mattresses and other devices that help reduce the pressure on dependent areas should be used when needed. Elevating areas of localized edema promotes increased venous and lymphatic drainage of interstitial fluid. The child's skin must be kept clean and dry, and all pressure areas should be inspected for signs of breakdown at least daily.

Ensuring appropriate nutritional intake is important and can be a challenge in the child who must receive a minimal amount of fluids but has high caloric needs. Daily calorie counts should be recorded. A dietitian can help devise meal plans that provide all necessary nutrients and are appealing to the child.

The child life specialist, social worker, nurse, parent, and other supportive personnel can help the child deal with any distortions of his or her normal body image. This can be a major issue to the child or adolescent with severe edema. Including on-site school personnel and the child's regular teacher in the plan of care can be beneficial. They may be able to provide routine, normalizing experiences for the child.

Parents and siblings, as appropriate, should be taught about disease management, administration of medications and side effects, skin care, positioning, and promoting appropriate nutritional intake.

Acid-Base Imbalances

Regulation and maintenance of acid-base balance is essential to the action of vital hormones, enzymes, and all basic physiologic functions. Normal acid-base balance is maintained through the interaction of a complex system of buffers, respiratory compensation, and the metabolic component of kidney function. When an alteration occurs, the body mobilizes these physiologic mechanisms to restore normal acid-base balance.

A buffer is a weak acid. It can facilitate a change in the pH of the blood when a stronger acid or base is added. The body's most effective buffer is the bicarbonate/carbonic acid system. Other effective buffers include proteins, hemoglobin, and phosphates.

In normal metabolism, all cells produce carbonic acid (H_2CO_3) and metabolic acids. Carbonic acid is excreted by the lungs in the form of carbon dioxide (CO_2). Metabolic acids are excreted through the kidneys. The effectiveness of the bicarbonate and carbonic acid buffering systems can be measured in the arterial blood gas values of pH, CO_2, and bicarbonate (HCO_3). See Table 16–4 for more information on these values.

Alterations in acid-base homeostasis are classified as either metabolic or respiratory, based on their cause. The imbalance is termed *respiratory* when it is primarily caused by a change in the partial pressure of carbon dioxide in arterial blood ($PaCO_2$); imbalances resulting from all other primary changes are classified as *metabolic*. An abnormally low pH is called *acidosis*, or acidemia. An abnormally high pH is termed *alkalosis*, or alkalemia. Severe acidosis (pH <7.0) and severe alkalosis (pH >7.55 with a HCO_3 >28) are life threatening if not corrected.

Respiratory compensation can be affected within minutes by any change in respiratory pattern. Any clinical condition that affects the respiratory system can also have an impact on respiratory compensation. If a child's respiratory rate is too slow or too shallow, CO_2 will increase, serum pH can decrease, and acidosis may occur. If a child's respiratory rate is too rapid, CO_2 will decrease, serum pH may increase, and alkalosis can occur.

The renal system regulates the excretion of hydrogen ions and bicarbonate (HCO_3). This compensatory mechanism is a slow, long-term response that can take days to restore acid-base balance.

Acid-base disorders are common in children. The causes are varied and cover a wide range of clinical conditions and exogenous pathologic processes. Arterial blood gas and serum electrolyte values are essential to diagnosing the imbalance's origin (metabolic or respiratory) and devising an effective plan of care.

Metabolic Acidosis

Possible causes of metabolic acidosis include hypovolemia, congenital heart disease, sepsis, cold stress, and inborn errors of metabolism. Acidosis affects the metabolism of all cells. It has the most significant effects on the cardiovascular and respiratory systems. When the pH is below 7.2, cardiac contractility is reduced. Blood pressure falls, dysrhythmias can occur, and collapse of the cardiovascular system typically follows.

Urine pH can be valuable to assess whether the renal compensatory mechanism is functioning. In metabolic acidosis, urine pH less than 6.0 indicates that the renal system is reabsorbing HCO_3 and excreting hydrogen ions, and thus compensation is occurring. Renal compensatory mechanisms to correct acidosis help protect the cells but do not change the underlying cause of the disorder.

Metabolic Alkalosis

Hydrogen ion loss, such as occurs with vomiting or nasogastric suctioning or HCO_3 retention from administration of sodium bicarbonate, massive blood transfusion, or milk-alkali syndrome (chronic ingestion of milk and antacids containing calcium carbonate, which generates HCO_3) may result in metabolic alkalosis.

The child with metabolic alkalosis may be asymptomatic or show signs similar to dehydration. Alkalotic tetany or hypertonicity may occur. The muscle hyperto-

Chart 17–11
Nursing Interventions Classification (NIC)

Acid-Base Monitoring

Definition

Collection and analysis of patient data to regulate acid-base balance

Activities

Draw ABGs, ensuring adequate circulation to the extremity before and after blood withdrawal.
Place ABGs on ice, as appropriate, and send to the lab.
Note patient's temperature and percent of oxygen administered at time of drawing ABG.
Note if arterial pH level is on the alkaline or acidotic side of the mean (7.4).
Note if $PaCO_2$ level shows respiratory acidosis, respiratory alkalosis, or normalcy.
Note if the HCO_3 level shows metabolic acidosis, metabolic alkalosis, or normalcy.
Examine the pH level in conjunction with the $PaCO_2$ and HCO_3 levels to determine whether the acidosis/alkalosis is compensated or uncompensated.
Note the PaO_2, SaO_2, and Hgb levels to determine the adequacy of arterial oxygenation.
Monitor end-tidal CO_2 level, as appropriate.
Monitor for an increase in the anion gap (>14 mEq/L), signaling an increased production or decreased excretion of acid products.
Monitor for signs and symptoms of HCO_3 deficit and metabolic acidosis: Kussmaul respirations, weakness, disorientation, headache, anorexia, coma, urinary pH level of <6, plasma HCO_3 level of <22 mEq/L, plasma pH level of <7.35, BE of <−2 mEq/L, associated hyperkalemia, and possible CO_2 deficit.
Monitor for causes of possible HCO_3 deficit, such as diarrhea, renal failure, tissue hypoxia, lactic acidosis, diabetic ketoacidosis, malnutrition, and salicylate overdose.
Administer oral or parenteral HCO_3 agents, if appropriate.
Administer prescribed insulin and potassium for treatment of diabetic ketoacidosis, as appropriate.
Monitor for signs and symptoms of HCO_3 excess and metabolic alkalosis: numbness and tingling of the extremities, muscular hypertonicity, shallow respirations with pause, bradycardia, tetany, urinary pH level of >7, plasma HCO_3 level of >26 mEq/L, plasma pH level of >7.45, BE of >2 mEq/L, associated hypokalemia, and possible CO_2 retention.
Monitor for possible causes of HCO_3 excess, such as vomiting, gastric suction, hyperaldosteronism, diuretic therapy, hypochloremia, and excessive ingestion of medications containing HCO_3.

nicity is secondary to alkalosis, which causes decreased ionized calcium.

Respiratory Acidosis

Respiratory acidosis results from events that depress the respiratory drive or interfere with ventilation (air moving in and out of the lungs), such as pulmonary diseases (e.g., pneumonia, asthma), central nervous system (CNS) disorders that affect the neuromuscular system (e.g., muscular dystrophy, Guillain-Barré syndrome, tumors, botulism), and ingestion of substances (e.g., opiates, barbiturates, alcohol). The result is a retention of CO_2 and a decrease in pH.

Hypoxia is a factor often seen in respiratory acidosis that can initiate and exacerbate the symptoms. CO_2 causes vasodilation. In addition to a red flush to the skin, vasodilation in the brain results in CNS signs. CNS disorders may depress the respiratory drive, and the associated muscle weakness may make ventilation ineffective. Chemical ingestion may also depress the respiratory drive.

Respiratory Alkalosis

The most common cause of respiratory alkalosis is hyperventilation (fast and deep breaths that excrete CO_2). Factors contributing to hyperventilation can include hypoxia, sepsis, anxiety, ingestions, and pulmonary disease (e.g., pneumonia, chronic lung disease).

Interdisciplinary Interventions

The goal of treatment for a child with an acid-base disorder is to correct the primary cause, such as administering oxygen and improving ventilation in a child who is hypoxic or administering insulin and fluid to a child with diabetic ketoacidosis. Most children who are acidotic and who have adequate circulation, renal function, and pulmonary function can be managed by treating the

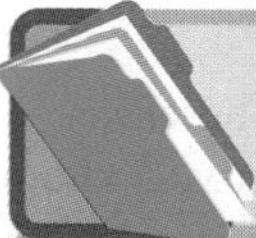

Chart 17–11
Nursing Interventions Classification (NIC) *Continued*

Acid-Base Monitoring

Activities

Teach patient to avoid excessive use of medications containing HCO_3, as appropriate.
Administer pharmacological agents to replace chloride, as appropriate.
Monitor for signs and symptoms of carbonic acid deficit and respiratory alkalosis: frequent sighing and yawning, tetany, paresthesia, muscular twitching, palpitations, tingling and numbness, dizziness, blurred vision, diaphoresis, dry mouth, convulsions, pH level of >7.45, $PaCO_2$ <35 mm Hg, associated hyperchloremia, and possible HCO_3 deficit.
Monitor for possible causes of carbonic acid deficits and associated hyperventilation, such as pain, CNS lesions, fever, and mechanical ventilation.
Sedate patient to reduce hyperventilation, if appropriate.
Administer pain medication, as appropriate.
Treat fever, as appropriate.
Administer parenteral chloride solutions to reduce HCO_3, while correcting the cause of respiratory alkalosis, as appropriate.
Monitor for signs and symptoms of carbonic acid excess and respiratory acidosis: hand tremor with extensions of arms, confusion, drowsiness progressing to coma, headache, slowed verbal response, nausea, vomiting, tachycardia, warm sweaty extremities, pH level of <7.35, $PaCO_2$ level of >45 mm Hg, associated hypochloremia, and possible HCO_3 excess.
Monitor for possible causes of carbonic acid excess and respiratory acidosis, such as airway obstruction, depressed ventilation, CNS depression, neurological disease, chronic lung disease, musculoskeletal disease, chest trauma, infection, ARDS, cardiac failure, and use of respiratory depressant drugs.
Support ventilation and airway patency in the presence of respiratory acidosis and rising $PaCO_2$ level, as appropriate.
Administer oxygen therapy, as appropriate.
Administer microbial agents and bronchodilators, as appropriate.
Administer low flow oxygen and monitor for CO_2 narcosis, in cases of chronic hypercapnia.

From McCloskey, J., & Bulechek, G. (Eds.). (1996). *Nursing interventions classification (NIC)* (2nd ed.). St. Louis: Mosby–Year Book. Reprinted with permission.

underlying cause of the acid-base imbalance. Many do not require alkali therapy such as with sodium bicarbonate (Finberg et al., 1993). If alkali therapy is used, dosage should always be based on measured serum bicarbonate levels (Behrman et al., 1996).

Alert: *It is imperative to correct any low blood pressure along with the acidosis that is present. Together, they present a life-threatening situation. Complete collapse of the cardiovascular and respiratory systems may be imminent.*

Nursing responsibilities include monitoring the child's status and adequacy of ventilation, including vital signs: heart rate and rhythm, respiration, blood pressure, and temperature (Chart 17–11). Maintaining a clear airway and ensuring adequate ventilation are other care priorities.

caREminder: *Observe the child's work of breathing and auscultate the lungs. Assess for actual air movement along with respiratory effort. Assist the child with positioning for maximum ventilation and minimum effort by elevating the head of the bed and not letting the child slouch, which will interfere with diaphragmatic excursion. Administer oxygen and perform suctioning, if necessary. Provide manual ventilation if the child does not appear to have adequate respiratory effort.*

If a child requires mechanical ventilation, the nurse and respiratory therapist must collaborate to perform frequent evaluation of ventilator settings. One iatrogenic cause of respiratory alkalosis is overventilation. Ongoing monitoring should include the appropriateness of ventilator parameters, the adequacy of ventilation, and the child's response to changes that are made.

caREminder: *Vital signs can be affected by anxiety as a result of being placed in an unfamiliar environment and the presence of unusual activity.*

The nurse compares vital signs to those obtained previously and observes for trends that indicate improvement or deterioration in the child's status. A normal temperature should be the goal, because body temperature alterations (hypothermia and hyperthermia) increase metabolic demands and cause further deterioration of acid-base balance. A child with hypothermia should be warmed with blankets and an external warming source, if necessary. A child with hyperthermia should have no bedcovers, or only a light cover, and the room temperature should be lowered, if possible. Antipyretics, such as acetaminophen and ibuprofen, may be ordered to decrease fever and thus decrease metabolic demands.

The nurse continuously monitors the child for changes in level of consciousness. Laboratory values are monitored closely, with the findings interpreted in light of the child's condition, and changes made in the treatment regimen accordingly. Findings that do not fall within normal parameters for the child's age or significant changes should be reported to the medical team.

Intake and output are carefully monitored. Parents and other family members that stay with the child can aid the nurse in obtaining this information. The method of fluid administration depends on the child's physical condition, level of consciousness, and age. The physician will order IV therapy, if indicated.

Electrolyte Imbalances

The body maintains a delicate balance of electrolytes, all which contribute to homeostasis and healthy functioning. Electrolyte imbalance has many causes. More than one electrolyte imbalance may occur simultaneously in a child in the clinical setting. It is important to assess all electrolytes and address each imbalance to provide complete, comprehensive treatment of the child.

Sodium Imbalance

Sodium is the principal cation in ECF. Therefore, it exerts the greatest proportion of ECF osmolarity. Sodium influences distribution of body water and helps maintain acid-base balance and neuromuscular function.

Hyponatremia

Hyponatremia is defined as a serum sodium level below 130 mEq/L. Clinical symptoms are more severe with a level below 120 mEq/L.

A variety of situations can cause hyponatremia that results in either a net sodium loss or net water excess. Net sodium loss can result from increased gastrointestinal output such as diarrhea, vomiting, nasogastric suction (a major cause of hyponatremia in children), diuretic therapy, excessive diaphoresis, and kidney disease. Net water excess can be caused by dilutional hyponatremia or sodium deprivation that results from increased water intake with a decreased sodium intake, administration of hypotonic IV solutions, administration of excessively diluted formulas, or syndrome of inappropriate antidiuretic hormone secretion (SIADH).

Important factors in the development of symptoms include the rate of the declining sodium level and the duration of the low level. Severe hyponatremia that occurs rapidly over a few hours is called *water intoxication* (Finberg et al., 1993). Neurologic consequences result from a too-rapid change in sodium balance, which causes massive fluid shifts into the cerebral space. The cranium of a child with a closed fontanelle is a fixed space. Normal cerebral contents (brain, cerebrospinal fluid, blood) occupy part of that space. Shifting of excess fluid into the cerebral compartment causes cerebral edema, which can produce seizures, coma, respiratory arrest, and brain damage (Chart 17–12).

Interdisciplinary Interventions

Treatment of hyponatremia varies depending on the cause. The low serum sodium level should be raised in a slow and controlled manner and then maintained within normal limits.

caREminder: *Hyponatremia can be prevented in the child receiving IV fluids by not infusing hypotonic solutions unless indicated by a documented elevated serum sodium level.*

When a net loss of sodium and body water is present, oral or IV sodium and fluid replacement may be ordered by the physician. Nursing assessments and interventions are similar to those for children with hyponatremic dehydration to prevent or treat hypovolemic shock. When a net water excess is present, treatment is directed toward reducing the ECF and ICF excess. This may involve water restriction or diuretic therapy. Nursing assessment and interventions are similar to those for the child with fluid overload and edema.

The nurse is responsible for implementing treatment, monitoring the child's response, and providing child and family teaching. Nursing care should include a close observation and documentation of the child's intake, output, and fluid balance.

Community Care

If hyponatremia is due to an excessive oral fluid intake, either directly or through diluted formula, it is important to assess the family's socioeconomic status. Parents experiencing financial hardship may dilute formula to make it last longer. They may not understand that prolonged feeding of overdiluted formula can lead to harmful consequences for their child. Basic education on formula preparation and delivery can help such families. Dietitians and social service case workers can also provide valuable assistance and resources to families in need.

Hypernatremia

Hypernatremia is a serum sodium level exceeding 150 mEq/L. The most severe clinical manifestations of hypernatremia occur when the serum sodium level exceeds 160 mEq/L.

Hypernatremia results from insufficient fluid intake or excessive fluid loss or from excessive salt intake or insufficient sodium excretion. This can be caused by an altered thirst mechanism or an inability to respond to thirst (as may occur, for example, in infants and disabled or comatose children), increased insensible water loss, increased gastrointestinal output, excessive solute intake (e.g., from incorrectly diluted formulas, boiled skim milk), renal immaturity (e.g., in premature infants), or such disorders as diabetes insipidus or renal medullary impairment.

Children with hypernatremia are almost always dehydrated (Finberg et al., 1993). Cellular dehydration results when water shifts out of the ICF, pulled by the now hyperosmolar ECF. Children with hypernatremia often do not have circulatory disturbances, because of the relative increase in vascular volume that occurs as fluid is pulled from the ICF into the ECF. Neurologic manifestations result when cerebral vessels shrink and tear as cellular dehydration occurs. The outcome is often a cerebral hemorrhage. Neurologic signs in children with hypernatremia may also include lethargy with irritability on stimulation and a high-pitched cry. Irritability may be a worrisome clinical sign, possibly indicating a cerebrovascular injury.

Interdisciplinary Interventions

The primary goals in treating hypernatremia are to restore adequate hydration and to bring the serum sodium level down to normal gradually, allowing the child's body to adjust to the change. A too-rapid change in sodium level can disrupt the cell membranes in the cerebral vessels, possibly causing cerebral hemorrhage. If fluid is replaced too rapidly, water quickly crosses into brain cells (sodium levels decrease more slowly because of the blood-brain barrier), causing swelling of the brain cells and increased intracranial pressure, a dangerous condition. Replacement of fluid deficit in hypernatremia should be done over at least 48 hours, to reduce the risk of increased intracranial pressure (Finberg et al., 1993). Fluid boluses of 20 mg/kg may be administered to a child in shock, however (see Chapter 30).

After fluid replacement therapy is initiated, the focus shifts to determining and treating the underlying cause of hypernatremia. Obtaining a complete nursing history helps evaluate the onset of clinical symptoms. This includes the child's normal weight and a dietary history, including the amount and types of intake and output. The nurse also records the child's daily weight and compares it with previous weights, to monitor fluid balance.

The nurse also monitors laboratory data, reporting any significant findings to the physician. Other nursing responsibilities may include administering prescribed IV fluids with the appropriate sodium content. The child with an altered level of consciousness should be positioned in the upright or side-lying position to allow for adequate ventilation and to decrease the risk of aspiration.

A nutrition consultation can help provide the optimum electrolyte concentration and the maximum calories

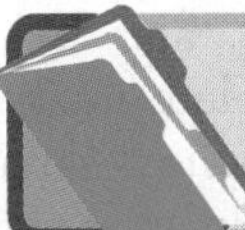

Chart 17–12
Nursing Interventions Classification (NIC)

Electrolyte Monitoring

Definition

Collection and analysis of patient data to regulate electrolyte balance

Activities

Monitor the serum level of electrolytes.
Monitor serum albumin and total protein levels, as indicated.
Monitor for associated acid-base imbalances.
Identify possible causes of electrolyte imbalances.
Recognize and report presence of electrolyte imbalances.
Monitor for fluid loss and associated loss of electrolytes, as appropriate.
Monitor for Chvostek and/or Trousseau sign.
Monitor for neurological manifestation of electrolyte imbalance (e.g., altered sensorium and weakness).
Monitor adequacy of ventilation.
Monitor serum and urine osmolality levels.
Monitor EKG tracings for changes related to abnormal K, Ca, and Mg levels.
Note changes in peripheral sensation, such as numbness and tremors.
Note muscle strength.
Monitor for nausea, vomiting, and diarrhea.
Identify treatments that can alter electrolyte status, such as GI suctioning, diuretics, antihypertensives, and calcium channel blockers.
Monitor for underlying medical disease that can lead to electrolyte imbalance.
Monitor for signs and symptoms of hypokalemia: muscular weakness, cardiac irregularities (PVC), prolonged QT interval, flattened or depressed T wave, depressed ST segment, presence of U wave, paresthesia, decreased reflexes, anorexia, decreased GI motility, dizziness, confusion, increased sensitivity to digitalis, and depressed respirations.
Monitor for signs/symptoms of hyperkalemia: irritability, restlessness, anxiety, nausea, vomiting, abdominal cramps, weakness, flaccid paralysis, circumoral numbness and tingling, tachycardia progressing to bradycardia, ventricular tachycardia/fibrillation, tall peaked T waves, flattened P wave, broad slurred QRS complex, and heart block progressing to asystole.

for the prescribed volume of fluid intake, whether administered orally or intravenously.

Potassium Imbalance

The primary intracellular ion, potassium (K^+) plays a major role in neuromuscular excitability. The ratio of intracellular potassium to extracellular potassium is a major determinant of cell membrane resting potential. Potassium also participates in cell metabolism through its action in protein and glycogen synthesis. Potassium is absorbed from the intestines and excreted in urine, feces, and sweat.

Blood pH affects serum potassium levels. When acidosis occurs, hydrogen ions (H^+) increase in number and are distributed equally in body compartments. To maintain electroneutrality, as H^+ moves into the cell, K^+ moves out of the cell. The result is an elevated serum potassium level with a concomitant decrease in serum pH.

caREminder: *If acidosis persists, total body potassium may be depleted even though the serum potassium level is elevated, because potassium is moving out of the ICF where it is most abundant.*

With alkalosis, this shift is reversed and changes in potassium levels are less pronounced.

Hypokalemia

Defined as serum potassium level below 3.5 mEq/L, hypokalemia has many possible causes. These include inadequate potassium intake and excessive renal potassium loss, as often occurs in a child receiving diuretic therapy.

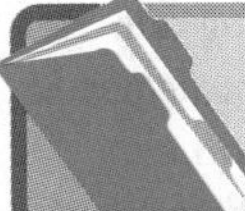

Chart 17–12
Nursing Interventions Classification (NIC) *Continued*

Electrolyte Monitoring

Activities

Monitor for signs/symptoms of hyponatremia: disorientation, muscle twitching, nausea and vomiting, abdominal cramps, headaches, seizures, lethargy and withdrawal, and coma
Monitor for signs and symptoms of hypernatremia: extreme thirst; fever; dry, sticky mucous membranes; altered mentation; seizures
Monitor for signs and symptoms of hypocalcemia: irritability, muscle tetany, muscle cramps, decreased cardiac output, prolonged ST segment and QT interval, bleeding, and fractures.
Monitor for signs and symptoms of hypercalcemia: deep bone pain, excessive thirst, anorexia, lethargy, weakened muscles, shortened QT segment, wide T wave, widened QRS complex, and prolonged PR interval.
Monitor for signs and symptoms of hypomagnesemia: respiratory muscle depression, mental apathy, confusion, facial tics, spasticity, and cardiac dysrhythmias.
Monitor for signs and symptoms of hypermagnesemia: muscle weakness, inability to swallow, hyporeflexia, hypotension, bradycardia, CNS depression, respiratory depression, lethargy, coma, and depression.
Monitor for signs and symptoms of hypophosphatemia: bleeding tendencies, muscular weakness, paresthesia, hemolytic anemia, depressed white cell function, nausea, vomiting, anorexia, and bone demineralization.
Monitor for signs and symptoms of hyperphosphatemia: tachycardia, nausea, diarrhea, abdominal cramps, muscle weakness, flaccid paralysis, and increased reflexes.
Monitor for signs and symptoms of hypochloremia: hyperirritability, tetany, muscular excitability, slow respirations, and hypotension.
Monitor for signs and symptoms of hyperchloremia: weakness; lethargy; deep, rapid breathing; and coma.
Administer prescribed supplemental electrolytes, as appropriate.
Provide diet appropriate for patient's electrolyte imbalance (e.g., potassium-rich foods or low-sodium diet).
Teach patient ways to prevent or minimize electrolyte imbalance.
Instruct patient and/or family on specific dietary modifications, as appropriate.
Consult physician, if signs and symptoms of fluid and/or electrolyte imbalance persist or worsen.

McCloskey, J., & Bulechek, G. (Eds.). (1996). *Nursing interventions classification (NIC)* (2nd ed.). St. Louis: Mosby–Year Book. Reprinted with permission.

(Many diuretics promote increased potassium excretion in the distal tubule of the kidney.) In diabetes, hyperglycemia typically produces an osmotic diuresis and high urine output, resulting in potassium loss. Because the child is acidotic, serum potassium levels may not decrease to reflect the total body deficit of potassium until the acidosis starts to resolve. Gastrointestinal potassium losses occur through vomiting and diarrhea. Integumentary loss of potassium, occurring in sweat and burns, can be dangerous if the loss is extreme and not treated appropriately.

Clinical manifestations of hypokalemia include general muscle dysfunction and dysrhythmias (see Chart 17–12).

Interdisciplinary Interventions

When the potassium level falls below normal values, IV or oral potassium replacement is needed to restore and maintain adequate intracellular potassium concentrations. The route and rate of potassium replacement depends on the child's serum potassium concentration and renal function. Moderate to severe hypokalemia may be treated with potassium supplements, administered either orally or intravenously.

▽ **Alert:** *Before administering a potassium supplement, ensure that the child is producing urine, which demonstrates renal function. Because potassium is excreted through the kidneys, if renal function is inadequate, potassium readily accumulates, which can lead to ventricular dysrhythmias and cardiac arrest.*

Mild hypokalemia usually can be resolved with dietary modifications. A dietitian can help the child and family increase potassium content in their diet based on the child's preferences and the family's resources and finances (Chart 17–13). For instance, salt substitutes that contain potassium can provide a low-cost potassium source. Social services should be involved to help low-

Chart 17–13

Good Food Sources of Potassium*

Fruits
Apricots Bananas Orange juice Peaches, dried Pomegranates Prunes, dried
Vegetables
Beans, lima Chard Plantain, green or ripe Potato, baked or boiled (skin on is better) Pumpkin Spinach Squash, winter Tomatoes, stewed Tomato juice, canned
Grains
100% bran cereal (check label)
Legumes
Black, brown, or red kidney beans Lentils Peas, split, green or yellow
Dairy Products
Milk Milk-based fruit drinks Yogurt
Meat and Fish (baked or broiled)
Pork and veal, lean cutlet or steak Carp, catfish, flounder, mullet, cod, croaker, pompano, trout

* More than 350 mg/serving.
USDA. (1990). *Good sources of nutrients*. Washington, DC: USDA.

income or at-risk families identify and utilize community resources.

Nursing responsibilities include ongoing assessment and monitoring. Because potassium influences cell membrane excitability, muscle weakness or dysfunction is often apparent. Observing the child's activity level can help detect generalized weakness and determine whether it is progressive.

Tip: *If the child is receiving a potassium-wasting diuretic or has other risk factors for hypokalemia, ask whether he or she is tired ("Can you do the things you normally do?"), or ask the parents about the child's activity level. Instruct the child to tell the parent or caretaker if he or she feels tired or otherwise "different."*

Assessment also includes respiratory effort, cardiac function, and the presence or absence of bowel sounds. Signs of compromise should be reported to the health care team. Positioning of the child with the head of the bed elevated optimizes respiratory effort, and manual ventilations should be provided as needed. Feedings are withheld when bowel sounds are absent.

The child receiving digoxin therapy should be assessed for signs of digoxin toxicity, because hypokalemia potentiates digoxin.

Community Care

Along with preparing the child for ongoing interventions, teaching should include how to administer prescribed medications and monitor for their side effects, as well as how to avoid potentially dangerous drug interactions. For example, if the child is taking a potassium-wasting diuretic and a potassium supplement, the child or parents need to remind the health care provider of this when changing medication regimens. (Hyperkalemia can occur if the diuretic is discontinued but not the potassium supplement.) Discuss with the family the benefit of obtaining all prescriptions from one pharmacy, or at least informing the pharmacist of other medications or food supplements that the child is receiving. Often the pharmacist monitors for drug interactions and alerts the physician and family to these.

If the family's access to medications or financial status is an issue, they can request that the physician prescribe a commercial salt substitute (KCl) rather than a more costly pharmaceutical preparation.

Hyperkalemia

A serum potassium level above 5.0 mEq/L can result from various conditions. Dehydration or renal disease can impair renal excretion of potassium. Because potassium is the primary intracellular ion, damage to cells or the cell membrane (as occurs in crush injuries and burns, for instance) releases potassium from the cells into the ECF. This may also occur with transfusion of stored blood when old, damaged red blood cells release their intracellular potassium.

Clinical manifestations of hyperkalemia vary with severity of the imbalance. The most serious manifestations are cardiovascular changes; neuromuscular and gastrointestinal affects may also occur (see Chart 17–12). Severe hyperkalemia is a life-threatening emergency requiring immediate treatment.

Alert: *Significant dysrhythmias and cardiac arrest may result when potassium levels rise above 6.0 mEq/L.*

Interdisciplinary Interventions

Treatment of hyperkalemia must be initiated promptly to prevent serious physiologic effects. Several measures can lower a dangerously high potassium level (Chart 17–14). During treatment, the nurse assesses for rebound hypokalemia that may result from the treatment.

Electrocardiogram (ECG) waveforms are continuously monitored for dysrhythmias. The nurse also assesses vital signs, including heart rate and rhythm and blood pressure, and intervenes to support optimal cardiorespiratory function, as needed. Emergency equipment should be readily accessible.

Serum potassium levels are carefully monitored. Blood specimen collection must be done by qualified nursing or laboratory personnel, because a hemolyzed blood sample can result in falsely elevated potassium levels.

caREminder: *Use caution when collecting blood specimens to avoid blood cell hemolysis: warm an extremity if blood is being obtained by skin puncture; do not excessively squeeze or milk an extremity to obtain blood; use blood that easily flows from skin puncture or vein; and do not use excessive pressure to force blood from syringe into specimen collecting device.*

Potassium intake and urine output, indicative of renal function, are also monitored. This involves calculating intake of potassium from IV fluids, medications, and foods. Many foods contain potassium. Foods low in potassium include pears, apples, pineapple, rice, green beans, and salads without tomatoes. Most servings of meat, poultry, and fish contain 200 to 349 mg of potassium (USDA, 1990). Ensuring adequate fluid intake helps increase output of potassium in urine. Because potassium is excreted through the kidneys, it is important to monitor renal function through urine output volume and related laboratory values such as BUN and creatinine levels.

A child receiving multiple blood transfusions or a child with renal dysfunction who requires blood administration also needs careful monitoring for hyperkalemia. To help prevent this complication, the freshest blood available should be transfused.

Community Care

For the child with hyperkalemia resulting from a chronic medical condition, teaching the family how to manage the child's condition at home successfully is an important nursing responsibility. Other members of the health care team, such as social service case workers and the dietitian, should be included in designing the teaching plan for the family.

The child and family should be instructed to avoid foods high in potassium and assisted to make dietary modifications that fit in with the family's lifestyle and dietary habits. Parents or other caregivers can be taught to keep potassium-containing salt substitutes away from children and to avoid their use in a child with renal problems.

Calcium Imbalance

Calcium is vital to cardiac, muscle, and nerve function and helps maintain normal cell membrane permeability. It also plays a role in the secretion of certain hormones (e.g., parathyroid hormone, calcitriol, calcitonin) and the activation of some enzymes (e.g., insulin and glucagon). Circulating calcium concentrations are maintained by interactions of vitamin D metabolism, calcitonin, and parathyroid hormone. Parathyroid hormone helps regulate calcium concentration by stimulating reabsorption of calcium from bone and glomerular filtrate (Root & Diamond, 1993).

The largest calcium stores in the body are in the bones and teeth. This calcium is not readily available for use by the body. A small amount of body calcium is found in the plasma as protein-bound calcium, bound to diffusible molecules such as phosphate and citrate, or as ionized calcium (Finberg et al., 1993). The level of ionized calcium, the physiologically active form of calcium, is about half that of total calcium (Finberg et al., 1993).

Serum calcium levels are affected by serum protein concentration, pH, and phosphorus. Because calcium binds to protein, hyperalbuminemia (elevated serum protein level) may result in hypocalcemia. pH affects the physiological availability of calcium. Acidosis causes hypercalcemia by decreasing calcium binding to serum proteins and increases the amount of calcium released from bone; alkalosis causes the opposite affect. Calcium and phosphorus normally have an inverse relationship; when the level of one rises, the level of the other falls.

Hypocalcemia

Defined as a total calcium concentration below 8.8 mEq/L, hypocalcemia can result from inadequate dietary intake, vitamin D deficiency, hyperalbuminemia, renal disease, or diuretic therapy. Transfusion of blood containing citrate as an anticoagulant, particularly large or rapid infusions, may cause hypocalcemia because the citrate binds with calcium and decreases the amount of available ionized calcium. In a newborn, ingestion of cow's milk, which is high in phosphate, may lead to hypocalcemia. This is due to the newborn's relatively high tubular absorption of

Chart 17–14
Nursing Interventions

Management of Hyperkalemia

Medical Treatment Option	Nursing Intervention
Create chemical antagonism to the membrane effects of potassium	
Administer calcium gluconate 10% IV to temporarily stabilize the cell membrane.	Ensure that IV is not infiltrated; monitor IV closely before and during infusion because calcium extravasation causes severe tissue necrosis. Administer calcium slowly, as ordered. Monitor ECG during infusion; report ECG changes, bradycardia immediately. If child is receiving digoxin, administer calcium slowly while monitoring for signs of digoxin toxicity, because hypercalcemia potentiates digoxin toxicity. Monitor effectiveness of therapy (decrease in signs of hyperkalemia) and for return of negative effects due to hyperkalemia, because effects of calcium are effective within minutes but short-lived.
Expand the extracellular fluid volume	
Decrease, by dilution, the extracellular potassium concentration.	Administer IV fluid as ordered. Monitor for change in signs of hyperkalemia that indicate effectiveness of therapy. Monitor for signs of fluid overload. Calculate fluid balance and intake and output.
Increase cellular uptake of potassium	
Administer insulin IV, which facilitates cellular potassium uptake; glucose is usually administered with insulin to prevent hypoglycemia.	Administer insulin and glucose as ordered. Monitor for signs of hypoglycemia. Monitor for changes in potassium levels; effects usually occur in 30 minutes and last several hours.
In the presence of metabolic acidosis, administer sodium bicarbonate to normalize pH and reverse the shifting of potassium out of the cell that occurs with acidosis.	Administer sodium bicarbonate as ordered Monitor for return of hyperkalemia because effects may only last 1 to 2 hours.
Remove potassium from body	
Administer potassium-wasting diuretics (e.g., furosemide) to increase renal excretion of potassium.	Administer diuretic as ordered. Monitor urine output. Monitor for signs of dehydration. Evaluate effectiveness of therapy based on clinical changes.
Administer a cation exchange resin (e.g., Kayexalate) that exchanges 1 mEq of potassium for 1 mEq of sodium; it is usually administered in a suspension with sorbitol.	Administer via nasogastric tube or by enema as ordered. Maximize effect of enema by having the child retain it for 2 to 3 hours. Monitor for signs of dehydration because sorbitol creates an osmotic load that pulls water into the gut. Monitor for change in potassium levels, which show a maximal decrease in 3 to 4 hours (other treatment options are usually used as interim measures to decrease the cardiotoxic effects of excess potassium, while waiting for removal techniques to have an effect). Monitor serum sodium and potassium levels. Monitor for fluid overload and hypernatremia due to sodium exchanging properties of resin.
Institute peritoneal dialysis or hemodialysis.	Prepare child for dialysis as appropriate. Implement interventions and monitoring as specific to type of dialysis.

phosphate and physiologically low glomerular filtration rate. Correction of acidosis may lead to hypocalcemia. This occurs because in an acidotic state the calcium that moves out of the bones may be lost through urine output. Restoration of normal pH causes calcium to reenter the bones, resulting in hypocalcemia.

Hypocalcemia causes increased cell membrane permeability. Thus, clinical manifestations are characterized by increased neuromuscular excitability, particularly affecting the neuromuscular and cardiovascular systems (see Chart 17–12). Common signs of hypocalcemia include positive Chvostek's sign (spasm of the cheek and corner of the mouth after percussion of the facial nerve in front of the ear) and Trousseau's sign (carpal spasm when blood flow is occluded to the hand for 3 minutes). The child may complain of numbness or tingling of the nose, ears, fingers, and toes. Laryngospasm may produce high-pitched inspiratory noises and may result in apnea. Severe hypocalcemia can cause seizures and cardiac arrest.

Interdisciplinary Interventions

Asymptomatic hypocalcemia can be treated with dietary modifications, involving increased intake of foods rich in calcium. These foods include dairy products, bony fish (e.g., sardines), and green leafy vegetables (see Chart 20–7). Calcium supplements and vitamin D may be administered. Treatment of symptomatic hypocalcemia typically includes IV administration of calcium.

▽ **Alert:** *Before administering IV calcium, take extra care to ensure that the IV is correctly placed with no signs of complications. Extravasation of calcium causes severe tissue necrosis. Administer IV calcium slowly and monitor the ECG during infusion for QRS changes and bradycardia.*

Seizure precautions should be maintained for a child with hypocalcemia. Emergency equipment to provide manual ventilation should be readily available.

Hypercalcemia

Hypercalcemia is defined as a total calcium level exceeding 10.8 mEq/L. Causes include increased resorption of calcium from bone due to a malignancy (see Chapter 22), immobility, hyperparathyroidism, or hyperthyroidism; increased gastrointestinal absorption of calcium from excessive oral intake of calcium or vitamin D; and decreased excretion of calcium due to renal failure or diuretic therapy. Acidotic states also cause an increase in physiologically available calcium.

Hypercalcemia decreases cell membrane permeability, with a resultant decrease in neuromuscular excitability. High calcium levels may be asymptomatic, an incidental finding when other laboratory values are obtained. Hypercalcemia may also have a nonspecific presentation such as bone pain, fatigue, or polyuria and polydipsia (Finberg et al., 1993). ECG changes may be present (see Chart 17–12). Deep tendon reflexes are usually hypoactive with diminished muscle tone and strength. Renal calculi and renal failure, caused by the increased excretion of calcium in urine, or pathologic fractures may occur. Decreased motility in the gastrointestinal tract may cause abdominal pain, anorexia, nausea, and vomiting.

Interdisciplinary Interventions

Hypercalcemia is often an indication of an underlying disease that requires treatment. Severe hypercalcemia is treated with forced diuresis, giving normal saline at 1.5 times maintenance fluid (Juppner, 1996). Generous fluid administration helps maintain vascular volume in the presence of dehydration and promotes calcium excretion. After ensuring adequate hydration, diuretics are often administered to further promote diuresis. Administration of phosphate binds the calcium and can rapidly lower serum calcium levels. Peritoneal or hemodialysis, with low-calcium dialysate, may be used if the child remains severely hypercalcemic (Juppner, 1996). Medications to decrease the absorption of calcium, such as calcitonin and glucocorticoids, may also be administered.

Nursing responsibilities include monitoring serum calcium levels and reporting any abnormal findings to the physician. Assessing neuromuscular and cardiac status (including ECG waveforms), maintaining fluid balance, and providing parent teaching are also important.

Monitoring fluid balance in hypercalcemia is important for several reasons. The child may be dehydrated on initial presentation or during the course of therapy, or administration of large fluid volumes may overload the vascular system. Moreover, two goals of treatment are to promote urinary calcium excretion and prevent renal damage from the deposits of calcium salts. Thus, intake and output must be monitored and balance evaluated as often as indicated by the child's status (e.g. every hour, every 12 hours, or every 24 hours). Other indicators of fluid balance (e.g., blood pressure, presence of edema or signs of dehydration, rales when auscultating breath sounds) must also be evaluated and interventions implemented as indicated. If the child's blood pressure is low or unstable, diuretics should be used with caution.

Mobilization is encouraged to prevent the development of hypercalcemia due to excessive resorption of calcium from the bones. If the child must be immobilized, the nurse needs to ensure adequate fluid intake to prevent renal damage and handle the child gently when moving to avoid fractures.

Community Care

Education is an important component of family care, particularly when the primary cause of the hypercalcemia is a chronic condition. The child and family are taught signs and symptoms of calcium imbalance and instructed to notify their health care provider if these occur. If medications are used in managing hypercalcemia, the child and family are taught about administration, side effects, and potential interactions with other medications or food.

Food sources of calcium and the degree to which these must be limited should be included in family teaching. A dietitian should be involved in assisting the family to adapt dietary restrictions into their lifestyle. Because excessive intake of vitamin D can cause hypercalcemia, parents are instructed to keep vitamin supplements out of children's reach and told about the hazards of excessive vitamin supplementation.

Magnesium Imbalance

Magnesium imbalance is less common than imbalances of other electrolytes, but it can be life threatening if severe. A neuromuscular depressant, magnesium is necessary for soft tissue and bone formation, along with the maintenance of normal cellular function and muscle and nerve activity. It is the second most abundant intracellular ion and is found in small amounts in the ECF. Normal plasma values in children are 1.5 to 2.3 mEq/L (Finberg et al., 1993).

Magnesium affects cell functions through its interactions with calcium. Calcium often opposes the actions of magnesium. Magnesium is excreted primarily in urine and in small amounts through the gastrointestinal tract. Absorption occurs primarily in the upper gastrointestinal tract. Food sources of magnesium include green vegetables, whole grains, legumes, nuts, meat, and dairy products.

Besides restoring magnesium balance, treatment also focuses on correcting the primary cause of the imbalance. Because magnesium imbalances are relatively rare compared with other electrolyte imbalances, they may be overlooked. The nurse assesses the child for conditions that may lead to imbalance, as well as for electrolyte imbalances associated with hypomagnesemia (e.g., hypokalemia, hypocalcemia, hypochloremic alkalosis) and hypermagnesemia (e.g., elevated BUN and creatinine levels). Ongoing assessment of the child's vital signs is imperative to detect hypotension, cardiac dysrhythmias, and respiratory impairment. Assessing muscle tone and monitoring serum electrolyte values are also important.

Hypomagnesemia

Defined as a serum magnesium level below 1.5 mEq/L, hypomagnesemia can be caused by inadequate intake (e.g., malnutrition, prolonged IV therapy without supplement), impaired absorption (e.g., in the presence of excessive calcium intake, diarrhea, vomiting, hypoparathyroidism, or bowel resection), or increased excretion (e.g., use of thiazide diuretics, aldosterone excess). Administration of citrated blood, which binds free magnesium, may also cause hypomagnesemia. Severe hypomagnesemia interferes with the release of parathyroid hormone; thus, hypomagnesemia and hypocalcemia often coexist. Parathyroid hormone stimulates intestinal absorption of magnesium and calcium release from bones. Hormones (e.g., calcitonin, aldosterone) that inhibit intestinal absorption of magnesium also stimulate calcium resorption into the bones.

caREminder: *Hypocalcemia that does not respond to treatment may be indicative of a concomitant hypomagnesemia that also requires treatment.*

Signs and symptoms of hypomagnesemia can be similar to those of hypocalcemia. Manifestations of increased neuromuscular irritability (hyperactive reflexes, tetany, seizures) and impaired cardiac function (hypotension, tachycardia, ECG changes and dysrhythmias) are of most concern.

Interdisciplinary Interventions

Mild hypomagnesemia can be corrected by increasing the child's intake of magnesium-rich foods. This may be supplemented by magnesium-based antacids (e.g., milk of magnesia). Moderate to severe hypomagnesemia may require IV administration of magnesium supplements. Renal function (which is necessary for excretion of excess magnesium) must be assessed before administration to prevent iatrogenic hypermagnesemia.

IV administration of magnesium requires close monitoring. Infiltration of magnesium into the tissues can lead to necrosis and sloughing of the surrounding area. Optimally, magnesium is administered into a central vein and is infused slowly to decrease discomfort caused by vasodilation (feeling hot, flushing). Rebound hypermagnesemia may result from magnesium infusion. Deep tendon reflexes are assessed during infusion to detect hyporeflexia, a relatively early sign of hypermagnesemia.

Nursing care also addresses symptom management. For instance, a child with muscle spasms needs reduced environmental stimuli (e.g., quiet speaking, dim lighting). The child must also be handled gently to avoid causing additional discomfort from neuromuscular excitability.

Hypermagnesemia

Hypermagnesemia, serum magnesium level exceeding 2.3 mEq/L, can be caused by impaired excretion (e.g., decreased renal function) or excessive intake (e.g., magnesium-containing antacids, IV supplementation, treatment of maternal eclampsia with magnesium, which crosses the placenta and can cause elevated magnesium levels in neonates). Signs and symptoms of hypermagnesemia reflect altered neuromuscular function (e.g., hyporeflexia, lethargy, respiratory depression) and cardiac function (e.g., flushing from vasodilatation, bradycardia, hypotension, dysrhythmias).

Interdisciplinary Interventions

If hypermagnesemia is detected, all medications and IV fluids containing magnesium are promptly discontinued, as ordered. Severe hypermagnesemia, or hypermagnesemia in the presence of renal failure, is treated with IV administration of calcium (usually calcium gluconate in children), which blocks the neuromuscular effects of magnesium. (See the section on hypocalcemia for discussion of hazards associated with IV calcium infusion.) Thiazide diuretics may be given to remove excess magnesium, and IV fluids may be given to increase urine output. Children with severe hypermagnesemia may require dialysis.

Nursing care focuses on carefully monitoring fluid balance. Fluid excess may occur because of impaired myocardial contractility due to effects of magnesium and/or impaired renal function. Signs of fluid overload include fluid intake greater than output, increased respiratory rate, and rales.

Phosphorus Imbalance

Although it is relatively rare, phosphorus imbalance can be life threatening when severe. Phosphorus is crucial to the integrity of cells and cell membranes and plays an important role in energy production for normal metabolic activity and growth. The majority of phosphorus, like calcium, is found in the bones. A small percentage is found in ECF. Children have higher serum phosphorus levels than adults because of their rapid skeletal growth. Normal serum phosphorus levels vary depending on age: birth to 5 days, 4.8 to 8.2 mg/dL; 1 to 3 years, 3.8 to 6.5 mg/dL; 4 to 11 years, 3.7 to 5.6 mg/dL; 12 to 15 years, 2.9 to 5.4 mg/dL (Behrman et al., 1996).

Renal excretion, intestinal absorption, and bone mineralization all affect serum phosphorus level. Parathyroid hormone inhibits reabsorption of phosphorus and increases its excretion in urine (Root & Diamond, 1993). The excretion and retention of phosphorus is closely related to glomerular filtration and general kidney function. In impaired renal function, the kidney retains phosphorus and elevated serum levels occur.

Increased serum phosphorus can lead to decreased serum calcium. Usually phosphorus and calcium vary inversely because parathyroid hormone, while inhibiting absorption of phosphate, promotes calcium uptake. In a child with malabsorption or malnutrition, levels of both electrolytes are low.

As with all electrolyte imbalances, in phosphorus imbalance, identifying and treating the underlying cause of the imbalance is the ultimate goal. Phosphorus levels are monitored along with associated electrolytes such as calcium and magnesium, as well as serum pH. Indicators of renal function, such as BUN and creatinine, are also monitored.

Hypophosphatemia

Hypophosphatemia may result from inadequate intake and impaired absorption. Inadequate phosphorus intake is particularly prevalent in preterm infants, who have high phosphorus needs because of rapid growth. Hypophosphatemia caused by "refeeding syndrome" may occur after carbohydrate administration in severely malnourished children. Phosphate shifts intracellularly when glucose enters the cell. Intracellular shifting of phosphate also occurs with alkalosis and after administration of corticosteroids or insulin. Antacids containing aluminum or magnesium hydroxide bind phosphate and can decrease serum phosphate levels. Hypophosphatemia also may result from increased urinary excretion of phosphorus due to decreased tubular reabsorption, administration of thiazide diuretics, ECF volume expansion, or hyperparathyroidism.

Because of phosphate's role in energy production for cellular metabolism, mild hypophosphatemia may manifest as weakness and tissue hypoxia. As the deficit becomes more severe, signs and symptoms similar to those of encephalopathy (irritability, confusion, seizures, coma, paresthesia) and other manifestations may appear (see Chart 17–12).

Interdisciplinary Interventions

Ensuring adequate phosphorus intake is the primary preventive measure in hypophosphatemia. This is especially important in preterm infants receiving TPN or breast milk, which does not adequately meet their phosphorus needs during rapid growth. Breast milk fortifier should be given as ordered. The physician and dietitian should collaborate in writing orders for TPN to ensure a balance of essential nutrients.

Treatment of mild hypophosphatemia typically involves increasing phosphorus intake to restore serum levels. Increased dietary intake of phosphorus may promote increased serum phosphorus levels (see Chart 20–7). Phosphorus supplements can be given orally, in the form of phosphate salts, or intravenously. The route of administration is based on the cause and severity of deficit. During IV phosphorus administration, renal function is carefully monitored to avoid hyperphosphatemia. Levels of other electrolytes are also monitored to detect any imbalances that may be associated with hypophosphatemia or its treatment.

The nurse teaches the child and family about treatment measures, how to increase intake of foods high in phosphorus, and the need to avoid phosphate-binding antacids and diuretics.

Hyperphosphatemia

Phosphorus excess is generally not of major concern unless renal excretion of phosphorus is impaired. Hyperphosphatemia most commonly results from decreased glomerular filtration of phosphorus, such as occurs in chronic renal disease. It can also be caused by excessive phosphorus intake, either orally, intravenously, or from administration of phosphate-containing enemas. Hyperphosphatemia also may develop in children receiving treatment for malignancies, especially lymphoma or leukemia, who have rapid cytolysis of cells with resultant release of intracellular phosphorus.

Because of the inverse relationship between phosphorus and calcium, hypocalcemia usually develops concurrently with hyperphosphatemia. Thus, signs and symptoms of hyperphosphatemia mimic those of hypocalcemia. These include hyperreflexia, tetany, tachycardia, nausea, abdominal cramps, and diarrhea.

Interdisciplinary Interventions

Treatment of hyperphosphatemia aims to increase phosphorus excretion and decrease phosphorus intake. Excretion is promoted by maintaining high urine output through the administration of oral and IV fluids. Dietary intake of high-phosphate foods is reduced (see Chart 20–7). Aluminum-containing antacids bind phosphorus, preventing gut absorption, and thus may be ordered. However, in children, phosphate binders that contain aluminum or magnesium may cause accumulation of heavy metals in the brain and bones (Heiliczer, 1996). Therefore, they must be used cautiously. Calcium carbonate can be used as an oral phosphate binder. Hypocalcemia should be treated concurrently. A child with severe hyperphosphatemia may need dialysis.

The nurse monitors for electrolyte imbalances associated with hyperphosphatemia (e.g., hypocalcemia, hypomagnesemia) and assesses urine output as an indicator of renal function. Seizure precautions are instituted to prevent injury caused by tetany. The nurse teaches the child and family about the treatment regimen and instructs them to avoid phosphate-containing foods.

Summary of Key Concepts

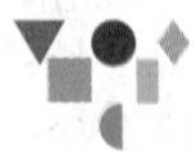

- Water and electrolytes are distributed in the ICF and ECF compartments. Water distribution varies with age; younger children have more total body water in the extracellular space. Water and electrolyte balance is regulated by hydrostatic, osmotic, and oncotic pressure; active and passive transport; and the kidneys, gastrointestinal tract, skin, and lungs.
- Because imbalances in fluid and electrolytes affect all body systems, usually at the cellular level, assessment must include all systems and must take into account the physiologic changes that occur with growth and maturation.
- Results of laboratory analysis of blood and urine must be evaluated in conjunction with the child's history and physical findings to diagnose the imbalance. IV therapy may be lifesaving but requires meticulous nursing care to avoid iatrogenic injury to the child.
- Children are more prone to dehydration because they have a greater proportion of body water in the extracellular space, have higher metabolic rates, and are more prone to diseases that impact fluid and electrolyte balance, such as vomiting, diarrhea, and febrile diseases.
- In children, sudden weight changes can be a fairly sensitive indicator of fluid balance. Sudden weight gain may indicate edema—excess fluid in the ECF compartment.
- Acid-base imbalance negatively affects functioning of all body systems. Respiratory compensation by the body can be effective within minutes; renal compensation may take days.
- Electrolytes affect body water distribution and nerve, cellular, hormone, and enzyme activity. Electrolytes within the ICF and ECF compartments are balanced; changes in one affect the others. Electrolyte imbalances can be life threatening.
- Sodium plays a primary role in influencing distribution of body water; water follows sodium.

- Potassium is a major determinant of cell membrane resting potential, influencing neuromuscular excitability. Deficit causes generalized muscle weakness and cardiac dysrhythmias. Potassium accumulates rapidly in the presence of inadequate renal function. Hyperkalemia can cause dysrhythmias and can rapidly progress to cardiac arrest.
- Calcium helps maintain normal cell membrane permeability. Deficit is characterized by increased permeability, resulting in neuromuscular excitability and tetany. Excess decreases neuromuscular excitability, causing hypotonia and decreased deep tendon reflexes.
- Magnesium is important for muscle and nerve activity. Deficit increases neuromuscular irritability, causing hyperactive reflexes and tetany, and impairs cardiac function, causing dysrhythmias, tachycardia, and hypotension. Excess acts as a neuromuscular depressant causing hyporeflexia, lethargy, respiratory depression, dysrhythmias, bradycardia, and hypotension.
- Phosphorus is crucial to energy production for normal metabolic activity and for growth. Hypophosphatemia may manifest as weakness, tissue hypoxia, and symptoms similar to those of encephalopathy. Usually, phosphorus and calcium levels vary inversely. Thus, manifestations of hyperphosphatemia mimic those of hypocalcemia.

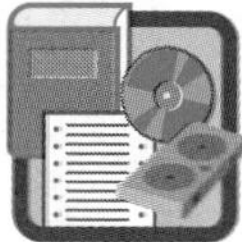

Resources

Organizations

American Society for Clinical Nutrition
9650 Rockville Pike, Room 3300
Bethesda, MD 20814
(301) 530-7710

American Society for Parenteral and Enteral Nutrition (ASPEN)
8630 Fenton Street, Suite 412
Silver Spring, MD 20910-3805
(800) 587-6315
E-mail: aspen@access.digex.net
Web: http://www.clinnutr.org

Catheter Technology Corporation
3385 West 1820 South
Salt Lake City, UT 94194
(800) 443-3385

Home Health Care of America
4340 Von Karman
Newport Beach, CA 92660

Intravenous Nurses Society
10 Fawcett Street
Cambridge, MA 02138
(617) 441-3008

Oley Foundation for Home Parenteral and Enteral Nutrition
214 Hun Memorial, A-23
Albany Medical Center
Albany, NY 12208
(518) 262-5079
This nonprofit research and educational foundation maintains a registry of home TPN patients and publishes a bimonthly newsletter.

Guideline/Position Statements

A.S.P.E.N. Board of Directors. (1996). Standards for hospitalized pediatric patients. *Nutrition in Clinical Practice, 11,* 217–228.

Computer Resources

Laboratory Values
Web: http://www.ghsl.nwu.edu/Norm.html
Gives normal laboratory values.

References

Acra, S. A., & Ghishan, F. K. (1996). Electrolyte fluxes in the gut and oral rehydration solutions. *Pediatric Clinics of North America, 43,* 433–449.

Behrman, R. E., Kliegman, R. M., & Arvin, A. M. (Eds.). (1996). *Nelson textbook of pediatrics* (15th ed.). Philadelphia: W. B. Saunders.

Bossert, E., & Beecroft, P. C. (1994). Peripheral intravenous lock irrigation in children: Current practice. *Pediatric Nursing, 20,* 346–349, 355.

Danek, G., & Noris, E. M. (1992). Pediatric IV catheters: Efficacy of saline flush. *Pediatric Nursing, 18,* 111–113.

Finberg, L., Kravath, R., & Hellerstein, S. (1993). *Water and electrolytes in pediatrics: Physiology, pathology, and Treatment* (2nd ed.). Philadelphia: W. B. Saunders.

Ford, E. G. (1996). Nutrition support of pediatric patients. *Nutrition in Clinical Practice, 11,* 183–191.

Freiberger, D. (1994). The use of Hibiclens in pediatric central venous line skin care. *Journal of Pediatric Nursing, 9*, 126–127.

Gyr, P., Smith, K., Pontious, S., Burroughs, T., Mahl, C., & Swerczek, L. (1995). Double blind comparison of heparin and saline flush solutions in maintenance of peripheral infusion devices. *Pediatric Nursing, 21*, 383–389, 366.

Hanrahan, K. S., Kleiber, C., & Fagan, C. L. (1994). Evaluation of saline for IV locks in children. *Pediatric Nursing, 20*, 549–552.

Hazinski, M. F. (1988). Understanding fluid balance in the seriously ill child. *Pediatric Nursing, 14*, 231–236.

Heiliczer, J. D. (1996). Acute renal failure. In F. D. Berg, J. R. Ingelfinger, E. R. Wald, & R. A. Polin (Eds.), *Gellis & Kagan's current pediatric therapy* (15th ed., pp. 452–456). Philadelphia: W. B. Saunders.

Holliday, M. (1996). The evolution of therapy for dehydration: Should deficit therapy still be taught? *Pediatrics, 98*, 171–177.

Hughes, W. T. (1996). Fluid and metabolic therapy. In H. W. Taeusch, R. O. Christiansen, & E. S. Buescher (Eds.), *Pediatric and neonatal tests and procedures* (pp. 253–294). Philadelphia: W. B. Saunders.

Juppner, H. (1996). Parathyroid disease. In F. D. Berg, J. R. Ingelfinger, E. R. Wald, & R. A. Polin (Eds.), *Gellis & Kagan's current pediatric therapy* (15th ed., pp. 336–338). Philadelphia: W. B. Saunders.

Keegan-Wells, D., & Stewart, J. L. (1992). The use of venous access devices in pediatric oncology nursing practice. *Journal of Pediatric Oncology Nursing, 9*, 159–169.

Kuhn, M. M. (1991). Crystalloid vs. colloid. *Critical Care Nurse, 11*(5), 37–44, 46–51.

Long, C. A., Byrnes, K., Leclair, J., Stashinko, E. E., & Molchan, E. (1996). Central line associated bacteremia in the pediatric patient. *Pediatric Nursing, 22*, 247–251.

Orlowski, J. P. (1994). Emergency alternatives to intravenous access intraosseous, intratracheal, sublingual, and other-site drug administration. *Pediatric Clinics of North America, 41*, 1183–1199.

Pickering, L. K., & Snyder, J. D. (1996). Gastroenteritis. In R. E. Behrman, R. M. Kliegman, & A. M. Arvin (Eds.), *Nelson textbook of pediatrics* (15th ed., pp. 721–724). Philadelphia: W. B. Saunders.

Root, A. W., & Diamond, F. B. (1993). Disorders of calcium and phosphorus metabolism in adolescents. *Endocrine and Metabolic Clinics of North America, 22*, 573–592.

Skaer, T. L. (1993). Total parenteral nutrition: Clinical considerations. *Clinical Therapeutics, 15*, 272–282.

Straughn, A., & English, B. (1996). Oral rehydration therapy: A neglected treatment for pediatric diarrhea. MCN, *21*, 144–147.

U.S. Department of Agriculture. (1990). *Good Sources of Nutrients*. Washington, DC: Author.

Bibliography

Alhimyary, A., Fernandez, C., Picard, M., Tierno, K., Pignatone, N., Chan, H-S., Malt, R., & Souba, W. (1996). Safety and efficacy of total parenteral nutrition delivered via a peripherally inserted central venous catheter. *Nutrition in Clinical Practice, 11*, 199–203.

Angeles, T. (1997). How to prevent phlebitis. *Nursing 97, 27*, 26.

Arieff, A. I., Ayus, J. C., & Fraser, C. L. (1992). Hyponatremia and death or permanent brain damage in healthy children. *British Journal of Medicine, 304*, 1218–1222.

Bjornson, H.S. (1993). Pathogenesis, prevention, and management of catheter-associated infections. *New Horizons, 1*, 271–278.

Bloch, A. S., & Brown, P. (1990). Methods of nutritional support in the home, *Journal of Pain and Symptom Management, 5*, 297–306.

Broner, C. W., Stidham, G. L., Westenkircher, D. F., & Tolley, E. A. (1990). Hypermagnesemia and hypocalcemia as predictors of high mortality in critically ill pediatric patients. *Critical Care Medicine, 18*, 921–928.

Davenport, M. (1996). Paediatric fluid balance. *Care of the Critically Ill, 12*(1), 26–28, 30–31.

DeBruin, W. J., Greenwald, B. M., & Notterman, D. A. (1992). Fluid resuscitation in pediatrics. *Critical Care Clinics, 8*, 423–438.

Farrington, E. (1991). Treatment of hyperkalemia. *Pediatric Nursing, 17*, 190–192.

Filston, H. C. (1992). Fluid and electrolyte management in the pediatric surgical patient. *Surgical Clinics of North America, 72*, 1189–1205.

Flemmer, L., & Chan, J. S. L. (1993). A pediatric protocol for management of extravasation injuries. *Pediatric Nursing, 19*, 355–358.

Grisanti, K. A., & Jaffee, D. M. (1991). Dehydration syndromes—oral rehydration and fluid replacement. *Emergency Medicine Clinics of North America, 9*, 565–585.

Gruskin, A. B., & Sarnaik, A. (1992). Hyponatremia: pathophysiology and treatment, a pediatric perspective. *Pediatric Nephrology, 6*, 280–286.

Herbst, S. F. (1993). Accumulation of blood products and drug precipitates in VADs: A set up for trouble. *Journal of Vascular Access, 3*(3), 9–13.

Keating, J. P., Shears, G. J. & Dodge, P. R. (1991). Oral water intoxication in infants, an American perspective. *American Journal of Diseases in Childhood, 145*, 985–990.

Keller, V. E. (1995). Management of nausea and vomiting in children. *Journal of Pediatric Nursing, 10*, 280–286.

Kotter, R. W. (1996). Heparin vs saline for intermittent intravenous device maintenance in neonates. *Neonatal Network, 15*(6), 43–47.

Lynch, R. E. (1990). Ionized calcium: Pediatric perspective. *Pediatric Clinics of North America, 37*, 373–389.

McAbee, R. R., Grupp, K., & Horn, B. (1991). Home intravenous therapy: Part 1—issues. *Home Health Care Services Quarterly, 12*(3), 55–119.

Meyers, A. (1994). Fluid and electrolyte therapy for children. *Current Opinion in Pediatrics, 6*, 303–309.

Micetic-Turk, D. (1995). Evaluation of five oral rehydration solutions for children with diarrhea. *Journal of Pediatric Gastroenterology and Nutrition, 20*, 358–360.

Mioneau, G., & Newman, J. (1990). Rapid intravenous rehydration in the pediatric emergency department. *Pediatric Emergency Care, 6*, 186–188.

Noerr, B. (1996). Urokinase. *Neonatal Network, 15*(8), 66–68.

Nursing Subcommittee of the Food and Drug Administration Central Venous Catheter Working Group. (1992). Central venous catheter complications: a nursing perspective. *Journal of Pediatric Oncology Nursing, 9*, 81–83.

Pascale, J. A., Brittian, L., Lenfestey, C. C., & Jarrett-Pulliam, C. (1996). Breastfeeding, dehydration, and shorter maternity stays. *Neonatal Network, 15*(7), 37–43.

Roper, M. (1996). Assessing orthostatic vital signs. *AJN*, 96(8), 43–46.

Ruble, K., Long, C., & Connor, K. (1994). Pharmacologic treatment of catheter-related thrombus in pediatrics. *Pediatric Nursing, 20*, 553–557.

Salzman, M. B., & Rubin, L. G. (1995). Intravenous catheter-related infections. *Advances in Pediatric Infectious Diseases, 10*, 337–368.

Satlin, L. M., & Schwartz, G. J. (1990). Disorders of potassium metabolism. In I. Ichikawa (Ed.). *Pediatric Textbook of Fluid and Electrolytes* (pp. 218–236). Baltimore: Williams & Wilkins.

Seaman, S. L. (1995). Renal physiology part II: fluid and electrolyte regulation. *Neonatal Network, 14*(5), 5–11.

Seigel, N. J., Carpenter, T., & Gaudio, K. M. (1994). Pathophysiology of body fluids. In C. D. DeAngelis, R. D. Feigin, J. A. McMillan, & J. B. Warshaw (Eds.). *Principles and Practice of Pediatrics* (pp. 60–78). Philadelphia: J. B. Lippincott.

Shiao, S. P. (1992). Fluid and electrolyte problems of infants of very low birth weight. *AACN Clinical Issues, 3*, 698–704.

Smith, A. B., & Wilkinson-Faulk, D. (1994). Factors affecting the life span of peripheral intravenous lines in hospitalized infants. *Pediatric Nursing, 20*, 543–547.

Statter, M. B. (1992). Fluid and electrolytes in infants and children. *Seminars in Pediatric Surgery, 1*(3), 208–221.

Thompson, V. (1994). An IV therapy teaching tool for children. *Pediatric Nursing, 20*, 351–355.

Walter, J. H. (1992). Metabolic acidosis in newborn infants. *Archives of Diseases in Childhood, 67*, 767–769.

Wattad, A., Chiang, M. L., & Hill, L. L. (1992). Hyponatremia in hospitalized children. *Pediatrics, 31*, 153–157.

Wickham, R., Purl, S., & Welker, D. (1992). Long-term central venous catheters: Issues for care. *Seminars in Oncology Nursing, 8*, 133–147.

Winskunas, C. A. (1990). A creative approach to comprehensive IV therapy documentation. *Journal of Intravenous Nursing, 13*, 115–118.

Workman, M. L. (1992). Magnesium and phosphorus: The neglected electrolytes. *AACN Clinical Issues, 3*, 655–663.

HEALTH CHALLENGE:

Alterations in Gastrointestinal Status

OUTLINE

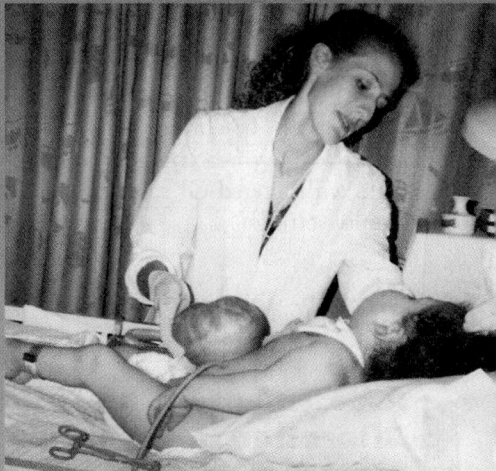

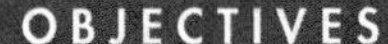

OBJECTIVES

- Discuss components of the history and physical assessment that are important to assess when evaluating a child with an alteration in gastrointestinal (GI) status.
- Identify specific tests and laboratory results that assist the health care team to identify alterations in GI status.
- Discuss diet modifications and alternative feeding methods used to treat alterations in GI status.
- Explain the etiology and expected patient outcomes of congenital and acquired GI disorders.
- Review the significant pathophysiologic principles that clarify the uniqueness of each GI disorder.

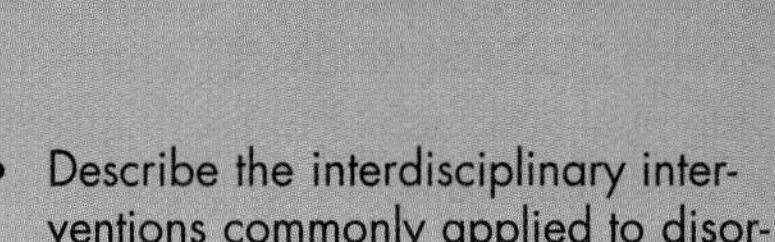

- Describe the interdisciplinary interventions commonly applied to disorders of the GI system.

KEY TERMS

ascites
cholestasis
dysphagia
ileus
regurgitation

CHAPTER

18

The gastrointestinal (GI) system is a complex organ system that extends from the mouth to the anus and includes the esophagus, stomach, small and large intestines, liver, and pancreas. The primary functions of the GI system are ingestion, digestion, and absorption of nutrients and excretion of solid waste. Proper function of the GI system is essential for normal growth and maintenance of fluid and electrolyte balance. This system also plays an important role in metabolic functions, such as protein synthesis and glucose homeostasis, as well as immunologic function.

Alterations in GI status may be congenital or acquired, acute or chronic, and may vary in severity from minor to life-threatening. The nurse may encounter the child with altered GI status in both acute care and community settings.

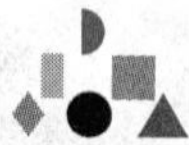

Assessment of the Child with an Alteration in Gastrointestinal Status

Focused Health History

The focused health history is an important part of the overall assessment of the child with GI tract dysfunction (Chart 18–1). Many GI diseases have relatively few observable physical findings, which makes the history of symptoms and factors impacting their onset and duration an important diagnostic tool. Conversely, a pathologic process that initially appears to be of GI origin may indicate a pathologic process in another system, such as pneumonia presenting as abdominal pain.

It is important to obtain information on the presence of pain, its location, characteristics, and exacerbating or relieving factors. Obtain information about feeding habits (what, when, how often, how prepared), changes in appetite and fluid intake (increased, decreased, type of intake), and bowel habits (frequency, appearance, use of aids such as laxatives or enemas). Ask about the relationship of symptoms to meals or specific food intake.

When obtaining the history, careful attention should be paid to the specifics of the timing and characteristics of the symptoms. The child should be included in the interview as much as possible and should be encouraged to describe symptoms in familiar terms. The interviewer should be careful to clarify the parent or child's reports so as to avoid underrepresentation or overrepresentation of symptoms. For example, if the parent reports that the child had "a lot of diarrhea last night," the interviewer should ask for an estimation of how many episodes of diarrhea the child has had in the previous 24 hours and at what times the episodes occurred. The parent should be questioned regarding the volume of the stool output using familiar measures such as a tablespoon, a cup, or number of saturated diapers to estimate the amount. Finally, the characteristics of the stool output should be defined, including color, consistency, and presence of blood or mucus.

Focused Physical Assessment

Physical assessment of the GI system must occur in the context of an overall comprehensive physical examination. Manifestations of altered GI function are varied and may be subtle. Children with conditions that result in alterations of intake, digestion, or absorption of nutrients may exhibit signs of growth failure or malnutrition. These children may have alterations in skin integrity or abnormal findings on neurologic or musculoskeletal examination. Children with conditions that result in excessive loss of fluid and electrolytes from the GI tract may present with the physical findings of acute dehydration. The child with gastroesophageal reflux may present with the physical findings of pneumonia secondary to aspiration of refluxed stomach contents.

Throughout the physical assessment of the child, it is important to keep in mind the potential relationships between the GI system and altered physical findings in other systems (Chart 18–2). Malnutrition may manifest in changes in hair or nails, lack of wound healing, and skin and oral lesions (see Chapter 25). Decreased protein level due to malnutrition causes a fluid shift out of the vascular space into the interstitial space, resulting in edema. Because infants and young children use their diaphragm as the primary muscle of respiration, abdominal distention caused by GI tract dysfunction may rapidly cause respiratory distress, which can lead to respiratory arrest if severe.

Because GI tract function may be reflected in growth and nutritional status, accurately measuring and recording growth parameters are important aspects of GI assessment. Children up to age 24 months should be weighed lying down or sitting on an infant scale. Very young infants should be undressed and the diaper removed while being weighed. Older children may be weighed on a standing scale wearing light clothing with their shoes off. Recumbent length should be measured on children up to age 24 to 36 months using an infant measuring board, if the growth chart for birth to 36 months is used. Standing height is measured in children age 24 to 36 months, and in older children, when the growth chart for age 2 to 18 years is used. Head circumference is measured in children up to age 3 years. (See Chapter 6 for further discussion of measuring growth parameters.)

The abdominal examination is a major part of GI system assessment. Assessment of the abdomen may

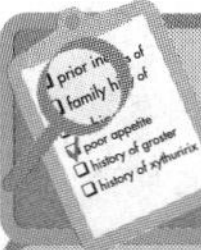

Chart 18–1
Focused Health History

Gastrointestinal System

Identifying Data	Child's age and sex Ethnic background Informant
Present Illness	Symptoms: onset, duration, character, aggravating or alleviating factors Recent weight loss or gain Recent change in diet, food intake Presence of: Nausea Vomiting, retching Abdominal pain Abdominal distention Bulges in abdominal or inguinal area with crying or straining Diarrhea Constipation Blood in emesis or stool Related systemic problems: Fever Fatigue Urinary tract symptoms (change in color, frequency, pain) Respiratory symptoms (cough, asthma) Skin lesions, rashes, pruritus, changes in hair or nails
Past Medical History	Birth history Birth weight, length History of prematurity Failure to pass meconium Feeding difficulties History of maternal prenatal infections Previous health challenges History of GI illness Problems with growth, weight gain History of other illnesses (e.g., recurrent respiratory or urinary tract infection, congenital heart disease) Childhood illnesses Immunization Status of current immunizations, including hepatitis B vaccine Allergies: describe reaction and how it resolves Formula, milk allergies Food allergies Medication allergies
Current Medications	List all systemic medications child has recently taken or is currently taking List any vitamins or food supplements the child is taking List homeopathic remedies being used Describe how the medication is taken (e.g., on empty stomach; with food or fluid, with what and how much; taken in conjunction with other medications; if tablets, are they swallowed or crushed) Describe any changes noted in GI tract function secondary to medication

Chart continued on following page

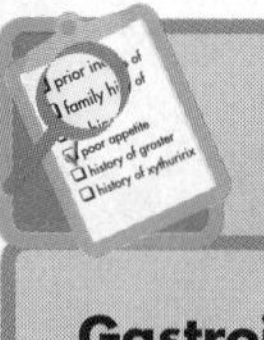

Chart 18–1
Focused Health History *Continued*

Gastrointestinal System	
Nutritional Assessment	Weight and height when well Recent weight loss or gain Current intake, usual intake Feeding method (breast, bottle, cup, tube fed) Method of formula preparation Vitamin, mineral supplements
Family Medical History	Family history of GI illness
Environmental History	Exposure to affected individuals (hepatitis, diarrhea)—home, daycare, school History of recent travel Recent exposure to food prepared outside home
Social History	Recent changes, stressors in family, lifestyle School attendance, performance Friends, hobbies
Growth and Development	Developmental milestones, especially feeding milestones Sleep patterns Play, hobbies, activities

present unique challenges in children. (See Chapter 6 for further discussion of physical examination techniques.)

caREminder: *The usual order of physical assessment techniques is altered during assessment of the abdomen. Auscultation must precede percussion and palpation to obtain a accurate assessment of bowel sounds.*

An infant may become distressed during the examination, crying and tensing the abdominal wall. This may interfere with the nurse's ability to see, hear, and feel changes in assessment parameters. Placing the infant in a parent's lap during the examination can help soothe the infant and facilitate the examination. Providing comfort measures, such as a pacifier or bottle, may also help calm the infant. The older child may become frightened or ticklish during the examination. Demonstrating parts of the examination on a doll or stuffed animal can help put the child at ease and enhance cooperation. Allowing the child to handle examination tools or distracting the child with toys or conversation about favorite activities also may be helpful. The adolescent may have privacy concerns and should be draped to avoid unnecessary exposure.

During *inspection*, the nurse observes the color, shape and contour of the abdomen. Any signs of distention or asymmetry are noted. Visible peristalsis may be seen in the thin, malnourished infant or in the infant with obstruction due to pyloric stenosis. The presence of any hernias is noted. A prominent venous pattern may be seen in children with cirrhosis of the liver.

Inspection of GI tract secretions, such as vomitus and stool, should be done if the opportunity presents itself. Mucus and blood may be present in the stool in various infectious and inflammatory conditions. Changes in stool color, consistency, or odor can point to GI tract dysfunction (Table 18–1). Accurate description of the appearance and characteristics of stool and other GI secretions is important not only in diagnosing alterations in function but also in evaluating the patient's response to treatment.

Auscultation of all four quadrants of the abdomen is done to assess bowel sounds, which represent peristaltic movement throughout the intestinal tract. Normal bowel sounds have a metallic, tinkling quality and may be heard every 10 to 30 seconds. The absence of bowel sounds indicates intestinal ileus. Increased, or hyperactive, bowel sounds may be heard in acute gastroenteritis. High-pitched, hyperactive bowel sounds may indicate partial intestinal obstruction.

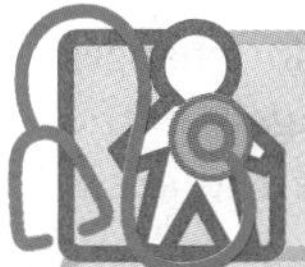

Chart 18–2
Focused Physical Assessment

Alteration in the Gastrointestinal System

Parameter	Abnormal findings
General appearance	Unwell Poor state of hygiene Overall nutritional status (obese, cachectic) Alterations in speech, motor development Disturbed/abnormal parent/child interaction
Skin	Color—jaundice, erythema, pallor Integrity—presence of lesions, rashes Turgor—tenting, edema
Hair	Color changes, depigmentation Texture—dry, coarse Distribution—sparse, easily plucked
Nails	Clubbing, ridges Pitting, spooning
Eyes	Periorbital edema Jaundiced sclera
Mouth	Perioral, oral lesions Cheilosis Glossitis Fetor
Chest	Increased respiratory rate Breath sounds—wheeze, rhonchi Gynecomastia
Abdomen	Inspection: Shape, contour—presence of distention, irregular contour Color—discoloration, redness Visible peristaltic waves Visible mass, hernia Prominent venous pattern Auscultation: Absent bowel sounds High-pitched, hyperactive high-pitched bowel sounds Vascular bruits, rushes Percussion: Presence of excessive gas, masses, fluid Enlarged liver span Palpation: Pain, tenderness Rigidity Enlarged liver, spleen margins Abdominal girth (circumference)
Inguinal region	Scrotal edema, ability to transilluminate Hernia
Anus, rectum, vagina	Fissures Lesions Excoriation Inflammation Skin tags Rectovaginal fistula

caREminder: *Listen for a full 5 minutes in all four abdominal quadrants to establish the absence of bowel sounds.*

Percussion of the abdomen is done to distinguish between solid organs or masses in the abdominal cavity versus the presence of fluid or gas. The abdomen is percussed in all four quadrants. Tympanic, drum-like sounds are heard over air-filled organs, particularly the stomach and intestines. When the abdomen is distended, increased tympanic sounds may be heard if gas has accumulated due to an ileus or obstruction. In some cases, an infant may have increased tympanic sounds due to air swallowing while feeding or crying. Flat, dull sounds on abdominal percussion may indicate an accumulation of fluid or a solid mass.

Liver size, or span, can be measured by percussing along the right midclavicular line. The normal liver span of the pediatric patient varies according to age. It averages 2.6 cm at 6 months, 3 cm at 12 months, 3.5 cm at 24 months, 4.4 cm at 4 years, 5 cm at 6 years, 5.4 cm at 8 years, and 5.8 cm at 10 years. Any enlargement of the liver is noted and reported to the advanced practice nurse or physician.

Palpation of the abdomen is done to assess for enlargement of solid organs and to detect the presence of masses. The character of the abdomen (soft or hard) and the presence of tenderness or pain are also assessed. To

Table 18–1
Abnormal Findings: Emesis and Stool

Parameter	Finding/Potential Pathology
Emesis	
Hematemesis	Emesis containing blood Bright red blood indicates acute upper GI hemorrhage Brown, "coffee ground" blood indicates ongoing or chronic process
Bilious vomiting	Emesis containing bile Green or yellow, indicative of GI obstruction
Feculent vomiting	Emesis containing stool Brown, foul smelling, indicative of GI obstruction
Stool	
Hematochezia	Bright red or maroon blood per rectum Usually associated with bleeding from lower GI tract or anal fissures
Melena	Dark, tarry stool Usually associated with bleeding from upper GI tract
Currant jelly stool	Stool with red blood and mucus Associated with intussusception
Steatorrhea	Fatty stools, may be pale, bulky, malodorous Associated with fat malabsorption, pancreatic insufficiency
Acholic stool	Clay-colored stool Occurs with biliary tract obstruction or bile deficiencies

promote relaxation of the abdominal muscles, the nurse has the child flex the knees before palpating the abdomen. Preschool and school-age children in particular may be ticklish, thus making palpation difficult.

Tip: *To reduce ticklishness in the child, the examiner should place the child's hand under his or her own, with the examiner's fingers extending beyond the child's, so the examiner can palpate with the child's fingerpads.*

When attempting to examine a crying child, the difference between a hard and soft abdomen can best be felt when palpating during the inspiratory phase of the respiratory cycle. In a child with reported abdominal pain, palpation should start in an area distant from the identified area of pain. In the case of the preverbal child or the child who has difficulty verbally identifying the exact location of the pain, the nurse observes for changes in facial expression or body posture or changes in the pitch of crying during palpation of the abdomen to assess for the location of pain.

Alert: *If a mass is identified in the area of the kidneys it should not be palpated. If the mass is a tumor, this can cause release of cells that are potentially metastatic.*

Infants and young children may normally have a palpable liver edge 1 to 2 cm below the right costal margin in the midclavicular line. The liver edge should not be palpable in the adolescent. Enlargement of the liver, known as hepatomegaly, is present when the liver is palpable more than 3 cm below the right costal margin.

Measuring abdominal girth is a fairly accurate way to monitor progressive abdominal distention in children. A paper tape measure is used; cloth tape measures (in addition to their associated infection control issues) stretch over time and provide inaccurate readings. If the tape measure is not long enough, two can be taped together to provide sufficient length. The abdomen is measured over the umbilicus (Fig. 18–1). The tape measure is pulled snug, but not tight, around the abdomen, and the reading is taken on expiration. When ostomies, tubes, or other devices prevent measuring over the umbilicus, the measurement is made over the same area each time to allow for comparison. When serial measurements are being taken, two small lines are marked with a marker or ball-point pen on each side of the tape measure and on the right and left sides of the abdomen, to indicate where to place the tape measure. If serial readings are being done and the child is uncomfortable with move-

Figure 18–1
Abdominal girth should be measured over the umbilicus whenever possible.

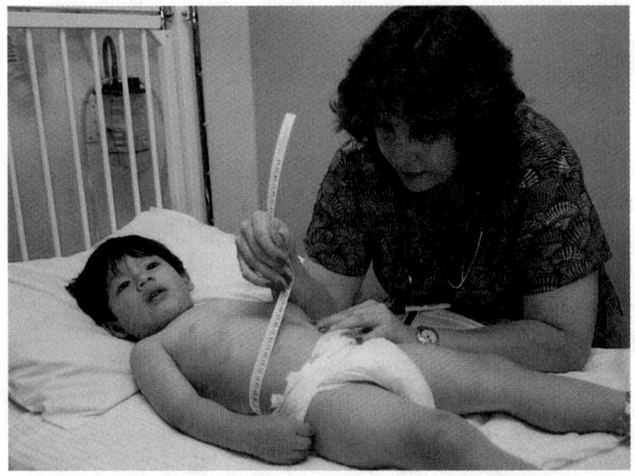

ment, the nurse leaves the tape measure in place under the child, making sure that it is smooth and not twisted.

Nursing Diagnoses and Outcomes

Analysis of assessment findings will identify nursing diagnoses pertinent to that child and family. Chapter 9 identifies nursing diagnoses commonly applicable to the psychosocial needs of the acutely ill child. Nursing diagnoses pertinent to the child with an alteration in GI status often reflect the alteration in nutrition or fluid and electrolyte status caused by GI conditions. Nursing diagnoses generally applicable to a child with altered GI status are listed in Chart 18–3. Nursing diagnoses more specific to a particular GI disorder are identified in the section covering that disorder.

Developmental and Biological Variances

Developmental and biological variances in the GI system are most pronounced during infancy and especially so in the preterm infant (see Chapter 8). The GI tract begins to develop during the fourth week of gestation. By the end of the second trimester, the organs of the GI tract are formed and have many of the structures in place that allow for some elementary physiologic function. During the third trimester, these structures become more developed and differentiated in their functions. Some functions—particularly those related to ingestion, digestion, and absorption of nutrients—are not fully developed at birth, accounting for the special feeding requirements of infants (Fig. 18–2, see Table 8–6).

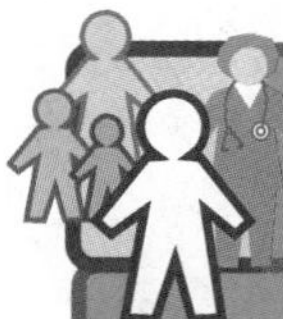

Chart 18–3
Nursing Diagnoses and Outcomes

Alteration in Gastrointestinal Function

Fluid volume deficit related to inadequate intake or excessive losses from GI tract

Outcomes: The child will achieve and maintain normal fluid and electrolyte balance.
The child and parents will identify signs of fluid imbalance and implement interventions to treat this.

Pain related to the effects of GI system dysfunction, procedures, and treatments

Outcomes: The child will not verbalize or exhibit behavioral signs of discomfort.
The child/family will describe interventions to be implemented if the child experiences pain.

Altered nutrition: less than body requirements related to effects of alteration in GI tract function

Outcomes: The child/family will identify ways to achieve appropriate nutritional intake.
The child will demonstrate appropriate nutritional intake.
The child will show maintenance of growth velocity along own growth curve.

Knowledge deficit: the child's GI condition and treatment

Outcomes: The child/family will be able to describe the illness and identify significant clinical manifestations and potential complications.
The child/family will be able to describe the treatment plan for the illness and demonstrate the ability to administer the necessary medications and treatments.

Altered family processes secondary to illness of child, demands of management, and stress

Outcomes: The child/family will show positive patterns of family functioning.
The child/family will receive support/referrals to assist them in maintaining family processes.

Altered growth and development related to restrictions imposed by condition, parents, or self; inability to participate in developmentally appropriate activities

Outcomes: The child will perform developmentally appropriate tasks.
The parents will identify normal developmental milestones for their child and ways to help their child achieve these milestones.

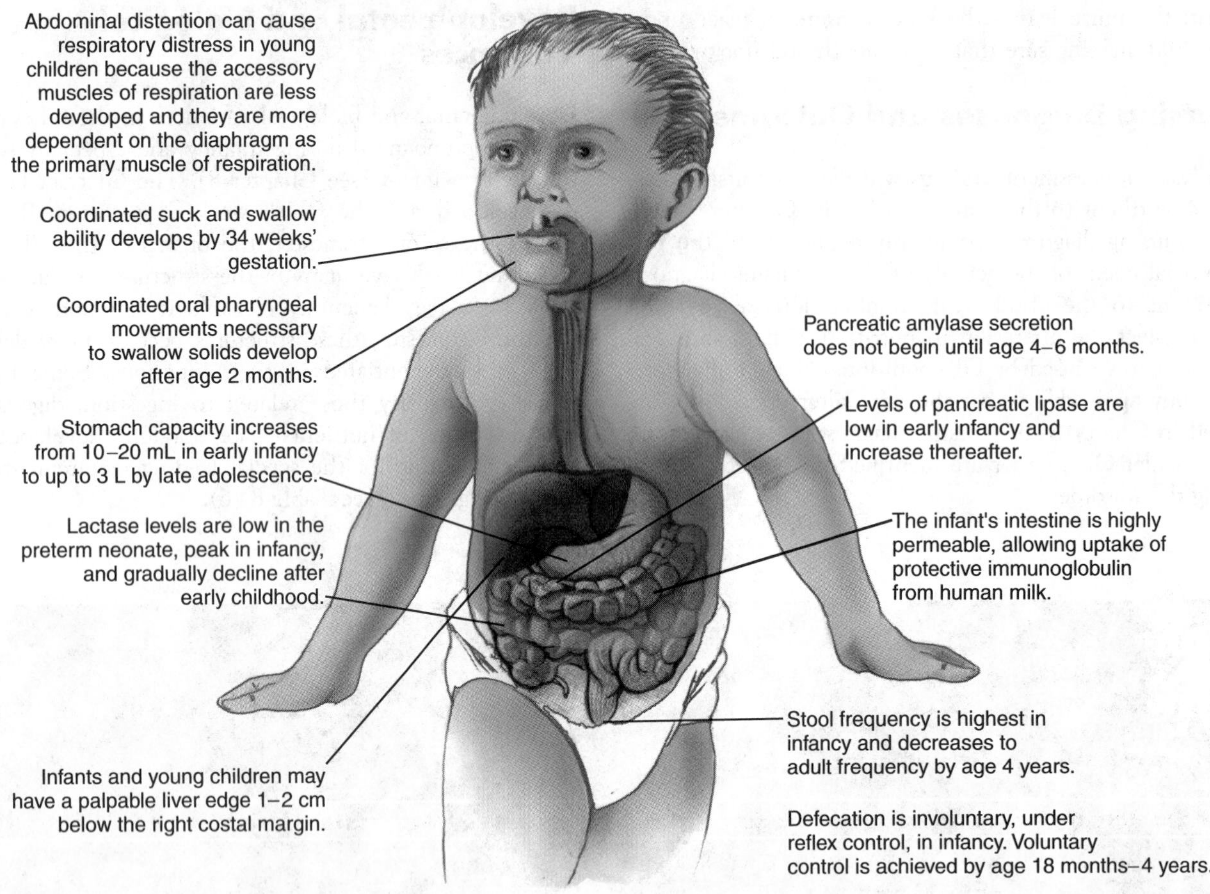

Abdominal distention can cause respiratory distress in young children because the accessory muscles of respiration are less developed and they are more dependent on the diaphragm as the primary muscle of respiration.
Coordinated suck and swallow ability develops by 34 weeks' gestation.
Coordinated oral pharyngeal movements necessary to swallow solids develop after age 2 months.
Stomach capacity increases from 10–20 mL in early infancy to up to 3 L by late adolescence.
Lactase levels are low in the preterm neonate, peak in infancy, and gradually decline after early childhood.
Infants and young children may have a palpable liver edge 1–2 cm below the right costal margin.
Pancreatic amylase secretion does not begin until age 4–6 months.
Levels of pancreatic lipase are low in early infancy and increase thereafter.
The infant's intestine is highly permeable, allowing uptake of protective immunoglobulin from human milk.
Stool frequency is highest in infancy and decreases to adult frequency by age 4 years.
Defecation is involuntary, under reflex control, in infancy. Voluntary control is achieved by age 18 months–4 years.

Figure 18–2
Developmental and biological variances: gastrointestinal system.

Ingestion of Nutrients

The coordinated suck and swallow pattern necessary for feeding develops around 34 weeks' gestation. The coordinated oropharyngeal movements necessary to swallow solid foods are not developed until after the second month of life. The stomach capacity of the newborn is quite small, holding only 10 to 20 mL, but expands rapidly to hold 30 to 90 mL by the end of the first week of life and reaches adult capacity of 2000 to 3000 mL by late adolescence. The small intestine, which is only 200 to 250 cm long at birth, lengthens to 350 to 600 cm by adulthood.

Food intake, along with calorie and nutrient requirements, varies from infancy to childhood to adolescence. During periods of rapid growth, such as infancy and adolescence, food intake is increased. During periods of slower growth, food intake may decrease. This may help to explain the behavior of the toddler or preschooler who has become a "picky eater."

Digestion and Absorption of Nutrients

The systems for digestion and absorption of major nutrients are not fully mature in the premature and term infant. In the older child and adult the initial breakdown or hydrolysis of *carbohydrates* depends on both salivary and pancreatic amylase. In the infant, carbohydrate hydrolysis is limited by the fact that although salivary amylase is present by 34 weeks' gestation, secretion of pancreatic amylase does not begin until age 4 to 6 months. Because of this, young infants are relatively intolerant of starches and may experience diarrhea if cereals are offered too early. Lactose is the primary source of carbohydrate in breast milk and most infant formulas. At the level of the intestinal villi, lactose is hydrolyzed by the enzyme lactase. Lactase levels are highest in early infancy and begin to decline during the first year of life. In some individuals, lactase levels may decline to the point where lactose intolerance occurs. This is especially common in Asian and African-American populations.

Digestion and absorption of *protein* is relatively efficient in the preterm and newborn infant. The infant's intestine is more permeable than that of the older child or adult, which allows for the uptake of protective immunoglobulin proteins from human milk. This same permeability allows passage of cow's milk protein and other potential allergens through the intestinal barrier into the bloodstream, making infants more susceptible to food protein allergies and GI infections.

Digestion and absorption of *fat* in infancy is limited by low levels of pancreatic lipase, one of the enzymes responsible for breaking down ingested fats, and low concentrations of bile acids. The breast-fed infant demonstrates more efficient absorption of fat than the formula-fed infant, owing to the uniqueness of the lipase contained in breast milk.

Elimination

Normal patterns of GI elimination vary throughout the life cycle. The number and consistency of stools, as well as the ability to control elimination of stool, change during the period from infancy to early childhood. Stool frequency in the infant may be highly variable. The newborn may have three to seven stools per day, depending on the type and amount of feeding given. The breast-fed infant may go up to a week without any stool, without any signs of discomfort or abdominal distention, owing to the low residue of breast milk. The color and consistency of stool also vary. A breast-fed infant's stools may have a yellow, "seedy" appearance and a somewhat runny consistency; a formula-fed infant's stools may have a yellow or brownish color and a more pasty consistency. As solid foods are introduced, stool color may be affected by the particular foods the child eats.

By age 4 years, stool frequency decreases to the adult level of one or two stools per day. Stool consistency is also comparable to the adult's.

In infancy, defecation takes place by reflex and is not under voluntary control. Voluntary control of defecation may be attained at age 18 months to 4 years. Cultural variations in toilet-training practices may account for this variability as much as physiologic variables.

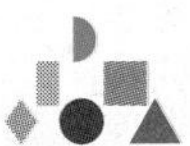

Diagnostic Criteria for Evaluating Alterations in Gastrointestinal Status

A wide variety of diagnostic tests and procedures are used to evaluate alterations in GI structure and function. Laboratory studies analyze blood, GI secretions, urine, and stool. Radiographic and nonradiographic imaging techniques visualize both the structure and the function of GI organs. Endoscopic examination directly visualizes the inner lumen of the GI tract. Biopsy techniques evaluate alterations in GI organs at the cellular level.

The nurse must be familiar with both the purpose of and the procedures involved in the various diagnostic tests and studies used to evaluate alterations in GI status. This is important so that the nurse can ensure appropriate preparation and support of both the patient and family before, during, and after each diagnostic procedure. Preparing the child and family includes providing age-appropriate explanations of the test's purpose, steps, and duration, as well as anticipatory guidance about sensations the child may experience during the test. Conscious sedation is commonly used for many endoscopic procedures, requiring vigilant monitoring of the child (see Chapter 13).

Diagnostic specimens are obtained and handled carefully. Many agents causing GI illness are highly infectious, such as viral and bacterial stool pathogens. Meticulous attention to standard precautions must be maintained when handling stool specimens, blood samples, and other GI tract secretions and tissues. Table 18–2 summarizes tests and procedures commonly used in the evaluation of alterations in the GI system.

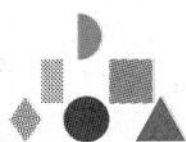

Treatment Modalities

The disease and child's clinical condition determine needed treatment. Treatment may include diet modification, nutritional support including enteral feeding, endoscopy, or surgical intervention.

Therapeutic Endoscopy

Therapeutic endoscopy involves the use of endoscopic techniques for the treatment of specific GI alterations. *Dilation* of strictured GI tract structures, most commonly the esophagus, may be accomplished endoscopically. *Foreign body removal* may be done by upper GI endoscopy. Endoscopic *sclerotherapy* is used in the treatment of the esophageal and gastric varices and dilated blood vessels, which can be a life-threatening source of GI bleeding in the child with end-stage liver disease. In sclerotherapy, a sclerosing agent that causes hardening of the blood vessel is injected into and around the varix to cause thrombosis and obliteration of the vein. *Excision* of GI polyps, most commonly found in the colon, may be done by endos-

Text continued on page 1041

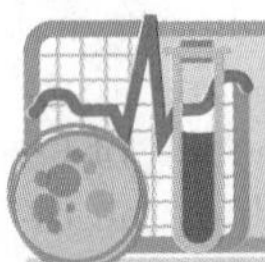

Table 18–2
Tests and Procedures for Evaluation of Alteration in the Gastrointestinal System

Test	Purpose	Health Care Provider Responsibility
Imaging Radiologic and Nonradiologic		
Flat plate abdominal x-ray	Used for initial evaluation for presence of obstruction, air-fluid levels, structural changes, and calcifications	Infants and younger children may require assistance with positioning and immobilization.
Barium swallow	Used to evaluate esophagus for presence of strictures, foreign bodies, ulcerations, varices, and motility disorders	NPO before examination
Upper gastrointestinal (UGI) series with small bowel follow-through	Radiographic evaluation of esophagus, stomach, and small intestine; may be used for diagnosis of strictures, obstruction, ulcers, inflammatory bowel disease, and motility disorders.	NPO before examination (infants 3 to 4 hours, older children after midnight for AM test). Children who are unable or unwilling to drink contrast medium used in examination; may require nasogastric administration. Younger children may require immobilization during examination.
Barium enema	Used for evaluation of colon. Structural and functional changes and polyps may be identified.	Contraindicated in patients with fulminant ulcerative colitis, or suspected perforation. Should be performed before upper GI studies to prevent contamination from previous contrast. No bowel prep for infants. Bowel prep for older children may include clear liquid diet, cathartics, or enema.
Gastric emptying study	Evaluates rates at which stomach empties after ingestion of radionuclide-labeled solid or liquid meal. Used in diagnosis of obstruction and motility disorders of stomach.	Child must be NPO before test. Prepare child and caregivers that child must ingest labeled meal in radiology department and images will be taken every 15 minutes for up to 3 hours.
Abdominal ultrasound	Used to visualize size, structure of liver, gallbladder, and biliary tract. Can be used to identify cysts, abscess, tumor, gallstones, and appendicitis.	Prepare child, family that test will take 20 to 30 minutes; lubricant gel will be used on skin over abdomen. Younger children may require assistance with positioning and immobilization.
Computed tomography (CT)	Used to identify tumors, presence of intra-abdominal or hepatic abscess or cyst, and obstruction of biliary ducts.	Child may be required to take oral contrast material before the test. If unable to take by mouth, may require nasogastric administration. Child must lie still for 30 to 90 minutes during test. May require sedation.
Liver biliary scan (HIDA scan)	Radionuclide scan used to visualize flow in the biliary ductal system, both uptake and excretion. Used in the diagnosis of biliary atresia and evaluation of biliary tract obstruction after liver transplant.	Child must be NPO before test. Requires an IV access for administration of contrast medium.
Cholangiogram	Used to evaluate biliary tract for presence and location of stones and other causes of obstruction. May be done intraoperatively or postoperatively with contrast medium injected via a T-tube. Contrast medium may also be given intravenously.	Document patient allergies before procedure. Contrast medium used in test is usually iodine based, so patients with history of iodine or seafood allergy or history of previous reaction to iodine-based contrast medium must be identified.

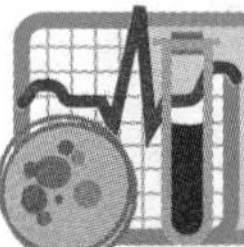

Table 18–2
Tests and Procedures for Evaluation of Alteration in the Gastrointestinal System *Continued*

Test	Purpose	Health Care Provider Responsibility
Endoscopic Examination		
Esophageal manometry	Used to diagnose and evaluate motility disorders of the esophagus. Used in the work-up of patients with dysphagia and reflux. A long, flexible catheter with pressure transducers is passed into the esophagus orally or transnasally and intraluminal pressures of the lower esophageal sphincter and esophageal body are measured.	The child must be NPO before the procedure. Sedation is usually required.
Upper gastrointestinal endoscopy	Using a fiberoptic endoscope, the lumen and mucosal lining of the esophagus, stomach and upper portion of the small intestine can be seen. Tissue abnormality, upper GI bleeding, ulcers can be identified and evaluated, biopsies may be done. Endoscopy may be used therapeutically for sclerosing of esophageal or gastric varices or placement of percutaneous endoscopic gastrostomy tube.	The child must be NPO before the procedure. Conscious sedation or general anesthesia will be used. Vital signs and oxygen saturation should be monitored during the procedure and afterward until the child is fully awake. Monitor for signs of pulmonary aspiration, perforation, or bleeding.
Lower gastrointestinal endoscopy (colonoscopy)	Endoscopic evaluation of colon and terminal ileum. May be used in diagnosis and evaluation of inflammatory bowel disease, gastrointestinal or rectal bleeding, and diarrhea. Biopsies may be done in conjunction with colonoscopy.	Bowel prep required pre-procedure. Infants may require only clear liquids 12 to 24 hours before the procedure. Older children's prep may include cathartics by mouth or nasogastric tube or enemas. Sedation usually required, although adolescents may tolerate procedure without. Patients should be monitored during and after procedure for abdominal pain, bleeding, and any change in vital signs.
Anorectal manometry	Used in the diagnosis and treatment of children with chronic constipation and fecal incontinence. May be used in the diagnosis of Hirschprung's disease. Pressure transducers record the response of the internal sphincter to distention of balloons on the manometry equipment.	Monitor patient for signs of rectal bleeding, abdominal distention, or perforation after procedure.
24-Hour pH probe	Used in the evaluation of gastroesophageal reflux. A pH probe is passed transnasally into the distal esophagus. The probe is attached to an external monitor that measures and records the intraesophageal pH. Reflux of acid stomach contents will result in pH readings <4.	The child must be NPO before the probe placement and must be off acid antagonists during the examination. pH probe placement must be maintained throughout the test. All activities must be recorded in a designated log—sleep, wake periods, start and stop of feedings, position and occurrence of any reflux symptoms: cough, choking, emesis, apnea, bradycardia, or cyanosis. Family members may participate in record keeping and should be instructed as to the above.

Table continued on following page

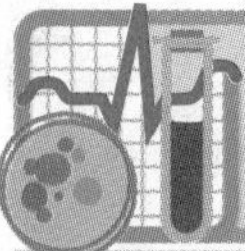

Table 18–2
Tests and Procedures for Evaluation of Alteration in the Gastrointestinal System *Continued*

Test	Purpose	Health Care Provider Responsibility
Biopsy		
Liver biopsy	Percutaneous needle aspiration of liver used for microscopic examination of tissue cells and structure. Used to diagnose and evaluate the extent of liver disease and evaluate graft function after liver transplant.	Child must be NPO for biopsy. Blood prothrombin time activated partial thromboplastin time, and platelet count should be done before the test and the physician notified regarding any abnormal levels. The procedure is most often done with conscious sedation so an IV access should be established for administration of the necessary medications. Vital signs and oxygen saturation should be monitored during the procedure and for 6 to 8 hours afterward. The child must remain positioned on the right side for 1 to 2 hours after the procedure. The child should be observed for any signs of bleeding, peritonitis, or pneumothorax after the procedure.
Esophagus, stomach, intestine	Used to diagnose mucosal abnormalities and evaluate response to therapy. Done in conjunction with endoscopic procedure.	Same as for endoscopic procedures.
Stool		
Occult blood (guaiac test)	Used to detect fecal occult blood from a GI source. May be positive in patients with gastritis, inflammatory bowel disease, peptic ulcer disease, malabsorption.	A small amount of stool is applied to guaiac paper; then 2 drops of developing solution are placed on the reverse side. Paper will turn blue in the presence of blood. Menstrual blood, anal fissures, and perianal skin breakdown may cause false-positive results. Instruct family members regarding collection of specimen if home testing is desired.
Stool pH	Bedside screening test for malabsorption of sugar, utilizing nitrazine pH paper.	Small amount of fresh liquid stool is applied to pH paper and resulting color is compared to pH color chart. A pH <6 is indicative of malabsorption.
Reducing substances	Screens for intestinal malabsorption of sugars as indicated by presence of reducing substances (sugars) in stool.	A Clinitest tablet is placed in 5 drops of fresh liquid stool mixed with 10 drops of water. Resulting color is compared to Clinitest color chart. A reading over 0.5% indicates malabsorption of sugars.
Fecal fat	72-Hour stool collection used to evaluate the ability of the GI tract to digest and absorb fat from dietary intake. Elevated levels of fat in the stool are found in patients with malabsorption syndromes, short bowel syndrome, and biliary tract obstruction.	All stool is collected for 72-hour period in one heavy plastic screw-cap container. Specimen must stay refrigerated during collection period. A concurrent diet record may be requested. Instruct child and family regarding collection procedure if home testing is desired.
Stool for white cells (methylene blue stain)	Rapid, nonspecific screening test used to detect the presence of polymorphonuclear leukocytes in the stool. Leukocytes may be present in diarrhea caused by invasive bacteria such as *Salmonella* or *Shigella* and in ulcerative or antibiotic-associated colitis.	Collect fresh stool specimen in clean, plastic container with a lid. Send immediately to the lab. Barium in the specimen may interfere with test results.

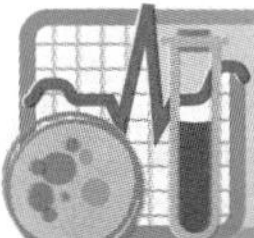

Table 18–2
Tests and Procedures for Evaluation of Alteration in the Gastrointestinal System *Continued*

Test	Purpose	Health Care Provider Responsibility
Stool *Continued*		
Ova and parasite	Used to identify the presence of specific parasites in GI tract.	Requires special specimen container with preservative. Fresh stool specimen is placed in designated container. Test may be repeated on 3 consecutive days.
Bacterial culture	Used to identify presence of bacterial organisms causing intestinal infections, commonly resulting in fever and diarrhea.	Specimen should be obtained before antibiotic therapy is started. Specimen should not be mixed with urine and should be transported directly to the lab.
Rotavirus	In cases of suspected viral gastroenteritis, used to identify presence of rotavirus, a viral infection that is a common cause of vomiting and diarrhea in infants and toddlers during the winter months.	Stool should be collected in sterile specimen container. Specimen should be refrigerated if immediate transport to lab is not available.
Alpha$_1$-antitrypsin	Used to identify protein loss in the stool, found in protein-losing enteropathies and diarrheal disease and characterized by excessive protein losses in the stool and hypoalbuminemia.	Send fresh stool specimen to lab in clean container.
Other		
Hydrogen breath test	Used in the diagnosis of carbohydrate malabsorption and bacterial overgrowth of the intestine. Uses gas-liquid chromatography to measure amount of hydrogen exhaled after ingestion of a carbohydrate solution, usually lactose based. Elevated levels of breath hydrogen may be found in patients with lactase deficiency, mucosal damage, delayed intestinal transit, or colonic flora in the small intestine.	Child must be NPO before the procedure. Expired air is collected before ingestion of carbohydrate drink and at 30-minute intervals for 3 hours after. Ask family to bring child's usual bottle or cup from home to facilitate intake of drink and a favorite toy or activity to provide distraction during waiting time.
Schilling test	Measures the ability of the small intestine to absorb vitamin B_{12}. Results may be decreased in patients with ileal resection, Crohn's disease, and celiac sprue.	After administration of radionuclide-labeled vitamin B_{12}, urine is collected in a designated container for 24 hours. Fecal contamination of urine will alter results. Instruct child and family in appropriate collection procedure for home collection.
Gastric pH	Used to assess pH of gastric secretions. Of importance in measuring levels of gastric acidity in patients who are at risk for or are being treated for gastritis.	Gastric secretions are aspirated from a nasogastric or gastrostomy tube. Secretions are placed on pH paper and resulting color is compared to color chart. Usual goal in treatment of gastritis is a gastric pH ≥ 4.
Blood Studies		
Hemoglobin (Hgb), hematocrit (Hct)	Used to detect anemia from blood loss from GI tract and inadequate nutrient intake. Hct may be increased with dehydration.	Explain procedure and support child during specimen collection.
Red cell indices (MCV, MCHC, RDW)	Used to determine cause of nutritional anemias. Indices decreased and iron-deficiency anemia and increased with vitamin B_{12} deficiency.	Explain procedure and support child during specimen collection. Obtain blood sample and send to lab in correct container.

Table continued on following page

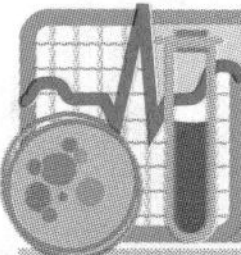

Table 18–2
Tests and Procedures for Evaluation of Alteration in the Gastrointestinal System *Continued*

Test	Purpose	Health Care Provider Responsibility
Blood Studies *Continued*		
WBC, differential	Used to evaluate for presence of infection and inflammation. Increased with bacterial infection and inflammatory bowel disease. May be decreased in cases of splenic sequestration in end-stage liver disease and immunosuppression after liver transplant.	
Platelet count	May increase with acute infection and inflammatory disease. Levels may decrease with liver disease.	
Prothrombin time (PT), activated partial thromboplastin time (APTT)	Used to evaluate efficacy of coagulation system. Reflects degree of liver dysfunction in patients with liver disease. Used to assess for Vitamin K deficiency in patients with impaired intake or absorption.	PTT may be falsely elevated when drawn from intravascular lines containing heparin.
Fibrinogen	Levels may be elevated in sepsis and inflammation. Levels are decreased in severe liver disease.	
Electrolytes: sodium (Na^+), potassium (K^+), chloride (Cl^-), carbon dioxide (CO_2)	Used to assess hydration status, acid-base balance. Of special importance in diseases characterized by excessive loss of fluid and electrolytes from GI tract due to diarrhea, vomiting, or gastric drainage.	
Blood urea nitrogen (BUN), creatinine (Cr)	Used to evaluate hydration status. Elevation seen in dehydration. BUN may be elevated with excessive protein intake, especially in parenterally fed children. ↑ BUN with concurrent ↑ Cr may suggest renal impairment.	
Glucose	Levels may be elevated with excess dextrose administration with TPN, corticosteroid therapy, or sepsis. Levels may be low in patients with impaired glycogen storage in liver disease.	
Alanine aminotransferase (ALT), aspartate aminotransferase (AST)	Used to assess the degree of hepatocellular damage in liver disease and graft function in liver transplantation. Also used to monitor liver function in children receiving hepatotoxic medications and total parenteral nutrition (TPN).	
Alkaline phosphatase	Used for assessment of liver function. May be elevated with liver disease or cholestasis. May also be elevated in children with rickets secondary to impaired intake or absorption of calcium and phosphorus.	
Ammonia	Used to monitor patients with severe liver failure. Levels are elevated in patients with hepatic encephalopathy.	
Bilirubin (total, direct, indirect)	Used for evaluation of liver function and determine cause of various forms of jaundice. Levels are elevated in many forms of liver disease.	

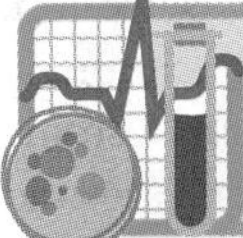

Table 18–2
Tests and Procedures for Evaluation of Alteration in the Gastrointestinal System *Continued*

Test	Purpose	Health Care Provider Responsibility
Blood Studies *Continued*		
Hepatitis antigens, antibodies	Used to detect causative agents of hepatitis infection. Specific antibodies and antigens help to determine whether infection is active, chronic, or resolved.	
Calcium	Used to evaluate acid-base balance, adequacy of calcium intake, and absorption. May be increased with excess intake (especially in the TPN dependent child), dehydration. Decreased values may be seen in malnutrition, vitamin D deficiency, and hypoalbuminemia.	
Magnesium	Abnormal levels may be seen with excessive or inadequate intake, especially in the TPN-dependent child. Low levels may be seen with excessive losses from gastric drainage or malabsorptive states.	
Phosphorus	Levels may be elevated with dehydration and cirrhosis. Absorption may be impaired and levels decreased in patients with malabsorptive diseases. Levels may also be decreased with excess fluid loss from GI tract, malnutrition, vitamin D deficiency.	
Total protein, albumin	Used to monitor nutritional status and liver function. Levels may be elevated with dehydration. Levels are decreased in patients with malnutrition, liver disease, and protein-losing enteropathies.	
Vitamins A, D, E	Absorption of fat-soluble vitamins A, D, and E may be impaired in children with malabsorption syndromes or liver disease. Levels are used to identify deficiencies and evaluate response to replacement therapy.	
Zinc	An important element in protein synthesis and wound healing. Zinc is normally excreted through the GI tract. Children with excess losses through the GI tract from diarrhea or prolonged nasogastric drainage may be at risk for deficiencies.	

copy. Gastrostomy tubes, used in the delivery of enteral nutrition, may be placed by endoscopy. *Percutaneous endoscopic gastrostomy* (PEG) eliminates the need for laparotomy and, in many cases, general anesthesia, which are used in traditional surgical gastrostomy.

Surgical Intervention

Surgical intervention is used to repair alterations in GI tract structures, remove diseased structures, or, in the case of liver transplant, replace nonfunctional structures. Surgical intervention may also be used to place medical devices, such as gastrostomy tubes and central venous catheters, used in the treatment of GI disorders. Surgical interventions specific to a particular GI disorder, along with the associated nursing care issues, are discussed in the section covering that disorder.

General care of the child undergoing surgery is discussed in Chapter 9. Pain control and promotion of deep breathing are particularly important in the child after abdominal surgery. Pain may prevent good lung excursion, increasing the risk of atelectasis.

Peristalsis takes longer to return after abdominal surgery than after surgery in other systems. This depends in part on the extent of bowel manipulation during surgery. The nurse monitors for the return of bowel sounds by auscultating the child's abdomen periodically. The child is kept NPO until peristalsis returns. Early ambulation is encouraged to promote lung excursion and the return of peristalsis.

Excess losses of fluid from the GI tract, such as occur with suction and diarrhea, hypoproteinemia, and malnutrition, may cause fluid and electrolyte imbalance. The nurse monitors the child's fluid and electrolyte status and administers appropriate replacement therapy as ordered.

Ostomy Care

An ostomy is a surgically created opening between the GI tract and the outside of the body (Fig. 18–3). Ostomies may be created at various sites in the GI tract and may be temporary or permanent, depending on the child's clinical condition. An *esophagostomy* communicates between the esophagus and an external site on the neck. A *gastrostomy* provides an opening between the stomach and the abdominal wall. Ostomies may be created at various sites in the small intestine (e.g., jejunostomy, ileostomy) or in the large intestine (e.g., colostomy). (See Chapter 19 for further discussion of stomal diversions.)

An *enterostomal therapist* is an RN with specialized training and certification in the management of ostomies and is an essential resource for the care of the child with an ostomy. The enterostomal therapist collaborates with the surgeon in ostomy site selection whenever possible and provides information regarding product selection, pouching techniques, and patient and family education.

Nursing management of the child with an ostomy includes both interventions that provide direct care and interventions that promote self-care or care by parents (Chart 18–4). Developmental issues are varied and should be addressed in the nursing plan of care and patient and family education. The parents of an infant with an ostomy may need tips regarding clothing options that protect the pouch system from the infant's exploring hands. School-age children, their parents, and school personnel may need help in dealing with the ostomy in the school setting. The adolescent may have concerns regarding body image and sexuality that need to be discussed. Referral to community support groups may provide children and their families additional support in dealing with adjustment issues surrounding the ostomy.

Nutritional Therapy

Modification of infant formulas, special oral diets, enteral and parenteral nutrition, and specialized feeding techniques are all used in the treatment of the child with altered GI status. Nutritional therapy is an interdisciplinary effort and requires the participation of many health care team members. The nurse plays an important role, not only in the delivery of the various nutritional therapies, but also in assessing the child's response to therapy and in teaching the child and family about the therapeutic regimen.

Infant Formulas

Infant formulas are available in a wide range of formulations designed to meet the variety of nutritional needs.

Figure 18–3
Note the reduction in stoma from shortly after establishment *(A)* to several weeks later *(B)*.

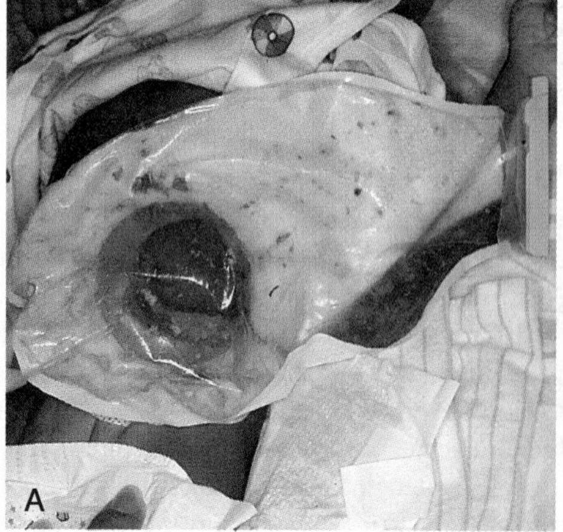

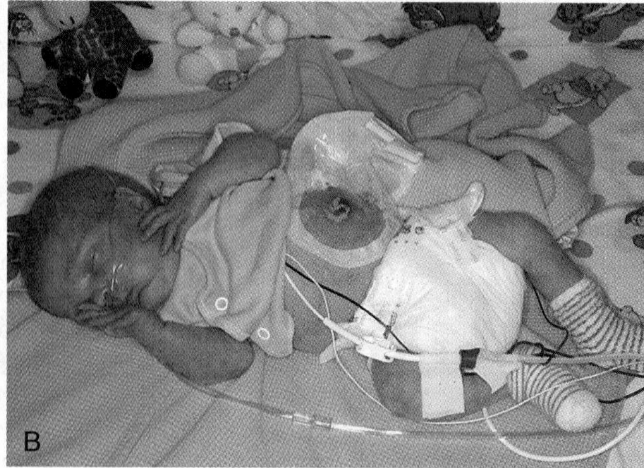

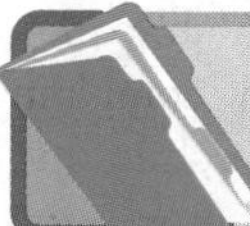

Chart 18–4
Nursing Interventions Classification (NIC)

Ostomy Care

Definition

Maintenance of elimination through a stoma and care of surrounding tissue

Activities

Mark the skin for stoma placement.
Instruct patient/significant other in the use of ileostomy/colostomy equipment.
Assist patient in providing ostomy/ileostomy self-care.
Have patient/significant other demonstrate use of equipment.
Apply appropriately fitting ostomy appliance, as needed.
Monitor for incision/stoma healing.
Encourage patient/significant other to express feelings and concerns about changes in body image.
Encourage visitation to client by persons from such support groups as ileostomy/colostomy clubs.
Irrigate colostomy, as appropriate.
Assist patient in obtaining ostomy/ileostomy equipment.
Instruct patient on mechanisms to reduce odor.
Instruct patient/significant other in appropriate diet and expected changes in elimination function.
Provide support and assistance, while client develops skill in caring for stoma/surrounding tissue.
Monitor stoma/surrounding tissue healing and adaptation to ostomy equipment.
Change/empty ostomy bag, as appropriate.
Encourage participation in ostomy support groups after hospital discharge.

From McCloskey, J., & Bulechek, G. (Eds.). (1996). *Nursing interventions classification (NIC)* (2nd ed.). St. Louis: Mosby–Year Book. Reprinted with permission.

Breast milk is the gold standard for infant feeding. The composition of breast milk is ideally suited to the infant's nutritional needs and the digestive and absorptive capabilities of the infant's GI system. When breast milk is fed to a preterm infant, it must be supplemented with a *human milk fortifier*. This supplements the caloric, protein, vitamin, and mineral content of the breast milk to meet the increased requirements of the preterm infant. *Standard cow's milk infant formulas* are designed to meet the nutrient needs of infants up to age 1 year. They are commonly available in powder, liquid concentrate, and ready-to-feed preparations. For home use, the powdered form is usually most economical. *Preterm infant formulas* contain increased concentrations of calories and proteins and have their fat and vitamin contents modified to meet the unique physiologic and nutritional needs of the premature infant's immature system. *Soy-based infant formulas* utilize a soy protein instead of cow's milk protein and are designed for infants with lactase deficiency or cow's milk protein intolerance. A significant number of infants with cow's milk intolerance also exhibit intolerance to soy proteins. For these infants, as well as infants with various disorders of digestion and absorption, *protein hydrolysate formulas* may be indicated. These formulas have the protein component broken down and have their fat and carbohydrate components modified to facilitate digestion and absorption. These formulas are commonly used for infants with short bowel syndrome. Portagen (Mead Johnson) is a *fat-modified formula* used in the care of infants with disorders that result in malabsorption of fat, such as biliary atresia or cystic fibrosis. This formula provides most fat as medium-chain triglycerides, which are more easily absorbed by the GI tract. *Modular components* can be added to the various infant formulas to increase the concentration of a specific component within the formulas. Individual fat (e.g., MCT oil), carbohydrate (e.g., Moducal, Polycose), and protein (e.g., Casec) supplements are available that may be used to increase the caloric or nutrient density of the formula.

The caloric density of infant formulas may also be altered by varying the amount of water used to mix the formula. Formulas may be diluted by mixing them with extra water. An infant who has increased calorie and nutrient requirements but is fluid restricted or cannot tolerate a large volume of formula may need a concentrated formula. Formula is concentrated by mixing less than the standard amount of water to formula in the powder or liquid concentrate form. Formulas may be concentrated up to as many as 30 calories per ounce in this manner.

Teaching parents and other caregivers about the proper use of infant formulas is an important nursing responsibility in both inpatient and ambulatory settings. Topics to cover include appropriate formula selection, proper technique for mixing and storing formula, and assistance with formula procurement (see Chapters 5 and 7). Parents may try to save money by diluting formula or attempt to "give better nutrition" by feeding concentrated formula. Parents need to be taught that altering caloric density by adding more or less water should be done only with the guidance of a health care provider. Parents are also taught never to mix powdered infant formula with oral electrolyte or rehydrating solutions. Doing so can cause electrolyte imbalance.

Special Oral Diets

Modified oral diets are another form of nutritional therapy used in the treatment of children with GI disorders. The consistency of oral diets may be altered to facilitate ingestion of food for children with oropharyngeal, esophageal, or neuromuscular (e.g., cerebral palsy) impairments that make ingestion of foods difficult. The nutrient composition of a child's diet may be altered to meet disease-specific requirements. Diet modification may be necessary to prevent or alleviate symptoms caused by GI disease or its treatment (Table 18–3).

Various oral supplements may be used to increase caloric and nutrient intake for a child unable to meet nutritional needs from usual dietary sources. Milk-based oral supplements may be added to cow's milk to supplement calories and protein. Clear liquid oral supplements are clear liquid or juice drinks supplemented with protein. Lactose-free oral supplements may be used as a supplement or as a sole source of nutrition. These formulas (e.g., Pediasure [Ross], Kindercal [Mead Johnson]) have 1 calorie/mL, are isotonic, and are formulated to meet the nutritional requirements of children 1 to 10 years of age. Adult lactose-free oral supplements may be used for older children and are available in a variety of preparations, including fiber-enriched, high-protein, and high-calorie formulas.

Although most oral supplements are available in a variety of flavors, many children may initially complain about their palatability. Collaboration with the child and parent, as well as creativity, are helpful in promoting acceptance of oral supplements.

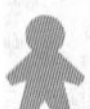

Tip: *Provide opportunities for the child to try different flavors. Altering the temperature and texture of the oral supplement to present them in "kid friendly" forms may also be helpful. Popsicles can be made by freezing the supplement, or a slushie drink can be made by blending the formula with ice.*

Enteral Nutrition

Children with functional GI tracts who are unable to meet their fluid or nutrient requirements by oral feeding may require enteral nutrition (Chart 18–5). Enteral feeding allows delivery of fluids and nutrients directly into the GI tract by means of an enteral feeding tube. Contraindications to enteral nutrition include complete intestinal obstruction, intractable vomiting, and severe enterocolitis.

Enteral Formulas

Various formulas are used for enteral feeding. Formula selection is dictated by the child's age, clinical condition,

Table 18–3
Modified Oral Diets

Diet	Description	Indication
Puree, mechanical soft	Blenderized, ground or chopped whole foods	Dysphagia, esophageal stricture
High fiber	Dietary fiber increased in soluble and nonsoluble forms	Constipation, irritable bowel syndrome
Lactose free	Milk, milk products, lactose-containing foods eliminated	Lactose intolerance
High protein, high calorie	Added portions of food sources of protein, fat provided to increase calorie, protein content of diet	Weight below ideal for age; increased calorie protein needs for wound healing
Fat controlled	Limits dietary fat	Fat malabsorption
Protein restricted	Limits protein intake to decrease nitrogenous waste products in blood stream	Advanced liver disease Renal dysfunction
Salt restricted	Sodium intake restricted to varying degrees depending to reduce sodium and/or fluid retention	Liver disease, children on corticosteroid therapy Renal dysfunction
Gluten restricted, gliaden free	Restricts gluten-containing foods; eliminates gliaden to reduce symptoms caused by sensitivity to gliaden from wheat, rye, oats, and barley	Celiac sprue

Chart 18–5

Indications for Enteral Nutrition

Gastrointestinal Disorders

Esophageal atresia, strictures
Gastroesophageal reflux
Inflammatory bowel disease
Liver disease
Malabsorption, chronic diarrhea
Motility disorders
Pancreatitis
Short bowel syndrome

Increased Metabolic Needs

Burns
Sepsis
Trauma
Congenital heart disease
Bronchopulmonary dysplasia
Cancer

Chronic Disease

Acquired immunodeficiency syndrome
Cystic fibrosis
Renal disease

Neurologic Disorders

Head injury, coma
Cerebral palsy with oral motor impairment
Dysphagia
Tumor

Prematurity

Psychiatric Disorders

Anorexia nervosa

and nutrient requirements. Children younger than age 1 may receive breast milk and standard or specialty infant formulas by enteral feeding tube. For older children, a number of enteral feeding formulas are available.

Standard tube feeding formulas are formulas that are nutritionally complete and designed for use in children with normal digestion and absorption. These formulas (e.g., Pediasure [Ross], Kindercal [Mead Johnson]) are lactose free, have 1 calorie/mL, are isotonic, and are formulated to meet the nutritional requirements of children 1 to 10 years of age. Both the pediatric and adult standard tube feeding formulas are available with or without fiber. Fiber may be indicated for children who experience constipation or diarrhea while on enteral feedings. The adult formulas are also available in a number of high-calorie and high-protein formulations.

Elemental formulas are designed for use in children who have impaired digestion and absorption. These formulas are partially predigested, with protein supplied as peptides or amino acids and a large proportion of fat supplied in the form of medium-chain triglyceride oils. Elemental formulas are available in both pediatric and adult formulations (e.g., Pediatric Vivonex, Peptamen Junior [Clinitec]). Occasionally, an elemental formula may be used as an oral supplement. Flavor packets are available to increase the palatability of the formula in this case. Some tube feeding formulas are designed for use in specific disease states such as renal failure or liver failure. *Modular components* may be added to tube feeding formulas to supplement the carbohydrate, fat, or protein concentration of the formula.

Enteral Feeding Methods

Enteral feedings are delivered into the stomach or, if the child is at risk for pulmonary aspiration, into the small intestine. Feedings may be delivered on a *continuous* or an *intermittent* schedule. *Continuous enteral nutrition* feedings are dripped in slowly over 12 to 24 hours using an enteral feeding pump. Continuous feedings are used when feedings are being delivered into the small intestine. They are also indicated whenever an enterally fed child is assessed to be at high risk for aspiration or has impaired digestion and absorption of nutrients. Continuous nighttime feedings may also be used to supplement the dietary intake in children with some chronic conditions who have increased nutritional needs (e.g., cystic fibrosis, inflammatory bowel disease). *Intermittent enteral nutrition* is administered by bolus or gravity drip method on an interval schedule. The frequency and volume of the feedings are determined by the patient's age, size, and nutritional requirements. A small infant may receive intermittent feedings every 2 to 3 hours, whereas an adolescent may require feedings only every 6 to 8 hours. Intermittent feedings more closely approximate the normal hunger-satiety and physiologic cycles of normal meals and do not require the specialized equipment used for continuous feedings.

Enteral Feeding Tubes

Various enteral feeding tubes may be used to deliver enteral nutrition. Tube selection depends on the child's age, clinical condition, nutrient requirements, desired feeding route, and the anticipated duration of therapy. *Nasoenteric feeding tubes* (nasogastric [NG] or nasojejunal [NJ] tubes) are small-bore feeding tubes passed transnasally through the esophagus into the stomach or small intestine. (See Chart 9–22 for details of NG tube placement.) They are used for short-term enteral nutrition when the anticipated length of therapy is less than 3 months (Mascarenhas, Redd, Bilodeau, Peck, & Liacouras, 1996). These tubes may stay in place continuously or may be placed intermittently as indicated by the child's feeding regimen.

Nasoenteric tubes for short-term or intermittent use are generally made of relatively stiff plastics such as polyvinyl chloride. These tubes have the advantage of being relatively easy to place but may stiffen when left in place for prolonged periods, causing irritation to mucous membranes. These tubes are also commonly used for *orogastric* feedings, where the feeding tube is passed through the mouth directly into the stomach. The orogastric feeding method is most commonly used for premature infants or infants younger than age 4 weeks, who are obligate nose breathers and might experience airway obstruction if the tube is passed transnasally.

Nasoenteric tubes made of softer, more biocompatible materials such as silicone are available. These tubes are less irritating and may stay in place for up to 4 to 6 weeks at a time. These tubes come with a wire stylet, which is inserted into the tube to stiffen it and facilitate placement. The stylet is removed before using the tube for feeding.

Alert: *If resistance is encountered during placement of a nasoenteric feeding tube, do not force the tube. Withdraw the tube and attempt placement again. Use of excessive force may cause perforation.*

Gastrostomy tubes are feeding tubes placed through the abdominal wall directly into the stomach. They are used for children who are anticipated to require enteral feedings for prolonged periods of time. Gastrostomy tubes may be placed surgically or by endoscopic methods (percutaneous endoscopic gastrostomy [PEG] tube). A skin-level gastrostomy tube, sometimes referred to as a "button" gastrostomy, may be placed into a well-healed gastrostomy tract. The skin-level gastrostomy lies flat against the abdominal wall and does not have an external tube (Fig. 18–4). A special feeding adapter is connected to the device when feedings are to be administered. Besides being more cosmetically appealing for many children and parents, this device may be easier to maintain because it is less likely to be subject to dislodgement from tugging or pulling by the child or during vigorous activity.

Jejunostomy tubes are surgically placed directly into the small intestine. They are indicated for long-term enteral nutrition in children with severely impaired gastric emptying because of mechanical obstruction or a motility disorder. Like nasojejunal tubes, feedings administered through a jejunostomy tube are given by the continuous method. Skin level devices may also be used for jejunostomy access. Combination *gastrojejunal tubes* are also available in both nasoenteric and gastrostomy designs.

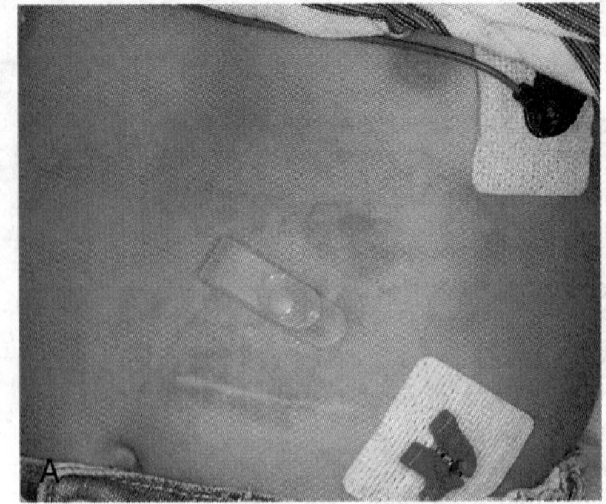

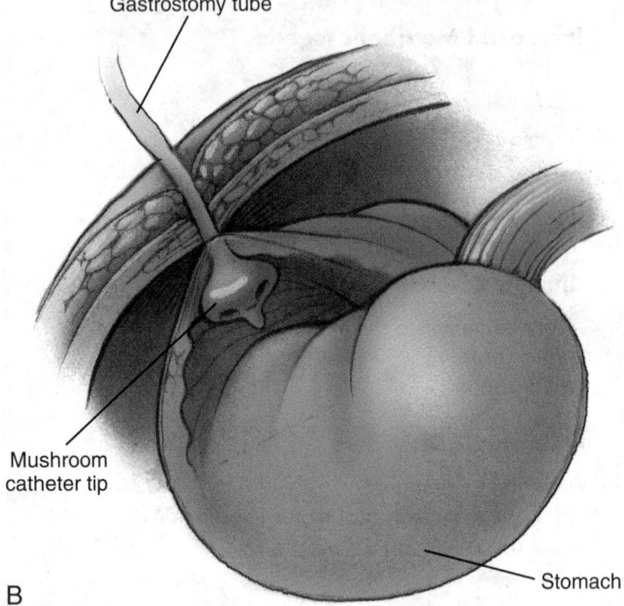

Figure 18–4
A, A skin level gastrostomy access device has a low profile and therefore is not as bulky or obvious as gastrostomy tubes. *B*, The gastrostomy mushroom tip prevents the tube from being pulled out.

These tubes have two lumens within the body of the tube. One lumen ends in the stomach, and the second lumen extends into the jejunum. These tubes are used for children who require simultaneous gastric decompression and jejunal feeding because of gastric outlet obstruction.

Interdisciplinary Interventions

Nursing care of the child receiving enteral nutrition involves the following:

- Managing the enteral feeding tube and enteral nutrition delivery system to ensure accurate delivery of fluid and nutrients and prevent system-related complications

TIP 18–1 A Teaching Intervention Plan for the Child with a Gastrostomy or Jejunostomy Tube

Nursing Diagnoses and Family Outcomes

- Knowledge deficit: care of enteral feeding tube; safety issues regarding enteral feeding
  Outcomes:
  Family and child, if developmentally appropriate, will demonstrate care of tube.
  Child will not develop complications associated with the presence of an enteral feeding tube (displacement, blockage, infection).
- Altered nutrition: less than body requirements related to effects of child's condition
  Outcomes:
  Child will demonstrate appropriate weight, height, and head circumference growth along own growth curve.
  Family and child will demonstrate appropriate feeding techniques.

Interventions

Teach the child, family, and caregivers:

Enteral Feeding Tube Care

Maintaining placement
- Monitor integrity of system used to secure tube. Resecure as necessary.
- Monitor position of gastrostomy tube before each feeding and with site care by pulling back gently on the tube to ensure inner balloon or retention device is snug against abdominal wall.
- If the tube becomes dislodged, cover site with clean gauze and tape; notify health care provider.

Maintaining patency
- Flush tube with water after each intermittent feeding or every 4 to 6 hours during continuous feedings, per facility protocol. Monitor total fluid volume of flushes to prevent fluid overload.
- Administer medications in liquid form. If medications must be crushed, consult with pharmacist regarding appropriate solution for dissolving medications. Never crush enteric-coated or time-release medications.
- Administer medications *one* at a time with a water flush before and after each medication.

Preventing infection
- Provide site care to enteral feeding tube every 24 hours or whenever area around tube is moist or crusted with secretions.
- Sterile saline may be used to clean around newly placed gastrostomy and jejunostomy tubes. Half-strength hydrogen peroxide may be used to remove dried blood or crusted secretions at tube exit sites.
- Soap and water may be used to clean around established tube sites.
- Dry site thoroughly after cleaning and apply external securing device as necessary for specific tubes.
- Avoid covering tube sites with ointments or occlusive dressings unless otherwise instructed. This may cause friction and moisture retention at the tube site and promote granuloma formation.
- Rotate gastrostomy and jejunostomy tube position every 24 hours with skin care. This helps to prevent erosion from pressure of the tube and prevents the tube from imbedding in the gastric mucosa.

Administration of Enteral Feedings

Administering feeding
- Prepare formula: type, concentration, amount

TIP continued on following page

TIP 18–1 A Teaching Intervention Plan for the Child with a Gastrostomy or Jejunostomy Tube *Continued*

- Check for gastric residual before starting feeding by aspirating from tube with a syringe.
- Position the child either upright in caregiver's lap, in infant seat (making sure infant does not slouch down, putting increased pressure on abdomen), lying on right side, or sitting.
- How to administer feeding
  - By enteral pump: connect tubing to enteral feeding tube; adjust flow rate.
  - By syringe: connect syringe barrel to tube, pour formula into syringe, and let it free flow slowly by gravity; it should take about as long as it would if the child was sucking or drinking the formula
- After feeding, flush tube with a small amount of water, unless contraindicated; leave gastrostomy tube open for 5 to 10 minutes after feeding to allow for escape of air.
- If formula does not flow freely, reposition child slightly and give brief gentle push to start the flow with syringe plunger; do not force, and do not use plunger to infuse entire feeding.

Preventing infection

- Change enteral feeding pump bags every 24 hours.
- Limit formula in enteral feeding bags to no more than 4 to 6 hours worth at a time.
- Refrigerate excess formula after opening and use within 24 to 48 hours.

Safety

- *Never* use parenteral infusion equipment for administration of enteral feedings. Inadvertent administration of enteral formulas through the parenteral route has been reported and has led to fatal complications.
- Keep the tube secured to the body to prevent dangling and accidental dislodgment.
- Elevate the child's head at least 30 degrees during feedings and for 30 to 60 minutes afterward to reduce the risk of aspiration.

Developmental issues

- Provide infant with pacifier during enteral feedings.
- Provide all children with developmentally appropriate social interaction during enteral feedings.
- Use developmentally appropriate safety precautions to ensure integrity and safety of enteral feeding system (e.g., cover site with a shirt so an infant cannot pull at tube; use longer feeding tubing when child is learning to walk; if child is on nighttime feedings, thread tubing through pajamas and out bottom of leg to avoid the child's getting tangled up in tubing).
- Normalize the child's routine so that the feeding can be administered during mealtimes with family.

Contact Health Care Provider if

- Feedings will not infuse.
- The tube may have moved (migrated) because the tube looks shorter, or the child has diarrhea or vomiting with no other signs of illness.
- Child has signs of infection such as increased amounts of or yellow or green drainage from skin exit site; tenderness, swelling, or increased redness around the skin exit site; fever.
- The child has vomiting, diarrhea, constipation, increasing abdominal distention, general discomfort, or signs of dehydration (decreased urination, lack of tears, dry mucous membranes) or fluid overload (shortness of breath, edema).
- The tube has leakage or redness around the tube or becomes displaced.

- Monitoring the child's response to enteral nutrition, including metabolic complications
- Supporting the child and family's educational and developmental needs in regard to the therapy

Care of the child receiving enteral nutrition is an interdisciplinary effort, and nursing interventions are enhanced through collaboration with other members of the health care team. The dietitian plays a key role in assessing nutritional status, calculating nutrient requirements, selecting formulas, monitoring response to therapy, and educating the patient and family. The occupational therapist may be involved in helping to promote oral feeding skills (see the discussion in Chapter 17 under total parenteral nutrition). The enterostomal therapist can be a resource for care of the enteral tube site. The pharmacist is a valuable consultant for drug/nutrient interactions when medications must be administered by enteral feeding tubes.

Nursing research indicates that aspiration and pH testing of aspirates is a more reliable way of verifying enteral feeding tube placement than the commonly used practice of auscultating the abdomen while insufflating air through the feeding tube (Metheny, 1993). Although the flushing of enteral feeding tubes with cranberry juice or carbonated cola beverages is frequently cited as the most effective method for maintaining tube patency, research has indicated that water is an equally effective flushing agent (Metheny, Eisenberg, & McSweeney, 1988).

Research has also demonstrated multiple benefits of the practice of providing infants with nonnutritive sucking experiences during enteral feedings. Improved weight gain, decreased heart rate and energy expenditure, decreased restlessness, and increased alert states have all been documented with nonnutritive sucking (Gill, Behnke, Conlon, & Anderson, 1992; Kimble, 1992; Miller & Anderson, 1993; Woodson & Hamilton, 1986).

Gastrointestinal, hydration, and nutritional status must be assessed. The nurse monitors the child for abdominal distention, nausea, or vomiting. Stool output, including signs of diarrhea, constipation, or malabsorption, is assessed. When the child's nutritional status and enteral intake are being stabilized, the nurse monitors gastric residuals before each intermittent feeding and every 4 to 6 hours during continuous feedings. The feeding is withheld and the physician or advanced practice nurse is notified if residuals exceed ordered parameters. The child is placed on his or her right side or prone after feeding to facilitate gastric emptying. The child's weight is obtained and documented daily and height and head circumference (in children younger than age 3 years) is checked weekly. Values are compared with previous ones to evaluate the child's growth pattern. The nurse also monitors for signs of dehydration or fluid overload, electrolyte imbalance, and vitamin, mineral, and trace element deficiencies.

Community Care

Most children with gastrostomy tubes are sent home with the tube in place, making parent education and planning for home care an important consideration in the nursing care of these children. The nurse must collaborate with discharge planning personnel to ensure that the child and family have appropriate formula, supplies, and equipment for home and to arrange necessary home and outpatient follow-up. The nurse must also educate the family and child, as developmentally appropriate, regarding care of enteral feeding tube, preparation and administration of enteral feedings, monitoring for complications, and developmental and safety issues (TIP 18–1). The nurse collaborates with the parents and school staff to facilitate transition back to school and the normal classroom (see Chapter 10).

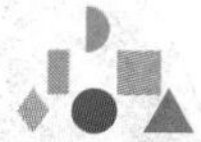

Alterations in Gastrointestinal Status

Malformations of the Upper Gastrointestinal Tract

Cleft Lip and Palate

Cleft lip and palate are the most common congenital craniofacial anomalies. Cleft lip, with or without cleft palate, occurs in approximately 1 in 700 live births (Eliason, 1991) and is more predominant in males than females by a ratio of 3 to 1. The incidence of cleft lip varies by ethnic group, with children of Asian descent having the highest reported rates. Cleft palate alone occurs in about 1 in 2000 births and is slightly more predominant in females. Multiple causes have been identified for cleft lip and palate. Familial patterns of inheritance have been established for cleft lip with or without cleft palate and, to a lesser extent, cleft palate alone. Environmental factors have also been identified in the etiology of cleft lip and palate (Litwak-Saleh, 1993). Drugs such as phenytoin, dietary factors such as folic acid and vitamin deficiencies, excess maternal intake of alcohol, and in utero irradiation have all been implicated.

Pathophysiology

Cleft lip results from the incomplete fusion of the embryologic structures surrounding the primitive oral cavity be-

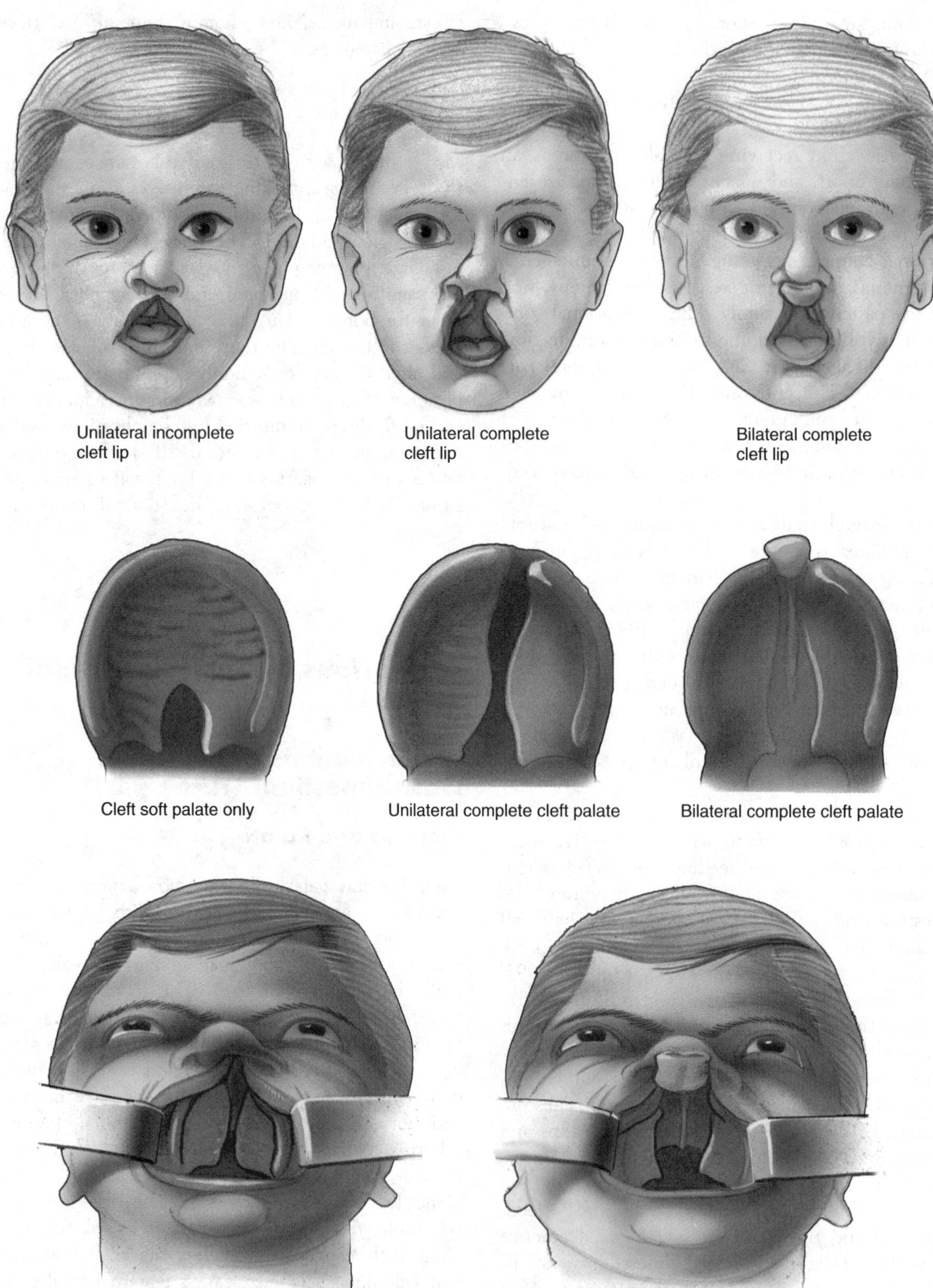

Figure 18–5
Variations of cleft lip and palate.

tween the 5th and 8th weeks of gestation. The cleft may be unilateral or bilateral and may vary from a small indentation in the lip to a wide, deep fissure that extends to the nostril (Figs. 18–5 and 18–6). Dental anomalies may also be present with missing, malpositioned, or deformed teeth.

Between the 7th and 12th week of gestation, the palate is formed by the migration and fusion of the palatine plates. Cleft palate occurs when the plates fail to migrate and fuse normally. The cleft may involve only the soft palate or may extend into the hard palate. Eustachian tube dysfunction is associated with cleft palate, leading to an increased risk of recurrent otitis media and the development of hearing impairment in affected children if not treated.

Children with cleft lip and palate may have other associated anomalies. Although some of the associated anomalies may be relatively minor, others, such as cardiac malformations, may be life threatening. More than 300 different syndromes that include cleft defects, particularly cleft palate, have been reported. Trisomy 13, Pierre Robin syndrome, and Treacher Collins syndrome are associated with a cleft palate. Because of familial patterns of inheritance and the many associated syndromes, genetic counseling is recommended for families after the birth of a child with cleft lip/palate.

Prognosis. The child with cleft lip and palate may have long-term problems with impaired facial growth and dental anomalies. The child with cleft palate may experience problems with speech disorders and hearing impairment. Mortality is related to the severity of associated syndromes.

Assessment

A diagnosis of cleft lip and/or palate may be made in utero by ultrasound. When diagnosis of the cleft is made in utero, the family is referred to the interdisciplinary cleft team even before the birth of the child. If not diagnosed in utero, cleft lip and, in most cases, cleft palate are immediately obvious at birth. Visual inspection and palpation of the palate all the way back to the soft palate should be done as part of every newborn examination. When cleft palate is not noted at birth, nasal regurgitation of fluids may alert the health care team to its presence.

Nursing Diagnoses and Outcomes

In addition to the nursing diagnoses and outcomes listed in Chart 18–3 and TIP 18–2, the following may be applicable for the child with a cleft lip and/or palate:

- **Altered parenting related to perception of an infant with a cleft lip/palate**
  Outcomes: The parents will receive psychosocial support and services to facilitate their coping and adjustment responses.

Figure 18–6
Child with cleft lip and palate at birth *(A)*, immediately after lip repair *(B)*, and at 3 years of age *(C)*.

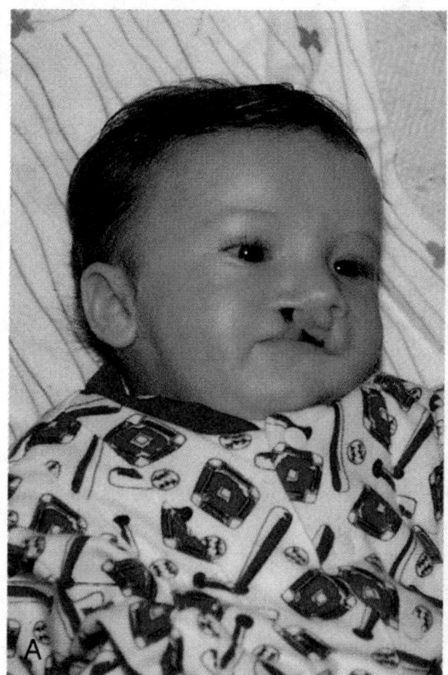

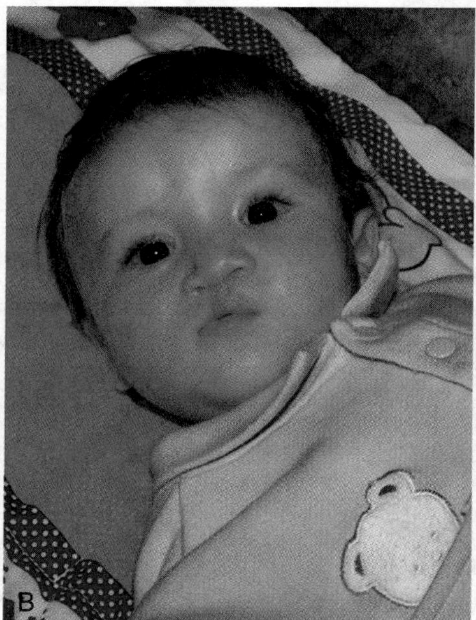

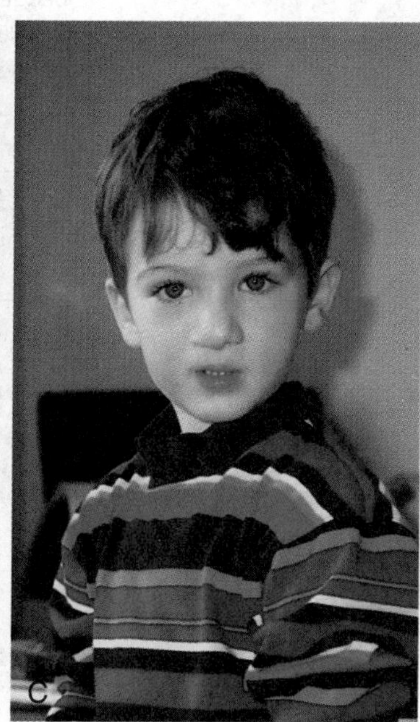

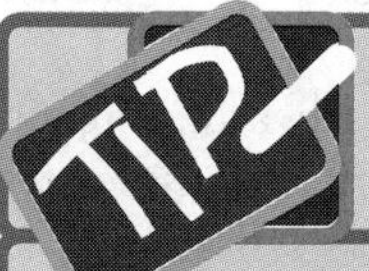

TIP 18–2 A Teaching Intervention Plan for the Family of the Child with Cleft Lip/Palate

Nursing Diagnoses and Family Outcomes

- Altered nutrition: less than body requirements related to impaired ingestion of nutrients
  Outcomes:
  Infant will take in adequate nutrients for normal growth and development.
  Infant will show weight/length increases along growth curve.
  Parents will demonstrate the ability to feed the infant in a manner that facilitates optimal intake of nutrients.
- Risk for infection related to effects of dysfunctional eustachian tubes, aspiration, or surgery
  Outcomes:
  Child is free from ear and respiratory infections, incisional infection postoperatively.
  Parents verbalize an understanding of the symptoms of infection and appropriate follow-up measures.
- Risk for injury related to potential trauma at operative site post cleft lip/palate repair
  Outcomes:
  Operative site will be protected from injury using developmentally appropriate measures.
  Family will demonstrate an understanding of how to prevent injury to the operative site.
- Knowledge deficit: cleft lip/palate pathology and treatment, feeding and suctioning techniques, surgical site care
  Outcomes:
  Child is free from complications associated with cleft lip/palate.
  Family is able to describe the pathology of cleft lip/palate, short- and long-term potential complications, and treatment plan.
  Family verbalizes the need for corrective surgery and possible later revisions.
  Family demonstrates appropriate feeding, suctioning, and restraint techniques and surgical site care.

Interventions

Teach the parents:

Preoperative Care

Feeding

- If mother wishes to breast-feed, teach her to manually extend nipple and place it in child's mouth.
- Because children with cleft palates in particular may have trouble generating enough pressure to breast-feed or use a regular nipple, teach the parents the ESSR Feeding Method:

	Action	Effect
E	*Enlarge* precut nipple hole by placing tip of sharp scissors into hole and cutting in four directions.	Allows infant to receive formula to the back of the throat for swallowing without relying on ineffective suction.
S	*Stimulate* the suck reflex by gently rubbing the nipple against lower lip. Insert, then invert bottle.	Prepares infant for feeding. Due to enlarged nipple, inverting after inserting prevents spillage and waste.
S	*Swallow* fluid normally.	The infant receives an adequate amount of formula without using excess energy and will meet nutritional requirements for proper weight gain.
R	*Rest* after signal (signal is when infant exhibits a facial expression indicating a short break in feeding is necessary).	Allows infant to finish swallowing formula already in back of throat and avoid uncomfortable gagging or nasal regurgitation.

TIP 18–2 A Teaching Intervention Plan for the Family of the Child with Cleft Lip/Palate *Continued*

Repeat the process until infant has eaten normal amount of formula in normal amount of time.

- Ensure that the nipple is in a normal feeding position, not the cleft; encourage sucking by stroking cheek or moving jaw; place the feeder's index finger lengthwise over the cleft in lip to help create suction.
- Feed the child slowly in an upright position; burp frequently but not so often that it frustrates the infant, causing increased distress.
- Hold and feed the infant in a relaxed manner to avoid communicating anxiety to the infant.
- Position the infant in an infant seat or on right side after feeding.

Oral hygiene

- Rinse the infant's mouth with water after every feeding.
- If the infant has a removable maxillary prosthesis, remove and clean it every day.

Preventing infection

- Monitor for signs of infection such as fever over 101°F, excessive mucus, coughing, rubbing ears, diarrhea, and irritability.
- Keep child away from persons with upper respiratory tract infections.
- Use good feeding techniques to prevent aspiration; suction oropharynx with bulb syringe as needed.
- Reposition the child every 2 hours.

Preparation for surgery

- Practice feeding technique that will be used postoperatively; check with surgeon to verify which technique will be used; some may allow breast-feeding or bottle feeding with enlarged nipple; others prefer a syringe with feeding tube at the end be used for feeding; it is helpful to teach this technique regardless so the child will be familiar with it, because pain may prevent the child from sucking postoperatively.

  Use rubber tubing or 8 French feeding tube cut to 1 inch, attach to 30-mL syringe, and pull formula into syringe; fill enough syringes for the feeding to avoid having to stop feeding and frustrating the infant.

  Hold infant upright as for normal feeding; direct tube to side of cheek away from surgical site.

  Drip feeding into mouth by gently pushing on the plunger.

  Burp after every 15 mL.

  Practice this until it is comfortable for parent and child; this may help avoid distress postoperatively.

- Apply elbow restraints for a few hours each day so the infant becomes used to wearing them.

  Secure restraints tight enough so they do not slip, but not so tight that they impair circulation; your index finger should be able to fit under the restraint; to make sure they are not too tight, check the child's hands to make sure they are warm and pink.

  Remove the restraints every hour, one at a time, so the child can exercise that arm; check the skin under the restraint at this time for signs of irritation.

Postoperative Care

Pain management

- Administer acetaminophen with codeine or acetaminophen, as prescribed, for pain; do not hesitate to use these agents because a comfortable child is less likely to cry and put stress on the suture line. Discomfort usually lasts 2 to 4 days after surgery.
- Use nonpharmacologic measures such as distraction, putting in swing, reading books, or playing music to comfort child.

TIP continued on following page

TIP 18–2 A Teaching Intervention Plan for the Family of the Child with Cleft Lip/Palate *Continued*

Positioning

- Position the child upright in infant seat, on side or back; do not put the infant on his or her abdomen after lip repair to avoid rubbing the incision on the sheets and injuring it.

Incision care

- Clean the lip incision three times a day with sterile water/half-strength hydrogen peroxide and apply thin layer of antibiotic ointment (how often to clean, solution, and ointment will be prescribed by the surgeon).

Feeding

- Use the feeding method practiced preoperatively; avoid touching or putting stress on the suture line. Usually for lip repairs breast- or bottle feeding is permitted; for palate repairs, use syringe with feeding tube at end.
- Avoid putting things into the child's mouth, such as pacifiers, feeding utensils, straws, or cups with a spout.
- Feed only liquids or pureed foods as ordered; do not give foods that need to be chewed or have chunks in them.
- Rinse the child's mouth with water after every feeding.

Restraints

- Keep the elbow restraints on at all times; to check fit use the same technique as practiced preoperatively; monitor for adequate circulation and skin irritation.
- Remove restraints every hour, one at a time, and closely monitor the child so nothing goes near the mouth.
- Offer a variety of developmentally appropriate distractions to keep the child content: holding, cuddling, looking at books, touching different textured objects, picking up small objects and putting them in a container, puzzles, clay, wagon rides.
- Use the restraints until the surgeon says to stop, usually 2 to 6 weeks.

Contact Health Care Provider if

Preoperatively

- The child has signs of infection: fever over 101°F, excessive mucus, coughing, rubbing ears, diarrhea, irritability.

Postoperatively

- There is bright red bleeding from mouth or nose.
- Above signs of infection, swelling, increasing redness, or pus around the suture line is present.
- Pain is not controlled with the prescribed medications and child cannot be comforted.
- The child refuses to eat.

Adapted from Richard, M. (1991). Feeding the newborn with cleft lip and/or palate: The enlargement, stimulate, swallow, rest (ESSR) method. *Journal of Pediatric Nursing, 6,* 317–321. Used with permission.

The parents will verbalize acceptance of the child and demonstrate appropriate nurturing behaviors.

▶ **Self-esteem disturbance related to perception of facial deformity and speech impediment**

Outcomes: The child verbalizes that others like or love him or her and that he or she likes himself or herself.

The child demonstrates no signs of depression, sleeps well, does well in school, and has appropriate appetite.

Interdisciplinary Interventions

Care of the child with cleft lip/palate involves a large interdisciplinary team, including the pediatrician, nurse, plastic surgeon, oral surgeon, ENT surgeon, audiologist, orthodontist, speech therapist, social worker, and geneticist. The nurse's role involves providing direct care to the child, along with parent support and education and coordination of services.

Psychological Support

When the diagnosis of cleft lip is made at birth, after the initial stabilization and assessment, the parents need information about their neonate's condition. Because of the obvious and disfiguring nature of the defect, its presence is often very distressing to the family. Information about the anomaly and anticipated care needs should be provided in simple, direct terms. Information may need to be repeated, because parents may become easily overwhelmed trying to process new information while dealing with the crisis of the birth of a child with a visible defect. Early involvement of a member of the cleft lip/palate team is recommended to provide the family with accurate information about the child's condition and treatment plan.

The family's emotional response to the birth of a child with cleft lip/palate may range from grief to anger to denial (see Chapters 8 and 10). The nurse should convey an open, nonjudgmental attitude to encourage the parents to express their feelings. The nurse may play a key role in supporting the family's adjustment to a child's condition by demonstrating an accepting, caring attitude toward the child and family and providing the parents with opportunities and support for normal infant–parent interactions.

caREminder: *Point out positive qualities in the infant, such as color of hair and eyes and turning toward the parent's voice.*

Feeding

The infant with cleft lip and palate presents special challenges in terms of feeding. Although the infant with cleft lip alone may do well with either breast or bottle feeding, the infant with a cleft palate may experience problems due to an inability to generate negative suction pressure in the oropharynx and regurgitation of milk into the nasal cavity. Breast feeding may be unsuccessful, and bottle feeding may require modification of the nipple.

Alert: *An infant with cleft lip and palate who is being breast-fed must be closely monitored for weight gain and hydration status.*

Many feeding methods have been described to facilitate feeding the infant with cleft palate, including use of various nipple designs, cross-cut nipples, and palatal obturators. The feeding method selected should be as simple as possible (Habel, Sell, & Mars, 1996). The enlarge, stimulate, swallow, rest (ESSR) feeding method uses readily available feeding equipment and provides a framework for educating parents. In an initial study, the ESSR method was more effective than traditional methods in promoting weight gain in infants with cleft palate (Richard, 1991).

Feeding methods that promote sucking are used whenever possible. Use of the orofacial muscles is necessary for muscle development, feeding, and speech skills. Rarely, feeding must be done using a large syringe with rubber tubing at the tip to squirt formula in the side of the infant's mouth or by NG tube. If these feeding methods are necessary, an occupational therapist and/or speech and language therapist should be involved to develop and maintain oral-motor skills.

Surgical Management

Operative repair of a cleft lip usually takes place at age 2 to 3 months. The goals of the surgery are to close the defect and achieve a balanced symmetrical appearance. The timing of cleft palate repair varies from age 6 months to 2 years, depending on the nature of the defect and surgeon preference. It is often done before age 1 to promote better speech outcomes. Cleft lip repair usually involves only a 24-hour hospital stay or is done as an outpatient procedure, whereas cleft palate repair typically involves a 2-day hospital stay. Preoperative preparation of the family focuses on information regarding the surgical procedure and the child's postoperative care needs both in the hospital and at home (see TIP 18–2).

Immediate postoperative care focuses on airway management, hemostasis, and pain control. The child is at risk for airway compromise due to laryngeal edema as a result of intubation during surgery and incisional edema. After palate repair, the child must learn to breathe through smaller nasal passages. Blood clots may also fall off the incision and obstruct the airway. Use of a high-humidity oxygen tent may be ordered. The nurse observes the child carefully for signs of respiratory distress, bleeding, and excess mucus in the mouth.

Alert: *Suction with a bulb syringe if necessary. Only in an emergency should a soft catheter or low suction be used, avoiding the suture lines. Remember that the roof of the mouth is also the floor of the nose.*

To prevent pooling of secretions in the oropharynx, the child is positioned in an infant seat or on his or her side. If only the palate has been repaired, the child is positioned on his or her abdomen.

Bleeding may occur at the suture line. Gentle pressure or ice may be applied to the lip incision, as ordered. If the child is bleeding from the palate repair, the nurse intervenes as needed for respiratory distress and notifies the physician.

Pain is not unusual during the first 24 to 48 hours postoperatively. Pain and discomfort from other sources (e.g., hunger, wet diaper, need for attention or repositioning) should be minimized to prevent crying, which puts tension on the suture line. Interventions to promote comfort are instituted. The nurse determines the need for analgesics and evaluates their effects after administration (see Chapter 13). The child's needs should be anticipated and met *before* the child becomes distressed.

Elbow restraints are used for the first 10 to 14 days postoperatively. The child's hands are still free, but the elbow restraints prevent the child from bending at the elbow and touching or injuring the operative site. The elbow restraints must be tight enough so they do not slide off the child but loose enough so a finger can slide underneath. Neurovascular checks must be performed and documented on a routine basis. The restraints are released every hour, one at a time, to allow range of motion movements. The child must be prevented from putting his or her hands near the mouth.

After cleft lip repair, the child will have sutures on the exterior portion of the lip that remain in place for up to a week. Wound care involves regular cleansing of the suture line with normal saline or dilute hydrogen peroxide and application of an antibiotic ointment. Clear liquids are usually offered after the child recovers from the anesthesia. The infant's usual breast or bottle feedings are commonly resumed within 6 to 24 hours of cleft lip repair. Resumption of oral feeding is usually delayed up to 48 hours after cleft palate repair. Care must be taken to avoid injury to the palatal suture line during the first 10 to 14 days postoperatively. During bottle feeding, the nipple must be positioned so that it does not touch the palatal suture line. The use of straws or cups with spouts is avoided. Pureed or soft foods may be carefully fed to the child through spoon or cup.

Community Care

After surgical repair, the child with cleft lip and/or palate faces various ongoing health challenges. The child with cleft palate is at risk for hearing loss due to recurrent otitis media from eustachian tube dysfunction. Speech impairments may be present due to inadequate function of the pharyngeal and palatal muscles after repair, requiring long-term speech therapy. Abnormal dental development and malocclusion require the ongoing involvement of pediatric dentists and orthodontists. Maxillofacial surgery may be required later in life to manage impaired midfacial growth. Alterations in appearance and speech impairment may have a negative impact on the child's self image. The involvement of social work or other mental health disciplines is important in dealing with these concerns.

Esophageal Atresia and Tracheoesophageal Fistula

Esophageal atresia (EA) is a congenital anomaly that results from the failure of the esophagus to recanalize normally between the fourth and sixth weeks of fetal development. The proximal esophagus ends in a blind pouch instead of communicating normally with the stomach. In most cases, EA is associated with tracheoesophageal fistula (TEF), an abnormal communication between the esophagus and trachea. TEF results from the failure of the separation of the trachea and esophagus that normally takes place between the sixth and seventh weeks of gestation.

TEF occurs in approximately 1 in 4000 births. Its etiology is unknown. In 50% to 70% of all cases, associated congenital anomalies are seen. Cardiac defects, such as ventral septal defects, patent ductus arteriosus, or tetralogy of Fallot, occur in up to 30% of all cases. GI abnormalities, such as imperforate anus, duodenal atresia, or malrotation, may occur in 10% of affected infants. Urinary tract and musculoskeletal anomalies may also occur. In approximately 25% of cases, TEF occurs as a part of VACTERL syndrome. Infants affected with VACTERL syndrome have three or more anomalies from a group that includes *v*ertebral defects, *a*norectal malformations, *c*ardiac anomalies, *t*racheoesophageal fistula, *e*sophageal atresia, *r*enal defects, and *l*imb defects.

Pathophysiology

The esophagus and trachea normally begin to develop from a common foregut between the third and fourth weeks of gestation. During the sixth to eighth weeks of embryologic development the mesodermal ridges form and separate the esophagus from the trachea. EA and TEF result when the trachea and esophagus fail to separate normally during this period. Epithelialization and recanalization of the esophagus also occur at this time. Failure of normal recanalization processes has been hypothesized as a cause of EA.

EA and TEF present in various ways (Fig. 18–7). In 80% of cases, the esophagus ends in a blind pouch with a fistula communicating between the distal esophagus and the trachea. EA without TEF is the next most common form, occurring in up to 8% of cases. TEF without EA occurs in approximately 4% of cases. Numerous other configurations of EA and TEF have been classified.

Prognosis. The overall survival of the child with EA/TEF is 85% to 90%. Mortality is usually due to associated congenital anomalies rather then the EA/TEF itself. Children with EA/TEF may experience long-term problems with esophageal dysmotility and gastroesophageal reflux. Esophageal stricture at the site of surgical repair may occur in up to 60% of children postoperatively, requiring recurrent esophageal dilatations.

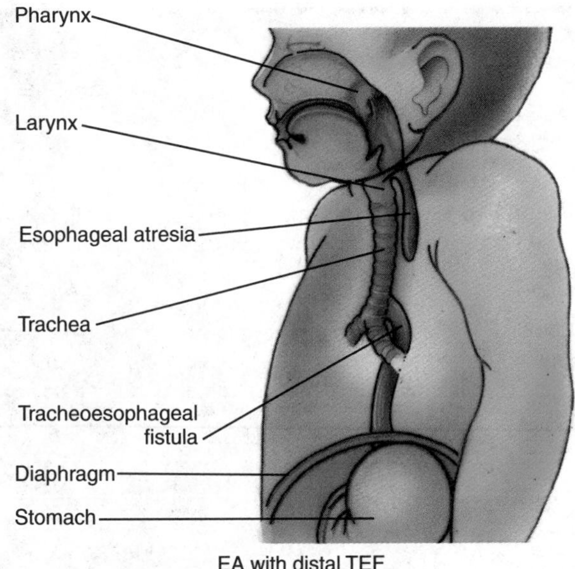

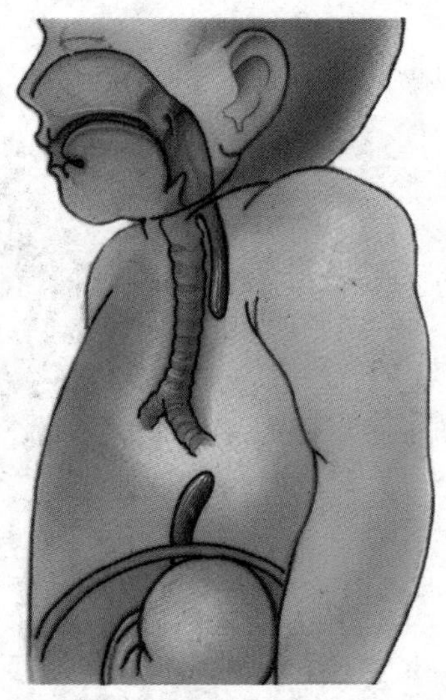

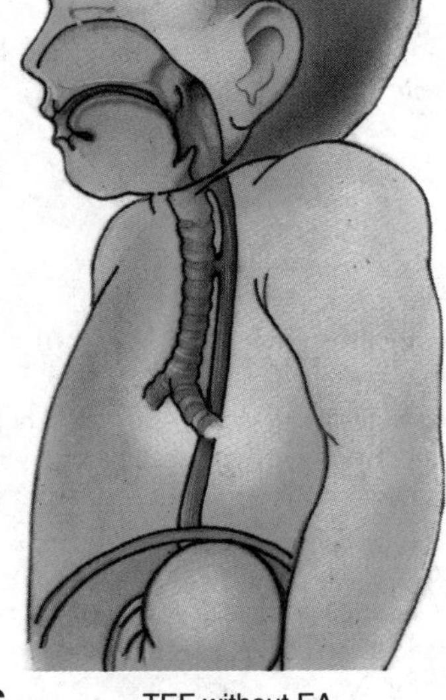

Figure 18–7
A, The esophagus ends in a blind pouch with a fistula between the distal esophagus and trachea. *B*, Esophageal atresia without fistula. C, Tracheoesophageal fistula without esophageal atresia.

Assessment

Clinical manifestations of EA/TEF may be noted prenatally. A maternal history of polyhydramnios is usually present in cases of EA and in some cases of TEF. In many cases the fetal stomach cannot be visualized on ultrasound because of the absence of gas.

At birth, the infant demonstrates excessive oral secretions accompanied by coughing, choking, and cyanosis, which become worse when feeding is attempted (Chart 18–6).

caREminder: *Excessive drooling of saliva may be the first symptom of TEF. When fed, the infant sucks well but then chokes and coughs as the feeding enters the lungs.*

Respiratory distress may ensue from aspiration of pooled secretions in the proximal esophageal pouch or from secretions passing through a proximal fistula. In the presence of distal TEF, gastric juices can reflux into the respiratory tract, causing a chemical pneumonitis. Overt clinical manifestations of cardiac, musculoskeletal, or other GI anomalies may also be present.

When TEF is present without EA, diagnosis may be difficult. The infant may choke during some feedings as the formula crosses the fistula and enters the lungs. Other feedings may proceed without symptoms.

Diagnostic Tests. The initial diagnosis of EA is established by passage of a small-bore NG tube into the esophagus. If EA is present, the tube will only pass a few centimeters before resistance is felt. The diagnosis is confirmed radiologically, with visualization of the chest and

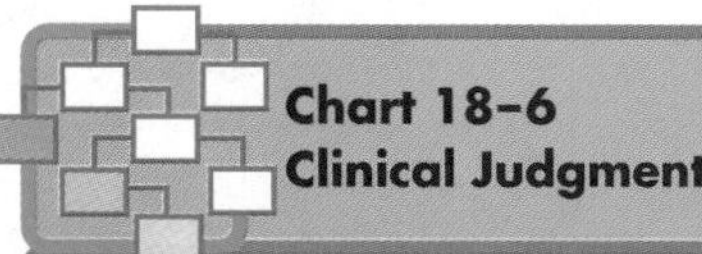

Chart 18–6
Clinical Judgment

An Infant with Tracheoesophageal Fistula

Maikhanh is a term newborn female, 2 hours old, APGARs 9 and 9 with no obvious congenital anomalies. The nurse had noted a large amount of mucus but, because the infant had a rapid descent through the birth canal, had attributed the excessive mucus to that.

Maikhanh's father is bottle-feeding her first feeding. Maikhanh started sucking and then turned extremely blue. The nurse suctioned Maikhanh with a bulb syringe, getting copious amounts of secretions, and gave free-flow oxygen. Maikhanh responded immediately and regained a pink color. The nurse tried to feed Maikhanh herself, to see if the cyanotic episode would be repeated. Maikhanh eagerly began sucking, then started coughing, and became extremely cyanotic. Again, Maikhanh responded promptly to suction and oxygen.

Questions

1. Is Maikhanh demonstrating normal newborn behavior?
2. What behaviors are of concern?
3. Are the symptoms that Maikhanh presents classic signs of tracheoesophageal fistula? What other pathologic process might be considered?
4. What should the nurse do?
5. Maikhanh is 36 hours postoperative tracheoesophageal fistula repair and has a chest tube in place. What should the nurse evaluate? What are signs of complications?

Answers

1. No.
2. Duskiness with feeding and excessive saliva during the first few hours after birth are not normal. Acrocyanosis is to be expected for the first few hours after birth; central cyanosis around the mouth and mucous membranes is not normal. A moderate amount of mucus is normal for the first 24 hours, as the infant goes through the transition to extrauterine life.
3. Maikhanh does present with classic tracheoesophageal fistula, particularly the *immediate* color change with feeding and swallowing of fluid. Cardiac or respiratory pathology manifests as cyanosis that does not respond as well to suctioning and oxygen administration; such cyanosis is prolonged after feedings, or continuous, and can be exacerbated by other things such as stress.
4. Position Maikhanh upright. Maintain a clear airway with intermittent or continuous suction as necessary. Notify the physician or advanced nurse practitioner. Continue to assess Maikhanh's cardiorespiratory status and maintain a neutral thermal environment during diagnostic testing such as chest radiography. Provide psychosocial support for Maikhanh's parents. Maintain NPO and IV fluids as ordered.
5. The nurse should evaluate respiratory status, functioning and integrity of chest tube, efficacy of pain management, fluid and electrolyte balance including nutritional support, incision site for integrity and infection, and parental coping. Signs of complications due to anastomosis leak include respiratory distress with tachypnea, cyanosis, the presence of saliva in the chest tube tubing, and signs of sepsis caused by the leak (e.g., temperature instability, hypoglycemia, apnea, bradycardia).

abdomen. The position of the tube in the proximal esophageal pouch is seen. The presence or absence of gas in the stomach on x-ray is also assessed. The presence of gas in a distended stomach indicates the presence of a distal TEF. The absence of gas in the stomach is associated with EA without TEF. Chest radiographs also screen for the presence of pneumonia, cardiac defects, or vertebral anomalies. Contrast studies, bronchoscopy, or endoscopy may also be used to establish the presence of TEF with or without EA. Contrast medium is used with caution because of the risk of aspiration.

Nursing Diagnoses and Outcomes

In addition to the nursing diagnoses and outcomes listed in Chart 18–3, the following may be applicable to the child with TEF:

Preoperatively

- **Ineffective airway clearance related to inability to swallow secretions**
  Outcome: The infant will maintain a clear airway

and will have signs of airway compromise recognized promptly and interventions implemented (e.g., suctioning, positioning) to facilitate clearance.

- **Risk for aspiration related to secretions or fluids entering respiratory tract secondary to structural defect**
  Outcomes: The infant will not aspirate.
  The infant will not develop infection secondary to aspiration.

Postoperatively

- **Risk for injury related to procedures disrupting integrity of suture line**
  Outcomes: The infant will not develop a disruption of the surgical anastomosis.
  The infant's NG tube will be secured and not be accidentally dislodged.
  The infant will be suctioned to a depth shorter than the position of the suture line.
- **Impaired swallowing related to presence of esophageal stricture or impaired peristalsis**
  Outcomes: The infant will be monitored for signs of stricture development and have dilatation performed as needed.
  The child will use methods to enhance effective swallowing, such as eating slowly, chewing foods well, and maintaining upright position.

Interdisciplinary Interventions

Surgical repair of EA/TEF is delayed until the infant is medically stable. The goal of preoperative care is to prevent and treat any complications that may arise from aspiration or reflux of secretions into the respiratory tract.

caREminder: *Maintain the infant with EA in an upright position preoperatively to reduce the risk of aspiration. Some surgeons prefer to have the infant positioned prone to facilitate drainage of the blind pouch by gravity.*

A sump catheter can be maintained in the upper esophageal pouch to provide continuous suction of pooled secretions. Respiratory support and broad-spectrum antibiotics are given as needed to treat aspiration pneumonia. In some cases, a gastrostomy may be performed to provide gastric decompression. Nutritional support with total parenteral nutrition (TPN) is initiated after the infant is stabilized.

The timing of definitive surgical repair of EA/TEF depends on the infant's condition. The infant who is close to term and is without other significant medical problems, such as aspiration pneumonia, may undergo repair within 24 to 72 hours of birth. Premature infants with significant respiratory distress or severe associated anomalies are maintained with proximal esophageal suction, gastric decompression, and TPN until medically stable enough to undergo definitive repair.

Surgical repair is done through a thoracotomy. The TEF is ligated, and then the proximal and distal segments of the esophagus are anastomosed. If primary anastomosis is not possible owing to inadequate length of the esophageal segments, then esophageal replacement through gastric interposition may be done. If the infant's condition does not permit esophageal replacement during the initial surgery, a cervical esophagostomy may be done, with subsequent esophageal replacement at age 6 months to 1 year by gastric or colonic interposition, in which a portion of the stomach or colon is used to replace the esophagus.

During the initial postoperative period the infant will have a chest tube, gastric decompression, and continued respiratory support. Ongoing attention to preventing aspiration is vital. A suction catheter with markings to indicate the distance from the infant's nose to the point just above the anastomosis may be kept at the bedside. This can be used as a guide so that when the infant is suctioned the catheter does not cause trauma at the site of the anastomosis.

Alert: *Insert suction catheters less than the distance to the anastomosis. Secure the NG tube well and use extreme caution to avoid displacement. If displacement occurs, do not reinsert the tube. Introducing catheters around the area of the suture line increases the risk of disrupting the suture line and causing leaks.*

Antibiotic coverage is continued, and nutritional support with TPN is maintained until full enteral feedings are tolerated. Enteral nutrition through an NG or gastrostomy tube may be started as early as the fourth postoperative day. Small-volume drip feedings are usually instituted because of the risk of gastroesophageal reflux with bolus feedings. A radiologic study with water-soluble contrast medium is done by postoperative day 7 to 10 to assess the patency of the esophageal anastomosis. If no leak is seen, the chest tube is removed and oral feedings are begun.

Ongoing assessment for anastomotic leak or stricture is essential. Anastomotic leaks occur in 5% to 15% of cases. The infant typically exhibits respiratory distress with tachypnea, cyanosis, and signs of sepsis. Continued NPO status and TPN support are required, along with antibiotics and respiratory care, until the leak heals. Most leaks heal spontaneously within 1 to 3 weeks. The infant with a stricture at the anastomotic site may demonstrate coughing, regurgitation, recurrent aspiration, and failure to thrive. A stricture may not be evident in an infant until after solid foods are introduced. The older child may complain of dysphagia or exhibit difficulties swallowing solid foods. Strictures are managed with esophageal dilations.

Tracheomalacia occurs in more than 25% of children with TEF. These children have a characteristic harsh cough and are at risk for frequent respiratory infections during infancy and early childhood. Gastroesophageal reflux may also be an ongoing problem for many children, requiring nonsurgical or, in severe cases, surgical management of symptoms. Infants with EA/TEF are at risk for oral feeding dysfunction related to their often prolonged NPO status, subsequent reliance on NG or gastrostomy feeds, and frequent problems with esophageal function. Early attention to oral-motor stimulation and involvement of occupational therapy in the infant's plan of care may help address this (see Chapter 17 for discussion under total parenteral nutrition).

Community Care

Nursing management of the infant with EA/TEF is challenging, not only in terms of the direct care of the child in the inpatient setting but also in the preparation of the child and family for the transition from hospital to home and in the ongoing care of the child in the outpatient setting. The child with EA/TEF frequently has other associated medical conditions that can make discharge teaching very complex. The child with EA/TEF as a part of VACTERL syndrome may require follow-up with numerous health care providers. The nurse can play a key role in case management of these children by promoting coordination of care and facilitating communication among the various health care providers as well as providing ongoing parent support and education.

Pyloric Stenosis

Pyloric stenosis is the most common cause of gastric outlet obstruction in infants. It occurs in 1:500 live births and is three to four times more common in males than females. The exact cause of pyloric stenosis is not known.

In pyloric stenosis, hypertrophy and hyperplasia of the circular smooth muscle of the pylorus of the stomach occurs (Fig. 18–8). The lumen of the pylorus narrows and lengthens, and progressive gastric outlet obstruction takes place.

Surgical correction of pyloric stenosis is curative. With prompt diagnosis and treatment, the operative mortality for treatment of pyloric stenosis is less than 1%.

Assessment

Typically, manifestations of pyloric stenosis become apparent at age 2 to 4 weeks. The infant usually presents with a history of regurgitation and nonbilious vomiting during or shortly after feeding. Within a week of onset of symptoms, the vomiting may become projectile. The vomitus usually consists of gastric contents but may become "coffee ground" in color secondary to esophagogastritis. Parents may describe the infant as irritable and

Figure 18–8
In pyloric stenosis, the pyloric muscle hypertrophies and obstructs the passage of stomach contents into the intestines. Surgically splitting the muscle relieves the obstruction.

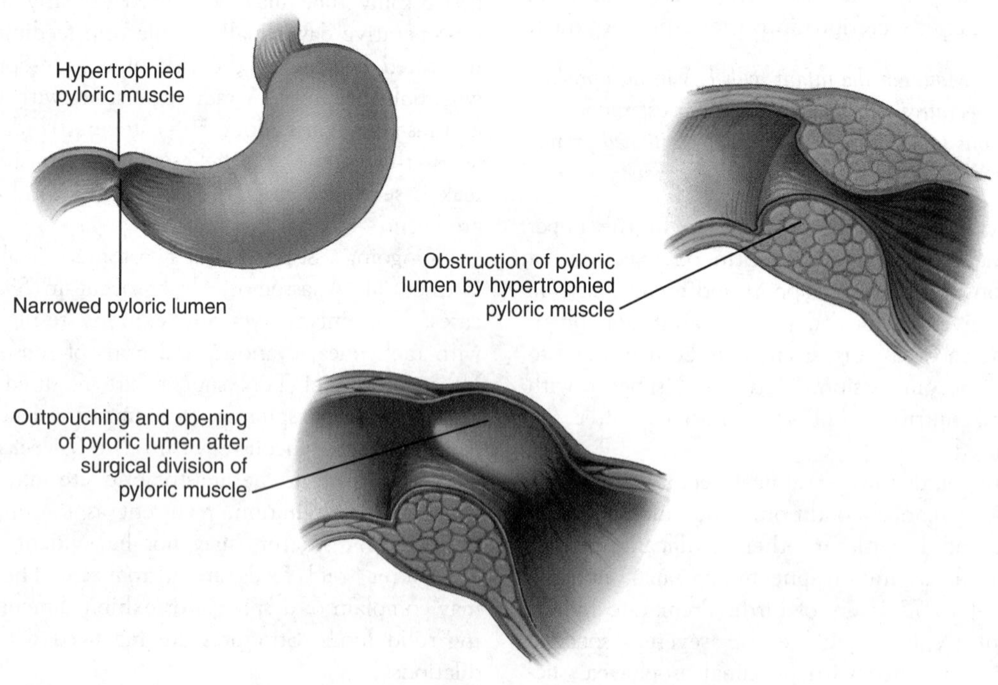

hungry all the time. Weight loss and failure to thrive may be noted. With progressive dehydration due to vomiting, the parents may report lethargy, decreased urine output, and constipation.

On physical examination, the infant may appear fussy and fretful. In severe dehydration, the infant may seem apathetic and even moribund. The upper abdomen is typically distended, and visible peristaltic waves may be seen moving from left to right across the upper abdomen (Fig. 18–9). On palpation of the abdomen, a mass can be felt in the epigastrium to the right of the midline. The mass is hard, mobile, nontender, and usually about the size of an olive.

Diagnostic Tests. Diagnosis of pyloric stenosis can usually be made based on health history and physical assessment findings. If the examiner is unable to palpate the olive-sized mass in the epigastrium, ultrasound or a barium study may be used to establish the diagnosis. On ultrasound evaluation the mass may be seen as a hypoechoic mass measuring 1.5 cm or more. The barium study will demonstrate the "string sign," which indicates a narrowed pyloric channel and retained gastric contents.

Because of persistent vomiting, the infant with pyloric stenosis presents with varying degrees of dehydration. A hypochloremic alkalosis is most typical, with decreased serum sodium, potassium, and chloride levels and increased serum bicarbonate level.

Interdisciplinary Interventions

After establishing the diagnosis of pyloric stenosis, the initial goal of therapy is to correct any fluid and electrolyte imbalances that the infant may have. The infant may be made NPO to prevent further losses from vomiting; IV therapy is initiated for rehydration and correction of electrolyte imbalances. Careful monitoring of IV fluid intake, along with accurate quantification and documentation of urine output and losses from emesis are important components of nursing management in this phase of treatment. Comfort measures for the infant, as well as reassurance and support for parents, are also important.

Figure 18–9
Visible peristaltic waves associated with pyloric stenosis. (From Liebert, P. S. [1996]. *Color atlas of pediatric surgery* [2nd ed., p. 129]. Philadelphia: W. B. Saunders. Reprinted with permission.)

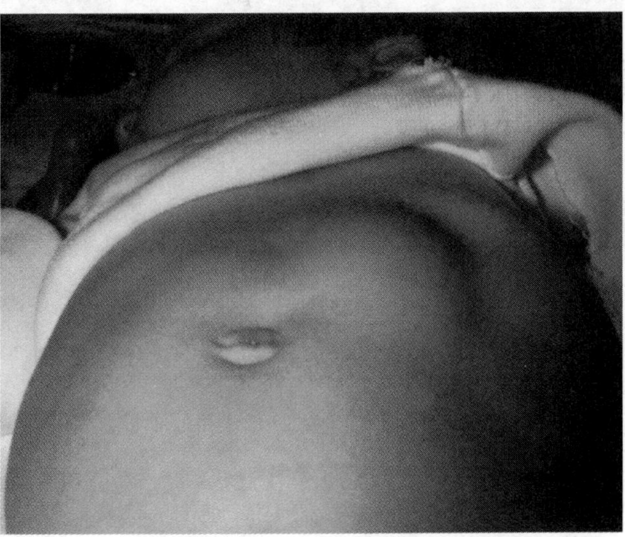

The definitive treatment of pyloric stenosis is surgical pyloromyotomy. After normal fluid and electrolyte balance is reestablished, the infant is taken to surgery. A small abdominal incision is made, and the pyloric mass is incised longitudinally, splitting the underlying muscle. This allows the gastric mucosa to bulge up between the split, relieving the obstruction.

Postoperatively, the infant is maintained on IV fluids until oral feedings are started, usually shortly after the child recovers from anesthesia. Small amounts of an oral electrolyte solution such as Pedialyte may be offered for the initial feedings. If this solution is tolerated, the volume and concentration of feedings are advanced until full feedings are achieved, usually from 24 to 48 hours postoperatively. Up to 50% of infants may have some vomiting postoperatively owing to persistent edema of the pylorus and inefficient gastric emptying (Care Path 18–1).

Community Care

Infants with pyloric stenosis may be discharged 24 to 48 hours postoperatively, once normal feedings are reestablished. Parents require instruction regarding the infant's feeding schedule and any necessary wound care for the abdominal incision. They also need to be taught signs of complications, such as recurrent vomiting, wound infection, and signs of dehydration. Follow-up referral to a community pediatric caregiver ensures that the infant will be monitored for resumption of normal growth and weight gain after surgery.

Malformations of the Lower Gastrointestinal Tract

Intestinal Atresia and Stenosis

Intestinal atresia is a congenital defect that results in complete obstruction of the bowel. *Duodenal atresia* accounts for approximately 50% of all atresias of the small intestine and is frequently associated with other congenital defects, including trisomy 21, intestinal malrotations, and congenital heart defects. Duodenal atresias are seen in 1 in 10,000 live births. *Jejunoileal atresia* results in the obstruction of one or multiple segments of the jejunum

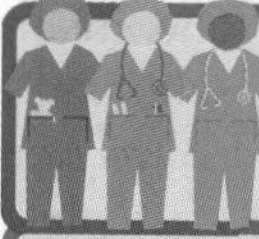

Care Path 18–1 An Interdisciplinary Plan of Care for the Child with Pyloric Stenosis

	Patient/Family Intermediate Outcomes		
Nursing Diagnosis	**Day: Admission**	**Day: Postop 1**	**Day: Postop 2**
Fluid volume deficit related to effects of persistent vomiting	Child shows improved fluid and electrolyte balance.	Child demonstrates normal fluid and electrolyte balance, as evidenced by normal urine output (1 mL/kg/hr), moist mucous membranes, good skin turgor, laboratory values within normal limits.	⟶
Altered nutrition: less than body requirements related to persistent vomiting	Child stops vomiting.	Child ingests and retains small amounts of formula.	Child ingests and retains sufficient nutrients to meet dietary needs.
Pain related to incision, muscle cutting and manipulation during surgery		Child has signs of pain recognized and interventions promptly implemented. Child experiences minimal levels of pain.	⟶
Knowledge deficit: treatments, surgery, postoperative care	Parents verbalize understanding of treatments and surgery.	Parents verbalize understanding of postoperative pain management, feeding, and incision care.	Parents verbalize understanding of home care and follow-up needs.
Care Intervention Categories			
Consults	Surgical consult		
Labs	CBC, electrolytes Repeat electrolytes prn to monitor Cl^- and CO_2 values		
Medications and IVs	IV fluids: maintenance and replacement Give acetaminophen with codeine or acetaminophen p.r.n. for pain	Heparin lock IV when tolerating PO fluids	Discontinue IV if tolerating PO fluids.

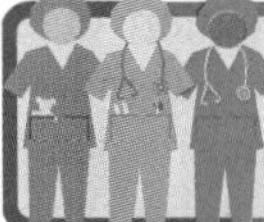

Care Path 18–1 An Interdisciplinary Plan of Care for the Child with Pyloric Stenosis *Continued*

Care Intervention Categories	Day: Admission	Day: Postop 1	Day: Postop 2
Nutrition	NPO	Give 10 mL oral electrolyte solution after recovered from anesthesia; start pyloric refeeding protocol (increasing feeding volumes from clear fluids to dilute to full-strength formula); repeat previous step if emesis × 1, notify surgeon if emesis × 2.	Give full-strength formula at normal feeding volumes.
Pain management	Give acetaminophen with codeine or plain (see medications above). Flex knees; position to avoid stretching abdominal muscles. Burp frequently to avoid abdominal distention.	⟶	⟶
Procedures	NG tube to gravity drainage	Discontinue NG tube before starting feedings.	
Radiology	Sonogram of abdomen and barium study p.r.n. to confirm diagnosis		
Teaching/discharge planning	Teach parents about preoperative care routines. Teach parents about surgical routines; review postoperative care.	Teach parents methods of pain assessment and management; reintroduce feedings; provide incision care. Assess what supplies will be needed at home (medications, dressings) and ability of parents to obtain them.	Evaluate parent's ability to manage pain, feed, and care for incision; review techniques p.r.n. Discharge child when full oral feedings are tolerated.
Vital signs/baseline parameters	Vital signs with blood pressure on admission and q 4 hr Daily weight Urine specific gravity each shift Intake and output	⟶ ⟶ ⟶ ⟶	⟶ ⟶ ⟶ ⟶

or ileum. It is not commonly associated with other congenital defects. The incidence of jejunoileal atresia varies from 1 in 300 to 1 in 3000 live births. *Stenosis* of the intestine results in a partial or incomplete obstruction.

Because of commonly associated congenital malformations, duodenal atresia is believed to occur very early in embryologic development, resulting from a failure of the lumen of the intestine to recanalize during the 8th to 10th week of gestation. Jejunoileal atresia is believed to occur at a much later stage of gestation, because of the observation that meconium is commonly present in the bowel distal to the atretic segment. A mesenteric vascular insult, resulting in ischemia of the affected portion of intestine, may be the causative factor in jejunoileal atresia. Clinical observations of children born with jejunoileal atresia and experimental findings using animal models support this hypothesis.

Pathophysiology

Various forms of duodenal and jejunoileal atresia result in intestinal obstruction. Type I atresia occurs when a mucosal membrane or web occludes the inner lumen of the bowel. In type II atresia the proximal intestine ends in a blind loop and is connected to the collapsed distal intestine by a fibrous cord. Type III atresia results in both the proximal and distal segments of intestine ending in blind loops with no connection. In cases of jejunoileal atresia, a type IV defect may also occur, resulting in multiple atretic segments of bowel, often described as having the appearance of a string of sausages.

Prognosis. The prognosis for duodenal atresia after surgical repair is excellent, with most patients experiencing no long-term sequelae. The prognosis for infants born with jejunoileal atresia is impacted by the amount of bowel involved and the birth weight of the infant. Overall survival rates are reported to be in the range of 90%. Infants who require massive resection of defective intestine resulting in short bowel syndrome and infants with very low birth weights may experience more complications and poorer long-term outcomes.

Assessment

Polyhydramnios is observed in many cases of both duodenal and jejunoileal atresia. Most infants become symptomatic within the first 24 hours of life. Bilious vomiting and abdominal distention occur in most cases. Failure to pass meconium and jaundice are also commonly observed.

Diagnostic Tests. Intestinal atresia may be diagnosed by ultrasound during the prenatal period. In cases of intestinal atresia the ultrasound examination demonstrates polyhydramnios during the third trimester, along with fluid-filled cysts in the abdomen of the fetus.

When undiagnosed in utero, initial evaluation of a symptomatic infant includes a flat plate abdominal radiograph. The infant with duodenal atresia customarily demonstrates a "double bubble" sign on radiography with both the stomach and duodenum dilated and filled with gas. The infant with jejunoileal atresia demonstrates distended loops of intestine with multiple air-fluid levels. In some cases of jejunoileal atresia when obstruction is evident in the distal intestine, a barium enema may be done.

Interdisciplinary Interventions

Prenatal diagnosis allows planning for the delivery of the infant in a facility where further diagnostic work-up and intervention can be done soon after delivery. The nurse may provide anticipatory guidance to the parents so that they have an understanding of the infant's condition and what to expect at the time of delivery.

At birth or when clinical symptoms otherwise become evident, the infant requires initial stabilization with intravenous fluids to ensure that maintenance needs are met and that ongoing losses are replaced. An NG tube is placed to provide gastric decompression and prevent aspiration of gastric contents. Serum electrolytes and blood cell counts are monitored, and any abnormalities are corrected. The infant's blood glucose levels are also closely monitored. Broad-spectrum intravenous antibiotics may be administered prophylactically. Respiratory support may be necessary.

Surgical correction of duodenal atresia involves resection of the atretic segment of duodenum and duodenoduodenal or duodenojejunal anastomosis. Resection and primary anastomosis are also commonly done in the surgical correction of jejunoileal atresia. In cases involving extensive resection of bowel, massive dilation of proximal bowel, or colonic atresia, a two-stage procedure is done. A jejunostomy or ileostomy is created initially to drain the proximal bowel, with final anastomosis to the remaining distal intestine done some months later. In all cases, the surgical goal is to preserve as much intestine as possible. Massive resection of the small intestine may leave the infant with a short bowel syndrome, leading to long-term problems with meeting fluid and nutrient requirements using the GI tract (see discussion of short bowel syndrome).

In infants with both duodenal and jejunoileal atresia, a gastrostomy tube may be placed at the time of surgery to facilitate gastric decompression during the initial postoperative period and to use for administration of enteral feedings if it is anticipated that oral feedings may not be well tolerated. If a large amount of bowel has been resected or a very proximal ostomy exists, a central venous catheter may be inserted for administration of parenteral nutrition.

Postoperative care continues many of the interventions begun in the preoperative period. Respiratory support may continue in the early postoperative period. Gastric decompression by NG tube or gastrostomy is continued until intestinal motility normalizes. This may take from 5 to 7 days up to 2 to 3 weeks, depending on the location and the extent of the atresia.

Nursing measures to maintain patency of the gastric drainage system and close monitoring of output are essential. Parenteral nutrition is begun to meet the infant's nutritional needs until enteral feedings are well tolerated. Careful monitoring of the infant's fluid and electrolyte status is necessary. Intravenous antibiotics are continued for 5 to 7 days postoperatively. Oral or enteral feedings are begun when the intestinal motility normalizes. Formula choice varies depending on the extent of bowel resected: infants with limited resection may be given breast milk or cow's milk infant formula, and infants with massive intestinal resection or an ostomy placed high in the intestinal tract will require a protein hydrolysate or elemental formula. As formula intake is advanced, parenteral nutrition is weaned. Careful monitoring to ensure adequate growth and weight gain, as well as GI tolerance, is important.

Nursing measures to monitor and support the infant's physiologic needs are important in the postoperative period. Assessment of fluid status, including careful documentation of all losses from gastric drainage and the ostomy, if present, is essential. Monitoring GI function, including gastric residuals and feeding tolerance, is a key aspect of care. Parent support and education are important nursing functions in the care of the infant with intestinal atresia. Hospitalization may be prolonged, and the parents may need support and guidance in establishing their parental role with their sick newborn. Social work involvement to provide support to the parents in dealing with the crisis of the birth of an infant with health problems and the stress of prolonged hospitalization is very important. Parent education regarding home care for their infant is incorporated into the plan of care from the start. Gastrostomy and ostomy care, administration of feedings, and signs of intestinal dysfunction are addressed. If parenteral nutrition will be required for a prolonged period, the parents will need extensive preparation to handle administration of parenteral nutrition and central venous catheter care at home (see Chapter 17).

Hernias and Hydroceles

A hernia is a protrusion of an organ, or part of an organ, or other structure through the wall of the cavity in which it is contained. A hernia in the abdominal region is considered *reducible* when its contents are easily manipulated back into the peritoneal cavity. An *incarcerated* hernia occurs when the abdominal contents become trapped and irreducible. A *strangulated* hernia occurs when the herniated intestines become twisted and edematous. Intestinal obstruction and ischemia may occur.

A hydrocele is a collection of peritoneal fluid in the tunica vaginalis. Omphalocele, gastroschisis, and diaphragmatic hernias are types of hernias that have special considerations; their care is discussed later.

An *umbilical hernia* results from imperfect closure or weakness of the umbilical ring allowing portions of intestine or omentum to protrude. It is more common in low-birth-weight, female, and black infants. It presents as a usually small bulging of the umbilicus. Umbilical hernias usually cause no problems and often regress spontaneously. Surgical repair is not indicated unless the hernia becomes strangulated, becomes incarcerated, persists beyond age 3 to 4, or continues to enlarge after age 2.

Worldview: *Parents should be taught that home remedies, such as using belly bands or taping a coin over the umbilicus, will not prevent or cure an umbilical hernia. If parents insist on using such remedies, encourage them to use a small coin and clean the umbilical area well.*

Inguinal hernias and *hydroceles* are among the most common congenital anomalies requiring surgical repair in infants. Inguinal hernias are caused by abdominal contents exiting the peritoneal cavity and protruding into the processus vaginalis, a peritoneal sac that normally closes early in infancy. Hydroceles are caused by peritoneal fluid communicating with the scrotal area through a patent processus vaginalis (Fig. 18–10).

Inguinal hernias occur in 9% to 11% of preterm infants and in 3.5% to 5% of term infants. They are nine times more common in males than in females. They may also occur in children with conditions characterized by increased intra-abdominal pressure, because this additional stress forces the abdominal contents into the processus vaginalis. These include children with ventriculoperitoneal shunts, children with chronic cough secondary to cystic fibrosis, and children receiving peritoneal dialysis. Inguinal hernias most often present as unilateral, with bilateral hernias occurring in only 15% of cases.

Pathophysiology

The processus vaginalis is an outpouching of the peritoneum that develops during the third month of gestation. In males, it descends along the inguinal canal to the area of the scrotum. In females, it terminates in the area of the labia majora. In the seventh month of gestation, the testes descend through the processus vaginalis into the scrotum. The processus vaginalis typically remains patent until birth and closes at birth or during early infancy. Protrusion of abdominal contents through the patent processus vaginalis into the inguinal area causes the hernia.

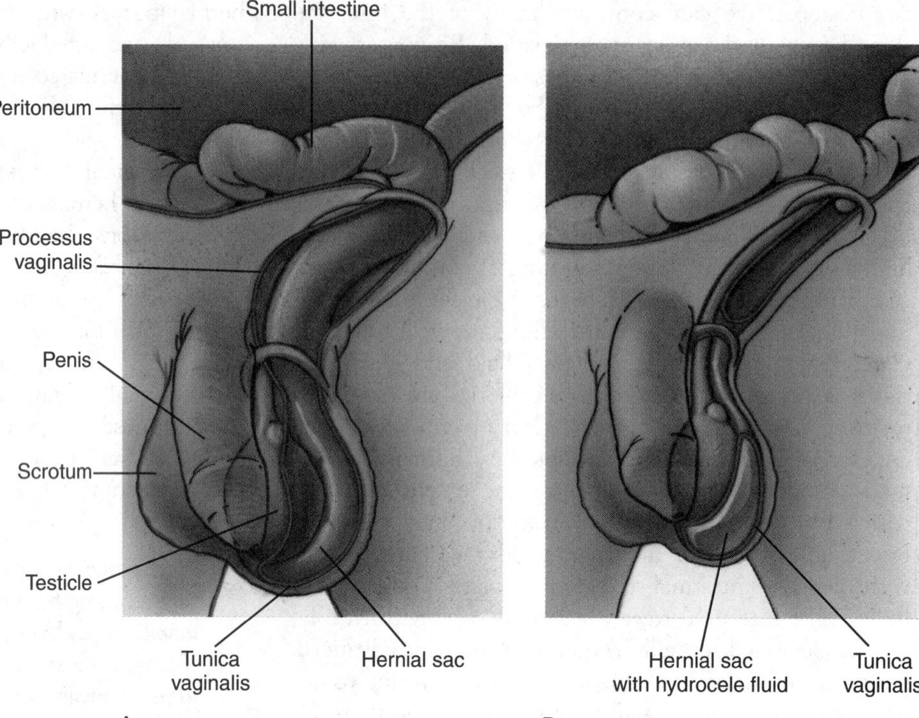

Figure 18–10
A, In an inguinal hernia, the bowel protrudes into the patent processus vaginalis. *B*, A noncommunicating hydrocele has no connection with the abdominal cavity, so the amount of scrotal swelling does not fluctuate with activity. In a communicating hydrocele, the processus vaginalis remains patent and the amount of scrotal swelling may vary with the infant's activity.

A hydrocele may be communicating or noncommunicating. A noncommunicating hydrocele results from complete obliteration of the processus vaginalis and is a collection of fluid in the scrotal area that does not increase in size and usually disappears by age 1 year. A communicating hydrocele occurs when the processus vaginalis remains patent and allows peritoneal fluid to cause intermittent scrotal swelling that waxes and wanes in relation to the infant's level of activity.

Prognosis. Inguinal hernias and communicating hydroceles are treated by surgical repair. Outcomes are generally good. Approximately 50% of children younger than age 1 who present with a unilateral inguinal hernia eventually develop a hernia on the opposite side.

Assessment

The parents of the child with an inguinal hernia typically report seeing a bulge in the groin area that occurs only when the child cries, strains, or coughs (Fig. 18–11). Pain is not typically reported unless the hernia becomes incarcerated or strangulated. In this case the child may be irritable, with cramping abdominal pain and vomiting that may progress from nonbilious to feculent as obstruction of the trapped bowel progresses. The child with a communicating hydrocele demonstrates a scrotal bulge or swelling that increases with crying or straining and decreases when the child is at rest.

The diagnosis of hernia or hydrocele is most commonly made by history and physical examination. Relevant history data includes the parent's observations as to onset of hernia, factors exacerbating the occurrence of the hernia, and any pain or obstructive symptoms associ-

Figure 18–11
Inguinal hernia in a male may occur only with crying and straining. (From Liebert, P. S. [1996]. *Color atlas of pediatric surgery* [2nd ed., p. 102]. Philadelphia: W. B. Saunders. Reprinted with permission.)

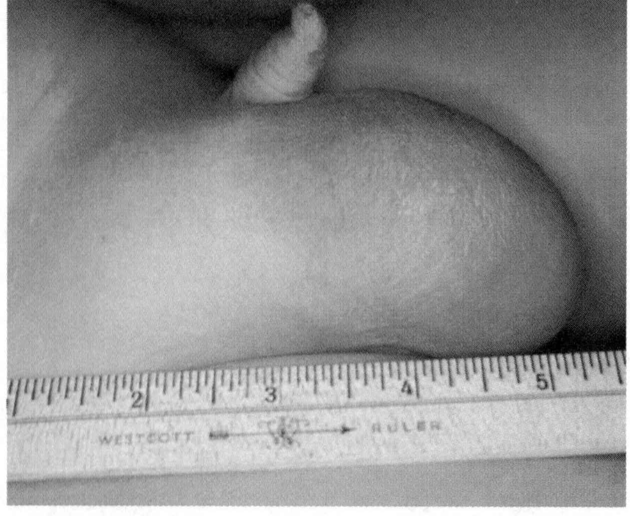

ated with the hernia. On physical examination, an inguinal hernia appears as a bulge in the inguinal or scrotal area. In an inguinal hernia, thickening of the structures of the inguinal canal may be felt with palpation.

Interdisciplinary Interventions

Nonoperative reduction of an incarcerated hernia is attempted before surgical repair. The child is sedated, the lower torso is elevated, and the incarcerated contents of the hernia are gently manipulated back into the peritoneal cavity. Application of an ice pack may also be utilized. If the reduction is successful, surgical repair of the hernia will take place 24 to 48 hours later. Delaying the surgery allows time for resolution of any edema of the bowel resulting from the incarceration. If nonoperative reduction is unsuccessful or the hernia shows evidence of strangulation, immediate surgical repair is indicated.

Surgical repair of the hernia, an inguinal herniorrhaphy, may be done as an outpatient surgery in term infants and children. Preterm infants may require 24-hour observation in the hospital postoperatively because of their increased risk of apnea with anesthesia. The herniorrhaphy is done through an incision through the inguinal crease. The processus vaginalis is identified and ligated. Bilateral exploration and herniorrhaphy are done in children younger than age 1 year who are at high risk for occurrence of "second side" hernia after repair of the initial hernia.

Preoperative nursing measures for the child with a hernia include careful assessment of the hernia site and the child's vital signs, being alert for signs of incarceration or strangulation.

caREminder: *Assessment of the skin condition in the inguinal area is important; diaper rash or skin breakdown may lead to poor wound healing or wound infection and necessitate delay of elective surgery.*

Postoperative nursing care is routine. The surgical site is assessed for bleeding or drainage, as well as any recurrence of the hernia and any vascular compromise to the gonads. Education of parents is an important nursing activity in both the preoperative and postoperative periods, especially in light of the short stay the child will have after the surgery. Information regarding the surgical procedure, preoperative routines, postoperative care, and signs and symptoms of recurrence or complications is provided.

Abdominal Wall Defects: Gastroschisis and Omphalocele

In these congenital defects, a defect of the anterior abdominal wall allows the bowel to eviscerate outside the abdominal cavity. *Gastroschisis* is a full-thickness defect of the abdominal wall, usually to the right of the umbilical cord, through which loops of bowel eviscerate. In *omphalocele*, the intestines herniate into the base of the umbilical cord and are covered with a large peritoneal sac.

The combined incidence of gastroschisis and omphalocele is reportedly 1 in 10,000 to 20,000 live births. The etiology of abdominal wall defects is poorly understood. A mechanical or teratogenic event early in fetal development is hypothesized.

Pathophysiology

The defect associated with gastroschisis is believed to occur between the fourth and eighth weeks of fetal development. Although the exact mechanism is unclear, gastroschisis may be the result of an early tear in the umbilical cord before closure of the umbilical ring. The bowel eviscerates into the amniotic cavity, where prolonged contact with amniotic fluid creates a fibrous peel over the exposed loops of bowel. The fibrous peel apparently contributes to the intestinal dysmotility often seen in infants with gastroschisis. Associated anomalies are usually confined to the GI tract, with intestinal atresia occurring in 5% to 15% of all cases. Intestinal malrotation may also be seen.

The pathophysiology that leads to the development of omphalocele is also poorly understood. An early defect in abdominal wall development may result in a disparity between the size of the abdominal cavity and the abdominal viscera, leaving inadequate space for the midgut to return to the abdominal cavity during the 10th week of gestation, after its normal exocoelomic phase of development. Omphalocele is often associated with other congenital defects. Cardiac anomalies are found in 30% to 50% of cases. Cloacal defects involving the bladder may also be associated.

Prognosis. Infants born with gastroschisis have a 90% survival rate. Long-term complications are associated with significant intestinal atresias that result in short bowel syndrome. Omphalocele carries a reported 80% survival rate. Mortality is usually related to chromosomal anomalies or life-threatening associated anomalies.

Assessment

Both gastroschisis and omphalocele may be seen in utero by ultrasound. Both defects are evident at birth, with abdominal viscera being visually obvious.

Nursing Diagnoses and Outcomes

In addition to the nursing diagnoses and outcomes listed in Chart 18–3, the following may apply to the child with an abdominal wall defect:

- **Ineffective breathing pattern related to the effects of diaphragm elevation by bowel**
  Outcome: The child will maintain adequate lung expansion and blood oxygenation.
- **Hypothermia related to effects of increased heat loss through exposed viscera**
  Outcomes: The child will be supported in a neutral thermal environment.
  The child will maintain body temperature within normal limits.
- **Risk of infection related to presence of exposed viscera**
  Outcome: The child will not develop an infection.
- **Risk for injury related to presence of exposed viscera and potential for torsion of bowel or supporting vessels**
  Outcome: The child will have bowel supported in therapeutic position and will maintain blood supply to the bowel.

Interdisciplinary Interventions

When abdominal wall defects are diagnosed prenatally, arrangements can be made for the mother to be delivered of the infant in a center with expertise in the care of infants with these defects. In some cases the infant with gastroschisis may be delivered electively at 36 weeks' gestation to reduce the exposed bowel's contact with amniotic fluid, thereby minimizing formation of the fibrous peel.

At birth, the exposed bowel or peritoneal sac must be handled carefully to prevent twisting or torsion of the mesentery. The exposed viscera are wrapped with warm saline–soaked gauze and covered with a plastic sheet or bag to prevent heat and fluid loss from the exposed viscera. IV access is obtained. Fluid resuscitation is given, and any electrolyte abnormalities are corrected. Broad-spectrum antibiotics are also administered as ordered. Hemodynamic and respiratory support, including mechanical ventilation, are given as needed. An orogastric tube is placed to prevent the accumulation of air in the bowel.

Surgical intervention is necessary to close the abdominal wall defect. Small defects may be treated with reduction of the eviscerated bowel into the abdominal cavity and primary closure of the abdominal wall. Larger defects require a staged repair. The exposed viscera have a Silastic silo placed around them (Fig. 18–12), and the protruding bowel is slowly reduced into the abdominal cavity over a period of up to 7 days. This allows for gradual expansion of the cavity to accommodate the bowel. After the bowel is fully reduced into the abdominal cavity, the abdominal wall is closed.

If a silo has been placed, the nurse must monitor for signs of hypothermia and for shock from fluid depletion due to heat and insensible water loss through the exposed viscera. The infant must be positioned and moved with extreme caution, to avoid tension on the wound or torsion of the mesentery. If a staged repair is necessary, the nurse monitors for respiratory distress, which may be caused by elevation of the diaphragm from returning too much bowel to a small abdominal cavity. The nurse also monitors for cyanosis of the lower extremities, which may indicate pressure on the descending aorta and its femoral branches. The infant is usually sedated to minimize movement, with pain medications administered before bowel reductions.

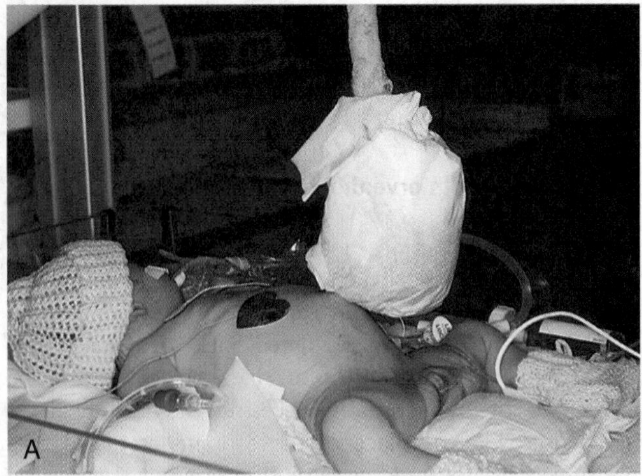

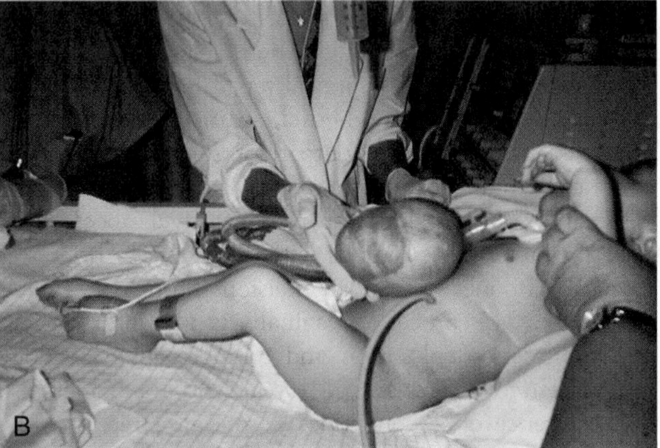

Figure 18–12
A, If an omphalocele or gastroschisis is too large to repair immediately, a Silastic silo is placed over the exposed viscera and the intestines are gradually reduced into the abdominal cavity over a period of days. *B*, A child with an omphalocele whose condition was too unstable to permit surgical reduction. The sac covering the intestines has toughened over time.

Supportive care is continued after the abdominal wall has been closed. Monitoring respiratory and hemodynamic status, pain management (see Chapter 13), and parenteral support are priorities. Nutritional support with TPN is usually initiated 1 or 2 days after surgery, once the infant's fluid and electrolyte balance has been stabilized. Feedings are given when the child is medically stable and bowel function has returned. The child with gastroschisis may have a prolonged postoperative ileus and may require parenteral support for several weeks before feedings can be initiated. In some cases, enteral drip feedings by NG or gastrostomy tube are necessary because of persistent intestinal dysmotility that causes intolerance to oral or bolus feedings. In cases in which intestinal atresias are associated with the gastroschisis, short bowel syndrome may be present, resulting in prolonged dependence on TPN, making discharge planning and parent education for home parenteral nutrition an additional nursing consideration (see Chapters 9, 11, and 17).

Congenital Diaphragmatic Hernia

Congenital diaphragmatic hernia (CDH) is the protrusion of abdominal contents into the chest cavity through a defect in the diaphragm. CDH results from the failure of the pleuroperitoneal canal (the opening between the chest and abdomen) to close completely during fetal development or from an early return of the intestines to the abdomen after the normal herniation into the umbilicus during fetal development. Exposure to teratogens, such as drugs, may disrupt the developing thoracic mesenchyme, from which portions of the diaphragm and pulmonary parenchyma develop (Hartman, 1996).

Reported incidence varies from 1 in 2000 to 1 in 5000 births. Associated anomalies such as esophageal atresia, omphalocele, and central nervous system and cardiovascular lesions occur in 20% to 30% of affected children (Hartman, 1996).

Pathophysiology

The defect in the diaphragm may be large or small, allowing proportional amounts of abdominal contents to herniate. The herniation is most commonly on the left side, through the posterolateral foramen of Bochdalek.

More threatening to the infant's survival are the associated effects on the pulmonary system. The lung on the side of the defect is usually hypoplastic with decreased numbers of airway generations, alveoli, and arterioles. The arterioles also show increased muscular mass. The contralateral lung has similar abnormalities, but to a lesser extent. Compression of the lungs by the herniated viscera during fetal development may contribute to the hypoplasia. Abnormal development of the mesenchyme is another possible cause.

Prognosis. Despite advances in neonatal medicine, CDH is associated with a significant mortality rate of 40% to 50%. Correction of the defect in utero has shown some promise for infants who have no other life-threatening anomalies. Children who survive often have long-term pulmonary, neurologic, and growth abnormalities (Hartman, 1996).

Assessment

Most infants with CDH experience respiratory distress within the first few hours of life. As the infant swallows air, the herniated segment distends and further compromises lung and diaphragm excursion. Breath sounds are decreased or absent on the affected side, although bowel sounds may be heard. If the defect is on the left, as is common, heart sounds are shifted to the right. Chest sounds are dull on percussion. Tachypnea and cyanosis are present. Blood gas analysis reveals acidosis.

The infant's chest appears barrel-like, particularly on the affected side. In contrast to the normal protruding abdomen, the abdomen of the infant with CDH looks scaphoid, or sunken, because of the absence of abdominal contents (Fig. 18–13).

Diagnostic Tests. CDH is often diagnosed in utero by ultrasound. After birth, chest radiography is usually diagnostic, showing gas-filled intestinal loops in the chest and displacement of the cardiac silhouette.

Nursing Diagnoses and Outcomes

In addition to the nursing diagnoses listed in Chart 18–3, the following nursing diagnoses and outcomes may be applicable to the infant with CDH:

Figure 18–13
The infant with congenital diaphragmatic hernia has a scaphoid abdomen because some of the abdominal contents are in the thoracic cavity. (From Liebert, P. S. [1996]. *Color atlas of pediatric surgery* [2nd ed., p. 76]. Philadelphia: W. B. Saunders. Reprinted with permission.)

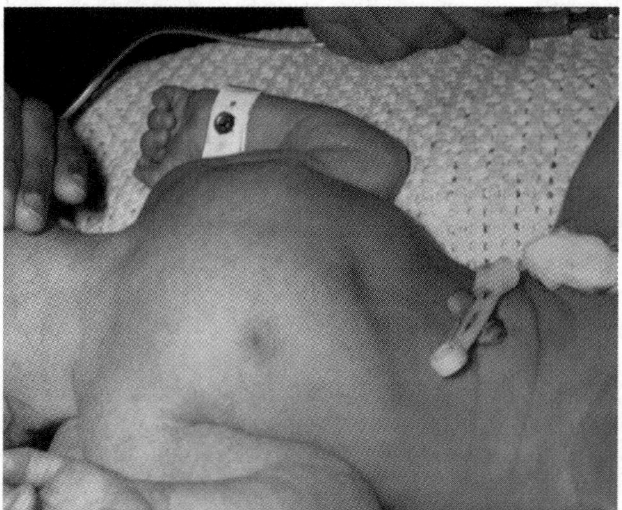

- **Impaired gas exchange related to effects of lung hypoplasia and lung compression**
  Outcome: The child will maintain adequate oxygen saturation levels to sustain life and prevent the sequelae of oxygen deprivation.
- **Risk for injury related to high ventilatory pressures needed to oxygenate causing pneumothorax**
  Outcomes: The child will not suffer iatrogenic injury. The child will have signs of pneumothorax recognized promptly and interventions implemented.
- **Anticipatory grieving (family) related to child's high risk of death**
  Outcomes: The family will be supported in coping with the child's condition.
  The family will spend as much time as possible with the child.
  The family will be given timely, honest information about the child's condition.

Interdisciplinary Interventions

CDH is a life-threatening emergency. Initially, the primary concern is the infant's respiratory status.

Alert: *Ventilatory support is usually required. This includes insertion of an endotracheal tube if the infant requires ventilatory assistance. Infants with CDH should not have bag and mask ventilatory support.*

Air insufflation causes further distention of the intestinal loops in the chest, causing further lung compression and thus decreasing the infant's ability to oxygenate. Rapid, gentle ventilation is used to optimize oxygenation while minimizing barotrauma. These infants have a high risk of pneumothorax. A chest tube may be placed prophylactically. An umbilical artery catheter or arterial line is usually placed to monitor blood gas values.

An NG tube must be inserted to decompress the stomach and intestines. The infant is placed in semi-Fowler's position to allow expansion of the thorax and prevent pressure on the lungs, diaphragm, and viscera. The infant is positioned on the affected side to promote expansion of the unaffected lung. Crying should be minimized as much as possible, to prevent increasing intrathoracic pressure and air swallowing.

The child is kept NPO, and IV fluids with prophylactic antibiotics are administered. The goal of initial stabilization is to address the cardiorespiratory compromise due to pulmonary hypertension and hypoplasia before surgery is attempted. Pharmacologic treatment of the pulmonary hypertension has proven to be of limited value. If the foregoing measures are unsuccessful, extracorporeal membrane oxygenation may be used.

The hernia is most commonly reduced using an abdominal approach. This permits the surgeon to address the intestinal malrotation that is usually present. The defect in the diaphragm is corrected using primary closure, if possible. If primary closure will cause excessive tension on the intestines, diaphragm, and large vessels, then a synthetic patch is used to close the defect.

Postoperatively, an infant with CDH usually remains critically ill and a challenge to manage. The infant's respiratory status continues to be of primary concern. The goal is to optimize oxygenation and avoid acidosis, which exacerbates the pulmonary hypertension. Oxygen therapy is continued; mechanical ventilation may be necessary. The infant remains at high risk for pneumothorax because of the pulmonary abnormalities and the high ventilatory pressures often required. The chest tube is left in place until the lung has expanded, until air has been evacuated from the chest, and often until high ventilatory pressures are no longer necessary.

The nurse constantly monitors chest tube function and assesses for signs of pneumothorax and notifies the physician or advanced nurse practitioner if they occur. Routine postoperative care includes closely monitoring for changes in the infant's status and administering IV fluids and antibiotics. An NG tube remains in place for gastric decompression. A gastrostomy tube may be placed during surgery to facilitate postoperative GI decompression and feeding.

The infant is positioned as was done preoperatively. Environmental stimuli are reduced (dim lights, decrease noise, gentle handling) to decrease stress on the infant. Social service case workers or clergy should be involved as appropriate, to help support the family.

When mechanical ventilation is no longer required and bowel function returns, feedings are initiated gradually. Infants with CDH frequently have gastroesophageal reflux (GER) (D'Agostino, 1997). The nurse must monitor for signs of GER and use appropriate positioning and feeding techniques. The infant may have problems sucking and swallowing or show aversive behaviors to oral stimulation, owing to being NPO for a prolonged period or after oral intubation. If this occurs, the occupational therapist should be involved to implement a program of oral motor stimulation. These problems may be prevented by involving the occupational therapist early in the infant's illness. The infant often gags and vomits easily. Feedings should be small and frequent; overfeeding must be avoided. The infant is fed in a semi-upright position and burped frequently.

Alert: *The infant with CDH is prone to abdominal obstruction. Vomiting, abdominal distention, or a change in bowel elimination pattern should be reported immediately.*

Community Care

The parents are involved in the infant's care to the greatest extent possible. Before discharge, the nurse ensures that the parents can demonstrate appropriate feeding techniques. The parents are also taught to recognize signs of respiratory distress, respiratory infection, and bowel obstruction and to notify their health care provider if such signs occur.

Meckel's Diverticulum

The most common congenital malformation of the GI tract, Meckel's diverticulum affects an estimated 2% to 3% of the population. Incidence is greater in males than females by a ratio of 3 : 1. Meckel's diverticulum is asymptomatic in most cases, but it may cause disease in approximately 4% of those affected. Most symptomatic cases present in children younger than age 2 years. With early identification and surgical intervention, Meckel's diverticulum is usually resolvable.

Pathophysiology

Meckel's diverticulum arises from a vestigial segment of the embryonic yolk sac that fails to separate from the primitive intestine during the sixth week of gestation. It is found on the antimesenteric border of the ileum, usually within 100 cm of the ileocecal valve. Ectopic tissue may be found in the distal tip of a Meckel diverticulum. In symptomatic children, gastric mucosal tissue is the most common tissue found. Secretion of acid and pepsin from the ectopic gastric tissue causes peptic ulceration and, ultimately, bleeding in the lower GI tract.

Assessment

Intermittent, painless rectal bleeding is the most common clinical manifestation of Meckel's diverticulum. The blood is most often bright red or maroon and may be passed independent of stool. Bleeding may be so severe as to cause severe anemia or hemorrhagic shock. Intestinal obstruction (secondary to intussusception or volvulus) and diverticulitis are less common than bleeding.

Diagnostic Tests. Depending on the degree of bleeding, complete blood cell counts may reveal severe anemia. Standard radiologic imaging and barium studies of the GI tract are of little value in identifying Meckel's diverticulum. Definitive diagnosis is most commonly made with a Meckel scan, which utilizes intravenous injection of a technetium isotope to visualize the ectopic gastric mucosa commonly found in bleeding Meckel's diverticulum. If the Meckel scan is not diagnostic, a tagged red blood cell study may be done to localize the bleeding site.

Interdisciplinary Interventions

Because rectal bleeding is the most common manifestation of Meckel's diverticulum, assessment and restoration of circulating fluid volume is the most important initial step in patient management. Physical assessment findings may include pallor, lethargy, and hemodynamic instability. Administration of intravenous fluids and transfusion of packed red blood cells are used to restore circulating fluid volume. Once the child is stabilized, further diagnostic work-up can take place.

An exploratory laparotomy is done to remove the Meckel's diverticulum. Under most circumstances, intestinal resection is not required and recovery is complete, with infrequent complications. Nursing measures to promote the child's comfort during both the preoperative and postoperative periods are an important aspect of care. Providing information and support to the child and family regarding diagnostic procedures and therapeutic interventions may help to allay anxiety during the course of the hospitalization.

Malrotation and Volvulus

Malrotation is the result of incomplete or deviated rotation of the midgut during embryologic development, causing incomplete fixation of the mesentery on the posterior abdominal wall. *Volvulus* is a life-threatening complication of malrotation in which the malrotated bowel twists on itself, causing vascular compromise and, ultimately, necrosis of the bowel.

Although the incidence of malrotation is reported to be approximately 1 in 500 live births, the true incidence is difficult to ascertain, because many affected infants are asymptomatic. Volvulus occurs within the first year of life in an estimated two thirds of all infants born with malrotation. Delayed presentation of volvulus, with onset in later childhood or adulthood, occurs in 10% to 15% of cases of malrotation.

Pathophysiology

The midgut comprises the duodenum distal to the entry of the bile duct, jejunum, ileum, appendix, cecum and colon up to the midtransverse segment. Between the 5th and 10th weeks of gestation, the midgut grows rapidly and, because of lack of space, is forced to rotate out of the abdominal cavity into the umbilical cord. Between the 10th and 11th weeks of gestation, the abdominal cavity enlarges to a point that allows the midgut to reenter the abdominal cavity. The midgut normally rotates 270 degrees counterclockwise as it returns to the abdominal cavity. Failure of the midgut to complete this rotation normally results in incomplete fixation of the mesentery on the posterior abdominal wall and formation of a foreshortened mesenteric base that allows the bowel to twist on itself, causing abdominal pain and intermittent intestinal obstruction. Bands of adhesions known as Ladd's bands are usually present. These bands extend from the right upper quadrant across the duodenum to the cecum and may cause duodenal obstruction. Midgut volvulus occurs when the malrotated bowel strangulates, causing vascular compromise and necrosis of the bowel.

Prognosis. The prognosis for the child with malrotation and volvulus depends on the extent of necrotic bowel present at the time of surgical correction. Massive resection of bowel may result in a short bowel syndrome and prolonged dependence on TPN. Death may result in cases where bowel necrosis is extensive. The mortality rate for midgut volvulus has been reported as high as 20%.

Assessment

The child with malrotation may present with signs of acute or intermittent intestinal obstruction. Young infants may exhibit bilious vomiting and abdominal distention. Older infants may have abdominal pain that mimics colic. Older children and adolescents may present with a history of recurrent vomiting, postprandial abdominal pain, and weight loss. Midgut volvulus is most commonly associated with acute onset of signs of intestinal obstruction, bilious vomiting, abdominal pain, and distention and must be treated as an emergent situation.

In some cases, physical assessment reveals no obvious abnormalities, whereas in other cases where volvulus and significant vascular compromise has occurred, the child may demonstrate abdominal distention and tenderness, signs of peritonitis, and hypovolemic shock.

Diagnostic Tests. Diagnosis of malrotation is supported by radiologic evaluation. A flat plate of the abdomen may demonstrate an air-filled stomach and duodenum with a proximal obstruction or gas-filled intestinal loops consistent with distal obstruction. Free air in the peritoneum may be seen if perforation has occurred. A flat plate alone may not be sufficient to diagnose malrotation. An upper GI contrast study may show abnormal position of the small bowel in the abdominal cavity or the presence of obstruction. Barium enema may reveal abnormal position of the cecum and colon.

Interdisciplinary Interventions

Surgical correction of malrotation is necessary in symptomatic infants. Preoperatively, an NG tube is placed for gastric decompression and IV fluids are administered to aggressively correct any fluid volume deficits. IV antibiotics are also administered. During surgery, the malrotation is identified and "untwisted." All adhesive bands are divided, and the cecum is placed in the left abdomen. In volvulus with intestinal necrosis, resection of nonviable bowel is necessary. If bowel necrosis is extensive, or the bowel is of questionable viability after the volvulus has been untwisted, "second-look" surgery may be done 24 to 36 hours after the initial surgery, to achieve maximal salvage of bowel.

Postoperative management is impacted by the degree of involvement of the intestine at the time of surgery. The child with a simple malrotation with no vascular compromise to the intestine may have a relatively uneventful postoperative course and experience no long-term sequelae. The child with midgut volvulus and extensive bowel necrosis may be critically ill during the immediate postoperative period and require prolonged hospitalization. The child who requires extensive resection of necrotic bowel may be left with a short bowel syndrome and long-term or life-long dependence on parenteral nutrition.

Nursing care for the child with a midgut volvulus takes place in the setting of what can be considered a catastrophic event for the child and family. Physiologic intervention and educational interventions must be provided within a framework of emotional support that recognizes and responds to the family's response to this acute and catastrophic change in the child's health. A social worker or psychologist may be of help to the child and family in dealing with the acute crisis of the child's illness and in long-term adjustment to alterations in the child's health and life style. Child development specialists may provide developmentally appropriate play experiences to help the child cope with the impact of hospitalization and changes in health and bodily function.

Intussusception

A common cause of acute bowel obstruction in infants and young children, intussusception occurs when a proximal segment of bowel prolapses into a distal segment of bowel. This prolapse results in vascular compromise, edema, and, eventually, mechanical obstruction. The ileocecal junction is a common site of intussusception (Fig. 18–14).

Although intussusception is idiopathic in most cases, it has been hypothesized that hypertrophied lymphoid tissue (Peyer's patches) in the bowel may serve as a lead point. In approximately 5% of cases a lead point can be identified, most commonly a Meckel's diverticulum, polyp, or hemangioma. The incidence of intussusception is estimated to be 1 in 4 per 1000 live births; 80% of cases occur in children age 3 to 24 months.

Pathophysiology

Edema develops within the intussuscepted bowel wall secondary to vascular and lymphatic compression. Bleeding occurs, resulting in the passage of blood and mucus in the stool. As the bowel becomes more edematous, mechanical obstruction of the bowel occurs. If left untreated, this may lead to perforation.

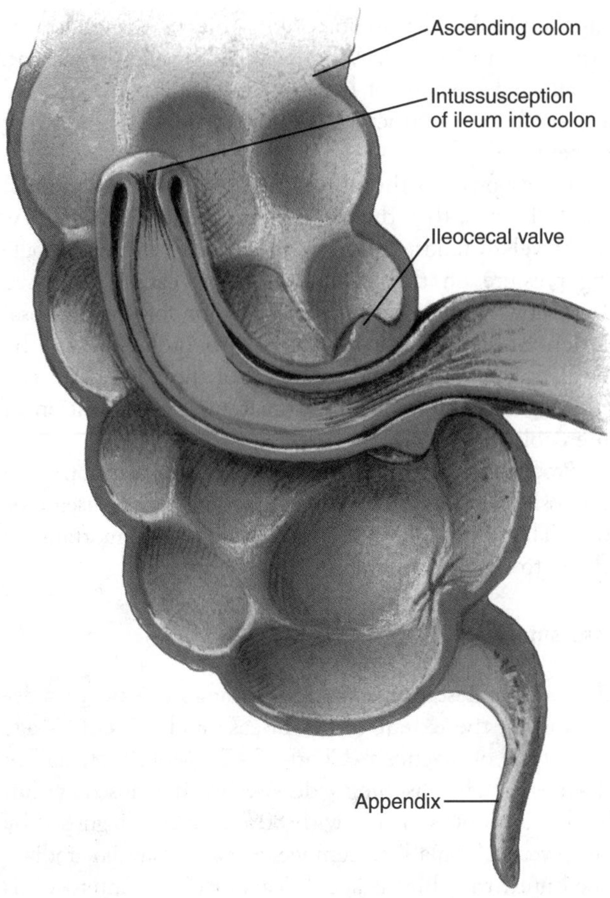

Figure 18–14
In intussusception, a portion of the bowel telescopes into itself, causing signs and symptoms of intestinal obstruction.

Prognosis. The prognosis for the child with intussusception is good with prompt detection and treatment. Recurrence occurs in 3% to 5% of cases after nonoperative correction, but long-term sequelae are uncommon. At highest risk for morbidity associated with intussusception are young infants whose symptoms were not recognized early and who developed intestinal perforation and peritonitis by the time of corrective surgery.

Assessment

The child with intussusception classically presents with severe abdominal pain that is crampy and intermittent, causing the child to draw in his or her knees to the chest. Vomiting is nonbilious at first but may progress to bilious as the disease progresses and complete intestinal obstruction occurs. Bright-red blood and mucus are passed through the rectum; this is commonly described as "currant jelly" stools (Fig. 18–15).

In the early stages of intussusception, physical examination may reveal no abnormalities other than episodic pain. As the disorder progresses, the child may appear more lethargic and listless. A low-grade fever may be present. The abdomen is usually soft and nontender. A sausage-shaped mass is commonly palpable in the upper right abdomen. With progressive obstruction, the abdomen may become more distended and the mass may become nonpalpable.

Diagnostic Tests. A complete blood cell count and electrolyte panel may be done as a part of the evaluation of the child with suspected intussusception. The complete blood cell count may show a slight increase in white blood cells, and the electrolyte panel may reflect some degree of dehydration if the child has had excessive fluid losses from vomiting.

Radiologic evaluation begins with a flat plate of the abdomen. This often reveals nonspecific findings but may demonstrate some density in the area of the intussusception. A contrast enema, done with air, barium, or water-soluble contrast medium, may be used as a diagnostic or therapeutic tool in the treatment of intussusception. The contrast enema is done after the child has received nasogastric decompression, fluid resuscitation, and IV antibiotics. A surgeon stands by in the event of bowel perforation during enema administration. The child is sedated before the procedure. The contrast material infused during the enema radiographically delineates the area of intussusception, which appears like a coiled spring within the lumen of the bowel. The pressure of the contrast material is maintained for up to 5 minutes, which causes reduction of the intussusception in up to 95% of cases. After radiologic reduction of an intussusception, the

Figure 18–15
"Currant jelly" stools are a classic sign of intussusception. (From Liebert, P. S. [1996]. *Color atlas of pediatric surgery* [2nd ed., p. 159]. Philadelphia: W. B. Saunders. Reprinted with permission.)

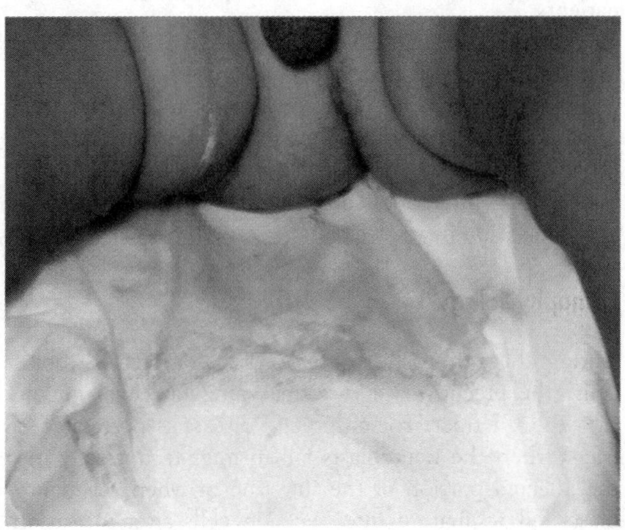

child is observed for 24 to 36 hours for signs of recurrence, which occurs in up to 12% of all cases.

Interdisciplinary Interventions

Surgical reduction of intussusception is required in cases in which overt signs of peritonitis, bowel perforation, or septic shock are present or when radiologic methods fail to resolve it. Fluid resuscitation and IV broad-spectrum antibiotics are given preoperatively. A laparotomy is performed through a transverse right lower quadrant incision. Manual reduction of the intussusception is attempted after the bowel is mobilized. If this is not successful, resection of the affected bowel with end-to-end anastomosis is performed. If bowel perforation is detected during surgery, a temporary ostomy may be created.

A key nursing intervention in the care of the child with intussusception is teaching the family about the signs and symptoms of recurrent intussusception. Recurrence may develop shortly after the initial reduction or months later. Early recognition and treatment are important in avoiding the increased morbidity that results from delayed diagnosis and intervention.

Hirschsprung's Disease

Hirschsprung's disease, or aganglionic megacolon, is among the most common causes of distal bowel obstruction in the newborn. Hirschsprung's disease is characterized by the absence of ganglion nerve cells in a defined portion of the rectum and colon, resulting in abnormal peristalsis and functional obstruction of the affected segment. The rectum and rectosigmoid colon are involved in as many as 85% of cases; the entire colon and portions of the small intestine are involved in 5% to 8% of cases. Ultra-short-segment Hirschsprung's disease, involving less than 5 cm of colon, occurs in a small number of patients.

Hirschsprung's disease occurs in 1 in 5000 live births and has a 4:1 predominance in males. Although the etiology of Hirschsprung's disease is not fully understood, genetic factors have been implicated in some cases. Up to 25% of children with Hirschsprung's disease have associated congenital anomalies, including Down syndrome and congenital heart defects.

Pathophysiology

During the 6th to 12th weeks of gestation, neuroblast cells (the precursors of intestinal ganglion cells) migrate into the GI tract. Hirschsprung's disease is postulated to occur when the neuroblasts fail to migrate normally into the affected portion of the intestine or when the neuroblasts fail to mature into ganglion cells after migration. Ganglion cells play an important role in the peristaltic activity of the bowel. When ganglion cells are absent, the affected segment of bowel maintains a constant state of contraction, obstructing the flow of stool through that segment.

In response to the obstruction, the proximal normal bowel distends; thus the term *megacolon* (Fig. 18–16). As the bowel distends, intraluminal pressure increases, putting pressure on the bowel wall. This causes decreased blood flow, ischemia, and deterioration of the mucosal barrier. Stasis also allows bacteria to proliferate in the bowel. Inflammation and infection of the bowel wall can result in the potentially life-threatening complication of enterocolitis.

Prognosis. With timely surgical intervention, the prognosis for the child with Hirschsprung's disease is good. The main risk factor for morbidity and mortality is related to sepsis from enterocolitis.

Assessment

Clinical manifestations of Hirschsprung's disease vary depending on the extent of the disease and the child's age at the time of diagnosis (Chart 18–7). More than half of all cases of Hirschsprung's disease are diagnosed within the first 3 months of life, with 80% of cases diagnosed by age 1 year. A small percentage of cases may go undiagnosed until the child is age 5 years or older. Enterocolitis is the presenting symptom in approximately 6% of newborns with Hirschsprung's disease. Risk factors for enterocolitis in this group include delay in diagnosis beyond age 1 week and Down syndrome. Physical examination of the child with Hirschsprung's disease is most often significant

Figure 18–16
In Hirschsprung's disease, dilation of the colon occurs proximal to the aganglionic section.

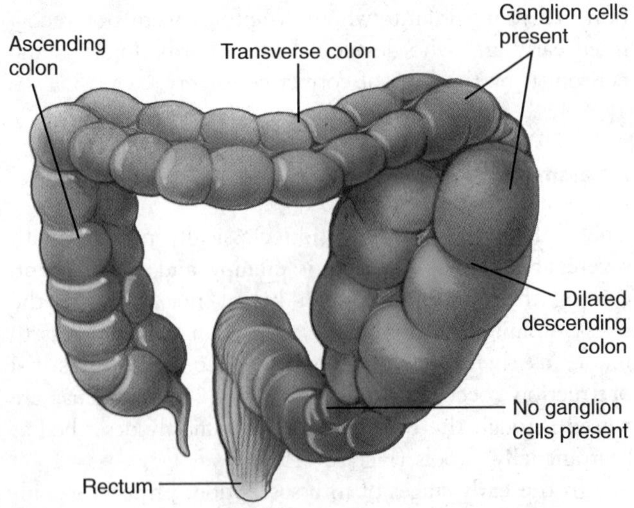

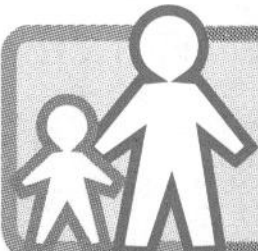

Chart 18-7
Developmental Considerations

Presentation of Hirschsprung's Disease

Newborn

Breast-fed infants may present with less severe manifestations.

- Failure to pass meconium within 48 hours after birth
- Abdominal distention
- Bilious vomiting
- Liquid stool (from seepage around fecal impaction—must be differentiated from diarrhea of enterocolitis)
- Enterocolitis
  - Abdominal distention
  - Diarrhea
  - Fever
  - Hematochezia

Older Infants and Children

- Chronic constipation
- Characteristic stools
  - Foul smelling
  - Consistency varies: small pellets, ribbon-like, or liquid (from seepage around fecal impaction—must be differentiated from diarrhea of enterocolitis)
- Abdominal distention
- Enterocolitis
  - Abdominal distention
  - Diarrhea
  - Fever
  - Hematochezia
- Failure to thrive

for the presence of a distended abdomen and the absence of stool in the rectum on digital rectal examination.

Diagnostic Tests. Barium enema is commonly the first step in establishing the diagnosis of Hirschsprung's disease. The child receives no bowel prep before the examination. In most cases, the study demonstrates the characteristic transition zone where the contracted aganglionic segment of bowel and the dilated proximal segment meet. Rectal manometry may be used as a diagnostic tool. In Hirschsprung's disease, the internal sphincter of the rectum contracts instead of relaxing normally in response to distention of the rectum. Definitive diagnosis is made by suction rectal biopsy demonstrating the absence of ganglion cells in the submucosa and myenteric plexus.

Nursing Diagnoses and Outcomes

In addition to the nursing diagnoses listed in Chart 18–3, the following nursing diagnoses and outcomes may be applicable to the infant with Hirschsprung's disease:

- **Constipation related to effects of aganglionic bowel**
  Outcomes: The child will demonstrate normal patterns of elimination.
  The child and family will verbalize understanding of signs of alterations in elimination and implement appropriate interventions.
- **Risk for infection related to potential of enterocolitis, postoperative incision, and atelectasis**
  Outcomes: The child will be free of infection.
  The child and family will recognize the signs of infectious complications and contact the health care provider when present.

Interdisciplinary Interventions

Preparation and support of the child for tests and procedures, as well as parent education and support, are important nursing activities throughout the diagnostic work-up. Treatment of Hirschsprung's disease requires surgical intervention to remove the aganglionic segment of bowel and anastomose the normal bowel to the rectum. This is often done as a two-stage procedure. At the time of diagnosis, the child undergoes a diverting colostomy just proximal to the transition zone. This allows the normal bowel to decompress and return to normal size. At a later date, usually when the child is 6 to 12 months old or has reached a body weight of 5 to 10 kg and is medically stable, a second-stage pull-through procedure can be done to reestablish bowel continuity. Various surgical approaches can be taken. The most common is the endorectal pull-through procedure, in which the aganglionic rectum is stripped of its mucosa and the normal colon is brought down within the muscular layer of the rectum and anastomosed 1.0 to 1.5 cm above the dentate line. Recently, some centers have reported treating Hirschsprung's disease with a primary corrective surgery of pull-through without a decompressing colostomy with satisfactory results (Allen, 1995).

Preoperative care of the child initially diagnosed with Hirschsprung's disease includes all the standard care of any child with suspected bowel obstruction. The child is kept NPO, and gastric decompression is instituted. IV fluids and electrolytes are administered to meet maintenance requirements and correct any deficits, along with IV antibiotics if enterocolitis is suspected. Neonates do not require a preoperative bowel prep, but older children may require extensive preparation. The involvement of the enterostomal therapist is important in the preoperative period so that the ostomy site is appropriately marked and the bedside nurse receives support while preparing the family for surgery.

The child will require routine postoperative care after surgery. The enterostomal therapist will collaborate with the bedside nurse in monitoring the appearance and function of the colostomy, as well as in selecting appropriate pouching appliances. After the endorectal pull-through, the child is monitored closely for signs of anastomotic leak or intraabdominal abscess such as fever, irritability, and abdominal distention. Long-term complications of endorectal pull-through include anastomotic stricture, resulting in constipation and obstruction. Enterocolitis occurs as a late complication of surgery in approximately 5% of all cases.

Alert: *Medications should not be administered by the rectal route for the first 2 to 3 weeks after an endorectal pull-through procedure.*

Community Care

The child with Hirschsprung's disease has special care needs at home after both first-stage and second-stage surgeries. The family's understanding of Hirschsprung's disease and the treatment plan are assessed. The family must be prepared to meet the child's anticipated care needs at home. After the first-stage surgery, the family will need instruction in colostomy care. The child is included in all teaching, as developmentally appropriate. Skin care, pouch application and management, and signs of complications are addressed. The enterostomal therapist will collaborate with the bedside nurse in the teaching process, as well as in referral to community resources for follow-up teaching and support. Referral to a home health nursing agency may be necessary for ongoing family education. The family should receive needed ostomy care supplies at discharge as well as referral to a community resource for obtaining further supplies.

After endorectal pull-through, the child and family will need teaching about postoperative complications. Signs of anastomotic stricture, bowel obstruction, and enterocolitis are emphasized, along with the appropriate follow-up contacts.

Long-term problems may include delays in toilet training, staining, fecal incontinence, and constipation (Diseth, Bjornland, Novik, & Emblem, 1997). Although many children attain satisfactory bowel function, parents need to be prepared for these problems, supported during toilet training of the child, and encouraged to have realistic expectations about the child's ability to achieve continence.

Children and families may benefit from peer support in dealing with Hirschsprung's disease. Community organizations such as the local ostomy association offer opportunities for children and families to interact with others who have been similarly affected.

Anorectal Malformations

Anorectal malformations encompass a number of defects in anal development resulting from alterations in prenatal development of the GI and genitourinary tracts during the 4th to 16th weeks of gestation. Anorectal agenesis (also referred to as imperforate anus), anal stenosis, and rectovaginal fistula or fistulas in females or rectourethral fistula in males are examples of anorectal malformations.

Anorectal malformations are classified as either high, when the rectum fails to descend through the pelvic musculature; intermediate; or low, when the rectum has descended through the pelvic musculature. Specific malformations are generally common to each classification (Table 18–4).

Anorectal malformations occur in 1 in 5000 live births and are slightly more common in males than females. Although their precise etiology is not known, anorectal malformations are frequently associated with the presence of other congenital anomalies, often as a part of VACTERL syndrome. Genitourinary anomalies, other than fistulas, are associated with low lesions in 20% of cases and with high lesions in 50% of cases.

Pathophysiology

During the 4th week of gestation, the cloaca (a transitory embryologic cavity) forms at the end of the primitive hindgut. The cloaca serves as the early common channel of the rectum and the urogenital structures. The urorectal septum develops at 4 to 6 weeks' gestation, descending in a cephalocaudal direction to unite with the cloacal membrane that divides the rectum from the urogenital structures. Rupture of the cloacal membranes at 8 weeks' gestation forms the urogenital and anal orifices. Further differentiation takes place over the next 8 weeks to form the bladder, the urethra and seminal vesicles in males, and the urethra and vagina in females. Failure of embryologic development at any point in this process can result in anorectal anomaly. The form of the anomaly is closely related to the timing of the disruption in embryologic development, with high anomalies occurring around the 4th week of gestation and low anomalies occurring between the 10th and 12th weeks.

Prognosis. The prognosis for a child with an anorectal malformation depends on the type of malformation and the presence of other congenital anomalies. Morbidity usually results from associated defects. After surgical repair, a child with a high lesion usually has long-term problems with fecal incontinence. A child with a low

Table 18–4
Classification of Anorectal Malformations

	Male	Female
High	Anorectal agenesis Anorectal agenesis with recto-urethral fistula Rectal atresia	Anorectal agenesis Anorectal agenesis with recto-vaginal fistula Rectal atresia
Intermediate	Rectobulbar urethral fistula Anal agenesis	Rectovestibular fistula Rectovaginal fistula Anal agenesis
Low	Anocutaneous fistula Anal stenosis	Anocutaneous fistula Anal stenosis Anovestibular fistula

lesion usually achieves fecal continence but may experience long-term problems with constipation.

Assessment

Anorectal malformations are usually immediately obvious at birth. On the initial physical examination the anus is absent or displaced (Fig. 18–17). Affected females may have a variable number and configuration of openings noted in the perineal area. The presence of a fistula may be noted when gas or stool is expelled from the urethra or vagina. In males, fistulas may be seen anywhere along the tract between the usual location of the anus and the tip of the penis, appearing as epithelial pearls or spots of meconium. Meconium may be seen in the urine in the presence of a fistula between the bowel and urinary tract. An anal malformation that is not immediately noted may present with signs of lower intestinal obstruction with abdominal distention and bilious vomiting.

Diagnostic Tests. Radiologic evaluation is necessary to determine the extent of the malformation. A cross-table lateral radiograph can be used to differentiate a high lesion from a low lesion. The presence of gas in the bladder or urethra can also be seen, indicating the presence of a fistulous connection with the bowel.

Computed tomography or magnetic resonance imaging may also be used to visualize the anorectal anatomy. Radiopaque dye studies of any obvious fistulous tracts may be done to determine the exact anatomy of the tract.

Interdisciplinary Interventions

The infant with anorectal malformation requires a careful physical examination to determine the presence of any other anomalies. Immediate stabilization focuses on relieving intestinal obstruction by nasogastric decompression. IV fluids and antibiotics are administered.

Surgical intervention depends on the nature of the malformation. Children with low lesions require anoplasty (creation of an anal opening). Three weeks after surgery, anal dilatations are begun for 2 to 3 months to prevent stenosis of the operative site. Children with high lesions require a diverting colostomy within the first 24 to 48 hours of life. Definitive repair is done in two subsequent stages. This first stage is done at age 3 to 6 months when the rectovaginal or rectourethral fistula tract (if present) is repaired and a posterior sagittal anorectoplasty procedure is done to create an anal opening. Dilations of the new anus begin 3 weeks after surgery and

Figure 18–17
An anal dimple may be present in low types of anal agenesis but not in high types.

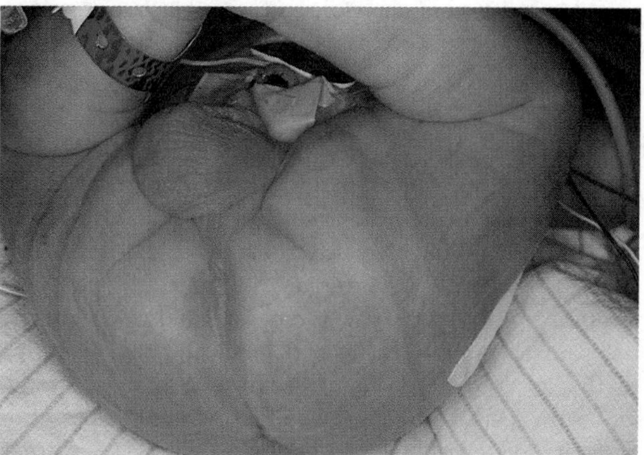

continue for approximately 6 weeks, at which time final closure of the colostomy is done.

Besides the usual preoperative and postoperative care, nursing management for the infant with anorectal malformation includes family education about colostomy care and anal dilation as appropriate. The family also may be referred for home care nursing follow-up as needed. Long-term follow-up concerns related to fecal incontinence have nursing implications in both the clinic and school settings. Anticipatory guidance for parents, along with support with bowel management programs, are key nursing interventions in this regard.

Inflammatory Disorders

Appendicitis

Appendicitis, the inflammation of the vermiform appendix at the end of the cecum, is the most common disease requiring emergency surgery in children. It occurs in 4 of 1000 children and is most common in children between age 6 and 14 years, with peak incidence at age 9 to 11 years. Appendicitis is rare in children younger than age 2 years.

Pathophysiology

Appendicitis begins with obstruction of the lumen of the appendix by a fecalith (a concrete mass of fecal material) or by lymphocytic hyperplasia. As the disease progresses, edema and vascular compromise of the appendix occur. Bacteria invade the walls of the appendix causing inflammation. Without prompt surgical intervention, gangrene and perforation of the appendix may take place.

Prognosis. The prognosis for appendicitis is good with early recognition and surgical intervention. Between 25% and 30% of cases may be perforated by the time of surgical intervention, resulting in increased complications of wound infection and intra-abdominal abscess formation. Mortality from appendicitis is rare but is reported to occur in 0.5% to 1% of cases.

Assessment

The health history and physical assessment provide valuable information in the diagnosis of appendicitis and often are the only tools needed to make the diagnosis. The history focuses on determining the time of onset and location of the pain. The parent or child may describe the pain as initially being periumbilical, then migrating to the lower right quadrant. Younger children may describe the pain as more generalized, whereas older children are better able to localize the pain. The pain is initially crampy as the appendix distends against obstruction, but becomes more constant as inflammation and distention of the appendix increases. Loss of appetite, vomiting, and low-grade fever may follow the onset of pain.

The history of fever and anorexia and vomiting is also elicited. In appendicitis, low-grade fever, anorexia, and vomiting typically occur *after* the onset of abdominal pain.

Alert: *With perforation of the appendix, abdominal pain is suddenly relieved; but as peritonitis develops, it returns, along with signs of a generalized acute abdomen.*

On physical examination, the child may appear to guard the area of pain and may wince with movement, such as walking or climbing onto the examination table. The child with unperforated appendicitis may have only mild temperature elevation. The temperature may rise to 101° to 104°F with perforation, and the child may appear dehydrated. Signs of shock may be present if peritonitis is advanced. The abdomen appears flat with unperforated appendicitis; abdominal distention may be present with perforation. On auscultation, bowel sounds are normal to hyperactive early in the course of appendicitis but become hypoactive with perforation. Percussion reveals irritation and pain in the right lower quadrant. Palpation demonstrates rebound tenderness in the right lower quadrant.

caREminder: *The right lower quadrant is palpated last during the physical assessment of the child with suspected appendicitis. This allows a more accurate assessment of the child's response in comparison with the quadrants that should be free of pain.*

Diagnostic Tests. A CBC and urinalysis are usually obtained as a part of the work-up of the child with suspected appendicitis. Although laboratory tests may not be helpful in establishing a definitive diagnosis of appendicitis, they are important tools in ruling out other potential causes of illness. White blood cell counts are elevated in 70% to 90% of patients with acute appendicitis (Graffeo & Counselman, 1996). These counts may be normal early in the course of the disease but rise as inflammation progresses. Therefore, a second complete blood cell count is often done for comparison. Urinalysis may reveal a small number of white blood cells in the urine as a result of urethral irritation from the proximity of the urethra to the inflamed appendix.

Radiologic evaluation is not a standard part of the work-up of the child with suspected appendicitis but may be useful if the diagnosis is uncertain. A flat plate of the abdomen or abdominal ultrasound are two of the most commonly used tools.

Interdisciplinary Interventions

Surgical appendectomy through a right lower quadrant transverse incision is the definitive treatment for appendicitis. In some centers, laparoscopic appendectomy may be a treatment option for the child with uncomplicated, unperforated appendicitis or occasionally with perforated appendicitis. The child with an uncomplicated appendectomy will usually receive antibiotics for 24 hours postoperatively, be able to resume oral intake within 24 hours of surgery, and be discharged home 24 to 72 hours postoperatively (Care Path 18–2).

Care Path 18–2 An Interdisciplinary Plan of Care for the Child with Nonperforated Appendicitis

	Patient/Family Intermediate Outcomes		
Nursing Diagnosis	**Day: Admission**	**Day: Postop 1**	**Day: Postop 2**
Fluid volume deficit related to inadequate intake, vomiting, diarrhea	Child will regain normal fluid and electrolyte balance.	Child will maintain normal fluid and electrolyte balance.	⟶
Risk for infection related to potential for rupture of the appendix preoperatively or postoperative wound infection	Child will be free of infection.	⟶	⟶
Pain related to effects of tissue ischemia, tissue damage, postoperative wound	Child will experience minimal amounts of pain. Child and family use objective (tool) and subjective methods to assess child's pain.	⟶ ⟶ Child and family identify interventions to implement when the child experiences pain.	⟶ ⟶ ⟶
Ineffective breathing pattern related to effects of abdominal pain	Child has clear breath sounds and maintains adequate tissue oxygenation. Child demonstrates effective lung excursion, coughing, and deep breathing.	⟶ ⟶	⟶ ⟶
Knowledge deficit: surgery, postoperative routines, home care	Child and family will verbalize understanding of need for surgery and preoperative routine.	Child and family perform postoperative routines: pain assessment, cough, deep breathing, ambulation.	⟶ Child and family demonstrate knowledge of home care: pain management, wound care, signs of complications.
Care Intervention Categories			
Consults	Surgical consult Social services as needed for high-risk family		

Care Path continued on following page

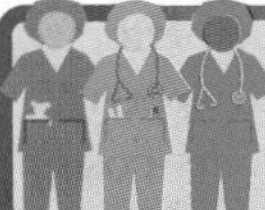

Care Path 18–2 An Interdisciplinary Plan of Care for the Child with Nonperforated Appendicitis *Continued*

Care Intervention Categories	Day: Admission	Day: Postop 1	Day: Postop 2
Labs	CBC, differential, repeat in 4 to 6 hours Urinalysis Pregnancy test as indicated	CBC, differential	
Medications and IVs	IV fluids: maintenance and replacement IV antibiotics IV morphine prn pain Give acetaminophen PO, PR p.r.n. for temperature of 101°F or discomfort	IV morphine PCA IV antibiotics × 24 hours IV maintenance fluids	IV heparin lock; discontinue if tolerating PO fluids and after last antibiotic dose. Give acetaminophen with codeine PO for pain.
Nutrition	NPO	Give clear liquids when bowel function returns.	Advance diet as tolerated.
Pain management	Medications as above Positioning (knees flexed) Distraction (videos, music, stories)	⟶	⟶
Procedures	I&O with urine specific gravity NG tube	Discontinue NG when bowel function returns.	
Radiology	As needed to confirm diagnosis: · Flat-plate of abdomen · Abdominal ultrasound · Computed tomography		

In the event of perforation, intraoperative debridement of necrotic material and lavage of the peritoneal cavity are performed. In some cases of perforation, the surgical wound may be closed only at the level of the fascia and allowed to heal by secondary intention to decrease the risk of wound infection. Broad-spectrum IV antibiotics are administered preoperatively and continued for up to 10 days after surgery. Intestinal ileus may persist for 3 to 5 days after surgery, making it necessary for the child to remain NPO and receive nasogastric decompression and IV fluids until oral intake can be resumed. In some cases, the child may be discharged early and allowed to complete the course of IV antibiotics at home.

Nursing management of the child with appendicitis during the preoperative period requires careful and ongo-

Care Path 18–2 An Interdisciplinary Plan of Care for the Child with Nonperforated Appendicitis *Continued*

Care Intervention Categories	Day: Admission	Day: Postop 1	Day: Postop 2
Safety and activity	As tolerated	Sit in chair, then ambulate as tolerated	⟶
Teaching/discharge planning	Teach child/family: preoperative routines, pain assessment methods, effective coughing, and deep breathing technique.	Teach child/family: postoperative routines, pain management, incision care, signs of complications, supplies needed at home.	Teach diet and activity restrictions, if any. Give written instructions and evaluate family's ability to · Manage pain, diet, activity (including return to school) · Perform incision care · Recognize signs of complications · Follow-up with health care provider. Discharge if afebrile, CBC within normal limits, tolerating PO intake, pain well managed, family meets above criteria.
Vital signs/baseline parameters	HR, RR, BP, temperature q 4 hr Weight, height	⟶ Weight	⟶

BP, blood pressure; CBC, complete blood count; HR, heart rate; I&O, intake and output; PCA, patient-controlled analgesia; PR, per rectum; RR, respiratory rate.

ing assessment of the child's vital signs, pain, and hydration status. Changes in vital signs and the character of the child's pain consistent with the onset of perforation and peritonitis must be promptly reported to the medical team. Pain medication may not be ordered until the diagnosis of appendicitis is firmly established, to avoid masking symptoms. Other comfort measures, including positioning (keeping the knees flexed prevents stretching of the abdominal muscles and avoids tension on the incision) and relaxation techniques may be used. The child will be made NPO and have access obtained to provide IV antibiotics and fluids.

Both the child and parent may be fearful and anxious about the child's pain, multiple procedures, and examinations and the impending surgery. Offering clear, developmentally appropriate explanations of all interventions and providing emotional support to the child and family may help alleviate this (Fig. 18–18) (see Chapter 9).

After surgery, the child requires routine postoperative care and comfort measures. The child with a perforated appendix should be monitored for signs of infection and should be assessed for return of bowel function, maintenance of nasogastric drainage, and delivery of IV fluids and antibiotics. A drain may be placed to promote excretion of infected peritoneal fluid (Fig. 18–19). Parents of

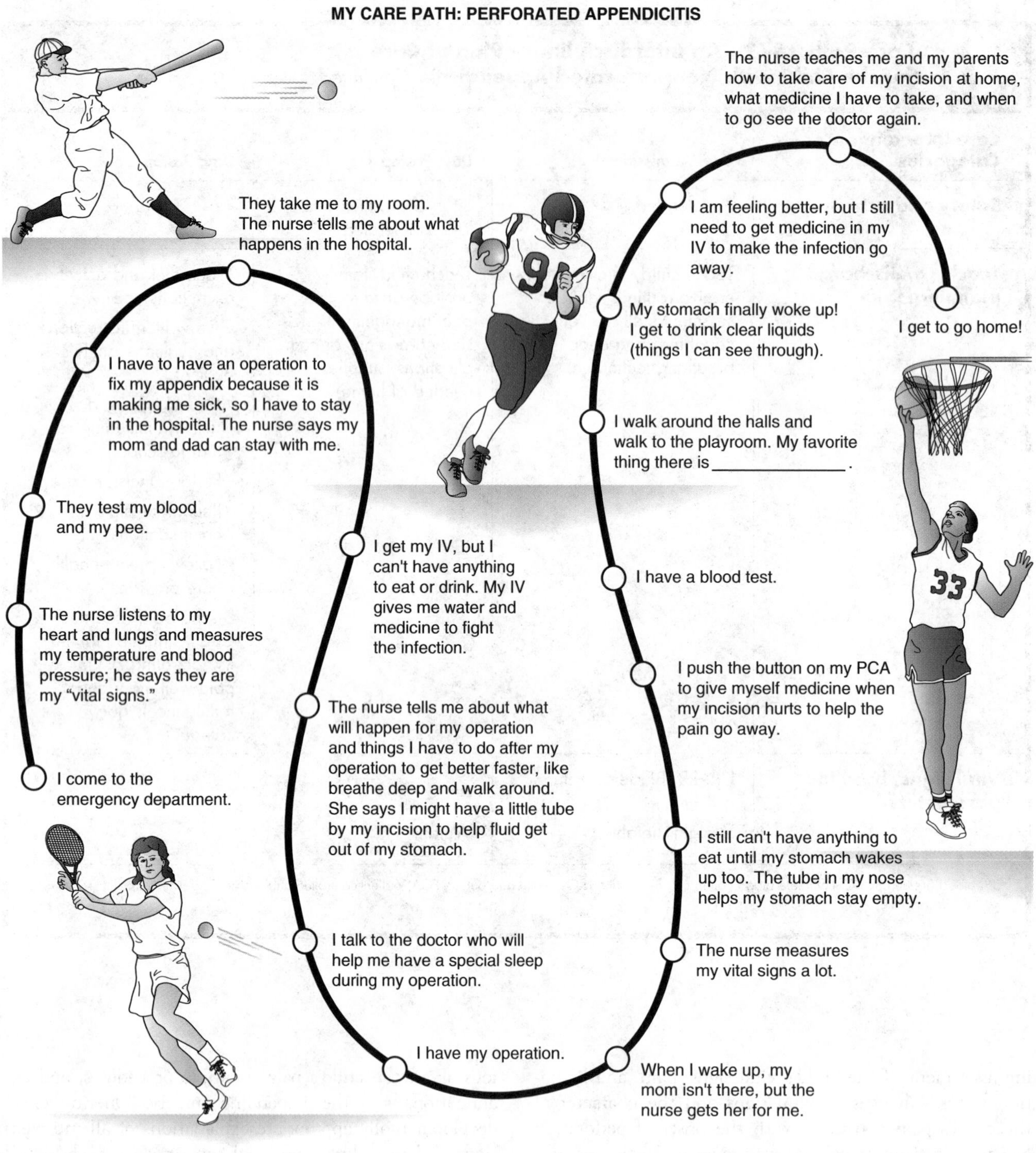

MY CARE PATH: PERFORATED APPENDICITIS

I come to the emergency department.

The nurse listens to my heart and lungs and measures my temperature and blood pressure; he says they are my "vital signs."

They test my blood and my pee.

I have to have an operation to fix my appendix because it is making me sick, so I have to stay in the hospital. The nurse says my mom and dad can stay with me.

They take me to my room. The nurse tells me about what happens in the hospital.

I get my IV, but I can't have anything to eat or drink. My IV gives me water and medicine to fight the infection.

The nurse tells me about what will happen for my operation and things I have to do after my operation to get better faster, like breathe deep and walk around. She says I might have a little tube by my incision to help fluid get out of my stomach.

I talk to the doctor who will help me have a special sleep during my operation.

I have my operation.

When I wake up, my mom isn't there, but the nurse gets her for me.

The nurse measures my vital signs a lot.

I still can't have anything to eat until my stomach wakes up too. The tube in my nose helps my stomach stay empty.

I push the button on my PCA to give myself medicine when my incision hurts to help the pain go away.

I have a blood test.

I walk around the halls and walk to the playroom. My favorite thing there is ______________.

My stomach finally woke up! I get to drink clear liquids (things I can see through).

I am feeling better, but I still need to get medicine in my IV to make the infection go away.

The nurse teaches me and my parents how to take care of my incision at home, what medicine I have to take, and when to go see the doctor again.

I get to go home!

Figure 18–18
A care path for a child with perforated appendicitis.

a child who is eligible for early discharge require instruction regarding wound care and administration of IV antibiotics. Referrals are made for home care nursing and home pharmacy services to support the family in this area.

Inflammatory Bowel Disease

Inflammatory bowel disease (IBD) refers to a group of diseases characterized by inflammation of the GI tract. Crohn's disease (CD) and ulcerative colitis (UC) are the

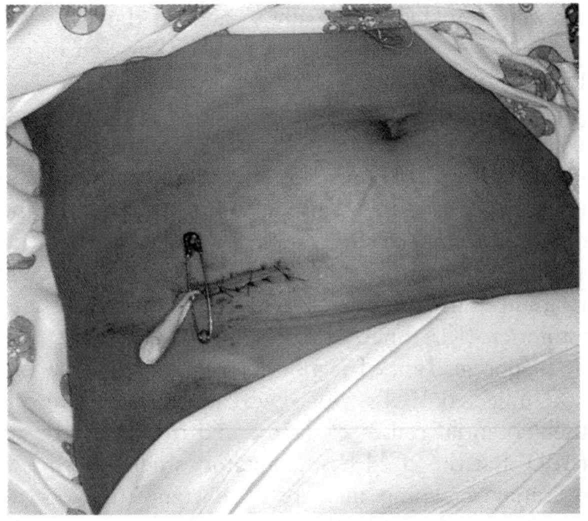

Figure 18–19
The presence of a surgical drain after appendectomy may be distressing for the child. The nurse should explain why the drain is necessary and reassure the child that it will be removed after just a few days.

most common forms of IBD and account for more than 80% of all cases. UC results in an inflammation of the mucosal layer of the large intestine and rectum. Inflammatory disease associated with CD can occur in any part of the GI tract from the mouth to the anus and is transmural.

The overall incidence of CD is 2 to 6 per 100,000, with approximately 25% of all new cases occurring in patients younger than 20. UC has an incidence of 2 to 14 per 100,000. Most children with IBD are diagnosed between ages 10 and 20, with less than 5% of cases occurring in children younger than age 5.

Genetic, immunologic, and environmental factors have been cited in the etiology of IBD. Although the precise interaction between these factors is not well understood, it is hypothesized that individuals with IBD have a genetic predisposition to an immunologically mediated inflammatory response to selected environmental triggers. The most significant risk factor for the development of IBD is having a close relative with the disease. IBD will develop in 10% of those individuals with a first-degree relative (mother, father, sibling) with the disease.

Pathophysiology

The exact pathophysiology of IBD is not known, but it is believed to involve defective regulation of the intestine's immune-mediated response to an environmental trigger that results in varying degrees of injury to the inner lumen of the GI tract. The patterns of injury vary by disease both grossly and histopathologically (Table 18–5). The inflammation associated with UC is confined to the rectum and large intestine. The inflammatory lesions are continuous and involve only the mucosal layer. The inflammation associated with CD may present in any part of the GI tract but commonly involves the terminal ileum and colon. Lesions are intermittent and transmural with areas of healthy tissue between areas of inflammation. Linear ulcerations, aphthous ulcers, and granulomatous lesions are all associated with CD.

Prognosis. The prognosis for all forms of IBD depends on the severity and extent of the disease and the response to medical therapy. Surgery is ultimately curative

Table 18–5
Characteristics of Inflammatory Bowel Disease

	Ulcerative Colitis	Crohn Disease
Gross Morphologic		
Areas of involvement	Rectum and variable length of colon	Any area of GI tract, terminal ileum, and colon are common sites
Distribution of lesions	Continuous, uniform	Intermittent, "skip" lesions with healthy tissue between areas of inflammation
Fistulas, strictures	Absent	May occur
Histologic		
Ulcerations	Shallow, limited to mucosal, submucosal layers	Transmural, penetrating all layers of GI tract
Granulomas	Absent	Present in >50% of histologic specimens

for UC. Over the long term, individuals affected with UC have demonstrated a higher risk of developing colorectal cancer and require ongoing monitoring for this. CD is a recurrent disease. Long-term complications may include stricture, fistula, and intra-abdominal abscess formation. Individuals with severe disease who require significant resection of diseased bowel may be left with a short bowel syndrome and long-term dependence on TPN. Although the risk of developing colorectal cancer is lower in persons with CD than UC, it is still higher than that of the general population.

Assessment

Clinical manifestations of IBD can be seen in not only the GI tract but systemically as well (Chart 18–8). The characteristic GI manifestation of UC is bloody diarrhea accompanied by crampy, typically left-sided lower abdominal pain. Disease severity is assessed based on stool frequency and the severity of abdominal pain, along with the degree of fever, weight loss, anemia, and hypoalbuminemia present. The diarrhea associated with CD is often watery, as opposed to bloody. Abdominal pain is a common complaint and is usually located in the right lower quadrant. Perianal disease with fistula, skin tags, or granulomas is often present.

Chart 18–8

Clinical Manifestations of Inflammatory Bowel Disease

Gastrointestinal

Weight loss
Diarrhea
Rectal bleeding
Abdominal pain
Malabsorption
Nutritional deficiencies

Systemic

Delayed growth
Delayed sexual maturation
Fever
Anorexia
Anemia
Fatigue

Extraintestinal

Arthritis, arthralgia
Rash
Mucocutaneous lesions (oral apthous ulcers)
Ocular manifestation (uveitis, iritis)
Hepatobiliary complications (sclerosing cholangitis)
Renal disease (stones)

Systemic symptoms such as delayed growth and anorexia may precede GI symptoms by months to years in many cases of IBD, making the initial diagnosis more difficult (Hyams, 1996; Kirschner, 1996). Delayed growth and weight loss in IBD arise from decreased nutrient intake secondary to anorexia and early satiety, as well as malabsorption of nutrients. Active UC may delay sexual maturation (Kirschner, 1996).

Diagnostic Tests. Diagnostic evaluation of the child with suspected IBD is done with the goal of ruling out other potential causes of disease and to classify the type of IBD that the child has. Laboratory studies are done as an initial screening measure. The complete blood cell count of the child with IBD frequently demonstrates leukocytosis and microcytic anemia. The erythrocyte sedimentation rate (ESR) is elevated in active CD but less often in UC. Low serum albumin and iron levels are also common. Stool samples are obtained, looking for gross or occult blood and to rule out the presence of enteric pathogens. Radiologic studies are done to visualize the pattern and extent of lesions as well as screen for the presence of strictures or fistulas. An abdominal flat plate radiograph, barium enema, and upper GI series with small bowel follow-through are usually done. Endoscopic evaluation and intestinal biopsy are done with the goal of definitively establishing the diagnosis of IBD during the initial evaluation. Subsequent endoscopic evaluation may be done during the course of treatment to assess the child's response to therapy.

Nursing Diagnoses and Outcomes

In addition to the nursing diagnoses and outcomes listed in Chart 18–3, the following may be applicable to the child with IBD:

- **Risk for impaired skin integrity related to effects of diarrhea**
  Outcome: The child has no perineal erythema or excoriation.
- **Body image disturbance related to perceptions of disease, effects of medications, retarded growth, delayed sexual maturation**
  Outcome: The child will verbalize a positive self-image.
- **Ineffective individual coping related to chronicity of the condition**
  Outcomes: The child will verbalize feelings and identify own strengths.
  The child will develop alternative coping strategies.
  The child will identify and use external resources.

Interdisciplinary Interventions

Interventions for the management of IBD may involve a variety of treatment modalities, including medical, nutritional, and surgical therapies. IBD is a chronic condition with symptoms that are frequently distressing and may cause alterations in the child's usual activities of daily living. Ongoing psychosocial assessment and support, as well as sensitivity to the stresses that the disease and its treatment place on the child and family, is essential.

Medical therapy for IBD uses various agents. Treatment regimens are individualized depending on the type, location, and severity of the disease. Patient and family education, as well as monitoring for response to therapy and side effects, are important nursing activities.

Pharmacologic Therapy. *Corticosteroids* are the mainstay of medical therapy in the treatment of both CD and moderate to severe UC. Although their specific mechanism of action in IBD is not precisely understood, the manner in which they modulate cell-mediated immunity produces an anti-inflammatory effect that can induce remission of IBD symptoms. Corticosteroids are administered as oral prednisone or IV methylprednisolone. In severe disease in which malabsorption may be present, corticosteroids are initiated in the IV form and then switched to the oral form when enteric absorption becomes more reliable. These agents are administered at high doses during the initial 4 to 6 weeks of treatment, then tapered slowly on a weekly basis until a maintenance dose is achieved. Children require ongoing monitoring for side effects while receiving corticosteroid therapy. Acute side effects during high-dose therapy include glucose instability, hypertension, fluid and sodium retention, and mood swings. Long-term side effects of special concern in children include growth impairment and bone demineralization. The cushingoid changes associated with corticosteroid use (moon facies, hirsutism, acne) may create body image concerns for the adolescent that impact compliance with drug therapy.

Sulfasalazine and other *aminosalicylate*-containing medications such as 5-aminosalicylic acid (5-ASA) are used in the treatment of mild to moderate UC and of colonic disease in CD. 5-ASA is the active agent in sulfasalazine and is primarily activated in the colon. 5-ASA inhibits prostaglandin synthesis, which leads to a localized anti-inflammatory effect in the colon. 5-ASA–containing products are available in oral, enema, or suppository form.

Immunosuppressive agents are used in the treatment of severe corticosteroid-resistant CD. They are also used to maintain remission in both CD and UC in conjunction with low-dose corticosteroids. 6-Mercaptopurine is commonly used for this. Therapy must be administered for at least 3 months before efficacy can be established. Close monitoring for side effects, including bone marrow suppression, pancreatitis, and hepatitis is necessary. Cyclosporine has been used in the treatment of both CD and UC when other agents fail to induce a remission of symptoms. Close monitoring for nephrotoxic side effects is necessary.

Metronidazole, an antibiotic with both antibacterial and antiprotozoal properties, has been used in the treatment of IBD. Its primary benefit is in the treatment of CD when perianal complications are present.

Nutritional Intervention. The goal of nutritional intervention in IBD is to provide adequate nutrient intake to promote normal growth and development and to prevent and correct nutrient deficiencies. Dietary management focuses on enhancing protein and calorie intake. In some cases, lactose intolerance may be present with IBD, making elimination of lactose-containing foods from the diet necessary. Iron and zinc deficiencies may be seen. The child is carefully monitored for deficiencies and given supplements as necessary.

Enteral supplementation through an NG or gastrostomy tube may be used in cases of growth failure or to support calorie requirements during the adolescent growth spurt. An elemental or semi-elemental formula is commonly used, because it is most easily absorbed. TPN may be used for children who require bowel rest to alleviate acute symptoms of disease. In children with CD who require prolonged bowel rest for the treatment of fistulas or who have lost significant amounts of intestine because of resection, long-term TPN in the home may be necessary (see Chapter 17).

Surgical Management. Indications for surgical intervention in IBD vary depending on the type of disease present. For the child with UC, surgery is indicated in the presence of the following:

- Colonic perforation or hemorrhage
- Toxic megacolon
- Growth failure morbidity from corticosteroids

Removal of the diseased colon is curative for UC. In the past, colectomy with standard ileostomy was the traditional operative approach. Over the past 15 years, the ileoanal pull-through procedure has become more common. With this approach, after colectomy, an internal pouch is constructed from the distal ileum and is anastomosed to the anus (Fig. 18–20). Complications of the ileoanal pull-through procedure include pouch stenosis, which results in the obstruction of the outflow of stool from the pouch, and pouchitis, an inflammation of the pouch, resulting from stool stasis. Although 90% of children achieve acceptable stool continence (Mascarenhas & Altschuler, 1997) and frequency after the surgery, a small number may experience soiling or nighttime fecal staining.

Surgical intervention is not curative for CD, because it is a recurrent disease. Surgical intervention is reserved

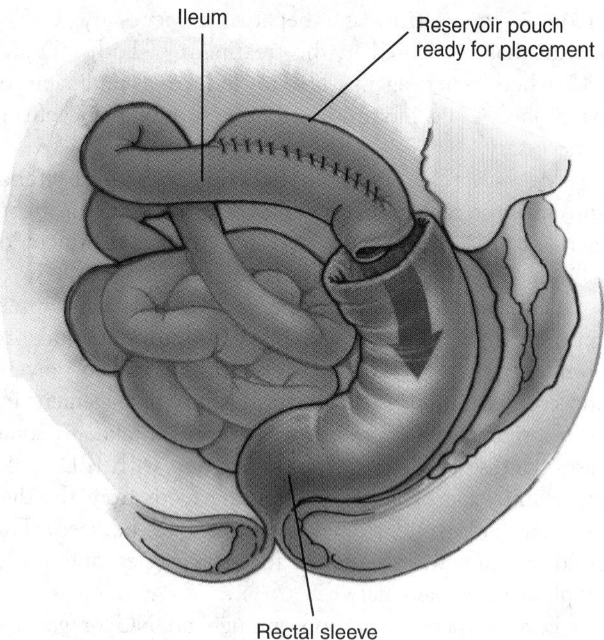

Figure 18–20
Ileoanal anastomosis with pouch reservoir is commonly used for ulcerative colitis.

for the treatment of complications of CD. As with UC, emergency surgical intervention is necessary in the case of bowel perforation or hemorrhage. Intestinal obstruction from chronic inflammation and fibrosis may be treated with bowel resection and primary anastomosis. Strictureplasty may be used in cases of partial obstruction. Surgical intervention may be indicated for the treatment of fistula or abscess that does not respond to medical therapy. If colectomy is required for intractable disease, a standard ileostomy is performed. The ileoanal pull-through is contraindicated for individuals with CD because of the risk of recurrent disease.

The symptoms of IBD, as well as the side effects of therapy, may significantly impact the daily life of the child. Shame and secrecy regarding GI symptoms, body image concerns, anxiety, and depression may all occur in the child with IBD. Supportive relationships with family, peers, and health care workers may be very therapeutic. Education and open discussion of concerns relating to symptoms, treatments, and side effects are necessary on an ongoing basis. Referral to community support organizations can provide further opportunities for education and support.

Peptic Ulcer Disease

Peptic ulcer disease (PUD) occurs when the normal protective barrier of the gastric mucosa is disrupted, allowing gastric acid and enzymes to eat through the mucosal layer into the submucosa.

Ulcers are categorized as primary or secondary. Primary ulcers occur in 5% to 10% of adults but are much less common in children (Bujanover, Reif, & Yahov, 1996). They are most common in older children or adolescents, and a positive family history is reported in 30% of cases. Primary ulcers occur most frequently in the duodenum. For many years the etiology of primary ulcers was not well understood, and a variety of factors, such as psychologic stress and diet, were cited as causes. In more than 80% of cases, primary ulcers are caused by infection with *Helicobacter pylori,* a gram-negative bacterium.

Secondary ulcers occur most frequently in children younger than age 10 and are usually associated with physiologic stress states such as trauma, sepsis, or shock (Sherman, 1994). Drugs may also play a role in the development of secondary ulcers. Aspirin, nonsteroidal anti-inflammatory agents (NSAIDs), and corticosteroids are frequently implicated. Secondary ulcers are also associated with conditions involving gastric hypersecretion, such as chronic renal failure.

Pathophysiology

Normally, the stomach maintains a balance between its digestive and protective elements. The stomach secretes hydrochloric acid and enzymes, including pepsin, that are essential to the gastric digestion of protein. The lining of the stomach is protected from autodigestion by a thick layer of bicarbonate-rich mucus that is continuously secreted by the gastric epithelial and pit cells. Prostaglandin secretion also contributes to these protective mechanisms.

Ulcers occur when the protective mucosal barrier is disrupted, allowing acid and pepsin to come into contact with the gastric mucosa and cause injury. Infection with *H. pylori* causes gastritis, an inflammation of the gastric mucosa, which in turn can lead to ulcer formation. Transmission of *H. pylori* is not fully understood. It is thought to be waterborne, and evidence exists for human-to-human transmission, which may explain the familial pattern of occurrence in PUD.

Secondary ulcers most often occur in the child who is experiencing profound physiologic stress such as trauma, shock, sepsis, or hypoxemia. In these situations, gastric acid secretion is increased, mucosal blood flow and prostaglandin secretion are decreased, and mucosal ischemia may be present. These factors all contribute to alter the resistance of the protective mucosal barrier and put the child at risk for ulcer formation. These ulcers are also known as stress ulcers. GI bleeding and perforation may be associated with PUD in the critically ill child. Aspirin and NSAIDs cause injury both by local inflammation and systemic effects that alter gastric secretion of acid and prostaglandins.

Prognosis. Treatment outcomes for both primary and secondary PUD are generally good. Children with *H.*

pylori infection have a 10% rate of ulcer recurrence after antibiotic therapy. Most children with secondary ulcers do not experience recurrence once their underlying medical condition has been treated. Morbidity or mortality is usually associated with the sequelae of GI hemorrhage or perforation.

Assessment

Typical clinical manifestations of primary ulcer disease include complaints of epigastric pain, discomfort, and fullness that are exacerbated by meals. The child may wake from sleep complaining of epigastric pain. Anorexia, nausea, frequent belching, vomiting, and weight loss may also be experienced. Younger children may not be able to localize their pain but may exhibit irritability and lack of appetite. Secondary or stress ulcers may not be associated with pain. Hematemesis, melena, or bloody output from gastric drainage tubes may be the first signs noted.

Diagnostic Tests. An upper GI barium study is sometimes done as the first step in evaluating the child with suspected primary PUD. The study may demonstrate the presence of an ulcer crater but cannot distinguish the presence of *H. pylori*-related gastritis. Definitive diagnosis of primary PUD is made by upper GI endoscopy. Besides allowing direct visualization of the ulcer, biopsies may be performed to confirm the diagnosis of *H. pylori* infection. Blood tests that screen for the presence of antigens to *H. pylori* are also available.

Interdisciplinary Interventions

Because the child with a stress ulcer often presents with GI bleeding or hemorrhage, emergent stabilization of the child's medical condition must take place before diagnostic evaluation. Restoration of circulating volume with blood products and colloids is an immediate priority (see Chapter 30). The child's hemodynamic stability must be carefully monitored. Nasogastric lavage is done to assess for the presence of active bleeding in the stomach and to prepare for endoscopy. Upper GI endoscopy can be both diagnostic and therapeutic for the child with a secondary ulcer. Besides visualizing the ulcer, hemostasis of obvious bleeding sites may be achieved through thermal coagulation or electrocoagulation. The child will be made NPO for 48 hours after the bleeding has been controlled because any recurrent bleeding is most likely to happen during that time period.

Treatment of both primary and secondary PUD is geared toward healing the mucosal injury and eliminating the precipitating agents that caused the injury. Histamine-2 blockers such as cimetidine, ranitidine, and famotidine are used to suppress acid production, which provides symptomatic relief as well as supports the healing process. In some cases, omeprazole, which blocks the proton pump of the parietal cell, may be used. Cytoprotective agents such as sucralfate may be used to protect the injured mucosa. Diet therapy has not been found to play a significant role in the treatment of ulcers. Antibiotic therapy for *H. pylori* infection is essential to the long-term resolution of the associated PUD.

Prevention is as important a consideration as treatment in the care of patients with stress ulcers. Nurses are in a key position to identify those children who may be at risk for secondary ulcers. In many cases, prophylactic therapy with histamine-2 blockers or cytoprotective agents will be given to children who are at high risk for ulcers related to physiologic stress states or drug therapy. Education of the child and family regarding medical therapy, along with signs and symptoms of PUD and associated complications, are important in both the treatment and prevention of PUD.

Disorders of Gastrointestinal Motility and Function

Functional Abdominal Pain

Functional abdominal pain, also referred to as recurrent abdominal pain, is one of the most common complaints of school-age children. Functional abdominal pain is defined as the occurrence of at least three episodes of abdominal pain reported over a period of at least 3 months. Abdominal pain that is severe enough to interfere with normal activities of daily living has a reported prevalence of 10% to 15% in children aged 5 to 14 years. In 90% to 95% of these cases, no organic cause of pain is found.

Although the etiology of functional abdominal pain is poorly understood, one must keep in mind that functional abdominal pain does not signify imaginary abdominal pain. The child's experience of pain is real. In cases of functional abdominal pain, physical or psychologic stressors may cause disturbances in GI tract motility that result in pain. In most cases, the prognosis for resolution of symptoms is very good.

Assessment

Functional abdominal pain typically manifests as episodic attacks of abdominal pain in children ages 5 to 14 that recur over periods of more than 3 months' duration. Pain episodes may cluster in the morning or the evening. They may delay the onset of sleep at night but typically do not awaken the child from sleep. The episodes are not consistently associated with activities such as meals or bowel movements. Pain is usually localized in the periumbilical area without radiation and is nonspecific in character.

Environmental stressors are frequently reported. Family stressors such as recent illness or death of a close family member, marital discord, or financial problems may be present. A recent geographic move or school change may be reported. A history of frequent school absences is common in functional abdominal pain. In some cases, physical, emotional, or sexual abuse may be associated with functional abdominal pain.

Physical assessment reveals no obvious abnormalities. Growth is not impaired, and weight loss is not seen.

The diagnosis of functional abdominal pain is based on typical health history data and normal physical assessment findings. The history should carefully assess the nature of the pain and associated factors. It should also investigate symptoms that point to organic disease such as fever, weight loss, pain localized away from the periumbilical area, emesis, or diarrhea. A thorough diet history assesses for food allergies or intolerances. The child is included in the interview in a developmentally appropriate manner to elicit his or her perceptions of the cause of pain, as well as exacerbating and alleviating factors.

Diagnostic Tests. A simple laboratory evaluation may be done to screen for organic disease. This includes a complete blood cell count, erythrocyte sedimentation rate, and urinalysis, because urinary tract infections can present as symptoms of abdominal pain. Stool specimens for ova and parasites and occult blood may be obtained. If lactose intolerance is suspected, a lactose breath hydrogen test may be done.

Interdisciplinary Interventions

Once organic disease is ruled out, education and reassurance of the child and parents are the key elements in treating functional abdominal pain. The nurse reassures the child and family that the symptoms are not due to an organic disease and explains the underlying mechanism of functional abdominal pain. Environmental stressors and ways to eliminate or modify them are discussed. The child and parent's specific perceptions and concerns about the pain are addressed (Chart 18–9).

If school absence has been an issue, a plan for school reentry and for handling episodes of pain in the school setting is made. The school nurse and teacher should be involved in the plan to ensure a consistent approach. The nurse in the office or clinic setting can serve as a valuable support and communication link for the family in the treatment of functional abdominal pain.

Colic

Colic is a term used to describe a constellation of infant behaviors characterized primarily by prolonged periods of inconsolable crying in an otherwise healthy, thriving infant. Although often interpreted by parents to be caused by GI distress, colic is actually a more multifactorial phenomenon.

Colic is reported to occur in 10% to 30% of infants. No differences in the incidence of colic by sex, cultural background, breast-feeding versus bottle-feeding, or birth weight have been proven.

The exact etiology of colic remains unclear, although many theories, both physiologic and psychologic, have been proposed. Physiologic factors that apparently play a role in colic include immaturity of the nervous system (making it difficult for the infant to screen out sensory stimuli), immaturity of the GI tract, hypermotility of the GI tract, and food allergies. Psychosocial factors that have been cited include parental anxiety and variances in infant temperament. Most cases of colic apparently result from some interaction between physiologic and psychosocial factors.

Pathophysiology

Like the etiology of colic, the pathophysiology of colic is also unclear. In most cases, crying is a normal physiologic response on the part of the infant to distress or discomfort and serves to communicate the infant's needs to the caregiver. The normal 6-week-old infant may cry up to 3 hours a day, decreasing to 1 hour per day by age 3 months (Brazelton, 1962). In the case of colic, crying will generally last more than 3 hours a day more than 3 days a week (Sferra & Heitlinger, 1996). The episodes usually occur around the same time of day, often in the evening. Most colic begins within the first 2 to 3 weeks of life and resolves by age 3 to 4 months. No long-term negative physiologic sequelae are associated with colic.

Assessment

The infant with colic has prolonged episodes of crying but appears otherwise healthy and demonstrates appropriate weight gain. The crying episodes are often accompanied by abdominal distention and flatus. The infant may be noted drawing the knees in to the chest. Parents may report that simple soothing measures are ineffective during the crying episodes.

Nursing Diagnoses and Outcomes

In addition to the nursing diagnoses and outcomes listed in Chart 18–3, the following may be applicable to the family of an infant with colic:

- **Risk for altered parent/infant attachment related to effects of prolonged, distressed crying**
  Outcomes: The parents will learn to read infant's cues and respond quickly and appropriately.
  The infant will have decreased amounts of daily crying.

Interdisciplinary Interventions

The first step in caring for an infant with colic is a thorough history and physical examination to rule out

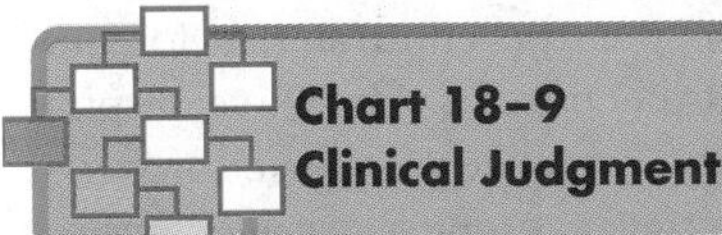

Chart 18–9
Clinical Judgment

A Child with Functional Abdominal Pain

Rose is a 9-year-old girl brought in by her mother to the clinic complaining of abdominal pain. This pain has occurred before.

Questions

1. What other history would the nurse want to obtain?
2. What factors in the history are significant?
3. Does Rose have symptoms of organic disease?
4. What is the next step in the evaluation?
5. All laboratory results are normal. Rose and her mother are taught about functional abdominal pain, pain relief interventions (warm baths, distraction, talking about stressors), and Rose is referred for counseling to help her cope with her parents' divorce. What are symptoms of organic disease that warrant further follow-up?

Answers

1. *Past medical history:* previous and current illnesses, immunizations, fever, allergies, food intolerances, normal weight, has Rose started puberty (occasional colds, otitis media, diarrhea, immunizations up-to-date, typical weight 62 pounds, she has not started puberty).
   Daily routines: patterns of elimination, describe number, amount, appearance; diet history, sleep patterns (voids four to six times per day, yellow urine, no dysuria, 1 stool every 1 to 2 days, brown, formed, no pain with evacuation, abdominal pain unrelated to stooling pattern, no change in sleep habits).
   Pain history: how long has the pain been occurring, how often, when does it occur (time of day, location such as school, home), where is it located, what is done when the pain occurs, does anything relieve or exacerbate it, has it been interfering with ADLs or school attendance or performance, Rose's and family's response to the pain, what does the family think is wrong (pain has been occurring one to two times per week for about 5 months, is crampy pain, located in the periumbilical region lasting 1 to 3 hours, usually in the evening, no medications are given, mother sits with Rose and distracts her with "talking about happy times" until the pain resolves, does not impact ADLs, Rose and her mother think Rose may have some disease).
   Family history: inflammatory bowel disease, ulcer disease, recurrent or chronic pain, anxiety disorders (unremarkable except mother suffers from occasional migraines).
   Psychosocial history: family functioning, school performance, peer relationships, previous stressors and typical coping style and response (parents are getting a divorce, Rose is doing her typical B and C work in school, has many friends, no major stressors previously, Rose usually reads or goes out to play when she is stressed).
2. History is predominately unremarkable except for recurrent abdominal pain, mother's history of migraines, and impending parental divorce.
3. No.
4. Explain to Rose and her mother that this type of pain may be caused by dysfunctional motility and things other than disease and that some laboratory tests will be done. A complete blood cell count, sedimentation rate, urinalysis, and possibly stool for hematest will be done. Extensive testing may indicate to Rose and mother that the health care team thinks something is seriously wrong and can increase their anxiety further.
5. Weight loss, fever, blood in emesis or stool, abdominal distention, or fatigue.

any organic sources of discomfort or distress. This is important to be able to reassure parents that there is nothing medically wrong with the infant. The history should elicit specific information about the crying episodes, associated behaviors, and feeding history. The parents' responses to episodes are also reviewed. Physical assessment includes the infant's length, weight, and head circumference to verify that growth is appropriate.

Parent education and counseling are the key interventions in the management of infant colic. Parent education is done regarding reading the infant's cues as to what need is being communicated, normal infant crying, and the importance of meeting the infant's needs in a timely fashion to avoid escalating the crying episode to where the infant cannot be consoled. Teaching regarding soothing techniques and ways to reduce sensory stimuli are beneficial. The parents should be reassured that too much holding will not spoil the infant.

Caring for the infant with colic can be very stressful and frustrating for the parent. Acknowledging the parents' feelings and providing support to the parents are very important. Assisting the parents in identifying family and community resources for respite may be helpful, along with emphasizing the time-limited nature of colic.

Gastroesophageal Reflux

Gastroesophageal reflux (GER) refers to the effortless passage of gastric contents into the lower esophagus. Postprandial GER is a normal physiologic phenomenon without negative sequelae in most cases. GER becomes pathologic when GI, pulmonary, or neuropsychiatric complications arise from reflux episodes.

GER occurs in an estimated 1 in 500 infants, with boys affected three times more frequently than girls. In infancy, GER is commonly associated with delays in the normal maturational process of the lower esophageal sphincter (LES). Other factors that may contribute to the development of GER include esophageal motor dysfunction, increased intragastric pressure, delayed gastric emptying, and central nervous system disorders.

Pathophysiology

The body has a natural barrier system at the gastroesophageal junction to prevent the reflux of gastric contents into the esophagus. The most important component of this barrier system is the LES. Under normal circumstances, the LES remains closed and prevents reflux. The LES relaxes and opens during swallowing, belching, and vomiting. Conditions that cause a decrease in basal LES pressure lead to the development of GER. Continuous LES hypotonia and inappropriate LES relaxation independent of swallowing are the most common mechanisms of decreased LES pressure. Esophageal motor dysfunction, increased intragastric pressure, and delayed gastric emptying are other contributing factors. Both intrinsic and extrinsic factors can cause decreased LES. Children with central nervous system disorders have demonstrated an increased incidence of LES hypotonia. Medications such as theophylline and foods containing fat, chocolate, or caffeine may cause transient decreases in LES pressure. Children who are fed enterally are at risk for reflux related either to gastric distention from bolus feedings or the presence of an NG tube.

When the esophagus is repeatedly exposed to gastric secretions, esophagitis ensues. The associated inflammation can cause pain (often referred to as heartburn), dysphagia, ulcerations, and chronic occult blood loss leading to anemia. Chronic esophagitis can result in alterations in esophageal motility and stricture formation.

Severe GER can cause vomiting, which over time may lead to inadequate nutrient intake and failure to thrive. Vomiting may also put the child at risk for pulmonary aspiration of gastric contents. Reflexive respiratory system responses to the presence of refluxed material in the esophagus may trigger bronchospasm, laryngospasm, and, in rare cases, apnea.

Prognosis. The prognosis for the child with GER is related to the severity of symptoms and the associated treatment. Some 80% of infants who present with symptoms of GER in the first months of life will experience resolution of symptoms by age 1 to 2 years with either conservative or pharmacologic management. Reported outcomes for children who require surgical intervention for GER are good, with recurrence of GER in only 5% to 10%.

Assessment

A thorough history and physical examination are essential to the evaluation of the child with suspected GER to assess for causative factors and severity of symptoms and to rule out other pathologic conditions. A careful feeding history and direct observation of feeding technique may be helpful in distinguishing GER from more benign problems, such as overfeeding or inadequate burping technique.

GER has numerous GI manifestations. Effortless regurgitation or vomiting after feeding is commonly reported in infants with GER. Vomiting may result in decreased nutrient intake and failure to thrive. The infant may appear irritable and refuse feedings. Older children may not experience vomiting but will have episodes of chest pain or heartburn associated with reflux. Dysphagia and anemia associated with esophagitis may occur in both infants and children.

Pulmonary manifestations of GER include chronic cough, frequently noted at night when the child is in a supine position, and recurrent bronchopulmonary infections. Bronchospasm, laryngospasm, apnea, and bradycardia have also been associated with reflux episodes.

Diagnostic Tests. Various diagnostic tools are used in evaluating GER. Radiologic evaluation commonly includes a barium swallow or upper GI series to assess for changes associated with reflux or esophagitis such as strictures or ulcerations. A gastric emptying study may be done to assess for reflux along with upper GI motility. Upper GI endoscopy may be done to assess for esophagitis.

Twenty-four-hour intraesophageal pH monitoring is the most sensitive diagnostic test for reflux. It is used to determine the frequency and duration of reflux episodes and their association with the child's activity and symptoms. The parent or nurse must maintain a thorough record of all the child's activities and symptoms during the study. The beginning and end of feedings, sleep/wake periods, position, and the occurrence of any GI or respiratory symptoms must all be recorded. The child must also be carefully observed to ensure that the pH probe is not dislodged during the study period. The study may be done in the hospital or in the outpatient setting. In either setting, the nurse plays an important role in educating and supporting parents as to their role in monitoring and recording their child's activity during the study period (Fig. 18–21).

Interdisciplinary Interventions

Various treatment strategies are used to manage GER. The choice of treatment depends on the severity of the child's symptoms and associated medical problems.

A conservative management approach is commonly taken for infants with mild GER symptoms. This involves positioning, dietary, and feeding modifications to ameliorate symptoms. Parents are advised to position the child in an upright, semiprone position after feeding to promote increased gravity resistance to reflux. Feedings may be thickened with cereal, and the feeding schedule may be altered to provide smaller feeding volumes at more frequent intervals to decrease gastric distention (Chart 18–10).

For more severe cases of GER, pharmacologic therapy is utilized in conjunction with conservative management strategies. Antacid preparations and histamine-2 blocking agents such as cimetidine are used to provide symptomatic relief of esophagitis and reduce the damaging effects of refluxed gastric contents on the esophageal mucosa (Hillemeier, 1996). Prokinetic agents such as cisapride or metaclopramide are used to enhance gastric emptying. Because metoclopramide can produce central nervous system side effects such as extrapyramidal reactions and dystonia, it is used less frequently. Only a few side effects are associated with cisapride. Cisapride may interact with some antibiotics and cause cardiac abnormalities. Accordingly, parents should receive verbal and written instructions regarding medication administration, drug interactions, and early recognition of untoward reactions.

Figure 18–21
During a pH study, a log must be kept of the child's activities and the child closely monitored to keep him or her from pulling at the probe.

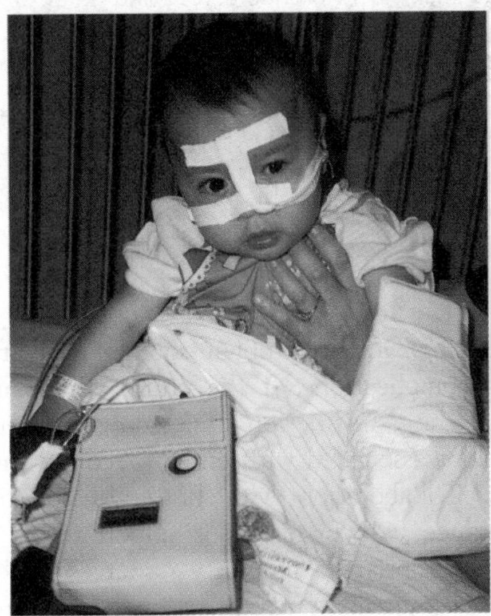

Surgical intervention for GER is indicated when GER symptoms are unresponsive to medical therapy, when significant complications of GER exist, or when GER episodes are life threatening. The goal of surgical intervention is to create an anatomic barrier to reflux. The most commonly used antireflux procedure in children is the Nissen fundoplication. The fundoplication creates a valve by wrapping the gastric fundus 360 degrees around the lower end of the esophagus. The fundoplication is traditionally done as an open operative procedure, requiring a 5- to 7-day hospitalization. In select cases, the laparoscopic approach has also been used for fundoplication.

After fundoplication, the junction between the stomach and esophagus is tight enough that belching and vomiting are initially impossible. A temporary gastrostomy is placed at the time of surgery to allow for venting of the stomach in the immediate postoperative period. The gastrostomy tube is usually removed approximately 6 weeks after surgery, unless the child has a continued need for gastrostomy access for enteral feedings.

Community Care

Discharge planning and family education are important nursing concerns no matter what management approach is being used in the treatment of the child with GER. The parents should receive initial and ongoing assessment to ensure that they have a solid understanding of the GI system alterations resulting from GER and the rationale and goals of therapeutic interventions. Preparation of the child and family for diagnostic tests and procedures is important. This is especially true for children undergoing 24-hour pH monitoring, in which parental participation in monitoring and record keeping contributes greatly to meaningful test outcomes.

Discharge planning and family education regarding treatment strategies must take into consideration any underlying disease the child may have. Families should receive instruction regarding dietary modifications, feeding techniques, positioning, and medication administration. Direct observation of the parents while feeding and positioning the child may help the nurse give more meaningful feedback. Home nursing follow-up may help support the parents in successfully transitioning their knowledge to the home setting.

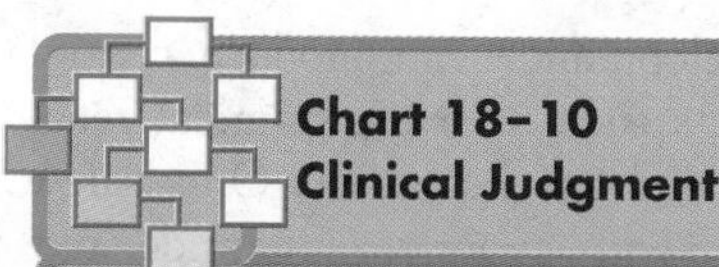

Chart 18–10
Clinical Judgment

The Infant with Gastroesophageal Reflux

Jorge is a 2-month-old male infant who parents describe as difficult to feed with choking during feedings and extremely fussy. He has demonstrated vomiting and poor weight gain since birth. He is being admitted for 24-hour esophageal pH probe monitoring to rule out GER.

Questions

1. When performing an admission history and physical examination, what aspects would be of particular importance for Jorge?
2. What findings are of concern?
3. During the pH study, what aspects of care are the physician and nurse responsible for?
4. Results of the pH study demonstrate GER. What care interventions should the nurse implement and teach the parents?
5. What signs will indicate that the interventions are effective in controlling the GER?

Answers

1. Respiratory assessment (respiratory rate, 70; occasional cyanosis with gagging; breath sounds moist; slight intercostal retractions).
   Hydration and growth assessment (skin turgor good, moist mucous membranes, capillary refill 2 seconds; weight at third percentile, length and head circumference at tenth percentile).
   Parental coping (parents state they are tired; they are dressed neatly with good hygiene and are attentive to Jorge and attempt to comfort him).
   When the opportunity presents, observe the parents feeding Jorge (good technique, positive parent–child interactions, responsive to each other's cues).
2. Respiratory assessment; cannot make a decision regarding growth parameters at 3rd and 10th percentiles unless previous measures are available to compare with.
3. The physician inserts the probe, determines correct placement, and interprets study findings. The nurse teaches the parents about the study and, in collaboration with them, monitors the child so that the pH probe is not dislodged during the study, maintains a record of the child's activities (feedings, sleep and wake periods, position) and symptoms (e.g., coughing, cyanosis, vomiting) during the study.
4. Position Jorge with head elevated 30 degrees in a right side-lying or prone position (supine or side lying is recommended to reduce the incidence of SIDS in healthy infants, but prone may be needed and recommended for infants with GER); if an infant seat is used, make sure Jorge does not slouch, thus increasing intra-abdominal pressure; when changing his diapers, elevate Jorge's head and trunk on a pillow or blanket roll. Head-up positioning is particularly important to maintain for 30 to 60 minutes after feedings. Feed frequently in small amounts, 2 to 3 ounces every 2 to 3 hours; burp frequently. Feedings thickened with rice cereal and medications may be given. Monitor for signs of complications—aspiration, respiratory infection, apnea, poor weight gain. Support the parents in coping with their child's condition and encourage them to have others learn Jorge's care needs and to take time for themselves.
5. Jorge has decreased vomiting, less fussiness, and demonstrates weight gain. No signs of respiratory infection, cyanosis, or aspiration are evident.

Education about medications, dosing schedules, and potential side effects is given verbally and in writing. Ongoing nursing monitoring of response to medical therapy is done in both the clinic and home settings. The child undergoing surgical intervention for GER will need instruction regarding gastrostomy tube management in addition to routine preoperative and postoperative instruction. The child and family should receive instruction in gastrostomy site care, in use of the gastrostomy for gastric venting, and in problem-solving mechanical and infectious complications. If the child will be using the tube for feeding, instruction on feeding techniques and complications associated with enteral feedings should also be given. Collaboration with hospital-based or health care insurance case managers is important to link the family to appropriate community resources for obtaining supplies and equipment necessary for home care. Home nursing follow-up may be necessary to support the family during the initial postoperative period. Instruction of child care and school personnel should be considered in the discharge plan. The school nurse is an important collaborator in this effort.

Constipation and Encopresis

Constipation is defined as an alteration in the frequency, size or consistency of passage of stool. Normal stool frequency varies developmentally, so the definition of constipation must be made relative to the expected developmental norm. Constipation may also be present when a child has normal stool frequency but stools are hard and difficult to pass. *Encopresis* is defined as fecal soiling as a result of functional constipation (constipation unrelated to an organic cause) that persists after age 4 years (Loening-Baucke, 1996).

Constipation and encopresis are common pediatric problems. Constipation is the presenting complaint in 3% of pediatric outpatient visits and in 25% of children referred to pediatric gastroenterologists. Constipation is more prevalent in males during early childhood. During adolescence it is more frequently reported in females. Encopresis is reported to occur in 2% to 3% of children 4 to 6 years old, decreasing to 1.5% in children older than age 7. Encopresis is more common in males than females.

Constipation may arise from a variety of disorders, both organic and nonorganic (Table 18–6). The most common etiology of constipation in children is related to

Table 18–6
Causes of Constipation in Children

Functional (Nonorganic)	
Toilet training (starting too early, routine, or coercive)	
Excessive parental intervention	
School bathroom avoidance	
Busy lifestyle	
Very sedentary lifestyle	
Immobility	
Sexual abuse	
Cognitive handicaps	
Depression	
Organic	
Genetic predisposition	Medications
Dietary	Opiates
Excessive dairy intake	Antacids
Low fiber diet	Antihypertensives
Dehydration	Anticholinergics
Malnutrition, underfeeding	Antidepressants
Anal malformations	NSAIDs
Imperforate anus	Diuretics
Anal stenosis	Developmental
Anterior anus	Cognitive handicaps
Intestinal motility disorder	Attention-deficit hyperactivity disorder
Intestinal pseudo-obstruction	Situational
Neurogenic	Febrile or prolonged illness
Hirschsprung's disease	Surgery or bed rest
Spina bifida	Anal fissure or diaper dermatitis
Tethered cord	Change in child's diet or routine
Hypotonia	Toilet phobia
Myelomeningocele	
Cerebral palsy	
Metabolic/endocrine disorders	
Hypothyroidism	
Hypercalcemia	
Diabetes mellitus	
Diabetes insipidus	
Lead poisoning	

functional or behavioral causes. Encopresis most commonly arises from functional constipation. Fecal incontinence, with or without constipation, arising from organic disease is rarer.

Pathophysiology

The process of defecation depends on the interaction between numerous sensory and motor mechanisms. The rectum forms a right angle with the anal canal. The urge to defecate is initiated by distention of the rectum with stool. This induces a reactive relaxation of the internal anal sphincter and contraction of the external anal sphincter. Squatting or sitting straightens out the angle between the rectum and the anal canal, allowing for easy passage of stool. Increasing intra-abdominal pressure with the Valsalva maneuver along with voluntary inhibition of the external anal sphincter permits feces to be expelled.

Constipation in children is commonly the result of voluntary fecal withholding, owing to or resulting in painful defecation. As previously noted, various factors can cause a predisposition to constipation. Painful lesions, such as fissures of the anal or perianal region or hardened stools secondary to inadequate dietary intake of fiber or free water, may result in pain when feces are passed, causing the child to withhold stool to avoid pain. Psychosocial or behavioral factors may contribute to constipation. Overly aggressive toilet training, childhood anxieties resulting in avoidance of school bathrooms, or intrusive parental interventions surrounding toileting habits may all result in stool withholding.

Once a pattern of withholding is begun, a vicious cycle develops. As defecation is delayed, progressively larger amounts of stool are built up in the rectum for longer periods of time, resulting in more pain and more withholding. Encopresis results when a large stool mass stretches the walls of the colon and rectum and involuntary leakage of semi-formed or liquid stool around the fecal mass occurs.

Prognosis. Reported outcomes for children with constipation and encopresis who have undergone a variety of treatment regimens demonstrate a 50% to 90% favorable response rate. Response to treatment may be influenced by child and family compliance with the prescribed treatment regimen and ongoing behavioral and psychosocial issues.

Assessment

The goals of the initial history and physical examination of the child with chronic constipation or encopresis are to look for causative factors and to rule out any potential organic causes. Information regarding stool frequency and size and associated symptoms, such as abdominal pain, distention or anorexia, is noted. A thorough diet history is obtained. The child's toilet training history is reviewed, as well as any pertinent psychosocial stressors.

The child with constipation will pass firm or hard stools of variable size. Small, hard stools may be passed at regular intervals or large, hard masses of stool may be passed at prolonged intervals of days to weeks. As stool accumulates, the child may become progressively more irritable. Complaints of abdominal pain may ensue, and abdominal distention may be noted. Palpable fecal masses may be noted on physical examination. Appetite may become poor. After passage of stool, parents may note that the child's mood and appetite improve. Encopresis is manifested by the leakage of liquid, often foul-smelling stools.

Urinary tract symptoms can be seen in the child with chronic constipation and encopresis. Recurrent urinary tract infections have been reported in 10% of affected children, usually related to ascending bacteria from fecal soiling. Urinary incontinence has been reported in 20% of encopretic children.

The child with chronic constipation and encopresis can experience many negative psychologic and social sequelae. Low self-esteem, poor school performance, and impaired peer relations have been reported. Family relationships can be negatively impacted. Parents who do not understand the physiologic mechanisms causing constipation and encopresis may become frustrated and angry with their child's recurrent soiling.

Diagnostic Tests. Barium enema or anorectal manometry may be done if the examiner strongly suspects an organic etiology such as Hirschsprung's disease.

Interdisciplinary Interventions

The treatment plan for the child with constipation and encopresis will be individualized depending on the severity of symptoms and on the child's developmental level. Mild symptoms of constipation may be treated with dietary measures or oral agents alone. For the child whose symptoms are more severe, the treatment plan is generally designed in three stages: (1) education, (2) bowel clean out, and (3) maintenance and reconditioning to normal bowel habits.

During the initial education phase, the child and parents receive information with the goal of "demystifying" the process of defecation and explaining the treatment plan. The normal process of defecation is explained, along with the pathophysiologic alterations associated with constipation. The purpose of each therapeutic intervention is explained, along with anticipated outcomes and potential problems. The education process is geared to help in decreasing feelings of guilt or blame that may exist on the part of the child and parents.

Colon clean out, or disimpaction, is necessary to eliminate any fecal mass that may be present. This may be achieved with large doses of lubricants such as mineral oil or, in severe cases, a colonic lavage solution. Some clinicians routinely use enemas for this purpose, although their use may be traumatic for both child and parent and can contribute to the cycle of aversive experiences associated with defecation.

The goal of the maintenance phase of treatment is to establish normal bowel habits. Cathartic agents are used at doses titrated to overcome the child's tendency to withhold stool. Various agents are used for this purpose, including lubricants such as mineral oil, osmotic agents such as milk of magnesia, and stimulants such as senna derivatives. Mineral oil should not be given to children at risk for pulmonary aspiration. Oral agents are usually continued until 4 to 6 months after the last painful stool. The child must be weaned off the laxative slowly.

Tip: *Give the child choices regarding how the mineral oil is taken. Serving it cold or mixing it with orange juice or carbonated beverages enhances palatability. It also goes well served on top of yogurt.*

Dietary interventions are also part of the maintenance phase of treatment. Increased dietary fiber and fluid intake are recommended to increase water retention in the stool. The child and parents should receive information regarding sources of dietary fiber such as fruits, vegetables, legumes, and whole grain breads and cereals.

A program to encourage regular toileting behaviors is also initiated at this time. Children are asked to attempt to defecate on the toilet for 5 to 10 minutes after every meal. This takes advantage of the natural gastrocolic reflex. A system of positive reinforcements, such as stickers, can be instituted to reward compliance with medications and toileting session. The treatment plan should be communicated to significant school and child care personnel to promote consistency. Psychologic and behavioral issues may present ongoing concerns for the child and family and may require intervention from a psychologist, social worker, or child development professional.

A collaborative effort between the child, family, and health care team is essential to successful outcomes in the treatment of constipation and encopresis. The nurse, in the clinic and school settings, plays an important role in the treatment plan. Child and family evaluation, education, and support along with phone and clinic follow-up to monitor progress and make necessary modifications in the treatment plan are key nursing activities.

Irritable Bowel Syndrome

Irritable bowel syndrome (IBS) is a GI disorder characterized by a constellation of symptoms:

- Abdominal pain, relieved with defecation or associated with a change in the frequency or consistency of stool
- Alterations in defecation, either altered stool frequency, altered stool form (hard or loose), or altered stool passage (straining, feeling of urgency, or sense of incomplete evacuation)
- Bloating and feelings of abdominal distention

IBS is a chronic recurrent disorder, the etiology of which is not well understood. In the past, psychogenic factors such as stress were thought to cause IBS. Currently, most believe that although psychogenic factors may exacerbate IBS symptoms, they do not cause symptoms.

The incidence of IBS has not been widely described in children. In the adult population, IBS has a reported prevalence of 15% to 30%. In two reported community-based studies of adolescents, symptoms that met the diagnostic criteria for IBS were reported in 6% of middle school students and 14% to 16% of high school students (Hyams, 1996; Thomson & Dancey, 1996). In adult studies, IBS is more prevalent in females. No such pattern has been found in the pediatric studies.

Pathophysiology

IBS was initially thought to be a functional disorder of the GI system with no identifiable organic cause. Studies have demonstrated differences in the physiologic responses of adults with IBS and their normal counterparts, which suggest that IBS may be a disorder of GI motility affecting both the upper and lower GI tract. In IBS, the intestine is thought to have an exaggerated motor response to agents that normally stimulate intestinal activity. Thus, factors such as foods, drugs, or stress may trigger or exacerbate symptoms of IBS.

Although IBS is not a life-threatening disease, it is chronic and recurrent and can have a negative impact on the lives of affected individuals. Depression and anxiety, as well as disruptions in school, family, and social relationships and activities have been reported in adolescents affected with IBS.

Assessment

IBS is diagnosed primarily by exclusion. The initial history and physical examination of the child with suspected IBS are important in ruling out any potential organic cause of disease. The health history includes a thorough diet history, including food allergies and food intolerances. In some cases, children with lactose intolerance may have symptoms that mimic IBS. A travel history is obtained, along with any other potential exposures to intestinal parasites, such as a *Giardia* infection, which may also cause IBS-like symptoms. The child is also assessed for symptoms of inflammatory bowel disease, and any recent stressful life events are noted. Physical assessment usually reveals no abnormalities.

Symptoms of IBS may differ among individuals. Reports of abdominal pain may vary in character. Pain may be described as crampy or sharp, dull, or burning. In some cases an overall feeling of fullness in the abdominal region may be reported. Abdominal pain is often not well localized, although the periumbilical area or lower abdomen is often cited. Pain may be precipitated by meals but rarely awakens the child from sleep. Pain is often relieved by defecation. Adults with IBS frequently report a sense of abdominal distention, accompanied by increased burping and flatulence.

Alterations in bowel habits are common in IBS, especially in adolescents. Diarrhea or constipation may occur. Constipation may be accompanied by a sense of incomplete evacuation after defecation. Diarrhea may consist of small, loose stools preceded by abdominal pain. Passage of excess mucus with stools is frequent.

Adults with IBS have demonstrated significantly higher levels of anxiety and depression than unaffected individuals. This has been corroborated in adolescent studies (Hyams, Burke, Davis, Rzepski, & Andrulonis, 1996). Although it is not felt that psychogenic factors cause IBS, these factors may potentially influence how the individual experiences and copes with IBS.

Diagnostic Tests. Several laboratory tests may be done to rule out other potential organic diseases. A complete blood cell count with sedimentation rate and urinalysis may be ordered, along with stool samples for ova and parasites. In children with suspected lactose intolerance, a lactose breath hydrogen test may be performed.

Interdisciplinary Interventions

The initial step in treating IBS is reassuring the child and parent that the child has no serious underlying disease. Treatment strategies are directed toward alleviating symptoms and controlling aggravating factors. Diet therapy focuses on increasing the fiber content of the child's diet, either from food sources or with fiber supplements. Increasing dietary fiber has been found to help with diarrheal symptoms of IBS by increasing stool transit time. Fiber also increases the water content of stool, which helps those who experience constipation.

The child and parents are also educated about potential dietary triggers for IBS symptoms and ways to avoid them. Medications, often anticholinergic drugs, may be used in the treatment of IBS, but their effectiveness remains questionable.

Counseling about psychosocial triggers that impact IBS symptoms is an important aspect of management. The nurse in both clinic and school-based settings may help the child and parents in identifying the child's individual triggers and in developing strategies to alleviate them. Psychotherapy may also be useful in supporting the child in this regard and in enhancing coping skills.

Disorders of Malabsorption

Chronic Diarrhea

Chronic diarrhea is defined as diarrhea that persists for more than 2 weeks. Because normal stool consistency and frequency varies developmentally, diarrhea is defined as an increase in stool frequency and alteration in stool consistency compared with the child's norm. Chronic diarrhea has numerous possible causes (Table 18–7). Infectious, immunologic, malabsorptive, mechanical, and dietary causes have all been identified. In Munchausen syndrome by proxy, a rare form of child abuse (see Chapter 30), diarrhea may be induced by the administration of laxatives. The incidence of chronic diarrhea varies depending on the etiology. Although some causes of chronic diarrhea are easily resolved, others may have serious, life-long consequences for the child.

Pathophysiology

The pathophysiology of chronic diarrhea depends on the cause of the diarrhea. Numerous physiologic mechanisms can result in diarrhea. An osmotic diarrhea results from malabsorption of an absorbable solute. This creates a solute load in the intestine that results in increased fluid losses. Malabsorption of carbohydrates, whether because of mucosal injury or congenital defects of carbohydrate absorption, will result in an osmotic diarrhea. Overfeeding or excess fruit juice consumption creates a high solute load in the intestine that also will result in an osmotic diarrhea.

Certain intestinal infections or tumors may result in secretory diarrhea, in which excessive secretions from the GI tract cause diarrhea to persist even when the child is NPO. In the case of mechanical obstruction, formed stool cannot pass past the area of blockage but liquid stool may leak around the blockage. Massive resection of intestine reduces the absorptive surface area of the bowel and decreases the bowel transit time, resulting in diarrhea.

Assessment

The child with chronic diarrhea requires a comprehensive diagnostic evaluation to establish the etiology of the illness. The history aims to identify risk factors for infection, family history of GI illness, and any history of illness that may indicate altered immune function. The child's diet history and history of growth and weight gain are carefully reviewed. Physical assessment focuses on

Table 18–7
Causes of Chronic Diarrhea

Infectious
Viral
Bacterial
Protozoal

Malabsorption
Congenital carbohydrate malabsorption
Lactase deficiency
Malabsorption secondary to mucosal damage
  Postinfectious enteropathy
  Cow's milk, soy protein intolerance
  Intractable diarrhea of infancy
  Celiac disease
Pancreatic insufficiency
  Cystic fibrosis
Short bowel syndrome
Malnutrition

Inflammatory bowel disease
Crohn's disease
Ulcerative colitis

Immune deficiency states
Acquired immunodeficiency syndrome
Severe combined immune deficiency

Oncology
Hormone-secreting tumors
Radiation enteritis
Graft-versus-host disease

Drugs
Antibiotic-associated diarrhea
Sorbitol-containing drugs

Dietary
Overfeeding
Fruit juice
Excessive sweets, sorbitol

Anatomic
Partial obstruction
Malrotation
Blind loop syndrome

Other
Toddler's diarrhea
Motility disorders
Encopresis
Bacterial overgrowth
Munchausen syndrome by proxy

signs of dehydration, as well as signs of malnutrition and GI dysfunction. Direct observation of the stool is also important.

Clinical manifestations of chronic diarrhea can vary depending on its etiology. The appearance, frequency, odor, and urgency of stool can provide clues as to the underlying cause. Blood in the stool and associated symptoms such as abdominal pain, fever, and vomiting are also significant. The child with chronic diarrhea secondary to pancreatic insufficiency will have the large, bulky, foul-smelling stools characteristic of fat malabsorption. The child with diarrhea secondary to an inflammatory illness, such as ulcerative colitis, may have liquid stool with mucus and bright-red blood.

Physical assessment findings also vary. Although some children may appear quite well, others may appear acutely or chronically ill. The child's pattern of growth and weight gain will reflect the duration and severity of the diarrhea. Some children do not exhibit any alteration in growth and weight gain, whereas others demonstrate delayed growth and significant weight loss. Overt signs of nutrient deficiencies may be present in these cases. If the child has experienced significant fluid and electrolyte losses from the diarrhea, dehydration and metabolic imbalances may be evident on physical examination.

Diagnostic Tests. Laboratory evaluation of the stool can help differentiate between infectious, inflammatory, or malabsorptive causes. Stool culture for bacteria and ova and parasites are obtained to assess for infection. Stool specimens for white blood cell counts, occult blood, and alpha$_1$-antitrypsin assess for inflammatory causes. Screening for malabsorptive disorders is done by measuring stool pH, reducing substances, and fecal fat.

Blood specimens are taken to evaluate for systemic disease, fluid and electrolyte imbalance, and nutritional status. A complete blood cell count with erythrocyte sedimentation rate, chemistry panel with electrolytes, liver and renal function tests, and serum protein level determination are done. Trace mineral and vitamin levels may be assessed if clinical evidence of deficiency is noted. A breath hydrogen study or D-xylose absorption test may be done if malabsorption is suggested.

Radiologic studies are usually used only in situations in which the results of the history and physical examination are suggestive of an anatomic defect, obstruction, or inflammatory bowel disease. Endoscopic evaluation with intestinal biopsy is reserved for the child with suspected inflammatory bowel disease or infection from a source not identified by stool culture or mucosal injury.

Nursing Diagnoses and Outcomes

In addition to the nursing diagnoses and outcomes listed in Chart 18–3, the following may be applicable to the child with chronic diarrhea:

- **Impaired skin integrity related to presence of diarrheal stools**
  Outcome: The child will have intact perineal skin and will suffer no skin breakdown.

Interdisciplinary Interventions

Treatment of the child with chronic diarrhea involves treating the underlying organic source of the diarrhea, along with nutritional intervention to optimize digestion and absorption of nutrients and foster growth and weight gain. For the child with chronic diarrhea related to overfeeding or excessive juice consumption, treatment consists of nutritional counseling to normalize the child's diet. Modification of formula or diet may be necessary in malabsorptive disorders. Casein hydrolysate formulas or elemental formulas are commonly used in these cases. In cases of severe mucosal injury, enteral or parenteral nutrition may be necessary to support the child's fluid and nutritional requirements until mucosal healing takes place. The child with secretory diarrhea may require complete bowel rest and support with parenteral nutrition until the cause of the diarrhea resolves.

Nursing management of the child with chronic diarrhea involves meticulous attention to fluid and electrolyte balance. Careful assessment and documentation of all the child's intake, both oral and IV, and all outputs is necessary. Stool volume and characteristics should be carefully assessed and documented.

caREminder: *Assess infant stool volumes by weighing diapers. If mixing of urine and stool makes accurate assessment difficult, stool and urine should be separated by use of an infant urine bag. To obtain a stool specimen, a disposable diaper can be applied inside out. The plastic barrier will not absorb the stool which can then be scraped off and placed in the specimen container.*

Replacement of stool losses should be considered when stool volumes exceed 15 to 20 mg/kg body weight per day. Careful assessment of hydration status and feeding tolerance should be made. Skin integrity may be impaired secondary to frequent diarrheal stools. Frequent diaper changes and meticulous skin care are important. Parent education regarding medical and dietary management of the child's diarrhea, along with instruction in specialized nutrition support techniques and home monitoring, is also necessary.

Short Bowel Syndrome

Short bowel syndrome (SBS) is a condition in which massive resection of small bowel results in malabsorption, fluid and electrolyte loss, and malnutrition.

SBS in neonates is associated with congenital anomalies of the GI tract such as jejunoileal atresia, gastroschisis, and omphalocele. Preterm infants with severe necrotizing enterocolitis may undergo intestinal resections that leave them with a short bowel. Infants and older children who experience malrotation with midgut volvulus may sustain severe ischemic injury to the small intestine and may require massive intestinal resection. Children with Crohn's disease who undergo repeated resections of diseased bowel also may be left with a short bowel.

The reported incidence of SBS varies from study to study. Many studies report necrotizing enterocolitis as the most common cause of SBS, whereas others cite jejunoileal atresia and gastroschisis as the most common causes. SBS has been reported to occur in 7% to 38% of neonates who have undergone surgery for necrotizing enterocolitis.

Pathophysiology

The small bowel is the primary site for digestion and absorption of nutrients. SBS occurs when massive resection of small bowel leads to reduced absorptive surface area and malabsorption of nutrients, fluid, and electrolytes. Intestinal adaptation is the process by which the remaining bowel develops the capability to do the work of digesting and absorbing adequate fluid and nutrients to support life. At 26 to 38 weeks' gestation, the small bowel undergoes extensive development, doubling in length. The full-term neonate is born with 200 to 300 cm of small bowel, which has an absorptive surface area of 950 cm. By adulthood, small bowel length grows to 600 to 900 cm with an absorptive surface area of 7500 cm. These facts are important in understanding the infant's response to massive small bowel loss.

Although the very small infant does not initially tolerate resection of large amounts of small bowel as well as the adult, over the long term the infant has greater potential for intestinal adaptation because of a greater capacity for growth and development of the small bowel. A number of factors affect the small intestine's ability to adapt. The length of remaining bowel, the site of the resection, and the presence of the ileocecal valve all play an important role in determining long-term outcomes. Reports in the medical literature have demonstrated that infants with as little as 25 cm of small bowel with no ileocecal valve and 11 cm of small intestine with an ileocecal valve have been able to achieve full intestinal adaptation.

Resection of the jejunum is less well tolerated than resection of the ileum, because the ileum has greater capacity for adaptation. The presence of the ileocecal valve is an important prognostic factor because it serves to slow intestinal transit time and prevent reflux of bacteria from the large bowel into the small bowel. The quality of the child's residual bowel is also an important factor, with residual disease and surgical complications such as strictures and fistulas having a negative influence.

Intestinal adaptation in SBS occurs through various mechanisms. The presence of nutrients in the lumen of the small intestine leads to dilation of the residual bowel and mucosal hyperplasia, which results in increased villous height and crypt depth. This results in an increased absorptive surface area in the small bowel. The very young neonate's inherent capacity for intestinal growth may also contribute to the process of adaptation. The process of adaptation can take from months to years. Provision of adequate nutrition support during the adaptation process is essential. Full or partial support with parenteral nutrition is required until intestinal adaptation to full enteral feedings takes place.

Prognosis. Reported survival rates for the child with SBS average around 82%. Full adaptation to enteral feeding with no reliance on TPN is reported in 60% to 70% of survivors. Morbidity and mortality are related to long-term complications associated with TPN use, underlying prematurity and disease states, and surgical complications. Small bowel transplant, alone or in combination with liver transplant, is a treatment option for children who have impending loss of further vascular access or who develop end-stage liver disease in conjunction with SBS. Five-year survival rates for children who have undergone small bowel transplant are reported at 50%.

Assessment

Clinical manifestations of untreated SBS include profuse watery diarrhea, malabsorption, and failure to thrive. Dehydration, electrolyte imbalances, and vitamin and mineral deficiencies may also occur. Skin breakdown may occur on the buttocks and perineum secondary to ongoing diarrheal stools. Infants with SBS may also be at risk for oral feeding aversions because of prolonged nutrition support with parenteral and enteral feedings.

Children with SBS are at risk for hepatobiliary complications. Cholestasis and cholelithiasis can result from malabsorption of bile salts and gallbladder stasis. Prolonged parenteral nutrition may put the child with SBS at risk for the development of cirrhosis. Liver disease in the parenterally fed child is believed to be multifactorial. Prematurity, amino acid toxicity, lack of enteral nutrition, and recurrent infection are all believed to play a role in the development of TPN-related liver disease. Diarrhea and malabsorption in the child with SBS may be exacerbated by bacterial overgrowth syndrome, a condition involving abnormal bacterial colonization of the small bowel. This can result from impaired motility secondary to adhesions or strictures and absence of the ileocecal valve.

Interdisciplinary Interventions

The basic principles of managing the child with SBS are early and aggressive use of enteral nutrition to facilitate small bowel adaptation and ongoing support with TPN until adaptation takes place. Careful management of fluids and electrolytes and prevention, early identification, and treatment of complications are also essential. Excellent nursing care of the child with SBS in hospital, clinic, and home settings contributes greatly to promoting optimal outcomes. Care of the child with SBS is a collaborative effort and, in addition to nurses in the aforementioned settings, involves the pediatrician, pediatric gastroenterologist, pediatric surgeon, dietitian, pharmacist, occupational therapist, and social worker.

The initial diagnosis of SBS is established at the time of operative intervention for the underlying intestinal anomaly or disease state. During the initial postoperative period, the immediate goal is stabilization of fluid and electrolytes. Accurate measurement and documentation of all output, including urine, stool, NG or gastrostomy tube drainage, and ostomy outputs, is essential at all times in the care of the child with SBS. Careful ongoing replacement of excess fluid losses is vital.

caREminder: *To monitor urine and stool output accurately, diapers should be weighed. If urine and stool are mixed and their relative quantities cannot be estimated, temporary separation of urine and stool with use of a urine bag or urinary catheter may be necessary.*

Gastric hypersecretion is typical in the early stages after intestinal resection and is treated with the administration of a histamine-2 blocker (e.g., Tagamet). Frequent laboratory evaluation of electrolyte balance is done. TPN is initiated after the initial postoperative stabilization and advanced gradually until the child's nutritional requirements are met (see Chapter 17). Baseline TPN laboratory values, including liver and renal function tests, calcium, magnesium, phosphorus, total protein, and albumin, are done at the time TPN is initiated and on a regular basis throughout the course of therapy.

When the child's GI function returns postoperatively, enteral feedings are started. The primary goal of enteral nutrition in the immediate postoperative period is not to provide significant nutrition support but rather to stimulate the intestine's adaptive response. Enteral feedings are usually initiated at low volumes by continuous drip through an NG or gastrostomy tube to promote optimal tolerance. Elemental or casein hydrolysate formulas are frequently used, although in some cases breast milk is given, if available. Maternal support in establishing and maintaining a breast milk supply while the infant is NPO or unable to feed by mouth is an important nursing consideration. Small-volume oral feedings and oral stimulation through a pacifier are established as early as possible to prevent oral feeding aversions.

Ongoing assessment of the infant's tolerance of parenteral and enteral feedings is done by careful evaluation of weight gain, fluid and electrolyte balance, and stool output. Stools are evaluated for malabsorption with testing for occult blood, pH, and reducing substances. Excess fluid losses are replaced with IV electrolyte solutions. Enteral feedings are advanced slowly, and parenteral nutrition is weaned proportionally as the child demonstrates progressive tolerance to enteral feeding.

When the child is medically stable, discharge home on parenteral and enteral nutrition can be considered. Meticulous technique in TPN administration and central venous catheter care is vital in both the hospital and home settings, as catheter-related infections are a common, but preventable, complication.

Celiac Disease

Celiac disease is a malabsorptive disorder caused by a permanent intolerance to dietary gluten. Injury to the mucosa of the small intestine and malabsorption is manifested after the introduction of gluten from wheat, oats, barley, or rye in the diet. Symptoms resolve when gluten is removed from the diet. Celiac disease is also known as *celiac sprue* or *gluten enteropathy*.

The incidence of celiac disease varies greatly geographically. In the United States, celiac disease is relatively rare, with an estimated prevalence of 1 in 3000. In European countries the reported prevalence is much higher, especially in Ireland, where incidence is 1 in 300.

Although descriptions of celiac disease can be found in medical literature of the late 19th century, the relationship between gluten and the development of celiac disease was not established until 1950. W. K. Dickie, a Dutch pediatrician, noted improvement in children with preexisting symptoms of celiac disease during World War II, when wheat bread was not widely available. After the war, wheat bread was reintroduced into the children's diets and celiac symptoms recurred. Dickie became convinced of the relationship between wheat products and celiac disease and went on to conduct research that established the role of gluten in the etiology of the disease.

Pathophysiology

The child with celiac disease demonstrates villous atrophy of the proximal small intestine. The mucosal layer of the small intestine appears "flat" instead of having the normal finger-like projections of healthy villi, which results in impaired digestion and absorption of nutrients. The damage to the intestinal mucosa is believed to be mediated by immunologic mechanisms, with mucosal injury arising from an adverse immunologic reaction to gliadin, a polypeptide protein fraction of gluten.

Prognosis. The prognosis for the child with celiac disease is good with the institution of a life-long gluten-free diet. Symptoms typically improve within the first week of starting the diet, with resolution of mucosal damage within 6 months. Over the long term, adults with celiac disease have demonstrated an increased risk of developing lymphoma of the small intestine.

Assessment

The clinical presentation of celiac disease may vary, depending on the child's age and the degree of injury to the intestinal mucosa. A young child, after demonstrating normal growth during the first months of life, typically presents with a history of failure to thrive when gluten products are introduced into the diet. Chronic diarrhea, with foul-smelling, bulky, greasy stools is usually present, although in some cases constipation accompanied by dilation of the colon and rectal prolapse are present. Abdominal distention, muscle wasting, and hypotonia are frequently present. Anorexia, irritability, and lassitude are also common. In severe cases, overt signs of nutritional deficiencies may be present on physical examination.

In adolescence, celiac disease may present as growth retardation with delayed menses or puberty. Anemia may also be present.

Diagnostic Tests. To conclusively establish the diagnosis of celiac disease, biopsy specimens of the small intestine must demonstrate the characteristic histologic appearance of celiac disease and the child must demonstrate a clinical response to a gluten-free diet. The work-up of the child with suspected celiac disease includes an initial history and physical examination that contains a detailed nutritional assessment evaluating the child's pattern of growth and diet history and looks for signs and symptoms of malabsorption and nutritional deficiencies.

Laboratory tests evaluate for malabsorption and nutritional deficiencies. Blood cell counts and serum iron, protein, mineral, and vitamin levels may all be decreased in chronic malabsorption. Immunologic assays screen for celiac disease. Tests for serum levels of antigliadin antibodies and antiendomysial antibodies are commonly ordered. Testing for malabsorption of dietary fat and xylose absorption may also be done. If there is a high suspicion of celiac disease after initial screening, an upper GI endoscopy with small bowel biopsy is performed.

Nursing Diagnoses and Outcomes

In addition to the nursing diagnoses and outcomes listed in Chart 18–3, the following may be applicable to the family of a child with celiac disease:

- **Ineffective individual management of therapeutic regimen related to life-long maintenance of dietary restrictions**
  Outcomes: The child will not ingest gluten-containing products.

The child will not demonstrate injury to intestinal mucosa.
The child and family will list palatable alternatives to gluten products.

Interdisciplinary Interventions

Treatment of celiac disease consists of a lifelong gluten-free diet. Education regarding the diet is an essential part of the treatment plan and is a collaborative endeavor including the physician, dietitian, nurse, patient, and family. The teaching plan includes information about obvious and hidden sources of gluten in the diet. Children and parents are taught to read the labels of processed foods carefully to look for gluten-containing additives, such as vegetable proteins. Referrals to community resources for gluten-free foods are helpful, along with referral to peer support organizations such as the Celiac Sprue Association (see Resources).

Ongoing monitoring is necessary to evaluate the child's response to therapy. Failure to respond to the gluten-free diet or exacerbation of symptoms may be due to noncompliance. Developmental factors in younger children and social pressure on older children and adolescents may make adherence to the diet difficult (Chart 18–11). Because of this, it is important to find develop-

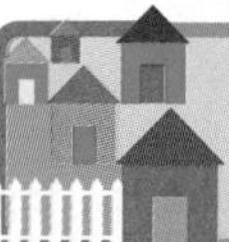

Chart 18–11
Community Care

Maintenance of a Gluten-Free Diet

- All forms of wheat, rye, barley, and usually oats (some people can tolerate) should be omitted.
- Other foods are permitted as desired or as specified by the physician.
- *Caution:* always read labels on commercially prepared foods; when in doubt contact the producer.

Foods	Allowed	Not allowed
Beverages	Milk Fruit juices Carbonated beverages Cocoa (read label to check that no wheat flour has been added) Coffee (ground, read label on instant) Tea	Malted milk Ovaltine Beer
Bread/cereal	Breads made from rice, corn, soybean, potato, tapioca, sago or gluten-free wheat flour Dry cereals made only with rice or corn; cornmeal, hominy	Breads, rolls, crackers, cakes, cookies, cereals, noodles, spaghetti, etc. made from wheat, rye, wheat germ, barley, bran, oats
Fruit	As desired	
Meat/fish/fowl/egg/cheese/nuts	As desired, plain Peanut butter	None with breading, cream sauce, thickened gravy Cold cuts (unless labeled all meat)
Vegetable	As desired	None with cream sauce or breading
Fats	Butter, margarine, oil, pure mayonnaise Salad dressing thickened with allowed flours	Commercial salad dressings (read label)
Condiments/sweets	Salt, pure spices Sugar, honey, molasses, syrup, jam, jelly, candy (read label) Gelatin, homemade ice cream, rice pudding, pudding thickened with allowed flours	Some candies are dusted with flour to prevent sticking, or made with flour Ice cream, sauce and gravy mixes may contain wheat flour without listing on label Soy sauce

mentally sensitive ways to include the child in all dietary counseling to increase their sense of involvement and responsibility in the treatment plan.

Lactose Intolerance

Lactose intolerance, also known as lactase deficiency, is the most common cause of carbohydrate malabsorption. The most common cause of lactose intolerance is adult-onset lactase deficiency, which results from the normal physiologic decline in lactase activity that usually begins after age 5. The incidence of adult-onset lactase deficiency varies greatly by ethnic group. Although only 15% of white adults experience lactose intolerance, up to 80% of black adults and 100% of Asian adults are affected. Symptoms may begin in early childhood.

Worldview: *In parts of the world such as Asia and Africa where adult-onset lactase deficiency is very common, milk products are not a large part of the usual adult diet, so symptoms of lactose intolerance are relatively rare.*

True congenital lactase deficiency, in which symptoms are present shortly after birth, is extremely rare. Premature infants may experience transient lactose intolerance related to immature lactase activity. Intestinal disease or inflammation can cause transient lactose intolerance.

Pathophysiology

Lactose is the primary carbohydrate found in mammalian milk. Lactase, an enzyme located on the brush border near the tip of the intestinal villi, breaks down lactose so that its component parts can be absorbed. When lactase activity is inadequate, lactose is malabsorbed. Premature infants have significantly lower levels of lactase activity than term infants. The 34-week premature infant has only 40% of the lactase activity of a term infant. Lactase levels begin to decline at varying rates after age 5.

GI disease can adversely affect lactase activity. Acute infectious gastroenteritis can cause partial villous atrophy, resulting in a transient lactase deficiency. Individuals with disease characterized by inflammation of the GI tract, such as Crohn's disease or ulcerative colitis, may also experience lactase deficiency.

Assessment

A thorough history is the initial step in the evaluation of the child with suspected lactose intolerance, including a detailed diet history and information regarding timing and quality of symptoms. The child with lactose intolerance will usually experience watery diarrhea and crampy abdominal pain after ingestion of lactose-containing food products. Abdominal distention, flatulence, and borborygmi may also be present. In some cases, complaints of recurrent abdominal pain may be the only presenting symptom.

Diagnostic Tests. The most reliable diagnostic tool in establishing the diagnosis of lactose intolerance is the lactose breath hydrogen test. After ingesting a concentrated solution of lactose, serial measurements of expired breath hydrogen are made. When lactose is malabsorbed, the bacterial flora in the colon produce hydrogen gas, which is absorbed across the colonic mucosa into the colon and expired through the respiratory system. A rise in breath hydrogen levels after ingestion of a load of lactose indicates lactose malabsorption.

Interdisciplinary Interventions

Lactose intolerance is treated by reducing or eliminating lactose-containing foods in the diet. Dietary counseling focuses on helping children and parents identify both obvious and hidden sources of lactose in processed foods. Milk products treated with a microbially derived lactase may be utilized. The lactase derivative is also available in tablet form, which may be ingested with lactose-containing foods to improve tolerance.

Dietary counseling also includes ensuring that daily calcium requirements are adequately met through other sources. The nurse, in collaboration with the dietitian, makes sure that counseling is developmentally and culturally sensitive to enhance compliance.

Hepatic Disorders

Biliary Atresia

Biliary atresia is characterized by obstruction of bile flow out of the liver due to the absence or progressive sclerosis of the extrahepatic bile ducts. This process begins during the prenatal period and, if untreated, will cause death by age 12 to 24 months. Advances in the surgical management of biliary atresia and liver transplantation have greatly improved the outlook for the child with biliary atresia. Biliary atresia is currently the most common indication for liver transplant in children.

Biliary atresia occurs in 1 in 15,000 births and is slightly more predominant in females than males. Its etiology remains unclear. Evidence suggests that it may result from an inflammatory process that starts during the prenatal period and causes progressive compression and obliteration of the bile ducts. A viral etiology has also been hypothesized. Approximately 13% of infants with biliary atresia have associated malformations (malrotation, polysplenia, absent inferior vena cava, congenital heart defects) that suggest a defect in early embryologic development.

Pathophysiology

The child with biliary atresia experiences a chronic obstruction of bile flow that results in progressive damage to the liver. Cholestasis leads to edema and inflammation of the portal tracts of the liver, destruction of the portal bile ducts with bile plugs, secondary proliferation of intralobular bile ducts, and inflammation of the parenchyma of the liver. Progressive fibrosis and, eventually, cirrhosis of the liver tissue result in end-stage liver disease (see the section on end-stage liver disease).

Prognosis. The prognosis for the child with biliary atresia is dependent on early recognition and treatment of the condition. If not treated, the child with biliary atresia will succumb to end-stage liver disease by age 12 to 24 months. Early surgical intervention to restore bile flow through a hepatic portoenterostomy improves the long-term outlook for the child if it is performed within the first 2 months life before extensive damage to the liver has been sustained.

Thirty percent of infants who undergo hepatic portoenterostomy before age 2 months do well and may never require liver transplant. An additional group will experience a stabilization in liver function after hepatic portoenterostomy that allows delay in liver transplantation until the child is older. The remainder will not experience any improvement in liver function after surgery and will require liver transplant within the first 2 years of life.

Infants who are diagnosed with biliary atresia after age 3 months are not considered candidates for hepatic portoenterostomy and are referred directly for liver transplant. The current 5-year survival rate for children with biliary atresia who undergo liver transplant is 75% to 80%.

Assessment

Roughly 75% of infants with biliary atresia present with jaundice at birth. The remainder develop jaundice within the first month of life. The jaundice is persistent and progressive. Stools appear acholic, and the urine may be dark. On physical examination, the liver feels large and firm. Splenomegaly may develop after the first 6 weeks. Infants with biliary atresia often thrive during the first month of life and then demonstrate progressive malnutrition and growth failure as the disease progresses. As liver function deteriorates, the child will demonstrate the manifestations of end-stage liver disease, including ascites, portal hypertension, and decrease in liver size.

Chart 18–12

Diagnostic Evaluation of the Child with Liver Dysfunction

Laboratory Evaluation

ALT, AST
Alkaline phosphatase
Bilirubin, total/direct
Hepatitis A, B, C serologies
"TORCH" titers
HIV screen
Alpha$_1$-antitrypsin
Metabolic screen
CBC
PT, PTT
Sweat chloride

Radiology

Abdominal ultrasound
HIDA scan
Cholangiogram (percutaneous or intraoperative)

Liver Biopsy (percutaneous or intraoperative)

Diagnostic Tests. Laboratory evaluation is used to rule out nonbiliary tract causes of jaundice and to establish the degree of damage that the liver has sustained (Chart 18–12). Radiologic studies are used to visualize the architecture and function of the biliary tract. Liver biopsy and cholangiography may be done percutaneously or intraoperatively as a means to definitively establish the diagnosis of biliary atresia.

Nursing Diagnoses and Outcomes

In addition to the nursing diagnoses and outcomes listed in Chart 18–3, the following may be applicable to the child with biliary atresia:

- **Risk for impaired skin integrity related to pruritus secondary to liver dysfunction**
  Outcomes: The child will have interventions implemented to decrease discomfort and scratching.
  The child will maintain intact skin.

Interdisciplinary Interventions

Because jaundice and liver failure have many possible causes (see the section on cirrhosis), a comprehensive evaluation is needed to establish the diagnosis of biliary atresia. Nursing care during the diagnostic period focuses on supporting the child's physiologic and psychosocial care needs, as well as on meeting the parent's information needs throughout the many diagnostic procedures.

Hepatic portoenterostomy, also known as the Kasai procedure, is the first-line operative intervention for infants diagnosed with biliary atresia before age 2 months. Infants diagnosed later in life have usually sustained a greater degree of damage to their liver, making it unlikely that they would substantially benefit from the procedure. These children are usually referred directly for liver transplantation.

The goal of hepatic portoenterostomy is to reestablish bile flow out of the liver. This is accomplished by dissecting away the atretic extrahepatic biliary ducts and then anastomosing a limb of jejunum, which acts as a conduit for bile flow, to the exposed porta hepatis. A transhepatic tube (T-tube) may be left in place for the first 4 to 6 weeks postoperatively to monitor the bile flow out of the liver.

caREminder: *Cover the T-tube with clothing so the infant does not pull at, or dislodge, it.*

Nursing measures to prevent infection of the drainage system as well as preventing obstruction or dislodgement of the tube are very important. Cholangitis is a frequent complication after hepatic portoenterostomy. Organisms ascending from the intestinal tract are frequently implicated. Prophylactic antibiotic therapy with trimethoprim-sulfamethoxazole may be given to prevent cholangitis. Fever, increased jaundice, and decreased bile flow are the overt clinical signs of cholangitis. Treatment is with broad-spectrum IV antibiotics. Parents are taught to recognize the signs and symptoms of cholangitis to ensure their child receives medical attention in a timely manner.

With or without operative intervention, the child with biliary atresia requires ongoing nutritional and medical intervention. The child is at high risk for failure to thrive and malnutrition secondary to malabsorption of dietary fat and fat-soluble vitamins because of decreased intraluminal concentrations of bile acids. Infant formulas that provide a higher percentage of fat as medium-chain triglycerides and thus are more readily absorbed (e.g., Portagen, Pregestimil) are used. Nasogastric feedings or supplements of IV fat emulsions may also be used to ensure adequate calorie intake. Supplements of the fat-soluble vitamins A, D, E, and K are given. Collaboration between the dietitian, nurse, physician, and family is essential in ongoing nutritional monitoring and intervention.

Medical therapy will depend on the degree of liver dysfunction (see the section on cirrhosis). Phenobarbital or ursodeoxycholic acid may be given to try to improve bile flow. Pruritus, stemming from jaundice, may be treated with rifampin, which increases bile flow.

Community Care

The family of the child with biliary atresia faces multiple psychosocial stressors owing to the chronic and often degenerative nature of the disease. Involved medical care in the home, multiple acute hospitalizations, and, for many, the prospect of liver transplant may present a source of ongoing anxiety, as well as stress family and personal relationships, work performance, and finances. The family's coping can be enhanced by ongoing involvement with a social worker or other mental health professional, as well as referral to peer support organizations.

Cirrhosis and End-Stage Liver Disease

Cirrhosis is defined by the World Health Organization as a diffuse liver process characterized by fibrosis and the conversion of normal liver tissue into structurally abnormal nodules. The end result of most forms of liver disease, cirrhosis has many possible causes (Table 18–8). The precise incidence of cirrhosis in children is difficult to ascertain.

Table 18–8
Diseases Leading to Cirrhosis

Etiology	Disease
Infectious	Viral hepatitis Herpesvirus
Metabolic disorders	Alpha$_1$-antitrypsin deficiency Cystic fibrosis Glycogen storage disease Hemochromatosis Wilson's disease
Biliary malformations	Biliary atresia Alagille syndrome Choledochal cyst
Toxic exposure	Acetaminophen Isoniazid Natural toxins (mushrooms)
Vascular disease	Budd-Chiari syndrome Congestive heart failure Veno-occlusive liver disease
Other	TPN liver disease Neonatal hepatitis Primary sclerosing cholangitis

Pathophysiology

Cirrhosis and end-stage liver disease are the end result of the liver's response to injury. The mechanisms of injury may vary, but the liver's response follows a typical pattern. Cell injury to the hepatocyte leads to cell necrosis. Cell necrosis releases factors that lead to fibrous connective tissue formation. Disruption of normal liver structures by fibrosis and nodule formation occurs, leading to compression and distortion of intrahepatic vascular structures. This, in turn, causes further ischemic and hypoxemic injury to the hepatocytes.

In compensated cirrhosis, cirrhosis presents without biochemical or clinical evidence of impairment in liver function. In active cirrhosis, the signs and symptoms of cirrhosis are manifest and progressive. In fulminant hepatic failure, sudden impairment in liver function leads to hepatic encephalopathy within 8 weeks of symptom onset (Pappas, 1995).

Prognosis. The long-term outlook for the child with cirrhosis varies depending on the nature and severity of the disease. Although the child with compensated cirrhosis may experience very little impairment, the child with active cirrhosis or fulminant hepatic failure will require liver transplant to achieve long-term survival.

Assessment

Clinical manifestations of cirrhosis and end-stage liver disease depend on the etiology of the injury to the liver and on how rapidly hepatic failure progresses. Children with compensated cirrhosis may have few findings on physical examination or laboratory evaluation. Children in fulminant hepatic failure demonstrate multiple alterations both physically and biochemically.

General manifestation of cirrhosis often mimic other systemic illnesses. A pattern of failure to thrive may be noted along with anorexia and easy fatigability. Jaundice may be present but is not always evident. Nausea, vomiting, and abdominal pain may occur.

On physical examination, muscle wasting may be noted. The liver may be large and tender during the early stages of cirrhosis but progress to becoming small and shrunken as it becomes increasingly nodular. A marked enlargement of the spleen and abdominal ascites is noted when portal hypertension is present. Ascites may also be noted when hypoalbuminemia is present. Deep tendon reflexes may be absent related to malabsorption of vitamin E (Sokol, 1994). Cyanosis and digital clubbing occur in the presence of chronic hypoxemia from pulmonary systemic collateral shunting. Easy bruisability or overt signs of bleeding may be seen related to clotting factor deficiencies and low platelets.

Diagnostic Tests. Laboratory evaluation is done to detect serologic evidence of causative factors (see Chart 18–12). Evaluation of liver function tests, blood indices, clotting parameters, and visceral protein status helps to establish the degree of impaired liver function. Radiologic evaluation detects any structural abnormalities within the liver and biliary duct system. Liver biopsy provides histologic evidence to confirm the diagnosis of cirrhosis.

Interdisciplinary Interventions

The goal of the initial diagnostic evaluation of the child with suspected cirrhosis is to establish the underlying cause of liver disease and to determine the degree of injury to the liver. As with nursing management of the child undergoing evaluation for suspected biliary atresia, the goal of nursing measures during the diagnostic phase is to support the child's physiologic and psychosocial care needs, as well as meet the parent's information needs throughout the many diagnostic procedures.

Care of the child with cirrhosis is geared toward preventing and treating the complications associated with cirrhosis and end-stage liver disease. Therapy to treat the underlying cause of the liver disease is undertaken with the goal of eliminating whatever agent or mechanism is causing injury to the liver.

Medical and nutritional therapies are similar to those discussed for biliary atresia. Nutritional therapy is geared toward optimizing calorie and protein intake without exacerbating the underlying symptoms of cirrhosis. Ascites is managed with fluid and sodium restrictions. Diuretics are commonly administered to enhance fluid excretion. Hypoalbuminemia can contribute to the accumulation of ascites and edema in the child with end-stage liver disease and may necessitate intermittent albumin transfusions. Bleeding complications may require transfusions with blood products. Portal hypertension can lead to the development of esophageal or gastric varices that can be potential sites of GI bleeding. Endoscopic sclerotherapy may be used to treat such varices. Hepatic encephalopathy is treated with reduction and modification of protein intake and administration of neomycin or lactulose.

Liver transplantation offers definitive treatment for the life-threatening complications of cirrhosis and end-stage liver disease. Liver transplantation is offered at specific tertiary care centers throughout the country (Ganley, 1995). The liver transplant team manages the child through all phases of transplant from evaluation to the ongoing follow-up care after surgery. The nurse coordinator on the team plays a vital role in coordinating the child's care and providing child and family education during the preoperative and postoperative periods.

Summary of Key Concepts

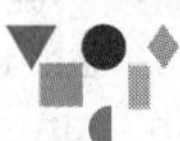

- Many GI diseases have relatively few observable physical findings. Thus, the history of symptoms and factors impacting their onset and duration is an important diagnostic tool.
- Endoscopic examination may be utilized for direct visualization of the inner lumen of the GI tract and as treatment for alterations in GI function.
- Altered GI function often affects nutritional status. Special formulas, oral diets, enteral and parenteral nutrition, and modification of feeding techniques may be used to maintain nutritional status.
- Use of the orofacial muscles is necessary for muscle development, feeding, and speech skills. Therefore, feeding methods that promote sucking, or nonnutritive sucking, should be used whenever possible.
- The hallmark symptom of esophageal atresia is excessive oral secretions.
- Polyhydramnios is observed in many cases of intestinal atresia.
- The child with an abdominal wall defects is at high risk for fluid deficit and hypothermia due to the exposed bowel.
- The infant with congenital diaphragmatic hernia has a scaphoid abdomen because of the absence of abdominal contents. An infant experiencing respiratory distress should be immediately intubated; bag and mask ventilation further compromises lung expansion and thus should be avoided.
- Anal malformations not noted at birth may present as signs of lower intestinal obstruction with abdominal distention and bilious vomiting.
- The pain of appendicitis is initially periumbilical and then migrates to the lower right quadrant.
- Functional abdominal pain is a common complaint of school-age children. Although not pathologic, the pain is real and is often associated with frequent school absences.
- Malabsorptive diseases may cause delayed growth, significant weight loss, and nutrient deficiencies.
- Cholangitis is a frequent complication after hepatic portoenterostomy for biliary atresia, often due to organisms ascending from the intestinal tract.

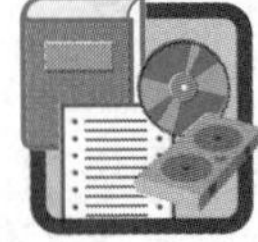

Resources

Organizations

American Liver Foundation
1425 Pompton Avenue
Cedar Grove, NJ 07009
(800) 223-0179
E-mail: info@liverfoundation.org

American Pseudo-Obstruction and Hirschsprung's Disease Society
158 Pleasant Street North
Andover, MA 01845-2797
(800) 394-APHS

Celiac Sprue Association/United States of America, Inc.
P.O. Box 31700
Omaha, NE 68131-0700
(402) 448-0600

C.L.A.S.S.—Children's Liver Association for Support Services
26444 Emerald Dove Drive
Valencia, CA 91355
E-mail: SupportSrv@aol.com

The Cleft Palate Foundation
1218 Grandview Avenue
Pittsburgh, PA 15211
(800) 24-CLEFT
(412) 418-1376
Web: http://www.cleft.com

Crohn's & Colitis Foundation of America
386 Park Avenue South, 17th Floor
New York, NY 10016-8804
(800) 932-2423

IFFGD (International Foundation for Functional Gastrointestinal Disorders)
P.O. Box 17864
Milwaukee, WI 53217
(414) 964-1799

National Digestive Diseases Information Clearinghouse
2 Information Way
Bethesda, MD 20892-3572
E-mail: nddic@aerie.com

Oley Foundation for Home Parenteral and Enteral Nutrition
214 Hun Memorial, A-23
Albany Medical Center
Albany, NY 12208-3478
(518) 262-5079

United Ostomy Association
36 Executive Park, Suite 120
Irvine, CA 92614
(800) 826-0826
E-mail: uoa@deltnet.com
Web: http://www.wocn.org

Guidelines/Position Statements

American Society for Parenteral and Enteral Nutrition. (1996). Standards for hospitalized pediatric patients. *Nutrition in Clinical Practice, 11,* 217–228.

American Cleft Palate Craniofacial Association. (1993). Parameters for evaluation and treatment of cleft lip/palate or other craniofacial anomalies. *The Cleft Palate-Craniofacial Journal, 30*(2), S1–S16.

Printed Material

Benkov, K., & Winter, H. (1996). *Managing your child's Crohn's disease or ulcerative colitis.* New York: Mastermedia Ltd.

Thomson, P. (1996). *Gluten-free cookery. The complete guide for gluten-free or wheat-free diets.* North Pomfret, VT: Trafalger Square.

Computer Resources

Web sites: Gluten-free diet
http://www.brookeline.com/nutrition/gluten/gluten.htm
http://www.wwwebguides.com/nutrition/diets/
glutenfree/index.html

References

Allen, K. D. (1995). Differential diagnosis: A case study. *Neontal Network, 14*(4), 41–45.

Brazelton, T. B. (1962). Crying in infancy. *Pediatrics, 29,* 579–588.

Bujanover, Y., Reif, S., & Yahov, J. (1996). *Heliocobacter pylori* and peptic disease in the pediatric patient. *Pediatric Clinics of North America, 43,* 213–234.

D'Agostino, J. A. (1997). Congenital diaphragmatic hernia: What happens after discharge? *MCN, 22,* 263–266.

Diseth, T. H., Bjornland, K., Novik, T. S., & Emblem, R. (1997). Bowel function, mental health, and psychosocial function in adolescents with Hirschsprung's disease. *Archives of Disease in Childhood, 76,* 100–106.

Eliason, M. (1991). Cleft lip and palate: Developmental effects. *Journal of Pediatric Nursing,* 6, 107–113.

Ganley, P. P. (1995). Living related liver transplantation (LRLT) in children: Focus on issues. *Pediatric Nursing, 21,* 532–525.

Gill, N. E., Behnke, M., Conlon, M., & Anderson, G. C. (1992). Nonnutritive sucking modulates behavioral state for preterm infants before feeding. *Scandinavian Journal of Caring Science,* 6(1), 3–7.

Graffeo, C. S., & Counselman, F. L. (1996). Appendicitis. *Emergency Medicine Clinics of North America, 14,* 653–671.

Habel, A., Sell, D., & Mars, M. (1996). Management of cleft lip and palate. *Archives of Disease in Childhood. 74,* 360–366.

Hartman, G. E. (1996). Diaphragmatic hernia. In R. E. Behrman, R. M. Kliegman, & A. M. Arvin (Eds.), *Nelson textbook of pediatrics* (15th ed., pp. 1161–1163). Philadelphia: W. B. Saunders.

Hillemeier, A. C. (1996). Gastroesophageal reflux diagnostic and therapeutic approaches. *Pediatric Clinics of North America, 43,* 197–212.

Hyams, J. S. (1996). Crohn's disease in children. *Pediatric Clinics of North America, 43,* 255–277.

Hyams, J. S., Burke, G., Davis, P., Rzepski, B., & Andrulonis, P.A. (1996). Abdominal pain and irritable bowel syndrome in adolescents: A community-based study. *Journal of Pediatrics, 129,* 220–225.

Kimble, C. (1992). Nonnutritive sucking: Adaptation and health for the neonate. *Neonatal Network, 11*(2), 29–33.

Kirschner, B. S. (1996). Ulcerative colitis in children. *Pediatric Clinics of North America, 43,* 235–254.

Litwack-Saleh, K. (1993). Practical points in the care of the patient post-cleft lip and palate repair. *Journal of Post Anesthesia Nursing,* 8(1), 35–37.

Loening-Baucke, V. (1996). Encopresis and soiling. *Pediatric Clinics of North America, 43,* 279–297.

Mascarenhas, M. R., & Altschuler, S. M. (1997). Treatment of inflammatory bowel disease. *Pediatrics in Review, 18*(3), 95–98.

Mascarenhas, M. R., Redd, D., Bilodeau, J., Peck, S., & Liacouras, C. A. (1996). Pediatric enteral access center: A multidisciplinary approach. *Nutrition in Clinical Practice, 11,* 193–198.

Metheny, N. (1993). Minimizing respiratory complications of nasoenteric tube feedings: State of the science. *Heart and Lung, 22,* 213–223.

Metheny, N., Eisenberg, P., & McSweeney, M. (1988). Effect of feeding tube properties and three irrigants on clogging rates. *Nursing Research, 37,* 165–169.

Miller, H. D., & Anderson, G. C. (1993). Nonnutritive sucking: Effects on crying and heart rate in intubated infants requiring assisted mechanical ventilation. *Nursing Research, 42,* 305–307.

Pappas, S. C. (1995). Fulminant viral hepatitis. *Gastroenterology Clinics of North America, 24,* 161–173.

Richard, M. (1991). Feeding the newborn with cleft lip and/or palate: The enlargement, stimulate, swallow, rest (ESSR) method. *Journal of Pediatric Nursing,* 6, 317–321.

Sferra, T. J., & Heitlinger, M. D. (1996). Gastrointestinal gas formation and infantile colic. *Pediatric Clinics of North America, 43,* 489–510.

Sherman, P. M. (1994). Peptic ulcer disease in children: Diagnosis, treatment and the implication of *Helicobacter pylori. Gastroenterology Clinics of North America, 25,* 707–725.

Sokol, R. J. (1994). Fat-soluble vitamins and their importance in patients with cholestatic liver diseases. *Gastroenterology Clinics of North America, 23,* 673–705.

Thomson, S., & Dancey, C. P. (1996). Symptoms of irritable bowel in school children: Prevalence and psychosocial effects. *Journal of Pediatric Health Care, 10*(6), 280–285.

Woodson, R., & Hamilton, C. (1986). Heart rate estimates of motor activity in preterm infants. *Infant Behavior and Development,* 9, 283–290.

Bibliography

Ament, M., & Vargas, J. (1994). Medical therapy for ulcerative colitis in childhood. *Seminars in Pediatric Surgery, 3*, 28–32.

Armentrout, D. (1995). Gastroesophageal reflux in infants. *Nurse Practitioner, 20*(5), 54–63.

Ascher, H. Krantz, I., Rydberg, L., Nordin, P., & Kristiansson, B. (1997). Influence of infant feeding and gluten intake on coeliac disease. *Archives of Diseases of Childhood, 76*, 113–117.

Baker, S. S. (1997). Enteral nutrition in pediatrics. In J. L. Rombeau & R. H. Rolandelli (Eds.), *Enteral and tube feeding*. Philadelphia: W. B. Saunders.

Belkengren, R., & Sapala, S. (1996). Pediatric management problems. *Pediatric Nursing, 22*, 444–445.

Berube, M. C., & Parrish, R. S. (1994). Home care of the infant with gastroesophageal reflux and respiratory disease. *Journal of Pediatric Health Care, 8*, 173–180.

Bilodeau, J. (1995). A home parenteral nutrition program for infants. *JOGNN, 24*, 72–76.

Borowski, S. (1994). Common pediatric surgical problems. *Nursing Clinics of North America, 29*, 551–562.

Branski, D., Lerner, A., & Lebenthal, E. (1996). Chronic diarrhea and malabsorption. *Pediatric Clinics of North America, 43*, 307–331.

Brydolf, M., & Segesten, K. (1996). "They feel your needs in the air": Experiences of supportive activities among adolescents with ulcerative colitis. *Journal of Pediatric Nursing, 11*, 71–78.

Chaet, M., Farrell, M., Ziegler, M., et al. (1994). Intensive nutritional support and remedial surgical intervention for extreme short bowel syndrome. *Journal of Pediatric Gastroenterology and Nutrition, 19*, 295–298.

Cervisi, J., Chapman, M., Niklas, B., & Yamaoka, C. (1991). Office management of the infant with colic. *Journal of Pediatric Health Care, 5*, 184–190.

Chaney, C. A. (1995). A collaborative protocol for encopresis management in school-aged children. *Journal of School Health, 65*, 360–363.

Coulsen, W. (1994). Pathological features in inflammatory bowel disease in children. *Seminars in Pediatric Surgery, 3*, 8–14.

Dennison, B., Rockwell, H., & Baker, S. (1997). Excess fruit juice consumption by preschool-aged children is associated with short stature and obesity. *Pediatrics, 99*, 15–22.

Dillon, P. W., & Cilley, R. E. (1993). Newborn surgical emergencies: Gastrointestinal anomalies, abdominal wall defects. *Pediatric Clinics of North America, 40*, 1289–1314.

Dumont, R. C., & Rudolph, C. D. (1994). Development of gastrointestinal motility in the infant and child. *Gastroenterology Clinics of North America, 23*, 655–671.

Ellett, M., Beckstrand, J., Welch, J., Dye, J., & Games, C. (1992). Predicting the distance for gavage tube placement in children. *Pediatric Nursing, 18*, 119–121.

Fonkalsrud, E. (1994). Surgical management of ulcerative colitis in childhood. *Seminars in Pediatric Surgery, 3*, 33–38.

Frost, G. (1992). Hirschsprung Disease in infants and children. *Gastroenterology Nursing, 15*(8), 45–48.

Garvin, G. (1994). Caring for children with ostomies. *Nursing Clinics of North America, 29*, 645–654.

Georgeson, K., & Breaux, C. (1992). Outcome and intestinal adaptation in neonatal short bowel syndrome. *Journal of Pediatric Surgery, 27*, 344–350.

Giese, L. A., & Terrell, L. (1996). Sexual health issues in inflammatory bowel disease. *Gastroenterology Nursing, 19*(1), 12–17.

Gitnick, G. (1994). Current views of the etiology of inflammatory bowel disease. *Seminars in Pediatric Surgery, 3*, 2–7.

Glassman, M., George, D., & Grill, B. (1995). Gastroesophageal reflux in children: Clinical manifestations, diagnosis, and therapy. *Gastroenterology Clinics of North America, 24*, 71–84.

Gorard, D. A., Libby, G. W., & Farthing, M. J. (1995). Effect of a tricyclic antidepressant on small intestinal motility in health and diarrhea-predominant irritable bowel syndrome. *Digestive Diseases and Sciences, 40*, 86–95.

Grant, D. (1996). Current results of intestinal transplantation. *Lancet, 347*, 1801–1803.

Gryboski, J. L. (1995). Crohn's disease in children 10 years old and younger: Comparison with ulcerative colitis. *Journal of Pediatric Gastroenterology and Nutrition, 18*, 174–182.

Haas-Beckert, B., & Heyman, M. B. (1993). Comparison of two skin-level gastrostomy feeding tubes for infants and children. *Pediatric Nursing, 19*, 351–354, 364.

Haddock, G., Davis, C., & Raine, P. (1995). Gastroschisis in the decade of prenatal diagnosis. *European Journal of Pediatric Surgery, 6*, 18–22.

Joachim, G., & Hassall, E. (1992). Familial inflammatory bowel disease in a pediatric population. *Journal of Advanced Nursing, 17*, 1310–1316.

Keller, V. E. (1995). Management of nausea and vomiting in children. *Journal of Pediatric Nursing, 10*, 280–286.

Khoshoo, V., Reifen, R., Neuman, M. G., Griffiths, A., & Pencharz, P. B. (1996). Effect of low- and high-fat, peptide based diets on body composition and disease activity in adolescents with active Crohn's disease. *Journal of Parenteral and Enteral Nutrition, 20*, 401–405.

Kirschner, B. (1995). Ulcerative colitis and Crohn's disease in children: Diagnosis and management. *Gastroenterology Clinics of North America, 24*, 99–117.

Kocoshis, S. A. (1994). Small bowel transplantation in infants and children. *Gastroenterology Clinics of North America, 23*, 727–742.

Kocoshis, S. A., Tzakis, A., Todo, S., Reyes, J., & Nour, B. (1993). Pediatric liver transplantation: History, recent innovations, and outlook for the future. *Clinical Pediatrics, 32*, 386–391.

LoBiondo-Wood, G., Bernier-Henn, M., & Williams, L. (1992). Impact of the child's liver transplant on the family: Maternal perspective. *Pediatric Nursing, 18*, 461–465.

MacDonald, C. A. (1991) Biliary atresia. *Journal of Pediatric Nursing, 6*, 374–383.

Martin, S. A. (1992). The ABC's of pediatric LFTs. *Pediatric Nursing 18*, 445–449.

McKenna, C. J. (1994). Gastrointestinal bleeding in children. *Nursing Clinics of North America, 29*, 599–613.

McWade, L. J. (1992). Irritable bowel syndrome: Diagnosis and management in school-aged children and adolescents. *Journal of Pediatric Health Care, 6*, 82–83.

Misra, S., & Ament, M. (1995). Diagnosis of coeliac sprue in 1994. *Gastroenterology Clinics of North America, 24*, 133–143.

Misra, S., Ament, M., & Reyen, L. (1997). Home parenteral nutrition. In R. Baker, S. Baker, & A. Davis (Eds.), *Pediatric Parenteral Nutrition* (pp. 354–369). New York: Chapman & Hall.

Moss, J. R., & Craft, M. J. (1990). Accurate assessment of infant emesis volume. *Pediatric Nursing, 16*, 455–457.

Moukarzel, A., & Ament, M. (1993). Home parenteral nutrition in infants and children. In J. L. Rombeau & M. D. Caldwell (Eds.), *Parenteral nutrition* (pp. 791–813). Philadelphia: W. B. Saunders.

Moukarzel, A., Reyen, L., & Ament, M. (1994). Home enteral feeding in children. In R. Baker, S. Baker, & A. Davis (Eds.), *Pediatric enteral nutrition* (pp. 157–168). New York: Chapman & Hall.

Muscari, M. E., & Milks, C. J. (1995). Assessing acute abdominal pain in adolescent females. *Pediatric Nursing, 21*, 215–220.

Orenstein, S. R., Shalaby, T. M., & Cohn, J. F. (1996). Reflux symptoms in 100 normal infants: Diagnostic validity of the Infant Gastroesophageal Reflux Questionnaire. *Clinical Pediatrics, 35*, 607.

Parrish, R. S., & Berube, M. C. (1995). Care of the infant with gastroesophageal reflux and respiratory disease: After the Nissen fundoplication. *Journal of Pediatric Health Care, 9*, 211–217.

Quinn, D., & Shannon, L. (1996). Congenital anomalies of the gastrointestinal tract: III. The colon and rectum. *Neonatal Network, 15*(2), 63–67.

Quinn, D., & Shannon, L. (1996). Congenital anomalies of the gastrointestinal tract: I. The stomach. *Neonatal Network, 14*(8), 63–66.

Rayhorn, N. (1992). Colonoscopy and the pediatric patient. *Gastroenterology Nursing, 15*(8), 18–22.

Repucci, A. H. (1996). Pediatric gastroenterology. In H. W. Taeusch, R. O. Christiansen, & E. S. Buescher, *Pediatric and neonatal tests and procedures* (pp. 477–552). Philadelphia: W. B. Saunders.

Richard, M. (1994). Common pediatric craniofacial reconstructions. *Nursing Clinics of North America, 29*, 791–799.

Richard, M. (1994). Weight comparison of infants with complete cleft lip and palate. *Journal of Pediatric Nursing, 20*, 191–196.

Roy, C., Silverman, A., & Alagille, D. (1995). *Pediatric clinical gastroenterology* (4th ed.). St. Louis: Mosby–Year Book.

Saunderlin, G. (1994). Celiac disease: A review. *Gastroenterology Nursing, 17*(3), 100–105.

Seth, R., & Heyman, M. (1994). Management of constipation and encopresis in infants and children. *Gastroenterology Clinics of North America, 23*, 621–636.

Shah, H. A., & Spival, W. (1994). Neonatal cholestasis: New approaches to diagnostic evaluation and therapy. *Pediatric Clinics of North America, 41*, 943–966.

Shannon, L. F., & Quinn, D. (1996). Congenital anomalies of the gastrointestinal tract: II. The small bowel. *Neonatal Network, 15*(1), 57–61.

Shannon, R. (1993). Gastroesophageal reflux in infancy: Review and update. *Journal of Pediatric Health Care, 7*, 71–76.

Sherkin-Langer, F., Langer, J. C., Zupancic, J., Winthrop, A., & Issenman, R. (1993). Home esophageal self-dilation in children. *Gastroenterology Nursing, 15*(11), 5–8.

Simon, N., & Smith, D. (1992). Living with chronic pediatric liver disease: The parent's experience. *Pediatric Nursing, 18*, 453–458.

Society of Gastroenterology Nurses and Associates. (1993). *Gastroenterology nursing: A core curriculum*. St. Louis: Mosby–Year Book.

Sterling, C. E., Schaffer, S., & Jolley, S. G. (1993). Home management related to medical treatment for childhood gastroesophageal reflux. *Pediatric Nursing, 19*, 167–173.

Takacs, L. F., & Kollman, C. E. (1994). An inflammatory bowel disease support group for teens and their parents. *Gastroenterology Nursing, 17*(1), 11–13.

Talley, N. (1994). Why do functional gastrointestinal disorders come and go? *Digestive Diseases and Sciences, 39*, 673–677.

Telander, R., & Schmeling, D. (1994). Current surgical management of Crohn's disease in childhood. *Seminars in Pediatric Surgery, 3*, 19–27.

Thobani, S., Molla, A., & Synder, J. (1994). Nutritional therapy for persistent diarrhea. In R. Baker, S. Baker, & A. Davis (Eds.), *Pediatric enteral nutrition* (pp. 291–304). New York: Chapman & Hall.

Todd, D., & Dozios, R. R. (1993). Ileoanal reservoirs: Construction and management. *Journal of ET Nursing, 20*(1), 26–35.

Treem, W. R. (1994). Infant colic: A pediatric gastroenterologist's perspective. *Pediatric Clinics of North America, 41*, 199–229.

Udall, J. N. (1996). Secretory diarrhea in children. *Pediatric Clinics of North America, 43*, 333–351.

Uzark, K. (1992). Caring for families of pediatric transplant recipients. *Critical Care Nursing Clinics of North America, 4*, 255–261.

Vandeplas, Y. (1993). The diagnosis and treatment of gastroesophageal reflux disease in infants and children. *Annals of Medicine, 25*, 323–328.

Vargas, J. (1994). Medical management of Crohn's disease in childhood. *Seminars in Pediatric Surgery, 3*, 15–18.

Warner, B., & Ziegler, M. (1993). Management of the short bowel syndrome in the pediatric population. *Pediatric Clinics of North America, 40*, 1335–1350.

Winch, A., & Ouverson, K. (1992). Nursing interventions for thromboembolic complications of chronic ulcerative colitis in children. *MCN, 17* (2), 86–90.

Wise, B. (1992). Neonatal short bowel syndrome. *Neonatal Network, 11*(7), 9–15.

Wylie, R., & Hyams, J. (1993). *Pediatric gastrointestinal disease: Pathophysiology, diagnosis, management*. Philadelphia: W. B. Saunders.

Young, R. J. (1996). Pediatric constipation. *Gastroenterology Nurse, 19*(3), 88–95.

Young, R., & Murray, N. (1993). *Helicobacter pylori:* A cause of chronic abdominal pain in children. *Gastroenterology Nursing, 15*, 247–251.

Zelasney, B. (1991). Techniques in performing continuous distal pH monitoring in infants. *Gastroenterology Nursing, 13*(8), 48–53.

HEALTH CHALLENGE:

Alterations in Genitourinary Status

OUTLINE

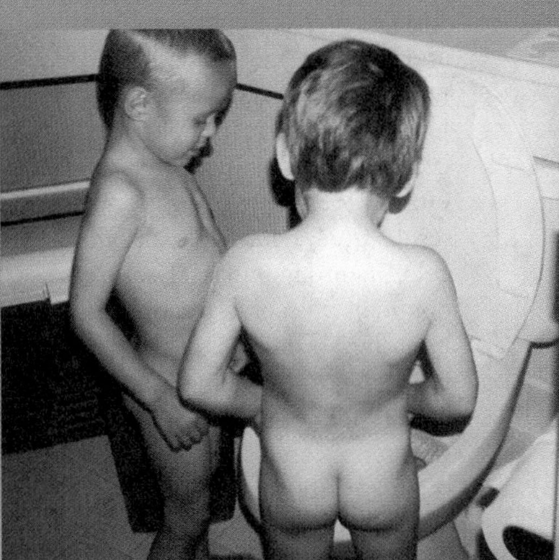

OBJECTIVES

- Correlate the child's history, symptoms, and physical signs as manifestations of genitourinary abnormalities.
- Identify various diagnostic procedures and their applications in genitourinary evaluation.
- Describe the treatment modalities available to children with alterations in genitourinary status.
- Describe common alterations in health patterns affecting the genitourinary system.
- Choose nursing interventions that support the interdisciplinary plan of care for the child with a genitourinary disorder.
- Identify the teaching needs of the child experiencing challenges related to urinary elimination.
- Describe the types of renal replacement therapies available for the child experiencing acute or chronic renal failure.

KEY TERMS

antidiuretic hormone (ADH)
anuria
bacteriuria
cystinuria
dialysate
dialysis
ectopia
hydronephrosis
lithotripsy
oliguria
osmosis
proteinuria
pyuria
renal parenchyma
third spacing
torsion
ultrafiltration
vesicoureteral reflux (VUR)

CHAPTER

19

Pediatric urology and nephrology are complementary disciplines that have emerged as distinct practice specialties over the past 30 years. Urology studies the structure and function of all parts of the urinary tract. Nephrology studies kidney function —how the kidneys regulate serum chemistries, maintain fluid balance, and produce hormones.

Urologic and nephrologic disorders in children run the gamut from such problems as hydrocele, proteinuria, and urinary tract infections (UTIs) to complex disorders including bladder exstrophy and renal failure. Recurrent UTIs and enuresis continue to be the most common genitourinary conditions affecting children (Hoyler-Grant, 1995b). Urologic and nephrologic sequelae often result from neurologic disorders such as myelomeningocele, neuromuscular dysfunction, or accompanying abdominal or sacral tumors, like rhabdosarcoma or sacral teratomy. Trauma to the genitourinary tract, or shock resulting from trauma, can cause renal or urologic problems. Malformations of the genitalia and urinary system structures can occur during fetal development. Although some of these malformations are life-threatening, many can be surgically corrected when the child is young.

Medical advances have led to development of more types of diagnostic tools, improvement in surgical techniques, and refinements in the equipment used to treat genitourinary abnormalities. As a result, the lives of many children have been prolonged and improved by treatment of these disorders (Hoyler-Grant, 1995b).

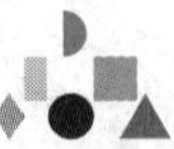

Assessment of the Child with Alterations in Genitourinary Status

Focused Health History

In the focused health history, the nurse collects data that may indicate a primary or secondary condition affecting genitourinary function (Chart 19–1). Many signs and symptoms of genitourinary and renal conditions are subtle, such as mild abdominal pain, low-grade fever, slow weight gain, and edema. It may be difficult to determine when symptoms began because clinical signs may have gone unnoted for some time before the current health care visit.

The nurse should obtain a detailed history of the child's voiding pattern. Solicit information about frequency of urination, presence of pain or burning during voiding, the color and odor of the urine, and the presence of enuresis, abdominal pain, or flank pain.

Any recent colds or other respiratory or dermatologic infections should be noted. Streptococcal infections can

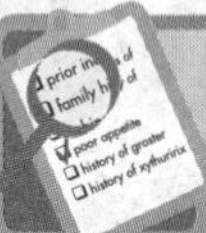

Chart 19–1
Focused Health History

Genitourinary

Identifying Data	Age and race
Present Illness	Chief complaint—reason for the visit Associated complaints Duration, intensity, frequency of symptoms Poor growth or weight gain Intermittent fevers, chronic infections Convulsions Changes in or abnormal voiding patterns, dysuria Edema Foul-smelling urine or discharge Hematuria, proteinuria, hypertension Enlargements, lumps, or masses in groin, abdomen, or scrotum Abdominal or flank pain

Past Medical History

Prenatal History	Maternal polyhydramnios or oligohydramnios Maternal diabetes or hypertension Toxemia Alcohol ingestion or cocaine exposure Use of nephrotoxic drugs

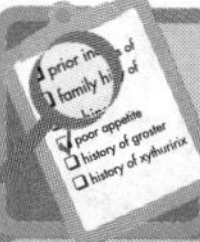

Chart 19–1
Focused Health History *Continued*

Genitourinary

Neonatal History	Birth weight Gestational age Asphyxia Presence of a single umbilical artery Abdominal mass Abnormal newborn screening test results Chromosome anomaly Malformations (spina bifida, cardiac, esophageal, rectal, pulmonary)
Childhood History	Congenital anomalies Bleeding disorders Toilet training
Childhood Illnesses	Streptococcal infections and treatment Varicella Hospitalizations or surgeries
Immunizations	Status of current immunizations, especially varicella
Allergies	Medications Latex sensitivity
Current Medications	Medications related to current treatment of any chronic genitourinary/renal disease Home remedies for current genitourinary/renal conditions
Family Medical History	Familial renal disease or uropathology Familial type I insulin-dependent diabetes Chronic urinary tract infections Renal or urinary tract calculi Parental enuresis and age at resolution
Social History	Psychosocial Educational Cultural
Growth and Development	Physical milestones Developmental milestones Habits: play, sleep

lead to antigen–antibody reactions that can affect renal function as much as 2 to 3 weeks after the infection has resolved, as seen in one type of acute glomerulonephritis or hemolytic-uremic syndrome (HUS).

A history of sudden weight gain may point to fluid retention. Reports of decreased appetite and frequent thirst may also be significant.

For a child with a history of a prior genitourinary or renal problem, information should be elicited about the condition, including any ongoing treatments, medications, or special appliances that the child is using as a result of the condition.

Family medical history is important; many genitourinary abnormalities in children are more likely to occur if other family members have had the same condition. For instance, enuresis, urinary tract anomalies, and renal calculi have familial dispositions.

Focused Physical Assessment

Although direct examination of the kidneys and urinary tract is difficult, the nurse can inspect, auscultate, percuss, and palpate parts of the genitourinary system and other body systems that may provide information about renal function (Chart 19–2). Genitourinary conditions, renal disease, and renal failure have particularly far-reaching effects on different body systems because of the critical role of the renal system in regulating fluid and elec-

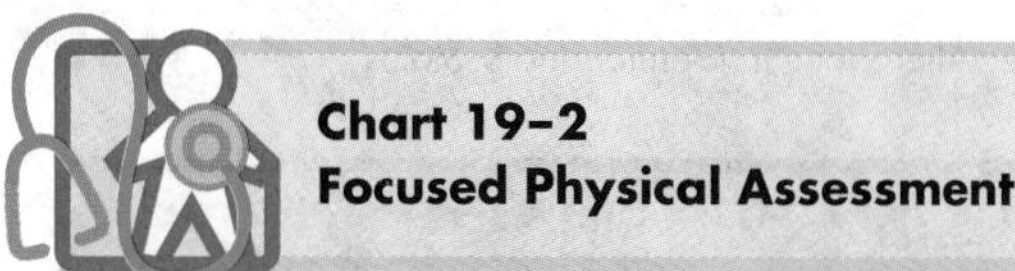

Chart 19–2
Focused Physical Assessment

Genitourinary

Assessment Parameters	Alterations and Clinical Significance
General appearance	Genitourinary abnormalities. Child may be listless or in pain. Blacks have low incidence of uropathologic disease; sickle cell disease may be associated with genitourinary complications (priapism, hematuria, renal failure); familial glomerulonephritis can occur in northern Europeans.
Temperature	Subnormal or elevated temperature may indicate infection.
Pulse	Rapid, irregular pulse may indicate fluid overload.
Respirations	Rapid or deep breathing may be a sign of respiratory compensation for acidosis. Rales may indicate fluid overload.
Blood pressure	Elevation can occur with renal failure or fluid overload. Be sure to use proper size cuff.
Weight and height	Chronic urinary tract infection (UTI) or renal failure may cause poor growth. Sudden weight gain may indicate fluid overload.
Head circumference	Microcephaly can be associated with obstructive uropathy or chronic renal failure in infants.
Skin	Pallor suggests anemia resulting from decreased erythropoietin. Dry, pruritic skin with petechiae can be caused by uremia. "Doughiness" can be due to poor nutrition or to fluid overload.
Face	Potter's facies can occur with renal agenesis. Periorbital edema is caused by fluid retention from UTI or renal failure. Low-set ears or high-arched palate may be indicators of multisystem syndrome with associated urologic abnormalities. Pale mucosa can indicate anemia. Circumoral cyanosis can indicate a heart defect with associated renal anomalies.
Neck	Webbed neck occurs with Turner's or Noonan's syndromes, which also have renal or gonadal malformations.
Cardiovascular	Murmurs are associated with anemia as well as cardiac defects. A friction rub can indicate pericarditis caused by uremia or inadequate dialysis. Hemodialysis access (catheters, grafts, fistulas) should be noted and examined for signs of infection.
Abdominal	Fluid overload can lead to edema, ascites, and descent of the liver margin. Exit sites for urinary drainage tubes and peritoneal dialysis catheters should be noted and examined for signs of infection. Hydronephrotic kidneys or distended bladder may be palpable.
Gastrointestinal	Nausea and vomiting are common signs of uremia. Some medications cause constipation; others cause diarrhea. Chronic constipation/encopresis correlates with UTI.
Neuromuscular	Fatigability, muscle wasting, and lethargy can occur with renal failure. Level of consciousness may be decreased in renal failure. Reflexes may be diminished. Very high levels of blood urea nitrogen can cause temporary psychosis with hallucinations. Gait can change as a result of fluid in abdomen for peritoneal dialysis. Check sacrum for deformed gluteal cleft, tuft of hair, vascular markings, a dimple, or lipomeningocele.
Genitourinary	Birth defects/anomalies affect genital appearance. Puberty is delayed in chronic renal failure. Amenorrhea, anovulation, impotence, and sterility are common in postpubertal young people with chronic renal failure. Palpate scrotal sac for testicular anomalies.
Skeletal	"Renal rickets" (changes to ribs and long bones of arms and legs) occurs with renal osteodystrophy in children. Bones can be so weakened from changes in calcium and phosphorus metabolism with renal failure that pathologic fractures happen frequently.
Growth and development	Chronic illness and its treatment may cause developmental delay. Alterations in body chemistry caused by renal failure can stunt growth. Children with end stage renal disease need more growth hormone than do normal children to achieve the same amount of growth. Fine/gross motor development delay may be associated with enuresis.

trolyte balance. Furthermore, abnormalities in other body systems, such as ears, eyes, or lungs, are often associated with genitourinary disorders because, during gestation, an insult that affects genitourinary development may also affect other developing systems.

A general impression of the child's renal health can be formulated while obtaining the health history. The nurse can observe for poor skin color, fatigability or lethargy, bony configurations, and abnormalities in speech patterns, all of which can occur in urinary conditions or renal failure. In particular, nurses use their assessment skills to note signs of fluid overload and electrolyte imbalance, including changes in vital signs and the presence of edema and ascites. Electrolyte imbalance can lead to skeletal and cardiac manifestations, such as fractures and murmurs. Chapter 17 presents more information on fluid and electrolyte imbalances and their effects on all body systems.

On physical examination, the child's abdomen should appear flat when the child is lying supine. A protuberant abdomen may suggest fluid retention, organomegaly, peritonitis, or ascites. Distended veins may indicate abdominal or vascular distention. Slack abdominal muscles may indicate prune belly syndrome.

Bowel sounds should be auscultated in all four quadrants and counted in each quadrant for one full minute. Absence of bowel sounds can indicate peritonitis.

On percussion, dullness or flatness should be heard along the right costal margin over the spleen and kidneys, and 1 to 3 cm below the left costal margin over the liver. Dullness heard above the symphysis pubis is indicative of a full bladder. Tympany is heard throughout the rest of the abdomen.

It is difficult to palpate most genitourinary organs. The kidneys are rarely palpable, except in neonates. A distended bladder may be palpated above the symphysis pubis. Palpation that elicits complaints of abdominal tenderness is common in UTI.

Genitalia should be examined for structural anomalies such as labial fusion in a female and hypospadias or epispadias in a male. In an uncircumcised male older than age 3, the foreskin of the penis is usually retractable without difficulty; inability to retract the foreskin may be a clinical indicator of phimosis. The testes should be palpated to ensure that they have descended. Chapter 6 presents a more detailed description of abdominal and genital assessment.

Nursing Diagnoses and Outcomes

The nursing diagnoses and outcomes that apply to the child with a genitourinary disorder should address the potentially dangerous alterations in fluid and electrolyte status that can result from these disorders. Adequate urinary and renal function is central to the efficient excretion of toxins from the body. Failure to remove waste products via urinary excretion can lead to dysfunction of other body systems, such as the cardiovascular and the musculoskeletal systems. Chart 19–3 lists common nursing diagnoses and desired outcomes for children with genitourinary disorders.

Most children and their families find it difficult and embarrassing to discuss conditions that affect elimination patterns and competency of the genitalia. If the condition is congenital, the parents may feel guilty and question whether they could have prevented the anomaly. If the condition is acquired, the family may feel frustrated because of their inability to determine what was wrong with their child and obtain effective treatment. The nurse plays a pivotal role in helping children and their

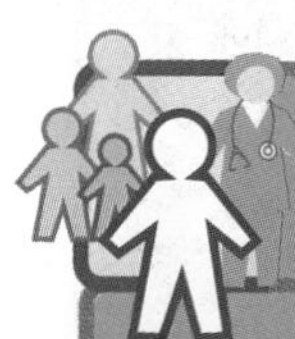

Chart 19–3
Nursing Diagnoses and Outcomes

The Child with Alterations in Genitourinary Status

Fluid volume excess related to effects of accumulation and retention of fluids, electrolytes, and waste products

Outcomes:
Child exhibits no evidence of fluid retention.
Child maintains normal electrolyte levels.
Signs and symptoms of fluid volume excess are recognized promptly and treatment is initiated.

Altered urinary elimination related to effects of disease process

Outcomes:
Child excretes .5 to 2 mL/kg of urine per hour.
Signs and symptoms of altered urinary output are recognized early and interventions are initiated promptly.

Chart continued on following page

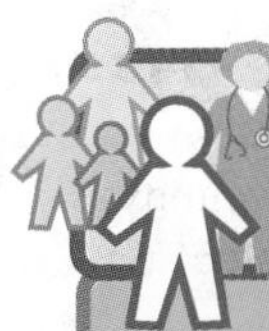

Chart 19–3
Nursing Diagnoses and Outcomes *Continued*

The Child with Alterations in Genitourinary Status

Altered nutrition: less than body requirements related to decreased intake of nutrients and increased metabolic needs resulting from disease state and general developmental needs

Outcomes: Child, assisted by the family, achieves and maintains the desired caloric intake and fluid balance.
Child maintains or gains weight along own growth curve.

Altered nutrition: more than body requirements related to poor adherence to dietary restrictions

Outcomes: Child and family are able to state which foods must be limited.
Child maintains nutritional intake that adheres to dietary plan needed to manage the child's condition.

Urinary elimination: altered patterns related to obstruction

Outcomes: Child maintains fluid balance with intake approximating output.
Child and family verbalize understanding of treatment measures to enhance urinary elimination patterns.
Child and family demonstrate skill in managing urinary elimination problem.

Urinary retention related to obstruction, sensory, or neuromuscular impairment

Outcomes: Child maintains fluid balance with intake equaling output.
Child does not experience bladder distention.
Child and family demonstrate interventions to avoid urinary retention.

Risk for infection related to effects of disease, chronic illness, medications, and invasive procedures or catheters

Outcomes: Infection does not develop.
Child has signs and symptoms of infection recognized early and interventions initiated in a timely manner.

Ineffective management of therapeutic regimen related to complex health care needs and lack of understanding of importance of regimen

Outcomes: Child and family show understanding of the child's health care needs and how to manage current needs.
Child and family develop plan to incorporate components of therapeutic regimen into their lifestyle (diet, medications, activities).
Child and family effectively manage the child's health care needs.

Knowledge deficit: care needed by child

Outcome: Child and family state rationale for care needed and demonstrate correct care behaviors.

Activity intolerance related to fatigue secondary to anemia

Outcomes: Child receives adequate rest.
Child participates in age-appropriate activities (school, play).
Family helps the child plan exercise and rest periods to be able to participate in desired activities.

Anxiety related to child's diagnosis and uncertainty of outcomes for the child

Outcome: Child and family verbalize their feelings of grief, loss, fear, powerlessness, or spiritual distress to an appropriate support source.

Chart 19–3
Nursing Diagnoses and Outcomes *Continued*

The Child with Alterations in Genitourinary Status

Altered family process related to presence of child with chronic or acute genitourinary disorder

Outcomes: Child and family verbalize their feelings to each other and to the health care team.
Child and family demonstrate effective decision-making and mutual support activities.
Child and family participate in treatment activities at developmentally appropriate levels.
Child and family implement effective coping mechanisms to work through problems associated with the illness.

Body image disturbance related to effects of illness

Outcomes: Child verbalizes positive self-concept.
Child and family are prepared for potential alterations in the child's appearance caused by the disease process and treatment interventions.
Child's peers are prepared for the child's altered appearance and provide support for the child.

families follow the treatment regimen that allows the children to live full and normal lives within any constraints imposed by their condition. The nurse can also work with the family to help the child feel self-confident and comfortable with any changes in appearance that may result from the condition. Various support organizations can provide information and other help to the child with a genitourinary condition (see Resources).

Developmental and Biological Variances

The genitourinary system begins to form in the first month of gestation with the rudimentary development of the kidneys. Between the 11th and 12th weeks of gestation, the fetal kidneys begin to produce urine. In utero, the placenta serves as a "pseudokidney," helping the fetus regulate fluid and electrolyte balance. The kidneys do not function independently until after birth, and they do not reach their maturity until age 2 years. Kidney size remains large in proportion to the abdomen throughout the childhood years, with less protection offered by the ribs and by fat padding (Fig. 19–1). Thus, children are more vulnerable than adults to kidney trauma from compressive force to the abdomen—for example, a bicycle accident in which the handlebars jam into the abdomen.

During fetal development, the failure of structures to form or the abnormal or duplicate formation of structures results in congenital genitourinary abnormalities (Table 19–1). Obstruction of urine flow as a result of misplaced vessels, or abnormal innervation can cause back pressure of urine and damage to renal tissue before birth. The cause of more than 90% of congenital abnormalities is not yet understood (Gilman & Frauman, 1997).

By age 2 years, the kidneys reach full functional maturity. In the young child, renal blood flow is slow, the reabsorption of amino acids is limited, autoregulation is not fully developed, and concentration of urine is not as effective as in an adult. Thus, during periods of fluid loss (such as is caused by diarrhea, fever, fluid restrictions, or reduced fluid intake), the child is at increased risk for dehydration. Renal function improves in collaboration with improved cardiac output and increased plasma protein levels.

Most children with genitourinary disorders are younger than 7 years old, because the most common disorders seen are usually congenital, with symptoms manifesting early in life. The most common noncongenital genitourinary condition is UTI. These infections are common in girls until they reach school age, dramatically decreasing in incidence either until puberty or the commencement of sexual activity.

Before age 5 years, diseases that result in end-stage renal disease (ESRD) are generally congenital in origin. Those leading to ESRD between age 6 and 12 years are usually the result of urologic abnormalities. The different forms of glomerulonephritis are the leading causes of ESRD in the teen years and beyond (Gilman & Frauman, 1997).

Although genitourinary abnormalities occur in males and females, certain disorders have a distinct gender-associated predisposition. For example, UTIs and VUR have a far greater prevalence in females. Structural de-

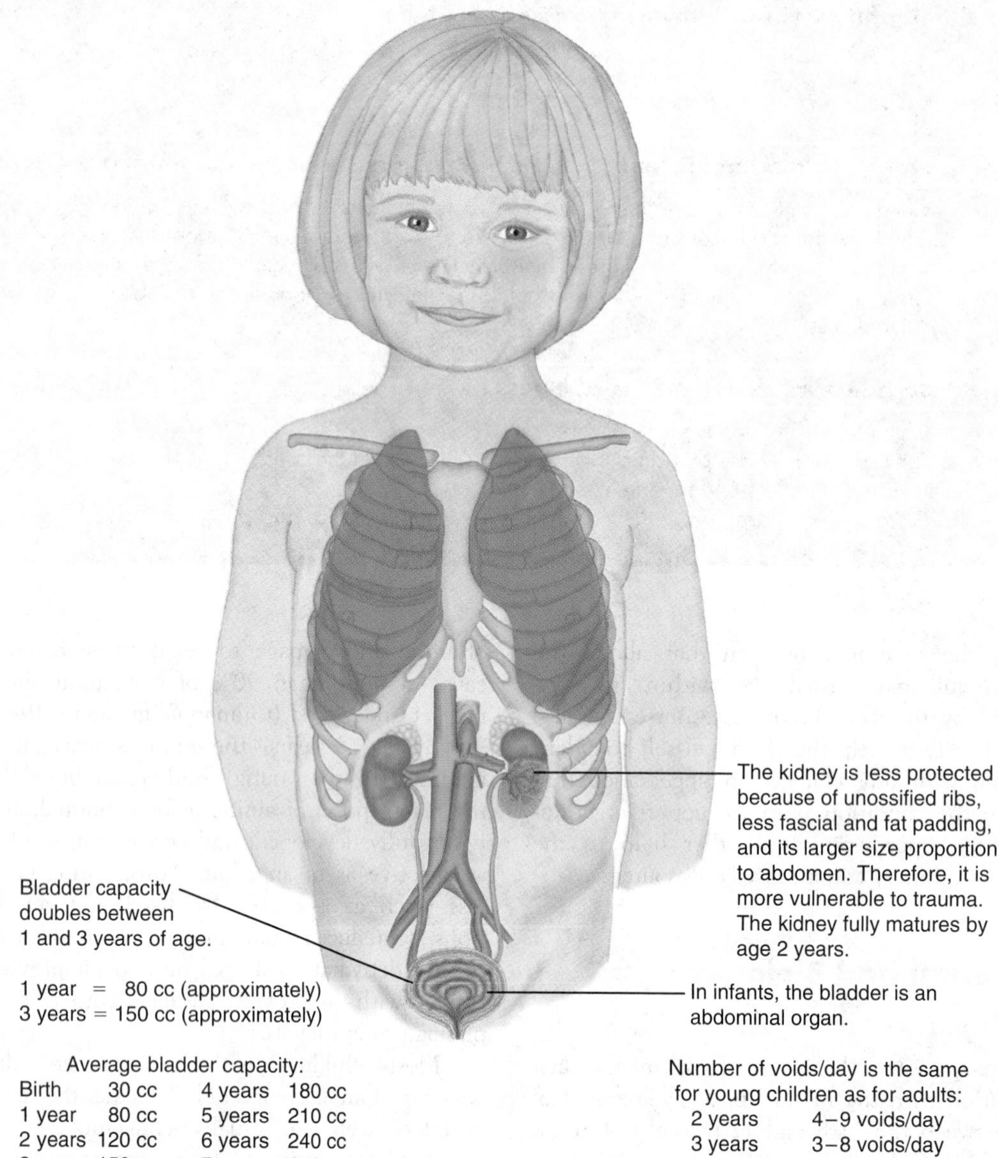
The kidney is less protected because of unossified ribs, less fascial and fat padding, and its larger size proportional to abdomen. Therefore, it is more vulnerable to trauma. The kidney fully matures by age 2 years.
Bladder capacity doubles between 1 and 3 years of age.
1 year = 80 cc (approximately)
3 years = 150 cc (approximately)
In infants, the bladder is an abdominal organ.
Average bladder capacity:
Birth 30 cc
1 year 80 cc
2 years 120 cc
3 years 150 cc
4 years 180 cc
5 years 210 cc
6 years 240 cc
7 years 270 cc
Number of voids/day is the same for young children as for adults:
2 years 4–9 voids/day
3 years 3–8 voids/day
> 18 years 3–8 voids/day
Daily urine output is high in infancy because of
1. Decreased ability to concentrate urine
2. High fluid intake
Newborn 15–60 cc/day
1 year 400–500 cc/day
3 years 500–600 cc/day
5 years 600–700 cc/day
8 years 650–1000 cc/day
14 years 800–1400 cc/day

Figure 19–1

Developmental and biologic variances: genitourinary system. (Illustration from Ashwill, J. W., & Droske, S. C. [Eds.]. [1997]. *Nursing care of children: Principles and practice* [p. 774]. Philadelphia: W. B. Saunders. Reprinted with permission.)

Table 19–1
Congenital Anomalies and Associated Genitourinary Defects

Anomaly	Associated Genitourinary Defect	Incidence of Association (%)
Genitourinary System		
Cryptorchidism	Upper tract defects, contralateral inguinal hernia	2–3
Hypospadias	Inguinal hernia, ureteral reflux, upper tract defects	3–25
Nongenitourinary System		
Congenital heart defects	Hydronephrosis, ureteral duplication Renal agenesis or dysplasia	7–28
Neonatal spontaneous pneumothorax or pneumomediastinum	Renal anomalies	19
Scoliosis or kyphosis	Upper tract defects	33
Femoral avascular necrosis	Upper tract defects	4
Polydactyly, oligodactyly	Renal agenesis, ureteral duplication	Unknown
Imperforate anus	Reflux	17–38
Supernumerary nipples	Ureteropelvic junction obstruction, bilateral polycystic kidneys, double collecting system	Male: 20–40 Female: 5–10
Facial anomalies, oligohydramnios, hypoplastic lungs (Potter's syndrome)	Renal agenesis or posterior ureteral valves	100
Low-set ears, malformed ears	Hydronephrosis, renal agenesis, duplication, hypospadias	Unknown
Single umbilical artery	Renal defects	Variable
Female genital anomalies—bifid or bicornuate uterus, vaginal septum or agenesis	Unilateral renal agenesis, renal fusion, ureteral ectopia	90

From Hoyler-Grant, C. (1995). Health assessment of the pediatric urology patient. In K. A. Karlowicz (Ed.), *Urologic nursing: Principles and practice.* Philadelphia: W B Saunders. Reprinted with permission.

fects of the genitourinary organs, however, are found almost exclusively in males. These include hypospadias, epispadias, cryptorchidism, inguinal hernia, hydrocele, varicocele, and posterior urethral web or valve.

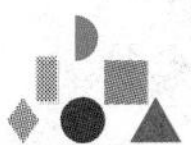

Diagnostic Criteria for Evaluating Alterations in Genitourinary Status

Various diagnostic tests are used to evaluate genitourinary function. These include laboratory studies of blood, laboratory studies of urine, radiographic and other imaging studies, microscopic study of biopsy samples, and direct observation of parts of the system using such techniques as endoscopy. Table 19–2 describes common diagnostic studies for evaluating the genitourinary system.

Urine Specimen Collection

Several methods are used to obtain urine samples (see Chapter 9 for further description of these techniques). The choice of method is based on the reason for testing the urine and on the child's ability to void. **Midstream urine samples** are the easiest samples to obtain and are satisfactory for most routine urinalysis studies. The child is asked to void normally, allowing the initial stream to be discarded. This washes away external debris. The specimen container is then held in place to capture 30 to 60 mL of urine. The remaining urine is excreted in the toilet.

caREminder: *Many children have difficulty voiding on command. When it is anticipated that a urine sample will be needed during an examination, the nurse should remind the parent to offer fluids to the child on the trip to the office or clinic or have the specimen collected at home using the appropriate collection technique.*

Text continued on page 1124

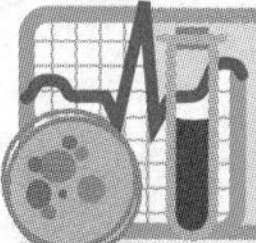

Table 19–2
Diagnostic Tests and Procedures for Evaluating Genitourinary Status

Diagnostic Test or Procedure	Purpose	Normal Findings	Abnormal Finding Indication	Health Care Provider Considerations
Blood Studies				
CBC-WBC	To determine number of white blood cells in blood	Newborn: 9000–30,000/mm³ 0–2 years: 6000–17,000/mm³ >2 years: 5000–10,000/mm³	Elevated in presence of infection or inflammation	Deliver specimen to laboratory within 4 hours of drawing blood
Hemoglobin	To determine total concentration of hemoglobin in peripheral blood; to test for anemia	Newborn: 14–24 g/dL Infant: 10–15 g/dL Child: 11–16 g/dL	Lower in presence of renal parenchymal disease, obstructive uropathy	None
Hematocrit	Percentage of red blood cells to total volume of blood	Newborn: 44–64% Infant: 30–40% Child: 31–43%	Lower in presence of renal parenchymal disease, obstructive uropathy	None
Clotting studies	To determine prothrombin and partial thromboplastin time, thus evaluating the extrinsic coagulation system	Prothrombin time (sec) Newborn: 12–17 Child: 11–13 Partial thromboplastin time (sec) Newborn: 25–45 Child: 30–45 Thrombin time (sec) Newborn: 12–16 Child: 7–12	Prolonged in children experiencing renal complications Thrombocytopenia	If insufficient blood is added to a citrate-containing tube, a falsely elevated prothrombin time may result. Do not obtain blood sample for test within 3 hours of a heparin dose.
Serum chemistries (blood urea nitrogen, creatinine, electrolytes, calcium, phosphorus, total protein, albumin, glucose, uric acid, and cholesterol)	To evaluate fluid and electrolyte status in presence of acute or chronic renal failure.	Elevated levels indicative of renal disease	None	
Triglycerides	To evaluate for hyperlipidemia, which is common in renal failure		Elevated in children with acute or chronic renal failure	Patient should fast 12 to 14 hours before sample is drawn.
Erythrocyte sedimentation rate (ESR)	A nonspecific test to detect inflammatory or infectious disease	Newborn: 0–2 mm/hr Child: 0–20 mm/hr	Elevated levels suggest urinary tract infection.	None
C-reactive protein	Nonspecific test to diagnose infection or inflammation	<0.8 mg/dL	Elevated levels indicate presence of disease.	None
Immunoglobulin A (IgA) Immunoglobulin G (IgG) Immunoglobulin M (IgM)	To evaluate quantity of individual immunoglobulin isotypes and to assess specific antibody responses to certain antigens	Normal range varies with child's age.	Immunoglobulin deficiencies or antibody response present to antigens such as *Haemophilus influenzae*, poliovirus, tetanus.	If samples containing macroglobulins or cold agglutins are handled at increased temperatures, false low values may result.

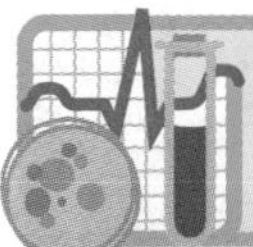

Table 19–2
Diagnostic Tests and Procedures for Evaluating Genitourinary Status *Continued*

Diagnostic Test or Procedure	Purpose	Normal Findings	Abnormal Finding Indication	Health Care Provider Considerations
Serology	To identify an infectious agent by demonstration of a specific humoral immune response (specific antibody formation)	Negative	Antibody formation present. Antibodies are produced in most group A streptococcal infections.	Whole blood is obtained and allowed to clot.
Urine Studies				
Urinalysis				
Blood	To determine presence of RBCs in urine	0–2 RBCs high-power field	Elevated levels indicate possible UTI, calculus, trauma, urethral obstruction, renal parenchymal disease.	When obtaining urine sample from adolescent females, question about presence of menstruation.
Glucose	To determine presence of sugar in urine	Negative	Presence of glucose may indicate diabetes mellitus, a potential cause for nocturnal enuresis.	None
Specific gravity (sp gr)	A measure of the concentration of particles in the urine to evaluates the concentrating and excretory ability of the kidneys	Newborn: 1.001–1.015 Child: 1.001–1.025	Low—diabetes insipidus, pyelonephritis, renal damage High—dehydration	To accurately determine sp gr, use first morning void. If not analyzed immediately, refrigerate the urine.
Leukocyte esterase (LE)	To detect leukocyte esterase, an enzyme which breaks down WBCs	Negative	Positive dipstick testing indicates probable UTI.	Obtain midstream, clean catch urine sample. Test may not be accurate for children. False-positive results in urine mixed with vaginal secretions. False-negative results in urine with high protein levels or raised ascorbic acid levels.
Nitrites	To indicate conversion of nitrate to nitrite by bacteria	Negative	Positive test may indicate bacteriuria.	False-negative result occurs often with children. Obtain midstream clean catch sample from adolescent females.
Protein	To indicate renal disease	Negative—<8 mg/dL	Positive test indicates renal disease.	False-positive result occurs after strenuous activity or stress. Obtain first morning void; keep refrigerated.

Table continued on following page

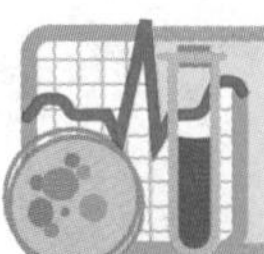

Table 19–2
Diagnostic Tests and Procedures for Evaluating Genitourinary Status *Continued*

Diagnostic Test or Procedure	Purpose	Normal Findings	Abnormal Finding Indication	Health Care Provider Considerations
pH	To indicate acid/base balance of patient	4.6–8.0 (average 6.0)	Increased in presence of bacteriuria	Urine becomes alkaline upon standing. Foods may affect pH: citrus fruits, dairy products, vegetables cause alkaline urine. Meat and fruits (e.g., cranberry) cause acidic urine.
Creatinine clearance	To assess glomerular filtration rate from timed (4–24 hour) urine collection and blood sampling.	Creatinine clearance values should be close to glomerular filtration rate values.	Increased levels indicate renal failure.	Refrigerate urine collection as retrieved. To the collection bottle, attach a sticker indicating the date and times urine collection started and stopped, and the child's height and weight.
Urine Microscopic Studies				
WBC	To detect WBCs in urine	0–4/high-power field	>5 indicates pyuria	Obtain midstream clean catch urine from females.
Bacteria	To detect UTI	Negative	Positive visible bacteria	Difficult to detect Obtain midstream clean catch sample to avoid contamination.
Microbiologic Studies				
Urine culture and sensitivity Peritoneal dialysate culture and sensitivity	To determine the presence of bacterial pathogens. To determine the type of bacteria. To determine how effectively various antibiotics will inhibit bacterial growth.	No growth <100,000 cfu/mL of dialysate	>100,000 cfu/mL Lower counts are diagnostic for certain urine specimens. Sensitivity reported by zone of inhibition or by degree of sensitivity/resistance per antibiotic	Obtain midstream, clean catch samples. Young or non–toilet-trained children may require suprapubic aspiration or catheterization. If unable to process urine within 30 minutes, refrigerate sample. Obtain sample before initiating antibiotic therapy. Obtain dialysate sample in sterile manner.
Radiologic Studies				
Kidney, ureter, and bladder (KUB, or flat plate)	Screening study to check for urinary calculi and to assess location, size, and shape of urinary organs.	Normal organ placement and size, no calculi, normal gas pattern	Abnormal findings require further testing.	Barium from other radiologic studies may interfere. No special preparation

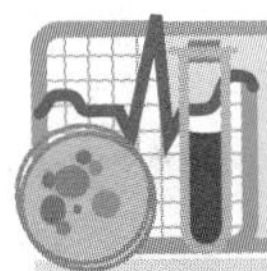

Table 19–2
Diagnostic Tests and Procedures for Evaluating Genitourinary Status *Continued*

Diagnostic Test or Procedure	Purpose	Normal Findings	Abnormal Finding Indication	Health Care Provider Considerations
Ultrasound (sonogram)	Use of reflected sound waves to evaluate kidney, bladder, ureters, and fetal urinary system	Normal structures	Useful initial study to evaluate urinary structures, abdominal masses, hydronephrosis, urinary calculi. Used during shock wave lithotripsy to focus on the urinary stone.	No preparation No radiation No contrast material used
Intravenous pyelogram (IVP) or excretory urogram	To evaluate kidneys and internal drainage structures. Renal function is demonstrated by contrast material being filtered and excreted by kidney.	Normal anatomy and normal function	Can diagnose multiple congenital anomalies, calculi, obstruction, tumors	Bowel preparation is required. Barium in bowel interferes with study. Contraindication is allergy to iodine or shellfish. Increase fluids after study.
Voiding cystourethrogram (VCUG)	To visualize bladder and urethra, evaluate urine flow during bladder emptying To evaluate effects of reflux on upper urinary tract	Complete emptying, no reflux, smooth bladder, no urethral anomalies	Vesicoureteral reflux, lower urinary tract trauma, tumors, pelvic masses, urethral obstruction	Not to be performed in the presence of a UTI Requires catheterization
Renal scan (scintigraphy)	Injected radioisotope to evaluate anatomy and function of renal parenchyma		Pyelonephritis, urinary obstruction, nonfunctioning kidney (which may not be visualized by an IVP), tumor, abscess, trauma	Do not schedule within 24 hours after IVP. Minimal radiation exposure Patient should be well hydrated. Radioactive tracer is excreted within 24 hours. Requires intravenous injection
Dimercaptosuccinic acid (DMSA)	Defines the parenchymal tissue and outlines defects in the cortex	Normal renal tissue		
Diethylenetriamine pentaacetic acid (DTPA)	Evaluates renal function; used to detect kidney obstruction when diuretic medication is included with the scan	Normal renal function, normal time to excrete dye		
Computed tomography (CT)	To visualize horizontal or vertical cross section of kidney; to determine nature of tissue material. Use of iodine contrast dye enhances the image.	Normal	Renal trauma, tumor, cyst, hematoma, calculi, congenital anomalies	Requires intravenous injection Patient must not move during procedure—child or infant is sedated. Inquire about allergy to shellfish or iodine. Equipment may induce feelings of claustrophobia.
Additional Tests				
Cystoscopy	To directly visualize urethra and bladder, bladder trigone, ureteral orifices	Normal structures	Urethral strictures, urethral webs, posterior urethral valves, cystitis, ectopic or displaced ureteral orifice, calculi	Requires anesthesia Preoperative preparation Dysuria noted up to 24 hours, may be intense with initial void

Table continued on following page

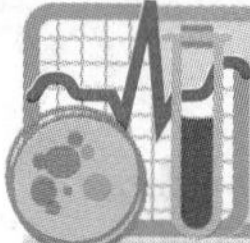

Table 19-2
Diagnostic Tests and Procedures for Evaluating Genitourinary Status *Continued*

Diagnostic Test or Procedure	Purpose	Normal Findings	Abnormal Finding Indication	Health Care Provider Considerations
Urodynamics	A series of tests to evaluate bladder and urethral function and innervation. · Cystometrogram—measures bladder capacity and pressure in the filling phase · Urinary flow rate—measures volume of urine voided in a specific time · Urethral pressure profile—measures urethral and sphincter competency · Electromyography—measures neurologic activity of sphincter · Postvoid residual	Normal	Detrusor sphincter, dyssynergia, urethral obstruction, hyperreflexia, hyporeflexia, uninhibited bladder contractions, neurogenic bladder, congenital sphincter anomaly (e.g., bladder exstrophy)	Requires externally placed perineal electrodes Requires catheterization Requires cooperation of child, who is asked to void on command and to lie still
Percutaneous renal biopsy	To determine exact type of kidney disease or cause of renal failure and likelihood of recovery or disease progression	Normal	Diseased or nonfunctioning kidneys	Conscious sedation required. Observe for signs of bleeding for 18 hours after biopsy.

When a urine sample is needed for culture and sensitivity tests, a **clean-catch midstream sample** is collected in a sterile container. Proper genital cleansing is imperative to avoid sample contamination. Boys are asked to retract the foreskin (if present), to wash the glans with an antibacterial solution, and to provide a midstream sample. Girls wipe each labial fold and then wipe the perineum with an antibacterial solution. Separating the labia and leaning slightly forward to redirect the urine stream away from the vagina, the girl provides a midstream sample. Menstruating females should use a tampon to avoid contaminating the urine specimen.

Obtaining a urine sample from a non–toilet-trained child presents a major challenge. The three most reliable methods for urine collection involve the use of a urine bag, urethral catheterization, and suprapubic aspiration. Urine may be obtained from an infant using an **adhesive urine-collection bag**. The technique is most appropriate for routine urine testing rather than for microbiologic studies, because there is a high incidence of sample contamination associated with this technique. The urine bag may not stick securely to the child's skin and it may cause skin irritation. Because adhesive urine-collection bags are irritating to the infant's skin, many nurses recover urine to be tested from diapers via the aspiration technique (see Chapter 9). However, since the advent of "ultra-absorbent" diapers, this testing method has elicited inaccurate results. Therefore the following recommendations have been made:

- Do not recover urine from diapers containing absorbent gelling material (AGM) for testing of specific gravity, pH, or protein.
- To recover urine for testing with Ultra Pampers, use a liner of 100% cotton balls.
- Use only urine from AGM-free diapers for accurate testing of specific gravity, pH, glucose, and protein (Kirkpatrick, Alexander & Cain, 1997).
- Cotton-ball aspiration is a safe and valid way to collect urine specimens from neonates for pH, specific gravity, and latex-particle agglutination (LPA) (Burke, 1995).

Catheterization involves the insertion of a polyurethane catheter into the bladder, using sterile technique. Urine may be collected in a sterile cup or in a syringe. Streamlined catheterization kits, which have a pre-placed 8-F feeding tube in a flip-top sterile test tube, are less cumbersome to use and reduce the risk of sample contamination or of introduction of bacteria into the bladder. Selection of the catheter should be based on the child's age and gender, the construction material of the catheter, and the internal and external diameter of the catheter. In general, the following sizes are suggested (Gray, 1997).

0 to 1 year	4 to 5 F, 15-inch feeding tube 6 F in-and-out catheter
13 months to 12 years	4 to 5 F, 15-inch feeding tube 6 to 10 F in-and-out catheter
12 to 18 years	8 F feeding tube (females) 8 to 12 F in-and-out catheter (females) 8 to 12 F straight or tipped catheter (males) 8 to 12 F coudé tipped catheter (males)

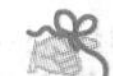
caREminder: *A sterile lubricant containing 2% Xylocaine should be used when obtaining a specimen or inserting an indwelling catheter.*

In males, the lubricant is gently inserted into the urethra and retained for 1 to 3 minutes by occluding the meatus. In females, 2 to 3 mL of the lubricant is applied to the mucosa immediately adjacent to the urethra. These measures provide temporary effective anesthesia

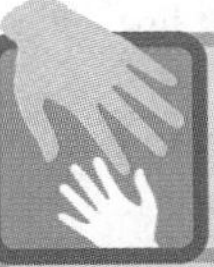

Chart 19–4
Nursing Interventions

Urine Culture Collection Methods

Method	Procedure	Advantages	Disadvantages	Comments
Midstream clean catch	Preparation–female • Wash hands. • Using front to back motion, clean labia with a towelette. • Swipe introitus with a towelette. • Seat girl on toilet with legs widely separated, leaning forward. • With one hand separate vulva, with other hand hold container. Preparation–male • Wash hands. • Retract foreskin if uncircumcised. • Wash glans of penis with towelette. Collection • Expel initial urinary stream into toilet to wash out urethra. • Position cup to capture urine. • Allow final volume of urine to drain in toilet. • Cover container. • Wash hands.	Non-invasive Parent can assist young child. Older children can perform without help if they understand how to obtain sample midstream.	Anxiety or genital manipulation may hamper urine flow. Increased rate of urine contamination if there is heavy vaginal discharge or during menses	Significant bacteriuria—10^5 cfu/mL Indicated for toilet-trained child Encourage urine flow in the apprehensive child by running water in sink or placing child's hands in warm water. Use of vaginal tampon reduces contamination during menses.

Chart continued on following page

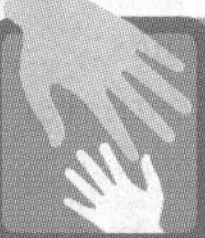

Chart 19–4
Nursing Interventions *Continued*

Urine Culture Collection Methods

Method	Procedure	Advantages	Disadvantages	Comments
Urinary catheterization	• Put on sterile gloves. • Either separate labia or retract foreskin to expose urinary meatus. • Insert a lubricated number 8 Fr feeding tube until urine flows. • Discard the first few milliliters of urine. • Use a sterile container or syringe to collect sample. • Encourage intake of extra fluids following procedure.	Not dependent on a full bladder Sample obtained quickly Low risk of contamination Prevents overdiagnosis of UTI and unnecessary urologic evaluation	Invasive procedure Requires sterile technique Child preparation time may be increased Difficult to perform if child has labial adhesions or phimosis	Significant bacteriuria—10^4 cfu/mL Indicated for child who is not toilet trained, who cannot void on command Locate meatus before preparing to catheterize: • Have child assume frog-leg position. • Hold labia with thumbs and first fingers. • Retract labia using a lateral downward motion. • Meatus should be visible. Garner child's cooperation by use of distraction (mobile, musical toy) or blow-type toy (pinwheel)
Suprapubic aspiration	Nurse practitioner or physician performs procedure. • Use sterile gloves. • Palpate abdomen for full bladder. • Cleanse suprapubic area with antibacterial. • Using 22-g, 1.5-inch needle, pierce skin 2 cm above pubic bone. • Direct needle slightly cephalad. • Apply negative pressure as soon as skin is punctured until needle is withdrawn. • Collect 1–2 mL of urine. • Cover site with adhesive bandage.	Most sterile method Useful if catheterization is difficult No risk of contamination	Most invasive procedure Requires full bladder Complications include bowel perforation, abdominal wall abscess. Requires sterile technique	Significant bacteriuria—10^4 cfu/mL Indicated for child who is not toilet trained and is unable or unwilling to be catheterized Bladder is an abdominal organ in early childhood

and pain relief for the urethra and surrounding mucosa (Gray, 1997).

Suprapubic aspiration uses a syringe to withdraw urine directly from the bladder. This method is best reserved for infants since the bladder, when full, protrudes into the abdominal cavity. Many institutions only allow specially trained personnel to perform this procedure. Bacterial count criteria used to establish the diagnosis of UTI are determined by the method used for sample collection. Nursing interventions related to the three methods of urine collection are summarized in Chart 19–4.

Freshly voided samples are preferred for routine urine

Chart 19–4
Nursing Interventions *Continued*

Urine Culture Collection Methods

Method	Procedure	Advantages	Disadvantages	Comments
Sterile urine bag	• Wash hands. • Cleanse genital area and dry. • Apply medical adhesive (benzoin) or ostomy skin preparation to help bag stick to the skin. • Remove backing from adhesive plate of sterile bag. • Place bag over urinary meatus. • In females, apply to posterior fourchette to exclude anal opening. • Remove after voiding and transfer to sterile container.	Non-invasive	High rate of contaminated samples, especially among females and uncircumcised males Positive sample does not diagnose UTI. Must be reapplied after 30 minutes if child does not void May cause perineal irritation	Significant bacteriuria—10^5 cfu/mL of single gram-negative organisms Indicated when sample contamination is not a concern (e.g., urinalysis) Negative sample excludes a diagnosis of UTI.

tests, and they are necessary for urine culture and sensitivity tests. If the sample cannot be sent to the laboratory within 30 minutes, it should be refrigerated or mixed with a preservative to arrest bacterial multiplication.

Radiologic Procedures

Radiologic procedures can be invasive and frightening, particularly for the young child who is only vaguely aware of internal body parts. Catheterization is especially feared because of the coinciding features of urologic function and sexual expression that shape the child's concept of the genital organs. Current teachings of "good touch/bad touch" sexual abuse programs further compound the child's apprehension.

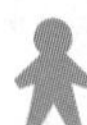

Tip: *Preprocedural preparation for the child and parents (who often welcome clarification of internal structures, too) is necessary. Helpful steps include giving demonstrations using anatomically correct dolls, showing pictures or giving tours of the radiology department, and describing the visual, auditory, and somatic experiences the child will encounter during the study or procedure.*

Child life specialists, radiology technicians, or nurse specialists and the child's nurse can teach the child coping skills (e.g., guided imagery, deep breathing, or distraction techniques) and can reinforce their use during the procedure.

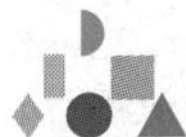

Treatment Modalities

The prime urologic functions of the genitourinary system are waste extraction from the blood stream, which is accomplished by two complex filtration centers, and waste removal from the body, through a system of free-flowing conduits and a collection reservoir. Liquefied waste (i.e., urine) is unidirectionally expelled from the body via the physical forces of gravity and muscular contraction. Conditions that impede regular urine flow act by interfering with these two forces. For example, neurologic compromise may cause voiding dysfunction by altering muscular innervation. VUR, a condition in which urine flows up the ureter during voiding, interferes with both ureteral gravitational forces and with muscular peristaltic action (secondary to dilatation and atony). Treatment for maintaining or restoring genitourinary function is aimed at compensating for alterations in gravity flow or muscular contraction and reestablishing the free flow of urine from the body. When renal failure is present, a number of treatment modalities must be initiated to rid the body of the toxins and perform the work of the nonfunctioning kidneys.

Urinary Diversion

Urine should flow unimpeded from the renal unit through the ureters and collect in the bladder. At a time that is physiologically and socially appropriate, the sphincter should relax to allow micturition by a bladder contraction (smooth muscle component of the bladder). Anomalies or conditions that restrict urine flow, such as ureteral strictures or kinking, massive VUR, or spinal cord trauma, may require urologic management by urinary diversion. Diversion techniques either incorporate the use of tubes or are tubeless. The time frame for urinary diversion is most often temporary, although some functional disabilities require permanent diversion.

Drainage Tubes

Various drainage tubes are used to divert urine flow. Foley catheters, ureteral stents, and nephrostomy or ureterostomy tubes provide an exit for urine from the body either proximal to an obstruction or through a section that may be occluded following surgical manipulation. In some cases, a stent or catheter is also used to create hemostasis within incised urinary mucosa or to act as a splint after ureteral reconstruction.

Advantages of externalized urinary drainage tubes are their uncomplicated design, their multiple applications, and their easy removal. However, drawbacks, such as increased risk for infection, mucous plugs, and urolithiasis, plus the potential for accidental dislodgment, favor the practice of intubated urinary diversion as a short-term management option only.

Nursing care for the child with tubed urinary diversion focuses on preventing infection, maintaining tube patency, avoiding dislodgment of the apparatus, and providing comfort measures (Chart 19–5). For a child with urinary drainage tubes, all aspects of home care should be taught and demonstrated to the parents before the child is discharged. The nurse should review the signs and symptoms of complications, emergency procedures, and methods of telephone contact in case of emergency. Home care nursing visits and telephone follow-up ensure consistency of care and provide additional reassurance to the family.

Chart 19–5
Nursing Interventions Classification (NIC)

Tube Care: Urinary

Definition

Management of a patient with urinary drainage equipment

Activities

Maintain a closed urinary drainage system.
Maintain patency of urinary catheter system.
Irrigate urinary catheter system using sterile technique, as appropriate.
Cleanse genital skin area at regular intervals.
Change the urinary catheter at regular intervals.
Change the urinary drainage apparatus at regular intervals.
Clean the urinary catheter externally at the meatus.
Note urinary drainage characteristics.
Clamp suprapubic or retention catheter, as ordered.
Position patient and urinary drainage system to promote urinary drainage.
Empty urinary drainage apparatus at specified intervals.
Empty leg bag at regular intervals.
Disconnect leg bag at night and connect to bedside drainage bag.
Check leg bag straps for constriction at regular intervals.
Maintain meticulous skin care for patients with a leg bag.
Cleanse leg bag daily.
Obtain urine specimen through closed urinary drainage system's port.
Monitor for bladder distention.
Remove catheter as soon as possible.

From McCloskey, J., & Bulechek, G. (1996). *Nursing interventions classification (NIC)* (2nd ed.). St. Louis: Mosby–Year Book. Reprinted with permission.

Stents

In contrast to tubes, which provide diversion of urine to an external collection device, an indwelling double-J stent facilitates continuous flow of urine within the ureter. A cystoscopic procedure is required to visualize the uretheral opening so the stent can be applied. Using a guidewire to straighten the curled segment at either end, the double-J stent is inserted into the ureter. Once positioned so that the stent ends protrude into the renal pelvis and the bladder, the wire is removed, and the stent is secured in place.

This form of urinary diversion may be used after corrective ureteral procedures or as an adjunct to shock wave lithotripsy in the treatment of large renal calculi. Children with internalized urinary diversion require no special care or activity restrictions, although a repeat cystoscopic procedure is necessary to remove the stent.

Nonintubated Urinary Diversion

Nonintubated diversion is accomplished by the externalization of a urinary structure, allowing urine to drain via a stoma. First introduced in the early 1950s, this technique quickly became the treatment of choice for long-term management of children with urologic malfunction secondary to neurologic compromise, trauma, or severe congenital outlet defects. Short-term tubeless urinary diversion is useful to quickly drain the hydronephrotic kidney and to stabilize renal function before definitive corrective surgery. The stoma is located proximal to the diseased, obstructed, or atonic urinary structure, most commonly as a *ureterostomy*, *pyelostomy*, or *vesicostomy* (Fig. 19–2).

Stomal Diversion in Infants

Stomal diversion for infants or toddlers requires minimal postprocedure skin care and urine collection management. The high volume of dilute urine produced by most of these children spares them from skin breakdown. Also, the usual stomal location in the suprapubic region or at the flank permits urine to drain into diapers, which are worn conventionally or girdle style. Tub bathing is allowed, but the water level is kept below the stoma (Montagnino, Welsh, & Hoyler-Grant, 1995).

Stomal Diversion for the Older Child

Older children requiring long-term or permanent nonintubated urinary diversion are managed with either an end ureterostomy or an intestinal conduit (ileal loop). In the case of an end ureterostomy, one ureter is anastomosed to the other and the remaining distal branch of ureter is brought to the abdomen. For an intestinal conduit, a segment of either the large or the small bowel is isolated and sutured at one end to form a sack, while the open end protrudes through the abdomen. The bowel is then reconnected. Using antirefluxing techniques, the ureters are anastomosed to the conduit. In most cases, the bladder and urethra are left undisturbed. Placement of the intestinal or ureteral stoma is carefully chosen to ensure adequate skin contact to an adhesive collection device.

The child who undergoes surgery for a permanent urinary diversion requires routine postoperative care and management of intestinal manipulation. Additional nursing responsibilities involve postoperative peristomal skin care and teaching the child and family to change the bag. The nurse periodically assesses the stoma for healing and tissue perfusion, and evaluates the site for early signs of peristomal breakdown.

The greatest challenge involved in performing faceplate changes is keeping the peristomal skin dry. Moisture prevents adherence and dramatically shortens attachment time. A meticulously applied faceplate on a well-positioned, healed stoma may last as long as 7 days. The urine drainage bag and faceplate need to be changed on a regular basis, preferably before the faceplate loses its adhesion. Over time, urine tends to "melt" the faceplate around the stoma, undermining the skin seal and possibly

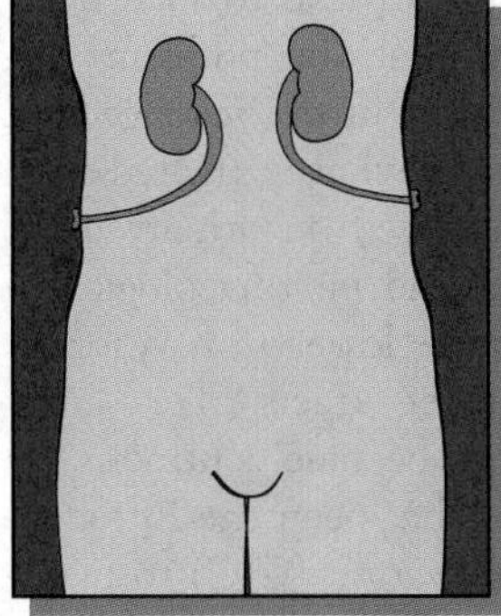

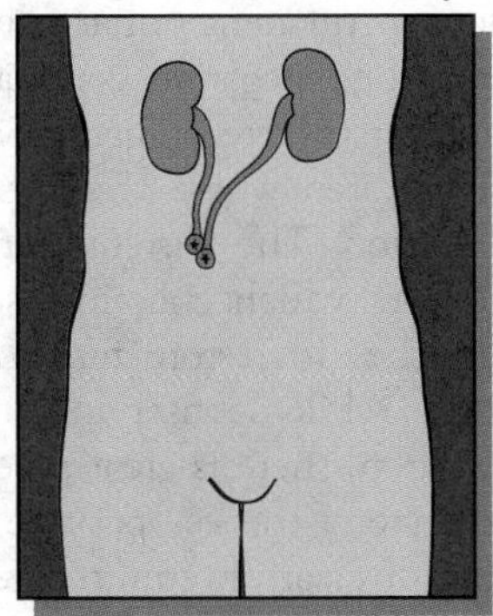

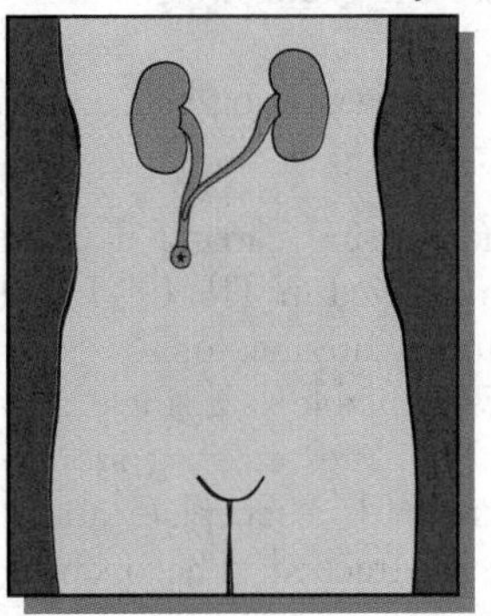

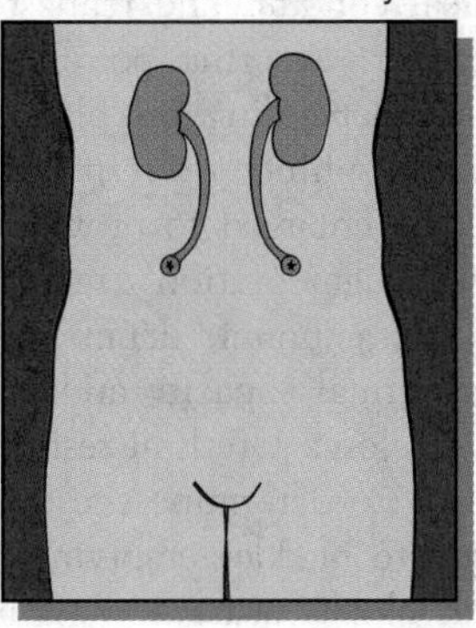

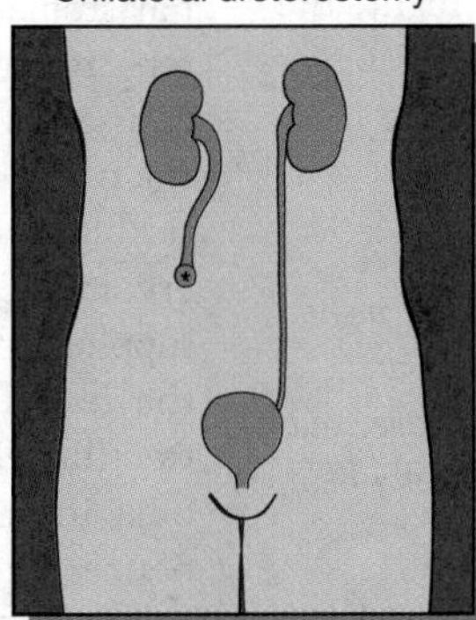

Figure 19–2
Various types of stomal diversion can be used to facilitate the excretion of urine.

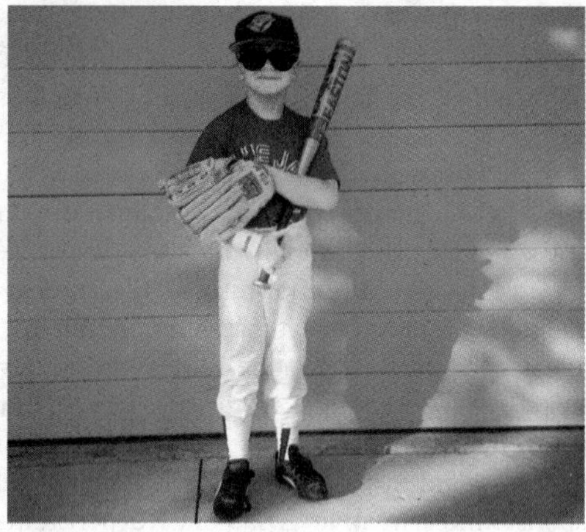

Figure 19–3
Children with stomas should be encouraged to participate in age-appropriate activities to promote positive self-concept.

leading to skin erosion. Some pointers for secure faceplate adherence include the following:

- Have all supplies ready to use before the old faceplate is removed.
- Place rolled 4- by 4-gauge pads on the stoma to wick urine during the change procedure (tampons work well for this step).
- A hair dryer set on "warm" helps to thoroughly dry the skin.
- Instruct the child or the parent to empty the bag when it fills halfway, because the excess weight may loosen the adhesion.
- Encourage the active child to wear a snug belt designed to attach to the bag.

Principles important to the nursing care of a child with a urinary diversion are summarized in TIP 19–1; see also Chart 18–5 for general ostomy care measures.

Urine collection devices are available as a single unit system, whereby the adhesive faceplate and bag are attached, or as a two-piece system with a faceplate and a rim to which the separate bag is attached. The opening on the faceplate should fit snugly, but not tightly, around the stoma to protect the skin. The bags are equipped with a spout mechanism for easy drainage. At night, the urine collection bag is connected via tubing to a larger collecting unit. This keeps the urine bag flush to the child's body, preventing leaks and increasing comfort during sleep.

Tip: *Older children may be too embarrassed by the night urine-collecting unit to participate in sleepovers at a friend's home or at camp. Placing the night drainage unit in a gym bag, knapsack, or duffel bag can discreetly hide the equipment.*

Discharge planning for the child with a urinary stoma includes arranging for the family to obtain ostomy supplies. A social worker can consult with the family to determine whether the child qualifies for supplemental state or federal subsidy. Personnel at the child's school or daycare should be notified about the child's condition and advised of any recommended activity modifications (Fig. 19–3).

Advantages of long-term stomal diversion include prevention of urinary stasis, deterred progression of renal damage, and potential reduction in the incidence of UTI. Disadvantages to stomal diversion are multiple and significant: long-term complications can be ravaging to the upper renal tracts. Disruption of the urinary tract produces extensive renal compromise secondary to the backwash of bacteria-rich urine from the collection bag into the ileal conduit, from which infection can easily ascend to the kidney. Ureteral reflux, mucus formation, and stomal stenosis are additional risks that can lead to hydronephrosis and renal calculi (Fernandes, Reinberg, Vernier, & Gonzalez, 1994; Hendren, 1990; Reilly, 1995).

The emotional effects of such a disfiguring change are often devastating, especially during adolescence. Many children remain in a constant state of anxiety, fearing urine leakage and persecution by peers. Also, the costs of lifelong stomal supplies can place a financial burden on the family (Hoyler-Grant, 1995c).

Urinary Undiversion

Although once holding promise as a life-saving procedure, permanent urinary diversion can lead to such overwhelming negative consequences that the problems encountered have brought about a shift in the management of children whose condition was previously treated with diversion. The current trend is focused on urinary undiversion, which combines surgical and pharmacologic approaches to restore function to the lower urinary structures while conserving the upper tracts. For many children, there is great potential to become continent. By far, one of the key positive factors has been the introduction of clean intermittent catheterization (CIC) to maintain regular and complete vesicle emptying.

The undiversion process entails removing the original stoma, or ileal conduit, and reanastomosing the ureters to the bladder. At this point, there are several courses of action, depending on bladder capacity, contraction ability, and sphincteric response. A small, inelastic bladder must be enlarged to provide an adequate reservoir. Bladder augmentation material is typically supplied by cecum, jejunum, ileum, or gastric tissue. If the bladder has normal capacity and good detrusor contractility, it is left alone. Urethral resistance is considered next in attempting to determine the capability for continence and complete bladder emptying. High sphincteric resistance, which blocks urine flow, is managed by CIC. Insufficient resistance, however, either requires a snug

TIP 19–1 A Teaching Intervention Plan for the Child with a Urinary Stoma

Nursing Diagnosis and Child/Family Outcomes

- Effective individual management of therapeutic regimen.
  Outcomes: Child/family will perform urinary bag changes proficiently.
  Child/family will change the urinary collection apparatus in a timely manner to prevent urine leakage and skin breakdown.
  Child/family will identify signs and symptoms of stomal stenosis.

Interventions

Teach Family to Change Stoma Bag

- Develop a schedule for bag changing to avoid the pressure of time constraints.
- Faceplate should be changed when the adhesive backing starts to deteriorate or loosen, but before leaking occurs.
- Assemble all supplies—faceplate, bag, unsterile 4 × 4 gauze pads or tampons, peristomal skin cleanser, belt, hair dryer, towel, other supplies as needed (e.g., adhesive remover, moisture cream, skin barrier, and peristomal paste).
- Empty bag, then remove bag and faceplate.
- Place rolled 4 × 4 gauze or tampons over the stoma to wick urine drainage.
- Remove faceplate residue with adhesive remover.
- Wash skin with peristomal skin cleanser. Avoid soap because it can leave a film that interferes with adhesion.
- Dry with towel or hair dryer.
- Apply peristomal moisture cream if skin is irritated. Do not use oil-based creams.
- If peristomal skin is uneven (e.g., from an incision), apply peristomal paste to even the skin surface.
- If skin is very sensitive, wipe on a thin coating of peristomal skin barrier. NOTE: Some skin barriers turn tacky during the drying process. Applying a faceplate at this point improves adherence.
- Remove the wick; carefully but quickly apply the faceplate.
- Snap on the bag, if using two-piece system.
- Clip on the belt.
- Apply warmth to increase the faceplate adherence, either by cupping faceplate with the hand, using a hair dryer, or briefly placing child on abdomen.

Teach Family to Monitor Urinary Function

- Evaluate amount of urine output; note consistent decrease in volume.
- Observe urine for mucus, odor, or discoloration.
- Check stoma for signs of irritation, bleeding, shrinkage, protrusion, or other change in appearance.

Teach Family to Contact Health Care Provider if

- Child has high temperature or persistent or unexplained fever.
- There is a foul odor, consistent discoloration, or excess mucus in urine.
- Child complains of flank pain or aching, extreme fatigue, or loss of appetite.
- Child has reduced urine output, despite high intake.
- Child has chronic peristomal skin irritation.

bladder neck reconstruction procedure or the surgical implantation of an artificial sphincter to prevent dribbling. A regimen of CIC may be instituted to ensure full voiding. Any impairment to catheterization, such as poor fine motor control or extreme skeletal deformity, may necessitate the creation of a new urethra with an end cutaneous stoma. Tubular tissue such as the appendix, a ureteral segment, or a fallopian tube is attached to the bladder and fashioned into a supple, narrow conduit with a flap-valve mechanism at the suprapubic exit site. This procedure also requires catheterization for voiding. Pharmacologic agents that mediate detrusor function may be administered as adjuncts to achieve the goal of continence (Cendron & Gearhart, 1991; Hendren, 1990b; Hensle & Ring, 1991; Reilly, 1995).

Benefits from reconstructing the urinary tract include less disfigurement, no need for an external collection device, improved preservation of the upper tracts, improved continence, and no expense of supplies. The disadvantages to urinary undiversion are either procedure dependent or related to poor patient compliance with the postoperative regimen or lax follow-up. Complications related to the augmented bladder, or the associated gastrointestinal resection, include electrolyte disturbances, chronic diarrhea, altered bile metabolism, formation of gallstones, mucous plugs, or calculi in the bladder reservoir, reservoir cancer, reflux, and ascending pyelonephritis (from chronically neglected catheterization). Stomal problems include stomal stenosis, conduit kinks or puncture, and obliteration of the flap-valve mechanism, causing incontinence (Cendron & Gearhart, 1991; Hensle & Ring, 1991). The success of urinary undiversion depends on strict adherence to the CIC protocol and vigilant medical follow-up.

Clean Intermittent Catheterization

CIC has revolutionized the management of voiding dysfunction related to neurogenic or congenital causes (Chart 19–6). By reversing the cycle of chronic bladder

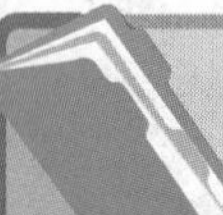

Chart 19–6
Nursing Interventions Classification (NIC)

Urinary Catheterization: Intermittent

Definition

Regular periodic use of a catheter to empty the bladder

Activities

Perform a comprehensive urinary assessment, focusing on causes of incontinence (e.g., urinary output, urinary voiding pattern, cognitive function, and preexistent urinary problems).
Teach patient/family purpose, supplies, method, and rationale of intermittent catheterization.
Teach patient/family clean intermittent catheterization technique.
Teach designated staff at child's daycare/school how to perform intermittent catheterization, as appropriate.
Monitor technique of staff who perform intermittent catheterization in daycare/school settings and document as required by state regulations.
Determine child's readiness and willingness to perform intermittent self-catheterization.
Instruct designated staff how to monitor and support child performing self-catheterization at school.
Provide quiet private room for procedure.
Provide child a private place at school to store catheterization supplies in a school bag or other carrying case that is acceptable to child.
Monitor child performing self-catheterization on a regular basis, and provide continued instruction and support, as needed.
Demonstrate procedure and have a return demonstration, as appropriate.
Assemble appropriate catheterization equipment.
Use clean or sterile technique for catheterization.
Determine catheterization schedule, based on a comprehensive urinary assessment.
Adjust frequency of catheterization to maintain output of 300 cc or less for adults.
Maintain patient on prophylactic antibacterial therapy for 2 to 3 wk at initiation of intermittent catheterization, as appropriate.
Complete a urinalysis about every 2 wk to 1 mo.
Establish a catheterization schedule based on individual needs.
Maintain a detailed record of catheterization schedule, fluid intake, and output.
Teach patient/family signs and symptoms of urinary tract infection.
Monitor color, odor, and clarity of urine.

From McCloskey, J., & Bulechek, G. (1996). *Nursing interventions classification (NIC)* (2nd ed.). St. Louis: Mosby–Year Book. Reprinted with permission.

distention, which creates mucosal ischemia, urinary stasis, and an environment conducive for bacterial colonization, CIC significantly lowers the rate of UTI. Additionally, CIC alleviates the persistently elevated intravesical pressure, a precursor for VUR and upper tract damage. An added benefit of CIC involves the therapeutic effects on detrusor function. A regularly emptied bladder, timed for drainage before distention occurs, maintains detrusor contractility and prevents overflow incontinence (Karlowicz & Meredith, 1995).

Technique

CIC can be performed on children of any age, using a catheter sized from 8 to 14 F diameter. Long or short red rubber catheters are a popular choice, along with plastic feeding tubes, although some children prefer the stability of a metal catheter. Metal catheters may be straight or have a coudé tip.

▽ **Alert:** *To prevent a possible urethral allergic reaction, latex catheters should not be used.*

The catheter should be prelubricated with a water-based gel and should be inserted only until urine begins to flow. Urine flows more readily when the child raises intra-abdominal pressure, using methods such as the Valsalva technique, laughing, or blowing (e.g., blowing bubbles or a pinwheel). The Credé maneuver to massage the vesical dome is employed only if the child has no VUR, per the physician's approval.

Sterile technique is originally used until the child and/or parents have mastered the procedure. However, UTI from catheterization therapy is rare, not because of the absence of bacterial introduction into the bladder, but because there is immediate drainage of pathogens before mucosal invasion begins. Timing of CIC should be every 3 to 4 hours, although more frequent drainage may be needed initially for continence (Lawrence, 1995).

Only minimal catheter care is required. Following catheterization, the tube is rinsed with soap and water, dried, and placed in a plastic zip-lock bag, toothbrush holder, or zipped case. Once a week, the tube can either be soaked in 1:1 solution of vinegar and water, rinsing well before use, or can be boiled for 5 to 10 minutes. Metal catheters should be cleaned internally with pipe cleaners, and the tip checked for abrasive sediment. Plastic tubes last for 2 to 4 weeks, red rubber catheters last for months, and metal tubes can last indefinitely. It is advisable to carry disposable towelettes and lubricant with the catheter for adequate meatal hygiene (Karlowicz & Meredith, 1995).

Patient Education

A preliminary step before teaching the child or parent how to perform CIC is to review the pelvic and perineal anatomy, clearly highlighting the urethral pathway. The nurse demonstrates how the normal male urethra is much straighter when held erect and perpendicular to the abdomen, whereas the female urethral tract is angled toward the umbilicus. The procedure should initially be performed on an anatomically correct doll until proficiency is achieved, before attempting the procedure on the child. Boys have little difficulty locating the external meatus, but girls often need to use a mirror affixed to the toilet seat. When the child is able to easily locate and enter the urethra with a tube, the mirror is removed.

The age to consider teaching a child self-catheterization depends on developmental and emotional factors, such as attention span, fine motor and manipulative control, family support, emotional readiness, and the ability to perform sequential behaviors. Age 3 to 4 years for the child with normal growth and development is a reasonable age to introduce the technique (Lawrence, 1995). Individualized judgment and procedural adaptation are required for children who are physically, emotionally, or developmentally challenged. Full independence with the procedure occurs later, when the child acquires a concept of time and record-keeping, typically around age 6 to 8 years.

Bearing in mind the importance of regular bladder drainage and the consequences of negligence, the nurse can strategize with the family to devise a workable voiding routine for the child. Contact with school officials may be necessary to solicit flexibility in the school day schedule and to provide privacy for the child who performs CIC at school. Because the child with a neurogenic bladder lacks sensory pathways to detect a full bladder, an alarm watch can be set to provide the needed cue for voiding.

Acceptance of Clean Intermittent Catheterization

The psychosocial chaos of adolescence may impinge on the teen's acceptance of CIC and on the teen's willingness to commit to a long-term bladder emptying routine. Driven to fit in with peers, teens who have never previously balked at the technique may refuse to perform CIC. Teens will often deny their need for assisted bladder emptying as there is a self-deceptive attempt to normalize the body and be like other teens. The nurse can offer parents anticipatory guidance about this problem as the child approaches puberty. The following suggestions can be given to enhance the teen's cooperation:

- Acknowledge and validate the teen's conflicting feelings about his or her body.
- Maintain privacy and confidentiality.
- Avoid shaming the teen, especially around peers.
- Assist the teen in creating a contract of responsibility.
- Offer either age-appropriate rewards or negative feedback to promote expected behavior.

Pharmacologic Management

Management of many genitourinary and renal conditions involves various pharmacologic agents as part of the therapeutic regimen. Medications may be used in a curative role, as in the administration of an antibiotic to treat UTI. Another approach is to use medications as adjuncts to other treatment modalities, such as in the management of voiding disorders. Thus, the nurse needs to be familiar with common genitourinary medications used in children and adolescents. Table 19–3 lists some of these medications and presents their urologic and renal applications. See Chapters 22 and 25 for information regarding steroid therapy. Steroid therapy is used in the treatment of several renal conditions.

These modalities are described under the section in Chronic Renal Failure.

Table 19–3
Medications Used to Manage Genitourinary Conditions

Medication	Mode of Action	Indication	Dosage	Side Effects	Special Considerations
Antibiotics					
Sulfamethoxazole-trimethoprim (SMZ/TMP)	Combination of antibacterial agents that block DNA and protein synthesis at differing stages.	Treatment for uncomplicated urinary tract infection (UTI). The following organisms are usually sensitive: *Escherichia coli, Klebsiella, Enterobacter* species, *Morganella morganii, Proteus mirabilis, Proteus vulgaris.*	>2 months: SMZ—40 mg/kg/day; TMP—8 mg/kg/day PO in 2 divided doses. Prophylactic dosage: SMZ—10 mg/kg/day; TMP—2 mg/kg/day PO single dose <2 months: contraindicated	Nausea, vomiting, thrombocytopenia, low white blood cell count, pruritus, urticaria, severe allergic reaction, Stevens-Johnson syndrome, drug chills, Henoch-Schönlein purpura, headache, peripheral neuritis, renal failure. *Avoid use in glucose-6-phosphate dehydrogenase (G6PD) deficiency.*	Increase fluids. Rarely, hypersensitivity reaction occurs, leading to death. Use drug with caution. Decrease dose with impaired renal failure.
Nitrofurantoin	Bactericidal agent that disrupts the cell wall and interferes with cellular metabolism.	Treatment of uncomplicated UTI. Destroys most gram-negative and gram-positive cocci associated with UTI: *E. coli, Klebsiella, Enterobacter* species, enterococci.	>1 month: 5–7 mg/kg/day PO in 4 divided doses Prophylactic dosage: 1–2 mg/kg/day PO in 1–2 doses <1 month: contraindicated.	Nausea, vomiting, abdominal distress, low white blood cell count, thrombocytopenia, peripheral neuropathy, allergic reaction. *Avoid use in G6PD deficiency.*	Taken with food or milk. May produce brown or yellow coloration in urine. Drug achieves high concentrations in urine. Prophylactic dose is best given late in day to achieve high nocturnal urine concentrations. Decrease dose with impaired renal function.

Table 19–3
Medications Used to Manage Genitourinary Conditions *Continued*

Medication	Mode of Action	Indication	Dosage	Side Effects	Special Considerations
Nalidixic acid	Antimicrobial effect resulting from interference with DNA action	Treatment of uncomplicated UTI due to susceptible gram-negative organisms: *Proteus* species, *Klebsiella, Enterobacter* sp., *E. coli.*	>3 months: 55 mg/kg/day PO in 4 divided doses Prophylactic dose: 33 mg/kg/day PO in 4 divided doses <3 months: contraindicated.	Headache, dizziness, increased intracranial pressure, nausea, vomiting, diarrhea, visual changes, skin rash, skin photosensitivity	Taken with food. May induce drowsiness. Avoid prolonged exposure to sunlight.
Methenamine mandelate	In acidic urine, drug is metabolized to form ammonia and formaldehyde. Both are bactericidal.	Treatment of uncomplicated UTI caused by susceptible gram-negative and gram-positive organisms and fungi: *E. coli,* enterococci, staphylococci, *Micrococcus pyogenes.* Well suited for chronic infection because resistance does not develop in susceptible organisms.	0.2 mg/kg q.i.d. PO. Add 25–50 mg ascorbic acid per dose.	Nausea, vomiting, diarrhea, stomatitis, bladder irritation, urticaria	Taken with food. Patients avoid alkalinizing foods (citrus fruits, milk products). Monitor urinary pH to ensure acidity. Increase fluids. Avoid concomitant use with sulfonamides.
Aminoglycosides Gentamicin Tobramycin Amikacin	Bactericidal agents that inhibit protein synthesis of pathogens.	Treatment of complicated UTI or gram-negative sepsis, effective on some gram-positive and most gram-negative organisms: *Staphylococcus* species, *Streptococcus* species, *Enterobacter* species, *Proteus* species, *E. coli, Pseudomonas aeruginosa, Klebsiella* species, *Serratia* species, *Citrobacter* species, *Providencia* species.	Gentamicin: 6–7 mg/kg/day IM/IV in 3 divided doses Tobramycin: 6–7 mg/kg/day IM/IV in 3 divided doses Amikacin: 15 mg/kg/day IM/IV in 3 divided doses Poor gastrointestinal absorption	NOTE: *All aminoglycocides are nephrotoxic and ototoxic. Renal function studies and audiograms are recommended during therapy.* Muscle weakness, elevated liver enzymes, vertigo, tinnitus, urticaria, nausea, pain at injection site, heart palpitations.	Therapeutic range is narrow. Administration requires peak and trough serum level monitoring to avoid toxicity. Avoid dual administration of beta-lactam antibiotics (penicillin and cephalosporins) by spacing doses. Synergistic effect noted during combined treatment with penicillin and cephalosporins, especially against *Pseudomonas* infection.

Table continued on following page

Table 19–3
Medications Used to Manage Genitourinary Conditions *Continued*

Medication	Mode of Action	Indication	Dosage	Side Effects	Special Considerations
Anticholinergic Agents					
Oxybutynin	Blockade of acetylcholine effects of smooth muscle, resulting in muscle relaxation and increased bladder volume	Management of urinary tract spasms secondary to intubation or surgical manipulation. Treatment for diurnal enuresis and detrusor sphincter dyssynergia by suppression of uninhibited bladder contractions.	<5 years: 1 mg/year of age PO b.i.d. >5 years: 5 mg PO b.i.d.–t.i.d.	Dry mouth, facial flushing, heat intolerance, moodiness, photosensitivity, blurred vision, peripheral neuropathy, urinary retention, tachycardia, cardiac palpitations	Patient should increase fluids during exercise or in hot weather, avoid use when febrile, start with low dose and increase gradually, avoid caffeine. Gum or hard candy may offset oral dryness.
Propantheline bromide	Inhibition of muscarinic effects of acetylcholine on smooth muscle, resulting in reduced urinary tract motility	Treatment of enuresis, urinary frequency and urgency, ureteral colic. Increased bladder capacity	0.5 mg/kg PO b.i.d.–q.i.d.	Dry mouth, facial flushing, heat intolerance, blurred vision, photosensitivity, dizziness, headache, excitability, heart palpitations, nausea, vomiting, constipation, urinary retention.	Patients should increase fluids during exercise or in hot weather, avoid use if febrile, use caution with concomitant administration of antihistamines, which may potentiate effects of anticholinergic drugs.
Belladonna and opium suppository	Belladonna—inhibition of acetylcholine action on smooth muscle with resultant antiperistaltic and antispasmodic effect Opium—narcotic analgesic	Suppression of bladder contractions following surgical intervention	>12 years: 1 suppository q 4–6 hr per rectum 5–12 years: 1/2 suppository q 4–6 hr NOTE: Dosage in children is not clearly established.	Respiratory depression, circulatory depression, shock, hallucinations, disorientation, constipation, hypotension, circulatory collapse, facial flushing, reduced gastrointestinal secretion	Potent narcotic should be used with caution. Monitor vital signs during administration. Switch to oral antispasmodic when medically indicated.
Sympathomimetics					
Pseudoephedrine	Stimulation of adrenergic receptors of bladder base, neck, and proximal urethra, creating increased muscular constriction and sphincteric competence	Treatment of nocturnal or urge incontinence	Dosage range: 6–12 years: 30 mg q 6 hr >12 years: 60 mg q 6 hr	Excitability, vertigo, insomnia, heart palpitations, photosensitivity, sweating, nausea and vomiting, urinary retention	Effects of drug may be increased with concomitant use of theophylline, tricyclic antidepressants, urinary alkalinizing agent.

Table 19–3
Medications Used to Manage Genitourinary Conditions *Continued*

Medication	Mode of Action	Indication	Dosage	Side Effects	Special Considerations
Imipramine	Unclear: may exert adrenergic effect on urinary sphincter, which increases muscle tone and functional bladder capacity	Treatment of nocturnal enuresis	1.2–2.5 μg/kg/day at bedtime.	Dry mouth, insomnia, mood changes, nervousness, mild gastrointestinal disturbances, increased diastolic blood pressure, cardiac arrhythmia, hypotension	High relapse rate. Evaluate effectiveness after 2- to 3-week trial. Restart therapy if relapse occurs. Avoid abrupt discontinuation of medication. Avoid overdose. *Monitor use. Keep in child-proof container. Prevent accidental ingestion by patient and siblings.*
Hormonal Supplements					
DDAVP	Synthetic analog of vasopressin (antidiuretic hormone). Directly affects renal tubule to resorb water, reducing urine volume.	Treatment of nocturnal enuresis	20–40 μg h.s., intranasal spray.	Nasal irritation, headache, or nausea (rare)	Quick response, high relapse rate; often used in combination with other therapeutic agents. Alternate nares with each dose.
Human chorionic gonadotropin (hCG)	Normally secreted by human placenta, hCG stimulates production of gonadal steroids (testosterone and progesterone) and gonadal hypertrophy. It may precipitate testicular descent.	Used preoperatively to stimulate testicular growth, increase gonadal size, and stimulate descent of nonobstructed testicle.	50 USP units/kg IM q 5 days × 5 doses.	Minimal with short-term use; may induce symptoms of precocious puberty, fluid retention, headache, pain at injection site, irritability	

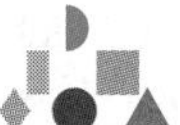

Alterations in Genitourinary Status

Urinary Tract Infections

The most common disorder of the genitourinary tract, UTI, is the inflammatory process resulting from bacterial invasion into the sterile urinary tract. The epithelial cells that line the urinary tract respond quickly to bacterial infiltration, flooding the area with pathogen-destroying leukocytes. Voiding rids the body of the substances; however, endotoxins released during bacterial breakdown cause irritation of mucosal nerve endings and localized inflammation. White blood cells (**pyuria**) and bacteria (**bacteriuria**) in the urine confirm the diagnosis of a UTI. Descriptive terminology used to classify UTI is presented in Chart 19–7.

Etiology and Incidence

Childhood bacterial UTI ranks second in prevalence after upper respiratory infections, affecting 3% to 5% of all

Chart 19–7

Terminology Used to Describe Urinary Tract Infections

Colony-forming units

Colony-forming units (cfu) per milliliter of urine
A measure to quantify bacteriuria

Significant bacteriuria

Minimum number of cfu present to diagnose a UTI
Differentiates true infection from sampling contamination
Dependent on method of sample collection
100,000 (10^5) cfu/mL for midstream clean catch urine sample

Asymptomatic bacteriuria

Significant bacteriuria in the absence of symptoms
Also called "covert" infection

Recurrent infection

Reinfection within 6 months of index infection

Relapsing infection

Return of symptoms during or shortly following treatment
Caused by inadequate treatment, bacterial resistance, multiple organisms, or medication noncompliance

Breakthrough infection

UTI that occurs while the child is on long-term suppressive therapy

girls and 1% of boys by age 11 years (Monfort, 1990; Rushton, 1995). The highest incidence of UTI is among white females 5 years old or younger; it occurs rarely in black children (Rushton, 1995). Hoberman and coworkers (1993) detected UTI at a rate of 17% for white female infants with temperature exceeding 39°C.

Escherichia coli, prevalent in the gastrointestinal tract, is recognized as the organism responsible for 80% of pediatric UTIs (Monfort, 1990). Other gram-negative enteric pathogens include *Klebsiella pneumoniae*, *Proteus vulgaris*, *Enterococcus*, and *Pseudomonas aeruginosa*. *Staphylococcus aureus* is a rare cause of UTI and only when it is the sole isolated pathogen; cultures that grow mixed flora or gram-positive organisms usually represent contamination (Monfort, 1990; Rushton, 1995; Khan, Schaeffer, & Evans, 1996).

UTI can occur anywhere along the urinary tract but is most often confined to the bladder (cystitis). Urethritis in children can result from haphazard perineal hygiene or from contact with various products, such as bubble bath solutions or soaps that irritate the child's urinary tract. Upper tract infections (pyelonephritis) are the most common serious infection of young children. They are associated with a high incidence of systemic toxicity and can result in renal scarring.

Risk factors for the development of UTI include anatomic and host factors. Anatomically, the female's short, straight urethra, situated in close proximity to the rectum, provides a convenient access route for invading bacteria. Female infants are especially vulnerable because of perineal colonization from fecal soiling. Urinary stasis is a prominent risk factor. Congenital anomalies such as VUR are a cofactor in approximately 33% of children with UTI (Hoberman, 1993; Monfort, 1990). UTIs are frequently associated with prostate problems in males (Khan et al., 1996). The rate of UTI among children with a neurogenic bladder was found to be nearly 50% (Liptak, Campbell, Stewart, & Hulbert, 1993). Numerous studies have correlated UTI with documented bowel dysfunction. This is believed to be due to pressure of the distended rectal segment and possibly from colonic seeding of bacteria via the hematogenic route.

Host-related risk factors include reduced immune response, bacterial adherence, and other unknown factors. In neonates, males with UTI outnumber females by 3 to 5:1, theoretically because of greater immune system immaturity and decreased resistance to pyelonephritis and septicemia (Rushton, 1995). The uncircumcised male infant has elevated preputial colonization, increasing his risk of UTI for the first 6 months of age, until the colony count drops. Breast-feeding, for reasons that are unclear, offers protective benefits against UTI, reducing the risk by 75% (Pisacane, 1992).

Pathophysiology

Normally, the urinary tract is a sterile system and the slightly acidic urine creates a hostile environment for most alkaline-favoring microorganisms. Bacteria that invade the urinary tract meet the first line of defense—expulsion via bladder flushing, or voiding. Anything that compromises the act of total and frequent voiding, such as an anatomic defect, constipation, or neurologic dysfunction, increases the risk of mucosal infiltration of the bladder.

Bacterial growth triggers an immune response. Within hours, leukocytes flood the area. The affected tissue becomes inflamed and edematous. Bacteria-released endotoxins, alkaline in nature, promote disease progression. Sensitized nerve endings respond with uninhibited, painful bladder spasms in an attempt to flush out the pathogens. Localized mucosal infiltration produces hemorrhagic areas. Distorted by tissue inflammation, the ureterovesicle junction (UVJ) may be temporarily incompetent.

If untreated, transient reflux permits the infection to ascend into the kidneys; the resulting pyelonephritis may cause irreversible renal involvement. More than 70% of children with pyelonephritis sustain renal parenchymal scarring with loss of glomeruli (Kimura, 1995; Shortliffe, 1995). The cycle from initial bacterial influx to pyelonephritis can be rapid, reaching completion in 48 hours or less.

Pyelonephritis in children younger than age 2 years seems to be especially troublesome. Bladder trigone instability promotes UVJ shifting during infection, magnifying the likelihood of reflux and renal involvement. Scarring of the renal tissue and frequency of UTI recurrence are more likely following initial infection. Infants acquire pyelonephritis at a rate of 7% and incur more extensive renal damage than children older than 4 years old. They have a 30% UTI recurrence rate after the first infection. Although many children maintain adequate renal function throughout life, others are at risk for hypertension, pregnancy complications, or renal compromise in adulthood (Hellerstein, 1994; Reynolds & Hoberman, 1995). Early detection and treatment, coupled with long-term surveillance, are paramount to improve the prognosis for these children.

Pyelonephritis may progress to gram-negative septic shock, a response to circulating bacterial endotoxins. The child appears moribund and may experience seizures, hypotension, subnormal temperature, and loss of consciousness. Gram-negative septic shock is a medical emergency that requires life-saving treatment. (See Chapter 30 for specific management.)

Pyelonephritis traditionally requires hospitalization for the administration of intravenous (IV) fluids and parenteral antibiotics. This regimen is designed to provide rapid, high-dose drug therapy and fluid replacement to reduce or prevent renal parenchymal infiltration. It is appropriate for the child who is acutely ill or who is unable to maintain a high fluid intake. Outpatient management of pyelonephritis among selected children has been cautiously considered. A recent study by Hoberman (1994) demonstrated comparable rates of response and upper urinary tract scarring following outpatient management.

Assessment

The classic symptoms of infection of the lower urinary tract include urinary frequency, urgency, and hesitancy, as well as dysuria, hematuria, and stranguria (stopping and starting the urinary stream). The urine may appear cloudy or blood-tinged, and may be malodorous.

When a toilet-trained child experiences incontinence, especially during the day, UTI should be suspected (Sorenson, Lose, & Nathan, 1988). Mild fever and suprapubic pain are common manifestations of UTI. Constitutional symptoms, such as high temperature (over 39°C), flank pain, vomiting, lethargy, and generalized malaise, are more serious and point to pyelonephritis.

In infants, however, the presenting symptoms are more generalized and often more subtle. Vomiting, diarrhea, irritability or crying, poor feeding, slow weight gain or weight loss, or persistent diaper rash should raise suspicion of UTI. Children with frequent, unexplained fevers or recurring infections of other systems (e.g., otitis media, bronchiolitis) may be coinfected with UTI, despite the apparent lack of typical symptoms (Hoberman, 1995).

Diagnostic Tests. When the child's symptoms suggest a UTI, the nurse is often responsible for properly collecting and handling a urine sample. Accurate diagnosis depends on selecting a collection method with the least risk of contamination (see Chart 19–4).

caREminder: *Urine cultures should either be processed within 30 minutes or be kept chilled until ready to be processed to prevent false-positive results.*

Positive findings of blood and protein in the urine, using a urine Chemstrip, are suggestive of a UTI. Leukocyte esterase and nitrate readings, although accurate in adults, are problematic in children. Leukocyte esterase is an enzyme that is released during white blood cell destruction. Positive findings are closely correlated to a UTI. However, negative findings are common even when an infection is present.

caREminder: *Leukocyte esterase and nitrate testing are often negative for the child with a UTI because of frequent voiding and lower esterase levels in the child's blood.*

Diagnostically, a UTI is identified by the presence of white blood cells in the urine (pyuria) and by a urine culture that grows bacteria (bacteriuria) of a significant number to exclude sample contamination (Reynolds & Hoberman, 1995; Miller, 1996).

Interdisciplinary Interventions

Prompt intervention for UTI is necessary to provide symptomatic relief, halt the spread of infection, eliminate systemic infiltration of bacteria, and preserve the kidney unit. Short-term interventions combine antibiotic therapy, increased fluid intake, and frequent voiding. Long-term management involves further urinary evaluation and monitoring for recurrence.

Antibiotic Therapy. Antibiotics used to treat infection of the lower urinary tract include combined sulfamethoxazole/trimethoprim, nitrofurantoin, penicillins, and cephalosporins administered orally for 7 to 10 days. The antibiotic regimen may be altered when the bacterial sensitivity results are available, generally 48 hours after inoculation of the culture medium. A repeat urine specimen should be collected 48 to 72 hours after initiation of medications. If the culture is sterile, antibiotics are continued. If no clinical improvement is seen, the urine should be analyzed for bacterial identification and sensitivities. An alternative broad-spectrum antibiotic is given until results of the culture are known.

Increased Fluid Intake. A high daily fluid intake (up to 1000 cc for the older child) dilutes and washes out endotoxins and tissue debris. Water is the recommended fluid, along with juice, soup, milk, ice cream, gelatin, and frozen liquid desserts. Bladder irritants such as chocolate and caffeine-rich beverages should be avoided. A recent study of adult women (Avorn et al., 1994) demonstrated

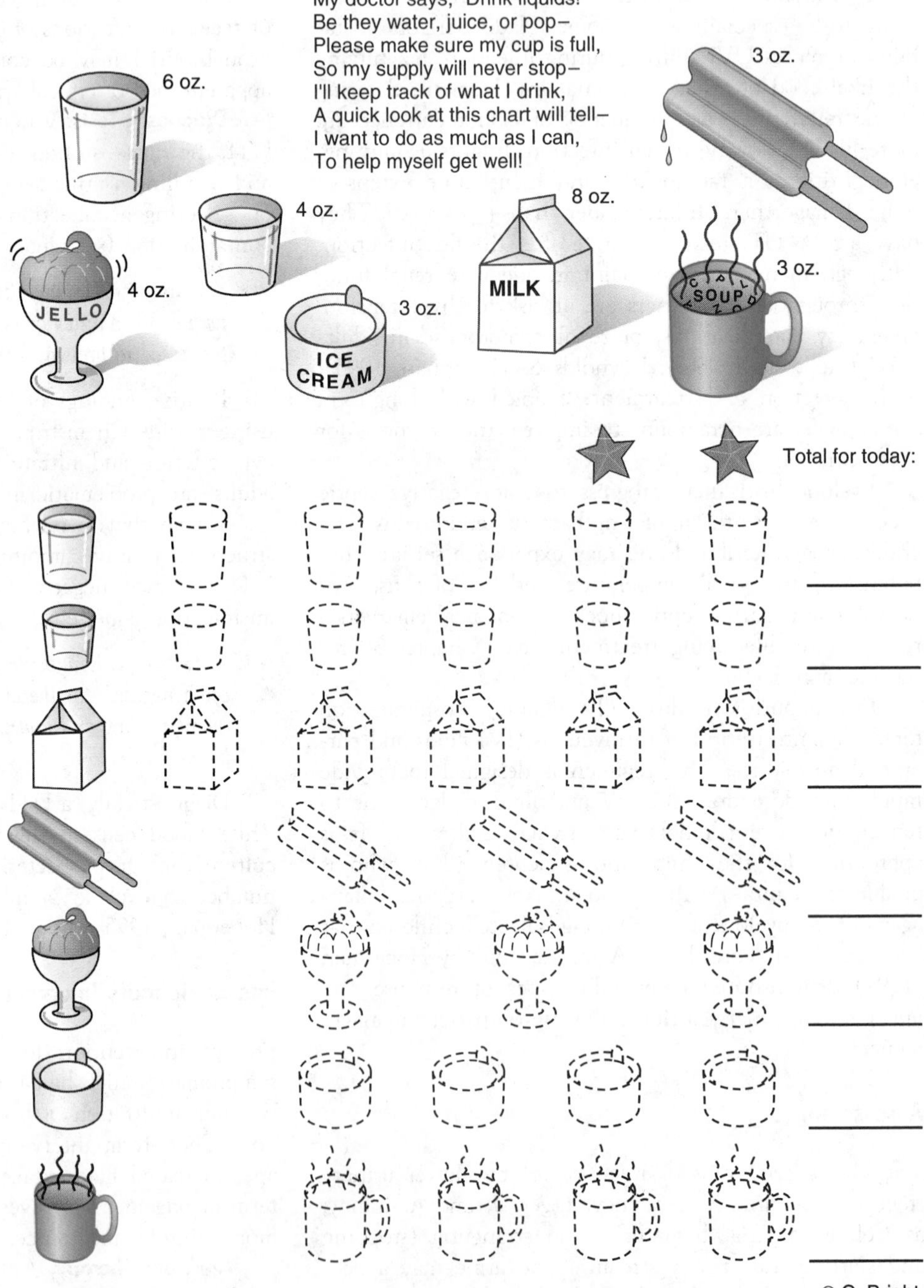

Figure 19–4
Having the child keep a fluid record may help motivate him or her to consume more fluids. (Redrawn from Hoyler-Grant, C. [1995]. Growing up with a urologic disorder: Developmental considerations. In K. A. Karlowicz [Ed.], *Urologic nursing: Principles and practice* [p. 475]. Philadelphia: W. B. Saunders. Used with permission.)

an antimicrobial effect from 8 ounces of cranberry juice daily. Although no studies have been replicated among the pediatric population, it seems wise to encourage the consumption of cranberry juice, either alone or mixed with other juices.

Frequent Voiding. Most children with UTI experience uncontrolled frequency of urination resulting from detrusor hypersensitivity. However, the accompanying dysuria and bladder spasm may cause some children to withhold urine. Localized relief can be afforded by a tub or sitz bath or with a perineal rinse during voiding. A mild analgesic, such as acetaminophen, is recommended every 3 to 4 hours for comfort.

Hospitalization. Nursing care for the hospitalized child is directed toward maintaining adequate fluid intake, either intravenously or orally, and documenting response to treatment. Vital signs, level of discomfort, and intake and output are carefully monitored. Maintaining a fluid record (Fig. 19–4) assists with this task and may help motivate the child to maintain a high daily intake during and after hospitalization. Children enjoy coloring the pictures and are proud to receive a reward sticker or star each day.

Community Care

When the diagnosis of UTI is confirmed, the nurse directs the child and the family teaching to include all aspects of disease progression and management. The nurse needs to review the importance of the consistent use, completion, safe storage, and handling of medication. The parents are instructed to develop a plan for medication administration while the child attends school, daycare, or other care situations. A home care instruction sheet is useful for the child undergoing treatment at home (TIP 19–2). It is important to discuss the risk factors that affect the child's potential for reinfection and recommended prevention techniques. Parents are encouraged to share this information with teachers, baby sitters, or other adult caregivers. Finally, the nurse needs to emphasize the importance of long-term follow-up to identify and reduce the impact of long-term sequelae.

Follow-Up Management. After the resolution of an infection, a radiologic evaluation of the urinary tract is standard practice. Females whose first UTI occurred before age 5 years and all males should have a renal ultrasound, voiding cystourethrogram (VCUG), and, if needed, an intravenous pyelogram (IVP). Abnormal findings that indicate obstructive lesions increase the child's risk of recurrence and renal involvement. Renal cortical scintigraphy (RCS) is performed during initial therapy for all infants with UTI and among children with presumed pyelonephritis. At age 3 to 6 months, the RCS is repeated to monitor for delayed renal changes (Benador, et al., 1994; Reynolds & Hoberman, 1995; Miller, 1996).

After completing the antibiotic therapy, a urine culture is obtained to ensure sterility of the urine. The child with a negative urine culture should undergo repeat cultures every 3 months over the ensuing year. If a UTI recurs, the child is placed on prophylactic therapy, using low-dose antibiotics. Nitrofurantoin or a combined sulfamethoxazole-trimethoprim preparation is the usual choice because of their low serum and high urine concentrations. Long-term suppressive therapy is recommended for the child with urologic anomalies until the defect is outgrown or surgically corrected.

Urethritis

Urethritis is a common problem among young girls. Sensitive urethral tissue is easily irritated by chemicals such as bubble bath, soap or shampoo residue in bath water, chlorine, tight or synthetic clothing, or haphazard hygiene measures following voiding or defecation. Mechanical factors such as genital manipulation in response to pinworm infestation or masturbation can likewise trigger this problem. Vaginal discharge could suggest vaginal washout resulting from the child's position during urination, or can signal a vaginal infection, or sexual abuse.

Chronic urethral and introital irritation causes some young girls to develop labial adhesions or synechiae, beginning at the posterior fourchette and advancing anteriorly. In severe cases, the vagina may be completely occluded. Labial adhesions appear as a translucent line of central fusion, acting as a hood that deflects urine into the vagina, producing dysuria (Smith, 1997).

Although benign, urethritis is alarming, because the symptoms may be similar to those of cystitis. Differentiating cystitis from a UTI is important to prevent misdiagnosis, unnecessary medication administration, and overaggressive urologic evaluation. A meticulous history and urine sample are obtained by the health care team to confirm this diagnosis.

The symptoms of urethritis can be distressing for the child and frightening to the parents. Nursing care begins with reassurance of the benign nature of this condition and is followed by guided questioning in search of the precipitating cause (e.g., bubble bath, pinworms, inadequate hygiene). Treatment of urethritis is directed toward symptom relief and eradication of the underlying irritant. Home management is summarized in TIP 19–2.

Voiding Disorders

The successful achievement of urinary bladder control is a highly anticipated childhood milestone. Delay or difficulty in achieving control after a socially acceptable age provokes a spectrum of negative responses from the child and parents—anxiety, disgrace, frustration, anger, insecurity, and lowered self-esteem. If uncorrected, a childhood

TIP 19–2 A Teaching Intervention Plan for the Child with a Urinary Tract Infection or Chemical ("Bubble Bath") Urethritis

Nursing Diagnoses and Child/Family Outcomes

Urinary Tract Infection

- Alteration in pattern of urinary elimination related to infection
  Outcomes: Child returns to normal voiding pattern.
  Child/family demonstrate skill in managing protocol to treat urinary tract infection (UTI).
  Parents verbalize signs and symptoms that indicate the child has a UTI.
- Pain with urination related to bladder spasms
  Outcomes: Family implements relief measures that ease urination.
  Child is free from pain.
- Health-seeking behavior related to prevention of UTI
  Outcome: Child/family will identify methods that decrease risk of reinfection.

Chemical Urethritis

- Impaired skin integrity related to chemical or mechanical irritation of the genital area
  Outcomes: Child/family identify irritants that precipitate or exacerbate the condition.
  Child's skin remains intact and free from secondary infection.
- Child/family pursue comfort measures which reduce urethral inflammation.

Interventions

Discuss Cause of Urinary Tract Infections and Urethritis

- UTIs are infections of the bladder or kidneys caused by bacteria (germs) that travel up the urethra and start to grow in the bladder.
- UTIs are more common in girls, possibly because they have a short, straight urethra.
- Constipation is commonly associated with UTI.
- Causes of UTI include:
  - Abnormalities of the urinary tract
  - Improper wiping after urination or bowel movement
  - Infrequent urination
  - Chemicals that irritate the urethra, including chlorine, bubble bath, soapy bath water.

Discuss Cause of Chemical Urethritis

- Exposure to harsh soaps or chemicals causes inflammation of urethral meatus
  - Bubble bath, chlorine, soapy bath water
  - Use of cleansing towelettes to clean perineal area
  - Inadequately rinsed laundry items
  - Poor genital hygiene
- Other causes
  - Itching from rectal pinworms (worse at night)
  - Wearing tight jeans or spandex pants
  - Masturbation
  - Presence of constant moisture in genital area if overweight
- Treatment delay may lead to infection of bladder

Review Signs and Symptoms of Urinary Tract Infection

- Bladder pressure/spasm before and after urinating
- Painful, frequent urination in small amounts
- Difficulty holding urine, or wetting the bed or underwear
- Cloudy, dark, or foul-smelling urine
- Stomachache
- Temperature over 100°F

TIP 19–2 A Teaching Intervention Plan for the Child with a Urinary Tract Infection or Chemical ("Bubble Bath") Urethritis *Continued*

Infants may also have

- Vomiting or weight loss, and decreased appetite
- Diarrhea or constant diaper rash
- Crankiness or listlessness
- Poor color to skin

Review Signs and Symptoms of Chemical Urethritis

- Painful urination
- Mild frequency or avoidance of urination
- Genital rash or burning
- May experience wetting or leaking of urine during daytime
- Bedwetting rare

Treatment of the Child with a UTI

Antibiotics

- Take ________________________________.
- Dose ______________________________—use proper measuring spoon.
- Give medicine ________ times a day for ________ days.
- The child should finish all medicine, even if feeling well.
- Do not skip doses. Instruct daycare, school personnel, or babysitter to give medication.

Fluids

- Encourage drinking of 6 to 8 glasses of fluid daily, especially water.
- Give 8 ounces of cranberry juice per day, which may be mixed with other juices.
- Do not give carbonated sodas, tea, and coffee.

Pain and Fever Control

- Give acetaminophen (Tylenol) at dose of ________ every 3–4 hours as needed.

Diet

- Increase child's fiber and bran intake.
- Increase child's intake of fresh fruits and vegetables daily.

Skin Care for Chemical Urethritis

- Soak two times a day in basin or bathtub for 15 to 20 minutes. Use plain water. Baking soda or vinegar may be added.
- OR, apply compresses of witch hazel three times a day.
- OR, apply boric acid compresses. Mix 1 teaspoon of boric acid powder in 2 cups of water; apply with paper towel or cotton balls three times a day.
- OR, apply hydrocortisone cream, A and D ointment, or zinc oxide two to three times a day; symptoms should be gone after 2 to 3 days.
- If pinworms are detected, further instructions will be given.

Preventive Care

- Continue high daily fluid intake.
- Monitor pattern of bowel movements.
- Teach daughters to wipe carefully from front to back after urinating or having a bowel movement.

TIP continued on following page

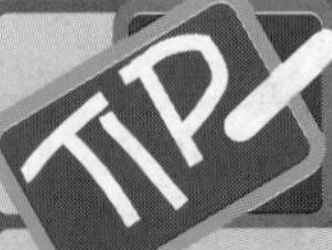

TIP 19–2 A Teaching Intervention Plan for the Child with a Urinary Tract Infection or Chemical ("Bubble Bath") Urethritis *Continued*

- Encourage showers; discourage bubble baths, soapy bath water.
- If baths are given, hair should be shampooed at end of bath and genital areas rinsed after bath.
- Genital areas should be rinsed after swimming in pool. Child should not sit in wet bathing suit.
- Encourage urination every 3 to 4 hours.
- Because the child has a high risk of another UTI, urine cultures must be checked every 3 months for 1 year.
- Child should not wear tight pants or nonbreathable materials, such as spandex and nylon.
- New clothes should be washed before the child wears them.
- Use of irritating laundry additives should be discontinued.
- Child's fingernails should be kept short and free from dirt buildup.

Contact Health Care Provider if

- Temperature of more than 38.0°C develops.
- Urine is pink or bloody.
- Child looks sick, has a seizure, or has chills.
- Child complains of back pain.
- There is no improvement in child's condition after 2 to 3 days of antibiotic therapy.

voiding disorder can lead to acting-out behaviors, childhood depression, dysfunctional family interactions, and a marked risk for child abuse. The health care team can help the child and family to manage and to cope with this condition (Butler, 1994).

Enuresis (urinary incontinence) is defined as involuntary expulsion of urine beyond the expected chronologic or developmental age when bladder control should be achieved, usually thought to be age 5 years (Willert, 1995). There are two general categories of incontinence: *functional* and *neurogenic/anatomic*.

Functional incontinence is a lack of urinary control secondary to a multitude of exogenous causes. Usually referred to as *enuresis*, functional incontinence implies mild or episodic urine leakage. *Nocturnal enuresis* is the term for nighttime wetting; *diurnal enuresis* occurs during the daytime. *Primary enuresis* refers to children who never achieve bladder control. In *secondary enuresis*, the child achieves total control for at least 6 months but then relapses.

Neurogenic, or anatomic, incontinence is a voiding disorder that results from a congenital anomaly of the bladder and the sphincter or from a disruption of the neurologic pathways that innervate the lower genitourinary tract. Examples include bladder exstrophy, myelomeningocele, and spinal cord trauma. Generally, children with this type of incontinence experience moderate to complete loss of bladder function.

Functional Enuresis

Incidence

The incidence of functional incontinence is age dependent. An estimated 15% to 20% of 5-year-olds have enuresis, whereas only 5% of 10-year-olds continue to experience functional incontinence. By puberty, that percentage dwindles to approximately 1% to 2%, where it remains throughout adulthood. Most of these children have nocturnal enuresis. Only 15% to 20% of enuretic children have a diurnal component, which is generally experienced as marked frequency, urgency, or urge incontinence (Riley, 1997; Rushton, 1995; Schneider, King, & Surwit, 1994). Most children are primary enuretics, and boys outnumber girls by a 3:2 margin. Because most children experience spontaneous resolution of functional enuresis, it only becomes a problem when the child or the parents become concerned about the interference that enuresis exerts on their lifestyle. Heredity is a factor in the development of enuresis, although the mechanism is unclear. The rate for one child to develop enuresis is only 15%, but that rate escalates to 50% if one parent experienced enuresis and to 66% if both parents were affected (Riley, 1997; Garber, 1996).

Etiology

Enuresis is thought to be precipitated or exacerbated by various interconnected factors, based on the perspective that enuresis is a symptomatic response, not a disease entity. The prevailing thinking interprets enuresis as a neuromaturational/developmental lag with superimposed familial, social, environmental, psychological, or organic mediating components. To appreciate the concept of neuromaturational lag requires the understanding of bladder physiology.

In infants, voiding occurs as a spontaneous response to the activation of stretch receptors, following the sensation of bladder filling. In spinal arc fashion, the stretch stimulus is carried to the spinal cord and rerouted along motor neurons back to the bladder and sphincter, bypassing higher neurologic centers. Micturition results from the simultaneous involuntary action of a bladder detrusor contraction and sphincter relaxation. Between age 2 and 4 years, myelination of the lumbosacral neural circuits is gradually accomplished, completing the neuromaturation of the detrusor and sphincter. This maturational process follows a recognizable sequence, whereby the child first identifies bladder fullness, but voids spontaneously, followed by the acquisition of voluntary control over sphincter constriction and relaxation, and the eventual ability to initiate or inhibit a detrusor contraction to delay voiding (Himsl & Hurwitz, 1991; Kramer, 1992; Sellinger, 1997).

The theory of *neuromaturational lag* proposes that enuretic children possess bladders with a small capacity and also experience a delay in myelination of the lower spinal nerves. The result is that these children respond with premature detrusor contractions during the filling state and cannot effectively contract the sphincter. Rather, they rely on forced bladder neck/sphincteric constriction to remain continent during the day, but they are unable to exert sphincter pressure at nighttime to prevent bed-wetting. Because most children with functional enuresis eventually acquire complete bladder control, even without treatment, the cause is believed to be a neuromaturational delay (Rushton, 1995).

Other physiologic factors may contribute to the development of enuresis. Bladder stretch receptors may be abnormal or dulled in early childhood. As the child acquires the ability to interpret bladder fullness, he or she acquires urinary control by the contraction of pelvic floor muscles or by waking to void (Butler, 1994). Numerous studies have discounted the presumption that enuretic children have sleeping disorders, based on the data that demonstrate that sleep patterns are similar for both enuretic and non-enuretic children. The sleep patterns of enuretic children do not vary between wet and dry nights, and enuretic episodes occur during all stages of sleep (Gillin et al., 1982; Norgaard, Hansen, & Neilson, 1985). Also, episodes of involuntary sphincter relaxation may allow urinary seepage (Kelleher, 1997).

Organic factors are also known to predispose a child to enuresis. Antidiuretic hormone (ADH) follows a circadian rhythm that peaks during sleep, reducing urine production by 50% (Norgaard, 1992). Research has demonstrated a flat nocturnal secretion level of ADH in some enuretic patients (Norgaard, Pedersen, & Djurhuus, 1985). Conditions that produce polyuria, such as diabetes mellitus or diabetes insipidus, may be underlying causes of enuresis.

Food allergens have been periodically identified as precipitating factors in enuresis, but few studies back up this phenomenon. Some children have experienced improvement or eradication of enuresis or urgency when chemical additives or artificial sweeteners were eliminated from the diet. It is possible that these additives may exert a diuretic effect that increases urine production. Children who responded favorably to the elimination of additives also had reduced sensation of bladder irritability.

UTI is another factor in enuresis, especially among females. It is estimated that, among 5- to 7-year-old girls with enuresis, 5% have bacteriuria with or without underlying symptoms of UTI. Eradication of bladder infection may stop bed-wetting in up to 30% of these girls (Rushton, 1995).

Psychosocial and developmental influences also can play a part in the incidence of enuresis. For example, enuresis is more common among children from lower social economic groups and deprived backgrounds, but this may be related to the disorganization that often is present in these children's daily life experiences. Although psychological factors that affect the child may affect the persistence of primary enuresis or incite secondary enuresis, no common psychopathologic disease has been demonstrated among enuretics. In a self-reported survey conducted by Butler (1994), similarities of mood and character traits between enuretic and non-enuretic children were noted. Notable exceptions, however, were that enuretic children expressed higher anxiety levels, were more self-conscious, and felt "different" from their peers. Numerous studies have shown that children with functional enuresis are more likely to exhibit immature behavior patterns or conduct disorders. After successful treatment, these children report greater self-esteem and happiness, improved appearance, and reduced acting-out behaviors, suggesting that emotional disorders are expressions of distress related to the inability to control their voiding function (Couchells, Johnson, Carter, & Walker, 1981; Moffatt, Kato, & Pless, 1987). Developmental delay, as determined by assessment of fine motor abilities and social skills, has also been cited to have predictive value for enuresis (Ferguson, Hons, & Horwood, 1986). Jarvelin (1989) collected data that correlated low birth weight and positive "soft signs" of neurologic compromise, such as clumsiness, delayed fine motor control, and perceptual dysfunction, with primary onset enuresis.

Neurogenic and Anatomic Incontinence

Neurologic control of the lower urinary tract (bladder, urinary sphincter, pelvic floor muscles, and urethra) involves the coordinated efforts of cerebral structures and spinal pathways. The urologic end result of lesions to these segments of the nervous system is a neurogenic bladder. Neurologic defects that have a detrimental effect on the urologic function are wide ranging. Included are congenital neuromuscular disorders, such as myelomeningocele, spina bifida, sacral agenesis, spinal lipoma, sacral teratoma, or tethered spinal cord, and acquired conditions, such as spinal trauma, transverse myelitis, osteomyelitis, muscular dystrophy, degenerative disorders, or residual sequelae from rectal or genital surgical procedures.

Some profound anomalies of the lower urinary tract may precipitate severe incontinence by distortion of the sphincter mechanism. These defects include bladder exstrophy, epispadias, posterior urethral valves (PUVs), ureterocele, and marked or multiple urethral strictures. Ureteral ectopia, whereby the ureter terminates at a site within, or distal to, the sphincter likewise causes constant dribbling.

There is no uniformity to the type of neurogenic bladder problems that children can manifest, even among those with similar neuromuscular deficits. Furthermore, the neurogenic effects may change in response to growth and developmental changes. Therefore, children with a neurogenic bladder must be monitored closely for accurate assessment of their bladder function and their response to treatment. Improper management of the child with a neurogenic bladder can have ominous consequences on the upper urinary tract. Renal damage or failure can develop from chronic ascending infection or reflux following bladder atony. In the past, 40% of patients with a neurogenic bladder died of renal failure; today this is a rare occurrence (Yalla & Fam, 1991).

Assessment

The evaluation of a child with a voiding disorder begins with a complete health history, social history, and developmental assessment or review. Then follows a detailed inquiry of the child's voiding function. Because parents are often unaware of "normal" voiding and age-appropriate bladder control, it is important to ask precise questions and to obtain explicit details.

Features to be assessed include age at onset of enuresis (primary versus secondary), type of enuresis (nocturnal, diurnal, or combined), history of UTI, associated daytime control problems, and presence of other health problems that induce polyuria. The creation of a multigenerational family tree may highlight a genetic predisposition for enuresis. The amount of urine voided during a typical enuretic episode can be estimated by evaluating the size of a wet spot or soaking of bed linens. Previous treatment measures are discussed as are the child's diet and any concomitant bowel problems, particularly chronic constipation. Encopresis, or stool incontinence, describes the paradoxical leakage of bowel contents around an impacted stool. When present, encopresis often indicates a neurologic component for the voiding disorder.

Psychosocial factors such as recent lifestyle changes, the effect of the voiding disorder on the child and family, and school performance are important topics to explore. The nurse can assess family dynamics by observing parent–child interactions for nonverbal clues. The parents' commitment, situations that may influence timing or choice of treatment, and factors that may impede compliance with a treatment regimen are ascertained. For example, if the child has several caregivers at home, it is imperative that they cooperate in the management plan and not send the child contradictory messages.

Voiding History. A thorough voiding history is the cornerstone in differentiating functional enuresis from more severe incontinence; it also directs the treatment regimen. Management of enuresis is aimed at controlling the symptoms, not necessarily producing a cure. The following tools are useful to ensure that all salient data are gathered:

- Voiding profile. This questionnaire is used to glean important facets of the child's voiding problem. Designed to be completed before the child's first visit, it also assists the parent in gaining a clear perspective of the child's problem (Chart 19–8).
- Voiding diary. This is a 2- to 3-week record of the child's drinking habits and voiding pattern, along with a brief description of daytime activities and the child's emotional state. The diary should include weekend days as well as school days.
- Child interview. Using age-appropriate wording, the nurse inquires about urinary habits, daytime symptoms, emotional response, and motivation level. Sample questions include the following: "Can you tell when you need to void during the day . . . usually, sometimes, never?" "At night?" "When you feel the urge to void, what do you do . . . ignore the sensation? Try to get to the bathroom? Assume a squat position, cross your legs, or press together your thighs to stop the urge or hold

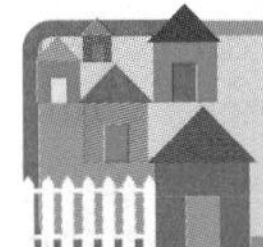

Chart 19–8
Community Care

A Voiding Profile

1. Do you feel your child has difficulty with bladder control? ________
2. Does your child feel there is a problem with bladder control? ________
3. Has there been a change in bladder control since the last visit? ________
4. List the times when your child urinates on an average day (e.g., immediately upon awakening, after lunch). _____
5. Does your child wet the bed? Yes ____ No ____ If yes, Nightly? ____ More than once a night? ____ Times a week? ____ Times a month? ____
6. Does your child wet during the day? Yes ____ No ____ If yes, Constantly? ____ Times a day? ____ Times a week? ____ At certain times during the day?
7. What has been your child's longest dry period (e.g., 1 month, 6 months, never)? ________
8. Have you tried to treat the wetting problem?
   Yes ____ No ____ How? ____
   ____
9. Does your child dribble urine? Yes ____ No ____ Before urinating? ____ After urinating? ____
10. Has your child ever had a urinary tract infection? Yes ____ No ____ How many? ____ Most recent? ____
11. Has your child ever experienced a fever that the doctor couldn't explain? Give details.
    ____
    ____
12. Does your child complain of any of the following symptoms during urination?
    ________ Burning?
    ________ Strains to start or maintain stream?
    ________ Urgency (cannot hold urine after feeling urge)?
    ________ Needs to urinate again shortly after completing urination (within 5 minutes)?
    ________ Frequency (more often than every 2 hours)?
13. Does your child have frequent stomachaches? ________
14. Does your child have lower abdominal pressure when urinating? ________
15. Does your child's urine ever look "red" or cloudy or have a bad odor? ________________
16. Is your child frequently constipated? ________________
    Other bowel problems? ________________
17. How much fluid does your child drink on an average day (including all liquids, such as milk, water, and soup)?
    ____
18. How often does your child drink flavored drinks (e.g., Kool-Aid), carbonated beverages, tea, or coffee (e.g., daily, on occasion)? ________________
19. If your child is a girl, does she usually take a bath, shower, or bubble bath? ________________

Adapted from Hoyler-Grant, C. (1995). Health assessment of the pediatric urology patient. In K. Karlowicz (Ed.), *Urologic nursing: Principles and practice*. Philadelphia: W. B. Saunders. Used with permision.

the urine?" "Is your underwear damp very often?" "How worried are you about this problem?" "What bothers you the most?" "What would change if you become dry?" "What are some good things about being wet?" A lack of motivation on the part of the child predisposes all initiatives to failure. In that case, the nurse counsels the family to delay treatment for 6 months, then reassesses the child's readiness.

- Voiding progress report. The child or parents can complete this form at designated intervals to monitor response to therapy. An increasing total score provides concrete positive reinforcement for the child and forms the basis of a reward and motivation system (see Fig. 19–4).

It is useful to observe the child while he or she is voiding. The observer should note a weak or intermittent stream, dribbling, or straining to initiate urination. These are signs that suggest organic involvement (Schmitt, 1990; Kellehor, 1997). Some girls who need to double-void, or who experience dampness, actually pool urine in the vagina. This problem can be detected if the girl leans backward or does not separate her legs during a void. The child's daytime urine volume can be determined by measuring the urine during a typical void. For the child older than 24 months, expected bladder capacity, in ounces, should equal the child's age in years, plus 2.

A careful physical examination is performed to detect signs of anatomic or neuromuscular abnormalities (see Focused Health History). The nurse specifically notes any genital abnormalities and palpates the abdomen for a distended bladder or for stool in the colon. Neurologic integrity can be checked by examining the lumbosacral spine for dimpling, a hairy patch, sinus tract, deviated or absent cephalad segment of the gluteal clef, or a flattened buttock. If any of these signs are present, the examiner assesses the peripheral pulses and the anal reflex. The child's gait is evaluated and a developmental assessment performed, when applicable (Chart 19–9).

Diagnostic Tests. A urine sample is collected to check levels of glucose and presence of blood or protein. Urine concentration of the first morning void is measured by specific gravity. A level above 1.015 excludes a diagnosis of diabetes insipidus (Schmitt, 1990). A urine culture is obtained to test for bacterial infection.

At this point, all data are scrutinized and compiled to determine a diagnosis and to consider the need for further studies. If a neurologic deficit is suspected, a VCUG, renal ultrasound, serum creatinine, and blood urea nitrogen (BUN) levels are obtained to define the lower urinary tract and screen for renal dysfunction. Sacral deformities are highlighted by magnetic resonance imaging of the lower spine. Urodynamic testing of the bladder is crucial to establish the specific type of bladder dysfunction (Fernandes et al., 1994).

Most children with voiding disorders are diagnosed with functional enuresis. An overwhelming proportion of

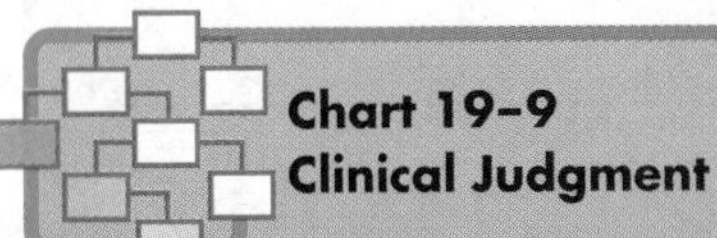

Chart 19–9
Clinical Judgment

The Child with Painful Urination

Mrs. Sternberg received a call from her daughter's teacher at preschool stating that 4-year-old Sally was complaining of vomiting, abdominal pain, and pain with urination and had a temperature of 38.3°C. Mrs. Sternberg immediately picked Sally up from daycare and brought her to the community clinic where you work. Mrs. Sternberg thinks Sally must have a stomachache from all of the candy she ate at a party the day before.

Questions

1. What assessment data would be important to collect?
2. Which of the data in the above vignette would suggest Sally has a stomachache?
3. Select a nursing diagnosis that reflects the family's need for information and home care regarding urinary tract infections.
4. Laboratory analysis reveals bacteria present in the urine, and the diagnosis of UTI is confirmed. Based on your assessment and nursing diagnosis, what is your next plan of action?
5. How would you determine whether Mrs. Sternberg understood the plan of care?

Answers

1. Did Mrs. Sternberg notice any of symptoms before today? Has Sally experienced any enuresis? Is anyone else sick at home? Weight and blood pressure should be assessed. A clean catch urine specimen or a urine specimen obtained by catheterization is needed.
2. Abdominal pain and vomiting. However, in light of the other symptoms such as fever and pain on urination, the health care team should suspect that the child has a urinary tract infection.
3. Knowledge deficit: management and prevention of urinary tract infections.
4. Teach Mrs. Sternberg the following:
   Importance of administering oral antibiotics for the full course of therapy.
   Need for follow-up urine culture 48 to 72 hours after initiating treatment.
   Need to monitor urine cultures every 3 months for a 1-year period.
   Need for radiologic evaluation to rule out other genitourinary conditions.
   Need to increase Sally's fluid intake, especially of water.
   Need for proper hygiene and avoidance of irritants such as bubble baths.
5. Mrs. Sternberg brings Sally in for repeat urine cultures as requested. She reports that Sally is drinking more fluids and that she is maintaining good perineal hygiene.

this group consists of children with uncomplicated nocturnal enuresis, meaning that they have no history of UTI and minimal daytime symptoms. No further diagnostic studies are recommended, because the rate of organic anomaly mirrors that of the general pediatric population.

However, children with a history of UTI, significant diurnal symptoms, or encopresis are at risk for a superimposed uropathologic condition and constitute a group with complicated enuresis. They should be evaluated with VCUG, renal sonogram, and spinal radiographs to screen for effects of lower tract dysfunction. Urodynamic or renal function studies are pursued if warranted (Rushton, 1995).

Nursing Diagnoses and Outcomes

Chart 19–3 presents nursing diagnoses generally applicable to the child with a genitourinary condition. The following diagnoses address some more specific care needs of the child with a voiding disorder:

- **Altered urinary elimination: urinary incontinence**
  Outcomes: The child and/or parents state their understanding of etiology of voiding disorders.
  The child achieves urinary continence.
- **Body image disturbance related to urinary incontinence**
  Outcomes: The child defines self, using expressions that indicate positive self-esteem.
  The child describes the voiding disorder as a physiologic process, rather than as a willful negative behavior.
  The child actively participates in age-appropriate social interactions.
- **Risk for altered parenting related to child's inability to achieve continence**
  Outcomes: The parents verbalize their acceptance of the child.
  The parents identify the stressors related to the voiding disorder.
  The parents use positive coping mechanisms in response to the child and the voiding disorder.
  The parents refrain from blaming the child for the voiding disorder, while encouraging responsibility in managing the consequences.
- **Health-seeking behaviors: managing urinary incontinence**
  Outcomes: The child and parents participate in a management protocol.
  The child and/or parents verbalize an understanding of the therapeutic goals of managing the voiding disorder.
  The child or parents demonstrate accurate and safe use of medications.
  The child and/or parents express realistic expectations and an appropriate time frame for the management protocol.

Interdisciplinary Interventions

Management of the child with a voiding disorder requires an interdisciplinary effort using medical, nursing, nutritional, and psychosocial health care professionals, whose skills are used as a combined approach to ameliorate the child's problem, guided by the child's acceptance and response to treatment. A summary of diagnostic studies and treatment approaches for the child with a voiding disorder is presented in Figure 19–5.

Surgical Management

Congenital anomalies detected during the diagnostic evaluation are assessed by a pediatric urologist to determine the appropriateness of corrective or reconstructive surgery. Various procedures include reimplantation of the ureters for VUR or ureteral ectopia, bladder neck reconstruction for defects of the sphincteric mechanism, and endoscopic fulguration (destruction with electric current) of urethral webs or strictures. Implantation of an artificial sphincter has been used to manage the neurogenic bladder. Bladder atrophy or a noncompliant, rigid detrusor may require bladder augmentation to increase urine capacity. Urinary diversion may be a temporary or a permanent choice in cases of massive obstructive uropathy, when the sphincteric reconstruction fails, or to provide bladder access for intermittent catheterization. For the child with a diagnosis of spinal agenesis or tethered spinal cord, neurosurgical intervention such as a laminectomy is used to release neural compression. Bladder function may return fully, or only partially; ongoing urodynamic evaluation is necessary to monitor progress (Lawrence, 1995).

Surgical techniques, even when successful at correcting urologic anomalies, do not always afford total eradication of incontinence. Supplemental techniques should be based on the residual symptoms.

Pharmacologic Management

Medications are used to treat UTI and to modify bladder activity that is detrimental to continence. Urinary antibacterials are administered when a UTI is documented; long-term suppressive therapy may be necessary for the child at risk of recurring infections. Medications that moderate neurotransmission to the lower urinary tract are used to treat urgency or to increase bladder capacity. The anticholinergic agent oxybutynin chloride (Ditropan) exerts an antispasmodic effect on the detrusor, counteracting uninhibited contractions. This is an effective treatment for an unstable or noncompliant bladder. Imipramine hydrochloride (Tofranil), an anticholinergic

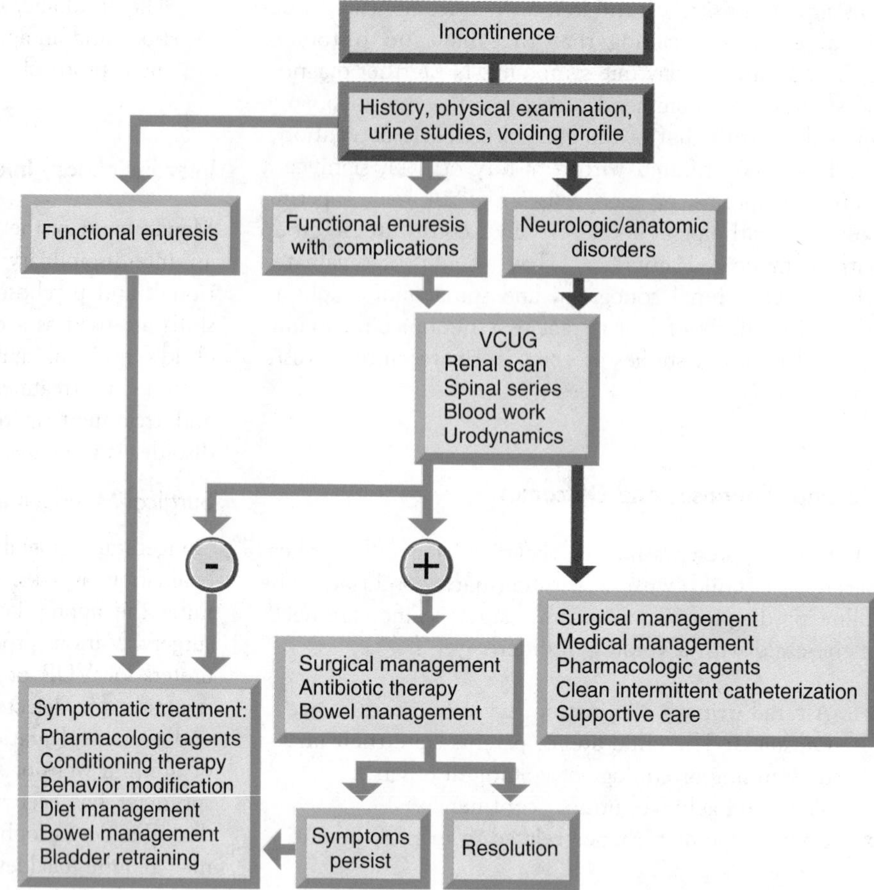

Figure 19–5
Management plan for the child with a voiding disorder. (Adapted from Himsl, K. K., & Hurwitz, R. S. [1991]. Pediatric urinary incontinence. *Urologic Clinics of North America, 18*(2), 287. Used with permission.)

and antidepressant drug, has mild sympathetic action on the detrusor and a significant effect on sphincteric constriction. It may also lower the sleep arousal threshold, making the child more responsive to the nocturnal filling sensation. Desmopressin acetate (DDAVP) is a derivative of ADH. Administered nightly intranasally, it reduces the volume of urine produced during sleep (Sellinger, 1997).

Numerous studies report initial high success rates for these pharmacologic agents, ranging from 50% to 90% for improvement or total cure. Relapse rates are also high and may approach 75% (Himsl and Hurwitz, 1991; Moffatt, Harlo, Kirshen, & Burd, 1993; Rushton, 1995). Many parents are reluctant to administer medications to their child on a long-term basis, fearing side effects or personality changes. Safety issues are a concern, particularly for imipramine, which has caused death in overdosed children. It appears that these medications are most effective as an adjunct to other enuretic therapies, to enhance the management of the neurogenic or unstable bladder, or to offer short-term alleviation of enuresis such as before camping or vacation experiences.

Conditioning Therapy

Moisture alarms work by the application of moisture-sensing devices to the child's bed or underwear. An alarm awakens the child as wetting occurs. The child is gradually conditioned to associate the sensation of a full bladder with arousal and learns to inhibit micturition. This system is highly effective (up to 70% cure rate), but requires a long-term commitment to therapy (Fitzwater & Macknin, 1992; Sellinger, 1997).

Motivational Counseling

Motivational counseling offers rewards for the accomplishment of predetermined goals or behaviors, such as dry nights, compliance with medication or diet changes, or appropriate responses to the alarm (Kelleher, 1997). Another component of motivational counseling is to encourage the child to demonstrate responsibility, for example, by changing bed linens.

This approach is often coupled with use of the moisture alarm for added improvement. The benefits derived from this intervention can be generalized to include enhanced self-esteem, improved outlook on life, and a positive sense of self-control.

Bladder Retraining

Kegel exercises are pelvic floor contractions that simulate the stopping and starting of urine flow. They can be performed as the child experiences urgency during bladder filling. Kegel exercises can be taught to children as young as 7 years, but require a great deal of practice and involved support. These maneuvers effectively suppress involuntary detrusor contractions and have been shown to be effective in improving nocturnal enuresis (Schneider et al., 1994).

Children with hyperextended bladders develop a pattern of delayed daytime voiding, up to 4 hours or longer, followed by urgency, or wetting, owing to the desensitization of the bladder during the fill stage. They require an opposite method of therapy. These children are encouraged to void every 2 hours, even before they sense bladder fullness, as a means to restore detrusor sensitivity. Multiple alarm watches are useful reminders to void on schedule.

Clean intermittant catheterization (CIC) permits regular, complete bladder emptying of an atonic bladder (see Treatment Modalities). In addition to preventing infection via urinary stasis, this procedure stops overflow incontinence. It also counteracts hydronephrosis, which results from a constantly filled bladder.

Bowel Management

Encopresis is a component of enuresis due to the constricting pressure of stool on the bladder. It is also a significant risk factor for UTI. Initial treatment of encopresis focuses on bowel evacuation using daily enemas for 1 week. Bran, fiber, fruit, and extra fluids are added to the diet. Some practitioners recommend the administration of 1 to 3 teaspoons of mineral oil daily until regular bowel function is established, although there is a concern about vitamin depletion using this regimen. Bulk laxatives also may be needed to ensure stool softness. Parents are encouraged to help devise a daily routine for defecation. These measures need to be maintained for a prolonged time span, perhaps for life, to prevent recurrence.

Dietary Manipulation

Along with the nutritional recommendations for improved bowel functioning, foods with dyes, preservatives, and, especially, artificial sweeteners can be eliminated. Caffeinated foods, such as cola, tea, and coffee, exert a diuretic effect and should be discouraged. Fluid intake for the 1 to 2 hours before bedtime can be reduced, and overall daily intake is best maintained at approximately 32 ounces (Himsl & Hurwitz, 1991; Willert, 1995; Riley, 1997).

Psychotherapy

Although most enuretic children do not manifest psychopathologic symptoms, concurrent distressing life circumstances, discipline problems, depression, and family conflicts warrant assistance from mental health professionals. Successful management of these issues is important to prevent complicating the already tenuous emotional climate for the enuretic child. Unresolved issues drain the family's ability to formulate and adhere to a long-term, often complex, management program.

Nursing Management

The nurse's role in the interventions for a child with a voiding disorder is varied (Chart 19–10). All aspects of therapy require comprehension and acceptance by the child and family; therefore, child and parent education is instrumental to the success of a chosen mode of therapy. When surgical intervention is indicated, the nurse provides preoperative, postoperative, and follow-up teaching. Medications must be fully described, including their dosage, expected results, side effects, and home safety mea-

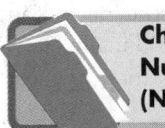

Chart 19–10
Nursing Interventions Classification (NIC)

Urinary Incontinence Care: Enuresis

Definition

Promotion of urinary continence in children

Activities

Assist with diagnostic evaluation (e.g., physical exam, cystogram, cystoscopy, and lab tests to rule out physical causation).
Interview parent to obtain data about toilet-training history, voiding pattern, urinary tract infections, and food sensitivities.
Determine frequency, duration, and circumstances of enuresis.
Discuss effective and ineffective methods of prior treatment.
Monitor family's and child's level of frustration and stress.
Perform physical exam.
Discuss techniques to use in reducing enuresis (e.g., night light, restricted fluid intake, scheduling nocturnal bathroom trips, and use of alarm system).
Encourage child to verbalize feelings.
Emphasize child's strengths.
Encourage parents to demonstrate love and acceptance at home to counteract peer ridicule.
Discuss psychosocial dynamics of enuresis with parents (e.g., familial patterns, family disruption, self-esteem issues, and self-limiting characteristic).
Administer medications as appropriate for short-term control.

From McCloskey, J., & Bulechek, G. (1996). *Nursing interventions classification (NIC)* (2nd ed.). St. Louis: Mosby–Year Book. Reprinted with permission.

sures. Developmental, temperamental, and motivational assessments provide the child and family with predictions as to the appropriateness of a subscribed therapeutic intervention. The nurse must be alert for expressions of intolerance that the parents direct toward the child and the problem of enuresis; this evaluation assesses the risk for child abuse and the potential for the family's participation in a long-term management regimen (Butler, 1994). Skin care and hygiene measures, such as the use of protective emollients and enzyme washing solutions, prevent chafing or skin breakdown related to chronic exposure to urine.

Changes in diet may require creative problem-solving to ensure the child's acceptance. The nurse can offer parenting and coping techniques gleaned from feedback of other parents or from personal experience. Through the role of a consistent resource person, the nurse can monitor progress and offer encouragement. Finally, it is reassuring to remind the child and parents that, in most cases, voiding disorders are self-limiting.

Obstructive Uropathy

Obstructive uropathy is a term used to describe organic damage caused by a congenital or acquired condition that impedes urine excretion. Common obstructive lesions within the tubular structures (urethra or ureters) include redundant tissue leaflets ("valves") or strictures at sites of segmental attachment. Insufficiently innervated ureteral segments halt the wavelike flow of muscular contractions from the renal pelvis to the bladder. Ureteral placement outside of the trigone affects compression of the ureteral orifice during voiding. Anomalous ureteral placement creates an ectopic orifice in the proximal urethra or in the vagina. Despite continuous dribbling, the ectopic ureteral opening is often too stenotic for complete urine drainage.

During early fetal development, the kidney originates in the pelvis. It gradually ascends to a retroperitoneal site, acquiring new vasculature while the outgrown vessels degenerate. An aberrant vessel remnant may constrict the ureter during the migratory process, causing obstruction. If the kidney fails to rise from the pelvis (the so-called pelvic kidney), the ureteral growth may become redundant and kink. Likewise, kinking or twisting may occur as a result of either a sharply angled ureteropelvic junction (UPJ) or following inadequate rotation of the renal unit shortly before birth.

Normal Urine Transport

Forces that maintain urinary excretion originate in the renal pelvis, because accumulated urine is propulsed through the ureter. Low-pressure peristaltic contractions, initiated within the pelvic musculature, transmit urine in a wavelike fashion past the UPJ to the ureter. The distal ureteral segment burrows into the bladder wall and is tunneled within the inner bladder mucosa. The ureteral orifice emerges within the bladder interior at the trigone. Initially, a bolus of urine spurts into the empty bladder sac unimpeded; as bladder distention stretches and thins the submucosal tunnel, increasing bladder pressure eventually collapses the ureteral lumen to prevent urine regurgitation. During micturition, the sphincter relaxation is coordinated with high-pressure detrusor (bladder muscle) contractions to expel urine.

Sequelae of Obstruction

Urinary tract obstruction interferes with the normal urine drainage process, resulting in pathophysiologic changes ranging from mild to severe (Fig. 19–6). Partial urethral blockage is initially compensated for by hypertrophy of the bladder wall, necessary to generate the elevated pressure for bladder emptying. Failure of this protective effect produces retrograde ureteral dilatation and progressive loss of tissue elasticity. The most serious insult from obstructive uropathy is the visceral destruction induced by hydronephrosis. Escalated pressures within the renal tubules and glomerular structures compromise the filtration process. Normal kidney function can be maintained until 75% of combined renal parenchymal tissue has been destroyed (Ashcraft, 1990b).

Posterior Urethral Valves

PUVs represent exaggerated intralumen folds of the anterior urethra, present almost exclusively in males. The incidence of PUVs is estimated at 1 in 5000 to 8000 live births. There is no genetic predisposition in the expression of this disease. Males with PUV occasionally manifest other congenital disorders of the urinary tract (Kaplan & Scherz, 1992).

The cause of PUVs is unknown, but it appears that they are redundant bits of embryologic structures. They may originate as thickened membranes proximal to the sphincter; the valvular tissue elongates and thins like a sail in response to increasing detrusor pressure (Kaplan & Scherz, 1992).

Because the configuration of the epithelial membrane that comprises PUV can vary from a leaflet arrangement to an almost full diaphragm, the degree of retrograde obstruction may vary dramatically. Severe obstruction is typically diagnosed prenatally or in early life, whereas mild effects from PUV may escape detection for years. The effects of chronic obstruction are insidious but progressive; PUV may become apparent only during an evaluation for renal failure (Sugar & Hoyler-Grant, 1995).

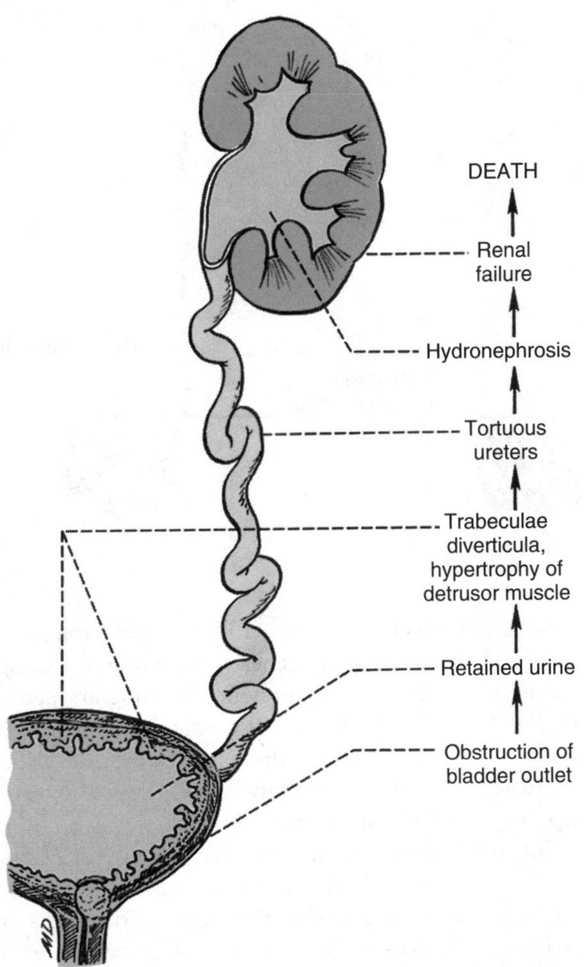

Figure 19–6
Urinary tract obstruction can occur anywhere in the upper or lower tract. This illustration shows some of the most common sites and their effects. (From Black, J. M., & Matassarin-Jacobs, E. [Eds.]. [1997]. *Medical-surgical nursing: Clinical management for continuity of care* [5th ed., p. 1600]. Philadelphia: W. B. Saunders. Reprinted with permission.)

Pathophysiology

The bladder initially responds to valvular obstruction with muscular hypertrophy. Complete voiding may necessitate intravesical pressures of up to 80 to 100 mmHg, an increase of three to four times the normal force (Hendren, 1990). In most instances, the sphincter remains unaffected and continence is maintained, but the widened bladder neck and coincidental UTI may precipitate loss of control.

Intrauterine production of amniotic fluid, which is dependent on fetal urine production, may be dangerously low in the presence of severe PUV disease. Oligohydramnios adversely compromises fetal respiratory development. The classic triad of Potter's syndrome, composed of oligohydramnios, pulmonary hypoplasia, and renal dysgenesis, is a particularly lethal outcome of severe PUV disease (Potter, 1946).

Prognosis. The prognosis for a male with PUV depends on the extent of renal parenchymal involvement. In most cases, the urethral obstruction is not life-threatening, and a satisfactory outcome follows surgical correction. At the opposite extreme, PUV can be fatal or result in ESRD. Multiple-stage reconstructive procedures may be necessary to ensure continuous urinary drainage and complete voiding.

Vesicoureteral Reflux

VUR occurs when an improperly placed ureteral orifice fails to close during micturition but rather remains open, allowing ascending regurgitation of urine. Because the reflux process is silent, the anomaly escapes detection until UTI prompts urologic evaluation. Using prenatal sonograms, researchers have discerned a preponderance of VUR among male neonates in a 6:1 ratio (Marra et al., 1994). By preschool age, VUR is more prominent among girls, however. Their high rate of UTI is a complicating factor that makes the girls vulnerable to pyelonephritis and renal parenchyma scarring.

The incidence of VUR among the general pediatric population is approximately 1%, whereas VUR is detected in 25% to 30% of children with UTI (Peeden & Noe, 1992; Shortliffe, 1995). Comparing the occurrence of VUR among groups of children with infection disclosed a 3:2 ratio for white versus black children (Skoog & Belman, 1991). Genetic factors play a role in reflux transmission; the exact mechanism is unclear but is suspected to result from multifactorial expression (Sugar & Hoyler-Grant, 1995). Although investigators have recognized a 30% to 50% risk of reflux among siblings of children with VUR, current data demonstrate a 60% to 70% rate of the phenomenon among patients' offspring (Ashcraft, 1990b; Dwoskin, 1978; Noe, Wyatt, Peeden, & Rivas, 1992; Peeden & Noe, 1992; Rushton, 1992).

Pathophysiology

Primary VUR, the most common variant of VUR, originates when a combination of anatomic factors inactivate the "valve" mechanism at the UVJ. These factors include the following (Fig. 19–7):

- Attachment of the distal ureter to bladder at a horizontal, not oblique angle
- Shortened submucosal tunnel
- Entrance of the ureteral orifice lateral to the trigone.

The extent of reflux is expressed by a five-point grading system (Kramer, 1992). Even though the grades

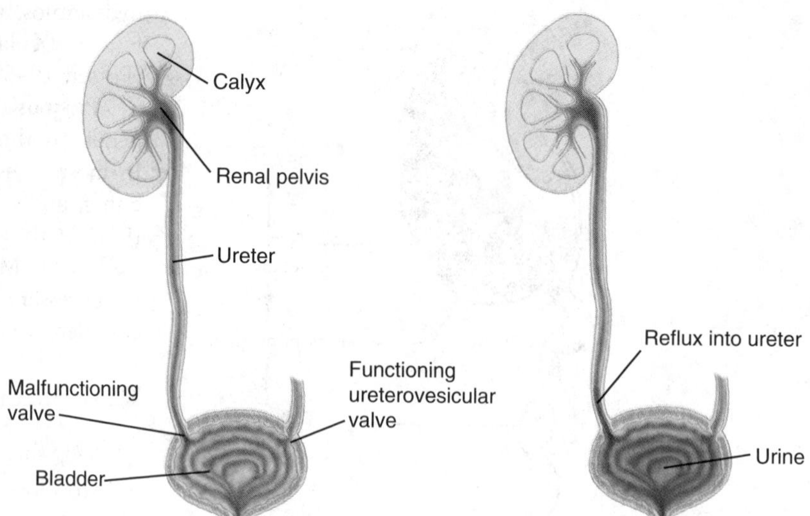

Figure 19–7
During voiding, a defect in the vesicoureteral junction allows urine to flow back into the ureter. After voiding, the urine leaves the ureter and returns to the bladder. This creates a pattern of incomplete emptying, which can lead to infection. (From Ashwill, J. W., & Droske, S. C. [Eds.]. [1997]. *Nursing care of children: Principles and practice* [p. 796]. Philadelphia: W. B. Saunders. Reprinted with permission.)

of reflux are only loosely correlated with renal compromise, the system offers long-term predictive value. Low-grade reflux (I or II) has an 80% likelihood of resolution in early childhood secondary to bladder maturation and linear growth of the ureters (Ashcraft, 1990b). Some instances of high-grade reflux (III to IV) may also be self-limiting, but children with this degree of disease are prone to deleterious renal sequelae from infection. The consequences of pyelonephritis can be especially destructive for children younger than 24 months (Ashcraft, 1990b; Hoberman, 1994).

Secondary reflux is an acquired condition that occurs as a consequence of bladder instability, or elevated intravesical pressures. It is most often seen in children with dysfunctional voiding, urethral obstruction, or a neurogenic bladder. The effect of these conditions is an alteration of the UVJ or a functional ureteral obstruction following bladder distention. Effective management of the underlying condition often eliminates reflux (Ashcraft, 1990b).

Ureteropelvic Junction Obstruction

Obstruction-related hydronephrosis most often originates as a malfunction of the UPJ. UPJ accounts for 40% of the cases of neonatal hydronephrosis and is the most common cause of infantile abdominal masses (Mann, 1990). Incidence of UPJ is 2 to 3 times greater in males than in females, and males have a more pathogenic degree of hydronephrosis than females. The condition is detected in the left kidney more often than the right (Mann, 1990).

Although UPJ obstruction may be an isolated defect, reflux in the adjacent ureter is present in 10% of children, and up to 25% of contralateral kidneys are also obstructed (King, 1995; Mann, 1990). Other urologic abnormalities, such as renal agenesis, malrotation, hypospadias, and calculi may be present (Montagnino et al., 1995). The widespread use of prenatal sonograms has significantly affected the timely diagnosis of UPJ obstruction, whereas, previously, many cases escaped detection unless the child had frank renal disease.

Intrinsic factors are the most likely cause of obstruction. Substitution of collagen for smooth muscle creates an inelastic ureteral segment that halts peristaltic activity. Ureteral valves, polyps, or fibroid growths are rare causes of obstruction (Mann, 1990). Remnants of aberrant fetal vasculature that band the proximal ureter are the usual extrinsic factor in UPJ obstruction. Kinking, which reduces urine flow, may result from adhesions between the upper ureter and the renal pelvis or from a sharply angled ureteropelvic insertion angle.

Pathophysiology

The intrapelvic pressure created by hydronephrosis exerts a direct negative effect on glomerular filtration. As pressures within the nephron exceed glomerular capillary pressure, reverse fluid and solute transport occurs. Concentration of urine is hampered because of restricted renal blood flow and long-standing distal tubular damage. The acceleration of fluid build-up provides a nourishing broth for bacterial colonization, and altered hydrogen excretion creates metabolic acidosis (Leaky, Ryan, McEndfee, Nelson, & Fitzpatrick, 1989).

In its most severe form, hydronephrosis leads to obliteration of the functional renal unit. However, factors such as degree and duration of obstruction, plus the presence or absence of calculi or infection, are mediating variables in the expression of renal involvement.

Assessment of Obstructive Uropathy

The most common sign leading to a diagnosis of obstructive uropathy is UTI; the second most common sign is the presence of a voiding disorder. Children with obstruction, particularly UPJ defects, experience flank pain either intermittently or after high fluid intake. Also, hematuria may occur after minimal trauma. Delayed growth and weight gain may occur in the child with VUR, even when reflux is low grade and without infection. Infants and young children with VUR are often colicky, lethargic, and appear "sickly" (Montagnino et al., 1995). Boys with mild to moderate PUV obstruction typically void infrequently, emptying their bladder with a weak intermittent stream or a thin, forceful one. Having experienced this abnormal voiding pattern since birth, these boys (and their parents) wrongly assume this to be normal micturition. Detection of this anomaly often requires meticulous attention to the voiding history and observation of the urinary stream.

The newborn with severe hydronephrosis is critically ill from metabolic acidosis, fluid overload, uremia, and, possibly, respiratory compromise. Prompt treatment is initiated to stabilize the child's condition before urologic reconstruction is begun.

Diagnostic Tests. Antenatal diagnosis of obstructive uropathy has become commonplace since the addition of ultrasonography in routine prenatal care. Hydronephrosis, ureteral enlargement, and a "keyhole" hypertrophic bladder are signs of a major urologic anomaly. A reduction of amniotic volume is pathognomonic for obstructive uropathy as well as for other genitourinary and gastrointestinal disorders. Since oligohydramnios is not apparent until 18 weeks of gestational age, a screening sonogram should be delayed until after that time. Prenatal findings suggestive of an obstructive lesion may be transient or idiopathic; therefore, radiologic evaluation should be repeated during the neonatal period to confirm the diagnosis. The value of prenatal detection rests not with its ability to predict the degree of renal function, but rather as a signal to facilitate early therapeutic intervention on a nonemergent basis (Reznick & Budorick, 1995).

Because VUR can cause delayed growth and weight gain, urologic studies should be a part of the diagnostic evaluation of a child with the syndrome known as failure to thrive. Uroradiologic techniques are used to thoroughly investigate the nature of obstructive uropathy. The basic work-up requires an IVP to define renal anatomy and function and a VCUG to outline the urethra and assess bladder anatomy during micturition. Using the two studies, most pathologic effects from PUV, VUR, and UPJ obstruction can be observed. Damaged kidneys or renal segments, however, may not be visualized. In those instances, renal function and parenchymal damage may best be demonstrated by RCS.

Current research has highlighted the concept that some infants incur benign hydronephrosis, which is stable and causes no impairment to renal function. Differentiating physiologic hydronephrosis from pathologic UPJ obstruction in the infant can be difficult. A diuretic renogram, which uses furosemide augmentation to induce high-volume urine, is the current study of choice to pinpoint which infants could benefit from surgical intervention (Hilton & Kaplan, 1995; King, 1995).

Kidney function and other tests may be done, including serum BUN, creatinine, pH, and electrolytes, complete blood count (CBC) with differential, and urinary pH, creatinine clearance, and electrolytes. Unless renal function is significantly impaired, these values will be in a normal range. Urinalysis, specific gravity, and urine culture complete the assessment.

Nursing Diagnoses and Outcomes

Chart 19–3 presents nursing diagnoses generally applicable to the child with a genitourinary condition. The following diagnoses address some more specific care needs of the child with obstructive uropathy.

- **Knowledge deficit: congenital urologic anomaly**
  Outcome: The child and/or family verbalize their understanding of the anomaly, its effect on urinary tract function, and its medical and surgical management.
- **High risk for infection related to urinary retention**
  Outcomes: The child and/or family identify the signs and symptoms of UTI.
  The child and/or family state the measures that decrease the likelihood of infection.
  The child and/or family express their understanding of the need for prompt medical intervention if an infection occurs.
- **Altered family processes related to caring for a child with a chronic condition**
  Outcomes: Parents verbalize their awareness of stressors that compromise their caregiving role.
  Parents express their feelings regarding their child's condition and the long-term management of it.
  Parents seek emotional, physical, and financial support from significant others, professionals, or other parents.
  Parents demonstrate parenting behaviors that are positive and appropriate for the age of their child.
- **Altered urinary elimination related to congenital anomaly and/or surgical intervention**
  Outcomes: The child and/or parents state their understanding of physiologic alterations in the child's voiding pattern.
  The child and/or parents participate in activities or adopt techniques aimed at normalizing the child's urinary elimination.

The child and/or parents demonstrate skill in self-care and hygiene measures in response to altered urinary elimination.

Interdisciplinary Interventions

Optimal care for children with obstructive uropathy combines a mixture of medical and surgical approaches, tailored to the degree of obstruction, the child's age, and the renal status.

Medical and Surgical Management

The primary goal of medical management is prevention of infection by adherence to a long-term antibacterial regimen. Medications of choice include nitrofurantoin (Furadantin, Macrodantin), trimethoprim-sulfamethoxazole (Septra), nalidixic acid (NegGram), or methenamine mandelate (Mandelamine) augmented by ascorbic acid. Breakthrough infections while on suppression therapy may direct a change in medical management toward surgical correction of the anomaly.

PUV can be obliterated by endoscopic ablation, using a pediatric-sized resectoscope to cauterize redundant tissue. Temporary insertion of a silicone rubber (Silastic) catheter is used in rare cases to reduce postoperative bleeding. In most cases, the child is discharged after postsurgical recovery and an initial voiding. When the child's condition is complicated by VUR, a reimplantation of the submucosal ureteral segment can be undertaken at the same time, or the child can be reevaluated several months later to detect unresolved reflux and undergo the procedure at that time. After surgical correction, any residual negative effects on voiding or urinary continence need further attention. Medical or surgical interventions can be implemented based on the remaining symptoms (see Voiding Disorders).

The infant with high-grade urethral valve disease and severely affected upper tracts demands immediate medical attention to correct metabolic acidosis and antibiotics to eradicate urosepsis. Surgical intervention for urinary tract decompression can be provided by bladder catheterization or temporary urinary diversion (see Treatment Modalities). Procedures such as loop-cutaneous pyelostomy, ureterostomy, or vesicostomy carry minimal surgical risk and are safe for the unstable infant. Definitive procedures such as reimplantation, bladder diverticulectomy, and valve ablation can be delayed to allow for renal rejuvenation, reduction of ureteral tortuosity, and improved bladder compliance.

Management of the child with VUR is less clear-cut than that for PUV. For grades I through III reflux among infants and young children, many pediatric urologists adhere to a protocol of radiologic surveillance in anticipation that the condition will resolve within 3 to 5 years (Kramer, 1992). It is improbable that high-grade reflux in the young child and any reflux in the child older than age 5 will be spontaneously outgrown. Episodes of breakthrough UTI compound the risk of renal parenchymal scarring and usually require surgical management. Severe reflux with massive hydronephrosis and aperistaltic megaureters may be initially treated with temporary urinary diversions (see Treatment Modalities). Because surgical correction of the reflux by an experienced pediatric urologist approaches 100%, many surgeons more readily choose to perform reimplantation. Surgical correction of VUR involves the separation of the ureter from the bladder and the creation of a tunnel between the layers of bladder mucosa. The ureter is threaded within the tunnel so that its opening into the bladder is within the trigone. Advantages of this aggressive approach include proven reduction of pyelonephritic episodes, lowered degree of radiologic exposure, and short-term use of chemoprophylaxis (Ashcraft, 1990b).

Hydronephrosis secondary to UPJ obstruction is most often treated with a pyeloplasty or ureteroplasty. The focus of these procedures is to dissect the obstructive ureteral component and either anastomose the ureteral segments or suture the remaining ureter to the renal pelvis. Best results are obtained when the surgical correction is performed before the child's first birthday, because renal function may improve markedly. When the initial renal scan demonstrates less than 10% of function, the diseased organ is excised to avoid the long-term manifestation of hypertension. For the infant with severe or bilateral UPJ obstruction, a temporary percutaneous pyeloplasty can be performed with the expectation that low-pressure urinary draining will improve function (Mann, 1990). Permanent surgical repair is done after the infant is 1 year old.

Nursing Management

The child with obstructive uropathy, will require health care support in the prenatal and hospital settings and continuing in the home, school, and camp settings. With a full understanding of disease etiology, management, and long-term precautions, the nurse working in these settings is uniquely positioned to support the child and family's decision-making and compliance with the treatment regimen.

During the evaluation phase, the nurse expands the family's knowledge base, clarifying and supplementing information presented by the physician. Diagnostic studies are explained and preprocedural preparation techniques are offered. Parents easily become overwhelmed by the shock that an apparently healthy child has a major organic anomaly that may undermine a vital body function. Siblings may likewise be affected. Basic facts of urologic anatomy and physiology require constant review.

Once a diagnosis has been made, the parents and the child are both in need of information and support to assist in acceptance of a management program. Medications are described thoroughly, including therapeutic effects, dosage, side effects, and safety precautions. If surgical intervention has been recommended, the nurse assists with preoperative preparation for the child and family and monitors the postoperative course.

Postoperative Care

Pain Management. Incisional pain is most prominent for the first 2 days after surgery. Relief can be afforded by parenteral administration of morphine sulfate or by extradural nerve blockage in the spinal canal. Patient-controlled analgesic (PAC) devices can be especially useful for the older child with a flank incision following pyeloplasty or ureteroplasty (Wilton, 1995). The child who has undergone reimplantation of the ureter needs medication to subdue bladder spasms until the urinary drainage tubing is removed and full bladder reexpansion occurs, approximately 1 to 2 days later.

Fluid Balance. Once the urologic obstruction is corrected, the child may experience postobstructive diuresis. In the immediate postoperative period, the nurse carefully monitors urine output and specific gravity, keeping in mind that these children have reduced concentrating ability.

> **Alert:** *Urine output that approaches the IV intake is an early indicator of diuresis, whereas an increasing specific gravity approaching 1.020 and dwindling urine output are later signs of dehydration from excessive fluid loss.*

An added bolus of IV fluids may be needed to compensate for the high urine output. Fluid balance stabilizes within 1 to 2 days, and, after removal of the IV fluids, oral intake is pushed. Normal daily urine output is approximately one third to one half of fluid intake (Stock, Packer, & Kaplan, 1995). Measuring urine output for the infant with a temporary urinary diversion requires weighing of stomal dressings and diapers. A bedside record showing dry and wet dressing weights accurately assesses output. Disposable diapers wrapped girdle fashion around pyelostomy or ureterostomy sites are often used over sterile dressings; their weight should also be recorded.

Urinary Tube Care. A ureteral stent, a urethral catheter, or a suprapubic tube may be used following uncomplicated reconstructive repairs of obstructive uropathy (Brandell & Brock, 1993). If the child's surgical repair is extensive or if it involves ureteral tapering, stents are necessary to prevent obstruction from postoperative edema (Chart 19–11).

> **Alert:** *In the postoperative child with ureteral, suprapubic, or urethral drainage tubes, bladder spasms may indicate a mucous plug in the tube. The nurse must monitor patency of the system, checking for urine flow and milking the tubes every 2 hours, or in accordance with the hospital's policy.*

Infection Prevention. The nurse must be cognizant of the risk for nosocomial infections that use of these tubes places on the child. Meticulous attention must be paid to incisional and urinary tube care. The child's urine is observed for cloudiness or foul odor, and any changes in vital signs that indicate infection are noted. Antibiotics are administered to prevent gram-negative infection.

To promote wound healing, the child's diet should be high in protein and fluids. Nutritious snacks such as milkshakes or Carnation Instant Breakfast are excellent ways to meet both dietary goals. The dietitian is consulted for the child with special dietary needs, lactose intolerance, or poor appetite.

Reconstructive surgery of the genitourinary tract can be psychologically traumatic to children of all ages. To alleviate negative responses to such emotionally charged concerns as body image, sexual identity, and modesty violation, the nurse may seek assistance from the child life specialist.

Community Care

Home care following surgical procedures to alleviate urologic obstructions is directed toward activity restriction, prevention of infection, maintenance of high fluid intake, and prevention of potential long-term complications. Any residual voiding discomfort dissipates more quickly with a high fluid intake by the child, which promotes bladder stretching. Mild analgesics are rarely needed after the child's first day or two at home. Vigorous activity, especially jumping or bouncing, is prohibited for the first week or until the first postoperative visit. The child may return to school when he or she feels comfortable, as long as activity is restricted. Baths and showers are permitted after wounds are healed. Following ureteral reimplantation, antibiotics may be continued for the immediate postoperative period or until a follow-up VCUG documents successful resolution of reflux (Montagnino et al., 1995).

The infant with ureterostomies or pyelostomies is generally comfortable at the time of discharge. The nurse should demonstrate girdle-style diapering, with the diaper ends overlapping and taped, to collect the urine. As the infant's abdomen grows, a second diaper may be added to extend the length. Another diaper is applied in the usual fashion for bowel movements and the occasional urine that may dribble from the bladder. This dribbling, although not harmful, may cause bladder spasms; mild analgesics, such as acetaminophen, offer adequate pain relief.

Stomal sites usually require minimal skin care. Soap and water cleansing is generally adequate. If irritation occurs, emollients such as zinc oxide or Vitamin A and D ointments usually suffice. Chronic irritation may signal a UTI and should be brought to the physician's atten-

Chart 19-11
Nursing Interventions

Postoperative Care of the Child with a Ureteral Stent

Plastic size 8 Fr feeding tubes are used during reconstructive urologic surgery to divert urine from the surgical site. These stents prevent urinary extravasation through the incision and prevent urine flow obstruction caused by edema. The stents exit the body through the incision and attach to external collection containers. Removal of the stent is readily accomplished shortly before the child's discharge from the hospital, and the ureteral exit site epithelializes quickly.

Nursing interventions to ensure tube patency include the following:

- Encourage high fluid intake.
- Observe tubes for mucous shreds or debris and check for kinking.
- Milk tubes every 2 hours by bending the tubing between the thumb and finger, then pinching the bent tubing together vigorously.
- Demonstrate this technique to the older sibling or parent and incorporate their participation in the child's care.

Nursing considerations to prevent infection include the following:

- Keep collection device below the level of incision.
- Observe urine for signs and symptoms of infection (e.g., foul odor, cloudiness).
- Monitor the child's temperature.
- Aspirate urine sample for culture.
- Apply antibacterial ointment to tube site.
- Maintain a closed urinary drainage system.

Nursing interventions to manage bladder spasms include the following:

- Ensure tube patency.
- Tape tubes securely to the leg or body.
- Medicate for spasms with oxybutynin or belladonna and opium suppositories per physician orders.
- Prevent bladder stimulation secondary to a full rectum by completing a preoperative bowel evacuation, encouraging a high fluid intake, promoting early ambulation postoperatively, and administering a stool softener or glycerin suppository postoperatively.

tion. Bathing is allowed as long as the water level is below the stoma. Occasional splashing of water over the stoma sites is not harmful.

The nurse prepares the child and family for ongoing urologic radiologic studies, which assess for unresolved obstruction and monitor renal function. If one kidney is severely compromised, restriction from contact sports is wise and may be mandated by the child's school system. The nurse can assist the physical education department in creating an adaptive sports program for the child. Parents often require emotional support in altering their expectations for their child and help in rechanneling the child's energies in other, less physical outlets.

Potential long-term ramifications of hydronephrosis include the risk of hypertension, urinary calculi, pregnancy-related infections or renal compromise, and genetic transmission of congenital defects to offspring. The nurse's role is to present parents with strategies to prevent these complications or allow for early detection, such as encouraging a lifelong habit of high fluid intake and frequent voiding and yearly blood pressure monitoring. The child must ensure that every health care provider is aware of the urologic history and that progeny are evaluated for congenital urologic anomalies shortly after birth (Montagnino et al., 1995).

Anomalies of the Bladder and Urethra

Exstrophy–Epispadias Complex

The bladder exstrophy–epispadias complex is a serious congenital anomaly affecting multiple organs of the urologic and musculoskeletal systems. Interrupted abdominal development in early fetal life produces an exposed bladder and urethra, pubic bone separation, and associated anal and genital abnormalities. The three variations of this complex seen are cloacal exstrophy, classic exstrophy, and epispadias.

Bladder exstrophy–epispadias complex is a rare

anomaly that occurs in approximately 3:100,000 live births, affecting males twice as frequently as females (Gearhart & Jeffs, 1990). The cause of the anomaly is unknown, but it appears to be unrelated to genetic or teratogenic exposure.

Pathophysiology

The three general variants of the exstrophy–epispadias complex share a common precipitating factor: persistence of the cloacal membrane beyond the point of expected resorption during embryologic development. In early gestational life, the embryo possesses an alimentary tract that terminates as an enlarged chamber, the *cloaca*. Its posterior border is the *cloacal membrane*, which runs from the umbilicus to the tail gut. A mound of tissue, the *urorectal septum*, protrudes into the upper cloacal chamber, migrating toward the cloacal membrane. The urorectal septum separates the cloaca into the anterior *urogenital sinus* and the posterior *anal canal*. Meanwhile, the cloacal membrane recedes as it is filled in with strong mesodermal tissue. In rare instances, the cloacal membrane becomes overly prominent and blocks the proliferation of mesodermal cells. Later, the membrane weakens and ruptures, leaving cloacal structures uncovered. The timing of cloacal membrane rupture determines which of the three exstrophy variations will occur (Bowers, Hannigan, & Kushner, 1995).

Cloacal Exstrophy. If the cloacal membrane disintegrates before the completed cloacal division of its anterior and posterior compartments, the exposed surface is a combined bladder and rectal structure. Both ureters are lateral and have an incompetent bladder junction, whereas the internal sphincter and urethra are split. This condition results in bilateral reflux and total incontinence after initial bladder closure. This version of the defect is rare and occurs between the fourth and sixth weeks of gestational life.

Classic Exstrophy. In classic exstrophy, rupture of the cloacal membrane occurs after the anterior-posterior separation has been completed, exposing the urinary structures only. An everted bladder with lateral ureteral orifices is noted, along with a splayed internal sphincter and urethra (Fig. 19–8). Bilateral reflux and total incontinence occur postoperatively to bladder closure. The incidence of classic exstrophy is 1:40,000 live births, and the defect occurs between the sixth and eighth gestational weeks (Gearhart & Jeffs, 1990).

Epispadias. The least involved presentation in the exstrophy–epispadias complex triad is epispadias, which results from cloacal membrane disintegration after the eighth fetal week. A urethral groove extends along the dorsal penile shaft or along the entire female urethra. If the internal sphincter is affected, total incontinence results (see Fig. 19–9).

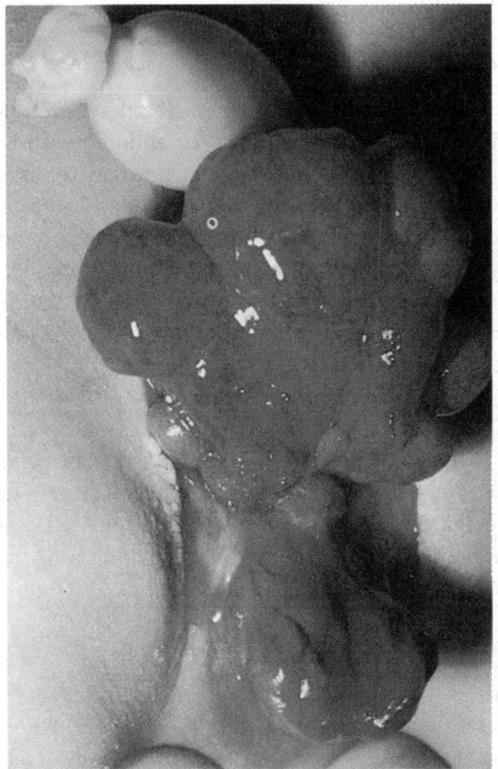

Figure 19–8
In classic exstrophy, the bladder is open and exposed on the abdomen. (From Liebert, P. S. [1996]. *Color atlas of pediatric surgery* [2nd ed., p. 261]. Philadelphia: W. B. Saunders. Reprinted with permission.)

Assessment

At birth, the infant with bladder exstrophy–epispadias complex is healthy and is physiologically normal, except for the affected structures. Classic bladder exstrophy is apparent at birth, with the exposed inner mucosal surface appearing red, shiny, and rugated. The bladder capacity is small, possibly only 5 mL after bladder closure in the neonatal period (Gearhart, 1992). When cloacal exstrophy is present, the rectal segment protrudes within the bladder mucosa. In males, the penis is short, splayed, and exhibits dorsal curvature (chordee). Cryptorchidism is often present. In females, the urethra and the vagina are short. When primary reconstruction has been delayed beyond infancy, the vagina may prolapse. Orthopedic manifestations are minimal following early pelvic ring closure. When surgery has been delayed, the child may ambulate with a waddle.

Diagnostic Tests. Renal structures are evaluated by a newborn ultrasound or by a renal scan. Beyond the neonatal period, an IVP may be substituted. A pubic computed tomography (CT) scan highlights the severity of pubic separation (Bowers et al., 1995).

Interdisciplinary Interventions

Surgical Management

Surgical advances over the past 2 decades have dramatically improved the management for children with bladder exstrophy–epispadias complex. Rather than resort to urinary diversion, the focus of care is on early surgical correction. Within days after birth, the bladder is covered with peripheral tissue and the pelvic ring is closed. Postoperatively, the infant is placed in Bryant's traction until fibrous healing of the symphysis pubic occurs, generally after 3 to 4 weeks.

Because postoperative edema of the bladder is expected, ureteral stents and a suprapubic tube are temporarily inserted to prevent urinary obstruction. Successive surgical procedures to correct reflux, reconstruct a sphincter mechanism, close the urethra, and repair the phallus are individualized, depending on the child's anatomy and response to previous surgery.

Nursing Management

Because of the physical disfigurement of the genitalia and the parents' unfamiliarity with this anomaly, parents often react to the child's birth with this disorder with horror, disbelief, and revulsion. The nurse not only provides emotional support, education, and reinforcement of the proposed medical management but also demonstrates skin care, diapering, and hygiene measures. Delicate bladder mucosa should be protected by a plastic wrap covering at all times. Gauze, either wet or coated with petroleum jelly, may denude the mucosal tissue and is not used. Ointments or creams may occlude the ureteral orifices and impede urine flow. Soaps and powders may be abrasive and can promote bacterial growth. Therefore, all of these hygiene products are contraindicated. Clear water is best for cleansing, and a hair dryer set on a low setting effectively keeps the surrounding skin surface dry. Loosely fastened diapers may be worn. Tub bathing is avoided. Postoperative nursing care depends on the child's specific surgical procedure and on the preference of the attending surgeon. Management of the child in Bryant's traction is discussed in Chapter 20.

Community Care

Regular evaluation studies to monitor reflux and to assess for UTI are required to conserve renal function. Urodynamic testing may be used to demonstrate bladder capacity and sphincteric activity. Urinary continence for the child with bladder exstrophy–epispadias complex may be an ongoing concern. Management of this problem often requires a multifaceted approach, incorporating pharmacologic agents, behavioral and motivational techniques, and skin care to provide optimal urine control. Pediatric-sized absorbent products and undergarments are available over-the-counter or in many specialty catalogues.

Negative emotional sequelae from repeated hospitalization, altered parenting response, or dysfunctional coping techniques may require psychological intervention. Because of frequent encounters with the child and the family, the nurse is ideally suited to recommend an appropriate referral source.

Patent Urachus

A patent urachus is a rare congenital defect of the bladder. The urachus is a passageway that connects the bladder dome to the umbilicus. During fetal development, this tubelike structure involutes to a solid cord. For unknown reasons, the involution process fails and the urachus remains patent, or open, allowing urine to leak from the umbilicus. Exact incidence of this defect is unknown, but males are affected more frequently than females by a 2:1 margin.

Patent urachus exerts minimal, if any, effect on renal function. The main concern is its potential to cause UTIs or vesical stones. Patent urachus may close spontaneously when the urinary drainage is intermittent or scant in volume, such as during infancy.

Assessment

The infant with a patent urachus can be recognized by a wet or leaking umbilicus, which may be more pronounced by straining or voiding. An associated umbilical hernia may also be present. Periumbilical excoriation and odor may be the only signs if fluid leakage is minimal. Patent urachus may be detected in an older child during a urologic evaluation for chronic UTI. A VCUG can effectively highlight the bladder defect as well as demonstrate a coexisting urethral obstruction. Pelvic ultrasound is useful in that it can define the bladder parameters.

Other conditions that produce umbilical leakage include an infected umbilical stump, delayed granulation at the umbilical site, omphalitis, and an enteroumbilical fistula. Analysis of the fluid for creatinine and urea confirm the diagnosis of patent urachus.

Interdisciplinary Interventions

Treatment for patent urachus is the surgical removal of the complete fistula via an abdominal approach. Nursing care is minimal, encompassing routine postoperative care for the child with an abdominal incision. Voiding function is unaltered by the surgical procedure, unless a coinciding urethral obstruction requires a cystoscopy and urethral dilation. In that case, the child will require analgesics and a high oral intake to ease the initial postoperative voidings.

Prune Belly Syndrome

Prune belly syndrome is a triad of congenital anomalies that comprises lax abdominal musculature, urinary tract defects, and cryptorchidism. The full expression of this syndrome occurs exclusively among males, with an incidence of 1:40,000 live births. A modified version of the syndrome occurs less frequently among females (Ashcraft, 1990a). The cause of prune belly syndrome is poorly understood but is thought to result from inadequate maturation of muscle tissue throughout the abdominal cavity. Further unidentified factors probably contribute to other aspects of this anomaly. This developmental insult appears during early embryologic life, probably around the fourth gestational week (Skoog, 1992). There appears to be no genetic determinant for the syndrome.

Pathophysiology

The physiologic ramifications of this disorder result from inadequate contractility of numerous abdominal and pelvic structures. The abdominal wall is protruding and offers little support to internal contents. Upward pressure of abdominal organs on the pleural cavity causes a flared lower rib cage. The ureters often have mixed musculature development, with the lower segments more atonic than the upper tracts. Bladder hypotonia produces incompetency at the UVJ, leading to VUR. The sphincter and the urethra are typically dilated, affecting urinary continence. The gastrointestinal tract may be segmentally aperistaltic, leading to Hirschsprung's disease or to chronic constipation (Skoog, 1992).

A spectrum of multisystem malformations is commonly associated with prune belly syndrome. Cryptorchidism is a hallmark of this disorder. The testes are typically intra-abdominal. Although the gonads are hormonally competent, the affected males are sterile. Damaging effects of prune belly syndrome include renal dysplasia and hydronephrosis, resulting in various degrees of renal compromise. Marked intrauterine renal dysfunction, with resultant oligohydramnios, may lead to life-threatening pulmonary hypoplasia. Imperforate anus is a common occurrence that complicates the medical management of these children. Congenital heart defects and orthopedic anomalies may also be present (Ashcraft, 1990a).

Assessment

The most obvious manifestations of prune belly syndrome involve the abdomen, which has a wrinkled, doughy appearance. The excessive flabby musculature exceeds the confines of the child's abdominal profile. When upright, the child has a pot belly appearance. Cryptorchia is also apparent.

When the physician performs the newborn examination, palpation of the abdomen detects distortion within the urinary and gastrointestinal tract. Abnormal findings include ureteral dilatation, bladder enlargement, and looped bowel segments. Urine may drain from the patent urachus, located at the umbilicus. Inspection of the rectal area, visually as well as digitally, is imperative to ensure rectal integrity. Genital defects should be documented. The infant is thoroughly evaluated for signs of respiratory, cardiac, or skeletal involvement (Montagnino et al., 1995).

Diagnostic evaluation of renal, pulmonary, and gastrointestinal function must be performed expeditiously to ensure the child's greatest chance for survival. Once the child's condition has stabilized, radiologic evaluation of urologic anatomy and functional defects can be pursued.

Interdisciplinary Interventions

The neonate with prune belly syndrome is typically under the care of a pediatric urologist, a nephrologist, and a pulmonologist during the early neonatal period. Stabilization of critical body systems is the immediate priority and may necessitate respiratory support and kidney dialysis.

Once viability seems assured, the neonate faces the prospect of numerous surgical procedures. Early urinary diversion is often established, and the urinary tract is monitored for signs of infection secondary to urinary stasis. As the child matures, urologic surgical procedures are performed to allow for urinary undiversion, penile reconstruction, and maximal testicular function. Because the bladder musculature has patchy areas of atony, long-term success following surgical manipulation cannot be assured. These children face a lifetime of vigilant renal surveillance (Ashcraft, 1990c).

The nurse's role in providing care for children with prune belly syndrome focuses on education. Ongoing family teaching is necessary in preparation for various surgical procedures. The family needs to be thoroughly educated for long-term management following specific procedures and to recognize signs and symptoms that indicate a complication of treatment failure. Nursing care following individual surgical procedures is discussed elsewhere in this chapter.

Prevention of UTI is critical for conservation of renal function. The nurse reviews the age-related presentations of UTI and ensures that the family is aware of the treatment regimen.

Respiratory infection is common, especially in the early years, and may be difficult to manage. The nurse reviews the impending signs of respiratory decompensation with the family and encourages communication with the primary health care provider.

Constipation is a continuous concern. The nurse can recommend dietary supplements and elimination routines that assist in regular bowel habits. It is important for the child and the family to be willing to make a lifelong commitment to these routines.

The overwhelming nature of prune belly syndrome places the child at a high risk for psychosexual maladjustment. The parents may find acceptance and bonding with the child to be an unending struggle. Developing positive self-esteem may be difficult because the child often feels ashamed and rejected by peers. Sexuality issues become pronounced at puberty and continue through adulthood when sexual dysfunction and infertility are acknowledged. Psychotherapeutic intervention and sexual counseling may be instrumental to ensure that the child is well adjusted, feels valued, and pursues a productive lifestyle.

Hypospadias

The most common anomaly of the male phallus, hypospadias, is the incomplete formation of the anterior urethral segment, either as a result of arrested fusion of the ventral urethral folds or of inadequate tubularization of the glanular urethra. The resulting urethral formation is a meatus that terminates at some point along the ventral fusion line, ranging from the perineum to the distal penile shaft, or a splayed glans with an ectopic meatus (Fig. 19–9). The ventral preputial segment is likewise separated and assumes a hooded appearance. The affected urethral pathway is commonly replaced with tight fibrous bands that produce a curvature called **chordee,** although either hypospadias or chordee may occur independently (Smith, 1990).

Associated genitourinary anomalies include cryptorchia (10% to 20%) and inguinal hernias (16% to 20%). Among males with more pronounced degrees of hypospadias, upper urinary tract defects may coexist (Smith, 1990). Because the hypospadias is distal to the urinary sphincter, continence remains intact. Spermatozoa transport to the urethra is unaffected, and any compromise to fertility is a function of testicular effects from cryptorchia.

Etiology and Incidence

The cause of hypospadias is not clear. Hereditary transmission is weakly correlated with the anomaly in that the sibling rate of recurrence when there is no family history of hypospadias is 12%, whereas the risk increases to 26% if the father had hypospadias (Stock et al., 1995). It is postulated that multigenetic factors interplay to cause the defect. An earlier study noted an association between paternal testicular defects (undescended testes, varicocele, or atrophy after mumps) and hypospadias among offspring, suggesting defective chromosome material within spermatozoa as a possible cause. Race is a minimal factor; the incidence is slightly lower for black than for white males (Smith, 1990).

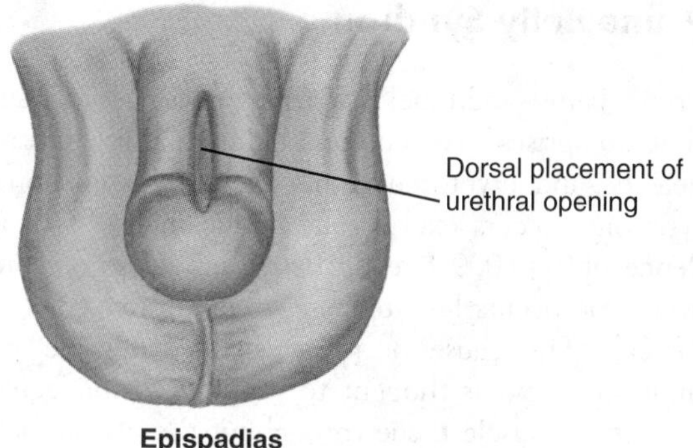

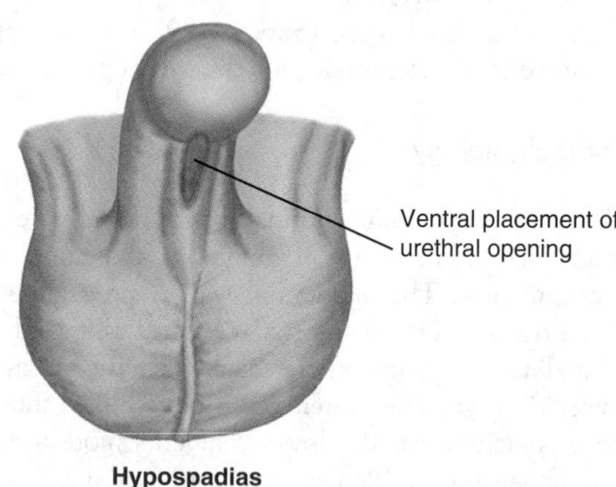

Figure 19–9
Possible locations of the urethral meatus in the child with hypospadias and penile chordee. (From Ashwill, J. W., & Droske, S. C. [Eds.]. [1997]. *Nursing care of children: Principles and practice* [p. 798]. Philadelphia: W. B. Saunders. Reprinted with permission.)

Exogenous factors influencing hypospadias include teratogens such as prenatal exposure to cocaine, alcohol, phenytoin, progestins, rubella virus, or gestational diabetes. Inadequate testosterone stimulation to the genital tissue may also negatively affect penile development. It has been hypothesized that either the penile tissue lacks sufficient hormone receptor sites or that embryologic testosterone levels are deficient. This second theory is particularly plausible in that up to 20% of affected males have undescended testes, a condition that can suppress exogenous hormone secretion (Smith, 1990; Stock, Scherz, & Kaplan, 1995; Stock et al., 1995).

Pathophysiology

Creation of the male urethra begins with the appearance of a urethral groove in the forming genital tubercle, at about the sixth fetal week. Fusion of the urogenital folds that border this groove is initiated during week 9, proceeding along the ventral line from the perineum toward the distal shaft. Simultaneously, a glanular dimple forms at the tip and carves a notch to the corona, splitting the glans. This groove then becomes contiguous with the penile urethra and undergoes ventral fusion. The prepuce develops during week 12, following completed urethral development; scrotal fusion also occurs at this time. Testicular descent into the scrotal sac is delayed until the fetus is almost full term (England, 1990).

Urethrogenesis may be arrested at any point along the fusion line; however, the ectopic meatus terminates at the corona or glans in 75% of cases (Stock et al., 1995). Perineal hypospadias may indicate an intersex condition, especially if the gonads are nonpalpable. Further studies are warranted for proper sex assignment. In the past, infants with extreme microphallus were surgically altered to female, in the hope of providing the child with safisfying sexual function as an adult. (At this time, the practice of sexual reassignment has been questioned as anecdotal reports of sexual maladjustment in these children are beginning to surface (Smith, 1990; Stock et al., 1995).

Assessment

Careful neonatal examination of the male genitalia should disclose hypospadias. The hooded prepuce without ventral attachment is noted, along with a splayed glans. Ventral curvature may be present. The aberrant urethral meatus can be buried, especially when chordee is marked. Accurate assessment of meatal location and patency is best accomplished by securely holding the glans and ventrally retracting the shaft tissue (Sugar & Hoyler-Grant, 1995). Chordee complicates the diagnosis of hypospadias because, after surgical correction, the resultant penile lengthening repositions the meatus proximally and makes the final repair more complex. Testicular descent should be assessed, along with signs of an inguinal hernia or hydrocele. Because of the potential for upper tract involvement, palpate the abdomen for bladder distention or renal enlargement. Parents of an older child are asked about the child's urine stream, voiding pattern, and signs and symptoms of a UTI.

It is important to assess the parents' emotional response to their son's anomaly. Parents mourn the "less than perfect" son and fear for his sexual ability and satisfaction, gender identity, and peer acceptance. The idea of delicate reconstructive surgery on a body part that is integral for urologic, sexual, and psychosocial response is abhorrent to many parents, especially fathers. The nurse can assist the parents by emphasizing that the genitalia, although definitely male, is incompletely formed rather than defective or inadequate. Presenting them with illustrations of surgical procedures and before-after photographs can allay their anxieties and promote bonding.

Diagnostic Tests. Infants with severe hypospadias and cryptorchia should undergo tissue karyotyping and cystoscopic or genitoscopic evaluation (Stock et al., 1995). Upper tract evaluation is controversial but may be considered in the following circumstances: family history of uropathology, anomaly of another body system, or symptoms suggestive of urinary infection or voiding disorder (see Obstructive Uropathology) (Smith, 1990).

▽ **Alert:** *The neonate with hypospadias must not be circumcised. Some corrective repairs require tissue grafts, and tissue of the foreskin is ideal for this purpose.*

Interdisciplinary Interventions

Surgical Management

Surgical correction for hypospadias is one of the major success stories in urologic care of children. Improved surgical materials and equipment, creative corrective procedures, skilled pediatric urologists and anesthesiologists, expertise of urologic nurse specialists, and the humanization of hospitalization, all allow for safe surgical reconstruction performed in early childhood with a minimal risk of psychodevelopmental trauma. Corrective surgery for hypospadias has a complication rate of less than 10%, and most residual problems are treated with minor procedures (Smith, 1990; Stock et al., 1995).

Corrective surgery is performed in one stage for distal hypospadias (glanular, coronal, and distal to mid-shaft). A two-stage procedure is necessary for proximal shaft and penoscrotal to perineal defects. The goals of surgical repair are the production of a sexually functional phallus by correction of chordee, meatal advancement to the glans for physiologically and socially appropriate ejaculation and voiding, urethral integrity unimpeded by residual stricture or stenosis, and cosmetic acceptability (Care Path 19–1).

Surgery is often performed between age 6 and 12 months, with many advantages to early initiation of the repair. First, penile length changes only slightly between late infancy and preschool age (Stock et al., 1995). Mobility restrictions are easier to maintain before toddlerhood. Psychic trauma is negligible because the child lacks a sense of modesty during postoperative care and has yet to acquire a sense of gender identity. If early intervention is not feasible, postponing the repair until after age 2½ years is advisable. By this age, the child can be prepared for hospitalization, can cooperate with postoperative care and restrictions, and can verbalize his needs or concerns. Two-stage procedures are often begun at age 6 to 12 months, followed by a final urethral advancement 3 to 6 months later (Smith, 1990; Sugar & Hoyler-Grant, 1995).

The most widely used procedures for distal to penile hypospadias are the MAGPI (meatal advancement and

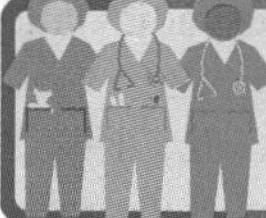

Care Path 19-1 An Interdisciplinary Plan of Care for the Child with Penoplasty—Surgical Correction of Hypospadias

Nursing Diagnosis	Patient/Family Intermediate Outcomes			
	Day: Surgery	Postoperative Day 1	Postoperative Day 2	Postoperative Days 3–7, Discharge date based on procedure
Knowledge deficit: Surgical procedure and postoperative care	Child/family express their understanding of specific operative procedure.	Child/family express their understanding for activity restriction and care of incision and tubing.	Parents state their understanding of home care and follow-up care.	⟶ Parents demonstrate appropriate care for urinary tubing. Discharge when all outcomes are met.
Pain related to surgical manipulation and apparatus	Child states relief from postoperative pain. Child displays pain-free demeanor.	⟶ ⟶	Child expresses minimal pain or bladder spasms (if catheterized). Parents identify signs of pain in child.	Child has no pain. Parents use measures to reduce child's pain.
Risk for injury related to urinary diversion equipment	Child does not exhibit signs of infection; temperature is normal, urine is clear with no odor. Urine output is 1–3 mL/kg/hr.	⟶ ⟶ Child maintains adequate urine output and drinks adequate fluids.	⟶ ⟶ ⟶ Parents state signs and symptoms that indicate urinary infection.	⟶ ⟶ ⟶ ⟶
Body image disturbance related to presence of urinary diversion apparatus	Child/family express acceptance of urinary drainage apparatus.	⟶	⟶	Child performs self-care within parameters of age and skill.
Care Intervention Categories				
Labs	Preoperative CBC, clotting studies, U/A		Urine culture, if indicated	
Medications and IVs	IV postoperatively until clear fluids are retained. Prophylactic antibiotics PO.	IV discontinued. Antibiotic ointment applied to urinary meatus	Antibiotic ointment applied to urinary meatus	⟶

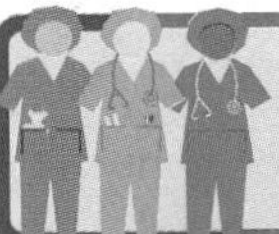

Care Path 19–1 An Interdisciplinary Plan of Care for the Child with Penoplasty—Surgical Correction of Hypospadias *Continued*

Care Intervention Categories	Day: Surgery	Postoperative Day 1	Postoperative Day 2	Postoperative Days 3–7, Discharge date based on procedure
Nutrition	NPO before surgery IV fluids Clear, full liquids as tolerated after surgery	Add full liquids to regular diet as tolerated. Increase fluids to 32–40 ounces per day.	Regular diet ⟶	⟶ ⟶
Pain management	Penile nerve block intraoperatively Analgesics as needed	Continued analgesics PO; antispasmodics if catheterized	⟶	Mild analgesics for dysuria after tubing is removed Antispasmodics during bladder reexpansion
Psychosocial	Preoperative preparation before admission for parents and child older than 18 months of age	Use anatomically correct doll Help older child maintain modesty.	Reassure parents and child that penis will look normal after edema resolves.	Reassure parents that child will have normal psychosexual maturation.
Safety and activity	Bed rest	Out of bed to chair Diversional play	May ambulate	No vigorous play or straddle toys
Special considerations	Preoperative bowel prep if ordered	Avoid restrictive diapers, bed clothes, sheets Sponge bath only	⟶	⟶
Teaching	Preoperative teaching Orient to hospital unit Immediate postoperative care	Acceptable activity level while catheterized Care of urinary tubing Pain relief	High fluid intake Care of penile incision Hygiene measures Medications	Follow-up care Signs of complications postoperatively Signs of long-term problems
Urinary drainage equipment	Monitor free flow of urine; check for mucous plugs	Maintain proper placement of tubing to collection device or use double diaper technique.	⟶	Tubing or penile stent removed when risk of urine extravasation and wound edema is decreased.
Vital signs/ baseline parameters	Vital signs every 2 hours Measure intake and output every 2 hours Monitor penile edema and dressing	Vital signs every 4 hours Measure intake and output every 4 hours ⟶	⟶ ⟶ ⟶	⟶ ⟶ ⟶

CBC, complete blood count; IV, intravenous; NPO, nothing by mouth; PO, by mouth; U/A, urinalysis.

glanuloplasty), the Mathieu flip-flap, the GAP (glans approximation procedure), and the Thiersch-Duplay repairs. Chordee, if present, is ablated by making a circumferential subglanular incision, degloving the penile shaft of its epidermal layer, and releasing the fibrous bands. Depending on the availability and adequacy of urethral tissue, the surgeon uses various techniques to isolate the urethral tissue and tubularize it. The new urethra is channeled within the penile core and then wrapped by glanular and penile epithelium. Preputial tissue can be used as a graft for urethral extension or rotated ventrally to form a collar, reinforcing the ventral penis and adding bulk (Smith, 1990; Stock et al., 1995). If repairs are complicated, surgery is repeated, or the prepuce is inadequate or absent, the buccal or bladder mucosa make satisfactory alternatives (Brock, 1994; Stock et al., 1995).

The first phase of a multistaged procedure involves correcting the chordee and creating a perineal urethrotomy. A subsequent procedure entails neourethral development with available non–hair-bearing tissue and penile reconstruction, similarly to the aforementioned processes.

In general, postoperative care for the child undergoing hypospadias repair focuses on urinary diversion, wound care, pain management, and activity restrictions. Several methods of bladder drainage systems may be used, including suprapubic cystotomy, Foley catheter, or urethral stent drainage. The drainage tube may be connected to a closed drainage unit or may remain as an open system, in which case the use of a "double diaper" technique shields the operative site from moisture. With this technique, the open drainage tube is sandwiched between two diapers. The bottom diaper, covering the penis, remains dry. Some urologists choose to insert a penile stent, a tube that is inserted within the penile urethra only. The stent diverts urine past the internal incision but spares the child from bladder catheterization and resultant bladder spasms. This type of stent, which only extends 2 to 3 mm past the meatus, is secured to the glans by sutures, which dissolve in 7 to 10 days. The child painlessly expels the tube during a normal voiding.

Nursing Management

Nursing care for the child undergoing hypospadias correction is guided by the specific surgical procedure and by the child's age. Depending on the degree of hypospadias, tissue adequacy, and the urologist's preference, the repair may require urinary diversion or may be completely tubeless. When present, the urinary drainage system may be open or closed, and hospitalization can vary from less than 24 hours to 5 days. Preoperative preparation and interventions to enhance postoperative healing and psychological adjustment must reflect the child's developmental level. Appropriate nursing interventions must be clarified by the attending urologist or urology nurse specialist.

Nursing care for the closed drainage catheter or stent follows the principles described for postoperative care following reimplantation. Careful taping of the tube to angle for ventral penile exposure is imperative to ensure that the fragile urethral incision remains free from tension. An oral antibiotic and a urine acidifying agent (such as ascorbic acid) are administered prophylactically to reduce the risk of infection. An antibiotic ointment is dabbed on the urethral meatus daily (Sugar & Hoyler-Grant, 1995).

A compression dressing is applied to the penis to reduce incisional edema and to control ecchymosis. The dressing remains undisturbed until the glanular edema visibly decreases, usually for 4 to 7 days, and is then removed. Dressing removal can be facilitated by a brief tub bath, which the child can undergo even if urinary apparatus remains in place.

Postoperative discomfort is surprisingly minimal following hypospadias repair. Single-dose spinal blockage, administered during the procedure, affords adequate analgesia for most children, but parenteral narcotics may occasionally be necessary for the first or second day after the procedure (Wilton, 1995). Bladder spasms in response to bladder intubation are controlled with medication to reduce detrusor contractility. Oxybutynin chloride (Ditropan) or belladonna-opium suppositories are commonly used agents. Bowel evacuation before surgery helps to lessen this problem.

The preschool-age child who remains hospitalized after hypospadias surgery has some degree of activity restriction. Because most boys feel alert and well postoperatively, diversional activities need to be provided. Gross motor activities and games, such as wheelchair kickball or rhythm movements, are especially important to dissipate stored energy in a constructive manner.

With the hospital stay typically limited to less than 48 hours, the nurse must provide discharge teaching expeditiously. The nurse should demonstrate how to care for urinary drainage systems, paying particular attention to tube anchoring and patency. One or both of the parents should perform a repeat demonstration of catheter irrigation to remove a mucous plug. The nurse must emphasize that the tubing should never be clamped or kinked and should also explain the "double-diaper" process. The child should be encouraged to eat a nutritious diet high in protein, with extra fluids. Prescribed medications should be thoroughly described. Bathing techniques should be reviewed, based on the surgeon's instructions. The child's parents must be prepared with instructions on how to care for postoperative wound edema and the process of normal ecchymosis resolution. The nurse should explicitly describe activities that need to be curtailed until healing is complete (usually 2 to 3 weeks)—rough play, swimming, and contact sports. The child must not play on any straddle-type toys for at least 2 to 3 weeks. Postdischarge visits to the surgeon should be planned.

Postoperative complications may develop years after the procedure, resulting from tissue shrinkage, infection, or inappropriate choice of corrective procedure. The most likely problems are stricture formation at the anastomosis site, meatal stenosis, meatal retraction to the original site, urethrocutaneous fistula, or urethral diverticulum (Stock et al., 1995; Smith, 1990). The nurse should discuss the potential for these complications and remind parents to observe the child's voiding pattern on a regular basis. Indicators of problems include a thin, forceful stream, infrequent voiding, a spray-type stream, dysuria, or ventral leaking during a void. These symptoms should be reported to the surgeon. Older children should be taught to recognize the signs and symptoms that indicate complications, and they should be encouraged to assume self-care.

Conditions Affecting the Male Genitalia

Cryptorchidism

In a normally developed male child, each testicle is secured within its sac in either side of the scrotum. Although the testicles are retractable by the action of the cremasteric muscle when needed for warmth or protection, the testicle should be palpable in its normal location outside the body of the child. Cryptorchia, "hidden testicle," refers to a testicle that occupies an anomalous position. Possible areas of displacement include the following:

- Canalicular—within the inguinal canal
- Intra-abdominal—above the internal inguinal ring
- Ectopic—perineal, femoral, or penopubic locations

A truly cryptorchid testis assumes a nonpalpable position within the abdomen, and 20% of children with this anomaly have either an absent gonad or one that is a rudimentary, nonfunctioning streak (Hazebroek & Molenaar, 1992).

Etiology and Incidence

An undescended testis is noted in 3% to 5% of male births. Spontaneous descent usually occurs during the first 3 months of life, reducing the rate of persistent cryptorchia to 1%. The risk of cryptorchia among offspring whose father had the defect is double that of the average population, although it is not clear how the inheritance mechanism affects the child. Cryptorchia is unilateral in 85% of males and most often affects the right testicle (Ellis, 1990). Risk for undescended testes include low birth weight and multiple births, with one of every three premature males demonstrating the defect (Sugar & Hoyler-Grant, 1995).

The cause is unknown, but several hypotheses have been presented. Hormonal causes include inadequate testosterone production or insufficient response to the androgenic hormone. Ineffective development of the inguinal canal, abnormal epididymal development, and reduced intra-abdominal pressure represent possible structural causes (Sugar & Hoyler-Grant, 1995).

Pathophysiology

Cryptorchidism represents a maldescent of the testicle, with etiologic roots in early fetal development. The testicular germ cells first appear along the mesonephric duct. Between 6 and 9 weeks after conception, hormones secreted by the structure stimulate cellular growth and maturation into an organized testicle. It remains in a perinephric position until a fibrous band exerts downward tension on the organ. By the end of the 12th week, the gonad has journeyed to the internal inguinal ring, resting there until the seventh month.

During the last trimester of the pregnancy, the inguinal canal opens and a hollow space is created into the scrotal sac. The testicle migrates into the scrotal sac, where it bonds to the scrotal lining. Closure of the internal ring of the inguinal canal concludes the process of testicular descent (Skoog & Conlin, 1995).

At birth, a vigorous cremasteric muscle allows for oscillating testicular movement. Up to 90% of newborns can easily retract the descended testicle into the distal portion of the inguinal canal. Progressive fusion of the inguinal canal eventually restricts the degree of retractility (Rozanski & Bloom, 1995).

An undescended testicle never assumes a scrotal location. The testis has less volume and density than normal (Ellis, 1990). The epididymal structure is abnormal. Spermatozoa production occurs in only 25% to 40% of these testes, although spermatozoa appear normal and mobile when analyzed microscopically (Farrer, Walker, & Rajfer, 1995). Current research suggests that these pathophysiologic features are malformations that developed during the embryonic stage of testicular development and are caused by inadequate stimulation from the pituitary gland. These pathophysiologic features are also affected by excessive heat because of their location within the child's abdomen. Early surgical correction does not reverse the underlying pathologic condition, but it does halt the progression of damage to the testicles (Huff, Hadziselimovic, & Snyder, 1993).

For reasons not clearly defined, undescended testes are subject to seven to nine times increased risk for metastatic cellular changes. A reported 6% to 10% of all malignant testicular tumors are found in men with congenital cryptorchia, and 20% of these cancers occur in a normally descended contralateral testis (Farrer et al., 1985; Huff et al., 1993).

Assessment

Assessment for testicular descent begins with the parental interview. Because the cremasteric reflex is weak during the neonatal period, the nurse should ask about the parents' observation of testicular descent during the first 3 months after birth (Rozanski & Bloom, 1995). Inquire whether the parents have noticed normal testicular descent when the child is relaxed, such as during a bath.

On visual inspection of the scrotum, a flaccid, nonpendulous scrotum suggests an absent testis. Associated inguinal hernias or hydroceles often coincide, increasing the difficulty of the scrotal examination.

Testicular retraction exerts tension on the scrotal attachment; therefore, a scrotal dimple or inversion are clues pointing to normal testicular descent. Scrotal palpation requires that the examiner have warm hands and that the child be relaxed. Relaxation can be encouraged if the toddler is placed in his parent's lap, assuming a frog-leg position. To counteract recoil of the testes, pressure may be applied at the external inguinal ring. Once the testicle is isolated, the examiner should use a milking action to coax it into the sac. Coating the finger with talc or soap may ease this process. Older boys may be examined as they sit cross-legged, leaning slightly forward to facilitate palpation.

The retractable, but normally descended, testis is equal in size to its contralateral mate, whereas the cryptorchid testis is small and softer. If no testicle can be discerned, the nurse should examine the lower abdomen, perineum, or femoral regions for an ectopic gonad.

Interdisciplinary Interventions

Medical and Surgical Management

Surgical manipulation of the undescended testis is the treatment of choice, preferably performed at age 3 to 12 months. Surgical placement accomplishes three goals: preserves as much testicular function as possible, offers the child a normal scrotal appearance, and permits regular testicular scrutiny. The orchidopexy procedure begins with a groin incision and an inguinal exploration to identify the testis, which is then dissected from its inguinal or abdominal attachment. The testicle and spermatic cord are next mobilized and extended, and the testis is inserted into a created scrotal pouch. Once the testis is in place, a scrotal incision is made to suture the testicle, preventing a possible torsion. Closure of the patent inguinal canal completes the procedure (Sugar & Hoyler-Grant, 1995).

Management of the child with a nonpalpable testis includes a presurgical laparoscopic evaluation to ascertain the presence and viability of the intra-abdominal organ. Laparoscopy allows for visualization of testicular tissue and spermatic vessels with a 90% to 100% accuracy rate. If the spermatic vessels are atretic, or undeveloped, the gonad will be absent and no surgery is required. A testicular prosthesis is surgically implanted when the child reaches puberty.

Intra-abdominal testes must be identified because of the risk of malignancy. Surgical options include gonadal excision or attempted orchidopexy. The choice is determined by physiologic potential (Moore, Peters, & Bauer, 1994).

In the past few decades, some practitioners have advocated hormonal intervention to encourage testicular descent or to facilitate surgical exploration by enlarging the gonad. Results have been disappointing for these purposes, but other benefits are emerging. Some urologists recommend the early administration of parenteral human chorionic gonadotropin or intranasal luteinizing hormone-releasing hormone to reinstate a therapeutic endocrine environment and to maximize fertility (Rozanski & Bloom, 1995).

Nursing Management

Nursing care for the child with an undescended testis and his family begins when the defect is first suspected. Parents need education regarding the importance of timely surgical correction and the endocrinologic consequence of cryptorchidism. The nurse is well suited to offer guidance related to hospitalization, preoperative and postoperative teaching, and age-appropriate coping techniques.

Once a management plan has been provided by the attending urologist or surgeon, the nursing focus is to reinforce teaching and to clarify any misconceptions held by the child or his family. If hormonal therapy is instituted, the nurse should explain all facets of the medication and emphasize the need for compliance. The nurse may use illustrations to explain the defect and the chosen medical/surgical regimen.

Postoperative nursing care following orchidopexy is usually provided in an outpatient surgical suite. The potential for nausea and vomiting is present because of the extensive abdominal exploration and, particularly, because of the spermatic cord traction. Consequently, intravenous replacement should be maintained until oral intake is ensured, and fluids are introduced slowly. High-dose intraoperative nerve blockade and caudal analgesia are given to control pain and nausea (Wilton, 1995).

Community Care

Discharge instructions encompass incisional care and activity restriction. Most surgeons either cover the operative site with a transparent dressing or leave it open to air. No special care is necessary other than inspection for signs of infection and prompt cleansing after bowel movements. The return to tub bathing depends on the surgeon's preference. Vigorous activity, straddle toys, and contact sports are restricted for 7 to 10 days.

Long-term follow-up care is imperative for the child with cryptorchia. The parents should be referred for endocrinologic consultation if infertility or hormonal dysfunction is suspected. Counseling with a psychoendocrinologist and, in time, a reproductive endocrinologist may be necessary when the boy reaches adulthood, becomes sexually active, or considers paternity.

Because of the potential for endocrinopathy and malignancy, many urologists continue to see the cryptorchid child on a yearly basis. Some physicians also recommend testicular sonograms after puberty at periodic intervals to monitor for early neoplastic changes (Lenz, Giwereman, & Skakkebaek, 1987).

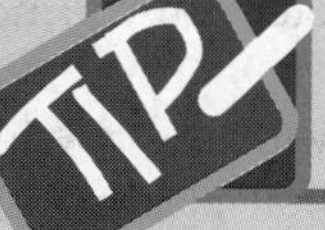

caREminder: *Monthly testicular self-examination (TSE) is recommended for all males beginning in puberty, but it is essential for the male with cryptorchia (TIP 19–3).*

As a part of discharge teaching, the nurse should provide the parents with an instructional brochure on testicular self-examination. The nurse can offer it to the child's father as an added reminder that he should also perform the procedure. Nurses who care for adolescents in any setting should be prepared to teach TSE as part of routine health maintenance. Also, nurses in clinic settings can display brochures on TSE in a prominent area with other health teaching publications.

Testicular Torsion

Torsion, or rotation, of the testicle constitutes one of the few urologic emergencies. This condition occurs when the testicular suspensory apparatus, the spermatic cord, twists and obstructs circulation to the testis. In such a case, emergency medical attention is needed to prevent tissue necrosis.

Testicular torsion occurs in 1 of every 400 males, and the peak incidence is in the second decade of life (Rabinowitz & Hulbert, 1995). The condition affects the left testicle more often that the right, possibly because it has a longer spermatic cord (Leape, 1990). No familial or racial tendencies toward the defect have been documented, nor is it associated with other congenital anomalies.

Scrotal examination of the child with testicular torsion invariably discloses a "bell-clapper" defect. Normally, the testis resides partially encased within a scrotal sheath,

TIP

TIP 19–3 A Teaching Intervention Plan for Testicular Self-Examination

Nursing Diagnosis and Child/Family Outcomes

- Health-seeking behavior related to risk for testicular malignancy

  Outcomes: Child receives demonstration of testicular self-examination (TSE).

  Child expresses comprehension of the importance of TSE and the mechanics of performing TSE.

  Child performs TSE monthly.

  Family supports the health habit of monthly TSE.

Interventions

Teach Child to Perform TSE

- Pick one day to perform TSE each month (e.g., birth date, age, house number).
- Perform TSE after bathing, when scrotal skin is moist and slippery.
- Gently roll testicle between thumb and first two fingers.
- Testicle should feel smooth and firm, like a hard-boiled egg.
- There should be no tenderness during palpation, except along the anterior border where blood vessels and nerves are attached.
- One testicle, usually the left one, is slightly larger and hangs lower than the other.

Contact Health Care Provider if

- There is tenderness.
- There are lumps or hard areas.
- The testicles have a softened texture.
- The testicles have a change in size.

and the exposed spermatic cord–epididymal layer is securely attached to the scrotal lining. This attachment stabilizes the testicle and places it in a vertical position.

In some boys, the scrotal sheath completely encases the testicle, epididymis, and spermatic cord, blocking adherence of these structures to the scrotum. This results in a loosely suspended gonad, which lies horizontally within the sac. The precipitating factor for testicular rotation is unknown, but a rising testosterone level with increased testis weight is a possible cause (Leape, 1990).

The number of males born with the "bell-clapper" defect is unknown, but it is estimated that less than 10% of affected males actually experience a torsion episode. Although the anomalous testicular attachment is bilateral in more than 50% of males, torsion is generally restricted to one testis (Bloom, Wan, & Key, 1992). Because an undescended testis can also become twisted, acute abdominal pain in the cryptorchid child should raise suspicion of torsion (Sugar & Hoyler-Grant, 1995).

A variation of testicular torsion involves the twisting of a testicular or epididymal appendix. Torsion of these congenital appendages usually occurs during preadolescence, but the condition may become manifest at any age. Damage is confined to the appendix, sparing the testicle (Rabinowitz & Hulbert, 1995).

A second form of testicular torsion occurs during testicular descent, either antenatally or within the neonatal period. This second form accounts for an estimated 5% to 10% of all torsion events (Bloom et al., 1992). Because the process is usually painless, the child undergoes treatment for cryptorchia. At the time of surgical exploration, however, testicular atrophy is evident. The "bell-clapper" deformity is often seen in the remaining testis, which is then secured to the scrotum as a precaution (Leape, 1990).

Pathophysiology

Twisting of the spermatic cord occludes testicular circulation. The initial response is tissue congestion and testicular edema; unrelieved obstruction leads to vascular thrombosis and necrosis. If the occlusion is complete and unrelieved, tissue death occurs swiftly, possibly within 2 hours and certainly after 12 hours (Leape, 1990). Intermittent or self-resolving episodes are possible and may cause varying degrees of tissue damage. The prognosis for adequate hormonal function is consequently unpredictable.

Assessment

Acute scrotal pain, often associated with nausea and vomiting, is the hallmark sign of this disorder. Because testicular torsion can occur in association with scrotal trauma, complaints of scrotal pain must always be evaluated to rule out a diagnosis of torsion.

▽ **Alert:** *The boy who complains of scrotal pain may be experiencing a testicular torsion. He* **must** *receive immediate medical attention to prevent infarction of the gland.*

A history of previous inguinal or scrotal surgery does not discount the potential for torsion (Rabinowitz & Hulbert, 1995).

Historical data should be obtained with the physical examination. The nurse should ask for details about the child's condition, such as onset and duration of pain, and any similar episodes of scrotal pain that resolved spontaneously. Persistent but mild scrotal discomfort is more suggestive of torsion of the testicular appendage. The nurse should question the adolescent male about sexual activity or urethral symptoms. Affirmative responses to these queries suggest epididymitis or orchitis.

During the history and the physical examination, it is important for the examiner to address psychosexual issues. The child should be reassured that the pain is not related to self-manipulation or to arousal from sexual fantasies. The examination must be conducted in privacy, and the child should be assured of the confidentiality of his responses. The nurse should explain that testicular torsion is a secondary effect from a congenital anomaly and that it is unrelated to sports or vigorous activity. Neither the child nor the parents should be blamed for any delay in seeking treatment. Teens typically ignore early signs of illness, and parents are frequently unaware that scrotal pain may have such serious consequences (Sugar & Hoyler-Grant, 1995).

The nurse begins the examination with the boy in a standing position to check for a horizontal placement of the opposite testis. With the boy lying down, the nurse can assess the abdomen for tenderness and pain or swelling in the inguinal area, especially if the boy has an undescended testis on the side corresponding to the pain.

The scrotum is inspected for edema. A blue dot suggesting torsion of the testicular appendix may be noted in light-skinned males (Rabinowitz & Hulbert, 1995). The nurse strokes the inner thigh of the affected side to elicit a cremasteric sign. Presence of this reflex excludes a diagnosis of testicular torsion. On palpation, the twisted testicle is exquisitely tender throughout the organ. A torsion of the appendix creates localized discomfort with a palpable upper pole nodule.

Diagnostic Tests. Microscopic urinalysis without evidence of pyuria and bacteriuria provides additional diagnostic confirmation. If the examination does not provide a clear diagnosis, high resolution sonograms with color Doppler are used to assess testicular perfusion and intrascrotal contents. This non-invasive technique has an accuracy rate that approaches 100%. Drawbacks to the color Doppler sonogram include the necessity of having an experienced radiologist available to perform the study and to confidently interpret the results, and the limited ability to assess the testicle of a prepubescent boy. The sonogram may be falsely negative if the torsion is intermittent (Atkinson, Patrick, Ball, Stevenson, & Broecker, 1992; Meza, Amundson, Aquilina, & Reitelman, 1992). If the physical examination and diagnostic studies do not conclusively exclude testicular torsion, the boy must undergo surgery.

Interdisciplinary Interventions

Suspected testicular torsion is a surgical emergency. Open exploration via a midline scrotal incision is performed, and the testis is derotated and surgically fixed to the scrotal wall. If infarction has occurred, the necrotic gland is removed to prevent detrimental effects to the remaining testis (Rabinowitz & Hulbert, 1995). A pinched testicular appendage is excised for the same reason.

Nursing care following correction of a testicular torsion is directed toward enabling the child and his parents to cope with the long-term effects of the condition. If the function of the affected testis has been severely impaired or if the organ was unsalvageable, the boy should be counseled to avoid high-impact contact sports. Many municipalities prohibit a child with only one of a paired organ set from participation in organized sports, and, for many adolescents, the forced redirection of their energy and skills may seem punitive and unfair. The nurse can facilitate a positive adjustment by candidly discussing the issue and providing referrals to counseling facilities if necessary.

Community Care

Nurses can exert the greatest effect on this disorder within the community health sphere. The best way to ensure an optimum outcome for boys with testicular torsion is by raising public awareness of the disorder. Numerous vehicles exist to educate the public about this condition, including boys' clubs, Boy Scout troops, parent groups, religious youth organizations, school health classes, and health publications in print and on the Internet.

Circumcision

Circumcision—surgical removal of the prepuce (or foreskin) of the penis—is the most common operative procedure performed on males in the United States; in 1990, an estimated 80% of male neonates were circumcised (Wiswell & Hachey, 1993). The procedure also represents one of the most controversial issues in modern pediatric health care. Until the early 1970s, circumcision was a standard practice, with approximately 90% of male infants undergoing the procedure immediately after birth. By the mid-1970s, debate arose regarding the efficacy of an elective procedure being performed on such a routine basis, usually without the compassion of pain relief. After consideration of the potential risks and cost, and without a clear indication of medical need, the American Academy of Pediatrics advised against routine circumcision in 1975, only to reverse its stance 14 years later following reports of adverse consequences for uncircumcised males (Schiff, 1989; Thompson, King, & Knox, 1975).

The rate of delayed circumcision (beyond the neonatal period) has been increasing steadily over the past 15 years in response to changing attitudes about the procedure and as a means to overcome negative consequences to the child's health (Ephgrone & Chang, 1983; Wiswell, Tencer, Welch, & Chamberlain, 1993).

Worldview: *The practice of neonatal circumcision varies dramatically worldwide. Approximately one ninth of all the male population is circumcised. North American countries have high circumcision rates. It is unlikely that male infants from Central and South America, Europe, or the Orient will experience the procedure.*

Pathophysiology

Creation of the foreskin is begun during the third fetal month. Originating at the base of the glans, the prepuce proceeds distally to envelop the penile tip, and the adjacent tissue layers become adherent. As fetal growth nears completion, clefts of cells resembling holes in a sponge develop within the preputial-glanular layer to begin the separation process. At birth, only 4% of males have a retractile prepuce, but by age 3 years, the foreskin is retractable in 90% of boys. Total preputial separation may not be accomplished until up to age 17 years (Niku, Stock, & Kaplan, 1995).

Smegma in the child is a byproduct of preputial separation. As the epithelial cells degenerate, they form white clumps, which are expelled normally during micturition. During puberty, sebaceous cell secretions mix with epithelial cells to lubricate the glans (Bloom et al., 1994).

It is surmised that the penile prepuce serves a protective function until the child is toilet trained, although its exact role is unclear. Meatitis, meatal stenosis, or glanular excoriation, which is common among circumcised infants, is almost nonexistent in uncircumcised male babies (Hoyler-Grant, 1995a).

Two pathologic conditions are related to foreskin development: phimosis and paraphimosis. **Phimosis** is defined as an unretractile foreskin. Because most infants exhibit physiologic phimosis, the description among young males is confined to foreskin constriction that obstructs urine flow. A foreskin that balloons during urination indicates phimosis. Ulceration of the glans resulting from this phenomenon may lead to balanoposthitis, an infectious condition of the glans.

Table 19–4
The Circumcision Debate

	Rationale
Pro	
Reduced risk of urinary tract infection (UTI)	· Multiple studies document rate of UTI among uncircumcised males 6 months or younger is 5 to 89 times the rate of circumcised males (Wiswell & Hachey, 1993; Wiswell et al., 1987; Hoberman et al., 1995). · There is a high incidence of systemic infection from UTI among uncircumcised male infants (Wiswell & Gischke, 1989). · Report by Craft et al. (1996) disclosed increased UTI risk for uncircumcised boys through 5 years of age.
Reduced rate of delayed circumcision when performed during neonatal period	· Rate of delayed circumcision is steadily increasing following the drop in neonatal circumcision. · Reasons for delayed circumcision include parental choice, procedure included with other surgery, history of UTI or balanoposthitis. · Requires general anesthesia, is costly and painful. · Complication rate following delayed circumcision is 1.7% (Wiswell & Hachey, 1993)
Treatment for phimosis, paraphimosis, and balanoposthitis	· These conditions are complications related to preputial retraction.
Prevention of penile cancer	· Risk is almost nonexistent in circumcised men. · Risk of cancer for uncircumcised males is 1:600; mortality rate is 25% (Niku et al., 1995).
Prevention of cervical cancer among partners	· Rate of squamous cell cancer among partners of circumcised males is low. · Human papilloma virus (HPV) types 16 and 18 are implicated in cervical cancer; their presence is more prevalent among uncircumcised males.
Special hygiene measures unnecessary	· Meatal or glanular irritation from diaper dermatitis is resolved when the child is toilet trained. · Uncircumcised males must commit to lifelong, diligent cleansing. · Increased risk of candidal infections among uncircumcised males.
Con	
Contraindicated in unstable or premature infant	· If desired, circumcision is performed before discharge.
Contraindicated for males with hypospadias or penile anomalies	· Prepuce may be needed for penile reconstruction. · Up to 38% of males with penile anomalies are inadvertently circumcised (Niku et al., 1995). · Infant with penile abnormality should be evaluated by pediatric urologist.
Infant with blood dyscrasia may have prolonged oozing after the procedure	· Circumcise with caution. · Administer coagulation therapy: silver nitrate, vitamin K, thrombin, fibrin.
Complication rate after neonatal circumcision is 0.2%–0.6%; mortality rate is 1–2 : 1 million infants (Hoyler-Grant, 1995a)	· Most complications are minor. · Complications include bleeding, wound infection, redundant foreskin from inadequate removal, penile-glanular tissue bridge. · Major complications include urethral fistula, concealed penis (excision of shaft epithelium with adhesions), penile necrosis, hypospadias, penile amputation.

Paraphimosis is the forced retraction of a tight or stenotic foreskin below the coronal ridge, usually occurring during an overzealous attempt to clean the glans before separation is complete. The resulting constriction creates distal edema, pain, and difficulty replacing the foreskin. Emergency medical intervention is needed to relieve the obstruction, and circumcision is generally recommended as a preventive measure (Hoyler-Grant, 1995a).

Assessment

Detailed scrutiny of the genitalia is necessary before neonatal circumcision is attempted. Signs that are suggestive of a congenital anomaly include chordee, a hooded prepuce, or meatus dislocation. A newborn with bilateral undescended testes and severe hypospadias should be evaluated for an intersex condition. A male infant with an apparently small phallus should also be examined by a urologist before a decision regarding circumcision is made. The nurse should palpate the bladder for distention and should assess voiding.

Alert: *The baby should be examined for signs of a bleeding dyscrasia, such as unexpected ecchymotic spots or prolonged bleeding after newborn testing.*

Vitamin K can be administered before the procedure to offset this complication. Also, the nurse should question the parents regarding a family history of coagulation disorders.

Interdisciplinary Interventions

With shortened hospital stays following delivery and intensive well-baby education condensed into that time span, many parents have little opportunity to make a thoughtful decision about circumcision. Nurses have ample opportunity to provide anticipatory guidance during prenatal visits and childbirth education programs. Offering objective information requires that the nurse be familiar with both the advantages and disadvantages of the procedure (Table 19–4). If the parents choose not to have their son circumcised, the nurse should provide instructions for proper genital care. Hygiene measures for uncircumcised males are discussed in TIP 19–4.

Circumcision is ideally performed within the first 48 hours after delivery, but it can also be performed anytime through the first month of life without anesthesia. The procedure begins with a thorough cleansing of the glans, then the inner preputial epithelium is separated from the glans. A dorsal slit is made through the foreskin, which allows a clamp mechanism to be applied over the glans. The prepuce covering the clamp is excised. Hemostasis is provided where needed, and a lubricated gauze pad is wrapped circumferentially over the raw edges. Circumcision for the older infant or child is similar, but sutures are needed to approximate the skin edges (Hoyler-Grant, 1995a).

Pain management during and following circumcision is advisable because current research has documented the ability of newborns to experience pain (Bozette, 1993; Dixon, Snyder, Holve, & Bromberger, 1984). Therapeutic options include caudal block, dorsal penile block, and eutectic mixture of local anesthetics (EMLA cream), all of which offer continued relief for 4 to 8 hours after the procedure (Niku et al., 1995; Wilton, 1995). Discomfort following circumcision may persist for 24 to 48 hours. Mild analgesics are generally adequate to extinguish pain. The need for analgesics in young infants can be determined using behavioral and physiologic parameters, such as the Neonatal Infant Pain Scale (NIPS) (Lawrence et al., 1993).

Following circumcision, the nurse should observe the child's penis for bleeding or for signs of infection. In many cases, the first sign of a blood dyscrasia is prolonged oozing after the procedure. Although most infants void within 6 hours after circumcision, an excessively tight dressing may induce urinary retention. The bandage should be reapplied to correct the problem.

Community Care

Discharge teaching includes providing parents with petroleum-coated gauze strips and giving instructions to reapply the dressing for 1 to 2 days. Parents can also use petroleum-coated gauze bandages and apply them to the tip of the penis. This dressing helps prevent the circumcised area from rubbing against the diaper or sticking to the diaper as the healing process is occurring. The older boy should avoid straddle toys or vigorous play for 3 to 4 days. Tub baths may be instituted after the fifth day to help the suture dissolve. The nurse should tell the parents that the penis will appear edematous and ecchymotic during the process of wound healing.

Worldview: *Religious and ceremonial circumcisions have been performed since ancient times. Early Egyptian art depicts the performance of a circumcision. The ritual "bris milah" is an integral part of the Jewish religion. Circumcision is also practiced by Muslims, black Africans, and Australian aborigines, frequently as a rite of passage for males in the society.*

Varicocele

A varicocele is a scrotal mass resulting from engorgement of the left spermatic vein and scrotal vasculature. Blood return from the scrotum into the left renal vein is impeded, producing antegrade vascular dilatation and stasis (Bates, 1995). The pooled blood raises the temperature

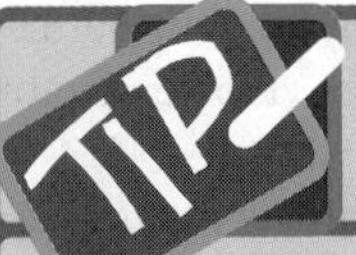

TIP 19–4 A Teaching Intervention Plan for a Boy Who Is Uncircumcised

Nursing Diagnoses and Child/Family Outcomes

- Knowledge deficit: normal preputial separation
  Outcome: Parents express an understanding of appropriate hygiene measures, which vary by age of the child.
- Potential for infection related to inappropriate hygiene measures
  Outcomes: Parents adhere to recommended hygiene measures and teach them to the child.
  Child gains independence in adopting a consistent hygiene regimen.

Hygiene Measures

Birth to 3 Years

- The foreskin and the glans (the end of the penis) are normally fused during these years.
- No specific care of the foreskin is recommended.
- Occasionally retract the foreskin to check for separation.
- The foreskin should *only* be retracted with gentle pressure until resistance is felt.

Following Complete Foreskin Separation

- Retract the foreskin fully to expose the glans.
- Cleanse the glans with a mild soap and water, dry completely.
- Return the foreskin to its normal position.
- Perform this routine daily.

Adolescence

- White discharge, called smegma, needs to be removed daily.
- Retained smegma can be irritating and may be a source of infection.
- When sanitation facilities are inadequate (such as long hiking trips) or in hot, humid climates, disposable wash towelettes may be used.

Contact Health Care Provider if

- The glans become sore or excoriated.
- There is an unusual odor, rash, or discharge around or from the penis.
- The foreskin cannot be retracted.

around the testicle, with potentially adverse effects on the organ.

Varicoceles are seldom evident before the second decade of life, reaching their peak incidence by the mid-teens. It is estimated that the rate of scrotal varicoceles may approach 15% of the adult male population; however, the defect is not palpable in most instances and may escape detection for years (Kass & Reitelman, 1995). No genetic, racial, or associated congenital risk factors are correlated with the phenomenon.

The etiologic basis for a varicocele rests with a discrepancy in the attachment angles of the right and left spermatic veins to their corresponding renal vein. The right spermatic renal junction is obliquely angled, allowing unobstructed circulation, whereas the left junction is a 90-degree angle, which reduces blood velocity. It is probable that anatomic changes in relative renal position and vascular configuration, secondary to the pubertal growth spurt, trigger the development of the varicosed venous network.

Pathophysiology

By the time the child reaches mid to late adolescence, the deleterious effects of a varicocele can be noted. Increased glandular volume, which normally occurs during puberty, is delayed in the affected left testicle. Histologic evaluation of the affected gonad demonstrates delayed maturation and decreased spermatogenesis. These changes are progressive into adulthood and eventually affect the contralateral testis (Kass, Chandra, & Belman, 1987). Semen analyses of adults with a varicocele have disclosed a reduction in density and motility of spermatozoa (Chehval & Purcell, 1992). The presence of a varicocele is a common cause for male factor infertility, and its effects are cumulative. The risk for infertility is 35% when the defect is corrected early, but increases to 80% when surgical repair is delayed beyond the third decade of life (Kass & Reitelman, 1995).

The youth's response to surgical correction of the varicocele seems to depend on the severity and duration of the condition. If correction is performed early in the disease process, the testis responds with catch-up growth and markedly improved semen quality. Testicular atrophy from long-standing or marked varicosities is irreversible (Kass & Reitelman, 1995).

Assessment

The cardinal sign of a varicocele is a palpable scrotal mass of veins, typically described as a "bag of worms." The defect is noted when the boy is in an upright position, and it resolves when the adolescent is examined in a supine position. Occasionally, boys describe a heavy or dragging sensation to the scrotum, but most varicoceles are asymptomatic. They are usually detected during a routine scrotal examination or when teaching the child to perform TSE.

When a varicocele is palpated, the examiner should determine testicular volume, monitoring for a discrepancy between the affected gland and its mate. Testicular volume should be measured on a regular basis with an orchidometer, which is a valid indicator of testicular damage.

Another test to determine testicular failure involves the injection of gonadotropin-releasing hormone (GnRH). Abnormally high levels of luteinizing hormone and follicle-stimulating hormone after injection represent positive indicators of reduced spermatozoa-producing capabilities (Kass, Freitas, Salisz, & Steinert, 1993).

Interdisciplinary Interventions

Early detection of the varicocele and vigilant monitoring for testicular changes are necessary to avoid testicular damage.

caREminder: *Thorough genital examinations should be instituted once the boy enters puberty, and they should be repeated yearly.*

Surgical correction is recommended when signs of testicular impairment are present, such as abnormal semen analysis, left testicular volume deficit as compared with the right gonad, or excessive response to the GnRH stimulation test. The recommended procedure is a ligation of the varicosity and removal of the spermatic vein, either as an open procedure or by laparoscopic approach (Kass & Reitelman, 1995).

Nursing care for the adolescent undergoing a varicocelectomy includes routine postoperative stabilization, relief from pain, and wound assessment. The hospital stay is minimal, and home instructions focus on activity restrictions for 10 to 14 days.

Community Care

Important components of discharge teaching by the nurse are to review the possible postoperative complications with the child and his family and to stress the necessity of performing monthly TSE to the boy himself. Long-term problems, although infrequent, include the development of a hydrocele or the recurrence of a varicocele arising from varicosed collateral vessels. A postoperative hydrocele is asymptomatic and is typically left unrepaired. A recurring varicocele requires additional surgery to ensure that the affected testicle will catch up to its contralateral mate in volume size.

Renal Disorders

The nephron is the basic structural and functional unit of the kidney; each kidney has about 1 million nephrons. Approximately one fourth of the output of each ventricular contraction goes through the kidneys, so that the body's total blood volume passes through the kidneys 12 times each hour.

Inside each nephron, the hydrostatic pressure of blood in the capillary tuft, or glomerulus, causes water and solutes to filter into Bowman's capsule. Although they are 100 to 500 times more permeable that other capillaries in the body, glomerular capillaries are selective about the types of molecules that pass through them. The three major layers of the glomerular capillaries—the endothelial layer, the basement membrane layer, and the podocytes on the inner layer of Bowman's capsule—regulate the size of molecules filtered by the size of their respective fenestrae, spaces, and slit pores. Molecules weighing less than 5000 daltons are easily filtered, but filtration decreases as molecular weight increases. Molecules heavier than 68,000 daltons filter poorly or not at all (Bergstein, 1996; Lancaster, 1995).

In addition, all three layers of the glomerular capillaries have negative electric charges, which repel the negatively charged plasma proteins and solutes. Thus, some molecules, such as albumin, which should filter well because of their size, are not usually found in glomerular filtrate because electrostatic forces inhibit their passage through the glomerular capillary layers (Bergstein, 1996; Lancaster, 1995).

As glomerular filtrate passes through the proximal convoluted tubule, the loop of Henle, and the distal convoluted tubule, additional solute is absorbed into or secreted from the peritubular capillaries into the tubular lumen. Once the modified glomerular filtrate has reached the collecting tubules, it has become urine (Lancaster, 1995).

Acute Renal Failure

Acute renal failure (ARF) is a condition that develops rapidly, over days or weeks. It can be classified according to the site of injury to the kidney:

- Prerenal, resulting from impaired blood flow to or oxygenation of the kidneys
- Renal (or parenchymal), resulting from injury to or malformation of the kidney tissue
- Postrenal, resulting from obstruction of the urinary flow at some level between the kidney and the urinary meatus (Frauman & Gilman, 1979)

Prerenal ARF is usually cured with early supportive treatment. Renal ARF may require dialysis. Postrenal ARF usually requires surgical removal of the obstruction (Guignard, Semama, John, & Huet, 1993).

Etiology

Prerenal causes of ARF are most common in newborns, and include hypotension, hypoxia, or complications of surgical treatment of congenital cardiac problems. Renal vein thrombosis is a less common cause of prerenal ARF. Drug toxicities and congenital renal malformations are causes of renal ARF in newborns (Evans, 1994). Postrenal ARF is due to obstruction somewhere in the urinary tract.

One form of ARF is called acute tubular necrosis (ATN) because the cells lining the kidney tubules die and slough off (Frauman & Gilman, 1979). ATN can be caused by either ischemia or nephrotoxicity (Kellen, Aronson, Roizen, Barnard, & Thisted, 1994).

Most commonly, ARF develops in infants and preschool children as a result of HUS. In older children and adolescents, ARF usually develops as a result of renal causes, such as rapidly progressive glomerulonephritis, the side effects of systemic lupus erythematosus, or other vascular diseases. However, some cases of HUS can occur in older children (Evans, 1994).

Pathophysiology

Prerenal ARF results from the kidneys' protective responses to diminished renal blood flow in an effort to regain normal intravascular volume, blood pressure, and renal perfusion. In the first response, the myogenic reflex, the glomerular afferent arteriole dilates to maintain glomerular blood flow. With the second response, glomerulotubular feedback, constriction or dilation of the afferent arteriole is further regulated by sodium and chloride delivery to the macula densa area of each nephron. Third, decreased blood pressure in the kidneys causes release of renin, which leads to production of angiotensin, a potent vasoconstrictor, and increased aldosterone synthesis, which increases sodium resorption from distal tubule. Also, vasopressin secretion is increased, which results in more water being resorbed from the distal tubule. However, these protective responses work for a limited time. Without volume replacement to correct hypotension, renal ARF or permanent renal damage can result (Bock, 1992).

In renal ARF, the kidney parenchyma is damaged by ischemia or nephrotoxic substances. Decreased renal blood flow, decreased glomerular filtration volume, and "back leak" of filtrate from tubular lumens to peritubular capillaries are the result of the tubular damage.

Renal ARF can also be caused by damaged glomeruli, as in HUS, acute glomerulonephritis, or renal vessel thrombosis in neonates. The endothelial cells in the microvasculature are damaged in renal ARF. Platelet-fibrin thrombi form, which damage passing red blood cells. Decreased or blocked glomerular capillary blood flow results, which decreases filtration surface area in the kidney (Bock, 1992).

UPJ stricture, PUVs, calculi, tumors, or compression of the ureters or the urethra may cause postrenal ARF. However, deposition of substances such as uric acid crystals, xanthines, or casts in the tubular lumens can also cause postrenal ARF. Renal blood flow increases in early hours after an obstruction occurs, but it slowly declines with prolonged obstruction from renal vasoconstriction (Bock, 1992).

Prognosis. If oliguria does not last long, if the blood chemistry values are not severely abnormal, and if the child's general condition is good, then the prognosis for regaining normal kidney function is good (Frauman & Gilman, 1979). Mortality rate in ARF can range from 37% to 80%, depending on associated complications (Chart 19–12). In children younger than 1 month, the requirement for mechanical ventilation, elevated serum creatinine levels, the need for dialysis, hypotension and cardiomyopathy significantly increase mortality rates. On the other hand, ARF resulting from renal causes has a very good prognosis; in one study, there were no deaths (Gallego et al., 1993).

Assessment

The symptoms of ARF have a sudden onset and are related directly to the lack of kidney function. The first sign may be oliguria, production of less than 1 mL of urine per kilogram of body weight per hour in infants or less than 0.5 mL/kg/hr in children (Gaudio, Devarajan, Boydstun, Van Why, & Siegel, 1994). Anuria, essentially no urine production, is a less common sign of ARF.

Volume overload resulting from retained fluid can cause hypertension, edema, or shortness of breath. Acido-

Chart 19–12

Systemic Effects of Renal Failure

Serum Chemistries Change

- Urea—increased
- Creatinine—increased
- Uric acid—increased
- Potassium—usually increased
- Sodium—increased or decreased
- Calcium—decreased
- Magnesium—increased
- Chloride—usually decreased
- Phosphate—increased
- Sulfate—increased

Metabolic Acidosis

- Decreased ability to excrete acid
- Decreased ability to resorb bicarbonate

Water Metabolism

- Decreased ability to concentrate urine
- Decreased ability to dilute urine

Cardiovascular

- Hypertension
- Congestive heart failure
- Pericarditis

Pulmonary

- Pulmonary edema

Hematopoietic

- Normocytic, normochromic anemia
- Decreased erythropoiesis
- Shortened red cell life span
- Tendency to bleed

Gastrointestinal

- Bleeding
- Anorexia, nausea, vomiting
- Parotitis or stomatitis

Skeletal

- Impaired growth
- Renal osteodystrophy
- Osteomalacia
- Osteitis fibrosa
- Osteosclerosis

Endocrine

- Delayed puberty
- Decreased libido
- Impotency in males
- Ovulation and menstruation suppressed in females

Psychological

- Lethargy
- Decreased mental acuity
- Impaired concentration
- Depression
- Psychosis with paranoid delusions and hallucinations

Neuromuscular

- Grand mal seizures
- Involuntary muscle twitching
- Peripheral neuropathy

Integumentary

- Dryness
- Scaliness
- Itching
- Yellow-gray-brown tint
- Bruises and petechiae
- Uremic frost

General

- Increased susceptibility to infection
- Hypothermia
- Slower wound healing

Adapted from Harrington, J. D., & Brener, E. R. (1973). *Patient care in renal failure.* Philadelphia: W. B. Saunders. Used with permission.

sis and serum electrolyte imbalance can cause gastrointestinal disturbances (anorexia, nausea, vomiting, diarrhea), cardiac arrhythmias, altered level of consciousness (lethargy, drowsiness, coma), or central nervous system disturbances (headache, seizures). Diuresis marked by polyuria is usually the first sign of recovery.

Diagnostic Tests. Renal failure can affect the results of various laboratory tests (see Chart 19–12). Prolonged alterations in serum chemistries can cause anemia resulting from shortened red blood cell life span as well as from bleeding diathesis. In addition, decreased renal production of erythropoietin impairs production of red blood cells, potentiating the anemia. Also, susceptibility to infection is increased in renal failure (Frauman & Gilman, 1979).

The oliguria of ARF lasts about 3 weeks. The polyuric recovery phase is heralded by a slow increase in urine volume, often greatly exceeding normal volumes, followed by slow decline in serum creatinine and BUN.

Alert: *Assessment for electrolyte imbalances and dehydration during the polyuric phase of ARF is important. Massive urine output can quickly place the child in electrolyte or fluid imbalance.*

Interdisciplinary Interventions

The goals in treating ARF are to reduce symptoms and to provide supportive care until renal function returns. Treatment can range from conservative management to some form of dialysis, depending on the severity of the symptoms (see Chronic Renal Failure). Medication, dietary restrictions, or dialysis may be needed to control fluid overload, acidosis, electrolyte imbalance, or central nervous system disturbances. Recombinant synthetic human erythropoietics (i.e., Epogen or Procrit) should be administered to prevent the anemia of renal failure. Good hygiene practices such as diligent handwashing and daily baths at home and in the health care setting are needed to prevent infections.

Chronic Renal Failure

Chronic renal failure (CRF) may develop slowly, over months to years. Its progress is usually divided into four stages: decreased renal reserve, chronic renal insufficiency, CRF, and ESRD.

In the first stage, decreased renal reserve, the kidney function is slightly impaired, but the body chemistries remain within the normal range. The glomerular filtration rate (GFR) is 50% to 80% of normal for age (Kher, 1992a). The second stage, chronic renal insufficiency, begins when the GFR declines below 50% of normal for age. Wastes accumulate in the blood, and the body is slow to cope with electrolyte disturbances (Frauman & Gilman, 1979; Kher, 1992a). The third stage, CRF, is defined by a GFR of 10% to 25% of normal for age, although it has been used to name all types of declining renal function (Kher, 1992a). The final stage of CRF is called uremia, azotemia, or ESRD. In this stage, the GFR is 10% or less of normal for age, insufficient to support life.

Pathophysiology

Although many different diseases can cause CRF, the morphologic changes associated with the progression to ESRD are somewhat standard. Sclerotic glomeruli with proliferative matrix changes as well as interstitial fibrosis are common. Chronic interstitial inflammation and tubular atrophy are also seen. The few remaining functional glomeruli may have hypertrophic tubules as the kidney attempts to compensate for lost function (Jacobson, 1991).

In children with CRF, some form of renal replacement therapy is required to avoid inevitable death. Kidney transplantation is the ultimate treatment goal for children with ESRD (Frauman & Gilman, 1979).

Assessment

There is no clearly defined change from health to illness as CRF develops. Symptoms of CRF are the same as in ARF, with the addition of delayed growth and sexual maturation, dry itchy skin, and renal osteodystrophy or bony changes—bone pain, slipped epiphyses, pathologic fractures, myopathy, and hyperparathyroidism (Frauman & Gilman, 1979; Kher, 1992a).

The clinical manifestations of CRF are caused by the build-up of metabolic wastes, fluid and electrolyte imbalance, and lack of hormones produced by the kidney. Anemia, metabolic acidosis, hyperkalemia, hypernatremia, the inability to concentrate or dilute urine, glucose intolerance, hyperlipidemia, hypertension, pericarditis, exercise intolerance, peripheral neuropathies, impaired platelet function, and impaired immune system function are common results of decreasing kidney function (Kher, 1992a).

The nurse must assess the child and the family for their response to CRF. Like any other chronic illness, the psychological effects of CRF on the child and family can be devastating (Frauman & Gilman, 1979). Both the diagnosis and the required treatment cause stress for all family members. Parents mourn the loss of their "normal, healthy" child and experience anger, denial, and hopelessness. (See Chapter 12 for information on the grieving family.) Even though they intellectually understand that ESRD means total, permanent loss of kidney function, parents still may repeatedly question the necessity of recommended treatments and ask for second opinions. Children, too, mourn the loss of their good health. If nephrectomy is necessary, they mourn the loss of this body part, even though there was no normal kidney function remaining. Some children believe that being "bad" has brought on the illness and that only being "good" will result in a cure. These children need frequent reassurance to decrease their fright and increase their sense of well-being.

If the cause is a hereditary disease, guilt is a common parental feeling. Parents who believe that the disease may result in the child's death may become distant and less supportive of the child because they are experiencing anticipatory grief.

Family or relationship problems are intensified by the stress of chronic illness. Strong families can draw closer together, but breakup is common in weaker ones. Sometimes, close parent–child relationships become pathologically overprotective. Children can respond to chronic renal disease in different ways. Some demonstrate maximal denial by withdrawing from the world and sleeping almost constantly. Others become dependent and demanding of attention from parents and caregivers. Children with personality maladjustments and behavior problems usually become worse owing to the stress of chronic illness.

Diagnostic Tests. Kidney function can be evaluated in various ways: urine volume, urine specific gravity, urine osmolality, serum creatinine and BUN, urine/plasma creatinine, urine/plasma urea, urinary sodium, fractional excretion of sodium, free water clearance, creatinine clearance, and renal blood flow. Serial creatinine clearance measurement is the most sensitive test for determining decreasing renal function. Such creatinine clearances require a 24-hour urine collection and a blood sample obtained at the end of the collection. Clearance is determined by multiplying urine creatinine by urine volume, then dividing by the plasma creatinine (Kellen et al., 1994).

Nursing Diagnoses and Outcomes

The slow onset of CRF and the anticipation of needing dialysis and transplantation at some future point in time govern the selection of diagnoses, which reflect the child's psychosocial needs. Nursing diagnoses and outcomes typically applicable to the child with renal disease are presented in Chart 19–3. The child and family require extensive teaching to prepare them for each different phase of the child's disease progression. Diagnoses that can be applied to direct the child's psychosocial care needs should be evaluated and include those related to activity intolerance and body image disturbance. In addition, the following nursing diagnoses may be applicable to reflect alterations in family and individual coping:

- **Compromised, ineffective family coping related to presence of chronic condition and ongoing care requirements of child**
  Outcomes: The child and/or family demonstrate effective decision-making and mutual support activities.
  The child and/or family share ongoing concerns with one another and with members of the health care team.
  The child and/or family participate in treatment activities at developmentally appropriate levels.
- **Anticipatory grieving related to loss of kidney function and restricted lifestyle**
  Outcomes: The child and/or family verbalize feelings of grief and accept these responses as appropriate to the situation.
  The child and/or family seek support from appropriate resources to assist in dealing with grief.

Interdisciplinary Interventions

Treatment for CRF or ESRD ranges from conservative medical management to dialysis or kidney transplantation. All treatment modalities for children require a major investment of parental time and energy as well as commitment from an interdisciplinary caregiver team. Each discipline tries to correct family members' knowledge deficits, and each supports the other disciplines in caring for the child and family. Because their work overlaps significantly, team members need to meet regularly to discuss care plans, which permits consistent care and a unified approach to the child and family.

In the child's early stages of renal failure, regular observation of the child's condition may be all that is required. However, when a child is first diagnosed with renal failure requiring some kind of treatment, all of the appropriate treatment modalities should be explained to the parents and to the child, if the child is old enough. Extended family or significant others who support the family and assist in caring for the child also should be included in the educational process.

Nursing care of the child with CRF includes teaching the child and family about the illness, the treatment options (do nothing, conservative management, peritoneal dialysis [PD], hemodialysis, and transplantation), and the long-term implications of the possible choices (TIP 19–5). It is important to assess family coping mechanisms and to enhance their function. Both the child and family should be aware of the results of noncompliance with the prescribed treatment regimen, and the nurse should focus on promoting the most normal lifestyle possible (Frauman & Gilman, 1979; Gilman & Frauman, 1997).

Conservative Management

Conservative management is commonly used for children with impaired renal function before dialysis is required. The main focus of conservative management is to treat the symptoms of renal failure. Conservative management is used to control symptoms and prevent their interfering with the child's lifestyle as much as possible.

The nurse caring for a child undergoing conservative management should be prepared to observe the child's affect, alertness, and energy level. Frequent blood pressure readings are necessary.

Alert: *When caring for a child undergoing conservative management, the nurse should observe affect, alertness, and energy level often. Changes in these areas can be the first signal that the disease is progressing and may require a different treatment modality.*

Frequent blood pressure readings are necessary during conservative management. Changes in the kidneys' ability to concentrate urine can lead to hypertension if fluid

TIP 19–5 A Teaching Intervention Plan for the Child with Renal Disease

Nursing Diagnoses and Child/Family Outcomes

- Risk for fluid volume excess related to excess fluid intake or excess sodium intake or retention
  Outcomes: Child maintains fluid intake within ordered parameters.
  Child maintains baseline weight.
  Child/family demonstrate skill in monitoring child's fluid intake and sodium intake.
- Risk for altered skin integrity related to delayed healing, pruritus, edema, and/or Tenckhoff catheter insertion
  Outcomes: Child's skin remains intact.
  Child/family institute measures to monitor and maintain skin integrity.
- Altered growth and development related to effects of disease and medications
  Outcome: Child demonstrates age-appropriate skills and behaviors to the extent possible.

Interventions

Fluid Intake

- If fluids need to be encouraged, offer small amounts (30 to 60 mL) of the child's favorite fluid every hour while the child is awake.
- Keep a chart of the fluids consumed to assist in monitoring intake.
- If fluids are restricted, pour out the day's fluid allotment in a single container to be kept in the refrigerator. Set aside enough fluid to consume with medications.
- Any food substance that melts (e.g., ice cream, ice, gelatin dessert) counts as liquid intake.
- Ensure that all fluids have some calories in them to maximize the number of calories that the child receives. Low-calorie and diet drinks should not be offered unless the child is significantly overweight.

Nutrition

- If the child is in renal failure, protein intake is restricted to 20 to 40 g/day.
- If the child is receiving peritoneal dialysis, protein intake may be up to 100 g/day.
- A potassium-restricted diet (2 g/day) is generally recommended. High-potassium foods include citrus fruits, dried fruits, bananas, potatoes, chocolate, nuts, and tomatoes.
- No-added-salt diet
  - No more than 4 g of sodium/day
  - Do not use table salt at all
- Low-salt diet
  - No more than 2 g of sodium/day
  - Do not use table salt at all
- Encourage intake of high-carbohydrate and/or high-fat foods, such as hard candy, bread, and butter, and adding Polycose or vegetable oil to formulas.
- Calcium supplements should be given to prevent bowing of the long bones and joint swelling (renal rickets).

Skin Care

- Because healing times are prolonged, monitor skin integrity daily and provide routine skin care.
- Clean the Tenckhoff catheter, hemodialysis access catheter, or urinary diversion tube site daily.
- Itching is common in renal failure. The child's nails should be kept trimmed to prevent scratching, and a moisturizing cream (e.g., Eucerin) should be used to help minimize itching.

TIP 19–5 A Teaching Intervention Plan for the Child with Renal Disease *Continued*

Health Maintenance

- Practice proper hand washing to prevent infections in the child with immunosuppression.
- Immunizations (especially chickenpox vaccine) should be current before kidney transplantation.
- Platelet function is decreased. Observe child for bleeding; if bleeding occurs, apply direct pressure to the site, elevate the affected area, and apply a dressing or ice to the site.
- Promote good dental hygiene to prevent cavity formation and the need for extensive dental work.

Developmental Considerations

- Encourage independence and activities appropriate to child's developmental level.
- Encourage school attendance.
- Set behavioral limits and reward desired behaviors.
- Give the child choices, allowing some participation in decisions about his or her care.

is retained or in hypotension in cases of high-output renal failure.

Although laboratory tests are a good means of monitoring serum chemistries, health care personnel should keep laboratory tests to a minimum and decrease the trauma associated with laboratory tests as much as possible. For instance, drawing blood from a child's heparin lock or implanted venous access device eliminates the need for multiple needle sticks.

Alert: *Renal failure affects the body's ability to form blood clots. Children who have been in renal failure for a while can be at risk for prolonged bleeding. Excessive bleeding with laboratory tests or injuries can be controlled with the application of ice and direct pressure.*

Nausea and vomiting are common symptoms of renal failure, particularly as the child gets closer to requiring dialysis. This is thought to be a result of the altered serum chemistries. If medications are vomited, the caregiver must give the dose again.

The child in renal failure is immunosuppressed by his or her disease. The nurse should help the child to avoid exposure to contagious disease, to avoid skin breakdown, and to take antibiotics as ordered (Frauman & Gilman, 1979).

Dietary Management

Each diet for a child with renal failure is individualized and designed to compensate for impaired kidney function. Although most diets are low in protein (1.5 to 2 g/kg of body weight), low in potassium (2 g), and low to moderate in sodium (1 to 2 g), the permitted levels may be modified depending on the child's requirements. To achieve fluid balance, the child's intake is usually restricted. However, early CRF can sometimes involve high output of urine, which is mostly water with few waste products excreted. In that event, fluid intake must be liberal.

The diet for a child with renal failure is essentially a balanced diet. No food is entirely forbidden, but total intake of each substance must be monitored. The family needs to know of any restrictions and should help the child comply with the regimen. Grandparents or friends, too, may inadvertently sabotage the diet by handing the child a candy bar or a banana if they are unaware of the scope of restrictions.

The child in renal failure should live as normal a life as possible. Attending school, after-school activities, sports, scouting, and camp are part of a normal lifestyle. The child, parents, and health care givers can explain the dietary limitations to school and camp personnel. Most institutions can adjust menus for children with dietary restrictions.

Family outings to amusement parks or restaurants can be planned for. Most eating establishments provide sample menus to allow choices to be made in advance. Diligent dietary compliance before and after a special event can allow leeway for more liberal intake during the event. Children on diets for renal failure can eat "junk food" along with their peers, but they must do it less frequently and in moderate amounts.

The child with renal failure should never be made to feel different or deprived because of dietary limitations. Having the whole family eat the diet for renal failure at home helps the child to feel more normal. In addition, the family's food preparer avoids the stress of preparing two different menus at each meal; salt, spices, or butter can be added to individual portions after they have been served.

The child on a limited potassium diet needs to limit his or her intake of citrus fruits, bananas, potatoes, chocolate, nuts, and tomatoes, which are all high in potassium. Dried fruits of all kinds are also high in potassium, because the dehydration process concentrates the substance.

Renal Replacement Therapies

When a child with ARF or CRF has insufficient kidney function to maintain reasonable fluid and electrolyte balance, or to prevent serious symptoms despite dietary restrictions and medication therapy, some form of renal replacement therapy must be instituted. If such therapy is not begun when kidney function is less than 10% of normal, death generally ensues within a week or two.

Renal replacement therapies are based on three processes: diffusion, osmosis, and ultrafiltration. Water removed from the body during dialysis is called ultrafiltrate. The process that removes it is called ultrafiltration. In hemodialysis, ultrafiltration results from hydrostatic pressures; in PD, it is due to osmotic forces.

In hemodialysis, osmosis and ultrafiltration take place outside of the body in the artificial kidney, or dialyzer, which is part of the extracorporeal circuit. In PD, these processes take place inside the child's peritoneal cavity.

Indications for Dialysis. Altered laboratory values or fluid imbalance that cannot be controlled with conservative measures, such as diet or medication, require dialysis. The child with severe hyperkalemia, hyponatremia, increased BUN levels, fluid retention, and metabolic acidosis is a candidate for dialysis. Symptoms or complications of uremia such as anorexia, nausea and vomiting, lethargy, and an inability to concentrate are also indications to begin dialysis (Evans, 1994).

Specific serum creatinine and creatinine clearance values and other criteria have been established as indications for dialysis in adult patients. However, such specific criteria have not been adopted for pediatric patients because serum creatinine levels depend on the child's muscle mass. Thus, a serum creatinine of 3.0 mg/dL in a newborn could demonstrate the same need for dialysis shown by a level of 8 mg/dL in an adolescent. As a result, creatinine clearance may be more useful in determining the need for dialysis in smaller children. Symptoms of ESRD are sufficient reason to begin dialysis even if laboratory values do not seem to indicate that it is needed. For children with ARF, the rapidity of onset,

Table 19–5
Comparison of Dialysis Modalities

Modality	Advantages	Disadvantages
Peritoneal dialysis	Easy to start Easy for staff to learn Liberal diet Liberal fluids Consistent therapy Most normal lifestyle No heparinization	Slow, gentle fluid removal and solute correction Not appropriate if recent abdominal surgery Unrelenting—7 days per week Risk of peritonitis, tunnel and exit site infections
Hemodialysis	Rapid fluid and solute chemistry correction	Expensive equipment Trained and experienced staff required Blood vessel access required Heparinization required Diet and fluid restrictions Intermittent therapy Extracorporeal circuit required
Continuous renal replacement therapy	Slow, gentle fluid removal and solute correction for the hemodynamically unstable patient	Blood vessel access required Requires high staff-to-patient ratio with highly trained and experienced staff Heparinization required Extracorporeal circuit required Continuous arteriovenous hemofiltration requires mean arterial pressure >60 mmHg

duration, severity of abnormalities, and symptoms govern the physician's decision to begin dialysis (Table 19–5) (Gaudio et al., 1994).

Peritoneal Dialysis. In PD, both osmosis and ultrafiltration take place inside the child's body. Sterile dialysate flows into the peritoneal cavity via the dialysis catheter. The dialysate stays in the peritoneal cavity for 2 to 12 hours (dwell) and then is drained out. Fresh dialysate is instilled to complete the cycle (Chart 19–13). In PD, the dialyzing membrane, the peritoneum, is exactly the right size compared to body surface area for each child.

The rate of osmosis in PD is determined by the amount of dialysate put into the child's abdomen; 30 to 50 mL of dialysate per kilogram of body weight is the usual amount. Frequency of exchanges also affects the osmosis rate. Very sick, catabolic children undergo hourly exchanges. Essentially healthy children on long-term PD receive four exchanges each day (Gilman & Frauman, 1997).

Commercially prepared dialysate is available in three dextrose concentrations: 1.5%, 2.5%, and 4.25%. The dextrose concentration governs the rate of ultrafiltration; the higher the dextrose concentration, the more fluid is removed during an exchange (Gilman & Frauman, 1997).

PD can be done in various ways. Intermittent peritoneal dialysis (IPD), continuous ambulatory peritoneal dialysis (CAPD), and continuous cycling peritoneal dialysis (CCPD) (sometimes called automated PD, or APD) are the methods commonly used for pediatric patients.

IPD is the usual method for the acutely ill child who requires a dialysis exchange every 1 to 2 hours. Such children are usually seriously ill and are in the intensive care unit. Their serum chemistries fluctuate and dictate frequent adjustments in the composition of their dialysate (Gilman & Frauman, 1997).

The IPD system is an open system; it has air vents and other openings in the tubing. This arrangement, along with recurrent breaks in the system caused by frequent dialysate bag changes, increases the likelihood of peritonitis. Peritonitis develops in most children on IPD for more than 4 to 5 days. Changing to a closed PD system as soon as the child's condition stabilizes helps prevent peritonitis (Gilman & Frauman, 1997).

CAPD is an excellent way to dialyze the pediatric patient. CAPD is performed at home, and just one clinic visit per month is required for the stable child. Children younger than 3 years may need more frequent clinic visits. Few dietary restrictions and medications are required. CAPD is easily incorporated into most lifestyles, so normal activities, such as full-time school attendance, are possible. Children on CAPD usually grow, feel well, and have time to engage in their preferred activities (Gilman & Frauman, 1997).

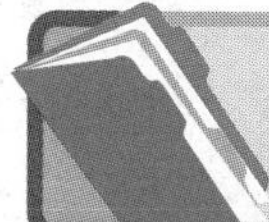

Chart 19–13
Nursing Interventions Classification (NIC)

Peritoneal Dialysis Therapy

Definition

Administration and monitoring of dialysis solution into and out of the peritoneal cavity

Activities

- Explain the selected peritoneal dialysis procedure and purpose.
- Warm the dialysis fluid before instillation.
- Assess patency of catheter, noting difficulty in inflow/outflow.
- Maintain record of inflow/outflow volumes and individual/cumulative fluid balance.
- Have patient empty bladder before peritoneal catheter insertion.
- Monitor blood pressure, pulse, respirations, temperature, and patient response during dialysis.
- Ensure aseptic handling of peritoneal catheter and connections.
- Draw laboratory samples and review blood chemistries (e.g., blood urea nitrogen, serum creatinine, and serum Na, K, and PO_4 levels).
- Obtain cell count cultures of peritoneal effluent, if indicated.
- Record baseline vital signs: weight, temperature, pulse, respirations, and blood pressure.
- Measure and record abdominal girth.
- Measure and record daily weight.
- Anchor connections and tubing securely.
- Check equipment and solutions, according to protocol.
- Administer dialysis exchanges (inflow, dwell, and outflow) according to protocol.
- Monitor for signs of infection (e.g., peritonitis and exit site inflammation/drainage).
- Monitor for signs of respiratory distress.
- Monitor for bowel perforation or fluid leaks.
- Work collaboratively with patient to adjust length of dialysis, diet regulations, and pain and diversion needs to achieve optimal benefit of the treatment.
- Teach patient to monitor self for signs and symptoms that indicate need for medical treatment (e.g., fever, bleeding, respiratory distress, irregular pulse, cloudy outflow, and abdominal pain).
- Teach procedure to patient requiring home dialysis.

From McCloskey, J., & Bulechek, G. (1996). *Nursing interventions classification (NIC)* (2nd ed.). St. Louis: Mosby–Year Book. Reprinted with permission.

Three to five exchanges per day of 30 to 50 mL of dialysate per kilogram of body weight are the norm in CAPD. The exchanges can be timed to fit into the family's daily schedule. A precise time schedule is not required; rather, completion of the correct number of exchanges each day is essential. A usual schedule is to do the exchanges upon arising, immediately after school, at mid-evening, and before bedtime. On weekends, the schedule may be adjusted to coincide with meals.

Dwell times (the time the fluid remains in the child's abdomen) should be a minimum of 2 hours, but they can be as long as 12 hours. The dextrose concentration is prescribed according to the child's fluid balance, oral intake, residual renal function, and blood pressure (Gilman & Frauman, 1997).

CAPD is a closed system. Many different types of commercial CAPD systems are available. Each system should be resistant to error and should be user-friendly. The choice of system depends on recommendations from the health care team, the patient support services offered by the vendor, the cost-effectiveness of the system, and the child and family's preference (Gilman & Frauman, 1997).

CCPD, or **APD**, works in the same way as CAPD. However, a machine delivers dialysate to the peritoneum, measures the dwell period, and ensures that all of the dialysate and ultrafiltrate is drained from the peritoneal cavity. Usually, CCPD is completed at night while the child sleeps (Gilman & Frauman, 1997).

Many medical facilities use CCPD exclusively for pediatric patients, believing that it lessens the burden of parental responsibility because the system is opened only twice a day—at bedtime and upon rising. Hernias are also less likely to develop in children on CCPD than on CAPD (Gilman & Frauman, 1997).

caREminder: *When the abdominal cavity is filled with a large volume of dialysate, less pressure is exerted on the abdominal wall and the inguinal canal when the patient is in a recumbent position than in a standing position; thus, hernias are less likely to occur.*

Other medical centers find that CCPD provides less dialysis than is required unless a CAPD exchange is also done during the day. Sometimes, two such exchanges are required to achieve optimal solute removal.

Child's Participation in Care. The responsibility of performing PD exchanges at home is approximately equivalent to that of driving a car. Therefore, a child should not be expected to perform PD without adult supervision unless the child is mature enough to accept the equivalent responsibility of driving (Chart 19–14). Usually, two parents of younger children or a teen patient and one parent are trained to perform PD treatments. However, it is not unusual to train several caregivers to support one child on PD. A child whose parents are divorced and/or remarried and who spends time in two different households may need to have both parents and both stepparents trained to perform PD. Extended family members or daycare providers may need to be trained as well. Each trained person should perform at least three exchanges a week so that their technique does not deteriorate through lack of use (Fig. 19–10).

Chart 19–14
Developmental Considerations

Participation in Peritoneal Dialysis at Home

Age	Age-Appropriate Activities
Infant	Wears a mask during sterile procedures without distress, and without removing it Tolerates catheter exit site care without undue distress Easily distracted by diversional activities during exchange procedure
Toddler	Same as Infant Does not attempt to pull on catheter tubing
Preschooler	Same as Toddler Assists in gathering supplies or preparing the room where an exchange will be performed Fully cooperates during an exchange procedure Assists in disposing of supplies after procedure
School-Age	Gathers supplies and prepares room where exchange will be performed Completes exchanges or sets up cyclers with parental or other adult supervision Examines effluent for cloudiness Disposes of supplies after procedure
Adolescent	Gathers supplies and prepares room where exchange will be performed Completes exchanges with minimal or no supervision Disposes of supplies after procedure Informs parents when supplies are low and need to be reordered Recognizes early signs of peritonitis

Tenckhoff Catheter. No matter which type of PD is done, access to the peritoneum is achieved with a Tenckhoff catheter. These catheters are available in different lengths, cuff arrangements (single or double), and

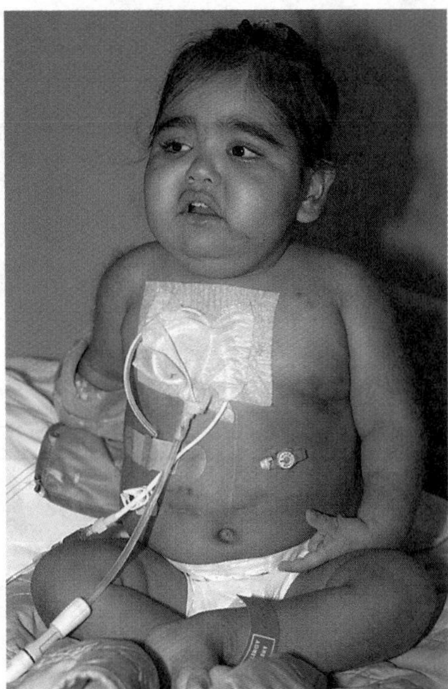

Figure 19–10
In peritoneal dialysis an implanted tube allows instillation of the dialysate fluid into the child's peritoneal cavity. (Courtesy of Children's Medical Center, Dallas, TX.)

configurations (straight or curly). The pediatric nephrologist or surgeon placing the catheter determines which type is used. The catheter is placed in the peritoneum through a midline incision below the umbilicus. The distal portion is tunneled to a lateral exit site on the abdomen where it does not interfere with the child's clothing (Fig. 19–11).

Catheter function can be compromised by poor catheter position, fibrin or omentum clogging the holes, abdominal adhesions from past surgeries, or constipation. If dialysate flows in slowly, the rate can be increased by raising the level of the inflow bag or by squeezing the bag gently to increase the rate of flow. Outflow problems are more difficult to overcome. Lowering the outflow bag by raising the child's height (e.g., picking up the child or seating the child on a taller piece of furniture) or having the child change position (roll from side to side, sit up, stand up, or walk around) are the only methods that are easily done at home. If outflow is still a problem, the physician may prescribe an oral medication, usually sorbitol, to induce diarrhea. The increased intestinal peristalsis may change the position of the Tenckhoff catheter to one that allows more flow. If none of these procedures is effective, the dialysis nurse may be asked to perform forceful flushes of the catheter with normal saline using sterile technique.

If forceful flushes do not correct the outflow problem, radiopaque dye is instilled under sterile conditions and its flow is followed with fluoroscopy. If these studies of the catheter show that a fibrin sheath has formed around the catheter, urokinase may be used to dissolve the fibrin. A volume sufficient to fill the catheter is instilled using sterile technique, allowed to dwell for 30 to 60 minutes, then aspirated out of the catheter. A dialysate exchange is done to check the catheter function. If outflow is still poor, surgical replacement of the catheter is the only option.

Exit site or tunnel infections are fairly common, particularly in children who are not toilet-trained. Contamination of the exit site by feces can happen if the child is still wearing diapers and has a loose, runny bowel movement. If fecal contamination occurs, the exit site dressing must be changed with each diaper change. An occlusive dressing helps prevent contamination and decreases the need for frequent dressing changes. Diligent exit site care can usually prevent infections. In some children, eosinophilia develops at the exit site or in the peritoneal cavity as a result of hypersensitivity to the silicone catheter (TIP 19–6) (Gilman & Frauman, 1997).

caREminder: *Some dialysis centers allow children with Tenckhoff catheters to swim; others do not. If swimming is permitted, the nurse should remind the child and family to swim only in well-chlorinated private pools or the ocean. Public pools, ponds, lakes, and rivers can have high bacteria counts, putting the child at risk for an exit site infection.*

Figure 19–11
The Tenckhoff catheter is inserted into the abdomen, with the distal end tunneled subcutaneously. The external tip of the catheter has a metal or plastic adaptor, which is used to connect the catheter to the dialysate tubing. (Modified from Black, J. M., & Matassarin-Jacobs, E. [Eds.]. [1997]. *Medical-surgical nursing: Clinical management for continuity of care* [5th ed., p. 1650]. Philadelphia: W. B. Saunders. Reprinted with permission.)

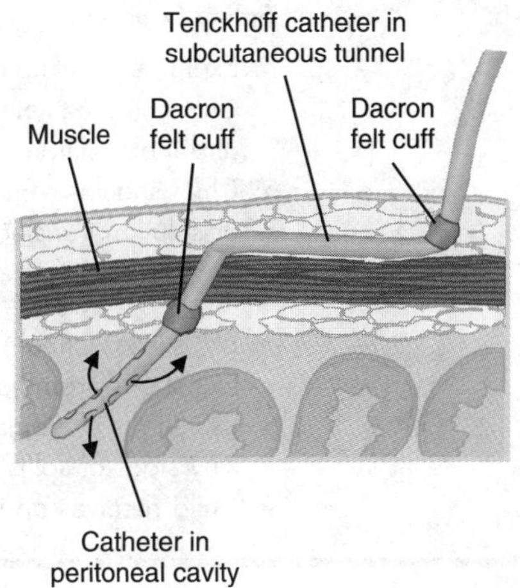

TIP 19–6 A Teaching Intervention Plan for the Child with a Tenckhoff Catheter

Nursing Diagnoses and Child/Family Outcomes

- Skin integrity impairment related to presence of catheter
  Outcomes: Skin at catheter entrance site remains intact and free from breakdown.
  Family performs cleaning and catheter maintenance procedures.
- High risk for infection related to catheter and dialysate exchange process
  Outcomes: Child/family protect catheter exit site from trauma.
  Family identifies signs and symptoms of infection.
  Family verbalizes measures to prevent infection.

Daily Care Interventions

Newly Placed Catheter (first 1 to 14 days after placement)

- Clean exit site daily (or as required if child is still wearing diapers).
  1. Wash hands well.
  2. Remove old dressing.
  3. Use hydrogen peroxide on sterile cotton swabs or sterile 4 × 4 dressings to remove scabs or crusts at exit site.
  4. Use povidone-iodine solution on sterile 4 × 4 dressings to clean exit site and surrounding area. Start at exit site and go outward in ever-increasing spiral, then discard 4 × 4 dressing.
  5. Dry area with sterile 4 × 4 in increasing spiral.
  6. Place one sterile 4 × 4 dressing under Tenckhoff catheter as it lies on skin. Place another overlapping the first one and the exit site. Use non-irritating tape or occlusive dressing (for children still in diapers). Rotate tape site daily.
  7. Tape solution transfer set to dressing to prevent pulling on exit site or secure with an expandable gauze net.

Well-Healed Catheter Site

- Dressing is optional.
- Daily exit site cleaning is still required.
  1. Child should shower daily and not bathe wherein the exit site soaks in dirty water.
  2. Use regular soap on washcloth to wash rest of body.
  3. Use povidone-iodine scrub to wash exit site.
  4. Rinse under shower.
  5. Dry rest of body with bath towel. Dry exit site with sterile 4 × 4 dressing.
  6. Apply dressing if desired.

Secure solution transfer set with tape to abdomen to prevent pulling on exit site, or secure with expandable gauze net.

Safety Concerns

- Examine Tenckhoff catheter and solution transfer set daily for signs of splits or cracks. Check that catheter adapter between Tenckhoff and solution transfer set is firmly seated and that solution transfer set is finger-tightly screwed on to adapter.
- Child should avoid contact sports or games likely to impact on exit site or pull on catheter or solution transfer set.

Contact Health Care Provider if

- Exit site or tunnel is hot, red, painful, or swollen.
- Exit site is draining or smells bad.
- Exit site is bleeding.
- Any signs of splits or cracks in the Tenckhoff catheter are observed.
- Child receives an injury to abdominal insertion site of catheter.

Chart 19–15

Clinical Indicators of Peritonitis

Cloudy dialysate outflow (effluent)
Abdominal pain
Rebound abdominal tenderness
Acute discomfort during fill phase of dialysis
Fever
General malaise
Nausea
Vomiting
Increased white blood cell count of dialysate outflow
Positive bacterial culture of dialysate outflow

Complications. The most serious complication of PD is **peritonitis** (Chart 19–15). Peritonitis can result from a break in sterile technique when changing the dialysate, from a break in the closed PD system, or from an exit site infection migrating along the tunnel and into the peritoneal cavity (Gilman & Frauman, 1997).

▽ **Alert:** *The caregiver should suspect peritonitis in a child receiving PD in whom abdominal pain, fever, and nausea or vomiting develop.*

Completing an exchange earlier than scheduled may be required to immediately evaluate the character of the dialysate. If the fluid is not cloudy and abdominal pain is not generalized, then peritonitis may be ruled out by the health care provider. Some older children who have had peritonitis several times may be able to recognize the prodromal symptoms before the dialysate is cloudy (Chart 19–16).

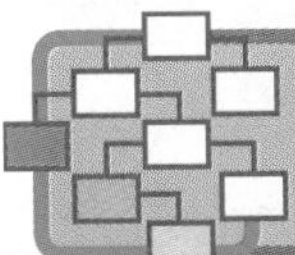

Chart 19–16
Clinical Judgment

A Child with Chronic Renal Failure

Neal is a 6-year-old boy who has been on home peritoneal dialysis for the past 6 weeks. His grandparents are the primary caregivers and have been responsible for managing all of his care at home. Over the weekend, Neal complained of abdominal pain, especially during infusion of the dialysate. He vomited once this morning and has a temperature of 101.6°F. Neal and his grandfather come to the outpatient renal clinic for evaluation.

Questions

1. What other assessment data would be important to elicit?
2. When a child has peritonitis, what would you expect the dialysate to look like after an exchange?
3. Does Neal need to be hospitalized?
4. What measures should be instituted to reduce Neal's pain and discomfort?
5. Two days later, the home health nurse visits Neal. What data would indicate that his peritonitis is improving and that the grandparents are taking measures to prevent another infection?

Answers

1. When was an exchange last completed? What did the dialysate look like after drainage from the abdomen? When does Neal experience pain? Do any specific events produce abdominal pain? What does the catheter exit site look like? Have the grandparents describe their technique for catheter site care and for connecting and disconnecting the child to the dialyzer.
2. The dialysate looks cloudy. A specimen of the dialysate should be evaluated for culture and sensitivity study. Gram stain and cell count of the fluid should also be completed to determine the infecting organisms.
3. No. If the child has not demonstrated severe weight loss or signs of dehydration, and if the grandparents feel they can manage the child's care at home with the assistance of home health care, then the child need not be hospitalized.
4. Begin antibiotic therapy immediately. Acetaminophen can be given to reduce fever and promote comfort. The dialysate should be warmed before instillation. A slow introduction of the fluid during inflow may also help reduce abdominal discomfort.
5. Neal has no fever. Complaints of abdominal pain are minimal. The dialysate fluid is clear after infusion. The grandparents demonstrate the use of aseptic techniques to clean the catheter site and to connect and disconnect the child for an infusion.

Frequent episodes of peritonitis can lead to thickening of the peritoneal membranes and reduced ability to ultrafiltrate or move solute. Inadequate peritoneal membrane function can mean that a child must be switched permanently from PD to hemodialysis (Andreoli et al., 1993).

Hemodialysis. Hemodialysis (HD) removes waste products and corrects serum chemistry values of the child's blood by circulating it through an extracorporeal circuit. The artificial kidney, or dialyzer, contains a blood compartment and a dialysate compartment. Substances in the blood but not in the dialysate, such as BUN or creatinine, cross the semipermeable membrane of the dialyzer into the dialysate via osmosis and are carried away as waste.

HD machines precisely measure the amount of water removed from the child's blood (Gilman & Frauman, 1997). Solute in the dialysate, such as sodium or potassium, is not removed completely from the blood. Instead, blood levels of these substances increase or decrease to equal the dialysate level. Commercially prepared dialysate concentrates are selected based on levels of component chemicals, or powdered additives can be added to increase selected solutes to desired levels if needed to meet the child's requirements (Gilman & Frauman, 1997).

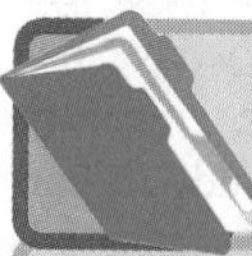

Chart 19–17
Nursing Interventions Classification (NIC)

Hemodialysis Therapy

Definition

Management of extracorporeal passage of the patient's blood through a dialyzer

Activities

Draw blood sample and review blood chemistries (e.g., blood urea nitrogen, serum creatinine, and serum Na, K, and PO_4 levels) pretreatment.
Record baseline vital signs: weight, temperature, pulse, respirations, and blood pressure.
Explain hemodialysis procedure and its purpose.
Monitor for AV fistula patency at frequent intervals (e.g., palpate for thrill and auscultate for a bruit).
Check equipment and solutions according to protocol.
Use sterile technique to initiate hemodialysis and for needle insertions and catheter connections.
Use gloves, eyeshield, and protective clothing to prevent direct contact with blood.
Initiate hemodialysis according to protocol.
Anchor connections and tubing securely.
Check system monitors (e.g., flow rate, pressure, temperature, pH level, conductivity, clots, air detector, negative pressure for ultrafiltration, and blood sensor) to ensure patient safety.
Monitor blood pressure, pulse, respirations, temperature, and patient response during dialysis.
Administer heparin, according to protocol.
Monitor clotting times and adjust heparin administration appropriately.
Adjust filtration pressures to remove an appropriate amount of fluid.
Institute appropriate protocol if patient becomes hypotensive.
Discontinue hemodialysis according to protocol.
Compare postdialysis vital signs and blood chemistries to predialysis values.
Avoid taking blood pressure or doing intravenous punctures in arm with fistula.
Provide catheter or fistula care according to protocol.
Work collaboratively with patient to adjust diet regulations, fluid limitations, and medications to regulate fluid and electrolyte shifts between treatments.
Teach patient to self-monitor signs and symptoms that indicate need for medical treatment (e.g., fever, bleeding, clotted fistula, thrombophlebitis, and irregular pulse).
Work collaboratively with patient to relieve discomfort from side effects of the disease and treatment (e.g., cramping, fatigue, headaches, itching, anemia, bone demineralization, body image changes, and role disruption).
Work collaboratively with patient to adjust length of dialysis, diet regulations, and pain and diversion needs to achieve optimal benefit of the treatment.

From McCloskey, J., & Bulechek, G. (1996). *Nursing interventions classification (NIC)* (2nd ed.). St. Louis: Mosby–Year Book. Reprinted with permission.

The HD machine mixes dialysate concentrate with treated water to make an isotonic dialysate solution. Most commonly, 34 parts of water are mixed with 1 part of dialysate concentrate. The HD machine also performs the following functions:

- Monitors the dialysate solute concentration
- Warms the dialysate to body temperature and monitors that temperature
- Pumps the dialysate and the child's blood through their respective compartments in the artificial kidney
- Infuses anticoagulant medication into the blood
- Monitors effluent (i.e., waste dialysate coming from the dialyzer) for the presence of red blood cells, which would indicate a leak in the semipermeable membrane
- Checks the cleansed blood returning to the child for air bubbles

Alarms and safety mechanisms alert the nephrology nurse or technician to problems arising in the circuit. Blood or dialysate flow shuts off if safety parameters are exceeded; this requires intervention by the nurse or technician (Gilman & Frauman, 1997) (Chart 19–17). Bloodlines must be selected carefully based on the volume of blood they hold.

caREminder: *The total volume of the extracorporeal circuit (bloodlines plus dialyzer) cannot exceed 10% of the child's circulating blood volume (Kjellstrand et al., 1971).*

The dialysate concentrate to be used is also selected by the physician. The numerous commercially prepared concentrates available contain varying levels of components (sodium, potassium, calcium, magnesium, chloride, dextrose, and bicarbonate or acetate). Sometimes, powdered potassium or calcium is added to the concentrate to increase the level of the substance in the dialysate if the child's serum level of that electrolyte is particularly low.

All dialysate used on pediatric patients should contain at least 200 to 250 mg% dextrose and should be buffered with bicarbonate. There are fewer side effects with such dialysis baths, and children receive extra energy from the calories in high-dextrose baths. Although children with healthy livers can metabolize acetate to bicarbonate, using dialysate buffered with acetate can cause extreme nausea and vomiting (Gilman & Frauman, 1997).

To prevent blood in an extracorporeal circuit from clotting, heparin is administered. Activated clotting times (ACTs) are performed just before the procedure and at regular intervals (every 30 to 120 minutes) during the procedure to monitor the effectiveness of the heparin infusion. The goal is to keep the ACT of the blood in the venous blood tubing between 180 and 200 seconds. ACTs are performed more frequently on acute or newly diagnosed chronic hemodialysis patients. Children's heparin requirements usually fluctuate more than an adult's. Thus, even long-term chronic hemodialysis patients require one or two ACTs per treatment. Infectious processes or exposure to cigarette smoke can markedly increase a child's heparin requirement.

CRF causes anemia and prolongs clotting time, but ARF does not. Therefore, children with ARF who are hemodialyzed need higher doses of heparin because they have not had renal failure long enough for their normal clotting factors to be affected (Gilman & Frauman, 1997).

Access to the bloodstream is a major problem in pediatric HD. Arteriovenous fistulas (AVFs) can be appropriate for teenagers on HD. However, dual-lumen catheters are more commonly used for acute and chronic pediatric hemodialysis patients.

Catheter Site. Catheters for acute HD can be placed in either the subclavian, jugular, or femoral veins, depending on the size of the child and the size of the veins (Fig. 19–12). Site selection is done by the surgeon or pediatric nephrologist at the time of catheter insertion. These catheters are designed to be removed after a time, usually after a few days to a month or so. However,

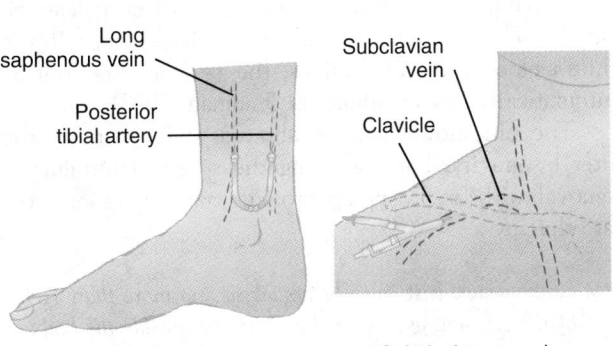

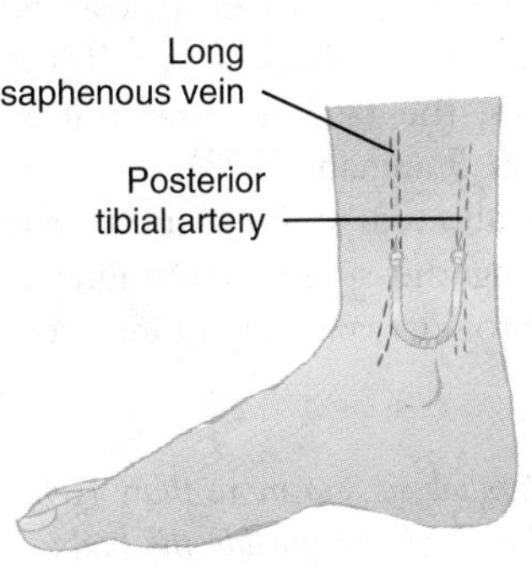

Figure 19–12
External sites for vascular access in hemodialysis include the internal jugular, subclavian, and femoral sites. (From Black, J. M., & Matassarin-Jacobs, E. [Eds.]. [1997]. *Medical-surgical nursing: Clinical management for continuity of care* [5th ed., p. 1653]. Philadelphia: W. B. Saunders. Reprinted with permission.)

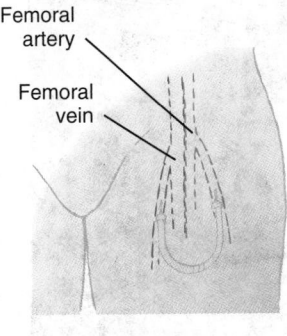

permanent catheters, most commonly placed in a subclavian vein or jugular vein, can last for many years. If other catheter sites are used for access, diligent attention to sterility is imperative when attaching the catheter to or detaching it from the hemodialysis circuit, or when performing exit site care. Adequate functioning of the catheter is often highly related to the position of the child's body. Sometimes children with subclavian catheters must assume and hold unusual body positions so that adequate blood flow through the catheter can continue (Gilman & Frauman, 1997).

Complications. As with any device passing through the skin, infection at the exit site is a possibility, as is septicemia if proper sterile technique is not observed during attachment or detachment for a treatment. Children with subclavian catheters should not swim, take showers, or bump or pull on the catheter or exit site. In addition, a sterile occlusive dressing should be kept in place over the exit site at all times (Gilman & Frauman, 1997).

Clotting can occur within the catheter lumen or around the catheter in the vein. Instilling heparin in the catheter between hemodialysis treatments helps prevent such clotting. Urokinase can be used to dissolve any intraluminal clots (Gilman & Frauman, 1997). Sometimes, injecting radiopaque dye under fluoroscopy is required to determine the reason for a nonfunctioning catheter. A sheath of fibrin around the catheter, for example, can be detected only in this way.

Children are more unstable than adults during HD (Fig. 19–13). The nurse must continuously monitor the child's weight (with a metabolic scale if the child's dry weight is less than 12 kg), check the blood pressure frequently (every 1 to 15 minutes), and constantly observe the child for changes in hydration status or for early signs of complications. These complications include fever, fluid overload, hyperkalemia, hypernatremia, hypocalcemia, and muscle cramps. In addition, machine malfunctions, blood leaks, and allergic reactions are concerns that the nurse must assess and address as these emergencies arise.

Figure 19–13
Hemodialysis must be performed at a specialized center where the child's status can be constantly monitored by the specialty nursing staff.

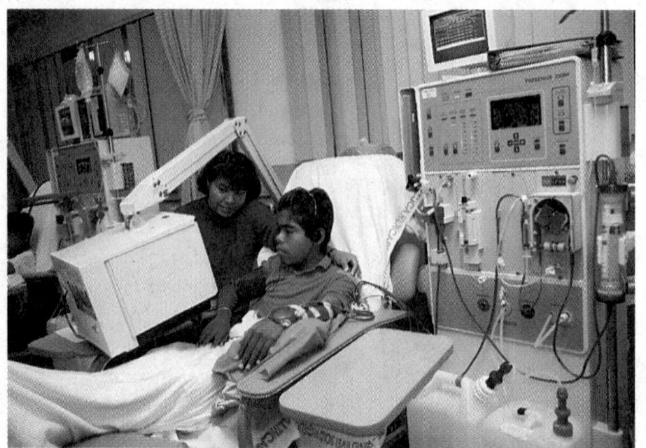

Continuous Renal Replacement Therapy. Continuous renal replacement therapies (CRRTs) are relatively new treatments for children with renal failure. Forms of CRRT commonly used on children include continuous arteriovenous hemofiltration (CAVH), continuous venovenous hemofiltration (CVVH), and continuous venovenous hemodiafiltration (CVVHD). CRRTs provide slow, continuous removal of fluid and solute, allowing safe, effective therapy for critically ill, hemodynamically unstable children. Pediatric patients receiving CRRTs must be monitored in the intensive care unit.

All CRRT methods work by removing plasma from the child's body, along with the solute dissolved in it, and replacing the plasma with fluid that has the correct levels of electrolytes. To illustrate, a large coffee urn contains very strong coffee. If a thin stream of coffee flows out the bottom of the urn, and an equally thin stream of water runs into the top, eventually the coffee urn has only clear water in it. It may take several days for the process to be complete. The overall fluid level in the urn may be raised or lowered by varying the rate at which water is put into the urn.

All CRRTs have an extracorporeal circuit with a hemofilter and blood tubing. Large amounts of plasma with dissolved solute flow out through the filter, but blood cells and proteins remain in circulation. Replacement fluids containing the correct amount of electrolytes are simultaneously put into the system. If the child is overloaded with fluid, slightly more water is removed than replaced; if the child is dehydrated, more water is replaced than removed. The system effectively removes waste products and maintains fluid and electrolyte balance.

Continuous Arteriovenous Hemofiltration. CAVH requires access to an artery and a vein. The pressure differential between the two vessels causes blood to flow through the system and fluid to cross the membrane in the filter. For the system to work effectively, the child must have a mean arterial pressure (MAP) of at least 60 mmHg. This provides a built-in feedback loop. If the child's blood pressure declines, the rate of ultrafiltration automatically slows (Gilman & Frauman, 1997).

The ultrafiltrate can be allowed to flow out of the filter by gravity, but regulating the speed of ultrafiltrate removal with an IV pump provides a much more accurate therapy.

caREminder: *Just as in hemodialysis, no more than 10% of the circulating blood volume can be outside the body for CAVH or CVVH.*

To prevent clotting and to ease the burden on the child's heart, the blood tubing segments should be kept as short as possible. The longer a blood tubing segment is, the greater its resistance and the harder the heart has to work to push blood through it. Heparin is infused into the system in the same way as in hemodialysis. The ACTs should be kept at 180 to 220 seconds.

The critically ill children who benefit most from CAVH may have problems receiving this therapy because of their inability to maintain an MAP of 60. In the past, some units compensated for this by adding a blood pump to the system and running it at 2 to 5 mL/min to assist the extracorporeal circulation (Bell, 1988). CVVH evolved from this technique.

Continuous Venovenous Hemofiltration. CVVH is essentially CAVH with a blood pump. An arterial access is not required, the child's MAP is not an issue, and adequate blood flow is not a problem. The reliable blood flow often means that decreased heparinization is required as well. However, the blood pump makes it easy to pull air in the system. Therefore, a venous drip chamber and foam detector must be added to the system to prevent air embolism. These additional system features also require longer bloodlines (the same ones as are used for hemodialysis). The longer bloodlines require more blood and may exceed the 10% limit for smaller children. Blood priming would then be necessary (Gilman & Frauman, 1997).

Another concern is that filtration can continue in CVVH even if the child's blood pressure is decreased. Thus, careful monitoring and system regulation by the intensive care unit nurse are crucial to successful CVVH.

Hemodiafiltration. CAVH or CVVH may not remove enough solute to control a highly catabolic child. In that event, solute removal can be increased by initiating continuous arteriovenous hemodiafiltration (CAVHD) or continuous venovenous hemodiafiltration (CVVHD). Sterile 1.5% dextrose peritoneal dialysate is pumped through the ultrafiltrate chamber of the filter in the opposite direction of the blood flow. The ultrafiltrate pump must be set at a high enough rate to remove the desired amount of ultrafiltrate along with the required amount of dialysate. The dialysate increases solute removal via osmosis, the same way it works in hemodialysis (Jenkins, Harrison, Jackson, & Funk, 1991).

The dialysate used for CAVHD or CVVHD must be sterile because of the large pores in the filter membranes. Bacteria could pass through these pores and cause septicemia if the dialysate used were not sterile.

Femoral or umbilical arteries, and femoral, umbilical, or subclavian veins are used for CAVH or CAVHD access. Femoral, subclavian, or jugular veins can be used for CVVH or CVVHD. As in all blood vessel access, there is risk of infection, clotting, or compromised circulation in the distal limb.

Kidney Transplantation. A successful kidney transplant is the ultimate treatment goal for each child with ESRD. Some centers try to accomplish this goal as quickly as possible. In some cases, preemptive transplants are performed before dialysis is needed.

Donor Considerations. The best possible kidney donor is an identical twin. The next best choice is a human lymphocyte antigen (HLA)–identical sibling. In a family, each sibling has a 25% chance of being HLA identical, a 50% chance of being a half-match, and a 25% chance of being a mismatch. Each child receives 50% of his or her genetic code from each parent; thus, parents are always half-matches. The prospective donor must also have a compatible blood type.

Siblings must be at least 18 years old to give legal consent to be a transplant donor. Parents are not usually allowed to give such consent. A donor nephrectomy is not medically necessary as are the other surgeries that parents can give consent for. Siblings younger than age 18 may sometimes be used as donors if the benefits of donation outweigh the risks. For example, an 8-year-old twin may be permitted to donate to an identical twin who is doing poorly on dialysis. A state may require a court order to permit a minor to donate a kidney for transplantation.

For children who do not have a living-related donor (LRD), a cadaver donor is the usual choice. Cadaver donors are patients who have been declared brain dead. The cadaver donor must have good kidney function and be free from infectious disease. Usually, cadaver kidneys are from adults; children's organs are seldom available as cadaveric donors. More recently, emotionally related living donors (ERDs) have been used if other donors are not available. These people are genetically unrelated to the recipient but have close emotional ties. Spouses, aunts, uncles, and adoptive parents have been ERDs. Kidneys from these donors have the same long-term graft survival as cadaveric donor kidneys. Living donors must go through extensive physiologic evaluation to ensure that they will not be harmed by the loss of one kidney and that they are in physical and mental health to endure the stresses of surgery.

An adult kidney may be transplanted into a child as long as the child weighs at least 10 kg. Fluid shifts, maintaining adequate blood pressure to perfuse the large kidney, and mechanical problems with crimped arteries or kinked ureters are concerns when using an adult donor for a child. The transplant surgeon decides whether a particular kidney will fit the child (Gilman & Frauman, 1997).

Medication Regimen. Immunosuppressive agents, such as azathioprine (Imuran), prednisone, cyclosporine (Sandimmune), muromonab (OKT3), and tacrolimus (FK506 or Prograf), are required to prevent rejection of the transplanted kidney. Some of the medications can be given by

IV infusion in the immediate postoperative period. By the time the recipient is discharged home, the medication can be taken orally. These medications must be taken in the exact amount prescribed for as long as the transplanted kidney is functioning. Adolescents are at particular risk for noncompliance with the medication regimen, because the side effects of immunosuppressants, such as cushingoid facies, acne, and hirsutism, may negatively affect their body image.

The child and caregiver need to learn which medications to take, the amounts prescribed, and the effects and side effects of each medication before discharge. In addition to preventing rejection of the transplanted organ, these medications increase the recipient's susceptibility to infection and can cause other side effects (Chart 19–18). Children who take immunosuppressants for many years have a higher incidence of cancer and other immune system disorders.

Community Care. Transplant patients are not "cured." These children never reach a point where they no longer require medical attention or drug therapy. However, a well-stabilized transplant patient requires only daily or every-other-day medication. Clinic visits are usually twice a week at the outset, but as the child continues to do well, the visits can slowly be decreased until they are necessary only every 3–4 months. Monthly checks of blood chemistries and CBCs are required to monitor kidney function and to detect signs of rejection.

Some centers recommend periodic biopsies of the transplanted kidney to detect rejection before it has caused enough damage to change laboratory values.

Transplanted kidneys last varying lengths of time. Hyperacute rejections cause the loss of the kidney in the operating room as the transplant is being performed. Acute rejections usually occur within the first 7 to 14 days after transplantation. Rejection can occur at any time after transplantation, particularly if the child stops taking the immunosuppressive medications. Even if medications are taken as prescribed, chronic rejection, a slow, insidious process, can result in the loss of the kidney. However, the longer the transplant remains in place without complications, the more likely it is that it will never be rejected.

caREminder: *Adolescents are particularly at risk for transplant medication noncompliance because the side effects of immunosuppressants, such as "chubby cheeks," acne, and hirsutism, may negatively affect their body image.*

Acute or chronic rejection can cause loss of transplant function. This is treated in the same manner as the initial loss of native kidney function: conservative management followed by dialysis. Retransplantation at a future date is usually an option, except when hyperacute rejection occurred for an unknown cause or when the likelihood of the basic disease recurring in the transplant is too great.

Despite the short-term risks and the long-term side effects, successful transplantation still offers the child with renal failure the best chance at the most normal lifestyle possible (Chart 19–19).

Chart 19–18

Side Effects of Immunosuppressant Therapy

- Leukopenia
- Hypertension
- Weight gain
- Posterior subcapsular cataracts
- Hirsutism
- Tremor
- Hepatotoxicity
- Nephrotoxicity
- Impaired growth
- Gum hyperplasia
- Neurologic disturbances
- Increased incidence of cancer
- Increased incidence of other immune system disorders

Congenital Renal Disease

Congenital renal disease results from improper embryonic development of urinary tract structures. It occurs in several forms. Agenesis is the complete absence of kidney tissue. If agenesis is unilateral, it may not be discovered until later in life, as long as there is normal renal function in the sole kidney. Usually, the left kidney is absent and the right kidney is normal. The condition predominates in males (Gilman, Mooney, & Andrews, 1994).

Bilateral renal agenesis, or Potter's syndrome, is incompatible with life outside the uterus. The syndrome, which involves facial abnormalities and pulmonary hypoplasia as well as kidney problems, occurs once in 3000 births. Forty percent of these infants are stillborn (Gilman et al., 1994; Gonzalez, 1996).

A small kidney with fewer than normal nephrons is called a hypoplastic kidney (Gilman et al., 1994). Like other congenital malformations, hypoplasia can be unilateral or bilateral. Children with bilateral hypoplastic kidneys usually reach ESRD by their early teenage years (Bergstein, 1992).

Dysplastic Kidneys

Aplastic and dysplastic are terms that are often used interchangeably to describe kidneys that have not devel-

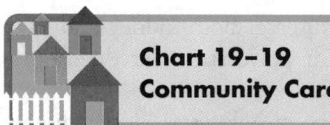

Chart 19–19
Community Care

Concerns of the Newly Transplanted Patient

Concern	Response
Can I go back to school soon and do all of the activities like the rest of the children?	You will not be able to return to school for 6 to 8 weeks. Immediately after transplantation, driving is not allowed and you cannot lift anything heavier than 10 pounds for 8 weeks. Once healing is complete, you can return to school. However, you are not allowed to participate in contact sports (e.g., tackle football, wrestling, or hockey) or sports that could severely jar the kidney (e.g., skydiving).
Can I be with all of my friends when I get out of the hospital?	For the first 4 to 6 weeks, you will need to stay away from places with large crowds of people to prevent infection. Your friends can come see you and you can visit some of them, as long as they do not have any signs of a cold or other illness.
Are there any restrictions on what I can eat?	Although protein and fluid intake can be liberal, sodium and calories need to be controlled to prevent hypertension and obesity. Remember, prednisone will increase your appetite, so be sure you eat healthy snacks and keep a close eye on your weight.
Do I have to take the medications every day?	All medications must be taken every day, on time, and in the correct amount. Your family will help you to remember to take these medications. When you go back to school, you will have to help remind the nurse that you need to take your medication every day. Failure to take immunosuppressives correctly can lead to infection or loss of the transplanted kidney.

oped normally. Aplastic/dysplastic kidneys can occur bilaterally or unilaterally in an individual. Dysplasia often occurs along with a functional obstruction of the collecting system, such as prune belly syndrome, PUVs, or ureterocele (Gilman et al., 1994).

Pathophysiology

Dysplastic kidneys show abnormal differentiation of renal tissues with primitive glomeruli and tubules, cysts, and nonrenal tissues, like cartilage, found in the kidneys (Gilman et al., 1994). The variations in the morphologic makeup of dysplastic kidneys suggest that the abnormalities can develop at many different times during embryonic development (Watkins & Avner, 1994).

Assessment

The function of dysplastic kidneys varies as widely as the types of anomalies do. Presenting signs and symptoms can be apparent (flank mass, urinary tract infections, hematuria, proteinuria) or can be somewhat concealed by other conditions, such as the syndrome known as failure to thrive (Watkins & Avner, 1994).

Children with dysplastic kidneys can show the signs and symptoms of CRF. The degree of renal impairment often progresses as the child grows. Dysplastic kidneys may have enough function to maintain a newborn but are not able to keep a larger child healthy.

Diagnostic Tests. Dysplastic kidneys can be seen on ultrasound, their size can be measured, and any scarring can be noted. However, a kidney biopsy is needed to differentiate between dysplastic and hypoplastic tissue.

Interdisciplinary Interventions

As the child with dysplastic kidneys progresses through the stages of CRF, first conservative management, then some form of renal replacement therapy will be required (see Chronic Renal Failure).

Polycystic Kidneys

Like dysplastic kidneys, polycystic (from the Greek *polys*, meaning many, and *kystis*, meaning cysts) disease also results from fetal developmental error. Polycystic kidneys result when the upper and lower collecting ducts fail to join properly (Frauman & Gilman, 1979). Urine is formed, but it has no way to leave the kidney, so it collects in many cysts throughout the kidney.

Pathophysiology

There are two types of polycystic kidney disease. In autosomal recessive (or infantile-type) polycystic kidney disease (ARPKD), 25% to 90% of the renal tubules are cystic (Frauman & Gilman, 1979). Symptoms can develop as early as the perinatal period or as late as late childhood or even adolescence. In general, the earlier the disease manifests, the greater the number of nephrons affected and the poorer the prognosis. Hepatic fibrosis is part of the disease; the degree of hepatic fibrosis is inversely proportional to the severity of renal disease. Pulmonary hypoplasia and pneumothorax are frequently found in neonates with ARPKD (Kher, 1992b).

Less than 10% of tubules are affected in the autosomal dominant (or adult-type) polycystic kidney disease (ADPKD). The disease may not become apparent until the fourth decade of life, but symptoms develop in approximately 10% of children or adolescents with this type of polycystic disease (Frauman & Gilman, 1979). Polycystic liver disease can accompany ADPKD.

Assessment

The signs of ARPKD are large, tense, symmetrical bilateral flank masses that do not transilluminate. There is variable urinary output, but oliguria is typical. Hypertension and the congestive heart failure triad (tachycardia, tachypnea, and hepatomegaly) are common problems. Respiratory distress can result from the large size of the kidneys or from associated pneumothorax or pneumomediastinum (Frauman & Gilman, 1979).

The manifestations of ADPKD in children may not appear until late childhood or even adolescence, but they are occasionally found affecting neonates. A flank mass, hematuria, hernias, hypertension, urinary tract infection, or headache may be the presenting symptom (Kher, 1992b). As the disease progresses, the signs and symptoms of CRF develop: slowly elevating BUN and creatinine levels, growth failure, renal osteodystrophy, and anemia. Additionally, esophageal and gastric varices and hematemesis can occur as a result of portacaval hypertension. Splenomegaly and hypersplenism including thrombocytopenia are also frequent findings (Frauman & Gilman, 1979).

Interdisciplinary Interventions

Children born with ARPKD may die at birth, especially if they have the associated pulmonary hypoplasia. Those with the adult type of polycystic disease (ADPKD) usually do well, although some deaths have been reported. If a child with ADPKD dies, the cause is usually attributed to cirrhosis, portal hypertension, or ruptured esophageal varices resulting from liver disease. Both kidney and liver transplantation are needed if polycystic liver disease accompanies ADPKD.

Treatment of either type of polycystic kidney disease is symptomatic. In addition to treatment of hypertension, congestive heart failure, respiratory distress, or other symptoms of CRF, surgical removal of the polycystic kidneys is often necessary. Maintenance dialysis is then required until renal transplantation is successful (see Chronic Renal Failure).

Because polycystic kidney disease is hereditary, older children with the disease and their parents should receive genetic counseling along with preparatory teaching about dialysis and transplantation. This permits them to make informed decisions about reproductive choices (Frauman & Gilman, 1979).

Glomerular Disorders

Nephrotic Syndrome

Nephrotic syndrome is a clinical entity produced by the loss of urinary protein, manifested by a complex of symptoms including proteinuria, hypoproteinemia, hyperlipidemia, and edema. It can develop during the course of several different renal or systemic diseases. In primary, or idiopathic, nephrotic syndrome, the kidney is the main, or only, involved organ. Secondary nephrotic syndrome is caused by systemic disease, drugs, or toxins (Bergstein, 1996; Gilman et al., 1994).

Most cases (90% to 95%) of nephrotic syndrome are primary, or idiopathic, usually developing in 2- to 3-year-old children. Nephrotic syndrome occurs rarely in children older than 8 years. The disease develops in approximately 3 in 100,000 children; boys are affected twice as often as girls (Bergstein, 1996; Gilman et al., 1994).

Pathophysiology

As nephrotic syndrome evolves, the glomerular capillaries become increasingly permeable to proteins, especially albumin. This is thought to be due to loss of the negative electric charge on the glomerular structures. Increased glomerular capillary pore size is another possible cause (Kher, 1992c).

Increased glomerular permeability causes proteinuria and decreases plasma oncotic pressure, which allows intravascular fluid to migrate to the interstitial space. Edema develops, and the lower intravascular volume stimulates the renin-angiotensin-aldosterone system as well as the release of ADH. Both of these cause the body to retain sodium and fluid, which are promptly lost to the interstitial space, exacerbating the edema (Bergstein, 1996; Kher, 1992c).

Minimal change nephrotic syndrome (MCNS) occurs in 80% to 85% of children with nephrotic syndrome. It is so named because of the lack of pathologic findings on renal biopsies of these children (Kher, 1992c).

Assessment

Typically, the first sign of nephrotic syndrome is periorbital edema. It is most noticeable on arising, but subsides as the child is upright during the day. Weight gain usually occurs, but parents may mistake it as being caused by growth. Urine becomes diminished, foamy, or frothy. Ascites, pleural effusion, and labial or scrotal swelling may develop. Blood pressure is usually normal to slightly decreased (Gilman et al., 1994).

The child is as edematous on the inside of the body as on the outside. Gastrointestinal edema can cause diarrhea, anorexia, and poor food absorption. If the protein loss is prolonged, signs of malnutrition, such as hair changes, pallor, or shiny skin with prominent veins, may ensue. The child is irritable, lethargic, fatigued, and increasingly susceptible to infection, especially pneumonia, peritonitis, cellulitis, and septicemia (Gilman et al., 1994).

Interdisciplinary Interventions

Treatment aims to decrease urinary protein loss (thus controlling edema), balance nutrition, restore normal metabolic function, and prevent or treat any infection (Care Path 19–2). The child is usually hospitalized for the first episode of nephrotic syndrome so that the diagnosis may be confirmed, therapy can be initiated, and the family can be taught about the disease and its management. Recurrences, in which edema is merely a cosmetic problem, can be managed at home, which allows for continued school attendance. However, severe edema with pleural effusion causing respiratory distress, ascites, or massive scrotal swelling requires hospitalization (Bergstein, 1996; Gilman et al., 1994).

The child may ambulate as tolerated and is given a low-sodium, well-balanced diet with fluid restriction only if the edema is severe. Glucocorticosteroids (prednisone) usually cause diuresis. However, diuretics (furosemide and metolazone) and, sometimes, immunosuppressants (Cytoxan, Imuran) may be required. (Bergstein, 1996; Gilman et al., 1994).

A child with nephrotic syndrome but not gross hematuria can receive corticosteroid therapy. A total of 2 mg/kg/day is given in divided doses, to a maximum of 80 mg/day. This continues for 4 weeks. The same dose is given once every other day for 4 weeks if the child's proteinuria still has not cleared. If there is still 2+ protein in the urine after 8 weeks of therapy, the child has failed the steroid trial.

Response to steroid therapy can be divided into three categories: steroid responsive, frequently relapsing, and steroid dependent. In steroid-responsive children, the amount of protein in the urine decreases to negative or trace amounts within 10 to 15 days after steroid therapy begins. Frequently relapsing children respond to steroid therapy, but then relapse at least two times within 6 months. Steroid-dependent children relapse when alternate-day therapy is begun or within 2 weeks after all steroid therapy has been discontinued (Kelsch & Sedman, 1993). Most children respond to the prednisone therapy within 2 weeks and have a complete remission with minimal to no residual renal pathologic findings (Bergstein, 1996).

Community Care

Immunization with live virus vaccines or viral illness may trigger relapses in affected children (Bergstein, 1996). Most children have had their childhood immunizations by the time nephrotic syndrome first develops. Booster immunizations with killed virus vaccine should not cause a relapse, but live virus vaccines should be delayed until the child enters school.

Viral illnesses, especially upper respiratory infections, are an unavoidable part of childhood. If a relapse occurs, owing to viral illness, parents should seek medical care again, so that steroid treatment can be reinitiated. Spontaneous resolution without further relapse usually occurs by the time the individual is 30 years old (Gilman et al., 1994).

Proteinuria

Many healthy children excrete protein in their urine; 150 mg every 24 hours is the upper limit of the normal range. Proteinuria in excess of that amount can be either nonpathologic or pathologic (Bergstein, 1992). The causes of proteinuria can be classified into three main categories. In **postural, or orthostatic, proteinuria**, a nonpathologic form, children excrete normal or slightly increased amounts of protein when they are recumbent. Upon arising, however, protein excretion may increase 10-fold or more (Bergstein, 1996). **Nonpathologic transient proteinuria** can occur with a temperature of 38.3°C or more, following vigorous exercise, with congestive heart failure, with seizures, following exposure to cold, with emotional stress, or associated with epinephrine infusions (Bergstein, 1996; Makker, 1992b). **Persistent proteinurias** are more likely to be pathologic. The abnormal proteinurias are due to glomerular or tubular disorders, overload of protein in the blood, and alterations in intrarenal blood flow (Makker, 1992b).

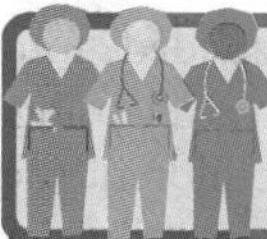

Care Path 19–2 An Interdisciplinary Plan of Care for the Child with Nephrotic Syndrome

	Patient/Family Intermediate Outcomes		
Nursing Diagnosis	**Day 1**	**Day 2**	**Days 3 to 5**
Fluid volume excess related to retention	Anasarca begins to decrease while electrolyte balance is maintained.	Anasarca continues to decrease while maintaining electrolyte balance.	Anasarca continues to decrease with electrolytes within normal ranges
Risk for infection related to placement of Tenckhoff catheter	Child shows no signs or symptoms of infection, particularly peritonitis.	→	→
Altered family processes related to situational crisis of illness	Child/family begin to recognize changes in family processes.	Child/family identify positive coping mechanisms.	→
Body image disturbance related to edema and side effects of medications	Child/family begin to adapt to body changes caused by illness/treatment.	Child/family can state expected body changes caused by illness/treatment.	Child/family state expected body changes and expected duration of change.
Care Intervention Categories			
Labs	CBC with platelets, Mg, Chem 17, C3. If an adolescent, ANA (to rule out SLE)	Chem 17 and Mg	Chem 17 and Mg daily with aggressive diuresis
Medications and IVs	Diuretics	Continue diuretics after negative PPD reading; start prednisone 60 mg/m^2/24 hr	Patients with significant edema get IV albumin slowly: Day 1: ½ g/kg over 4 hr Day 2: 1 g/kg over 4 hr Day 3: 1.5 g/kg over 4 hr Day 4: 2 g/kg over 4 hr until diuresis begins
Nutrition	NPO if Ileus is present. If not, diet: 1 g sodium, no potassium or protein restriction, fluid limit 1000 mL/m^2/day.	Advance diet as tolerated or continue diet restrictions if edema remains severe	→
Pain management	Acetaminophen p.r.n. for pain. Elevate swollen body parts.	→ →	→ →
Radiology	Chest radiograph if pulmonary edema is present		

Care Path 19–2 An Interdisciplinary Plan of Care for the Child with Nephrotic Syndrome *Continued*

Care Intervention Categories	Day 1	Day 2	Days 3 to 5
Safety and activity	Activity as tolerated according to degree of edema	→	→
		Attend play sessions as interested	→
Self-care		Save all urine to be tested; perform dipstick test if child is old enough	→
Teaching	Disease and its treatment	How to test urine with dipstick; effects of medications	When to call physician; possibility of relapse
Tests	Dipstick all urine voids for protein; 24-hour urine for creatinine clearance and protein.	→	→
Vital signs/baseline parameters	VS q 4 hr	→	→
	Strict monitoring of intake and output.	→	→

ANA, anti-nuclear antibodies; CBC, complete blood count; IV, intravenous; Mg, magnesium; NPO, nothing by mouth; p.r.n., as needed; PPD, purified protein derivative; SLE, systemic lupus erythematosus; VS, vital signs.

Pathophysiology

Glomerular proteinuria results from changes in the electrostatic charge or size of the pores of the glomerular capillary membranes, which increase membrane permeability. Increased levels of plasma proteins in the filtrate result (Makker, 1992b). In tubular proteinuria, normal levels of smaller molecular weight proteins are filtered but are not reabsorbed from the proximal tubule as they should be (Makker, 1992b).

Overload proteinuria occurs when excessive amounts of low molecular weight proteins, present because of a disease process, are present in glomerular filtrate. The levels exceed the resorptive capacity of the proximal tubules. The compensatory changes in a single functioning kidney give rise to altered blood flow within that kidney and can lead to proteinuria (Makker, 1992b).

Assessment

Protein in urine can sometimes be detected by a "foamy" appearance, but this is an unreliable indicator. A dipstick test, a turbidimetric test with sulfosalicylic acid, or both types of tests are required for accurate detection. However, both tests can give false-negative or false-positive results, so repeat urinalysis may be necessary (Makker, 1992b).

Interdisciplinary Interventions

There is no treatment for proteinuria. Children with symptoms of pathologic proteinuria should have a physical examination, urinalysis, urine culture, 24-hour urine collection for creatinine clearance and protein excretion, serum albumin and C3 levels, and IVP. If hematuria, hypertension, or impaired renal function is found, a kidney biopsy is necessary. These children should be reevaluated annually (Bergstein, 1996).

If a child loses less than 1 g of protein in the urine every 24 hours, no treatment is required. The child should have a repeat 24-hour urine collection every 2 years to check for changes in the degree of proteinuria.

A child who excretes more than 1 g of protein every 24 hours, in whom the cause is not orthostatic proteinuria, should have a kidney biopsy to determine whether a kidney disease (e.g., occult glomerulonephritis) is the cause. If the tissue obtained on biopsy is normal, the child should be followed up with a 24-hour urine collection every 2 years. If the amount of protein lost in the urine increases or if other signs and symptoms of decreased kidney function are found, a repeat biopsy should be performed (see Table 19–2).

Hemolytic-Uremic Syndrome

Although HUS is the most common cause of ARF in children younger than age 4 years, its precise cause is unknown. In association with a bacterial or viral infection and endotoxins, the initiating event of HUS appears to be injury to endothelial cells of the glomerular arterioles. The endothelial cells swell and pull away from the glomerular basement membrane, creating a subendothelial space where fibrin, lipids, and platelet fragments collect. Glomerular blood flow is impaired because of the narrowing or thrombosis of blood vessels. Ischemia or necrosis can result (Geller, 1990; Neumann & Urizar, 1994).

RBCs are damaged as they pass through damaged vessels. The damaged RBCs are removed from circulation by the spleen, causing hemolytic anemia. Platelets adhere to the injured vessels, or they are also damaged and removed by the spleen, causing thrombocytopenia (Bergstein, 1996; Gilman et al., 1994).

Assessment

The prodromal illness in HUS is usually gastrointestinal (fever, vomiting, and diarrhea, which is sometimes bloody), but it can be an upper respiratory infection. From 5 to 10 days after onset of the prodromal illness, HUS begins, with the child manifesting a sudden onset of pallor, bruising or purpura, irritability, and oliguria. The child usually has a slight fever, anorexia, abdominal pain, vomiting, watery and blood-stained diarrhea, and mild jaundice. Signs of circulatory overload also may occur. Lethargy and seizures develop with central nervous system involvement (Chart 19–20). In the first few days of the illness, an increasing number of glomeruli are damaged, leading to renal damage that ranges from mild renal insufficiency to ARF that requires dialysis (Bergstein, 1996; Gilman et al., 1994).

Alert: *A child in whom vomiting and watery, bloody diarrhea develops along with purpura and/or pallor should be brought to a hospital immediately for work-up for HUS.*

Interdisciplinary Interventions

Supportive therapy should begin early (Care Path 19–3). Frequent PD exchanges and transfusions of packed RBCs

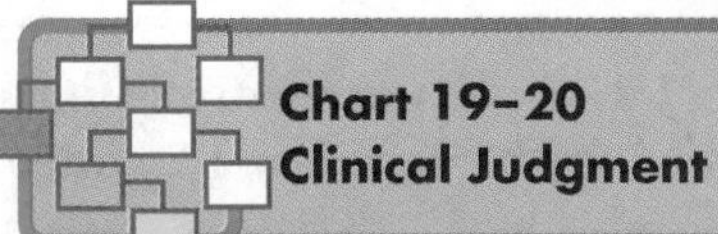

Chart 19–20
Clinical Judgment

The Child with Hemolytic-Uremic Syndrome

Leo is a 3-year-old with hemolytic-uremic syndrome. He presented in the emergency room with a temperature of 100.9°F, lethargy, vomiting, abdominal pain, and watery, blood-stained diarrhea. His skin is pale, slightly jaundiced, and bruises easily. Within several hours after admission to the hospital, a decision is made to initiate peritoneal dialysis. The physician explained the purpose of dialysis and the need for surgery to place a Tenckhoff catheter. As you enter the child's room, the mother is crying and asks "Is my baby going to die?"

Questions

1. During your health assessment, what additional information would be beneficial to elicit to clarify the diagnosis?
2. Why does Leo's skin appear pale, with slight jaundice and have evidence of bruising?
3. What should be the focus of your nursing plan of care at this time?
4. What actions would you take to implement your plan?
5. How would you determine that the parents understood the treatment plan?

Answers

1. Has Leo recently had a bacterial or viral illness? HUS is commonly associated with these conditions.
2. Leo is pale due to anemia, which is a result of damaged red blood cells. The jaundice and easy bruising are a result of thrombocytopenia.
3. Providing comfort to the parents, addressing the parents' concerns by reemphasizing and clarifying the plan of care as explained by the physician, and determining what other concerns the parents may have.
4. Show parents pictures of the Tenckhoff catheter and peritoneal dialysis process. Discuss how they can help support their child and hold him during dialysis. Help parents select diversionary activities for their child. Review with parents the clinical indicators that the health care team will be evaluating to determine when kidney function is returning.
5. Parents verbalize that they understand the plan of care, they are able to discuss the plan of care with their child and other family members, and they select activities to keep the child calm and content during dialysis treatments.

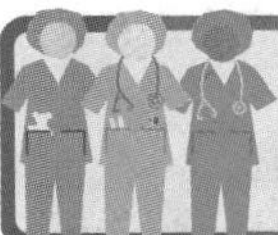

Care Path 19–3 An Interdisciplinary Plan of Care for the Child with Acute Renal Failure Due to Hemolytic-Uremic Syndrome

Nursing Diagnosis	Patient/Family Intermediate Outcomes		
	Days 1–3, Acute phase	**Days 3–15, Beginning recovery**	**Days 16–18, Recovery phase**
Fluid volume excess related to renal insufficiency	Child has beginning control of fluid and electrolyte balance.	Fluid balance is maintained and electrolytes are within normal ranges with treatment.	Fluid balance is maintained and electrolytes are within normal ranges without treatment.
Decreased cardiac output related to renal insufficiency and fluid overload	Child's BP is controlled with medications and IPD exchanges.	Child's BP is controlled with PD exchanges and medications p.r.n.	Child's BP is under control with medications or PD.
Altered tissue perfusion (renal) related to decreased cellular exchange	Child's Hgb is ≥7 with treatment.		Child maintains Hgb ≥7 without treatment.
Risk for infection related to Tenckhoff catheter placement and peritoneal dialysis	IPD effluent is clear, with no signs of infection at Tenckhoff exit site.	PD effluent is clear, with no signs of infection at Tenckhoff exit site.	Tenckhoff catheter is removed. Exit site heals without signs of infection.
Care Intervention Categories			
Consults	Surgery (Tenckhoff catheter placement)	Nutrition	Surgery (Tenckhoff catheter removal)
Labs	Daily CBC with differential and platelets; PT and PTT; Chem 17; Mg; if child is voiding, U/A, C&S, electrolytes. Check stool for *Escherichia coli*.	Daily CBC with differential and platelets, Chem 17, Mg	
Medications and IVs	IV fluids Antihypertensives p.r.n., calcium carbonate; PIV without potassium	Heparin lock	Oral iron; discontinue IV
Monitors	Cardiac monitor if child is hyperkalemic	→	DC cardiac monitor
Nutrition	NPO; advance to low potassium, clear liquid	Advance to regular diet for age; restrict protein, potassium, and fluid if necessary	Regular diet for age
Pain management	Morphine p.r.n.	→	Acetaminophen p.r.n.
Procedures (diagnostics)	Transfuse for Hgb ≤7.0; Tenckhoff catheter placed; IPD exchanges q 1 hr	Advance from IPD to PD with closed system and q.i.d. exchanges On day 3, start daily Tenckhoff dressing changes	Tenckhoff removed before discharge

Care Path continued on following page

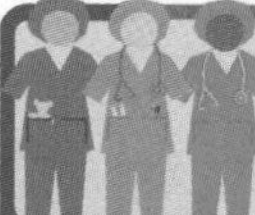

Care Path 19–3 An Interdisciplinary Plan of Care for the Child with Acute Renal Failure Due to Hemolytic-Uremic Syndrome *Continued*

Care Intervention Categories	Days 1–3, Acute phase	Days 3–15, Beginning recovery	Days 16–18, Recovery phase
Radiology	Chest radiograph; KUB in OR for Tenckhoff location		
Safety and activity	Bed rest in ICU	Participate in play therapy activities and school activities as tolerated	Increase as tolerated on inpatient unit
Self-care	Cooperate with care	Continue to cooperate and participate in care as able	
Social service			Arrange transportation for clinic visits if required
Teaching	Disease and its treatment	Dietary/fluid restrictions	Return visit appointment made; when to call physician; home medication regimen
Vital signs/baseline parameters	VS and BP q 1–2 hr Daily weight Document I & O Assess skin turgor	VS and BP q 4 hr daily ⟶ ⟶ ⟶	⟶ ⟶ ⟶ ⟶

BP, blood pressure; CBC, complete blood count; C&S, culture and sensitivity; Hgb, hemoglobin; ICU, intensive care unit; I & O, input and output; IPD, intraperitoneal dialysis; IV, intravenous; KUB, Kidney-ureter-bladder; Mg, magnesium; NPO, nothing by mouth; OR, operating room; PD, peritoneal dialysis; PIV, peripheral intravenous; p.r.n., as needed; PT, prothrombin time; PTT, partial thromboplastin time; U/A, urinalysis; VS, vital signs.

to maintain the hemoglobin level usually result in recovery. More than 90% of affected children survive. Most recover normal renal function, but all should be evaluated by a nephrologist at least biennially to observe for development of hypertension or CRD (Bergstein, 1996; Gilman et al., 1994). See Chronic Renal Failure for more information regarding management of the renal sequelae of this condition.

Acute Poststreptococcal Glomerulonephritis

Various renal disorders are called glomerulonephritis. All are caused by proliferation and inflammation of the glomeruli, usually as a result of an immune mechanism. A kidney biopsy is the only way to identify the type of glomerulonephritis (Chart 19–21).

Having a specific diagnosis is useful in determining treatment for the basic disease, in assessing the likelihood of retaining or regaining normal renal function, or in assessing the probability of the disease recurring in a transplanted kidney. However, the need for renal replacement therapy is the same once the disease progresses to ESRD, no matter which kind of glomerulonephritis is the cause.

Acute poststreptococcal glomerulonephritis is one of the most common acute renal syndromes. The child has symptoms of varying severity 1 to 2 weeks after a throat or skin infection with certain nephrogenetic strains of group A beta-hemolytic streptococci. In cold weather, the precipitating infection is most likely to be pharyngeal; in warm weather, skin infections (impetigo, infected insect bites or varicella sores) predominate (Bergstein, 1996).

Pathophysiology

Biopsy specimens from children with poststreptococcal glomerulonephritis show that pathologic findings vary with the severity of the disease. Mild cases show minimal to moderate proliferation of mesangial cells and matrix.

Chart 19–21

Causes of Glomerulonephritis

Congenital or Inherited

Alport's syndrome
Congenital nephrotic syndrome (Finnish type)
Familial hematuria
Nail patella syndrome

Acquired

Primary or idiopathic

Minimal change disease
Mesangial proliferative glomerulonephritis
Focal segmental glomerulosclerosis
Membranoproliferative glomerulonephritis
Membranous glomerulopathy
IgA nephropathy
Rapidly progressive glomerulonephritis
Focal proliferative glomerulonephritis
Diffuse proliferative glomerulonephritis
Unclassified chronic glomerulonephritis

Secondary

Infection related
- Poststreptococcal glomerulonephritis
- Hepatitis B
- Subacute bacterial endocarditis
- Shunt nephritis
- Postpneumococcal glomerulonephritis
- Congenital syphilis
- Malaria, leprosy, schistosomiasis, filariasis
- Acquired immunodeficiency syndrome

Associated with a multisystem disease
- Henoch-Schönlein purpura
- Systemic lupus erythematosus
- Hemolytic-uremic syndrome
- Diabetes mellitus
- Other collagen vascular diseases
- Goodpasture's syndrome
- Amyloidosis

Pharmaceutical agents
- Penicillamine
- Nonsteroidal anti-inflammatory drugs
- Captopril, gold salts, "street" heroin
- Trimethadione, lithium, mercury

Neoplasia
- Leukemia, lymphoma, carcinoma

Miscellaneous
- Chronic transplant rejection
- Reflux nephropathy
- Sickle cell disease

From Makker, S. P. (1992). Glomerular diseases. In K. K. Kher & S. P. Makker (Eds.), *Clinical pediatric nephrology* (p. 181). New York: McGraw-Hill. Reprinted with permission.

In severe cases, mesangial cell, matrix, and endothelial cell proliferation, as well as infiltration with polymorphonuclear cells and monocytes, can be so extensive that the capillary lumens are occluded. In fact, severe disease is called diffuse endocapillary exudative proliferative glomerulonephritis (Makker, 1992a).

Prognosis. The disease usually runs its course in about 1 month. Up to 95% of children recover completely, but some may have abnormal urinalysis for up to a year. In some children with oliguria, rapidly progressive glomerulonephritis develops; in others, chronic glomerulonephritis develops more slowly. In general, children with prolonged proteinuria and an abnormal glomerular filtration rate have a poor prognosis (Bergstein, 1996; Gilman et al., 1994).

Assessment

Severe clinical manifestations may include ARF with sudden onset of gross hematuria, edema, hypertension, and renal insufficiency. However, up to half of the children are asymptomatic with only microscopic hematuria. A typical case might show the sudden onset of mild proteinuria, hematuria, and periorbital edema. The urine is smoky brown or cola colored from the presence of red blood cells. The child is usually irritable and complains of flank or midabdominal pain, general malaise, and fever. Acute hypertension can cause headache, vomiting, somnolence, other central nervous system symptoms, including seizures. Fluid overload can cause cardiovascular symptoms such as dyspnea and tachypnea as well as an enlarged, tender liver (Bergstein, 1996; Gilman et al., 1994).

Diagnostic Tests. Although frequent blood pressure readings and 24-hour urine collections for creatinine clearance and protein excretion help indicate the severity of the disease, a kidney biopsy is the only way to distinguish between the various types of glomerulonephritis. The biopsy specimen is examined by both light microscopy and electron microscopy, and it is stained for immunofluorescence.

Interdisciplinary Interventions

Treatment of acute poststreptococcal glomerulonephritis is symptom specific. Dietary restrictions of fluid, sodium, and potassium are recommended. Bed rest, antihypertensives, and diuretics are also helpful in treatment of this condition. Early treatment of streptococcal infections with antibiotics does not always prevent the development of the disease, but the affected child and all other family members with positive cultures should undergo treatment for 10 to 14 days (Chart 19–22) (Gilman et al., 1994). See Chronic Renal Failure for information on supportive care for renal sequelae.

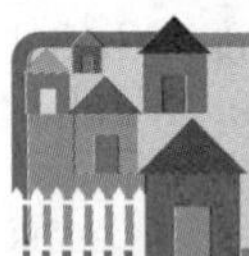

Chart 19–22
Community Care

Preventing Acute Poststreptococcal Glomerulonephritis

When a child is diagnosed with acute poststreptococcal glomerulonephritis (APSGN):

- All people living in the home should have throat cultures completed to evaluate for the presence of streptococci.
- Any individual who has a positive throat culture should have a course of penicillin therapy. It can be given by mouth for 10 days, or benzathine penicillin can be administered intramuscularly once.
- Community contacts generally do not need to be tested for streptococcal infection.
- Prophylactic therapy with penicillin to prevent further streptococcal infections is not necessary because APSGN tends not to recur with subsequent infections.

Prevention or early effective treatment of APSGN can be accomplished by the following:

- All children who have had a sore throat, tonsillitis, otitis media, or impetigo caused by streptococcus should have a urinalysis 2 weeks after the infection.
- Encourage children who are prescribed penicillin or other antibiotics for a streptococcal infection to complete the entire course of the treatment regimen.

Familial Glomerulopathy (Alport's Syndrome)

Of the several types of hereditary glomerulonephritis, Alport's syndrome is the most common, accounting for approximately 3% of cases of CRF in children (Makker, 1992a). The disease seems to be an X-linked dominant genetic disorder, because it tends to be more severe in males than in females. However, up to 20% of children with the syndrome have no prior family history, which seems to indicate a high spontaneous mutation rate (Bergstein, 1996).

Pathophysiology

In children younger than age 5 years with Alport's syndrome, biopsies are normal except for a few fetal glomeruli. As the child grows older, microscopic changes occur in the glomeruli: mesangial cells and matrix proliferate, capillary walls thicken, and tubules atrophy or dilate. Electron microscopy shows a typical basket-weave appearance in the glomerular basement membrane (Makker, 1992a). These changes usually start to occur in the teenage years, but presentation of the disease can vary widely. Progression to renal failure may or may not occur (Bergstein, 1996).

Assessment

The presenting symptom of Alport's syndrome may be a persistent asymptomatic microscopic hematuria or an episode of gross hematuria after an upper respiratory infection (Makker, 1992a). If renal failure occurs, hypertension and UTI are among the first signs (Bergstein, 1996). Some children with Alport's syndrome have progressive sensorineural hearing loss that begins in the high frequencies and progresses to total deafness. Approximately 10% of children also have eye disorders such as cataracts, macular lesions, and anterior lenticonus (Bergstein, 1996).

Interdisciplinary Interventions

Children with hearing or vision loss associated with Alport's syndrome should be given hearing aids and glasses as needed. Genetic counseling helps both the parents and the child make informed reproductive choices in the face of this hereditary disease. If Alport's syndrome progresses to ESRD, as it generally does in males, then dialysis and transplantation are the usual treatments (Bergstein, 1996; Makker, 1992a).

Renal Calculi

Renal calculi (urolithiasis) are uncommon in children. Although the exact incidence is unknown, urolithiasis is estimated to account for less than five new admissions to major pediatric centers per year (Smith & Segura, 1992). Premature infants are at particular risk for stone formation resulting from the furosemide (iron), intravenous calcium gluconate, total parenteral nutrition, and vitamin D supplements that they may receive over the course of their hospitalization (Levin & Hensle, 1990).

Diet and heredity play a part in calculi formation. For example, bladder stones are endemic in countries where the diet is high in grains and low in milk. In developed countries, however, this type of stone is nonexistent (Levin & Hensle, 1990). Metabolic disorders, a common basis for urinary calculi, also display genetic tendencies.

Urolithiasis can be broadly classified into three categories, defined by the precipitating condition:

- Infection-related calculi
- Calculi resulting from a metabolic imbalance
- Pharmacologically induced calculi

Distinguishing characteristics identify each type (Table 19–6).

Infection-Related Calculi. Infection-related stones are usually composed of struvite crystals, and their incidence peaks at a mean age of 4 years. Infection-related calculi are a complication of urinary stasis. Conditions that predispose a child to urinary stasis include congenital obstructive uropathy and neuromuscular disorders, such as myelomeningocele or spinal cord injury. UTI is a major risk factor for stone formation. Bacteria react with urinary urea to produce ammonium, which is a buffer. The elevated ammonium levels increase the urinary pH above 6.8, inducing the precipitation of struvite (magnesium ammonium phosphate) crystals in urine. The causative organisms—*Klebsiella, Proteus, Pseudomonas, Streptococcus, Providencia, Mycoplasma,* and some *E. coli* strains—then become embedded in the stone matrix, where they are immune to the effects of antibiotics (Drach, 1995).

Calculi Resulting from Metabolic Imbalance. Stones resulting from metabolic dysfunction are high in calcium, oxalate, cystine, or uric acid. These types of stones are most often manifested during adolescence or later. Elevated levels of calcium suggest hyperparathyroidism as an underlying cause of stone formation. Numerous enteric

Table 19–6
Presentation of Renal Calculi

Peak Age of Onset	Causative Factor in Stone Formation	Prevalence	Stone Analysis	Urinary pH	Treatment Approach
Neonatal or infancy	Secondary to pharmacologic agents	Rare	Calcium Uric acid Xanthine	—	Discontinue offending pharmaceutical agent
Preschool	Infection-related urinary stasis	40%	Struvite (Magnesium-ammonium-phosphate)	Alkaline (>6.8)	Stone removal Antibiotic therapy Prevention of urinary stasis Increase fluids Add acidifying agents
Adolescence	Metabolic imbalance	50%	Calcium Oxalate Uric acid	Normal or acidic	Parathyroidectomy
	Parathyroidism				Pyridoxine Magnesium gluconate Allopurinol
	Renal disease				Alkalizing agents Thiazide therapy Management of underlying cause Increase fluid intake
	Enteric disease				Calcium-restricted diet Oxalate-restricted diet Restricted purine intake
	Immobilization				Exercise Weight-bearing activity Increased fluids Calcium intake at recommended daily allowance level

conditions create metabolic imbalances, which enhance the risk of renal stones. Bowel malabsorption syndrome, small bowel resection, cystic fibrosis, inflammatory biliary disorders, or hereditary errors of metabolism are associated with excessive oxalate levels in the urine, creating calcium-oxalate stones (Drach, 1995). Hyperabsorption of calcium within the intestinal tract can progress to hypercalciuria and calcium stones. Uric acid and cystine calculi may result from abnormal bowel function or an inborn error of metabolism, and are often found in the presence of acidic urine. Conditions that compromise renal glomerular or tubular function predispose the child to urolithiasis. Chief among these conditions are renal tubular acidosis, cystinuria, renal hypercalcemia, and primary hyperoxaluria, all of which may occur as autosomal recessive disorders (Levin & Hensle, 1990). Diet is another metabolic factor to consider. Excessive ingestion of calcium or protein, or diets rich in oxalate-containing foods such as rhubarb, strawberries, cola, spinach, citrus, or tea promote calculi formation (Levin & Hensle, 1990).

Recurrence rates for calculi resulting from infection, immobility, or medication are low, following correction of the underlying condition, whereas metabolic associated urolithiasis tends to be a lifelong condition (Drach, 1995).

Pharmacologically Induced Calculi. The necessary use of various pharmacologic agents among high-risk neonates and infants has introduced urolithiasis into this population. Hypercalcemia and metabolic alkalosis occur secondary to the long-term administration of furosemide in the treatment of bronchopulmonary dysplasia or cardiac disease (Hufnagle, Khan, Penn, Cacciarelli & Williams, 1982). The use of total parenteral nutrition (TPN), vitamin D therapy, and IV calcium gluconate can also elevate serum calcium levels. Allopurinol (Zyloprim), acetazolamide (Diamox), triamterene-hydrochlorothiazide (Dyazide), corticosteroids, and chemotherapeutic agents have all been implicated in renal stone disease (Levin & Hensle, 1990).

Assessment

Urolithiasis generally becomes evident when the child experiences an acute attack of colicky flank pain, nausea and vomiting, hematuria and dysuria, indicating sudden urine blockage or stone movement. Signs of systemic infection, such as fever, malaise, abdominal pain, and septicemia, warrant consideration of urinary calculi as part of the investigational evaluation. Suspicions of urinary calculi should be heightened if the child has other predisposing factors, such as neuromuscular disease. The child's diet should be evaluated for unusual or extreme nutrient ingestion. Hydration status, especially water intake, should be determined.

Diagnostic Tests. The preliminary evaluation of the child with urolithiasis may include plain abdominal films or an ultrasound; however, a CT scan most clearly highlights stones (Nimkin, Lebowitz, Share, & Teele, 1992). An excretory urogram (IVP) and VCUG are useful to determine the extent of damage to the urinary tract and as initial diagnostic tools to detect congenital urologic anomalies.

The next step is to strain the urine to capture stone matter, because the stone analysis directs further evaluation and treatment. Other urologic tests include a urine culture, urinalysis for cells, pH, protein, and crystals, and measurement of urine volume. An overnight urine collection is analyzed for creatinine to calcium ratio, and other urine samples measure uric acid, calcium, oxalate, creatinine and phosphate, magnesium, and citrate. Serum is collected to measure calcium, uric acid, creatinine, electrolytes, and pH balance. Thyroid and parathyroid hormone levels are also obtained (Drach, 1995).

Nursing Diagnoses and Outcomes

Chart 19–3 presents nursing diagnoses generally applicable to the child with a genitourinary/renal condition. The following diagnoses address some more specific care needs of the child with renal calculi:

- **Pain related to obstruction of urinary tract by calculi**
  Outcome: The child's pain is controlled by use of pharmaceutical and nonpharmaceutical interventions.
- **Knowledge deficit: Fluid requirements and dietary modifications**
  Outcomes: The child and/or family express the benefits of dietary changes and adequate fluid intake to prevent calculi formation.
  The child and/or family make appropriate dietary selections to help prevent calculi formation.

Interdisciplinary Interventions

Initial treatment involves intravenous hydration and pain relief. Symptoms of UTI or septicemia require immediate antibiotic and supportive therapy. Therapy following resolution of the acute phase is determined by the nature of the primary problem that caused the stone formation. Stones are removed by surgical excision or are dissolved via extracorporeal shock wave lithotripsy if feasible. The underlying urologic anomaly or cause of urinary stasis is then corrected surgically. Techniques such as timed voiding and CIC may be used to ensure regular, complete emptying of the bladder, reducing the risk of UTI.

Stones that are the end products of a metabolic imbalance require treatment to correct the underlying condition. Alkaline urine is acidified by the administration of ascorbic acid. Mild metabolic acidosis and the attendant acidic urine are balanced by alkalizing agents such as soda bicarbonate or potassium citrate. The child may be placed on allopurinol or D-penicillamine to bind with excessive serum cystine.

Long-term immobilization of the child is discouraged. Regular weight-bearing exercise and a physical therapy program individualized to the child's capabilities are important adjuncts to the medical protocol.

Nutritional Management

Nutritional services assist parents in providing a nutritionally balanced diet. The Dietary Reference Intake (DRI) for calcium recommends that daily intake should be maintained at 500 mg for children up to 3 years, 800 mg for school-age children, and 1300 mg for adolescents (Institute of Medicine). Moderate sodium restriction, moderate intake of animal protein, and avoidance of high doses of vitamin C also help prevent stone formation.

caREminder: *Limiting dietary calcium in children can inhibit their ability to form new bone, thus limiting their growth.*

Further nutritional counseling may be required to help parents add or restrict nutrients that contribute to specific types of stone formation and to monitor the child's general health status while on a particular dietary plan.

Adequate daily water intake (enough to cause a urine output of more than 2000 to 3000 mL/day in the older child) is the mainstay of therapy for all children with urinary calculi. It is believed that children have established their drinking habits by age 3 years. An important role for the nurse is to develop a plan with the parents for creative techniques to encourage adequate water intake. The use of positive reinforcement and age-appropriate rewards is influential in modifying the child's learned drinking pattern and choices. The daycare provider or school nurse, teacher, and lunchroom staff should be incorporated into this plan to ensure proper hydration of the child during the school day.

Surgical Management

Historically, operative management of urinary calculi was accomplished by nephrolithotomy or ureterolithotomy, whereby an open flank or abdominal incision was made and the stone was directly extracted from its site. Although effective for total stone eradication, the open procedure carried negative consequences: anesthesia risks, potential for postoperative complications, discomfort, extended hospitalization, trauma to urinary structures, and potential obstruction secondary to operative site scarring.

Since 1980, several new techniques have emerged that have drastically altered the treatment of urinary stones. These techniques are percutaneous lithotripsy (PL), shock wave lithotripsy (SWL), and ureteroscopy (US). Used individually or in combination, the successful use of these new modalities has reduced the incidence of open stone extraction to 1% to 2% (Smith & Segura, 1992). Table 19–7 summarizes the uses, advantages, and disadvantages of these three procedures.

Percutaneous Lithotripsy. PL creates a nephrostomy tract by the insertion of a percutaneous catheter into the renal pelvis. Fluoroscopic observation is used to ensure proper catheter placement and to monitor the stone extraction. A variety of instruments can be placed within this percutaneous tract, including a nephroscope, a stone retrieval basket, and laser, ultrasonic, or electrolysis equipment for calculus disintegration. Small calculi are removed intact by the basket, whereas larger stones are fragmented and then either extracted by the basket or flushed through the urinary tract. The nephrostomy tube is left in place for urinary drainage until postoperative edema resolves (Bruton, Einhorn, Reardon, Snyder, & Williams, 1995).

Nursing care for the child undergoing PL focuses on preventing infection, ensuring adequate urine flow, controlling pain and/or ureteral spasm, providing wound care, and maintaining nephrostomy tube placement and patency. High fluid intake is required to flush stone fragments, tissue debris, and mucoid shreds from the operative site and to prevent tube obstruction. The percutaneous tube is a temporary, nonretention tube that must be well secured to prevent dislodgment or inadvertent removal. The tube exit site is cleansed, an antiseptic ointment is administered, and a dry sterile dressing is applied daily. The child's vital signs, wound site, and urinary drainage are monitored for signs of infection. Prophylactic antibiotics are usually ordered. If the child is discharged with a percutaneous tube in place, parents need instruction in tube management. Home visits by a community health nurse are useful to oversee the child's condition and to supplement the care provided by the parents.

Shock Wave Lithotripsy. Treatment of urolithiasis was revolutionized by the introduction of SWL during the 1980s. Also known as extracorporeal shock wave lithotripsy, the procedure entails the use of shock waves, generated by an electronic or electromagnetic source, which are discharged and transmitted via a water bath or a water cushion to the site of the calculus. Cross-directional sources simultaneously emit a charge, directed toward the stone as a focal point. Fluoroscopic or ultrasound guidance is used to ensure that shock waves converge on the stone and to minimize trauma to surrounding tissue.

Because the resulting calculi sludge requires a high urine volume for excretion, IV fluids are administered both during and after the procedure. General anesthesia, epidural anesthesia, or IV sedation is used to prevent the

Table 19-7
Surgical Treatment Options for Renal Calculi

Technique	Indications/Advantages	Contraindications/Disadvantages
Percutaneous lithotripsy (PL)	High rate (85%–90%) of complete stone removal (Patterson et al., 1987) Indicated in presence of urinary tract obstruction or stenosis distal to calculus Treatment of choice for · Large stones (>2–3 cm) · Cystine or brushite stones · Lower calyceal stones Used if SWL fails to pulverize calculus or if stone cannot be placed in focal point.	Requires incision to ureter or renal pelvis —discomfort and risk of infection Potential for secondary urologic obstruction caused by scarring at the site Hospitalization is often required, home care may be needed.
Shock wave lithotripsy (SWL)	Outpatient procedure No external access to urinary tract Well tolerated, minimal trauma to urologic structures or adjacent organs Treatment of choice for · Upper and midcalyceal stones · Upper and midureteral stones Lower radiation exposure than PL; may use ultrasound to monitor procedure May be used in conjunction with PL to remove residual calculi fragments	Contraindicated in pregnancy or with coagulopathy Release of stone-encased bacteria during treatment of struvite stones Large stone fragments or high volume of stone sediment may occlude ureter. An indwelling double "J" stent is inserted before the procedure to prevent obstruction. Stones composed of hard matrix (e.g., cystine, brushite) may not fragment. Requires shielding of lung fields Transient hemoptysis/hematuria
Ureteroscope (US)	Treatment of choice for calculi in lower ureteral segment Newer "miniscopes" have expanded the use of this technique among small children. No external entry site needed to access calculus	Potential for trauma to vesicoureteral junction, leading to reflux Limited access to small or stenotic ureters

child from moving, and the shock waves are discharged in coordination with the child's respiration to keep the calculus in focus (McCullough, 1992). Numerous studies have documented the effectiveness of SWL in removing obstructing calculi with minimal negative consequences for children, although residual nonobstructing stone fragments are common (Kroovand, Harrison, & McCullough, 1987; Newman et al., 1986).

SWL is generally performed as an outpatient procedure, with the possibility of an overnight stay. Preprocedural evaluation includes an IVP to assess for degree of obstruction, calculi position and additional urinary tract anomaly, a CBC and clotting studies, renal and liver function studies, and a urinalysis and urine culture. Antibiotic coverage is used to treat existing UTI or in the presence of struvite calculi (Kroovand, Harrison, & McCullough, 1987; Newman et al., 1986). If indicated, a double "J" stent is inserted via cystoscopy before the start of SWL.

Following SWL, the child requires routine postoperative care. Hemoptysis and hematuria are expected and are transient. Flank ecchymosis is common. The nurse should monitor the degree of the child's discomfort and should provide pain relief with acetaminophen as needed. Because discomfort is mild, extreme pain may indicate ureteral blockage and should be reported to the urologist.

High-volume IV fluids are maintained to ease the flushing of calculus sludge. The child with an indwelling double "J" stent requires no special nursing care or discharge teaching, because the tube is well tolerated and has no effect on urinary function. The stent is removed via cystoscopy at a later date.

Ureteroscopy. Access to ureteral calculi can be obtained by inserting an endoscope through the vesicoureteral segment during a cystoscopic procedure. Although commonly used among adults, US in children has been limited by the need to use large caliper endoscopes to manipulate calculi. Several ureteroscopes designed for pediatric use are currently available, making US extraction of lower tract calculi a viable treatment option. Because of the potential for damage to the vesicoureteral junction, possibly resulting in reflux, urologists remain cautious in their choice of US management for urinary calculi (Smith & Segura, 1992).

Nursing care for the child undergoing US is minimal. The procedure is performed on an outpatient basis, and the child is discharged when stable after voiding. High fluid intake for several days is advised and prophylactic antibiotics may be ordered. Mild analgesics such as acetaminophen are given to control ureteral spasms related to endoscopic manipulation.

Renal Trauma

Renal injury usually occurs in conjunction with abdominal trauma, although it can occur as an isolated event. Damage to the kidney is a component of 3% of all pediatric trauma cases. The overwhelming majority of injuries occur after blunt force trauma such as passenger or pedestrian motor vehicle accidents or sports injuries. Penetrating wounds resulting from gunshots or stabbing account for less than 10% of all renal injuries, but are increasing significantly, mirroring increasing trends of violence involving children (McAleer & Kaplan, 1995). Renal trauma rarely causes death, but may compound the effects of other life-threatening injuries.

Certain characteristics of the child's renal structure increase its susceptibility to damage. The child's kidney fills proportionately more space in the abdomen compared with the adult organ. Its position is lower in the retroperitoneum and less protected by fat and fascia. Supporting structures have greater elasticity, which allows for excessive renal motion following bodily force. Immature ossification of the encircling ribs further compromise protection to the kidney. Congenital anomalies or an aberrant renal location (e.g., hydronephrosis, fused kidneys, or a pelvic kidney) increase the potential for damage following even minimal force.

Pathophysiology

Blunt abdominal trauma can compress the renal unit against skeletal structures (i.e., ribs or vertebrae), causing a rupture of its surrounding renal capsule or a subcapsular hematoma. In situations such as a bicycle–automobile accident, the child's increased kidney motility can create an **acceleration–deceleration injury**, which can shear or thrombose the vascular attachment site or can disrupt the UPJ. **Penetrating forces**, such as a bullet, a knife, or a rib, can cause injury by puncturing or shattering a renal segment. **Iatrogenic injuries** can occur during invasive procedures such as biopsy, tube placement, or stone manipulation (Murphy, 1990).

Most children who sustain renal trauma heal completely, with little or no residual negative sequelae. The child's long-term prognosis is more closely dependent on the severity of other wounds.

Assessment

Any child who sustains a compressing, penetrating, or blunt wound to the abdomen, chest, flank, or spine should be assessed for renal trauma. Hematuria may be gross or microscopic, but is not always diagnostic of renal trauma. Careful evaluation should be given to the liver or spleen, additional potential sources of hematuria (Taylor, Eichelberger, & Potter, 1988). Other indications of renal trauma include tenderness or pain to the flank or upper abdomen, ecchymosis of the trunk, palpable abdominal mass, nausea and vomiting, and hypotension (McAleer, Kaplan, & Scherz, 1993). Elevated BUN and creatinine, oliguria, and anuria that accompany a history of trauma are also indications of severe renal injury (Smith, 1990).

Diagnosis of renal trauma is best determined by CT scan, which provides detailed views highlighting organ involvement (McAleer & Kaplan, 1995). Based on the accuracy of CT evaluation for renal injuries, a classification system has evolved that not only describes the extent of damage but also has useful predictive value for management, need for surgical intervention, and follow-up care. This system distinguishes renal injury as minor, major, or critical (Fig. 19–14).

Interdisciplinary Interventions

Emergency care and stabilization must be the first priority for the child with multiorgan trauma. Once this is accomplished, results of the renal CT scan direct management of this injury. Reattachment of renal vessels or the ureter, evacuation of blood clots, and closure of renal lacerations are surgical goals for critical or selected major injuries.

Conservative treatment, the management of choice for minor injuries and certain major injuries, necessitates strict bed rest. The child is hospitalized and fluids are increased via IV therapy or by mouth if tolerated. Urine is monitored for volume and degree of hematuria. Vital signs are monitored frequently for indications of hemorrhage and shock. Fever can be treated with increased fluids, sponge baths, and antipyretics. Pain medications, positioning the child off the affected site, and application of ice packs to the affected area can be used to help control discomfort. Diversional activities are extremely important during this phase, because resolution of gross hematuria may require confinement of a week or longer. Healing progress is monitored by CT scans, and hospital discharge is considered when gross hematuria fades. Out-

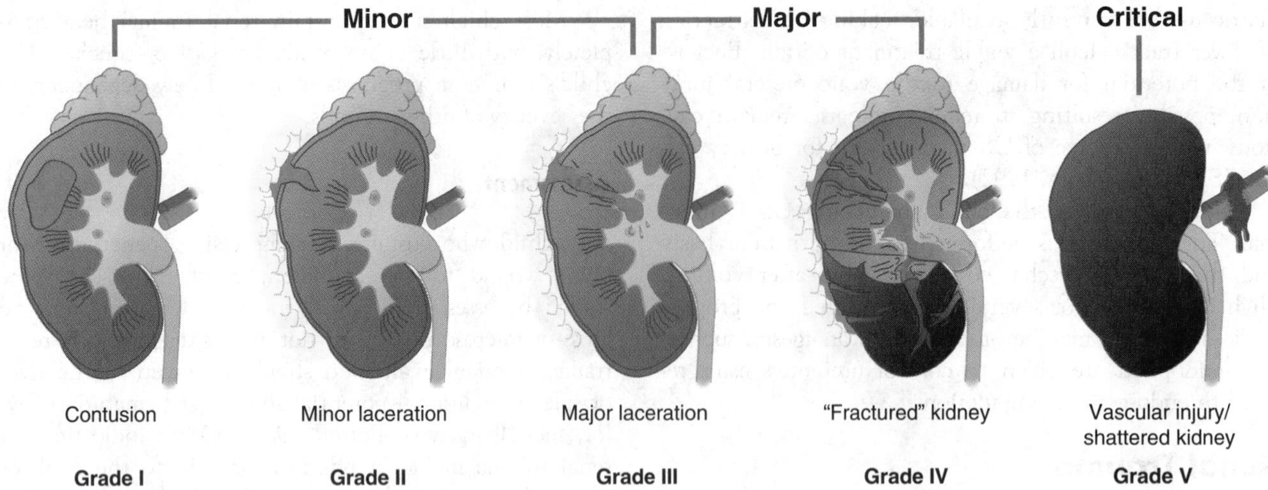

Figure 19–14
Classification of renal trauma injuries. Minor injury includes grades I through III as follows: grade I, contusion or subcapsular hematoma; grade II, shallow cortical laceration, confined perirenal hematoma; grade III, deep cortical injury without extension into medulla. Grade IV injury is a major injury, which includes laceration extending into the medulla and collection system or a vascular pedicle tear or hematoma. Critical injury is grade V, which is a shattered kidney or vascular pedicle avulsion. (Modified from Black, J. M., & Matassarin-Jacobs, E. [Eds.]. [1997]. Medical-surgical nursing [5th ed., p. 1675]. Philadelphia: W. B. Saunders. Reprinted with permission.)

patient follow-up with activity restrictions continues until microscopic hematuria disappears.

When conservative treatment is chosen for major renal injuries, the child should be monitored for the following complications: infection, persistent or recurring bleeding, perirenal bleeding or hematuria, urinary leakage or obstruction, or renal necrosis. The nurse should be alert for changes in vital signs, decreased urine output, increasing level of hematuria, or increased flank or abdominal pain, all clues to potential problems.

Community Care

At discharge from the hospital, the nurse should review with the parents the need for long-term follow-up. Late complications include hydronephrosis, hypertension, renal atrophy, or arteriovenous fistula or aneurysm, conditions that generally develop slowly and silently (Abdalati et al., 1994; Murphy, 1990). Blood pressure monitoring should occur periodically during the ensuing year to monitor for hypertension (Gonzalez, 1996). For the child who underwent a nephrectomy or who has a severely compromised residual kidney, restriction from contact sports may be prudent as well as legally mandated. The nurse should focus patient and family counseling around acceptable low-impact sports and assist in the planning of the child's physical education program at school, in day-care, or in extracurricular sports settings.

Summary of Key Concepts

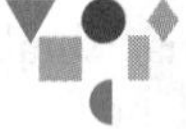

- Genitourinary conditions are often characterized by a history of changes in the child's voiding patterns, a history of recent respiratory or dermatologic, complaints of abdominal pain, a weight gain, or edema.
- During a physical assessment of the child with a suspected or actual genitourinary condition, the nurse should observe the child for poor skin color, lethargy, bony configurations, abnormalities in speech, or a protuberent abdomen, all of which can occur in urinary conditions or renal failure.
- The child's kidneys do not reach full functional maturity until age 2 years.
- Midstream urine samples or urine absorbed from AGM-free diapers are

the easiest methods of specimens collection for routine urinalysis. When a urine sample is needed for culture and sensitivity tests a clean-catch midstream sample, or samples extracted via a urine bag, uretheral catheterization, or suprapubic aspiration, must be used.

- Treatment modalities such as urinary diversion, drainage tubes, stents, and catheterization are aimed at compensations for alterations in gravity flow or muscular contraction and reestablishing the free flow of urine from the body.
- The child with urinary tract infection is managed with a combination of antibiotic therapy, increased fluid intake, frequent voiding, and teaching hygienic techniques to clean the genital area.
- Urethritis is common among young girls because the sensitive uretheral tissue is easily irritated by chemicals, such as bubble bath, soap, or shampoo residue in bath water; chlorine; tight or synthetic clothes; and poor hygienic techniques.
- Management of the child with a voiding disorder requires an interdisciplinary effort using medical, nursing, nutritional, and psychosocial health care professionals. Surgical and pharmacologic treatment measures are usually combined with dietary, bladder retraining, and/or motivational programs to achieve full-day and nighttime continence.
- The child with obstructive uropathy will have pathophysiologic changes, ranging from mild to severe, that have been caused by the congenital or acquired condition that has impeded urine excretion.
- Children with anomalies of the bladder or urethra generally require one or more surgical procedures to correct the defect or provide long-term urinary diversion.
- Undescended testes are noted in 3% to 5% of male babies at birth. Surgical manipulation is required, preferably performed at 3 to 12 months of age.
- Testicular torsion is considered a urologic emergency. Acute scrotal pain, often associated with nausea and vomiting, is the hallmark sign of this disorder.
- Discharge teaching for the family of a circumcised male includes application of a petroleum-coated gauze bandage, avoidance of vigorous play activities and tub baths for 3 to 5 days, and observation of the penis for edema or bleeding.
- Males should perform testicular self-examination once a month after bathing, when the scrotal skin is moist and slippery.
- Acute renal failure develops rapidly over days or weeks. The first sign may be oliguria. Retained fluid subsequently causes other systemic manifestations, such as hypertension, edema, and shortness of breath. Acidosis and serum electrolyte imbalances can cause gastrointestinal or central nervous system disturbances.
- There are many treatment modalities available for the pediatric patient with temporary or permanently impaired renal function. Conservative management, hemodialysis, PD, CRRT, renal transplantation, or a combination of these therapies is selected based on the underlying illness, the degree of renal damage, the likelihood of recovering renal function, the signs and symptoms experienced, and the child and the family's preference.
- The dietary plan for the child with renal failure is individualized and designed to compensate for impaired kidney function. Most diets are low in protein, low in potassium, and low to moderate in sodium. No food is entirely forbidden, but total intake of each substance must be monitored.
- Patient education is extensive for the child receiving renal replacement

therapy. The family is instructed about the body's natural osmotic and filtration process and the manner in which the therapy will carry out these processes for the body. Catheter site care is demonstrated, and the family is taught to assess the child for signs and symptoms of catheter site complications or complications of the dialysis process.

- Nephrotic syndrome is characterized by periorbital edema, weight gain, and foamy or frothy urine. Treatment aims to decrease urinary protein loss, balance nutrition, restore normal metabolic function, and prevent or treat any infection.
- The prodromal illness in hemolytic-uremic syndrome is usually gastrointestinal distress or an upper respiratory tract infection. Symptoms of this appear 5 to 10 days after onset of the prodromal illness.
- Early treatment of streptococcal infection with antibiotics will not always prevent the development of acute poststreptococcal glomerulonephritis. However, the risk of occurrence can be reduced by ensuring that all children with a streptococcal infection undergo antibiotic therapy for 10 to 14 days.
- Renal calculi are uncommon in children. If present, a combination of nutritional and surgical therapies are used to remove the calculi and to decrease the incidence of subsequent stone formation.
- Children are more susceptible to renal trauma because of the lower position of the kidneys in the retroperitoneum; the kidneys are also less protected by fat and fascia.

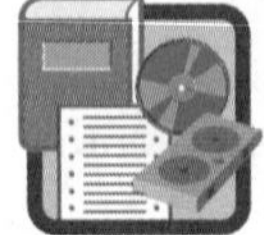

Resources

Organizations

American Academy of Nephrology
2221 University Avenue SE
Suite 335
Minneapolis, MN 55414
(612) 623-8115

American Association of Kidney Patients
100 South Ashley Drive
Suite 280
Tampa, FL 33602
(800) 749-2257

American Kidney Fund
6110 Executive Boulevard
Suite 1010
Rockville, MD 20852
(800) 638-8294
(301) 881-3052
Web: http://aztec.asc.edu/cins/alpha/50275.html

American Nephrology Nurses' Association
East Holly Avenue
P.O. Box 56
Pitman, NJ 08071-0056
(609) 256-2320
E-mail: anna©mail.ajj.com
Web: http://www.inurse.com/-anna

American Organ Transplant Association
P.O. Box 277
Missouri City, Texas 77459
(713) 261-2682

American Urologic Association, Allied
11512 Allecingie Parkway
Richmond, VA 23235
(804) 379-1306

Childrens Organ Transplant Association
2501 Cota Drive
Bloomington, IN 47403
(800) 366-2682

International Continence Society
11 West Graham St.
Glasgow, Scotland 649LF

International Transplant Nurses Society
Foster Plaza
Building 5
Suite 300
651 Holiday Drive
Pittsburgh, PA 15220
(412) 928-3667

National Kidney Foundation
30 East 33rd Street
New York, NY 10016
(800) 622-9010

North American Transplant Coordinators Organization
P.O. Box 15384
Lenexa, KS 66215
(913) 268-9830

Polycystic Kidney Disease Research Foundation
922 Walnut Street
Suite 411
Kansas City, MO 64106
(800) 753-2873

Society of Urologic Nurses & Associates
P.O. Box 56
Pitman, NJ 08071
(609) 256-2335
E-mail: suna©mail.ajj.com

United Network for Organ Sharing (UNOS)
P.O. Box 13770
Richmond, VA 23225
800-24-DONOR

Urodynamics Society
2916 TC/Box D330
University of Michigan Medical Center
1500 East Medical Center Drive
Ann Arbor, MI 48109
(313) 936-5775

Wound, Ostomy and Continence Nurses Society
2755 Bristol Street
Suite 110
Costa Mesa, CA 92626
(714) 476-0268

Books and Printed Materials

Ahlstrom, T. (1991). *The Kidney Patient's Book*. Delran, NJ: Great Issues Press.

Daugirdas & Ing. *The Handbook of Dialysis*. Little Brown and Company.

Kidney Transplant Patient Partnering Program.
(800) 893-1995
Free newsletter to all pre- and post-transplant recipients.

National Kidney Foundation Council on Renal Nutrition. *Living Well on Dialysis: A cookbook for patients and their families*. New York: Global Medical Communications, Inc.

U.S. Department of Agriculture. *Handbook of the Nutritional Contents of Foods*. New York: Doric Publications, Inc.

Computer Resources

National Kidney and Urologic Information Clearinghouse
Web: http:///www.aerie.com/nihdb/nkudic/kudbase.html

NutriGenie Renal Diet
Web: http://pages.prodigy.com/nutrisoft/ngrd41.html
Computer program based on U.S. Surgeon General's and National Institutes of Health's guidelines for kidney disease dietary management

Renal Help Books
Web: http://cybermart.com/aakpaz/guides.html

References

Abdalati, H., Bulas, D. I., Sivit, C. J., Majd, M., Rushton, H. G., & Eichelberger, M. R. (1994). Blunt renal trauma in children: Healing of renal injuries and recommendations for imaging follow-up. *Pediatric Radiology, 24*, 573–576.

Andreoli, S. P., Langefeld, C. D., Stadler, S., Smith, P., Sears, A., & West, K. (1993). Risks of peritoneal membrane failure in children undergoing long-term peritoneal dialysis. *Pediatric Nephrology, 7*, 543–547.

Ashcraft, K. W. (1990a). Prune belly syndrome. In K. W. Ashcraft (Ed.), *Pediatric urology*, (pp. 257–268), Philadelphia: W. B. Saunders.

Ashcraft, K. W. (1990b). Vesicoureteral reflux. In K. W. Ashcraft (Ed.), *Pediatric urology* (pp. 151–167). Philadelphia: W. B. Saunders.

Atkinson, G. O., Jr., Patrick, L. E., Ball, T. I., Jr., Stevenson, C. A., & Broecker, B. H. (1992). The normal and abnormal scrotum in children: Evaluation with color Doppler sonography. *American Journal of Radiology, 158*, 613–617.

Avorn, J., Monane, M., Gurwitz, G. H., Glynn, R. J., Chodnovsky, I., & Lipsitz, L. A. (1994). Reduction of bacteriuria and pyuria after ingestion of cranberry juice. *Journal of the American Medical Association, 271*(10), 751–754.

Bates, P. (1995). External genital disorders. In K. A. Karlowicz (Ed.), *Urologic nursing: Principles and practice* (p. 322). Philadelphia: W. B. Saunders.

Bell, S. B. (1988). CAVH in pediatrics: Meeting the challenge. *ANNA Journal, 15*(1), 25–26.

Benador, D., Benador, N., Slosman, D., Nussle, D., Mermillod, B., & Gurardin, E. (1994). Cortical scintigraphy in the evaluation of renal parenchymal changes in children with pyelonephritis. *Journal of Pediatrics, 124*, 17–20.

Bergstein, J. (1996). Nephrology. In R. Behrman, R. Kliegman, & A. Aruin (Eds.), *Nelson textbook of pediatrics* (pp. 1480–1506). Philadelphia: W. B. Saunders.

Bloom, D. A., Wan, J., & Key, D. W. (1992). Disorders of male external genitalia and inguinal canal. In P. P. Kalalis, L. R. King, & A. B. Belman (Eds.), *Clinical pediatric urology* (3rd ed., pp. 1015–1049). Philadelphia: W. B. Saunders.

Bock, G. H. (1992). Acute renal failure. In K. K. Kher, & S. P. Makker (Eds.), *Clinical pediatric nephrology* (pp. 469–497). New York: McGraw-Hill.

Bowers, V., Hannigan, K. F., Kushner, K. L. (1995). Bladder exstrophy and epispadias. In K. A. Karlowicz (Ed.), *Urologic nursing: Principles and practice* (pp. 565–592). Philadelphia: W. B. Saunders.

Bozette, M. (1993). Observation of pain behavior in the NICU: An exploratory study. *Journal of Perinatal-Neonatal Nursing, 7*, 76–87.

Brandell, R. A., & Brock, J. W. (1993). Postoperative management of bilateral reimplantation without catheters. *Urology, 42*(6), 705–707.

Brock, J. (1994). Autologous buccal mucosal graft for urethral reconstruction. *Urology, 44*(5), 753–755.

Bruton, D. S., Einhorn, C., Reardon, L. M., Snyder, J. M., Williams, A. (1995). Urinary calculi. In K. A. Karlowicz (Ed.), *Urologic nursing: Principles and practice* (pp. 177–198). Philadelphia: W. B. Saunders.

Burke, N. (1995). Alternative methods for newborn urine sample collection. *Pediatric Nursing, 21*(6), 546–549.

Butler, R. J. (1994). *Enuresis: The child's experience*. Oxford, England: Butterworth-Heinemann.

Cendron, M., & Gearhart, J. P. (1991). The Mitrofanoff principle. Technique and application to continent urinary diversion. *Urologic Clinics of North America*, 18(4), 615–621.

Chehval, M. J., & Purcell, M. H. (1992). Deterioration of semen parameters over time in men with untreated varicocele: Evidence of progressive testicular damage. *Fertility and Sterility, 57*(1), 174–177.

Couchells, S. M., Johnson, S. B., Carter, R., & Walker, D. (1981). Behavioral and environmental characteristics of treated and untreated enuretic children and non-enuretic controls. *Journal of Pediatrics*, 99(6), 812–816.

Craig, J., Knight, J., Sureshkumar, P., Mantz, E., & Roy, L. (1996). Effect of circumcision on incidence of urinary tract infection in preschool boys. *Journal of Pediatrics, 128*(1), 23–27.

Dixon, S., Snyder, J., Holve, R., & Bromberger, P. (1984). Behavioral effects of circumcision with and without anesthesia. *Journal of Developmental and Behavioral Pediatrics, 5*, 246.

Drach, G. W. (1995). Metabolic evaluation of pediatric patients with stones. *Urology Clinics of North America, 22*(1), 95–100.

Ellis, D. G. (1990). Undescended testis: Cryptorchidism. In K. W. Ashcraft (Ed.), *Pediatric urology* (pp. 415–428). Philadelphia: W. B. Saunders.

England, M. A. (1990). *Color atlas of life before birth: Normal fetal development.* London: Wolfe Medical Publications.

Ephgrone, K., & Chang, J. (1983). Pediatric circumcision revisited. *Texas Medicine, 79*, 62–65.

Evans, J. H. C. (1994). Acute renal failure in children. *British Journal of Hospital Medicine, 52*(4), 159–161.

Farrer, J. H., Walker, A. H., & Rajfer, J. (1985). Management of the postpubertal cryptorchid testis: A statistical review. *Journal of Urology, 134*, 1071.

Ferguson, D. M., Hons, B. A., & Horwood, L. J. (1986). Factors related to the age of attainment of nocturnal bladder control: An 8 year longitudinal study. *Pediatrics, 78*, 884–890.

Fernandes, E. T., Reinberg, Y., Vernier, R., & Gonzalez, R. (1994). Neurogenic bladder dysfunction in children: Review of pathyphysiology and current management. *Journal of Pediatrics, 124*, 1–7.

Fitzwater, D., & Macknin, M. L. (1992). Risk/benefit ratio in enuresis therapy [Editorial]. *Clinical Pediatrics, 31*, 308–310.

Frauman, A. C., & Gilman, C. M. (1979). The urinary system. In M. E. Armstrong, E. J. Dickason, J. Howe, D. A. Jones, & M. J. Snider (Eds.), *McGraw-Hill handbook of clinical nursing* (pp. 436–462). New York: McGraw Hill.

Gallego, N., Gallego, A., Pascual, J., Liano, F., Estepa, R., & Ortuno, J. (1993). Prognosis of children with acute renal failure: A study of 138 cases. *Nephron, 64*, 399–404.

Garber, K. (1996). Enuresis: An update on diagnosis and management. *Journal of Pediatric Health Care, 10*(5), 202–208.

Gaudio, K. M., Devarajan, P., Boydstun, I. I., Van Why, S. K., & Siegel, N. J. (1994). Acute renal failure. In M. A. Holliday, T. M. Barratt, & E. D. Avner (Eds.), *Pediatric nephrology* (3rd ed., pp. 1176–1203). Baltimore: Williams & Wilkins.

Gearhart, J. P. (1992). Bladder and urachal abnormalities: The extrophy-espadias complex. In P. P. Kelalis, L. R. King, & A. B. Belman (Eds.), *Clinical pediatric urology* (3rd Ed., pp. 579–618). Philadelphia: W. B. Saunders.

Gearhart, J. P., & Jeffs, R. D. (1990). Management and treatment of classic bladder extrophy. In K. W. Ashcraft (Ed.), *Pediatric urology*, (pp. 269–300). Philadelphia: W. B. Saunders.

Geller, M. (1990). Multisystem failure in a child with HUS. *Critical Care Nurse, 10*(4), 56–64.

Gillen, J. C., Rapoport, J. C., Mikkelsen, E. J., Langer, D., Vonskiver, C., & Mendelson, W. (1982). EEG sleep patterns in enuresis: A further analysis and comparison with normal controls. Biological Psychology, 17, 947–953.

Gillenwater, J. Y., Grayhack, J. T., Howards, S. S., & Duckett, J. W. (Eds.) (1996). *Adult and pediatric urology* (2nd Ed.). St. Louis: Mosby–Year Book.

Gilman, C. M., & Frauman, A. C. (1997). The pediatric patient. In J. Parker (Ed.), *Contemporary nephrology nursing*. In press.

Gilman, C. M., Mooney, K. H., & Andrews, M. M. (1994). Alterations of renal and urinary tract function in children. In K. L. McCance & S. E. Huether (Eds.), *Pathophysiology: The biologic basis for disease in adults and children* (2nd ed., pp. 1265–1279). St. Louis: Mosby.

Gonzalez, R. (1996). Urologic disorders in infants and children. In R. Behrman, R. Kliegman, & A. Aruin (Eds.), *Nelson textbook of pediatrics* (pp. 1527–1553). Philadelphia: W. B. Saunders.

Gray, M. (1996). Atraumatic urethral catheterization of children. *Pediatric Nursing, 22*(4), 306–310.

Guignard, J-P., Semama, D., John, E., & Huet, F. (1993). Acute renal failure. *Critical Care Medicine, 21*(Suppl. 9), S349–351.

Hazebroek, R. W., & Molenaar, J. C. (1992). The management of the impalpable testis by surgery alone. *Journal of Urology, 148*, 629.

Hellerstein, S. (1994). Evolving concepts in the evaluation of the child with a urinary tract infection. *Journal of Pediatrics, 124*, 589–592.

Hendren, W. H. (1990). Posterior urethral valves. In K. W. Ashcraft (Ed.), *Pediatric urology* (pp. 313–335). Philadelphia: W. B. Saunders.

Hensle, T. W., & Ring, K. S. (1991). Urinary tract reconstruction in children. *Urologic Clinics of North America, 18*(4), 701–715.

Herzog, L. (1989). Urinary tract infections and circumcision: A case control study. *American Journal of Disease in Childhood*, 143, 348–352.

Hilton, S. V. W., & Kaplan, G. W. (1995). Imaging of common problems in pediatric urology. *Urologic Clinics of North America, 22*(1), 1–20.

Himsl, K. K., & Hurwitz, R. S. (1991). Pediatric urinary incontinence. *Urologic Clinics of North America, 18*(2), 283–293.

Hoberman, A. (1994). *Oral vs. intravenous therapy for acute pyelonephritis in children 1–24 months.* Poster presented at the meeting of the Ambulatory Pediatric Association, Seattle, WA.

Hoberman, A., Chao, H. P., Keller, D. M., Hickey, R., Davis, H. W., & Ellis, D. (1993). Prevalence of urinary tract infection in febrile infants. *Pediatrics, 123*, 17–23.

Hoyler-Grant, C. (1995a). Circumcision. In K. Karlowicz (Ed.), *Urologic nursing: Principles and practice* (pp. 499–502). Philadelphia: W. B. Saunders.

Hoyler-Grant, C. (1995b). Health assessment of the pediatric urology patient. In K. A. Karlowicz (Ed.), *Urologic nursing: Principles and practice* (pp. 439–463). Philadelphia: W. B. Saunders.

Hoyler-Grant, C. (1995c). Growing up with a urologic disorder: Developmental considerations. In K. A. Karlowicz (Ed.), *Urologic nursing: Principles and practice* (pp. 464–482). Philadelphia: W. B. Saunders.

Huff, D. S., Hadziselimovic, F., & Snyder, H. M. (1993). Histologic maldevelopment of unilaterally cryptorchid testes and their descended partners. *European Journal of Pediatrics, 152*, 510–513.

Hufnagle, K. G., Khan, S. N., Penn, D., Cacciarelli, A., & Williams, P. (1982). Renal calcification: A complication of long-term furosemide therapy in preterm infants. *Pediatrics, 70*, 360–363.

Institute of Medicine (1997 in press). *Dietary reference intake*. Washington, DC: National Academy Press.

Jacobson, H. R. (1991). Chronic renal failure: Pathophysiology. *The Lancet, 338*, 419–423.

Jarvelin, M. R. (1989). Developmental history and neurologic findings in enuretic children. *Developmental Medicine and Child Neurology*, 31, 728–736.

Jenkins, R. D., Harrison, H. L., Jackson, E. C., & Funk, J. E. (1991). Continuous renal replacement in infants and toddlers. *Contributions to Nephrology, 93*, 245–249.

Kaplan, G. W., & Scherz, H. C. (1992). Intravesical obstruction. In P. P. Kelalis, L. R. King, & A. B. Belman (Eds.), *Clinical pediatric urology* (3rd ed., pp. 821–864). Philadelphia: W. B. Saunders.

Karlowicz, K. A., & Meredith, C. E. (1995). Adult voiding dysfunction. In K. A. Karlowicz (Ed.), *Urologic nursing: Principles and practice* (pp. 377–407). Philadelphia: W. B. Saunders.

Kass, E. J., Chandra, R. S., & Belman, A. B. (1987). Testicular histology in the adolescent with a variocele. *Pediatrics, 79*(6), 996–998.

Kass, E. J., Freitas, J. E., Salisz, J. A., & Steinert, B. W. (1993). Pituitary gonadal dysfunction in adolescents with varicocele. *Urology, 42*(2), 179–182.

Kass, E. J., & Reitelman, C. (1995). Adolescent varicocele. *Urologic Clinics of North America, 22*(1), 151–159.

Kelleher, R. (1997). Daytime and nighttime wetting in children: A review of management. *Journal of the Society of Pediatric Nurses, 2*(2), 73–82.

Kellen, M., Aronson, S., Roizen, M. F., Barnard, J., & Thisted, R. A. (1994). Predictive and diagnostic tests of renal failure: A review. *Anesthesia and Analgesia, 78*, 134–142.

Kelly, M. (1997). Acute renal failure. *American Journal of Nursing, 97*(3), 32–33.

Kelsch, R. C., & Sedman, A. B. (1993). Nephrotic syndrome. *Pediatrics in Review, 14*(1), 30–38.

Khan, A., Schaeffer, H., & Evans, H. (1996). Urinary tract infection in boys. *Journal of the National Medical Association, 88*(1), 25–26.

Kher, K. K. (1992a). Chronic renal failure. In K. K. Kher & S. P. Makker (Eds.), *Clinical pediatric nephrology* (pp. 501–541). New York: McGraw-Hill.

Kher, K. K. (1992b). Cystic renal diseases. In K. K. Kher & S. P. Makker (Eds.), *Clinical pediatric nephrology* (pp. 421–446). New York: McGraw-Hill.

Kher, K. K. (1992c). Nephrotic syndrome. In K. K. Kher & S. P. Makker (Eds.), *Clinical pediatric nephrology* (pp. 137–174). New York: McGraw-Hill.

Kimura, D. Y. (1995). Urinary tract infections in children. In K. Karlowicz, (Ed.), *Urologic nursing: Principles and practice* (pp. 483–497). Philadelphia: W. B. Saunders.

King, L. R. (1995). Hydronephrosis: When is obstruction not obstruction? *Urologic Clinics of North America, 22*(1), 31–42.

Kirkpatrick, J., Alexander, J., & Cain, R. (1997). Recovering urine from diapers: Are test results accurate? *MCN, 22*, 96–102.

Kjellstrand, C. M., Shideman, J. R., Santiago, E. A., Mauer, S. M., Simmons, R. L., & Buselmeier, T. J. (1971). Technical advances in hemodialysis of very small pediatric patients. *Proceedings of the Dialysis and Transplant Forum*, 124–132.

Kramer, S. A. (1992). Vesicoureteral reflux. In P. P. Kelalis, L. R. King, & A. B. Belman (Eds.), *Clinical pediatric urology* (3rd ed., pp. 441–499). Philadelphia: W. B. Saunders.

Kroovand, R. L., Harrison, L. H., & McCullough, D. L. (1987). Extracorporeal shock wave lithotripsy in childhood. *Journal of Urology, 138*(4 Pt 2), 1106–1108.

Lancaster, L. E. (1995). Renal anatomy and physiology. In L. E. Lancaster (Ed.). *ANNA Core Curriculum for Nephrology Nursing* (3rd ed., pp. 1–32). Pitman, NJ: American Nephrology Nurses' Association.

Lawrence, C. A. (1995). Pediatric voiding disorder. In K. Karlowicz (Ed.), *Urologic nursing principles* (pp. 593–619). Philadelphia: W. B. Saunders.

Lawrence, J., Alcock. D., McGrath, P., Kay, J., MacMurray, S. B., & Dulberg, C. (1993). Development of a tool to assess neonatal pain. *Neonatal Network, 12*(6), 59–66.

Leaky, A. L., Ryan, P. C., McEndfee, G. M., Nelson, A. C., & Fitzpatrick, J. M. (1989). Renal injury and recovery in partial ureteric obstruction. *Journal of Urology, 142*, 199–203.

Leape, L. L. (1990). Testicular torsion. In K. W. Ashcraft (Ed.), *Pediatric urology* (pp. 429–436). Philadelphia: W. B. Saunders.

Lenz, S., Giwereman, A., & Skakkebaek, N. E. (1987). Ultrasound in detection of early neoplasia of the testis. *International Journal of Andrology, 10*, 187.

Levin, R. K., & Hensle, T. W. (1990). Pediatric urolithiasis. In K. W. Ashcraft (Ed.), *Pediatric urology* (pp. 461–487). Philadelphia: W. B. Saunders.

Liptak, G. S., Campbell, J., Stewart, R., & Hulbert, W. C., Jr. (1993). Screening for urinary tract infection in children with neurogenic bladders. *American Journal of Physical Medicine and Rehabilitation, 72*, 122–126.

MacDonald, H. (1995). Chronic renal disease: The mother's experience. *Pediatric Nursing, 21*(6), 503–507, 574.

Makker, S. P. (1992a). Glomerular diseases. In K. K. Kher & S. P. Makker (Eds.). *Clinical pediatric nephrology* (pp. 175–276). New York: McGraw-Hill.

Makker, S. P. (1992b). Proteinuria. In K. K. Kher & S. P. Makker (Eds.). *Clinical pediatric nephrology* (pp. 117–136). New York: McGraw-Hill.

Mann, C. M. (1990). Ureteropelvic junction obstruction. In K. W. Ashcraft (Ed.), *Pediatric urology* (pp. 117–124). Philadelphia: W. B. Saunders.

Marra, G., Barbieri, G., Dell'Agnola, C. A., Caccumo, M. L., Castellani, M. R., & Assael, B. M. (1994). Congenital renal damage associated with primary vesicoureteral reflux detected prenatally in male infants. *Journal of Pediatrics, 124*, 726–730.

McAleer, I. M., & Kaplan, G. W. (1995). Pediatric genitourinary trauma. *Urologic Clinics of North America, 22*(1), 177–188.

McAleer, I. M., Kaplan, G. W., & Scherz, H. C. (1993). Genitourinary trauma in the pediatric patient. *Urology, 42*, 563–568.

McCullough, D. L. (1992). Extracorporeal shock wave lithotripsy. In P. C. Walsh, A. B. Retik, T. A. Stamey, E. D. Vaughan (Eds.), *Campbell's urology* (6th ed., pp. 2157–2180). Philadelphia: W. B. Saunders.

Meza, M. P., Amundson, G. M., Aquilina, J. W., & Reitelman, C. (1992). Color flow imaging in children with clinically suspected testicular torsion. *Pediatric Radiology, 22*, 360–373.

Miller, K. (1996). Urinary tract infections: Children are not little adults. *Pediatric Nursing, 22*(6), 473–480, 544.

Moffatt, M. E. K., Harlo, S., Kirshen, A. J., & Burd, L. (1993). Desmopressin acetate and nocturnal enuresis: How much do we know? *Pediatrics, 92*, 420–425.

Moffatt, M. E. K., Kato, C., & Pless, I. B. (1987). Self concept after treatment for nocturnal enuresis. *Journal of Pediatrics, 110*(4), 647–652.

Monfort, G. J. (1990). Management of patients with urinary tract infections. In K. W. Ashcraft (Ed.), *Pediatric urology* (pp. 35–47). Philadelphia: W. B. Saunders.

Montagnino, B., Welsh, V. W., Hoyler-Grant, C. (1995). Congenital anomalies that affect the kidney, ureter and bladder. In K. A. Karlowicz (Ed.), *Urologic nursing: Principles and practice* (pp. 526–565). Philadelphia: W. B. Saunders.

Moore, R. G., Peters, C. A., & Bauer, S. A. (1994). Laparoscopic evaluation of the non-palpable testis: A prospective assessment of accuracy. *Journal of Urology, 151*, 728.

Murphy, J. P. (1990). Genitourinary trauma. In K. W. Ashcraft (Ed.), *Pediatric urology* (pp. 437–445). Philadelphia: W. B. Saunders.

Neumann, M., & Urizar, R. (1994). Hemolytic uremic syndrome: Current pathophysiology and management. *ANNA Journal, 21*(2), 137–143.

Newman, D. M., Coury, T., Lingeman, J. E., Mertz, J. H. O., Mosbargh, P. G., Steele, R. E., Knapp, P. M. (1986). Extracorporeal shock wave lithotripsy experience in children. *Journal of Urology, 136*, 238–240.

Niku, S. D., Stock, J. A., & Kaplan, G. W. (1995). Neonatal circumcision. *Urologic Clinics of North America, 22*(1), 57–65.

Nimkin, K., Lebowitz, R. L., Share, J. C., & Teele, R. L. (1992). Urolithiasis in a children's hospital: 1985–1990. *Urologic Radiology, 14*, 139–143.

Noe, H. N., Wyatt, R. J., Peeden, J. N., Jr., & Rivas, M. L. (1992). Transmission of vesicoureteral reflux from parent to child. *Journal of Urology, 148*, 1869–1871.

Norgaard, J. P. (1992). A pathogenesis-based approach to enuresis. *Dialogues in Pediatric Urology, 15*, 5–6.

Norgaard, J. P., Hansen, J. M., & Neilsen, J. B. (1985). Simultaneous registration of sleep stages and bladder activity in enuresis. *Urology*, 26, 316.

Norgaard, J. P., Pedersen, E. B., & Djurhuus, J. C. (1985). Diurinal antidiuretic hormone levels in enuretics. *Journal of Urology, 134*, 1029–1031.

Peeden, N. J., & Noe, H. N. (1992). Is it practical to screen for familial vesicoureteral reflux within a private pediatric practice? *Pediatrics, 89*, 758–760.

Perlmutter, A. D. (1985). Enuresis. In P. P. Kalalis, L. R. King, & A. B. Belman (Eds.), *Clinical pediatric urology* (2nd ed., pp. 311–325). Philadelphia: W. B. Saunders.

Pisacane, J. (1992). Breastfeeding and urinary tract infections. *Journal of Pediatrics, 120*(1), 87–89.

Potter, E. L. (1946). Bilateral renal agenesis. *Journal of Pediatrics, 29* 68–76.

Rabinowitz, R., & Hulbert, W. C., Jr. (1995). Acute scrotal swelling. *Urologic Clinics of North America, 22*(1), 101–106.

Reilly, N. J. (1995). Cancer of the bladder. In K. A. Karlowicz (Ed.), *Urologic nursing: Principles and practice* (pp. 243–270). Philadelphia: W. B. Saunders.

Reynolds, E., & Hoberman, A. (1995). Diagnosis and management of pyelonephritis in infants. *Maternal-Child Nursing Journal, 20*(2), 78–84.

Reznik, V. M., & Budorick, N. E. (1995). Prenatal detection of congenital renal disease. *Urologic Clinics of North America, 22*(1), 21–30.

Ribby, K., & Cox, K. (1997). Organization and development of a pediatric end state renal disease teaching protocol for peritoneal dialysis. *Pediatric Nursing, 23*(4), 393–399.

Riley, K. (1997). Evaluation and management of primary nocturnal enuresis. *Journal of the American Academy of Nurse Practitioners, 9*(1), 33–39.

Ring, K. S., & Hensle, T. W. (1992). Urinary diversion. In P. P. Kelalis, L. R. King, & A. B. Belman (Eds.), *Clinical pediatric urology* (3rd ed., pp. 865–903). Philadelphia: W. B. Saunders.

Rozanski, T. A., & Bloom, D. A. (1995). The undescended testis: Theory and management. *Urologic Clinics of North America, 22*(1), 107–118.

Rushton, H. G. (1992). Genitourinary infections: Non-specific infections. In P. P. Kelalis, L. R. King, & A. B. Belman (Eds.), *Clinical pediatric urology* (3rd ed., pp. 286–331). Philadelphia: W. B. Saunders.

Rushton, H. G. (1995). Wetting and functional voiding disorders. *Urologic Clinics of North America, 22*(1), 75–91.

Schiff, D. (1989). *AAP member alert.* Elk Grove Village, IL: American Academy of Pediatrics.

Schmitt, B. D. (1990). Efficacy and safety of drugs available for treatment of nocturnal enuresis. *Drug Investigations, 2(Suppl. 5), 9–16.*

Schneider, M. S., King, L. R., & Surwit, R. S. (1994). Kegel exercises and childhood incontinence: A new role for an old treatment. *Journal of Pediatrics, 124*, 91–92.

Sellinger, V. (1997). Urinary dilemmas in pediatrics. *Advances for Nurse Practitioners, 5*(4), 34–40.

Shortliffe, L. (1995). Management of urinary tract infection in children without urinary tract abnormalities. *Urologic Clinics of North America, 22*(1), 67–73.

Skoog, S. J. (1992). Prune-belly syndrome. In P. P. Kelalis, L. R. King, & A. B. Belman (Eds.), *Clinical pediatric urology* (3rd ed., pp. 943–976). Philadelphia: W. B. Saunders.

Skoog, S. J., & Belman, A. B. (1991). Primary vesicoureteral reflux in the black child. *Pediatrics, 87*, 538–543.

Skoog, S. J., & Conlin, M. J. (1995). Pediatric hernias and hydroceles: The urologist's perspective. *Urologic Clinics of North America, 22*(1), 119–130.

Smith, L. H., & Segura, J. W. (1992). Urolithiasis. In P. P. Kelalis, L. R. King, & A. B. Belman (Eds.), *Clinical pediatric urology* (3rd. ed., pp. 1327–1352). Philadelphia: W. B. Saunders.

Smith, M. F. (1990). Renal trauma—Adult and pediatric considerations. *Critical Care Nursing Clinics of North America, 2*(1), 67–77.

Sorenson, K., Lose, G., & Nathen, E. (1988). Urinary tract infections and diurinal enuresis in girls. *European Journal of Pediatrics, 148*, 146–147.

Stock, J. A., Packer, M. G., & Kaplan, G. W. (1995). Pediatric urology facts and figures. *Urologic Clinics of North America, 22*(1), 205–219.

Stock, J. A., Scherz, H. C., & Kaplan, G. W. (1995). Distal hypospadias. *Urologic Clinics of North America, 22*(1), 205–219.

Sugar, E., & Hoyler-Grant, C. (1995). Disorders of the external genitalia in children. In K. A. Karlowica (Ed.), *Urologic nursing: Principles and practice* (pp. 498–525). Philadelphia: W. B. Saunders.

Taylor, G. A., Eichelberger, M. R., & Potter, B. M. (1988). Hematuria: A marker of abdominal injury in children after blunt trauma. *Annals of Surgery, 208*, 688–693.

Taylor, J. (1996). End stage renal disease in children: Diagnosis, management and interventions. *Pediatric Nursing, 22*(6), 481–490.

Thompson, H. C., King, L. R., & Knox, E. (1975). Report of the *ad hoc* task force on circumcision. *Pediatrics, 55*, 610–611.

Walther, P. C., Lamm, D., & Kaplan, G. W. (1980). Pediatric lithiasis: A 10 year review. *Pediatrics, 65*, 1068.

Watkins, S. L., & Avner, E. D. (1994). Renal dysplasia and cystic disease. In M. A. Holliday, T. M. Barratt, & E. D. Avner (Eds.), *Pediatric nephrology* (3rd ed., pp. 467–490). Baltimore: Williams & Wilkins.

Willert, D. D. (1995). Nocturnal enuresis: How nurses can help. *Nursing Spectrum*, 4(22), 12–13.

Wilton, N. C. T. (1995). Postoperative pain management for pediatric urologic surgery. *Urologic Clinics of North America, 22*(1), 189–204.

Wiswell, T. E., & Gischke, D. W. (1989). Risks from circumcision during the first month of life compared with those for uncircumcised boys. *Pediatrics, 83*, 1011–1015.

Wiswell, T. E., & Hachey, W. W. (1993). Urinary tract infections and the uncircumcised state: An update. *Clinical Pediatrics, 32*, 130–134.

Wiswell, T. E., Tencer, M. L., Welch, C. A., & Chamberlain, J. L. (1993). Circumcision on children beyond the neonatal period. *Pediatrics, 92*, 791–793.

Yalla, S. Y., & Fam, B. A. (1991). Spinal cord injury. In R. J. Krane & M. B. Sikorsky (Eds.), *Clinical neurourology* (pp. 319–331). Boston: Little, Brown Co.

Bibliography

Ashcraft, K. W. (Ed.). (1990). *Pediatric urology*. Philadelphia: W. B. Saunders.

Brown, W. W., & Wolfson, M. (1993). Diet as culprit or therapy. *Medical Clinics of North America, 77*(4), 783–794.

Cianflocco, A. J. (1992). Renal complications of exercise. *Clinics in Sports Medicine, 11*(2), 437–451.

Cohen, B., Kagan, L., Richter, B., Topor, M., & Saveedra M. (1991). Children's compliance to dialysis. *Pediatric Nursing, 17*(4), 359–365, 420.

Curry, N. (1995). Renal imaging and congenital lesions. In D. Sutton & J. Young (Eds.), *A concise textbook of clinical imaging* (pp. 621–636). St. Louis: Mosby–Year Book.

Grimm, P. C., & Ogborn, M. R. (1994). Hemolytic uremic syndrome: The most common cause of acute renal failure in childhood. *Pediatric Annals, 23*(9), 505–511.

Harrington, J. D., & Brener, E. R. (1973). *Patient care in renal failure*. Philadelphia: W. B. Saunders.

Health Care Financing Administration. (1993). End-stage renal disease medical evidence report—Medicare entitlement and/or patient registration (Form HCFA-2728-U4). Washington, DC: U.S. Government Printing Office.

Hendrix, W. (1992). Dialysis therapies in critically ill children. *AACN Clinical Issues, 3*(3), 605–613.

Jantausch, B. A., Criss, V. R., O'Donnell, R. O., Wiedermann, B. L., Maja, A. M., Rushton, H. G., Shireij, R. S., & Luban, N. L. (1994). Association of Lewis blood group phenotypes with urinary tract infection in children. *Journal of Pediatrics, 124*, 863–868.

Kalowicz, M. G., & Adelman, R. D. (1992). Acute renal failure in the neonate. *Clinics in Perinatology, 19*(1), 139–158.

Reinburg, Y., Fleming, T., & Gonzalez, R. (1994). Renal rupture after the crede maneuver. *Journal of Pediatrics, 124*(2), 279–280.

Sommers, M. S. (1990). Blunt renal trauma. *Critical Care Nurse, 10*(3), 38–48.

VanGool, J. D., Vejverberg, M. A. W., & Messer, A. P. (1992). Functional daytime incontinence: Non-pharmacologic treatment. *Scandinavian Journal of Urology and Nephrology, 141*, 93–103.

Warody, B. A., Alon, U., & Hellerstein, S. (1991). Primary nocturnal enuresis: Current concepts to an old problem. *Paediatric Annals, 20*, 246–255.

HEALTH CHALLENGE:

Alterations in Musculoskeletal Status

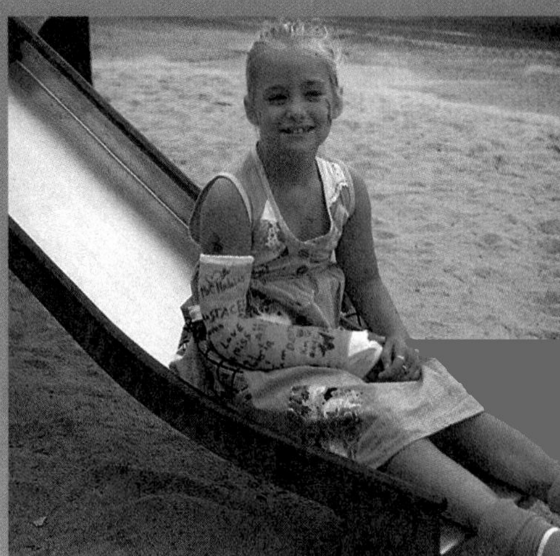

OUTLINE

Assessment of the Child with an Alteration in Musculoskeletal Status
- Focused Health History
- Focused Physical Assessment
- Nursing Diagnoses and Outcomes
- Developmental and Biological Variances

Diagnostic Criteria for Evaluating Alterations in Musculoskeletal Status

Treatment Modalities
- Heat and Cold Applications
- Braces and Splints
- Serial Manipulation
- Casts
- Traction
- External Fixation
- Surgical Interventions
- Continuous Passive Motion
- Ambulatory Devices
- Prosthetic Devices
- Complications of Immobilization
- Nutrition
- Pain Management

Alterations in Musculoskeletal Status
- Congenital and Hereditary Disorders
  - Metatarsus Adductus
  - Clubfoot
  - Developmental Dysplasia of the Hip
  - Congenital Limb Defects
  - Osteogenesis Imperfecta
  - Cerebral Palsy
  - Muscular Dystrophy
- Growth-Related Disorders
  - Torsional Deformity: Femoral Anteversion
  - Torsional Deformity: Tibial Torsion
  - Legg-Calvé-Perthes Disease
  - Slipped Capital Femoral Epiphysis
  - Osteochondritis Dissecans
  - Osgood-Schlatter Disease
  - Scoliosis
  - Kyphosis and Lordosis
- Inflammatory and Infectious Disorders
  - Osteomyelitis
  - Septic Arthritis
  - Juvenile Arthritis
  - Systemic Lupus Erythematosus
- Traumatic Injuries: Fractures and Skeletal Trauma
- Sports Injuries
  - Overuse Injuries
  - Sprains and Strains
  - Dislocations

OBJECTIVES

- Recognize clinical signs and symptoms that would indicate a musculoskeletal disorder.
- Explain nursing care interventions to prevent skin breakdown and promote healing in the child receiving treatment for a musculoskeletal disorder or injury.
- Explain nursing care interventions for the child hospitalized with a musculoskeletal disorder.
- Provide family education regarding home care, activity, and dietary modifications for the child with a musculoskeletal disorder.
- Describe measures to protect children from musculoskeletal injury.
- State the interdisciplinary interventions that are commonly applied to each musculoskeletal disorder.

KEY TERMS

ankylosis
apophysis
arthrotomy
articular cartilage
dislocation
epiphysis
iridocyclitis
osteotomy
physis
quadriplegia
sprain
strain
subluxation
synovitis
tenotomy
varus

CHAPTER

20

The musculoskeletal system provides the framework for the human body. The symmetry of muscle and bone propelling a body through space is apparent in elite athletes. Not as visible to the naked eye is the force it takes for a child to walk across a room for the first time. Bone is resilient and, particularly in children, has a remarkable ability to remodel itself. Just as children should not be treated as "little adults," children's bones cannot be treated like "little adult bones."

This chapter focuses on various congenital and hereditary disorders that cause an alteration in this balance. Trauma, infection, sports injuries, and growth-related disorders specific to pediatrics are also explored.

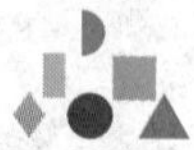

Assessment of the Child with an Alteration in Musculoskeletal Status

Focused Health History

Assessment of the musculoskeletal system begins with a history of the child's past health concerns from the prenatal period to the present (Chart 20–1). Certain orthopedic problems are congenital (e.g., polydactyly and limb deformities), developing in utero as the fetus matures. Orthopedic injuries (e.g., a brachial plexus injury or a fractured clavicle) may develop during the birthing process. Other orthopedic disorders may be noted only as the child grows physically during the early childhood years or may be acquired as a complication of another primary illness such as polio, tetanus, or an infection in a bone.

Developmental milestones that the child has reached are important to note (see Chapter 5). Missed milestones may be the first clue that a child has a musculoskeletal disorder such as cerebral palsy (CP), or some other degenerative disease. Family history should be explored for any hereditary disorders. For instance, a family history of genetic bone disease is significant for a child with a history of repeated fractures.

A thorough history of the present problem is obtained. This includes onset and duration of symptoms, extent of the disability, and the home remedies or medical treatments that have already been used.

Alert: *Children who have had repeated exposures to latex during hospitalizations and surgery are at higher risk for latex allergies. The possibility of a latex allergy should be investigated in all children with a suspected musculoskeletal disorder, especially those who have had surgical procedures.*

Focused Physical Assessment

Physical assessment of the musculoskeletal system includes the techniques of inspection and palpation to evaluate how the child looks and functions (Chart 20–2). The assessment is best accomplished with the child unclothed except for undergarments to allow the best visualization of all aspects of the musculoskeletal system. During inspection, symmetry of size between limbs and configuration, as well as ability to move, should be noted. Unequal growth, paralysis, or spasticity in a limb may be subtle. Important observations include absence of parts, duplication of parts, or abnormal swelling. Range of motion of all joints, either passively or actively, should be assessed. Gait analysis is done by asking the child to walk down a hall or to follow a parent who is walking and noting any limp, tiptoeing, or foot drop (Chart 20–3).

Palpation is done to detect any areas of tenderness or inflammation and to evaluate muscle strength. The examination begins at the most distal joints (e.g., begin with the toes and work up to the hip joint or begin with the fingers and work up to the shoulders). The size of any bony or soft tissue masses is estimated.

caREminder: *If injury has occurred, examine that area last and be gentle when palpating the injury site.*

The spine is palpated and observed for any dimples or hairy patches, which may be indicative of spina bifida. Also, the general contour of the spine, as well as hip or shoulder asymmetry, is noted. Alignment is altered in children with kyphosis, lordosis, or scoliosis. Neurovascular status of each extremity is assessed for sensation, motion, capillary refill, and temperature (Chart 20–4). The affected extremity should be compared with the unaffected extremity in terms of neurovascular status and strength (Table 20–1).

The child's muscle strength is assessed whenever a muscular weakness is suspected. The nurse does this by asking the child to bend his or her arm and push and pull against the nurse's hand; then, using his or her foot, the child pushes down and pulls up against the nurse's hand. Superficial and deep tendon reflexes are tested in each extremity. The child is observed as he or she stands up from a sitting or lying position. The child should be referred to a neurologist for a complete diagnostic evaluation if abnormal reflexes or muscle weakness is apparent.

Nursing Diagnoses and Outcomes

The child with a musculoskeletal disorder or injury faces challenges in mobility and movement. Such challenges may require long-term adaptation by the child and family to change the environment, their daily living activities, and their developmental expectations to complement the child's abilities. When temporary injury has occurred, al-

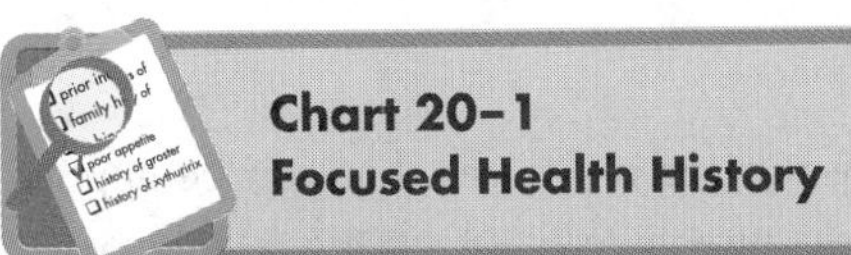

Chart 20–1
Focused Health History

Musculoskeletal System

Identifying Data

Age, gender, and ethnic background

Present Illness

When did the pain start? Does anything make it better or worse? Does it wake up the child at night? Is there any noticeable deformity? Is there any stiffness or swelling of the joint or extremity? Does the child limp? Obtain a detailed history of the accident, if one occurred, including the speed of the car or bicycle. Report any snapping sensation felt or heard by the child before or after the fall.

Past Medical History

Birth History	Maternal exposure to teratogens, infections, medications, or illegal drugs or alcohol Type of delivery (vaginal or cesarean) and complications Positioning of the child in utero, presentation (e.g., cephalic, breech) Neonatal history (e.g., Apgar scores, periods of anoxia)
Previous Health Challenges	Any chronic conditions or congenital anomalies History of surgery, hospitalizations, fractures, or bone and joint infections
Childhood Illnesses	Polio Tuberculosis Conditions that can affect the spine
Immunizations	Status of current immunizations, especially polio and Hib Date of last tetanus shot
Allergies	Medications Latex, especially in myelomeningocele children or children with indwelling shunts
Current Medications	Note medications that may affect bone density, wound healing, or bleeding time. Is the child taking medications for calcium deficiency or rickets?
Nutritional Assessment	Recent weight change or decreased appetite. Does the child take vitamin supplements? Does the child eat foods containing calcium?
Family Medical History	History of developmental dislocated hip, clubfoot, or other skeletal or neurologic disorders in the family
Environmental History	Safety issues: Has there been any exposure to unsafe physical or structural settings? Do the parents own a child's car seat, and do they use it consistently and properly? Does the child wear a helmet when bicycling? Does the child use wrist supports, knee pads, and elbow pads when skateboarding or roller blading?
Social History	Psychosocial—Does the child have many friends? Is the child a risk taker? History of thrill-seeking behavior? Is the child hyperactive, or does he or she have attention deficit disorder? Cultural—What cultural practices may influence musculoskeletal development? (e.g., binding of feet or use of papoose board)
Growth and Development	Physical milestones—When did the child first crawl, walk, run? Developmental milestones—What grade is the child in? Is the child participating in activities that are age appropriate? Habits—What does the child do when not in school? What kinds of games does the child like to play? What time does the child go to sleep and wake up? What sports activities is the child involved with? How many hours a week does the child practice or compete in sports? Are there any previously achieved developmental milestones that the child is no longer able to accomplish?

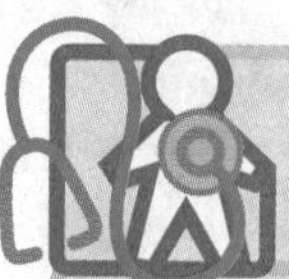

Chart 20–2
Focused Physical Assessment

Musculoskeletal System

Inspection

Observe child undressed except for diapers or underclothes
- Posture
- Truncal alignment
- Symmetry of the extremities
- Absence or duplication of any part
- Abnormal swelling
- Cutaneous lesions
- Café au lait spots indicative of neurofibromatosis
- Maculopapular rash indicative of juvenile arthritis
- Hairy patches on the spinal area

Gait
- Normal gait per developmental age
- Limping
- Torsional variations (in-toeing and out-toeing)
- Toe walking
- Footdrop

Spinal alignment
- Scoliosis screening

Sensory assessment

Palpation

Range of motion of joints
- Symmetry
- Presence of limited or hyperextended range of motion

Muscle strength testing
Evaluation of deep tendon reflexes
- Presence of reflexes after age at which they should have been extinguished (e.g., Babinski and tonic neck)

Spinal alignment
Joint or area of extremity or trunk that is of concern
- Tenderness
- Muscle spasm
- Masses
- Soft tissue swelling
- Increased warmth
- Synovial thickening

terations in the child's lifestyle usually only require short-term lifestyle modifications. However, the active young child or the adolescent concerned with body image issues may have difficulty meeting the demands of the treatment regimen. The nursing diagnoses that can be applied to the child with a musculoskeletal disorder address the impaired or altered mobility and movement that the child may experience. In addition, concerns regarding body image and achieving optimal levels of growth and development are likely to emerge during assessment. The nursing diagnoses and the interdisciplinary plan of care should reflect these concerns. Most musculoskeletal disorders or injuries are managed in the home. Nursing diagnoses may need to be formulated to address the teaching, family support, and resources that will be required to manage the child's illness at home, in school, and as the child participates in community activities (Chart 20–5).

Developmental and Biological Variances

Many anatomic and physiologic differences exist in the musculoskeletal systems of children, both throughout the

Chart 20–3

Differential Diagnosis of a Limp in Children

Toddlers (1–3 years)

Infection
Developmental dysplasia of the hip
Mild cerebral palsy
Toddler's fracture of the tibia
Neuromuscular disease (cerebral palsy)
Diskitis

Childhood (4–10 years)

Infection
Legg-Calvé-Perthes disease
Osteomyelitis
Synovitis of the hip
Septic hip or knee
Developmental dysplasia of the hip
Neuromuscular disease (cerebral palsy)
Leg length discrepancy
Rheumatic disorder (juvenile arthritis)
Trauma

Adolescence (11–16 years)

Slipped capital femoral epiphysis
Hip dysplasia
Tumor
Tarsal coalition
Rheumatologic disorder (juvenile arthritis)
Trauma

Sources: Thompson & Scoles, 1996; Wenger & Rang, 1993.

Chart 20-4
Nursing Interventions

Neurovascular Assessment

Assessing circulation to an extremity is done frequently for the first 24 hours after a cast has been applied, after surgery has been performed on an extremity, or when nerve injury is suspected. After that time, assessment every 4 to 8 hours is sufficient if there is no neurovascular compromise. The categories for assessment include the following:

- *Pain*—Is the child complaining of pain in the extremity? Pain is common at the injury site. If the pain is not relieved by narcotics, or pain becomes worse when the fingers or toes are flexed, the child may have compartment syndrome and the physician should be notified immediately.
- *Sensation*—Can the child feel touch on the extremity? Two-point discrimination is decreased when there is neurovascular compromise.
- *Motion*—Ask the child to move his or her fingers or toes. Lack of movement may signal nerve damage.
- *Temperature*—Does the extremity feel warm or cool? A cool extremity may become warm if a blanket is placed over it and the extremity is elevated. If these actions do not warm the extremity, there is poor circulation.
- *Capillary refill*—Apply brief pressure to the nail beds and note how quickly pinkness returns. Sluggish capillary refill signals poor circulation.
- *Color*—Note the color of the extremity and compare the color of the injured extremity with the other one.
- *Pulses*—Check pulses distal to the injury or cast. This may not be possible if the cast covers the foot or hand. If the pulse is difficult to locate, check it with a Doppler machine and mark it with an "X."

various stages of childhood and in comparison to adults. The variances affect both the types of musculoskeletal illnesses seen in children and the treatment modalities used (Fig. 20–1). Anatomically, much of an infant and young child's skeleton consists of preosseous cartilage and physes. The child's bones are more flexible, have a higher porosity, and have a lower mineral count. The osteogenic periosteum is thick and strong, producing callus more rapidly and in greater amounts than in adults (McCullough, 1989; Thompson & Scoles, 1996). Because of these structural differences, a child's bone absorbs more energy before breaking, and may even bow rather than fracture when trauma occurs. When fractures do occur, the thick periosteum is likely to remain intact. Fractures in children younger than age 1 are unusual because of the large amount of force necessary to produce a break.

Alert: *A child younger than age 1 who presents with a fracture should be evaluated for possible physical abuse or an underlying musculoskeletal disorder that would cause spontaneous bone injury.*

The young bone can bend to a 45-degree angle and straighten out when the bending force is removed. This accounts, in part, for the high incidence of greenstick fractures seen in young children. As the child matures, the type of fracture reflects the porosity and strength of the affected bone (Mason, 1989).

Young children have an active growth area at each end of the long bones (humerus, radius-ulna, femur, and tibia-fibula) known as physeal or epiphyseal plates. Longitudinal growth of the long bones takes place through a process known as endochondral ossification. The epiphyses at the ends of each bone are cartilaginous in infants and become more ossified with time.

caREminder: *The calcium deposits in bones make them appear white in radiographs. Cartilage, unlike many soft tissues, is not visualized on radiograph. Thus, fractures may be difficult to detect in young children because of the cartilaginous nature of their skeletal systems.*

Table 20-1
Normal Versus Abnormal Findings of the Neurovascular Assessment

	Pulses	Color	Sensation	Motion	Temperature
Normal findings					
	+2—Strong	Pink	Pinpoint discrimination	Able to move extremity	Warm
Abnormal findings					
Compartment syndrome	0—Absent +1—Weak	Pale Dusky Flushed	Numbness Tingling	Unable to move extremity	Cool

These findings may differ for children who are paralyzed or who have spina bifida.

Chart 20–5
Nursing Diagnoses and Outcomes

Alterations in Musculoskeletal Status

Knowledge deficit regarding the child's illness, disorder, or injury

Outcome: Child and family will describe the illness, identifying the child's specific manifestations and the planned treatment regimen.

Potential for altered peripheral tissue perfusion related to the effects of the musculoskeletal disorder

Outcome: Tissue damage due to decreased circulation will be prevented by frequent monitoring of neurovascular status.

Skin integrity impairment related to surgical incision, wounds, or application of treatment devices such as casts, braces, and external fixators

Outcomes: Child exhibits no signs of skin breakdown.
Child regains skin integrity.
Child or family demonstrates skill in care of wound, incision, or treatment devices to enhance skin integrity.

High risk for infection related to wound, invasive appliances, or decreased mobility

Outcomes: Child will be free from infection.
Child's vital signs, temperature, and laboratory values remain within normal limits.
Incisions, wounds, or other breaks in the skin remain free from signs and symptoms of infection.

Potential for impaired physical mobility related to the effects of disease, traction, deformity, or brace

Outcomes: Child will maintain muscle strength, endurance, and joint flexibility of unaffected extremities.
Child will be as mobile as possible, using assistive devices if needed.

Constipation related to decreased activity level and impairments in neuromuscular status

Outcomes: Child's elimination pattern is within normal limits.
Child increases fluid and fiber intake.
Child reports easy and complete elimination of stool.

The process of converting cartilage to bone continues until skeletal maturity is completed during adolescence. At that time, increasing levels of androgenic hormones produced during puberty cause the growth plates to gradually stop functioning.

Bones without epiphyseal plates grow by appositional bone growth from their surrounding perichondrium and periosteum. This includes such bones as the pelvis, scapulae, and carpal and tarsal bones. Other bones in the hands, feet, and spine grow by a combination of appositional and endochondral growth. Alterations in the growth of a child's bones can occur as a result of trauma, nutritional deficits, metabolic disorders, and soft tissue disorders (Thompson & Scoles, 1996).

The ephyseal plate is an area of vulnerability and structural weakness in the bone. The physes are not as strong as metaphyseal or diaphyseal bone (mature calcified bone). Ligaments frequently insert into the epiphyses. Thus, traumatic forces that are applied to an extremity may be transferred to the physes, causing injury. Trauma to the growth plate can result in complete or partial closure. Consequently, angular deformities or shortening of the bone can occur, depending on the physes involved and the amount of remaining growth (Thompson & Scoles, 1996).

When a child injures a bone, healing follows the same processes as in adults. In a child, however, the thick periosteum has an abundant blood and nutrient supply. The metabolically active periosteum, combined with the child's growth potential, creates a more rapid

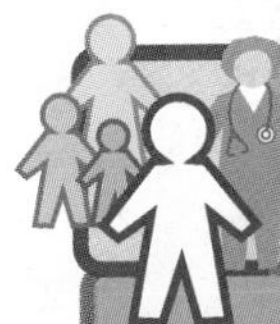

Chart 20–5
Nursing Diagnoses and Outcomes *Continued*

Alterations in Musculoskeletal Status

Chronic pain related to effects of the disease process or treatment regimen

Outcome: Child will be free from discomfort or will have a decrease in pain symptoms as evidenced by verbalization of pain relief and no behavioral pain indicators.

Potential for altered growth and development secondary to effects of an alteration in musculoskeletal status

Outcomes: Child will have prompt treatment to decrease potential alteration in physical growth.
Measures are instituted to optimize child's growth and development.
Family members demonstrate understanding of child's special needs.

Potential for body image disturbance related to physical manifestations and limitations of the child's illness

Outcomes: Child will develop a positive body image.
Child will discuss concerns related to body image.

Diversional activity deficit related to immobility, hospitalization, or separation from friends and family

Outcomes: Child will perform age-appropriate activities that do not compromise his or her physical condition.
Child maintains social contacts with friends and family members during acute phases of the illness.

Potential for self-care deficit related to physical and cognitive capabilities

Outcomes: The child will be able to perform as many activities of daily living as possible.
As child matures, child will accept more responsibility for maintaining the treatment regimen.

Alteration in family processes related to the impact of a chronic illness and/or hospitalization

Outcomes: Child and family will make use of appropriate sources of support.
Family members identify measures to meet each others' emotional and spiritual needs.
Family members develop strategies to cope with exacerbations of the child's illness.

healing process in the child (McCullough, 1989). During adolescence and with further skeletal maturity, the rate of healing slows to that of the adult. In children younger than age 10, overgrowth of 1 to 3 cm is common because of the increased circulation to a fracture and the growth plates of a bone.

Remodeling is the process in which correction of the fracture site occurs through a combination of periosteal reabsorption and new bone formation. Factors that affect remodeling include the child's age, proximity of the fracture to a joint, and relationship of the angular deformity to the plane of the joint axis of motion. If the child is young, the fracture occurred adjacent to a physes, and the deformity is in the plane of motion, then the remodeling potential is great. Thus, for certain pediatric fractures, anatomic alignment through reduction techniques is not necessary (Thompson & Scoles, 1996).

Children often outgrow many of the abnormalities in structure seen in the young, immature skeleton. For instance, in utero positioning may cause physiologic alterations in the child's musculoskeletal status that may take up to 3 to 4 years to completely resolve. Normal newborns have 20- to 30-degree hip and knee contractures, which usually resolve by age 4 to 6 months. The infant frequently has inward rotation of the lower leg, creating a bowed appearance. The feet may be in a mild equinus and inverted position as a result of being tucked close to the body. Metatarsus adductus (in-toeing) is a common finding in infants and toddlers. For some children, medical management is used to correct the malformation if

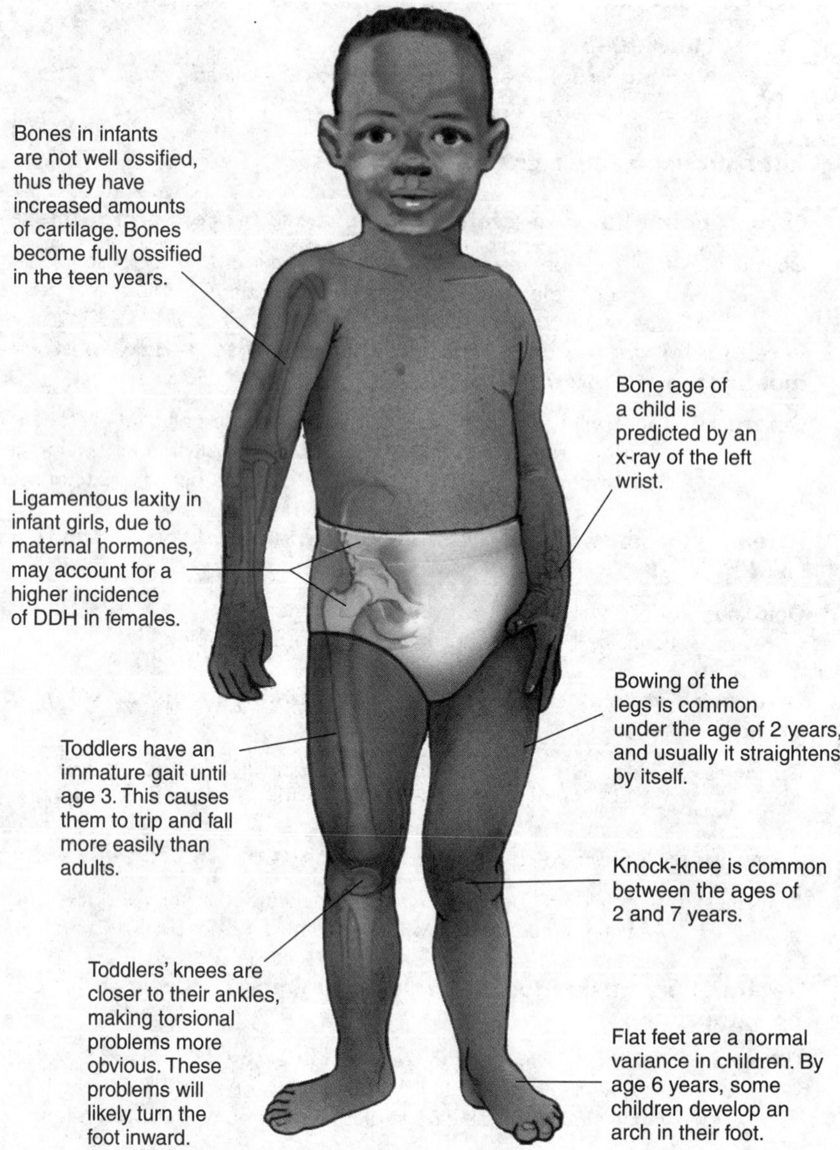

Bones in infants are not well ossified, thus they have increased amounts of cartilage. Bones become fully ossified in the teen years.
Bone age of a child is predicted by an x-ray of the left wrist.
Ligamentous laxity in infant girls, due to maternal hormones, may account for a higher incidence of DDH in females.
Bowing of the legs is common under the age of 2 years, and usually it straightens by itself.
Toddlers have an immature gait until age 3. This causes them to trip and fall more easily than adults.
Knock-knee is common between the ages of 2 and 7 years.
Toddlers' knees are closer to their ankles, making torsional problems more obvious. These problems will likely turn the foot inward.
Flat feet are a normal variance in children. By age 6 years, some children develop an arch in their foot.

Figure 20–1
Developmental and biological variances: musculoskeletal system.

spontaneous resolution does not occur as the child's bones and muscles grow (Mason, 1989; Thompson & Scoles, 1996). At birth, the child's spine has a C-shaped appearance. Spinal curvature undergoes several changes as the child gains the ability to first hold the head erect, then sit, and finally stand and bear weight. The child's weak abdominal musculature contributes to a "pot-bellied" or hyperlordosis appearance that is common in young toddlers (Mason, 1989).

Voluntary muscle control changes as the child's overall development proceeds in a cephalocaudal fashion. The primary protective reflexes seen in the infant (e.g., rooting, palmar grasp, stepping) are replaced by the purposeful movements associated with an intact, growing nervous system and an increasing muscle mass. The infant's muscles account for only 25% of total body weight, whereas they account for 40% to 45% in an adult (Mason, 1989). Muscle mass increases with use and with innervation by an intact nervous system. Muscle development is not normal in children with CP or other conditions in which connections between nerve fibers and muscle fibers are abnormal. Muscle atrophy and contractures are common. During adolescence, muscle growth is influenced by hormonal changes, primarily the increased production of androgenic hormones. Higher levels of androgen and testosterone are partly responsible for the more extensive muscle growth in males. Androgen excess, as seen in young athletes taking anabolic steroids, can accelerate muscle development and skeletal maturation. This can result in short stature, interfere with normal testosterone levels, and impair spermatozoa production (Mason, 1989).

The incidence of sports injuries increases dramatically in adolescents. The young child has resilient soft tissue, and dislocations and sprains are unusual occurrences. However, an adolescent's increased participation in athletics increases the opportunity for fractures, dislocation, and ligamentous tears. In addition, rapid bone and muscle growth may contribute to the appearance of "clumsy" and awkward motions of the adolescent who is trying to adjust to new body dimensions. These factors, combined with the "risk-taking" attitude of many adolescents, can lead to a higher rate of personal injury.

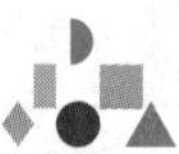

Diagnostic Criteria for Evaluating Alterations in Musculoskeletal Status

Two primary types of diagnostics are used in orthopedic medicine. The first type is blood or body fluid analysis (Chart 20–6). These studies include bone biopsies and fluid aspiration from joints to establish the presence of malignancy or infection. The physician performs a joint aspiration under local anesthesia with a long needle. A bone biopsy also requires general anesthesia. In this case, a piece of bone is excised and sent for pathologic analysis.

The second type of diagnostics—imaging techniques—is very useful in orthopedic medicine (Chart 20–7).

Alert: *If the child has a history of trauma, cervical spine precautions must be maintained during diagnostic testing until the physician rules out a cervical spine injury.*

The sensitivity and specificity of each test may vary with the disease process and the child's age. For example, a regular radiograph is sensitive and specific for a femur fracture in an infant. The radiograph shows the fracture and pinpoints its location. On the other hand, if the practitioner suspects a fracture of the spine be-

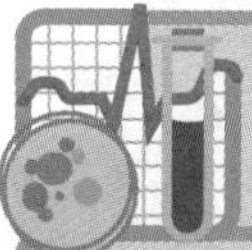

Chart 20–6
Diagnostic Tests and Procedures

Blood and Body Fluid Analysis

Diagnostic Test	Purpose	Findings and Indications	Normal Findings
CBC (complete blood count)	Blood sample analysis to evaluate several indicators	↑ WBC—Infection Septic arthritis ↓ Platelets—Bleeding disorder	6000–17,000/μL 150,000–400,000/μL
CRP (C-reactive protein)	To measure a protein in the blood that is released when infection is present	Level above .9 is indicative of infection, septic arthritis.	<1.0 mg/dL
Calcium and phosphorus	To test amount of minerals in blood sample	Low levels may indicate rickets.	Calcium 8.5–11 mg Phosphorus 3.0–4.5 mg/dL
Rh (rheumatoid factor)	To measure the body's autoimmune response to an antigen	May indicate JA if positive but not all children with JA have Rh factor.	Negative
Erythrocyte sedimentation rate	To measure how fast red blood cells settle out in solution	Elevated with septic arthritis; also can be indicative of infection.	0–10 mm/hr
Blood cultures	To see whether organisms grow from blood samples put in Petri dishes	Children with septic arthritis have a positive blood culture in 40% of cases. This can identify the causative organism.	No growth
Bone biopsies	To diagnose tumor or infection of the bone	Infection Malignant tissue	Normal bone cells
Fluid aspirations from joints	To diagnose infection or to relieve pressure in joint space	Purulent drainage Positive fluid culture	Clear fluid No growth from culture

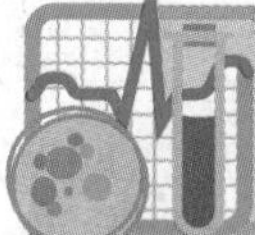

Chart 20-7
Diagnostic Tests and Procedures

Orthopedic Imaging Tests

Imaging Test	Advantages	Disadvantages
Plain film, radiograph	Easily available Inexpensive No sedation needed Visualizes fractures well	Radiation exposure Two-dimensional Does not visualize cartilage and other soft tissues well Patient must be positioned properly
Fluoroscopy	Real-time radiography Inexpensive Provides guidance for many orthopedic procedures Can be used with contrast	Radiation exposure
Arthrography	Good visualization of joints	Radiation exposure Quality and accuracy depend on skill of the arthrographer Risk of reaction to contrast
Computed tomography (CT)	Cross-sectional anatomic display Greater clarity than plain films CT software programs can reconstruct new images in various planes Can use contrast Three-dimensional imaging is available	Radiation exposure High cost May require sedation Risk of reaction from contrast
Nuclear medicine studies (bone scan)	High sensitivity in finding changes in bone resulting from infection, trauma, or tumor Directs attention to areas of the skeleton that may need further study	Not very specific; does not distinguish benign and malignant process Cannot always be done emergently Some radiation exposure to entire body Takes 4 hours to complete Intravenous access required
Ultrasound	No radiation Easily available No sedation needed Good for looking at soft tissue masses and cysts Inexpensive Painless	Limited use Results are dependent on skill of the technician
MRI (Magnetic resonance imaging)	No radiation Visualizes hard and soft tissue and bone marrow	Metal may produce artifact Experience needed to read MRIs Not readily available Often child needs sedation to lie still

cause of the condition of the cartilage in the infant's spine, radiographic imaging is not an appropriate diagnostic tool. Cartilage and other soft tissues are not clearly visible on radiographs, which are neither sensitive nor specific for a spinal fracture in an infant. A combination of tests is the best way to ensure a sensitive and specific diagnosis.

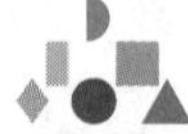

Treatment Modalities

Among the treatment modalities unique to orthopedic medicine are heat and cold application, brace and splint application, casting, traction, external fixation, and surgical intervention. To implement these orthopedic interventions, the nurse must understand the principles and mechanics of these treatment modalities. Also, the child should be involved in his or her own care as much as possible. For a child too young to manage self-care, other family members or caretakers should be prepared to manage or assist in meeting these needs. In doing so, the health care team can generally achieve better cooperation and compliance from the child and family in regard to the treatment regimen (Chart 20–8).

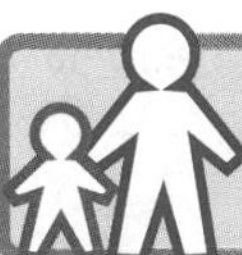

Chart 20–8
Developmental Considerations

Age-Appropriate Self-Care Activities for the Child with a Musculoskeletal Condition

Infants and Toddlers

Parents or caregivers provide all self-care needs.
Diversionary activities may be needed to prevent infants from pulling at straps, pins, wires.
Child indicates pain and discomfort in a manner recognizable to primary caregivers.

Preschooler

Wears or uses supportive devices without disturbing integrity and safety of the device
Uses walker, crutches, or wheel chair to assist in mobility
Takes medications as instructed
Indicates pain and discomfort in manner recognizable to primary caregivers

School-Age Child

Uses walker, crutches, or wheelchair to assist in mobility
Verbalizes feelings of pain and discomfort related to condition
Takes medications as instructed
Selects nonpharmacologic methods to manage pain and discomfort
Performs pin care
Selects foods to eat that provide a well-balanced diet
Wears clothes that are easy to put on and take off given the restrictions of his or her condition

Adolescent

Uses walker, crutches, or wheelchair to assist in mobility
Administers own medications
Verbalizes feelings of pain and discomfort related to condition and independently implements or seeks assistance in implementing non-pharmacologic methods to manage pain and discomfort
Selects activities that enhance mobility and do not cause additional pain or discomfort
Performs pin care
Selects foods to eat that provide a well-balanced diet
Monitors diet to prevent weight gain
Selects clothes that enhance body image and self-esteem

Heat and Cold Applications

Application of heat and cold is used in a variety of musculoskeletal disorders to minimize pain, increase joint range of motion, reduce swelling, and improve exercise performance. The choice of heat or cold application is often guided by the patient's preference. Most children prefer heat therapy because it seems less painful to them than cold therapy.

Heat Application

In general, heat is used for subacute or chronic conditions to warm muscle groups, cause vasodilation, relieve inflammation, and relieve pain from muscle stiffness or spasm. The application of heat allows the muscles to stretch further and increases the circulation of oxygenated blood to muscles and joints. Heat therapy is used by some athletes as part of their warm-up routine before exercising.

Heat therapy can be used in a dry or wet form. Dry heat is provided by means of infrared lamps, heating pads, electric heating blanket, and commercial hot packs. Tub baths, immersion in a hot tub, and hot water bottles are sources of wet heat. Heat should not be applied for more than 20 to 30 minutes at a time. After an hour of heat therapy, capillary vasoconstriction occurs as a secondary effect, making the therapy more destructive than beneficial. For this reason, reapplication of heat should be done no sooner than 1 hour after the initial application.

During heat therapy, the skin is evaluated for changes in color, integrity, and sensation. In addition, the child should be monitored for profuse sweating or an increase in respirations or pulse rate, indicating the need to immediately stop the therapy. Electric sources of heat should not be allowed to become wet, nor should the child be allowed to go to bed with a heating pad in place.

Tip: *When using electrical sources of heat, the caretaker should not make a point of showing the child how plugging in the apparatus makes the light come on or the dial* *glow. A young child is likely to consider this a game and want to play with the plug after the caretaker leaves the room.*

If hot moist compresses are applied, the bedding underneath the compress should be protected to prevent it from becoming cool, wet, and uncomfortable. Most importantly, the temperature of the heat application should be no hotter than is comfortable against the inner wrist or forearm.

caREminder: *Heat lamps are not recommended for home use with children, because of the risk of burns. When a warm or tepid therapeutic tub bath is given, the child should never be left unattended during the bath. A child who is feeling weak, ill, or lethargic may not be able to support himself or herself adequately in the tub.*

Cold Application

Cold applications cause vasoconstriction and the narrowing of surface capillaries. Cutaneous blood flow and cell perfusion are reduced, and metabolic function is slower at the site. Cold applications are used to prevent swelling and edema, reduce pain by reducing nerve impulse conduction, and reduce oxygen needs of the tissue by reducing circulation to the area. After an acute injury, such as a sprain or fracture, the application of cold or ice is recommended for 24 to 48 hours.

Cold applications reach their maximum effect after 30 to 60 minutes. After this time, a secondary effect of vasodilation occurs. At least 1 hour should elapse between applications of cold to prevent secondary effects from occurring. Treatment should be discontinued when numbness occurs. Moist cold applications include cold compresses and tepid or ice water baths. Dry cold therapy includes the use of commercial cold packs and ice bags. Cold therapy is not recommended for persons with a hypersensitivity to cold or with impaired circulation. The child's skin should be assessed for injury before and after cold application. After the treatment, the skin should be dried well. When applying an ice pack or cold compress, a towel or cloth should be placed between the compress and the skin to prevent injury to the skin.

Braces and Splints

Braces or splints are fabricated devices made from a solid material such as molded plastic. Straps consisting of Velcro or leather with buckles hold the splint or brace in place. A trained orthotist or therapist makes the splint or brace. The device is either custom fitted to the child or is a standard-sized device that is fitted onto the child and adjusted to fit. The purpose of a splint or brace is to immobilize a body part, to provide support for weak limbs, or to prevent deformities by maintaining optimal functional position of the joints.

The primary difference between a brace or splint and a cast is that the brace or splint can be removed for bathing, sleeping, or certain exercise regimens. The amount of time each day that the child must wear the brace or splint is dictated by the type of device and the medical reasons for the treatment. For instance, a child with scoliosis may have a Milwaukee brace or Boston brace. The plastic brace must be worn between 16 and 23 hours a day. For some children, the brace is only removed for bathing. The Pavlik harness is a cloth brace used in children with developmental dysplasia of the hip (DDH). This brace must be worn at all times for 4 to 6 weeks. A wrist or knee splint may be applied to immobilize an area during the acute phase of an arthritic condition or after an athletic injury. In these cases, the child may select not to wear the splint during periods of inactivity.

Primary care associated with a splint or brace focuses on maintaining skin integrity and ensuring that the device is used correctly to achieve its maximal effects. If the device does not fit properly, irritation and subsequent breakdown of the skin can occur. Wearing cotton clothing underneath the brace or splint can minimize skin irritation. Daily baths or skin care followed by thorough drying of the skin assists in maintaining cleanliness, stimulating the skin, and minimizing skin irritation. The child or the child's parents should be given verbal and written instructions regarding how and when the device is to be applied, how it should look on the child, what activities may be prohibited during the treatment, and how to care for and clean the device.

The child who wears a splint or brace may feel self-conscious about his or her physical appearance. This may negatively impact adjustment to and compliance with the treatment regimen. The child should be encouraged to participate in all care decisions surrounding brace or splint wear. Assisting the child to select appropriate and attractive clothes to wear over the brace is helpful. The child should be encouraged to verbalize his or her feelings associated with brace or splint wear and be directed toward positive coping behaviors and the positive eventual outcomes of therapy.

Serial Manipulation

In serial manipulation, passive range-of-motion exercises are used to manipulate a joint or muscle group. The purpose of serial manipulation is to restore joint alignment or to maintain functional mobility of a joint. Serial manipulation of a joint or muscle group is not recommended for all musculoskeletal disorders. The treatment is usually taught to the family by a physical therapist. The passive movements to the joint should not cause pain. Parents should be aware that the treatment may not be successful, thereby requiring the initiation of other therapies such as a brace or casting. An example of serial manipulation is its use on the child with metatarsus adductus. Passive manipulation during diaper changes is used to attempt to straighten the child's forefoot.

Casts

Casts hold a fractured extremity in alignment, prevent or reduce contracture, or provide postoperative immobilization. Casts can be made to fit an extremity or the trunk (Table 20–2). The location of the orthopedic problem and the degree of immobility needed to achieve healing or correction determine the type of cast to be applied. Casts are made from either of two types of materials: plaster or synthetic (Table 20–3). A trained physician or orthopedic technician applies and removes the cast.

Tip: *Fiberglass casts are available in a variety of colors and designs such as neon stripe and camouflage. The child or parents should be asked what design they prefer before the cast is placed.*

Neurovascular compromise, skin breakdown, and malalignment of a fracture can occur if the cast is not properly fitted. Careful assessment aids in prompt recog-

Table 20–2
Types of Casts

Type	Illustration	Body Part Covered	Uses
Short leg cast		Foot to below knee	Fracture of the foot, ankle, or distal tibia or fibula Severe sprain or strain Postoperative immobilization after open reduction and internal fixation Correction of deformity, such as talipes equinovarus
Leg cylinder cast		Ankle to upper thigh	Fracture or dislocation of the knee Soft tissue injury to the knee Postoperative immobilization after tibial valgus osteotomy Correction of varus or valgus deformity of the knee
Long leg cast		Foot to upper thigh	Fracture of the distal femur, knee, or lower leg Soft tissue injury to the knee or knee dislocation Postoperative immobilization after arthrodesis of the knee

Table continued on following page

Table 20–2
Types of Casts *Continued*

Type	Illustration	Body Part Covered	Uses
Abduction boots	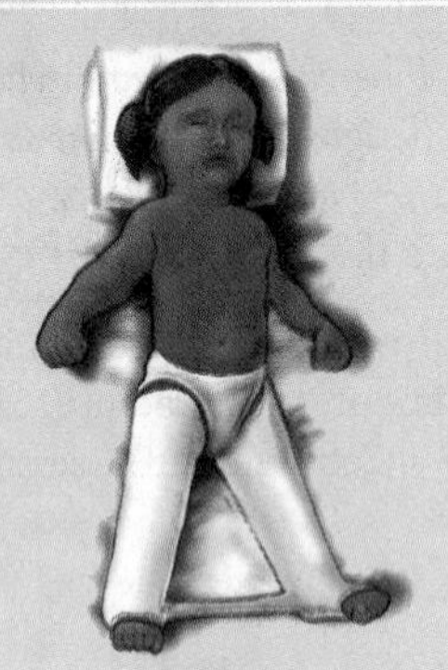	Feet to below knee or upper thigh	Postoperative immobilization after hip abductor release Maintenance of abduction
Unilateral hip spica cast	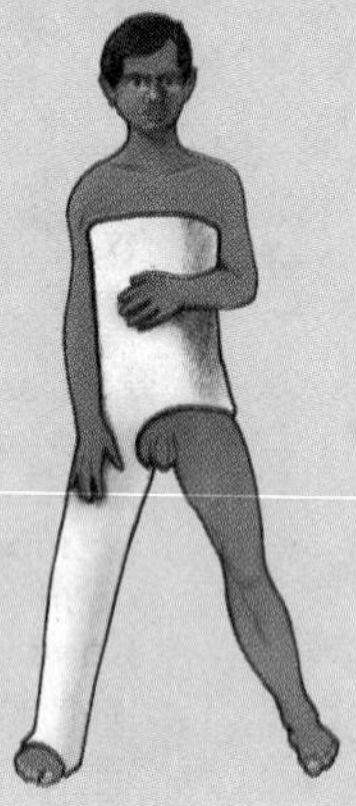	Entire leg and trunk to waist or nipple line	Fracture of the femur Postoperative immobilization after open reduction and internal fixation Correction of deformity, such as congenital soft tissue injury after hip dislocation
One and one-half hip spica cast	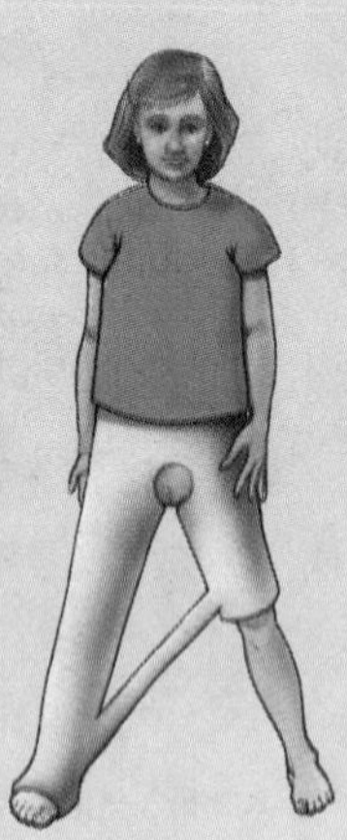	Entire leg, opposite leg to knee, and trunk to waist or nipple line	Fracture of the femur Postoperative immobilization after open reduction and internal fixation of the pelvis

Table 20–2
Types of Casts *Continued*

Type	Illustration	Body Part Covered	Uses
Bilateral long-leg hip spica cast	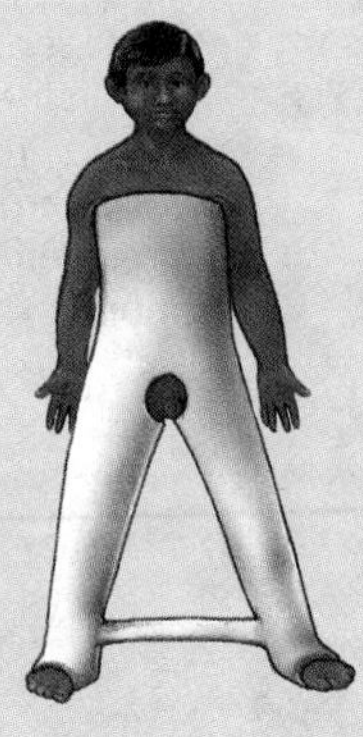	Entire leg bilaterally to waist or nipple line	Fracture of the femur, acetabulum, or pelvis Postoperative immobilization after open reduction and internal fixation
Short leg hip spica cast	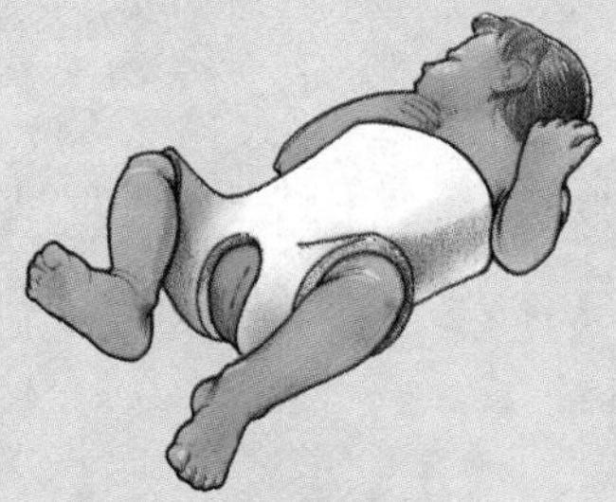	Knees or thighs bilaterally to waist or nipple line	Developmental hip dysplasia
Short arm cast	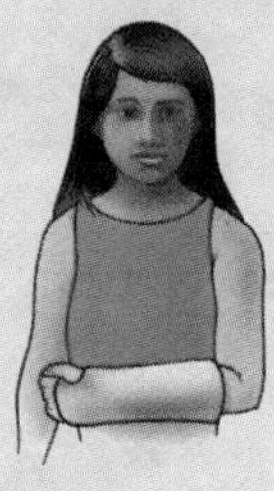	Hand to below elbow	Fracture of the hand or wrist Postoperative immobilization after open reduction and internal fixation
Long arm cast	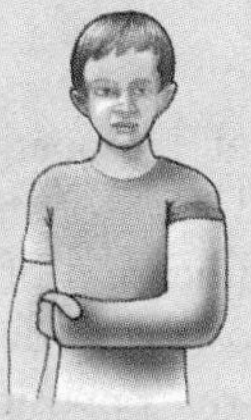	Hand to upper arm	Fracture of the forearm, elbow, or humerus Postoperative immobilization after open reduction and internal fixation
Arm cylinder cast	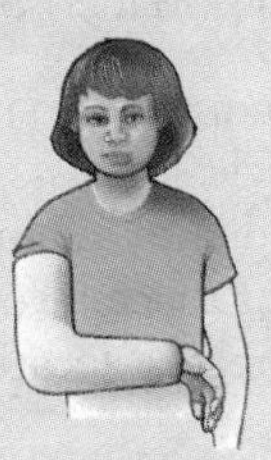	Wrist to upper arm	Elbow dislocation Postoperative immobilization after open reduction and internal fixation

Table continued on following page

Table 20–2
Types of Casts *Continued*

Type	Illustration	Body Part Covered	Uses
Shoulder spica cast		Trunk and shoulder, arm, and hand	Shoulder dislocation Soft tissue injury to the shoulder, such as rotator cuff tear Postoperative immobilization following open reduction and internal fixation
Minerva cast		Neck and trunk	Postoperative immobilization after cervical spine fusion or high thoracic spine fusion

Adapted from Maher, A. B., Salmond, S. W., & Pelerno, T. A. (1994). *Orthopaedic nursing.* Philadelphia: W. B. Saunders. Used with permission.

nition and treatment of these complications. Nursing interventions specific to wet and dry cast care should be implemented to ensure the cleanliness and integrity of the cast itself and of the child's skin (Fig. 20–2; Charts 20–9 and 20–10).

Casts are generally applied in an acute care setting or specialized outpatient clinic. Unless the child has an illness or injury that requires extensive hospitalization, after cast application the child promptly returns home, where cast care must be managed by the child and family. TIP 20–1 summarizes the important components to teach for the child with a cast. As discussed previously, maintaining skin integrity and noting any other complications of the treatment are important points to cover. Family members need to learn neurovascular assessment and cast maintenance techniques. Other aspects of home care include maintaining good nutrition and modifying activities as needed to promote the healing process (Adkins, 1997).

Traction

Since the time of Hippocrates (350 B.C.), traction has been an accepted form of medical treatment. Traction is defined as the application of a pulling force to an injured or diseased part of the body or extremity while countertraction pulls in the opposite direction. Traction is used to do the following (Maher, Salmond, & Pellino, 1994):

- Reduce, realign, and promote healing of fractures
- Decrease muscle spasms
- Relieve pain due to fractures
- Expand a joint space before surgery
- Reduce and treat dislocations

Several basic traction principles must be maintained to enable the traction to work effectively. First, *countertraction* is provided as sandbags, metal weights, or the child's body weight. Second, the prescribed *line of pull* is maintained. This requires a child to lie still in one posi-

Text continued on page 1237

Table 20–3
Advantages and Disadvantages of Types of Casts

Type	Advantages	Disadvantages
Plaster	Easily molded to hold fracture in alignment Inexpensive Smooth exterior, does not snag clothes or furniture easily Strong	If wet, it falls apart Heavy Takes 24 hours or more to dry Increased possibility that shape will change if it becomes wet Difficult to keep clean
Fiberglass	Lightweight, less bulky Water-resistant Washable Dries quickly Comes in a wide variety of colors and patterns	Not as easily molded as plaster casts, thus not suitable for small children or severely displaced fractures More expensive Increased possibility that activity may displace the fracture Rough exterior, can snag clothes and furniture
Fiberglass free Latex free	Lightweight, less bulky Water-resistant Washable Dries quickly Comes in a wide variety of colors and patterns Easily molded Latex and fiberglass free	Not as easily molded as plaster casts, thus not suitable for small children or severely displaced fractures More expensive Increased possibility that activity may displace the fracture Rough exterior, can snag clothes and furniture
Thermoplastic	Can remold with heat application Water-resistant Dries quickly	Difficult to mold Requires heat-activated application Can soften with inadvertent heat exposure Expensive

Figure 20–2
Diagram and instructions for "petaling" a cast.

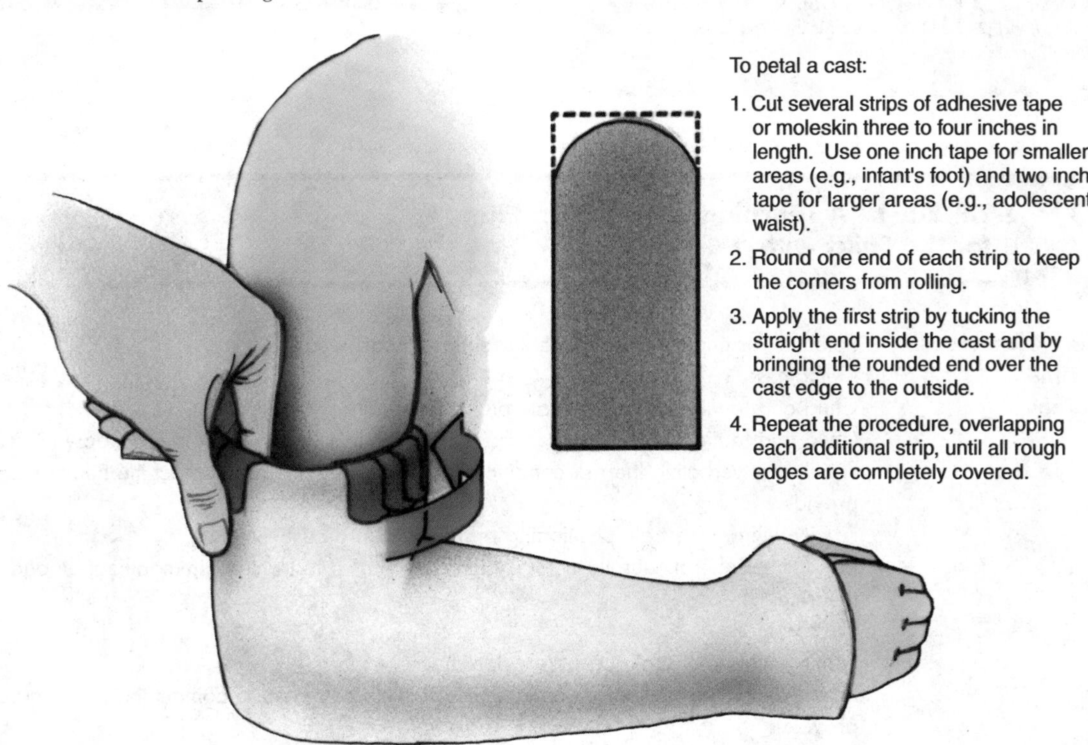

To petal a cast:
1. Cut several strips of adhesive tape or moleskin three to four inches in length. Use one inch tape for smaller areas (e.g., infant's foot) and two inch tape for larger areas (e.g., adolescent's waist).
2. Round one end of each strip to keep the corners from rolling.
3. Apply the first strip by tucking the straight end inside the cast and by bringing the rounded end over the cast edge to the outside.
4. Repeat the procedure, overlapping each additional strip, until all rough edges are completely covered.

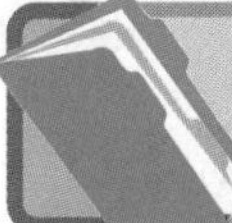

Chart 20–9
Nursing Interventions Classification (NIC)

Cast Care: Wet Cast

Definition

Care of a new cast during the drying period

Activities

Expose the drying cast to air.
Monitor circulation and color of fingers/toes on injured extremity.
Support the cast with pillows during the drying period.
Inform the patient that the cast will feel warm as the cast dries.
Monitor capillary refill by applying pressure to a fingernail or toenail.
Apply plastic to cast if close to groin.
Maintain the angles of the cast during the drying period.
Inspect cast for signs of drainage from wounds under the cast.
Mark the circumference of any drainage as a gauge for future assessments.
Explain the need for limited activity while cast dries.
Identify any change in sensation or increased pain at the fracture site.

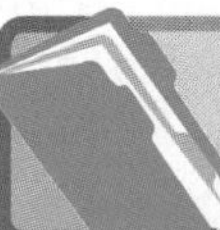

Chart 20–10
Nursing Interventions Classification (NIC)

Cast Care: Maintenance

Definition

Care of a cast after the drying period

Activities

Apply sodium bicarbonate (baking soda) to an odiferous cast.
Inspect cast for signs of drainage from wounds under the cast.
Mark the circumference of any drainage as a gauge for future assessments.
Apply plastic to cast if close to groin.
Instruct patient not to scratch skin under the cast with any objects.
Avoid getting a plaster cast wet.
Position cast on pillows to lessen strain on other body parts.
Check for cracking or breaks in the cast.
Apply an arm sling for support, if appropriate.
Pad rough cast edges and traction edges, as appropriate.

TIP 20–1 A Teaching Intervention Plan for the Child with a Cast

Nursing Diagnoses and Family Outcomes

- Potential for impaired skin integrity related to cast wearing
  Outcomes:
  Child and family will demonstrate proper cast care.
  Child and family will demonstrate care of the child's skin to prevent breakdown.
  Family will verbalize the risk conditions in which they need to contact the health care provider.
  Family will demonstrate positioning of the child in a cast.
- Risk for peripheral neurovascular dysfunction related to fracture, immobilization and cast wearing
  Outcomes:
  Family will demonstrate neurovascular checks.
  Family will verbalize the risk conditions in which they need to contact the health care provider.

TIP 20–1 A Teaching Intervention Plan for the Child with a Cast *Continued*

- Effective individual management of therapeutic regimen
  Outcomes:
  Child and family will verbalize safety measures to prevent further injury to the child and prevent damage to the cast.
  Child and family will verbalize comfort measures to institute when itching, muscle spasms, or minor aches occur.
  Child will be dressed appropriately to minimize sweating and maintain warmth of the extremities.
  Child and family will explain child's dietary needs.
- Diversional activity deficit related to altered mobility
  Outcomes:
  Child will perform age-appropriate activities that do not compromise his or her physical condition.
  Child will maintain social contacts with friends.
  Child will maintain school activities.

Interventions

Teach the Child and Family

- Cast Care
  Cast must be kept dry. If a Gore-Tex lining is used to make cast, the child can get the cast wet. Water may cause the cast to soften and lose its shape. If an area of the cast becomes wet, a blowdryer set on the "cool" setting will help dry the cast.
  To keep genitalia area of cast dry, tuck small diaper inside groin opening. At night a sanitary napkin may be added inside the diaper to prevent leakage. Do not cut a diaper to make it fit the groin opening of the cast; the cut unfinished edges of the diaper give off debris that can get under the cast and irritate the skin.
  Cover the edges of the cast with clothing to prevent crumbs, toys, and other articles from getting inside the cast.
  The child should not scratch inside the cast with anything.
  Clean soiled areas of the cast with a barely damp cloth. A small amount of white shoe polish can touch up a soiled white cast.
  A plastic bag may be taped over the cast to protect the cast while bathing.
  The child should not paint or write on the entire surface of the cast, because the cast needs to breathe.
- Skin Care
  To decrease skin irritation and protect the edges of the cast from excessive wear, petal the cast around the edges with moleskin, and cover edges around the perineal area with waterproof tape. A fiberglass cast should have the perineal area petaled with moleskin first, then covered with waterproof tape.
  A persistent foul odor could indicate an infection. Other signs include warmth over an area of the cast, drainage onto the cast, or development of a fever, lethargy, or discomfort.
  A daily tub bath or sponge bath is recommended to keep accessible skin areas clean.
  If itching occurs, try to divert the child's attention.
  Do not use lotion or powders on the skin around the cast edges or inside the cast.
  Inspect the skin daily for irritations.
  Alcohol applied 2 to 3 times a day under the edges of the cast can help toughen the child's skin. Do not use alcohol if the skin becomes cracked.

TIP continued on following page

TIP 20–1 A Teaching Intervention Plan for the Child with a Cast *Continued*

- Toileting
  - A bedpan or urinal may need to be used by the immobilized child.
  - For girls, placing toilet paper inside the bedpan is helpful to prevent splashing of urine onto the cast.
  - Plastic wrap can be tucked under the edges of the cast and funneled into the bedpan to prevent soiling of the perineal cast edges while using the bedpan.
  - The neck of the urinal can be extended by placing a paper cup with the bottom cut out into the neck of the urinal.
- Positioning
  - Change the child's position at least every 4 hours while he or she is awake.
  - The child in a body cast can be on his or her stomach with pillow under the legs, or propped up on the side or on the back at an angle of about 30 degrees with head up.
  - The abduction stabilizer bar between the legs of the spica cast should not be used as a handle to help turn the child unleess otherwise instructed by the orthotic technician who has constructed the cast.
  - Pillow or rolled blankets can be used to support the body and cast.
  - Keep casted extremity elevated and supported with a pillow when the child is not ambulating.
- Neurovascular Checks
  - Note color, sensation, motion and temperature of involved extremities at least twice a day.
  - Fingers and toes should be warm and pink.
  - Squeeze the finger or toe until it turns white and then watch to see if it immediately turns pink after you release it.
  - Ask the child if there is any tingling, numbness, or pain in the extremity.
  - Notify the health care provider if there is a change in the neurovascular status.
- Mobility and Transportation
  - Keep toys, throw rugs, and small pets out of the child's path.
  - Have the child use crutches as ordered to assist in ambulation.
  - To allow play, the child in a spica cast can be seated in a bean bag chair with toys placed within reach.
  - A reclining wheel chair can be used to allow the child with a spica cast to sit up or be transported.
  - A prone cart or scooter can be used as a means of transportation for the child in a spica cast.
  - The child weighing less than 40 pounds must be restrained in a car seat. Special car seats can be ordered to accommodate the child in a cast.
  - For the older child, a safety rest for the car restraint may be rented.
  - Special wide ambulances may be needed to transport children in abduction casts.
- Comfort
  - Benadryl may be ordered for severe itching.
  - Children with cerebral palsy may need Valium as needed for muscle spasms that occur during cast wear.
  - Acetaminophen can be administered to the child for discomfort.
  - The child should not be extremely uncomfortable in the cast. If the child complains of pain in one spot, it may indicate a pressure sore, and it should be evaluated by a health care provider.

TIP 20–1 A Teaching Intervention Plan for the Child with a Cast *Continued*

- Clothing

  When in a body cast, girls can wear dresses or skirts. Boys can wear boxer shorts and pants, which are cut down the side seam to accommodate the cast. The shorts can be pinned or fastened with Velcro strips.

  Clothing should be loose fitting (approximately two sizes larger than normal) and not have elastic around the hem, wrist, or ankle area.

  Clothing should be chosen to help the child stay as cool as possible because the cast will make the child's skin more sweaty.

  The lower extremities can be kept warm by wearing large socks over the feet and cast.
- Nutrition

  Diet should be high in fiber, with fresh fruits and vegetables to prevent constipation.

  Small, frequent meals decrease discomfort from abdominal distention.

  Fluid intake should be increased to prevent kidney stones and constipation.
- Diversional Activities and Schooling

  Child can return to school if mobile and the cast is dry.

  A home tutor should be arranged for the child in a body cast.

  A daily schedule should include age-appropriate diversional activities.

  Visitors are encouraged.

Call Health Care Provider if

Cast starts to fall apart or gets cracked or broken.

Child experiences pain, tingling, or numbness in the affected extremity.

Child complains of discomfort.

Fever or lethargy develops.

The cast has a persistent foul odor.

There is marked coolness of the skin on the affected side compared with the normal side.

There is warmth over an area of the cast or drainage onto the cast.

There is increased swelling above or below the cast.

tion, a challenging task. Third, the traction is *continuously applied.* Although the traction may be released for short periods (most commonly, in skin traction), the basic premise is that the traction is applied at all times for a period of several days or weeks. Fourth, there must be *prevention or reduction of friction* that interferes with the effectiveness of the traction (Styrcula, 1994).

Three types of traction are used: manual, skin, and skeletal. Chart 20–11 summarizes the nursing interventions associated with caring for a child in traction. During *manual traction,* force is applied to the bones by a physician, nurse, or technician to keep them in alignment. Manual traction is performed during casting, splinting, or application of skin or skeletal traction.

Skin traction is the pull achieved by using a variety of soft materials (moleskin or foam boot), bandages, and wraps that are applied directly to the skin (Table 20–4). Because the traction is used on the skin, the amount of weight that can be used is limited. The risk of skin breakdown precludes the long-term use of this modality. Nursing interventions to decrease skin irritation include making skin and neurovascular assessments every 4 hours, applying wraps over intact or protected skin, and careful wrapping to avoid wrinkling of the materials used to wrap the skin.

Skeletal traction applies force directly to the bone by using aseptically inserted pins, wires, or tongs. Table 20–5 describes and illustrates various types of skeletal traction. This traction is suitable for long-term use and unstable fractures. Weights are adjusted as necessary to

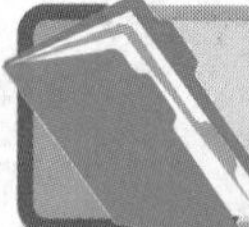

Chart 20–11
Nursing Interventions Classification (NIC)

Traction/Immobilization Care

Definition

Management of a patient who has traction and/or a stabilizing device to immobilize and stabilize a body part

Activities

Position in proper body alignment.
Maintain proper position in bed to enhance traction.
Ensure that proper weights are being applied.
Ensure that the ropes and pulleys hang freely.
Ensure that the pull of ropes and weights remains along the axis of the fractured bone.
Brace traction weights while moving patient.
Maintain traction at all times.
Monitor self-care ability while in traction.
Monitor external fixation device.
Monitor pin insertion sites.
Monitor skin and bony prominences for signs of skin breakdown.
Monitor circulation, movement, and sensation of affected extremity.
Monitor for complications of immobility.
Perform pin insertion site care.
Administer appropriate skin care at friction points.
Provide trapeze for movement in bed, as appropriate.
Instruct on bracing device care, as needed.
Instruct on external fixation device care, as needed.
Instruct on pin site care, as needed.
Instruct in importance of adequate nutrition for bone healing.

From McCloskey, J., & Bulechek, G. (1996). *Nursing interventions classification (NIC)* (2nd ed.). St. Louis: Mosby–Year Book. Reprinted with permission.

keep the bones in alignment. Skeletal traction carries a risk of pin tract infection and osteomyelitis. Aggressive pin care and frequent skin and neurovascular assessments are important components of care for a child in skeletal traction (Chart 20–12).

Before a child is admitted to the hospital for traction or surgery, a preadmission tour of the facilities is helpful in alleviating the parents' anxiety. On the child's admission to the hospital, the nurse reviews care of the child in traction, including skin care, neurovascular assessment, proper positioning, and developmental activities. The child life therapist can assist in providing age-appropriate toys to place around the bed. Children should be provided with a playroom setting, when possible. Photographs of family members or the child's favorite characters can be taped to the crib and traction bars to provide visual stimulation. Social services personnel can provide parking and meal passes for needful parents who stay with their child during the hospitalization and they can assist with the family's anticipated needs on discharge.

External Fixation

External fixation uses a system of percutaneous pins and wires connected to a rigid frame to hold the two fragments of a fracture together. This allows for immobilization after fracture reduction when a cast cannot be used because there is extensive soft tissue damage or open wounds. Using an external fixator also permits early ambulation.

An external fixator may also be used to lengthen bones or correct angular or rotational defects. In these cases, the wires, rings, and telescoping rods allow limb lengthening to occur by the process of distraction when two opposing bone ends are separated, and new bone regeneration occurs to fill in the gap (Carlino, 1991). Various types and sizes of external fixators are available; the type used depends on the physician preference and the underlying musculoskeletal problem.

Care of the child with an external fixator device

Chart 20–12
Nursing Interventions

Pin Care

The presence of skeletal pins increases the risk of infection. Opinions vary as to the method that most effectively reduces this risk. Some methods of delivering skin care to the pin site follow the protocol of the specific institution and should be followed. Whatever method is used, careful assessment should be done routinely to detect infection early.

1. Betadine-soaked gauze is wrapped around the pin and left to dry. Some protocols have this done 2 to 3 times/day; others leave the gauze in place until removed by a physician.
2. Half-strength hydrogen peroxide is applied 2 to 3 times/day. Sterile technique is used to remove all crusting around the site.
3. Do not clean site; let crusts form. The rationale is to prevent frequent moistening and tissue damage from frequent cleansing, both of which may increase bacterial invasion.

Table 20–4
Types of Skin Traction

Type	Illustration	Uses	Nursing Considerations
Cervical skin		Neck sprains or strains Torticollis Cervical nerve trauma Nerve root compression	There is a 5–7 pound limit of weights. Avoid compressing the throat or ears with the chin strap.
Side-arm 90-90		Fractures and dislocations of the upper arm or shoulder	Hand may feel cool because of its elevation. Hand can be covered with sock or mitten if desired.
Dunlop		Supracondylar elbow fracture of the humerus	Avoid pressure over bony prominences or nerves.
Pelvis sling		Pelvic fractures	There is a 10–25 pound limit of weights. Ensure proper size of belt and apply it just over iliac crest.
Bryant's traction		Infant with a femur fracture or developmental dislocated hip	Supply plenty of diversional activities. If child flips over, a sheet or Posey restraint may be used. Avoid pressure over dorsum of foot and heel.

Table continued on following page

Table 20–4
Types of Skin Traction *Continued*

Type	Illustration	Uses	Nursing Considerations
Buck's traction		Hip and knee contracture Legg-Calvé-Perthes disease Slipped capital femoral epiphysis (SCFE)	Remove boot every 8 hours and assess skin. Leg may be slightly abducted.
Russell's traction		Supracondylar femur fracture Hip and knee contracture	Sling may need to be repositioned often; mark leg to ensure proper placement.
Split Russell's		Femur fracture SCFE Legg-Calvé-Perthes disease	Avoid pressure over bony prominences or nerves. Weights are not added or removed without a physician's order.

involves maintaining skin integrity and preventing infection or injury. Skin and neurovascular assessments are needed. Skin care is similar to that for a child in skeletal traction. Pin care must be completed daily to prevent infection. To prevent dryness, lotions can be applied to skin away from the entry sites of pins and wires. Activities in which the fixator might be hit or bumped are restricted during the treatment. In some cases, the child may be able to bear weight on the affected limb. The child should be taught not to pick at or manipulate any of the wires or pins. The child may wear baggy sweat pants or skirts over the device. Velcro can be sewn into the seams of pants to allow them to easily slip over the fixator device.

Surgical Interventions

Pediatric orthopedic surgery is performed for two main reasons: to correct a musculoskeletal deformity or break of the bone and to prevent a deformity. The goal in either case is to enable the child to live a functional life. In some instances, a deformity that is mild can be observed closely with minor adaptations made to the child's life. For other children, the deformity interferes with their ability to sit, walk, sleep, or breathe, and surgery is indicated. Surgical interventions aim to restore mechanical balance to the body through bone fusions, bone lengthenings or shortenings, muscle realignments or releases, joint reconstruction, or even amputations. An orthopedic surgeon may use a variety of "hardware" such as pins, screws, wires, bolts, hooks, and rods to achieve the purpose of the surgery.

Nursing care of the postoperative child is discussed in Chapter 9. Range-of-motion exercises or restrictions on movement may be instituted to guard the area that was surgically treated. For instance, log-rolling is used to turn the child who has had a spinal fusion, whereas continuous passive range-of-motion machines may be used on the adolescent who has had knee surgery. Postoperatively, the child is likely to experience a great deal of pain. The assessment and management of pain in children is discussed in Chapter 13.

Continuous Passive Motion

Continuous passive motion (CPM) therapy maintains motion and decreases soft tissue adhesions and muscle stiffness after surgery, such as that for ligament recon-

Table 20–5
Types of Skeletal Traction

Type	Illustration	Uses	Nursing Considerations
Cervical skeletal tongs		Preoperative spine distraction Fractures or dislocations of cervical or high thoracic vertebrae	A special bed may be used to assist with turning patient. Logroll patient.
Halo cast or vest		Postoperative immobilization after cervical fusion Fracture or dislocation of cervical or high thoracic vertebrae	A small wrench is taped to the front of the brace to remove front panel in case of emergency. If patient is in halo cast, a cast saw must be with her or him in case of emergency. Balance is altered with a halo cast; patients ambulating need close supervision.
Dunlop's side-arm 00-90		Fractures of upper arm	Turn patient toward the affected side only. Hand may feel cool despite intact neurovascular status; cover hand with mitten or sock if desired.
Knee 90-90		Femur fractures	Encourage child to dorsiflex foot often to prevent foot drop; apply splint if necessary. Ensure weights do not catch on bottom of the bed.
Thomas ring with Pearson attachment (balanced suspension)		Femur fracture Hip fracture Tibial fracture	Avoid pressure to the area behind the knee, which could cause popliteal nerve injury. If the system is truly balanced, the splint can be placed at any height and it will remain there.

struction or joint replacement. The CPM machine takes a joint through a specified range of motion. CPM machines can be used for elbows, knees, hips, ankles, and fingers, and some are adaptable for use in children.

The physician specifies how many hours the patient must use the machine, the range of motion (both extension and flexion), and the speed of the cycle. Most machines have a small, handheld keypad that is programmed either by the nurse or physical therapist. The nurse places the patient in the machine with the joint properly aligned. The nurse also monitors patient compliance and skin integrity, and adjusts the settings as ordered. When the CPM machine is used at home, the patient and family must be taught how to properly position the joint in the machine and how to adjust the range-of-motion settings.

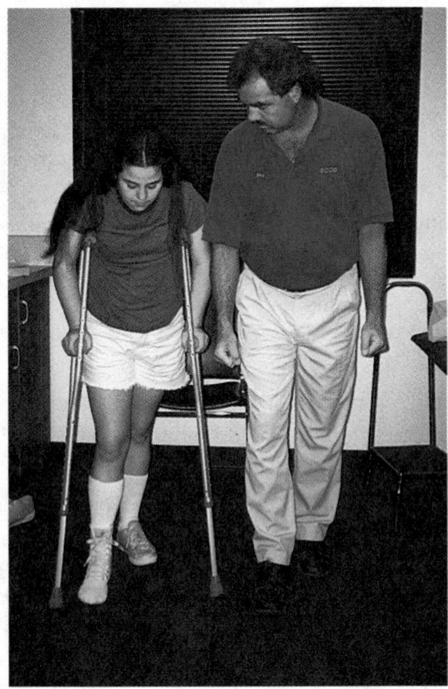

Figure 20–3
Crutches are placed under the child's arms. To avoid shoulder nerve injury, the child should not lean on the crutches. The crutches are placed approximately 1 foot in front of the child, and the child's legs should swing up to, but not beyond, the crutches.

Ambulatory Devices

Assistance with ambulation may be needed after surgery, injury, or immobilization of a lower extremity. The ambulatory device transfers a portion of the body weight to the arms and provides additional support during walking. The device can also assist the child to get up and down from a sitting position. The type of device selected is based on the child's age, overall functional ability, degree of strength in the arms and legs, balance, and ability to maintain an upright position. A physical therapist works with the child and family to choose the most appropriate device. Instructions are given regarding correct use of the device and how the child can best achieve an effective gait pattern.

The types of ambulatory devices that children can use include a cane, crutches, and a walker. A *cane* is used to widen the base of support to the side of the affected limb. The cane is held on the same side as the affected leg and is moved in coordination with the affected leg. A regular cane has a single base; a quad cane has a four-pronged base of support. When a cane is used, the affected leg experiences partial weight-bearing. Canes are more effective in school-age and older children who have good gait and upper extremity coordination.

Crutches relieve weight-bearing from the affected limb by transferring body weight and gait control to the arms and hands. The muscles of the arms, shoulders, back, and chest are all used during crutch walking. Exercises may be initiated before crutch use to strengthen these muscles. Instruction regarding the position and proper manipulation of the crutches is essential to prevent further injury to the child. To prevent nerve palsy, the top of the crutches should be between two and three finger-breadths below the axilla. The position of the crutches during periods of rest and movement is important to ensure that stability is maintained and gait is not compromised (Fig. 20–3). The term "point" refers to the number of points in contact with the floor. For instance a three-point gait occurs when the two crutches and the unaffected limb are touching the floor.

Walkers are useful ambulatory devices for young children and those with limited functional abilities. A walker uses a four-legged base to provide support during ambulation. A parallel stationary walker requires the child to lift and advance the entire walker when ambulating. This may be difficult for the child with more severe musculoskeletal challenges. The rolling walker has two to four wheels attached to the base, requiring the child to gently push the device to assist in ambulation. This type of walker is less stable, especially on wet or slippery surfaces.

Figure 20–4
The immobilized child should be provided with age-appropriate toys and diversional activities.

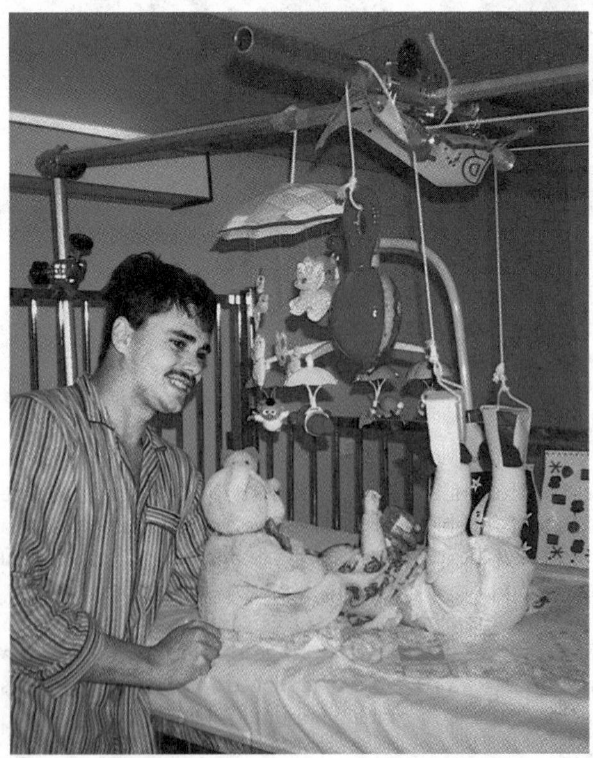

Prosthetic Devices

Children with limb deformities and those who have experienced permanent loss of a body part may elect to use a prosthetic device to enhance mobility and body image. Prostheses are individually fitted to the contour of the remaining body part. If the child has had an amputation or if a limb deformity is surgically prepared to correctly fit a prosthesis, the stump must be completely healed before prosthetic wear is fitted.

The prosthetic device can be a completely formed body part such as a hand or foot, or it can be a device with myoelectric controls to allow movement and use of the extremity. Myoelectric controls were previously believed not to be beneficial for children younger than adolescence. It has more recently been demonstrated to have positive effects for children as young as 18 months and is strongly recommended by age 3 to 4 years (Hubbard, Bush, Kurtz, & Naumann, 1991). Benefits include an integration to psychomotor development, decreased muscle atrophy, and improved development of fine motor movement when the prosthesis is introduced before other compensatory patterns develop. Early introduction also has a more positive effect on the child's acceptance of the prosthesis and on his or her body image.

Complications of Immobilization

The conditions affecting a child's muscles, bones, or connective tissues generally lead to immobility. A primary focus of the interdisciplinary team is to prevent the formation of contractures, the loss of muscle tone, or the fixation of joints of the child who is immobilized. The immobilized area may be limited to a specific body part or immobilization may affect every aspect of the child's activities and mobility. Immobilization may be instituted using splints, casts, and traction devices to safeguard an injured area and to promote healing. Immobility can also be hazardous to the child if the health care team and the family do not take measures to prevent systemic complications and disability. Table 20–6 summarizes the hazards of immobility and the interventions to prevent these hazards.

When a child is immobilized, passive and active range-of-motion exercises should be completed three or four times a day to maintain functional ability. The child's physical activities are based on the amount of motion allowed and the child's need for stimulation, peer interaction, and opportunities to promote normal development (Fig. 20–4). Attendance at school is strongly encouraged when possible. The school nurse can work with the family to adapt the child's environment, schedule, and physical activities as necessary. If the child is unable to attend school, diversionary activities in the home or in the acute care setting must be incorporated into the daily plan of care. The child can become easily bored and regress in social, personal, and academic skills. Providing age-appropriate activities and encouraging visits from friends can assist the child in adapting to the immobilized state.

Table 20–6
Hazards of Immobility

Body System	Pathophysiology	Clinical Manifestations	Nursing Interventions
Respiratory	Decreased chest and lung expansion Decreased respiratory effort and effects of gravity	Slower and more shallow respirations Pooling of secretions Decreased cough reflex	Encourage turning, coughing, and deep breathing. Apply incentive spirometer. Monitor vital signs. Apply chest physiotherapy/vibration. Mobilize patient as soon as possible.
Cardiovascular	Vasodilatation and impaired venous return Muscular inactivity Decreased respiratory effort and gravity Redistribution of body fluids	Circulatory stasis Venous dilation in dependent parts Decreased thoracic and abdominal pressures Decreased cardiac rate, circulatory volume, and arterial pressure	Turn patient. Encourage active/passive range-of-motion activities. Apply elastic stockings to lower extremities. Mobilize patient as soon as possible.

Table continued on following page

Table 20–6
Hazards of Immobility *Continued*

Body System	Pathophysiology	Clinical Manifestations	Nursing Interventions
Musculoskeletal	Decreased bone stress and muscle tension Imbalance between osteoblastic and osteoclastic activity leads to calcium and phosphorus loss Decreased muscle tone	Decreased muscle mass and strength Decreased bone mass and strength	Encourage active/passive range-of-motion activities. Encourage isometric/isotonic exercises. Mobilize patient as soon as possible.
Metabolic	Decreased basal metabolic rate and oxygen consumption Nitrogen loss and negative nitrogen balance due to protein loss from loss of muscle mass	Decreased efficiency in using nutrients Increased potassium and calcium excretion Decreased appetite	Give small, frequent meals. Give increased fiber, protein, vitamin C, acidifying foods. Limit calcium intake. Mobilize patient as soon as possible.
Skin	Negative nitrogen balance Continuous pressure on bone prominences	Increased potential for skin breakdown	Avoid positions that put pressure on bony prominences. Turn patient regularly. Keep patient's skin clean and dry. Apply lotion to dry skin areas. Apply pressure-equalizing and pressure-reducing devices.
Elimination	General muscle weakness and atrophy Slowed peristalsis from inactivity Urinary stasis in renal pelvis	Constipation Urinary retention Renal calculi Anorexia	Establish baseline for elimination pattern. Encourage adequate fluid intake. Monitor urine characteristics. Give stool softeners or suppositories to facilitate bowel elimination.

From Betz, C., Hunsberger, M., & Wright, S. (1994). *Family-centered nursing care of children.* Philadelphia: W. B. Saunders. Reprinted with permission.

Nutrition

Children with musculoskeletal disorders do not generally require any special dietary considerations. A healthy, well-balanced, age-appropriate diet provides for the nutritional needs of the child (see Chapter 5). Foods high in calcium and phosphorus are of particular importance in promoting the development of strong bones and teeth (Table 20–7). Also, adequate calcium intake during childhood and adolescence is a key strategy in preventing osteoporosis and skeletal fractures in later life (Gallo, 1996). Vitamins A and D are also needed to regulate absorption and deposition of calcium and phosphorus, thus aiding bone growth and contributing to bone strength.

When the child is immobile and has a low caloric expenditure, weight gain may become a concern. The child's diet can be modified to reduce the number of calories taken in while continuing to provide vitamins and minerals to promote growth.

Children who have experienced an acute injury to the bone, skin tissues, or muscle may require increased intakes of calcium, phosphorus, vitamins, and minerals. Calcium and phosphorus promote bone formation and growth to damaged areas. Vitamin A is needed for creation of collagen, for scar formation, and for the growth of new epithelial cells. Vitamin C is necessary for collagen synthesis, to improve resistance to infection, and to form capillaries to bring blood to the damaged musculoskeletal areas. Minerals such as zinc, copper, and iron also assist in the synthesis of collagen (DeWit, 1992).

Table 20-7
Important Nutrients to Promote Strong Bones and Teeth

Nutrient	Food Sources	Results of Deficiency on Musculoskeletal Status
Calcium	Milk, cheese Yogurt Cottage cheese Mustard and turnip greens Clams, oysters Broccoli, cauliflower, cabbage Molasses	Improper bone growth such as rickets, bowed legs, osteomalacia, and osteoporosis Porous bones Tetany and muscle spasm Poor tooth formation
Phosphorus	Milk, cheese Meat Egg yolk Fish Nuts Whole-grain cereals Legumes	Rickets Porous bones Bowed legs Stunted growth Poor tooth formation
Vitamin A	Liver and liver sausage Butter, cream, whole milk Egg yolks Green and yellow vegetables Yellow fruits Ripe tomatoes Fortified margarine Fish liver oils	Poor tooth and bone formation
Vitamin D	Vitamin D–fortified milk Small amounts in butter, egg yolk, liver, and saltwater fish Fish liver oils	Soft bones Bowed legs Poor tooth development Poor posture

Pain Management

Sources of pain and discomfort for the child with a musculoskeletal disorder include diagnostic and surgical procedures, muscle spasms, development of contractures, injury to the bone and tissues, joint inflammation, swelling, stiffness, and the processes of healing. Children by nature want to move and explore their world. Even in the presence of a painful illness, children are likely to find ways to adapt their movements and motion to remain as active as possible. Important interventions of the health care team are to provide pharmacologic and nonpharmacologic measures that make the child as comfortable as possible, to maintain the integrity of the child's musculoskeletal status, and to promote continuing achievement of developmental milestones. Chapter 13 provides a summary of the numerous pain management techniques effective in children. Because motion is so critical to the child, measures must be instituted to ensure that the child's mobility is not negatively affected by high levels of pain.

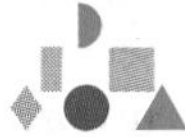

Alterations in Musculoskeletal Status

Congenital and Hereditary Disorders

Disorders that are caused by an inherited gene or that occur within the intrauterine environment are referred to as hereditary or congenital disorders. The child is born with the disorder, although it may not be apparent at birth. For example, a clubfoot is visible, whereas children with mild osteogenesis imperfecta (OI) may escape detection until they become active and experience numerous fractures.

Metatarsus Adductus

Metatarsus adductus, also known as metatarsus varus or in-toeing, is a mild deformity in which the bones of the forefoot turn inward. It is a common congenital problem that occurs in approximately 1 per 1000 live births (Morrissy, 1990). It occurs in both males and females and presents bilaterally in 50% of the cases. The cause of metatarsus adductus is unknown, although incidence apparently has a genetic component. Positioning in utero is also a factor, in that breech presentation may contribute to metatarsus adductus. The condition is further exacerbated by placing the infant in a sleeping prone position with the feet turned inward. Children with metatarsus adductus have an increased incidence of hip dysplasia.

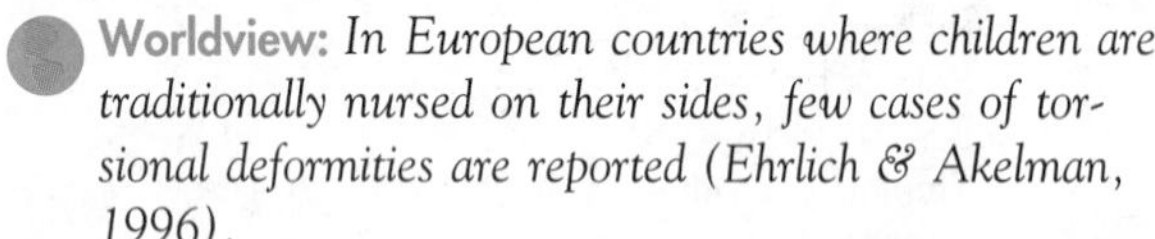

Worldview: *In European countries where children are traditionally nursed on their sides, few cases of torsional deformities are reported (Ehrlich & Akelman, 1996).*

Prognosis. The prognosis is usually good, depending on the flexibility of the deformity. The ultimate goal is to straighten the forefoot so that it is aligned with the heel. This position facilitates normal development of the foot as the child grows. Older children with metatarsus adductus may be ridiculed as being "pigeon-toed" if this deformity is not corrected at an early age.

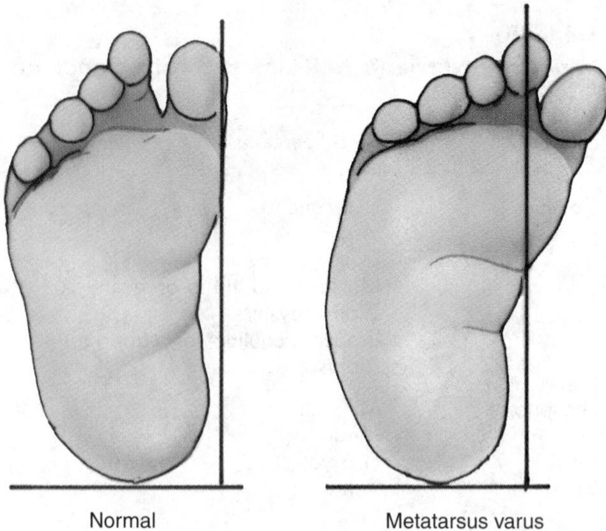

Figure 20–5
Metatarsus varus is graded according to the degree of inward toeing that passes beyond the medial border of the foot. Here, the left foot has normal alignment. In the right foot, the great toe is widely separated from the other toes and the foot angle turns inward, demonstrating metatarsus adductus.

Assessment

Physical characteristics of metatarsus adductus are a high arch and a great toe that is widely separated from the others (Fig. 20–5). The condition usually becomes more apparent when the child is placed in a weight-bearing position, such as when the child is first learning to walk. Metatarsus adductus can be diagnosed by pressing on the sole of the foot. The heel should align with the second metatarsal bone. If the second metatarsal faces inward and can easily be reduced by gentle pressure on the first metatarsal, it is considered supple. If passive correction with hand pressure is more difficult and if a prominent midfoot soft tissue vertical crease is present, the deformity is structural and rigid (Ehrlich & Akelman, 1996; Huurman, 1992).

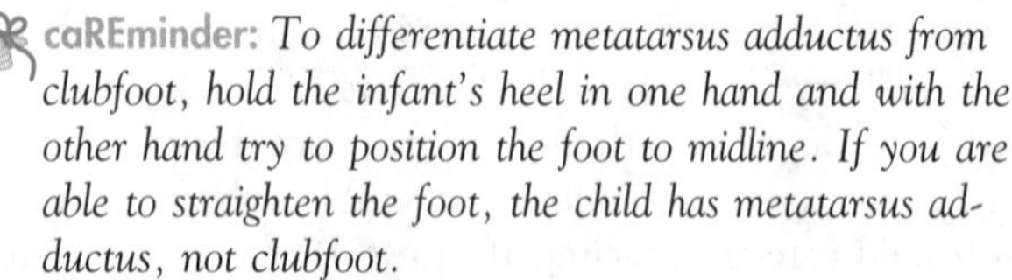

caREminder: *To differentiate metatarsus adductus from clubfoot, hold the infant's heel in one hand and with the other hand try to position the foot to midline. If you are able to straighten the foot, the child has metatarsus adductus, not clubfoot.*

Interdisciplinary Interventions

Treatment of supple metatarsus adductus in the infant consists of gentle *passive manipulation* performed during diaper changes by the parent. The parent holds the child's heel still with one hand while attempting to straighten the forefoot with the other hand. Often, metatarsus adductus corrects spontaneously, but this manipulation does not hurt the child. The parents may want to perform this manipulation during diaper changes to help them remember to do this activity routinely.

In addition to passive manipulation, alteration of sleeping habits should be instituted. The goal is to prevent the infant from assuming a prone position in which the hip and knees are flexed and internally rotated. A pair of soft shoes, laced together at the heel and worn during sleep hours can help the infant externally rotate the feet (Huurman, 1992). The older child may be instructed to wear exercise or outflare shoes at night that have a bar between them to face the feet out about 45 degrees.

At the time of follow-up, if the child's foot has not improved, serial plaster cast correction is initiated for several weeks. The foot is not forced into the correct position. Rather, as the cast is changed weekly, the stretching of the soft tissues allows the physician to gradually mold the foot into the anatomically correct plane. Plaster is the preferred type of casting material because it allows for molding, unlike the fiberglass cast. After casting is completed, some physicians recommend straight-last shoes. A straight-last shoe does not have a curve on the bottom of the shoe. However, most children have a normal appearance to the foot after casting and do not require special shoes or splints. Untreated metatarsus adductus rarely causes persistent problems in adult life other than abnormal shoe wear and pressure points.

Nursing care for a child with metatarsus adductus begins with teaching the family passive manipulation, correct infant sleeping positions, or cast care, if indicated (see Charts 20–9 and 20–10). The nurse may reinforce to the parents that metatarsus adductus is a common problem that can be corrected, and that weekly follow-up visits to the physician's office will be necessary.

Clubfoot

Also known as talipes equinovarus (TEV), clubfoot is a common congenital anomaly that occurs in 1.24 per 1000 live births (Morrissy, 1990). It occurs twice as often in males as in females. The exact cause of idiopathic clubfoot is unclear, although there is some genetic predisposition. Numerous theories have been proposed, but the most likely cause is multifactorial. Both positioning in utero and inherited genes play a part in the development of idiopathic clubfoot. Clubfoot also can be seen as part of a syndrome complex or in a child with a neuromuscular disorder such as myelomeningocele.

Pathophysiology

Clubfoot, usually obvious at birth, can be unilateral or bilateral. The main anatomic components of clubfoot are a flexed ankle, a turning in of the heel, and adduction of the forefoot (Fig. 20–6). If clubfoot is left untreated and the child tries to walk, the parent describes the effort as "walking on the side of his foot." Atrophy of muscles in the lower leg and contractures of the joint capsules in the foot occur.

Figure 20–6
The child with clubfoot has a flexed ankle, a turned heel, and an adducted forefoot.

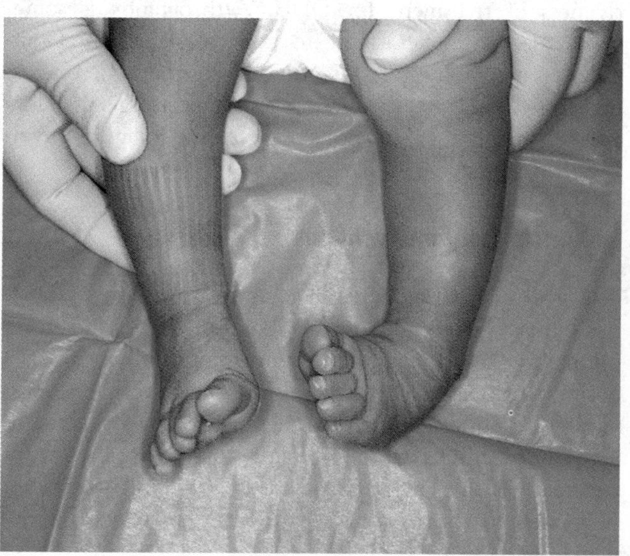

Prognosis. Regardless of the degree of severity of the clubfoot, starting treatment shortly after birth improves prognosis. The desired outcome for a child with clubfoot is to straighten the foot so that it can develop normally. However, the child's foot and lower leg are never entirely "normal," because the anatomic abnormalities result in a slightly smaller foot and underdeveloped calf muscles.

Interdisciplinary Interventions

Successful treatment of clubfoot may require only serial manipulation and casting in the physician's office. The ligaments of the foot in a newborn are elastic and easily stretch with gentle pressure. Serial casting consists of holding the foot in the most correct position possible and maintaining that position by the application of a plaster cast. Plaster is preferred over fiberglass because it molds easily. Treatment begins immediately after the diagnosis of clubfoot. The child has weekly cast changes for 1 month, then every 2 weeks until the foot is straight. This process usually takes months to achieve correction. If the child's foot reaches a point where it does not continue to improve, surgery is suggested.

Several surgical techniques can be used to correct clubfoot. Most involve cutting tight tendons and ligaments. Pins are also placed in the foot to keep it in alignment until it is healed. This is preferably a one-stage procedure performed before the child starts to walk (at about age 6 to 8 months). Surgery requires a brief hospitalization. Nursing care includes postoperative pain management, neurovascular assessment of the involved foot, and cast care teaching for the parents. After surgery, a cast is applied for 6 weeks, then the physician removes the cast and the pins and applies a new cast for 6 more weeks. After the last cast is removed, further treatment is not required if the surgery has been successful.

Developmental Dysplasia of the Hip

For many years, the term "congenital dislocated hip" (CDH), or congenital hip dysplasia, was used to describe a child with various abnormalities of the hip. More recently, the term "developmental dysplasia of the hip," or DDH, has been used to more accurately describe a problem that may result in a hip that is not normal (Jonides, Rudy, & Walsh, 1996; Wenger & Rang, 1993). The hip may be dislocated, dislocatable, or subluxable. In the case of hip subluxation, the head of the femur is in the socket but it is not concentrically located. A hip that is dislocatable can be displaced outside of the acetabulum or hip socket when placing the hip in certain positions. Hip dislocation occurs when the head of the femur lies outside of the acetabulum. Hip dislocation can occur in neonates or in the first few months of life; thus, the term "congenital" can be misleading. Also, "dislocated" does not describe hips that are merely unstable, nor does it indicate the presentation of a malformed acetabulum.

Etiology and Incidence

The etiology of DDH is multifactorial. Both environmental and genetic factors play a role in the development of DDH. Ligamentous laxity, either familial or induced by the maternal hormone estrogen, makes a definite contribution to DDH. Positioning in utero, especially the breech position, is a risk factor for DDH.

Worldview: *Another causal factor for DDH is postnatal positioning of the baby in a cradle board with the legs extended, such as is the custom in some Native American Indian and Canadian Eskimo cultures. In cultures in which babies are held on a person's backs or hips in a wide, abducted straddle position (the Far East and Africa), the incidence of DDH is rare (Speers & Speers, 1992).*

The incidence of DDH in live births is 1 in 1000, and it occurs more frequently in females. Postnatally, neonates are screened in the hospital before they go home. However, DDH is not always detectable at birth, or it may go undetected if the birth occurred without the presence of a skilled health care practitioner. Also, screening for this condition is highly dependent on the practitioner's skill. Early detection and treatment of DDH improve the odds for successful management.

Pathophysiology

In the newborn phase of DDH, the hips can be easily dislocated and then reduced back into position by the examiner or simply by the baby's spontaneous movements. At this stage, anatomic changes or muscle contractures do not occur. As the child grows with a dislocated hip, changes in the developing bones and muscles around the hip evolve. The result of a long-standing dislocation is the formation of degenerative changes in the head of the femur and the acetabulum. These children usually walk with a pronounced limp and have a leg-length discrepancy. However, this can be avoided with early recognition and prompt treatment.

Assessment

During early infancy, the physical findings for DDH may vary widely, depending on whether the hip is dysplastic, subluxable, or dislocated. The two classic assessment maneuvers for DDH are the Barlow and the Ortolani maneuvers. Both maneuvers are difficult to perform on a crying, tense infant and, even in the best of circumstances, an unstable hip can be missed (see Chapter 6 for illustration and explanation of these maneuvers). In children between ages 3 and 12 months, the Ortolani and Barlow signs are lost because of the tightening of soft tissue structures (Masear, 1996). During this period of time, hips that are well reduced stay in position, and those that are dislocated are fixed in their dislocated position.

caREminder: *If a child's hip is known to be dislocated, do not repeatedly assess it because there is an increased risk of causing vascular compromise.*

Other presumptive physical signs suggest DDH in a neonate. These include asymmetrical lower extremity skin creases, an apparent discrepancy in limb length (Galeazzi sign, Allis' sign), and limited abduction of the flexed thigh on either side. Skin creases can best be visualized by laying the infant on his or her back and holding the legs straight up in the air.

Radiologic evaluation of the newborn hip can be misleading and inconclusive. The newborn pelvis consists largely of cartilage and thus cannot be visualized well on a routine x-ray examination. However, because radiographs may show abnormalities and serve to establish a baseline, they are routinely performed.

Recently, ultrasound of the newborn hip has come into the forefront as a diagnostic tool. It is more sensitive in detecting subluxations and dislocations than a traditional radiograph (Rudy, 1996). In infants up to age 6 months, the lack of ossification centers in the bone makes it difficult to visualize the head of the femur with radiography. At approximately age 6 months, secondary ossification centers develop in the hip. Once these appear, radiography can be used as the standard diagnostic tool to confirm a diagnosis or monitor progress of DDH. Clinician manual assessment is still the most reliable indicator of hip positioning.

Other technologies can be used to assess the effectiveness of treatment for DDH. Arthrography is sometimes used intraoperatively to confirm reduction. Computed tomography (CT) scans and magnetic resonance imaging (MRI) are useful to confirm postsurgical reduction, although they are not cost-effective for initial evaluations (Shoppee, 1992).

Interdisciplinary Interventions

The goal of treatment of DDH is to reduce the femoral head into the acetabulum so that the hip can develop normally. This is facilitated by maintaining the hips in a position of flexion and abduction, usually with one of a variety of splints. When the diagnosis of DDH is made in a newborn child, the splint most commonly chosen for treatment is the Pavlik harness (Fig. 20–7). This harness is applied to the hips at 90 degrees flexion and 70 de-

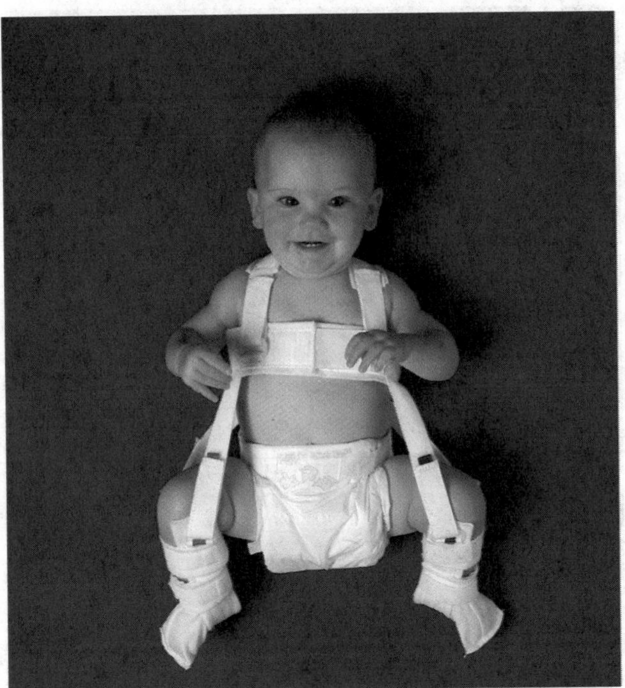

Figure 20–7
The Pavlik harness is used to maintain the hips in a position of flexion and abduction. (Wheaton Pavlik Harness. Courtesy of Wheaton Brace Co.)

grees abduction (Speers & Speers, 1992). In the abducted position, the weight of the lower extremities works to stretch the adductor muscles and consequently allow the dislocated femoral head to slide anteriorly over the acetabular rim and into the acetabulum (Speers & Speers, 1992). The child wears the Pavlik harness continually for 3 to 6 months, gradually decreasing wearing time to nighttime use only. Some physicians allow parents to remove the harness for bathing. The decision to allow this alteration in care is based on the severity of the child's dislocation and the ability of the parents to learn how to correctly reapply the harness.

The Pavlik harness not only maintains the position of the hip but also allows some movement of the lower extremities. A potential complication of the harness is avascular necrosis of the femoral head. Positioning the femoral head in extreme flexion or abduction restricts the blood supply to the femoral head. This complication can be avoided by properly fitting the harness, educating parents, and providing weekly or biweekly checkups in the physician's office.

If the Pavlik harness is not successful in reducing the hip, or if the child is between ages 2 and 6 months when diagnosed, the next step in treatment is traction. Bryant's traction aims to stretch some of the soft tissues around the hip so that it can be reduced (see Table 20–4). After 1 to 3 weeks in traction, the child is taken to the operating room, where the hip is reduced manually and a hip spica cast is applied (see Table 20–3). Often an arthrogram is done at the same time to confirm reduction of the hip. A percutaneous adductor tenotomy can be done at this time. This consists of cutting an adductor tendon of the hip to decrease the risk of avascular necrosis and increase range of motion of the hip. Pain management after the tenotomy consists of a narcotic given as needed for the first day; thereafter, acetaminophen is usually sufficient for discomfort. The incision from the tenotomy is short and is covered by the cast.

The physician reapplies the hip spica cast every 6 to 8 weeks because of the child's growth and softening of the cast.

caREminder: *Unless the crossbar (as found in some spica casts) has been specifically reinforced so that it can be used for lifting or turning, do not use it for these purposes. Check with the physician or orthopedic technician if you are unsure about the safety of using the crossbar.*

The total time for cast treatment usually ranges from 3 to 6 months (see Treatment Modalities for information regarding cast care). Afterward, the child is maintained in an abduction brace until the hip is clinically and radiologically normal.

Despite early diagnosis and treatment with the Pavlik harness, traction, and closed reduction, some children require an open hip procedure. Older children need open hip reduction, because their dislocation produces secondary changes in the shape of the hip. These changes are only corrected with a surgical procedure to recreate a socket that is similar to a normal hip joint.

An open reduction of the hip consists of an osteotomy of the acetabulum or femur and removal of soft tissues. This operation cuts the bone and realigns it, allowing the hip to be concentrically placed so that it can continue to grow correctly as the child ages. After an open reduction, the child is placed in a hip spica cast for 6 to 8 weeks and then in an abduction splint for up to 3 more months. This type of surgery is painful and children generally are in the hospital for 2 to 3 days after surgery. Intravenous narcotics are required for the first day after surgery and oral narcotics are often needed for several days after surgery. The nurse can reassure the parent that the incision will heal although it is under the cast.

Although they are rare, complications from DDH and its treatment do occur. One common complication is lack of concentric reduction that necessitates further operative procedures. Avascular necrosis, or loss of blood supply to all or part of the head of the femur, is another complication that can be caused by forced reduction and abduction.

Community Care

Beginning in the outpatient setting, the nurse's key concerns are educating and supporting the parents. After diagnosis, the family often expresses shock and denial because the baby looks "fine" to them. Parents are reluctant to hold the baby or change a diaper for fear of hurting the hip. Also, mothers tend to blame themselves for causing the dislocated hip. Seeing a small baby placed in a Pavlik harness for the first time can be upsetting. Once the parents realize that the harness does not hurt the child and the baby can still move, they feel better (Chart 20–13).

If the diagnosis of DDH is made when the child is older, the parents often become angry with their health care provider for not finding the disorder earlier. The stress may be compounded by hospitalization of the child for 2 weeks in Bryant's traction, followed by surgery and a body cast for up to 6 months.

Once the plan of treatment is established, the nurse instructs the parent on proper placement of the Pavlik harness, skin care, and other activities of daily living such as diaper changing (TIP 20–2). Community resources may be enlisted to help the family with frequent transportation between the home and clinic, if needed. Children do not need specialized transportation unless they cannot fit into a car.

Additional parental education and modifications to the home environment are necessary if the child is placed in a spica cast. Before surgery, the parents need to be prepared for how the child's lower extremities are placed and how the cast is applied to ensure abduction of the hips. Other elements that are taught include handling the child in a cast, petaling or waterproofing the cast, and feeding, dressing, and bathing the child in a cast (see TIP 20–1). Car seats and high chairs may be unusable or may need modification for a child with a spica cast. For infants, a bouncing seat can be used as a feeding chair and car seats can be purchased or rented that have been adapted for children in hip spica casts (see Resources). Strollers, wagons, or reclining wheelchairs provide mobility for the child.

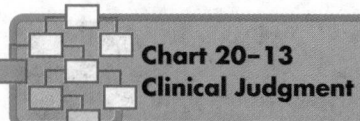

Chart 20–13
Clinical Judgment

The Child with Developmental Dysplasia of the Hip

Lauren is a 2-month-old female who comes to the community health clinic with her mother for her immunizations. During her physical examination, you note that the fat folds in her thighs are not even. When interviewing the mother for the birth history, she says that Lauren is her first child and that she was delivered via cesarean section because of her breech presentation.

Questions

1. During your assessment, what other information would help you to determine the problem?
2. What diagnostic studies would help you to determine the problem?
3. The mother is upset that the condition has not been noted sooner. What could you say to her at this time?
4. How can developmental dysplasia of the hip (DDH) be treated?
5. How would you determine that the harness is keeping the hip in the correct position?

Answers

1. Is there any family history of DDH or of joint laxity? Were Lauren's hips examined at birth or at any other time before this visit?
2. Ultrasound of the hip, possibly a plain radiograph. Ortolani and Barlow maneuvers would help to confirm the diagnosis.
3. The condition can be missed in the initial assessment of the child. Now that it has been noted, corrective therapy can begin, and the child should have very good outcome.
4. Use the Pavlik harness for a few months. If this does not work, traction and casting, or possibly surgery, may be needed.
5. Ultrasound of the hip or a plain radiograph of the child while she is in the Pavlik harness.

Congenital Limb Defects

Congenital malformations of the limbs are typically classified into seven categories (Table 20–8). The incidence of congenital limb defects varies with the disorder. Syndactyly, or webbing of two digits, is common, as is polydactyly (Tachdjian, 1990) (Fig. 20–8). These malformations have been associated with other syndromes, such as trisomy 13, trisomy 18, trisomy 21, Carpenter's syndrome, and orofaciodigital syndrome, to name a few. Some deformations are rare. For example, proximal femoral focal deficiency (PFFD), a localized absence of the proximal end of the femur that occurs bilaterally or unilaterally, is very rare. The severity of PFFD ranges from a short femur to absence of a femoral head. A high incidence of other anomalies is associated with PFFD.

Interdisciplinary Interventions

No standard interventions or treatments have been identified for congenital limb defects. If the child is function-

TIP 20–2 A Teaching Intervention Plan for the Child with a Pavlik Harness

Nursing Diagnoses and Family Outcomes

- Knowledge deficit: home care of the child wearing a Pavlik harness
  Outcome:
  Parents will demonstrate measures to care for the child wearing a Pavlik harness.
- Potential impairment of skin integrity related to the presence of the Pavlik harness
  Outcomes:
  Parents will demonstrate skin care techniques appropriate for use with the Pavlik harness.
  Child will have no skin breakdown.

Interventions

Teach the Family

- Positioning of the Harness
  - Explain the purpose and function of Pavlik harness.
  - The harness must be kept on the child at all times until the hip is stable (unless otherwise instructed by the physician). For this reason, only one harness is distributed and it is applied at the physician's office or clinic.
  - Buckles may loosen or become detached. Demonstrate how to correctly reattach the buckles and straps of harness.
  - Use indelible ink to make black lines to show where the straps should pass through the buckles.
  - Letter-code matching straps to their respective buckles.
  - Fasten diaper tapes under the straps to prevent any pull on the straps.
- Care of the Harness
  - Sponge the harness clean with mild soap if it becomes soiled.
  - If needed, the harness can be placed in the washing machine for cleaning on cold water/gentle cycle and then line-dried. This necessitates that a second harness be obtained and placed on the child by a person trained to do so.
  - The harness should not be removed by the family members unless otherwise instructed by a health care provider.
- Skin Care
  - Give the child a daily sponge bath, paying close attention to the skin under the straps and stirrups.
  - Check the skin under the harness daily for irritation, and gently massage the skin to stimulate circulation.
  - Do not use powders or lotions that will cake and irritate the skin.
  - Padding beneath the shoulder straps can be used to prevent discomfort at pressure points.
  - Shoulder straps can be unfastened to slip a shirt on the child. This should not affect hip position.
  - The harness does not affect perineal care because there are no straps covering that area. The legs should not be pulled when the diapers are changed because of the possibility of forced dislocation. Instead the child should be lifted from under the buttocks with the diaper slid under the bottom.
  - The use of disposable diapers with elastic around the legs is recommended to prevent the brace from becoming wet or soiled.

Contact Health Care Provider if

The harness becomes heavily soiled and needs to be replaced.
The skin underneath the harness becomes red or swollen or if areas of skin breakdown are noted.
The child appears to be in pain.
The harness comes off.

Table 20–8
Classification of Congenital Limb Malformations

Disorders	Example
Failure of formation of parts (arrest of development)	Absent right upper limb Absent femur Absent skull bones (or dysplastic)
Failure of differentiation (separation of parts)	Syndactyly Sprengel's deformity (congenital high scapula)
Duplication	Polydactyly Macrodactyly
Overgrowth (gigantism)	All or part of a finger is much larger than the other
Undergrowth	Small limb Skull bones
Congenital constriction band syndrome	Limb appears to have a rubber band tied tightly around it
Generalized skeletal abnormalities	Unique to each syndrome (e.g., Apert's syndrome results in webbing of toes and fingers)

Adapted from Tachdjian, M. O. (1990). *Pediatric orthopedics.* Philadelphia: W. B. Saunders. Used with permission.

ing well, no treatment interventions may be instituted. Many children with limb deformities learn to adapt to their condition and do not consider themselves limited in performing any normal developmental skills and abilities (Fig. 20–9). A limb deformity does not necessarily prohibit a child from participating in any age-appropriate activities. As the child matures, parents should be encouraged to support the child's independence and self-care abilities.

Figure 20–8
This infant with polydactyly has additional toes on each foot.

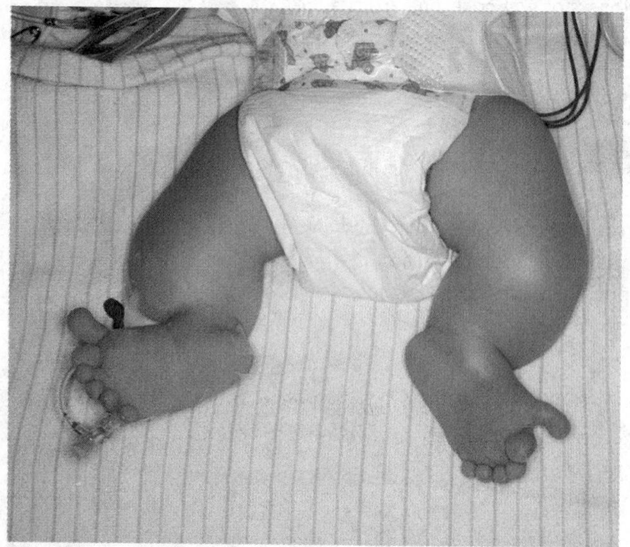

Prosthetics may be selected to equalize limb lengths, correct malrotation, and improve body mechanics. A prosthesis is expensive and requires maintenance. In the growing child, the prosthetic device must be replaced every year until age 5. Thereafter, annual assessment determines when the size of the prosthesis needs to be altered again. Some families choose not to obtain the prosthesis and to teach the child to function without it.

Surgical procedures are used to create a stump that is amenable to prosthetic fitting, to lengthen a deficient bone, or to improve limb function. In some cases, the defect can be repaired with a minor surgical procedure. Children with more severe defects may need several corrective procedures over a span of time. The ultimate goal of surgery is to provide the child with a limb that has good function and appearance. Function usually takes precedence: a hand that looks good but does not work correctly is of little help to the child. Rehabilitative services will be used to optimize function of the limb after surgery.

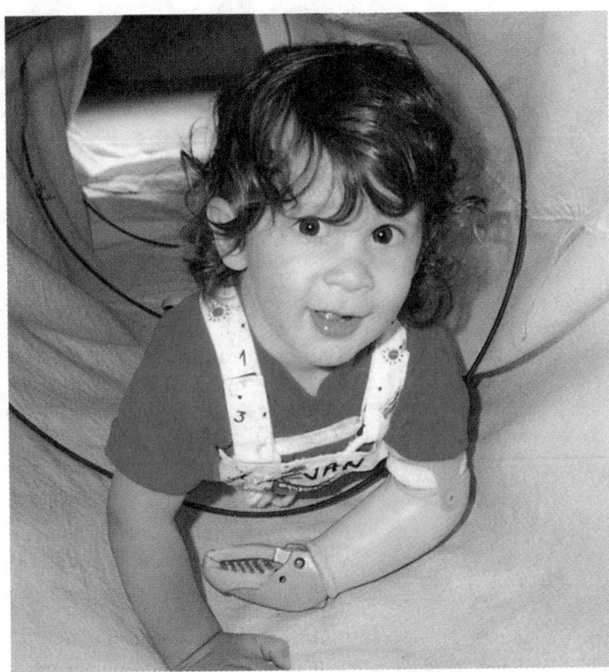

Figure 20–9
The child with a limb deformity should be encouraged to participate in age-appropriate activities to the limit of his or her abilities.

Community Care

The nurse helps to coordinate needed health care services and provide teaching to the family regarding the child's care. If the child has a prosthesis, the family must learn to assess the skin for signs of redness and irritation. The child is most likely to experience these complications when a new brace or prosthesis is being worn. If a particular area of the skin becomes irritated, the brace or prosthesis should be adjusted. Wear may need to be discontinued for a period of time in cases of severe skin breakdown. Lotions or oils should not be applied to the stump. Rubbing alcohol can be applied to toughen the skin. The child is encouraged to wear a cotton sock or other piece of clothing underneath the brace or prosthesis to absorb the moisture from perspiration.

Physical and occupational therapy can assist the child to become independent in activities of daily living and in the use of a prosthesis. Social services can provide the family with information regarding where to obtain assistive devices, alternative funding opportunities, and support groups.

Osteogenesis Imperfecta

Often referred to as "brittle bone disease," OI is the most common genetic disorder of the bone. OI is not just one disorder; rather, it is a group of similar hereditary diseases characterized by excessive bone fragility with an increased tendency to fracture (Gertner & Root, 1990). OI occurs in all races and is equally prevalent in males and females. The incidence per live births ranges from 1 in 20,000 to 1 in 50,000, varying with the type of OI (Stoltz, Dietrich, & Marshall, 1989).

Etiology

Workers in biochemical research are investigating the origin of OI, which is still unclear. In most cases, inheritance is autosomal dominant, although in some cases it is a result of new mutation.

Pathophysiology

In OI, a biochemical defect causes a reduction in the synthesis of collagen (Bender, 1991). It affects all connective tissues in the body, resulting in lax joints and small, weak muscles; this leads to an increased incidence of fractures whenever undue stress is placed on the bone. Fractures heal within the normal range of time, but without normal strength. Bone deformities occur as a result of fractures or as a result of bowing and growth pattern disturbances. Some affected newborns die of complications caused by the extreme fragility of the bones. Other children may have severe bone involvement during childhood that spontaneously improves during the adolescent years.

Assessment

Reliable prenatal diagnosis of OI is not available. Assessment and subsequent diagnosis is usually based on the severity of the clinical signs and the level of disability. OI is classified into four types, based on the severity and mode of genetic transmission (Table 20–9). A unique feature of a fracture in a child with OI is lack of bruising or swelling at the fracture site. However, the child has tenderness at the site of the fracture. Laboratory studies are not useful in diagnosing OI, although a skin biopsy can confirm the diagnosis. Radiographs reveal multiple normal callus formations at new fracture sites, generalized osteopenia (insufficiency of the bone), evidence of previous fractures, and skeletal deformities.

caREminder: *When the child is first noted to have multiple fractures, accusations of child abuse may be made by people who are not familiar with OI. Health care providers must be sensitive to this differential diagnosis if a young child is admitted with frequent fractures.*

As they grow older, many children are disabled by their severe deformities. Social development may be delayed because of increased dependence on parents and

Table 20–9
Characteristics of Osteogenesis Imperfecta

Type	Genetic Transmission	Blue Sclerae	Bone Fragility and Skeletal Deformities	Hearing Loss	Yellow or Gray-Blue Transparent Teeth	Other Characteristics
I	Autosomal dominant	Present	Severe with marked spontaneous reduction in fractures during adolescence	Onset between ages 20 and 30	Present in some cases	Genu valgum Flat feet with metatarsus varus Kyphosis in adults Excessive hyperlaxity of ligaments Mild short stature
II	Autosomal dominant mutations Some autosomal recessive	Unknown	Lethal	Absent	Unknown	Stillbirth in 50% Thin and fragile skin Multiple rib fractures Diffuse osteopenia in face and skull Beaklike nose Limbs short, bent, and deformed
III	Autosomal recessive	Blue at birth and less blue with age	Severe	Absent	Absent	Death in childhood Fractures present at birth Development of kyphoscoliosis during childhood Skull deformity Short stature Generalized osteopenia Diaphoresis
IV	Autosomal dominant	Blue at birth and less blue with age	Variable age of onset of fractures and degree of deformity Spontaneous improvement during adolescence	Less common	Present	Bowing of lower limbs Generalized osteopenia

decreased social interactions. Children with OI have normal intelligence.

Interdisciplinary Interventions

There is no effective intervention for the child with OI II. In all other cases, the management goals focus on preventing injury and providing prompt and aggressive orthopedic management. Interventions focus on early treatment and correction of fractures or bowing and bending of the bones to maximize mobility and prevent deformities. Fractures are a part of life for these children and complete elimination of them is not realistic. Acute management of a fracture consists of precise alignment to prevent deformity and application of lightweight immobilization. Early return to weight-bearing activity is crucial to stimulate formation of new bone. Often, splints and braces are used on the lower extremities to assist with ambulation and to protect against fractures (see Treatment Modalities for brace and splint care).

Children with OI often require surgery to reduce fractures, correct spinal deformities, and straighten long bones. A common procedure is intramedullary rodding. These rods can be solid or telescoping rods. Solid rods are easier to insert but they do not "grow" with the child and must be replaced every 2 to 4 years. Telescoping rods require more extensive surgery but they can be adjusted as the child grows. Placement of the rods is not a perfect solution. However, intramedullary rodding can provide stability to a deformed bone and assist in the prevention of progressive deformities.

Postoperative care includes pain management, neuro-

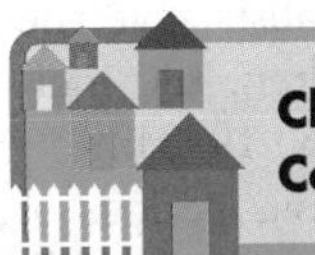

Chart 20–14
Community Care

Recommendations to Promote Health and Safety for the Child with Osteogenesis Imperfecta

In the Home

Active range-of-motion exercises are encouraged for children of all ages.
When moving the child, no jerking or pulling should be used. The child should be allowed to move independently whenever possible.
Watch for signs of a fracture, which include pain, swelling, or deformity at the site.
The child should wear rubber-soled shoes to assist with traction while ambulating.
Throw rugs should be removed from the floors to help prevent falls.
Toys placed on the floor should be monitored to prevent the child from tripping on them.
If a wheelchair is needed, the home may need ramps installed to permit easy transportation.
The child should be encouraged to do as much as possible.
The Osteogenesis Imperfecta Foundation has literature, support groups, social gatherings, and conferences for the children and their family members.

In the School

Children should attend regular school if possible.
Home tutors should be arranged during periods of hospitalization and home recovery.
Contact sports should be strongly discouraged.
Swimming, arts, crafts, and computer activities should be recommended.
Body image disturbances are common. School staff can assist in evaluating the child's acceptance of self and acceptance by others and provide interventions to support positive peer interactions.
Hearing should be evaluated annually to ensure that no loss has occurred, which may affect school performance.

After an Injury

If the parent or child suspects a fracture, the child should see a health care provider immediately.
Before transportation of the child, the suspected affected area should be immobilized.
Treatment measures instituted by the health care team (e.g., splinting, braces) should be used until follow-up care reveals no further need for these interventions.
Acetaminophen may be ordered for pain after an injury.

Dietary Needs

Inactivity and short stature may lead to obesity. Therefore, a low-fat, high-fiber diet, with reduced number of calories, may be recommended.
Adequate fluid intake should be encouraged to prevent dehydration from increased diaphoresis.

Oral Care

Yearly dental checkups are imperative. Teeth are frequently prematurely eroded or broken. Teeth may need to be capped.
Dental care should be provided after every meal.

Skin Care

Because of the problems with diaphoresis, the child should wear lightweight clothes that allow ventilation.
A sheepskin or softly padded mattress is suggested.

vascular checks, and special attention to hydration. Children with OI have excessive loss of fluid through the skin. Preoperative intravenous fluids must be administered and adequate hydration must be ensured throughout hospitalization.

Physical therapy is a mainstay of treatment for children with OI. On diagnosis, physical therapy focuses on range-of-motion and muscle-strengthening exercises. After a fracture has occurred or after surgical intervention, the physical therapist assists the child to regain mobility of the affected skeletal area. The presence of deformities may necessitate the child's use of ambulatory devices such as a walker or a wheelchair. The physical therapist ensures that the child can use the device safely.

Community Care

Most families are unaware of the different types of OI, of the prognosis for the disorder, and of the special care needs of a child with OI. Genetic counseling is aimed at primary prevention (Hall, 1996). Parents are anxious about the possibility of causing a fracture in their child. Information given to parents should be specific to the child's type of OI. Specific instructions on how to hold, change, and position the infant to reduce fractures help to decrease anxiety. Parents of children with OI must achieve a delicate balance between protecting the child and allowing the child to have normal life experiences (Chart 20–14).

caREminder: *Signs of a fracture, especially in an infant, are important items to teach caregivers. In a baby, these signs are general symptoms such as fever, irritability, and refusal to eat (Bender, 1991).*

Older children with OI become aware that if they injure themselves, they need to be evaluated for a possible fracture. Symptoms of a fracture in an older child include pain, swelling, and possibly deformity at the site.

Cerebral Palsy

CP is a term used to describe a group of disorders of movement and posture that are caused by a non-progressive abnormality or injury occurring to the developing brain. The injury may occur before, during, or after birth, usually before age 5 years. CP results in disturbances of voluntary muscle movement and posture, and may be accompanied by mental retardation of varying degrees (Davis, 1997; Maher et al., 1994).

The incidence of CP is between 1.2 and 2.7 per 1000 live births, with an increase of CP noted in the past decade in very-low-birth-weight babies (Davis, 1997; Palmer & Hoon, 1995). As the birth weight of the baby increases, the risk of CP decreases. Whereas some statistics indicate a decreased incidence of CP with improved neonatal and perinatal care, other factors indicate that, as pediatric and neonatal health care specialists save the lives of more seriously ill infants and children, the incidence of CP is increasing (Eicher & Batshaw, 1993).

Causes of CP can be identified at various periods of development, including prenatal, perinatal, and early childhood (Chart 20–15). Many cases of CP have no known cause.

Pathophysiology

The precise pathophysiology of CP is not known. In some cases, a specific lesion or area of infarct in the

Chart 20–15

Etiology of Cerebral Palsy

Prenatal

Teratogen
Genetic syndromes/chromosomal abnormalities
Brain malformation
Intrauterine infections (i.e., toxoplasmosis, syphilis, rubella, cytomegalovirus)
Problems in fetal/placental function
Maternal factors (e.g., Rh incompatibility, diabetes, anoxia, anemia, hypotension, toxemia, trauma)

Labor and Delivery

Pre-eclampsia
Complications of labor and delivery (e.g., prolapsed cord, placental abruption)

Perinatal

Sepsis/central nervous system infection
Asphyxia
Prematurity

Childhood

Meningitis/encephalitis
Traumatic brain injury
Carbon monoxide poisoning/toxins
Respiratory distress syndrome
Respiratory obstruction/foreign body
Drowning
Insulin reaction
Brain abscess
Granuloma
Hemorrhage
Embolus/thrombus

Data from Hagberg, B., & Hagberg, G. (1984). Prenatal and perinatal risk factors in a survey of 681 Swedish cases. In F. Stanley & E. Alberman (Eds.), *The epidemiology of the cerebral palsied* (pp. 116–134). Philadelphia: J. B. Lippincott.

brain cannot be found. Often, no specific pathophysiology can be demonstrated. The patterns of dysfunction seen in the child are related to whether damage is limited to one area of the brain, is scattered in multiple areas, or is unilateral or bilateral. Dysfunction is also related to the cause of the damage and the stage of development of the brain at the time of injury. In all cases, the lesion cannot be repaired, although it does not worsen. However, as the child grows, motor and nonmotor manifestations such as scoliosis and muscle contractures may become more disabling.

The essential motor problem in CP is lack of control of the muscles. The lack of control is usually related to a failure to inhibit specific reflexes of the central nervous system (CNS). The reflexes involving muscle movement are stretch, crossed extension, long spinal, symmetrical tonic neck, asymmetrical tonic neck, vestibular, and startle. Each of these is normally present in infancy. As development progresses, these reflexes normally fade or are inhibited. Injury to an area of the brain may cause these reflexes to persist, barring control of muscle movement. Without control of these movements, functional ability is lost or cannot be attained.

Children with CP are classified by the area most affected and by description of involvement (Table 20–10). The area of involvement refers to the extremity that is affected. Children with CP often have other physical abnormalities such as seizures; vision, hearing, or speech deficits; difficulty with feeding; and learning difficulties (Chart 20–16). Intelligence may be average or below average. These associated deficits reflect the fact that motor areas of the brain work together, and rarely is a specific area affected in isolation (Palmer & Hoon, 1995).

Assessment

Developmental surveillance is a key part of the assessment of a child with CP. Often, CP cannot be diagnosed until the child is 6 to 12 months old, a time when the

Table 20–10
Types of Cerebral Palsy

Type	Incidence	Characteristics
Spastic type	65%	Increased muscle tone with clasp knife character Increased deep tendon reflexes Pathologic reflexes Spastic weakness Difficulty with fine and gross motor skills Muscle contractures common Scoliosis
Hemiplegia	30%	Primary unilateral involvement, often with the arm more involved than the leg
Quadriplegia	5%	Four-limb involvement, with legs more involved than arms, although legs still show substantial involvement
Diplegia	30%	Four-limb involvement, with legs more involved than arms; arms may have only minimal impairment and no functional handicaps
Athetoid type	20%	Purposeless, involuntary, uncontrollable movements of face and extremities Fluctuating muscle tone Deep tendon reflexes and movements increase with stress and voluntary movements; deep tendon reflexes are absent during sleep. Symmetrical four-limb involvement
Ataxic type	5%	Disturbed coordination Unsteady gait Hypotonic muscles Slurred speech In general, good motor prognosis
Mixed type	10%	Usually a mixture of spastic athetoid types

Chart 20–16

Deficits Associated with Cerebral Palsy

Musculoskeletal and Reflexive Deficits

Hypotonia
Spastic hypertonia
Hypertonus—lead-pipe rigidity that can be "shaken out" by rapid movements of the extremities
Persistent primitive reflexes
Contractures
Osteoporosis
Scoliosis

Neurologic Deficits

Mental retardation (30% to 77%)
Language disorder (approximately 40%)
Learning disability (approximately 40%)
Range of neurobehavioral disorders (up to 50%)—attention deficit hyperactivity, autism, hyperkinetic or distractable behavior
Visual disorders (50% to 90%)
Hearing disorders (10%)
Somatosensation (up to 50% of hemiplegia)
Seizures (30% to 40%)

Gastrointestinal and Nutritional Problems

Drooling
Malnutrition
Bowel and bladder incontinence
Constipation

Other Systemic Complications

Growth failure
Genitourinary complaints
Respiratory infections
Fatigue

child's inability to achieve a developmental milestone becomes more evident.

The physical examination concentrates on range of motion, evaluation of muscle strength and tone, and presence of abnormal movements and contractures.

caREminder: *Reflexes that persist beyond the expected age of disappearance (e.g., tonic neck reflex) or the absence of expected reflexes is highly suggestive of CP.*

Presenting concerns may include poor hand control, generalized hypotonia, hypertonia (especially during activities such as bathing), early preferential hand use, absent weight-bearing activity, and feeding difficulties (Palmer & Hoon, 1995). Other causes, such as a metabolic disturbance or a brain or spinal cord lesion, must be ruled out before a definitive diagnosis of CP is made. These causes are likely to show evidence of the child's condition becoming progressively worse, as opposed to CP, in which the child's status seems static.

Diagnostic Tests. Neuroimaging tests can be performed on the child with CP to determine the site of the brain impairment and to give clues as to the potential cause. The results of these tests do not affect the child's treatment. Other diagnostic tests may be performed to rule out other potential causes of the child's current condition. These tests include cytogenic studies (genetic evaluation of the child and other family members) and metabolic studies.

Nursing Diagnoses and Outcomes

Nursing diagnoses applicable to the child with a musculoskeletal disorder are presented in Chart 20–5. The physical disabilities and impaired neuromuscular status of the child with CP can be recognized through diagnoses that focus on impaired physical mobility, skin integrity, and neurovascular function. Additionally, the child with CP experiences difficulty in self-care activities as a result of physical and cognitive limitations. The nursing diagnosis should also reflect the strain and stress on family members as they relate to a child with a lifelong disability. In addition to these considerations, the following diagnoses could apply to the child with CP:

- **Impaired verbal communication**
  Outcomes: The child will communicate and express his or her needs as much as possible.
  The child will communicate needs and desires without undue frustration.
  The child will use alternative means of communicating, including the use of adaptive equipment, as needed and as able.
- **Altered nutrition: Less than body requirements related to inability to ingest food or retain food in the presence of gastroesophageal reflux**
  Outcomes: The child will receive optimal nutrition to maintain ideal body weight.
  The child will tolerate gastrostomy tube feedings if needed to maintain ideal body weight.

Interdisciplinary Interventions

CP is not a correctable disorder; thus, interventions focus on preventing or minimizing deformities and maximizing the child's functioning in the home, school, and community. This is accomplished by providing the child and the family with an integrated health care plan using the expertise of a variety of professionals. The health care team works to maximize the child's potential, considering neurologic and other impairments. The child is encouraged to learn to function independently. The team also assists the parents in dealing with their child's limitations and learning methods to support their child's unique needs.

Orthopedic Management

Orthopedic evaluation is needed in any child with limited range of motion. Orthopedic treatment generally consists of conservative measures such as bracing. Braces provide support for ambulation and discourage contractures. If contractures do develop, orthopedic surgery may be indicated. Various muscle releases and tendon transfers can be done to correct or to relieve the contracture. For example, because of muscle pull imbalances, a subluxated or dislocated hip frequently develops in children with CP. This can lead to pain and problems with sitting. To correct this problem, a hip osteotomy and release of soft tissues and tight tendons may be performed to hold the hip in place. Scoliosis is another result of muscle pull imbalances in children with CP. If not treated, scoliosis may cause lung compression, loss of ambulation, or inability to sit. Spinal stabilization with instrumentation can greatly improve or stop the progression of scoliosis.

Neurosurgical Interventions

Selective dorsal rhizotomy is a recently developed surgical procedure for children with CP and lower extremity spasticity. A neurosurgeon identifies and selectively divides certain sensory nerve rootlets that cause spasticity. After cutting the rootlets, the child should have decreased tone, less chance of contractures, and increased normal movements. Rhizotomy is not a cure for CP, but it can improve the gait of those children who are ambulatory, and it can ease sitting, positioning, and other activities of daily living for those children who are wheelchair-bound. "Ideal" candidates for rhizotomy are 3 to 6 years old, have no contractures or deformities, are age-appropriate mentally, and have little or no ataxic or athetoid components to their CP (Philichi & Brunn, 1990). The family's ability to follow through with frequent physical therapy is another important factor to consider. Rhizotomy requires extensive physical therapy for 1 year, and long-term outcomes are not yet known. Complications may include paralysis, incontinence, poor muscle tone, and infection.

Pain Management

Pain management is a complex area in the care of the child with CP. Although narcotics are useful for incisional pain after surgery, they do not ease muscle spasms. Because of positioning and immobilization in casts, children with CP have more problems with muscle spasms than other children. Muscle relaxants, such as diazepam or other benzodiazepines (e.g., clonazepam), can be administered along with narcotics to relieve discomfort.

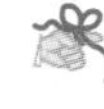
caREminder: *Undermedication of children with CP is common because of their communication difficulties. Careful assessment of non-verbal pain cues is necessary (see Chapter 13). Epidural analgesia is a good option for pain management in children with CP who have had lower extremity surgery. Administration of a constant infusion maintains a steady level of analgesia. Epidurals are helpful in non-verbal children with CP.*

Community Care

Acute care of the child with CP is usually only necessary during initial evaluation, to perform surgical procedures to deal with mobility or nutritional issues, or to provide supportive care during serious illnesses such as pneumonia, dehydration, or systemic infection. To optimize the child's level of functioning and provide for the child's basic health care needs, orthopedic and neurosurgical services collaborate with a variety of other professionals in outpatient and community settings. These services continue throughout the child's life, with modifications in the treatment goals made as the child grows and matures.

Physical and Occupational Therapy

The interventions provided by the physical and occupational therapist are essential in helping to reduce the risk of contractures and promote the optimal use of motor function. The child is likely to have difficult or inefficient ambulation. Formal gait analysis and ongoing therapy can assist the child to ambulate. Abnormalities of tone and reflexes can interfere with the child's abilities to perform daily functions. The therapist can introduce techniques or adaptive equipment to help the child achieve activities of daily living that they are cognitively capable of completing.

Nutritional Management

The nutritional status of children with CP needs to be addressed. Poor swallowing and the presence of gastroesophageal reflux is common in severe CP. The child with spastic quadriplegia may have difficulty eating because there is incoordination of the jaw muscles and an inability to self-feed. The child may be at risk for aspiration. Inadequate nutrition affects wound healing and increases the risk of skin breakdown for the child with decreased mobility. Food must be easy to swallow and jaw support must be given to help the child chew. Gavage or gastrostomy feedings may be needed to meet the child's caloric requirements or if risk of aspiration is severe. A nutritionist can provide the family with suggestions to increase the caloric intake, including giving high-calorie milkshakes and formulas.

Speech and Language

Special consideration must be given to those children who have difficulty communicating. At times, it is difficult to assess whether the child is in pain, anxious, agitated, or just frustrated. Some children with CP have difficulty speaking even though receptive language skills may be quite good, and alternative forms of expressive communication (e.g., computer, "touch-talker," communication board, sign language, or facial gestures) should be used. Parents or other caregivers are usually adept at interpreting their child's needs and can help decrease the child's frustration at his or her inability to communicate. Speech therapy is important for children with CP, because therapists can help devise innovative ways for the child to communicate.

Audiology Support

Children with CP are prone to hearing loss, which is often not detected. Failure to follow directions or be attentive to sounds can be wrongly associated with the child's level of mental retardation. Thus, all children with CP should have their hearing assessed. Referral to an audiologist is essential to ensure accurate and sensitive assessment of the child's hearing. In most cases, an amplification device (hearing aid) is recommended. (See Chapter 28 for more information on hearing loss and treatment.) The early treatment of hearing loss can significantly improve the child's overall outcomes.

Psychosocial Resources

A child with CP puts great demands on the parents' emotional, physical, and financial resources. Social services can assist the family with finding support groups, respite care, and other community resources for needed equipment. (See Chapters 7 and 10 for more information on chronic illness and community care.) Ramps, vans, electric wheelchairs, computers, and mechanical feeders are just a few devices that can make the child more independent. The United Cerebral Palsy Association can help parents dealing with the problems of children with CP (see Resources).

Special Education

Children with CP who have a normal intellect can be mainstreamed into regular schools. If the child has some degree of mental retardation, assessment for special educational programs is necessary. Included in the special programs may be therapies for the child such as physical therapy, occupational therapy, or speech therapy. An interdisciplinary health care team collaborates with school officials to develop an Individualized Educational Plan (IEP) for the child. This plan may be implemented as based in the home, special school or center, or regular school. The health team's goal is to integrate the child into normal school activities as much as possible and to provide a learning environment that is structured to meet the child's unique learning and developmental needs. Chapters 7 and 10 contain more information about IEPs and the nurse's role in implementing them. Every effort should be made to allow the child the intellectual and social stimulation that school provides. Chapter 11 also provides more detailed descriptions of the rehabilitative and home care measures that can be provided for the child with CP.

Table 20–11
Types of Muscular Dystrophy

Clinical Diagnosis	Inheritance	Age at Onset	Pattern of Muscle Involvement	Rate of Progression
Pseudohypertrophic (Duchenne's)	X-linked recessive	Early childhood, usually by age 3	Pelvic and shoulder muscles affected early Spreads to periphery of limbs late in the course of the disease	Steady rapid progression
Limb-girdle	Autosomal recessive; occasionally autosomal dominant	Variable, usually after childhood	Weakness of pelvic and shoulder girdles Spreads to periphery late in the course	Slow, variable progression
Facioscapulohumeral	Autosomal dominant	Variable, usually occurs in second decade	Face and shoulder girdle affected early Later spreads to pelvic girdles	Very slow

Muscular Dystrophy

Muscular dystrophy refers not to one specific disease but to a group of genetically transmitted disorders of muscle. These disorders vary in age of onset, hereditary pattern, and area of weakness. Most dystrophies begin during childhood or adolescence and all are progressive to some degree (Table 20–11). The most common type of muscular dystrophy is Duchenne's (DMD), also known as pseudohypertrophic dystrophy.

Etiology

The etiology of DMD is a defect on the short arm of the X chromosome. Because it is sex-linked, DMD affects males almost exclusively. One in 3500 live-born males is affected with DMD. This disease has a high mutation rate. As many as one third of children with DMD have no family history of the disease. When DMD affects a female, the disorder seems to be less severe and more slowly progressive than in males. Females are the carriers of DMD and there is a genetic test that determines whether the female is a carrier. Genetic counseling should be considered for females in the family.

Pathophysiology

In DMD, the defect on the X chromosome results in a lack of production of dystrophin (Wenger & Rang, 1993). Dystrophin can be found on the surface membrane of muscles and in the brain. The actual function of dystrophin is unclear, but its absence results in the breakdown of muscle fibers with replacement of fatty deposits and fibrosis.

Usually, the onset of symptoms of DMD begins before age 5. The symptoms become more noticeable after a child begins to walk, because children with DMD appear clumsy and have difficulty climbing stairs. The weakness involves the shoulder and pelvic muscles first. The classic finding for DMD is Gowers' sign (Fig. 20–10). Because of the muscular weakness in the pelvis and legs, children must use one or both hands to brace the lower extremi-

Figure 20–10
Gowers' sign. The adolescent must use one or both hands to brace the legs and then raise himself off the floor to a standing position.

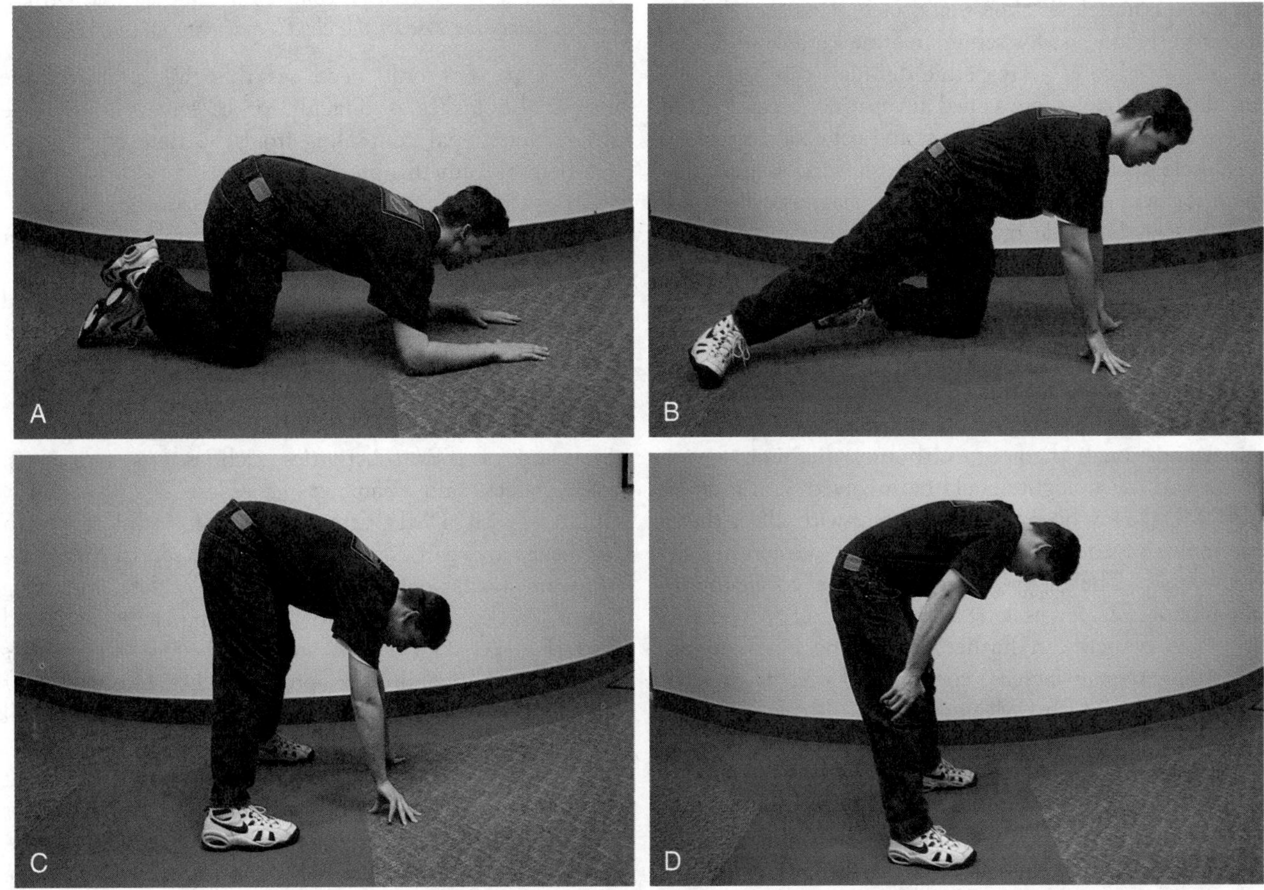

ties and to raise themselves off the floor from a sitting or prone position. Tiptoe walking is also common.

Apparent hypertrophy of the calf muscles marks the progression of DMD. This is the reason for the term "pseudohypertrophic" muscular dystrophy. Although the calf muscles look big and strong, fat and fibrous tissue have infiltrated the muscle, actually making it weaker. Deep tendon reflexes eventually diminish or disappear. However, the child with DMD does not lose sensation to the extremity.

Prognosis. The usual course of DMD is a steady progression of weakness and increasing disability. Walking becomes increasingly difficult, and many children resort to crawling. On average, most children with DMD are wheelchair-dependent by age 10 to 12 years. As the trunk muscles continue to atrophy, scoliosis often occurs. The scoliosis exacerbates already poor respiratory function caused by thoracic muscle weakness. Death results from cardiac or respiratory failure sometime in the late teens or early twenties. Currently, DMD has no cure. Gene therapy techniques are being investigated as a technique to prevent muscle degeneration (Heydemann, 1996).

Assessment

Clinical diagnosis of DMD is made by observation of gait, specific muscle weakness, and lack of sensory deficit. Laboratory blood test for serum creatine kinase, which at high levels indicates a myopathic disorder, can be useful. Muscular dystrophies are called myopathic because they involve muscle wasting, weakness, and cellular changes in the muscle tissue. A muscle biopsy showing muscle degeneration with fiber loss confirms the diagnosis. Prenatal diagnosis can be made by chorionic villus sampling and by amniocentesis.

Interdisciplinary Interventions

An interdisciplinary team consisting of a nurse, orthopedist, neurologist, pediatrician, geneticist, physical therapist, occupational therapist, orthotist, dietitian, social worker, and psychologist should be involved with a child with DMD. Many hospitals have clinics with all of these personnel and they provide services on a monthly or weekly basis. The goals of treatment are to maintain daily functioning for as long as possible and to prevent deformities, which can further disable the child. Good supportive care can increase comfort and the life expectancy of the child with DMD.

Conservative treatment for DMD generally begins with lightweight bracing to stabilize the knee and ankle. Despite adequate care, contractures may develop in the legs and feet. To maintain the child's ability to stand or walk, a surgical release of the contracture may be needed. Scoliosis, a frequent occurrence in DMD, is treated aggressively. Surgical stabilization of the spine is necessary before the child has a decrease in respiratory capacity. Delayed treatment may result in the child's respiratory status being unsafe for surgery. Care of the child with DMD who requires surgical intervention involves helping the child return to his previous level of activity.

Community Care

The impact of the diagnosis of DMD on a family cannot be underestimated. (See Chapter 10 for more information on intervening for a family of a child with a chronic illness.) Families experience a grief process that begins with recognition that a normal life is not possible. Next is a stage of working through the disease as family members adapt and their world becomes smaller. Finally, the family members reach the stage of resolution when they identify with others with disabilities and realize that life must go on (Gagliardi, 1991).

Letting children with DMD be as independent as possible is important to their self-esteem. Children with DMD often have problems with pressure sores, particularly if they are obese and wheelchair dependent. An enterostomal therapy nurse can be consulted for specific cases. Nutritional counseling is also important.

caREminder: *Obesity is common in the child with DMD, probably because of the child's inactivity and boredom.*

Obesity not only decreases the child's functioning but it also makes it difficult for caregivers to lift the child. Nutritional counseling from the time of diagnosis can help prevent this problem.

Appropriately selected activities can boost self-esteem, provide social interaction, and normalize life for the child with DMD. Children attend school until they are not able to sit up. When the child cannot attend school, a home-bound tutor can be arranged. School personnel meet with the family and selected members of the health care team to develop an IEP to meet the child's educational needs. (See Chapters 7 and 10 for more discussion of IEPs.) Activities such as arts and crafts, board games, and computer games are favorites. Many children with DMD attend camps for children with handicaps and participate in wheelchair sports. Many options are available for the wheelchair athlete, including tennis, track, swimming, rowing, skiing, and track and field (Fig. 20–11). Teams are organized on state levels and through rehabilitation programs. Local tournaments and national championships provide opportunities for all levels of athletes to participate.

Physical and occupational therapy are an important part of the life of a child with DMD. The need for assistive devices increases as the child becomes weaker. Types of aids that help the family and child include

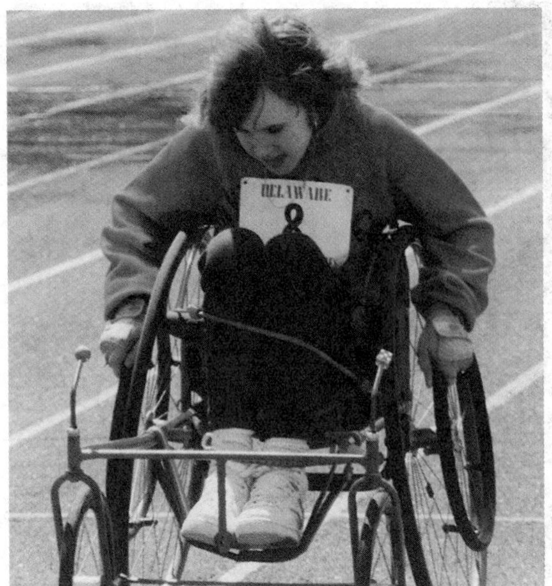

Figure 20–11
Wheelchair sports provide an opportunity for the child with muscular dystrophy to enjoy physical activity and interact with peers.

electric feeding devices, elevated toilet seats, bath chairs, and lifts. An electric-powered wheelchair, although expensive, provides the child with some independence. The Muscular Dystrophy Association can be a great social and financial support to families (see Resources).

As the child's status deteriorates, some families decide to use ventilatory support, especially at night. A tracheostomy also may be required but this is a decision that should be made after careful consideration by the family. The nurse, clergy, and ethics committees can help support the family as they deal with quality of life issues and impending death.

Growth-Related Disorders

Growth-related disorders become evident as the musculoskeletal system matures. In this section, eight types of growth-related disorders are discussed. Many of these disorders are self-limiting, meaning that, as the child grows, the disorder resolves itself. In other cases, such as with Legg-Calvé-Perthes (LCP) disease or scoliosis, destruction of a joint can occur or the child is left with a permanent disfigurement. In all of these cases, the cause is either not known or not fully understood.

Torsional Deformity: Femoral Anteversion

A torsional deformity describes an orthopedic condition in which the bone is "twisted." This can occur in the femur or tibia. In femoral anteversion, or internal femoral torsion, the femur is medially rotated. It is often associated with metatarsus adductus, neuromuscular disorders, LCP disease, and DDH. Torsional deformities affect females twice as often as males, and a familial tendency has been noted.

The rotational and angular alignment of the legs changes during a child's growing years. Children begin life with the femurs anteverted; with growth, they gradually derotate. In a child with a neuromuscular problem, the derotation may not occur. However, in most children, femoral anteversion resolves spontaneously with growth, and no treatment is needed.

Assessment

Assessment of femoral anteversion frequently begins with a subjective complaint that the child is walking "pigeon-toed." The child or parent may also complain of a clumsy gait that can be a source of ridicule. The child's thighs medially rotate, and the knees and patellae turn inward (Fig. 20–12). The legs appear bowed when the feet are pointed straight ahead. Clinical measurements determine medial and lateral rotation of the hip. In children with femoral anteversion, lateral rotation of the femur is de-

Figure 20–12
In femoral anteversion, the thighs rotate medially and the knees and patellae turn inward. Braces can be used to correct this problem. (Wheaton Bracing System. Courtesy of Wheaton Brace Co.)

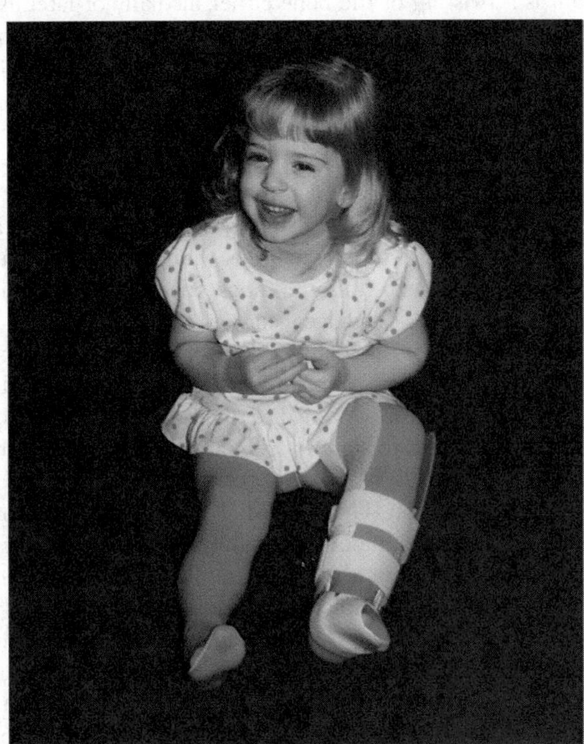

creased and medial rotation appears increased on measurement. Traditional radiographs are not helpful in diagnosing femoral anteversion, but they can rule out other causes of in-toeing. CT and MRI can be useful but are usually not necessary.

Interdisciplinary Interventions

Orthotic devices such as braces have not proven effective for the correction of femoral anteversion. After the initial diagnosis, the child is evaluated at 6-month intervals. The condition in most children spontaneously corrects by age 8 to 10 years. If the child has a severe problem or a neuromuscular disorder, a derotation femoral osteotomy may be done to correct alignment after age 8. An osteotomy is cut through the femur, the bone is rotated to the desired position, and screws are placed to hold it until the bone heals. A hip spica cast is then applied for approximately 6 weeks (see TIP 20–1).

Nursing interventions begin with assuring the parents and child that this problem often resolves on its own. Only approximately 1% of children with femoral anteversion require surgery (Morrissy, 1990). When surgery is necessary, the nurse educates the family on the care of the hip spica cast and arranges for a wheelchair rental as well as a home tutor. In most cases, postoperative physical therapy is not needed.

Torsional Deformity: Tibial Torsion

Another common type of torsional deformity, tibial torsion, is a twisting of the bone either medially or laterally. Medial torsion causes an in-toeing gait; lateral torsion causes an out-toeing gait (Fig. 20–13). The degree of tibial torsion varies with the child's age. At birth, the tibia rotates medially, but with normal growth and development, it spontaneously derotates.

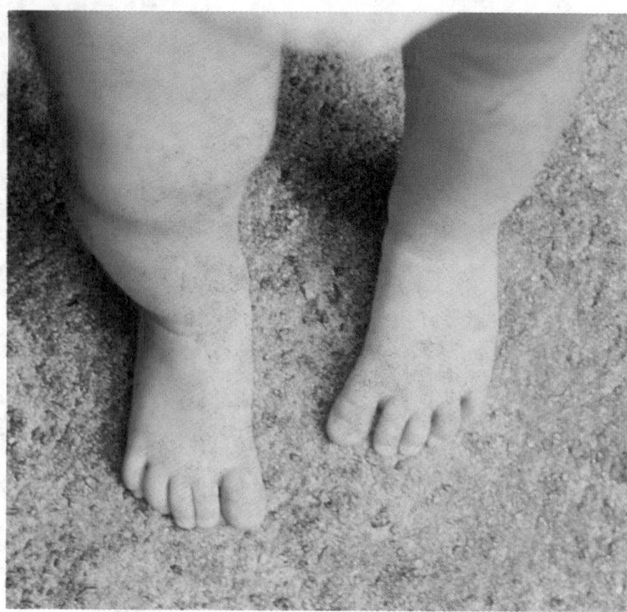

Figure 20–13
In tibial torsion, the hips, thighs, and knees are normally oriented, and the lower leg and foot turn inward (medial) or outward (lateral).

Abnormal medial tibial torsion rarely occurs as a single deformity. It is commonly associated with femoral anteversion, congenital metatarsus varus (in-toeing), or developmental genu varum (knock-knees). It occurs in approximately 5% of adult females and 3% of adult males (Maher et al., 1994). The child with medial tibial torsion usually presents with a history of being "pigeon-toed." Often, a family history of medial tibial torsion is noted.

Lateral tibial torsion is seen as an out-toeing gait. Children usually do not have a positive family history for lateral tibial torsion. Unlike medial torsion that may improve during late childhood, lateral torsion usually worsens. This results from a contracture of the iliotibial band, a congenital deformity that has caused the torsion.

Radiographs are not very useful in the diagnosis of tibial torsion in young children. The diagnosis is made on clinical examination. Two methods can be used to screen for tibial torsion. First, the child sits with the knees at a 90-degree angle and the examiner palpates the malleoli. Normally, the medial malleolus lies farther forward than the lateral malleolus. Second, with the child lying prone, the examiner measures the thigh-foot angle.

Prognosis for correction of tibial torsion is very good. Many practitioners do not treat tibial torsion but follow up the cases in the office every 6 to 12 months. Other practitioners try conservative measures such as passive stretching exercises or splints. Surgical correction with a derotational osteotomy is reserved for children older than age 8 years with severe medial torsion and age 10 for children with abnormal lateral torsion. Most cases spontaneously correct without treatment.

Legg-Calvé-Perthes Disease

Also known as coxa plana, LCP disease is a self-limiting disease of the hip in which the femoral head loses its blood supply. The precise cause is unknown and the treatment is controversial.

LCP disease has an incidence of 1 per 1200 live births with some hereditary factors influencing incidence. LCP occurs four times more often in males than in females and rarely occurs in blacks. LCP also occurs more frequently in lower socioeconomic groups (Wenger & Rang, 1993). The peak age for occurrence is age 4 to 7 years, although the range is from age 3 to age 12. Generally, LCP occurs unilaterally; however, 10% to 12% of cases are bilateral (Herring, 1989).

Table 20-12
Phases of Legg-Calvé-Perthes Disease

Phase	Physiologic Process	Time Span
Avascularity	Blood supply to femoral head is interrupted. Bone growth ceases. Bone density does not change. Surface cartilage is intact.	Several months to a year
Revascularization	Blood supply returns to femoral head. Dead bone is reabsorbed and immature new bone is laid down. Femoral head may remodel in a deformed position.	1–3 years
Reossification	New bone is laid down. Remodeling continues.	1–3 years
Residual deformity	Healing is complete. Hip is either normal or deformed forever (oval shaped rather than round).	Ongoing

The progression of LCP is well defined into four distinctive phases (Table 20–12). Diagnosis of LCP usually occurs in the second phase when the child begins to have symptoms such as pain. The earlier that treatment begins, the less risk there is of residual deformity to the hip joint. Also, children whose LCP disease is diagnosed at a younger age tend to have fewer long-term problems. Approximately 80% of children have a good recovery, although they may have difficulty later in life with hip degeneration (Morrissy, 1990).

Assessment

The first symptoms of LCP are pain, limp, and decreased range of motion in the affected hip. These symptoms usually have been plaguing the child for months, although some children present with a traumatic injury. Occasionally, pain is referred to the knee or thigh and the diagnosis can be missed. Usually, the child reports that rest relieves the pain.

On physical examination, the child may hold the leg in slight flexion and a hip contracture may be present. Limited hip motion, especially internal rotation and abduction, is a classic sign of LCP disease. Most children walk with a limp that becomes more pronounced in later stages of the disease.

Radiographs are the standard technique for diagnosis and evaluation of treatment of LCP disease. The two basic classification systems for LCP are based on radiography (Table 20–13). The Catterall system is used retrospectively; the Salter-Thompson classification system tries to predict outcome.

Bone scans are particularly useful in diagnosing early cases of LCP when radiographic changes may not be evident. A bone scan shows decreased uptake of dye in an affected femoral head and more clearly demarcates the area of avascularity than can be done by standard radiographic techniques. MRI and arthrography also may be performed. There are no relevant laboratory studies for LCP disease.

Interdisciplinary Interventions

The goals of treatment of LCP are to keep the femoral head as round as possible and to prevent deformity while the disease runs its course. Opinions differ as to the best way to achieve these goals.

The first step in treatment is to regain motion around the hip joint and relieve pain. This pain is a result of synovitis or muscle spasm around the hip. Nonsteroidal anti-inflammatory drugs (NSAIDs) help decrease inflammation and pain. Some physicians place the child in Buck's traction until range of motion improves and pain diminishes (approximately 1 to 2 weeks). The child must be on strict bed rest, and even sitting in bed (except to eat meals) is discouraged. This traction can be done at home or in the hospital. When the child is placed on home traction, a home care company provides the traction equipment, trains the parent to set up traction, and sends nurses or physical therapists to the home periodically. Home traction requires an enormous time commitment from the family, and the child will need home tutoring. Also, compliance to staying in traction may be an issue for some children at home. Children who are younger or whose disease is detected early may require only observation and follow-up with radiographs obtained every 2 to 4 months.

After the inflammation in the hip has decreased and

Table 20–13
Classification of Legg-Calvé-Perthes Disease Based on Radiographic Appearance

Salter-Thompson Classification	Catterall Classification	Description
A	I	Anterior porition of the epiphysis is involved. The epiphysis on the involved side is smaller. Prognosis is good.
	II	Anterior superior and posterior portion of the epiphysis is involved. The medial and latera margins are not involved. Prognosis remains good because the lateral margin is intact.
B	III	There is a loss of the lateral margin, which increases the risk of collapse and subsequent deformity. The prognosis is less favorable.
	IV	The entire epiphysis involved. The prognosis is poor because growth plate is often severely damaged, further increasing the risk of residual deformity.

range of motion has improved, the next goal, containment, can be addressed. Containment involves holding the femoral head in abduction to prevent the edge of the acetabulum from denting the head. However, some movement of the hip is desirable to mold the soft head round.

Containment can be achieved in a variety of ways and the choice of the treatment depends on the stage of the disease and physician preference. Nonsurgical options for containment include braces and Petrie casts. The most commonly used brace is the Atlanta–Scottish Rite orthosis. A child may be placed in Petrie casts for a few weeks and then braced, or the child may be put in a brace immediately. Both options have advantages and disadvantages, but both maintain the hips in abduction. To be effective, bracing must be used for 6 to 18 months. The brace is worn constantly, except for bathing. Children can wear the brace over regular clothes and some can even participate in other activities, such as baseball, while wearing the brace. The child must be followed up every 3 months. In recent medical literature, the efficacy of the Atlanta orthosis has been questioned (Meehan, Angel, & Nelson, 1992). Some physicians prefer to treat the child with physical therapy or no brace at all.

Surgical options for containment of the hip are reserved for children with severe deformity. Surgical options achieve containment with an osteotomy of the femur, acetabulum, or both. The child is hospitalized for approximately 3 days and is discharged home in a hip spica cast for 6 to 8 weeks. When the cast is removed, no further treatment is needed. The advantages of this treatment method are that the child is restricted in a cast for only 2 months and the hip containment is permanent. The disadvantages are those related to any surgery and the possibility of a leg length discrepancy as a result of the osteotomy.

Community Care

Nursing interventions for the child with LCP start with education regarding the disease process and the use of corrective devices (i.e., traction, casting, or bracing). Despite the healthy appearance of the affected child, parents and other caretakers must come to understand the seriousness of this disease and the importance of compliance in regard to the treatment regimen. The treatment for LCP can span a few years. This can be a stressful time for families emotionally as well as financially. Because LCP is more prevalent in lower socioeconomic groups, these problems may be compounded. Social services can help families find the resources they need.

If home traction is required, the parent must learn the principles of traction and immobilization (see Chart 20–11). Home health care services can be arranged to monitor the child's progress and evaluate the family's ability to manage the traction device. If both parents work, the home health agency may be able to assist in locating a daytime caregiver for the child. Home tutoring arrangements should be made with the child's school so that the child does not fall behind in school work.

Principles of cast care are listed in TIP 20–2. The cast placed on these children is very wide. Fitting through a door of a house or car may be impossible unless the child turns sideways. A reclining wheelchair allows some mobility, although it is limited. Special transportation services in a van or ambulance can be arranged by social services or the home care nurse if required.

If the child is in a brace, he or she may attend school and participate in many of the activities with other children. The child is given specific instructions regarding how and when to wear the brace. If the brace becomes dirty, it can be washed with a damp cloth. If the brace breaks, the company that issued the brace should be contacted immediately to provide an immediate replacement.

Slipped Capital Femoral Epiphysis

In slipped capital femoral epiphysis (SCFE), the top of the femur—the capital femoral epiphysis—slips through the growth plate in a posterior direction (Fig. 20–14). It can be likened to slippage of a scoop of ice cream on the top of a cone.

Although it is the most common hip disorder of adolescence, SCFE is rare, affecting only 2 to 10 per 100,000 children. It occurs primarily in the teenage years, with a peak incidence at age 10 to 14 in girls and age 10 to 16 in boys. Incidence is two to five times higher in males than in females and is greatest in the eastern United States and in blacks. A high proportion of children with SCFE are obese (Morrissy & Selman, 1991).

Figure 20–14
In slipped capital femoral epiphysis, the femoral head moves upward and forward while the capital epiphysis becomes displaced backward and downward.

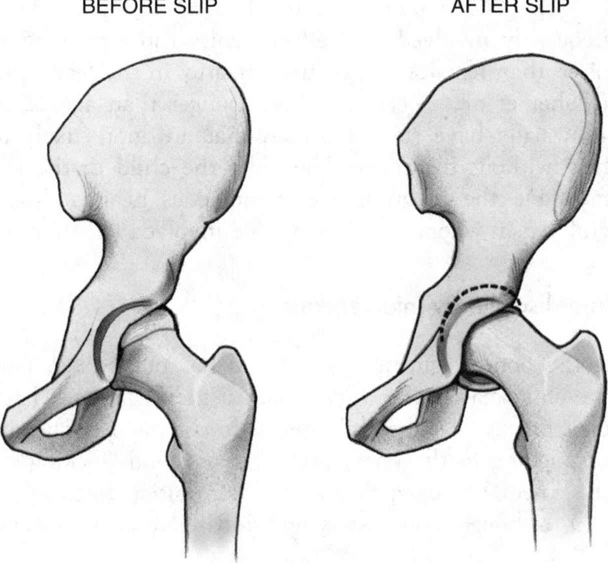

Etiology

The exact cause of SCFE is unknown. Numerous theories have been proposed, but none has been proven. A genetic component has been noted, and the most plausible theory is that SCFE is related to an endocrine abnormality. During the adolescent growth spurt, the growth plate in the femur weakens and is less resistant to shear stresses. This fact, combined with an assumed imbalance between growth and sex hormones, may precipitate a "slip."

Trauma also has a role in the development of a slip. If the growth plate is already weak and then a heavy child falls on his or her hip, an SCFE may result. Other conditions associated with SCFE include hypothyroidism, renal osteodystrophy, and postradiation therapy.

Pathophysiology

The classification of SCFE is determined by the stage and the severity of the disease, which, in turn, influence prognosis (Table 20–14). Complications that can occur as a result of SCFE are chondrolysis, or acute necrosis of

Table 20–14
Classification of Slipped Capital Femoral Epiphysis

Stage	Severity
Preslip phase The child complains of weakness in the leg and pain in the hip or knee when standing or walking for prolonged periods of time.	**Grade I (preslip)** The physis widens without actual displacement of the epiphysis.
Acute slip A child falls and then reports hip pain.	**Grade II (minimal slip)** The femoral neck is displaced from the femoral head by up to one third.
Chronic slip The femoral head gradually slips off the femoral neck and remodels.	**Grade III (moderate slip)** The femoral neck is displaced by more than one third, but less than one half of the femoral head.
Acute on chronic slip Slow progressive slippage becomes more displaced when a child falls.	**Grade IV (severe slip)** The epiphysis is displaced by greater than 50%.

the cartilage of the hip, and avascular necrosis, or loss of blood supply, of all or part of the femoral head. With prompt treatment, many children do well after a slip, although degenerative arthritis may develop later in life.

Assessment

The primary presenting complaint of a child with SCFE is pain. This pain can either be in the groin area or can be referred to the thigh or the knee. The child usually walks with a limp and with the affected limb externally rotated. Duration of complaint depends on the stage of the disease. In an acute slip, the symptoms are present for less than 3 weeks; in a chronic slip, they are present for weeks or months. In an acute or in a chronic slip, the child reports weeks or months of discomfort followed by a recent episode of severe pain.

On physical examination, the hip does not fully internally rotate and abduction is limited. The affected leg also may be shorter in a moderate or severe slip.

Alert: *Range of motion should not be attempted in a child with a suspected acute slip—this could worsen displacement.*

Radiographs of the pelvis are the best tool for diagnosing SCFE. Occasionally, a CT scan may be used to determine the degree of slip or the amount of healing, but routine use is expensive and is not necessary.

Interdisciplinary Interventions

The goal of treatment for SCFE is to prevent further slippage. Surgery is the intervention of choice. Once SCFE is diagnosed, the child is not allowed to bear weight. For an acute slip, some practitioners place the child in split Russell's traction (see Treatment Modalities), with a minimal amount of weight, for a few days before surgery. This forced bed rest in traction decreases the synovitis in the hip. Other practitioners choose to operate on the hip immediately. The hip cannot be reduced manually because this further damages the blood supply to the femoral head.

The most common surgical procedure for a mild to moderate SCFE is in situ pinning. In situ pinning is the percutaneous placement of a large screw or pin into the femoral head to hold it in place. This requires a small incision and the child can be discharged, with crutches, on the day of surgery or the next day. After 1 week, the child can fully bear weight on the affected leg. The pin is removed later.

For a severe slip, an osteotomy of the hip may be the treatment of choice. This procedure not only prevents further slipping but also restores hip motion to a normal range. An osteotomy requires more extensive surgery than percutaneous pinning, requiring a longer hospital stay and prolonged immobilization.

Nursing intervention for a child with a recent diagnosis of SCFE begins with assisting the family in adjusting to sudden hospitalization, no weight-bearing, and surgery. Postoperative pain should be managed with oral or intravenous narcotics. Neurovascular status of the affected extremity should be closely monitored by the nurse (see Chart 20–4). The physical therapist instructs the child in crutch walking. The child can be discharged from the hospital when he or she can ambulate safely with crutches and when the pain is well controlled with an oral narcotic such as acetaminophen with codeine.

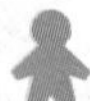

Tip: *Instruct the child that safe crutch walking starts with wearing low-heeled, rubber-soled shoes (sneakers are ideal). The child should not try to go fast on crutches or a fall may result.*

Osteochondritis Dissecans

Osteochondritis dissecans (OD) refers to a process in which a part of the femoral condyle (a rounded projection at the end of the bone) loses its blood supply, is damaged, and sometimes completely breaks free and floats around in the knee joint. This fragment varies in size and can permanently damage the cartilage surface in the joint if it remains there. The fragment also causes painful symptoms that can debilitate an active person.

The cause of OD is unclear. Most likely it occurs when the foot plants on the ground, the femur twists, and the top of the tibia cuts into the cartilage of the femoral condyle. In some cases, repetitive activity may disrupt the blood supply to the femoral condyle, weakening it and making it more susceptible to trauma. In other cases, it may be a primary blood supply deficiency of the femoral condyle.

The lateral portion of the femoral condyle is most frequently involved. OD affects males three times more often than females and occurs primarily in the teen years (Maher et al., 1994). Children younger than age 12 or 13 usually have smaller lesions that are more likely to heal without treatment. The older the child is, the less favorable the prognosis for spontaneous healing. Many children in whom OD develops are involved in athletics.

Interdisciplinary Interventions

If the bone fragment is small and has not broken free, the child may have no symptoms. If the fragment is large or it breaks free, the child begins to complain of clicking or popping in the knee, swelling, pain, and "locking" of the knee. Radiographs are used for initial diagnosis of OD, although bone scans and MRI give more specific information on the size of the lesion and its potential to separate.

Treatment of OD varies with age of onset and displacement status. In a young child with a nondisplaced lesion, conservative treatment consists of limiting activities that require running and turning, and wearing a knee immobilizer if the area is tender. This allows the lesion to heal itself and be held in place with scar tissue. An older child with a nondisplaced fragment is usually given the same treatment. However, some physicians prophylactically pin the fragment so that it does not break free and cause damage.

A displaced fragment necessitates surgical intervention. Using arthroscopic techniques, the surgeon removes small fragments. In larger lesions, the fragment is replaced, sometimes along with bone graft, and held with absorbable pins or wires.

Postoperatively, nursing care of the child with a repair of OD includes obtaining vital signs and assessing neurovascular status of the affected extremity. Pain management consists of intravenous or oral medications. A CPM machine placed on the leg immediately after surgery maintains motion and prevents stiffness (see Treatment Modalities). The CPM machine may also be used at home for 3 to 4 weeks postoperatively. Arrangements for outpatient physical therapy are made before discharge. Therapy focuses on range-of-motion exercises and hamstring and quadriceps strengthening. After approximately 4 to 6 months, the child can resume prior activities.

Osgood-Schlatter Disease

Osgood-Schlatter disease, a painful prominence of the tibial tubercle, or top of the tibia, is a common problem in active older school-agers or teenagers, but it is usually self-limiting. Females age 8 to 13 years and males age 10 to 15 years are the most commonly affected. It is more prevalent in males, perhaps because of their greater participation in sports. It can occur unilaterally or bilaterally.

The cause of Osgood-Schlatter disease is not completely understood. The most popular theory suggests that the lesion is caused by repetitive injury and repair to the tibial tubercle where the patellar tendon inserts. A strong quadriceps contraction, such as occurs when running, jumping, or stair climbing, coupled with an immature ossification center, can result in inflammation and small avulsions of the bone at the site of the tendon insertion. This cycle continues, with new bone forming each time the injury occurs, as the body attempts to heal itself.

The prognosis for Osgood-Schlatter disease is very good. Symptoms can be expected to resolve about the time that the child's skeletal growth ceases. This condition does not result in long-term complications.

Assessment

Pain below the kneecap is the most frequent complaint in Osgood-Schlatter disease. Symptoms are usually aggravated by activity and relieved by rest. Many children affected with this condition are active in sports such as basketball, gymnastics, soccer, and ballet. Physical examination reveals swelling, tenderness, and a firm mass at the patellar insertion site.

Tip: *Asking the child to squat or extend his or her knee against resistance usually elicits pain and is a good indicator of Osgood-Schlatter disease.*

When Osgood-Schlatter disease is suspected, knee radiographs are obtained to rule out other serious disorders, such as a tumor, which could have a similar appearance. Diagnosis is made by analysis of presenting symptoms and history.

Interdisciplinary Interventions

Treatment of Osgood-Schlatter disease begins with controlling the pain by limiting the activities that aggravate the condition. If the child is upset by not participating in sports, then he or she should be permitted to choose one or two sports that are the most important. However, the child should not participate in activities that cause pain, but once the symptoms have improved, he or she can return to those activities (Dyment, 1997; Zachazewski, Magee, & Quillen, 1996). Sports that involve running or jumping are particularly stressful on the knee and may cause more symptoms.

Other conservative methods of treatment include applying an ice pack on the affected area after activity and administering over-the-counter NSAIDs when pain occurs. Some physicians also advocate the use of an elastic wrap or neoprene sleeve over the knee during activities for the child's comfort. Kneepads are helpful in sports that involve direct knee contact.

Surgical management is rarely indicated unless a piece of bone has completely torn free from the tibial tubercle (a nodule on the bone). Surgery consists of excision of the fragment to relieve the symptoms. This should be done only after the child has reached skeletal maturity, because the growth plate could be injured.

Activity restrictions are frustrating for the child, and the child's social interactions may be impaired because of the restrictions. The nurse can help by teaching the child ways to reduce pain by using prescribed analgesics and ice after exercise. The child should not be pushed to do more physical activity if he or she is experiencing pain. The physical therapist provides instructions on exercises to strengthen the upper body and on lower extremity isometrics. The fact that this disease is self-limiting and will eventually improve should be stressed.

Scoliosis

Scoliosis is a term that describes a spine that has a lateral curve. Often, rotation of the vertebral body as well as kyphosis or lordosis is seen; thus, scoliosis occurs in three planes.

Etiology

Of the many different causes of scoliosis, the most common is idiopathic, meaning that there is no known cause for the deformity that occurs in otherwise healthy individuals. Possible theories that are suggested as the cause of idiopathic scoliosis range from genetic origin to postural dysequilibrium; however, none of these theories has been proven. Other known causes of scoliosis include congenital malformations, Marfan's syndrome, neurofibromatosis, neuromuscular disorders, spina bifida, and spinal cord tumor.

Children age 10 to 16 are at the highest risk for scoliosis. The incidence of scoliosis in the general population is 2% to 3% (Weinstein, 1991). Females are affected more often than males, and their curves tend to progress more severely than in males. However, of all children with the diagnosis of scoliosis, fewer than 10% require treatment.

Pathophysiology

Although the cause of scoliosis is not known, the natural history is well documented. The age at onset and location of the curve have significant impact on the prognosis. Four major curve patterns occur in children with idiopathic scoliosis: thoracic, lumbar, thoracolumbar, and double major (Fig. 20–15). The younger the child at the time of diagnosis, the higher the degree of curvature. A double-curve pattern as well as a high degree of curvature increases the risk for progression of a curve.

Prognosis. Progression of a curve is a basis for the decision on whether the child will need treatment. If a curve is untreated and progresses, pain, decreased pulmonary function, and psychosocial problems from an altered self-image may develop.

Congenital scoliosis, caused by a malformation of the vertebrae, occurs with less frequency than idiopathic scoliosis. However, congenital curves are more likely to progress and cause respiratory compromise, and they are noticeable at an earlier age.

Assessment

A thorough medical history of a child with scoliosis helps to ascertain the cause for the curvature. Some children with idiopathic scoliosis may have no prior history of health problems. Conversely, children with CP or spina bifida have an extensive health history. Questions about medical illnesses may reveal conditions that caution the practitioner to exclude idiopathic scoliosis as a diagnosis. These conditions include congenital heart disease, neurofibromatosis, and Marfan's syndrome. A family history of idiopathic scoliosis increases the likelihood of the child also having idiopathic scoliosis.

Important facts to include in the health history include the date that the curve was first noticed and by whom. Also, the history of progression of the curve is crucial. A slowly progressing curve is less worrisome than a sudden increase in severity of a curve.

Alert: *If pain is a reported symptom of the child's scoliosis, it should be investigated immediately. Pain is not a normal finding for idiopathic scoliosis, and the presence of this particular symptom could be signaling an underlying condition such as a tumor of the spinal cord.*

Also, if neurologic signs such as a limp, weakness, or change in gait pattern are evident, a full neurologic work-up should be pursued.

When examining a child for scoliosis, the examiner should observe gait, measure leg length, and assess overall physical maturity (Fig. 20–16). A scoliometer may be used during the screening to obtain a rough measurement of the curvature.

Diagnostic Tests. The diagnosis of scoliosis is confirmed by standing posteroanterior and lateral radiographs. The physician calculates the angle of curvature from the radiograph. A curve greater than 10 degrees is considered scoliosis. A number of studies have demonstrated a degree of error in this measurement technique of between 5 and 10 degrees, even when measured by experts (Bunnell, 1991). A radiograph may also identify rib or vertebral anomalies that could reveal the cause of the scoliosis.

Nursing Diagnoses and Outcomes

Nursing diagnoses and outcomes for the child with a musculoskeletal disorder are presented in Chart 20–5, and many of these are applicable to the child with curvature of the spine. In addition, the following nursing diagnoses may be applicable for the child with scoliosis:

- **Ineffective breathing pattern related to impact of curvature on ventilation and mobility**
  Outcome: The child will achieve maximal lung expansion with adequate ventilation.
- **Potential for noncompliance: brace-wearing**
  Outcome: The child will wear the brace for the prescribed amount of time daily.

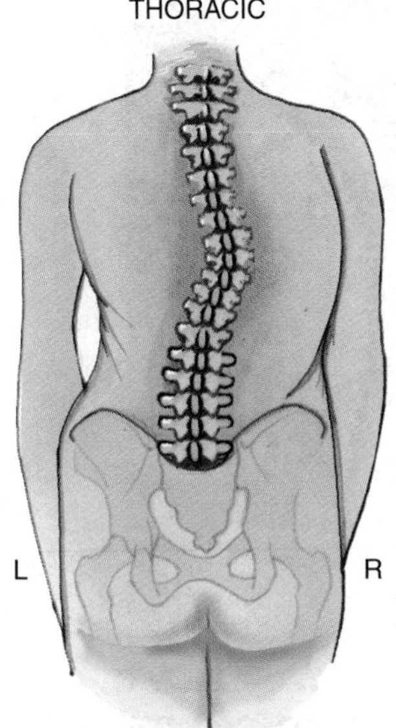
THORACIC
L
R
90% occur on the right side above T-11

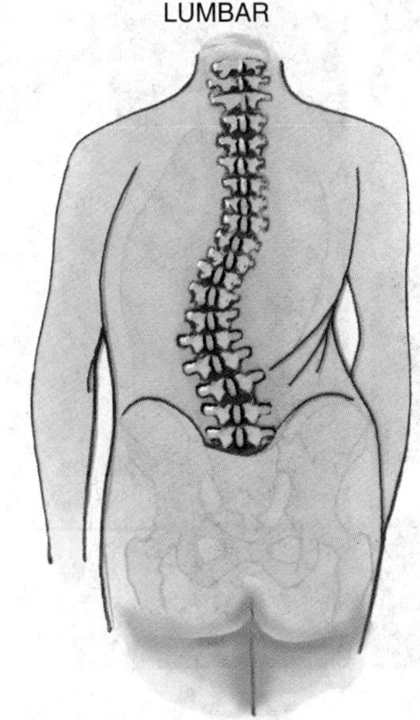
LUMBAR
70% occur on the left side at L-1 or lower

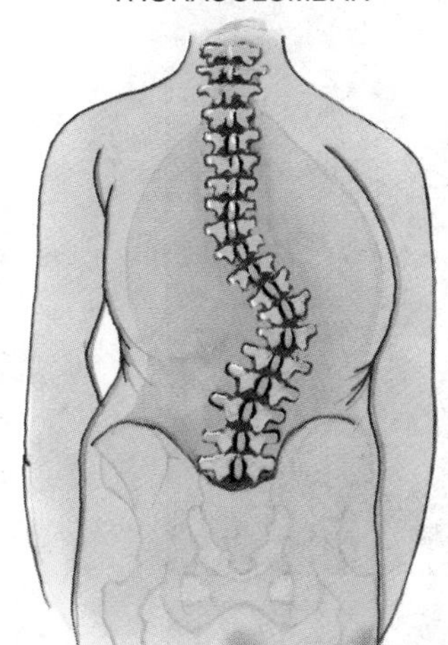
THORACOLUMBAR
80% occur on the right side at T-11 – T-12

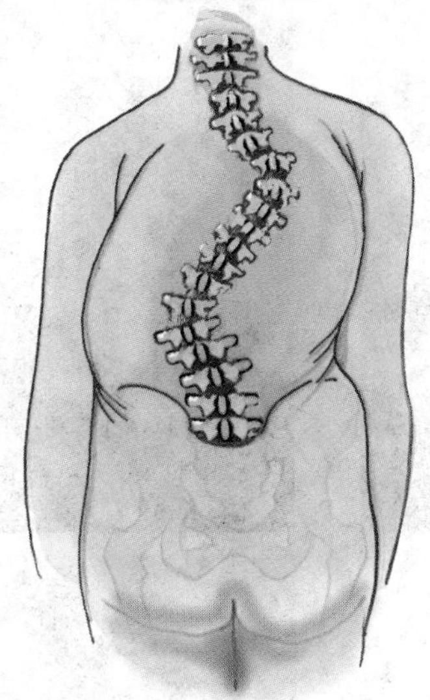
DOUBLE MAJOR
Usually involves right-sided and left-sided lumbar curves

Curve location is determined by the level of the apical vertebra

Figure 20–15
The four major curve patterns in idiopathic scoliosis.

- **Altered health maintenance related to management of diet, skin care, and wearing brace as needed for treatment of scoliosis**
  Outcomes: The child will perform activities of daily living with the aid of assistive devices or a family member.
  The child will accept responsibility for managing self-care activities that optimize the medical treatment regimen.
- **Risk for impaired skin integrity related to brace wear**
  Outcomes: The child will be properly fitted for a brace with adjustments made as needed to ensure comfort.
  The child and parents will manage the child's skin to prevent areas of breakdown under the brace.
- **Pain related to surgical intervention to treat scoliosis**
  Outcomes: The child will experience pain relief during the postsurgical recovery period.
  The child will identify measures effective in relieving pain.

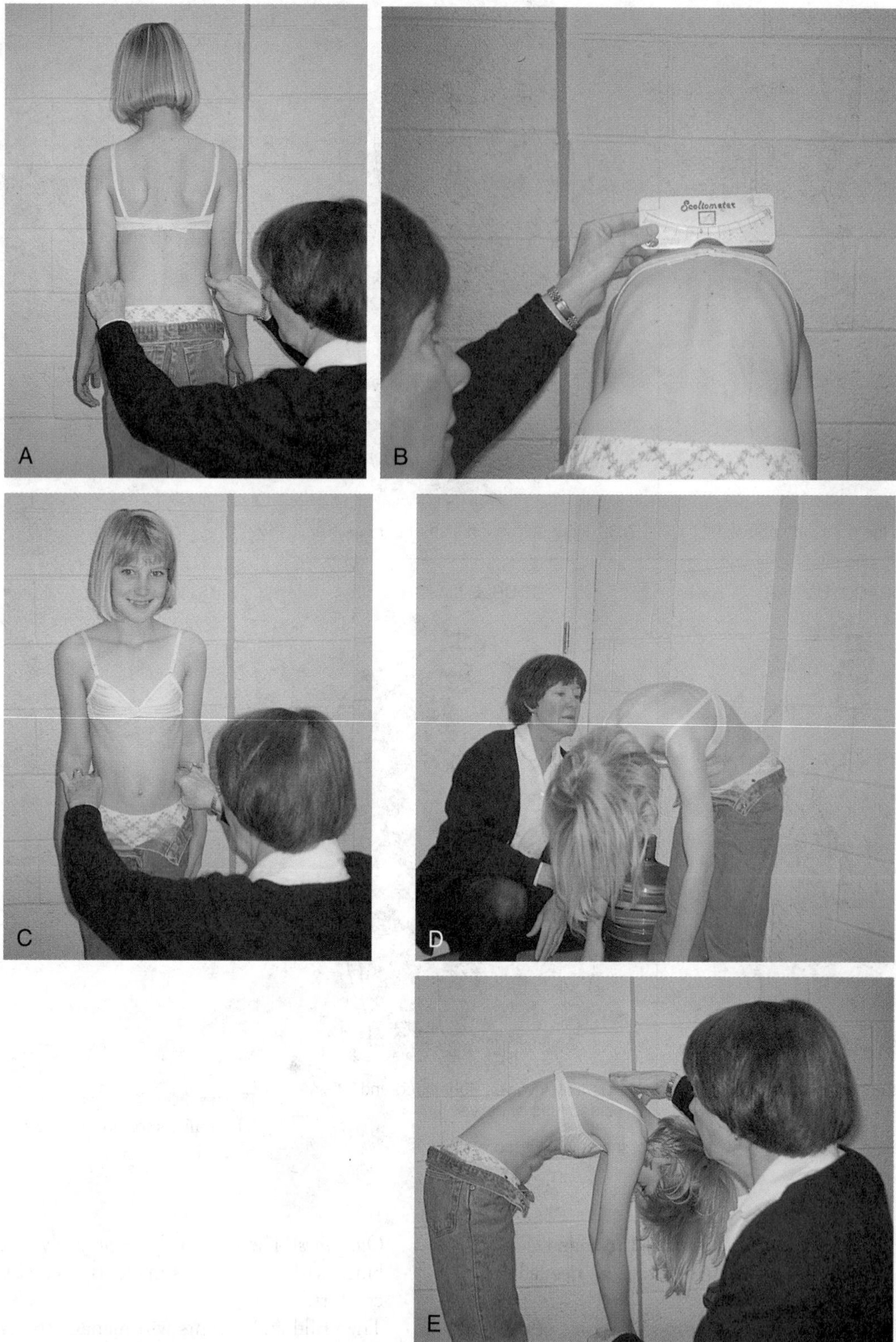

Figure 20–16
Scoliosis screening is performed by the school nurse. *A*, The examiner begins by viewing the child from the back, looking for symmetry of the shoulders, scapulae, and waist creases. *B*, Next, the child is asked to place her hands together and bend forward. The examiner uses a scoliometer to obtain a rough estimate of the degree of spinal curvature. *C*, The examiner looks from the front for anterior chest deformity or asymmetry. *D*, When the child bends forward toward the examiner, particular curves may become more visible. *E*, Observing the child from the side allows the examiner to assess for kyphosis and lordosis.

The parents will express awareness of the child's pain and perform measures to comfort the child.

▶ **Body image disturbance related to poor posture, presence of visible brace, or scars from surgical intervention**
Outcomes: The child will select clothing that enhances body image.
The child will express positive feelings about self.

Interdisciplinary Interventions

Education is an important component of the care for a child with scoliosis. At the time of diagnosis, many children and families are often upset and scared. Basic explanations and truthfulness are the best approach with teenagers. The selected treatment regimen is based on the child's age, the degree of curvature, and the child's willingness to comply with the treatment program. The treatment options for scoliosis fall into two groups: nonsurgical interventions and surgical interventions.

Nonsurgical Interventions

Nonsurgical treatments are primarily those of observation and bracing. In the past, traction and special exercises have not proven effective in preventing progression of the curve (Roach, 1991). The lateral electric surface stimulator (LESS) is another type of nonsurgical treatment that has been used for a number of years. Electrodes are strategically placed over the region of the thoracic curvature. The electric stimulation causes the underlying muscles to contract and push against the ribs. The corrective force against the spine causes it to straighten. The treatment may be considered painful at first; however, the child usually grows accustomed to the sensations. The therapy is usually completed over an 8-hour period while the child is sleeping. Therapy continues until skeletal maturity is obtained. The treatment has not been proven to be consistently effective and thus its use has declined dramatically.

If the curve of the child's scoliosis is less than 20 degrees, most physicians observe the child for any further progression of the curve. The child is assessed approximately every 6 months on an outpatient basis until the physician determines either that the curve is not worsening or that more aggressive treatment is needed.

When the scoliosis measures between 20 and 39 degrees of curvature and evidence of progression exists, bracing is generally the next course of action. Over the past 50 years, a variety of braces, or orthoses, have been developed to treat scoliosis. The Milwaukee brace is the most familiar, although in recent years the Boston brace has become more popular. This is most likely a result of its acceptance by teenagers because it is not visible when worn under clothing. However, the Boston brace is not effective for high thoracic curves. A brace also may be custom designed specifically for a child (Fig. 20–17).

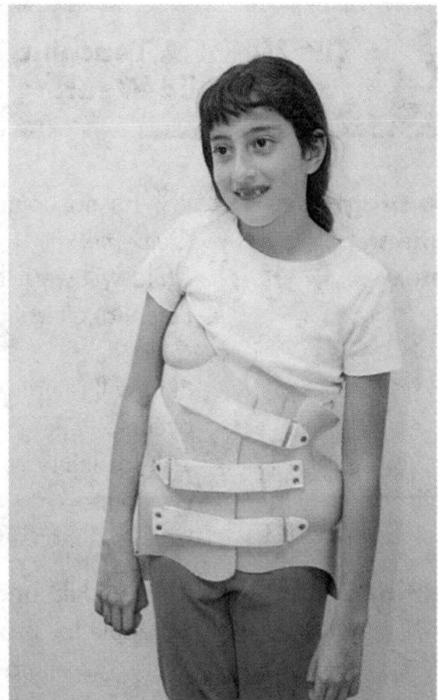

Figure 20–17
A brace can be custom designed to meet the child's specific corrective needs. This child wears her fitted brace only while sleeping.

Tip: *If the child expresses strong resistance to the idea of wearing a brace, it may not be worth the expense to have one fabricated.*

If the child must wear a brace, the schedule for brace wearing should be fit into a time slot that is convenient yet fulfills the required number of hours for brace wearing. Brace wearing is generally recommended for at least 16 hours a day. During brace treatment, children are seen in the physician's office every 4 to 6 months. Once the child reaches skeletal maturity, brace wearing is tapered off. When braces work, they prevent progression of the curve by holding it in place until the child reaches skeletal maturity. The ideal candidate for a brace is the child who is immature skeletally and has a curve with a high risk for progression. TIP 20–3 summarizes a teaching intervention plan for the child with a brace. Despite compliance with a bracing regimen, however, the curve does progress in some children, necessitating surgical intervention at some point.

Surgical Interventions

Most experts believe that if a spinal curve reaches 40 degrees or more, surgery should be considered because there is a great possibility that the curve will worsen. With a curve measurement of greater than 50 degrees, surgery is almost always needed. Each case is considered for neurologic status, bone age, diagnosis, curve size, physical and psychological impact of the deformity, and readiness for a major surgical intervention.

The goals of scoliosis surgery are to prevent further deformity and to correct the curve, if possible. The surgi-

TIP 20–3 A Teaching Intervention Plan for the Child Wearing a Brace for a Back Condition

Nursing Diagnoses and Patient Outcomes

- Risk for noncompliance related to discomfort, alteration in body image from brace
  Outcome:
  Child will wear brace for prescribed period of time.
- Potential alteration in skin integrity related to presence of brace
  Outcome:
  Skin will remain intact, pressure areas will be recognized early before skin breakdown occurs.
- Risk for injury related to the presence of a brace
  Outcome:
  Child will not sustain injury.

Interventions

Teach the Child and Family

- Schedule for Brace Wear
  The number of hours the brace must be worn depends on the type of brace.
  The child should wear the brace during sleep to use up the most hours.
- Skin Care and Comfort
  With a new brace, gradually increase wearing time so that the skin can develop tolerance for the pressure of the brace.
  Wear a 100% cotton T-shirt underneath the brace to absorb moisture.
  Do not use powders or lotions under the brace.
  Watch for areas of redness that do not disappear in 20 minutes, tingling, numbness.
  Cover the chin pad (if present) with a smooth cloth to preserve skin integrity.
  Fit and comfort are important factors. If the brace does not seem to fit well, consult the orthotist who made the brace.
  The brace may be loosened during meals.
  Avoid sitting in one position for long periods of time.
- Appearance
  Select loose clothing that will camouflage the brace.

Activity and Safety

Normal defense mechanisms and mobility are altered in a brace. Look for environmental hazards, and either remove them or find ways to avoid them.
Use safety precautions (e.g., handrail when using stairs).
Exercises and athletic activities for general conditioning can be done both in and out of the brace.
Child may ride a bicycle while in the brace.
No swimming, gymnastics, skating, skiing, or contact sports while in the brace.

Contact Health Care Provider if

Signs of skin redness, numbness, or tingling persists under or around the brace.
The brace seems to become uncomfortable, despite having fit well in the past.
The child is not wearing the brace for the prescribed amount of time each day.

cal procedure is a spinal fusion, usually with instrumentation. The most common surgical approach for idiopathic scoliosis is posterior. This consists of a long, straight midline incision extending to two levels above and below the segments of the spine to be fused. Iliac crest bone graft is used to augment the fusion. Care Path 20–1 outlines the preoperative and postoperative care for a child with a posterior spinal fusion.

Various types of instrumentation can stabilize and correct the spinal deformity (Table 20–15). The Texas

Table 20–15
Comparison of Types of Instrumentation Used for Posterior Spinal Fusion

Type of Instrumentation	Description	Indications	Area of Fixation	Early Postoperative Positioning	Brace Needed	Advantages	Disadvantages
Harrington	Single rod with two hooks	Scoliosis; not commonly used	Top and bottom of curve	Logroll and bed rest for 1 week until casted; do not logroll to convex side of thoracic curve	Yes; or cast	Inexpensive Highly adaptable Relatively simple technique	Minimal derotation Less cosmetic results—flat back
TSR/CD (Texas Scottish Rite Hospital/ Cotrel-Dubousset)	Double rod with multiple hooks and crossbars	Idiopathic scoliosis; lordosis	Segmental	Head of bed up 30–45 degrees Hip flexion over crease of bed Logroll until ambulating Bed flat when on side No overhead frame	No	Stable Three-dimensional correction	Technically difficult procedure Bulky hardware Adequate bone surface needed Expensive
Luque	Double rod with wires	Neuromuscular disease (scoliosis, muscular dystrophy, cerebral palsy)	Segmental	Logroll Head of bed up 30 degrees	Sometimes	Rigid fixation Inexpensive Adaptable No anterior instrumentation	Increased operating time Demanding technique Increased blood loss

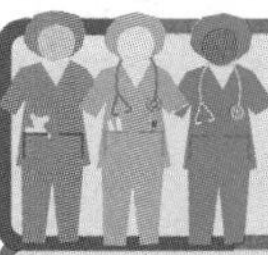

Care Path 20–1 An Interdisciplinary Plan of Care for the Child with Posterior Spinal Fusion

	Patient/Family Intermediate Outcomes		
Nursing Diagnosis	**Day 1**	**Day 2**	**Day 3**
Knowledge deficit related to preoperative teaching and postoperative routines	Child/family will verbalize understanding of surgical procedure. Orient them to the unit.	Child/family will verbalize understanding of logrolling technique, the need for various tubes, and the diet regimen.	⟶
Pain related to surgical maneuvers and surgical incision	Child will experience relief of pain as evidenced by verbalization of relief, HR and RR WNL, and uninterrupted sleep.	⟶	⟶
Ineffective breathing pattern related to lower lung expansion, pain, and analgesics	Child will maintain adequate aeration as evidenced by clear BS, absence of cyanosis, RR WNL.	⟶	⟶
Self-care deficit related to altered body mechanics	Child will remain on bedrest and be log rolled with assistance.	⟶	Child will demonstrate increased participation in ADLs.
Care Intervention Categories			
Consults	Anesthesia	Physical therapy Brace company, if indicated	
Discharge Planning	Arrange for homebound tutor, if indicated.	Discuss discharge needs with physician. Assess equipment needs.	Order equipment if needed. Assess home environment.
Labs	CBC with differential PT/PTT UA Chem #20 Type and cross for 4 units of blood	H & H Electrolytes	H & H Electrolytes

Day 4	Day 5 or 6
Child/family will verbalize understanding of discharge activity instructions and wound care.	⟶ Child is discharged when outcomes are met.
Child will experience relief of pain from PO medications.	Child will verbalize understanding of when and how to take pain medications at home.
⟶	⟶ Child is discharged when breath sounds are clear and no alterations are noted in breathing pattern.
⟶	Child will require minimal assistance with ADLs. Child can be discharged home.
Arrange for transportation if needed.	Ensure that needed equipment is delivered.
H & H Electrolytes	

Care Path continued on following page

Scottish Rite Hospital, Cotrel-Dubousset, and Luque rod instrumentations have an advantage in that they usually do not require bracing after the surgery. This allows the patient to be ambulatory within 1 to 2 days after surgery. When bone quality is poor, it may not be feasible to place any type of instrumentation. In those cases, a bony fusion is performed and a body cast must be worn until the fusion heals (approximately 4 to 6 months).

Occasionally, a child with severe scoliosis (greater than 90 degrees), is placed in halo traction before surgery. This stretches the spine and the musculature to allow a greater degree of correction of the spine. Halo traction can be used for 1 week before spinal surgery or in the week between an anterior and posterior spinal fusion.

If the child has a questionable or known decrease in pulmonary function, evaluation of whether the child is healthy enough to withstand surgery is needed. For children with intact sensation in their lower extremities, spinal cord impulses are monitored during surgery. This involves having electrodes attached to the scalp the morning of surgery. Spinal cord monitoring allows the surgeon to be immediately aware of any alteration in spinal cord transmission. To correct the situation, an instrument may need to be removed or replaced.

Before surgery, the health care team reviews the surgical plan with the family. The family is given information explaining postoperative activity restrictions (Table 20–16). Preoperative teaching focuses on what the patient and family can expect after surgery including pain management preferences, logrolling, and other daily care issues. A hospital tour helps prepare the child and family for the surgical experience. The nurse also assists the family in making arrangements for autologous and directed donor blood if they are concerned about bloodborne infections.

After surgery, children may go either to the intensive care unit for 1 night or to the pediatric unit. Nursing concerns for the first 24 to 48 hours focus on respiratory status, fluid volume shifts, and pain management. Occasionally, the child needs to be on a ventilator for a brief period of time to assist with breathing and optimize respiratory status. Preventive pulmonary care is essential, whether the child is mechanically ventilated or not, to avoid pneumonia. Patients are turned, using a logroll technique (Fig. 20–18), every 2 hours to decrease pooling of secretions in the lungs, and coughing and deep breathing are encouraged. Use of the incentive spirometer and early ambulation also help prevent pulmonary complications.

Ongoing nursing assessments in the care of a postoperative spinal fusion include evaluating fluid balance (intake and output), monitoring wound healing and drains, assessing neurovascular status of the extremities, and facilitating ambulation. Additionally, the child should be

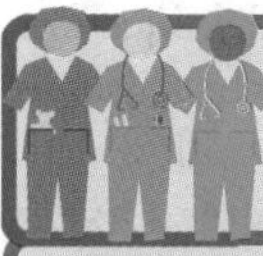

Care Path 20–1 An Interdisciplinary Plan of Care for the Child with Posterior Spinal Fusion *Continued*

Care Intervention Categories	Day 1	Day 2	Day 3
Medications	IV antibiotics (Ancef) IV fluids	→ →	→ IV to hep lock Laxative if needed
Monitors	Cardiac monitor Monitor if in ICU or on epidural infusion of morphine Arterial line Pulse oximetry	Discontinue monitors	
Nutrition	NPO	Begin clear liquids if bowel sounds are present.	Advance to regular diet as tolerated.
Pain management	PCA, morphine epidural, or IV infusion Pain assessment q 2 hr	→	→ Assessment q 4 hr
Play therapy/school	NA	Provide diversional activities such as movies	School teacher called
Procedures (diagnostics)	Posterior spinal fusion with TSRH instrumentation		
Psychosocial	Provide regular reports from OR to help relieve parental anxiety		Child can call family/friends on the telephone.
Radiology	PA radiograph in post-anesthesia unit	CXR	CXR if still on O_2
Rehabilitation		Active ROM to all extremities PT b.i.d.	PT b.i.d.
Respiratory	Extubate in OR. Wean O_2 to maintain $FiO_2 \geq 95\%$ Incentive spirometer q 1 hour while awake	Discontinue O_2 if FiO_2 $>95\%$	
Safety and activity	Bed rest HOB 30 degrees Log roll q 2 hr	Begin to get OOB to chair if no brace needed b.i.d. as tolerated	OOB b.i.d. ambulating in halls
Self-care	Foley catheter care		Using bedpan or bathroom
Social service	Consult social worker for family support, meal tickets		

Day 4	Day 5 or 6
⟶ ⟶	To PO antibiotics Discontinue IV
Regular diet	Regular diet
Tylenol with codeine p.r.n. Assessment q 4 hr	⟶
Encourage child to go to playroom	⟶
	Standing PA and lateral radiograph of the spine
PT b.i.d.	Discharge from PT when ambulating without assistance and able to climb stairs
OOB ambulating ad lib Practice on stairs	⟶
Using bathroom	⟶

Care Path continued on following page

encouraged to cough and deep breathe every 2 hours to avoid pulmonary complications. Bowel sounds should be assessed, with progression of fluids and diet made gradually to ensure that bowel motility is fully restored. Care of the postsurgical child is discussed in detail in Chapter 9.

The wound from a spinal fusion is closed with dissolvable sutures on the inside and Steri-Strips or staples on the outside. It is then covered with gauze bandages, and a pressure dressing is applied. The incision is kept covered with the dressing for 2 to 3 days. The nurse assesses the area for bleeding and notes any unusual drainage on the dressing. A Hemovac or similar surgical drain may be used to help evacuate excess blood from under the skin. The Hemovac generally has the most output in the first 24 hours, gradually tapering off over the next few days, and it is discontinued at about postoperative day 2 or 3. The nurse should monitor the amount of accumulated drainage. The child should also be assessed for infection at the incision site. The administration of prophylactic antibiotics for the first 72 hours postoperatively is a common practice to prevent infection.

Syndrome of inappropriate antidiuretic hormone (SIADH) is common in spinal fusion patients after surgery. This is due to a number of factors, including change in blood volume, anesthetic medications, and the physical and emotional stress of the surgical procedure itself (Bell, Gurd, Orlowski, & Andrish, 1986). SIADH causes low postoperative urinary output. The urine is concentrated but the serum is dilute. The treatment for SIADH is restriction of fluid. It resolves spontaneously in 2 to 3 days and the patient starts diuresis.

Pain after a spinal fusion cannot be eliminated but it can and should be controlled (see Chapter 13). For some patients, a continuous intravenous infusion of opioids works well, especially for non-verbal patients. Patient-controlled analgesia (PCA) is very effective in managing pain and is a common method of pain treatment. Other children benefit from an epidural, placed in the incision during surgery, which uses an infusion of a local anesthetic or opioid to block transmission of pain impulses. After approximately postoperative day 3, the child can be switched to oral pain medications such as acetaminophen with codeine (Chart 20–17).

Early mobilization is encouraged to prevent pulmonary emboli, phlebitis, and skin breakdown. Children are encouraged to move their extremities while they are on bed rest. The child should be turned using the logrolling technique every 2 hours. The child's level of pain should be assessed and pain relief provided as needed before turning or ambulation. On approximately postoperative day 5, the child is ambulated. Physical therapy after surgery assists the child in ambulation training, including teaching how to step and make transfers. Caregivers are

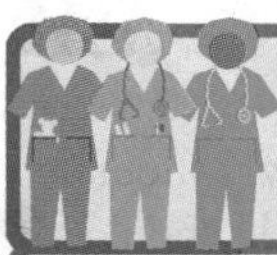

Care Path 20–1 An Interdisciplinary Plan of Care for the Child with Posterior Spinal Fusion *Continued*

Care Interventions Categories	Day 1	Day 2	Day 3
Teaching	Discuss postoperative expectations and routine. Give tour of unit.	Reinforce logrolling techniques. Use of incentive spirometer and appropriate use of pain medications.	Instruct child on proper body mechanics when getting OOB.
Visitors	Limit visitors	Visitors allowed as desired by patient	⟶
Vital signs/baseline parameters	Postoperative routine VS NV checks q 1 hr for 24 hours I&O q 4 hr Height and weight Monitor dressing for drainage and bleeding q 1–2 hr	I&O q 8 hr VS q 4 hr NV check q 4 hr	I&O q 8 hr VS q 4 hr NV check q 8 hr Dressing check q 4 hr

ADL, activity of daily living; b.i.d., twice daily; BS, breath sounds; CBC, complete blood count; Chem #20, blood chemistry test for 20 items; CXR, chest radiograph; H & H, hemoglobin and hematocrit; HOB, head of bed; HR, heart rate; ICU, intensive care unit; I&O, intake and output; NPO, nothing by mouth; NV, neurovascular; OOB, out of bed; OR, operating room; PA, posteroanterior; PCA, patient-controlled analgesia; PO, oral; PT, physical therapy; PT/PTT, prothrombin time/partial thromboplastin time; ROM, range of motion; RR, respiratory rate; TSRH, Texas Scottish Rite Hospital; UA, urinalysis; VS, vital signs; WNL, within normal limits.

Table 20–16
Activity Guidelines for Children After Back Surgery

Time Frame	Activities Encouraged	Activities Not Encouraged	Activities Restricted
Discharge from hospital to 4–6 weeks	Walking Quiet activities Study with homebound tutor; may start back to school in 3–4 weeks Riding in car, but not driving Swimming	Lifting more than 5 pounds Running Diving in a pool Playing contact sports Riding dirt bikes, all-terrain vehicles, or mountain bikes	Gymnastics Parachuting Bungee jumping Motorcycle riding Trampoline jumping
6 weeks to 3 months	Same as above, but driving is allowed	Same as above	Same as above
3–6 months	Riding a bike Light jogging Lifting 5–10 pounds	Same as above	Same as above
6 months to 1 year	Return to most of the normal activities done before surgery Bowling, skiing, skating, aerobics, golfing, horseback riding, diving, and racquet sports Lifting weights	Playing contact sports until 1 year from surgery Water park amusement rides or roller coasters until 1 year after surgery	Same as above unless approved by physician

Day 4	Day 5 or 6
Instruct child on PO pain medications. Instruct family on wound care.	Instruct child/family on care of cast/brace if needed. Discharge teaching completed.
⟶	⟶
VS q 4 hr NV check q 8 hr	⟶ Dressing or wound check q 4 hr

Figure 20–18
The logrolling technique is used after back surgery to prevent a child from flexing the back while being turned from side to side in bed.

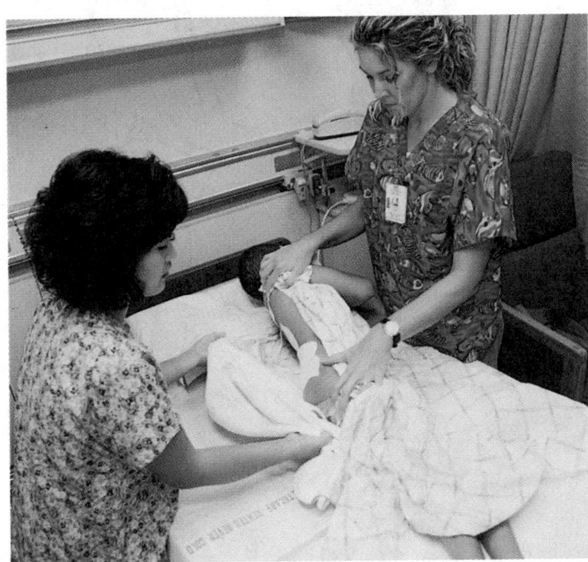

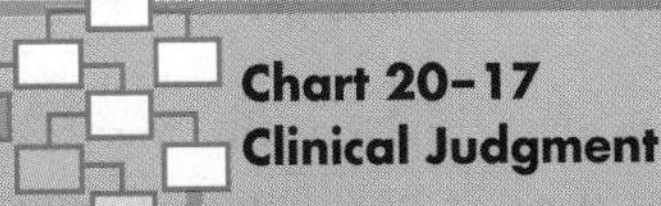

Chart 20–17
Clinical Judgment

The Child After Spinal Fusion

Whitney is a 13-year-old black female who is admitted to the hospital for a posterior spinal fusion for idiopathic scoliosis. She is brought to your unit from the post-anesthesia care unit (PACU) after her surgery. She has an intravenous line in her left hand, a nasogastric tube to low intermittent suction, and a Foley catheter. Her orders state that she is NPO, on strict intake and output, and must logroll every 2 hours. Her vital signs are as follows: temperature, 99.5°F; pulse rate, 90; respiratory rate, 28; blood pressure, 135/78. She is moaning.

Questions

1. During your assessment, what other data would be important to elicit from the PACU nurse who is giving you the report?
2. What are some of the important aspects of care you will want to evaluate in this postsurgical child?
3. Is Whitney in pain currently?
4. How can her pain be managed?
5. What factors would indicate that her pain is well controlled?

Answers

1. How much blood was lost in the operating room and how much blood did Whitney receive? How much fluid did she receive in the operating room? Assess the appearance of the wound and the amount of drainage in the Hemovac. Note the type of procedure that was done and any complications that occurred in the operating room. Also, check pain medication orders. When was the last pain medication given, and is the dose appropriate for her weight?
2. Fluid balance, pain management, and respiratory status.
3. Yes, she is probably in pain as evidenced by increased pulse, respirations, and blood pressure. Whitney should be asked to rate her pain to validate your assessment.
4. Intravenous or epidural infusion of opioids via patient-controlled analgesia pump or bolus.
5. Whitney is able to logroll easily, she is sleeping, she verbalizes relief of pain, and her vital signs return to baseline.

encouraged to accompany the child to therapy. The physical therapist can also teach strengthening and isometric exercises to the child who is bedridden. Children who are wheelchair-bound may need their wheelchair adjusted to conform to their new shape. If the child has a brace or cast after the surgery, care of the brace or cast and general skin care are reviewed before discharge. Parents must correctly demonstrate how to apply the brace. Brace adjustments should be made before the child goes home.

Community Care

Although special equipment is usually not needed after a spinal fusion, some children require an elevated toilet seat, hospital bed, or a shower chair in their home after discharge. These needs can be assessed in the hospital as the child's activity progresses. Plans need to be made regarding who will watch the child at home and provisions made to ensure that the child is able to continue with school studies during the recovery period at home. The child can usually return to school within 4 to 6 weeks.

During the home recovery period, children should avoid twisting or bending activities and not lift heavy objects. The child should not participate in contact or high-impact sports for up to 2 years. Swimming and cycling are encouraged and can be resumed within 3 to 4 months.

Good nutrition is an important aspect of wound healing and general health. By the time of discharge, children are eating a regular diet. Some children need iron supplementation after surgery to augment anemia caused by blood loss during surgery. Vitamin C and protein are important for healing, and eating foods containing those dietary elements should be encouraged. Extra calcium intake is not needed if the diet is well balanced. If the child has constipation caused by decreased activity and medication regimens, eating foods high in fiber and increasing fluid intake should be encouraged. A stool softener such as Colace may also be necessary.

The diagnosis of scoliosis often happens at a vulnerable time in a child's life—the teenage years. Body image is at the forefront of a teenager's mind and, to him or her, the hump on his or her back is enormous. Anything that makes a teenager different from his or her peers is stressful. Putting the child in contact with someone who is undergoing the same problems can be helpful. Parents also need to be supported with counseling, because they can be frightened by the unfamiliar situation as well. Difficulties can arise when the parents and teenager disagree on the type of treatment to be undertaken. Most teenagers comprehend what is happening to their bodies and they should be included in decision-making from the start. (See Chapter 2 for more information on informed consent, autonomy, and self-determination issues.) The National Scoliosis Foundation is a good resource for families seeking more information or support groups (see Resources).

Kyphosis and Lordosis

Kyphosis and lordosis are two terms used to describe a spinal curvature in the sagittal plane. Kyphosis is commonly described as a "humpback" or excessive forward concavity of the spine. Lordosis is a "swayback" or excessive backward concavity of the spine (Fig. 20–19). Both curves are present in the normal spine, but, when they become excessive, families may seek treatment. Lordosis, usually of the lumbar spine, is not a major deformity in children.

Most cases of kyphosis occur in the thoracic region of the spine. The normal range of kyphosis in a growing child is from 20 to 45 degrees (Bradford, Lonstein, Moe, Ogilvie, & Winter, 1987). Greater than 45 degrees is considered abnormal. Females are affected slightly more often than males. Kyphosis can be a congenital or acquired condition. Common causes of kyphosis include ankylosing spondylitis, metabolic disorders, neuromuscular conditions, OI, Paget's disease, Scheuermann's disease, and spina bifida.

Figure 20–19
A, A child with kyphosis. *B*, A child with lordosis.

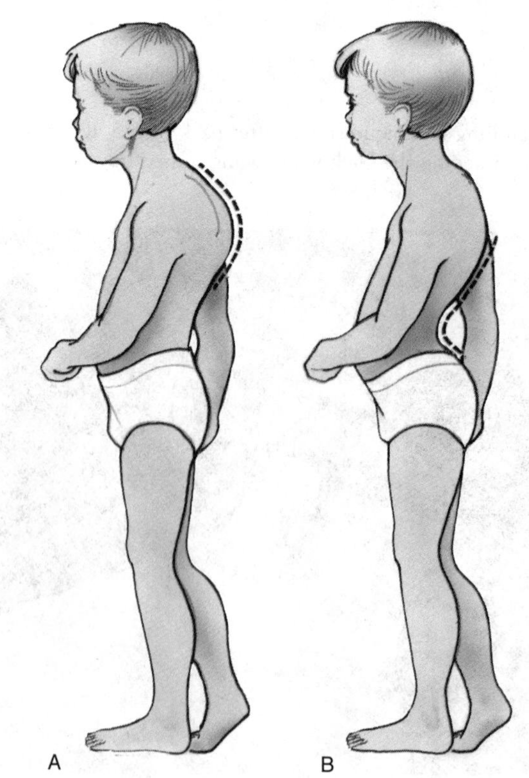

Kyphosis may also be an acquired postural problem. This is seen in the child who can voluntarily bend the spine to correct the curvature and in whom no underlying evidence of structural changes is seen.

Assessment

Kyphosis and lordosis are most commonly noted for the first time during the teenage years. Evaluation of the child during an in-school back screening program may be the first time the appearance of the back deformity is assessed. Parents may notice a curve or uneven shoulders when the child is trying on clothes or a bathing suit. Some children complain of back pain in the thoracic area, especially with Scheuermann's disease. Scheuermann's disease, also called juvenile or adolescent kyphosis, results from wedge-shaped vertebrae in the thoracic region of the spine.

The evaluation for kyphosis should include a full orthopedic and neurologic examination. This examination helps distinguish the cause for the kyphosis and rule out intraspinal problems such as cysts or tumors. Physical examination reveals a sharp angulation of the thoracic spine when the child bends over and is viewed from the side (see Fig. 20–16). Radiographs should be obtained to diagnose and follow up the progression of kyphosis.

Interdisciplinary Interventions

A nonsurgical treatment program is used for a child with kyphosis of 50 to 70 degrees. Depending on the physician and the case, this program can range from observation to bracing to thoracic hyperextension exercises. The most common type of brace used for treatment of kyphosis is the Milwaukee brace. The child wears the brace for at least 16 hours a day until skeletal maturity develops. The child may wear a lightweight cotton shirt under the brace to absorb moisture and decrease chafing. After the child has reached skeletal maturity, the risk of curve progression is small. If the child is having back pain, the physician also may prescribe back strengthening and thoracic hyperextension exercises.

Despite compliance with nonsurgical treatments, some curves do progress. Other children may present with a kyphosis greater than 70 degrees. Physicians recommend surgical treatment in either case. The goal of surgery is to prevent further progression of the curve that could cause respiratory compromise or spinal cord compression if left unchecked. An added benefit of the surgery is correction of the curve to a normal degree.

If a child has a congenital kyphosis, the treatment plan is different. Congenital kyphosis does not respond well to bracing. The curve tends to be worse and to progress earlier in the child's life. Most orthopedists observe these children until the curve reaches 65 to 70 degrees, and then they proceed with surgery. The higher the degree of curvature, the more respiratory compromise the child exhibits.

The standard surgical procedure for kyphosis is an anterior–posterior spinal fusion. This approach allows the surgeon to release the disks on the front of the spine, thereby making it more flexible and easier to achieve correction of the curve. In addition, the surgeon fuses the spine posteriorly to stop growth and progression of the curve. A spinal fusion fuses one vertebra to another, stopping motion between them. Metal fixation consisting of hooks and rods holds the spine in place until the bones fuse. After the spine heals in 4 to 6 months, the metal fixation is no longer necessary, but it remains in place unless it causes pain.

An anterior–posterior spinal fusion can be done in one operation, or it can be completed in two separate operations. Some children cannot tolerate the one-step operation because of their medical condition. The most common type of instrumentation used for kyphosis surgery is segmental fixation, or the Texas Scottish Rite Hospital and Cotrel-Dubousset systems. Care of the child after spinal fusion is discussed in the previous section on scoliosis.

Inflammatory and Infectious Disorders

Inflammatory and infectious diseases in orthopedics are generally caused by bacteria that invade bone or joints. The bacteria alarms the immune system, which sends white blood cells to the area to fight the infection. The resulting pus formation, edema, and vascular congestion cause destruction of not only the bacteria but also the bone or membranes in the joint. Additionally, rheumatic disorders such as systemic lupus erythematosus (SLE) cause inflammation of connective tissue, thereby altering a child's musculoskeletal status. This section describes the most commonly seen inflammatory and infectious diseases.

Osteomyelitis

Osteomyelitis is an infection of the bone and of the tissues around the bone. The two most common types in children are acute and subacute hematogenous osteomyelitis.

Alert: *All types of osteomyelitis require immediate treatment if suspected, because they can cause massive bone destruction and life-threatening sepsis.*

Osteomyelitis most often involves the long bones of the lower limb, although it can occur in any bone of the body. Many kinds of organisms cause osteomyelitis but the most common is *Staphylococcus aureus*. Osteomyelitis can arise through a variety of routes. These include an open fracture or penetration of the skin by a contaminated object, spread from a septic joint or infected wound, or spread from a bacterial infection somewhere in the body, such as dental caries. Blunt trauma also may precede osteomyelitis because the hematoma formed from the trauma acts as an entry port for microorganisms. Premature babies and infants with birth complications are at a higher risk for osteomyelitis in the first year of life, although it usually occurs in healthy children.

Pathophysiology

In the acute phase of osteomyelitis, bacteria lodge and multiply in the middle of the bone where the circulation is sluggish. The infection then spreads to the ends of the bone if not treated, and it can destroy the growth plate in children. The body's inflammatory response produces pus formation, edema, and vascular congestion in the area of infection. If this process continues, pressure in the bone increases and eventually cuts off the blood supply, causing necrosis. The body attempts to lay down new bone over the old dead bone, but this process causes a pocket of dead tissue (sequestrum) to form. Sequestra are a medium for more microorganism growth. The sequestra can grow and extrude through the bone into soft tissues, causing further problems.

Prognosis. If osteomyelitis is treated promptly with intravenous antibiotics, prognosis is good. Before antibiotics became available, children either lived with chronic osteomyelitis or they had the extremity amputated to prevent sepsis.

Assessment

Children with acute osteomyelitis often present in the emergency room complaining of pain in a bone. Some children have fever; however, affected neonates usually do not exhibit a fever. The child is irritable and will not use the painful limb. When obtaining a history, the parent may report a recent infection, such as a cold or otitis media in the child. Alternatively, the child may have a history of falling or bumping an extremity.

Physical examination of the affected area reveals localized tenderness, redness, warmth, and pain on palpation of the area. Occasionally, children have soft tissue swelling around the area. Radiographs and a bone scan assist with the diagnosis.

Nursing Diagnoses and Outcomes

Nursing diagnoses and desired patient outcomes for the child with a musculoskeletal disorder are presented in Chart 20–5. Based on the assessment data, the following nursing diagnoses may also apply to the child with osteomyelitis:

- **Impaired tissue integrity related to the infectious process**
  Outcomes: The child will maintain the affected extremity in proper alignment.
  The child will not bear weight on the affected extremity.
  Wound and skin isolation precautions will be maintained to minimize infection transmission.
- **Risk for altered body temperature related to the infectious process**
  Outcomes: The child's body temperature remains within normal range.
  Measures are instituted to decrease hyperthermia.

Interdisciplinary Interventions

A child with suspected osteomyelitis is started on broad-spectrum parenteral antibiotics after blood cultures are drawn. After the patient demonstrates a response to parenteral antibiotics (usually in 2 to 3 days) and final blood cultures are obtained, the parenteral medication is stopped and the patient is started on oral antibiotics. Children who do not respond well initially to intravenous antibiotics may remain on intravenous antibiotic therapy much longer. The length of oral therapy ranges from 4 to 8 weeks. Monitoring the response to antibiotic therapy consists of erythrocyte sedimentation rate (ESR) measurements once a week. As the infectious process resolves, the ESR decreases.

caREminder: *The antibiotics used to treat osteomyelitis are caustic to veins. The nurse must be diligent about diluting the medication and infusing it slowly.*

The intravenous site should be monitored closely for signs of infiltration. Usually, long-term antibiotic therapy is given to the child with osteomyelitis. Whenever possible, the nurse can advocate for the patient to have an intravenous line such as a peripherally inserted central catheter (PICC) line placed that can stay in for an extended period. Frequent laboratory tests can also be drawn from this line. Thus, placement of a PICC line is extremely helpful in decreasing the number of needle sticks the child will receive. (See Chapter 17 for a more complete discussion of care of the PICC line.)

Nursing interventions for a child with suspected or known osteomyelitis include making the child comfortable and ensuring relief from pain. Splinting the involved extremity may be helpful in the first few days of treatment (see Treatment Modalities). Splints should not be used indefinitely or use of the affected extremity may be discouraged. If required, oral medications such as acetaminophen, ibuprofen, or narcotic analgesics can be given to relieve pain. After antibiotics have been administered for at least 24 hours, bone and tissue pain should start to subside.

The hospitalized child may become easily bored and frustrated by the limitations imposed by the lengthy intravenous therapy. The involvement of a child life therapist can be extremely helpful in providing age-appropriate diversions and activities that do not compromise the intravenous site or cause the child pain in the affected limb.

Community Care

Many children with osteomyelitis are discharged on a regimen of home intravenous antibiotics. This option should be discussed with the family at the start of treatment. Home intravenous antibiotic administration requires a large commitment from the family. The nurse helps in assessing whether a family can maintain a child on home intravenous antibiotics. If the antibiotics can be scheduled every 8 to 12 hours, compliance increases. A parent who is administering one or two antibiotics every 4 to 6 hours can easily become sleep deprived. Some children may return to school while they are on home intravenous antibiotics, if the medicine is given every 12 hours. Other children use a home-bound tutor until they have completed the medications.

The child with chronic osteomyelitis may benefit from increased psychological support to help deal with depression associated with physical limitations and frequent hospitalizations. Although symptoms of chronic osteomyelitis are similar to those of acute osteomyelitis, the child has a history of symptoms persisting for longer than 3 weeks. Other children may have a history of prior (by weeks or months) bone infection after surgery or trauma. Treatment is prolonged, painful, and frustrating for the child and family. However, with the increased awareness of the need for prompt, aggressive treatment, the incidence of chronic osteomyelitis in children is decreasing.

Septic Arthritis

Septic arthritis is an infection within a joint or synovial membrane. Bacterial organisms enter into a joint and begin an infectious process through a variety of ways. These include hematogenous seeding (transmitted by the bloodstream), by extension of an adjacent bone infection, or by a penetrating wound or foreign body in the joint. Septic arthritis occurs in all age groups, although the most common age of occurrence is 1 to 2 years. *S. aureus* is the most common causative organism.

Pathophysiology

The process of septic arthritis begins when bacteria enter the joint space. This causes an inflammatory reaction that results in fluid and white cells entering the joint. These white blood cells release an enzyme that breaks down the surface of the articular cartilage. Scar tissue then replaces the articular cartilage, restricting joint motion. If not treated promptly and aggressively, septic arthritis results in permanent loss of function. Before antibiotics became available, septic arthritis often was fatal. Children died of septicemia resulting from inoculation from the joint infection.

Assessment

The symptoms of septic arthritis in a child are pain, fever, motion limitation, and joint swelling. It usually involves only one joint that is red, warm, and tender when palpated. Common sites for septic arthritis, in decreasing order of prevalence, are as follows:

- Knee
- Hip
- Ankle
- Elbow
- Wrist
- Shoulder
- Pelvis

When asked to move the joint, the child may resist or guard the joint. The parent usually reports that the child will not walk or crawl if the hip or lower extremities are involved.

In giving a health history, the parent frequently reports a recent ear infection, cold, or joint trauma. Any history of a bite or penetrating wound, such as with a needle or thorn, is also important in trying to ascertain the cause for the septic arthritis.

Diagnostic Tests. Radiologic tests for septic arthritis include a traditional radiograph, ultrasound, and bone scan. The radiograph can rule out any lesions and detect soft tissue swelling. An ultrasound may be done, especially if the hip is affected, to look for fluid in the joint. A bone scan is helpful in identifying osteomyelitis, but it does not show septic arthritis.

The definitive test for septic arthritis is a needle aspiration of joint fluid. The physician can often identify infected fluid by looking for the "no string sign." Infected joint fluid is less viscous than normal joint fluid. Thus, if the physician puts a drop of the fluid between two fingers and pulls them apart, no strings of mucus stretch between the fingers. Also, infected joint fluid is cloudy rather than clear. On joint aspiration, cultures of the fluid are obtained to identify the causative organism.

Interdisciplinary Interventions

In septic arthritis, the inflammatory process, not the bacteria itself, causes damage to the joint. Thus, the inflammatory exudate that causes the damage to articular surfaces must be released. The physician may aspirate the fluid with a needle. If the fluid continues to accumulate, then arthroscopy can be used to clean out the joint and obtain a synovial biopsy. In certain joints such as the hip or shoulder, an arthrotomy, or surgical opening into the joint, is needed. The fluid and biopsy samples are sent for laboratory examination to ascertain the causative organism.

The administration of antibiotics for a 4- to 6-week period is an important aspect of the treatment plan. Broad-spectrum parenteral antibiotics are started after a culture has been obtained. Once an organism has been identified, the type of antibiotic is changed to one that is specific for the causative organism. If the causative agent is not identified, intravenous antibiotics are continued for the entire course of therapy. Children who require continuing parenteral therapy need not be hospitalized for the entire course of therapy. Intravenous antibiotics can be administered in the home by a home care nurse.

If the causative agent is identified and if the child has a good response to the treatment regimen, oral antibiotics may be given to replace intravenous antibiotics and the child may be discharged. A good response includes decreased pain and swelling, laboratory values on a downward trend, and fever resolution. The child takes oral antibiotics for 3 to 6 weeks or for the length of time it takes for the erythrocyte sedimentation rate (ESR) to return to normal. Antibiotic levels are monitored throughout treatment to ensure a therapeutic dosage range of antibiotics at all times.

Nursing care for the child with septic arthritis includes managing pain, reducing body temperature, and ensuring that consistent administration of the medication is given. If the child is uncomfortable, oral pain medications are administered and their effectiveness monitored. Analgesics should be given before beginning daily activities or treatments that may cause discomfort.

The affected limb or joint may be splinted initially for comfort. The splint may be removed after a few days. The child should be observed to note the extent of joint mobility, voluntary movement, and weight-bearing capabilities. Children should be encouraged to participate in daily activities as they feel able to do so. Assistive devices such as crutches or a walker may be needed to support ambulation. Wound management of an open arthrotomy site consists of securing the dressing, noting the color and amount of secretions, and changing the dressing if necessary.

The child's temperature should be monitored frequently. Antipyretics are administered as ordered by the physician to reduce temperature if the child is febrile. Other cooling measures such as a tepid sponge bath and removing blankets or clothing should be implemented. To prevent dehydration secondary to the fever, fluids are encouraged.

Families require support during the acute phase of the illness. With a diagnosis of septic arthritis, concern about loss of joint function is paramount. If treatment was delayed, the parent may feel guilty about not seeking medical attention earlier. The nurse can encourage the parent to seek support from family members, social services, clergy, and friends.

Before discharge, the family is taught about medication administration. Important points include the importance of not missing scheduled doses and the need to continue administering the medication until the prescription is gone, even if the child feels better. Insufficient treatment can result in permanent damage to the articular cartilage or in chronic osteomyelitis. Follow-up care is needed to assess the effectiveness of the treatment.

Juvenile Arthritis

Juvenile rheumatoid arthritis (JRA) is a common chronic inflammatory condition of the joints and connective tissue. "Arthritis" is defined as swelling or both pain and limitation of motion in at least one joint (Jacobs, 1992). The term juvenile arthritis (JA) is gradually replacing the term JRA to better express the differences between juvenile arthritis and the rheumatoid arthritis found more commonly in adults. The diagnostic label of JA is given when onset occurs before age 16 years and duration exceeds 6 weeks without any other obvious cause. In addition, swelling or effusion in one or more joints; the presence of limited of range of motion, tenderness, or pain on motion; or increased periods of fever are indicative of JA. Joint symptoms in children can be caused by other sources including strenuous activity, trauma, or viral and bacterial illnesses. However, these problems rarely persist for an extended period.

JA is classified according to one of three types based on the mode of onset: pauciarticular, polyarticular, and systemic (Table 20–17). A further division of polyarticular JA into seronegative and seropositive groups refers to the presence or absence of the rheumatoid factor (RF) in the blood. RFs are autoantibodies that have formed in the body after long-term exposure to an antigen (Hughes & D'Ambrosia, 1993). Pauciarticular JA is also further divided into an early (before age 6) and late (age 10 to 16) onset group.

Incidence

The prevalence of JA is estimated to be 1 per 1000 school-age children, with Asian-American and black children less affected than white children (Jacobs, 1992). Onset of JA may occur as early as age 6 weeks; however, peak incidence of onset is at age 2 to 16 years. Each type has its own characteristic incidence (see Table 20–17).

Etiology

The cause of JA and the mechanisms that lead to the perpetuation of chronic synovial inflammation are unknown. It has been hypothesized that JA may be an inappropriate immune response to an unidentified antigen (Hughes & D'Ambrosia, 1993). Many inconclusive attempts have been made to link infectious agents to the onset of JA (Schaller, 1996a). Although the clinical onset of JA may follow an acute systemic infection or physical trauma to a joint, no research can support a direct cause and effect mechanism.

Some familial tendencies have been demonstrated in pauciarticular JA type I and RF-positive polyarthritis. Siblings appear to be at increased risk for development of JA. Some genetic markers (e.g., HLA-B27, HLA-DR5, HLA-DR8, HLA-DR4) can be linked to certain types of JA. However, more research is needed in this area.

Pathophysiology

JA starts with an inflamed synovial membrane and adjacent joint capsule. The inflammation of the synovial tissues produces increased amounts of fluid that are secreted into the joint. The increased fluid volume causes the joint to become swollen and boggy, termed joint effusion. The joint feels edematous and warm to touch. The synovial membranes become infiltrated with lymphocytes and plasma cells. This causes the normally clear joint fluid to become cloudy. Prolonged synovitis can result in the erosion of joint structures and narrowing of joint spaces. Eventually, bone deformity, subluxation, and ankylosis of joints occur. Growth disturbances adjacent to the affected joint can cause overgrowth or undergrowth of the affected part (Schaller, 1996a).

The joint pain and stiffness associated with JA are initially due to the pressure applied to sensory nerves in the area of the edematous membranes. As the disease progresses, pain and discomfort may also be a result of joint destruction or contractures, which lead to stiffness and immobility.

The inflammatory process may affect other systems. Carditis, pleurisy, pneumonia, and organomegaly are typically manifestations of progressive illness. Inflammation of the iris and ciliary body, termed anterior uveitis, iritis, or iridocyclitis may occur. This complication is most typically seen in young girls with pauciarticular onset. The inflammation can cause eye pain and diminished vision. In some cases, permanent blindness occurs. Ocular changes can be noted using slit-lamp examination. Early detection and treatment can assist in the preservation of the child's vision.

Assessment

Physical manifestations of JA vary according to the type (see Table 20–17). Most commonly, family members state that the child has become "cranky" or "irritable." The child may tire easily, have a poor appetite with poor weight gain, and demonstrate some growth delays. Questions should be asked regarding the child's daily activities and comfort. Children with JA have a difficult time getting out of bed in the morning because of joint stiffness. They may not participate in play activities or sports that are painful to them. The child's gait may be altered to avoid putting pressure on a distal joint. The child assumes a position of comfort, that of flexion, to protect the inflamed joint and avoid pain.

With systemic-onset JA, the child usually has a history of spiking fevers with temperatures greater than 39.5°C daily for 2 weeks in association with arthritis of two or more joints. The child with RF-negative polyarticular JA has temperatures below 39.5°C. An evanescent, pale red, non-pruritic macular rash is commonly associated with systemic onset of JA. It is present during febrile periods and may appear when the skin is irritated from scratching, heat, or trauma. The rash usually decreases or disappears during afebrile periods. When present, the rash typically appears over the trunk and extremities (except soles and palms).

During physical assessment, the examiner should inspect and palpate each joint for redness, swelling, warmth, and tenderness and should note any nodules on the joints that may be present in polyarticular-onset JA. To assess for limping or guarding behavior, the child should be observed while walking down a hall. Children with JA tend to keep their joints flexed, which can cause contractures. Accurate measurement of height and weight is also essential, because JA can retard growth.

In addition to examining the musculoskeletal system, the child should be assessed for other systemic changes. If pauciarticular-onset JA is suspected, an ophthalmologist should examine the child for iridocyclitis using slit-lamp examination. Also, a child with systemic-onset JA may have pleuritis or myocarditis. An enlarged liver, spleen, and lymph nodes are other common physical findings.

Diagnostic Tests. No laboratory test is diagnostic for JA. However, the presence of RFs, antinuclear antibodies, and certain human leukocyte antigens assist in classifying patients. The ESR is usually elevated in the child with JA. Anemia is common, the white blood cell count is frequently elevated, and any or all of the serum immunoglobulins may be elevated.

Baseline radiographs are obtained when JA is suspected. Radiographs do not show any changes until late in the disease course but they are useful to compare bone growth or damage from the time of diagnosis onward.

Table 20–17
Types of Juvenile Arthritis

Type	Age at Onset	Gender Predominance	% Affected	Systemic Manifestations	Laboratory Tests	Chronic Systemic Involvement	Prognosis
Pauciarticular Four or fewer joints for the first 6 months after disease onset; only affects the knee in some patients				Irritable, tired, poor appetite, poor weight gain, chronic eye inflammation, joints appear swollen and warm but not red			
Type I	Early onset: 2–6 years	Female	30%–40%		Less than 5% have positive RF ANA present in 90% HLA-DR8, -DR5 and -DR6	Chronic iridocyclitis Modest hepatosplenomegaly Lymphadenopathy Mild anemia	At least 60% go into remission. 10%–50% will have ocular damage from iridocyclitis.
Type II	Late onset: 10–15 years	Male	10%–15%		RF negative ANA negative HLA-B27	Self-limiting, acute iridocyclitis Ankylosing spondylitis Inflammatory bowel disease	Disease responds well to therapy. Patients generally will not have crippling disease.

Polyarticular 5 or more joints involving both upper and lower extremities, especially cervical spine				Temperature less than 39.5°C Malaise, organomegaly, adenopathy, anemia, weight loss, delayed growth			
Subtype I	RF-positive disease occurs at any age during childhood.	90% girls	20%–30%	Swollen and tender joints Child walks with shuffle, or assumes a position of comfort (flexion) to relieve or avoid joint pain	RF positive ANA present HLA-DR4	Rheumatoid nodules Adenopathy Weight loss Fatigue Growth retardation Vasculitis	50% will have disabling arthritis.
Subtype II	RF-positive disease occurs later in childhood.	80% girls	5%–10%		RF negative ANA may be present		10%–15% will have disabling arthritis.
Systemic Any joint affected	Occurs at any age during childhood (median age, 5 years).	60% males	10%–20%	Temperature greater than 39.5°C, spikes one or two times daily Evanescent, pale red, nonpruritic, macular rash present Leukocytosis, severe anemia Joint problems may be mild at onset	RF positive in 5% Elevated ESR Rarely positive ANA	Myalgia Pleuritis Enlarged spleen Enlarged liver Enlarged lymph nodes Severe anemia	50% will completely recover. 50% will have severe, chronic arthritis.

RF, rheumatic factor; ANA, antinuclear antibody; HLA-B27, histocompatability antigen-B27; ESR, erythrocyte sedimentation rate.

The diagnosis of JA can be made by physical examination. Other radiologic tests such as MRI, CT, or bone scan may be performed to rule out other diagnoses.

Nursing Diagnoses and Outcomes

The child with juvenile arthritis can be managed primarily in the home environment. The health care team in the acute setting may encounter the child when he or she is experiencing a severe illness exacerbation that requires intense physical therapy and nutritional support, when an alteration in medications is required, or when surgical intervention is needed to treat severe musculoskeletal complications such as muscle or tendon releases. Clinic, home health, and school nurses are primarily responsible for collaborating with the health care team to monitor and manage the needs of the child with this condition. Issues of impaired physical mobility, altered nutrition, potential for impaired skin integrity, and chronic pain need to be managed on a daily basis. The child also faces challenges related to altered growth and development and potential for body image disturbances caused by the debilitating nature and sometimes disfiguring outcomes of the child's arthritic condition (TIP 20–4).

The following nursing diagnoses should also be considered for the child with juvenile arthritis. These diagnoses are applicable to those children with a subtype of JA in which fever is a frequent occurrence.

- **Risk for injury related to fever**
  Outcome: The child will maintain normal body temperature.
- **Risk for fluid volume deficit related to fever and hypermetabolic state**
  Outcome: The child will maintain normal fluid volume as evidenced by good skin turgor, moist mucous membranes, and adequate urine output.
- **Altered nutrition: less than body requirements related to anorexia, dietary inadequacies, drug/nutrient interactions, limitations in physical activity, and mechanical feeding difficulties**
  Outcomes: The child will exhibit weight gain appropriate to his or her age, height, and physique.
  The child and family will implement measures to ensure that the child consumes adequate amounts of nutritious food.

Interdisciplinary Interventions

The desired outcomes for children affected with JA are to prevent deformities, keep discomfort to a minimum, allow little or no restriction of mobility, and preserve the ability to perform activities of daily living. Drug therapy and physical therapy are mainstays of treatment for JA. The interdisciplinary team works collaboratively to ensure that the child is managed in a consistent manner whether they are at home, at school, or in the acute care setting. An interdisciplinary teaching plan should be implemented to provide family members with the knowledge and skills needed to attend to the child's care needs at home (see TIP 20–3). The plan should be reviewed with the child periodically so that, as the child grows and matures, he or she can continue to learn more about the condition and accept increasing responsibility for managing self-care.

Drug Therapy

The primary pharmacologic approach to managing the child with JA begins with the administration of medications that reduce inflammation. These include salicylates, NSAIDs, and slow-acting antirheumatic drugs (SAARDs) such as gold and antimalarials. The milder the disease, the less medication is required. Some children may not require drug therapy because they do not experience joint pain, stiffness, or immobility.

Alert: *The use of aspirin has been highly associated with the development of Reye's syndrome in children who have had chickenpox or the flu. Because aspirin may be an ongoing part of the regimen of the arthritic child, parents should be warned of the relationship between viral illnesses and aspirin, and they should be taught to identify the symptoms of Reye's syndrome.*

Salicylates

The association between aspirin and Reye's syndrome is leading practitioners to make a gradual change away from salicylates to NSAIDs to manage inflammatory effects of JA. When aspirin is used, the dosage must be sufficient to maintain blood levels of 20 to 30 mg/dL to alleviate the arthritic and systemic manifestations of the disease. Because metabolism of aspirin varies among children, all children must be assessed for salicylate toxicity. Hyperventilation, heavy breathing, drowsiness, nausea, vomiting, bruising, tinnitus, and hearing loss may be noted. The salicylate should be given with food to avoid gastric irritation.

Other NSAIDs

Several other NSAID agents have been approved for use in children. These agents include tolmetin, naproxen, and ibuprofen. Indomethacin can be used but is not recommended for children younger than age 14 unless other drugs have not been effective, because its efficacy has not been determined in children. NSAIDs are used to reduce inflammation, pain, and fever. They are more expensive than aspirin; however, they are administered less frequently and are likely to cause fewer gastric side effects.

TIP 20-4 A Teaching Intervention Plan for the Child with Juvenile Arthritis

Nursing Diagnoses and Family Outcomes

- High risk for impaired physical mobility related to joint inflammation, swelling, and pain
  Outcomes:
  Child will take medications as ordered.
  Child will follow daily exercise program.
  Child will moderate activity with adequate periods of rest and relaxation.
- Chronic pain related to joint inflammation and contracture
  Outcomes:
  Child and family members will describe interventions to reduce pain and discomfort associated with child's condition.
  Child will experience no pain or acceptable levels of reduced pain as evidenced by play and participation in daily self-care actvities.
- Potential for altered growth and development related to physical limitations, discomfort, and clinical progression of the child's condition
  Outcomes:
  Child will maintain a normal weight for age and height.
  Child and family will acknowledge the importance of well-balanced meals and rest periods.
  Child will participate in age-appropriate activities that are modified as needed based on the child's current status.

Interventions

Teach the Child and Family

- Medications
  - Anti-inflammatory and analgesic medications must be taken per physician's order.
  - Medications must be given as ordered to maintain a therapeutic blood level and to reduce the likelihood of joint pain and swelling.
  - To prevent side effects of the medications, salicylates should be taken with food or milk to reduce gastric irritation. The physician will monitor serum salicylate levels on a routine basis to assess for toxicity. Toxic side effects of salicylates include headaches, dizziness, gastric distress, tinnitus, confusion, and signs of bleeding such as nosebleeds and excessive bruising.
  - Toxic side effects of SAARDs include rash, thrombocytopenia, neurotoxicity, photosensitivity, proteinuria, and damage to the mucous membranes, skin, kidney, and bone marrow.
- Activity and Safety
  - Encourage the child to participate in low-impact exercises, especially swimming.
  - Avoid overexercising and stimulating swollen joints, which aggravate the pain.
  - Complete exercise program daily.
  - Determine whether this program will be completed at home, at school, or at another community location.
  - Develop a daily routine to complete the exercise program.
  - Incorporate exercise program into daily play activities such as throwing a ball, riding a bike, or molding clay.
  - The use of splints, sandbags, or casts may be necessary to maintain position of function and to prevent muscle contractions.
  - Encourage child to attend regular school.
  - Schedule daily rest periods for the child.
  - Encourage the child to participate in daily self-care activities and tasks around the home.

TIP continued on following page

TIP 20–4 A Teaching Intervention Plan for the Child with Juvenile Arthritis *Continued*

Assistive devices such as elevated commodes and handrails may be helpful to aid in body mechanics.
The child should wear clothing that is easy for her or him to put on and take off.
Eating utensils, brushes, combs, and toothbrushes may need to be modified for easier grasp.
Child should be evaluated by an ophthalmologist for slit-lamp examination and routine eye care.

- Pain Management

If possible, the child should take a warm bath for 20 minutes upon awakening in the morning. An electric blanket may also be used if bath is not feasible.
Warm moist packs and heating pads can be used as needed to relieve joint discomfort.
Paraffin baths can be used to reduce joint pain.
The child should use a firm mattress and lie flat in bed to reduce flexion deformity.

- Nutrition

Provide well-balanced diet to avoid weight gain or weight loss.
Select foods high in iron if anemia is a concern.
Monitor weight on a weekly basis. If the child becomes overweight, an extra burden can be put on weight-bearing joints.
The child's hematocrit should be monitored on a regular basis to assess for anemia, which can be associated with the inflammatory process.
During febrile periods, monitor the child for adequate hydration and encourage intake of fluids.

- Psychosocial

Encourage the child to ventilate his or her feelings regarding the condition.
Encourage the child to meet other children with juvenile arthritis.
Encourage independence. Do not do for the child what the child can do for himself or herself.
Include the child in therapy and treatment decisions to promote self-care, sense of autonomy, and control over the situation.
Encourage the child to engage in activities in which he or she can be successful and thus promote positive self-esteem.

Contact Health Care Provider if

Joint pain and inflammation worsen despite current medication regimen.
Child spikes a temperature greater than 39.5°C, which is not reduced by such measures as medication, tepid baths, and cool clothes.
The child appears to be dehydrated. Lips are dry and cracked, no tearing is present, urine output is low.
The child has signs of drug toxicity.
Child's vision appears to be impaired.

Slow-Acting Antirheumatic Drugs

SAARDs, also known as disease-modifying or remittive agents, are administered to children at risk for crippling or disability caused by their multijoint disease state. SAARDs include gold salts and antimalarials (e.g., penicillamine, hydroxychloroquine). These medications are not effective in achieving remission of the disease; rather, they modify disease activity to improve joint function, reduce pain and stiffness, and permit more endurance. It may take up to 6 months for the beneficial effects to be noted. These medications are quite toxic and thus children must be monitored carefully for side effects. A rash, mucosal ulcers, leukopenia, thrombocytopenia, anemia, and proteinuria are signs of toxicity. Toxicity of hydroxychloroquine can lead to ocular damage; thus, while taking the medication the child should be examined every 6 months by an ophthalmologist (Szer, 1996).

Immunosuppressive Drugs

If the child does not respond to conventional medications, immunosuppressive agents may be used. These include cyclophosphamide (Cytoxan), chlorambucil (Leukeran), azathioprine (Imuran), and methotrexate. Children taking these medications need to be monitored for bone marrow, liver, gonadal, and renal toxicity.

Steroids

The use of corticosteroids is not generally considered unless warranted by the presence of severe systemic complications of JA that are not responding to other drug therapies. These agents suppress the symptoms of JA but do not induce remission of the disease or prevent joint damage. Additionally, the side effects of steroid use may lead to even more physical complications for the child. If steroids such as prednisone are used, the dosage of the medication should be reduced and gradually discontinued as soon as symptoms have been suppressed.

Physical Therapy

Providing physical and occupational therapy to the child with JA is an important measure to promote optimal musculoskeletal development. A key part of the interdisciplinary treatment of JA is the design of a therapeutic exercise program. The program includes providing posture assessment; implementing measures to prevent contractures (fixed flexion of a muscle); teaching exercises to increase strength, endurance, and range of motion; and selecting methods to deal with joint stiffness and discomfort. Although physicians prescribe the program, physical or occupational therapists design it to fit the child's needs. The clinical nurse specialist educates the child and family regarding these techniques and evaluates the child's progress with the program.

Splints, braces, and casts are important components of the physical program for the child with JA (see Treatment Modalities). During an illness flare-up, an inflamed joint can be continually maintained in a neutral position by the use of an immobilization device. Once the disease is under control, the splint or brace may be worn only at night. Wrist and knee splints are commonly used to prevent contractures. Serial casting is a treatment for a contracture that has already formed. Casts are placed on the extremity to hold it in extension, and the cast is replaced every week. Each time it is replaced, more extension should be possible. This process is continued until the contracture has resolved.

Passive, active, and resistive exercises are carried out daily by the child to preserve range of motion, muscle strength, and gross motor activity (Szer, 1996). Exercises can be completed at home, at school, in an acute care setting, or at a local health club. Age-appropriate activities are encouraged and modified as needed based on the severity of the child's symptoms. Children with JA can participate in normal school and family activities. Gymnastics and high-impact contact sports are the few exceptions. Swimming is an excellent exercise for children with JA. Other therapeutic exercises include playing with clay, bicycling, playing the piano, and softball. Extreme stress and fatigue may trigger exacerbations of JA. Rest, relaxation, leisure activities, and relief from emotional distress should be encouraged to reduce the risk of exacerbations.

For children with progressive debilitation caused by their arthritic condition, occupational therapy can be beneficial. Measures are taken to adapt the child's environment and to train the child to use assistive devices to continue to perform independent daily tasks and activities.

Children and families should be taught several measures to promote comfort and reduce generalized body stiffness. Heat therapy to alleviate pain and stiffness is important for the child with JA. Other treatments include warm baths, moist warm packs, and paraffin (wax) baths for the small joints of the hands once a day (see Treatment Modalities). Getting out of bed in the morning is often a difficult task for a child with JA because of early morning stiffness. A warm morning bath is helpful but it may be impractical for busy families. An alternative is to have the child use a sleeping bag at night to stay warm. Another alternative is to have an electric blanket with a timer that turns on 1 hour before the child awakens (Page-Goertz, 1989). Use of a waterbed is another option for easing stiffness.

Surgical Interventions

Orthopedic surgery for the treatment of JA is rare. Arthroscopic synovectomy may be performed to decrease pain. Occasionally, some patients require or request a total joint replacement. This should be performed only on older children, because joint replacements wear out in about 20 years.

Nutritional Support

Children with JA are at nutritional risk from factors such as anorexia, dietary inadequacies, drug/food interactions, limitations in physical activity, mechanical feeding difficulties, and susceptibilities to food fads and quackery. Stiffness combined with decreased activity increases the tendency to gain weight, thus exacerbating the problems with mobility. Arthritis of the temporomandibular joint can impact the child's ability to chew, causing pain and limitations of jaw movement. Undernutrition and wasting can contribute to poor linear growth and a low lean body and muscle mass. Anorexia can lead to acute or chronic undernutrition as a result of an inadequate intake of both calories and protein. Many of the medications taken by the child with JA have potential adverse effects on nutritional status. These effects include anorexia, constipation, nausea, fatigue, diarrhea, and gastrointestinal distress. Additionally, parents of children with JA may select unconventional dietary remedies to "treat" their child. These therapies can interfere with the child's medical therapy and may be a source of malnutrition (Purdy, Dwyer, Holland, Goldberg, & Dinardo, 1996).

Several measures can be instituted to enhance the child's growth and development by addressing dietary concerns (Chart 20–18). Frequent assessment of the child's nutritional status should be an integral part of the contacts between the child and the health care team. Height and weight measurements should be obtained on a regular basis. The child and family should be questioned regarding side effects of any medications, appetite and appetite changes, frequency of meals and snacks, types of foods eaten on a day-to-day basis, and the presence of discomfort or any mechanical difficulties when chewing (Purdy et al., 1996).

Promoting Normal Development

Chronic illness has a great effect on a child's psychosocial well-being (see Chapter 10). Normal developmental milestones such as starting school, socialization, and independence in activities of daily living may be delayed. The family may "overprotect" the child and restrict play activities for fear of injury. To promote the child's growth and development, the child should be encouraged to interact with peers in school and social settings by participating in age-appropriate activities as much as the child's physical condition allows. Modifications to the child's environment and schedule should be implemented to decrease the likelihood of fatigue and account for the child's physical limitations (Hughes & D'Ambrosia, 1993).

The child may be at risk for self-esteem or body image disturbances because of the limitations imposed by illness and any physical manifestations. Family members should encourage the child to speak openly about his or her condition and to feel comfortable asking others for assistance when needed. Support organizations can provide educational materials, specialized services, and financial aid for qualified children and their families (see Resources). Important measures that promote adaptation to the disease and enhance development are encouraging the child's natural skills and characteristics and creating an atmosphere in which the child has realistic perceptions and expectations.

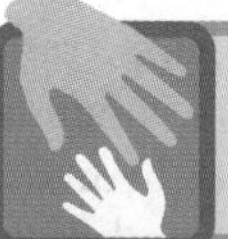

Chart 20–18
Nursing Interventions

Measures to Promote Adequate Dietary Intake for the Child with Juvenile Arthritis

- Encourage children with poor appetites to eat higher calorie, nutrient-dense tasty foods such as nuts, peanut butter sandwiches, milk shakes, and cheese.
- Encourage children with small appetites to eat small frequent meals throughout the day.
- Make meal time a pleasant event. Nagging and food battles only serve to decrease the child's appetite.
- Provide calcium and vitamin D supplementation under the guidance of a dietitian.
- Choose iron-fortified cereals and other products.
- Follow the standards of the Food Guide Pyramid to plan meals with serving sizes appropriate to the child's age.
- If mechanical feeding difficulties are present, provide the child with a soft diet and teach him or her to take small bites. If eating difficulties persist, referral to an occupational therapist may be necessary.
- Assist the child to select activities that will keep him or her mobile and active without causing undue pain and joint problems.
- Assess and treat the side effects of drug/food interactions (e.g., constipation, diarrhea, nausea).
- Discourage children and their parents from using unconventional remedies to treat their child's condition.
- Refer the child to a registered dietitian if dietary issues continue to be an ongoing threat to the child's growth and development.

Systemic Lupus Erythematosus

SLE is a systemic inflammatory disease that affects many organs in the body. The disease may scar the skin and cause disfigurement, hence the name "lupus" for "the wolf." Lupus is an autoimmune disorder that may involve any organ system, but most commonly involves skin, joints, and kidneys. The onset may be sudden, affecting one or more major organ systems, or it may be insidious in nature, with nonspecific symptoms such as fever, fatigue, or joint and muscle pain. When the onset is insidious, diagnosis is often delayed for weeks or months. The cause of SLE is unknown, but genetic, hormonal, environmental, and immunologic factors are believed to interact and to lead to disease expression.

Childhood SLE accounts for 20% of all cases. The incidence of SLE in the United States is approximately 0.6 cases per 100,000 total population. The incidence in the United States is higher in African-American, Asian, and Hispanic populations. Girls are affected more frequently than boys in a ratio of 3 to 1. In adults, that ratio approaches 10 to 1. Childhood SLE is diagnosed most frequently during adolescence. The mortality rate has decreased with the evolution of newer treatment options; the 10-year survival rate approximates 85%. Infection is currently the leading cause of death. Previously, end-stage renal disease was the primary cause of death.

Pathophysiology

SLE is characterized by the development of antibodies against nuclear antigens such as DNA and RNA. Production of autoantibodies that affect the red blood cells, neutrophils, platelets, lymphocytes, and other tissues and organs can also occur. When the autoantibody–antigen complexes lodge in tissue and organ sites, a local inflammatory reaction is produced that leads to additional tissue injury (Peck, 1995). Alterations in humoral immunity typify SLE. Autoantibody production changes T-cell function, making them less effective. This leads to increased levels of antinuclear, anti-DNA, antiplatelet, and antilymphocyte antibodies and a positive Coombs test. Circulating immune complexes are elevated and are directly associated with the vasculitis, synovitis, rash, glomerulonephritis, and myositis characteristic of SLE. Kidney involvement is associated with nephritis and glomerulonephritis. Skin symptoms include rash, purpura, alopecia, mucosal ulcerations, subcutaneous nodules, and splinter hemorrhages. Symptoms of arthritis may be present. Thrombocytopenia and anemia can occur. Retinal changes, gastrointestinal ulceration, and CNS involvement such as seizures and neuritis may be present (Allen, 1988; Copstead, 1995).

Assessment

Eleven disease manifestations are included in the criteria established by the American College of Rheumatology to distinguish SLE from other connective tissue diseases (Chart 20–19). The presence of four manifestations in the absence of other definable disease entities is sufficient for the diagnosis of SLE. Nonspecific findings that may be present at the onset of the disease include fever, malaise, weight loss, recurrent abdominal pain, anorexia, and fatigue. Headaches are present in more than 10% of children at the time of diagnosis. Conjunctivitis is a common early manifestation.

Arthritis is the most common symptom of SLE. The child may complain of morning stiffness and joint pain or swelling. The arthritis of SLE is usually symmetrical and affects both small and large joints. Commonly affected joints are hands, wrists, and knees. Joint deformities or erosions are rarely seen. Rheumatoid nodules may appear during periods of disease exacerbations, disappearing as the disease activity diminishes.

The next most common physical manifestations of SLE are dermatologic. Skin findings may include maculopapular and vasculitic rashes and periungual erythema. Many acutely affected individuals may have a butterfly rash across the bridge of the nose and on the cheeks. The rash may be photosensitive and may spread to the face, scalp, neck, chest, and extremities. Photosensitivity is a classical dermatologic sign of SLE, especially if it occurs in the presence of arthritis (Peck, 1995). The rash may become bullous and a secondary infection may develop.

Other skin eruptions may include vasculitic lesions with ulceration, purpuric lesions, and subcutaneous nodules on the palms, fingertips, soles, extremities, or trunk. Vasculitic rashes, livedo reticularis, and nail bed changes may occur. Macular and painless ulcerative lesions in the mouth and nose may be present. Alopecia caused by inflammation around the hair follicles may lead to patchy or generalized loss of hair and may cause the hair to be coarse, dry, and brittle (Schaller, 1996b).

Polyserositis, inflammation of several mucous membranes, is another clinical manifestation of SLE. Pericarditis, peritonitis, or pleuritis may be present. Cardiovascular symptoms that may develop over time include pericarditis, substernal or precordial pain, murmurs, persistent tachycardia, transient dysrhythmias, and pleural and pericardial effusions. Raynaud's phenomenon, in which vasoconstriction causes blanching, cyanosis, and erythema in the toes and fingers in response to cold or stress, may be present.

Renal involvement is common in children. Nephrotic syndrome and acute glomerulonephritis may develop and are considered life-threatening occurrences. Renal insufficiency is indicated in the presence of weight gain, hypertension, edema, increased serum creatinine levels, and decreased creatinine clearance. Additionally, urinalysis reveals hematuria, proteinuria, and increased urinary sediment.

Almost all children with SLE have one or more hematologic abnormalities including anemia, leukopenia, and thrombocytopenia. Lymphoid involvement may be noted in the form of generalized lymphadenopathy and hepatomegaly.

CNS symptoms may arise as indications of the CNS vasculitis, as toxic symptoms resulting from the medication regimen, or as behavioral outcomes of this chronic illness. CNS vasculitis can lead to irritability, depression, headache, lethargy, dizziness, seizures, ataxia, and hallucinations. Ongoing use of corticosteroids lowers the threshold for seizure activity and may cause personality changes

Chart 20–19

Revised Criteria for Diagnosis of Systemic Lupus Erythematosus*

1. Malar rash—fixed erythema, flat or raised, over the malar eminences, tending to spare the nasolabial folds
2. Discoid rash—erythematous raised patches with adherent keratotic scaling and follicular plugging; atrophic scarring may occur in older lesions
3. Photosensitivity—skin rash as a result of unusual reaction to sunlight, by patient history or by physician observation
4. Oral ulcers—oral or nasopharyngeal ulceration, usually painless, observed by a physician
5. Arthritis—non-erosive arthritis involving two or more peripheral joints, characterized by tenderness, swelling, or effusion
6. Serositis
   a. Pleuritis—convincing history of pleuritic pain or rub heard by a physician or evidence of pleural effusion
   OR
   b. Pericarditis—documented by electrocardiogram or rub or evidence of pericardial effusion
7. Renal disorder
   a. Persistent proteinuria >0.5 g/day or greater than 3+ if quantitation is not performed
   OR
   b. Cellular casts—may be red blood cell, hemoglobin, granular, tubular, or mixed
8. Neurologic disorder
   a. Seizures—in the absence of offending drugs or known metabolic derangements (e.g., uremia, ketoacidosis, or electrolyte imbalance)
   OR
   b. Psychosis—in the absence of offending drugs or known metabolic derangements (e.g., uremia, ketoacidosis, or electrolyte imbalance)
9. Hematologic disorder
   a. Hemolytic anemia—with reticulocytosis
   OR
   b. Leukopenia—<4000/mm^3 total on two or more occasions
   OR
   c. Lymphopenia—<1500/mm^3 on two or more occasions
   OR
   d. Thrombocytopenia—<100,000/mm^3 in the absence of offending drugs
10. Immunologic disorder
    a. Positive LE cell preparation
    OR
    b. Anti-DNA: antibody to native DNA in abnormal titer
    OR
    c. Anti-Sm: presence of antibody to Sm nuclear antigen
    OR
    d. False-positive serologic test for syphilis known to be positive for at least 6 months and confirmed by *Treponema pallidum* immobilization or fluorescent treponemal antibody absorption test
11. Antinuclear antibody
    An abnormal titer of antinuclear antibody by immunofluorescence or an equivalent assay at any time and in the absence of drugs known to be associated with "drug-induced lupus" syndrome

* For the purpose of identifying patients in clinical studies, a person shall be said to have systemic lupus erythematosus if any four or more of the 11 criteria are present, serially or simultaneously, during any interval of observation.

From Tan, E. M., et al. (1982). The 1982 revised criteria for the classification of systemic lupus erythematosus. *Arthritis and Rheumatism, 25*(11), 1271–1274. Reprinted with permission.

such as depression or euphoria. Depression can also occur as a result of learning that one has SLE or from coping with the issues associated with acute disease activity that limit the child's activities.

The course of SLE is characterized by exacerbations and remissions varying in severity, depending on the particular organ system involved. The disease only rarely involves previously unaffected organ systems after the first

2 years. Distinguishing the symptoms of disease exacerbation from those of infectious complications may be difficult. Onset of fever, coughing, shortness of breath, chest pain, and changes in behavior and visual acuity should be considered to be of possible infectious origin until proven otherwise.

Diagnostic Tests. Initial screening of suspected SLE includes the following tests: a complete blood count with differential, ESR, C-reactive protein measurement, antinuclear antibody count, RF test, Venereal Disease Research Laboratory screen, Lyme titer, thyroid function test, chemistry panel 20, and a monospot to rule out other conditions that may present with similar clinical findings (Peck, 1995).

Interdisciplinary Interventions

Treatment of SLE is dictated by the extent and the severity of the disease, and must be directed by a desire to allow the child to maintain a normal lifestyle. Medical management is tailored to meet the individual child's needs based on organ system involvement and on the severity of inflammation at the time of evaluation. The goal of therapy is to control both the acute exacerbations of the illness and the ongoing chronic disease manifestations to enable optimal functioning, to prevent scarring in any organ system, and to prevent intolerable side effects of the therapy. Cooperation among a number of health care professions may be required to adequately treat renal disease complications, hypertension, neurologic disease, hematologic disease, and arthritis. Child life specialists in the hospital setting and a variety of allied health professionals in outpatient settings, including social workers and psychologists, may help the family and child to cope with issues (e.g., body image concerns related to disease and medications) in a positive manner.

Joint Involvement

If the child has isolated joint involvement (arthralgia/arthritis), NSAIDs, such as naproxen, salicylates, indomethacin, or tolmetin sodium alone or with hydroxychloroquine are recommended.

Alert: *Ibuprofen has been associated with an aseptic meningitis syndrome in SLE; thus, it should not be administered to children with SLE (Athreya, 1996).*

Medications must be taken daily to maintain adequate blood levels. NSAID therapy requires careful monitoring of renal function, because these agents decrease glomerular blood flow and can precipitate acute renal failure in children with SLE.

A physical therapy program can be implemented to assist the child in dealing with joint pain, enhancing range-of-motion activities, and preventing injury and contractures. Periods of rest should be incorporated into the child's daily routine, especially during active disease periods.

Skin Involvement

The rash of SLE is generally treated with an antimalarial drug, preferably hydroxychloroquine. Topical steroids may also be used for limited cutaneous involvement. An eye examination should be performed every 6 months in patients receiving hydroxychloroquine because of the risk of retinal damage.

Rashes and lesions need to be monitored carefully for signs of infection. Additionally, vascular compromise should be assessed in the toes and fingers. During cold weather, extremities should be kept warm using socks, gloves, and layered clothes. Tight clothing should be avoided.

Skin disease in children with SLE can be well controlled by the use of sunscreens, the practice of sun avoidance, and the use of steroid therapy. When the child is exposed to the sun, the importance of protection against sun exposure through the use of sunscreens that block both ultraviolet A and B rays (SPF 15 or higher), avoidance of long-term sun exposure, and the use of long-sleeved clothing, pants, large-brimmed hats, and sunglasses should be emphasized. Not only can sun exposure exacerbate skin rash, but it may also precipitate systemic exacerbations.

Systemic Involvement

Major organ system involvement in SLE usually necessitates the use of corticosteroids. Symptoms such as fever, skin manifestations, pleuropericarditis, and lymphadenopathy can usually be effectively treated with low-dose prednisone or hydroxychloroquine. Alternate-day steroid therapy is currently being used to minimize the linear growth and sexual maturation problems associated with steroid use (Kredich, 1988).

Tip: *A child with SLE should wear a Medic Alert bracelet to alert emergency personnel to his or her dependence on steroids.*

High-dose oral prednisone for a period of 4 to 6 weeks may be indicated for the child with CNS and renal involvement. Long-term use of high-dose prednisone is avoided whenever possible because of the serious complications (e.g., cataracts, fractures, hypertension, and metabolic disturbances) that may occur. Once the child's condition has been stabilized, the high-dose steroids are tapered off. This prevents the effects of sudden withdrawal of the medications. The aim of therapy is to have the child on the lowest possible dose of prednisone needed to control activity of the disease. To aid in this process, steroid-sparing agents such as azathioprine, methotrexate, and hydroxychloroquine may be used.

Antihypertensives, anticonvulsants, and antipsychotic drugs may be indicated in patients with thrombotic complications to prevent recurrent thromboembolic events. Intravenous human gamma immunoglobulin (IVGg) is also useful for the treatment of thrombocytopenia and, to some extent, hemolytic anemia (Athreya, 1996).

An ophthalmic evaluation for retinal damage should be performed within the first 30 to 60 days after initiating drug therapy and every 6 months thereafter (Peck, 1995). These evaluations are done to evaluate and prevent the onset of macular inflammatory problems.

Periodic blood work for evaluation of drug toxicity and disease activity must also be discussed with the patients and caregivers.

Nutritional Support

The child receiving steroid therapy needs to be monitored for weight gain and fluid retention. If renal involvement is a concern, a low-sodium, low-protein diet may be instituted. Increased calcium should be given to adolescent females on steroid therapy.

Pregnancy

Sexually active adolescent girls must be made aware that SLE can become more active during pregnancy and that a fetus could be harmed both by the mother's disease and by the side effects of the drugs required to treat the mother's disease (Chart 20–20).

Enhancing Growth and Development

Attention must be given to helping the child deal with any problems that he or she may have related to self-image and self-esteem. The undesirable effects of medication therapy such as weight gain and "moonface," the restrictions related to skin photosensitivity, and the increased risk for depression are among the factors that can affect the child's self-concept. The child may refuse to follow preventive measures, thereby precipitating an acute episode of the condition (Chart 20–21). The health care team and family members should strive to help the child achieve as normal a lifestyle as possible within the constraints of the illness. Independence in decision-making should be encouraged while still monitoring for safety and wellness. Social workers or psychologists trained to deal with chronic illness in children may be helpful in assisting them to learn to cope with their frustrations. Support groups are useful for some children, allowing them to meet others with SLE and to discuss common concerns. Several resource organizations offer written information about SLE and can direct families to local support groups and activities in their community (see Resources).

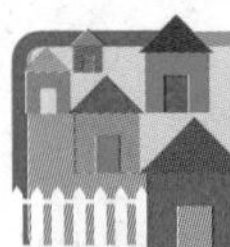

Chart 20–20
Community Care

Pregnancy and the Adolescent with Systemic Lupus Erythematosus

Pregnancy is not contraindicated in the patient with systemic lupus erythematosus (SLE). However, pregnancy and delivery can precipitate a flare-up of the disease. The incidence of spontaneous abortions and premature deliveries is higher than normal in patients with SLE. Infants of these mothers have a slightly higher incidence of congenital heart block and an increased chance of fetal distress, which has been linked to high maternal anticardiolipin antibody titers.

Some oral contraceptives, especially high-dose estrogen-containing preparations, can exacerbate SLE. It is usually recommended that a diaphragm and spermicide be used for birth control because they do not have adverse side effects. However, low-dose oral contraceptives may be used if the patient is carefully monitored, especially if compliance with barrier contraception is poor.

Health care providers in community settings should counsel the female SLE patient regarding the health concerns associated with pregnancy and the postpartum period. The sexually active teenager should receive education regarding the birth control measures that do not precipitate further disease crises. If the teenager becomes pregnant, progress through the pregnancy should be closely monitored by a health care professional familiar with the SLE and its disease process.

Traumatic Injuries: Fractures and Skeletal Trauma

Childhood trauma has been the leading cause of death in children for nearly 50 years, and it has been the second leading cause of morbidity. The most common childhood injuries are sprains, followed by lacerations, fractures (excluding the skull), intracranial injuries, and internal injuries. The most serious injuries tend to be the fractures and intracranial injuries. This section describes the care of children with fractures and sprains; however, the best medicine is to prevent the injury altogether.

A fracture occurs when the bone receives more stress than it can absorb. Skeletal trauma accounts for 10% to 15% of all childhood injuries (Rockwood, Wilkins, & King, 1991). The most common reasons for fractures in

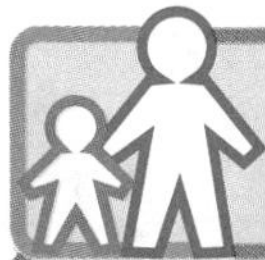

Chart 20–21
Developmental Considerations

Management Issues for Children with Systemic Lupus Erythematosus

Concerns of the Child	Actions Demonstrated by Child	Health Care Provider and Family Interventions
"I do not want to be different than other children."	Refuses to take medications while at school	Arrange medication schedule to eliminate or minimize need to take medications during school and social activities.
"I do not like the effects of medications on appearance."	Avoids taking medication	Have parent unobtrusively monitor child taking medication.
"I want to participate in summer activities in the sun."	Refuses to avoid the sun	Help child select hats, clothing, lotions, and other protective gear that can be used to protect against overexposure to the sun.
"Applying sunscreen is messy and not cool."	Does not use sunscreen consistently each day when out in the sun	Review with the child the importance of using sunscreen. Have child select a favorite type of sunscreen to use. Have child apply sunscreen at home before meeting friends.
"Rashes make me look funny."	Does not want to socialize with others or go out in public	Encourage child to use hypoallergenic cosmetics to cover rashes.
"I cannot do anything. I cannot be like my other friends."	Feels depression	Assist parents to emphasize child's positive attributes and accomplishments. Encourage participation in counseling or support group.
"I look fat."	Feels depression; cries	Help child select clothes that camouflage weight gain.
"I am too tired to participate in activities with other kids."	Wants to be excused from school activities and extracurricular activities because of fatigue	Assist child to pace activities and periods of rest to minimize fatigue. Assist child to select activities that are not as physically demanding such as piano playing, art work, and computer activities.

children are falls, motor vehicle accidents, and bicycle accidents.

Some important variables affect the care of fractures in children as compared with that in adults. First, a child's bone heals faster than an adult's bone. The younger the child, the faster the bone heals because younger children have a proportionately higher metabolic rate. Children's bones are also softer than an adult's bones, and their bones may bend or buckle rather than break. Another crucial difference in the management of adult versus pediatric fractures is that children's bones have an open growth plate or epiphysis. Any damage to the growth plate can result in limb length discrepancy, joint incongruity, and progressive angular deformity of the limb. Approximately 15% of fractures in children involve the growth plate (Maher et al., 1994).

During the birthing process, fractures may occur in the newborn. In general, fractures are rare in the first year of life because the child has limited mobility. Multiple, severe fractures in an infant may be an indication of a metabolic bone disease, such as OI. In the first 2 years of life, many fractures in children are the result of physical abuse.

Table 20–18
Classification of Open Fractures

Type	Size of Wound	Amount of Contamination	Type of Fracture	Amount of Soft Tissue Damage
Type I	Less than 1 cm	Minimal	Simple transverse Oblique with skin pierced by bone spike	Minimal
Type II	Greater than 1 cm	Moderate	Moderate comminution or crush injuries	Moderate
Type III*	Large; traumatic amputations	High degree	Severe comminution and instability	Extensive

* Type III open fractures are further divided into groups A, B, and C based on soft tissue coverage and arterial injury.
Adapted from Maher, A. B., Salmond, S. W., & Pellino, T. A. (1994). *Orthopaedic nursing*. Philadelphia: W. B. Saunders. Used with permission.

Alert: *In a non-ambulatory child, the accidental occurrence of a spiral fracture is rare. Thus, spiral fractures in young children are most often the result of twisting of the extremity by an abusive adult.*

When the child starts to walk, the clavicle and radius are the most commonly fractured bones (Rockwood et al., 1991). Fractures can occur from trauma, sudden twisting of a limb, or a force applied to the limb, such as a kick. Pathologic fractures occur when preexisting diseases weaken a bone, such as with bone tumors.

A fracture is either open or closed. An open fracture occurs when a portion of the bone protrudes through the skin or when an external wound connects to the fracture site. Open fractures are classified as type I, II, or III depending on the degree and severity of the soft tissue damage or loss, the size of the wound, and the amount of wound contamination (Table 20–18). A closed fracture involves no break in the skin. One fracture type is not more complicated than the other, but the potential for infection is greater with an open fracture.

Classification of fractures also involves identifying the location and descriptive nature of the fracture. The location refers to where the fracture occurs along the shaft of the bone (Fig. 20–20). Fractures can also be described in terms of the amount of injury that has occurred (Table 20–19). Familiarity with these terms enables caregivers to communicate accurately and concisely. For example, "closed transverse femur fracture" indicates the type and location of the fracture.

Pathophysiology

The amount of force required to fracture a bone depends on the strength of the bone, the size of the bone, and other extrinsic factors, such as the direction of the force. Once the fracture occurs, inflammation develops at the site. Osteoblasts (bone-forming cells) activate within 24 hours to begin making new bone. Over the ensuing few weeks, callus forms and knits together into compact bone. This process takes 4 to 12 weeks in children, de-

Figure 20–20
Classification of fracture by location.

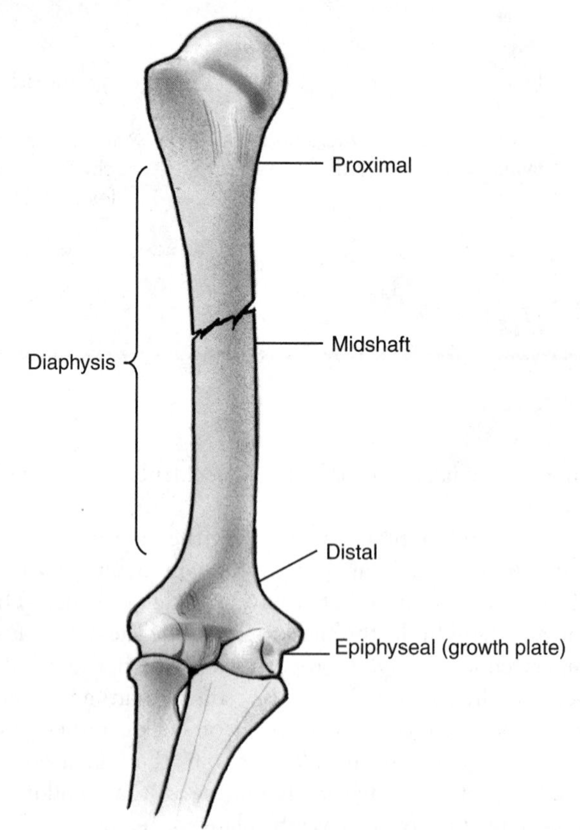

pending on their skeletal age. Remodeling, a process that rounds off angles and fills in hollows, continues for up to 1 year after the fracture. Because the ability of bone to remodel is enhanced in children, the ends of the fracture do not have to be aligned perfectly, as they do in adults.

Prognosis. In general, fractures in children heal without complications. Possible complications such as limping, decreased range of motion, and nerve deficits rarely occur. The prognosis varies according to the type of fracture and its location. If the injury involves the growth

Table 20–19
Classification of Fractures by Description of the Type of Break

Type	Illustration	Description
Transverse	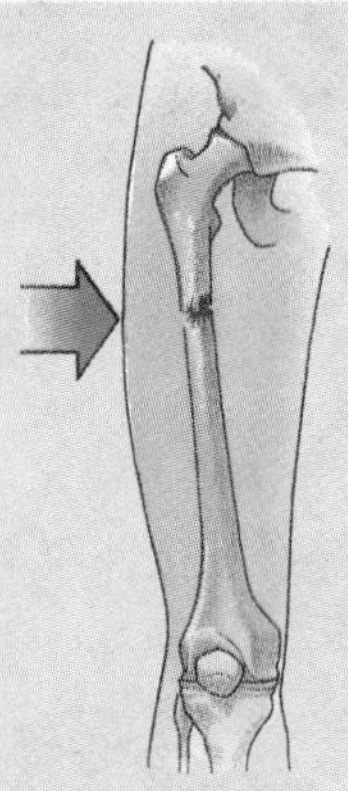	Line crosses the shaft at a 90-degree angle.
Spiral	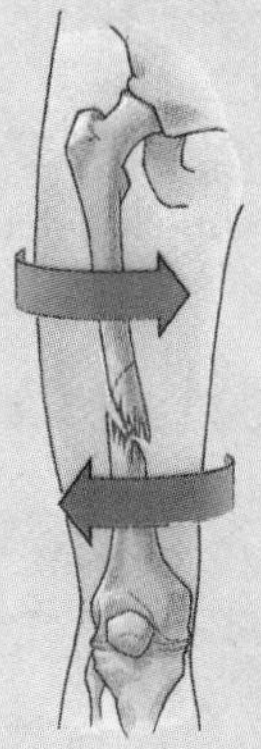	A diagonal line coils around the bone; caused by a twisting force
Oblique	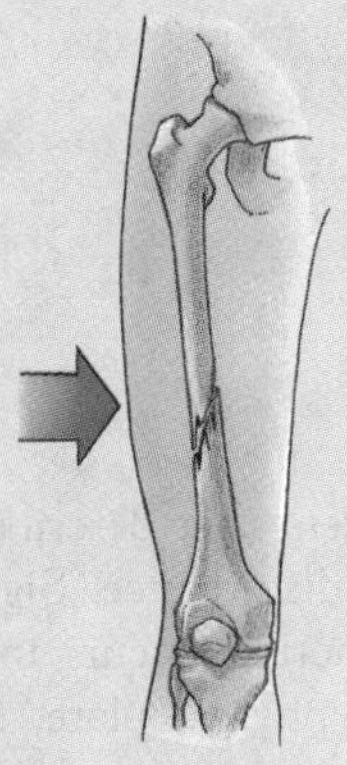	A diagonal line across the bone

Table continued on following page

Table 20–19
Classification of Fractures by Description of the Type of Break *Continued*

Type	Illustration	Description
Greenstick	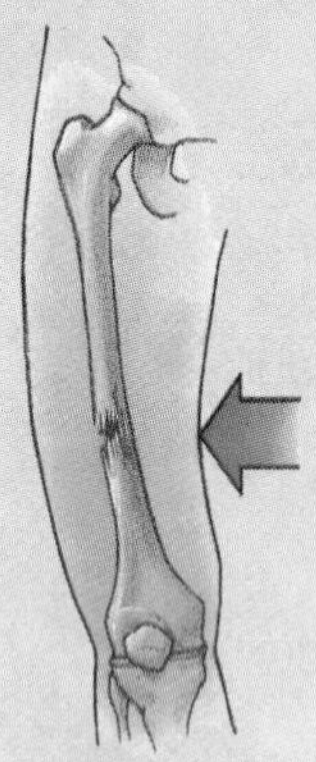	Bone is bent, but not broken; more common in children than adults
Comminuted	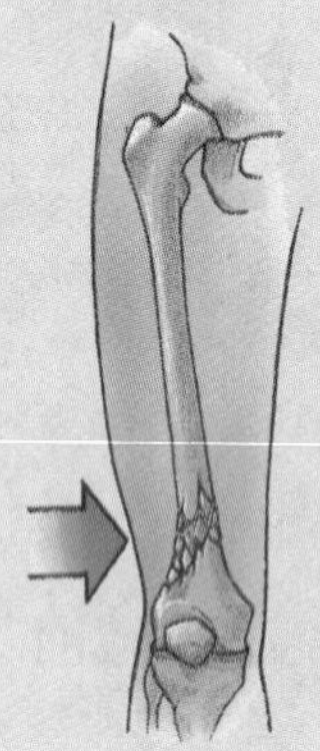	Three or more fracture fragments
Compression	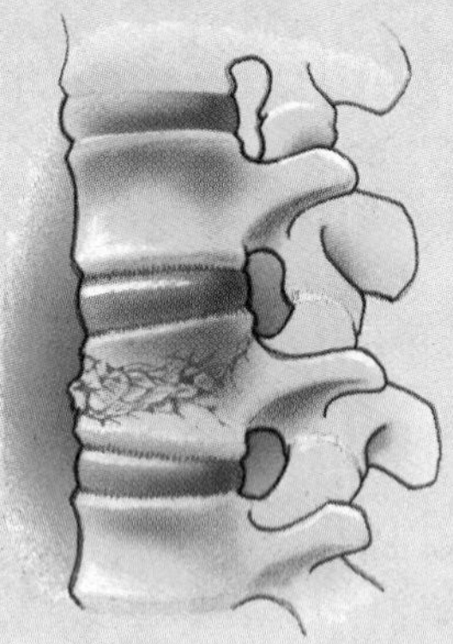	Bone becomes wider and more flat; usually seen in the spine.

plate in an immature bone, growth disturbance may follow. The growth plates of the lower extremities are primarily responsible for determining the height of the child. Disturbance of their function may result in slow growth, overgrowth, or cessation of growth. Table 20–20 is a classification system that describes the injury and the potential for growth disturbance. Significant alteration in the growth plate function occurs in approximately 10% of injuries to the epiphyseal plate, but the frequency of minor disturbances is high (Maher et al., 1994).

Table 20–20
Salter-Harris Classification of Epiphyseal Fractures

Classification	Illustration	Description
Type I		Separation of the epiphysis May be mistaken for a sprain Does not usually affect growth
Type II		Fracture separation of the epiphysis Circulation remains intact; growth usually not affected
Type III		Fracture through the epiphysis into the joint Does not usually affect growth if reduced properly
Type IV		Fracture of the epiphysis extending into the joint and the metaphysis Open reduction and internal fixation usually necessary to prevent growth disturbance
Type V		Crush injury to the epiphyseal plate Results in premature closure of the epiphyseal plate and growth arrest (occurrence is rare)

Assessment

Assessment for fractures is part of the emergency trauma care of a patient after initial stabilization. Obtaining a history of the accident helps determine the nature and extent of the injuries. Motor vehicle accidents and falls have a high index of suspicion for fractures, especially if the child was unrestrained in the vehicle.

Tip: *Ask the child to tell in his or her own words how the fracture occurred. If possible, ask this question without the caregivers present if abuse is suspected and an honest response is desired from the child.*

The child may complain of pain, numbness, or tingling in an extremity. All clothing should be removed to facilitate assessment. Open fractures may be obvious, or a closed fracture can make the limb grossly distorted. However, some fractures, such as of the spine or pelvis, are not as evident. The cervical spine in all trauma patients is protected by a cervical collar until radiographs rule out a fracture.

Other abnormal physical findings with a fracture include shortening of the limb, swelling, muscle spasm, crepitus, and discoloration of the limb. The child may refuse to move the limb, or a change in neurovascular status may be apparent. A fracture always causes pain, although the intensity and severity of the pain vary among children (Rockwood et al., 1991). Asking the parent or caregiver about the child's normal response to pain or previous experience with pain assists in defining the pain associated with a possible fracture. In non-verbal children, facial grimacing, whimpering, or crying may be elicited when the child is repositioned or when articles of clothing are removed.

The diagnosis of a fracture is based on the patient's symptoms, trauma history, physical examination, and radiologic deformity (Maher et al., 1994). Radiographs are the primary method used to evaluate fractures. However, a radiograph is a two-dimensional representation of a three-dimensional object. Thus, at least two views, anteroposterior and lateral, are usually needed for adequate evaluation of a suspected fracture. The joints above and below the suspected fracture also need to be included to evaluate potential associated injuries. If child abuse if suspected, radiographs are used to evaluate the presence of old fractures and to determine the extent of healing that has taken place at other fracture sites. In certain cases, other tests can be ordered to evaluate a suspected fracture. These include CT scans, MRI, fluoroscopy, and myelograms.

Interdisciplinary Interventions

Medical Management

The choice of treatment for a fracture depends on the type, the location, and other associated injuries. A general treatment principle is to allow the child to mobilize as quickly as possible while the fracture is reduced and the bone is immobilized. For the bone to heal, the edges of the fracture must be close together or aligned, and relatively immobile. Although bone healing is important, restoring the use and appearance of the extremity is also crucial. Fracture treatment involves one of two main methods: closed reduction or open treatment.

Closed Reduction

Closed reduction aligns the fracture fragments by manually manipulating the extremity or applying traction. The child is given conscious sedation (see Chapter 13) or general anesthesia before attempting a closed reduction. Ideally, the fracture is reduced as soon as possible. However, certain situations, such as there being a large amount of swelling at the site or when the child's life is in danger, make immediate reduction impossible. In those cases, the physician may have to delay reducing the fracture for a few days. If fractures are not displaced, they do not need to be reduced.

An orthopedist uses open reduction when a fracture cannot be reduced by closed methods or when torn muscles or ligaments need to be repaired. Usually, some type of internal fixation stabilizes the fracture until it is healed. A variety of pins, screws, plates, and rods are available for fixation depending on the type of fracture and the age of the child (see Treatment Modalities). Pins are used percutaneously or through an open incision for supracondylar elbow fractures in children. Internal fixation with screws, plates, or rods is standard treatment with older children. Intramedullary fixation places a rod in the shaft of the femur to provide stabilization. After the bone has healed, the rods are removed. Telescoping rods can be lengthened to grow with the child. These rods are ideal for children who have a chronic bone disease such as OI, but they are not indicated for the treatment of femur fractures in otherwise healthy children.

After reduction, the fracture is immobilized. This can be done using a variety of different methods including splints, braces, casts, external fixators, or traction (see Treatment Modalities). Immobilization is used to prevent rotation and shearing of the fracture site, to maintain the position of the fracture after reduction, and to permit active muscle contraction. Also, keeping the site in good alignment relieves pain and allows more ease in movement of the adjacent unaffected areas of the body.

Open Fractures

The treatment of open fractures differs from that of closed fractures. The potential for infection from contamination in the wound is great. The child receives antibiotics in the emergency room and for a minimum of 3 days thereafter. The child then goes to the operating room for wound cleaning, debridement, and stabilization of the fracture. If the wound is small it may be closed, but often the physician leaves it open and draining until the infection has cleared. The child is then returned to the operating room for more debridement or closure of the wound. Either external or internal fixation can be used to treat open fractures.

Complications

Early complications from a fracture can occur despite prompt treatment and careful observation (Table 20–21). Late complications often can be prevented or their effects minimized by aggressive treatment and proper evaluation.

Compartment syndrome is one of the most feared complications of orthopedic surgery and trauma. The syndrome occurs when the non-elastic fascia that covers bone, muscle, nerves, blood vessels, and soft tissue cannot expand enough to compensate for the bleeding or swelling from trauma or the pressure from splints or casts (Monk, 1993). As the pressure increases, circulation slows, and, if the pressure is unchecked, the tissues and nerves may die. The compartments of the lower leg and forearm are most commonly affected.

▽ **Alert:** *The color and pulses of a limb with compartment syndrome remain intact at first. The classic sign of com-*

Table 20–21
Early and Late Complications of Fractures

Type	Complication
Early	Shock Fat emboli Compartment syndrome Deep vein thrombosis Pulmonary embolism Infection
Late	Malunion Non-union Refracture Joint stiffness Reflex sympathetic dystrophy Loss of reduction Post-traumatic arthritis Delayed union Pseudoarthrosis

partment syndrome is unrelenting pain that is not relieved by narcotics. Notify the physician immediately.

If the child in a cast has compartment syndrome, the first step the physician takes is to bivalve, or split, one side of the cast. If that does not relieve the symptoms, the child needs a fasciotomy. A fasciotomy is a surgical incision made through the fascia to release the pressure. It remains open but wrapped with a sterile dressing for a few days. At that point, either the physician closes the fasciotomy site or allows it to heal by itself. The best treatment for this complication is prevention of excessive swelling and early detection of neurovascular compromise.

Nursing Management

The goals of nursing care for a child with a fracture are to prevent complications and to restore function. Any fracture has the potential to interfere with neurovascular function, which, if unchecked, can lead to loss of feeling in an extremity. The nurse assesses neurovascular status frequently and notifies the physician of any change. Other nursing measures to prevent neurovascular compromise include elevating the extremity above the level of the heart to decrease swelling and applying cold packs in the first 24 hours.

Children with fractures do not have extra nutritional needs if they eat a well-balanced diet containing sufficient amounts of protein, calcium, and iron to promote the healing process. A child in a body cast should eat small, frequent meals to avoid abdominal distention. The diet should have increased amounts of fluid and fiber to prevent constipation. A laxative or stool softener is helpful for some children who are in traction or a body cast. A decrease in appetite may be seen because of the inactivity.

Children with open fractures, open reductions, or skeletal traction are at higher risk for infection. They receive antibiotics for a minimum of 3 days after surgery. If the wound culture is positive, antibiotic therapy continues for a few weeks. The protocol for skeletal traction pin care differs among practitioners (see Chart 20–12). If pin care is very uncomfortable for the patient, pain medications should be given an hour before the procedure. Older children should be encouraged to assist with pin care, even if they only open the packages of cotton applicators. This gives them some control over a frightening situation.

Pain management for a fracture is essential. Intravenous opioids such as morphine provide relief for the first 24 hours. After the fracture is set and immobilized, the nurse administers oral narcotics such as acetaminophen with codeine to control discomfort. Muscle spasms, especially with a femur fracture, can be extremely painful. The best treatment for spasms is diazepam, which relaxes the muscle. Muscle spasms generally subside after the first week.

The child who enters the acute care setting for treatment of a fracture probably has not had any preparation for the experience and has most likely undergone some sort of trauma. The family may also be in a state of shock. Crisis intervention for both the child and family is essential. If the family was part of a motor vehicle accident or community disaster, multiple family members or friends may be hospitalized. Siblings are encouraged to visit, especially if they witnessed the accident or causal event. A visit helps to reassure siblings that their brother or sister is alive.

Children often regress when hospitalized. Given no preparation for a stressful event, they use coping mechanisms previously learned, such as thumb sucking. Also, separation from a parent can be difficult for a young child. The nurse should encourage the use of security objects such as a favorite blanket or stuffed animal to help ease the separation. Parents should be encouraged to stay with the child in the hospital, if possible.

The hospital-based teacher can see any child who is in the hospital for an extended period. For example, children in traction for a femur fracture may be in the hospital for 3 to 4 weeks. The teacher obtains homework assignments from the child's school and assists the child with completing the work. When the child returns home in a hip spica cast, a home tutor should be arranged for. Many children can return to school with a cast.

Child life specialists are an integral part of the interdisciplinary team. Children with fractures or any kind of trauma often experience nightmares. Pin care and other

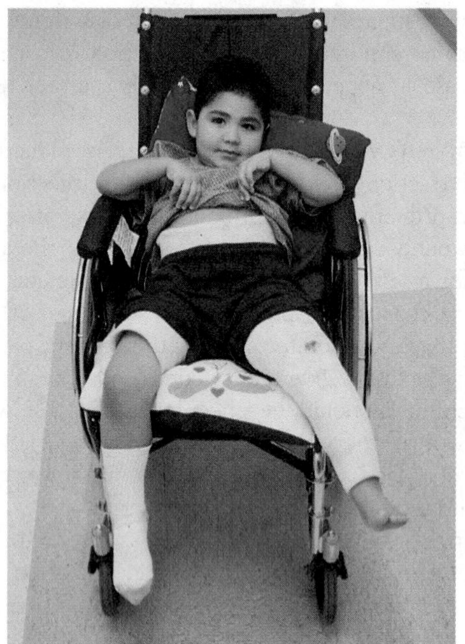

Figure 20–21
The child in a spica cast cannot sit up straight. If the child is small enough, a wheelchair with pillow supports can be used to place the child in a comfortable position. For a larger child, a reclining wheelchair may be necessary.

uncomfortable procedures can cause the child to act out. Child life specialists or nurses can assist children in working through their fears or frustrations by using medical play and art therapy. Computers, movies, and video games can help a normally active child stay busy. To control behavior, star charts and countdown calendars are ideal for children.

Social services personnel assist the family on admission to the hospital. Ideally, the social worker first meets the family in the emergency room. Social services personnel help with handling crisis situations, arranging transportation, and identifying community resources. The nurse or social worker can also arrange for home equipment such as a wheelchair or hospital bed.

Community Care

Teaching is an important component of the care of a child with a fracture. Instructions on the treatment plan, basic principles of bone healing, neurovascular assessments, and cast care by the nurse can help parents feel more confident about caring for their child in the home (see Charts 20–9 and 20–10 and TIP 20–1).

Depending on the type of fracture, the child's physical mobility may be limited after he or she returns home. Adaptations to the home environment may be needed to accommodate the child in a cast or in traction. A child in a hip spica cast may use a reclining wheelchair to get around (Fig. 20–21). Crutches and walkers are other aids used to restore mobility. Wagons for small children are fun and useful. A physical therapist can assist the family in learning methods of transfer and use of assistive devices. The nurse should demonstrate good body mechanics and safety practices to the child to prevent further injury.

A primary role of the health care team is to promote public awareness of measures that can prevent accidental injury and trauma to children. Safety fairs held at malls and other public places educate parents and children about ways to prevent accidents, child-proof the home, and develop a family escape plan for fires. Programs can also be taken into schools to educate children directly by use of puppets and other interactive displays. The programs focus on street safety, fire safety, and emergency routines, as well as seat belt and helmet use. In recent years, legislation has been passed in many states that requires certain safety precautions for children, such as the mandatory use of helmets when bike riding and of car safety restraint devices (Fig. 20–22). The National Safe Kids Campaign is one example of a nationwide program that has local coalitions in every state to focus on community education about the prevention of accidents (see Resources).

Sports Injuries

Organized sport activities are a popular mode of recreation in the pediatric and adolescent population. Com-

Figure 20–22
Children should be introduced at a young age to wearing protective gear to prevent physical injury.

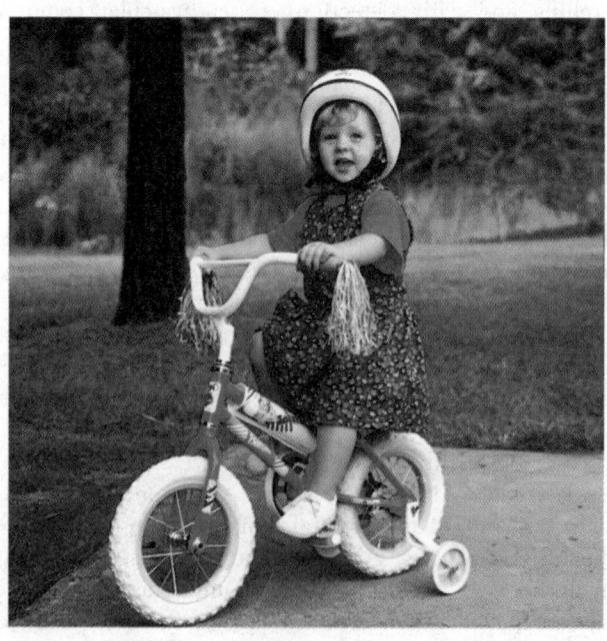

petitive sport programs are found in three fourths of all junior high and middle schools in the United States. An estimated one half of boys and one fourth of girls ages 8 to 16 participate in these programs. In addition, 20% of those same children are also involved in a community sport organization (Pecina & Bojanic, 1993). The increase in popularity of competitive sports, recreational sports, and cheerleading has brought a corollary increase in overuse injuries, sprains, strains, and dislocations. It is estimated that 22% to 39% of high school athletes sustain a significant injury and as many as 20% of these injuries are preventable (Krowchuk, 1997). Causative factors in sport-related injuries include inadequate health physicals before participation in sport activities, hazardous practice and play areas, training and practice errors, improper safety equipment, improper nutrition in athletes, overtiredness while performing sport activities, and limited awareness or concern for possible risk factors (Gottlieb, 1994).

Overuse Injuries

Overuse injuries stem from repetitive microtrauma to areas of the body, resulting in pain and inflammation (Table 20–22). There is usually a history of increased physical activity before the onset of symptoms. No traumatic injury is generally reported (Dyment, 1997). A 9-year review of more than 3000 children found the knee to be the most common site of overuse injury in two thirds of children ages 0 to 12 years and in more than one half of 13- to 18-year-olds (Garrick & Van Pelt, 1989).

Table 20–22
Common Overuse Injuries

Type	Cause	Physical Findings
Jumper's knee (patellar tendonitis)	Repetitive pulling action on the distal pole of the patellar tendon	Point tenderness at proximal aspect of tibia associated with tendonitis
Little Leaguer's elbow	Repetitive valgus stress Common in adolescent pitchers	Osteochondral injuries Damage to proximal radial epiphysis and growth plate
Little Leaguer's shoulder	Repetitive overhead throwing	Stress fracture of proximal humeral growth plate
Osgood-Schlatter disease	Irritation of tibial tubercle from excessive running or jumping exercises	Point tenderness to proximal tibia Inflammation Possible avulsion injury
Osteochondritis dissecans	Cause unknown May be familial or result of metabolic bone problem	Knee pain Inflammation Swelling Portion of articular cartilage separates
Sever's disease	Activities that include vigorous running or jumping resulting in heel pain	Limp Apophysitis of the calcaneous Point tender heel pain Tight achilles tendon
Shin splints	Excessive running Improper shoewear Running on hard surfaces	Pain Inflammation in anterior aspect of the tibia
Sinding-Larsen-Johansson disease	Excessive extension action on the patellar tendon associated with jumping activities	Knee pain Diagnosed radiographically Avulsion fracture of the lower pole of patella
Spondylolisthesis	Excessive flexion and extension activities; commonly seen in gymnasts, skaters, and football linemen	Back pain Diagnosed radiographically; anterior displacement of L_5 on S_1
Spondylolysis	Excessive flexion and extension activities	Back pain Diagnosed radiographically

A common area of injury is the apophysis, the articular cartilage of the bone. In apophyseal injuries, as seen in Osgood-Schlatter disease, the cartilaginous area near the end of a long bone, where a musculotendinous unit inserts, becomes inflamed with activity. Damage to the articular cartilage occurs secondary to the serial trauma to the layer of cartilage that covers the joint surface at the end of a bone, as discussed previously (see Osteochondritis Dissecans).

Overuse injuries can also produce various stress fractures. For example, the repetitive overhead throwing maneuver that leads to microfractures in the proximal humeral physis is known as "Little Leaguer's shoulder" (American Academy of Orthopaedic Surgeons, 1991). Shin splints are usually associated with running activities, improper footwear, and running on hard surfaces. Athletes with shin splints describe pain in the anterior aspect of the tibia. The pain is produced by microscopic tearing of tendons away from the tibia, resulting in inflammation and point tenderness (Maher et al., 1994). If untreated or ignored, shin splints can lead to stress fractures. Stress fractures can also occur in the vertebrae. Spondylolysis is a stress fracture of the pars interarticularis of the vertebrae, usually occurring in the area of L5–S1. Actual anterior displacement of L5 onto S1 is called spondylolisthesis. These fractures are frequently seen in gymnasts, ice skaters, and football linemen, who are prone to flexion and hyperextension activities.

Interdisciplinary Interventions

Overuse injuries generally have a good prognosis. Treatment aims to restore as much function as possible in the shortest time and to enable the athlete to return to preinjury performance (Tipton, 1990). Children experience pressure from coaches, peers, and even parents when they are absent from a sport. Emphasis needs to be placed on the player's personal capabilities, because serious injuries result when the child returns prematurely.

Initially, the nurse documents a baseline neurovascular assessment of the injured extremity. Diagnosis is made by clinical examination and by a history consistent with the mechanism of injury. Radiographs may depict soft tissue swelling avulsion injuries; however, acute stress fractures may not be recognized. Stress fractures may not be seen on a radiograph for 4 to 6 weeks until periosteal reaction (new bone formation) indicates that healing has begun. Bone scans are the preferred diagnostic test to help localize the injury.

Conservative treatment modalities for the child with an overuse injury include avoiding the causative activity for 6 to 8 weeks. NSAIDs are used for inflammation and pain control. A stretching and strengthening program is instituted by a physical therapist for the appropriate muscle groups.

The goals for a child's return to play are at the discretion of the health care team. The physician and the nurse should discuss realistic expectations of the treatment plan with the patient and the family.

caREminder: *Parents and coaches may not understand that the level of activity that causes overuse symptoms varies from child to child. To relay information to the child's coach, notes or telephone conversations from the physician or nurse can clarify any misconceptions of what is expected during the recovery and recuperative periods.*

The physical therapist also plays an important role. Vital facts regarding the athlete's rehabilitative progress and potential can determine outcome. Nurses can link the chain of communication in this interdisciplinary approach (Wenger & Rang, 1993).

Sprains and Strains

A *sprain* is a tear or a stretch in a ligament resulting from a pulling or twisting injury to a joint. A *strain* is a tear to the musculotendinous unit. Sprains and strains are uncommon in younger children and are usually seen in the adolescent age group. The growth plate, or physis, is weaker than the ligaments in younger children, because this is an area of new bone formation and, as a result, is prone to fracture. When children reach puberty, skeletal growth declines and the growth plates begin to close. Thus, the growth plate is less susceptible to injury, and the ligaments and tendons are more vulnerable to sprains and strains. The ankle is the most frequently sprained or strained joint (Bernhardt, 1997; Maher et al., 1994).

Pathophysiology

Ankle sprains and strains are usually the product of an inversion injury, in which the lateral aspect of the ankle joint is thrust outward and the foot is turned inward as if stepping on its side. This mechanism of injury causes insult to the anterior talofibular ligament and, in severe cases, involves the posterior talofibular ligament (Fig. 20–23) (American Academy of Orthopaedic Surgeons, 1991).

Sprains are classified according to severity. *First degree*, or mild, sprains result when the ligament is stretched and the affected joint is stable. *Second degree*, or moderate, sprains occur when the ligament is partially torn and joint laxity is noted on examination. *Third degree*, or severe, sprains are produced when the ligament is completely torn and the injured joint is unstable (American Academy of Orthopaedic Surgeons, 1991; Onieal, 1996).

Prognosis. The prognosis is favorable for first- and second-degree sprains. However, severe sprains carry an increased risk of recurrent injury, persistent instability,

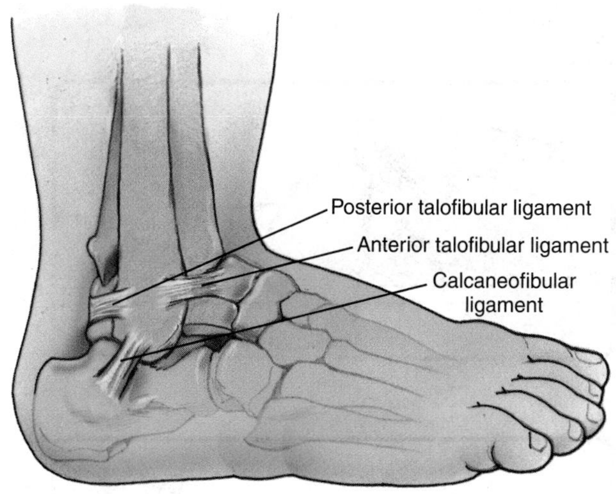

Figure 20–23
Ankle sprains occur when the foot is suddenly turned inward, causing tearing of the outside ligaments.

and traumatic arthritis, particularly if the athlete does not comply with the rehabilitation regimen.

Assessment

Obtaining a history of the event that caused the injury is helpful in determining the extent of the injury. The timing of swelling and local hemorrhage at the injury site indicates the amount of joint injury sustained. The presence of an audible sound at the time of injury may also indicate the severity of the problem.

The affected area and the surrounding structures should be palpated to determine the site of injury and the ligaments injured. The most painful areas should be palpated last. A first-degree sprain is characterized by minimal pain, swelling, and ecchymosis. Full range of motion of the joint and weight-bearing are possible. The joint is stable, with mild tenderness noted over the point of injury. The child with a second-degree sprain has moderate pain, swelling, and ecchymosis. Motion of the extremity is slightly limited and painful. Mild joint laxity is present with tenderness noted over the joint. The child may be unable to bear weight or perform daily activities with the extremity. When a third-degree sprain has occurred, significant swelling and severe ecchymosis occur rapidly, usually within the first 30 minutes after the injury. Severe pain over the joint may make it difficult for the health care provider to examine the injury and evaluate the extent of immobility. The child cannot bear weight on or otherwise use the extremity (Onieal, 1996).

A radiograph of the injured extremity is obtained if an obvious fracture or misalignment is noted or if physical examination reveals a third-degree sprain. Fractures may not be easily noted due to the cartilaginous nature of the young child's bones. The child who does not show improvement within 4 days of therapy should be reevaluated for a potential fracture at the site (Newland, 1996).

Nursing Diagnoses and Outcomes

The nursing diagnoses for a child with a musculoskeletal condition are presented in Chart 20–5. In addition, because a sprain or strain can severely limit the mobility of an active youth, the following diagnosis may be applicable:

- **Noncompliance related to degree of mobility restrictions over an extended period**
  Outcomes: The child will demonstrate compliance with treatment regimen as demonstrated by use of elastic wraps, braces, crutches, or other orthopedic supportive devices.
  The child will refrain from weight-bearing and sports activities as prescribed.

Interdisciplinary Interventions

Initially, all sprains and strains are treated with a period of rest, ice packs, compression, and elevation (RICE), and early motion of the limb is also encouraged (Fig. 20–24). This can be done immediately at the location in which the child was injured.

caREminder: *In an injury to the foot or ankle, be sure to keep the player's shoe in place to help control swelling and until any fractures are ruled out radiographically.*

The severity and location of injury guide further management decisions. External support can be provided with the application of an elastic bandage, brace, or ankle lacer in mild sprains. In moderate sprains, a posterior splint or cast may be used for 2 to 3 weeks in conjunction with crutches. Severe sprains may be treated conservatively or surgically, requiring a cast for 4 to 6 weeks and no weight-bearing activities (American Academy of Orthopaedic Surgeons, 1991).

Early motion after acute injury of the soft tissue will help the child make a more rapid recovery (Bernhardt, 1997; Chorley & Hergenroeder, 1997). A stretching and strengthening program is instrumental in returning the child to full function. Physical therapists instruct the patient in quadriceps and hamstring exercises for knee sprains and strains. For ankle injuries, a range-of-motion program is implemented. Crutch walking can be taught by the nurse or physical therapist. In crutch walking, the child should bear weight on the hands and not the underarms to avoid nerve damage (see Fig. 20–3).

Community Care

Home care instructions vary based on the injury and on the treatment indicated. To decrease the potential for

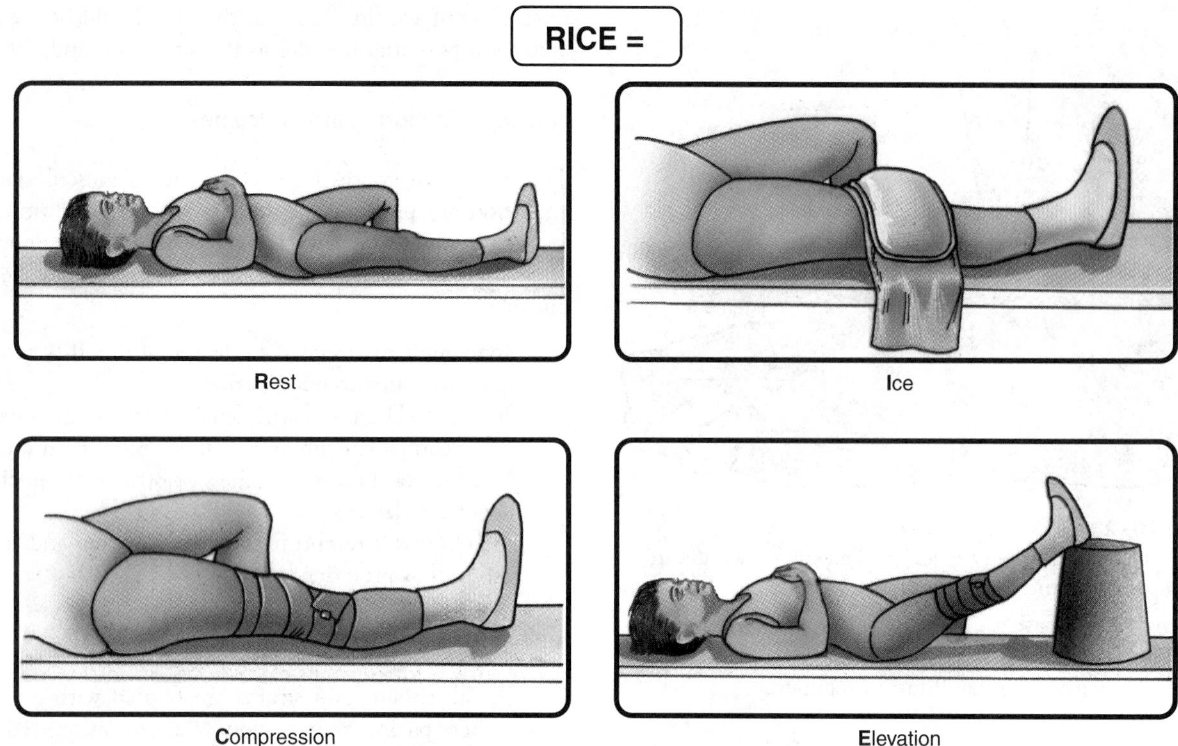

Figure 20–24
Rest, ice, compression, and elevation.

swelling, the patient and the family are taught the proper technique for wrapping the injured extremity. The wrap should be started distal from the affected area. If the joint is located below the level of the heart, swelling is alleviated by elevating the limb. If anti-inflammatory medicines are used, advise the patient and family of the proper route, action, dosage, and side effects of the agent.

Notes to the physical education teacher or coach provide an explanation of the extent of the injury and list any restrictions the child may have. The note can also state what the child is permitted to do. For example, if the patient sustained a knee strain and is walking with the assistance of crutches, upper body strengthening exercises can continue. The child with a first-degree injury can return to sport activities within 2 to 3 weeks with support of the affected joint. The child with a second-degree sprain can do partial weight-bearing activities using crutches. A return to full weight-bearing and sport activities should be done gradually. When a complete tear of the ligaments has occurred, a return to sport activities should not occur for 4 to 8 weeks after the injury.

Dislocations

A dislocation occurs when extreme force is placed on a ligament, causing partial or complete displacement of two bone ends or dislodgment of the head of the bone from its socket. The child experiences pain with decreased movement of the extremity, and obvious deformity may be seen. Dislocations can occur alone or can be accompanied by an avulsion or growth plate fracture. As in sprain and strain injuries, dislocations are not as common in younger children because the epiphysis is less susceptible to stress and more likely to fracture. However, dislocations are commonly associated in children with ligamentous laxity, as is seen in patients with trisomy 21 who are prone to subluxation (partial displacement) or dislocation of the hips. Nursemaid's elbow, dislocation of the proximal radial head, is commonly seen in 1- to 4-year-olds. This dislocation occurs when the child is lifted, jerked, or swung with the arm extended and the forearm pronated (Flynn & Zink, 1993).

Pathophysiology

Most dislocations result from one acute incident that ruptures the surrounding soft tissues and ligaments around a joint. Insult to vascular and neurovascular structures are possible. Whereas simple dislocations can be reduced quickly, manipulation may be more difficult for unreduced joints because of the swelling and possible interposed tissue. Radiographs are recommended before reduction to rule out any fractures. If the injury did not involve a fracture through the growth plate, which can disturb or arrest the growth potential of the bone, the patient should recover with full function and range of motion of the involved joint.

Interdisciplinary Interventions

The patient experiences pain immediately after the injury accompanied by swelling, bruising, and possible deformity. On clinical examination, the opposite joint is first evaluated for a baseline comparison. Radiographs may be obtained before reduction. Conscious sedation or a general anesthetic is used before relocation.

Dislocations are treated conservatively by physicians. Acute dislocations are treated with RICE and immobilization. Slings, splints, or casts are used for 3 weeks after reduction for patient comfort and to allow healing of the capsular structures. Recurrent dislocations require possible surgical intervention.

Frequent neurovascular evaluations by the nurse detect any variations of normal physiology secondary to the injury or swelling. Parents are instructed on normal and abnormal neurovascular findings. Dosage, route, action, and side effects of pain medication and cast care instructions need to be reviewed.

Mobilization of the joint begins approximately 3 weeks after the injury has occurred to prevent joint stiffness. The physical therapist instructs the patient and parents on a home exercise program to aid the patient in returning to full range of motion with joint stability. As previously discussed, written notes to coaches and teachers should detail permitted and non-permitted activities.

Summary of Key Concepts

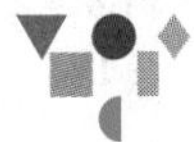

- The orthopedic care of a child differs from that of the adult in that the tissues and bones are still growing. This results in special treatment techniques to protect the growth areas and promote optimal development of the musculoskeletal system.
- Treatment for the child with an alteration in musculoskeletal status includes use of heat and cold applications, braces and splints, serial manipulation, casts, traction, external fixators, surgery, and CPM. These modalities may be used in a variety of combinations to restore the damaged area or to prevent further injury.
- Many orthopedic treatment modalities are implemented in the home. The health care team needs to provide the child and family with the knowledge and skills to manage the child's health care needs for the duration of the healing process or to promote adaptation to a chronic condition.
- The child in a brace or splint must receive instruction regarding the proper way to apply the appliance to ensure it fits correctly and comfortably. Home maintenance of the brace and the child's skin and compliance with the treatment regimen are also aspects of family teaching.
- Care of children in a cast includes preparing them for the sensations associated with cast placement and removal and monitoring circulatory status, neuromuscular status, and skin integrity. Family teaching focuses on prevention of skin breakdown, prevention of further injury, control of pain and muscle spasms, and prevention of complications such as infection.
- When traction is used, the nurse must assess the extremities for color, sensation, and motion. Providing skin care to the immobilized area and any pin sites is essential. Releasing traction to provide skin care is not allowed with skeletal traction.
- Complications of musculoskeletal surgery include phlebitis, infection, alterations in pulmonary function, alterations in skin integrity, and pain. Providing adequate pain relief measures and encouraging early mobility can prevent many of these potential complications.
- The nutritional requirements for a child with a musculoskeletal disorder include adequate intake of foods high in protein to promote healing, adequate intake of vitamins C and D, calcium, and phosphorus, and intake of plenty of fluids and food high in fiber to prevent constipation.

- Musculoskeletal disorders can be particularly challenging to children because of the limitations imposed on their activities and mobility. The health care team should encourage the use of age-appropriate activities that prevent developmental delay and do not interfere with the treatment regimen. Contacts with family members and peers should be encouraged. Measures should be instituted to ensure that school work can be completed during the entire course of the child's therapy.
- Children with chronic conditions are a large portion of the pediatric orthopedic population. Although their disorder cannot be cured, deformities can be corrected or minimized to enable the child to live a productive life.
- Infections in the bone or joint can be destructive and difficult to treat if not detected early. Recent advances in antibiotic therapy and immunizations are helping to decrease the number and severity of bone and joint infections seen in children.
- Fractures heal faster in the young. At approximately age 10 years, children's fractures are treated in the same manner as adults'.
- Overuse injuries are a common problem in the pediatric athlete. Primary treatment involves the principles of rest, ice, compression, and elevation.
- The most difficult challenge regarding care of the child with an overuse injury, sprain, strain, or dislocation is to prevent recurrent trauma. The nurse needs to relay the importance of rest and healing of the affected area to the child, family, sports coaches, and school teachers.

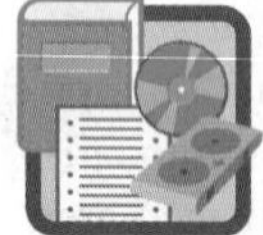

Resources

Organizations

American Academy for Cerebral Palsy and Developmental Medicine
P.O. Box 11086
Richmond, VA 23230-1086
(804) 282-0036

American Juvenile Arthritis Foundation
1314 Spring Street, NW
Atlanta, GA 30309
(404) 872-7100

Arthritis Consulting Services
4620 North State Road 7
Suite 206
Ft. Lauderdale, FL 33319
(800) 327-3027

Arthritis Foundation
1314 Spring Street, NW
Atlanta, GA 30309
(800) 283-7800

Canadian Cerebral Palsy Association
40 Dundaj Street West
Suite 222
Toronto, Ontario, Canada M5G 2C2
(416) 979-7923

Council for Disability Rights
343 South Dearborn #1503
Chicago, IL 60604
(312) 922-1093

March of Dimes Birth Defects Foundation
1275 Manaroneck Avenue
White Plains, NY 10605
(914) 428-7100

Muscular Dystrophy Association
3300 East Sunrise Drive
Tucson, AZ 85718
(602) 529-2000

National Association of Orthopaedic Nurses
East Holly Avenue
Box 56
Pitman, NJ 08071
(609) 256-2310

National Handicapped Sports and Recreation Association
1145 19th Street, NW
Suite 717
Washington, DC 20036
(202) 393-7505

National Information Center for Handicapped Children and Youth
1555 Wilson Boulevard
Suite 700
Rosslyn, VA 22209
(703) 893-6061

National Safe Kids Campaign
111 Michigan Avenue, NW
Washington, DC 20010
(202) 884-4993

National Scoliosis Foundation
72 Mount Auburn Street
Watertown, MA 02172
(617) 926-0397

Osteogenesis Imperfecta Foundation, Inc.
5005 West Laurel Street
Suite 210
Tampa, FL 33607
(813) 282-1161

Spina Bifida Association of America
4590 MacArthur Boulevard, NW
Suite 250
Washington, DC 20007
(800) 621-3141

Spina Bifida Association of Canada
633 Wellington Crescent
Winnipeg, Manitoba
Canada R3M0A8
(204) 452-7580

United Cerebral Palsy Association
1660 L Street, NW
Washington, DC 20036
(800) 872-5827

Wheelchair Sports, U.S.A.
3595 East Fountain Boulevard
Suite L-1
Colorado Springs, CO 80910
(719) 574-1150

Printed Materials

Exceptional Parent (*A magazine for parents of handicapped children*)
1170 Commonwealth Avenue
Brighton, MA 02134

A Reader's Guide: For Parents of Children with Physical or Emotional Disabilities Publication (HSA) 77-5290. Washington, DC: US Government Printing Office.

Hotlines

Aerobics and Fitness Association of America
(818) 904-0040
FAX (818) 990-5468

Shriners Hospital Referral Line
(800) 237-5055
Free orthopedic or burn care for children

Car Safety Restraint Options for Children with Orthopedic Disorders

Infants

Dream Ride by Cosco, Inc. *Can be used for infants who must lie prone; fits infants up to 17 pounds.*

Cosco Eurosport car seat. *Accommodates infants in hip spica casts; fits children up to 40 pounds.*

Children

Modified E-Z-On Vest. *Allows small child or teen to lie prone or supine on the back seat of the car; available in a variety of sizes; works well for children in hip spica casts.*

EZ Products
500 Commerce Way West
Jupiter, FL 33458
(800) 323-6598

References

Adkins, L. (1997). Cast changes: Synthetic versus plaster. *Pediatric Nursing, 23*(4), 422–427.

Allen, N. (1988). Rheumatology. In J. Crapo, M. Hamilton, & S. Edgman (Eds.), *Medicine and pediatrics* (pp. 369–418). St. Louis: Mosby–Year Book.

American Academy of Orthopaedic Surgeons. (1991). *Athletic training and sports medicine*. Park Ridge, IL: American Academy of Orthopaedic Surgeons.

Athreya, B. (1996). Systemic lupus erythematosus. In F. Burg, J Ingelfinger, E. Wald, & R. Polin (Eds.), *Current pediatric therapy 15* (pp. 388–389). Philadelphia: W. B. Saunders.

Bell, G. R., Gurd, A. R., Orlowski, J. P., & Andrish, J. T. (1986). The syndrome of inappropriate antidiuretic hormone secretion following spinal fusion. *The Journal of Bone and Joint Surgery*, 68-A(5), 720–723.

Bender, L. H. (1991). Osteogenesis imperfecta. *Orthopaedic Nursing, 10*(4), 23–31.

Bernhardt, D. (1997). General principles in treating soft-tissue injuries. *Pediatric Annals 26*(1), 20–25.

Bradford, D. S., Lonstein, J. E., Moe, J. H., Ogilvie, J. W., & Winter, R. B. (1987). *Moe's textbook of scoliosis and other spinal deformities* (2nd ed.) Philadelphia: W. B. Saunders.

Bunnell, W. P. (1991). Adolescent idiopathic scoliosis: Patient evaluation. *Seminars in Spine Surgery, 3*(40), 202–211.

Carlino, H. 1991. The child with an Ilizarov external fixator. *Pediatric Nursing, 17*(4), 355–358.

Chorley, J., & Hergenroeder, A. (1997). Management of ankle sprains. *Pediatric Annals, 26*(1), 56–64.

Copstead, L. (1995). *Perspectives on pathophysiology*. Philadelphia: W. B. Saunders.

Davis, D. (1997). Review of cerebral palsy, Part I: Description, incidence, and etiology. *Neonatal Network, 16*(3), 7–12.

DeWit, S. (1992). *Keane's essentials of medical-surgical nursing*. Philadelphia: W. B. Saunders.

Dyment, P. (1997). Apophyseal injuries. *Pediatric Annals*. 26(1), 28–30.

Ehrlich, M., & Akelman, E. (1996). Orthopedic problems of the extremities. In F. Burg, J. Ingelfinger, E. Wald, & R. Polin (Eds.), *Current pediatric therapy 15* (pp. 479–483). Philadelphia: W. B. Saunders.

Eicher, P., & Batshaw, M. (1993). Cerebral palsy. *The Pediatric Clinics of North America, 40*(3), 537–551.

Flynn, J., & Zink, W. (1993). Fractures and dislocations of the elbow. In G. MacEwen, J. Kasser, & S. Heinrich (Eds.), *Pediatric fractures a practical approach to assessment and treatment* (pp. 133–164). Baltimore: Williams & Wilkins.

Gagliardi, B. A. (1991). The impact of Duchenne muscular dystrophy on families. *Orthopaedic Nursing, 10*(5), 41–48.

Gallo, A. (1996). Building strong bones in childhood and adolescence: Reducing the risk of fractures in later life. *Pediatric Nursing, 22*(5), 369–374 & 422.

Garrick, J., & Van Pelt, S. (1989). Management of anterior knee pain in pediatric sports medicine. *Pediatric Basics, 52*, 9–12.

Gertner, J. M., & Root, L. (1990). Osteogenesis imperfecta. *The Orthopaedic Clinics of North America. 21*(1), 151–162.

Gottlieb, A. (1994). *Cheerleaders are athletes too*. Pediatric Nursing, 20(6), 630–633.

Hall, B. (1996). Inherited osteoporoses. In R. Behrman, R. Kliegman, & A. Arvin (Eds.), *Nelson textbook of pediatrics* (pp. 1978–1980). Philadelphia: W. B. Saunders.

Herring, J. A. (1989). Legg-Calve-Perthes disease: A review of current knowledge. In J. Barr (Ed.), American Academy of Orthopaedic Surgeons *Instructional course lectures*, XXXVIII (pp. 309–315). Park Ridge, IL: American Academy of Orthopaedic Surgeons.

Heydemann, P. (1996). Muscular dystrophy and related myopathies. In F. Burg, J. Ingelfinger, E. Wald, & R. Polin (Eds.), *Current pediatric therapy 15* (pp. 510–511). Philadelphia: W. B. Saunders.

Hubbard, S., Bush, G., Kurtz, I., & Naumann, S. (1991). Myoelectric prostheses for the limb deficient child. *Physical Medicine and Rehabilitation Clinics of North America, 2*(4), 854.

Hughes, R. B., & D'Ambrosia, K. D. (1993). Nursing management of a child with juvenile rheumatoid arthritis. *Orthopaedic Nursing, 12*(5), 17–22.

Huurman, W. (1992). Orthopaedics in infancy and childhood: Lower extremity torsional deformities. *Pediatric Basics*, 60, 2–7.

Jacobs, J. C. (1992). *Pediatric rheumatology for the practitioner*. New York: Springer-Verlag.

Jonides, L., Rudy, C., & Walsh, S. (1996). Developmental dysplasia of the hip: What's new in the 1990's? *Journal of Pediatric Health Care, 10,* 85.

Kredich, D. (1988). Pediatric rheumatology. In J. Crapo, M. Hamilton, & S. Edgman (Eds.), *Medicine & pediatrics—In one book* (pp. 419–424). St. Louis: Mosby–Year Book.

Krowchuck, D. (1997). The preparticipation athletic examination: A closer look. *Pediatric Annals.* 26(1), 37–49.

Maher, A., Salmond, S., & Pellino, T. (1994). *Orthopaedic nursing.* Philadelphia: W. B. Saunders.

Masear, V. (1996). *Primary care orthopedics.* Philadelphia: W. B. Saunders.

Mason, K. (1989). Pediatric orthopedics: Developmental norms. *Orthopedic Nursing,* 8(4), 45–50.

McCullough, F. L. (1989). Skeletal trauma in children. *Orthopaedic Nursing,* 8(2), 41–46.

Meehan, P. L., Angel, D., & Nelson, J. M. (1992). The Scottish Rite abduction orthosis for the treatment of Legg Calve Perthes. *Journal of Bone and Joint Surgery, 63*-A(1), 85–95.

Monk, H. L. (1993). Fractures are never simple. *RN, 56*(4), 30–36.

Morrissy, R. T. (Ed.). (1990). *Lovell and Winter's pediatric orthopaedics.* Philadelphia: J. B. Lippincott.

Morrissy, R. T., & Selman, S. (1991). Slipped capital femoral epiphysis. *Orthopaedic Nursing, 10*(1), 11–20.

Newland, J. (1996). Ankle injuries. *AJN,* 96(7), 16E.

Onieal, M. E. (1996). Common wrist and ankle injuries. *Advance for Nurse Practitioners,* August, 31–36.

Page-Goertz, S. S. (1989). Even children have arthritis. *Pediatric Nursing, 15*(1), 11–16, 30.

Palmer, F., & Hoon, A. (1995). Cerebral palsy. In S. Parker & B. Zuckerman (Eds.), *Behavioral and Developmental Pediatrics* (pp. 88–94). Boston: Little, Brown and Company.

Pecina, M., & Bojanic, I. (1993). *Overuse injuries of the musculoskeletal system.* Boca Raton: CRC Press.

Peck, B. (1995). *Systemic lupus erythematosus. Advance for Nurse Practitioners,* 3(10), 24–29.

Philichi, L. M., & Brunn, V. (1990). Rhizotomy surgery to relieve spasticity in young children. *Maternal Child Nursing, 15*(6), 367–370.

Purdy, K., Dwyer, J., Holland, M., Goldberg, D., & Dinardo, J. (1996). You are what you eat: Healthy food choices, nutrition, and the child with juvenile rheumatoid arthritis. *Pediatric Nursing, 22*(5), 391–398.

Roach, J. W. (1991). The non-operative treatment of scoliosis. *Seminars in Spine Surgery,* 3(4), 202–211.

Rockwood, C. A., Wilkins, K. E., & King, R. E., 3rd (Eds.). (1991). *Fractures in children.* Philadelphia: J. B. Lippincott.

Rudy, C. (1996). Developmental dysplasia of the hip: What's new in the 1990's. *Journal of Pediatric Health Care, 10,* 85, 95, 96.

Schaller, J. (1996a). Juvenile rheumatoid arthritis. In R. Behrman, R. Kliegman, & A. Arvin (Eds.), *Nelson textbook of pediatrics* (pp. 661–670). Philadelphia: W. B. Saunders.

Schaller, J. (1996b). Systemic lupus erythematosus. In R. Behrman, R. Kliegman, & A. Arvin (Eds.), *Nelson textbook of pediatrics* (pp. 673–676). Philadelphia: W. B. Saunders

Shoppee, K. (1992). Developmental dysplasia of the hip. *Orthopaedic Nursing, 11*(5), 30–36.

Speers, A., & Speers, M. (1992). Care of the infant in a Pavlik harness. *Pediatric Nursing, 18*(3), 229–232.

Stoltz, M. R., Dietrich, S. L., & Marshall, G. J. (1989). Osteogenesis imperfecta: Perspectives. *Clinical Orthopaedics and Related Research, 242*(5), 120–134.

Styrcula, L. (1994). Traction basics: Part I. *Orthopaedic Nursing, 13*(2), 71–74.

Szer, I. (1996). Juvenile rheumatoid arthritis and spondyloarthropathy syndromes. In F. Burg, J. Ingelfinger, E. Wald, & R. Polin (Eds.), *Current pediatric therapy 15* (pp. 383–386). Philadelphia: W. B. Saunders.

Tachdjian, M. O. (1990). *Pediatric orthopaedics.* Philadelphia: W. B. Saunders.

Thompson, G., & Scoles, P. (1996). Bone and joint disorders. In R. Behrman, R. Kliegman, & A. Arvin (Eds.), *Nelson textbook of pediatrics* (pp. 1915–1990). Philadelphia: W. B. Saunders.

Tipton, D. (1990). A therapist's view of rehabilitation in the pediatric athlete. In J. Sullivan, & W. Grana (Eds.), *The pediatric athlete* (pp. 249–252). Park Ridge, IL: American Academy of Orthopaedic Surgeons.

Weinstein, S. L. (1991). Natural history of adolescent idiopathic scoliosis. *Seminars in Spine Surgery,* 3(4), 196–201.

Wenger, D., & Rang, M. (1993). *The art and practice of children's orthopaedics.* New York: Raven Press.

Zachazewski, J. E., Magee, D. J., & Quillen, W. S. (1996). *Athletic injuries and rehabilitation.* Philadelphia: W. B. Saunders.

Bibliography

Batshaw, M., & Perret, Y. (1992). *Children with disabilities: A medical primer.* Baltimore: Paul H. Brooks.

Bleck. E. (1987). *Orthopaedic management of cerebral palsy.* Philadelphia: J. B. Lippincott.

Francis, E. (1987). Lateral electrical surface stimulation treatment for scoliosis. *Pediatric Nursing, 13*(3), 157–160.

Gartland, J. J. (1987). *Fundamentals of orthopaedics.* (4th ed.). Philadelphia: W. B. Saunders.

Hauser Holland, S. (1983). Up-to-date home care of a baby in a hip spica cast. *Pediatric Nursing,* 9(2), 114–115.

Ibrahim, K. (1984). An overview of childhood fractures. *Pediatric Nursing, 10*(1), 57–65.

Jacobs-Zacny, J. M., & Horn, M. J. (1988). Nursing care of adolescents having posterior spinal fusion with Cotrel-Dubousset instrumentation. *Orthopaedic Nursing,* 7(1), 17–21.

Kling, T. F., Jr. (1991). Current theories of the etiology of adolescent idiopathic scoliosis. *Seminars in Spine Surgery,* 3(4), 186–195.

Kyzer, S. P. (1991). Congenital idiopathic clubfoot. *Orthopaedic Nursing, 10*(4), 11–18.

McCarty, D. J., & Koopman, W. J. (1993). *Arthritis and allied conditions.* Philadelphia: Lea & Febiger.

Mulley, D. A. (1984). Harnessing babies' dysplastic hips. *American Journal of Nursing,* 8(84), 1006–1008.

Paneth, N. (1986). Etiologic factors in cerebral palsy. *Pediatric Annals, 15,* 191–201.

Pecina, M. M., & Bojanic, A. (1993). *Overuse injuries of the musculoskeletal system.* Boca Raton: CRC Press.

Schumacher, H. R. (1993). *Primer on rheumatic diseases.* Atlanta: Arthritis Foundation.

Sillence, D. (1981). Osteogenesis imperfecta: An expanding panorama of variants. *Clinical Orthopaedics and Related Research, 159*(11), 11–24.

Sprague, J. B. (1992). Surgical management of cerebral palsy. *Orthopaedic Nursing, 11*(4), 11–18.

Thompson, D., Blanke, K., Fueyo, L., Griffin, C., Hunter, S., Moellering, J., & Sturner, S. (1991). Traction. In S. Salmond, N. Mooney, & L. Verdisco (Eds.), *Core curriculum for orthopaedic nursing.* (pp. 168–170, 173–177). Pitman, N. J.: National Association of Orthopaedic Nurses.

Varni, N. A., & Jaffe, M. (1984). Osteogenesis imperfecta: The basics. *Pediatric Nursing, 10*(1), 29–33.

Wise, L. B. (1986). A comparison of orthopaedic casts: Breaking the mold. *Maternal Child Nursing, 11,* 174–176.

HEALTH CHALLENGE:

Alterations in Neurologic Status

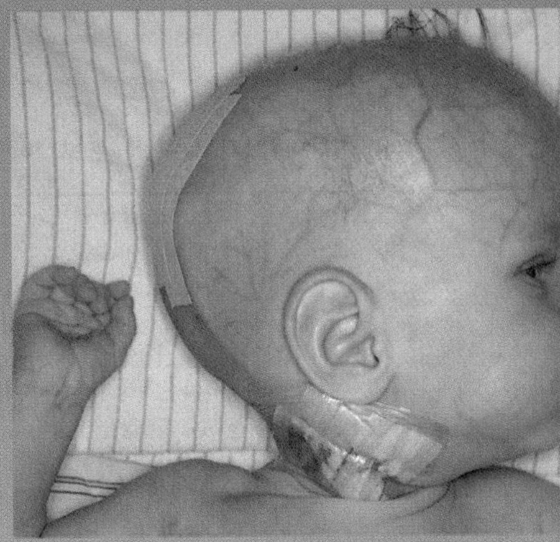

OUTLINE

OBJECTIVES

- Identify components of the neurologic assessment.
- Explain the ways in which neurologic assessment and evaluation differ between children and adults.
- Explain the purposes of diagnostic tests used in the assessment of the child with altered neurologic status.
- Examine the impact of alterations in embryonic development on neurologic functioning of the child.
- Discuss the treatment modalities that can be selected to therapeutically manage the needs of the child with altered neurologic status.
- Identify common neurologic conditions, causes, and defining characteristics of neurologic alterations that children may experience.

KEY TERMS

areflexia
decerebrate posturing
decorticate posturing
fasciculations
level of consciousness
oculocephalic reflex
opisthotonos
otorrhea
postictal
rhinorrhea

CHAPTER

21

The child with an alteration in neurologic status presents a variety of complex and challenging health care concerns. This chapter highlights some of the more common disorders and offers guidelines for comprehensive health care management. From assessment to evaluation, the nurse must provide developmentally appropriate interventions that take into account the pediatric patient's physiologic, emotional, and social needs. The family is an integral part of the health care system and must be included in all areas of care delivery to the child.

Nurses are often in the best position to coordinate the interdisciplinary teams that manage children with neurologic and neurosurgical problems. Depending on the size and setting of the pediatric facility, personnel available to the child and family may include physicians, advanced practice nurses, nurses, psychologists, social workers, child life specialists, physical therapists, occupational therapists, pastoral care staff, recreation specialists, nutritionists, and speech therapists. In addition, support groups and national organizations can provide assistance, education, and networking for specifically affected populations. Organization of these resources requires critically important nursing skills to provide families with the highest level of professional health care available. When these services are unavailable to a family whose child has a complex neurologic problem, referral to a regional medical center for evaluation is indicated.

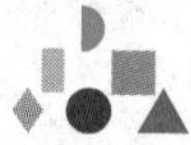

Assessment of the Child with Alterations in Neurologic Status

Focused Health History

The most important factor in evaluating a child with altered neurologic status is the history (Chart 21–1). The health history is gathered by interviewing the child and the parents, by interviewing other caregivers, and by reviewing medical records. The focused health history is guided by the acuity of the child's problem, the age of the child, and the availability of reliable historians.

The history begins with the parents' or child's description of the reason for the visit or hospitalization. In emergency or critical care areas, this history may be given by emergency or transport personnel. Once the problem is identified, inquiry into the duration, fre-

Chart 21–1
Focused Health History

Neurologic	
Identifying Data	Age Gender Ethnicity
Present Illness	Duration, frequency, and character of presenting problem Precipitating or related factors Relief measures or home remedies Interference with daily activities, such as missed school days Static or progressive nature of condition Recent changes in ability to meet developmental milestones Weakness of any body part Trembling, shakiness, or abnormal movements Any loss of consciousness, vomiting, visual disturbances, or changes in breathing patterns Significant lethargy or irritability
Birth History	Gestational age at birth Apgar scores Birth weight Results of alpha-fetoprotein, amniocentesis, or chorionic villi sampling Any significant pre-, peri-, or postnatal events causing asphyxia, trauma, jaundice, apnea Need for ventilator support in neonatal period

Chart 21–1
Focused Health History *Continued*

Neurologic	
Previous Health Challenges	Previous hospitalizations, serious illness, injury, or surgeries History of child abuse Recent infection, i.e., upper respiratory, ear, and sinus Metabolic disorder Past neurologic or developmental testing Psychological disorders
Childhood Illnesses	Chickenpox or any type of herpes infection
Immunizations	Are immunizations up-to-date Any recent immunizations Previous responses to immunizations
Allergies	Any known allergies (latex, food, medications)
Current Medications	Home remedies Prescription and nonprescription medications Use of illicit drugs
Nutritional Assessment	History of height and weight parameters Recent weight loss or gain History of pica or lead poisoning
Family Medical History	Seizures/epilepsy Headaches/migraines Mental retardation Hypotonia Learning problems Neurocutaneous lesions Problems similar to those for which the child is being evaluated Early deaths in family
Environmental History	Exposure to radiation
Social History	Perceived stressors for the child or among other family members Changes in lifestyle Changes in academic performance
Growth and Development	Sleep patterns Ability to meet developmental milestones

quency, and character of the presenting problem must occur. Although the focus of the health interview is on the child's presenting neurologic signs, evaluation of non-neurologic signs and symptoms can also provide useful information. For example, neurologic disorders may initially present with nonspecific viral illnesses, failure to thrive, or developmental delay or regression or they may occur at the same time as other systemic diseases.

Aspects of the past medical history aid in placing the current problem in perspective. Premature infants are likely to have a history of intracranial bleeding, seizure activity, or episodes of apnea that can significantly affect neurologic functioning. Nutritional status is an important aspect of the history. Poor nutritional intake can affect the child's attention span and ability to concentrate. Ingestion of nonfood substances (pica) can cause harmful toxicities that may effect neurologic function. For instance, the ingestion of lead (e.g., lead-based paint chips or lead in the water source) can cause permanent brain damage in proportion to the amount ingested. Lead is poorly excreted from the body and crosses the blood–brain barrier. No assessment is complete without evaluating the child's achievement of certain specific developmental and biological milestones. These parameters can be used to determine normal, delayed, or regressed patterns. Developmental milestones include activities such as when the infant/child first rolled over, sat unsupported, took steps, and rode a tricycle. The ages at which babbling, first words, and putting words together began are also important cognitive milestones to evaluate. When these parameters are integrated into the neurologic assessment, the nurse can use such information to adapt standard assessment criteria to the individual child. Before conducting a neurologic examination, the nurse must first assess the child's emotional state and cognitive ability. Documentation should reflect any factors that may alter optimal responses, such as anxiety, pain, limited mobility, or influence of medication.

Chart 21–2
Focused Physical Assessment

Neurologic Status

Focus Area	Parameters to Assess
Consciousness	Arousal Response to stimuli
Mentation	Attention Thinking/language Ability to name and define objects (should be age-appropriate) Short- and long-term memory Ability to eat, drink, bathe, and dress self Toileting skills
Movement	Eye movements Facial expressions Movement of head, trunk, and extremities Fine motor skills Gait Coordination Reflexes
Sensory	Blinking Vision Hearing Tasting Touch and feeling Response to painful stimuli
Regulatory functions	Breathing Circulation Temperature Digestion Bowel function Bladder function
Head circumference	Children younger than 2

Focused Physical Assessment

Various types of assessments may be conducted depending on the severity, location, and nature of the child's neurologic problem. From infancy to adolescence, children progress through stages of growth that share common characteristics. Aspects of the general physical examination should be considered. In particular, a thorough examination of the skin should be performed to allow the examiner to check for evidence of neurocutaneous disorders; to observe the spine for curvatures, hairy patches, or sacral dimples; and to palpate the abdomen to note an enlarged liver or spleen and growth parameters (Chart 21–2).

During routine check-ups, the primary care provider should obtain serial measurements of head circumference. Head size is plotted on a graph and compared with other growth parameters such as height and weight. (See Chapter 6 for standard growth parameter charts, including head circumference from the National Center for Health Statistics [NCHS]. The chart is easy to understand and provides valuable ongoing data during the early period of the child's development by comparing the child to his or her own growth as well as standardized and normalized growth patterns of thousands of other children in the United States.) The child's head should be inspected for cranial shape and for the presence of any cranial or facial asymmetry (Fig. 21–1). The fontanelles are palpated and observed for size and for presence of bulging or sunkenness.

The neurologic examination should follow a systematic approach to include the cranial nerves, motor skills, sensory responses, and cerebellar function. In infants, reflexes should also be checked. A large portion of the neurologic examination in children can be accomplished by careful observation. Often the child's motor and cog-

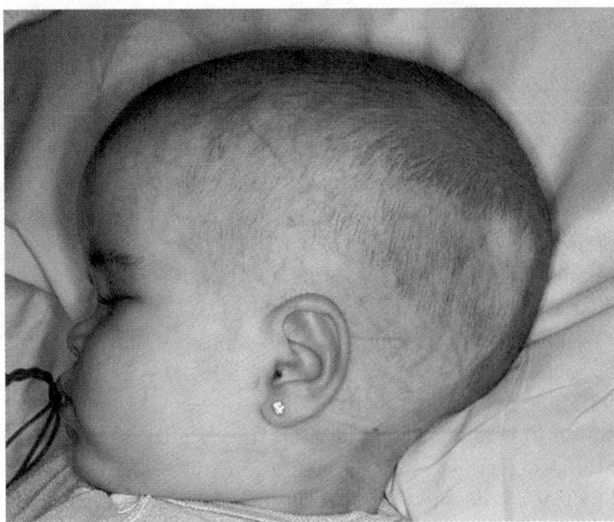

Figure 21–1
The head of an infant with hydrocephalus is larger than normal.

nitive skills can be observed as he plays in the examination room or climbs on his parents lap. Many children, particularly older infants and toddlers, will be unwilling to cooperate with a formal examination but can be engaged in play after they have become accustomed to the examiner.

Tip: *The nurse should incorporate developmentally appropriate toys or games as part of the assessment.*

The following are examples of familiar and inexpensive items that may be helpful in assessment of the child:

- To assess dexterity, handedness, and grip strength, use blocks, crayons and paper, and play dough.
- To assess cerebellar functions such as CN VIII gait and balance, use pull toys, jump rope, and a ball.
- To assess visual acuity and eye movement of CN III, IV, and VI, use brightly colored picture books and bean bag toss toys.
- To assess CN I and sensory portion of CN VII and IX, use salty snacks, lemon juice, sugar, and tonic water.
- To assess language skills, use books, magazines, and flash cards.

Assessment of the child's neurologic system can be divided into three common forms: the brief screening examination, acute neurologic checks, and the comprehensive examination. It is common to use combined portions of these examinations, depending on the child's status and on the nature of the problem. Brief screening examinations are usually performed in emergency situations. The neurologic assessment is limited in scope. The brief screening examination includes:

- Cerebral function, vital signs, level of consciousness, mental status, and verbal response
- Cranial nerves: usually CN II, III, IV, and VI for pupil reactivity, cardinal fields of gaze, and eye movement
- Motor system: strength, movement, and symmetry
- Sensory system: tactile and pain sensation in extremities
- Reflexes: deep tendon reflexes (DTRs) and superficial reflexes

Once cardiac and respiratory status are deemed stable, level of consciousness, cranial nerve function, reflexes, and motor, sensory and cerebellar responses should be assessed.

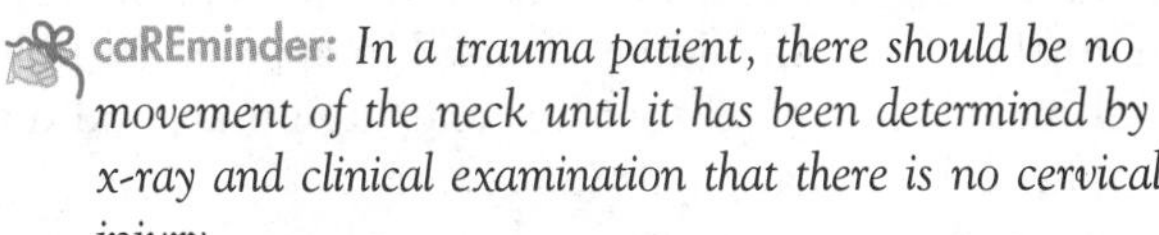

caREminder: *In a trauma patient, there should be no movement of the neck until it has been determined by x-ray and clinical examination that there is no cervical injury.*

The purpose of this screening examination is to triage neurologic deficits, to establish baseline data for later evaluation, and to develop an initial plan of care.

Acute neurologic checks are performed to monitor the child's status in the following areas:

- Level of consciousness
- Pupil size and reactivity
- Eye movements
- Motor function
- Verbal responses
- Respiratory pattern
- Vital signs, especially blood pressure and pulse

Close monitoring of at-risk patients is required because subtle changes in neurologic function may lead to rapid deterioration. The acute examination is often done repeatedly and frequently, and is documented in a serial fashion. Early intervention is indicated to avoid potential life-threatening situations. The frequency of assessments is based on the child's acuity level; the type of injury, illness, or surgery; nursing judgment; and physician's orders. A high degree of skill and accuracy is required to correctly assess deficits in all components of the acute neurologic examination. Nursing diagnoses and interventions should reflect knowledge of age-specific biological and developmental variations in the pediatric population.

The child's level of consciousness is assessed by answering three questions:

1. What stimulus was needed to achieve a response (voice, light touch, deep pain)?
2. What is the quality of the response (arousal with ability to answer questions appropriately; arousal with momentary eye opening and no meaningful verbalizations; no response)?
3. What is the length of the response (e.g., awake

and conversant for 15 to 20 minutes after arousal, awake and able to maintain alertness for only 1 to 2 minutes)?

Sequential assessments are compared with the baseline to determine deterioration or improvement. Some institutions use the Glasgow Coma Scale (GCS) in addition to acute neurologic checks to evaluate the child with a depressed level of consciousness (Table 21–1).

Assessment of the pupils is done by first observing the pupils in an indirect light and then by applying the bright light stimulus. There should be prompt constriction of the pupils. Description of this response is usually recorded as nonreactive, sluggish, or brisk. Extremely small pupils may be a side effect of narcotic medications used during anesthesia or for pain control postoperatively. Abnormalities that should be reported to appropriate personnel include any pupil that was reacting briskly and no longer is, and unequal pupils (anisocoria).

Eye movements are assessed as indicated in Table 6–9 or in the comatose patient by use of the oculocephalic maneuver. Motor function is assessed by the ability to move the extremities spontaneously or only in response to stimuli. The overall level of tone of the extremities should also be noted. Terms used include flaccid, normal, and spastic. Ankle clonus is a repetitive movement seen after quick flexion of the foot, which is felt to be indicative of motor pathway abnormalities.

Verbal responses evaluate age-appropriate abilities to use language. In the infant or nonverbal child, age-appropriate sounds are used. The GCS for verbal response in infants (Table 21–2) can be used to more specifically define changes in the very young.

The comprehensive neurologic assessment, used in nonacute situations or after the child's status has been stabilized, is described in Chapter 6. Aspects of this examination include conducting the health history and evaluating consciousness, mentation, movement, sensory function, integrated regulatory functions, head circumference, and fontanelles.

Nursing Diagnoses and Outcomes

Conditions affecting the child's neurologic status are of special concern to the health care team because there is

Table 21–1
Pediatric Coma Scale*

		Age	
	Score	>1 Year	<1 Year
Eyes opening	4	Spontaneously	Spontaneously
	3	To verbal command	To shout
	2	To pain	To pain
	1	No response	No response
Best motor response	6	Obeys	Localizes pain
	5	Localizes pain	Flexion withdrawal
	4	Flexion withdrawal (decorticate rigidity)	Flexion abnormal (decorticate rigidity)
	2	Extension (decerebrate rigidity)	Extension (decerebrate rigidity)
	1	No response	No response
		>5 Years	2–5 Years
Best verbal response	5	Oriented and converses	Appropriate word and phrases
	4	Disoriented and talks	Inappropriate words
	3	Inappropriate words	Cries and/or screams
	2	Incomprehensible sounds	Grunts
	1	No response	No response
Total	3–15		

* Modification of Glasgow Coma Scale.

Table 21-2
Glasgow Coma Scale: Verbal Response of Infants

Score Given	Response	Score Given	Response
	1 Month		**5 and 6 Months**
1	None	1	None
2	Crying to stimuli	2	Crying to stimuli (moans)
3	Crying spontaneously	3	Localizes general direction of sound
4	Blinks when eyelashes touched	4	Discrimination of family members
5	Throaty noises	5	Babbles to people, toys
	2 Months		**7 and 8 Months**
1	None	1	None
2	Crying to stimuli	2	Crying to stimuli (moans)
3	Shuts eyes to light	3	Recognizes familiar voices and family
4	Smiles when caressed	4	Babbles
5	Babbles single vowel sounds voices	5	"Ba," "Ma," "Da"
	3 Months		**9 and 10 months**
1	None	1	None
2	Crying to stimuli (moans)	2	Crying to stimuli
3	Stares at response and looks at environment	3	Recognizes (smiles or laughs)
4	Smiles to sound stimulation	4	Babbles
5	Chuckles vowels in prolonged manner	5	"Mama," "Dada"
	4 Months		**10 Months to 1 Year**
1	None	1	None
2	Crying to stimuli (moans)	2	Crying to stimuli
3	Turns head to sound	3	Recognizes (smiles)
4	Smiles spontaneously or laughs when socially stimulated	4	Babbles
5	Modulating voice and perfect vocalization of vowels	5	Words (specifically "Mama" and "Dada")

Courtesy of Dr. Kenneth Shapiro, Department of Neurosurgery, Albert Einstein College of Medicine, New York. Adapted from Zimmerman, S. S., Gildea, J. H. (1985). *Critical care pediatrics* (p. 370). Philadelphia: W. B. Saunders.

potential for long-term sequelae that can impact the child's cognitive and motor functioning. Additionally, the child's social and personal development may become impaired because of activity limitations, isolation from peers, and challenges to self-esteem. Therefore, the goals of health care management are to immediately intervene to prevent progression of neurologic insult while simultaneously treating, if possible, the underlying condition. During these early critical stages of the child's care, nursing interventions are focused on monitoring and maintaining physiologic functioning of all body systems because the brain and its functions are vitally linked to other systemic body functions. Nursing personnel play an important role in supporting the family as the child is stabilized, a diagnosis is reached, and treatment interventions are initiated. As the child responds to the interdisciplinary interventions, the goals of the health care team become directed toward optimizing the child's outcomes through rehabilitation activities. The nurse in the home, the school, and the rehabilitation center assists the family in evaluating the child's capabilities and assists the child in meeting his or her highest level of growth and development. Chart 21–3 summarizes the numerous nursing diagnoses that can be applied to children experiencing a neurologic disorder. These diagnoses reflect the broad scope of problems that confront the child and family as they deal with both the emergent and long-term issues surrounding the child's condition.

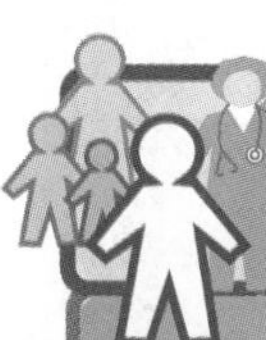

Chart 21–3
Nursing Diagnoses and Outcomes

The Child with Alterations in Neurologic Status

High risk for altered tissue perfusion: cerebral, related to brain injury or seizure activity

Outcomes: Child maintains or improves current level of consciousness.
Intercranial pressure remains in normal range.
Risk factors for altered cerebral perfusion and complications are reduced as much as possible.

Confusion related to altered level of consciousness

Outcomes: Child remains oriented.
Child responds to environmental stimuli.
Child's safety is maintained in environment.

Thought process alteration related to neurologic injury or illness

Outcomes: Child receives treatment for physiologic causes, resulting in restoration of thought processes.
Child's safety is maintained and child is protected from injury.

High risk for infection related to presence of surgical incision, head trauma, or bacteria infecting the neurologic system

Outcomes: Child receives prompt treatment for infectious process.
Child remains afebrile.
Child's infectious process resolves without complications to neurologic integrity.

High risk for injury related to sensory and motor deficits

Outcomes: Child and family identify factors that increase potential for injury.
Family assists in identifying and implementing safety measures to prevent injury.
Child increases self-care activities within parameters posed by sensorimotor limitations.

Ineffective breathing pattern related to neurotrauma and central nervous system damage

Outcomes: Child's respiratory rate remains within age-appropriate parameters.
Arterial blood gases remain in normal range.
Child maintains respirations without ventilatory support.

Ineffective thermoregulation related to neurologic trauma or illness

Outcome: Child's body temperature remains within normothermic levels.

Diversional activity deficit related to long-term hospitalization or isolation

Outcomes: Child selects and participates in age-appropriate play.
Child and family adopt age-appropriate play activities with consideration to child's level of fatigue, neurologic irritability, and level of pain.

Growth and development alteration related to physical or neurologic impairment

Outcomes: Child demonstrates age-appropriate skills as able, given sensorimotor limitations.
Parents express understanding of norms for growth and development.
Parents express understanding of their child's growth and developmental potential as defined by the child's condition.
Child and parents participate in activities to enhance child's achievement of developmental milestones.

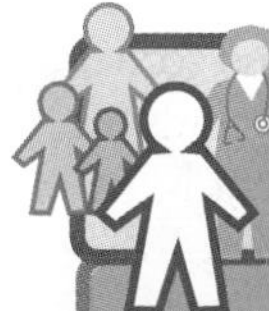

Chart 21–3
Nursing Diagnoses and Outcomes *Continued*

The Child with Alterations in Neurologic Status

Body image disturbance related to altered physical capabilities, lifestyle changes, or physical appearance following neurologic injury or illness

Outcomes:
Child discusses feelings about change in body image.
Child expresses positive feelings about self.
Child implements positive coping skills to deal with change in body image.

Knowledge deficit: child's condition, treatment plan, and home care requirements

Outcomes:
Child and family express interest in learning about child's condition.
Child and family participate in teaching sessions to learn about child's condition.
Child and family demonstrate health care behaviors needed to manage child's care at home.

Ineffective, compromised family coping related to severity of child's illness and potential or actual long-term disability

Outcomes:
Family members express their concerns about coping with child's illness.
Family members are able to identify their needs.
Family members seek resources and sources of emotional and spiritual support.
Family members are able to meet their needs as well as the child's to their mutual satisfaction.

High risk for altered health maintenance after discharge related to parental knowledge deficit

Outcomes:
Family manages child's health care in the home.
Family obtains financial and physical resources to manage child's care in the home.
Family verbalizes confidence in caring for child's ongoing health needs.

Developmental and Biological Variances

Development of the nervous system in utero and after birth follows distinct patterns. The development of the spinal cord and brain, myelinzation, cranial bone development, cerebrospinal fluid circulation, and cerebral blood flow will be addressed briefly.

Embryology of CNS Development. The initial development of the fetal nervous system begins at approximately 18 days of gestation (postconceptual age). The neural tissue begins to differentiate, and the neural plate and tube down to the upper lumbar region are formed in what is referred to as *primary neurulation*. Closure of the anterior and posterior end of the neural tube is generally completed by 26 days. If it fails to close at this stage of development, there are alterations of the axial skeleton as well as of meningovascular and dermal coverings (Volpe, 1995).

Formation of the lower lumbar and sacral segments of the spinal cord is described as **secondary neurulation**. Many neurologic conditions may occur at either developmental phase, as a result of teratogenic influences. These conditions are discussed later in this chapter. Antenatal testing procedures can be used for early detection of some chromosomal aberrations such as Down syndrome and neural tube defects. (See Chapter 9 for a discussion of these testing procedures.)

After the neural tube has elongated and the brain has developed at the rostral end of the tube, further development of the brain takes place in the form of ventricular formation and eventually neuronal cell proliferation and migration. In the second to fourth month of gestation, the neurons (gray matter) proliferate. Abnormalities at this stage can result in too few neurons (microcephaly) or in too many neurons (macrocephaly). Once the neurons have proliferated, they must migrate (from 3 to 6 months' gestation) to their final location in the central nervous system. Effects on migration are multifactorial. Interference with this phase results in abnormalities of structure including lissencephaly (absent or few gyri) and pachygyria (few, broad gyri) or neuronal heterotopia (collections of nerve cells in white matter). Regardless of difficulties with neurulation, proliferation, and migration, all neurons are present at birth.

Myelination of the central nervous system (CNS), on the other hand, begins in utero and continues in a cephalocaudal fashion until approximately 10 years of age. At birth, it is not clear how mature all parts of the CNS are, but the major structures and cranial nerves are developed at that time (Hazinski, 1995). Many sensory functions are in place at birth, with continued maturation occurring throughout the early childhood years.

For instance, vision is central in neonates, with peripheral vision developing later in time. At birth, infants can establish locked eye contact in the en face position or they can fix on objects 8 to 12 inches from their eyes. They prefer stark contrasts, for example, black and white, and they respond better to arrangements similar to the human face rather than to random, free-form shapes. Newborns respond slowly to all auditory stimuli, but they are more receptive to (and more comforted by) high-pitched voice tones, including female voices. Sweet tastes are preferred by most neonates, whereas bitter, salty, and sour tastes are rejected. When awake and offered noxious olfactory stimuli (e.g., an alcohol swab), the neonate expresses displeasure. Further olfactory discrimination was reported in a classic study by Klaus and Kennel (1976), who noted that breast-fed babies indicate preference for the breast pads of their own mothers over those of other women by day 5 of extrauterine life.

Most of the behaviors and responses of the newborn are subcortical, and, for the most part, reflexive in nature. Normal neonatal reflexes in the term and premature neonate occur in a logical sequence of tonic neck, to roll over to tripod sit, and so on.

A newborn's cranial bones are soft and movable to facilitate passage of the head through the birth canal. This initial abnormal skull shape in children of a vaginal vertex delivery is referred to as *molding* and is only a temporary condition. The head should appear normocephalic within a few hours to a day. In some cases, molding may be evident for several days following prolonged labor or after deliveries requiring forceps or vacuum-assisted extraction. Complete ossification of the skull does not occur until the child is approximately 12 years old.

During the first two years of life, the brain grows to 80% of its adult size (Fig. 21–2). The size and shape of a child's head should follow proportional dimensions and should grow somewhat proportionately with the rest of the child's body.

The best way to evaluate cranial growth patterns is to obtain serial head circumferences and plot them on an NCHS growth chart for head circumference at each well-child visit (see Chapter 6 for this technique). For example, it is not normal for head circumference to gradually increase in percentile growth while height and weight remain stable along the same percentiles since birth. The child's parents should keep a copy of this and other growth parameter charts with their personal records in case they change primary care providers or records become lost. Simple inspection of the child's head for disproportionate growth and unusual shape is also done. Children have proportionately large and heavy heads. This makes them prime candidates for cerebrospinal trauma secondary to decreased head control. For example, toddlers learning to ambulate are clumsy and top heavy. An awkward lurch in the direction of something attractive may send them tumbling "headlong," possibly down a flight of stairs or over a crib railing. Because children have distensible skulls before the fontanelles and sutures are completely fused (up to about 18 months to 2 years of age), they are at higher risk for more serious consequences of head injury than older children and adults. Aspects of head trauma are discussed in more depth later in the chapter.

In children, the ventricular system plays an important part in the overall function of the CNS. The ventricles are interconnected cavities in the brain where 90% of the body's cerebrospinal fluid (CSF) is produced (Shiminski-Maher & Disabato, 1944). After CSF is made in the lateral ventricles by the choroid plexus, it flows through a small passageway called the intraventricular foramina of Monro to the third ventricle. From there it travels through the aqueduct of Sylvius to the fourth ventricle, exiting to the subarachnoid space around the brain stem via the foramina of Luschka or the foramen of Magendie (Greif & Miller, 1991). It then circulates up over the surface of the brain and downward around the spinal cord (see Fig. 21–5). Reabsorption of CSF occurs in the arachnoid villi located in the subarachnoid space and through the walls of capillaries of the CNS and pia mater (Swaiman, 1994).

CSF bathes the brain and acts as a liquid shock absorber, decreasing the force of impact to the head on the brain. It also carries away waste products from tissues in and around the brain. Normally, the rate of CSF production, approximately 0.35 mL/min, equals the rate of absorption. The circulating volume of CSF in children is approximately 65 to 140 mL and for adults is 90 to 150 mL (Swaiman, 1994).

Cerebral blood flow (CBF) is estimated and averaged in various age groups. In adults, it is thought to be 50 mL per 100 g of brain tissue per minute. The rate in newborns is similar to that in adults, with normal CBF estimated at 40 mL per 100 g of brain tissue per minute. These values are by contrast physiologically different from those in young children, in whom CBF is estimated at 75 to 100 mL per 100 g of brain tissue per minute (Hazinski, 1995). Such differences may be attributed to the rapid metabolism of young children combined with their very busy activity levels. Newborns and infants, by contrast, are more sedentary.

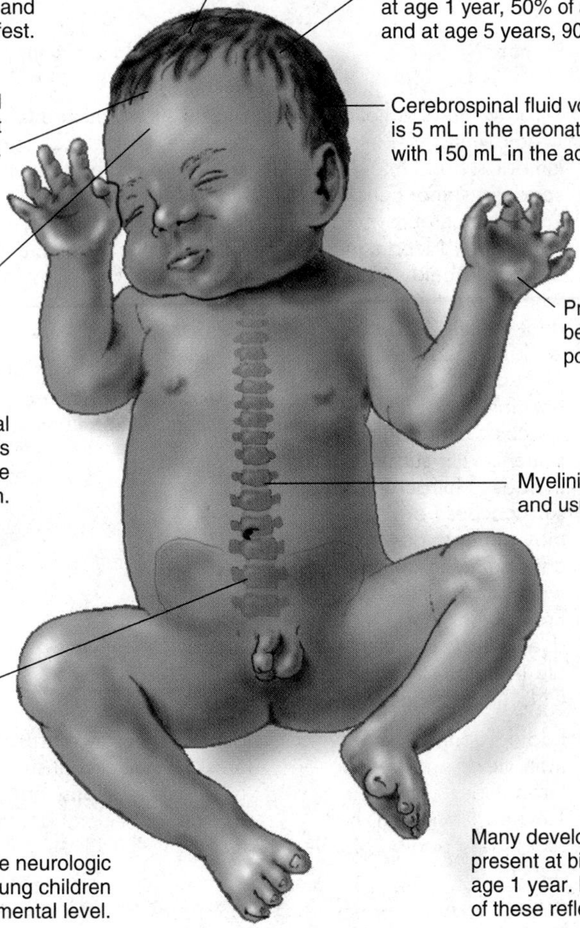

Open sutures and fontanelles in infants and toddlers help compensate for increases in ICP.

The child's brain is constantly undergoing organization of function and myelinization; thus, the full implications of a neurologic insult or injury may not be immediately apparent and may take up to several years to manifest.

At birth, the brain is about 25% of adult size; at age 1 year, 50% of adult size; and at age 5 years, 90% of adult size.

A child may exhibit focal or generalized electrical discharges on an EEG that would be considered abnormal in an adult.

Cerebrospinal fluid volume is 5 mL in the neonate, compared with 150 mL in the adult.

Increased intracranial pressure (ICP) may separate the sutures, especially the sagittal suture, until age 10–12 years.

Premature development of handedness before age 1 year is not usual and may point to a focal neurologic lesion.

A neonate's neurodevelopmental age is calculated to be the neonate's chronological age minus the number of weeks born before term.

Myelinization begins in the third fetal month and usually is complete by puberty.

In the neonate, the spinal cord terminates at L3, compared with an adult, where it terminates at L1–L2. This affects the site of needle insertion for lumbar puncture.

Accurate and complete neurologic assessment of infants and young children is limited by their developmental level.

Many developmental reflexes are present at birth and disappear by age 1 year. Persistence or asymmetry of these reflexes may indicate an abnormality.

Figure 21–2
Developmental and biological variances: neurologic system.

Diagnostic Criteria for Evaluating Neurologic Status

The 1990s have been declared "the Decade of the Brain," and much of modern scientific study is focused on improving the understanding of the complex function of the brain and its associated neuropathologic processes. Numerous diagnostic studies are available to assist health care practitioners with diagnosis of neurologic dysfunction. Table 21–3 describes various invasive and noninvasive procedures, and lists specific preparations for each test. The nurse's role in helping children and their families who are undergoing these tests includes:

- Teaching
- Physical preparation
- Conveying awareness of risk factors
- Implementing specific interventions based on patient needs before and after each study

For children, any diagnostic procedure can be frightening, especially if the child is separated from family members for any length of time.

Preparation must take into account the child's developmental level, cognitive ability, and physical status, including level of consciousness and pain threshold. In emergency situations, there may be little time to provide teaching; therefore, the nurse must offer the patient comfort measures during the study, and be able to support the family until the child is stabilized. Every effort should

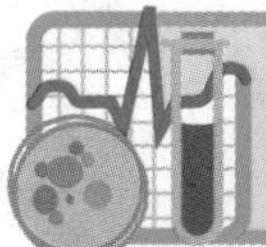

Table 21-3
Diagnostic Tests and Procedures for Evaluating Neurologic Status

Diagnostic Test or Procedure	Purpose	Findings and Indications	Health Care Provider Responsibilities
Lumbar puncture (LP)	Introduction of a hollow needle with stylet into the lumbar subarachnoid space of spinal canal to withdraw cerebrospinal fluid (CSF). Needle must be placed below the area where cord terminates (age dependent). Strict asepsis is maintained. Child is placed in lateral knee-chest position to open vertebral spaces. Contraindicated in patients with substantially increased intracranial pressure because brain stem may herniate downward, causing tissue compression, which may lead to death. Presence of blood may be due to trauma during needle insertion or may signal CNS hemorrhage.	Diagnostic: Measure CSF pressure, collect CSF sample for laboratory tests for blood or microorganisms, injection of contrast dye for radiographic studies, evaluation of CSF flow dynamics. Therapeutic: Injection site for spinal anesthesia or intrathecal medications.	Nurse may need to assist with positioning, securing, and calming child. Encourage fluids before and after LP. Empty bladder before LP, because child must remain supine for 4–6 hours after procedure. Premedicate for pain and monitor for signs and symptoms of headache related to decreased amount of CSF.
Radiography	Radiographic films. Common views are P/A (posteroanterior), lateral, Towne's (semiaxial, half axial), any portion of spinal column.	Identifies presence of fractures, widened skull sutures, calcifications, bone erosion, or skeletal anomalies.	Child must be still during procedure. Support person must wear protective apron.
Ultrasound	Pulsed ultrasonic beam (Doppler) locates midline brain structures. Probe is placed at vertical angle, reflecting sound waves off structures. Images are created on a screen and produce measurable pictures. Sometimes called an echoencephalogram.	Diagnoses intracranial abnormalities such as mass lesions and enlarged ventricles. Measures two tables of the skull and the third ventricle. May be used in prenatal testing for fetal anomalies such as spina bifida.	Child must have open fontanelle. Child must remain still for the study. Conductive gel may feel cold or warm. Ultrasound is a painless procedure and usually takes 15 minutes.
Computed tomography (CT) scan	Radiographic study to view the brain in three dimensions. Patient is supine, on movable table, with head immobilized. X-ray beam scans cranium in successive layers (cuts), and computer digitizes image. Differentiates density of bone (lighter) and air (darker). Test becomes invasive if radioisotope dye is injected to enhance views of blood vessels, vascular lesions, and localized changes in blood–brain barrier.	Effective visualization of tumors, ventricles, brain tissue, CSF, hematomas, and cysts.	If CT is enhanced, child must have intravenous (IV) access. Motion destroys clarity of scan; child may require sedation. CT takes about 20–30 minutes. Noncontrast study is painless.

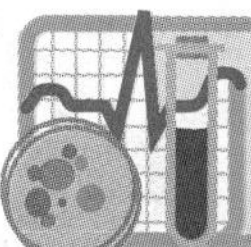

Table 21–3
Diagnostic Tests and Procedures for Evaluating Neurologic Status *Continued*

Diagnostic Test or Procedure	Purpose	Findings and Indications	Health Care Provider Responsibilities
Magnetic resonance imaging (MRI)	Imaging without radiation by radio frequency emissions that are converted to computer images. Child is supine and placed in a cylindrical opening that encases a strong magnet. MRIs make loud humming and intermittent tapping noises. MRI produces images that differentiate between gray and white matter.	MRI provides sharp anatomic detail and information about the chemistry of living tissue. Useful in tumor identification. T_1-weighted images may be done to determine hydrogen-tissue density. T_2 images detect changes in tissue biochemistry, indicating early disease.	Contrast MRI requires IV access. Sedation is indicated if child is restless or dislikes confined spaces. Most children under 6–7 years of age require sedation. Remove all metal/magnetic items; surgical implants such as pacemakers, bone pins, or cerebral clips are contraindications. Noncontrast study is painless. Ear plugs or headphones may be used to dampen noise. Use music as distraction. If age appropriate, child may benefit from seeing MRI before study. Depending on scanner, study takes 45–60 minutes. Avoidance of motion is critical.
Positron emission tomography (PET) scan	On-line cyclotron creates positron-emitting radionuclides. Patient is injected with or inhales radioactive tracer (such as carbon 11, nitrogen, or oxygen), which crosses the blood–brain barrier. The positron reacts to electrons, creating gamma rays. The biochemical and physiologic function of living tissue is studied as gamma rays are measured and coded by a computer. Cross-sectional tissue images are created in areas of tracer concentration. PET images are more clear than conventional radionuclide scans.	PET scans can measure cellular processes, cerebral metabolism, cerebral blood flow, membrane transport, synthesis, and receptor binding. They identify specific areas of the brain that are functioning or malfunctioning.	Consent must be obtained because of the nature of radioactive tracer substance. Child may need sedation to remain still.

Table continued on following page

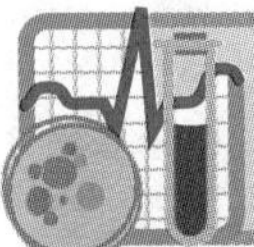

Table 21-3
Diagnostic Tests and Procedures for Evaluating Neurologic Status *Continued*

Diagnostic Test or Procedure	Purpose	Findings and Indications	Health Care Provider Responsibilities
Myelography	Water-based contrast media such as metrizamide (Amipaque), iohexol (Omnipaque), or iopamidol (Isovue, Isovue-M) have replaced oil-based media in most hospitals. Once in the CSF, all three enter nerve tissue by upward diffusion. This eliminates the need to reposition the patient. The rate of uptake is reduced by maintaining the child in a sitting position. If water-based media enter the cranial vault, seizures are likely to occur. There is no need to remove contrast fluid when the myelogram is completed because it is absorbed and excreted in the urine. Metrizamide can cause extreme diuresis.	Visualization of any or all of the spinal axis for diagnosis of tumor, congenital lesions, or bony changes. Images are produced via radiographs, fluoroscopy, or CT. Significant risk factors include: 1. Allergic reaction to iodine 2. Headache 3. Aseptic meningitis/infection 4. Seizures	Obtain detailed history of iodine allergy. Give nothing by mouth (NPO) 4 hours before myelogram. Obtain frequent neurologic assessment and vital signs. Maintain seizure precautions. Minimize activity. Strictly monitor intake and output. Water-based medium: Discontinue all neuroleptic drugs, monoamine oxidase inhibitors, and psychostimulants 48 hours before myelogram. After study: Avoid administration of phenothiazines, maintain a quiet environment, and keep child supine with head of bed elevated 30–45 degrees for 12–24 hours. Oil-based medium: Premedication such as Demerol or atropine may be ordered. After study: keep patient flat in bed for 6–24 hours per physician's order.
Electroencephalogram (EEG)	Graphic recording of electrical activity of the brain via 17–21 electrodes glued to the scalp. Differences in electrical activity between electrodes create brain wave patterns, which are classified based on the number of cycles per second (cps). Four frequency bands are identified: · Delta (1–4 cps) · Theta (4–8 cps) · Alpha (8–13 cps) · Beta (13–35 cps) Brain waves are usually recorded at rest, after hyperventilation, during photic (flashing light) stimulation, and during sleep.	EEG detects and locates abnormal electrical discharges produced in the brain. It is used to detect seizure activity, monitor patients with head injury, stroke, metabolic coma, and some psychologic illness, and to assist with brain death determination. EEG may also be used during intracranial surgery for intractable seizures. EEG strips "map" electrical activity on the surface and guide the extent of cortical resection. Abnormal findings are epileptiform activity, slowing of normal waves, abnormal amplitude, or disorders of age-specific patterns.	Medications or foods known to alter brain wave activity may be withheld (per physican's order) such as 1. Stimulants 2. Depressants 3. Anticonvulsants 4. Tranquilizers 5. Chocolate, colas, tea Child's hair must be clean, without oils, sprays, or lotion. Alleviate common fears such as that the EEG will cause electrical shock and reads minds. EEGs are painless proceudures and usually take 45–60 minutes. After the EEG, clean hair of glue and gel, and resume medication.

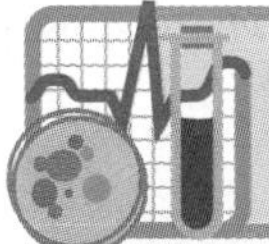

Table 21–3
Diagnostic Tests and Procedures for Evaluating Neurologic Status *Continued*

Diagnostic Test or Procedure	Purpose	Findings and Indications	Health Care Provider Responsibilities
Evoked potential studies (EVP)	Small electrodes attached to a wire and placed over the skull and a visual or auditory stimulus is given (visual auditory). Electrodes are placed on either arm or leg and stimulus is given (somatosensory).	*Visual EVP:* Determines that visual pathway is intact. In infants, light-emitting diode goggles are used. *Auditory EVP:* Determines that auditory pathway is intact. Earphones are used. *Somatosensory EVP:* Determines both spinal cord and critical appreciation of electrical stimulus. These can be obtained in the upper extremities by stimulation of midarm nerve and in lower extremities by stimulation of popliteal nerve.	Complete cooperation and immobility are required. In young or uncooperative children, NPO status is maintained for 4 hours, and sedation may be required.
Electromyography (EMG) and Nerve conduction velocity (NCV)	Small Teflon-coated needles attached to a wire are inserted into muscle, and the brief electrical discharge is recorded. Patient contracts muscle, causing electrical activity, and motor unit action potential is studied. NCV can slow if child is hypothermic. Electrodes are placed over a peripheral nerve in two locations, reclining and sending. An electrical impulse is sent from sending to receiving with the speed and amplitude of the response measured.	Analyzes electrical events associated with skeletal muscle fiber contraction. EMG and NCV are usually ordered together to diagnose and differentiate between peripheral nerve and muscle disorders.	

be made to minimize painful interventions, including premedicating the child (if allowed) to reduce anxiety (Fig. 21–3). Many neurologic diagnostic procedures though not painful, may be considered uncomfortable to the child because he must remain still or be positioned in an awkward manner. The nurse can employ measures to help the child relax during procedures such as CT and MRI. Effective interventions include using guided imagery, use of music therapy, and use of audiotapes to tell stories to the child during the procedure. Such methods have been documented to help minimize the use of sedatives to assist the child in remaining calm (Smith, 1997).

Children with acute, grossly abnormal neurologic findings may be in imminent danger of rapid deterioration and possible permanent morbidity or death. It is critical that nurses identify these children and engage in appropriate caregiving, especially in children younger than 2 years of age. Many nurses have used their knowledge to prevent serious complications in neurologically fragile children simply by investigating findings that "didn't look right."

In the expanding field of biomedical electronic engineering (BMEE), more sophisticated and less invasive diagnostic procedures have been developed, including computed tomography (CT) scans, magnetic resonance imaging (MRI), and positron emission transaxial tomography (PET) scans.

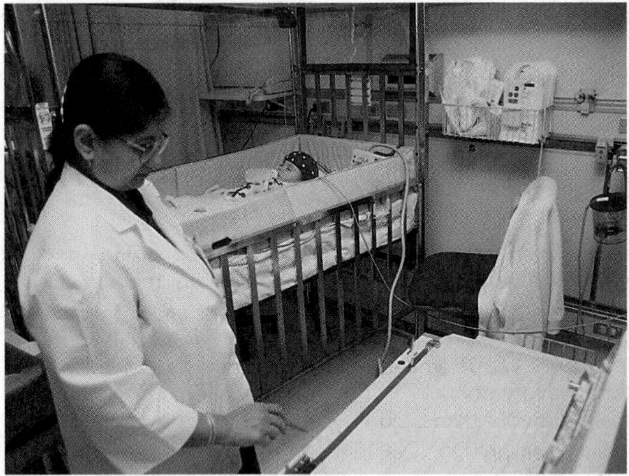

Figure 21–3
A child undergoing electroencephalography.

caREminder: *In some cases, hair ornaments (e.g., beads) may cause artifact on CT or MRI. The family should be informed by the nurse about the specific requirements of the radiology department in regard to specific diagnostic tests. Children with head lice should be treated prior to undergoing an electroencephalogram (EEG).*

Treatment Modalities

Pharmacotherapy

Pharmacologic agents are used for a variety of reasons in the treatment of neurologic conditions. **Antibiotics** are used to treat known or suspected infectious disease processes. In general, if there is any suspicion that an infectious process may be occurring or that the child is at risk for infection that would alter the structural integrity of the neurologic system, broad-spectrum antibiotic therapy is initiated until CSF, blood, and wound cultures indicate that no infection exists or that the type of antibiotics used needs to be changed in response to sensitivities. Antibiotics are started after CSF, blood, and wound samples are obtained. Acetaminophen is given concurrently to reduce fever associated with the infectious process.

Anticonvulsants are used to prevent seizures. **Glucocorticoids** and **diuretics** are used to reduce cerebral edema. **Paralytic agents** may be used if the child is mechanically ventilated to control restlessness and agitation in children at risk for increased intracranial pressure (ICP). **Pain medications** mediate the response elicited by meningeal irritation, surgical interventions, invasive procedures, and immobility. Sedatives are given to relieve anxiety and agitation. They should be administered only if the child is in an intensive care setting where close monitoring of neurologic status is available.

Cranial Surgery

The treatment of many neurosurgical injuries or problems requires direct access to the brain through the bony structures of the skull. The following discussion addresses the general care given to children having cranial surgery involving craniotomy and craniectomy.

A **craniotomy** refers to a "flap" opening of the skull in which the bone is removed and then the bone is replaced at the completion of surgery. If part of the cranium (skull) is excised and not replaced, the procedure is termed a **craniectomy**. These surgical procedures are indicated to relieve ICP from cerebral edema or as a means of removing abnormal suture in infants with cranial bone deformities. When large portions of bone are not replaced, a **cranioplasty** may be done to repair the cranial defect and to protect the brain by inserting a molded piece of synthetic material, usually Silastic, or autologous or donor bone over the opening.

Anatomically, the brain can be divided into two regions for surgical access to tumors, hematomas, or abscess formations. The **tentorium cerebelli** is a double fold of the dura mater that forms a separation between the upper brain structure (the cerebrum), or **supratentorial** region, and the lower **infratentorial** area of the cerebellum and brain stem (which includes the midbrain, pons, and medulla). Most surgical procedures in the **supratentorial** region of the brain are indicated for

- Resection or biopsy of tumors or cysts
- Resection of eleptogenic cortex (seizure foci)
- Placement of ventricular catheters to drain CSF
- Draining collected blood following head injury
- Placement of ICP monitors

Surgical procedures in the infratentorial region are usually indicated for tumor or cyst resection. (Care of the child with a tumor is discussed in Chapter 22.)

Preoperative Care

It is not always possible to prepare children and families for intracranial surgery. If the child is admitted following trauma or other emergency situation, little time is available for teaching. In these cases, the physician's priority is to obtain informed consent from the parents by discussing the purpose of the surgery, the possibility of alternative treatment or lack of treatment, the potential risks, and the expected outcomes (Hickey, 1992).

Ideally, the nurse should be present during the physician's discussion with the family to reinforce and clarify the information presented. If the admission is planned, education should begin in the time before surgery. Assessment of the family's ability to comprehend the diagnosis and planned treatment is the first step of nursing management. Parents are often overwhelmed with fear and anxiety; therefore, the nurse must incorporate the family's coping mechanisms into the teaching plan and must review information as needed. Emotional support is essential from the first contact with the family and throughout the child's recovery period. Along with general perioperative preparation, including laboratory tests, scans or x-rays, an anesthesia consult, and tours of the intensive care unit and hospital, the nurse should address specific topics pertaining to the child undergoing a neurosurgical surgery as outlined in Chart 21–4.

The preparation for neurologic surgery may involve shaving hair from the operative area. The amount and area of hair removed as well as the shape and size of the incision are determined by the surgeon. The shave and the skin preparation are usually done after the child is anesthetized. Recently there has been a trend in adult and pediatric neurosurgery toward not shaving or clipping any hair for surgery (Winston, 1992).

Some of the child's preoperative anxiety and fear of mutilation can be related to shaving the hair and worrying about visible scars. The child and the family need to understand that the child's hair will grow back, and they may consider the use of a wig, a scarf, or a cap after surgery. Neurologic surgery that involves the frontal or temporal bones often results in marked periorbital edema for several days after surgery. Often the child and the family understand the reasons for the after effects of surgery and they simply need the nurse's presence for support, reassurance, and as a sounding board to express their feelings or to begin an anticipatory grief process.

An accurate, well-documented preoperative neurologic baseline assessment becomes essential in monitoring the child's postoperative functioning for potential complications. Problems with vision, hearing, communication, and any other preexisting neurologic deficits or developmental delays should be carefully documented.

If the child has seizures preoperatively, the events should be well described, and the side rails of the bed should be padded to prevent injuries. If the patient has been taking anticonvulsant medications, these are usually given before surgery with a sip of water so that serum levels remain constant.

Intraoperative Procedure

During the surgical procedure, the child's head position is usually secured well with pins. Various operative positions may be used, depending on the nature and location of the surgery. The scalp is incised, muscles are stripped, and usually 4 to 5 burr holes are drilled at the borders of the planned skull opening. A craniotome is used to cut across the bone and to lift off the skull. After the skull is

Chart 21–4
Nursing Interventions

Teaching Needs of the Child and Family Experiencing Cranial Surgery

Preoperative Care

- Complete or partial head shave possible
- Where the incision will be, how it will look, and its visual ramifications
- What kinds of dressings to expect, and their maintenance
- *Neurologic monitoring* and vital sign checks
- Length of the surgery (i.e., number of hours) and postanesthesia recovery
- Intensive care stay, if known
- Reinforce knowledge; clarify misconceptions related to child's surgery
- Parent participation/visitation after surgery

Postoperative Care

- Postoperative cerebral edema (when appropriate)
- Incision—hair loss if applicable
- Necessity for assessments and their frequency
- Necessity for and types of tests and medications
- Necessity for and types of monitors, access lines, catheters, etc.
- Anticipated child's response related to surgery and/or neurologic deficit
- Progression in diet and activity orders
- Pain management
- Transitions in nursing care (routines, shift changes, unit transfers)

Home Maintenance

- Incisional care (staple or stitch removal)
- Restriction/precaution associated with activities; returning to school; resumption of leisure and recreational activities
- Signs and symptoms of potential complications
- Medications
- Diet
- Clinic appointments and scheduled tests or scans
- Specific therapies
- Contacts and telephone numbers for information about concerns and questions
- Anticipatory guidance about pertinent anatomy and physiology of neurologic deficits, safety measures, and adaptations
- Home health care or public health care referrals as appropriate
- Support network information as appropriate
- Social service referrals as appropriate

Adapted from Betz, C. L., Hunsberger, M., & Wright, S. (Eds.). (1994). *Family-centered nursing care of children* (2nd ed., p. 1745). Philadelphia: W. B. Saunders. Used with permission.

opened, the meninges are peeled back and secured. Hemostasis must be meticulously attended to during cranial surgery, to avoid excessive bleeding and irritation to the brain.

Following the surgical procedure, all anatomic layers, starting with the meninges, are closed. During a craniotomy, the skull is sutured or wired back into place. Muscles and scalp layers are closed and a pressure dressing is applied for 1 to 2 days. A drain may be used for the first 24 hours. Postoperatively, sutures or staples are usually removed in 7 to 10 days.

Worldview: *If hair is shaved it is not discarded during the surgery, but is returned to the postoperative unit where the child is managed in case the parents or family request its return. In some cultures, this is a very important request because loss of the hair is considered to be a serious loss to the child's spiritual well-being.*

The type and location of surgery done will affect the postoperative nursing assessments. Surgery in the *supratentorial* area (above the tentorium cerebelli) is more likely to be associated with postoperative seizures, focal motor deficits, or confusion. One type of *infratentorial* surgery involves entry to the area from a midline incision at the back of the skull. Because entry into the cranial vault is so close to the medulla oblongata, which contains the major respiratory center of the brain, there is a much greater chance of respiratory compromise caused by edema after this surgery. The patient may remain intubated for a longer period of time, especially if the reason for surgery was to remove a tumor of the spinal cord, cerebellum, or brain stem. Perioperative monitoring for air embolus is imperative in this type of surgery.

Another type of infratentorial craniectomy is a transsphenoidal approach. This is done through the nasal tissue and sphenoid bones of the skull. Most often, this approach is to remove tumors of the pituitary or hypothalamus. One of the major postoperative concerns is syndrome of inappropriate antidiuretic hormone secretion (SIADH), which may occur when the posterior pituitary is gone or malfunctioning. SIADH is managed by hormone replacement with desmopressin, also known as DDAVP, which is snorted or sprayed into the patient's nasal passage, crossing the mucous membranes. Other posterior pituitary hormone replacement is given as managed by collaboration of the neurosurgery and endocrinology teams.

Postoperative Care

The nursing role after cranial surgery involves frequent acute neurologic monitoring and assessment of vital signs, intake and output, and dressing and drainage to monitor the child for any potential complications. These complications include

- Increased ICP
- Seizures
- Hemorrhage
- CSF leakage
- Local tissue hypoxia
- Hyperthermia
- Hydrocephalus
- Hypovolemic shock (diabetes insipidus)
- Infection
- Respiratory compromise caused by edema in the respiratory centers

The nurse accurately and frequently assesses the child's neurologic status to identify even the most subtle changes. Close monitoring of acute findings as well as potential long-term complications begins as soon as the child is in the postoperative setting. Complications of immobility include pneumonia, deep vein thrombosis, constipation, and skin breakdown. These should not be totally overlooked even in the acute monitoring phase. The pediatric critical care nurse is skilled in determining potential life-threatening neurologic changes and must always be prepared for rapid emergency interventions.

Along with making frequent neurologic assessments, the nurse should note and should report to the physician any significant drainage on the dressing. It is a common practice to gently outline the border of the fluid with a surgical marker, indicating the time and change in amount. Strict infection control measures must be followed because the patient is more vulnerable to infection with a healing surgical wound.

Alert: *Drainage from the dressing, incision, nose, or ears after neurosurgery should be monitored closely for its similarity to CSF. If there is a tear in the dura during surgery, CSF can leak into the ear or nose.*

Suspicion of CSF drainage is higher when the surgery is done after a traumatic injury in which a skull fracture may have occurred or after skull base surgery for tumor. Drainage that is suspect should be collected in a sterile test tube for CSF glucose determination. Children should be discouraged from touching, or should be instructed not to touch, the drainage, and they should be told not to blow their nose. To minimize sources of infection, these areas should not be packed, suctioned, or disturbed until the drainage is identified. The child should be encouraged to remain quiet. Table 21–4 summarizes the guidelines for immediate postoperative nursing management of the child after intracranial surgery.

Recent Neurologic Developments

The advances in neuroscience care have been impressive since the early 1970s. The practice of neurosurgery requires highly technical and precise equipment in all areas

Table 21–4
Assessment and Interventions After Cranial Surgery

System	Assessment	Interdisciplinary Interventions
Neurologic	Level of consciousness Pupillary reaction Corneal reflex Ocular movement Gag reflex Motor function Sensory function Vital signs including ICP Reflexes Monitor for seizures	Monitor frequently. Test cranial nerve function. Note medications that may affect pupillary response. Maintain ICP <20 mmHg. Note widening pulse pressure, bradycardia, and altered respirations (Cushing's triad) and report immediately. Maintain neutral position of head and neck. Elevate head of bed 30 degrees. Palpate infant fontanelle. Provide safe environment with side rails up. Minimize activity. Consult: neurology and ophthalmology as needed.
Respiratory	Breath sounds Oxygen saturation Cyanosis Respiratory rate Airway patency Blood gases	Turn child q 2 hr to promote postural drainage. Adjust ventilator settings per physician's order. Gently suction secretions. Provide humidified oxygen per physician's order. Encourage deep breathing exercises. Consult: respiratory therapy.
Elimination	Urine output 0.7 mL/kg/hr Foley catheter intact Constipation Monitor blood urea nitrogen, creatinine, specific gravity	Ensure strict input and output. Provide Foley care to prevent infection. Give daily stool softener to reduce hard stools or straining (Valsalva maneuver), which increases ICP. Consult: nutritionist.
Fluid and electrolytes	Mucous membranes and eyes for dryness	Restrict fluids per physician's orders. Provide hydration/medication. Use intravenous pump to avoid fluid bolus. Use artificial tears in eyes. Use glycerin swabs for mouth and lips.
Musculoskeletal	Pressure sores Flexibility of joints	Provide range-of-motion exercises QID. Provide skin care/sheepskin pad on bed. Consult: physical therapy.
Psychosocial	Level of pain Level of fear or anxiety	Administer pain medication to decrease discomfort. Provide emotional support. Encourage parental visitation. Explain all interventions before touching child. Anticipate and answer questions. Consult: child life specialist.

of patient care. The less invasive diagnostic procedures (e.g., CT, PET, and MRI) are completed before any surgical intervention. In the operating room, recent advances in microsurgery, updated stereotactic frames, laser surgery, and the use of gamma knife radiation have vastly improved access to previously inoperable lesions. The neurosurgeon can perform more aggressive tumor resection with less risk or damage to delicate surrounding tissue. This preserves neurologic function and decreases the incidence of complications (Arbour, 1993).

The child undergoing intracranial surgery benefits from these improvements by

- Greater diagnostic imaging accuracy, safety, and comfort
- Less invasive surgical techniques
- Shorter hospital stays and costs, with reduced postoperative complications
- Increased chances of survival

Supportive Care

The child who has experienced an alteration in neurologic status is at high risk for experiencing altered responsiveness during the course of his or her condition. Responsiveness refers to the child's ability to

- *Receive input,* that is, to select and prioritize stimuli for response. This process requires conscious awareness, attention span, orientation, and the ability to focus beyond self.
- *Complete throughput,* that is, to process, analyze, and integrate input.
- *Produce output,* that is, to produce a response, or end product, to stimuli. This is expressed by thoughts, verbalizations, facial or body expression, movement, and changes in mood or behavior.

Responsiveness is affected by developmental age and by the current level of maturity of the nervous system.

Altered responsiveness involves the loss of one or more of the components of input, throughput, or output. For example, input may be altered in a child with congenital blindness or deafness by decreasing the availability of external stimuli. Throughput may be altered in a child with a perceptual problem such as a visual motor deficit or a child who experiences delays in processing time after a severe head injury. Output is altered in a child who experiences paralysis, sensory motor deficits, or speech impairment.

Altered responsiveness may appear as an acute, self-limiting process for one child (e.g., following head injury) or may be a daily, long-term reality for other children (e.g., inoperable brain tumor). If the child is immobilized because of decreased responsiveness, the hazards of immobility also become a problem. The mobile child with sensory and perceptual deficits is at increased risk for physical injury.

Health care varies according to the nature of altered responsiveness. In general, goals for nursing care are to continue assessment for health care problems, especially those of a life-threatening nature, to protect the child from additional injury, and to assist the family in adapting to the child's needs.

The following discussion reviews the supportive care measures that are implemented to reduce the risk of injury and disuse syndrome and to promote health maintenance over the course of the illness. Chapter 11 presents information that is applicable to the child who is experiencing altered responsiveness due to a chronic illness or disability.

Risk of Injury

The child with altered responsiveness must be protected against further physiologic injury, including additional neurologic complications, and against physical injury from falls.

Monitoring for changes in neurologic status that may signal either progress toward recovery or deterioration of the child's condition includes acute neurologic checks (Chart 21–5) and observation for potential complications, such as increasing ICP. The nurse must assess ease of arousal, pupil size and reactivity, eye movements, motor function, respiratory pattern, and vital signs of the child.

Physical safety is a concern for the child with altered responsiveness. To prevent falls from the bed, the nurse must keep the side rails up at all times. When the child is positioned in a chair while out of bed, the nurse must ensure that restraints help maintain the child comfortably in an upright position and that there is no chance that the child will slip from the chair to the floor or become tangled in the restraints. Even with these precautions, the child who is positioned out of bed must always be closely monitored. The mobile child may be prone to falls because of altered spatial perception and altered motor ability. Altered mental processing can lead to impulsive behavior. Protective helmets can be used to protect the mobile child's head from further injury. Toys and equipment in the child's room or in a playroom should be confined as much as possible to allow a clear path for the child to move around. Gates can also be used to keep the child safe.

Risk for Disuse Syndrome

Complications from lack of responsiveness and immobility can include stasis of pulmonary secretions, musculoskeletal problems, gastrointestinal problems, aspiration, stimulus deprivation, urinary tract problems, skin integrity problems, and conjunctival problems. These complications place the child at risk for disuse syndrome, a state in which the child is at risk for deterioration of a body system as a result of his or her prescribed or acquired musculoskeletal inactivity or immobility. Disuse syndrome may affect children with myelomeningocele, akinetic mutism, and various types of coma. The syndrome may also pertain to children in a drug-induced coma. Emphasis is placed on preventing the hazards of immobility.

Preventing Respiratory Complications

The bedridden child has a decreased lung capacity because inspiratory muscles are not aided by gravitational

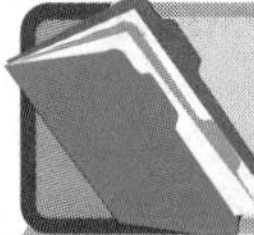

Chart 21–5
Nursing Interventions Classification (NIC)

Neurologic Monitoring

Definition

Collection and analysis of patient data to prevent or minimize neurologic complications

Activities

Monitor pupillary size, shape, symmetry, and reactivity.
Monitor level of consciousness.
Monitor level of orientation.
Monitor trend of Glasgow Coma Scale.
Monitor recent memory, attention span, past memory, mood, affect, and behaviors.
Monitor vital signs: temperature, blood pressure, pulse, and respirations.
Monitor respiratory status: ABG levels, pulse oximetry, depth, pattern, rate, and effort.
Monitor invasive hemodynamic parameters, as appropriate.
Monitor ICP and CPP.
Monitor corneal reflex.
Monitor cough and gag reflex.
Monitor muscle tone, motor movement, gait, and proprioception.
Monitor for pronator drift.
Monitor grip strength.
Monitor for tremor.
Monitor facial symmetry.
Monitor tongue protrusion.
Monitor for tracking response.
Monitor EOMs and gaze characteristics.
Monitor for visual disturbance: diplopia, nystagmus, visual field cuts, blurred vision, and visual acuity.
Note complaint of headache.
Monitor speech characteristics: fluency, presence of aphasias, or word-finding difficulty.
Monitor response to stimuli: verbal, tactile, and noxious.
Monitor sharp/dull or hot/cold discrimination.
Monitor for paresthesia: numbness and tingling.
Monitor sense of smell.
Monitor sweating patterns.
Monitor Babinski response.
Monitor for Cushing response.
Monitor craniotomy/laminectomy dressing for drainage.
Monitor response to medications.
Consult with coworkers to confirm data, as appropriate.
Identify emerging patterns in data.
Increase frequency of neurological monitoring, as appropriate.
Avoid activities that increase intracranial pressure.
Space required nursing activities that increase intracranial pressure.
Notify physician of change in patient condition.
Institute emergency protocols, as needed.

From McCloskey, J., & Bulechek, G. (1996). *Nursing interventions classification (NIC)* (2nd ed.). St. Louis: Mosby–Year Book. Reprinted with permission.

pull, chest expansion is limited by the weight of the body against one aspect of the chest, and, when the child is in a horizontal position, the abdominal contents push against the diaphragm. Furthermore, there is little stimulus for fully expanding the lungs when there is little or no muscular activity. Pooling of secretions within the lungs and exposure to microorganisms may lead to serious respiratory infection. The nurse should include respiratory monitoring in the plan of care for the unresponsive or immobilized child.

Although chest physiotherapy for the unresponsive child cannot include voluntary deep breathing and coughing, turning the child from side to side at least every 2 hours helps to expand different areas of the lungs and reduces the pooling of secretions in the lungs. The head of the child's bed should be elevated periodically, if the child can tolerate it, and the child should be positioned in a sitting posture for short periods, if the physician's orders permit. For health care personnel in contact with the unresponsive child, careful hand washing and avoidance of persons with active respiratory infections are imperative.

Airway management through attention to gentle suctioning of nasal and oral secretions and attention to hygiene of oral and nasal mucous membranes also helps to prevent infection in the child. The child's mucous membranes should be kept free of dried secretions and should be lubricated regularly to prevent breaks in membrane integrity. Oral health maintenance is often complicated by the bite reflex in children with neurologic damage.

caREminder: *The nurse should never insert his or her fingers in the child's mouth, and care should be taken not to insert anything in the child's mouth that could damage the teeth or gums in case the child's jaws close unexpectedly.*

Preventing Musculoskeletal Complications

Muscles that are not used regularly lose strength, tone, and mass rapidly. Also, contractures may form at unused joints, permanently limiting the child's musculoskeletal functions. Exercise therapy, including passive range-of-motion exercises (unless contraindicated by volatile ICP), and attention to body alignment in positioning the child can prevent these complications. The heavier the child, the more care is needed in positioning him or her, because the weight of the limbs pulls against major joints, causing strain on muscles, ligaments, and tendons. Pillows placed under the arms and between the legs can greatly minimize the stress. Shoulder supports can help to prevent dislocation. The hands and the feet also must be protected. Washcloths, small gauze rolls, or hand splints can help keep the fingers in functional alignment.

Tip: *High-top tennis shoes or ankle-foot orthoses can help prevent footdrop.*

When the child begins to recover, weight bearing should be reinstituted as soon as it can be tolerated. Physical therapy regimens include range-of-motion exercises and use of a tilt table, a standing frame, and parallel bars to help gradually restore weight bearing and active range of motion.

Preventing Gastrointestinal Complications of Immobility

The unresponsive child is usually fed through a nasogastric tube, a jejunostomy tube, or a gastrostomy tube. Posturing or seizures during feeding can cause reflux of food. If enteral tube feedings are used, elevating the head of the child's bed may help prevent aspiration of food particles.

caREminder: *Oral feedings should not be attempted unless the child's gag and swallow reflexes are intact.*

Nutritional monitoring, including careful calculation of caloric needs, must be carried out to ensure that the child is receiving adequate nutrition to prevent muscle wasting. Because metabolism decreases with inactivity, care must also be taken not to overfeed the unresponsive child. Infants who retain a sucking reflex should be given a pacifier during gavage feedings. The suck reflex is rapidly lost if it is not stimulated in this manner.

Infants and small children can usually be held for feedings to preserve the social contact and caring interactions they have previously associated with feeding. Holding, rocking, and other caring interactions with the family and with the nursing staff are equally important for older children. The child's incapacity for output does not necessarily rule out his or her ability for benefit from input and throughput. If the child's condition contraindicates being held, techniques such as massage (tactile stimulus), singing to the child (auditory stimulus), and frequent contact that keeps the nurse's face in the child's line of vision (visual stimulus) may be appropriate substitutions.

Bowel function can be assessed by auscultating bowel sounds in all abdominal quadrants and by maintaining a record of the child's bowel movements. Diarrhea and constipation are common for unresponsive children, and they may alternate because of variable peristaltic action. Diarrhea may accompany a change in the feeding regimen and may be a sign that the feeding is not being tolerated. Diarrhea management may therefore involve adjustments in enteral volume, rate, or formulation.

Constipation, however, may be a sign of inadequate fluid intake, as well as a sign of sluggish peristalsis related to the child's immobility. Lack of bowel movements, passage of hard balls of stool, or abdominal palpation for firm, full intestines can help to confirm suspicions of inadequate bowel evacuation. Constipation and impaction management includes prompt assessment of this condition by the nurse. The nurse can request an order for bulk fiber additives, stool softeners, glycerin suppositories, mild laxatives, or enemas for the child. A good bowel management program can promote regularity and can prevent constipation and diarrhea in the unresponsive child.

Preventing Urinary Tract Complications

Bladder tone and bladder emptying are also affected by the child's immobility. Intermittent straight catheterization is usually instituted for the unresponsive child. Urine output provides an indication of whether the child's fluid intake is adequate to maintain a healthy urinary tract. Some children may have an indwelling catheter for a short period. Meticulous catheter care helps to reduce the risk of infection for the child.

Maintaining Skin Integrity

Bed rest is a major assault to the child's integumentary system. Constant rubbing on bed linens, body pressure against wrinkled garments, pressure of body weight on delicate tissues, reduced blood flow in pressure areas, mechanical irritation from tubing, and chemical irritation from wet and soiled diapers all contribute to the need for skin integrity vigilance and thorough skin care by the nurse for the unresponsive child. General body hygiene is much easier for the nurse to provide for the infant than for the heavier school-age child or adolescent. Help should be obtained as needed for bathing, washing hair, and positioning the child for skin massage. The perineum should be cleansed after each diaper change or each episode of incontinence.

The child's skin should be protected from mechanical irritation. Pressure-relieving mattresses should be used as available. Linen wrinkles are kept to a minimum, and no small objects (e.g., plastic sheaths from disposable needles) are to be left in the child's bed. Opposing skin surfaces and pressure points are to be protected with pillows and foam supports. The skin is inspected thoroughly for any areas of redness during regular care. Nonred, bony prominences are repositioned and massaged to increase circulation. Reddened areas of the child's skin should not be further irritated with massage.

Unresponsiveness sometimes includes the loss of motor function of the eyelids. In such a case, the eyes should be protected with eye moisture shields or with protective taping to prevent corneal abrasions. Tarsorrhaphy, suturing either a portion or the entire upper and lower eyelids, can be done to keep the child's eyes closed to protect the eye.

Promoting Health Maintenance

For some children, altered responsiveness may be either a long-term or a permanent condition, and discharge teaching should begin as soon as possible. Involving the parent and the family members who will help care for the child at home as early as possible helps to ensure that they have time to develop the skills that are needed for procedures. The child should be included in teaching and in self-care to the extent possible.

The family needs explanations of how the illness or disorder affects the child, including the anatomy and physiology of neurologic processes. Familiarity with responsiveness in terms of input, throughput, and output may help the family to understand and cope with alterations in the child's response as well as to recognize the capabilities for response that have been retained by the child. The family needs to know about treatment modalities and how to provide or monitor the child's response to treatment.

If the child has reflex movements, the family needs to be able to distinguish these from voluntary movements so that movements such as posturing are not mistaken for purposeful responses or seizures. The family should have a list of signs and symptoms that indicate the need for medical intervention so they know when to call the physician.

Special care techniques are taught through procedure or treatment teaching. Such techniques may involve feeding the child through a nasogastric tube, tracheostomy care, eye care, oral care, positioning, use of various types of equipment (e.g., suction machine), passive range-of-motion exercises, skin care, and safety concerns. If the child with altered responses is mobile, parents often appreciate discussing behavior modification and discipline with the nurse.

The family also needs information about the availability of physical and financial support for the child's care after discharge. They should be counseled about the physical and emotional hazards associated with full-time care of the disabled child. Family members should be encouraged to take advantage of respite care offered by friends and relatives. Caring for a child with altered responsiveness has a tremendous impact on the family. Sensitivity, presence, communication skills, and knowledge help the nurse provide support to the family. Family members may need to deal with the loss of closeness that results from the child's altered ability to communicate and to respond to affection. They may question the child's ability to hear or to feel in the absence of normal output responses.

Family members often have concerns about the child's prognosis and questions about whether to seek additional opinions from other health care professionals. Such discussions call for sensitivity on the part of the nurse. It takes time for the family to understand and to accept the reality of a neurologic deficit, whether temporary or permanent. The nurse can help the family obtain needed information by being present for discussions with the physicians and ensuring that their questions are adequately addressed. In many cases, arranging a meeting for the family with the multidisciplinary team will allow many concerns to be dealt with while all the care providers are present. Often, the presence of a social worker who has been involved with the family is very helpful in the running of the meeting.

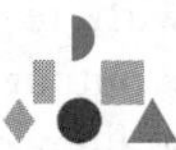

Alterations in Neurologic Status

Adverse Outcomes of Neurologic Conditions

Increased Intracranial Pressure

Intracranial pressure (ICP) is determined by the space occupied by the three intracranial components: **brain**, **blood**, and **CSF**. Once the fontanelles are closed and the cranial sutures are fused, the skull acts as a rigid container with a fixed volume. For the ICP to remain constant in the presence of an increase in one of the components, the other components must decrease in volume. These components, the brain, blood, and CSF, can alter their volume to maintain normal ICP in a mechanism known as **compensation**. When an increase in volume occurs, compensatory mechanisms allow for the maintenance of a normal volume-pressure relationship for as long as possible. If these mechanisms become exhausted, an imbalance occurs, volume increases, and increased ICP results.

In infants and young children, open sutures allow for growth of the head in the initial phases of increased ICP, especially when the build-up of pressure is slow or chronic. In instances of acute increased ICP, the skull may not change as readily to compensate for the added volume. Because of this phenomenon, the signs and symptoms of acute and chronic increased ICP in infants and young children vary.

When an acute increase in the overall volume of the intracranial contents occurs, the brain begins a complex series of metabolic and vascular activities aimed at decreasing the overall intracranial pressure and perfusing the sensitive brain tissue as much as possible. In tissue injury and hypoxia, glutamate and glyceine are released. Intra- and extracellular shifts of sodium, potassium, and calcium occur. The end result is cerebral edema and ultimately cell death (Bullock & Fujisawa, 1992). A more detailed description of the processes of initial compensation and autoregulation follows.

Pathophysiology

Cerebral Blood Flow. CBF is essential for oxygenation of the brain and for transportation of metabolic nutrients to and from the cell. CO_2 is a potent vasodilator of cerebral blood vessels. Vasodilation causes increased blood volume and, therefore, increased ICP. Reducing the $Paco_2$ by controlled hyperventilation causes vasoconstriction of cerebral blood vessels, which, in turn, decreases ICP. Controlled hyperventilation is routinely used in the management of increased ICP because of this unique phenomenon. Oxygen content can also affect ICP, although to a much lesser degree. Profound hypoxia (Pao_2 less than 50 mmHg) can lead to cerebral vasodilation as the body tries to send more oxygen to the brain tissue. For these reasons, airway management for the child at risk for, or currently experiencing, increased ICP is paramount.

Cerebral Perfusion Pressure. A major concept related to CBF is cerebral perfusion pressure (CPP). CPP is the gradient of blood flow and oxygenation to the brain tissue. It is calculated by subtracting the ICP value (known by using an ICP monitor) from the mean arterial blood pressure. CPP is affected by changes in arterial blood pressure as well as by changes in ICP. A normal CPP is approximately 80 mmHg with values over 60 mmHg considered acceptable in children with an acute increase in ICP secondary to trauma.

Initial Compensatory Mechanisms. Several compensatory mechanisms serve to maintain ICP in the face of increasing volume within the skull. These include (1) a displacement of CSF from within the cranial cavity to the distensible subarachnoid space around the spinal cord, (2) an increase in the rate of CSF absorption secondary to the pressure gradient across the venous system, and (3) a reduction in cerebral blood volume resulting from compression of the low pressure venous system.

Autoregulation. *Autoregulation* is defined as a mechanism by which the cerebral blood vessels alter their diameter to maintain a constant blood supply to brain tissue, despite fluctuation in the arterial blood pressure. When the initial compensatory measures are no longer effective in reducing increased ICP, autoregulation of blood flow is another mechanism for maintaining cerebral perfusion. This is accomplished by constriction and dilation of the cerebral blood vessels. When arterial pressure rises, vasoconstriction occurs; when arterial pressure falls, vasodilation occurs. Dramatic changes in arterial blood pressure (less than 50 mmHg or greater than 150 mmHg) impair cerebral autoregulation and blood flow to the brain. When the systemic blood pressure declines below this level, cerebral ischemia occurs and cell function is impaired. When severe hypertension occurs, cerebral edema results secondary to the breakdown of the blood–brain barrier. When autoregulation is impaired, CBF and CPP become passively dependent on systemic arterial pressure (American Association of Neuroscience Nurses, 1996).

Herniation of Brain Tissue. Herniation can be described as a physical displacement of a portion of the brain through and into other brain structures, usually because of an increase in the volume of brain, blood, or CSF. When pressure in one area is excessive, brain may displace to an area of less resistance, causing serious and potentially life-threatening consequences. The best treatment is to prevent a situation in which these events would occur, by early management of increased ICP. The most common type of supratentorial (above the tentorium) herniation is uncal herniation. As the uncus of the temporal lobe pushes into midline structures, it puts pressure on the oculomotor nerve (CN III), causing pupil dilatation and sluggish or absent response to light ("fixed and dilated"). Uncal herniation can be unilateral or bilateral.

Infratentorial herniation (beneath the tentorium) is less common and can involve herniation of the cerebellar tonsils up through the tentorium putting pressure on the midbrain, or down through the foramen magnum putting pressure on the medulla. The brain stem can also herniate down through the foramen magnum. There are a wide range of symptom possibilities with infratentorial herniation syndromes. Medullary compression can result in death from cardiac or respiratory arrest. The nurse needs to be astute to detect possible mechanisms of herniation and potential signs and symptoms (Hickey, 1992).

Mechanisms That Increase Intracranial Pressure. Several mechanisms are known to increase ICP. These mechanisms include increased brain mass, increased cerebral blood volume, increased CSF volume, and obstruction to CSF flow. Increased brain mass can result from brain tissue edema secondary to cell anoxia after head injury, brain surgery, infections, and inflammatory diseases such as encephalitis (Table 21–5).

Growths within the brain, including tumors, abscesses, cysts, and vascular abnormalities (e.g., aneurysms or arteriovenous malformations) also increase brain mass. Increased cerebral blood volume is secondary to vasodilation, which occurs for numerous reasons, including oxygen deprivation and increased systemic blood pressure. Decreased venous outflow and increased intrathoracic pressure are also factors that increase cerebral blood volume.

Increased CSF volume secondary to congenital or acquired hydrocephalus or meningitis is common in children. All of these processes result in obstruction of the CSF pathways. CSF production also increases in the presence of a tumor called a choroid plexus papilloma, but this occurrence is rare.

For the child experiencing increased ICP, several of these mechanisms may occur simultaneously. This development can lead to a confusing, yet challenging, task for the nurse. The clinical picture is made clearer by a well-thought-out, thorough diagnostic assessment done in a timely manner.

Table 21–5
Causes of Increased Intracranial Pressure

Causes	Common Treatments
Increased Brain Mass	
Edema from cell anoxia secondary to head injury, brain surgery, infectious and inflammatory diseases (e.g., encephalitis) Increased mass resulting from growths (cysts, tumors) and large anteriovenous malformations	Surgery (mass lesions, hematomas) Corticosteroids (for edema around mass lesions) Osmotic diuretics (mannitol, glycerol)
Increased Cerebral Blood Volume	
Vasodilation (e.g., with oxygen deprivation resulting in increased $PaCO_2$, decreased PaO_2) Decreased venous outflow (e.g., head position restricting jugular venous flow) Increased thoracic pressure (Valsalva, positive end-expiratory pressure) Increased systemic blood pressure	Hyperventilation Elevating head of bed Maintaining alignment of head and neck Maintaining normothermia Diuretics (furosemide, acetazolamide, ethacrynic acid) Pancuronium to decrease muscular response to stimuli
Increased Cerebrospinal Fluid (CSF) Volume	
Decreased CSF absorption (e.g., from debris clogging arachnoid villi in meningitis)	Shunting of trapped CSF to a resorptive body cavity
Obstruction to CSF Flow (e.g., Infratentorial Tumor, Brain Cyst)	
Increased CSF production from choroid plexus tumors (rare)	Surgery to remove obstruction Closed ventricular drainage for short-term treatment

From Betz, C., Hunsberger, M., & Wright, S. (Eds.). (1994). *Family-centered nursing care of children* (2nd ed., p. 1760). Philadelphia: W. B. Saunders. Reprinted with permission.

Assessment

Differences in the signs and symptoms of increased ICP vary depending on the age of the child. Open fontanelles and unfused sutures are present in infants allowing for some expansibility for compensation; the skulls of older children are less accommodating to changes in ICP. Differences in the signs and symptoms are also related to whether the underlying process is acute or chronic as well as to the child's developmental level and ability to communicate subjective symptoms. Early recognition of these manifestations can lead to prompt treatment and more favorable outcomes for children with increased ICP.

A complete assessment of factors in the child's history, including changes in behavior, attainment of developmental milestones, or level of alertness or responsiveness, is vital. Any history of headache, vomiting, or visual problems is also salient. After a baseline is established, the nurse should carry out *neurologic monitoring* and should monitor vital signs with a frequency relative to the child's condition and to the physician's orders. This may be as frequently as every 15 minutes for an unstable child whose condition is changing rapidly, or it may be several times daily for a more stable patient (see previous discussion of neurologic assessment).

Diagnostic Tests. Diagnostic studies are obtained to identify the specific cause of increased ICP. These tests may include skull radiographs, CT and MRI scans, CBF studies, EEG, evoked potentials, and laboratory tests.

Intracranial Pressure Measurement. ICP is measured in millimeters of mercury (mmHg) or in centimeters of water (cm H_2O). Monitoring devices range from a noninvasive transducer that may be placed over a fontanelle to more commonly used invasive devices, such as an epidural transducer, a subarachnoid bolt or screw, and an intraventricular catheter transducer. Fiberoptic technology has led to greater accuracy of these measuring devices and increased ease of care, because the transducer is in the tip of the catheter, which eliminates the need to "zero" the catheter with the child's movement. Placement of an ICP monitor will be made by a neurosurgeon either at the bedside or in the operating room. Systemic and local analgesia should be administered. After a small scalp incision is made off the midline in the anterior aspect of the skull, a burr hole is made through which the catheter is placed and secured. The nurse will assist in gathering supplies, ensuring strict asepsis during the procedure, and supporting the family with information as needed.

Normal ICP ranges from 0 to 15 mmHg under normal conditions. The ICP is usually stable, although temporary elevations to as high as 100 mmHg can occur with activities such as coughing and the Valsalva maneuver. Increased ICP may be moderate (20 to 40 mmHg) or severe (greater than 40 mmHg). The placement of an ICP monitor allows for the calculation of CPP, which is a more accurate predictor of long-term outcome for children with increased ICP.

Nursing Diagnoses and Outcomes

Chart 21–3 presents a variety of nursing diagnoses that can be applied to the child with a neurologic condition. The following diagnoses are also specifically applicable to the child with increased ICP:

- **High risk for altered cerebral tissue perfusion related to increase in volume of brain tissue mass, cerebral blood volume, or CSF volume**
  Outcomes: Child maintains adequate cerebral perfusion.
  Child achieves adequate oxygenation and nutrition at the cellular level.
- **Hyperthermia related to neurologic insult or infection**
  Outcome: Child's temperature is less than 38.5°C.
- **Impaired gas exchange related to pooling of pulmonary secretions, ineffective cough, and altered breathing pattern secondary to decreased level of consciousness**
  Outcomes: Child is free from respiratory infection and atelectasis.
  Child maintains adequate arterial blood gas values.

Interdisciplinary Interventions

The treatment of increased ICP may involve both surgical and medical modalities. Generally, medical measures are instituted while the diagnostic assessment is being done to ascertain the need for surgery and to direct further care. In many instances, surgical and medical management occur simultaneously.

Surgery. Surgery to relieve rapidly increasing ICP may be acutely needed in cases of severe head injury resulting in epidural or large intraparenchymal (within brain tissue) hemorrhages. Open wounds, large lacerations, and skull fractures also require immediate surgical attention because of the risk of serious infection. Clinical conditions of a more chronic nature may present as a surgical emergency, especially if they go undiagnosed for a long period of time: for example, children with brain tumors or infants with subdural hematomas secondary to nonaccidental trauma in the form of "shaken baby syndrome." In these latter cases in particular, medical management is optimized before surgery begins to lessen the risk of significant operative morbidity or mortality during surgery on a highly pressurized brain; in some cases, this risk cannot be avoided. In most cases, an ICP monitor is inserted during surgery to assist in postoperative management of ICP. A neurosurgeon may also be called on to place an ICP monitor in children with closed head injuries not requiring surgery. This procedure can be done at the child's bedside in the critical care area with appropriate attention to asepsis, analgesia, sedation, and nursing care.

Closed Ventricular Drainage/Ventriculostomy. In cases of increased ICP in which ventricular access is obtained to measure ICP, controlled drainage of CSF may be used as an adjunctive measure during the acute phase of treatment. Newer, sterile closed drainage systems allow for close monitoring of CSF drainage and for a "pop-off" level to be set, at which CSF drains independently. These systems also allow for easy access to in-line ports for drawing CSF specimens to follow up infection and other CSF parameters.

In either case, the ventricular drainage tube has an exit point through the scalp and is connected to a closed, sterile drainage system. The physician may order continual drainage at a specific pop-off level or intermittent drainage when the ICP reaches a specific level. Nursing care for these systems includes careful recording of the color and amount of drainage (Chart 21–6). Proper leveling and setting of the ordered pop-off level and awareness of the effects of positioning on the system are essential. Close scrutiny of electrolytes and monitoring of the need for CSF replacement with intravenous fluids are also important nursing measures.

Monitoring ICP and Drainage System. If the child's ICP is being monitored, the goal is usually to keep the ICP at less than 15 to 20 mmHg and the CPP at greater than 50 mmHg. This goal necessitates that mean arterial blood pressure be 70 mmHg or greater. If sudden increases occur in ICP, the nurse should quickly assess the patient to note any change in vital signs or in neurologic checks (Chart 21–7).

A close scrutiny of the monitoring or drainage system should also take place to ensure proper functioning. Some reasons for a sudden increase in ICP include a change in head and neck positioning, a partially obstructed airway, hyperthermia, and increased patient agitation secondary to noxious external stimuli. The nurse must also be aware of stroke, intracranial hemorrhage, and impending herniation as potential causes of a change in ICP.

The nurse needs to assess the child for hypercapnia and hypoxia by means of blood gas analysis and pulse oximetry. Suctioning may be necessary and should be limited to short intervals to prevent suction-induced hypoxia. When *ventilation assistance* by mechanical ventilator support is used, parameters for a Pco_2 between 24 and 30 torr and a Po_2 greater than 85 torr are adhered to for control of ICP. When positive end-expiratory pressure is used for pulmonary hypoxia, attention must be given to excessively high intrathoracic pressure that may also contribute to high ICP. Manual hyperventilation (bagging) may be used as a short-term treatment for increased ICP in the critical care setting.

Neurologic Positioning. Head and neck position should be kept neutral with regard to the shoulders and upper trunk. Nurse researchers have found that neck flexion and head rotation appear to increase ICP. Maintenance of a neutral head position can be accomplished with head elevation to 10 to 20 degrees and with extra support to prevent the child from sliding down in bed. Pillows may be used to support the neutral position in a side-lying manner. The child's head should be supported in a neutral position during turning and lifting. Increases in ICP have also been seen in response to lateral and prone positioning. The prone positions should be avoided in increased ICP.

Temperature Regulation. Normothermia is maintained by keeping body temperature at 36.5° to 38.0°C (97.7° to 100.4°F) without using cooling devices or antipyretics. Fever causes vasodilation and increased CBF. The administration of antipyretics and the use of tepid water sponge baths and cooling blankets are recommended.

Hypothermia as a treatment modality in increased ICP has fallen out of favor and is rarely instituted; normothermia is preferred.

Medications. Administering and monitoring the effects of medications are a major focus of medical management. A common treatment is the use of intravenous mannitol, which, when present in cerebral blood vessels, increases the osmotic pressure, thereby causing water to move from the brain tissue to the vascular space. The administration of mannitol requires frequent monitoring of neurologic status, urinary output, and fluid and electrolyte balance, and awareness of potential hypovolemia.

Chart 21–6
Nursing Interventions Classification (NIC)

Tube Care: Ventriculostomy/ Lumbar Drain

Definition

Management of a patient with an external cerebrospinal fluid drainage system

Activities

Monitor drainage trends.
Monitor amount/rate of cerebrospinal fluid drainage.
Monitor CSF drainage characteristics: color, clarity, and consistency.
Record CSF drainage.
Change or empty drainage bag, as needed.
Administer antibiotics.
Monitor insertion site for infection.
Reinforce an insertion site dressing, as needed.
Restrain patient, as needed.
Explain and reinforce mobility restrictions to patient.
Monitor for CSF rhinorrhea/otorrhea.

From McCloskey, J., & Bulechek, G. (1996). *Nursing interventions classification (NIC)* (2nd ed.). St. Louis: Mosby–Year Book. Reprinted with permission.

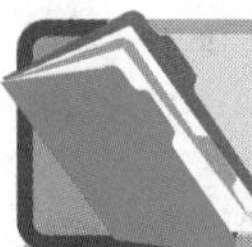

Chart 21–7
Nursing Interventions Classification (NIC)

Cerebral Edema Management

Definition

Limitation of secondary cerebral injury resulting from swelling of brain tissue

Activities

Assess for confusion, changes in mentation, complaints of dizziness, and syncope.
Establish means of communication: ask yes or no questions; provide magic slate, paper and pencil, picture board, flashcards, and vocaid device.
Monitor neurologic status closely and compare to baseline.
Monitor CSF drainage characteristics: color, clarity, and consistency.
Record CSF drainage.
Decrease stimuli in patient's environment.
Give sedation, as needed.
Note patient's change in response to stimuli.
Monitor respiratory status: rate, rhythm, and depth of respirations; PaO_2, PCO_2, pH, and bicarbonate levels.
Allow ICP to return to baseline between nursing activities.
Screen conversation within patient's hearing.
Administer anticonvulsants, as appropriate.
Avoid neck flexion or extreme hip/knee flexion.
Avoid Valsalva maneuvers.
Administer stool softeners.
Hyperventilate patient.
Position with head of bed up 30 degrees or greater.
Avoid use of PEEP.
Analyze ICP waveform.
Plan nursing care to provide rest periods.
Monitor patient's ICP and neurological response to care activities.
Administer paralyzing agent.
Encourage family/significant other to talk to patient.
Restrict fluids.
Avoid hypotonic IV fluids.
Adjust ventilator settings to keep $PaCO_2$ at prescribed level.
Limit suction passes to less than 15 seconds.
Monitor for CSF rhinorrhea/otorrhea.
Monitor lab values: serum and urine osmolality, sodium, and potassium levels.
Monitor volume pressure indices.
Perform passive range of motion.
Monitor CVP.
Monitor ICP and CPP.
Monitor PAWP and PAP.
Monitor P and BP.
Monitor intake and output.
Drain CSF, according to standing orders.
Hyperventilate before suctioning.
Maintain normothermia.
Administer loop active or osmotic diuretics.
Implement seizure precautions.
Titrate barbiturate to achieve suppression or burst-suppression of EEG, as ordered.

From McCloskey, J., & Bulechek, G. (1996). *Nursing interventions classification (NIC)*. (2nd ed.). St. Louis: Mosby–Year Book. Reprinted with permission.

The drug may be most effective during the first 48 hours of its use.

Other non-osmotic diuretics may be given to decrease total body water, thereby reducing the amount of water in the intracranial space. The persistent administration of these diuretics, such as furosemide (Lasix) is associated with significant potassium depletion.

The use of barbiturate-induced coma to reduce cerebral metabolic activity has significantly decreased in the past several years. The lack of an ability to obtain consistent neurologic examinations and the side effects of these drugs have led many medical professionals to abandon this practice in favor of sedation with newer, shorter-acting agents such as midazolam. The intravenous drip may be increased or decreased, depending on the child's level of agitation and ICP. Antianxiety agents should never take the place of appropriate analgesics, such as morphine or fentanyl.

Pancuronium (Pavulon), a paralyzing agent, may be used in the initial phases of management to decrease muscle responses to voluntary, central, and environmental stimuli (e.g., mechanical ventilation). Although the child has no movement or response to stimuli, sensory functions are not altered, so the child may still be able to hear, feel, and touch. Nursing care includes meticulous skin care, the application of artificial tears and eye lubricant, and frequent neurologic assessments.

Anticonvulsants such as phenobarbital or phenytoin (Dilantin) may be ordered if the child has a history of seizures. Avoidance of toxicity should be monitored with frequent levels. There is some controversy about giving head-injured patients an anticonvulsant on a prophylactic basis if a seizure has not occurred. Prophylactic antibiotics are ordered for the child with an ICP monitor in place and peak and trough levels should be monitored to prevent toxicity and to optimize their effect.

Steroids such as dexamethasone are used primarily in patients with neoplastic lesions. Antacids must be given concurrently to minimize side effects, including gastritis and stress ulcer.

Nursing care should focus on reducing the child's pain, crying, and agitation. Unnecessary stimuli that increase ICP should be avoided. The timely administration of analgesics and sedatives serves as an effective intervention to meet these goals. In addition, the parents' help should be enlisted to provide nonpharmacologic comfort measures. (See Chapter 13 for a review of these measures.) The presence of family members at the child's bedside should be encouraged. In some cases parental presence will lead to more agitation and further increased ICP. If this occurs the parents will need frequent explanations and support through the acute phase of treatment. Security objects can be brought from home to comfort the child. Care activities should be planned to allow for uninterrupted periods of rest and sleep for the child, and medical personnel can avoid performing too many nursing activities at any one time.

Treatment begins with prevention of the cause of increased ICP (e.g., use of helmets, use of seat belts, avoidance of aspirin, use of water access barriers). Once the cascade leading to increased ICP has begun, treatments are based on interrupting the cycle.

In summary the treatment of increased ICP is complex and specific to the causative factors. Prevention programs focus on the use of helmets, seatbelts, and water access barriers. More recently, programs have also focused on prevention of high-risk behaviors and violence as a means to decrease the number of children who suffer brain injury every year. Standard therapies once an injury has occurred include osmotic and loop diuretics and fluid restriction, aggressive ventilatory management, and surgical intervention where indicated. Monitoring of ICP is routinely done. The type of monitoring device will depend on the type of injury and the ability to access the ventricular space. More recently, blockage of the metabolic effects of glutamate/glyceine has been investigated. Although medications studied to date have had numerous side effects preventing their use, research is ongoing in an effort to develop new therapies. Frequent neurologic assessments and monitoring of vital functions and complications of immobility are critical. Finally, support for the family during this crisis is vital. Nurses, social workers, and hospital chaplains are often the key individuals who assist the family in coping with the loss of the child they knew and in some cases the ultimate death of the child.

Seizures

A seizure is a paroxysmal, uncontrolled episode of behavior that results from an abnormal electrical discharge from the brain. This episode may affect the child in any one or combination of the following ways:

- Altered responsiveness
- Altered sensation, perception, or both
- Altered movements, mobility, or muscle tone

What happens to the child during the seizure depends on the characteristic of the abnormal electrical discharge and what part of the brain is involved. Children may have a single seizure, perhaps related to a febrile illness or to an electrolyte imbalance. Some children may continue to have repeated seizures for an unidentifiable reason (idiopathic), and others may have seizures resulting from an acquired cause. The discussion in this chapter includes care of the child experiencing a seizure, regardless of circumstances, cause, and seizure type. Additionally, status epilepticus seizure disorder and epilepsy are reviewed. Febrile seizures are discussed briefly here and in more detail in Chapter 30.

The incidence of seizures is much higher during the first year of life and after age 55 (Hauser, 1990). Studies have shown that 1 of every 11 people (9%) will have experienced a seizure sometime in his or her life (Hauser, 1990). Most seizures occur before the age of 18 years.

Etiology

The cause of seizures ranges from neuronal migrational disorders to head trauma and includes brain tumors, metabolic disturbances, and cerebrovascular disease (Chart 21–8). Several factors may contribute to the propensity of the brain to have seizures. Many of these relate to the normal developmental process of synapse formation in infants and children. These include the following:

- A relative increase in the number of synapses in children, leading to the potential for increased risk for seizure activity
- Stimulation of enhanced receptors at synapses by neurotransmitters
- Involvement of more neurons, with continuous firing present during seizure activity
- Reduced threshold to activate seizures

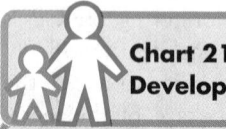

Chart 21–8
Developmental Considerations

Common Causes of Seizures in Different Age Groups

Neonatal (Birth to 28 Days)

Asphyxia
Intracranial hemorrhage
  Subarachnoid hemorrhage
  Periventricular-intraventricular hemorrhage
  Subdural hemorrhage
Hypocalcemia
Hypomagnesemia
Hypoglycemia
Hyponatremia/hypernatremia
Infection
  Intrauterine
  Postnatal
Congenital central nervous system malformations
Inborn errors of metabolism
Drug withdrawal
Accidental injection of anesthetic

Infancy to Adolescence

Chronic conditions continuing from neonatal period
Infection
  Brain abscess
  Meningitis
  Encephalitis
Trauma
Neoplasms
Degenerative disorders
Idiopathic
Genetic disorders

From Holmes, G. (1987). *Diagnosis and management of seizures in children*. Philadelphia: W. B. Saunders. Reprinted with permission.

In normal brain activity, certain groups of neurons are active (firing) in the process of thinking, hearing, moving, or doing other activities, whereas other groups of neurons are less active, and still others are inactive at any given moment. During a seizure, for reasons that are poorly understood, groups of neurons all activate at the same time, causing a sudden burst of electrical activity in the brain and disrupting normal brain function. In a partial seizure, this burst of activity is initially confined to one hemisphere of the brain, and the effect on brain function is limited, or "focal." In a generalized seizure, however, the abnormal electrical activity occurs throughout the brain, and some cortical functions are disrupted (Vining, 1994).

There are many paroxysmal events that occur in childhood that can be mistaken for seizure activity. These events can range from the benign (e.g., breath-holding spells, hyperventilation, night terrors, gastrointestinal attacks) to those of a life-threatening nature (e.g., cardiogenic syncope, hypoglycemic attack). Tourette's syndrome and other related tic disorders are inherited disorders characterized by involuntary, sudden, rapid, brief, repetitive, nonrhythmic stereotyped movements or vocalizations. They are not the same as seizures and require different medical management (Singer, 1993). Careful observation of the child and provision of interventions to reduce the risk of injury to the child are essential nursing skills.

Classification of Seizures

Several types of seizures can be characterized in children. These types include partial seizures, generalized seizures, and unclassified seizures.

The term *seizure* or *convulsion* should not be confused with, or used interchangeably with, epilepsy. Epilepsy is a state of recurrent seizures that are not related to fever or to any type of acute cerebral insult. Epilepsy may develop as a result of a chronic neurologic problem, or may be considered idiopathic, without known cause.

Partial Seizures. In partial seizures, the group of neurons involved in abnormal firing is initially localized to one or more areas within the same hemisphere of the brain. The abnormal electrical activity may spread to involve the entire brain. Partial seizures are further classified according to whether consciousness is lost during the attack. In a simple partial seizure, consciousness is not impaired, whereas a complex partial seizure involves decreased consciousness or awareness.

Simple partial seizures are usually brief, often lasting less than 1 minute (Holmes, 1996). Clinical manifestations are determined by the area of the brain involved. For example, if the neuronal burst occurs in the occipital region, vision is altered. Motor involvement is the most common type of partial seizure; this type of seizure was formerly called a *focal motor* (or jacksonian) seizure. Clonic seizure activity is typically limited to one muscle group (such as the fingers) or to a contiguous group of muscles (as in an arm or a leg). Involvement may spread from this initial site to involve all of the muscles on one side of the body, a phenomenon formerly labeled "jacksonian march." Transient paralysis of the involved muscle groups (lasting up to 24 hours) may follow a simple partial seizure, especially in young children.

Simple partial seizures that begin in the parietal lobe are associated with sensory symptoms, such as a "needles and pins" sensation or a feeling of numbness. Autonomic symptoms, which may occur with either simple or complex partial seizures, include vomiting, pallor, flushing, sweating, dizziness, erection of body hairs, pupillary dilation, tachycardia, incontinence, and other autonomic functions (Holmes, 1996).

Complex partial seizures are the most common type of seizure to occur in children. The focus of these seizures often arises in the temporal lobe, an area concerned with memory and emotion. Clinical symptoms may be complex and variable, and may include a wide range of behaviors.

Some children with complex partial seizures experience a *prodrome*; that is, they are aware of an impending seizure days or hours before it occurs. A prodrome differs from an aura in that a prodrome is not part of the actual seizure (*ictal*) event. An aura is an ictal phenomenon; it is part of the actual seizure activity. It is the portion of the seizure that occurs before consciousness is lost and for which memory is retained when consciousness is regained (Holmes, 1996). Auras vary considerably among individuals; children may experience sensory (e.g., visual, auditory, olfactory, gustatory) symptoms, visceral sensations, or complex subjective experiences such as fear, embarrassment, or dizziness. Following the loss of consciousness, various types of automatic behavior (automatisms) may occur, such as chewing, gagging, choking, lip smacking, spitting, waving, clapping, scratching, masturbating, walking, skipping, running, screaming, crying, or laughing. Because of the bizarre behavior associated with this type of seizure, it was formerly termed a "psychomotor seizure." On regaining consciousness (the *postictal period*), the child often feels tired and falls asleep. If the attack is brief, however, normal alertness may return quickly.

Generalized Seizures. Generalized seizures involve both hemispheres and there is loss of consciousness. Seizures that begin partially can become generalized. There are several types of generalized seizures:

- Generalized tonic-clonic (GTC): rigid extension followed by generalized jerking movements
- Myoclonic: sudden flexor jerk resembling Moro reflex
- Atonic: sudden loss of postural tone
- Absence: eye blinking, altered awareness, and occasionally mouth or facial movements (Haslam, 1997)

GTC seizures were formerly called "grand mal seizures." These seizures may be preceded by both a prodromal phase and an aura. An aura indicates that the seizure began focally (as a partial seizure) and then spread throughout the brain. In this case, the seizure is referred to as *secondarily generalized.* Typically, GTC seizures involve five recognizable phases: flexion, extension, tremor, clonic, and postictal (Holmes, 1996).

Consciousness is lost during the brief (5-second) flexion phase. Seizure activity usually begins in the face with the eyes rolling upward and the mouth opening with jaw muscles rigid. Flexion of the extremities follows. The extension (tonic) phase (lasting 10 to 30 seconds) begins with extension of the back and the neck and includes extension of the legs. The jaws clamp together tightly and tongue biting can occur. Apnea may begin with the rigid extension of the thoracic and abdominal muscles and may persist through the clonic phase. The tremor phase (5 to 10 seconds) marks the transition between the tonic and clonic phases. Fine tremors usually begin in the extremities and spread proximally. The clonic phase may last 30 to 50 seconds. The characteristic rhythmic jerking is produced by the rapid contraction and relaxation of opposing muscle groups. The jerking decreases in frequency as this phase nears completion. Apnea frequently lasts through the clonic phase, causing increasing cyanosis. Secretions pool in the mouth and throat, leading to noisy respirations. This can be a difficult stage for observers because the child appears to be in great distress, yet nothing can interrupt the seizure. After the last clonic jerk is finished, the bladder sphincter relaxes and incontinence may occur. In the immediate postictal phase, the child is still unconscious, but relaxation of muscles results in a flaccid posture. Cyanosis resolves as breathing returns to normal, but pallor often lingers. The child may either gradually awaken or progress directly into a sleeping state.

The term *myoclonus* means a quick movement of a muscle. **Myoclonic seizures,** then, are characterized by sudden, brief jerks of muscle groups. Flexor muscles are often involved on both sides of the body, resulting in sudden falls for older children or infantile spasms for infants. Consciousness is lost only momentarily, and may go unobserved. Myoclonic seizures may occur in clusters, either occurring several in a row or several during a day.

Infantile spasms are an age-dependent form of myoclonic epilepsy. They occur in infants from 3 to 12 months of age and consist of sudden flexor or extensor movements of neck, trunk, and extremities. The EEG usually demonstrates a characteristic pattern called hypsarrhythmia. Infantile spasms most frequently occur upon awakening or going to sleep and can number 100 or more daily (Kolodgie, 1994). Infantile spasms are classified as symptomatic (cause known) or cryptogenic (cause unknown). Prognosis depends on the cause. The goal of therapy is to begin treatment within the first 4 weeks after onset of spasms.

Atonic seizures involve a sudden loss of muscle tone and loss of consciousness. During a brief attack, the child's head may drop suddenly or the child may fall. These are often referred to as "drop attacks." More prolonged attacks may begin with a fall, but then continue with the child lying limp and unresponsive for seconds, or for minutes (Holmes, 1996). Longer attacks are usually followed by a period of postictal drowsiness.

Absence seizures are a type of generalized seizure that were formerly called "petit mal." Occurrence of these seizures is uncommon; they consist of a sudden, brief (usually no longer than 30 seconds) arrest of the child's motor activity accompanied by a blank stare and loss of awareness. The child's posture is maintained. At the end of the seizure, the child returns to the activity that was in progress as though nothing had happened. Interruption of mental activity may be incomplete, allowing the child to continue simple or automatic behavior during the lapse of full mental function. There is no memory of the seizure, but the child may be aware of a "time loss."

Febrile Seizures. Between 2% and 5% of all children in the United States experience a seizure provoked by fever. These seizures most frequently occur in children from 6 months to 6 years of age (Berg et al., 1990). Simple febrile seizures are less than 15 minutes in length, are generalized, and occur in a child without neurologic disability. Complex febrile seizures have the risk factors of being longer than 15 minutes, having a focal component, and occurring in children with a neurologic disability.

The concern with febrile seizures is their recurrence and potential development of epilepsy. The younger the child, the more likely that febrile seizures will recur. In addition, a family history of febrile seizures has a 20% risk of recurrence of febrile seizures (Berg, Skinnar, Hauser, & Leventhal, 1990). When children are neurologically normal, there is a slight association of epilepsy development after febrile seizures (Berg et al., 1990).

The potential for prevention of further febrile seizures forms the basis for treatment decisions. Each decision is made on an individual basis after consideration of the various risk factors. Medications that are effective in the treatment of febrile seizures include phenobarbital, valproic acid, and diazepam. Febrile seizures are discussed in greater depth in Chapter 30.

Neonatal Seizures

Metabolic, toxic, structural, and infectious disease processes place the newborn at risk for seizures. **Neonatal seizures** do not resemble the seizures of infants or older children. In the newborn, generalized tonic-clonic convulsions do not usually occur during the first months of life. Myelinization of the CNS is incomplete in the neonatal period. This seizure activity is not transmitted well in the neonate's brain. As a result, partial or fragmentary motor events or subtle behavioral changes such as apnea may be manifestations of seizures. Types of seizures that are recognizable in the infant include

- Focal seizures: rhythmic twitching of muscle groups (e.g., extremities and face)
- Multifocal clonic seizures: simultaneous involvement of multiple muscle groups
- Tonic seizures: rigid posturing of the extremities and trunk, fixed deviation of eyes may be present
- Myoclonic seizures: brief focal or generalized jerk of the extremities or the body
- Subtle seizures: consist of chewing motions, excessive salivation, apneas, blinking nystagmus, bicycling or pedaling movements, and changes in skin color (Haslam, 1996)

Seizure activities in neonates may be difficult to distinguish (Chart 21–9). Correlation with EEG may or may not be helpful. Focal clonic and focal tonic seizures are the most likely to be picked up with EEG evaluation. Interictal EEG patterns (activity in between seizures) are helpful in predicting outcome. Normal interictal patterns are associated with a good prognosis, whereas abnormal

Chart 21–9

Distinguishing Seizure Activity from Nonepileptic Movements

Seizure Activity	Nonepileptic Movements
Tachycardia and increased blood pressure may occur	No changes in vital signs
Movement not suppressed by general restraint	Gentle restraint easily suppresses movements
Sensory stimuli do not change seizure activity	Sensory stimuli enhance nonepileptic movements

patterns are associated with poor prognosis. Observation of the neonate is crucial for appropriate diagnosis (Ballweg, 1991).

Status Epilepticus

Seizures lasting longer than 30 minutes, or serial seizures without return to baseline function between seizures, are known as *status epilepticus*. It is one of the most common neurologic emergencies in the pediatric population (Mitchell, 1996). The causes of status epilepticus can range from acute CNS disorders to idiopathic or unknown factors. Acute CNS disorders may include meningitis, encephalitis, head injury, subarachnoid hemorrhage, subdural hematoma, metabolic encephalopathy, toxin exposures, tumors, degenerative disease, and cerebrovascular accidents. The most likely cause of status epilepticus for a child with a history of epilepsy or seizure disorder is poor adherence to taking medications or acute antiepileptic drug withdrawal. Morbidity and mortality from status epilepticus remain high despite advances in treatment (Holmes, 1996).

Assessment

One difficulty with providing seizure observation and first aid is recognizing when a seizure is occurring. Seizure detection is difficult when there is no preexisting history of seizures and when nurses are relatively inexperienced observers of seizure. For example, a nurse may enter the room to find the child staring and unresponsive, yet sitting in the bed holding a puzzle piece. Thinking that the child is simply daydreaming, the nurse may continue with activities. The nurse may be concerned about the child's lack of responsiveness and may question the event as a possible seizure, but repeated observations may be needed. In another example, the nurse may hear a crash and enter the room to find the child lying on the floor in a rigid posture. In this case, the nurse recognizes the event as a seizure and immediately proceeds with seizure first aid and observation.

Documentation of seizure events should include:

- When and where the seizure began (date, time of day, preseizure activity of child)
- Duration
- Any warning signs that the seizure was about to happen (aura)
- Clinical characteristics (specific description of movements and behaviors)
- Level of consciousness
- Signs and symptoms after the seizure stopped (postictal events)

The nurse needs to specify in the written description whether the onset of the seizure was observed. The details surrounding the onset of the seizure may be highly significant in seizure classification. Clinical manifestations of the seizure depend on the area of the brain that is involved. If the seizure was observed, an accurate description of the event assists the interdisciplinary health care team in making an accurate diagnosis and selecting an appropriate treatment regimen (Chart 21–10).

Diagnostic Tests. An EEG helps in differentiating epileptic from nonepileptic events, because each seizure type has characteristic EEG findings.

Ancillary studies such as blood analysis to check for electrolyte imbalances, CSF examinations, and neuroimaging provide information about the cause of the seizures.

Interdisciplinary Interventions

The approach to care of the child with a seizure is multifaceted and involves providing primary first aid, treatment to terminate the seizure, and simultaneous investigation of the cause. Additionally, measures are taken to reduce the potential for injury to the child if another seizure occurs. General care measures are also provided until the child is able to care for himself or herself.

First Aid. Basic first aid can be divided into four parts, regardless of the seizure type:

- Remain calm and stay with the child.
- Protect the child from any additional injury; use common sense.
- Provide time for the child to recover after the seizure stops.
- Reassure and provide support to the child and to others.

Protecting the child from injury depends on what happens during the seizure. Individuals experiencing only staring or altered responsiveness may require no first aid other than to have the nurse stand by to make sure that the child does not fall or lose balance. The nurse should speak softly, if at all, to the child with altered responsiveness. Shouting and shaking may only agitate or confuse the child.

If the child is having altered sensations or perceptions, these states should be acknowledged. The child should be reassured that he or she is safe and that the experience will soon be over.

If altered movements occur, the child's movements should not be restrained or restricted. Any harmful objects should be moved away from the child. If the child is walking during the seizure and is headed for a dangerous situation, such as open stairs, the nurse should attempt to steer the child in a safe direction.

If a child begins a seizure with movements in a standing position, it may be prudent to assist or to move the child into a lying position on the floor. When the event is finished, the nurse should turn the child to a semiprone or side-lying position with the head turned toward the floor. This positioning prevents choking and

Chart 21–10
Nursing Interventions

Seizure Observations and Documentation

Describing the Beginning

- What were the circumstances?
- Were there any precipitating factors?
- Was the seizure onset observed?
- Did child state or give any indication that the seizure was beginning? (An aura is the beginning of the seizure, expressed before altered responsiveness occurs.)
- Did child attempt to continue, stop, or slow down in their activities?
- What happened first? Then, describe in order, how the rest occurred.

Assessing Responsiveness

- Describe patient's observed response to you, self, environment.
- Describe whether responses were rote or more complex and how much they were affected (e.g., partially, totally).
- Assess response to tactile stimuli (blow on face, light touch, tickle, a mild shake of an extremity, ice, attempt to open eyes or move extremities).
- Assess response to auditory stimuli (clap hands, call name, give a command, state a word, and ask for recall later).
- Assess response to visual stimuli (note visual flinch: throw an object to child unexpectedly). Check pupil reactions.

Assessing Movements, Mobility, or Tone

- Was there any movement or change in posture? Give location and description: be as specific as possible. Consider a head-to-toe approach.
- Did this affect one or both sides of body? If both sides involved, did they look the same or different?
- Assess whether tone is increased (tonic, spastic, rigid), decreased (flaccid, limp), or normal.
- Were there any automatisms (repetitive, purposeless movements)? Were there any purposeful movements?

Assessing Sensation and Perception

- What does child describe or state? Ask child during or after seizure for a detailed description if possible.
- Are there any autonomic signs and symptoms (e.g., skin temperature change, change in color, sweating)?
- Did child say or do anything strange (mumbling, speaking inappropriately, cursing, wandering, climbing up or under objects, fumbling, resisting or combatting touch, agitation, and so on)?

Assessing Postictal Responses

- What was child like after the seizure? Describe child's behavior.
- How long did it take before resumption of previous activities?
- Could child recall the event in general or remember what happened at the beginning or throughout the seizure?
- Were there any temporary deficits (memory loss, aphasia, paresis)?
- Was there any confusion or disorientation? Describe and give duration.

From Betz, C., Hunsberger, M., & Wright, S. (1994). *Family-centered nursing care of children*. Philadelphia: W. B. Saunders. Reprinted with permission.

aspiration on saliva that may have pooled in the child's mouth during the seizure. If the child is lying on the floor, something soft may be placed under the child's head. No tongue blade or similar object should be inserted into the child's mouth, because it may only cause injuries. The child is given nothing to eat or drink until he or she has clearly recovered from the seizure. The child's recovery time after a seizure can vary. Some children can immediately return to activities. Other children may be confused or may fall deeply asleep for several hours. Chart 21–11 summarizes the nursing interventions that should be implemented when a child has a seizure.

Reassurance and psychosocial support during and after a seizure are important for the child and for others who may have observed the seizure.

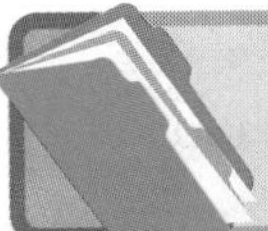

Chart 21-11
Nursing Interventions Classification (NIC)

Seizure Management

Definition

Care of a patient during a seizure and the postictal state.

Activities

Guide movements to prevent injury.
Monitor direction of head and eyes during seizure.
Loosen clothing.
Remain with patient during seizure.
Maintain airway.
Establish IV access, as appropriate.
Apply oxygen, as appropriate.
Monitor neurologic status.
Monitor vital signs.
Reorient after seizure.
Record length of seizure.
Record seizure characteristics: body parts involved, motor activity, and seizure progression.
Document information about seizure.
Administer medication, as appropriate.
Administer anticonvulsants, as appropriate.
Monitor antiepileptic drug levels, as appropriate.
Monitor postictal period duration and characteristics.

From McCloskey, J., & Bulechek, G. (1996). *Nursing interventions classification (NIC)* (2nd ed.). St. Louis: Mosby–Year Book. Reprinted with permission.

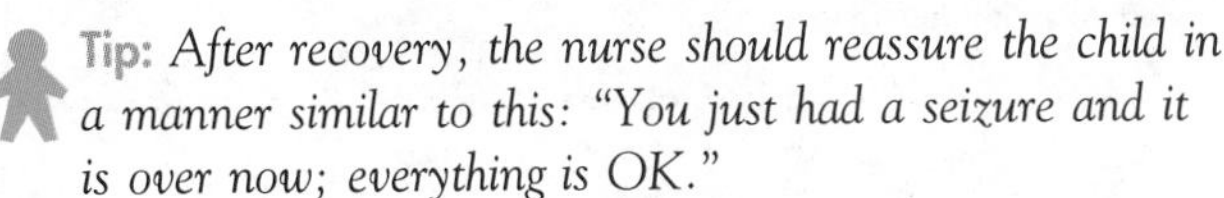

Tip: *After recovery, the nurse should reassure the child in a manner similar to this: "You just had a seizure and it is over now; everything is OK."*

The child's questions determine whether more information is needed. Children who have missed instructions or information because of altered responsiveness may need to have instructions repeated when they have recovered. Young children witnessing a seizure may think that the child is dying, having a tantrum, choking, or misbehaving. Adults often think the same thing. Again, simple explanations are helpful. Simple statements such as "It's OK, he's having a seizure; it will be over soon" can be tremendously reassuring if delivered in a calm, confident manner by the nurse.

Terminating the Seizure. It may not be necessary to call for emergency help during a seizure because the event is self-limiting and, by itself, does not cause damage to the child. The following situations indicate times when emergency help should be sought:

- The child does not start breathing after the seizure, in which case the nurse should initiate mouth-to-mouth resuscitation or bag and mask ventilation if available.
- The seizure activity continues for longer than 5 minutes.
- The child has one seizure after another without a return of consciousness between the seizures.
- The child has sustained serious injuries.

If this is the child's first seizure, emergency help is usually obtained. If the child is experiencing status epilepticus, emergency care is warranted to treat the child, to monitor the child, and to stabilize the child's condition.

Almost simultaneously in an emergency setting, an airway is secured, cardiac status is evaluated, vital signs are measured, an intravenous line is established, blood is drawn, antiepileptic drugs are given, and diagnostic tests are completed. Blood is usually drawn to obtain glucose level, complete blood count, sequential multiple analysis-12 (SMA-12) (includes electrolytes, calcium, magnesium, and phosphorus), and antiepileptic drug levels (if appropriate), as well as blood culture. At this point, intravenous glucose is injected by using a 2 mL/kg of 25% glucose in children, and in infants less than 6 months, 5 mL/kg of 10% glucose.

Medication Administration. The most common mistake in treating status epilepticus is the failure to give a sufficient amount of drug early enough. Typically, either intravenous diazepam or lorazepam is initially given to the child, followed by phenytoin or fosphenytoin sodium (Voytko & Farrington, 1997). If the seizures persist, an infusion of phenobarbital may be started. After early aggressive treatment has brought status epilepticus under control, maintenance therapy is initiated. Further information on maintenance antiepileptic drug therapy can be found in the discussion of epilepsy. If status epilepticus does not resolve, the use of a barbiturate-induced coma may be considered.

The dosages of antiepileptic drugs used in the treatment of status epilepticus cause decreased responsiveness, with the potential for ineffective breathing patterns and ineffective airway clearance. Less common but more serious reactions may include allergic and other idiosyncratic responses. The nurse may administer or may assist in administering the medications, and may provide early identification and treatment of side effects. Nursing care involves monitoring serum antiepileptic drug levels and seizure activity; laboratory testing; monitoring oxygenation, vital signs, and lung sounds; assessing the adequacy of breathing patterns; and airway clearance. To minimize aspiration and airway problems, the child should not be in a supine position with the child's head flexed. The child should be positioned in a side-lying position and should be turned every 2 hours.

Investigation of the Cause. As previously discussed, several diagnostic tests involving the evaluation of urine, blood, and CSF fluid are conducted to determine causative factors in children experiencing seizures. Additionally, assessment for otitis media should be conducted because this condition can lead to febrile seizures. Neuroimaging is completed once the child is stabilized.

Preventing Injury. Activities to protect the child having seizure activity include preventing seizure-related falls and injuries, aspiration pneumonia, hyperthermia, and drug side effects. Children with seizure-related falls and injuries may have fractures, dislocations, lacerations, or hematomas. There is also a risk for injury secondary to continued seizure activity. Nursing care includes continuous observation of the child and the use of side rails with adequate protective padding (Chart 21–12). The nurse must remove any harmful objects from the child's bedside. Health care providers should never force open a child's clenched jaw to insert an endotracheal tube, because this may injure the child. Nasal intubation may be preferred in this situation. Padded tongue blades are no longer used.

Aspiration pneumonia can occur during status epilepticus secondary to choking on food or other objects in the child's mouth or from the child vomiting stomach contents. Nursing care may include suctioning, adequate positioning of the child in a semiprone or side-lying position, monitoring vital signs and lung sounds, placing a nasogastric tube, and maintaining the child in a nothing-by-mouth (NPO) status until the child has recovered from status epilepticus and from the depressant side effects of antiepileptic drugs, and until the child has adequate gag and swallow reflexes.

Hyperthermia may occur as a symptom of CNS infection, or it may occur as a result of continued status epilepticus, especially when motor symptoms are involved. Nursing care may include keeping the child in minimal, light clothing; giving the child tepid sponge baths; monitoring the child's temperature; and using cooling devices.

Supportive Care. The level of self-care deficit depends on the type of status epilepticus and how consciousness and responsiveness are affected. For example, status epilepticus of the GTC or absence seizures type involves total self-care deficits, whereas status epilepticus of a partial seizure (epilepsia partialis continua) may vary from partial to total self-care deficits, depending on how consciousness and responsiveness are affected. If the child is unconscious, nursing care includes the provision of adequate fluids and nutrition, starting with NPO status, intravenous fluids, and enteric feeding until the child recovers, then progressing to oral food and fluids, as tolerated by the child. The child may also require attention to maintenance of skin integrity, turning and positioning, hygiene related to urine and bowel incontinence, eye care if the eyelids do not shut, and oral hygiene.

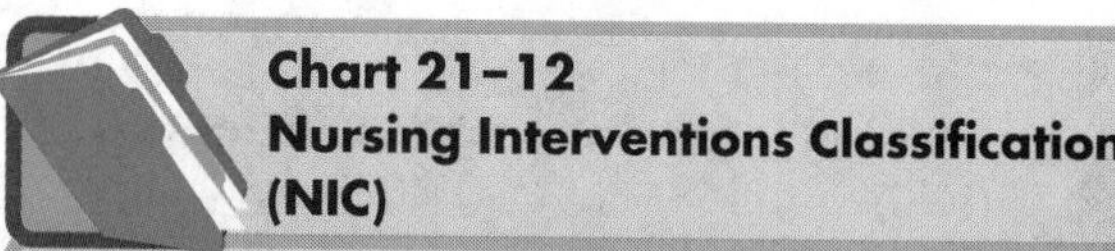

Chart 21–12
Nursing Interventions Classification (NIC)

Seizure Precautions

Definition

Prevention or minimization of potential injuries sustained by a patient with a known seizure disorder.

Activities

Provide low-height bed, as appropriate.
Escort patient during off-ward activities, as appropriate.
Monitor drug regimen.
Monitor compliance in taking antiepileptic medications.
Have patient/significant other keep record of medications taken and occurrence of seizure activity.
Instruct patient not to drive.
Instruct patient about medications and side effects.
Instruct family/significant other about seizure first aid.
Monitor antiepileptic drug levels, as appropriate.
Instruct patient to carry medication alert card.
Remove potentially harmful objects from the environment.
Keep suction at bedside.
Keep Ambu bag at bedside.
Keep oral or nasopharyngeal airway at bedside.
Use padded siderails.
Keep siderails up.
Instruct patient on potential precipitating factors.
Instruct patient to call if aura occurs.

From McCloskey, J., & Bulechek, G. (1996). *Nursing interventions classification (NIC)* (2nd ed.). St. Louis: Mosby–Year Book. Reprinted with permission.

Community Care

Parents and caretakers may need information about status epilepticus, antiepileptic drugs, diagnostic tests, cause, seizure recognition, and first aid. The nurse becomes involved with assessment, provision, and evaluation of instruction. Parents need specific information about the drugs used and need to have a basic understanding of how they work. Parents should know why the medicine must be given consistently and why it cannot be stopped abruptly. They should also be familiar with common and uncommon side effects and what to do if side effects occur. It may be unknown whether seizures will recur, but it is usually appropriate to discuss seizure recognition and first aid measures. The parents should know what to do for the child if status epilepticus recurs. Written material can be helpful to reinforce verbal information. Teaching should include safety measures that will protect the child from harm if another seizure occurs (Chart 21–13).

Epilepsy

A seizure is a sudden, involuntary, time-limited alteration in function occurring as the result of an abnormal discharge of neurons in the CNS (Holmes, 1996). The terms *seizure* and *epilepsy* are not synonymous. Epilepsy is a chronic condition characterized by seizures. Many types of seizures do not fall under the classification of epilepsy.

Although epilepsy indicates a chronic seizure disorder, it does not necessarily mean that the disease will last for the child's lifetime. Remissions of childhood epilepsy occur frequently (Holmes, 1996). Epilepsy is not a single disease entity; rather it is an indication of underlying brain dysfunction.

The child with a seizure disorder (epilepsy) requires intervention from nearly every member of the interdisciplinary health team. From acute to chronic care, nurses are often the best resource for organizing, planning, and evaluating the complex nature of seizure management. The physical manifestations of this neurologic symptom are frightening, yet most pediatric seizure disorders can be successfully controlled. A commitment from family members to maintain close medical follow-up in outpatient clinic visits, to consent for periodic diagnostic evaluations, and to comply with recommended drug therapy is required.

Families must cope with the emotional, social, financial, and medical impact of their child's illness. Education should be an ongoing process and should be tailored to meet the needs of individual cases. Because of the chronic nature of seizures, the plan of care must allow for changes based on physical growth and emotional maturation. Because siblings and extended family are an integral part of the child's life, they may provide valuable support if they are included in the overall treatment regimen.

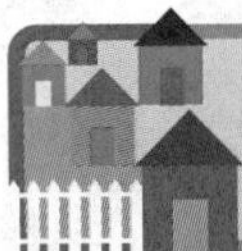

Chart 21–13
Community Care

Promoting Safety for the Child Who Has Refractory Seizures

To prevent seizure-related falls and injuries
- May use helmets—extra protection where likely to strike head; consider least restrictive helmet possible.
- Use stairs with supervision; instruct to use rail, consider elevator.
- Use chairs with arms to prevent falls off chair.
- Provide a safe environment, carpeting, protected stairs; remove breakable glass.

To promote water safety
- Bathe child with supervision (showers preferable, baths in few inches of water—consider foam protectors for fixtures; for teens, bathe when someone responsible is in house; keep bathroom doors unlocked).
- Swim with direct supervision (pool safer than lake).

To promote sleeping safety
- Consider room changes rather than allowing child to sleep with parents or parent with child.
- Use side rails or mattress on floor; remove nearby furniture.
- Avoid excess pillows and numerous stuffed animals in bed.
- Protect open stairways.

Adapted from Betz, C. L., Hunsberger, M., & Wright, S. (Eds.). (1994). *Family-centered nursing care of children* (2nd ed., p. 1750). Philadelphia: W. B. Saunders. Used with permission.

Etiology and Incidence

The incidence of epilepsy is 73 to 86 per 100,000 in children younger than 9 years of age, and 46 to 83 per 100,000 in children younger than 14 years of age (Holmes, 1996.) Information regarding the frequency and distribution of epilepsy is difficult to obtain, probably because of the discrepancies in defining the disease. There are numerous causes of epilepsy. It may be the only evidence of an underlying brain abnormality or it may be one of many symptoms. The younger the child at the onset of symptoms, the greater is the likelihood that the cause of the disorder will be identified. There does appear to be a familial predisposition to epilepsy. Evidence from siblings, offspring, and twin studies points to a genetic component, although it is poorly defined. The pathophysiology of this condition is described in the section on seizures.

A diagnosis of epilepsy is made on the basis of clinical data and historical information. A specific history obtained from a parent or the individual who witnessed the seizure is extremely helpful in establishing the diagnosis. A complete developmental examination also helps in understanding the disease. An EEG can provide supportive evidence and can aid in classification, location of the seizure focus, and choice of treatment for the seizure disorder (Holmes, 1996).

In most cases, epilepsy is idiopathic, or without an

identifiable cause. Indications for further work-up may include failure of medications to control the seizures or specific focal findings on the neurologic examination that indicate an underlying brain abnormality. If a structural abnormality is found, antiepileptic medications are still administered, but they may be gradually discontinued at a later date if other treatment measures are able to control or eliminate the seizure activity. Diagnostic testing varies, depending on the nature of the structural or metabolic problem leading to epilepsy.

Interdisciplinary Interventions

Management of the child with epilepsy includes the use of anticonvulsant drugs, education of the family and the child, and attention to associated emotional or learning disabilities. The goal of drug therapy is to control the seizures with as few drug side effects as possible (Chart 21–14). Surgery may be an option for the child with seizures that are unresponsive to drug therapy. Supportive care is discussed in the section on seizures.

Medications. The drug of choice for absence seizures is ethosuximide (Zarontin). The major anticonvulsants used in epilepsy are phenobarbital, phenytoin (Dilantin), carbamazepine (Tegretol), and valproic acid (Depakene) (Table 21–6) (Crumrine, 1996). Drug treatment typically begins with one anticonvulsant agent, with the dosage being increased gradually until seizures are controlled, clinical manifestation of toxicity is experienced, or serum drug levels reach the high end of the therapeutic range without controlling the seizures. If the first drug is ineffective, a second is added or another drug is tried. During

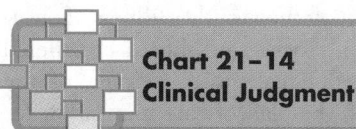

Chart 21–14
Clinical Judgment

The Child Who Presents with Seizures

Four-year-old Dwayne is brought to the clinic by his mother because he had a seizure earlier in the morning. His mother describes the seizure as jerking movements of the arms and legs with drooling from the mouth. Dwayne was very tired after the seizure and fell asleep. Dwayne has had three similar episodes in the past so his mother decided to wait until he awoke to come to the clinic. His previous seizures occurred when he was 1 year, 2½ years, and 3½ years old. All of these were associated with a fever and illness. Dwayne has had a cold for the past 4 days. His mother has not taken his temperature but has been giving him acetaminophen because he felt warm.

Questions

1. What other information would you collect from the mother at this time?
2. What type of seizure might Dwayne be exhibiting?
3. Dwayne has an electroencephalogram that reveals consistent findings for the diagnosis of epilepsy. He will be placed on an anticonvulsant medication. What is a nursing diagnosis you could select to reflect the family's teaching needs at this time?
4. When Dwayne returns to the clinic 1 month later, what data should be reviewed with the family?
5. What information would help you determine that Dwayne and his family are responding well to his treatment plan?

Answers

1. More information regarding diagnostic tests and treatment measures that occurred when Dwayne had other seizures; family history of seizures; Dwayne's ability to meet age-appropriate developmental milestones; history of recent ear infections, other illnesses, or immunizations; medications he is taking at home. Ask mother to provide more details of when the seizure occurred, how long it lasted, the child's responsiveness during and after seizure, and behaviors seen during the seizure.
2. Simple febrile seizure, complex febrile seizure, exposure to medications or toxins or epilepsy.
3. Knowledge deficit: management of epilepsy, or health seeking behaviors: management of epilepsy.
4. Go over parent and child's perception and understanding of diagnosis, treatment plan, and future course of illness; discuss the importance of monitoring child's development; review medication schedule, dosage, and side effects; review parental interventions if Dwayne has another seizure; determine whether other child care providers are prepared to assist Dwayne if he has a seizure when in their care.
5. Family reports medications are given as scheduled with no difficulty encountered in refilling the prescription as needed. Family attends all scheduled clinic visits. Dwayne has no seizure activity and continues to progress well developmentally.

Table 21-6
Antiepileptic Medications

Drug	Indication	Route of Administration	Side Effects
Carbamazepine (Tegretol)	Complex partial Generalized tonic-clonic	PO	Liver toxicity Granulocytopenia
Valproic acid (VPA, Depakene, Depakote)	Myoclonic Absence Generalized tonic-clonic	PO	Hepatic failure Thrombocytopenia Hair loss Increased appetite
Phenytoin (Dilantin)	Complex partial Generalized tonic-clonic	PO IV	Hirsutism, ataxia Gum hyperplasia Cardiac (related to rate of administration)
Fosphenytoin (Cerebyx)	Status epilepticus	IM IV	Ataxia Nystagmus
Primidone (Mysoline)	Generalized tonic-clonic	PO	Sedation
Ethosuximide (Zarontin)	Absence	PO	Rash Decreased WBC
Gabapentin (Neurontin)	Partial seizures as adjunct therapy Secondarily generalized	PO	Ataxia Sleepiness Dizziness
Lamotrigine (Lamictal)	Partial seizures as adjunct therapy Secondarily generalized	PO	Rash Dizziness Tremor
Felbamate (Felbatol)	Partial Secondarily Generalized	PO	Hepatotoxicity Aplastic anemia Insomnia
Topiramate (Topamax)	Partial seizures as adjunct therapy	PO	Cognitive difficulties Tremor Ataxia
Clonazepam (Klonopin)	Myoclonic Infantile spasms	PO	Sedation Increased secretions
Clorazepate (Tranxene)	Myoclonic	PO	Sedation Increased secretions
Phenobarbital	Generalized tonic-clonic Status epilepticus	PO IM IV	Sedation Irritability Cognitive
Diazepam (Valium)	Status epilepticus	IV	Sedation Respiratory arrest

PO, by mouth; IV, intravenously; IM, intramuscularly; WBC, white blood cell count.

this process, it is essential that the child and family be aware of the need to report changes in sensation and behavior that may signal a toxic reaction, and they must understand the importance of close follow-up care. Serum blood levels are drawn frequently until it is determined how a particular drug is metabolized by the child.

Anticonvulsant therapy is usually continued until the child has been seizure-free for 2 or 3 years (Holmes, 1996). Anticonvulsant drugs are always tapered in dosage to the point of complete withdrawal; the drug should not be stopped suddenly.

Diet. Alternative therapies such as the ketogenic diet have been used in the treatment of refractory epilepsy. The diet is high in fat and low in carbohydrates. Careful monitoring of the patient for hypoglycemia and ketonuria is essential. The diet requires commitment by the family because it is a very restrictive diet and must be maintained for at least 3 months (unless severe side effects are noted) (Batchelor, Nance, & Short 1997; McDonald, 1997).

Surgery. In recent years, some children whose epilepsy is intractable to drug therapy have been candidates for a complex surgical procedure to remove the area of seizure focus, and those children more severely affected have undergone a hemispherectomy of the brain. In the first instance, the child undergoes a craniotomy to implant a grid on the subdural surface. This grid allows mapping of critical brain areas that are involved in vision, speech, sensation, and memory, as well as identification of the seizure focus (Lannon, 1997). After surgery, leads extend from the implanted grid to computerized video and EEG monitoring. After a period of monitoring and extensive testing, a second surgery is performed to excise the seizure focus (Rutkowski, 1990; Lannon, 1997). In cases of intractable seizures with infantile hemiplegia, a hemispherectomy may be the procedure of choice (Tatum & Wang, 1990). These procedures are complex and are done only in certain major medical centers. Appropriate medical selection of the children who may benefit from this procedure is essential. Seizures must be focal, intractable to medical management, and arising from an area of the brain that could be removed without significant neurologic deficit (Rutkowski, 1990).

Epilepsy surgery may be indicated for children with intractable or uncontrolled seizures who have failed to gain seizure control after therapeutic trials with the most appropriate antiepileptic drugs. Children would be referred to a medical center for a comprehensive epilepsy evaluation. Diagnostic evaluation includes careful review of medication and seizure history and previous diagnostic

TIP 21–1 A Teaching Intervention Plan for the Child with a Seizure Disorder

Nursing Diagnoses and Family Outcomes

- High risk for injury related to hypoxia, aspiration, and loss of or impaired consciousness
  Outcomes:
  Child will not experience seizure activity.
  Child will remain free from injury, aspiration or respiratory distress during a seizure.
- Knowledge deficit: medications, diet, and management of child during a seizure
  Outcomes: Family administers medications safely to the child.
  Family verbalizes side effects of medications.
  Family identifies when treatment plan is not controlling child's seizures.

Teach the Family

Management of the Child During a Seizure

- Assist child to side-lying position.
- Remain with child.
- Remove sharp objects and hazards from area around the child.
- Loosen tight clothing.
- Do not restrain child or put anything into child's mouth.
- Remove child's eyeglasses to prevent injury to face.
- Prevent child from hitting hard objects.
- Allow seizure to end without interference.
- After the seizure, position child in side-lying position with head in midline position. Do not hyperextend the neck. If child vomits, carefully turn child to right side to prevent aspiration.
- Observe and document details of child's seizure including activity before, during, and after; date, time, and length of episode; child's physical status during seizure (e.g., incontinence, difficulty breathing, paralysis, loss of consciousness).
- Observe child's respiratory status during seizure. If breathing becomes impaired, call for emergency medical assistance.

Preventing Seizures

- Give medications as ordered. Consistent drug therapy is critical.

tests. The child may have intense EEG monitoring with surgical implantation of either depth electrodes or an electrode grid in an effort to define more clearly the epileptogenic focus. Potential candidates for lobectomy may also have a Wada angiogram to localize the speech center. Neuropsychological testing as well as evaluations with psychologists and speech, physical, and occupational therapists are usually completed.

Community Care

Education of children and their parents is crucial to promote compliance and seizure control (Martin, 1990). This education should include information about the child's seizure type, trigger events to the seizures, and medications (TIP 21–1).

Nursing research has documented the parents' (Austin, 1995) and teachers' (Bannon, Weldig, & Jones, 1992) need for clear information about the child's seizures and their treatment. In addition, Austin and coworkers (1994) noted a compromised quality of life in psychosocial and educational areas for children with epilepsy when compared with children with asthma. Institutions in practices treating children with epilepsy frequently have developed specific teaching materials. The Epilepsy Foundation of America also has numerous information sheets and videos in both English and Spanish.

Although most children with epilepsy have normal intelligence, some have cognitive and developmental delays. The school nurse and teacher need to be involved in understanding the disease and associated treatment. The school-age child may be at risk for absenteeism if seizures are not controlled. A staff conference may be held to identify the child's specific needs and to alert the school staff of any potential side effects of medications. The nurse should encourage the family to provide a

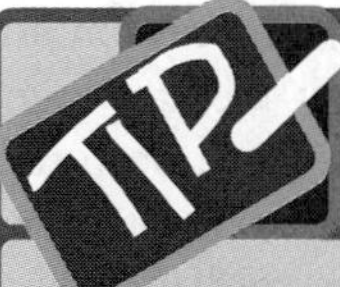

TIP 21–1 A Teaching Intervention Plan for the Child with a Seizure Disorder *Continued*

- Avoid events, activities, or stimuli that trigger seizure activity.
- Inform teachers or daycare providers about child's condition and how to intervene if a seizure occurs.

Medications

- Ensure that family knows names of drugs, amount, time to be administered, and possible side effects.
- Monitor for side effects such as drowsiness, lethargy, ataxia, nystagmus, gastrointestinal upset.
- Take child to health care provider for scheduled evaluations of therapeutic drug levels and blood counts.

Nutrition

- Provide instructions regarding ketogenic diet if used for seizure control.
- Encourage adequate intake of vitamin D and folic acid if child is taking phenytoin or phenobarbital.

Activity

- Child may have some activity restrictions depending on frequency of seizures and degree of seizure control that is maintained.
- Provide companionship during activities such as swimming or bicycle riding.
- Avoid having the child become overtired.

Contact Health Care Provider if

- Child experiences a seizure.
- Child is lethargic or listless.
- Child has a high fever.
- Child is experiencing depression or negative feelings about self because of seizure disorder.
- Child experiences breathing difficulties during a seizure.

Medic Alert bracelet for the child to wear at all times. A helmet may be necessary only for children with kinetic, or "drop," seizures or for those children with significant delays in motor development. Parents should be encouraged to focus attention on well siblings who may have unexpressed fears about the disease or may harbor guilt or anger toward the affected sibling. Most children with epilepsy are effectively managed in the outpatient setting.

Breathholding Spells

A number of nonepileptic paroxysmal events may resemble seizures but are not epileptic. Breathholding spells are the voluntary cessation of breathing, which occurs in response to a painful, noxious, or frustrating stimulus. Although dramatic, breathholding spells are considered to be benign. If prolonged, breathholding spells can lead to unconsciousness of the child or seizures. They are also referred to as vasovagal syncope or reflex anoxic events. Breathholding spells are most common in children 1 to 3 years of age. In the child older than 6 years of age, breathholding spells are an unusual occurrence, and further investigation of causative factors is warranted. Breathholding spells occur equally in males and females. Twenty-five percent of all children who have a breathholding spell have a positive family history of this behavior (Zuckerman, 1995).

Assessment

There are two types of breathholding spells: pallid and cyanotic. **Pallid breathholding spells** are vagally mediated events following a trivial, unpleasant stimulus such as the bumping of the leg or a mild injury to the head. A sudden collapse, pallid color, diaphoresis, and rigid posture with a few extremity jerks are noted. Following the precipitating event, loss of consciousness may occur. The hyperresponsive vagal response also results in bradycardia and, sometimes, asystole. Crying is usually not noted (Breningstall, 1996). Sleep may follow the episode.

Cyanotic breathholding spells are more complex events precipitated by anger or frustration. In the midst of crying, the child holds his or her breath to the point of cyanosis. The breathholding spells occur during expiration. There is a decrease in cerebral oxygenation and loss of consciousness occurs. There may be associated clonic movements of the extremities.

Both types of breathholding spells, therefore, may resemble seizures. Differentiating factors are triggers for the event, for time of occurrence (never during sleep), and for the progression of events (Table 21–7). An EEG may not be completed unless it is not possible to identify the precipitating events. If an EEG is performed, bradycardia or asystole is noted with ocular compression for pallid breathholding spells. The EEG may indicate signs of anoxia if cyanotic breathholding spells have occurred. In both types, cardiac evaluation may be warranted because prolonged QT syndrome or other cardiac events may be the cause (Breningstall, 1996; Sharp, 1997).

Interdisciplinary Interventions

There is usually no treatment for breathholding spells, and spontaneous resolution without sequelae is usually seen (Breningstall, 1996). For witnessed cyanotic spells, an intense stimulus such as a cold cloth held on the

Table 21–7
Characteristics of Breathholding Spells Versus Seizures

	Breathholding Spell	Seizure
Precipitating Factor	Anger, frustration, fright, or minor trauma	None noted
Time of Occurrence	Never during sleep	May occur anytime
Crying	Present prior to spell	Not usually present
Cyanosis	Present, occurs before unconsciousness	Not generally present; may occur if seizure is prolonged
Unconsciousness	Present	Present
Twitching or seizure movements	Occasionally present	Present
Electroencephalogram	Usually normal	Usually abnormal

Adapted from Zuckerman, B. (1995). Breath Holding. In S. Parker & B. Zuckerman (Eds.). *Behavioral and developmental pediatrics* (pp. 86–87). Boston: Little, Brown and Company. Used with permission.

child's face may cause the child to stop the breathholding spell (Zuckerman, 1995). If unconsciousness occurs during either type of breathholding spell, the child should be carefully placed on the floor on his or her side to prevent aspiration. If seizure activity occurs, medical evaluation should be sought.

Family interventions should focus on behavior modification and assisting the child to express anger and frustration in other ways. Families may benefit from an understanding of normal developmental parameters. Parents should be advised not to give undue attention to the child after the breathholding event because this may unintentionally reinforce continued demonstration of these behaviors.

Headaches

Headaches are a common neurologic symptom in childhood with 40% of 7-year-old and 75% of 15-year-old children having experienced a headache (Shinnar, 1991). Headaches affect children of all nationalities, races, ages, and both genders equally (Divertie, 1996).

The incidence of migraine headaches is approximately 10% of the population of the United States. Female to male ratio for classic migraine (with aura) is reported as 2:1 and for common migraine (without aura) is 7:1. Tension headaches, however, occur more frequently than migraine by 5:1 (Pearce, 1994).

Etiology

In general, the term *headache* is used to describe pain or discomfort in the skull or facial structures, because the brain has no pain receptors. The pain is referred from dura, from blood vessels (traction), from dilation of blood vessels, or from sustained contraction of muscles (Cohen, 1995).

Headaches may be single events or may be repetitive in nature. Four types of headaches are acute, acute recurrent, chronic progressive, and chronic nonprogressive (Table 21–8) (Rothner, 1995; Burns, 1996). Acute headaches are caused by an acute illness such as meningitis or subarachnoid hemorrhage. Acute recurrent headaches are caused by migraine. Chronic progressive headaches are caused by intracranial hypertension or tumor, and chronic nonprogressive headaches may be caused by muscle contraction (tension). The acute or chronic progressive headaches are of the most concern as potential causes of neurologic problems. Characterization of the headaches aids in defining the cause (e.g., tumor, tension,

Table 21–8
Characteristics of Types of Headaches

	Acute	Acute Recurrent	Chronic Progressive	Chronic Nonprogressive
Etiology	Acute illness (e.g., meningitis) Subarachnoid hemorrhage	Migraine	Intracranial hypertension Tumor	Muscle contractions Tension Psychogenic
Description	Diffuse, often localized to one area (e.g., occipital)	Intense, pulsating, front temporal, unilateral in older children	Diffuse, often localized to one area (e.g., occipital)	Diffuse, bandlike, tight, dull, bifrontal or occipital, mild to moderate intensity
Prodrome	No	Most likely to occur in older children	No	No
Associated findings	Positive neurologic sign Photophobia Fever	Transient neurologic signs Relieved by sleep Nausea and vomiting Visual changes in older children	Positive neurologic signs Papilledema	Depression Feelings of inadequacy, anxiety School avoidance common
History	Recent illness Head trauma	Positive family history for migraine Head trauma	Head trauma Gradual increase in head circumference	Problems at home, school, or with peers

Adapted from Burns, C. (1996). Neurological disorders. In C. Burns, N. Barber, M. Brady, & A. Dunn (Eds.), *Pediatric primary care* (pp. 551–572). Philadelphia: W. B. Saunders. Used with permission.

migraine). In children, documentation of a specific cause such as tumor or stroke is infrequent (Frishberg, 1994).

Prognosis. Studies of the prognosis of migraine in childhood demonstrate that two thirds of children become improved or symptom-free by long-term follow-up. Eighty-eight percent of children with nonmigrainous headaches were improved or symptom-free at a 6-year follow up in one study (Pearce, 1994).

Assessment

A complete clinical history and examination provide the basis for determining the specific characteristics of the headaches to determine their cause. Headaches associated with meningitis or subarachnoid hemorrhage are described as bursting with a rapid progression of pain that radiates down the neck and spine. The chronic-progressive headache of intracranial hypertension usually presents as aching and throbbing, which is increased by coughing or straining and which is present on arising in the morning. Both acute headaches and those associated with intracranial hypertension have other associated neurologic symptoms such as papilledema or alterations of consciousness. Muscle contraction headaches are described as bilateral, manifesting diffuse tightness or pressure in a bandlike distribution.

The acute, recurrent headache is most commonly manifested as migraine. Fifty percent of all children who will have migraine headaches have their first attack before 20 years of age (Lewis, 1995). Migraine headaches are paroxysmal episodes of a pounding pain (may be hemicranial) accompanied by nausea, vomiting, photophobia, and an intense desire to sleep. There may occasionally be vertigo, acute confusion, or hemiparesis. The interval between headaches is pain free.

Migraine headaches may occur with or without aura. The aura, if present, is described as unusual spots in front of the eyes or loss of visual fields (scintillating scotomata). Initially thought to be vascular in origin, migraine is currently considered to be an inherited sensitivity of the trigeminovascular system. Stimulation of brain structures produces norepinephrine and serotonin. A cascade of reactions results from this stimulation and leads to inflammation of pial and dural blood vessels, stimulation of the trigeminal nerve, and pain. Assessment of the child begins with a detailed history of the child's condition (Chart 21–15). The purpose of the history is to evaluate the characteristics of the headaches, and, most important, to distinguish any findings that may indicate serious pathologic abnormality.

Alert: *During the history taking, the following data may indicate a serious underlying condition that requires immediate, extensive evaluation:*

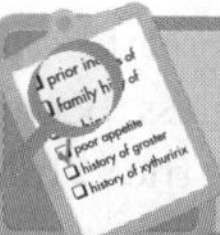

Chart 21–15
Focused Health History

Headaches

Chronic History

Pertinent past history of illness, infection, developmental abnormalities, dental problems, alcohol or drug use, allergies, visual disturbances or corrections, surgery, sleep patterns, family history of migraine or other disorders

Acute History

Recent illness, injury, change in sensory perception or mobility, diet or weight change, new medication or oral contraceptive use, level of activity, onset of puberty or menses

Psychosocial Factors

Perceived stressors, scholastic ability, feelings of depression or sadness, changes in lifestyle, concept of self, affect, appearance, relationship with family and friends, social activities and hobbies, nonverbal cues, family history of headache and effect on patient, patient's perception of significance of headache (e.g., fear of cause, outcome, diagnosis), past experience with hospitals or health care providers, identification of other person in the patient's confidence

Headache Data

Location, duration, frequency, quality, time of occurrence, severity, accompanying symptoms, treatment attempts, outcome of treatment, documentation of headache pattern, presence or lack of prodromal warning (aura)

Pain Assessment

Type of pain, pattern of progression or intensity, identification of factors that make pain worse or better, specific causes related to headache pain (e.g., bright lights, foods), nonpharmacologic therapy and effectiveness, medication and effectiveness, patient's experience with other types of pain

Identification of Headache Triggers

What factors seem to start headache: activity, foods, medication, menses, specific stressors, change in environment or seasons, work or school atmosphere

- *Recent onset or recent increase in frequency and severity*
- *Occipital or consistently localized headaches*
- *Changes in gait, personality, or behavior that do not occur at the same time as the headache*
- *Head trauma associated with headache*
- *Headaches that interrupt sleep*
- *Headaches that occur on arising, then fade*
- *Headaches that are exacerbated by changes in position*
- *Headaches in children younger than 3 years of age*

Clinical examination of the child with headaches includes a thorough neurologic assessment, percussion of the sinuses, and notation of blood pressure. Visual acuity is evaluated, and cranial bruits are listened for. The presence of a bruit is indicative of a serious pathologic abnormality and warrants further investigation. Children with tension or migraine headaches usually have a normal physical examination.

Extensive laboratory investigation is required in acute and chronic progressive headaches. Disorders such as brain tumors or meningitis must be eliminated as a cause for these headaches. This investigation would include neuroimaging and possibly CSF examination.

Nursing Diagnoses and Outcomes

Chart 21–3 presents a variety of nursing diagnoses that can be applied to the child with a neurologic condition. The following diagnosis is also specifically applicable to the child with headaches:

► **Pain related to cerebral discomfort**
Outcomes: Child does not experience pain from headaches.
Child/family uses measures to reduce factors that precipitate onset of headaches.
Child/family implements pain control measures to reduce child's discomfort.

Interdisciplinary Interventions

The goal of therapy is cessation of the headaches. Treatment for acute or chronic progressive headaches focuses on treating the underlying organic cause and most likely requires hospitalization to provide health care interventions such as surgery, ICP management, or intravenous antibiotic therapy. Health care management of chronic, nonprogressive headaches usually includes the administration of mild analgesics and stress management.

Treatment of migraines involves the use of a number of medications, as well as dietary manipulation and behavioral management. Use of medications is based on the pathophysiology of altered neurotransmitter responses in migraine. Persistent or acute attacks may respond to sumatriptan (Imitrex) or dihydroergotamine (DHE) with Reglan and steroids.

Medications. Three approaches to migraine therapy have been described. **Abortive** medications modify changes in blood vessels and are usually ergot alkaloid preparations. Cafergot is an ergotamine titrate medication. The most common side effect is nausea and vomiting, which can be treated with antiemetics. Midrin is a medication that combines a vasoconstrictive agent, a mild sedative, and acetaminophen; it creates less nausea than ergotamine but is available only in oral form. Sumatriptan is a serotonin agonist that can be administered subcutaneously, orally, or as a nasal spray for acute attacks.

Rescue medications are the most popular analgesics because they are available in both over-the-counter and prescription form. Caution must be exercised if only acetaminophen or aspirin is given to the child. Tylenol (acetaminophen) has been linked to changes in liver function if taken for extended periods of time. Salicylates, such as aspirin, are documented to be a factor in causing Reye's syndrome. Perhaps the most important educational point for parents is to read medication labels.

Preventive therapy includes use of daily doses of medications in the category of tricyclic antidepressants, calcium channel blockers, beta-blockers, alpha-agonists, monoamine oxidase inhibitors, and ergotamine derivatives. It generally takes 7 to 10 days to achieve therapeutic serum levels and resultant relief of pain.

Diet. A migraine elimination diet may be suggested before or concomitant with initiation of medications (Chart 21–16). Not all of the foods presented on Chart 21–16 trigger headaches in all children; therefore, children should carefully monitor any foods eaten before onset of a headache. A headache calendar or diary may be used to assist in determining which foods are acting as triggers. Elimination of these foods may prevent recurring headaches. A dietary consult may assist the child and family in identifying foods to avoid.

Behavior Management. Headache pain can be incapacitating and may be associated with nausea, vision changes, loss of equilibrium, and emotional lability. If these symptoms are not treated, children may lose valuable time in school and social activities. The patient or family may need assistance to identify potential causes for migraine attacks. If stress is a major factor triggering headaches, supportive counseling should be made available through hospital, school, community, or even religious resources. School counselors are often able to provide observations of the child. School attendance should be mandatory. If the child needs to remain at home, bed rest should be encouraged. A return to school the same day should be made if the headache recedes. Attention to the headache should be minimized so as not to create a situation in which the headaches are used to draw

Chart 21–16

Foods and Products Associated with the Onset of Migraine

Beverages
Any beverage containing chocolate, alcohol, or caffeine

Meat, Fish, Poultry
Cured or processed meat, liver, pickled herring, sardines, bacon, spiced dishes, smoked sausages, salami, chicken liver, and hot dogs

Vegetables
Sauerkraut, beets, and legumes including broad beans, lima beans, lentils, navy beans, fava beans, snow peas, and garbanzo beans

Fruits
Avocado, strawberries, figs, raisins, papaya, red plums, canned fruit

Bread
Yeast breads, cakes, doughnuts, sourdough bread

Dairy
Aged cheeses such as cheddar, blue cheese, Brie, Camembert, Parmesan, Gouda, Swiss, and mozzarella; cultured dairy such as sour cream, yogurt, and buttermilk

Snacks
Pickles, olives, peanuts, sunflower and pumpkin seeds, nuts, cheese crackers, pizza, any foods with monosodium glutamate (MSG), such as Chinese food

Sweets
Chocolate, mincemeat pie

Additives
Spices, MSG, meat tenderizers, soy sauce, and any foods containing nitrites or yeast

Other
Vapors from perfume, solvents, paint, nail polish, and cleansers

Drugs
Oral contraceptives and over-the-counter cold remedies

unnecessary attention to the child or to serve as a means to avoid school.

Other interventions in the treatment of headaches include provision of a dark, quiet environment (especially if the patient experiences photophobia). Therapeutic touch or massage therapy may help. The use of biofeedback mechanisms is also useful to try to help avoid the heavy use of pharmaceuticals. Migraine headache usually diminishes during pregnancy because of the vasodilating effects of placental hormones.

The nurse can provide education to the child and parents regarding types of headaches, combinations of preventive measures (including avoidance of known triggers), and judicious use of medication. It is also critical that, if the child requires acute pain management, pharmacologic interventions should precede implementation of the longer term strategies.

Congenital Disorders

The most CNS anomalies present at birth are those that result from abnormalities in the formation of the neural tube and orderly development and movement of the neurons in the fetal brain. Others result from abnormal formation of the bony covering of the nervous system. Genetic syndromes can be associated with many of these CNS anomalies. The most serious defects involve large portions of the spinal column and brain. Smaller defects may be limited to specific areas. Severity of the anomaly is related to its location, size, and degree of involvement of the nerve tissue.

Besides those children with outwardly obvious nervous system abnormalities, there are a number of children with neurodevelopment anomalies such as mental retardation and learning disabilities. Until recently, most of these children were thought to have idiopathic causes of their disorders. New evidence suggests that barely detectable abnormalities of brain development (cerebral dysgenesis) comprise the inherent pathophysiology (Schaefer, Sheth, & Bodensteiner, 1994).

The congenital disorders discussed in this chapter include anencephaly, spina bifida, hydrocephalus, Chiari malformation, microcephaly, and craniosynostosis (Table 21–9). Of these listed, anencephaly, spina bifida, and encephalocele are classified under the broader term *neural tube defects* (NTDs).

Incidence

The incidence of NTDs is 1 in 1000 births and is more common in females than males. It occurs six times more frequently in whites than blacks. Epidemiologic studies demonstrate a striking variety in prevalence rates. The highest incidence is in Great Britain and Ireland, and the lowest incidence occurs in Asia (Swaiman, 1994). There is also a higher incidence of such defects in children whose parents are of Celtic genetic descent. For example, in Dublin, Ireland, the incidence of neural tube defects is approximately twice as high as it is in the United States (Raloff, 1995).

Table 21-9
Commonly Seen Neural Tube Defects

Type	Description	Outcomes
Anencephaly	Absence of brain tissue above a rudimentary brain stem and basal ganglia	Sustained extrauterine life is virtually impossible.
Encephalocele	An external sac or mass that may occur at any point over the vertex or base of the skull. May be covered with either scalp or a transparent membrane	Dependent on presence of hydrocephalus, infection, actual rupture of the encephalocele, and amount of neural tissue in sac.
Spina bifida cystica	Incomplete fusion of one or more vertebral laminae, resulting in an external protrusion of the spinal tissue. Occurs most commonly in lumbosacral area	
	Myelomeningocele: protruding saclike structure contains meninges, spinal fluid, and neural tissue	Spinal roots may terminate in sac, which significantly affects motor and sensory function below that point.
	Meningocele: protruding sac contains meninges and cerebrospinal fluid	Neurologic complications are less severe than in myelomeningocele.
Spina bifida occulta	Incomplete fusion of vertebra at one level that may be signaled only by an overlying dimple or tuft of hair	Usually there is no evidence of dermatologic, neurologic, or musculoskeletal disorders. It may present with some of these problems in late childhood.

Etiology

The causes of many neural tube defects are unknown (Schaefer, Sheth, & Bodensteiner, 1994). Although genetics play an integral part of the normal or abnormal development of a fetus, exposure to some potential hazards or lack of essential nutrients has been directly linked with neurologic deficits.

It is difficult for researchers to define specific causes of neural tube defects because maternal exposure to many possible teratogens may occur during any given pregnancy (Werler & Mitchell, 1993). Especially deleterious risks are poor maternal nutrition and fetal hypoxia secondary to placental insufficiency or poor maternal oxygenation. Maternal alcohol consumption creates a number of problems in neurologic and biological organization (Werler, Mitchell, Rosenberg, & Lammer, 1991). In addition, research on prescription drugs, such as ovulation induction drugs (Werler, Louik, Shapiro, & Mitchell, 1994) and phenylhydantoins (Buehler, Rao, & Finnell, 1994; Yerby, 1994) has documented a role in congenital CNS birth defects. Effects of over-the-counter and recreational drug ingestion are less well documented, but they can nonetheless create serious defects if ingested by the mother at a critical period during her pregnancy, usually weeks 3 through 8 postconception for the serious deformities. (See Chapter 9 for further discussion of teratogens.) Other factors associated with increased risk of neural tube defects include environmental teratogens, perinatal infections, maternal hypothermia, and maternal obesity (Graham, 1992; Shaw, Velie, & Schaffer, 1996; Swaiman, 1994).

New evidence suggests that the interaction of a specific genome with the environment may influence how needed nutrients are metabolized into normal neural tissue or defects (Scott, 1995). Fifteen percent to 20% of children with neural tube defects were found to have two abnormal copies of a gene that metabolizes homocysteine (a short chain polypeptide or amino acid). The function of this gene is to make an enzyme that uses folic acid as a coenzyme. Therefore, if the mother's pregnancy develops under conditions in which she does not have a strong dietary source of folic acid and vitamin B_{12}, a developing embryo with such a genotype would be at higher risk for development of a neural tube defect than in the general population. The lack of folic acid (folate) and vitamin B_{12} before and during early pregnancy is a well-documented nutritional deficit related to the development of neural tube defects (Laurence, James, Miller, Tennent, & Campbell, 1991; Werler & Mitchell, 1993). The nurse should counsel all women contemplating pregnancy to take supplemental B vitamins with folate in the months before planned conception.

Pathophysiology

If the neural tube fails to close at the stage of development between approximately 18 and 26 days after conception, there are alterations of the axial skeleton as well as of the meningovascular and dermal coverings. Disorders of **primary neurulation** include anencephaly, myeloschisis, encephalocele, myelomeningocele, and Chiari malformation. Myelomeningocele and meningocele fall under the heading of spina bifida *cystica*.

Formation of the lower lumbar and sacral segments of the spinal cord is described as **secondary neurulation**. Development of spina bifida *occulta* can occur from day 28 of gestation through the end of the fetal period. This differs from the cystic form in that neither meninges, neural tissue, nor CSF herniate through the malformed structures of the spine. Myelocystocele, lipomas, dermoid cysts, and spinal cord tethering are the disorders that fall into the "occult" classification.

Hydrocephalus is often associated with myelomeningocele and Chiari malformation; these are also discussed in this section.

Anencephaly

Anencephaly is defined as a failure of anterior neural tube closure, resulting in only rudimentary development of the brain and no bony covering of the dorsal skull area. The primitive brain consists of portions of connective tissue, vessels, and neuroglia, with no cerebral hemispheres or cerebellum usually being present. The brain stem is difficult to identify, the pituitary gland is hypoplastic, and the spinal cord pyramidal tracts are missing. It is one of the most severe congenital neurologic anomalies. There is no specific treatment. Approximately 75% of the infants with anencephaly are stillborn; the remaining percentage of infants die in the neonatal period.

Assessment

As with many neural tube defects, prenatal diagnosis of anencephaly is possible using assays of fetal amniotic fluid, ultrasonography, or maternal serum to check for elevated alpha fetoprotein (MSAFP) concentrations (see Chapter 9). There are a number of false-positive results with MSAFP assays that may result in high, possibly unnecessary, prenatal anxiety for parents who understand the full implications of a child possibly born with a neural tube defect.

Clinical presentation involves portions of the forebrain and parts of the brain stem appearing to have little definable structure. The exposed neural tissue resembles a mass of hemorrhagic, fibrotic, degenerated neural tissue, and the frontal, parietal, and parts of the occipital bone structure are usually absent. The physical appearance of the infant is grossly abnormal. Additional anomalies that may be present include folding of the ears, cleft palate, and congenital heart defects. Health care professionals must be particularly sensitive in handling the postpartum experience with involved family members.

Interdisciplinary Interventions

Supportive care is given to the infant until all body functions cease. Social work and pastoral care may provide the most beneficial interventions in the acute time period; parents will likely require medical and nursing services to answer genetic and physiologic questions. Each family responds to the situation in different ways and it is important to approach their needs individually.

United States regulations do not permit organ donation from anencephalic infants because brain death criteria as established by the 1981 President's Commission are not fulfilled. This policy is controversial. In a California study, nurses wrestled with their beliefs and values to provide quality care for anencephalic infants. They felt challenged by the ethical issues of organ donation to assist viable recipients, yet wanted to preserve the rights of the affected baby to die with dignity.

Spina Bifida

Spina bifida refers to incomplete closure of the primary neural tube. The term *myelodysplasia* is often used interchangeably with spina bifida. The Spina bifida condition is one of several malformations of the neural tube that are often referred to as neural tube defects. The most commonly seen neural tube defects include anencephaly, encephalocele, spina bifida cystica (myelomeningocele and meningocele), and spina bifida occulta (see Table 21–9 and Fig. 21–4). Of the group of defects collec-

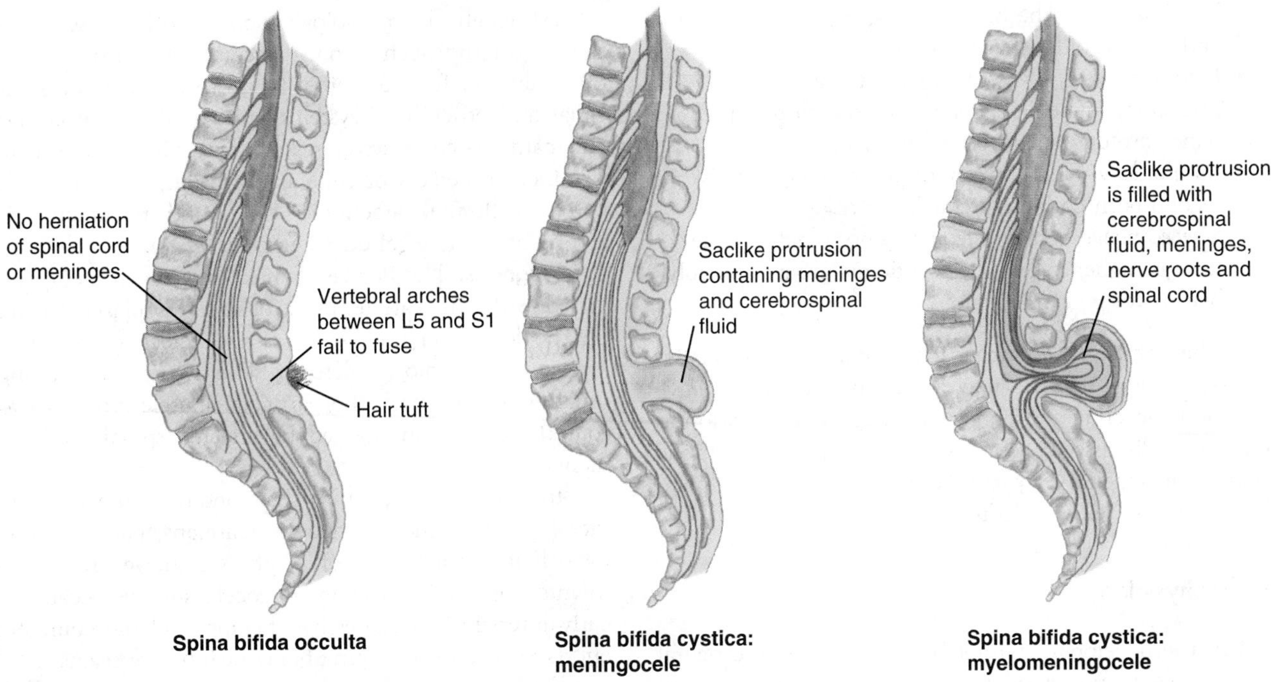

Figure 21–4
Malformations of the spine. (From Ashwill, J. W., & Droske, S. C. [1997]. *Nursing care of children: principles and practice* [p. 1233]. Philadelphia: W. B. Saunders.)

tively termed spina bifida cystica, 95% are myelomeningoceles, the most severe form of spina bifida. The remaining 5% are meningoceles, and because they do not involve the spinal cord, they may be easier to repair and are often asymptomatic.

Incidence

In the United States, the incidence of open neural tube defects is approximately 5 per 10,000 live births. The range of occurrences varies among states from 30 per 10,000 in Washington to 7.8 in Arkansas (Centers for Disease Control, 1992). Many countries, such as Ireland, report higher rates, with 4.2 cases per 1000 deliveries (CDC, 1992). The risk of having a second child with this disorder is approximately 5%, increasing to nearly 12% to 15% for a third child.

A number of anomalies are associated with myelodysplasia. These anomalies include cardiac defects, intestinal tract malformations, orthopedic deformities, and urogenital defects. Clinically, 85% to 90% of children with spina bifida have hydrocephalus and all affected children have a Chiari type II malformation. These children may also have sensory loss below the level of the lesion, neurogenic bowel and bladder, congenital hip dislocation, lower limb flaccidity, and a protuberant abdomen.

Etiology

There is no one identified cause of neural tube defects, and most occur as isolated malformations. The exact reasons for abnormal closure of the neural tube remain unclear. Neural tube defects may occur as a part of various chromosomal aberrations or after fetal exposure to teratogenic drugs. Isolated, nonsyndromic neural tube defects are recognized as being caused by many factors. This means that a combination of both genetic and environmental factors may interact in the development of the malformation (Reigel & Rotenstein, 1994). For example, if an individual had a genetic predisposition for a neural tube defect, an environmental trigger could act to manifest such a defect in that person's children. One or more trigger mechanisms can be involved, and they may vary among populations. Genetic and environmental components are considered to be additive, increasing a particular couple's risk for producing a child with neural tube defects (Reigel & Rotenstein, 1994). Many epidemiologic studies have been carried out to identify etiologic agents and to promote prevention of these defects. A variety of factors thought to contribute to the development of neural tube defects are as follows:

- *Poor nutrition*—Zinc, folate, and generalized vitamin deficiencies are particularly thought to be contributing factors.

- *Maternal age*—The highest risk groups are teenagers and women older than 35 years.
- *Pregnancy history*—Women who miscarry in the pregnancy immediately preceding the current pregnancy are thought to be at higher risk.
- *Birth order*—First-born children are at highest risk; second-born children are at lower risk.
- *Socioeconomic status*—Frequency of neural tube defects is higher in low socioeconomic groups, possibly because of poor nutrition.

The increased incidence of neural tube defects in siblings underscores the importance for families to have genetic counseling and proper periconceptual nutrition as previously discussed. Dietary sources of supplemental folic acid seem imperative, particularly in genetically vulnerable groups of families (Scott, 1995).

Pathophysiology

All of the developmental anomalies involving the neural tube are best understood by considering the normal embryologic development of the brain and spinal cord. At approximately 18 days of gestation, the nervous system begins to develop a thickened area of embryonic ectoderm called the neural plate. By the 22nd day of gestation, the neural plate begins to fold into the neural tube. This folding initially occurs centrally, and then proceeds in a somewhat irregular fashion superiorly and inferiorly. The upper opening of the neural tube is called the *rostral neuropore*, and the lower spinal opening is called the *caudal neuropore*. These neuropores close on the 25th and 27th days of embryonic life, respectively. The central lumen of the neural tube eventually becomes the ventricular system of the brain superiorly, and the central canal of the spinal cord inferiorly (Moore & Persaud, 1993).

Malformations of the neural tube usually involve malformations of the laminae and pedicles of the vertebral column (Moore & Persaud, 1993). The formation of the bony vertebral column occurs simultaneously with the formation of the neural tube, except that it originates from mesodermal, rather than ectodermal, cells. If the neural tube either fails to close properly on either end or becomes overdistended and ruptures after initial normal closure, then a neural tube defect of the varieties described earlier occurs.

The most common site of involvement in the spine is the lower thoracic lumbar or sacral area. Approximately 85% of lesions are located in that region, and the remaining 15% are located in the upper thoracic and cervical regions. The anterior aspects of the spinal cord are frequently intact, and varying degrees of destruction of the dorsal columns may exist (Reigel & Rotenstein, 1994).

Although the pathologic abnormalities observed at the site of the open spinal defect are the most obvious, other abnormalities are often found throughout the spinal canal and other body systems, such as the genitourinary and cardiovascular systems. Associated brain abnormalities include defects of cellular migration, agenesis of the corpus callosum, arachnoid cysts, and polymicrogyria, among others (Reigel & Rotenstein, 1994).

Prognosis. The degree of functional impairment associated with the various types of myelodysplasia depends on the level and the extent of the defect as well as of associated neurologic defects. The neurologic findings usually correlate with the particular muscle groups (myotomes) that are innervated by affected spinal cord segments.

In children affected by this condition, the mortality rate is high in the absence of treatment, particularly by overwhelming infection of a split sac; however, 90% of infants born with myelomeningocele survive because of early intervention, aggressive therapy, and the combined efforts of parents and spina bifida health care teams.

Except in cases of severe myeloschisis, extremely high myelomeningoceles, or concurrent serious medical problems, it is recommended that the lesion be surgically closed. In years past, families may have been told that without surgery these severely affected lesions would become infected, causing meningitis and rapid demise of the infant. This was a choice some parents made to avoid prolonging a severely limited life. Many of the infants who were expected to die lived despite infection. Therefore, except in rare cases, most children have operations to close the open lesion, even when overall prognosis may not appear favorable.

Assessment

Prenatal Diagnosis. Modern ultrasound and laboratory techniques have made possible the prenatal diagnosis of open spina bifida. In the early 1970s, an association between an elevated serum alpha-fetoprotein (AFP) level and the presence of an open neural tube defect was discovered. Many health care providers have since relied on AFP levels drawn between 16 and 18 weeks of gestation as a screening tool for open neural tube defects.

Initially, amniocentesis can detect elevated levels of MSAFP in the amniotic fluid. Alpha-fetoprotein and acetylcholinesterase are proteins found in large amounts in fetal CSF. MSAFP is detectable 30 days after conception, but peak levels occur at 10 to 13 weeks' gestation (Volpe, 1995). At this time, an open neural tube defect leaks CSF into surrounding amniotic fluid with concentrations four to five times those of normal pregnancies (Cotton, 1984). According to one report, the rate of false-positive findings using this procedure is less than 0.5% (Swaiman, 1994). Diagnosis is even more accurate when the amniotic fluid is screened for high acetylcholinesterase levels. Level II ultrasonography by qualified tertiary centers usually accompanies positive MSAFP levels discovered by amniocentesis and can be helpful in determining structural defects.

In the case of fetal myelomeningocele, MSAFP levels increase by 16 to 18 weeks of pregnancy. Although not as accurate as amniocentesis (80% detection rate), this screening measure is less invasive and more cost-effective, especially for low-risk mothers. Awareness that it is a ***screening*** measure leading to a complete diagnostic evaluation helps the nurse give appropriate knowledge to families who find themselves in this extreme situation (Swaiman, 1994).

Early detection of neural tube deformities can present moral and ethical dilemmas for parents. Any decision regarding the pregnancy is a highly charged issue, and great care must be exercised to support the family's choice. Education and counseling are vital parts of the process.

Postpartum Assessment. Immediately following the delivery of an infant with myelomeningocele, a comprehensive evaluation of the lesion, of the nerve involvement, and of the degree of hydrocephalus must be determined by a team of specialists. This evaluation is best accomplished in medical centers offering spina bifida teams and may require transportation of the infant to a tertiary care hospital. It is a time of major crisis for parents as they deal with an unexpected outcome of the pregnancy; their expectations of a perfect baby are shattered by the reality of the birth defect, by separation from the infant if the infant is transported, and by the need for critical medical intervention.

caREminder: *In addition to the appropriate delivery room routines, care is taken to protect the child's spinal or cranial lesion from injury and infection.*

As soon as possible, the infant is brought from the delivery room to the specialty care nursery to be monitored closely and to be examined by a neonatologist or pediatrician. A complete physical examination with attention to the neural tube defect itself, the presence or absence of hydrocephalus, and motor and sensory functional capacities is carried out. The possibility of associated cardiac, renal, or gastrointestinal conditions that might interfere with early surgery is ruled out.

The defect is examined in regard to size, level, and nature of tissue covering. Any leakage of CSF is noted. Palpation of the cranial sutures and fontanelles and a measurement of head circumference are performed. Development and movement of upper and lower extremities are assessed. Infants with thoracic or high lumbar lesions are often born with atrophied lower extremities. An initial evaluation of bowel and bladder function is also carried out. Because 90% of children with myelomeningocele have a form of neurogenic bladder, it is difficult to predict long-term function at the time of the newborn examination. Once an assessment of the infant is completed, a discussion with the family in regard to long-term prognosis should take place. The nurse must emphasize to the parents that surgery does not restore normal neurologic function, but only preserves existing function (Reigel & Rotenstein, 1994).

Ongoing Assessment. The dysfunction secondary to spina bifida can range from complete paralysis to minimal involvement, but is most often somewhere in between. A lesion at the middle thoracic level causes total paralysis of the lower extremities. The more common lumbosacral lesions generally leave the child with some degree of hip, knee, or ankle flexion, allowing for walking with either braces and crutches or with minimal assistive devices, depending on the functional level of the lesion. The closed or nonvisible lesions (spina bifida occulta) often go undiagnosed until later in childhood and are frequently not associated with any degree of impairment.

In most lumbosacral lesions, the muscles of the legs are affected, and the electrical responses of these muscles may vary. Sensory disturbances are usually symmetric but patchy. The sensory level is determined with a dermatome chart, which is used to delineate areas of skin innervated by each sensory spinal nerve. Club feet, scoliosis, contractures, and dislocated hips are common in children born with lesions of the lumbosacral area. Bowel and bladder dysfunction are almost always apparent, because the nerves that supply these organs are located in the sacral area. Bowel problems commonly include constipation or incontinence. The neurogenic bladder can make the child susceptible to retention of urine and resultant urinary tract infections, or the child may have problems with incontinence. Nursing assessment and care strategies are addressed separately after the discussion of therapeutic management. The clinical manifestations associated with all of the myelodysplastic lesions are only as clear as the diagnostic assessment of functional capacity. As in most instances of congenital CNS disorders, the true extent of dysfunction is often apparent only as the child grows and a clearer assessment of function is obtained. Recently, children with spina bifida were found to have a higher incidence of allergy to latex products than the general public. Repeated exposure to latex occurs through multiple surgical procedures, repeat daily catheterizations, exposure to latex gloves, and wheelchair tires. Nurses are in key positions to assist the family to understand this risk and to supply them with educational materials and non-latex equipment.

Nursing Diagnoses and Outcomes

Chart 21–3 presents a variety of nursing diagnoses that can be applied to the child with a neurologic condition. The following diagnoses are also specifically applicable to the child with spina bifida:

- **High risk for infection: meningitis, urinary tract infection, and decubitus**
  Outcomes: Child's lesion or incision remains protected to prevent infection.
  Child is free from urinary stasis.
  Child is free from breaks in skin integrity.
- **Risk for injury related to latex allergy**
  Outcomes: Child/family is able to identify and avoid substances containing latex.
  Latex precautions are implemented during all health care encounters.
- **Bowel incontinence related to decreased innervation to lower intestinal tract**
  Outcomes: Child is not constipated.
  Child learns measures to control bowel function.
  When appropriate for age, child participates in bowel training program.
- **Altered urinary elimination related to urinary retention associated with decreased innervation of bladder and sphincter**
  Outcomes: Child remains free from urinary tract infection.
  Child's bladder is emptied at regular intervals.
  When appropriate for age, child participates in bladder training program.

Interdisciplinary Interventions

Early neurosurgical treatment for the child is aimed at preventing infection such as meningitis (particularly if the myelomeningocele sac is leaking CSF) by surgical reduction and closure of the open lesion. The infant undergoes ultrasound or CT studies of the head to determine the degree of hydrocephalus present. In most cases, a ventriculoperitoneal shunt is placed to aid CSF drainage and to reduce intracranial pressure (Cotton, 1984). The treatment plan, therefore, is multifaceted, including both surgical and medical management.

Surgical Management. The goals of early operative care of spina bifida cystica are to preserve all neural tissue, to provide a normal anatomic barrier, and to control early progressive hydrocephalus. A sterile, constantly moistened saline dressing is maintained on the sac until the surgery is performed. The surgical procedure involves dissection of the exposed sac and closure of the dura mater and skin over the preserved neural tissue. When the defect is large, the assistance of a plastic surgeon is called for to perform skin grafting over the lesion. If hydrocephalus is present at birth, a ventriculoperitoneal shunting device may be placed at the time of initial closure. If the clinical features of hydrocephalus are not apparent initially, the child is assessed for this condition frequently. Hydrocephalus eventually develops in 80% to 90% of children with myelomeningocele (Reigel & Rotenstein, 1994).

Surgical repair of symptomatic spina bifida occulta, regardless of the specific anomaly, is undertaken relatively soon after diagnosis, although it need not be an "emergency procedure." The primary surgical aim in these cases is to free up the tethered or tied spinal cord so that progressive deterioration of function is arrested.

In cases of encephalocele, the timing of surgical intervention may vary, depending on the size, location, and extent of nervous tissue involvement. In severe cases, early death is common, usually related to complications of hydrocephalus, infection, or actual rupture of the encephalocele. In any of the aforementioned cases, when surgery is performed, the primary concerns of the neurosurgeon relate to wound integrity, prevention of infection and CSF leaks, and timely healing of the repair (Reigel & Rotenstein, 1994). Meticulous postoperative care is essential.

Medical Management. Once the neurosurgeon has repaired the cranial or spinal defect and has placed a ventriculoperitoneal shunt (if necessary), the neonatologist or the pediatrician becomes involved in postoperative management. Cardiopulmonary function and adequate nutrition are essential to wound healing. The child must lie prone for several days postoperatively to avoid pressure on the wound and to avoid possible CSF leaks that invite infection. Once the infant is less restricted in positioning and is allowed to be supine, then orthopedic, rehabilitative, and urologic consultations are obtained to better understand the child's functional capacity. Hip and spine roentgenographs, renal ultrasound, electrical muscle testing, and auditory testing are commonly done before discharge from the hospital. Close follow-up of fontanelle size and head circumference is also important. Normal well-child care routines and infant development are followed up as they would be for any child and should not be overshadowed by the special care requirements of these children. As the child heals from the surgery and discharge is planned, an assessment of the family's coping skills and available resources is essential to ensure a successful transition to home. It is normal for parents to still be grieving the birth of a defective child even as they feel relief that their child has recovered from surgery.

Postoperative Nursing Care. Postoperative evaluation of the child entails a determination of functional abilities, including motor performance and sensory deficits. Skin assessment, including observation of incisions from surgical closure or shunt placement and any pressure points or areas of breakdown, is essential. Bowel and bladder function, including patterns of elimination and problems secondary to poor function, such as urinary tract infection or bowel obstruction, should also be addressed. Other important elements of assessment include nutrition, mobility, and psychosocial adjustment of the child and the family to the disease and to its associated problems.

Postoperatively, the nurse is responsible for preventing infection of the repair site, observing for shunt malfunction, and observing for symptoms of infection. Monitoring for signs and symptoms of increased ICP includes obtaining serial daily head circumference measurements, checking for bulging fontanelles, and noting changes in the child's level of consciousness.

Preventing Infections. In the neonatal period, care of the protruding sac is extremely important. For an encephalocele covered with skin, the infant is positioned to avoid pressure on the lesion. If the encephalocele is in the occipital area, a foam "half donut" may be useful in positioning. The more common lumbosacral spinal myelomeningoceles are usually protected only by a thin membrane. A sterile, saline-soaked dressing is applied after the sac is examined for gross tears or leakage. Rather than being changed frequently, the dressing is usually kept moist with a sterile saline solution at regular intervals. The infant may be placed on a prophylactic broad-spectrum antibiotic if the defect appears to be infected, and meticulous care is taken to avoid any contamination of the sac by the child's stool and urine. Surveillance for signs and symptoms of meningitis should be carried out by the nurse. These signs and symptoms may include irritability, fever, feeding intolerance, and seizures. The physician should be alerted if any of these symptoms become apparent.

Postoperatively, the wound is treated aseptically, and the child is maintained in the prone position for several days to avoid both pressure on the incision and CSF leak. A protective barrier drape is used to prevent contamination by stool or urine, and must be changed when necessary. The neurosurgeon should be notified of any potential contamination. Frequent diaper changes may be necessary, because these children may be stool incontinent and void continuously.

Urinary tract infections are prevented by a bladder program that includes intermittent catheterization or, in more severe cases, surgical diversion techniques to protect the kidneys from infection. Nursing interventions include teaching children (when they are old enough) and parents how to perform intermittent catheterization and how to recognize urinary tract infections. Odorous or cloudy urine, pain on urination, increased irritability, and hematuria are common symptoms. The nurse should educate the family and should alert the urologic specialist about changes in bladder function throughout the child's developing years.

Pressure ulcer prevention can be accomplished with skin care geared toward optimizing skin integrity and toward avoiding pressure on any at-risk area. Areas requiring special attention include the spinal defect area, perianal area, sacrum, knees, elbows, ankles, and any area where sensation is diminished. If frequent dressing changes are required with the initial closure, the use of stomadhesive in two parallel strips around the incision can prevent skin breakdown from continual tape removal. After the dressing is changed, a barrier drape is pulled over the dressing to prevent contamination from stool below the closure. Often the best nursing care for skin breakdown in the anal area is to leave the child's buttocks exposed to air or to safely use a heat lamp to promote drying of the area. Another important factor in optimizing skin integrity is ensuring adequate nutrition for the child. As children grow, they should be taught to inspect their skin routinely and to avoid skin contact with potentially abrasive or thermal sources to prevent unnoticed skin breakdown secondary to decreased sensation.

Preventing Latex Allergy. It has recently become recognized that sensitivity to latex products such as gloves and urinary catheters poses a life-threatening health risk for patients with myelomeningocele. Although allergic reactions to latex are reported in only 1% of the general population, it has been estimated that between 18% and 40% of spina bifida patients may be affected.

caREminder: *Careful screening for latex and rubber allergies in the patient and family is an important part of the nursing history.*

The incidence of allergic reactions increases with age, because the older child has exposure over time to latex products like urinary catheters, latex gloves, and multiple surgical procedures (Leger & Meeropol, 1992).

The child with latex sensitivity should be premedicated with steroids or Benadryl before surgery or diagnostic testing. Caregivers should have nonlatex products available in operating rooms, emergency departments, and all other settings where care is likely to be given to latex-sensitive children.

Alert: *Prevention of anaphylactic shock by avoiding latex products (including toys, balloons, sports equipment, stethoscope tubing, and even adhesive tape) is the only effective mode of therapy (Vessey et al., 1993).*

All personnel who come into contact with the child (e.g., the nursing assistant who bathes the child or changes the child's diaper) must be educated to avoid exposure to latex products. Vinyl gloves are an acceptable alternative to latex gloves, which may trigger the anaphylactic response through contact with the skin. Finally, the child with latex allergy should be encouraged to wear a latex allergy alert bracelet to alert others to the risk of exposing the child to latex. Chapter 9 discusses the management of latex allergies.

Preventing Neurologic Injury. Rupture of the fluid-filled sac could lead to immediate death as a result of sudden decompression of CSF from the cranial cavity. Correct positioning for children with spinal lesions is in either the prone or side-lying position, depending on the function of the child's lower extremities. A flat position to decrease the pressure in the sac is also favored. A cloth roll under the infant's hips in the prone position is helpful in allowing for proper alignment of the lower extremities and for a downward flow of stool and urine away from the open lesion.

Between 80% and 90% of children with spina bifida manifest clinically significant hydrocephalus. Many children are shunted during the time of the back closure, whereas others are followed with serial ultrasound examinations and have a shunt placed, if needed, at a later date. Most children require shunting within the first few months of life (Reigel & Rotenstein, 1994). Nursing care includes surveillance of the appearance and the nature of the fontanelle, the sutures, and the child's head circumference. Infants who are not yet shunted should be placed on a cardiorespiratory monitor to watch for signs of apnea and bradycardia secondary to increased ICP. Lethargy, feeding intolerance, and seizures are also evidence of increasing ICP and of the need for shunt placement.

Preventing Orthopedic Injury. Neuromuscular and sensory deficits can lead to orthopedic problems, including scoliosis, kyphosis, hip dislocation, and ankle deformities. Joint stability may be affected by contractures, muscle control, and altered sensation (Rudy & Woodside, 1991). Nursing care to prevent injury includes teaching parents and children about safe activities and potentially risky ones. As children with this condition become more mobile, parents need to pay close attention to any changes in the child's use of or function of his or her limbs. Hip dislocation and limb fractures may go unnoticed for long periods of time, secondary to decreased sensation. The nurse should encourage routine orthopedic follow-up.

Promoting Optimal Bowel Elimination. More than 90% of children with spina bifida have a neurogenic colon. Fecal incontinence and constipation are the two most common problems and are related to the loss of parasympathetic innervation to the colon and the pelvic floor, to the loss of sensation to the rectum, and to the loss of motor innervation to the external anal sphincter (Rudy & Woodside, 1991). The nurse should encourage institution of a bowel program by toddlerhood. The five key elements to training the colon are timing, diet, exercise, posture, and rectal stimulation. The parents and the child should be taught to plan bowel evacuation following a meal and the child should eat a well-balanced diet that is high in fiber and low in carbohydrates. Exercising the lower portion of the body after the meal and adopting a knee-chest position to put pressure on the abdomen are measures known to aid in bowel evacuation. Finally, rectal stimulation with a suppository or by digital stimulation should be encouraged to initiate or to sustain the defecation reflex (Rudy & Woodside, 1991).

Managing the Neurogenic Bladder. The Credé maneuver (manual pressure applied from the umbilicus toward the symphysis pubis to express urine) has generally been replaced by clean intermittent catheterization. Drug therapy with anticholinergic drugs and surgical procedures, including bladder augmentation and placement of an artificial sphincter, are also common. Nursing care includes maintaining bladder programs in outpatient or inpatient settings, teaching parents signs of urinary tract infection, and addressing the psychosocial issues about bladder elimination.

Promoting Family Coping. The initial crisis following the birth of a "not-perfect" child must be effectively resolved if the family is to function well as a unit. Appropriate nursing strategies include grief work facilitation, that is, allowing the parents to grieve by being with them and listening to them. An example of a phrase that might be helpful in eliciting some of their feelings is "This isn't really what you expected, is it?" or "This whole event must be so overwhelming to you." Truth telling is another important intervention. The family needs to have honest information about the most immediate aspects of medical care—specifically, closure of the defect or potential for ventriculoperitoneal shunting, or both—if a procedure is to be done imminently.

The nurse is often the one person who has the knowledge, the skill, and the time to clarify any misconceptions, to repeat any information as necessary, and to assess the family values and perceptions about neural tube defects. Another important nursing intervention is to assess the support system enhancement and availability of resources. The parents may need assistance in mobilizing resources to help them care for a child with special needs.

Community Care

Caring for the child with spina bifida is a life-long commitment for families. The impact of medical costs as well as social and emotional concerns can be overwhelming. Management of the many stressors is difficult, but nurses can be instrumental in assisting families to cope with concerns and in directing care toward maximizing the child's abilities rather than focusing on disabilities (Chart 21–17; TIP 21–2).

Cognitively, the most consistent finding in children with myelomeningocele has been an overall reduction in intelligence quotient (IQ) and specific weaknesses of per-

Chart 21-17
Developmental Considerations

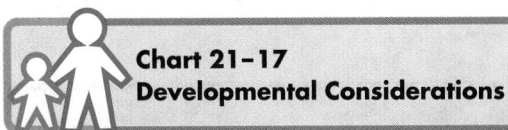

Teaching Needs of the Child with Spina Bifida

Infants (0–18 Months)

Focus teaching toward parents, siblings, relatives:

Teach skin care.
Teach bowel and bladder function.
Discuss nutrition.
Discuss signs of increased intracranial pressure.
Discuss activity and mobility.
Demonstrate methods to promote achievement of developmental milestones.
Select methods to promote family coping.

Toddlers (18–36 Months)

Continue teaching with family, begin including child:

Continue bowel and bladder program training.
Teach diet and weight management.
Identify behavioral concerns.
Teach activities to allow independence and autonomy.
Consult specialists to maximize mobility (braces, wheelchair).
Discuss availability of preschool or daycare.
Discuss behavior management.
Encourage socialization with other toddlers.
Encourage age-appropriate activities.
Teach skills to adapt home environment for child safety and mobility.

Preschoolers (3–5 Years)

Teaching directed toward family and child:

Continue with content identified for toddler years.
Discuss child's concept of spina bifida.
Obtain "Handicapped" tags for cars.
Encourage use of developmental toys and games.
Perform baseline intellectual function testing.

School-Age (5–12 Years)

Teaching more advanced concepts to child and parents:

Discuss body image.
Begin to use more medically correct terminology.
Encourage discussion of emotions and social supports.
Encourage peer interaction via summer camp and school groups.
Plan activities to promote sense of achievement.
Discuss accomplishments as well as failures.
Provide teaching and consults to school staff.
Begin teaching intermittent bladder catheterization.

Parental involvement:

Outline self-care activities within the child's ability level.
Assist parents with the child's psychosocial changes.
Discuss parent's concept of child's progress and needs.

Adolescence (12–18 Years)

Focus teaching on the adolescent:

Discuss issues of body image, sexuality, social interactions.
Teach self-care regarding bladder emptying, hygiene, skin care.
Encourage peer interaction to develop group identity.
Refer to nutritionist for diet and weight management.
Discuss theory of personal identity within family structure.
Suggest patient begin a journal for questions and concerns.

Parental involvement:

Stress importance of the child's need to be included in decisions.
Discuss methods to promote independence at home and school.
Begin transition to adult health care facility.

TIP 21–2 A Teaching Intervention Plan for the Child with a Repaired Neural Tube Defect

Nursing Diagnoses and Family Outcomes

- High risk for infection related to surgical incision, shunt infection, urinary retention, and immobility
  Outcomes: Child's incision site remains free from infection.
  Child remains free from urinary tract infections.
  Child's skin remains intact.
- Chronic urinary retention related to lack of innervation of bladder and sphincter
  Outcomes: Child remains free of urinary tract infection.
  Child remains free of constipation.
  Child participates in bowel and bladder training program when age appropriate.
- High risk for orthopedic injury related to neuromuscular and sensory deficits
  Outcome: Child remains free of contracture, alterations in skin integrity, and trauma to extremities with altered sensation.
- Altered growth and development related to sensorimotor limitations
  Outcomes: Parents participate in activities to promote child's developmental outcomes.
  Child achieves developmental milestones to highest level of ability given the sensorimotor limitations.

Teach the Family

Skin Care

- Examine skin daily for areas of redness or a break in the skin integrity.
- Provide wound care and dressing changes (if necessary).
- Turn child every 2 hours.
- Use sheepskin or air mattresses on areas of bony prominence.
- When removing splints and braces, assess skin for reddened areas.

Promoting Bowel and Bladder Function

- Establish routine and regular bowel program with suppository and stimulations.
- Credé bladder as needed.
- Institute bowel and bladder training program when age appropriate.

Nutrition

- Maintain good fluid intake to prevent constipation.
- Provide diet high in fiber to prevent constipation.
- Encourage intake of fluids such as cranberry, grape, and prune juices or those high in vitamin C to prevent urinary tract infections.
- Monitor child's weight.
- A low-calorie diet may be necessary.

Activity and Mobility

- Observe child's movements for signs of loss of sensation of lower extremities.
- Consult specialist to maximize mobility as child grows (braces, wheelchair).
- Perform passive range-of-motion exercises.
- Use proper positioning with pillows, pads, and rolls, as needed.
- Have child ambulate or sit in wheelchair whenever possible.
- Periodically evaluate adaptive equipment for damage, loose screws, alignment, or similar faults.

Growth and Development

- Modify home environment as child grows to ensure child's safety.
- Encourage stimulation with age-appropriate activities.

TIP 21-2 A Teaching Intervention Plan for the Child with a Repaired Neural Tube Defect *Continued*

- Encourage child to be as independent as possible.
- Teach alternative methods for personal hygiene and mobility.
- Praise child's independent behaviors.
- Allow child to ventilate feelings about self and interactions with peers.

Monitoring for Complications

- Monitor for signs of increased intracranial pressure (changed level of consciousness, changes in behavior, headache, vomiting, fever) that may be signs of shunt malformation.

Health Maintenance

- Organize and maintain child's medical records.
- Access community resources and support groups.
- Seek financial assistance as needed.
- Discuss babysitting and child care options.

Contact Health Care Provider If

- Redness or discharge is noted from site of surgical incision(s).
- Areas of the child's skin become reddened or there is a break in the skin surface.
- Urine becomes cloudy or foul smelling.
- Child displays changes in neurologic status as demonstrated by changes in level of consciousness, lethargy, irritability, vomiting, fontanelle seeming to be full.
- Child has fever.

ceptual motor function. Many children with spina bifida are able to attend regular schools and, with proper evaluation, are able to maintain attendance in age-appropriate classes (Tew, 1991).

Many factors affect the self-esteem of a child with spina bifida. These factors include mobility; physical appearance, including weight; family support; and experiences within the health care system. Nurses can promote healthy eating habits at an early age in accordance with the child's activities of daily living. Obesity is a common problem, particularly in adolescents with spina bifida. Involvement in wheelchair sports activities should be encouraged. Activities for improving self-esteem may have a direct impact on the child's desire to maintain a normal weight. Involving the whole family in these activities is paramount, because, to be truly successful, a program of weight maintenance or reduction must be a family-centered project.

Because children with spina bifida may have many operative procedures throughout their lives, providing for a successful operative experience is essential. Preoperative preparation should include age-appropriate play activities, and honest, but not scary, information about the procedure. Many of the orthopedic procedures required for these children involve long periods of rehabilitation in order to achieve the best results. Continual support and positive reinforcement from the nursing staff are important to the child's optimal recovery and function.

The collective goals for the interdisciplinary spina bifida team should be to provide ongoing support, understanding, and information, and to involve both the parents and the child in the decision-making process throughout childhood and into adulthood.

Hydrocephalus

The term *hydrocephalus* is derived from the Greek terms *hydro*, meaning water, and *cephalo*, meaning brain. Hydrocephalus is defined as a dilation of the ventricles inside the brain caused by an imbalance in the rate of production and rate of absorption of CSF. The two primary causes of congenital or acquired hydrocephalus are (1) a blockage of the flow of CSF and (2) impaired venous absorption of CSF in the subarachnoid space. A third and rare cause is the overproduction of CSF caused by a tumor identified as a choroid plexus papilloma. The clinical manifestations of this disease vary with the precise cause and duration of hydrocephalus, with the age of the child, and with the ability of the skull to expand (Kaney & Park, 1993).

Incidence

Congenital hydrocephalus occurs in approximately 0.5 to 1 per 1000 live births, and is usually readily apparent at birth or in the first 2 to 4 months of life (Carey, Tullous, & Walker 1994). Congenital etiologies include the following: Chiari malformations, congenital arachnoid cysts, congenital stenosis of the aqueduct of Sylvius, Dandy-Walker cyst, and other intracranial masses, including congenital tumors.

Acquired hydrocephalus occurs secondary to mass lesions, such as tumors, vascular malformations, or cysts, and scarring of CSF pathways occurs from infection of intracranial hemorrhage (Kaney & Park, 1993). Acquired lesions in infancy are more commonly a result of intracranial bleeding, meningitis, or both, resulting in fibrosis of the meninges, thus preventing reabsorption of CSF by the arachnoid villi. Infants born prematurely are at increased risk of intraventricular hemorrhage (Carey, Tullous, & Walker, 1994).

Pathophysiology

CSF is primarily manufactured in, and secreted by, the choroid plexus. This structure lines the base of the lateral ventricles and the roof of the third and fourth ventricles. CSF is produced at the approximate rate of 0.3 to 0.4 mL/min, or 25 mL/hr (Carey, Tullous, & Walker, 1994). From the paired lateral ventricles, CSF is propelled in a pulsatile fashion through the foramen of Monro to the third ventricle and then through the aqueduct of Sylvius into the fourth ventricle. From the fourth ventricle, the CSF flows through the foramen of Magendie and the paired foramina of Luschka into the subarachnoid space around the brain and spinal cord. The CSF is then reabsorbed by the arachnoid villi located in the dural sinuses, which are the large blood vessels draining the venous blood from the head. Small amounts of CSF are absorbed in the cells lining the ventricles and through the lymphatic system of the spinal cord (Fig. 21–5).

The terminology used to describe hydrocephalus has been confusing and unclear. Many of the terms used were useful before the era of modern diagnostic testing, when the site of the blockage may have been implied rather than precisely identified. The terms *communicating* and *noncommunicating* hydrocephalus are still used occasionally to describe the status of the ventricles in this disease. Communicating hydrocephalus describes a blockage "outside" of the ventricular system (e.g., meninges, arachnoid villi). The implication is that the ventricles communicate. Noncommunicating hydrocephalus implies a blockage somewhere in the ventricular system that prevents CSF from reaching the subarachnoid space for reabsorp-

Figure 21–5
Normal cerebrospinal fluid circulation and alterations that can cause hydrocephalus. (From Ashwill, J. W., & Droske, S. C. [1997]. *Nursing care of children: principles and practice* [p. 1238]. Philadelphia: W. B. Saunders.)

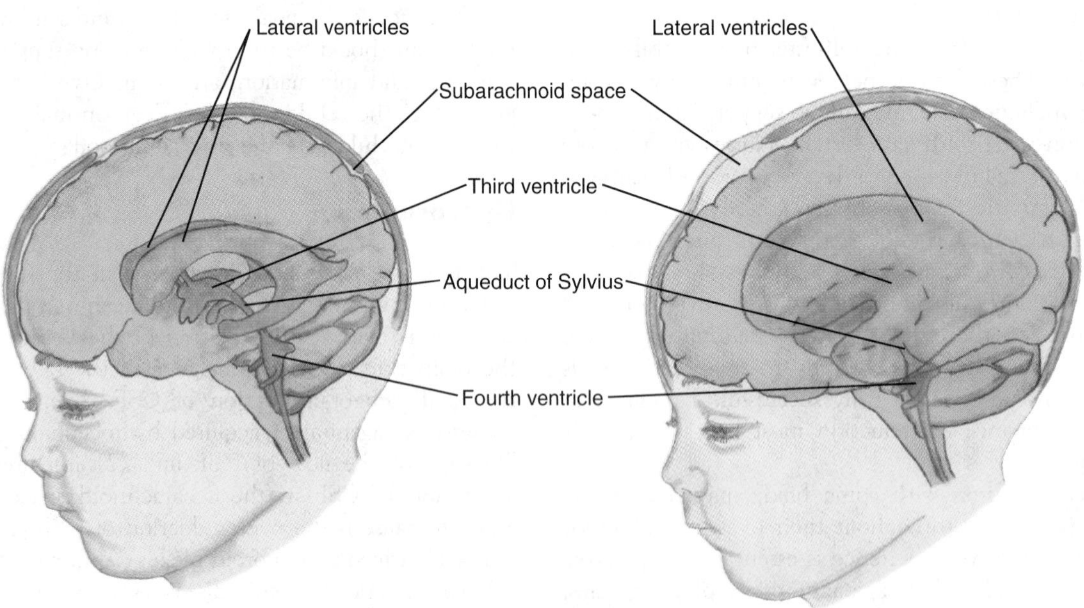

tion (Kaney & Park, 1993; Swaiman, 1994). Another way to classify hydrocephalus is to delineate when and how the hydrocephalus developed and to categorize the disorder as either *congenital* or *acquired* as described earlier. Most authors believe that it is best to classify hydrocephalus by the site of the blockage, by the cause, and by the state of progression.

Assessment

It is important for the nurse to begin assessment by collecting information on any history of trauma, CNS infection, familial megalencephaly, birth injury, or prematurity. The onset and duration of symptoms should be noted. A head circumference measurement is completed. An abnormal increase in head circumference above the established growth curve or a circumference that begins above the 95th percentile at birth should always raise suspicion of hydrocephalus. A full or bulging fontanelle, especially one that is nonpulsatile, indicating high pressure, should be noted. Other clinical signs and symptoms that become apparent as hydrocephalus progresses include increased motor tone, irritability, poor feeding, projectile vomiting, high-pitched cry, and cranial nerve palsies, resulting in the classic "sunset" (or "setting sun") appearance of the eyes, in which the sclera are visible above the iris and the infant is unable to look upward with the head facing forward (Chart 21–18). Collier's sign, upper eyelid retraction, may also be present and may occur with third ventricle lesions (Swaiman, 1994). Developmental delays or lack of acquisition of milestones is also common in children under 2 years of age.

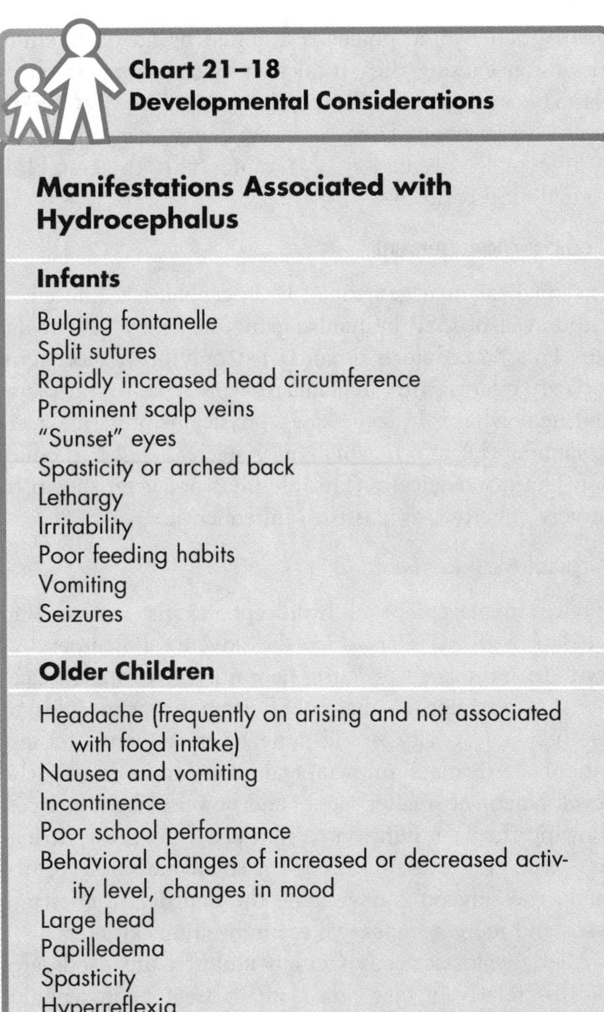

Chart 21–18
Developmental Considerations

Manifestations Associated with Hydrocephalus

Infants

Bulging fontanelle
Split sutures
Rapidly increased head circumference
Prominent scalp veins
"Sunset" eyes
Spasticity or arched back
Lethargy
Irritability
Poor feeding habits
Vomiting
Seizures

Older Children

Headache (frequently on arising and not associated with food intake)
Nausea and vomiting
Incontinence
Poor school performance
Behavioral changes of increased or decreased activity level, changes in mood
Large head
Papilledema
Spasticity
Hyperreflexia
New onset seizures, change in seizure pattern

In the older child with a fused cranium, signs and symptoms of hydrocephalus may develop either slowly or rapidly. Rapid development leads to acute neurologic deterioration. Signs of increased ICP in these children include frontal headache, nausea, and vomiting that may be projectile. If these symptoms occur on awakening, increased ICP should be suspected and the cause investigated. While asleep, the child retains CO_2, which, in turn, dilates cerebral vasculature. On awakening, the child's symptoms are exacerbated. Once the child is awake and CO_2 has decreased, the symptoms may temporarily subside. Decreased venous drainage while the child is lying flat may also contribute to morning symptoms. Other signs and symptoms include diplopia (double vision), restlessness, personality change, and ataxia. In later stages, bradycardia or altered respirations and seizures are life-threatening if not treated.

Diagnostic Tests. Early diagnosis of hydrocephalus may be done prenatally by level II ultrasonography of the fetus. This condition is not always detected by a screening ultrasound. Transuterine placement of ventriculoamniotic shunts during late pregnancy is being developed, but the technique remains controversial (Swaiman, 1994). Risks of this procedure include fetal demise and the same surgical and anesthesia risks of any surgical procedure for the mother.

In infants and children, radiographic evidence of hydrocephalus is most frequently obtained with a CT scan. In infants with an open fontanelle, ultrasound may be used. When a complex lesion is suspected, MRI may be used initially. Skull x-ray films may show widened or split sutures, and the skull may have a "beaten silver" appearance, characteristic of chronically increased ICP. Other rarely used radiographic tests include isotope cisternography or ventriculography to obtain a more accurate assessment of how CSF flows in the brain.

Interdisciplinary Interventions

Once hydrocephalus is identified, treatment is directed toward resolving the cause of obstruction. Resolution of the problem may be impossible for congenital hydrocephalus. When hydrocephalus is acquired by an older child, the lesion causing the obstruction (most frequently neoplasm) can be removed to allow the flow of CSF to return to normal. There are cases, however, in which even complete resection of a tumor fails to reestablish normal CSF pathways.

Medical Management

The medical management of hydrocephalus is limited to withdrawal of CSF by lumbar puncture or by ventricular tap. This procedure is usually tried only on a short-term basis in infants with inflammatory processes or intracranial hemorrhage. In some cases, physicians prescribe acetazolamide (Diamox), which may decrease CSF production pharmacologically. This drug has not been shown to be very effective, so it is tried infrequently.

Surgical Management

Surgical management of hydrocephalus has changed in the last 5 to 10 years since the advent of neuroendoscopy. In most large pediatric neurosurgery centers, placement of a shunt to drain CSF from the ventricles to another body cavity is still done to treat many of these patients. Advances in neuroendoscopy have led to the development of smaller scopes and powerful light sources, allowing the neurosurgeon to gain access to the ventricular space in the brain through a small burr hole. Once there, the surgeon can visualize the ventricles, fenestrate cysts, and more accurately place indwelling catheters.

IIIrd Ventriculostomy. Certain children are candidates for this relatively new procedure to treat hydrocephalus without the need to place a shunt. Criteria for selection include large ventricles at baseline, no evidence of abnormal absorption of CSF in the subarachnoid space (communicating hydrocephalus), and absence of previous infection and bleeding into the brain. Older children with acquired obstructive hydrocephalus are often appropriate candidates. The procedure is done under general anesthesia with a small incision. The scope is placed into the lateral ventricles and moved into the IIIrd ventricle where a small hole is punctured to create a natural opening for CSF to flow into the subarachnoid space. The recovery time is 1 to 2 days. The size of the ventricles on postoperative CT does not change rapidly as is sometimes the case with a shunt. Some of these children fail this procedure and eventually require the placement of a shunt (Walker & Meijer, 1995).

Mechanical Shunting Devices. The most common treatment for hydrocephalus is to reduce the intracranial pressure by surgically shunting the CSF from the ventricles to be absorbed in another body cavity. The most commonly chosen distal site is the peritoneal shunt, followed by either atrial or direct cardiac shunts, and, less frequently, pleural shunts.

The three main components of mechanical shunting devices are (1) ventricular catheter, (2) reservoir and valve to regulate flow of CSF and ICP (placed directly under the scalp on the skull bones) and (3) distal tubing (peritoneal, vascular, pleural). The CSF is drained by the distal catheter to the distal site where the CSF is resorbed into the body's fluids. The soft shunt tubing is palpable under the skin of the scalp and travels along the neck, where it is then placed into the distal site.

Ventriculoperitoneal Shunt. The ventriculoperitoneal location is chosen for most mechanical shunts (Fig. 21–6). After insertion of the ventricular tube through a cranial burr hole, the length of the shunt is tunneled subcutaneously to the upper quadrant of the abdomen. A small incision is made, and the shunt is guided into the peritoneal cavity with plenty of extra tubing to allow for the child's growth without having to perform further surgery to lengthen the shunt. Specific risks of this procedure include bowel perforation and ascites if the CSF is poorly absorbed.

Ventriculoatrial Shunt. The ventriculoatrial shunt is rare and is chosen only if a concurrent abdominal problem exists, precluding the insertion of a ventriculoperitoneal shunt. This shunt can be inserted into the right atrium of the heart by passage through the jugular vein, or, in more extensive cases, directly into the heart. Specific risks include catheter movement, dysrhythmias, operative risks associated with more extensive surgery, endocarditis, septicemia, and congestive heart failure (Greif & Miller, 1991; Marlin & Gaskill, 1994).

Ventriculopleural Shunt. Used very infrequently, the ventriculopleural shunt is chosen if either peritoneal or cardiac access is unobtainable. Children under the age of 8 to 10 years are not candidates. Because of the variable absorptive properties of the pleura, ventriculopleural shunts may not be as effective as the ventriculoperitoneal shunt. Specific risks include pleural effusion, resulting in respiratory compromise or infection, or both, from stasis of respiratory secretions. The child will require frequent chest x-rays to monitor expected pleural effusion.

Preoperative Care. The head of the child's bed should be elevated to 30 degrees. Cardiorespiratory monitoring and frequent monitoring of pupil size, motor movements, and level of consciousness are essential. Changes in status should be reported immediately, and medications (diuretics, analgesics) should be administered as ordered. If needed, the nurse should be ready to assist in the event of a ventricular shunt tap. Bulging or flatness of fontanelles should be recorded regularly. If the child is vomiting, intravenous hydration may be necessary. This should be administered at a rate of no more than 75% to 80% of *maintenance* fluid requirements. Other nursing interventions include decreasing external stimuli and having O_2 and suction ready at the bedside in case the patient has a seizure. In some centers a preoperative dose of IV antibiotics may be ordered as prophylaxis against infec-

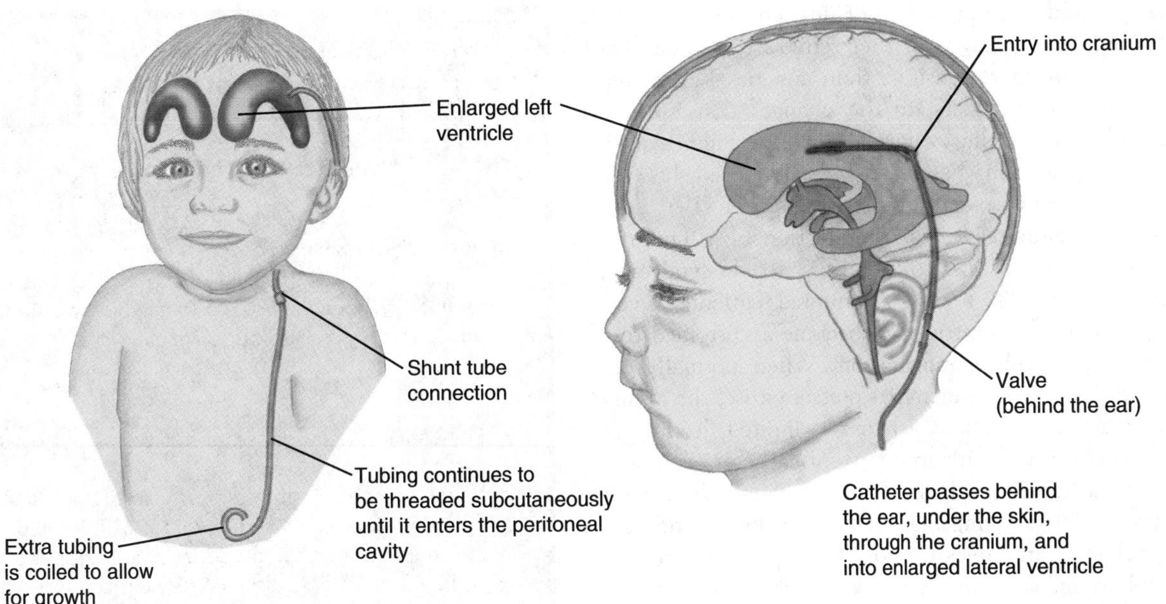
Enlarged left ventricle
Shunt tube connection
Tubing continues to be threaded subcutaneously until it enters the peritoneal cavity
Extra tubing is coiled to allow for growth
Entry into cranium
Valve (behind the ear)
Catheter passes behind the ear, under the skin, through the cranium, and into enlarged lateral ventricle

Figure 21-6
Placement of ventriculoperitoneal and ventriculoatrial shunts. (From Ashwill, J. W., & Droske, S. C. [1997]. *Nursing care of children: principles and practice* [p. 1239]. Philadelphia: W. B. Saunders.)

tion. Individual surgeon preferences for laboratory work or skin shampoo prep should be followed. Preoperative teaching and preparation of the child and family for the procedure should begin as soon as the decision to place a shunt is made.

Postoperative Care

Care of the Shunt. In caring for the shunt, the nurse may be responsible for teaching families and children about the shunt, its function, and how to manage follow-up care. Written handouts, preprinted booklets, and a structured teaching session should be a part of the preoperative plan.

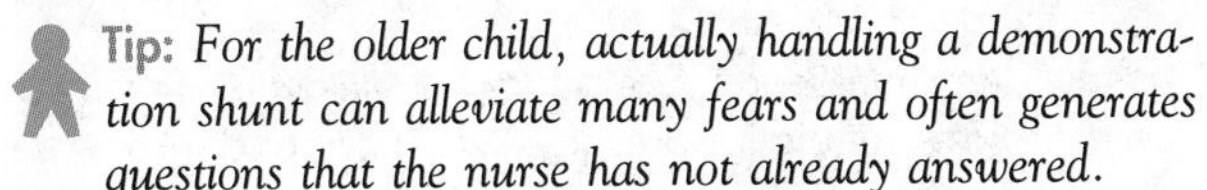
Tip: *For the older child, actually handling a demonstration shunt can alleviate many fears and often generates questions that the nurse has not already answered.*

Photographs of normal CT scans and those showing hydrocephalus are compelling comparisons, especially for parents. A brief overview can prove helpful in assisting families to understand the terminology and the equipment used.

Complications. Complications after shunt insertion include infection, shunt malfunction, and overdrainage of CSF. Infection rates vary from 2% to 40% and are largely dependent upon neurosurgical technique and duration of postoperative follow-up (Greif & Miller, 1991). The organisms most commonly isolated from infected shunts are *Staphylococcus epidermidis* and *Staphylococcus aureus*.

After the infecting organism is determined, intravenous antibiotic therapy is instituted. In organisms that are difficult to eradicate, intraventricular instillation of antibiotics may be useful. In most cases of shunt infection, the distal end of the shunt is externalized to a CSF collecting system until the bacteria are eradicated and a new shunt is placed. In nearly all cases of shunt infection, the shunt must be completely removed and replaced to achieve a "cure."

Shunt malfunctions may be hardware related (e.g., malposition or disconnection of the catheter). Obstructions of the tubing are often caused by infection or a build-up of fibrin debris and protein substances.

Alert: *Signs and symptoms of shunt infection or malfunction can be acute or chronic in nature, depending on the reason for it and the individual variables of the child's brain abnormality and compliance. Acute presentation includes rapid onset of vomiting, severe headaches, irritability, lethargy, fever, redness along the shunt tract, and fluid around the shunt valve.*

The child should be evaluated immediately to determine the extent of the problem and the need for possible shunt revision, so as to prevent further neurologic deterioration. Some children present with more insidious symptoms of shunt failure from infection or malfunction over a longer period. Occasional changes in school performance, intermittent headaches, and mild behavior changes are noted by those around the child, leading to eventual evaluation and determination of malfunction. Because parents are usually aware of their child's day-to-day behavior, they are more sensitive than anyone else, including health care providers, to the changes that indicate shunt malfunction. Nurses must listen to a parent's intuition, even if a shunt has recently been placed, because shunts may require several revisions (Chart 21–19).

Shunt overdrainage is a complication of a functioning shunt. This may lead to the **slit ventricle syndrome,** which occurs in 4% to 6% of shunted patients. Overdrainage causes the ventricles to become accustomed to a very small or slitlike configuration. When normally occurring variations in intracranial pressure arise, the ability of the ventricles to act as a buffer is limited, leading to symptoms consistent with intermittent catheter occlusion, like such as headache, dizziness, and nausea. These children present challenging management problems and may require changes in valves to more finely regulate pressure and siphoning. In rare cases, skull expansion may be recommended to deal with this problem.

Preventing Neurologic Compromise. Nursing interventions to prevent neurologic compromise are the same as those for increased ICP. Children who experience a rapid decrease in ventricular size are susceptible to the development of subdural fluid collections after shunting. Nursing assessment for this problem as well as blockage of a newly placed shunt includes watching for signs of neurologic deterioration after an initial period of recovery or signs of slow and incomplete recovery. Any of these trends should be reported to the physician so that appropriate radiographic tests can be ordered.

Preventing Skin Breakdown. Many children who require ventricular shunting have fragile infant skin. Nursing interventions include avoiding the application of cardiac lead patches, temperature probes, or unnecessary tape over the shunt site. Careful attention should be given to the scalp, because it is often stretched and is therefore more susceptible to breakdown. A small, newborn infant may be placed on a waterbed during the initial postoperative phase to prevent pressure on the skin around the shunt.

Providing Pain Relief. Both pharmacologic and nonpharmacologic comfort measures should be used to keep the child comfortable during the postoperative period. Analgesics should be carefully titrated to provide relief for the child while allowing for adequate neurologic assessment.

Preventing Infection. The nurse must pay close attention to the integrity of the surgical incisions and must ensure that the child keeps his or her hands away from the fresh incision. A stockinet cap may be useful. Appropriate administration of antibiotics is essential, if they are ordered postoperatively. Close monitoring of the child's temperature postoperatively is also essential.

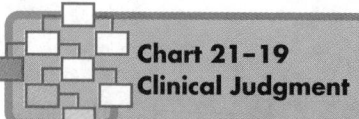

Chart 21–19
Clinical Judgment

The Child with a Ventriculoperitoneal Shunt

Three-month-old Shila had a ventriculoperitoneal shunt placed 2 weeks ago following a diagnosis of congenital hydrocephalus. The family has returned to the clinic for a follow-up appointment.

Questions

1. How could the diagnosis of hydrocephalus be assessed in one so young?
2. What concerns might parents have at this time?
3. Shila has a fever of 101° F and it is noted that the shunt incision site is reddened and not healing well. What nursing diagnosis would be appropriate for the child with a shunt infection?
4. What health care interventions are appropriate to treat Shila's ventriculitis?
5. Family teaching is given regarding management of the child's shunt. What information should the family be able to relate back to the nurse to indicate that effective teaching has taken place?

Answers

1. During well-child visits at 1 and 2 months of age, an abnormal increase in head circumference may be noted. Other findings that are suspicious include a full or bulging fontanelle, increased motor tone, developmental delays, irritability, high-pitched cry, poor feeding, projectile vomiting, and cranial nerve palsies resulting in the classic "sunset" appearance of the eyes.
2. Is the shunt working? How can they tell if it is working? Will their child be normal?
3. High risk for infection related to placement of ventriculoperitoneal shunt.
4. First the shunt is tapped to look for suspected bacteria. Antibiotics are given correctly and in a timely manner. Vancomycin in conjunction with gentamicin or a broad-spectrum cephalosporin is initially given. Antibiotics are readjusted based on the determination of the cultures and susceptibility outcomes. Acetaminophen is given for fever. Monitor for signs of improvement or worsening. Provide comfort measures.
5. Family knows signs and symptoms of increased intracranial pressure and shunt malfunction, proper handling of child with new shunt, home safety measures, and indications for calling the health care provider if problems occur.

Community Care

Home care instructions for parents include monitoring for signs and symptoms of shunt malfunction, proper handling of the infant with a new shunt, home safety, and indications for calling the physician if problems occur (Chart 21–20).

It is imperative that the health care team and the family establish trust and good communication. Maintenance of a therapeutic relationship involves ongoing education, mutual decision-making, and the creation of a supportive atmosphere for verbalizing questions and concerns. Nurses facilitate this process by teaching, initiating care conferences, and organizing resources to assist families.

Children should be closely followed up with developmental screening either in the school setting or with routine medical checkups. Most parents are concerned with the effect that hydrocephalus may have on their child's intelligence and development. The degree of disability depends on several factors, including the severity of hydrocephalus, the presence of other brain anomalies, and the presence of conditions such as intraventricular hemorrhage, infection, and hypoxia (Swaiman, 1994). It is generally agreed that normal intelligence is enhanced if shunts are placed early, proper function is maintained, and infection is avoided.

Chart 21–20
Community Care

Home Care of the Child with a New Shunt

Positioning

Physician may recommend placing child on unoperated side to prevent pressure on the shunt valve.
Elevate head of bed to enhance gravity flow through the shunt.

Skin Care

Observe operative site for redness, puffiness, or oozing of fluid.

Care of Shunt

Pump shunt *only* if instructed by physician.
Depress valve area firmly and quickly with forefinger. Leave finger on pump to feel it refilling. If it is difficult to depress, do not force. Call health care provider.
Observe for blockage or infection: increasing drowsiness, vomiting, headache, irritability, restlessness, swelling around pump, persistent bulging of fontanelle, fever, poor feeding, seizure activity.

Chiari Malformation

Chiari malformations are congenital anomalies of the structures at the junction of the brain and the spinal cord. This anatomic area is often referred to as the cervicomedullary junction. The condition was first described by Chiari in 1891, with insight to this particular problem further described by Arnold. In 1907, Arnold's colleagues coined the term *Arnold-Chiari malformation* to label the hindbrain malformations. Historical investigation of this anomaly by Oakes (1985) revealed that very little insight into the problem was actually added by Arnold; therefore the term *Chiari malformations* is more commonly accepted.

Two other diagnoses associated with Chiari malformations are *syringomyelia*, or *syrinx*, and *hydromyelia*. The former describes a cavity lying outside the central canal area of the spinal cord that is not lined by ependymal cells, and the latter is a cavity within the spinal cord that is partially or completely lined with ependyma. All three diagnoses are frequently discussed in conjunction with each other because of their similar clinical presentations and their probably common pathophysiologic development (Oakes, 1985).

Pathophysiology

Chiari malformation is characterized by abnormalities of anatomy and physiology (Fig. 21–7). Primary anomalies of the hindbrain and skeletal structures, in turn, produce mechanical deformities (Menkes, 1995).

Four variations of the Chiari malformation exist, the most common being type II (Swaiman, 1994). Each type is defined by associated structural anomalies and by the symptoms they produce. Chiari type I presents most often in adolescents and adults. The condition is characterized by a displacement of the cerebellar tonsils into the cervical canal. The clinical features of Chiari type I malformation include malformation of the base of the skull and upper cervical spine. Klippel-Feil syndrome, hydromyelia, syringomyelia, and diastematomyelia are frequently present (Menkes, 1995). Because the progression of symptoms is often slow, it may go undetected for many years (Dauser, DiPetro, & Venes, 1988).

Chiari type II is found in infants and is the most common of the malformations. Chiari type II is characterized by downward displacement of the cerebellar tonsils and medulla through the foramen magnum. As the cerebellar tonsils at the base of the spine protrude downward into the foramen magnum of the cervical spine,

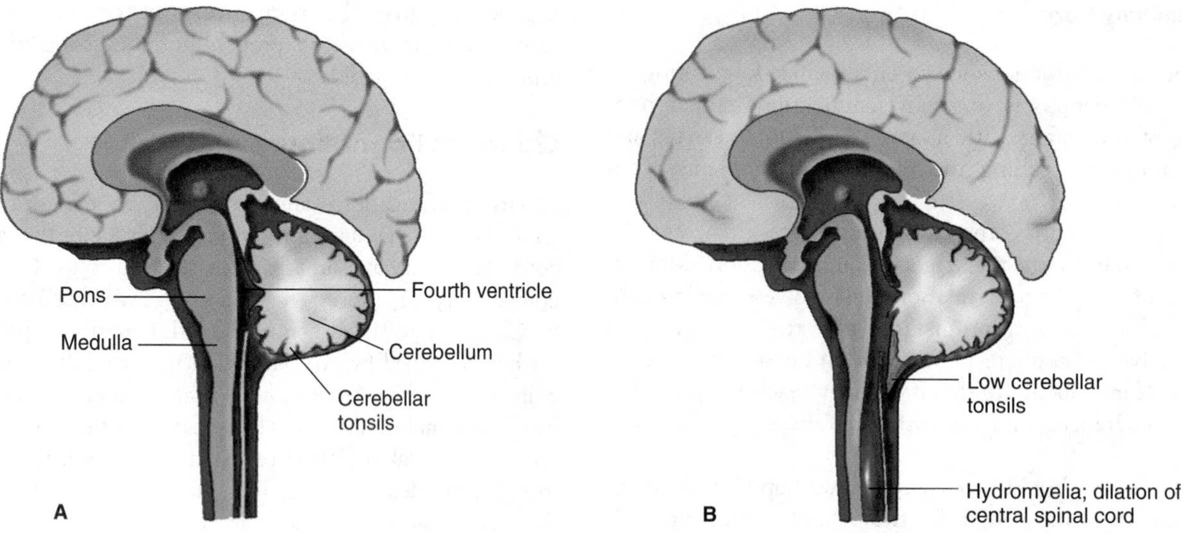

Figure 21–7
Normal posterior fossa *(A)* and Chiari malformation with hydromyelia *(B)*.

there is blockage of normal CSF pathways, and the fourth ventricle becomes dilated with CSF. Signs and symptoms of hydrocephalus occur. It is theorized that aqueductal stenosis, when associated with myelomeningocele, does not cause hydrocephalus, but rather results from compression caused by expansion of the fourth ventricle. Nearly every case of thoracolumbar, lumbar, and lumbosacral myelomeningocele is accompanied by the Chiari type II malformation. Hydrocephalus is also associated with type II in 80% to 90% of cases. In addition to the complications of the myelomeningocele lesion, other common problems occur, including apnea, laryngeal stridor, and feeding disturbances such as reflux and aspiration. Functional compromise of lower cranial nerves may occur. Ataxia and nystagmus indicate cerebellar impairment, and there may be increased deep tendon reflexes, loss of vibration and position sense, and recurrent occipital and frontal headaches (Swaiman, 1994). Despite careful treatment of the myelomeningocele lesion and hydrocephalus, research has indicated that approximately one half of the deaths of infants with myelomeningocele can be attributed to hindbrain anomalies that affect vital physiologic processes (Volpe, 1995). The age of presentation of symptoms of Chiari type II has implications regarding prognosis. The earlier the symptoms appear, the more likely it is that brain stem nuclei are hypoplastic and the poorer the prognosis.

Type III Chiari malformation is essentially an occipital encephalocele, and consists of an opening of the skull and cervical area with protrusion of the cerebellum through the opening. Type IV consists of a single abnormality, failure of the cerebellum to develop, and may be a variation in the Dandy-Walker syndrome (Swaiman, 1994).

Assessment

The clinical examination focuses on the most common signs and symptoms of the Chiari type II malformations. These include nystagmus, nuchal rigidity, poor suck reflex, drooling, difficulty swallowing, vomiting, weak or absent cry, and inspiratory stridor during agitation. In more severe cases, episodes of apnea may be reported. In older children, decreased strength in upper extremities with increased tone and exaggerated deep tendon reflexes may also be present. The adolescent with Chiari type I malformation is likely to have occipital headaches, neck pain, urinary infrequency, and progressive lower limb spasticity and scoliosis.

Diagnostic Tests. Radiographic techniques are used to demonstrate the type and extent of the lesion, including the presence of hydromyelia or hydrocephalus. Plain roentgenographs of the skull and spine are obtained. MRI is being used to replace other more invasive techniques for imaging this disease. MRI is particularly useful in identifying the anatomy in this area and in providing for accurate diagnosis.

Interdisciplinary Interventions

Management of infants and children with a Chiari malformation requires careful monitoring by MRI scans and by reporting of clinical signs and symptoms to determine the extent of neurologic involvement associated with the condition. Surgery may be recommended to decompress the suboccipital and cervical area.

Surgical decompression involves removing the posterior aspect of the foramen magnum and excising the upper cervical vertebral arches. This decompression alleviates the pressure on the fourth ventricle and the affected cranial nerves, hopefully allowing for an arrest of symptom progression. Beside bony decompression of the area, many surgeons incise the dura and place a graft to allow further decompression of the anatomic structures. The grafts are commercially available products like bovine pericardium. Postoperatively, some of these children who have received grafts develop symptoms of meningeal irritation, which is self-limiting but bears close watching to rule out infection. Some children show only little objective improvement, and existing preoperative deficits may be permanent. The goal of the surgery is to prevent further symptoms, rather than to relieve existing ones, although the latter usually occur to some degree. Ventriculoperitoneal shunts are placed to treat hydrocephalus, and as they are rarely removed, patients are followed up by a neurosurgery team throughout their life.

If signs and symptoms are not life threatening, a conservative approach is undertaken in the hope that the child will stabilize and outgrow the symptoms.

Nursing measures postoperatively are the same as those described for cranial surgery. Special attention is given to avoiding respiratory distress and respiratory infection. Airway function and protection may be altered owing to preexisting symptoms and compromise during surgery. Placement on a cardiorespiratory monitor is warranted, with oxygen and suction available at the bedside of the child to be used as needed. Infants or children with poor gag and swallow reflexes should be fed slowly and should be placed in an upright position after feeding to avoid aspiration and pneumonia.

The nurse should ensure that adequate control of postoperative pain is provided to the child. Neurologic assessments assist in determining whether overmedication or postoperative complications have occurred. Parents should be taught to assess changes in their child's neurologic status and to recognize impending signs of respiratory problems. Parents should also report any signs of incisional redness or irritation. The need for occupational therapy to adapt feeding or stimulation programs to meet the child's functional capacity should be addressed before discharge if the child will later require a referral.

Craniofacial Abnormalities

Craniofacial malformations may occur as a result of genetic influences, multifactorial prenatal influences, acute craniofacial trauma, and disfigurement associated with cranial or facial tumor resection. Advances in imaging techniques and three-dimensional reconstructive surgery techniques have resulted in improved methods to enhance the physical appearance of affected children. Recent developments in fetal surgery offer the potential of treating selected anomalies in utero. This section discusses some of the most common craniofacial malformations seen in the pediatric population that occur as a result of alterations in normal development.

Microcephaly

Microcephaly is defined as a head circumference that measures three standard deviations (SD) below the mean for the child's age and gender (Haslam, 1996). Primary microcephaly (genetic) refers to a small head circumference caused by a genetic inheritance pattern or associated with a specific genetic syndrome. Inheritance may be autosomal recessive or autosomal dominant. Associated genetic syndromes include trisomy 21, trisomy 18, cri du chat, and Cornelia de Lange. Infants with these conditions are usually identified at birth because of their small head circumference.

Secondary microcephaly (nongenetic) can occur as a result of a variety of noxious agents that may affect the fetus in utero or during times of rapid brain growth (most commonly in the first 2 years of life). Teratogenic agents include radiation, congenital infections (such as with cytomegalovirus, rubella, and toxoplasmosis), maternal ingestion of drugs or alcohol, meningitis or encephalitis, malnutrition, maternal diabetes, hyperthermia, and hypoxic-ischemic encephalopathy.

Assessment

Measurement of head circumference and visual inspection of the newborn may reveal a very small head. This indicates that the microcephalic process began early in fetal development. Serial head circumference measurements of neonates performed as a part of health care visits to complete developmental surveillance may also reveal small head circumference. The head circumference of parents and siblings should be recorded to evaluate for familial tendencies.

The child is assessed for other physical and congenital abnormalities, such as abnormal facies, short stature, deformities of the hands, and congenital heart disease.

Diagnostic Tests. Karyotypes are obtained if a chromosomal syndrome is suspected. CT or MRI scanning may be performed to assess for structural abnormalities of the brain or intracerebral calcifications. Additional blood and urine analyses are completed to determine specific causative agents such as infection with cytomegalovirus, rubella, or herpes simplex.

Interdisciplinary Interventions

There is no treatment to alter or reverse the child's small head circumference. Care for the child and family is based on treatment of the causative agent (if known) to minimize further body system involvement. Most children with microcephaly experience some degree of mental retardation. The health care team must work in collaboration with the family to help optimize the child's developmental outcomes in light of the existing neurologic damage. Chapter 29 presents more information regarding care of the mentally retarded child.

Craniosynostosis

Craniosynostosis is a term that describes the absence of, or the premature fusion of, one or more cranial sutures that join the bony plates in the skull. The term *craniostenosis* is often used synonymously with craniosynostosis. Craniostenosis describes the deformity that results from the early fusion of the sutures. Craniosynostosis refers to the process of early suture closure.

Craniosynostosis is classified as primary, secondary, or syndromic. Primary craniosynostosis may be either simple or compound. *Simple synostosis* refers to the involvement of one suture, whereas *compound synostosis* refers to the absence or to the early fusion of two or more of the cranial sutures. Most cases of primary craniosynostosis present as an isolated problem and are not associated with any other syndromes or anomalies (Chart 21–21).

Chart 21–21

Genetic Disorders Associated with Craniosynostosis

Disorder	Characteristics
Crouzon's syndrome	Inherited autosomal dominant trait Premature craniosynostosis Most often, head shape is compressed back-to-front diameter (brachycephalic) Bilateral closure of coronal sutures Orbits underdeveloped with ocular proptosis Hypoplasia of maxilla Increase in interocular distance
Apert's syndrome	Inherited autosomal dominant trait Premature fusion of multiple sutures, including coronal sagittal, squamosal, and lambdoid Symmetrical face Less displacement of the eyes Complex syndactyly of the fingers and toes Progressive calcification and fusion of bones in hands, feet, and cervical spine
Carpenter's syndrome	Inherited autosomal recessive trait Multiple suture fusion to create kleeblattschädel skull deformity Soft tissue syndactyly of hands and feet Mental retardation common May have presence of other abnormalities: congenital heart disease, corneal opacities, coxa valga, and genu valgum
Chotzen's syndrome	Inherited autosomal dominant trait Asymmetric craniosynostosis and distortion of head shape Facial asymmetry Ptosis of eyelids Shortened fingers Soft tissue syndactyly of second and third fingers
Pfeiffer's syndrome	Inherited autosomal dominant trait Turricephalic (oxycephalic) shaped head Prominent and widely spread eyes Thumbs and great toes short and broad

Secondary craniosynostosis occurs as a result of a known disorder that results in failure of brain growth and expansion. Various metabolic and hematologic disorders such as hyperthyroidism and thalassemia may lead to early fusion. The failure of brain growth that occurs in microcephaly may also lead to early suture closure.

Syndromic craniosynostosis involves closure of multiple sutures and occurs in conjunction with other morphologic syndromes or developmental anomalies (see Chart 21–21). In these cases, development of facial bones is also affected and increased ICP can be a serious secondary complication.

Etiology and Incidence

The etiology of craniosynostosis is unknown. It is generally believed that the cause is multifactorial. Genetic syndromes account for 10% to 20% of all cases. The incidence is 1 per 2000 live births, with males being affected twice as often as females (Haslam, 1996).

Pathophysiology

Figure 21–8 shows a superior view of the normal infant head. Five cranial sutures allow the rapidly developing brain to grow at a normal rate. Three of these sutures—the coronal, lambdoidal, and squamosal—are paired. The posterior and anterior fontanelles close at approximately 2 to 3 months and 12 to 18 months, respectively.

Cranial Bone Development. The cranial bones originate as a series of ossification centers that emerge from the fibrous embryologic cerebral capsule. At a later point, the cerebral capsule actually develops into the outer and inner layers of the dura mater. In early fetal life, the brain and cranial bones expand rapidly, although their borders (eventual suture sites) are widely separated. When the rate of brain growth slows down later in fetal life, the bones become more closely approximated, allowing for the eventual formation of a suture. The suture itself is not thought to have potential for actual cell proliferation, but rather it acts as a site of adaptation during growth by allowing for new bone generated from the cerebral capsule to be deposited and resorbed in a continuous and progressive fashion. In essence, the sutures grow in response to the changes and needs of the developing brain, particularly its fibrous covering.

The cranial bones grow perpendicular to each of the cranial sutures. For example, the sagittal suture allows for growth of the parietal skull bones in a lateral fashion, thereby adding to the width of the skull. When this suture is absent or closed, growth is inhibited in the lateral direction, and instead, growth occurs parallel to the ossified suture.

Cranial asymmetry in the presence of craniosynostosis is determined by the number of sutures involved and the rate and degree of fusion. The rule of thumb in remembering how head shape will appear is that growth is inhibited at right angles to the fused suture with compensatory expansion occurring at the sutures that are functional. When diagnosing craniosynostosis, the Greek terminology may be used to classify the synostosis; however, it is more important that a clear description of the suture or sutures involved and the degree of fusion be thoroughly described (Cohen, 1986). The earlier in fetal or infant life that synostosis occurs, the more dramatic is the effect in cranial growth and appearance; the later synostosis occurs, the less dramatic is the child's appearance.

Assessment

Craniosynostosis may be suspected at birth or may be detected at later visits to health care providers. In many cases, parents are the first to notice abnormalities in the shape of the infant's head.

When a diagnosis of craniosynostosis is suspected, a thorough "hands-on" assessment of the child's cranium is necessary. Palpation of the head for suture location and mobility is essential. Bony ridges along suture lines and any facial or cranial asymmetry are noted. Asymmetry can be evaluated by comparing the location of the external ear canals and the outer canthi of the eyes from right to left. This comparison is best made with the examiner looking down on the infant or child from a superior position. The examiner should move the child's hair away from the child's forehead during examination, especially when synostosis of the metopic or either coronal suture is suspected.

Measurement of the child's head circumference is vital. Many infants with craniosynostosis initially have a mild to moderate fall-off in this measurement. Height and weight parameters and head circumference need to be measured simultaneously to ensure that the child is not failing to grow on all parameters for other reasons.

A complete neurologic examination is an essential component of the assessment. Included in this examination are evaluation of sensory and motor function, cranial nerve findings, and the presence of chronic increased ICP. A developmental evaluation is completed to determine cognitive function, achievement of age-appropriate gross and fine motor skills, and speech and language development. The family history may reveal genetic or syndromic findings in other family members, living or dead.

Diagnostic Tests. Once the primary health care provider suspects a diagnosis of craniosynostosis, a referral to a neurologist or neurosurgeon is made. Diagnostic evaluation continues with the completion of radiographic studies and a CT scan. CT studies should include "bone windows" along with coronal and axial views. Bone win-

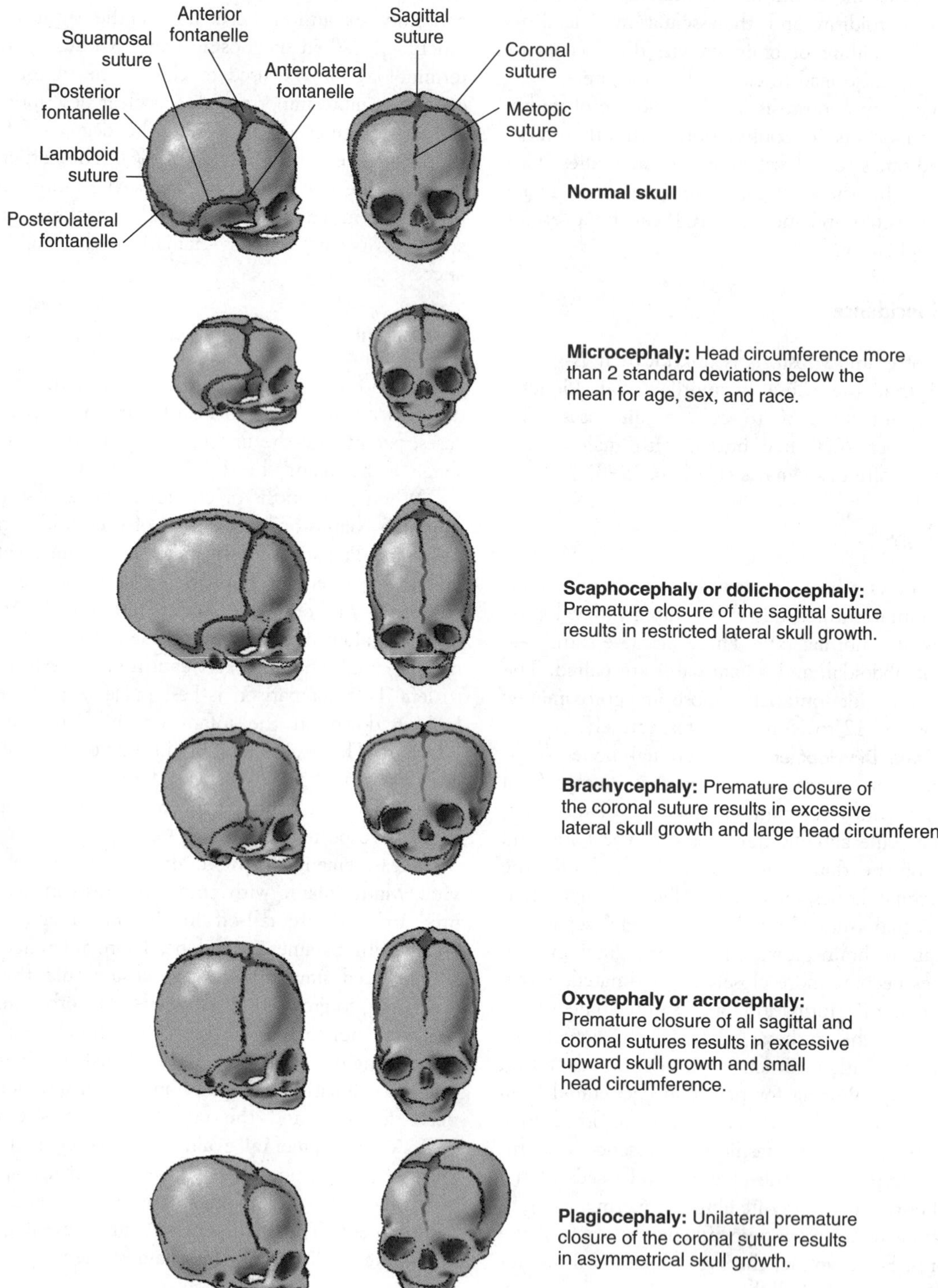
Anterior fontanelle
Squamosal suture
Sagittal suture
Coronal suture
Anterolateral fontanelle
Posterior fontanelle
Metopic suture
Lambdoid suture
Posterolateral fontanelle
Normal skull
Microcephaly: Head circumference more than 2 standard deviations below the mean for age, sex, and race.
Scaphocephaly or dolichocephaly: Premature closure of the sagittal suture results in restricted lateral skull growth.
Brachycephaly: Premature closure of the coronal suture results in excessive lateral skull growth and large head circumference.
Oxycephaly or acrocephaly: Premature closure of all sagittal and coronal sutures results in excessive upward skull growth and small head circumference.
Plagiocephaly: Unilateral premature closure of the coronal suture results in asymmetrical skull growth.

Figure 21–8
Normal skull and variations that result from premature closure of cranial sutures.

dow images highlight the outline of the skull bones, in contrast to the dark, solid presence of cortical tissue.

Interdisciplinary Interventions

Before therapeutic management begins, it is essential to assess the family's goals and concerns. Despite the child's physical appearance, family members may not think that treatment is indicated. The physician must clearly delineate whether intervention is indicated for purely cosmetic correction or, more importantly, whether the child requires treatment to reduce the risk of neurologic impairment. If the cranial bones are not able to expand with the brain's growth, the child may experience increased intracranial pressure. The symptoms are progressive papilledema, impairment of vision, and changes in mental status such as increased irritability or lethargy.

Surgical Management. The goals of surgical management for the child with craniosynostosis are to prevent development of increased intracranial pressure and to correct the cosmetic deformity of the skull and facial bones. The decision to correct craniosynostosis surgically is based on the severity of the deformity, on the number of sutures thought to be synostosed, and on the child's present neurologic and developmental condition. Surgical interventions are usually undertaken between 3 months and 1 year of age when the child's bone is still pliable and easy to work with.

The choice of surgical technique depends primarily on the individual surgeon and his or her philosophy and experience. Techniques among surgical centers vary and range from aggressive reconstruction to placement of synthetic materials to recreate symmetry. Techniques include the removal of strips or large portions of bone alone and/or reconstruction of the removed bone to reshape the skull. In other instances, synthetic materials are placed along cut bone edges around the affected suture to prevent reclosure after surgery. Acrylic onlays to correct an asymmetric appearance of the skull and plication or incision of the dura mater to reshape the underlying brain are also techniques used at various surgical centers. There has been a trend toward combining neurosurgical and plastic surgery techniques and forming interdisciplinary craniofacial teams to provide care for children with craniosynostosis.

Before surgery, parents should be made aware of the potential for blood loss in the child. The family may wish to donate blood to be used as needed during the procedure. Family members should receive instruction regarding skull anatomy and the changes that will occur in their child's bony structure as a result of surgery. It is helpful for parents to see "before and after" photographs of children who have undergone similar corrective surgery. Parents must be prepared for the physical appearance of their child in the postsurgical period. A turban-style head dressing will cover the child's cranium, and the child will be irritable the first few days. Orbital edema is common and may cause the child's eyelids to swell shut for 24 to 48 hours.

Postoperative nursing assessment of the child undergoing craniofacial surgery entails *neurologic monitoring*, including level of consciousness, pupillary responses (not done if the eyes are swollen shut), and monitoring of vital signs and indicators of increased ICP (see discussion of ICP). Assessment of surgical dressings and drains and of fluid and electrolyte balance is necessary because children undergoing this surgery often have mild to moderate cerebral edema. Facial swelling and severe eye and periorbital swelling require *skin surveillance* and prevention of further trauma, skin breakdown, or infection of this area.

Preventing Decreased Cerebral Perfusion. The infant or child usually returns from surgery with the head of the bed elevated at least 20 to 30 degrees. It is necessary to ensure proper body alignment in relation to the elevation desired. Increased intrathoracic pressure, a result of torso elevation, has been known to increase ICP. For this reason, children recovering from surgery for craniosynostosis are maintained on moderate fluid restrictions. Assessment and documentation of neurologic status are vital.

Preventing Infection. Some surgeons may order prophylactic antibiotics for a few postoperative days. Once the head dressing is removed, preventing the child from putting his or her hands on the incision is essential. This may require the use of elbow splints. Prolonged eye swelling puts the child at risk for conjunctival infections or ulcers. If such swelling is noted, the physician should be notified to allow consideration of the administration of prophylactic eye drops or ointments. The child should be monitored for CSF leak.

Pain Management. To assist in the management of postoperative headaches, to minimize pain, and to promote comfort and rest, the physician's orders may frequently include narcotic analgesics, such as morphine, and non-narcotic pain medications, such as acetaminophen (Tylenol). Sedatives are rarely ordered, because they may mask the assessment of true neurologic status. Easing the fear and anxiety of a young child who cannot see is a nursing challenge. Often parents are the experts at the nonpharmacologic measures that help their child to cope. Maximizing the use of the senses of touch, taste, smell, and hearing is usually the best way to assure infants or children that their familiar and comforting world has not disappeared. Adequate periods of rest are also vital, even as the child appears to get back to normal activity.

Nonsurgical Management. In some cases, nonsurgical intervention can be selected. Nonsurgical intervention incorporates the use of specially designed hard-shell helmets. These can be designed by orthotic technicians or by physical therapists. The helmets have internal inserts that place gentle pressure on the skull, aligned opposite to the affected area. The helmet is worn 24 hours a day, generally for 3 to 6 months.

This therapy is referred to as *dynamic orthotic cranioplasty* (DOC) and is offered at several centers throughout the country. This treatment is generally reserved for patients who have what is referred to as *positional plagiocephaly*. This is a nonsynostosis disorder that results from molding from repeat positioning on the same side of the head (Ripley et al., 1994). Some controversy exists over whether the helmets are really beneficial, as many children outgrow this deformity over time.

Nursing education for the child and the family undergoing helmet therapy includes providing instructions as to the maintenance of the skin under the helmet. This maintenance includes a daily assessment of the scalp for redness or abrasions and providing good hygiene to the scalp. As the child adjusts to the helmet, the use of acetaminophen (Tylenol) may be needed to decrease irritability and to promote overall comfort.

It is important that the family maintain follow-up evaluations and that the helmet design is adjusted according to the progression of the therapy.

Supporting the Family. Many families have difficulty understanding the procedures necessary to correct craniosynostosis. It is hard for the parent of an otherwise healthy-appearing child to consent to surgery of this magnitude, even when the child is obviously deformed. Often what parents need most is *presence*, including someone to listen to their concerns and to provide positive reinforcement for their participation in, and coping with, hospitalization. In some circumstances, other families who have been through the surgery are helpful. Anxiety on the part of the parents is often sensed by children and contributes to their fear. Family members may feel guilt if they leave the child's side. They need to be encouraged to spend time away from the child so that their time with the child is a helpful, rather than a draining, experience. For all of these reasons, a family-centered approach to the nursing care of these children is essential to the creation of a positive hospitalization experience.

Infectious Processes

Meningitis

By definition, the term *meningitis* refers to the pathologic condition of *inflammation of the membranes* of the brain and/or spinal cord. The three meningeal layers that can be affected include (1) the dura mater (pachymeningitis), (2) the subarachnoid mater, and (3) the pia mater (leptomeningitis). The etiologic agents involved in meningitis include bacterial, viral, and fungal organisms. In addition, chemical toxins such as lead and arsenic, contrast media used in myelography, and metastatic malignant cells can trigger an inflammatory process that, although not infectious, is similar in clinical appearance. The following discussion presents sequelae and health care management associated with bacterial, tuberculous, and aseptic meningitis.

Bacterial Meningitis

Bacterial meningitis is a pyogenic or purulent infection that involves the pia mater and arachnoid mater layers of the meninges and the subdural space, including the CSF (Hickey, 1992). Most cases of community-acquired bacterial meningitis are caused by *Neisseria meningitidis* (meningococcal meningitis), *Haemophilus influenzae type B* (*H. influenzae* meningitis), and *Streptococcus pneumoniae* (pneumococcal meningitis) (Table 21–10). Other types of meningitis and pathogens less commonly seen include the following:

- Nosocomial bacterial meningitis, which is associated with ventriculoatrial or ventriculoperitoneal shunts that are used for children with hydrocephalus
- Neonatal nosocomial meningitis resulting from exposure to group B streptococci or gram-negative bacteria in the birth canal
- Meningitis resulting from infection with *Listeria monocytogenes*
- Meningitis resulting from infection with *Mycoplasma pneumoniae*

After head trauma and neurosurgery, organisms can include *S. epidermidis*, *S. aureus*, *Klebsiella*, and *Pseudomonas*.

Bacterial meningitis appears most frequently among children between 1 month and 5 years of age, with 95% of cases occurring during these developmental years. Because of infant immunizations, the incidence of some types of bacterial meningitis has decreased. For example, *H. influenzae* meningitis has decreased dramatically due to the *H. influenzae* type B vaccine protocol for neonates starting at 24 or 18 months of age. Outbreaks of *H. influenzae* meningitis, however, can occur in unvaccinated populations, such as in immigrants, various religious sects, and immunocompromised children (Saez-Llorens & McCracken, 1992).

Pathophysiology

The pathogens responsible for meningitis usually disseminate from a distant site of infection and then into the meninges. Bacterial colonization and subsequent infiltration of the meninges most commonly occur following an upper respiratory infection or accompanying bacteremia of otitis media, sinusitis, or mastoiditis. Pathogens can also enter through penetrating wounds, such as skull fractures or operative incisions, or through the skin in the presence of a structural defect, such as a meningomyelocele. In the neonate, additional risk factors include maternal infection, premature rupture of amniotic membranes, premature birth, low birth weight, and prolonged labor. The immune system of the neonate is less mature. Once the pathogen is implanted, it proliferates and spreads into CSF and through perivascular channels and meningeal folds to brain parenchyma. Later, clumps of purulent exudate collect around the base of the brain to cause obstruction of CSF with possible hydrocephalus and cranial nerve palsies. Blood vessel walls and endothelium become involved and cerebral perfusion may be compromised, leading to cerebral edema. Vasculitis associated with thrombosis can cause infarctions (strokes), seizures, and focal deficits. Continued necrosis of cells in the brain cortex and hydrocephalus can lead to permanent damage, increased ICP, and death.

Prognosis. Major factors in predicting unfavorable outcome of bacterial meningitis are young age, delay in treatment, coma, or focal neurologic signs on admission and a poor clinical course. Neurologic sequelae can range considerably, from mild learning disabilities to severe physical and mental disabilities. Deafness and alteration in vision may result. Seizures occur in approximately 20% to 50% of all meningitis patients, presumably in response to cerebral edema, fever, or cortical irritation and damage (Prober, 1996).

Other complications include hydrocephalus, cranial nerve dysfunctions, peripheral circulatory collapse, arthritis (especially after meningococcal meningitis), arteritis, phlebitis, and abscess. Subdural effusion and empyema should be suspected in infants who do not respond to treatment and who have prolonged fever, bulging tense fontanelles, increasing head circumference, seizures, and other focal deficits.

Assessment

In neonates, the symptoms of infection and meningeal irritation may be minimal or absent. Bacterial meningitis should be considered in any newborn who fails to thrive and who exhibits irritability, apnea, seizures, a tendency of opisthotonos, poor feeding, emesis, hypothermia, hyperthermia, hypotonia, hypertonia, a gray appearance, jaundice, or other evidence of sepsis. The neonate may simply be "fussy" and refuse to feed. Bulging fontanelles are present as ICP rises.

The infant may have few striking symptoms. The parents may notice only the infant's resistance to being cuddled or diapered, irritability, and mild fever. The infant may have a high-pitched cry, a transient vacant stare, and anorexia. A bulging tense fontanelle is a frequent symptom and may indicate increased ICP.

Older children may have nonspecific complaints, such as high fever, vomiting, and fatigue. Severe headache, altered consciousness, stiff neck (nuchal rigidity), and convulsions are often present and suggest neurologic involvement.

Tip: *Ask the child to try to touch the chin to the chest. If pain prevents the child from doing this, nuchal rigidity due to inflamed meninges may be present.*

The Kernig sign (the inability to extend the legs fully when lying supine) and the Brudzinski sign (flexion of the hips when the neck is flexed from a supine position) are frequently present.

Both *H. influenzae* meningitis and *meningococcal* meningitis can cause a petechial rash. As the rash rapidly progresses, darker purpuric eruptions occur. These eruptions are associated with meningococcemia septic shock known as the Waterhouse-Friderichsen syndrome (Fig. 21–9) (Saez-Llorens & McCracken, 1992).

Alert: *Any parent inquiring about a "purple rash," especially if associated with other symptoms such as fatigue, fever, and vomiting, should be advised to have the child be seen by a health care provider immediately.*

Meningococcemia, an overwhelming septic infection, may develop in 10% of patients with *N. meningitidis* meningitis (Hickey, 1992). The high fevers, purpuric lesions, and circulatory collapse from adrenal insufficiency constitute a medical emergency. The accompanying inflammatory response is marked by disseminated intravascular coagulation, encephalitis, lung abscess, and organ hemorrhage leading to tissue necrosis. This collection of symptoms may result in death only hours after the onset of fever. Accurate diagnostic studies and rapid institution of antibiotic therapy can be lifesaving.

Diagnostic Tests. Characteristic signs and symptoms, plus a positive spinal fluid examination and culture, are diagnostic for bacterial meningitis. Spinal fluid is obtained by a lumbar puncture and sent immediately to the

Figure 21–9
This child's legs exhibit the characteristic purpuric lesions of meningococcal meningitis.

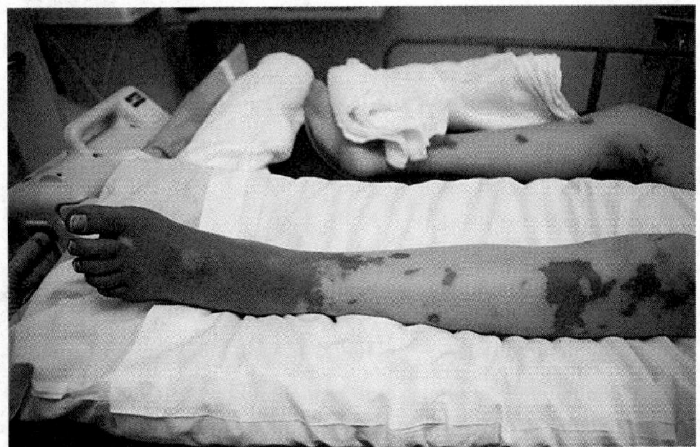

Table 21–10
Predisposing Factors for Bacterial Meningitis

Pathogen	Predisposing Factors	Considerations	Recommended Antibacterial Agent	Prevention
Pneumococcus (*Streptococcus pneumoniae*)	Otitis media, mastoiditis, basilar skull fracture, sickle cell disease, asplenia	Accounts for 25% of all cases and has a 25% mortality rate with treatment. A pneumococcal vaccine is available for immunosuppressed children.	**Cefotaxime:** 200 mg/kg/24 hr IV, 4 divided doses **Ceftriaxone:** 100–150 mg/kg/24 hr IV, 2 divided doses **Ampicillin:** 300 mg/kg/24 hr, 6 divided doses **Chloramphenicol:** 100 mg/kg/d, 4 divided doses **Aqueous penicillin 6:** 500,000 U/kg/24 hr, 6 divided doses **Vancomycin:** 40–60 mg/kg/24 hr, 4 divided doses (for multiple resistant organisms)	Vaccination available for children >2 years of age
Meningococcus (*Neisseria meningitidis*)	Close contact with a previous case at daycare center, nursery school, or college dorm	Accounts for 25% of all cases. Has a 5%–10% mortality rate with treatment.	**Penicillin:** 500,000 U/kg/24 hr, 6 divided doses	**Rifampin** for all close contacts: 10 mg/kg/dose every 12 hours for 4 doses for all nonpregnant contacts Meningococcal quadrivalent vaccine against serogroups A, C, Y, and W135 recommended for high-risk children >2 years

Haemophilus influenzae	Otitis media, pharyngitis, sickle cell anemia, asplenia	Accounts for 10%–15% of cases. Has a 5% mortality rate with treatment.	**Ampicillin** plus **ceftriaxone** or **cefotaxime:** 300 mg/kg/24 hr, 6 divided doses DC above if strain is sensitive to ampicillin	**Rifampin:** 20 mg/kg/24 hr for 4 days for **all** household contacts *H. influenzae* type B conjugated vaccine is available.
Gram-negative enteric bacteria	Maternal vaginal or perineal colonization, congenital dural defects (meningomyelocele)	Accounts for 10% of cases. Has a 50%–75% mortality rate with treatment.	**Cefotaxime** or **ceftriaxone** plus **aminoglycoside:** DC above if strain is sensitive to ampicillin	No chemoprophylaxis or vaccine is available.
Group B streptococcus	Maternal vaginal or perineal colonization	In twin delivery, requires treatment of both twins even if only one is symptomatic.	**Penicillin G:** 300,000–500,000 U/kg/day	No chemoprophylaxis or vaccination is required. Intrapartum administration of ampicillin by mother may prevent infection of newborn.
Listeria monocytogenes	Maternal vaginal or perineal colonization. Maternal infection from consuming contaminated dairy products.	Pregnant women should avoid unpasteurized milk and soft cheeses, such as goat cheese.	**Penicillin** or **ampicillin:** 500,000 U/kg/24 hr, 6 divided doses	No chemoprophylaxis or vaccine is available.
Shunt-associated meningitis (coagulase-negative or coagulase-positive *Staphylococcus,* gram-negative rods, enterococci)	Ventriculoatrial or ventriculoperitoneal shunt	Requires scrupulous technique. Requires adequate skin asepsis when accessing shunt.	Based on causative pathogen	Based on causative pathogen

IV, intravenous; DC, discontinue.

laboratory for microscopic examination and culture. Spinal fluid is examined for cloudiness, blood cell counts, white blood cell differential, and protein and glucose levels (Table 21–11).

caREminder: *A low glucose level and high protein count in spinal fluid indicate bacterial meningitis. In viral meningitis, the spinal fluid typically shows a normal to high glucose level and a normal to low protein count.*

Common microbiological tests for bacterial meningitis include a Gram stain, culture of the spinal fluid, and a blood culture. These microbiological tests are positive in 80% to 90% of infected patients for spinal fluid and 30% to 60% for blood specimens. Counter-immunoelectrophoresis and latex agglutination tests can detect bacterial antigen in spinal fluid, urine, or blood in less than 1 hour. These rapid tests are helpful when children have been pretreated with antibiotics before the lumbar puncture or blood culture and evaluation for meningitis. Although these rapid diagnostic tests are available for meningococci, pneumococci, group B streptococci, and *H. influenzae*, they cannot be used as the sole basis of diagnosis because false-positive and false-negative tests can occur.

The limulus test detects endotoxins from gram-negative bacteria in the spinal fluid. This test is not available in many laboratories because the results are difficult to interpret. An elevated lactic acid level in spinal fluid suggests bacterial meningitis but is not pathogen specific.

Other laboratory tests may include cultures of blood, urine, nasopharynx, and CSF leaks to identify the source of septicemia. Complete blood cell counts may show an increase in total white blood cells with an increase in immature granulocytes. Serum C-reactive protein increases acutely to more than 40 mg/dL with bacterial infection.

CT or MRI imaging may help to monitor the course of the illness and to determine the need for specific interventions.

Nursing Diagnoses and Outcomes

Chart 21–3 presents a variety of nursing diagnoses that can be applied to the child with a neurologic condition. The following diagnoses are also specifically applicable to the child with meningitis:

- **Pain related to meningeal irritation**
  Outcomes: Child is free from pain.
  Child rests in environment in which stimuli are reduced and activities are minimized so as to promote comfort and rest.
- **Activity intolerance related to immobility**
  Outcomes: Child regains and maintains muscle mass and strength.
  Child is able to participate in play and self-care activities.
- **Diversional activity deficit related to prolonged hospitalization**
  Outcome: Child selects and participates in age-appropriate play within limits of his or her physical tolerance and ability.

Interdisciplinary Interventions

Medical Management. Treatment for bacterial meningitis calls for aggressive intervention with appropriate intravenous antibiotics given for 7 to 14 days (Care Path 21–1). Antibiotic therapy is initiated before the results

Table 21–11
Analysis of Cerebrospinal Fluid for Central Nervous System Infections

	Pressure (mm H_2O)	Appearance	Leukocytes (mm^3)	Protein (mg/dL)	Sugar (mg/dL)
Normal cerebrospinal fluid	60–200 (5–15 mm Hg)	Clear	0–5	10–30	40–80
Bacterial meningitis	Elevated	Turbid, cloudy	Elevated, 100–60,000, polymorphonuclear cells predominate	Elevated, 100–500	Decreased
Aseptic meningitis	Normal or slight elevation	Clear	10–1000	Not greater than 100	Normal to low, <40
Tuberculosis meningitis	Elevated	Clear	25–100	100–200	<50
Brain abscess	Elevated	Clear	Elevated, 10–200	Elevated, 75–500	>50

of CSF cultures are obtained. The empiric drugs of choice are third generation cephalosporins such as ceftriaxone or cefotaxime. After organism sensitivities are available, antibiotic therapy is further selected and modified. The choice of antibiotic should show consideration of any allergies that the patient may have. Dosages are adjusted to maintain therapeutic serum antibiotic levels, when appropriate. Intravenous steroids, such as dexamethasone, may be used as an adjunct to antibiotic therapy to decrease meningeal inflammation and prevent hearing loss. (American Academy of Pediatrics, 1990; Pohl, 1993; and Bell, 1992).

Supportive care includes management of fever, hydration, and monitoring response to treatment. Overhydration is carefully avoided to prevent the onset of SIADH. This syndrome is characterized by further exacerbation of cerebral edema that can lead to life-threatening compromise of cerebral tissues. Fluids are often restricted to an oral and intravenous total of one half to two thirds of maintenance fluids. Care Path 21–1 provides a summary of health care interventions for the child with bacterial meningitis. Supportive care may also include recognition and treatment of increased ICP, seizures, cerebral edema, hydrocephalus, subdural effusion, and empyema.

If seizures have occurred, the child may receive a loading dose of phenobarbital, phenytoin (Dilantin), or fosphenytoin sodium (Cerebyx), followed by maintenance doses (Voytko & Farrington, 1997). If seizure activity persists beyond 4 days, there is greater risk of residual damage and chronic seizure disorders. Surgical treatment may be necessary for infants or children with severe problems, increased ICP, ventriculomegaly, hydrocephalus, subdural effusion, or empyema. Treatment may include ventriculostomy for drainage of infected or obstructed fluid. If hydrocephalus persists after appropriate antibiotic treatment, a shunt may be necessary. Some organisms, such as *Klebsiella* and *Pseudomonas*, may require careful intraventricular administration of antibiotics. Subdural effusions may be treated with subdural antibiotic irrigation and sump drainage.

Nursing Management. Droplet precautions, until at least 24 hours of effective antibiotic therapy have elapsed, are recommended. Generally, continuing isolation is not recommended for any of the forms of bacterial meningitis except *H. influenzae* and *N. meningitidis*.

Nursing assessment includes acute *neurologic monitoring*, checking vital signs and head circumference, palpating the anterior fontanelle, measuring daily weight, measuring intake and output, and assessing the intravenous site (Chart 21–22). The infant or child can also be assessed for discomfort, irritability, behavioral problems, seizures, vomiting, appetite, thirst, and a variety of potential complications. The child is at risk for seizure activity, so bedside rails are kept up. Someone should stay with

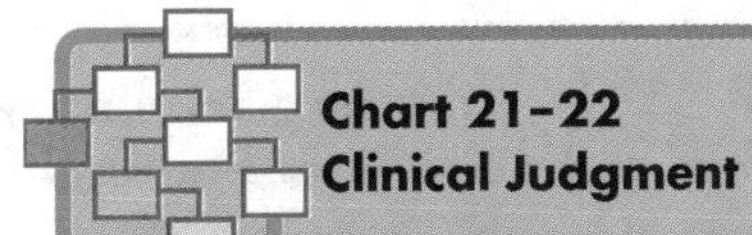

Chart 21–22
Clinical Judgment

The Child with Meningitis

Kara is 9 years old and is brought to the emergency department (ED) by her guardian because of severe headaches and a stiff neck for the past 24 hours. Kara did not want to go to school today. Upon arrival in the ED, she vomited. She has had no history of a recent cold or other illness. Her temperature is 102° F.

Questions

1. To determine whether Kara has meningitis, what diagnostic tests and procedures should be completed?
2. What clinical finding is classically associated with meningococcal meningitis?
3. The CSF fluid is cloudy with an increased white blood count, low glucose level, and elevated protein level. What nursing diagnosis could be selected to reflect Kara's potential for neurologic dysfunction?
4. Kara is transferred to the pediatric unit. What nursing measures should be taken to make Kara comfortable and free from pain?
5. Twenty-four hours later, Kara demonstrates no improvement. She remains febrile, continues to vomit, has become very irritable and lethargic. What action should the nurse take?

Answers

1. Lumbar puncture; cultures of blood, urine, and nasopharynx; CT scan or MRI of the head for child with symptoms of increased ICP.
2. Rapidly spreading purpuric skin lesions.
3. High risk for injury: complications of meningitis including increased intracranial pressure, seizures, and hearing loss.
4. Analgesics should be given as ordered; head of bed should be elevated; room should be kept quiet with subdued lighting; health care activities should be arranged so as to cause least amount of disturbance to Kara; comfort objects should be provided.
5. Report these findings immediately to the physician. The antibiotics may need to be changed. New spinal tap and blood cultures may be performed.

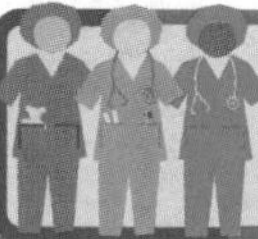

Care Path 21-1 An Interdisciplinary Plan of Care for the Child with Bacterial Meningitis Without Complications

	Patient/Family Intermediate Outcomes		
Nursing Diagnosis	**Day 1: Admission**	**Day 2**	**Day 3**
Pain related to meningeal irritation	Child's pain will be optimally managed using pharmacologic and nonpharmacologic measures.	→	→
High risk for injury related to complications of meningitis including increased intracranial pressure, seizures, hearing loss, arthritis, and stress ulcers	Child will have signs of increased ICP recognized immediately and treatment initiated.	→	→
	Child experiences no seizure activity.	→	→
	Child experiences no loss of hearing.	→	→
	Child does not experience arthritis or stress ulcers.	→	→
Family fear, related to concerns about potential effect of child's condition on brain functioning	Family members express their fears to the health care team.	→	→
	Family members receive support from others as needed to cope with their fears.	→	→
Knowledge deficit: disease process, interdisciplinary plan of care and home care	Family members verbalize understanding of etiology of disease and purpose of diagnostic tests.	Family members verbalize understanding of interdisciplinary plan of care.	Family will describe signs and symptoms of increased ICP
		Family members participate in measures to increase child's level of comfort.	→
Care Intervention Categories			
Labs	CSF analysis, Gram's stain, culture, cell count with differential, glucose and protein, CBC, serum electrolytes, serum osmolality, urine osmolality, blood cultures, urine specific gravity	→	→

Days 4–5	Days 6–10 Hospital or Home Care Setting
Child is free from pain.	⟶
Child remains afebrile.	⟶
⟶	⟶
⟶	⟶
⟶	⟶
⟶	Family members express comfort in managing the child's care at home.
⟶	
Family members participate in medication administration and care of IV access site.	⟶
Family members describe signs and symptoms that require immediate referral to a health care provider.	⟶
DC Dexamethasone after 16th dose	DC medication if child is afebrile for 5 days, or continue course for 7–10 days.

Care Path continued on following page

the child in the bathroom because there is potential for the child to experience seizures. If a seizure occurs, the nurse provides appropriate first aid, observes and documents seizures, and gives antiepileptic medications, as ordered by the physician. Family members and the child should be taught about seizure observation, first aid, and medications.

The nurse should monitor the child for potential hearing loss caused by meningitis or ototoxic side effects of aminoglycoside antibiotics and diuretics by assessing the child's response to auditory stimuli and the ability to localize sounds. If hearing loss is suspected, the physician is notified for appropriate testing of the child (e.g., brain stem auditory evoked potentials, audiometry testing). An otologist can be consulted for treatment considerations and ongoing follow-up.

Assessment for potential arthritis and stress ulcer is also indicated in the child with meningitis.

Pain Management. The child with meningitis is likely to experience pain related to meningeal irritation. In addition, discomfort may be associated with diagnostic tests such as the lumbar punctures and blood draws, the administration of intravenous fluids and antibiotics, and immobility associated with bed rest. Although complete relief of pain and discomfort may not be possible, available pharmacologic and nonpharmacologic measures can be used to maximize the success of pain relief interventions (Chart 21–23). The nurse should have a truthful conversation with the child about pain, including how much a procedure will hurt, how long it will last, and what will help to lessen the pain. Care should be taken to ensure that the child understands that pain is *not* a punishment.

Community Care

Prevention. Preventive measures for bacterial meningitis include prompt treatment for upper respiratory infections, otitis media, sinusitis, mastoiditis, and other infections, especially in younger infants and children. Immunization with *H. influenzae* type B vaccine prevents bacteremia, thus preventing meningitis. This vaccine is recommended at 24 or 18 months of age for children who attend daycare centers.

For family members and exposed staff, chemoprophylaxis is only necessary in cases of exposure to meningococcus or *H. influenzae*. Family members who share the same household with the infected child should receive rifampin prophylaxis, or adults can receive a single dose of ciprofloxacin. Any daycare or school contacts should also receive prophylaxis because the duration and extent of contact with the child may be difficult to determine. Generally, if there has been close intimate mouth-to-mouth contact, then prophylaxis is necessary. However, many parents of children in the same classroom or school

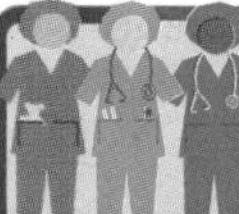

Care Path 21-1 An Interdisciplinary Plan of Care for the Child with Bacterial Meningitis Without Complications *Continued*

Care Intervention Categories	Day 1: Admission	Day 2	Day 3
Medications and IVs	Cefotaxime or ceftriaxone IV Acetaminophen p.r.n. for fever Dexamethasone IV D5½ NS ½ to ⅓ maintenance	→ Increase fluids if child is dehydrated or hypotensive.	Antibiotics changed based on sensitivity results Increase fluids when serum sodium levels are normal.
Monitors	Cardiac monitor	→	→
Nutrition	Nothing by mouth	Clear liquid as tolerated. Advance diet as tolerated.	→
Play therapy/school	Bed rest	→	Quiet activities in room
Procedures (diagnostics)	Lumbar puncture (LP)		Repeat LP if child shows lack of improvement.
Special considerations	Rifampin prophylaxis for at-risk contacts is initiated.		
Tests		CT or MRI if abnormal neurologic signs persist	
Vital signs/baseline parameters	q 15 min until child is stable, then q 1–2 hr based on status Neurologic assessment q 4 hr Head circumference if 3 years or younger Weight Intake and output	Vital signs q 2–4 hr based on status → → →	Vital signs q 4 hr → → →

CBC, complete blood count; CSF, cerebrospinal fluid; CT, computed tomography; DC, discontinue; MRI, magnetic resonance imaging.

demand prophylaxis because meningitis is so devastating. Rifampin is relatively inexpensive and causes few side effects. Thus, most health departments give prophylaxis generously. Ciprofloxacin is an attractive alternative to rifampin for persons older than 18 years because it is given as a single dose.

caREminder: *Unless a health care worker has unprotected, intimate contact with the patient, prophylaxis is not indicated. Intimate contact involves face-to-face encounters, such as in intubating the child, assisting with a lumbar puncture, or giving mouth-to-mouth resuscitation without using a mask.*

Many employee health and infection-control programs offer prophylaxis to health care workers regardless of the extent of the exposure. However, the American Academy of Pediatrics and the Centers for Disease Con-

Days 4–5	Days 6–10 Hospital or Home Care Setting
DC cardiac monitor	
⟶	⟶
Activities as tolerated	⟶
Discharge home if afebrile 48–72 hours	
	Audiologic studies at time of discharge or at first clinic visit
⟶	DC if afebrile for 48–72 hours
Neurologic assessment every shift ⟶ ⟶	

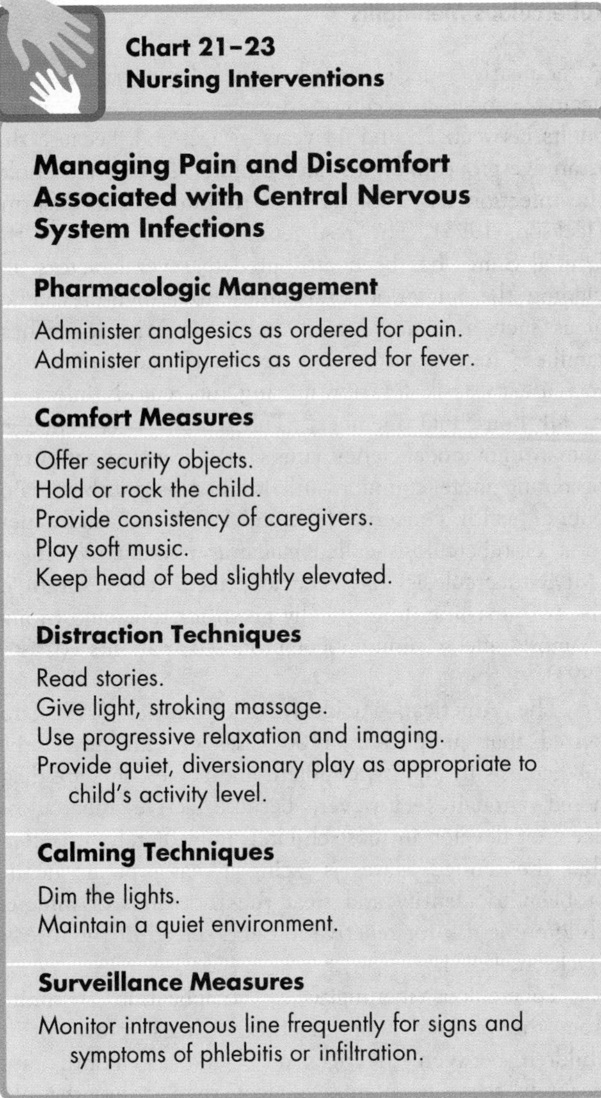

Chart 21–23
Nursing Interventions

Managing Pain and Discomfort Associated with Central Nervous System Infections

Pharmacologic Management

Administer analgesics as ordered for pain.
Administer antipyretics as ordered for fever.

Comfort Measures

Offer security objects.
Hold or rock the child.
Provide consistency of caregivers.
Play soft music.
Keep head of bed slightly elevated.

Distraction Techniques

Read stories.
Give light, stroking massage.
Use progressive relaxation and imaging.
Provide quiet, diversionary play as appropriate to child's activity level.

Calming Techniques

Dim the lights.
Maintain a quiet environment.

Surveillance Measures

Monitor intravenous line frequently for signs and symptoms of phlebitis or infiltration.

trol (CDC) recommend prophylaxis for health care workers based on exposure rather than heightened concern.

Home care and rehabilitation is based on the residual effects of the disease and varies for each child. Bacterial meningitis can be a devastating illness because of the systemic involvement and severity of its clinical course. It is clear that rapid diagnosis and early treatment contribute to the most favorable recovery. The child may be discharged while still on intravenous antibiotic therapy. Arrangements with the home health nurse are made before discharge to ensure a smooth transition of care from acute to home care settings. Parents are instructed to assess neurologic status and to evaluate changes in vital signs. Throughout the child's recuperation, the parents collaborate with the health care team to monitor the child's progress on developmental tasks. Findings are compared with previously recorded assessments to evaluate developmental delays. Additionally, the health care team works with the family to provide rehabilitation as needed to address problems that resulted from system involvement during the course of the illness. Before discharge, brain stem auditory evoked potentials or audiometry for older children is usually done. When hearing loss occurs, early intervention is possible. Careful follow-up with developmental testing and information about appropriate infant stimulation is advisable. Early detection of delays allows for early intervention.

Tuberculous Meningitis

After nearly 3 decades of decline, tuberculosis has once again become a common disease. It primarily affects adults between 25 and 44 years of age, and, because this is an age group likely to have children in the household, the infection has a high risk of transmission to offspring (Jackson, 1993). The resurgence of tuberculosis in the United States has been attributed to several factors, including the migration of families from high-prevalence areas such as Asia, Africa, and Latin America. These families often live in overly crowded conditions, which increase the risk for transmitting tuberculosis infections to all household members. Tuberculosis occurrence in human immunodeficiency virus (HIV) infected patients is becoming more common and is cited as another major public health concern (Jackson, 1993). A deadly new form of tuberculosis called *multidrug resistant tuberculosis* (MDR-tuberculosis) has been identified. It is resistant to the two first-line drugs usually given for tuberculosis, and it most affects immunocompromised patients (Casey, 1993).

The American Academy of Pediatrics (1992) reported that more than 1100 cases of clinically active tuberculosis in infants, children, and adolescents are diagnosed annually. However, because active tuberculosis does not develop in most children immediately, it is clear that the United States is facing a major public health problem to identify and treat the thousands of infected children at risk for reactivation and spread of the disease (Jackson, 1993).

Tuberculous meningitis, a complication stemming from the primary lung infection, is most prevalent in children between the ages of 6 and 24 months and is rarely seen in infants younger than 3 months old. Congenital cases are rare. Occasionally, tuberculous meningitis may occur many years after the primary infection resulting from the rupture of one or more tubercles, which discharge bacilli into the subarachnoid space.

Pathophysiology

Mycobacterium tuberculosis is the organism responsible for tuberculosis infections. It most often occurs in the adult respiratory system and is easily transmitted to children. When an infected person coughs or sneezes, the susceptible child may inhale minute airborne droplets, and thus tubercle bacilli begin their cycle of disease again. In children younger than 20 years of age, the lungs are the predominant site for **primary** tuberculosis infections, followed by the lymph nodes, pleural space, and meningeal covers of the brain (Feigin & Cherry, 1992). **Secondary** infection occurs as M. *tuberculosis* bacteria enter the lungs and rapidly spread throughout the body via the lymphatic system and bloodstream. When organisms reach the highly vascular meningeal covering of the brain, the child becomes at risk for development of tuberculous meningitis; therefore, it may be classified as either a primary or secondary infection.

Assessment

The onset of tuberculous meningitis is gradual, with mild prodromal symptoms of fever, lethargy, headache, or vomiting. Within 7 to 10 days, positive meningeal signs (nuchal rigidity, Kerning's sign, severe headache) develop. If untreated, the child deteriorates into a comatose state and dies.

Analysis of CSF fluid may show little abnormality because the fluid is obtained from a site proximal to the inflammation and obstruction (see Table 21–11). CT or MRI scans are usually normal during the early stages of the illness.

Complications of tuberculous meningitis are related to the effectiveness of treatment and the time at which the child is diagnosed. Long-term sequelae can include hearing loss, communicating hydrocephalus, intellectual and emotional disturbances, seizures, and muscle spasticity. As with other forms of meningitis, if diagnosed and treated in the early stage of infection, more favorable outcomes may be predicted for the child.

The preventive drug treatment course for this population spans 9 months; for HIV infected children, 12 months is recommended. Daily doses of oral isoniazid (INH) are given, based on the child's weight (10 mg/kg, not exceeding 300 mg). If long-term drug therapy is contraindicated because of concern of noncompliance or immunosuppression, infants and children may receive the bacillus of Calmette-Guérin vaccination. Treatment of clinically active tuberculosis involves a 6-month regimen of INH, rifampin (10 to 20 mg/kg/d), and pyrazinamide (20 to 40 mg/kg/d) in the first 2 months, and INH and rifampin for the remaining 4 months (American Academy of Pediatrics, 1991). If MDR-tuberculosis is suspected, second-line drugs may be needed to combat the infection. These medications include kanamycin (Kantrex), capreomycin (Capastat), ethionamide (Trecator-SC), and cycloserine (Seromycin) (Casey, 1993).

Perhaps the most challenging aspect of this disease is to determine how health care practitioners can maximize compliance over the several months, especially because tuberculosis is most prevalent in depressed communities of the homeless, poor, and ethnic minorities who may be medically underserved. Approximately one third of tuberculosis cases in the United States occur in middle and upper income socioeconomic groups, refuting the myth that tuberculosis is a disease only of the poor (American Thoracic Society, 1992).

The treatment goals for the hospitalized child with active tuberculosis are to

- Identify the pathogen causing symptoms
- Contain the illness and prevent further infection such as meningitis
- Begin aggressive drug therapy
- Evaluate all family members for the absence or presence of tuberculosis via history and skin testing

Isolation is indicated if the patient's sputum contains acid-fast bacilli or if MDR-tuberculosis is suspected. The child may be admitted to a hospital room with special ventilation flow, if available. If family members also have clinically active tuberculosis, there is no need to prevent visitation, but health care workers should maintain universal precautions during all interactions.

The CDC has recommended that health care workers wear small-micron, fitted filtration masks or particulate respirators because airborne droplets containing the nuclei of tuberculosis organisms easily pass around or through ordinary surgical masks (Nardell, 1990). By law, cases of tuberculosis must be reported to local health departments (Jackson, 1993). Evaluation of family and close contacts is essential to identify the source of infection, initiate medical therapy, and break the cycle of reinfection.

Aseptic Meningitis

Aseptic meningitis is also known as acute benign lymphocytic meningitis and acute viral meningitis or serous meningitis (Hickey, 1992). Enteroviruses such as ECHO and coxsackievirus, mumps, and polio are the most common causes of aseptic meningitis. Herpes simplex types I and II may cause aseptic meningitis in adolescents and life-threatening encephalitis in neonates and children (Prendergast, 1987). Less common pathogens include cytomegalovirus, arbovirus, parasites, and Epstein-Barr virus (Givner, 1996). Aseptic meningitis is usually not fatal and most children recover completely within 3 to 14 days.

Pathophysiology

Viruses gain access to the CNS through systemic circulation. They enter cells in the meninges for obligatory growth and reproduction, causing inflammation and edema. Enteroviruses are probably transmitted by the enteric-oral pathway and have the greatest incidence during the summer months. Lymphocytic choriomeningitis virus is transmitted by the bite of infected mice or by vectors such as mosquitoes and ticks that transmit the virus to humans.

Assessment

The clinical manifestations are similar to those of bacterial meningitis; however, they do not progress as rapidly and are usually less severe. Clinical symptoms include fever, headache, vomiting, and stiff neck. Seizures are seen less frequently in aseptic meningitis than in bacterial meningitis. Irritability, drowsiness, and lethargy may occur but are mild, compared with encephalitis. The child's history usually reveals the presence of a recent or concurrent viral illness.

When aseptic meningitis occurs with or follows a discrete, red, maculopapular rash, enterovirus or coxsackievirus infection may be likely. When coxsackievirus is the offending pathogen, symptoms may also include the appearance of vesicles and ulcers on the soft palate, paroxysmal pain in the intercostal muscles caused by irritation of pleural surfaces, and symptoms of pericarditis. If aseptic meningitis is caused by mumps virus, parotiditis may also occur.

Diagnostic Tests. Lumbar puncture is completed to examine the CSF and to differentiate aseptic meningitis from bacterial meningitis. The CSF in aseptic meningitis usually contains a greater amount of white blood cells than normal, but fewer than in bacterial disease. CSF glucose may be normal, and protein may be only mildly elevated (see Table 21–11). Virus or virus antibodies may be isolated from CSF, blood, sputum, stool, or other specimens. The lumbar puncture may help to alleviate symptoms of increased ICP.

Interdisciplinary Interventions

Health care interventions for aseptic meningitis are primarily symptomatic. The child may be hospitalized to monitor and manage neurologic status, to monitor fluid and electrolyte balance, to control hyperthermia, to give supportive body care, to control pain, to maintain adequate nutrition, and to treat seizures, if they occur.

Young infants are routinely hospitalized because of the risk of meningitis caused by *L. monocytogenes* infection. Young infants should receive broad-spectrum antibiotics (ampicillin and cefotaxime) until CSF cultures for bacteria are negative.

Older and less severely affected children may be managed on an outpatient basis with analgesics and antipyretics administered as needed.

Encephalitis

Encephalitis is defined as an inflammation of the brain. When there is simultaneous involvement of the meninges, the term *meningoencephalitis* is used. If there is involvement of the spinal cord, the term *myelitis* or *encephalomyelitis* is used. Although encephalitis closely resembles meningitis in origin and presentation, the clinical course may be more severe because there is involvement of actual brain tissue.

Etiology

A wide variety of infectious agents may cause encephalitis. Viral encephalitis is most commonly seen in children.

The viruses most frequently identified as causative agents are enteroviruses (echoviruses, coxsackievirus A and B, enterovirus 71, and poliovirus), arboviruses, and herpes simplex virus. Viral encephalitis is more common in children who are immunosuppressed. The advent and widespread use of measles, mumps, rubella, and chickenpox vaccines have significantly decreased the incidence of viral encephalitis.

Nonviral causes of encephalitis include bacteria (e.g., *H. influenzae*, *Neisseria* meningitis, spirochetal infections, cat-scratch disease), parasites, fungi, rickettsial infections, protozoa, and helminths (Hickey, 1992). Introduction of these organisms into the body may be through the administration of certain chemotherapeutic agents, diagnostic imaging dyes, detergents, or alcohol into the CSF.

Pathophysiology

It is believed that CNS involvement is secondary to an infectious process occurring elsewhere in the body. The virus or other causative agent enters the body and subsequently infects the blood. Proliferation of the virus occurs (viremia) and the CNS becomes infected. As the brain tissue becomes inflamed, fever, headache, seizure, agitation, and alterations in state of awareness result from increasing cerebral or cerebellar dysfunction.

Prognosis. The prognosis of encephalitis depends on the degree and duration of cerebral and CNS involvement, and the ability to successfully manage secondary complications. Mortality rate is highest in those children with herpes simplex encephalitis. Severe permanent neurologic sequelae is present in approximately 25% of children with encephalitis.

Assessment

The onset of symptoms may be acute or gradual, with complaints of general muscle pain, fever, gastrointestinal distress, and mild respiratory symptoms. Clinically, the neurologic presentation is similar to meningitis. Headache, photophobia, changes in arousal and consciousness, and persistent seizures may be present. The CNS may be severely affected, with associated dysfunctions as seen in Guillain-Barré syndrome and Reye's syndrome (Krywanio, 1991). As the condition progresses, increased ICP and cerebral edema may lead to coma and death.

Diagnostic Tests. After a thorough history is completed to evaluate any recent viral illnesses or exposures that may identify the causative organism, the child undergoes diagnostic tests. Laboratory evaluation includes examination of CSF, blood, stool, and sputum to help establish the cause of the disease. In many cases, CSF values are unspecific (see Table 21–11). Lymphocyte count may be increased, glucose is usually normal, and a mild elevation in protein is often seen. If localized CNS hemorrhage has occurred, red blood cells and hemoglobin may be present in the CSF fluid. CSF fluid should also be examined for acid-fast organisms, parasites, and bacteria. Fourteen to 21 days after the onset of encephalitis, the CSF fluid should again be evaluated and tested for antibody against specific causative agents (McMillan, 1996).

CT and MRI tests may show cerebral edema, hydrocephalus, or lesions. An EEG may show abnormalities consistent with seizure activity.

Interdisciplinary Intervention

The care of the child with encephalitis is directed toward management and prevention of secondary complications such as seizures, increased ICP, and respiratory involvement. Severely affected children are managed in the intensive care setting, with the need for mechanical ventilation, ICP monitoring, and ventriculostomy care implemented as warranted by the child's condition. (See the discussion on increased ICP.)

If a causative organism is identified, appropriate antibacterial and antifungal medications are prescribed. Few antiviral medications are available. Herpes simplex encephalitis should be treated with intravenous acyclovir for 10 days. Children with fever and acute encephalic symptoms are generally given acyclovir and an antibacterial agent until the blood, CSF, sputum, or stool cultures reveal a specific etiologic agent. Antimicrobial therapy is then adjusted to treat the identified infectious agent.

If seizures have occurred, treatment is initiated by administering intravenous diazepam. The nurse needs to evaluate the child for efficacy of the medication and for the potential side effects of hypoventilation and lethargy. Characteristically, the seizures associated with encephalitis are difficult to control. If diazepam is ineffective, intravenous phenytoin is administered. Further demonstration of seizure activity may call for the use of phenobarbital. The aggressive and prolonged use of antiseizure medications creates the need for mechanical ventilation to support the child's respiratory status and cardiac monitoring to assess for cardiac conduction defects.

Nursing care involves the assessment and management of alterations in a variety of systems including respiratory, neurologic, cardiac, and fluid and electrolyte status. As discussed previously, the child's status may warrant treatment for seizures, increased ICP, and respiratory complications. The child's precarious condition and the lack of a definitive treatment for the child's illness is likely to cause the family a great deal of stress and fear. The nurse should assist in providing frequent communication to the family regarding the child's status. Support services should be accessed to assist with alterations in family processes. Parents should be encouraged to assist in providing for the child's care and should be given ample opportunity to participate in care decisions.

Brain Abscess

A brain abscess is defined as a localized infection that extends into the brain parenchyma. Within 2 weeks of initial microbial entry, the abscess becomes an encapsulated lesion filled with pus (Twomey, 1992). Brain abscess can be multiple or single and is most often located in the frontal and temporal lobes.

Etiology

The origin of brain abscesses can usually be traced to one of three situations:

1. Extension of local infections of the middle ear, mastoid, or sinuses (20% to 50%)
2. Distal infections in the chest or lungs, or spread through bloodstream in immunocompromised host (metastatic abscess)
3. Direct infection as a result of open head trauma, intracranial surgery, bacterial meningitis, or cranial traction (Hickey, 1992; Hinkle, 1990)

The extension of local infections includes complications from dental procedures, otitis media, mastoiditis, and frontal or sphenoidal sinusitis.

Extension of Local Infections. The nursing assessment for brain abscess should elicit any history of otitis media and subsequent mastoiditis, which are common childhood illnesses. Various strains of anaerobic streptococci are responsible for 60% of these infections, but they may also be caused by staphylococci and species of bacteroides (Twomey, 1992). Distal infective causes were previously attributed to congenital heart defects; more recent reports also implicate pulmonary infection and immunocompromised status (e.g., transplant patients or patients with leukemia, lymphoma, or HIV infection) (Mampalam & Rosenbluth, 1988). Bloodborne spread of organisms is likely to cause multiple abscess formation, whereas other mechanisms generally result in single lesions (Hinkle, 1990).

Distal Infections. Four agents known to cause brain abscess are bacteria, yeast, fungi, and parasites. The bacterial agents most often cultured from distal infections are *Clostridium*, *Nocardia*, and *L. monocytogenes* (Scheld & Winn, 1990; Twomey, 1992). Immunosuppressed patients are at risk for development of fungal and yeast infections from *Candida* or *Cryptococcus neoformans*, which can result in abscess formation. The parasite *Toxoplasma gondii* has been linked with 30% of cases of patients with acquired immunodeficiency syndrome who have CNS infections.

Direct Infection. In the third source of infection (direct entry), compound or depressed skull fractures provide immediate entry routes for microorganisms to meningeal and brain tissue. It is rare to find neurosurgical interventions as the sole cause of brain abscess. *Staphylococcus aureus* is the etiologic agent in 10% to 15% of abscesses, and is the primary cause of infection following head trauma or intracranial procedures (Twomey, 1992).

Assessment

Brain abscesses are more frequent in adults, but they may occur in children. Symptoms occur in two stages and vary according to the location of abscess. At the onset of infection, the child may complain of earache, fever, or vomiting. Mild neurologic changes such as drowsiness and sensory deficits may be present but unnoticed. Organization and enlargement of the abscess leads to compression of brain tissue, causing signs of increased ICP. Severe headaches, changes in ocular function, seizures, and ataxia may occur, signaling parents to seek medical attention.

Diagnostic Tests. Diagnosis is confirmed by CT scan and MRI. In infants with an open fontanelle, cranial ultrasonography may also be used for diagnostic purposes. Radiographs of the chest and skull assist in locating the primary source of infection, such as an object aspirated into the lungs.

▽ **Alert:** *Lumbar puncture is contraindicated because there is risk of cerebral herniation from increased ICP.*

Blood analysis is usually inconclusive. Blood cultures reveal the causative organism in only 10% of all cases. White blood cell count may be normal and an elevated erythrocyte sedimentation rate is not consistently present (Sutton & Pomeroy, 1996).

Interdisciplinary Interventions

Management of brain abscess involves both intravenous antibiotic therapy and surgical draining of the lesion. The type of antibiotic used depends on the causative organism, the site of the abscess, and the child's state of health. Initial antibiotic therapy usually includes cefotaxime or ceftazidime and nafcillin or vancomycin. Antibiotic therapy is adjusted after culture sensitivities of the abscess drainage are obtained. Antibiotic therapy continues for 4 to 8 weeks.

Surgical excision and drainage of the abscess remains the definitive treatment for brain abscess. Children should be postoperatively monitored for increased ICP and drainage or bleeding from the incision site.

In some cases, if the child is medically stable, conservative treatment with antibiotics only, administered in the home or outpatient setting, may be scheduled. The child's progress is monitored by follow-up CT scans and by careful clinical examinations.

With the widespread use of antibiotics and development of more precise diagnostic imaging tools, the mortality rate associated with brain abscess has decreased from 40% to 60% to only 15% to 20%. Favorable outcome is enhanced by rapid diagnosis, antimicrobial medications, and diligent monitoring. Interdisciplinary management improves the overall quality of care by providing an organized approach to treatment.

Community Care

Once fever is reduced and the aspiration or excision of the abscess has reduced intracranial pressure, the child can be discharged home to complete the course of antibiotics. A central line is usually placed before discharge to avoid needless repeat punctures of the child's skin. Parents can be taught to administer intravenous antibiotics and to assess the child for changes in neurologic status. If the family feels uncomfortable administering the medications, a home care nurse can be employed to complete the task and to monitor the child's progress.

Tetanus

Tetanus is an acute infectious process caused by the exotoxin *Clostridium tetani*, a gram-positive anaerobic rod. The infectious process leads to a spastic, paralytic illness. The illness has been reported to occur following penetrating or crushing wounds, burn injury, pregnancy, and general surgery and in neonates with umbilical stump infections. The incidence is worldwide, except in polar regions, and it is prevalent in nonimmunized populations or in regions with poor aseptic conditions. The mortality rate is high, with infants and the elderly being most at risk. The disease is preventable with proper health care and a series of vaccinations.

Pathophysiology

C. *tetani* spores are found in soil contaminated by horse and cattle feces. The spores are harmless until entering a susceptible host. Once introduced, the incubation period from time of injury to onset of symptoms is usually between 7 and 14 days. Prognosis is worse when symptoms manifest in 2 to 3 days, because up to 75% of tetanus-related deaths occur within the first week of symptoms (Lutkus, Hirsh, & Wood, 1984). Any patient who has been exposed to high levels of bacterial contamination from an injury, and whose injury is not thoroughly cleansed and prophylactically treated for infection within 24 hours, is at high risk for tetanus (Angelucci & Todaro, 1990).

Following injury, there is local production of exotoxins in the wound, which are then carried centrally via neural pathways. The primary sites affected are the spinal cord and brain stem. Tetanus toxin blocks normal inhibition of antagonist muscles, thus affecting voluntary coordinated movement. This causes affected muscles to sustain maximal contraction. The autonomic nervous system also becomes unstable as a result of the infectious process (Arnon, 1996). Neonatal tetanus is likely to be seen in infants whose birth occurred outside a medical facility, whose mothers were not immunized for tetanus, and when sterile umbilical cord care was not adequately provided.

Worldview: *Tetanus neonatorum is more common in developing countries where women are not immunized against it, where contaminated instruments are used to cut the umbilical cord, or where native poultices such as cow dung or fermented milk are used for umbilical cord care.*

Early signs of tetanus vary but may include low back pain, stiffness in the jaw and lower limbs, and dysphasia. As the disease progresses, the classic "lockjaw" or trismus is seen, which is spasm of the masticatory (chewing) muscles. As the facial muscles become more rigid, the corners of the mouth are drawn up and outward. This condition is referred to as *risus sardonicus* and is a result of intractable spasm of facial and buccal muscles. Airway obstruction and asphyxiation can occur as a result of laryngeal and respiratory muscle spasm. Paralysis extending into the abdomen, lumbar spine, hip, and thigh muscles can cause the child to assume an arched posture (opisthotonus) in which only the back of the head and the heels touch the ground.

The seizures associated with tetanus appear suddenly and are characterized by tonic contractions of muscles with clenched fists, flexion and abduction of the arms, and hyperextension of the legs. Seizures last a few seconds to a few minutes, with intervening periods of rest. As the illness progresses, the seizures become sustained and exhausting. Seizure activity may be triggered by disturbances of sight, sound, or touch.

Dysuria and urinary retention occur from bladder sphincter spasm. Bowel incontinence may occur during seizures. Temperature as high as 40°C is generally present as a result of the sustained metabolic energy generated by spastic muscles. Tachycardia, arrhythmias, labile hypertension, diaphoresis, and cutaneous vasoconstriction occur as the autonomic nervous system becomes involved. The child does not lose consciousness and experiences extreme pain. The seizure activities are likely to be very frightening to the child (Arnon, 1996).

The paralysis of tetanus rapidly becomes severe in the first week of onset, stabilizes during the second week, and gradually recedes over an ensuing 1- to 4-week period.

Neonatal tetanus is characterized by poor suck, abnormal cry, intermittent muscular spasms, and fever. Symptoms usually appear 3 to 12 days after birth. The umbilical cord may hold remnants of dirt, dried blood, or animal dung.

Diagnosis of tetanus is based on the clinical presentation, because there are no characteristic laboratory findings.

Interdisciplinary Interventions

The most critical goals of interdisciplinary management of tetanus include maintaining a patent airway, controlling seizures, and eradicating the C. *tetani*.

Respiratory Support. Endotracheal intubation may be required to prevent aspiration and respiratory arrest resulting from laryngospasm. In many cases, oxygen therapy and suctioning to manage oral secretions is sufficient. Suctioning should be approached cautiously because manipulation of the airway can provoke muscle spasm and seizures. In severe cases, a tracheostomy may be performed.

Seizure Control. Diazepam is considered to be the most effective sedative for control of tetanic activity. The medication is given by continuous intravenous infusion and is titrated as needed to control spasms. The dosage is slowly reduced as the child's symptoms recede. Additionally, phenobarbital may be used to control seizures. Apnea can occur as a result of high doses of these medications; thus, mechanical respiratory support may be needed.

Eradicating the Toxin. In tetanus, the neurotoxin must be killed to halt continuation of the infectious process, and the toxin within the child's system must be neutralized. Penicillin G given intravenously for 10 to 14 days remains the antibiotic of choice. Erythromycin and tetracycline can be given if the child is allergic to penicillin.

To neutralize toxin that is diffusing from the wound, human tetanus immune globulin (TIG) is administered as a single intramuscular dose. If TIG is not available, human intravenous immune globulin (IVIG) or equine tetanus antitoxin (TAT) can be administered. In addition, once the child is actively recovering from the disease, immunization with DT (diphtheria-tetanus) or DPT (diphtheria-tetanus-pertussis) can be given if

- Five years have lapsed since the child's last tetanus shot.
- The child is younger than 6 years of age.
- Immunizations have never been initiated for tetanus.

Wound debridement is essential to the healing process. Meticulous care of the umbilical cord site or wound site is needed to ensure no further growth of spores.

Supportive Care. Care should be provided to minimize stimulation of the child. A quiet, darkened setting is preferred. Sedating the child is necessary to manage pain and prevent seizure activity. Cardiorespiratory monitoring is needed. Nursing care includes monitoring respiratory status and initiating suctioning as needed.

Fluid and electrolyte status is monitored, as is bowel and bladder function. Seizure, sustained rigid paralysis of the muscles, and instability of the autonomic nervous system predispose the child to many complications. The child is likely to be hemodynamically unstable and thermoregulation may be difficult to manage. When the child's condition becomes more stabilized, physical therapy personnel should be consulted to begin rehabilitation of affected muscle groups. Long-term sequelae may include cerebral palsy, hypoxic brain injury, diminished mental capabilities, and behavioral problems.

Community Care

Prevention. Tetanus is preventable through active immunization. Chapter 6 summarized the pediatric immunization schedule. Immunization of pregnant women with tetanus toxoid can prevent neonatal tetanus.

Tetanus prophylaxis should be followed as a part of wound management. Tetanus toxoid should always be given after a dog or other animal bite. Treatment of all wounds, except those experienced by fully immunized patients, should include administration of human TIG. If immunization status of the child is unclear or if the child is injured by a tetanus-prone wound (i.e., crush or projectile wound, contaminated wound), TIG should be administered intramuscularly. The wound itself should be immediately cleaned and debrided. A tetanus toxoid booster (Td) is given to all persons with a wound if their immunization status is

- Unknown
- Incomplete
- The wound is clean but more than 10 years have passed since the last booster
- The wound is serious and more than 5 years have passed since the last booster (Arnon, 1996)

Nurses play an important role in ensuring that a child's immunization status is up to date. Providing education to high-risk communities with limited health care resources is a valuable activity to be pursued by nursing personnel. Parents should be encouraged to keep organized immunization records that are easily accessed by family members if the child should ever become injured.

Parainfectious Processes

Reye's Syndrome

Reye's syndrome is an acute, noninflammatory encephalopathy with fatty degenerative changes in the liver, brain, and kidneys. Early diagnosis and intervention are critical because the disease can have a rapid onset, leading to coma or death within hours. First described in 1963 by Reye and colleagues, the cause of Reye's syndrome still remains unclear.

Etiology

Three types of antecedent viral illnesses are frequently associated with the onset of Reye's syndrome: approximately 60% to 75% of children have respiratory infections, 15% to 30% have varicella (chickenpox), and 10% to 15% have diarrhea (Budd & Hobdell, 1983). Research has linked Reye's syndrome with ingestion of salicylates, acetaminophen, chemical toxins, and antiemetic drugs (Lovejoy, 1996). Strong warnings were issued from the CDC and the American Academy of Pediatrics in the early 1980s when studies confirmed a relationship between aspirin administration during viral illnesses and the onset of Reye's syndrome. Warning labels continue to be placed on salicylate containers. It is thought that the subsequent decreased use of salicylates by children has markedly reduced the incidence of this disease.

Pathophysiology

The pathophysiology of Reye's syndrome is complex and appears to involve a defect in mitochondrial function. Chemical metabolic imbalances are a hallmark feature of Reye's syndrome. Examples include hyperammonemia from a decrease in the enzymes that convert ammonia to urea, hypoglycemia and lactic acidosis from prolonged vomiting, and increased short chain fatty acids. Any combination of these metabolic dysfunctions can generate cerebral edema and increased ICP (Budd & Hobdell, 1983).

Prognosis. Poor outcomes are seen in children who deteriorate rapidly with severe cerebral edema, who have a blood ammonia level greater than 300 μ/dL, who have a prothrombin time two times greater than control time, and who experience an increase in liver and skeletal creatinine phosphokinase (Lovejoy, 1996). Early diagnosis and the early implementation of supportive care can prevent the progression of the syndrome. Full neurologic recovery is usually noted if cerebral edema does not progress.

Assessment

Evaluation of the child's clinical history generally reveals an antecedent factor of mild respiratory or gastric illness. Abnormalities in hepatic function are present (Table 21–12). Clinical signs and symptoms include persistent vomiting and diarrhea in the recovery phase of a viral illness, and alterations in level of consciousness such as lethargy, agitation, combativeness, or seizures. A liver biopsy, completed only if the diagnosis is unclear, reveals microvascular fat and mitochondrial alterations. A staging system is used to describe the clinical course and the severity of the syndrome (Table 21–13).

Interdisciplinary Interventions

Children with Reye's syndrome are cared for in an intensive care setting because of the high risk for increased ICP and liver dysfunction. There is no specific treatment

Table 21–12
Laboratory Tests for Diagnostic Evaluation of Reye's Syndrome

Test	Values in Reye's Syndrome
Liver function tests: AST, ACT, LDH	Elevated
Bilirubin	Usually normal
Ammonia level	May be elevated as much as 3 times as normal
Arterial blood gases	Decreased CO_2, elevated pH
Clotting factors: PT, PTT, platelets	Decreased with prolonged PT
Blood urea nitrogen (BUN)/creatinine	Normal-increased
Serum electrolytes	Varies
Blood glucose	Decreased-normal
Osmolarity	Normal-increased
Salicylate and acetaminophen levels	May have positive screen

AST, aspartate transaminase; ACT, activated clotting time; LDH, lactate dehydrogenase; PT, prothrombin time; PTT, partial thromboplastin time.

Table 21-13
Stages and Treatment of Reye's Syndrome

Stage	Symptoms	Treatment
Stage I	Vomiting, lethargy, sleepiness, mild confusion, elevated serum liver enzymes, normal blood ammonia level, grade I EEG	Baseline, monitor vital signs ⅓ Maintenance fluids Diuretics given Vitamin K Monitor serum ammonia/glucose/osmolarity
Stage II	Disorientation, delirium, combativeness, hyperventilation, hyperreflexia, appropriate response to noxious stimuli, elevation in blood ammonia and serum liver enzymes, grade II or III EEG	Continue baseline Give anticonvulsants Arterial line CVP (central venous pressure) line Neurologic monitor
Stage III	Coma, decorticate posturing, preservation of pupillary light reflexes, pupils dilated, persistent elevation in blood ammonia and serum liver enzymes, grade III or IV EEG	Monitor intracranial pressure Mechanical ventilation Treat increasing serum osmolarity All previous care activities
Stage IV	Deepening coma, decerebrate rigidity and posturing to painful stimuli, oculocephalic response, fixed pupils, hypoventilation, decreased blood ammonia and serum liver activity, grade III or IV EEG	Barbiturate coma All previous care activities
Stage V	Coma, seizures, absent deep tendon reflexes, respiratory arrest, flaccidity, hypotension, decreased blood ammonia and serum liver enzyme activity, grade IV or electrocerebral silence on EEG	Supportive care All previous care activities

for Reye's syndrome. Supportive care is directed toward monitoring and managing cerebral edema (see discussion on increased ICP). Care interventions include nasotracheal intubation with ventilatory control to maintain low PCO_2 levels and to decrease CPP. Mannitol is administered to decrease elevated serum osmolarity. A barbiturate-induced coma may be used if cerebral edema is uncontrolled. Fluid intake is restricted while cerebral edema is present. Vitamin K may be administered to correct prolonged prothrombin time. Phenytoin may be given to control seizures (see Table 21–13).

The rapid deterioration of the child and the intensity of health care interventions are frightening experiences for the family. The nurse has an important role in ensuring that frequent and open communications are maintained between the health care team and the family. All equipment and treatment measures should be fully explained. Parents may desire social services or clerical support to assist them to access coping strategies that can help them to deal with this unexpected crisis.

To prevent Reye's syndrome, all adults should be aware that salicylate products should not be given to children, especially if the child is demonstrating respiratory or gastrointestinal symptoms. Salicylate can be found in over-the-counter products such as Pepto-Bismol (an antacid) and in several cold preparations. Parents should be warned to carefully read the labels on all medications or other preparations before they administer any of them to the child.

Guillain-Barré Syndrome

Guillain-Barré syndrome (GBS) is an acute, demyelinating polyneuropathy of primarily peripheral nerves which occurs as a postinfectious process. The incidence is approximately 0.8 per 100,000 persons in children younger than 17 years of age (Jones, 1996). GBS affects all ages, races, and socioeconomic groups (Anderson, 1992; Hickey, 1992). It is unusual in infants younger than 6 months of age.

Pathophysiology

Although the exact etiology is unknown, research has suggested an immune-mediated process triggered by a viral illness. During the viral illness, the myelin sheath surrounding the peripheral nerves is altered. Myelin is responsible for rapid nerve conduction. The altered myelin in GBS is perceived as a foreign protein. Sensitized lymphocytes attack the myelin, leading to edema, destruction, and nerve-root compression. Normal nerve conduction is interrupted and symmetric ascending weakness is noted. Sensory and autonomic symptoms may accompany the weakness. Progression of weakness occurs over 7 to 14 days. A plateau of function at maximal weakness may then last from 5 to 46 days, with full recovery noted in 2.5 to 15 months (Shahar et al., 1997).

Prognosis. It is estimated that 75% to 90% of GBS patients recover with no residual disabilities (Anderson, 1992; Hickey, 1992). GBS is a reversible disease with a good prognosis for most children. Poor outcomes are seen in those children in whom respiratory complications secondary to muscle weakness develop; these children, therefore, require prolonged ventilator support.

Assessment

Criteria for diagnosis of GBS include a progressive motor weakness of more than one limb and areflexia. The clinical examination focuses on motor, sensory, cranial nerve, and autonomic functions (Chart 21–24). Of concern is rapid progression of symptoms, leading to respiratory failure, loss of swallow and gag, and need for ventilatory support. Respiratory failure may be preceded by progressive involvement of truncal musculature and cranial nerves, as well as sensory impairment (Shahar et al., 1997). The child's immunization status should be determined to eliminate the possibility of poliomyelitis.

Diagnostic Tests. Blood and urine cultures are completed to search for a causative agent and underlying systemic or immune-mediated disorders. Analysis of CSF reveals few white blood cells, with elevation of protein. Peripheral nerve conduction time studies and electromyogram demonstrate decreased nerve velocities.

Chart 21–24

Clinical Manifestations of Guillain-Barré Syndrome

- Progressive, ascending motor weakness of more than one limb
- Areflexia (absence of reflexes)
- May have initial excruciating pain in upper legs and back
- Mild sensory symptoms
- History of upper respiratory tract infection a few weeks prior to visit
- Absence of fever when neurologic symptoms develop
- Bilateral facial nerve involvement
- Cranial nerve involvement

Interdisciplinary Interventions

The treatment of GBS is primarily supportive. Because of the potential for rapid deterioration and respiratory failure, admission to a high observation area is necessary. Rapid transfer to an intensive care unit should occur at the first sign of increasing respiratory dysfunction. During the acute phase of the disease, frequent assessment of respiratory function by pulmonary function studies, cranial nerve function, and blood pressure is imperative so that rapid intervention may be implemented if deterioration occurs.

The postulated immune basis for GBS suggests use of intravenous immune globulins or plasmapheresis to prevent demyelination. Either therapy should be used early in the acute phase. The goal is to prevent respiratory compromise and the need for ventilatory support, therefore promoting a shorter recovery course. Research in either therapy has demonstrated a shorter acute phase with no or less ventilatory support needed and, in one study, a shorter recovery time (Shahar et al., 1997).

Nursing Management. Early prevention of the complications of immobility are of paramount importance and should be initiated during the acute phase. The child is at risk for mobility problems such as joint contractures, skin breakdown, and deep vein thromboses. Passive range-of-motion exercises, frequent repositioning, and meticulous skin care minimize these complications. Total parenteral nutrition is provided if the child is intubated. Extubated solid foods are introduced once it is assured that the child's ability to swallow is fully intact. If severe pain is present in the initial stages of the disease, both pharmacologic and nonpharmacologic comfort measures are indicated. Pain medications should not interfere with the child's respiratory function or ability to cough.

Nursing care differs with each phase of the disease. In the acute period, the nurse provides supportive measures to sustain life, to prevent complications, and to promote comfort. If children have severe respiratory insufficiency, they may be intubated and placed on a ventilator. Alternate methods for communication must be established because the child will no longer be able to verbalize needs. Such dramatic changes and loss of bodily functions are frightening to the child and the family. Parents may feel helpless in the busy surroundings of an intensive care setting. The child becomes isolated from his or her normal world of play, friends, and activities. Nursing diagnoses and care paths should incorporate developmental assessments and psychosocial support measures throughout the acute course.

In the static phase, nerve conduction to the bladder may be poor; therefore, an indwelling or intermittent catheter is indicated to relieve urinary retention. Tachycardia and arrhythmias may occur and cardiac monitoring should continue. Sleep disturbances are common and are caused by pain, lack of scheduled rest periods, noisiness, and treatment interventions. The nurse can organize care and create a schedule to provide quiet time for the child. Unless all health care team members adhere to the plan, it is ineffective.

During recovery, children slowly regain muscle strength and sensation, and they are in less pain. Emotionally, there is a sense of relief as functional abilities return. Comprehensive care is still vitally important in the five most commonly affected areas: respiration, mobility, nutrition, autonomic nervous system, and psychologic response. The early phases of the recovery program must balance activities with adequate rest. Fatigue or exhaustion can cause symptoms to return, which may be devastating for the child. The nurse should provide support and encouragement as progress is made in each area.

Community Care

Relatives and friends can help by caring for siblings, preparing meals, assisting with transportation, or providing parents respite by staying with the affected child for a few hours. Before the child's discharge, parents should receive and should become comfortable with instructions for exercise, diet, and measures to provide psychosocial support to their child. Ideally, discharge planning begins with the child's admission to the care facility. A variety of resources outside the acute care setting should be explored to assist the child and the family's return to normal life. For the school-age child or adolescent, the illness creates an abrupt interruption of established routines. The family may require home health nursing services. Good communication between the acute care setting and outreach teams facilitates high-quality continuity of care. GBS is an illness that requires a highly skilled, interdisciplinary health care team to manage the many facets of patient care. The nurse's role includes not only the provision of clinical skills but also expertise as an educator, patient advocate, supportive listener, and coordinator of resources. This holistic approach to care minimizes the stressors affecting both the child and family and provides the best chance for optimal recovery. If mentally and physically able, some children are able to continue their education using home-bound teaching sessions. Child life therapists may offer suggestions for developmentally appropriate activities to alleviate boredom. The stress of becoming dependent and being in pain, and the lack of social interaction may cause feelings of anger or depression. It is likely that the child will regress to previous developmental stages to meet needs for security. When parents are aware of these natural responses, they can provide better support throughout each phase of the disease.

Neuromuscular Disorders

Spinal Muscular Atrophy

Spinal muscular atrophy is a degenerative disorder of the anterior horn cell of the spinal cord and some cranial nerve nuclei, resulting in weakness and wasting of voluntary muscles. It is the most common recessive genetic disorder that is lethal in infants (Crawford, 1996) and, in the milder forms, is the second most common neuromuscular disorder of childhood (Crawford, 1996; Russman et al., 1992). Recently, research has indicated that spinal muscular atrophy may not be a degenerative disease and that an abnormality on chromosome 5 is consistent across all forms of the disorder (Russman et al., 1992). The different forms are expressed by full or partial dysfunction of the gene. A high rate of spontaneous mutation has been noted (Crawford, 1996). Prevalence at birth is approximately 1 in 25,000 live births (Russman et al., 1992).

Pathophysiology

The basic problem in spinal muscular atrophy is in the function of the motor neurons. Loss of function in one motor neuron results in abnormalities and loss of function in the muscles supplied by the motor neuron. As deterioration or loss of motor neuron function increases, loss of muscle fibers and function also occurs. The most common mode of inheritance for spinal muscular atrophy is autosomal recessive, although sex-linked and autosomal dominant forms have been documented.

Assessment

Historically, three forms of spinal muscular atrophy have been described. Although a new classification has not been developed, recent research indicates that the current classification system may not adequately describe characteristics of affected children to assist in prognosis or in planning an effective rehabilitation program (Russman et al., 1992). Common to all forms is the presence of more proximal, lower extremity weakness. Spinal muscular atrophy type I, also known as Werdnig-Hoffmann disease, is the most severe form and begins in utero or early infancy. These infants have few spontaneous movements, an inability to lift the head, difficulty with sucking and swallowing, and loss of deep tendon reflexes. Initial examination may also document fasciculations, continuous intermittent "worm-like" movements of the tongue. These movements are best observed in the tongue, but they may also be present in the child's deltoid, biceps, and quadriceps muscles. Intercostal muscles are affected and death usually occurs in the first 2 to 3 years secondary to respiratory insufficiency. Presentation at birth or early infancy usually decreases life expectancy to less than 1 year.

Spinal muscular atrophy type II is the late infantile form. Less initial weakness and a later onset (6 to 24 months) are noted. These infants may achieve sitting and, with orthotic support, may achieve ambulation (Fidzianska, 1996). On clinical examination, deep tendon reflexes are absent and fasciculations may be present. Life expectancy is to the second or third decade of life (Russman et al., 1992).

Type III spinal muscular atrophy, also called Kugelberg-Welander disease, is the juvenile form of the disease, with onset occurring between 3 and 17 years of age. Early symptoms are nonspecific and include delayed developmental milestones and motor clumsiness. Atrophy of proximal muscles may be present. The course is usually mild. In most cases, there is little tendency to deterioration (Fidzianska, 1996). Patients may live well into their adult years.

A variant of the spinal muscular atrophies, called Fazio-Londe disease, is a condition resulting from motor neuron degeneration, which occurs more in the brain stem than in the spinal cord.

Diagnosis of spinal muscular atrophy is made by clinical evaluation (including family history), testing for chromosomal deletion, electromyogram (EMG), and possibly muscle biopsy. Notation of early infant deaths within the family, family members with similar problems, and maternal observation of decreased fetal movements are suggestive. The clinical evaluation focuses on assessment of the motor system and cranial nerves. Hypotonia, generalized weakness, thin muscle mass, the presence of fasciculations, and alterations in tendon stretch reflexes are characteristics of spinal muscular atrophy. Inability to meet normal gross and fine motor developmental milestones are some of the first diagnostic clues that are of concern to family members. There is no cardiac involvement. Intelligence is normal.

Diagnostic Tests. Once the diagnosis is suspected, the specific gene deletion study by blood sample should be performed. Documentation of the defect in chromosome 5 eliminates the need for muscle biopsy. However, there are many potential causes for weakness and hypotonia in infants. Therefore, an EMG is usually performed to document specific muscle responses. The EMG results vary by type of spinal muscular atrophy in the quantity and character of fibrillations and fasciculations.

When the blood deletion study is negative and the EMG suggests spinal muscular atrophy, a muscle biopsy is performed. The histologic specimens differentiate spinal muscular atrophy from other intrinsic muscle diseases. Specifically, large group muscle atrophy is seen in spinal muscular atrophy.

Interdisciplinary Interventions

Treatment of spinal muscular atrophy is supportive. In all forms of the disorder, the evaluation of respiratory and nutritional status is critical. The muscle weakness leads to ineffective airway clearance of secretions and diminished vital capacity. In type I spinal muscular atrophy, the most common cause of death is loss of respiratory function. Involvement of cranial nerve nuclei and swallowing problems lead to inadequate nutrition. Alternative feeding methods may be required.

In types II and III spinal muscular atrophy, loss of function may also occur but is usually not as rapid as is seen in type I. Careful developmental surveillance of the child is necessary. As the child grows and continues to have weakness, contractures and scoliosis may occur secondary to immobility. Orthopedic care is instituted to provide support to muscle groups and to maintain strength of functional muscles. Evaluation and treatment of the skin become necessary as immobility increases.

This condition presents many challenges for the child and family. The rapid deterioration characteristic of type I spinal muscular atrophy requires the family to make many decisions regarding the extent and the degree of medical intervention that should be instituted. Measures taken may prolong the child's life, although quality of life may not be impacted. The child with type II or III spinal muscular atrophy should be encouraged to participate in age-appropriate activities to the extent that he or she is able. Monitoring is needed to ensure that nutritional intake is adequate and that immobility of a muscle group does not lead to further musculoskeletal alterations. Chapter 10 discusses care of the child with a chronic condition, and the concepts therein should be reviewed to ensure that the family's psychosocial, emotional, cognitive, and interpersonal needs are all being addressed.

Myasthenia Gravis

Myasthenia gravis (MG) is a neuromuscular disease caused by immunologic neuromuscular blockade. The disease is characterized by progressive weakness of certain voluntary muscles. The disease most commonly affects the oculomotor, facial, laryngeal, pharyngeal, and respiratory muscles (Chipps, Clanin, & Campbell, 1992; Drachman, 1994).

Etiology

The cause of MG is an antibody-mediated autoimmune attack directed against acetylcholine receptors (Drachman, 1994). In affected children, antibodies destroy acetylcholine receptor sites, resulting in diminished muscle response and weakness. The condition may be acquired (autoimmune) or congenital (genetic). Acquired MG includes *transient neonatal* MG and *juvenile* MG. The genetic forms of MG are rare.

Assessment

Transient neonatal MG occurs in approximately 15% of infants born to mothers with MG (Drachman, 1994). The infants acquire maternal acetylcholine receptor antibodies transplacentally, and symptoms occur shortly after birth. Low Apgar scores for respiratory effort, muscle tone, and reflex irritability should immediately alert perinatal nurses to the possibility of MG. The baby may appear cyanotic, "floppy," expressionless, and too weak to cry. Initial attempts to feed are marked by poor sucking and rapid fatigue. Within 2 to 4 weeks, the symptoms of transient neonatal MG disappear without residual neurologic or developmental complications. These infants are not at risk for developing MG later in life.

Diagnosis of MG is confirmed by injection of edrophonium chloride in age-determined dosage. An initial administration of 20% of the dose is followed by a full dose once no adverse effects have been noted. Immediate, but brief improvement in muscle tone should be noted. This is known as the Tensilon test. The test also assists in the diagnosis of MG in older patients.

Twenty percent of patients with MG are seen in childhood or adolescence with *juvenile* MG. The incidence in prepubertal white patients is equal for males and females, with an increase in incidence in females after puberty. In black patients, there is a 2:1 female to male ratio. Symptoms are less severe in peripubertal and postpubertal males compared with females (Spiro, 1996). Most cases begin after 1 year of age, with the mean onset at 8 years of age. The pathophysiology for juvenile MG demonstrates a decrease of acetylcholine receptors secondary to antibody depletion of the receptors.

Juvenile MG resembles the adult form in its onset, treatment, and progress. Initial symptoms of juvenile MG include unilateral or bilateral ptosis or diplopia in a diurnal pattern. Patients who experience muscle weakness only in the extraocular and facial muscles generally have a milder course. Permanent, spontaneous remission of symptoms is inversely proportional to the severity of the symptoms. For more severely affected children, dysarthria, dysphagia, skeletal muscle weakness, and respiratory problems can occur. The onset of these symptoms may develop over years or as quickly as 24 hours.

Congenital (genetic) MG is a familial abnormality of neuromuscular transmission (Roach, Buono, McLean, & Weaver, 1985). It differs from the transient form in that

- It is not immunologically mediated.
- Mothers do not have MG.
- Symptoms appear from birth to age 12 months.
- Extraocular muscles are more severely affected.
- Response to medication or surgery (thymectomy) is limited.
- Symptoms are present throughout life.

There are currently many research studies to define the pathophysiology of this form of MG. The defect may be either presynaptic or postsynaptic and may involve calcium and sodium channels.

Diagnostic Tests. Electrodiagnostic evaluation of muscle response identifies the defect at the myoneural junction, indicating myasthenic disease. In 80% to 90% of older patients, serum acetylcholine receptor antibodies are elevated (Hickey, 1992) and the Tensilon test is positive.

Interdisciplinary Interventions

Treatment is based on the type of MG, the child's age, and the severity of symptoms. In all cases of MG, supportive care is essential to ensure that airway protection and adequate oxygenation are maintained. For the newborn with transient MG, intubation, mechanical ventilation, and enteral feedings may be necessary until natural resolution of the condition takes place. Nurses should promote bonding by encouraging parents to hold their infant, assist with daily care activities, and spend time alone with their infant. If the mother wishes to nurse her infant and the infant shows no signs of respiratory distress, she can attempt short periods of breast-feeding. She may also express milk and freeze it for later use. Supplemental nutrition should be administered via nasogastric or oral gastric feeding tube to conserve the infant's energy.

Short-term use of anticholinesterase drugs is effective in transient neonatal MG. The drug of choice in neonatal MG is Mestinon.

Nurses need to monitor the infant's respiratory function by assessing breath sounds, rate, and oxygen saturation (especially during feedings). Suction equipment should be available at the bedside if the airway becomes blocked with secretions. Continuous pulse oximetry is a useful tool in ongoing evaluation of the infant's oxygenation status. Controversy still exists as to the most effective management of MG, but any combination of anticholinesterase agents, thymectomy, or immune suppression may be used. Anticholinesterase drugs, usually pyridostigmine (Mestinon), are the first line of treatment to control symptoms. The dosage of medication is closely monitored to ensure symptom control without causing significant toxicity.

If symptoms are disabling, steroid therapy (prednisone) is used. When long-term steroid therapy is initiated, potassium supplements, antacids, or H_2-blocking agents, vitamin D, and calcium supplements may be required to promote healthy bone development and healing.

Performing a thymectomy remains a controversial therapy in the pediatric population. The entire thymus and mediastinal fat are removed during the procedure. If removal of the thymus gland is indicated, the nurse must prepare the child for surgery and must manage postoperative care.

The nurse must be knowledgeable about drug therapy, side effects, and disease course to develop a teaching plan for the child and family. Health teaching involves reducing factors that may cause exacerbation of the disease to the point of myasthenic crisis, a life-threatening event. These precipitants include stress, infection, or prolonged physical activity. Emergency situations may also arise with elevations of acetylcholinesterase drugs (cholinergic crisis) with need for intubation and ventilatory support. The Tensilon test is used to differentiate between myasthenic and cholinergic crisis (Table 21–14).

Alert: *Certain medications can exacerbate weakness in the child with MG. These drugs include aminoglycosides, procainamide, quinidine, curare, succinylcholine, and possibly channel blockers and beta-blockers. Sedatives, antibiotics, and cold remedies that contain these products should be avoided.*

As previously discussed, if the injection of edrophonium causes improvement in muscle strength, the likely diagnosis is myasthenic crisis. More medication is then needed for treatment. If there is no improvement or there is worsening with the Tensilon test, the most likely cause is cholinergic crisis. Temporary withholding of the medication is then indicated.

Because of the chronic nature of persistent and juvenile MG, teaching is a lifelong part of the treatment

Table 21–14
Myasthenic versus Cholinergic Crisis

Myasthenic	Cholinergic
Etiology	
Severe weakness with bulbar and respiratory compromise occurring during natural course of disease May be preceded by an infection Symptoms may lead to an overdose of anticholinesterase drugs	Anticholinergic drug (ACED) toxicity
Symptoms	
Anoxia Cyanosis Bowel and bladder incontinence Decreased urinary output Absence of swallow reflex and cough	Hypotension Nausea Vomiting Diarrhea Abdominal cramps Pallor Blurred vision Facial muscle twitching
Tensilon Test	
Produces temporary improvement	Produces no improvement or worsening of symptoms
Treatment	
Early detection Managing respiratory function Medical support of other body functions Plasmapheresis Discontinue anticholinesterase medications	Discontinue ACEDs and gradually reinstate medications as symptoms improve Manage respiratory function

plan. As children grow older, they should assume appropriate responsibility for management of the disease to foster independence through self-care.

Neurocutaneous Syndromes

The most frequently occurring neurocutaneous syndromes are collectively called *phakomatoses*. These diseases are characterized by their tendency toward tumor formation in the CNS, skin, and visceral linings of various organ systems, and by their recognizable cutaneous manifestations. Because of the rarity of these diseases, only the three most common phakomatoses are addressed here; they are tuberous sclerosis, neurofibromatosis, and Sturge-Weber disease.

Tuberous Sclerosis

Tuberous sclerosis is an autosomal dominant disease affecting many organ systems. A wide variety of clinical findings are associated with this disease, the most common being mental retardation, seizures, and adenoma sebaceum. The major organ systems that may be affected in tuberous sclerosis are the brain, skin, kidneys, heart, lungs, and skeleton. Growths called "tubers" may invade the brain and the retina. Other types of tumors may invade the heart and the kidneys (Berg, 1996).

Neurofibromatosis

Neurofibromatosis is also referred to as "von Recklinghausen disease," named for the man who identified it. Like tuberous sclerosis, neurofibromatosis is an autosomal dominant trait disease. Its main characteristics are areas of increased skin pigmentation (café au lait spots), central and peripheral nervous system tumors, and other skeletal, endocrine, and vascular findings. This disease is characterized by multiple tumors called neurofibromas that may occur in only a few organ systems or in many organ systems of the affected child. Peripheral nerve tumors are the most common, and a higher incidence of brain tumors in these children has been documented. Neurofibromatosis is more common in males. The first symptoms are usually cutaneous changes rather than the neurologic symptoms that often occur in later stages of the disease (Berg, 1996).

Sturge-Weber Disease

Sturge-Weber disease (encephalofacial angiomatosis) is the only phakomatosis without a recognizable hereditary pattern. The characteristic features are a port wine stain (facial nevus), focal or generalized seizures, intracranial calcification, hemiparesis, and, often, mental retardation. Abnormalities of the dura mater over the occipital lobe are common, as are calcification and necrosis of underlying brain tissue. The facial nevus is usually apparent at birth, and often it is associated with congenital glaucoma. Seizures usually begin before 1 year of age and are difficult to treat. Behavior problems, mental retardation, and hemiparesis can also occur (Berg, 1996).

Assessment

The diagnosis of neurocutaneous diseases is often made on the characteristic clinical findings of each disease. A thorough genetic and family history is helpful in the diagnosis of tuberous sclerosis and neurofibromatosis. Nursing assessment of children with neurocutaneous disorders should be focused on developmental, behavioral, and psychosocial issues. Physical assessment should be focused on obtaining a neurologic baseline and on other systems that are known to be affected by tumors, tubers, or other findings associated with these disorders for the individual child.

Diagnostic Tests. In these diseases, a confirmed diagnosis is made through a tissue sample of one of the characteristic lesions or tumors. Because of the wide variability of manifestations of these diseases, the diagnostic assessment may range from minimal to extensive. Some possibilities include the need for EEG, CT scan, MRI, skin biopsy, ophthalmologic examinations, and various other tests, depending on the organ systems involved.

Interdisciplinary Interventions

Care for children with these disorders is individualized and depends on the clinical characteristics of the specific disease. Health care management of neurocutaneous disease in childhood is aimed at alleviating symptoms, because there are no cures for these conditions. Many neurocutaneous diseases manifest with convulsive disorders; therefore, when seizures are present, anticonvulsant regimens may be tried until control is achieved. In some cases of Sturge-Weber disease, surgical removal of the lobes of the brain causing the seizures is attempted. Any lesions of the brain (tumors, tubers, or neurofibromas) may be surgically excised, especially if they cause increased ICP.

When these children are hospitalized, seizure precautions may be necessary. The child may also display behavior that is difficult to control or an element of retardation. The child's safety should be guarded at all times, with modifications made in the plan of care to adapt to the child's special behavioral needs.

Health care is also directed toward helping the family to cope with the diagnosis and the provision of expert genetic counseling to assess the probability of future children manifesting such abnormalities.

Information given to families should be geared

toward their level of understanding. Nurses should rely on principles of teaching and learning to plan a teaching strategy for parents. It is important to accept the initial denial and guilt that may manifest shortly after diagnosis and to allow for its expression.

Families facing these seemingly unexplainable and incurable diseases require ongoing support. This is especially true when the family is faced with many hospitalizations. In some instances, the nurse may need to encourage the family to explore long-term resources. Because of the wide variety of symptoms of these diseases, an individual assessment of each family is necessary, because some children may have few outward signs of illness. A nurse may interact with the same child several times during many hospitalizations. Continuity of nursing care can promote trust and a more positive view of the health care system for the child.

Neurologic Trauma

Head Injuries

Head injury in the pediatric population is one of the most common causes of death and disability. Nearly 250,000 children are admitted annually to United States hospitals for evaluation or treatment of minor or major head trauma. The spectrum of injury ranges from minor concussion requiring a few hours of observation to major trauma necessitating heroic efforts by the health care team and resulting in dismal, long-term consequences for the child (Thomas & Taylor, 1997).

The incidence of head injury in boys is twice that for girls. The age group affected most frequently is the adolescent population. Head injuries occur most frequently in the spring and summer, on weekends, and in the late afternoon or early evening (American Association of Neuroscience Nurses, 1996). *Head injury* is the general term for several different types of injury. Scalp injuries, skull fractures, concussions, contusions and lacerations, vascular injuries and hematomas, and cranial nerve and diffuse brain tissue injuries are each addressed in this section.

Etiology

The common causes of head trauma in infants and children are falls, child abuse, and motor vehicle accidents. Infants may have head trauma as a result of a difficult delivery with forceps or a prolonged, traumatic labor and delivery. Infants or toddlers may sustain a head injury because of a fall from a caretaker's arms, from a loft or balcony, in walkers, out of windows, or down stairs. These children are also at the age when they may be victims of child abuse, particularly shaking injuries. Preschool children may be hurt in a vehicular accident as either a passenger or a pedestrian. The preschooler is susceptible to being injured while playing or climbing outside. School-age children may be hurt in playground accidents or, more commonly, in accidents involving bicycles, skateboards, or athletic activities. Vehicular accidents and athletic injuries are the most common causes of head trauma in adolescents. Other factors that may predispose a child to head injury are seizure disorders, gait instability, alcohol or drug ingestion, and cognitive delays, including poor judgment.

Pathophysiology

The pathophysiology of head injuries is complex in that the extent of the visible injury may not be indicative of the extent of actual brain injury. A head injury may involve any or all of the cranial and skull layers, including scalp, skull, dura, brain, and blood vessels, as well as neurons and supportive glial cells. Injuries can be classified as *primary*, meaning they result from the actual traumatic event, or as *secondary*, indicating that the damage is caused by pathologic processes (such as cerebral edema or anoxia) that occurred as a result of the initial injury. Secondary injury may be related to the rapidity of treatment once the injury has occurred.

There are several mechanisms of injury in pediatric head trauma. An injury may be either blunt or nonpenetrating, causing the distortion of brain tissue and shearing of neurons, even without outward evidence of injury or trauma. Penetrating or open injuries can produce either focal or diffuse damage, depending on the velocity and the type of penetration. Compression injuries are the result of the skull being compressed between two forces, causing the brain integrity to be crushed. Other commonly used terms are *coup* (pronounced *coo*) and *contrecoup* injuries. These terms are used to describe an injury to brain tissue that results when a blow to the head causes the brain to hit the skull at the location of impact (*coup*), and then rebound to the opposite side of the skull where injury can also occur (*contrecoup*) (Fig. 21–10).

Scalp Injuries. The scalp is composed of five layers, including connective tissue and vascular structures. Together these layers offer tremendous protection to the skull. Scalp injuries include abrasions and lacerations. For these injuries, gentle cleaning followed by hemostasis, conservative debridement of dead tissue, and suturing without tension is the recommended approach to management (Swaiman, 1994).

Skull Fractures. The human skull is composed of two layers—the inner and outer tables—separated by a spongy tissue called the diploic space. In a head injury, a fracture may occur at the site of impact or in areas of the skull with less tensile strength. Skull fractures are found in more than one fourth of children who are seen at

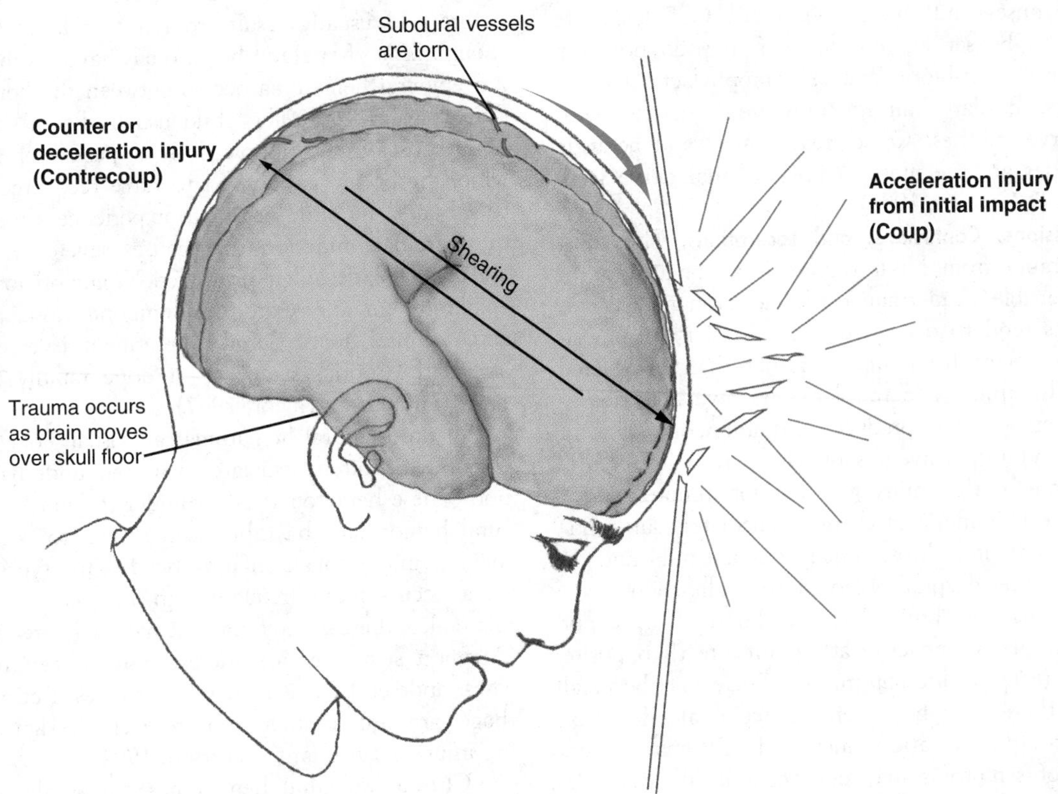

Figure 21–10
Mechanisms of coup–contrecoup injury. (From Ashwill, J. W., & Droske, S. C. [1997]. *Nursing care of children: principles and practice* [p. 1260]. Philadelphia: W. B. Saunders.)

hospitals with head injuries. There are five types of skull fractures. Nearly 70% of skull fractures are *linear* and involve the cranial vault. Fracture lines may be simple or complex and follow no predictable pattern. Children with uncomplicated linear fractures are usually admitted to the hospital for a short period of observation and are likely to resume normal activities within a few days. The bone heals on its own, and the fracture is not likely to be evident on skull radiographs 6 months to 1 year after the injury (Raffel & Litofsky, 1994). There are two concerns with linear fractures. First, there may be an unrecognized tear in a layer of meninges permitting escape of CSF. If unrepaired, a "growing fracture of childhood" may occur as the CSF collects and begins pulsating outward. The fracture widens and a small lump is seen over the area of the fracture. The second concern is the presence of a linear fracture over the middle meningeal artery in the temporal region. The artery is closely adherent to bone in this area. A linear fracture can result in a tear of the artery. The end result is an epidural hematoma.

Depressed skull fractures are often associated with scalp lacerations. The exception is "Ping-Pong" fractures or other fractures of the infant skull. A fracture is considered depressed when the inner table is displaced by more than the thickness of the skull. Compound depressed skull fractures (those with lacerations) should be debrided and elevated as soon as possible after the injury. Surgical elevation of the fragments is considered in closed injuries in which fragments are depressed more than 0.5 to 1.0 cm. Depressed fractures with many fragments are referred to as *comminuted* (Raffel & Litofsky, 1994).

Diastatic skull fractures occur along the suture line. The separation is usually visible on skull roentgenograph. These fractures often do not occur at the site of impact; they are seen most frequently in newborn babies and infants.

The most serious type of skull fracture is a *basilar skull fracture*. These fractures involve a break in the basal portions of the frontal, ethmoid, sphenoid, temporal, or occipital bones. Two classic findings associated with this type of skull fracture are the Battle sign and "raccoon eyes." The first is the presence of bruising or ecchymosis behind the ear caused by leakage of blood into the mastoid sinus. "Raccoon eyes" are caused by blood leaking into the frontal sinuses, causing an edematous and bruised periorbital area. Patients with these fractures may also have CSF leakage from the nose (rhinorrhea) or ears (otorrhea) secondary to tears in the meninges near the paranasal sinuses and the petrous bone. CSF leaks are rare and can be serious, especially if they do not stop spontaneously. Antibiotics are used prophylactically if a leak occurs. Basilar skull fractures are associated with cranial nerve injuries. Optic, extraocular, and acoustic nerve injuries are the most common cranial nerve injuries (Raffel & Litofsky, 1994).

Concussions, Contusions, and Lacerations. The most common injury from blunt trauma is a concussion. In minor, reversible head trauma, a concussion may occur. Concussions tend to occur when the head is in a position of movement from impact, rather than in a fixed position. This injury is a transient and reversible neuronal dysfunction that produces instantaneous loss of awareness and responsiveness on the part of the child. This response to the injury may last for minutes or for hours. There is amnesia of events immediately surrounding the head trauma. Most concussions are mild and do not require either hospital observation or admission.

Contusions are "bruises" to the brain. They occur either at the site of impact or at a point directly opposite the impact (*coup, contrecoup* injury). There may be focal edema, or there may be generalized cerebral edema or bleeding at either location; increased ICP may occur. The peak of symptoms may not occur until 48 to 72 hours after the injury, and complications from the edema last for days.

Lacerations are discontinuity of brain tissue. They are caused by penetrating craniocerebral trauma like gunshot wounds. Lacerations are considered to be serious because of the significant intracerebral bleeding that can be caused by this type of injury.

Vascular Injuries and Hematomas. Subdural and epidural hematomas occur in approximately 6% to 7% of pediatric head injuries. The shearing force created by the impact can cause the tearing of bridging vessels that supply blood to the various layers of the dura mater. Epidural hematomas are more likely to be of an acute nature and usually result from a tear in an artery, although 25% of epidural hematomas have a venous origin. An epidural hematoma occurs between the bone and the dura (Fig. 21–11). The child usually has a short period of unconsciousness followed by a period of lucidity in which he or she is believed to have recovered; within 4 to 8 hours, the child begins to experience a rapid decline in neurologic function that causes severe cerebral shift and even death if left untreated. Common locations for epidural hematomas are the temporal fossa, subfrontal, and occipital areas. Surgical treatment is emergent and arrests the serious symptoms if done rapidly (Swaiman, 1994; Thomas & Taylor, 1997).

Acute subdural hematomas are usually of venous origin and are often associated with an underlying contusion. These hematomas occur under the dura mater. Subdural hemorrhage has also been shown to occur from a shaking injury to an infant's head. This type of hematoma occurs more frequently in infants and is usually bilateral, whereas epidural hematomas are unilateral. Common symptoms are increased ICP, seen in 60% of cases, and seizures, seen in 40% of cases. Retinal hemorrhages are also common and are a classic sign of a shaking injury in an infant (Leurrsen, 1994).

Chronic subdural hematomas are usually related to trauma, but they may be identified at a much later date, usually after skull growth has accelerated beyond normal level. The characteristic symptoms are irritability, full nonpulsatile fontanelle, failure to thrive, and low hematocrit levels.

Alert: *Infants and small children have a proportionately larger CBF than adults; therefore, intracranial hemorrhage or bleeding may go undetected for a longer period of time.*

Cranial Nerve and Brain Tissue Injury. As discussed, basilar skull fractures are the most common cause of

Figure 21–11
Subdural hematoma and epidural hematoma. (From Ashwill, J. W., & Droske, S. C. [1997]. *Nursing care of children: principles and practice* [p. 1261]. Philadelphia: W. B. Saunders.)

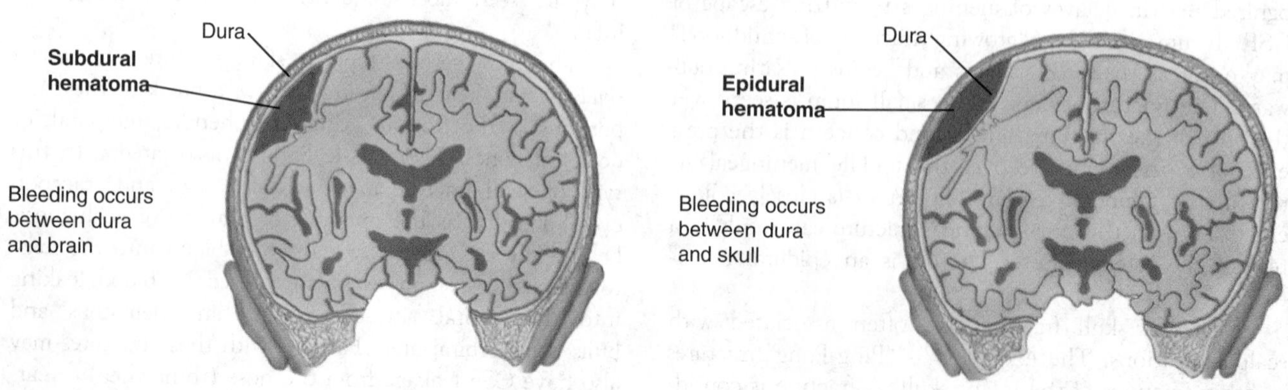
Dura
Subdural hematoma
Bleeding occurs between dura and brain
Dura
Epidural hematoma
Bleeding occurs between dura and skull

cranial nerve injury. Compression, stretching, or severe laceration can also cause cranial nerve damage. The most common cranial nerve injuries are to CN I (loss of smell), VII (facial paralysis), V and VI (eye movements), II (optic fields), and VIII.

Injury to actual brain tissue occurs in the form of a concussion, contusion, or laceration, as discussed. Damage of neurons is referred to as *diffuse axonal injury* (also called *shearing*). The mechanism for this injury is the difference in densities of the gray and white matter in the brain. When the head is subjected to impact, there is more displacement of the gray matter on the cortical surface than there is of the deep white matter. As a result, the axons degenerate and their ability to transmit impulses effectively diminishes. The course and outcome for the child depend on the extent of the injury (Leurrsen, 1994; Thomas & Taylor, 1997).

Assessment

The two primary components of the diagnostic assessment are a thorough history and physical examination and appropriate radiographic studies. A complete history of the traumatic event or injury is particularly important in cases of head injury. The actual mechanism of injury or state of consciousness after the injury, or both, can be a useful tool in diagnosing the type of trauma. Another major aspect of history taking is to determine whether there has been post-traumatic amnesia, as in concussion injuries, or a seizure at the time of injury, predisposing the child to injury. Family history of bleeding disorders should also be noted.

Once the family history and the history of the event have been gathered, a complete neurologic assessment should be carried out. Testing of cognitive and mental functions, as well as cranial nerve testing and assessment of signs and symptoms of increased ICP, is vital. If the injured child arrives at the health care facility in a state of rapid neurologic decompensation, assessment and interventions are often done simultaneously. If there is any evidence of a pressure build-up great enough to threaten herniation of the cerebral lobes, immediate action must be taken to alleviate the pressure. More in-depth coverage of this type of assessment and management is found in the discussion of increased ICP.

Level of consciousness, ability to follow commands, presence of confusion or irritability, pupil responsiveness, extraocular eye movements, and generalized strength and tone of extremities should be determined and well documented. In severe cases of neurologic trauma, posturing may be present (Fig. 21–12). Each assessment should start with the same degree of stimuli to the patient so that a comparison of responses can be made over time. Nursing assessment should also include observation of

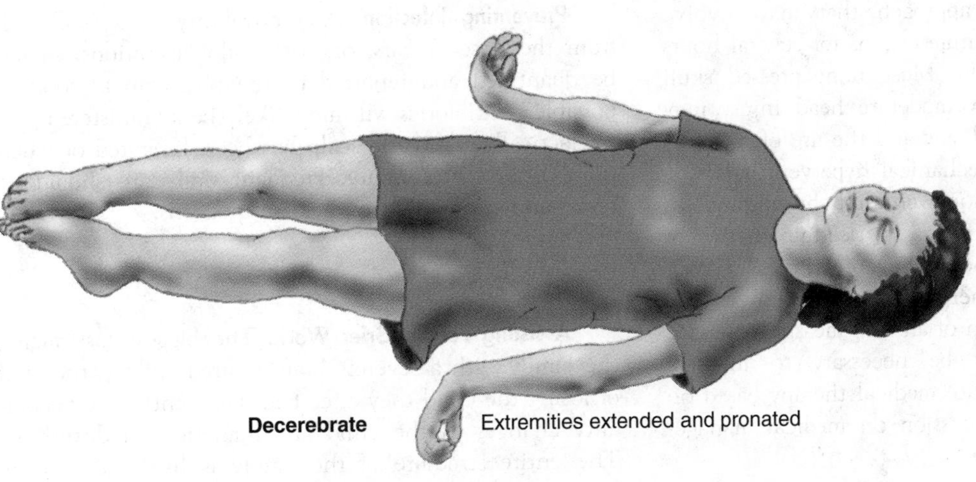

Figure 21–12
Decorticate and decerebrate posturing.

any potential CSF leak from the ear canals or nares, or changes in external findings (increased swelling or tenderness over scalp abrasions or wounds). Any abnormal motor movements or potential seizure activity should be observed and recorded. Finally, close scrutiny of cardiorespiratory and vital sign parameters is essential, because evidence of increasing ICP should be reported immediately (see discussion of increased ICP).

Diagnostic Tests. Radiographic studies for head injury are basically skull and cervical spine films and a CT scan. If the injury is minor and the child appears to be neurologically intact, a CT scan may not be necessary, although plain skull films are usually obtained to rule out a skull fracture. MRI scans are being used more frequently, particularly in children with more severe injuries as a way to follow white and gray matter changes over time.

If there has been seizure activity after the injury, an EEG is necessary. Injuries involving the cranial nerves may be followed with brain stem auditory evoked responses or with visual evoked responses, or both. A child with long-term cognitive deficits may require a neuropsychological evaluation to assess functional, learning, and vocational abilities.

Interdisciplinary Interventions

Care of the child with head trauma varies by the mechanism of injury, location of injury, and association with multisystem injuries (e.g., fracture of ribs, femur, laceration of liver).

Surgical Management. Surgical management is necessary in a few instances of head injury. The elevation of a depressed skull fracture and the removal of an acute epidural or subdural hematoma are the most common reasons for surgical intervention in the head-injured child. Chronic subdural hematomas may require mechanical shunting to the peritoneal space. Aggressive medical and pharmacologic management is usually the therapy of choice for moderately to severely injured children.

The treatment for mild head injury is generally a conservative observational approach that may involve following up the clinical manifestations for several hours before discharging the child. Most nondepressed skull fractures heal over time. A moderate head injury may involve a prolonged hospital stay and the use of methods to decrease ICP short of mechanical hyperventilation. It may be necessary to keep some children hospitalized to follow cranial nerve functions and to ascertain that there is no worsening disease process. Severe injuries necessitate a critical care environment with close monitoring of vital functions. The insertion of an ICP measuring device by the neurosurgeon may be necessary to monitor changes in ICP and to initiate medical therapy based on these changes. (See the discussion on medical management for increased ICP.)

The child with head injury is at high risk for altered cerebral perfusion. Nursing care for the child with threatened cerebral tissue perfusion includes careful monitoring of oxygen saturation with pulse oximetry and administration of oxygen as necessary. It is preferable to administer oxygen when a child's oxygenation status is questionable, even before a pulse oximetry reading is obtained. The nurse should also be aware of, and closely follow, the child's hemoglobin and hematocrit levels to ensure adequate oxygen-carrying capacity within the blood. Other nursing interventions aimed at promoting optimal cerebral tissue perfusion include close monitoring of systemic perfusion parameters, such as blood pressure and other vital signs. Close scrutiny of fluid and electrolyte status is also warranted to avoid fluid overload and resultant cerebral edema. Anticonvulsants should be administered as ordered, and any seizure activity should be well documented.

Avoiding Airway Compromise. Slight elevation of the head of the child's bed is important in managing potential or actual increases in ICP, and it is useful in optimizing airway position. Slight hyperextension can be achieved by placing a towel roll underneath the child's shoulders. This should never be attempted until cervical spine injury has been ruled out. Oral or deep suction may be necessary every 2 to 4 hours to clear secretions and to stimulate a cough. An appropriate-size bag and mask should always be available at the bedside for emergency use, as needed.

Ongoing Assessments. Ongoing assessments of the child's neurologic function, including assessment of the level of awareness or responsiveness and the presence of confusion, should be done initially every 1 to 2 hours following the injury. The bedside nurse must document any changes in the child's condition and assess the child more frequently, if warranted. Changes in level of consciousness are frequently the first indication of changes in ICP and cerebral perfusion. Confusion can lead to safety risks, if the child is not being closely watched or properly restrained.

Preventing Infection. Any possibility of a CSF leak from the nose or ears, or from scalp lacerations, should be quantified and reported to the physician as soon as possible. Antibiotics will most likely be administered prophylactically when the scalp has been lacerated or when there is an open injury. Frequent oral care should be given and extra attention paid to incisions.

Community Care

Assisting Family Grief Work. The biggest task facing the family with a severely brain-injured child is the grief of losing the child they once had. Frequently, the personality changes in the child are dramatic and disturbing. The entire structure of the family is likely to change.

Initially, when progress seems to occur daily, families have a lot of hope for a complete recovery for their child. As the family realizes their loss, depression can set in. Stress also has its effect on the marital and sibling relationships. The nurse's role is to offer the family realistic expectations and support through their grief work. Referring the family for further counseling is also an important role. The family needs to be encouraged to take part in their child's care, but they also need to be given permission to take occasional breaks for themselves.

Preventing Injury. For the head-injured child, a major component of nursing care may be to provide assistance in making sounder judgments in his or her daily activities. Comprehensive rehabilitation programs that involve a component of behavior modification are usually effective in helping children become aware of their own safety. Wearing a protective helmet is often necessary.

The family's ability to adapt is affected by the extent of the injury, the family's involvement in the incident, and the chance (or lack thereof) for full recovery.

For children with any long-term sensory deficits (vision, hearing, smell), the nurse should address the need for adaptations to prevent further injury from lack of sensory input. Family members should be educated about seizure precautions, if they are needed. Toxic side effects of anticonvulsants should also be discussed with patients and families, as appropriate.

The sequelae from a head injury in the pediatric years can become a lifetime burden. Seizure activity becomes post-traumatic epilepsy. Postconcussion syndrome can be apparent for a year or more after the injury. Hydrocephalus can occur as the result of an infectious process. The most difficult aspects of long-term outcome are the ensuing personality and behavior changes that can prevent a completely independent lifestyle for the child. Persistent physical difficulties may affect independence. Nevertheless, most pediatric head injuries are minor occurrences that require no hospitalization and engender no long-term damage.

Acute Spinal Cord Injury

Although acute spinal cord injury (SCI) is an infrequent occurrence in the general pediatric population, the incidence of these injuries does increase significantly in middle and late adolescence. The most common causes are vehicular accidents, falls, athletic injuries, or violent penetrating wounds.

caREminder: *All injured children should be treated as if an SCI has occurred until the potential for this problem has been eliminated. This includes immediate immobilization of the head and spine on a "spine board" before transfer from the scene of the injury.*

The emotional and psychological sequelae of these potentially devastating injuries are overwhelming. The need for excellent acute care management and comprehensive long-range planning for these children or adolescents and their families cannot be overstated. The changes affecting a child and family after an SCI are significant and long lasting.

Incidence

A large proportion of spinal fractures results in no neurologic deficit. However, SCI with no evidence of radiographic abnormality is well documented in children. Birth injuries affect the cervical spine. After the neonatal period, 60% to 75% of injuries occur in the cervical region, 20% in the thoracic region, and the remainder in the lumbar area.

Etiology

SCIs are often described in the relationship to the mechanism and anatomic location of injury. Flexion-dislocation, hyperextension, vertical compression, and rotation are the major mechanisms of injury. Flexion-dislocation injuries are common in motor vehicle accidents, whereas vertical compression injuries are associated with diving or trampoline injuries. The location and classification of an SCI is usually referred to as the level of injury below which sensory and motor function are impaired (Table 21–15).

Quadriplegia results from injuries at the cervical level and implies complete loss of leg function and limited, if any, use of the arms. Paraplegia results from thoracic or high lumbar injury and is characterized by a loss of leg function alone. Most SCIs are incomplete and result in variable degrees of motor and sensory loss below the level of the lesion. Complete lesions are rare.

Several factors influence the severity of the actual injury to the spinal cord. The mechanism for cellular damage and functional impairment is usually compression and contusion, rather than actual transection. In the first hours after injury, decreased blood flow and ischemia result in extensive tissue destruction. Compression injuries may result from spinal epidural or subdural hematomas that can be surgically alleviated.

A common physiologic consequence of SCI is a phenomenon referred to as *central cord necrosis*. As further edema and ischemia develop, vascular stasis and thrombosis occur, propagating the vicious circle; the eventual outcome is necrosis of gray matter.

Assessment

Immediate signs and symptoms of SCI vary, depending on whether the cord transection is complete or partial.

Table 21–15
American Spinal Injury Association (ASIA) Impairment Scale

A = Complete: No motor or sensory function is preserved in the sacral segments S_4–S_5.
B = Incomplete: Sensory but not motor function is preserved below the neurologic level and includes the sacral segments of S_4–S_5.
C = Incomplete: Motor function is preserved below the neurologic level, and more than half of key muscles below the neurologic level have a muscle grade less than 3.
D = Incomplete: Motor function is preserved below the neurologic level, and at least half of key muscles below the neurologic level have a muscle grade of 3 or more.
E = Normal: Motor and sensory function is normal.

From American Spinal Injury Association. (1996). *International standards for neurological and functional classification of spinal cord injury.* Chicago: Author. Reprinted with permission.

Partial transection is seen most commonly and is discussed here. A symmetric flaccid paralysis and loss of reflexes below the portion of damaged cord occur. There may be some preservation of pain, temperature, and proprioception below the level of the injury. Moderate vasomotor instability and lowering of the blood pressure usually occur. Cervical cord injury is characterized by respiratory insufficiency secondary to disruption of innervation to the diaphragm. Another condition that occurs immediately after injury is referred to as *neurogenic shock.* This condition is characterized by hypotension caused by vasodilation of the vascular bed below the level of injury, bradycardia, and loss of the ability to sweat below the level of injury.

During the recovery period from the acute phase, hyperreflexia and spasticity may appear. Clinical manifestations in chronic SCI are related to the degree of recovery and functional return after the initial injury. Complications, such as autonomic dysreflexia and bladder dysfunction, occur in the postacute phase.

The immediate response to SCI is referred to as *spinal shock.* This phenomenon is the temporary suppression of reflexes controlled below the level of the injury. Spinal shock can last from a few hours to many months. The appearance of perianal reflexes signifies the end of spinal shock and the beginning of recovery. Functional loss from SCI is determined by the level and degree of injury.

Diagnostic Tests. Once the clinical examination has been carried out, a thorough roentgenographic examination should be made. Anteroposterior, lateral, and oblique views of the spine down to the suspected level of injury are obtained. Routine films of the spine and pelvis below the level of the injury are necessary to rule out any other hidden fractures. Spinal CT scans and MRI, may each be useful, depending on the type of injury and information desired. It is important to avoid further injury to the child when radiographs or scans are being obtained.

Interdisciplinary Interventions

Treatment of acute SCI begins immediately. Initial management at the scene of the trauma should include stabilization of the spine and establishment of an adequate airway. Other appropriate medical measures during the acute phase include the administration of intravenous dexamethasone to reduce swelling around the spinal cord and aggressive pulmonary hygiene measures to prevent pneumonia. Stress ulcer is common and is often prevented by administering antacids. Frequent repositioning is ordered, and the patient may be placed in a special frame or bed for turning. Urinary catheterization is also necessary until a determination of bladder function can be made.

Throughout the acute care phase, rehabilitative measures are instituted to ensure the best possible outcome for the child. Safe and early mobilization is attempted by using a variety of stabilizing devices. Cardiovascular complications include *orthostatic hypotension* and *autonomic hyperreflexia* (also called dysreflexia). The latter occurs when there is an uncontrolled increase in sympathetic activity that cannot be inhibited because of the SCI. It is usually caused by overdistention of the bladder or bowel, and it can be a serious complication if not managed.

Health care during the rehabilitative phase following acute SCI is multifaceted. These children are at risk for thromboembolism and respiratory compromise. Many children with cervical lesions require a tracheostomy. Bowel and bladder care need to be adapted as mobility increases. A bladder program geared toward prevention of urinary tract infection is vital. Prevention of skin breakdown is a task assumed by all personnel who provide care for the child with SCI. Physical, occupational, and speech therapy, as well as an assessment of learning and nutritional and psychosocial needs, are essential. The complex and emotional medical care of these children is best managed in a interdisciplinary rehabilitative center. Reintegrating the disabled child into the family requires a group of individuals committed to the ultimate goal of providing the child with the best possible quality of life. Chapter 11 provides more information regarding the rehabilitation needs of these children.

Summary of Key Concepts

- ◆ Emergency neurologic assessment of the infant and child includes evaluation of level of consciousness, cranial nerve function, pupil reactivity, and reflexes.
- ◆ Aspects of the normal assessment of neurologic functioning include head size, shape, and symmetry; achievement of motor and social milestones; presence, absence, and symmetry of developmental reflexes; vision and hearing examination; and assessment of cranial nerve functioning.
- ◆ Neurologic development of the child is not complete at birth. Maturational changes continue into the early childhood years, which affects myelinization, skull ossification, elongation of the spinal cord and the cranial and peripheral nerves, and CSF production. These changes ultimately improve the child's ability to respond to neurologic stimuli.
- ◆ The two primary treatment modalities for the neurologic disorders are use of medications and cranial surgery. The nurse should be aware of the use, side effects, and potential drug interactions of medications used. The principles of preoperative and postoperative care for the neurologic patient are similar to those for children with other surgical conditions; however, the child is at great risk for increased intracranial pressure and hemorrhage.
- ◆ Nursing care for the child with increased ICP is focused on assessing ICP, maintaining the integrity of the monitoring system, and assessing the child for signs of infection, hemorrhage, CSF leakage, and neurologic deterioration.
- ◆ A seizure is a sudden, involuntary, time-limited alteration in function occurring as a result of an abnormal discharge of neurons in the CNS. The child experiencing a seizure should be provided immediate first aid to prevent injury. After the seizure has resolved, care is focused on determining the underlying cause of the seizure and thereby preventing its recurrence.
- ◆ Children with epilepsy must be continually evaluated by the health care team to ensure that pharmacotherapy is achieving suppression of seizure activity and that health maintenance activities are being promoted in the home and community to prevent seizure activity and to protect the child.
- ◆ Many children experience headaches. Even though stress can be a cause of headaches, it is important to determine the type of headache that the child is having in case the causative agent is life-threatening.
- ◆ The child with anencephaly has an absence of brain tissue above a rudimentary brain stem and basal ganglia. Sustained extrauterine life is virtually impossible for these children.
- ◆ Major health care priorities for the child with spina bifida are to prevent infection, prevent neurologic injury, prevent injury to the limbs secondary to disuse, promote optimal bowel elimination, manage neurogenic bladder, promote skin integrity, promote family coping, and promote the child's positive self-concept.

- Hydrocephalus may be congenital or acquired. Management involves the placement of a shunt to promote drainage of CSF into another body cavity. Families need to be prepared to care for the child with a shunt through knowledge of the signs of increased ICP, shunt infection, and shunt malfunction.
- Chiari malformation is a type of hindbrain herniation. Some children outgrow the symptoms of this condition and require no medical intervention. Other children may have severe difficulties with respiratory and neurologic complications, which require immediate posterior fossa decompression to prevent further symptoms.
- Two conditions that impact cranial ossification are microcephaly and craniosynostosis. The child with microcephaly has a small skull and may have mental retardation due to inadequate brain growth. The child with craniosynostosis has early closure of the sutures, which need not affect cognitive functioning if diagnosed and treated in a timely manner.
- Meningitis can be caused by bacterial, viral, and fungal organisms. Nursing care of the child with meningitis is directed toward providing comfort, relieving pain, assessing for possible complications, and supporting the family.
- The child with encephalitis has symptoms that may be acute or may be gradual, with complaints of general muscle pain, fever, gastrointestinal distress, and mild respiratory symptoms. Clinically, the neurologic presentation is similar to meningitis. The prognosis for encephalitis depends on the degree and duration of cerebral and CNS involvement, and on the ability to successfully manage secondary complications.
- Brain abscesses may be a result of extension of local infections of the middle ear, mastoid, or sinuses; distal infections in the chest or lungs; or spread through the bloodstream in immunocompromised hosts (metastatic abscess). Direct infection occurs as a result of open head trauma, intracranial surgery, bacterial meningitis, or cranial traction.
- To prevent tetanus in children, they should be inoculated with DT or DPT immunization.
- To reduce the incidence of Reye's syndrome, acetaminophen should not be administered to children who have a viral illness.
- Guillain-Barré syndrome is an acute, demyelinating polyneuropathy of primarily peripheral nerves, occurring as a postinfectious process. It is a reversible condition that has a good prognosis for most children affected.
- Neuromuscular disorders such as spinal muscular atrophy and myasthenia gravis result in progressive weakness of neurologic functions. Nursing care is directed toward optimizing functions that are not compromised and assisting the family to modify their care of the child in relation to the degree of impairment that occurs during the various stages of the child's condition.
- Neurocutaneous syndromes are characterized by their tendency toward tumor formation in the CNS, skin, and visceral linings of various organ systems, and by their recognizable cutaneous manifestations.
- Nursing care for the child with a head injury includes promoting optimal cerebral perfusion, avoiding airway compromise, responding to altered sensorium and changes in level of consciousness, preventing infection, and facilitating rehabilitation and home care.
- All injured children should be treated as if an SCI has occurred until the potential for this problem has been eliminated. This includes immediate immobilization of the head and spine on a "spine board" before transfer from the scene of the injury.

Resources

Organizations

American Association of Neuroscience Nurses
224 North Des Plaines
Suite 601
Chicago, IL 60661
(312) 993-0043
Web: http: //www.aann.org

American Neurological Association
5841 Cedar Lake Road
Suite 108
Minneapolis, MN 55416
(612) 545-6284
Web: http: //trooft.rbdc.com/ana/ana.html

American Trauma Society
8903 Presidential Parkway, Suite 512
Upper Marlboro, MD 20772
(800) 556-7890

Children's Craniofacial Association
10210 North Central Expressway
Suite 230
Dallas, TX 75231
(800) 535-3643

Epilepsy Foundation of America
4351 Garden City Drive
Suite 406
Landover, MD 20785
(301) 459-3700
(800) 332-1000

Epilepsy Information Center
Bowman Gray School of Medicine
Medical Center Blvd.
Winston-Salem, NC 27157-1078
(800) 642-0500

International Rett Syndrome Foundation
9121 Piscataway Road
No. 2B
Clinton, MD 20735
(301) 856-3334

Myasthenia Gravis Foundation
222 South Riverside Plaza
Suite 1540
Chicago, IL 60606
(800) 541-5454

National Association for the Craniofacially Handicapped
P. O. Box 11082
Chattanooga, TN 37401
(800) 3FACES3 (332-2373)

National Headache Foundation
5252 North Western Avenue
Chicago, IL 60625
(800)-444-NHIF

National Head Injury Foundation
1176 Massachusetts Avenue NW
Suite 100
Washington, DC 20036-1904
(800) 444-6443

National Institute of Neurologic Disorders and Stroke (NINDS)
P. O. Box 5801
Bethesda, MD 20824
(800) 352-9424

National Reye's Syndrome Foundation, Inc.
P. O. Box 829
Bryan, OH 43506
(800) 233-7393

National Spinal Cord Injury Association
8300 Colesville
Suite 551
Silver Spring, MD 20910
(800) 962-9629
E-mail: NSCIAZ@aol.com
Web: http: //www.spinalcord.org

National Spinal Cord Injury Association
545 Concord Avenue
Suite 29
Cambridge, MA 02138
(800) 962-9629

Spina Bifida Association of America
4590 MacArthur Boulevard
Suite 250
Washington, DC 20007
(800) 621-3141
Web: http: //www.sbaa.org

Spina Bifida Association of Canada
220-388 Donald Street
Winnipeg, MB Canada R3B 2J4
(204) 957-1784

Spinal Cord Injury Hotline
2201 Argonne Drive
Baltimore, MD 21218
(800) 526-3456

Computer Resources

Spina Bifida Information Resources
Web: http: //www.waisman.wisc edu/rowley/sb-kids/sb_sourc.htm

✏ In Touch With Kids Program
Web: http: //www.spinalcord.org/resource/infoitwk.html
Free program for children with spinal cord injury.

Books and Printed Materials

Sandler, A. (1977). *Living with spina bifida: A guide for families and professionals.* Chapel Hill, NC: University of North Carolina Press.

✏ Panzarino, C. *Rebecca finds a new way.* Available from National Spinal Cord Injury Association.

SCI Life
Magazine for people with spinal cord injury. Available from National Spinal Cord Injury Association.

✏ Resources specifically for children.

References

American Academy of Pediatrics, Committee on Infectious Diseases. (1990). Dexamethasone therapy for bacterial meningitis in infants and children. *Pediatrics*, 86(1), 130–133.

American Academy of Pediatrics. (1991). *Report to the Committee on Infectious Diseases* (22nd ed.). Elk Grove Village, IL: Author.

American Academy of Pediatrics Committee on Infectious Diseases (1992). Update. *Pediatrics, 89*, 161–165.

American Association of Neuroscience Nurses (1996). *Core curriculum for neuroscience nursing*. Des Plaines, IL: Author.

American Thoracic Society (1992). Control of tuberculosis in the United States. *American Review of Respiratory Diseases, 142*, 725–735.

Anderson, S. (1992). Guillain-Barré syndrome: Giving the patient control. *Journal of Neurosurgical Nursing, 124*(3), 158–162.

Angelucci, D., & Todaro, A. (1990). Action stat! Tetanus. *Nursing, 20*(8), 33.

Arbour, R. B. (1993). Stereotactic localization and resection of intracranial tumors. *Journal of Neuroscience Nursing, 25*(1), 14–21.

Arnon, S. (1996). Tetanus. In R. Behrman, R. Kliegman, & A. Arvin (Eds.), *Nelson textbook of pediatrics* (pp. 815–817). Philadelphia: W. B. Saunders.

Austin, J. K., Smith, M. S., Risinger, M. W., & McNeles, A. M. (1994). Childhood epilepsy and asthma: Comparison of quality of life. *Epilepsia, 35*, 608–615.

Austin, J. K. (1995). New onset childhood seizures: Parents' concerns and needs. *Clinical Nursing Practice in Epilepsy*, Winter, 8–10.

Ballweg, D. (1991). Neonatal seizures: An overview. *Neonatal Network, 10*, 15–21.

Bannon, M. J., Weldig, C., & Jones, P. W. (1992). Teacher's perception of epilepsy. *Archives of Diseases in Childhood, 67*, 1467–1471.

Batchelor, L., Nance, J., & Short, B. (1997). An interdisciplinary team approach to implementing the ketogenic diet for the treatment of seizures. *Pediatric Nursing, 23*(5), 465–471.

Bell, W. (1992). Bacterial meningitis in children: Selected aspects. *Pediatric Clinics of North America, 39*(4), 651–658.

Bell, W. E., & McCormick, W. F. (Eds.). (1981). *Neurologic infections in children* (2nd ed.). Philadelphia: W. B. Saunders.

Berg, A. T., Skinnar, S., Hauser, E., & Leventhal, J. M. (1990). Predictions of recurrent febrile seizures: A meta analytic review. *Journal of Pediatrics, 116*, 329–336.

Berg, B. (1996). *Principles of child neurology*. New York: McGraw-Hill.

Breningstall, G. N. (1996). Breathholding spells. *Pediatric Neurology, 14*, 91–97.

Budd, R. A., & Hobdell, E. F. (1983). Reyes syndrome. *Critical Care Nurse, 3*(2), 94–97.

Buehler, B. A., Rao, V., & Finnell, R. H. (1994). Biochemical and molecular teratology of fetal hydantoin syndrome. *Neurologic Clinics, 12*(4), 741–748.

Bullock, R., & Fujisawa, H. (1992). The role of glutamate antagonists for treatment of CNS injury. *Journal of Neurotrauma, 9*, S443–S458.

Burns, C. (1996). Neurological disorders. In C. Burns, N. Barber, M. Brady, & A. Dunn (Eds.). *Pediatric primary care* (pp. 551–572). Philadelphia: W. B. Saunders.

Carey, C. M., Tullous, M. W., & Walker, M. L. (1994). Hydrocephalus: Etiology, pathologic effects diagnosis and maternal history. In W. Cheek (Ed.), *Pediatric neurosurgery: Surgery of the developing nervous system* (3rd ed., pp. 185–201). Philadelphia: W. B. Saunders.

Casey, K. M. (1993). Fighting MDR-TB. *RN, 56*(9), 26–30.

Centers for Disease Control. (1992). Spina bifida incidence at birth—United States, 1983–1990. *Morbidity and Mortality Weekly Report, 41*, 497–500.

Chipps, E. M., Clanin, N. J., & Campbell, V. G. (1992). *Neurologic disorders*. St. Louis: Mosby–Year Book.

Cohen, B. H. (1995). Headaches as a symptom of neurological disease. *Seminars in Pediatric Neurology, 2*, 144–150.

Cohen, M. (1986). *Craniosynostosis: Diagnosis, evaluation, and management*. New York: Raven Press.

Cotton, J. M. (1984). A comprehensive nursing approach to the neonate with myelomeningocele. *Neonatal Network, 3*, 7–16.

Crawford, T. O. (1996). From enigmatic to problematic: The new molecular genetics of childhood spinal muscular atrophy. *Neurology, 46*, 335–340.

Crumrine, P. (1996). Seizure therapy. In F. Burg, J. Ingelfender, E. Wald, & R. Polin (Eds.), *Current pediatric therapy* (pp. 97–104). Philadelphia: W. B. Saunders.

Dauser, R. C., DiPetro, M. A., & Venes, J. L. (1988). Symptomatic Chiari I malformations in childhood: A report of 7 cases. *Pediatric Neuroscience, 14*, 184–190.

Divertie, V. C. (1996). Recurrent headaches in children. *MCN, 21*, 235–240.

Drachman, D. B. (1994). Myasthenia gravis. *New England Journal of Medicine, 330*, 1797–1810.

Feigin, R. D., & Cherry, J. D. (1992). *Textbook of pediatric infectious diseases* (3rd ed.). Philadelphia: W. B. Saunders.

Fidzianska, F. (1996). Spinal muscular atrophy in childhood. *Seminars in Pediatric Neurology, 3*, 53–58.

Frishberg, B. M. (1994). The utility of neuroimaging in the evaluation of headache in patients with normal neurologic examinations. *Neurology, 44*, 1191–1197.

Givner, L. (1996). Aseptic meningitis. In F. Berg, J. Ingelfinder, E. Wald, & R. Polin (Eds.), *Current pediatric therapy* (p. 637). Philadelphia: W. B. Saunders.

Graham, J. M. (1992). Congenital anomalies. In M. D. Levine, W. B. Carey, & A. C. Crocker (Eds.), *Developmental-behavioral pediatrics* (pp. 229–243). Philadelphia: W. B. Saunders.

Greif, L., & Miller, C. L. (1991). Shunt lengthening: A descriptive review. *Journal of Neuroscience Nursing, 23*(2), 120–124.

Haslam, R. (1996). Craniosynostosis. In R. Behrman, R. Kleigman, & A. Arvin (Eds.). *Nelson textbook of pediatrics* (pp. 1685–1686). Philadelphia: W. B. Saunders.

Haslam, R. H. A. (1997). Nonfebrile seizures. *Pediatrics in Review, 18*, 39–49.

Hauser, W. (1990). *Epilepsy: Frequency, causes and consequences*. New York: Demos.

Hazinski, M. F. (1995). Systematic assessment of the critically ill or injured child: The nine point check. *Nursing Care of Children and Their Families, Changing Practice, Changing Roles and Changing Environments, The Fifth Annual Meeting of the Society of Pediatric Nurses, USA*, 43–56.

Hickey, J. V. (1992). *The clinical practice of neurological and neurosurgical nursing*. Philadelphia: J. B. Lippincott.

Hinkle, J. L. (1990). Home antibiotic therapy for brain abscess. *Journal of Intravenous Therapy, 13*(3), 172–176.

Hobdell, E. F. (1988). Infantile spasms. *Pediatric Nursing, 14*, 207–209.

Holmes, G. L. (1996). Epilepsy and other seizure disorders. In B. Berg (Ed.), *Principles of child neurology*. New York: McGraw-Hill.

Jackson, M. M. (1993). Tuberculosis in infants, children and adolescents: New dilemmas with an old disease. *Pediatric Nursing, 19*(5), 437–442.

Jones, H. R. (1996). Childhood Guillain-Barré syndrome: Clinical presentation, diagnosis, and therapy. *Journal of Child Neurology, 11*, 4–12.

Kanev, P. M., & Park, T. S. (1993). The treatment of hydrocephalus. *Neurosurgery Clinics of North America, 4*(4), 611–620.

Klaus, M., & Kennel, J. (1976). *Maternal-infant bonding*. St. Louis: C. V. Mosby.

Kolodgie, M. J. (1994). Home care management of the child with infantile spasms. *Pediatric Nursing, 2*, 270–273.

Krywanio, M. L. (1991). Varicella encephalitis. *Journal of Neuroscience Nursing, 23*(6), 363–368.

Lannon, S. (1997). Epilepsy surgery for partial seizures. *Pediatric Nursing, 23*(5), 453–459.

Laurence, K. J., James, N., Miller, M. H., Tennent, G. B., & Campbell, H. (1991). Double blind randomised controlled trial of folate treatment before and after conception to prevent recurrence of neural tube defects. *British Medicine Journal, 282*, 1509.

Leger, R., & Meeropol, E. (1992). Children at risk: Latex allergy and spina bifida. *Journal of Pediatric Nursing, 7*, 371–376.

Leurrsen, T. G. (1994). Acute traumatic cerebral injuries. In W. Cheek (Ed.), *Pediatric neurosurgery: Surgery of the developing nervous system* (3rd ed., pp. 266–278). Philadelphia: W. B. Saunders.

Lewis, D. W. (1995). Migraine and migraine variants in childhood and adolescence. *Seminars in Pediatric Neurology, 2*, 127–143.

Lovejoy, F. (1996) Reye syndrome. In F. Burg, J. Ingelfinger, Z. Wald, & R. Polin (Eds.). *Current pediatric therapy, 15* (pp. 112–113). Philadelphia: W. B. Saunders.

Lutkus, E. R., Hirsch, A. F., & Wood, J. P. (1984). Tetanus. *Annals of Emergency Medicine, 13*, 186–188.

Mampalam, T., & Rosenbluth, M. (1988). Trends in the management of brain abscesses: A review of 102 cases. *Neurosurgery, 4*(23), 451–557.

Marlin, E. D., & Gaskill, S. J. (1994). Cerebrospinal fluid shunts: Complications and results. In W. Cheek (Ed.), *Pediatric neurosurgery: Surgery of the developing nervous system* (3rd ed., pp. 221–233). Philadelphia: W. B. Saunders.

Martin, J. (1990). Pediatric management problems. *Pediatric Nursing, 16*, 394–396.

McDonald, M. (1997). Use of the ketogenic diet in treating children with seizures. *Pediatric Nursing, 23*(5), 461–464.

McMillan, J. (1996). Encephalitis. In F. Burg, J. Ingelfinger, E. Wald, & R. Polin (Eds.). *Current pediatric therapy, 15* (pp. 632–634). Philadelphia: W. B. Saunders.

Menkes, J. H. (1995). *Textbook of child neurology* (4th ed.). Philadelphia: Lea and Febiger.

Mitchell, W. G. (1996). Status epilepticus and acute repetitive seizures in children, adolescents, and young adults: Etiology, outcome, and treatment. *Epilepsia, 37*(Suppl.), 574–580.

Moore, K., & Persaud, T. (1993). *The developing human*. Philadelphia: W. B. Saunders.

Nardell, E. A. (1990). Dodging droplet nuclei—Reducing the possibility of nosocomial tuberculosis transmission in the AIDS era [Letter]. *American Review of Respiratory Diseases, 142*(3), 501.

Oakes, W. (1985). Chiari malformations, hydromyelia, syringomyelia. In R. Wilkins & S. Rengachary (Eds). *Neurosurgery* (vol. 3, pp. 2102–2115). New York: McGraw-Hill.

Pearce, J. M. S. (1994). Headache. *Journal of Neurology, Neurosurgery, and Psychiatry, 57*, 134–143.

Pohl, C. (1993). Practical approach to bacterial meningitis in childhood. *American Family Physicians, 47*(7), 1595–1603.

Prendergast, V. (1987). Bacterial meningitis update. *Journal of Neuroscience Nursing, 19*(2), 95–99.

Prober, C. (1996). *Infections of the central nervous system*. In R. Behrman, R. Kliegman, & A. Arvin (Eds.), *Nelson textbook of pediatrics* (pp. 707–716). Philadelphia: W. B. Saunders.

Raffel, C., & Litofsky, N. S. (1994). Skull fractures. In W. Cheek (Ed.), *Pediatric neurosurgery: Surgery of the developing nervous system* (3rd ed., pp. 257–265). Philadelphia: W. B. Saunders.

Raloff, J. (1995). Enzyme error behind neural tube defects. *Science News, 157*, 53.

Reigel, D. H., & Rotenstein, D. (1994). Spina bifida. In W. Cheek (Ed.), *Pediatric neurosurgery: Surgery of the developing nervous system* (3rd ed., pp. 51–76). Philadelphia: W. B. Saunders.

Ripley, C., Pomatto, J., Beals, S., Joganic, E., Manwaring, K., & Moss, D. (1994). Treatment of positional plagiocephaly with dynamic orthotic cranioplasty, *Journal of Craniofacial Surgery, 5*(3), 150–156.

Roach, E. S., Buono, G., McLean, W. T., & Weaver, R. G. (1985). Early onset myasthenia gravis. *Journal of Pediatrics, 108*(2), 193–197.

Rothner, A. D. (1995). The evaluation of headaches in children and adolescents. *Seminars in Pediatric Neurology, 2*, 109–118.

Rowe, P. C. (1987). *The Harriet Lane handbook* (11th ed.). Chicago: Year Book Medical Publishers.

Rudy, D. C., & Woodside, J. R. (1991). The incontinent myelodysplastic patient. *Urology Clinics of North America, 18*, 295–300.

Russman, B. S., Iannacone, S. T., Buncher, C. R., Samaha, F. S., White, M., Perkins, B., Zimmerman, L., Smith, C., Burhans, K., & Barker, L. (1992). Spinal muscular atrophy: New thoughts on the pathogenesis and classification schema. *Journal of Child Neurology, 7*, 347–353.

Rutkowski, K. (1990). Grid implantation in seizure patients. *AORNS Journal, 52(5)*, 953–975.

Saez-Llorens, X., & McCracken, G. H. (1992). Meningitis. In S. Krugman, S. Katz, A. Gershon, & C. Wilfert (Eds.), *Infectious diseases of children* (9th ed., 246–259). St. Louis: Mosby.

Schaefer, G. B., Sheth, R. D., & Bodensteiner, J. B. (1994). Cerebral dysgenesis: An overview. *Neurologic Clinics, 12*(4), 773–788.

Scheld, M., & Winn, R. (1990). *Principles and practices of infectious diseases*. New York: John Wiley.

Scott, J. M. (1995). November *Quarterly Journal of Medicine*. NEURAL TUBE DEFECTS.

Shahar, E., Shorer, Z., Raifman, C. M., Levi, Y., Brand, N., Ravid, S., & Murphy, E. G. (1997). Immune globulins are effective in severe pediatric Guillain-Barré syndrome. *Pediatric Neurology, 16*, 32–36.

Shaw, G. M., Velie, E. M., & Schaffer, D. (1996). Risk of neural tube defect—Affected pregnancies among obese women. *JAMA 275*(14), 1093–1096.

Shiminski-Maher, T., & Disabato, J. (1994). Current trends in the diagnosis and management of hydrocephalus in children. *Journal of Pediatric Nursing*, 9(4), 74–82.

Shinnar, S. S. (1991). An approach to the child with headaches. *International Pediatrics*, 6, 140–148.

Singer, H. (1993). Tic disorders. *Pediatric Annals, 22*(1), 22–29.

Smith, G. (1997). Helping children relax during magnetic resonance imaging. *MCN, 22*, 237–241.

Spiro, A. J. (1996). Disorders of the myoneural junction. In B. Berg (Ed.), *Principles of child neurology*. New York: McGraw Hill.

Sutton, M., & Pomeroy, S. (1996). Brain abscess. In F. Burg, J. Ingelfinger, E. Wald, & R. Polin (Eds.), *Current pediatric therapy 15* (pp. 68–69). Philadelphia: W. B. Saunders.

Swaiman, K. F. (1994). *Pediatric neurology: Principles and practice* (2nd ed.). St. Louis: C. V. Mosby.

Tatum, S., & Wang, A. (1990). Hemispherectomy—A radical solution. *Today's OR Nurse, 12*(3), 9–12.

Tew, B. (1991). The effect of spina bifida and hydrocephalus upon learning and behavior. In C. M. Bannister & B. Tew (Eds.), *Current concepts in spina bifida and hydrocephalus*. New York: Cambridge University Press.

Thomas, R., & Taylor, K. (1997). Assessing head injuries in children. MCN, *22*, 198–202.

Twomey, C. R. (1992). Brain abscess: An update. *Journal of Neuroscience Nursing, 24*(1), 34–39.

Vessey, J., Holland, C., McVay, C., Williams, S., & McNatt, S. (1993). Latex allergy: A threat to you and your patients. *Pediatric Nursing, 19*(5), 517–520.

Vining, E. (1994). Pediatric Seizures. *Emergency Medicine Clinics of North America, 12*(4), 973–988.

Volpe, J. J. (1995). *Neurology of the newborn* (3rd ed.). Philadelphia: W. B. Saunders.

Voytko, S., & Farrington, E. (1997). Fosphenytoin sodium: New drug to replace intravenous phenytonin sodium. *Pediatric Nursing, 23*(5), 503–506.

Walker, J., & Meijer, J. (1995). Neuroendoscopic third ventriculostomy: A nursing perspective. *Journal of Neuroscience Nursing, 27*(2), 78–82.

Werler, M. M., Louik, C., Shapiro, S., & Mitchell, A. A. (1994). Ovulation induction and risk of neural tube defects. *The Lancet, 344*, 445–446.

Werler, M. M., Mitchell, A. A., Rosenberg, L., & Lammer, E. J. (1991). Maternal alcohol use in relation to selected birth defects. *American Journal of Epidemiology, 134*, 691–698.

Werler, M. M., & Mitchell, A. A. (1993). Case-control study of vitamin supplementation and neural tube defects: Consideration of potential confounding by lifestyle factors. *Annals of the New York Academy of Sciences, 678*, 276–283.

Werler, M. M., Shapiro, S., & Mitchell, A. A. (1993). Periconceptual folic acid exposure and risk of occurrent neural tube defects. *Journal of the American Medical Association, 269*, 1257–1261.

Winston, K. (1992). Hair and neurosurgery. *Neurosurgery, 31*(2), 320–329.

Yerby, M. S. (1994). Pregnancy, teratogenesis and epilepsy. *Neurologic Clinics, 12*(4), 749–772.

Zuckerman, B. (1995). Breath holding. In S. Parker & B. Zuckerman (Eds.), *Behavioral and developmental pediatrics* (pp. 86–87). Boston: Little, Brown.

Bibliography

Jackson, P. L., & Vessey, J. A. (1996). *Primary care of the child with a chronic condition* (2nd ed.). St. Louis: C. V. Mosby.

Menkes, J. H. (1990). *Textbook of child neurology* (4th ed.). Philadelphia: Lea and Febiger.

O'Flaherty, J. E., & Pirie, P. L. (1997). Prevention of pediatric drowning and near-drowning: A survey of members of the American Academy of Pediatrics. *Pediatrics, 99*, 169.

Swaiman, K. F. (1994). *Pediatric neurology: Principles and practice* (2nd ed.). St. Louis: C. V. Mosby.

HEALTH CHALLENGE:

Pediatric Malignancies

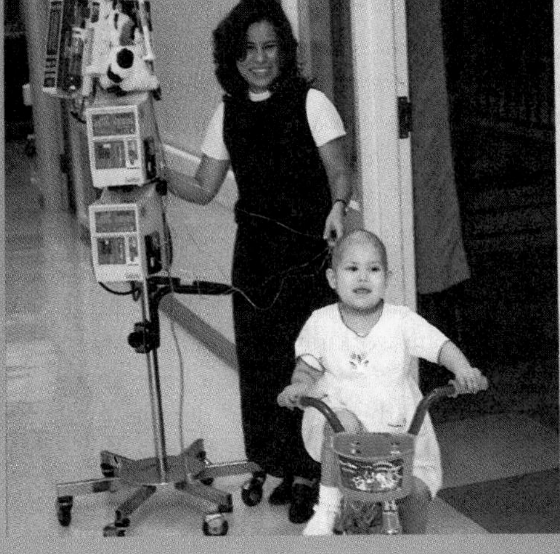

OUTLINE

Assessment of the Child with a Malignancy
- Focused Health History
- Focused Physical Assessment
- Nursing Diagnoses and Outcomes
- Developmental and Biological Variances

Diagnostic Criteria for Evaluating Pediatric Malignancies

Treatment Modalities
- Surgery
- Chemotherapy
- Radiation Therapy
- Biotherapy
- Bone Marrow Transplantation
- Supportive Care

Pediatric Malignancies
- Childhood Leukemia
  - Acute Lymphocytic Leukemia
  - Acute Myelogenous Leukemia
  - Chronic Myelocytic Leukemia
- Central Nervous System Tumors
  - Cerebellar Astrocytoma
  - Cerebral Astrocytoma
  - Medulloblastoma
  - Brain Stem Glioma
  - Ependymoma
  - Optic Nerve Glioma
- Lymphomas
  - Hodgkin's Disease
  - Non-Hodgkin's Lymphoma
- Neuroblastoma
- Wilms' Tumor (Nephroblastoma)
- Rhabdomyosarcoma
- Bone Tumors
  - Osteogenic Sarcoma
  - Ewing's Sarcoma
- Retinoblastoma

OBJECTIVES

- Detect abnormal findings that can be found on physical assessment of a child with cancer.
- Describe the nursing care for children undergoing diagnostic tests for the detection and diagnosis of pediatric malignancies.
- Describe the treatment options used in children with cancer.
- Differentiate the types of malignancies commonly found in the pediatric population.
- Describe the interdisciplinary interventions to minimize the harmful effects of the treatment regimen associated with each type of malignancy.
- Identify the psychosocial needs of children with cancer and their families.

KEY TERMS

biotherapy
bone marrow aspirate
immunosuppression
infratentorial
ionizing radiation
leukopenia
metastasis
multimodal
myelosuppression
nadir
neutropenia
pancytopenia
proptosis
relapse
remission
staging
stomatitis
supratentorial
thrombocytopenia
tumor burden
tumor grading
tumor lysis syndrome
venous access device (VAD)

CHAPTER

22

Cancer is the second leading cause of death in children, exceeded only by accidents. In the United States, approximately 8300 new cases of childhood cancer were reported in 1996, with cancer being accountable for an estimated 1700 deaths (American Cancer Society, 1996; National Cancer Institute, 1996). Recent incidence rates (1990 to 1991) of cancer among children younger than age 15 were 14.4 per 100,000 among whites and 11.8 per 100,000 among black children in the United States (National Cancer Institute, 1996).

Caring for children with cancer presents the health care provider with unique challenges and opportunities. The challenge of pediatric oncology is to provide the aggressive multimodal therapy needed to eradicate the disease or slow its progress, while at the same time minimizing toxicities and improving long-term quality of life by decreasing long-term sequelae. The opportunities arise from working in a field that has demonstrated dramatic advances in the treatment and cure of childhood cancer over the past few decades. The mortality rate among children with cancer has decreased by 42% since the 1960s. The 5-year survival rate for all childhood cancers combined has increased from less than 30% to nearly 70% (National Cancer Institute, 1996). The increasing survival rate is the result of aggressive multimodal treatment and improved supportive care. Multimodal therapy is accomplished by providing various combinations of therapies such as multiagent chemotherapy, radiation, surgery, bone marrow transplantation, and biotherapy to the child. The combination of therapies depends on the type of malignancy and extent of disease at the time of diagnosis.

Various health care personnel are involved in the short- and long-term care of the child with cancer. The success of complex cancer treatment depends on experienced team members collaborating and communicating effectively with one another and with the child and his or her family. Team members must strive to complement each other's role and to coordinate the optimal plan of treatment to become true advocates for the child and the family. Only then will the child and the family be able to establish trusting therapeutic relationships with, and be able to use the expertise available from, designated team members.

The interdisciplinary team involved in the care of the child with cancer may include physicians, nurses, nurse practitioners, social workers, psychologists, child life specialists, teachers, pharmacists, dietitians, religious advisors, and the rehabilitation team. The field of pediatric oncology can be as emotionally draining as it is challenging and exhilarating. The interdisciplinary team must work in harmony, demonstrating support and confidence in the plan of care that is selected for each child.

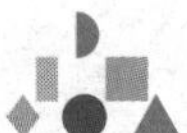

Assessment of the Child with a Malignancy

Childhood cancers may present rapidly or be diagnosed after symptoms have been present for several weeks or months. The delay in diagnosis may be due to the vagueness and nonspecificity of symptoms or to a lack of experience and knowledge of childhood cancers. In some cases, a child may have recently been under the care of a physician and there was no suspicion of a malignancy. Yet, within a few weeks, the fast-growing nature of the cancer may completely alter the child's previous healthy status. In other cases, the child may have already undergone treatment for vague symptoms that characterize many common childhood illnesses such as the flu, gastroenteritis, or headaches. In most instances, the child's health history and physical examination are limited to the chief complaint. For example, a child complaining of headaches and blurred vision may appear to have eye strain requiring glasses and is referred to an optometrist for follow-up.

Cancer is usually not suspected until the physician has ruled out a variety of different diagnoses based on clinical presentation. The completion of diagnostic tests may reveal an abnormal complete blood count, or a mass detected on plain x-ray films may cause the health care provider to suspect cancer. At this point, the child is usually referred to an oncologist for a diagnostic work-up.

The signs and symptoms of childhood cancer are different from those associated with cancer in adults. Adult cancers are generally detected as a result of changes in bowel or bladder habits, rectal bleeding, an unusual lump, a chronic cough, a non-healing wound, a nosebleed, or complaints of pain when certain body areas are palpated. In contrast, the signs and symptoms of cancer in children are primarily the result of one or more of the following factors:

- Compression, infiltration, or obstruction caused by the tumor (e.g., bone pain, abdominal pain)
- Changes in blood cell production such as decreased hemoglobin, hematocrit, white blood count, or platelets (e.g., the child is pale, tired, bruises easily, and has petechiae)
- Secretion by the tumor of a substance that interferes with normal organ functioning
- Metabolic, electrolyte, hormonal, or immunologic alterations caused by tumor metabolism or cell death (e.g., increased frequency of infections, hypercalcemia)

A limited health history and physical assessment can lead to delays in the detection and diagnosis of cancer in children. Conversely, a systematic health history and complete physical examination can assist in the early detection and diagnosis of a suspected malignancy.

Focused Health History

A systematic approach to obtaining a focused health history is necessary to elicit the most relevant data for detecting a possible malignancy in a child (Chart 22–1). The presenting signs and symptoms and the chief complaint, as stated by the child or parent, provide the most important clues as to the type of cancer that should be suspected (Table 22–1). For instance, it is important to elicit information specific to the sequence of events related to the present illness, such as the date the symptoms appeared, the sequence and duration of symptoms, and any diagnosis or treatment that was prescribed by another practitioner. It is also helpful to determine whether culturally based remedies were tried before conventional medical treatment was sought. For example, some remedies from other cultures might be vitamins, Laetrile, shark cartilage, organic compounds, holy water, or herbs.

Pertinent questions are asked about each body system to elicit additional symptoms that the parent has not recognized or considered important. The child's past medical history may assist in identifying symptoms that were clinically significant even though the family or other health care providers may not have associated them with the current diagnostic evaluation. Often parents downplay or self-diagnose certain symptoms and attribute them to normal childhood findings (e.g., "growing pains," frequent colds, "finicky eater"). Information regarding past medical history should include the child's prenatal and neonatal history, allergies, immunizations, childhood illnesses, and previous hospitalizations.

If the child has a positive history for a previous malignancy, it is especially important to obtain information regarding the malignancy and therapeutic treatments that were used. This information is significant in identifying the presence of a secondary malignancy. Chemotherapy and radiotherapy have been proven to be powerful carcinogens. In children who survive 5 years after the diagnosis of cancer, another cancer is 10 to 20 times more likely to develop than is expected in children without a previous cancer history (Meadows, 1985; National Cancer Institute, 1996). Certain childhood cancers are associated with an increased incidence of a secondary cancer site. Children with Hodgkin's disease, leukemia, ovarian cancer, retinoblastoma, or the genetic form of Wilms' tumor, and children who received radiation or alkylating agents are among those at particularly high risk (National Cancer Institute, 1996; Pizzo & Poplack,

Table 22–1
Common Chief Complaints That Suggest a Pediatric Cancer

Chief Complaints	Suggested Cancer
Chronic drainage from ear	Rhabdomyosarcoma
Recurrent fever with bone pain	Ewing's sarcoma, leukemia
Morning headache with vomiting	Brain tumor
Lump in neck that does not respond to antibiotics	Hodgkin's or non-Hodgkin's lymphomas
White dot in eye	Retinoblastoma
Swollen face and neck	Non-Hodgkin's lymphoma, leukemia
Mass in abdomen	Wilms' tumor, neuroblastoma
Paleness and fatigue	Leukemia, lymphoma
Limping	Osteosarcoma, other bone tumors
Bone pain	Leukemia, Ewing's sarcoma, neuroblastoma
Bleeding from vagina	Rhabdomyosarcoma
Weight loss	Hodgkin's disease

From Pizzo, P. A., & Poplack, D. G. (Eds.). (1997). *Principles and practice of pediatric oncology* (3rd ed.). Philadelphia: J. B. Lippincott. Reprinted with permission.

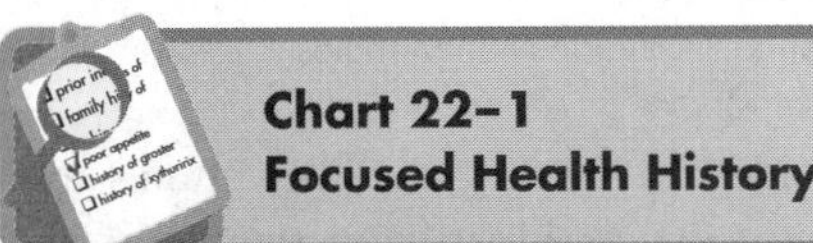

Chart 22–1
Focused Health History

Pediatric Malignancies

Identifying Data	Birthdate and place Gender Race Religion
Current History	Recurrent fever, bruising, fatigue, pallor, nausea, vomiting, constipation, morning headache with vomiting, masses, swollen or tender lymph nodes, unsteady gait, limping, bone pain, visual disturbances, decreased appetite resulting in weight loss, chronic drainage from ear, alterations in bowel or bladder habits
Birth History	Maternal drug or substance use, infection or mass at birth, maternal history of miscarriage, fetal death Parental exposure to chemicals, radiation, alkylating agents
Previous Health Challenges	History of persistent occurrence of infections, nontraumatic bone fractures, unusual bleeding (nose, mouth, rectum), unusual bruising, failure to thrive, anemia
Childhood Illnesses	Chickenpox, measles Previous contagious exposure Recent contagious exposure
Immunizations	Up-to-date
Allergies	Drugs, food, other
Current Medications	Prescription, non-prescription, home remedies
Nutritional Assessment	Weight loss, decreased appetite, nausea, vomiting, constipation
Family Medical History	Family history of cancer, especially childhood malignancies, immune disorders Family history of genetic abnormalities, e.g., Down syndrome, neurofibromatosis
Environmental History	Exposure to drugs containing radioisotopes and immunosuppressive agents during fetal life or childhood Exposure to toxic chemicals, fumes, aerosols, smoke, radiation Exposure to household members' smoking behaviors Exposure to environmental risks, e.g., power lines, chemical treatment plants, waste dumps
Social History	Primary cultural group of the family, including the child's personality and temperament, relationship with other family members and friends, and behavioral manifestations that parents do not consider consistent with other children of the child's age School performance Recent out-of-country travel
Growth and Development	Any achievement of or variation from significant normal growth and developmental patterns The child's habits, including toileting, sleeping, pediatric rituals, speech patterns, and daily activities Previous exposures to and coping mechanisms for stress and illness

1997). Hodgkin's disease is the most common tumor preceding both hematologic and non-hematologic secondary tumors. A secondary malignancy may also be associated with the treatment of the primary tumor, or there may be a genetic connection between the primary and secondary cancer (e.g., children with retinoblastoma are at risk for secondary development of an osteosarcoma) (Donaldson, Egbert, & Lee, 1993).

The family medical history is a very important aspect of history taking when cancer is suspected. Familial and genetic diseases such as autoimmune diseases, immune deficiencies, Down syndrome, and neurofibromatosis have been linked to various types of cancer in children.

Worldview: *There are notable differences in the incidence of certain cancers among ethnic groups from different geographic locations. For instance, acute lymphocytic leukemia (ALL) is the most frequently occurring cancer in white children in the western countries. The incidence of ALL is low among black children in the United States and in Africa, and among Arab and Indian children. In tropical Africa, Burkitt's lymphoma accounts for more than half of all cases of childhood cancer. In Ankara, Turkey, acute myelomonocytic leukemia accounts for more than half of the childhood cases of cancer (National Cancer Institute, 1996).*

A family genogram is helpful in plotting health problems of parents, grandparents, aunts, uncles, siblings, and first cousins. The information collected should include ages, a list of serious illnesses, and, if deceased, the cause of death. Special attention is given to a family history of malignancies.

A history of environmental exposures may be significant whenever there is a suspicion of cancer. Information should include exposures to hazardous materials, pollutants, ionizing radiation, insecticides, or unsafe physical or structural environmental settings. Environmental factors have long been implicated in the increased risk of certain cancers. Among the most common environmental factors believed to be associated with cancer are ionizing radiation, electromagnetic fields, radon, drugs, viruses, and alkylating agents. Exposures to these elements by parents before conception, by the mother during fetal development, or by the child once born have all been associated with cancer development. Some cancers are more prevalent in certain geographic regions (National Cancer Institute, 1996).

A social history provides the practitioner with important information about family functioning and support systems. It includes psychosocial and cultural aspects such as parents' race, marital status, age, socioeconomic status, names and ages of all children and their familial relationship to the ill child, and cultural beliefs. In addition, the strengths and weaknesses of each family member must be assessed to determine the impact of the diagnosis, previous experience with stressors, and ability to cope with the stress. It is also necessary to assess the group dynamics within the family and to determine whether there are other stressors present (e.g., financial difficulty, divorce). Cancer is a chronic illness that affects the entire family. Over time, family relationships and dynamics change as the family adjusts to the varying demands of the child's illness. An early understanding of family roles, strengths, and coping mechanisms assists the health care team in helping the family to deal with the ramifications of the illness.

Worldview: *Korean and Japanese mothers provide most of the care of the children and may be held responsible for not protecting their child from cancer. In contrast, Chinese fathers care for the ill child and remain with the child during the entire hospitalization (Martinson et al., 1995).*

A baseline of physical and developmental milestones, as well as the child's eating, sleeping, and toileting habits, is documented. Also noted are any recent regressions in behavior that may be related to the current illness. For example, a 14-month-old who has been walking and drinking from a cup may regress to crawling and have difficulty sitting unsupported or holding a bottle. These regressions are not uncommon in young children with brain tumors.

Focused Physical Assessment

When cancer is suspected in a child, a head-to-toe assessment should be performed with special attention to areas related to symptoms. Chart 22–2 provides a detailed review of findings that should be evaluated during the physical assessment when a malignancy is suspected. The practitioner should begin the assessment by observing the child's overall appearance. Observations should include skin color, presence of ecchymoses or petechiae, nutritional status, asymmetry of facial features or extremities, and level of activity. A child with cancer often appears pale and thin, with symptoms of lethargy and generalized malaise. The presence of pallor, ecchymoses, and petechiae may indicate that the cancer has invaded the bone marrow and is interrupting the normal production of red blood cells and platelets, such as in the case of leukemia.

The child may have experienced recent weight loss and appear malnourished. This is often secondary to a loss of appetite or nausea and vomiting caused by a malignancy. Asymmetry of facial features may indicate a retinoblastoma or nasopharyngeal rhabdomyosarcoma. Asymmetry of an extremity may indicate a bone tumor or soft tissue sarcoma.

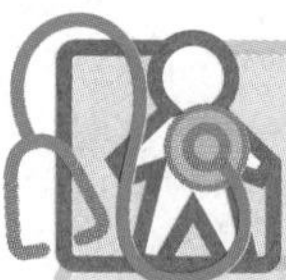

Chart 22–2
Focused Physical Assessment

Pediatric Malignancies

Head and Neck Region

Masses on cranium
Drainage from ear
Asymmetry of face
Bruising or swelling around eyes (proptosis)
Bleeding gums
Enlarged or tender cervical lymph nodes
Presence of white reflection in pupil of the eye

Thoracic and Axillary Region

Asymmetry
Mediastinal mass (may only be seen on x-ray film)
Difficulty breathing or respiratory distress
Enlarged or tender axillary lymph nodes

Abdominal Region

Asymmetry
Palpable mass
Rectal bleeding
Vaginal discharge
Hepatomegaly
Splenomegaly
Petechiae, bruises, hemorrhage
Rashes, lesions
Pallor

Extremities

Bone pain or tenderness
Limited range of motion
Palpable bone or soft tissue mass
Asymmetry
Gait, limp

Neurologic Findings

Cranial nerve abnormalities
Ataxia
Level of consciousness
Altered reflexes

Other

Anemia
Infection
Sepsis
Neutropenia
Fever

The presence of fever is a frequent finding when a child is ill. It can be caused by many common childhood illnesses, including cancer. Fever is most often caused by an infectious process secondary to the cancer but can also be caused by the tumor itself.

Swollen lymph nodes are a common finding in children. In children with enlarged lymph nodes that are firm and painful on palpation and that are associated with weight loss, fever, and an abnormal chest x-ray film, however, the clinician may suspect a lymphoma, such as Hodgkin's disease or non-Hodgkin's lymphoma (NHL).

The presence of pain, limping, or decreased range of motion should be further investigated. The practitioner should obtain a thorough history of the location, onset, duration, frequency, and intensity of the pain, as well as precipitating and alleviating factors. Headaches, especially when associated with vomiting, should be further evaluated for a possible brain tumor.

An abdominal mass is often the first presenting sign in Wilms' tumor and neuroblastoma. It is usually detected by a parent who then brings the child in for evaluation.

A white reflection in the pupil of a child's eye (cat's eye reflex) as opposed to the normal red pupillary reflex is an abnormal finding and is a classic sign in retinoblastoma. The presence of blurred or decreased vision, squinting, strabismus, or swelling can also be the result of other solid tumors of the eye.

Nursing Diagnoses and Outcomes

The nursing diagnoses that can be applied to the child with cancer and the child's family reflect the complex nature of the disease and the need to implement creative care strategies (Chart 22–3). Whenever possible, the child's treatment should be guided by an interdisciplinary team at a specialized facility with the technology to quickly diagnosis and treat the child's disease. The plan of care is focused on eradicating the cancer and minimizing and treating the effects of the multimodal treatment regimen. The nurse plays an instrumental role in humanizing the cancer experience to enhance the dignity, strengths, and uniqueness of each child and his or her family. Providing education to the family is an ongoing part of the plan of care. Concerns for the child's ability to achieve developmental goals and for the family to maintain effective levels of coping must be addressed during all phases of the child's treatment program.

Developmental and Biological Variances

Cancers in children differ significantly from those in adults (Chart 22–4). Most childhood cancers arise from

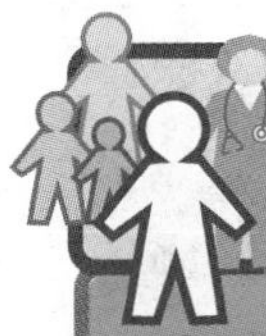

Chart 22–3
Nursing Diagnoses and Outcomes

The Child with a Malignancy

Knowledge deficit: diagnosis, treatment plan, and health care needs of the child

Outcomes: Child/family will verbalize understanding of diagnosis, treatment, and child's health care needs.
Child/family will participate in the decision-making process and care of the child based on their understanding of the child's illness and treatment options.

Pain related to disease process, diagnostic procedures, or treatment modalities

Outcomes: Child will experience minimal discomfort during and after procedure.
Child will state that adequate pain relief has been obtained.
Pain behaviors are not demonstrated by the child.
Child/family will demonstrate effective pain relief measures.

High risk for infection related to neutropenia, immunosuppressive therapy, and presence of vascular access device

Outcomes: Child will remain free from infection.
Child/family will recognize and report signs and symptoms of infection to their health care providers.
Child/family will verbalize measures to reduce risk of infection.
Child/family will demonstrate measures to reduce incidence of infection from the vascular access device.

High risk for injury: bleeding related to thrombocytopenia

Outcomes: Child will remain free from bleeding.
Child/family will state signs and symptoms of bleeding.
Child/family will demonstrate knowledge of measures to prevent bleeding.

Urinary elimination pattern alteration related to chemotherapy or disease process

Outcome: Renal function remains adequate during course of therapy.

High risk for impaired skin integrity related to radiation therapy, presence of a venous access device, graft-versus-host disease, and immobility

Outcomes: Child/family will demonstrate measures to prevent or minimize skin breakdown.
Child's skin will remain intact and free from infection.

High risk for fluid volume deficit related to nausea, vomiting, or oral mucositis

Outcomes: Mucous membranes remain moist.
Skin turgor is good with no signs of dehydration.
Child is able or assisted to maintain adequate fluid intake by oral, nasogastric, or intravenous access.

Altered nutrition: less than body requirements related to disease process and medication-induced vomiting, anorexia, changed taste sensations, depression, or changes in intestinal epithelium

Outcomes: Child is able to eat frequent, small nutritious meals.
Child's caloric intake is adequate for age.
Child is able to maintain weight that is normal for age.

Altered oral mucous membrane related to effects of mucositis

Outcomes: Child will demonstrate measures to preserve and restore mucosal integrity.
Signs of oral ulceration are not present.

Chart continued on following page

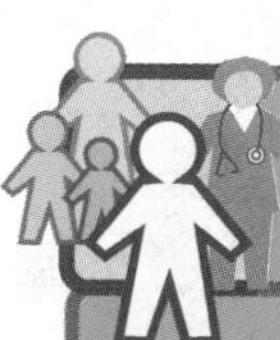

Chart 22–3
Nursing Diagnoses and Outcomes *Continued*

The Child with a Malignancy

Constipation related to effects of chemotherapeutic agents

Outcomes: Child/family use measures to prevent or minimize constipation.
Child has no evidence of hard or dry stools.
Child maintains normal pattern of bowel elimination.

Diarrhea related to effects of chemotherapeutic agents

Outcomes: Child/family use measures to prevent or minimize diarrhea.
Child has no evidence of loose, fluid, or unformed stools.
Child maintains normal pattern of bowel elimination.

Anxiety related to unfamiliar environment, procedures, and uncertainty of future outcomes

Outcomes: Through the use of coping mechanisms, child will have increased psychological and physiologic comfort.
Parents verbalize methods to support their child during therapy.

Anticipatory grieving related to anticipation of loss of child through death, loss of a child's physical attributes, or loss of hoped-for expectations of the child's future

Outcomes: Child/caregiver will verbalize feelings related to losses experienced during the course of the child's illness.
Child/family will seek appropriate support and comfort from significant others during time of grief.
Child/family will be able to accept the necessity of medications, surgery, or radiation, which may alter the child's appearance.
Child/family will seek to develop new realistic expectations of the child's future.

Ineffective or compromised family coping related to situational crisis

Outcome: Family demonstrates effective coping strategies.

Altered growth and development related to repeated hospitalizations (e.g., regression, isolation) and treatment modalities (e.g., radiation)

Outcomes: Child will demonstrate continued progress in meeting normal growth and developmental norms.
Child will continue to participate in age-appropriate activities as condition permits.

Self-esteem disturbance related to changes in physical appearance caused by chemotherapy, medications, radiation, or surgery

Outcomes: Child will verbalize positive feelings about self.
Child will select interventions to enhance self-esteem.

Altered parenting related to role changes necessary to care for child

Outcome: Parents will adapt parenting skills to meet demands of their child's ongoing health needs.

Home maintenance management impairment related to insufficient resources available to care for child's needs safely in the home

Outcomes: Family demonstrates adjustments to home environment and routine to help manage the child's condition.
Family utilizes individuals or organizations to provide health care services, equipment, and resources in the home.

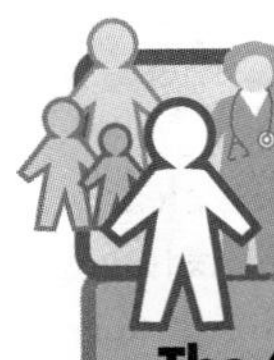

Chart 22–3
Nursing Diagnoses and Outcomes *Continued*

The Child with a Malignancy

Health-seeking behaviors related to completion of treatment regimen and long-term sequelae of cancer

Outcomes: Child will participate in regular physical examinations to evaluate for long-term effects.
Child will participate in rehabilitation activities as needed.
Child will select activities and a lifestyle that will reduce the chances of acquiring a preventable cancer in the future.
Child/family will seek support resources as needed to deal with issues surrounding survivorship.

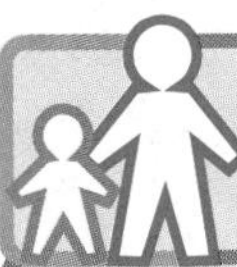

Chart 22–4
Developmental Considerations

Comparison of Childhood and Adult Cancers

Factor	Childhood Cancers	Adult Cancers
Incidence	Rare; <1% of all cancers	Common; >99% of all cancers
Sites	Involves tissue (e.g., reticuloendothelial system, central nervous system, muscle, bone)	Involves organs (e.g., lung, breast, colon, prostate)
Histology	Most common type: non-epithelial sarcomas, embryonal, leukemia, lymphoma	Most common type: epithelial carcinomas
Latency (from initiation to diagnosis)	Relatively short period	Long period; can be well over 20 years
Influence of environmental factors in causation	Some environmental factors; few lifestyle factors; overall, no strong influence shown; more likely interaction of genetic alterations and environmental factors (i.e., ecogenetics)	Strong relationship to environmental exposures and lifestyle factors
Prevention	Minimal strategies known	80% estimated to be preventable
Early detection	Generally accidental; small percentage known as genetically at high risk can be followed more closely	Possible with adherence to early detection screening tests and examination recommendations
Stage at diagnosis	Metastatic disease present in 80%	Local or regional disease
Response to treatment	Very responsive to chemotherapy; higher doses tolerated	Less responsive to chemotherapy
Treatment of side effects	Less difficulty with acute toxicity but more significant long-term consequences	More difficulty with acute toxicity but fewer long-term consequences
Prognosis	>60% cure	<60% cure

From Fernbach, D. G., & Vietti, T. J. (1991). General aspects of childhood cancer. In D. G. Fernbach & T. J. Vietti (Eds.), *Clinical pediatric oncology* (4th ed.). St. Louis: Mosby. Reprinted with permission.

the mesodermal germ layer, which, in the embryo, becomes connective tissue, muscle, bone, cartilage, kidneys, sex organs, blood, blood vessels, lymphatic, and lymphoid organs. As a result, 92% of childhood cancers are made up of primitive embryonal tissue, sarcomas, leukemias, and lymphomas. The remaining 8% of childhood cancers arise from neuroectodermal tissue and give rise to central nervous system (CNS) tumors (Hardin-Mooney, 1993). In contrast, most adult cancers involve the epithelial tissue and are called carcinomas. These epithelial cancers are quite rare in children younger than 15 years.

Tumors derived from mesectodermal and neuroectodermal tissue are more deep-seated than epithelial tumors and, thus, are not easily detected until they are quite large. In almost 80% of pediatric oncology cases, there is distant metastasis at the time of diagnosis.

Occurrence of certain pediatric malignancies clearly coincides with peak times of physical growth and cellular maturation (Fig. 22–1). This concept is key in understanding the mechanism of cancer in children and suggests that cellular development and growth are central to the development of cancer in children. In contrast, environmental exposures are a primary component of carcinogenesis in adults.

Data gathered by the Surveillance, Epidemiology, and End Results (SEER) Program from 1986 to 1991 have clearly demonstrated age-, sex-, race-, and site-specific incidence rates of cancer for persons younger than

Figure 22–1
Developmental and biological variances: pediatric malignancies.

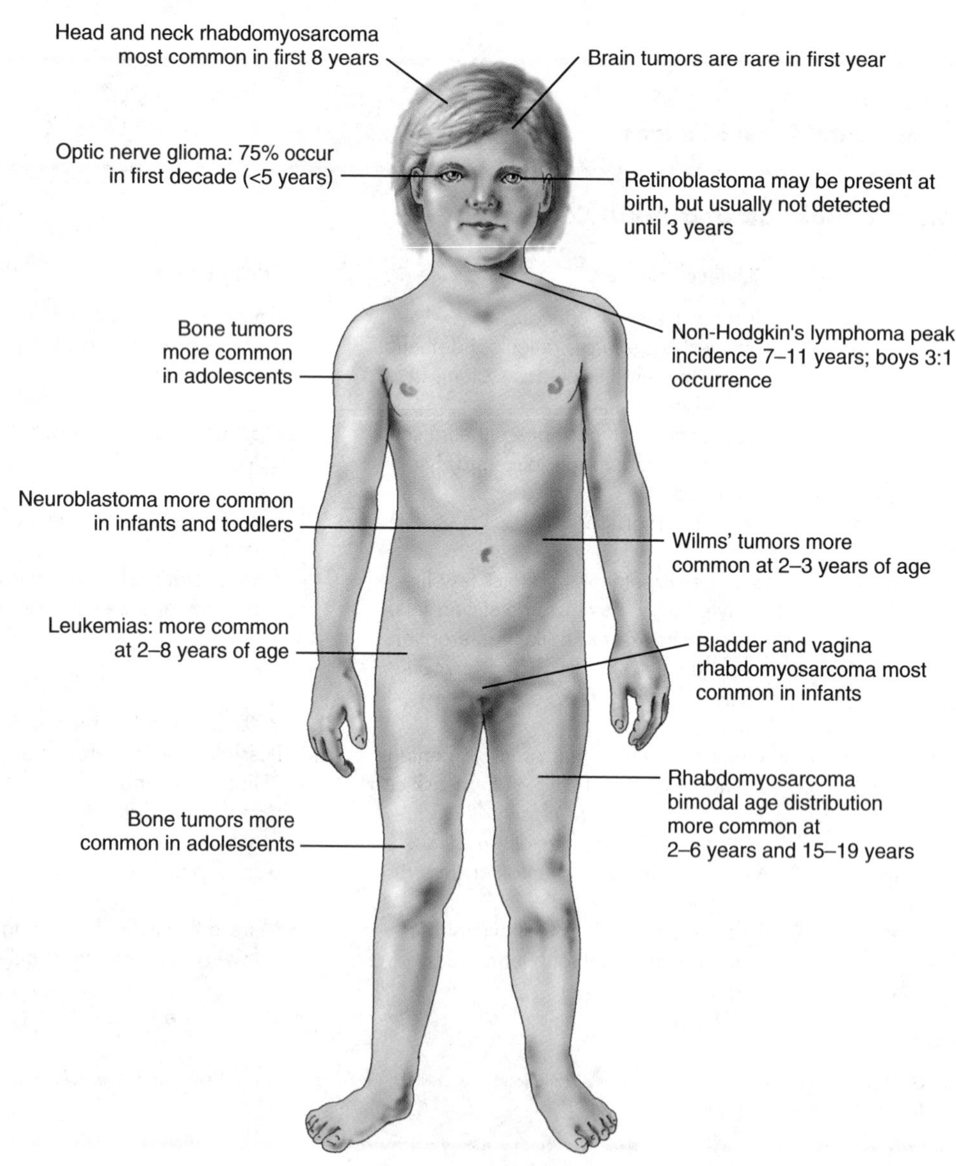
Head and neck rhabdomyosarcoma most common in first 8 years
Brain tumors are rare in first year
Optic nerve glioma: 75% occur in first decade (<5 years)
Retinoblastoma may be present at birth, but usually not detected until 3 years
Bone tumors more common in adolescents
Non-Hodgkin's lymphoma peak incidence 7–11 years; boys 3:1 occurrence
Neuroblastoma more common in infants and toddlers
Wilms' tumors more common at 2–3 years of age
Leukemias: more common at 2–8 years of age
Bladder and vagina rhabdomyosarcoma most common in infants
Rhabdomyosarcoma bimodal age distribution more common at 2–6 years and 15–19 years
Bone tumors more common in adolescents

20 years (National Cancer Institute, 1996). A classic peak incidence occurs in the 0- to 4-year age group for many childhood cancers (e.g., leukemia; cancer of the CNS, eye, and kidney; and sarcoma) and there is an increasing incidence with age in others (e.g., bone tumors and lymphomas). Age is also an important factor because some histologically identical cancers have a different prognosis based on the age at onset. For example, acute lymphocytic leukemia (ALL) has a favorable prognosis in children age 1 to 10 years and a very poor prognosis for infants younger than 1 year and children 10 years and older. Differences in the higher incidences of certain cancers in males than females is apparent in cases of NHL, ALL, and medulloblastoma. Overall, the cancer rate in the United States for white children is 10% to 25% higher than for black children (Fernbach & Vietti, 1991). This is accounted for by lower rates in black children of ALL (53% in whites), lymphomas (41% in whites), and Ewing's sarcoma (89% in whites).

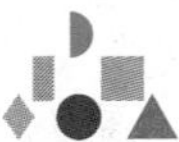

Diagnostic Criteria for Evaluating Pediatric Malignancies

The nurse caring for children suspected of having cancer is in a unique position to offer support and guidance to the child and the family as they undergo the numerous diagnostic and staging procedures. It is important for the nurse to possess a thorough understanding of these procedures and the usual sequence in which they are completed. In most instances, the child's nurse plays a key role in preparing the child and family for tests and procedures and for ensuring the child's safety.

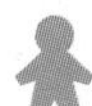

Tip: *It is important to establish an open, honest nurse–child relationship. One of the easiest ways to do this is to give a simple, honest answer when children ask a question. If the procedure is going to hurt, the child should be told and prepared for it. Let the child know that it is all right to be afraid and cry. Do not tell the child to "act like a big boy" or "big girl."*

It is helpful to children undergoing tests for the nurse to provide them with an age-appropriate explanation of the procedure and why it is necessary. Children are more apt to cooperate if they understand what is being done and why the test or procedure is necessary. During diagnostic tests, it is better not to restrain the child if possible. If children have some freedom of movement, they feel they have some control over the situation.

Children undergoing evaluation and treatment for cancer frequently encounter painful procedures such as needle sticks, lumbar punctures, bone marrow aspirations, and biopsies. The nurse caring for children with cancer must intervene to prevent or minimize the child's pain experiences when possible. When the child must undergo a painful procedure or experiences pain as a result of the cancer itself, pharmacologic and nonpharmacologic interventions can be implemented to maximize the child's comfort. Pharmacologic interventions include conscious sedation for invasive procedures (e.g., lumbar punctures and bone marrow aspirations/biopsies), the use of EMLA, a topical anesthetic, for injections and venipunctures, and nonsteroidal anti-inflammatory drugs (NSAIDs) to decrease cancer pain (Nagengast, 1993). Nonpharmacologic interventions such as age-appropriate preparation, reassurance, diversion, relaxation, breathing exercises, music therapy, and imagery have been cited as effective measures to reduce a child's pain during invasive procedures (Pederson, 1996). These interventions can easily be taught to the parents and to the child or adolescent, thereby increasing their sense of control. (See Chapter 13 for a comprehensive discussion of pain management techniques.)

Diagnostic and staging procedures are used to detect the presence of cancer, to identify the type of cancer, to localize the cancer, and to determine the extent of disease. Once cancer is suspected, these procedures are usually carried out expeditiously so that the appropriate treatment plan can be initiated quickly. The cancer evaluation process includes clinical assessment, laboratory and roentgenographic tests, and, most importantly, a biopsy of tissue or fluid for pathologic confirmation (Table 22–2). Recent advances in radiologic techniques have dramatically improved the ability to diagnose cancer. Non-invasive imaging studies such as computed tomography (CT), ultrasonography, and magnetic resonance imaging (MRI) enable earlier detection of a malignant growth (Table 22–3). However, a definitive diagnosis of cancer cannot be made without pathologic confirmation. Additionally, the use of radio-labeled isotopes and monoclonal antibodies is making scanning procedures more thorough and cancer specific. These techniques provide a method for the oncologist to follow up treatment response or disease progression.

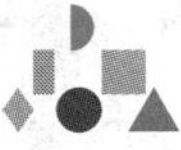

Treatment Modalities

The diagnosis of cancer may include more than 100 different disease presentations. Choosing the best treatment to eradicate or control the disease is a complex task. Decisions made on the course of treatment for cancer are based on the type of cancer, the location of the cancer, and the extent of the disease. The major goal of treat-

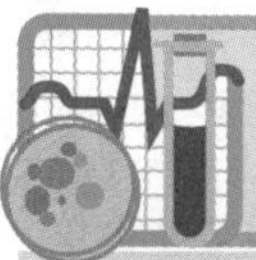

Table 22–2
Diagnostic Tests and Procedures for Evaluating Pediatric Malignancies

Diagnostic Test or Procedure	Purpose	Health Care Provider Responsibilities
Chest x-ray film	Obtained for every patient either as baseline or for diagnosis. Used to examine soft tissue and bony structures of thorax.	Determine whether adolescent female patients may be pregnant. It is very important that the child hold very still. Age-appropriate explanations of the x-ray machine being a "camera" that takes pictures of "your insides" may help a child cooperate. Reassurance that parents are waiting outside the door provides comfort. Infants and very young children may require assistance with positioning and restraints.
Skeletal survey	Collection of plain x-ray films of the entire skeletal system. Used in detecting bony lesions. Continues to be the procedure of choice for evaluating complications of therapy such as drug reactions and pulmonary infections.	Same as above
Computed tomography (CT)	Used in children with known or suspected solid tumors. Represents a cross-sectional view of a structure to detect masses, locate lesions, and evaluate response to treatment.	The child must be very still for 30–90 minutes. Immobilization or sedation in young children is usually required. NPO status should be maintained 3–4 hours before the test to reduce the risk of aspiration if vomiting occurs.
	IV contrast is often used during brain CT scans if a tumor is present or suspected.	Inform the child that he or she may experience a temporary flush or warmth sensation or an unusual metallic or bitter taste. IV access is usually required.
	CT scanning of the abdomen and pelvis is enhanced by oral contrast material. For the medium to work effectively, the child must drink the entire volume within 45–60 minutes.	Parent education is necessary if the scan is done on an outpatient basis. The parents may mix the material in a palatable drink such as fruit juice or 7-Up. The volume of contrast depends on the child's age. If the child is unable to tolerate the contrast by mouth, the oral contrast may be administered via NG tube.
Bone scan	Highly sensitive method of detecting bony lesions. However, it does not distinguish between malignancy and inflammatory processes.	The scan lasts 30–60 minutes and requires the child to lie still. Sedatives are often used.
Ultrasound	Non-invasive process used to visualize body structures. Images are made by sound waves reflected from body tissues. Often, ultrasound is the initial screening test for the child with a palpable mass.	Parent can stay with child during the procedure. Inform the child that the transducer may "tickle." Infants may be given a juice bottle during the procedure to alleviate crying. A full bladder may be needed to differentiate organs. Verbal praise and encouragement often help, but the child should not be scolded if he or she urinates before the procedure is completed.

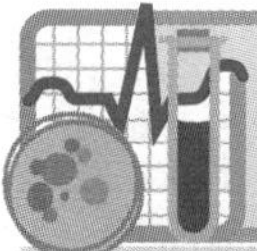

Table 22–2
Diagnostic Tests and Procedures for Evaluating Pediatric Malignancies *Continued*

Diagnostic Test or Procedure	Purpose	Health Care Provider Responsibilities
Magnetic resonance imaging (MRI)	Scan of choice for brain stem and bone tumors. MRI pictures are extremely precise and can provide as much information as direct visualization of tissue. The strong magnetic field precludes MRI study of persons who have any implanted metallic objects in their body.	The MRI scan lasts about 60 minutes and the child must lie very still. Children who cannot do so, or who may become frightened by the loud noise made by the machine, or become claustrophobic because of the close quarters are sedated before the scan. Patients who are sedated require continuous pulse oximetry and heart rate monitoring throughout the scan and until child is awake. Jewelry and other metallic objects must be removed.
Bone marrow aspiration and biopsy	Detection of leukemia as well as many solid tumors. An adequate specimen can usually be obtained through the aspiration method.	Assist and position. Place pillows or folded blanket under the child's abdomen to elevate the hips. Allow parents to stay in the room during the procedure. Position the parent at the head of the table, allowing the parent to provide verbal and physical support. The parent should not assist in restraining. Conscious sedation monitoring is required for patients receiving sedatives and analgesics in a treatment room. The procedure can also be done while the child is in the operating room for biopsy, resection, or line placement. Apply pressure dressing. Dressing should be removed and the site inspected after 24 hours.
Lumbar puncture	Detection of malignant cells in the CSF. Used for introduction of chemotherapeutic agents into the spinal canal and circulating CSF. Diagnostic or staging workup in children with leukemia, lymphoma, parameningeal rhabdomyosarcoma, and medulloblastoma.	Assist in positioning. Explain the procedure to the child and parent. Emphasize the importance of correct positioning. Encourage parents to stay with the child. Properly label specimens. Bandage should be removed and site inspected after 24 hours.
CBC with differential	Used for detection of anemia, increased or decreased WBC, and thrombocytopenia, and as a prognostic factor of acute lymphocytic leukemia.	Inform the child and family about the purpose of the test. Children requiring numerous venipunctures may become fearful and uncooperative. These reactions can be lessened by providing good explanations and by using EMLA cream before initiating a venipuncture, and by using a Hep-Lock for venous blood sampling.
Urine catecholamines VMA, HVA (catecholamine metabolites)	Detection of neuroblastoma.	Obtain sample before CT scan because the contrast medium affects the results.
Alpha-fetoprotein (AFP)	AFP is found in high concentrations in the serum of children with hepatoblastoma, hepatocellular cancer, and teratocarcinomas.	—

Table continued on following page

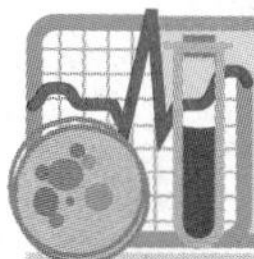

Table 22-2
Diagnostic Tests and Procedures for Evaluating Pediatric Malignancies *Continued*

Diagnostic Test or Procedure	Purpose	Health Care Provider Responsibilities
Serum chemistries	May be elevated in certain oncologic diseases. Also important as prognostic indicators and as treatment response and management tools.	Ensure proper tubes are used and amounts obtained. Monitor results.
Pathology (fluid and tissue specimens)	Identifies specimen type of tumor cells for initiating optimal treatment.	Ensure proper labeling and handling.

CBC, complete blood count; CSF, cerebrospinal fluid; HVA, homovanillic acid; IV, intravenous; NG, nasogastric; NPO, nothing by mouth; VMA, vanillylmandelic acid; WBC, white blood cell count.

ment is to *cure* the child with cancer without causing significant harm or impairment.

Advances have been made over the past decade in understanding cancer, and technological advances have aided in multimodal therapy that is considered the "gold standard," or the best possible treatment. A therapeutic plan is developed for each child using multimodal therapy to offer the best chance of survival. The modes of therapy at present include surgery, chemotherapy, radiation therapy, biotherapy, and bone marrow transplantation.

Two national groups of interdisciplinary health care professionals collaborate with one another, as well as with other national and international treatment groups, to continue to provide optimal diagnostic, acute, long-term, and supportive care for children with cancer. The Children's Cancer Group (CCG) and the Pediatric Oncology Group (POG) are the two main groups of health care professionals involved in pediatric oncology (Pizzo & Poplack, 1997). The therapeutic plan developed includes initial and ongoing treatment for the child with cancer as well as supportive care guidelines, all using an interdisciplinary approach. One or more therapies are selected based on the child's unique presentation of the disease.

Surgery

Surgery is the oldest form of cancer treatment. The primary goal of surgery in pediatric oncology is to remove all evidence of disease while maintaining or restoring normal body function. The best prognosis is related to the early detection and removal of disease. Thus, surgery

Table 22-3
Advantages and Disadvantages of MRI Versus CT Scan

Advantages of MRI Versus CT Scan	Disadvantages of MRI Versus CT Scan
No radiation exposure	More sensitive to movement artifact
No requirements for IV contrast	Requires longer scanning time in a confined space
Images obtainable in multiple planes	Differentiation of tumor from edema difficult because of sensitivity
Avoidance of bone artifacts	Does not image calcification unless it is quite extensive
Shorter imaging time	Loud clanking noise frightening to child
	Difficulty in monitoring unstable child during imaging

CT, computed tomography; IV, intravenous; MRI, magnetic resonance imaging.

is considered a definitive treatment in more than half of all cancer patients (Eilber, 1985). Surgery may also be used for diagnosis (biopsy), rehabilitation, or palliation.

Recent advances in surgical oncology have provided major improvements in the surgical management of children with cancer. These improvements have allowed a better quality of life for the child, both physically and psychosocially. Surgery is most frequently combined with chemotherapy, radiation therapy, or biotherapy. Surgery and adjuvant therapy can lengthen disease-free and long-term survival for children with cancer. Nursing care of the child with cancer following surgical treatment is similar to the care given to any child who undergoes surgery. (See Chapter 9 for an in-depth discussion of presurgical and postsurgical care.)

Chemotherapy

Chemotherapy is a systemic mode of cancer treatment. This approach for treating cancer in children has been extremely effective, especially with certain diseases that cannot be managed effectively by surgery or radiation therapy alone. The development of new drugs and administration techniques has resulted in advanced treatment regimens and increasing survival rates. Children with cancer undergo chemotherapy regimens for periods ranging from a few months to years. Side effects experienced by children range from minimal to severe. The nurse plays a key role in providing children and their families with the appropriate information and support throughout their treatment course (Chart 22–5).

To understand how chemotherapy works, it is important to review the cell cycle. Cells go through four phases to complete a cell growth cycle: G1 (the first "gap"), S (synthesis phase), G2 (the second "gap"), and M (mitosis). Cells move into G0 (the resting phase) after mitosis when they are not actively dividing (Fig. 22–2). The G1 phase is the most variable in time (8 to 48 hours) and is the phase in which DNA synthesis is beginning and active RNA and protein synthesis occurs. Cells then enter the S phase, in which DNA synthesis occurs. This phase takes from 10 to 30 hours, during which time the DNA content of the cell doubles. After the S phase, cells move into G2. In this phase, the RNA

Figure 22–2
Cell life cycle.

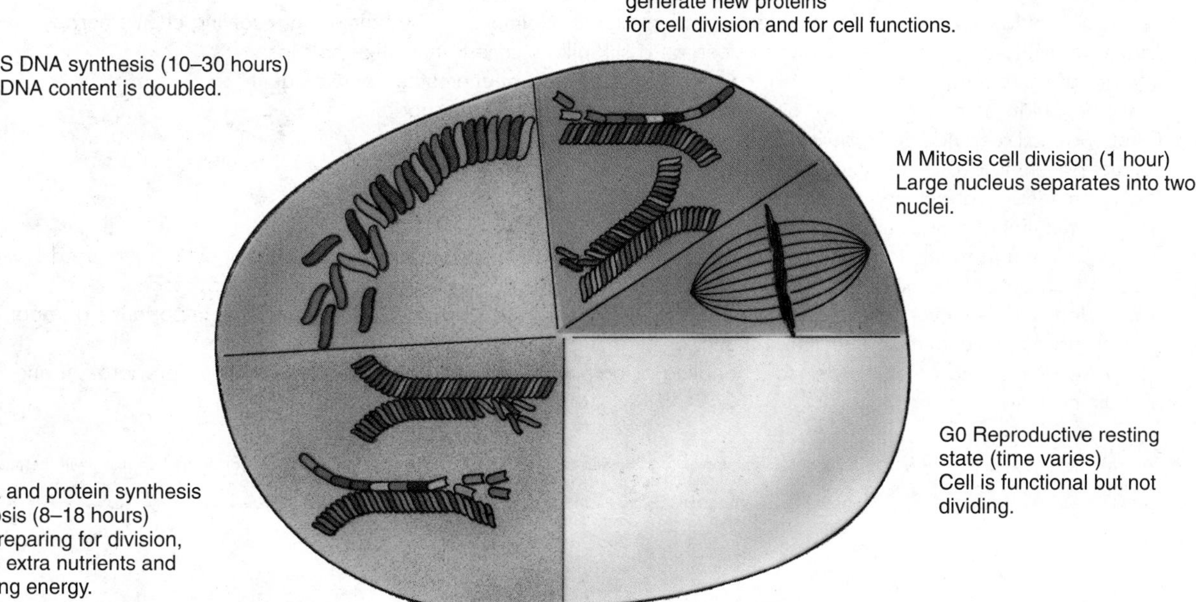
G2 RNA and protein synthesis
generate new proteins
for cell division and for cell functions.
S DNA synthesis (10–30 hours)
DNA content is doubled.
M Mitosis cell division (1 hour)
Large nucleus separates into two nuclei.
G0 Reproductive resting state (time varies)
Cell is functional but not dividing.
G1 RNA and protein synthesis postmitosis (8–18 hours)
Cell is preparing for division, taking in extra nutrients and generating energy.
Cell cycle phase specific chemotherapy agents:
Antimetabolites
Plant alkaloids
Miscellaneous agents
Cell cycle phase nonspecific chemotherapy agents:
Alkylating agents
Antitumor antibiotics
Nitrosoureas
Miscellaneous agents

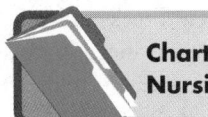

Chart 22-5
Nursing Interventions Classification (NIC)

Chemotherapy Management

Definition

Assisting the patient and family to understand the action and minimize side effects of antineoplastic agents

Activities

Monitor for side effects and toxic effects of chemotherapeutic agents.
Provide information to patient and family on how antineoplastic drugs work on cancer cells.
Teach patient and family about the effects of chemotherapy on bone marrow functioning.
Instruct patient and family on ways to prevent infection, such as avoiding crowds and using good hygiene and handwashing techniques.
Instruct patient to promptly report fevers, chills, nosebleeds, excessive bruising, and tarry stools.
Instruct patient and family to avoid the use of aspirin products.
Institute neutropenic and bleeding precautions.
Determine the patient's previous experience with chemotherapy-related nausea and vomiting.
Administer antiemetic drugs for nausea and vomiting.
Minimize stimuli from noises, light, and odors, especially food.
Teach the patient relaxation and imagery techniques to use before, during, and after treatments, as appropriate.
Offer the patient a bland and easily digested diet.
Administer chemotherapeutic drugs in the late evening, so the patient may sleep at the time emetic effects are greatest.
Ensure adequate fluid intake to prevent dehydration and electrolyte imbalance.
Monitor the effectiveness of measures to control nausea and vomiting.
Teach patient and family to monitor for signs and symptoms of stomatitis.
Instruct patient on proper oral hygiene techniques.
Teach patient to use oral nystatin suspension to control fungal infection, as appropriate.
Teach patient to avoid temperature extremes and chemical treatments of the hair while receiving chemotherapy.
Teach patient to comb hair gently and to sleep on a silk pillow case to minimize hair loss.
Inform patient that hair loss is expected, as determined by type of chemotherapeutic agent used.
Assist patient in obtaining a wig or other head-covering device, as appropriate.
Offer six small feedings daily, as tolerated.
Instruct patient to avoid hot, spicy foods.
Provide nutritious, appetizing foods of patient's choice.
Monitor nutritional status and weight.
Teach patient and family to monitor for organ toxicity, as determined by type of chemotherapeutic agent used.
Discuss with patient the possibility of sterility and other reproductive system impairments, as appropriate.
Instruct long-term survivors and their families of the possibility of second malignancies and the importance of reporting increased susceptibility to infection, fatigue, or bleeding.
Follow recommended guidelines for safe handling of parenteral antineoplastic drugs during drug preparation and administration.

From McCloskey, J., & Bulechek, G. (1996). *Nursing interventions classification (NIC)* (2nd ed.). St. Louis: Mosby–Year Book. Reprinted with permission.

and protein necessary for mitosis are synthesized. This process takes 1 to 12 hours. In the last phase of the cell cycle—the M phase—mitosis takes place. This phase is the time of actual cell division and takes approximately 1 hour. Mitosis is a four-step process (prophase, metaphase, anaphase, and telophase) that results in two identical daughter cells. Cancer cells are difficult to treat in the G0 phase because the cell is not dividing. It is believed that malignant cells have a shorter cell cycle time and grow at a faster rate because of their uncontrolled, erratic growth patterns (Renick-Ettinger, 1993).

Generally, chemotherapeutic agents fall into one of two classifications: *cell cycle–specific* or *cell cycle–nonspecific*. Cell cycle–specific agents have their maximal effect during a specific phase of the cell cycle. Cell cycle–nonspecific agents act on cells regardless of their phase.

The maximal amount of cell destruction is directly proportional to the doses of drug given and to the combination of drugs given. Combining drugs that act at different phases of the cell cycle allows for optimal cell cycle disruption and for the destruction of cancer cells. The combination of drugs also helps prevent drug resistance that occurs when a cancer cell builds up a tolerance to a single agent, thus rendering therapy ineffective. Finally, combination therapy allows multiple drugs to be given at safe dosages to help minimize toxic side effects while maximizing cancer cell destruction.

Chemotherapeutic agents are pharmacologically classified into seven categories (Balis, Holcenberg, & Poplack, 1993):

- Alkylating agents
- Nitrosoureas
- Antitumor antibiotics
- Antimetabolites
- Plant alkaloids
- Hormones and corticosteroids
- Miscellaneous agents

Common chemotherapeutic agents and their classification, route of administration, and side effects, as well as some special nursing considerations are summarized in Table 22–4.

Alkylating agents are cell cycle–nonspecific, destroying both resting and dividing cells. During alkylation, the hydrogen atoms of some molecules within the cell are replaced by an alkyl group. This group interferes with DNA replication and RNA transcription (Brown & Hogan, 1992). Nitrogen mustard, one of the first effective chemotherapeutic agents to be discovered, is an alkylating agent that is still used and is the prototype for all alkylating agents.

Nitrosoureas are similar to the alkylating agents in that they cause cross-linking and breaks in DNA strands, inhibiting DNA formation (Brown & Hogan, 1992). These agents are lipid soluble and cross the blood–brain barrier, which is helpful in treatment of cancer in the CNS by allowing the agents to penetrate through the natural protective barrier of the brain.

Antitumor antibiotics are synthesized naturally by various bacteria and fungal species. They interfere with cellular metabolism, thereby blocking DNA transcription, RNA transcription, or both (Brown & Hogan, 1992). They apparently are cell cycle–nonspecific agents.

Antimetabolites are similar to normal cellular metabolites that are necessary for cell function and replication. These drugs damage cells by acting as a substitute for a natural metabolite in an important molecule, thereby altering the function of the molecule (Brown & Hogan, 1992). They are cell cycle–specific and are most active in the S phase.

Plant alkaloids are derived from the periwinkle plant (*Vinca rosea*) and are sometimes called vinca alkaloids. These drugs are cell cycle–specific because they crystallize microtubular proteins and arrest mitosis (Brown & Hogan, 1992).

Hormones and corticosteroids are not chemotherapeutic drugs but are effective in treating cancers that arise in tissues that are dependent on hormones for cellular proliferation. The hormonal environment of the cancer cell can be altered, thereby affecting cancer cell division. Hormones and corticosteroids can interfere with protein synthesis and modify the DNA transcription process (Renick-Ettinger, 1993).

Miscellaneous agents are medications whose mechanism of action is not fully understood, or their action is not like any of the other categories described. Examples include hydroxyurea, procarbazine, asparaginase, cisplatin, and carboplatin.

Chemotherapy agents do not distinguish between cancer cells and other rapidly dividing normal cells, and, as such, cause predictable side effects. The hematopoietic system, the gastrointestinal tract (GI), and the integumentary system are composed of rapidly dividing cells and are highly susceptible to toxic effects (Lilley, 1990). Nursing care of these side effects is discussed in the section of this chapter on supportive care. Bone marrow depression, nausea, vomiting, diarrhea, hair loss, and skin problems are common side effects in children receiving chemotherapy. Some agents cause more severe side effects than others.

A chemotherapy regimen is composed of several phases. During the initial phase, *induction*, intensive therapy is given to kill enough cancerous cells to induce a remission. Remission occurs when a temporary or permanent response to therapy causes a decrease or absence of the primary malignancy. In the next phase, *consolidation*, intensive therapy is given to destroy remaining cancer cells. The *maintenance* phase is a designated period of time in which treatment is continued to destroy any residual cancer cells. This phase can continue for several years. During the *observation* phase, therapy has ended and the child is followed up for recurrent or late effects of the disease (Renick-Ettinger, 1993). During any of these phases, the child may relapse. In these cases, the treatment protocol is changed and the child goes through each of the phases again, beginning with induction. A child is considered to be a survivor of cancer when he or she has been disease free for 5 years past the end of the maintenance phase.

Chemotherapy doses for children are most often calculated by the child's weight in kilograms or according to the child's body surface area to minimize toxic effects to tissues and organs. Chemotherapeutic agents are administered intrathecally, into the veins via central venous access devices (VADs), into the lateral ventricle using the Ommaya reservoir, or into intraperitoneal, intracavitary,

Text continued on page 1446

Table 22-4
Commonly Used Chemotherapy Agents

Drug	Classification	Route	Side Effects	Special Considerations
Asparaginase (L-asparaginase, Elspar) Erwinia and PEG-L-asparaginase (long-acting form of *Escherichia coli* L-asparaginase with less risk for serious hypersensitivity reactions) are investigational	Enzyme from *Escherichia coli* or *Erwinia carotovora* Cell cycle–nonspecific	Intramuscular (IM) IV May be reconstituted with 1 cc for 10,000 U/mL or 2 cc for 5000 U/mL Use within 8 hr Refrigerate	Coagulation abnormalities A, N—mild Pancreatitis, hyperglycemia, transient diabetes mellitus Convulsions Abnormal liver function test (LFT) results Somnolence, lethargy Allergic reactions ranging from mild urticaria to anaphylaxis	IV administration is associated with increased risk of anaphylaxis. Have emergency equipment and drugs available. Observe patient for at least 30 min after dose. Dipstick urine for glucose before each dose (treat with insulin if ordered for hyperglycemia).
5-Azacytidine (5-AC, 5-AZA)	Antimetabolite	IV infusion Refrigerate Dilution in Ringer's lactate only	Myelosuppression Neutropenia—dose dependent, with nadir from 2–3 wk N, V, D—severe with IV or subcutaneous (SQ) pulse dosing; less severe with continuous infusion Skin rash Liver damage rare but severe Rare and dose-dependent muscle pain, weakness, lethargy Fever during and for 24 hr after administration	Administer carefully to patients with liver disease or decreased serum albumin level (<3.8 g/dL) Continuous infusions should be changed every 3 hr.
Bleomycin sulfate (Blenoxane)	Antibiotic	IV IM SQ Intracavitary Intratumor Refrigerate May be diluted with as little as 0.5 mL of sterile water, sodium chloride, 5% dextrose, or bacteriostatic water	N, V, A Pneumonitis with dry cough, dyspnea, rales, progressive pulmonary fibrosis—total cumulative lifetime dose of 400 U Fever with or without chills Skin rash, cutaneous hyperpigmentation, discolorations—dose related Mild stomatitis	Rare, lethal anaphylactoid reactions can occur—have emergency equipment available. Administer test dose 1–2 U IM; wait 1 hr and give remaining dose. Lower dose may be given when pulmonary radiotherapy is used. Pulmonary function tests are done as baseline, throughout the course of therapy, and for a period of time after therapy; pneumonitis can progress to fatal fibrosis.
Busulfan (Myleran)	Alkylating agent	By mouth (PO) 2-mg tablets	Myelosuppression, pancytopenia with nadir from 11–30 days and recovery at 25–54 days Hyperpigmentation Gynecomastia—rare Gastrointestinal (GI) disturbances—mild	Interstitial pulmonary fibrosis within a year of starting therapy is rare and can occur after long-term therapy.
Carboplatin (Paraplatin)	Heavy metal	IV infusion Room temperature Discard after 8 hr Protect from light	Myelosuppression N, V Renal impairment, electrolyte wasting Peripheral neuropathies Ototoxicity Liver function abnormalities	IV infusion is given over 15–60 min or longer. Aluminum reacts with carboplatin, causing precipitate formation and loss of potency; therefore, do not allow needles or IV sets containing aluminum parts to come in contact with the drug.
Carmustine (BCNU, BiCNU)	Nitrosourea Lipid-soluble alkylating agent that crosses blood–brain barrier	IV infusion Refrigerate Reconstitute with absolute alcohol diluent	Delayed myelosuppression—leukopenia, thrombocytopenia (nadir 3–4 wk and resolving slowly) N, V appearing within 2 hr of administration and lasting up to 6 hr Liver and renal dysfunction Alopecia Pulmonary fibrosis with long-term use Hypotension	Drug is an irritant and may cause pain and phlebitis at the injection site, facial flushing, and hypotension from alcohol diluent, especially with rapid infusion. Solution may be further diluted, IV rate slowed, and ice or warm pack applied to extremity to decrease pain. Drug infusion may cause pain and brown staining of skin.

Table 22–4
Commonly Used Chemotherapy Agents *Continued*

Drug	Classification	Route	Side Effects	Special Considerations
Cisplatin (*cis*-platinum, Platinol)	Heavy metal	IV infusion Do not refrigerate reconstituted solution Protect from light Diluted solutions must contain at least 0.45% sodium chloride (NaCl)	Severe and often protracted N, V Myelosuppression Nephrotoxicity during second week after dose, becoming more severe with repeated courses of drug Ototoxicity, especially high-frequency hearing loss and tinnitus Electrolyte wasting, especially calcium and magnesium Hypomagnesemia may be protracted, requiring magnesium replacement therapy Allergic reactions—rare Hyperuricemia Peripheral neuropathy	Aluminum reacts with cisplatin, causing precipitate formation and loss of potency; therefore, do not allow needles or IV sets containing aluminum parts to come in contact with drug. Premedicate the child with antiemetics and continue throughout the course of therapy. It may be necessary to replace emesis "mL for mL." Monitor creatinine clearance, blood urea nitrogen (BUN), and creatinine levels before each dose is given. During the course of therapy, carefully monitor input and output. Urinary output should be maintained at least at 1–2 mL/kg/hr. Administer furosemide (Lasix) or mannitol as ordered to ensure adequate urinary output Drug intensifies aminoglycoside toxicity and should be used with caution when administered concurrently.
Corticosteroids Prednisone (Deltasone, Liquid Pred syrup) Dexamethasone (Decadron) Hydrocortisone (Solu-Cortef) Methylprednisolone (Solu-Medrol)	Lympholytic (effective in the treatment of acute lymphocytic leukemia [ALL], non-Hodgkin's lymphoma [NHL], and certain other malignancies) Decreases edema produced by tumor or caused by tumor necrosis	PO IV Intrathecal (IT) For IT use, mix with saline, lactated Ringer's, or Elliott's B solution	Salt or fluid retention, electrolyte depletion, hypertension, cushingoid appearance, increased appetite, obesity Hyperglycemia, diabetes Muscle weakness, osteoporosis Gastritis, gastric and peptic ulcers, gastrointestinal (GI) bleeding Immunosuppression, impaired wound healing Personality and mood changes Acne Growth retardation with long-term high-dose use Sterile arachnoiditis with IT use	Decrease salt intake; protect from infection; observe for hyperglycemia. To decrease or prevent GI upset, give with meals or snacks. Histamine H_2 receptor antagonist such as cimetidine or ranitidine may be needed. Drug may mask infection.
Cyclophosphamide (Cytoxan, CTX)	Alkylating agent	IV push or infusion PO tablets May be difficult to dissolve when diluted Observe for any particulate matter Store at room temperature once reconstituted and discard in 24 hr Reconstitute with preserved diluent Oral liquid preparation may be made from parenteral solution mixed in aromatic elixir	Hemorrhagic cystitis resulting from chemical irritation of bladder by metabolites of CTX N, V—may be severe, beginning 4–8 hr after administration and lasting 8–10 hr Leukopenia is dose-limiting, toxicity reaching nadir at 7–10 days; recovery in 14–24 days Syndrome of inappropriate antidiuretic hormone secretion (SIADH; water intoxication) with seizures Alopecia Sterility related to dose and pubertal status Cardiac toxicity and pulmonary fibrosis—rare May be carcinogenic (second malignant neoplasms)	Ensure adequate hydration, urinary output, urinary specific gravity <1.010 before giving high dose; administer drug in morning or early afternoon. Check urine for blood before, during, and after giving drug. Encourage patient to urinate before going to bed for the night to empty bladder completely. With high dose, ensure urinary output at 1500 mL/m²/12 hr and measure q 2 hr for 12 hr. Furosemide may be given to maintain urinary output (0.5 mg/kg; maximum 40 mg IV).

Table continued on following page

Table 22–4
Commonly Used Chemotherapy Agents *Continued*

Drug	Classification	Route	Side Effects	Special Considerations
Cytarabine (ara-C, cytosine arabinoside, Cytosar-U)	Antimetabolite	IV, SQ, IM, IT Reconstituted solution is stable at room temperature for 48 hr May be diluted with 1–2 mL for SQ or IM use Do not use diluent that is packaged with drug for IT use because it contains benzyl alcohol	A, N, V—may be severe at high doses or with IT use Myelosuppression with nadir of 7–14 days Ara-C syndrome—flulike symptoms, conjunctivitis, fever, maculopapular rash occurring 6–12 hr after administration Alopecia IT—headache, vomiting, pleocytosis; rare convulsions and paresis High-dose ara-C regimens may result in severe myelosuppression lasting at least 28 days	Anticipate vomiting immediately or within 2 hr after IT dose. Administer steroid eye drops to prevent conjunctivitis with high dose.
Dacarbazine (DTIC-Dome)	Alkylating agent	IV push, infusion	Myelosuppression with nadir of 21–25 days N, V can be severe Diarrhea—rare Alopecia Flulike syndrome Facial flushing Facial paresthesias Erythematous and urticarial rashes—rare	Drug is an irritant causing severe local pain and burning at injection site and long vein; it is thought to be caused by degradation of drug by light. Give slow infusion; apply cold pack to arm. Drug is extremely light sensitive. Tissue necrosis can occur if drug is extravasated.
Dactinomycin (actinomycin D, ACT-D, Cosmegen)	Antibiotic	IV push Golden colored Protect vial from light	Myelosuppression—nadir in 2–3 wk N, V—severe Diarrhea Alopecia Skin eruptions, acne Radiosensitizer—recall phenomenon at prior radiation site Flare-up of erythema or increased pigmentation of previously irradiated skin	Drug is vesicant—severe tissue damage can result from extravasation. Do not use with 0.2-μm filters. Toxicity may be enhanced if liver damage is present, especially with concomitant radiation to or near liver.
Daunomycin *and* Doxorubicin (Adriamycin)	Anthracycline antibiotic	IV push or infusion Continuous infusion Red color	Myelosuppression with nadir of 10–14 days; recovery in approximately 1 wk after nadir N, V Alopecia Cardiomyopathy—total lifetime dose of 550 mg/m^2, less if cardiac radiation was given Hyperpigmentation of nailbeds Radiosensitizer—recall phenomenon at prior radiation or infiltration site Increased sensitivity to sunlight Stomatitis—may be severe	Drug is vesicant—severe tissue damage can result from extravasation. Continuous infusions should be done through patent central line. Erythematous streak may appear up the vein of injection or hives at or near the injection site. Cardiac studies with echocardiogram or multiple-gated arteriography (MUGA) scan should be done periodically to monitor cardiac function. Patient must have acceptable cardiac ejection fraction. Cardiac toxicity may be less with continuous infusions. Urine may have red-orange tinge.
Etoposide (VP-16 VePesid)	Plant alkaloid—semisynthetic derivative of podophyllotoxin	IV infusion over 30–60 min Do not refrigerate reconstituted solution	Myelosuppression with nadir of 7–14 days and recovery by 10–16 days Hypersensitivity reactions, including bronchospasm, fever, erythema, pruritus N, V—mild Headache Neurotoxicity Alopecia Hypotension	Drug is an irritant; severe hypotension can occur with rapid infusion. Look for precipitates in dextrose solutions.

Table 22–4
Commonly Used Chemotherapy Agents *Continued*

Drug	Classification	Route	Side Effects	Special Considerations
5-Fluorouracil (5-FU, fluorouracil, Adrucil)	Antimetabolite	IV push, infusion PO (parenteral form may be given orally) Intrahepatic artery Protect from light Store at room temperature Clear, light yellow	Myelosuppression—leukopenia with nadir of 9–14 days; thrombocytopenia with nadir of 7–14 days N, V, D Stomatitis beginning at 5–8 days and can be severe Esophagitis Alopecia Dermatitis Hyperpigmentation of nail beds	For oral administration, mix parenteral solution of 5-FU with flavored water or carbonated beverage; avoid acidic fruit juices. Give on empty stomach (at least 2 hr before or after food).
Hydroxyurea (Hydrea, HU, HUR)	Antimetabolite	PO 500-mg capsules	Myelosuppression with rapid decrease in white blood cell (WBC) count N, V, D—mild Stomatitis Rash or facial erythema	Renal impairment enhances toxicity.
Idarubicin, Idamycin	Anthracycline	IV slow push or infusion	See doxorubicin	Drug is vesicant—severe tissue damage occurs with extravasation. See doxorubicin. Drug has perhaps less cardiotoxicity than doxorubicin and daunorubicin.
Ifosfamide (isophosphamide, IFEX)	Alkylating agent Analogue of cyclophosphamide	IV infusion	Myelosuppression with nadir in 7–10 days; recovery in 16–21 days Renal tubular damage (Fanconi's syndrome) Alopecia N, V—mild Mild, transient abnormal liver and renal function Encephalopathy Peripheral neuropathy	There is risk of hemorrhagic cystitis. Drug can be mixed with mesna. More severe symptoms may occur at higher doses and after rapid injection. Patient must receive PO or IV hydration for 24 hr after dose. Monitor I & O and urinary specific gravity.
Lomustine (CCNU) (CeeNU)	Nitrosourea	PO—10-, 40-, 100-mg capsules	Myelosuppression—delayed and persistent N, V—3–6 hr or longer after administration Alopecia Pulmonary fibrosis—rare Confusion, lethargy, ataxia	Give on empty stomach.
Mechlorethamine hydrochloride (nitrogen mustard, Mustargen, HN_2)	Alkylating agent	IV push	Myelosuppression with nadir in 10–14 days Leukopenia can occur within 24 hr and thrombocytopenia at 6–8 days N, V—severe Sterility, infertility Hyperuricemia Rash Alopecia May cause second malignant neoplasm	Drug is vesicant—can also cause skin irritation with local contact. Use within 1 hr after reconstitution. Drug may cause thrombosis, phlebitis, and discoloration of vein.
Melphalan (Alkeran, L-PAM) 1-Sarcolysin	Alkylating agent	PO—2-mg tablets IV agent available with diluent	Severe myelosuppression with nadir in 14–21 days, lasting 5–6 wk Anorexia Alopecia Profuse diarrhea Dermatitis Stomatitis, mucositis IV—serious hypersensitivity reactions Pulmonary fibrosis	Infuse over 15–30 min. Administer within 1 hr after reconstitution. Give daily dose at one time. Give on empty stomach. Ensure good hydration for 24 hr after dose. Furosemide may be given to maintain urinary output.

Table continued on following page

Table 22-4
Commonly Used Chemotherapy Agents *Continued*

Drug	Classification	Route	Side Effects	Special Considerations
Mercaptopurine (Purinethol, 6-MP)	Antimetabolite	PO—50-mg tablets IV (investigational) IT (investigational)	Hepatic dysfunction Atopic dermatitis Myelosuppression A, N, V—rare Stomatitis, mucositis Fever—rare	Reduce dose if given with allopurinol. Give daily dose at one time, preferably at bedtime. Avoid extravasation of IV form. Hematuria and crystalluria may occur with high IV doses.
Methotrexate (amethopterin, MTX)	Antimetabolite	PO—2.5-mg tablets IV push, infusion IM IT (mix with preservative-free diluent)	Ulcerative stomatitis, glossitis, gingivitis N, V, A, D Myelosuppression Hepatic toxicity Malaise Rash Alopecia Arachnoiditis or leukoencephalopathy after IT use Renal failure (with high-dose administration) Photosensitivity	Renal impairment enhances toxicity. Advise patients to use sunscreen; severe sunburn can occur even with low weekly doses. When intermediate or high-dose methotrexate is given, leucovorin is administered as ordered as a rescue agent. Give oral dose at one time. Avoid giving vitamins containing folic acid in order not to bypass the metabolic block caused by methotrexate. Many agents adversely interact with methotrexate (consult *Physicians' Desk Reference*).
Mitoxantrone (Novantrone)	Anthracycline analogue	IV infusion Dark blue solution	N, V Cardiomyopathy Mucositis, stomatitis Myelosuppression with nadir in 7–14 days Transient elevations in liver enzymes Alopecia Radiation recall dermatitis	Drug is vesicant—severe tissue damage occurs with extravasation. Drug is not recommended for patients who have received full doses of anthracyclines. Monitor cardiac status. Urine, serum, and sclera may appear green; there may be bluish discoloration of veins and nails. Phlebitis may occur at injection site. Do not give IV push.
Paclitaxel (Taxol)	Plant product isolated from the stem bark of the western yew, *Taxus brevifolia*	Intact ampules are kept dry and refrigerated until reconstituted Dilute paclitaxel to final concentration of 0.3 mg/mL–1.2 mg/mL, which is stable for 12 hr in D5W or normal saline solution All solutions exhibit a slight haze A small number of fibers (within acceptable levels of the USP Particulate Matter Test) have been observed after dilution	Acute hypersensitivity reactions characterized by cutaneous flushing, bronchospasm, tachypnea, bradycardia, hypotension within minutes of administration secondary to dilution vehicles Myelosuppression with WBC count nadir at 10 days and normalization within 18 days Sensory neuropathy Mucositis and ulcerations occurring on day 3–7 and resolving within 5–7 days Joint discomforts and myalgias occurring 2–3 days after administration and resolving within 4–7 days Alopecia Bradycardia N, V during infusion Diarrhea occurring within 1 week after infusion	Premedicate with corticosteroids, H_1 and H_2 antagonists, diphenhydramine, ranitidine. Monitor patient frequently, using cardiac monitor, pulse oximetry, if necessary. Slow continuous IV infusion decreases risk of serious anaphylactic reactions. 0.2 μm inline filters must be used. Solutions exhibiting excessive particulate formation should not be used. PVC bags and sets should be avoided.

Table 22–4
Commonly Used Chemotherapy Agents *Continued*

Drug	Classification	Route	Side Effects	Special Considerations
Procarbazine (Matulane) Investigational in parenteral form	Alkylating agent	PO—50-mg capsules Keep bottle tightly closed; moisture causes decomposition IV—use immediately after reconstitution	Myelosuppression—protracted nadir for thrombocytopenia at 4 wk Stomatitis A, N, V, D Alopecia Rash, pruritus Azoospermia, cessation of menses Myalgia, flulike syndrome CNS reactions—headache, paralysis, nervousness, nightmares, dizziness, hallucinations, confusion, coma, or convulsions May induce second malignant neoplasms	Hypertension or central nervous system (CNS) depression may occur in the presence of alcohol, monoamine oxidase (MAO) inhibitors, phenothiazines, phenytoin (Dilantin), tricyclic antidepressants, barbiturates, and tyramine-rich foods such as aged cheese, wine, bananas, yogurt, chocolate.
Retinoic acid (13-*cis*-retinoic acid, isotretinoin, Accutane) All *trans*-retinoic acids are investigational	Vitamin A and its derivatives Stimulate clonal proliferation of erythroid and myeloid progenitor cells and play a role in growth, reproduction, epithelial cell differentiation, and immune function; functions as a maturation agent in diseases such as neuroblastoma, rhabdomyosarcoma, acute promyelocytic leukemia (APL), and osteosarcoma	Accutane commercially available as soft gelatin capsules in 10-, 20-, and 40-mg sizes Store at room temperature in light-resistant container	Adverse mucocutaneous effects, primarily cheilitis, xerosis, and conjuctivitis Hypertriglyceridemia Transient increase in LFTs May produce birth malformations and should not be administered during pregnancy or to women who may become pregnant while undergoing treatment	Capsules can be swallowed directly or opened with a large needle and contents mixed with food.
Teniposide (VM-26)	Plant alkaloid Epipodophyllotoxin	IV infusion over 60 min	Allergic reactions Myelosuppression with nadir in 3–14 days Hypotension with rapid infusions Chemical phlebitis Fever, chills Alopecia	Drug is irritant—avoid extravasation. Anaphylaxis may occur with rapid infusions. Drug may appear "oily" or foamy when mixed, but this effect disappears quickly.
Thioguanine (6-thioguanine, 6-TG)	Antimetabolite	PO—40-mg tablets IV—investigational in parenteral form	Myelosuppression A, N, V, D—mild Hepatic toxicity Atopic dermatitis Stomatitis	Give oral dose at one time. Refrigerate after IV reconstitution; precipitate forms if stored at room temperature.
Thiotepa (Triethylene thiophosphoramide, TESPA)	Alkylating agent	IV infusion IT IM SQ Intracavitary Intratumor	Myelosuppression N, V Dizziness, headache Stomatitis Pain at injection site Alopecia Rash	Reconstitute to hypertonic or isotonic solution. Solution must be clear; discard otherwise.
Vinblastine (Velban, VBL)	Plant alkaloid	IV push Reconstituted to concentration 1 mg/mL Stable for 4 wk in refrigerator	Myelosuppression Stomatitis Alopecia A, N, D, or constipation Neurotoxicity—loss of deep tendon reflexes, paresthesias, peripheral neuropathy, hoarseness, ptosis, double vision	Drug is vesicant—severe tissue damage occurs with extravasation. Administer stool softeners; increase bulk and fiber in diet.

Table continued on following page

Table 22-4
Commonly Used Chemotherapy Agents *Continued*

Drug	Classification	Route	Side Effects	Special Considerations
Vincristine (Oncovin)	Plant alkaloid	IV push 1 mg/mL	Minimal myelosuppression Alopecia SIADH Peripheral neuropathies such as numbness and tingling of distal extremities, myalgias, cramping, foot drop, jaw pain, seizures, constipation, paralytic ileus, ptosis, vocal cord paralysis, cranial nerve palsies, absent deep tendon reflexes	Drug is vesicant—severe tissue damage occurs with extravasation. Stool softeners may be given prophylactically or for constipation. Liver dysfunction may enhance toxicity. Infants may have difficulty sucking because of jaw pain. Maximal single dose is 2 mg, regardless of body surface area.

A, anorexia; D, diarrhea; N, nausea; V, vomiting.
Modified from Renick-Ettinger, A. (1993). Chemotherapy. In G. Foley, D. Fochtman, & K. Hardin-Mooney (Eds.), *Nursing care of the child with cancer* (pp. 81–116). Philadelphia: W. B. Saunders. Used with permission.

or intra-arterial sites using implantable pumps. Portable infusion pumps deliver continuous therapy to children in ambulatory settings. The administration of chemotherapy necessitates that safety precautions be taken for both the child and the nurse or caregiver administering the medication (Table 22–5). The United States Occupational Safety and Health Administration (OSHA) has developed guidelines to protect health care workers from unwarranted exposure to cytotoxic agents caused by accidental absorption, inhalation, or ingestion (U.S. Department of Labor, 1986).

Radiation Therapy

Radiation therapy is used frequently in conjunction with chemotherapy or surgery to treat cancer in children. It can be used for curative treatment or as a palliative measure to reduce the size of a tumor so as to relieve symptoms. New advances in the delivery of radiation have led to less acute and long-term side effects and to better targeted sites of delivery (Hilderley, 1992).

Radiation is cytotoxic by damaging the synthesis of nucleic acids, causing breaks in the DNA or RNA molecule, or causing double stranded breaks in the molecules (Hall & Cox, 1989; Korinko & Yurick, 1997). The tumor cells become impaired. They cannot divide, or the cells lose their function and die during division. The cells may not die until they divide. Thus, normal and malignant cells that divide frequently are most susceptible to the effects of radiation. Many of the acute side effects of radiation are the result of damage to normal cells that divide frequently. These include the cells of the mucous membranes, hair follicles, and bone marrow. Acute side effects are usually anticipated 7 to 10 days after treatment has been initiated and may last for several weeks or even several months after therapy is completed (Chart 22–6).

Nursing responsibilities for the child receiving radiation treatments include providing concrete explanations to the child and the child's family regarding the radiation procedure and its side effects. Before the procedure, inked lines are drawn on the child's body to define the radiation field. During the procedure, the child must lie still and not change position. Plastic casts and molds may be used to immobilize the child during the treatment. Shielding devices made of lead are used to protect surrounding healthy tissues and organs against unnecessary radiation exposure. These shields may feel heavy to the child. The machinery involved in the treatment can create a variety of noises that may frighten the child. The child is alone in the treatment room, although he or she can communicate verbally with the staff. All of these sensations can make the child feel uncomfortable, claustrophobic, anxious, or bored. Young children may need to receive a mild sedative. Older children can be taught distraction techniques. Parents, who are located outside the room, can talk or read to the child to focus attention away from the procedure. After radiation treatment, nursing and family interventions focus on managing the side effects of the therapy and preventing further complications (see Chart 22–6).

Biotherapy

For many years, researchers have studied the complex functions of the immune system as it is related to cancer.

Table 22–5
Safety Guidelines for Chemotherapy Administration

	Guidelines
Extravasation Minor to severe tissue damage resulting from the leakage of certain chemotherapy drugs outside of the designated vein for administration	Use a central vascular access device for administration whenever possible. The peripheral vascular access site should be selected and the catheter placed by a health care provider who is competent in peripheral intravenous access. A physician should be notified immediately if a suspected or definite extravasation is identified. Institutional extravasation guidelines should be performed immediately for an identified extravasation (i.e., elevate extremity, apply ice, apply topical or injectable antidotes).
Preparation	Chemotherapy agents should be mixed and prepared in a biological safety cabinet by a health care provider wearing protective gear (i.e., latex gloves, gown, face shield) using sterile techniques. The health care provider administering chemotherapy should also wear protective gear, ensure IV connections have a Luer-Lok and are secured, and use a plastic-backed absorbent pad under the site of administration to catch any leakage.
Disposal	Equipment that has contained chemotherapy drugs or body excretions after chemotherapy administration is considered hazardous waste. Hazardous waste should be disposed of in designated containers that are properly labeled. Linens and clothing contaminated with chemotherapy or body excretions should be considered hazardous waste and should be handled appropriately. Chemotherapy may be excreted in the urine for up to 48 hr after administration.
Spills	Accidental spills of chemotherapy drugs should be cleaned up immediately. Spills should be confined and the area should be restricted until appropriate cleaning procedures have been completed.
Family teaching	Family members should be taught safety procedures for home chemotherapy administration and disposal to be used for a minimum of 48 hr after administration.

Through research and technological advances, biotherapy has emerged as a modality of cancer treatment. Biotherapy, sometimes called immunotherapy, may be prescribed for some children with cancer as a part of their initial treatment plan, or it may be used later in their treatment plan. Researchers have long known that certain substances in the body can influence the immune system, thereby helping to fight cancer or the side effects of cancer treatment. These substances, referred to as biological response modifiers (BRMs), include a host of naturally occurring or synthetic agents that elicit clinical responses in cancer patients (Chart 22–7).

The exact mechanism of action of BRMs is unclear. However, they apparently do the following:

Chart 22–6
Nursing Interventions

The Side Effects of Radiation Therapy

Site	Response	Nursing Intervention
Skin	Loss of epidermal layer Erythema, dryness Wet desquamation	Keep skin clean with daily baths. Avoid applying creams, perfumes or lotions during radiation treatments. Help child to avoid sun exposure and to use sunscreen with minimum SPF 30. Do not remove radiation markings. Contact skin care specialist for severe skin toxicities. Avoid applying tape adhesives when radiation is to be delivered.
Gastrointestinal tract	Mucositis Pain Dysphagia Ulceration Nausea, vomiting Diarrhea	Provide daily oral and dental care. Give antiemetics before and during radiation treatments. Encourage oral fluid intake. Encourage small, freqent meals. Assess for dehydration. Give analgesics as needed.
Salivary glands and parotid glands	Decreased formation of saliva Dryness of mucous membranes Taste disorder Parotiditis	Encourage daily oral hygiene. Give analgesics as needed. Encourage oral fluid intake.
Kidney or bladder	Cystitis Ulceration	Encourage fluid intake. Assess for blood in urine.
Bone marrow	Myelosuppression Anemia Thrombocytopenia	Exercise infection precautions. Observe for temperature >38°C and notify physician. Observe for signs of bleeding. Teach avoidance of large crowds. Observe for any signs of inflammation or infection.
Hair follicle	Alopecia	Recommend wigs or hair accessories. Help with skin hygiene.
Lungs	Pneumonitis Pulmonary fibrosis	Assess respiratory status, both long and short term.
Heart	Myocarditis or pericarditis	Assess cardiac status, both long and short term.
Brain or spinal cord	Edema	Assess neurologic status, both long and short term.
Ovary	Permanent sterility possible	Give patient/family education on sterility possibilities.
Testes	Mature spermatozoa: radioresistant Immature spermatozoa: permanent sterility	Provide sperm banking option when appropriate.

Modified from McGuire, P. (1993). Radiation therapy. In G. Foley, D. Fochtman, & K. Hardin Mooney (Eds.), *Nursing care of the child with cancer* (p. 122). Philadelphia: W. B. Saunders. Used with permission.

- Enhance a cancer patient's immune system to fight growth of cancer cells
- Eliminate or suppress body responses that allow cancer growth
- Make the cancer cells more susceptible to destruction by the immune system
- Stimulate cancer cells to grow and mature in ways that are less harmful to normal cells

Chart 22–7

Types of Biotherapy

Colony-Stimulating Factors

A family of glycoproteins responsible for stimulating and regulating hematopoiesis

Colony-stimulating factors (CSFs) stimulate cells or colonies within the blood-forming elements of the body to proliferate, prolong cell survival, stimulate cell maturation, and stimulate functional activity of mature cells (Betcher & Burnham, 1991). Five factors have been purified and manufactured including erythropoietin, granulocyte-macrophage CSF, granulocyte CSF, macrophage CSF, and interleukin-11.

Interleukins

Cytokines that relay information between leukocytes to modulate their activities. IL-11 is a recombinant growth factor that activates the body's immune system.

Tumor Necrosis Factor

A lymphokine protein that causes antitumor activity by disrupting the vascular endothelium of the cancer cell, resulting in hemorrhagic necrosis

Monoclonal Antibodies

A cancer-specific antibody produced in a laboratory for a target antigen; used to detect the presence of tumors and linked with chemotherapy as a treatment measure

Interferons

Members of the cytokine network, capable of inhibiting viral replication, modulating immune responses, and altering cellular proliferation

- Block the processes that change a normal cell into a cancerous cell
- Enhance the body's ability to repair normal cells that my be damaged from other cancer treatment modalities (Haynes, 1990)

Management of children receiving biotherapy is a challenge, because each individual is biologically different and may experience different reactions or side effects from receiving biotherapy. Some side effects associated with biotherapy are general flu-like symptoms, fluid retention, low-grade fevers, bone pain, chills, rash, and neuropathic pain. Nursing interventions are aimed at minimizing the discomfort associated with these side effects.

Bone Marrow Transplantation

Current advances in bone marrow transplantation (BMT) and technological progress have benefited many children with cancer by providing BMT as a viable treatment option. The bone marrow is the liquid portion of the bone. Its primary functions are to produce and maintain all blood cells in the body and maintain immune cell function. BMT is a therapy not only used to treat solid tumors but also used to treat diseases that affect the hematopoietic systems, the immune system, and metabolism.

Two sources of bone marrow can be used for transplantation: autologous (auto-BMT), which uses the child's own bone marrow, and allogeneic (allo-BMT), which uses a matched donor's bone marrow. The donor for an allo-BMT comes primarily from a sibling, sometimes from a twin (syngeneic BMT); however, it can also come from a parent or an unrelated donor (UBMT). Healthy blood cells for reinfusion can also be donated from cord blood from the child's newborn sibling or from an unrelated donor cord from the cord blood bank. The goal is to provide the child with the most genetically compatible bone marrow donor. This is achieved by determining the histocompatibility typing of the potential donor. Human leukocyte antigen (HLA) and DNA analyses are completed using a blood test to determine the type. HLAs are protein antigens located on the cell surfaces of all nucleated cells. In the body, the HLA system recognizes foreign tissues and activates the immune system to fight foreign tissue. The donor and recipient need to have matched tissue types to prevent the recipient from rejecting the donor marrow or have an increased potential for developing graft-versus-host disease (GVHD).

Before undergoing BMT, the child undergoes extensive physical and psychosocial evaluation to confirm that he or she is eligible for this procedure. During the BMT process, the child is monitored, isolated, and hospitalized, sometimes for several weeks, or possibly for several months. The initial phase of BMT is called *conditioning*. Conditioning involves a 7- to 10-day period during which the child receives very high (lethal) doses of chemotherapy or total body irradiation, depending on the child's diagnosis and type of bone marrow he or she is to receive. This therapy causes bone marrow ablation and attempts to eliminate any remaining disease and to prepare the child's body to accept the new, healthy bone marrow. During this time, the child is at high risk for infection. Measures are instituted to protect the child from infection, including placing the child in a protective environment with the use of laminar air flow rooms or HEPA-filtered positive-pressure rooms. Administration of intravenous gamma-globulins and acyclovir may also be used to prevent infection (Bryant & Guinan, 1992). Antibiotics are used as needed in the presence of infection.

Table 22–6
Complications of Bone Marrow Transplantation

Complication	Manifestation	Health Care Interventions
Alterations in nutrition	Nausea Vomiting Mouth ulcerations	Administer total parenteral nutrition. Provide meticulous oral care. Provide diet to maximize caloric intake. Administer antiemetic.
Infection	Neutropenia	Provide isolation. Administer prophylactic medications. Use irradiated blood products. Obtain cultures when clinically indicated. Supply routine hygiene. Ensure good skin integrity. Avoid rectal medications or temperature measurements.
Hematologic complications	Thrombocytopenia Anemia Hemorrhage	Administer blood products. Ensure safety precautions so as to avoid injury.
Mucositis	Deterioration of mucosa and gastrointestinal tract Excessive secretions Difficulty swallowing and breathing Anorexia Difficulty eating Abdominal cramping Watery diarrhea	Provide meticulous oral care. Intubation facilitates breathing. Provide measures to control pain. Treat diarrhea.
Veno-occlusive disease (VOD)	Sudden unexpected weight gain Thrombocytopenia refractory to platelet infusions Jaundice Hepatomegaly Right upper quadrant pain Ascites Encephalopathy	Observe oral and intravenous fluid restrictions. Obtain daily weights and abdominal girth. Elevate head of bed. Monitor hepatic function. Assess mental status.

After conditioning, there is 1 day of rest. On the following day, the *harvesting phase* occurs in which the donor bone marrow is obtained and infused into the recipient using a process similar to a blood transfusion. These healthy blood cells migrate into the child's empty spaces in the bone marrow, take root, grow, and attempt to repopulate into a healthy, new bone marrow. The *rescue, engraftment,* or *post-BMT phase* is a critical time when the child is at high risk for complications until new blood cells and immune cells are present (Frederick & Hanigan, 1993; Hathaway & McCord, 1988). An effective transplant produces new, cancer-free hematopoietic and immune systems in the recipient.

The complications associated with BMT are weighed against the benefits to cure the child's disease (Table 22–6). The acute toxicities can be life-threatening; thus, the nurse must assess the child daily for any organ toxicities, infections, bleeding complications, fluid and electrolyte imbalances, and skin and mucous membrane toxicities. Management of these side effects is addressed under the supportive care section of this chapter.

Table 22–6
Complications of Bone Marrow Transplantation *Continued*

Complication	Manifestation	Health Care Interventions
Interstitial pneumonia	Non-productive dry cough Fever Tachypnea Nasal flaring Dyspnea Hypoxia	Assess respiratory and ventilation status. Provide respiratory treatments as needed. Administer oxygen. Promote rest.
Renal complications	Dehydration Third spacing Hemorrhage Hypovolemia Septic shock Hypoproteinemia	Assess fluid and electrolyte status. Maintain adequate intravascular volume and renal perfusion. Correct fluid and electrolyte imbalances. Minimize use of nephrotoxic agents.
Graft-versus-host disease (GVHD)	Maculopapular rash on the palmar and plantar surfaces of the hand and feet evolving into erythematous rash over most of body Diarrhea (guaiac positive) Fever Jaundice Hepatomegaly Hypertension Infection	Ensure daily evaluation of blood counts. Provide platelet infusion. Provide packed red cell transfusion. Administer immunosuppressive/anti-GVHD medications.
Graft rejection or failure	Fever Infection Decrease in blood counts	Reinfuse source of blood stem cells into child.
Long-term effects	Short stature Delayed puberty Cataracts Growth hormone deficiency Pulmonary or cardiac toxicities	Interventions vary depending on exact effect. Provide supportive care.

Graft-Versus-Host Disease

GVHD from the donor source is a minor, or possibly severe, immune reaction that occurs in the immunosuppressed child receiving donor-immunocompetent cells. The reaction is usually restricted to certain organs such as the skin, liver, and GI tract. The child may have slight redness of the skin, particularly on the palms and soles, or complete skin desquamation (Fig. 22–3). The child may also experience diarrhea, possibly up to 2 to 3 L per day. The level of elevation of the total bilirubin is the direct indicator of GVHD of the liver. If these symptoms occur within the first 100 days after BMT, it is usually referred to as "acute GVHD." Chronic GVHD may develop after 100 days after BMT. The occurrence of GVHD is lessened according to how closely the HLA matches between the donor and the child. Infectious complications, especially fungal and viral, are a major problem for children with chronic GVHD. Respiratory complications can also lead to serious compromises in the child's health (Fidler, Roell, & Wiley, 1993; Hanigan, 1990).

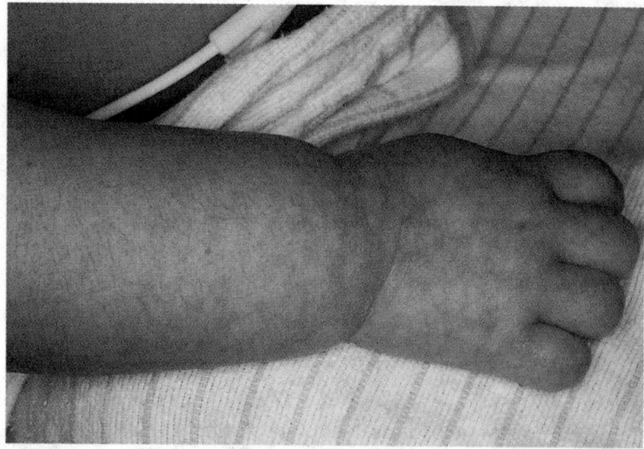

Figure 22–3
Graft-versus-host disease typically presents as a maculopapular rash that starts on the palms and soles and evolves to an erythematous rash over most of the body.

Supportive Care

Although cancer treatment has become more effective in children, the damage to normal cells and organs remains a concern. Optimal, ongoing use of supportive care measures by the interdisciplinary team is a vital component in the prolonged, intensive treatments that children with cancer undergo (Chart 22–8). Not all children have the same needs or interventions required in relation to their response to treatment of their cancer, and each case must be viewed individually.

Patient and Family Education

All health care interventions for the child and the child's family must incorporate the intervention of providing education so as to bring about positive actions that can benefit the child's health status. Patient and family education includes planned learning experiences that use a combination of techniques such as teaching, counseling, and behavior modification. Patient education also involves imparting information and interpreting information as the situation warrants. The purpose of the education process is to influence behavior and produce changes in knowledge, skills, and attitudes. Each encounter with the child and the child's family must be viewed as an opportunity to participate in the education process.

The educational process for families dealing with childhood cancer begins at the time of diagnosis, continues through each phase of the child's treatment, and must be maintained to assist the child in the postsurvival years or to assist the family after the death of the child. From the moment that cancer is suspected, the family is thrown into a new world in which they must learn new medical terms, procedures, and methods to care for the needs of their child. Through education, most families become sophisticated in their base and depth of knowledge of pediatric oncology. All members of the health care team play a critical role in providing information to help the child and family cope and make informed decisions.

TIP 22–1 provides an overview of the topics that are included in the long-term educational process with the child and family. The topics are not discussed at a single visit; rather they are subjects whose content is reviewed over and over again as the need arises. As the child grows and develops new levels of cognitive understanding, topics should be revisited to ensure that the child has an age-appropriate understanding.

Worldview: *In some cultures, children's autonomy is not encouraged. Parents and children are not likely to discuss difficult issues. Full disclosure of information about the child's illness may be filtered or not discussed at all among family members. The health care team should share their beliefs about the importance of disclosing information to the child. The family may agree to have the health care provider discuss the illness and treatment with the child, but they may choose not to participate in these discussions (Munet-Vilaró & Vessey, 1990).*

Chart 22–8

Supportive Care for the Child with a Malignancy

- Patient and family education
- Pain management
- Prevention of infection
- Management of fever and sepsis
- Administration of blood products
- Provision and maintenance of vascular access
- Drug toxicity evaluations
- Management of oncologic emergencies
- Prevention and management of nausea and vomiting
- Nutritional support
- Oral hygiene care
- Prevention and management of constipation
- Prevention and management of diarrhea
- Psychosocial support
- Promotion of normal childhood growth and development
- Provision of home care services
- Management of long-term sequelae

TIP 22–1 A Teaching Intervention Plan for the Child with a Malignancy

Nursing Diagnosis and Outcomes

- Knowledge deficit: diagnosis, treatment plan, and health care needs of the child

Outcomes:

Child and family will verbalize understanding of diagnosis, treatment plan, and child's health care needs.

Child and family will participate in the decision-making process and care of the child based on their understanding of the child's illness and treatment options.

Interventions

The educational plan for the child and family should contain the following content:

- Pathophysiology of diagnosis
- Signs and symptoms of the malignancy
- Purpose and methods of diagnostic testing
- Interpretation of blood counts
- Treatment options and outcomes
- Prognosis
- Pain management techniques
- Prevention of infection
- Temperature taking
- Signs and symptoms of infection
- Care of the venous access device
- Treatment-induced side effects
- Management of nausea and vomiting
- Oral hygiene care
- Management of stomatitis
- Dealing with alopecia and other changes in body appearance
- Management of constipation
- Management of diarrhea
- Nutritional needs of the child
- Signs and symptoms of dehydration
- Developmental needs of the child
- Activities at home and school
- Home management of medications
- Home management of medical equipment and assistive devices
- Coping techniques
- Needs of parents and siblings
- Management of long-term sequelae

Pain Management

Children with cancer may experience pain for a variety of reasons. Initially, children may experience pain caused by the disease itself, for example, bone pain in leukemia, headaches in brain tumors, abdominal pain for abdominal tumors. Disease-related pain is more prevalent in adults than children (Patterson, 1992). More commonly, children with cancer experience pain from the numerous procedures and tests that are done at the time of diagnosis and throughout the treatment course. Pain is also associated with side effects of the various treatment modalities, such as postoperative pain, oral mucositis, skin irritation and breakdown, and esophageal and abdominal pain from GI irritation or ulcerations. Pediatric cancer pain has not been well researched. The primary body of literature has focused on the pain and discomfort associated with certain biopsy diagnostic procedures such as bone marrow aspiration and lumbar puncture, although, even in this area, pain management techniques vary significantly among practitioners (Bossert, Van Cleve, & Savedra, 1996; Klein, 1992). Areas in need of further research include describing the trajectory of a child's pain over the course of the illness, the late effects of pain, the reported incidence of pain after the disease has been eradicated, and evaluating traditional and non-traditional pain management approaches that can be effective before, during, and after procedures and treatments (Heiney, Goon-Johnson, Ettinger, & Ettinger, 1990; Sutters & Miaskowski, 1992).

Pain management is a challenge in caring for children, because not all children can describe their symptoms completely or even verbalize that they have pain. Parents and health care providers may have fears and misconceptions concerning the use of pain medications and thus avoid administering these agents to the child. Parents may fear that the child will become addicted to the medications. A general concern holds that narcotics, "drugs," are bad for children. Some health care providers fear that the narcotics will depress the child's respirations and thus should not be given. The child's lack of verbal expression about the pain and a child's quiet demeanor may cause misinterpretations between the health care provider and the child regarding the existence of pain and the need for medication (Klein, 1992). Many helpful nonpharmacologic techniques are frequently not used because they require greater time commitments with the child, separate training sessions for staff, family members, and the child to learn the techniques, and practice on the part of the family and child (McCarthy, Cool, Petersen, & Bruene, 1996).

Both pharmacologic and nonpharmacologic interventions are important in managing pediatric pain. Mild analgesics, topical anesthetics, and narcotics can be used to treat pain. Sedation or anesthetic medications such as Versed or ketamine may be used to assist children undergoing painful procedures that are required routinely during their cancer treatment.

Chronic or terminal pain may be managed in the home with the use of continuous administration of narcotics. The method of narcotic administration may be oral, bolus intravenous (IV), or continuous IV infusion (see Chapter 13). Management of pain in the home setting is a collaborative effort among the child and family, home health nurse, home care pharmacist, and oncologist.

Several nonpharmacologic pain management strategies have been successful in dealing with the pain associated with procedures. These interventions include music therapy, hand-holding, imagery, hypnosis, relaxation, diversion, rest and sleep, massaging, heat, breathing exercises, and biofeedback (Bossert et al., 1996; Rasco, 1992). Chapter 13 discusses in detail these pain management techniques. A variety of techniques can be taught to the child and the child's family to provide a repertoire of coping skills and an effective alternative or adjunct to the administration of pain medications.

Infection Prevention

Children receiving cancer treatment are immunosuppressed and at increased risk for infection, particularly 7 to 10 days after receiving chemotherapy (nadir). Prevention is essential during the management of these children because any infection can become serious and could lead to death.

caREminder: *In the home, a focus on infection precautions is encouraged by instituting thorough hand washing, allowing no "ill" visitors, encouraging excellent daily hygiene, avoiding crowds, particularly when the child is neutropenic (white blood cell count decrease), and scheduling follow-up appointments to monitor blood counts.*

Children receiving chemotherapy may also receive prophylactic medications to help prevent certain opportunistic infections. For example, trimethoprim-sulfamethoxazole (Bactrim) is administered to prevent severe respiratory infections such as with *Pneumocystis carinii*, acyclovir may be administered to prevent herpes virus infections, and fluconazole or ketoconazole may be administered to prevent fungal infections. Another preventive medication to help minimize risks of infection is the use of granulocyte–colony stimulating factor (G-CSF). This biotherapy agent is administered by subcutaneous injection or IV route for up to 14 days after chemotherapy. This agent helps stimulate the bone marrow to repopulate granulocytes more quickly and efficiently, which decreases the length of time that the child remains neutropenic, thereby decreasing the risk of infection.

Alert: *Varicella-zoster infection (chickenpox) can be life-threatening to the immunosuppressed child. The child with cancer who is exposed to chickenpox should receive varicella-zoster immune globulin (VZIG) within 5 days of exposure if the child has not had this communicable disease before. The varicella vaccine has not yet been approved for use in children with cancer.*

The immunosuppressed child can receive childhood immunizations under certain circumstances. The child can be receiving maintenance chemotherapy but must have been in remission for at least 1 full year. Chemotherapy is stopped for 1 week before administration of the first vaccine dose. Steroids are withheld for 2 weeks after vaccine administration. After immunization, antibody titers are evaluated to assess for seroconversion. A second dose of the vaccine may be necessary. Administration is contraindicated for children with acquired immunodeficiency syndrome (AIDS) (Braun, 1996).

Exposure to measles has become a growing concern for children with a malignancy. The incidence of measles in the United States has increased, thus placing the immunosuppressed child at increased risk for exposure. Regardless of vaccination status, administration of intramuscular IgG is recommended within 6 days of a measles exposure for all immunocompromised children. The child is isolated for 7 to 18 days and, if infection occurs, isolation continues for the full course of the illness. To prevent measles, live measles vaccine can be administered when the child has been off immunosuppressive therapy for a minimum of 3 months (Meeske, Chamberlin, Cipkala-Gaffin, Harlander, & Reed, 1991).

Management of Fever and Sepsis

Sepsis is a common complication of chemotherapy treatment. Fever can be the first sign of sepsis; thus, the family and the nurse must monitor the child for the occurrence of fever and must recognize and prevent the progression of septic shock (TIP 22–2). Symptoms can be subtle in the immunosuppressed child.

Alert: *If a child's temperature is 100.5°F or higher for 4 hours or longer or the temperature is 101.5°F, the child must be evaluated by a physician immediately.*

Rectal temperatures should not be obtained to avoid damaging the rectal mucosa, which can cause bleeding or infection. Blood and other specimen cultures (e.g., urine,

TIP 22–2 A Teaching Intervention Plan for the Oncology Patient Who Gets Sick at Home

Nursing Diagnosis and Family Outcomes

- High risk for infection related to neutropenia, immunosuppressive therapy, and presence of vascular access device
  Outcome: Child/family will recognize and report signs of infection to their health care provider.

Interventions

Teach the Family

If the child appears to be sick:

- Check child's temperature any time that he or she feels warm to touch or is uncomfortable.
- Obtain temperature measurement under the arm or by mouth.
- Do not give the child medication for fever unless instructed by physician.
- Administer acetaminophen as prescribed by physician; never give aspirin.
- Encourage intake of fluids and small, frequent offerings of nutritious food.
- Observe the child's skin for pallor or bruising.
- Give antiemetics as prescribed.
- Observe whether the child's urine or stool appears bloody.
- Observe venous access device site for signs of infection or leaking.

Contact Health Care Provider if

- Child has a temperature of 101.5°F or higher or has a temperature of 100.5° to 101.4°F lasting more than 4 hours.
- Child appears seriously ill without a fever.
- Child has shaking chills.
- Child has fever, shaking chills, or both, after flushing his or her vascular access device.
- Child is confused, has slurred speech, or is difficult to arouse.
- Child is extremely weak, is pale or has bruising or bleeding.
- Child has repeated excessive vomiting or diarrhea.
- Child has decreased urinary output or blood in urine.
- Vascular access device cracks, leaks, pulls out, or does not flush, or if redness, swelling, or damage appears at the site.

wound drainage) are obtained from all possible sources, including the VAD. In the presence of fever, broad-spectrum antibiotics are administered immediately and close monitoring of the child is necessary until the origin of the fever is established. If no source of fever is identified, the child receives medication for approximately 48 to 72 hours and then is reevaluated for continuing treatment (Care Path 22–1). If an organism is isolated, more specific antibacterial agents are given. Intravenous fluids are given to prevent dehydration and prevent further complications of septic shock. (See Chapter 30 for more information about septic shock.) The child is at risk for

Care Path 22–1 An Interdisciplinary Plan of Care for the Child with Neutropenia and Fever

	Patient/Family Intermediate Outcomes			
Nursing Diagnosis	**Day 1**	**Day 2**	**Day 3**	**Day 4 Inpatient or Outpatient Setting**
High risk for infection related to neutropenia and fever	Child is admitted to acute care if T >101.5°F or 100.4°F × 3 days or ANC <1000. Urine output remains ≥1 cc/kg/hr.		Child remains free from signs of infection. Child has less than 3 temperature spikes of T >100.4°F per day.	Child is afebrile; vital signs and weight are stable. Hospitalization continues and this care path is exited if cultures are positive and child requires continuing IV and antibiotic support *or* child is evaluated in outpatient setting.
High risk for injury related to effects of overwhelming infection	Child will maintain O_2 saturation >95%, and heart rate, respiration, and blood pressure are normal for age.	⟶	Child maintains good hydration and nutrition. Child has no signs of oral mucosa or skin breakdown.	⟶ ⟶
Knowledge deficit: care of the child with neutropenia and fever	Child and family verbalize concerns and understand risk of infection. Child and family demonstrate good hand washing.	Family verbalizes when to contact health care personnel if infection is suspected.	Child and family demonstrate infection precautions.	⟶
Care Intervention Categories				
Consults	System-specific consults for areas of involvement Social service assessment visit to address any identified needs	Infectious disease consult if child remains febrile with no positive C/S		

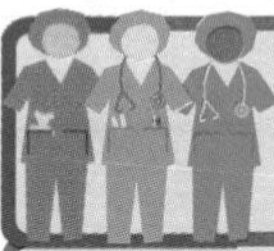

Care Path 22–1 An Interdisciplinary Plan of Care for the Child with Neutropenia and Fever *Continued*

Care Intervention Categories	Day 1	Day 2	Day 3	Day 4 Inpatient or Outpatient Setting
Discharge planning		Anticipate length of stay based on continuing presence of fever spikes, positive C/S, and home support.		If child is afebrile and C/S negative, discharge home. If child remains febrile, continue treatment plan.
Labs	CBC, with differential and platelet Blood chemistries PT/PTT, DIC screen Blood C/S (central line and peripherally) U/A, urine C/S Stool C/S if diarrhea is present C/S of any suspected areas of involvement including skin and oral cavity	Blood cultures daily if fever is present CBC with differential until ANC >500 Antibiotic peak and trough levels	Blood and urine culture for fungal infection and cytomegalovirus if fever persists	
Medications and IVs	Fluid bolus on admission (20 cc/kg over 30 minutes) Repeat fluid bolus × 2 if diastolic BP is less than 10% norm. Start maintenance IV fluids. Broad-spectrum antibiotics as indicated (ceftazidime, tobramycin, vancomycin) Acetaminophen as needed Chemotherapy regimen may require modification. Nystatin, Peridex, Bactrim continued if mucositis or GI involvement noted.	Reevaluate antibiotics based on clinical signs. Decrease IV fluids if taking PO.	If C/S is positive, select antibiotic therapy with sensitivity to known infectious agent. IV to heparin lock if PO intake is good	If fever persists, consider IV amphotericin. Discontinue all IV fluids if cultures are negative. Antibiotics may be continued in the home.

Care Path continued on following page

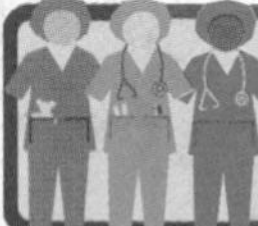

Care Path 22–1 An Interdisciplinary Plan of Care for the Child with Neutropenia and Fever *Continued*

Care Intervention Categories	Day 1	Day 2	Day 3	Day 4 Inpatient or Outpatient Setting
Monitors	Pulse oximetry	Discontinue pulse oximetry if O_2 saturation >95%.		
Nutrition	Regular diet as tolerated	⟶	⟶	⟶
Play therapy/ school	Child must stay in room if febrile.	Child may visit playroom if afebrile after 24 hr, regardless of ANC.	⟶ Arrange for hospital tutor.	⟶
Radiology	Chest radiograph if pulmonary symptoms are present			
Respiratory	O_2 per nasal mask or cannula to keep O_2 saturation >95%	Discontinue O_2 if O_2 saturation >95%.		
Safety and activity	Bleeding precautions Place child in single room. Enforce strict hand washing. Limit visitors for infection prevention.	⟶ ⟶ ⟶ ⟶	⟶ ⟶ ⟶ ⟶	⟶ ⟶ ⟶ ⟶
Self-care	Daily bath Oral care VAD dressing change per institution policy	⟶ ⟶ ⟶	⟶ ⟶ ⟶	⟶ ⟶ ⟶

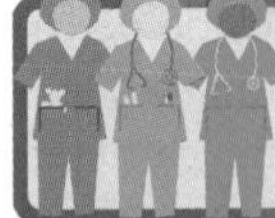

Care Path 22–1 An Interdisciplinary Plan of Care for the Child with Neutropenia and Fever *Continued*

Care Intervention Categories	Day 1	Day 2	Day 3	Day 4 Inpatient or Outpatient Setting
Teaching	Provide information related to diagnostic procedures. Discuss sources of infection at home and in hospital. Discuss need for strict hand washing.	Teach family how to monitor child for infection at home. Notify health care team if signs of infection are present or if temperature is increased.	Discuss measures to prevent introduction of infectious organisms (e.g., good oral care, good nutrition, proper VAD care).	
Vital signs/ baseline parameters	Every 2 hr Input and output Peripheral pulses and capillary refill Assess oral cavity and skin for signs of infection Respiratory status GI and GU status	Vital signs routine ⟶	⟶ ⟶	⟶ ⟶

ANC, absolute neutrophil count; CBC, complete blood count; C/S, cultures and sensitivity; DIC, disseminated intravascular coagulation; GI, gastrointestinal; GU, genitourinary; IV, intravenous; PO, by mouth; PT, prothrombin time; PTT, partial thromboplastin time; T, temperature; U/A, urinalysis; VAD, venous access device.

development of disseminated intravascular coagulation and liver failure in severe cases of septic shock (DeSwarte, 1991).

Administration of Blood Products

Anemia, neutropenia, and thrombocytopenia are common results of bone marrow suppression following chemotherapy. Blood counts are monitored closely, a minimum of once a week, or more frequently if clinically indicated.

▽ **Alert:** *Spontaneous bleeding may occur at platelet counts of less than 20,000 μL.*

Red blood cells and platelet transfusions are given to maintain a hemoglobin of at least 7.0 g/dL and a platelet count of 20,000 K/μL or more. Some oncologists advocate that children with brain tumors should maintain their platelet counts at greater than 50,000 to minimize the risk of intracranial bleeding (Chart 22–9).

Certain chemotherapy drugs may alter the blood coagulation studies and children may need to receive fresh-frozen plasma, cryoprecipitate, or factor VIII to correct coagulopathy. For example, the drug L-asparaginase, which is used to treat acute leukemia, may decrease the fibrinogen level. Fibrinogen levels should be checked once a week when a child is receiving L-asparaginase.

Provision and Maintenance of Vascular Access

Vascular access devices (VADs), also called "central lines," are placed in children undergoing cancer treatment to allow ease of delivery of chemotherapy, blood products, nutrition, IV fluids, and IV medications and to

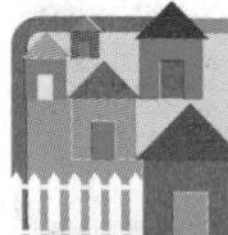

Chart 22–9
Community Care

Precautions for Children with Thrombocytopenia

- Avoid aspirin and products containing aspirin.
- Perform mouth care with a soft toothbrush or sponge.
- Avoid contact sports, rough play, and amusement park rides with increased centrifugal force.
- Postpone elective invasive procedures, such as dental work.
- Avoid intramuscular injections, rectal temperature measurement, or enemas.
- Increase intake of roughage and fluids to avoid constipation and straining.

obtain blood samples. The types of devices include percutaneous central venous catheters, Silastic catheters, implanted ports, and peripherally inserted central catheters (Keegan-Wells & Stewart, 1992). Primary caretakers are given thorough instruction on how to manage these devices at home. School officials should be notified when a child has a VAD (Chart 22–10). Use and maintenance of the external device at home includes dressing changes, cap changes, heparin flushes, blood draws, medication administration, and emergency care guidelines (Marcoux, Fisher, & Wong, 1990). In addition to nursing instruction, aids such as booklets, videos, and hands-on demonstration with a doll should be used to support teaching interventions (Fig. 22–4). A thorough discussion of these devices is presented in Chapter 17, including information regarding home management of the child with a central line and developmental considerations when securing the VAD.

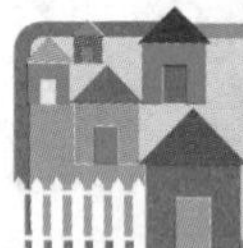

Chart 22–10
Community Care

Teacher Information Letter for the Child with a VAD

Date __________

To the Teacher(s) of ____________________:

This letter is to inform you about a common surgical procedure that ______________ recently had done. As you are aware, this student has a condition that necessitates frequent administration of chemotherapy and/or medication. For this reason, a rubber-like tube has been placed in a major blood vessel in the upper part of the chest. This is a semi-permanent tube that is used to administer therapy. When not in use, the tube is capped and covered with a small dressing. This special tube (called a ____________) will be cared for by the family and/or student at home.

We would like to make it clear that this tube should not interfere with the student's normal activities, e.g., gym class. At first, the child must avoid getting this area wet. Trauma to the area should be avoided, e.g., other children pulling at it. Contact sports should be avoided. Usually, this tubing is undetectable under clothing worn to school.

We do not expect that there will be any problems with the tube when the child is at school. There is a remote possibility that the small cap could come off the end of the tubing. If this did occur, it would be necessary to pinch off the tubing with one's fingers or the special clamp that is on the tube. The student would then need to have the school notify the parents for further directions. If the small dressing over the tube loosens during the day, it can be reinforced with some tape until the child finishes school for the day. Most of the children and all of the families are very knowledgeable about the tube. Please discuss any concerns you have with them.

Again, it is very unlikely that problems will occur. If you have any concerns or questions, please feel free to contact us. We appreciate your support.

Sincerely,

Pediatric Hematology/Oncology Nurse

Phone -

Parent's Signature ______________________
Work Phone ____________
Home Phone ____________

From Dufour, D. (1990). Information for teachers of children with central venous catheters. *Journal of Pediatric Oncology Nursing, 7*(1), 37–38. Reprinted with permission.

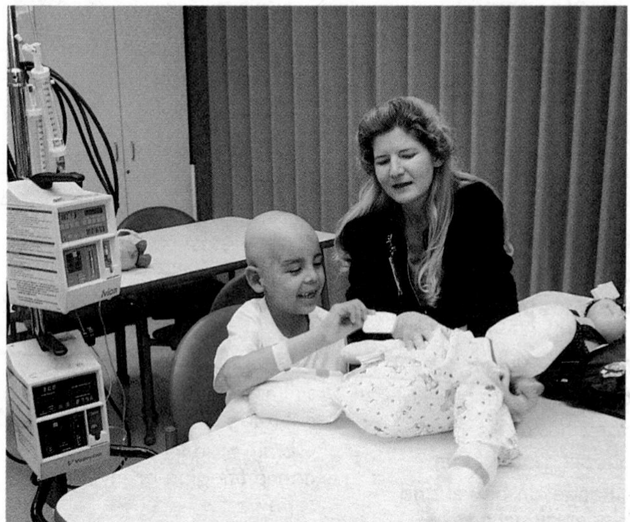

Figure 22-4
The child life specialist uses a doll and medical equipment to help this child learn to care for her venous access device.

It is not uncommon for the VAD to become infected, either at the exit site from the body or hematogenously from sepsis (Freiberger, Bryant, & Marino, 1992) (Chart 22-11). The primary portal for entry of microorganisms is at the catheter exit site. Thus, careful local skin care is imperative to reduce the incidence of infection and sepsis. Institutions vary in their approach to VAD site maintenance. In general, an antiseptic solution is used to clean the site, followed by the placement of a sterile occlusive dressing. The length of time between dressing changes also varies with institutional policy and with the condition of the site itself.

Extravasation occurs when chemotherapy administered peripherally or through a VAD or an implantable access device leaks into surrounding tissue areas, causing cellular tissue damage. The extent of damage may range from a small area of redness to a large lesion that becomes necrotic and requires plastic surgery. Most extravasations are preventable by maintaining good assessment techniques before, during, and after chemotherapy administration. The vein size, location, and patency should all be noted. If areas of redness or ulceration occur at the administration site during the infusion, the chemotherapy should be stopped and patency further assessed. The child may also complain of burning or loss of sensation or movement. If extravasation does occur, prompt intervention using an antidote identified for the particular vesicant is indicated (Lavezzo, 1990).

Drug Toxicity Evaluations

In response to the metabolism, detoxification, and excretion of many chemotherapy agents, certain organs may succumb to potential toxic side effects. Every child must be evaluated for organ function as a baseline before chemotherapy administration. Liver and renal function blood tests (i.e., blood urea nitrogen, creatinine clearance tests, bilirubin levels) are obtained and evaluated to ensure normal function of the liver and kidneys. An electrocardiogram or echocardiogram may be indicated to evaluate the heart function. Pulmonary function tests are used to evaluate the presence of decreased lung elasticity. Neurologic examinations indicate the loss of deep tendon reflexes or sensory loss. The findings of increased creatinine, the presence of proteins, or hematuria through urine analysis indicate drug toxicity. Appropriate drug modifications, deletions of doses, or modification of the timing of delivery are based on the changes in organ function or laboratory values. The decision to modify therapy is complex because the goal of eradicating the cancer must always be maintained while supporting the child through the toxic side effects.

Management of Oncologic Emergencies

At the time of diagnosis and during cancer treatment, certain emergencies may arise that must be swiftly recognized and treated by the health care team (Table 22-7). These emergencies can arise due to secondary effects of the cancer or from toxicities of chemotherapy administration. The size of the tumor mass can cause severe complications by compressing other vital internal struc-

Chart 22-11

Sources of Infection from the Venous Access Device

- Surgical incision made by placement of the venous access device (VAD) allows normal flora in the body's exterior surface to penetrate the interior surface and enter the bloodstream.
- Catheters used for more than one purpose have a higher infection rate than those used for one purpose.
- Newly placed catheters have a higher infection rate than those in place for longer periods of time.
- Children may tamper with dressings.
- Children may transport vomit or stool onto the dressing via contaminated hands.
- Children may have more severe allergic reactions to tape, antiseptic solutions, or dressings placed on the VAD.
- Children are often neutropenic at the time of VAD placement.

Table 22-7
Oncologic Emergencies

Emergency	Etiology	Clinical Presentation	Health Care Interventions
Superior vena cava syndrome (SVCS)	Mediastinal compression of the superior vena cava caused by size and location of tumor mass	Airway obstruction Respiratory distress Edema Changes in mental status	Apply emergency radiation or steroids to reduce tumor mass from vena cava. Emergency radiation consult
Spinal cord compression	Compression of the spinal cord caused by tumor mass on or near the spinal cord; can be a result of primary tumor of the spine or from spinal metastases	Motor weakness Difficulty bearing weight Paresthesia Shooting back pain Changes in bowel and bladder function	Obtain neurosurgical consult to determine extent of neurologic impairment. Obtain magnetic resonance imaging or myelography. If indicated, perform emergency surgery to relieve compression.
Syndrome of inappropriate antidiuretic hormone secretion (SIADH)	Vincristine and cyclophosphamide administration can precipitate SIADH	Hyponatremia Low serum osmolarity High urinary specific gravity and osmolarity Decreased urinary output	Ensure fluid restriction to below maintenance levels. Monitor intake and output. Monitor specific gravity of each void. Monitor serum sodium. Administer diuretics. Monitor for seizure activity.
Hypercalcemia	Caused by certain malignancies and/or chemotherapy agents	Irregular heart rate Arrhythmias	Monitor blood calcium levels. Delete calcium and phosphorus from intravenous (IV) and total parenteral nutrition fluids. Monitor heart rate and rhythm.
Tumor lysis syndrome	Caused by rapid release of metabolites from the cancer cells during induction of chemotherapy	Hyperuricemia Hyperkalemia Hyperphosphatemia Hypocalcemia Renal failure	Provide IV hydration ($3\ L/m^2/day$) to flush cell by-products through the kidneys. Add $NaHCO_3$ to IV fluids to keep urine alkalotic. Administer allopurinol to reduce uric acid production. Monitor serum chemistries. Monitor intake and output. Provide dialysis if renal failure occurs.

tures. Superior vena cava syndrome occurs when the tumor mass (usually a lymphoma) compresses the vena cava. Spinal cord compression can be a result of a tumor mass on or near the spinal cord. Alterations in fluid and electrolyte status can occur as a result of the malignancy or secondary to chemotherapy. Syndrome of inappropriate antidiuretic hormone secretion (SIADH) and hypercalcemia are two of the most critical conditions that can occur. Tumor lysis syndrome is caused by a rapid release of metabolites from the breakdown of cancer cells during the initial induction of chemotherapy. This syndrome is most often associated with acute leukemias and lymphomas. The accumulation of these metabolites can cause severe renal impairment. Critical ongoing nursing assessment and immediate expert medical attention are required to treat and minimize deleterious outcomes of these emergencies.

Prevention and Management of Nausea and Vomiting

Nausea and vomiting may be mild to severe, depending on the chemotherapeutic drug being administered and the tolerance of the child receiving the drugs. The key to optimal prevention and control of chemotherapy-induced nausea and vomiting is the timing of the antiemetic that is given (Chart 22–12).

caREminder: *It is vital that antiemetic therapy be given orally or intravenously before the start of chemotherapy and that it be continued on a regularly scheduled basis. This treatment plan provides the maximal effect to minimize nausea and vomiting.*

Ondansetron (Zofran) is a common antiemetic drug that is administered to children receiving chemotherapy. Metoclopramide (Reglan), diphenhydramine (Benadryl), lorazepam (Ativan), promethazine (Phenergan), dexamethasone (Decadron), and granisetron (Kytril) are some other agents used to prevent and control chemotherapy-induced nausea and vomiting. A combination of drugs and modifications of timing are useful in individualizing a child's antiemetic regimen.

Nonpharmacologic measures can be used to control nausea and vomiting. Distraction, relaxation, and guided imagery are methods the nurse can use to help the child. Manipulation of the environment to remove sights, sounds, and smells that may contribute to the child's feelings of nausea may also be helpful. The child who is unable to tolerate minimal, if any, oral intake may require supplemental IV fluid to ensure adequate hydration. The child should be offered clear fluids or bland foods as tolerated. Salty dry foods such as soda crackers and toast can be offered. Carbonated beverages that are drunk through a straw to ensure slow uptake may be acceptable to the child. The child may have specific food preferences as he or she begins to feel less nauseous. Every effort should be made to provide food and fluid for the child that is palatable to the child and that provides optimal nutrition (Veninga, 1985).

The child experiencing vomiting must have accurate records maintained of his or her intake and output. Emesis should be measured and tested for the presence of blood using guaiac measures. A guaiac-positive result can result from irritation of the GI tract from vomiting. These results should be discussed with the physician, because a more effective antiemetic regimen may be needed.

The child and parents should be prepared to handle post-treatment nausea and vomiting that may occur at home. TIP 22–3 summarizes the content to cover in discussions with the family about home management of nausea and vomiting.

Chart 22–12
Nursing Interventions

Minimizing and Managing Nausea and Vomiting

- Encourage fluids and small, frequent meals as tolerated. The child should avoid spicy or strong, odorous food.
- Assist the child in using relaxation techniques such as guided imagery and distraction (videos, video games, games, reading) to focus thoughts away from physical discomforts.
- Control environmental sights, smells, and sounds that may heighten feelings of nausea.
- Administer antiemetic agents 30 minutes before initiating chemotherapy, and on a regularly scheduled basis for up to 24 hours after the chemotherapy ends.
- As needed, provide antiemetics to be administered at home the night before and again on the morning of a clinic visit.
- Keep accurate records of intake and output.
- Test all emesis for blood.
- Give intravenous fluids as ordered to maintain hydration.

Nutritional Support

Many factors contribute to appetite suppression and decreased food intake in the child undergoing cancer treatment. Anorexia and weight loss may result from anorexia-inducing substances secreted by the tumor cells, pain, nausea, vomiting, stomatitis, metabolic disturbances, and alterations in taste. A child may experience increased appetite, fluid retention, and weight gain with the use of steroids. Nutritional problems may also be psychosocially related. The child may feel apathetic, depressed, or fearful and not wish to eat. These children may use eating or drinking as a way to manipulate parental behavior and responses to them and to feel some control over the events occurring to them (Hanigan & Walter, 1992; Veninga, 1985).

Maintenance of the child's nutritional status is im-

TIP 22–3 An Interdisciplinary Teaching Plan for Gastrointestinal Complications

Nursing Diagnoses and Outcomes

- High risk for fluid volume deficit related to nausea, vomiting, oral mucositis
  Outcome: Child is able or assisted to maintain adequate fluid intake by mouth or by nasogastric or intravenous access.
- Altered nutrition: less than body requirements related to disease process and medication-induced vomiting, anorexia, changed taste sensations, depression, or changes in intestinal epithelium.
  Outcomes:
  Child is able to eat frequent, small, nutritious meals.
  Child's caloric intake is adequate for age.
  Child is able to maintain weight that is normal for age.
- Altered oral mucous membrane related to effects of mucositis
  Outcome: Child will demonstrate measures to preserve and restore mucosal integrity.
- Constipation related to effects of chemotherapeutic agents
  Outcome: Child and family use measures to prevent or minimize constipation.
- Diarrhea related to effects of chemotherapeutic agents
  Outcome: Child and family use measures to prevent or minimize diarrhea.

Interventions

Management of Nausea and Vomiting

- Implement diet measures such as eating small, frequent, bland meals, avoiding noxious smells, eating food high in protein, providing plenty of fluids.
- Administer antiemetic as ordered.
- Recognize side effects of antiemetic.
- Recognize signs and symptoms of dehydration.
- Stress importance of oral hygiene.

Management of Stomatitis

- Encourage intake of soft, bland, cool foods when ulcerations are present.
- Stress importance of meticulous oral hygiene.
- Recognize signs and symptoms of dehydration.
- Recognize signs and symptoms of fungal infection.
- Use comfort measures such as topical rinses, toothettes to clean teeth, ice chips.
- Avoid irritants such as spicy foods and alcohol-based rinses.

Management of Constipation

- Maintain toileting routines.
- Increase fiber and fluids in diet.
- Avoid rectal manipulation and medications.
- Promote physical activity.

Management of Diarrhea

- Recognize signs and symptoms of diarrhea.
- Maintain accurate records of stool patterns.
- Recognize signs and symptoms of fecal impaction.
- Institute meticulous perianal hygiene and strict hand washing.

Adapted from Aitken, T. (1992). Gastrointestinal manifestations in the child with cancer. *Journal of Pediatric Oncology Nursing, 9*(3), 99–109. Used with permission.

portant because it allows the body to better tolerate the cancer treatment. A child who is malnourished generally does not handle the treatment regimen well and tends to have more complications than the child who receives aggressive nutritional support.

Nutritional assessment should include daily weighing, intake and output records, calorie count, and laboratory values of such elements as sodium, potassium, albumin, calcium, magnesium, glucose, and protein. The nurse should also assess the child for factors that may be contributing to the anorexia such as pain, nausea, diarrhea, or stomatitis.

It is necessary to prevent, alleviate, or minimize the side effects associated with the treatment regimen before the child's nutritional status can be improved. It is always preferable to use the oral route for supplemental nutrition.

Tip: *Supplemental nutrition given orally can be achieved by providing small, frequent meals, high-protein shakes, and nutritional supplements such as Ensure or Sustacal, and by allowing the child to eat whatever he or she desires and can tolerate.*

If increasing oral intake is not possible, the enteral route (tube feedings) is the second choice in children whose GI tract is intact and can tolerate it. Nasogastric or nasojejunal tubes are used on a short-term basis and gastrostomy tubes should be considered if prolonged support is required. Parenteral nutrition is indicated if the child cannot tolerate the oral or enteral route.

The dietitian can be an excellent resource to work with the child and the family in selecting the child's diet plan based on the child's health problems. For the child experiencing weight gain related to steroid therapy, a plan must be implemented to meet the child's nutritional needs and to prevent fluid retention. Foods low in sodium and adherence to a no-added-salt diet are recommended. The child may be experiencing an increase in appetite; thus, meals and snacks should be offered that are satisfying, but not overly high in calories. If rapid weight loss is a problem, then foods high in protein and carbohydrates are recommended.

Oral Hygiene Care

The oral cavity is a common site of stomatitis, mucositis, infections, or bleeding. The terms stomatitis and mucositis are often used interchangeably. Some clinicians distinguish between the two by clarifying that stomatitis can be any oral mucosal reaction to local factors (e.g., infection, injury, poor oral care). Mucositis refers to the mucosal reaction that can occur throughout the GI system as a side effect of systemic chemotherapeutic agent administration (Gross & Johnson, 1994).

The rapidly dividing mucosal epithelial cells lining the oral cavity and the GI tract are easily damaged by chemotherapeutic agents, with mucosal changes appearing within 2 to 3 days after chemotherapy administration. Changes in the oral mucosa can also be a result of anorexia, radiation to the oral cavity, and poor oral care. Radiation to the oral cavity causes decreased saliva production. Saliva is needed to provide a natural defense against tooth decay. Poor nutritional status and dental care can indirectly affect the oral cavity and the integrity of the mucous membranes (Fig. 22–5). In addition, children who are neutropenic are more at risk for development of oral infections such as with *Candida*, herpes simplex, herpes zoster, gram-negative organisms (*Pseudomonas*), and gram-positive organisms (*Streptococcus*) (Aitken, 1992).

A baseline assessment of the child's oral cavity should include evaluation of the integrity and color of the lips, tongue, gingivae, and mucous membranes. The child's ability to salivate, swallow, and eat should be determined. Dental examinations should be performed as a baseline before beginning therapy and on a routine basis to assess and treat any dental problems. Oral assessments should be performed on a daily basis during chemotherapy treatments, when radiation to the head or neck regions has been given, or when the child has undergone BMT.

caREminder: *An ulcerated or inflamed oral area can cause emotional distress to the infant and toddler who use sucking on a thumb or pacifier as a form of coping (Aitken, 1992). Diligent assessment of the oral cavity to prevent stomatitis is important.*

Figure 22–5
Ulceration around the lips and in the mouth causes great discomfort and makes it difficult for the child to open the mouth, eat, and swallow.

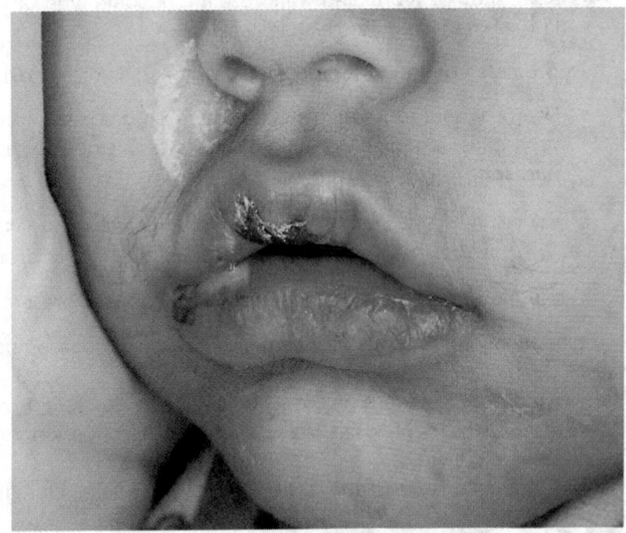

The goals of oral care interventions are to preserve the integrity of the oral cavity, to promote oral comfort, and to rapidly treat any oral problems that occur. Meticulous oral care is taught to the family and must be instituted in the home, school, and hospital settings (see TIP 22–3). Measures to treat the discomfort caused by tender gums or oral lesions can be used to ensure that the child can speak, eat, and swallow (Chart 22–13). If oral infections occur, appropriate medications specific to the organism suspected should be prescribed for the child. Children with severe mucositis may be hospitalized because the effects are likely to involve other parts of the GI tract such as the esophagus, stomach, or intestines. Severe mucositis with excessive secretions may cause localized swelling, which, in turn, can place the child at risk for airway occlusion and aspiration.

Prevention and Management of Constipation

Certain chemotherapeutic agents, particularly vincristine, and certain narcotics cause constipation. In addition, tumor growth, decreased mobility, and altered fluid and nutritional intake can cause the child to have difficulty with elimination. Complications of constipation include the development of hemorrhoids and the aggravation of rectal fissures or perineal abscesses.

The child or parent should be questioned regarding his or her normal pattern of bowel elimination. In the acute care setting, accurate intake and output records should be maintained, noting the number, amount, color, and consistency of the stool (Panzarella & Duncan, 1993). If changes have been noted in the child's elimina-

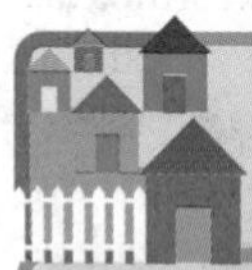

Chart 22–13
Community Care

Oral Hygiene for the Child with Cancer

Oral hygiene should be completed by the child 3 to 4 times a day and as needed whether the child is hospitalized, at home, or participating in activities away from home.

To promote healthy oral mucosa, the child needs to do the following:

- Brush with soft toothettes to prevent bleeding of the gums.
- Use floss when there are no mouth sores or bleeding.
- Rinse and spit with 0.1% chlorhexidine mouthwash (Peridex), saline, or sodium bicarbonate. These solutions should not be swallowed so as to prevent them from killing the normal flora of the gastrointestinal tract.
- Swish and swallow with nystatin, as ordered. Oral intake should be restricted for 30 minutes afterward to promote absorption of the medication into the mucosa.
- Avoid hard foods that can cause abrasions to the gum line.
- Avoid acidic foods that can irritate tender or sore areas in the mouth.
- Maintain a good fluid intake to keep mucous membranes moist.
- Keep the lips lubricated with Vaseline or some type of lip balm to prevent cracking.
- Participate in regular dental checkups.

To promote comfort in the presence of stomatitis or mucositis, the child may:

- Use oral analgesic agents that contain an antacid, diphenhydramine (Benadryl), and a topical anesthetic (Dyclone or viscous lidocaine) for mild discomfort. This agent can be applied directly to sore areas of the mouth or swished and spit.

Alert: *The side effects of viscous lidocaine include a decreased gag reflex, tingling, and seizures. The child must be instructed not to swallow a solution containing this agent.*

When moderate to severe stomatitis or mucositis is present:

- Continue meticulous oral hygiene. Oral rinses can be used to clean the teeth, with a toothette used to remove debris loosened by the rinse.
- Moderate to severe mucositis pain may be controlled with intravenous opioids (e.g., morphine or fentanyl).
- When severe mucositis is present, premedication to manage pain control may be necessary before oral care can be completed.
- If the child is unable to eat or swallow, supplemental intravenous fluids and nutrition must be administered.

tion patterns in the home, parents should be instructed to keep a record of the child's elimination pattern (see TIP 22–3). The stool can be tested for occult blood as an indication of bowel integrity.

Abdominal girth should be evaluated daily in the presence of constipation. In palpating the abdomen, areas of tenderness, swelling, or rigidity should be identified. Inspection of the genitalia and buttocks area is required to note the presence of redness, skin breakdown, hemorrhoids, fissures, or abscesses.

For the constipated child a stool softener such as docusate sodium (Colace) can be administered.

caREminder: *The use of enemas, suppositories, digital manipulation, or rectal thermometers should be avoided so as not to cause trauma to the rectal mucosa.*

A sitz bath or perineal irrigations can be used to treat abscesses or fissures to the perineal and rectal area. Eating a diet that is high in fiber, maintaining an active lifestyle, and maintaining good perineal and rectal hygiene can prevent the onset of complications. Reducing distractions and allowing ample private quiet time for bowel elimination are important (Aitken, 1992).

Tip: *Foods high in fiber that may entice the older child include granola bars, cookies with raisins, popcorn, and apple slices.*

Prevention and Management of Diarrhea

Diarrhea may occur as a side effect of surgery, radiation therapy, or chemotherapy. The use of antibiotics and nutritional supplements can cause diarrhea. Tumor growth, infections, and stress may also cause diarrhea. Prolonged diarrhea can lead to fluid and electrolyte imbalances, dehydration, and perineal discomfort.

Assessment of bowel elimination patterns should follow guidelines presented in the preceding section. The child's weight should be evaluated, noting any significant losses. Signs of dehydration include dry mucous membranes and sunken fontanelle, and poor skin turgor should be noted. Fluid and electrolyte imbalances may be assessed by laboratory analysis of the child's blood. Stool cultures may be obtained to determine the presence of infectious agents.

In the presence of severe dehydration or electrolyte imbalances, IV fluids are administered. Medications may be administered to thicken the child's stool, decrease peristalsis, or treat infection (Panzarella & Duncan, 1993). A bland, low-residue diet or a lactose-free diet may be instituted to curb further elimination problems. Meticulous skin care is needed to the perineal and rectal area to prevent skin irritation and breakdown. Parents should be taught the signs and symptoms of dehydration. Additionally, the importance of good hand washing techniques when handling stools should be emphasized (see TIP 22–3).

Psychosocial Support

Children with cancer and their families are placed in stressful situations throughout the course of the child's illness. Stressors include the diagnosis itself, chemotherapy or radiation treatments, unplanned hospitalizations, added financial demands, unexpected complications, involvement of other family members (or lack of involvement), relapse or progression of the disease, completion of therapy, awareness of other children's deaths, and possibly the impending death and actual death of the child. Peer support groups and assistance from health care workers such as recreational therapists, social workers, and psychologists can assist with stress management and coping strategies (Fig. 22–6).

Establishing open communication and trust with the child and family is key to providing optimal psychosocial support for the child with cancer and the child's family. At the time of diagnosis, family members are often in a state of shock or denial and are unable to accept or comprehend the vast amount of information that is given to them. After the initial family conference, at which time the diagnosis and treatment plan are discussed with the family, it is necessary to review and clarify the information. When the child is hospitalized, daily contact with a consistent oncology team member allows for ongoing guidance, education, and support. It also provides an opportunity for the family to ask questions and to verbalize concerns as well as allows them to be an integral part

Figure 22–6
Summer camps and other planned social activities provide opportunities to build relationships with other children who have cancer. These friendships provide sources of support, understanding, and encouragement. (Courtesy of Camp Ronald McDonald for Good Times.)

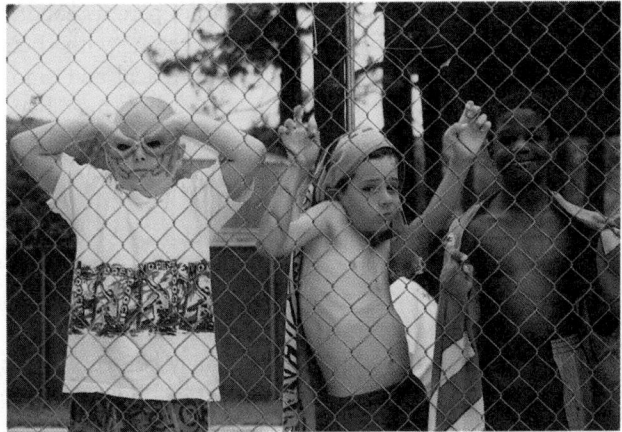

of the daily decision-making about the treatment plan for their child with cancer.

The nurse is the health care worker who has the most direct contact with the child and thus plays a key role in providing psychosocial support. Strategies that the nurse can use include establishing a trusting relationship with the child by communicating honestly and answering questions directly. In addition to providing age-appropriate explanations for daily routines and procedures, the nurse should encourage the child to verbalize fears and concerns regarding his or her disease and treatment.

Tip: *Children age 7 years and older have a right to give their assent to participate in clinical research studies. The nurse caring for these children should assess the child's understanding of the clinical research study and provide adequate time for the child to ask questions regarding his or her treatment. Equally important is the nurse's role as the child's advocate if the child refuses to participate (Thurber, Deatrich, & Grey, 1992).*

Special attention should be given to adolescents because they sometimes experience greater difficulties following their treatment regimen and grappling with the consequences of their disease (Chart 22–14). The social isolation from their peers as a result of hospitalization or home-bound illnesses can make the child feel lonely and depressed. Non-compliance, excessive anxiety, moodiness, depression, and fear of changes in body image are common reactions expressed by adolescents who delay, modify, or stop their treatment (Ellis, 1991; Overbaugh & Sawin, 1992).

Strategies used by health care personnel to help children cope with their chronic condition include therapeutic play, art therapy, music therapy, story telling, guided imagery, relaxation, biofeedback, and social interaction with other children. Chapter 10 provides a detailed discussion of the needs of the child with a chronic illness. This information is applicable to the child with a malignancy who faces several years of therapy and the potential long-term effects of the treatment regimen.

When cancer is diagnosed in a child, parents experience overwhelming stress as a result of coping with their own feelings and needs, and with the physical and emotional needs of the ill child and other family members, especially those of the siblings. Stressors include the following:

- The shock of the diagnosis of cancer
- Role changes necessary to meet the demands of caring for a chronically ill child
- The financial burden caused by medical costs and a possible loss of income because it may be necessary for one parent to stay home with the child
- Fear of losing the child
- Marital discord
- Feelings of guilt related to spending less time with the siblings and with one's spouse
- The need to learn technical and medical information to better understand the child's disease and its treatment

Many of these stressors continue throughout the course of the child's illness and postsurvival period. Although parents know that there will be periods of exacerbations and remissions during the child's illness, additional stress comes from constantly being on the alert for the situation to get worse. Chapter 10 provides an in-depth discussion of the effects of a child's chronic condition on the family and gives practical interventions to assist family members as they cope with these stressors. The nurse is often the health care team member who initially provides psychosocial support for the parents as well as facilitating consultations with other health care team members.

Siblings must also adjust to the diagnosis of cancer. The major stressors experienced by siblings include short- or long-term separation from one or both parents, decreased attention from the parents even in the presence of the ill child, the need to assume additional household responsibilities, fear of losing their brother or sister, and guilt that their thoughts or wishes may be responsible in some way for causing the cancer. These stressors may become evident through changes in the sibling's behavior both at home and in school. (See Chapter 10 for more information about supporting siblings of the ill child.)

The child and the family members also experience grieving. Grieving may be a result of the actual death of the child. Grieving and disappointments may also occur along various points of the child's treatment regimen. The loss of hair or a limb, the inability to achieve remission using a certain combination of chemotherapeutic agents, and the missed school dances and plays caused by an unexpected hospitalization are a few of the events that can intensify the child's or family's sense of grief. It is important for members of the health care team to be cognizant and sensitive to the issues that may cause great disappointment to a particular child or member of the child's family. Chapter 12 summarizes interventions to help the family deal with losses and progress through the grieving process.

Promoting Growth and Development

Children with cancer face challenges to their physical, social, emotional, and intellectual growth. The treatment regimen and its side effects may inhibit normal physical development. For instance, chemotherapy and steroids can cause delays in pubertal development. Radiation can impair bone growth and growth hormone production.

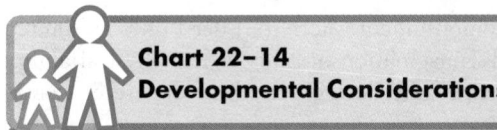

Chart 22–14
Developmental Considerations

Concerns of the Adolescent with Cancer

Concern	Family and Health Care Provider Interventions
Peer acceptance	Use school reentry program to educate peers about child's condition.
Changes in friendships	Assist adolescent to find new supportive relationships. Encourage relationships with other adolescents who have cancer. Encourage participation in activities such as summer camps and rap sessions with other adolescents with cancer. Be a friend.
Physical changes	Help adolescent to maintain normal appearance by using wigs and wearing loose clothing. Stress the temporary nature of many of the side effects of therapy.
Desire to be "normal"	Encourage adolescent to engage in usual activities. Control the amount of information given out about the adolescent's condition.
Desire to be independent and have sense of control	Respect the adolescent's privacy during physical care. Assist the adolescent to learn measures to control anxiety and pain related to procedures or treatment modalities (e.g., biofeedback, self-hypnosis, progressive muscle relaxation, guided imagery). Encourage participation in decision-making regarding care. Do not encourage adolescent to be overly dependent on nurses and family for physical care.
Poor self-esteem	Communicate confidence in the adolescent's ability to succeed. Assist the adolescent to participate in activities in which they will be successful. Plan for the adolescent to return to school as soon as possible after an illness or hospitalization. Assist the adolescent to develop effective mechanisms to cope with stress. Ensure that parents' expectations for the adolescent and how the adolescent sees such expectations are congruent and realistic.
Future life expectations	Encourage the adolescent to make plans for the future. Openly discuss the long-term sequelae of cancer.

Chronic malnutrition, anorexia, and lethargy can affect weight gain and development of muscles.

The child's social, emotional, and intellectual development may be impaired because of frequent hospitalizations and chronic health problems that restrict the child's activities to the home. Absence from school and social activities can impair the child's ability to sustain meaningful relationships with peers. Overprotection by well-meaning parents can prohibit the child from learning self-care and how to make decisions.

Many measures can be used to promote age-appropriate development for the child with cancer. Children of all ages should be allowed to maintain a sense of control by providing them choices in their daily care whenever possible. This can be accomplished by establishing a schedule of daily activities with the child. The schedule incorporates the health care interventions that the child must participate in as well as the child's normal activity schedule (such as attending school). If the child is hospitalized, the schedule should provide opportunities for the child to visit with school friends and enjoy activities with other hospitalized children. If the child is on isolation, visitors can be screened and activities and schoolwork can be brought to the child's room to maintain the child's social and intellectual development.

School reentry may be difficult for the child who is returning after a prolonged absence or who returns with notable changes in his or her appearance. These children may be afraid that other children will make fun of them, try to pull off their wig, or gossip about them. Classmates may be afraid that they will "catch" cancer, or they may wonder whether the child is going to die. Chart 22–15 summarizes interventions that can be used to help children rejoin their classmates. These interventions focus on easing the transition to the classroom through peer programs and by providing medical information to key school officials.

Children returning to the classroom should be encouraged to participate in sports and in musical and artistic activities that they enjoy and in which they find a sense of accomplishment. Activities need only be limited by the child's imagination and his or her physical ability to perform, especially during periods of disease exacerbation.

Home Care

Given the current demands of managed care as well as the technological advances related to medical and nursing care, there has been a significant increase in the delivery of home care and hospice services for the child with cancer. Professional home care services may be requested by a family when a child becomes terminal. Hospice care provides psychosocial support and interdisciplinary health care for the dying child and family. Home care and hospice services allow the child to remain with the family in familiar surroundings while continuing to receive interventions that make him or her comfortable and that minimize visits to the hospital (Martinson, 1993).

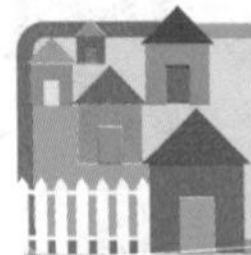

Chart 22–15
Community Care

School Reentry

The child with a malignancy may experience problems that can impact school attendance and performance. These problems include periods of absenteeism, increased school anxiety, negative attitudes by school officials, taunting by peers, social isolation, and illness- or treatment-induced learning difficulties. Reentering the classroom can be emotionally, physically, and mentally difficult for the child, the teacher, and the other students.

To facilitate successful reentry of the child into the classroom, the following measures can be undertaken:

- Contact the school nurse and child's teacher to discuss the child's reentry, providing teachers and school officials with adequate information regarding the child's condition.
- Use federally mandated education planning for students with special needs (Individualized Education Plan, or IEP) to establish educational goals and mechanisms to achieve these goals for the child.
- Provide teachers with books and other resources about cancer.
- Provide teachers with a toll-free number so they can contact a health care provider regarding any questions or concerns they may have about the child with cancer in their classroom.
- Upon agreement by the child, the family, and school officials, a nurse can attend the child's classroom before reentry. Discussion with classmates should include causes of cancer and the physical changes caused by the treatment program. Classmates should be allowed to ask questions, with respect given to the child's privacy at all times.
- Use skits or puppet shows to educate peers and gain their support.
- Film the child with cancer in the hospital setting. Include a tour of the hospital, a view of the child's room and place where procedures are done, and footage of the child. Take the movie to the child's class for viewing before the child's reentry. Use the video as a means to discuss the child's cancer.
- Provide homebound instruction until the child is able to return to school.
- During homebound instruction, encourage the child to remain in contact with peers and teachers through pictures, letters, electronic mail, and visits.
- Refer family to counseling if school phobia or truancy persists as a problem for the child.
- Evaluate on an ongoing basis the existence of any problems related to school performance or relationships with teachers or peers at school.

The scope of pediatric oncology home care ranges from a single intervention such as antibiotic administration to a complex plan of care requiring multiple services. Infusion therapy is a common regimen that can be provided in the home. Total parenteral nutrition, pain medications, chemotherapeutic agents, antimicrobials, and blood products can be delivered to the child in the home setting. Routine home care that may be provided by the family with little or no assistance from a home care nurse include care and maintenance of the VAD, daily oral hygiene, daily skin care, administration of oral medications, administration of medications via subcutaneous or intravenous routes, total parenteral nutrition, pain management, and vigilance for signs and symptoms of infection.

The role of the home care nurse is to conduct ongoing assessments of the family's ability to care for the ill child in the home, assist in the procurement of medical equipment and supplies, provide needed health care interventions, and coordinate the delivery of home care services by other members of the team. Collaboration with the home care pharmacist, primary oncologist, physical and occupational therapist, nutritionist, speech therapist, and respiratory therapist is essential to ensure that all aspects of the child's development are supported. (See Chapter 11 for more detailed information regarding the nurse's role in home care.)

Long-Term Sequelae

At least 60% to 70% of children with cancer become long-term survivors, defined as being disease free for at least 5 years (Morris-Jones & Craft, 1990). Survival rates have increased dramatically over the past 2 decades because of increases in medical and technological care related to surgery, radiation therapy, chemotherapy, immunotherapy, and supportive care. As a result of increased long-term survival, significantly more long-term effects are being observed. Pediatric oncology nurses need to be knowledgeable about the possible long-term effects of cancer treatment. Only then can nurses provide information to the child and family to help them monitor and identify potential late complications. Pediatric nurses have a great responsibility and opportunity to provide this family education and to reinforce the importance of follow-up examinations for both the short and the long term (Rogers, 1992). Additionally, guidance regarding health care decisions and risk-taking behaviors (e.g., smoking, drug use) needs to be provided to the child. The child's treatment history and long-term physiologic effects place the child at higher risk for injury from risk-taking behaviors (Hollen & Hobbie, 1996).

Long-term effects may be caused by direct care or by tissue injury, scar tissue formation, or impaired cell growth as a direct result of single or combination cancer treatments. All cells and organs of the body can suffer some long-term effects. Some of the more common systems or organs likely to suffer from long-term effects are listed in Table 22–8. The nurse should always reinforce that complications are risks that occur as an inevitable aftermath of the cancer "cure."

Long-term psychosocial issues may also occur in childhood survivors. Interruptions in the child's developmental trajectory, alterations in family dynamics, con-

Table 22–8
Long-Term Effects of Cancer Therapy

System/Organ	Long-Term Effect	Associated Cause	Nursing Considerations
Endocrine			
Ovaries/testes	Dysfunction	Procarbazine, Cytoxan, nitrogen mustard, radiation therapy 400–800 cGy	Refer patient to endocrinologist. Refer patient for counseling, sperm banking before treatment, and replacement hormones.
Thyroid, hypothalamus	Hypothyroidism Hypothalamic dysfunction	Radiation >2000 cGy Radiation >2400 cGy	Refer patient to endocrinologist and for replacement hormones. Prepare patient for short stature.

Table continued on following page

Table 22–8
Long-Term Effects of Cancer Therapy *Continued*

System/Organ	Long-Term Effect	Associated Cause	Nursing Considerations
Cardiovascular	Cardiomyopathy Pericardial damage Early coronary athero-sclerosis Ventricular arrhythmias	Anthracyclines, e.g., Adria-mycin Mediastinal radiation	Monitor cumulative lifetime anthracycline dosages. Refer patient to cardiologist. Digoxin, diuretics, sodium restriction, anti-inflammatory drugs may be necessary.
Musculoskeletal	Scoliosis Kyphosis Spinal shortening Facial asymmetry Dental problems	Radiation therapy to abdo-men, vertebrae, spine, long bones, maxilla Surgery to head and neck, bones	Refer patient for rehabilita-tion services. Encourage nutritional bal-ance and maintenance. Prepare patient for short-ened growth of bones. Refer patient to orthopedic surgeon. Advise patient to avoid rough sports. Encourage frequent dental evaluations.
Vision	Cataracts	Cranial radiation Long-time steroid dosage	Refer patient to ophthalmol-ogist. Prepare patient for surgical removal.
Hearing	Hearing loss	Cisplatin Recurrent ear infections Ototoxic antibiotics	Hearing aid may be needed. Refer patient for speech ther-apy consult.
Respiratory	Pulmonary fibrosis	Radiation to lung fields Bleomycin	Encourage smoking pre-vention. Provide immediate care for respiratory infections. Encourage yearly flu vac-cines.
Gastrointestinal	Chronic enteritis Cirrhosis or fibrosis of the liver	Radiation therapy Previous abdominal surgery Some chemotherapy agents	Refer patient for nutrition consults. Dietary modifications may be needed.
Kidney/urinary tract	Chronic nephritis Chronic hemorrhagic cystitis Nephrectomy	Radiation to pelvis Cytoxan Inadequate hydration during therapy	Refer patient to nephrologist. Dialysis may be needed. Ensure adequate hydration. Bladder irrigations and anti-biotics may be needed.
Hematopoietic	Prolonged immunosup-pression	Prolonged or high-dose chemotherapy or radiation	Encourage infection precau-tions. Administer adequate antibi-otic therapy. Give prophylactic anti-biotics. Monitor blood count.

cerns regarding return of the malignancy, defining a new identity, and coping with long-term physical complications are issues that need to be addressed to ease the psychosocial rehabilitation of the survivor (Chesler, 1990; Hockenberry, Coody, & Bennett, 1990; Koocher, 1985). The nurse plays a pivotal role in providing anticipatory guidance for the child and the family to assist them in coping with uncertainty, living with compromised health and possible disabilities, and fear of discrimination due to the disease.

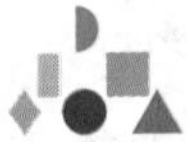

Pediatric Malignancies

Childhood Leukemia

Leukemia is the most common childhood malignancy. Annually, leukemia occurs in 4 in 100,000 children younger than age 15 years (Poplack, 1997). Peak incidence is at age 4 years. Leukemia occurs more frequently in white children and in males (National Cancer Institute, 1996). Approximately 90% of acute lymphocytic leukemia (ALL) cases and more than 80% of acute myelogenous leukemia (AML) cases have been linked to chromosomal disorders (National Cancer Institute, 1996). The survival rate for childhood leukemia has improved dramatically over the past few decades owing to the introduction of new treatment regimens and the ability to better control the harmful side effects of chemotherapy and radiation.

Acute Lymphocytic Leukemia

ALL accounts for approximately 78% of childhood leukemia in the United States. Genetic factors are presumed to play a significant role in the origin of ALL. Some chromosomal abnormalities are associated with the development of childhood leukemia. For example, leukemia is 15 times more likely to develop in children with trisomy 21 (Down syndrome) than in normal children. Leukemia has been reported to develop in children with other autosomal recessive disorders (e.g., Fanconi's anemia). Other less common chromosomal abnormalities as well as familial tendencies (identical twins and siblings) have also been reported to have a higher risk for development of childhood leukemia (Cohen, 1993; National Cancer Institute, 1996; Neglia & Robinson, 1988).

In addition to genetics, environmental factors (e.g., exposure to radiation, toxic chemicals, electromagnetic fields, and chemotherapy), viral infections (e.g., with Epstein-Barr virus or human immunodeficiency virus), and immunodeficiencies or abnormalities of the immune system have been linked as causative factors in children with leukemia (Crist & Pui, 1996; Gibson, Broiss, Graham, et al., 1986; National Cancer Institute, 1996). In summary, the reason for leukemia to develop in any one child in particular is rarely known, but tendencies or similarities that have been documented remain of interest to health care providers.

Pathophysiology

ALL refers to the extreme proliferation of immature lymphocytes. These immature lymphocytes are referred to as blast cells. The French-American-British (FAB) cooperative group has established a classification system for acute leukemia based on the form, structure, and chemistry (morphology) of the blast cells. Lymphoblasts occur in three types: L1, L2, and L3. The cell type most commonly found in ALL is L1, which is seen in 84% of children with ALL (Poplack, 1997).

Immunobiological study of ALL determines which lymphocytes have been transformed into leukemia and identifies the stage of cellular development in which the leukemia occurred. B-lymphocytic leukemia is more prevalent (80% to 85%) than T-lymphocytic leukemia (10% to 15%) (Borowitz, 1990). Abnormalities in chromosomal numbers and structures are also examined to assist in predicting long-term prognosis.

Extramedullary disease (systemic disease outside the blood and bone marrow) is a common feature of ALL. Extramedullary spread may be easily detected by diagnostic procedures and clinical assessment of the child. The pattern or evidence of spread of leukemia is significant in predicting long-term prognosis. The most common sites of extramedullary spread (also called "sanctuary sites") are the CNS, testes, liver, kidneys, and spleen. Extramedullary disease can be present at time of diagnosis or occur later in the disease process. The presence of CNS disease at diagnosis occurs in less than 5% of cases. CNS metastasis is diagnosed by lumbar puncture, which detects circulating lymphoblasts in the cerebrospinal fluid. Testicular disease found at diagnosis is rare; however, relapse of leukemia occurring in the testicles has an incidence of approximately 10%. Leukemia can also infiltrate other organs such as the liver, spleen, lymph nodes, or kidneys. In addition to establishing the extent or spread of the disease at diagnosis, other factors (such as age, sex, and race) aid in predicting long-term disease-free survival.

Prognosis. The initial white blood cell count (WBC) is perhaps the most significant prognostic factor. Children presenting with WBCs greater than 50,000 tend to have a poorer prognosis. WBCs greater than 100,000 have a particularly poor prognosis. Children younger than age 2 years and older than age 10 years at diagnosis have a relatively poor prognosis. The least favorable prognosis

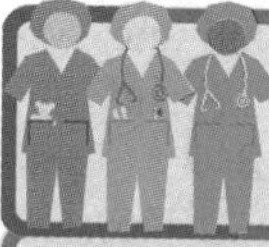

Care Path 22–2 An Interdisciplinary Plan of Care for the Child with Newly Diagnosed Leukemia

Nursing Diagnosis	Patient/Family Intermediate Outcomes		
	Day 1 Admission for R/O Leukemia	Days 2–3 Diagnosis Confirmed	Day 4
Knowledge deficit: hospitalization, diagnostic procedures, diagnosis, and treatment regimen	Child and family are knowledgeable regarding procedures, orientation of unit.	→ Child and family begin establishing trusting and therapeutic relationships for gaining information. Child and family have knowledge of disease process, treatment regimen, side effects, and blood counts.	Child and family verbalize understanding of blood counts. Child and family participate in VAD care.
High risk for infection related to neutropenia	Child and family verbalize concerns and understand risk of infection.	→ Child and family demonstrate infection precautions. Child remains free from infection.	
High risk for injury: bleeding related to thrombocytopenia	Child and family understand risk of bleeding complications.	→ Child and family demonstrate bleeding precautions. Child has no signs of bleeding. White blood cell (WBC) and platelet counts remain within normal limits.	→ → →
High risk for altered nutrition	Child is able to eat frequent, small, nutritious meals. Child's calorie intake is adequate for age. Child is able to maintain normal weight for age.	→ → →	Child and family verbalize measures to maintain good nutritional status and appropriate weight for age.

Day 5	Days 6–8 Inpatient or Outpatient Setting
→ →	Child and family verbalize their understanding of the disease process and treatment regimen. Child and family demonstrate VAD care. Parents demonstrate temperature-taking technique. Child and family verbalize management techniques to deal with side effects of treatment regimen. Family states when to call health care providers.
Child can demonstrate measures to preserve mucosal integrity.	Child and family verbalize measures to reduce risk of infection at home.
→ →	Child and family verbalize measures to prevent bleeding at home. → →
→	→

Care Path continued on following page

is for children younger than age 1 year. In most reports, girls have a better prognosis than boys. Current statistics indicate that three fourths of all children with ALL survive the disease at least 5 years past diagnosis (National Cancer Institute, 1996).

Assessment

Most children diagnosed with leukemia have usually been symptomatic for approximately 2 weeks. Very few children report being "sick" for several weeks or months. Signs and symptoms of childhood leukemia are directly related to the degree of bone marrow infiltration and the spread of the disease. A complete blood count followed by a bone marrow aspiration and biopsy are the first diagnostic procedures completed to confirm the diagnosis of leukemia (Chart 22–16).

Interdisciplinary Interventions

Treatment for children with ALL is governed by the child's symptoms, age, chromosomal abnormalities, and type of disease. Once all factors have been evaluated, a risk category is determined and combination therapy is initiated as indicated. The first goal is to induce a remission with combination chemotherapy. Children with ALL achieve remission 98% of the time with induction therapy. Once remission is attained, children receive further intensive administration of chemotherapy as well as maintenance chemotherapy over a 2- to 3-year period. Chemotherapy and possibly radiation therapy to the

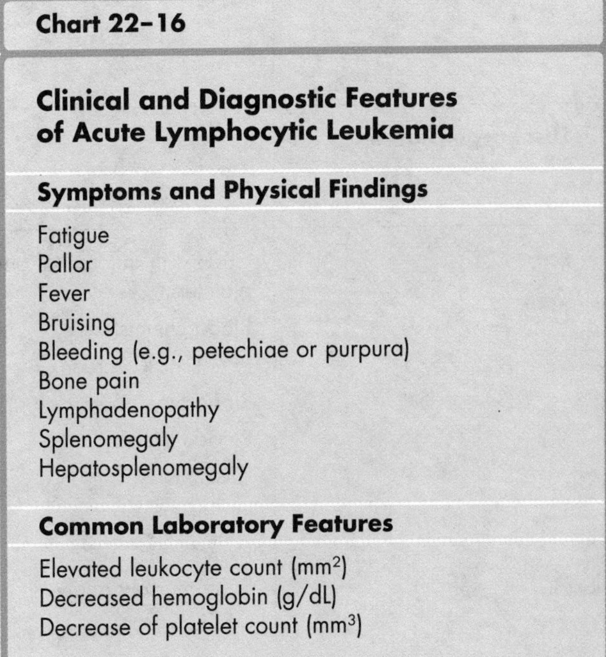

Chart 22–16

Clinical and Diagnostic Features of Acute Lymphocytic Leukemia

Symptoms and Physical Findings

Fatigue
Pallor
Fever
Bruising
Bleeding (e.g., petechiae or purpura)
Bone pain
Lymphadenopathy
Splenomegaly
Hepatosplenomegaly

Common Laboratory Features

Elevated leukocyte count (mm^2)
Decreased hemoglobin (g/dL)
Decrease of platelet count (mm^3)

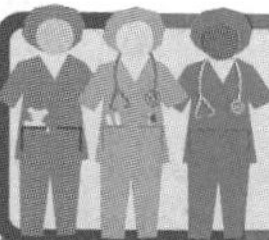

Care Path 22–2 An Interdisciplinary Plan of Care for the Child with Newly Diagnosed Leukemia *Continued*

Nursing Diagnosis	Patient/Family Intermediate Outcomes Day 1 Admission for R/O Leukemia	Days 2–3 Diagnosis Confirmed	Day 4
Pain related to diagnostic procedures	Child experiences minimal discomfort during and after procedures. Child states that adequate pain relief has been obtained.	→ →	Child selects nonpharmacologic pain relief measures to implement during periods of discomfort and pain.
Anxiety related to unfamiliar environment, procedures, and uncertainty of future outcomes.	Child and family verbalize feelings of anxiety.	→ Child and family identify coping mechanisms and use resources to deal with anxiety of diagnosis.	→
Care Intervention Categories			
Consults	Hematology/oncology Social services Clinical nurse specialist	Recreational therapy Pediatric surgery for placement of VAD Chaplain or clergy, as per family request Pharmacy Radiation oncology, if needed Dentist	Nutrition Psychology School teacher
Discharge planning		Notify case manager Interdisciplinary/patient care conference	Order VAD supplies for home
Labs	CBC, with differential and platelets Blood chemistries PT/PTT, DIC screen Blood type and cross Blood cultures CMV titer HIV titer U/A Bone marrow analysis	→ → Lumbar puncture with chemotherapy Quantitative immunoglobulin IgGs Varicella titer Hepatitis screen HLA typing	→ →

Day 5	Days 6–8 Inpatient or Outpatient Setting
⟶	Child uses nonpharmacologic measures to deal with pain and discomfort.
⟶	Parents verbalize measures to support the child during therapy. Child and family verbalize readiness to return home and care for child's health care needs.
	Home health
Interdisciplinary conference	
CBC, with differential	⟶

Care Path continued on following page

CNS may also be used to ensure that no leukemia cells are present in, or return in, the cerebrospinal fluid, because the cerebrospinal fluid is considered a hidden sanctuary for leukemia. Supportive care is ongoing to prevent acute bleeding or infectious complications throughout treatment.

▽ **Alert:** *Acute bleeding can be a potentially life-threatening emergency for children with leukemia. The platelet count should be greater than 20,000 μL at all times, and the child should be transfused with platelets when there is evidence of bleeding or extreme bruising.*

Thorough hand washing, limited visitors and exposure to germs, and prophylactic antibiotics are key components for the care of the child with leukemia.

Children with "ultra" high-risk prognostic factors at diagnosis, children who fail to achieve remission, or children who relapse receive more intensive combination chemotherapy and possibly a BMT. This aggressive approach has proved to be valuable in increasing disease-free long-term survival rates. Supportive care and child observation is more prolonged and intense for this group of children. Care Path 22–2 provides an overview of the interdisciplinary interventions involved in the care of a child with newly diagnosed leukemia.

Acute Myelogenous Leukemia

AML, also called acute non-lymphocytic leukemia (ANLL) or acute myeloid leukemia, represents approximately 15% to 20% of all cases of childhood leukemia. AML is equally distributed among races and sexes. Although much progress has been made in the past decade in treating this disease, the 5-year survival rate for children younger than age 15 is only 29.4% (National Cancer Institute, 1996). The exact cause of AML is unknown; however, certain risk factors are associated with the development of this disease, including radiation exposure in utero, treatment with alkylating agents, maternal cigarette or marijuana use during pregnancy, history of a previous malignancy, trisomy 21, Fanconi's anemia, and environmental exposure to chemicals (especially benzene) and pesticides (National Cancer Institute, 1996; Wiley, 1993).

Pathophysiology

Most cases of AML are believed to result from a malignant transformation of a single blood stem cell. Most often, this transformation occurs on a non-lymphocytic cell line, which is why it is called acute non-lymphocytic leukemia. AML develops in the bone marrow. The malignant clone causes a proliferation of immature, relatively undifferentiated cells that replace healthy bone marrow elements. The immature cells accumulate in the

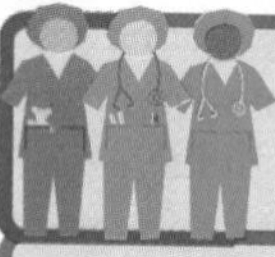

Care Path 22–2 An Interdisciplinary Plan of Care for the Child with Newly Diagnosed Leukemia *Continued*

Care Intervention Categories	Day 1 Admission for R/O Leukemia	Days 2–3 Diagnosis Confirmed	Day 4
Medications and IVs	Maintenance fluids Broad-spectrum antibiotics as indicated Hydration with $NaHCO_3$ if indicated Transfuse packed red blood cells if needed	→ → Chemotherapy regimen begins per road map: vincristine, prednisone, others Stool softener Transfuse platelets as needed Allopurinol if needed	→ Begin supportive care: nystatin, Peridex, Bactrim Hepatitis vaccine #1
Nutrition	NPO 3–4 hr before bone marrow aspiration and biopsy Regular diet as tolerated Identify child's preferences and eating patterns	NPO for operation. Progress from clear liquids to regular diet postoperatively Calorie counts	→
Pain management	Acetaminophen p.r.n. Opioids p.r.n. EMLA for venipuncture and bone marrow aspirate/lumbar puncture	→ →	→ →
Play therapy/school	Activity ad lib Playroom	→ →	Playroom if afebrile Set up program for school
Procedures (diagnostics)	Bone marrow aspirate and biopsy Lumbar puncture Peripheral IV	Echo/ECG if needed	
Radiology	Chest radiograph		
Self-care	Age-appropriate participation in care and daily hygiene	→	→
Social service	Daily visits Insurance verification	Address insurance concerns Attend family conference	
Special considerations	If possible, designate blood donor program		

Day 5	Days 6–8 Inpatient or Outpatient Setting
→ →	→ →
→	→
→ →	→ →
Play therapy for VAD care	
→	→

Care Path continued on following page

marrow and in extramedullary sites, causing bone marrow failure.

The term AML refers to a heterogeneous group of malignancies that have been classified into subtypes according to the morphologic and cytochemical characteristics of the malignant cells. The FAB system is the standard classification used to describe the eight subtypes of AML (Kalwinsky et al., 1990) (Chart 22–17).

Prognosis. Most research supports that children with a high WBC count at diagnosis have a poorer outcome. Children younger than age 2 years have a poor prognosis. Long-term outcome for this disease may be more directly related to the intensity of therapy rather than to the prognostic factors. Approximately 75% of children diagnosed with AML achieve remission (Baehner, Kennedy, Sather, Chard, & Hammond, 1981).

Assessment

Children with AML may present with a few, seemingly benign flu-like symptoms, or they may have severe symptoms that may be life-threatening. Bleeding or severe hemorrhaging, as well as extremely high white blood counts (greater than 100,000), is often seen in these children. Extramedullary spread of disease, particularly in the CNS at diagnosis, may occur in as many as 25% of cases (Holmes et al., 1985). Initially, the same diagnostic procedures and nursing assessment are done as for the child with ALL, including bone marrow aspiration biopsy and a lumbar puncture.

Interdisciplinary Interventions

Initial treatment of AML is targeted at preventing life-threatening complications and achieving remission (see Care Path 22–2). Immediate blood product support, infection prevention, and initiation of combination chemo-

Chart 22–17

French-American-British (FAB) Subtypes of Myeloid Leukemia

Acute myeloblastic leukemia without differentiation:	M0 and M1
Acute myeloblastic leukemia with differentiation:	M2
Acute promyelocytic leukemia:	M3
Acute myelomonocytic leukemia:	M4
Acute monocytic leukemia:	M5
Erythroleukemia:	M6
Acute megakaryoblastic leukemia:	M7

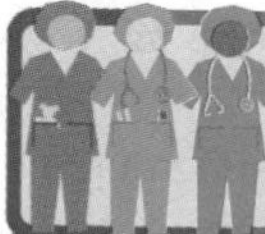

Care Path 22–2 An Interdisciplinary Plan of Care for the Child with Newly Diagnosed Leukemia *Continued*

Care Intervention Categories	Day 1 Admission for R/O Leukemia	Days 2–3 Diagnosis Confirmed	Day 4
Surgical procedures		To OR, VAD placement	
Teaching	Provide information related to diagnostic procedures Explain transfusion and blood counts Orient to hospital routine and environment	Provide information related to diagnosis results and treatment plan Discuss VAD options Infection precautions VAD care Managing side effects of treatment regimen	Blood counts Nutrition
Visitors	Limited for infection prevention	⟶	⟶
Vital signs/baseline parameters	VS q 4 hr and p.r.n. Input and output Daily weights Check all urine for blood and pH	⟶ ⟶ ⟶ ⟶ Assess bone marrow site every shift.	⟶ ⟶ ⟶ ⟶ Assess bone marrow site once per day.

CBC, complete blood count; CMV, cytomegalovirus; DIC, disseminated intravascular coagulation; ECG, electrocardiogram; Echo, echocardiogram; HIV, human immunodeficiency virus; HLA, human leukocyte antigen; NPO, nothing by mouth; OR, operating room; p.r.n., as needed; PT, prothrombin time; PTT, partial thromboplastin time; q, every; R/O, rule out; U/A, urinalysis; VAD, venous access device; VS, vital signs.

therapy drugs to reduce leukemia burden are crucial treatments (Chart 22–18).

Once remission is achieved and complications are no longer life-threatening, treatment of the CNS with more intensive chemotherapy is recommended. BMT may be indicated. Five-year survival rates have been as high as 50% to 70% with the use of BMT (Sanders et al., 1985). Children are often hospitalized for extended periods of time to undergo aggressive treatment and for treatment of subsequent infections that require vigilant supportive care (Fig. 22–7).

Chronic Myelocytic Leukemia

Chronic myelocytic leukemia (CML) is a proliferation of mature myelocytic cells in which mutation can begin years before the onset of symptoms. This disease appears to have more chronic activity and clinically may present at different phases. A hallmark chromosomal abnormality is the translocation of chromosome 9;22, identified as the Philadelphia chromosome (Castro-Malespina et al., 1983; Wiley, 1993). CML presents as a hyperproduction of myeloid cells up to 100-fold times normal.

Little is known about the cause of CML. It is a rare disease in children, accounting for 1% to 3% of all cases of childhood leukemia (Altman, 1993; National Cancer Institute, 1996). There are no significant differences in incidence among race or sexes. Ionizing radiation exposure may be the only environmental risk factor associated with this disease (Altman, 1993).

Prognosis. The extreme elevation of the WBC as well as the degree of organ and lymph node involvement

Day 5	Days 6–8 Inpatient or Outpatient Setting
Oral care	Temperature taking Measures to reduce risk of infection and prevent bleeding When to call health care provider
→	→
→ → → →	→ → → →

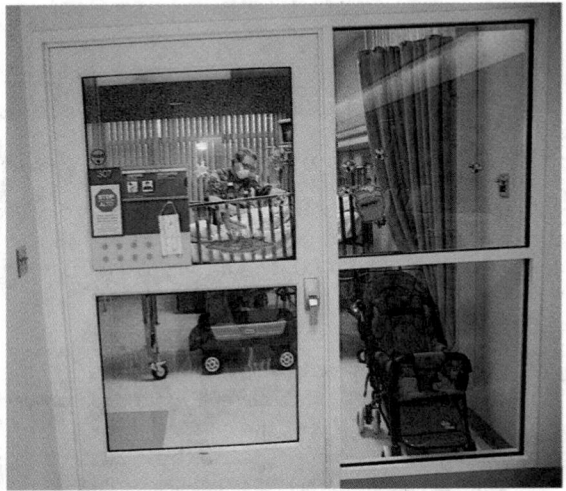

Figure 22–7
For the child who undergoes bone marrow transplantation, the isolation room becomes home for 100 or more days.

reflects a poor prognosis. The phase of the disease at the time of clinical presentation also determines the outlook. Currently, the only curative treatment is allogenic bone marrow transplantation. Among children with CML, the long-term survival rate varies between 50% and 80%, depending on the ability to receive an allograft from an HLA-identical sibling, and the phase of the illness. Children in the early, chronic phase are likely to have a higher survival rate (Heslop, 1996).

Assessment

Children with CML may present in the chronic phase or the blast phase of the disease. In many cases, the onset of the disease is slow and not easily detected. The diagnosis may be made when a blood count is performed for another reason. In the chronic phase, children may present with non-specific symptoms of pallor, low-grade fever, weight loss, anorexia, and night sweats. The chronic phase can last up to 3 to 4 years before progression to a myeloid or lymphoid blast crisis is noted. In this case, the blast phase symptoms appear more like acute leukemia, with the presence of splenomegaly, bone marrow depression, and lymphadenopathy (Heslop, 1996).

Interdisciplinary Interventions

The initial goal of therapy is to achieve remission of the disease in the child. Chemotherapy and biotherapy (interferon) are used during the induction treatment. The chance of achieving remission is 80% to 85%, with as many as 5% to 10% of children dying during the induction phase because of infection (Britfeld, 1996).

Once remission is achieved, an allogeneic BMT is recommended if an HLA-identical sibling is identified. GVHD is a common complication in the child who has had a transplant. If no donor is available, the child continues to receive intensive chemotherapy treatments with an expected cure rate of 40% to 50%. For those children who experience a relapse, the remission rate is only about 50% (Britfeld, 1996). Thus, the best chance of survival for a child with CML lies in receiving the allogeneic BMT.

Central Nervous System Tumors

Tumors of the CNS are the second most common malignancy in childhood. The annual age-adjusted incidence in children younger than age 15 years is 3.4 per 100,000. In the United States, approximately 1000 to 1500 newly

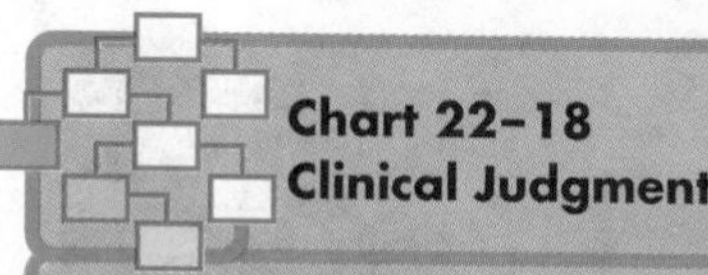

Chart 22–18
Clinical Judgment

The Immunosuppressed Child with Fever

Jasmine is a 4-year-old girl with the diagnosis of leukemia. She completed her most recent course of chemotherapy 7 days ago. She is now being admitted to the hospital with a fever of 101.8°F, chills, white blood cell count of 0.7, platelet count of 59,000, and hemoglobin of 8.8.

Questions

1. What additional assessment data should be obtained at this time by members of the health care team?
2. The father states that Jasmine has not been around any sick people. He is confused as to how she could have gotten ill. What should the nurse tell him?
3. The physician orders include blood cultures, a chest x-ray film, urine and throat cultures, intravenous fluids, and administration of antibiotics. Which of these orders should be completed first?
4. What precautions should be taken to protect the child who is neutropenic?
5. Jasmine's 6-year-old brother is standing outside the room crying. He says, "It is all my fault she is sick, I spit on her." What should he be told about his sister's current situation?

Answers

1. Vital signs, type of chemotherapy last received, presence of mouth sores, redness or irritation at the venous access device site, intake and output history, absolute neutrophil count, and O_2 saturation measured using a pulse oximeter.
2. Most infections are from commonly occurring bacteria in the child's system and are harmful to Jasmine only because of her depressed immune system.
3. Cultures of the blood, urine, and throat should be taken before starting antibiotics. As soon as these tests are completed, the intravenous fluids should be started and antibiotics given immediately. Vital signs should be carefully monitored. Chest x-ray film can be obtained once antibiotic therapy has been initiated.
4. Good hand washing by all who come in contact with Jasmine. Protective precautions. Placement in a single room. No rectal temperature measurements.
5. Reassure the boy that his spitting did not cause his sister to be sick. Encourage him to go in the room and be with his sister. Instruct him on good hand washing techniques to help protect his sister from getting sicker and explain how he can do this at home to help her not get an infection.

diagnosed pediatric cases occur each year (National Cancer Institute, 1996). Brain tumors, although rare in the first year of life, tend to occur more frequently in children younger than age 10 years. Incidence is roughly equal in males and females. Approximately 62% of all children with CNS tumors demonstrate a 5-year survival rate (National Cancer Institute, 1996).

Of all pediatric CNS tumors, astrocytomas are the most common (approximately 50% of cases), followed by medulloblastomas (25%), brain stem gliomas (10%), ependymomas (9%), and others (9%) (Finlay, Goins, Uteg, & Giese, 1987; Petriccione, 1993). There are important differences between the types and locations of tumors in children and adults. Gliomas account for 75% of intracranial tumors in children compared with 45% in adults. In children, 50% to 60% of brain tumors are infratentorial (located in the cerebellum, fourth ventricle, or brain stem), whereas in adults they are primarily supratentorial (located in the cerebrum). Also, 75% or more of brain tumors in children occur in the midline (third and fourth ventricles, optic chiasm, and brain stem). The high incidence of medulloblastomas and astrocytomas in children accounts for many of these differences (Chutorian, 1987). Brain tumor is a general term for many histologic categories. Each type has distinctly different clinical manifestations, treatment modalities, and outcomes.

Pathophysiology

The cause of CNS tumors remains unknown. There appears to be a strong link between hereditary and environmental factors and the occurrence of certain brain tumors. Direct correlations exist between certain hereditary and familial syndromes (e.g., neurofibromatosis, tuberous sclerosis, von Hippel-Lindau disease, retinoblastoma) and CNS tumors (Cohen & Duffner, 1984; National Cancer Institute, 1996). Children with neurofibromatosis have a significantly increased risk of CNS tumor development (Baptiste et al., 1989; Petriccione, 1993). There have been several reports of families with development of CNS tumors in more than one child.

Environmental factors related to the incidence of CNS tumors include industrial and chemical toxins, ionizing radiation, and exogenous immunosuppression as is seen in transplant recipients. Studies have investigated prenatal and perinatal exposures to these risk factors that may correlate with the increased incidence of brain tumors in children. Association has been made between the incidence of brain tumors and certain parental occupations, particularly those in which there was exposure to electromagnetic fields or ionizing radiation (Giuffre, Liccardo, Pastrol, Spallone, & Vagnozzi, 1990; National Cancer Institute, 1996).

Various types of ionizing radiation exposures have been associated with the occurrence of CNS tumors in children. These include exposure to x-rays, radioisotopic contrast media, ultraviolet radiation, and nuclear bomb fallout. Several reports document the development of a second primary brain tumor after receiving cranial irradiation for a prior malignancy such as ALL (National Cancer Institute, 1996; Shapiro, Mealey, & Sartorius, 1989).

CNS tumors are frequently described as low grade or high grade. Low-grade tumors are slow growing, contain a few mitotic cells, and show no evidence of necrosis or vascular proliferation. Their progress may go undetected for some time, causing major damage to adjacent tissue. High-grade tumors are faster growing, contain multiple mitotic cells on histologic analysis, and show evidence of necrosis and endothelial and vascular proliferation (McGuire, 1990).

Assessment

The clinical presentation of a child with a CNS tumor depends on the size and location of the tumor and the child's age and developmental stage. Most brain tumors in children arise in the posterior fossa and result in initial symptoms associated with increased intracranial pressure (ICP) and hydrocephalus caused by a compression of the fourth ventricle (Chart 22–19). The most common complaint in children older than age 2 years associated with increased ICP is headache. Characteristically, the headache is worse in the morning and is relieved by vomiting or gradually lessens during the day. Activities such as straining with a bowel movement, coughing, or, in severe cases, changing the position of the head cause the headache to worsen. However, the occurrence of a headache does not always fit the "classic" picture of a headache associated with increased ICP. The head pain may be more vague and non-specific.

Chart 22–19

Clinical Manifestations of Increased Intracranial Pressure and Focal Neurologic Signs

Increased Intracranial Pressure

Headache in the morning that decreases with vomiting or lessens throughout day
Cranial enlargement secondary to hydrocephalus
Vomiting
Diplopia
Papilledema
Lethargy and somnolence (late signs)

Increased ICP in a Child Younger Than 3 Years

Marked irritability
Disrupted sleep patterns
Resistance to being held or comforted
Decreased appetite
Developmental delays or loss of acquired milestones
Increased head circumference
Delayed closure of anterior fontanelle (usually between 8 and 18 months of age)
Bulging fontanelle

Focal Neurologic Signs

Nystagmus
Impaired vision
Cranial neuropathy
Head tilt
Personality changes
Ataxia
Focal pyramidal deficits (subtle changes in handedness, posture, and dexterity)
Seizures
Hypothalamic and endocrine dysfunction

Alert: *Any headache associated with vomiting or lethargy should be evaluated immediately by a physician to rule out increased ICP.*

An array of symptoms specific to certain tumor locations (Chart 22–20) assists the health care team in localizing the particular tumor region in the brain. Cerebellar tumors can cause symptoms such as gait ataxia, truncal ataxia, head tilt, hypotonia, abnormal reflexes and speech, and increased ICP. Brain stem tumors present with multiple cranial nerve deficits, a spastic gait, hemiparesis, and a positive Babinski sign. Tumors in the

Chart 22–20

Signs and Symptoms of Brain Tumors

Infratentorial Tumors (Brain Stem and Cerebellar)

Increased intracranial pressure
Ataxia
Nystagmus
Head tilt
Diplopia
Cranial nerve deficits

Supratentorial Tumors

Headaches
Seizures
Hemiparesis
Hyperreflexia
Sensory losses
Visual disturbances
Aphasia
Personality changes
Growth failure

temporal lobe can cause focal seizures, and temporoparietal tumors in the dominant hemisphere may cause aphasia. Lesions in the frontal lobe can produce personality changes, and occipital lesions affect vision. Midline tumors can lead to visual loss or multiple endocrine dysfunctions such as thyroid dysfunction, diabetes insipidus, and precocious puberty.

Diagnostic Tests. Children with suspected CNS tumor require a thorough physical and neurologic examination. CT is one diagnostic tool used for children with CNS tumors. When performed with and without contrast, CT can detect 95% of such lesions. MRI is another important diagnostic tool in the diagnosis and follow-up evaluation of CNS tumors. Because of its ability to image in three planes, MRI is particularly useful in diagnosing infiltrative tumors of the brain stem. The presence of calcification, hemorrhage, or cysts may assist in identifying certain types of tumors (Finlay et al., 1987; Haslam, 1996).

Initial evaluation for a child with a suspected brain tumor can be achieved by either CT or MRI. A CT scan is more appropriate for children in whom sedatives are contraindicated, for example, children with increased ICP, a history of seizures, or changes in neurologic status. The MRI is the scan of choice for a medically stable and cooperative child because of its safety and its ability to collect detailed information. Conscious sedation may be used to keep the infant or younger child quiet and calm during the procedure. Positron emission tomography (PET), where available, is also used to image the tumor and assess its level of activity (McGuire, 1990).

A lumbar puncture is usually performed to obtain cerebrospinal fluid for analysis when there are no signs of obstructive hydrocephalus or increased intracranial pressure (Fig. 22–8). The fluid is tested for the presence of tumor cells as well as for cytologic study, decreased sugar, increased protein, and increased enzymes.

Nursing Diagnoses and Outcomes

General nursing diagnoses and desired outcomes are presented in Chart 22–3. In addition, the following diagnosis may be applicable to the child with a brain tumor:

- **High risk for injury related to seizure activity**
  Outcome: The child will not experience injury during a seizure.

Interdisciplinary Interventions

When possible, complete surgical resection is the treatment of choice for children with brain tumors. The location of the brain tumor is the determining factor as to the surgical approach and resectability of the mass and surrounding brain tissue. In some instances, a resection is too risky and a biopsy is done for histologic confirmation.

The child usually requires monitoring in a pediatric intensive care unit for 48 to 72 hours postoperatively. Frequent assessment of vital signs, neurologic status, and mental status is crucial in identifying early signs of increased ICP secondary to cerebral edema. Intravenous

Figure 22–8
During a lumbar puncture, the nurse holds the child in a side-lying position with the head flexed and the knees drawn upward toward the chest. This position enlarges the spaces between the vertebral spines, thereby improving access to the spinal fluid spaces.

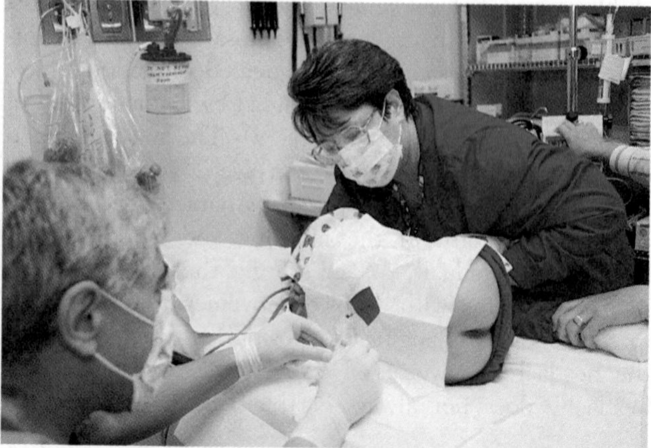

steroids are used intraoperatively to minimize edema of the brain tissue. Anticonvulsants may also be ordered prophylactically to prevent seizures. Children who have hypothalamic, pituitary, or other suprasellar tumors are at high risk for development of SIADH or diabetes insipidus, and should be managed in collaboration with an endocrinologist.

Radiation therapy may be used alone or in combination with surgery. The success of radiation therapy depends on the location and radiosensitivity of the tumor and on the expertise of the radiation oncologist. Young children are at high risk for the development of significant sequelae associated with the radiation of immature brains (learning disorders, varying degrees of retardation). Thus, radiotherapy is not recommended in children younger than age 3 years.

The nurse plays a key role in the education of the child and family and in the management of side effects related to radiotherapy, such as nausea, hair loss, and anorexia. It is extremely important that the child lie still during the entire radiotherapy session. Precision is required to maximize the dose of irradiation to the tumor and to minimize the effects in surrounding tissue. Very young children require sedation or general anesthesia for each therapy session. Special devices such as soft blocks, Styrofoam molds, tape, and Velcro straps may also be used to immobilize the head and neck (Fig. 22–9). The nurse is responsible for preparing the child for sedation and for monitoring the child's status during sedation and during the recovery period. (See Chapter 13 for an in-depth discussion of sedatives and nursing responsibilities associated with conscious sedation.)

The efficacy of chemotherapy in the treatment of brain tumors requires further investigation. Many studies have demonstrated either regression of symptoms or tumor regression with the use of several chemotherapeutic agents that are capable of penetrating the blood–brain barrier. Care of children undergoing treatment for a brain tumor with either one or a combination of the modalities discussed requires collaboration among many disciplines. The interdisciplinary team includes an oncologist, neurosurgeon, endocrinologist, radiation oncologist, nurse, occupational therapist, physical therapist, speech therapist, psychiatrist, social worker, and child life specialist. When an interdisciplinary team is composed of so many members, it may be difficult to coordinate care and communicate effectively with the family. It is usually the role of the primary nurse to act as a liaison with all disciplines and to discuss the treatment plan with the child and the family. Table 22–9 summarizes the treatment modalities used for each type of tumor.

Figure 22–9
During radiation treatment, the child is immobilized and instructed to lie still. The position may be uncomfortable and frightening. Parents are encouraged to have the child practice at home by lying still for a short, timed period on a hard surface such as a table.

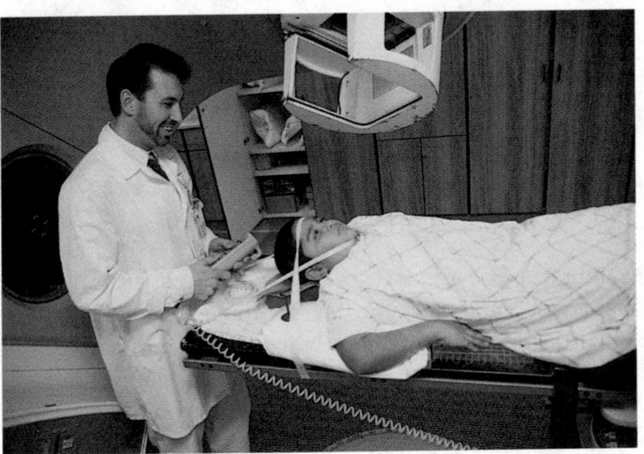

Cerebellar Astrocytoma

Astrocytomas, including cerebellar, cerebral, and brain stem sites, constitute the largest category of CNS tumors occurring in childhood. Cerebellar astrocytomas represent 13% of all pediatric brain tumors. They occur most commonly during the first decade of life, with a peak incidence at age 5 to 8 years.

The two types of cerebellar astrocytomas are graded based on degree of malignancy. The classic, or pilocytic, astrocytoma accounts for 80% to 85% of these tumors. Children with this type of tumor have a projected long-term survival rate (more than 25 years) of 94%. The second type of tumor, fibrillary astrocytoma, accounts for 15% of these tumors. These tumors are diffuse and thus carry a much lower long-term survival rate of 38% (Gjerris & Klinken, 1978; Petriccione, 1993).

Assessment

The course of symptoms in children with an astrocytoma is insidious in onset and slow in progression. Most affected children are symptomatic for 2 to 7 months before diagnosis—some for as long as several years. Ninety percent of children with these tumors present with symptoms associated with increased ICP. They also have focal neurologic signs such as ataxia, nystagmus, and head tilt. Decreased muscle tone, abnormal reflexes, and speech that is characterized by pauses between syllables (scanning speech) may also be present.

Interdisciplinary Interventions

With advanced neurosurgical techniques, as many as 90% of all children with astrocytomas have total resections. Complete surgical resection is clearly associated with an improved long-term and disease-free survival. If the resec-

Table 22-9
Treatment Modalities for Central Nervous System Tumors

Tumor	Surgery	Radiation	Chemotherapy
Cerebellar astrocytoma	Complete resection is clearly associated with long-term, disease-free survival.	Not necessary unless there is evidence of residual tumor	Not useful
Cerebral astrocytoma	Complete surgical resection is very difficult.	Dependent on extent of tumor resection	Uncertain role in initial therapy. Patients with recurrent disease are generally treated with the same chemotherapy regimens as are used for high-grade tumors.
Medulloblastoma	Complete resection is goal of surgery and is associated with improved outcomes.	One of the most radiosensitive CNS tumors in childhood. Irradiation of the entire craniospinal axis is standard therapy for all patients.	One of the most chemosensitive of all CNS tumors. Chemotherapy is used in patients with poor prognosis.
Brain stem glioma	Vast majority are not resectable because of the location in the vital area of the brain. Surgery is generally considered an unacceptably high risk.	Only routinely used treatment modality. Almost all patients show a significant response to radiation after 3–6 wk. Response may include improvement in CNS palsies, pyramidal signs, and ataxia.	—
Ependymoma	Complete resection when possible, followed by radiation. Total and near-total resections are more commonly achieved in supratentorial lesions. Such resections are more difficult in the post-fossa where infiltration of the brain stem is common and operative morbidity is higher.	Post-fossa lesions receive craniospinal (neuraxis) irradiation. Supratentorial lesions receive focal irradiation.	Not used initially. Used in recurrent disease.
Optic nerve glioma	Surgical intervention is done for cosmetic reasons, intractible pain, jeopardy to the integrity of the globe or the cornea, severe proptosis.	May be initial choice for patients with isolated optic nerve tumors.	Chemotherapy is an alternative to radiation in the treatment of progressive disease.

tion is complete, no further treatment is necessary. If complete resection is not achieved, the tumor is observed and a second surgery may be performed if there is recurrence. Radiation therapy may be used in cases of residual tumor. Chemotherapy is reserved for recurrent or progressive tumor growth or as adjunct therapy for children with high-grade astrocytomas.

Cerebral Astrocytoma

Cerebral astrocytomas can be low or high grade (highly malignant) and account for approximately 22% of all pediatric brain tumors. Cerebral astrocytomas are located in the cerebrum and are infiltrative in nature. Several favorable prognostic indicators include young age, minimal neurologic deficits following surgery, low grade, and slow onset of symptoms. Cerebral astrocytomas tend to have a poorer prognosis than cerebellar astrocytomas because of their infiltrative nature. Five-year survival rates for low-grade tumors range from 58% to 88%, and from 0% to 40% for high-grade tumors.

Assessment

The initial symptoms vary with the specific location of the tumor within the cerebrum. Symptoms are progressive and increase over months, and, in some cases, years. Non-specific and non-localizing signs of increased ICP occur in 75% of children regardless of tumor location. Papilledema (edema of the optic nerve) is commonly present at diagnosis. Seizures, which occur in 25% of children, are usually grand mal type. More specific clinical manifestations are related to the location of the tumor within the cerebrum (see Chart 22–20).

Interdisciplinary Interventions

Complete surgical resection is extremely difficult if the tumor has infiltrated other areas of the brain, especially the brain stem. The location of the tumor dictates the extent of surgical resection possible. For example, motor and speech areas are not readily amenable to surgical intervention, whereas frontal lobe tumors can be resected more easily. Complete resection is the best indicator for long-term survival. Anticonvulsant therapy is instituted preoperatively due to the high incidence of seizures associated with tumors.

Adjunct therapy may include radiation or chemotherapy. The role of radiation in children with low-grade astrocytomas depends on the degree of tumor resection. The role of chemotherapy is still being investigated in national clinical trials. Early reports demonstrate tumor shrinkage and prolonged stabilization of progressive low-grade astrocytomas with chemotherapy regimens using carboplatin and vincristine. It is not generally used as part of the initial therapy except for young children in whom the risk of radiation therapy is unacceptable. For most children, especially those younger than age 5 years, it is reasonable to consider delaying radiation until evidence of recurrence appears.

Medulloblastoma

A medulloblastoma is a cerebellar tumor composed of medulloblasts. Medulloblasts are undifferentiated cells of the neural tube. Medulloblastomas are usually located in the midline of the cerebellum but may occur in the cerebellar hemispheres. Medulloblastomas are the most common primary posterior fossa tumor in children, constituting approximately 25% of all brain tumors in children younger than age 15 years. Peak incidence occurs at age 3 to 5 years. Incidence in males is double that in females (Chutorian, 1987; Haslam, 1996).

Prognosis. Prognosis is related to tumor size, extent of disease, cerebrospinal fluid findings, extent of resection, histologic make-up, and age at the time of diagnosis. Children younger than age 2 years frequently have a poorer prognosis than older children. Children older than 2 years who undergo surgery and total neuraxis (brain and spine) irradiation have a 5-year survival rate of approximately 50% (Chutorian, 1987; Haslam, 1996).

Assessment

Medulloblastomas are rapidly growing tumors; thus, the child may have a short duration of symptoms before diagnosis. Most affected children are symptomatic for less than 2 months before diagnosis. Symptoms occur as a result of the tumor's location in the posterior fossa. Initial symptoms are those associated with increased ICP. As the tumor enlarges and displaces surrounding brain tissue, more characteristic signs appear such as progressive lower extremity ataxia. Pressure and tumor infiltration at the brain stem may cause diplopia and multiple other cranial nerve deficits.

Interdisciplinary Interventions

Complete resection of the tumor is the ultimate goal of surgical intervention (Care Path 22–3). A CT or MRI should be completed at 72 hours postoperatively to evaluate tumor resection. Once postoperative swelling has diminished, a lumbar puncture for cerebrospinal fluid studies is performed to establish extent of disease. Medulloblastomas are highly radiosensitive tumors. Because of the likelihood of the tumors spreading into the cerebral spinal fluid, radiotherapy is routinely directed to the entire brain and spine. Chemotherapy may also be used in high-risk cases, such as when the child has recurrent disease, and in very young children (younger than age 2–3 years) to delay the use of radiation to the brain (Chart 22–21).

Brain Stem Glioma

Brain stem gliomas occur almost exclusively in children and represent 10% of all CNS tumors. The median age of occurrence is 5 to 9 years. The pons is the most common site (78%) of occurrence, although tumors can also arise in the medulla (14%) or midbrain (8%).

Prognosis. Because of the location of the tumor, the overall prognosis for brain stem tumors remains poor, with no significant improvements in the past several decades. The overall survival rate is 20%, with a median survival time of 15 months. The tumor grade has a signif-

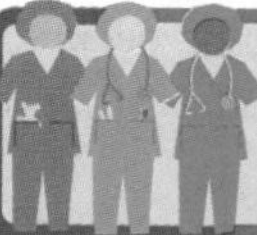

Care Path 22–3 An Interdisciplinary Plan of Care for the Child with Medulloblastoma

Nursing Diagnosis	Patient/Family Intermediate Outcomes			
	Day 1 Admission	**Day 2 Surgery and Biopsy**	**Days 3–4**	**Day 5 to Discharge**
Knowledge deficit: hospitalization, diagnostic procedures, disease process	Child and family are knowledgeable about unit routines, diagnostic procedures.	Child and family verbalize need for PICU admission, ventilator, hemodynamic monitoring, and possible external ventriculostomy.	Child and family observe care of the VAD if placed.	Child and family demonstrate care of the VAD if placed.
Pain related to operative procedure	Child and family verbalize measures to decrease pain postoperatively.	Child is medicated around the clock per physician order with minimal pain behaviors demonstrated.	Child experiences minimal postoperative pain.	Child is free from postoperative pain.
Care Intervention Categories				
Consults	Neurologist Neurosurgeon Social services	Pediatric intensivist Case manager	Occupational therapist/physical therapist Speech therapist Oncologist Clinical nurse specialist Radiation oncologist Dietitian	⟶
Discharge planning			Interdisciplinary patient care conference	
Labs	CBC with differential, electrolytes, platelets, type and crossmatch, LFTs, renal function	In OR: CSF and biopsy specimens obtained	Culture and sensitivity if fever is present (blood, urine, and ventricular fluid)	GFR or creatinine clearance
Medications and IVs	Maintenance IV fluids Anticonvulsant therapy, usually Dilantin (4–8 mg/kg/day) Corticosteroids	⟶ ⟶ ⟶	Plan for steroid taper Antibiotics if needed	Begin to plan chemotherapy regimen (to begin in 1 month).

Care Path 22–3 An Interdisciplinary Plan of Care for the Child with Medulloblastoma *Continued*

Care Intervention Categories	Day 1 Admission	Day 2 Surgery and Biopsy	Days 3–4	Day 5 to Discharge
Monitors	Cardiorespiratory Apnea	⟶ ⟶ ICP monitor	⟶ ⟶ ⟶	Discontinue all monitors as child stabilizes.
Nutrition	As tolerated NPO for surgery	NPO during recovery period Advance diet as tolerated	⟶ Nasogastric tube placed, if needed	⟶ Discontinue nasogastric tube if taking PO well.
Pain management	Acetaminophen p.r.n. for headaches	IV analgesics	Patient-controlled analgesics	PO analgesics
Play therapy/ school			Set up recreational program Bedside activities	⟶ Playroom
Procedures (diagnostics)	EEG MRI/CT scan Lumbar puncture	Brain biopsy or resection Placement of external ventriculostomy	Postoperative CT and MRI to rule out metastasis Placement of VAD if needed Shunt placement Lumbar puncture Bone marrow aspiration to rule out metastasis	Baseline audiogram Baseline ECG
Psychosocial	Crisis intervention	Family conference Spiritual care	Relief periods for parents	
Radiology		Chest radiograph for line placement		Radiation therapy planned
Safety and activity	Bed rest	⟶	Out of bed with assistance	Progressive activity
Social service	Meet with family Needs assessment	Daily visits	⟶ Attend family conference	⟶

Care Path continued on following page

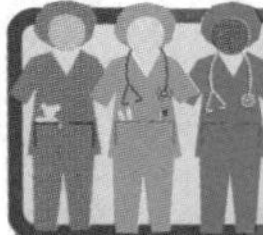

Care Path 22–3 An Interdisciplinary Plan of Care for the Child with Medulloblastoma *Continued*

Care Intervention Categories	Day 1 Admission	Day 2 Surgery and Biopsy	Days 3–4	Day 5 to Discharge
Special considerations		Admit to PICU postoperatively	Transfer to oncology unit	
Teaching	Provide information related to diagnostic procedure Preoperative teaching Orient family to hospital environment and routine	Orient to PICU Explain reason for ventilator, lines, and tubes	VAD care	General oncology home care Chemotherapy regimen Radiation regimen
Visitors		Per PICU policy	Minimize visits	⟶
Vital signs/ baseline parameters	Vital signs and neurologic checks every 2 hr Head circumference every day if child is younger than 2 years old	Vital signs every 1 hr with neurologic checks ⟶	Vital signs routine postoperatively, then every 4 hr ⟶	⟶ ⟶

CBC, complete blood count; CSF, cerebrospinal fluid; CT, computed tomography; ECG, electrocardiogram; EEG, electroencephalogram; GFR, glomerular filtration rate; ICP, intracranial pressure; IV, intravenous; LFT, liver function test; MRI, magnetic resonance imaging; NPO, nothing by mouth; OR, operating room; PICU, pediatric intensive care unit; PO, by mouth; p.r.n., as needed; VAD, venous access device.

icant correlation with the survival rate. Children with low-grade (I–II) tumors have a 2-year survival rate of 55% to 66% versus 0% to 14% for those with high-grade (III–IV) tumors. Tumor location has also been correlated with prognosis. The duration of symptoms before diagnosis and the presence of cranial nerve deficits are also significant prognostic factors. Tumors that are present for a shorter duration (1 to 2 months) and are causing cranial nerve deficits are associated with poorer prognosis.

Assessment

The onset of neurologic symptoms is usually insidious, with a duration of approximately 3 to 5 months. Brain stem gliomas present with one of the most characteristic clinical pictures, a characteristic triad of signs and symptoms arises from early interference with the functioning of the cranial nerve nuclei (cranial nerve deficits, paresis of conjugate gaze), pyramidal tracts (subtle change in gait or handedness, hemiparesis, bilateral reflex changes), and cerebellar pathways (ataxia, horizontal nystagmus).

A single cranial nerve deficit may occur early; later, multiple cranial nerve involvement is more common. As a result of the infiltrative nature of the tumor, "skip lesions" are common, and bilateral involvement of different cranial nerves is seen. Paresis of conjugate gaze (eye movement not in unison), the most important sign for localizing the lesion within the brain stem, occurs in more than 50% of these children.

Signs of pyramidal tract involvement are present in 80% to 90% of these children. The signs may be masked by the more obvious ataxia or may present chiefly as subtle changes in gait, handedness, or posture of an extremity. Hemiparesis and bilateral reflex changes are also present.

Cerebellar pathway signs include ataxia and nystagmus. Both truncal and extremity ataxia are present in most affected children, indicating involvement of cortico-

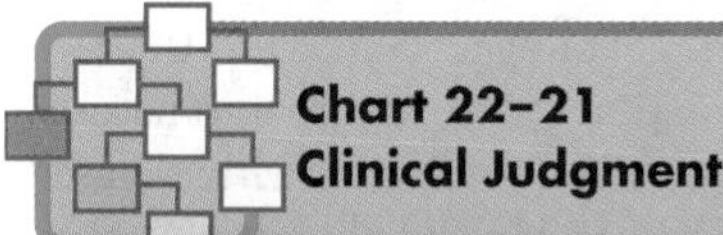

Chart 22–21
Clinical Judgment

Postoperative Care of a Child with a Central Nervous System Tumor

Remus, a 4-year-old boy, was brought to his pediatrician with complaints of irritability, headaches, morning vomiting, and clumsiness. Examination of the child revealed papilledema, photophobia, and ataxia. A computed tomography (CT) scan was performed, revealing a large mass in the fourth ventricle with significant hydrocephalus. The child was begun on steroids overnight and had a craniotomy the next day. The pathologic diagnosis was medulloblastoma. You are caring for the child 3 days after surgery on the pediatric hematology/oncology unit.

Questions

1. What aspects of the physical assessment are of particular importance?
2. Which information might reveal the presence of neurologic compromise?
3. The grandparents come to visit Remus and are overheard to tell the mother that no therapy will do any good and she should just take him home to die. Using your knowledge of medulloblastoma treatment and outcomes, how would you intervene?
4. Considering that this child will need a postoperative CT scan, magnetic resonance image (MRI) of the spine, placement of a venous access device (VAD), lumbar puncture, and bone marrow aspiration and biopsy, what would be your priority in scheduling these procedures?
5. Based on the treatment plan of chemotherapy and radiation therapy, what teaching elements will be necessary for the family before discharge?

Answers

1. Neurovital signs, signs of infection, drainage from surgical or external ventriculostomy site, intake and output
2. Decrease in level of consciousness, vomiting, ataxia, major variations between intake and output
3. Reassure the grandparents that successful treatments are available for children with brain tumors and invite them to the patient care conference where the plan for determining the spread of disease with accompanying treatment plan will be discussed.
4. Usually, by working with the surgeon who will place the VAD, the bone marrow and lumbar puncture can be done in the operating room and the child taken for MRI and CT under the same anesthesia, accomplishing all procedures with one anesthetic exposure.
5. The same as for all oncology patients, with increased emphasis on nutrition and provision of nutrition because many of these children experience prolonged anorexia and weight loss

pontocerebellar fibers running through the brain stem. Horizontal nystagmus is found in almost one third of these cases.

Interdisciplinary Interventions

Due to their location in the vital area of the brain, the vast majority of brain stem gliomas are not resectable. Surgical intervention is considered an unacceptably high risk. Radiation is the only routinely used treatment. One or more courses of radiotherapy have been associated with an average survival time of 1 year. Almost all children show a significant clinical response to radiation after 3 to 6 weeks. Typically, cranial nerve palsies, pyramidal signs, and ataxia resolve. Improvement may be dramatic, or the child may demonstrate only slight improvement.

Ependymoma

The third most common infratentorial tumor is the ependymoma, which accounts for 10% of posterior fossa tumors in children. Incidence is twice as high in males as in females. These tumors occur at an early age, with more than 50% of children younger than age 5 years at the time of diagnosis, and as many as 25% to 40% younger than age 2 years.

Ependymomas arise from ependymal cells and are divided histologically into two types: low grade and high grade. Low-grade ependymomas are highly cellular, with a diagnostic pattern of rosettes around blood vessels. High-grade, or anaplastic ependymomas, have the rosette formation but also reveal necrosis, mitoses, and increased cellularity.

Prognosis. The overall survival rate depends on histologic grade, degree of dissemination (spread of the disease), and age. Survival varies from several months to 10 years or longer. One third to one half of patients survive for 5 years.

Assessment

Clinically, ependymoma tumors resemble medulloblastomas more than astrocytomas. The average duration of symptoms is 2 to 3 months and varies according to tumor location. If the tumor is located in the posterior fossa, the child presents with increased ICP, with papilledema being the most common finding. Supratentorial tumors usually cause local motor weakness, visual disturbances, and seizures.

Interdisciplinary Interventions

Complete resection, when possible, followed by radiation is the optimal therapy. Total and near-total resections are more easily achieved in supratentorial tumors; such resections are less common in the posterior fossa where infiltration of the brain stem is common and operative morbidity is higher (Fig. 22–10).

Optic Nerve Glioma

Optic nerve gliomas account for 5% of intracranial tumors in children younger than age 16 years, with most (75%) occurring in children younger than age 10 years. There is a strong association with neurofibromatosis, which is present in 50% to 70% of children with isolated optic nerve gliomas (Haslam, 1996; Oxenhandler & Sayers, 1978).

Tumors of the optic nerve and chiasm (junction of the optic nerves) consist almost entirely of astrocytomas, of which more than 95% occur in children. They are mainly confined to structures of the visual pathways, but they may also extend into the frontal lobes, hypothalamus, thalamus, and other midline structures.

Prognosis. In general, children with proptosis (a forward or downward displacement of the eyeball), which reflects the origin of a very slow-growing tumor in the optic nerve, seem to fare better than children with tumors in other locations. Children with isolated optic nerve glioma can almost always achieve long-term survival.

Figure 22–10
A school-ager wears a bandanna to conceal his lack of hair.

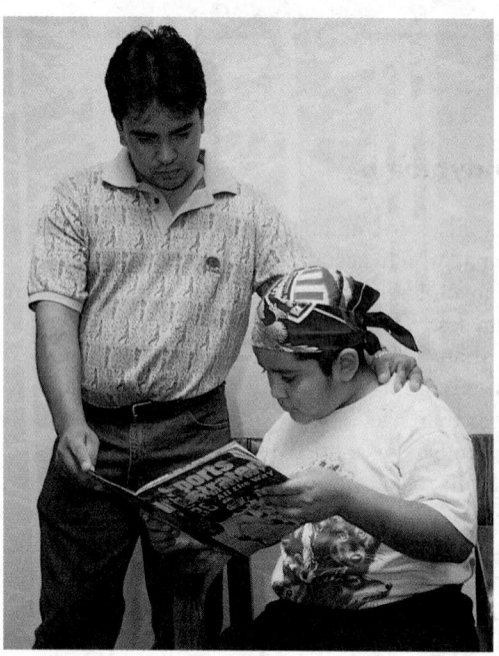

Assessment

Symptoms of optic nerve gliomas depend on the location of the tumor and the age of the child. Symptoms include diminished visual acuity, exophthalmos (forward protrusion or bulging of the eyes), nystagmus, optic atrophy, and multiple café au lait spots. Almost all children with optic nerve glioma have diminished visual acuity, but it is not recognized early because children rarely complain about the slow, progressive loss of vision that is characteristic of these tumors. More commonly, children younger than 3 years old are brought to medical attention because of strabismus, proptosis, or developmental difficulties. Exophthalmos is a particularly frequent (96%) and early sign when the tumor is confined to a single optic nerve. Nystagmus is chiefly a result of severe visual deficit before age 4 years, more particularly before age 2. Optic atrophy and pallor may be found on funduscopic examination. Multiple café au lait spots, the most common manifestation of neurofibromatosis, are present in approximately 25% of these children.

Interdisciplinary Interventions

CT and MRI scans are highly reliable for making a clinical diagnosis of optic nerve glioma. Biopsy is usually reserved for unusual clinical or radiologic circumstances because it may further compromise vision in as many as 75% of cases (Dosoretz, Blitzer, & Wang, 1980; Haslam, 1996). If it is suspected that an optic nerve glioma is confined to a single optic nerve, a complete resection is performed. In many cases, the tumor can be removed with preservation of the globe (Tenny, Laws, Younge, & Rush, 1982).

Radiation may be the best initial therapeutic choice for children with isolated tumors and a functioning eye.

Nine percent to 44% of children reported improved vision with radiation therapy, and as many as 90% show at least stabilization of visual decline. Chemotherapy is an alternative to radiation in the treatment of progressive disease.

Lymphomas

Malignant lymphomas represent the third most common type of childhood cancer (National Cancer Institute, 1996). These neoplasms occur in the lymphoid and reticuloendothelial systems, which are widely distributed throughout the body. Thus, most lymphomas are generalized diseases from the onset. Hodgkin's disease is generally more localized and can be treated as a solid tumor (Table 22–10). NHLs are often disseminated and must be treated as systemic disease.

Hodgkin's Disease

Hodgkin's disease is a lymphoid malignancy that arises from a single lymph node or lymph node region. The disease spreads by extending to contiguous (connected) lymph node areas. In advanced disease, it disseminates and may involve any organ in the body, but particularly involves the spleen, liver, bones, lung, and bone marrow.

Hodgkin's disease accounts for 5% of pediatric malignancies diagnosed in the United States. The annual incidence in the United States is 7.3 per million white children and 5.2 per million black children younger than age 15 years. The exact cause is unknown, but epidemiologic studies suggest an infectious agent. This finding is based on the occurrence of a bimodal age incidence as well as geographic location and socioeconomic factors. In children and young adults, age distribution patterns vary with geographic location and socioeconomic condition. For example, in developed countries, the overall incidence of childhood Hodgkin's disease is higher (National Cancer Institute, 1996). The most frequent histologic type seen in these populations is nodular sclerosis. In underdeveloped countries or lower socioeconomic groups, the overall incidence of Hodgkin's disease is lower but peaks before age 15 years. Mixed cellularity and lymphocytic depletion are the most frequent histologic types in these populations (Liebhauser, 1993). These patterns suggest an infectious cause with social class factors affecting the age when exposure occurs (Gutensohn & Shapiro, 1982).

Studies have reported an increased risk of Hodgkin's disease in close relatives, particularly same-sex siblings (Grufferman, Cole, Smith, & Lukes, 1977). This higher risk may be linked to genetic or environmental factors associated with immunocompetence. Hodgkin's disease is more prevalent in persons with immunodeficiency diseases such as ataxia-telangiectasia, Wiskott-Aldrich syndrome, and AIDS (Leventhal & Donaldson, 1993).

Pathophysiology

The histologic diagnosis of Hodgkin's disease is determined by the presence of the Reed-Sternberg cells. The presence of these cells alone is not diagnostic because similar cells can be seen in infectious mononucleosis, other reactive lymphoid hyperplasias, and other neoplasms. Hodgkin's disease is classified by the predominating cells. The most common classification system for Hodgkin's disease, the Rye classification, lists four types of Hodgkin's disease: lymphocytic predominance (LP), nodular sclerosis (NS), mixed cellularity (MC), and lymphocytic depletion (LD). They are listed in relative prognostic order from best to worst.

Prognosis. Sixty percent of children with Hodgkin's disease are determined to be stage I–II at the time of diagnosis, 30% at stage III, and 10% have already advanced to stage IV (Leventhal & Donaldson, 1993). Children with stage I and II disease have 10-year survival rates of more than 90% and relapse-free survival rates of 70% to 90%. Children with stage III disease have 5-year survival rates of 80%. The prognosis for children with

Table 22–10
Differences Between Hodgkin's Disease and Non-Hodgkin's Lymphoma

Hodgkin's Disease	Non-Hodgkin's Lymphoma
Malignant cells are more differentiated	Malignant cells appear undifferentiated
Reed-Sternberg cells	
Pattern of infiltration is more specific	Pattern of infiltration is diffuse
Subacute onset	Rapid onset
Localized disease at diagnosis	Presents with widespread involvement at diagnosis
Slower response to therapy	Responds quickly to treatment

stage IV disease continues to improve, with a 5-year survival rate of 70% (Tan, 1989).

Assessment

Characteristically, the first sign of Hodgkin's disease is painless, progressive lymph node enlargement. Other signs and symptoms vary according to the sites of the enlarged nodes, resulting in local tissue compression. For example, mediastinal lymphadenopathy may produce a persistent non-productive cough. The primary nodal site of Hodgkin's disease is above the diaphragm in two thirds of cases, and below it in one third. Signs and symptoms of Hodgkin's disease include the following:

- Cervical or supraclavicular lymphadenopathy in 60% to 90% of cases
- Painless, firm nodes that are movable in surrounding tissue
- Hepatomegaly, splenomegaly, or both in generalized disease
- Anorexia
- Weight loss
- Malaise
- Lethargy
- Night sweats
- Fever in 30% of cases; intermittent elevations of 1°C to 2°C above normal

Certain systemic symptoms are considered prognostically significant. Children with unexplained weight loss of more than 10% in the past 6 months, unexplained fever with temperatures of more than 38°C, or night sweats are classified "B" in the staging procedure. The absence of these symptoms places the child in the "A" classification (Lister et al., 1989). The percentage of children with B classification increases in advanced disease (Thompson, 1991).

Diagnostic Tests and Staging Studies. Diagnostic evaluation of the child with suspected Hodgkin's disease involves many tests and studies (Chart 22–22). Staging is the determination of the extent of disease at the time of diagnosis. The standardized staging system for Hodgkin's disease is shown in Figure 22–11. Accurate clinical, laboratory, and diagnostic imaging evaluations are necessary for precise staging of disease extent. The use of staging laparotomy with splenectomy is controversial. Staging laparotomy is the only reliable technique for determining the presence and extent of abdominal disease. With this procedure, as many as one third of children thought to have stage I–II disease based on clinical stage were found to have stage III–IV disease. The risk of inadequate staging and inadequate or excessive therapy must be weighed against the trauma, surgical risk, and long-term risk of fulminating sepsis following splenectomy. In many centers, the procedure is performed in all cases except those in which therapy would not be changed based on findings.

Chart 22–22

Components of Diagnostic Evaluation for Hodgkin's Disease

- Physical examination with measurement of enlarged nodal areas
- Posteroanterior and lateral chest radiographs
- Complete blood count, erythrocyte sedimentation rate, serum copper, liver and renal function tests, alkaline phosphatase assay, baseline thyroid-stimulating hormone, and free T_4 measurement
- Lymph node biopsy to establish diagnosis
- Chest computed tomography (CT) scan
- Gallium scan (optional)
- Abdominal and pelvic CT scan and magnetic resonance image
- Staging laparotomy
  - Splenectomy
  - Sampling of splenic hilum, celiac axis and portal area, mesenteric, iliac, and para-aortic lymph nodes
  - Wedge biopsies of both lobes of liver
- Bone marrow biopsy
- Bone scan (optional)

Interdisciplinary Interventions

The goal of treatment is to cure the child of the disease with minimal treatment-related toxicities. Children with localized disease may be treated with radiation therapy alone. However, most children are treated with a combined treatment modality using radiation and chemotherapy. Radiation may be involved-field for localized disease or extended-field for advanced disease. Involved-field focuses the radiation treatment to those areas in which disease involvement has been positively identified. Extended-field radiotherapy treats adjacent uninvolved lymph node regions. In unfavorable or advanced disease, the child may receive total nodal irradiation. Radiotherapy may be delayed until the child is 8 years old whenever possible to prevent retardation of bone growth and soft tissue development. Chemotherapy is the primary treatment in advanced disease.

Non-Hodgkin's Lymphoma

NHL is a malignant disorder of the lymphocytes, differing significantly from Hodgkin's disease. In NHL, the malig-

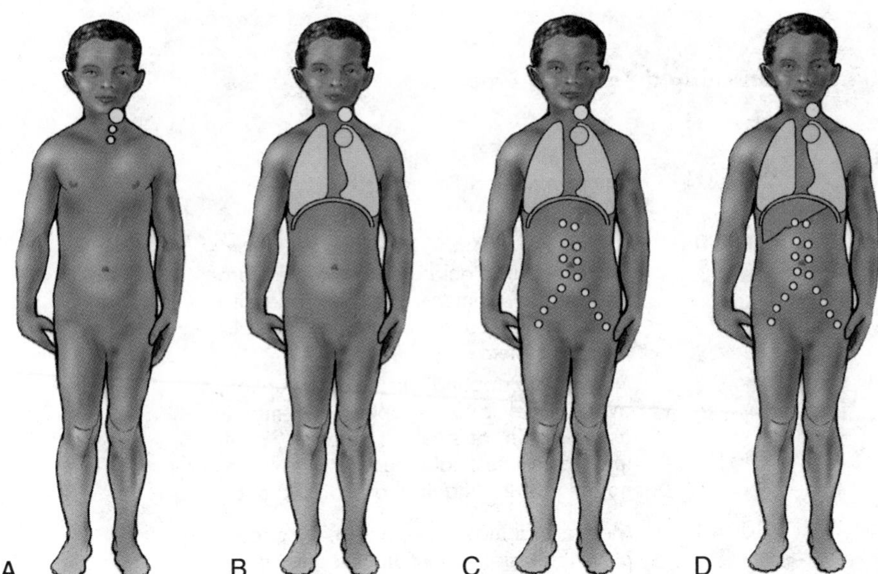

Figure 22–11
Staging of Hodgkin's disease.

nant cells appear undifferentiated, and the pattern of infiltration is diffuse. The disease has a rapid onset and presents with widespread involvement. NHL is 1½ times as prevalent as Hodgkin's disease in children. Peak incidence occurs at age 7 to 11 years. Incidence in boys is three times that in girls (Graham, 1988; Quinlan, 1993). The highest incidence rates of NHL exist in the United States and Canada (National Cancer Institute, 1996). A higher incidence of NHL has been noted in several population groups, specifically individuals with human immunodeficiency virus, Epstein-Barr virus, and congenital immunodeficiency syndromes such as Wiskott-Aldrich syndrome, Bloom syndrome, and severe combined immunodeficiency syndrome. Additionally, patients whose immune systems were suppressed with medications for other illnesses have a higher risk for development of this cancer (National Cancer Institute, 1996).

Pathophysiology

Two classification systems can be applied to childhood NHL: the modified Rappaport classification schema and the Working Formulation for Clinical Uses. In this chapter, the terminology of the Working Formulation for Clinical Uses is used. Within this classification system are three categories of NHL: lymphoblastic, small non-cleaved (Burkitt's or non-Burkitt's), and large cell lymphomas (Burke, 1990). The categories are derived from the actual appearance of each type of tumor cell in terms of appearance and differentiation.

Prognosis. Tumor burden at the time of presentation is believed by many to be the most significant prognostic factor. Current staging systems do not accurately reflect the amount of tumor burden. Tumor burden is determined by laboratory analysis of lactate dehydrogenase (LDH), uric acid, and lactic acid. Localized versus advanced disease also demonstrates prognostic significance; for instance, CNS involvement is thought to be a poor prognostic indicator. The 5-year survival rate is 72% in children (National Cancer Institute, 1996).

Assessment

Because the lymph system is widely distributed throughout the body, most lymphomas are generalized at the time of diagnosis. This means that most children have stage III or IV disease at diagnosis. The course of symptoms is generally short in duration, ranging from a few days to a few weeks (Graham, 1988; Quinlan, 1993). Signs and symptoms vary, based on the cell type or histologic appearance and the specific organs involved (Table 22–11).

The most common sites are intra-abdominal, mediastinal, peripheral nodal, and nasopharyngeal. Intra-abdominal disease accounts for one third of childhood NHLs. The primary site closely correlates with the specific cell type. Children with small, non-cleaved cell lymphomas present with abdominal tumors with or without ascites in approximately 90% of cases (Magrath & Sariban, 1985; Sandlund, 1996). The child with intra-abdominal lymphoma may present with signs and symptoms that mimic those of appendicitis, such as pain, intestinal obstruction, right lower quadrant tenderness, and fever.

Alert: *Intussusception (telescoping of the bowel) may be caused by lymphoma. As a rule, symptoms of intussusception in children older than age 5 years are highly suspicious of NHL.*

Table 22–11
Clinical Presentation of Non-Hodgkin's Lymphoma

Working Formulation Classification	Cases (%)	Common Clinical Presentation
Small non-cleaved cell (Burkitt's or non-Burkitt's)	40–50	Abdominal primary; tumor lysis syndrome (increased uric acid and lactate dehydrogenase); jaw tumor (African); propensity for spread to bone marrow and central nervous system May mimic appendicitis; intussusception; ovarian, pelvic, or retroperitoneal masses; ascites, pain, or swelling; nausea, vomiting, gastrointestinal bleeding; lymphadenopathy of the inguinal or iliac regions
Lymphoblastic	30–40	Mediastinal mass, dysphagia, dyspnea, pleural effusion, supradiaphragmatic lymphadenopathy; superior vena cava syndrome (swelling in the back, neck, and upper extremities); respiratory distress; propensity for rapid spread to bone marrow, CNS, and gonads
Large cell	15	Extranodal site common (lung, face, brain, skin, bone)

Intra-abdominal disease may also present as ovarian, pelvic, or retroperitoneal masses, or as nausea, vomiting, GI bleeding, ascites, swelling, pain, and lymphadenopathy of the inguinal or iliac regions. Signs of massive tumor burden often develop in these children, and they are prone to tumor lysis syndrome, particularly during the initial phase of therapy. Children with intra-abdominal NHL also tend to have CNS disease and bone marrow involvement.

Children with lymphoblastic lymphomas most commonly manifest intrathoracic tumors, particularly a mediastinal mass in 50% to 70% of cases (Magrath, 1993). The usual presentation of mediastinal disease is acute respiratory distress. These children have pleural effusion or tracheal compression, causing pain, tachypnea, cough, wheezing, or dyspnea. A phenomenon known as superior vena caval syndrome may cause increased blood flow to the neck and face, edema of the upper extremities and face, conjunctivitis, or mental status changes. This disease process tends to grow rapidly, causing severe respiratory compromise. These children often require admission to a pediatric intensive care unit. Primary mediastinal disease can also have extensive disease outside the thoracic cavity such as abdominal, bone marrow, and CNS involvement.

Children with large cell lymphomas frequently have a similar distribution of tumor sites as those with small, non-cleaved cell lymphomas, but they also have unusual sites of involvement (i.e., skin, lung, face, brain, and bone).

Diagnostic Tests. Diagnostic studies include complete blood count; renal and liver function studies; serum electrolytes, calcium, phosphorus, magnesium, LDH, and uric acid determinations; Epstein-Barr virus titers; urinalysis; chest x-ray; bone marrow aspirate; cerebrospinal fluid cytologic study; and diagnostic images of the involved tumor sites, in particular, CT studies of the head and neck, chest, or abdomen. The stage of disease has important implications, both for prognosis and for selecting optimal therapy.

Staging. Accurate staging of lymphomas is extremely important in determining the extent of disease and ensuring that the appropriate treatment regimen is used. Staging systems in childhood NHL generally reflect the tumor burden (Table 22–12). The systems are applicable to all histologic types and separate children with limited stage disease from those with extensive intrathoracic or intra-abdominal disease. Stages I, II, and III have relatively clear-cut definitions, whereas stage IV is more complicated because of differentiation of bone marrow

Table 22-12
Clinical Staging Systems for Childhood Lymphomas

Stage	Memorial Sloan-Kettering Cancer Center	St. Jude Children's Research Hospital	Stage	National Cancer Institute
I	One single site	Single tumor (extranodal) or single anatomic area (nodal) with the exclusion of mediastinum or abdomen	A	Single solitary extra-abdominal site
II	Two or more sites on same side of diaphragm	Single tumor (extranodal) with regional node involvement Two or more nodal areas on the same side of the diaphragm Two single (extranodal) tumors, with or without regional node involvement, on the same side of the diaphragm Primary GI tract tumor, usually in the ileocecal area, with or without involvement of associated mesenteric nodes only	B	Multiple extra-abdominal sites
III	Disseminated disease without marrow or CNS involvement	Two single tumors (extranodal) on opposite sides of the diaphragm Two or more nodal areas above and below the diaphragm All the primary intrathoracic tumors (mediastinal, pleural, thymic) All extensive primary intra-abdominal disease All paraspinal or epidural tumors, regardless of other tumor site(s)	C	Intra-abdominal tumor
IV	Any of above with bone marrow and/or CNS involvement	Any of the above, with initial CNS or bone marrow involvement (<25% blasts)	D	Intra-abdominal tumor with involvement of one or more extra-abdominal sites
IVA	Bone marrow with <25% blasts		AR	Intra-abdominal tumor with more than 90% of tumor surgically resected
IVB	Bone marrow with >25% blasts			

CNS, central nervous system; GI, gastrointestinal.
From Quinlan, N. (1993). Non-Hodgkin's lymphoma. In G. Foley, D. Fochtman, & K. Hardin-Mooney (Eds.), *Nursing care of the child with cancer* (p. 267). Philadelphia: W. B. Saunders. Used with permission.

involvement. Much controversy surrounds the extent of bone marrow involvement present in stage IV lymphoma and the potential for making the diagnosis of leukemia in children with greater than 25% blasts. Stage IV NHL is commonly defined as bulky disease with less than 25% blasts in the bone marrow. More than 25% blasts in the bone marrow is classified as ALL rather than lymphoma.

Nursing Diagnoses and Outcomes

Nursing diagnoses applicable to the child with cancer are presented in Chart 22–3. In addition, the following may be applicable to the child with NHL:

- **Altered urinary elimination related to the effects of tumor lysis syndrome**
  Outcome: The child will be free from complications of fluid and electrolyte imbalance and renal failure related to tumor lysis syndrome.

Interdisciplinary Interventions

With the advent of aggressive multiagent chemotherapy and available supportive therapy, most cases of NHL are curable. The survival rate for children with localized disease is currently near 90%, and it is 60% to 70% for children with advanced disease (Magrath, 1993). Improved response rates, sustained remissions, and higher cure rates are achieved by accurately determining the immunohistologic cell type and extent of disease and by initiating aggressive combination chemotherapy.

The intensity and duration of therapy are directly related to the extent of disease. Children in stages I and II with a lower tumor burden generally require less intense and shorter duration therapy. Children in stages III and IV with a higher tumor burden require more aggressive and longer therapy.

Alert: *As tumor burden increases, as in advanced disease, so does the likelihood of spontaneous or therapy-induced tumor lysis syndrome.*

Tumor lysis syndrome may present before the initiation of therapy and often worsens once chemotherapy is begun. The syndrome results from rapid lysis (breakdown) of tumor cells, either by intrinsic cell death or in response to chemotherapeutic agents. The dead cells release large quantities of electrolytes and metabolites into the blood stream, resulting in hyperuricemia, hyperkalemia, hyperphosphatemia, and hypocalcemia. This sudden alteration in serum chemistries may produce an electrolyte imbalance that can lead to renal failure or even death. (See Table 22–7 for a summary of the management of tumor lysis syndrome.) To prevent this complication, the nurse must initiate prophylactic therapy, as ordered, and must continuously monitor the child for signs of fluid and electrolyte imbalance and renal failure. Intensive hydration (3 L/m^2/day) is required to flush the cell by-products through the kidneys. Allopurinol therapy and urinary alkalinization (by adding sodium bicarbonate to the IV fluid) is started before initiating chemotherapy. Serum chemistries and urinary output must be monitored closely. Dialysis may be necessary if renal failure occurs before or during therapy.

Neuroblastoma

Neuroblastoma is a solid tumor occurring in infants and young children. Composed of cells that are very similar to those of the sympathetic nervous system, the tumor can be found anywhere that sympathetic nervous tissue is present.

Incidence and Etiology

Neuroblastoma is the fourth most common childhood cancer. It is the most common tumor found in children younger than 1 year of age (Brodeur & Castleberry, 1993). Neuroblastoma occurs slightly more in males than females and more frequently in white children. The true incidence of neuroblastoma is unknown. In neonates, a phenomenon occurs in which the newborn presents with this tumor and, within a relatively short period of time, the tumor spontaneously regresses.

The cause of neuroblastoma remains unknown. Some familial causes have been proposed; however, the risk of development of neuroblastoma in siblings or offspring is less than 6% (Kushner, Gilbert, & Helson, 1986; Santana, 1996). Oncogene *n-myc* (a cancer-causing gene) has been identified in cell lines of human neuroblastoma. The higher the number of copies of this oncogene that are present, the poorer is the child's prognosis (Look et al., 1991).

Pathophysiology

Neuroblastoma is a solid tumor that is usually encapsulated. The tumor is usually composed of small round cells (rosettes) surrounding a region of neural or ganglion cells (Santana, 1996). The neuroblastoma may occur at a primary site only, or it may spread to other metastatic sites, including the bone marrow. Neuroblastomas often secrete two catecholamine metabolites, homovanillic acid (HVA) and vanillylmandelic acid (VMA). These metabolites can be found in the child's urine.

Worldview: *In Japan, research has been conducted involving screening of infants for the preclinical detection of neuroblastoma by analyzing urine samples. These studies have indicated that screening was effective in determining the presence of neuroblastoma in many children before the presentation of any other clinical signs (Woods, 1993).*

Prognosis. Two well-known factors predict a favorable prognosis for children with neuroblastoma. Children younger than 1 year and who are in stage I, II, or IVS (see Staging later) have a favorable prognosis. Children with these stages characteristically demonstrate disease-free survival ranges from 70% to 100% (Kushner et al., 1986; Santana, 1996; Sullivan, 1993).

Children with greater than 10 copies of the n-*myc* oncogene and stage III and IV (see Staging later) disease and those with serum ferritin levels greater than 150 mg/mL are associated with a poor prognosis (Altman, 1993). With an intensive treatment approach (surgery, chemotherapy, radiation), disease-free survival or initial response rates for these children may be greater than 40%.

Assessment

The signs and symptoms of neuroblastoma depend primarily on the site or the spread of tumor. The most common site is the abdomen. Less common sites are the thorax, neck, and pelvis. Metastases are found in approximately 70% of newly diagnosed children, accounting for the poor prognosis rates associated with this disease (Moss et al., 1991). Bone pain, spinal cord compression, neurologic deficits, and abdominal pain may all be present based on tumor size and location. Sphenoid bone and retro-orbital involvement can cause ecchymosis of the eyelids and proptosis. The child has a "raccoon-eyed" presentation and may appear to be abused. Manifestations of other bone involvement may cause limping or refusal to walk.

Diagnostic Tests. Neuroblastoma causes overproduction of the catecholamine metabolites vanillylmandelic acid and homovanillic acid. These metabolites are excreted in excessive amounts in the urine. Analysis of the urine for these metabolites is useful in the diagnosis of neuroblastoma (Santana, 1996).

Staging. A major staging system used internationally to standardize the definition of diagnosis and better assist in treatment of the disease is the International Staging System for Neuroblastoma. Stage I refers to localized minimal disease. Disseminated disease to the bone, lymph nodes, bone marrow, liver, and perhaps organs is referred to as stage IV. Stage IVS refers to the neuroblastoma that is disseminated to all areas except the bone and occurs in neonates with subsequent spontaneous regression.

Interdisciplinary Interventions

To provide an optimal chance of cure, multimodal treatment is used based on the stage and significant prognostic indicators at diagnosis. Surgery plays a major role in treatment, as does diagnosis. When the tumor is localized, complete surgical resection may be feasible and is often curative. Children with disseminated disease are poor candidates for surgery. In these cases, chemotherapy is the primary treatment modality. Chemotherapy may render a large tumor resectable, allowing for the possibility of a delayed or second-look surgery to remove the remaining tumor. Irradiation may be used for local control of the tumor or for local palliation of metastatic disease. Children with more advanced neuroblastoma (unresectable or metastatic disease) undergo aggressive chemotherapy and radiation, as well as autologous BMT (Fig. 22–12).

Nursing considerations for the child with neuroblastoma include general oncology supportive care, similar to that previously discussed. This includes psychosocial support, teaching, and physical preparation for procedures, surgery, side effects of chemotherapy, and radiation therapy in standard doses or in higher doses associated with BMT. This tumor most often has a poor prognosis; thus, every treatment modality option is offered to the child and the family.

Figure 22–12
High-dose corticosteroid therapy for this child after bone marrow transplantation has produced a characteristic "moon face" appearance.

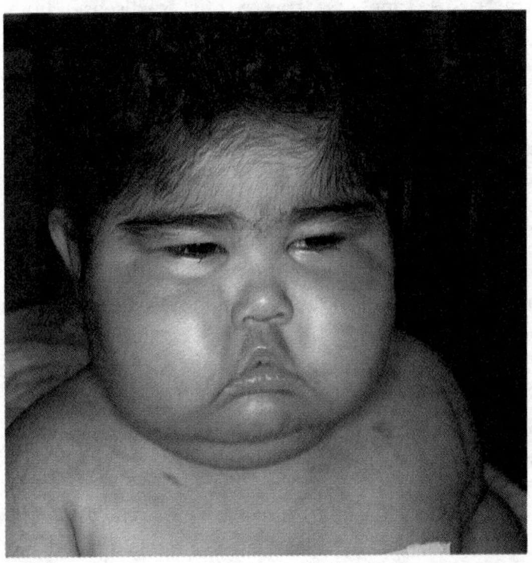

Wilms' Tumor (Nephroblastoma)

A primary tumor of the kidney, Wilms' tumor, or nephroblastoma, accounts for 6% of cancers in children younger than age 15 (Crist, 1991; National Cancer Institute, 1996). The average age at diagnosis is 2 to 3 years. Approximately 400 new cases of Wilms' tumor occur each year, with a slightly higher than average incidence in black children and females.

Most cases of Wilms' occur without any genetic predisposition. A very small number of cases exhibit some familial tendency. Some children are born with large deletions of the short arm of chromosome 11. These children often have other congenital anomalies such as microcephaly, mental retardation, and genitourinary tract problems (National Cancer Institute, 1996; Reeve, Sih, Raizis, & Feinberg, 1989; Shearer & Wilimas, 1996). It is suggested that children with these anomalies be screened routinely for development of Wilms' tumor.

Pathophysiology

Wilms' tumor is usually a large, rapidly growing tumor and is often very soft and vascular. After surgical resection, the composition of the tumor cells is examined microscopically and determined to be either a favorable or an unfavorable tissue type (Drigan & Androkites, 1993). The tumor may be present in one or both kidneys, which is a very important prognostic factor. The pathologic staging for Wilms' tumor ranges from stage I, in which disease is limited to the kidney and allows for complete removal, to stage V, in which bilateral kidney involvement occurs. This staging system is currently recommended by the National Wilms' Tumor Study Group (Green et al., 1993).

Prognosis. The most promising prognostic factors rely on the tissue type and the extent of disease. Five-year survival rate is 87% of all children with the disease (National Cancer Institute, 1996). Recurrence of disease is possible and most often occurs in the lungs.

Assessment

An abdominal mass is the most common sign in the otherwise asymptomatic child at the time of diagnosis. Some children may experience abdominal pain, hematuria, or hypertension. The tumor is confined to one side, not crossing the midline, as is seen with neuroblastoma. The mass is firm and non-tender. The presence of distended abdominal veins may indicate occlusion of the inferior vena cava by the mass.

caREminder: *If Wilms' tumor is suspected, palpation of the abdomen should be* avoided. *Palpating the abdomen may cause rupture of the tumor capsule, resulting in tumor "spillage." Tumor spillage can change the tumor from stage I to stage II or III depending on the amount of spillage occurring.*

Interdisciplinary Interventions

Multimodal therapy is recommended for the child with Wilms' tumor. It is imperative to have immediate surgical removal of the affected kidney, even if pulmonary metastasis is present (Shearer & Wilimas, 1996). The goals of surgery are to remove the tumor without producing hematogenous spread, to prevent rupture of the tumor capsule and subsequent spillage of tumor cells, and to provide a tissue sample for pathologic evaluation to determine spread and staging (Drigan & Androkites, 1993). Members of the health care team have an opportunity to provide preoperative education for the child and the family while they await surgical intervention. Preoperative teaching should include a discussion of the other treatment modalities that may be used such as radiation and chemotherapy.

Postoperative care involves pain management and ongoing abdominal assessment to observe for intestinal obstruction and signs of infection, bleeding, or fluid and electrolyte imbalance. This care also involves frequent monitoring of the child's blood pressure because manipulation or pressure on the kidney or the removal of a kidney may alter renin production and cause hypertension. Postoperatively, the tumor site is highly sensitive to radiation therapy and adjuvant chemotherapy regimens improve overall survival rates. The intensity and longevity of chemotherapy treatment protocols are determined by the completeness of the surgical resection and the extent or staging of the tumor (Green et al., 1993). Most children can be cured of this tumor, and ongoing investigations continue to improve outcomes for children with unfavorable and metastatic Wilms' tumor.

Rhabdomyosarcoma

Incidence and Etiology

Rhabdomyosarcoma is the most common soft tissue tumor in children, accounting for 5% to 8% of all childhood cancers (Crist, 1996). It mainly affects persons younger than age 21 and is slightly more common in males. A bimodal incidence distribution seems to occur, with peak incidences at age 2 to 6 years and again at 15 to 19 years (Lanzkowsky, 1989).

Rhabdomyosarcomas occur in four anatomic sites: the head and neck (35% to 40% of cases), the genitourinary tract (20%), the extremities (15% to 20%), and the trunk (10% to 15%). Rhabdomyosarcomas of the head and neck can occur throughout childhood but most commonly occur before age 8 years (Maurer & Ragab, 1991). Rhabdomyosarcomas of the bladder and vagina occur most frequently in infants and are histologically different than those of the trunk and extremities, which are more common in older children.

The cause of rhabdomyosarcoma is unknown. However, rhabdomyosarcoma has been associated with familial cancer syndromes and with neurofibromatosis (Crist, 1996; Li & Fraumeni, 1982; McKeen, Bodurtha, Meadows, Douglass, & Mulvihill, 1978). An increased incidence of adrenocortical cancer and brain tumors has been reported in first-degree relatives of children with rhabdomyosarcoma (Li & Fraumeni, 1969; National Cancer Institute, 1996). Epidemiologic studies of rhabdomyosarcoma have demonstrated an increased incidence of parental smoking and exposure to environmental chemicals, as well as an increased ingestion of animal organs in families of children with rhabdomyosarcoma (Grufferman, Wang, & Delong, 1982).

Pathophysiology

All sarcomas originate in primitive mesenchymal cells. Mesoderm cells form tissue known as mesenchyme. The mesenchyme cells give rise to fibrous and adipose connective tissue, blood vessels, lymphatic structures, and smooth and striated muscles (Crist, 1996). Thus, sarcomas can arise in many sites throughout the body. Sarcomas differ histologically and are identified by the mature cell type that they most closely resemble. Rhabdomyosarcomas arise from tissue resembling striated muscle tissue, which contains rhabdomyoblasts, or primitive muscle cells. Because striated muscles are located throughout the body, these tumors occur in many sites.

Rhabdomyosarcoma can be classified into four histologic types:

- The embryonal type is the most common; it predominantly affects children younger than 15 years of age in the head and neck region and genitourinary tract.
- The botryoid type is a variant of the embryonal type and is most often seen in the vagina, uterus, bladder, nasopharynx, and middle ear.
- The alveolar type carries the poorest prognosis. This type commonly involves muscles of the extremities and trunk.
- The pleomorphic type is the least common, usually arising in muscles of the extremities.

The histologic diagnosis of rhabdomyosarcoma is based on the overall cellular pattern and the presence of rhabdomyoblasts with or without characteristic cytoplasmic cross striations. Embryonal, botryoid, and pleomorphic are considered favorable histologic types and alveolar is considered an unfavorable histologic type.

Prognosis. Several prognostically significant variables have been identified and are of major importance in determining treatment regimens. The most important factors appear to be the location and the extent of disease at the time of diagnosis. Children with no detectable metastases at diagnosis (group I) have much better outcomes than those with widespread disease (group IV). Children with tumors of the head and neck have a better prognosis than do those with genitourinary tumors. Tumors of the extremities tend to have a high relapse rate and a lower survival rate (Hayes et al., 1989).

The primary site is an important prognostic variable for several reasons. First, the location of a tumor determines the symptoms that lead to diagnosis. Deeply situated tumors are often large and have presumably been in place and with the potential to spread over a longer period of time than superficial, easily visible tumors. Second, the likelihood of lymphatic spread and hematogenous spread varies with primary site. Third, the location has implications for therapy (i.e., surgical resectability). The histopathologic type of tumor is another important variable; children with embryonal and botryoid rhabdomyosarcoma have a better survival rate than those with alveolar or undifferentiated types. The most meaningful prognostic variable is the response to treatment. Early response to treatment appears to correlate with higher survival rates for these children.

Assessment

Signs and symptoms of rhabdomyosarcoma vary according the location of the primary site and the presence and extent of metastasis. Presenting symptoms can be caused by the primary tumor, by metastases, or by both (Maurer & Ragab, 1991). The signs and symptoms are usually attributed to the mass lesion or to obstructive phenomena.

Rhabdomyosarcoma in the head and neck occurs predominantly in the orbit, nasopharynx, maxillary antrum, middle ear, and soft tissues of the scalp, face, and neck. Approximately one fourth of head and neck rhabdomyosarcomas occur in the orbit (Raney et al., 1993). Tumors in the orbit grow rapidly and are usually detected early because of the obvious changes they produce. Symptoms include ptosis, with or without lid swelling, exophthalmos, orbital cellulitis, or cranial nerve deficits.

Approximately one half of head and neck rhabdomyosarcomas and undifferentiated sarcomas arise in nonorbital parameningeal sites (paranasal sinuses, nasopharynx, middle ear, and pterygoid-infratemporal fossae). Tumors originating in the paranasal sinuses can cause nasal obstruction, chronic sinusitis, epistaxis, swelling, or local pain. Symptoms of nasopharyngeal tumors include hypernasal speech, nasal obstruction, discharge, visible polypoid masses in the nasopharyngeal cavity, and serous otitis. Middle ear rhabdomyosarcoma can present as chronic otitis media. Symptoms may include mucopurulent or sanguinous drainage from the affected ear, facial nerve palsy, conduction types of hearing loss, or a polypoid mass seen in the external ear canal.

Parameningeal tumors have a high probability of direct extension into the meninges. Multiple cranial nerve palsies occur as the tumor invades the neurovascular sheath. As the tumor extends, it may cross multiple foramina and fissures and invade the epidural space. Intracranial spread can produce symptoms associated with increased ICP, such as headache with vomiting or diplopia. Overall survival rates are drastically reduced when intracranial extension is present.

Within the genitourinary tract, rhabdomyosarcoma in younger children presents in the urinary bladder, prostate, and vagina. In adolescent males, the tumor occurs in the paratesticular soft tissue or spermatic cord. Tumors of the retroperitoneal area are usually asymptomatic until their growth is quite extensive. At the diagnosis, the child may complain of vague abdominal pain or genitourinary or bowel obstruction. A palpable mass may be present. Local lymph nodes are commonly affected. A tumor arising in the bladder may cause urinary retention, straining to void, hematuria, or passage of tissue in urine. Paratesticular tumors usually present as asymptomatic non-tender masses in the scrotum, lying above and separate from the testes. They may be associated with abdominal or pelvic masses resulting from metastasis. Half of all vaginal rhabdomyosarcomas are associated with abnormal vaginal bleeding and the other half are associated with a protruding polypoid mass.

Tumors originating in the extremities are usually deep-seated, palpable masses with soft to firm consistency that may be mistaken for a traumatic hematoma, especially in school-age children (Ghavimi, Mondell, Heller, Hajdu, & Exelby, 1989). Tumors are relatively fixed to the underlying musculature and occasionally involve the skin. Sarcomas of the extremity are recognized by swelling in the affected limb. Pain, tenderness, and redness may be present. Tumors of the trunk are similar to those of the extremities in exhibiting all histologic types and in their tendency for local recurrence and for distant spread despite wide local excision. Tumors of the trunk are of relatively large diameter compared with head and neck and bladder tumors.

Rhabdomyosarcoma involving the bone can produce pain, swelling, and limited functioning of the child's affected body part. Bone marrow metastasis can result in symptoms of pancytopenia such as anemia, bleeding, or infection. Most children with bone marrow involvement have extremity or truncal rhabdomyosarcoma and have concomitant metastases to bone, lung, or lymph nodes. Primary lesions of the prostate and maxillary sinus are also frequently associated with bone marrow metastasis.

Staging. Local, regional, and distant disease extent are used to determine the tumor stage or group. The most commonly used staging system (Table 22–13) for rhabdomyosarcoma in the United States was developed in 1972 by the Intergroup Rhabdomyosarcoma Study Group (IRS). The Intergroup Rhabdomyosarcoma staging system is based on disease extent and resectability, defining groups I to IV by local disease status, the involvement of regional lymph nodes, and the extent of residual tumor after primary surgery (Kun & Etcubanas, 1987). Approximately 15% of children have resected, localized disease (group I) at diagnosis, 25% have residual microscopic disease with or without associated lymph node

Table 22–13
Rhabdomyosarcoma Clinical Grouping System (IRS-I and IRS-II)

Group	Description
I	A. Localized, completely resected, confined to site of origin B. Localized, completely resected
II	A. Localized, grossly resected with microscopic residual B. Regional disease, involved lymph nodes, completely resected C. Regional disease, involved lymph nodes, grossly resected with microscopic residual
III	A. Local or regional grossly visible disease after biopsy only B. Grossly visible disease after greater than 50% resection of primary tumor
IV	Distant metastases present at diagnosis

involvement (group II), 40% have gross residual local-regional disease (group III), and 20% have metastases at diagnosis (group IV).

Interdisciplinary Interventions

Combined modality treatment of rhabdomyosarcoma has greatly improved long-term survival rates. Surgical resection of the primary tumor usually offers the best prospect for local tumor control in limited disease cases. The addition of radiotherapy and multiagent chemotherapy has decreased indications for radical surgery, allowing more limited surgical intervention or potentially eliminating the need for surgery.

The goal of surgical intervention is complete tumor resection whenever possible. It is always desirable to preserve the child's vital or functionally useful structures or organs. In many cases, however, the location of the tumor, the degree of metastasis, and infiltration of adjacent organs prohibit complete tumor excision. In combined modality treatment, surgery includes the initial incisional biopsy and evaluation of disease extent. Gross total resection is the most rapid way to eradicate the disease and should always be used if subsequent function or cosmesis (cosmetic appearance) will not be greatly impaired.

Bone Tumors

Malignant bone tumors account for approximately 5% of all childhood malignancies (Betcher, 1993; Hayes et al., 1989). Most of these tumors occur in adolescence. The two most common bone tumors are osteogenic sarcoma and Ewing's sarcoma. The cause of most bone cancers is unknown.

Osteogenic Sarcoma

Osteogenic sarcoma (OS), also called osteosarcoma, is a malignant tumor of the bone derived from osteoid tissue. The most common sites are in the long bones such as the distal femur, proximal tibia, and proximal humerus. OS accounts for approximately 60% of malignant bone tumors in children (Link & Eilber, 1993). Peak incidence occurs between age 10 and 20 years, coinciding with the time of rapid bone growth.

A genetic predisposition for OS has been suggested. In some cases, OS has developed in multiple members of the same family, and children with a history of hereditary retinoblastoma have an increased risk for development of OS (Newton, Meadows, Shimada, Bunin, & Vawter, 1991). Involvement of the p53 gene has been associated with this tumor development (Meyers, 1987).

Pathophysiology

The malignant bone growth of OS is detected at the time of rapid growth of bone-forming tissue during the adolescent years. Five distinct tissue types of OS have been described: conventional (most common), periosteal, telangiectatic, multifocal, and miscellaneous. Some of these types are more common and some are more aggressive, factors that assist the health care professional in determining the chances for the patient's long-term survival.

Prognosis. The prognosis for OS continues to improve. With aggressive multimodal therapy, approximately two thirds of children without metastases can be cured (Link & Eilber, 1993). The most significant prognostic factor for OS is the extent of the disease. Ten percent to 20% of children present with metastatic disease to other bony structures or to the lungs. Their outcome is poor. Many die within 2 years after diagnosis (Betcher, 1993; Meyers, 1987). Primary tumor sites that are inoperable are associated with poor prognosis. It also appears that children younger than age 10 years who have elevated LDH levels have a poor prognosis.

Assessment

Most children present with pain in the affected limb that increases with activity or weight bearing. Refusal to walk and limited range of motion are common. Tenderness and the presence of local edema or redness may also be presenting symptoms. The older child should be able to specify the location of the pain. In the younger child, irritability, crying, and decreased movement or locomotion may be the only indicators of a problem. Ten percent to 20% of children have metastatic disease at time of diagnosis, most commonly in the lung (Link & Eilber, 1993). Many times, the diagnosis is made after a traumatic injury for which x-ray films are obtained. The x-ray films may reveal the presence of a previously unknown tumor site.

Interdisciplinary Interventions

Once diagnosis has been confirmed, surgical intervention is a vital component for children with OS. Tumor removal, limb salvage procedures, and amputation are all viable surgical options at this time. Limb salvage procedures provide tumor removal while preventing the physical and psychosocial complications that occur with amputation (Fig. 22–13).

Historically, surgery alone was used as the primary treatment modality, but the results in 5-year survival rates were less than 20% (Meyer & Marina, 1996). Chemotherapy is currently used for all patients, and it plays a significant role in providing survival rates of 65%

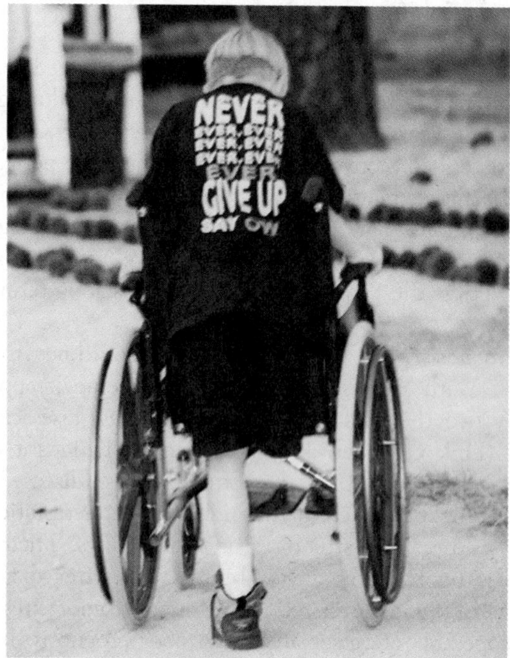

Figure 22–13
One child's strategy to deal with his cancer: "Never ever give up, say ow." (Courtesy of Camp Ronald McDonald for Good Times.)

(Eilber & Rosen, 1989). Preoperative and postoperative multiagent chemotherapy is used to prevent metastasis. Additional limb salvage procedures have been demonstrated to be more successful if performed after tumor viability and extent are modified by chemotherapy (Betcher, 1991). OS is highly resistant to radiation. If radiation is considered as a treatment option, it must be delivered in high doses. Radiation is more often used for pain control and palliation. Most children with OS require intensive physical and psychosocial management postoperatively and during their intense therapy.

Good pain assessment and effective management are vital components of nursing care for children with OS. (See Chapter 13 for further discussion of pain management.) Children may experience specific bone pain and tenderness before or during treatment as well as "phantom" limb pain postoperatively. It is important to provide pain management without hesitation to promote physical as well as psychosocial well-being for these children (Chart 22–23). An intensive and structured rehabilitation program is also highly recommended for these children. Once the surgeon has "cleared" the child postoperatively, physical therapy and occupational therapy are instituted as soon as possible to maintain and improve the child's motor function and quality of life. Because most of these patients are adolescents, body image is a major issue. Social and psychosocial intervention from peers and health care workers is a vital component of the child's plan of care (Fig. 22–14).

Ewing's Sarcoma

Ewing's sarcoma is a highly malignant tumor of the bone. These tumors may arise in any bone, but are most often located in flat bones (pelvis, chest wall, and vertebrae) and the diaphyseal region of the long bones (Meyer & Marina, 1996). It is often seen in the extremities with soft tissue involvement. Ewing's sarcoma is rare in chil-

Chart 22–23
Nursing Interventions

Support for the Child Diagnosed with Osteosarcoma

Nursing interventions for the child diagnosed with osteosarcoma include the following:

- Assist the child in making informed decisions about treatment options, in understanding the surgery planned, and in knowing what to expect from postoperative routines and treatments. Prepare the child for the possibility of amputation or limb salvage.
- Allow the child to verbalize fears or concerns about the loss of a limb.
- Allow the child to examine an actual prosthesis and to see other children with amputated limbs or who have undergone limb salvage procedures.
- Discuss the options for managing hair loss caused by chemotherapy, especially with adolescents whose appearance and self-image are crucial to them. These options include wearing wigs, hats, bows, scarves, and other items of apparel.
- Prepare the child for the possibility of phantom limb pain. Explain that the child might feel itching, tingling, or pain sensation even though the limb is no longer there. Discuss the drugs, such as antidepressants, that are used to treat these symptoms.
- Discharge teaching should include follow-up rehabilitation programs and help and support addressing the child's emotional readiness to face peers and family members.
- Encourage the child to wear loose clothing to distract attention from the deformity or the prosthesis.
- Give information on peer support groups and camps.
- Review the risks and complications associated with chemotherapy and radiation that accompany surgical intervention for the osteosarcoma.

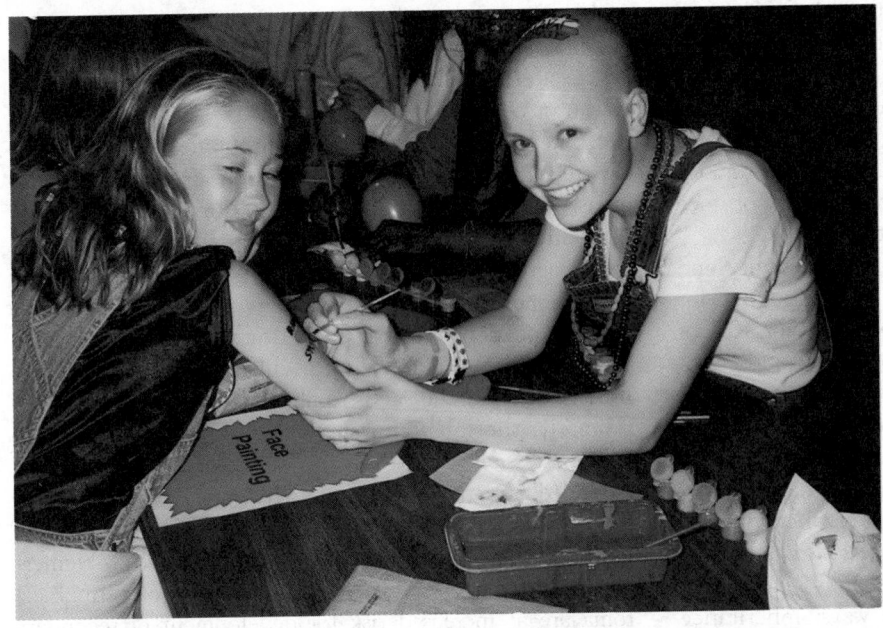

Figure 22–14
The adolescent undergoing treatment for cancer can grow to accept changes in her appearance and continue to develop a positive self-image. (Courtesy of Camp Ronald McDonald for Good Times.)

dren younger than age 5 years. Seventy percent of all children with Ewing's sarcoma are diagnosed before age 20 years (Horowitz, Delaney, Malawer, & Tsokos, 1993). In males, Ewing's sarcoma accounts for 30% of pediatric bone cancers (Crist, 1996). It is very rare in black children. There is no known hereditary factor.

Pathophysiology

Ewing's sarcoma is a tumor composed of small round cells, comparable to other childhood solid tumors. A comprehensive initial diagnostic evaluation is crucial because 10% to 30% of children have metastases at diagnosis (Betcher, 1993; Sauer, Jurgens, & Burger, 1987). Ewing's sarcoma commonly occurs in the pelvis, tibia, fibula, and femur.

Prognosis. The extent of the disease at the time of diagnosis is most important in determining outcome. Children with metastatic disease to the bone, bone marrow, or lungs have a poorer prognosis.

Assessment

Pain and a soft tissue mass around the affected bone are the common clinical presentations of Ewing's sarcoma. The signs may be misdiagnosed for some time as an injury related to sports or other physical activities. Children who have metastasis of their disease may present with anorexia, malaise, fever, fatigue, and weight loss. Other clinical signs depend on the location of the site of the sarcoma.

Interdisciplinary Interventions

Children who receive multimodal treatment have demonstrated improved long-term survival and control of Ewing's sarcoma. Surgery, radiation, and chemotherapy are used for primary lesions. Surgery is used to resect the primary tumor while maintaining an intact limb. Amputation is rarely indicated. Local radiation is given to primary and metastatic sites. The use of multiagent chemotherapy has been found to improve survival rates and has become the mainstay of therapy. Treatment advances for bone tumors result in more long-term survivors as well as long-term effects. Skeletal impairments and the risks of secondary malignancies are concerns that reinforce the necessity for long-term patient follow-up.

The psychosocial adjustments related to Ewing's sarcoma are usually less traumatic than those seen with osteosarcoma, because, usually, the affected limb remains preserved. A thorough explanation of the side effects of chemotherapy and radiation therapy is still a vital component to the child and family's plan of care. A physical therapy program is often needed to strengthen the affected limb or to assist recovery from orthopedic reconstructive surgery that may be required after the removal or shrinkage of the tumor.

Retinoblastoma

Retinoblastoma is a malignant tumor composed of embryonal retinal cells. It is the most common intraocular tumor in childhood. The incidence is 1 in 16,000 live births in the United States, constituting only 2.5% of all childhood cancers (National Cancer Institute, 1996). The tumor may be present at birth, although most tumors are not detected before age 3 years. The average age at diagnosis is 11 months for children with bilateral tumors and 22 months for those with unilateral tumors. Incidence does not vary significantly with sex or race (National Cancer Institute, 1996; Pratt, 1996).

Retinoblastoma occurs in two types: hereditary and non-hereditary. The non-hereditary type accounts for 60% of cases and the hereditary type accounts for 40% of cases (National Cancer Institute, 1996). The non-hereditary type of tumor arises by spontaneous mutation in somatic cells such as retinoblasts. Children with non-hereditary retinoblastoma have unilateral disease and no family history or increased risk of other malignancies.

Hereditary retinoblastoma is suspected when there is a positive family history or, in the case of sporadic disease, when the child is affected bilaterally. Hereditary retinoblastoma arises in one of three ways: inheritance from an affected parent by autosomal dominant transmission, inheritance from a non-affected gene carrier parent, or acquired as a new germinal mutation from a normal parent (Donaldson et al., 1993). Children with the hereditary type of retinoblastoma are at higher risk for development of other malignancies.

The strong hereditary nature of retinoblastoma underscores the extreme importance of genetic counseling. Unilateral disease with a positive family history and all bilateral cases are autosomal dominant genetic disorders. As with all autosomal dominant disorders, male or female carriers of the gene have an equal chance of transmitting the defective or mutated gene to offspring of either sex. Every child of an affected parent has a 50% chance of inheriting the mutated gene. Of the children inheriting the mutated gene, retinoblastoma develops in 60% to 98%.

caREminder: *Because of the strong hereditary influence of retinoblastoma and its curability in early stages, children with a positive family history should be monitored very closely. The child should receive a complete eye examination a few days after birth, at age 6 weeks, every 2 to 3 months until age 2 years, and then every 4 months until age 3 years.*

Pathophysiology

Retinoblastoma usually develops in the posterior portion of the retina (Pratt, 1996). The malignancy may appear as a single tumor in the retina, appearing in a rosette formation. The tumor can also have multiple foci extending locally to adjacent structures or spreading distantly. Local extension usually occurs within the intraocular space before invading the structures surrounding the globe. Distant spread, or metastasis, occurs when tumor cells grow along the optic nerve, enter the subarachnoid space, and spread to the CNS. Intracranial extension is the most common cause of death.

The tumor has a tendency to outgrow its blood supply, resulting in necrosis. Calcification appears in necrotic areas, especially in large tumors. The intraocular calcium is readily detected on radiographic study and is an important diagnostic sign.

Prognosis. The prognosis in retinoblastoma depends on the location and size of the tumor and the presence and degree of ocular or extraocular involvement. If the tumor is unilateral and small and the eye is treated promptly, the long-term survival rate is more than 90% (National Cancer Institute, 1996). Once the tumor has extended into the optic nerve, the cure rate decreases to 50%. Children with extraocular extension fare poorly, with a 25% survival rate (Apt & Gaffney, 1987). Numerous studies have indicated that survivors of retinoblastoma are at increased risk for development of secondary malignant tumors. These tumors are not associated with the ocular disease but are primary tumors of other organs (Berro, 1993).

Assessment

The signs and symptoms of retinoblastoma vary according to the stage at the time of diagnosis. When the tumor is small, the child may initially present with strabismus secondary to impaired vision. As the tumor enlarges, a creamy white pupillary reflex, known as leukocoria, or "cat's eye," develops, and the tumor may be visualized easily. Leukocoria is present in 60% of cases (Lanzkowsky, 1989). Children with red, painful eyes demonstrate late symptoms, resulting from inflammation, uveitis, or vitreous hemorrhage.

Early detection and diagnosis is extremely important because early intervention is effective and may preserve the child's vision. Without pathologic confirmation, the diagnosis must be made by the ophthalmoscopic, ultrasonographic, and radiographic appearance. A definitive diagnosis of retinoblastoma can usually be made during a complete funduscopic examination. Pupillary dilation and examination under sedation or general anesthesia are necessary to evaluate the retina fully. The tumors appear as creamy pink or white masses, but they may be obscured by retinal detachment, hemorrhage, or cloudy fluid in the anterior chamber.

Diagnostic Tests. Ultrasonography is a particularly valuable diagnostic tool in demonstrating the presence of a mass in the posterior segment of the eye when the fundus may be obscured by retinal detachment or hemorrhage. Radiographic identification of intraocular calcium is strongly suggestive of retinoblastoma because it is extremely rare for any other ocular disorder of childhood to produce such a finding. CT of the orbit is more sensitive than plain x-ray film in detecting the presence of calcium. MRI is usually not necessary but may be helpful in confirming the diagnosis in the absence of calcium.

Staging. The treatment of retinoblastoma depends on the size of the tumor and the extent of the disease. Thus, accurate staging is important. The Reese-Ellsworth staging classification is the standard system for prognostic evaluation of retinoblastoma (Chart 22–24). The Reese-Ellsworth classification system predicts the likelihood of tumor control and preservation of vision, but it does not predict survival. It divides children with retinoblastoma according to classifications of "very favorable," "favorable," "doubtful," and "unfavorable likelihood of preservation of vision" following radiotherapy on the basis of tumor size, number and location of tumors, and presence of vitreous seeding. No standard staging system exists for disease that has extended beyond the orbit of the eye.

Chart 22–24

Reese-Ellsworth Staging Classification of Retinoblastoma

Group I. Very Favorable Prognosis

A. Solitary tumor, smaller than 4 disk diameters,* at or behind the equator
B. Multiple tumors, none larger than 4 disk diameters, all at or behind the equator

Group II. Favorable Prognosis

A. Solitary tumor, 4–10 disk diameters, at or behind the equator
B. Multiple tumors, 4–10 disk diameters, behind the equator

Group III. Doubtful Prognosis

A. Any lesion anterior to the equator
B. Solitary tumors, larger than 10 disk diameters, behind the equator

Group IV. Unfavorable Prognosis

A. Multiple tumors, some larger than 10 disk diameters
B. Any lesion extending anteriorly to the ora serrata

Group V. Very Unfavorable Prognosis

A. Tumors involving more than half the retina
B. Vitreous seeding

*1 disk diameter = 1.5 mm.

Nursing Diagnoses and Outcomes

Nursing diagnoses applicable to the child with cancer are presented in Chart 22–3. In addition, the following nursing diagnosis may be applicable to the child with retinoblastoma:

- **Sensory and perceptual alterations of vision related to effects of the loss of vision or of the eye**
  Outcome: The child will adapt to receiving visual input from one eye or to blindness if severe bilateral involvement has occurred.

Interdisciplinary Interventions

The treatment plan for retinoblastoma is tailored to each individual case and is based on the extent of disease. Several considerations must be taken into account when planning treatment: whether involvement is unilateral or bilateral, whether the child has vision or any potential for vision, whether the tumor is confined to the globe or has extended to the optic nerve, and whether orbital, CNS, or distant metastases have occurred. Treatment modalities include surgery, radiotherapy, phototherapy, and cryotherapy.

The surgical intervention in the treatment of retinoblastoma is enucleation, or removal of the eye. Enucleation must be considered in children with severe retinal disruption with no possibility of restoration of sight, extension of the tumor into the anterior chamber, painful glaucoma with permanent loss of vision, or unresponsiveness to other forms of treatment. A cosmetic disadvantage for children younger than age 3 years is that the orbit ceases to grow normally after an eye is removed. As the face continues to grow, the orbit appears increasingly sunken. External beam radiation produces the same appearance because it interferes with bone growth. The surgeon and the nurse must prepare the parents for the child's appearance after surgery or radiation. Initially, the child has an eye patch in place that is changed regularly by the ophthalmologist. The orbit and the face are edematous in the postoperative period, making it difficult to fit the prosthesis until the edema subsides. Fitting for the prosthesis can usually take place 3 weeks after surgery unless complications occur.

Radiotherapy is used to control local disease while attempting to preserve vision. Retinoblastoma is known to be highly radiosensitive. Radiotherapy can be administered in one of two methods: external beam or application of radioactive applicators. Radioactive surface applicators (plaques) are indicated if recurring small tumors remain after external beam therapy or as initial therapy for small solitary tumors. A surgical procedure is performed to suture the radioactive applicators to the sclera. The device is left in place for 7 days. The child is placed under general anesthesia for the application and removal of the radioactive devices.

caREminder: *The child with radioactive devices is placed alone in a single room to prevent radiation exposure to other children and staff. Staff members wear radiation-sensitive badges to ensure that their exposure is minimal and within the guidelines determined by the National Council on Radiation Protection and Measurements.*

Photocoagulation therapy destroys the blood vessels supplying the tumor. It is generally used in conjunction with external beam radiation in tumors in the posterior part of the eye that fail to respond after 4 to 6 weeks of radiation or that recur after radiation therapy. Photocoagulation must be performed under direct visualization and is appropriate for tumors located posterior to the equator. It may also be used for small tumors that are located away from the optic nerve and macula. Photocoagulation is performed with the child under general anesthesia.

Cryotherapy destroys the tumor cells by forming intracellular ice crystals that interfere with the microcirculation of the tumor and results in cell death. Cryotherapy may also be used in conjunction with external beam radiation. The treatment is indicated for small primary or recurrent tumors in the anterior part of the retina or for small recurrences of the disease after radiotherapy has been administered. Cryotherapy does not require direct visualization of the tumor. Cryotherapy is performed with the child under general anesthesia.

Chemotherapy may be used in cases of metastatic disease. It is administered intravenously or intrathecally. Despite chemotherapeutic treatment, prognosis is poor in the presence of metastatic involvement.

Nursing care of the child who has an eye removed includes providing support to the child and family, postoperative care of the socket, discharge teaching, and providing information about the prosthesis.

The child's family needs support and counseling because of the genetic aspect of retinoblastoma. They may feel guilty for transmitting the defect to their child. The child and family need preparation for the prospect of the child losing vision in the affected eye as well as loss of the affected eyeball. The nurse should emphasize that the vision in the affected eye is probably already lost and that the child can still have a normal life with one functioning eye. It is also helpful to show the child pictures of a child with a prosthetic eye. Doing this helps the child and family to picture how the prosthetic eye will look.

Care of the socket includes maintaining a clean, dry dressing or eye pad. The eye pad should be changed daily until the socket is healed. The parents may need additional discharge instructions on cleansing of the socket or application of an antibiotic ointment if one is prescribed by the physician.

Initial instructions for care of the prosthesis are given by the ocularist, who fits and manufactures the device. The prosthesis is only removed when cleaning is necessary. It is cleaned by placing the prosthetic eyeball in room temperature, slightly warm water and soaking for several minutes. Parents are instructed in the removal and replacement of the prosthesis by the ocularist.

Summary of Key Concepts

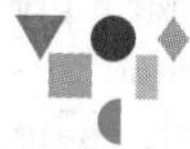

- The causes of most childhood cancers are unknown. Research is ongoing to determine linkages between environmental, genetic, and hereditary factors and the incidence of cancer in children.
- A thorough health history and physical examination are imperative if childhood cancer is suspected. In many cases, these cancers go undetected for long periods because the symptoms were misdiagnosed and associated with a different source, such as the flu or a cold.
- The treatment of cancer in children depends on the type of cancer and the location and extent of disease. Treatment options include surgery, chemotherapy, radiation, biotherapy, and bone marrow transplantation.
- Treatment of the cancer may also cause damage to normal cells and organs. Optimal ongoing use of supportive measures is vital for the treatment of cancer in children. These supportive measures include providing adequate nutritional support, management of fever, oral hygiene care, blood products support, management of nausea and vomiting, pain management, and maintenance of vascular access devices.
- The diagnostic evaluations to determine the presence of cancer can be painful and frightening for a child. Pain management and stress reduction measures should be an important part of the nurse's intervention during this phase of the diagnosis.

- Leukemia is the most common childhood malignancy, with acute lymphocytic leukemia accounting for 80% of these cases.
- The most common complaints associated with a CNS tumor are headaches and vomiting. Headaches in children are not a usual or normal occurrence.
- Hodgkin's disease is a lymphoid malignancy arising from a single lymph node or lymph node region. The disease spreads by extending to contiguous lymph node areas.
- Non-Hodgkin's lymphoma is a malignant disorder of the lymphocytes, differing significantly from Hodgkin's disease.
- Neuroblastoma, a solid tumor affecting infants and young children, is composed of cells that are very similar to those of the sympathetic nervous system and can be found anywhere that sympathetic nervous tissue is present.
- Wilms' tumor (nephroblastoma) is a primary tumor of the kidney in childhood.
- Rhabdomyosarcoma is the most common soft tissue tumor in children. Four anatomic sites in which rhabdomyosarcoma occurs are the head and neck region, the genitourinary tract, the extremities, and the trunk.
- Osteosarcoma is a malignant tumor of the bone derived from osteoid tissue. The most common sites are in the long bones such as the distal femur, proximal tibia, and proximal humerus.
- Ewing's sarcoma is a tumor composed of small round cells, comparable to other childhood solid tumors. Ewing's sarcoma occurs in the pelvis, tibia, fibula, and femur.
- Retinoblastoma is a malignant tumor composed of embryonal retinal cells. The prognosis in retinoblastoma depends on the location and size of the tumor and the presence and degree of ocular or extraocular involvement.

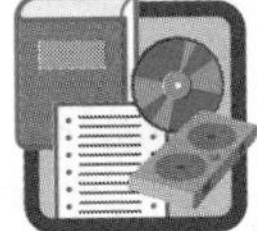

Resources

Organizations

American Brain Tumor Association
2720 River Road
Des Plaines, IL 60018
(708) 827-9910

American Cancer Society
1599 Clifton Road, NE
Atlanta, GA 30329
(800) ACS-2345
Web: http:www.cancer.org
Provides information about cancer and support groups; helps with transportation, limited financial assistance, and some in-home equipment.

✎ Candlelighter's Childhood Cancer Foundation
7910 Woodmont Avenue
Suite 460
Bethesda, MD 20814
(800) 366-2223
Web: http://www.candlelighter.org
National organization made up of families of children with cancer. A good source of support and educational material. Also provides a periodic newsletter free of charge.

Leukemia Society of America
National Headquarters
600 3rd Avenue
New York, NY 10016
(212) 573-8484
(800) 955-4572
May provide financial assistance (up to $750 per year) to children with leukemia, lymphoma, multiple myeloma, and preleukemia. Provides referral services to other community resources. May provide transportation and fees related to some drugs, blood transfusions, and x-ray therapy. Conducts a monthly support group for children, families, and friends. Provides written materials for children with leukemia, lymphoma, and bone marrow transplant.

✎ Make-a-Wish Foundation of America
100 W. Claredon
Phoenix, AZ 85013-3518
(800) 722-9474
May provide a special wish for a child (through age 17 years) with a life-threatening illness. Holds special events and holiday parties for the entire family.

National Cancer Institute
Cancer Information Service
Bethesda, MD 21227
(800) 4-CANCER

Provides many handouts, pamphlets, and written materials on a variety of diagnoses, treatments, and psychosocial issues for children with cancer and their families.

National Children's Cancer Society
1015 Locust Street
Suite 1040
St. Louis, MO 63101
(314) 241-1600

Assists qualifying families with ancillary expenses related to their child's bone marrow transplant and other ancology treatment.

National Marrow Donor Program
3422 Broadway Street, NE
Suite 400
Minneapolis, MN 55413-1762
(800) 627-7692

✏ Starlight Children's Foundation
1900 Avenue of the Stars
Suite 739
Los Angeles, CA 90067
(310) 286-0271
(800) 950-9474

May provide special wish for a child with a life-threatening illness.

Hotlines

American Institute for Cancer Research Nutrition Hotline
(800) 843-8114

Books and Printed Materials

✏ Baker, L. (1988). *You and leukemia: One day at a time*. Philadelphia: W. B. Saunders.

✏ Berglund, R. (1994). *An alphabet about kids with cancer*. Denver, CO. The children's legacy.

✏ Resources specifically for children.

✏ Cangelosi, J., Miceli, T., Siede, B., & Fineberg, B. (1994). *The radiation therapy coloring and activity book: A child's eye view of radiation therapy*. New Orleans: The Ochsner Center for Radiation Oncology.

✏ Chamberlain, S. (1994). *My ABC book of cancer*. San Francisco: Synergistic Press.

Chesler, M., & Barbarin, O. (1987). *Childhood cancer and the family*. New York: Brunner/Mazel.

✏ Friends Funletter Network
955 La Paz Road
Santa Barbara, CA 93108

Provides a national activities letter for kids and families living with cancer. An excellent tool for discussion regarding cancer and treatment. A nominal fee for subscription for those families who can afford it. Recommended for ages 5 through 12.

✏ Gaes, J. (1987). *My book for kids with cancer*. Pierre, SD: Melius and Peterson.

✏ Kuntz, N., & Secola, R. (1993). *G-CSF teaching booklets, Children's Hospital of Orange County*. Thousand Oaks, CA: AmGen, Inc.

✏ Landier, W., & Scott, T. (1996). *My central line book*. Salt Lake City, UT: Bard.

✏ Murray, S. (1991). *Fuzzy and Frankie*. (Ronald McDonald characters). Washington, DC: Goet Printing.

✏ Roloff, T. A. (1995). *Navigating through a strange land: A book for brain tumor patients and their families*. San Francisco: Indigo Press.

✏ Schultz, C. (1990, March). *Why, Charlie Brown, why?* (Animated commentary). Available from the American Cancer Society.

U.S. Department of Health and Human Services (1994, March). *Management of cancer pain: Clinical practice guideline*. Washington, DC: Public Health Service.

Audiovisuals

✏ *My hair is falling out . . . Am I still pretty?* 22-minute video available from the Association for the Care of Children's Health. (800) 808-ACCH.

Computer Resources

American Brain Tumor Society
http://neurosurgery.mgh.harvard.edu/abta
American Leukemia Society
http://www.leukemia.org
APON (Association of Pediatric Oncology Nurses)
http://www.apon.org
Cancer Guide
http://bcn.boulder.co.us/health/cancer
Cancerlink
http://dialin.ind.net/-rmarriag/rcancer.html
Case Studies (multiple different cases)
http://www-medlib.med.utah.edu/WebPath/webpath.htm
Family Support Group
http://www.squirreltales.com
National Childhood Cancer Foundation
http://www.nccf.org
Oncolink
http://www.oncolink.org
http://oncolink.upenn.edu/specialty/ped_onc *(specific to pediatric oncology)*
PedInfo (general pediatric information)
http://www.UAB.EDU/pedinfo
POG (Pediatric Oncology Group) Research Foundation for Cancer Treatment Protocols)
http://www.pog.ufl.edu
Virtual Hospital
http://vh.radiology.uiowa.edu
Virtual Patient
http://musom.marshall.edu/medicus.htm

References

Aitken, T. (1992). Gastrointestinal manifestations in the child with cancer. *Journal of Pediatric Oncology Nursing, 9*(3), 99–109.

Altman, A. J. (1993). Chronic leukemias of childhood. In P. A. Pizzo & D. G. Poplack (Eds.), *Principles and practice of pediatric oncology* (2nd ed., pp. 501–518). Philadelphia: J. B. Lippincott.

American Cancer Society. (1996). *Cancer facts and figures—1996*. Atlanta, GA: Author.

Apt, L., & Gaffney, W. L. (1987). The eyes. In A. M. Rudolph (Ed.), *Pediatrics* (18th ed., pp. 1782–1783). Norwalk, CT: Appleton & Lange.

Baehner, R. L., Kennedy, A., Sather, H., Chard, R. L., & Hammond, D. (1981). Characteristics of children with ANLL in long term continuous remission: A report from the Children's Cancer Group. *Pediatric Oncology, 9*, 393–394.

Balis, F. M., Holcenberg, J. S., & Poplack, D. G. (1993). General principles of chemotherapy. In P. A. Pizzo & D. G. Poplack (Eds.), *Principles and practice of pediatric oncology* (2nd ed., pp. 197–245). Philadelphia: J. B. Lippincott.

Baptiste, M., Nasca, P., Metzger, B., Field, N., MacCubbin, P., Greenwald, P., Armbrustmacher, V., Waldman, J., & Carlton, K. (1989). Neurofibromatosis and other disorders among children with CNS tumors and their families. *Neurology, 39,* 487–492.

Berro, E. (1993). *Retinoblastoma.* In G. Foley, D. Fochtman, & K. Hardin-Mooney (Eds.), *Nursing care of the child with cancer* (pp. 310–318). Philadelphia: W. B. Saunders.

Betcher, D. (1991). New trends in osteogenic sarcoma. *Journal of Pediatric Oncology Nursing,* 8(2), 70.

Betcher, D. (1993). *Bone tumors.* In G. Foley, D. Fochtman, & K. Hardin-Mooney (Eds.), *Nursing care of the child with cancer* (pp. 300–309). Philadelphia: W. B. Saunders.

Betcher, D., & Burnham, N. (1991). Granulocyte-macrophage colony-stimulating factor. *Journal of Pediatric Oncology Nursing,* 8(3), 134–135.

Borowitz, M. (1990). Immunologic markers in childhood acute lymphoblastic leukemia. *Hematology/Oncology Clinics of North America, 4,* 743–765.

Bossert, E., Van Cleve, L., & Savedra, M. (1996). Children with cancer: The pain experience away from the health care setting. *Journal of Pediatric Oncology Nursing, 13*(3), 109–120.

Braun, I. (1996). Varicella zoster virus: Trends and treatment. MCN, *21,* 187–190.

Britfeld, P. (1996). Acute leukemia. In F. Burg, J. Ingelfinger, E. Wald, & R. Polin (Eds.), *Current pediatric therapy 15* (pp. 303–306). Philadelphia: W. B. Saunders.

Brodeur, G. M., & Castleberry, R. P. (1993). Neuroblastoma. In P. A. Pizzo & D. G. Poplack (Eds.), *Principles and practice of pediatric oncology* (2nd ed., pp. 739–767). Philadelphia: J. B. Lippincott.

Brown, J. K., & Hogan, C. M. (1992). Chemotherapy treatment modalities, part III. In S. L. Groenwald (Ed.), *Cancer nursing* (pp. 230–271). Sudbury, MA: Jones & Bartlett.

Bryant, J., & Guinan, E. (1992). Bone marrow transplantation from A to Z. *Journal of Pediatric Oncology Nursing,* 9(2), 49.

Burke, J. (1990). The histopathologic classification for non-Hodgkin's lymphomas: Ambiguities in the working formulation and two newly reported categories. *Seminars in Oncology, 17,* 3–10.

Castro-Malespina, H., Schaison, G., Briere, J., Passe, S., Briere, J., Pasquier, A., Tanzer, J., Jacquillat, C., & Bernard, J. (1983). Philadelphia chromosome–positive CML in children: Survival and prognostic features. *Cancer, 52,* 721–727.

Chesler, M. (1990). Surviving childhood cancer: The struggle goes on. *Journal of Pediatric Oncology Nursing, 7*(2), 57–59.

Chutorian, A. M. (1987). Tumors of the central nervous system. In A. M. Rudolph (Ed.), *Pediatrics* (18th ed., pp. 1603–1616). Los Altos, CA: Appleton & Lange.

Cohen, D. (1993). Leukemia in children and adolescents. In G. Foley, D. Fochtman, & K. Hardin-Mooney (Eds.), *Nursing care of the child with cancer* (pp. 208–234). Philadelphia: W. B. Saunders.

Cohen, M. E., & Duffner, P. K. (1984). Introduction. In *Brain tumors in children: Principles of diagnosis and treatment* (International Review of Child Neurology Series). New York: Raven Press.

Crist, W. (1996). Soft tissue sarcomas. In R. Behrman, R. Kliegman, & A. Arvin (Eds.), *Nelson Textbook of Pediatrics* (pp. 1465–1467). Philadelphia: W. B. Saunders.

Crist, W., & Pui, C. (1996). The leukemias. In R. Behrman, R. Kliegman, & A. Arvin (Eds.), *Nelson Textbook of Pediatrics* (pp. 1452–1455). Philadelphia: W. B. Saunders.

D'Angio, G. J., Breslow, N., Beckwith, J. B., Evans, A., Baum, E., DeLorimer, A., Fernbach, D., Hraborsky, E., Jones, B., Kelalis, P., Otherson, B., Tefft, M., & Thomas, P. (1989). Treatment of Wilms' tumor. *Cancer, 64,* 349–360.

DeSwarte, J. (1991). Septic shock: Oncological emergency. *Journal of Pediatric Oncology Nursing,* 8(2), 66–68.

Donaldson, S. S., Egbert, P. R., & Lee, W. H. (1993). Retinoblastoma. In P. A. Pizzo & D. G. Poplack (Eds.), *Principles and practice of pediatric oncology* (2nd ed., pp. 683–696). Philadelphia: J. B. Lippincott.

Dosoretz, D. E., Blitzer, P. H., & Wang, C. L. (1980). Management of gliomas of the optic nerve and/or chiasm. *Cancer, 45,* 1467.

Drigan, R., & Androkites, A. (1993). Wilms' tumor. In G. Foley, D. Fochtman, & K. Hardin-Mooney (Eds.), *Nursing care of the child with cancer* (pp. 272–277). Philadelphia: W. B. Saunders.

Eilber, F. R. (1985). *Principles of cancer surgery.* Philadelphia: W. B. Saunders.

Eilber, F. R., & Rosen, G. (1989). Adjuvant chemotherapy for osteosarcoma. *Seminars in Oncology, 16,* 312–322.

Ellis, J. (1991). Coping with adolescent cancer: It's a matter of adaptation. *Journal of Pediatric Oncology Nursing,* 8(1), 10–17.

Fernbach, D. J., & Vietti, T. J. (1991). General aspects of childhood cancer. In D. J. Fernbach & T. J. Vietti (Eds.), *Clinical pediatric oncology* (4th ed.). St. Louis: Mosby–Year Book.

Fidler, P., Roell, S., & Wiley, F. (1993). Issues in bone marrow transplant. *Journal of Pediatric Oncology Nursing, 10*(2), 48.

Finlay, J. L., Goins, S. C., Uteg, R., & Giese, W. L. (1987). Progress in the management of childhood brain tumors. *Hematology/Oncology Clinics of North America, 1,* 753–776.

Frederick, B., & Hanigan, M. (1993). Bone marrow transplantation. In G. Foley, D. Fochtman, & K. Hardin-Mooney (Eds.), *Nursing care of the child with cancer* (pp. 130–178). Philadelphia: W. B. Saunders.

Freiberger, D., Bryant, J., & Marino, B. (1992). The effects of different central venous line dressing changes on bacterial growth in a pediatric oncology population. *Journal of Pediatric Oncology Nursing,* 9(1), 3–7.

Ghavimi, F., Mondell, L. R., Heller, G., Hajdu, S. I., & Exelby, P. (1989). Prognosis in childhood rhabdomyosarcoma of the extremity. *Cancer, 64,* 2233–2237.

Gibson, R., Broiss, I., Graham, S., et al. (1986). Leukemia in children exposed to multiple risk factors. *New England Journal of Medicine. 279,* 906–909.

Giuffre, R., Liccardo, G., Pastrol, F. S., Spallone, A., & Vagnozzi, R. (1990). Potential risk factors for brain tumors in children: An analysis of 200 cases. *Child's Nervous System,* 6, 8–12.

Gjerris, F., & Klinken, L. (1978). Long-term prognosis in children with benign cerebellar astrocytoma. *Journal of Neurosurgery, 49,* 179–184.

Graham, M. (1988). Non-Hodgkin's lymphoma. *Pediatric Annual, 17,* 192–203.

Green, D. M., D'Angio, G. J., Finklestein, J. Z., Beckwith, J. B., Breslow, N. E., Kelalis, P., & Thomas, P. R. M. (1993). Wilms' tumor (nephroblastoma, renal embryoma). In P. A. Pizzo & D. G. Poplack (Eds.), *Principles and practice of pediatric oncology* (2nd ed., pp. 483–500). Philadelphia: J. B. Lippincott.

Gross, J., & Johnson, B. (Eds.). (1994). *Handbook of oncology nursing.* Sudbury, MA: Jones & Bartlett.

Grufferman, S., Cole, P., Smith, P. G., & Lukes, R. J. (1977). Hodgkin's disease in siblings. *New England Journal of Medicine, 296,* 248–250.

Grufferman, S., Wang, H. H., & Delong, E. R. (1982). Environmental factors in the etiology of rhabdomyosarcoma in childhood. *Journal of the National Cancer Institutes, 68,* 107–113.

Gutensohn, N. M., & Shapiro, D. S. (1982). Social class risk factors among children with Hodgkin's disease. *International Journal of Cancer, 30,* 433–435.

Hall, E. J., & Cox, J. D. (1989). Physical and biologic basis of radiation therapy. In W. T. Moss & J. D. Cox (Eds.), *Radiation oncology* (pp. 1–57). St. Louis: Mosby.

Hanigan, M. (1990). Complex problems of children following allogenic bone marrow transplantation. *Journal of Pediatric Oncology Nursing, 7*(2), 73–75.

Hanigan, M., & Walter, G. (1992). Nutritional support of the child with cancer. *Journal of Pediatric Oncology Nursing,* 9(3), 110–118.

Hardin-Mooney, K. (1993). Biologic basis of childhood cancer. In G. V. Foley, D. Fochtman, & K. Hardin-Mooney (Eds.), *Nursing care of the child with cancer* (2nd ed., pp. 25–55). Philadelphia: W. B. Saunders.

Haslam, R. (1996). Brain tumors in children. In R. Behrman, R. Kliegman, & A. Arvin (Eds.), *Nelson textbook of pediatrics* (pp. 1731–1735). Philadelphia: W. B. Saunders.

Hathaway, G., & McCord, D. (1988). Autologous bone marrow transplantation in childhood cancer. *Pediatric Nursing, 14*(6), 454–456.

Hayes, F. A., Thompson, E. I., Meyer, W. H., Kun, L., Parham, D., Rao, B., Kumar, M., Hancock, M., Parvey, L., Magill, L., et al. (1989). Therapy for localized Ewing's sarcoma of bone. *Journal of Clinical Oncology,* 7, 208–213.

Haynes, A. (1990). Clinical uses of interferons, interleukins, tumor necrosis factor, monoclonal antibodies, and growth factors in patients with cancer. *Journal of Pediatric Oncology Nursing, 7*(2), 54–55.

Heiney, S., Goon-Johnson, K., Ettinger, R., & Ettinger, S. (1990). The effects of group therapy on siblings of pediatric oncology patients. *Journal of Pediatric Oncology Nursing, 7*(3), 95–100.

Heslop, H. (1996). Chronic myelogenous leukemia. In R. Behrman, R. Kliegman, & A. Arvin (Eds.), *Nelson textbook of pediatrics* (pp. 1456–1457). Philadelphia: W. B. Saunders.

Hilderley, L. J. (1992). Radiotherapy treatment modalities, part III. In S. L. Groenwald (Ed.), *Cancer nursing.* Sudbury, MA: Jones & Bartlett.

Hockenberry, M. J., Coody, D. K., & Bennett, B. S. (1990). Childhood cancers: Incidence, etiology, diagnosis and treatment. *Pediatric Nursing, 16*(3), 239–246.

Hollen, P., & Hobbie, W. (1996). Decision-making and risk behaviors of cancer-surviving adolescents and their peers. *Journal of Pediatric Oncology Nursing, 13*(3), 121–134.

Holmes, R., Keating, M. J., Cork, A., Broach, Y., Trujillo, J., Dalton, W. T., Jr., McCredie, K. B., & Freireich, E. J. (1985). A unique pattern of central nervous system leukemia in acute myelomonocytic leukemia. *Blood, 65,* 1071–1072.

Horowitz, M. E., Delaney, T. F., Malawer, M. M., & Tsokos, M. G. (1993). Ewing's sarcoma family of tumors: Ewing's sarcoma of bone and soft tissue and the peripheral primitive neuroectodermal tumors. In P. A. Pizzo & D. G. Poplack (Eds.), *Principles and practice of pediatric oncology* (2nd ed., pp. 795–821). Philadelphia: J. B. Lippincott.

Kalwinsky, D. K., Raimondy, S. C., Schell, M. J., Mirro, J., Santana, V. M., Behm, F., Danl, G., & Williams, D. (1990). Prognostic importance of cytogenetic subgroups in de novo pediatric acute nonlymphocytic leukemia. *Journal of Clinical Oncology, 8,* 75–83.

Keegan-Wells, D., & Stewart, J. (1992). The use of venous access devices in pediatric oncology nursing practice. *Journal of Pediatric Oncology Nursing,* 9(4), 159–169.

Klein, E. (1992). Premedicating children for painful invasive procedures. *Journal of Pediatric Oncology Nursing,* 9(4), 170–179.

Koocher, G. (1985). Psychological care of the child cured of cancer. *Pediatric Nursing, 11*(2), 91–93.

Korinko, A., & Yurick, A. (1997). Maintaining skin integrity during radiation therapy. *American Journal of Nursing,* 97(2), 40–44.

Kun, L. E., & Etcubanas, E. (1987). Rhabdomyosarcoma. In A. M. Rudolph (Ed.), *Pediatrics* (18th ed., pp. 1121–1123). Norwalk, CT: Appleton & Lange.

Kushner, B. H., Gilbert, F., & Helson, L. (1986). Familial neuroblastoma: Case reports, literature review, and etiologic considerations. *Cancer, 57,* 1887–1889.

Lanzkowsky, P. (1989). *Manual of pediatric hematology and oncology.* New York: Churchill Livingstone.

Lavezzo, S. (1990). Assessment and intervention of acute side effects of chemotherapy. *Journal of Pediatric Oncology Nursing,* 7(2), 66–67.

Leventhal, B. G., & Donaldson, S. S. (1993). Hodgkin's disease. In P. A. Pizzo & D. G. Poplack (Eds.), *Principles and practice of pediatric oncology* (2nd ed., pp. 577–594). Philadelphia: J. B. Lippincott.

Li, F. P., & Fraumeni, T. F., Jr. (1969). Rhabdomyosarcoma in children: Epidemiologic study and identification of familial cancer syndrome. *Journal of the National Cancer Institutes, 43,* 1365–1373.

Li, F. P., & Fraumeni, T. F., Jr. (1982). Prospective study of a family cancer syndrome. *Journal of the American Medical Association, 247,* 2692–2694.

Liebhauser, P. (1993). Hodgkin's disease. In G. V. Foley, D. Fochtman, & K. Hardin-Mooney (Eds.), *Nursing care of the child with cancer* (2nd ed., pp. 254–263). Philadelphia: W. B. Saunders.

Lilley, L. (1990). Side effects associated with pediatric chemotherapy: Management and patient education issues. *Pediatric Nursing, 16*(3), 252–255, 272.

Link, M. P., & Eilber, F. (1993). Osteosarcoma. In P. A. Pizzo & D. G. Poplack (Eds.), *Principles and practice of pediatric oncology* (2nd ed., pp. 841–866). Philadelphia: J. B. Lippincott.

Lister, T. A., Crowther, D., Sutcliffe, S. B., Glatstein, E., Canellos, G. P., Young, R. C., Rosenberg, S. A., Coltman, C. A., & Tubiana, M. (1989). Report of a committee convened to discuss the evaluation and staging of patients with Hodgkin's disease: Cotswold meetings. *Journal of Clinical Oncology, 7,* 1630–1636.

Look, A. T., Hayes, F. A., Shuster, J. J., Douglass, E. C., Castleberry, R. P., Bowman, L. C., Smith, I. E., & Brodeur, G. (1991). Clinical relevance of tumor cell ploidy and n-*myc* gene amplification in childhood neuroblastoma. *Journal of Clinical Oncology,* 9, 581–582.

Magrath, I. (1993). Malignant non-Hodgkin's lymphomas in children. In P. A. Pizzo & D. G. Poplack (Eds.), *Principles and practice of pediatric oncology* (2nd ed., pp. 537–575). Philadelphia: J. B. Lippincott.

Magrath, I. T., & Sariban, E. (1985). Clinical features of Burkitt's lymphoma in the USA. *Proceedings. Burkitt's lymphoma: A human cancer model* (pp. 119–127). Lyon, France: IARC Publications.

Marcoux, C., Fisher, S., & Wong, D. (1990). Central venous access devices in children. *Pediatric Nursing, 16*(2), 123–133.

Martinson, I. (1993). Hospice care for children: Past, present, and future. *Journal of Pediatric Oncology Nursing, 10*(3), 93–98.

Martinson, I., Davis, A., Liu-Chiang, C., Yi-Hua, L., Quia, J., & Gan, M. (1995). Chinese mothers' reactions to their child's chronic illness. *Health Care Women International, 16*(4), 365–375.

Maurer, H. M., & Ragab, A. H. (1991). Rhabdomyosarcoma. In D. J. Fernbach & T. J. Vietti (Eds.), *Clinical pediatric oncology* (4th ed.). St. Louis: Mosby–Year Book.

McCarthy, A., Cool, V., Patersen, M., & Bruene, D. (1996). Cognitive behavioral pain and anxiety interventions in pediatric oncology centers and bone marrow transplant units. *Journal of Pediatric Oncology Nursing, 13*(1), 3–12.

McGuire, P. (1990). New approaches in the treatment of children with central nervous system tumors. *Journal of Pediatric Oncology Nursing, 7*(2), 59–61.

McKeen, E. A., Bodurtha, J., Meadows, A. T., Douglass, E. C., & Mulvihill, J. J. (1978). Rhabdomyosarcoma complicating multiple neurofibromatosis. *Journal of Pediatrics, 93,* 992–993.

Meadows, A. (1985). Second malignant neoplasms. *Clinical Oncology,* 4, 247–261.

Meeske, K., Chamberlin, K., Cipkala-Gaffin, J., Harlander, C., & Reed, K. (1991). Measles epidemic: Impact on pediatric oncology patients. *Journal of Pediatric Oncology Nursing,* 8(4), 151–158.

Meyer, W. (1996). Neoplasms of the bone. In R. Behrman, R. Kliegman, & A. Arvin (Eds.), *Nelson textbook of pediatrics* (pp. 1467–1468). Philadelphia: W. B. Saunders.

Meyer, W., & Marina, N. (1996). Ewing sarcoma/peripheral neuroepithelioma. In R. Behrman, R. Kliegman, & A. Arvin (Eds.), *Nelson textbook of pediatrics* (pp. 1468–1470). Philadelphia: W. B. Saunders.

Meyers, P. (1987). Malignant bone tumors in children: Osteosarcoma. *Hematology/Oncology Clinics of North America, 1,* 655–665.

Morris-Jones, P. H., & Craft, A. W. (1990). Childhood cancer: Cure at what cost? *Archives of Disease in Childhood, 65,* 638–640.

Moss, T. J., Reynolds, C. P., Sather, H. N., Romansky, S. G., Hammond, G. D., & Seeger, R. C. (1991). Prognostic value of immunologic detection of bone marrow metastasis in neuroblastoma. *New England Journal of Medicine, 324,* 219.

Munet-Vilaró, F., & Vessey, J. (1990). Children's explanation of leukemia: A Hispanic perspective. *Journal of Pediatric Nursing,* 5(4), 274–282.

Nagengast, S. (1993). The use of Emla cream to reduce and/or eliminate procedural pain in children. *Journal of Pediatric Nursing,* 8(6), 406–407.

National Cancer Institute. (1996). *Cancer rates and risks* (NIH Publication No. 96–691). Bethesda, MD: Author.

Neglia, J. P., & Robinson, L. L. (1988). Epidemiology of childhood acute leukemia. *Pediatric Clinics of North America, 35,* 675–692.

Newton, W. A., Meadows, A. T., Shimada, H., Bunin, G. R., & Vawter, G. F. (1991). Bone sarcomas as second malignant neoplasms following childhood cancer. *Cancer, 67,* 193–201.

Overbaugh, K., & Sawin, K. (1992). Future life expectations and self-esteem of the adolescent survivor of childhood cancer. *Journal of Pediatric Oncology Nursing,* 9(1), 8–16.

Oxenhandler, D. C., & Sayers, M. P. (1978). The dilemma of childhood optic gliomas. *Journal of Neurosurgery, 48,* 34.

Panzarella, C., & Duncan, J. (1993). Nursing management of physical care needs. In G. Foley, D. Fochtman, & K. Hardin-Mooney (Eds.), *Nursing care of the child with cancer* (pp. 335–352). Philadelphia: W. B. Saunders.

Patterson, K. (1992). Pain in the pediatric oncology patient. *Journal of Pediatric Oncology Nursing,* 9(3), 119–130.

Pederson, C. (1996). Promoting parental use of nonpharmacologic techniques with children during a lumbar puncture. *Journal of Pediatric Oncology Nursing, 13(1),* 21–30.

Petriccione, M. (1993). Central nervous system tumors. In G. Foley, D. Fochtman, & K. Hardin Mooney (Eds.), *Nursing care of the child with cancer* (pp. 239–253). Philadelphia: W. B. Saunders.

Pizzo, P. A., & Poplack, D. G. (Eds.). (1997). *Principles and practice of pediatric oncology* (3rd ed.). Philadelphia: J. B. Lippincott.

Poplack, D. G. (1997). Acute lymphoblastic leukemia. In P. A. Pizzo & D. G. Poplack (Eds.), *Principles and practice of pediatric oncology* (3rd ed., pp. 431–481). Philadelphia: J. B. Lippincott.

Pratt, C. (1996). Retinoblastoma. In R. Behrman, R. Kliegman, & A. Arvin (Eds.), *Nelson textbook of pediatrics* (pp. 1470–1471). Philadelphia: W. B. Saunders.

Quinlan, N. (1993). Non-Hodgkin's lymphoma. In G. Foley, D. Fochtman, & K. Hardin-Mooney (Eds.), *Nursing care of the child with cancer.* (2nd ed., pp. 264–271). Philadelphia: W. B. Saunders.

Raney, R. B., Hays, D. M., Tefft, M., & Triche, T. J. (1993). Rhabdomyosarcoma and the undifferentiated sarcomas. In P. A. Pizzo & D. G. Poplack (Eds.), *Principles and practice of pediatric oncology* (2nd ed., pp. 769–791). Philadelphia: J. B. Lippincott.

Rasco, C. (1992). Using music therapy as distraction during lumbar punctures. *Journal of Pediatric Oncology Nursing,* 9(1), 33–34.

Reeve, A. E., Sih, S. A., Raizis, A. M., & Feinberg, A. P. (1989). Loss of allelic heterozygosity at a second locus on chromosome 11 in sporadic Wilms' tumor cells. *Molecular Cellular Biology, 9,* 1799–1803.

Renick-Ettinger, A. (1993). Chemotherapy. In G. Foley, D. Fochtman, & K. Hardin-Mooney (Eds.), *Nursing care of the child with cancer* (pp. 81–116). Philadelphia: W. B. Saunders.

Rogers, P. (1992). Late effects in childhood cancer survivors. *Journal of Pediatric Nursing, 7*(5), 364–366.

Sanders, J. E., Thomas, E. D., Buckner, C. D., Flournoy, N., Stewart, P. S., Clift, R. A., Lum, L., Bensinger, W. I., Storb, R., Applebaum, F. R., & Sullivan, K. M. (1985). Marrow transplantation of children in first remission of ANLL: An update. *Blood, 66,* 460–461.

Sandlund, J. (1996). Non-Hodgkins lymphoma. In R. Behrman, R. Kliegman, & A. Arvin (Eds.), *Nelson textbook of pediatrics* (pp. 1459–1460). Philadelphia: W. B. Saunders.

Santana, V. (1996). Neuroblastoma. In R. Behrman, R. Kliegman, & A. Arvin (Eds.), *Nelson textbook of pediatrics* (pp. 1460–1463). Philadelphia: W. B. Saunders.

Sauer, R., Jurgens, H., & Burger, J. M. V. (1987). Prognostic factors in the treatment of Ewing's sarcoma. *Radiotherapy Oncology, 10,* 101.

Shapiro, S., Mealey, J., Jr., & Sartorius, C. (1989). Radiation-induced intracranial malignant gliomas. *Journal of Neurosurgery, 71,* 77–82.

Shearer, P., & Wilimas, J. (1996). Neoplasms of the kidney. In R. Behrman, R. Kliegman, & A. Arvin (Eds.), *Nelson textbook of pediatrics* (pp. 1463–1465). Philadelphia: W. B. Saunders.

Sullivan, M. (1993). Neuroblastoma. In G. Foley, D. Fochtman, & K. Hardin-Mooney (Eds.), *Nursing care of the child with cancer* (pp. 278–287). Philadelphia: W. B. Saunders.

Sutters, K., & Miaskowski, C. (1992). The problem of pain in children with cancer: A research review. *Oncology Nurses Foundation,* 19(3), 465–471.

Tan, C. T. C. (1989). Hodgkin's disease in children and adolescents: Experiences from Memorial Sloan-Kettering Cancer Center, New York. In W. A. Kamps, G. B. Humphrey, & S. Poppema (Eds.), *Hodgkin's disease in children: Controversial and current practice* (pp. 291–302). Boston: Kluwer Academic.

Tenny, R. T., Laws, E. R., Younge, B. R., & Rush, J. A. (1982). The neurosurgical management of optic glioma. *Journal of Neurosurgery, 57,* 452.

Thompson, E. I. (1991). Hodgkin's disease. In D. J. Fernbach & T. J. Vietti (Eds.), *Clinical pediatric oncology* (4th ed.) (pp. 355–375). St. Louis: Mosby–Year Book.

Thurber, F. W., Deatrich, J. A., & Grey, M. (1992). Children's participation in research: Their right to consent. *Journal of Pediatric Nursing,* 7(3), 165–170.

U.S. Department of Labor, Office of Occupational Medicine: Occupational Safety and Health Administration. (1986). *Work practice guidelines for personnel dealing with cytotoxic (antineoplastic) drugs* (OSHA Publication No. 8-1.1). Washington, DC: U.S. Government Printing Office.

Veninga, K. (1985). Improving nutrition in children with cancer. *Pediatric Nursing, 11*(1), 18–20.

Wiley, F. (1993). Acute myelogenous leukemia. In G. Foley, D. Fochtman, & K. Hardin-Mooney (Eds.), *Nursing care of the child with cancer* (pp. 226–234). Philadelphia: W. B. Saunders.

Woods, W. (1993). Neuroblastoma screening. *Journal of Pediatric Oncology Nursing, 10*(2), 53–54.

Bibliography

Ablin, A. (1993). *Supportive care of children with cancer: Current therapy and guidelines from the Children's Cancer Group.* Baltimore: Johns Hopkins University Press.

Baysinger, M., Heiney, S., Creed, J., & Ettinger, R. (1993). A trajectory approach for education of the child/adolescent with cancer. *Journal of Pediatric Oncology Nursing, 10*(4), 133–138.

Cornwell, C. (1990). The Ommaya reservoir: Implications for pediatric oncology. *Pediatric Nursing, 16*(3), 249–251.

Crist, W. M., & Kun, L. E. (1991). Common solid tumors of childhood. *New England Journal of Medicine, 324,* 1295.

Dufour, D. (1990). Information for teachers of children with central venous catheters. *Journal of Pediatric Oncology Nursing, 7*(1), 37–38.

Foley, G., Fochtman, D., & Hardin-Mooney, K. (1993). *Nursing care of the child with cancer* (2nd ed.). Association of Pediatric Nurses. Philadelphia: W. B. Saunders.

Frierdich, S. (1991). Back to the future: Biologic response modifiers and colony-stimulating factors. *Journal of Pediatric Oncology Nursing,* 8(2), 72–75.

Hanigan, M. (1991). Unrelated bone marrow transplantation: Past, present and future. *Journal of Pediatric Oncology Nursing,* 8(2), 80–81.

Hanigan, M. (1992). Unrelated bone marrow transplantation and the national marrow donor program: An update. *Journal of Pediatric Oncology Nursing,* 9(2), 71–75.

Lee, L. (1991). Ethical issues related to research involving children. *Journal of Pediatric Oncology Nursing,* 8(1), 24–29.

Murray, J. S. (1995). Social support for siblings of children with cancer. *Journal of Pediatric Oncology Nursing, 12(2),* 62–70.

Rechner, M. (1990). Adolescents with cancer: Getting on with life. *Journal of Pediatric Oncology Nursing, 7*(4), 139–144.

Ruccione, K. S. (1994). Informed consent in pediatric oncology: A nursing perspective. *Journal of Pediatric Oncology Nursing, 11*(3), 128–133.

Weekes, D., Kagan, S., James, K., & Seboni, N. (1993). The phenomenon of hand holding as a coping strategy in adolescents experiencing treatment-related pain. *Journal of Pediatric Oncology Nursing, 10*(1), 19–25.

Wofford, L. (1987). "Cured" . . . now what? *Pediatric Nursing, 13*(4), 252–254.

HEALTH CHALLENGE:

Alterations in Hematologic Status

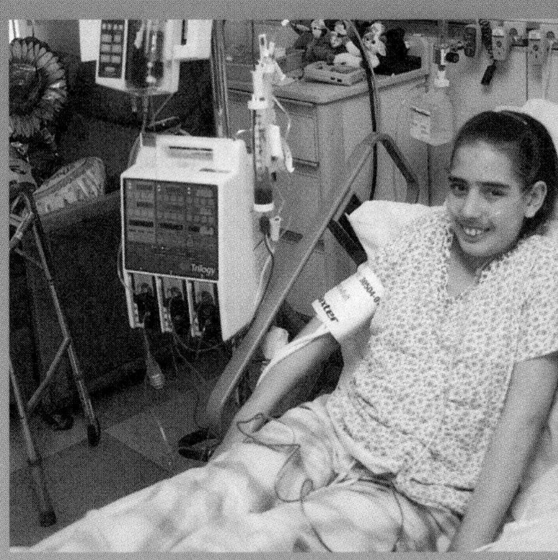

OUTLINE

OBJECTIVES

- Describe how assessment data are used to identify and manage bleeding disorders, hemoglobinopathies, and anemias in children.
- Discuss the role of the health care team in preparing children and families for various diagnostic studies that aid in identification and management of hematologic disorders.
- Summarize the interventions of the health care team during transfusion therapy.
- Discuss the rationale for the interdisciplinary interventions used in managing pediatric hematologic alterations.
- Describe the nursing care of children with bleeding disorders, hemoglobinopathies, and anemias.

KEY TERMS

Absolute neutrophil count (ANC)
anemia
coagulopathy
erythropoiesis
Heinz bodies
hematemesis
hematochezia
hematocrit
hematoma
hematopoiesis
hematuria
hemoglobin
hemoglobin A
hemoglobin A_2
hemoglobin F
hemolysis
Howell-Jolly bodies
neutropenia
pancytopenia
polycythemia
stem cell
thrombocytopenia

CHAPTER

23

A healthy hematologic system is essential to overall well-being. Conversely, alterations in hematologic status may result in serious illness and death. Composed of blood-forming organs, plasma, blood cells, and blood vessels, the hematologic system is responsible for transporting essential elements to, and waste products from, cells throughout the body. The hematologic system has a significant role in hemostasis (blood clotting), immunity, and heat regulation.

There are a number of ways in which the hematologic system may deviate from normal among children and adolescents. This chapter discusses the more significant hematologic alterations that can affect the young. In addition, this chapter provides information to enhance the nurse's role in collaborating with the interdisciplinary health care team as, together, they work toward patient and family outcomes that will correct or minimize the effects of pediatric hematologic disorders.

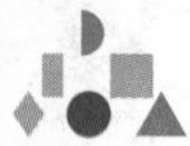

Assessment of Hematologic Status

Alterations in hematologic status can affect the function of multiple body systems, besides the hematologic system. Thus, when acquiring the health history and physical assessment data, consider not only the hematologic abnormalities but also how these abnormalities may alter other physiologic processes. In addition, be aware of normal hematologic developmental and biological variances when assessing children and adolescents, because what is normal at one age may be abnormal at another age.

Focused Health History

A focused health history contributes significant information for making a diagnosis of a particular hematologic disorder. Components of this health history are identified in Chart 23–1.

Worldview: *The child's identifying data are important because some hematologic diagnoses are more commonly associated with a certain age group, sex, race, or geographic location. Examples include, respectively, iron deficiency anemia during late infancy and adolescence, hemophilia in males, sickle cell disease among blacks, and thalassemia among those whose ancestral roots are in the Mediterranean part of the world. In addition, knowledge of the child's religious background is important because some religious groups may not consent to health care, or they may refuse specific recommended interventions. Jehovah's Witnesses, for example, may not consent to the use of blood or blood products, even in life-threatening situations. In the absence of parental consent, a court order is required to permit the health care team to give needed transfusions to a minor.*

Hematologic alterations may affect multiple body sites. Thus, in addition to obtaining a description of the perceived health problem from the child and family, ask the family for information that may identify abnormalities involving the integumentary, respiratory, cardiovascular, gastrointestinal, genitourinary, reproductive, musculoskeletal, and neurologic systems.

The past health history is of great importance in identifying factors that may point to, or rule out, specific hematologic disorders. Begin with the birth history and proceed on to the child's current age. Ask about bleeding, anemia, and infection. For each occurrence of these health alterations, identify the child's age, prescribed treatment, and subsequent course of events. When inquiring about previous health challenges, especially note instances of abnormal bleeding and delayed wound healing associated with accidental and surgical wounds. In addition, note normal wound healing after scalp lacerations, extraction of teeth, tonsillectomy, and adenoidectomy because normal healing of these wounds is highly dependent on efficient hemostasis. In contrast, surgical wounds resulting from herniorrhaphy and appendectomy tend to be less taxing to the coagulative processes (Grabowski & Corrigan, 1995).

When reviewing childhood illnesses, make particular note of infections, as these are frequently responsible for hematologic alterations in children. Also note the child's immunization history, because vaccines have been associated with hematologic disorders on occasion. In addition, note the presence of allergies, as these may cause hematologic alterations, particularly eosinophilia.

The child's nutritional status and dietary habits provide helpful data for assessing and managing hematologic disorders that may be associated with nutritional deficiencies. Examples include iron deficiency anemia and megaloblastic anemia. In addition, the child's environmental history may be significant. For examples, exposure to certain chemicals may precede the onset of aplastic anemia; pica with the ingestion of lead-containing products may result in lead poisoning and subsequent anemia; decreased humidification in the home may lead to epistaxis. Also, if the child has lived in or visited other countries, there may have been exposure to infectious agents not common in the United States. The dengue virus, for example, found in Southeast Asia, Central America, and South America, may interfere with normal hematopoiesis (Miller & O'Reilly, 1995).

The family medical history and the social history provide data that may be significant in establishing the diagnosis of a hereditary hematologic disorder. Family history data may indicate familial predispositions to certain hematologic alterations such as hemophilia, von Willebrand's disease, sickle cell disease, thalassemia, and hereditary spherocytosis. Inquire about the presence of hematologic abnormalities in parents, siblings, aunts, uncles, cousins, and relatives from preceding generations. Note the name or description of the hematologic disorder and the relationship of the affected family member to the child. In addition, note if the child is the offspring of a consanguineous relationship. Consanguinity is associated with a higher incidence of certain hematologic disorders such as aplastic anemia (Miller & O'Reilly, 1995).

When a chronic hematologic disorder such as hemophilia or sickle cell disease has been diagnosed, the ongoing health care history should be carefully noted with regard to compliance with, and response to, the recommended interdisciplinary interventions. Also, note the development and management of long-term sequelae, as well as the incidence and course of events associated with acute health problems.

Chart 23-1
Focused Health History

Hematologic Status	
Identifying Data	Birthdate Place of birth Sex Race Religion
Present Illness	Description of current health problem and time of onset
Past Medical History	Birth history Abnormal blood tests • Coombs' test • Blood cell profile (CBC) Bleeding problems • Umbilical cord • Circumcision site Infection Jaundice Hemolytic anemia Prematurity Previous health challenges Epistaxis or other bleeding episodes and their precipitating event Surgical procedures, including dental extractions Soft tissue abscesses Traumatic injuries HIV or immunologic disorder Leukemia or malignant tumor
	Receipt of blood or blood products • Note any adverse reactions • Note use of premedication

Chart continued on following page

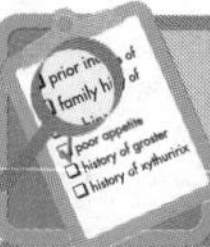

Chart 23–1
Focused Health History *Continued*

Hematologic Status

Past Medical History *Continued*	Childhood illnesses Influenza, chickenpox, hepatitis, mononucleosis, or other infectious diseases Helminth infestation Immunizations Are immunizations up to date? Date and type of most recent immunization Allergies Allergies to food, drugs, plants, animals, and so on
Current Medications	All medications child currently takes • Prescribed medications • Over-the-counter medications • Folk remedies • "Street" drugs Particularly note the use of aspirin, aspirin-containing medications, nonsteroidal anti-inflammatory drugs (NSAIDs), anticoagulants, or other medications that may alter the hematologic status
Nutritional Assessment	Decreased weight Decreased appetite Dietary habits; particularly note amount of milk, meat, and vegetables Vitamin and mineral dietary supplements; particularly note ascorbic acid
Family Medical History	Family history of bruising, bleeding, anemia, thrombosis, neutropenia, immune disorder Family history of specific hematologic disorder such as hemophilia, von Willebrand's disease, immune (idiopathic) thrombocytopenia purpura (ITP), or sickle cell disease Pregnancy history of mother, especially when pregnant with this child; note infections, anemia, nutritional deficiencies, and medications

Chart 23-1
Focused Health History *Continued*

Hematologic Status	
Environmental History	Exposure to chemicals, insects, animals, or helminths Ingestion of lead from laundry starch, lead paint, and so on Lead-based paint in home Decreased humidification in home
Social History	Ethnicity and geographic origin of ancestors Consanguinous marriages or partnerships Name of home town and previous places of residence Recent travel; especially note travel to other countries Beliefs about health care; especially note beliefs related to the use of blood and blood products
Growth and Development	Daily activities • Play • Sleep • School • Social Child's activities for a typical day and any recent changes in these activities

Focused Physical Assessment

Although a specific hematologic disorder is usually identified or confirmed by laboratory studies, the physical assessment contributes significant information for determining which laboratory studies are needed. Physical assessment data aid in the management of the child with a hematologic disorder.

Pediatric hematologic alterations are usually characterized by:

- Atypical hemostasis
- Anemia
- Neutropenia

These abnormalities may occur separately or together, and because they can affect multiple body systems, physical assessment must include multiple body sites. Physical alterations may be associated with bleeding disorders, anemia, and neutropenia (Chart 23–2).

The skin is a primary source of information about the hematologic system. Often it is the first site to provide clinical evidence of a hematologic alteration. Documenting normal findings and noting the location and description of abnormal findings provide data that help to rule out or identify specific hematologic alterations. For example, random areas of ecchymoses are typical of a platelet disorder, whereas severe bruising to specific areas, such as the head or buttocks, indicates the need to evaluate the child for possible abuse.

The complete documentation of physical findings provides information that may point to, or rule out, specific hematologic disorders. Follow-up physical assessment findings are important as well. They provide information for evaluating the response to treatment and contribute data that are helpful in planning for ongoing health care needs.

For the child with a chronic hematologic disorder, be alert for changes that may occur with disease or long-term treatment. For example, document the onset and development of cardiac abnormalities in the child with chronic anemia secondary to sickle cell disease or thalassemia. Also, document cardiac abnormalities in the child who has acquired iron overload secondary to blood transfusion therapy.

Text continued on page 1525

Chart 23–2
Focused Physical Assessment

Hematologic Status

Children may be at increased risk for physical alterations in various body systems secondary to bleeding disorders, anemia, and neutropenia.

Body System	Bleeding Disorders	Anemia	Neutropenia
Integumentary	Easy bruising • Petechiae • Ecchymoses • Purpura Bleeding from: • Wounds • Line sites • Invasive procedure sites Bleeding from: • Telangiectatic lesions • Hemorrhagic bullae	Pallor Jaundice Bronzed skin Waxy skin "Spoon nails" Lower extremity ulcers Hyperpigmentation	Skin lesions Skin breakdown at: • Skin folds • Perianal area Cutaneous cellulitis Abscesses Wound infections at: • Line sites • Procedure sites • Surgical sites • Trauma sites
Respiratory	Epistaxis Hemoptysis Dyspnea Wet cough	Tachypnea Dyspnea	Tachypnea Sinusitis Pharyngitis Bronchitis Pneumonia
Cardiovascular	Tachycardia Hypotension	Tachycardia Decreased diastolic blood pressure Palpitations Arrhythmias Murmurs Ankle edema Enlarged heart Congestive heart failure Hypoxia	Tachycardia Septicemia Septic shock Endovascular infections, for example, at site of central venous access device

Gastrointestinal	Oral petechiae Bleeding from mouth lesions Hematemesis Hematochezia Melena	Anorexia Angular stomatitis Glossitis Hepatomegaly	Stomatitis Periodontal disease Esophagitis Hepatitis Enterocolitis
Genitourinary	Hematuria Hemorrhagic cystitis		Urinary tract infection
Reproductive	Menorrhagia	Delayed secondary sex characteristics	
Musculoskeletal	Hematoma Hemarthroses leading to: • Joint deformities • Decreased range of motion • Muscular atrophy	Fatigue Weakness Decreased activity Skeletal abnormalities Abnormal facies • Frontal bossing • Prominence of malar and maxillary bones	Abscesses
Neurologic	Headache Scleral or conjunctival bleeding Retinal hemorrhage Intracranial hemorrhage Focal neurologic changes Seizures Altered level of consciousness	Headache Dizziness Retinal pallor Decreased concentration Irritability Listlessness Confusion Altered sleep pattern Altered level of consciousness	Otitis media Meningitis Encephalitis Brain abscess Altered level of consciousness

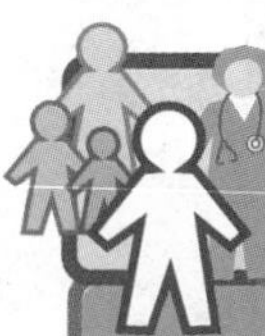

Chart 23–3
Nursing Diagnoses and Outcomes

Disorders in Hemostasis

- Knowledge deficit related to bleeding disorder
  Outcome: Child/family identify the child's specific bleeding disorder, its clinical manifestations, and its management.
- Risk for injury related to bleeding
  Outcomes: Child/family identify common types of bleeding associated with the child's particular bleeding disorder.
  Child/family identify signs and symptoms associated with overt and covert bleeding.
  Child/family describe interventions needed for bleeding episodes.
  Child maintains normal tissue perfusion to all body systems.
  Child maintains laboratory values consistent with normal hemostasis.
  Child/family state the importance of notifying health care workers about the child's bleeding disorder before surgery or other procedures.
  Child/family select activities for the child that are unlikely to cause bleeding.
  Child/family notify school and child care personnel of any limitations in the child's activities.
  Child/family inform school and child care personnel of appropriate interventions to use if the child has a bleeding episode.
- Fear related to blood loss and possible impairment of body functions
  Outcome: Child/family verbalize concerns regarding blood loss and impaired body functions, and receive informational and emotional support.
- Risk for altered parenting related to child's chronic bleeding disorder
  Outcomes: Parents identify normal developmental milestones and their role in helping the child achieve these milestones.
  Parents use nonphysical disciplinary measures for the child.

Anemias

- Knowledge deficit related to anemia
  Outcomes: Child/family define anemia.
  Child/family identify the reason for the child's anemia and describe the clinical management of the particular disorder.
- Risk for injury related to anemia
  Outcomes: Child/family identify short-term and long-term effects of impaired tissue oxygenation caused by anemia.
  Child/family identify measures to correct and prevent anemia, in general, and the child's anemia, in particular.
  Child/family select activities for the child that help to conserve energy during times of anemia.
  Child responds to measures to correct anemia.
  Child/family identify signs and symptoms of anemia and the need to report these promptly.
- Risk for injury related to receiving transfused blood
  Outcomes: Child receives blood that is compatible with his or her blood type.
  Child does not experience hemolytic, febrile, or allergic reactions.
  Child requiring an ongoing transfusion program does not acquire cardiac abnormalities secondary to iron overload.
- Risk for altered parenting when child has chronic anemia
  Outcomes: Parents identify normal developmental milestones and their role in helping the child achieve these milestones.
  Parents use appropriate disciplinary measures for the child.

Figure 23–1
Developmental and biological variances: hematologic system.

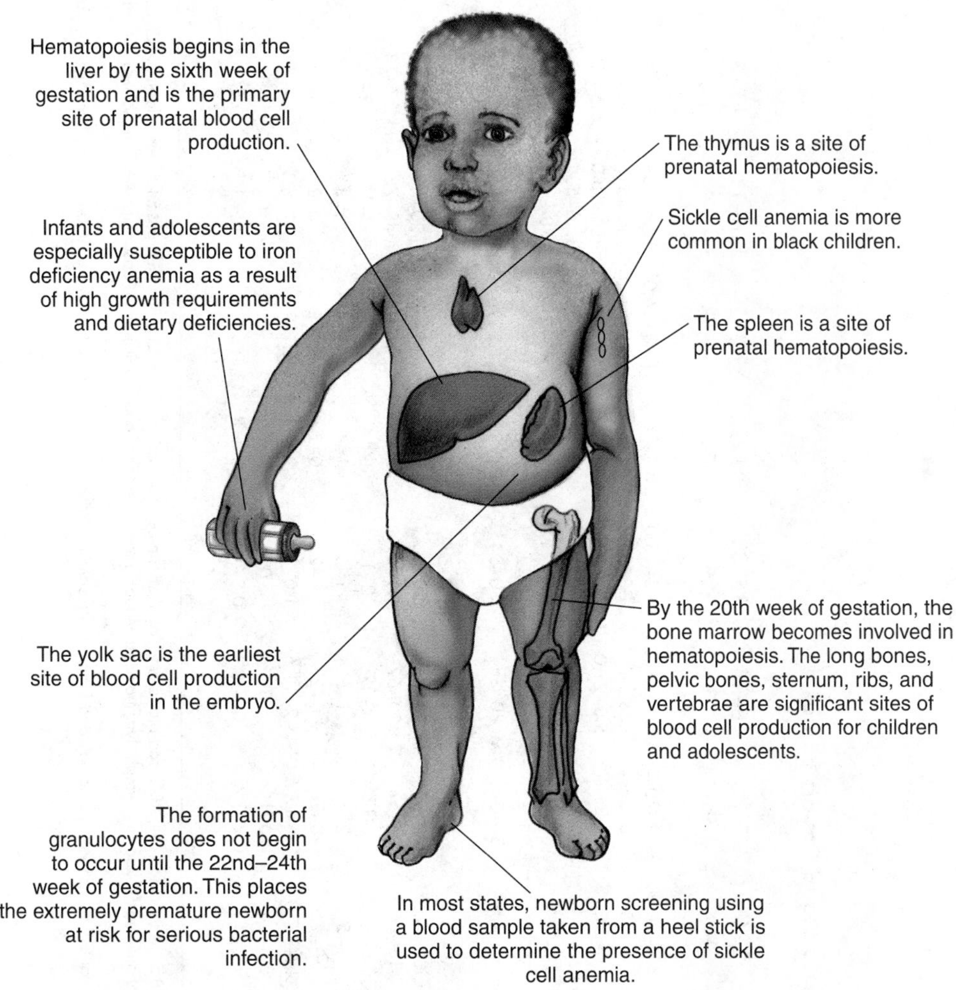

Hematopoiesis begins in the liver by the sixth week of gestation and is the primary site of prenatal blood cell production.
The thymus is a site of prenatal hematopoiesis.
Infants and adolescents are especially susceptible to iron deficiency anemia as a result of high growth requirements and dietary deficiencies.
Sickle cell anemia is more common in black children.
The spleen is a site of prenatal hematopoiesis.
By the 20th week of gestation, the bone marrow becomes involved in hematopoiesis. The long bones, pelvic bones, sternum, ribs, and vertebrae are significant sites of blood cell production for children and adolescents.
The yolk sac is the earliest site of blood cell production in the embryo.
The formation of granulocytes does not begin to occur until the 22nd–24th week of gestation. This places the extremely premature newborn at risk for serious bacterial infection.
In most states, newborn screening using a blood sample taken from a heel stick is used to determine the presence of sickle cell anemia.

Table 23–1
Blood Cell Profile (Complete Blood Count) Values

Test/Units	0–1 d	2–4 d	5–7 d	8–14 d	15–30 d	1–2 mo	3–5 mo	6–11 mo	1–3 y	4–7 y	8–13 y	Adult female	Adult male
Hgb (g/dL)	16.5–21.5	16.4–20.8	15.2–20.4	15.0–19.6	12.2–18.0	10.6–16.4	10.4–16.0	10.4–15.6	9.6–15.6	10.2–15.2	12.0–15.0	12.0–15.0	14.0–18.0
Hct (%)	48–68	48–68	50–64	46–62	38–53	32–50	35–51	35–51	34–48	34–48	35–49	35–49	40–54
WBC (× 10^3/mm^3)	9.0–37.0	8.0–24.0	5.0–21.0	5.0–21.0	5.0–21.0	6.0–18.0	6.0–18.0	6.0–18.0	5.5–17.5	5.0–17.0	4.5–13.5	4.5–11.5	4.5–11.5
RBC (× 10^6/mm^3)	4.10–6.10	4.36–5.96	4.20–5.80	4.00–5.60	3.20–5.00	3.40–5.00	3.65–5.05	3.60–5.20	3.40–5.20	4.00–5.20	4.00–5.40	4.00–5.40	4.60–6.00
MCV (fL)	95–125	98–118	100–120	95–115	93–113	83–107	83–107	78–102	76–92	78–94	80–94	80–94	80–94
MCH (pg)	30–42	30–42	30–42	30–42	28–40	27–37	25–35	23–31	23–31	23–31	26–32	26–32	26–32
MCHC (%)	30–34	30–34	30–34	30–34	30–34	31–37	32–36	32–36	32–36	32–36	32–36	32–36	32–36
RDW							11.5%–14.5%						
Bands (%)	4–14	3–11	3–9	1–9	0–5	0–5	0–5	0–5	0–5	0–5	0–5	0–5	0–5
Polys (%)	37–67	30–60	27–51	22–46	20–40	20–40	18–38	20–40	22–46	30–60	35–65	50–70	50–70
Lymph (%)	18–38	16–46	24–54	30–62	41–61	42–72	45–75	48–78	37–73	29–65	23–53	18–42	18–42
Monos (%)	1–12	3–14	4–17	4–17	2–15	3–14	2–11	2–11	2–11	2–11	2–11	2–11	2–11
Eos (%)	1–4	1–5	2–6	1–5	1–5	1–4	1–4	1–4	1–4	1–4	1–4	1–3	1–3
Baso (%)	0–2	0–2	0–2	0–2	0–2	0–2	0–2	0–2	0–2	0–2	0–2	0–2	0–2
ANC × 10^3	3.7–30.0	2.6–17.0	1.5–12.6	1.2–11.6	1.0–9.5	1.2–8.1	1.1–7.7	1.2–8.1	1.2–8.9	1.5–11.0	1.6–9.5	2.3–8.6	2.3–8.6
NRBC/100 WBC	2–24	5–9	0–1	0	0	0	0	0	0	0	0	0	0
Retic (%)	1.8–5.8	1.3–4.7	0.2–1.4	0–1.0	0.2–1.0	0.8–2.8	0.5–1.5	0.5–1.5	0.5–1.5	0.5–1.5	0.5–1.5	0.5–1.5	0.5–1.5
Plts (× 10^3/mm^3)							150–450						

Hgb, hemoglobin; Hct, hematocrit; WBC, white blood cell; RBC, red blood cell; MCV, mean corpuscular volume; MCH, mean corpuscular hemoglobin; MCHC, mean corpuscular hemoglobin concentration; RDW, red cell distribution width; Polys, polymorphonuclear leukocytes; Lymph, lymphocytes; Monos, monocytes; Eos, eosinophils; Baso, basophils; ANC, absolute neutrophil count; NRBC, nucleated red blood cell; Retic, reticulocytes; Plts, platelets.

Adapted from Indiana University Medical Center. (1994). *Pathology and laboratory medicine: Handbook of services.* Hudson, OH: Lexi-Comp. Used with permission.

Nursing Diagnoses and Outcomes

The primary foci of health care interventions for pediatric hematologic alterations are (1) to prevent injury to the affected child, and (2) to provide the child and family with a strong knowledge base about the disorder, crisis prevention, and supportive measures. Chart 23–3 summarizes the nursing diagnoses and outcomes that might be applicable to the child experiencing a disorder of hemostasis or a form of anemia.

Developmental and Biological Variances

The hematologic system begins early in fetal development. By the third week of gestation, blood islands are evident in the yolk sac. The peripheral cells of the blood islands become blood vessel walls in the developing embryo, while the central cells of the blood islands become the embryo's primitive blood cells. By the fourth week of gestation, circulation is evident.

The liver shows evidence of hematopoiesis by the sixth week of gestation and becomes the major site of blood cell production during the prenatal period. Also, the spleen, thymus, and lymph nodes engage in hematopoiesis in the developing fetus.

About the 20th week of gestation, the bone marrow becomes involved in blood cell production. It is the primary site of hematopoiesis during the childhood and adult years (Fig. 23–1).

Stem Cell

The stem cell is the earliest stage in the development of all blood cells. Hematopoiesis depends on the stem cell for two major reasons: (1) The stem cell can differentiate to form progenitor (or precursor) cells for red blood cells, white blood cells, and platelets, and (2) the stem cell is capable of self-renewal, providing a continuous supply of the cells required for hematopoiesis. Fetal blood and umbilical cord blood are rich sources of stem cells (Broxmeyer, 1991).

Red Blood Cell

The red blood cell undergoes several developmental changes as it progresses through the prenatal period to infancy and childhood. These include changes in production rate, life span, appearance, and type of hemoglobin.

The red blood cell production rate is relatively high as gestation draws to a close. It decreases after birth, reaching its low point during the neonatal period. There is some increase in red blood cell production during infancy, again during the preschool years, and, for males, during the adolescent years (Table 23–1). Those living in high-altitude environments generally produce a higher number of red blood cells and develop a physiologic polycythemia.

Worldview: *The literature refers to ethnic variations in red blood cell indices. In particular, it notes that African Americans tend to have lower hemoglobin and hematocrit values than European Americans (Beard, 1994; Feroli & Hobson, 1995; Perry, Byers, Yip, & Margen, 1992). However, further research is necessary to determine whether or not these differences represent normal physiologic variance (Hegenauer & Saltman, 1993; Jackson & Jackson, 1991; Perry et al., 1992). Even if race-specific standards could be established, their clinical application would be difficult, because children who appear to be of one race may be genetically biracial or triracial (Berti & Leonard, 1995).*

The life span of red blood cells gradually increases with gestational age, and by the end of the neonatal period it reaches the normal life span of 100 to 120 days. Red blood cell survival time at birth for a full-term baby is 60 to 70 days. For a premature infant, the red blood cell survival time is less, with the amount of decrease positively correlated with the degree of the infant's immaturity.

The appearance of the newborn's red blood cells shows variance with regard to size and shape. These cells are larger in size, and they are more likely to show irregularity in shape than the red blood cells of older children and adults.

Hemoglobin is the major component of red blood cells. Normally, it consists of two pairs of globin polypeptide chains. There are various types of globin chains, differing with respect to their amino acid composition. Hemoglobin F, hemoglobin A_2, and hemoglobin A are the most significant among the pediatric and adult populations.

Hemoglobin F is composed of alpha and gamma globin chains. It is the predominant hemoglobin during the fetal stage of development and at birth. During the first 6 months after birth it gradually declines, but it continues to be present in trace amounts throughout the remainder of the child's life. An increased amount of hemoglobin F may be associated with hemoglobinopathies and certain other disorders.

Hemoglobin A_2 is composed of alpha and delta globin chains. It is a minor hemoglobin, constituting approximately 2.5% of hemoglobin. Its increase or decrease may contribute information important in the diagnosis of hematologic disorders such as thalassemia.

Hemoglobin A is composed of alpha and beta globin chains. It is the predominant hemoglobin after early infancy, constituting more than 95% of hemoglobin. A deficiency of hemoglobin A is associated with certain forms of sickle cell disease and thalassemia.

Red blood cells experience several phases in their

maturation process. Initially, erythropoietin (a hormone) stimulates certain stem cells to commit to the red blood cell lineage. The committed stem cells then proceed on in their development, sequentially becoming erythroblasts, normoblasts, reticulocytes, and red blood cells. Reticulocytes and red blood cells are present in the peripheral circulation, and they are non-nucleated cells, in contrast to red blood cells in earlier stages of development.

White Blood Cell

Although white blood cell production can be detected in the liver during fetal development, red blood cell development predominates until the neonatal period. As with red blood cell development, there are stem cells that commit to the various white blood cell lineages: myeloid, monocytic, and lymphoid.

Myeloid Lineage. Stem cells that commit to the myeloid lineage sequentially progress in their development to myeloblasts, promyelocytes, myelocytes, metamyelocytes, bands, and granulocytes. The mature granulocyte cells appear as neutrophils, eosinophils, or basophils in the peripheral circulation. A few bands may appear in the peripheral circulation as well. Circulating granulocytes have a short life span of approximately 12 to 14 hours (Sieff & Nathan, 1993).

After declining during infancy, the white blood cell differential shows a steadily increasing percentage of neutrophils (also known as "polys" or "segs"). The peak level is achieved during adolescence and continues into the adult years. The percentage of eosinophils and basophils in the differential remains fairly constant over the life span.

Monocytic Lineage. Stem cells that commit to the monocytic lineage sequentially proceed in their development to monoblasts, promonocytes, and monocytes. Mature monocytes appear in the peripheral circulation for about 12 hours before entering body tissues. Although monocytes engage in phagocytosis, they do so more slowly than neutrophils (Miller, 1995). Apart from minor changes during infancy, the percentage of monocytes in the white blood cell differential remains quite steady over the life span.

Lymphoid Lineage. Stem cells that commit to the lymphoid lineage sequentially progress in their development from lymphoblasts, to prolymphocytes, and then to mature lymphocytes. The life span of lymphocytes is variable, ranging from a few days to months or years. After increasing during infancy, the white blood cell differential shows the percentage of lymphocytes gradually decreasing throughout childhood. A plateau occurs during adolescence and remains through the adult years.

There are two major types of lymphocytes: T cells and B cells. T cells, or thymus-derived lymphocytes, are involved in cell-mediated immunity. B cells, or bone marrow–derived lymphocytes, are involved in humoral immunity.

Platelet

Platelets develop from stem cells that commit to the platelet lineage. These committed stem cells sequentially proceed on in their development to become megakaryoblasts, promegakaryocytes, and then mature megakaryocytes or platelets. The number of circulating platelets is relatively constant over the life span and ranges from 150,000 to 450,000 per mm^3.

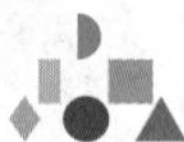

Diagnostic Criteria for Evaluating Hematologic Status

Laboratory studies provide significant data for assessing the physical status of the child with a hematologic disorder. Three common hematologic laboratory studies are:

- Coagulation profile
- Blood cell profile (complete blood count or CBC)
- Bone marrow examination (aspiration and biopsy)

The coagulation profile furnishes initial data regarding the body's blood clotting status. The blood cell profile provides information related to the cellular components of the circulating blood. The bone marrow sample yields data on the bone marrow's cellularity and identifies the presence or absence of cells that are precursors of cells that are normally found in the vascular circulation.

caREminder: *Assessment of the hematologic system depends on scrupulous techniques for obtaining, transporting, and testing blood or bone marrow specimens. Pay careful attention to the instructions for acquiring such samples so that:*

- *The correct technique is employed to obtain the desired specimen, including the use of universal precautions*
- *The correct sample amount is secured*
- *The specimen is appropriately smeared on a slide or placed in the correct specimen receptacle (e.g., blood tube, Microtainer)*
- *The sample is correctly labeled with the patient's name and other identifying data.*

A number of laboratory studies provide information related to the hematologic system (Table 23–2).

The nurse may be responsible for the acquisition of certain blood samples. However, for more specialized procedures such as bone marrow aspiration, the staff nurse usually assists specially prepared physicians, nurse practitioners, and clinical laboratory personnel in acquiring the needed specimens. Also, the nurse provides ongoing monitoring of the child, particularly when sedation is used.

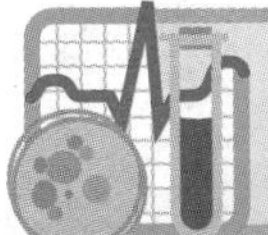

Table 23–2
Diagnostic Tests and Procedures for Evaluating Hematologic Status

Diagnostic Test or Procedure	Purpose	Health Care Provider Responsibilities
Antithrombin III	Measures antithrombin III level Helps to identify coagulation disorders such as DIC	Contraindicated for patients receiving anticoagulant therapy When more than one blood sample is being obtained, draw blood for antithrombin III last Discard first 1–2 mL of blood when other blood samples are not needed at the same time Gently, but thoroughly, mix blood sample with anticoagulant in specimen tube to prevent clotting Place specimen tubes on ice Transport to laboratory immediately
Bilirubin fractions	Evaluates liver function Measures direct (conjugated) bilirubin Measures indirect (unconjugated) bilirubin Evaluates hemolytic anemia	Protect specimen from prolonged exposure to light Handle specimen gently to avoid hemolysis
Bleeding time	Measures bleeding time after a standard skin incision Screens for platelet function disorders and von Willebrand's disease Measures ability of platelets to adhere to blood vessel wall and form a platelet plug	Note use of aspirin, anticoagulants, anti-inflammatory drugs, and any other medications that may cause prolonged bleeding time Apply butterfly closure to wound for 24 hr
Blood cell profile with differential and platelet count (complete blood count; CBC)	Provides quantitative data for peripheral blood cells Hemoglobin Hematocrit Red blood cell count White blood count Platelet count Identifies size and hemoglobin content of red blood cells MCV MCH MCHC Quantifies the various types of peripheral white blood cells, helping to distinguish among infection, leukemia, and other disorders Identifies presence of anemia, neutropenia, and thrombocytopenia	Be aware that specimens obtained when a child is upset may show an increased white blood cell count Gently mix blood sample with anticoagulant in specimen tube to prevent clotting Avoid rough handling of blood specimen to prevent hemolysis Keep specimen at room temperature

Table continued on following page

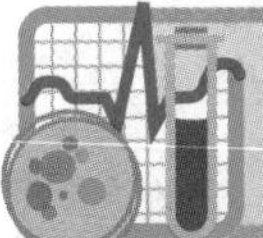

Table 23-2
Diagnostic Tests and Procedures for Evaluating Hematologic Status *Continued*

Diagnostic Test or Procedure	Purpose	Health Care Provider Responsibilities
Bone marrow aspirate (fluid specimen) and Bone marrow biopsy (tissue specimen)	Distinguishes normal from abnormal hematopoiesis Identifies and evaluates specific hematologic disorders Identifies and evaluates primary and metastatic malignancies in bone marrow Evaluates status of bone marrow iron stores (biopsy)	Evaluate platelet count before procedure Administer prescribed sedation Monitor for bleeding and infection at aspirate/biopsy site Monitor for side effects of sedation
Coagulation profile	Provides data for various indicators of coagulation status Prothrombin time (PT) Partial thromboplastin time (PTT) Fibrinogen Platelet count Thrombin clotting time	Note use of medications that may interfere with normal coagulation Draw blood for coagulation studies last when more than one blood sample is being obtained Discard first 1–2 mL of blood when other blood samples are not needed at the same time Gently mix blood sample with anticoagulant in specimen tube to prevent clotting
Coombs' test, direct (antiglobulin test, direct)	Detects antibody attached to red blood cells Tests for hemolytic disease of the newborn	Handle specimen gently to prevent hemolysis Transport to laboratory immediately
DIC profile (disseminated intravascular coagulation profile)	Provides data for various indicators of DIC PT PTT Fibrinogen Platelet count Thrombin clotting time D-dimer assay for fibrin derivatives (FDP)	Note use of medications that may interfere with normal coagulation Draw blood for coagulation studies last when more than one blood sample is being obtained Discard first 1–2 mL of blood when other blood samples are not needed at the same time Gently mix blood sample with anticoagulant in specimen tube to prevent clotting
Factor assays	Detects specific factor deficiency in those with prolonged PT or PTT	Contraindicated for patients receiving anticoagulant therapy Draw blood for factor assays last, when more than one blood sample is being obtained Discard first 1–2 mL of blood when other blood samples are not needed at the same time Gently mix blood sample with anticoagulant in specimen tube to prevent clotting Place specimen tubes on ice Transport to laboratory immediately Apply pressure to venipuncture site for at least 10 min after venipuncture

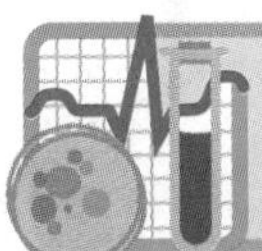

Table 23–2
Diagnostic Tests and Procedures for Evaluating Hematologic Status *Continued*

Diagnostic Test or Procedure	Purpose	Health Care Provider Responsibilities
Folate, red blood cell	Evaluates megaloblastic anemias	Place specimen tubes on ice Protect specimen from light
Folate, serum	Tests for folate deficiency	Handle specimen gently to avoid hemolysis Protect from light
Hemoglobin electrophoresis	Measures quantity of hemoglobins Identifies abnormal hemoglobins found in sickle cell disease	Gently mix blood sample with anticoagulant in specimen tubes Note that test result may be inaccurate, if blood sample obtained within 4 mo after a blood transfusion
Osmotic fragility test	Tests for spherocytic red blood cells	Handle specimen gently to prevent hemolysis Deliver specimen to laboratory within 1 hr Note that test results may be abnormal, if severe anemia present
Peripheral blood smear	Determines morphologic alterations in red blood cells, white blood cells, and platelets	Request test with blood cell profile Gently mix blood sample with anticoagulant in specimen tubes to prevent clotting
Plasminogen	Measures plasminogen activity in plasma Helps identify disorders associated with decreased plasminogen, such as DIC and thrombosis	When more than one blood sample is being obtained draw blood for plasminogen last Discard first 1–2 mL of blood when other blood samples are not needed at the same time Gently but thoroughly mix blood sample with anticoagulant in specimen tubes to prevent clotting Place specimen tubes on ice Transport to laboratory immediately
Protoporphyrin, free erythrocyte (FEP)	Tests for iron deficiency anemia Adjunct test for lead poisoning	Note current hematocrit on test requisition Avoid exposure of specimen to direct light
Reticulocyte count	Evaluates red blood cell production Contributes diagnostic information for various disorders associated with decreased production or increased destruction of red blood cells	Request test together with blood cell profile Gently mix blood sample with anticoagulant in specimen tube to prevent clotting Transport to laboratory promptly
Ristocetin cofactor assay	Indicates level of von Willebrand's factor activity Helps differentiate von Willebrand's disease from hemophilia A	Discard first 1–2 mL of blood to avoid contamination of specimen with tissue thromboplastin Place specimen tubes on ice Transport to laboratory immediately

Table continued on following page

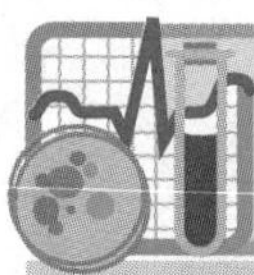

Table 23–2
Diagnostic Tests and Procedures for Evaluating Hematologic Status *Continued*

Diagnostic Test or Procedure	Purpose	Health Care Provider Responsibilities
Serum ferritin	Tests for iron deficiency anemia Tests for iron overload Measures iron stores	Place specimen on ice
Serum iron and total iron binding capacity	Evaluates iron binding capacity Evaluates iron toxicity	Handle specimen gently to avoid hemolysis Transport specimen to laboratory immediately
Sickle solubility test	Identifies presence of a sickling hemoglobin	Note that when positive, this test does *not* distinguish between sickle cell trait and sickle cell disease If test is positive, perform a hemoglobin electrophoresis test to identify type of abnormal hemoglobin and to identify whether sickle cell trait or sickle cell disease is present
Transferrin	Tests for iron deficiency anemia	Handle specimen gently Transport specimen to laboratory immediately
Type and crossmatch	Identifies blood type, Rh factor, and antibodies to red blood cell antigens Crossmatches donor red blood cells with those of recipient to check for compatibility	Document that patient identification verified Handle specimen gently to prevent hemolysis
von Willebrand's factor antigen assay	Measures quantity of von Willebrand's factor antigen Helps differentiate von Willebrand's disease from hemophilia A	Discard first 1–2 mL of blood when other blood samples not needed at same time, to avoid contamination of specimen with tissue thromboplastin Place specimen tubes on ice Transport to laboratory immediately
von Willebrand's factor multimer analysis	Identifies multimer structure of von Willebrand's factor Helps identify specific type of von Willebrand's disease	Discard first 1–2 mL of blood when other blood samples not needed at same time, to avoid contamination of specimen with tissue thromboplastin Place specimen tubes on ice Transport to laboratory immediately
Vitamin B_{12}	Tests for vitamin B_{12} deficiency Evaluates megaloblastic anemia	Protect specimen from light

Alert: *Children with a known or suspected hematologic disorder should be monitored for prolonged bleeding after a blood draw, bone marrow aspiration, or other invasive procedure.*

Transporting blood samples requires attention to preserving the specimens so that accurate test results can be secured. Gentle handling helps to preserve blood cells and prevent laboratory rejection of specimens because of hemolysis. Some specimens need to be transported on ice for preservation. Other specimens need to be transported to the laboratory immediately to ensure that the quality of the blood sample does not deteriorate over time.

Laboratory testing of blood samples is conducted by specific criteria to provide reliable test results. However, normal values for certain hematologic tests, such as coagulation studies, may vary from laboratory to laboratory, depending on the specific test methodology and the reagents used in testing. Thus, to evaluate test results, acquire the normal values from the laboratory performing the test. Although it is best to use the same laboratory for each child for consistency in test results, this may not always be feasible. For example, a child may travel many miles to receive health care at a regional center specializing in pediatric hematologic disorders. Follow-up studies are often done by a laboratory closer to the child's home, with test results sent to both the pediatric hematologist and the child's local physician.

Whenever blood or bone marrow sampling is required, the nurse has a significant role in preparing the child and family. Accurate information about the test's purpose and procedure and honest responses to questions such as "Will it hurt?" help the child and family know what to expect before, during, and after the procedure. In addition, developmentally appropriate play activities that simulate the test procedure often help the child prepare for the test and cope with it.

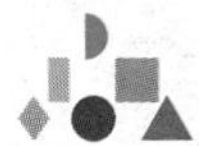

Treatment Modalities

Transfusion Therapy

Transfusion therapy refers to the transfer of blood or a blood component from a healthy donor to a recipient whose blood has a specific quantitative or qualitative deficiency. Although it is possible to transfuse whole blood, it is more common to transfuse specific components of blood. This decreases the risk of circulatory overload and allows the donor blood to benefit more than one person in need.

The primary concern associated with transfusion therapy is safety. Meticulous care is required when obtaining, processing, typing, and crossmatching blood to ensure compatibility between donor and recipient and to prevent the transmission of diseases such as hepatitis and acquired immunodeficiency syndrome (AIDS).

The most frequently transfused blood components are packed red blood cells (PRBCs), platelets, and fresh frozen plasma (FFP) (Table 23–3).

Before administration, blood products may be irradiated. This interferes with lymphocyte proliferation and prevents transfusion-associated graft-versus-host disease in the recipient who is immunodeficient. Also, blood products are often purposely leukocyte depleted, by means of special microaggregate filters, to minimize the probability of febrile reactions and to decrease the incidence of alloimmunization. When packed red blood cells are to be transfused, they are occasionally washed to remove residual leukocytes.

It is essential for the nurse to ensure that the right patient is the recipient of any transfused blood product.

caREminder: *To prevent a potentially fatal reaction, blood compatibility data, patient identification number, and patient name must be verified before administering blood products. Be especially careful to distinguish among children with the same or similar names. Also, be aware that surnames of children and their parents may differ.*

The nurse who is preparing to give blood products should educate the child and family regarding the purpose and procedure of the transfusion. Other common nursing activities associated with blood product administration are outlined in Chart 23–4. In addition, the nurse must adhere to specific institutional policies and procedures when administering blood products.

The first 15 minutes of transfusion are particularly significant because this is when most transfusion reactions occur. Thus, during this time, the rate of infusion is slower and the recipient is monitored closely. If no transfusion reactions are apparent, the infusion rate is increased to that which is appropriate for the specific blood

Table 23–3
Commonly Transfused Blood Components

Product	Indications For Use
Packed red blood cells (PRBCs)	Symptomatic anemia Replacement therapy (e.g., during surgery)
Platelets	Bleeding associated with thrombocytopenia or platelet dysfunction Preoperatively when thrombocytopenia present High risk for bleeding related to severe thrombocytopenia
Fresh frozen plasma (FFP)	Replacement of noncellular coagulation factors

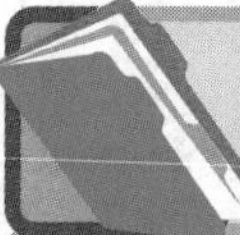

Chart 23–4
Nursing Interventions Classification (NIC)

Blood Product Administration

Definition

Administration of blood or blood products and monitoring of patient's response

Activities

Verify physician's orders.
Obtain or verify parent or guardian's informed consent.
Verify that blood product has been prepared, typed, and crossmatched (if applicable) for the recipient.
Instruct patient and family about signs and symptoms of transfusion reactions.
Assemble administration system with filter appropriate for blood product and recipient's immune status.
Prime administration system with isotonic saline.
Prepare an IV pump approved for blood product administration, if indicated.
Perform venipuncture, using appropriate technique, if central venous access device is not in place.
Avoid transfusion of more than one unit of blood or blood product at a time, unless necessitated by recipient's condition.
Monitor IV site for signs and symptoms of infiltration, phlebitis, and local infection.
Monitor vital signs (e.g., baseline and throughout and after transfusion).
Monitor for fluid overload and transfusion reactions.
Monitor and regulate flow rate during transfusion.
Refrain from administering IV medications or fluids, other than isotonic saline, into blood or blood product lines.
Refrain from transfusing product removed from controlled refrigeration for more than 4 hours.
Change filter and administration set at least every 4 hours.
Administer saline when transfusion is complete.
Document time frame of transfusion.
Document volume infused.
Stop transfusion if blood reaction occurs and keep veins open with saline.
Obtain blood sample and first voided urine specimen after a transfusion reaction.
Coordinate the return of the blood container to the laboratory after a blood reaction.
Notify physician and laboratory immediately, in the event of a blood reaction.
Maintain universal precautions.

From McCloskey, J., & Bulechek, G. (1996). *Nursing interventions classification (NIC)* (2nd ed.). St. Louis: Mosby–Year Book. Reprinted with permission.

product and the recipient's condition. Regular monitoring continues throughout the transfusion.

When packed red blood cells are given, children usually receive 10 to 15 mL/kg. This is generally transfused over 2 to 3 hours, with 4 hours being the maximum infusion time. Children who are severely anemic are at particular risk for congestive heart failure if packed red blood cells are given too rapidly. Thus, they must receive blood more slowly than usual and have their anemic state gradually corrected over time with separate transfusions. Platelets and fresh frozen plasma are given as quickly as can be tolerated by the recipient, usually over 20 to 30 minutes (Coffland & Shelton, 1993; Foley, 1993).

During, as well as after, the administration of blood products, it is important for the nurse to be alert for signs and symptoms of a transfusion reaction. There are three major types of transfusion reaction:

- Hemolytic reaction
- Febrile reaction
- Allergic reaction

When transfusion reactions take place, stop the transfusion immediately, monitor the child closely, and notify the physician. Additional interventions depend on the nature and severity of the reaction.

Hemolytic reactions cause red blood cell destruction and occur when the blood product is not compatible with the recipient's blood type. Also, hemolytic reactions may occur when the donor blood contains minor blood group antigens to which the recipient has been previously sensitized (alloimmunized). This is most likely to happen in children who have previously received multiple blood transfusions and been exposed to allogeneic antigens. Hemolytic reactions may be immediate or delayed.

Hemolytic reactions may lead to significant cardiovascular and renal alterations. Fluids, as well as corticosteroids, vasopressors, and mannitol, may be required to maintain circulation and urinary output (Kevy, 1993).

Febrile reactions, not associated with hemolysis, generally occur when the recipient has developed antibodies to leukocyte, platelet, or plasma protein antigens in the donor blood. This is more likely to occur in children who have previously received blood products.

Febrile reactions are usually treated with acetaminophen and corticosteroids.

Allergic reactions are nonhemolytic reactions that occur when the donor blood contains plasma proteins or other antigens to which the recipient is hypersensitive. Signs and symptoms of the primary transfusion reactions, as well as preventive measures, are outlined in Table 23–4.

Allergic reactions, such as rash and pruritus, usually respond to the antihistamine diphenhydramine. However, severe allergic reactions characterized by bronchospasm, hypotension, and shock require treatment with epinephrine. If the child is in shock, the nurse helps to provide intravenous fluids, airway protection, oxygen, vasopressors, and other interventions as needed (Kevy, 1993).

Experiencing transfusion reactions, especially when they are more severe, is likely to be stressful for the child and family. The nurse needs to be sure they receive emotional support, as well as ongoing progress reports about the child's state.

Exchange Transfusion

Exchange transfusion involves the substitution of donor red blood cells for recipient red blood cells. During an exchange transfusion, small quantities of the recipient's blood are alternately removed and replaced with donor

Table 23–4
Transfusion Reactions

	Hemolytic Reaction	Febrile Reaction	Allergic Reaction
Signs and symptoms	Fever Chills Urticaria Restlessness Headache Chest pain Abdominal/lower back pain Tachycardia Hypotension Oliguria Shock Laboratory findings Anemia Spherocytosis Disseminated intravascular coagulation (DIC) Hemoglobinemia Hemoglobinuria Positive Coombs' test	Fever Chills Diaphoresis	Rash Hives Urticaria Swelling Respiratory distress Anaphylaxis
Preventive measures	Type and crossmatch accurately Use leukocyte-depleted blood products to help prevent alloimmunization	Pretreat with antipyretic and corticosteroid Use leukocyte-depleted blood products	Pretreat with antihistamine and corticosteroid Wash red blood cells

blood until the desired volume of blood has been exchanged.

The following clinical situations illustrate instances in which exchange transfusions may be prescribed.

- Exchange transfusions may be indicated when there is concern that the increased blood volume from a simple transfusion will not be tolerated. Examples include the newborn who is at risk for fluid overload and the child with severe anemia who is at risk for congestive heart failure.
- Exchange transfusions may be used to decrease the quantity of an abnormal element in the blood and to remove an excessive amount of a normal blood component. Examples include the child with a severe sickle cell crisis secondary to a significant number of sickled red blood cells and the child with polycythemia.

Exchange transfusion is discussed further in the section on hemolytic diseases of the newborn (HDN).

Hypertransfusion

Hypertransfusion refers to an ongoing program in which blood transfusions are given at regularly scheduled intervals (usually about every 3 weeks). The purpose of hypertransfusion is to suppress erythropoiesis in children who have severe chronic anemia secondary to the production of abnormal red blood cells. By providing normal red blood cells through hypertransfusion, production of abnormal erythrocytes is suppressed. Beta-thalassemia major (Cooley's anemia) and certain severe vaso-occlusive crises associated with sickle cell disease exemplify clinical situations in which a hypertransfusion program may be prescribed. Children receiving such a program are at increased risk for infection from blood-borne viruses, and they should be immunized against hepatitis B.

Goals of a hypertransfusion program for children with severe chronic anemia include:

- To decrease tissue hypoxia.
- To decrease the workload of the heart.
- To increase the hemoglobin content of the blood. During the years when the children are growing, the desired hemoglobin level is 10 to 12 g/dL. When growth is complete, a lower hemoglobin level of 8 to 9 g/dL may be acceptable (McDonagh & Nienhuis, 1993).
- To inhibit overstimulation of erythropoiesis in the bone marrow. This suppresses expansion of the bone marrow cavity and the concomitant development of bone abnormalities such as the abnormal facies associated with beta-thalassemia major. Also, it is thought to decrease the enhanced gastrointestinal absorption of iron that may occur with severe chronic anemia.
- To promote normal growth and development. During the preadolescent years, normal growth is a good indicator of an adequate transfusion program. However, during adolescence, delayed growth may be indicative of endocrine deficits rather than an inadequate transfusion program (McDonagh & Nienhuis, 1993).
- To delay the onset of splenomegaly with hypersplenism (see Fig. 23–12) and the accompanying need for splenectomy. It is beneficial to delay a splenectomy when children are younger than 5 years because young children are at greater risk than older children for developing life-threatening postsplenectomy sepsis. However, splenectomy is indicated when the annual transfusion requirement exceeds 200 to 250 mL/kg (Giardina & Hilgartner, 1992; McDonagh & Nienhuis, 1993). The risk of postsplenectomy sepsis and its management are discussed later in the section on immune thrombocytopenia purpura (ITP).

The major complication of an ongoing transfusion therapy program is the development of toxic iron overload. This leads to pathologic changes in various body systems, including the hepatic, endocrine, and cardiac systems.

Hepatic changes are among the earliest to occur and include fibrosis and cirrhosis.

Endocrine changes include pancreatic destruction with the onset of insulin-dependent diabetes mellitus, as well as hormone deficiencies that impair growth and delay the appearance of secondary sex characteristics.

Cardiac changes include arrhythmias and congestive heart failure. Without the addition of iron chelation therapy during early childhood, the cardiac alterations become severe and often lead to death during the teenage years.

Prevention of Iron Overload. To prevent iron overload among children who are participating in a transfusion therapy program, iron chelation therapy is required. This is usually started before the age of 5 years or when iron stores become excessive. Iron chelation is accomplished with the use of deferoxamine (Chart 23–5). The prolonged, painful nature of chelation therapy makes it difficult for many children and adolescents to adhere to it. This is of concern to those who provide their health care and a reason for the significant interest in current research on orally administered iron chelating agents.

Tip: *Measures to improve compliance with parenterally administered chelation include the use of behavioral contracts with the child. One such contract provides token rewards upon the return of the contracted number of empty deferoxamine vials (Koch, Giardina, Ryan, MacQueen, & Hilgartner, 1993).*

Chart 23–5
Nursing Interventions

Administering Deferoxamine (Desferal)

Deferoxamine (Desferal) is an iron antidote used for the child with acute iron toxicity or chronic iron overload secondary to multiple blood transfusions. The drug binds to ferric ions, forming ferrioxamine, which is excreted by the kidneys. Deferoxamine is contraindicated for children with severe renal disease.

Nursing considerations include the following:

1. Protect deferoxamine from light.
2. Administer deferoxamine subcutaneously or intravenously.
   a. Subcutaneous administration via portable pump
      (1) 20 to 40 mg/kg/day over 8 to 12 hours.
      (2) Give at least five times per week.
      (3) Higher doses may be necessary for older children and adolescents who have a large iron overload.
   b. Intravenous infusion
      (1) Up to 15 mg/kg/hr.
      (2) Maximum daily dose is 6 g.
3. Instruct child/family regarding subcutaneous home administration of deferoxamine.
   a. Use of portable infusion pump
   b. Preparation and administration of medication
   c. Need to alternate infusion sites in abdomen and lateral thighs
   d. Importance of regular use of medication
   e. Possible side effects
      (1) Irritation or pain at infusion site
      (2) Visual changes
      (3) Sensorineural hearing loss
      (4) Cardiac complications with excessive intake of vitamin C
      (5) Reddish urine
      (6) Abdominal discomfort; diarrhea
      (7) Leg cramps
      (8) Hypersensitivity reactions
         (a) Rash
         (b) Erythema
         (c) Pruritus
         (d) Fever
         (e) Hypotension; shock
         (f) Anaphylaxis

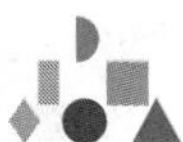

Alterations in Hematologic Status

Disorders of Hemostasis

Hemostasis is a complex process designed to prevent hemorrhage. Effective hemostasis requires ongoing interaction among the vascular wall, platelets, and certain plasma factors. Injury to a blood vessel evokes a vasoconstrictive response that slows down blood loss from the damaged vessel. Platelets adhere to the exposed vascular subendothelium, and subsequent platelet aggregation leads to the formation of a platelet plug at the site of injury. Platelet plugs are usually adequate to seal off tiny ruptures in blood vessels, but clot formation is necessary to close larger vascular injuries.

Plasma factors consist of various clotting factors (Table 23–5) and clot dissolution factors. Shortly after damage to a blood vessel, the clotting cascade is activated. The clotting cascade consists of an intrinsic pathway, an extrinsic pathway, and a common pathway (Fig. 23–2), and its activation leads to clot formation at the injured site. Subsequently, when bleeding is controlled, the degrading action of plasmin leads to clot dissolution and release of fibrin degradation products.

Rapid, excessive blood loss is of particular concern because it can quickly place the child in a life-threatening situation. Prompt interventions to control hemorrhage are necessary, as outlined in Chart 23–6. Bleeding precautions, as delineated in Chart 23–7, are indicated whenever children are at increased risk for bleeding.

Following is a discussion of some disorders in hemostasis that are seen in children. These include hemophilia, von Willebrand's disease, disseminated intravascular coagulation, immune thrombocytopenic purpura, Henoch-Schönlein purpura, and the symptom of epistaxis.

Hemophilia

Hemophilia is a serious bleeding disorder, affecting an estimated 1 in 5000 males (Hoyer, 1994; Montgomery & Scott, 1993). The most prevalent forms—hemophilia A (classic hemophilia) and hemophilia B (Christmas disease)—are usually inherited in a recessive manner via a genetic defect on the X chromosome. In general, sons inherit hemophilia from their mothers, and daughters inherit the carrier status for hemophilia from their fathers (Fig. 23–3). Some females who are carriers have an increased tendency to bleed and, although it is rare, females can actually have hemophilia if their fathers have the disorder and their mothers are carriers of the genetic defect. Also, hemophilia may occur as a result of a spon-

Table 23–5
Clotting Factors

Clotting Factor	Name
Factor I	Fibrinogen
Factor II	Prothrombin
Factor III	Tissue thromboplastin
Factor IV	Calcium
Factor V (no factor VI)	Proaccelerin
Factor VII	Proconvertin
Factor VIII	Antihemophilic factor
Factor IX	Plasma thromboplastin component; Christmas factor
Factor X	Stuart's factor
Factor XI	Plasma thromboplastin antecedent
Factor XII	Hageman's factor
Factor XIII	Fibrin-stabilizing factor
—	Prekallikrein; Fletcher's factor
—	High-molecular-weight kininogen (HMWK); Fitzgerald's factor
—	Platelets

Chart 23–6
Nursing Interventions Classification (NIC)

Hemorrhage Control

Definition

Reduction or elimination of rapid and excessive blood loss

Activities

Apply a pressure dressing, as indicated.
Identify the cause of the bleeding.
Monitor the amount and nature of blood loss.
Apply manual pressure over the bleeding or the potential bleeding area.
Apply ice pack to affected area.
Note hemoglobin/hematocrit level before and after blood loss, as indicated.
Evaluate patient's and family's psychological response to hemorrhage and perception of events.
Inspect for bleeding from mucous membranes, bruising after minimal trauma, oozing from puncture sites, and presence of petechiae.
Monitor for signs and symptoms of persistent bleeding (e.g., check all secretions for frank or occult blood).
Hematest all excretions and observe for blood in emesis, sputum, feces, urine, nasogastric drainage, and wound drainage, as appropriate.
Monitor neurologic functioning.
Maintain standard precautions.

From McCloskey, J., & Bulechek, G. (1996). *Nursing interventions classification (NIC)* (2nd ed.). St. Louis: Mosby–Year Book. Reprinted with permission.

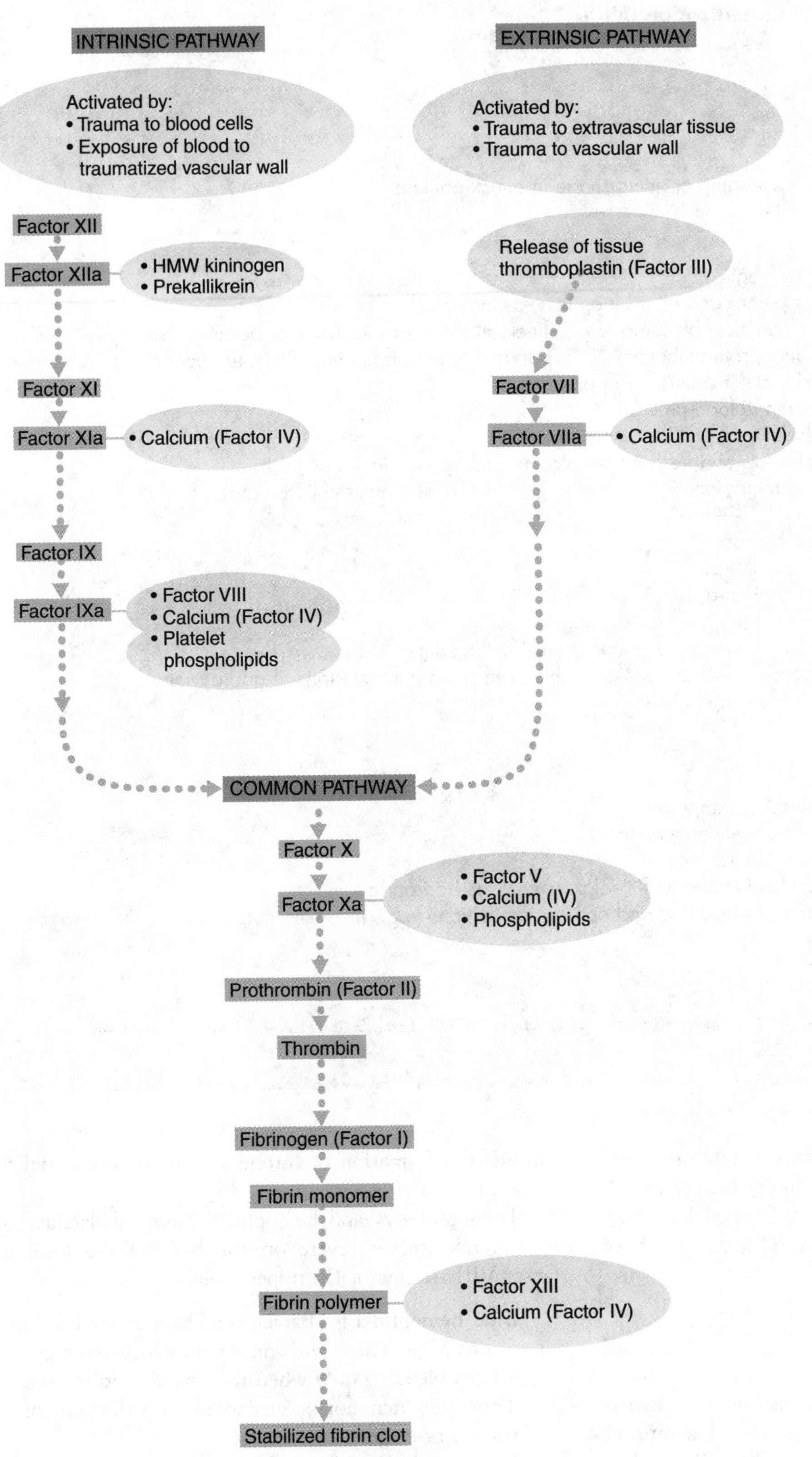

Figure 23–2
The clotting cascade.

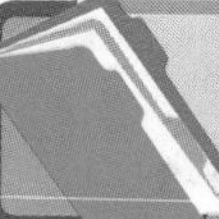

Chart 23–7
Nursing Interventions Classification (NIC)

Bleeding Precautions

Definition

Reduction of stimuli that may induce bleeding or hemorrhage in at-risk patients

Activities

Monitor the patient closely for hemorrhage.
Note hemoglobin/hematocrit levels before and after blood loss, as indicated.
Monitor for signs and symptoms of persistent bleeding (e.g., check all secretions for frank or occult blood).
Monitor coagulation studies, including prothrombin time (PT), partial thromboplastin time (PTT), fibrinogen, fibrin degradation/split products, and platelet counts, as appropriate.
Monitor orthostatic vital signs, including blood pressure.
Maintain bed rest during active bleeding.
Administer blood products (e.g., platelets and fresh frozen plasma), as appropriate.
Protect the patient from trauma, which may cause bleeding (e.g., toddlers and other children at risk for falls should wear a helmet).
Avoid injections (IV, IM, or SQ), as appropriate.
Instruct the ambulating patient to wear shoes.
Use soft toothbrush or toothettes for oral care.
Use electric razor, instead of straight-edge razor, for shaving.
Avoid invasive procedures: if they are necessary, monitor closely for bleeding.
Coordinate timing of invasive procedures with platelet or fresh frozen plasma transfusions, if appropriate.
Refrain from inserting objects into a bleeding orifice.
Avoid taking rectal temperatures.
Avoid lifting heavy objects.
Avoid contact sports and rough activity.
Administer medications (e.g., antacids), as appropriate.
Instruct patient to avoid aspirin or other anticoagulants.
Use therapeutic mattress to minimize skin trauma.
Avoid constipation (e.g., encourage fluid intake and stool softeners), as appropriate.
Instruct the patient and family on signs of bleeding and appropriate actions (e.g., notify the nurse), should bleeding occur.
Maintain standard precautions.

Adapted from McCloskey, J., & Bulechek, G. (1996). *Nursing interventions classification (NIC)* (2nd ed.). St. Louis: Mosby–Year Book. Used with permission.

taneous genetic mutation, with approximately one third of the affected children having no family history of this disorder (Bell, Canty, & Audet, 1995; DiMichele, 1996). Among those who have hemophilia, 80% to 85% have hemophilia A.

Pathophysiology

Hemophilia A and hemophilia B are distinguished by the particular procoagulant factor that is decreased, absent, or dysfunctional. In hemophilia A it is factor VIII, and in hemophilia B it is factor IX. A disorder in either factor inhibits the formation of thrombin, which is essential to normal coagulation.

Hemophilia A and hemophilia B are subclassified as mild, moderate, or severe on the basis of the level of factor VIII and factor IX, respectively.

- **Mild hemophilia** is characterized by a factor level of 5% to 50%. Those with mild hemophilia have prolonged bleeding only when they have been injured. Thus, they may not be diagnosed until the time of trauma or surgery.
- **Moderate hemophilia** is distinguished by a factor level of 1% to 5%. Those with moderate hemophilia

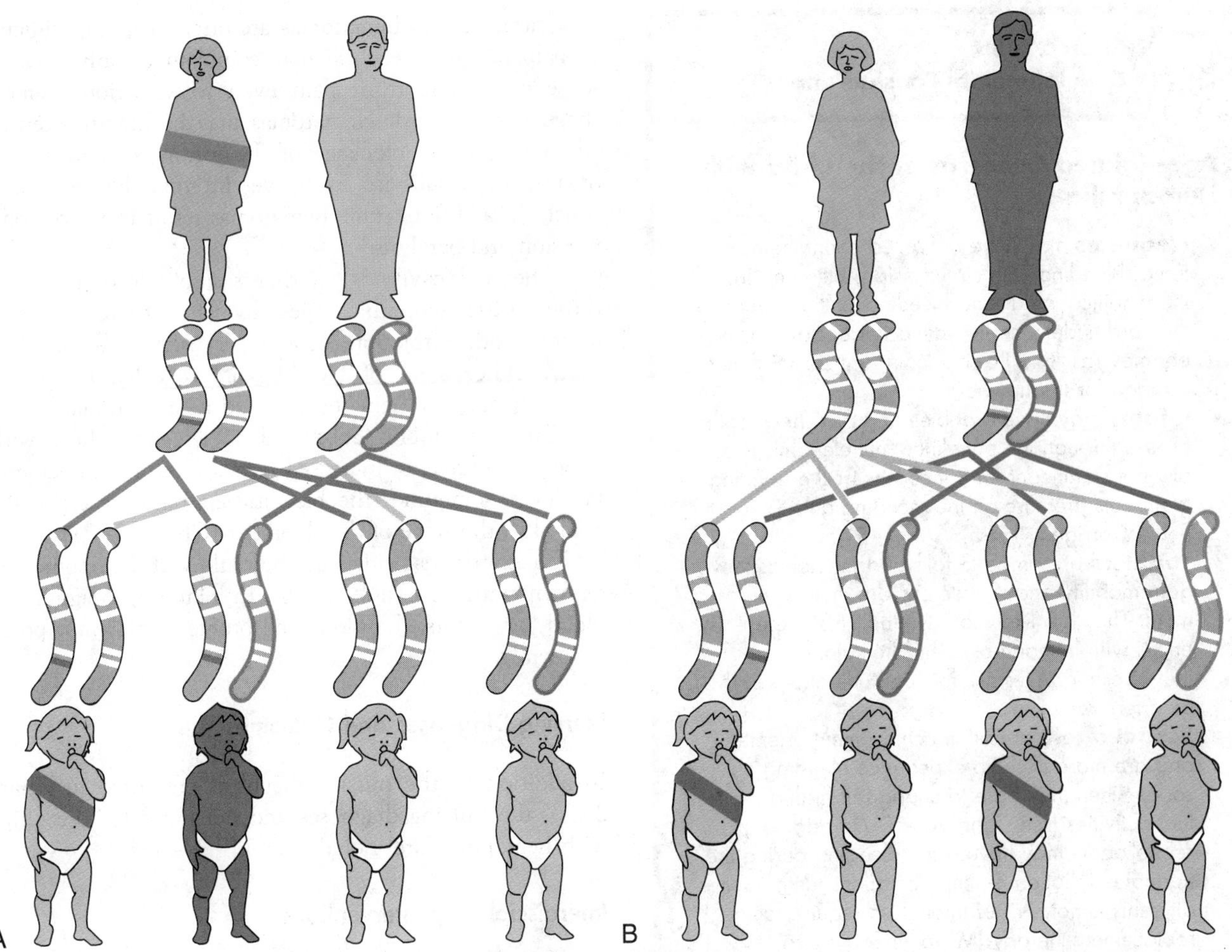

Figure 23-3
Genetic inheritance of hemophilia. A, Among the offspring of a carrier female and a normal male, half of the daughters are carriers of hemophilia and half are normal. Half of the sons have hemophilia and half are normal. B, Among the offspring of a normal female and a male with hemophilia, all of the daughters are carriers of hemophilia; all of the sons are normal.

usually have prolonged bleeding only at times of trauma or surgery, but they may experience occasions of spontaneous bleeding as well.

- **Severe hemophilia** is characterized by a factor level that is less than 1%. Those with severe hemophilia have prolonged bleeding at times of trauma or surgery. In addition, they tend to have frequent episodes of spontaneous bleeding, that is, bleeding that occurs in the absence of injury.

Although bleeding may occur in any area of the body, the classic type of bleeding identified with hemophilia is **hemarthrosis** (bleeding into a joint cavity). Frequently, the person with hemophilia develops a "target" joint—a particular joint that is repeatedly the site of bleeding episodes. If bleeding is not effectively treated, target joints are particularly at risk for deterioration and the development of chronic, disabling arthropathy (joint disease). Other common types of bleeding connected with hemophilia are intramuscular hematomas and oral cavity bleeding.

Bleeding associated with hemophilia may be life threatening. This is especially true of bleeding into the central nervous system, iliopsoas intramuscular hemorrhage, as well as any incident of extensive internal or external blood loss.

Prognosis. The prognosis for hemophilia has improved significantly. The development of comprehensive treatment centers and the availability of improved factor replacement therapy have reduced the disorder's disabling consequences. They have also decreased the premature death rate that, historically, has been associated with hemophilia. However, there is now deep concern for those with hemophilia who received factor concentrates

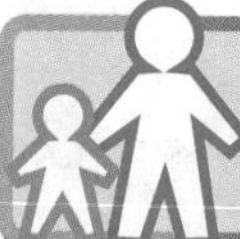

Chart 23–8
Developmental Considerations

Age-Related Concerns of the Child with Hemophilia

- **Neonates** may have a marked cephalhematoma, bleeding with circumcision, bleeding from the umbilical cord, and bleeding at the navel after the cord is detached. A difficult labor and delivery may result in life-threatening intracranial hemorrhage for the newborn.
- **Infants** may have oral bleeding as a new tooth breaks through the gum line. This bleeding is usually not significant, and it ceases as the erupting tooth puts pressure on the receding gum (Hilgartner & Corrigan, 1995).
- **Toddlers** are prone to falls and injuries as they gain mobility and seek to explore their environment. They are likely to have their first experiences with hemarthroses and hematomas, and they are at greater risk for oral lacerations such as a torn frenulum.
- **School-agers** are often achievement oriented and are more likely to experience bleeding episodes when they dare to engage in high-risk physical activities (see Chart 23–10). In addition, school-agers may have some bleeding during the normal exfoliation of their deciduous teeth. Generally, this is not serious enough to require factor replacement therapy (McKown & Shapiro, 1991).
- **Adolescents** are at greater risk for bleeding incidents when they yield to peer pressure and participate in high-risk physical activities that are not recommended for them.

contaminated with the human immunodeficiency virus (HIV) during the late 1970s and first half of the 1980s. Many children with hemophilia have acquired AIDS and face, or have already experienced, an untimely death. Factor concentrates used since 1985 have received heat or chemical treatment to kill the virus and prevent AIDS among those with hemophilia.

Assessment

The clinical hallmark of hemophilia A or hemophilia B is deep bleeding into joints and muscles (Hoyer, 1994; Montgomery & Scott, 1993). **Hemarthrosis** most often affects the knee, elbow, and ankle joints and causes tingling, tenderness, pain, warmth, swelling, and decreased mobility. As a target joint undergoes cartilage erosion and joint space tapering, its range of motion decreases, its proximal muscles weaken, and it becomes chronically disabled.

Intramuscular **hematomas** are often deep and difficult to palpate, and the child may complain of only a vague sense of discomfort or pain even when serious hemorrhage has occurred. Hematomas may be life threatening when they cause blockage of the airway, compress vital organs, or result in extensive internal bleeding and shock. In addition, some hematomas result in nerve compression and paralysis.

The oral cavity is another site of bleeding among those with hemophilia, especially when there has been injury, tooth extraction, or a surgery such as a tonsillectomy. Other areas of bleeding are revealed by ecchymoses, hematuria, hematemesis, and hematochezia.

Throughout childhood and adolescence, those with hemophilia have an increased risk of bleeding, in general. However, sometimes the bleeding episodes are especially related to the stage of development (Chart 23–8).

Laboratory data identify the child with hemophilia A or hemophilia B (Table 23–6). In addition, if significant blood loss occurs, the blood cell profile (CBC) may point to anemia.

Nursing Diagnoses and Outcomes

In addition to the nursing diagnosis presented in Chart 23–3, the nursing diagnoses and outcomes for the child with hemophilia are included in TIP 23–1.

Interdisciplinary Interventions

Management of the child with hemophilia is multifaceted. This is reflected in the comprehensive programs of regional hemophilia centers. These centers are staffed by professionals from various disciplines who work together to provide complete health care for children with hemophilia.

Table 23–6
Laboratory Data Commonly Associated with Hemophilia

Laboratory Test	Result in Hemophilia A	Result in Hemophilia B
Bleeding time	Normal	Normal
Factor VIII	Decreased	Normal
Factor IX	Normal	Decreased
Fibrinogen	Normal	Normal
Partial thromboplastin time (PTT)	Prolonged	Prolonged
Platelet count	Normal	Normal
Prothrombin time (PT)	Normal	Normal

TIP 23–1 A Teaching Intervention Plan for the Child with Hemophilia

Nursing Diagnoses and Outcomes

- Knowledge deficit related to hemophilia
  Outcome:
  Child and/or family describes hemophilia, identifying the child's specific factor deficit and the severity of that deficit
- Risk for injury related to bleeding
  Outcomes:
  Child/family identifies common sites of bleeding associated with hemophilia
  Child/family describes interventions needed to stop bleeding episodes
  Child/family states the importance of notifying health care workers about hemophilia prior to surgery or other invasive procedures
  Child/family selects activities for the child which are unlikely to cause bleeding
- Risk for injury related to long-term complications of hemophilia and its treatment
  Outcomes:
  Child/family identifies common long-term complications of hemophilia and its treatment
  Child receives ongoing health care to prevent and manage long-term complications associated with hemophilia and its treatment
- Risk for altered parenting related to child's chronic physical disorder
  Outcome:
  Parents identify normal developmental milestones, and their role in helping their child achieve these milestones

Interventions

- Instruct regarding hemophilia: bleeding disorder; deficiency of a blood clotting factor.
- Educate concerning major types of hemophilia: factor VIII deficiency; factor IX deficiency.
- Teach regarding severity of hemophilia: mild hemophilia; moderate hemophilia; severe hemophilia.
- Inform about child's type of hemophilia, its degree of severity, and its usual clinical course.
- Instruct concerning the etiology of hemophilia and the risk of future children having hemophilia or being a carrier for the disorder.
- Educate regarding measures to prevent bleeding:
  1. Selection of daily activities with low risk for injury
  2. Use of preventive measures
     - Protective equipment, such as helmets for toddlers and other children prone to falls
     - Notification of health care workers about hemophilia prior to invasive procedures
     - Prophylactic factor prior to invasive procedures
- Teach concerning common bleeding sites:
  Joints
  Muscles
  Oral cavity
- Instruct regarding signs and symptoms of bleeding:
  Tingling
  Tenderness
  Pain
  Warmth
  Swelling
  Decreased mobility

TIP continued on following page

TIP 23–1 A Teaching Intervention Plan for the Child with Hemophilia *Continued*

- Educate concerning home factor replacement therapy:
  - Advantage of home treatment for bleeding episodes
  - Home storage of factor
  - Procedure for home administration of factor
  - Procedure to contact home care agency for additional factor and needed supplies
- Instruct regarding long-term complications of hemophilia and its treatment:
  - Joint deformity
  - Muscle weakness
  - Inhibitor (antibody to factor VIII or factor IX)
  - Viral diseases
- Advise about the importance of ongoing health care to prevent and manage long-term complications associated with hemophilia and its treatment.
- Teach measures that promote normal growth and development:
  - Safety
  - Nutrition
  - Exercise
  - Dental care
  - Stress management
  - Avoidance of tobacco, alcohol, and unprescribed drugs
  - Immunizations (including hepatitis B vaccine for those who have not been previously exposed to the virus)
- Provide guidelines for activities that are appropriate for the child's physical state and developmental level.
- Discuss nonphysical disciplinary measures; encourage balance between overprotective and overly permissive parental behaviors.
- Coach concerning communication with siblings and affected child about hemophilia.
- Advise regarding communication with school and child care personnel about child's needs.

The most important aspect of management for the child with hemophilia is **prompt** factor replacement as needed for the treatment of specific bleeding episodes.

Alert: *Factor replacement should begin as soon as an injury occurs or the child indicates that bleeding has started, even when bleeding is not clinically evident.*

Prompt therapy is so essential that treatment usually precedes diagnostic testing to assess fully the current injury or bleeding episode. Replacement therapy comes first so that the factor level is raised as quickly as possible, thereby shortening the bleeding episode and decreasing the probability of long-term complications.

Factor Replacement Therapy

Factor replacement therapy has evolved significantly since the 1960s. Prior to that time, plasma was the primary treatment for bleeding episodes among those with hemophilia. Although plasma provides factor VIII, factor IX, and other clotting factors, volume limitations generally prevent the administration of plasma in the amount required to correct a factor deficit for the child with moderate or severe hemophilia.

Shortly after the discovery in 1964 that factor VIII is concentrated in plasma cryoprecipitate (Hoyer, 1994; Montgomery & Scott, 1993), cryoprecipitate and, subsequently, **factor VIII concentrates** became available for replacement therapy. It became possible to increase the factor VIII level to the point required for adequate control of particular bleeding incidents among those with hemophilia A.

For hemophilia B, **factor IX concentrates** became commercially available in 1969 in the form of prothrombin complex concentrates (Roberts & Eberst, 1993). This made it possible for those with hemophilia B to receive factor to control bleeding episodes. However, high doses and prolonged use of prothrombin complex concentrates are associated with an increased risk for thrombosis.

Thromboses have not been reported for the newer highly purified factor IX concentrates, AlphaNine and Mononine (Roberts & Eberst, 1993).

Recombinant DNA technology led to the production of recombinant factor VIII during the late 1980s. Unlike the other factor replacement products, recombinant factor VIII is not derived from human plasma and, thus, there is no risk of transmitting HIV, hepatitis, or other viruses that may be present in human plasma (Hoyer, 1994). Recombinant factor IX is expected to be available soon (DiMichele, 1996).

For those with mild or moderate hemophilia A, **desmopressin acetate (DDAVP)** may be used to promote the release of factor VIII from its endogenous storage sites and thereby increase the level of factor VIII. DDAVP is used only for those who have previously demonstrated a satisfactory increase in factor VIII levels in response to it. For these children, DDAVP is the treatment of choice when they experience mild to moderate hemorrhage (see Chart 23–13). DDAVP is **not** prescribed for those with hemophilia B.

The level of factor correction required to achieve hemostasis depends on the nature of the injury or specific bleeding episode. Mild to moderate hemorrhage requires factor correction to 30% to 50% of the normal factor level (DiMichele, 1996; Montgomery & Scott, 1993). This is often achieved with a one-time infusion of factor VIII or factor IX for hemophilia A and hemophilia B, respectively, but at times an additional one or two doses may be needed. Severe or life-threatening hemorrhage necessitates an immediate factor correction to 100%, followed by the maintenance of a 50% to 100% factor level for a number of days (DiMichele, 1996; Montgomery & Scott, 1993). Similar factor correction and maintenance are prescribed when surgical procedures are required. Maintenance levels are achieved by intermittent infusions or by continuous infusion of the appropriate factor.

Future Treatment Options

Neither factor replacement nor factor-releasing therapy is curative. However, the genes for factor VIII and factor IX have been cloned, and **gene transfer** methods are currently being developed that are likely to have future clinical application. The goal of gene transfer therapy is to facilitate the endogenous production of factor VIII and factor IX in quantities that will cure hemophilia or at least decrease its severity (DiMichele, 1996; Lozier & Brinkhous, 1994).

Management of Complications

In addition to treatment for bleeding episodes, the child with hemophilia requires management for complications that are secondary to replacement therapy or bleeding.

Inhibitors. A significant complication associated with the various replacement therapies is the development of an inhibitor (antibody) by approximately 15% of those who receive factor replacement. Factor VIII inhibitors are most common, but factor IX inhibitors may occur. The presence of an inhibitor is suspected when a child does not achieve the expected factor level after replacement therapy.

Most children with inhibitors receive the same factor replacement as children without inhibitors. However, they may need a larger dose to attain the desired factor level. Some children with inhibitors require individualized alternative therapy.

Viral Diseases. The transmission of viral diseases is a major concern among those who received factor VIII or factor IX concentrates before the mid-1980s. Hepatitis and HIV are of particular significance. However, since 1985, factor replacement concentrates have been treated with heat or chemicals to inactivate HIV and significantly reduce the risk of hepatitis and other viral diseases. For children with hemophilia A, the factor VIII concentrates of today are generally safer than cryoprecipitate unless the latter has been obtained from a carefully screened, single donor (Gill, 1993).

Bleeding Episodes. Complications associated with bleeding most often involve joints, muscles, and the oral cavity. Management of hemarthroses requires infusion of factor replacement at the first indication of bleeding. This is the best way to prevent joint deterioration. Adjunct measures include splinting, ice packs, and, with severe bleeding, joint aspiration. In children who are HIV negative, corticosteroids may be used to reduce inflammation at the joint site. Hemarthroses in target joints frequently lead to weakness and dysfunction in adjoining musculature. Thus, muscle strengthening exercises that do not cause tissue damage or bleeding are likely to be incorporated into a rehabilitation program for those with hemophilia (Pietri, Frontera, Pratts, & Suarez, 1992).

Management of hematomas in the child with hemophilia is aimed at reducing the size of the hematoma and preventing muscular fibrosis and contractures (Montgomery & Scott, 1993). Two measures are particularly significant in achieving these goals:

- The prompt infusion of factor replacement
- A physical therapy program designed to maintain normal range of motion

At times, a hematoma may quickly lead to life-threatening hemorrhage or paralysis without advance warning. The child, parents, family, and health care personnel need to know how to access and provide emergency care in these situations.

Appropriate factor replacement is the mainstay of treatment for oral cavity bleeding. In addition, antifibrinolytic agents (Chart 23–9) provide important adjunct therapy. They often decrease the amount of factor re-

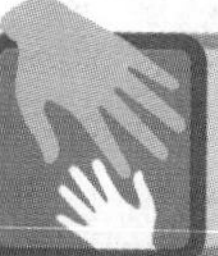

Chart 23–9
Nursing Interventions

Administering Aminocaproic Acid (Amicar)

Amicar is an antifibrinolytic agent that provides adjunct therapy for the control of oral bleeding. It is used for children with hemophilia and von Willebrand's disease when there is increased risk of oral bleeding (e.g., with oral surgical procedures, such as tooth extractions). The drug interferes with fibrinolysis by inhibiting the activation of plasminogen.

Amicar is contraindicated for children with disseminated intravascular coagulation (DIC) and renal bleeding. It should be used cautiously in those with cardiovascular, renal, and hepatic disease, as well as those receiving estrogen therapy.

Nursing considerations include:

1. Store at room temperature.
2. Administer orally or intravenously, as prescribed; it is usually given for 5 to 10 days.
   a. Oral administration
      (1) Loading dose is 100 to 200 mg/kg.
      (2) Maintenance dose is 100 mg/kg every 6 hours.
      (3) Maximum daily dose is 30 g.
   b. Intravenous administration
      (1) Infuse slowly.
      (2) Loading dose is 100 mg/kg or 3 g/m^2.
      (3) Continuous infusion dose is 33.3 mg/kg/hr or 1 g/m^2/hr.
      (4) Maximum daily dose is 18 g/m^2.
3. Monitor blood pressure and pulse during infusion.
4. Monitor intake and output.
5. Be alert for coagulation abnormalities in laboratory reports.
6. Instruct child/family regarding possible side effects.
   a. Rash
   b. Nasal congestion
   c. Ringing or buzzing in ears
   d. Bloodshot eyes
   e. Low blood pressure
   f. Slow or irregular pulse
   g. Nausea; vomiting; diarrhea
   h. Abdominal cramps
   i. Decreased urine output
   j. Muscle weakness
   k. Dizziness
   l. Headache
   m. Hallucinations
   n. Thrombosis

placement that is required and help to maintain oral clots until wound healing is complete.

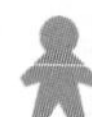

Tip: *During antifibrinolytic therapy, children should not use drinking straws, baby bottles, or pacifiers; they should not suck on hard candy, eat chips, or place any hard objects in their mouths. These measures help to avoid clot dislodgment.*

Community Care

Health care of the child with hemophilia is a coordinated effort between parents, school nurses, and the child's outpatient health care team. Major points of focus include preventing bleeding, providing support to the child and parents, ensuring smooth transitions from inpatient to outpatient care, and providing education about the disease and its course.

Prevention of Bleeding

The potential for serious, life-threatening bleeding underscores the need for prudence in the selection of daily activities. Decisions regarding sports participation may be especially challenging. Such decisions should be made in consultation with the comprehensive health care team and must consider the child's developmental level and physical ability, as well as the severity of the hemophilia (Chart 23–10). Even children who do not participate in sports need to engage in a regular exercise program. This helps them develop a strong musculature to support their joints and decrease the risk of bleeding.

It is important that parents, as well as older children and adolescents, be instructed by the nurse to notify health care providers of the presence of hemophilia prior to any invasive procedures. This allows the incorporation of specific prophylactic measures to prevent bleeding. Such measures include the application of pressure for at least 10 minutes after a procedure such as a venipuncture, the use of antifibrinolytics for dental work, and the use of factor replacement therapy for surgical procedures (Chart 23–11).

Fever and pain in the child with hemophilia are often managed with acetaminophen or acetaminophen with codeine.

caREminder: *Aspirin and aspirin-containing medications, such as Excedrin and Percodan, are contraindicated in children with bleeding disorders because they interfere with normal platelet function.*

Psychosocial Needs

Management of the child with hemophilia requires attention to the psychosocial needs of the child and the family.

Child. Initially, the child is usually too young to be aware of the diagnosis and its significance. However, as growth and development proceed, the child increasingly

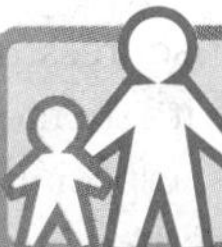

Chart 23–10
Developmental Considerations

Sports Guidelines for Children with Hemophilia

Category I	Category II	Category III
Archery	Baseball	Boxing
Badminton	Basketball	Diving
Fishing	Bicycling	Football
Golf	Bowling	Hockey
Hiking	Cross-country skiing	Motorcycling
Ping-Pong	Frisbee play	Racquetball
Swimming	Gymnastics	Rugby
Walking	Horseback riding	Skateboarding
	Ice skating	Wrestling
	Jogging	
	Roller skating	
	Running	
	Soccer	
	Tennis	
	Volleyball	
	Waterskiing	
	Weight lifting	

Category I sports are usually safe for those with hemophilia.

Category II sports are riskier and may be discouraged for some. However, for the majority of those with hemophilia, the physical and psychosocial benefits are likely to outweigh the risks.

Category III sports are those in which the risks outweigh the benefits, and they are *not* recommended for those with hemophilia.

Data from *Hemophilia and sports* (1985) and from *The hemophilia handbook* (1988).

learns about the disorder and is affected by the realization that not everyone has hemophilia.

Helping children with hemophilia acquire accurate knowledge about the disorder, its management, and its complications is important for their physical and psychological well-being. As children progress developmentally, teaching must be an ongoing process that assesses each child's previous knowledge and expands on it. The need for such education is supported by the results of a nursing research study (Spitzer, 1992a) that found that a number of school-age children with hemophilia have misperceptions or knowledge deficits related to the nature of the disorder, its cause, and its management.

Children with hemophilia need to develop effective coping skills for dealing with both physical and psychosocial concerns. They may fear bleeding. They may wonder

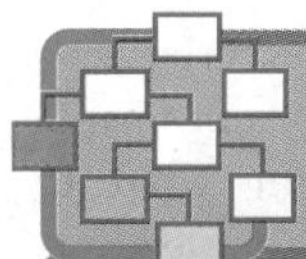

Chart 23–11
Clinical Judgment

A School-Ager with Hemophilia A

Jason is a 7-year-old male with severe hemophilia A. He is admitted to the hospital this morning for a scheduled tonsillectomy later today. The health history reveals that hemophilia was diagnosed during infancy shortly after prolonged bleeding occurred with circumcision. Recently, he experienced a tonsillar bleeding episode in conjunction with pharyngitis. Today's physical examination findings are within normal limits. There is no evidence of bleeding or pharyngitis. Admission laboratory studies are within normal limits except for a prolonged partial thromboplastin time (PTT) of 74.2 seconds and a factor VIII level of less than 1%.

Questions

1. What additional information would you elicit to assess Jason's readiness for surgery?
2. Is Jason's hemophilia classified as mild, moderate, or severe? Why?
3. Why is Jason a candidate for a tonsillectomy?
4. How can Jason's bleeding be controlled after surgery?
5. Identify two significant clinical findings associated with post-tonsillectomy bleeding.

Answers

1. Inquire about what Jason has been told regarding his surgery and what to expect after surgery. Ask whether or not he has attended a preoperative class for children and, if so, ask about his response to it. Ask what Jason knows about the precautions that will be taken to control bleeding during and after surgery, that is, continuous infusion of factor VIII and close monitoring by nursing staff for signs and symptoms of bleeding.
2. Jason has severe hemophilia because his uncorrected factor VIII level is less than 1%.
3. A history of a tonsillar bleeding episode together with severe hemophilia places Jason at increased risk for another tonsillar bleeding episode, particularly if there is recurrent pharyngitis.
4. Jason's bleeding can be controlled after surgery by
   - Factor VIII infusion
   - Antifibrinolytic medication
   - Avoidance of hard or sharp foods and objects in the mouth
   - Soft diet with no hot or spicy foods and beverages
5. Two significant clinical findings associated with post-tonsillectomy bleeding are
   - Bleeding at the surgical site
   - Rapid pulse rate

what will happen to them when they do experience a bleeding episode. Knowing the signs and symptoms of bleeding, knowing what to do, and knowing what to expect others to do help children cope with bleeding. Children should notify their parents, teachers, or other caregivers when they experience bleeding, so that measures to stop bleeding can be promptly implemented. These measures usually include factor replacement. Older children and adolescents have probably learned how to prepare and administer their own factor, whereas parents usually perform this procedure for younger children.

Children may be concerned about pain associated with obtaining blood for laboratory studies. A common coping strategy during such procedures is the use of distraction. Parents or health care staff help the children focus their attention elsewhere, or the children themselves learn to direct their thoughts to more pleasant things.

Children with hemophilia are involved in establishing their identities as individuals with a particular chronic disorder. A nurse researcher (Spitzer, 1992b) reported that these children tend to minimize their personal experiences with hemophilia. Nevertheless, the stories they tell in response to pictorial stimuli involving other children indicate that hemophilia is a significant part of their own personal identities. They actually are concerned about being different from other children. There are times when they feel left out because they cannot participate in all activities with their peers. It is important to help children with hemophilia identify their positive qualities, help them see what they can do, help them develop healthy self-images, and help them formulate realistic goals for their future.

Parents. Parents of a child with hemophilia are likely to have psychosocial concerns. A significant role for members of the comprehensive health care team is to provide informational and emotional support in response to parental needs.

Informational support refers to providing parents with timely information. It is helpful for nurses to have a teaching outline that covers areas in which parents commonly need informational support (see TIP 23–1). However, such a plan must be adapted in response to the specific needs of parents at any given point in time.

Although the desired outcomes of providing information include improved parental coping and the ability to parent a child with hemophilia effectively, the information received is likely to be emotionally disturbing at first. It is stressful for parents to learn that their child has hemophilia and faces a lifetime of living with a chronic disorder. As they begin to learn about hemophilia, its management, and its complications, parents may be concerned that they will not recognize a bleeding episode or will not respond appropriately to it. The diagnosis of hemophilia, the early bleeding episodes thereafter, and any painful or serious bleeding episodes are all sources of emotional stress for most parents of a child with hemophilia. Also, there is likely to be parental guilt, especially for the mother, when the hemophilia is inherited and the mother is a carrier of the abnormal chromosome.

As time progresses, health care expenses may generate stress, especially if the child has severe hemophilia and frequently requires costly factor replacement therapy. For parents whose children received treatment before the middle 1980s, a major stressor is likely to be the presence of or the fear of hepatitis and HIV.

Emotional support for the parents of a child with hemophilia includes listening, identifying previously effective coping skills, providing positive reinforcement, and offering practical information when appropriate.

Listening attentively to parents is a significant means of emotional support. Even when the situation of having a child with hemophilia cannot be changed, parents are likely to feel support when they are given the opportunity to express their feelings, needs, concerns, and hopes. Support groups provide an opportunity for parents to share, learn from others, and encourage one another.

Identifying coping skills that have been used effectively in the past may enable the parents to transfer these skills to the issues they face in having a child with hemophilia.

Providing positive reinforcement encourages parents. For example, when they effectively manage their child's first bleeding episode at home, the nurse can let them know they responded appropriately to that situation.

When concerns arise for which practical help is available, let the parents know about the resources for this help. For example, when they express a concern about lack of money for health care expenses, direct them to a financial counselor. The counselor can advise them of benefits for which they may qualify and develop a payment plan suitable to the family's financial resources.

Siblings. As in other chronic disorders, the siblings of children with hemophilia need attention. Sometimes they feel left out, or they may feel guilty because they are well and do not experience the health problems they observe in the child with hemophilia. Siblings need a sense of belonging within the family. They need to feel that their parents have time for them and value them just as much as the child with hemophilia. Also, siblings need accurate knowledge about hemophilia, its etiology, its management, and its complications, as well as information about how they can help during bleeding episodes or other complications in the child with hemophilia.

Discharge Planning

For children with hemophilia, the nurse may view discharge planning from two perspectives. One involves discharge planning related to specific events such as bleeding episodes, surgical procedures, and dental work. The second relates to discharge planning associated with scheduled outpatient appointments designed for the ongoing assessment and management of children with hemophilia. In both situations, the nurse needs to identify desired outcomes, and plan and provide appropriate interventions to facilitate attainment of these outcomes by the end of a hospital stay or an outpatient visit.

Discharge planning for episodic events takes into account the needs related to the particular event, in addition to the needs associated with hemophilia. Often there is referral to a home care company to provide factor replacement therapy, as well as the various supplies needed at home.

Teaching is a significant part of discharge planning. The nurse needs to start teaching as early as possible and plan time for review. Teaching may encompass a variety of topics, depending on the specific situation. For example, when a child with hemophilia has lower extremity orthopedic surgery, teaching is likely to include cast care, crutch walking, pain management, signs and symptoms of bleeding at the surgical site, administration of factor replacement therapy at home, schedule for outpatient follow-up appointments, and need to call the physician for bleeding, fever, increased pain, or other complications. An important component of the teaching process is an assessment of the family's understanding of the child's home care needs and their ability to care for the child at home.

Care Path 23–1 illustrates how, even with a com-

Care Path 23–1 An Interdisciplinary Plan of Care for a Child with Hemophilia A Undergoing Tonsillectomy

	Patient/Family Outcomes		
Nursing Diagnosis	**Day: Admission**	**Day 2**	**Day 3**
Risk for fluid volume deficit related to potential bleeding	Factor level corrected to 100% Pulse normal for age No evidence of bleeding	Factor level corrected to 60% Pulse normal for age No evidence of bleeding Child/parents verbalize need to avoid hard/sharp foods and objects in mouth	Factor level corrected to 60% Pulse normal for age No evidence of bleeding Child/parents verbalize signs and symptoms of bleeding Parents verbalize plan for home factor VIII infusions and antifibrinolytics
Pain related to surgery	Ice collar and analgesic effective in relieving pain Vital signs stable and within normal limits	Ice collar and analgesic effective in relieving pain Vital signs stable and within normal limits	Ice collar and analgesic effective in relieving pain Vital signs stable and within normal limits Parents identify home pain relief measures Parents verbalize need to notify health care provider, if pain relief measures are ineffective
Altered nutrition: less than body requirements related to throat pain and difficulty swallowing	Tolerating sips of oral fluids	Tolerating oral fluids in adequate amounts	Tolerating oral fluids in adequate amounts Parents verbalize signs and symptoms of dehydration Parents verbalize need to notify health care provider if fluid intake is inadequate or signs and symptoms of dehydration are present

Care Path continued on following page

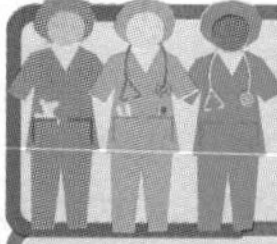

Care Path 23–1 An Interdisciplinary Plan of Care for a Child with Hemophilia A Undergoing Tonsillectomy *Continued*

Nursing Diagnosis	Day: Admission	Day 2	Day 3
Risk for injury related to infection	Child's temperature < 38.0°C No evidence of infection	Child's temperature <38.0°C No evidence of infection	Child's temperature < 38.0°C No evidence of infection Parents verbalize importance of notifying health care provider, if fever occurs
Care Intervention Categories			
Consults	Ear, nose, and throat specialist (ENT)	⟶	⟶
Discharge planning	Home Care Company Name: ____________ Phone: ____________	Plan for home administration of factor VIII	Discharge day Prescriptions for home medications
Labs	PT, PTT, fibrinogen, FSP, TCT CBC with differential Platelet count Bleeding time Factor VIII level 1 hr after initial preoperative factor VIII infusion Chem 17, SGPT Factor VIII level postoperatively Review preadmission laboratory results · Factor VIII level · Factor VIII inhibitor level · HIV · Hepatitis screen	PT, PTT, fibrinogen CBC with differential Platelet count Factor VIII level	⟶ ⟶ ⟶ ⟶
Medications and IVs	IV fluids Factor VIII drip Analgesic Antibiotic Antifibrinolytic	IV heparin lock ⟶ ⟶ ⟶ ⟶	Discontinue IV ⟶ ⟶ ⟶ ⟶
Nutrition	Preoperatively: NPO Postoperatively: Tonsil diet **Avoid sharp foods** **Do not use straws**	Soft diet as tolerated ⟶ ⟶	⟶ ⟶ ⟶

Care Path 23–1 An Interdisciplinary Plan of Care for a Child with Hemophilia A Undergoing Tonsillectomy *Continued*

Care Intervention Categories	Day: Admission	Day 2	Day 3
Pain management	Ice collar p.r.n. Analgesic	→ →	→ →
Play therapy or school	Preoperatively: Play to simulate preoperative, perioperative, and postoperative experiences	Quiet play or study activities appropriate for developmental level	→
Procedures	Tonsillectomy		
Psychosocial	Parents encouraged to be with child pre- and postoperatively Informational and emotional support	Parents or significant others encouraged to be present Informational and emotional support	→ →
Safety and activity	Elevate head of bed 30 degrees post-op	Out of bed as tolerated	Ambulatory
Social service	Notify social worker for hemophilia of child's admission	Assess family's ability to care for child at home postoperatively	
Special considerations	Observe closely for signs of hemorrhage and airway obstruction	→	→
Teaching	Pre-, peri-, and postoperative management of hemophilia Tonsil diet Need to avoid sharp foods and objects in mouth	Soft diet Home administration of factor VIII Discharge instructions	Review signs and symptoms of late bleeding
Vital signs	Preoperatively: Vital signs q 4 hr Postoperatively: · Bleeding check q 2 hr · Pulse q 2 hr · Temperature q 4 hr · Respirations q 4 hr · Blood pressure q 4 hr · Continuous pulse oximetry	Vital signs q 4 hr	→

CBC, complete blood count; FSP, fibrin split products; NPO, nothing by mouth; PT, prothrombin time; PTT, partial thromboplastin time; SGPT, serum glutamate pyruvate transaminase; TCT, thrombin-clotting time.

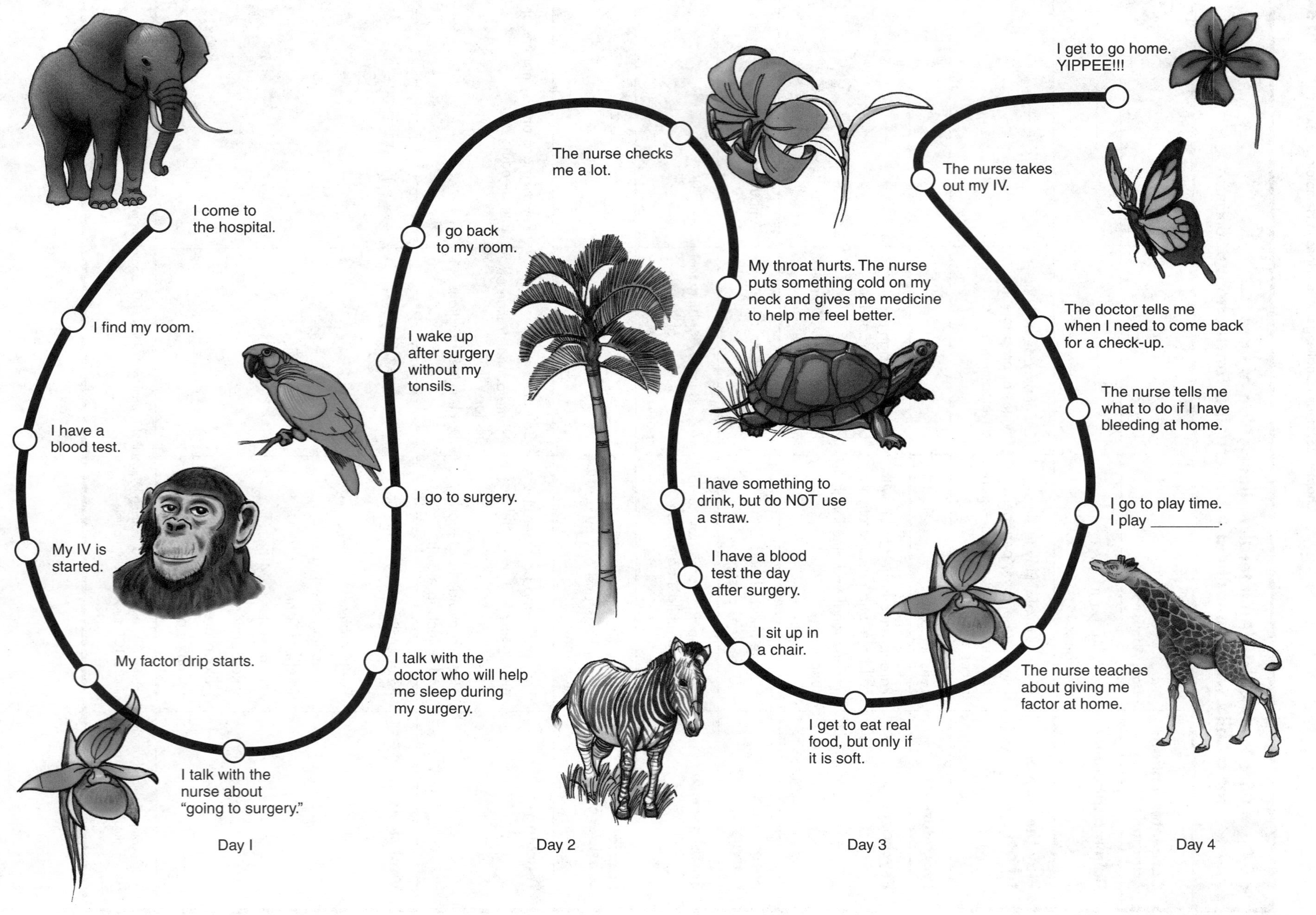

Figure 23–4
A care path for a child with hemophilia undergoing tonsillectomy. (Adapted with permission from Susan P. Kyzer, M.S., R.N., C.P.N., Shriners Hospitals for Children, Greenville Unit, Greenville, SC.)

mon surgical procedure, nursing care and discharge planning need to be adapted to account for increased bleeding tendencies in the child with hemophilia.

When working with children, it is important to include them as partners in the teaching plan. The use of a more simplified care path (Fig. 23–4) can assist in this process. The child may color the pictures. In addition, the child may color the circles or place small stickers in the circles as each event occurs.

Outpatient visits for the ongoing assessment and management of children with hemophilia generally occur at a comprehensive treatment center at least once per year. Desired outcomes for these visits are related to physical and psychosocial needs on the basis of an updated history and current physical assessment.

Be alert for the developing child's readiness to learn more about hemophilia, as well as the need to correct misperceptions the child and family may have about the disorder, its effect, and its management. Also, as the child and family reach new developmental milestones, be alert for the need to discuss the child's activities and specific concerns associated with each developmental phase.

Discharge planning for outpatient visits may include referral or follow-up information to a local physician, a home care company, and a community health agency. It may entail contact with community groups, such as the child's daycare center or school (Chart 23–12). It may involve assisting a family with planning for camp or vacation by arranging for a source of health care for the child while away from home and by identifying an appropriate storage place for the child's particular type of factor replacement. In addition, discharge planning may include a referral to The National Hemophilia Foundation for literature, as well as for information about the services and local chapters of this organization (see Resources).

von Willebrand's Disease

von Willebrand's disease (vWD) is the most common hereditary bleeding disorder (Rick, 1994; Vosburgh, 1993;

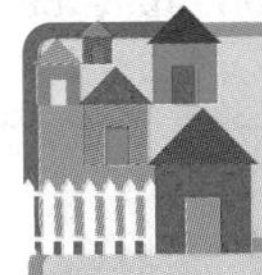

Chart 23–12
Community Care

The Child with Hemophilia in School

Children with hemophilia usually attend school on a regular basis when they are not having active bleeding. It is important that their teachers know they have a bleeding disorder. Also, the teaching staff should know the guidelines that have been established to prevent and manage an individual child's bleeding episodes and to promote the child's normal growth and development.

The school nurse collaborates with the comprehensive health care team and joins the child and family in providing information to the teaching staff. Outcome objectives for teachers and teaching assistants include the following:

- State the type and severity of the child's hemophilia, and correlate an increased severity with an increased risk of bleeding, including spontaneous bleeding.
- Identify body joints and muscle tissue as the hallmark sites of bleeding for the child with hemophilia.
- Describe signs and symptoms associated with covert bleeding, such as tingling, tenderness, pain, warmth, and altered motor function of the affected body site (e.g., refusal to walk or to participate in usual physical activities).
- Discuss the need for prompt factor replacement for bleeding episodes to prevent joint injury, tissue damage, and possible life-threatening hemorrhage.
- State the rationale for not giving aspirin to the child with a bleeding disorder.
- Discuss the importance of the child's participation in physical activities except for activities that are identified as high risk and inappropriate for the child. School personnel should be informed of the activities in which the child is not to participate.
- Explain the importance of telephoning the designated family member whenever the child is injured or says he is bleeding, *even when there are no signs and symptoms of bleeding*. Parents may advise school personnel that it is not necessary to telephone them regarding small, superficial cuts and scrapes because factor replacement is usually not required in such situations.
- Describe the significance of treating the child as the classmates are treated. Although there is a need to be aware of the bleeding disorder, the teaching staff should not focus on it or single the child out for special attention or privileges.

Note: If the child with hemophilia has acquired the human immunodeficiency virus (is HIV positive), it is important that the school nurse discuss this with the teaching staff (see Chapter 24).

Werner, 1996). It results from a quantitative, structural, or functional abnormality of the von Willebrand's factor.

In general, vWD is inherited in an autosomal dominant fashion via a genetic defect on chromosome 12. The exact incidence of vWD is not known because, in its mild form, it may not be diagnosed until there is an episode of prolonged bleeding at a time of surgery or trauma. The estimated incidence is close to 1% of the population (Montgomery & Scott, 1993; Rick, 1994). Males and females and the various racial groups are affected in equal numbers.

In addition, vWD may be acquired with certain clinical disorders such as hypothyroidism, disseminated intravascular coagulation (DIC), and congenital heart disease (Montgomery & Scott, 1993; Werner, 1996). Acquired vWD usually resolves when the accompanying clinical disorder has been treated.

Pathophysiology

von Willebrand's factor has two primary functions with regard to hemostasis. First, it acts as an adhesive bridge between platelets and injured vascular subendothelium (Montgomery & Scott, 1993; Rick, 1994). Platelet adhesion is necessary for normal platelet aggregation and fibrin clot formation (Fig. 23–5).

Second, von Willebrand's factor serves as a carrier protein for the procoagulant factor VIII. Without von Willebrand's factor, factor VIII has a markedly decreased survival time, which may decrease the level of factor VIII (Montgomery & Scott, 1993; Rick, 1994; Werner, 1996).

There are three major categories of vWD: type I, type II, and type III (Table 23–7). Types I and III are characterized primarily by a quantitative deficiency in von Willebrand's factor. Type II is characterized primarily by structural and functional abnormalities of the factor.

In general, the prognosis for children with vWD is good, particularly because most of them have a milder form of the disease.

Assessment

The primary clinical manifestations of vWD are bruising and mucous membrane bleeding from the nose, mouth, and gastrointestinal tract. Prolonged bleeding after trauma and surgery, including tooth extraction, may be

Table 23–7
Major Types of von Willebrand's Disease (vWD)

	Type I	Type II		Type III
Percentage affected among those with vWD	70%–80%	15%–20%		1%–10%
		Type IIA	Type IIB	
Degree of bleeding	Mild to moderate	Mild to moderate	Moderate to severe	Severe*
Distinctive characteristics	All sizes of von Willebrand's factor multimers are present but in decreased quantity Decreased von Willebrand's factor activity	Intermediate-size and large von Willebrand's factor multimers are absent Small von Willebrand's factor multimers are increased von Willebrand's factor activity is decreased and may be disproportionate with quantity of von Willebrand's factor	von Willebrand's factor has an abnormal attraction to platelets Large von Willebrand's factor multimers bind to platelet surfaces, leaving von Willebrand's factor with only small and intermediate-size multimers Platelet agglutination increases Thrombocytopenia may be present	All sizes of von Willebrand's factor multimers are absent or almost absent von Willebrand's factor activity is absent or minimal Factor VIII level is low

* In addition to ecchymoses and mucous membrane bleeding, which are characteristic of von Willebrand's disease in general, those with type III disease may have deep bleeding into joints and muscles similar to that associated with hemophilia.

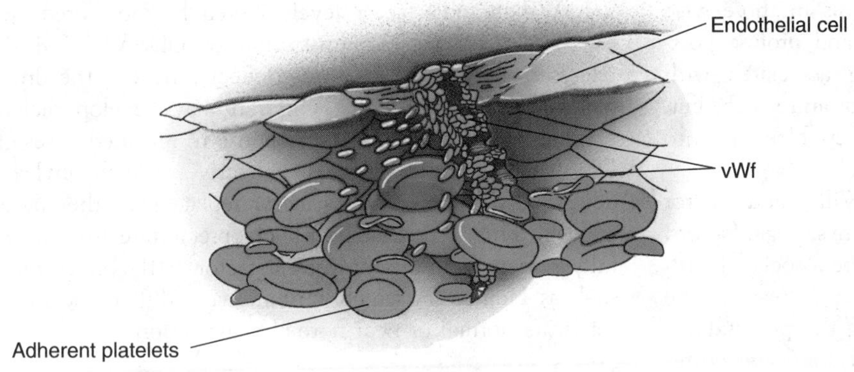

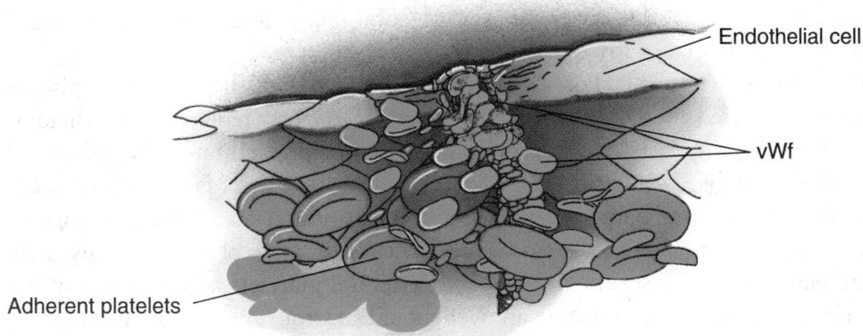

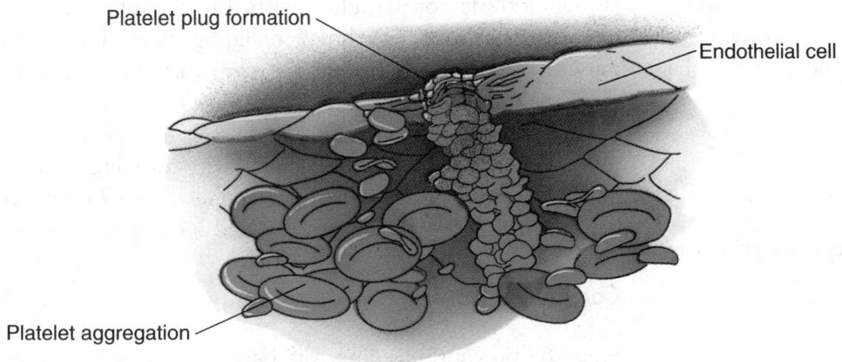

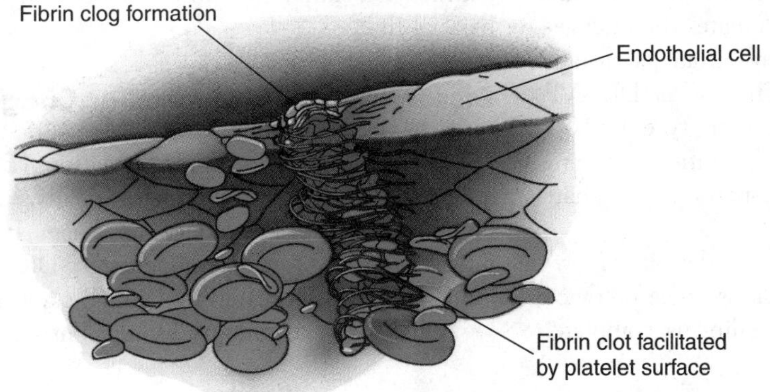

Figure 23–5
After vessel injury, plasma von Willebrand's factor binds to the endothelium and supports platelet adherence. The adhered platelets recruit more platelets and promote fibrin clot formation.

the first evidence of abnormal hemostasis in those with mild vWD. For females, menorrhagia and profuse postpartum bleeding may occur. Bleeding associated with vWD may be severe and lead to anemia and shock, but, unlike the situation in hemophilia, deep bleeding into joints and muscles is rare.

Diagnostic Tests. The level of von Willebrand's factor may vary in conjunction with certain physiologic factors. High estrogen levels during pregnancy are associated with higher von Willebrand's factor levels, decreasing the probability of prolonged bleeding during the prenatal period. Also, inflammation, exercise, and stress are correlated with increased levels of von Willebrand's factor. If blood samples are drawn at these times, or if the children experience particular stress from the venipuncture procedure itself, the presence of vWD may be masked.

Fluctuating levels of von Willebrand's factor may make it difficult to diagnose vWD, especially in its milder form. Initial screening studies may document a prolonged activated partial thromboplastin time (APTT) and a prolonged bleeding time, but results of these tests may be within normal limits. Factor VIII levels may be decreased or within normal limits. The von Willebrand's factor antigen level is usually decreased or absent but may be borderline in mild vWD. The ristocetin cofactor level generally reflects decreased von Willebrand's factor activity, but this, too, may be borderline in mild vWD. A von Willebrand's factor analysis is helpful in distinguishing among the various types of vWD.

A diagnosis of vWD cannot be ruled out by normal laboratory values alone. When the child's history indicates the possibility of vWD, laboratory studies should be repeated periodically.

Interdisciplinary Interventions

Management of the child with vWD depends primarily on the classification of the disease.

Type I

Type I vWD is the most common type, and bleeding episodes associated with it are generally easy to treat. Most children with type I vWD respond well to **desmopressin acetate (DDAVP)**, which stimulates the endogenous release of von Willebrand's factor from its storage sites (Gill & Montgomery, 1993). The use of DDAVP is the treatment of choice for those with type I vWD who have previously demonstrated a satisfactory increase in von Willebrand's factor in response to it (Chart 23–13).

Often a single dose of DDAVP is adequate. However, for major surgery, repeated infusions, once or twice a day, are generally required until healing is complete. von Willebrand's factor levels should be monitored before and after the administration of DDAVP. This is necessary to confirm continued effectiveness of the drug, particularly because some children may develop tachyphylaxis, a rapidly declining response to repeated doses of DDAVP. When DDAVP is ineffective or tachyphylaxis develops, von Willebrand's factor replacement therapy is needed. This is provided with cryoprecipitate from carefully screened donors or with a factor VIII concentrate, such as Humate-P, which contains von Willebrand's factor in its normal or near-normal composition.

Type II

Bleeding episodes and surgery associated with type IIA vWD are generally managed by replacement therapy. However, minor bleeding may sometimes be managed with DDAVP.

For children with type IIB vWD, bleeding episodes and surgery are managed by replacement therapy. DDAVP is not used because it facilitates the release of additional abnormal von Willebrand's factor, thereby enhancing the platelet agglutination and thrombocytopenia that are associated with this type of vWD. Only with severe thrombocytopenia are platelets administered in addition to von Willebrand's factor replacement therapy.

Type III

Type III vWD is managed primarily with replacement therapy with factor VIII concentrates that contain von Willebrand's factor. Children with this type of vWD may have spontaneous bleeding, including deep joint and muscle bleeding. Their ongoing care may be similar to that of children with severe hemophilia.

Antifibrinolytic agents (see Chart 23–9) provide significant adjunct therapy for oral cavity bleeding among children with vWD. As with hemophilia, antifibrinolytics help to maintain oral clots until wound healing is achieved.

Community Care

Steps to prevent bleeding, discharge planning for home care and return to school, and measures to provide for the psychosocial needs of children with vWD and their families are similar to those described in the section on hemophilia.

Disseminated Intravascular Coagulation

Disseminated intravascular coagulation (DIC) is an acquired coagulopathy that, paradoxically, is characterized by both thrombosis and hemorrhage. Its acuity level ranges from low-grade compensated DIC to fulminant, multisystem, life-threatening DIC (Bick, 1994).

DIC is **not** a primary disorder but occurs as a result

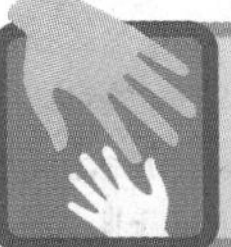

Chart 23-13
Nursing Interventions

Administering Desmopressin Acetate (DDAVP)

In addition to being an antidiuretic hormone, desmopressin acetate (DDAVP) is an antihemorrhagic agent. It can be effective in the management of mild hemophilia A and type I von Willebrand disease. DDAVP promotes higher levels of both factor VIII activity and von Willebrand factor activity by releasing endogenous factor VIII and von Willebrand factor from their storage sites. DDAVP is contraindicated for children with hemophilia B, severe hemophilia A, and type IIB and type III von Willebrand disease. The intranasal route of administration is contraindicated with nasal mucosa alterations such as rhinorrhea, edema, and scarring.

Nursing considerations include the following:

1. Refrigerate DDAVP; avoid freezing.
2. Note that doses of DDAVP for hemophilia A and von Willebrand's disease are higher than those for nocturnal enuresis and diabetes insipidus.
3. Administer DDAVP intravenously or intranasally.
   a. Intravenous infusion
      (1) Dosage is 0.3 μg/kg diluted in normal saline.
      (2) Give slowly over 15 to 30 minutes.
      (3) Monitor blood pressure and pulse during infusion.
   b. Intranasal spray
      (1) Use high concentration spray, 1.5 mg/mL.
      (2) Give via metered-dose spray pump.
      (3) Dosage:
         (a) Children <50 kg: 150 μg (one metered-dose spray in one nostril)
         (b) Children >50 kg: 300 μg (one metered-dose spray in each nostril)
4. Monitor intake and output; avoid overhydration.
5. Be alert for hyponatremia in laboratory reports.
6. Be alert for inadequate levels of factor VIII or von Willebrands factor in laboratory reports.
7. Instruct child/family regarding side effects of DDAVP:
   a. Facial flushing
   b. Nasal congestion
   c. Increased blood pressure
   d. Nausea
   e. Abdominal cramps
   f. Decreased urination
   g. Vulval pain
   h. Signs and symptoms of water intoxication
      (1) Headache
      (2) Drowsiness
      (3) Confusion
      (4) Weight gain
      (5) Seizures
      (6) Coma

of a variety of alterations in health status (Chart 23–14). Conditions that precipitate DIC may, in turn, be complicated by DIC.

The etiology of DIC is not well understood. In general, it appears that damaged, diseased, or necrotic body tissue and certain enzymes and toxins enter the circulation and excessively activate elements in the normal coagulation system (Bick, 1994; Hilgartner & Corrigan, 1995). In addition, DIC may be triggered when blood comes in contact with the foreign surfaces of implanted prosthetic devices (Bick, 1994).

Pathophysiology

Although DIC may be precipitated by different disorders, its basic pathophysiology is the same and leads to the development of both thrombosis and hemorrhage.

Thrombosis in DIC occurs when the coagulation

Chart 23–14

Conditions That May Precipitate Disseminated Intravascular Coagulation (DIC)

- Burns
- Traumatic injuries
- Hypoxia
- Severe shock
- Hemolytic transfusion reactions
- Cardiovascular disorders
- Acute myelogenous leukemias
- Metastatic malignancies
- Infections
- Septic abortion
- Pregnancy complications
- Venomous bites and stings
- Inflammatory bowel disease
- Liver disease
- Reye's syndrome
- Hypothermia or hyperthermia
- Implanted prosthetic devices

system is overstimulated by a primary triggering disorder (Fig. 23–6). This leads to an excessive amount of circulating thrombin which, in turn, leads to increased fibrin clot formation. Microvascular and, at times, macrovascular thrombosis occurs. This hinders normal blood flow and may result in ischemia and organ damage.

Also, red blood cells become fragmented as they circulate among the numerous fibrin deposits in the vasculature, and a hemolytic anemia may develop.

Hemorrhage associated with DIC may occur as a consequence of various pathophysiologic events (Fig. 23–7). First, the intravascular thrombi, which form as a result of excessive thrombin in the circulation, are a trap for platelets. This results in hemorrhage secondary to thrombocytopenia.

Second, excessive amounts of circulating plasmin are produced. This leads to excessive fibrinolysis and an abnormally high amount of circulating fibrin degradation (split) products (FDPs or FSPs). FDPs function as anticoagulants, thereby contributing to hemorrhage. Also, FDPs cover platelet membranes, making the platelets dysfunctional and leading to hemorrhage.

Third, the clotting factors involved in normal coagulation are significantly decreased or absent in DIC, resulting in hemorrhage.

Prognosis. The prognosis for DIC is variable. It depends primarily on the prognosis for the underlying disorder, as well as the severity of the DIC. Fulminant DIC can be life threatening.

Assessment

The most obvious clinical feature of DIC is bleeding. However, it is equally important to be alert for clinical manifestations of the other major pathophysiologic event in DIC: thrombosis. Bleeding and thrombosis may occur in multiple, unrelated anatomic locations. The most common sites of DIC include the kidneys, lungs, skin, gastrointestinal tract, and central nervous system.

- **Renal** involvement with DIC may be manifested by hematuria, oliguria, and anuria.
- **Pulmonary** involvement with DIC may be evidenced by hemoptysis, tachypnea, dyspnea, and chest pain.
- **Cutaneous** involvement with DIC may be characterized by petechiae, ecchymoses, hemorrhagic bullae, pallor, jaundice, acrocyanosis, and gangrene. In addition, there may be bleeding from surgical or traumatic wounds and from invasive procedure sites.

Figure 23–6
Pathophysiology of thrombosis in DIC.

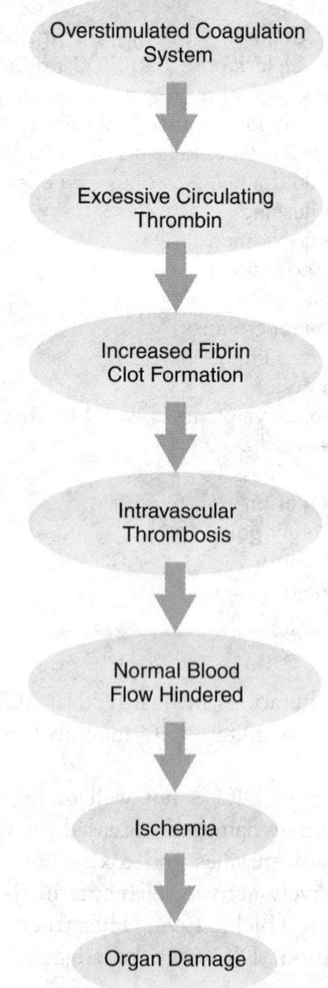

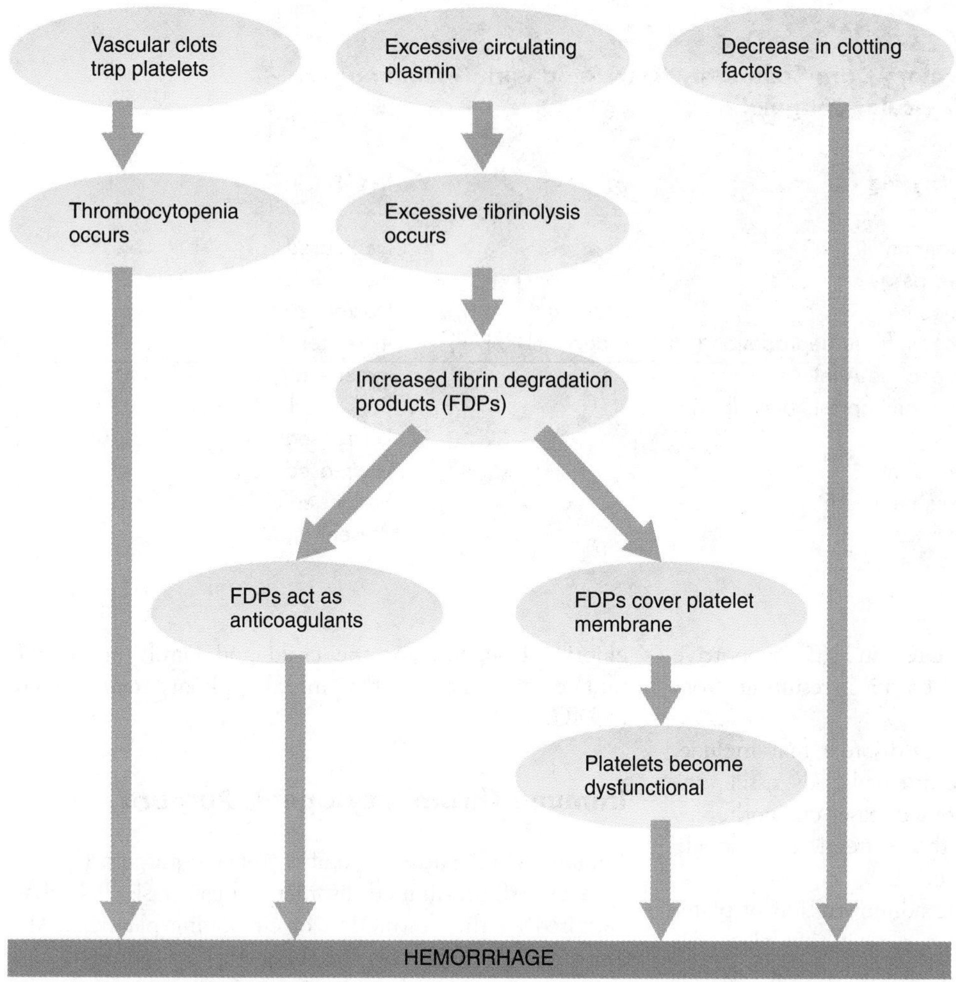

Figure 23–7
DIC leads to hemorrhage by various mechanisms as illustrated in this diagram.

- **Gastrointestinal** involvement with DIC may be manifested by hematemesis, hematochezia, and absent or hypo- or hyperactive bowel sounds.
- **Central nervous system** involvement with DIC may be suspected when there are headaches, increased intracranial pressure, sensory deficits, seizures, altered mental status, and decreased level of consciousness.

DIC may have systemic manifestations, as well. These include fever, hypotension, acidosis, and hypoxia. In addition, all anatomic sites affected by DIC are at risk for ischemia, tissue damage, organ failure, and necrosis.

Diagnostic Tests

Although there is not a test that is specifically diagnostic for DIC, certain alterations in hematologic laboratory data can contribute to its identification (Table 23–8). Such laboratory data, however, must be assessed within the context of the child's history, underlying disorder, and general clinical state. In addition, note that the absence of laboratory findings commonly associated with DIC does not necessarily exclude its presence.

Nursing Diagnoses and Outcomes

Nursing diagnoses and outcomes for the child with a bleeding disorder are presented in Chart 23–3. In addition, the following nursing diagnosis and outcome pertain to the child with DIC:

▶ **Altered tissue perfusion related to intravascular thrombosis and hemorrhage**
Outcome: The child maintains normal function of all body systems affected by DIC and regains normal laboratory values for hemostasis.

Interdisciplinary Interventions

Management of the child with DIC is individualized on the basis of the underlying disorder, as well as the degree of DIC. Thus, specific treatment may vary from no treatment in the absence of clinical manifestations to intensive treatment in the presence of fulminant DIC.

When clinical manifestations are present, primary interventions are directed toward (1) effective treatment of

Table 23-8
Laboratory Data Commonly Associated with Disseminated Intravascular Coagulation

Laboratory Test	Result
Antithrombin III	Decreased
D-Dimer assay	Increased
Fibrinogen	Decreased
Fibrinogen/fibrin degradation (split) products (FDP/FSP)	Increased
Fibrinopeptide A level	Increased
Partial thromboplastin time (PTT)	Prolonged
Plasminogen	Decreased
Platelet count	Decreased
Prothrombin time (PT)	Prolonged
Schistocytes	Present

the disorder that precipitated DIC and (2) supportive care to correct physiologic alterations resulting from DIC.

Treatment of the precipitating disorder may include, for examples, surgery to remove diseased body tissue, antibiotic therapy to treat infectious disease, chemotherapy to destroy malignancies, and the correction of shock, hypoxia, and acid-base imbalance.

Supportive care includes the administration of platelet concentrates and fresh frozen plasma to replace depleted platelets and coagulation factors, respectively. At times, exchange transfusion may be done, especially with neonates. This removes FDPs, in addition to replacing clotting factors (Gill & Montgomery, 1993). Exchange transfusion is discussed earlier in the section on treatment modalities and later in the section on hemolytic disease of the newborn.

In some situations, treatment of DIC may include administration of the anticoagulant heparin. Heparin potentiates antithrombin III, which, in turn, inhibits thrombin and the further development of intravascular thrombosis (Chart 23–15).

Nurses collaborate with the health care team to plan and provide for the therapeutic and supportive measures that are needed by the child with DIC. A key aspect of the nurse's role is to assess the child for signs and symptoms of impaired tissue perfusion in the various body systems that may be affected by DIC. Significant outcome objectives for the child and related nursing interventions are delineated in Chart 23–16.

Concerns about bleeding, clotting, and organ failure with serious DIC are likely to produce significant emotional stress in both the child and family. It is important that the health care team be sensitive to this stress. Education about DIC, ongoing progress reports, and emotional support for the child and family are important components of the interdisciplinary management of DIC.

Immune Thrombocytopenic Purpura

Immune or idiopathic thrombocytopenic purpura (ITP) is an acquired, self-limited disorder of hemostasis. It is characterized by the destruction of circulating platelets. Also known as autoimmune thrombocytopenic purpura, it is the most common thrombocytopenic disorder in the pediatric population.

Frequently, within 1 month of its onset, ITP is preceded by a viral illness. Most often this is an upper respiratory infection, but it may be another infection such as varicella or infectious mononucleosis. Also, ITP has occurred after vaccination for smallpox and measles.

ITP may be acute or chronic. Acute ITP, the predominant form among children, is characterized by a sudden onset of thrombocytopenia, which resolves within 6 months. Typically, acute ITP occurs between 2 and 6 years of age and affects males and females in equal numbers.

Chronic ITP is characterized by thrombocytopenia that exists for more than 6 months in either a continuous or recurrent form. It is more likely to affect older children and adolescents and to affect females more than males.

Pathophysiology

The accelerated destruction of circulating platelets in ITP is mediated by platelet autoantibodies. These antibodies

Chart 23–15
Nursing Interventions

Administering Heparin

Heparin is an anticoagulant used to prevent fibrin clot formation in children at risk for thrombosis. The drug enhances the action of antithrombin III, inactivates thrombin, and prevents the conversion of fibrinogen to fibrin. Heparin is **not** effective in dissolving existing blood clots. Although heparin may be used in the management of disseminated intravascular coagulation (DIC), it is generally contraindicated for children with hemorrhage, severe thrombocytopenia, severe hypotension, and hypersensitivity to the drug.

Nursing considerations include the following:

1. Administer heparin subcutaneously or intravenously, as prescribed.
   a. Subcutaneous route—may be used for mini doses
      (1) Give dose slowly.
      (2) Do not massage injection site.
      (3) Rotate injection sites.
   b. Intravenous route
      (1) Intermittent IV: initially 50 U/kg, then 50 to 100 U/kg q 4 hr
      (2) Continuous IV: initially 50 U/kg, then 20,000 U/m^2 for 24 hours
   c. Ongoing dosage is dependent on PTT results—goal is a PTT that is 1.5 to 2.5 times normal.
2. Anticipate the use of protamine, if a heparin antidote is needed.
3. Monitor PTT and platelet count.
4. For an accurate PTT, do not draw blood sample from IV tubing or vein that is receiving heparin infusion.
5. Avoid aspirin and nonsteroidal anti-inflammatory drugs (NSAIDs).
6. Avoid activities with increased risk of injury.
7. Use with caution during menstrual and postpartum periods.
8. Instruct child/family regarding side effects of heparin:
   a. Easy bruising and bleeding
   b. Hemorrhage
   c. Irritation at injection site
   d. Hypersensitivity reactions
      (1) Rash
      (2) Headache
      (3) Hyperemia
      (4) Hypotension
      (5) Fever; chills
      (6) Nausea; vomiting
      (7) Itching, burning sensations
      (8) Anaphylactoid reaction

coat the platelets and, thereby, facilitate platelet trapping and destruction in the spleen (Souid & Sadowitz, 1995). It is not known why these autoantibodies are produced after a viral infection or other event. Neither is it known what causes the production of these autoantibodies to cease when ITP resolves (Beardsley, 1993).

Prognosis. The prognosis for ITP is good, especially for those who have had a preceding viral illness. Remission often occurs within 1 month. Within 6 months, most children with ITP experience complete resolution. Ultimately, even with chronic ITP, more than 90% of children have complete resolution of this disorder.

Assessment

The hallmark of ITP is random purpura in the presence of an otherwise normal physical examination. The extent of purpura is usually related to the degree of thrombocytopenia. When the platelet count is below 20,000 cells per mm^3, spontaneous bleeding is more likely and may occur as epistaxis, hematuria, hematemesis, hematochezia, and menorrhagia. In addition to the cutaneous petechiae and ecchymoses, there may be petechiae and hemorrhagic bullae of the mouth and pharynx.

Intracranial hemorrhage, although rare, is a life-threatening form of spontaneous bleeding that is associated with ITP. It is evidenced by headaches, vomiting, retinal hemorrhage, irritability, seizures, lethargy, and coma.

Diagnostic Tests. The laboratory manifestation of ITP is the presence of a low platelet count, usually less than 50,000 cells per mm^3. Thrombocytopenia is the only laboratory abnormality expected with ITP. However, if there has been significant blood loss, there may be evidence of anemia in the blood cell profile (CBC).

If a bone marrow examination is performed, the results with ITP show a normal or increased number of megakaryocytes, the precursors of platelets. This indicates that the thrombocytopenia is secondary to a destructive process rather than failure of the bone marrow to produce an adequate number of platelet precursor cells. Also, with ITP the bone marrow examination rules out aplastic anemia, leukemia, the presence of malignant tumor cells, and other bone marrow disorders.

Interdisciplinary Interventions

Management of the child with ITP is directed toward preventing serious, life-threatening bleeding. This involves supportive care, possible pharmaceutical intervention, and, occasionally, splenectomy. It is not customary to give platelet transfusions because of the destructive process that affects platelets in ITP. However, at times of

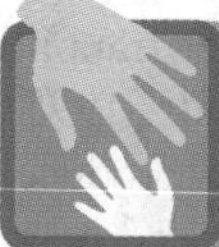

Chart 23–16
Nursing Interventions

Objectives and Interventions for the Child with Disseminated Intravascular Coagulation

Outcome Objectives	Nursing Interventions
Maintain normal renal function	Measure intake and output accurately Report the following: • Intake greater than output • Hematuria • Oliguria, anuria
Maintain normal pulmonary function	Assess breath sounds for all lobes of the lungs Report the following: • Abnormal breath sounds • Tachypnea • Dyspnea • Chest pain • Hemoptysis • Abnormal pulse oximetry readings
Maintain cutaneous integrity	Inspect the skin Report the following: • Overt bleeding • Pallor; jaundice • Petechiae; ecchymoses • Hemorrhagic bullae • Acrocyanosis • Poor healing at sites of injury or invasive procedures
Maintain normal gastrointestinal function	Assess bowel sounds in all quadrants Report the following: • Absent or hypo- or hyperactive bowel sounds • Blood in emesis or stool
Maintain normal neurological function	Assess neurological status Report the following: • Unstable or abnormal blood pressure, temperature, pulse, and respiratory rates • Unequal size of pupils • Absent or unequal pupillary responses to light • Headaches • Seizures • Changes in sensory perception, such as altered vision or hearing; numbness • Changes in motor function, such as altered speech or mobility • Irritability • Changes in behavior • Decreased level of consciousness • Rigid posturing

surgery or life-threatening bleeding, platelets are likely to be used.

Supportive care is indicated for all children with ITP and includes the following:

- Observe closely for evidence of bleeding, especially life-threatening bleeding.
- Instruct the child's parents and the older child about overt and covert signs of bleeding. Instruct them to report these promptly (TIP 23–2).

Alert: *The child with evidence of intracranial hemorrhage requires immediate medical attention.*

- Restrict from contact sports and rough activities.
- Ban medications that can interfere with normal platelet function. These include aspirin and aspirin-containing drugs, nonsteroidal anti-inflammatory drugs (NSAIDs), and certain antihistamines and cough medicines.

TIP 23–2 A Teaching Intervention Plan for the Child with Immune Thrombocytopenic Purpura (ITP)

Nursing Diagnoses and Outcomes

- Knowledge deficit related to ITP
  Outcome:
  Child/family describes ITP, and identify it as a blood disorder that is *not* malignant.
- Risk for injury related to bleeding
  Outcomes:
  Child/family selects activities which are unlikely to result in bleeding for the child.
  Child/family identifies signs and symptoms associated with overt and covert bleeding.

Interventions

- Teach regarding primary features of ITP:
  - Autoimmune disorder in which the body makes antibodies against its own platelets
  - Bleeding disorder related to premature destruction of platelets
  - Two forms of the disorder:
    - Acute ITP—resolves within 6 months; most common form among children
    - Chronic ITP—continues for more than 6 months, but usually resolves
- Inform about the absence of treatment for ITP; it resolves spontaneously.
- Instruct concerning the role of corticosteroids and immune globulin in raising the platelet count to prevent bleeding during ITP.
- Advise that ITP is *not* a leukemia, cancer or infection.
- Educate regarding the increased risk of bleeding when the platelet count is less than 50,000/mm^3.
- Teach concerning activity restrictions when the platelet count is less than 50,000/mm^3:
  - Do not take aspirin, ibuprofen, or other medicines that decrease platelet function and increase the risk for bleeding.
  - Do not receive injections such as vaccinations and allergy shots.
  - Do not use enemas or suppositories.
  - Do not blow nose forcefully.
  - Do not participate in contact sports such as wrestling, football, or soccer.
  - Do not bicycle ride, skate, climb trees, or dive.
  - Do not participate in rough activities.
- Instruct regarding signs and symptoms of bleeding:
  - Bruising
  - Bleeding from a cut or other wound
  - Reddish pinpoint rash on skin or in mouth
  - Bleeding from nose or mouth
  - Blood in sputum
  - Blood in vomit
  - Blood in stool
  - Black, tarry stool
  - Blood in urine (urine may appear tea or coke colored)
  - Increase in bleeding with menstrual period
  - Signs and symptoms of *possible* bleeding in the head:
    - Headache
    - Vomiting
    - Irritability
    - Seizure
    - Sleeping more than usual
    - Difficult to wake up
- Discuss the importance of emergency care when there is significant bleeding, and whenever there is a blow to the head, a head injury, or any indication of bleeding in the head.

- Do not give vaccinations or allergy desensitization injections, as these may further lower the platelet count (Beardsley, 1993).
- Check the platelet count. When severe thrombocytopenia is present, the platelet count may be checked daily. As the platelet count improves, gradually decrease the frequency with which it is checked.
- Check the bleeding time in chronic ITP because it may not correlate with the platelet count. For example, the bleeding time may be normal when the platelet count is low, or the bleeding time may be prolonged when the platelet count is nearly normal (Beardsley, 1993).

Pharmaceutical intervention with corticosteroids or immune globulin is indicated when there is significant bleeding or risk of life-threatening bleeding related to severe thrombocytopenia (platelet count less than 20,000 cells per mm^3).

Corticosteroid therapy is usually with oral prednisone given daily for 2 to 3 weeks. At times, high-dose corticosteroid therapy is given for the first few days. This consists of a daily dose of intravenous methylprednisolone (Beardsley, 1993; Souid & Sadowitz, 1995). Corticosteroids enhance vascular stability, decrease production of antiplatelet antibodies, and decrease clearance of opsonized platelets, thereby improving platelet survival, increasing the platelet count, and decreasing bleeding. However, prolonged use of corticosteroids is not considered beneficial and may actually suppress platelet production. If there is recurrence of severe thrombocytopenia or significant bleeding, alternative therapy is recommended.

Intravenous immune globulin (IVIG) therapy is given daily for up to 5 days and is usually effective in bringing about a quick increase in the platelet count. IVIG is thought to act by interfering with the attachment of antibody-coated platelets to Fc receptors on the macrophage cells of the reticuloendothelial system (Souid & Sadowitz, 1995; Taketomo, Hodding, & Kraus, 1997). IVIG is expensive, but if it decreases hospitalization time and decreases the likelihood of splenectomy, it can be a cost-effective intervention for ITP (Beardsley, 1993).

It is important for children and their parents to know that neither corticosteroids nor IVIG shortens the duration of ITP. The primary purpose of these agents is to increase the number of circulating platelets and, thereby, reduce the risk of life-threatening bleeding. If severe thrombocytopenia recurs, intermittent pharmaceutical intervention may be employed with the goal of keeping the platelet count from being dangerously low until the ITP spontaneously resolves.

Splenectomy with ITP is usually reserved for children with life-threatening bleeding or for those with chronic ITP who are at risk for serious bleeding despite supportive care and pharmaceutical intervention. The purpose of splenectomy is twofold: (1) to remove the primary site of antiplatelet antibody production and (2) to remove the major site for the destruction of antibody-coated platelets.

When possible, it is best to delay splenectomy in children younger than 5 years because they are at greater risk than older children for developing life-threatening postsplenectomy sepsis. When splenectomy is planned, certain vaccines are given to help decrease the risk of postoperative sepsis. The polyvalent pneumococcal vaccine is given at least 2 weeks before surgery to allow time for an effective antibody response. The vaccine for *Haemophilus influenzae* may be given, as well. In addition, the nurse should expect prophylactic antibiotics to be initiated.

For children who are receiving or who recently received corticosteroids, there is a need to receive steroids during the pre-, peri-, and postoperative periods. Surgery is a time of increased stress during which the adrenal gland would normally be stimulated to release increased amounts of corticosteroids. When these hormones are or have recently been supplied from exogenous sources, the release of adrenocorticotropic hormone (ACTH) is inhibited. Without ACTH, the adrenal gland is not stimulated to produce corticosteroids. Thus, the nurse must be sure the child receives stress doses of corticosteroid medication to prevent life-threatening complications such as hypotension and cardiovascular collapse during and after surgery.

Postsplenectomy fever and systemic illness are taken quite seriously. The nurse instructs the child and parents on the increased risk of rapidly progressing, life-threatening sepsis in the asplenic individual and the importance of immediately calling the physician in the event of fever or illness. The family should be told to anticipate a septic work-up, including physical examination, blood culture, and blood counts, as well as the initiation of intravenous antibiotics. Therapeutic antibiotics are continued at least until the blood culture is known to be negative and any sepsis has been treated. Thereafter, postsplenectomy antibiotic prophylaxis is resumed.

▽ **Alert:** *The child with fever and systemic illness after splenectomy requires immediate evaluation for sepsis.*

Postoperatively, there is often a prompt resolution of the ITP. There may even be a reactive thrombocytosis with the platelet count greater than 500,000 and even exceeding 1 million cells per mm^3. A high platelet count may continue for several months before returning to normal, but this is viewed as a favorable prognostic indicator, and it does not put the child at increased risk for thrombosis (Beardsley, 1993). On the other hand, postoperative thrombocytopenia may indicate that the ITP is not yet in remission.

Bleeding and the fear of bleeding are generally stressful for children with ITP and their families. It is important that health care providers be sensitive to this stress. Education about ITP (see TIP 23–2)and the provision of ongoing physical assessment data and emotional support are important parts of the interdisciplinary management of ITP.

Henoch-Schönlein Purpura

Henoch-Schönlein purpura (HSP) is an acquired, nonthrombocytopenic vasculitis that may involve multiple body organs. Also known as allergic purpura or anaphylactoid purpura, HSP is the most common vasculitis of childhood. HSP usually occurs in children younger than 7 years, and it is three times more likely to occur in boys than in girls.

The etiology of HSP is unknown. However, the predominant hypothesis is that the disease is initiated by an abnormal immunologic response to any one of a number of antigens. These antigens include viruses, bacteria, vaccines, medications, insect bites, and various foods (Bussel & Corrigan, 1995; Szer, 1994).

Pathophysiology

HSP is characterized by an aseptic inflammation of small blood vessels. The lesions accompanying this vasculitis are distinguished by:

- **Erythema**, secondary to vasodilation
- **Urticarial edema**, secondary to increased vascular permeability
- **Purpura**, secondary to extravasation of blood

HSP may be recurrent or chronic but, generally, it is an acute disease. The prognosis for complete recovery is usually good.

Assessment

The hallmark diagnostic feature of HSP is **nonthrombocytopenic palpable purpura,** which tends to occur in a symmetric pattern and is visible primarily below the waistline (Fig. 23–8). It may be noted on the face and on extensor surfaces of the upper extremities as well. For some children, the rash of HSP may include petechiae, wheals, and erythematous maculopapules besides the classic purpura.

In addition to the skin, other anatomic locations may be affected by HSP, and these sites may show evidence of disease before the appearance of the characteristic palpable purpura. Common noncutaneous sites of involvement are the joints, gastrointestinal tract, and kidneys. Less common sites of involvement are the central nervous system, lungs, and, for males, scrotum.

Joint involvement with HSP is characterized by periarticular inflammation. Multiple joints may be affected but, most commonly, the arthritic effects are noted in larger joints. As swelling, tenderness, and pain increase, the children are likely to disengage from activities that require them to use the affected joints. For example, they may refuse to walk when their knee joints are painful. Unlike hemophilia, the joint involvement associated with HSP resolves without permanent injury. This is because it is periarticular in nature, in contrast to the intraarticular joint involvement associated with hemophilia (Bussel & Corrigan, 1995).

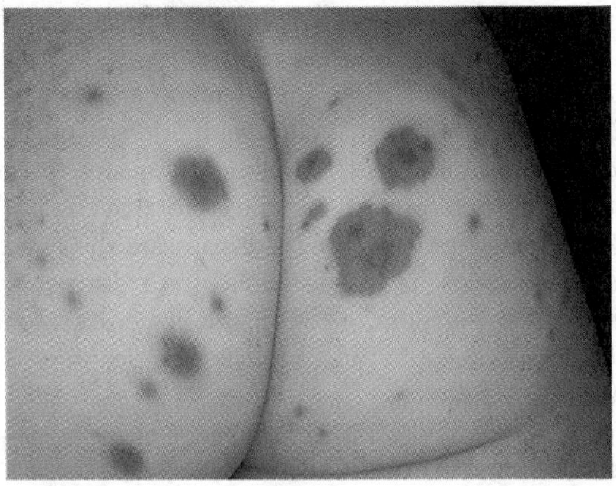

Figure 23–8
Henoch-Schönlein purpura produces hemorrhagic and erythematous lesions on the buttocks, legs, and other sites. (From Hurwitz, S. [1993]. *Clinical pediatric dermatology* [2nd ed., p. 540]. Philadelphia: W. B. Saunders. Reprinted with permission.)

Gastrointestinal involvement with HSP is manifested by vomiting, hematemesis, diarrhea, and melena. The most frequent complaint is abdominal pain, which may be severe and colicky in nature. This pain is secondary to mucosal edema and hemorrhage of the bowel wall. Also, the pain may be due to intermittent ischemia associated with diseased arterioles (Bussel & Corrigan, 1995). Potential complications involving the gastrointestinal tract include intussusception and, rarely, intestinal obstruction and bowel perforation.

Renal involvement with HSP is evidenced by urinalysis findings of hematuria, proteinuria, and casts. Hypertension may be present as well. Most children with HSP involving the kidneys recover normal kidney function. However, some may develop chronic glomerulonephritis and subsequent renal failure.

Central nervous system involvement with HSP may be suspected when there are headaches, irritability, sensory deficits, seizures, and altered levels of consciousness. Although involvement of the central nervous system occurs less frequently and is usually temporary, there is the potential for a fatal intracranial hemorrhage.

Pulmonary involvement with HSP is usually not clinically apparent. However, some children may have hemoptysis and, occasionally, there is life-threatening or fatal pulmonary hemorrhage.

Scrotal and testicular involvement may occur with HSP. Indicators of such include purpuric scrotal lesions, testicular pain, and scrotal swelling secondary to inflammation and hemorrhage of the scrotal vessels (Szer, 1994). When scrotal swelling and pain are the first clinical manifestations, it may be difficult to distinguish between HSP and torsion of the spermatic cord without the use of ultrasonography and radionuclear scanning (Szer, 1994).

Nursing Diagnoses and Outcomes

In addition to the nursing diagnoses provided in Chart 23–3, the nursing diagnoses and outcomes for the child with HSP include the following:

- **Knowledge deficit related to HSP**
  Outcome: The child/family identify HSP as a noncontagious, nonmalignant disorder that involves the skin and that may involve internal body organs.
- **Risk for impaired physical mobility, if joint involvement occurs**
  Outcomes: The child maintains or regains normal physical mobility.
  The child does not have joint swelling, tenderness, or pain.
- **Risk for fluid volume deficit, if vomiting, diarrhea, and bleeding occur**
  Outcomes: The child maintains normal fluid and electrolyte balance.
  The child has no vomiting or diarrhea.
  The child has no evidence of bleeding.
- **Risk for altered urinary elimination, if renal involvement occurs**
  Outcomes: The child maintains or regains normal urinary elimination.
  The child's urinalysis is normal.
  The child's blood pressure is normal.
- **Body image disturbance related to HSP**
  Outcome: The child/family verbalize concerns related to altered body appearance and receive informational and emotional support.

Interdisciplinary Interventions

Management of the child with HSP requires careful, ongoing assessment, particularly noting any evidence of increased severity of the disease. Treatment for HSP is primarily supportive, based on its specific clinical manifestations. When these are severe, corticosteroids may be prescribed (Jonides, 1996).

The **skin** is assessed for progressive purpura and the presence of edema and pruritus. Antihistamines may be helpful in relieving severe itching (Tapson, 1993).

Joints are evaluated by observing the child's activities and specifically noting range of motion at joint sites. Nonsteroidal anti-inflammatory medications may be prescribed to relieve pain.

Assessment of the **gastrointestinal tract** is done by noting verbal and nonverbal manifestations of abdominal pain, incidents of vomiting, hematemesis, diarrhea, and hematochezia. Normal bowel movements should be noted as well. If any foods are suspected of triggering HSP, they are eliminated from the diet. Severe gastrointestinal involvement may require that the gut be rested. Dehydration and inadequate nutrition generally require parenteral fluid support. Occasionally, surgery may be required to correct gastrointestinal tract complications in the child with HSP.

Renal function is evaluated primarily by monitoring blood pressure and by checking urine specimens for abnormalities. Family members are taught to use a dipstick to check the child's urine for hematuria and proteinuria.

The neurologic system is assessed for **central nervous system** involvement. Note the presence of headaches, irritability, sensory deficits, seizures, and altered levels of consciousness.

Pulmonary function is evaluated by assessing breath sounds for all lobes of the lungs. Note abnormal breath sounds and any signs of respiratory distress. Examine sputum for blood.

The **scrotum** is examined for purpuric lesions, swelling, and tenderness.

Community Care

The nurse has a significant role in providing instruction about HSP and the multiple body systems that may be affected by this disorder. Children with HSP are frequently outpatients. By educating family members and highlighting for them the signs and symptoms that require immediate notification of the physician, the nurse prepares the family to be key participants in helping the child with HSP achieve desired outcomes.

The abnormal body appearance and the potential for serious complications with HSP are likely to be stressful for the child and family. It is important that the health care team show sensitivity to this stress. Education about HSP and the provision of ongoing physical assessment data and emotional support to the child and family are significant elements of the interdisciplinary management of HSP.

Hemoglobinopathies

Hemoglobinopathies are disorders in which there is a structural or quantitative abnormality involving hemoglobin. These alterations range in severity from clinically insignificant to profound and life-threatening disease.

Sickling disorders are hemoglobinopathies in which there is a structural alteration in the hemoglobin molecule, causing the red blood cell to assume a sickle shape under certain circumstances. This sickling may be reversible or irreversible. Hemoglobin S is an example of a structurally abnormal hemoglobin. It is present instead of the normal hemoglobin A and is associated with the most common sickling disorder, hemoglobin SS disease.

Thalassemia disorders are hemoglobinopathies in which there is a deficiency or absence of one or more of the globin chains necessary for the synthesis of hemoglobin. The normal hemoglobin A molecule is composed of paired alpha and beta globin chains. A deficiency in the alpha chain results in alpha-thalassemia, whereas a deficiency in the beta chain is associated with beta-thalassemia.

Sickle Cell Disease

Sickle cell disease is a hereditary disorder characterized by any one of a number of structural abnormalities in the beta globin chains of the hemoglobin molecule. These abnormalities may be clinically insignificant or may result in serious overt disease. The most common form of sickle cell disease is hemoglobin SS disease.

The inheritance pattern for sickle cell disease is autosomal recessive, with the genetic defect present on chromosome number 11. When children have sickle cell disease, each of their parents is at least heterozygous for the abnormal gene (Fig. 23–9). Most children with sickle cell disease are homozygous, having inherited the same abnormal beta globin gene from each parent. However, approximately 35% have a double heterozygous

Figure 23–9

Genetic inheritance of sickle cell disease. A, When both parents are heterozygous for the hemoglobin S gene, there is a 25% probability that each child will have hemoglobin SS disease, and a 50% probability that each child will have the sickle cell trait. In addition, there is a 25% probability that each child will have normal hemoglobin. *B*, When one parent is heterozygous and the other parent is homozygous for the hemoglobin S gene, there is a 50% probability that each child will have hemoglobin SS disease. Children who do not have hemoglobin SS disease will have the sickle cell trait.

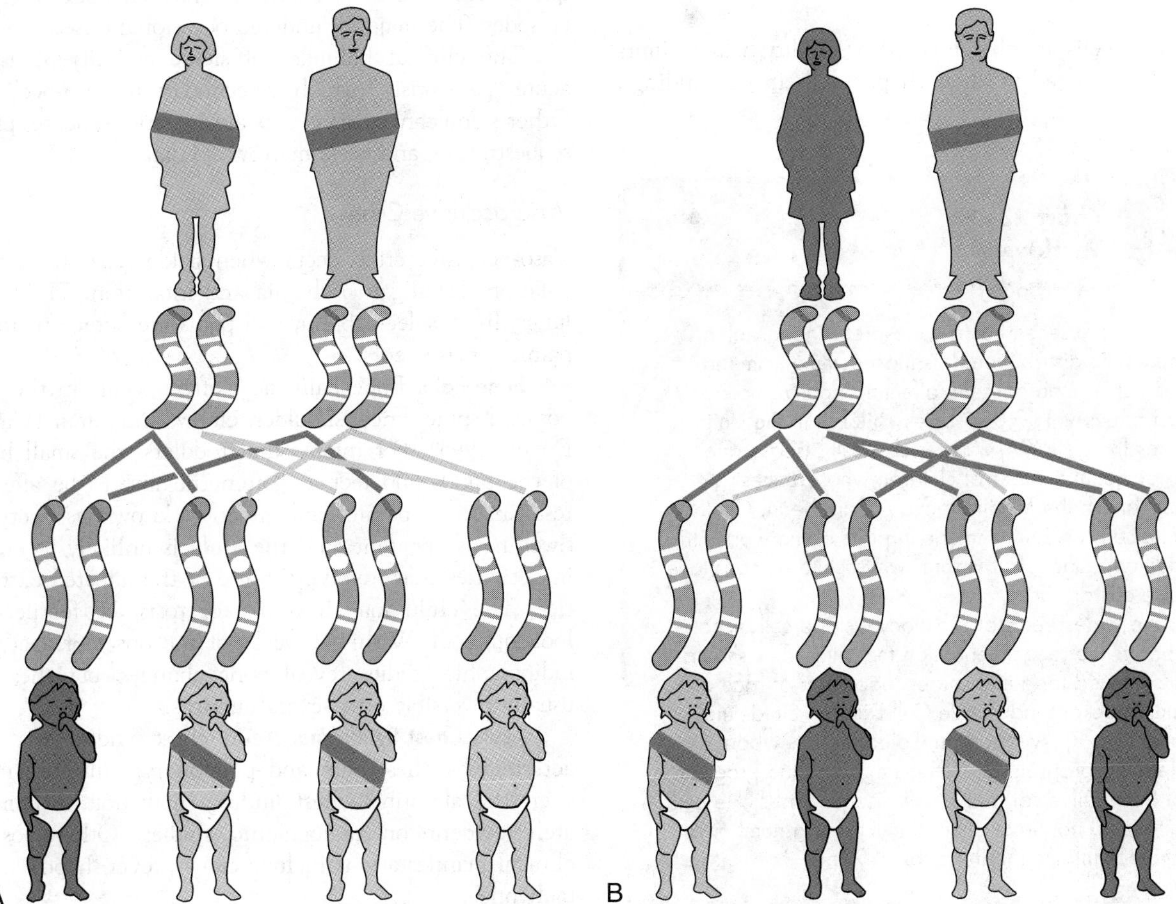

sickling disorder (Mankad, 1995); they have inherited a different abnormal gene from each parent. Hemoglobin SC disease, the second most common form of sickle cell disease, is an example of a double heterozygous sickling disorder. Children with hemoglobin SC disease have inherited a gene for hemoglobin S from one parent and a gene for hemoglobin C from the other parent (Chart 23–17). The widespread distribution of sickle cell disease has led to neonatal screening programs to identify children with this disorder.

The following discussion of sickle cell disease centers on the primary form of this disorder, hemoglobin SS disease.

Pathophysiology

The red blood cells of children with hemoglobin SS disease are prone to become sickle shaped and fail to function in a normal manner. Circumstances such as increased body temperature, high hemoglobin concentration, decreased oxygen level, decreased pH, and dehydration enhance the sickling process.

Sickle-shaped erythrocytes may be reversibly sickled cells or irreversibly sickled cells. The former lose their sickle shape with reoxygenation, whereas the latter remain sickled despite their return to an oxygenated environment.

Sickle cells are characterized by rigidity, which limits their ability to adapt their shape to their surroundings, particularly in the microvasculature. Sickle cells undergo premature hemolysis, accounting for the chronic anemia seen in children with hemoglobin SS disease. In addition, sickle cells enhance blood viscosity, and their increased adherence to the vascular endothelium is a significant factor in the intricate process of vaso-occlusion, which is commonly associated with sickle cell disease.

Prognosis. The prognosis for sickle cell disease among children has significantly improved since the 1980s, when a research study showed that the prophylactic use of penicillin was effective in decreasing the incidence of pneumococcal sepsis (Gaston et al., 1986). Children with sickle cell disease who are younger than 5 years are at particular risk for this infection, and it is the most common cause of death among these young children. Splenic sequestration and stroke are other causes of death in this population of patients. The long-term prognosis for sickle cell disease is variable, depending on its type and clinical severity. In general, the average life expectancy is about 45 years, with some living beyond 60 years.

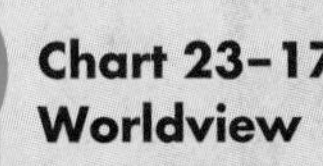

Chart 23–17
Worldview

Sickle cell disease has a widespread geographic and ethnic distribution. It is most common among those of African descent, affecting approximately 265 of every 100,000 black children in the United States (Berg, 1994). Also, sickle cell disease affects a significant number of children whose ancestral roots are in the Mediterranean, Caribbean, Central American, or South American parts of the world. In addition, although it is rare, white children can have sickle cell disease.

The widespread distribution of sickle cell disease supports the recommendation that all infants should be screened for this disorder regardless of race or ethnic background (Sickle Cell Disease Guideline Panel, 1993). A report on California's newborn screening program documents that had the program not been universal, sickle cell disease and sickle cell trait would not have been identified in a number of nonblack infants (Shafer et al., 1996).

Assessment

The clinical manifestations of hemoglobin SS disease vary significantly, with some children experiencing frequent crisis events and others rarely encountering such episodes. The majority undergo occasional crises.

The clinical hallmark of sickle cell disease is the acute "pain crisis," which is secondary to vaso-occlusion. Other significant crisis events are infections, acute splenic sequestration, and bone marrow aplasia.

Vaso-occlusive Crises

Vaso-occlusive crises occur when sickle cells obstruct circulation, leading to ischemia and infarction. The bones, lungs, liver, spleen, brain, and penis are common sites of painful crisis events.

Bone Pain. Bone pain most often occurs in the lumbosacral spine, knee, shoulder, elbow, and femur (Platt & Dover, 1993). For infants and toddlers, the small bones of the hands and feet are often the first to be affected, resulting in a painful inflammation known as dactylitis. Swelling is apparent, and the child is unlikely to engage in activities that involve the use of the affected extremities. The child may have leukocytosis, be febrile, and look quite ill. Within 2 weeks of the onset of dactylitis, radiographic studies reveal bone changes, but these are usually reversible over several months.

Acute Chest Syndrome. Acute chest syndrome is characterized by chest pain and pulmonary infiltrates. However, the abnormal chest findings may not be immediately evident on radiographic studies. Other possible clinical manifestations include cough, fever, hypoxia, and tachypnea.

Alert: *Respiratory failure may occur* rapidly *with acute chest syndrome.*

It is usually difficult to distinguish between pulmonary infarction and infection. Often, they exist simultaneously, and the child with acute chest syndrome is treated for both disorders. Pneumonia in children with sickle cell disease may be more extensive and slower to resolve than in children with normal hematologic status (Platt & Dover, 1993).

Laboratory studies associated with acute chest syndrome frequently show a decreased hemoglobin and an increased reticulocyte count in comparison with the child's baseline values. Also, leukocytosis is generally present.

Acute Abdominal Pain. Acute abdominal pain crises occur with vaso-occlusion involving one or more organs of the abdomen. Clinical manifestations include distention of the abdomen with enlargement of the liver, spleen, or other organ experiencing vaso-occlusion. Guarding and tenderness, including rebound tenderness, may be present, and at times it is difficult to discriminate between an acute abdominal pain crisis and a "surgical" abdomen (in the child who may have an appendicitis or other abdominal crisis requiring surgery). Although the body temperature and white blood cell count may be increased in both situations, the elevation tends to be less significant with pain crises. Also, the condition of the child experiencing an abdominal pain crisis tends to stabilize or improve, in contrast to that of the child with a surgical abdomen. School-age children and adolescents who have undergone pain crises previously can help to distinguish between an abdominal pain crisis and a surgical abdomen, if they recognize their current pain as typical or nontypical of pain crises associated with sickle cell disease.

Cerebrovascular Accidents. Vaso-occlusion in the brain is associated with cerebrovascular accidents. The clinical manifestations are those commonly associated with strokes, such as hemiparesis, hemiplegia, impaired speech, impaired comprehension, visual disturbances, severe headache, seizures, and coma. Diagnostic studies generally include angiography to identify sites of sickling and vaso-occlusion. Although children who sustain cerebrovascular accidents may experience only transient neurologic abnormalities, a significant concern is that there may be chronic impairment of motor function and decreased IQ. Another major concern is the high rate of stroke recurrence among these children.

Priapism. Priapism is a painful nonsexual erection of the penis. It may occur for an extended time, more than 24 hours, or it may occur as a short episode. Repetitive brief episodes are referred to as "stuttering" priapism. Prolonged episodes of priapism may be accompanied by urine retention.

Infections

Infections occur more frequently and tend to be more severe, even life threatening, among children with sickle cell disease. This is due to alterations in immune status. A primary factor is the development of a nonfunctional spleen. Generally, this occurs early in life among children with hemoglobin SS disease and places them at high risk for sepsis, meningitis, pneumonia, and other infections.

Alert: *Even in the absence of other clinical manifestations of infection, febrile children with sickle cell disease require emergency health care.*

Acute Splenic Sequestration

Acute splenic sequestration results from the trapping of sickled red blood cells and the accumulation of a large amount of blood within the spleen. It occurs among those whose spleen is still functional. With hemoglobin SS disease, the spleen generally ceases to function during early childhood. Thus, the incidence of acute splenic sequestration decreases when children with hemoglobin SS disease reach the preschool years.

Clinical manifestations of acute splenic sequestration may suddenly appear and quickly progress. These manifestations include splenic enlargement, abdominal distention, pallor, weakness, dyspnea, tachycardia, and hypotension. At times, left upper quadrant abdominal pain and vomiting may be present.

Alert: *Acute splenic sequestration can rapidly progress to cardiovascular collapse and death.*

Laboratory alterations associated with acute splenic sequestration include decreased hemoglobin, hematocrit, and platelet count; increased reticulocyte count; and the presence of nucleated red blood cells.

Aplastic Crises

Aplastic crises are transient episodes of bone marrow suppression in which red blood cell production is markedly decreased. Normally, children with sickle cell disease have increased bone marrow activity and produce an above-average number of red blood cells to compensate for the shortened survival time of their atypical erythrocytes. In hemoglobin SS disease, red blood cells live for approximately 10 to 20 days (Mankad, 1995), in contrast to the 120-day average in the general population.

Aplastic crises associated with sickle cell disease may occur in conjunction with bacterial and viral infections. Parvovirus B19 is of particular concern in children with a hemolytic anemia, such as that associated with sickle cell disease. This viral agent can interfere with normal erythropoiesis, triggering erythroid aplasia.

Laboratory alterations associated with aplastic crises include absence of reticulocytes, decreased hemoglobin and hematocrit, and decreased red blood cell precursors in the bone marrow.

Chronic Complications

In addition to acute complications, the chronic complications of hemoglobin SS disease may be multiple. They can involve the heart, kidneys, liver, bones, lungs, eyes, ears, and skin. General growth and development are often delayed.

Heart. When sickle cell disease is associated with severe chronic anemia, the heart responds with greater cardiac output. This leads to enlargement of the heart, as well as cardiac murmurs.

Kidneys. The renal environment increases the probability of sickling, and some degree of renal impairment is generally present among those with sickle cell disease. Most common among children is hyposthenuria, the inability to produce urine with high specific gravity. This results in the excretion of large amounts of dilute urine and accounts for the common occurrence of nocturia and enuresis. Hematuria and nephrotic syndrome are infrequent.

Liver and Biliary System. It is not unusual for children with sickle cell disease to have abnormalities of the liver and biliary system. Intrahepatic sickling can lead to hyperbilirubinemia and high liver enzyme levels. Hepatomegaly is likely to appear during early childhood. Gallstones are common, with the incidence increasing as the children advance in age.

Bones. Skeletal changes associated with sickle cell disease are usually due to expansion of the bone marrow cavity, as well as bone infarction. Common bone changes include frontal bossing (prominence of the frontal bone), maxillary overgrowth, and flattened vertebrae. Avascular necrosis of the femoral head is a painful disability that occurs after repeated bone infarctions. It is more likely to occur among adolescents than children.

Lungs. Although uncommon in children, chronic lung disease may become apparent in the adolescent or young adult with sickle cell disease after repeated episodes of pulmonary infarction and pneumonia.

Eyes. Children with sickle cell disease often have vascular changes in their eyes. Most of these are not harmful. However, proliferative retinopathy is especially significant because it may lead to blindness.

Blunt trauma to the eye requires emergency care. Such trauma may cause bleeding in the anterior chamber, where the environment is highly conducive to the sickling of hemoglobin S erythrocytes. The sickled cells may cause obstructive glaucoma and blindness (Platt & Dover, 1993).

Ears. Sensorineural hearing loss occurs in some children with sickle cell disease. This is most likely due to hair cell destruction in the inner ear secondary to sickling (Platt & Dover, 1993).

Skin. Although uncommon in younger children, skin ulcerations may become a chronic problem for adolescents with sickle cell disease. The ankles and lower legs are the primary sites for these ulcerations. At first small, the lesions can increase in size and involve a significant portion of the lower leg.

Growth and Development. Children with sickle cell disease appear normal in size at birth. However, their subsequent growth and development pattern is altered. Increases in standing and sitting height occur more slowly than usual. Weight gain is delayed. Although full height is generally achieved by the completion of adolescence, weight gain frequently continues to be less than normal. It is thought that the delay in weight gain among those with sickle cell anemia may be secondary to the body's need for increased calories to support increased bone marrow activity and cardiovascular compensation (Platt & Dover, 1993).

In addition, slow weight gain among those with sickle cell disease is associated with a delay in the development of secondary sexual characteristics. When sexual maturity is attained, fertility is generally normal for females. However, among males with sickle cell disease, fertility may be decreased.

Diagnostic Tests. The diagnostic process for identifying sickle cell disease and discriminating among its various forms often begins with screening tests during the neonatal period. Such tests, now mandatory in most states, may be performed by different methods. The most common are:

- Isoelectric focusing (IEF)
- High-performance liquid chromatography
- Cellulose acetate electrophoresis
- Citrate agar electrophoresis

Sickle solubility testing may be used in an adjunctive manner for older children and adults. However, this is not reliable for neonatal screening because newborns have a high level of hemoglobin F, which inhibits the polymerization of sickle hemoglobin. Also, the sickle solubility test does not discriminate among the various forms of sickle cell disease, and it does not reliably distinguish between sickle cell disease and sickle cell trait (Adams, 1994).

Alterations in laboratory studies may differ among the various forms of sickle cell disease. With hemoglobin SS disease, anemia is generally evident by 4 months of age. Reticulocytosis is present, and baseline hemoglobin levels usually range between 6.0 and 10.0 g/dL. By the time the child reaches preschool age, the peripheral blood smear typically shows the presence of abnormal red blood cells, such as sickle cells and target cells. In addition, when the spleen is nonfunctional or absent, red blood cells may contain inclusions such as Howell-Jolly bodies and Heinz bodies.

Nursing Diagnoses and Outcomes

General nursing diagnoses and outcomes for the child with sickle cell disease are presented in TIP 23–3. Nursing diagnoses and outcomes for a particular sickle cell crisis event (acute chest syndrome) are illustrated in Care Path 23–2.

Interdisciplinary Interventions

Whenever possible, management of the child with sickle cell disease is directed by an interdisciplinary professional team that is affiliated with a comprehensive center for the treatment of pediatric hematologic disorders. This team collaborates with health care providers in the child's home community to ensure complete health care for the child.

An ongoing health maintenance program is essential to the effective management of the child with sickle cell disease. Such a program begins with an accurate diagnosis of the specific type of sickle cell disease. Thereafter, it includes regular visits to the health care center, at which time the health history and physical assessment data are updated and needed interventions provided. Current baseline data are especially helpful in the management of crisis events. For example, a hemoglobin level of 6.5 g/dL is more significant for a child whose baseline hemoglobin

TIP 23–3 A Teaching Intervention Plan for the Child with Sickle Cell Disease

Nursing Diagnoses and Outcomes

- Knowledge deficit related to sickle cell disease
  Outcome:
  Child/family describes sickle cell disease in general and the child's hemoglobinopathy in particular.
- Risk for injury related to sickle cell crises
  Outcomes:
  Child/family identifies signs and symptoms of the following types of crisis events:
  - Vaso-occlusion
  - Infection
  - Acute splenic sequestration
  - Bone marrow aplasia

  Child/family seeks emergency health care when there is fever and when there are signs and symptoms of life-threatening or severely painful crisis events.
- Pain related to crisis events
  Outcomes:
  Child is well-hydrated.
  Child receives prescribed analgesics.
  Child experiences relief from pain.
  Child/family identifies pain relief measures that may be used at home.
- Risk for injury related to chronic complications of sickle cell disease
  Outcomes:
  Child/family identifies common chronic disorders that may develop with sickle cell disease.
  Child receives ongoing health care to identify and manage chronic complications associated with sickle cell disease and, when possible, to prevent such complications.
- Body image disturbance related to physical alterations associated with sickle cell disease
  Outcome:
  Child/family verbalizes concerns regarding physical alterations and receive informational and emotional support.
- Risk for altered parenting related to child's chronic physical disorder
  Outcome:
  Parents identify normal developmental milestones and their role in helping their child achieve these milestones.

TIP 23–3 A Teaching Intervention Plan for the Child with Sickle Cell Disease *Continued*

Interventions

- Teach regarding characteristics of sickle cell disease:
  - Abnormal hemoglobin
  - Sickling of red blood cells
  - Abnormal function of sickled cells
- Inform about child's type of sickle cell disease and its usual clinical course.
- Instruct concerning the etiology of sickle cell disease and the risk of future children having sickle cell disease or sickle cell trait.
- Advise about factors that may precipitate sickling of red blood cells:
  - Fever
  - Infection
  - Dehydration
  - Hot and/or humid environment
  - Cold air and/or water temperature
  - High altitude
  - Excessive physical activity
- Educate regarding crisis events:
  - Vaso-occlusion
    - Bone pain
    - Acute chest syndrome
    - Acute abdominal pain
    - Cerebrovascular accidents
    - Priapism
  - Infection
  - Acute splenic sequestration
  - Aplastic crises
- Inform about signs and symptoms of sickle cell crises:
  - Fever
  - Pain
  - Respiratory distress
  - Abdominal distention
  - Pallor
  - Weakness
  - Penile erection
  - Neurologic deficits
    - Impaired vision or speech
    - Impaired motor function or paralysis
    - Seizures
- Instruct regarding the need for emergency health care for fever, severe pain, and other signs and symptoms of crisis events.
- Teach concerning measures to relieve pain associated with sickle cell crises:
  - Rest
  - Increased fluid intake
  - Analgesic medication

TIP 23–3 A Teaching Intervention Plan for the Child with Sickle Cell Disease *Continued*

- Educate regarding chronic complications of sickle cell disease:
  - Cardiac complications
  - Renal complications
  - Hepatic complications
  - Skeletal complications
  - Pulmonary complications
  - Visual complications
  - Auditory complications
  - Dermatologic complications
  - Delayed growth and development
- Inform about the importance of ongoing health care to identify and manage chronic complications associated with sickle cell disease.
- Facilitate expression of concerns regarding altered body image related to sickle cell disease; follow up with emotional support and additional information, as needed.
- Teach measures which promote normal growth and development:
  - Safety
  - Nutrition
  - Extra fluid intake
  - Exercise
  - Dental care
  - Stress management
  - Avoidance of tobacco, alcohol, and unprescribed drugs
  - Immunizations, including hepatitis B, *Haemophilus influenzae* B, and pneumococcal vaccines
- Provide guidelines for activities that are appropriate for the child's physical state and developmental level.
- Discuss nonphysical disciplinary measures; encourage balance between overprotective and overly permissive parental behaviors.
- Coach regarding communication with siblings and affected child about sickle cell disease.
- Advise concerning communication with school and child care personnel about child's needs.

is 8.8 g/dL than it is for a child whose baseline hemoglobin is 6.8 g/dL.

Monitor the child with sickle cell disease for signs and symptoms of crisis events and chronic complications referred to earlier. Note current laboratory data for hematologic status, liver function, and renal function. Review the results of special studies such as arterial blood gas studies, pulmonary function tests, electrocardiography, and radiographic studies.

Clinical practice guidelines for the management of young children with sickle cell disease have been prepared by the Agency for Health Care Policy and Research (Sickle Cell Disease Guideline Panel, 1993). These guidelines include recommendations for

- Newborn screening
- Health maintenance measures
- Parent education
- Assessment of the child who presents for emergency care

An algorithm incorporating recommended guidelines is presented in Figure 23–10.

Surgical procedures for children with sickle cell disease require perioperative measures to prevent sickling. Preoperative transfusion corrects anemia and provides an increased number of hemoglobin A erythrocytes. Also,

Text continued on page 1577

Care Path 23–2 An Interdisciplinary Plan of Care for a Child with Hemoglobin SS Disease and Acute Chest Syndrome

Nursing Diagnosis	Patient/Family Outcomes				
	Day: Admission	Day 2	Day 3	Day 4	Day 5
Impaired gas exchange related to acute chest syndrome	Child's oxygen saturation 95% with supplemental oxygen	⟶	⟶	Child's oxygen saturation maintained at >95% during weaning of supplemental oxygen	⟶
	Child's respiratory rate stable and within normal limits	⟶	⟶	⟶	⟶
					Parents verbalize signs and symptoms of respiratory distress Parents verbalize importance of notifying health care provider, if respiratory distress occurs
Pain related to crisis events	IV analgesic effective in relieving child's pain	⟶	⟶	Oral analgesic effective in relieving pain	⟶
	Child's vital signs stable and within normal limits	⟶	⟶	⟶	⟶
					Parents state home pain relief measures Parents verbalize signs and symptoms of ineffective pain relief measures Parents verbalize need to notify health care provider, if pain relief measures are ineffective

Risk for injury related to fluid volume deficit and hyperthermia	Child receives IV fluids to restore normal hydration status Child afebrile with antipyretic	Child receives IV and oral fluids to maintain normal hydration status ⟶	⟶ Child afebrile without antipyretic	⟶ ⟶	Child receives oral fluids to maintain normal hydration status ⟶ Parents verbalize signs and symptoms of dehydration Parents verbalize importance of immediately notifying health care provider, if fever occurs
Risk for constipation related to narcotic analgesic	Child has normal bowel movement with or without use of stool softener	⟶	⟶	⟶	⟶ Parents verbalize signs and symptoms of constipation Parents verbalize need to notify health care provider, if constipation occurs
Care Intervention Categories					
Consults	Hematology-oncology specialty nurse if available				
Discharge planning	Notify case manager of admission	Assess family's ability to care for child after discharge from hospital			Discharge day Prescriptions for home medications · Antibiotic · Analgesic · Folic acid Follow-up outpatient appointment

Care Path continued on following page

Care Path 23–2 An Interdisciplinary Plan of Care for a Child with Hemoglobin SS Disease and Acute Chest Syndrome *Continued*

Care Intervention Categories	Day: Admission	Day 2	Day 3	Day 4	Day 5
Laboratory	CBC with differential	→	→	→	→
	Platelet count	→	→	→	→
	Reticulocyte count	→	→	→	→
	Chem 17	Chem 7	→	→	→
	Hemoglobin electrophoresis				
	Type and crossmatch				
	Cultures				
	· Blood				
	· Sputum				
	Cold agglutinins				
	ESR				
Medications and IVs	IV fluids	→	→	Decrease IV fluids	Discontinue IV fluids
	IV antibiotic	→	→	→	→
	IV analgesic	→	→	Oral analgesic	→
	Folic acid	→	→	→	→
	Antipyretic	→			
Monitors	Pulse oximetry	→	→	→	→
	Cardiac/apnea monitor	→	→	→	

Nutrition	Regular diet for age, as tolerated	⟶	⟶	⟶ Encourage oral fluid intake as IV fluids are weaned	⟶ Encourage to continue good oral fluid intake after discharge
Pain management	IV analgesic IV fluids	⟶ IV and oral fluids	⟶ ⟶	Oral analgesic ⟶	⟶ Oral fluids
Play therapy or school		Quiet activities appropriate for developmental level	⟶	⟶	⟶
Procedures	Oxygen Arterial blood gases Blood transfusion	⟶ ⟶ ⟶	⟶	Wean oxygen—keep oxygen saturation >95%	Discontinue oxygen Arterial blood gases
Psychosocial	Parents encouraged to be with child Informational and emotional support Notify social worker for sickle cell disease of child's admission	Parents or significant others encouraged to be with child ⟶	⟶ ⟶	⟶ ⟶	⟶ ⟶
Radiology	Chest x-ray		Chest x-ray		Chest x-ray
Safety and activity	Bed rest	⟶	Out of bed in wagon	⟶	Ambulatory
Special considerations	Observe closely for signs of respiratory distress	⟶	⟶	⟶	⟶

Care Path continued on following page

Care Path 23–2 An Interdisciplinary Plan of Care for a Child with Hemoglobin SS Disease and Acute Chest Syndrome *Continued*

Care Intervention Categories	Day: Admission	Day 2	Day 3	Day 4	Day 5
Teaching	Acute chest syndrome with sickle cell disease	Management of acute chest syndrome with sickle cell disease	Measures to decrease risk of acute chest syndrome and other sickle cell crises	Discharge instructions Pain management at home	Review signs and symptoms of respiratory distress Review signs and symptoms of sickle cell crisis events Review signs and symptoms of dehydration Review signs and symptoms of constipation Review plan for pain management at home Review signs and symptoms of ineffective pain relief measures
Vital signs	Vital signs q 4 hr	→	→	→	→
	Continuous pulse oximetry	→	Continuous pulse oximetry except when out of bed	→	
	Accurate intake and output (I & O)	→	→	→	→
	Weight	→	→	→	→
	Height				

CBC, complete blood count; ESR, erythrocyte sedimentation rate.

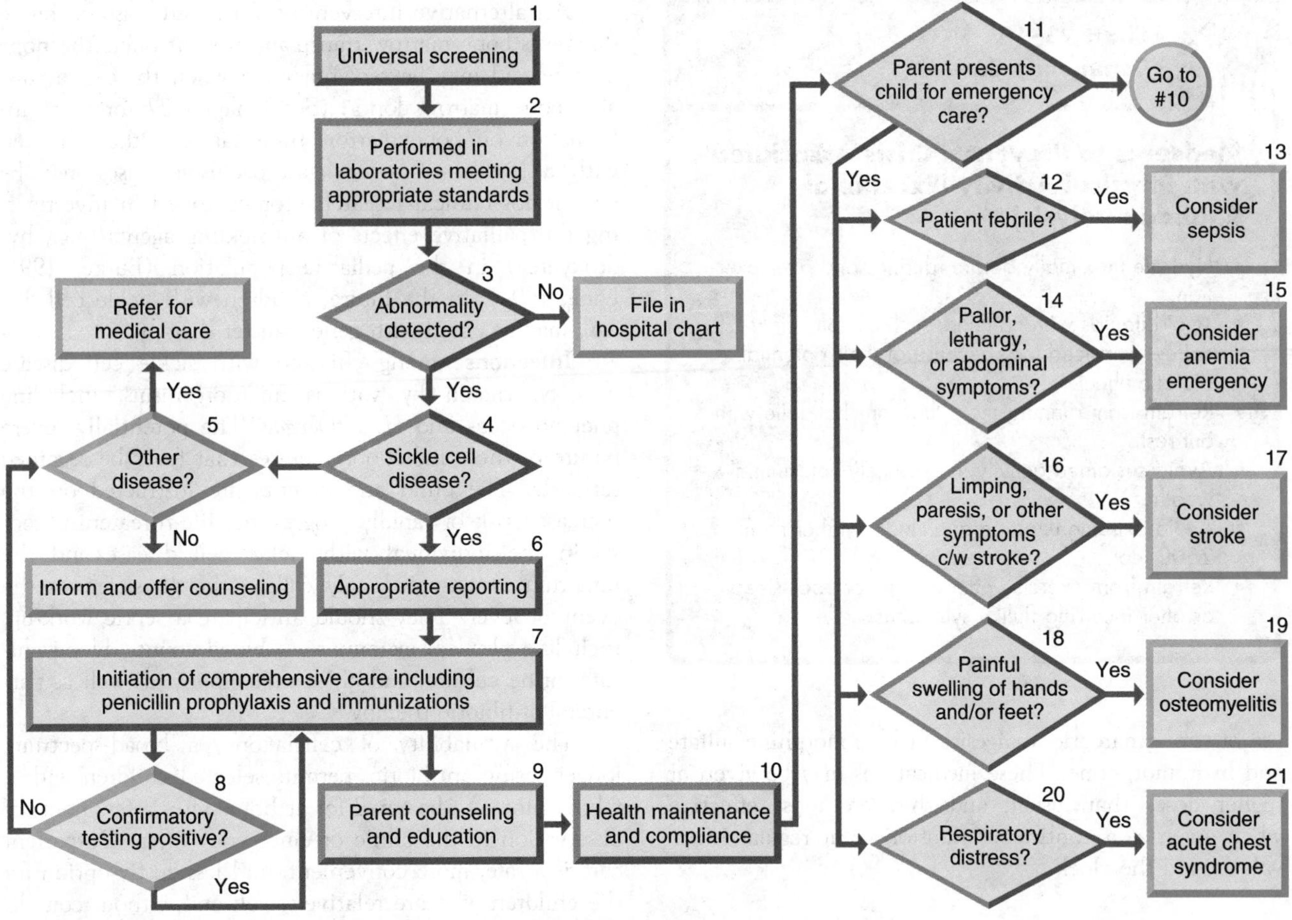

Figure 23–10
Detection and management of sickle cell disease: an algorithm. (From U.S. Department of Health and Human Services, Public Health Service, Agency for Health Care Policy and Research [1993]. Sickle Cell Disease: Screening, Diagnosis, Management, and Counseling in Newborns and Infants [AHCPR Publication No. 93-0562]. Rockville, MD: Author.)

transfusion decreases the body's need to engage in erythropoiesis, thereby reducing the number of hemoglobin S erythrocytes entering the circulation. Other common measures that help prevent sickling during the perioperative period are adequate fluid support, oxygenation, and environmental warmth, as well as prevention of acidosis (Ware & Filston, 1992).

Although sickle cell trait is not generally associated with health problems, health maintenance measures are important for those with the trait. An area of particular concern is intense physical activity. Those with sickle cell trait who are involved in competitive sports or strenuous exercise programs are at risk for exertional rhabdomyolysis, a potentially life-threatening syndrome characterized by the disintegration and death of muscle cells. Dehydration and hypoxia contribute to the onset of this syndrome. Browne & Gillespie (1993) identify several measures to prevent this crisis (Chart 23–18).

Management of Crisis Events

Vaso-occlusive pain crises, which are mild to moderate, can frequently be managed at home with increased fluid intake, analgesics, and nonpharmacologic measures such as relaxation and bed rest. However, with persistent and severe pain, the child is hospitalized to receive intravenous fluids, intravenous analgesics, and other interventions appropriate to the particular crisis event (Chart 23–19). Supplemental oxygen is usually reserved for those who demonstrate hypoxia. Blood transfusions may be indicated for those with continuing hypoxia and those with cerebral hyperemia. (See the section on treatment modalities for a discussion of blood transfusions.)

Pain associated with sickle cell crises can be excruciating, and adequate analgesia is necessary to provide relief. Management of severe pain generally includes the

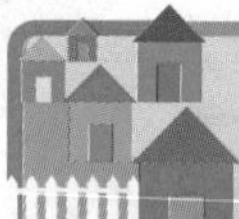

Chart 23–18
Community Care

Measures to Prevent a Crisis Associated with Physical Activity (Exertional Rhabdomyolysis)

- Hydrate maximally before, during, and after exertion.
- Avoid liquids with caffeine, such as soft drinks, coffee, and iced tea, because of their potential diuretic effect.
- Refrain from running more than one-half mile without rest.
- Avoid sustained activity in extremely hot, humid weather.
- Avoid extreme exertion at altitudes higher than 2500 feet.
- Refrain from exercise after a night of poor sleep or after incurring flulike symptoms.

use of strong narcotic analgesics such as morphine sulfate and hydromorphone. These medications may be given at higher doses than usual, and they are most effective when given as a continuous infusion or at regular intervals around the clock.

caREminder: *Meperidine is contraindicated for ongoing pain management because of the increased risk of seizures.*

As the child improves, weaker narcotics alone or in combination with non-narcotic analgesics (e.g., acetaminophen with codeine) are substituted and subsequently weaned as the painful crisis resolves.

Nursing responsibilities associated with pain management include (1) assessment of the child for verbal and nonverbal indicators of pain (e.g., crying, grimacing) and (2) collaboration with the interdisciplinary health care team to ensure interventions that provide pain relief for children with sickle cell crises. (See Chapter 13 regarding pain management in children.)

Repeated episodes of severe vaso-occlusive crises or the history of a cerebrovascular accident may lead to the implementation of an ongoing transfusion program to suppress the production of sickled red blood cells. However, such a transfusion program is not without the risks typically associated with blood transfusions. In addition, a long-term transfusion program eventually results in iron overload and the need for iron chelation therapy with deferoxamine. This is discussed in the section on treatment modalities.

An alternative intervention for severe vaso-occlusive disease is bone marrow transplantation. It offers the hope of cure and may be recommended when there is a suitable bone marrow donor. (See Chapter 22 for more information on bone marrow transplants.) Other children with a history of severe vaso-occlusive crises may be eligible for clinical research protocols used in investigating the palliative effects of antisickling agents (e.g., hydroxyurea) in the pediatric population (Burke, 1996; Lane, 1996). In the future, children with sickle cell disease may be cured with gene transfer therapy.

Infections among children with sickle cell disease may be caused by various microorganisms, including pneumococcus and *H. influenzae.* The potentially severe nature of these infections requires that fever be regarded seriously. The child and parents are instructed on the increased risk of rapidly progressing, life-threatening sepsis in the individual with sickle cell disease and the importance of immediately calling the physician in the event of fever. They should anticipate a septic work-up, including physical examination, blood counts, blood culture, urine culture, and chest radiography, as well as parenteral antibiotic therapy.

The availability of ceftriaxone, a broad-spectrum, longer-acting antibiotic, permits selected children with a febrile illness to be cared for at home after a few hours of observation in the clinic or emergency room. Outpatient care is a safe, more convenient, and less costly option for the children who are relatively well and without complications, and whose caretakers are reliable in providing the prescribed follow-up health care. Febrile children who are quite young, especially infants, and children with severe illness and complications are generally hospitalized (Lane, 1996).

Therapeutic antibiotics are continued at least until cultures are known to be negative and any infection has been treated. Thereafter, antibiotic prophylaxis is resumed. Other measures to prevent serious infection in children with sickle cell disease include the administration of pneumococcal vaccine and *H. influenzae* vaccine.

Acute splenic sequestration requires emergency intervention to restore normal blood volume to the general circulation and normal oxygenation to body tissues. Most often, this is achieved with blood transfusions. As normal cardiovascular status is restored, blood trapped in the spleen is again mobilized and the sequestration episode resolves.

Children who have experienced splenic sequestration crises may subsequently have an elective splenectomy. However, this surgical procedure is not indicated during times of acute splenic sequestration.

Aplastic crises are generally transient. Although the resulting anemia may become severe and the child may

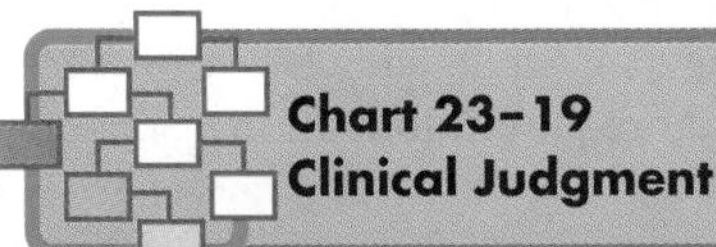

Chart 23–19
Clinical Judgment

A Toddler with Sickle Cell Disease

Shauna is a 2-year-old female with hemoglobin SS disease. Last evening she was admitted to the hospital via the emergency room after an acute onset of chest pain. The pain was not relieved at home by increased fluid intake and acetaminophen with codeine. Pertinent findings from the admitting physical examination include fever with a temperature to 39.4°C, irritability, mild nasal flaring, tachypnea, and decreased breath sounds. Shauna's oxygen saturation on room air was 89%. Her chest radiograph shows bilateral pulmonary infiltrates. Admitting laboratory studies include

- Hemoglobin 5.7 g/dL
- Reticulocytes at 24%
- White blood cell count of 26,000 mm^3
- Arterial blood gases: 78 mmHg (PaO_2); 35 mmHg ($PaCO_2$), 7.44 (pH)

Questions

1. What additional information would you elicit to assess Shauna's present illness?
2. What data from Shauna's medical record will help you interpret her admitting laboratory test results?
3. What is most likely to be Shauna's current health problem?
4. How can Shauna's pain be managed?
5. What assessment data would indicate that Shauna's physical condition has improved?

Answers

1. Seek additional information about Shauna's symptoms and the time of their onset. Ask for further detail about home interventions, particularly the amount of fluid intake and the dose and frequency of analgesic medication. Inquire about conditions that may have precipitated sickling in Shauna, such as inadequate fluid intake, exposure to heat and/or humidity or cold, excessive physical activity, travel to high altitude, exposure to infectious organisms. NOTE: There are many times when the precipitating factor cannot be identified.
2. Shauna's baseline laboratory values help to interpret her current laboratory values. With certain crisis events, it is not unusual to note a fall in hemoglobin and a rise in reticulocyte count. Also, the white blood cell count may be elevated above its baseline value.
3. Children with sickle cell disease who present with respiratory symptoms, chest pain, and fever are generally diagnosed with acute chest syndrome. Its etiology is usually difficult to identify with certainty, and it is assumed that both sickling and infection are present.
4. Because Shauna's pain was not relieved by oral fluids and oral analgesics at home, she should receive intravenous fluids and an intravenous narcotic, such as morphine sulfate, on a regular schedule around the clock. As her condition improves, oral fluids and a weaker analgesic will be substituted. The analgesic will be discontinued when the painful crisis resolves.
5. The following assessment data would indicate that Shauna's physical condition has improved:
   Afebrile
   No nasal flaring
   No evidence of chest pain
   Normal respiratory rate and rhythm
   Normal breath sounds
   Tolerating oral fluids
   Normal sleep pattern
   Not irritable
   More talkative
   More playful

require blood transfusion and other supportive interventions, aplastic crises usually resolve spontaneously. Adequate folic acid intake is especially important for the child who is recovering from an aplastic crisis (Platt & Dover, 1993). Normally, a sufficient amount of folic acid is absorbed from the diet. However, to ensure adequate intake for the child with hemoglobin SS disease, folic acid supplements may be prescribed.

Community Care

Psychosocial Needs

Management of the child with sickle cell disease requires attention to the psychosocial needs of the child and the family.

Child. At first, the child is too young to be aware of the diagnosis and its significance. However, as growth and development progress, the child increasingly learns about the disorder and is affected by the realization that not everyone has sickle cell disease.

Helping children with sickle cell disease acquire accurate knowledge about the disorder, its management, its crisis events, and chronic complications is important for their physical and psychological well-being. As children move forward in their development, teaching must be an ongoing process that assesses their previous knowledge and expands upon it.

Children with sickle cell disease need to develop effective coping skills for dealing with both physical and psychosocial concerns. They may fear painful crisis events. They may wonder what will take place when they experience a crisis event. Knowing the signs and symptoms of crises, knowing what to do, and knowing what to expect others to do help children cope with crisis events. Children should notify their parents or caretaker when they experience pain or other indicators of sickle cell crises, and measures should be taken promptly to abate crisis events.

Like their peers, children with sickle cell disease are involved in establishing their identities. It is important to help them identify their positive qualities, help them recognize what they can do, and help them develop realistic, healthy self-concepts despite the presence of a chronic disorder. This is particularly important for adolescents, whose peers achieve physical growth and develop secondary sex characteristics sooner than those with sickle cell disease.

Parents. Parents of a child with sickle cell disease are likely to experience a number of psychosocial concerns. A significant role for members of the comprehensive health care team is to provide informational and emotional support in response to parental needs.

Informational support refers to providing parents with timely information regarding sickle cell disease and its impact on their child. It is helpful for the nurse to have an ongoing teaching plan that addresses the areas in which parents commonly require informational support (see TIP 23–3).

Although the desired outcomes of providing information include enhanced parental coping and the ability to parent effectively a child with sickle cell disease, the information received may be emotionally disturbing at first. Often, it is stressful for parents to learn that their child has sickle cell disease and faces a lifetime of living with a chronic disorder. As they begin to learn about sickle cell disease, its management, and its complications, parents may be concerned that they will not recognize the occurrence of a crisis event and will fail to respond appropriately to it. The diagnosis of sickle cell disease, the crisis events, and the subsequent chronic complications are common sources of emotional stress for parents of a child with sickle cell disease. In addition, there may be parental guilt because of the hereditary etiology of the disorder.

Emotional support for the parents of a child with sickle cell disease goes beyond the provision of information. It includes listening, identifying coping skills that have been used effectively in the past, providing positive reinforcement, and offering practical information when appropriate.

Siblings. As in other situations in which there is a chronic disorder, the siblings of the children need attention. Siblings need a sense of belonging within the family. They need to feel that their parents have time for them and value them just as much as the child with sickle cell disease. Also, siblings require accurate knowledge about sickle cell disease, its etiology, its management, and its complications, as well as information about how they can be helpful during times of crisis events and other complications in the child with sickle cell disease.

Siblings should know whether or not they have sickle cell trait. As discussed earlier, those who have sickle cell trait need to take extra precautions with strenuous physical activities. In addition, as they reach adolescence, siblings should receive information on the probability that their own children of the future will be born with sickle cell trait or sickle cell disease.

Discharge Planning

For children with sickle cell disease, the nurse may view discharge planning from two perspectives. One involves discharge planning related to specific events such as vasoocclusive crises, infections, and surgical procedures. The second relates to discharge planning associated with scheduled outpatient appointments designed for the ongoing assessment and management of children with sickle cell disease. In both situations, the nurse needs to identify desired outcomes and plan and provide appropriate interventions to facilitate attainment of these outcomes by the end of a hospital stay or an outpatient visit.

Discharge planning for episodic events takes into account the needs related to the particular event, in addition to the needs associated with sickle cell disease. When special supplies and services are required, a referral to a home care company may be necessary.

Teaching is a significant part of discharge planning. The nurse needs to start teaching as early as possible and plan time for review. Teaching may encompass a variety of topics, depending on the specific situation. For example, when a toddler with sickle cell disease has an elective splenectomy after two earlier episodes of splenic sequestration, teaching is likely to include measures to promote good hydration, signs of abnormal wound healing, signs of wound infection, identification of nonverbal cues of pain, pain management, schedule for outpatient follow-up appointments, and need to call the physician for bleeding, fever, increased pain, or other complications. An important component of the teaching process is an assessment of the family's understanding of the child's home care needs and their ability to care for the child at home.

Outpatient visits for the ongoing assessment and management of children with sickle cell disease generally occur at least two times per year. These visits occur more frequently when the children are newly diagnosed or quite young and when they have health needs that require more frequent monitoring. Desired outcomes for these visits are related to physical and psychosocial needs on the basis of an updated history and a current physical assessment.

Be alert for the developing child's readiness to learn more about sickle cell disease, as well as the need to correct misperceptions that the child and family may have about the disorder, its effect, its complications, and its management. Also, as the child and family reach new developmental milestones, be alert for the need to discuss the child's activities and specific concerns associated with each developmental phase.

Discharge planning for outpatient visits may include referral or follow-up information to a local physician, a home care company, and a community health agency. It may involve contact with community groups such as the child's school or daycare center (Chart 23–20). It may entail helping a family with planning for camp or vacation by providing a letter concerning the child's need for emergency health care if a crisis event occurs. It may incorporate a referral to the Sickle Cell Disease Association of America for literature, as well as for information about the services and local chapters of this and related organizations (see Resources).

Beta-Thalassemia

Thalassemia refers to a variety of microcytic hemolytic anemias that are characterized by a decrease or absence of one or more of the normal globin chains in the hemoglobin molecule. A primary example is beta-thalassemia, in which there is inadequate production of beta globin chains. The classification of thalassemia ranges from clinically insignificant thalassemia minima to clinically severe thalassemia major (Cooley's anemia).

Beta-thalassemia is a hereditary disorder. Its inheritance pattern is autosomal recessive, with the genetic defect present on chromosome number 11. The disorder affects equal numbers of females and males. Children who are heterozygous for the defective gene usually do not show clinically significant disease. In contrast, those who are homozygous for the defective gene tend to have serious disease, especially if the disorder is not diagnosed and if appropriate interventions are not implemented.

In addition, some children inherit a gene for hemoglobin S from one parent and a gene for beta-thalassemia from the other parent. This results in sickle beta-thalassemia. The severity of this disorder depends on the extent to which the beta-thalassemia gene is contributing to the production of hemoglobin A. When no hemoglobin A is present in the red blood cells, the disorder tends to be more severe. When some hemoglobin A is present in the red blood cells, the disorder is usually milder.

Worldview: *Beta-thalassemia is most common among those of Mediterranean descent. Also, it affects a significant number of people whose ancestral roots are in the Middle East, Asia, and Africa. In the United States, thalassemia major affects approximately 1400 people (Martin & Butler, 1993). Screening programs are common in Europe and Asia, where the incidence of thalassemia is greater. In the United States, hemoglobin electrophoresis is recommended for at-risk populations to identify those with thalassemia and thalassemia trait.*

Genograms for thalassemia are similar to those for sickle cell disease (see Fig. 23–9).

Pathophysiology

Beta-thalassemia stems from a defect in the beta globin gene. The result is inadequate production of the beta globin chains, which are required for the synthesis of hemoglobin A.

Those who are heterozygous for beta-thalassemia generate about half the normal quantity of beta globin chains. Those who are homozygous for beta-thalassemia are subclassified as having beta^{+}-thalassemia and beta^{0}-thalassemia. Those in the beta^{+} group synthesize up to one third of the normal quantity of beta globin chains, whereas those in the beta^{0} group produce no beta globin chains.

Alpha globin chains, which are also required for the synthesis of hemoglobin A, continue to be produced in their normal quantity. However, the lack of beta globin

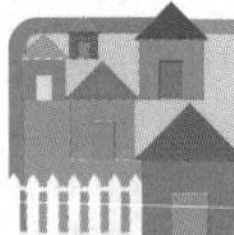

Chart 23–20
Community Care

The Child with Sickle Cell Disease at a Daycare Center

Children with sickle cell disease are likely to be among those who attend community daycare centers. It is important for their caretakers to know that they have sickle cell disease. Also, staff at daycare centers should know the guidelines that have been established to prevent and manage crisis events and to promote normal growth and development in children with sickle cell disease.

The nurse may assist the child's family in providing information to the daycare center staff. Outcome objectives for the child's caretakers include the following:

- Describe sickle cell disease, in general, and how it affects the child who will be cared for at the daycare center, in particular.
- State factors that may precipitate crisis events in the child with sickle cell disease, such as humidity, heat, cold, and excessive physical activity.
- Describe common types of crisis events associated with sickle cell disease:
  - Vaso-occlusive crises
  - Infections
  - Acute splenic sequestration
  - Aplastic crises
- Discuss common signs and symptoms associated with "crisis" events:
  - Pain
  - Fever
  - Pale color
  - Difficulty breathing
  - Enlarged abdomen
  - Vomiting, diarrhea
  - Refusal to eat or drink
  - Irritability
  - Increased somnolence
  - Weakness or numbness of arms or legs
  - Swelling of hands or feet
- Discuss the need for prompt medical care for "crisis" events associated with sickle cell disease.
- Discuss the importance of the child receiving extra fluids and pausing for rest periods during times of physical activity. Daycare center personnel should be informed of any activities in which the child is not to participate, such as swimming in cold water.
- Relate the child's more frequent use of restroom facilities to the effect of sickle cell disease on kidney function.
- Describe the significance of treating the child as other children are treated. Although there is a need to be aware of sickle cell disease and what to do if a crisis event occurs, the daycare center staff should not focus on it or single the child out for special attention or privileges.

chains with which they may be paired leads to an excess amount of free alpha globin chains. These free alpha globin chains precipitate and appear as inclusion bodies within developing red blood cells. The inclusion bodies have a destructive effect, leading to the demise of the majority of red blood cells while they are still maturing in the bone marrow.

The red blood cells that enter the peripheral circulation in decreased number are characterized by microcytosis (small size), hypochromia (decreased hemoglobin), abnormal shape (poikilocytosis), and the presence of inclusion bodies. Their life span is usually limited to a few hours or a few days, with damaged cells being removed from circulation by the spleen and liver. If the red blood cells contain a significant amount of hemoglobin F, their survival time is longer. Those with thalassemia may produce an increased amount of hemoglobin F in an effort to compensate for the deficiency of hemoglobin A.

In response to the severe anemia associated with thalassemia major, the bone marrow greatly expands and produces an increased number of erythroid precursor cells. However, these cells meet an early demise, just like their predecessors, and erythropoiesis is ineffective.

Prognosis. The prognosis for beta-thalassemia depends on its severity. Thalassemia major is of particular concern. When this is untreated, the majority of children die during their first year of life from septicemia or heart failure. With a regular transfusion program and the timely addition of iron chelation therapy, those with thalassemia major can be expected to live into their fourth decade.

Assessment

The clinical manifestations of beta-thalassemia vary significantly, depending on its severity. Thus, the disorder is classified in terms of its clinical intensity as *thalassemia minima*, *thalassemia minor*, *thalassemia intermedia*, and *thalassemia major* (Table 23–9).

Thalassemia minima is referred to as "silent" because there are no significant hematologic abnormalities. **Thalassemia minor** is associated with some abnormal hematologic findings, but the majority of these children are asymptomatic on physical examination.

Thalassemia intermedia usually becomes apparent during the toddler or preschool years. In addition to hematologic abnormalities, the classic findings include hyperbilirubinemia, splenomegaly, hepatomegaly, delayed growth, and abnormal facial appearance (Giardina & Hilgartner, 1992).

Thalassemia major, also known as **Cooley's anemia**, is the most severe form of this disorder. Clinical manifestations generally become apparent during the first year of life. Pallor, fatigue, weakness, and poor feeding are commonly observed. Failure to thrive and delayed growth and development are also apparent. When untreated, the severe anemia progresses and becomes incompatible with life.

Classic facial changes begin to develop during infancy, including frontal bossing, prominent cheek bones, depression of the nasal bridge, maxillary overbite, and mandibular prominence. This "thalassemic" facies is secondary to the expanding bone marrow. Other bone changes appear on radiographic studies, including a thinning of long bone cortices, which makes these bones fragile and prone to pathologic fractures.

Extramedullary areas of hematopoiesis develop as the body attempts to compensate for ineffective erythropoiesis in the bone marrow. These sites may appear on radiographic studies as masses in the chest, for example, or they may be evident on physical examination as enlargements of involved anatomic sites, such as the liver, spleen, and lymph nodes.

Table 23–9 identifies common hematologic findings associated with thalassemia major. In addition, dark tea-colored urine may be present and the bilirubin may be increased as a result of red blood cell hemolysis. When

Table 23–9
Laboratory Data Commonly Associated with Beta-Thalassemia

	Thalassemia Minima	Thalassemia Minor	Thalassemia Intermedia	Thalassemia Major
Hemoglobin	Normal	Normal in general May have anemia during pregnancy	Anemia Hemoglobin >7 g/dL	Severe anemia Hemoglobin <7 g/dL
Mean corpuscular volume (MCV)	Normal	Decreased	Decreased	Decreased
Mean corpuscular hemoglobin (MCH)	Normal	Decreased	Decreased	Decreased
Red blood cell count	Normal	Increased	Increased	Decreased
Red blood cell morphology	Normal	Normal or abnormal	Abnormal	Abnormal
Hemoglobin electrophoresis	Normal	Abnormal Decreased Hgb A Increased Hgb A_2	Abnormal Decreased Hgb A Increased Hgb A_2 Increased Hgb F	Abnormal Decreased Hgb A Increased Hgb A_2 Increased Hgb F
Beta-globin synthesis	Decreased	Decreased	Decreased	Decreased
Alpha-to-beta globin chain ratio	Increased	Increased	Increased	Increased

leukocytosis is present, a normal differential distinguishes it from the leukocytosis associated with infection (McDonagh & Nienhuis, 1993).

Although the clinical manifestations of beta-thalassemia can be severe, they are less frequently seen today because of the use of transfusion therapy.

Diagnostic Tests. Diagnosis of beta-thalassemia is generally made after the third month of life, when the normal switch from predominantly hemoglobin F to predominantly hemoglobin A fails to occur and the child becomes anemic. Hemoglobin electrophoresis shows decreased to absent hemoglobin A, normal or increased hemoglobin A_2, and increased hemoglobin F.

Nursing Diagnoses and Outcomes

Nursing diagnoses and outcomes for the child with anemia appear in Chart 23–3. In addition, the following nursing diagnoses and outcomes are applicable to the child with beta-thalassemia:

- **Risk for injury related to iron overload**
  Outcomes: Child/family identify the etiology of iron overload.
  Child/family identify the physical changes associated with iron overload and their life-threatening potential.
  Child/family identify the importance of iron chelation therapy in preventing severe iron overload.
- **Fear of chronic physical impairment and premature death related to severe anemia and iron overload**
  Outcomes: Child/family verbalize fears concerning chronic physical impairment and the potential for early death when the child has severe beta-thalassemia.
  Child/family receive informational and emotional support.

Interdisciplinary Interventions

Management of the child with beta-thalassemia varies, depending on its severity. In general, children with thalassemia minima or thalassemia minor do not require blood transfusion therapy because they do not tend to have anemia. An exception occurs during pregnancy, when transfusion support may be necessary.

It is important to recognize the beta-thalassemia trait so that microcytic, hypochromic red blood cells are not erroneously attributed to other causes such as iron deficiency anemia. When children with beta-thalassemia are suspected of having iron deficiency anemia as well, appropriate laboratory studies are required to confirm the latter diagnosis. Iron therapy in the absence of iron deficiency anemia may lead to iron overload.

When beta-thalassemia results in severe anemia, the primary intervention is a hypertransfusion program (discussed in the section on treatment modalities). Such a transfusion program facilitates adequate oxygenation of body tissues and practically eliminates all symptoms of thalassemia (Piomelli, 1995).

Children with mild to moderate beta-thalassemia, who do not require an ongoing transfusion program, may need supportive transfusions during times of infection and other events that trigger hemolytic or aplastic crises. Oral folic acid supplements may be prescribed to maintain adequate folate stores.

A newer mode of treatment for severe beta-thalassemia is bone marrow transplantation (see Chapter 22 for more information on this treatment modality). When successful, it offers the hope of cure. Although it is not an option for every child with severe beta-thalassemia, bone marrow transplantation may be recommended when there is a suitable bone marrow donor.

Current investigations include the use of medications to stimulate increased synthesis of hemoglobin F, as well as the development of curative gene transfer therapy.

Community Care

Interdisciplinary management of the child with beta-thalassemia requires ongoing physical assessment and laboratory studies to monitor for anemia and its sequelae. Although children in a hypertransfusion program often lead nearly normal lives, they need to be assessed regularly for iron overload and the physical alterations with which it is associated. The psychosocial interventions for children with beta-thalassemia and their families are similar to those described in the section on sickle cell disease.

The nurse and other members of the health care team have a significant role with respect to beta-thalassemia. In addition to family-centered patient care and education, they provide community education concerning the disorder and its management, as well as genetic counseling concerning the probability of having a child with heterozygous or homozygous beta-thalassemia. The Cooley Anemia Foundation is an additional source of information (see Resources).

Anemias

Although the anemias of childhood have distinguishing features, they share a common characteristic. For each, laboratory values show that the hemoglobin concentration or the red blood cell count is less than normal. Severe anemia is present when the hemoglobin falls below 8 g/dL. Both moderate and severe anemias lead to decreased oxygenation of body tissues. When symptomatic and life-threatening anemia is present, red blood cell transfusions provide increased hemoglobin and improved oxygenation.

There are two major methods for classifying the anemias: (1) by morphologic features and (2) by physiologic characteristics. Red blood cell size (mean corpuscular volume, MCV) is the most significant morphologic classification. Herein the anemias are described as microcytic (small cell size), normocytic (normal cell size), and macrocytic (large cell size). Disorders of red blood cell production and red blood cell destruction are the two primary categories for the physiologic classification of anemia. Iron deficiency anemia, megaloblastic anemia, lead poisoning, and aplastic anemia are examples of disorders that interfere with normal red blood cell production. Abnormalities involving the red blood cell membrane, such as hereditary spherocytosis, together with the various hemolytic anemias, exemplify disorders of red blood cell destruction. In addition to productive and destructive physiologic disorders, anemia may result when there is significant internal and external bleeding.

Iron Deficiency Anemia

Iron deficiency anemia (IDA) is the most common nutritional anemia during childhood. It is a microcytic, hypochromic anemia that occurs after depletion of the body's iron stores. Severe IDA is present when the hemoglobin is less than 8 g/dL (Dallman, Yip, & Oski, 1993).

IDA is most likely to occur when children experience:

- Rapid physical growth
- Low iron intake
- Inadequate iron absorption
- Loss of blood

Development of IDA is more prevalent during infancy and adolescence, when physical growth is rapid and iron intake is frequently insufficient.

Iron fortification of food products, greater use of iron-fortified infant formulas, and an increase in breastfeeding have contributed to a significant decrease in the incidence of IDA in the United States. However, IDA is still the most common cause of anemia in infants and children who are otherwise in good health (Dallman et al., 1993).

Worldview: *In developing countries of the world, it is estimated that half of the children are iron deficient (Yip, 1994). This deficiency is due to poor diets, lack of iron fortification, infections such as malaria, and parasitic infestations such as hookworm. IDA in developing countries is frequently associated with deficiencies in other nutrients such as folic acid, vitamin C, and vitamin A (Yip, 1994). Thus, when children with nutritional anemia come to the United States, health care providers need to consider that lack of iron may not be the only nutrient deficiency.*

Pathophysiology

Iron deficiency is described in three stages.

- **Stage one** is characterized by depletion of ferritin, hemosiderin, and other iron storage compounds in the liver, spleen, and bone marrow. Anemia is not present during this stage.
- **Stage two** is characterized by a lack of transport iron. Iron saturation of transferrin decreases and, although anemia is generally not yet present, the hemoglobin concentration trends toward low normal.
- **Stage three** is characterized by a marked deficit in transport iron that inhibits normal production of hemoglobin. Erythrocyte protoporphyrin increases because there is inadequate iron with which it may combine to form heme. Transferrin receptors, located on cell surface membranes in various body tissues, become more numerous in response to the iron-poor environment. A microcytic, hypochromic anemia develops during this stage of iron deficiency.

In addition to inadequate dietary intake, impaired iron absorption may lead to IDA. The intestinal mucosal cells are particularly important because they act as a holding zone and gatekeeper for iron. When the body does not need iron, it is lost with desquamation of intestinal mucosal cells. However, when the body needs iron, it enters the circulation via the intestinal mucosa.

Alert: *The intestinal mucosa is not a barrier against large quantities of iron. Fatal poisoning in young children can result from acute iron intoxication (Dallman et al., 1993).*

Impairment of the intestinal mucosa may inhibit adequate iron absorption. Also, iron malabsorption may occur in conjunction with inflammatory and infectious disorders.

Prognosis. IDA is easily treated and, thus, its prognosis is good. When IDA is not corrected, or when it recurs, consider the possibilities of (1) a continuing inadequacy of iron intake, (2) a continuing inadequacy of iron absorption, and (3) a continuing site of blood loss. When untreated, severe IDA may lead to loss of life, particularly when it occurs in conjunction with increased physiologic stress (e.g., an acute febrile illness) (Yip, 1994).

Assessment

IDA may not be readily apparent when the anemia is mild. However, as it progresses, pallor, fatigue, shortness of breath, irritability, and decreased tolerance of physical work and exercise become increasingly apparent. There may be a decreased ability to resist infection, fissures at corners of the mouth, inflammation of the tongue, and spoon-shaped nails. Heart murmurs and congestive heart failure can occur with severe anemia. Skeletal abnormalities may appear as well.

Children with iron deficiency absorb greater amounts of lead and, thus, they are at greater risk of developing lead poisoning. In addition, iron deficiency may impair cognitive and psychomotor development. These deficits can occur even with moderate anemia, and they may remain despite correction of the IDA (Barness, 1993; Dallman et al., 1993; Lozoff, Jimenez, & Wolf, 1991; Yip, 1994).

Diagnostic Tests. As the child progresses through the three stages of iron deficiency, there is increasing laboratory evidence of this deficiency (Table 23–10). During the first stage, the depletion of iron stores is most commonly identified by a decrease in serum ferritin. However, it should be noted that a normal serum ferritin does not rule out IDA, especially during times of inflammation and infection. A less practical means of evaluating storage iron is by testing a sample of bone marrow for hemosiderin, which is decreased in IDA.

During the second stage of iron deficiency, the lack of transport iron is identified primarily by a decrease in transferrin saturation. A decrease in serum iron and an increase in total iron-binding capacity are likely to be evident as well. However, these tests individually are not as reliable as transferrin saturation in assessing the status of iron transport (Dallman et al., 1993). In addition, during this stage, early red blood cell changes may be noted, with the hemoglobin falling to low normal.

Laboratory manifestations of the third stage of iron deficiency include changes in red blood cell indices. These include an increase in erythrocyte protoporphyrin and transferrin receptors and a decrease in hemoglobin, hematocrit, mean corpuscular volume (MCV), mean corpuscular hemoglobin (MCH), and mean corpuscular hemoglobin concentration (MCHC). Generally, a hemoglobin test is used when children are initially screened for IDA.

Nursing Diagnoses and Outcomes

In addition to the nursing diagnoses presented in Chart 23–3, specific nursing diagnoses and outcomes for the child with IDA are incorporated in TIP 23–4.

Community Care

Management of the child with IDA is aimed at correcting the anemia, replenishing the depleted iron stores, and preventing further iron deficiency. These goals are achieved primarily with iron supplementation and nutritional counseling.

Iron Supplementation

Iron supplementation frequently begins as a therapeutic trial in the child with suspected but unconfirmed IDA who is otherwise healthy. Anemia in such children is

Table 23–10
Pathophysiologic and Laboratory Alterations Associated with Iron Deficiency Anemia

Stage of Iron Deficiency	Pathophysiologic Alterations	Laboratory Alterations
Stage I	Depletion of iron storage compounds	Decreased serum ferritin
Stage II	Lack of transport iron	Decreased transferrin saturation Decreased serum iron Increased total iron binding capacity
Stage III	Increased erythrocyte protoporphyrin Increased transferrin receptors Microcytic, hypochromic anemia	Increased erythrocyte protoporphyrin Increased transferrin receptors Decreased hemoglobin Decreased hematocrit Decreased MCV Decreased MCH Decreased MCHC

TIP 23-4 A Teaching Intervention Plan for the Child with Iron Deficiency Anemia

Nursing Diagnoses and Outcomes

- Knowledge deficit related to iron deficiency anemia
  Outcome:
  Child/family describe iron deficiency anemia and the need for adequate dietary iron to prevent this anemia.
- Knowledge deficit related to sources of dietary iron
  Outcomes:
  Child/family identify sources of dietary iron.
  Child/family identify dietary habits that enhance bioavailability of iron intake.
- Risk for injury related to anemia
  Outcomes:
  Child/family identify short-term and long-term effects of impaired tissue oxygenation caused by iron deficiency anemia.
  Child/family identify child's need for iron supplements to correct anemia and replenish iron stores.

Interventions

- Instruct regarding iron deficiency anemia.
  - Inadequate iron
  - Decreased hemoglobin in red blood cells
  - Decreased oxygenation of body tissues
- Inform about causes of iron deficiency anemia:
  - Inadequate iron intake, especially during times of rapid physical growth:
    - Infancy
    - Adolescence
  - Malabsorption of iron
  - Iron loss related to excessive bleeding
- Educate concerning dietary sources of iron; distinguish between heme iron and nonheme iron
  - Heme iron—easy for the body to absorb. Dietary sources include:
    - Meat
    - Poultry
    - Fish
  - Nonheme iron—harder for the body to absorb. Dietary sources include:
    - Vegetables
    - Fruits
    - Cereals
    - Breads
  - Dietary habits that facilitate absorption of nonheme iron:
    - **Include** meat, poultry, fish, and foods or beverages with vitamin C in the same meal.
    - **Exclude** bran foods, milk, tea, and coffee in the same meal.
  - *Note:* Milk is *not* a dietary source of iron.
- Teach regarding dietary sources of iron for infants:
  - Iron-fortified formula
  - Iron-fortified cereal
  - Breast milk—avoid solid foods near breast-feeding time to enhance bioavailability of the limited amount of iron in human milk.
  - *Note:* Breast-fed babies need iron supplements or iron-fortified infant foods because the amount of iron in breast milk is insufficient.

TIP continued on following page

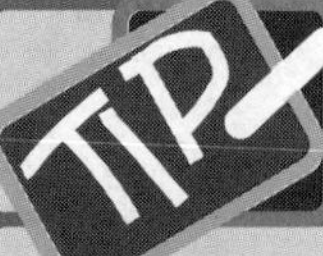

TIP 23-4 A Teaching Intervention Plan for the Child with Iron Deficiency Anemia *Continued*

- Coach concerning meals that provide adequate iron intake within the context of the family's ethnic group and budget limitations.
- Instruct regarding signs and symptoms of iron deficiency anemia in children:
  - Less active
  - Less playful
  - Sleeping more
  - Pale in color
  - Short of breath
  - Irritable
  - More prone to infection
  - Heart murmurs
  - Congestive heart failure
  - Abnormal growth and development
  - *Note:* Children often adapt to a gradual decline in hemoglobin. Thus, signs and symptoms of anemia may not be readily apparent at first.
- Teach concerning iron supplements, when prescribed.
  - For best absorption, give iron with water or juice between meals; do *not* give with antacids, milk, bran foods, tea, or coffee.
  - To avoid staining of teeth, give liquid iron with a straw or use syringe to place toward back of child's mouth.
  - Give full dose of iron, but do *not* overdose.
  - Expect color of child's stools to become dark while iron is supplemented.
  - Report constipation or other gastrointestinal changes to physician or nurse practitioner.
  - Store iron medicine where children cannot reach it.
  - If child takes too much iron, emergency care is needed; *immediately* call physician or poison control center for your community.

most often caused by iron deficiency, and a therapeutic trial of iron is less costly than a series of tests to determine that the anemia is definitely due to deficiency of iron. The trial period is usually 1 month. If the hemoglobin concentration rises significantly during this period, the presumed diagnosis of IDA is supported. Iron supplementation continues for up to 4 additional months to complete the correction of anemia and to replenish the iron stores. To avoid iron overload, therapeutic iron supplementation should not continue longer.

Supplements of iron are generally given orally as elemental iron in the form of ferrous sulfate, a well-absorbed and less expensive iron preparation. The therapeutic dose is 3 mg/kg per day (Barness, 1993). A higher dose may be prescribed when IDA is seen.

caREminder: *Iron is absorbed better on an empty stomach, and it is most often given to infants as a single dose before breakfast. For older children, the daily amount of iron supplementation is usually divided into two or three doses and given between meals. Children receiving oral iron supplements have dark-colored stools, and they may experience gastrointestinal side effects such as nausea and constipation. Also, although it is temporary, teeth may be stained by contact with liquid iron preparations. To avoid staining of teeth, give liquid iron using a straw or a syringe to place the medication toward the back of the child's mouth.*

Parenteral forms of iron supplementation are available, but they can cause significant side effects and their use is rarely necessary.

During infancy, iron deficiency is especially common after depletion of the iron stores that are present at birth. Thus, special care must be taken to ensure that infants have an adequate supply of iron. Full-term infants require an iron intake of 1 mg/kg per day, starting at 4 to 6 months of age. Formula-fed infants receive iron-fortified formula, whereas babies continuing to breast-feed receive iron-fortified infant cereal two times per day.

Preterm infants require an iron intake of 1 to 2 mg/kg per day, starting at 1 to 2 months of age. As with the full-term infant, iron-fortified formula may be given. For breast-fed infants or infants receiving human milk, iron supplementation is indicated, at least until the babies are old enough to receive iron-fortified infant cereal.

In general, prophylactic iron supplementation is given whenever an infant's dietary intake is inadequate to provide the needed iron. When supplemental iron is used, it should be stored out of the reach of children to guard against accidental poisoning. Children between infancy and adolescence who are provided with sufficient food usually have their iron needs adequately met without supplementation. However, iron supplements may be needed during adolescence, especially among teenagers who are prone to fad diets and poor nutrition while experiencing rapid physical growth. Also, teenage girls who are pregnant, lactating, or heavily menstruating require iron supplements because their total iron need is not provided by diet alone.

Nutritional Counseling

Nutritional counseling is an important intervention in both the treatment and prevention of IDA. Certain dietary habits enhance iron intake and increase the bioavailability of iron.

For infants, iron intake is improved with the use of iron-fortified infant formula instead of fresh cow's milk. In addition to being poor in iron content, fresh cow's milk is associated with intestinal blood loss and, thus, contributes to iron deficiency, especially during the first 6 months of infancy. The distribution of iron-fortified infant formula in the federal Special Supplemental Food Program for Women, Infants and Children (WIC) is a significant factor in the decreased incidence of IDA in the United States.

Iron intake is enhanced with the use of iron-fortified infant cereal. The inclusion of meat for infants, as well as foods and juices fortified with ascorbic acid, promotes the absorption of iron from a meal. Also, the avoidance of solid foods at or near the time of breast-feeding enhances the bioavailability of the limited amount of iron in human milk.

Although many foods for children and adolescents contain iron, this iron may be in different forms. Heme iron is found primarily in foods from animal sources and is readily absorbed by the intestinal mucosa. In contrast, nonheme iron is found mainly in foods derived from nonanimal sources, and it must be changed from the ferric to the ferrous form to facilitate absorption.

Meat, poultry, and fish are excellent sources of heme iron, and their incorporation into a meal enhances the bioavailability of nonheme iron. In addition, the inclusion of dietary sources of ascorbic acid promotes the absorption of nonheme iron. Nonheme iron is found in varying amounts in vegetables, fruits, cereals, and breads.

Just as the absorption of nonheme iron can be facilitated in combination with certain foods, it can be hindered in the presence of other dietary components. Inhibitors of nonheme iron absorption include bran foods, milk, and tannin-containing beverages such as tea and coffee. In addition, certain antacids and antibiotics may impede the absorption of nonheme iron.

Those with vegetarian diets consume iron that is mainly nonheme in form. When planning meals, they need to be aware of the role of ascorbic acid in facilitating the absorption of nonheme iron and to note particularly those foods and beverages that decrease the bioavailability of their iron intake.

Education

The nurse has a significant role in providing education concerning the treatment and prevention of IDA (see TIP 23–4). In addition to providing education to children and families in the health care setting, the nurse reaches out into the community. By arranging for educational programs at schools, daycare centers, health fairs, and so forth, the nurse can make an important contribution to the prevention of IDA. Children and families who develop dietary habits that facilitate iron intake and absorption, and who receive prophylactic iron supplements during times of increased iron need, are less likely to experience IDA (Chart 23–21).

Megaloblastic Anemia

Megaloblastic anemia is a nutritional anemia that most often results from a deficiency of either vitamin B_{12} or folate (folic acid). Bone marrow and peripheral blood samples show immature red cells that appear nucleated and macrocytic and fail to engage normally in the reproductive process. Not all occurrences of vitamin B_{12} or folate deficiency result in megaloblastic anemia.

Vitamin B_{12} and folate deficiencies may be due to

- Inadequate intake
- Malabsorption
- Metabolic disorder

Vitamin B_{12} Deficiency. Inadequate vitamin B_{12} intake is more likely to occur among those who are strictly vegetarian, in contrast to those who include meat and other animal products in their diet. Also, the newborn may have inadequate vitamin B_{12} as a result of maternal vitamin B_{12} deficiency. Malabsorption is associated with pernicious anemia, in which the intrinsic factor, which is required for absorption of vitamin B_{12}, is either absent or dysfunctional. Also, malabsorption of vitamin B_{12} may stem from gastric and intestinal disorders such as necrotizing enterocolitis, as well as from infection with the

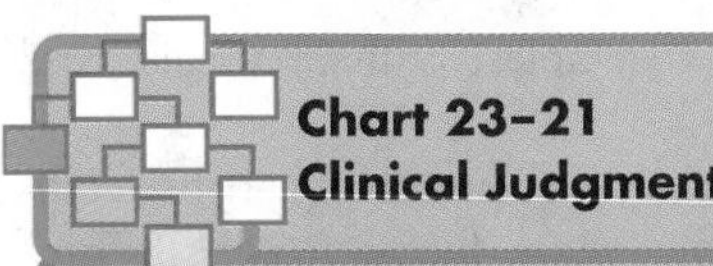

Chart 23–21
Clinical Judgment

A Toddler with Anemia

Cody is a 15-month-old male who comes to clinic. His mother reports that he was doing well until about 1 week ago. Since then, he has been less playful and sleeping more than usual. His past history is negative for hematologic disorders and other abnormalities. There is no history of recent illness, injury, or foreign travel, and his mother has not noted any blood loss. Apart from skin pallor and decreased activity, Cody's physical examination is unremarkable. His laboratory results include the following:

- Hemoglobin = 7.7 g/dL
- Mean corpuscular volume (MCV) = 54 fL
- Mean corpuscular hemoglobin (MCH) = 17 pg

Questions

1. What additional information would you elicit concerning Cody?
2. Assuming that Cody's diagnosis is iron deficiency anemia, at what stage is it?
3. Why is iron deficiency the most probable reason for Cody's anemia?
4. How is iron deficiency anemia managed?
5. What data would indicate that an iron deficiency anemia is resolving?

Answers

1. Obtain a diet history for Cody. Particularly elicit information to help assess Cody's intake of dietary iron. For examples:
   Does Cody drink formula or cow's milk? If formula, is it iron fortified? If cow's milk, is Cody taking iron supplements?
   How many ounces of milk or formula does Cody drink on a typical day? (Too much may interfere with Cody's appetite for solid foods.)
   Does Cody eat solid foods? If yes, are they a source of iron?
2. The iron deficiency anemia would be stage three because Cody is anemic (hemoglobin 7.7 g/dL), and his red blood cells are small in size and decreased in hemoglobin content (MCV = 54 fL; MCH = 17 pg). These changes are not characteristic of the first two stages of iron deficiency anemia.
3. Iron deficiency anemia is the most frequent reason for microcytic, hypochromic anemia in older infants and toddlers. Generally, it is due to an inadequate intake of dietary iron coupled with depletion of the iron stores that are present at birth.
4. When iron deficiency anemia appears to be due to a dietary deficiency, it is managed with the following:
   Iron supplementation to correct anemia and replenish iron stores
   Nutritional counseling to promote an adequate dietary intake of iron and prevent further iron deficiency
   If these measures are not effective, further studies are needed to assess for malabsorption of iron or loss of iron through bleeding.
5. Data that indicate that iron deficiency anemia is resolving include a decrease in the signs and symptoms that are present at diagnosis and a return to normal hematologic laboratory values. With Cody, look for increased activity and playfulness and the return of normal skin color and normal sleep pattern. Also, note the return of normal-for-age hematologic values. For a 15-month-old, these are as follows:
   Hemoglobin = 9.6 to 15.6 g/dL
   MCV = 76 to 92 fL
   MCH = 23 to 31 pg

human immunodeficiency virus (HIV). In addition, vitamin B_{12} deficiency may be due to an inborn error of vitamin B_{12} metabolism.

Folate Deficiency. Insufficient folate intake may occur at any age. However, it is more likely to occur among infants, especially among premature infants who are experiencing rapid physical growth and have an increased folate need. Also, there is an increased demand for folate with pregnancy, lactation, alcoholism, sickle cell disease, and infections such as hepatitis and HIV. Malabsorption of folate can occur with intestinal disorders such as chronic diarrhea. In addition, folate deficiency may stem from an alteration in folate metabolism. For example, such an alteration has been reported with the ongoing use of anticonvulsant medication (e.g., phenytoin) (Cooper, Rosenblatt, & Whitehead, 1993; Griffith, 1996; Pipes & Glass, 1993).

Pathophysiology

Although megaloblastic anemia can develop with both vitamin B_{12} deficiency and folate deficiency, it takes longer for the anemia to occur with vitamin B_{12} deficiency. This is because the body's stores of vitamin B_{12} are greater than its stores of folate. The liver is the primary site for both vitamin B_{12} and folate stores.

A deficit of vitamin B_{12} or folate interferes with normal DNA synthesis within the red blood cells. The deficient cells fail to synthesize enough DNA for normal erythropoiesis, resulting in slow reproduction and red blood cells that are immature and reduced in number.

The prolonged reproductive process does not interfere with RNA formation, but the cells acquire more RNA than normal. This appears to increase the amount of hemoglobin and other cellular components, which, in turn, results in the cellular enlargement commonly associated with megaloblastic anemia (Guyton & Hall, 1996).

Megaloblasts evidence immaturity, showing the presence of nuclei and the absence of the biconcave disks that characterize mature red blood cells. In addition, their fragility is a significant reason for a life span that is one half to one third that of normal red blood cells. Despite these alterations, circulating megaloblastic cells are capable of transporting oxygen normally (Guyton & Hall, 1996).

Prognosis. In general, vitamin B_{12} and folate deficiencies are readily treated. Thus, the prognosis for megaloblastic anemia is good. When treatment is ineffective, consider the possibilities of (1) an incorrect identification of the deficient nutrient, (2) a continuing inadequacy of vitamin B_{12} or folate intake, and (3) a continuing inadequacy of vitamin B_{12} or folate absorption.

Assessment

Megaloblastic anemia is not an early manifestation of vitamin B_{12} deficiency or folate deficiency; it appears after these deficiencies have been present for a period of time.

Children with megaloblastic anemia are likely to show pallor, weakness, unsteady gait, irritability, poor feeding, failure to thrive, and developmental delay. They may experience abnormal sensations and, with severe anemia, there may be evidence of heart failure and inflammation of the tongue. With vitamin B_{12} deficiency, in particular, there may be neurologic and gastrointestinal disturbances that occur in the absence of or before the onset of megaloblastic anemia.

Diagnostic Tests. Laboratory evidence of megaloblastic anemia may be categorized as follows: (1) evidence that shows the presence of megaloblastic anemia, (2) evidence that identifies or rules out vitamin B_{12} or folate deficiency, and (3) evidence that points to the etiology of vitamin B_{12} or folate deficiency.

Megaloblastic anemia is characterized by typical changes in the bone marrow and blood cell profile. Bone marrow shows the presence of megaloblasts, a hallmark feature of megaloblastic anemia. Blood cell profile changes include decreased hemoglobin and hematocrit and increased mean corpuscular volume (MCV) and mean corpuscular hemoglobin (MCH). In addition to oval, macrocytic red blood cells, there are hypersegmented neutrophils. With severe anemia, neutropenia and thrombocytopenia may be observed as well.

Vitamin B_{12} deficiency may be identified by a low vitamin B_{12} level. A distinction is made between serum vitamin B_{12} and tissue vitamin B_{12}, and it is possible for either to be low while the other is within normal limits. In megaloblastic anemia the serum vitamin B_{12} level is usually low before megaloblasts become evident. Tissue vitamin B_{12} deficiency is better indicated by elevated levels of urinary methylmalonic acid, serum methylmalonic acid, and total homocysteine. Tissue deficiency may be evident in those with neurologic and gastrointestinal disturbances in the absence of megaloblastic anemia. When vitamin B_{12} deficiency is identified or suspected, the Schilling test is helpful in determining a malabsorptive etiology such as pernicious anemia. Note that a vitamin B_{12} deficiency is not ruled out by either a normal vitamin B_{12} level or a normal Schilling test.

Folate deficiency is likely to be recognized by a low folate level. A distinction is made between serum folate and red cell folate. A decrease in serum folate usually becomes apparent before there is evidence of a reduced level of red cell folate and the onset of megaloblastic anemia.

caREminder: *Folate deficiency may be masked by a normal serum folate level when the folate deficiency exists simultaneously with a vitamin B_{12} deficiency.*

Nursing Diagnoses and Outcomes

Nursing diagnoses and outcomes for the child with anemia are given in Chart 23–3. In addition, the following nursing diagnosis and outcome pertain to the child with megaloblastic anemia:

▶ **Knowledge deficit regarding sources of dietary vitamin B_{12} and folate**
Outcome: The child/family identify sources of dietary vitamin B_{12} and folate.

Community Care

Management of the child with megaloblastic anemia is directed at (1) identification of the cause of the anemia, (2) correction of the anemia, (3) replenishment of vitamin B_{12} and folate stores, and (4) prevention of further deficiency and anemia.

Identification of the etiology of megaloblastic anemia is achieved by careful evaluation of the child's history and clinical presentation, as well as the results of pertinent laboratory studies (referred to in the section on clinical manifestations). It is necessary to consider that there may be a deficit of both vitamin B_{12} and folate, rather than deficiency of just a single nutrient. It is especially important not to treat a folate deficiency while overlooking a vitamin B_{12} deficiency and the possible neurologic alterations associated with the latter type of deficiency.

Correction of the anemia, replenishment of vitamin B_{12} and folate stores, and prevention of further deficiency and anemia are attained by supplementation with vitamin B_{12} and folate, as well as by nutritional counseling regarding dietary sources of these nutrients. Follow-up care includes physical assessment and laboratory studies to ascertain that the anemia is corrected and that the stores of vitamin B_{12} and folate are replete.

Vitamin B_{12} supplementation is given orally when the vitamin B_{12} deficiency is due to inadequate intake. When the deficiency is secondary to malabsorption, parenteral injections of vitamin B_{12} are likely to be prescribed, although oral and intranasal routes are being investigated (Cooper et al., 1993). Children with congenital alterations in vitamin B_{12} metabolism may receive injections or large doses of oral vitamin B_{12}.

Folate supplementation is given orally. Even when folate deficiency is due to malabsorption, some folate is absorbed when it is given orally in large doses. However, those with vitamin B_{12} deficiency who are receiving oral vitamin B_{12} therapy should avoid large doses of folate, because if vitamin B_{12} supplements are ineffective in correcting the vitamin B_{12} deficiency, the folate may protect against megaloblastic anemia but fail to prevent the neurologic impairment associated with vitamin B_{12} deficiency.

Nutritional counseling is important, particularly when megaloblastic anemia is due to inadequate intake of vitamin B_{12} or folate. The nurse has a key role in ensuring that the child and family receive information concerning dietary sources of these nutrients (Chart 23–22). In addition, the nurse can instruct staff in daycare centers, schools, and other community groups about the importance of including foods with vitamin B_{12} and folate in the diets of children and adolescents.

Chart 23–22

Dietary Sources of Vitamin B_{12} and Folate

Vitamin B_{12}

Dietary sources of vitamin B_{12} are primarily:

- Meat
- Eggs
- Milk
- Milk products

Note that plant foods do *not* provide this vitamin. Thus, those who are strictly vegetarian need to include vitamin B_{12}-fortified foods in their diet or take vitamin B_{12} supplements.

Folate

Dietary sources of folate include:

- Leafy green vegetables
- Whole-grain cereals
- Wheat germ
- Legumes

Hemolytic Disease of the Newborn

Hemolytic disease of the newborn (HDN), also known as erythroblastosis, refers to the destruction of red blood cells in the neonate whose blood is not compatible with the mother's blood. HDN can result from any one of a number of red blood cell antigen incompatibilities. The most common of these are related to the Rh factor and to the ABO blood groups.

When the Rh factor is involved, the neonate's red blood cells are Rh positive and the mother's red blood cells are Rh negative. When the ABO blood groups are involved, the neonate's erythrocytes are positive for the A and/or B antigens and the mother's erythrocytes are usually negative for both of these antigens. HDN is rare when the mother possesses the A antigen and the newborn possesses the B antigen or vice versa. Although the incidence of blood group incompatibility is greater than that of Rh factor incompatibility, the latter is more likely to result in significant physical alterations for the neonate.

Red blood cell antigen incompatibilities may result in the generation of maternal isoantibodies that can subsequently enter the fetal circulation and destroy fetal erythrocytes. However, even when there is incompatibility between the blood of the newborn and that of the mother, HDN does not necessarily occur, because some mothers at risk do not actually develop and transfer isoantibodies to the neonate.

Worldview: *The potential for HDN varies among racial and ethnic populations according to the extent to which the different red blood cell antigens are present or absent. For example, the possibility of HDN secondary to Rh factor incompatibility is greater among whites because approximately 15% of the white population is Rh negative. About 5% of the black population is Rh negative and, thus, there is less potential for Rh factor incompatibility within this group. Among Chinese, Japanese, and Native Americans, it is unusual to find Rh factor incompatibility because it is rare to find individuals in these populations who are Rh negative.*

The incidence of HDN has decreased remarkably since the 1960s, when Rh immunoprophylaxis became available. Rh immunoprophylaxis provides a means of preventing the generation of Rh isoantibodies in the mother who is Rh negative and whose baby is Rh positive.

Pathophysiology

Generally, HDN stemming from Rh factor incompatibility is more serious than that which results from ABO incompatibility. Thus, Rh factor incompatibility is the primary focus in this discussion.

Although a number of antigens are present in the Rh system, the common terms Rh positive and Rh negative refer to the D antigen. Rh-positive erythrocytes have the D antigen, whereas Rh-negative erythrocytes do not have the D antigen.

HDN develops during pregnancy when maternal anti-D antibodies cross the placenta and coat Rh-positive fetal erythrocytes. This results in destruction of fetal red blood cells, primarily by the reticuloendothelial cells of the spleen.

Maternal anti-D antibodies are produced after the mother's exposure to fetal Rh-positive blood. Most frequently, such exposure occurs via transplacental hemorrhage during pregnancy and via bleeding at the time of childbirth. Maternal anti-D antibodies remain with the mother and tend to have a greater impact on subsequent pregnancies in which the fetus is Rh positive.

With regard to ABO incompatibility, anti-A and anti-B antibodies occur naturally in those who lack the A and/or B antigens. Formation of these antibodies stems from stimulation of the immune system by the A and B matter found in food and bacteria (Zipursky & Bowman, 1993).

The two primary pathophysiologic alterations associated with HDN are:

- Anemia
- Hyperbilirubinemia

Anemia. Anemia is a concern both before and after the birth of the affected child. It occurs when red blood cell production cannot keep pace with red blood cell destruction. Initially, the body responds by increasing red blood cell production in the bone marrow. Also, extramedullary sites of erythropoiesis develop in the liver and spleen.

As anemia progresses, the increased effort of the heart to provide adequate circulation eventually fails. Subsequent hypoxia of body tissues can lead to metabolic acidosis and hydrops fetalis, a syndrome characterized by massive edema. Ultimately, death may occur.

Hyperbilirubinemia. Before birth, hyperbilirubinemia usually does not occur because bilirubin is removed from the fetus via the placenta. After birth, however, hyperbilirubinemia presents as a major concern because it can result in kernicterus, a condition in which there is yellow staining of brain cells in the basal ganglia and cerebellum. Kernicterus can lead to brain damage including severe, irreversible neurologic deficits and even death. The greater the amount of unconjugated free bilirubin in the blood, the greater the probability of brain damage secondary to kernicterus.

Hyperbilirubinemia associated with HDN results from the increased red blood cell destruction accompanying this disorder, as well as from the normally decreased ability of the neonate's liver to conjugate and excrete bilirubin efficiently from the body.

Hypoglycemia. In addition to anemia and hyperbilirubinemia, hypoglycemia is a concern in HDN. The hypoglycemia is associated with hypertrophy of pancreatic islet cells and increased levels of insulin. The occurrence of hypoglycemia is significant because it can have a harmful effect on the central nervous system and enhance bilirubin toxicity (Klemperer, 1995).

Prognosis. The prognosis for HDN has improved with the use of advanced diagnostic and therapeutic measures. In particular, intrauterine diagnosis and treatment have contributed significantly to the decreased morbidity and mortality associated with severe HDN. The most noteworthy advance with regard to HDN has been the ability to prevent the formation of maternal anti-D antibodies by Rh immunoprophylaxis and, thereby, prevent HDN in the neonate who is Rh positive and whose mother is Rh negative.

Assessment

The hallmark of HDN is jaundice secondary to hyperbilirubinemia. Unlike physiologic jaundice of the neonate,

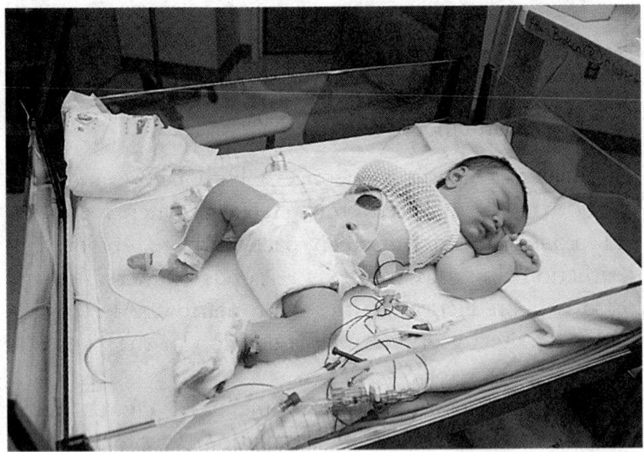

Figure 23–11
The skin of the newborn with hemolytic disease will appear yellow.

jaundice associated with HDN usually appears within 24 hours of birth. In addition to the skin appearing yellow, the sclerae and mucous membranes may appear jaundiced (Fig. 23–11).

Kernicterus is a particular risk for newborns with serum bilirubin levels of 20 mg/dL or greater. Brain damage associated with kernicterus may evidence itself in poor feeding, hypotonia, and lethargy. More severe brain damage may reveal itself in high-pitched crying, spasticity, opisthotonos, and seizures. There may be long-term neurologic deficits such as deafness, altered gait, and decreased mental ability. In its most severe form, kernicterus may impair the body's vital functions and lead to death.

Manifestations of anemia may or may not be present, depending on the neonate's ability to produce the number of red blood cells needed to compensate for the increased rate of erythrocyte destruction. Efforts to maintain a balance between production and destruction of red blood cells usually lead to some degree of hepatosplenomegaly. When balance is not achieved, the neonate becomes anemic and manifests pallor, lethargy, and other signs of anemia. Severe anemia can occur. Note that the severe anemia may have a delayed onset, developing over the first few weeks of life. Thus, it is necessary to continue to be alert for signs of anemia in the neonate with HDN, even when such signs are not initially present.

▽ **Alert:** *Severe anemia may have a delayed onset in hemolytic disease of the newborn.*

Diagnostic Tests. Laboratory manifestations of HDN during the prenatal period are generally those of an increasing concentration of bilirubin in the amniotic fluid and the presence of anemia in the fetal blood. When the maternal pregnancy history and the maternal anti-D titer indicate that the fetus is at risk for HDN, amniocentesis and fetal blood sampling procedures may be employed as early as the 18th week of gestation to identify the presence and severity of HDN.

Amniocentesis is performed to obtain a sample of amniotic fluid. The concentration of bilirubin in the fluid is measured with a spectrophotometer. The amniotic fluid's optical density at a wavelength of 450 nm is determined, and the fluid may then be classified by Liley's zone (Chart 23–23). Depending on the initial optical density, amniocentesis is repeated every 1 to 4 weeks to determine whether the optical density is rising. Severe HDN is associated with a rising optical density.

Fetal blood sampling provides a more accurate means of assessing HDN during the prenatal period. However, it involves considerable risk for fetal-maternal hemorrhage. Thus, it is usually reserved for the fetus whose amniotic fluid bilirubin concentration indicates severe HDN. Also, it is used when amniocentesis is contraindicated.

After birth, the primary laboratory manifestation of HDN is an elevated level of indirect (unconjugated) bilirubin. This laboratory value may be somewhat elevated during the first week of life with physiologic jaundice. However, in HDN, there are pathologic levels of 10 mg/dL or greater, and the bilirubin level may rise quickly. Also, HDN is associated with a positive direct antiglobulin (direct Coombs') test, indicating attachment of the maternal anti-D antibody to the neonate's red blood cells.

Perinatal and postnatal blood counts with HDN usually show an increase in reticulocytes and nucleated red blood cells, signs of increased erythrocyte production. Hemoglobin is decreased when anemia is present.

Nursing Diagnoses and Outcomes

Nursing diagnoses and outcomes for a child with anemia appear in Chart 23–3. In addition, the following nursing diagnoses and outcomes are applicable to a newborn with HDN:

Chart 23–23

Liley Zone Classification of Amniotic Fluid Bilirubin Levels

Zone I: absent or mild HDN
Zone II: mild to moderate HDN
Zone III: severe HDN

- **Risk for injury related to hyperbilirubinemia**
  Outcomes: Family identifies signs and symptoms of hyperbilirubinemia.
  Family identifies signs and symptoms of neurologic deficits.
  Neonate responds to measures to correct hyperbilirubinemia.
- **Risk for eye injury related to phototherapy**
  Outcomes: Family identifies need to protect neonate's eyes from intense light during phototherapy.
  Neonate has eye shields correctly in place when under phototherapy light.
  Neonate wrapped in fiberoptic blanket has it securely in place to prevent light radiating to eyes.
  Neonate's eyes show no evidence of irritation.
- **Fear that neonate will incur chronic impairment or die as a result of HDN**
  Outcomes: Family verbalizes fears concerning potential for chronic impairment, stillbirth, or death of neonate with severe HDN.
  Family receives informational and emotional support.

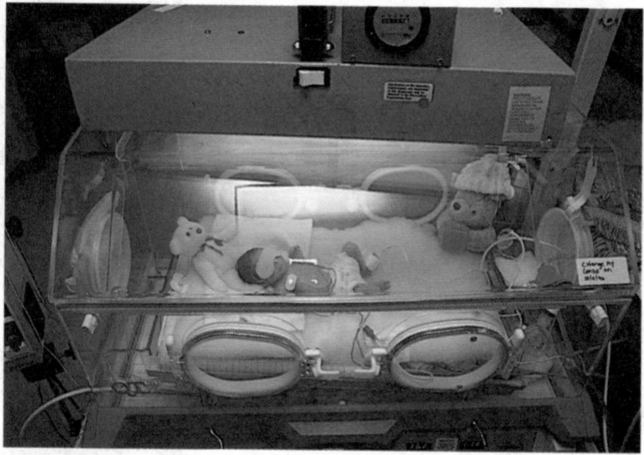

Figure 23–12
Phototherapy light used in treatment of neonatal jaundice. Note that the infant's eyes must be covered to prevent retinal damage.

Interdisciplinary Interventions

Management of the neonate with HDN requires close monitoring of the red blood cell profile and bilirubin to note increasing severity of anemia and hyperbilirubinemia. Also, these laboratory values provide evidence of resolving anemia and hyperbilirubinemia in response to therapeutic interventions.

Two primary interventions are associated with the management of HDN:

- Phototherapy
- Exchange transfusion

Phototherapy

Phototherapy is beneficial in the treatment of unconjugated hyperbilirubinemia. It involves exposure of the infant's skin to a source of light. Tissue bilirubin in the skin then absorbs light energy and undergoes a photodynamic reaction in which the bilirubin is altered to form water-soluble substances that can be excreted by the liver and kidney without conjugation.

Phototherapy may be delivered by conventional means in which the newborn is placed under fluorescent phototherapy light (Fig. 23–12). Also, phototherapy may be conveyed by wrapping the neonate in a fiberoptic blanket. Light travels to this blanket via a cable attached to an illuminator box. A disposable blanket cover directs the radiating light to the skin (Fig. 23–13). Neither heat nor electricity is transmitted to the infant (McFadden, 1991; Rose, 1990). In addition to artificial light delivered by phototherapy, natural sunlight aids in altering the structure of bilirubin so that it can be excreted from the body.

A neonate who is placed under a phototherapy light is unclothed, except for the genital area. Frequent turning of the infant allows the light to reach as much of the skin as possible. Eye shields must be used to prevent retinal damage by the intense light. To prevent eye injury, in general, care must be taken so that when the eye shields are secured in place, they are neither too loose nor too tight for the baby. Also, the environmental temperature should be appropriate to protect the infant from hyperthermia and hypothermia.

When a fiberoptic blanket is used, it is placed below the armpits, wrapped around the torso, and secured in place so that the light cannot reach the infant's eyes. A significant advantage of the fiberoptic blanket is that it permits greater opportunity for parent-infant bonding. Parents can pick up, hold, and feed their infant while phototherapy is in progress (Fig. 23–14). Also, the fiberoptic blanket allows greater environmental stimulation because the infant is not restricted to the phototherapy light location and does not need to wear eye shields. In contrast, conventional phototherapy requires that the infant remain in an isolette or crib while under the phototherapy light. Usually this limits opportunities for parent-infant bonding to times when the baby is removed from the phototherapy light for feeding.

In general, phototherapy is well tolerated. However, there may be an increased number of stools and, for some, diarrhea may occur. This may be due to increased intestinal secretion in response to the greater quantity of unconjugated bilirubin entering the intestines (Whittington & Gartner, 1993). Also, with phototherapy there may be an increased amount of insensible water loss that

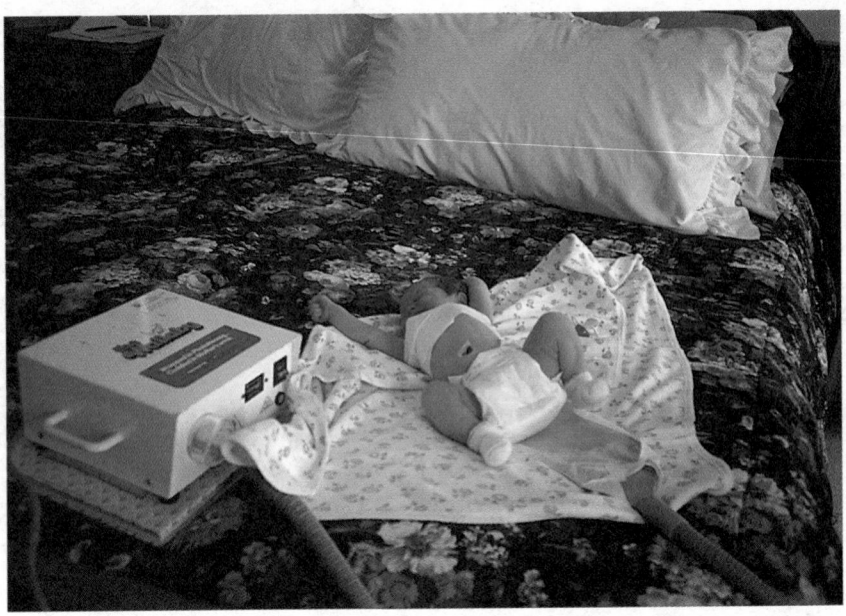

Figure 23–13
The fiberoptic blanket is wrapped around the infant to direct radiating light to the skin.

adds to the risk of dehydration. It is necessary to monitor the infant's weight, body temperature, intake, and output and to observe for clinical manifestations of dehydration. Frequent feedings help prevent dehydration and enhance the effectiveness of the phototherapy in reducing the level of serum bilirubin.

Home Phototherapy. Phototherapy can be set up in the home using the phototherapy light or, more commonly, the fiberoptic blanket (Chart 23–24). Generally, this therapy continues until the serum bilirubin falls to less than 10 mg/dL.

Figure 23–14
A parent can hold the child while he or she is receiving phototherapy via the fiberoptic blanket.

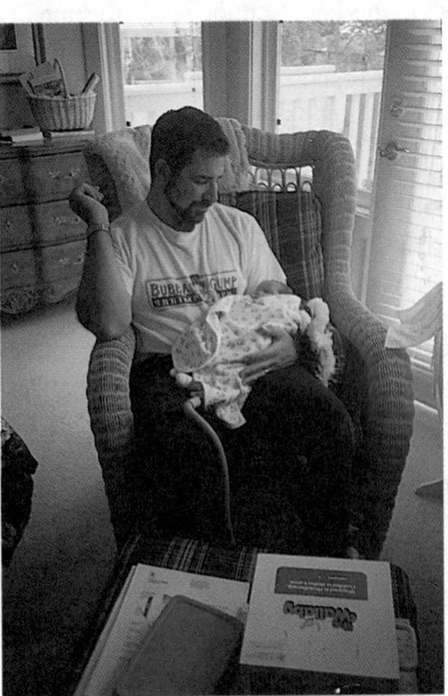

Exchange Transfusion

Exchange transfusion is indicated for neonates with moderate to severe HDN and for those with rapidly rising bilirubin levels. Low-birth-weight and high-risk infants receive their first exchange transfusion sooner than other neonates with HDN. Exchange transfusion helps to correct both anemia and hyperbilirubinemia.

Exchange transfusion involves the substitution of donor red blood cells for the neonate's sensitized red blood cells. When exchange transfusion occurs in conjunction with Rh incompatibility, the donor blood is Rh negative. With ABO incompatibility, the donor blood is group O. This prevents infusion of red blood cells with the antigen that would attract the respective maternal antibody and be prematurely destroyed.

During an exchange transfusion small quantities (5 to 20 mL) of the neonate's blood are alternately removed and replaced with donor blood until the desired total volume is infused. The total volume of exchange is usually twice the neonate's blood volume (about 170 mL per kilogram of body weight). Caution is exercised to avoid fluid overload, and aseptic technique is maintained throughout exchange transfusions. Generally, an exchange transfusion is via arterial and venous umbilical catheters. Thus, neonates at risk for HDN have moist dressings applied to the umbilical cord shortly after birth to prevent drying of the cord. This allows the umbilical vessels to remain suitable for access if an exchange transfusion becomes necessary.

During and after an exchange transfusion, the

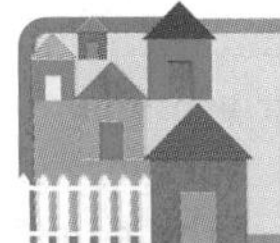

Chart 23–24
Community Care

The Newborn Receiving Fiberoptic Phototherapy at Home

Home phototherapy for neonatal jaundice is a safe, cost-effective alternative to extended hospitalization when the newborn meets certain criteria (Ryan, 1996). These criteria include

- No health problems other than neonatal hyperbilirubinemia.
- Gestational age of more than 37 weeks.
- Birth weight greater than 2500 g.
- Apgar score at 5 minutes of 7 or higher.
- Age between 2 and 7 days at start of home phototherapy.
- Safe home environment with grounded electric outlet.
- Child's caretaker willing and able to follow through on instructions for using the home phototherapy system.
- Child's caretaker willing and able to monitor key indicators of the newborn's physical state.
- Child's caretaker agrees to permit daily nursing assessment and drawing of necessary blood specimens.

The fiberoptic system is a common means of home phototherapy and, generally, the nurse is responsible for teaching the child's caretakers about its use. In addition, the nurse provides instruction on care of the newborn who is receiving phototherapy at home. Outcome objectives for the child's caretakers include the following:

- Identify components of the fiberoptic system: illuminator box, cable connector, and fiberoptic blanket with disposable cover.
- Set up fiberoptic system and be sure it is working.
- Wrap newborn in fiberoptic blanket, placing it below the armpits and securing it around the torso, so that light cannot reach the neonate's eyes and gonads.
- Diaper newborn to protect gonads further from light.
- Provide newborn with frequent feedings to help prevent dehydration and enhance the effectiveness of phototherapy.
- Monitor newborn's body temperature.
- Monitor newborn's output.
  - Frequency and description of voidings
  - Frequency and description of bowel movements
- Monitor newborn for signs of dehydration.
  - Decreased urine output
  - Decreased body weight
  - Decreased skin turgor
  - Dry mucous membranes
  - Sunken eyeballs
  - Sunken fontanelles
  - Irritability
  - Lethargy
- Pick up, hold, and interact with newborn while phototherapy is in progress.
- Discuss importance of ongoing blood tests and nursing assessments for the newborn receiving phototherapy at home.
- State telephone number to call for concerns about the newborn or the fiberoptic system during home phototherapy.

neonate requires close observation by the nurse to identify and respond quickly to complications that may occur.

- Note vital signs frequently, monitoring for arrhythmic, hypotensive, respiratory, and body temperature alterations.
- Obtain blood samples, particularly checking for hypoglycemia, electrolyte alterations, and acid-base imbalance.
- Note seizure activity that may occur secondary to hypocalcemia.
- Measure intake and output accurately, noting imbalance between these measurements.
- Note adverse reactions to blood transfused to the neonate.
- Inspect umbilical cord site, monitoring for hemorrhage.

Despite an effective exchange transfusion, "rebound" hyperbilirubinemia may occur as the concentration of tissue bilirubin equilibrates with that of serum bilirubin. Additional exchange transfusions may be required when there is continuing or increasing hyperbilirubinemia.

HDN in the Unborn Child

When amniocentesis or fetal blood sampling results indicate severe HDN in the unborn child, intervention is necessary to prevent stillbirth. Induction of premature birth is likely when fetal development reaches the point at which survival outside the uterine environment can be expected. This is usually at a gestational age of 32 weeks or more.

When it is too early to induce premature birth, severe HDN is managed by intrauterine blood transfusion under the guidance of ultrasonography. Traditionally, the blood has been given by injection into the fetal peritoneal cavity. A newer method is intravascular transfusion via the umbilical vein.

HDN is likely to provoke stress for parents and other family members. Particularly with severe HDN, there may be fear that the baby will die or live with chronic impairment. It is important that health care providers be sensitive to the family's stress. Education about HDN, ongoing provision of information about the baby's physical state, and emotional support for the family are significant components of the interdisciplinary management of HDN.

Community Care

Despite the increased ability to diagnose, monitor, and treat HDN, significant interdisciplinary interventions are directed toward the prevention of this disorder. Prevention is possible via immunoprophylaxis when HDN is due to Rh factor incompatibility.

Generally, Rh immunoprophylaxis is provided by giving anti-D gamma globulin, within 72 hours of childbirth, to mothers who are Rh negative and whose babies are Rh positive. Rh immunoprophylaxis is recommended after spontaneous and induced abortions and may be given to women who experience vaginal bleeding during the first trimester of pregnancy (Gibble & Ness, 1992). In addition, Rh immunoprophylaxis may be administered to women during pregnancy, usually in the 28th week of gestation.

Rh immunoprophylaxis is effective in most women who receive it and, as a result, the incidence of HDN has remarkably decreased. It is important that women at risk for anti-D antibody formation be identified so that Rh immunoprophylaxis can be given in a timely manner.

The nurse and other members of the interdisciplinary health care team have a significant role in the prevention and early treatment of HDN. In addition to patient care and family education, they provide community education that underscores the importance of early prenatal care. Through prenatal care, women at risk for giving birth to children with HDN are identified and their unborn children are monitored for evidence of HDN.

Hereditary Spherocytosis

Hereditary spherocytosis (HS) is characterized by loss of red blood cell membrane surface area. The spherocytic erythrocytes are prone to premature destruction, placing the child at risk for hemolytic anemia, especially with severe HS.

Most often HS becomes evident during childhood, but it can be discovered during any phase of life. HS affects an estimated 1 in 5000 people. However, the actual incidence is probably higher, because those who are asymptomatic or mildly affected may not yet have been diagnosed with the disorder. Although HS may occur in various racial and ethnic groups, its highest incidence is among those of Northern European heritage.

For 75% of those with HS, there is an autosomal dominant pattern of inheritance. For others, the inheritance pattern of HS is autosomal recessive. Also, HS may occur as a result of a spontaneous genetic mutation in individuals who have no family history of this abnormality.

Pathophysiology

The normal red blood cell membrane has a large surface area relative to the cell's volume. This permits red blood cells to adapt their shape to their environment and safely navigate through the vascular system, even the narrow capillaries. In contrast, spherocytic erythrocytes have a diminished membrane surface area with a reduced surface-to-volume ratio. This decreases their ability to adapt their shape to their environment. Also, spherocytes are osmotically fragile, which leads to their premature rupture and a life span that is considerably shorter than that of normal red blood cells.

The spleen poses the greatest challenge for erythrocytes. Whereas normal erythrocytes can contort themselves to pass through spaces that are narrower than they are, spherocytic red blood cells are more likely to be trapped in the splenic cords or to rupture as they journey through the venous sinus walls.

Prognosis. In general, the prognosis for HS is good. However, life-threatening complications, such as severe hemolytic anemia and aplastic crises, are possible, especially among those with severe HS. Also, the risk of postsplenectomy sepsis is of concern, particularly in children who require removal of the spleen before 5 years of age.

Assessment

Although the clinical presentation can be quite varied, with some children even being asymptomatic, the primary manifestations of HS are anemia, splenomegaly, and jaundice.

The degree of anemia tends to parallel the severity of spherocytosis. The greater the degree of spherocytosis, the greater the degree of anemia and the more likely the children are to show pallor, fatigue, weakness, and other manifestations of anemia. Chronic anemia may interfere with normal growth and development.

Splenomegaly is a common physical finding in children with HS and may be associated with abdominal distention as well as abdominal tenderness and pain. Although the degree of splenomegaly may range from minimal to marked, the size of the spleen does not necessarily correlate with the severity of the spherocytosis (Becker & Lux, 1993).

Most children with HS intermittently manifest acholuric jaundice, that is, jaundice without bilirubin in the urine. Jaundice in the neonate with undiagnosed HS can pose a particular challenge, because neonatal jaundice may occur in conjunction with a variety of other disorders such as sepsis and hemolytic disease of the newborn.

Anemia, splenomegaly, and jaundice are often accelerated during times of infection. Children who are otherwise asymptomatic are likely to show these manifestations when viral illnesses and other infections occur.

In addition, children with HS may experience indigestion and biliary colic secondary to gallstone formation. This cholelithiasis is more likely to occur in older children and adolescents than in younger children.

Diagnostic Tests. The primary laboratory evidence for HS consists of (1) a positive osmotic fragility test, (2) an elevated reticulocyte count (usually greater than 6%), and (3) the presence of spherocytes on the peripheral blood smear. In addition, the bilirubin is usually elevated, and the red blood cell indices are likely to exhibit low normal or abnormal hemoglobin and hematocrit, with an increased mean corpuscular hemoglobin concentration (MCHC). The mean corpuscular volume (MCV) and mean corpuscular hemoglobin (MCH) are generally within normal limits.

Interdisciplinary Interventions

Splenectomy is the most effective intervention for symptomatic HS. Although spherocytic erythrocytes are still present in the blood after removal of the spleen, their life span generally improves to about 80% of normal as hemolysis decreases. Anemia and jaundice usually disappear soon after splenectomy. In addition, removal of the spleen is associated with a reduction in symptomatic galbladder disease among children and adolescents with HS.

The benefits of splenectomy must be balanced with the potential complications. The risk of life-threatening sepsis is a particular concern for asplenic individuals, especially young children. Thus, every effort is made to delay splenectomy until the child is at least 5 years of age. When young children with HS experience marked hemolytic anemia, they are generally supported with red blood cell transfusions until they reach the age at which the postsplenectomy course is safer. The risk of postsplenectomy sepsis and its management have been discussed in the section on ITP.

Children with HS are likely to have an increased need for folic acid. Folic acid supplements may be required to maintain adequate folate stores and prevent the megaloblastic crises that can complicate HS.

The nurse should instruct children with HS and their families to notify their physician or nurse practitioner when signs and symptoms of anemia, splenomegaly, or infection develop. They should report such things as

- Pallor
- Fatigue
- Weakness
- Jaundice
- Abdominal distention
- Abdominal tenderness or pain
- Fever
- Viral illness or other infection

Even with mild HS, severe hemolysis and splenomegaly can occur with infections. Red blood cell transfusions may be required at such times even though, generally, the child is not transfusion dependent.

Also, children with HS and their families should be instructed with regard to appropriate physical activities. It is best to avoid contact sports and strenuous physical activities because, even with mild HS, these may increase red blood cell hemolysis (Becker & Lux, 1993) and lead to anemia.

Aplastic Anemia

Aplastic anemia is a disorder in which the normal production of blood cells in the bone marrow is absent or decreased. This leads to altered peripheral blood counts that reflect pancytopenia and not merely the presence of anemia.

There are two primary classifications for aplastic anemia:

- Acquired aplastic anemia
- Inherited aplastic anemia (Fanconi's anemia)

The former may occur at any age, and the latter may not be evident until some years after birth.

Aplastic anemia is categorized as mild, moderate, or severe. Severe aplastic anemia is characterized by marked pancytopenia and is specifically defined as having at least two of the following three peripheral blood cell alterations (Alter & Young, 1993; Miller & O'Reilly, 1995):

- Absolute neutrophil count (ANC) less than $500/mm^3$
- Platelet count less than $20,000/mm^3$
- Reticulocytes less than 1% after correction for hematocrit

In addition, the bone marrow is hypocellular. With mild to moderate aplastic anemia, the pancytopenia and bone marrow hypocellularity are less pronounced.

When a child is diagnosed with aplastic anemia, it is important to determine its classification and degree of severity so that accurate information is provided to the family and appropriate treatment is prescribed for the child.

Acquired Aplastic Anemia

Acquired aplastic anemia (AAA) is a bone marrow disorder. The bone marrow is characterized by a lack of precursor cells for the platelets, red blood cells, and white blood cells that are normally present in the peripheral circulation. As a result, the blood cell profile typically shows thrombocytopenia, anemia, and neutropenia.

The cause of AAA is often unknown, particularly in children. However, in a number of cases it is associated with a history of

- Exposure to drugs (e.g., chloramphenicol)
- Exposure to chemicals (e.g., benzene)
- Exposure to toxins (e.g., ionizing radiation)
- Infection (e.g., hepatitis)

Occasionally, AAA has been diagnosed during pregnancy, and it is hypothesized that increased estrogen levels may contribute to the onset of this disorder during the antepartum period (Alter & Young, 1993). In addition, genetic factors may play a role in one's susceptibility to AAA. The incidence of consanguinity and familial aplastic anemia is higher among those with AAA than among those in the general population (Miller & O'Reilly, 1995).

The overall annual incidence of AAA is estimated as 2 to 6 cases per million people (Alter & Young, 1993). However, the incidence for specific populations throughout the world is somewhat variable depending on environmental factors, genetic predisposition, diagnostic criteria, and reporting practices (Miller & O'Reilly, 1995). In general, the disorder affects all racial groups, and its incidence among females and males is similar.

Pathophysiology

Much remains unknown about the pathophysiology of AAA. However, it appears that the stem cells of the bone marrow are affected and that these cells incur both qualitative and quantitative deficits. This leads to pancytopenia in the peripheral blood, placing the child at increased risk for

- Bleeding, secondary to thrombocytopenia
- Tissue hypoxia, secondary to anemia
- Infection, secondary to neutropenia

Prognosis. The prognosis for AAA is related to the severity of the disorder. Generally, mild to moderate disease can be easily managed and has a good prognosis. However, those with severe disease require more aggressive treatment and, even then, approximately one of five children with severe AAA does not survive.

Assessment

The primary clinical manifestations of AAA are related to bone marrow failure and pancytopenia. With mild to moderate disease, AAA may not be identified except by laboratory data. However, with severe AAA, abnormal findings are usually noted on physical examination as well. These findings are likely to include signs and symptoms of bleeding, tissue hypoxia, and infection (see Chart 23–2).

Diagnostic Tests. Thrombocytopenia, anemia, and neutropenia are revealed by respective abnormalities in the blood cell profile. These deficits are especially pronounced when severe aplastic anemia is diagnosed (Table 23–11). The anemia associated with AAA is most often normocytic but, at times, the red blood cells appear macrocytic. Bone marrow aspirations and biopsies reveal hypocellular and fatty marrow. Tests on the bone marrow sample are particularly important, not only in diagnosing

Table 23–11
Laboratory Data Commonly Associated with Severe Aplastic Anemia

Laboratory Test	Result
Absolute neutrophil count (ANC)	Less than $500/mm^3$
Hemoglobin	Less than 7 g/dL
Platelet count	Less than $20,000/mm^3$
Reticulocytes	Less than 1%

AAA but also in ruling out other possible reasons for pancytopenia, such as leukemia.

Nursing Diagnoses and Outcomes

Nursing diagnoses and outcomes for children with bleeding and anemia are given in Chart 23–3. In addition, the following nursing diagnoses and outcomes apply when the child has neutropenia:

- **Risk for injury related to infection**
  Outcomes: The child/family identify the need to report promptly fever and other signs and symptoms of infection.
  The child/family identify measures to decrease the risk of infection associated with neutropenia.
  The child responds to measures to treat infection.
- **Fear of child's death related to severe aplastic anemia**
  Outcomes: The child/family verbalize fears concerning potential for premature death of child.
  The child/family receive informational and emotional support.

Interdisciplinary Interventions

In addition to necessary supportive care, management of the child with AAA centers on the restoration of normal hematopoiesis. Children with mild or moderate disease may require only supportive care. However, for those with severe AAA, bone marrow transplantation is the treatment of choice when a suitable donor is available. When such transplantation is not feasible, immunosuppressive therapy is the primary treatment modality.

Bone Marrow Transplantation

Bone marrow transplantation is a complex process. Children receiving such transplants are hospitalized in an environmentally controlled, intensive care setting to prepare for, receive, and await marrow engraftment of donor stem cells. They require intensive prophylactic and supportive therapy, particularly while they await the restoration of hematopoiesis and the resolution of pancytopenia. Their care is provided by specially prepared physicians, nurses, social workers, dietitians, pharmacists, and others. The reader is referred to Chapter 22 and to the specialty literature for information on care of the child, donor, and family involved in bone marrow transplantation.

Immunosuppressive Therapy

Children with severe AAA who are not candidates for bone marrow transplantation are given immunosuppressive therapy. Antithymocyte globulin (ATG) is often the first line of such treatment. Although this cytotoxic agent is effective in about one third of those who receive it, its mode of action in the treatment of AAA is unclear. Generally, ATG is administered intravenously, once a day, for about 4 days. Before the first dose, a test dose is recommended to identify those with hypersensitivity to the drug. Children receiving ATG should be observed for adverse reactions such as fever, chills, rash, urticaria, pruritus, dyspnea, chest pain, nausea, vomiting, leukopenia, and thrombocytopenia. Other side effects that happen less frequently but that are life threatening include hypotension, pulmonary edema, laryngospasm, and anaphylaxis. Also, serum sickness may occur. In addition to ATG, corticosteroids and cyclosporine may be incorporated into the treatment plan for severe AAA.

Generally, those who respond to immunosuppressive therapy do so within 3 months. However, they may continue to have some degree of abnormal hematopoiesis. This is in contrast to the complete restoration of bone marrow function that usually follows successful bone marrow transplantation.

Supportive Care

Supportive care for children with AAA involves close monitoring of blood counts for evidence of thrombocytopenia, anemia, and neutropenia, as well as close observation for indicators of bleeding, tissue hypoxia, and infection. Although blood product support is sometimes necessary, every effort is made to refrain from such transfusions.

Transfusions place one at risk for becoming sensitized to the surface antigens on donor blood cells (alloimmunization). This decreases the probability of marrow engraftment and increases the probability of graft-versus-host disease (GVHD) among bone marrow transplant recipients. When a suitable marrow donor is available, it is likely to be a family member. Thus, to decrease the risk of alloimmunization when pretransplantation blood products are necessary, it is important that the blood products not be from family members. In addition, required blood products are usually irradiated and then filtered during administration to the child. This decreases the number of white blood cells and, in turn, reduces the risk of alloimmunization.

Supportive Care for Thrombocytopenia. Therapeutic platelet support is given when there is evidence of bleeding. In addition, antifibrinolytic agents and topical agents are used to control bleeding. Prophylactic platelet support may be considered for children whose platelet count falls below 5000/mm^3. The primary purpose of such prophylaxis is to decrease the risk of intracranial hemorrhage. During times of thrombocytopenia, the child and family should be instructed to observe certain precautions (see TIP 23–2).

caREminder: *For children with thrombocytopenia, firm pressure must be applied to venipuncture and intramus-*

cular injection sites for 15 minutes immediately after each procedure.

Supportive Care for Anemia. Packed red blood cells are given when transfusion support is required for symptomatic anemia and dangerously low hemoglobin levels. However, children often adapt to chronic anemia, and when they can tolerate hemoglobin levels as low as 6 g/dL, they should be allowed to do so (Alter & Young, 1993).

If red blood cell transfusion therapy is required for a long time, monitor the child for iron overload. When the serum ferritin level is greater than 500 ng/mL, iron chelation therapy is usually initiated (Alter & Young, 1993).

The child and family should be instructed to identify activities that are tolerated by the child with anemia. In general, these are activities that are less strenuous, help the child conserve energy, and provide adequate oxygenation to support the child's vital body functions and activities of daily living. The child and family should be alert for and report signs that indicate that the child is not tolerating the anemic state, such as dyspnea, irritability, listlessness, and marked fatigue.

Supportive Care for Neutropenia. Neutropenia places the child at increased risk for infection, especially when the absolute neutrophil count (ANC) is less than 500/mm^3. Fever in the child with neutropenia is taken seriously and is presumed to indicate sepsis until proved otherwise. Common inflammatory responses associated with infection are likely to be absent in those with neutropenia.

The child and family are instructed on the increased risk of rapidly progressing, life-threatening sepsis in the neutropenic individual and the importance of notifying the physician immediately when there is a fever with a temperature of 38.3°C (101°F) or greater.

Alert: *The child with fever and neutropenia requires immediate evaluation for sepsis, even if the child looks well.*

The child with fever and neutropenia should receive a septic work-up, including physical examination, blood cultures, and blood counts, as well as the initiation of intravenous antibiotics. Antibiotics are continued at least until the child is afebrile, blood cultures are known to be negative, and any sepsis has been treated. In general, prophylactic antibiotics are not given to the child with neutropenia associated with aplastic anemia. Neither are granulocyte transfusions used, except in the presence of life-threatening sepsis that is not responding well to intravenous, broad-spectrum antibiotic therapy.

It is not always possible to prevent infection in the child with neutropenia, especially sepsis caused by endogenous microorganisms. However, the child and family should be instructed on measures that help prevent infection in those with neutropenia (Chart 23–25).

Chart 23–25

Neutropenic Precautions

- Practice good hand-washing habits.
- Do not share eating utensils, drinking glasses, baby bottles, pacifiers, and so on.
- Eat a well-balanced diet.
  - Avoid unpeeled raw vegetables and fruits.
  - Avoid salad bars.
- Brush teeth after each meal, using a soft toothbrush.
- Avoid crowds and people with communicable diseases.
- Provide good personal hygiene, with particular attention to keeping the perineum and other skin-fold areas clean.
- Include fiber foods and good fluid intake in the diet to prevent constipation; notify the physician if constipation occurs.
- To prevent perianal fissures and infection, do not insert anything into the rectum (e.g., no rectal thermometers, no suppositories, no enemas).
- Do not use tampons.
- Avoid fresh flowers and plants.
- Postpone immunizations until AAA resolves.

Experiencing a life-threatening disorder is usually stressful for children with aplastic anemia and their families. It is important that health care providers are sensitive to this stress. Education about aplastic anemia and its treatment and the ongoing provision of laboratory data, physical assessment data, and emotional support are important components of the interdisciplinary management of aplastic anemia. The Aplastic Anemia Foundation of America is an additional source of support (see Resources).

Fanconi's Anemia

Fanconi's anemia (FA) is an inherited form of aplastic anemia that is associated with an autosomal recessive inheritance pattern. Children with this disorder may be recognized before the development of bone marrow failure and pancytopenia if they have physical anomalies that are associated with the disorder. However, the hematologic abnormalities may occur with or without other physical alterations.

Generally, FA is diagnosed during childhood or adolescence, with the median age being 8 years for females and 6.5 years for males (Alter & Young, 1993). Those with characteristic abnormal physical features are likely to be diagnosed earlier. Also, siblings without apparent physical anomalies may have chromosomal studies performed and be diagnosed with FA before the onset of hematologic alterations.

Pathophysiology

Much is unknown about the pathophysiology associated with the onset of bone marrow failure in FA. However, as with acquired aplastic anemia, it appears that the stem cells become qualitatively and quantitatively deficient, leading to pancytopenia and increased risk of bleeding, tissue hypoxia, and infection. In addition, FA is associated with an increased number of chromosomal breaks.

Prognosis. Although current treatment of bone marrow failure associated with FA has improved the prognosis for children with this disorder, the majority do not live beyond the third decade of life. In addition to developing resistance to therapy, those with FA are at increased risk for developing a malignancy, especially myeloid leukemia (Miller & O'Reilly, 1995).

Assessment

The development of bone marrow failure in FA may occur over a period of time. When it becomes severe, signs and symptoms of bleeding, tissue hypoxia, and infection appear. In addition to hematologic alterations, multiple physical anomalies may be present. The most common anomalies include:

- Café au lait spots and other areas of hyperpigmentation or hypopigmentation
- Short stature, frequently because of a short trunk
- Anomalies of the hands and forearms, such as absent thumb
- Renal anomalies
- Hypogonadism, particularly in males
- Microcephaly
- Characteristic facial appearance, including a broad nasal base, epicanthal folds, small eyes, and small jaws

Diagnostic Tests. The hematologic laboratory alterations reported for the blood cell profile and the bone marrow samples are similar for both FA and acquired aplastic anemia, and they cannot be used to discriminate between the two disorders. To make this distinction, especially in the absence of physical anomalies, chromosome breakage studies are performed on peripheral blood lymphocytes. With FA, an increased number of chromosome breaks is noted, particularly after stress with a clastogenic agent. Other physical alterations associated with FA may be identified or ruled out with additional diagnostic studies such as a skeletal survey or renal ultrasonography.

Interdisciplinary Interventions

As in acquired aplastic anemia, management of bone marrow failure in the child with FA is directed at the restoration of normal hematopoiesis. However, in FA, androgen therapy is usually the treatment prescribed.

Androgen therapy may be used alone or in combination with corticosteroids to stimulate hematopoiesis. To be effective, it must be given continuously. However, the beneficial effects may not be evident in laboratory tests for several weeks.

When androgen therapy is no longer helpful, bone marrow transplantation may be possible. In addition to the usual tests to identify a suitable marrow donor, the potential donor must be evaluated for covert FA. When bone marrow transplantation is successful, it offers the hope of cure for aplastic anemia associated with FA.

Supportive care is provided, as needed, during times of thrombocytopenia, anemia, and neutropenia. This care is discussed in the section on acquired aplastic anemia.

In addition to the management of aplastic anemia, the interdisciplinary team is involved in identifying and treating nonhematologic health problems that may be present. Ongoing informational and emotional support and genetic counseling are significant interventions for the child and family experiencing FA.

Summary of Key Concepts

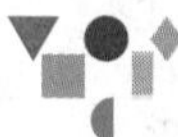

- ◆ Hematologic disorders may be acute or chronic, common or rare. They range from those that are mild to those that are life threatening and those that lead to premature death.
- ◆ Hemophilia is a genetic bleeding disorder. The most common types involve a deficiency or dysfunction of factor VIII or factor IX.
- ◆ von Willebrand's disease is a genetic bleeding disorder characterized by a deficiency or dysfunction of von Willebrand's factor.
- ◆ Disseminated intravascular coagulation (DIC) is a coagulopathy characterized by both thrombosis and hemorrhage. It is secondary to primary health problems such as infections and malignancies.

- Immune thrombocytopenic purpura (ITP) is a bleeding disorder characterized by destruction of circulating platelets.
- Henoch-Schönlein purpura (HSP) is a nonthrombocytopenic vasculitis that may affect multiple organs of the body.
- Sickle cell disease is a genetic sickling disorder caused by a structural defect in the beta chains of the hemoglobin molecule.
- Thalassemia is a genetic disorder characterized by a deficiency of beta chains in the hemoglobin molecule.
- Iron deficiency anemia is a nutritional anemia that is secondary to depletion of the body's iron stores.
- Megaloblastic anemia is a nutritional anemia that is usually secondary to vitamin B_{12} or folate deficiency.
- Hemolytic disease of the newborn is a hemolytic disorder that may occur when the newborn's blood is not compatible with the mother's blood.
- Hereditary spherocytosis is a hemolytic disorder characterized by spherocytic, osmotically fragile red blood cells.
- Aplastic anemia is an acquired or hereditary disorder that is characterized by pancytopenia.

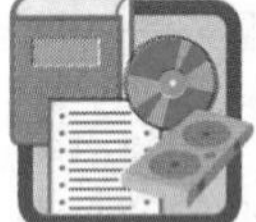

Resources

Organizations

Aplastic Anemia Foundation of America
P.O. Box 613
Annapolis, MD 21404
(800) 747-2820
Email: AAFACENTER@aol.com

Cooley's Anemia Foundation (Thalassemia)
129-09 26th Avenue
Suite 203
Flushing, NY 11354
(718) 321-2873; (800) 522-7222
Email: NCAF@aol.com

The National Hemophilia Foundation
110 Greene Street, Suite 303
New York, NY 10012
(212) 219-8180

Sickle Cell Disease Association of America
200 Corporate Point, Suite 495
Culver City, CA 90230
(310) 216-6363; (800) 421-8453

Sickle Cell Disease Foundation of Greater New York
127 West 127th Street, Suite 421
New York, NY 10027
(212) 865-1500

Print Materials

Hemophilia

Beiersdorfer, W. A., Clements, M. J., & Weisman, C. *The student with hemophilia: A resource for the educator*. New York: National Hemophilia Foundation.

Hemophilia of Georgia. *The hemophilia handbook*. Atlanta, GA: Author. (770)-671-1223.

National Hemophilia Foundation. *What you should know about hemophilia*. New York: Author.

National Hemophilia Foundation and American Red Cross. *Hemophilia and sports*. New York: National Hemophilia Foundation.

von Willebrand's Disease

LaFon, J. *Exploring von Willebrand disease*. New York: National Hemophilia Foundation.

Montgomery, R. R., & Hilgartner, M. W. *Understanding von Willebrand disease*. New York: National Hemophilia Foundation.

Zimmerman, C. *von Willebrand disease*. Nashville, TN: Hemophilia Health Services. (800) 800-6606.

Sickle Cell Disease

Agency for Health Care Policy and Research. *Sickle cell disease in newborns and infants: A guide for parents*. Rockville, MD: U.S. Department of Health and Human Services.

Earles, A., Lessing, S. & Vichinsky, E. (Eds.). *A parents' handbook for sickle cell disease, part II, six to eighteen years of age*. Oakland, CA: Sickle Cell Center at Children's Hospital. (Request publication from National Maternal and Child Health Clearinghouse, 2070 Chain Bridge Road, Suite 450, Vienna, VA, 22182-2536).

Lessing, S. & Vichinsky, E. (Eds.). *A parents' handbook for sickle cell disease, part I, birth to six years of age*. Oakland, CA: Sickle Cell Center at Children's Hospital. (Request publication from National Maternal and Child Health Clearinghouse, 2070 Chain Bridge Road, Suite 450, Vienna, VA, 22182-2536.)

Sickle Cell Disease Association of America. *Answers to questions about sickle cell disease*. Culver City, CA: Author.

Thalassemia (Cooley's Anemia)

Cooley's Anemia Foundation. *All you need to know about being a carrier of thalassemia*. Flushing, NY: Author.

Cooley's Anemia Foundation. *What is Cooley's anemia?* Flushing, NY: Author.

Cooley's Anemia Foundation. *What is Cooley's anemia?—Basic facts*. Flushing, NY: Author.

Aplastic Anemia

Aplastic Anemia Foundation of America. *Aplastic anemia answer book*. Annapolis, MD: Aplastic Anemia Foundation of America.

Aplastic Anemia Foundation of America. *Families coping with hospital life: Aplastic anemia and myelodysplastic syndrome*. Annapolis, MD: Aplastic Anemia Foundation of America.

Aplastic Anemia Foundation of America. *What to do after the diagnosis*. Annapolis, MD: Aplastic Anemia Foundation of America.

References

Adams, J. G., III. (1994). Clinical laboratory diagnosis. In S. H. Embury, R. P. Hebbel, N. Mohandas, & M. H. Steinberg (Eds.), *Sickle cell disease: Basic principles and clinical practice* (pp. 457–468). New York: Raven Press.

Alter, B. P., & Young, N. S. (1993). The bone marrow failure syndromes. In D. G. Nathan & F. A. Oski (Eds.), *Hematology of infancy and childhood* (4th ed., pp. 216–316). Philadelphia: W. B. Saunders.

Barness, L. A. (Ed.). (1993). *Pediatric nutrition handbook* (3rd ed.). Elk Grove Village, IL: American Academy of Pediatrics.

Beard, J. L. (1994). Iron deficiency: Assessment during pregnancy and its importance in pregnant adolescents. *American Journal of Clinical Nutrition, 59*(Suppl.), 502S–510S.

Beardsley, D. S. (1993). Platelet abnormalities in infancy and childhood. In D. G. Nathan & F. A. Oski (Eds.), *Hematology of infancy and childhood* (4th ed., pp. 1561–1604). Philadelphia: W. B. Saunders.

Becker, P. S., & Lux, S. E. (1993). Disorders of the red cell membrane. In D. G. Nathan & F. A. Oski (Eds.), *Hematology of infancy and childhood* (4th ed., pp. 529–633). Philadelphia: W. B. Saunders.

Bell, B., Canty, D., & Audet, M. (1995). Hemophilia: An updated review. *Pediatrics in Review, 16*(8), 290–298.

Berg, A. O. (1994). Sickle cell disease: Screening, diagnosis, management, and counseling in newborns and infants. *Journal of the American Board of Family Practice, 7*(2), 134–140.

Berti, P., & Leonard W. R. (1995). The merits of race-specific standards [Letter to the editor]. *American Journal of Clinical Nutrition, 61*(3), 616.

Bick, R. L. (1994). Disseminated intravascular coagulation: Objective criteria for diagnosis and management. *Medical Clinics of North America, 78*(3), 511–543.

Browne, R. J., & Gillespie, C. A. (1993). Sickle cell trait: A risk factor for life-threatening rhabdomyolysis? *Physician and Sportsmedicine, 21*(6), 80–88.

Broxmeyer, H. E. (1991). Self-renewal and migration of stem cells during embryonic and fetal hematopoiesis: Important, but poorly understood events. *Blood Cells, 17*, 282–286.

Burke, S. M. (1996). Hydroxyurea in sickle cell disease. *MCN American Journal of Maternal/Child Nursing, 21*(4), 210.

Bussel, J. B., & Corrigan, J. J., Jr. (1995). Platelet and vascular disorders. In D. R. Miller & R. L. Baehner (Eds.), *Blood diseases of infancy and childhood* (7th ed., pp. 866–923). St. Louis: Mosby–Year Book.

Coffland, F. I., & Shelton, D. M. (1993). Blood component replacement therapy. *Critical Care Nursing Clinics of North America, 5*(3), 543–556.

Cooper, B. A., Rosenblatt, D. S., & Whitehead, V. M. (1993). Megaloblastic anemia. In D. G. Nathan & F. A. Oski (Eds.), *Hematology of infancy and childhood* (4th ed., pp. 354–390). Philadelphia: W. B. Saunders.

Dallman, P. R., Yip, R., & Oski, F. A. (1993). Iron deficiency and related nutritional anemias. In D. G. Nathan & F. A. Oski (Eds.), *Hematology of infancy and childhood* (4th ed., pp. 413–450). Philadelphia: W. B. Saunders.

DiMichele, D. (1996). Hemophilia 1996: New approach to an old disease. *Pediatric Clinics of North America, 43*(3), 709–736.

Feroli, K., & Hobson, S. (1995). Defining anemia in a preadolescent African American population. *Journal of Pediatric Health Care,* 9(5), 199–204.

Foley, M. K. (1993). Nursing management of the child or adolescent with blood component deficiencies. In G. V. Foley, D. Fochtman, & K. H. Mooney (Eds.), *Nursing care of the child with cancer* (2nd ed., pp. 385–396). Philadelphia: W. B. Saunders.

Gaston, M. H., Verter, J. I., Woods, G., Pegelow, C., Kelleher, J., Presbury, G., Zarkowsky, H., Vichinsky, E., Iyer, R., Lobel, J. S., Diamond, S., Holbrook, C. T., Gill, F. M., Ritchey, K., & Falletta, J. M. (1986). Prophylaxis with oral penicillin in children with sickle cell anemia. *New England Journal of Medicine, 314*(25), 1593–1599.

Giardina, P. J., & Hilgartner, M. W. (1992). Update on thalassemia. *Pediatrics in Review, 13*(2), 55–63.

Gibble, J. W., & Ness, P. M. (1992). Maternal immunity to red cell antigens and fetal transfusion. *Clinics in Laboratory Medicine, 12*(3), 553–576.

Gill, J. C. (1993). Therapy of factor VIII deficiency. *Seminars in Thrombosis and Hemostasis, 19*(1), 1–12.

Gill, J. C., & Montgomery, R. R. (1993). Principles of therapy for hemostasis factor deficiencies. In D. G. Nathan & F. A. Oski (Eds.), *Hematology of infancy and childhood* (4th ed., pp. 1796–1818). Philadelphia: W. B. Saunders.

Grabowski, E. F., & Corrigan, J. J., Jr. (1995). Hemostasis: General considerations. In D. R. Miller & R. L. Baehner (Eds.), *Blood diseases of infancy and childhood* (7th ed., pp. 849–865). St. Louis: Mosby–Year Book.

Griffith, C. (1996). Evaluation and management of anemia. *Advance for Nurse Practitioners, 4*(5), 29–35.

Guyton, A. C., & Hall, J. E. (1996). *Textbook of medical physiology* (9th ed.). Philadelphia: W. B. Saunders.

Hegenauer, J., & Saltman, P. (1993). Comment on the paper by Perry et al. (1992): Hemoglobin differences between blacks and whites. *Journal of Nutrition, 123*(3), 597–598.

The hemophilia handbook. (1988). Atlanta: Hemophilia of Georgia.

Hemophilia and sports. (1985; reprinted 1994). New York: National Hemophilia Foundation and American Red Cross.

Hilgartner, M. W., & Corrigan, J. J., Jr. (1995). Coagulation disorders. In D. R. Miller & R. L. Baehner (Eds.), *Blood diseases of infancy and childhood* (7th ed., pp. 924–986). St. Louis: Mosby–Year Book.

Hoyer, L. W. (1994). Hemophilia A. *New England Journal of Medicine, 330*(1), 38–47.

Jackson, R. T., & Jackson, F. L. C. (1991). Reassessing 'hereditary' interethnic differences in anemia status. *Ethnicity and Disease, 1*(1), 26–41.

Jonides, L. (1996). Infant with a purpuric rash. *Journal of Pediatric Health Care, 10*, 139–140; 147–148.

Kevy, S. V. (1993). Red cell transfusion. In D. G. Nathan & F. A. Oski (Eds.), *Hematology of infancy and childhood* (4th ed., pp. 1769–1780). Philadelphia: W. B. Saunders.

Klemperer, M. R. (1995). Hemolytic anemias: Immune defects. In D. R. Miller & R. L. Baehner (Eds.), *Blood diseases of infancy and childhood* (7th ed., pp. 241–271). St. Louis: Mosby–Year Book.

Koch, D. A., Giardina, P. J., Ryan, M., MacQueen, M., & Hilgartner, M. W. (1993). Behavioral contracting to improve adherence in patients with thalassemia. *Journal of Pediatric Nursing, 8*(2), 106–111.

Lane, P. A. (1996). Sickle cell disease. *Pediatric Clinics of North America, 43*(3), 639–664.

Lozier, J. N., & Brinkhous, K. M. (1994). Gene therapy and the hemophilias. *Journal of the American Medical Association, 271*(1), 47–51.

Lozoff, B., Jimenez, E., & Wolf, A. W. (1991). Long-term developmental outcome of infants with iron deficiency. *New England Journal of Medicine, 325*(10), 687–694.

Mankad, V. N. (1995). Sickle cell disease and other disorders of abnormal hemoglobin. In D. R. Miller & R. L. Baehner (Eds.), *Blood diseases of infancy and childhood* (7th ed., pp. 415–459). St. Louis: Mosby–Year Book.

Manning, S. C., & Culbertson, M. C., Jr. (1996). Epistaxis. In C. D. Bluestone, S. E. Stool, & M. A. Kenna (Eds.), *Pediatric otolaryngology* (3rd ed., pp. 781–786). Philadelphia: W. B. Saunders.

Martin, M. B., & Butler, R. B. (1993). Understanding the basics of β thalassemia major. *Pediatric Nursing, 19*(2), 143–145.

McDonagh, K. T., & Nienhuis, A. W. (1993). The thalassemias. In D. G. Nathan & F. A. Oski (Eds.), *Hematology of infancy and childhood* (4th ed., pp. 783–879). Philadelphia: W. B. Saunders.

McFadden, E. A. (1991). The Wallaby Phototherapy System: A new approach to phototherapy. *Journal of Pediatric Nursing, 6*(3), 206–208.

McKown, C. G., & Shapiro, A. D. (1991). Oral management of patients with bleeding disorders: Dental considerations. *Journal of the Indiana Dental Association, 70*(2), 16–21.

Miller, D. R. (1995). Normal blood values from birth through adolescence. In D. R. Miller & R. L. Baehner (Eds.), *Blood diseases of infancy and childhood* (7th ed., pp. 30–53). St. Louis: Mosby–Year Book.

Miller, D. R., & O'Reilly, R. J. (1995). Aplastic anemia. In D. R. Miller & R. L. Baehner (Eds.), *Blood diseases of infancy and childhood* (7th ed., pp. 499–538). St. Louis: Mosby–Year Book.

Montgomery, R. R., & Scott, J. P. (1993). Hemostasis: Diseases of the fluid phase. In D. G. Nathan & F. A. Oski (Eds.), *Hematology of infancy and childhood* (4th ed., pp. 1605–1650). Philadelphia: W. B. Saunders.

O'Sullivan, T. J. (1990). Epistaxis in children. In G. B. Healy (Ed.), *Common problems in pediatric otolaryngology* (pp. 267–273). Chicago: Year Book Medical.

Perry, G. S., Byers, T., Yip, R., & Margen, S. (1992). Iron nutrition does not account for the hemoglobin differences between blacks and whites. *Journal of Nutrition, 122*(7), 1417–1424.

Pietri, M. M., Frontera, W. R., Pratts, I. S., & Suarez, E. L. (1992). Skeletal muscle function in patients with hemophilia A and unilateral hemarthrosis of the knee. *Archives of Physical Medicine and Rehabilitation, 73*(1), 22–28.

Piomelli, S. (1995). The management of patients with Cooley's anemia: Transfusions and splenectomy. *Seminars in Hematology, 32*(4), 262–268.

Pipes, P. L., & Glass, R. P. (1993). Developmental disabilities and other special health care needs. In P. L. Pipes & C. M. Trahms (Eds.), *Nutrition in infancy and childhood* (5th ed., pp. 344–373). St. Louis: Mosby.

Platt, O. S., & Dover, G. J. (1993). Sickle cell disease. In D. G. Nathan & F. A. Oski (Eds.), *Hematology of infancy and childhood* (4th ed., pp. 732–782). Philadelphia: W. B. Saunders.

Rick, M. E. (1994). Diagnosis and management of von Willebrand's syndrome. *Medical Clinics of North America, 78*(3), 609–623.

Roberts, H. R., & Eberst, M. E. (1993). Current management of hemophilia B. *Hematology/Oncology Clinics of North America, 7*(6), 1269–1280.

Rose, B. S. (1990). Phototherapy: All wrapped up? *Pediatric Nursing, 16*(1), 57–58, 72.

Ryan, M. M. (1996). Home phototherapy. *SPN News, 5*(3), 6.

Shafer, F. E., Lorey, F., Cunningham, G. C., Klumpp, C., Vichinsky, E., & Lubin, B. (1996). Newborn screening for sickle cell disease: 4 years of experience from California's newborn screening program. *Journal of Pediatric Hematology/Oncology, 18*(1), 36–41.

Sickle Cell Disease Guideline Panel. (1993). *Sickle cell disease: Screening, diagnosis, management, and counseling in newborns and infants.* Rockville, MD: Agency for Health Care Policy and Research, U.S. Department of Health and Human Services.

Sieff, C. A., & Nathan, D. G. (1993). The anatomy and physiology of hematopoiesis. In D. G. Nathan & F. A. Oski (Eds.), *Hematology of infancy and childhood* (4th ed., pp. 156–215). Philadelphia: W. B. Saunders.

Souid, A.-K., & Sadowitz, P. D. (1995). Acute childhood immune thrombocytopenic purpura: Diagnosis and treatment. *Clinical Pediatrics, 34*(9), 487–494.

Spitzer, A. (1992a). Children's knowledge of illness and treatment experiences in hemophilia. *Journal of Pediatric Nursing, 7*(1), 43–51.

Spitzer, A. (1992b). Coping processes of school-age children with hemophilia. *Western Journal of Nursing Research, 14*(2), 157–169.

Szer, I. S. (1994). Henoch-Schönlein purpura. *Current Opinion in Rheumatology, 6*(1), 25–31.

Taketomo, C. K., Hodding, J. H., & Kraus, D. M. (1997). *Pediatric dosage handbook* (4th ed.). Hudson, OH: Lexi-Comp.

Tapson, K. M. P. (1993). Henoch-Schönlein purpura. *American Family Physician, 47*(3), 633–638.

Vosburgh, E. (1993). Rational intervention in von Willebrand's disease. *Hospital Practice, 28*(3A), 31–41, 45–48.

Ware, R. E., & Filston, H. C. (1992). Surgical management of children with hemoglobinopathies. *Surgical Clinics of North America, 72*(6), 1223–1236.

Werner, E. J. (1996). von Willebrand disease in children and adolescents. *Pediatric Clinics of North America, 43*(3), 683–707.

Whitington, P. F., & Gartner, L. M. (1993). Disorders of bilirubin metabolism. In D. G. Nathan & F. A. Oski (Eds.), *Hematology of infancy and childhood* (4th ed., pp. 74–114). Philadelphia: W. B. Saunders.

Yip, R. (1994). Iron deficiency: Contemporary scientific issues and international programmatic approaches. *Journal of Nutrition, 124*(Suppl. 8), 1479S–1490S.

Zipursky, A., & Bowman, J. M. (1993). Isoimmune hemolytic diseases. In D. G. Nathan & F. A. Oski (Eds.), *Hematology of infancy and childhood* (4th ed., pp. 44–73). Philadelphia: W. B. Saunders.

Bibliography

Abramovitz, L. Z., & Senner, A. M. (1995). Pediatric bone marrow transplantation update. *Oncology Nursing Forum, 22*(1), 107–117.

Aledort, L. (1994). Inhibitors in hemophilia patients: Current status and management. *American Journal of Hematology, 47*(3), 208–217.

Allen, L. H. (1993). Iron deficiency anemia increases risk of preterm delivery. *Nutrition Reviews, 51*(2), 49–52.

Alter, B. P. (1992). Fanconi's anemia: Current concepts. *American Journal of Pediatric Hematology/Oncology, 14*(2), 170–176.

Armstrong, F. D., Lemanek, K. L., Pegelow, C. H., Gonzalez, J. C., & Martinez, A. (1993). Impact of lifestyle disruption on parental discipline in children with sickle cell anemia. *Children's Health Care, 22*(3), 189–203.

Auerbach, A. D. (1995). Fanconi anemia. *Dermatologic Clinics, 13*(1), 41–49.

Bale, J. F., Contant, C. F., Garg, B., Tilton, A., Kaufman, D. M., & Wasiewski, W. (1993). Neurologic history and examination results and their relationship to human immunodeficiency virus type 1 serostatus in hemophilic subjects: Results from the hemophilia growth and development study. *Pediatrics, 91*(4), 736–741.

Bastian, H. M. (1995). Hematologic disorders including sickle-cell syndromes, hemophilia, and beta-thalassemia. *Current Opinion in Rheumatology, 7*(1), 70–72.

Beck, W. S. (1991). Diagnosis of megaloblastic anemia. *Annual Review of Medicine, 42*, 311–322.

Behrman, R. E., Kliegman, R. M., Nelson, W. E., & Vaughan, V. C., III (Eds.). (1992). Acquired disorders of the nose. In *Nelson textbook of pediatrics* (14th ed., pp. 1053–1054). Philadelphia: W. B. Saunders.

Bell, T. N. (1993). Disseminated intravascular coagulation: Clinical complexities of aberrant coagulation. *Critical Care Nursing Clinics of North America, 5*(3), 389–410.

Benz, E. J., & Giardina, P. J. V. (1995). Thalassemia syndromes. In D. R. Miller & R. L. Baehner (Eds.), *Blood diseases of infancy and childhood* (7th ed., pp. 460–498). St. Louis: Mosby–Year Book.

Blanchette, V., Imbach, P., Andrew, M., Adams, M., McMillan, J., Wang, E., Milner, R., Ali, K., Barnard, D., Bernstein, M., Chan, K. W., Esseltine, D., deVeber, B., Israels, S., Kobrinsky, N., & Luke, B. (1994). Randomised trial of intravenous immunoglobulin G, intravenous anti-D, and oral prednisone in childhood acute immune thrombocytopenic purpura. *Lancet, 344*(8924), 703–707.

Brigden, M. L. (1993). Iron deficiency anemia. Every case is instructive. *Postgraduate Medicine, 93*(4), 181–192.

Brown, B. A. (1993). *Hematology: Principles and procedures* (6th ed.). Philadelphia: Lea & Febiger.

Brown, L. K., & DeMaio, D. M. (1992). The impact of secrets in hemophilia and HIV disorders. *Journal of Psychosocial Oncology, 10*(3), 91–101.

Brown, R. T., Armstrong, F. D., & Eckman, J. R. (1993). Neurocognitive aspects of pediatric sickle cell disease. *Journal of Learning Disabilities, 26*(1), 33–45.

Buchanan, G. R. (1993). Sickle cell disease: Recent advances. *Current Problems in Pediatrics, 23*, 219–229.

Bushnell, F. K. L. (1992). A guide to primary care of iron-deficiency anemia. *Nurse Practitioner, 17*(11), 68, 71–74.

Butler, R. B., Cecil, R., Ettinger, J. L., & Martin, M. B. (1991). β-Thalassemia major and sickle cell disease. *NAACOGS Clinical Issues in Perinatal and Womens Health Nursing, 2*(3), 349–356.

Buzby, M. (1991). Assessment of hyperbilirubinemia in full-term infants: Part I. *Journal of Pediatric Health Care, 5*(2), 94–96.

Buzby, M. (1991). Assessment of hyperbilirubinemia in full-term infants: Part II. *Journal of Pediatric Health Care, 5*(4), 210–212.

Cahill, M. (1996). Hematologic problems in pediatric patients. *Seminars in Oncology Nursing, 12*(1), 38–50.

Causey, A. L., Woodall, B. N., Wahl, N. G., Voelker, C. L., & Pollack, E. S. (1994). Henoch-Schönlein purpura: Four cases and a review. *Journal of Emergency Medicine, 12*(3), 331–341.

Chorba, T. L., Holman, R. C., & Evatt, B. L. (1993). Heterosexual and mother-to-child transmission of AIDS in the hemophilia community. *Public Health Reports, 108*(1), 99–105.

Cook, L. S. (1995). An overview of leukocyte depletion in blood transfusion. *Journal of Intravenous Nursing, 18*(1), 11–15.

Corbett, J. V. (1995). Accidental poisoning with iron supplements. *MCN American Journal of Maternal/Child Nursing, 20*(4), 234.

Corbett, J. V., & Fonteyn, M. E. (1995). Treating disseminated intravascular coagulation. *MCN American Journal of Maternal/Child Nursing, 20*(5), 290.

Day, S., Brunson, G., & Wang, W. (1992). A successful education program for parents of infants with newly diagnosed sickle cell disease. *Journal of Pediatric Nursing, 7*(1), 52–57.

Day, S., Dancy, R., Kelly, K., & Wang, W. (1993). Iron overload? In sickle cell disease? *MCN American Journal of Maternal/Child Nursing, 18*(6), 330–335.

De Alarcon, P. A. (1991). Diagnosis and treatment of sickle cell anemia and other hemoglobinopathies. *Comprehensive Therapy, 17*(11), 10–15.

Doheny, M. O., Sedlak, C., Broome, B., & Murphy, L. (1992). Caring for the orthopaedic patient with sickle cell disease. *Orthopaedic Nursing, 11*(1), 41–48.

Drummond, S. B. (1992). Disseminated intravascular coagulation. *NAACOGS Clinical Issues in Perinatal and Womens Health Nursing, 3*(3), 530–537.

Dunn, P. A., Bhutani, V., Weiner, S., & Ludomirski, A. (1988). Care of the neonate with erythroblastosis fetalis. *Journal of Obstetric, Gynecologic, and Neonatal Nursing, 17*(6), 382–386.

Earles, A., & Dorn, L. (1994). Nursing considerations. In S. H. Embury, R. P. Hebbel, N. Mohandas, & M. H. Steinberg (Eds.), *Sickle cell disease: Basic principles and clinical practice* (pp. 773–780). New York: Raven Press.

Eber, S. W., Armbrust, R., & Schroter, W. (1990). Variable clinical severity of hereditary spherocytosis: Relation to erythrocytic spectrin concentration, osmotic fragility, and autohemolysis. *Journal of Pediatrics, 117*(3), 409–416.

Edlestein, D. R. (1997). Epistaxis. In R. A. Hoekelman, S. B. Friedman, N. M. Nelson, H. M. Seidel, & M. L. Weitzman (Eds.) *Primary pediatric care* (3rd ed., pp. 936–939). St. Louis: Mosby–Year Book.

Emery, M. L. (1992). Disseminated intravascular coagulation in the neonate. *Neonatal Network, 11*(8), 5–13.

Esposito, N. W. (1992). Thalassemias: Simple screening for hereditary anemias. *Nurse Practitioner, 17*(2), 50–61.

Filer, L. J., Jr. (1990). Iron needs during rapid growth and mental development. *Journal of Pediatrics, 117*, S143–S146.

Fithian, J. H. (1992). Sickle cell disease education at the Children's Hospital of Philadelphia. *Journal of School Health, 62*(8), 388–391.

Fricke, W. A., & Lamb, M. A. (1993). Viral safety of clotting factor concentrates. *Seminars in Thrombosis and Hemostasis, 19*(1), 54–61.

Gallagher, P. G., Tse, W. T., & Forget, B. G. (1990). Clinical and molecular aspects of disorders of erythrocyte membrane skeleton. *Seminars in Perinatology, 14*(5), 351–367.

Garmel, S. H., Craigo, S. D., Morin, L. M., Crowley, J. M., & D'Alton, M. E. (1995). The role of percutaneous umbilical blood sampling in the management of immune thrombocytopenic purpura. *Prenatal Diagnosis, 15*(5), 439–445.

Gollin, Y. G., & Copel, J. A. (1995). Management of the Rh-sensitized mother. *Clinics in Perinatology, 22*(3), 545–559.

Grabowski, E. F., & Corrigan, J. J., Jr. (1995). Hemostasis: General considerations. In D. R. Miller & R. L. Baehner (Eds.), *Blood diseases of infancy and childhood* (7th ed., pp. 849–865), St. Louis: Mosby–Year Book.

Gribbons, D., Zahr, L. K., & Opas, S. R. (1995). Nursing management of children with sickle cell disease: An update. *Journal of Pediatric Nursing, 10*(4), 232–242.

Hawiger, J., & Handin, R. I. (1993). Physiology of hemostasis: Cellular aspects. In D. G. Nathan & F. A. Oski (Eds.), *Hematology of infancy and childhood* (4th ed., pp. 1494–1533). Philadelphia: W. B. Saunders.

Hill, A. S., Cochran, C. K., & Dickerson, C. (1989). Nursing care of the infant with erythroblastosis fetalis. *Journal of Pediatric Nursing, 4*(6), 395–402.

Jones, M. B. (1990). A physiologic approach to identifying neonates at risk for kernicterus. *Journal of Obstetric, Gynecologic, and Neonatal Nursing, 19*(4), 313–318.

Kamen, B. A., & Meyers, P. A. (1995). Megaloblastic anemias. In D. R. Miller & R. L. Baehner (Eds.), *Blood diseases of infancy and childhood* (7th ed., pp. 220–240). St. Louis: Mosby–Year Book.

Kark, J. A., & Ward, F. T. (1994). Exercise and hemoglobin S. *Seminars in Hematology, 31*(3), 181–225.

Khatib, Z., Wilimas, J., & Wang, W. (1994). Outcome of moderate aplastic anemia in children. *American Journal of Pediatric Hematology/Oncology, 16*(1), 80–85.

Kirchner, J. T. (1992). Acute and chronic immune thrombocytopenic purpura. *Postgraduate Medicine, 92*(6), 112–118, 125–126.

Kleinert, D., Cahill-Bordas, M., & Hilgartner, M. W. (1990). Hemophiliac patients in surgery. *AORN Journal, 52*(4), 743–752.

Kline, N. E. (1996). A practical approach to the child with anemia. *Journal of Pediatric Health Care, 10*(3), 99–105.

Korones, D. N., & Cohen, H. J. (1997). Anemia and pallor. In R. A. Hoekelman, S. B. Friedman, N. M. Nelson, H. M. Seidel, & M. L. Weitzman (Eds.), *Primary pediatric care* (3rd ed., pp. 865–876). St. Louis: Mosby–Year Book.

Koshy, M., & Burd, L. (1991). Management of pregnancy in sickle cell syndromes. *Hematology/Oncology Clinics of North America, 5*(3), 585–596.

Limentani, S. A., Roth, D. A., Furie, B. C., & Furie, B. (1993). Recombinant blood clotting proteins for hemophilia therapy. *Seminars in Thrombosis and Hemostasis, 19*(1), 62–72.

Listianingsih, M. F. H., Griffith, E. R., Hurtig, A. L., & Keehn, M. T. (1991). Functional outcomes of children with sickle-cell disease affected by stroke. *Archives of Physical Medicine and Rehabilitation, 72*, 498–502.

Loosli, A. R. (1993). Reversing sports-related iron and zinc deficiencies. *Physician and Sportsmedicine, 21*(6), 70–78.

Luban, N. L. C. (1995). Blood groups and blood component transfusion. In D. R. Miller & R. L. Baehner (Eds.), *Blood diseases of infancy and childhood* (7th ed., pp. 54–108). St. Louis: Mosby–Year Book.

Ludwig, M. A. (1990). Phototherapy in the home setting. *Journal of Pediatric Health Care, 4*(6), 304–308.

Lukens, J. N. (1995). Iron metabolism and iron deficiency. In D. R. Miller & R. L. Baehner (Eds.), *Blood diseases of infancy and childhood* (7th ed., pp. 193–219). St. Louis: Mosby.

Lusher, J. M. (1994). Response to 1-deamino-8-D-arginine vasopressin [DDAVP] in von Willebrand disease. *Haemostasis, 24*(5), 276–284.

Macik, B. G. (1993). Treatment of factor VIII inhibitors: Products and strategies. *Seminars in Thrombosis and Hemostasis, 19*(1), 13–24.

Manno, C. S. (1996). What's new in transfusion medicine? *Pediatric Clinics of North America, 43*(3), 793–808.

Martinelli, A. M. (1991). Sickle cell disease: Etiology, symptoms, patient care. *AORN Journal, 53*(3), 716–724.

McGuigan, M. A. (1996). Acute iron poisoning. *Pediatric Annals, 25*(1), 33–38.

Medeiros, D., & Buchanan, G. R. (1996). Current controversies in the management of idiopathic thrombocytopenic purpura during childhood. *Pediatric Clinics of North America, 43*(3), 757–772.

Miller, D. R. (1995). Anemias: General considerations. In D. R. Miller & R. L. Baehner (Eds.), *Blood diseases of infancy and childhood* (7th ed., pp. 111–139). St. Louis: Mosby–Year Book.

Miller, D. R. (1995). Hemolytic anemias: Membrane defects. In D. R. Miller & R. L. Baehner (Eds.), *Blood diseases of infancy and childhood* (7th ed., pp. 272–315). St. Louis: Mosby–Year Book.

Montgomery, K. S. (1996). Caring for the pregnant woman with sickle cell disease. *MCN: The American Journal of Maternal/Child Nursing, 21*(5), 224–228.

Nash, K. B. (1990). A psychosocial perspective: Growing up with thalassemia, a chronic disorder. *Annals of the New York Academy of Sciences, 612*, 442–449.

Niedbala, B., & Ekvall, S. W. (1993). Postnatal growth in infancy. In S. W. Ekvall (Ed.), *Pediatric nutrition in chronic diseases and developmental disorders* (pp. 19–28). New York: Oxford University Press.

Nilsson, I. M., Berntorp, E., & Freiburghaus, C. (1993). Treatment of patients with factor VIII and IX inhibitors. *Thrombosis and Haemostasis, 70*(1), 56–59.

Nugent, D. J. (1993). Platelet transfusion. In D. G. Nathan & F. A. Oski (Eds.), *Hematology of infancy and childhood* (4th ed., pp. 1781–1795). Philadelphia: W. B. Saunders.

Oliver, C. (1994). Triage decisions: A 4-year-old with petechial rash. *Journal of Emergency Nursing, 20*(2), 164.

Oski, F. A. (1993). Differential diagnosis of anemia. In D. G. Nathan & F. A. Oski (Eds.), *Hematology of infancy and childhood* (4th ed., pp. 346–353). Philadelphia: W. B. Saunders.

Patrignelli, R., Sheikh, S. H., & Shaw-Stiffel, T. A. (1995). Henoch-Schönlein purpura: A multisystem disease also seen in adults. *Postgraduate Medicine*, *97*(5), 123–134.

Peterec, S. M. (1995). Management of neonatal Rh disease. *Clinics in Perinatology*, *22*(3), 561–592.

Pipes, P. L., & Trahms, C. M. (1993). Nutrient needs of infants and children. In P. L. Pipes & C. M. Trahms (Eds.), *Nutrition in infancy and childhood* (5th ed., pp. 30–58). St. Louis: Mosby.

Pollack, C. V., Jr. (1993). Emergencies in sickle cell disease. *Emergency Medicine Clinics of North America*, *11*(2), 365–378.

Ranney, H. M. (1992). The spectrum of sickle cell disease. *Hospital Practice*, *27*(1), 133–163.

Raunikar, R. A., & Sabio, H. (1992). Anemia in the adolescent athlete. *American Journal of Diseases of Children*, *146*(10), 1201–1205.

Rick, M. E. (1994). Laboratory diagnosis of von Willebrand's disease. *Clinics in Laboratory Medicine*, *14*(4), 781–794.

Ritchey, A. K. (1990). Anemia. In M. Green & R. J. Haggerty (Eds.), *Ambulatory pediatrics* (4th ed., pp. 376–383). Philadelphia: W. B. Saunders.

Ruggeri, Z. M. (1994). Pathogenesis and classification of von Willebrand disease. *Haemostasis*, *24*(5), 265–275.

Sanders, J. E., Storb, R., Anasetti, C., Deeg, H. J., Doney, K., Sullivan, K. M., Witherspoon, R. P., & Hansen, J. (1994). Marrow transplant experience for children with severe aplastic anemia. *American Journal of Pediatric Hematology/Oncology*, *16*(1), 43–49.

Scott, J. P., & Montgomery, R. R. (1993). Therapy of von Willebrand disease. *Seminars in Thrombosis and Hemostasis*, *19*(1), 37–47.

Shapiro, A. D. (1990). Hemophilia. In M. Green & R. J. Haggerty (Eds.), *Ambulatory pediatrics* (4th ed., pp. 372–375). Philadelphia: W. B. Saunders.

Shapiro, A. D. (1990). Purpura. In M. Green & R. J. Haggerty (Eds.), *Ambulatory pediatrics* (4th ed., pp. 261–264). Philadelphia: W. B. Saunders.

Selekman, J. (1993). Update: New guidelines for the treatment of infants with sickle cell disease. *Pediatric Nursing*, *19*(6), 600–605.

Shapiro, A. D., & McKown, C. G. (1991). Oral management of patients with bleeding disorders: Medical considerations. *Journal of the Indiana Dental Association*, *70*(2), 28–31.

Smith, J. A., & Wethers, D. L. (1994). Health care maintenance. In S. H. Embury, R. P. Hebbel, N. Mohandas, & M. H. Steinberg (Eds.), *Sickle cell disease: Basic principles and clinical practice* (pp. 739–744). New York: Raven Press.

Soff, G. A., & Rosenberg, R. D. (1993). Physiology of hemostasis: The fluid phase. In D. G. Nathan & F. A. Oski (Eds.), *Hematology of infancy and childhood* (4th ed., pp. 1534–1560). Philadelphia: W. B. Saunders.

Tavassoli, M. (1991). Embryonic and fetal hematopoiesis: An overview. *Blood Cells*, *17*, 269–281.

Thomas, D. O. (1991). Ear, eye, nose, and throat problems. In D. O. Thomas (Ed.), *Quick reference to pediatric emergency nursing* (pp. 309–318). Gaithersburg, MD: Aspen.

Thompson, A. R. (1993). Factor IX concentrates for clinical use. *Seminars in Thrombosis and Hemostasis*, *19*(1), 25–36.

Vlachos, A., & Lipton, J. M. (1996). Bone marrow failure in children. *Current Opinion in Pediatrics*, *8*(1), 33–41.

Walters, M. C., & Abelson, H. T. (1996). Interpretation of the complete blood count. *Pediatric Clinics of North America*, *43*(3), 599–622.

Ward, C. L. (1992). Hemorrhaging at menarche: A case report. *Journal of Family Practice*, *34*(3), 351–354.

Waters, E., & Fister, S. (1991). Pediatric management problems. *Pediatric Nursing*, *17*(1), 72–73.

Wilson, D. A., Nelson, M. D., Jr., Fenstermacher, M. J., Bohan, T. P., Hopper, K. D., Tilton, A., Mitchell, W. G., Contant, C. F., Jr., Maeder, M. A., Donfield, S. M., & the Hemophilia Growth and Development Study Group. (1992). Brain abnormalities in male children and adolescents with hemophilia: Detection with MR imaging. *Radiology*, *185*(2), 553–558.

Young, N. S., & Barrett, A. J. (1995). The treatment of severe acquired aplastic anemia. *Blood*, *85*(12), 3367–3377.

HEALTH CHALLENGE:

Pediatric Infections

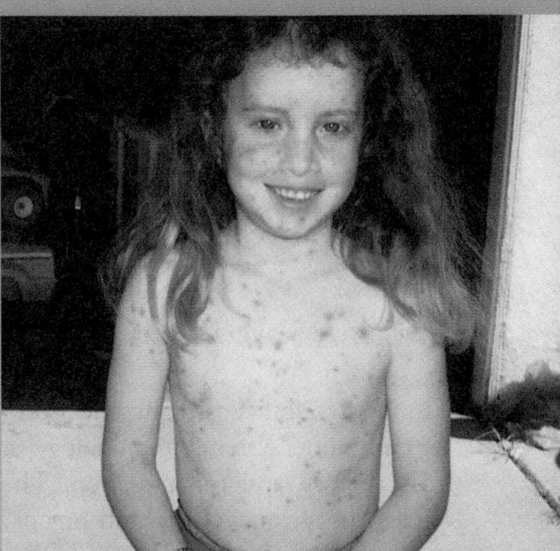

OUTLINE

OBJECTIVES

- Discuss interventions that disrupt the chain of infection.
- Identify assessment findings specific to pediatric infections and diagnostic criteria used to confirm diagnosis.
- Discuss nursing interventions to comply with the three types of transmission-based isolation.
- Describe two ways to prevent the spread of resistant organisms.
- Identify the symptoms of at least three tick-borne fevers and teaching needed to reduce transmission of tick-borne fevers.
- Describe at least one key intervention to decrease the risk of transmission of human immunodeficiency virus from a pregnant female to her fetus.
- Compare the six herpesviruses and discuss the nursing care for each.
- Name the diseases that constitute the TORCH syndrome and the nursing care for congenitally infected infants.
- Name three sexually transmitted diseases and interventions to prevent transmission.
- Discuss how the local health department follows up on contact tracing for infectious diseases.

KEY TERMS

antibiotic
antibody
antigen
catarrh
Centers for Disease Control and Prevention (CDC)
communicable disease
contamination
immunity
incubation period
infectious agents
isolation precautions
lymphadenopathy
nosocomial infection
prodromal period
virulence

CHAPTER

24

Microorganisms are as ancient as life itself. They are essential to life. Yet, they can be a great nemesis worthy of annihilation. Some organisms cause devastating disease and acute illness. Others live quietly in a symbiotic relationship with the body, benefiting the organism and the human host. Disease-producing microorganisms, such as bacteria, viruses, fungi, and parasites, are often referred to as infectious agents (Table 24–1). This chapter explores these infectious agents and the diseases they produce, their period of communicability (incubation period), and their assessment and related nursing interventions.

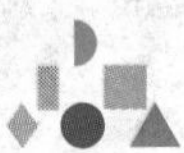

Epidemiology of Infections

The body's ability to fight infection depends on a competent immune system. Immunology is the basic science of host defense and inflammation. The immune system includes the primary lymphoid organs, which are the bone marrow (where hematopoiesis and B cell maturation and differentiation occur) and the thymus (where maturation and differentiation of T cells occur), and the secondary lymphoid organs, the lymph nodes, spleen (filters the blood and traps antigens so they can be destroyed by B and T cells), and mucosa-associated lymphoid tissue found close to potential sites of invasion (e.g., submucosal areas of the gastrointestinal tract, including the tonsils and respiratory and urogenital tracts).

Lymphocytes mediate the specificity of the immune system through identification of, and memory for, specific antigens. B lymphocytes mediate **humoral immunity** through differentiation into immunoglobulin (antibody) secreting plasma cells. When antibodies recognize their specific antigen they bind to it and either neutralize the antigen or enable other immune system cells to destroy it. T lymphocytes play a central role in **cell-mediated immunity**. T lymphocytes directly carry out important immunologic functions and also modulate the activity of most other immune effector cells. Generation of a specific immune response requires complex interactions between T cells, B cells, and macrophages. In addition, full expression of most defense capabilities is dependent on maturation of effector mechanisms involving other cell lines (neutrophils, eosinophils, basophils, and mast cells) and serum proteins, such as complement and properdin. After the lymphocytes, primarily T cells, recognize an invader as foreign, complement, neutrophils, and macrophages play roles in completing the antigen destruction. After primary exposure to an antigen, memory cells are left in the host. Upon subsequent exposure to that antigen, these memory cells serve to generate a more rapid reaction with higher antibody titers produced in response to smaller quantities of antigen as compared with the primary exposure (Rosenthal-Dichter & Allen, 1996).

Infection occurs when the body's defenses fail. Infectious diseases are those that cause acute or chronic infections. *Communicable diseases* are infectious diseases that have the potential to spread within a given community. Some communicable diseases are preventable through immunization (see Chapter 6). Immunization has become such an excellent method for preventing transmission of communicable diseases that most school systems now require certain immunizations before a child begins school. The ultimate goal of immunization is to eradicate a disease. A more immediate goal of immunization is to decrease disease transmission.

Table 24–1
Summary of Infectious Agents

Agent	Description	Examples
Bacteria	Free-living, single-celled microorganisms that occur in nature and the body.	*Salmonella* *Staphylococcus* *Rickettsia* *Mycobacterium*
Viruses	Obligate intracellular parasitic organism that takes over the genetic mechanism of an infected cell to reproduce itself. Viruses have either DNA or RNA but not both.	Herpes Hepatitis Influenza Polio
Fungi	Free-living microscopic organisms of the class to which molds and yeasts belong.	*Candida* *Tinea* *Malassezia furfur*
Parasites	An organism deriving its nutrition from another living organism.	Lice Scabies Mosquitoes

The Chain of Infection

For any infection to develop, certain conditions must be met in the *host* (usually the patient), the *environment* (the social, biological, and physical environment), and the *agent* (the organism). Changes in the equilibrium increase or decrease the frequency of disease.

The infectious disease process involves six components. These are often referred to as the "chain of infection" (Fig. 24–1). Disease-producing characteristics can be organism related or host related (Chart 24–1). A thorough assessment and good detective work may be needed to identify the cause of illness.

Figure 24–1
The chain of infection is only as strong as its weakest link. All components must be present for the disease process to progress.

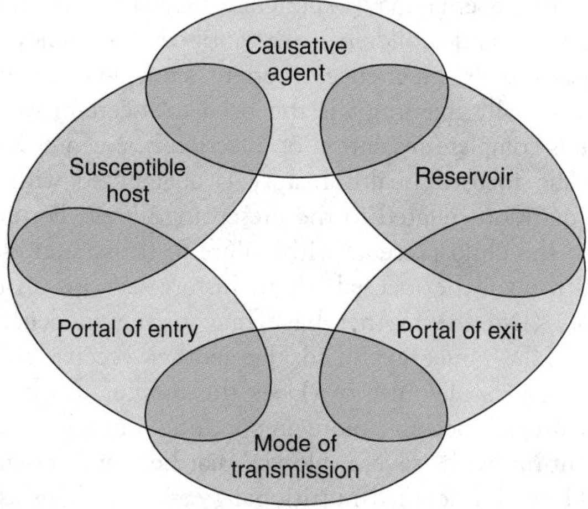

The chain of infection is only as strong as its weakest link. All six components must be present for the disease process to progress:

- **Causative agent**: Bacteria, viruses, fungi, protozoa, or helminths (worms) must be present in large enough numbers to cause infection.
- **Reservoir**: The organisms must have a place where they can survive but do not multiply. Common reservoirs include humans, animals, and environment (inanimate objects).
- **Portal of exit**: The organisms must have a way to leave the reservoir. Respiratory tract organisms may leave through sneezing, coughing, or talking. GU tract organisms may leave in urine. GI tract organisms may leave in vomitus or feces. Other portals of exit include blood or placenta.
- **Mode of transmission**: The organism must have a mechanism of transfer from the reservoir to a susceptible host. There are four chief modes of transmission:
  - **Contact.** Direct: Person to person, touching, kissing
    Indirect: Contact with an inanimate object
    Droplet: Brief passage through air for a short distance (3 feet) from sneezing or coughing.
  - **Vehicular.** A common vehicle such as food, blood, or water transports organisms to the new host.
  - **Airborne.** Organisms travel suspended in the air for long distances on droplet nuclei (tuberculosis).
  - **Vector.** Organisms use another species (usually insects) for transmission. For example, mosquitos carry *P. falciparum*, which causes malaria.
- **Portal of entry**: The organism must have a way to gain entry into the body. Examples would be the respiratory tract, GU tract, GI tract, skin/mucous membranes, blood, and transplacental.
- **Susceptible host**: The host must not be immune to the disease. A person who has an altered immune system or is extremely young or old is likely to be susceptible.

Chart 24–1

Disease-Producing Characteristics

Microorganism Characteristics

- Virulence: The capacity of the organism to produce disease.
- Infectious dose: The amount of organisms needed to produce disease.
- Adherence characteristics: Pathogen attaches to the site of infection (e.g., streptococcus and heart valves).
- Eluding host defense: The ability of the organism to attack the host defense system (as in HIV) or develop physical attributes to avoid detection (e.g., the polysaccharide capsule of pneumococcus).
- Host specificity: Organisms causing disease in specific species (e.g., the measles virus causes disease in humans only).

Host Characteristics

- Age: Diseases seen in the early years of life are referred to as childhood diseases.
- Sex: Reproductive diseases are sex specific.
- Socioeconomic status: The ability to purchase health care services, housing, and food is related to economic status.
- Disease history, underlying disease: Children with diabetes are at increased risk for infection.
- Lifestyle: IV drug abusers may share needles and infect each other with blood-borne pathogens.
- Immunization status: Children who are not immunized against vaccine-preventable diseases are at risk for these diseases.
- Ethnicity: Some religious groups prohibit outside medical intervention, such as immunization.
- Medications: Steroids and other drugs are known to increase the risk of infection.

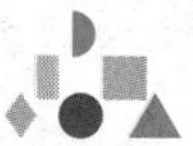

Assessment of the Child with an Infectious Disease

It is difficult to focus on one system when discussing infectious diseases. The infection may be localized to one system, or it may be systemic. Infections may have a rapid onset or occur long after exposure to the infectious agent. Infections may also mimic other diseases. Thus, astute questioning and assessment skills are needed. Infections occur when the immune system does not function properly; thus, an underlying immunodeficiency must be considered when features of this are present (Chart 24–2).

History of response to previous infections and of the present illness, as well as meticulous documentation of physical findings, is essential for the health care team to diagnose the child accurately and to decide on effective therapy.

Depending on the causative organism and resulting disease, infectious illness may be manifest in different ways. A deviation from normal behavior may be the first sign, such as sleep pattern alteration, irritability, or increasing lethargy. One may also see inflammation, fever, and/or rash as a general sign. More system-specific signs of infection include rhinitis, cough, diarrhea, and jaundice.

Focused Health History

Infectious disease processes cover such a wide range of health concerns that the nurse must start with a broad systems approach when obtaining a health history. Responses to general questions should lead to a more focused assessment (Chart 24–3).

The assessment should strive to determine whether the child has features suggestive of impaired host defense.

Chart 24–2

Features of Immunodeficiency

Features Frequently Present and Highly Suspicious

Chronic infection
Recurrent infection
Unusual infecting agents: *Pneumocystis carinii, Candida*
Incomplete clearing between episodes of infection
Incomplete response to treatment

Features Frequently Present and Moderately Suspicious

Skin (eczema, *Candida*)
Diarrhea
Growth failure
Hepatosplenomegaly
Recurrent abscesses
Recurrent osteomylitis

The practitioner should determine whether the child has infections that are too frequent, too severe, or rare in nature. For example, five to six upper respiratory infections each year can be expected in the preschool and school-age child. However, more than one pneumonia in a 5-year period would be unusual in children without asthma, cystic fibrosis, or another underlying pulmonary pathology. The time required to clear infections may be prolonged in children with compromised immune function.

A history of infection with an unusual pathogen (e.g., *Aspergillus, Serratia, Pneumocystis carinii*) suggests a defect in immune surveillance. The site of infection may also imply specific immune deficits. For example, children with neutropenia may experience frequent dermatologic infections, and children with antibody deficiency syndromes usually experience recurrent sinopulmonary infections. Equally important is the need to ascertain whether there is complete resolution of infection between episodes.

The focused health history is augmented with specific questions related to the presenting illness. For example, if the child presents with failure to thrive and esophageal thrush, the focused health history sections on birth history (Did the mother have human immunodeficiency virus [HIV] infection? Did the mother receive zidovudine?) and social history (Does the mother use intravenous drugs?) become more important. Similarly, a child presenting with severe bloody diarrhea and cramping would need a detailed nutritional assessment. This assessment could focus on the names and locations of restaurants where the child has eaten or the name of the infant formula and how the formula is prepared in the home.

Worldview: *Different infectious agents are prevalent in different parts of the world. To uncover clues about the causative agent, ask about recent travel abroad or exposure to people who have traveled abroad.*

Focused Physical Assessment

After a thorough history, examine the child, reviewing each major system. Children with severe immunodeficiency often have growth failure, which can be an important indicator of disease severity. Weight is typically impaired first, so low weight for height may be an early indicator of failure to thrive.

In children with competent immune systems, the infectious process may be localized to one system but often has systemic effects (Chart 24–4).

caREminder: *If one child in the family has symptoms of an infection, assess the siblings for infection also.*

Most children cannot produce sputum or mucus when they cough. What little is produced, they usually

Chart 24-3
Focused Health History

The Child with an Infectious Disease

Demographic Data	Child's age, height, weight Source of data (historian)
Present Illness	Time and site of onset Known infectious contacts Presence of: Neuromuscular symptoms: headache, stiff neck, ataxia, joint pain (describe) Eyes, ear, nose, throat: change in vision, drainage, conjunctivitis, otitis media, rhinitis, sore throat, cough Skin: rash (describe), pruritis (describe) Gastrointestinal symptoms: vomiting, diarrhea (frequency, appearance) Genitourinary symptoms: discharge (describe), pain on urination, rash or lesions (describe)
Past Medical History	Birth history: maternal infectious disease history, method of infant feeding, prematurity, neonatal illnesses, skin lesions noted at birth Previous health challenges: recurrent or chronic illness, prior hospitalizations, transfusion, surgery, evidence of complete resolution of infection between episodes Childhood illnesses: previous communicable diseases, recent exposure to disease Immunizations: immunizations received, dates, any rashes, unusual responses to live vaccines Allergies: allergic reactions to drugs, antibiotics, food, or plants (describe reaction)
Current Medications	All medications the child is currently taking (e.g., oral, topical), prescription and nonprescription
Nutritional Assessment	Recent changes in food or fluids consumed; recent weight change; formula preparation (describe); ingestion of honey, raw or undercooked meats, or seafood; fast food or restaurant food
Environmental History	History of pica; animal or insect bites or scratches; living or playing near or recent visit in wooded area, pond, lake, or farm
Family History	Family history of early infant mortality, immunodeficiency, autoimmune disease, or malignancy History of child's presenting illness in other family members (describe)
Social History	Recent changes in family lifestyle, daycare or school attendance (name and location), living arrangements (home, apartment, homeless, number of family and extended family living there), family pets (list), travel history (domestic and foreign) General hygiene, hand washing routines of child and caregivers, bathing
Growth and Development	Child's growth plotted along own height and weight growth curves, head circumference in children younger than 3 years Achievement of age-appropriate developmental milestones

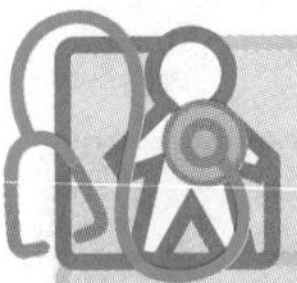

Chart 24–4
Focused Physical Assessment

The Child with an Infectious Disease

System	Abnormal Findings, Potential Pathology
Integument	Color: erythema (on cheeks—fifth disease, scarlet fever); jaundice (hepatitis); pallor (generalized—some chronic infections, e.g., intestinal parasites; circumoral—scarlet fever). Rash: appearance—macular (rubella, rubeola), papular, vesicular, pustular (varicella), crusts (impetigo), blanches with light pressure (roseola), petechial (meningococcemia); location and distribution—on trunk, extremities, face (e.g., varicella starts on trunk and spreads to face and extremities); eczema may be present in immunodeficiency syndrome; lymphadenopathy often present during infection.
EENT (eyes, ears, nose, throat)	Throat and mouth: presence and size of tonsils; oral ulcers; adherent white patches on tongue, palate, inner cheeks (candidiasis); membrane in pharynx, adherent, gray-white (diphtheria, scarlet fever); Koplik's spots on buccal mucosa opposite molars (rubeola); white strawberry tongue (white coat on tongue with red, edematous papillae projecting through) or later red strawberry tongue (white coat desquamates leaving red, edematous papillae projecting [scarlet fever]). Ears and neck: earache, parotid swelling and tenderness (mumps). Eyes: conjunctivitis (rubella, rubeola, adenovirus).
Neuromuscular	Change in level of consciousness, sluggish pupillary response (meningitis, encephalitis), Brudzinski's or Kernig's sign (meningitis). Limited range of motion: arthritis, arthralgia (rheumatic fever, fifth disease, Lyme disease).
Cardiovascular	Tachycardia above expected for fever (diphtheria, scarlet fever, rheumatic fever).
Respiratory	Cough (rubeola, TB, pertussis, diphtheria); note whether cough is productive, associated with cyanosis, vomiting (pertussis).
Gastrointestinal	Appearance: distention (intestinal parasites); pain with palpation; hepatomegaly (hepatitis, visceral larva migrans, mononucleosis, congestive heart failure resulting from rheumatic heart disease); splenomegaly (mononucleosis).
Genitourinary	Pain with abdominal palpation. Vaginal or urethral discharge (sexually transmitted diseases).

swallow. In contrast to the typical appearance of diseases such as tuberculosis in adults, there may be few diagnostic symptoms in children.

Jaundice is rare in childhood hepatitis. In many cases of hepatitis, the child does not have the appearance of being "ill." Thus, a well-documented history along with physical assessment assists the practitioner in analysis of the infectious process.

Nursing Diagnoses and Outcomes

The history and physical assessment should identify health issues that need to be addressed. Applicable nursing diagnoses depend on specific assessment findings. General nursing diagnoses may apply to the child suffering from an infection (Chart 24–5). More specific diagnoses depend on the specific pathology and its effect on the child's health.

Developmental and Biological Variances

Children experience higher incidences of infections because of physiologic and immunologic immaturity (Fig. 24–2). Changing social trends indicate that an increasing number of children, especially infants and toddlers,

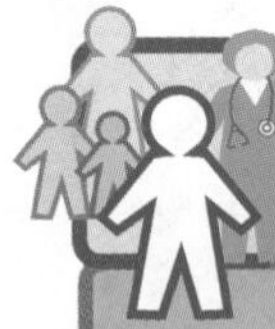

Chart 24–5
Nursing Diagnoses and Outcomes

The Child with an Infectious Disease

Hyperthermia related to effects of pathogen

Outcomes: Child will report or evidence minimal discomfort related to fever.
Child will suffer no injury if febrile seizure occurs.

Altered nutrition: less than body requirements related to effects of decreased intake and increased metabolic demands.

Outcome: Child will have adequate calorie and nutrient intake (oral, enteral, or IV) to meet maintenance and growth needs.

Diversional activity deficit related to effects of isolation, fatigue

Outcome: Child will engage in situation and developmentally appropriate activities:
If fatigued will engage in sedentary activities such as painting, reading, watching television.
If pruritic rash present, will distract from scratching.

Knowledge deficit: disease process

Outcome: Child and family will demonstrate an accurate understanding of the infection and its signs and symptoms, transmission, isolation, treatment, and complications.

Risk for infection related to potential for exposure

Outcomes: Child and siblings will have age-appropriate immunizations.
Family will be educated with regard to importance of immunizations.
Child will not expose others to the disease.

Noncompliance (with drug regimen)

Outcome: Child (and family, if applicable) will complete prescribed course and will verbalize the importance of continuing medications even after symptoms disappear.

attend daycare. Infections that were commonly seen in school-age children 25 years ago are now seen in infants, toddlers, and preschoolers.

Some infections are particularly prevalent in specific age groups:

- Infants: upper respiratory infections, enteric infections, vaccine-preventable diseases such as pertussis because of incomplete immunity, gastroenteritis, and other diseases transmitted by the oral-fecal route
- Toddlers: upper respiratory infections, enteric infections (in those not toilet trained), communicable diseases transmitted by adults and other caregivers, soil-borne diseases (parasites)
- Preschool-age children: upper respiratory infections, food-borne illness
- School-age children: ectoparasites (lice), food-borne illness, upper respiratory illness, pharyngitis
- Adolescents: sexually transmitted diseases, mononucleosis ("kissing disease")

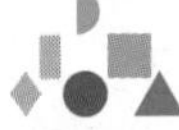

Diagnostic Criteria for Evaluating Pediatric Infections

Numerous methods can be used to analyze immune system function and identify causative organisms of infectious diseases (Table 24–2). Prudent use of laboratory tests requires that they be selected on the basis of history and physical examination findings. Rapid and accurate identification of causative organisms facilitates initiation of appropriate therapy and improves outcomes.

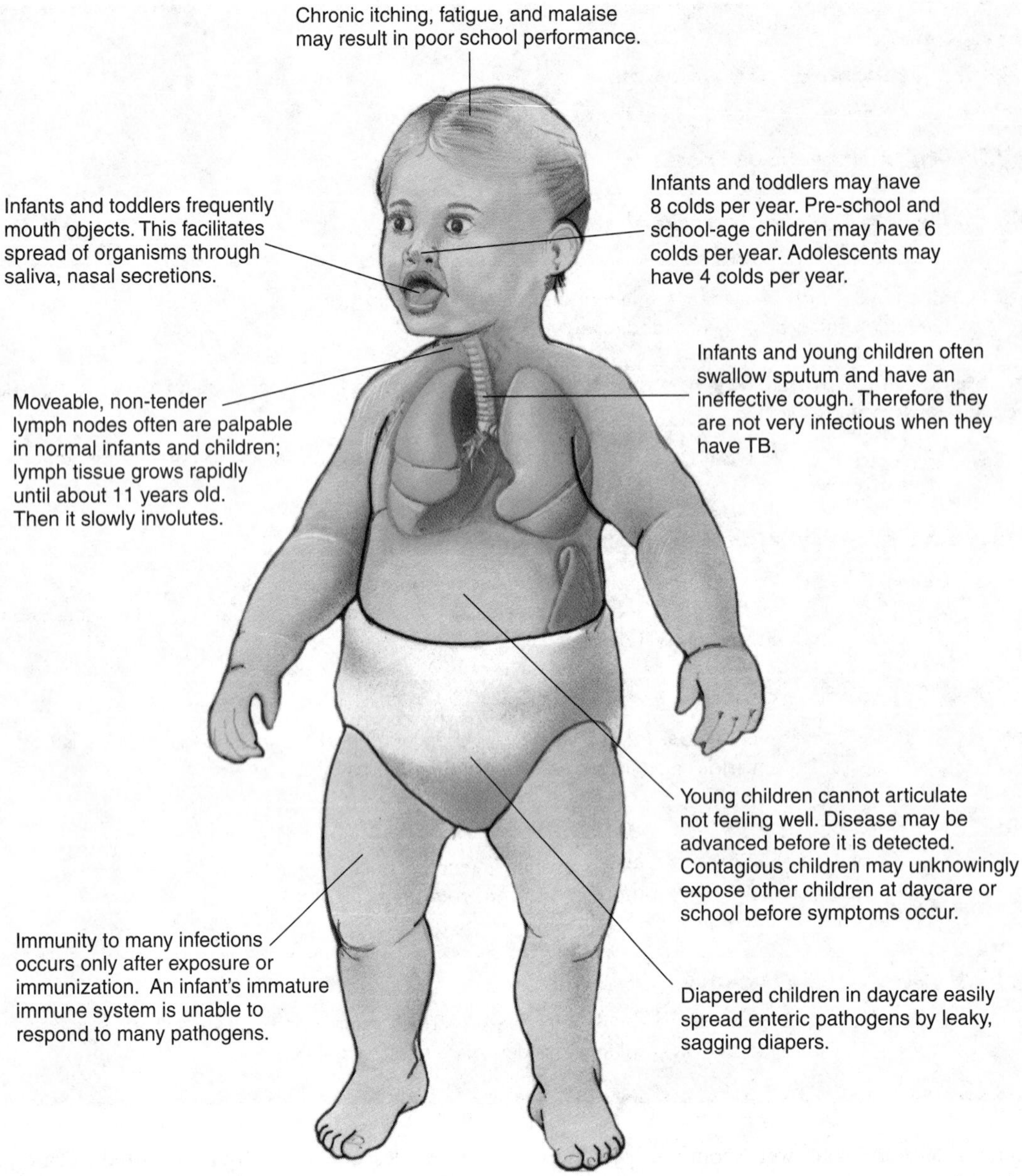

Chronic itching, fatigue, and malaise may result in poor school performance.

Infants and toddlers frequently mouth objects. This facilitates spread of organisms through saliva, nasal secretions.

Infants and toddlers may have 8 colds per year. Pre-school and school-age children may have 6 colds per year. Adolescents may have 4 colds per year.

Infants and young children often swallow sputum and have an ineffective cough. Therefore they are not very infectious when they have TB.

Moveable, non-tender lymph nodes often are palpable in normal infants and children; lymph tissue grows rapidly until about 11 years old. Then it slowly involutes.

Young children cannot articulate not feeling well. Disease may be advanced before it is detected. Contagious children may unknowingly expose other children at daycare or school before symptoms occur.

Immunity to many infections occurs only after exposure or immunization. An infant's immature immune system is unable to respond to many pathogens.

Diapered children in daycare easily spread enteric pathogens by leaky, sagging diapers.

Figure 24–2
Developmental and biological variances: infection in children.

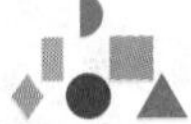

Treatment Modalities

The primary treatment modality for infectious disease is prevention (Chart 24–6). Standard precautions must be used and additional patient isolation as indicated. Individual treatment of the child depends on the disease process.

Children with immunodeficiencies are treated with prophylactic antibiotics. A variety of other treatment modalities may be used depending on the specific deficiency. These include intravenous gamma globulin, enzyme replacement, gene therapy, interleukin-2 infusions, and bone marrow transplantation.

Infectious diseases are generally classified into five major categories on the basis of causative agents: bacteria, viruses, fungi, parasites, and rickettsiae. Regardless of the causative agent, certain standard precautions must be taken to prevent disease transmission (Chart 24–7).

Some health care workers may refuse to comply with standard precautions (treating all body fluids from all patients as if contaminated) and may insist on knowing which children have what infection. In turn, these health care workers might take extra precautions (use

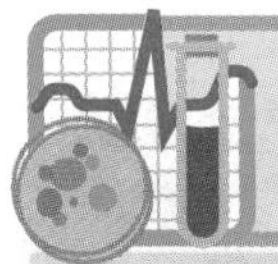

Table 24–2
Diagnostic Tests and Procedures for Evaluating the Child with an Infection

Diagnostic Test or Procedure	Purpose	Findings	Health Care Provider Responsibilities
Complete blood count (CBC) with differential	To compare the status of specific blood elements; a detailed evaluation of the white blood cell (WBC) count and morphology may help to detect infection.	Values outside age-appropriate laboratory reference ranges indicate how the body is responding to the infection and adequacy of response. Infection usually causes leukocytosis. Neutropenia in a neonate often indicates sepsis. Neutrophilia after the neonatal period indicates an infectious process. An increase in bands (immature neutrophils) may indicate bacterial infection. Immunocompromised patients may not be able to mount a response that is reflected in an increased WBC count or change in the differential.	Provide psychosocial support. Obtain specimen, appropriately label, and send to laboratory. Obtain results, notify physician or advanced nurse practitioner.
Serum C-reactive protein (CRP)	To detect elevated levels of CRP, normally present in trace amounts; production is increased after tissue injury or destruction.	Levels of 10 to 19 mg/L suggest viral infection or noninvasive bacterial infection* Levels above 19 mg/L suggest invasive bacterial infection or fungal septicemia.* In neonates, levels above 10 mg/L suggest sepsis or meningitis.*	Provide psychosocial support. Obtain specimen, appropriately label, and send to laboratory. Obtain results, notify physician or advanced nurse practitioner.
Erythrocyte sedimentation rate (ESR)	A screening procedure to identify children who may have an infectious or inflammatory process.	An elevated ESR is generally indicative of the presence of infection or an inflammatory process; it is nonspecific (not diagnostic for any particular pathology).	Provide psychosocial support. Obtain specimen, appropriately label, and send to laboratory. Obtain results, notify physician or advanced nurse practitioner.
Urine culture	To diagnose a urinary tract infection. To monitor microbial colonization after urinary catheter insertion.	Cultures are reported as "no growth" if urine is sterile (no infection). Bacterial count of greater than 100,000 organisms per mL of a single species is indicative of infection. Counts less than 10,000 organisms per mL are indicative of contamination.	Use gloves when handling all specimens. Obtain a sterile catheterized specimen (preferred) or a clean-catch specimen. Collect at least 3 mL of urine and send to the laboratory immediately or store in a specimen refrigerator until transport to the laboratory.
Stool culture	To identify pathogenic bacteria.	Normal fecal flora consists of gram-negative aerobic and anaerobic bacteria. Pathogenic bacteria include *Salmonella, Shigella, Campylobacter, E. coli* O157:H7, *Clostridium difficile, Clostridium botulinum, Yersinia,* and *Vibrio.*	Send a fresh specimen collected from a bedpan or diaper. Use a tongue blade to transfer it to a sterile container. If a rectal swab is used, insert the swab into the anus just past the anal sphincter. Rotate the swab gently. Withdraw it and place it in a transport tube.

Table continued on following page

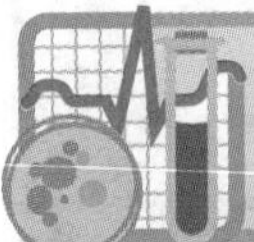

Table 24–2
Diagnostic Tests and Procedures for Evaluating the Child with an Infection *Continued*

Diagnostic Test or Procedure	Purpose	Findings	Health Care Provider Responsibilities
Sputum culture	To identify the cause of pulmonary infection.	Expectorated sputum has normal flora (alpha streptococci and *Neisseria*) and is Gram stained before processing to determine the quality of the specimen. The presence of the following organisms is usually significant: *Mycobacterium tuberculosis, Haemophilus influenzae, Klebsiella* spp., *Staphylococcus aureus, Pseudomonas* spp.	Send early morning specimen (before eating breakfast) for TB. Have the child rinse or gargle with water and then cough deeply into a sterile container. Transport specimen to laboratory within 2 hr. Small children may not be able to produce sputum. Consider using gastric lavage as an alternative.
Blood culture	To confirm sepsis. To identify the microorganism in bacteremia and sepsis.	The presence of any organism is usually indicative of infection. Common skin contaminants (coagulase-negative *Staphylococcus, Bacillus, Corynebacterium*) isolated from a single bottle nearly always represent contamination.	Disinfect blood culture bottles (two in a set) with 70% isopropyl alcohol. Clean venipuncture site with 70% alcohol followed by iodophor. Allow to dry. For endocarditis, send two specimen sets from two sites over 2 hr.
Gastric lavage	To identify TB in a child when bronchoscopy cannot be performed. Often gives better results than bronchoscopy in children.	The presence of TB in the specimen by acid-fast staining and culture techniques is indicative of infection.	In the early morning, before eating, introduce a nasogastric tube. Lavage 50 mL of chilled, sterile water. Withdraw a sample and place in a sterile container. Transport to the laboratory within 15 min at room temperature.
Enzyme linked immunosorbent assay (ELISA) Enzyme immunosorbent assay (EIA)	Direct detection of viral antigens in body fluids.	Specific viral antigens are tested and are either positive or negative.	Obtain a blood specimen for most tests. Obtain a nasal wash for respiratory syncytial virus or influenza testing.
Nucleic acid probes (GYN-Probe, GEN-Probe) Polymerase chain reaction	Screening test that can detect specific viral or bacterial DNA or RNA.	Some tests, such as GYN-Probe, detect the nucleic acid of *Neisseria gonorrhoeae* and chlamydia. The test is positive for either or both. Probes are also available for detecting various strains of *Mycobacterium*. This rapid test method can determine whether *M. tuberculosis* is present versus an atypical strain. Genetic probes are available for various viruses including hepatitis C virus.	Send throat, urogenital, or rectal swabs to the laboratory. Other specimen sources include blood and CSF.

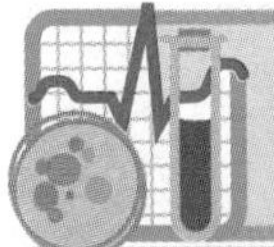

Table 24–2
Diagnostic Tests and Procedures for Evaluating the Child with an Infection *Continued*

Diagnostic Test or Procedure	Purpose	Findings	Health Care Provider Responsibilities
Direct fluorescent antibody (DFA)	Detection of specific enzyme-labeled antibodies. Usually used for respiratory viruses, herpes, rabies, some respiratory bacteria (pertussis).	Results are virus and bacteria specific and are positive.	Send throat swabs on transport medium to the laboratory.
Western blot	Lysate of concentrated virions is placed on specialized gel. Viral proteins separate by molecular weight. Used as a confirmatory test with ELISA for HIV but can be specific for other viruses.	Positive results are reported as bands. The specimen has bands in specific molecular weight ranges for the virus being tested. For example, HIV has p24, gp120, and so on.	Send a blood specimen. If a patient has a positive ELISA for HIV, perform a confirmatory Western blot test before explaining the results to the patient.
Rapid antigen extraction	To test rapidly for the presence of group A streptococci (antigen).	Result is positive if group A streptococci are present. Negative tests require a 24-hr incubation for conventional growth on agar.	Send a throat swab to the laboratory. Swab both tonsillar pillars. Have the child take a deep breath to reduce gagging.
Delayed hypersensitivity skin testing	To test for certain diseases (e.g., coccidioidomycosis, tuberculosis). To serve as a positive control when conducting these tests; two or more antigens (e.g., *Trichophyton,* tetanus, *Candida,* mumps) are injected intradermally at the same time; if the child responds to any of them, it demonstrates effective T cell function and results of the others can be considered valid. Sometimes used to test T cell–mediated immunity, although it has limited value in the HIV era.	A positive reaction (induration at site) to the antigens indicates the body has mounted a T cell–mediated immune response. Findings depend on antigens injected. All children older than 1 yr should demonstrate a reaction to *Candida,* which is ubiquitous, as well as tetanus, mumps, and diphtheria, to which they have been exposed via routine immunizations. A positive reaction to PPD indicates a history of infection with TB. Immunocompromised or chronically ill children or those with severe nutritional deficiencies may not demonstrate a response (anergy).	Review the child's history for hypersensitivity to the test antigens. Observe the child for signs of anaphylaxis. Each antigen is injected intradermally to the forearm using a separate needle for each antigen; a control antigen must be used. Use a pen to circle each site and label appropriately. Teach the child and family that the test involves injecting small doses of antigens under the skin; that the area needs to be monitored at 24, 48, and 72 hr after the test; and that the circles should not be washed off until the test has been completed. A negative reaction may require placement of additional or stronger antigens. When reading the test, record erythema and induration in millimeters.

* Singer, J. I., Vest, J., & Prints, A. (1995). Occult bacteremia and septicemia in the febrile child younger than two years. *Emergency Medicine Clinics of North America, 13,* 381–415.

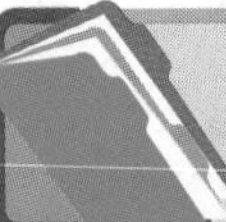

Chart 24–6
Nursing Interventions Classification (NIC)

Infection Control

Definition

Minimizing the acquisition and transmission of infectious agents

Activities

Allocate the appropriate square feet per patient, as indicated by CDC guidelines.
Clean the environment appropriately after each patient's use.
Change patient care equipment per agency protocol.
Isolate persons exposed to communicable disease.
Place on designated isolation precautions, as appropriate.
Maintain isolation techniques, as appropriate.
Limit the number of visitors, as appropriate.
Teach improved hand washing to health care personnel.
Instruct patient on appropriate hand washing techniques.
Instruct visitors to wash hands on entering and leaving the patient's room.
Use antimicrobial soap for hand washing, as appropriate.
Wash hands before and after each patient care activity.
Institute universal precautions.
Wear gloves as mandated by universal precaution policy.
Wear scrub clothes or gown when handling infectious material.
Wear sterile gloves, as appropriate.
Scrub the patient's skin with an antibacterial agent, as appropriate.
Shave and prepare the area, as indicated in preparation for invasive procedures and/or surgery.
Maintain an optimal aseptic environment during bedside insertion of central lines.
Maintain an aseptic environment while changing TPN tubing and bottles.
Maintain a closed system while doing invasive hemodynamic monitoring.
Change peripheral IV and central line sites and dressings according to current CDC guidelines.
Ensure aseptic handling of all IV lines.
Ensure appropriate wound care technique.
Use intermittent catheterization to reduce the incidence of bladder infection.
Teach patient to obtain midstream urine specimens at first sign of return of symptoms, as appropriate.
Encourage deep breathing and coughing, as appropriate.
Promote appropriate nutritional intake.
Encourage fluid intake, as appropriate.
Encourage rest.
Administer antibiotic therapy, as appropriate.
Administer an immunizing agent, as appropriate.
Instruct patient to take antibiotics, as prescribed.
Teach patient and family about signs and symptoms of infection and when to report them to the health care provider.
Teach patient and family members how to avoid infections.
Promote safe food preservation and preparation.

From McCloskey, J. & Bulechek, G. (1996). *Nursing interventions classification (NIC)* (2nd ed.). St. Louis: Mosby–Year Book. Reprinted with permission.

gloves, gown, mask) with the children they know are infected. This approach is flawed because many children are treated for reasons other than infections, such as a broken leg, yet may be infected. In the course of treatment, it may *never* be discovered that the child has hepatitis B or C or HIV infection.

Alert: *It is essential that all body fluids be handled carefully at all times to prevent infection transmission.*

In addition to standard precautions, children who have known or suspected infections transmitted by airborne,

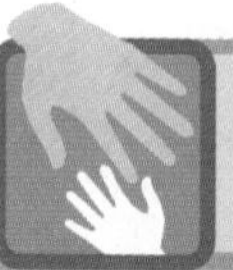

Chart 24-7
Nursing Interventions

Standard Precautions

Use Standard Precautions for the Care of All Patients

Hand washing: Wash hands between patients, after removing gloves, and if hands are contaminated with body fluids.
Gloves: Wear gloves when handling body fluids. Change gloves between patients or before touching environmental surfaces. Wash hands after gloves are removed.
Mask, face shield, eye protection: Wear a mask, face shield, or eye protection whenever fluid splashing to the face is likely.
Gown or apron: Wear a fluid-resistant cover gown or apron to protect uniforms or clothing if contamination is likely. Change the gown between patients.
Equipment: Properly process critical patient care equipment, equipment that must be sterile (such as surgical instruments), and semicritical equipment (equipment that can be disinfected); clean, disinfect, and/or sterilize it as appropriate. Send contaminated equipment for reprocessing in bags or containers in such a way that leakage or accidental injury (to receiving department) is minimized.
Linen: Place soiled linen in leakproof containers.
Occupational health: Never recap needles. Place needles in puncture-proof containers. Use mouthpieces or resuscitation bags instead of traditional mouth-to-mouth resuscitation whenever possible. Report all injuries regardless of perceived significance.

droplet, or contact methods may require special precautions (Table 24–3).

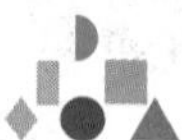

caREminder: *Most communicable diseases must be reported to the local health department. Check local regulations; they vary in terms of which communicable diseases are reported.*

Pediatric Infections

Bacterial Infections

Bacteria are single-celled microorganisms that are classified according to their shape and ability to retain various stains. These organisms can occur in round forms (cocci) that cluster or form long chains when stained. Bacilli are the rod-shaped forms, and spirilla are the spiral forms. Gram staining and acid-fast staining further define the classes of bacteria.

Serious bacterial infections include diphtheria, mycoplasmal pneumonia, pertussis, pneumonic plague, and streptococcal pharyngitis. Vaccination programs have virtually eliminated diphtheria. However, another vaccine-preventable disease, pertussis, is regaining a foothold because of poor compliance and public misunderstanding of the vaccine. Fortunately, the pneumonic form of bubonic plague is geographically limited to the western states, mainly Arizona.

Sepsis

"Rule out sepsis" is a common diagnosis for infants admitted to the hospital. The reason is that, because of their immature immune systems, infants can rapidly be

Table 24–3
Special Precautions

Type	Protective Equipment	Patient Placement	Patient Transport
Airborne precautions: measles, varicella, tuberculosis. Health care workers who are not immune to measles or varicella should be reassigned.	Measles and varicella: Wear an N95 respirator if not immune to measles or varicella and must enter room. Tuberculosis: Wear an N95 respirator when entering the room of a patient with known or suspected pulmonary tuberculosis.	Private room with monitored negative pressure, 6–12 air changes per hour, and discharge of air outdoors or through HEPA filtration if air is recirculated.	Limit transport of patient from room to essential purposes only. Have patient wear a surgical mask during transport.

Table continued on following page

Table 24–3
Special Precautions *Continued*

Type	Protective Equipment	Patient Placement	Patient Transport
Droplet precautions: adenovirus, influenza, invasive *Haemophilus influenzae* type B disease, invasive *Neisseria meningitidis* disease, diphtheria (pharyngeal), mumps, *Mycoplasma* pneumonia, parvovirus B19, pertussis, pneumonic plague, rubella (German measles), and streptococcal pharyngitis, pneumonia, or scarlet fever in infants and young children.	Wear a surgical mask when working within 3 feet of the patient (or upon entering the room).	Use a private room. Patients with the same disease may share a room and be separated by 3 feet.	Limit transport of the patient to essential purposes only. Have patient wear a surgical mask during transport.
Contact precautions: use contact precautions for patients known or suspected to have serious illnesses easily transmitted by direct patient contact or contact with items in the patient's environment. Examples of such diseases include gastrointestinal, respiratory, skin, or wound infections or colonization with multidrug-resistant bacteria, enteric organisms that exhibit prolonged environmental survival, respiratory syncytial virus, parainfluenza virus, or enteroviral infections in infants and young children, skin infections that are highly contagious, viral hemorrhagic conjunctivitis, and viral hemorrhagic infections.	Wear gloves when entering room. Change gloves after having contact with infective material that may contain high concentrations of microorganisms. Remove gloves before leaving the patient's room. Wear gown when entering the room and it is anticipated that clothing will become soiled. Wear a gown if uniform or clothing will come into substantial contact with the patient or items in the patient's room. Remove gown before leaving room and ensure that clothing does not come in contact with potentially contaminated environmental surfaces. Wash hands after removing gloves with an antimicrobial soap and again after exiting the room. Patient care equipment: dedicate the use of noncritical patient care equipment (e.g., stethoscope, bedside commode, thermometer) to a single patient.	Private room. Patients with the same disease may share a room.	Limit transport to essential purposes.

In addition to standard precautions, use these precautions for patients with known or suspected diseases listed. For all isolation precautions, visitors should report to the nurses' station before entering the child's room.

made critically ill by bacterial invasion, resulting in overwhelming sepsis (Witek-Janusek & Cusack, 1994). Aggressive treatment must begin immediately.

Children with certain congenital or acquired defects are at particular risk for sepsis. Infants with skin defects, such as aplasia cutis, epidermolysis bullosa, or ichthyosis, often have breaks in the skin that provide an opening for bacteria to invade. Secondary blood stream infections result from superficial skin infections in these infants. Defects in skin closure, as with gastroschisis or exstrophy of the bladder, expose underlying tissues and organs to outside microbial contamination and invasion resulting in sepsis. Children who are immunocompromised (e.g., because of chemotherapy, steroid therapy, asplenia, or immune cell dysfunction) or who have invasive devices such as central lines are also at increased risk for sepsis.

The incidence of neonatal sepsis has been followed by the National Nosocomial Infection Surveillance (NNIS) section of the Centers for Disease Control and Prevention (CDC) for more than two decades. To participate in NNIS, hospitals must use stringent guidelines for defining neonatal sepsis (Chart 24–8).

Neonatal sepsis can be caused by viruses such as herpes simplex or enteroviruses and by protozoa (*Toxoplasma gondii*). Typically, bacteria are the culprits. The infants are infected during the birthing process or by transplacental transmission. Events such as prolonged rupture of the membranes (longer than 18 to 24 hours) and amnionitis contribute to contamination at birth or ascending infections. Hospitalized neonates, especially premature infants, run an extremely high risk for sepsis because of invasive devices, endotracheal tubes, and central venous catheters. Fungi also play a role in sepsis, particularly in the hospitalized neonate. Multiple antibiotics may be used, killing the infant's normal flora and leaving the infant susceptible to opportunistic organisms such as fungi. Common skin fungi, such as *Candida* spp., are often important causes of sepsis.

Chart 24–8

CDC Definition of Sepsis

Laboratory-confirmed blood stream infection must meet one of the following criteria:

Criterion 1

Patient has a recognized pathogen cultured from one or more blood cultures *and* the organism cultured from blood is not related to an infection at another site.

Criterion 2

Patient has at least *one* of the following signs and symptoms: fever, chills, hypotension, *and* at least one of the following:

- Common skin contaminant in two or more blood cultures
- Common skin contaminant in one blood culture and physician begins appropriate antibiotics
- Positive antigen test on blood

Criterion 3

Patient is younger than 1 year and has one of the following signs and symptoms: fever, hypothermia, apnea, bradycardia, *and* one of the following:

- Common skin contaminant from two blood cultures
- Common skin contaminant from one blood culture and physician begins appropriate antibiotic therapy
- Positive antigen test on blood

Group B Streptococcal Infections

One bacterium stands out as a major contributor to neonatal sepsis, group B streptococcus (GBS). Colonization of the lower genitourinary tract occurs in approximately 20% to 25% of pregnant women (Crossley, 1996). Infants acquire the bacteria as they descend through the birth canal. Within 24 hours after birth, signs and symptoms of sepsis occur. Some infants have a late onset of GBS disease. These infants are typically 1 to 3 months of age. For infants with GBS neonatal sepsis, the mortality rate is 25% (Crossley, 1996).

Assessment

An early onset of GBS disease often begins as an overwhelming septic event. The infection has a sudden onset within the first few days of life. Meningitis and pneumonia are often present with sepsis. Fever or hypothermia can be present. The infant may show signs of apnea and bradycardia. Conversely, tachypnea and tachycardia may be observed. These symptoms are similar for all infants with sepsis (Chart 24–9).

Late-onset disease with GBS often presents with meningitis, osteomyelitis, septic arthritis, or cellulitis. A certain type of streptococci, type III, is associated with 90% of cases of late-onset neonatal sepsis (Crossley, 1996).

A positive culture of blood from the infant with gram-positive cocci in chains can provide a presumptive diagnosis of GBS infection. Cultures from any sterile body site, such as spinal or pleural fluid, are also diagnostic. Rapid antigen test kits, which test for the presence of GBS in cerebrospinal fluid (CSF), blood, or urine, are available and offer quick and accurate results. Positive cultures for the infant are not required to diagnose clinical sepsis. Positive maternal cultures and the signs and symptoms of sepsis in the neonate are evidence of infection.

Nursing Diagnoses and Outcomes

Common nursing diagnoses and outcomes for the child with an infection are identified in Chart 24–5. In addition, the following may be applicable to the child with sepsis:

Chart 24–9

Symptoms of Neonatal Sepsis

General

Temperature instability
Hypothermia (more common) or fever
Irritability, lethargy, or coma
Decreased urine output
Floppiness (hypotonia)
Feeding intolerance
Hypoglycemia

Cardiac

Bradycardia or tachycardia
Mottling or pallor
Poor capillary refill
Hypotension
Cyanosis

Pulmonary

Apnea or tachypnea
Sternal retractions
Grunting
Nasal flaring
Irregular respirations

▶ **Ineffective breathing pattern related to increased energy demand and fatigue**
Outcome: The child will maintain adequate tissue oxygenation.

Interdisciplinary Interventions

Treatment for GBS requires penicillin or ampicillin and an aminoglycoside. This combination of antibiotics is often used to treat suspected bacterial infections empirically when the organism has not been identified. Antibiotic therapy for all forms of sepsis is summarized in Table 24–4.

Maintaining aseptic technique and good nutrition and decreasing stress for the infant may help promote immunocompetence, thus bolstering the infant's ability to resist infection. Close observation of the child for subtle changes in vital signs, behavior, feeding tolerance, and physical assessment is critical for prompt detection of signs of sepsis. When sepsis is suspected, maintenance of intravenous (IV) antibiotic therapy is necessary. Isolation is not necessary for GBS disease but may be needed for other organisms such as methicillin-resistant *Staphylococcus aureus* (MRSA) or varicella (requiring airborne precautions). Frequent updates to the family are appreciated and critical in communicating information that may be difficult for a layperson to understand (Chart 24–10).

The length of hospitalization for an infant admitted with GBS sepsis can vary from 3 to 5 days to 1 to 3 weeks (see Care Path 30–1). The infant may be sent home with oral antibiotics. The nurse must instruct the parents on how to give oral antibiotics to the infant as well as the importance of finishing all the medication. Parents must also be taught signs of infection and when to call their health care provider.

Staphylococcal Infections

Staphylococcus is a gram-positive coccus that appears in clusters similar to grapes when stained. The name *Staphy-*

Table 24–4
Summary of Antimicrobial Therapy for Sepsis

Microorganism	Antimicrobial Agent
Group B *Streptococcus*	Penicillin
Enterococcus	Ampicillin and aminoglycoside
Listeria	Ampicillin
Staphylococcus	Nafcillin and oxacillin
(MRSA, MRSE*)	Vancomycin
Enterobacteria (e.g., *E. coli, Klebsiella*)	Ampicillin and aminoglycoside or cefotaxime
Pseudomonas species	Ceftazidime and ticarcillin
Herpes simplex	Acyclovir
Candida species	Amphotericin B

* Methicillin-resistant *Staphylococcus aureus*, methicillin-resistant *Staphylococcus epidermidis*.

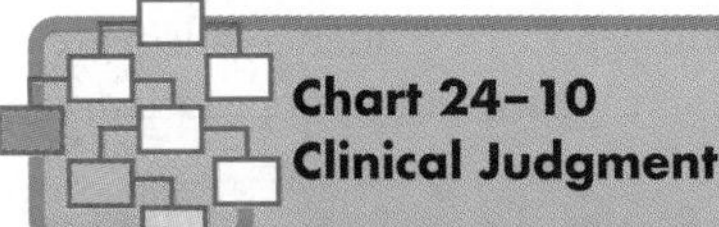

Chart 24–10
Clinical Judgment

Infant with Sepsis

Melissa is a 4-day-old infant who was admitted to the pediatric intensive care unit after an episode of cyanosis and difficulty in breathing. Her mother states that she has not been "doing well." The mother describes Melissa as fussy, irritable, and not nursing well. Admitting vital signs showed tachycardia and tachypnea with grunting and sternal retractions. She was intubated and given mechanical ventilation and a cardiac monitor. Baseline laboratory tests included blood cultures, complete blood count with differential, arterial blood gas, and spinal fluid for cultures and cell counts.

Questions

1. During your assessment, what other information would it be important to have concerning Melissa's present illness?
2. What is the current problem?
3. What is the best way to support the family during this crisis?
4. Why was Melissa having difficulty feeding?
5. What nursing consultations might be considered?

Answers

1. The birth history is always important, along with information concerning other sick family members or siblings. If she was born at your facility, request that the old medical record be sent to the nursing unit.
2. Respiratory distress, behavioral changes, and poor feeding, which are signs of sepsis. Melissa is admitted with a diagnosis of suspected sepsis. The culture results revealed group B streptococcus as the causative organism.
3. Keep the family informed. Explain all tests and procedures. Provide paper and pencils so that the parents can write down questions for the nurses or the physicians. Offer to call the hospital-based clergy for support.
4. Melissa has a respiratory infection resulting in blocked nares and tachypnea. Neonates are obligate nose breathers, and feeding is difficult when they cannot breathe through their nose. To suckle, an infant must coordinate breathing with sucking and swallowing, which is difficult when the infant is tachypneic.
5. Consult a lactation specialist to assist the mother with expression during the current crisis and help with any problems when the infant begins to breast-feed again.

lococcus comes from the Greek word meaning a bunch of grapes. *S. aureus* (coagulase-positive staphylococcus) and *Staphylococcus epidermidis* (coagulase-negative staphylococcus) are normal flora of the skin. It is when the staphylococcus enters normally sterile body fluids that infection results. *S. aureus* can produce toxins that contribute to its virulence. Some toxins can cause skin desquamation (blistering and peeling); others cause toxic shock syndrome (hypotension, skin desquamation, fever, and multiple system involvement).

MRSA is common in hospitals, especially large teaching hospitals and in the community. The major reservoir for MRSA is the lower part of the nose (anterior nares). Hands become contaminated by touching or rubbing the nose. Then health care workers, colonized with MRSA in their noses, spread the organism unwittingly from patient to patient on their hands. Children can easily become colonized with MRSA if they frequently encounter health care workers in inpatient, outpatient, or home settings. Children can also develop MRSA as a result of antibiotic therapy for persistent infections such as chronic otitis media or lung infections.

Because staphylococcus is commonly found on the skin, skin and wound infections of infants and children make up 5% to 44% of these infections (Schutze & Yamauchi, 1996). Indeed, impetigo is a hallmark example of such staphylococcal infections (Fig. 24–3).

Toxic shock syndrome gained national attention in 1989, when women who used superabsorbent tampons became quite ill with fever, vomiting, a desquamating rash, and hypotension (John & Barg, 1996). Later, a toxic shock–like syndrome was observed in nonmenstruating women and children who had one thing in common: positive cultures for *S. aureus*.

Staphylococcus can infect the blood, pulmonary system (pneumonia), bones, joints, skin, and surgical wounds. The major complication of a staphylococcal blood infection is endocarditis. Although it is common in IV drug abusers, children with congenital heart disease can also develop staphylococcal endocarditis. Artificial heart valves, grafts, and patches, which are often used in pediatric heart surgery, can become the foci of staphylococcal lesions. The lesions may break off later to form emboli.

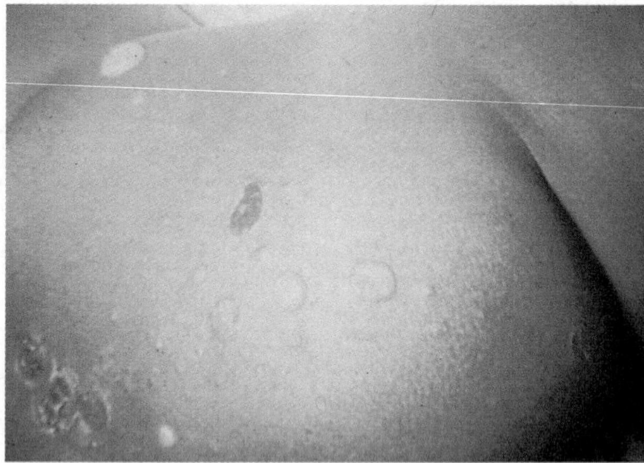

Figure 24–3
In impetigo, small breaks in the skin can evolve to pus-filled abscesses. (Courtesy of the Centers for Disease Control and Prevention.)

Assessment

Species of staphylococcus that produce exfoliating toxins can cause scalded skin syndrome. In this syndrome, bullae form on the skin and evolve into generalized desquamation. The child's skin can be painful to touch, and even the slightest touch can lead to skin peeling.

Bone and joint infections resulting in septic arthritis or osteomyelitis often begin as a blood stream infection. These infections often begin in the metaphyseal portions of the long bones. Symptoms of painful joints, crepitus and heat, may first appear as the child refuses to move a limb. Soft tissue swelling is evident either on physical examination or radiography.

Surgical wound infections and device-related infections produce yellow, foul-smelling pus at the operative site or device insertion site. The wound becomes red, inflamed, and hot to touch. Pus oozes from the suture line, or the nurse can express pus by applying gentle pressure along the sides of the suture line. Areas of fluctuance are often palpable.

Diagnostic Tests. Diagnosis is confirmed by a Gram's stain of the infected body fluids. Cultures determine whether the gram-positive cocci in clusters are coagulase-positive or coagulase-negative staphylococci.

Nursing Diagnoses and Outcomes

Nursing diagnoses and outcomes for the child with an infection are identified in Chart 24–5. Additional nursing diagnoses most commonly associated with staphylococcal infections include:

- **Activity intolerance related to effects of joint pain in septic arthritis**
  Outcome: The child will report or evidence adequate pain control and will participate in age-appropriate activities.
- **Impaired skin integrity related to effects of staphylococcus causing desquamation**
  Outcomes: The child will not develop secondary infection.
  Skin integrity will be restored.

Interdisciplinary Interventions

Most staphylococci are resistant to penicillin. Vancomycin is the drug of choice for serious infections involving multiply drug-resistant strains. However, sensitive strains respond to most antibiotics including oxacillin, nafcillin, methicillin, most cephalosporins, erythromycin, and clindamycin.

Methicillin-resistant *S. aureus* infections are no more virulent than infections with a more sensitive strain. However, the only drug to which many strains of MRSA are sensitive is vancomycin. Typically, MRSA infections may have a slow response to vancomycin therapy simply because methicillin and other antistaphylococcal drugs are more active.

Nursing care for patients with staphylococcal infections should focus on scrupulous hand washing. Staphylococcus is present in the normal flora on the patient's and nurse's skin. Provide wound care wearing gloves. Wear a gown if there is any risk that your uniform, clothing, or scrub clothes may become soiled.

Implement contact precautions for children with MRSA infections or those who are colonized with MRSA. Contact precautions should be continued until antibiotic therapy is discontinued and repeated cultures are negative.

During outbreaks of MRSA infection, cultures may be taken of health care workers' anterior nares, axilla, and groin as part of an epidemiologic work-up. The infection control practitioner can use the results to determine a common source of the outbreak. Individuals found to be positive may undergo decolonization by taking daily showers with chlorhexidine gluconate, applying mupirocin ointment to the anterior nares, or taking oral ciprofloxacin for 10 to 14 days. Some studies show that outbreaks of MRSA in large intensive care units can be controlled using these three measures (Black, Linnemann, Staneck, & Kotagal, 1996).

Tuberculosis

Before 1985, pulmonary tuberculosis (TB) was a disease on the decline (CDC, 1994). However, the rapid rise in acquired immunodeficiency syndrome (AIDS), cutbacks in public health funding, and increased numbers of homeless people and of immigrants from TB-endemic countries contributed to a rise in TB cases in the early 1990s.

Worldview: *In some areas of the world, tuberculosis is an endemic disease. Large percentages of the populations in Africa, Central and South America, Asia and Southeast Asia, and India have been infected. Poverty, poor nutrition, and overcrowded living conditions contribute to high infection rates in these countries.*

The CDC and the Occupational Safety and Health Administration (OSHA) have issued stringent guidelines to prevent TB transmission in health care facilities (CDC, 1994). These guidelines focus on early diagnosis and appropriate isolation of hospitalized patients. With more attention focused on TB, cases began to decline again in 1994.

In the early 1990s, outbreaks of a strain of TB that was resistant to many familiar antitubercular drugs were documented in New York, New Jersey, Atlanta, and Miami (CDC, 1994). Resistant stains of TB continue to be an increasing problem because of patients not finishing all of the TB drugs as ordered and decreased funding for public health clinics used to distribute the TB drugs and monitor patients.

Assessment

In children, TB presents a great diagnostic challenge. Unlike adults, children, especially younger children, are usually asymptomatic when the TB skin test is positive. History of exposure is often the most vital piece of information obtained. Chest radiographs are seldom useful.

Children often manifest tuberculosis in forms other than the traditional pulmonary symptoms (persistent cough that is productive and often bloody, night sweats, weight loss, fatigue, and chest pain). Up to 50% of childhood tuberculosis patients are free of symptoms (Peloquin & Berning, 1995). Notable exceptions include children with HIV infection and infants. Children with HIV infection usually present with fever, weight loss, anorexia, and a cough. In infants, tuberculosis manifests with fever, cough, wheezing, rales, and failure to thrive (Peloquin & Berning, 1995). The first obvious signs and symptoms of tuberculosis after an asymptomatic pulmonary infection may be meningitis, bone infection, and miliary tuberculosis.

TB in children is more likely to result in lymphadenitis (enlarged lymph nodes) than in adults. In infants and some children, the lymph nodes continue to enlarge to the point that bronchial obstruction results (Starke, 1993). Miliary tuberculosis is also more common in childhood tuberculosis. Miliary tuberculosis is a form of extrapulmonary tuberculosis (tuberculosis that occurs outside the lungs). In miliary tuberculosis, massive numbers of tubercle bacilli are released into the blood stream and then disseminate to other organs. Central nervous system involvement, tuberculous meningitis, is a serious and often fatal complication seen almost exclusively in children younger than age 4. TB meningitis usually develops gradually 3 to 6 months after the primary infection. Older children complain of headache, irritability, and insomnia. Infants and younger children lose developmental milestones.

Alert: *An abrupt onset of lethargy, convulsions, and nuchal rigidity precedes the development of hydrocephalus and increasing intracranial pressure. Coma and irregular pulse and respiration may follow, culminating in death. Constantly assess neurologic signs and notify the attending physician of changes.*

Diagnostic Tests. The tuberculin skin test (or Mantoux's test) is the primary method used for determining TB exposure. Intradermal administration of purified protein derivative (PPD) is the most accurate and reliable test method. The skin test must be read in 48 to 72 hours and the reaction (induration) measured. Control tests may be performed at the same time the PPD test is placed. These control skin tests are usually for mumps, *Candida*, or tetanus. Two are chosen and administered on the opposite forearm. Because most children have had exposure to *Candida* in the form of diaper rash and exposure to tetanus and mumps through vaccination, no reaction in the control tests indicates that the child is **anergic**. Anergy means that the immune system is so deficient that it cannot mount a reaction to the skin tests. Thus, TB cannot be ruled out in a child with a negative tuberculin skin test and negative control tests.

Chest radiographs are of little diagnostic value because they usually appear normal. Children also have great difficulty in producing sufficient sputum and coughing productively. They often swallow their secretions. Trying to obtain a sputum specimen for an acid-fast bacteriologic culture and smear from a young child may be difficult. Often, gastric washings, in place of sputum samples, and stool specimens are used. The tubercle bacilli pass through the digestive system completely intact and unharmed by stomach acid and other digestive processes. Hence, sputum smears may be negative for tuberculosis, but gastric washings or a stool culture will be positive.

The standard for diagnosis is still a positive culture for *Mycobacterium tuberculosis*. Acid-fast smears are helpful but cannot be specific for *M. tuberculosis*.

Interdisciplinary Interventions

Because *M. tuberculosis* takes up to 6 weeks to grow in the laboratory, therapy is started on the basis of a positive smear or strong clinical evidence of pulmonary, meningeal, or extrapulmonary infection. Standard drug therapy consists of isoniazid, rifampin, and pyrazinamide

Table 24–5
Common Pediatric Dosages for Antitubercular Drugs

Drug	Route	Dose (mg/kg)	Nursing Interventions
Isoniazid (INH)	PO, daily	10–15	Potential liver toxicity—monitor liver function tests, watch for jaundice.
Rifampin (Rif)	PO, daily	10–20	Orange discoloration of secretions or urine. Could stain contact lenses. Teach parents about discoloration.
Pyrazinamide (PZA)	PO, daily	20–40	Potential liver toxicity. Monitor liver function tests.
Streptomycin	IM	20–40	Usually given only in meningitis because of ototoxicity. Conduct hearing screens at initiation of therapy, midway, and at the end of therapy. Observe for skin rashes.
Ethambutol (EMB)	PO, daily	15–25	Use for older children only. Can cause reversible optic neuritis. Check visual acuity, visual fields, and red-green color discrimination daily.

given for 2 months, followed by isoniazid and rifampin for 4 months (Table 24–5). However, specific drug therapy is based on the organism's drug sensitivity.

Preventive therapy is given to children with positive skin tests (PPD) and no clinical evidence of disease. It consists of isoniazid for 9 months. For children with HIV infection, preventive therapy may be extended to 12 months. Rifampin is given as preventive therapy in known cases of exposure to multiply drug-resistant TB.

Nursing care of children with known or suspected pulmonary tuberculosis must be individualized (Fig. 24–4). Because young children are often asymptomatic, their relative infectiousness is variable. If hospitalized, most children do not need airborne precautions in a negative-pressure isolation room. Infants and small children with pulmonary tuberculosis rarely cough up phlegm. What little sputum they do manage to cough up has few tubercle bacilli. This is because their cavitary lung lesions have few bacilli. As these cavitary lesions break open, few or no bacilli escape into the bronchi to be coughed up.

As children mature, especially into adolescents, the ability to cough and infect others increases (Starke, 1993). Place adolescents and children with positive sputum smears in negative air pressure rooms (in which air flows into the room from the hallway and is exhausted by a separate, filtered exhaust to the outside). Wear an N95 respirator or a high-efficiency particulate air (HEPA) respirator before entering the room.

Frequently, the TB source for the child is a parent or close relative. Thus, the child may not pose an isolation risk, but the parents or visitors may. Refer infected relatives to the local health department (Chart 24–11) for testing and treatment.

Children need their parents, especially when they are ill and in the strange surroundings of a hospital. Parents or close relatives with pulmonary TB can wear a mask to and from the isolation room when visiting. Other accommodating strategies can also be arranged, including having food trays for the parents delivered to the child's room.

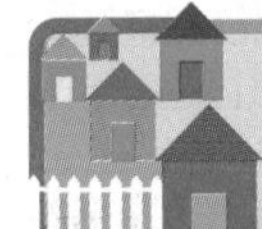

Chart 24–11
Community Care

Tuberculosis Follow-up

The attending physician, diagnosing laboratory, and treating institution (clinic, hospital, or private physician's office) are legally responsible for informing the local health department of all cases of tuberculosis. The local health department then initiates contact investigations. Contacts are persons exposed to the child with pulmonary tuberculosis and could be in many locations, such as church, school, or daycare center. The health department:

- Determines who in the community has been exposed to the child.
- Performs screening tests (skin tests) on exposed individuals, such as family members, neighbors, and schoolmates.
- Provides preventive drug therapy (isoniazid).
- Provides drug treatment and follow-up laboratory work and radiographs.
- Provides for directly observed therapy to families who may be noncompliant because of homelessness, parental drug abuse, or other reason.
- Assists with arranging temporary placement in halfway housing or other state-run facilities.

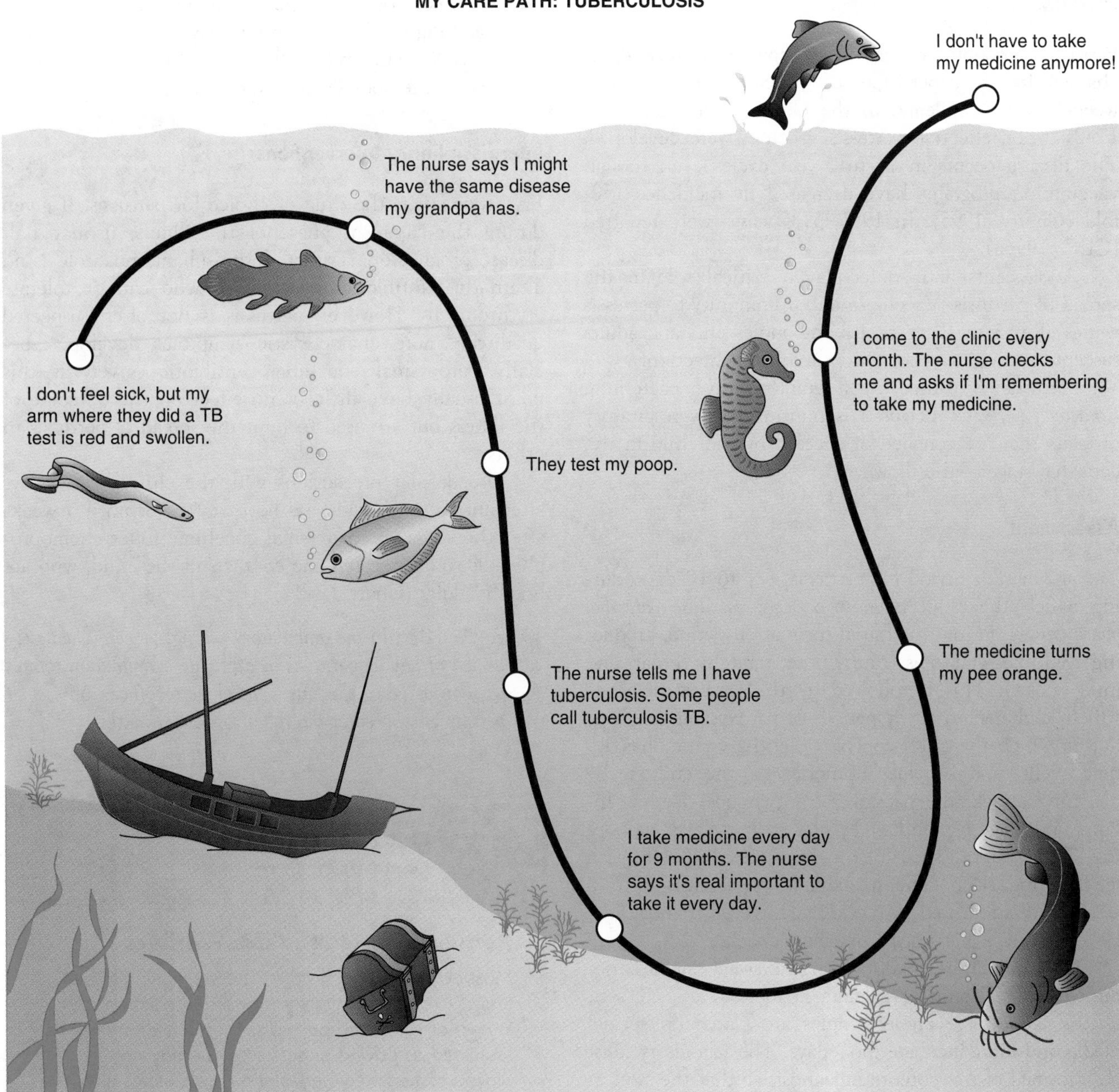

Figure 24–4
A care path for a child with tuberculosis.

Community Care

Long-term follow-up of the child with TB is particularly important because of the potential for noncompliance in completing the typically lengthy treatment regimen. Strains of TB that are resistant to common antitubercular drugs arise as a result of partial treatment. Patients should be monitored by the community health nurse for the presence of drug side effects and compliance with therapy. If noncompliance is an issue, directly observed therapy may need to be implemented, where the medication is taken in the presence of the nurse.

Nutritional status should also be assessed and diet counseling given if needed to prevent poor healing due to inadequate nutrition affecting immune function. Social services may be involved if poor intake is related to inadequate finances.

Pertussis

Pertussis (whooping cough) is an upper respiratory illness characterized by a persistent cough (lasting more than 2 weeks). It was endemic in the United States until the 1940s, when effective pertussis vaccines were developed. The disease occurs in 2- to 5-year cycles even though vaccination programs have decreased its incidence 150-fold (Cherry, 1995). In 1995, 5137 cases were reported (CDC, 1996a).

Adolescents and adults play a critical role in the spread of pertussis. Vaccine-induced immunity to pertussis wanes after 5 to 10 years, leaving adolescents and adults susceptible and an important reservoir for infection.

Pertussis is caused by a gram-negative bacterium, *Bordetella pertussis*. Pertussis is transmitted by respiratory droplets that are coughed or sneezed by the child in the catarrhal stage of the illness.

Assessment

The incubation period for pertussis is 7 to 10 days, during which the child is most contagious. The *catarrhal phase* occurs during this initial incubation period, producing cold-like symptoms (runny nose, scratchy throat, and mild cough). This is followed by the *paroxysmal phase*, which is characterized by periods of paroxysmal coughing during which the child coughs violently, vomits, has apneic spells, and becomes cyanotic. At the end of the coughing attack, the patient gasps (whoops) for air. Infants under age 6 months may not exhibit classic whooping. These intense spells of coughing often interfere with feeding and sleep. The paroxysmal phase lasts 2 to 6 weeks and is followed by a *convalescent stage* characterized by a persistent (but not paroxysmal) cough.

Diagnostic Tests. Nasopharyngeal swab samples, obtained using Dacron or calcium alginate swabs, are sent to the laboratory. These samples are plated on special media and must incubate for 7 days. The laboratory must be informed of the potential diagnosis so that the swab is appropriately handled. A positive culture is diagnostic for pertussis, but the organism is not likely to grow if obtained 3 weeks or longer after the onset of coughing or if antibiotics have already been started.

Nursing Diagnoses and Outcomes

Common nursing diagnoses and outcomes for the child with an infection are identified in Chart 24–5. Additional diagnoses for infants with pertussis may include the following:

- **Altered tissue perfusion: cardiopulmonary and cerebral related to prolonged coughing attacks**
  Outcome: The child will maintain adequate tissue perfusion and oxygenation.
- **Sleep pattern disturbance related to effects of coughing spells interrupting rest**
  Outcome: The child will obtain adequate sleep and resume previous sleep patterns.

Interdisciplinary Interventions

Erythromycin is the drug of choice for pertussis. If given during the catarrhal phase of the illness, it may halt disease progression. Trimethoprim-sulfamethoxazole is an alternative antibiotic for children who cannot tolerate erythromycin. However, pertussis is not often suspected until the more characteristic symptoms develop, especially paroxysmal coughing. Antibiotics given at this point usually have little or no effect on the outcome of the illness but are used to limit the spread of pertussis to others.

Use droplet precautions with the child until 5 days after antibiotic therapy has been started or until 3 weeks after the onset of paroxysmal coughing. Offer chemoprophylaxis to all nonimmune contacts of the child, who are usually adults (Chart 24–12).

caREminder: *In the ambulatory setting, place a child suspected of having pertussis in a private examination room as soon as he or she enters the clinic or office. Advise personnel who enter the room to wear a mask.*

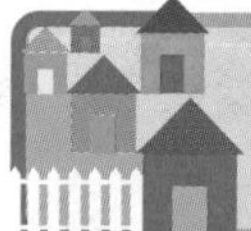

Chart 24–12
Community Care

Pertussis in Health Care Workers

Most adolescents and adults are susceptible to pertussis. They are frequently exposed to children with known or suspected pertussis. These children may be identified as having pertussis late or may not be placed immediately on isolation precautions, thus exposing health care workers who may be susceptible. The CDC recommends the following measures:

- Health care workers exposed to known or suspected pertussis should receive erythromycin prophylaxis (40 to 60 mg/kg per day) in four doses for 14 days.
- Health care workers with unexplained rhinitis and persistent cough should report to the occupational health clinic for evaluation. If these workers have pertussis, they should be removed from patient care activities. They may return to work after 7 days of antibiotic therapy.
- Erythromycin-intolerant health care workers may take trimethoprim-sulfamethoxazole as an alternative.

During the paroxysmal phase, the child can have up to 20 coughing attacks a day and may vomit after the attacks. Avoid stimulating the child, which may precipitate a coughing paroxysm. Maintain a calm manner while supporting the child and parents during coughing paroxysms, which are quite frightening. Such coughing also disturbs sleep and nutrition. Nursing care should focus on keeping the child adequately hydrated and nourished and alleviating coughing episodes with antitussives. Gentle suctioning after coughing may be needed to maintain a patent airway. Maintenance of ventilatory support by the nursing staff and the respiratory care staff is a priority (see Chapter 16).

Pneumococcal Disease

Incidence

Pneumococcal infections are common in the extremes of life (very young and very old). Because pneumococcal disease is not normally reported to the health department, the CDC can only estimate disease occurrence on the basis of several sentinel states. The CDC has estimated that in 1995, pneumococcus was responsible for 7 million cases of otitis media, 500,000 cases of pneumonia, 50,000 cases of sepsis, and 3000 cases of meningitis.

Pathophysiology

Streptococcus pneumoniae is a gram-positive diplococcus commonly found in the upper respiratory tract of many asymptomatic persons. If the organism itself is protected by a capsule, it is virulent. Pneumococci without capsules are not virulent.

Many children and adults are colonized with pneumococcus in the upper respiratory tract. Transmission is person to person by respiratory droplets. The progression from pneumococcal colonization to invasive disease is multifactorial. Preceding viral infections lower resistance to disease and may contribute to invasive disease. Agents and diseases that decrease the normal self-cleaning functions of the respiratory system, such as bronchial obstruction, irritants, or allergens that decrease ciliary function, can also push colonization toward invasive disease. Errors in immune response in such conditions as AIDS, splenectomy, agammaglobulinemia, leukemia, and sickle cell disease inhibit the body's natural defenses and lead to invasive disease (Table 24–6). Epidemics of pneumococcal pneumonia occur most frequently in the winter in overcrowded situations. Finally, infants have immature immune systems and thus are prone to develop invasive disease.

Pneumococcal meningitis usually results from the bacteria crossing the blood-brain barrier into the central nervous system and seeding the meninges. This may happen as the result of trauma, such as a basilar skull fracture with a slow CSF leak, or by direct extension from a pneumococcal infection in the mastoid or paranasal sinuses to the meninges.

Pneumococcal disease occurs in many forms, including meningitis, sinusitis, otitis media, occult bacteremia, and pneumonia. Because pneumococci commonly colonize the upper respiratory tract, pneumonia, otitis media,

Table 24–6
Risk for Pneumococcal Disease Associated with Altered Immune Function

Immune Defect	Reason for Increased Risk	Interventions
Immature immune system (premature infant or term neonate) response	Decreased phagocytic activity Varying levels of protective maternal antibodies (IgG) Decreased response to polysaccharide antigen	Antibiotic therapy Proper nutrition to increase infant's response to infection Hand washing in hospitals, clinics, daycare centers, and other child care settings
Asplenic infants, children, adolescents	Diminished or absent neutrophil function	Pneumococcal vaccine for children of age 2 yr and older Daily prophylaxis with oral penicillin until adulthood
Acquired or congenital immunodeficiency (such as in HIV infection or agammaglobulinemia)	Dysfunctional immune system Increased respiratory infections	Antibiotic therapy Pneumococcal vaccine in children older than 2 yr
Sickle cell disease	Decreased immune function related to functional asplenia	Daily prophylaxis with oral penicillin starting at age 4 mo Pneumococcal vaccine

sinusitis, and mastoiditis are a direct result of this colonization.

Assessment

Pneumococcal pneumonia often occurs abruptly with the child exhibiting a temperature of 102° to 103°F, chills, productive cough, and otitis media. Rales are heard on auscultation of the lungs, and there is dullness to percussion. Assess sinuses by pressing the fingers along the sinus tracts of the face and ask the child if the pressure is painful.

Children with bacteremia or meningitis may exhibit a fever and irritability. In cases of meningitis, neck stiffness, or nuchal rigidity, may occur.

caREminder: *Ask the child to try to touch the chin to the chest. If pain prevents the child from doing this, it may be from nuchal rigidity caused by inflamed meninges.*

Diagnostic Tests. In pneumococcal pneumonia, chest radiographs reveal subsegmental lobar consolidation. Bacteriologic cultures of blood, spinal fluid, and other body fluids are commonly collected to reveal pneumococcus. These body fluids are usually Gram stained. Elevated white blood cell counts are helpful in assisting with the diagnosis but are not conclusive. Counterimmunoelectrophoresis or rapid antigen tests can detect pneumococcal capsular antigen in urine, spinal fluid, pleural fluid, and blood. These tests are of great value if the child has been pretreated with an antibiotic. However, a negative rapid antigen test does not preclude pneumococcal disease.

Nursing Diagnoses and Outcomes

Common nursing diagnoses and outcomes for the child experiencing an infection are listed in Chart 24–5. The following may also be applicable for a child with pneumococcal disease:

- **Ineffective airway clearance related to effects of excessive mucus production**
  Outcome: The child will maintain a patent airway.

Interdisciplinary Interventions

The drug of choice is penicillin. Because of increasingly resistant pneumococcal strains, vancomycin or chloramphenicol may be used as an alternative for treatment of serious infections, such as meningitis or bacteremia. Erythromycin and trimethoprim-sulfamethoxazole are effective alternative antibiotics for mild to moderate infections, such as otitis media. Extended-spectrum cephalosporins such as cefotaxime and ceftriaxone are also useful, especially in cases of penicillin allergy.

Children with pneumococcal pneumonia need to be isolated only if the organism is penicillin resistant (Gar-

Table 24–7
Types of Streptococcal Infections

Infection	Clinical Manifestations	Complications
Streptococcal pharyngitis	Sore throat, malaise, fever, enlarged tonsils studded with gray-white exudate, enlarged lymph nodes	Peritonsillar abscess Scarlet fever Rheumatic fever Damage to mitral valve that may necessitate replacement in midlife
Erysipelas	Red, edematous, warm, raised lesions with sharply demarcated margins Edema that advances rapidly	Bullae that leave open weeping lesions that can develop secondary infection
Streptococcal impetigo	Fragile vesicles that evolve into pustules Pustules that enlarge and erode	Secondary bacterial infection Streptococcal toxic shock Glomerulonephritis
Streptococcal cellulitis	Warm, erythematous, painful, edematous lesion with ill-defined margins that rapidly spreads History of trauma, varicella lesions, burns, or surgery	Invasion of lymph nodes and blood stream Streptococcal toxic shock
Necrotizing fasciitis (invasive group A streptococcal disease)	Within 24 hr of trauma, site swelling and cellulitis that spreads to surrounding tissue Deep infection of subcutaneous tissue that destroys fascia and fat Frank gangrene that develops by 4–5 days	Life-threatening infection Need for surgical drainage or amputation

ner & HICPAC, 1996). Contact precautions should be used until cultures are negative and antibiotic therapy is complete.

Prevention of pneumococcal disease has two mainstays. The first regimen offers prophylactic low-dose antibiotic therapy to high-risk patients. High-risk patients are those with an underlying disease that would predispose them to invasive disease, such as leukemia, AIDS, or sickle cell disease. Otherwise, a pneumococcal vaccine is available for children who are age 2 or older. Children younger than 2 years do not respond to the vaccine. Refer to the specific disease forms caused by pneumococcus for other nursing care (e.g., otitis media; see Chapter 28).

Group A Streptococcal Disease

Etiology and Incidence

Group A streptococcal disease is probably one of the most common diseases of childhood (streptococcal pharyngitis). Because it is so common and not reportable to the health department, it is impossible to estimate the true incidence of the disease. The organism inhabits the upper respiratory tract in 15% to 30% of asymptomatic children. Pharyngitis is spread primarily through droplets as the infected child coughs or sneezes. Food can be a vehicle of transmission if handled by an individual who is infected or colonized with group A streptococci (Farley et al., 1993). In daycare centers and nursery schools, hand-to-hand-to-mouth transmission may occur, especially among toddlers. The incubation period is 2 to 5 days.

Group A streptococcus produces various disorders including pharyngitis, pneumonia, scarlet fever, tonsillitis, erysipelas (a superficial cellulitis), toxic shock–like syndrome, acute glomerulonephritis, rheumatic fever, and invasive disease (Table 24–7).

Before the antibiotic era, scarlet fever, rheumatic fever, and glomerulonephritis were common complications of group A streptococcal disease. The incidence of all three complications has decreased since World War II. They are now relatively preventable with appropriate antibiotic therapy. Rheumatic fever typically occurs a week after the onset of pharyngitis with the development of fever, polyarthritis, and carditis. Nephritis is more common after streptococcal skin infections than after pharyngitis. Long-term renal disease is seldom seen in children as a sequel. Invasive group A streptococci have received media attention as "flesh-eating" bacteria. However, they have existed for decades but have not received much publicity. Approximately 10,000 to 15,000 cases of invasive group A streptococcal disease occur in the United States each year, with 2000 to 3000 deaths (CDC/NCID Focus, 1995). The severity of the illness is determined in part by the susceptibility of the host and the serotype of group A streptococci.

Assessment

Tonsillitis is scarlet fever without a rash, because the same symptoms characterize both disease entities except for the rash. The nurse should look for fever, malaise, and a sore throat. Lymph nodes in the neck are palpable. The tongue at first appears white, then within 2 days becomes red (strawberry tongue). The rash of scarlet fever appears 12 hours after onset of the disease. It has been compared to a "sunburn with goose pimples" (Kaplan & Krugman, 1992). The rash follows an ordered progression (Fig. 24–5).

Invasive group A streptococcal disease begins as a mild infection such as strep throat and progresses to a severe illness characterized by bacteremia (blood infection), toxic shock–like syndrome, multisystem organ failure, a rapid drop in blood pressure, and necrotizing fasciitis that destroys fat and underlying tissue. It may lead to death.

Figure 24–5
Progression of rash in scarlet fever. Scarlet fever begins with flushed cheeks, a white-coated tongue, and a central rash. By the third day, the rash becomes more generalized, with increased density in the groin and axilla. (Courtesy of the Centers for Disease Control and Prevention.)

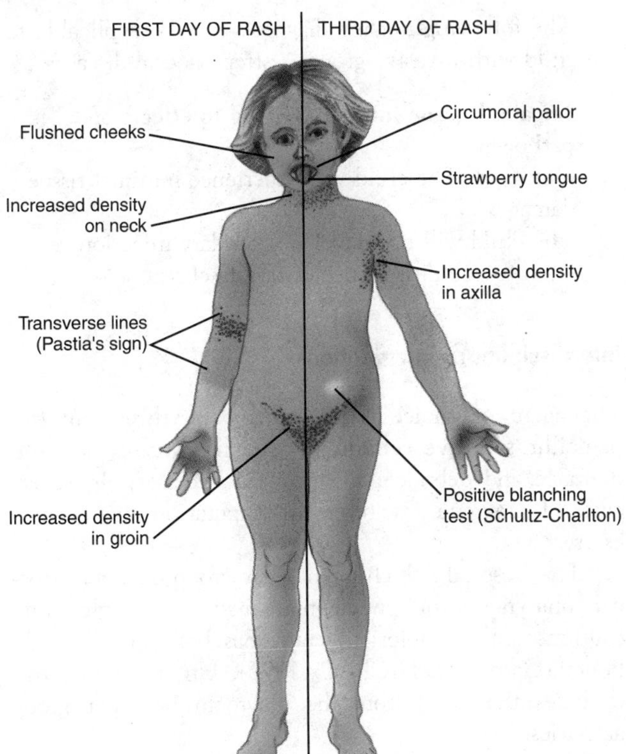

Diagnostic Tests. A positive throat culture for group A streptococcus makes the definitive diagnosis for streptococcal pharyngitis. However, rapid antigen tests have proved useful in diagnosing patients quickly in order to begin antibiotic therapy. Because these tests are not as sensitive as a throat culture, a negative test must be confirmed by a culture.

Common serologic tests used for diagnosis include antistreptolysin-O (ASO) and a latex agglutination test (Streptozyme). These serologic tests are frequently used to diagnose rheumatic fever. The nurse expects a positive result if group A streptococcus is present.

Skin infections are usually diagnosed by skin or wound cultures. Invasive group A streptococcal infections are diagnosed by positive cultures of CSF or synovial, peritoneal, or pleural fluid. Tissue biopsies may be performed in cases of suspected gangrene.

Nursing Diagnoses and Outcomes

In addition to the common nursing diagnoses and outcomes listed in Chart 24–5, the following may be applicable to the child with group A streptococcal pharyngitis:

- **Impaired swallowing related to painful sore throat**
  Outcomes: The child will experience minimal throat pain.
  The child will maintain adequate fluid and nutritional intake.

The following nursing diagnosis may be applicable to the child with invasive group A streptococcal disease:

- **Impaired tissue integrity related to effects of pathogen**
  Outcomes: The child will experience minimal tissue damage.
  The child will not develop secondary infection related to cellulitis or necrotizing fasciitis.

Interdisciplinary Interventions

The agent of choice is penicillin or erythromycin (for penicillin-sensitive children). In necrotizing fasciitis, drainage and débridement are often necessary. In severe cases of gangrene, fasciotomy or amputation may be necessary.

For hospitalized children with group A streptococcal pharyngitis or pneumonia, maintain droplet precautions until antibiotic therapy has been given for 24 hours (Garner & HICPAC, 1996). Unfortunately, this excludes the child from the playroom or other group activities.

Community Care

Nurses should advise parents of nonhospitalized children with group A pharyngitis to exclude the child from daycare or school until after 24 hours of effective therapy.

caREminder: *Instruct parents to discard the toothbrush of the child with group A pharyngitis. The organism can survive on the toothbrush and is a source of reinfection to the child after antibiotic therapy is completed.*

Observe strict hand washing between patients and adhere to aseptic techniques to prevent nosocomial spread of infection. In outbreaks, cohort (group) the patients with group A streptococcal infection. Have the same nurse or nurses care for only the infected patients.

Gastroenteritis

Second only to upper respiratory tract infections, acute gastroenteritis causes significant illness in children worldwide (Committee on Infectious Diseases, American Academy of Pediatrics, 1994). It is caused by gastrointestinal irritants, such as bacteria, viruses, and toxins produced by fish, mushrooms, and chemicals (food additives). Infants are particularly vulnerable to gastroenteritis and the dehydration it causes. Death claims 15% of affected children in developing countries (Committee on Infectious Diseases, American Academy of Pediatrics, 1994).

Life-threatening gastroenteritis seldom occurs in the United States. Outbreaks of gastroenteritis occur in daycare centers, schools, institutions for the handicapped, and other places where overcrowding is prevalent and hygiene is inadequate. Food-borne outbreaks occur fairly regularly. Nosocomial gastroenteritis involves two main organisms: rotavirus and *Clostridium difficile*. Both organisms can linger in the environment for a long time and can be easily transmitted from child to child on the unwashed hands of health care workers. The microorganisms and food-borne agents associated with gastroenteritis are summarized in Table 24–8.

Pathophysiology

Microbes that cause gastroenteritis are transmitted by the fecal-oral route. Hands are contaminated with stool by not washing them after toileting or changing an infant's diapers. These contaminated hands are then placed directly into the mouth or on foods. Then the contaminated food is consumed. The bacteria or viruses either remain unchanged in the food or continue to grow and multiply, possibly producing toxins.

Table 24–8
Causes of Gastroenteritis

Microorganisms		
Bacteria	**Viruses**	**Parasites**
Campylobacter	Adenovirus	*Cryptosporidium*
Clostridium difficile	Astrovirus	*Entamoeba histolytica*
Clostridium perfringens	Calcivirus	*Giardia lamblia*
E. coli (four types)	Norwalk virus	*Isospora*
Salmonella		
Shigella		
Staphylococcus aureus		
Vibrio cholerae		
Yersinia		
Nonmicrobial Food-Borne Agents		
Agent	**Food**	
Anatoxin	Poisonous mushrooms *(Amanita phalloides)*	
Ciguatera fish neurotoxin	Barracuda, snapper, amberjack, grouper, oysters, mollusks	
Histamine—scombroid (fish)	Tuna, mackerel, bonito, mahi-mahi	
Monosodium glutamate	Chinese food	

Assessment

Typical signs and symptoms include diarrhea, nausea, vomiting, and abdominal pain. However, specific findings vary with the causative organism. For example, some organisms produce watery diarrhea; others produce bloody diarrhea. Fever, nausea, and vomiting may be present with some and missing with others. Signs and symptoms may also vary with the organism.

Diagnostic Tests. Examination of the stool both physically (noting color, consistency, odor, and volume) and microscopically (leukocytes, ova or parasites, culture) is essential. Fresh stool is sent to the laboratory for culture. The laboratory plates the stool on differential and selective media that inhibit the growth of normal bowel flora while allowing the pathogenic bacteria to grow. The laboratory reports positive culture results for *Salmonella*, *Shigella*, *Campylobacter*, or hemorrhagic *Escherichia coli*. Other tests include enzyme immunoassay for *C. difficile* toxins and rotavirus as well as neutralizing antibody for other viral agents. Some laboratories can use DNA probes and polymerase chain reaction for certain organisms.

Nursing Diagnoses and Outcomes

In addition to the common nursing diagnoses and outcomes listed in Chart 24–5, the following may be applicable to the child with gastroenteritis:

- **Fluid volume deficit related to effects of diarrhea**
  Outcome: The child will maintain adequate intravascular fluid volume and tissue perfusion.
- **Risk for impaired skin integrity related to effects of liquid stool on skin**
  Outcome: The child will maintain skin integrity.

Interdisciplinary Interventions

Treatment consists of rehydration and correcting any electrolyte imbalances. Antibiotic therapy depends on the severity of the illness. Often, antibiotics do not alter the course of the illness significantly and contribute to the development of resistant strains. However, they may be useful for life-threatening infections.

Assess and monitor the child for signs of fluid and electrolyte imbalance (see Chapter 17 for an in-depth discussion of assessment and treatment). Oral rehydration therapy (ORT) is the method of choice for treatment of children with gastroenteritis who are dehydrated. ORT does not necessitate hospitalization, so it is advantageous in reducing this threat to family cohesion. The parents need detailed teaching about how to implement ORT: what fluid to use, how long to continue, how to advance the child's diet, signs of worsening status in the child, and when to notify the health care provider. If the child is severely dehydrated, hospitalization may be necessary for IV hydration (Care Path 24–1). Observe standard precautions by wearing gloves when handling stool or stool-contaminated items.

Diarrheal stools are irritating to the perianal area. Instruct the older child to wipe gently but thoroughly. If the area is excoriated, use moist towelettes. If not toilet trained, children should have their diapers changed as soon as possible after stooling. Wash with a moist cloth and apply a thick layer of petroleum jelly or zinc oxide ointment.

Community Care

Because 30% to 100% of randomly checked poultry at processing plants are positive for *Campylobacter* and *Salmonella,* teach parents and others to wash their hands and cooking implements thoroughly after handling poultry. Often, daycare centers are sources of outbreaks for *Campylobacter*, *Salmonella*, and rotaviral gastroenteritis. Again, teach effective hand washing, especially after diapering infants. Emphasize that food preparation areas and diaper changing areas should be separated. Serve as a liaison between the daycare center and the parents by providing accurate information. Advise parents to keep infants not yet toilet trained out of the daycare center until diarrhea stops.

Food-borne outbreaks of gastroenteritis should be reported to the local health department to prevent further cases of food poisoning.

Infantile Botulism

Infantile botulism results after an infant, usually younger than 6 months, ingests vegetative cells or spores of *Clostridium botulinum*. The spores are found in honey and various fruits and vegetables. When the infant ingests the spores, the bacteria multiply in the child's intestine, producing the botulinum toxin. Infantile botulism is not transmissible from person to person.

Assessment

The parents may report feeding the infant honey. The infant is constipated for 3 days or longer. This is followed by lethargy, floppiness, poor head control, poor sucking, and slow feeding. Because the suck reflex is diminished, oral secretions pool and swallowing is difficult. Physical findings are summarized in Chart 24–13. The infant may exhibit a descending paralysis that could lead to respiratory failure. Respiratory arrest has been observed in infants with this infection, prompting many physicians to hospitalize the infant in an intensive care unit for possible intubation. Because symptoms are general and infants cannot verbalize, the diagnosis of infantile botulism may be missed. Many infants are admitted for suspected sepsis. A high index of suspicion must be maintained, particularly with a history of constipation followed by the other symptoms.

Diagnostic Tests. In infected infants, stool cultures may grow *C. botulinum*. Serum may show toxins. Either positive result confirms infantile botulism.

Nursing Diagnoses and Outcomes

In addition to the common nursing diagnoses and outcomes listed in Chart 24–5, nursing diagnoses for infant botulism may include:

- **Impaired gas exchange related to effects of botulism toxin**
  Outcome: The infant will maintain adequate gas exchange and oxygenation, either spontaneously or via assisted ventilation.
- **Constipation related to the effects of the botulism toxin (descending paralysis)**
  Outcomes: The infant will be assisted to evacuate his or her bowels.
  The infant will resume a normal bowel elimination pattern.

Interdisciplinary Interventions

For infantile botulism, antibiotics are not useful. However, penicillin is sometimes given to eradicate the organism from the intestinal tract.

Chart 24–13

Physical Findings in Infantile Botulism

Constipation	Ptosis (eyelid)
Poor sucking	Ophthalmoplegia
Slow feeding	Shallow respirations
Decreased gag reflex	Facial paresis
Lethargy and weakness	Decreased deep tendon reflexes
Floppiness (hypotonia)	Weak cry
Loss of head control	
Pupillary dilation	

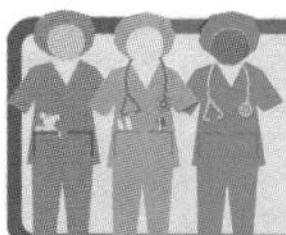

Care Path 24-1 An Interdisciplinary Plan of Care for the Child with Gastroenteritis

Nursing Diagnosis	**Patient/Family Intermediate Outcomes**			
	Day: Admission	**Day 1**	**Day 2**	**Day 3**
Fluid volume deficit related to excessive output, inadequate intake	The child will maintain adequate fluid intake and output. The family will express adequate understanding of the treatment plan.	The child will maintain body weight within normal parameters. The child will tolerate oral fluid intake.	⟶ ⟶	The child will tolerate a solid diet. The family will demonstrate the ability to meet the child's care needs.
Impaired skin integrity related to excoriation caused by diarrhea	The child will maintain intact skin in the perianal area.	The child will exhibit improvement in excoriation with the use of a drying agent such as zinc oxide.	The family will demonstrate the ability to assess for excoriation and apply a drying agent.	The child will exhibit intact skin integrity. The family will demonstrate proper skin care measures.
Risk for infection (for siblings) related to exposure	The family will express adequate understanding of standard infection precautions.	The family will demonstrate proper hand washing technique.	The family will demonstrate proper laundry practices and diaper disposal techniques.	
Care Intervention Categories				
Consults	Consult with the referring physician for assessment findings, treatment plan, and specific infection control measures.	Consult with infection control to report pathogens to health department.	Send water and/or formula samples to health department, as requested.	
Labs	Obtain SMA6 (Sequential Multiple Analyzer, six tests), BUN, complete blood count (CBC) with differential, platelet count, creatinine clearance, urinalysis with microscopic stool for fecal leukocytes, urine culture, stool culture, blood culture. Consider testing stool for ova and parasites and a viral work-up.	Monitor laboratory results.		

Care Path continued on following page

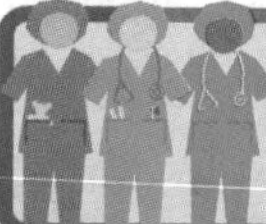

Care Path 24–1 An Interdisciplinary Plan of Care for the Child with Gastroenteritis *Continued*

Care Intervention Categories	Day: Admission	Day 1	Day 2	Day 3
Medications and IVs	Administer IV fluids: $D_5W\frac{1}{4}NS$ until laboratory data are available. Consider administering potassium when appropriate.	Decrease the IV infusion rate as the child's oral fluid intake increases.		Discontinue IV fluid administration.
Nutrition	Keep the child with nothing by mouth (NPO) if he or she is unable to tolerate oral fluids. Consider oral rehydration.	Reintroduce oral fluids as tolerated. Give an infant an oral electrolyte solution and/or breast milk or formula.	Slowly advance oral intake as tolerated.	Advance diet as tolerated; specify diet.
Safety and activity	Impose strict hand washing by all care workers. Keep the child in his or her room until diarrhea subsides. Allow only washable toys.			
Teaching/ discharge planning	Provide family teaching about hospital and unit policies, the etiology of diarrhea, and the treatment plan.		Teach family signs of dehydration and early treatment to decrease severity. Review dietary restrictions.	Schedule follow-up appointment with physician.
Vital signs/ baseline parameters	Assess vital signs every 4–8 hours. Monitor daily weight and intake and output. Check stool for blood, mucus, and parasites.			Discharge when · Signs of adequate hydration · Tolerating oral intake

Alert: *Avoid aminoglycosides in infants with botulism. These drugs tend to exacerbate the effects of the toxin.*

A human-derived botulinum antitoxin (botulism immune globulin) is undergoing clinical trials in California as part of the Infant Botulism Prevention Program.

Infants may be prophylactically intubated to support respiratory effort and prevent aspiration.

Nursing care includes meticulous respiratory and nutritional support. This disease has an extremely long recovery period, which varies with each infant. The family often needs emotional support to help them through this prolonged period.

Proper positioning supports airway patency and respiratory mechanics. The infant should be placed supine on a rigid crib or bed with the head elevated to 30 degrees.

caREminder: *Because the child is hypotonic, ensure that the child does not slouch into a position in which the thorax is resting on the abdomen. This position limits diaphragmatic excursion and compromises respiratory effort.*

Place a small cloth roll under the neck to facilitate drainage of secretions away from the airway. Suctioning pooled secretions should be done if needed. Standard care protocols should be followed if the child requires mechanical ventilation.

Because the infant is hypotonic, sucking and swallowing may be difficult and the child is prone to aspiration. Tube feeding is preferable to parenteral alimentation because using the gut stimulates peristalsis. Feeding should be done via nasogastric or nasojejunal tube until the infant demonstrates sufficient strength and coordination for adequate nutrient ingestion. Breast milk is the preferred food because of its immunologic components (e.g., immunoglobulin A [IgA], leukocytes).

Stool and urine output patterns must be monitored. Stool softeners are often helpful for the constipation that is present. Gentle suprapubic pressure may be needed to assist with bladder emptying.

Community Care

Referrals for physical therapy help the infant maintain any remaining muscle tone and regain the strength that is lost. The physical therapist can teach the parents or other caregivers how to perform the various muscle strengthening exercises.

Respiratory therapists can help the nursing staff and parents maintain adequate airway clearance through various nebulizer therapies and percussion therapies. The therapist can instruct the parents on how to perform chest percussion. The respiratory therapist is also a key team member if the infant requires mechanical ventilation.

Evaluation of nutritional needs by a dietitian and methods for meeting these needs can be of great value. The dietitian should instruct parents to avoid giving honey to children younger than 12 months.

Tick-Borne Infections

Many organisms produce tick-borne infections in humans. Most organisms belong to the Rickettsiaceae family of bacteria. Because Rocky Mountain spotted fever (RMSF), ehrlichiosis, and Lyme disease are the most common tick-borne infections, they are described in detail in this section. The incidence of tick-borne disease follows the seasonal pattern of tick exposures: incidence is generally highest in the spring and summer. Most cases of tick-borne infections occur in children between ages 2 and 15. This is generally due to the fact that children play outdoors in tick-infested areas. Most ticks live in grasses and plants, especially in heavily wooded areas. As a child brushes past the grass or plant, the tick crawls onto the child and attaches. Unattached ticks on a family pet may climb onto the child who is playing with or grooming the animal.

Not every tick is infected. The total number of organisms in a tick varies. The severity of the resulting disease is dose related. As the tick ingests blood, the warmth of that blood activates the bacteria. After the tick feeds for 6 to 10 hours, the organisms are released from the tick's salivary glands.

Assessment

In all three of these tick-borne diseases, the child may present with fever, headache, and malaise.

The rickettsiae in the spotted fever group of diseases cause a vasculitis that involves the skin (as a rash) and major organ systems. This rash begins on the sixth day of illness, typically on the wrists and ankles, and spreads within hours to the trunk (Fig. 24–6). With prompt treatment, complications are rare. However, untreated cases with high numbers of organisms can present as overwhelming meningitis, multisystem organ failure, disseminated intravascular coagulopathy, and death.

Ehrlichiosis symptomatically resembles RMSF. It usually presents with fever, headache, chills, and malaise but rarely a rash. Rare reported complications include renal failure, meningitis, encephalopathy, and respiratory failure. Some deaths have been reported.

Lyme disease usually presents in three distinct stages: early localized, early disseminated, and late persistent. Some patients are totally asymptomatic. Most patients do not have all three stages. In the early localized stage, a

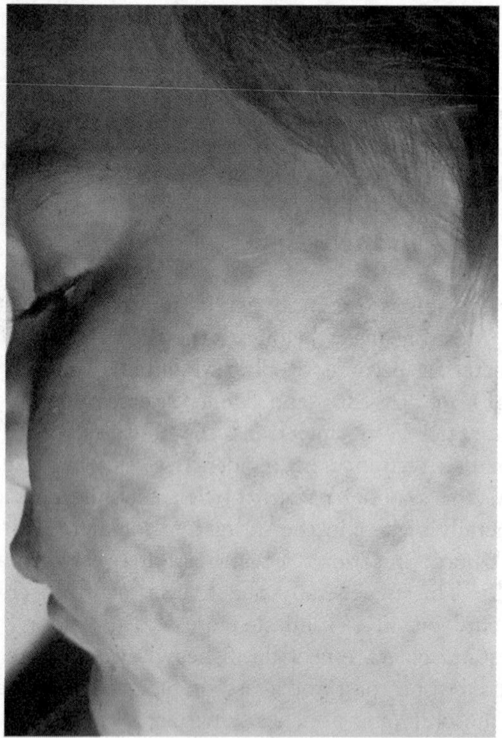

Figure 24–6
The rash of Rocky Mountain spotted fever begins on the wrists and ankles, then spreads to become more generalized. (Courtesy of the Centers for Disease Control and Prevention.)

distinctive rash known as *erythema migrans* (EM) appears (Fig. 24–7). It begins at the site of the tick bite as a reddened area. Then it expands as circular waves of erythema with a central area of clearing. Early treatment of EM should prevent other manifestations, including later stages of the disease.

The early disseminated stage is characterized by secondary EM rashes that are much smaller than the original lesion. Headache, fever, and neck stiffness along with other symptoms occur (Table 24–9). The late disseminated stage involves neurologic dysfunction including seizures, ocular lesions including panuveitis and retinal vasculitis, and severe chronic arthritis that can become erosive and unresponsive to treatment.

Diagnostic Tests. Diagnosis is based primarily on the history of a tick bite (especially with attachment of the tick) and specific serologic tests for each of the three organisms. Acute and convalescent antibody titers for RMSF, Lyme, and ehrlichiosis show a fourfold increase in the indirect fluorescent antibody (IFA) test. These titers are usually accurate 7 to 10 days after the onset of the illness and are diagnostic at 1:64 (Committee on Infectious Diseases, American Academy of Pediatrics, 1994). IgM and IgG antibodies for each of the specific organisms can be measured by enzyme immunoassay (EIA).

Interdisciplinary Interventions

Treatment usually begins empirically while waiting for the test results. For a child who requires hospitalization, the treatment of choice for RMSF is intravenous tetracycline, 10 to 25 mg/kg in two to four doses (adult dose is 1 to 2 g), or intravenous chloramphenicol, 50 to 100 mg/kg in four divided doses (adult dose is 2 to 4 g). Doxycycline is usually given as an oral alternative during convalescence or in less severe cases. The course of therapy is 6 to 10 days.

Alert: *Administration of tetracycline to children younger than 9 years is typically avoided because of the risk of permanently staining developing teeth. However, some experts consider tetracycline to be the drug of choice at any age in acute life-threatening cases of rickettsial infection (Committee on Infectious Diseases, American Academy of Pediatrics, 1994).*

For Lyme disease, the treatment is similar to that for RMSF. For erythema migrans and early disease, oral doxycycline or amoxicillin is given for 10 to 21 days. Erythromycin is the alternative for children younger than 9 years who are allergic to penicillin. Lyme carditis (inflammation of the heart) is treated with doxycycline in mild cases. For severe cases, intravenous penicillin or ceftriaxone is used for 14 to 21 days.

For ehrlichiosis, tetracycline is the drug of choice. Chloramphenicol may also be effective.

Children with tick-borne illnesses are not contagious and therefore do not need isolation. Prevention is paramount; tick attachment should be avoided (TIP 24–1).

Figure 24–7
The erythema migrans of Lyme disease begins as a small circular, reddened area and then expands with a central zone of clearing. (Courtesy of the Centers for Disease Control and Prevention.)

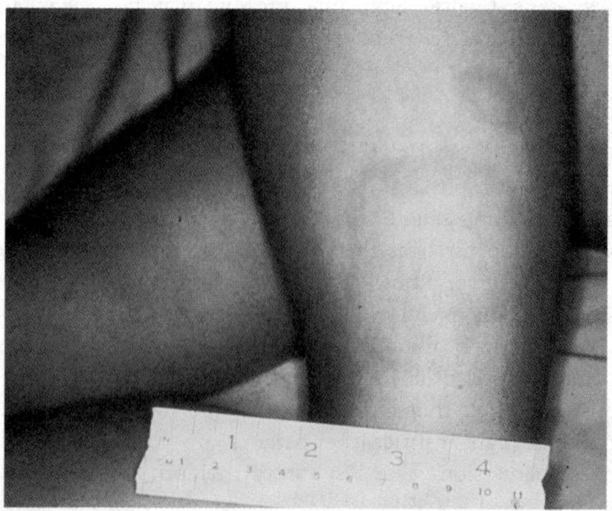

Table 24-9
Clinical Features of Selected Tick-Borne Diseases

Disease	Bacterial Agent	Vector	Clinical Manifestations
Rocky Mountain spotted fever	*Rickettsia rickettsii*	Dog tick Lone star tick Wood tick	Fever, headache, malaise. Rash: occurs before sixth day of illness. Begins on wrists and ankles, then spreads to legs, abdomen, chest, and so on; 10%–15% of cases have no rash (spotless fever). Severe case: disseminated intravascular coagulopathy (DIC), organ failure, and death.
Ehrlichiosis	*Ehrlichia chaffeensis*	Deer tick	Fever, headache, chills, malaise. Severe: renal failure, meningitis, encephalopathy, respiratory failure.
Lyme disease	*Borrelia burgdorferi*	Deer tick	Early localized stage: erythema, migraine. Early disseminated stage: headache, fever, chills, malaise, hepatosplenomegaly, sore throat with a nonproductive cough, testicular swelling, conjunctivitis, lymphadenopathy, carditis. Late disseminated: seizures, ataxia, chronic fatigue, numerous ocular lesions, chronic arthritis.

TIP 24-1 A Teaching Intervention Plan to Avoid Tick-Borne Disease

Nursing Diagnosis and Family Outcomes

- Risk for injury related to environmental conditions (tick-infested areas)
  Outcomes: Child and family will state and implement preventive measures to avoid tick attachment. Child will not become infected with rickettsial disease.

Interventions

Teach parents and child:

Preventive Measures to Avoid Tick Attachment

- Spray clothing and exposed skin with tick repellent containing permethrin or DEET. In young children, use products containing DEET sparingly. Do not use products with greater than 35% DEET. Do not put DEET on a young child's hands (to prevent getting the product in the mouth or eyes). Do not apply to skin with sunburn or rash (absorbed more readily). Products with DEET last 4 to 8 hours; do not apply more than twice daily. Wash repellent off skin after child comes indoors.
- Wear light colors and long sleeves, long pants, socks, and shoes. Tuck shirt or blouse into pants and pants into socks.
- Check skin and scalp for ticks every 2 to 3 hours, when leaving infested areas, after playing with outdoor pets, and when coming indoors.
- Inspect pets daily for ticks.

Tick Removal Techniques

- Inspect and detect promptly; ticks are easier to pull off when not firmly attached.
- Grasp the tick (try to get its head) with tweezers as close to the skin as possible.
- Apply steady upward pull. Do not twist or exert enough pressure to crush.
- If the head remains in the skin, remove similarly to a sliver (splinter).
- Wash the site and your hands with soap and water.

Contact Health Care Provider if

- Tick, or parts of it, cannot be removed.
- Child develops a rash or fever in the week after the bite.

Nurses and other health care workers can remind parents to use insect repellents and visually inspect their children for ticks.

Alert: *Skin repellents used to prevent tick infestation contain N,N-diethyl-m-toluamide (DEET). Products with greater than 35% DEET should not be used on young children because of systemic toxicity (seizures, coma).*

Report all tick-borne infections to the state and local health departments. Although the child is not contagious, notify school officials or the school nurse when a school-age child is being treated to dispel unwarranted fear among classmates.

Viral Infections

Viral infections account for the majority of upper respiratory tract infections. They are caused by such viruses as respiratory syncytial virus, parainfluenza virus, influenza virus, coronavirus, various enteroviruses, rhinovirus, and adenovirus. These viruses and their serotypes are summarized in Table 24–10. (See Chapter 16 for information on respiratory syncytial virus infection and influenza.) Vaccines have been developed for many common and easily transmissible viral infections. These vaccines, coupled with new antiviral agents, have contributed to the development of new viral treatment modalities.

Adenovirus Infection

Adenovirus causes croup, a common respiratory ailment in young children during the winter months. It also causes other disorders, including conjunctivitis, severe respiratory infections, and gastroenteritis. It has been associated with a pertussis-like syndrome and hemorrhagic cystitis.

Incidence and Etiology

Adenovirus infection is common in all pediatric age groups; however, immunosuppressed children are at greatest risk for complications. In bone marrow transplant recipients, adenovirus may cause pneumonia, hepatitis, or renal insufficiency.

Transmission of respiratory infections is by direct contact through exposure to respiratory secretions (as in coughing or sneezing). Enteric strains are transmitted by the oral-fecal route. Eye infections result from swimming in pools that are not properly chlorinated, from direct contact with the conjunctiva with contaminated fingers, or from ophthalmologic equipment that has not been properly disinfected. The incubation period for adenovirus is 2 to 14 days.

Assessment

Respiratory tract infections can present as pharyngitis, bronchiolitis, croup, or severe pneumonia. (See Chapter 16 for specific signs and symptoms of these respiratory disorders.) The pharyngitis is typically exudative and often confused with streptococcal pharyngitis. The nurse can differentiate adenoviral pharyngitis from group A streptococcal pharyngitis only if conjunctivitis is present with the adenovirus infection. Adenoviral upper respiratory tract infections often mimic pertussis, with prolonged episodes of paroxysmal coughing.

Eye infections (epidemic keratoconjunctivitis [EKC]) present as a red, granular appearance of the conjunctiva with clear drainage. The child has frequent tearing and photophobia. Eye irritation and redness can last for 1 to 2 weeks. Superficial erosion of the cornea and subepithelial corneal infiltrates can be seen by ophthalmologic examination.

caREminder: *Adenovirus is not inactivated by ethanol, commonly used in eye clinics to disinfect equipment. Immerse instruments in a 75°C water bath for 5 minutes or 1% chloramine-T for 15 minutes.*

Gastroenteritis infections caused by enteric strains of adenovirus are second only to rotavirus in frequency. Symptoms include diarrhea that lasts for 6 to 9 days accompanied by vomiting.

Table 24–10
Viral Serotypes and Diseases Produced

Virus	Types	Diseases
Adenovirus	42	Croup, bronchiolitis, pertussis-like syndrome
Influenza virus	3	Influenza, croup, pneumonia
Nonpolio enteroviruses	65	Pharyngitis
Parainfluenza virus	4	Croup, bronchiolitis, pneumonia
Respiratory syncytial virus	2	Bronchiolitis, pneumonia
Rhinovirus	100+	Common cold

Hemorrhagic cystitis caused by adenovirus occurs more often in males than females. The child excretes grossly bloody urine for 1 to 2 weeks.

Diagnostic Tests. Viral cultures of samples from pharyngeal swabs or rectal swabs, urine, or eye drainage all yield adenovirus. Serologic tests by complement fixation (CF) can detect adenovirus if acute and convalescent sera are used.

Nursing Diagnoses and Outcomes

In addition to the common nursing diagnoses and outcomes listed in Chart 24–5, the following may be applicable for the child with EKC:

- **Pain related to effects of conjunctivitis**
  Outcome: The child will report or evidence only minimal discomfort.

The following may be applicable for the child with adenovirus gastroenteritis:

- **Risk for impaired skin integrity related to effects of diarrheal stool in contact with perianal skin**
  Outcome: The child will maintain intact perianal skin.
- **Fluid volume deficit related to excessive diarrheal output and decreased intake**
  Outcome: The child will maintain adequate fluid volume and tissue perfusion.

Interdisciplinary Interventions

There is no effective treatment for adenovirus. A vaccine is being developed that appears to be effective against adenovirus types 4 and 7 (types associated with respiratory infections).

If soothing saline eye drops are used for conjunctivitis, nurses should instruct the parents to wash their own hands after instilling the drops to avoid infecting themselves. Hand washing after diapering an infant with diarrhea is essential to prevent further spread in the family.

Children with croup seem to benefit from cool mist humidifiers. During acute exacerbations, it is often helpful for the child to breathe the water vapor created by running hot water in the shower or the cool night air (see Chapter 16).

Community Care

Children in daycare centers are at increased risk for respiratory and enteric infections with adenovirus. Parents should be encouraged to exclude their child from daycare if diarrhea, conjunctivitis, or respiratory infection symptoms are present.

Acquired Immunodeficiency Syndrome (AIDS)

Etiology and Incidence

Human immunodeficiency virus type 1 is a retrovirus that attacks the immune system by destroying T lymphocytes (cells that are critical to fighting infection and developing immunity). HIV renders the immune system useless, and the child is unable to fight even the most benign infection.

From 1982 to December 1995, 6948 children younger than 13 years with AIDS or HIV infection were reported to the CDC (HIV/AIDS Surveillance Report, 1996). The majority of these cases occurred in black (57%) or Hispanic (23%) children. As with adult cases, ethnic minority groups constitute the majority of the AIDS cases but not the majority of the population at large.

The number of HIV or AIDS cases in children is a direct reflection of the number of AIDS cases in females of childbearing age. The proportion of women who are infected with HIV or who have AIDS increased from 7% in 1985 to 18% in 1994 (HIV/AIDS Surveillance Report, 1996). Through June 1995, 2184 cases of AIDS were reported to the CDC in persons aged 13 to 19 years.

Babies born to HIV-positive women test positive for HIV antibody. This is actually a measure of maternal antibody and not indicative of true infection. Usually, 13% to 39% or one in four babies born to HIV-positive mothers are actually infected. Thus, HIV-infected children are a reflection of HIV-infected women. Infants may remain HIV positive for as long as 18 months because of the slow rate of decay of maternal HIV antibody. Therefore, true infections in infants are confirmed by the detection of HIV (p24 antigen assay, culture of HIV, or polymerase chain reaction [PCR]). In the presence of HIV antibodies and in the setting of immunosuppression, infected infants meet the CDC definition for pediatric AIDS. HIV cultures can take up to 4 weeks to grow.

caREminder: *Routinely offer HIV testing to all pregnant adolescents. Administration of zidovudine can decrease the likelihood of perinatal transmission (from 25% to 8%).*

There are three chief modes of transmission for HIV (Chart 24–14). Blood transfusions and administration of clotting factors are rarely modes of transmission because donated blood is tested and clotting factors are heat treated.

In maternal-infant transmission of HIV, timing is the key. Transmission to the fetus may occur during the intrauterine, intrapartum, or postpartum period (see Chart 24–14). Yet, transmission of HIV to the infant occurs in one out of every four births to HIV-positive women.

Chart 24–14

Modes and Timing of Transmission for Human Immunodeficiency Virus

Modes of Transmission

- Sexual contact (both homosexual and heterosexual)
- Percutaneous or mucous membrane exposure to needles or other sharp instruments contaminated with blood or bloody body fluids
- Mother-to-infant transmission before or around the time of birth

Timing of Transmission

- Intrauterine: HIV can be detected in aborted fetal tissue as early as 8 weeks.
- Intrapartum: In a twin pregnancy, there is a higher incidence of infection in the first twin born.
- Postpartum: HIV-negative mothers receive a blood transfusion after delivery that is contaminated with HIV. These women then breast-feed the infant and the infant acquires HIV infection from the breast milk.

Several maternal factors determine the likelihood of HIV transmission to the infant (Chart 24–15). Clearly, pregnant women with advanced HIV disease and therefore more circulating virus in their blood are more likely to transmit HIV to the fetus (Dickover et al., 1996). The main goal in prenatal care of the pregnant woman with AIDS is to decrease her viral load by giving her antiretroviral drugs such as zidovudine during the pregnancy. Furthermore, the presence of diseases such as syphilis in the pregnant female with HIV infection can tax the immune system and compromise the placental barrier by causing placental inflammation. Diagnosis of occult sexually transmitted disease and prompt treatment are necessary.

One study suggested that women whose membranes ruptured more than 4 hours before delivery were 26 times more likely to transmit HIV to their infants (Minkoff et al., 1995). The study suggested that in these cases, cesarean section may be of benefit in lessening the risk of HIV transmission.

Pathophysiology

The sole purpose of HIV is to replicate or make copies of itself. It enters a cell, basically takes over the DNA, and commandeers the cell to make copies of HIV. Although HIV selects T4 lymphocytes as the preferred cells, it invades many other cells as well. However, T4 cell invasion is significant because T4 lymphocytes defend the body against invading pathogens. HIV either renders T4 cells dysfunctional or creates "holes" in the membrane of T4 cells that result in osmotic pressure differences (outside cell versus inside cell) that literally cause the cells to destroy themselves. Thus, T4 cells are depleted in number and cannot signal B cells to form protective antibodies to fight off the invading virus. In short, HIV targets the immune system to leave the body defenseless.

Prognosis. The prognosis for an HIV-infected child who has the first AIDS-defining illness in the first year of life is usually grim. This is especially true if the first illness is *P. carinii* pneumonia (PCP). Children who can fend off the first AIDS-defining illness have the best prognosis. Adjunctive therapies include antiviral therapies and PCP prophylaxis.

Assessment

Most children infected with HIV develop symptoms within the first 9 months of life. The remainder become symptomatic sometime before age 3. Children, with their immature immune systems, have a much shorter incubation period than adults. Opportunistic infections in children with HIV are summarized in Chart 24–16. Children with HIV infection present with a host of health problems, including chronic pneumonitis, encephalopathy, chronic diarrhea, wasting, developmental delay, numerous opportunistic infections, and various malignancies.

PCP is one of the most common diseases indicative of AIDS in children. Along with PCP, children may experience at least two serious bacterial infections in 2 years. These infections are sepsis, otitis media, chronic sinusitis, meningitis, gastroenteritis, and pneumonia (Care Path 24–2). The causative organism varies, although *S. pneumoniae* is a common cause.

Lymphoid interstitial pneumonia (LIP) is a form of

Chart 24–15

Maternal Factors That Determine Transmission of Human Immunodeficiency Virus

- Low maternal $CD4^+$ lymphocyte counts (<100): advanced HIV disease
- High maternal viral load
- Presence of STDs, such as syphilis, causing placental inflammation
- Zidovudine therapy during pregnancy: reduces transmission of HIV to the baby by 67%

Chart 24–16

AIDS-Defining Illnesses in Children with Human Immunodeficiency Virus Infection

Candidiasis: esophagus, tracheal, bronchi, or lungs
Coccidiodomycosis: disseminated or extrapulmonary
Cryptococcoses: extrapulmonary
Cryptosporidiosis: chronic intestinal
Cytomegalovirus (CMV) disease: (other than liver, spleen, lymph nodes) in children older than 1 month
CMV retinitis: with loss of vision
Chronic herpes simplex: ulcer (longer than 1 month), pneumonitis, esophagitis in children older than 1 month
Histoplasmosis: disseminated or extrapulmonary
HIV encephalopathy
Isosporosis: chronic (greater than 1 month)
Kaposi's sarcoma: rare in young children
Lymphoid interstitial pneumonitis
Lymphoma, primary brain
Lymphoma (Burkitt's or immunoblastic sarcoma)
Mycobacterium avium complex or *Mycobacterium kansasii* (disseminated or extrapulmonary)
Mycobacterium tuberculosis: disseminated or extrapulmonary
Pneumocystis carinii pneumonia
Progressive multifocal leukoencephalopathy
Toxoplasmosis of brain: onset in child older than 1 month
Wasting syndrome caused by HIV

chronic pneumonitis. These children usually have acquired HIV infection perinatally. Beginning as an asymptomatic infiltrate, LIP can progress to severe respiratory compromise.

Developmental delay is often seen in HIV-infected children with or without central nervous system (CNS) involvement. Infants normally have an immature CNS. Therefore, they are particularly susceptible to neurologic impairment and delayed or impaired brain growth.

Differential diagnosis in children with HIV is often difficult. Many conditions mimic HIV and the failure to thrive that it causes (Chart 24–17). For example, children born with congenital heart defects often fail to thrive because of the severity of their lesions. Inborn errors of metabolism and genetic causes of immunodeficiency must also be ruled out. Typical TORCH infections could be opportunistic infections in the HIV-infected child.

Diagnostic Tests. Because the infant has positive enzyme-linked immunosorbent assay (ELISA) and Western blot tests for HIV as a result of maternal antibody, these tests are not diagnostic. A presumptive diagnosis of HIV can be made on the basis of a single positive HIV culture, PCR, or p24 antigen test. Additional laboratory or imaging studies are performed to evaluate the presence of other manifestations of HIV disease, such as chest radiography for PCP or magnetic resonance imaging (MRI) for toxoplasmosis brain lesions.

Interdisciplinary Interventions

Maternal treatment consists of oral zidovudine (azidothymidine [AZT]) during the pregnancy and intravenously during delivery. Zidovudine reduces the likelihood of transmission without harming the fetus. The newborn receives zidovudine for 6 weeks after birth.

The goal of treatment is to keep the child as healthy as possible for as long as possible. Zidovudine, or AZT, effectively interferes with HIV replication but can cause bone marrow suppression and nausea. If it fails or the

Chart 24–17

Conditions That Mimic Pediatric Acquired Immunodeficiency Syndrome

Syndrome	Description
Cardiac syndrome	Poor contractility Myocarditis Congestive heart failure
Chronic pneumonitis	Lymphoid interstitial pneumonitis Pulmonary lymphoid hyperplasia
Encephalopathy or myelopathy	Progressive encephalopathy Subcortical dementia Impaired brain growth Neoplasm Stroke
Hematologic syndrome	Idiopathic thrombocytopenic purpura Lymphadenopathy
Hepatitis syndrome	Hepatosplenomegaly Hyperbilirubinemia
Malignancies	Lymphoreticular tumors Burkitt's lymphoma Leiomyosarcomas
Opportunistic infections	PCP See Chart 24–16
Renal syndrome	Progressive glomerulopathy
Wasting syndrome	Failure to thrive Wasting

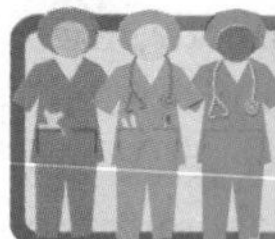

Care Path 24–2 An Interdisciplinary Plan of Care for the Child with AIDS—Pneumonia

	Patient/Family Intermediate Outcomes		
Nursing Diagnosis	**Day: Admission**	**Day 1**	**Day 2**
Impaired gas exchange related to effects of pneumonia	The child will exhibit improved oxygenation.	⟶	⟶
Altered nutrition: less than body requirements, related to decreased intake and increased metabolic demands	The child will undergo a complete nutritional assessment.	The child will receive adequate daily caloric intake (IV or PO).	⟶
Ineffective family coping: compromised, related to the effects of the child's serious illness and hospital isolation	The family's strengths and weaknesses will be evaluated and appropriate interventions identified.	⟶	⟶
Care Intervention Categories			
Consults	Pediatric infectious disease Infection control Social services Consult a dietitian for TPN therapy if the child's nutritional status is poor. Home health	Infection control to report case (if newly diagnosed AIDS) to health department.	Home health to arrange for home IV therapy.
Labs	Obtain CBC with differential; HIV ELISA with p24 antigen; $CD4^+$ and $CD8^+$ cell counts; immunoglobulin levels.	Consider SMA6 if the child is dehydrated.	
Medications and IVs	IV fluid p.r.n. Administer antibiotics, third-generation cephalosporin or vancomycin. Continue AZT or DDI or protocol medications. Give acetaminophen for fever. Continue trimethoprim-sulfamethoxazole prophylaxis.	Readjust antibiotic dosage according to laboratory results. Provide central line care. Place a heparin lock on the IV.	

Day 3	Day 4: Discharge
The child will demonstrate no signs of respiratory compromise.	
	The child will maintain adequate body weight.
The family will verbalize adequate understanding of the child's treatment plan and knowledge of available resources.	
	Discharge the child on IV antibiotics and oral AZT or DDI and Bactrim prophylaxis.

Care Path continued on following page

child cannot tolerate it, the physician usually selects another drug, such as dideoxyinosine (DDI) or dideoxycytidine (DDC).

PCP prophylaxis with trimethoprim-sulfamethoxazole (Septra or Bactrim) should begin when age-adjusted T4 cell counts start to drop. Age-appropriate immunizations are given on schedule with only one substitution: inactivated polio vaccine is given instead of oral polio vaccine.

Nursing care of HIV-positive infants and children involves using standard precautions. Because these children have many needs and the mothers of HIV-positive infants may not have health insurance because of homelessness, IV drug abuse, or unemployment, notify social services as soon as possible. Refer mothers and infants to the dietitian for counseling to prevent the general decline in nutritional status of HIV-positive children. Explain all current medications, especially antiviral (AZT, DDI, DDC) drugs, and PCP prophylaxis to the primary caregiver.

Community Care

Many educators and top government officials believe that education and prevention are the best ways to manage AIDS. Recommend safer sex practices. Although the only safe sex practice is abstinence, safer sex can be achieved through latex condom use, a monogamous relationship, and avoidance of substances such as drugs and alcohol that cloud judgment.

Children cope with the diagnosis of AIDS in different ways at different ages (Chart 24–18). Assist the family by listening to their concerns and make appropriate referrals to the various agencies and organizations that can offer both moral and financial support.

Measles

Incidence and Etiology

The measles vaccine has dramatically decreased the incidence of measles (rubeola). In 1995, 301 confirmed cases of measles were reported to the CDC, the lowest number of cases since 1912. The few cases that do occur appear in preschoolers, especially those 15 months of age or younger. Because the measles-mumps-rubella (MMR) vaccine is typically given at age 12 to 15 months, infants older than 6 months but younger than 12 to 15 months are susceptible to measles. The protection of maternal antibodies transferred to the infant during pregnancy wanes in about 6 months after birth.

Worldview: *Underimmunized populations, especially in large urban areas, are also at risk for measles. Immigrants, members of religious groups that prohibit vaccination, and homeless or impoverished people may have un-*

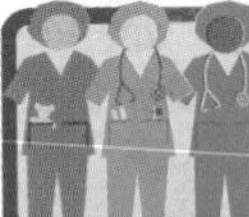

Care Path 24–2 An Interdisciplinary Plan of Care for the Child with AIDS—Pneumonia *Continued*

Care Intervention Categories	Day: Admission	Day 1	Day 2
Procedures (diagnostics)	Arrange for chest radiograph and possible chest CT scan.	Consider broncheoalveolar lavage for suspected PCP.	
Psychosocial	Encourage parental involvement in the child's care. Assess status of siblings. Refer the family to available community pediatric AIDS resources.	Developmentally appropriate play/school activities	Refer the family to hospital-based parent support groups.
Safety and activity	Reinforce safety measures with the family; for example, keep side rails up. Maintain standard precautions.		
Teaching/discharge planning	Assess the child's discharge needs. Implement parent teaching as needed. Begin teaching the family home IV therapy skills.	Have the dietitian meet with the family to plan for discharge. Have the family observe the nurse giving IV care.	Observe family giving return demonstration of IV care and medication administration.
Vital signs/baseline parameters	Monitor temperature, pulse, and blood pressure every 4 hours; respirations, every 2 hours. Use pulse oximetry if the child is in acute respiratory distress.		

CBC, complete blood count; CT, computed tomography; ELISA, enzyme-linked immunosorbent assay; PCP, *Pneumocystis carinii* pneumonia; PO, by mouth; p.r.n., as needed; SMA6, Sequential Multiple Analyzer, six tests; TPN, total parenteral nutrition.

vaccinated children. Some of these people have limited access to health care. Others lack adequate knowledge of the health care system.

Measles is a seasonal disease. Outbreaks peak in the winter and spring. It is highly contagious and is transmitted by the airborne route. It can be spread directly by coughing or sneezing or indirectly by airborne suspended droplets. The child harbors the virus in nasopharyngeal secretions during the acute stage of the illness. The typical incubation period is 8 to 12 days. Children are contagious from 1 to 2 days before the rash appears until 4 days after the onset of the rash.

Assessment

The hallmark of measles is the appearance of Koplik's spots. These first appear as red spots along the inside of the cheek (Fig. 24–8A). They evolve over time to form pinpoint white papules on a rose red base. Two days after

Day 3	Day 4: Discharge
Arrange for home IV therapy equipment delivery. Have the family demonstrate giving IV care.	Review the child's diet with the family. Give them printed diet plan samples.
Discontinue pulse oximetry if the child shows no signs of respiratory distress.	

the appearance of Koplik's spots, a red maculopapular rash appears with fever (Fig. 24–8*B*). The rash first appears on the face and neck and then progresses down the body.

Other typical symptoms include fever, conjunctivitis, and a cough. Between the second and third days, symptoms peak. The rash generally begins to fade by the third day. By the fourth day, symptoms begin to resolve with the fever decreasing and conjunctiva clearing.

Occasional complications include otitis media, mastoiditis, pneumonia, encephalomyelitis, and rarely subacute sclerosing panencephalitis (SSPE). SSPE is a degenerative central nervous system process associated with progressive behavioral and intellectual deterioration followed by convulsions, coma, and death. Measles vaccination programs have reduced the incidence of SSPE to nearly zero.

Diagnostic Tests. Diagnosis is typically made by the presenting clinical features. The measles virus can be isolated in tissue culture from nasopharyngeal secretions, blood, urine, and conjunctival fluid. However, viral cultures are generally not used because many laboratories are not equipped to cultivate viruses.

The most useful antibody test is a paired sera test comparing the rise in titers of an acute specimen and a convalescent specimen taken 2 to 4 weeks later. IgM antibodies can be detected in a single specimen if collected after the second day of the rash but before 30 days after the onset of illness.

Nursing Diagnoses and Outcomes

In addition to the common nursing diagnoses and outcomes listed in Chart 24–5, the following may be applicable to the child with measles:

- **Sensory-perceptual alteration: visual related to effects of measles photophobia**
  Outcome: The child will have interventions implemented to decrease the discomfort associated with photophobia.
- **Hyperthermia related to effects of measles**
  Outcome: The child will experience minimal discomfort and no injury associated with fever.

Interdisciplinary Interventions

No specific antiviral treatment is available. Uncomplicated measles is self-limiting and usually requires only supportive care.

If the child is hospitalized with measles, use airborne precautions for the duration of the illness. Provide care that includes supportive therapy and fluids. Coughs are sometimes difficult to control, and common cough suppressants seem inadequate. Therefore, encourage fluid intake to lubricate the mucous membranes. Do not treat associated conjunctivitis with antibacterial drops or ointments. The virus is unaffected by the antibacterial medication. If photophobia is present, dim the lights. However, avoid completely darkening the room because it may be depressing to a child whose activity is already curtailed. Provide quiet, diversionary activities.

Alert: *As with all viral illnesses, avoid aspirin products because of the increased risk of Reye's syndrome.*

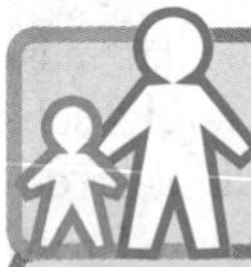

Chart 24–18
Developmental Considerations

Psychosocial Issues Related to Pediatric Human Immunodeficiency Virus Infection

Children	Families
Birth through 2 Years	
Unable to grasp concept of illness and death. Infant and toddler have immediate concern about physical trauma and parent separation.	Trauma of diagnosis falls on the caretaker. Biological mother may have found out her status upon diagnosis of child. Guilt: regardless of mode of acquisition all parents experience some degree of guilt.
Preschool	
Begin to conceptualize death process involving physical harm. Concerns center around medical tests and procedures.	Anger: against medical system if contracted through a transfusion, against themselves if prenatal. Families tend to move past this phase when reassured of ongoing comprehensive family care.
School-age	
Children begin to understand "something is wrong." By age 10 or 11, understand death is permanent and universal. Fear of ostracism and rejection. Guilt regarding origin of illness.	Task overload, whether due to scarce resources, lack of support, or burden of secrecy. Caring for a child with HIV infection is overwhelming.
Adolescents	
Diagnosis often produces denial, fear, withdrawal, fear of being rejected by peers. Disruption of forming relationships outside the family. Anxieties may lead to poor school performance, depression, isolation, and acting-out behavior.	Isolation: most parents unwilling to share child's diagnosis. Therefore, the traditional supports available to families of a child with a life-threatening illness are not available from friends, community, and clergy. Medical home may be only source of support for these families. Depression: reactive depression may result from facing HIV infection of the family and parents may also have chronic depressive state that is a result of the coexistence of multiple problems. Fears of multiple losses. Parents begin to mourn loss of other family members, lifestyle, trust of friends, self-esteem.

Community Care

Susceptible persons exposed to measles may be given the measles vaccine to prevent disease. This is possible because the body's immune response to the measles vaccine is elicited in 7 days, whereas the incubation period of natural measles is 8 to 12 days. Vaccination is certainly the method of choice in outbreaks in schools or daycare centers. In daycare centers, the vaccination age may be lowered to 6 months. These children can then resume the normal vaccination schedule of 15 months and again before school entry or at age 11 or 12, depending on local school requirements. Pregnancy is a contraindication for the measles vaccine or the MMR vaccine. Measles is not known to cause congenital birth defects. However, it has been associated with increased risk of spontaneous abortion and premature labor (Krugman, 1992a). Administration of MMR vaccine is not harmful if it is given to a person who is already immune to one or more of the viruses.

Mumps

Mumps is a vaccine-preventable disease that occasionally occurs in outbreaks in undervaccinated populations. Known as infectious parotitis, it is an acute inflammation

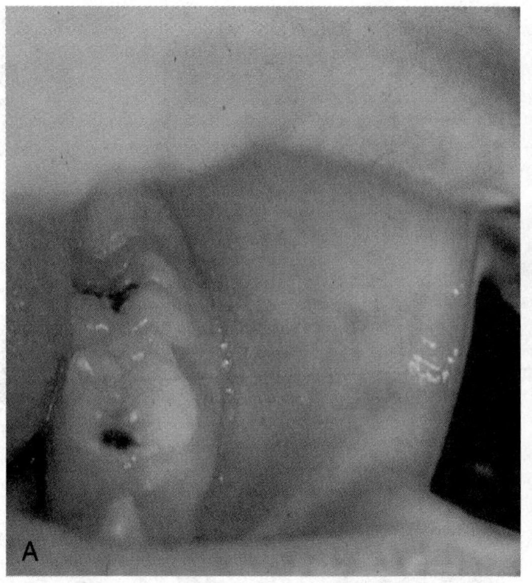

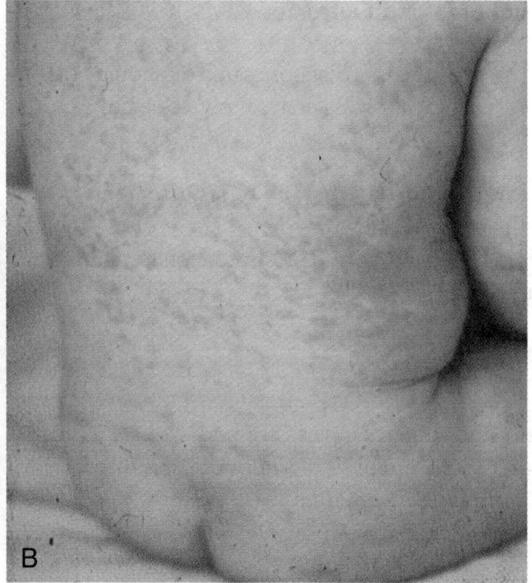

Figure 24–8
The rashes of measles. *A*, Koplik's spots appear as red spots along the inside of the cheek. *B*, The typical rash of measles has confluent maculopapular lesions. (Courtesy of the Centers for Disease Control and Prevention.)

of the salivary glands, particularly the parotid glands (Fig. 24–9). It is seasonal in its occurrence, with most cases arising in late winter and spring.

In the past, vaccination for mumps implied permanent immunity. However, outbreaks of mumps among high school and college students in the late 1980s and early 1990s suggest that waning immunity is a possibility. In 1994, the Advisory Committee on Immunization Practices of the CDC recommended a second MMR vaccine dose for persons born after 1957 (Committee on Infectious Diseases, American Academy of Pediatrics, 1994).

Figure 24–9
In mumps, the parotid glands swell and obscure the angle of the jaw. (Courtesy of the Centers for Disease Control and Prevention.)

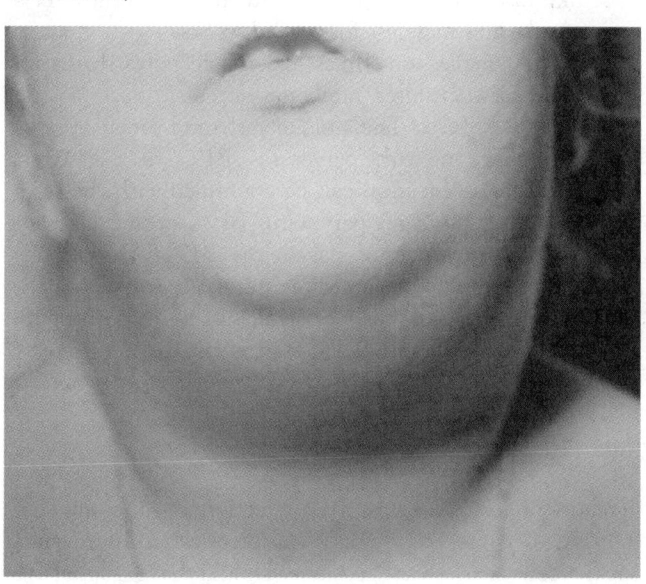

Complications of mumps are rare. Occasionally, adolescent or adult males experience orchitis (inflammation of the testis), but sterility rarely occurs (Committee on Infectious Diseases, American Academy of Pediatrics, 1994). Mumps during pregnancy does not result in birth defects. However, it increases the rate of spontaneous abortion by 27%. Pregnancy is a contraindication for the mumps vaccine or MMR vaccine.

Assessment

Swelling of the salivary glands is the hallmark of mumps. In the classic illness, the child complains of an earache made worse by chewing. Fever, headache, and generalized malaise are often accompanying symptoms. Other causes of parotid swelling must be ruled out. Such causes include stones that block Stensen's ducts, coxsackievirus or parainfluenza 3 virus infections, and various tumors, hemangiomas, and lymphangiomas of the parotid gland.

Diagnostic Tests. Mumps can be diagnosed by isolation of the mumps virus from throat swabs, urine, and spinal fluid. Specific mumps serologic tests include mumps hemagglutination inhibition test, complement fixation, and enzyme immunoassay.

Nursing Diagnoses and Outcomes

In addition to the nursing diagnoses and outcomes listed in Chart 24–5, the following may apply to a child with mumps:

- **Altered nutrition: less than body requirements related to pain with chewing**
  Outcome: The child will maintain adequate fluid and food intake.

Interdisciplinary Interventions

There are no antiviral therapies. Supportive care is indicated. Children with mumps are seldom hospitalized.

When hospitalized, children with mumps should be placed in a private room with droplet precautions until 9 days after the onset of swelling. In an outbreak, when two or more children with mumps are admitted, they may share a room.

Community Care

In the home, the child with mumps should not attend school, nursery school, or daycare until 9 days after the onset of swelling. The home health nurse can arrange for home teachers for school-age children.

Nursing care of children with mumps should be supportive. Swollen parotid glands may cause discomfort while eating. Because the child often complains of increased pain upon chewing, a soft diet is recommended. Citrus foods and some sour candies or foods may elicit pain and increased salivation. They should be avoided.

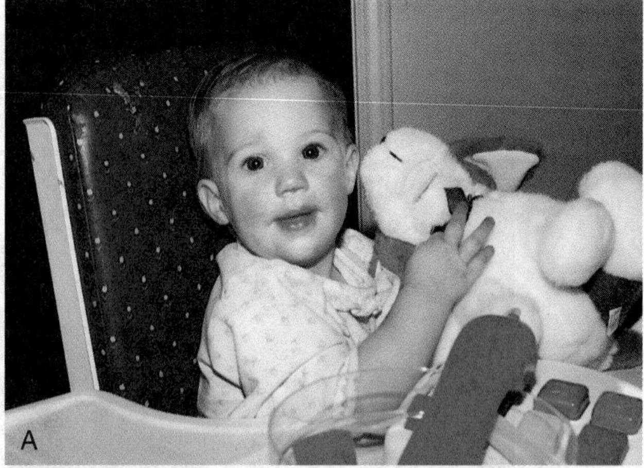

Figure 24–10
Rashes of parvovirus B19. *A*, The hallmark sign is the "slapped cheek" appearance of the face. *B*, The lace-like rash. (*B*, Courtesy of the Centers for Disease Control and Prevention.)

Parvovirus B19 Infection

Parvovirus B19 infection is also known as erythema infectiosum or fifth disease. It is called fifth disease because it was the fifth childhood disease recognized to cause a rash-like illness in children. The other four diseases are measles, rubella, varicella, and scarlet fever. The mode of transmission is through respiratory secretions. It is contagious upon close contact with the infected individual. Outbreaks among elementary and middle school classmates are often demonstrated. Secondary transmission among family members accounts for 50% of new cases. The incubation period is 4 to 14 days. Complications are rare in children.

Assessment

Known mainly for the "slapped cheek" appearance of the face, parvovirus B19 infection also produces a lace-like rash on the abdomen and extremities (Fig. 24–10). The lace-like rash increases in color with heat, such as after a warm bath, and may last for several weeks.

Adult females sometimes experience polyarthritis for several months; children rarely develop arthritis.

Diagnostic Tests. The unique rash and facial appearance in children with parvovirus B19 are diagnostic. However, acute infection can be confirmed with the serologic test that measures parvovirus B19–specific IgM antibody. The presence of parvovirus B19 IgG antibody indicates past infection and immunity. Viral detection by PCR is also helpful but not available in most hospital laboratories. Parvovirus B19 antigens can be detected by radioimmunoassay (RIA) or by enzyme assay.

Interdisciplinary Interventions

Treatment for parvovirus B19 infection is generally supportive. Because parvovirus B19 infections can trigger a sickle cell crisis, these patients should have supportive care as indicated. Intravenous immunoglobulin can be used for the immunocompromised patient, who could develop severe anemia. In such patients, transfusion with red cells is often necessary.

By the time the rash appears, most children are no longer infectious, so isolation is unnecessary. However, in individuals with sickle cell disease and other chronic hemolytic conditions, parvovirus B19 infection causes aplastic crisis, rendering them infectious over the entire course of the illness. For these individuals, droplet precautions are needed. Fetal infection can result in fatal nonimmune hydrops. Thus, pregnant employees and visitors must observe droplet precautions.

Because only about half of the population has had parvovirus B19, health care personnel could be susceptible. For children managed with droplet precautions, arrange for play therapy, video games, and other diversions because trips to the playroom are not possible.

Rubella

Rubella (German measles) is a vaccine-preventable disease. In 1995, 146 cases and 7 cases of congenital rubella occurred. It is also referred to as "3-day measles" because it produces a rash that lasts approximately 3 days. It has an incubation period of 14 to 21 days.

Rubella is a relatively mild disease but is important in nonimmune pregnant females. If maternal infection occurs in the first trimester, transplacental infection can have disastrous effects on the fetus. Rubella is part of the TORCH syndrome of infections affecting fetal development. In the pregnant woman, rubella is a relatively mild disease. In 25% to 50% of the cases, the woman has no symptoms at all. The rash occurs as an immune response to viral invasion, which occurs at the end of the incubation period. Much of the fetal damage occurs in the viremic stage, when the viable virus is circulating in the maternal blood. As the pregnancy progresses, risk of fetal damage declines (Table 24–11).

Table 24–11
Risk of Fetal Damage in Congenital Rubella

Gestational Month*	Fetal Damage
1–2	35%–60% multiple defects
3	30%–35% single defect
4	10% single defect

* Fetal exposure after the fourth month of gestation rarely causes birth defects.

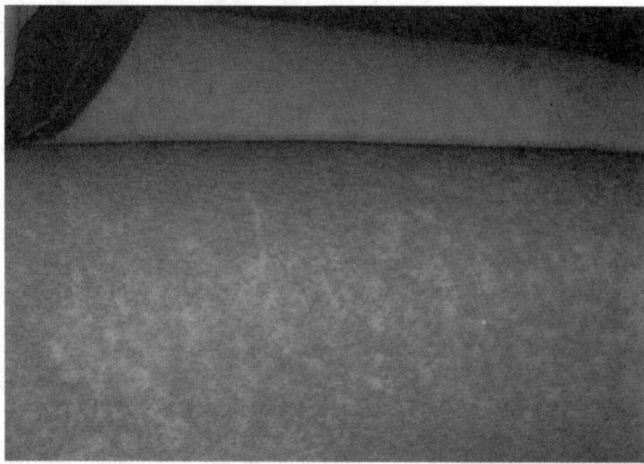

Figure 24–11
The rash of rubella is fine and diffuse. (Courtesy of the Centers for Disease Control and Prevention.)

Assessment

In children with acquired rubella, a fine rash appears (Fig. 24–11). There can be a slight fever and generalized lymphadenopathy (enlarged lymph nodes), particularly in the suboccipital, postauricular, and cervical areas. In infants with congenital rubella, skin lesions, such as a "blueberry muffin" rash (Fig. 24–12), and major organ system defects (Chart 24–19) are the hallmarks.

Figure 24–12
"Blueberry muffin" syndrome in congenital rubella. The rash is so deep in color that it acquires a blue hue. (Courtesy of the Centers for Disease Control and Prevention.)

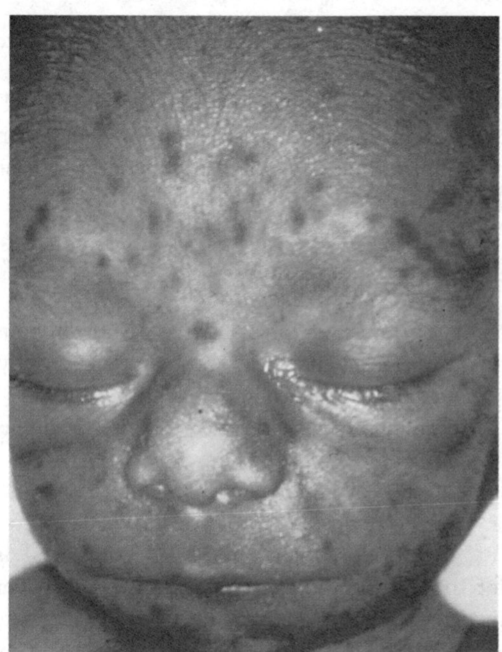

Chart 24–19

Effects of Congenital Rubella

- Intrauterine growth retardation
- Hepatosplenomegaly
- Thrombocytopenia
- "Blueberry muffin" rash
- "Celery stalking" (radiographic lines through long bones)
- Cataracts, salt-and-pepper retinopathy, glaucoma, microphthalmia
- Mental retardation, microcephaly, encephalitis, seizures, hearing loss
- Pneumonitis
- Ventricular septal defect, valvular stenosis, myocardial stenosis

Diagnostic Tests. Most virology laboratories can perform serologic tests that isolate rubella virus from blood, urine, throat, and spinal fluid. Observing a fourfold rise in antibody titer in paired sera (acute and convalescent) is a common test for determining immunity versus acute infection. Detection of rubella-specific IgM and IgG antibodies is especially useful for confirming congenital infection.

Nursing Diagnoses and Outcomes

In addition to the common nursing diagnoses and outcomes listed in Chart 24–5, the following may be applicable to the child with congenital rubella:

▶ **Sensory-perceptual alterations: visual and auditory related to effects of rubella**
Outcome: The child will have sensory-perceptual deficits recognized early and interventions implemented to minimize their deleterious effects on growth and development.

Interdisciplinary Interventions

Treatment is considered supportive. Rubella immune globulin (RIG) is available for postexposure prophylaxis for pregnant women in whom pregnancy termination is not an option. RIG may prevent or limit the disease in these women.

Nursing care of children with rubella is largely supportive. Maintain contact precautions for 7 days after the onset of the rash or, for a child with congenital infection, for the duration of the hospital stay. Teach parents to maintain these precautions. Provide specific care related to the number and type of defects the child exhibits. Discharge planning along with parent teaching eases the transition from the hospital to the home.

All health care personnel should be vaccinated with rubella vaccine (or MMR vaccine) or demonstrate immunity via titer. Most individuals born before 1957 have had rubella, ensuring immunity. Those born after 1957 need a second MMR vaccination to guard against waning immunity.

Community Care

Infants with congenital rubella can shed rubella virus in urine and nasopharyngeal secretions for up to 1 year or longer. Congenitally infected infants must be excluded for this time period from large groups, such as in daycare and church nurseries. Passive maternal antibodies wane after 4 to 6 months. Because the MMR vaccine is usually given at ages 12 to 15 months, all infants in the infant room of a daycare center (usually ages 6 weeks to 12 months) are susceptible.

Herpes Infections

Seven herpesviruses produce significant infection in humans:

- Varicella-zoster virus (VZV)
- Herpes simplex virus type 1 (HSV-1)
- Herpes simplex virus type 2 (HSV-2)
- Cytomegalovirus (CMV)
- Epstein-Barr virus (EBV)
- Human herpesvirus type 6 (HHV-6)
- Human herpesvirus type 7 (HHV-7)

All herpesviruses can remain dormant in the body after the primary infection has subsided, producing periodic, recurrent, or latent infections. Recurrent infections are usually not as severe as the primary infection.

Varicella-Zoster Virus Infection

Primary VZV infection is commonly known as chickenpox; the recurrent form is known as shingles. Varicella or chickenpox is a common, relatively benign childhood illness. Once a person is infected with varicella, the virus remains in the body hidden among the dorsal root and trigeminal nerve ganglia. Reactivation of varicella causes shingles, which can occur years to decades later and can produce painful lesions along ganglia (nerve pathways). Reactivation is triggered by exposure to a stressor, such as excessive sunlight, extreme cold, labor, the loss of a loved one, job loss, or chemotherapy or other forms of immune suppression.

In 1995, the Food and Drug Administration (FDA) approved the release of the first vaccine to prevent varicella. The vaccine and its ramifications are discussed in Chapter 6.

Assessment

Varicella is transmitted by direct contact with the vesicles and by the airborne route (Valenti, 1992). After an incubation period of 10 to 21 days, the illness begins with a low-grade fever and malaise. The vesicular lesions that characterize the disease usually begin as superficial vesicular lesions that resemble dewdrops on the skin. A red base develops, followed by pustules. The rash is extremely pruritic. The lesions appear in three successive crops over 3 days and affect the trunk, scalp, face, and extremities. Lesions can appear on the mucous membranes of the eyes, vaginal mucosa, rectal mucosa, mouth, and throat. As the child talks, coughs, sneezes, and so forth, viral particles can become airborne. Sunburned skin and diapered areas have significantly more lesions, but they are smaller than in other areas. Between 5 to 7 days after onset, the lesions begin to crust (Fig. 24–13).

Although 95% of all adults are immune to varicella because of a history of the disease, maternal varicella can occur, leading to fetal infection. Fetal infection in the first or second trimester can cause limb atrophy, scarring of the arms and legs, and eye and central nervous system disorders.

Diagnostic Tests. The enzyme-linked immunosorbent assay is the most common antibody test used to determine immunity. Paired sera for acute and convalescent antibodies can be used to determine acute infection. Collecting the virus using skin scrapings and then staining with immunofluorescent monoclonal antibodies can rule out herpes simplex. Because the tests are specific for VZV, test results are positive for an infected child.

Figure 24–13
A soothing oatmeal bath can help relieve the pruritus associated with chickenpox.

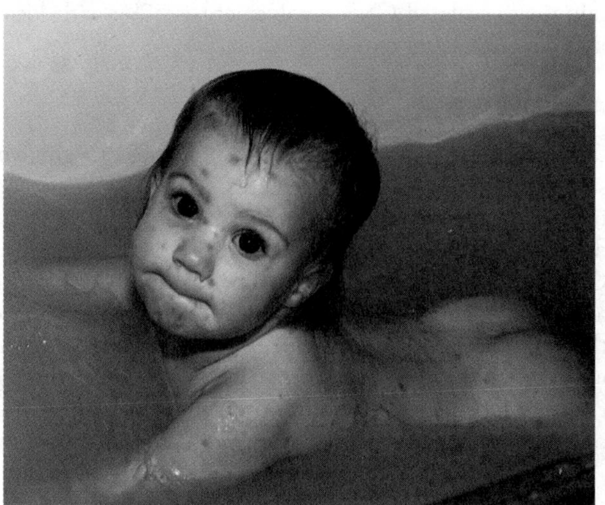

Interdisciplinary Interventions

Varicella-zoster immune globulin (VZIG) is given to immunosuppressed children immediately after exposure to someone with varicella. The VZIG is given in the hope of preventing varicella, because varicella infection in an immunosuppressed child can be life threatening. VZIG decreases the infection's effects on the already weakened immune system. For hospitalized children who receive VZIG prophylactically, airborne isolation precautions must be used from day 10 to 28 after the exposure occurred.

Treatment for immunocompromised patients and pregnant patients with severe complications involves administration of intravenous acyclovir.

Children with active varicella are rarely hospitalized. If a child with varicella is hospitalized, maintain isolation precautions. Place the child in a private room, preferably a negative-pressure room. If the child must leave the room for tests or procedures, ensure that the child wears a mask. Examine the child's skin for new lesions daily. When lesions have begun to crust and no new lesions appear, isolation precautions can be discontinued. To relieve the child's boredom on being confined in an isolation room, ask the child life specialist to bring washable toys, videotapes, or games into the room.

The most common complication of varicella is secondary bacterial infection caused by the child scratching the lesions. Teach the child and parents interventions that promote comfort and prevent infection or scarring caused by scratching the lesions (TIP 24–2).

Parents may sometimes need to bring a child with active varicella to the pediatrician or family practitioner's office. Teach parents to alert the office staff about the child's potential diagnosis. Many physicians' offices have an alternative entrance for contagious children.

Community Care

The largest impact varicella has on families is on those who use daycare centers and dual-income families. Because the child is highly contagious, a parent must often stay home with the sick child. Home care nurses can often assist parents by exploring alternative baby-sitting arrangements with agencies that accommodate sick children.

Herpes Simplex Types 1 and 2

HSV-1 and HSV-2 produce similar clinical syndromes. Generally, HSV-1 is associated with oral lesions and HSV-2 is associated with genital lesions. However, HSV-1 infections can occur in the genital area and HSV-2 infections can occur orally. Lesions of HSV-1 and HSV-2 appear to be identical: vesicular lesions on an erythematous base.

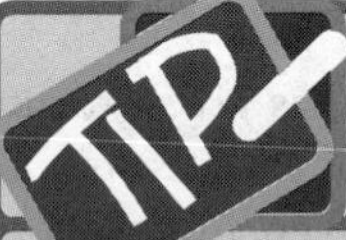

TIP 24–2 A Teaching Intervention Plan for the Child with Varicella

Nursing Diagnoses and Family Outcomes

- Risk for impaired skin integrity related to effects of pruritic skin lesions
- Risk for infection related to effects of scratching

Outcomes: Child will not develop secondary infection.
Child will experience minimal discomfort from pruritus.

Interventions

Teach parents and child how to manage discomfort and rash

- The best treatment for skin discomfort is a cool bath with soothing oatmeal (Aveeno) every 3 to 4 hours for the first few days. Calamine lotion may help decrease itching. If the itching becomes severe or interferes with sleep, give the child a nonprescription antihistamine (diphenhydramine HCl [Benadryl]).
- Keep fingernails short. Wash child's hands frequently with antibacterial soap to reduce bacterial colonization.
- Remind child not to scratch lesions. If young child scratches at lesion, consider applying mittens or cotton socks over hands.
- If urination becomes painful, apply some 2½% lidocaine (Xylocaine) or 1% dibucaine (Nupercainal) ointment (nonprescription) to the genital lesions every 2 to 3 hours to relieve pain.
- Administer acetaminophen for fever. Aspirin should be avoided in children and adolescents with varicella because of the link with Reye's syndrome.
- If child is uncomfortable because of oral lesions, offer cool fluids, ice pops, or soft, bland food. Avoid citrus, spicy, or salty foods. If mouth ulcers become troublesome, have the child gargle or swallow 1 teaspoon to 1 tablespoon of an antacid solution four times a day after meals.

Contact Health Care Provider if

- Red, tender areas are noted on skin, or a speckled, fine rash develops.
- Child seems very sick or develops the following: difficulty awakening, stiff neck, trouble walking, difficulty breathing or rapid breathing, or vomiting more than three times.
- Scabs become soft and drain pus.
- Fever lasts more than 4 days.

Incidence

Disseminated herpes simplex infection in the newborn has a high mortality rate. Fifty percent of the survivors experience neurologic impairment (Hensleigh & Nguyen, 1994). Still, the incidence of infection remains low, ranging from 1 in 3000 live births to 1 in 20,000 live births. Relative risk of infection is greater in infants born to mothers with primary infection (33% to 50%) and much lower in infants of mothers with recurrent infection (3% to 5%).

Prognosis. Neonatal herpes presents in three distinct groups: disseminated disease, isolated CNS involvement, and localized infection. Mortality among neonates with disseminated disease is 85%. Surviving infants face the lifelong sequelae of neurologic impairment, blindness, and recurrent skin lesions (Hensleigh & Nguyen, 1994). Mortality with isolated CNS involvement is 50%; with localized disease, nearly zero.

Assessment

Oral infections range from mild "cold sores" to gingivostomatitis (Fig. 24–14). Shedding of herpesvirus occurs in the saliva. Severe gingivostomatitis can result in dehydration because the mouth becomes intolerably sore (see Chapter 22 for interventions). Illness usually begins with a fever, sore mouth, and anorexia. Lesions can extend to the entire mouth area, tongue, gums, and inside of the cheek (buccal mucosa). Infants who suck their thumbs can develop herpetic whitlow (herpetic lesion appearing on the fingers or thumb).

Primary infections begin with an "aura" or tingling sensation. Then, 24 to 48 hours later, painful vesicular

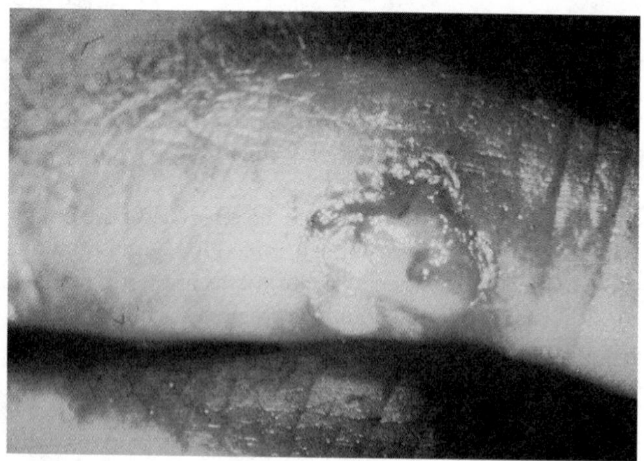

Figure 24–14
Cold sores of herpes simplex often begin with a tingling sensation 1 to 2 days before the outbreak of lesions. (Courtesy of the Burroughs Wellcome Corporation.)

lesions with an erythematous base erupt. The lesions last 10 to 14 days.

Primary genital infections often involve painful labial lesions (Fig. 24–15) and cervical lesions. Recurrent infections are less severe and, in females, may be limited to the cervix, which has few nerve endings for pain. Thus, a recurrent infection could be asymptomatic. For this reason, pregnant females with a history of genital herpes should have weekly cervical smears from 36 weeks' gestation until delivery. Maternal transmission to the fetus occurs via passage through an infected birth canal or as an ascending infection with prolonged (greater than 6 hours) rupture of amniotic membranes (Eutropius, Overall, & Spruance, 1996). Occasionally, during a maternal primary infection, the virus crosses the placenta during the maternal viremic phase, when a high volume of virus is circulating in the maternal blood.

Figure 24–15
The primary lesions of genital herpes simplex infections occur in the genital area, as in these labial lesions. (Courtesy of the Burroughs Wellcome Corporation.)

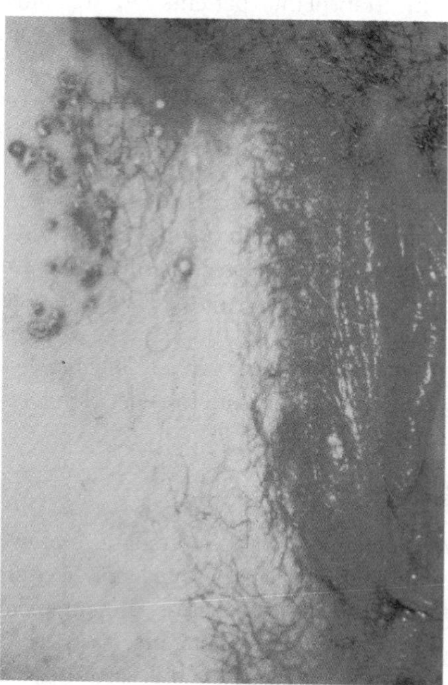

The pregnant female may experience painful recurrent genital lesions or relatively painless recurrent cervical lesions. Babies born through this infected vaginal canal acquire HSV. Approximately 1 week after birth, vesicular lesions erupt on the infant's trunk and extremities, and fever, jaundice, and hepatosplenomegaly occur. Other symptoms can follow (Chart 24–20), leading to circulatory collapse and death in untreated infants.

The infant with disseminated neonatal herpes presents with hypothermia, progressive jaundice, hepatosplenomegaly, and vesicular lesions in the first 2 weeks of life (Fig. 24–16). Anorexia, vomiting, and respiratory and circulatory collapse soon follow. Isolated CNS involvement is manifest as encephalitis. Localized disease affects the eye, mouth, or skin.

Diagnostic Tests. HSV is easily cultured from skin lesions; 1 to 3 days are required for viral detection. Rapid diagnosis is made with detection of HSV antigens in lesion swabs using commercially available ELISA kits. Commercially available ELISA antibody blood test kits can be used to identify recent (IgM) or past (IgG) HSV infection. A Western blot for HSV can distinguish between HSV-1 and HSV-2 but is available only in research facilities.

Because neonatal herpes is linked with passage through an infected birth canal, pregnant women with a history of genital herpes have Papanicolaou smears performed during the last month of pregnancy. Cervical cells

Chart 24–20

Effects of Congenital Herpes Simplex Virus Infection

- Intrauterine growth retardation
- Jaundice, hepatitis, hepatosplenomegaly
- Anemia, thrombocytopenia, disseminated intravascular coagulopathy
- Vesicular lesions
- Chorioretinitis
- Meningoencephalitis, cerebral calcifications, mental retardation, microcephaly, seizures
- Pneumonitis

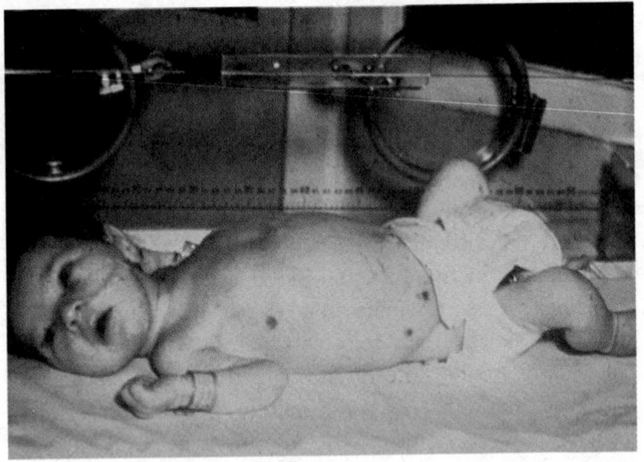

Figure 24–16
Lesions in congenital herpes simplex. (Courtesy of the Burroughs Wellcome Corporation.)

that are infected with herpes enlarge greatly, indicating infection with herpes.

Nursing Diagnoses and Outcomes

The common nursing diagnoses and outcomes listed in Chart 24–5 are applicable to the infant with congenital herpes simplex infection. Depending on the disease manifestations in the child, other diagnoses may be applicable. For the child with acquired herpes simplex disease, the following may be applicable:

- **Impaired skin integrity related to effects of herpesvirus**
  Outcome: The child and family will implement interventions to minimize discomfort and speed healing.
- **Altered oral mucous membrane related to effects of herpesvirus**
  Outcome: The child will ingest sufficient fluid to prevent dehydration.

Interdisciplinary Interventions

Treatment for congenital infection is with intravenous acyclovir. Topical treatment for eye involvement is usually with trifluridine, idoxuridine, or vidarabine. Topical acyclovir ointment on oral or genital lesions can decrease viral shedding and encourage faster resolution of the lesions.

Because the lesions of varicella and herpes simplex resemble each other, varicella infection is considered in the differential diagnosis for an infant who may have a congenital herpes infection.

Postpartum women with active herpes lesions should be educated in the value of hand washing. Transmission of HSV to the infant can occur if the mother touches the baby with contaminated hands. HSV transmitted to the mother's hands after postpartum pericare can be washed off with soap and water. Mothers, fathers, grandparents, or any visitor who has active oral HSV lesions should not kiss the infant, because transmission to the infant can occur.

Contact precautions should be used with the infant with congenital herpes simplex infection. Because infants are confined to bassinets, private rooms are not necessary. Health care workers should wear gloves while handling the infant because the lesions contain active virus.

Advise parents to exclude their child with cold sores from daycare only if the child *cannot* control oral secretions (drooling). Ensure that health care workers with active oral lesions wear a surgical mask to cover the lesions, avoid touching the lesions, and pay scrupulous attention to hand washing.

Cytomegalovirus Infections

Etiology and Incidence

Cytomegalovirus belongs to the herpes family of viruses. Like all herpesviruses, it can be reactivated after primary infection. Almost everyone encounters CMV eventually. However, the infection is usually asymptomatic and of little consequence, except in immunosuppressed individuals, such as those undergoing organ transplantation.

Reactivation of CMV after transplantation could cause organ rejection. Some researchers suggest that CMV is itself immunosuppressive (Grundy, 1990). It suppresses the activity of natural killer cells and may contribute to immunosuppression in children with HIV infection. Yet CMV is also frequently associated with graft rejection in transplant patients. It remains unclear whether CMV causes the rejection or is activated by the treatment (immunosuppressive therapy).

Transmission of CMV is by direct contact with virus-containing secretions, such as urine or saliva. This can occur in daycare centers or nurseries when drooling, teething babies share toys that they bite or gum. Adolescents may acquire CMV through sexual intercourse and kissing (saliva). Transmission from an infected mother to her infant may occur by transplacental passage of the virus in utero, passage of the neonate through an infected birth canal, or ingestion of infected breast milk. Other modes of transmission include blood transfusions and solid organ transplants.

Assessment

Most CMV infections are asymptomatic. A few individuals may exhibit a vague mononucleosis-like illness with fatigue, fever, and mild hepatitis. Immunocompromised children may experience pneumonia, gastritis, colitis, arthralgia, arthritis, encephalopathy, retinitis, fever, and lymphadenopathy. AIDS patients with reactivated CMV typically develop vision loss caused by CMV retinitis.

Most infants with congenital CMV infection (95%) are asymptomatic. However, 5% or less of them have significant manifestations of fetal damage, as summarized in Chart 24–21. Approximately 10% to 20% of these infants suffer mental retardation or deafness. Although the risk for a profoundly affected infant is low (less than 5%), the results are usually devastating (Fig. 26–17).

Diagnostic Tests. The diagnosis of congenital CMV is difficult. An infected newborn typically presents with liver and spleen enlargement, jaundice, a blueberry muffin rash (deep, bluish, purpuric lesions), microcephaly, thrombocytopenia, and cerebral calcifications as evidenced on radiographs. Despite this physical evidence, viral culture or serologic testing is still needed to confirm the diagnosis. Viral culture specimens can be obtained from urine or pharyngeal or cervical secretions. CMV can also be isolated from human milk, semen, and leukocytes. In addition, the presence of IgM CMV antibodies in cord blood can identify congenitally infected infants. The shell vial assay is the standard rapid culture method for detecting CMV infections. Newer methods for CMV detection include a CMV antigenemia assay, which detects a viral protein in the infant's white cells, and the polymerase chain reaction, which detects CMV DNA in blood.

Nursing Diagnoses and Outcomes

In addition to the common nursing diagnoses and outcomes listed in Chart 24–5, the following may be applicable to the infant affected with congenital CMV:

- **Altered family processes related to extremely ill infant**
  Outcome: The parents will express concerns regarding the infant's treatments and prognosis.

Chart 24–21

Effects of Congenital Cytomegalovirus Infection

- Intrauterine growth retardation
- Jaundice, hepatitis, hepatosplenomegaly
- Anemia
- "Blueberry muffin" rash
- "Celery stalking" (radiographic lines in the long bones)
- Chorioretinitis
- Cerebral calcifications, mental retardation, microcephaly, seizures, hearing loss

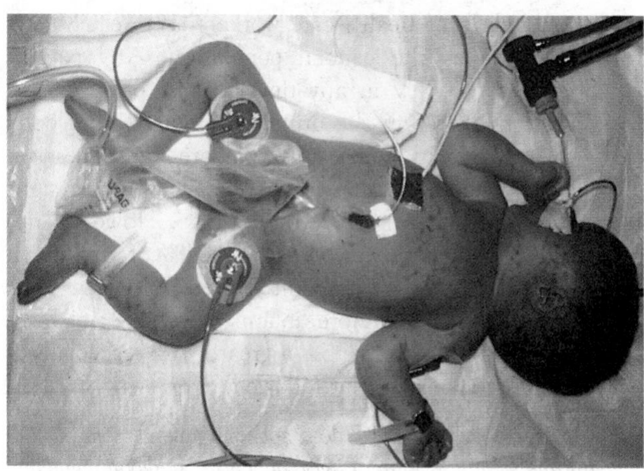

Figure 24–17
A dark rash resembling the blueberry muffin rash of rubella is also seen in congenital CMV infection. (Courtesy of Dr. William Gruber.)

- **Ineffective breathing pattern related to the disease process**
  Outcome: The child will maintain adequate oxygenation.

Interdisciplinary Interventions

Treatment for CMV, especially retinitis, is with ganciclovir or foscarnet. Antiviral drugs are given by induction therapy (dosages that gradually increase over 3 weeks to the therapeutic dose). Limited studies show that ganciclovir is beneficial in children. However, more studies are needed to verify its safety in children (Committee on Infectious Diseases, American Academy of Pediatrics, 1994). After therapeutic levels are reached, some HIV-infected children and bone marrow transplant recipients are given 6 to 12 weeks of maintenance therapy with reduced dosages. Even with reduced dosages, ganciclovir and foscarnet are highly toxic. Ganciclovir may induce bone marrow toxicity, and foscarnet can trigger renal tubular dysfunction.

Nursing care of infants or children who may have congenital CMV syndrome or who may be shedding CMV should focus on supportive care and good hand washing. The risk of acquiring CMV infection during pregnancy can provoke anxiety among health care workers who are pregnant or planning to become pregnant, because of the risk of congenital CMV syndrome. Infection in the pregnant female is typically asymptomatic. However, when women experience their first or primary infection during pregnancy, CMV is transmitted to the fetus 40% of the time (Valenti, 1992). Nevertheless, it is a common misconception that nurses and other health care workers are at increased risk for acquiring CMV from pediatric or neonatal patients (Valenti, 1993). Many studies of CMV transmission in health care settings conclude that health care workers acquire CMV at the same rate as the general population. Any patient could reactivate CMV at any time because of stress and could shed the virus in the urine, saliva, and other body fluids. Neonates with CMV infection are sometimes isolated by the nursing staff with handmade warning signs stating NO PREGNANT CAREGIVERS. However, approximately 1% of *all* newborns and 14% of infants in the neonatal intensive care unit excrete CMV in their urine (Zaia, 1996). Therefore, infants who have not been identified as infected may pose a greater risk, especially if standard precautions are not followed.

caREminder: *The CDC does not recommend isolating infants with congenital CMV infection. It recommends educating health care workers about hand washing, especially pregnant health care workers, and using standard precautions.*

Epstein-Barr Virus Infection (Mononucleosis)

Epstein-Barr virus was discovered as the causative agent in a common adolescent and young adult disease, mononucleosis. Also known as the kissing disease, mononucleosis is transmitted primarily by oral-salivary spread in young children and close intimate contact (kissing) in adolescents and young adults. The highest incidence is in adolescents. EBV is also associated with Burkitt's lymphoma, nasopharyngeal cancer, Hodgkin's disease, and some autoimmune disorders such as Sjögren's syndrome.

Assessment

Three symptoms of mononucleosis present as a triad: sore throat (exudative pharyngitis), fever, and lymphadenopathy. Other common symptoms include fatigue, headache, and an enlarged liver and/or spleen. In some rare cases, the spleen enlarges and ruptures, leading to hemorrhage, shock, and death. In other rare cases, severe involvement of the central nervous system results in encephalitis.

Although a rash is not typical, a central rash may occur during the first few days of the illness. Jaundice occurs in conjunction if EBV induces hepatitis, which happens in only 5% of cases.

The disease can begin insidiously over 30 to 50 days after the 4- to 6-week incubation period, or it may begin abruptly after the incubation period. In general, symptoms are more pronounced in adolescents than in children. A simultaneous throat infection with group A streptococcus could mask the symptoms and lead the health care practitioner to believe the child has streptococcal pharyngitis and overlook the mononucleosis.

Diagnostic Tests. The total number of atypical lymphocytes in the blood characteristically increases along with a high titer of heterophil antibody. Monocytes constitute 50% of the total white cell count. The overall leukocytosis that is present early in the disease can be so elevated that leukemia is suspected.

Diagnosis is based on a blood count showing lymphocytosis and at least 10% atypical lymphocyte formation, symptoms, and testing for heterophil antibody. In young children, the heterophil antibody test is usually negative.

Viral cultures can be obtained from saliva, blood, or lymph tissue but can take up to 6 to 8 weeks. Polymerase chain reaction is also useful in determining the presence of EBV DNA. A positive test is indicative of infection.

Newer tests measure EBV-specific antibodies. During the course of mononucleosis, EBV produces an initial anti–viral capsid antigen (VCA) IgM. This VCA IgM declines to barely detectable levels over time. As VCA IgM starts to decline, there is a detectable rise in anti-VCA immunoglobulin G (VCA IgG). This VCA IgG persists for life.

Nursing Diagnoses and Outcomes

In addition to the common nursing diagnoses and outcomes listed in Chart 24–5, the following may be applicable to the child with EBV:

- **Fatigue related to effects of disease process**
  Outcome: The child will obtain adequate rest and perform age-appropriate quiet activities as tolerated.

Interdisciplinary Interventions

In general, no current therapy is recommended for EBV. Steroids may be used to control swelling if enlarged tonsils block the airway. Acyclovir seems to be active against EBV in the laboratory but is not effective clinically.

caREminder: *Avoid ampicillin if concomitant streptococcal pharyngitis is present. Use of ampicillin causes a rash in most individuals with mononucleosis.*

No isolation precautions are recommended for the hospitalized patient. Most otherwise healthy children and adolescents recover with no sequelae. Nursing care is supportive and consists of acetaminophen for fever reduction and pain relief.

Suggest a soft or liquid diet for patients with throat pain. Encourage enough liquids to prevent dehydration. Because of their chronic fatigue, children and adolescents usually self-limit their activity; thus bed rest is not necessary. Recommend home teachers for children with prolonged fatigue who cannot attend school.

Tip: *Advise children with enlarged spleens to avoid contact sports until splenomegaly resolves.*

Teach children and parents to notify the health care provider if abdominal pain, especially in the left upper quadrant, or left shoulder pain occurs (may indicate splenic rupture).

Human Herpesvirus Type 6 Infection

This infection is also known as sixth disease, roseola, because it is the sixth childhood disease that produces a rash. Roseola is typically characterized by a high fever that often leads to febrile convulsions. The virus is thought to be transmitted primarily through the respiratory secretions of infected children (Committee on Infectious Diseases, American Academy of Pediatrics, 1994). Incidence is highest at age 6 to 24 months. Viral shedding continues after the rash and fever subside. The incubation period is approximately 9 days (Committee on Infectious Diseases, American Academy of Pediatrics, 1994).

Assessment

The disease begins with 3 to 4 days of high fever (103° and 104°F). The child does not appear ill and typically is quite playful. A rash appears briefly after the fever subsides. The rash begins centrally (on the trunk) and then spreads to the face, arms, and legs. The rash is rose colored and blanches under pressure. It can disappear within hours of its initial appearance.

Diagnostic Tests. The diagnosis of roseola is based on the clinical presentation. Some research virology laboratories may be able to isolate the virus from blood. There are currently no commercially available tests to confirm antibodies or titers.

Nursing Diagnoses and Outcomes

In addition to the common nursing diagnoses and outcomes listed in Chart 24–5, the following may be applicable to the child with roseola:

- **Risk for injury related to the effects of the fever (febrile seizures)**

  Outcomes: The parents will implement fever management interventions.

  The child will suffer no sequelae of the fever.

Interdisciplinary Interventions

Isolation of the infant is not necessary if the infant is hospitalized. Nursing care consists of standard precautions and supportive care. Acetaminophen or ibuprofen is given for fever reduction. Seizure precautions and anticonvulsants, such as phenobarbital, can be used for children with a history of febrile convulsions (Committee on Infectious Diseases, American Academy of Pediatrics, 1994). Tepid baths can be given to augment the antipyretic agents.

Viral Hepatitis

The hepatitis group of viruses (hepatitis A [HAV], hepatitis B [HBV], hepatitis C [HCV], hepatitis D or delta [HDV], and hepatitis E [HEV]) are related in name only. For example, hepatitis A virus is an RNA virus and hepatitis B virus is a DNA virus, but they share a common pathology: infection of the liver. These viruses are summarized in Table 24–12. Hepatitis can cause liver inflammation, jaundice, a rise in liver enzymes, and liver failure.

Etiology

Hepatitis A viral infection was formerly known as infectious hepatitis. HAV is transmitted via the oral-fecal route by eating food contaminated with HAV. Infected children shed HAV and HEV in the stool. Transmission can occur in children and caregivers in daycare centers. For example, a daycare worker could change the diaper

Table 24–12
Common Hepatitis Viruses

Name	Mode of Transmission	Incubation Period (wk)	Clinical Features
Hepatitis A virus (HAV)	Oral-fecal Food and/or water	2–6	Symptoms are mild or absent in children.
Hepatitis B virus (HBV)	Sexual Parenteral Perinatal	7–26	Symptoms are mild or absent in children.
Hepatitis C virus (HCV)	Parenteral Sexual Perinatal	2–24	Symptoms are mild or absent in children.
Hepatitis D virus (HDV)	Sexual Parenteral Perinatal	3–12	Concurrent infection with hepatitis B. Fulminant hepatitis.
Hepatitis E virus (HEV)	Water-borne	2–9	Similar to HAV. Rare in children.

of an infant who is shedding HAV. Then the worker might prepare food without washing the hands first.

Hepatitis B was once known as serum hepatitis. Maternal transmission of HBV to the fetus occurs during delivery. HCV is known as transfusion-associated hepatitis because blood transfusions account for 90% of cases (Krugman, 1992b). HDV is a defective RNA virus that requires HBV to complete its life cycle. Finally, HEV is associated with water-borne outbreaks in India, Africa, Central America, and South America. Fulminant hepatitis occurs in rare cases. This highly fatal complication of hepatitis infection leads to hepatic coma and death.

Assessment

Symptoms can have an abrupt onset as in HAV and HEV or can be more insidious. Generally, children have mild symptoms without jaundice or are asymptomatic.

There are two stages of disease in hepatitis: the prejaundice stage and the jaundice stage. The prejaundice stage is characterized by headache, malaise, anorexia, nausea, vomiting, and abdominal pain. The jaundice stage is marked by dark urine, clay-colored (light) stools, and yellowish skin (jaundice) and sclera.

The clinical signs and symptoms of congenital hepatitis B are described in Chart 24–22 for infants born to hepatitis B antigen–positive pregnant females.

The symptoms and modes of transmission for hepatitis D are similar to those in hepatitis B infection. However, the symptoms of HDV infection can be more severe. HDV infections are more likely to be found in IV drug abusers, people with hemophilia, or immigrants from countries in which HDV infection is endemic, such as eastern Europe, the Middle East, South America, and Africa (Committee on Infectious Diseases, American Academy of Pediatrics, 1994).

Diagnostic Tests. In hepatitis, liver enzymes are elevated, including lactate dehydrogenase (LDH), serum glutamic-oxaloacetic transaminase (SGOT), and serum glutamic-pyruvic transaminase (SGPT). Serologic tests for specific hepatitis viruses and their corresponding IgM and IgG antibodies confirm the diagnosis. In acute hepatitis, IgM antibodies are present. Later in the infection, IgG antibodies are present. The presence of IgG antibodies alone suggests that hepatitis occurred sometime in the past and that the patient is no longer infectious. Tests for hepatitis are summarized in Table 24–13.

Serologic tests for hepatitis B can help confirm the diagnosis. Generally, the presence of any hepatitis B **antigen** always indicates that circulating virus is present and that the child's blood and body fluids are infectious. The presence of hepatitis B **antibody** means that the body is responding to the infection and that immunity is beginning.

Tests for HCV are constantly evolving. The current HCV antibody test does not differentiate between IgM or IgG antibodies. It is difficult to ascertain whether the HCV infection is current or occurred in the past. The recombinant immunoblot assay (RIBA) detects antibodies and several HCV proteins and is therefore more specific.

Tests for HEV are mainly exclusion tests. If the child has negative tests for all other known hepatitis sources and has traveled to a country in which HEV is endemic, the diagnosis of HEV is assumed. Tests for HEV antigen and antibody are not yet available.

Chart 24–22

Effects of Congenital Hepatitis

- Nausea, vomiting, abdominal pain, and clay-colored stools
- Jaundice, lymphadenopathy, thrombocytopenia, disseminated intravascular coagulopathy, coma, and death (rare)
- Ninety percent of infants born to mothers with active hepatitis are 275 times more likely to develop liver cancer when they reach age 30 to 40 years

Nursing Diagnoses and Outcomes

In addition to the common nursing diagnoses and outcomes listed in Chart 24–5, the following may be applicable to the older child or adolescent with hepatitis:

- **Activity intolerance related to fatigue**
  Outcome: The child will have increasing activity tolerance and maintain school requirements.

Interdisciplinary Interventions

There are basically no treatment and no cure for acute hepatitis infection. Vaccines have been developed for some of the hepatitis viruses (Table 24–14).

Antiviral therapy for HBV infection has been evaluated. Some patients with chronic hepatitis B and hepatitis C infection respond to interferon alfa-2b therapy (Katov & Dienstag, 1991). High-dose interferon therapy for hepatitis D is currently undergoing clinical trials.

caREminder: *Liver transplantation has been used as a treatment for end-stage liver disease resulting from hepatitis B infection. However, because other body tissues still harbor HBV, the new liver may also become infected.*

Nursing care for children with hepatitis A and E infection should focus on teaching preventive measures,

Table 24–13
Tests for Viral Hepatitis

Virus	Tests	Positive Findings	Interpretation
HAV	Anti-HAV	Antibody to HAV	Acute infection
	IgM anti-HAV	IgM antibody to HAV	Acute infection
	IgG anti-HAV	IgG antibody to HAV	Past infection
HBV	HB_sAg	Hepatitis B surface antigen	Acute or chronic infection
	Anti-HB_s	Antibody to hepatitis B surface antigen	Vaccinated or past HBV
	HB_eAg	Hepatitis B little e antigen	Highly contagious
	Anti-HB_e	Antibody to HBV little e antigen	Resolving HBV infection
	Anti-HB_c	Antibody to HBV core antigen	Acute or past infection
	IgM anti-HB_c	IgM antibody to core antigen	Acute infection
	HBV-DNA	Hybridization test	Acute or chronic HBV
HCV	Anti-HCV	Antibody to hepatitis C	Acute or past infection
	RIBA	Recombinant immunoblot assay	Acute infection
	PCR-HCV	Polymerase chain reaction to HCV	Under research
HDV	Anti-HDV	Antibody to HDV	Chronic infection
	PCR-HDV	Polymerase chain reaction for HDV	Acute infection
HEV	Tests are negative for HAV, HBV and HCV		Diagnosis by exclusion

good sanitation, and careful hand washing. Through family hygiene instruction, nurses can help prevent outbreaks in families. This instruction should include teaching family members about cooking shellfish and avoiding raw shellfish. Finally, hand washing after toileting or diaper changing is essential to hygiene but specific in preventing HAV infection.

Adolescents may be educated about sexual activity during the acute phase of HBV, HCV, or HDV infection, when transmission may be likely. Health care workers should advise abstinence or the use of condoms.

Nursing care of an infant born to a hepatitis B antigen–positive mother should focus on standard precautions. Nurses and other health care workers should wear gloves when handling the infant after delivery and until all amniotic fluid is wiped off. Because hepatitis B has a long incubation period (up to 6 months), the infant of a chronic carrier or a woman with active HBV infection should receive hepatitis B immune globulin (HBIG). Active immunization with hepatitis B vaccine is also initiated. Giving hepatitis B vaccine to the child along with HBIG can prevent disease in 95% of the infants.

Community Care

The Immunization Practices Advisory Committee of the CDC recommends routine testing of *all* pregnant women for hepatitis B surface antigen (HB_sAg). Infants born

Table 24–14
Vaccines and Immunoprophylaxis for Viral Hepatitis

Virus	Immunoprophylaxis	Vaccine	Vaccine Recipients
HAV	Immune globulin	Yes	International travelers, members of the military, daycare workers, laboratory workers
HBV	Hepatitis B immune globulin	Yes	All infants, health care workers, public safety workers, hemodialysis patients, institutionalized individuals (mentally disabled, prisoners), hemophiliacs, household and sexual partners of HBV carriers, IV drug abusers, nonmonogamous sexually active individuals
HCV	None	None	Not applicable
HDV	Hepatitis B immune globulin	See HBV	See HBV
HEV	None	None	Not applicable

with congenital hepatitis B have a 90% likelihood of developing liver cancer. Because hepatitis B infection is preventable in these infants with the administration of HBIG and hepatitis B vaccine, the CDC recommended the vaccine universally for all newborns (CDC, 1991).

caREminder: *Pregnant patients should ideally be tested for hepatitis B early in pregnancy and before delivery (in patients at high risk) so that infants who need immediate prophylaxis at birth can be identified.*

In general, preventing and controlling viral hepatitis transmission include hand washing after toileting or diapering infants, giving immunoprophylaxis after exposure (immune globulin), and active immunization. Limiting environmental contamination and water sanitation can decrease the potential for exposure to hepatitis A and E. The inability to identify children who are infected because of lack of symptoms emphasizes the importance of routine infection control procedures such as hand washing, sterilization of medical equipment, and standard precautions.

TORCH Infections

TORCH (*toxoplasmosis, other, rubella, cytomegalovirus, herpes simplex virus*) is the acronym used for several infectious diseases that can affect the fetus and cause developmental and physical damage. In most cases, the infant fails to thrive and exhibits physical disorders such as blindness, hydrocephalus, and mental retardation. To rule out a TORCH infection in infants, a careful maternal history must be obtained along with a serologic blood panel of tests for toxoplasmosis, rubella, CMV, and herpes. A Venereal Disease Research Laboratory (VDRL) test is useful for syphilis, and a hepatitis profile can rule out hepatitis B.

Because rubella, CMV, hepatitis B, and herpes simplex infections were previously discussed, this section focuses on toxoplasmosis and syphilis.

Toxoplasmosis

Etiology and Incidence

Toxoplasmosis is a disease caused by a parasite, *Toxoplasma gondii*, that lives in the intestinal tract of many animals including domestic cats. The parasite occurs in three forms: tachyzoites (an ameba-like form), bradyzoites (a cast form), and highly infectious oocysts. Transmission occurs by eating foods contaminated with *T. gondii* cysts or inhaling dust that contains oocysts from cat feces. Eating fruits or vegetables harvested in countries that use fecal fertilizer sprays, drinking unpasteurized milk, and eating unfrozen or undercooked lamb, pork, or beef are the principal ways in which transmission occurs. Pregnant women who empty cat litter boxes can inhale oocysts from the litter dust. The woman may then develop toxoplasmosis and transmit the parasite to her fetus.

Congenital toxoplasmosis occurs when a pregnant woman contracts toxoplasmosis for the first time during pregnancy. The organism can cross the placenta. However, the incidence of fetal infection is only 40% (McLeod, Wisner, & Boyer, 1992).

Prognosis. Damage to the fetus depends on the trimester in which the infection occurred. Maternal infection during the first trimester causes the most fetal damage. Although the incidence of transmission is low (17%), the severity of fetal damage is great. If maternal infection occurs in the second trimester, 25% of the fetuses are infected and suffer intermediate fetal damage. Conversely, last trimester maternal infection results in 100% transmission to the fetus but little or no fetal damage.

Assessment

The signs and symptoms of congenital toxoplasmosis are summarized in Chart 24–23. Maternal symptoms are vague, usually consisting of fatigue. Acquired toxoplasmosis in otherwise healthy children is usually asymptomatic. Ocular *Toxoplasma* infection can result from congenital or acquired infection. It can cause tissue necrosis in the retina, vitritis, iridocyclitis, and cataracts. Undetected and therefore untreated congenital infections usually become manifest during adolescence as ocular disease (chorioretinitis).

Diagnostic Tests. A positive result for maternal IgM antibody to *T. gondii* is diagnostic. Fetal blood samples can be tested for the presence of IgM specific antibodies. A polymerase chain reaction specific for *T. gondii* is becoming available to more laboratories; results are promising, and it can be performed on blood from the fetus, infant, or mother.

Chart 24–23

Effects of Congenital Toxoplasmosis

- Intrauterine growth retardation
- Jaundice, hepatitis, hepatosplenomegaly
- Anemia, thrombocytopenia, disseminated intravascular coagulopathy
- "Blueberry muffin" rash
- Chorioretinitis, microphthalmia, optic atrophy, blindness
- Intracranial calcifications, seizures, hydrocephalus, microcephaly, severe retardation, developmental delay

Fetal ultrasonography can show the presence of cerebral calcifications. After birth, ophthalmologic and neurologic examinations of the infant can be performed to look for chorioretinitis, hydrocephalus, microcephaly, and meningoencephalitis. A computed tomographic scan of the infant's head can show calcified brain lesions indicative of congenital toxoplasmosis.

Nursing Diagnoses and Outcomes

In addition to the common nursing diagnoses and outcomes listed in Chart 24–5, the following is applicable to a severely affected infant who may be in the neonatal intensive care unit and require mechanical ventilation:

- **Ineffective breathing pattern related to effects of disease process**
  Outcome: The child will have breathing pattern supported to maintain adequate tissue oxygenation.

Interdisciplinary Interventions

Treatment for maternal infection and infected children is with pyrimethamine and sulfadiazine. These two agents act together (synergistically) and, along with leucovorin (folinic acid), serve as standard therapy. Pyrimethamine causes severe bone marrow depression; leucovorin is given to counteract the suppression.

Spiramycin is an experimental drug used with special permission of the Food and Drug Administration (FDA). Some investigators have reported decreased maternal transmission with spiramycin treatment (McLeod et al., 1992).

Because the infection cannot be transmitted from human to human, no special isolation precautions are observed. Explaining ophthalmologic examinations and the various diagnostic laboratory tests (e.g., TORCH titers, *Toxoplasma* titer) to the parents helps them cope with an adverse outcome of pregnancy (see Chapter 8).

Preconception and prenatal teaching includes washing all fruits and vegetables and freezing all meats and then cooking them thoroughly before consuming them. Avoid steak tartare and other raw meat pâté. Nurses should encourage cat owners to have someone other than the pregnant woman empty the cat litter box daily. It takes 1 to 5 days before the oocyst can turn into the highly infectious spore form; thus, daily attention to the litter box is a must. Nurses must teach patients and their families to use disposable plastic litter box liners or disinfect the box with boiling water for 5 minutes.

Syphilis

The overall incidence of congenital syphilis is increasing. Any increase in congenital syphilis reflects a rise in rates of women who are infected. The disease is caused by a spirochete, *Treponema pallidum*. The incubation period is typically 3 weeks but ranges from 10 to 90 days after exposure. *T. pallidum* is transmitted by direct contact with the lesions (usually involving sexual intercourse) or transplacental transmission from an infected mother to her fetus.

Prognosis. The disease is treatable, even in pregnancy, with penicillin. Lack of treatment or late treatment in pregnancy often results in stillbirth (Committee on Infectious Diseases, American Academy of Pediatrics, 1994). In liveborn infants, congenital syphilis can affect many body systems (Chart 24–24).

Assessment

Maternally acquired syphilis occurs in three stages—primary, secondary, and tertiary—each of which has distinct clinical characteristics (Table 24–15).

Diagnostic Tests. The spirochete can be visualized using darkfield microscopy on smears taken from maternal primary lesions. Serologic tests include the VDRL slide test or the rapid plasma reagin (RPR) test, the fluorescent treponemal antibody absorption (FTA-ABS) test, and the microhemagglutination test for *T. pallidum* (MHA-TP). All women seeking prenatal care are screened for syphilis with a VDRL or RPR test early in pregnancy and again at delivery. The FTA-ABS or the MHA-TP test is used as a confirmatory test and remains positive for life.

Diagnosis in the newborn is confirmed by persistent or rising VDRL titers. Radiographs of long bones in the legs and arms show metaphysitis (inflammation of the growing end of the bone). Spinal fluid of the newborn is

Chart 24–24

Effects of Congenital Syphilis

- Intrauterine growth retardation
- Jaundice, lymphadenopathy, thrombocytopenia
- Severe, sometimes bloody rhinitis, associated with hoarse cry
- Macropapular rash covered by a fine silvery scale followed by desquamation
- Osteochondritis, periostitis (both painful), saber shins (long bones at lower leg are broad at the knee and narrow at the ankle, resembling a saber), perforated hard palate, saddle nose (cartilage in the nose is deformed so that it has a saddle-like appearance), mulberry molars (molars are deformed and take on the appearance of a cluster of mulberries), Hutchinson's teeth (teeth are malformed and small, resembling shoe peg corn)
- Interstitial keratitis
- Hearing loss, neurosyphilis

Table 24–15
Stages of Syphilis: Symptoms, Diagnosis, and Nursing Precautions

Stage	Symptoms	Diagnosis	Nursing Precautions
Primary	Painless chancre lasting 3–6 wk	Positive darkfield examination Reactive VDRL or RPR Positive MHA-TP or FTA-ABS	Wear gloves during examination of lesion (lesion contains organisms).
Secondary	Primary lesion healed or absent Generalized maculopapular rash that includes palms and soles of feet and lasts 3–12 wk	Reactive VDRL or RPR (usually >1 : 16) Positive MHA-TP, FTA-ABS	Wear gloves when handling blood or body fluids (standard precautions).
Tertiary	Obliterative endarteritis with tissue necrosis Optic atrophy Meningitis Parenchymatous neurosyphilis, which may range from personality changes to psychosis Cardiovascular syphilis caused by aortic necrosis Gummas (granulomatous-like lesions on skin or bone)	Positive CSF-VDRL	Observe standard precautions.

also sent for a VDRL test. A positive result is indicative of infection.

Interdisciplinary Interventions

Maternal treatment consists of intramuscular (IM) or IV penicillin G, even in individuals who are allergic to it. Women with penicillin allergy are desensitized to penicillin and then receive penicillin therapy. Desensitization is accomplished while the woman is hospitalized to ensure adequate emergency care should a severe reaction occur. Alternatives to penicillin include erythromycin and tetracycline or doxycycline. These alternatives are less effective. The infant receives IV crystalline penicillin G.

Alert: *Tetracycline drugs (including doxycycline) are avoided in pregnant women because they can produce dental staining in the fetus.*

Nursing care for the infant with congenital syphilis consists of careful hand washing and handling all secretions (even nasal) with gloves. Syphilitic infants have chronic, bloody nasal drainage containing *T. pallidum*. Observe glove precautions for at least 24 hours after antimicrobial therapy has started.

Report syphilis and congenital syphilis to the local health department. For pregnant women with syphilis, offer testing for HIV. Also, instruct them about the intensive follow-up health care visits for their infants. For infants with congenital syphilis, expect the VDRL or RPR test to be rechecked at 3, 6, and 12 months after treatment or until the test is negative.

Congenital syphilis is preventable. Consistent prenatal care and education are essential.

Rabies

Human rabies is an acute life-threatening illness involving the central nervous system. A rabid animal bites the child. The rabies virus gains access to the central nervous system through the blood stream via the bite. Human rabies was once common in the United States because of the prevalence of rabid dogs with the canine rabies strain. Beginning in the 1950s, vaccination programs for dogs and cats reduced the incidence of animal rabies. Five thousand cases of animal rabies were reported in 1995 (CDC, 1996a). Since 1980, 29 cases of human rabies have been reported to the CDC (CDC, 1996a). Exposure to dogs and bats accounts for most of the cases; however, any small wild animal, especially raccoons, skunks, and foxes, can be rabid. In many of the human rabies cases, a documented bite is never found. Once the exposure has occurred, the incubation period can range from 5 days to 1 year (an average of 2 months post exposure). Human infection is universally fatal.

Assessment

Symptoms of rabies develop over 7 to 14 days. The disease presents in three stages: prodromal, acute, and coma and death. In the prodromal stage, the child typically complains of headache, fever, and malaise. Other symptoms include a sore throat, dysphagia, nausea, vomiting, and anorexia. Drowsiness, irritability, and restlessness soon follow. The bite area may become numb or hypersensitive.

In the acute stage, the virus progresses throughout the central nervous system. The child displays either the furious form or the paralytic form. In the furious form, the child experiences increased anxiety and hyperexcitability, followed by increasing bouts of fever and delirium. Involuntary twitching and generalized convulsions occur and are seen as neurons and cranial nerves necrose. The child experiences spasmodic contractions of the larynx and pharynx when attempting to drink or if water is even seen. These painful spasms associated with water give rabies its common name, hydrophobia. Children with rabies avoid swallowing, even saliva, and may drool.

In the paralytic form, the child experiences paralysis in the bitten extremity or as an ascending, diffuse paralysis. The child's mental status deteriorates much more slowly than in the furious form of the disease. There is no treatment, and the disease process terminates in 7 to 14 days with coma followed by death.

Diagnostic Tests. Encephalitis after an animal bite along with the classic hydrophobic syndrome is clinically diagnostic. Antemortem diagnostic tests include staining of corneal impressions for direct fluorescent antibody (DFA) to rabies virus. The corneal impressions are made by taking a slide and gently pressing it against the cornea. Infected superficial corneal cells cling to the slide. The DFA test can also be performed with brain, nuchal (back of the neck), or lip biopsy tissue. These samples are stained for DFA to rabies virus.

Postmortem testing includes inoculation of suckling mice with the infected brain tissue. The mice die in a few days, and the mouse brain is sent to the CDC for gene sequencing.

Nursing Diagnoses and Outcomes

The following nursing diagnoses and outcomes may be applicable to the child with rabies:

- **Anticipatory grieving related to the child's fatal prognosis**
  Outcome: The family will be informed of all changes in the child's status and individually supported in their grieving.
- **Ineffective airway clearance related to effects of disease process**
  Outcome: The child will have comfort measures provided.
- **Impaired physical mobility related to effects of disease process**
  Outcome: The child will have supportive care and comfort measures implemented.

Interdisciplinary Interventions

There is no treatment for human rabies; only three people with human rabies have survived (CDC, 1995). Therefore, treatment centers on prevention. Animal bites are taken seriously by all physicians and emergency departments. After an animal bite, if the animal is captured, it is evaluated for rabies. Two products for rabies postexposure prophylaxis are given concurrently within 24 hours of the bite: rabies immune globulin (RIG) and rabies vaccine (Table 24–16). RIG provides rapid protec-

Table 24–16
Rabies Postexposure Prophylaxis Guide

Animal Type	Disposition	Recommendation
Dogs and cats	Check for vaccination records of animal. Observe animal for 10 days.	Do not vaccinate the child unless the animal develops rabies. If rabid, give RIG and begin vaccination.
Wild animals	Capture animal and test for rabies. If animal not captured, assume the animal is rabid.	Begin vaccination.
Farm animals	Observe for 10 days for signs of rabies.	Vaccinate the child if the animal is rabid.

From CDC guidelines for rabies postexposure prophylaxis. *MMWR 44*(14), 269–272.

tion, boosting the immune system for 21 days. Rabies vaccine provides an antibody response in 7 to 10 days and lasts 2 years (see Chapter 30).

Alert: *To decrease the likelihood of infection, clean bite wounds immediately with soap and water. The virus is inactivated by soap and other local disinfectants, such as isopropyl alcohol or povidone-iodine.*

Because human rabies is almost always fatal, family support is essential. Keep family members informed and allow them to visit without restriction. Place the hospitalized child in contact isolation. Explain the isolation precautions and the reason for them. Human transmission of rabies to health care workers or other close contacts has never been documented. However, a human rabies case always raises concern among those who had close contact with the patient's oral secretions. Wear gowns, gloves, and a mask with eye protection for adequate protection of health care workers during procedures.

The child is likely to be in an intensive care unit, preferably in a private room. If this is impossible, provide a private, quiet atmosphere. Minimize stimuli as much as possible. If the child survives, make referrals for intensive rehabilitative services.

Parasitic Infections

Parasites have infested humans worldwide throughout the centuries. Parasites can range in size from the microscopic *Plasmodium* spp. that cause malaria to the guinea worm, which can measure up to 3 m. Parasites have one aspect in common: they are free-living organisms. In many instances, humans are merely incidental hosts. In other cases, humans are a vital part of an elaborate life cycle that could include other animals or insects.

Of all the infectious and parasitic diseases, few cause more distress to nursing staff than lice and scabies. These parasites are discussed in detail in Chapter 25.

Giardiasis

Giardia lamblia is a protozoal organism that lives in freshwater streams. It infects both humans and wildlife. It exists as a trophozoite and as a cyst. The cyst form is infectious. Transmission is via ingestion of cyst-contaminated water or direct hand-to-mouth inoculation from cyst-contaminated hands. Infection with this organism causes giardiasis.

Assessment

Acute watery, foul-smelling diarrhea with abdominal pain is the hallmark of the disease. Watery stools are often accompanied by flatulence and abdominal distention. Anorexia is often seen, leading to weight loss and failure to thrive.

Diagnostic Tests. Identification of trophozoites or cysts in a direct stool smear is diagnostic. These smears can be observed directly (wet mount) or after being stained with iodine. Enzyme immunoassay tests for *Giardia* are commercially available that give a positive result if the child is infected.

Interdisciplinary Interventions

Treatment with quinacrine hydrochloride is 95% effective. However, this medication is extremely bitter and children are reluctant to finish the therapy (usually 1 week). An alternative medication, furazolidone, is 80% effective and available in a liquid form. Because of the ease of transmission within households, all family members should be treated simultaneously.

Community Care

Because outbreaks of giardiasis have occurred in daycare centers, instruct the parents to withdraw their infected child from daycare until the diarrhea resolves. If more than one child is involved, notify local health department officials, who should investigate. To avoid infection, family members should wash their hands after diapering infants and toileting.

Advise families who camp and hike that the pristine appearance of cool mountain water may be deceiving. Beavers and other wildlife can harbor *Giardia* cysts and contaminate streams. Therefore, advise families who enjoy camping to boil all water and avoid drinking from streams.

Hookworm Infection

Hookworm infection is rare in the United States. In the past, it was prevalent in the Southeast, where the larvae flourished in the warm, moist soil. However, as farming decreased and sanitation improved, hookworm infection decreased in frequency. It remains a problem in tropical developing countries.

Hookworm infection is caused by two species of worms with similar life cycles: *Ancylostoma duodenale* and *Necator americanus*. *N. americanus* is isolated most frequently in the United States. Worm larvae reside in warm, loose soil contaminated by human feces. Transmission is by larval penetration of the skin of the feet when children walk barefoot. The incubation period is 4 to 6 weeks from the time of exposure to the appearance of eggs in the stool.

Assessment

The clinical manifestations of hookworm infection can be divided into three phases: invasion, migration, and intestinal establishment.

Invasion occurs when the larvae penetrate the skin of the foot. Local stinging, burning, and rash (ground itch) accompany this phase, which lasts 1 to 2 weeks.

The migration phase begins as the larvae move up the blood stream to the lungs. There, the larvae leave the capillaries, enter the alveoli, and progress up the bronchi to the throat. This phase can be accompanied by hemoptysis and sore throat.

The child swallows the worms as they migrate up the throat. The worms then pass through the gastrointestinal tract to the small intestine. This begins the intestinal establishment phase. There, the worms embed in the mucosa of the small intestine and feed on capillary blood. They continue to mature and eventually lay eggs. It is the eggs, not the adult worms, that are excreted with the stool.

Severe infestations can lead to anemia. The child can become lethargic, exhibit anorexia, and have a distended abdomen.

Diagnostic Tests. Observing the distinctive hookworm egg in the stool is diagnostic. Often, a direct stool smear on a slide and special staining reveal the egg. The egg is oval and has a short hook at its apex.

Nursing Diagnoses and Outcomes

In addition to the common nursing diagnoses and outcomes listed in Chart 24–5, the following may be applicable to the child with hookworm infestation:

- **Anxiety related to the presence of worms in stool or vomitus**
  Outcome: The child and family will verbalize anxiety and the understanding that the worms will disappear after treatment.

Interdisciplinary Interventions

Treatment is with mebendazole or pyrantel pamoate. Infected pregnant women are treated after delivery. This therapy has not been sufficiently evaluated in children younger than 2 years.

Maintain excellent nutrition to help avoid many complications of hookworm disease, such as malabsorption and nutritional deficiencies. Two weeks after treatment, collect another stool specimen to verify the efficacy of treatment.

No isolation is necessary. Use standard precautions when handling stools and items contaminated with stool.

Teach the family ways to prevent hookworm infection. Wearing shoes can reduce the incidence of infection. The sanitary disposal of feces in endemic areas is helpful but not always possible.

 **caREminder:** *Dogs can also become infected with hookworm. Teach parents to dispose of dog feces properly, especially in areas where children play.*

Malaria

Malaria is rarely seen in the United States, except in individuals returning from malaria-endemic areas. Vigorous mosquito eradication, proper use of insecticides, and elimination of mosquito breeding sites have drastically reduced malaria worldwide since the 1960s. Malaria remains a problem in equatorial Africa, India, southern Asia, and parts of Central America and South America.

Malaria is caused by one of four parasites of the *Plasmodium* species: *P. vivax, P. malariae, P. ovale, P. falciparum*. It is transmitted by the female *Anopheles* mosquito, which feeds on blood. The parasites have a complex life cycle that involves the midgut and salivary glands of the *Anopheles* mosquito and the hepatic and peripheral circulatory system of humans.

Pathophysiology

As the mosquito feeds on a child, it injects saliva that contains an anticoagulant and houses malaria parasites. The organisms travel in the child's blood stream to the liver. There, they undergo changes to enable them to invade erythrocytes. At this point, the trophozoites (as they are now called) can be identified in a stained thin smear of peripheral blood. The trophozoites burst out of the erythrocyte and are carried in the blood stream. The disease can now be transmitted to another person when a mosquito takes a blood meal from the infected child.

Assessment

Infection caused by *P. falciparum* is more pathogenic than infections with the other three species. However, the classic symptoms of malaria infection are similar for all species. Classic symptoms include high fever, shaking chills, sweats, and headache. The fever occurs in a cyclic pattern, appearing every other day or every third day. Infection with *P. falciparum* and *P. malariae* can lead to signs and symptoms of numerous complications (Table 24–17).

Diagnostic Tests. Identification of the parasite in peripheral blood smears is diagnostic. Thick and thin smears are examined. Thick smears allow visualization of parasites present even in small numbers. Thin smears allow visualization of the trophozoite stage (ring forms).

Table 24–17
Complications of Malaria

Complications and Usual Cause	Clinical Manifestations
Cerebral malaria *P. falciparum*	Seizures Increased intracranial pressure Confusion Stupor Coma Death
Pulmonary edema *P. falciparum*	Pulmonary edema unresponsive to drug therapy Death
Renal failure *P. falciparum*	Acute tubular necrosis
Vascular collapse *P. falciparum*	Hypothermia Adrenal insuffiency
Black water fever *P. falciparum*	Hemoglobinuria after massive hemolysis and renal failure
Tropical splenomegaly *P. malariae*	Enlarged spleen Hemolytic anemia
Nephrotic syndrome *P. malariae*	Deposition of immune complexes in the kidneys
Congenital malaria *P. malariae*	Neonatal sepsis-like syndrome Poor appetite Restlessness Fever Lethargy

The actual parasite is seen inside a red blood cell in the shape of a signet ring. Other tests are specific for malaria, such as the quantitative buffy coat (QBC) test, a rapid test used in conjunction with peripheral blood smears. These tests are positive in a malaria-infected child. Newer tests in the developmental stage include PCR, DNA probes, and tests that detect malarial ribosomal RNA.

Interdisciplinary Interventions

Treatment is with oral chloroquine or parenteral quinidine gluconate. Some species of *P. falciparum* are resistant to chloroquine. For these infections, quinine sulfate is given with oral doxycycline, clindamycin, or pyrimethamine-sulfadoxine (Fansidar). As always, when choosing tetracycline therapy, the benefits of therapy should be weighed against the possibilities of dental staining.

In areas of the world where chloroquine-resistant malaria is present, the oral drugs of choice for treatment are quinine sulfate and doxycycline. For a child younger than 9 years, clindamycin or Fansidar is recommended (Committee on Infectious Diseases, American Academy of Pediatrics, 1994). Alternative regimens include mefloquine or parenteral quinine.

Alert: *Mefloquine is contraindicated for children who weigh less than 15 kg, pregnant women in the first trimester, patients receiving beta-blockers or other cardiac conduction–type drugs, those who have epilepsy or psychosis, and those who need fine motor control. Keep all antimalarial drugs in childproof containers. Overdosage can be fatal.*

Community Care

The key to controlling malaria worldwide is prevention. Adequate prophylaxis for travelers to malaria-endemic countries is essential. Prophylaxis with mefloquine or chloroquine begins 1 week before leaving and continues weekly while in the country and for 4 weeks after returning. Drugs are prescribed on the basis of the traveler's destination. The nursing responsibility is to teach the traveler accordingly. Alternatives include doxycycline or chloroquine with or without proguanil. Although proguanil is not available in the United States, it can be purchased in Canada, Europe, and many African countries.

Teach travelers to malaria-endemic countries about the importance of the prophylaxis. Instruct them on using insect repellents containing DEET, using mosquito netting impregnated with insecticide while sleeping, and remaining in screened-in areas. Advise them to reapply insect repellents according to package instructions. Use the lowest possible strength on younger children to avoid neurotoxicity. Spray clothing as well as skin.

Pinworm Infection (Enterobiasis)

Pinworm infestation occurs frequently in preschoolers and in those who attend daycare centers. The causative agent is the pinworm, *Enterobius vermicularis*. Clusters of infection are known to occur in families. In the past, up to 15% of the United States population was infested with pinworm. The incidence has been declining, however (Committee on Infectious Diseases, American Academy of Pediatrics, 1994).

Pathophysiology

The mode of transmission is oral-fecal. The gravid female pinworm lays eggs at the child's perianal region at night. It usually dies after depositing the eggs. Rectal itching leads to scratching. Autoinoculation results if the child scratches the rectal area and then puts the hand in his or her mouth (e.g., thumb sucking). Eggs can remain viable and infective on inanimate objects for 2 to 3 weeks. Eggs are swallowed and then hatched in the duodenum. The larvae live and grow, then slowly make their way toward the colon. Molting twice, adults mature in 1 to 1½ months. Then gravid females once again migrate to the anus to lay eggs.

Assessment

Perianal itching and localized irritation are hallmarks of pinworm infections. Children heavily infested may exhibit sleeplessness, hyperactivity, weight loss, tooth grinding, abdominal pain, and vomiting.

Aberrant migration of gravid female worms to the vagina may cause vaginitis. Subsequent aberrant migration from the perineum can contribute to salpingitis and pelvic peritonitis in female children (Committee on Infectious Diseases, American Academy of Pediatrics, 1994).

Diagnostic Tests. Diagnosis is confirmed by direct visualization of worms by the parents or via microscopy. Parents can view the sleeping child's anus with a flashlight. The worm is white, thin, about ½ inch long, and moves. A simple technique, the cellophane tape slide method, is used to capture worms and eggs. Transparent adhesive tape is lightly touched to the anus and then applied to a slide. The tape is examined under low power for worms and eggs. The best specimens are obtained as the patient awakens, before toileting or bathing.

Nursing Diagnoses and Outcomes

In addition to the common nursing diagnoses and outcomes listed in Chart 24–5, the following may apply to the child with pinworm infestation:

- **Impaired skin integrity related to scratching perianal region from pruritus caused by pinworm**
  Outcomes: The child will receive treatment to eradicate pinworm, thus pruritus.
  The child will maintain intact skin.

Interdisciplinary Interventions

Treatment is with a single dose of pyrantel pamoate or mebendazole. A repeated treatment is given 2 weeks later. Entire families or daycare groups should be treated simultaneously. Retreatment is often necessary.

Children infested with pinworm are rarely hospitalized. Nursing care centers on teaching parents and children appropriate eradication techniques. Linens and bedclothes can harbor eggs that remain infective for 2 to 3 weeks. Therefore, the nurse should emphasize rigorous hand washing after contact with the child, linens, or clothes. Teach parents to wash all linens and contaminated clothing using the hot cycle of the washing machine.

Community Care

Educating family members, schools, and daycare centers that recurrence is common can reduce some anxiety. Control of infections in schools and daycare centers can be difficult. Keeping fingernails clipped short and emphasizing hand washing seem to help.

Roundworm Infection (Toxocariasis)

Roundworm infections cause two conditions in children: visceral larva migrans and ocular larva migrans. The infection is caused by second-stage larval migration of roundworms to the liver, lungs, central nervous system, and eyes of humans, usually children. The adult worms are common roundworms found in dogs and cats, *Toxocara canis* and *Toxocara cati*. Young children are accidental hosts. These children ingest soil contaminated by infective eggs or play with infected puppies. Approximately 98% of all puppies younger than 10 weeks are congenitally infected with *T. canis* and excrete eggs in their feces (Glickman & Magnuval, 1993).

Pathophysiology

A child ingests the eggs, which can exist in the soil for years. The eggs hatch in the intestine, and the larvae penetrate the intestinal wall. Using the intestinal capillary system, the larvae gain access to the blood stream and migrate to the liver. Most of the larvae remain in the liver, but some pass on to the lungs, central nervous system, and eyes. Eventually, the larvae gravitate to a single location (either the liver or the eyes). The incubation period in humans is unknown.

Assessment

A history of exposure to puppies or a history of pica (eating dirt) is useful in establishing the diagnosis. The degree of symptoms depends on the number of eggs ingested. Most infections are asymptomatic. Fever, increased white blood cell count, persistent eosinophilia, hypergammaglobulinemia, and hepatomegaly are typical. Malaise, anemia, and cough are sometimes present. Rare manifestations include myocarditis, encephalitis, and pneumonia.

Ocular manifestations occur as a visual decrease or even total visual loss in one eye. The retinal damage goes unnoticed until the child (now adolescent) applies for a driver's license and fails the eye examination.

Diagnostic Tests. Eosinophilia and hypergammaglobulinemia, along with high titers of isohemagglutinin to the A and B blood groups, are suggestive of *T. canis* infection. Antibody titers for *T. canis* are positive in infected children.

Liver biopsies and retinal examinations can reveal larvae either by histological preparation and staining of biopsy specimens or by direct visualization of the larvae in the eye. Other eye damage, such as retinal detachment, can also be directly observed.

Nursing Diagnoses and Outcomes

In addition to the common nursing diagnoses and outcomes listed in Chart 24–5, the following may be applicable to the child with ocular larva migrans:

- **Sensory-perceptual alterations: vision related to effects of eye infestation**
  Outcome: The affected child will be identified early and corrective visual aids prescribed, if applicable.

Interdisciplinary Interventions

Treatment is with corticosteroids to reduce the allergic, inflammatory reaction and with anti-helminthic drugs, such as thiabendazole or diethylcarbamazine, to destroy the parasite. Some physicians are reluctant to treat ocular larva migrans with anthelmintic drugs because dying larvae and their metabolites can cause an increased hypersensitivity reaction in the retina (Glickman & Magnuval, 1993).

Community Care

Roundworm infection is preventable. Parents should be instructed to cover sandboxes when not in use, to keep cats from using them as litter boxes. Puppies should be dewormed at age 2, 4, 6, and 8 weeks, and children's play areas should be kept free of dog and cat feces.

Parents may need to administer eye drops to a child with ocular larva migrans. Because some types of drops are administered hourly, the parents of a school-age child may need to discuss eye drop administration with the school nurse. Parents may need to arrange for a home teacher if their child's school does not have a school nurse.

Fungal Infections

Fungal infections often occur when the child's immune system has been suppressed because of chemotherapy, radiation, or a disease. Fungi are opportunists: they take advantage of a vacated ecologic niche. When antibiotics are used to kill pathogenic strains of bacteria, they often kill useful bacteria (normal flora) as well. These useful bacteria normally keep fungi in check. When they are gone, fungi can take over and cause serious infections.

Aspergillosis

Aspergillosis is an infection of the lungs, central nervous system, and other major organ systems. Spore-forming *Aspergillus* spp. are environmental fungi found in the soil and on live or decaying plants. The spores are on our clothing, in our hair, and in the air we breathe. The rarity of aspergillosis is a testament to the proper functioning of an intact immune system. High-dose chemotherapy, radiation therapy, various leukemias, and lymphomas result in prolonged neutropenia and severe immunosuppression. Under these circumstances, fungi emerge as opportunists.

The mode of transmission of *Aspergillus* spp. is inhalation of airborne spores, which causes pulmonary infection. The incubation period is unknown.

Pathophysiology

Aspergillus can colonize the upper respiratory tract, resulting in bronchial inflammation, or it can form aspergillomas (fungus balls in previously formed cavities in the lungs). The cavities can be produced by other diseases such as tuberculosis or sarcoidosis. The patients experience hemoptysis.

Assessment

Most children manifest either allergic bronchopulmonary aspergillosis or invasive disease. Children with HIV infection, bone marrow transplants, and other severely immunosuppressive childhood cancers are at the greatest risk for infection with aspergillus. Asthmatic children are at risk for allergic aspergillosis and exhibit signs of bronchial obstruction, eosinophilia, and persistent pulmonary infiltrates.

Invasive disease involves pulmonary erosion and ulceration followed by necrotizing pneumonia or hemorrhagic infarction. Signs and symptoms of invasive disease include productive cough with or without hemoptysis. It can spread to other body systems, such as the central nervous system, gastrointestinal tract, liver, kidneys, heart, and skin. Invasive disease is usually fatal.

Diagnostic Tests. A positive culture for *Aspergillus* in the sputum or bronchial washings coupled with a lung biopsy is diagnostic for aspergillosis. The lung tissue is processed and stained for *Aspergillus*. Some children with invasive aspergillosis are too ill for a lung biopsy procedure and other criteria must be used, including the following:

- Aspergillomas on a chest radiograph and a positive sputum culture for *Aspergillus*
- Unexplained fever, pulmonary infiltrates, and a positive nasal swab for *Aspergillus* in an immunocompromised child
- Unexplained pulmonary infiltrates in an immunosuppressed child without a history of lung disease and a positive sputum culture for *Aspergillus*

A computed tomographic (CT) scan of the lung reveals a halo sign around the suspected aspergilloma. The aspergilloma appears with a highlighted rim. Magnetic resonance imaging (MRI) reveals a target-like appearance of the nodular lung infiltrates.

Nursing Diagnoses and Outcomes

In addition to the common nursing diagnoses and outcomes listed in Chart 24–5, the following may be applicable to the child with aspergillosis:

▶ **Impaired gas exchange related to effects of pneumonia**
Outcome: The child will maintain adequate tissue oxygenation.

Interdisciplinary Interventions

Treatment is with amphotericin B, which is usually administered first in a test dose to detect the child's response to it. Nephrotoxicity is the major complication of amphotericin therapy. Commonly observed side effects include fever with shaking chills, nausea, vomiting, and phlebitis at the IV site.

Care of the child receiving amphotericin B centers around careful monitoring of vital signs (temperature, pulse, respiration, and blood pressure) every 20 minutes for 4 hours. Observe the IV site at least hourly for redness and swelling. Check laboratory values for signs of renal dysfunction (hypokalemia, elevated blood urea nitrogen [BUN], and serum creatinine) frequently while therapy continues. Administration of an antipyretic (acetaminophen) before therapy begins decreases the incidence of fever and chills. Antihistamines are given before therapy to decrease allergic reactions. Because antihistamines induce drowsiness, amphotericin is often administered during the evening hours. Also, sleeping during treatment helps reduce the perceived discomfort.

Use high-efficiency particulate air filtration in bone marrow–myelosuppression units to remove *Aspergillus* spores from the air handling system. However, remember that children may be colonized before admission to the special unit and may develop community-acquired aspergillosis.

In a hospital that includes oncology or severely immunosuppressed patients, renovation and construction projects should be carefully orchestrated. Use of plastic barriers and judicious air monitoring can reduce high levels of airborne aspergillus.

Histoplasmosis

Histoplasmosis is an infection primarily involving the lungs. Acute pulmonary histoplasmosis resembles influenza in intensity. Chronic pulmonary histoplasmosis resembles tuberculosis.

Disseminated disease most frequently affects children younger than 2 years and children of all ages who are severely immunosuppressed.

The disease is caused by *Histoplasma capsulatum*, spores of which are found in dust and soil contaminated by bird droppings or in caves contaminated by bat guano (feces). The fungus resides on bird feathers, but bats are actually infected. It is endemic in the central and eastern United States, especially areas along the Ohio River valley. The disease is not communicable from person to person. Transmission is via inhalation of airborne spores. The incubation period is variable.

Assessment

Histoplasmosis is usually asymptomatic in immunocompetent persons. The initial pulmonary infection is usually benign. A caseating (necrotic tissue resembling crumbly cheese) granuloma forms, usually in the lower lobes of the lung. In TB, it forms in the upper lobes. The child may experience flu-like symptoms, including fever, cough, headache, and pleuritic pain.

Children at greatest risk are those with preexisting malignancies or HIV infection. However, invasive histoplasmosis occurs primarily in children younger than 2 years and older men. Children with AIDS and infants have dysfunctional or immature immune systems that allow the fungus to disseminate to other areas of the body. These children have symptoms such as fever, anemia, weight loss, malaise, hepatosplenomegaly, and lymphadenopathy. Painful mouth ulcers inhibit adequate nutrition. Gastrointestinal ulcers can bleed or perforate. CNS involvement may be indicated by a chronic meningitis (high fever and headache).

Diagnostic Tests. The chest radiograph shows a distinctive "buckshot" pattern of pulmonary calcifications. Skin tests yield a positive reaction to histoplasmin. However, because most of the population in endemic areas have been exposed to *H. capsulatum*, a positive skin test does not indicate an acute infection. *H. capsulatum* can be cultured from sputum, pulmonary specimens such as bronchial washings, lung biopsy specimens, blood, spinal fluid, bone marrow, and skin.

Interdisciplinary Interventions

Treatment of uncomplicated pulmonary infection is not necessary. Treatment of invasive disease usually requires amphotericin B. Outbreaks after the demolition of chicken coops, barns, or other structures housing birds or bats may trigger an acute pulmonary reaction. These massive fungal exposures are generally treated with corticosteroids.

No isolation precautions are indicated for hospitalized children. Nursing care for histoplasmosis is the same as that for aspergillosis (see p. 1675).

Coccidioidomycosis

This airborne pulmonary infection caused by *Coccidioides immitis* is endemic to the southwestern United States. This organism requires specific climatic conditions: hot summers; little frost; alkaline, dry soil; and low rainfall. It lives in soil and dust and is carried by the wind. Acute infection occurs mainly in newcomers (people moving from nonendemic areas) to the Southwest.

Assessment

Most infections are asymptomatic and are indistinguishable from any other upper respiratory infection. In some children, primary pulmonary infection resembles influenza, causing cough, fever, headache, muscle aches, and pleuritic pain. Erythema nodosum (tender enlarged nodules under the skin) can occur. A rash resembling measles can occur and is usually referred to as toxic erythema.

Children rarely have coccidioidomas (fungus balls, similar to aspergillomas). However, dissemination in younger children often occurs, producing plaque-like skin lesions, osteomyelitis, meningitis, and hydrocephalus. Meningitis can be fatal if left untreated. Other extrapulmonary sites include lymph nodes, joints, bones, and abdominal organs. Bones, joints, and tendons become swollen, warm, and painful.

Diagnostic Tests. A high eosinophil count is common in coccidioidomycosis. The chest radiograph reveals thin-walled cavitary lesions. Tuberculosis must be ruled out because of the similar presentation and the cavitary lesions. The organism is easily cultured on standard fungal media. However, laboratory personnel must handle cultures under a laminar flow hood because they can be a source of infection. Skin tests are available and useful for children who are newcomers to the Southwest. A positive reaction in a skin test (red, indurated area) appears 10 to 21 days after infection, but there is no reaction in disseminated cases. Serologic tests include *Coccidioides*-specific immunoglobulins M and G. A positive test indicates infection.

Spinal fluid titers are used to predict the outcome of current therapy. Rising titers of antibody to *C. immitis* suggest progression of disease, whereas decreasing titers suggest improvement.

Interdisciplinary Interventions

Treatment is not usually recommended, except in acute pulmonary infection, dissemination, or meningitis. Amphotericin B is the treatment of choice. Cases of meningitis that do not respond to intravenous amphotericin B administration must often be treated with intrathecal administration. This is accomplished through an implanted cisternal Ommaya reservoir.

Alert: *Amphotericin B must contain no preservatives if given intrathecally.*

No isolation precautions are necessary for hospitalized children. Nurses are advised to use masks when changing and discarding dressings on deep wounds or skin lesions and when changing casts. This is to prevent inhalation of spores that may be released when the dressing is disturbed. See the section on aspergillosis for nursing care considerations when administering amphotericin B.

Malassezia furfur

Malassezia furfur is a lipid-dependent yeast. It is found primarily in premature infants or other infants who require total parenteral nutrition (TPN) that includes lipid therapy (fat emulsions). Because of this close association with a central line and hospitalization, M. *furfur* infections are considered hospital acquired.

The organism colonizes the skin of the infant, but usually does not cause skin infection. Instead, it migrates down the central line from the catheter site and then colonizes the central line.

Assessment

Sometimes fungus balls clog the catheter and a new catheter must be inserted. More often, a fungemia (blood infection with a fungus) results, leading to apnea spells, bradycardia, and pneumonia.

Diagnostic Tests. To grow M. *furfur*, the laboratory must layer the blood culture bottle with sterile olive oil. This oil supplies the lipids necessary to identify the organism. The organism can then be stained and plated by the laboratory worker for observation of the colony morphology and biochemical reactions.

caREminder: *Inform the laboratory if* M. furfur *is suspected. Most laboratories do not routinely add olive oil to a blood culture.*

Interdisciplinary Interventions

Treatment involves removing the central venous catheter. This action in and of itself is usually curative. However, antifungal agents along with catheter removal are sometimes necessary. The need for further therapy with antifungal agents, such as amphotericin B, is determined by the child's response to central catheter removal. Thus, children are evaluated on a case-by-case basis.

Nursing care focuses on strict adherence to hand washing and scrupulous aseptic techniques when handling the central venous line. This becomes even more crucial when the child is receiving TPN and lipids.

Sexually Transmitted Diseases

Genital infections in sexually transmitted diseases (STDs) typically affect adults or sexually active teenagers. Females usually exhibit vaginitis, and males display urethritis. An STD in a child (other than a newborn) suggests sexual abuse, which the nursing or medical staff must report to the appropriate authorities. Some forms of vulvovaginitis, especially in infants and toddlers, result from chemical irritation rather than infection. This is true for vulvar irritation induced by ammonia (from wet diapers) and allergic or chemical irritation of the vulva resulting from the use of harsh soaps or bubble baths.

The typical causative agents for STDs are summarized in Table 24–18. The classic STDs, gonorrhea and syphilis, have been joined by such entities as chlamydia, venereal warts, genital herpes, hepatitis B, and HIV infection. Herpes, hepatitis B, syphilis, and HIV infection have been previously discussed in this chapter. Venereal warts are caused by human papillomavirus and are discussed in Chapter 25. The other STDs are discussed in this section.

The sexual activity leading to infection includes genital-genital, oral-genital, oral-anal, and genital-anal contact between heterosexuals or homosexuals. Adolescence is the prime time for STD acquisition.

Gonorrhea

Gonorrhea is caused by a gram-negative diplococcus, *Neisseria gonorrhoeae*. In 1995, 392,848 cases of gonorrhea infection were reported to the CDC (CDC, 1996a). Like its cousin, *Neisseria meningitidis*, N. *gonorrhoeae* is a fragile organism with strict growth requirements. It rapidly dies on inanimate objects, such as toilets. Transmission occurs during vaginal, anal, or oral intercourse. Transmission to the neonate (neonatal eye infection) occurs when the infant descends through an infected birth canal. The incubation period is usually 2 to 7 days.

Assessment

Gonorrhea infections occur in three distinct age groups: neonates, adolescents, and adults. Neonates typically develop an eye infection (*ophthalmia neonatorum*), which formerly was a leading cause of neonatal blindness. Young girls may exhibit a vulvovaginitis as a result of sexual abuse by an infected individual.

caREminder: *Sexual abuse is reportable to the local Department of Health and Human Services.*

Sexually active adolescent girls tend to exhibit vaginitis, which may progress to pelvic inflammatory disease (PID). Some infected persons remain asymptomatic. However, hallmark symptoms include a thick yellow or white vaginal or urethral discharge, painful or burning urination, and, in females, abdominal cramping or pain.

In males, the infection is often limited to urethritis. However, some males exhibit acute epididymitis and prostatitis. In females, the infection could extend beyond vulvovaginitis to include abscesses of Bartholin's glands, salpingitis, and perihepatitis. The organism could gain access to the circulatory system through traumatic sexual intercourse, causing sepsis, arthritis, endocarditis, and meningitis.

Diagnostic Tests. The standard for diagnosis is a culture of eye drainage, cervical secretions, urethral discharge, or a rectal or throat swab sample that is positive for N. *gonorrhoeae*. Smears with Gram's stains of these

Table 24–18
Sexually Transmitted Diseases

Sexually Transmitted Disease	Symptoms	Treatment	Nursing Precautions
Chlamydia	Incubation for 7 to 21 days Sometimes no symptoms *Girls:* · Vaginal discharge · Abnormal vaginal discharge or bleeding · Painful urination · Abdominal pain · Fever · Nausea *Boys:* · Watery, white or yellow penile discharge · Burning or painful urination	Doxycycline PO for 7 days or Azithromycin PO in a single 1-g dose Erythromycin PO for 7 days (small children or pregnant patients)	Good hand washing. Standard precautions. Retest patients receiving erythromycin after 2 weeks.
Genital warts (papilloma virus)	Incubation for 1 to 8 mo Small bumpy warts on labia, vagina, penis, or anus Burning or itching in pubic area	Laser vaporization Electrocautery Surgery Intravaginal fluorouracil instillation Trichloracetic acid application Intralesional interferon application *Note:* Treatment does not eradicate the virus. Recurrences are common.	Operating room team should wear laser masks during surgery, cautery, or vaporization because viable virus can be in laser plume (smoke). Good hand washing. Standard precautions.
Gonorrhea	Incubation for 2 to 21 days Sometimes no symptoms *Girls:* · Thick yellow or white vaginal discharge · Painful urination · Abnormal vaginal bleeding · Abdominal cramps *Boys:* · Thick yellow or white penile discharge · Painful urination	Ceftriaxone IM Cefixime or ofloxacin in single oral dose It is recommended to treat for chlamydia simultaneously because both infections often occur together.	Good hand washing. Standard precautions.

fluids can also be helpful in making the diagnosis. The smears are positive for gram-negative diplococci.

caREminder: *The laboratory must be notified for the possible diagnosis of gonorrhea pharyngitis when throat swabs are submitted. A throat swab in most laboratories is evaluated for group A streptococcus. Additional methods are used to isolate gonorrhea.*

The laboratory should differentiate the gonococci from other *Neisseria* species, especially meningococci. Both appear as gram-negative diplococci. Individuals with disseminated gonorrhea often appear clinically as if they have infection with *N. meningitidis*.

Nursing Diagnoses and Outcomes

Refer to Chart 24–5 for general nursing diagnoses and outcomes for the child with an infection. Nursing diagnosis and outcomes for the child with gonorrhea depend on how the child or adolescent acquired the infection and clinical manifestations. If rape was involved, the following may be applicable:

- **Rape-trauma syndrome related to forced sexual activity**
  Outcome: The child will verbalize feelings and have interventions implemented to assist with coping.

If pelvic inflammatory disease is present, the following may apply:

- **Pain related to effects of disease**
  Outcome: The child will experience minimal discomfort.
- **Knowledge deficit: STD prevention**
  Outcome: The adolescent will state and implement methods for preventing STDs (e.g., abstinence, condoms).

Interdisciplinary Interventions

Gonorrhea can be treated in the emergency room or ambulatory setting. Single-dose therapy with intramuscular ceftriaxone or oral ofloxacin is effective. On occasion, the infection spreads to the cervix and fallopian tubes. PID ensues, requiring intravenous antibiotic therapy that includes either cefoxitin and doxycycline or clindamycin and gentamicin followed by oral doxycycline. Conditions such as appendicitis, cystitis, and pyelonephritis must be ruled out in the differential diagnosis.

The current practice of applying prophylactic eye drops (erythromycin) at birth decreases the incidence of ophthalmia neonatorum drastically. For children older than 1 month, the drug therapy of choice is ceftriaxone IM as a single dose, because of the increasing incidence of penicillin-resistant gonorrhea. Patients should be treated simultaneously for chlamydia, because these two infections frequently occur together.

Community Care

Condoms effectively prevent transmission of gonorrhea and most other STDs. Teaching sexually active teenagers about using condoms can occur in the clinic, schools (controversial), and at centers such as Planned Parenthood.

Report gonorrhea in children over age 1 month to the local Department of Health and Human Services because of suspected sexual abuse. Also report gonorrhea to the local health department to initiate contact tracing and treatment.

Chlamydia

Chlamydia trachomatis infection of the genital tract often accompanies a gonorrhea infection, requiring treatment of both diseases at once. The CDC recorded 477,638 cases of chlamydia reported in 1995 (CDC, 1996a). Genital infection is sexually transmitted. Neonatal infection is acquired as the infant passes through an infected birth canal. The untreated infection can last for years. The incubation period is variable but is generally 1 week.

Assessment

Chlamydia can be asymptomatic or can produce urethritis in both sexes, vaginitis in girls, cervicitis in adolescent girls, and epididymitis in boys. In girls, the infections may ascend the vaginal tract and progress to PID that may ultimately lead to infertility or ectopic pregnancy.

Infants may acquire neonatal chlamydial conjunctivitis or pneumonia. The conjunctivitis appears as a keratoconjunctivitis with purulent discharge. The risk of chlamydial conjunctivitis in the neonate is 25% to 50%. The infant may also have an asymptomatic infection of the pharynx, rectum, or vagina that can persist for 2 years (Committee on Infectious Diseases, American Academy of Pediatrics, 1994). The risk of pneumonia in the neonate is 20%. The symptoms of pneumonia include a staccato cough without fever and hyperinflation of the chest on radiography.

Diagnostic Tests. *C. trachomatis*, the causative agent, can be grown in tissue culture cells. Rapid antigen detection includes direct fluorescent antibody, enzyme immunoassay, and genetic probe testing, the results of which are positive for chlamydia. The DNA probe methods can rapidly and accurately test for the presence of both gonorrhea and chlamydia.

Nursing Diagnoses and Outcomes

Nursing diagnoses and outcomes for adolescents with sexually transmitted chlamydial infections are similar to those for gonorrhea. For the infant or child with chlamydia pneumonia, the following may apply:

- **Ineffective breathing pattern related to effects of disease**
  Outcome: The child will be assisted to maintain an effective breathing pattern and tissue oxygenation.
- **Sleep pattern disturbance related to coughing**
  Outcome: The child will have cough controlled to obtain adequate sleep.

Interdisciplinary Interventions

Treatment of adolescents usually involves doxycycline or erythromycin for 7 days. Sexual partners should also be treated. Conjunctivitis in the newborn is treated with oral erythromycin to ensure that asymptomatic carriage is eradicated. Topical application with erythromycin eye drops is ineffective.

Nurses who work with adolescents may have the opportunity to discuss STD prevention with adolescents who have already been infected or are sexually active. If so, explain abstinence and the use of latex condoms as ways to prevent transmission. Teaching must include instruction to finish the prescribed dose of medication completely and when to return for follow-up care.

Bacterial Vaginosis

Bacterial vaginosis (BV) is a syndrome of infections caused by *Gardnerella vaginalis* and other vaginal anaerobes. In adolescent girls and adults, BV is usually an STD. BV may occur with other vaginal infections such as cervicitis or trichomoniasis. In prepubescent girls, the etiology is unknown.

It is unclear whether G. *vaginalis* is part of the normal vaginal flora of children and prepubescent girls. Few studies have addressed what constitutes normal vaginal flora in young children. Because G. *vaginalis* could be part of the normal flora, cultures are not helpful in making a diagnosis.

Assessment

Sexually active adolescent girls report increased vaginal discharge with a yellow or gray-white color. This discharge irritates the vulva, causing inflammation, itching, and pain. It often has a fishy odor. In other cases, the infection is asymptomatic.

Bacterial vaginosis in prepubescent girls is more likely to be caused by other bacteria, such as group A streptococcus, *Shigella* species, or *Trichomonas vaginalis*. The symptoms are the same as in older girls.

Diagnostic Tests. Diagnosis is made by excluding other causes of vaginitis, such as candidiasis and gonorrhea. A wet mount of a vaginal swab reveals "clue" cells, which are vaginal epithelial cells covered with bacteria. Clue cells are present only if the child has bacterial vaginosis. The "whiff" test is also positive. The whiff test is performed by dropping 10% KOH onto the slide. An unpleasant fishy odor develops on positive slides.

Nursing Diagnoses and Outcomes

Applicable nursing diagnoses and outcomes for a child with bacterial vaginosis may include:

- **Risk for impaired skin integrity related to pruritus, vaginal discharge**
  Outcome: The child will maintain intact perineal skin and remain comfortable.

Interdisciplinary Interventions

Treatment is with oral metronidazole for 7 days. Vaginal creams are effective alternative forms of treatment. These creams are metronidazole or clindamycin based. Treatment of the male partner does not seem to influence recurrence rates and is therefore unnecessary.

Teach the child and parents, as appropriate, good perineal hygiene techniques, such as wiping front to back after toileting, good hand washing, using mild soap and nonperfumed powder products for prepubescent girls, and avoiding bubble baths and getting shampoo in the bath water. White cotton underpants should be worn because they are more absorbent than nylon and free of dyes.

Tip: *Tell pregnant adolescents to avoid metronidazole because of possible teratogenic effects. Teach adolescents to avoid latex condoms during therapy with the vaginal clindamycin cream and for 72 hours afterward. This cream has an oil base and weakens the latex.*

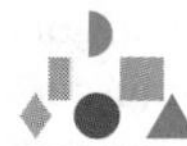

Future Infectious Disease Challenges

Some human infections result from ecologic changes in the environment. For instance, deforestation and encroachment on the deer habitat in Connecticut contributed to the introduction of Lyme disease in 1975. Air travel has made outbreaks of exotic tropical diseases a concern in most towns in the United States. Insects and animals once confined to distant islands can travel on freighters or airplanes and arrive anywhere in the world.

Unusually dry weather in the southwestern United States may have contributed to the outbreak of hantavirus pulmonary syndrome in 1994 (Butler & Peters, 1994). Hantavirus was spread by inhaling aerosolized rodent droppings. The drought forced the rodents into closer contact with humans as they searched for food. The virus produces a severe pulmonary hemorrhagic fever with a renal syndrome. It involves a 10% to 15% mortality rate and a risk of permanent kidney damage (Butler & Peters, 1994).

In 1985, the tiger mosquito was introduced from Asia in a shipment of tires to Texas. This mosquito has a voracious appetite and can transmit dengue and yellow fever. Tiger mosquitoes thrive in areas where environmental sanitation is lax. In the United States, mosquito extermination is minimal because malaria was eradicated in this country. Even more alarming, this mosquito is becoming resistant to some insect repellents.

Dengue hemorrhagic fever has worldwide outbreaks every 15 to 40 years. Known as breakbone fever, it causes fever, joint pain, epistaxis, and a macular rash. Most cases occur in children because they play outdoors and receive many insect bites. Most domestic cases are imported from countries where dengue fever is endemic.

However, two cases were reported in Texas that were not imported. The tiger mosquito was blamed (CDC, 1996b).

Finally, one of the most deadly human viruses, the Ebola virus, demonstrated that what happens in a small village in Africa could affect the average United States citizen. Outbreaks of Ebola in Virginia and Texas research facilities, along with movies and popular books, have heightened public awareness.

Ebola hemorrhagic fever has a 2- to 15-day incubation period. The patient becomes acutely ill with a flu-like illness that rapidly progresses to gross hemorrhage from all body orifices. Hypovolemic shock and death follow 6 to 9 days after the onset of the illness. There is no treatment or cure.

Modern medicine has seen many advances in technology, such as PCR testing and DNA or RNA tracking of bacteria and viruses. It has also seen some surprises, such as HIV and reencounters with old foes as in the resurgence of TB. Emerging infections, such as *E. coli* O157:H7 or Ebola virus, will continue to challenge modern medicine. Nurses must strive to learn of these new diseases, their modes of transmission, their effects on humans, and the associated nursing care.

Summary of Key Concepts

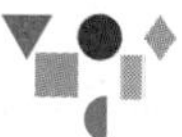

- Children experience infections and infectious diseases more frequently than adults.
- The bacteria, viruses, and parasites that cause the infections affect all races, sexes, and economic levels.
- Nurses must be a constant resource to the parents and caregivers concerning isolation, modes of transmission, and treatment needed to prevent secondary cases.
- Conventional sputum cultures for children with pulmonary tuberculosis are of little value because children have difficulty producing sputum to confirm the diagnosis.
- Tick-borne infections can be avoided by using insect repellent and following commonsense tips.
- Many virus-based infectious diseases are vaccine preventable.
- All herpes infections share the characteristic of latency: the ability to recur.
- Parasitic infections are seen more in underdeveloped countries.
- Sexually transmitted diseases can be prevented by using abstinence or latex condoms.

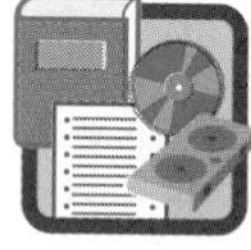

Resources

Organizations

Association for Professionals in Infection Control and Epidemiology
1016 16th Street NW, Sixth Floor
Washington, DC 20036
(202) 296-2742

Association of Nurses in AIDS Care
1555 Connecticut Avenue NW, Suite 200
Washington, DC 20036
(215) 321-2371

Immune Deficiency Foundation
3565 Ellicott Mills Drive, Unit B2
Ellicott City, MD 21043
(410) 321-6647

National Pediatric HIV Resource Center
Children's Hospital of New Jersey
15 South Ninth Street
Newark, NJ 07107
(201) 268-8251

Pediatric AIDS Coalition
1331 Pennsylvania Avenue, NW
Suite 721 North
Washington, DC 20001
(202) 638-2952

Books and Printed Materials

AIDS Information Sourcebook
Oryx Press
4041 North Central Avenue, Suite 700
Phoenix, AZ 85004
(800) 279-6799

American Red Cross HIV/AIDS Education
National Capital Chapter
2025 E Street NW
Washington, DC 20006

Recommendations for the School Health Nurse in Addressing HIV/AIDS with Adolescents
American Nurses' Association
600 Maryland Ave SW
Suite 100 West
Washington, DC 20024
(202) 651-7079

Children with AIDS
Newsletter of the Foundation for Children with AIDS
401 Wythe Street
Alexandria, VA 22314
(703) 684-1355

Department of Health and Human Services, Public Health Service
National AIDS Clearinghouse
PO Box 6003
Rockville, MD 20850
(800) 458-5231

Materials Catalog America Responds to AIDS
Department of Health and Human Services
Public Health Service/CDC
Atlanta, GA 30333

National Institute of Allergy and Infectious Diseases
31 Center Drive, Building 31
Suite 7A50
Bethesda, MD 20892
(301) 496-5717
E-mail: niaidoc@/flash.niaid.nih.gov

Hotlines

National HIV/AIDS Hotline
(800) 342-AIDS
Spanish: (800) 344-SIDA
Hearing Impaired: (800) AIDS-TTY

National Pediatric HIV Resource Center
(800) 362-0071

National STD Hotline
(800) 227-8922

Pediatric AIDS Coalition
(800) 336-5475

Computer Resources

Association for Professionals in Infection Control (http://www.apic.org).
The APIC home page provides a variety of information on infection control–related issues.

CDC/NCID Focus (http://www.tdh.state.tx.us/phpep.dpnhome.htm).
Disease Prevention News is a biweekly publication from the Texas Department of Health covering various topics on disease prevention.

CDC (http://www.cdc.gov/inpho/inpho.htm).
This Web site provides coverage of public health issues and the Morbidity and Mortality Weekly Report (MMWR).

Medscape (http://www.medscape.com.home/medscape-id/medscape-id.html).
Medscape is produced by SCP Communications, Inc., providing an interactive, multispecialty Internet journal.

References

Black, N. A., Linnemann, C. C., Staneck, J. L., & Kotagal, U. R. (1996). Control of methicillin resistant *Staphylococcus aureus* in a neonatal intensive care unit: Use of microbiologic surveillance and mupirocin. *Infection Control and Hospital Epidemiology, 17,* 227–231.

Butler, J. C., & Peters, C. J. (1994). Hantavirus and the hantavirus pulmonary syndrome. *Clinical Infectious Diseases, 19,* 387–395.

Centers for Disease Control and Prevention. (1991). The hepatitis B virus: A comprehensive strategy for eliminating transmission in the United States through universal childhood vaccination. *MMWR Morbidity and Mortality Weekly Report,* 40(RR13), 1–25.

Centers for Disease Control and Prevention. (1994). Guidelines for preventing the transmissions of tuberculosis in health care facilities. *MMWR Morbidity and Mortality Weekly Report, 43,* 1–132; *Federal Register* 1994, *59,* 54242–54303.

Centers for Disease Control and Prevention. (1995). Human rabies—Alabama, Tennessee, and Texas, 1994. *MMWR Morbidity and Mortality Weekly Report,* 44(14), 269–272.

Centers for Disease Control and Prevention. (1996a). Table II. Provisional cases of selected notifiable diseases, United States, weeks ending October 26, 1996, and October 28, 1995 (43rd week). *MMWR Morbidity and Mortality Weekly Report, 45,* 954–958.

Centers for Disease Control and Prevention. (1996b). Imported dengue—United States, 1995. *MMWR Morbidity and Mortality Weekly Report, 45,* 988–991.

Centers for Disease Control and Prevention and National Center for Infectious Diseases. (1995). Group A streptococcus outbreak in Virginia. *CDC/NCID Focus,* 5, 1–4.

Cherry, J. D. (1995). Nosocomial pertussis in the nineties. *Infection Control and Hospital Epidemiology, 16,* 553–554.

Committee on Infectious Diseases, American Academy of Pediatrics. (1994). *1994 Red Book: Report of the Committee on Infectious Diseases* (23rd ed.). Grove Village, IL: American Academy of Pediatrics.

Crossley, K. (1996). Streptococci. In G. Mayhall (Ed.), *Hospital epidemiology and infection control* (pp. 330–334). Baltimore: Williams & Wilkins.

Dickover, R. E., Garratty, E. M., Herman, S. A., Sims, M. S., Plaeger, S., Boyer, P. J., Keller, M., Deveikis, A., Stiehm, E. R., & Bryson, Y. J. (1996). Identification of levels of maternal HIV-1 RNA associated with risk of perinatal transmission. *JAMA, 275,* 599–605.

Eutropius, L. J., Overall, J. C., & Spruance, S. L. (1996). Herpes simplex virus. In R. Olmstead (Ed.), *Infection control and applied epidemiology, principles and practice* (pp. 67.7–61.14). St. Louis: Mosby–Year Book.

Farley, T. A., Wilson, S. A., Mahoney, F., Kelso, K. Y., Johnson, D. R., & Kaplan, E. L. (1993). Direct inoculation of food as the cause of an outbreak of group A streptococcal pharyngitis. *Journal of Infectious Diseases, 167,* 1232–1235.

Garner, J., & The Hospital Infection Control Practices Advisory Committee. (1996). Guidelines for isolation precautions in hospitals. *American Journal of Infection Control, 24,* 24–52.

Glickman, L. T., & Magnuval, J. F. (1993). Zoonotic roundworm infections. *Infectious Disease Clinics of North America, 7,* 717–726.

Grundy, J. E. (1990). Virologic and pathogenic aspects of cytomegalovirus infection. *Reviews of Infectious Diseases,* 12(Suppl. 7), S117–S119.

Hensleigh, P. A., & Nguyen, L. K. (1994). Genital herpes simplex virus. In B. Gonik (Ed.), *Viral diseases in pregnancy* (pp. 50–63). New York: Springer-Verlag.

HIV/AIDS Surveillance Report, 1995. (1996). Rockville, MD: National AIDS Clearinghouse. NACFAX (800) 458-5231.

John, J. F., & Barg, N. L. (1996). *Staphylococcus aureus.* In G. Mayhall (Ed.), *Hospital epidemiology and infection control* (pp. 271–289). Baltimore: Williams & Wilkins.

Kaplan, E. L., & Krugman, S. (1992). Streptococcal infections, group A. In S. Krugman, S. L. Katz, A. A. Gershon, & C. M. Wilfert (Eds.), *Infectious diseases of children* (9th ed., pp. 474–486). St. Louis: Mosby–Year Book.

Katov, W. N., & Dienstag, J. L. (1991). Prevention and therapy of viral hepatitis. *Seminars in Liver Disease, 11,* 165–174.

Krugman, S. (1992a). Measles (rubeola). In S. Krugman, S. L. Katz, A. A. Gershon, & C. M. Wilfert (Eds.), *Infectious diseases of children* (9th ed., pp. 223–245). St. Louis: Mosby–Year Book.

Krugman, S. (1992b). Hepatitis. In S. Krugman, S. L. Katz, A. A. Gershon, & C. M. Wilfert (Eds.), *Infectious diseases of children* (9th ed., pp. 143–174). St. Louis: Mosby–Year Book.

McLeod, R., Wisner, J., & Boyer, K. (1992). Toxoplasmosis. In S. Krugman, S. L. Katz, A. A. Gershon, & C. M. Wilfert (Eds.), *Infectious diseases of children* (9th ed., pp. 518–550). St. Louis: Mosby–Year Book.

Minkoff, H., Burns, D. N., Landesman, S., Youchah, J., Goedert, J. J., Nugent, R. P., Muenz, L. R., & Willoughby, A. D. (1995). The relationship of the duration of ruptured membranes to vertical transmission of human immunodeficiency virus. *American Journal of Obstetrics and Gynecology, 173,* 585–589.

Peloquin, C. A., and Berning, S. E. (1995). Tuberculosis and multi-drug resistant tuberculosis in children. *Pediatric Nursing, 21,* 566–572.

Rosenthal-Dichter, C., & Allen, M. (1996). Host defenses. In M. A. Q. Curley, J. B. Smith, & P. A. Moloney-Harmon (Eds.), *Critical care nursing of infants and children* (pp. 468–509). Philadelphia: W. B. Saunders.

Schutze, G. E., and Yamauchi, T. (1996). Nosocomial bacterial infections of the central nervous system, upper respiratory tracts, and the skin in pediatric patients. In G. Mayhall (Ed.), *Hospital epidemiology and infection control* (pp. 493–505). Baltimore: Williams & Wilkins.

Starke, J. R. (1993). Tuberculosis in children. In L. Reichman & E. Hershfield (Eds.), *Tuberculosis* (pp. 329–367). New York: Marcel Dekker.

Valenti, W. (1992). Selected viruses of nosocomial importance. In J. Bennett & P. Brachman (Eds.), *Hospital infections* (pp. 789–821). Boston: Little, Brown.

Valenti, W. M. (1993). Infection control and the pregnant health care worker. *Nursing Clinics of North America, 28,* 673–686.

Witek-Janusek, L., & Cusack, C. (1994). Neonatal sepsis: confronting the challenge. *Critical Care Nursing Clinics of North America, 6,* 405–419.

Zaia, J. (1996). Cytomegalovirus (CMV). In R. Olmstead (Ed.), *APIC infection control and applied epidemiology: Principles and practice* (pp. 61.1–61.4). St. Louis: Mosby–Year Book.

Bibliography

Abernathy, R. S. (1997). Tuberculosis: An update. *Pediatrics in Review, 18*(2), 50–58.

Abraham, E. (Ed.). (1993). Sepsis: Cellular and physiologic mechanisms. *New Horizons, 1,* 1–159.

American College of Chest Physicians/Society of Critical Care Medicine Consensus Conference. (1992). Definitions for sepsis and organ failure and guidelines for the use of innovative therapies in sepsis. *Critical Care Medicine, 20,* 864–874.

Biddle, C. (1996). A review of the transmission of viral hepatitis for gastroenterology nurses. *Gastroenterology Nursing, 19*(1), 2–6.

Bone, R. C. (1996). Toward a theory regarding the pathogenesis of the systemic inflammatory response syndrome; what we do and do not know about cytokine regulation. *Critical Care Medicine, 24,* 163–172.

Brinsko, V. (Ed.). (1993). Infection control. *Nursing Clinics of North America, 28,* 597–709.

Buchanan, J. C. (1996). Lumbar puncture and evaluation of cerebrospinal fluid. *Neonatal Network, 15*(7), 59–61.

Committee on Infectious Diseases. (1997). Therapy for children with invasive pneumococcal infections. *Pediatrics, 99,* 289.

Department of Labor. Occupational Safety and Health Administration. (1991). Occupational Exposure to bloodborne pathogens: Final rule. *Federal Register, 56,* 64175–64182.

Fishman, L. N., Jonas, M. M., & Lavine, J. E. (1996). Update on viral hepatitis in children. *Pediatric Clinics of North America, 43,* 57–74.

Gordon, S. L. (1994). Lyme disease in children. *Pediatric Nursing, 20,* 415–418.

Hazinski, M. F., Iberti, T. J., MacIntyre, N. R., Parker, M. M., Tribett, D., Prion, S., & Chmel, H. (1993). Epidemiology, pathophysiology, and clinical presentation of gram-negative sepsis. *American Journal of Critical Care, 2,* 224–235.

Hogan, D. E. (1996). The emergency department approach to diarrhea. *Emergency Medicine Clinics of North America, 14,* 673–694.

Jones, C. L. (1996). Herpes simplex virus infection in the neonate: Clinical presentation and management. *Neonatal Network, 15*(8), 11–15.

Krugman, S., Katz, S. L., Gershon, A. A., & Wilfert, C. M. (Eds.). (1992). *Infectious diseases of children* (9th ed.). St. Louis: Mosby–Year Book.

Lambert, R. B., & Lambert, N. K. (1995). The effects of humor on secretory immunoglobulin A levels in school-age children. *Pediatric Nursing, 21,* 16–19.

Lofgren, M. A. (1996). The significance of the neutrophil in the diagnosis of neonatal sepsis: Using a metaphor. *Mother Baby Journal, 1*(3), 31–32.

Lumb, T. M. (1994). Group B streptococcus revisited. *Pediatric Nursing, 20,* 578–580.

Peterson, K. (1995). Iatrogenic immune suppression. *Pediatric Nursing, 21,* 11–15.

Polinski, C. (1996). The value of the white blood cell count and differential in the prediction of neonatal sepsis. *Neonatal Network, 15*(7), 13–23.

Rangel-Frausto, M. S., Pittet, D., Costigan, M., Hwang, T., Davis, C. S., & Wenzel, R. P. (1995). The natural history of the systemic inflammatory response syndrome (SIRS); a prospective study. *Journal of the American Medical Association, 273,* 117–123.

Singer, J. I., Vest, J., & Prints, A. (1995). Occult bacteremia and septicemia in the febrile child younger than two years. *Emergency Medicine Clinics of North America, 13,* 381–415.

Stevenson, L., & Brooke, D. S. (1995). Vulvovaginitis in the prepubertal child. *Journal of Pediatric Health Care, 9,* 227–228.

Alterations in Skin Integrity

OUTLINE

OBJECTIVES

- Identify characteristics of the child's skin that make the child more susceptible to injury.
- Perform a health history and physical examination that includes a complete evaluation of the skin, hair, and nails.
- Select nursing diagnoses that articulate the needs of the child, family, and community for the child who has a skin condition.
- Describe the presenting signs and symptoms of skin conditions frequently seen in the pediatric population.
- Use strategies to prevent further spread of a skin condition or further damage to tissue that has an alteration in skin integrity.
- Discuss therapies that are effective in treating conditions of the skin.

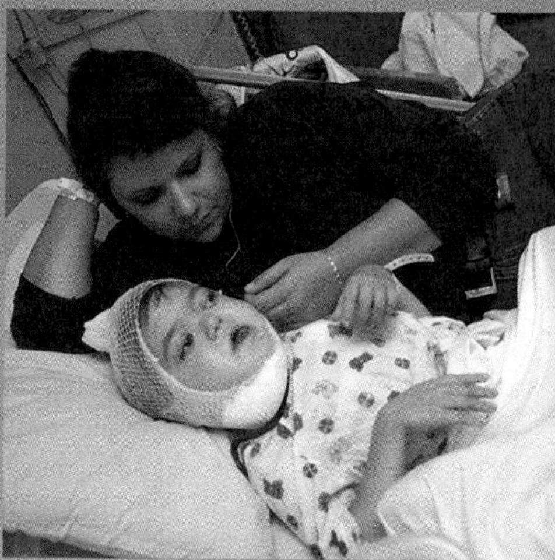

KEY TERMS

acrocyanosis
autograft
cutis marmorata
debridement
eschar
erythema
fomites
heterograft
homograft
hydrotherapy
keloid
pruritus
Tzanck smear
urticaria
Wood's lamp

CHAPTER

25

The skin is a most important, yet undervalued organ. It is constantly exposed to a changing environment, yet it still manages to provide an effective line of defense against disease and to promote homeostasis. To perform these functions, however, the skin must remain intact. This chapter explores various disorders that breach the skin's defense system including infections, noninfectious conditions, and trauma.

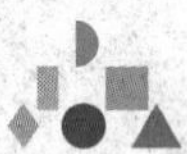

Assessment of the Child with an Alteration in Skin Integrity

The appearance of the skin, hair, and nails plays an important role in the child's body image and self-esteem. In the same manner, the ability of the skin, hair, and nails to perform their key functions is vital to maintaining health and in preventing the threat of illness from environmental factors. Even though the many layers of the surface of the skin cannot be seen (Fig. 25–1), assessment data can generate information to confirm the ongoing ability of the skin to perform its key functions (Chart 25–1). The health history and physical assessment serve as the clinician's tools to evaluate the potential and actual threats to the function, integrity, and cosmetic appearance of the skin and its appendages.

Focused Health History

The purpose of the health history is to collect data about the skin changes as reported by the child's caregiver or by the older child, and to successfully elicit information that will serve as indicators of the primary source of the skin eruption. The clinical findings from skin rashes, lesions, and infestations often lack specificity, and the etiologic agents may be elusive (Brimhall & Esterly, 1993). Discussing problems of the skin can be a source of acute embarrassment. Also, assessment of some highly contagious skin disorders requires complete openness from the family and sensitivity from the caregiver to ensure that all individuals possibly affected by the illness are identified and notified to limit further spread of the disorder.

The verbal history encourages both the child and the parent to subjectively evaluate the current status of the skin as compared with its past condition. Chart 25–2 specifies the dimensions of the health history specific to the identification of skin disorders. Because the skin yields rich information about the child's general health, hygiene practices, and nutritional status, it is essential to incorporate components of the skin assessment into all health interviews with the family. The skin also serves as a mirror to many complex systemic pathologic processes. In these situations, the skin history may serve as the preliminary screen, prior to a more in-depth review of a particular system.

Evaluating a particular skin disorder can be made easier by noting the child's age and ethnicity. For instance, distinguishing a bruise from a birthmark or, more specifically, a Mongolian spot would be easier by recognizing that the patient was a 7-day-old black child. Interview questions should also provide a mechanism to elicit culturally based attempts at self-remedy of the current problem and to assess typical health promotion practices in the home (Chart 25–3).

Chart 25–1

Key Functions of the Skin

Protection

Shields the body from internal injury from aqueous, chemical, mechanical, bacterial, and viral assaults and from ultraviolet radiation

Immunity

Contains cells (Langerhans, macrophages, mast cells) that ingest bacteria and other substances

Thermoregulation

Promotes heat regulation through sweating, shivering, and subcutaneous insulation

Communication

Allows for personal identification and portrayal of emotions (especially skin of the face), vascular responses (e.g., blushing), and signaling of emotions

Sensation

Allows for sensitivity to pain, touch, temperature, and pressure

Metabolism/Secretion

Synthesizes vitamin D; regulates excretion of waste products such as uric acid, sugars, minerals, electrolytes, and fluids from the body

Regeneration

Constantly undergoes shedding of old cells with replacement by newer cells; activates wound healing processes after injury to generate new tissue

Figure 25–1
The skin and its structures. (Illustration from Jarvis, C. [1996]. *Physical examination and health assessment* [2nd ed., p. 214]. Philadelphia: W. B. Saunders. Reprinted with permission.)

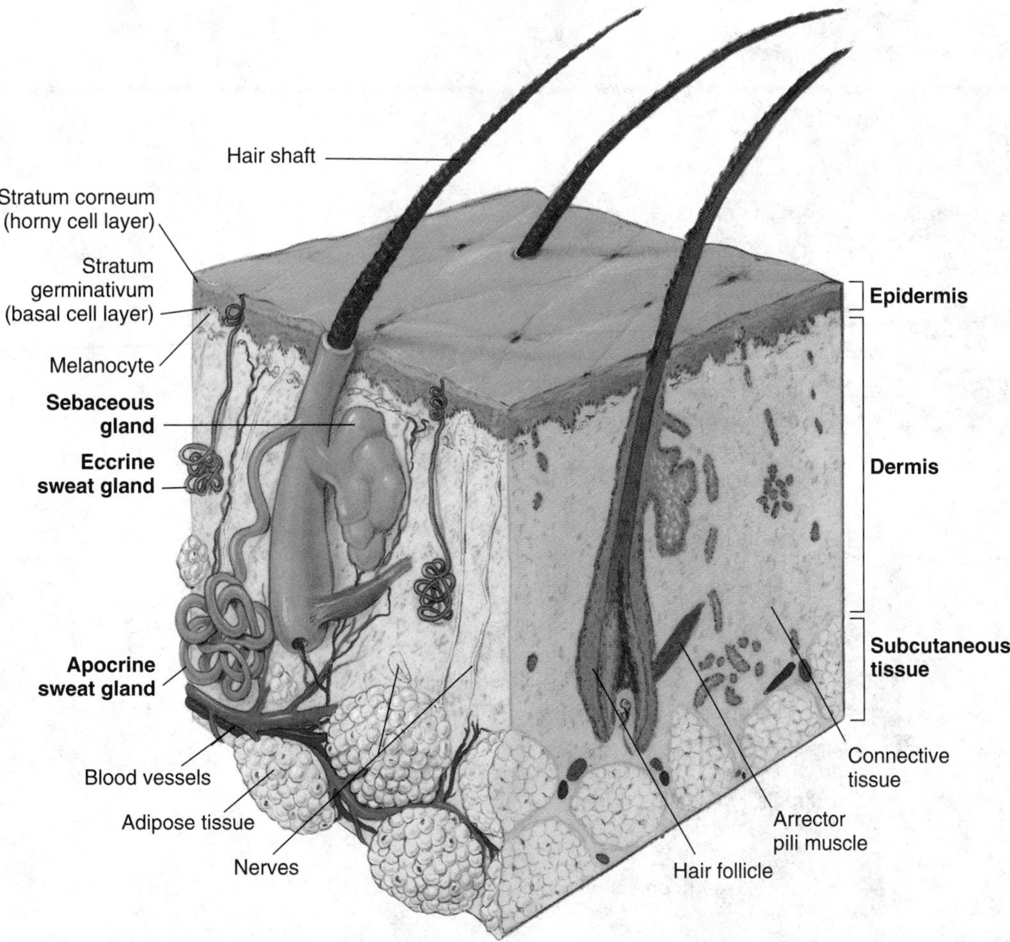

Epidermis: Outer, tough, avascular layer that depends entirely on the dermis for its blood supply and nourishment. Provides a barrier against physical injury, intense light, and infectious organisms. Comprises four layers:

- Stratum corneum—the top layer of skin composed of dead cells tightly joined, which are shed during bathing and rubbing of the skin
- Basal cell layer—produces melanin, which provides the skin color and helps to protect the body from ultraviolet rays of the sun
- Stratum spinosum—contains Langerhans cells, skin macrophages that respond or attack microorganisms that penetrate the stratum corneum
- Stratum granulosum—the layer in which skin cells begin their nuclear breakdown and are pushed upward to form the stratum corneum and eventually be shed

Dermis: Inner, supportive layer that is highly vascular. Provides a tough, elastic support system for body tissues. Contains connective tissue, elastic fibers, blood vessels, lymphatic vessels, hair follicles, and nerves.

Subcutaneous: The layer of adipose or "fat" tissue beneath the dermis. Insulates the body from cold and serves as a cushion that absorbs trauma to the body.

Sebaceous glands: Attached to hair follicles. Produce a protective lipid called sebum into the hair follicle. Present everywhere on the body except the palms, soles, and dorsa of the feet.

Eccrine glands: The sweat glands. Distributed all over the body, these glands fulfill a role in thermoregulation through evaporative heat loss of eccrine sweat.

Apocrine glands: Sweat glands that open into hair follicles. They become fully active during puberty to produce a fluid containing carbohydrates, lipids, and proteins that have a very characteristic odor.

Hair: Consists of two types: *terminal hair*, relatively long and coarse (on the scalp, axilla, pubic area, eyelashes, and eyebrows); and *vellus hair*, a soft hair that covers the rest of the body.

Nails: Composed of keratin, the child's nails are normally thin, flexible, and transparent with a smooth, shiny, and almost flat surface.

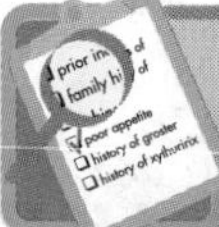

Chart 25–2
Focused Health History

The Skin

Identifying Data	Specifically note child's Age Informant source Race Religion
Present Illness	Time of onset Evolution of skin lesion Site of onset Normal appearance of the skin Presence of Itching Areas of wetness or dryness Cuts Rash—flat versus raised Changes in color, shape, contour of nails Change in skin color—localized or generalized Areas of skin thinning or thickening Bruises Hair loss or excessive growth, change in texture Related systemic problems: Pyrexia Sore limbs Recent contact with other persons who have skin disorders
Past Medical History	Birth history Skin lesions noted at birth Skin color changes after birth Breast-feeding Childhood illnesses Previous communicable diseases Recent exposure to a communicable illness Immunizations Any immunizations recently given? Previous postimmunization rashes/responses Allergies Allergic reactions to drugs, plants, medications, or food Recent changes in food, diaper products, laundry detergents, soap, or other skin products
Current Medications or Treatments	Any medications child is taking—topical and systemic, prescribed and over-the-counter Length of time on medication Recent changes in dosage Home remedies to treat current condition Cultural or religious practices that may have caused the condition
Nutritional Assessment	Recent changes in food or fluids Recent weight loss Weight within normal limits

Chart 25–2
Focused Health History *Continued*

The Skin	
Family Medical History	Family history of acne, psoriasis, impetigo, eczema, allergic reactions
Environmental History	Exposures to any household chemicals How much exposure to sun on routine basis Presence of insects/animals that may have bitten or scratched the child
Social History	Any recent changes in family lifestyle? School attendance—note the name of the child's school or daycare, because communication with a teacher may be necessary. Any recent travel abroad
Growth and Development	Health promotion activities: Concerns of child in relation to their skin Products used to care for child's hair, nails, and skin Frequency of bathing/hair washing Use of sunscreens

The informant should be an individual who can describe the evolution of the child's skin eruption, factors that may be related to the skin condition, and measures taken to relieve the condition. Older children may serve as their own informant and may be particularly helpful in delineating aspects of the present illness. However, the older child may be unable to relate information regarding immunization status, childhood illnesses, and family medical history.

Data about the present illness focus on the course, characteristics, and related systemic problems of the skin condition. The parent or child is asked to describe the site, size, configuration, distribution, and color of the lesion. Parents may identify contacts with other persons having a skin disorder.

caREminder: *The name of the child's school or daycare center should be noted, because communication with the teacher may be necessary if the child's diagnosis proves to be contagious.*

The past medical history elicits information that may specify origins of the skin eruption. In the infant, events occurring in the prenatal, natal, and neonatal periods are investigated. In all children, changes in medication, diet, environment, and lifestyle may be causative factors. Brief encounters with animals, insects, plants, and even the child's best friend may be key elements to explain the source of the skin condition.

Focused Physical Assessment

Skin

Physical assessment of the skin involves two basic techniques: inspection and palpation. Chart 25–4 summarizes the key data to assess during the examination. Ideally, the environment for the physical assessment is a well-lit room with white walls. Bright white fluorescent ceiling lighting is optimal, because it does not cast a yellow hue on the skin.

caREminder: *Gloves do not necessarily have to be worn to perform the skin assessment. If the examiner suspects a contagious disorder, if body fluids are present on the skin, or if lesions are moist, then gloves must be worn. Vinyl gloves should be used if there is any possibility that the child may have a latex allergy. In such a child, touching the skin with latex may precipitate urticaria and airway edema.*

The child should be placed in a warm room and should be wearing an examination gown to provide easy access to all areas of the skin. The infant's diaper should be removed at the time of inspection and palpation of the genital area.

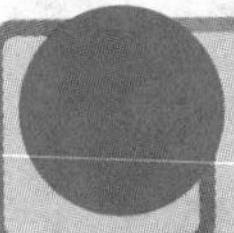

Chart 25–3
Worldview

Chinese Folk Practices

Skin lesions and irregular markings on the child's body may be a result of folk practices used by the family to treat a specific illness. For instance, in the Chinese culture, the practice of cupping, skin scraping, and moxibustion can injure the child's skin. Cupping is when a vacuum is created in a cup by placing a heated material in the cup. The cup is then placed on the child's skin until easily removed. The treatment leaves a burn mark. Skin scraping is the process of applying oil to an area of the skin then scraping the area with a coin repeatedly, leaving linear bruising on the skin. In the folk practice of moxibustion, the ignited moxa plant is applied to specific areas of the body to treat diseases that are caused from an excess of yin. This causes burn marks on the child. The nurse should emphasize to the parents that, although these practices are meaningful, they can further injure the child. In addition, the burns and lesions on the skin caused by this folk practice can become infected.

From Chang, K. (1995). Chinese Americans. In J. Giger & R. Davidhizar (Eds.), *Transcultural nursing: Assessment and intervention* (pp. 395–416). St. Louis: Mosby–Year Book. Reprinted with permission.

Chart 25–4
Focused Physical Assessment

Skin, Hair, and Nails

Inspection

Skin and Mucous Membranes
Generalized color and condition of the skin versus local changes in skin color (pallor, cyanosis, jaundice, erythema)
Pigmentation
Complexion
Lesions (distribution, configuration, primary versus secondary or both)
Vascular changes (telangiectasia, hemangiomas)

Hair
Color
Distribution
Quantity
Scalp lesions
Scalp condition and hygiene

Nails
Color
Shape
Angle
Condition (biting, infection, skin picking)

Palpation

Skin and Mucous Membranes
Turgor and mobility
Moisture
Temperature
Hygiene and odor
Texture
Thickness
Lesions (location, distribution, grouping pattern, type)

Hair
Texture
Dryness/oiliness
Brittleness

Nails
Consistency
Adherence to nail bed
Capillary refill

Tip: *Allow the child and the adolescent to wear underclothes during most of the examination to prevent any undue embarrassment and to protect the child's emerging sense of modesty.*

Skin assessment begins with a general inspection of the total skin surface before proceeding to a focused assessment of a specific lesion noted during the health history. This method provides an opportunity to validate the scope of the problem identified by the child and family. This also enables assessment of any premalignant changes and general fitness of the skin, which can serve as key points of dialogue during the health promotion and disease prevention discussions that conclude the health visit.

Skin color is an important assessment parameter. The child's pigmentation should be consistent with genetic background and age. For instance, the newborn's nail beds and extremities may be blue for up to 7 to 10 days after birth (acrocyanosis), during episodes of intense crying or breath-holding, and when exposed to cold environments. These changes in pigmentation in newborns are a result of vascular differences, which mature as the newborns adapt to extrauterine life. The white neonate generally has pink skin, whereas neonates of other races such as those of black, Asian, or Hispanic descent have a creamy tan complexion. The appearance of freckles and moles in young children is a function of aging. The presence of birthmarks such as Mongolian spots represent age-related changes that fade with further maturation of melanocytes in the dermis. Variations in skin color must be differentiated between transient changes (associated with crying, acne, sunburn) or reflections of pathologic processes (Table 25–1).

During inspection, the examiner uses the sense of smell to detect skin odors. Odors from sweat may be present in the adolescent and may be caused by hormonal changes in apocrine gland secretions. In the younger child, body odors may be a sign of poor hygiene. Intense odors may also signify an infection and should be further evaluated.

Throughout the assessment process, the child's verbal and nonverbal cues should be integrated into the examination findings. Older children may communicate and respond to the examiner's inquiries through verbal means. However, younger children and those who speak a different language than the examiner may be unable to offer verbal confirmation. In all cases, observation of behavioral cues may add important data to the assessment. For example, consistent scratching of the skin, persistent pulling of the clothes away from the body, and attempts to discreetly cover certain body areas with the hands may indicate a skin condition. Allowing the child to verbalize freely during the physical examination may yield pertinent information regarding the cause of the skin disorder, areas of pain or intense irritation, and the child's perception of the current health alteration.

Inspection and palpation yield information regarding skin moisture, color, thickness, temperature, and texture. The shape, color, size, consistency, and distribution of any lesions or birthmarks should be noted. Patterns of distribution are specific in many skin disorders. For example, candidiasis is usually found in the moist, dark intertriginous folds of the groin, axillae, and neck; warts and herpes lesions are most often located on mucous membranes. Eruptions appearing on previously healthy skin as a response to disease or trauma are called primary lesions (Table 25–2). Secondary lesions result from changes over time in the primary lesion, usually related to the progression of the disease process, scratching, or secondary infection (Table 25–3). Skin lesions may have characteristic shapes that clearly differentiates the diagnosis (Table 25–4). For example, the skin lesions of ringworm (tinea corporis) are circular and can be called "annular." Contact dermatitis usually forms in cluster shapes, whereas chickenpox appears as distinct, individual lesions.

Table 25–1
Changes in Skin Color Associated with Illness

Skin Color	Associated Illness
Yellow or jaundiced	Liver disease Hemolytic disease Renal failure Myxedema Anorexia nervosa
Red or red-blue	Alcoholism Local inflammatory process Fever Venous stasis
Blue	Heart conditions Lung disease Disorder of hemoglobin Disorder of circulation
Pallor or loss of color	Syncope Albinism Vitiligo Tinea versicolor Anemia Nephrosis Arterial insufficiency Anxiety states

Hair and Nails

The condition of the hair and nails serves as an indicator to help evaluate general hygiene, dietary patterns, responses to stress, and disease progression. Chart 25–5 summarizes the normal and abnormal findings of the hair and nail examination. Hair that is matted and dirty or nail beds that contain dirt may signify poor hygienic practices. Further inspection of the hair shafts may detect the presence of white nits (lice). Nutritional deficits are manifested in the child with dry, brittle, or depigmented hair and brittle nails. Children coping with a great deal of stress may exhibit chronic nail biting or pulling of the hair (trichotillomania). Diseases of the scalp and nails are not common in children, except in cases of infestations (e.g., lice and scabies), which spread easily in home, school, and daycare environments.

Nursing Diagnoses and Outcomes

The data from the focused health history and physical assessment yield information of concern regarding the

Table 25–2
Primary Skin Lesions

Type	Description	Example
Macule	Circumscribed change in skin color without elevation or depression, less than 1 cm	Freckle Petechia Flat nevi Measles Scarlet fever
Papule	Solid, elevated, circumscribed area, less than 1 cm	Mole Wart Lichen planus
Nodule	Solid, elevated, hard or soft lesion in the dermal or subcutaneous tissue, larger than 1 cm	Fibroma Intradermal nevi
Tumor	Solid, raised mass, firm or soft, benign or malignant, larger than 1–2 cm	Hemangioma Osteosarcoma
Wheal	Superficial raised area of localized skin edema, irregular, transient, and erythematous	Mosquito bite Allergic reaction Hive

Table 25–2
Primary Skin Lesions *Continued*

Type	Description	Example
Vesicle	Circumscribed elevated lesion containing serous fluid, less than 1 cm	Herpes simplex Early varicella (chickenpox) Contact dermatitis
Bulla	Circumscribed elevated lesion containing serous fluid, greater than 1 cm	Second-degree burn Blisters Contact dermatitis
Pustule	Vesicle containing pus	Impetigo Acne
Cyst	Encapsulated, fluid-filled cavity of dermis or subcutaneous layer	Sebaceous cyst Epidermal cyst

Illustrations from Jarvis, C. (1996). *Physical examination and health assessment* (2nd ed., pp. 249–250). Philadelphia: W. B. Saunders. Reprinted with permission.

child's skin, hair, or nails. Nursing diagnoses are formulated to direct the interdisciplinary team in a plan of action that addresses alterations in skin integrity (Chart 25–6). The immediate goals for the child include providing treatment of the skin condition (if possible) and providing comfort measures to relieve pain or itching. In addition, if the condition is contagious, measures must be taken to prevent the spread of the illness to children and adults who have had contact with the affected child. When the condition causes a limitation in physical mobility or alterations in body image, the interdisciplinary team must identify these concerns and provide measures to support the child and his or her family. Certain skin lesions are a secondary symptom of a primary condition that affects many other organs. In these cases, health care must encompass a plan to treat other systemic problems that may be occurring. Finally, nursing diagnoses must articulate the need for family education to prevent exacerbations of the skin condition and to manage the child's health needs in the home and at school.

Table 25-3
Secondary Skin Lesions

Type	Description	Example
Crust 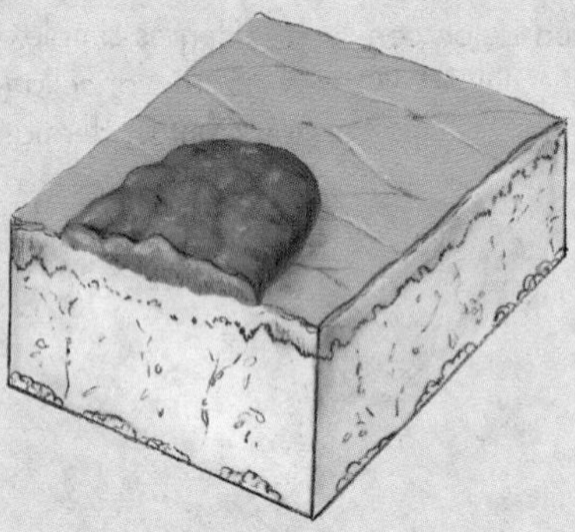	Thickened, dried-out area formed when serum, blood, or purulent exudate dries on the skin	Impetigo Scab formed following abrasion
Scale 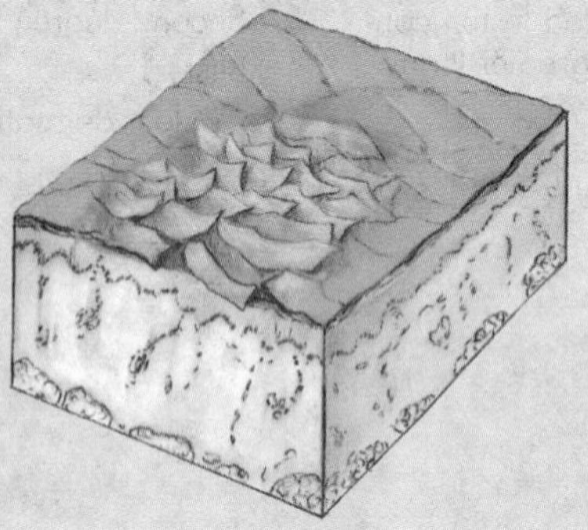	Thin, dry, or greasy flakes of skin, silvery or white in color	Psoriasis Drug reaction Seborrheic dermatitis Eczema Dry skin
Excoriation 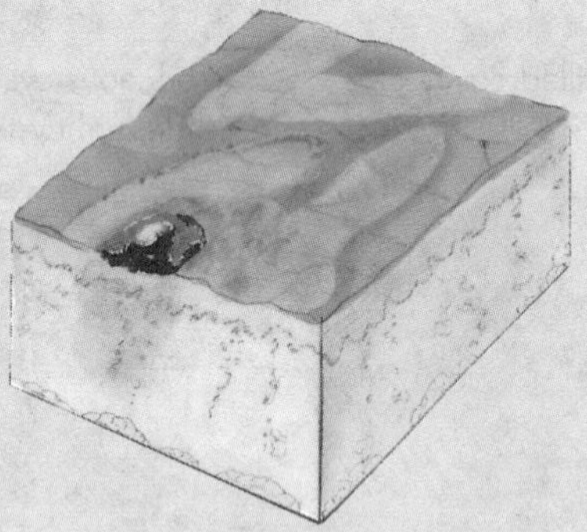	Superficial, self-inflicted abrasion or a scratch from intense itching	Insect bites Poison ivy Scabies Chickenpox
Fissure 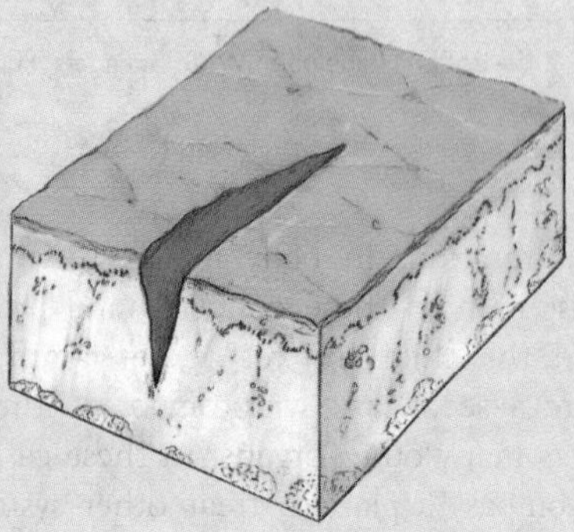	Linear crack with abrupt edges, extends into the dermis	Athlete's foot

Table 25–3
Secondary Skin Lesions *Continued*

Type	Description	Example
Erosion 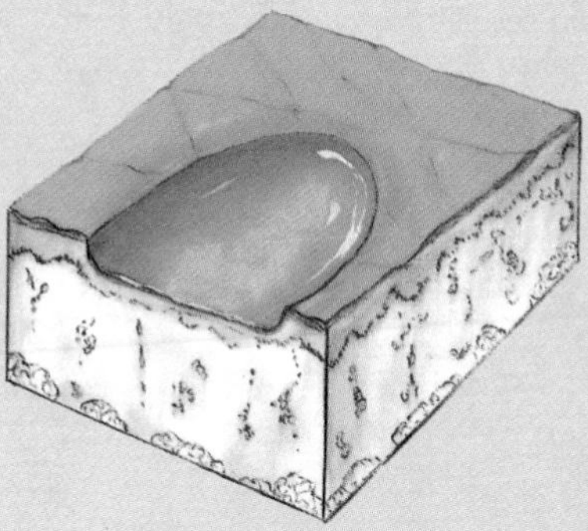	Moist, circumscribed depressed lesion that does not extend into dermis	Ruptured varicella lesion
Ulcer 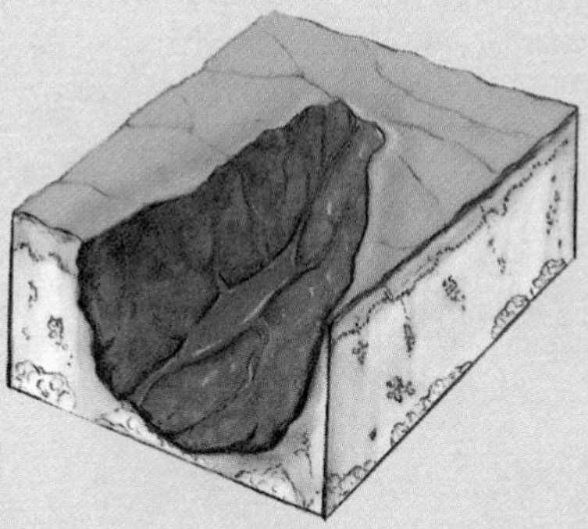	Deep depression that extends into the dermis, irregular shape, may bleed	Pressure sore Chancre
Scar 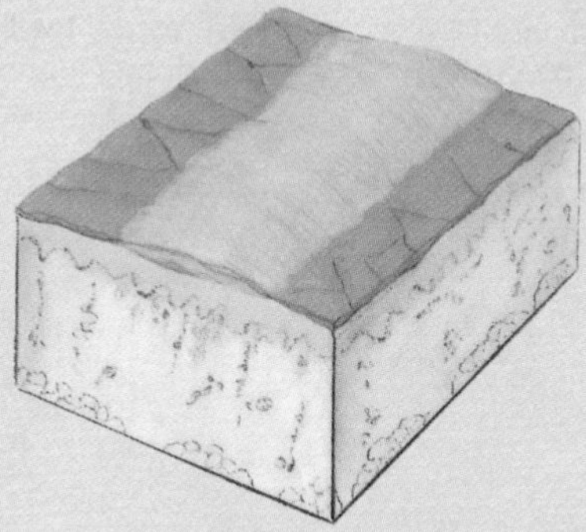	Fibrotic change resulting from the wound-healing process, normal tissue replaced with connective tissue (collagen)	Healed incision site or injury site Acne
Atrophic scar 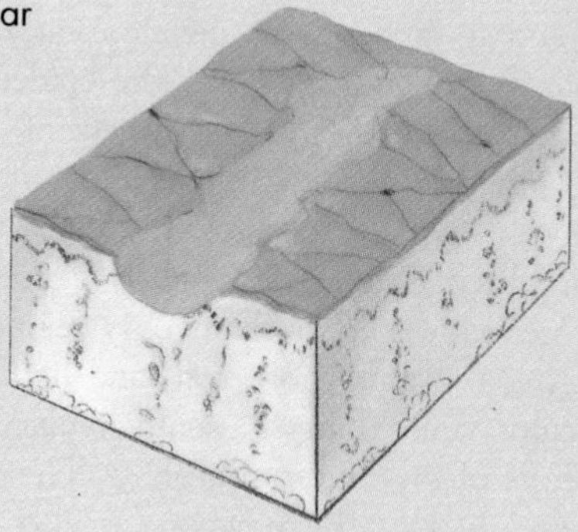	Thinning of the epidermis, which results in skin level depression	Striae associated with pregnancy or weight gain

Table continued on following page

Table 25–3
Secondary Skin Lesions *Continued*

Type	Description	Example
Lichenification	Thickened skin area resulting from prolonged intense scratching	Eczema
Keloid	Hypertrophic scar area that has built up tissue far greater than the size of the original injury	Site of multiple injuries or incisions
Petechia	Small, flat, nonblanchable vascular lesions caused by capillary hemorrhage	Rash evident with meningococcal meningitis Soft tissue injury
Ecchymosis	Large areas of hemorrhage that change in color over time	Bruise caused by a fall or abuse

Illustrations from Jarvis, C. (1996). *Physical examination and health assessment* (2nd ed., pp. 251–252). Philadelphia: W. B. Saunders. Reprinted with permission.

Developmental and Biological Variances

The integumentary system begins to develop by the eighth week of gestation and continues to undergo many metamorphic events over the course of the individual's life. Skin, hair, and nail cells are constantly moving through stages of growth, replication, and maturation. The most pronounced events can be witnessed as the infant's fragile skin transforms into an impermeable barrier of protection against a toddler's many falls (Fig. 25–2). Continuing toward adolescence, hormonal changes trigger changes in skin appearance, contour, and smell. In addition, biological variances (most noticeably, skin color) are more pronounced in the integumentary system than in most other body systems.

Infants

The skin and its appendages develop early in gestation. At less than 8 weeks of fetal life, the epidermis begins to form. Between the 14th and 16th weeks of gestation, nail and hair formation is established. By midgestation (approximately 20 weeks), most of the fetal skin is covered by lanugo, which is fine, soft, lightly pigmented hair. In the early neonatal period, lanugo is replaced by vellus hair, which is also fine, short, soft, and lightly pigmented. On the scalp, vellus hair is usually replaced within the first 6 months of life by terminal hair. The vellus hair on the arms and legs of the newborn is also replaced over time with terminal hair growth. Many other body areas continue to be covered with vellus hair until puberty.

Immediately after birth, vernix caseosa is seen cling-

Table 25–4
Common Configurations of Skin Lesions

Shape	Description	Example
Annular 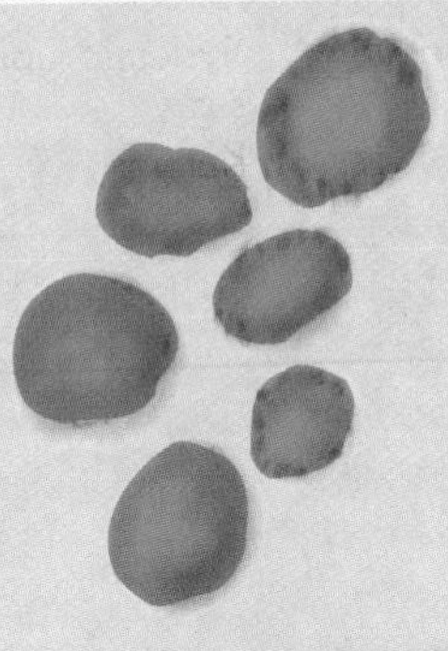	Ringlike with raised borders around flat clear centers of normal skin	Ringworm Tinea versicolor Pityriasis rosea
Polycyclic 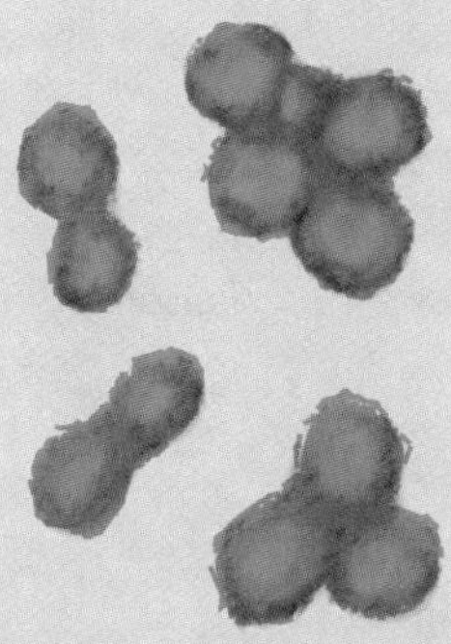	Annular lesions that have grown or merged with each other	Ringworm Tinea versicolor Pityriasis rosea
Confluent or coalesced 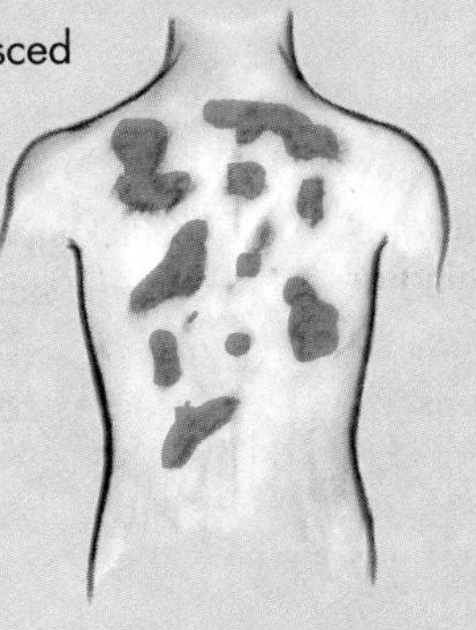	Lesions that merge with one another	Urticaria
Grouped or clustered 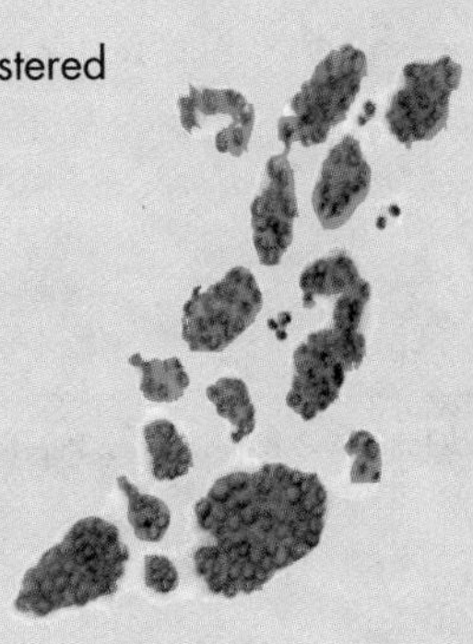	Several lesions grouped together	Vesicles of contact dermatitis

Table continued on following page

Table 25–4
Common Configurations of Skin Lesions *Continued*

Shape	Description	Example
Gyrate or serpiginous 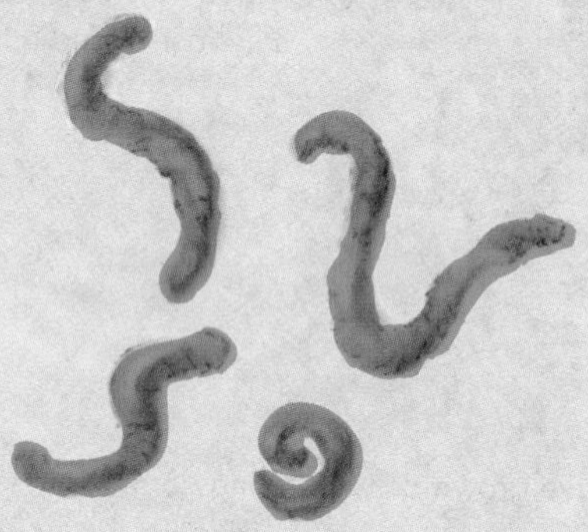	Wavy borders with twisted, coiled, or snakelike appearance	Systemic lupus erythematosus Keloids
Linear 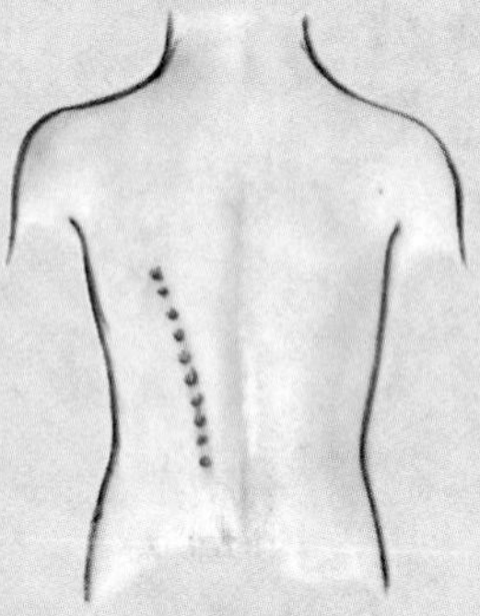	Occur in a straight line	Scratch Incision Poison ivy
Diffuse	Generalized widespread distribution of lesions with intervening areas of normal skin	Chickenpox Atopic eczema
Zosteriform 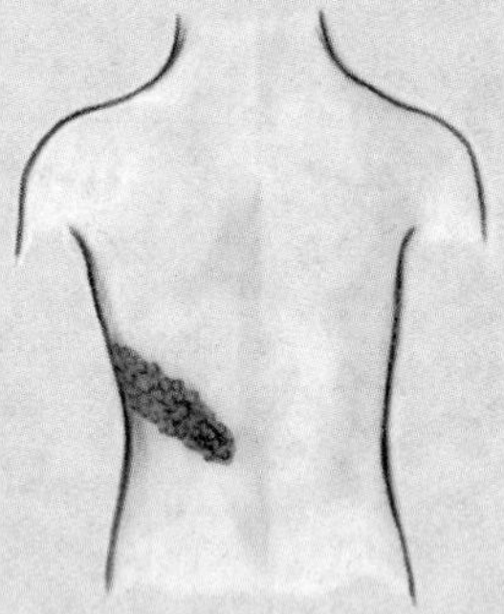	Linear arrangement of lesions formed along a nerve route	Herpes zoster

Illustrations from Jarvis, C. (1996). *Physical examination and health assessment* (2nd ed., p. 248). Philadelphia: W. B. Saunders. Reprinted with permission.

ing to the neonate's skin, especially on the neck, groin, and genital regions. Vernix caseosa is a white cheeselike substance produced in utero by the sebaceous glands. Following the 20th week of gestation, this substance begins to form to protect the delicate fetal skin from abrasions, chapping, and hardening as a result of continuous exposure to amniotic fluid.

Pigmentation is not well developed, with skin tones

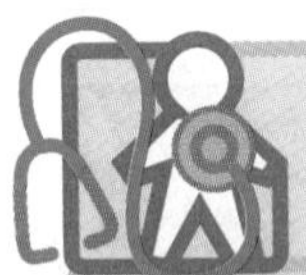

Chart 25–5
Focused Physical Assessment

Hair and Nails

Normal Findings	Abnormal Findings
Hair	
Scalp hair is shiny, silky, and strong; may look straight, curly, or kinky. Hair covers all other body surfaces except palms, soles, inner labial surfaces (girls), and prepuce and glans penis (boys). Hair distribution is appropriate to sex and age (puberty) of child.	Dry, brittle, or depigmented hair Areas of hair loss (alopecia) or balding Presence of white eggs (nits) on hair shaft Presence of lesions or scaling of skin on the head
Nails	
Nail surface is slightly curved or flat (spoon-shaped in the newborn–3 years of age). Nail surface in infant may appear translucent. Nail edges are smooth, rounded, and clean. Nails are clipped and clean, suggesting good hygiene practices.	Convex or curving nails Signs of nail biting Clubbing Presence of hangnail Signs of infection such as tenderness of nail beds, swelling of the cutaneous area, pus or blood underneath the nail Discoloration of the nail or nail bed such as cyanosis or yellowing

of pink being noted in white neonates and creamy tan noted in black, Asian, and Hispanic newborns. Pigmentation of the neonate's nail beds, ears, and scrotal areas are generally noted to be darker than the generalized appearance of the skin. Milia (white papules) secondary to blocked sebaceous ducts appear over the nose, cheeks, and chin. These disappear within a few weeks after birth. Because the vasomotor control of the skin in neonates is immature, a mottled appearance (cutis marmorata) may be observed in response to cooling. In addition, the hands and feet may appear blue (acrocyanosis). This is a transient color change. Prolonged cyanosis must be investigated further.

The neonate's skin is structurally similar to an adult's, but its functions are immature. The neonate's vascular and neuralgic integument structures are immature, and melanin production and eccrine gland function are reduced; therefore, the skin has yet to develop all of its protective, metabolic, and interactive functions. Skin pH is more alkaline in the first few weeks of life, making it a better host for harboring microorganisms that can cause infection. As the pH becomes more acidic, the skin's capacity to fight infection improves.

The full-term neonate has well-developed brown fat stores, some internal (e.g., on the neck, behind the sternum) and some found over the scapular area in the connective tissue. The skin of the newborn has a greater ratio of body surface area to body weight than does that of the older child or adult. As a result, chemicals placed on the skin can be absorbed systemically at higher doses than might be desired.

The premature neonate's skin is not equipped to handle the demands of thermoregulation, homeostasis, and protection (Chart 25–7). The premature neonate has very thin, permeable skin. This places the neonate at a greater risk for both fluid loss and heat loss. In addition, diminished cohesion between the epidermis and dermis and the dearth of sebaceous lubrication after the first few weeks compound to make the skin more susceptible to tearing and blistering (Gordon & Montgomery, 1996). The preterm infant's skin begins a rapid process of maturation immediately after birth; by 21 days of life, the

Chart 25–6
Nursing Diagnoses and Outcomes

The Child with Alterations in Skin Integrity

Impaired skin integrity related to primary break in the skin's surface

Outcomes: Child has improvement in skin integrity.
Child and family follow advised course of therapy to manage the child's skin condition.

Impaired tissue integrity related to physical, chemical, or environmental hazards

Outcomes: Child remains free from alteration in tissue related to physical, chemical, or environmental hazards.
Areas of impaired tissue integrity heal.
Child maintains tissue integrity in presence of other systemic conditions.
Child maintains adequate circulation and nutrients to the wound site or lesion.
Child's skin color and temperature remains within normal parameters.

Pain related to skin disorder, healing process, diagnostic and treatment measures

Outcomes: Child expresses a feeling of improved comfort or demonstrates pain relief through playful, smiling responsive behaviors.
Child and family perform measures to relieve pain and comfort child.

Risk for infection related to wound or open lesion

Outcomes: Vital signs, temperature, and laboratory values remain within normal parameters for the child.
Wound or lesion site remains free of signs and symptoms of infection.

Body image disturbance related to real and or perceived disfigurement caused by a skin condition

Outcomes: Child verbalizes concerns regarding changes in body appearance or function.
Child expresses positive feeling about self.
Family members acknowledge variations or changes in child's appearance and verbalize acceptance of child.
Child and family institute measures to positively impact child's appearance (makeup, selection of clothing).

Effective individual management of therapeutic regimen

Outcomes: Child and family recognize child's need for ongoing management of skin condition.
Child and family take measures to prevent spread of skin condition to other children and adults.
Child and family institute measures to alter environmental factors that may exacerbate the child's skin condition.

skin reaches the maturity of that of a full-term infant (Strickland, 1997). The premature neonate has lighter skin tones than a full-term neonate. This skin can be so translucent that it appears to have a "roadmap" quality resulting from the bluish veins beneath its surface. In addition, the premature neonate has notably less fat stores and more prominent vernix caseosa and lanugo. The skin of postmature and small-for-gestational-age neonates is thicker in comparison, and it appears dry and cracked, and may be meconium stained (Harper, 1990).

Young Children

As the child grows, both physical and developmental changes are manifested in the skin and its appendages. The skin thickens, hair grows at a faster rate, and sebaceous glands provide sebum, which lubricates the skin. Darker pigmentation is noted. Young skin is elastic in the well-nourished child. The skin of young children and infants who eat an abundance of yellow vegetables, such as carrots and squash, may take on a yellowish cast (carotenemia). This is generally considered harmless.

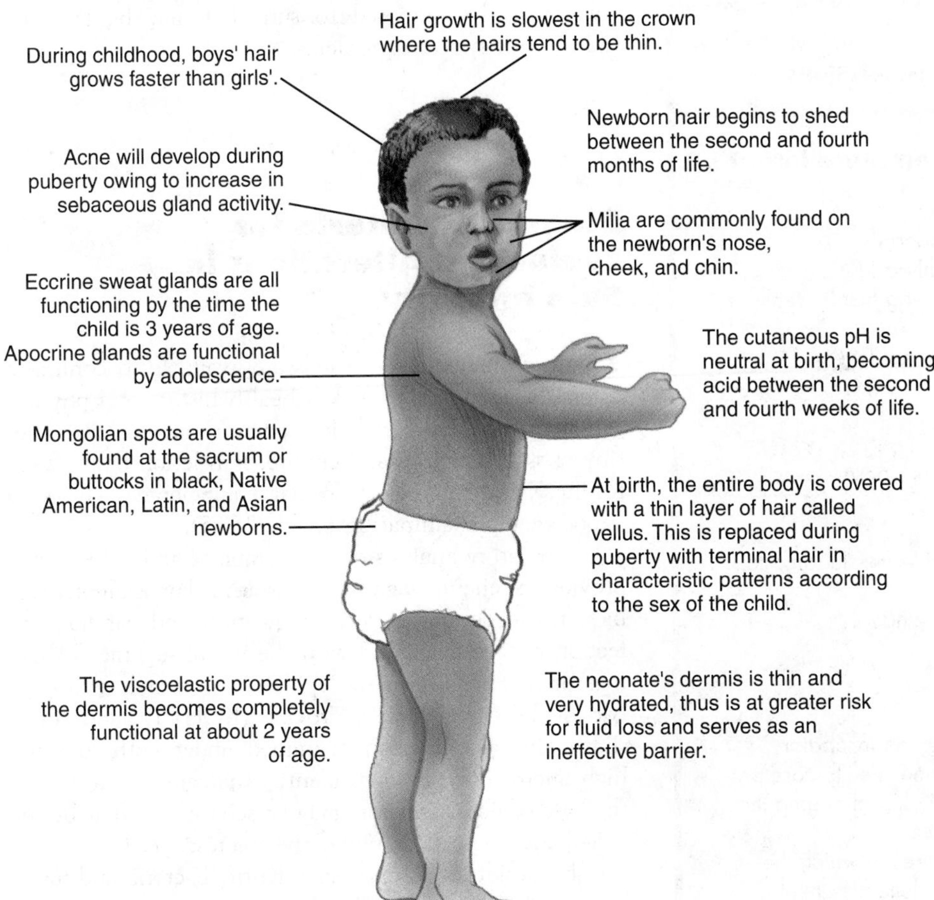

Hair growth is slowest in the crown where the hairs tend to be thin.
During childhood, boys' hair grows faster than girls'.
Newborn hair begins to shed between the second and fourth months of life.
Acne will develop during puberty owing to increase in sebaceous gland activity.
Milia are commonly found on the newborn's nose, cheek, and chin.
Eccrine sweat glands are all functioning by the time the child is 3 years of age. Apocrine glands are functional by adolescence.
The cutaneous pH is neutral at birth, becoming acid between the second and fourth weeks of life.
Mongolian spots are usually found at the sacrum or buttocks in black, Native American, Latin, and Asian newborns.
At birth, the entire body is covered with a thin layer of hair called vellus. This is replaced during puberty with terminal hair in characteristic patterns according to the sex of the child.
The viscoelastic property of the dermis becomes completely functional at about 2 years of age.
The neonate's dermis is thin and very hydrated, thus is at greater risk for fluid loss and serves as an ineffective barrier.

Figure 25–2
Developmental and biological variances: the skin and hair.

Older Children and Adolescents

As the child matures, significant skin changes occur in both boys and girls. Most of these changes represent the onset of puberty. The apocrine and sebaceous glands increase in activity, causing more pronounced body odor and oily skin in blacks and whites. This change in body function can generate problems with self-image in teenagers who are unaccustomed to dealing with body odor and acne problems.

Secondary sex characteristics appear in response to hormonal release, which also stimulates integumentary alterations. For example, in the male, there is growth of pubic and axillary hair, and facial hair starts to darken and grow. In the female, the areola of the breast darkens and enlarges, and pubic and axillary hair appears. Hair on the trunk and limbs increases through, and after, puberty, most noticeably in males. These changes occur as vellus hair converts to terminal hair in specific body regions. Concurrently, in the occipital and bifrontal areas of the male's scalp, some terminal hair converts back to vellus hair, resulting in a receding hair line.

Racial Variations

Differences in the hair and, as discussed earlier, skin pigmentation of children can be seen in persons of differing races. For example, there can be significant variation in the hair of black persons, ranging from long and straight, to thick, curly, and fragile. Asians and Native Americans generally have straight, silky hair, but this may not be true in all cases. Although there are many skin system similarities among members of the same racial and ethnic groups, variations are likely, especially with acculturation and commingling of the gene pool.

Skin eruptions are not generally associated with specific racial differences. The most commonly cited biologic difference is in the appearance of Mongolian spots in black, Native American, Latin, and Asian newborns. Identifying skin lesions and assessing the degree of redness, jaundice, cyanosis, or pallor may be more challenging in children with darker skin tones. In these cases, observing for color changes in the mucous membranes, earlobes, conjunctivae, nails, palms, abdomen, and trunk

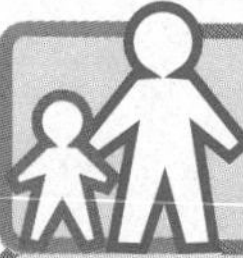

Chart 25-7
Developmental Considerations

Characteristics of the Premature Infant's Skin

Thin and poorly keratinized epidermis
Epidermal layer consisting of only a few layers of stratum corneum during first 3 weeks of life
Less cohesive epidermal and dermal layers
Immature acid mantle
Enhanced permeability of the skin
Little subcutaneous fat
Wrinkled, gelatinous skin hanging loosely over limbs
Lanugo covering the body
Increased loss of transepidermal water, leading to difficulty in fluid balance
Nonfunctional apocrine sweat glands

Implications for Care

Neonate is prone to hypothermia.
- Keep the baby warm using an incubator
- Minimize the number of times health care providers enter the Isolette, thus changing the ambient temperature.
- During bathing or procedures in which the neonate is out of the Isolette, use heat lamps to keep the child warm.

Neonate is prone to skin breakdown.
- Turn the neonate frequently to prevent skin breakdown.
- Minimize use of adhesive-based products on the skin.
- Use pectin-based barrier products to protect the skin.
- Remove adhesives with water and diluted soap.
- Do not bathe the neonate on a frequent basis.
- Prevent intravenous catheter infiltration.

Neonate is at risk for fluid and electrolyte losses.
- Monitor fluid and electrolyte status diligently.
- Provide fluid and electrolytes as needed via intravenous administration.

Neonate is at risk for potentially lethal topical absorption of chemicals.
- Minimize use of pharmacologic and cleansing compounds to the skin, such as neomycin, soap compounds, and lotions.

(two areas less exposed to sunlight) may be the best indicator of systemic problems.

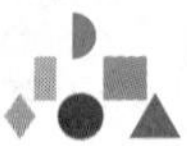

Diagnostic Criteria for Evaluating Alterations in Skin Integrity

A limited number of methods are available to confirm a diagnosis generated by a skin health history and physical examination. These include laboratory analysis via scrutiny of skin scrapings and culture, skin lesion biopsy, skin testing, and the use of special equipment, such as in Wood's lamp examination (Table 25–5).

Laboratory analysis of skin scrapings and cultures can provide excellent diagnostic assistance. For example, scabies, tinea, dermatophytes (ringworm), and candidal infection can be diagnosed with the use of superficial shavings or scrapings from the epidermis to which a drop or two of 20% potassium hydroxide (KOH) is added on a slide. The slide is then examined under both low and high microscope power to identify the causative agent. In the case of lice, adult nits may be seen in the hair by the naked eye, as well as under the microscope. Cultures of the skin lesion or wound may identify bacteria and fungi. Suspected staphylococcal and streptococcal organisms are easily collected from the integument with a polyester-tipped swab. After collection, suspected candidal and dermatophytes cultures must be placed in special media.

Skin biopsies can establish whether lesions are malignant or benign. Some minor biopsies can be completed in outpatient settings. A shave biopsy is performed for superficial lesions; a punch biopsy is used for deeper lesions. The tissue is fixed and stained on a slide before examination under the microscope. Biopsy of the skin by excision is rarely required for diagnosis in children. When it is necessary, special consent is required, and the child may need to be physically restrained during the biopsy procedure.

Skin testing is helpful in detecting the cause of an allergic contact dermatitis. It is performed in one of three ways: intracutaneous, scratch, or patch testing. Patch testing is highly standardized and is the most frequently used test. During patch testing, a small patch or swatch of the suspected cause of the allergy (often rubber in children) is taped in place for 48 hours. The patches are removed, and the tests are read 72 hours after the initial application. Erythema and vesiculation similar to that found during earlier periods of contact dermatitis indicate positive allergic responses. Other methods of skin testing (intracutaneous and scratch testing) involve injecting allergic substances under the skin or irritating the skin

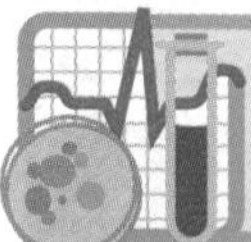

Table 25–5
Diagnostic Tests and Procedures for Evaluating Alterations of the Skin, Hair, and Nails

Diagnostic Test or Procedure	Purpose	Health Care Provider Responsibilities
Cultures Skin Wound Nails Hair	Samples of exudate, scales, and crusts are cultured to identify the bacterial, viral, or fungal causes of redness, irritation, or visible lesions.	Skin · Use polyester-tipped swabs to collect all skin and wound cultures. Cotton-tipped swabs are unsatisfactory because they may be treated with bacteriostatic solutions · Wash affected site with 70% isopropanol or sterile water, allow to dry, and culture several lesion sites, swabbing the edges of the lesion. Wound · All superficial debris adjacent to the lesion and the wound itself must be gently wiped with a 70% isopropanol solution before culture is obtained. · Specimens collected from the wound edge are not very accurate. · Specimens should be delivered to the laboratory immediately so that testing can begin within 60 minutes of collection. Hair · Obtain hair and hair stubs or scrapings from areas of hair loss or infection sites without cleansing the scalp. · Both shaft and infected root or suspicious hairs are clipped or plucked with sterile forceps and sent to the laboratory in Petri dish.
Scrapings for microscopic analysis	Samples of skin scraping, nail clippings, or plucked hairs are stained and evaluated under the microscope to identify the bacterial, viral, or fungal causes of redness, scaling, irritation, or visible lesions.	Same considerations as for cultures.
Potassium hydroxide. (KOH) stain	Test identifies fungi or yeast.	
Tzanck preparation Giemsa method Wright stain	Smears are useful in the diagnosis of some viral infections (herpes simplex, varicella, herpes zoster, and eczema herpeticum) and to examine the white cell morphology of pustular disorders (erythema toxicum neonatorum, candidiasis).	
Gram stain for bacteria	Stain identifies bacterial growth from a skin lesion.	
Scabies preparation	Test identifies presence of scabies.	Scrape intact vesicles, papules, or burrows with a #15 blade coated with immersion oil. Sample as many primary lesions as possible to have a greater chance of having a positive scabies preparation.
Skin biopsy Punch biopsy Shave biopsy	Technique is used to determine the histopathologic diagnosis of any skin tumor, palpable purpura, or persistent dermatitis	A local anesthetic using 1% to 2% plain lidocaine should be given prior to biopsy. After the punch biopsy, bleeding may occur at the site. Firm pressure should be applied until bleeding stops. Suturing is optional.

Table continued on following page

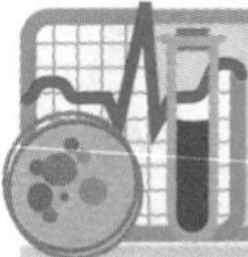

Table 25–5
Diagnostic Tests and Procedures for Evaluating Alterations of the Skin, Hair, and Nails *Continued*

Diagnostic Test or Procedure	Purpose	Health Care Provider Responsibilities
Skin testing Intracutaneous Scratch Patch	Testing identifies the offending allergen, which may be the cause of allergic dermatitis responses.	Conduct the test after the allergic dermatitis has subsided. The patches should not be allowed to become wet while taped on the skin. Testing should be performed by a physician experienced in the interpretation and potential hazards of the procedures.
Wood's lamp	Ultraviolet light is useful in diagnosis of certain superficial pigmentary or infectious skin lesions.	Test must be performed in a darkened room. Procedure is noninvasive. No pain is associated with testing. Infected hair follicles have a grayish appearance in normal light, but exhibit a yellow-green fluorescent appearance under Wood's light.

surface with the allergen. Both immediate and delayed reactions are monitored.

The Wood's lamp is a type of ultraviolet (UV) light used to fluoresce certain strains of tinea infestations of the scalp (Fig. 25–3). In a darkened room, the lamp is turned on and held up to the child's skin. This noninvasive procedure provides a quick, easy method to visualize the source of skin lesions in such cases as tinea capitis, tuberous sclerosis, and body lice.

Figure 25–3
A Wood's lamp uses ultraviolet light to fluoresce specific skin lesions.

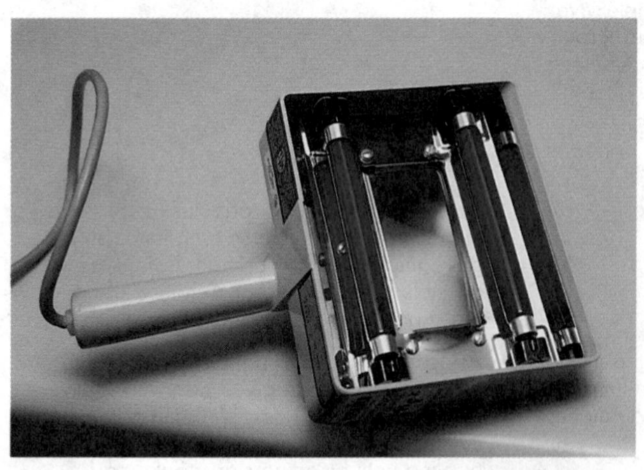

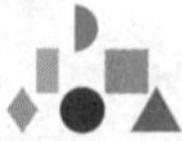

Treatment Modalities

Various treatments can enhance the healing of skin eruptions, lesions, and wounds in children. The nurse is responsible for performing many of these interventions or teaching family members how to do so. The nurse is also responsible for completing skin surveillance measures to monitor skin condition and implementing actions to maintain skin integrity (Chart 25–8). Additionally, the nurse is responsible for teaching children and their families hygienic practices that promote healthy skin and hair and that help prevent the spread of a contagion (Chart 25–9).

Providing optimal skin care is an interdisciplinary effort. Collaboration with the dietitian is critical to proper healing of the child's skin. The dietitian can assist in calculating the child's caloric needs. If the child is unable to meet these caloric needs orally, parenteral or enteral nutrition may be required to ensure adequate nutrition to support the healing process.

The physical therapist plays a role in skin care if debridement is necessary or if physical mobility has become restricted secondary to changes in elasticity of the skin or to immobility. The physical therapist can assist with whirlpool treatments for the child. The whirlpool enhances wound debridement and cleaning. It is generally soothing as well. As the wound continues to heal, it

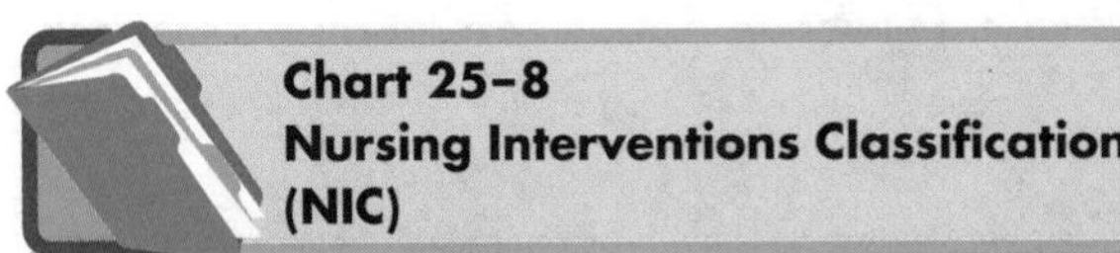

Chart 25–8
Nursing Interventions Classification (NIC)

Skin Surveillance

Definition

Collection and analysis of patient data to maintain skin and mucous membrane integrity

Activities

Inspect condition of surgical incision, as appropriate.
Observe extremities for color, warmth, swelling, pulses, texture, edema, and ulcerations.
Inspect skin and mucous membranes for redness, extreme warmth, or drainage.
Monitor skin for areas of redness and breakdown.
Monitor for sources of pressure and friction.
Monitor for infection, especially of edematous areas.
Monitor skin and mucous membranes for areas of discoloration and bruising.
Monitor skin for rashes and abrasions.
Monitor skin for excessive dryness and moistness.
Inspect clothing for tightness.
Monitor skin color.
Monitor skin temperature.
Note skin or mucous membrane changes.
Institute measures to prevent further deterioration, as needed.
Instruct family member/caregiver about signs of skin breakdown, as appropriate.

From McCloskey, J., & Bulechek, G. (1996). *Nursing interventions classification (NIC)* (2nd ed.). St. Louis: Mosby–Year Book. Reprinted with permission.

is important that scarring does not decrease the mobility and the function of the impaired body area. The physical therapist is skilled in techniques to facilitate elasticity of the affected area while maintaining the integrity of the healing wound.

Depending on the cause of the child's skin condition, the degree of systemic involvement, and the progression of healing, a social worker consult and visits by a home care nurse may be beneficial to ensure continuity of care in the home setting. In addition, these personnel can assist families in connecting with community support groups that can provide educational resources and social support for family members.

Amidst the many interventions of the health care team, the psychological and cognitive needs of the child must be met. It is vital for the nurse to approach each child, each situation as unique. The cause and nature of the skin condition itself may pose challenging issues for the child and the family. Approaches to skin care should account for the child's developmental stage and associated perception of the events surrounding the encounter with the health care team (Chart 25–10).

Finally, it is important to remember that the child with a skin condition may be in pain. The pain may be transient, chronic, or acute. Managing the pain may be as simple as wiping away some tears or as complex as implementing the use of patient-controlled analgesia. (See Chapter 13 for a thorough discussion of pain management options.)

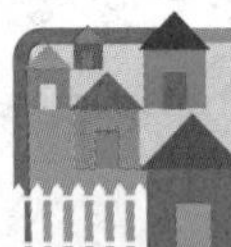

Chart 25–9
Community Care

Measures to Promote Skin Hygiene

Personal Care

Child is bathed and hair is washed on a regular basis.
Child's nails are trimmed and kept short.
Child's teeth and tongue are brushed at least twice daily.
Protective agents such as sunscreen and diaper rash ointments are used to protect the child's skin from injury.
Cuts and scrapes are cleaned immediately and covered with an appropriate type of dressing.

Home, Daycare, and School

New foods are introduced gradually and the skin is monitored for a reaction.
The presence of an unusual rash is noted and reported to a health care provider.
Clothing and other personal items such as hats, toothbrushes, and drinking cups are not shared.
Children with an unusual rash are separated from other children until the causative agent can be determined.
Care providers and teachers wash their hands frequently to prevent spread of infectious agents from one child to another.
Costumes used in play activities are washed frequently in hot water.
Care providers wear gloves when changing diapers, applying topical ointments, or treating wounds.

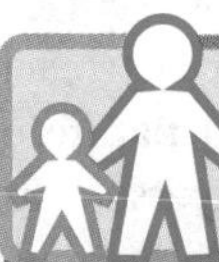

Chart 25-10
Developmental Considerations

Skin Care

Age	Developmental Principles	Nursing Strategies
Infant	Exploration of the body is occurring. Infants are acutely aware of attitudes portrayed by caregivers. Pain response may be difficult to interpret. There is high need for comfort by a person who is familiar to the infant.	Involve the primary caregiver in the skin care. Distract the infant with toys during the procedure. Ensure that the infant is free from pain during procedures. Decrease the pain caused by frequent dressing changes by using Montgomery straps or protecting the skin with a skin barrier.
Toddler	Child's thinking is egocentric, magical, and concrete. Child believes that two events contiguous in time are usually related. Child perceives injury or hospitalization as a result of a misbehavior. Limited experiences make it difficult to understand complicated explanations of events.	Use diversional play such as clay, crayons, or a favorite video during the procedure. Convey an attitude to the child that skin care is a process performed *with* them, not *to* them. Elicit cooperation and assistance when possible from the child; give choices. Provide careful, simple, present-oriented explanations.
Preschooler	Child learns about self and environment through play. Child is able to perform simple self-care tasks. Child follows rules or directions given by those in authority.	Use therapeutic play to foster expression of feelings and child's knowledge of the skin care activities. Allow child to perform skin care on a doll. Allow child to help with skin care. The child may want to place the bandage on or assist in putting on the tape. Explain that the dressing should not be touched, picked at, pulled off, or gotten wet by the child.
School-age	Child is able to apply logical reasoning skills to familiar situations. Child comprehends cause-and-effect relationships. Memory is improved. One of the major fears is loss of control.	Use of rules and limits are important. Explain all aspects of the procedure including the concept of sterile technique and germ transmission. Give specific guidelines regarding the degree of participation by the child and family in skin care. When medicating the child for pain, avoid drugs or doses that may make the child feel a loss of control.
Adolescent	Abstract through processes develop. Body image is paramount. Privacy is important. Child is developing independence from parents.	Teach the adolescent to manage their skin care independently as appropriate. Parents should be included in care for support and as wanted by the adolescent. Address issues about body image in a positive, thorough, and honest manner. Consider the adolescent's body image concerns as important if not more important than the actual skin care.

Measures to Promote Skin Hydration

Bathing

Bathing promotes good daily hygiene in children. Bathing is also often recommended to enhance hydration of the skin in dry climates or if the child has a condition in which the skin is very dry. Bathing can be used to promote comfort and reduce itching. Lukewarm (not hot) water should be used. The bath should not last long enough for the skin to become supersaturated. Soaps and oils may be used during the bath to cleanse and moisturize the skin. Mild soaps that can be used on the child's skin include Dove, Aveeno, Neutrogena, Basis, Alpha Keri, and Lubriderm. Bath oils include Alpha Keri and Domol. Aveeno is an acceptable colloid (Barber, 1996). The child with a skin condition should avoid bubble baths because they can further irritate the skin. After the bath, the child should be gently dried. Children with skin conditions such as atopic dermatitis (AD) should immediately apply an emollient to the skin to maintain the skin's hydration.

Environmental Considerations

Environmental humidity affects skin hydration. Excessive humidity (>90%) or deficient humidity (<10%) can lead to alterations in skin integrity. Children with dry skin are especially susceptible to discomfort when the humidity is low. Use of a vaporizer, humidifier, and humidified heating during the winter months may help relieve itching. In warmer weather, air conditioning may help alleviate discomfort and itching.

Skin hydration is also affected by the child's fluid intake. To promote good skin hydration, the child should be encouraged to drink plenty of water, especially if the skin will be exposed to dry-hot or dry-cold conditions.

Topical Agents

Several types of topical agents may be used on the child's skin to provide daily care, to promote hygiene, to moisturize and lubricate the skin, and to provide medication to areas in which skin integrity has been compromised. The use of soaps has been discussed in the previous section. Moisturizers and lubricants are composed of petrolatum or a mixture of petrolatum and lanolin. These agents assist the child's skin to retain water and are most effective when applied to wet skin. These agents are used for children whose skin appears very dry or is unable to maintain hydration such as in AD.

caREminder: *Moisturizers and lubricants should not be applied to the infant's or toddler's diaper area because these products are likely to enhance the incidence of skin breakdown. The agents cause the skin to become overhydrated and act as a friction agent between the diaper and the baby's skin.*

Petrolatum-based agents include Vaseline pure petrolatum jelly and Moisturel. Petrolatum and lanolin combination agents include Aquaphor ointment, Eucerin cream and lotion, Lubriderm, and Keri Creme (Barber, 1996).

Topical medications can be used to treat skin conditions or prevent alterations in skin integrity. A topical medication consists of an "active" agent contained in a vehicle, or base. Additionally, the topical application may contain an "accelerant," which increases skin permeability, thus enhancing the mechanisms for medication absorption (Balthrop & Brueton, 1991). Topical agents are widely used because of their ability to deliver an optimum concentration of a medication to the exact site where it is needed (Table 25–6).

The nurse applying a skin care agent to the child is responsible for monitoring the skin for effectiveness of the therapy. The child may have a sensitization to the agent that aggravates rather than relieves the symptoms or that creates new skin problems. Application of the agents should follow the frequency and dosage requirements recommended by the manufacturer or a pharmacist. The family must be instructed where and how to apply the agent. After application of the agent, parents should be advised to wash their hands to cleanse the agent off of their skin. If the child's skin becomes wet after application of a topical agent, reapplication may be necessary and, in some cases, such as with sunscreens and sunblocks, is highly recommended to continue the therapeutic action of the agent.

Systemic Drug Therapy

Many of the skin conditions that occur in the pediatric population are a result of infection or immune responses within the body. In these cases, the primary cause of the skin condition must be treated using some type of systemic therapy. Medications are given orally or intravenously to relieve pain, reduce inflammation, and combat viral, bacterial, or fungal invasions. Table 25–7 lists common systemic medications used to treat skin problems in children.

If systemic therapy is initiated, the nurse must assess the family's understanding of the need for this treatment and their ability to continue the course of therapy for the entire treatment. Some of the products are expensive, and reimbursement may not be adequately covered under the family's health care plan. Abrupt cessation of some of the agents may be hazardous to the child. For instance, discontinuing the use of steroid therapy should be done in a tapered fashion. To prevent reinfection, the entire course of antifungal, antiviral, or antibacterial agents

Table 25-6
Topical Agents

Agent	Purpose	Key Points
Emollients	To lubricate and hydrate skin for dry, scaly skin conditions As a bath additive to dry skin As a soap substitute, to cleanse the skin in treatment of all the inflammatory dermatoses	Apply with clean hands to avoid contaminating the contents of the container. Each family member should have a separate supply to avoid cross-contamination.
Barrier creams	To protect against irritation or repeated hydration To serve as water-repellent substance	In the diaper area, barrier creams should not be wiped away completely after each wet or dirty diaper. Such actions can cause further skin breakdown. Only clearly dirty or stained areas of cream should be removed. Additional cream may need to be applied with each diaper change.
Antiseptics and astringents	To cleanse skin To cleanse wounds	Povidone-iodine and hexachlorophene should not be used in neonates or those with badly burned or excoriated skin because of the risk of toxicity from absorption.
Keratolytics	To remove thickening of the surface of the skin (hyperkeratosis) in conditions with dry, scaling skin, such as ichthyosis, psoriasis, and eczema For acne, to relieve follicular obstruction by promoting peeling of the skin and inhibition of bacteria	The agent may leave a greasy feeling on skin. Generally agent needs to be used only every 12 hours.
Topical steroids	To treat inflammatory conditions of the skin, particularly eczematous disorders	The more potent the steroid, the higher the incidence of side effects, including adrenal suppression and cushingoid effects. *In children, the risk is increased:* · By prolonged application · Under occluded areas, such as those covered by disposable diapers · On areas of thin skin Local side effects include skin atrophy, telangiectasia, purpura, and striae. Topical steroids may mask signs of infection.
Coal tar	To treat eczema and psoriasis, although the mechanism for its therapeutic effect is unknown	Coal tar can be used alone, in ointment, or paste base. Scalp preparations and shampoos are also available.
Topical antibiotics, antifungals, and antivirals	To treat localized infections	Prolonged use may promote bacterial resistance and sensitization reactions. This treatment should be aimed at minor skin problems for 5–7 days only.
Antiparasitic preparations	To treat lice and scabies infestations	Give written instructions to the family to increase the likelihood of observing correct application procedure.
Sunscreens and sunblocks	To protect skin from effects of ultraviolet light	The higher the skin protection factor, the more efficient the preparation is in preventing burning. There is no internationally agreed standard of photoprotection.

Table 25–7
Systemic Drug Therapy

Agent	Purpose	Example of Condition
Antihistamines	To relieve itching and provide some sedation effect	Insect bites and stings Atopic dermatitis
Antibiotics	To treat known bacterial causes of skin disorders	Primary cellulitis Impetigo
	To treat potential or known secondary bacterial infections, which are a result of a preexisting skin condition	Secondary infections of atopic dermatitis
Antifungal agents	To treat fungal causes of skin disorders	Candidal infection Dermatophytes
Antiviral agents	To treat certain viral causes of skin disorders	Herpes Eczema herpeticum
Oral glucocorticosteroids	To reduce inflammation and decrease itching	Drug reactions

must be completed. Acute exacerbations of the child's condition may require periods of hospitalization. The family should also be informed of the side effects of the medications. If intravenous administration is required, hospitalization may be necessary.

Dressings

Various wet, dry, and occlusive dressings may be used to treat a skin condition or wound (Table 25–8). Dressings serve several functions, including to

- Reduce pain
- Provide a barrier to infection
- Help clean the wound or lesion via debridement
- Promote a moist environment
- Absorb drainage from the wound or lesion
- Provide an aesthetic barrier while maintaining easy access to view the wound or lesion site

Wet Dressings

Wet dressings help moisturize the skin, decrease itching, and remove crusts. The dressing should be wet with lukewarm water and applied for 10 to 20 minutes, four to six times per day for up to 1 week. During the treatment, the dressing should not be allowed to dry. The dressing should be rewetted or removed, with a new wet dressing being placed on the area. Creams or ointments are usually applied after the wet dressing therapy to promote hydration. In some cases, following the application of a cream or ointment, another wet dressing, followed by a dry dressing may be applied. For instance, in the treatment regimen for a child with psoriasis, a wet dressing is applied for 20 minutes followed by application of a moisturizing agent. This is then followed by covering the body with a wet sleeper pajama or long john, which is then covered by a dry sleeper or long john. The dressing and clothing are changed every 6 hours for a 24- to 72-hour period, or they may be used overnight for 5 to 10 hours (Barber, 1996).

caREminder: *Avoid chilling the child by making sure the room is warm, but not hot. Also make sure the damp dressing remains damp and does not dry out. Change the dry dressing as needed to ensure that it remains dry and to help prevent chilling.*

Dry Dressings

Dry dressings are most commonly used to cover a surgical wound or other break in the surface of the skin. A dry dressing may be as simple as a Band-Aid placed over scraped knee.

Tip: *Many children do not like bandages placed on their "owies." To gain the child's cooperation, allow the child to place the bandage on himself or herself. The use of bandages with cartoon characters on them or placing a*

Table 25-8
Types of Dressings for Skin Care

Type	Advantages	Disadvantages
Traditional gauze	Has good absorbency Is relatively inexpensive	Is bulky Can macerate surrounding skin if applied wet outside wound margins Debridement is nonselective Must be changed often
Nonadherent (Telfa, Adaptic, Vaseline gauze)	Occludes wound Is atraumatic to wound bed	Provides little absorption May contain antimicrobials, which can slow healing
Synthetic transparent films (Op-Site, Tegaderm, Bioclusive)	Provides easy wound assessment Promotes moist environment Is water resistant Conforms to body Speeds autolysis Has good adhesion Decreases friction	Provides little or no absorption Needs careful application Is not for infected or draining wounds
Hydrocolloids (Duoderm, Tegasorb, Restore)	Promotes moist wound environment Conforms to body Is occlusive Provides bacterial barrier Needs no secondary dressing Needs infrequent changing	Dressing melts with absorption Is not transparent Needs dressing to be flushed away Is not for infected wounds
Hydrogels (Carrington Wound Gel, Intrasite Gel)	Promotes moist wound environment Provides cooling; less pain Provides easy wound viewing Is usable in infection	Must be changed if there is leakage
Foams (Lyofoam, Allevyn)	Retains moisture Is absorbent Increases patient comfort	Needs a cover dressing
Exudate absorbers (Mesalt, Sorbsan)	Is highly absorbent Promotes moist wound environment Is excellent for infected wound	None identified

Adapted from Krasner, D. (1991). Resolving the dressing dilemma: Selecting wound dressings by category. *Ostomy/Wound Management, 35,* 62, 64–70; Krasner, D. (1992). The 12 commandments of wound care. *Nursing 92, 22*(12), 34–42.

sticker or pen-drawn smiling face on the outer aspect of the dressing before placing it on the child's skin may make wearing the bandage more acceptable to the child.

The dressings used to cover surgical wounds are used to protect the wound from microorganisms, reduce tension on the wound edges, and absorb drainage from the wound.

Prior to placement of a dressing, the wound should be cleansed gently with normal saline or other nontoxic wound cleanser. Surrounding normal skin should be treated in the same gentle fashion as the affected site to protect the healthy area from deterioration. When removing an old dressing, it should be taken off the skin carefully: never pulled off forcefully. Wetting the dressing and tape may be necessary to ease removal.

Alert: *The neonate's skin has weak intracellular attachments. Rapid removal of tape can cause separation of skin layers (epidermal stripping) and blister formation (Gordon & Montgomery, 1996; Strickland, 1997).*

Occlusive Dressings

Occlusive dressings enhance hydration of the skin, promote the absorption of topical medications, and prevent exposure of the area to microorganisms. Occlusive dressings are also effective in preventing epidermal stripping in preterm infants by eliminating the need for tape to be used and in preventing skin irritation by functioning as an artificial barrier (Strickland, 1997). Recently, the effectiveness of polyurethane dressings as a barrier to prevent microorganism growth on the excoriated skin of the preterm infant has been questioned. Data remain inconclusive, with some research indicating that high concentrations of bacterial growth under the dressings placed the neonate at risk for infection (Strickland, 1997; Vernon, Lane, Wischerath, David, & Menegus, 1990).

Occlusive dressings are used in a variety of ways. For instance, plastic wraps may be placed on the skin after hydrating the skin and applying a moisturizing agent. This type of occlusive dressing is left on for no longer than 8 hours. Occlusive dressings are also used to protect the entry site of a vascular access device, to promote absorption of a topical agent such as EMLA cream, and to protect an open area of the skin from fecal contamination (e.g., in the child with myelomeningocele).

Wound Care

A wound is a disruption of the normal skin integrity. Wounds occur traumatically from an accident or burn injury. Wounds may arise as an outcome of medical interventions such as a biopsy or surgery. Wounds can also occur in response to infectious or environmental agents that lead to a break in the surface of the skin. The nurse is responsible for completing regular, accurate assessment of a wound and the surrounding tissue. These observations are important as baseline data from which the clinician can make judgments about the nature or type of wound, progression of healing, and course of treatment (Chart 25–11).

Alert: *Signs of infection at the wound site may include a red streak running from the wound, a wound that progressively becomes more tender, dehiscing of the wound site, or a suture that comes out too early.*

Many options for treating wounds are available to the health care team. The physician or nurse practitioner can choose to treat the wound either surgically or medically. Surgical interventions involve debridement and closure of the open wound with sutures or staples. Medical intervention entails the use of medications (antibiotics, antiseptics, debriding enzymes, and vitamins) and special dressings. If antiseptics (e.g., Betadine, hydrogen peroxide) are applied topically to cleanse the wound area, they should be used only briefly and in low concentrations with the appropriate dressings.

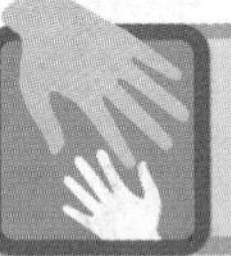

Chart 25–11
Nursing Interventions

Wound Assessment

Wound Dimensions

The indices of healing can be easily assessed with the naked eye by the observant nurse. Healing is generally considered to be progressing if the wound is shrinking in both width and depth and if the layer of damage becomes more superficial as the bottom of the wound heals.

Presence of Undermining Tracts

Wounds heal faster if no undermining tracts or spaces in the tissue are present. The presence of tracts can be assessed by using a sterile applicator to gently probe the wound site to find holes in the tissue. Bony prominences present a challenge to wound healing. Lesions over the distal extremities often heal slower than wounds in the upper body. If dead or desiccated tissue is present at the base of a wound, it can be removed with either sharp or blunt debridement or chemical debridement by a physician or nurse practitioner.

Color and Odor of Wound and Exudate

Wound color is also a crucial parameter. Clean wounds are usually beefy-red and shiny. The amount, color, odor, and consistency of the exudate must be observed. Malodorous, purulent exudate is suggestive of infection.

Condition of Wound Edges

Wound edges must be flat and not curled under. Curled wound edges will not allow for migration of skin cells to replace epithelial cells.

Presence of Foreign Bodies

Foreign bodies impede healing. A suture that is not removed, for example, can affect wound integrity.

Condition of Surrounding Skin

The condition of the surrounding skin can provide the nurse with a wealth of information about the wound itself, because it reveals the child's health status. The skin surrounding a wound should be intact and unmacerated if a wound is to heal.

Miscellaneous Treatments

Various physical and surgical interventions can be used to remove skin lesions or alter the appearance of the skin. For instance, camouflage makeup may be used to cover disfiguring birthmarks and scars. UV light therapy is used to treat psoriasis and acne. Repeated laser therapy treatments can remove vascular malformations such as a port wine stain. Liquid nitrogen is used to remove warts. Disfiguring or irritating lumps or bumps can be removed from the skin surgically. All of these therapies require the health care team to ensure that the child and family are well acquainted with the treatment options. The treatment options may be painful and may themselves cause some disfigurement between the time of treatment and the complete healing of the skin.

Nutritional Management

When managing skin conditions that affect children, the importance of nutrition cannot be overlooked. Nutritional deficiencies may be manifested by slow or insufficient wound healing, as well as by the presence of skin disorders such as dermatitis or hair loss (Goskowicz & Eichenfield, 1993). Poor nutrition is clearly related to improper or slowed healing. Protein deficiencies retard the formation of collagen. Vitamins and minerals are necessary for various metabolic processes and for epithelial tissue and collagen formation (Table 25–9).

Children can challenge the clinician's ability to provide sufficient nutrition. Certain developmentally appropriate behaviors place the child at risk for nutritional deficits. For example, a 4-year-old is nutritionally chal-

Table 25–9
Nutrients and Wound Healing

Nutrient	Effect on Wound Healing
Carbohydrates	
Glucose	Provides energy for leukocytes and fibroblasts
Protein	
Amino acids	Are necessary for neovascularization and fibroblast production, lymphocyte formation, synthesis of collagen, phagocytosis, and wound remodeling
Albumin	Is necessary to prevent edema by controlling oncotic pressure
Fats	
Essential fatty acids	Are metabolized in prostaglandins and form cell membranes; primary energy source for infants
Vitamins	
Ascorbic acid	Is necessary to collagen synthesis; improves immune response to infection
B complex	Is a cofactor of enzyme system
A	Promotes epithelialization and collagen synthesis
D	Is necessary for calcium metabolism
E	May protect vitamin A oxidation during digestion
K	Is necessary for synthesis of prothrombin and other clotting factors
Minerals	
Zinc	Stabilizes cell membrane; promotes cell mitosis; helps with epithelialization
Iron	Is necessary for collagen synthesis; enhances bactericidal action of leukocytes
Copper	Promotes formation of a stable collagen tissue
Magnesium	Is important for protein synthesis

lenged when he or she experience periods of physiologic anorexia, marked by swings from ravenous hunger to refusing all food offered. Young children especially can demonstrate a degree of stubbornness regarding which foods they will eat. The toddler is visually stimulated by food, selecting those that look the most pleasing and are familiar. Creating a balanced diet to promote healing of the skin may be difficult.

Metabolic and congenital disorders can make the challenge of meeting energy requirements difficult. In a severely debilitated child, wound healing is often compromised, because the nutrients crucial to the healing process are not available for metabolic purposes. For example, if albumin levels are below normal, protein depletion and edema impair wound healing. Parenteral protein and nutrients may be needed if the child is unable to ingest and digest foods taken orally.

Nutritional management may also be of concern to the child who has to avoid certain foods that cause a localized or systemic skin reaction. In these cases, consultation with a nutritional specialist is imperative. The specialist can assist the family in identifying all of the foods that may contain the allergic substance. In addition, a dietary plan must be established that ensures that, even though certain foods are avoided, a well-balanced diet is maintained. (See Chapter 5 for information on the nutritional needs of healthy children.)

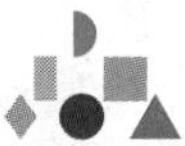

Alterations in Skin Integrity

Neonatal Skin Lesions

Skin lesions unique to neonates may be congenital or acquired. Acquired skin disorders include transient skin rashes, infestations, and infections. Acquired lesions usually have a short, benign course, although some neonates may be critically ill if there is overwhelming involvement of other body systems.

Congenital abnormalities include hemangiomas, vascular malformations, and disorders of pigmentation. Congenital lesions may pose specific problems because of their location on the body, their relation to other associated developmental defects, and their disfiguring appearance.

This section reviews the congenital lesions and common transient rashes found in the newborn population. Infestations and infections such as scabies, candidiasis, herpes simplex, and impetigo are discussed in subsequent paragraphs and are not unique to newborns.

Vascular Birthmarks and Pigment Abnormalities. Vascular birthmarks occur in 35% to 50% of newborn infants (Esterly, 1996). Affecting vascular or epidermal tissue, birthmarks can vary in the degree to which they cause more serious physical problems. Vascular lesions in infants and children are broadly classified as hemangiomas and vascular malformations (Table 25–10).

Hemangiomas are benign tumors of vascular epithelium characterized by a period of rapid growth followed by gradual disappearance of the lesions. Vascular malformations are developmental anomalies of blood and/or lymphatic vessel formation. These lesions do not have a rapid growth phase, rather they grow proportionally with the child and do not fade or disappear over time (Esterly, 1996). Pigment abnormalities occur as a result of underproduction or overproduction of melanin. Hypopigmentation, as is seen in albinism, or hyperpigmentation, as is seen in café au lait spots and Mongolian spots, may be seen as localized or generalized skin changes and may be congenital or acquired.

Vascular birthmarks and pigmentary disorders may range from relatively minor conditions, causing little if any disfigurement and pathologic consequences, to severe and potentially life-threatening conditions with visible skin alterations. The child's self-concept and development of body image may be negatively impacted based on how parents and others respond to the child's condition and how the child perceives they are valued by others (Dieterich-Miller, Cohen, & Liggett, 1992). Many of the conditions may regress spontaneously over time. Several treatment measures are available to help remove the lesion and cope with associated complications such as visual impairment and pulmonary obstruction. Response to therapy is slow. Parents may need assistance in learning how to deal with the uncomplimentary comments made by others and with strategies to build their child's self esteem.

Hemangiomas

Hemangiomas occur in approximately 10% to 12% of infants and children and in up to 30% of premature infants born before 30 weeks' gestation or who have birth weights less than 1500 g (Silverman, 1991). Only 20% of hemangiomas are present at birth; the remaining 80% arise at age 2 to 4 weeks (Weston, Lane, & Morelli, 1996). There are three major types of presentation: superficial, mixed, and deep (see Table 25–10). The superficial hemangiomas are bright-red papular lesions, often called strawberry hemangioma (Fig. 25–4). Blue nodular lesions characterize the deep (cavernous) hemangiomas. Most hemangiomas contain both a superficial and a deep component and are labeled as mixed hemangiomas.

Hemangiomas undergo a rapid growth phase at age 4 to 8 weeks. This growth phase continues for up to 10 months. After the rapid growth phase, the lesion grows more slowly, approximating the general growth of the child. The growth phase is followed by spontaneous

Table 25–10
Characteristics of Hemangiomas and Vascular Malformations

	Hemangiomas	Vascular Malformations
Types	Superficial (capillary or strawberry hemangioma) Mixed (capillary-cavernous) Deep (cavernous)	Capillary (port wine stain) Telangiectatic (salmon patch) Hypertrophic capillary (angiokeratoma) Venous Arteriovenous Lymphatic Cutis marmorata telangiectatica Mixed
Etiology	Tumor of endothelial cells	Developmental anomaly
Growth	Rapid growth phase lasts several months (up to age 1), followed by spontaneous regression by ages 6 to 9. Lesions usually do not more than double in size.	Slow, stable growth as child grows
Incidence	Female predominance 3 : 1	Male : female 1 : 1
Presence at birth	Only 20% of lesions are seen at birth as blanched or erythematous macule; most appear at about 1 month of age.	Always present at birth, but may not be entirely evident
Clinical presentation	Lesion has a well-demarcated, hypopigmented flat area. Small telangiectatic vessels may course across the lesion. Color may be erythematous or white. During involution, lesion becomes pale centrally with lacy gray regions within the lesion.	Flat, cutaneous vascular lesion, possibly with a subcutaneous component
Associated complications and syndromes	Obstruction of vision Obstruction of respiration Thrombocytopenia Disseminated intravascular coagulation Infection Congestive heart failure Kasabach-Merritt syndrome Diffuse neonatal hemangiomatosis Maffucci's syndrome Gorham syndrome Blue rubber bleb nevus syndrome Bannayan-Riley-Ruvalcaba syndrome	Glaucoma Sturge-Weber syndrome Beckwith-Wiedemann syndrome Klippel-Trenaunay syndrome Parkes-Weber syndrome Cobb syndrome
Treatment	Observation (most regress spontaneously) Corticosteroids (for visual or respiratory obstruction) Interferon-α Surgical resection Embolization (for arteriovenous complications) Vascular-specific pulsed dye laser therapy	Observation Cosmetics Tattooing (with flesh-colored insoluble pigments) Vascular-specific pulsed dye laser therapy

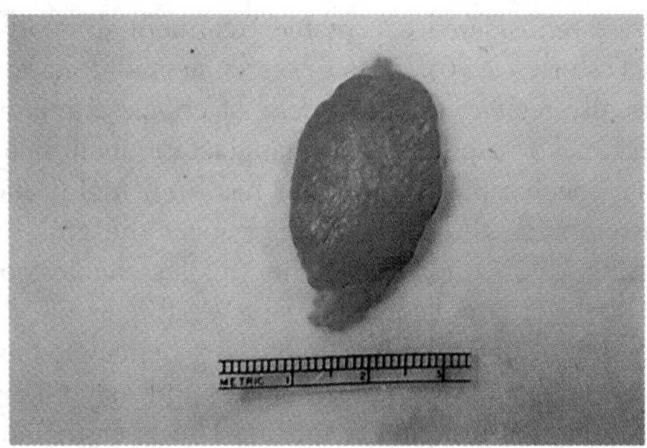

Figure 25–4
Strawberry hemangioma. (Lookingbill, D. P., & Marks, J. G. [1993]. *Principles of dermatology* [2nd ed., p. 102]. Philadelphia: W. B. Saunders.)

regression of the hemangioma, which begins in the second year of life and continues for several more years. By age 5 years, 50% of hemangiomas reach maximal regression and, by age 10, 90% have completed their regression phase (Silverman, 1991). The site of the lesion does not return to "normal skin"; rather, hypopigmentation, telangiectasia, and scarring may be present.

Most hemangiomas have a benign course. However, certain types, particularly deep hemangiomas, can cause airway obstruction, visual disturbance, or cardiac problems, depending on their location (e.g., subglottic, periorbital). Additionally, during the rapid growth phase, ulceration and subsequent infection are common complications.

Alert: *Platelet trapping with consumption coagulopathy can also occur during the rapid growth phase. Laboratory evaluation of the blood reveals a decreased platelet count and abnormal blood clotting. Although the condition is rare, it is a medical emergency (Silverman, 1991).*

Interdisciplinary Interventions

In most cases, hemangiomas require no treatment. The child is observed for complications and parents are instructed as to the natural course of the lesion. If the hemangioma interferes with vital function, such as obstruction of vision or the airway, then the treatment of choice is corticosteroids to reduce capillary cell division in the lesion (Fitzpatrick, Eisen, Wolff, Freedberg, & Austen, 1993). A combination of long-acting and rapid-acting steroids is given orally or injected directly into the lesion (intralesional) (Esterly, 1992). Recently, interferon-alpha-2a has been used to treat hemangiomas that are unresponsive to corticosteroid therapy. Fever is a common side effect of this medication.

Other treatment modalities include the administration of heparin and fresh-frozen plasma if needed to control bleeding in children experiencing coagulation abnormalities. Vascular-specific pulsed dye laser is very effective for the treatment of ulcerated hemangiomas. This type of therapy should be considered for facial and diaper area hemangiomas to reduce the risk of ulceration and secondary infection and scarring. The therapy is fast and has minimal side effects. The laser therapy is painful and few children tolerate the procedure well without anesthesia.

To manage the pain, local, regional, and topical anesthesia, general anesthesia, hypnosis, and distraction techniques have been used. Recently, the use of EMLA cream, a topical anesthetic, has been used successfully to decrease the pain associated with the procedure (Esterly, 1996).

Some families worry that laser therapy is "radioactive" and that treatment of hemangiomas is long term. The nurse can correct these misconceptions and provide counseling by allowing parents and the child to verbalize any feelings of anger, frustration, and sadness over the child's altered body image and the treatment that may be necessary.

Vascular Malformations

Vascular malformations differ from hemangiomas in that they are always present at birth and they do not experience a rapid growth phase. Rather, the lesion grows proportionally to the child's physical growth. Several types of vascular malformations exist; most common are the capillary malformations salmon patch and port wine stain.

Salmon patch occurs in more than 30% to 44% of neonates (Silverman, 1991). This flat, pink lesion is commonly found on the nape of the neck (stork bite), glabella, or eyelids (angel's kiss) (Fig. 25–5). Salmon patch lesions that appear on the face generally clear by age 1 to 2 years.

Port wine stains (nervus flammeus) occur in less than 1% of infants (Fitzpatrick et al., 1993). These dark-red lesions may cover large areas of the skin (Fig. 25–6). They occur most commonly on the face, followed by the extremities. As the malformation matures, it deepens in color and nodules and blebs develop. Overgrowth into underlying soft tissue and bone is possible. A more serious potential complication is Sturge-Weber syndrome, characterized by central nervous system abnormalities such as seizures, mental retardation, and hemiplegia, and ophthalmologic complications such as glaucoma. This condition occurs in approximately 8% of persons who have large facial port wine stains.

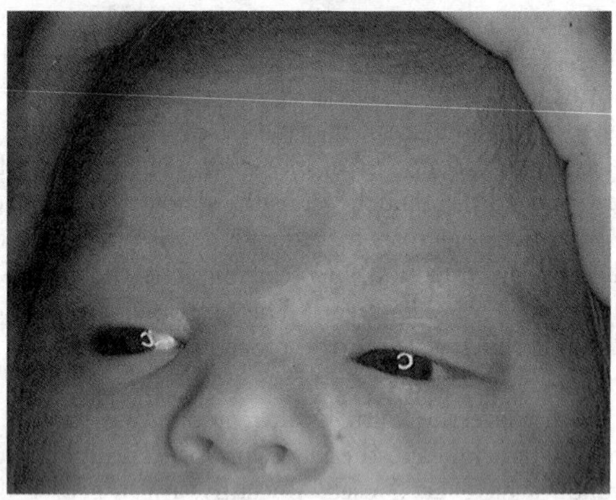

Figure 25–5
Salmon patch. (From Jarvis, C. [1996]. *Physical examination and health assessment* [2nd ed., p. 238]. Philadelphia: W. B. Saunders. Reprinted with permission.)

Interdisciplinary Interventions

Children with vascular malformations must be observed carefully for neurologic and ophthalmologic complications. In some cases, no treatment is required if the lesion is not in a prominent location and if complications are not present. Cosmetic camouflage can be used to cover the lesion. Cosmetics can be purchased that are water resistant and provide some degree of protection against the sun. Tattooing with flesh-colored insoluble pigments has also been a treatment option, although it is no longer considered acceptable treatment for port wine stains (Esterly, 1996). Because vascular malformations do not usually regress, the treatment of choice is removal of the lesion. For capillary and telangiectatic malformations, vascular-specific pulsed dye laser has been highly successful in removing the lesion. The younger the child at the beginning of treatment and the smaller the lesion, the more likely is complete removal (Weston et al., 1996). Unlike the response of treatment for hemangiomas, the response to treatment is much slower and may take up to 1 to 3 years for complete removal. The laser therapy has minimal side effects, although the treatment is painful. The use of EMLA cream, a topical anesthetic, has been successful in reducing pain associated with the procedure.

Figure 25–6
Port wine stain. (From Jarvis, C. [1996]. *Physical examination and health assessment* [2nd ed., p. 253]. Philadelphia: W. B. Saunders. Reprinted with permission.)

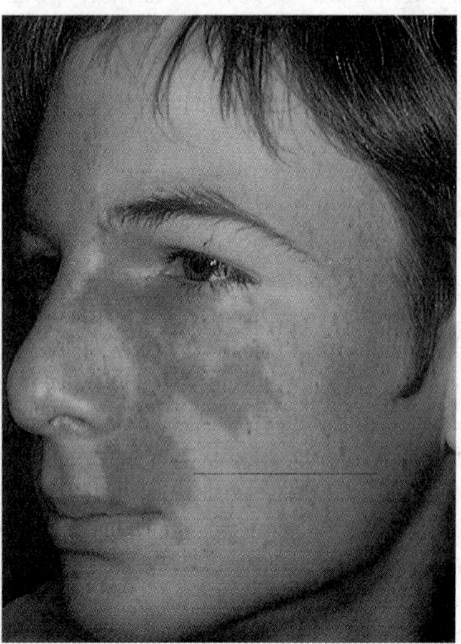

Pigment Abnormalities

The amount and distribution of melanin in the epidermis accounts for the color of a person's skin. Excessive melanin production results in hyperpigmentation; insufficient melanin production results in hypopigmentation. An alteration in melanin production generally cannot be treated. Other systemic clinical manifestations of the underlying condition may be treated if their sequelae are threatening to the well-being of the child.

Hyperpigmentation may be marked by the presence of Mongolian spots, café au lait spots, and freckles (Fig. 25–7). Mongolian spots are blue-black macules or

Figure 25–7
Mongolian spots are blue-black macules located on the lumbosacral area. Café au lait spots are light brown oval macules that may appear anywhere on the body.

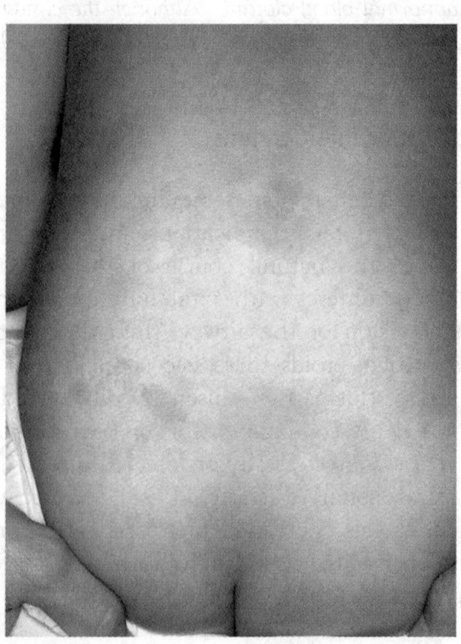

patches, poorly circumscribed lesions commonly located on the lumbosacral area. They are most common in Asian, black, and Hispanic infants. The spots are occasionally noted on the shoulders and back and may extend over the buttocks and lower extremities. Mongolian spots generally fade by age 2 to 3 years, although some traces of the lesions may persist into adulthood.

Café au lait spots are well circumscribed, light brown oval macules that may appear anywhere on the body. On black skin, the color of the spots may appear more dark brown. Black infants are more likely to have café au lait spots than white infants. The spots persist through childhood and may increase in number. Café au lait spots are a feature of several systemic disorders such as polyostotic fibrous dysplasia (large, usually solitary spot) and neurofibromatosis (greater than five spots). Familial café au lait is a rare, autosomal dominant pigmentary disorder associated with neurofibromatosis type 1 (Arnsmeier, Riccardi, & Paller, 1994).

Hypopigmentation occurs in newborns with phenylketonuria. These newborns have blond hair, blue eyes, and light-colored skin. The hypopigmentation is caused by the tight binding of the amino acid phenylalanine to the receptor sites of tyrosinase, which then does not allow the enzyme to oxidize phenylalanine to melanin (Weston et al., 1996).

Pigment loss is also a significant feature of *albinism*, a group of 14 syndromes characterized by congenital pigment loss in the skin, hair, iris, and retina. Most of these conditions have an autosomal recessive inheritance pattern. Nystagmus, strabismus, photophobia, decreased visual acuity, and presence of red reflex are common ocular findings. Blindness and skin cancer may occur in severe forms of albinism.

Neonatal Acne

Acne that is similar in distribution and appearance to adolescent acne develops in approximately 30% of all newborns. The acne begins at age 3 to 4 weeks, with eruptions extending until age 4 to 6 months. Small red bumps (papules and pustules) appear on the face, trunk, and proximal upper extremities. The face may have whiteheads that are 1 to 3 mm in diameter and that are skin colored to whitish colored (Johr & Schachner, 1997). The lesions are a result of blocked hair follicle (follicular comedones). Transfer of maternal androgens (hormones) to the fetus immediately before birth is believed to be the cause.

No treatment is usually required because the condition is self-limiting. Anti-acne medications are not recommended because the infant is more highly susceptible to the irritant effects of these topical agents. Parents are cautioned not to apply baby oil or other ointments to the skin as a curative measure. It is unknown what, if any, relationship exists between severe neonatal acne and severe adolescent acne later in the child's life.

Milia

Milia are multiple, white or yellow, 1- to 2-mm papules appearing on the infant's cheeks, nose, chin, forehead, and occasionally the upper trunks, and limbs. They can also appear on the midline of the palate where they are called *Epstein pearls*. These superficial epidermal cysts are caused by the blockage of the pilosebaceous glands by keratin and sebaceous materials. Although milia that appear on the face and limbs look like pimples, they are not infected.

▽ **Alert:** *If blisters or pimples appear on the infant's skin, they should be examined immediately; the cause may be herpes simplex.*

Milia usually spontaneously disappear at age 1 to 2 months. Parents should be advised not to apply cream or lotion to the lesion sites, and not to squeeze or pick the lesions with a sharp instrument.

Drooling Rash

It is not uncommon for a transient rash to develop on the chin or cheeks of an infant. The rash is similar to that seen in other cases of contact dermatitis in that erythema is noted, with edema and vesicles likely to develop. Two factors may cause the dermatologic changes. The first may be contact of the child's delicate skin with his or her own vomitus. The young infant is prone to wet burps, in which the food and the acid from the stomach contents may erupt and drool down the chin or, during sleep, may be absorbed into bed linen, resting against the cheeks. Some of this contact between the fluid and the skin may be averted by placing an absorbent diaper under the infant's face during naps and by rinsing the infant's face after feedings.

A drooling rash can also be caused by contact between the infant's cheek and the mother's breast during nursing, producing a rash. Changing the infant's position frequently and placing a cool washcloth on the infant's cheek will help to decrease the incidence of this rash.

Erythema Toxicum Neonatorum

Erythema toxicum neonatorum (ETN), or neonatal erythema, is a benign condition of the neonatal period that is self-limited in nature. It affects 20% to 60% of term neonates weighing more than 2500 g. The condition is rare in premature neonates. ETN occurs worldwide with no apparent gender, ethnic, racial, or seasonal predisposition (Johr & Shachner, 1997; Schwartz & Janniger, 1996).

Etiology

Most cases of ETN occur within 24 to 72 hours after birth, although lesions can erupt any time in the first 2 weeks of life. The cause of ETN is unknown. Medications and the mode of feeding and skin care do not correlate with the emergence of the condition. Several theories have been suggested to explain the cause of this condition. One study found a higher incidence of ETN in neonates from families with a history of atopy. It has also been suggested that the condition is an allergic manifestation of the "toxins of pregnancy" from mother to fetus, a reaction to colostrum, or perhaps an acute graft versus host reaction induced by maternal lymphocytes (Schwartz & Janniger, 1996).

Assessment

Within a the first few days after birth, ETN manifests as combinations of erythematous macules, papules with a central vesicle, or pustules, ranging in size from a few millimeters to several centimeters, found anywhere on the body except the soles of the feet and the palms of the hands (Fig. 25–8). Common locations include the face, trunk, buttocks, and extremities. Lesions are discrete but can become confluent. Lesions that begin as macules often turn into pustules. Individual lesions may appear for a few days then disappear. The rash usually remits within 1 week, although persistence beyond this period has been seen in some cases. In up to 11% of the cases, recurrences may occur within 5 to 11 days after the initial eruption. The secondary eruption is not as extensive as the original rash (Schwartz & Janniger, 1996).

Diagnostic Tests. Diagnosis of ETN depends on microscopic examination of the lesions. In the diagnostic test of choice, scrapings of pustules are stained with Wright's solution. If ETN is present, large numbers of eosinophils are detected. Also, microscopic examination of macules shows an accumulation of eosinophils in the dermis. However, neutrophils are rarely present. Cultures of lesions are sterile. A crucial factor differentiating ETN from other skin disorders is that, aside from eruption of the lesions, the neonate displays no other systemic involvement such as fever, lethargy, or poor feeding.

Figure 25–8
Erythema toxicum neonatorum. (From Jarvis, C. [1996]. *Physical examination and health assessment* [2nd ed., p. 236]. Philadelphia: W. B. Saunders. Reprinted with permission.)

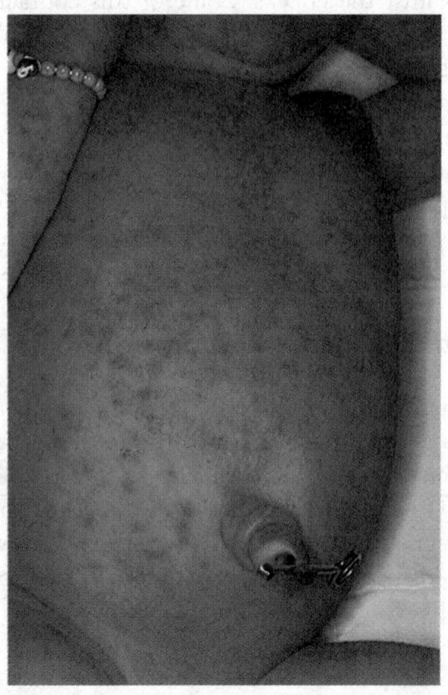

Interdisciplinary Interventions

Treatment of ETN is usually unnecessary, and lesions usually fade within 1 week. The nurse shares responsibility in monitoring the affected neonate to ensure that the rash fades within 1 week. The persistence of lesions beyond this period could indicate the presence of another skin disorder such as transient neonatal pustular melanosis, herpes simplex virus, *Staphylococcus aureus* infections, or candidiasis.

Inflammatory Skin Disorders

Dermatitis is a general term for skin conditions that present with erythema or with erythema accompanied by scaling, vesicles, or crusting. Four common types of dermatitis are discussed: diaper, contact, atopic, and seborrheic. Each type involves different causes, characteristics, and treatment plans.

Diaper Dermatitis

Diaper dermatitis, or "diaper rash," is one of the most common dermatoses of infancy. Diaper dermatitis is a type of irritant contact dermatitis. Because of its prevalence and specificity of interventions, the condition is discussed separately from contact dermatitis.

Etiology and Incidence

The exact incidence of diaper dermatitis is difficult to specify. It is a rare child who has not had at least one episode of "diaper rash" in infancy, especially during a bout of gastroenteritis. The incidence generally appears to be equal between the sexes, peaking at age 6 to 9 months because of the change in dietary intake. The cause of diaper dermatitis is multifactorial (Fig. 25–9).

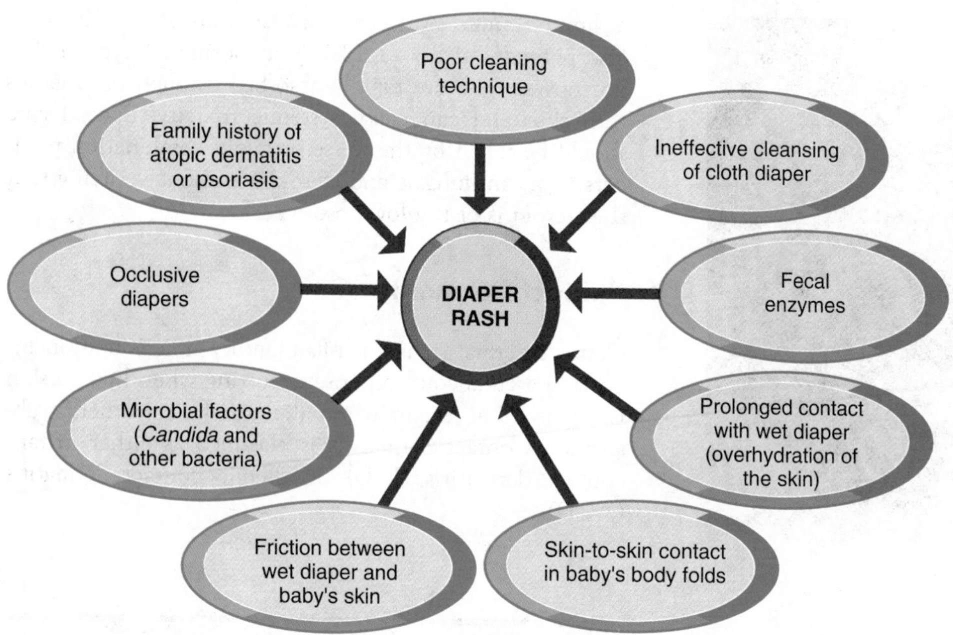

Figure 25–9
Causes of diaper dermatitis (diaper rash).

Pathophysiology

Prolonged contact with an irritant, most commonly, feces, urine, soaps, detergents, ointments, or friction, is a major contributing factor in diaper dermatitis. However, an irritant alone does not cause the problem; rather, diaper dermatitis results from a combination of factors generated by the presence of the diaper. Urinary ammonia once was believed to be the primary etiologic factor for diaper dermatitis, but recent research has indicated that urine itself is not detrimental. It was found that urine and fecal enzymes interact to liberate ammonia and increase pH. Excessive alkalinity makes fecal protease and lipase even more irritating to the infant's skin, contributing to diaper dermatitis.

Wet skin also plays a role in the pathogenesis of diaper dermatitis. Wet skin is more easily abraded and more permeable, and it has an increased microbial count. This situation can be exacerbated by alkaline soaps used to clean cloth diapers. The wet diaper also increases friction with the wet skin. The average newborn urinates approximately 20 times in one day, greatly increasing the likelihood of creating an environment in which wet skin rubs against a wet diaper.

Irritated, cut, or chapped skin is a contributing factor to diaper dermatitis. Skin breaks that breach the stratum corneum are even more susceptible to the combination of previously mentioned deleterious factors. When lesions or open wounds become infected, candidiasis may be a major culprit. *Candida albicans* can be cultured or recovered from the skin of 40% to 75% of infants with diaper dermatitis. It is rarely found in infants with healthy, unbroken skin.

Assessment

The affected skin over the diaper area can take various configurations. In general, it is bright red, swollen, and sharply marginated; however, it may also have a glazed and wrinkled appearance (Fig. 25–10). There may be papular-vesicular or bullous lesions, fissures, and erosions. If candidiasis develops, the rash consists of erythematous papular eruptions with satellite lesions. Diaper dermatitis rarely occurs in groin creases.

An infant with diaper dermatitis acts fussy and exhibits trouble sleeping and, in severe cases, even has difficulty with eating. Diaper changes can be extremely painful, especially if commercial diaper wipes are used for cleansing the genital area. Commercial wipes may contain alcohol and allergenic substances that may further irritate the child's skin. If dealt with promptly, the condition is usually self-limiting. However, severe diaper dermatitis may be one sign of poor care at home or in the daycare setting, indicating the possible need for further assessment and for intervention to improve the caregiver's child care practices.

Interdisciplinary Interventions

Successful management of diaper dermatitis requires identification and management of the causative agents. Interventions associated with diaper dermatitis focus on two major components: treatment and prevention. Treatment strategies involve differentiating irritant dermatitis versus candidiasis or staphylococcal infections. For mild irritant dermatitis, cleansing the soiled diaper area with a mild

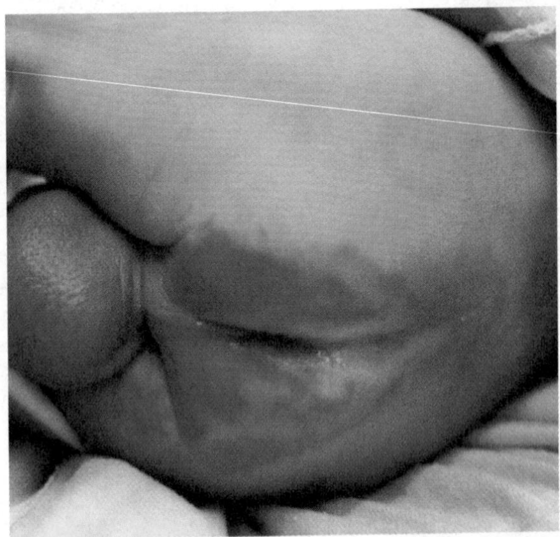

Figure 25–10
Diaper dermatitis.

cleanser and protecting the skin with a barrier cream (e.g., petrolatum, zinc oxide) is sufficient (Chart 25–12).

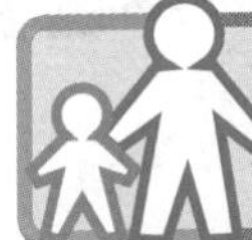

caREminder: *If the skin underlying the cream is clean, the cream does not have to be completely removed with each diaper change; rather, lightly wiping the area with a washcloth and mild cleanser is sufficient. The ointment prevents maceration and protects the skin from urine and feces.*

Wrapping the diaper loosely also helps clear up the lesions. Plastic pants should not be used. A waterproof pad can be placed under the sleeping child wearing cloth diapers to protect underlying materials and surfaces. Home laundering of cloth diapers should be done with mild soap, without the use of either bleach or fabric softeners (liquid or sheets). The diapers should be rinsed at least twice, using vinegar (1 ounce per gallon of water) in the final rinse. If the child wears disposable diapers, holes should be torn in the plastic to decrease the humidity, and the plastic edges should be folded away from the infant's body. The child's primary caregiver should receive detailed instructions regarding treatment and prevention measures (TIP 25–1). Early recognition and prompt response to any redness noted in the diaper area may help to avoid diaper dermatitis.

Medical therapy is not usually required for diaper dermatitis, unless secondary infections develop. If candidiasis is suspected, a topical antifungal agent is prescribed, such as nystatin, clotrimazole (Lotrimin), ketoconazole (Nizoral), and miconazole (Micatin). When the diaper dermatitis is severe, topical hydrocortisone ointment or other low-dose topical steroid can be used for a limited time. All prescribed steroids should be of a low potency (0.5% to 1%), nonfluorinated type. High-potency steroids are rapidly absorbed through the infant's thin skin and can cause systemic toxicity. Special care should be taken by the nurse to avoid combination products (e.g., antifungals and steroids) without verifying that the steroid is of the low-dose type.

Contact Dermatitis

Contact dermatitis is an inflammatory skin condition involving a cutaneous response occurring when human skin is exposed to certain external natural or synthetic substances. Contact dermatitis is classified as either irritant contact dermatitis (ICD) or allergic contact dermatitis (ACD).

Chart 25–12
Developmental Considerations

The Hazards of Baby Powder

Key Concepts

- Use of baby powders containing "talc" or known as "talcum powder" can cause accidental aspiration, pneumonia, and death.
- Aspiration is predominantly caused when the baby receives a "puff of smoke" when the powder is shaken from the container directly onto the baby's skin.

Guidelines

- Babies generally *do not* need any powders on their diaper area.
- If the parent wants to use a powder, cornstarch is an acceptable alternative to reduce friction in the diaper area.
- If the parent still desires to use talcum powder, *it should be applied by shaking it on the parent's hands first, as far away from the baby's head as possible.*
- All talcum powder containers should be closed and in a safe place, away from curious infants and toddlers.
- Lotions or creams (not alcohol-based products) should be substituted for powder to reduce diaper rash or other skin irritations.
- The parent should not self-administer talcum powder in an infant's or toddler's presence.
- Use of baby powder should be discouraged by all individuals with asthma or reactive airway disease.

TIP 25-1 A Teaching Intervention Plan for the Child with Diaper Dermatitis

Nursing Diagnoses and Family Outcomes

- Impaired skin integrity related to irritation of the diaper area
  Outcomes:
  Child regains skin integrity.
  Child exhibits no further evidence of skin breakdown.
- Knowledge deficit: prevention and treatment of rash
  Outcomes:
  Parents demonstrate skin care techniques to promote healing and prevent further skin breakdown.
  Parents verbalize measures to prevent diaper dermatitis.

Instructional Interventions

Medications

- If *candidal infection is present*—Topical anticandidal agent (Nystatin, Lotrimin, Micatin, Nizoral) is applied to diaper area.
- *If severe inflammation is present*—Apply a topical low-potency, nonfluorinated 1% hydrocortisone cream to rash site for 7 to 10 days.
- Children with recurrent diarrhea may be prescribed an oral anticandidal agent (Nystatin) to sterilize the gastrointestinal (GI) tract and prevent systemic infection.

Diaper Changes

- Change diaper frequently.
- Check diaper every 1 to 2 hours for wetness or soiling, and change immediately.
- Use superabsorbent diapers if affordable.
- With each wet diaper change, wipe the skin gently with a plain water or a diaper wipe (nonallergenic, nonscented).
- With each soiled diaper:
  Wash the skin with water and a gentle, pH-neutral soap. Rinse well.
  Pay particular attention to cleaning areas of skin folds.
- Pat the baby's bottom dry—*do not use a hair dryer to dry.*
- Avoid air-tight occlusive diapers or diaper covers.
  Do not use plastic pants.
  Fasten the disposable diaper loosely.
  Brand-name disposable diapers can be altered to breathe better by snipping the elastic bands around the legs in a few places, and cutting a few slits in the plastic diaper cover.
- Leave the baby's bottom exposed to air as much as possible:
  Put a towel or diaper open under the baby during nap time.
  Let the toddler be "diaper-free" for periods of time.

Creams, Lotions, and Powders

- Do not use on most babies.
- Do not use talcum powder
- Apply a simple barrier cream (such as zinc oxide paste) to the noninfected diaper rash.
  Do not remove the paste with every diaper change as long as a layer of paste remains on the skin, and the skin underneath is clean.
  If the paste must be removed, use minimal amount of oil.
- Cornstarch can be applied on areas in which friction might occur. When wet, however, the cornstarch can clump and retain moisture on the skin. There is some controversy regarding cornstarch. Some sources recommend not using it because microorganisms metabolize the cornstarch.

TIP continued on following page

TIP 25–1 A Teaching Intervention Plan for the Child with Diaper Dermatitis *Continued*

Nutrition

If the child has diarrhea, the child should be evaluated for dehydration. Dietary restrictions and hydration measures may be needed to stop the diarrhea and prevent dehydration.

Nighttime Care

- Apply creams liberally on diaper area before bedtime.
- Avoid plastic pants at night.
- Until rash improves, awaken the child at least once a night to change the diaper.

Cloth Diapers

- Cloth diapers should always be washed in hot water with a mild soap and double rinsed. Wash, rinse, let the diaper soak in water with ammonia added for a half hour, then rinse again.
- Use fabric softener in wash of cloth diapers to help prevent skin friction and chafing. Be aware that some fabric softeners make fabrics nonabsorbent, and thus should not be used.

Prevention

- After the child's bath, let child be "diaper free" for a period of time.
- Change diapers frequently. *Never leave a child in a soiled diaper.*
- Wash cloth diapers appropriately (see above).

Contact Health Care Provider if

- Rash develops big blisters (more than 1 inch across), open sores, or boils.
- Rash does not look better in 3 days.
- Rash becomes solid and bright red.
- Rash becomes raw and bleeds.
- The child is male and circumcised, and a sore or scab develops at the end of the penis.
- Rash causes enough pain to disrupt sleep.
- Child develops temperature over 100°F.

Etiology and Incidence

In older children and adults, ICD most commonly results from exposure to occupational or recreational irritants such as manufacturing processes, insecticides, or hobby supplies. In infants and toddlers, ICD is most commonly associated with saliva that causes a drooling rash or contact with abrasive soap and irritating detergents (Chart 25–13).

ACD results from a T-cell–mediated hypersensitivity reaction. The allergic reaction is commonly caused by exposure to plants (e.g., poison ivy, sumac, oak), nickel (in jewelry), rubber (latex) in shoes, animal fur, feathers, vegetables oils, synthetic fabrics, cosmetics, and perfumes or scented soaps that contain the offending allergen. Although uncommon, ACD can occur in neonates, because sensitization to an allergen and dermatitis can occur in as few as 10 days (Johr & Schachner, 1997). Common offending agents in this age group include fragrances in soaps or body lotions, rubber in the elastic of diaper products, and topical medications. Pierced earrings and metal pajama snaps may also be sources of metal allergy. The incidence of ACD is greatly increased after age 8 years (Wilkowska, Grubska-Suchanek, Karwacka, & Szarmach, 1996). Children at high risk for ACD reactions include those with a personal or family history of hay fever, AD (eczema), and asthma. Other risk factors include preexisting skin diseases, poor personal hygiene, and very dry-hot or dry-cold environmental conditions.

Pathophysiology

In ICD, the irritating substance causes a nonspecific inflammatory reaction in the skin. Individual skin strength,

Chart 25–13

Common Causes of Contact Dermatitis

Irritant Contact Dermatitis

Saliva
Citrus juices
Bubble bath
Detergents
Abrasive materials
Strong soaps
Occlusive shoes
Hobby supplies
Insecticides
Manufacturing agents

Allergic Contact Dermatitis

Poison oak, poison ivy, and poison sumac
Nickel (jewelry, buckles, clothing snaps)
Potassium dichromate (shoes, tanning agent)
Neomycin
Thimerosal, formaldehyde, and Quaternium 15 (preservatives and topical agents)
Balsam of Peru (fragrance)
Wood alcohol (lanolin)
Colophony (rosin from wood)

concentration (dose) of the offending substance, and length of contact all contribute to the severity of reaction. Prolonged or repeated exposure to an irritating substance results in erythema and the potential for skin breakdown and lesions. A detailed health history, evaluation of the involved sites, and the child's age all can provide clues as to the nature of irritating substance.

ACD is caused by an allergen that penetrates the epidermis from the skin surface. An interaction between the T-lymphocyte component of the cellular immune system is mediated by antigen-presenting epidermal cells (Langerhans cells) (Hogan & Weston, 1993; Lane & Darmstadt, 1996). When the antigen penetrates the skin, it is conjugated with a cutaneous protein and transported to the regional lymph nodes by Langerhans cells. A primary immunologic response occurs locally in the nodes as the sensitized T cells circulate throughout the body. This process is called the sensitization phase. The duration of this phase depends on the potency of the allergen. For example, the oil, urushiol, the offending agent in poison ivy, penetrates the epidermis, bonds with the dermis, and initiates the immune response usually after only one exposure. (Poison oak, poison ivy, and sumac are discussed in more detail in subsequent paragraphs of this chapter.)

Once sensitization occurs, children who are exposed to repeated contact by the same antigen experience an inflammatory reaction (ACD) within 8 to 24 hours (Hogan & Weston, 1993; Lane & Darmstadt, 1996). Children can remain sensitized to a certain allergen for many years.

Prognosis. The prognosis for contact dermatitis is very good if the offending substance is identified and exposure to the substance is prohibited. If the offending agent is removed, the skin's recuperative powers produce healing without treatment within 1 to 2 weeks. In more severe cases of ACD, the untreated dermatitis persists for 3 to 4 weeks. Any time a child has a break in the skin, there is risk for secondary infections. Therefore, prompt attention to the dermatitis and measures to stop exposure to offending agents should be instituted to prevent further alterations in skin integrity.

Assessment

Nurses are often the first to identify contact dermatitis during the history-taking process or physical examination. For example, skin breakdown and irritation in the vicinity of jewelry, clothing, or undergarments suggests local contact reactions. If more generalized skin involvement is noted, this is often due to spread of the offending allergen during a bubble bath or using bar soap that has not been well rinsed after each use.

Contact dermatitis usually occurs in exposed skin areas: the face, neck, hands, forearms, legs, and feet. A characteristic inflamed response varies from erythema to large bullae on a reddened base and edema. The lesions may be well demarcated, exactly resembling the shape and size of the offending substance (e.g., red marks on the abdomen the size and shape of pajama snaps). Itching is intense and constant.

Diagnosis of contact dermatitis depends heavily on patch testing and on a thorough history. During patch testing, the suspected trigger agent is applied to the skin and occluded by hypoallergenic tape. The site is evaluated for a reaction 48 to 72 hours later, using standardized results for interpretation. Children should avoid bathing and strenuous activity while the patches are in place. In addition to testing for the suspected allergen, the child undergoes testing with a standardized tested group of allergens that have been recognized by several medical associations as the most frequent causes of ACD (Hogan & Weston, 1993). The classic positive patch test consists of erythema, edema, and small vesicles that do not extend beyond the border of the patch. Results must be examined within the context of the history and of the physical examination. A positive test does not necessarily mean that the identified allergen is responsible for the child's current dermatitis, although it does indicate that the child has a sensitivity to a particular allergen. Skin cultures and biopsy may be used to rule out herpes simplex virus and staphylococcal infections.

Interdisciplinary Interventions

Untreated ACD slowly resolves over a 3- to 4-week period if contact with the allergen is avoided. Treatment for the itching and edema may include the use of Aveeno baths, calamine lotion, or Burow solution compresses. Mild (0.5% to 1%) to medium potency (0.1% to 0.2%) topical glucocorticoid may relieve inflammation and hasten the healing process. Oral corticosteroids may be prescribed for more severe reactions. Benadryl may be ordered to decrease itching. If infected lesions are present, antibiotic therapy is usually initiated.

Community Care

Nurses also have the responsibility of teaching children and parents about prevention of contact dermatitis. The initial treatment consists of the removal of the irritating and allergic substance from the home and school environment. Second, protective clothing minimizes exposure to irritants, especially with plant allergies and caustic materials. When a contact allergen is confirmed by patch testing, all products or substances containing that allergen should be avoided. Lists of products that contain the offending agents are usually available from a dermatologist and the family should be instructed regarding how to read product labels to ensure that the allergen is not present.

Children and families should be taught proper skin hygiene and that the use of mild antibacterial soaps and moisturizers can help to prevent painful scaling and cracking of the skin which can lead to the eruption of a secondary infection such as impetigo. The presence of a skin allergy may necessitate some restrictions of the child's activities to prevent contact with the offending agent. Young children may not understand or tolerate well the limitations on their activities. Parents can assist by providing enjoyable play alternatives for the child and by reinforcing the cause and effect relationship between the child's exposure to the irritant and the eruption of the skin rash.

Atopic Dermatitis

AD is a chronic, relapsing inflammation of the dermis and epidermis characterized by itching, edema, papules, erythema, excoriation, serous discharge, and crusting (Romeo, 1995). The term "atopic" refers to the fact that patients exhibit a heightened reaction to a variety of allergens. To the lay public the condition is commonly known as *eczema.* The term eczema describes the combination of erythema, scaling vesicles, and crusts. Eczema-like lesions occur in several skin diseases; hence, the term atopic dermatitis is used to refer to the condition described herein.

AD is categorized into three stages according to the child's age (Chart 25–14). The infantile stage begins at age 2 to 6 months and resolves in half of affected children between age 2 and 3 years. The childhood stage occurs at age 4 to 10 years and may represent a continuation of the infantile stage. The adolescent stage begins at age 11 to 12 years and may last into adulthood.

AD is a fairly common health problem. Research has indicated that as many as 20% of boys and 19% of girls have some form of atopy (Romeo, 1995). Males and females are equally affected, and AD is more common in industrialized cities and in white and Chinese populations (Su, Kemp, Varigos, & Nolan, 1997). AD is often inher-

Chart 25–14

Stages of Atopic Dermatitis

Infantile Stage

Age 2 to 6 months, resolving in half of children between ages 2 and 3 years

Characteristics

Pruritus
Erythema
Exudate and crusts
Common sites: cheeks, forehead, scalp, extensor surfaces of arms and legs
Diaper area not usually involved

Childhood Stage

Age 4 to 10 years or following on continuously from infancy stage

Characteristics

Less exudate than in previous stage
Dry, itchy patches of skin
Common sites: wrists, ankles, antecubital and popliteal spaces

Adolescent and Adult Stage

Age 10 years and older

Characteristics

Exudation caused by external irritation or secondary infection
Dry, itchy patches of skin
Common sites: flexor folds, face, neck, back, upper arms, and dorsal aspects of the hands, feet, fingers, and toes

ited, with an 80% chance of some atopy in a child if both parents are affected. Although AD is often seen with asthma, the two conditions are not inherited on the same gene pathways.

Etiology

Three theories have been proposed to describe the origin of AD: the inborn error of metabolism theory, the immunologic theory, and the psychosomatic theory. The first theory postulates that AD patients have a metabolic skin defect that causes excessive itching. The immunologic theory suggests that AD is just one component of the larger atopic pattern, because asthma develops in approximately 25% to 50% of affected children and allergic rhinitis develops in 30% (Su et al., 1997). The psychosomatic model holds that AD is caused by underlying stress and psychological dysfunctioning in the life of the child.

A number of factors exacerbate AD. These include sudden changes and extremes of temperature, irritating fabrics such as wool, excessive exercise that induces sweating, and direct contact with irritants such as detergents and perfumes.

Prognosis. Prognosis for this condition is optimistic. Spontaneous resolution of the condition occurs in 40% to 50% of affected children, especially in those children with milder cases (Romeo, 1995). Freedom from secondary complications depends on strict adherence to the treatment plan. In general, the exacerbations become less frequent after adolescence and most of these children can enjoy long periods of time in which they experience no symptoms.

Assessment

Diagnosis of AD depends on a review of history and dermatologic and behavioral findings. Most children have a family history of allergy (e.g., asthma, allergic rhinitis). AD distributions manifest differently, depending on age. The infantile form has lesions that are generalized on the trunk, scalp, cheeks, and extremities. The disorder spares the perioral and nasal areas. In childhood, the lesions occur in body creases such as the wrists, ankles, feet, and antecubital, flexural surfaces, and popliteal fossae. In the adolescent form, the face, feet, hands, flexural surfaces, and neck are affected.

The type of AD lesions also vary related to age. In the infantile form of the disorder, they include scaling, crusting, weeping, erythema, vesicles, papules, and oozing. In the childhood form, symmetric distribution of small erythematous papules or patches occurs along with lichenification (hardening of the skin) and hyperpigmentation. For adolescents, there is a pattern similar to the childhood form, except that dry, thick plaques are more common.

Other accompanying symptoms that produce the most distressing components of AD including intense itching, drying of the unaffected skin areas, restlessness, irritability, lymphadenopathy, and other signs of allergic response (such as a bluish discoloration under the eyes).

Many authorities believe that the intense itching and the resultant scratching are the main conditions that generate the lesions. Infants and young children scratch and rub their bodies against objects, generating more lesions. If scratching is controlled, the lesions heal. No laboratory tests are diagnostic for AD, although increased eosinophil counts and serum IgE are common findings.

Interdisciplinary Interventions

The major goals of therapy are to control itching, reduce inflammation, hydrate the skin, and prevent secondary infection (TIP 25–2). Medical treatment does not cure this condition, but effective palliation can be achieved. By carefully controlling or reducing the exacerbations, and by diligent management of inflammation and pruritus, the child or adolescent can have a normal lifestyle. Because the underlying cause is unknown, all therapy is symptomatic.

Controlling Itching. Itching, the most distressing symptom, is controlled through a variety of interventions such as topical cool compresses, colloid baths, and application of corticosteroid creams or ointments, or tar ointments. The nurse must ensure that the medical regimen is implemented and must teach caregivers to follow it meticulously. The child's nails must be kept short. During periods of intense itching, gloves and cotton stockings may have to be placed over the child's hands. Hand and elbow restraints are necessary to prevent generation of lesions and should not be removed during naps or sleep.

Items of clothing and bedding that increase itching should be removed. Parents should not use fabric softeners in the wash cycle and should double rinse the child's clothing to remove all detergent. Soaks and compresses must be applied as directed. Family members should schedule skin care activities at the best time of day for the child and for the family.

Children with AD have been noted to have disrupted sleep patterns and daytime behavioral difficulties that are associated with the lack of sleep (Dahl, Bernhisel-Broadbent, Scanlon-Holdford, Sampson, & Lupo, 1995). Treatments during the day must be timed to promote optimal rest periods. Regular sleep and awake schedules should be maintained. Caffeinated beverages should be avoided.

The use of antihistamines is not widely supported because the benefit to control itching is uncertain. The antihistamines cause drowsiness and may be used at night to reduce itching by promoting sleep. Recently, cyclosporine and interferon have been used successfully in

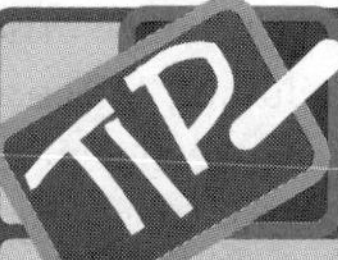

TIP 25–2 A Teaching Intervention Plan for the Child with Atopic Dermatitis

Nursing Diagnoses and Family Outcomes

- Impaired skin integrity related to chronic occurrence of dry skin, intense itching, erythema, and excoriation.
  Outcomes:
  Child exhibits improved skin integrity.
  Child/family demonstrate skin care regimen.
- Potential for infection related to presence of lesions, higher concentration of flora on atopic skin, and decreased integrity of skin barrier.
  Outcomes:
  Child/family demonstrate measures to prevent infection.
  Child/family identify signs and symptoms of skin infection.
  Child/family verbalize the actions to take if an infection is suspected or confirmed.
- Altered family processes related to child's discomfort and increased health care requirements.
  Outcomes:
  Child reports increased comfort.
  Child/family correlate precipitating factors with appropriate skin are regimen.
  Child/family verbalize confidence in their ability to manage the child's care.

Interventions

Treatment of the Child

Skin Care and General Hygiene

- Bathe child nightly for 15 to 20 minutes.
- Provide creative toys for water play, or encourage the older child to read a book while soaking.
- Do not use bath additives such as oatmeal or baking soda, bubble bath, soaps, or bath oils.
- For adolescents with mild symptoms, a daily shower may be sufficient.
- Pat, rather than rub, the skin dry.
- Follow bath with *immediate* application of occlusive emollient such as Eucerin or Lubriderm.
- Choose preparations with little artificial fragrance and chemical stabilizer additives that may cause further skin irritation.
- Wet wraps can be used on severely affected skin. Apply after soaking and after applying topical medications.
- For total body wrap, use wet pajamas, long underwear, or tube socks (for hands and feet). Layer dry clothing on top.
- Wet wraps of gauze or Kerlix with stockinette or surginet can be applied to smaller areas.
- Do not allow the wrap to dry.
- Chilling may occur if outer layer becomes wet.
- Use antibacterial soaps for hand washing.
- Keep child's nails clean and cut short.

Medications

Topical Steroids

- Medicine is used to control acute exacerbation.

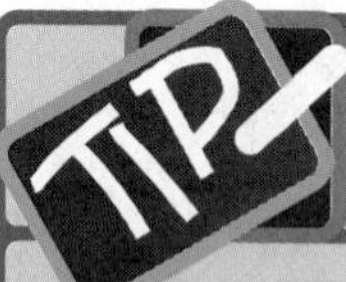

TIP 25–2 A Teaching Intervention Plan for the Child with Atopic Dermatitis *Continued*

- The potency of the medication is determined by the body area that it is applied to and the severity of the child's condition. In general, as low a level of potency as possible is used to achieve good effects.
- Side effects include thinning of the skin, hypopigmentation acne, secondary infection, and stretch marks.

Tar Preparations

- Preparations are used to control acute exacerbation; they have a slower inflammatory action than do topical steroids.
- Tar preparations should only be used when symptoms are mild.
- Tar preparations may cause burning and irritation if applied to skin areas with severe symptoms.

Antihistamines

- Medicine is used to reduce itching, primarily by causing drowsiness.
- Medicine may be taken at night to aid in comfort while sleeping.

Oral Antibiotics

- Medicine may be ordered if there is widespread skin breakdown or infection.

Nutrition

- Identify foods that exacerbate rash, and avoid these foods.
- Identify "hidden" ingredients in foods (e.g., eggs in baked goods) that might exacerbate the child's condition, and avoid these foods.

Safety and Activity

- Outdoor activities are encouraged.
- Child should avoid getting sunburned.
- Swimming is permitted if followed by a shower to remove chlorine from skin, and then occlusive emollient is applied to skin.

Comfort Measures

- Use antihistamines at night if scratching or rubbing of affected areas inhibits sleep.
- Use mittens to prevent scratching during sleep.
- Maintain good skin care at all times to maintain optimal skin integrity and decrease pain.

Special Considerations

- Avoid known or suspected sensitivities to contact allergens, pets, or other environmental factors.
- If infection occurs
  - Use antibiotic creams as ordered.
  - Use systemic antibiotics as ordered.
  - Continue daily skin care.

Contact Health Care Provider if

- Your child is in such discomfort that sleep and the ability to concentrate are affected.
- Your child spikes a temperature of 101.5°F or greater.
- An area of the child's skin has a colored discharge, is warm to touch, or has a foul smell.

adults with severe AD to diminish the extent of a flare-up (Romeo, 1995). These drugs may have promise as effective treatment modalities for the pediatric population.

Reducing Inflammation. To reduce inflammation, topical low-dose corticosteroids are administered to the affected area. Systemic corticosteroids are rarely used. Long-term consequences of the therapy can include thinning of the skin, hypopigmentation, acne, secondary infection, and stretch marks.

Tar preparations can also be applied to the skin. These agents have a slower anti-inflammatory action and have fewer side effects than do corticosteroid therapy. However, application of the tar preparations is messy and they have a bad smell, thus many children are not interested in this treatment.

Hydrating the Skin. To maintain healthy skin in the child with AD, hydration practices should be implemented to replace moisture in the stratum corneum and prevent transdermal water losses. Some dermatologists believe that frequent baths (three to four per day) followed by application of a moisturizer helps keep the skin moist. After the bath, the skin is patted dry, not rubbed vigorously, and a moisturizing occlusive agent is applied within 3 minutes to prevent evaporation of skin moisture.

Worldview: *In very humid or tropical climates, frequent emollient use is not recommended because the occlusive agent may cause malaria-like symptoms.*

Use of a room humidifier or vaporizer may help provide moisture to the skin. Other dermatologists prefer the "dry method" in which baths are infrequent and a nonsoap cleaner is used. Drying soaps, bath oils, and perfumes are avoided.

Preventing Infection. Another major nursing intervention is to prevent infection. The skin is kept clean with tepid baths of nonirritating hydrophilic cleaners. Skin folds and diaper areas need frequent cleaning with plain water. Topical and oral antibiotics are used for secondary infections.

Nurses can help parents by letting them vent their frustration. Parents can alternately be angry and then guilty about the demands of the child's care. Caregivers need to be given emotional support and to be made aware of community sources of help.

Food allergy has not been clearly related to AD. If a food substance is an identified allergen, then it is removed from the diet. However, the dietitian must reassure the parents that a hypoallergenic diet does not always give immediate relief. In addition, the dietitian should recommend that children at "atopic risk" should be breast-fed for at least 6 months. Cow's milk–based formula is avoided, and soy-based or other special formulas are recommended.

Community Care

AD causes much physical suffering, disability, and anguish for the child and the family. Prolonged discomfort and cosmetic disfigurement disrupt the activities of daily living. Infants and children with AD often have a characteristic sad facial appearance and exhibit significant scratching behaviors. The child and the family need intense emotional support and assurance that lesions do not produce scarring unless secondarily infected. The stress present in the family during an exacerbation of AD is to be expected. Parents need to be taught that feeling overwhelmed by the disorder is a common experience. Reducing anxiety has to be a major goal in dealing with the psychological repercussions of the disease. The vicious cycle of scratching-irritation-irritability-frustration can place severe strain on the family system unless the cycle can be broken.

Older children and teenagers can be badly affected by AD because they are often rejected by peers who are offended by their skin condition. These children and teenagers may be sullen and unsmiling because of the alteration in their self-concept.

The personal financial costs of managing this condition can be excessive for the family. One study estimated the costs to families of children with moderate or severe atopic eczema to be greater than costs to families of diabetic children or asthmatic children (Su et al., 1997). In these cases, social workers can provide assistance in several substantive ways. They can interview the child and family, assess needs, and identify available community resources. The social worker can assist with improvement of the home environment and lifestyle, especially for impoverished children. If psychotherapy is necessary because of poor self-concept and associated behaviors, social service may be able to generate financial support for the family.

School performance can be adversely affected by severe AD. Children may be unable to concentrate because of the scratching and this may cause their school achievement to be poor. The school nurse can act as a liaison with health care personnel to notify caregivers if they observe that the child's condition is worsening and affecting school performance. The school nurse's office can also be used by children with AD as a place where they can undress to apply moisturizing solutions to the skin. The nurse can assist them with this treatment and can simultaneously assess the status of the condition. The school nurse may also have to educate teachers and administrators about the nature of the disease itself and the environmental conditions that need to be considered as the atopic child participates in school activities. For example, physical education (which generates sweating) and art class (exposure to paint and thinning agents) may have to be eliminated if they cause the dermatitis to worsen. Adolescents who wish to find employment should be guided to find work conditions that do not aggravate or activate their skin condition. The school can also work with the student to help support a good self-concept. The nurse can educate classmates to help provide compassionate care of their peer.

Seborrheic Dermatitis

Seborrheic dermatitis is a common, chronic, noncontagious dermatitis of unknown cause. Characterized by scaling and redness, seborrheic dermatitis lesions usually develop on the face, eyelids, scalp, body folds, external ears, and diaper area.

Etiology and Incidence

The incidence of seborrheic dermatitis in the general population is 2% to 5%. Seborrheic dermatitis is most common in infancy, and 50% of cases occur before 5 weeks of age. A seasonal fluctuation of the disease occurs, with most cases being reported during the spring and summer when there is increased sebaceous gland activity caused by sweating. However, the child with an existing condition also has more symptoms in colder weather because of the low indoor humidity and lack of sunlight. A seborrhea-like dermatitis is common in children and adolescents infected with human immunodeficiency virus (HIV).

The cause of seborrheic dermatitis is unknown. Stressful situations, poor hygiene, and excessive perspiration have all been identified as conditions that can reactivate seborrheic dermatitis. In contrast to AD, seborrheic dermatitis is not genetically predisposed. Several theories have been suggested. It is noteworthy that the localized patches of seborrhea are usually found in areas of high sebaceous gland concentration, although the role of sebaceous glands in this disease is unclear. Occlusion of a skin area (e.g., diaper area), maceration, and moisture may also play distinct exacerbating roles. Some researchers believe that a yeast, *Pityrosporum ovale*, which grows in the hair follicles, is the causative agent (Peters, 1997a).

The presence of secondary bacterial infection or candidiasis is not uncommon. Patients with neurologic problems, such as mental retardation or Parkinson's syndrome, often have varying degrees of seborrhea, suggesting some neural relationship to onset of the condition (Lane & Darmstadt, 1996; Peters, 1997a).

Pathophysiology

Seborrhea is similar to psoriasis in that white blood cells migrate into the skin plaque. A hyperkeratosing process generates plaque formation (scaling). It may be difficult to distinguish psoriasis from seborrheic dermatitis.

Prognosis. The prognosis for infantile seborrheic dermatitis is excellent. Most cases clear up within 1 month, even without therapy. In the adolescent form, long-term prognosis is good if the treatment plan is adhered to faithfully.

Assessment

Seborrheic dermatitis has different manifestations in various age groups. In infants, yellow, waxy adherent scales occur over the fontanelle, scalp (cradle cap), and diaper area. In older children, seborrheic dermatitis manifests as erythematous, oily plaques and patches of vesicles and papules occurring on the forehead, eyebrows, and symmetrically on the nasolabial folds. Seborrhea may also cause scaling and erythema on the eyelids (blepharitis), on the external ears (otitis externa), and retroauricular areas. Blepharitis is often accompanied by styes. In severe cases, other affected areas include the intertriginous folds of the trunk, under the breasts in women, and the gluteal cleft.

Mild cases may involve no more than dealing with the nuisance of dandruff. However, severe cases can be extremely deleterious to body image and self-concept. Seborrheic dermatitis does not cause hair loss, so the child with a scalp condition can be reassured of this fact. Stress can activate an exacerbation in some children. No laboratory test or consistent pattern of laboratory abnormalities is associated with seborrheic dermatitis.

Interdisciplinary Interventions

Infantile seborrheic dermatitis usually responds well to cleansing the scalp with a mild shampoo. The thick, scaling lesions on the child's scalp can be treated by applying baby oil, salicylic acid in mineral oil, or a corticosteroid gel on the scalp for 10 to 15 minutes. The area is gently massaged with a soft toothbrush, then the scales can be rinsed away. A fine-toothed comb helps rid the hair of scale debris.

In the older child and adolescent, an antiseborrheic shampoo (selenium sulfide, sulfur, salicylic acid, zinc pyrithione, tar) should be used daily to control scaling. Common names for these shampoos include Sebulex, Selsun, and Head & Shoulders. When severe inflammation is present, a low-potency corticosteroid medication (0.5% to 1% hydrocortisone) may be administered two to four times a day. Scaling may be so severe that a tar gel preparation is prescribed that is left on the scalp all night. However, children are usually reluctant to have this applied because it is difficult to remove and has an offensive smell.

A major responsibility of the nurse is to teach parents how to prevent seborrheic dermatitis of the scalp.

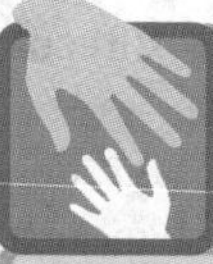

Chart 25–15
Nursing Interventions

Application of Topical Corticosteroids

Action

Topical corticosteroids are effective anti-inflammatory agents that reduce inflammation of the skin by promoting vasoconstriction of the blood vessels in the skin and preventing the shedding of inflammatory cells from the blood stream to tissue sites. These medications reduce redness (erythema) and itching (pruritus) associated with inflammatory and hyperproliferation skin diseases.

Potency

- Potency is determined by the amount of skin blanching (vasoconstriction that correlates with the anti-inflammatory effects of the agent). Four categories exist: low potency, moderate or midpotency, high potency, and highest potency. Steroids are also categorized as **nonfluorinated**, having less potent and fewer side effects, and **fluorinated**, which are rarely used in pediatric practice.
- Potency may be increased by the vehicle (agent) with which the steroid is combined to create a gel or cream form of the medication.
- Corticosteroids are available in several forms: creams, gels, ointments, lotions, powders, aerosols, and tapes.

Administration

- At home, parents should apply corticosteroids for their children.
- A thin layer is applied over the affected area; creams, lotions, and gels are rubbed in until no longer visible.
- Unaffected areas should be avoided.
- The agent may be applied with bare hands, although hands should be washed thoroughly after application.
- A tongue depressor can be used to scoop the ointment out of a large container.
- On the face and scrotum, only low-potency glucocorticosteroids should be used. The epidermis is thin in these areas and side effects may be severe.
- Occlusive dressings or coverings (plastic pants covering a cloth diaper) should not be placed over an area in which a corticosteroid has been applied because this increases the absorption of the steroid and may lead to toxic side effects.
- The agents should not be used with conditions such as acne, rosacea, and some fungal infections or on severely eroded skin.
- Treatment is usually begun using a low-potency steroid. If lesions do not respond to therapy, the potency may be increased.
- Steroid therapy should be used for as short a time period as possible to achieve the desired effects.

Side Effects

Striae
Persistent erythema and telangiectasis
Increased skin fragility
Hypopigmentation
Secondary infection
Acneform eruption (steroid rosacea)
Folliculitis, miliaria
Allergic contact dermatitis
Steroid addiction syndrome

Systemic Effects

Cataracts
Glaucoma
Glycosuria
Cushing's syndrome
Stunted growth in children (rare)

Good scalp hygiene with a mild shampoo and gentle rubbing prevents the situation. If crusts are present, the nurse should teach parents how to remove the crusts with mild shampoo and a soft toothbrush or a fine-toothed comb. Generally, topical ointments are not required, but, if they are prescribed, the nurse should teach the caregivers how to apply the ointments appropriately (Chart 25–15). Parents should be taught to avoid using greasy ointments or creams on the affected child.

Psoriasis

Psoriasis is an inherited scaling skin disorder affecting both males and females. Characterized by flare-ups and remissions, psoriasis can occur at any age.

Etiology and Incidence

Incidence of psoriasis peaks in adolescence and young adulthood and again in older adulthood. Psoriasis affects 1% to 3% of the population, and 35% of children experience the first flare-up before age 20 (Burdette-Taylor, 1995). Psoriasis is much more common in white children and is seen twice as often in females. Psoriasis is rare in neonates.

The causes of psoriasis are unknown, but several hereditary and environmental mechanisms have been suggested. These include genetic inheritance (one third of children have a family history), problems in cell division, and alterations in immune response. Other suggested causes are streptococcal and viral infections, hormones, contact with animal skins, increased weight, seasonal change (especially cold), drugs (lithium, indomethacin, and some beta blockers), stress, and inflammatory bowel disease.

Pathophysiology

The pathogenesis of psoriasis is not fully understood. In psoriasis lesions, basal cell layers reproduce cells too quickly, and these cells move upward in the skin in 3 to 5 days, instead of in 2 to 4 weeks. Normally, skin cells die as they move upward; in psoriasis, the quickly migrating cells do not. The partially living skin builds on the skin surface instead of being desquamated. As the heaped-up skin dries, it becomes brittle and cracks. Underlying this hyperactive epidermis is a swollen dermis congested with blood vessels and leukocytes; these conditions form minute abscesses that become pustules.

Protein malnutrition, failure to thrive, and fluid and electrolyte imbalances are significant risks for the child with psoriasis. The child has an increased need for protein resulting from the rapid production of keratin. Additional nitrogen may be needed to meet protein requirements. Protein malnutrition is also responsible for the loss of nails and hair. Fluid and electrolyte imbalances can also result from the fissuring and shedding of large sheets of skin. This process leaves a tender, denuded base where water loss can lead to dehydration, hypernatremia, and discomfort (Burdette-Taylor, 1995). The exposed skin areas can easily become infected, with overwhelming septicemia being a severe complication of this disorder.

Prognosis. The prognosis is good for children with limited disease, but remissions and exacerbations are expected. If psoriasis persists to adolescence, it becomes a lifelong disease. Arthritis can be a noncutaneous complication. Patient outcomes focus on normalizing skin physiology as much as possible. The promotion of normal activities of daily living is most important.

Assessment

The physical signs of psoriasis are varied. In some children, psoriasis is annoying; in others, it is a debilitating, devastating experience. Sharply demarcated red plaques covered in a silvery white, thick, adherent scale occur at the elbows, knees, scalp, back, genitals, and sacrum.

caREminder: *Psoriasis closely resembles AD. The nurse should ask the child if the lesions are greasy. Psoriasis scales are erythematous and are not oily.*

Facial psoriasis is rare, although facial lesions are more common in children than in adults. Affected skin over the palms of the hands and the soles of the feet thickens. Nail changes include pits, ridges, and brittleness. When the scales are peeled off, pinhead-sized bleeding can be seen (Auspitz' sign). As the plaques clear, the skin beneath may show either increased or decreased pigmentation. Another characteristic sign is exacerbation of eruptions in the winter.

Interdisciplinary Interventions

Treatment options for children with psoriasis are varied but can be divided into the topical and the systemic focus of treatment that normalize epidermal cell proliferation and keratinization. Contemporary treatment seeks to promote a hydrated, nonirritated skin that decreases discomfort and prevents formation of fissures (Chart 25–16). The goals of therapy include the following:

- Rehydration of the skin
- Removal of scales
- Prevention of infection
- Inhibition of the pathologic process and suppression of the immune response
- Promotion of acceptance of the child's condition

Rehydrating the Skin. To hydrate the skin, children are asked to use daily bath emollients, moisturizers, topi-

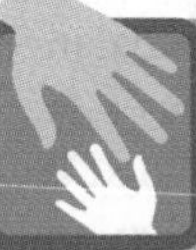

Chart 25–16
Nursing Interventions

Psoriasis Therapy

Goal	Action
Rehydrate epidermis. Risk for impaired skin integrity Fluid volume deficit	Apply moisturizers. Apply topical emollients. Use soap substitutes. Protect from overexposure to sun. Maintain good fluid intake.
Remove scales. Impaired skin integrity	Apply keratolytic preparations.
Prevent infection. Risk for infection	Protect against injury. Maintain hydrated skin. Monitor for infection. Administer systemic and topical antibiotics. Maintain protein-rich diet.
Reduce epidermal cell division and suppress immune response. Impaired skin integrity Altered tissue perfusion: peripheral	Administer PUVA, a combination of psoralen medication and ultraviolet light (has serious drawbacks; rarely used for children). Administer retinoid, a vitamin derivative, which can dramatically decrease scaling (has serious side effects). Administer methotrexate, an antimetabolite (serious side effects; rarely used for children). Avoid "triggers": cold, stress, trauma to skin, infections of skin.
Promote acceptance of the child's condition Alterations in parenting Ineffective family coping Body image disturbance Altered growth and development	Allow family and child to verbalize concerns. Encourage activities that promote child's self-esteem and achievement of normal growth and developmental milestones. Refer child or family to support services and agencies.

cal emollients, and soap substitutes. The importance of hydrating the skin by constantly applying some type of lubrication cannot be overemphasized. The skin must be moisturized several times during the day and must be moisturized after each washing and again at bedtime. The use of soap, talcum powder, and perfumed products should be avoided.

Even though sun exposure in moderate amounts alleviates lesions, the child should be protected from direct heat and sunlight in hot-dry weather to prevent drying of the skin. Maintaining a body temperature between 36.5°C and 37°C helps the child remain comfortable and hydrated. Systemic hydration is also important because of the potential of fluid and electrolyte loss during the shedding process. The child should be encouraged to drink plenty of fluids and eat a protein-rich diet.

Removing Scales. Some degree of scale removal is required. Descaling is effected by applying keratolytic preparations containing coal tar, salicylic acid, or dithranol. Mineral oil and warm towel soaks can also be used to remove thick plaques. When tar products are used, the family should wear latex gloves when applying the products. Tar products should not be used on inflamed skin. The healthy skin surrounding affected sites should be protected with petrolatum ointment during a tar treatment. All topical agents must be kept away from the eyes. Clothing and linen should be kept away from tar products because they will become stained.

Preventing Infection. When caring for the child's skin, aseptic technique should be used to minimize the risk for infection. Additional family members should be taught to regularly assess and identify early signs and symptoms of local and systemic infection. Maintaining the skin in a hydrated state assists in preventing infection. Fissures are less likely to develop in well-lubricated skin. Even though the daily skin protocol is tedious and time consuming, meticulous attention to this aspect of the child's care can prevent the complication of infection. If infection occurs, systemic and topical antibiotics are administered.

Inhibiting the Pathologic Process and Suppressing the Immune Response. Topical steroids (triamcinolone 0.025% to 0.1% twice daily or fluocinolone (Synalar) 0.025% twice daily) can help to decrease inflammatory responses. They work quickly, but can give a false sense of permanent improvement. Steroids are not curative and can promote fast rebound or flare-up symptoms. The side effects of the topical steroids are so deleterious that children must be educated about long-term use and cautioned against overuse (see Chart 25–15).

Some of the aims of therapy can also be accomplished by systemic therapy. For example, PUVA is a form of photochemotherapy in which the client receives special tablets (Psoralen) and then is exposed to long-wave UV light therapy. The pills act as a photosensitizer. The combination therapy reduces epidermal cell division. The treatment is not without side effects in that the tablets cause nausea and malaise, and can affect the kidney, liver, and heart. Protective goggles must be worn to prevent retinal damage during the treatment. The medication cannot be taken during pregnancy. PUVA is used rarely in children and sparingly in adolescents.

Although rarely used in young children, methotrexate can be used for severe psoriasis because of its antimetabolite activity. The child or adolescent given this medication becomes susceptible to infections, and blood tests should be done periodically to monitor for liver dysfunction and blood dyscrasias. Another intervention that can help in the treatment of psoriasis is the avoidance of "triggers." Exposure to cold, stress, and skin trauma should be minimized. Also, skin infections, such as with streptococcal organisms, should be diagnosed and treated promptly.

Promoting Acceptance of the Child's Condition. The care of a child with psoriasis is demanding. Treatment exacerbates the emotional effects of this disfiguring disorder. Bathing and cream application are time consuming, and topical treatments may stain clothes. The nurse can educate parents that psoriasis is not contagious and that the child should be encouraged to pursue normal activities, with vigilance being maintained toward keeping the child's skin hydrated. Neither overprotecting the child nor ignoring the problem is beneficial. Organizations such as the National Psoriasis Foundation are excellent resources for parents.

The most detrimental effect for the child is psychological pressure. Children fear being labeled and are embarrassed about their appearance caused by the scaling of the disease. Because the child's skin is prone to infection or because of the child's appearance, limits are often placed on the child's lifestyle. A child finds it hard to understand why special precautions must be instituted to sunbathe on the beach and play outdoors on a hot sunny day. Adolescents who are dealing with age-appropriate concerns regarding their self-esteem and body image may experience feelings of shame, anxiety, and depression because of their condition and its disfiguring qualities.

Community Care

Care of the child with psoriasis can be challenging for the nurse and the family. Children and their families may experience a great deal of stress owing to the meticulous, time-consuming skin care measures that must be followed, the restrictions on the child's activities, and the unsightly appearance of the lesions. It is important that the nurse help the family understand the long-term nature of the psoriasis treatment. Additionally, the family needs information regarding the side effects of the medications, how to monitor for fluid and electrolyte imbalances and for infection, and how to monitor the status of the skin (Vernon, 1997).

Epidermolysis Bullosa

Although many skin disorders and infections can generate vesicles and bullae, the phrase "bullous skin disease" is usually reserved for the condition called epidermolysis bullosa (EB). EB describes a family of inherited disorders characterized by exceptional skin fragility and the formation of bullae at the site of mechanical trauma. The disorders range in severity from mild (subtle small lesions) to severe (large, mutilating lesions with internal organ involvement). EB affects all races and both sexes equally.

Pathophysiology

EB is classified into three major types depending on the layer of skin in which blistering occurs. **EB simplex (EBS)** is the most superficial type, in which mechanical trauma causes splitting of the epidermis within the basal layer. The most common forms of EBS are autosomal dominant. Although the lesions can be widespread, they occur predominantly on the extremities. The lesions heal without scarring. Fingernails may detach, but they grow back. There is no involvement of the mucous membranes. By adolescence, blistering tends to lessen, and the child has the potential for a normal life span (Eichenfield & Honig, 1991).

Junctional epidermolysis bullosa (JEB) is predominantly an autosomal dominant inherited disease. The condition is characterized by bullae and erosions occurring on mucosal surfaces as a result of splitting within the lamina lucida, which is at the junction of the epidermis and dermis. This is considered a severe and life-threatening condition because the erosions can lead to infection, sepsis, anemia, dehydration, and malnutrition. The mucous membranes of the respiratory, gastrointestinal, and genitourinary systems may all be involved.

Dystrophic epidermolysis bullosa (DEB) has both autosomal dominant and recessive types, which are characterized by blistering in the dermis below the lamina densa. At birth, the child has large, dense bullae that heal slowly, leaving scars, fusion of scarred digits, and residual mucosal trauma. Blistering of the oral mucosa and larynx impacts the child's ability to have good nutritional intake. Intake and output is further compromised by increased protein loss through the skin, anemia, and chronic constipation (Eichenfield & Honig, 1991). Dystrophic and dermatolytic EB have the poorest prognosis, the greatest degree of scarring, and most contracture development.

Assessment

Diagnosis of EB is made by evaluating the family history and the child's clinical course and by completing a skin biopsy. Development of bullae in response to a minor trauma is characteristic and diagnostic.

EB usually manifests in neonates when blisters caused by delivery trauma appear. Lesions are clearly related to areas of handling or occur at sites of pressure or motion. The number and amount of blisters, scarring, and affected sites depend on the type of EB. Specific areas of the body commonly affected include the hands, feet, extremities, nails, and mouth. If the oral mucosa and larynx are involved, as in JEB, the child may have a hoarse cry. Involvement of other mucosal surfaces of the respiratory, gastrointestinal, and genitourinary tracts can lead to respiratory distress, severe dehydration, anemia, and chronic constipation. Musculoskeletal and eye involvement may be present as a result of scar formation.

Diagnostic Tests. A special maneuver called the Nikolsky technique is used to aid diagnosis. This procedure involves rubbing or rotating a portion of the child's skin with the examiner's fingers. Bullae that develop after this procedure are then sampled for standard light microscopy, transmission electron microscopy, and immunofluorescence mapping. Skin cultures may be assessed to rule out the presence of herpes simplex. Fetoscopy, a technique in which fetal skin samples are obtained between 18 and 21 weeks' gestation, can be used to elicit a prenatal diagnosis of this inherited condition.

Interdisciplinary Interventions

Therapy is supportive and is aimed at optimizing nutrition and growth and development. To prevent and treat infections, antibacterial baths and soaks, topical antibiotics, and, occasionally, systemic antibiotics may be ordered. Open wounds are treated with nontraumatizing dressings such as hydrogels (e.g., Vigilon), transparent dressings (e.g., Op-Site), and petrolatum gauze.

All nursing care is directed at minimizing trauma to external skin and internal mucous membrane surfaces. The child should be handled very carefully with measures taken to avoid rubbing or chafing the skin. Wearing a hospital armband may cause enough irritation for blistering to develop. The child should wear loose, soft clothing. Pressure reduction devices such as overlays and special mattresses can be used to reduce skin friction. The skin should be washed by soaking rather than by rubbing it with a washcloth.

To provide adequate nutrition, the health care team must consider deficits resulting from both poor intake and losses caused by leaking of protein and body fluids from the blistering lesions. Breast-feeding is encouraged. If bottle-fed, the infant should have only cool formula with a soft nipple that does not irritate the oral mucosa. If severe nutritional problems exist, gastrostomy tubes can be used to administer feedings. Nasogastric intubation should be avoided to prevent possible irritation of the mucous membranes.

Acne Vulgaris

Acne vulgaris is a chronic, inflammatory process of the pilosebaceous follicles. It is a skin condition that is nearly universal in adolescence. It is so prevalent that some parents and health professionals dismiss it as unimportant. However, acne can affect an adolescent physically by scarring the skin or psychologically by damaging self-esteem.

Etiology and Incidence

Acne accounts for one fourth of all skin diseases reported in the United States. Thirty-five million Americans suffer with acne, with the prevalence in teenagers aged 15 to 17 years approaching 85% (Novotny, 1989; Weston et al., 1996). Acne may develop in children on corticosteroid therapy, anticonvulsant drugs, or antituberculosis drugs. External agents such as suntan oils, heavy makeup bases, or grooming agents can cause acne-like eruptions. In rare instances, acne may be seen in infants. This infantile form requires no treatment.

Acne is more common in females than in males, usually beginning 1 to 2 years before the onset of puberty as a result of androgenic stimulation of the sebaceous glands (Hurwitz, 1994). It occurs more often in southern and western regions of the United States. Other factors that precipitate appearance of the lesions include stress, lack of sleep, and premenstrual hormone activity. Acne tends to be improved in the summer months. In general, the individual's choice of food and the level of cleanliness seem to play no specific roles (Hurwitz, 1994).

There is a recognized familial trend, with the disease often present in first-degree relatives. Ethnic variations also exist. Acne is more prevalent in American whites than in either African or Asian Americans.

Pathophysiology

The development of acne is attributed to an abnormal keratinization process that results in obstruction of the sebaceous follicle, an increase in sebum production, proliferation of ordinarily harmless bacteria, and inflammation (Hurwitz, 1996). When the normal flow of sebum of the skin is obstructed by the keratinization process, two types of comedones are formed. The open comedone (blackhead) is a firm, noninflammatory lesion filled with keratin and lipid, which block the mouth of the follicle. It has a blackened tip that is the result of oxidized melanin. Blackheads are easily managed except when traumatized or manipulated by the child. Inflammation rarely occurs with blackheads because the contents of the comedone easily escape to the skin surface.

The closed comedone (whitehead) is responsible for most of the problems seen in acne. This semisoft, noninflammatory lesion is caused by blockage at the neck of the follicle. It has a microscopic opening that does not allow easy escape of keratin and lipid. Therefore, as these substances build up, they rupture the follicular wall and expel sebum into surrounding dermis tissue. This begins the inflammatory process that results in the presence of inflammatory papules, pustules, or nodules depending upon the location of, and the extent of, the inflammatory reaction.

It is hypothesized that the overgrowth of certain bacteria on the skin, such as *Propionibacterium acnes* or *Staphylococcus epidermis* produce peptides or enzymes that exacerbate the inflammatory process. Additionally, an overproduction of sebum, although not the cause of inflammation, does promote the generation of comedones. Acne vulgaris is an inflammatory process in which sebum, bacteria, and a variety of other factors (stress, hormones, menses) interact to precipitate the eruption of these lesions.

Prognosis. Prognosis is individual, in that no two children with acne react to treatment identically. The ultimate goal for all children is the avoidance of the associated scarring. Acne is treatable, but treatment takes time and good self-care.

Assessment

Acne lesions include comedones (blackheads, whiteheads), papules, pustules, nodules, cysts, and scars (Fig. 25–11). Lesions usually occur on the face, back, chest, and shoulders. As the condition resolves, the lesion site may appear red and hyperpigmented. In more severe forms of acne, scar formation can occur. Atrophic scars appear as shallow, broad-based depressions or deep, steep-sided pits with irregular outlines (icepick scars). Hypertrophic or keloid scars most often appear on the back or chest as elevated thick fibrotic plaques. Black adolescents have a greater propensity for this type of scarring. Other epidermal structures (e.g., hair and mucous membranes) are normal; however, facial lesions may extend into the scalp, with scarring alopecia (loss of hair) occurring as a result.

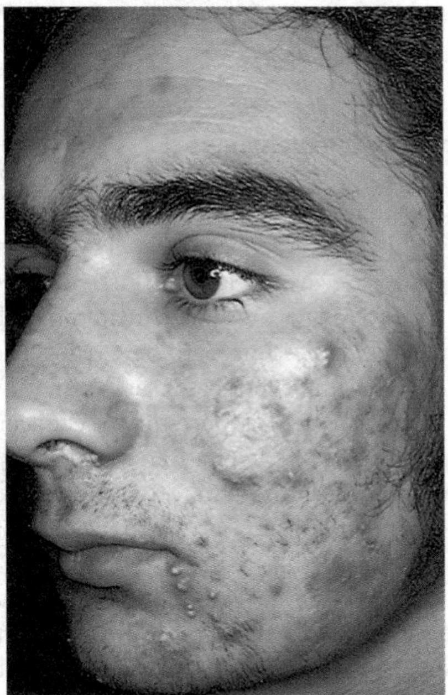

Figure 25–11
An adolescent with acne vulgaris. (From Jarvis, C. [1996]. *Physical examination and health assessment* [2nd ed., p. 239]. Philadelphia: W. B. Saunders. Reprinted with permission.)

The nursing assessment includes an evaluation of the factors that may exacerbate the onset of acne. The child's age should be determined because the appearance of acne usually occurs from 1 to 2 years before the onset of puberty.

caREminder: *Very young children with acne and other signs of pubertal maturity should be evaluated for precocious puberty.*

The adolescent should be questioned regarding his or her use of medications, suntan or sunscreen preparations, makeup, and grooming products. Additionally, information regarding contact with oils, greases, and waxes derived from petroleum and animal or vegetable oils should be noted. Affected adolescents may work at gas stations, garages, or restaurants that serve fast foods.

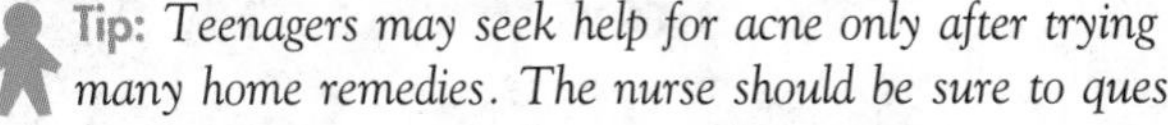

Tip: *Teenagers may seek help for acne only after trying many home remedies. The nurse should be sure to ques-*

tion the adolescent about previous treatments, hygiene habits, stress, and diet.

Interdisciplinary Interventions

The child or adolescent with acne may have serious concerns about his or her appearance. These concerns are the usual triggering events for the first health care visit. Although the disease is not life-threatening, the impact of acne on the adolescent can be great. Taunting by peers can be cruel in severe cases, and sometimes professional psychological help is necessary. Teenagers need to feel free to discuss their feelings and problems with self-esteem and relationships with others. Acne may even exert a profound influence on health beliefs. Saltzer and Saltzer (1987) found that college students with moderate to severe acne reported an external locus of control. That is, the sufferers believed that controlling their health was out of their personal ability and they were less likely to take personal responsibility for pursuing healthy behaviors.

Early intervention does not prevent acne, but it does help control scarring. Treatment usually revolves around medications, both topical and systemic (Chart 25–17). Systemic and topical treatments are often combined because no single agent has proven effective against acne. The dermatologist may also perform comedone extraction or incision and drainage of cystic lesions. Therapy is targeted at controlling the inflammatory process by altering bacterial flora around the sebaceous glands with antibiotics and reducing the obstruction of sebaceous skin glands by use of topical agents. The ultimate aim of treatment is to prevent a permanently altered appearance. The health care provider should discuss the possible side effects of these treatments with the teenager before prescribing them.

Topical Medications. Topical therapy has a more rapid effect and few systemic side effects, but it is less effective than systemic drugs and can cause local irritation of the skin. Topical therapy includes use of benzoyl peroxide, retinoid preparations, and antibiotics. The therapeutic success of these agents is enhanced through combination therapy. In particular, benzoyl peroxide or tretinoin is used in combination with a topical antibiotic agent. The adolescent should be instructed to clean the skin with a mild soap before applying the topical agent. Abrasive soaps and astringents should not be used, because these products only serve to cause drying and peeling of the skin and fail to prevent the lesions from appearing. These over-the-counter products may also interfere with the proper use of known effective topical agents.

Tip: *Advise the adolescent not to "pop" pimples because this can cause further inflammation at the site and scarring at sites of larger lesions. If teenagers are compelled to do it anyway, advise them to never open the pimple before it has come to a head. The hands and face should*

Chart 25–17
Nursing Interventions

Use of Acne Medications

Name	Form	Action	Side Effects	Special Instructions
Topical Medications				
Benzoyl peroxide (Clearasil, Oxy 5)	Gel Lotion	· Acts as bactericidal for *Propioni bacterium acnes* · Acts as comedolytic agent by reversing the formation of follicles that become compacted and clogged · Reduces levels of free fatty acids · Inhibits triglyceride hydrolysis · Decreases inflammation of acne lesions	Bleaching of clothes Skin irritation Occasional contact dermatitis Dryness of skin	· Agent should not be used with abrasive soaps or astringents because this dries out the skin and leads to irritation. · Therapy should be individualized and introduced gradually, especially for fair-skinned adolescents or atopic cases.

Chart 25–17
Nursing Interventions *Continued*

Use of Acne Medications

Name	Form	Action	Side Effects	Special Instructions
Topical retinoid preparations Tretinoin retinoic acid (Retin-A)	Cream Gel Liquid	· Used to treat open and closed comedones · Encourages cell turnover · Helps to eliminate existing comedones and stop formation of new ones · Decreases thickness of stratum corneum, thus aiding in absorption of other topical antibiotic agents	Erythema Desquamation Occasional Hyperpigmentation Susceptible to sunburn Teratogenic to fetus	· Agent initially should not be applied daily because it causes skin irritation and peeling. · Agent may cause some worsening of the condition in the first 1 to 2 months of use. · Start with low potency creams and progress to higher potency gel or liquid formulas as needed. · To minimize skin irritation, wash skin with a mild soap 2 to 3 times a day and wait 20 to 30 minutes after washing before applying agent. · When sun exposure is anticipated, use a noncomedogenic sunscreen with skin protection factor (SPF) of 15 or greater.
Azelaic acid		· Contains a comedolytic agent with an anti-inflammatory agent. · Useful in mild to moderate acne	Skin irritation Susceptible to sunburn	
Topical antibiotics (clindamycin, erythromycin, tetracycline)	Lotion Gel Liquid	· Acts as a bactericidal for *P. acnes* · Treats mild to moderate acne that is resistant to benzoyl peroxide	Fewer side effects than same medications given systemically Skin irritation Gastrointestinal (GI) upset	· Erythromycin solution is safest product to use during pregnancy. · Often used in combination with other products · Cleanse skin with a mild soap before use. · Wash hands immediately after application. · Avoid application while smoking or near heat or flame. Some of these agents are flammable (vehicle is isopropyl alcohol).

Chart continued on following page

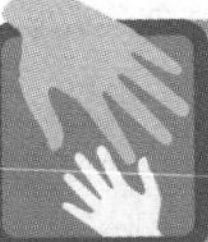

Chart 25–17
Nursing Interventions *Continued*

Use of Acne Medications

Name	Form	Action	Side Effects	Special Instructions
Systemic Medications				
Erythromycin	Oral pills	· Suppresses *P. acnes* · Inhibits bacterial lipases · Reduces concentration of free fatty acids · Inhibits follicular inflammation	GI upset Ototoxicity Rashes	· Therapy takes several weeks for improvement. · Agent is least expensive and has fewest side effects.
Tetracycline	Oral pills	· Suppresses *P. acnes* · Inhibits bacterial lipases · Reduces concentration of free fatty acids · Inhibits follicular inflammation	GI upset Vaginal yeast infections Photosensitivity Folliculitis Hyperpigmentation Teeth staining in children younger than 8 due to the presence of immature enamel formation	· Agent should be taken on an empty stomach, 1 to 2 hours before or after mealtimes. Absorption may be impaired by food, milk, iron supplements, aluminum hydroxide gel, and calcium-magnesium salts. · Therapy takes several weeks to demonstrate improvement. · Oral antibiotics may decrease the effectiveness of contraceptive pills. · Tetracycline should not be used at the same time as Accutane because the combination can cause benign intracranial hypertension.
Minocycline	Oral pills	· Suppresses *P. acnes* · Inhibits bacterial lipases · Reduces concentration of free fatty acids · Inhibits follicular inflammation	Dizziness Headaches Appearance of blue-gray spots on the skin and mucous membranes Photosensitivity	· Therapy takes several weeks to demonstrate improvement. · If side effects occur, drug should be discontinued. · Do not take drug within 1 to 3 hours of other medications. · Avoid use of calcium salts, antacids, magnesium-containing medications, or iron supplements within 1 to 3 hours of taking this medication.

Chart 25–17
Nursing Interventions *Continued*

Use of Acne Medications

Name	Form	Action	Side Effects	Special Instructions
Hormonal therapy Oral contraceptives containing cyoterone acetate Bromocriptine, spironolactone, and gonadotropin-releasing hormone antagonists	Oral pills	· Inhibits sebum production · Useful for women with acne who have hormonal abnormalities, are unresponsive to antibiotic therapy, or are candidates for Accutane therapy	Fluid retention Thromboembolitic problems Depression	· It is important to maintain dosage schedule. · It is not administered to girls before the onset of menses.
Isotretinoin (Accutane)	Oral pills	· Decreases oil production · Reverses the abnormal skin cell-shedding process · Decreases population of *P. acnes*	Dry skin and lips Frequent nosebleeds Hypertriglyceridemia Hypercholesterolemia Altered hepatic function Redness or irritation of the eyes Temporary worsening of the acne Myalgia Arthralgia Muscle pain and stiffness Elevated blood sugar in diabetics Photosensitivity Balding Teratogenic to fetus Premature bone closure	· Agent is teratogenic and cannot be used in pregnancy. Pregnancy test should be done before administration begins. · Contraceptives must be used 1 month before, during, and 1 month after therapy if the adolescent is sexually active. · Drug is not given to children younger than 12 years of age. · Dry mouth can be relieved by sucking on hard candy or chewing gum. · Dry skin can be relieved by using nonalcohol-based skin lotion and drinking 8 to 12 glasses of water a day. · Most of the side effects are reversible after discontinuing the medication. · Drug should not be used at the same time as tetracycline because the combination can cause benign intracranial hypertension.

be washed first and a sterile needle should be used to nick the surface of the yellow pimple. The pimple should not be squeezed, rather the pus should be allowed to run out and then be washed away with soap and water (Schmitt, 1994).

Systemic Medications. Systemic antibiotic therapy is used to treat moderate to severe papulopustular and cystic acne. Tetracycline, erythromycin, and minocycline are most often used. The medications must be used for a minimum of 3 to 4 weeks to achieve an effective level in the skin to produce significant results. The systemic agents may produce side effects (see Table 25–7). The patient should be instructed to stop taking the antibiotic and call the health care provider immediately if side effects occur.

Used only in severe acne, isotretinoin (Accutane) promotes a dramatic reduction in the activity of the sebaceous glands and sebum production and reduces bacteria (Peters, 1997b). This drug has numerous side effects and is recommended only for adolescents and adults who have severe cystic acne and for whom at least two courses of oral antibiotics have proven ineffective. The drug should not be given to children younger than age 12 years because of the risk of premature bone closure. Isotretinoin can also cause severe birth defects in a developing fetus. Adolescents taking the drug must not be pregnant and must use oral contraceptives 1 month before beginning the therapy, during the entire course of drug therapy, and for 1 month after stopping therapy (Peters, 1997b). A blood pregnancy test is usually required of a female adolescent before isotretinoin is prescribed. Written, informed consent by the girl and her parents is also generally required.

Community Care

Nurses in the school, physician's office, or clinic often serve as the initial contact for adolescents who are affected by acne. Nurses can be instrumental in the life of a teen seeking professional advice by helping to decrease the fears of treatment and by offering hope about positive outcomes. The nurse can provide significant counseling related to the many myths about appropriate treatment. The nurse can also teach about general lifestyle, hygiene, and appropriate medication use (Chart 25–18).

Dietary restrictions are no longer considered crucial to the progress and prognosis of acne care (Hurwitz, 1994). If any instruction is given by the dietitian, it is generally in reference to improving general dietary habits. However, there is still evidence that certain fatty acids may contribute to the different kinds of sebum production and that restriction of fatty foods might be reasonable. If a teenager believes that certain foods predispose him or her to acne flare-ups, then he or she should be counseled to avoid them.

Parasitic Infestations

Skin infestations are common in children. The growing incidence of these "unwelcome guests" is of concern to parents, daycare providers, school officials, and health care providers. In the United States, the most common infestations affecting children are pediculosis (lice) and scabies (mites). Often misdiagnosed because of their appearance on healthy, "clean" children, these pesky insects are highly contagious and can be a source of embarrassment to the infected child and family. Eradication is possible when parents closely follow prescribed instructions for treating the lice and mites, clean the home environment, and monitor those who have been in close contact with the infected child.

Pediculosis

Pediculosis (lice) infestations have been identified for thousands of years. In ancient Egypt, lice infestation was a status symbol; in the Dark Ages, it was considered a sign of sainthood, known as the "pearls of poverty" (Clore, 1983). Eventually, lice infestation came to be known as a sign of poor hygiene, with the only known cure being a complete head shave.

Lice have been known to transmit certain diseases, including typhus, trench fever, and relapsing fever. In the United States, none of these diseases has been transmitted by lice for decades. Improved hygiene, better ability to wash and change clothes, immunizations, and the development of pediculicides and antibiotics have all played roles in decreasing the threat of disease transference. However, lice infestation remains a major community health problem throughout the world, with prevalence rates ranging between 1% and 40% of all elementary school children in a given country (Chunge, Scott, Underwood, & Zavarella, 1991).

Etiology

Humans can be infested with three types of lice, each having its own unique set of characteristics and occupying a specific segment of the body: the head louse (*Pediculus humanus capitis*), the pubic or crab louse (*Phthirius pubis*), and the body louse (*Pediculus humanus corporis*). Head lice are the most common type seen in children. The increase in adolescent sexual activity has contributed to the increased incidence of pubic lice in this population.

Head Lice (*Pediculus humanus capitis*). A familiar malady in schools and child care centers, head lice infestation occurs in all regions of United States. In some areas,

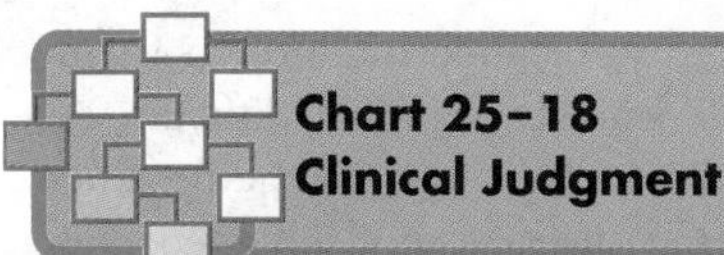

Chart 25-18
Clinical Judgment

The Adolescent with Acne

Maggie is a 14-year-old who was admitted to the hospital with status asthmaticus. She is being discharged today. As you enter her room, you find her standing near a mirror, squeezing the pimples on her face. When she sees you she says, "I just hate all of these zits. My face looks like frog skin. It is so embarrassing. My friend Kim has this neat medicine called 'Acu-something,' and when I am at home I use some of that to clear up my face."

Questions

1. What questions should you ask Maggie regarding the comments she has just made?
2. What data in the above scenario illustrate some poor health practices by Maggie?
3. What would be an appropriate nursing diagnosis based on the data you have collected?
4. What should be your plan of action regarding Maggie's concern about her acne?
5. As you discuss Accutane therapy with Maggie, what outcomes could you tell her can happen if she continues to squeeze her pimples and take her friend's medication?

Answers

1. Tell me more about this medicine you have been using (how often, how much, how long have you been using this). Have you been having any dry skin and lips, nosebleeds, muscle pain or stiffness, eye irritation, feel that your skin burns easily? Who knows that you are using this medicine?
2. Squeezing her pimples and taking someone else's medication. Further data would be needed to determine whether current hospital admission was related to poor home management of asthmatic condition.
3. Body image disturbance related to presence of skin lesions
   Knowledge deficit: skin care and management of acne
   Risk for injury related to use of friend's medication
4. Discuss the importance of not squeezing the acne lesions. Discuss some of the treatment options for acne. Discuss the extreme hazards of taking someone else's medication and the hazards associated with use of Accutane. Tell Maggie you would like to share her concerns with her parents and the doctor so that arrangements might be made for her to see a dermatologist. Tell Maggie's primary health care provider about her use of the Accutane. Unmonitored use of this medication places her at risk for injury, especially in light of her asthmatic condition.
5. She may have further inflammation of the facial lesions. Scarring is more likely to occur if she continues to manipulate the lesions. Accutane is a prescription medication, and the person given the medication must be carefully monitored by a physician or nurse practitioner when it is being used. It has several hazardous side effects that could be harmful to Maggie's general health.

incidence is as high as 40% among non-black school-age children. Head lice are less common in blacks, because the shape of the hair shaft is different and lice do not attach easily to tight, curly hair. Head lice can infest both adults and children, but the incidence is greatest in children between ages 5 and 12.

Transmission of head lice occurs by direct contact with an infested person or indirect contact with personal articles, clothing, or grooming materials. Carpeting, pillows, bed linens, hats, brushes, and ribbons from infested children are all possible sources of transmission.

Pubic Lice *(Phthirus pubis)*. Pubic lice have a more rounded body and prominent pincers than do head lice. These lice generally infest the pubic region, although infestation may also involve the eyebrows, facial hair, and axillary hair. Up to half of all patients with pubic lice have a sexually transmitted disease (Hogan, Schachner, & Tanglertsampan, 1991). Pubic lice are most commonly transmitted through intimate bodily contact, although they also may be transferred by fomites (combs, brushes, clothing). Infestation occurs most commonly in adolescents or adults; infestation in a younger child should raise the suspicion of sexual activity or abuse.

Body Lice *(Pediculus humanus corporis)*. The least common form of pediculosis in the United States is body lice. The lice attach to infested clothing and bedding, living in the seams of these materials. The lice attach to the skin only long enough to feed.

Pathophysiology

Lice are parasitic insects that infest humans and can have an effect on the host. Their bites are relatively painless and may be felt as a slight tickling sensation. The signs and symptoms of pediculosis infestation are due to the reactions of the host to the saliva or anticoagulants injected by the lice into the dermis. Intense itching may occur on the affected body part or in the scalp. Generally, the severity of symptoms is proportional to the degree of infestation.

Prognosis. Once treatment has begun, and if it is completed in a thorough fashion, eradication of these parasites can be successful. Most often, resurgence of lice occurs because caregivers fail to be meticulous in their efforts to follow the treatment plan and eradicate the nits in all of the environments in which the child has contact with other carriers or fomites. In addition, no pediculicide is 100% effective or ovicidal, and improper application of the pediculicide and poor nit removal combing techniques can influence the reinfestation rate (Clore & Longyear, 1993).

Assessment

Parents and clinicians alike often confuse pediculosis with scabies (mites). Both infestations are caused by organisms that primarily choose the scalp as their feeding ground. Lice and scabies may occur in some of the same areas such as the axillary, cubital, popliteal, and inguinal areas. Both lice and mites cause pruritus, although mite infestation is characterized by nocturnal itching as opposed to the continuous pruritus associated with lice. Both infestations are transmitted by close personal contact. Examination of the affected area and microscopic examination of the lice or nits are the classic discerning methods of analysis. Nits fluoresce white under Wood's light. Mites are not visible using this examination technique; rather, scrapings from infected skin must be examined under a microscope to discern the presence of scabies.

The hallmark of pediculosis is intense itching, at all times of the day or night. Any body area, including the scalp, may show signs of the child's intense scratching, such as erythema, scaling, and excoriation of the skin. Head lice infestation is commonly first suspected when children are observed scratching their heads vigorously. Listlessness or poor school performance may also be clues, indicating the child's high level of distraction. On inspection, the examiner observes whitish to sandy colored eggs, known as nits, on the hair shafts. Adult lice may be visualized under a microscope or a magnifying glass. They range in color from light beige to black and have six clawlike appendages.

Brown or cream-colored pubic lice nits attach themselves firmly to hair shafts, making removal difficult. As discussed earlier, pubic lice are often seen in the presence of other sexually transmitted diseases, and affected children must be examined for signs of other such diseases, particularly gonorrhea and syphilis.

Interdisciplinary Interventions

Nurses play a crucial role in assessing children for lice and in obtaining a detailed health history of the child and other family members who might be affected. Parents need to be taught the signs of lice infestation. As mentioned, an infested child typically scratches the infested area, most commonly the scalp, ears, and neck. Parents should examine the child's head in natural light near a window. The most readily identifiable sign is the presence of nits or eggs. Nits can easily be mistaken for dandruff, but the critical difference is that nits must be picked off to be removed.

When lice are detected, the nurse coordinates care to ensure that treatment of the child and affected family members begins immediately. Treatment of lice involves a three-step process: application of a pediculicidal agent, nit removal, and the thorough cleansing (delousing) of the environment. All three steps are crucial to preventing recurrence (TIP 25–3). All potentially exposed persons should be examined and treated if infested. Parents may react to the diagnosis of head lice with a strong emotional response owing to the many myths that surround lice infestation (Table 25–11). The nurse should take time to correct any such misconceptions as necessary.

Pediculicidal agents include lindane, permethrin, and pyrethrins; common brand names include Kwell, Nix, Rid, and Pronto. Parents must be taught how to use the agent, how to apply it, and when to repeat the application if necessary. Toxic side effects, most often seen with Kwell, may include nausea, vomiting, aplastic anemia, hypoplastic bone marrow, convulsions, and death. These serious side effects usually occur after repeated applications. With respect to the pediculicide treatment, parents must be taught that more is not better. Directions for application must be strictly followed. Overuse and misuse may lead to absorption into the blood stream and the possibility of adverse effects. The child's eyes must be carefully protected, and the parent should wear rubber gloves. Pediculicides cannot be used on eyebrows or eyelashes because they are irritating. Rather, lice infestation in these areas is treated by applying petrolatum to the lashes and brows three to four times a day for 2 weeks. The petrolatum seems to suffocate the insects. The nits can then be removed with a fine-toothed comb or tweezers. Lindane should not be used in children younger than 2 years of age or by pregnant women.

TIP 25–3 A Teaching Intervention Plan for the Child with Pediculosis or Scabies

Nursing Diagnoses and Family Outcomes

- Pain related to pruritus.
  Outcomes:
  Child verbalizes a decrease in itching.
  Child is able to concentrate and rest comfortably.
- Health seeking behaviors related to prevention of further infestations
  Outcomes:
  Family completes home treatment regimen to rid the child of the lice or mites, and to treat itching.
  Family cleans the house to rid the home of all lice and mites.
  Family notifies others in close contact with the child of the contagious nature of the infestation.
- Risk for infection related to itching and potential breakdown of the skin
  Outcomes:
  Child will remains free from infection.
  Parents notify health care provide promptly if lesions appear infected or if a fever develops.

Interventions

Treatment of the Child

Pediculosis (Lice)

- Antilice shampoo
  Pour about 2 ounces of the antilice shampoo onto the hair, adding warm water to lather. Scrub the hair and scalp for 10 minutes. Rinse the hair thoroughly and dry.
  Some shampoos require repeat application in 7 to 10 days.
- Removal of nits
  Divide the child's towel-dried hair into four parts and insert the comb at the top of the head first. If nits fall into the lower hair, they will be removed with combing of the inferior areas. Use a fine-toothed comb.

Scabies

- Scabies cream or lotion
  Apply the cream or lotion to every inch of the child's body from the head down. Pay special attention to the navel, between the toes, and in body folds or creases. Leave some under the fingernails. Six to 8 hours later, give the child a bath and remove the cream or lotion.
  Repeat application in 1 week may be recommended.

Cleaning the House

- Wash in hot water all of the child's sheets, blankets, pillowcases, pajamas, underwear, and recently worn clothes. Dry in hot dryer for at least 20 minutes.
- Items that cannot be washed should be set aside in plastic bags for 3 days (for mites) or 3 weeks (for lice/nits) before being used again.
- Vacuum all floors, rugs, play, and sleep areas, and furniture.
- *For lice*—Combs and brushes should be soaked for 1 hour in a solution made from antilice shampoo or in a solution of 1½ tablespoons of Lysol and 1 quart water.
- It is not necessary to have the house sprayed or fumigated.

Contagiousness

- Children can return to school after one treatment with the shampoo or medicine.

TIP continued on following page

TIP 25-3 A Teaching Intervention Plan for the Child with Pediculosis or Scabies *Continued*

- *Pediculosis*—Check the heads of everyone else in the home and treat any scalp rashes, sores, or itching with the antilice shampoo.
- *Sexual partners should be notified of the diagnosis.*
- *Scabies*—Everyone living in the house should be treated preventively with one application of the scabies medicine. Close contacts of the infected child (friends, babysitter, daycare provider) should also be treated.
- Encourage children not to share hats, coats, combs, and similar personal items.
- The child's school or daycare facility should be notified of the diagnosis, and close contacts should be examined and treated prophylactically.
- Promote good general personal hygiene measures.

Contact Health Care Provider if

- Itching interferes with sleep. Teach parents that the rash or the itch may continue for 2 to 3 weeks after treatment.
- The rash is not cleared within 1 week after treatment.
- The rash clears, then returns.
- The rash or sores begin to look reddened, warm to touch, or oozing secretions.
- Fever develops.
- New nits or burrows appear.

Infestation in infants should never be treated with pediculicidal products. Rather, the lice and nits should be manually removed or hand combed. Pregnant women and persons allergic to pediculicidal agents should never apply treatment with these agents.

Community Care

Parents must be instructed to follow the treatment plan faithfully, carefully reading the instructions for the prescribed pediculicide. They also must be taught how to remove nits properly. A fine-toothed comb, usually provided with the medication, is used to remove all nits. The nurse should explain that this is a time-consuming procedure that may be uncomfortable for the child. Hair should be towel dried and not sopping wet, because the nits may otherwise slip through the comb. Special attention should be given to the area around the ears and the nape of the neck, which are heavy infestation areas.

Parents should be warned to avoid treating lice infestation with home remedies. Dog shampoo or kerosene have not been clinically proven to be effective against lice. The latter substance is highly flammable. Furthermore, vinegar applied to the hair root (another common practice) has not been proven to loosen nits from the hair shaft.

Finally, the environment must be thoroughly cleaned. Laundry should be done in hot water or dry cleaned, and placed in plastic bags for 35 days. The home or daycare must be thoroughly vacuumed and dusted with a damp cloth. Pediculicide sprays are not recommended, because they can be toxic to humans and pets.

A social worker or visiting nurse may need to be called to investigate home conditions if lice infestation becomes recurrent or chronic resulting from lack of attention by the child's caregivers. The school nurse plays an important role in preventing and managing head lice epidemics. The school nurse should educate teachers, officials, and parents to do the following:

- Have carpeted areas frequently vacuumed.
- Discourage body contact and sharing of personal items between children.
- Know how to examine for and identify lice.
- Notify the nurse if a case is found.
- Store nap-time supplies in a clean area and send them home for frequent cleaning.
- Have student clothes storage areas (lockers) be separated adequately by space and not be shared.

Schools and daycare facilities should have administrative policies that protect other children (Clore & Longyear, 1990). Parents should be notified about the

Table 25–11
Seven Myths About Lice

Myth	Fact	Action
#1: Lice prefer long hair.	Short-haired children are equally vulnerable.	Female head lice lay eggs near the root of the hair shaft. Therefore, the junction of the hair shaft and the scalp at the nape of the neck and behind the ears should be checked.
#2: The infested person always experiences persistent itching.	A person may be infested and feel no discomfort.	Itching is only one symptom of lice infestation. Other symptoms include swollen glands and pruritus. Therefore, lymph glands should be examined for swelling.
#3: Children primarily get lice from classroom contacts.	The school classroom and daycare are sources of infestation, but a higher risk of contact exists in the home.	All siblings should be checked for infestation. In addition, fellow students, teachers, and daycare providers should be checked for lice.
#4: Lice infest only young children.	Lice can, and do, affect anyone: adults, adolescents, and young children.	When a child is infested, notifying those who have been in close contact with the child and recommending a visit to the family physician may help prevent the lice from spreading to siblings, friends, and adults.
#5: Pets carry lice and transfer them from person to person.	Pets are not a host for lice. Transmission occurs from direct contact (body to body, hair to hair) or indirect contact (clothing, brushes, hair-apparel).	Lice cannot live more than 72 hours off the human body. Therefore the house should be vacuumed thoroughly, combs and brushes should be soaked in antilice shampoo, and all clothing and sheets should be washed in hot water.
#6: Lice only affect those in low socioeconomic groups.	Lice infest individuals from all age groups and socioeconomic strata. If there is higher incidence among the poor, it is most likely due to overcrowded living conditions, a lack of information about the problem, or lack of access to services for help in treatment.	Children should be discouraged from sharing coats, caps, hats, combs, and other personal items with other children at school.
#7: When a person has lice, it means they have poor hygiene and live in a dirty home environment.	Lice infestation is a communicable disease, and everybody, no matter how "nice and clean," is susceptible to infestation.	During bath time, parents should check their child's skin, especially their scalp.

prevention, detection, and treatment program. Parents should clearly understand under what conditions their child may be sent home and when, following treatment, they may return. Children at school who are found to be infested should be sent home immediately. In addition, a treated child's hair must be examined upon return to school for the presence of residual eggs, which could signal reinfestation. Screening programs for lice should be instituted periodically, with parental notification given in advance. The National Pediculosis Association has free guidelines available for controlling head lice in child care environments and schools (see Resources).

Scabies

A contagious skin condition caused by the human skin mite *Sarcoptes scabiei*, or scabies, affects children regardless of gender, age, or socioeconomic strata. Scabies occurs worldwide, with outbreaks occurring in association with crowded conditions, poor hygiene, and malnutrition. In North America, the prevalence of the condition has increased, affecting persons from all socioeconomic levels with no regard for age, gender, or personal hygiene (Sargent & Martin, 1992). It is transmitted by close personal contact. The scabies mite cannot survive for more then 3 days away from human skin. Therefore, it is not carried by fomites (combs, brushes, toys) as often as pediculosis is, although some cases have been documented.

Pathophysiology

The human skin mite (*Sarcoptes scabiei*) present on an infested person is attracted to the warmth and odor of an uninfested host. Once transmitted to the new host, the mite secretes a fluid that allows it to burrow into the stratum corneum, rarely penetrating through the epidermis. The mite sucks human tissue fluids for nourishment. The female mite lays one to three eggs per day for 15 to 30 days. The larvae mature and hatch in 10 days, emerging on the surface of the skin as eight-legged mites. After mating, the males die and the females begin to burrow under the skin to continue the reproduction cycle (Rasmussen, 1994). The host's body begins to respond to the secretions of the mite or its feces, which are highly antigenic. This sensitivity response (itching, scratching) usually begins within a month of infestation.

Prognosis. The prognosis for scabies is excellent. The currently available agents are strong scabicides with minimal toxic side effects. Treatment failure, which does occur, may be due to inadequate education and improperly applied treatment of the child and the environment. Underlying serious immune suppression (as in acquired immunodeficiency syndrome [AIDS]) can delay eradication of the mite infestation.

Assessment

The most common presenting symptom of scabies is pruritus, which is especially profound at night and at nap time. Younger children and infants who cannot scratch effectively respond to the constant itching by crankiness, fitful sleeping, rubbing their feet and hands together, and even refusing to eat. Severe cases can cause significant interference with the mood of the child and with the activities of daily living.

The primary lesion of scabies is the burrow, although vesicles, papules, nodules, and wheals also may appear. The linear, grayish burrows are present in 90% to 95% of all patients with scabies and are easy to find (Rasmussen, 1994). Difficulty detecting the burrows may occur in the presence of excoriation and secondary infections with impetigo. Infestation sites differ by age group. In infants and young children, the lesions may be generalized with distribution on the palms, soles, and axillae being most common. The head and neck may also be affected. In older children, lesions are more often localized, being seen in finger webs, the axillae, body creases, the beltline, genitalia, and nipples.

Diagnostic Tests. Scabies is diagnosed by skin scrapings. A few drops of mineral oil are applied to a burrow, vesicle, or papule, and a dull edge of a scalpel is used to scrape the lesion. Scrapings are best obtained from interdigital areas or from flexor surfaces of the wrist. It may be possible to detect a mite itself moving in the oil. The ova or feces of the mites may be visible. Sometimes it is not possible to find either the ova or feces, leaving the clinician the responsibility of treating the infestation based on the clinical history alone.

Interdisciplinary Interventions

As with pediculosis, treatment of scabies involves not only the affected infant or child but also the family and close caregivers (e.g., baby sitter). Scabicidal agents available include permethrin (Elimite), lindane (Kwell), sulfur 6% in petrolatum, and crotamiton (Eurax). Permethrin 5% in cream is the drug of choice, especially in young children aged 2 months and older, because of its high efficacy and low toxicity (Johr & Schachner, 1997). It is applied once for 8 to 12 hours and removed, then reapplied 1 week later. Lindane 1% lotion is also a good agent, especially for older children. It is applied for 8 to 12 hours and then washed off. A second application is given in 1 week. Lindane can be used on anyone except premature infants younger than 2 months of age and patients with a preexisting seizure disorder (Rasmussen, 1994). The medication can cause convulsions if used improperly.

Sulfur 6% in petrolatum continues to be the scabicidal agent of choice by many physicians for infants (including those younger than 2 months of age), children, and pregnant or lactating women. It is applied nightly for 3 nights and washed off thoroughly 24 hours after the last application. Crotamiton 10% lotion or cream, the least effective scabicidal agent, is applied for 2 days per manufacturer's recommendation. However, studies have revealed that using this treatment regimen yields only a 40% to 50% cure rate (Rasmussen, 1994); thus, it must be given daily for 5 consecutive days. The lotion is malodorous and stains clothing. Topical steroids and antihistamines, such as diphenhydramine (Benadryl), may be administered to help reduce pruritus in older children.

Community Care

Nurses have a major responsibility in the treatment and prevention of scabies. The nurse needs to educate the family to apply the scabicidal agent, strictly following the manufacturer's directions. Most deleterious side effects result from overzealous application of these agents. Parents must be taught to apply the agent to the whole body in infants and children (including the scalp and face), with special attention given to the ears, gluteal clefts, and toe and finger webs. Before application, the child should be given a tepid bath and be dried with a towel. Then the agent should be applied evenly but thinly over the body. In older children, the scabicidal is applied from the neck down. The caregiver should wear rubber gloves during application.

Not all lesions clear immediately. Pruritus may persist after treatment, and postscabietic nodules may persist for months, even after eradication of the mites. The child should not be bathed too aggressively, because the resultant skin dryness can result in excoriation of the skin. The child with excoriated skin is at risk for secondary infection caused by impetigo.

Parents should also be taught that, because a latent period of 1 month occurs following infestation, there may be other, asymptomatic carriers present in the home or child's school. Clothing, bedding, and other contact items should be washed in hot water. Furniture, carpets, and mattresses should be vacuumed. Items that cannot be washed can be placed in plastic bags for 7 days (see TIP 25–3).

Worldview: *Sargent and Martin (1992) recommend that uniform and effective strategies be developed to prevent and control outbreaks of scabies in daycare settings. In one setting, an outbreak of scabies ultimately involved treatment of more than 600 people over a 4-month period at a cost of $16,000. All of the parents were health care workers, further emphasizing that acquiring scabies is unrelated to socioeconomic status and personal hygiene practices. However, effective eradication of the infestation was possible because the daycare staff, parents, and health care team worked collaboratively to use all measures possible to prevent further spread and reinfestation.*

The nurse can help prevent reinfestation by instructing the family in good personal hygiene practices. Other important family teaching topics include how to recognize the signs and symptoms of infestation and the need to make checking the child's skin for mites a regular bath time activity.

Bacterial Skin Disorders

Infections of the skin are so common that few individuals escape without having had at least one bacterial skin infection during the childhood years. Most of these skin problems are easily handled and are benign in course. However, some can evolve into major illnesses if not promptly diagnosed and treated. Cutaneous bacterial infections are among the most frequent inflammatory skin disorders. They can affect the comfort and health of infants and children.

Carbuncles and Furuncles

Carbuncles and furuncles are primary cutaneous abscesses caused by a follicular infectious (usually bacterial) agent, most commonly *S. aureus.* With furuncles, the infecting organism invades the hair follicle and goes deeper into surrounding subcutaneous tissue. When the organism goes deeper and spreads more extensively, it is called a carbuncle. Furuncles and carbuncles occur more often in males than females.

Furuncles and carbuncles have a distinct occurrence pattern. Furuncles occur on the face, neck, armpit, breasts, buttocks, forearms, and thighs, and not on areas with little hair, such as the palms. Carbuncles usually occur on the upper back, nape of the neck, buttocks, and thighs.

Pathophysiology

Furuncles and carbuncles develop when bacteria breach the natural barrier of the skin. Because the hair follicle creates an opening in the skin, bacteria enter it and the body responds to the pathogen in a classic inflammatory pattern (pain, swelling, exudate, fever).

Factors predisposing the patient to furuncles and carbuncles include folliculitis, secondarily infected dermatoses such as scabies, pediculosis, severe acne, obesity, diabetes mellitus, hematologic and immunologic conditions, poor nutrition, poor hygiene, chronic exposure to grease or oils, or trauma such as insect bites or after a drug injection (Ben-Amitai & Ashkenazi, 1993).

Assessment

A child with a furuncle or carbuncle complains of malaise, chills, fever, and adenopathy. The child complains of extreme pain over the area of infection, particularly if the lesions are situated in an area where the skin is fixed, such as the ear canal. The child may guard the affected area from movement to decrease pain.

A furuncle usually manifests as a 1- to 5-cm tender, reddened nodule in 2 to 4 days and develops a yellowish point ("head"). The furuncle may or may not spontaneously rupture at this point. Carbuncles are usually 3 to 10 cm in diameter, develop more slowly, and are extremely painful. Laboratory analysis of the blood or lesions reveals the presence of staphylococci. Bacteremia may also occur in a child with a carbuncle.

Interdisciplinary Interventions

In mild cases, furuncles and carbuncles may resolve without pharmaceutical interventions. Warm soaks can be used to relieve discomfort, and good hygiene measures should be encouraged to prevent spread of the bacteria. The child and parents should be told not to rupture the lesion. Most lesions rupture spontaneously, discharging an odorless, thick pus, tinged with blood. The pain subsides after rupture of the lesion and healing occurs over several days.

In some cases, the lesion has to be incised to release the pus-filled contents. Treatment with a topical antibiotic ointment such as mupirocin (Bactroban) three times per day may be ordered. Soaks and dressings to the lesion site may also be prescribed. Severe infection usually requires oral systemic antibiotics such as erythromycin, sodium dicloxacillin, or minocycline.

The nurse teaches the child and parents that the best protection against this and other skin infection is handwashing with an antibacterial soap. Any infected area should not be touched, and carbuncles and furuncles should not be squeezed. The child should have a daily shower rather than a bath. Clothing and towels touching the lesions should be thoroughly laundered after daily use. The affected child should not share clothing or bedding with other family members.

Impetigo

A superficial skin infection that most often occurs on the face, the arms, and the legs, impetigo is the most common bacterial skin infection in children, accounting for 10% of all childhood skin disorders (Darmstadt & Lane, 1994). Impetigo contagiosa (nonbullous impetigo) and bullous impetigo (staphylococcal impetigo) are the two most common types of impetigo recognized (Table 25–12).

In nonbullous impetigo, small vesicles with crusting develop. In bullous impetigo, large transparent bullae develop on the face, buttocks, trunk, and extremities. Impetigo neonatorum is a form similar to bullous impetigo found specifically in the newborn. Common or secondary impetigo refers to the form that occurs as a complication of a systemic condition or secondary to another dermatologic problem (Shriner, Schwartz, & Janniger, 1995). A child may have the characteristics of more than one type of impetigo at the same time.

Etiology

The cause of impetigo and its characteristic appearance is related to the particular type of impetigo present. Impetigo contagiosa is primarily caused by group A beta-hemolytic streptococcal (GABHS) and *S. aureus* organisms. Bullous impetigo is always caused by *S. aureus*.

Pathophysiology

The causative bacteria are carried in the nasal area and may pass onto the skin. The bacteria invade the superficial skin, causing a characteristic vesicular and pustular response and crusting. Areas most susceptible are those in which a break in the skin has occurred. The infection may be disseminated after scratching an infected site. The infection can also be acquired through contact with other infected children, or through contact with fomites such as combs, brushes, toys, or books that come into contact with areas of the skin that have been compromised by abrasions or minor trauma. Impetigo is more easily spread when such factors exist as crowded conditions, poor hygiene, and play situations in which children have skin to skin contact (e.g., contact sports). *S. aureus* is more prevalent in warm humid climes, whereas GABHS is more prevalent in temperate zones.

Impetigo neonatorum is the form of the skin condition that appears in the neonate as early as the second or third day of life. The neonate may be infected during the delivery or from fomites or people who come into contact with the newborn. Lesions can be few or many, and are most frequently found in moist areas such as the groin, axilla, neck, and umbilicus.

Common or secondary impetigo is a complication of a systemic disease or of a break in the skin caused by another dermatologic condition. For instance, the child with an abrasion or an insect bite is at risk for impetigo because *S. aureus* can easily become colonized in these areas.

Prognosis. Prognosis for uncomplicated impetigo is usually excellent because the lesions are shallow and usually heal without scarring. Transient pigmentation changes can occur in children with dark complexions. Lesions usually remain superficial, but organisms may invade deeper areas, causing cellulitis, lymphangitis, and more serious systemic infections. Bacterial endocarditis has been associated with impetigo. Acute poststreptococcal glomerulonephritis is a rare complication of impetigo. Early intervention with antibiotic therapy does not alter the risk of acquiring acute glomerulonephritis (Shriner et al., 1995).

Assessment

Impetigo lesions are rarely painful. Thus, the family may delay seeking medical attention. Most commonly, secondary symptoms, such as regional lymphadenitis, bring the child to the health care provider's attention. During this

Table 25–12
Types of Impetigo

	Cause	Characteristics of Lesions	Common Site of Lesions	Other Symptoms
Impetigo contagiosa (nonbullous impetigo)	Group A beta-hemolytic streptococcus *Staphylococcus aureus*	Lesions start with a single 2 to 4 mm erythematous macule that rapidly evolves to a vesicle or pustule. Vesicles are fragile and rupture easily, leaving a typical "honey-colored" yellow crusted exudate over the superficial erosion. Lesions spread rapidly to adjacent skin. There is often linear distribution, showing how patients scratched themselves	Skin surfaces exposed to environmental trauma Periorbital area Nares Face Extremities	Mild lymphadenopathy
Bullous impetigo (staphylococcal impetigo)	*S. aureus*	Flaccid and transparent bullae are usually less than 3 cm in diameter on previously untraumatized skin. When the blisters rupture, they leave a "varnish-like" superficial erosion with scant crusting.	Buttocks Trunk Perineum Extremities	Weakness Fever Diarrhea
Impetigo neonatorum	Acquired during delivery, from fomites, or from people *S. aureus* and *Streptococcus* most common	Lesions can range from bullous impetigo to the scaled skin syndrome. Bullae are tense, rupture easily, and leave red, glazed, oozing areas. Classic honey-colored crusting may be present. Lesions spread peripherally and clear centrally. Scale and satellite lesions are present.	Lesions may be few or many, favoring moist surfaces such as the groin, axilla, neck, and umbilicus.	Fever Adenopathy
Common or secondary impetigo	Complication of systemic diseases such as diabetes mellitus, acquired immunodeficiency syndrome Dermatologic conditions that cause a break in the skin may lead to secondary impetigo (e.g., scabies, pediculosis, herpes simplex, insect bites).	Similar to impetigo contagiosa	Site of primary lesions	Mild lymphadenopathy Symptoms of primary condition

time, the infection may have been spread to other members of the household or the child's peers (Chart 25–19).

Classic, nonbullous impetigo begins as a red macule that rapidly forms as a vesicopustule. When the vesicle ruptures, it leaves red, glazed, oozing areas. The drainage dries, forming a thick yellow "honey-colored" crust on the skin (Fig. 25–12).

The bullous form is characterized by pustular blisters that rupture, leaving a thin varnish-like coating. Often, only the remnants of the bullae are present, which can

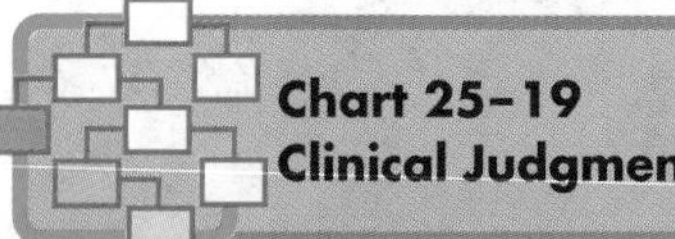

Chart 25–19
Clinical Judgment

The Child with a Rash

When Mrs. Sanchez picked up her daughter Ally from preschool, the teacher told her that Ally had a skin rash on her face that looked like impetigo. Ally could not come back to preschool until she had been seen by her health care provider, with treatment initiated if needed.

Questions

1. If Ally has impetigo, how would you expect the lesions to look?
2. What other characteristics of the lesions and history of this situation could help you confirm the presence of impetigo?
3. The nurse practitioner agrees with the evaluation of the lesions and tells Mrs. Sanchez that Ally has impetigo. What are the primary goals of care at this time?
4. What interventions should be implemented to treat the lesions?
5. What information should Mrs. Sanchez repeat to you to demonstrate her understanding of how to prevent spread of this skin condition?

Answers

1. Nonbullous lesions are vesicles that rupture, leaving moist, honey-colored, crusty lesions on erythematous eroded skin. Bullous lesions are pustular blisters that rupture, leaving a varnish-like coating.
2. The most common site is the face, as seen in Ally's situation. Satellite lesions may occur near the primary site and on other body parts, especially the extremities or perineum. Impetigo is most often seen in children younger than 6 years. A history of pruritus and an earlier skin disruption at the site also confirm the current physical findings. Determine whether any other children at school have impetigo.
3. Treat the bacterial infection and prevent spread of the disease.
4. Gently clean and remove the crusts on the skin. Use topical antibiotics (mupirocin) three times a day for 5 to 14 days. If there is no improvement in 3 days, the child should be seen again by a health care provider, and oral antibiotics would be started and administered for a 10-day period.
5. Ally should be discouraged from touching or picking at the lesions. She should wash her hands frequently throughout the day. If she or anyone else touches the lesions, they should wash their hands immediately with antibacterial soap and water. Ally's fingernails should be cut short. Other members of the family should not use Ally's towel or washcloth. Ally can return to school after she has used the topical antibiotics for 48 hours.

Figure 25–12
A child with impetigo. (From Jarvis, C. [1996]. *Physical examination and health assessment* [2nd ed., p. 256]. Philadelphia: W. B. Saunders. Reprinted with permission.)

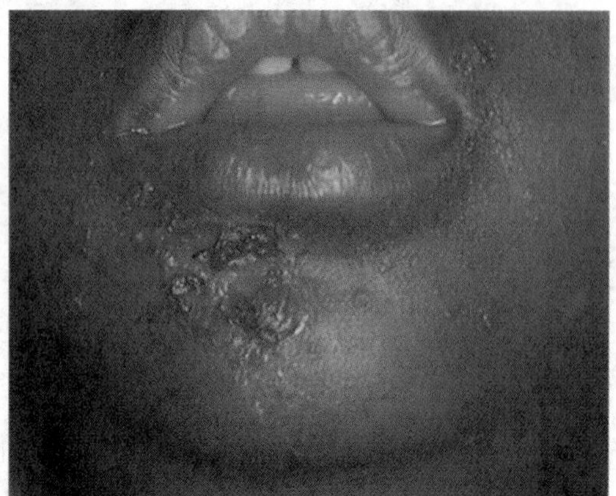

be noted by a narrow rim of scale observed around the edge of the crusted area (Dagan, 1993). The bullae are usually less than 3 cm in diameter on previously untraumatized skin. Impetigo spreads peripherally, and has sharply marginated, irregular borders. When the crusts are removed, a red or pink surface appears.

Diagnostic Tests. Laboratory studies often reveal a slight increase in leukocytes in the blood stream. Gram stains of scrapings from the lesions show gram-positive cocci in clusters, with neutrophils. Cultures and sensitivities are completed to guide therapy because there is an increasing number of methicillin-resistant and erythromycin-resistant strains of *S. aureus*.

Alert: *Some children are chronic carriers of* S. aureus. *Children with recurrent impetigo should be cultured for the organism in nares, perineum, and axillae.*

Interdisciplinary Interventions

Prompt therapy is crucial so that the impetigo does not spread to other children. Treatment of the child with impetigo involves performing daily hygiene to the affected areas, administering oral or topical antibiotic therapy, and instituting measures to prevent further spread. Topical therapies available include Neosporin, Polysporin, and Bacitracin applied four times daily. Mupirocin (Bactroban) is a newer topical agent that is applied three times daily to the skin for 5 to 14 days. The medication is not systemically absorbed. Topical antibiotics are effective if there is good hygiene, general good health, and the lesions are not widespread.

Although many physicians treat impetigo only topically, others prefer to use systemic therapy for neonates and young children at risk for widespread disease and if no improvement is seen within 3 days of initiating topical therapy (Johr & Schachner, 1997; Woolridge, 1991). For systemic therapy, oral dicloxacillin, cloxacillin, cephalexin, or cefaclor may be ordered. Erythromycin has been used effectively for children who are allergic to penicillin; however, S. *aureus* may become resistant to erythromycin during therapy (Kahn & Goldstein, 1993). Also, erythromycin should not be used if there is a widespread erythromycin resistance in the community.

Nursing responsibilities focus on providing education to the family about the treatment plan and helping the family to recognize the infection in case it recurs (TIP 25–4). When a child has a break in his or her skin surface from a cut, bite, or scratch, thorough cleansing of the area can help prevent impetigo.

Cellulitis

A full-thickness, nonsuppurative skin infection involving dermis and underlying connective tissue, cellulitis is fairly common in children. It affects slightly more males than females and occurs in all age groups. Any part of the body can be affected, but the most prevalent location is the legs. Cellulitis around the eyes (orbital cellulitis) is usually an extension of a sinus infection. In children younger than age 3 years, facial cellulitis is commonly associated with otitis media.

Pathophysiology

Most cases of cellulitis develop in skin that has been traumatized or compromised in some way. Predisposing factors include debilitating disease, trauma (e.g., puncture wounds), lymphatic damage, pressure ulcers, immune compromise, and tinea infections. In some hospitalized children, complex nosocomial cellulitis develops at intravenous infusion sites, surgery wound sites, and joint replacement sites. Periorbital cellulitis is often precipitated by infecting organisms from wounds, bites, and sinusitis (Powell, 1995). *Haemophilus influenzae* facial cellulitis has a violaceous hue that is commonly associated with otitis media.

The most common causative agents of cellulitis are GABHS and S. *aureus*, acting solo or in combination. Other microbes that have been implicated include *Escherichia coli*, *Proteus mirabilis*, group B streptococci, and anaerobes. *H. influenzae* and *Staphylococcus pneumoniae* also can cause cellulitis, especially in children (Kahn & Goldstein, 1993). The infecting agents, especially the streptococci, create a large amount of enzymatic spreading factors called hyaluronidase. These substances break down the fibrin network and other subcutaneous barriers that normally localize an infection. In addition, the hyaluronidase can also travel through the lymphatic system. As a result, severe cellulitis can rapidly progress to a life-threatening situation in a child if interventions are not prompt.

Prognosis. Prognosis for cellulitis depends on the promptness and efficacy of treatment as well as on the child's general health status. If not eradicated, persistent cellulitis can lead to necrotizing fasciitis, bacteremia, or osteomyelitis.

Assessment

Characteristic health history and physical examination findings suggest the clinical diagnosis of cellulitis. Other signs include increased white blood cell count, positive blood culture (especially in facial cellulitis), and culturing of an organism from lesion aspirate. In children, 50% of aspirates yield positive cultures, and 10% to 40% of the cases are accompanied by extensive bacteremia (Kahn & Goldstein, 1993).

Cellulitis is characterized by reddened or lilac-colored, swollen skin that pits when pressed by the fingertips (Fig. 25–13). The skin texture may resemble an orange peel, and the borders are usually indistinct and not palpable. Superficial blistering of the area is a common finding. Systemic symptoms include fever, chills, malaise, tachycardia, hypotension, and headache. Regional lymphadenopathy and lymphangitis may occur. The child may appear prostrate and listless and may complain of severe pain over the affected area.

Interdisciplinary Interventions

Hospitalization is required for children with large areas of cellulitis or cellulitis of the face, systemic toxicity, high fever, or hypotension. If the skin ruptures or tears, the physician may order treatment with various types of dressings, for example, a nonocclusive dressing such as with saline-dampened gauze. Moisture-retaining dressings, such as Tegasorb, are contraindicated in active cellulitis

TIP 25–4 A Teaching Intervention Plan for the Child with Impetigo

Nursing Diagnoses and Family Outcomes

- Impaired skin integrity related to presence of vesicles, erosions and exudates.
  Outcome:
  Child's skin shows evidence of healing within 42 to 78 hours of initiation of therapy.
- Risk for infection related to transfer of skin lesions from child to others during close personal contact with family/peers
  Outcomes:
  Child remains free from systemic infection.
  Family members and peers do not contract the skin infection.
- Knowledge deficit: treatment and prevention of impetigo
  Outcomes:
  Family demonstrates measures to treat the child's skin condition.
  Family members participate in measures to prevent spread of the infection.

Instructional Interventions

- Treat lesions as recommended by physician.
  Apply warm water compresses to areas of lesions to remove crust and exudate several times daily.
  Clean lesions gently with mild soap to prevent secondary infection.
  Apply topical antibiotics or give oral antibiotics as ordered.
  Observe for treatment effectiveness such as decreased erythema and drainage.
  Follow-up appointment should be scheduled in 48 to 72 hours if there is no improvement and in 10 to 14 days.
- Prevent spread of infection in affected child and others.
  Observe skin carefully for signs of new infection (erythema, vesicles, erosions, exudate).
  Wash hands before and after caring for lesions, using antimicrobial soap.
  Trim the child's nails and keep them clean.
  Keep the child out of school or daycare activities until after 24 hours of treatment with oral antibiotics or 48 hours with topical ointments.
  Keep child's personal care items (towel, washcloth) separate from other family items until the lesions disappear.

Contact Health Care Provider if

- Presence of lesions does not diminish within 48 to 72 hours of initiating treatment.
- Fever develops.
- Lesions begin to appear infected.
- Other members of the household exhibit the presence of similar lesions.

because they may contribute to the development of secondary infections.

Treatment of cellulitis typically involves administration of antibiotic therapy. The medication used depends on the infecting organism, the child's condition, and the site of infection. A common regimen involves 10 or more days of intravenous therapy with a broad-spectrum antibiotic, such as dicloxacillin, cefotaxime, ceftriaxone, or nafcillin. Once the infection subsides, the antibiotic is typically changed to an oral anti-infective agent, such as oxacillin, Augmentin, or trimethoprim-sulfamethoxazole. Parents should be kept informed of the medication regimen in preparation for continuing treatment of the child in the home following discharge from the acute care facility. Care Path 25–1 summarizes the typical plan of care for the child with periorbital cellulitis.

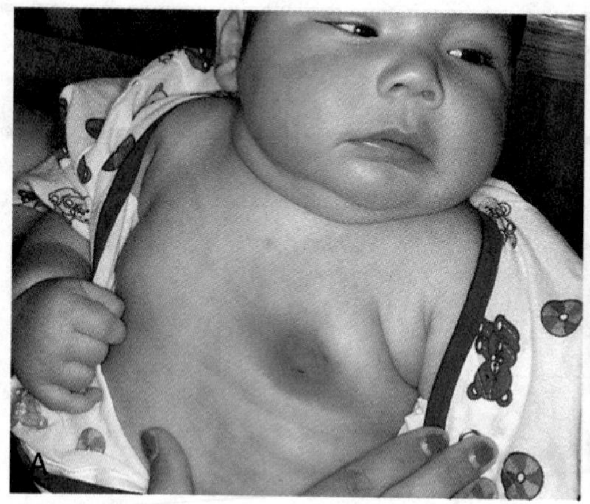

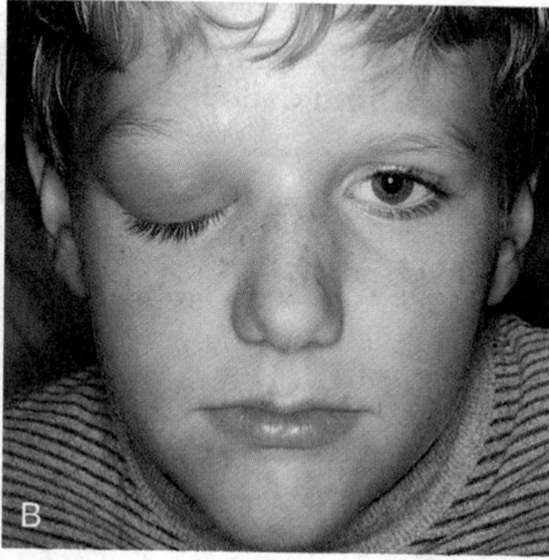

Figure 25–13
A, Cellulitis. *B*, Periorbital cellulitis.

Members of the interdisciplinary team can assist in monitoring and in facilitating the healing process. If the child is debilitated or unable to take foods orally, consultation with a dietitian may be necessary to plan ways to ensure adequate nutritional intake to support tissue healing. In a severely ill child, total parenteral nutrition (hyperalimentation) may be warranted.

During hospitalization, a play therapist or child life specialist can assist in providing diversionary activities for the child. Additionally, children may need to verbalize their feelings associated with the hospitalization and any pain they may be experiencing. The child life specialist can provide play experiences that encourage expression of the child's feelings. Chapter 9 discusses this aspect of the child's care in more detail.

Community Care

The hospital discharge team must be involved in coordinating the child's smooth transition to the home or to the extended care facility. If the child needs help with self-care as a result of hospitalization and debilitation, the discharge planner should arrange for visiting nursing care at home.

Family teaching before discharge should include the expected course or resolution of the cellulitis, the prescribed treatment regimen, and the coordination of home care and return clinic visits. Family members and, possibly, the child may need to learn aspects of dressing care and sterile technique. Caregivers should be instructed to bring the child for scheduled outpatient visits so that the health care team can monitor the healing process, and to promptly call the health care provider if signs of progressing infection develop, such as increased body temperature, or increased swelling or pain at the lesion site or adjacent skin areas.

Cat Scratch Disease

Transmitted by asymptomatic young cats, cat scratch disease (CSD) is caused by a small gram-negative bacillus, *Bartonella henselae*. The condition is characterized by a benign subacute, chronic course of lymphadenopathy that usually resolves spontaneously in 2 to 3 months. Occasionally, CSD causes severe systemic sequelae; this is seen more often in immunosuppressed children. CSD affects primarily children and adolescents; 80% of patients are younger than 20 years old.

Pathophysiology

In 80% of cases, contact with a young cat is reported (Weston et al., 1996). In particular, it has been found that patients with CSD have had close contact with flea-infested, symptom-free kittens, with *B. henselae* bacteremia (Demers et al., 1995). The organism is believed to be spread from kitten to kitten. As the kittens age, they retain antibodies for *B. henselae* and the bacteremia subsides, which is why adult cats are less likely to be the culprits in transmission of this disease. The inoculation site may be a scratch, puncture, or abrasion and is usually nonpruritic and nonscarring.

Assessment

Symptoms of CSD manifest in a classic sequence. Usually, 3 to 10 days after cat contact, maculopapular lesions appear on the skin in the inoculation area and progress to vesicles and pustules. Fourteen to 50 days after the contact, the lymph nodes draining the site of the cat scratch become swollen. The nodes are tender, warm, reddened, and indurated, and they remain enlarged for up to a year.

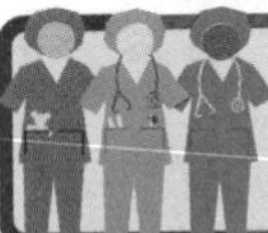

Care Path 25-1 An Interdisciplinary Plan of Care for the Child with Periorbital Cellulitis

Nursing Diagnoses	Patient/Family Intermediate Outcomes		
	Day 1: Admission	**Day 2**	**Day 3**
Impaired tissue integrity related to bacterial infection near the eye and possible sinusitis	Child regains tissue integrity of periorbital area. Child remains free of complications associated with spread of the infection (e.g., meningitis, visual impairment).	→ → Swelling of periorbital area is reduced.	→ → → Parents verbalize and demonstrate periorbital care interventions.
Pain related to periorbital swelling and possible sinusitis	Child experiences minimal levels of pain.	→	→
Sensory/perceptual alterations: visual related to unilateral eyelid swelling and risk for corneal trauma.	Child regains visual functioning. Child and family compensate for visual loss by modifying activities and environment to ensure safety.	→ →	→ →
Care Intervention Categories			
Consults	Ophthalmologic evaluation Otolaryngology	Surgery if trauma is severe	Ophthalmologic evaluation
Discharge planning		Notify home care agency of need for follow-up visits to administer and monitor medication administration.	
Labs	CBC with differential ESR Wound culture of eye Blood culture CSF analysis and culture if needed to rule out meningitis Lumbar puncture in child younger than 1 year of age or if meningitis is suspected in older child		CBC with differential

Day 4	Day 5
→ → → Parents verbalize understanding of home medication regimen.	→ → → Child is discharged home to continue therapy.
→	→
→ →	→ → Child is scheduled for follow-up visits with primary health care provider and with ophthalmologist.
	Ophthalmologic evaluation
Discuss discharge plans with family.	Give family written instructions for home care: medications, signs of complications, follow-up visits. Introduce family members to home care personnel.

Care Path continued on following page

Mild systemic symptoms also occur, including malaise, anorexia, headache, aching, sore throat, conjunctivitis, nausea, vomiting, abdominal pain, rashes, and arthralgia. Fever occurs in only about 25% of affected children. More severe symptoms, such as central nervous system involvement, rarely occur. These symptoms include seizures, myelitis, blindness, radiculitis, encephalitis, encephalopathy, paraplegia, cerebral arteritis, and coma. In severe cases, hospitalization and a critical care stay is necessary.

Diagnosis is based on a history of contact with a young kitten, the presence of lymphadenopathy, positive skin test for *B. henselae*, and identified *B. henselae* organisms cultured from lymph nodes.

Interdisciplinary Interventions

In most children, CSD resolves spontaneously in 2 to 4 months. Antibacterial therapy such as trimethoprim-sulfamethoxazole, gentamicin sulfate, ciprofloxacin, or rifampin may be used to treat the disease. Bed rest and analgesics may be ordered if fever is present. Treatment of local lesions includes warm, moist soaks. Nursing care is supportive and children are rarely hospitalized.

Viral Skin Disorders

Viruses affect the skin as a result of a systemic viral infection that causes viral replication in the skin (viral exanthem) or by producing a virus-induced skin tumor. Any skin eruption associated with an acute viral syndrome is called a viral exanthem (Weston et al., 1996). If the mucosa is involved, it is called a viral enanthem. Viral exanthems include measles, rubella, enteroviral and adenoviral exanthems, roseola, the mononucleosis syndromes, herpes simplex, and herpes zoster. These conditions are discussed in Chapter 24. The discussion in this chapter is limited to warts (nongenital and venereal), which are caused by the human papillomavirus (HPV), and hand, foot, and mouth disease, which is caused primarily by the coxsackievirus.

Warts (Verrucae)

Small epidermal tumors of the skin, verrucae or warts, are one of the most common skin problems seen in children. Caused by HPV, warts have different growth rates and sizes and shapes and can occur singly or in groups. Numerous "old-wives" tales for cures exist.

The warts affecting humans include the common wart (verruca vulgaris), flat warts (verruca plana), plantar warts, and "moist warts" or genital warts (condylomata acuminata).

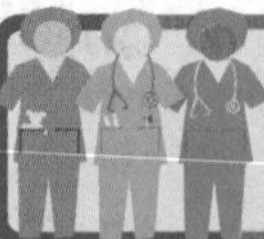

Care Path 25–1 An Interdisciplinary Plan of Care for the Child with Periorbital Cellulitis *Continued*

Care Intervention Categories	Day 1: Admission	Day 2	Day 3
Medications and IVs	Heparin lock IV fluids if unable to drink PO well Broad-spectrum IV antibiotics (cefotamine, ceftriaxime, or cefuroxine plus nafcillin or oxacillin) Acetaminophen p.r.n. for fever or pain Ibuprofen p.r.n. pain	→ *or* Convert IV to heparin lock if taking PO fluids well. → →	→ Change antibiotics as needed based on results of susceptibility testing. →
Nutrition	Diet as tolerated	→	→
Radiology	Radiograph of head to rule out sinusitis	Computed tomography scan of orbital area	
Safety and activity	Bed rest with crib or side rails up HOB elevated 45 degrees at all times Modify activity to adapt to child's visual limitations.	Room restriction if open drainage from wound site → →	To playroom. Continue to modify activities to accommodate child's visual limitations. →
Visitors	Encourage parents or significant others to be present.	Grandparents and other significant others	Encourage sibling visitation.
Teaching	Orient family to hospital and expected events. Discuss safety issues with parents regarding child's visual limitations. Discuss hand washing and other principles of standard precautions.		Wound care of periorbital area Assess and reinforce parent's ability to monitor child's temperature at home.
Treatments	Warm soaks to affected eye three times per day Clean wound site every shift and as needed based on drainage.	→ →	→ →

Day 4	Day 5
⟶	Discontinue Heparin lock
⟶	Change to PO antibiotics. Continue at home to complete 7- to 10-day course of therapy.
⟶	Discontinue pain medications if no longer needed.
⟶	⟶
⟶ ⟶	Discharge to home. Continue to modify child's activities related to visual limitations. Return to school based on visual limitations and recommendations of primary care provider
⟶	⟶
Discuss signs and symptoms of complications (fever, altered level of consciousness, visual disturbances. Oral administration of medications	Date and time of follow-up visits
⟶ Parents complete wound care every day and as needed	⟶ ⟶

Care Path continued on following page

Pathophysiology

More than 70 types of HPV exist that can produce a broad spectrum of conditions ranging from asymptomatic warts to squamous cell carcinoma of the skin (Beutner, 1993; O'Brien, 1995). The clinical manifestations of HPV depend on the type of HPV, the host, and the anatomic site affected.

HPV transmission is through direct contact. Incubation periods range from 1 to 8 months. The virus invades the skin or the mucous membranes, and then skin changes occur. Children who are immunocompromised either by disease or pharmacologic treatment are at greater risk for development of the disease because HPV is known to be a latent asymptomatic infection. That is, once infected, the virus may remain latent in the basal layers of the epidermis, demonstrating manifestations when the child has a weakened immune system.

Most warts resolve spontaneously within 1 to 2 years. Some may require extensive treatment to remove them if they are considered unsightly or occur in an area in which they are constantly irritated by friction against clothing. The therapy should eradicate the problem without causing scarring.

Assessment

Slightly raised above the skin surface, *common warts* are growths that can be very small, or they can be large and clustering. Warts usually occur on the hands, but they can also be seen on the face, knees, and elbows. *Plantar warts* occur on the soles of the feet. They are often surrounded by a collar of hardened skin, and they can cause pain with walking. Warts that are not raised or rough are called *flat warts* and are often seen on the face.

Genital "moist" warts (condylomata acuminata) are single or multiple soft masses that usually appear around the anus, the vagina, or the penis. Occasionally, they can obstruct the urethral meatus or vaginal introitus. The incubation period for genital warts ranges between 6 weeks to 6 months, although much longer periods are possible. The virus is transmitted predominantly through sexual contact, although other nonsexual modes of transmission are possible (Beutner, 1993). These warts are usually asymptomatic, but they can itch, burn, or cause local pain. When untreated, venereal warts resemble cauliflower-like masses. Warts of the genitalia in young children often signal sexual abuse. Strong evidence supports the hypotheses that cervical HPV infection is a major risk factor for development of cervical cancer (Beutner, 1993).

Care Path 25-1 An Interdisciplinary Plan of Care for the Child with Periorbital Cellulitis *Continued*

Care Intervention Categories	Day 1: Admission	Day 2	Day 3
Vital signs/baseline parameters	Vital signs every 4 hours with BP and temperature every 1 to 2 hours if febrile Neurochecks Input and output Height, weight, head circumference on admission	⟶ ⟶ ⟶	⟶ ⟶ ⟶

BP, blood pressure; CBC, complete blood count; CSF, cerebrospinal fluid; ESR, erythrocyte sedimentation rate; HOB, head of bed; PO, by mouth; p.r.n., as needed.

Interdisciplinary Interventions

Management that kills the warts virus has not been uniformly successful. Several treatment modalities may be used to treat warts because no single treatment has been found to be effective. Treatment usually involves freezing the wart or applying chemicals to the wart with the goal of killing the skin that contains the wart virus. It may take several treatments to eliminate the warts.

To freeze the warts, liquid nitrogen (cryotherapy) is applied to the site, followed by electrosurgery to remove the wart. A blister or blood blister may develop at the site within 1 to 2 days. The blistered skin should be soaked in warm soapy water and then the blister can be gently opened (Weston et al., 1996).

Caustic solutions such as lactic acid and salicylic acid are chemical agents that can be applied to eradicate the wart. Chemical solutions may turn the skin white. Every 2 to 3 days, the wart should be soaked in warm water for 30 to 60 minutes. The dead white skin is then gently rubbed off with a washcloth. Warts that are cut off are likely to spread.

Alert: *Concentrated drug store preparations of salicylic acid (e.g., wart removers, plantar wart removers) should never be used on venereal warts.*

Children and families need education about the cause and recurrence of warts. Parents need to know that warts can disappear spontaneously but, even when treated, the course of the disorder can be unpredictable. It is also important for nurses to teach that the spread of warts to other body parts is possible. The nurse should teach that repeated irritation of the wart usually causes enlargement. The nurse should also discuss the transmission of genital warts. Educating adolescents about the cancer risk associated with condylomata and the necessity of prompt treatment is essential.

The psychological and social issues associated with wart infection depend on the severity and location of the disease. Children and teenagers may be especially self-conscious about multiple warts present on the hands or other highly visible areas of the skin. Genital warts can be a cause of profound psychological and sexual dysfunction. Not only are the lesions cosmetically disfiguring, the affected adolescent has the responsibility of protecting his or her sexual partner from infection. There may also be fear of cancer development if the child is aware of the oncogenic link.

Hand, Foot, and Mouth Disease

Hand, foot, and mouth disease is a highly contagious viral syndrome seen most frequently in children during the summer and fall months. It is transferred from person to person by the fecal–oral route and possibly by the oral–oral route. Children younger than age 5 years are most commonly affected. There is also a higher incidence among close contacts in the same household, and outbreaks within a family are not uncommon (Thomas & Janniger, 1993).

Etiology

Hand, foot, and mouth disease is usually caused by the coxsackievirus A16. However, several other serotypes of

Day 4	Day 5
⟶	⟶
Discontinue neurochecks	
⟶	⟶

enteroviruses such as A5, A7, A9, A10, B2, B5, and enterovirus 71 have been linked to outbreaks of the disease (Kushner & Caldwell, 1996). Humans are the only known host of these viruses. The condition has been reported worldwide.

Pathophysiology

As discussed, the spread of hand, foot, and mouth disease is from child to child through the fecal–oral route or possibly the oral–oral route. The virus implants on the mucosa of the throat and ileum, followed by multiplication and extension of the virus to the lymph nodes within 24 hours. By the day 3, lesions on the oral mucosa appear, followed by extension of the disease to other secondary infection sites. Antibodies appear by day 7, with few newer lesions erupting at this time. The incubation period is from 3 to 6 days. Most cases completely resolve within 10 days (Kushner & Caldwell, 1996).

Prognosis. Hand, foot, and mouth disease generally causes only mild difficulties for the child and is self-limiting. However, central nervous system involvement (paralysis, encephalitis, and meningitis) has been noted to occur as a result of the disease. The condition may be dangerous to the newborn and has been associated with spontaneous abortions (Thomas & Janniger, 1993). The lesions of the coxsackievirus A16 may be chronic, reappearing at later dates.

Assessment

Hand, foot, and mouth disease manifests with a mild prodrome consisting of malaise and a low-grade fever. Symptoms of a cold, abdominal pain, and mild diarrhea may also be present.

The appearance of lesions on the oral mucosa is the most dramatic sign. The family generally seeks health care intervention for the child because the mouth and throat are painful, making it difficult for the child to eat. The oral lesions are 3 to 6 mm in diameter, irregularly distributed on the buccal mucosa, tongue, gums, palate, and pharynx. Eruptions of lesions on other body surface areas occurs within 48 hours of the appearance of the oral lesions. Maculopapular eruptions, which may progress to vesicles 3 to 7 mm in diameter, are most frequently seen on the palms, soles, fingers, and toes. Lesions on the buttocks, extremities, and face are more likely to be evident in young children. These lesions are painless.

Diagnosis is made based on the clinical presentation and distribution of the lesions. The virus can be cultured from the cutaneous vesicles or the oral lesions.

Interdisciplinary Interventions

Symptomatic treatment is all that is usually required. Young children may need to be monitored for dehydration and fluid and electrolyte imbalance if the lesions interfere with their ability to eat and drink. The child should avoid citrus, salty, and spicy foods that irritate the sensitive mouth ulcers. A soft diet for a few days and plenty of cool, clear fluids help prevent dehydration and food refusal. After meals, the child should rinse the mouth with warm water to prevent secondary infection of the oral lesions (Schmitt, 1994). Fever and discomfort can be managed with acetaminophen. Liquid Benadryl may be prescribed for the secondary lesion sites on the body if the child is particularly uncomfortable.

Community Care

Because hand, foot, and mouth disease is highly contagious, other family members and children who have had close contact with the affected child should be evaluated for signs of the condition. Spread of the disease is extremely difficult to prevent; therefore, children are not forbidden to return to their daycare or school once their fever has subsided. If the child becomes confused or delirious, has a fever that persists for more than 3 days, refuses to eat, and shows signs of dehydration (dry oral mucosa, decreased urination, listlessness, poor skin turgor, sunken fontanelle), then the child should be seen immediately by a health care provider.

Prevention is possible by teaching families, daycare providers and teachers to use good hygiene practices. In child care settings in which caregivers are changing diapers, gloves should be worn during the diaper change, and hands should be washed with antibacterial soap following disposal of the diaper. To dispose of the diaper, the nurse can instruct the caregiver to pull his or her glove off and over the diaper and diaper wipes, thus encasing the dirty diaper with the glove. The dirty diapers should be placed in a trash receptacle inaccessible to the young children. Children should be taught to wash their hands with antibacterial soap before ingesting any food. For children with pacifiers or bottle feeding, nipples that drop to the ground or are touched by other children should be cleansed thoroughly before being used again by the child.

Fungal Skin Disorders

Infections caused by fungi are common throughout the world, especially in areas where general hygiene measures are poor. Nearly everyone is colonized with some form of fungi. Fungal infections account for a large portion of pediatric outpatient visits. During childhood, infections of the scalp, hair, and body surfaces are common; fungal infections of the hands, feet, and nails are rare before adolescence. Fungal skin infections are not life-threaten-

Table 25–13
Forms of Tinea Infections

Name	Appearance of Lesions	Common Location	Treatment
Tinea capitis	Round patches of hair loss that increase in size Broken hair shafts at surface, leaving a black-dot, stubbled appearance Scaling of scalp Mild itching Usually affects children age 2 to 10 years	Hair and scalp	Apply oral antifungal medication (Griseofulvin) for 6 to 8 weeks. Use antifungal cream twice a week for 8 weeks; at other times, regular shampoo can be used. There is no need to shave or cut hair to prevent spread; hair regrowth is slow. Lesions are mildly contagious. The child can return to school once medications and antifungal shampoos have been started. Affected children should not share combs, brushes, or headwear.
Tinea corporis	Round, pruritic, expanding red lesions with well-circumscribed borders and central clearing Scaling on lesions borders Single or multiple lesions Annular lesions Uncommon after puberty	Entire body, especially face and extremities	Apply topical antifungal cream twice daily for 2 to 4 weeks. Continue application of cream for 2 weeks after the lesions have disappeared. Lesions are mildly contagious. The child can return to school after treatment with topical medication has been started. To control spread, direct contact with infected children and animals should be avoided.
Tinea faciei	Erythematous, scaly lesions that commonly have a "butterfly" distribution	Face	Apply topical antifungal cream twice daily for 2 to 4 weeks.
Tinea cruris (jock itch)	Erythematous, scaly eruption Not usually seen before adolescence	Inner thighs and inguinal creases	Apply topical antifungal cream twice daily for 2 to 4 weeks. Keep area dry. Wear loose-fitting cotton shorts. Cleanse area daily with water and carefully dry. Lesions are mildly contagious and will not affect dry, normal skin.

Table 25–13
Forms of Tinea Infections *Continued*

Name	Appearance of Lesions	Common Location	Treatment
Tinea pedis (athlete's foot)	Vesicles and erosions on the instep of one or both feet Fissuring between the toes, with scaling and erythema Itchy and burning rash Unpleasant foot odor Most forms found exclusively in the postpubertal adolescent	Feet	Apply topical antifungal cream twice daily for 2 to 4 weeks to clean feet. Keep feet dry by wearing sandals, thongs, or no shoes. Wear cotton socks only and change them twice daily. Thoroughly dry feet after bath or shower. Lesions are not contagious.
Tinea versicolor	Multiple annular to oval macules or patches with a fine scale On well-tanned or darkly pigmented children, lesions are hypopigmented.	Neck, upper back, shoulders, upper arms	Wash affected areas with prescribed medicated shampoo of 1% selenium sulfide or 2½% selenium blue over-the-counter shampoo (Selsun Blue) daily for 2 to 3 weeks. Apply topical imidazole antifungal agent twice daily for a week then tapering may be ordered. Not contagious Recurrence is likely. Monthly treatment with the shampoo can prevent recurrence. Normal skin color does not return for 6 to 12 months.
Tinea unguium (onychomycosis)	Distal thickening and yellowing of the nail plate caused by separation of nail plate from bed and entrapment of air between the two structures. Usually found in adolescents.	Fingernails, toenails	Topical agents have not proven effective as a cure. Oral antifungal agents may be used.

ing except when the child is depleted nutritionally or is immunocompromised.

Dermatophytoses (Tinea)

Formally called dermatophytoses, fungal skin infections are caused by the filamentous dermatophytes belonging to the classes *Trichophyton, Microsporum, and Epidermophyton.* These infections are commonly called either "ringworm" or, by the Latin term, "*tinea.*" Dermatophytoses, or tinea infections, are seen in several forms, depending on the body (Table 25–13) (Goldgeier, 1993; Lesh, 1996).

Pathophysiology

Dermatophytes infect the keratin, that is, the stratum corneum layer of the skin, the hair, or nails. Because keratin is shed constantly, fungi must multiply rapidly to keep pace with keratin production. As a result, tinea infections spread rapidly. These superficial fungi form an enzyme that enables them to digest keratin, causing scaling skin, crumbling nails, and breaking hairs. Inflammation associated with tinea infections is the result of an allergic response to fungal antigens that diffuse through the keratin to underlying living skin cells.

Tinea infections are usually transmitted from one infected person to another, either directly or indirectly.

caREminder: *Dermatophytes do not depend solely on humans for growth. Transmission can also occur from infected pets and items such as combs, towels, hats, and pillows.*

Prognosis. Prognosis for tinea infections is excellent because current medical therapy usually eradicates the problem; some forms, however, are resistant to therapy (tinea unguium). Underlying immune suppression, as occurs in AIDS, can make treatment more difficult.

Assessment

Because dermatophytes infect keratin, the superficial skin, nails, and hair are most commonly affected. Tinea lesions are circular or annular (hence the name "ringworm") with an active border that exhibits erythema and scaling. Table 25–13 summarizes the characteristics and treatment of the more common forms of tinea.

Diagnostic Tests. Diagnosis of a tinea infection can be confirmed by potassium hydroxide (KOH) preparation treatment of lesion scrapings and then completing microscopic examination to confirm the presence of fungi. In some cases, cultures of the lesions or a skin biopsy may be necessary to confirm the diagnosis. Some dermatophyte species fluoresce under Wood's lamp (Lesh, 1996).

Community Care

Nursing care focuses on educating children and their families how to follow the prescribed treatment plan (see Table 25–13). The lesion sites should be cleansed thoroughly with water before application of any medicated creams, solutions, or shampoos. Oral antifungal medications must be taken appropriately and any side effects reported to the health care provider. Griseofulvin, the treatment of choice for tinea corporis and tinea capitis, is best absorbed when taken with a fatty meal or glass of milk. To prevent recurrence, all medications must be taken for the entire prescribed period, even if the lesions have faded.

The school nurse can assist in periodic screening of sports participants, such as examining wrestlers for tinea corporis, to decrease the incidence of spread of the condition (Lesh, 1996). Students participating in athletics should be encouraged to change their socks and shoes immediately after a sports activity and expose their feet to warm, dry air by wearing sandals or thongs.

Children with tinea infections should refrain from applying oils or petroleum jelly to their skin or scalp because these agents act as an occlusive medium and can promote more fungal growth. All affected children should be advised not to share hairbrushes, combs, clothing, bedding, and headgear to prevent transfer of the fungi (Chart 25–20).

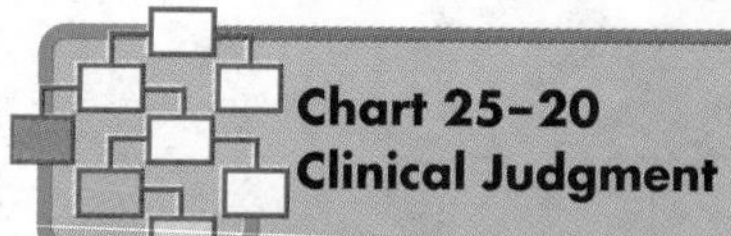

Chart 25–20
Clinical Judgment

The Adolescent with Tinea Cruris

Mrs. Law brings her 16-year-old son, Kevin, to the clinic because he is complaining that he has a pink rash on his inner thigh and groin areas. Kevin is embarrassed about being at the clinic for this problem. When his mother leaves the room during the examination, he asks you whether he got the rash from going skinny dipping in a neighbor's lake with some of his buddies.

Questions

1. As you complete a physical examination, what characteristics of the lesions would indicate that Kevin has tinea cruris (jock itch)?
2. Is Kevin's age a significant factor in confirming this condition?
3. Is the fact that Kevin was skinny dipping significant to the history of this skin condition?
4. What interventions should Kevin take to clear up the rash?
5. Kevin asks, "What do I do if this stuff doesn't go away?" What is your response?

Answers

1. The lesions should be symmetrical, scaly with raised borders, erythematous, and slightly brown or pink. The penis and scrotum should have no lesions on them.
2. Yes. Tinea cruris is unusual before adolescence.
3. No. Tinea cruris is most associated with hot, humid weather and wearing tight clothing.
4. Keep the groin area dry. Wear loose-fitting cotton shorts. Wash clothes, towels, and athletic supporter daily. Using plain water, wash and carefully dry the rash site daily. Apply topical antifungal cream to the site as ordered.
5. If the rash does not begin to improve within 1 week or if it is not completely cured within 1 month, return to the clinic to be reevaluated. To prevent a reinfection, be sure to use the topical ointment for 1 to 2 weeks after the rash has vanished.

Candidiasis

Caused by the yeast *Candida albicans*, candidiasis (candidosis or moniliasis) is an infection that is manifested in the mouth, eyes, and anywhere on the skin. When the yeast is present in the oral cavity, it is commonly called thrush. Candida is a normal flora, but overgrowth can occur on the skin and mucous membranes. Most susceptible are newborns infected during the birthing process, chronically ill children, those receiving antibiotic therapy, and immunocompromised children.

Children with an immunologic deficit are at even greater risk for development of chronic mucocutaneous candidiasis, a progressive infection characterized by large polycystic plaques, resembling ringworm or psoriasis but with thick hyperkeratotic crusts. A defective cell-mediated immunity is a feature of this syndrome. Once immunity is restored to normal, the cutaneous lesions resolve.

Pathophysiology

Congenital candidiasis is acquired in utero, affecting 1% of newborns. The infection is present at birth, characterized by pustular and vesiculopustular lesions that progress to a drying exfoliative stage (Johr & Schachner, 1997). The lesions often clear within a few weeks. Lesions can be found anywhere, including the nails, oral mucosa (thrush), palms, and soles.

Neonatal candidiasis is acquired by the child during the birthing process by delivery through an infected birth canal. The mother usually has a history of a past or present vaginal yeast infection. Neonatal candidiasis is seen in 1% to 4% of neonates (Johr & Schachner, 1997). A classic sign of the condition is the presence of a beefy, red, glazed, weeping dermatitis in the genitalia area. The lesions are well demarcated with raised borders and have slight scaling. Erythematous papules or vesiculopustular satellite lesions surround the periphery of the primary rash.

In infants and young children, candidal infections can develop as either an acute or chronic skin infection, and may be either generalized or localized. In a young child, it is not uncommon for a candidal infection of the diaper area to develop that transfers to other areas of the body, most commonly the oral mucosa (thrush). In the oral cavity, the lesions appear as white plaques on an erythematous base that adhere to the tongue and other oral surfaces tightly and that bleed when scraped. The outer lips appear chapped and cracked. The breast-feeding infant can transfer this infection to the mother's nipples if good hygiene is not promoted.

Candidiasis is often an opportunistic infection made possible by the weakened defense system of the child who is immunocompromised. At risk are children with HIV, children receiving immunosuppressive agents (e.g., steroids, chemotherapy), and children who are compromised by other systemic illnesses. Other contributing factors include trauma, malnutrition, and administration of broad-spectrum antibiotics. Eruption of the lesions has also been associated with excess perspiration or metabolic dysfunction. Local predisposing factors are moisture, macerated folds of skin, and warmth. The fact that infants and toddlers must wear diapers makes them particularly vulnerable to this infection. The prognosis is excellent, given the efficacy of antifungal agents. Systemic involvement must be considered if any of the following conditions are present: immunodeficient sates (HIV or cancer), prematurity with low birth weight, pneumonia or sepsis, or previous treatment with a broad-spectrum antibiotic.

Assessment

Candidiasis presents as a deep, livid, red area of macerated skin with small satellite papules and pustules along the margin. Warm, moist body folds such as the axilla or the genital areas are the most common site of the rash (Fig. 25–14). Diagnosis of candidiasis is confirmed by KOH (potassium hydroxide) slide examination showing budding yeasts and pseudohyphae. A positive fungus culture demonstrates white mucoid growth within 48 to 72 hours.

Older children with candidiasis may complain of discomfort and itching. Children who are too young to express themselves verbally may display fretful behavior and may have trouble sleeping.

Interdisciplinary Interventions

Treatment involves two primary interventions: (1) administering topical or oral antifungal agents and (2) keeping the affected area dry. Commonly used medications include topical anticandidal agents such as nystatin, miconazole, clotrimazole, and ketoconazole. Improvement should be noted within 3 to 5 days. Application of a low-potency corticosteroid cream may be required if inflammation is severe.

Oral infections are treated with nystatin oral solution four times a day for 1 to 2 weeks or with gentian violet 1% to 2% aqueous solution applied twice a day. The solutions should be swabbed onto the mucous membranes using a cotton-tipped applicator (Chart 25–21). Systemic infections are treated with intravenous amphotericin B for 4 to 6 weeks.

The affected area must be kept dry. Frequent diaper changes in infants and toddlers are recommended if candidal infection is in the groin area (see Diaper Dermatitis). The nurse and parents can assist the healing process by leaving the child's diaper off at times, thereby exposing the candidal lesions to the air, which helps them to dry. If topical antifungal agents are ordered, they should

Figure 25–14
An infant with candidiasis.

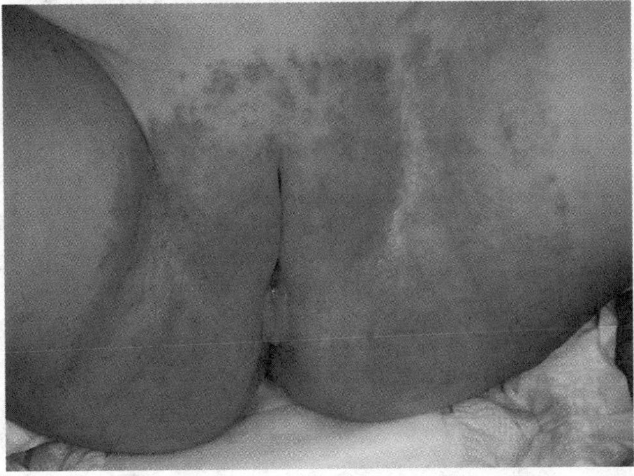

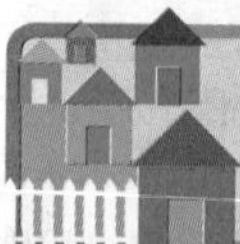

Chart 25-21
Community Care

Care of the Child with Thrush at Home

Medication Administration

- The prescribed solution is applied to the oral mucous membranes.
- A calibrated measuring device should be used to measure the amount of oral solution to be applied. One half of the dose is placed in each side of the mouth.
- A cotton-tipped applicator can be used to apply the solution to the oral mucosa of the young infant.
- Older children should be instructed to hold the suspension in their mouth or swish it throughout their mouth for several minutes.
- The solution is applied after feeding and cleaning of the mouth.
- The child should not drink immediately after application of the solution.
- The infant may swallow some of the solution. This is expected and does not harm the infant.
- If a dose is missed, the medication should be taken as soon as it is remembered, but not if it is almost time for the next dose. Doses should never be doubled.

Medication Storage

- Nystatin must be kept refrigerated.
- The solutions should be kept away from small children to prevent accidental ingestion.

Preventive Measures

- If the infant is bottle-fed, all nipples and pacifiers should be sterilized after each use.
- If breast-feeding, the mother should apply the solution or antifungal cream, as ordered, to her nipples to eliminate reinfection.
- The child's toothbrush should be cleansed thoroughly in hot water after each use.
- The infected child should not share drinking cups or eating utensils with others.

Notify Health Care Provider if

- Irritation of the mucous membrane increases.
- The child refuses to eat or drink.
- The child shows signs of dehydration (poor urine output, lethargy, sunken eyes, sunken fontanelle, poor skin turgor).
- The child shows other signs of illness (e.g., lethargy, fever, cold symptoms).

be applied after each washing or each diaper change. The nurse should teach caregivers to recognize the characteristic lesions indicative of a new candidal infection, especially if the child is receiving antibiotic therapy or is immunocompromised.

Reactions to Environmental Substances

Pressure Ulcers

Pressure areas are localized areas of tissue destruction that occur when the tissue is compressed between a bony prominence and an external surface for an extended period (Quigley & Curley, 1996). Pressure ulcers occur in children and adolescents whose mobility, activity, or sensory perception is severely restricted because of prolonged immobilization or conditions that may impede movement (e.g., a child with myelomeningocele).

Pathophysiology

A pressure ulcer arises secondary to tissue hypoxia caused by the prolonged pressure over a certain area. A critical relationship exists between time and pressure; a lower pressure over a longer period of time can generate an area of skin breakdown as easily as an area of high pressure for a short period of time. Preterm infants and children who are immobilized are two groups of children at high risk for pressure ulcers.

The high-risk areas for ulcer formation are the bony prominences all over the body, such as the sacrum, heel, and elbow, because subcutaneous fat and superficial fascia are thinner and higher pressures are generated. Pressure ulcer locations differ in children according to age. In infants, the occiput is the most likely spot; in older children, sacral pressure is greatest. The scapula is the area of least involvement (Quigley & Curley, 1996).

Assessment

The primary focus of the nursing assessment is to prevent alterations in skin integrity. Quigley & Curley (1996) present a skin care algorithm to establish daily practices that focus on assessment and prevention of skin alterations (Fig. 25–15). Most important is that the intrinsic and extrinsic factors that can precipitate a skin alteration are constantly evaluated. Immediate action should be taken to eliminate these factors or minimize their impact on the integrity of the skin.

If an ulcer has developed, the lesion must be continuously assessed for color, exudate, odor, and dimensions. Pressure ulcers are staged according to their severity (Agency for Health Care Policy and Research, 1992):

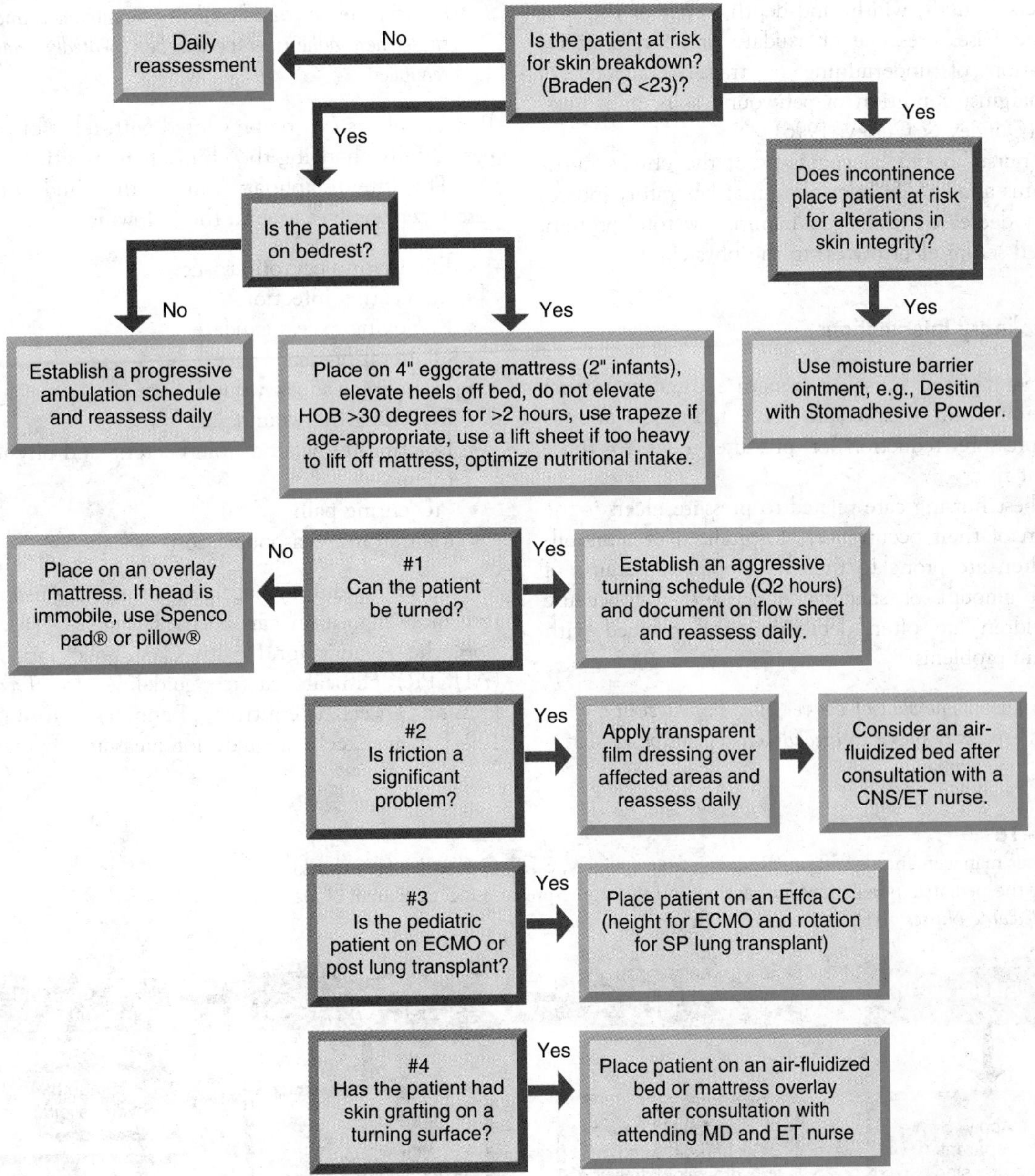

Figure 25–15
Skin care algorithm. (Redrawn from Quigley, S., & Curley, M. [1997]. Skin integrity in the pediatric population: Preventing and managing pressure ulcers. *Journal of the Society of Pediatric Nurses*, *1*[1], 7–18. Used with permission.)

Stage I. Nonblanchable erythema of intact skin, the heralding lesion of skin ulceration. Reactive hyperemia normally persists one half to three fourths as long as the pressure occluded blood flow to the area; it should not be confused with a stage I pressure ulcer.

Stage II. Partial thickness skin loss involving epidermis or dermis. The ulcer is superficial and presents clinically as an abrasion, a blister, or a shallow crater.

Stage III. Full-thickness skin loss involving damage or necrosis of subcutaneous tissue that may extend down to, but not through, underlying fascia. The ulcer presents clinically as a deep crater with or without undermining of adjacent tissue.

Stage IV. Full-thickness skin loss with extensive destruction, tissue necrosis, or damage to muscle, bone, or supporting structures (e.g., tendon or joint capsule). Undermining and sinus tracts may also be associated with stage IV pressure ulcers.

Assessment of the child includes noting anatomic location of the wound, staging (I through IV), size in centimeters (length, width, and depth), type of tissue at the wound base, presence of exudate or odor, presence and location of undermining or tracts, character of wound margins, condition of periwound skin, and dressing type (Quigley & Curley, 1996).

The nurse should be cognizant of the child's nutritional status and should relay abnormal laboratory indices (especially decreased levels of albumin, low total protein, and altered serum electrolytes) to the physician.

Interdisciplinary Interventions

It is crucial for the nurse to recognize the factors that predispose a child to pressure ulcer formation and to provide pressure reduction or pressure relief to those children at risk.

The best nursing care related to pressure ulcers is the prevention of their occurrence. Hospitalized or immobilized children are prone to their development because of the small amount of subcutaneous tissue and because these children are often debilitated and plagued with multisystem problems.

caREminder: *The skin of the very-low-birth-weight infant is especially prone to breakdown. Pectin-based skin barriers can be placed on bony prominences and under sites where adhesive tape will be repeatedly removed and reapplied.*

Pressure ulcers can be prevented with relief of pressure by periodically changing the child's body position.

The interdisciplinary care of the child with a pressure ulcer revolves around the following principles:

- Eliminating necrotic tissue
- Eradicating infection
- Removing excess exudate
- Obliterating dead space
- Providing a moist wound space
- Insulating the wound
- Isolating the wound from bacteria and physical trauma
- Preventing pain
- Maintaining reasonable costs of care

To standardize management of pressure ulcers, a pressure ulcer algorithm can be used (Fig. 25–16). In addition, the Agency for Health Care Policy and Research (AHCPR) clinical practice guidelines for *Treatment of Pressure Ulcers* (Bergstrom, Bennett, Carlson, et al., 1994) is an excellent guide for measures to prevent and

Figure 25–16
Pressure ulcer management algorithm. (Redrawn from Quigley, S., & Curley, M. [1997]. Skin integrity in the pediatric population: Preventing and managing pressure ulcers. *Journal of the Society of Pediatric Nurses, 1*[1], 7–18. Used with permission.)

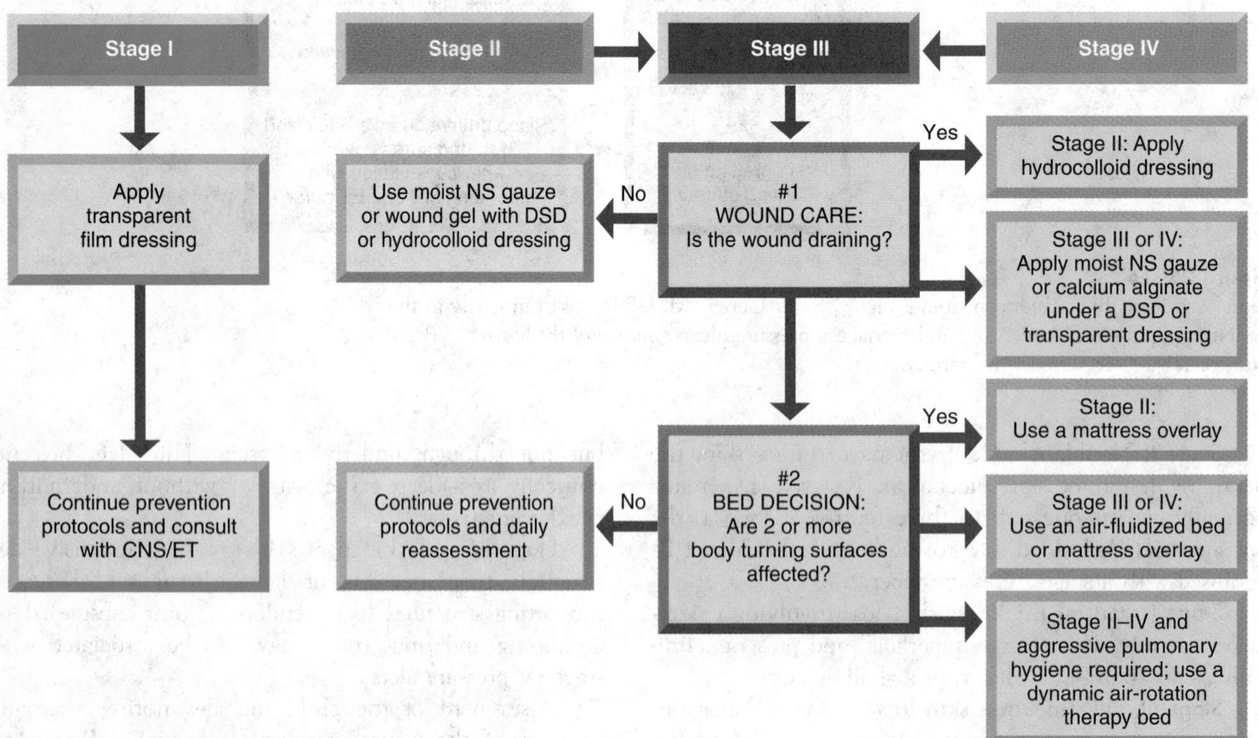

manage pressure ulcers. Although the document addresses the adult population, the principles of staging and the use of dressing options remains applicable to the pediatric population.

Devitalized tissue and exudate can be removed in several ways. Fine mesh gauze with saline dampening can be used on the ulcer in a "wet to damp" method. When removed, the dressing removes necrotic tissue. Another method that can be used is whirlpool therapy.

Special dressings can be used that absorb exudate, insulate the wound, and provide a moist treatment surface. These include the transparent dressings (Op-Site, Tegaderm) and the hydrocolloids (Tegasorb, DuoDerm). Special wound debriding enzymes may also be used to clean up wounds. Toxicity issues must be considered before choosing such an agent, as should be the age and general condition of the child. A final choice is sharp dissection done by the surgeon or by a specially prepared enterostomal therapy nurse.

Tip: *Children resist a painful wound cleansing and dressing change. Avoid using any painful cleansers and, if necessary, premedicate the child with pain relievers before the dressing change.*

If breakdown is present on several body surfaces, special pressure reduction surfaces are available. Special beds that provide pressure relief may be prescribed. These beds are costly, and clinical evidence has suggested that they are often overprescribed when less costly pressure relief devices would be just as effective.

For pressure ulcers that are not responding to any other interventions, a major treatment is the surgical creation of a myocutaneous flap. In this procedure, a piece of muscle near the pressure ulcer site is partially dissected from its original site and is swung over to cover the wound. Because the muscle is not fully removed from its blood supply, the healing process is hastened. Not commonly used in young children, muscle flaps are more common in school-age children and adolescents with mobility problems.

Poison Ivy, Oak, and Sumac

Poison ivy, poison oak, and poison sumac are three potent antigens that characteristically produce an intense dermatologic inflammatory reaction when contact is made between the skin and the allergens contained in the plants. The source of the allergen is *urushiol,* a saplike oil, present on live or dead leaves. Sensitization to one plant produces cross-reactions with other plants containing urushiol.

The skin eruption is a form of contact dermatitis known as **rhus dermatitis.** The rash begins 1 to 2 days after skin contact. The affected skin is characterized by erythema, edema, and vesiculobullous lesions in a streak or patchlike shape, representing the path in which the plant brushed across the skin. The vesicles and blisters rupture, leaking fluid that forms a crust over the lesion site. Fluid from the ruptured vesicles does not spread the eruption. However, antigen retained under fingernails and on clothing initiates new eruptions if not removed by washing with soap and water. The offending antigen may also be carried on animal fur that came into contact with the plants. The sap left on fur, clothing, or shoes is contagious for approximately 1 week if not cleansed properly (Hogan & Weston, 1993; Lane & Darmstadt, 1996).

Learning to recognize the plants and avoid contact with them is an important aspect of education for families, school classes, and youth groups who participate in activities in wooded or swampy areas. Chart 25–22 describes the plants and summarizes the care that should be initiated if the child or other family member comes into contact with poison ivy, poison oak, or poison sumac. Washing thoroughly with soap and water immediately after skin contact is essential because, after 1 hour, the oil is almost completely absorbed into the skin.

Adverse Drug Reactions

Adverse drug reactions (ADRs) are undesired effects arising from the appropriate use of medications (Gupta & Waldhauser, 1997). Although more than 50,000 drug products are available in the United States, the actual incidence of ADRs is not known. In general, 1 in 20 courses of drug therapy is complicated by some adverse drug response (Murray, 1988). The sudden eruption of skin lesions is the most common clinical feature of an ADR (Fig. 25–17).

Several factors have been associated with a higher risk for ADRs in children. These include age younger than 12 months, the presence of serious, concomitant disease, the use of multiple drugs, and an increase in the amount of dose previously prescribed. In many cases, ADRs are preventable by more carefully monitoring the administration of harmful drug–drug combinations and drug–food combinations.

Pathophysiology

Mechanisms that cause ADRs include dose-related reactions, drug interaction reactions, idiosyncratic reactions, and allergic or immune-mediated reactions. *Dose-related reactions* are those experienced by a child because the dose ingested was either below or above the therapeutic level desired. A child may also have a dose-related toxic effect of a drug that is being given at a therapeutic level (e.g., hair loss with Accutane therapy) (Knight, 1993). *Drug interaction reactions* are those caused by the combined use of certain medications that produces toxicity or

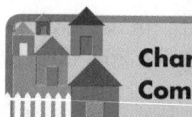

Chart 25–22
Community Care

Protecting Children Against Poison Ivy, Poison Oak, and Poison Sumac

Recognize the Plant

Poison Ivy
Small plant, vine, or low shrub with three shiny green leaflets that grow in groups of three. The leaf stems have waxy, yellow-green flowers, and, later, greenish berries. In the autumn months, the leaves turn red. Poison ivy grows all over the United States, except California and parts of adjacent states.

Poison Oak
Shrubs or vines with oak-shaped leaves that have a hairy, light green underside and darker green surface. The leaves grow in groups of three. Some shrubs or vines have clusters of greenish or creamy white berries. The plant grows on the west coast of the United States and from Mexico to Colombia.

Poison Sumac
Colorful woody shrubs that grow from 5 to 25 feet tall, most commonly found in the eastern United States in swampy areas. A branch of the shrub contains 7 to 13 long, smooth, paired leaves, topped with a single velvety leaf. The plant is bright orange in the spring months, which then turn to a glossy dark green with a pale underside, and then to a reddish orange color in the fall. Poison sumac has dropping clusters of green berries. The nonpoisonous variety has upright red berries.

Protect the Child from Exposure

- Children should wear long pants and enclosed shoes with socks when walking in the woods or swampy areas.

If the Child is Exposed

- Immediately wash and rewash the affected area with yellow or brown laundry soap or nonperfumed bath soap and cold water. Do not use a brush on the skin to avoid scratching the skin surface.
- Wash and rewash any clothes that came into contact with the plants.
- Wash any pets that came into contact with the plants. Wear gloves and do not touch the animal's fur with bare hands. Dispose of the gloves afterward.

To Help with Itching

- Soak the involved area in cool water or apply cool compresses to the skin. Then let it dry.
- Apply calamine lotion to the rash.
- Apply topical steroid creams as ordered by the health care provider.

Call Health Care Provider if

- Face, eyes, or lips become involved
- Signs of infection appear, such as redness, oozing, or pus at lesion sites
- Rash begins to blister
- Itching interferes with child's sleep

combined lethal side effects. For instance, morphine and diazepam used together place a child at higher risk for apnea than if the drugs were used alone. *Idiosyncratic reactions* are attributed to an unusual characteristic about a particular child that causes him or her to have an adverse response to a certain medication. Allergic or immune-mediated reactions are created by immunologic mechanisms that produce a wide variety of systemic responses to the drug, including anaphylaxis reactions, Stevens-Johnson syndrome (SJS), neutropenia, and thrombocytopenia (Knight, 1993).

Infants and children are at great risk for ADRs for several reasons:

- The child's neurologic system may respond and is susceptible to impairment because it is still develop-

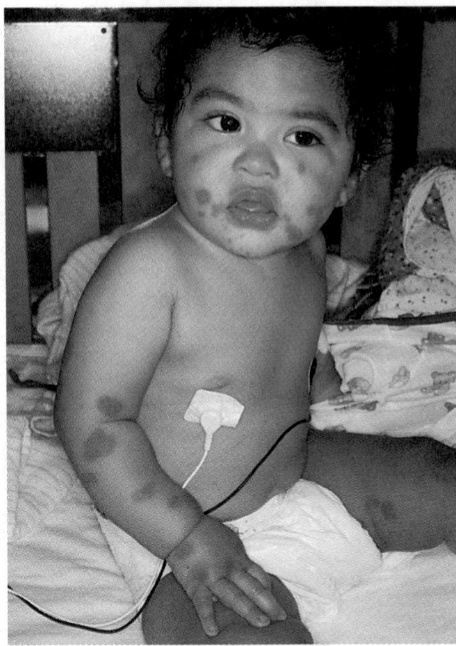

Figure 25–17
Adverse drug reactions can manifest in various skin eruptions.

ing after birth (e.g., first-generation antihistamines are sedating in adults but are associated with paradoxic excitation in some children).

- Drugs given to mothers during pregnancy, delivery, and lactation can lead to adverse reactions for the child owing to their teratogenic, pharmacologic, and toxic processes.
- Topical absorption of medications is enhanced in neonates and young children because of the increased permeability of their skin.
- The sick neonate and children with chronic conditions (e.g., cancer, asthma) are exposed to a large number of medications, thereby increasing their risk of an ADR.
- Symptoms of an adverse reaction may go undetected because the child's condition masks the side effects or are similar to those of an ADR.
- Premature infants and full-term neonates have a lesser capacity for renal elimination of drugs because of decreased glomerular filtration and tubular secretion.
- Many medications for children are in liquid form and contain excipients designed to improve the stability and tested acceptability of the medication. These additives can cause adverse side effects (Gupta & Walhauser, 1997).

Assessment

Skin eruptions caused by a drug reaction are diverse in nature, and it may be difficult to identify the exact cause. For example, in the seriously ill child, the appearance of an unusual rash may be an allergic response to a drug or may be the result of a newly acquired viral infection.

Questions that can help detect a drug reaction include

- What drugs or over-the-counter medications is the child receiving?
- Has the child ever had an allergic reaction to a medication in the past?
- Has there been a recent change in the child's dose of medication?
- Are any of the agents being taken by the child known to commonly cause drug reactions in children?
- What other agents or processes could be causing the skin lesions?
- What chronology of events occurred that led to the eruption of the lesions?
- Does the child have any chronic conditions?

Morbilliform (measles-like) rashes are the most common type of skin manifestation seen in children in response to an ADR. However, drug reaction rashes can also assume several other forms (Table 25–14). The lesions may be accompanied by itching, malaise, fever, nausea, vomiting, and liver or kidney damage. Severe anaphylactic reactions can occur as characterized by severe skin involvement, respiratory compromise, and shock. Anaphylaxis is discussed in more detail in Chapter 30. Any acutely occurring rash should be evaluated for a drug reaction. Common drug offenders include ampicillin, penicillin, cephalosporins, phenytoin, barbiturates, and diazepam.

Interdisciplinary Interventions

The most immediate measure to take when an ADR occurs is to stop using the suspected drug. Treatment is individualized and may vary from simply monitoring the child with no special interventions provided, to treating the severe manifestation of anaphylaxis. Most children do not require hospitalization. If itching and rash formation are severe, oral antihistamines, oral steroids, or both may be ordered. If blistering occurs, the child's fluid and electrolyte status should be monitored. The child with blisters is at risk for infection of the open lesions.

The nurse plays an important role in providing education to the family to help prevent future ADRs. Reviewing signs of an ADR with the family can assist in the early identification of problems that may reoccur. Medication derivatives from the same family as the agent that caused the adverse reaction should be avoided. It should be recommended that the child wear a Medic Alert bracelet to notify others that the child has a medication allergy.

Table 25-14
Clinical Features of Drug Reactions

Type of Drug Eruptions	Drugs Associated with the Reaction	Clinical Signs	Treatment
Morbilliform	Allopurinol Amoxicillin Ampicillin Barbiturates Carbamazepine Cephalosporins Chloramphenicol Erythromycin Gentamicin sulfate Gold Isoniazid Nonsteroidal anti-inflammatory drugs (NSAIDs) Penicillins Phenytoin Sulfonamides Trimethoprim	Measles-like (morbilliform) or exanthematous lesions that start on the trunk and move to extremities Areas of normal skin may surround areas of eruption. Initial lesions become papular and then form plaques from joining of several individual lesions Fever Malaise Arthralgia	Remove offending drug. Rash may fade with time, requiring no treatment. Give antihistamine therapy.
Urticarial	Acetylsalicylic acid Amoxicillin Ampicillin Cephalosporins Horse serum Penicillins Sulfonamides	Edematous, flat, erythematous papules that last less than 24 hours As lesions resolve, they may leave a macular brown bruised appearance. Angioedema of mucous membranes	Remove offending drug. Give antihistamine therapy. If needed, give systemic steroids to maintain airway and diminish swelling associated with angioedema.
Serum-sickness–like reaction	Cephalosporins Hydantoins Penicillins Sulfonamides Streptomycin	Fever Malaise Large urticarial plaques that resolve, leaving the skin areas with a dusky or bruised appearance	Remove offending drug. Take fever reduction measures. Apply symptomatic treatment using combination of analgesics, glucocorticoids, and antihistamines.

Genetic and Immune-Related Disorders with Dermatologic Manifestations

Several skin conditions appear linked to genetic susceptibility or a systemic immunologic response. The conditions discussed in this chapter include urticaria and angioedema, dermatomyositis, Stevens-Johnson syndrome, and Wiskott-Aldrich syndrome. In many cases, the exact mechanisms that trigger the dermatologic clinical features are unknown. The underlying insult that causes skin injury is likely to produce other clinical manifestations that can be severe. The child is cared for by an interdisciplinary team that includes support from dermatology, rheumatology, physical therapy, and nutrition specialists. Treatment is aimed at controlling skin lesions, preventing or reversing other systemic manifestations, and supporting the child and family through the course of long-term therapy if required.

Urticaria and Angioedema

Urticaria is manifested by well-demarcated, raised erythematous lesions that blanch with pressure. The lesions are usually pruritic and involve the superficial layer of the dermis. Urticaria is a symptom that might be triggered by several disease states (Charlesworth, 1995). In many cases, the exact causative source may not be known.

Table 25–14
Clinical Features of Drug Reactions *Continued*

Type of Drug Eruptions	Drugs Associated with the Reaction	Clinical Signs	Treatment
Serum-sickness–like reaction *Continued*	Thiouracils	Lesions may be accompanied by angioedema. Arthralgia Lymphadenopathy Edema Albuminuria	
Fixed	Barbiturates Carbamazepine Phenazone derivatives Phenolphthalein Sulfonamides Tetracycline Trimethoprim	Solitary or multiple sharply demarcated erythematous lesions that may look like urticaria or become bullous As lesions fade, skin remains hyperpigmented with residual sharply demarcated outlines of the lesions.	Remove offending drug. Give antihistamine therapy.
Vasculitis	Allopurinol Barbiturates Gold Penicillins Sulfonamides Thiazide derivatives	Soft, small erythematous papules or urticarial papules that blanch when pressure is applied Over several hours to several days, lesions become firm and dark red or purple.	Remove offending drug. Give antihistamine therapy.
Exfoliative dermatitis (Lyell's syndrome)	Allopurinol Barbiturates Hydantoin derivatives Penicillins Phenazone derivatives Sulfonamides Sulindac	Diffuse erythema followed by bullae and loss of large portions of epidermis tissue	Remove offending drug. Give cyclosporine therapy Give intensive, specialized care similar to that given to a child with severe burns.

Data from Weston, W., Lane, A., & Morelli, J. (1996). *Color textbook of pediatric dermatology*. St. Louis: Mosby–Year Book.

When the urticaria extends deep into the dermis (subcutaneous or submucosal layers), it is known as *angioedema*. Angioedema is usually characterized by normal-appearing skin with overlying swelling. Rather than pruritus, a tingling or burning sensation accompanies angioedema.

Urticaria and angioedema may occur at any age, although incidence is higher in young adults. Approximately 15% to 25% of the population has a history of one or more episodes of urticaria (Charlesworth, 1995). Most of these cases are acute and self-limiting, not extending beyond a 6-week period. Acute or transient urticaria is more common in children and young adults. In some cases, the urticaria extends beyond the 6 weeks and may display periods of exacerbation for years. This chronic or persistent form of urticaria most commonly affects older women.

Pathophysiology

The cause and effect relationship between a trigger agent and the development of urticaria and angioedema cannot always be established. In some cases, the reactions can be attributed to an allergic trigger or an infection. Urticaria may be the result of an immune-mediated reaction, a complement-mediated reaction, or a non–immunologic-mediated mechanism (Chart 25–23). In most cases, the urticaric response is caused by mast cell histamine release as a result of the trigger agent or toxin. The histamine release causes vasodilatation and edema of the skin and

Chart 25–23

Mechanisms That Cause Urticaria

Immune-Mediated Urticaria

Allergic reactions (drugs, food, insect venom)
hysical urticaria (cold, heat, pressure, vibration, solar exposure, exercise)
Atopic diathesis

Complement-Mediated Urticaria

Collagen vascular diseases
Transfusion-related reactions
Hereditary angioedema
Acquired angioedema
Serum sickness (type III)
Necrotizing vasculitis

Non–Immunologic-Mediated Urticaria

Direct mast cell–releasing agents (opiates, muscle relaxants, radio contrast media)
Histamine-releasing agents
Intolerance reactions (aspirin, nonsteroidal anti-inflammatory medications)

mucous membranes. In the physical urticarias (those caused by cold, heat, and so on), histamine levels appear normal. The chemical mediator of physical urticarias appears to occur through cholinergic fibers of the autonomic nervous system (Weston et al., 1996).

Assessment

Evaluation of the child must begin with a thorough history eliciting information that specifically identifies when the lesions occur, how long the lesions last, and the events that might precipitate a flare-up. In particular, the association between some type of food or medication (such as aspirin) that might trigger the occurrence of the lesions should be noted.

Acute urticaria and angioedema are defined by the sudden appearance of lesions or attacks of sensation (tingling). The lesions are pruritic with erythematous raised wheals, 2 to 15 mm in diameter, scattered over the body. The center of the lesion is pale in color and has tense edema.

The wheals usually persist for 20 minutes to 3 hours, disappear, and then reappear at another location. An episode generally lasts 24 to 48 hours, although it may extend up to 6 weeks. When lesions appear for longer than 6 weeks, the urticaria is considered to be chronic. The subcutaneous extensions of the lesions, or angioedema, appear as large swellings around the eyelids, lips, face, trunk, genitalia, and extremities.

The physical urticarias are characterized by large (10 to 20 mm) blotchy erythema areas surrounded by small (1 to 3 mm) central wheals. Heat, exposure to cold, ingestion of hot or spicy foods, a febrile illness, hot baths, and exercise sufficient to raise the body temperature 0.5°C induce an attack. Delayed-pressure urticaria can cause angioedema beginning 4 to 6 hours after the pressure and lasting up to 24 hours. This is most commonly seen in adolescents who wear backpacks to carry their schoolbooks and personal items.

The physical examination includes tests for physical urticaria. For instance, light stroking of the skin with a blunt object may cause an intense wheal and flare reaction known as *dermatographism*. The application of a warm or cold stimulus that causes the appearance of wheals and intense itching can be used to diagnose cold- or heat-induced urticaria. An exercise challenge may be used to help elicit exercised-induced urticaria.

Interdisciplinary Interventions

Interventions for the child experiencing an acute attack of angioedema includes treatment with oral antihistamines for 3 to 4 weeks until the antigen is eliminated. Hydroxyzine hydrochloride or diphenhydramine hydrochloride are most commonly used. Severe acute cases may require the use of subcutaneous or intramuscular epinephrine; in a few, systemic corticosteroids may also be needed.

If airway involvement results from angioedema, close monitoring in an acute care facility is indicated until the attack has been resolved. Narcotics may be required for relief of abdominal pain and nasogastric suction may be needed if the child has emesis. H_2 receptor antagonist may be useful in some children in controlling airway or bowel reactions.

Pharmacotherapy may include H_1 antihistamines. A prolonged course (3 months or longer) may be needed to suppress the condition and induce a remission. Failure to induce a remission may indicate inadequate dosage or the need to change to a different antihistamine. Medication withdrawal must be completed gradually to prevent a rebound effect. If the urticaria recurs, the medication must be restarted at full strength.

Community Care

Long-term treatment for the child should include avoidance measures to reduce the likelihood of another outbreak. These measures include excluding certain foods from the diet and avoiding medications that contain aspirin or related compounds. If no precipitating event is obvious, a daily diet and symptom record can be initiated to help elicit this information. If a clear precipitating factor is not found, an elimination diet consisting of lamb, chicken, rice, and water for 2 to 4 weeks may be tried. If the child's symptoms do not improve, it is unlikely that the urticaria was caused by a food substance. If improvement is seen, foods can gradually be reintroduced until a normal diet is achieved. A dietitian may provide assistance to families by providing them with suggestions for how nutritional requirements may be met through the diet phase and whether certain foods should be avoided for a long-term period.

If the child has urticaria triggered by physical factors, these factors should be avoided. For example, thermal protection is important for children with cold-induced urticaria and the generous use of sunscreens is helpful for the child with solar urticaria. The child with exercise-induced symptoms should be encouraged to decrease or stop the activity at the first sign of symptoms. Exercise-induced urticaria has been reported to be more pronounced in individuals who exercise after ingestion of certain foods such as shellfish, celery, peaches, grapes, and wheat. Therefore, it is important for some children to avoid exercise for 4 to 6 hours after ingesting a known offending food or medication.

Dermatomyositis

Childhood dermatomyositis is a multisystem inflammatory disease of uncertain origin that affects primarily skin and muscles. It is characterized by a nonsuppurative (without pus) inflammation of striated muscle and skin, which causes symmetrical proximal muscle pain and progressive weakness, and a rash of the hands, face, and trunk. Swallowing difficulties from pharyngeal and upper esophageal muscle involvement is common, as is palatal dysfunction. This typically results in nasal speech.

Etiology and Incidence

The frequency of dermatomyositis in the United States appears to be 1 per 200,000 people according to a hospital survey (Weston et al., 1996). In children, the prevalence rate is 1.1 per 1,000,000 whites and 7 per 1,000,000 blacks. Data suggest that the peak age of onset of childhood dermatomyositis occurs between the ages of 10 and 14. The average age of onset in childhood is 7 years of age. There is a concentration of symptoms in February, March, and April in 55% of the children with dermatomyositis. Girls are affected slightly more often than boys in a ratio of 1.7 : 1.0 (Warren, Perez, Wilking, & Myones, 1994).

Although there may be a relationship between several viruses and dermatomyositis, the cause is not completely clear. Coxsackievirus antibodies, influenza, echovirus, and hepatitis have been suggested as possible viral triggers for dermatomyositis (Pachman, 1990).

Pathophysiology

The primary process is a vasculitis that may cause ulceration of the skin or gastrointestinal tract in addition to affecting small blood vessels in the musculature. It may also involve both the respiratory system, leading to interstitial pneumonitis or hemorrhage, and the myocardium, resulting in congestive heart failure (Ansell, 1991). The disease may be monocyclic (occur once), chronic polycyclic (more than once occurrence), or chronic continuous in nature.

Prognosis. The overall prognosis for individuals with dermatomyositis has improved with the use of high-dose corticosteroids and steroid-sparing agents. The prognosis is related to the degree of vasculitis in the child and the length of time inflammation is present before therapy is initiated.

▽ **Alert:** *Evidence indicates that long-term prognosis is directly related to the rapidity of diagnosis and the treatment. In a child with dermatomyositis, progressive muscle weakness may slowly develop. This is often unnoticed until fever, rash, or muscle pain develops.*

Death may occur and is usually related to myocarditis, unresponsive myositis, pulmonary vasculitis, or acute gastrointestinal ulceration and bleeding. Death may also be caused by overwhelming infection during the course of treatment.

Assessment

The onset of juvenile dermatomyositis is acute in one half of cases, with a rapid development of muscle weakness and rash. In the other half of cases, the onset is more insidious. Muscle disease is usually marked by weakness and tenderness, which are most prominent in the proximal muscles of the lower extremities. Children may exhibit the Gowers' sign (an inability to walk, rise from the floor, or dress) (see Fig. 20–10).

The skin may exhibit signs of diffuse vasculitis. The child may have a heliotrope (sun-seeking) rash on the eyelids and periorbital edema. The child may also have cutaneous ulcers involving axillae, pressure points, digits, or oral mucosa. An erythematous dermatitis called Gottren's papules is often present over the knuckles of the hands, knees, elbows, and ankles. Calcinosis (deposits of calcium in the skin) can occur in children with chronic active disease.

The examiner must ascertain whether the child has had any difficulty swallowing as a result of pharyngeal or palatal weakness or experienced a change in voice (dysphonia). Muscle involvement of the upper esophagus may contribute to dysphagia.

Other clinical findings may include respiratory muscle weakness, hypertension, hematuria, myocarditis, vasculitis of the gastrointestinal tract with mucosal ulceration and bleeding, Raynaud's phenomenon, and pulmonary vasculitis, which may cause pulmonary hemorrhage or lead to interstitial fibrosis. In a small percentage of children, there may also be evidence of arthritis.

Diagnostic Tests. Laboratory evaluation usually demonstrates elevated erythrocyte sedimentation rate (ESR) and elevation of serum glutamic oxaloacetic transaminase greater than serum glutamic pyruvic transaminase. Aldolase is typically elevated with a normal gamma-glutamyltransferase, and elevations of muscle-specific enzymes are present. The levels of these enzymes should start to normalize after 3 to 4 weeks of treatment. Electromyography of affected muscles is abnormal. Muscle biopsy may be needed to confirm the diagnosis, especially when skin findings are absent or minimal.

Nursing Diagnoses and Outcomes

The child with dermatomyositis requires care that focuses primarily on the clinical features of the skin lesions, muscle weakness, and dysphagia. In addition to the nursing diagnoses presented in Chart 25–6, the following diagnoses may be applicable:

- **Impaired mobility related to muscle weakness with or without pain**
  Outcomes: The child exhibits increased mobility.
  The child shows no evidence of complications such as contractures, thrombus formation, or skin breakdown.
  The child attains highest degree of mobility within confines of the disease.
  Parents and other caregivers participate in mobility regimen with the child.
- **Impaired swallowing related to pharyngeal muscle weakness**
  Outcomes: The child maintains adequate nutritional intake.
  The child maintains weight within acceptable age parameters.
  The child shows no evidence of aspiration pneumonia.
  The child and parents demonstrate correct feeding techniques to maximize swallowing.

Interdisciplinary Interventions

The aims of therapy are to control inflammation, return ESR and muscle enzymes to normal, control skin lesions, promote restoration of muscular function, and maintain the child's nutritional status.

Medical Management

Medications. With active inflammation, corticosteroids have been the mainstay of medical management for several decades. Administration of oral prednisone with slow tapering over 6 to 12 months is the classic approach to therapy. More recent regimens aimed at decreasing steroid side effects and improving control of the disease and patient outcomes are replacing this regimen at many pediatric rheumatology centers. Infusion of intravenous methylprednisolone usually elicits improvement over the first 4 weeks of therapy. The nurse must monitor muscle strength, presence of rash, vasculitic lesions, dysphagia, diplopia, dyspnea, and myocarditis in children receiving this therapy. Attention must be given to gastrointestinal or respiratory hemorrhage. Complications of steroid therapy, including weight gain, salt retention, and elevated serum cholesterol and triglyceride levels, must also be monitored. Corticosteroids can also arrest linear growth. Therefore, the dose of corticosteroids and the time span that these drugs are used should be kept to a minimum while still achieving clinical improvement.

The addition of another medication such as cyclosporine or methotrexate must be considered in children who continue to have difficulty swallowing, vision problems, dyspnea, or steroid toxicity. If these medications do not bring about improvement over several weeks, the addition of still other cytotoxic agents such as azathioprine may be necessary to improve outcome. Cytotoxic medications have fewer side effects than steroids for long-term therapy and appear to be steroid sparing in their activity. A persistent rash can often be controlled with the addition of hydroxychloroquine to the medical regimen. Health care providers must be vigilant in monitoring both the disease process itself and the side effects related to the medical therapy. Early recognition of adverse effects may help prevent serious complications that can result in adverse patient outcomes.

Skin Care. Dermal vasculitis may be photosensitive, so sun avoidance is critical in its control. Hydroxychloroquine is often effective in healing the skin rash. Skin ulcerations pose a risk for secondary infections and require meticulous wound care to prevent extensive scarring. The therapeutic agents required to control the vasculitis may cause immune suppression, so care must be taken to prevent ulcerations and, if necessary, to treat them early.

Restoration of Muscular Function. Disability in affected children is not only related to the muscle weakness associated with active myositis but also to the severity of flexion contractures and the degree of calcinosis experienced by the child. Therefore, clinical management should be focused on these areas. Restoration of strength may require significant physical therapy and occupational therapy.

Once the diagnosis of acute disease is made, promoting rest is a primary intervention. Initially, when the muscles are actively inflamed, attention should be given to preventing the loss of muscle range through gentle stretching and passive range-of-motion exercises. A physical therapist may be helpful in ensuring that the correct posture is maintained while the child is on bed rest. The child should have straight hips and knees, and have his or her feet at a 90-degree angle. Splinting of the affected body part may be required in cases of severe weakness. The trunk and upper limbs may be supported by pillows, sandbags, or other devices as appropriate. If the child is to be placed in a sitting position, splints may be necessary to support the child's lower extremities and a soft neck collar may be needed to provide nuchal support and stability. Trunk support in a well-fitted wheelchair may be needed later in the course of the disease. The physical therapy program should focus on normalizing function as much as possible and preventing the formation of muscle contractures.

Nursing interventions to support the child's physical therapy progress include diligent skin care (prevention of skin ulcerations and checking for any redness or indentation that is indicative of pressure points). While the child is hospitalized, the splints should be removed every hour initially, progressing to at least once per shift or as otherwise recommended by physician or physical therapist. The nurse should explain the rationale for the program to the child before executing exercises.

Nutritional Management

Nutritional management includes ensuring that children receive a diet appropriate for their age and ability to swallow. For example, liquids may need to be thickened and pureed food may be required. A dietitian may help develop a diet that is low in lipids and salts but high in protein; this type of diet helps to decrease the child's development of weight gain and hypertension. Antacids may be used to relieve gastritis. Antacids that are low in sodium and contain both aluminum and magnesium hydroxide have advantages over others. However, because muscle weakness is a rare side effect of magnesium hydroxide, it may be necessary to alternate it with another agent (e.g., calcium carbonate).

Children who require long-term high-dose steroid therapy are at risk for osteopenia and compression fractures. The degree to which supplementation with dietary calcium and vitamin D is useful in preventing osteopenia is still uncertain. Excessive calcium supplementation may lead to hypercalciuria, which can predispose the child to calculus formation or increased blood pressure (Ansell, 1991).

As the child's overall status improves, the nurse should consult with the dietitian and physician to slowly normalize the consistency of the food. In conjunction with the dietitian, the nurse may instruct the family regarding necessary dietary restrictions and assist families to accommodate the diet while making the diet as palatable as possible.

Community Care

The nurse should educate the children and families about the disease and the medications used in its treatment. Parents should be taught how to appropriately administer the medications. Having this knowledge can empower families, leading to a more positive outcome for the child.

All children with dermatomyositis should be encouraged toward independence in all activities of daily living and physical activities. Children should participate in sports to the extent that they are able. Nurses should encourage the children and parents to set realistic goals, slowly progressing to normalization of activities. Children must be taught to heed warning signs such as joint pain and muscle fatigue and to stop activity accordingly. Again, when participating in outdoor activities, children should wear sunscreen.

The nurse should also provide both the child and the family with opportunities to discuss their concerns in an environment in which they can freely share their emotions. All health care providers should make families aware of educational resources (e.g., Arthritis Foundation, Muscular Dystrophy Association) and support networks within their community.

Stevens-Johnson Syndrome

SJS is a severe bullous form of erythema multiforme characterized by lesions of the skin and mucous membranes, fever, and systemic toxic effects.

SJS occurs in children and young adults and affects males more frequently than females. Onset often follows an upper respiratory infection. The association of SJS with patchy pneumonia, increased titers or cold agglutinins, and the isolation of *Mycoplasma pneumoniae* has suggested a relation to mycoplasma infection.

SJS is most often noted in association with ingestion of sulfonamides, anticonvulsants, penicillin, and barbiturates (Birdsall & Gabasan, 1993). There is increasing evidence that SJS may be the result of genetic susceptibility to this injury (Weston et al., 1996).

The mortality rate of SJS may be as high as 10% during the acute phase, particularly in children with pulmonary involvement. Subsequently, the disease is self-limiting: skin lesions gradually subside without scarring in 1 to 4 weeks; mucous membrane lesions may persist for months.

Assessment

Most children with SJS have a prodrome of fever and malaise, a nonspecific respiratory infection, and possible petechial rash. The hallmark of the syndrome is the development of an erythematous papular skin lesion that enlarges by peripheral expansion and usually develops a central vesicle. This eruption may involve cutaneous surfaces, including the palms and soles. Lesions may be scattered or confluent, and new lesions appear for 1 to 2 weeks after onset. Rupture of cutaneous lesions tends to occur, leaving the child at risk for fluid loss, anemia, bacterial superinfection, and sepsis. Vesiculobullous lesions also occur on mucous membranes of the conjunctivae, nares, mouth, anorectal junction, vulvovaginal region, and urethral meatus. Lesions have been described in the larynx, trachea, bronchi, bladder, and gastrointestinal tract (Barnes & Dire, 1994). Esophageal stricture or visual impairment from corneal scarring may produce long-term sequelae such as eating difficulties and impaired vision. The diagnosis of SJS is made by history, presence of vascular lesions on at least two mucous membranes, fever, presence of systemic toxic effects, and appearance of classic cutaneous iris or target lesions.

Diagnostic Tests. Laboratory diagnosis is not helpful in SJS because diagnosis is made clinically. However, complete blood count with differential, blood urea nitrogen, creatinine, electrolytes, urinalysis, and culture of lesions, blood, and urine are useful in supportive evaluation and management of systemic effects (Edwards & Ridder, 1985).

Interdisciplinary Interventions

The goals of therapy are to provide supportive care while the epidermis regenerates and to minimize the potential for subsequent morbidity. An interdisciplinary specialty team of health care providers is required to adequately assess and manage SJS. Consultants include intensivist and ophthalmologists to minimize morbidity and mortality. Nursing care is aimed at supportive measures in the acute phase of the illness and includes meticulous skin care, early detection and treatment of infection, careful attention to fluid balance, nutritional support, and alleviation of symptoms.

Skin Care. The intensivist is responsible for supportive care for children who are potentially unstable, particularly those with hypovolemia. Surgical consultation is required for children with severe skin lesions; treatment is similar to that for a child with burns, and the child may be managed in a burn unit or a pediatric intensive care unit. Therapy includes daily bathing with saline, antibiotic ointments applied to eroded areas, and antibiotic mesh gauze applied to denuded areas. For severe damage, operative wound debridement and xenografts may be required, but are rarely necessary. Pain management should be a critical part of wound management (Rasmussen, 1995). The nurse should use age-appropriate pain assessment tools such as Faces or numerical scale to monitor pain relief and adequacy of comfort measures (see Chapter 13).

Skin care includes use of sheepskin or air-fluid beds to reduce pressure on blistering or eroding skin. Lesions should be bathed daily with normal saline or Burow's solution compress and dressed with antibiotic or mesh gauze, depending on the extent of lesions. The child should be positioned frequently. Children with extensive lesions should be placed in reverse isolation. Mucous membranes should also be cleansed with normal saline, followed by application of petroleum jelly ointment. Viscous lidocaine may be used on oral mucosa. The nurse must be alert to early symptoms of infections such as elevated temperature, positive blood culture, change in vital signs, or increased irritability.

▽ **Alert:** *Viscous lidocaine should be applied with a cotton-tipped swab sparingly to the oral cavity. Swallowing viscous lidocaine interferes with the gag reflex and swallowing.*

Viscous lidocaine jelly can be used in the perineal area for pain relief, and saline compresses can be used on eyes to reduce crusting of eyelid margins.

Treatment of Infection. Antibiotic therapy is only indicated when sepsis is diagnosed or strongly suggested by the child's clinical condition or positive blood cultures. Neutropenia has been suggested as a criteria for prophylactic antibiotic therapy, because this finding has been shown to indicate a poor prognosis. Systemic steroid use is not indicated and may increase risk of complications such as sepsis and gastrointestinal hemorrhage.

Nutrition. Nutrition management is based on severity of clinical symptoms, ranging from a soft or liquid diet in mild cases to intravenous fluid management in moderate to severe cases. The child may require parenteral nutrition, or hyperalimentation, during acute phases of the illness.

Careful monitoring of fluid balance is required as it is in a burn patient. Fluid resuscitation with colloids or crystalloids may be required for hypovolemia or sepsis-induced hypotension. Urine output should equal 1 mL/kg/hr. A Foley catheter may be required for children with difficulty voiding or with urethritis.

Eye Care. The ophthalmologist should examine the child's eyes daily, mechanically separating the lids and the palpebral from bulbar conjunctiva, if necessary. Children may need systemic as well as topical analgesia for this procedure. Pseudomembranes obstructing vision may require removal. Topical antibiotics are prescribed for children with positive eye cultures. Upon the child's discharge, a follow-up appointment should be made with the ophthalmologist to ensure that no permanent visual impairment has occurred.

Community Care

If the onset of SJS is thought to be linked with a particular drug, an important aspect of patient education is to teach the child and family to avoid ingestion of that agent in the future. Long-term follow-up is necessary for children in whom complications develop as a result of mucosal or skin scarring. As discussed, ophthalmologic consultation is an important aspect of the overall plan of care, and further evaluation for visual impairment should be completed once the child is discharged form the acute care facility.

Wiskott-Aldrich Syndrome

Wiskott-Aldrich syndrome (WAS), an X-linked recessive immunodeficiency disorder, is characterized by eczema, thrombocytopenia, and recurrent infections. The immune abnormalities in these children include defective T-cell function, poor antibody response to polysaccharide antigens, and altered serum immunoglobulin levels (normal IgG, high IgA, high IgE, and low IgM levels). Platelets are small and have shortened survival. Affected children rarely survive to adulthood because of bleeding or serious infection.

Assessment

Boys with WAS usually are seen in infancy with petechiae or bleeding. Prolonged bleeding from the circumcision site may be noted. They typically have an eczematoid rash involving the antecubital and popliteal fossae. Superinfection of AD may lead to cellulitis, furunculosis, and abscess formation.

Eventually, recurrent infections such as sinusitis, otitis media, and pneumonia develop in most affected boys. Both gram-negative and gram-positive bacteria can cause disease. Children with this disorder are unable to form antibodies to bacterial polysaccharide antigens, resulting in a high incidence of bacterial infections. These children may also have severe periodontal disease. Children with WAS have increased susceptibility to infections with herpes simplex, varicella, and cytomegalovirus. Overwhelming sepsis or meningitis can be fatal in affected children. Splenectomy may be required for thrombocytopenia, but it can increase risk of septicemia and requires long-term antibiotic prophylaxis. Reactions to vaccines with polysaccharide antigens may exacerbate petechiae, eczema, and purpura in these children. They may also have asthma, autoimmune hemolytic anemia, arthritis, and glomerulonephritis. There is an increased risk for malignancy (primarily lymphomas and leukemias) during the second and third decades of life, which are often fatal.

Interdisciplinary Interventions

Topical or oral steroids may be required to treat AD in children with WAS. If the skin is superinfected, it should be cultured and treated aggressively with an antibiotic to which the organism is sensitive. Infections need to be treated immediately with antibiotics to prevent sepsis from developing. The nurse can educate parents to use the same skin care regimen used with a child with AD to maintain optimal skin integrity. The most common organisms to cause infection are *S. pneumoniae* and *H. influenzae*.

Biopsies are contraindicated in children with thrombocytopenia, even when they have chronic renal disease, because of the high risk for bleeding. Acute episodes of bleeding that may occur in WAS usually respond to transfusions with fresh platelets; the platelets must be irradiated before use to prevent graft-versus-host disease.

Splenectomy elevates platelet counts, increases platelet size, and may significantly reduce the risk of morbidity through bleeding. Milder thrombocytopenia can occur even after splenectomy. There is increased risk for severe bacterial infections occurring after splenectomy, which may be decreased through pre-splenectomy pneumococcal vaccination and the use of long-term prophylactic antibiotic therapy (daily penicillin). Preventing infection is, therefore, an important component in the care of children with WAS. The nurse can aid the child and family to formulate a plan for infection control measures (e.g., promoting good hygiene, screening visitors for infection). Even with the most stringent care, infection may still develop, and nurses must educate parents that the development of an opportunistic infection is in no way related to poor infection control.

Intravenous immune serum globulin (IVIg) may be used in these children to replace antibodies if the child's immunoglobulins are either deficient or absent. Otherwise, its use is primarily as an additional protection or barrier to infection. IVIg is usually given every 3 to 4 weeks because its half-life ranges from 21 to 28 days. It may be given in an outpatient or clinic setting or in the child's home. A nurse involved with these infusions must monitor the child's vital signs closely for the duration of the infusion. Most reactions to IVIg are rate dependent in nature; however, a small percentage of patients may experience anaphylaxis. Children with total IgA deficiency (<7 mg/dL) are at high risk for anaphylaxis during IVIg infusion because they can have anti-IgA antibodies that react with the IgA contaminating the IVIg preparations. If a rate-dependent reaction (i.e., fever, chills, back pain, arthralgia, myalgia, hypotension, or respiratory distress) develops, the infusion rate must be decreased. A mild reaction may simply require stopping the infusion briefly and then restarting it at a slower rate. A severe reaction may necessitate the use of epinephrine and Benadryl. For this reason, infusions must be administered in a setting where they can be closely monitored and emergency equipment is readily available until the child's tolerance for the infusions can be ascertained.

Bone marrow transplantation has been used successfully in WAS. Successful transplantation may completely reverse both the platelet and immune dysfunction, and, in many cases, completely eradicate the eczema as well.

Thermal Injuries

Thermal injuries are caused by hot and cold environmental forces that can result in alterations ranging from redness of the dermis to loss of circulation and cellular functioning in an extremity or other part of the body.

Severe burns are among the most debilitating and disfiguring of all skin alterations. The third most common accidental injury in children, burns can have a traumatic impact on the child and the family as they attempt to cope with the deleterious effects of the injury. All but the most minor burns may impact a child's self-image and can cause discomfort. Although it is substantially less ominous than major burns, sunburn, a type of minor burn, may have long-term carcinogenic effects in children.

Cold injury can also cause disfigurement and long-term discomfort to the child if exposure to cold-wet or cold-dry conditions is prolonged in the presence of inadequate protection against these elements.

The most important interdisciplinary management strategy for thermal injuries is to teach prevention. Wearing proper attire, using protective skin creams and lotions, and regulating the time exposed to very hot or very cold weather conditions are important interventions to prevent thermal injury.

Sunburn

One of the most common skin injuries, sunburn results from excessive exposure to UV radiation in the sun's rays. Human skin has several defenses against UV radiation, including the stratum corneum, which absorbs some of the UV rays, and melanin, which increases pigmentation in the skin and protects against UV damage. Generally, children with greater amounts of skin pigmentation (i.e., those with darker complexions) do not burn as quickly as fair-skinned children. Nonetheless, any child can be sunburned with sufficient sun exposure.

Pathophysiology

The cutaneous photosensitivity in sunburn is a result of overexposure to UV radiation, particularly to the radiation of the UVB wavelength. The UVA wavelength can also cause burns, but does so only after much longer exposure. The exact cause of UV radiation damage is unknown. It is thought to result from a combination of direct effects, generation of toxic oxygen species, and the production of inflammatory mediators (Weston et al., 1996). Most children respond to UV radiation with increased skin pigmentation (tanning). Thus, tanning is a sign of UV injury to the skin. UV effects are cumulative. Cutaneous cells may demonstrate the additive effects of radiation exposure many years later as demonstrated by fine and deep wrinkling of the skin, scaly red patches, and the potential for skin cancer formation.

Acute UV radiation exposure induces erythema secondary to vasodilation and increased blood volume in the dermis. Metabolic changes within the epidermis cause the cells to change shape and morphologic makeup. The symptoms of sunburn begin 30 minutes to 4 hours after sun exposure. Peak reactions to sunburn occur 24 to 36 hours after the initial symptoms and may last up to 72 hours. Symptoms fade within 4 or 5 days.

Worldview: *Approximately 15% of white children have skin that never tans. These fair-skinned children with their freckles, blond or red hair, and blue or green eyes are at increased risk for sunburn and skin cancer. These children should be taught to wear sunscreen throughout the summer and to avoid direct sun exposure whenever possible.*

Prognosis. The prognosis is good for sunburn, as long as the child is removed from sun exposure and he or she receives prompt treatment. The more serious issue related to chronic sunburn is the increased risk of skin cancer. UV radiation is the primary cause of skin cancer. UV radiation also damages the connective tissue of the dermis, causing premature skin sagging and wrinkling later in life. In most persons, nearly 50% of such skin damage occurs before age 18. Furthermore, it has been recognized that chronic UV-induced damage actually causes changes in the skin's immune function (Nicol & Fenske, 1993). Although acute sunburn may be treated adequately, parents and older children must be made aware of the aging and carcinogenic effects of chronic sun damage.

Assessment

Sunburned skin appears tender, reddened, and possibly slightly swollen. Severe sunburn may produce tense edema, vesicles, and bullae. On the head, the most prominent areas affected include the nose, cheeks, forehead, and ear lobes. On the extremities and trunk, skin areas unprotected by clothing are most effected.

Children with sunburn may have difficulty sleeping because of their discomfort. Sunburn over large areas of the body may result in systemic symptoms such as vomiting, headache, fever, chills, and malaise. In severe cases, extensive sunburn causes a reduction in the child's ability to sweat and may contribute to collapse from heat stroke.

Nursing Diagnoses and Outcomes

In addition to the nursing diagnoses presented in Chart 25–6, the following diagnoses may be applicable:

- **Altered tissue integrity related to reddened, tender, and swollen responses of the epidermis to overexposure to the sun**
  Outcome: The child experiences comfort and healing to areas that have been sunburned.
- **Health-seeking behaviors regarding sun exposure protection and prevention**
  Outcome: The parents and child initiate preventive measures to protect the child's skin from excessive exposure to the sun.

Interdisciplinary Interventions

Cool water soaks or wet dressings can be used to reduce the pain and erythema of sunburn. Aspirin or indomethacin are inhibitors of prostaglandin synthesis that may modify the intense epidermal response of sunburn if given within 48 hours of exposure. There is no evidence to suggest that topical glucocorticosteroids are beneficial in relieving pain or inflammation. When skin peeling occurs, a moisturizing cream may be applied.

Community Care

The best treatment of sunburn is prevention through limiting sun exposure and through using an effective sunscreening agent on exposed skin (Fig. 25–18).

caREminder: *Children younger than 6 months of age should not be exposed to direct sunlight because their sensitive skin and decreased sweating rate places them more at risk for heat stroke.*

Most sunscreens contain some combination of para-aminobenzoic acid (PABA), cinnamate, salicylates, and anthralin. A broad-spectrum sunscreen that protects against both UVA and UVB radiation should be used because it has been determined that both UVA and UVB can cause acute and chronic damage to the skin. Sunscreens protect the skin through absorption, reflection, and scattering of the UV radiation. The quantifiable effectiveness of the sunscreen is expressed as "sun protection factor," or SPF. SPF is based on the UV-absorbing properties of the active chemical ingredient in the sunscreen. In general, the higher the SPF number of a sunscreen, the greater the protection provided to prevent UV radiation damage to the skin. For example, if a child normally burns within 15 minutes of exposure to the sun without sunscreen, use of a sunscreen with SPF 15 allows the child to stay in the sun 15 times 15 minutes or 225 minutes (3 hours and 45 minutes) before achieving the same degree of erythema or burn (Nicol, 1989). Reapplication of the sunscreen does not prolong this time period. The SPF 15 sunscreen only protects the child for 225 minutes, no matter how many times it is applied during that period. Sunscreen agents that are waterproof with SPF of 15 or greater are recommended for children.

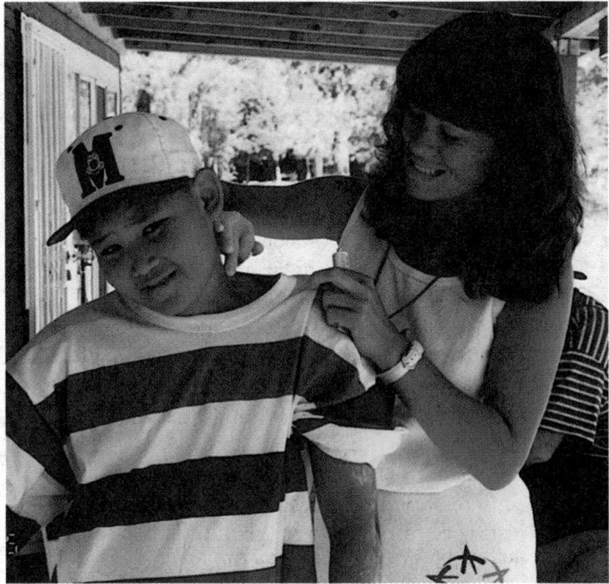

Figure 25–18
Sunscreens can be used to protect the skin through absorption, reflection, and scattering of the ultraviolet radiation. (Courtesy of Camp Ronald McDonald for Good Times.)

The nurse instructs parents and older children on how to treat acute sunburn and on how to prevent sunburn in the future (Chart 25–24). Recent research suggests that, although most parents are fairly knowledgeable about the relationship of sun exposure to skin cancer, many do not have a solid understanding of practical preventive strategies, such as how to choose the best sunscreen (Foltz, 1993). In addition, many parents have poor sun protection practices themselves, and their own degree of protection has been found to positively relate to degree of protection practiced for their children (Buller, Callister, & Reichert, 1995; Zinman, Schwartz, Gordon, Fitzpatrick, & Camfield, 1995). Thus, the nurse needs to teach parents to protect themselves and serve as an example of how to implement safe practices to their children. The nurse should point out that sunscreens do not protect the child's skin from all UV radiation; even with their use, tanning or burning will occur if exposure is of sufficient duration. Proper skin protection requires

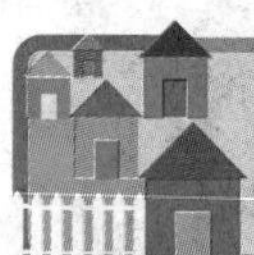

Chart 25-24
Community Care

Fun-in-the-Sun Safety: A Checklist

1. Choose a sunscreen that blocks both ultraviolet (UV) A and UVB radiation.
2. Choose a product that includes a sun protection factor (SPF) rating of 15 or greater.
3. Do not use sunscreens on children younger than 6 months of age. Instead, use hats, bonnets, and light-colored clothes to protect the skin, and keep the infant away from direct exposure to the sun.
4. For children older than age 2 years, choose a sunscreen product based on the child's previous history of response to sun exposure. Sun-sensitive children should not remain outdoors for a long period of time, and an SPF product of 39 or 50 should be used to protect them.
5. Apply the sunscreen indoors, before exposure to sun (some product labels recommend at least 30 minutes, and others recommend up to 2 hours).
6. Reapply sunscreen after bathing, swimming, or perspiring if exposure to the sun is resumed. However, reapplication does not prolong the time frame of initial protection, which is provided by the selected SPF.
7. Some sunscreen products are labeled to denote that they offer protection in special circumstances:
   Sweat-resistant—protects for up to 30 minutes of continuous heavy perspiration then must be reapplied
   Water-resistant—protects for up to 40 minutes of continuous water exposure then must be reapplied
   Waterproof—protects for up to 80 minutes of continuous water exposure then must be reapplied
8. Minimize exposure to the sun near the hour of noon.
9. Know whether any medication the child is taking causes photosensitivity.
10. Encourage children to wear lightweight, long-sleeved shirts and broad-brimmed hats during prolonged sun exposure.
11. If the child's skin feels warm, it is.
12. Take one or more of the following actions to protect the child's skin:
    Cover the skin.
    Apply sunscreen.
    Remove the child from sun exposure.

using a sunscreen and exercising good judgment in limiting sun exposure.

Fire and Burn Injuries

Burn injury to children may be accidental or may be nonaccidental. Nonaccidental injury involves child abuse by burning or by neglect in adult supervision that results in harm to the child. Accidental burns in children younger than 5 years of age are likely to occur as a result of environmental situations that are not controlled by caretakers. Natural curiosity and increasing mobility in the child at this age contribute to the risk. Scald injury is the cause of many burn injuries in infants and toddlers (Finkelstein, Schwartz, Madden, Marano, & Goodwin, 1992) (Table 25–15). Approximately 16% of burn injuries are related to child abuse (Herrin & Antoon, 1996a).

Incidence

Fire and burn injuries are a leading cause of accidental deaths in children ages 1 to 14 years. In the United States, one third of burn victims are children (Gordon & Goodwin, 1997). Eighty-five percent of all burns are related to scalds; flame burns cause 13% of injuries; and the remainder of burns are electrical and chemical. The total number of reported burn injuries has decreased since the mid-1970s. Of the approximately 50,000 children treated in hospitals for burns, about 45% are treated in one of the 120 burn centers in the United States. There are 15 pediatric burn centers in the United States.

Table 25–15
Scald Burns—Time of Exposure Versus Temperature

Water Temperature (°F)	Time (Seconds)
120°	>300
125°	120
130°	30
135°	10
140°	5
145°	3
150°	1.5
155°	1.0

From Tarnowski, K. (Ed.) (1994). *Behavioral aspects of pediatric burns.* New York: Plenum Press. Reprinted with permission.

Electrical Injury and Associated Conditions

Electrical injury is a major injury that often results in instant death as the electrical current disrupts the electrical rhythm of the child's heart, causing lethal arrhythmias. The child who does not die instantly is at risk for four major complications during the acute phase. These complications include cardiac arrest or arrhythmia, tissue damage due to interrupted blood flow, myoglobinuria (globulin from muscle serum), and metabolic acidosis.

Interdisciplinary Interventions

Cardiac Arrest/Arrhythmia. The immediate risk to the child is cardiac arrest or arrhythmia secondary to damage to the heart's electrical conduction system. If cardiac arrest occurs, standard cardiac life support measures are initiated.

Tissue Damage. The electrical current follows the path of least resistance through the body. Entering through the skin, electricity causes heat damage to the skin layers, bone, nerves, tendons, and blood vessels. The heat of the electrical current coagulates blood vessels and leaves the affected area without a blood supply. Gangrene develops in necrotic tissue unless it is removed. Amputation is required in more than 90% of children who sustain electrical injuries.

The location of the damage depends on the child's position and exposure. Electricity may enter one hand and exit from the other, for example; or it may travel through the body and exit from one or both legs. The greatest damage occurs at the entrance and exit sites.

Myoglobinuria. Myoglobinuria develops as a result of the release of products that are found in normal muscle but that are released into the blood after electrical injury. Myoglobin is a large molecule that mechanically obstructs the renal tubules and leads to acute tubular necrosis unless large amounts of IV fluid are administered to flush the myoglobin out of the kidney. Osmotic diuretics may be administered to promote increased urine volume. IV fluid is administered at a rate that maintains urine output at 2 mL/kg/hr until the myoglobinuria resolves.

Metabolic Acidosis. Metabolic acidosis follows electrical injury because of the associated cellular destruction and hypovolemic shock. Ringer's lactate, the fluid used for fluid resuscitation, contains sufficient bicarbonate to manage the acidosis that accompanies burn shock, but not enough to correct the acidosis associated with shock after electrical injury (i.e., pathophysiologic hypovolemic shock, not a "shock" from the electrical current). Thus, sodium bicarbonate is added to the intravenous infusion to maintain pH balance.

Other Complications. The four complications just described usually resolve within 24 hours after the injury. Other complications that follow electrical injury include loss of short-term memory and altered emotional states. The child can usually remember events up to the time of injury, including the names of family members and his or her address, telephone number, and personal information, but is unable to recall more recent events. This loss of memory can be distressing to the child and frustrating to the family. For example, the child may be unable to remember visits by the family and may feel abandoned by them. It is difficult for the child to follow instructions because of the inability to retain instructions, and this may lead to difficulty with planning care. Altered emotional states may include an absence of affect and blank stares or may include the opposite type of emotional response, such as hyperactivity and feelings of paranoia. Emotional responses usually become normal after about a week, but they may persist longer in some children. The electrical injury need not be to the head for these altered states to occur.

Community Care

Long-term sequelae to electrical injury include gait-pattern instability and development of ocular cataracts. In addition to adaptation to any amputations, neurologic deficits may lead to gait-pattern instability and alterations in depth perception and other spatial orientation. Ocular cataracts may occur in one or both eyes at varying times from within 3 months to 18 months after the injury. The very young child may not notice changes in visual acuity; therefore, regular eye examinations should be scheduled every 3 months for the first year after the injury.

Major and Minor Burns

Pathophysiology

Respiratory Compromise. Inhalation injury is a primary determinant of morbidity and mortality in burn patients. Pulmonary complications of burn injuries account for 60% to 70% of patient deaths in burn centers (Carrougher, 1993). As with all trauma patients, the first priority in management of the pediatric burn patient is assessment of airway and breathing. There are three types of respiratory system injury that may occur with a burn: upper respiratory tract injury, pulmonary injury, and carbon monoxide inhalation/hypoxia injury (Table 25–16).

Upper respiratory injury leads to swelling of the tissues in the throat and the upper airway, resulting in mechanical obstruction of the airway. Swelling starts within a few minutes of the injury, and the airway may occlude within a few minutes to a few hours. The edema remains in the tissues until it is slowly reabsorbed over a period of 2 to 5 days. Respiratory distress may be exhibited by abdominal breathing, head bobbing with respiratory efforts, nasal flaring, coughing, stridor, or wheezing. The young child may exhibit paradoxical inspiratory ef-

Table 25-16
Types of Respiratory Injury

Type of Injury	Cause	At Risk For	Treatment
Upper airway obstruction	Edema of upper airway secondary to direct burn injury from inhaling superheated air, swallowing extremely hot liquids, or as consequence of massive tissue swelling associated with extensive burns and burn shock therapy	Mechanical obstruction of upper airway	Intubation of airway; administration of warm, moist mist with oxygen as needed
Inhalation injury	Inhalation of toxic products of combustion (smoke), resulting in chemical irritation and trauma to lung tissue	Impaired gas exchange related to acute pulmonary failure 24–48 hours after burn injury	Early diagnosis of inhalation injury by bronchoscopy, or xenon-133 ventilation/perfusion scan, followed by intubation of airway and ventilatory support using a mechanical ventilator and oxygen as needed
Carbon monoxide	Carbon monoxide released as a by-product of combustion (especially common in structure fires). Carbon monoxide replaces oxygen on the hemoglobin molecule, leading to cellular hypoxia.	Systemic hypoxia; brain damage; death	Administration of 100% oxygen by mask if the child is awake, alert, and able to protect the airway until carboxyhemoglobin level returns to normal range; otherwise, intubation and ventilatory support as required. Continued monitoring of blood oxygen levels and oxygen administration until hypoxia resolves.

forts, which draw the chest wall inward while thrusting out the abdomen. The small size of the pediatric airway may become occluded by mechanical obstruction related to tissue edema or to mucous plugs.

Burn Shock. Burn shock is a type of hypovolemic shock that begins to develop shortly after a burn injury of more than 15% to 20% TBSA in children. Mechanisms of burn shock are not well understood, but the sequence of major burn injury followed by massive capillary leakage of circulating fluid into the surrounding tissues is well recognized.

caREminder: *Untreated burn shock leads to death from hypovolemia. The larger the total body surface burned, the greater and more rapid is the amount of fluid loss.*

Within minutes of a major burn injury, all of the capillaries in the circulatory system—not just those in the area of the burn—lose their capillary seal, resulting in leakage of intravascular body fluid into the interstitial spaces. Erythrocytes and leukocytes remain in the circulation and produce an elevated hematocrit and leukocyte count. The process of burn shock continues for approximately 24 to 48 hours, at which time the capillary seal is restored.

As with any other trauma patient in hypovolemic shock, concurrent systemic changes also occur, including the following:

- Ileus, which persists for about 48 hours after the burn
- Decreased blood flow to the stomach and intestines, resulting in bacterial translocation into the peritoneum
- Increased heart rate to increase cardiac preload
- Increased respiratory rate to meet the increased metabolic needs of the stressed body

Fluid and Electrolyte Deficits. In addition to the large amount of intravascular fluid volume lost during burn shock, a child has a relatively larger body surface area in relation to weight than an adult, thus increasing the extent of heat and evaporative water loss (Helvig, 1993). After the first 24 hours, even though the capillary seal is restored and circulating volume is maintained, major fluid and electrolyte losses continue to occur through the burn wound until wound closure is achieved. Fluid loss through the skin after burn injury peaks after the fourth day but continues to be a concern until the area heals. Fluid and electrolyte imbalances can occur rapidly. Whenever hypotension develops in burn patients, the body's ability to fight infection at the tissue level is compromised by inadequate tissue perfusion to the skin. Infection quickly develops, and infected wounds lead to more tissue destruction. In the event of overwhelming infection, sepsis develops rapidly.

Metabolic Alterations. The major metabolic responses to burn injury include hypermetabolism, elevated catecholamine levels, hyperglycemia, increased nutritional needs, and growth delay. These pathophysiologic responses are discussed below.

Hypermetabolism. Hypermetabolism characterizes the metabolic response to burn injury and occurs in proportion to the extent of the burn. Energy expenditures may increase from 40% to 100% above basal levels in children with burns of more than 30% TBSA. Core body temperature for a child with a major burn injury will reset at about 37.5° to 38°C, or 99°F, and will remain at that level or higher until skin coverage is achieved. When exposed to cooler temperatures, the child begins to shiver, increasing the oxygen and energy demands of the body tremendously. A warm environment minimizes the hemodynamic and metabolic stresses associated with major burn injury (Cortiella & Marvin, 1997).

Elevated Catecholamine Levels. Increased core temperature and metabolic rate are accompanied by an increase in catecholamine release. In addition, the stress associated with treatments, including the surface water evaporation that occurs with exposure of the child to room temperature air, increases catecholamine release, metabolic stress, and energy demands.

Hyperglycemia. Glucose metabolism is also altered after burn injury. Hyperglycemia is a common occurrence; the elevation of fasting blood glucose levels above normal is related to the severity of the injury or to the presence of systemic infection. Young children may quickly deplete their glucose stores and may become hypoglycemic unless they receive adequate nutritional support.

Increased Nutritional Needs. The increased need for nutritional intake associated with major burn injury is related to increased energy demands associated with the hypermetabolic state of the child and to the need to heal a major wound. Major injury and infections can lead to weight loss and severe alterations in body composition, even when calories and protein are supplied in substantial amounts. Nitrogen imbalance is associated with failure to meet the increased nutritional needs of a major burn injury. Wound healing cannot occur when the child is in negative nitrogen balance; thus, the provision of adequate nutrition is essential to recovery. However, overfeeding results in increased carbon dioxide production that requires increasing respiratory rates to clear and, in addition, can cause fatty liver and other hepatic dysfunction. Thus, the goal of nursing care is to provide sufficient nutritional support to help the child heal the burn injury (Cortiella & Marvin, 1997).

Growth Delay. Growth hormone levels are depressed after major burn injury. The child will not increase in height for many months after the injury, while the body focuses on restoring and healing damaged tissue. A growth spurt is usually noted about a year after the recovery phase.

Infection and Sepsis. Major burn wounds are an ideal location for bacterial growth because bacteria replicate rapidly in the warm, moist burn wound environment. If bacterial levels increase to the extent that invasion into the underlying tissue occurs, infection results. Bacteria then gain entrance into the systemic circulation and spread into other organs, causing sepsis.

Wound Infection. Conditions that predispose the child with a burn to the development of wound infection include a source of organisms capable of producing disease, a mode of transmission, and a susceptible host. The most common bacteria are found in the burn wound patient's own body, especially those bacteria normally present on the skin and in the gastrointestinal tract. Other bacteria can easily be spread to the patient by staff members who do not wash their hands after caring for other patients (nosocomial infection). Topical burn creams are used because the local blood supply to the area of burn injury is destroyed with the burn, thus systemic antibiotics are not delivered to the burn wound.

Infection in partial-thickness burn wounds converts the area to a full-thickness injury, which then requires skin grafting. Hypovolemia for any reason, especially in children, greatly increases the incidence of wound conversion.

Systemic Infection. In addition to the risk of wound infection, the burned child is susceptible to infection from aspiration of gastrointestinal fluid into the lungs, which may lead to pneumonia. The interface between the burn wound and healthy tissue is a potential location for anaerobic bacteria to develop.

Pediatric diseases, such as chickenpox or measles, that happen at the same time that the child is recovering from a major burn injury often prove lethal to the child. This is especially true for chickenpox and its virus, herpes zoster.

The child's immune system is impaired after major burn injury and cannot protect the child from infection and sepsis caused by previously benign bacteria (Kravitz, 1993). Monocyte and macrophage components of the immune system are not functioning well, nor are white blood cells such as neutrophils, granulocytes, and basophils. Phagocytosis, the normal mechanism for removing debris from a wound, does not occur, allowing pockets of infection to develop.

Assessment

The extent of injury refers to the percentage of the total body surface area (TBSA) that has been burned. The use of the adult rule of nines gives an inaccurate estimate of burn size in a child because of differences in body proportion between children and adults. When using the rule of nines in children, 9% is taken from the legs and is added to the percentage for the head for a child up to 1 year of age. For each subsequent year of age, 1% is returned to the legs, until, at approximately age 9 years, the child's head is in proportion to that of an adult (Miller, Richard, & Staley, 1994). Many burn facilities use the Lund and Browder chart, which is a body surface chart corrected for age (Fig. 25–19). The burn is also described according to the depth of the burn (Table 25–17).

Nursing Diagnosis and Outcomes

The following nursing diagnoses are appropriate for the child with a burn injury.

- **Impaired skin integrity related to burn**
  Outcome: The child's skin will heal without infection, as evidenced by restoration of the epithelial layer in partial-thickness injury or adherence of skin graft to area of full-thickness injury.
- **Pain related to thermal injury and related procedures**
  Outcome: Pain relief will be achieved as evidenced by age-appropriate behaviors, adequate nutritional intake, and appropriate sleep patterns.
- **Ineffective airway clearance/impaired gas exchange related to upper airway edema, smoke inhalation injury, or carbon monoxide/hypoxia**
  Outcome: The child will maintain normal oxygen saturation, will have unlabored respirations at a rate appropriate for age, and will have clear bilateral breath sounds.
- **Altered tissue perfusion (peripheral) related to burn shock**
  Outcome: The child will maintain a urine output of 1 to 2 mL/kg/hr for the first 24 hours after the burn and will remain alert and oriented.
- **Risk for fluid volume deficit related to loss of skin integrity in the area of the burn and systemic shifting of plasma and plasma components from the circulatory system into interstitial and intracellular spaces secondary to impaired capillary integrity**
  Outcome: The child will maintain normal fluid and electrolyte balance as evidenced by intake and output measurements and serum electrolyte values that are within normal limits.
- **Risk for infection related to burn wound contamination or to pulmonary complications**
  Outcome: The child will achieve wound closure without developing burn wound infection, systemic sepsis, or pneumonia.
- **Altered nutrition: less than body requirements, related to hypermetabolism and the increased energy requirements of wound healing**
  Outcomes: The child will maintain muscle mass and protein stores appropriate for age.

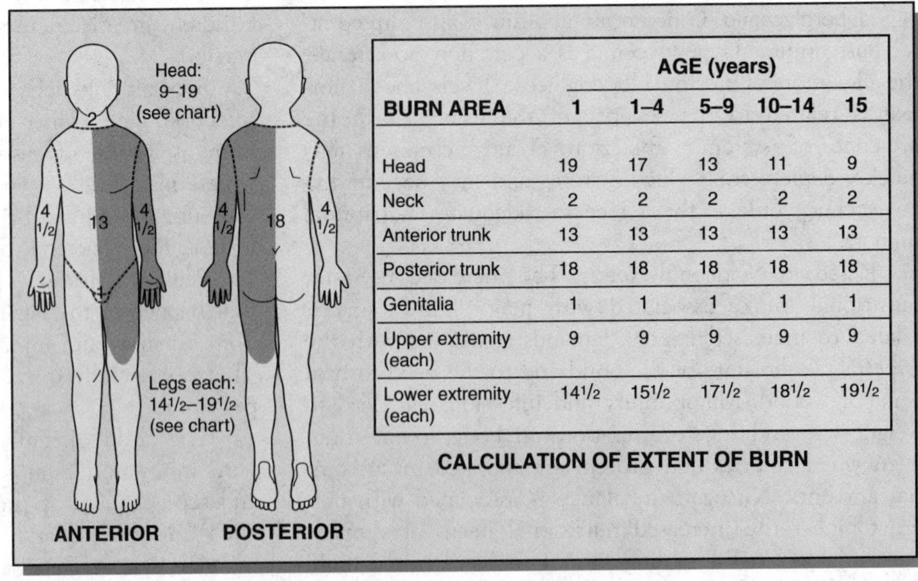

BURN AREA	AGE (years) 1	1–4	5–9	10–14	15
Head	19	17	13	11	9
Neck	2	2	2	2	2
Anterior trunk	13	13	13	13	13
Posterior trunk	18	18	18	18	18
Genitalia	1	1	1	1	1
Upper extremity (each)	9	9	9	9	9
Lower extremity (each)	14 1/2	15 1/2	17 1/2	18 1/2	19 1/2

CALCULATION OF EXTENT OF BURN

Figure 25–19
Child burn size estimation table. (Table from Lund, C. C., & Browder, N. C. [1944]. Estimation of burn size. *Surgery, Gynecology, and Obstetrics, 79,* 352–358. By permission of *Surgery, Gynecology, and Obstetrics,* now known as *Journal of the American College of Surgeons.*)

Table 25–17
Severity of Burns

Depth of Burn	Thickness	Appearance of Burn	Sensation	Example of Cause
First degree	Superficial epithelium	Erythema	Painful	Sunburn
Second degree	Partial thickness Destruction into, but not through, epidermis	Blisters Peeling epidermis Swelling White or red mottling Weeping, wet	Painful Hypersensitive to air, touch	Very deep sunburn Scalds
Third degree	Full-thickness destruction of skin into hypodermis Death to all skin appendages and subcutaneous tissue	Translucent Mottled white or tan Waxy Leathery Basically dry	Painless (initially)	Fire Prolonged exposure to hot liquid Electricity

From Himes, C., & Kuntz, K. (In press). Pediatric burn rehabilitation. In P. Edwards, D. Hertzberg, and N. Youngblood. (Eds.), *Pediatric rehabilitation.* Philadelphia: W. B. Saunders. Reprinted with permission.

The child's nitrogen balance and energy expenditure studies will consistently yield balanced results.

- **Body image disturbance related to appearance**
  Outcomes: The child will re-enter previous social settings and will express a feeling of comfort in these areas.
  The family will provide emotional support for the child.
  The child will discuss feelings related to reactions of others to the child's change in appearance.

Interdisciplinary Interventions for Minor Burn Injuries

In general, children with a minor burn injury are treated as outpatients in a physician's office, clinic, or hospital physical therapy department. Therapy is aimed at promoting wound healing, preventing infection, and providing pain relief. In addition, because anaerobic and aerobic bacteria can grow at the interface between burned and healthy tissue, tetanus toxoid is given to children whose immunizations are not up to date.

The wound is cleansed with mild soap and tepid water. The area is debrided of loose debris and necrotic tissue. The debridement of blisters is controversial. Some researchers believe that all blisters should be opened and debrided because they can become a culture medium for bacteria (Saffle & Schnebly, 1994). Other researchers contend that intact blisters should not be debrided because they form a moist, sterile, plasmatic environment that promotes wound healing and reepithelialization (Zuker, 1988). However, all agree that broken blisters should be debrided. The burned area is covered with an antimicrobial ointment (usually bacitracin or Silvadene) (Table 25–18). A nonadherent dressing and light gauze is applied over the ointment. Dressings are usually changed twice daily.

caREminder: *The meticulous and regular performance of debridement is the cornerstone of successful burn wound management (Saffle & Schnebly, 1994).*

The nurse should teach the parents or the child to wash the burned area with mild soap and tepid water, to apply the prescribed ointment and a light dressing, and to promote use of the affected area. The parents should be instructed to soak the dressing in tepid water before its removal in order to loosen the dressing and to decrease the child's discomfort. Acetaminophen is usually effective as an analgesic for the pain associated with minor burn injury, but the actual wound care will be very painful until healing is well established. Completing the wound care as quickly as possible reduces the pain, because the contact of air and water on the exposed wound causes much of the pain. Burns of the face are usually left exposed, and antimicrobial ointment is applied twice daily. Parents are informed of the importance of returning for follow-up visits.

The nurse should also provide instructions on meeting the child's nutritional needs, support, and methods of increasing caloric and protein intake. If the child is still receiving tube feedings, the nurse should instruct the family on the procedures of tube feedings, on checking residuals, and on recognizing and reporting any complications. It would probably be helpful to the family to be

Table 25-18
Topical Antimicrobial Agents Commonly Used for Burns

	Advantages	Side Effects/Disadvantages	Nursing Considerations
Silver sulfadiazine cream (Silvadene)	Effective against a wide range of gram-positive and gram-negative organisms Soothing on application Softens eschar and increases joint mobility Absorbed slowly, reducing the possibility of nephrotoxicity	May cause hypersensitivity reaction in 5–7% of patients Associated with initial decrease in leukocyte count	Applied to cleansed wound 1–3 times a day. Wound may be left open or may be covered with a light dressing.
Mafenide acetate cream (Sulfamylon)	Effective against a wide range of gram-positive and gram-negative organisms Rapidly diffuses through eschar (improved effectiveness in established infections) Permits open treatment of wound, thus increasing mobility	Painful on application May cause hypersensitivity reaction in 5–7% of patients Associated with acid-base derangements	Applied to cleansed wound 1–2 times a day. Treated area left open because wrapping causes maceration.
Silver nitrate solution	Effective against most gram-positive and some gram-negative organisms	Hyponatremia, hypokalemia, hypochloremia Decreased penetration of eschar Not effective against established infection Requires large, bulky dressings that limit mobility	0.5% solution in distilled water applied to wet dressing q 2 hr. Dressing changes twice daily.

Adapted from Marvin, J. (1991). Burn injuries and skin trauma. In M. L. Patrick, S. L. Woods, R. F. Craven, J. S. Robosky, & P. M. Bruno (Eds.), *Medical-surgical nursing: Pathophysiological concepts* (2nd ed., p. 1854). Philadelphia: J. B. Lippincott.

told of support groups for burn victims and their families. The nurse should be sure that the family members clearly understand the instructions for the administration of medications that the physician may have prescribed. The parents should also be instructed on the signs and symptoms that should be reported to the physician, the home health care nurse, or the clinic. To promote the child's normal growth and development, the parents should be assessed for their understanding of the normal parameters for their child's age. If the parents are not able to provide needed care, community and hospital resources are indicated.

Interdisciplinary Interventions for Major Burn Injuries

Respiratory Compromise. Children who are burned and who do not have other injuries are awake, alert, and oriented. Initial treatment consists of establishing an airway and administering a high concentration (40%) of oxygen until an assessment and treatment plan are completed. Assessment of actual or potential pulmonary injury in children with flame injury involves measurement of arterial blood gas and carbon monoxide levels.

▽ **Alert:** *If a child with burn injuries is unconscious, this condition is the result of factors other than the burn itself. The most common cause of unconsciousness in flame injury is hypoxia associated with smoke inhalation.*

Upper airway edema is managed by airway intubation and administration of humidified oxygen until the edema subsides, usually about 2 to 5 days later. When the assessment indicates that airway edema is accumulating and will lead to airway compromise or to occlusion, early planned intubation is preferred over emergency intubation. Inhalation injury is managed by airway intubation and ventilation support at settings appropriate to the child's lung size. A full-thickness burn encircling the chest may limit full expansion of the lungs. In such cases, it may be necessary to perform an escharotomy of the chest to allow for chest wall expansion.

Carbon monoxide inhalation and hypoxia are treated by administering high concentrations of oxygen by mask until the condition is resolved. Pure carbon monoxide intoxication resolves within 30 minutes of 100% oxygen therapy. No further treatment is needed for the hypoxia, although there may be other related problems, such as neurologic damage secondary to hypoxia.

Burn Shock. Therapy for burn shock is aimed at supporting the child through the period of hypovolemic shock until capillary integrity is restored. Fluids are administered intravenously at a rate greater than the rate of fluid loss in order to maintain adequate circulating volume. Many formulas can be used to calculate the rate of fluid administration, the most common of which is the Parkland formula of fluid resuscitation (Chart 25–25). Because urine output reflects end-organ tissue perfusion, IV fluids are administered at a rate sufficient to keep the child's urine output at 1 mL/kg of body weight per hour, thus reflecting adequate tissue perfusion. A Foley catheter is inserted into the child's bladder, and urine output is measured hourly. Ringer's lactate is the IV fluid of choice because it most closely approximates the composition of the extracellular fluid being lost. Children younger than 5 years of age handle free water poorly, making them susceptible to pulmonary and cerebral edema.

If a child does not have adequate urine output during burn shock, the reason is insufficient administration of resuscitative fluids. Renal failure is not a component of burn shock if an adequate volume of IV fluids is administered for burn shock resuscitation. It should be recognized that the Parkland formula and other burn shock fluid resuscitation formulas are only guidelines, and that individual children may require more than 4 mL/kg per percent of TBSA burn during the first 24 hours after the burn.

Sensorium is an important guide to the adequacy of fluid resuscitation. The burn injury itself does not affect the sensorium, so the child should be alert and oriented. Any alteration in sensorium should be evaluated further. When burn shock fluid resuscitation is delayed, cerebral hypoperfusion and hypoxia may occur, predisposing the child to development of cerebral edema upon initiation of massive fluid infusion.

caREminder: *Elevating the head of the child's bed 10 to 15 degrees to decrease cerebral edema fluid accumulation, along with monitoring for clinical signs of increased intracranial pressure, is essential to diminish the amount of cerebral edema during shock resuscitation.*

Placing the head of the bed on wheel blocks in order to elevate the entire bed on a slant is preferable to elevating only the head of the bed, which results in edema accumulating in the groin and legs.

Chart 25–25

Parkland Formula of Fluid Resuscitation for Burn Shock

4 mL Ringer's lactate solution
× kg of body weight
× % total body surface area (TBSA) burn

One half of total is administered in the first 8 hours post burn.
One fourth of total is administered in the second 8 hours post burn.
One fourth of total is administered in the third 8 hours post burn.

During the first 24 hours post burn, Ringer's lactate solution is administered IV using the formula as a guideline. The criterion for successful burn shock fluid resuscitation is based on an hourly urine output of 1 mL/kg/hr in children. Time is calculated from the time of injury, not from the time of admission.

Example: A 10-kg child with a 50% TBSA burn

4 mL × 10 kg × 50% TBSA burn
= 2000 mL or 2 L of Ringer's lactate in 24 hours

Administer: 1000 mL in first 8 hours at 125 mL/hr
500 mL in second 8 hours at 62 mL/hr
500 mL in third 8 hours at 62 mL/hr

In the event that fluid resuscitation is delayed, one half of the amount is still administered by 8 hours post burn. For example, if fluids are not started until 2 hours after the injury, one half of the fluids are administered in the next 6 hours.

From Baxter, C. R. (1974). Fluid volume and electrolyte changes of the early postburn period. *Clinics in Plastic Surgery, 1*, 693–709. Reprinted with permission.

In certain cases, children may require fluid in excess of the calculated amount. Some of these exceptions include an underestimation of burn size, pulmonary injury that sequesters fluid in the lungs, electrical injury with more tissue destruction than is visible, extremely deep injury, and delayed initiation of fluid resuscitation.

Once burn shock has resolved, the child is given a colloid-containing solution, such as plasma or albumin, to replace the loss of plasma from the circulating volume.

Fluid and Electrolyte Deficits. When burn shock resuscitation is completed, a maintenance fluid plan is initiated using formulas based on normal basal fluid requirements plus calculated evaporative water loss from the burn wound. The fluid infused is changed from Ringer's lactate to an electrolyte-free solution of 5% dextrose, with or without saline, depending on the patient's electrolyte status. A dextrose solution is used to meet some of the caloric needs of the hypermetabolic burn patient. One L of 5% dextrose solution contains 200 calories. Potassium may be added to the IV infusion as indicated for hypokalemia. The child's intake, output, and serum electrolyte balance are monitored closely. Fluids are administered in amounts equally divided throughout each 24-hour period. IV fluids are administered until the child's bowel function returns, usually within 48 hours after the burn. The child can then be started on oral fluids. The child must continue to maintain adequate fluid intake, either by IV infusion or orally, until wound closure is achieved.

At times during the clinical course, fluid losses may increase. This is especially true when the child's core body temperature exceeds 39°C (102.2°F), when tracheal intubation is required, when a paralytic ileus necessitates prolonged nasogastric suction, when perioperative procedures are accompanied by massive blood loss, and when diarrhea occurs.

Alert: *Fluid and electrolyte imbalance lasting for only a few hours can lead to sepsis, seizures, and death in burned children.*

Metabolic Alterations. The hypermetabolism of burn injury requires aggressive nutritional support. In addition, healing cannot occur in the presence of negative nitrogen balance. Therefore, establishing and maintaining adequate nutritional intake to meet the caloric needs of the child is essential to survival. Caloric requirements are two to three times the normal basal requirements in the child with major burn injury.

A number of formulas have been proposed for estimating caloric requirements (Chart 25–26). Correct estimates are important, because too little nutritional intake causes protein mobilization from muscle and weight loss, whereas administration of excess calories can cause hyperglycemia, liver abnormalities, and increased carbon dioxide production. Weight, calorie and protein counts, and nitrogen balance are monitored daily; when possible, indirect calorimetric measurements of resting energy expenditure are obtained.

caREminder: *Healing of burn wounds cannot occur if the child is in negative nitrogen balance. Nutritional support is essential.*

Most children with burns in excess of 25% of the TBSA are unable to consume an oral diet sufficient to meet their nutritional requirements. The child may refuse to eat because of the unfamiliarity of hospital food, because of pain, or in an effort to gain control over the environment. Many children require the placement of enteral feeding tubes and tube feeding with supplemental liquid nutrition. In addition, vitamins (C, A, E, B, and B_5) and trace elements (iron, zinc, copper, and magnesium) are provided to promote wound healing. If the enteral route does not meet all of the child's nutritional needs, parenteral hyperalimentation can be used as a last resort to supplement intake. This route is used only when necessary because of the risk of catheter-related infection and the desire to maintain intestinal integrity.

Care of the Burn Wound. Burn wound closure and prevention of infection are the goals of burn wound management. Wound closure is accomplished either by supporting spontaneous healing or by initiating surgical repair. The method used is determined by the depth, extent, and location of the burn wounds. Burns to areas designated as special care areas are treated in specific ways (Chart 25–27). Tetanus toxoid immunizations are administered as indicated to provide coverage appropriate for the child's age.

Application of Antimicrobial Agents and Dressings. Burn wounds receive daily care until closure is achieved. Wounds are cleansed using mild soap and then are covered with topical antimicrobial agents (see Table 25–18). Topical antibacterial agents are placed on burn wounds to penetrate the eschar and to reduce bacterial growth in and around the burn wound. Systemic antibiotics are not used to control burn wound bacteria because there is no blood supply to the burn wound to deliver the drug (Table 25–19). When systemic sepsis is diagnosed, systemic antibiotics are administered, and if possible, the source of the sepsis is eliminated.

caREminder: *If systemic sepsis occurs, children exhibit all the signs of hypovolemic shock, but the actual timing of the symptoms depends on the volume status of the child at the time of onset of sepsis.*

Silver sulfadiazine (Silvadene) is the topical agent that is most commonly used, but it is not typically used on the face or on electrical burns. Facial burns are covered with a light layer of antimicrobial ointment. Mafenide (Sulfamylon) is the topical agent of choice for burns to the ear or for electrical burns because of its deep penetration into the eschar. Sulfamylon should not be

Chart 25–26

Estimating Caloric Requirements in Burned Children Using the Galveston Formula

Children younger than 12 years of age:
1800 kcal/m²/BSA plus 1300 kcal/m²/BSA burned

Adolescents:
1500 kcal/m²/BSA plus 1500 kcal/m²/BSA burned

From Hildreth, M. A., Herndon, D. N., Desai, M. H., & Broemeling, L. D. (1990). Current treatment reduces calories required to maintain weight in pediatric patients with burns. *Journal of Burn Care and Rehabilitation, 11*, 405–409.

Chart 25–27

Treatment of Burns in Special Care Areas

Eyes

On admission, irrigate the eyes with sterile solution. Eyelids will swell shut for 3–5 days. Cleanse the area gently; do not attempt to force the eyes open. After the edema resolves, wash the area every 8 hours and apply ointment and eye drops per physician's order. Inform the child that vision may be blurred owing to application of medications.

Ears

On admission, remove blisters and secure hair away from the burned area. Position the child without using a pillow to prevent further trauma to the ears, because wounds tend to adhere to pillows or bed linens. Apply Sulfamylon ointment every 12 hours as ordered by the physician.

Face

On admission, remove blisters and shave face (if age appropriate), except for eyebrows, as indicated. Apply bacitracin or other ointments per physician's order. Cleanse the area every 8 hours, and reapply topical ointment. The area will heal quickly (7–10 days) if it is a superficial burn because of an abundant blood supply. Deeper burns are skin grafted early to decrease scarring. Pillows are not used with anterior neck burns so as to minimize scarring from chin to neck.

Hands

On admission, remove rings or other jewelry. Remove blisters and apply a topical antibiotic ointment (silver sulfadiazine), wrapping each finger individually and wrapping the entire hand in a manner that permits full range of motion. Cleanse the area every 8 hours, and reapply ointment and dressings. Encourage full range of motion and use of the hand. Elevate the child's hand above the level of the heart to promote edema reabsorption. Administer pain medication to facilitate use of the hand. The area will heal quickly (7–10 days) if it is a superficial burn because of abundant blood supply. Deeper burns should be skin grafted early to decrease scarring.

Feet

On admission, remove blisters. Apply topical antibiotic ointment (silver sulfadiazine) per physician's order. Wrap the toes individually; wrap the foot so that full range of motion is possible; and apply an elastic bandage, distal to proximal, over the dressing to promote comfort and reduce dependent edema. The patient should ambulate at least every 4 hours during the day unless contraindicated; pain medication should be administered so as to be effective at ambulation times. Elevate the patient's lower extremities when at rest.

Joints

On admission, remove blisters and shave areas with hair. Apply topical ointment per physician's order. Wrap the area to permit full range of motion. Cleanse the area every 8 hours, and reapply ointment and dressings. Shave areas of hair growth every 3–4 days. Encourage full range of motion. When at rest, joints should be kept in extension to prevent contracture formation.

Perineum

On admission, remove blisters and shave the area. Insert a bladder catheter before edema accumulates. Apply silver sulfadiazine, per physician's order, directly to the perineum or onto diapers before application. Maintain the bladder catheter until the edema subsides. Cleanse the area after each stool/voiding, and reapply silver sulfadiazine. Scrotal edema can accumulate and may impair walking until resolved.

Circumferential Burns

On admission, identify areas of full-thickness circumferential burn. Cleanse the area, remove blisters, and shave as needed. Monitor distal pulses every 15 minutes using a Doppler monitor. If distal pulses diminish or disappear, notify the physician immediately and prepare for escharotomy or fasciotomy. After the procedure, check for pulses every 15 minutes for 24 hours post burn. If pulses diminish or disappear again, notify the physician. Apply silver sulfadiazine and dressings to the area. Cleanse the area and change dressings every 8 hours.

Table 25–19
Functions of Skin Altered by Burn Injury

	Status After Burn Injury			
		Partial Thickness (2nd Degree)		
Normal Function	Superficial (1st Degree)	*Superficial*	*Deep*	Full Thickness (3rd Degree)
Protective barrier against infection and injury	Intact	Altered	Absent	Absent
Epidermis impermeable to most substances	Intact	Altered	Absent	Absent
Sensation from nerve endings	Intact	Intact	Absent	Absent
Vitamin D synthesis	Intact	Intact	Absent	Absent
Water vapor barrier to prevent water and electrolyte loss/absorption	Intact	Altered	Absent	Absent
Regulation of core body temperature	Intact	Altered	Absent	Absent
Immune components of skin present at dermal–epidermal junction	Intact	Altered	Absent	Absent
Local circulation	Intact	Altered	Absent	Absent
Elasticity of dermis	Intact	Intact	Altered	Absent
Ability to grow new skin	Intact	Intact	Altered	Absent

applied to the face. In a small number of burn units, the established protocol calls for ointments to be placed on the wounds without a protective dressing. However, in most burn units, dressings are applied over the wound to keep the area moist and the topical agents in place.

Dressings are changed one to three times daily, depending on the agents used and on specific wound care protocols. Dressing changes may take place in hydrotherapy tanks, in bathtubs, in showers, or, if the child is too ill to be moved, at the bedside. Placing the burned area in water facilitates cleansing of the area and softens the eschar, thereby promoting range of motion of the affected areas (see the section on hydrotherapy). Debris and previously applied topical agents are removed, and the wounds are re-dressed (see the section on debridement).

Aseptic technique is used during dressing changes. After dressings are applied to burn wounds, isolation is not necessary, and the child does not need to be restricted to a room or to an area of the hospital.

Pain medications are administered 20 to 30 minutes before dressing changes so that maximal effect can be achieved to control pain at the time of the procedure. In addition to pain control, measures to maintain the child's core body temperature, to minimize shivering, and to conserve energy must be implemented as part of wound care activities. To the degree possible, the child's capacity for self-care should be optimized.

Debridement. Burn injury produces necrotic skin and subcutaneous tissue called eschar. Eschar releases chemical mediators that stimulate leukocytes to digest debris, but this also damages capillaries and skin elements. Necrotic tissue within a wound prolongs inflammation and slows healing and epidermal coverage (Saffle & Schnebly, 1994).

Debridement is the removal of dead material from a wound in order to promote healing. Initial debridement may be performed in the emergency department or on the unit in the hydrotherapy treatment room. Burns are cleansed and debrided at least every 12 hours. Old creams and ointments must be removed as part of the debridement, and loose tissue is trimmed from around the wound (Fig. 25–20).

Hydrotherapy. Hydrotherapy is used to cleanse the wound and the child. During this cleansing process, active range of motion exercises may also be performed. The hydrotherapy can take place in a tank, in a tub, or in a shower. Some facilities use disposable plastic liners to prevent cross-contamination between patients. Hydrotherapy should last no longer than 20 minutes so as to prevent electrolyte loss through the skin into the water secondary to osmosis. The room's temperature should be very warm, and the child should be covered and should be dried immediately after cleansing.

Skin Grafts and Donor Sites. Full-thickness burn injuries and most deep partial-thickness burn injuries are managed surgically. The procedure to remove the burn tissue is excision. Wound coverage is achieved over healthy, unburned tissue. The skin used to cover the burn wound is harvested from an unburned area (donor site) of the child's own skin in a procedure called an

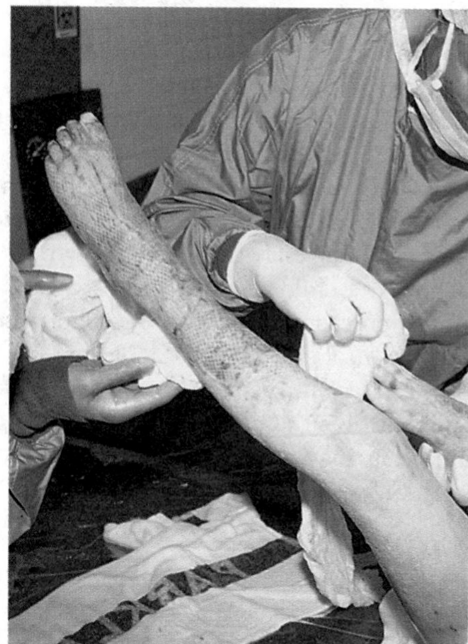

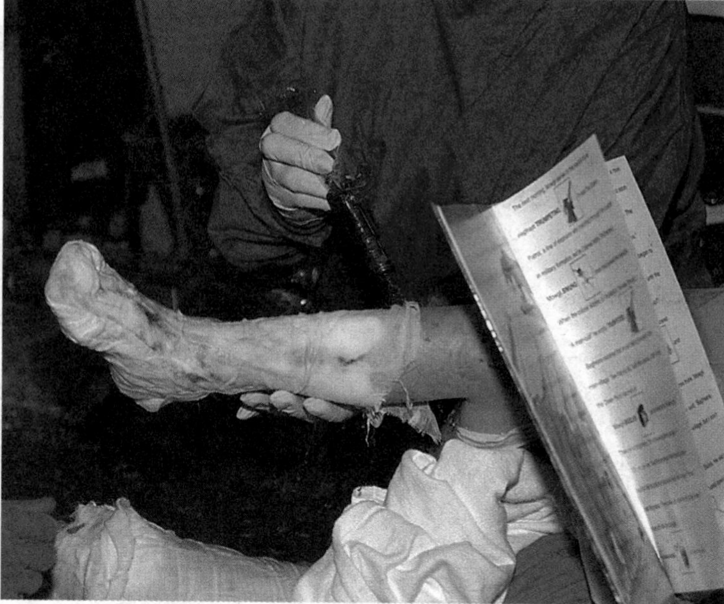

Figure 25–20
During hydrotherapy, water is used to cleanse the wound. Gauze pads are used to debride the wound by removing exudate and the previously applied medication. (Courtesy of Parkland Memorial Hospital, Dallas, TX.)

autograft. The skin that is surgically removed is a paper-thin section of the upper layers of the skin (split-thickness skin graft). In order to cover a greater area, autograft skin is usually prepared with a skin mesher. The mesher, which has variable settings, cuts small slits into the skin, allowing it to be stretched to cover a graft area from 1.5 to 9 times larger than the original size of the graft. The slit pattern disappears as the graft heals. If the child does not have sufficient unburned skin to cover the wound, temporary coverage can be achieved by using a homograft (cadaver skin) or xenograft (pig skin) that has been specially prepared for that use.

In some burn units, the burn eschar is removed in a two-stage excision and grafting procedure. On the first day, the burn is surgically excised and the area is covered with antibiotic-soaked dressings, after which the child is allowed to recover from anesthesia. On the second day, the child is returned to surgery for a procedure that involves removing a paper-thin layer of unburned skin from the child's body and applying that skin to the previously excised burn areas. In other burn units, excision and skin grafting are accomplished in one procedure, with an interval in between excision of the burn and application of the new skin to allow for control of blood loss. If blood collects between the excised area and the skin graft, the skin graft will not adhere. Infection can also cause loss of skin grafts.

Blood loss with excision of large burns is massive and may require replacement of as much as one half of the child's circulating blood volume. Burn patients receive many blood transfusions during their hospital course to replace blood lost during surgical wound management.

Scarring. Burn scars form in areas of healed burn, including those areas that received skin grafts. Scarring starts at the time healing starts and continues for about 8 to 12 months. Hypertrophic scarring results in an elevated, raised, reddened, and painful area that is very susceptible to traumatic injury from routine daily activities. Prevention of hypertrophic scarring is essential for optimal cosmetic and functional recovery. Keloid scars form in the area of the burn and then expand onto unburned tissue.

Within 1 or 2 weeks after a wound is closed by either skin grafting or healing, scarring is minimized by the application of pressure to the area using specially made anti-scarring compression garments. Garments such as gloves, shirts, pants, or face masks are individually measured and fitted to the burn area. They are worn 24 hours a day, except during bathing, for about 10 to 12 months after the burn (Kravitz, 1988). Some children wear the special garments for shorter or for longer periods of time, depending on the rate of scar maturity. Although these garments have been available only in tan for many years, several manufacturers are now creating them in bright, interesting colors with attractive appliqued figures and designs. As donning and wearing these garments can be a difficult and painful process, compliance is often an issue, and the child's level of cooperation is almost totally dependent on the attitude of the adult supervisor. Facial burns may be treated with masks of more rigid construction in order to restore a normal contour to the central face and chin.

Physical Therapy. Areas of burn become stiff, and range of motion is severely limited unless active range-of-motion therapy is initiated at the time of admission and is continued for several months until the scars mature. Muscles tend to shorten, and skin contracts in burn areas involving the joints. Extension muscles are not as strong as flexor muscles, and injured areas over joints (especially the elbows, axillae, and knees) tend to become permanently fixed in the flexed position. Frequent physical therapy exercise is required to prevent flexion contractures, which severely limit mobility and may require surgical correction. If the child is able and willing to cooperate, active range of motion and use of the burned areas promote optimal functional recovery. If the child is unable or is unwilling to cooperate, passive range of motion, performed by all staff, will help maintain function. The parents and the child will be taught the physical therapy exercises before the child's discharge from the hospital, because therapy must continue for about 12 to 18 months after the burn, or until scar formation has peaked.

Management of Pain and Itching. Pain and itching are both active components of recovery from a burn injury. With partial-thickness burns and in areas used for donor sites, nerve endings are exposed. Newly healed areas and those that have received skin grafts are highly sensitive to pressure pain, and the joints underneath develop an arthritic type of pain that is activated with movement. Burn patients awaken each day with chronic pain, stiffness, and aching in the burned areas for many months after the burn is healed.

Itching occurs in all healing areas and causes great distress unless it is relieved with medication. Itching persists for several months after burns heal, as new nerve endings and dermal elements reestablish themselves. Alterations in sweat glands after burning result in excessive sweat production, which leads to dry skin and itching, adding to the problem.

The perception of pain in the burned child varies widely, but it is usually related to procedural pain from burn dressing changes or physical therapy or background pain from attempting to remain still to avoid the pain of movement. Chronically abused children learn not to verbalize pain and often withdraw into a trancelike state when painful procedures occur. Other children in pain protest against every procedure with every bit of volume and energy available to them. The amount of protest a child manifests in response to painful procedures should not be the criterion for pain management.

Procedural pain is real and can be minimized with a pain management program that involves the administration of adequate analgesia 20 to 30 minutes before initiation of the procedure, additional analgesia as the procedure continues, and analgesia at the completion of the procedure to allow the child rest and recovery time. For especially painful procedures, the use of short-acting, memory-altering medications may be indicated so that the child does not recall the procedure. One effective method of pain control is the patient-controlled analgesia pump, a method that may be used for children as young as 6 years of age (Schumann, 1991).

caREminder: *Pain medication should be administered in anticipation of painful procedures as that maximal effectiveness coincides with the timing of the procedure. When the child undergoes a procedure that is known to produce prolonged pain, such as a skin grafting, pain medication should be administered on a scheduled basis, rather than as needed once pain is reported.*

Morphine is the drug of choice. It should be administered by the IV route rather than the intramuscular route because it will not be rapidly or evenly absorbed if it is injected into edematous tissue. To diminish pain between dressing changes, oral medications such as acetaminophen with codeine may be used.

In older children, anxiety and anticipatory stress may be factors that respond to anti-anxiety medications. Ensuring adequate sleep and uninterrupted quiet time is essential to allow the child to restore inner resources. Parental visiting should be unrestricted and individualized to the child's needs and to those of the family. The child's pain is also a source of great distress to the family.

Itching can be controlled by medications, such as diphenhydramine hydrochloride (Benadryl), and by the application of soothing lotions, such as Nivea or Eucerin, to healing skin.

Psychosocial Support for the Burn-Injured Child. The long-term effects of an accidental burn injury may be related to physical changes resulting from the healing and scarring process, the developmental differences associated with burns in young children, or to the psychosocial alterations in the relationship between the child and family members (Molter, 1993) (Chart 25–28).

The immediate psychosocial stresses for the burned child include separation from parents and from the home environment, as well as all of the known psychological traumas associated with hospitalization. Children who are intubated cannot speak or cry out, and often their arms and legs are restrained to prevent pulling on IV lines and tubes. Physical restraint is terrifying to a young child who cannot understand the reason for the restraint. Older

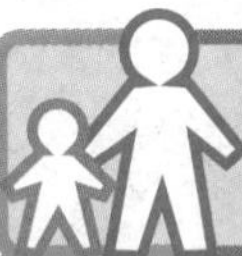

Chart 25–28
Developmental Considerations

Pediatric Differences in the Effects of Burn Injury

- Very young children who have been severely burned have a higher mortality rate than do older children and adults with comparable burns.
- Because a child's skin is thinner than an adult's, lower burn temperatures and shorter exposure to heat or chemicals can cause a deeper burn.
- A larger body surface area as compared with adults places severely burned children at increased risk for fluid and heat loss. Children are also at increased risk for dehydration and metabolic acidosis secondary to diarrhea, evaporative water loss, and increased fluid requirements.
- The highest proportion of body fluid to mass in children increases the risk of cardiovascular problems owing to their less effective cardiovascular response to changing intravascular volume.
- Burns involving more than 10% TBSA require some form of fluid resuscitation (Reeves, et al., 1994).
- Infants and children are at increased risk for protein and calorie deficiency because they have smaller muscle mass and lower body fat reserves than do adults. If they are not eating and their metabolism is increased, their protein and calorie needs will not be met.
- Hypertrophic scarring is more severe and scar maturation is prolonged (Reeves, Warden, & Staley, 1994).
- An immature immune system means an increased risk of infection for infants and young children.
- A delay in growth may follow extensive burns.
- In children, Curling's ulcer occurs in the third or fourth week post burn, which is later than in adults.

children, who may be able to understand the rationale for restraint, may experience anger and a lack of trust.

Tip: *Children must be allowed "safe time" during the day when no medical procedure, painful or not, is performed (Helvig, 1993). The period should be identified by the nurse as "safe" through a statement, such as "I am going to sit and read to you for the next 15 minutes, and nothing else will happen during that time."*

Periods of uninterrupted sleep must be planned into the day so that the child has time to rest and regain strength, both mentally and physically.

Infants manage stress by sucking. If the child cannot take liquids by mouth, a pacifier should be provided so that the child can achieve stress reduction and comfort from sucking. Children who have recently given up bottles or pacifiers tend to regress during hospitalization, and these items should be made available to them if desired. The feelings of safety and comfort afforded by their use far exceed any problems associated with weaning after discharge from the hospital.

Recently mastered toileting skills will be lost with the stress of a major burn injury, so children should be placed in diapers until they are once again able to invest the emotional and physical work required to resume independent toileting. The child must be reassured that this behavior is acceptable during the burn injury, that punishment will not occur, and that diapering is not intended as a punishment. After discharge at home, at a time that the child and the parents feel is appropriate, toilet training can begin again.

After the acute crisis of burn injury is over and the child is nearing the time of discharge, short trips may be taken to nearby parks or shops to help the child and the parents adjust to public reactions to the burn injury. The child may never look unburned, but the location of the burn and whether it can easily be covered with clothing during daily activities are factors that have a bearing on the child's and the family's adjustment. Depending on the age of the child, peer pressure may also be a factor. Some severely burned children lose all facial features, including ears, and going out in public becomes an ordeal that they and their family avoid. Other children lead well-adjusted lives despite major disfigurement. The inner strengths of the family and the value ascribed to the child by the family both before and after the burn appear to be deciding factors in the level of adjustment. More specifically, children appear to respond to the burn and to give it a meaning in a manner similar to the mother's reaction. Nevertheless, extensive, disfiguring burn scars have a tremendous long-term impact on the child and the family. Occasionally, family members will not be able to accept the child and will request foster placement.

Community Care

Involving the family early in the care of the child facilitates acceptance and eases the transition to the provision of care in the community. As soon as possible after discharge from the hospital, the child and the family should resume normal daily activities. Most burn units have a formal program designed to facilitate the child's return to school. A staff member may accompany the child on the first day back to school in order to explain what has happened to him or her and to describe the purpose of pressure garments or other therapeutic interventions. Age-related issues of intimacy and sexuality will eventually arise, as will self-image and self-esteem issues. Social workers and psychologists monitor the child's and the family's adjustment during return clinic visits the first year after burn injury.

In the case of nonaccidental burn injuries, the child's placement after hospital discharge is determined by the legal system. Nurses should be prepared for the fact that the child may be returned to the home environment if it is believed that the child's safety can be ensured. The younger child does not understand the concept of child abuse and loves and depends on the parents just as much as any other child. Separation of a child and parent carries significant psychosocial implications, and the goal of protective services is always to restore and to maintain the family unit if the child's safety can be ensured by close supervision by the agency.

Prevention. Children can be taught to evacuate the house in the event of a fire using fire drills that identify two or more exits from each room and a location for the family to meet outside the house. Other measures, such as the "stop, drop, and roll" program, can greatly decrease the severity of a burn injury by stopping the burning process and by decreasing the amount of smoke inhalation and facial burns that occur (Powell, 1986). Public campaigns to educate adults to turn hot water heater thermostats down to 120°F can also reduce the number of accidental scald burns (Malay & Achauer, 1987). Many of these programs are taught in schools and youth groups, but nurses can implement these programs by contacting their local fire department or burn center. Public education regarding the presence of a working smoke detector can also significantly decrease the incidence of burns.

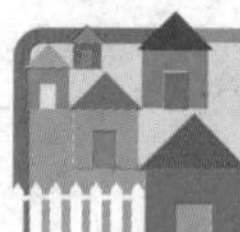

Chart 25–29
Community Care

Preventing Cold Injury

Parents and older children, especially those living in cold climates, must be educated about the hazards of cold injury. *The best treatment for cold injury is prevention.*

- Children should wear several layers of clothing under appropriate outerwear garments (including two pairs of socks, mittens, and a hat that covers the ears) to ensure warmth when playing outdoors.
- Outer garments should be waterproof, insulated, and offer protection against the wind.
- Children should wear well-fitted, insulated, waterproof, nonconstricting footwear in cold weather.
- If the child's hands, feet, or other body parts become wet while outdoors, a change to dry clothing or footwear should be made immediately.
- Children should rub their hands together or scrunch up their face when they are feeling cold to help warm up their bodies.
- Ample food and fluid should be provided during the time of outdoor activities.
- The child's exposure to extremely cold temperatures should be monitored and supervised by an adult.
- An adult who is feeling cold can be certain that children are also feeling cold, and should bring them indoors.
- Children who participate in outdoor sports activities should be alert to the presence of numbing of body parts, particularly the nose, ears, fingers, and toes.

Cold Injury

In cold-dry and cold-wet weather, children who play outdoors and participate in outdoor sports activities are at risk for cold injury and hypothermia (Chart 25–29). **Frostnip** is a superficial cold injury that causes no damage to the skin tissue. **Frostbite** may be superficial or deep and can cause significant tissue damage or even tissue death. Exposed areas of the face (nose, cheek, chin, ear) are at greatest risk. **Immersion foot (trench foot)** occurs in cold weather when the feet are exposed to damp or wet, poorly ventilated shoes, causing tissue maceration and infection. **Hypothermia** is defined as a core body temperature of less than 35°C. A decrease in body temperature can be caused by immersion in icy water or prolonged exposure to cold temperatures. Hypothermia is discussed in more detail in Chapter 30.

Extreme cold is an external force that freezes the cells of the skin layers. Ice crystals may form between or within cells, interfering with the activities of the normal sodium pump. This leads to rupture of the cell membranes (Herrin & Antoon, 1996b). Red cells or platelets may clump at the damaged site, causing microemboli or thrombosis. Blood may be shunted from the injured area, eventually causing cell death if not treated. The offending agent is not only the cold temperature but also the rapid motion of the surrounding wind or the presence of damp cold conditions; together, these forces combine to damage the skin by conduction and convection.

Alert: *Butane and propane propellants that are widely used in spray aerosols (e.g., hair spray, air fresheners) can cause moderately severe frostbite when sprayed directly on the skin at close range (Lacour & Le Coultre, 1991). Spray aerosols are a source of a variety of injuries and should be kept safely out of reach of children.*

Susceptibility to cold injury may be increased by dehydration, fatigue, hunger, anemia, ingestion of alcohol or illicit substances, and the presence of other illnesses. Therapy for any type of cold injury should begin as soon the injury is noticed.

Frostnip

Frostnip lesions are usually manifested as firm white patches on the face, ears, and extremities that are numb. As the body is warmed, erythema develops with no blistering at the time. Over the ensuing 24 to 72 hours, blistering and peeling may occur. The affected area may have a residual hypersensitivity to cold that lasts for several days to weeks.

Care for the child with mild frostnip primarily involves providing first aid and teaching prevention measures. The child should be removed to a warm area as soon as possible and the affected areas examined for the possibility of more serious damage.

Tip: *As the affected area rewarms, it may cause a stinging sensation, which may frighten the child. Explain to the child the sensations that he or she can expect. A good analogy may be to compare it to when a hand or foot "falls asleep." As the foot "wakes up," it tingles, almost to the point of hurting. The feeling does go away.*

Frostbite

Frostbite first develops as an initial erythema of the skin, which progresses to cold, hard, white, waxlike areas. The ears, fingers, and toes are some of the most common sites of frostbite. The skin sensation of cold progresses from numbness or warmth, followed by a burning feeling. Eventually, immobility of the joints and extremities occurs. If tissue damage is severe enough, even prompt treatment will not avert amputation of the diseased area.

Frostbite is more involved and usually requires more aggressive therapy. Rubbing the affected area may cause further damage. While the child is being transported to an acute care facility or clinic, the affected area can be warmed against an unaffected hand, abdomen, or axilla area. Dry heat should not be applied, rather, the affected area needs more rapid warming provided by a bath of warm water (approximately 42°C) (Herrin & Antoon, 1996b). A return of pink color should be observed. Blisters may develop on the affected area once thawing is initiated. The extremity should be kept elevated to avoid swelling, and the affected area should be aseptically wrapped to avoid secondary infection. If infection occurs, affected areas must be debrided by the health care provider. Anesthetics may be necessary if the area is painful and swelling occurs. Vasodilating agents such as prazosin and phenoxybenzamine have been used to improve circulation to the affected area.

Prognosis can be very good, especially if secondary infection does not occur. Amputation of tissue may be necessary if prolonged conservative management demonstrates no signs of vascular improvement.

Immersion Foot (Trench Foot)

When the feet, covered by poorly ventilated shoes, become damp or wet in cold weather, the extremity can become cold and numb. The foot becomes pale, edematous, and clammy. Tissue maceration and infection can occur, as can long-term hypersensitivity to temperature changes. As soon as it is known that the child's feet (or shoes) are wet, the child's footwear should be changed to more appropriate dry and well-fitting footwear. Treatment includes drying the skin, keeping the area well ventilated, and preventing or treating infection.

Disorders of the Hair and Nails

Disorders of the hair and nails may result from such diverse causes as growth pattern disturbances, hereditary or biological variances, localized or systemic diseases, nutritional deficits, or trauma. A hair or nail problem is rarely the primary reason for a child to seek health care; rather, the problem is usually discovered by an astute nurse during routine or focused assessment.

Hair Disorders

The nurse should inspect the hair for distribution, color, texture, amount, and quality. Hair is distributed over all parts of the body except the palms, soles, inner labial surfaces in girls, and the prepuce and glans penis in boys (Engel, 1997). The hair on the scalp is normally strong, shiny, and silky. Hair over other parts of the body varies in texture and color. For instance, pubic hair on the mature adolescent is dark in color and very coarse.

Hair color changes in response to certain dietary changes, ingested substances, or disease processes. For instance, kwashiorkor and zinc deficiencies can cause depigmented hair. Ingestion of copper can turn the hair green, and ingestion of cobalt can turn the hair blue. Discoloration can also be due to the dithranol therapy for treatment of psoriasis. Premature graying (before age 20) can be an early sign of pernicious anemia or thrombosis.

Delayed or absent hair growth may indicate an ectodermal dysplasia. Alopecia (loss of hair) may occur for a variety of reasons, including hair pulling, tinea capitis, and the use of chemotherapeutic agents. Hair disorders, including hair loss (alopecia) and structural anomalies of the hair shafts, are briefly described in Table 25–20. In most cases, disorders of the hair can be corrected by addressing or treating the underlying cause.

Table 25–20
Disorders of the Hair

Disorder	Definition
Hypertrichosis	Excessive hair growth in inappropriate locations
Hirsutism	Male-type secondary sexual hair growth in the female
Hypotrichosis	Deficient hair growth
Alopecia	Partial or complete hair loss, which may be hereditary or acquired, diffuse or patchy, scarring or nonscarring
Occipital alopecia of the newborn	Hair loss on the occipital area of the scalp due to friction between the child's head and, for example, a mattress or sheets
Telogen effluvium	Loss of scalp hair due to the premature conversion of hair loss in · The newborn during the first few years of life · Postpartum women · After an acute febrile illness · After discontinuation of oral contraceptives
Congenital circumscribed alopecia	Localized areas of hair loss present at birth, usually overlying a birthmark or a sebaceous or epidermal nevus
Friction alopecia	Patchy hair loss caused by a variety of hairstyles: ponytails, curlers, rollers, tight braids
Toxic alopecia	Hair loss as a side effect of radiation therapy and certain drugs, such as chemotherapeutic agents
Trichotillomania	Hair loss with broken hairs due to the habit of pulling or twisting the hair
Alopecia areata	Rapid and complete loss of hair in round or oval patches on the scalp. The cause is unknown; 20% of patients have a family history of the illness. There is increased incidence in patients with Down syndrome.
Trichorrhexis nodosa	Structural defect that appears as a node or swelling on the high shaft. The defect is caused by a fracture of the hair shaft with derangement of the cells in the cortex.
Monilethrix	Autosomal dominant hair shaft defect in which the hair appears dry, lusterless, and brittle and fractures spontaneously or with mild trauma. Eyebrows, lashes, body, and sexual hair may be affected. Spontaneous improvement may occur at puberty.
Trichorrhexis infaginata (bamboo hair)	Feature of Netherton's syndrome. Hair is dry and fragile with no apparent growth. It is thought to result from a transient defect in keratinization. Hair growth may improve significantly at puberty.
Trichoschisis	Hair shaft defect in which affected children have brittle hair. The hair shaft is actually fractured.
Pili torti	Autosomal dominant condition in which a structural defect of the hair shaft causes it to be twisted on its own axis. The hair is normal at birth, but is replaced by abnormal hair that becomes evident between ages 2 and 3 years. The affected hairs have a spangled appearance, are fragile, and are often ash-blonde in color.
Pili annulati	Ringed hair that is characterized by hair shafts banded with bright rings when viewed in reflected light. The hair is not fragile. It can be a familial or a sporadic defect.
Wooly hair disease	Tightly curled, abnormal hair seen at birth. It may occur as an autosomal dominant condition in which most other hair is normal, as an autosomal recessive condition in which all hair is affected and appears short and pale, or in sporadic form (wooly hair nevus) in which localized areas of the scalp are affected.

Table 25–20
Disorders of the Hair *Continued*

Disorder	Definition
Menkes' kinky hair syndrome	X-linked recessive disorder in which twisting of the hair is a result of a copper deficiency
Pityriasis aminatacea	Thick mat of scale on the scalp. It is a reaction pattern of the scalp to inflammation, infection, or trauma.
Tinea capitis	Fungal infection of the scalp caused by *Microsporum canis* or *Trichophyton tonsurans.* It produces thick white scaling, broken-off hairs, and areas of alopecia.

Table 25–21
Nail Abnormalities

Name	Definition
Anonychia	Absence of the nail plate
Koilonychia	Flattening and concavity of the nail plate with loss of normal contour
Macronychia	Abnormally large nail
Micronychia	Unusually small nail
Leukonychia	White opacity of the nail plate, which may involve the entire nail plate, may be punctuated, or may be striated. Can be due to trauma, infection, dermatosis, malnutrition, anemia, heavy metal poisoning, or a benign hereditary defect.
Onychogryposis	Acquired nail defect in which the nail plate is thick, overgrown, and distorted
Onycholysis	Separation of the nail plate from the nail bed resulting from trauma, psoriasis, fungal infection, contact dermatitis, porphyria, drugs, or drug-induced phototoxicity
Beau lines	Transverse grooves in the nail plate that represent an inability of the nail matrix to produce a nail plate of normal thickness owing to periodic trauma or secondary to systemic disease
Yellow nail syndrome	Nails are yellow and slow to grow. Associated with congenital abnormalities of the lymphatic vessels and chylothorax.
Pachyonychia congenita	Autosomal dominant disorder characterized by gross nail thickening
Pigmented naevi of the nail	Longitudinal band of pigment in the nail plate that is common in dark-skinned individuals
Lichen planus	Common longitudinal ridging of the nail plate. Nail thinning and pterygium formation may occur.
Twenty nail dystrophy	Characterized by longitudinal ridging, fragility, distal notching, and opalescent discoloration of all the nails. Tends to be self-limiting and reversible; eventually affects all 20 nails.
Paronychia	Acute infection of the nail fold, which can be very painful, and is seen commonly in thumb or finger suckers. Usually caused by staphylococcal, streptococcal, or pseudomonal infections. Usually requires removal of the nail bed.
Herpetic whitlow	Primary infection of the nail fold with herpes simplex
Ingrown toenail	Caused by incorrect cutting of toenail or ill-fitting footwear. Produces pain, bacterial paronychia, and overgrowth of granulation tissue around the soft, pliable nail plate

Nail Disorders

Disorders of the nails can cause changes in normal nail color, shape, texture, and size. The nurse inspects the nails for these changes and for the presence of nail biting, skin picking, and infection. Nails can become discolored from antimalarial agents and certain other drugs, bacterial or fungal infections, and skin disorders such as alopecia areata, lichen planus, and psoriasis. Nail discoloration can also occur secondary to a systemic problem such as jaundice or cyanosis. Clubbing of nails may indicate chronic respiratory or cardiac disease. The curve of the nail in a convex or concave fashion may simply be hereditary or indicate injury, iron deficiency, or infection (Engel, 1997). Nail abnormalities in children that may reflect generalized skin diseases, systemic disease, bacterial or fungal infections, or trauma are reviewed in Table 25–21.

Summary of Key Concepts

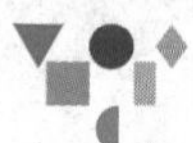

- The condition of the skin, hair, and nails serves as an indicator to help monitor general hygiene, dietary patterns, responses to stress, and the presence of systemic disease processes.
- Problems of the skin can be an acute source of embarrassment for the child and the family; therefore, the physical assessment should be conducted with great tact and discretion.
- The newborn's skin is structurally similar to an adult's, but it has yet to develop all of its protective, metabolic, and interactive functions.
- Wound healing in children involves the same physiologic responses as in adults; however, the responses are modified by the functioning of the child's immature, developing organ system.
- The best treatment for many pediatric skin disorders is for the child and family to use thorough preventive measures. By determining the causative factors of the disorder, the nurse can teach the child and the family to avoid potential irritants, to improve personal hygiene, and to protect the skin from unnecessary personal and environmental trauma.
- When a child has an alteration in skin integrity, a variety of treatment options may be used. It is important for the nurse to spend considerable time providing education to the family because most of the treatment modalities are carried out in the home by the family members. Both oral and written instructions must be given.
- Bacterial, viral, and fungal infections of the skin can be highly contagious. The nurse should assist the family to identify close contacts of the child, and to provide instructions for treatment or referral to minimize the continuing spread of the contagion.
- Drug allergies and drug hypersensitivity often manifest through changes in the skin. The nurse should educate parents to notify their health care provider immediately if a skin rash appears following the administration or application of a medication.

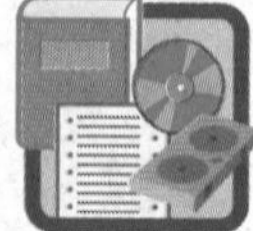

Resources

Organizations

American Academy of Dermatology
930 North Meacham Road
P. O. Box 4014
Schaumberg, IL 60168-4014

Canadian Psoriasis Foundation
1565 Carling Avenue
Suite 400
Ottawa, Ontario, Canada K 1Z8R1

Dermatology Nurses' Association
Box 56
Pitman, NJ 08071-0056
(609) 256-2330

Dystrophic Epidermolysis Bullosa Research Association (DEBRA)
141 Fifth Avenue
New York, NY 10010

Eczema Association for Science and Education
1221 S.W. Yamhill
Suite 303
Portland, OR 97205

Foundation for Ichthyosis and Related Skin Types (FIRST)
P. O. Box 20921
Raleigh, NC 27619-0921
(919) 782-5728

Herpes Resource Center
c/o American Social Health Association
P. O. Box 13827
Research Triangle Park, NC 27704

Ichthyosis Foundation of America
710 Laurel Avenue
Suite B-8
San Mateo, CA 94401

Large Congenital Nevocytic Nevi Registry
Oncology Section, Skin and Cancer Unit
New York University Medical Center
562 First Avenue
New York, NY 10016

Melanoma Foundation
750 Menlo Avenue
#250
Menlo Park, CA 94205

National Alopecia Areata Foundation
714 "C" Street
Suite 216
San Rafael, CA 94901

National Cancer Institute
National Institutes of Health
NIH 31
9000 Rockville Pike
Bethesda, MD 20892

National Congenital Port Wine Stain Foundation
125 East 63rd Street
New York, NY 10021

National Pediculosis Association
P.O. Box 149
Newton, MA 02161
(800) 446-4672

National Psoriasis Foundation
6600 SW 92nd Avenue
Suite 300
Portland, OR 97223
(800) 248-0886
Web: http://www.psoriasis.org

National Vitiligo Foundation
Box 6337
Tyler, TX 75711

Skin Cancer Foundation
245 Fifth Avenue
#2402
New York, NY 10016

Skin Phototrauma Foundation
P. O. Box 6312
Parsippany, NJ 07054

United Scleroderma Foundation, Inc.
P. O. Box 399
Watsonville, CA 95077-0399
(800) 722-4673
Web: http://www.scleroderma.com

Wound Ostomy and Continence Nurses Society
2755 Bristol Street
Suite 110
Costa Mesa, CA 92626
(714) 476-0268
Web: http://www.wocn.org

References

Agency for Health Care Policy and Research. (1992). *Pressure ulcers in adults: Prediction and prevention* (DHHS Publication No. 92-0050). Washington, DC: U.S. Government Printing Office.

Ansell, B. (1991). Juvenile dermatomyositis. *Rheumatology Disease Clinics of North America, 17*(4), 931–942.

Arnsmeier, S., Riccardi, V., & Paller, A. (1994). Familial multiple cafe au lait spots. *Archives of Dermatology, 130*, 1425–1426.

Balthrop, D., & Brueton, M. (1991). *Paediatric therapeutics*. London: Butterworth-Heinemann.

Barber, N. (1996). Dermatological diseases. In C. Burns, N. Barber, M. Brady, & A. Dunn (Eds.), *Pediatric primary care* (pp. 737–768). Philadelphia: W. B. Saunders.

Barnes, S., & Dire, D. (1994). What's your diagnosis? Answer: Stevens-Johnson syndrome. *Consultant, 34*(12), 1721–1723.

Ben-Amitai, D., & Ashkenazi, S. (1993). Common bacterial infections in childhood. *Pediatric Annals, 22*(4), 225–233.

Bergstrom, N., Bennett, M.A., Carlson, C. E., et al. (December, 1994). Treatment of pressure ulcers (Clinical practice guideline no. 15. Public Health Service, Agency for Health Care Policy and Research, publication no. 95-0652). Rockville, MD: U.S. Department of Health and Human Services.

Beutner, K. (1993). Cutaneous viral infections. *Pediatric Annals, 22*(4), 247–252.

Birdsall, C., & Gabasan, A. (1993). Preventing complications in severe exfoliative skin diseases. *Dimensions of Critical Care Nursing, 12*(3), 138–148.

Brimhall, C., & Esterly, N. (1993). Scabies, lice, and other unwelcome guests. *Contemporary Pediatrics, 2*, 10–19.

Buller, D., Callister, M., & Reichert, T. (1995). Skin cancer prevention by parents of young children: Health information sources, skin cancer knowledge, and sun-protection practices. *Oncology Nursing Forum, 22*(10), 1559–1566.

Burdette-Taylor, S. (1995). Eczema, ichthyosis, psoriasis: Conditions of cornification. *Ostomy/Wound Management, 41*(7), 36–42.

Carrougher, G. J. (1993). Inhalation injury. *AACN Clinical Issues in Critical Care Nursing, 4*, 367–377.

Chang, K. (1995). Chinese Americans. In J. Giger & R. Davidhizar (Eds.), *Transcultural nursing: Assessment and intervention* (pp. 395–416). St. Louis: Mosby.

Charlesworth, E. (1995). The spectrum of urticaria. *Immunology and Allergy Clinics of North America, 15*(4), 641–657.

Chunge, R., Scott, F., Underwood, J., & Zavarella, K. (1991). A review of the epidemiology, public health importance, treatment and control of head lice. *Canadian Journal of Public Health, 82*(3), 196–199.

Clore, E. (1983). Lice: Ancient pest with new resistance. *Pediatric Nursing, 9*(5), 347–350.

Clore, E., & Longyear, L. (1990). Comprehensive pediculosis screening programs for elementry schools. *Journal of School Health, 60*(5), 212–214.

Clore, E., & Longyear, L. (1993). A comparative study of seven pediculicides and their packaged nit removal combs. *Journal of Pediatric Health Care, 7*(2), 55–60.

Cortiella, J., & Marvin, J. A. (1997). Management of the pediatric burn patient. *Nursing Clinics of North America, 32*, 311–329.

Cuthbertson, G., & Grose, C. (1987). Antimicrobial chemotherapy in the adolescent. *Journal of Adolescent Health Care, 8*, 113–120.

Dagan, R. (1993). Impetigo in childhood: Changing epidemiology and new treatments. *Pediatric Annals, 22*(4), 235–240.

Dahl, R., Bernhisel-Broadbent, J., Scanlon-Holdford, S., Sampson, H., & Lupo, M. (1995). Sleep disturbances in children with atopic dermatitis. *Archives of Pediatric and Adolescent Medicine, 149*, 856–860.

Darmstadt, G. L., & Lane, A. T. (1994). Impetigo: An overview. *Pediatric Dermatology, 11*(4), 293–303.

Demers, D., Bass, J., Vincent, J., Person, D., Noyes, D., Staege, C., Samlaska, C., Lockwood, N., Regnery, R., & Anderson, B. (1995). Cat-scratch disease in Hawaii: Etiology and seroepidemiology. *The Journal of Pediatrics, 124*, 23–26.

Dieterich-Miller, C., Cohen, B., & Liggett, J. (1992). Behavioral adjustment and self-concept of young children with hemangiomas. *Pediatric Dermatology*, 9(3), 241–245.

Edwards, R., & Ridder, M. (1985). Stevens-Johnson syndrome: A multisystem case. *Dimensions of Critical Care Nursing*, 4(6), 335–348.

Eichenfield, L., & Honig, P. (1991). Blistering disorders in childhood. *Pediatric Clinics of North America*, 38(4), 959–976.

Engel, J. (1997). *Pocket guide to pediatric assessment*. St. Louis: Mosby–Year Book.

Esterly, N. (1992). Hemangiomas in infants and children: Clinical observations. *Pediatric Dermatology*, 9(4), 353–355.

Esterly, N. (1996). Cutaneous hemangiomas, vascular stains and malformations, and associated syndromes. *Current Problems in Pediatrics, 26*(1), 3–39.

Finkelstein, J., Schwartz, S., Madden, M., Marano, M., & Goodwin, C. (1992). Pediatric burns. *Pediatric Clinics of North America*, 39(5), 1145–1163.

Fitzpatrick, T. B., Eisen, A. Z., Wolff, K., Freedberg, I. M., & Austen, K. F. (1993). *Dermatology in general medicine* (vol. II). New York: McGraw-Hill.

Foltz, A. T. (1993). Parental knowledge and practices of skin cancer prevention: A pilot study. *Journal of Pediatric Health Care*, 7(5), 220–225.

Goldgeier, M. (1993). Fungal infections of the skin, hair, and nails. *Pediatric Annals, 22*(4), 253–259.

Gordon, M., & Goodwin, C. (1997). Initial assessment, management and stabilization. *Nursing Clinics of North America, 32*, 237–249.

Gordon, M., & Montgomery, L. (1996). Minimizing epidermal stripping in the very low birth weight infant: Integrating research and practice to affect infant outcome. *Neonatal Network, 15*(1), 37–44.

Goskowicz, M., & Eichenfield, L. F. (1993). Cutaneous findings of nutritional deficiencies in children. *Current Opinion in Pediatrics*, 5(4), 441–445.

Gupta, A., & Waldhauser, L. (1997). Adverse drug reactions from birth to early childhood. *Pediatric Clinics of North America*, 44(1), 79–93.

Harper, I. (1990). *Handbook of paediatrics*. London: Butterworth-Heinemann.

Helvig, E. (1993). Pediatric burn injuries. *AACN Clinical Issues in Critical Care Nursing, 4*, 433–442.

Herrin, J. T., & Antoon, A. Y. (1996a). Burn injuries. In R. Behrman, R. Kleigman, & A. Arvin (Eds.), *Nelson textbook of pediatrics* (15th ed., pp. 270–277). Philadelphia: W. B. Saunders.

Herrin, J., & Antoon, A. (1996b). Cold injuries. In R. Behrman, R. Kliegman, & A. Arvin (Eds.), *Nelson textbook of pediatrics* (pp. 277–278). Philadelphia: W. B. Saunders.

Hogan, D., Schachner, L., & Tanglertsampan, C. (1991). Diagnosis and treatment of childhood scabies and pediculosis. *Pediatric Clinics of North America*, 38(4), 941–957.

Hogan, P., & Weston, W. (1993). Allergic contact dermatitis in children. *Pediatrics in Review, 14*(6), 240–243.

Hurwitz, S. (1994). Acne vulgaris: Pathogenesis and management. *Pediatrics in Review, 15*(2), 47–51.

Johr, R., & Schachner, L. (1997). Neonatal dermatologic challenges. *Pediatrics in Review, 18*(3), 86–94.

Kahn, R., & Goldstein, E. (1993). Common bacterial skin infections. *Postgraduate Medicine*, 93(6), 175–182.

Knight, M. (1993). Adverse drug reactions. In F. Burg, J. Ingelfinger, & E. Wald (Eds.), *Current pediatric therapy 14* (pp. 681–683). Philadelphia: W. B. Saunders.

Kravitz, M. (1988). Thermal injuries. In V. D. Cardona, P. D. Hurn, A. M. Scanlon-Schipp, & S. W. Veise-Berry (Eds.), *Trauma nursing: From resuscitation through rehabilitation* (pp. 707–745). Philadelphia: W. B. Saunders.

Kravitz, M. (1993). Immune consequences of burn injury. *AACN Clinical Issues in Critical Care Nursing, 4*, 399–413.

Kushner, D., & Caldwell, B. (1996). Hand-foot-and-mouth disease. *Journal of the American Podiatric Medical Association*, 86(6), 257–259.

Lacour, M., & Le Coultre, C. (1991). Spray-induced frostbite in a child: A new hazard with novel aerosol propellants. *Pediatric Dermatology*, 8(3), 207–209.

Lane, A., & Darmstadt, G. (1996). Eczema. In R. Behrman, R. Kliegman, & A. Arvin (Eds.), *Nelson textbook of pediatrics* (pp. 1856–1860). Philadelphia: W. B. Saunders.

LaVoo, E., & Paller, A. (1994). Common skin problems during the first year of life. *Pediatric Clinics of North America, 41*, 1105–1119.

Lesh, D. (1996). Dermatophytosis. *Journal of the American Academy of Nurse Practitioners*, 8(6), 289–292.

Maley, M. P., & Achauer, B. M. (1987). Prevention of tap water scald burns. *Journal of Burn Care and Rehabilitation*, 8, 62.

Miller, S., Richard, R., & Staley, M. (1994). Triage and resuscitation of the burn patient. In R. Richard & M. Staley (Eds.), *Burn care and rehabilitation: Principles and practice* (pp. 105–118). Philadelphia: F. A. Davis.

Molter, N. (1993). When is a burn injury healed? Psychosocial implications of care. *AACN Clinical Issues in Critical Care Nursing, 4*, 424–432.

Murray, J. (1988). Dermatology. In J. D. Crapo, M. A. Hamilton, & S. Edgman (Eds.), *Medicine and pediatrics in one book* (pp. 478–509). Philadelphia: Hanley & Belfus.

Nicol, N. (1989). What's new with sunscreens? Choices–choices–choices. *Pediatric Nursing, 15*(4), 417–418.

Nicol, N. H., & Fenske, N. A. (1993). Photodamage: Cause, clinical manifestations, and prevention. *Dermatology Nursing*, 5(4), 263–275.

Novotny, J. (1989). Adolescents, acne, and the side effects of Accutane. *Pediatric Nursing, 15*(3), 247–248.

O'Brien, J. (1995). Common skin problems of infancy, childhood, and adolescence. *Primary Care, 22*(1), 99–115.

Pachman, L. (1990). Juvenile dermatomyositis: Natural history and susceptibility factors. In P. Woo, P. White, & B. Ansell (Eds.), *Paediatric rheumatology update* (pp. 171–181). Oxford: Oxford University Press.

Pappas, P. G., & Lipsky, B. A. (1983). Cellulitis: Recognition and management. *Hospital Medicine, 19*(7), 145–155.

Peters, S. (1997a). Treating dermatitis in children: The role of topical corticoste roids. *Advance for Nurse Practitioners*, 5(2), 50–51.

Peters, S. (1997b). Saving face: Treating adolescents affected by acne vulgaris. *Advance for Nurse Practitioners*, 5(3), 43–49 & 64.

Powell, K. (1995). Orbital and periorbital cellulitis. *Pediatrics in Review, 16*(5), 163–167.

Powell, P. A. (1986). Learn Not to Burn Foundation. *Fire Journal, 80*, 12–16.

Quigley, S., & Curley, M. (1996). Skin integrity in the pediatric population: Preventing and managing pressure ulcers. *Journal of the Society of Pediatric Nurses, 1*(1), 7–18.

Rasmussen, J. (1994). Scabies. *Pediatrics in Review, 15*(3), 110–114.

Rasmussen, S. (1995). Erythema multiforme, Steven's Johnson syndrome and toxic epidermal necrolysis. *Dermatology Nursing, 74*, 37–43.

Reeves, S., Warden, G., & Staley, M. (1994). Management of the pediatric burn patient. In R. Richard & M. Staley (Eds.), *Burn care and rehabilitation: Principles and practice* (pp. 499–530). Philadelphia: F. A. Davis.

Romeo, S. (1995). Atopic dermatitis: The itch that rashes. *Pediatric Nursing*, 21(2), 157–163.

Saffle, J., & Schnebly, W. A. (1994). Burn wound care. In R. Richard & M. Staley (Eds.), *Burn care and rehabilitation: Principles and practice* (pp. 119–176). Philadelphia: F. A. Davis.

Saltzer, E. B., & Saltzer, E. I. (1987). Internal control and health: Which comes first? *Western Journal of Nursing Research*, 9(4), 542–554.

Sargent, S., & Martin, J. (1992). Scabies outbreak in a day-care center. *Pediatrics*, 94(6), 1012–1013.

Schmitt, B. (1994). *Instructions for pediatric patients*. Philadelphia: W. B. Saunders.

Schumann, L. L. (1991). Care of the patient with major burns. In R. B. Trofino (Ed.), *Nursing care of the burn injured patient* (pp. 135–181). Philadelphia: F. A. Davis.

Schwartz, R., & Janniger, C. (1996). Erythema toxicum neonatorum. *Cutis, 58*, 153–155.

Sexton, D. J., & Corey, G. R. (1992). Rocky Mountain "spotless" and "almost spotless" fever: A wolf in sheep's clothing. *Clinical Infectious Diseases, 15*, 439–448.

Shriner, D., Schwartz, R., & Janniger, C. (1995). Impetigo. *Cutis, 56*(1), 30–32.

Silverman, R. (1991). Hemangiomas and vascular malformations, *Pediatric Clinics of North America, 38*(4), 811–833.

Strickland, M. (1997). Evaluation of bacterial growth with occlusive dressing use on excoriated skin in the premature infant. *Neonatal Network, 16*(2), 29–35.

Su, J., Kemp, A., Varigos, G., & Nolan, T. (1997). Atopic eczema: Its impact on the child and financial costs. *Archives of Disease in Childhood, 76*, 159–162.

Thomas, I., & Janniger, C. (1993). Hand, foot, and mouth disease. *Cutis, 52*, 265–266.

Vernon, H. J., Lane, A. T., Wischerath, L. J., Davis, J. M., & Menegus, M. A. (1990). Semipermeable dressing and transdermal water loss in premature infants. *Pediatrics, 86*(3), 357–362.

Vernon, P. (1997). The heartbreak of psoriasis: No laughing matter. *Journal of Pediatric Health Care, 11*, 32–33

Warren, R., Perez, M., Wilking, Q., & Myones, B. (1994). Pediatric rheumatology diseases. *Pediatric Clinics of North America, 41*(4), 783.

Weston, W., Lane, A., & Morelli, J. (1996). *Color textbook of pediatric dermatology*. St Louis: Mosby.

Wilkowska, A., Grubska-Suchanek, E., Karwacka, J., & Szarmach, H. (1996). Contact allergy in children. *Cutis, 58*, 176–180.

Woolridge, W. E. (1991). Managing skin infections in children. *Postgraduate Medicine, 89*(4), 109–112.

Zinman, R., Schwartz, S., Gordon, K., Fitzpatrick, E., & Camfield, C. (1995). Predictors of sunscreen use in childhood. *Archives of Pediatric Adolescent Medicine, 149*, 804–807.

Zuker, R. M. (1988). Initial management of the burn wound. In H. Carvajal & D. Parks (Eds.), *Burns in children: Pediatric burn management* (pp. 99–105). Chicago: Year Book Medical Publishers.

Bibliography

Abdullah, A., Blakeny, P., Hunt, R., Broemeling, L., Phillips, L., Herndon, D., & Robson, M. (1994). Visible scars and self-esteem in pediatric patients with burns. *Journal of Burn Care and Rehabilitation, 15*(2), 164–168.

Adams, R. (1993). Hand eczema: The atopic subject and work. *Cutis, 52*(5), 267–269.

Bass, J. W. (1992). Treatment of skin and skin structure infections. *Pediatric Infectious Disease Journal, 11*, 152–155.

Bates, B. (1991). *A guide to physical examination*. Philadelphia: J. B. Lippincott.

Berg, R. W., Milligan, M. C., & Sarbough, F. C. (1994). Association of skin wetness and pH with diaper dermatitis. *Pediatric Dermatology, 11*(1), 18–20.

Bergus, G. R., & Johnson, J. S. (1993). Superficial tinea infections. *American Family Physician, 48*(2), 259–268.

Black, J. (1994). Surgical management of pressure ulcers. *Nursing Clinics of North America, 29*(4), 801–809.

Bryant, R. A. (1992). *Acute and chronic wounds: Nursing management*. St. Louis: Mosby.

Cioffi, W. G., & Rue, L. W. (1991). Diagnosis and treatment of inhalation injury. *Critical Care Clinics of North America, 3*, 191–198.

East, M. K., Jones, C. A., Feller, I., Saxon, M. I., & Wolfe, R. (1988). Epidemiology of burns in children. In H. F. Carvajal & D. H. Parks (Eds.), *Burns in children: Pediatric burn management* (pp. 3–10). Chicago: Year Book Publishers.

Eichenfield, L. F., & Honig, P. J. (1991). Blistering disorders in childhood. *Pediatric Clinics of North America, 38*(4), 959–975.

Engelhardt, V., & Clark, S. (1994). Early enteral feeding of a severely burned pediatric patient. *Journal of Burn Care and Rehabilitation, 15*(3), 293–297.

Enjolras, O., & Mulliken, J. B. (1993). The current management of vascular birthmarks. *Pediatric Dermatology, 10*(4), 311–333.

Fairchild, S. (1993). *Perioperative nursing principles and practice*. Boston: Jones & Bartlett.

Faldmo, L., & Kravitz, M. (1993). Management of acute burns and burn shock resuscitation. *AACN Clinical Issues in Critical Care Nursing, 4*, 351–366.

Fallat, M. E., & Rengers, S. J. (1993). The effect of education and safety devices on scald burn prevention. *Journal of Trauma, 34*(4), 560–563.

Farrington, E. (1992). Diaper dermatitis. *Pediatric Nursing, 18*(1), 81–82.

Garvin, G. (1990). Wound healing in pediatrics. *Nursing Clinics of North America, 25*(1), 181–192.

Givens, T., Murray, M., & Baker, R. (1995). Comparison of 1% and 2.5% selenium sulfide in the treatment of tinea capitis. *Archives of Pediatric and Adolescent Medicine, 149*, 808–811.

Hagan, D. J., Schachner, L., & Tanglertsampan, C. (1991). Diagnosis and treatment of childhood scabies and pediculosis. *Pediatric Clinics of North America, 38*(4), 941–956.

Hanifin, J. M. (1991). Atopic dermatitis in infants and children. *Pediatric Clinics of North America, 38*(4), 763–787.

Hendricks, W. M. (1990). The classification of burns. *Journal of the American Academy of Dermatology, 22*, 838–839.

Herndon, D., Rutan, R., & Rutan, T. (1993). Management of the pediatric patient with burns. *Journal of Burn Care and Rehabilitation, 14*(1), 3–8.

Hotter, A. (1990). Wound healing and immunocompromise. *Nursing Clinics of North America, 25*(1), 193.

Kamper, C. (1991). Treatment of Lyme disease. *Journal of Pediatric Health Care, 5*(2), 99–105.

Konop, D. J. (1991). General local treatment. In R. B. Trofino (Ed.), *Nursing care of the burn injured patient* (pp. 42–67). Philadelphia: F. A. Davis.

Krasner, D. (1991). Resolving the dressing dilemma: Selecting wound dressings by category. *Ostomy/Wound Management, 35*(62), 64–70.

Krasner, D. (1992). The twelve commandments of wound care. *Nursing 95*(22), 34–42.

Kravitz, M. (Ed.). (1993). Burn care. *AACN Clinical Issues in Critical Care Nursing, 4*, 349–442.

Krowchuk, D. P., Tunnessen, W. W., & Hurwitz, S. (1990). Pediatric dermatology update. *Pediatrics, 86*(1), 125–129.

Levy, M. (1991). Disorders of the hair and scalp in children. *Pediatric Clinics of North America, 38*(4), 905–919.

LoPresti, L. (1992). Case study: Enhancing compliance in an adolescent with atopic dermatitis. *Dermatology Nursing, 4*(3), 198–200.

Mallory, S. B. (1991). Neonatal skin disorders. *Pediatric Clinics of North America, 38*(4), 745–789.

Malloy-Woods, M. B. (1991). Neonatal skin care: Prevention of skin breakdown. *Pediatric Nursing, 17*(1), 41–48.

Malinow, I., & Powell, K. (1993). Periorbital cellulitis. *Pediatric Annals, 22*(4), 241–246.

Marks, R. (1995). Summer in Australia: Skin cancer and the great SPDF debate. *Archives of Dermatology, 131*, 462–464.

Marrs, R. (1991). Coping with psoriasis. *Professional Nurse, 6*(11), 654–657.

Marrs, R. (1991). Motivation—The key to control: Nurses' role in the treatment of psoriasis. *Professional Nurse, 7*(2), 103–108.

Martin, M. T., & Seligman, R. (1991). Psychosocial care of the burn patient and significant others. In R. B. Trofino (Ed.), *Nursing care of the burn injured patient* (pp. 87–119). Philadelphia: F. A. Davis.

Martinez, S. (1992). Ambulatory management of burns in children. *Journal of Pediatric Health Care, 6*(1), 32–37.

Mayes, T., Gottschlich, M., Khoury, J., & Warden, G. (1996). Evaluation of predicted and measured energy requirements in burned children. *Journal of the American Dietetic Association, 96*(1), 24–29.

Meyer, W., Blakeney, P., Moore, P., Murphy, L., Robson, M., & Herndon, D. (1994). Parental well-being and behavioral adjustment of pediatric survivors of burns. *Journal of Burn Care and Rehabilitation, 15*(1), 62–68.

Morelli, J. (1993). On the treatment of hemangiomas. *Pediatric Dermatology, 10*(1), 84.

Nebraska Burn Institute. (1992). *Advanced burn life support course instructor's manual.* Lincoln, NE: Author.

Pagana, K., & Pagana, T. (1990). *Diagnostic testing & nursing implications.* St. Louis: Mosby.

Pappert, A., Scher, R., & Cohen, J. (1991). Nail disorders in children. *Pediatric Clinics of North America, 38*(4), 921–940.

Patrizi, A., DiLernia, A., Neri, I., DeGiorgi, L. B., & Masi, M. (1994). Epidermolysis bullosa simplex associated with muscular dystrophy: A new case. *Pediatric Dermatology, 11*(4), 342–345.

Reynolds, E. M., Ryan, D. P., & Doody, D. P. (1993). Mortality and respiratory failure in a pediatric burn population. *Journal of Pediatric Surgery, 28*(10), 1326–1331.

Rieg, L. S. (1993). Metabolic alterations and nutritional management. *AACN Clinical Issues in Critical Care Nursing, 4*, 388–398.

Ritchie, S. R., & Thompson, P. J. (1992). Primary bacterial skin infections. *Dermatology Nursing, 4*(4), 261–267.

Rivers, J. K. (1994). Too much sun: A tempest in a teapot? *Pediatric Dermatology, 11*(4), 351–353.

Sampson, L. J. (1990). The development of a discharge planning index for use in a pediatric acute burn unit. *Journal of Burn Care and Rehabilitation, 11*, 365–371.

Scarpa, C., Trevison, G., & Stinco, G. (1994). Lyme borreliosis. *Dermatologic Clinics, 12*(4), 669–683.

Slota, M. C., & O'Connor, K. O. (1992). Recognizing and treating cat scratch disease with encephalopathy in children. *Critical Care Nurse, 12*(6), 39–42.

Spraker, M. (1991). Diaper dermatitis. *Pediatric Basics, 56*, 2–5, 8.

Stewart, L. A., Engelken, G. J., & Nicol, N. H. (1992). Essentials of occupational contact dermatitis. *Dermatology Nursing, 4*(3), 175–183.

Uitlugt, N., & Ledbetter, D. (1995). Treatment of pediatric burns. In R. Arensman (Ed.), *Pediatric trauma* (pp. 173–199). New York: Raven Press.

Weber, J. M., & Tompkins, D. M. (1993). Improving survival: Infection control and burns. *AACN Clinical Issues in Critical Care Nursing, 4*, 414–423.

Weber, D. J., & Walker, D. H. (1991). Rocky Mountain spotted fever. *Infectious Disease Clinics of North America, 5*(1), 19–35.

Winston, M. H., & Shalita, A. R. (1991). Acne vulgaris: Pathogenesis and treatment. *Pediatric Clinics of North America, 38*(4), 889–901.

HEALTH CHALLENGE:

Alterations in Endocrine Status

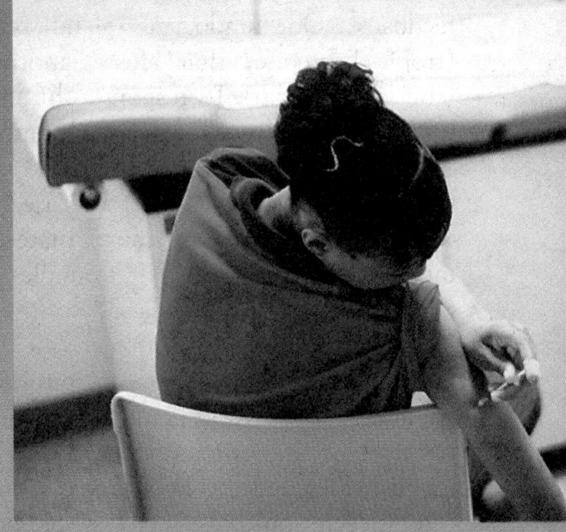

OUTLINE

Assessment of the Child with an Alteration in Endocrine Status
- Focused Health History
- Focused Physical Assessment
- Nursing Diagnoses and Outcomes
- Developmental and Biological Variances

Diagnostic Criteria for Evaluating Alterations in Endocrine Status

Treatment Modalities

Alterations in Endocrine Status
- Disorders of the Pituitary Gland
  - Diabetes Insipidus
  - Syndrome of Inappropriate Antidiuretic Hormone Secretion
  - Growth Hormone Deficiency (Hypopituitarism)
  - Precocious Puberty
  - Delayed Puberty
  - Other Pituitary Disorders
- Alterations in the Thyroid Gland
  - Hypothyroidism
  - Hyperthyroidism
- Alterations in Parathyroid Function
  - Hypoparathyroidism
  - Hyperparathyroidism
- Disorders of the Pancreas
  - Diabetes Mellitus
  - Hyperinsulinism
  - Ketotic Hypoglycemia
- Alterations in Function of the Adrenal Glands
  - Adrenocortical Insufficiency
  - Congenital Adrenal Hyperplasia
  - Cushing's Syndrome
  - Pheochromocytoma
  - Premature Adrenarche
- Gonadal Disorders
  - Ambiguous Genitalia
  - Gynecomastia
  - Premature Thelarche

OBJECTIVES

- Describe the functions of the endocrine system.
- Describe the symptoms associated with disorders of each endocrine gland.
- Identify diagnostic tests used to assess the disorders associated with each endocrine gland.
- Discuss the interdisciplinary plan of care for a child with an endocrine disorder.
- Describe the educational plan for a child with newly diagnosed insulin-dependent diabetes mellitus.

KEY TERMS

adrenarche
autoimmunity
delayed puberty
hormones
hyperfunction
hypofunction
ketoacidosis
menarche
precocious puberty

CHAPTER

26

The endocrine system is a network of six glands that regulate metabolic processes: pituitary, thyroid, parathyroids, adrenals, pancreas, and ovaries or testes (Fig. 26–1). Endocrine (or ductless) glands discharge their secretions (hormones) directly into the blood stream. These hormones exert physiologic effects on target cells in other endocrine glands, organs, or tissues.

Endocrine function is regulated largely by negative feedback. One endocrine gland produces a hormone (tropic hormone) that affects another endocrine gland (the target organ). In response, the target gland hormone inhibits the release of tropic hormone. The reverse is seen when the first endocrine gland detects low levels of target gland hormone. In that case, tropic hormone secretion increases, which causes increased secretion of the target gland hormone. For example, the pituitary gland (hypophysis or master gland) controls the release of at least seven different hormones, including thyroid-stimulating hormone (TSH). This pituitary tropic hormone stimulates the thyroid gland (target gland) to release thyroxine (T_4) and triiodothyronine (T_3) (target gland hormones). Elevated levels of these hormones then, in turn, inhibit secretion of TSH, the tropic hormone.

The hypothalamus regulates secretion of pituitary hormones. For each pituitary hormone there is a corresponding hypothalamic-releasing hormone. For some pituitary hormones there are hypothalamic-inhibiting hormones as well. The interrelationship between the hypothalamus and pituitary is called the hypothalamic-pituitary axis (Fig. 26–2). The hypothalamus is stimulated by other parts of the central nervous system (CNS), particularly in times of stress.

Regulation is not primarily by the hypothalamic-pituitary axis in the parathyroid glands, the adrenal medulla, the pancreas, and the hormones aldosterone and vasopressin. The mechanisms that regulate each of these glands and hormones are discussed in the section on the physiology of the specific gland.

Endocrine disorders are mainly two types: hypofunction and hyperfunction. Hypofunction causes deficient hormone secretion, and hyperfunction causes excessive hormone secretion. Normal levels of hormones vary widely, and the range of normalcy may overlap deficient and excessive hormonal blood levels. Several hormone determinations at various times may be necessary to establish glandular hypofunction or hyperfunction. Endocrine gland dysfunction may be due to disease of the gland itself (primary defect) or to increased or decreased secretion of its tropic hormone (secondary defect). A summary of the endocrine glands and their hormones is given in Table 26–1.

Figure 26–1
Developmental and biological variances: endocrine system.

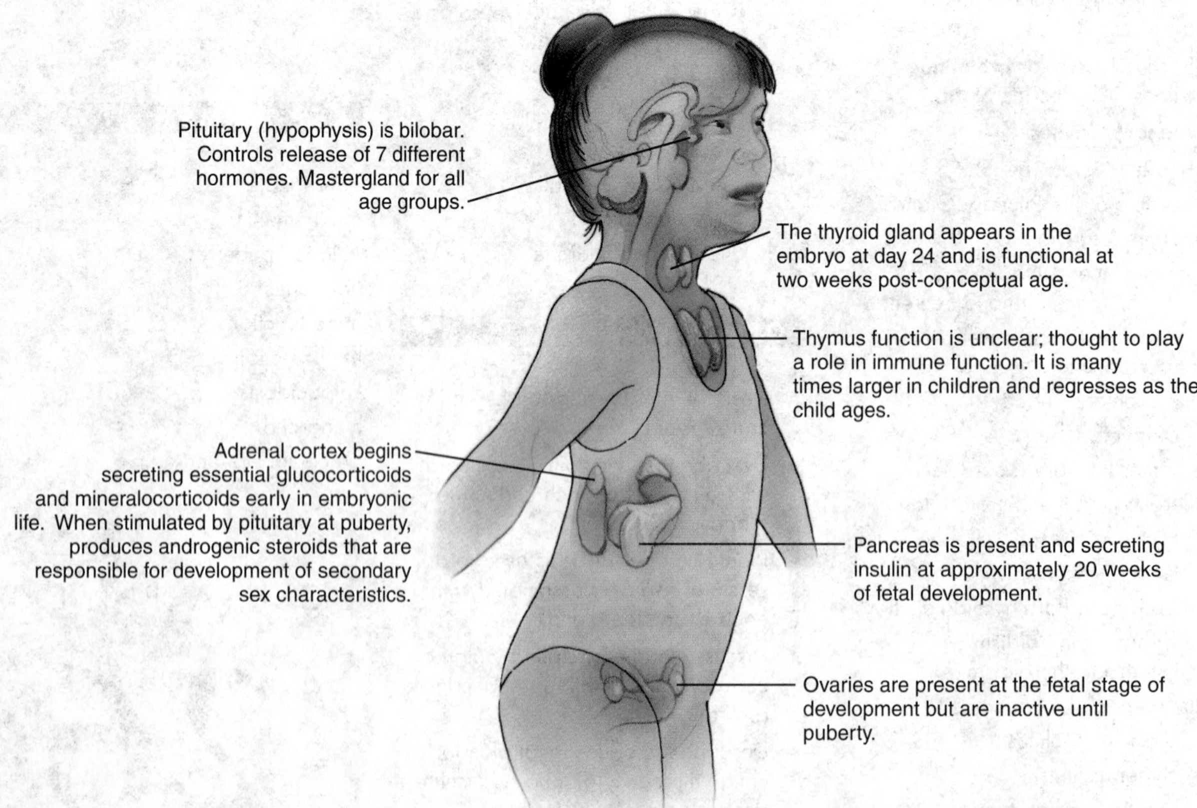

Pituitary (hypophysis) is bilobar. Controls release of 7 different hormones. Mastergland for all age groups.
The thyroid gland appears in the embryo at day 24 and is functional at two weeks post-conceptual age.
Thymus function is unclear; thought to play a role in immune function. It is many times larger in children and regresses as the child ages.
Adrenal cortex begins secreting essential glucocorticoids and mineralocorticoids early in embryonic life. When stimulated by pituitary at puberty, produces androgenic steroids that are responsible for development of secondary sex characteristics.
Pancreas is present and secreting insulin at approximately 20 weeks of fetal development.
Ovaries are present at the fetal stage of development but are inactive until puberty.

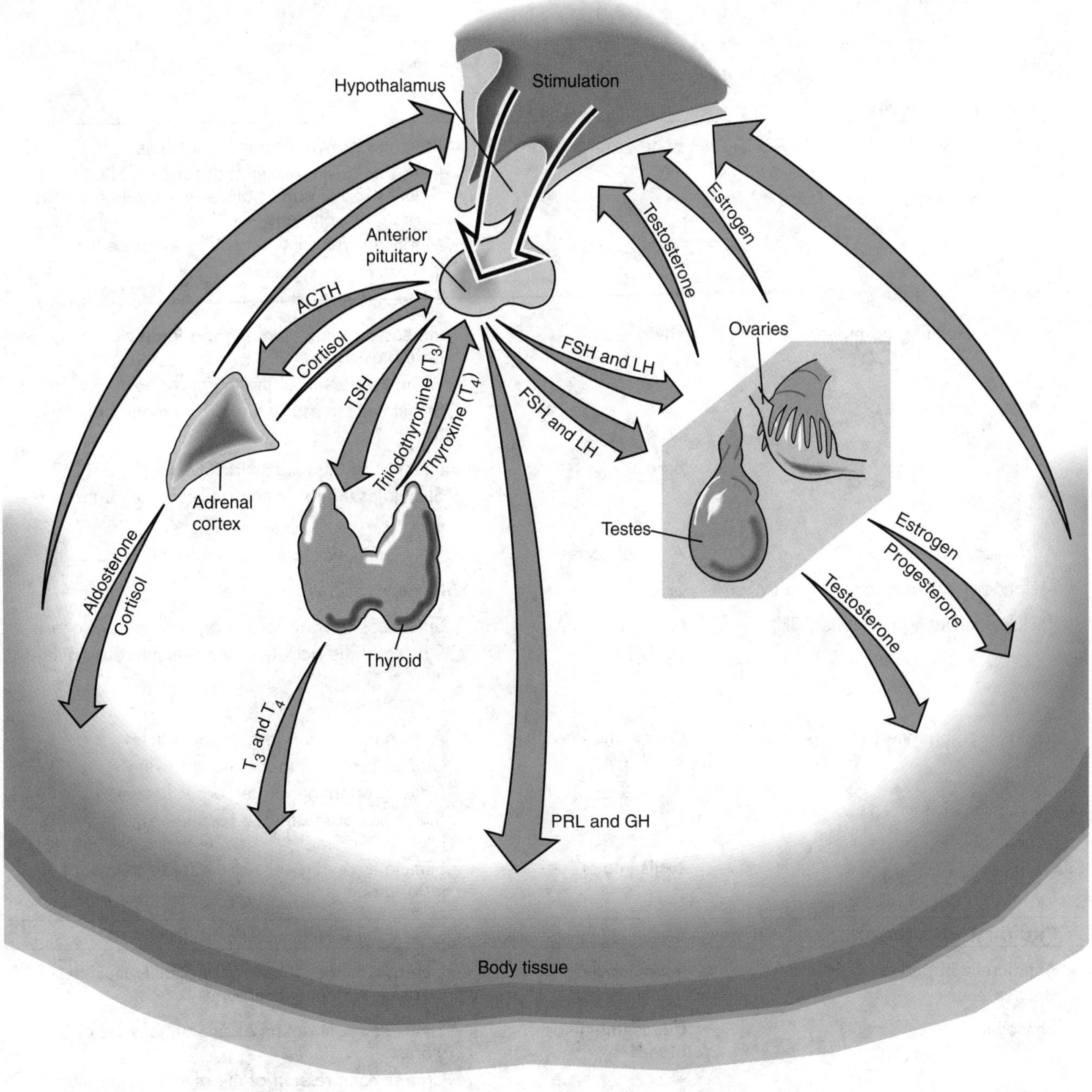

Figure 26–2
The hypothalamic-pituitary axis controls hormone secretion through a negative feedback mechanism.

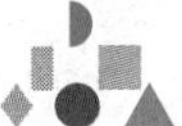

Assessment of the Child with an Alteration in Endocrine Status

Because the endocrine system varies greatly in its structures and functions, each gland requires its own specific assessment. The embryology, physiology, assessment, and disorders of each gland are discussed specifically and separately in this chapter, owing to the unique nature of the conditions that occur as a result of health challenges to specific organs in a variety of anatomic locations.

Focused Health History

Endocrine disorders are not generally suspected as a primary clinical condition when a child presents with

Table 26–1
Hormones and Their Actions

Gland and Hormone	Major Target Organ	Effect
Pituitary—Anterior		
Growth hormone (GH)	Bones, muscles, organs	Promotes growth of bone soft tissue Increases gastrointestinal absorption of calcium, reduces sodium and potassium excretion, raises plasma phosphate levels Mobilizes free fatty acids from adipose tissue Induces hyperglycemia Stimulates milk secretion
Thyroid-stimulating hormone (TSH)	Thyroid	Increases iodine uptake and iodide clearance from plasma Promotes growth of the thyroid Stimulates release of thyroid hormone from thyroid
Prolactin	Breasts	Initiates and maintains lactation Stimulates the formation and function of the corpus luteum
Adrenocorticotropin (ACTH)	Adrenal cortex	Stimulates release of cortisol from the adrenal
Melanocyte-stimulating hormone (MSH)	Skin	Promotes skin pigmentation
Follicle stimulating hormone (FSH)	Ovary (female) Testis (male)	Stimulates ovarian follicle growth and oogenesis Stimulates the activity of the seminiferous epithelium Controls spermatogenesis
Luteinizing hormone (LH)	Ovary and corpus luteum (female)	Aids in maturation in ovarian follicles Causes ovulation in the mature ovum Causes formation of the corpus luteum Stimulates progesterone secretion by the corpus luteum
	Testis (male)	Stimulates Leydig cells of the testes to produce testosterone
Pituitary—Posterior		
Antidiuretic hormone (ADH)	Renal tubules	Increases kidney tubule permeability thus increasing water reabsorption
Oxytocin	Uterus, mammary glands	Stimulates contraction of smooth muscles of the uterus Causes compression of the alveoli of the mammary glands (milk letdown reflex)
Thyroid		
Thyroxine (T_4) and triiodothyronine (T_3)	All tissues	Accelerates cell metabolism Works with growth hormone to stimulate growth (very essential to development of nervous tissue) Increases glucose uptake by cells Increases rate of cholesterol removal by liver
Calcitonin	Bone and renal tubules	Lowers serum levels of calcium and phosphorus; decreases kidney excretion of calcium and phosphorus Increases calcium and phosphorus deposition in bone

Table 26–1
Hormones and Their Actions *Continued*

Gland and Hormone	Major Target Organ	Effect
Parathyroid		
Parathyroid hormone (PTH)	Gastrointestinal tract, bone, renal proximal tubules	Increases absorption of calcium, phosphorus, and magnesium from the intestine Promotes reabsorption of bony tissue and release of calcium into the blood stream
Adrenal Glands—Cortex		
Aldosterone	Primarily renal distal tubules	Increases the reabsorption of sodium from distal tubule of the kidney Promotes water retention and potassium loss
Cortisol	All tissues	Increases protein catabolism, gluconeogenesis, and glycogenesis Is antagonistic to insulin and androgens Aids in erythrocyte formation and in maintenance of normal brain activity
Androgens	Many tissues, especially gonads and muscles	Increases retention of nitrogen, potassium, phosphorus, and sulfur Promotes growth and the development of male secondary sex characteristics Promotes axillary and pubic hair development in females
Adrenal Glands—Medulla		
Norepinephrine	Adrenergic receptors	Increases rate and strength of heart activity Dilates coronary vessels; constricts vessels in other organs (increases blood pressure) Stimulates alertness Mobilizes fatty acids from storage areas
Epinephrine	Heart, liver, lungs, brain, kidneys, and arteries	Dilates vessels to skeletal muscle Stimulates glycogenesis
Pancreas—Islets of Langerhans		
Insulin	Liver, muscle, adipose tissue	Increases glucose uptake by cells Stimulates the conversion of glucose to glycogen Promotes fatty acids and amino acid transport into cells Promotes lipogenesis and protein synthesis
Glucagon	Liver	Increases glycogenesis in the liver, thereby increasing blood glucose
Somatostatin	Alpha and beta cells in pancreas	Inhibits insulin and glucogen release

Table continued on following page

Table 26-1
Hormones and Their Actions *Continued*

Gland and Hormone	Major Target Organ	Effect
Ovaries		
Estrogen	Uterus, breasts, and bone	Causes initial stages of uterine regrowth during menstrual cycles Increases mammary duct growth Stimulates contraction of the uterus and uterine tubes Promotes development of female secondary sex characteristics Accelerates epiphyseal closure Increases fat deposition in subcutaneous tissues Causes salt and water retention
Progesterone	Uterus	Prepares the uterus for implantation of fertilized ovum Develops the secretory potential of the mammary gland Increases basal body temperature Promotes retention of salt and water
Relaxin	Pelvis	Softens pelvic ligaments before labor Creates sleepiness during pregnancy
Testes		
Testosterone	Spermatogenic tubules, penis, bone, and many other tissues	Ensures development of the male reproductive organs Promotes development of secondary sex characteristics Increases protein anabolism and calcium retention Increases rate of bone growth and epiphyseal closure

complaints of gastrointestinal, neurologic, or musculoskeletal problems. However, because endocrine dysfunction can affect all aspects of the child's growth, development, and physiologic functions, the health care provider must always keep a high index of suspicion for the possibility of endocrine dysfunction, especially in cases in which no other acute condition appears to be present.

Endocrine disorders often cause changes in normal growth and activity patterns. Good records of general health assessment, including serial recording of growth parameters according to the National Center for Health Statistics (NCHS), are especially helpful in making a diagnosis of endocrine dysfunction (Chart 26–1). Most general health assessment records in primary care note the child's height and weight but neglect to compare the individual child's growth parameters to norms. Parents' memories are often foggy and incomplete, but careful and thorough questioning by an expert in the field of pediatric endocrinology, as well as having the family bring in photographs of the child at various developmental ages, can help pinpoint the origin and timing of the problems with presenting symptoms. In addition, symptoms can be localized to individual glandular dysfunction more easily. Neonatal growth parameters, including weight, length, head and chest circumferences, and appearance at birth, are also useful to know when reconstructing a health history focused on possible endocrine dysfunction. They will also aid in avoiding misdiagnoses, which are common and can lead to ultimately life-threatening problems when undetected. When an endocrine dysfunction is suspected, it is time to go beyond primary care providers and seek the help of experts in the field of pediatric endocrinology.

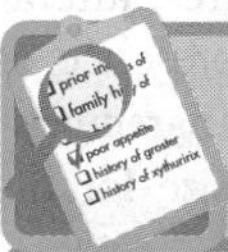

Chart 26–1
Focused Health History

Endocrine

Demographic Data	Age, height, weight, gender
Present Illness	Did the symptoms occur gradually, or was the onset sudden? Have the symptoms interfered with or affected the child's lifestyle? Has the family noted any changes in the child's physical appearance or general affect? Recent changes in growth velocity or weight gain or loss Changes in sleep patterns Changes in appetite or thirst Changes in vision Changes in voiding or stooling patterns
Past Medical History	Birth history Neonatal screening completed? What were the results? Feeding difficulties noted at birth and in infancy? Child's size at birth Maternal factors that may have affected weight and height of growing fetus (e.g., tobacco or alcohol use) Previous health history Has the child been treated for these problems in the past? Any recent minor illness such as gastroenteritis or a viral syndrome? Immunizations Current immunization status Allergies Any allergies to medications, food products, milk, or formula products?
Current Medications	All medications the child is currently taking (prescribed, over the counter, or home remedies)
Environment	Exposure to exogenous steroids or gonadotropins
Family History	Family history of any endocrine disorders (e.g., thyroid disorders, diabetes mellitus) Family members who have had growth or development difficulties (e.g., very short or very tall)
Social History	Describe the child's normal daily activities Describe the child's activity level (note fatigue versus hyperactivity) Does family have resources to maintain a healthy diet, purchase needed medications, continue with consistent health care follow-up?
Growth and Development	Growth and development plotted on height and weight growth curves Achievement of age-appropriate developmental tasks Presence of learning disabilities or cognitive delays

Focused Physical Assessment

Dysfunctions of the endocrine system can result in a variety of physical changes because of the influence circulating hormones have on growth and development, fluid and electrolyte balance, use of nutrients, and regulation of sex hormone levels. To pinpoint the exact systems affected by the dysfunction and thereby more accurately determine the actual endocrine disorder, a systematic physical assessment is performed (see Chapter 6). Inspection, palpation, and auscultation reveal specific findings that are indicative of certain conditions (Chart 26–2).

The child's general appearance should be inspected for abnormalities of facial structures and features; alterations in the appearance of the skin; and the presence of abnormal, premature, or late secondary sexual characteristics; and an evaluation of the child's general size for his or her age should be performed.

Further evaluation of the child's respiratory, cardiac, gastrointestinal, and urinary functions is likely to reveal dysfunctions consistent with specific endocrine disorders. Serial serum hormone assays are performed for most endocrine conditions, and blood levels of these hormones often pinpoint the problems. These can then be treated with hormone replacement or other interventions as needed.

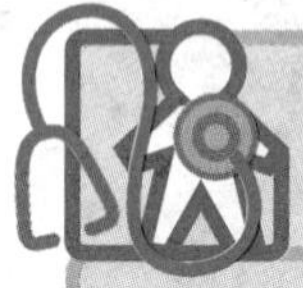

Chart 26–2
Focused Physical Assessment

Endocrine

Area	Finding	Potential Dysfunction
Stature	Abnormal growth velocity	Hypopituitarism
	Short	Pituitary disorders
	Tall/large	Pituitary disorders
Weight changes	Loss	Pancreatic disorders
		Thyroid disorders
		Adrenal disorders
	Gain or obesity	Thyroid disorders
		SIADH
Skin	Cold intolerance or cold extremities	Hypothyroidism
	Change in color or texture	Pituitary disorders
		Adrenal disorders
		Thyroid disorders
		Cushing's syndrome
	Easy bruising	Cushing's syndrome
	Striae	Adrenal disorders
	Enlargement in anterior neck	Goiter
	Brittle hair	Hypothyroidism
	Hirsutism (abnormal growth of hair)	Cortisol or androgen excesses
Eyes	Changes in vision	Pituitary tumor
		Pancreatic disorders
		Precocious puberty
Mouth	Delay in dentition	Hypocalcemia
		Hypopituitarism
Face	Rounded face	Cushing's syndrome
	Deformities or abnormal features	Hypoparathyroidism
		Hypothyroidism
Respiratory	Fruity odor to breath	Ketoacidosis
	Kussmaul respirations	Diabetes mellitus
Cardiovascular	Palpitations	Thyroid disorders
	Sweating	Thyroid disorders
	Tachycardia	Hyperthyroidism
	Hypertension	Cushing's syndrome

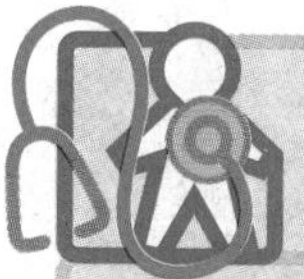

Chart 26–2
Focused Physical Assessment *Continued*

Endocrine

Area	Finding	Potential Dysfunction
Gastrointestinal	Nausea	Parathyroid disorders
		Diabetes mellitus
	Vomiting	Parathyroid disorders
		Diabetes insipidus
	Change in bowel habits (constipation or diarrhea)	Thyroid disorders
		Diabetes insipidus
		Parathyroid disorders
		Diabetes mellitus
	Polydipsia	Diabetes insipidus
	Dehydration	Diabetes insipidus
Musculoskeletal	Muscle weakness or lethargy	SIADH
		Hypothyroidism
		Parathyroid disorders
		Hyperinsulinism
		CAH
	Hyperactivity	Hyperthyroidism
	Pathologic bone fractures	Adrenal disorders
	Pain	Hyperparathyroidism
	Cramps	Parathyroid disorders
		Parathyroid disorders
	Gait disturbances	Hyperparathyroidism
	Diminished deep tendon reflexes	Hypercalcemia
	Hyperflexia/twitching	Hypocalcemia
		Parathyroid disorders
Nervous system	Confusion	Parathyroid disorders
	Increased irritability/behavioral changes	Diabetes insipidus
		SIADH
		Precocious puberty
	Headaches	Diabetes mellitus
		Adrenal insufficiency
		Cushing's syndrome
	Changes in sleep patterns	Pituitary disorders
Urinary	Polyuria	Pancreatic disorders
	Hematuria	Parathyroid disorders
Genital	Onset, timing, deviation of menses	Gonadal disorders, thyroid disorders
	Testicular mass or pain	Gonadal disorders
	Small genitalia	Hypopituitarism
	Ambiguous genitalia	CAH
		Ambiguous genitalia
	Presence of early pubertal changes or abnormal pubertal changes	Precocious puberty
		Premature thelarche
		Gynecomastia
	Delayed pubertal changes	Delayed puberty
		Adrenal insufficiency

CAH, congenital adrenal hyperplasia; SIADH, syndrome of inappropriate antidiuretic hormone.

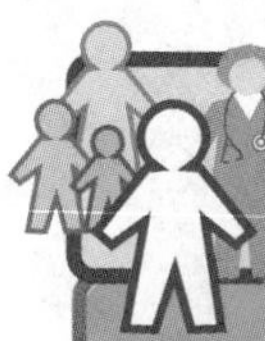

Chart 26–3
Nursing Diagnoses and Outcomes

The Child with an Endocrine Disorder

Impaired adjustment, related to major lifestyle changes to manage chronic conditions

Outcomes: Child and family report ability to cope and adjust adequately.
Child and family show ability to accept and adapt to new health status and integrate learning.

Body image disturbance related to changes in physical appearance due to hormonal imbalances

Outcome: Child expresses positive feelings about self.

Ineffective family coping compromised

Outcomes: Family members express their concerns about coping with the child's illness.
Family members identify their needs.
Family members seek appropriate resources and sources of support to assist in meeting their needs.

Risk for fluid volume excess or deficit, related to altered endocrine function

Outcomes: Child will remain well hydrated.
Child will have normal serum hormone or electrolyte levels.
Child and family understand the need for either replacement hormone or other medical therapy and long-term follow-up.
Child and family will administer the hormone therapy as prescribed.
Child and family will seek intervention when fluid volume excess or deficit occurs.

Altered growth and development, related to glandular hypo- or hyperfunction

Outcomes: Child and family understand the need for either replacement hormone or other medical therapy and long-term follow-up.
Child and family will administer hormone therapy as prescribed.
Child will demonstrate age-appropriate behaviors and skills to the extent possible.
Child will progress in physical development in age-appropriate manner.

Knowledge deficit: pathology, signs and symptoms of complications, home care, and long-term management

Outcome: Child and family will state understanding of disease pathology, signs and symptoms of complications, home care, and long-term management.

Noncompliance related to management of the specific health challenge

Outcomes: Child and family identify factors that influence noncompliance.
Child demonstrates a level of compliance that promotes physiologic safety.

Altered nutrition: potential for more or less than body requirements

Outcomes: Child and family understand the need for specific nutritional therapy and long-term follow-up.
Child adheres to prescribed diet.
Child maintains weight within parameters for age and gender.

High risk for altered parenting, related to health and life-threatening condition of the child

Outcomes: Parents communicate feelings about current situation.
Parents participate in daily care of the child.
Parents communicate understanding of child's needs.
Parents express feelings of control in present situation.

Nursing Diagnoses and Outcomes

Fortunately, with modern science and pharmacotherapy, most endocrine dysfunctions may be treated. Although the child and family with an endocrine condition may have to manage the problem on a chronic basis, the outcomes of management are generally successful when treatment regimens are carefully adhered to. General nursing diagnoses for a child experiencing health challenges with the endocrine system are presented in Chart 26–3.

Developmental and Biological Variances

As expected, the endocrine disorders most prevalent in infancy are those that are congenital: hypopituitarism, congenital hypothyroidism, congenital adrenal hyperplasia, aplasia of the parathyroid glands, and nesidioblastosis (see Fig. 26–1). Although diabetes is rare in children younger than 1 year of age, it does occur and the diagnosis is often delayed. Because diabetes requires that painful procedures be administered by parents, the infant's trust may waiver, and the parents may experience a great deal of guilt.

Growth disorders are most commonly manifested in the toddler age group. Children who are walking are compared with their peers in height, and discrepancies become evident. The toddler with diabetes must be allowed to explore the environment and begin to develop a sense of self.

Preschoolers may present with a growth disorder or with signs of early puberty. The preschooler with diabetes can begin to be involved in self-care, and the parents of this child must deal with difficult dietary issues in this age group.

School-age children most commonly present with growth disorders. These children are measured in school, and children not growing normally are referred. The ages of 6 to 7 years represent a peak for the development of type I diabetes. Developmental issues involve school, peer identification, and self-care.

Many endocrine disorders manifest during adolescence. Normal adolescents begin pubertal development with development of breasts, growth of pubic and axillary hair, and menarche in girls and with enlargement of the testes and growth of pubic and axillary hair in boys. Girls with irregular menses may present to the gynecologist or to an endocrinologist. Frequently, adolescents are evaluated because of early or delayed puberty. Autoimmune disorders rarely occur before adolescence. Therefore, a variety of autoimmune endocrine disorders appear at this time, including Hashimoto's thyroiditis, Graves' disease, autoimmune hypoparathyroidism, Addison's disease, and type I diabetes. Diabetes represents difficult problems for the adolescent who wants to be like his or her peers and eat the same foods and not have to adhere to a schedule of medication and self-care.

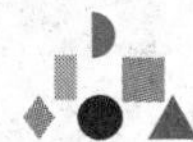

Diagnostic Criteria for Evaluating Alterations in Endocrine Status

Like a focused physical assessment, there are no specific diagnostic criteria for general health challenges to the endocrine system. Members of the pediatric endocrine team work backward from the child's presenting symptoms once a referral has been made. Tables 26–1 and 26–2 summarize the hormones of the endocrine system and the diagnostic tests used to determine whether the presenting symptoms are endocrine or some other clinical problem.

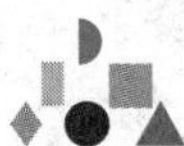

Treatment Modalities

Treatment modalities are concerned with replacing or blocking the hormonal hypofunction or hyperfunction that is occurring within the child's body. They are exquisitely calculated based on the child's own serum blood levels of the hormones in question and on the child's physical appearance, for example, short stature or premature development of secondary sex characteristics.

Treatment may also involve surgical removal of a gland or portion of a gland that is oversecreting a hormone. If a tumor is causing endocrine dysfunction, surgical removal of the tumor is completed.

Treatment of most pediatric endocrine conditions requires the expertise of a team that is well versed in handling numerous cases. The child's ability to reach full growth and development hangs in the balance and should not be left to health care providers who are not conversant with the problems on a large scale. Normal well-child health care is often administered by a primary care clinician, with oversight by the pediatric endocrine team.

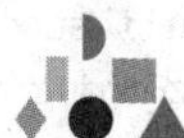

Alterations in Endocrine Status

Disorders of the Pituitary Gland

Disorders of the pituitary gland depend on the location of the lesion or physiologic abnormality. The posterior lobe is called the neurohypophysis because it is formed of

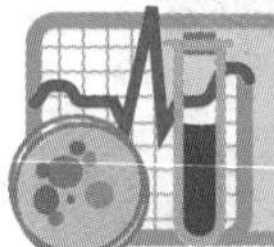

Table 26–2
Diagnostic Tests and Procedures to Evaluate Alterations in Endocrine Status

Diagnostic Test or Procedure	Purpose	Finding and Indications	Health Care Provider Responsibilities
Random hormone levels	To assess function of endocrine glands	High levels indicate hyperfunctions. Low levels indicate hypofunction.	Prepare child for needlesticks.
Stimulation studies	To stimulate the hypothalamic-pituitary axis with drug to evaluate hormone secretion To assess growth hormone level	Low levels indicate hormone deficiency.	Advise parents to keep child NPO. Explain procedure to child. Establish venous access. Obtain blood samples at precise times.
Urinalysis	To look for glucosuria, ketonuria, or dilute urine	May indicate diabetes, ketonuria, or diabetes insipidus	Describe procedure to child. Attach urine bag to a child who is not toilet trained.
Bone age radiographs	To compare radiographs of wrists and knees against standards for age To evaluate skeletal maturation	Delayed maturation indicates growth will continue for a longer period of time than normal. Accelerated maturation indicates growth will continue for a shorter period of time than normal.	Explain procedure to child.
Magnetic resonance imaging	To evaluate growth hormone deficiency or precocious puberty	May detect a brain lesion as the cause of growth hormone deficiency or precocious puberty	Explain procedure to child. Administer sedation if ordered.
Nuclear medicine studies	To assess contrast media uptake with serial radiographs usually to assess thyroid placement	Could indicate ectopic, enlarged, absent, or nodular thyroid	Explain procedure to child. Inquire about allergy to iodine substances.
Ultrasonography	To assess thyroid placement	Could indicate ectopic, enlarged, absent, or nodular thyroid	Explain procedure to child.

neural tissue. It secretes antidiuretic hormone (ADH; vasopressin) and oxytocin. The anterior pituitary, or adenohypophysis, is made up of endocrine glandular tissue and secretes growth hormone (GH), adrenocorticotropic hormone (ACTH), TSH, follicle-stimulating hormone (FSH), luteinizing hormone (LH), and prolactin. Usually several target organs are affected when there is a disorder of the pituitary gland, especially the adenohypophysis. Specific disorders are discussed with respect to their anatomic locations of origin and the effects of hyperfunction and hypofunction on target organs and the child as a whole.

The pituitary gland develops from the fusion of two ectodermal processes: an upgrowth from the ectoderm of the stomodeum and a downgrowth from the neuroectoderm of the diencephalon (Moore & Persaud, 1993). The double origin explains why the pituitary gland is composed of two completely different types of tissue. The adenohypophysis (a glandular portion) arises from the oral ectoderm, and the neurohypophysis (a nervous portion) originates from the neuroectoderm (Moore & Persaud, 1993).

At 24 days' gestation a diverticulum, Rathke's pouch, arises from the roof of the stomodeum (a primitive mouth cavity) and grows toward the brain to meet an outgrowth of the floor of the third ventricle (the future posterior pituitary). Rathke's pouch undergoes further proliferation to form the anterior lobe. The connection between the posterior lobe of the pituitary and the brain persists, but the lumen of Rathke's pouch disappears. The infundibulum (stem) becomes embedded in the sella turcica (Recker, 1993). The pituitary gland takes its permanent shape and location within the bony cavity of the sphenoid bone between the third and fourth months of gestation. Secretory granules appear in the fetal pituitary, and measurable amounts of hormones can be detected toward the end of the first trimester. The pituitary gland appears to synthesize GH and ACTH first, and these are followed by TSH, FSH, LH, and prolactin at approximately 20 weeks' gestation.

Diabetes Insipidus

Diabetes insipidus (DI), also known as neurogenic DI or hypothalamic DI, is a disorder of the posterior pituitary. It is the result of the deficiency in the secretion of ADH. The purpose of ADH is to concentrate the urine from the kidneys and to conserve water. ADH maintains normal osmolality by determining the amount of water to conserve. Consequently, if there is a deficiency in ADH there will be massive renal losses of fluid. It is important to distinguish the difference between neurogenic DI and nephrogenic DI. In contrast to neurogenic DI, nephrogenic DI is a rare sex-linked hereditary disorder characterized by unresponsiveness of the renal tubules to ADH. Hypothalamic DI may result from many different causes. Half the patients with hypothalamic DI are believed to have a primary hypothalamic lesion, one fourth of the cases occur after craniotomy, and the rest are idiopathic or familial (Fjellestad-Paulsen, Paulsen, d'Agay-Abensour, Lundin & Czernichow, 1993). Batcheller (1992) reports that familial or idiopathic causes make up 30% to 50% of the total cases of neurogenic DI. Trauma (accidental or surgical), tumors (craniopharyngiomas), granulomatous disease, infections (meningitis or encephalitis), or vascular anomalies cause the remainder of the cases.

Pathophysiology

Antidiuretic hormone works directly on the renal collecting ducts and distal tubules to increase membrane permeability for water and urea. A deficiency in ADH will cause the failure of the kidney to reabsorb water. The water will then diffuse into the urine. Subsequently, a decrease in ADH secretion will allow massive water loss and sodium retention in the serum.

Prognosis. The prognosis of children with DI depends on the cause; most children with proper treatment and follow-up can live fairly normal lives. DI is a permanent condition, and treatment must be continued for life.

Assessment

The most common symptoms of neurogenic DI are polyuria (excessive urination) and polydipsia (excessive thirst). Children with DI typically excrete 4 to 15 L/day of urine despite the fluid intake. The onset of these symptoms is usually sudden and abrupt. Repeated trips to the bathroom, nocturia, and enuresis are common. Other symptoms may include dehydration, fever, weight loss, increased irritability, vomiting, constipation, and, potentially, hypovolemic shock.

caREminder: *The first symptoms of diabetes insipidus seen in children, especially in infants, are irritability and incessant crying that can only be alleviated with feedings of water and not formula or breast milk.*

The child with diabetes mellitus also has polydipsia, which is satisfied with any type of fluid. With DI, the child's urine is extremely dilute and often colorless with a specific gravity usually not more than 1.005. Neurogenic DI may often be confused with diabetes mellitus because of the symptoms; however, in DI there is no glycosuria. Diagnosis of DI is usually confirmed with low urine specific gravity, excessive urination despite fluid restriction, and elevated serum sodium levels when fluid is withheld. Other tests may be done (Table 26–3).

Nursing Diagnoses and Outcomes

The following nursing diagnoses may apply to a child with DI:

- **Fluid volume deficit related to the inability of the renal tubules to concentrate urine in the absence of ADH**
  Outcome: The child will remain well hydrated.
- **Fluid volume excess related to excessive desmopressin (DDAVP) medication or excessive fluid intake**
  Outcome: The child will have normal serum sodium levels.
- **Activity intolerance related to dehydration, excessive thirst, and frequent need to urinate**
  Outcome: The child will regain strength and desire to have increased level of activity.

Interdisciplinary Interventions

Several treatment modalities are available for the child with DI. Treatment usually involves the administration of desmopressin, a synthetic analogue of ADH. It is usually administered by the nurse and then by the parents through nasal insufflation given every day or twice a day.

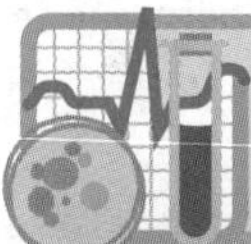

Table 26–3
Diagnostic Tests or Procedures for Evaluating Diabetes Insipidus

Diagnostic Test or Procedure	Purpose	Finding and Indications	Health Care Provider Responsibilities
Serum tests: Electrolytes, blood urea nitrogen, creatinine, sodium, glucose, osmolality	To screen urine and serum and assess renal function and dehydration	Hypernatremia	Obtain proper specimens and send to the laboratory promptly.
Urine tests: sodium, osmolality, specific gravity, glucose	To rule out diabetes mellitus (normal serum glucose and negative urine glucose)		Explain the purpose of the tests to the child and family.
Water deprivation study	To evaluate the effect of fluid restriction on urine concentration, specific gravity, and urine volume To monitor serum sodium and osmolality		Monitor I&O carefully. Assess vital signs every hour (blood pressure and pulse). Measure urine specific gravity and osmolality with each void. Obtain serum specimens for sodium, ADH hematocrit, and osmolality. Monitor the child's weight closely (twice daily in some). Terminate the test and give desmopressin (DDAVP) if the patient loses more than 3% of the baseline body weight or if tachycardia and significant hypotension occur.
Magnetic resonance imaging or computed tomography	To determine the underlying cause of diabetes insipidus (central vs. renal basis)		Explain the purpose of the test to the child and family.

The physician orders small doses and increases the dose as needed. Desmopressin has immediate action and lasts between 8 and 24 hours. Headaches, nasal congestion, and abdominal discomfort are rare side effects. The parents will interrupt treatment regularly or the dose is reduced over some months, per physician orders, to confirm the persistence of DI (Blizzard & Johanson, 1994). Fjellestad and colleagues (1993) reported the development of an oral form of desmopressin as an alternative for children. The dose, however, is much larger than the nasal dose and can be quite expensive. Parenteral desmopressin solution is also used postoperatively because of its shorter action. Lysine vasopressin nasal spray is available for use in severe, transient, or permanent neurogenic DI. Pitressin tannate in oil is often suggested for permanent DI and is administered intramuscularly. Patients with acute DI often use aqueous pitressin, which can be given intravenously, intramuscularly, or subcutaneously.

The nurse continues to monitor the child with DI for signs and symptoms of dehydration (poor skin turgor, dry mucous membranes, sunken fontanelles, weight loss, absence of tears, tachycardia, and decreased urine specific gravity) and hypernatremia (tachycardia, poor skin turgor, weak pulses, low blood pressure, cool skin, increased body temperature, dry mucous membranes, and changes in mental status). The physician orders and the nurse provides sufficient fluids to maintain balanced intake and output per 24 hours. The nurse records strict intake and output and specific gravity. The nurse notifies a physician if the urine output is greater than 100 mL/hr for 2 consecutive voids. The child is weighed on the same scale every day. The nurse should educate the child and parents in the administration of desmopressin (TIP 26–1).

The nurse and parents should give high caloric beverages such as milk and juice to children with DI who are underweight secondary to inadequate calorie consumption. The nurse instructs parents to note drinking patterns at home and to report changes to the physician. Parents need to understand the symptoms of water intoxication and dehydration to maintain good home records

TIP 26-1 A Teaching Intervention Plan for Administering Desmopressin (DDAVP)

Nursing Diagnoses and Outcomes

- Knowledge deficit: desmopressin (DDAVP) administration

  Outcomes: The parents and child understand the need for replacement hormone therapy and long-term follow-up.

  The parents/child demonstrate how to give DDAVP.

Teach the Family

Storage

- Keep DDAVP refrigerated at all times.

Medication Administration

- Clear the nostrils before giving medication.
- Insert measured tubing into the bottle of DDAVP.
- Fill the tube to the proper dosage.
- Hold the top of the tube closed.
- Insert the medication-filled end into the nostril.
- Blow the liquid out of the tubing and into the nostril.

Precautions

- Do not repeat doses that have been swallowed or poorly absorbed.
- The medication is poorly absorbed if the child has nasal congestion. Consult the health care provider.
- The dose may need to be repeated if the child sneezes immediately after the administration of the medication.
- Have an extra bottle of medication in case of breakage.

(see Chapter 17 for a discussion of fluid and electrolyte status). Adequate replacement fluid is needed during increased physical activity or in extremely hot weather.

Community Care

The parents should inform teachers and coaches that their child needs liberal bathroom privileges and extra fluids to prevent embarrassing accidents or dehydration.

caREminder: *The parents must educate teachers thoroughly on the symptoms of dehydration or hypernatremia so they do not mistake these signs as bad or unruly behavior. A teaching session with the school nurse can prevent this mistake.*

All children should be encouraged to wear Medic Alert tags that indicate that they have DI.

Syndrome of Inappropriate Antidiuretic Hormone Secretion

The syndrome of inappropriate antidiuretic hormone (SIADH) results from hypersecretion of ADH. In SIADH, the negative feedback mechanism fails to regulate ADH release and inhibition. SIADH may result from various conditions, such as tumors, central nervous system disease (meningitis), trauma to the central nervous system, or after certain surgical procedures on the brain. It may also stem from the use of certain medications, such as chlorpropamide, carbamazepine, analgesics, phenothiazines, nicotine, barbiturates, vincristine, and cyclophosphamide (Gray, St. Dennis-Feezle, Clark, & Parker, 1993).

Pathophysiology

Normally, ADH is not secreted when excess fluid is in circulation because the fluid needs to be excreted. When ADH is hypersecreted, it shuts down the normal kidney function of water filtration and loss. Water remains in circulation, diluting all blood components. Metabolic toxins accumulate in the blood instead of being excreted. Increased intracranial pressure results from the increased fluid volume.

Alert: *SIADH is a transient, but life-threatening, emergency that is usually treated in the intensive-care setting after head trauma or intracranial surgery.*

Once the underlying disorder is corrected, there should no longer be any risks to the child and the symptoms will usually disappear. Without immediate and effective interventions, CNS damage from the disorder can impair the child permanently.

Assessment

The child with SIADH gains weight and has decreased urine output as fluids are retained. Weakness, lethargy, anorexia, nausea, vomiting, and behavioral changes will develop as the fluid and electrolyte balance deteriorates. Confusion, convulsions, coma, and death may then occur if treatment is not immediate and aggressive.

Diagnostic Tests. Laboratory studies reveal low serum osmolality and elevated urine osmolality as well as low serum sodium levels with high urine sodium concentrations. Decreased serum urea, creatinine, uric acid, and albumin levels are also present.

Nursing Diagnoses and Outcomes

In addition to the nursing diagnoses presented in Chart 26–3, the following nursing diagnoses may apply to a child with SIADH:

- **High risk for injury related to altered level of consciousness, confusion, and the possibility of seizures**
  Outcomes: The child will remain alert and oriented.
  The child will not have seizure activity.
- **Fluid volume excess related to compromised regulatory mechanism and excess antidiuretic hormone**
  Outcomes: The child will remain well hydrated, as evidenced by good skin turgor and moist mucous membranes.
  The child's sodium levels will be within normal ranges.

Interdisciplinary Interventions

The nurse analyzes intake, output, and weight records carefully. The nurse places an indwelling urinary catheter to monitor hourly urine volume and specific gravity. The nurse assesses the child's level of consciousness related to the fluid and electrolyte imbalances. Any exposure to precipitating factors should be noted in the history.

Treatment consists of reducing the fluid overload and raising the serum sodium level and osmolality. The physician orders a restriction of fluids and usually orders that the intravenous fluids be maintained at a keep-open rate. The physician may order that the child be treated with 3% normal saline intravenously and given a diuretic, such as furosemide (Gray et al., 1993).

Growth Hormone Deficiency (Hypopituitarism)

Classic GH deficiency is the failure of the pituitary to produce sufficient GH to sustain normal growth in childhood or to produce minimally measurable GH after stimulation with two or more pharmacologic agents. The prevalence of GH deficiency in the United States is approximately 1 in 10,000 children (Gray et al., 1993).

The cause is usually not known in approximately 80% of children (idiopathic) with GH deficiency. Idiopathic GH deficiency is highly associated with prolonged or precipitous labor and births, breech presentation, and cesarean births (Gray et al., 1993). It occurs sporadically, but familial patterns may be noted. Males are four times more likely than females to be referred for idiopathic GH deficiency (Blizzard & Johanson, 1994). Males are referred more often, owing to the societal expectation for males to be taller. Girls may have as high an incidence of GH deficiency but may not be referred because short stature is more acceptable in females. Children with idiopathic GH deficiency usually have decreased length at birth but normal birth weights.

Beyond idiopathic GH deficiency, other causes of GH deficiency include tumors (craniopharyngiomas, optic glioma, adenoma, astrocytoma, and germinoma), septic-optic dysplasia (optic nerve hypoplasia, absence of septum pellucidum, and pituitary hormone deficiencies), empty sella (absent or small pituitary gland that does not fill sella foramen), and radiation therapy or trauma (Gray et al., 1993).

GH stimulates the growth of all organs and tissues in the body, particularly the long bones. The synthesis of insulin-like growth factor (IGF-1) in many tissues, especially the liver, is stimulated by GH. IGF-1, also known as somatomedin C, stimulates somatic growth. Blizzard and Johanson (1994) note that IGF-1 concentrations depend on the concentration of several IGF-binding proteins, particularly $IGFBP_3$, which increase directly in relation to increased GH production.

The child with GH deficiency usually attains an acceptable height with proper interventions and with compliance with the medication treatment plan.

Assessment

The child with GH deficiency may present to the health care team at any time from birth to adolescence. A complete evaluation includes a family history, the child's birth history, previous and current growth patterns, physical examination, bone age films, and specific endocrine studies.

Information about the family history of short stature is noted, as well as the specific heights and weights of both parents and siblings. These measurements may need to be obtained at the time of the initial visit. The birth history should include any history of maternal illness, infections, tobacco or alcohol use, or malnutrition that would affect the weight and height of the growing fetus. Growth charts should be obtained, and growth velocity is calculated. Growth velocity should be greater than 4 cm (about a half inch) per year (Styne, 1993).

The physical examination is extremely valuable and informative when diagnosing the child with GH deficiency. Physical findings vary somewhat depending on the age of the child.

The neonate with GH deficiency usually presents with seizures secondary to severe hypoglycemia and may also be cortisol deficient. Prolonged hyperbilirubinemia may also be present. The male can have small testes and micropenis. Infants usually have a cherubic facial appearance, frontal bossing (prominence of the forehead) is common, and the eyes appear prominent. The nasal bridge is not fully developed, the nose is small, and the infant may have micrognathia (abnormal smallness of the jaw). Truncal adiposity (excessive fat over the trunk area of the body) is common, along with small hands and feet. Dentition is often delayed. Growth velocity is decreased, which eventually leads to short stature.

The older child with GH deficiency will have a similar appearance to the infant. The child will appear much younger than the chronologic age. Developmental skills are normal because cognitive development is unaffected. The adolescent with GH deficiency may have a significant delay of puberty in addition to short stature (Chart 26–4).

Emotional difficulties related to small stature are common. The short child is often treated as if younger by teachers and coaches, is teased by peers, and may become shy and withdrawn toward others. Body image is altered, and the child may dress as a younger child.

Diagnostic Tests. The child with GH deficiency usually has normal results of renal and liver function tests as well as normal results of thyroid function tests. The sedimentation rate will be normal, indicating the absence of a chronic illness causing the short stature. IGF-1 and $IGFBP_3$ levels are usually below normal. Bone age, determined by radiography, is usually interpreted as below 2 or more standard deviations from normal. Computed tomography (CT) or magnetic resonance imaging (MRI) of the head will reveal no abnormalities. Overnight sleep studies evaluating GH secretion reveal less than three peaks of GH above 10 ng/mL. GH stimulation studies using at least two GH stimulants, such as arginine, clonidine, insulin, glucagon, or levodopa/propranolol will reveal GH levels less than 10 ng/mL.

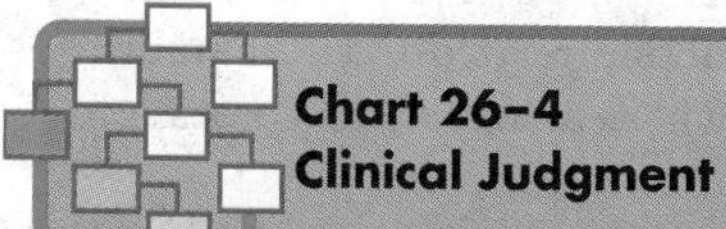

Chart 26–4
Clinical Judgment

The Child with Growth Hormone Deficiency

Ten-year-old Wallace has been diagnosed with growth hormone deficiency. As the nurse at his school, you have been working with Wallace and his family to help them adjust to the diagnosis and follow the treatment plan.

Questions

1. If left untreated, how would this condition manifest itself?
2. What therapy would you anticipate is being provided for Wallace by his primary care provider?
3. Based on Wallace's age and diagnosis, what are some important aspects of nursing care for him?
4. You have noted that other kids at school are teasing Wallace and have nicknamed him "Fly" because he is so little. How should you intervene?
5. How would you evaluate whether Wallace's parents and teachers are responding appropriately to his condition?

Answers

1. Child would continue to appear younger than chronological age.
2. Intramuscular injections of growth hormone.
3. Recognizing that Wallace may be experiencing threats to his self-esteem and body image. Assisting Wallace to cope with these feelings.
4. Discuss the situation with Wallace's teachers and ask them to intervene to stop and redirect the kids who are teasing Wallace. If Wallace feels comfortable with the idea, you could give a presentation about growth hormone deficiency to his classmates.
5. Assess if the parents and teachers are interacting with Wallace according to his age rather than to his size.

Nursing Diagnoses and Outcomes

In addition to the nursing diagnoses presented in Chart 26–3, the following nursing diagnoses may apply to a child with GH deficiency:

▶ **Body image disturbance related to altered growth**
Outcome: The child will verbalize positive feelings about his or her body image.

▶ **Impaired social interaction related to short stature**
Outcome: The child will demonstrate an increase in age-appropriate activities with peers.

Interdisciplinary Interventions

Therapy with GH is the treatment of choice for the child with GH deficiency. A nurse instructs the parent and child on the proper reconstitution and administration of the GH. The nurse may need to periodically evaluate the family on the proper techniques of administering the injection. The parent or the child gives recombinant DNA-derived GH by subcutaneous injection usually 6 to 7 days per week. The dose ranges from 0.18 to 0.3 mg/kg/wk. The growth is usually excellent in the first year of therapy as compared with later years. If GH therapy is initiated in the first years after birth, the GH-deficient child will often reach a height close to the genetic potential (Styne, 1993). Presently, GH injections are given until the bone fuses or until the child ceases to respond to treatment. Some endocrinologists believe adults with GH deficiency diagnosed in childhood may need continued treatment.

The possible side effects of GH need to be discussed with the child and family. These include an increase in blood glucose level, an increased incidence of slipped capital femoral epiphysis, local infection at the injection site, and pseudotumor cerebri. Rarely, leukemia without any predisposing causes has been noted in a small number of children and adults treated with GH (Blethen, 1995). The nurse needs to emphasize the importance of strict compliance with the medication.

Tip: *The child who has needle phobia may need extra attention by the nurse. The child can help by selecting the injection sites, using an injector pen, and by participating in preparing the equipment. Psychological counseling may be necessary.*

The nurse obtains precise heights and weights every 3 months and carefully plots them on the growth chart. The child has a bone age study performed at least every year after therapy has been initiated to monitor advancing bone age. GH is very expensive ($20,000 to $30,000/yr); however, many insurance companies will cover 80% to 100% of the expense in the case of classic GH deficiency.

Precocious Puberty

Precocious puberty is development of sexual characteristics before the usual age at onset of puberty. In girls, breast development beginning before the age of 7.5 years, sexual pubic hair before the age of 8.5 years, and menses before the age of 9.5 years is considered precocious. In the male child, secondary sexual development before the age of 9 years is considered precocious. In the United States, 1 of every 5,000 to 10,000 children begins puberty early (Parker, 1993). Girls are more commonly affected than boys.

Pathophysiology

Precocious puberty may be gonadotropin dependent, gonadotropin independent, or a combination of the two. Gonadotropin-dependent precocious puberty is initiated by hypothalamic-pituitary gonadal activation and is similar to the mechanism seen in normal puberty. It is often referred to as central precocious puberty. LH-releasing hormone (LHRH) is secreted by the hypothalamus in periodic bursts that stimulate the pituitary to release the gonadotropins LH and FSH. These gonadotropins stimulate the gonads to produce sex hormones, causing sexual maturation. Gonadotropin-dependent precocious puberty is idiopathic in more than 75% of girls (Goodpasture, Ghai, Cara, & Rosenfield, 1993). In boys, precocious puberty is most often due to a brain lesion.

Gonadotropin-independent precocious puberty does not involve the activation of the hypothalamic-pituitary gonadal activation (Chart 26–5). It is the result of the production of sex hormones by the adrenal gland or gonads or from exogenous exposure to steroids (Parker, 1993).

Combination precocious puberty is rare and is the result of secondary activation of the hypothalamic-pituitary-gonadal axis by elevated sex steroid levels from a peripheral source.

Prognosis. The prognosis for a child with precocious puberty depends on the age at diagnosis and immediate treatment. Appropriate treatment can halt, and sometimes even reverse, sexual development and can stop the rapid growth that results in severe short adult stature due to premature closure of the epiphysis. Treatment for precocious puberty allows the child to achieve the maximum growth potential possible.

Assessment

A comprehensive history and physical examination is essential in the diagnosis of precocious puberty. The nurse should obtain and properly graph on the growth charts the previous height and weight measurements. Growth spurts should be noted. Growth spurts during puberty are mediated by an interaction between gonadal sex steroids and GH. Increased sex steroids are associated with increased endogenous and stimulated GH secretion. IGF-1 levels are also increased at the time of puberty (Breyer, Haider, & Pescovitz, 1993). The history should include the chronologic timing of pubertal events, such as breast budding, phallic enlargement, body hair, acne, body odor, and deepening of the voice. Changes in behavior may

Chart 26–5

Causes of Precocious Puberty

Gonadotropin-Dependent Precocious Puberty

- Idiopathic
- Congenital anomalies
  - Septo-optic dysplasia
  - Hydrocephalus
- Tumors of the central nervous system
  - Glioma of optic nerve or hypothalamus
  - Astrocytoma
  - Ependymoma
  - Germinoma
  - Teratoma (HCG-producing)
  - Hamartoma (most common)
  - Craniopharyngioma
  - Suprasellar cysts
  - Sarcoid granuloma
  - Pinealoma
- Inflammatory conditions
  - Meningitis
  - Encephalitis
  - Brain abscess
- Trauma

Gonadotropin-Independent Precocious Puberty

- HCG-secreting tumors
  - Hepatoma
  - Chorioepithelioma
  - Teratoma
- Gonadal conditions
  - Ovarian conditions
    - Granulosa or theca cell tumor
    - Follicular luteal cysts
  - Testicular conditions
    - Leydig cell tumor or hyperplasia
    - Adrenal rest tumor
    - Familial male precocious puberty (testotoxicosis)
- Adrenal disorders
  - Congenital adrenal hyperplasia
  - Adrenal neoplasm
- Exogenous ingestion or absorption of steroids
- Other causes
  - McCune-Albright syndrome
  - Tuberous sclerosis
  - Male limited familial
  - Premature thelarche
  - Premature adrenarche
  - Premature menses
  - Russell-Silver syndrome
  - Primary hypothyroidism
  - Isolated luteinizing hormone secretion

Combined Gonadotropin-Dependent and Gonadotropin-Independent Precocious Puberty

- Congenital adrenal hyperplasia and gonadotropin-dependent precocious puberty
- Adrenal tumor and gonadotropin-dependent precocious puberty
- Ovarian tumor and gonadotropin-dependent precocious puberty
- McCune-Albright syndrome and gonadotropin-dependent precocious puberty

From Diamond, F., & Root, A. W. (1985). Delayed sexual maturation and sexual precocity. In R. B. Conn (Ed.), *Current diagnosis* (7th ed.). Philadelphia: W. B. Saunders. Reprinted with permission.

occur with increased moodiness, irritability, or aggressiveness. An extensive family history should include parental and sibling pubertal history, incidence of precocious puberty, congenital adrenal hyperplasia, neurofibromatosis, thyroid disease, and hypothyroidism. Exposure to exogenous steroids or gonadotropins should be noted along with any perinatal abnormalities or previous head trauma. Signs or symptoms of neurologic involvement are also noted, such as headaches, visual disturbances, or motor incoordination.

A current height and weight is properly graphed on the growth chart. The stage of sexual development according to Tanner classification (see Chapter 4) is noted. Testicular and phallic size and breast size are noted for gynecomastia and galactorrhea. The external genitalia are examined for signs of labial fusion, estrogenization, or enlarged clitoris. The skin should be examined for café au lait spots of neurofibromatosis, or McCune-Albright syndrome, and the presence of neurofibromas. Neurologic evaluation is essential with special attention paid to visual fields, optic disks, and signs of increased intracranial pressure. The child will have a bone age determination. A normal bone age is most consistent with premature adrenarche, premature thelarche, or exogenous ingestion of sex steroids. An accelerated bone age is more suggestive of gonadotropin-dependent precocious puberty, an adrenal or ovarian disorder, McCune-Albright syndrome, or familial male precocious puberty (Table 26–4).

Mental development in children with precocious puberty is normal, and the developmental milestones are not affected; however, the behavior may change to that of a typical adolescence. Girls may have episodes of moodiness and irritability, whereas boys may become more aggressive. School-age children with precocious puberty may become very self-conscious about their bodies around their peers and families. The child with precocious puberty may also have adverse psychological effects. The most difficult aspect for the child to endure may be teasing from other children about advanced sexual development. The child may feel isolated and rejected socially. Behavioral changes seen in boys and girls may cause problems in socializing with children in their own age group. Expectations may be higher for the child with precocious puberty because the physical appearance is older than the actual age. Teachers, relatives, and neighbors often expect the child to behave older than the chronologic age, causing frustration for the child who cannot live up to the expectations.

Nursing Diagnoses and Outcomes

In addition to the nursing diagnoses presented in Chart 26–3, the following nursing diagnoses may apply to a child with precocious puberty:

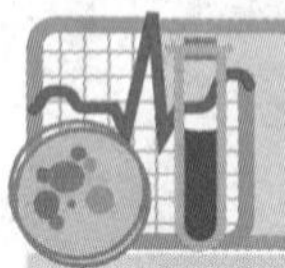

Table 26–4
Diagnostic Tests and Procedures for Evaluating Precocious Puberty

Diagnostic Test or Procedure	Purpose	Findings and Indications	Health Care Provider Responsibilities
Baseline serum studies: Luteinizing hormone (LH), follicle-stimulating hormone (FSH), dehydroepiandrostendione sulfate, estradiol, testosterone 17-OH progesterone, 17-OH pregnenolone, human chorionic gonadotropin, T_3RIA, T_4, thyroid-stimulating hormone	To assess pubertal status To evaluate adrenal androgen secretion To rule out congenital adrenal To rule out hypothyroidism		Obtain specimens and send them promptly to the laboratory. Explain the test and its purpose to the child and family.
Bone age (radiographs) of the left hand, wrist, and knee	To compare skeletal age with chronological age	Skeletal age will be more advanced than chronological age.	Explain the test and its purpose to the child and family.
Pelvic ultrasonography	To evaluate ovarian size and symmetry	Cysts or lesions may be seen.	Explain the test and its purpose to the child and family. Ensure that the child has a full bladder before the test.
Adrenal ultrasonography	To rule out adrenal mass	Adrenal lesion may be seen.	Explain the test and its purpose to the child and family.
Magnetic resonance imaging or computed tomography	To evaluate presence of lesion	Pituitary or hypothalamic lesion may be seen.	Explain the test and its purpose to the child and family. Give appropriate sedation to uncooperative young children.

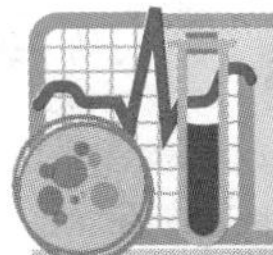

Table 26–4
Diagnostic Tests and Procedures for Evaluating Precocious Puberty *Continued*

Diagnostic Test or Procedure	Purpose	Findings and Indications	Health Care Provider Responsibilities
Gonadotropin-releasing hormone stimulation test (GnRH)	To determine whether the hypothalamic-pituitary gonadal axis is activated	LH and FSH levels may be elevated.	Explain that an intravenous needle is placed in the arm or hand and that GnRH is given and serum samples are obtained at timed intervals. Obtain baseline serum specimens. Administer medication by intravenous access. Maintain intravenous access throughout study. Nausea and/or vomiting are potential side effects of medication. Child should remain NPO 8 hours before testing.
Adrenocorticotropic hormone stimulation test	To determine whether the hypothalamic-pituitary adrenal axis is activated	Adrenal hormones may be elevated, indicating an enzymatic blockage.	Explain that an intravenous needle is placed in the arm or hand and that ACTH is given and serum samples are obtained at time intervals. Obtain baseline serum specimens. Give medication via intravenous access. Maintain intravenous access throughout study. Nausea and/or vomiting are potential side effects of medication. Child should remain NPO 8 hours before testing.

- **Alteration in body image related to maturing body and early presence of secondary sex characteristics**
  Outcomes: The child will verbalize concerns about bodily changes to the health care team.
  The child expresses acceptance of changes in body image.
- **Knowledge deficit: diagnosis of precocious puberty and its cause**
  Outcomes: The parents and/or child will verbalize the physical, emotional, and social changes that may occur. The parents and child will discuss the options for treatment and verbalize their feelings concerning their choices with the health care team.
- **Social isolation related to child and others' perception of child's age and developmental abilities**
  Outcome: The child will report acceptable peer relationships.

Interdisciplinary Interventions

Interventions and treatments vary depending on the cause of the precocious puberty. When a CNS tumor is detected, surgery, irradiation, chemotherapy, or a combination of these treatment modalities is recommended. In the absence of a CNS lesion, several treatment options may be contemplated. Long-acting gonadotropin-releasing hormone (GnRH) agonists are effective treatment for gonadotropin-dependent precocious puberty (Wheeler & Styne, 1991). The GnRh agonist inhibits the release of LH and FSH, reduces gonadotropins and sex steroids to prepubertal levels, causes regression of secondary sex characteristics, retards sexual maturation, and slows the linear growth velocity and skeletal maturation (Table 26–5). The ultimate goal of therapy is to restore normal growth potential while allowing puberty to occur at the normal age with subsequent normal reproductive potential. After the physician prescribes the specific dose of Lupron Depot, the nurse either instructs the parent to give the intramuscular injection or the child's primary care provider will administer the injection. Once treatment is initiated, GnRH testing is performed every 3 to 4 months to assess the effectiveness of the treatment.

Besides the medical treatment that may be needed, the child with precocious puberty needs psychosocial support. Parents need clear and concise explanations concerning the causes of precocious puberty and treatment options. The child also needs explanations in age-appropriate terms about what is happening to his or her body.

Community Care

Parents, teachers, and friends should be encouraged to interact with the child in an age-appropriate manner, and expectations for the child should be realistic. Parents should encourage the child to participate in activities with same-age children. Clothing should also be age appropriate, and parents may need assistance concerning how to minimize the appearance of breast development. Parents should realize that intellectual, emotional, and social maturation does not keep pace with physical and hormonal changes. The child must be treated according to chronological age and guarded against sexual abuse from older children or adults (Williams, 1995). Heterosexual curiosity is not usually advanced beyond the child's chronological age. Parents and their precocious girls should be educated for the potential of the onset of menarche if this has not yet occurred. Menstrual hygiene becomes an important concern for the child in elemen-

Table 26–5
Treatment of Precocious Puberty

Medication	Dosage	Action	Side Effects
Leuprolide acetate (Lupron Depot)	0.3 mg/kg SC daily for 28 days or IM sustained-released once every 28 days	Slows child's growth to pubertal level Gonadotropin and sex hormone levels decrease to prepubertal levels	Local tenderness Erythema Cellulitis Abscess
Nafarelin (Syneral)	1600–1800 μg/day intranasally (2 or 3 sprays morning and evening)	Stimulates high level of luteinizing hormone and follicle-stimulating hormone to generate ovarian steroidogenesis	Uneven absorption Nasal irritation
Histrelin (Supprelin)	10 μg/kg SC daily in a single dose given same time each day	Decreases release of gonadotropins by desensitizing the gonadotropins in the pituitary Decreases testosterone and estrogen levels Has decelerating effect on skeletal maturation	Local tenderness Erythema Vaginal bleeding Headache
Ketoconazole	400–600 mg PO daily	In familial male precocious puberty, inhibits several biosynthetic steps in the synthesis of both adrenal and gonadal steroids Decreases testosterone	Hepatotoxicity Impaired adrenal function
Combined therapy with			
Spironolactone	70–150 mg/m² PO daily	Antagonizes the action of androgen at its receptor	Gynecomastia
Testolactone	0–40 mg/kg PO daily	Blocks the conversion of androgen to estrogen	Impaired adrenal function

tary school and should be addressed with the teachers and the nurses in the school. Most children who have precocious puberty adapt well, with some assistance; however, some may encounter serious problems adapting to their premature development. Children who experience any signs of significant psychological effects, such as depression, withdrawal, or aggressive behavior should receive counseling.

Delayed Puberty

Delayed puberty is the failure to develop sexually at an appropriate age or over the normal 3- to 5-year period at the normal age at onset. In girls who have not developed breasts by 13 years of age, or if more than 5 years have passed between the initiation of breast development and menarche, delayed puberty is considered. Boys are considered to have delayed puberty if secondary sexual development has not started by 14 years of age.

Etiology and Incidence

Delayed puberty is more common in boys than girls and occurs in 2% to 3% of all adolescents. Constitutional growth delay is the most common cause. The serum gonadotropins are typically normal, and the bone age, determined by radiography, is moderately delayed. The child also has a history of small stature during infancy and early childhood. The two other major categories of delayed puberty are hypogonadotropic hypogonadism and hypergonadotropic hypogonadism. In hypogonadotropic hypogonadism, delayed puberty is associated with low serum gonadotropin levels secondary to abnormalities of the hypothalamus or the pituitary. These abnormalities include craniopharyngiomas, Kallmann's syndrome, idiopathic hypopituitarism, autoimmune disease, fertile eunuch syndrome, isolated FSH deficiency, and hyperprolactinemia.

In hypergonadotropic hypogonadism, delayed puberty is associated with elevated serum gonadotropin levels. In girls, the most common abnormality is Turner's syndrome. Girls with Turner's syndrome have delayed puberty, short stature, webbed neck, and cubitus valgus (deformity of the arm in which the forearm deviates laterally). The karyotype in the girls with Turner's syndrome is 46XO. In boys, abnormalities include Klinefelter's syndrome; bilateral gonadal failure secondary to trauma, autoimmune destruction, infection or radiation; and congenital anorchia.

Assessment

The assessment of the child with delayed puberty includes a detailed family history as well as the child's history, physical examination, and laboratory studies.

The family history includes the onset of puberty; the patterns of growth and sexual development of the mother, father, and siblings; a history of consanguinity; and any history of infertility. Growth charts documenting previous heights and weights are obtained. A child's history of chronic illness, nutritional disorders, birth trauma, and head trauma should be noted.

The physical examination of the child with delayed puberty includes an accurate height and weight, the arm span, and the upper to lower segment ratio. Any signs of puberty are documented, noting breast development and presence of axillary hair and/or pubic hair. Testicular size and penile length are measured carefully. The sense of smell is assessed to eliminate Kallmann's syndrome as a cause of delayed puberty. In Kallmann's syndrome, the sense of smell is absent. The child with delayed puberty may tend to withdraw from age-appropriate activities and have decreased academic performance and altered self-concept. The school-age child becomes self-conscious about his or her body. As in the child with precocious puberty, one difficult aspect may be teasing from peers about the delay in puberty. Boys tend to be more distressed about their short stature and lack of physical maturation.

Diagnostic Tests. Many laboratory studies are needed. Gonadotropin concentrations (LH and FSH) are usually significantly higher than normal. Electrolytes should be normal. Thyroid levels may indicate hypothyroidism, prolactin levels may be elevated indicating a pituitary adenoma, and estradiol levels and testosterone levels may be decreased. A bone age, which is usually delayed, is performed along with an MRI or CT scan (hypothalamic or pituitary lesion needs to be ruled out).

A GnRH stimulation test can also be performed to distinguish between constitutional delay of growth and hypogonadotropic hypogonadism. A human chorionic gonadotropin stimulation test can also assist in the diagnosis. Some endocrinologists believe that these last two studies are not helpful in making the diagnosis and may be far too expensive to be of any value and that the physical examination is sufficient.

Nursing Diagnoses and Outcomes

In addition to the nursing diagnoses presented in Chart 26–3, the following nursing diagnoses may apply to a child with precocious puberty:

- **Alteration in body image related to delayed maturation of secondary sex characteristics**
  Outcomes: The child will verbalize concerns about body image to the health care team.
  The child expresses acceptance of changes in body image.

▶ **Knowledge deficit: Delayed puberty and its causes**
Outcomes: The parents and/or child will verbalize the physical, emotional, and social changes that may occur.
The parents and/or child will discuss the options for treatment and verbalize their feelings concerning their choices with the health care team.

Interdisciplinary Interventions

The treatment of the child with delayed puberty depends on the specific cause of the problem and whether the delay in development will be temporary or permanent. When the diagnosis is constitutional delay of growth, the health care team should reassure the child and family that there is no serious problem and that pubertal development will occur with time. It is important to explain to the family that medical intervention will not affect final adult height. Medical intervention has been used in the boy who is older than age 14 years and whose emotional well-being is adversely affected, as evidenced by a decrease in school performance and a withdrawal from his social circle. A 3- to 6-month course of low-dose testosterone (100 to 150 mg testosterone enanthate) given intramuscularly every 4 weeks is recommended (Solomon, Khadir, & Asfour, 1995). Larger doses of testosterone were found to cause premature closure of the epiphysis and decrease the final height (Bergada & Bergada, 1995). Spontaneous growth velocity and sexual maturation usually follows, and therapy is no longer needed. Reassurance, close observation, and assistance with clothes selection is usually sufficient for girls with delayed puberty.

The child with hypogonadotropin hypogonadism or hypergonadotropic hypogonadism requires replacement therapy with sex steroids. In boys, testosterone needs to be replaced; and in girls, estrogen and progesterone need to be replaced. Testosterone enanthate is also given intramuscularly every 4 weeks and is started when puberty would normally begin in boys. The dose will start at 100 mg and increase by 50 mg every 6 months to a final dose of 200 to 300 mg (Styne, 1993). Oral therapy or synthetic androgens do not stimulate complete pubertal development and are not an adequate therapy. Oral ethinyl estradiol is the replacement therapy of choice for girls. The usual dose is 0.02 to 0.1 mg/day for the first 21 days of every month. This is combined with medroxyprogesterone, 10 mg/day from day 14 to day 21 of each month (Hung, 1992). See Organizations in the resources list at the end of this chapter.

Other Pituitary Disorders

Panhypopituitarism is the lack of all anterior pituitary function resulting in the deficiency of TSH, GH, ACTH, LH, and FSH. The posterior pituitary may also be affected and ADH may be deficient. The incidence is 1 in 100,000 live births (Gray et al., 1993). Causes of panhypopituitarism include tumors, radiation therapy, encephalitis, or head trauma.

Pituitary gigantism is an extremely rare disorder resulting from the hypersecretion of GH by the pituitary gland. Few cases of gigantism have been confirmed by appropriate hormonal testing and/or pathologic data. Hypersecretion of GH usually occurs as a result of a pituitary adenoma. Tumors of the hypothalamus may also produce an overabundance of GH. About 20% of the cases of gigantism have been associated with the McCune-Albright syndrome that have other features, including café au lait pigmentation of the skin and polyostotic fibrous dysplasia. Gigantism has also been associated with acanthosis, hyperinsulinism, obesity, and hyperandrogenism without elevated GH levels.

Alterations in the Thyroid Gland

The thyroid gland is the first endocrine gland to appear in embryonic development. It begins to develop at about day 24 of gestation just behind the future site of the tongue. It forms from a thickening in the floor of the pharynx. As the embryo elongates, the primordia of the thyroid descends into the neck and is connected to the tongue by the thyroglossal duct. By 7 weeks of development the thyroid has divided into two lobes. It has reached its final site in the neck, and the thyroglossal duct has closed.

The thyroid gland is located in the lower anterior neck below the larynx. It consists of two lateral lobes, each measuring about 4 cm in length and 2 cm in width. An isthmus connects the two lobes in the middle and lies below the cricoid cartilage. The gland is surrounded by a fibrous capsule and is fixed to the trachea by loose connective tissue.

Various congenital defects of the thyroid are due to developmental malformations. This is called thyroid dysgenesis. The failure of the thyroid to descend to its proper position will be manifested by the thyroid developing at the base of the tongue (a lingual thyroid) or in the upper part of the neck (a sublingual thyroid). If remnants of the thyroglossal duct remain, they may give rise to thyroglossal duct cysts.

Normally, the thyroid gland synthesizes sufficient T_4 and T_3. These hormones regulate metabolism, increase oxygen consumption, stimulate protein synthesis, affect carbohydrate and lipid metabolism, and promote growth and development. The thyroid also contains parafollicular or C cells. These cells secrete calcitonin, which helps to maintain blood calcium levels. This hormone inhibits skeletal demineralization and promotes calcium deposition in the bone.

Thyroid hormone synthesis is regulated by TSH, which is secreted by the anterior pituitary. The secretion of TSH is under the control of thyrotropin-releasing hormone (TRH), which is synthesized in the hypothalamus.

When thyroid hormone production decreases, as in primary hypothyroidism, there is a compensatory increase in levels of TSH. Therefore, thyroid hypofunction or hyperfunction may be due to a defect in the thyroid gland (primary defect) or a defect in the pituitary or hypothalamus (secondary defect).

Assessment of the child with a thyroid disorder includes a comprehensive history, physical examination, laboratory studies, and a scan of the thyroid. The history should include questions about other family members with thyroid disease, growth and development, level of activity, the integumentary system (temperature and moistness of skin; texture of hair), gastrointestinal problems (diarrhea or constipation), calorigenesis, feeding problems, and weight gain or loss. The physical examination should include accurate measurements of height and weight, heart rate, and blood pressure; assessment of skin temperature and moisture; palpation of the neck for a goiter; neurologic evaluation (presence of tremors or hypoactive or hyperactive reflexes); and a developmental assessment.

Diagnostic studies include measurements of levels of T_4 (normal = 6.5 to 13 μg/dL), T_3 (normal = 100 to 210 ng/dL), and TSH (normal less than 6 μU/mL), and titration of antimicrosomal thyroid antibody levels in serum (DiGeorge & LaFranchi, 1996a). The administration of TRH is a stimulation test that distinguishes hypothalamic deficiency from pituitary deficiency as a cause of thyroid disease. Thyroid scanning is performed by giving a radionuclide intravenously and then measuring the uptake by the thyroid gland. Technetium (^{99m}Tc) is the preferred radionuclide in children because it has the advantage of low radiation exposure.

Hypothyroidism

Hypothyroidism is one of the most common endocrine disorders of childhood. Hypothyroidism in children may be congenital, acquired, or secondary. Acquired hypothyroidism usually refers to thyroid deficiency that becomes evident after a period of apparently normal thyroid function. However, this deficiency could be due to a congenital defect.

Pathophysiology

Congenital Hypothyroidism

Congenital hypothyroidism, deficient thyroid hormone production that is caused by a congenital defect and is manifest in the newborn period, has a prevalence of 1 in 4000 newborns (Hoekelman, 1992). Congenital hypothyroidism is most commonly caused by defective embryonic development of the gland. The thyroid gland may be ectopic (present in a site higher than the normal position in the neck), aplastic, or hypoplastic. Such defective glands often produce insufficient hormone to meet physiologic requirements. Congenital hypothyroidism may also be due to maternal ingestion of goitrogens (substances that produce a goiter) such as excessive amounts of iodide or antithyroid drugs.

A relatively infrequent but important cause of congenital hypothyroidism is an enzymatic defect interfering with the synthesis of thyroid hormone. This type of congenital hypothyroidism appears to have an autosomal recessive form of inheritance and usually presents as a goiter.

A deficiency of thyroid hormone causes decreased oxygen consumption, decreased metabolic rate, and decrease of protein synthesis. Therefore, the child who is hypothyroid grows poorly and has a decreased metabolic rate.

caREminder: *Early diagnosis and prompt treatment of congenital hypothyroidism is essential for normal growth and brain development. The greater the delay in treatment of congenital hypothyroidism, the greater is the degree of mental retardation that will result. With early diagnosis and treatment children with congenital hypothyroidism can be normal.*

Acquired Hypothyroidism

Acquired hypothyroidism may result from a variety of causes. It may be due to a congenitally defective thyroid gland that furnishes sufficient amounts of hormone early in life but that is inadequate later in childhood. A thyroid gland that is ectopically located at the base of the tongue (lingual thyroid or sublingual thyroid) may be the cause of acquired hypothyroidism in children.

The most common cause of acquired hypothyroidism is lymphocytic thyroiditis (also called Hashimoto's or autoimmune thyroiditis). The prevalence may be as high as 1% in school children (Rallison, Dobyns, Keating, Rall, & Tyler, 1975). This is an autoimmune disorder, and antithyroid antibodies are present. Lymphocytic thyroiditis is often associated with other endocrine disorders, such as diabetes mellitus, and with certain chromosomal disorders, such as Down and Turner's syndromes. Lymphocytic thyroiditis is the most common cause of goiter in children and occurs much more frequently in girls than in boys.

With prompt diagnosis and treatment, children with acquired hypothyroidism will be completely normal. Delay or noncompliance with treatment can cause severe growth delay, learning difficulties, and other symptoms caused by decreased rate of metabolism.

Secondary Hypothyroidism

When hypothyroidism is due to a defect of either the hypothalamus or pituitary, it is termed *secondary hypothyroidism*. For a discussion of secondary hypothyroidism, see the section on panhypopituitarism.

Assessment

Congenital Hypothyroidism

Since the establishment of a nationwide program of neonatal screening for congenital hypothyroidism, the diagnosis is formulated within the first few weeks of life and neonates are treated before symptoms of hypothyroidism occur.

Rarely, the diagnosis is missed or delayed and symptoms occur. Symptoms of congenital hypothyroidism appear in the bottle-fed infant before they appear in the breast-fed baby. This is because breast milk contains small amounts of thyroid hormone. Affected infants have a history of feeding difficulties, inactivity, and constipation. They cry little and are often characterized as "good" babies.

On physical examination they may have a characteristic facies that includes a dull appearance, pallor, a flat nasal bridge, puffy eyelids, a thick protuberant tongue, and low hairline (Fig. 26–3). Growth is stunted, and the fontanelles are widely open. A large posterior fontanelle indicates hypothyroidism. Prolonged jaundice, carotenemia, and anemia are common. The skin is cool, dry, and mottled; and the infant may be hypothermic. Cardiovascular manifestations consist of bradycardia and decreased pulse pressure. The muscles are hypotonic, and there are abnormal deep tendon reflexes because of delayed relaxation after the reflex response. Congenital hypothyroidism has been associated with speech delay and sensorineural hearing loss.

Complications become more severe when treatment is delayed. Without treatment, children may die of respiratory obstruction because of macroglossia. Other severe effects of lack of treatment include dwarfism and severe mental retardation.

Acquired Hypothyroidism

The physical manifestations of acquired hypothyroidism depend on the age of the child. Impairment of mental development may occur in the very young child as it does in congenital hypothyroidism. A deceleration of growth rate is often the first sign of acquired hypothyroidism in children. The child may or may not have an enlarged thyroid, which is called a goiter. Children may also present with cold intolerance, constipation, weight gain, and lethargy.

Diagnostic Tests. Diagnosis of congenital or acquired hypothyroidism is based on a positive health history and physical examination for hypothyroidism. Definitive laboratory findings are low levels of T_3 and T_4 and high levels of TSH. However, in very mild hypothyroidism, T_3 and T_4 levels may be normal whereas TSH levels are elevated.

Neonatal screening for congenital hypothyroidism is mandatory; the assay usually consists of radioimmunoassay for T_4 on a drop of blood on filter paper. Neonatal screening has been extremely important in early detection and prevention of mental retardation (Fisher, 1987). Blood specimens for neonatal screening can be obtained by heelstick at the time screening for phenylketonuria is performed.

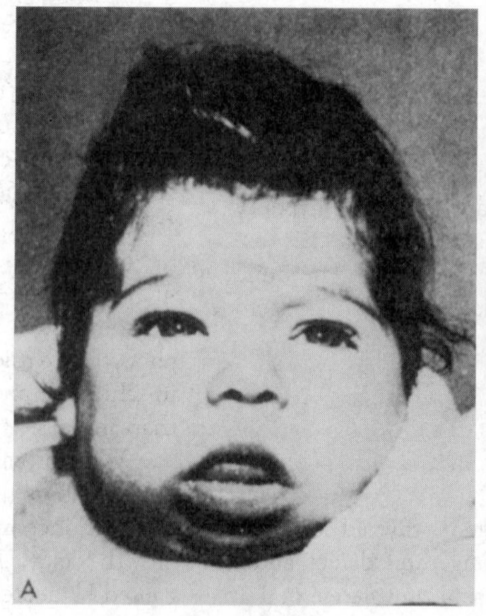

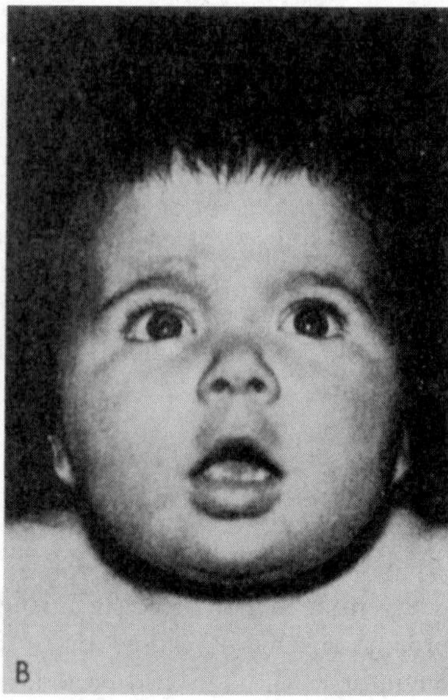

Figure 26–3
A, Congenital hypothyroidism in an infant produces facial puffiness, large tongue, and a dull expression. B, After treatment, the infant exhibits reduced puffiness and increased alertness. (From Behrman, R. E., Kliegman, R. M., & Arvin, A. M. [1996]. *Nelson textbook of pediatrics* [15th ed., p. 1592]. Philadelphia: W. B. Saunders.)

Thyroid scans are done to identify thyroid location, size, and function. Positive antithyroid antibodies are diagnostic of autoimmune thyroid disease.

Nursing Diagnoses and Outcomes

In addition to the nursing diagnoses presented in Chart 26–3, the following diagnoses may apply to the child with hypothyrodism:

- **Altered growth and development related to deficient thyroid hormone**
  Outcome: The child will grow and develop within normal age-appropriate parameters.
- **Constipation related to decreased motility of the gastrointestinal tract**
  Outcome: The child's bowel habits will normalize with thyroid hormone treatment.
- **Hypothermia related to decreased metabolic rate**
  Outcome: The child will remain normothermic.
- **Impaired physical mobility related to fatigue and decreased strength and endurance**
  Outcome: The child's excessive fatigue will resolve with thyroid hormone treatment.
  The child will regain physical strength and endurance.
- **Altered nutrition: more than body requirements, related to decreased metabolic need**
  Outcome: The child's appetite will improve and excessive weight gain will diminish.

Interdisciplinary Interventions

Treatment of hypothyroidism consists of replacement with sodium-L-thyroxine (Synthroid) (Dallas & Foley, 1996). Serum levels of thyroid hormones and TSH must be monitored by the physician or the nurse practitioner to ensure that the proper dose is administered and that compliance is adequate. Once therapy is instituted, growth rate and developmental levels are continually monitored.

Because of the importance of thyroid hormone for normal growth and development, it is essential that nurses promptly identify signs of hypothyroidism (Chart 26–6). Once hypothyroidism is diagnosed, families are instructed on the importance of administering thyroid hormone as ordered (see Chart 26–7).

caREminder: *Because children and adolescents do not "feel different" if they miss a dose or two of thyroid hormone they may forget to take the medication.*

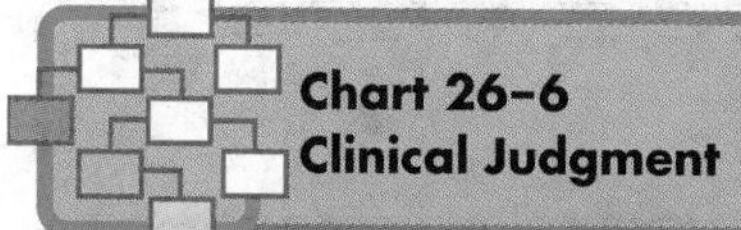

Chart 26–6
Clinical Judgment

The Child with Hypothyroidism

Denise is a newborn diagnosed with hypothyroidism. Her parents, Mr. and Mrs. Brown, are very concerned about her disease and about managing her care at home.

Questions

1. What diagnostic tests are used to assess for hypothyroidism in the newborn?
2. What clinical characteristics would be indicative of hypothyroidism?
3. What would be a major complication if Denise's condition had not been recognized and treated?
4. What steps should be included in the teaching plan for this family?
5. After your teaching is complete, what information would Mr. and Mrs. Brown be able to share with you to validate that they understand Denise's home care needs?

Answers

1. A simple blood test done via heelstick to diagnose hypothyroidism is required as part of the newborn screening tests in most states.
2. Feeding difficulties, prolonged physiologic jaundice, lethargy, constipation.
3. Mental retardation.
4. Teach family how to administer medications. Teach family importance of lifelong therapy and need for continual developmental surveillance.
5. Administration of sodium-L-thyroxine for life.

Community Care

Since the advent of thyroid screening, hypothyroidism that occurs early in life remains undiagnosed in very few children, and fewer suffer irreversible developmental delay. In the event developmental delay occurs, these children must be referred to early intervention programs to help them achieve their maximum potential. In the case of the child with acquired hypothyroidism, the quality of school work may have declined before the diagnosis and treatment of hypothyroidism. The diagnosis should be discussed with teachers to apprise them of the effect of hypothyroidism in learning ability and that treatment with thyroid hormone should return the child to the previous level of ability in school.

Hyperthyroidism

Hyperthyroidism (thyrotoxicosis) is characterized by excessive secretion of thyroid hormone. Hyperthyroidism in children is almost always caused by Graves' disease. Uncommon causes include functional adenoma (Plummer's

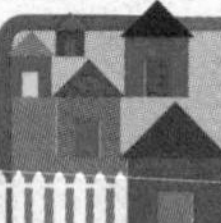

Chart 26-7
Community Care

Administration of Thyroid Hormone

- No liquid preparation of thyroid hormone exists.
- Thyroid pills must be crushed for very young children. Crush them in a shot glass. Mix with a medicine dropper. Add fluid to the glass and draw it into the dropper until no residue remains.
- Give thyroid hormone on an empty stomach to avoid the possibility of vomiting it.
- Give approximately 30 minutes before a feeding.
- Give the medicine at the same time each day (easier to remember).
- Parents must supervise to ensure that thyroid hormone is taken as ordered.

disease), polyostotic fibrous dysplasia (McCune-Albright syndrome), thyroid carcinoma, acute suppurative thyroiditis, or pituitary tumor, which secretes excessive TSH.

Hyperthyroidism occurs less often in children than hypothyroidism. It is five times more common in females, and the peak incidence occurs during adolescence (Zimmerman & Gan-Gaisano, 1992). The incidence is increased in Down syndrome, diabetes mellitus, and Addison's disease. There is an association with Hashimoto's thyroiditis.

Pathophysiology

Graves' disease, the most common cause of hyperthyroidism, is characterized by the triad of hypersecretion of thyroid hormone, presence of a goiter, and exophthalmos (bulging of the eyeballs). In this autoimmune disorder, thyroid-stimulating immunoglobins affect the thyroid gland in much the same fashion as TSH. There is evidence for genetic and immunologic components to Graves' disease. The disorder occurs frequently in families.

If the child is euthyroid after 2 to 3 years of therapy, and the thyroid is normal to slightly enlarged, therapy should be discontinued. The likelihood of permanent remission is great. However, if the thyroid is enlarged two times or greater, it is unlikely that remission has occurred and therapy may be continued or total thyroidectomy may be performed. Exophthalmos does not always resolve when hyperthyroidism is controlled.

Assessment

The signs and symptoms of hyperthyroidism are manifested in a variety of body systems. The onset is often insidious, with symptoms developing gradually. The most common early symptoms are related to emotional disturbances and increased motor activity.

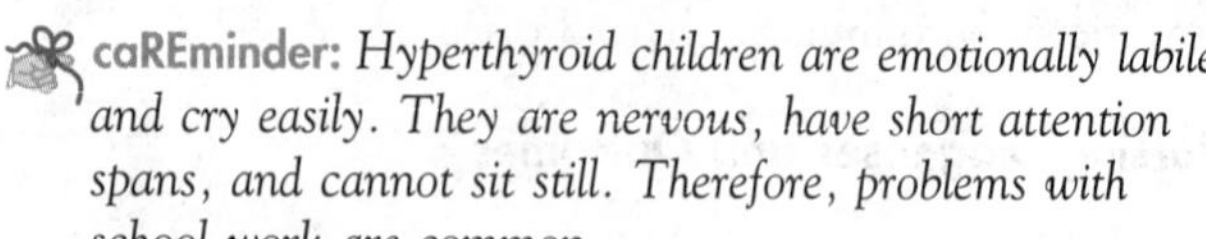

caREminder: *Hyperthyroid children are emotionally labile and cry easily. They are nervous, have short attention spans, and cannot sit still. Therefore, problems with school work are common.*

These children are hyperactive and have tremors and insomnia. Weight loss, in spite of polyphagia, is frequent. In addition, increased motility of the gastrointestinal tract may cause diarrhea. Cardiac manifestations include tachycardia with palpitations, increased systolic blood pressure yielding an increased pulse pressure, cardiomegaly, and systolic murmurs. The skin may be flushed, warm, sweaty, and very smooth. Heat intolerance can be mild or severe.

The thyroid gland is usually enlarged by two to four times, making it visible and easily palpable. The gland is most commonly symmetric, and smooth and systolic bruits may be auscultated over it. Exophthalmos varies in severity and may progress to the point that the child is unable to completely close his or her eyes. There is little correlation between the degree of exophthalmos and the severity of the hyperthyroidism. The most common ocular manifestations are lid retraction with the appearance of staring. Growth rate may be accelerated, and hyperthyroid children are frequently tall with slightly advanced osseous development.

Complications of hyperthyroidism include atrial fibrillation and thyroid "storm." Thyroid crisis or storm is rare in children, but it may be fatal. It is precipitated by stress, such as infection, trauma, and surgical emergencies, or by discontinuation of antithyroid therapy.

Alert: *The onset of thyroid storm is abrupt, and the symptoms are severe tachycardia, vomiting, diarrhea, hyperpyrexia, and confusion. If thyroid storm is not treated promptly, death may ensue.*

Diagnostic Tests. Diagnosis of hyperthyroidism is based on the history and the results of the physical examination and diagnostic studies. Levels of T_4 and T_3 are increased. Levels of TSH are very low because the high levels of thyroid hormone suppress the pituitary. If a thyroid nodule is present, a thyroid scan should be performed to differentiate between a malignant nodule and a thyroid-secreting adenoma. A malignant nodule is usually a "cold" nodule (a lesion with decreased concentration of radioisotope). A thyroid-secreting adenoma is usually "hot" (increased concentration of radioisotope).

Nursing Diagnoses and Outcomes

In addition to the nursing diagnoses presented in Chart 26–3, the following diagnoses may apply to the child with hyperthyroidism.

- **Diarrhea related to increased metabolic activity**
  Outcomes: The child's bowel habits will normalize.
  The child will not experience diarrhea.

- **Sleep pattern disturbance related to increased metabolic energy production**
  Outcome: The child's insomnia and restlessness will resolve.

- **Altered nutrition: less than body requirements related to the effects of a hypercatabolic state**
  Outcome: The child will gain an appropriate amount of weight with antithyroid hormone treatment.

- **Risk for decreased cardiac output related to atrial fibrillations**
  Outcomes: The child will maintain normal cardiac output.
  The child will receive prompt treatment for thyroid "storm."

Interdisciplinary Interventions

Medical treatment for children with hyperthyroidism includes antithyroid drugs to block T_4 synthesis, subtotal thyroidectomy, or radioiodine therapy (Castiglia, 1997). The drugs used to treat hyperthyroidism are propylthiouracil (PTU) and methimazole (Tapazole). Improvement is usually noticed in 2 weeks, and the patient becomes euthyroid in 1 to 3 months. Treatment may extend over long periods; therefore, compliance with the therapy may become a concern (Castiglia, 1997). Most side effects of antithyroid medications are mild and include pruritus, rash, and mild leukopenia. Severe leukopenia or agranulocytosis manifested by sore throat and sudden onset of high fever is an indication for discontinuation of the antithyroid medication. Beta-adrenergic blocking agents, such as propranolol, may be used with antithyroid drugs to control tachycardia, tremors, and hyperactivity in the severely toxic patient (Dallas & Foley, 1996). It is essential to administer antithyroid medications as ordered. If the medication is ordered three times a day, it is helpful to suggest that the second dose be given as soon as the child returns from school because that dose is the easiest to forget.

In children in whom drug therapy is not possible, or in whom medical management has been unsuccessful, subtotal thyroidectomy is indicated. The child must be euthyroid before surgery and is therefore treated with antithyroid medication. In addition, approximately 2 weeks before surgery, Lugol solution (potassium iodide), five drops twice a day, is added to the treatment regimen to decrease thyroid vascularity. Complications of thyroid surgery are uncommon but include hemorrhage, vocal cord paralysis, hypoparathyroidism, and hypothyroidism.

Worldview: *Radioactive iodine (^{131}I) therapy is used in the United States as an effective treatment for affected older children and adults. This treatment is not widely accepted in Europe. There is a theoretical risk of carcinoma and leukemia from radioactive isotope therapy. Therefore, this treatment modality remains controversial in the world community.*

Some symptoms of hyperthyroidism disease may be insidious, such as mood swings, poor attention span, and insomnia. It is crucial that nurses are alerted to these symptoms as signs of hyperthyroidism. Although the appropriate dose of antithyroid medication will cause a resolution of symptoms, there may be a time lag of a few weeks between the start of therapy and the end of symptoms.

Community Care

Exophthalmos and a large goiter may cause alterations in body image. Children with significant exophthalmos may have altered visual acuity. They may require surgery and should be referred to an ophthalmologist.

Tip: *For children and adolescents, suggest the use of high-necked clothing to mask the goiter. Girls can use scarves to hide the goiter and makeup to minimize exophthalmos.*

During the transition from the start of therapy until the disappearance of symptoms, parents must be educated about the child's need for small, frequent nutritious meals while polyphagic; lightweight clothing and good ventilation because of increased calorigenesis; and a low-pressure, nonstressful environment.

Teachers should be educated that excess thyroid hormone causes hyperactivity and poor attention span. School work should be structured accordingly until the child reaches a euthyroid state.

Alterations in Parathyroid Function

The parathyroid glands are derivations of the pharyngeal pouches. The third pharyngeal pouch expands into a dorsal bulbar portion. By the sixth week of development, each dorsal bulbar portion begins to differentiate into an inferior parathyroid gland. The parathyroid gland migrates caudally with the primordia of the thymus gland. At a later time, the parathyroids separate from the thymus and come to lie on the dorsal surface of the thyroid gland.

The fourth pharyngeal pouch also expands into a dorsal bulbar portion. By the sixth week of development, each dorsal portion develops in a superior parathyroid gland. These primordia of parathyroids migrate caudally and come to lie on the dorsal surface of the thyroid gland.

Located on the posterior surface of the thyroid gland, four parathyroid glands secrete parathyroid hormone (PTH), which maintains calcium homeostasis. PTH increases bone resorption, thereby increasing the level of calcium in the serum. In the kidneys, PTH decreases urinary excretion of calcium and increases urinary excretion of phosphate. PTH also increases calcium absorption from the intestine. The release of PTH depends on negative feedback relationship between the level of calcium in the serum and the level of PTH. A decreased level of serum calcium stimulates increased secretion of PTH. An elevated serum level of calcium causes decreased secretion of PTH.

Parathyroid disorder occurs if the PTH level is too low (hypoparathyroidism) or too high (hyperparathyroidism). Assessment of the child with a disorder of the parathyroid glands includes a health history, a physical examination, and laboratory studies. The history may reveal a child who has been asymptomatic or has had significant symptomatology. A review of systems should emphasize questions on neurologic status (twitching, convulsions, lethargy); musculoskeletal abnormalities (muscle cramp, muscle weakness, fractures); gastrointestinal disturbances (nausea, vomiting, diarrhea, constipation); and urologic problems (renal colic, hematuria). Questions should also include a history of weight loss or fever.

On physical examination, integumentary status must be assessed with attention to nails, hair, and skin. The ophthalmologic examination is essential in disorders of the parathyroid glands. Determination of skeletal growth, skeletal deformities, and dentition is important. Lastly, the child must be assessed for the presence of positive Chvostek or Trousseau signs.

caREminder: *To test for the Chvostek sign, an indication of hypocalcemia, tap sharply over the facial nerve below the temple and anteriorly to the ear. The sign is positive when twitching of the mouth (contraction of the lateral facial muscles) occurs. To check for the Trousseau sign, apply a blood pressure cuff to the patient's upper arm. Inflate the cuff until the blood supply is occluded. If this causes carpal spasm (the fingers contract and the patient is unable to open the hand), the Trousseau sign is positive, which indicates hypocalcemia.*

Diagnostic studies include measurement of serum levels of calcium, phosphorus, alkaline phosphatase, magnesium, PTH, and, in some instances, vitamin D. Renal function studies may be necessary to rule out renal insufficiency. Radiographs of the bones, skull, and/or abdomen, an electrocardiogram, and an electroencephalogram may be helpful.

Hypoparathyroidism

Hypoparathyroidism can be congenital or acquired. Familial congenital hypoparathyroidism, transmitted by an X-linked recessive gene, has been reported only a few times. Sporadic occurrence of aplasia or hypoplasia of the parathyroid glands is a more frequent cause of congenital hypoparathyroidism. Absence of the parathyroids is usually coupled with absence of the thymus gland. The absence of these glands is frequently associated with congenital heart defects, especially anomalies of the aortic arch. This constellation of defects is known as the DiGeorge syndrome and is associated with a deletion of the short arm of chromosome 22 (Greenberg, Elder, Hafner, Northrup, & Ledbetter, 1988).

Acquired hypoparathyroidism may be caused by autoimmune destruction of the glands or by inadvertent removal of the parathyroid glands during surgical thyroidectomy. Autoimmune hypoparathyroidism may be associated with Addison's disease, mucocutaneous candidiasis, and alopecia.

Pathophysiology

Hypoparathyroidism results in hypocalcemia and hyperphosphatemia. Low serum calcium levels cause twitching and tingling and, when severe, can induce tetany.

Prognosis. The prognosis of hypoparathyroidism depends on the severity of the disorder. Children with mild hypoparathyroidism usually do very well with calcium and vitamin D therapy. When ill, the child's calcium requirements may increase and require increased doses of medication. Children with severe hypoparathyroidism require higher doses of medication, and their condition is more precarious. If doses of medication are missed, severe hypocalcemia may ensue.

Assessment

Physical signs of hypoparathyroidism consist primarily of neurologic manifestations and include twitching, tingling and convulsions, muscular pain, and cramps. Severe hypocalcemia can induce tetany, which is a state of hyperexcitability of the central and peripheral nervous systems. Tetany is manifested by carpopedal spasms, laryngospasms, paresthesias, and/or convulsions.

Diagnosis is based on a positive history of the above signs and symptoms and on the physical examination. Children with DiGeorge syndrome may have severe midline facial defects (cleft lip/palate), have a particular facies (micrognathia, low-set ears), or look completely normal. Physical examination may demonstrate a positive Chvostek and/or Trousseau sign or laryngeal and carpopedal spasms.

Diagnostic Tests. Laboratory studies reveal low serum levels of calcium and PTH and an elevated serum level of phosphorus. Patients with long-standing hypocalcemia may exhibit cataracts and calcifications in the basal ganglia, which may be apparent in radiographs of the skull.

The electrocardiogram shows prolongation of the QT interval, and the electroencephalographic tracings usually show widespread slow activity. Infants with tetany should have radiographs of the chest. DiGeorge syndrome must be part of the differential diagnosis in these infants, and visualization of the thymus on the chest radiograph will rule out this syndrome. Chromosomal analysis looking specifically at chromosome 22 with fluorescence in-situ hybridization should be ordered when considering the diagnosis of DiGeorge syndrome (Budarf et al., 1995).

Nursing Diagnoses and Outcomes

In addition to the nursing diagnoses presented in Chart 26–3, the following diagnoses are applicable for the child with hypocalcemia:

- **Risk for injury related to seizures secondary to hypocalcemia**
  Outcome: The child will be seizure free when treated with calcium supplementation.
- **Ineffective airway clearance related to laryngospasm secondary to hypocalcemia**
  Outcome: The child will have no breathing impairment when treated with calcium supplementation.
- **Impaired skin integrity related to infiltration of calcium infusion**
  Outcome: The child will have no sloughing of skin during or after calcium infusion.
- **Altered cardiopulmonary tissue perfusion related to rapid infusion of calcium**
  Outcome: The child's heart rate and rhythm will remain normal while the calcium infusion is given.

Interdisciplinary Interventions

Medical treatment is aimed at correcting hypocalcemia and maintaining a normal serum calcium level (9 to 11 mg/dL). One must guard against hypercalcemia. Treatment consists of calcium and vitamin D. Calcium replacement is in the form of calcium gluconate or calcium lactate. For the child with tetany or seizures, the calcium should be given intravenously. It can later be administered orally. Vitamin D in the form of vitamin D_2 is also necessary to maintain normocalcemia and serves as a suitable alternative for PTH. Frequent monitoring of serum levels of calcium and phosphorus are indicated, particularly in the early stages of treatment.

Alert: *Early identification of the child with hypoparathyroidism is crucial in preventing severe hypocalcemia, which can cause tetany, resulting in laryngospasm and death.*

Children with severe hypocalcemia may require treatment with intravenous calcium gluconate, which the nurse must administer slowly over 5 to 10 minutes while monitoring the heart rate because this medication may cause bradycardia and circulatory collapse. Because calcium gluconate is caustic to tissue and infiltration causes sloughing, the nurse must administer this drug with extreme caution, making sure that the intravenous line does not become infiltrated. Other forms of intravenous calcium, such as calcium chloride, are given safely only through a central line.

The nurse should educate parents on the proper administration of calcium and vitamin D.

Tip: *Rocaltrol (vitamin D_3) is supplied in gelatinous capsules, and parents are taught to aspirate the contents of the capsule with a syringe and needle, separate the syringe from the needles, and squirt the medication into the mouth of a child too young to swallow a capsule.*

Community Care

The child with DiGeorge syndrome requires interdisciplinary, multisubspecialty follow-up. If the child has "classic" DiGeorge syndrome, referrals should include the cardiology, immunology, and genetics services. The cardiology service will evaluate for a conotrunchal defect, and the immunology service will assess the child's T-cell function. If the child is developmentally delayed, referral to an early intervention program is essential.

Hyperparathyroidism

Hyperparathyroidism (PTH hypersecretion by one or more of the parathyroid glands) may be primary or secondary. Primary hyperparathyroidism may be due to a defect of the parathyroid gland such as an adenoma or idiopathic hyperplasia of the parathyroid glands. Familial hyperparathyroidism has been described, and both autosomal recessive and autosomal dominant patterns of transmission have been documented in families of children with parathyroid hyperplasia (DiGeorge & LaFranchi, 1996b). Primary hyperparathyroidism is generally a disease of adults and is rare in children.

Secondary hyperparathyroidism is a compensatory increase in PTH in response to hypocalcemia that may be caused by a variety of disorders. Some causes of hypocalcemia that induce compensatory hyperparathyroidism include maternal hypoparathyroidism, vitamin D deficiency, and certain forms of rickets. The most common cause of secondary hyperparathyroidism is chronic renal failure.

Pathophysiology

Hyperparathyroidism resulting in hypercalcemia affects many body tissues and organs. Hypercalcemia may cause gastrointestinal, CNS, neuromuscular, skeletal, and renal disorders.

Prognosis. The prognosis of hyperparathyroidism depends on the disorder's etiology and severity. Some children with mild disease do very well. The major complication of hyperparathyroidism is hypercalcemic crisis.

Alert: *Signs of hypercalcemic crisis include lethargy, muscle weakness, coma, and oliguria. Their early detection and treatment can help prevent sequelae including mental retardation, convulsions, and blindness.*

Assessment

Physical manifestations of primary hyperparathyroidism are largely due to hypercalcemia. The systems affected in primary hyperparathyroidism are gastrointestinal, CNS, neuromuscular, skeletal, and renal. Gastrointestinal symptoms include anorexia, nausea, vomiting, pancreatitis, and constipation. CNS disturbances due to hypercalcemia are confusion, impaired memory, and an altered level of consciousness. Neuromuscular manifestations are weakness, muscle atrophy, paresthesias of the extremities, bradycardia, and cardiac irregularities. There may be bone pain, fractures, gait disturbance, and compression of the vertebrae. Renal changes related to increased urinary calcium loss are polyuria and polydipsia; in addition, renal calculi, hypertension, and renal colic have been described in children. Calcification in the cornea of the eye (band keratopathy) is an additional sign of hypercalcemia.

Signs and symptoms of secondary hyperparathyroidism depend on the disorder that induces the parathyroids to hypersecrete PTH. Children with secondary hyperparathyroidism usually have some degree of hypocalcemia. Signs and symptoms related to the direct action of excess PTH are bone demineralization (bone pain, fractures), renal damage (hypertension, renal calculi), and pancreatitis.

Diagnostic Tests. The diagnosis of hyperparathyroidism is based on history, physical examination, and laboratory studies. In patients with primary hyperparathyroidism, the level of calcium in the serum is elevated (greater than 10.8 mg/dL), the phosphorus level is decreased, and the magnesium level is low. PTH levels are elevated. Radiographs show demineralization of bone, subperiosteal resorption in the phalanges, and granular appearance of the skull. Abdominal films may show renal calculi. In secondary hypoparathyroidism the serum level of calcium is decreased, whereas serum levels of phosphorus and PTH are elevated. Additional tests must be done to determine the cause of secondary hyperparathyroidism, for example, renal function studies.

Interdisciplinary Interventions

Treatment of primary hyperparathyroidism consists of either surgical removal of the parathyroid adenoma or of subtotal or a total parathyroidectomy depending on where the glands are hyperplastic. In secondary hyperparathyroidism the underlying cause must be treated. In patients with renal disease, treatment of secondary hyperparathyroidism includes oral administration of vitamin D, phosphate binders, and calcium. In addition, a low phosphorus diet is prescribed. If secondary hyperparathyroidism is severe, parathyroidectomy may be necessary.

The nurse must identify signs of hyperparathyroidism early, because early recognition and treatment of hyperparathyroidism may prevent serious complications.

caREminder: *Hypercalcemia can affect cardiac muscle contractility. Therefore, children with hyperparathyroidism should be assessed for signs of bradycardia or cardiac arrhythmia.*

Parents should be instructed on the administration of vitamin D, phosphate binders, and calcium. Intervention by a nutritionist is required to instruct the family on a low-phosphate diet to decrease hyperphosphatemia. In addition, instruction is needed on the importance of giving large amounts of fluids, particularly acidic fluids such as cranberry juice, to help prevent renal calculi.

Because the child with hyperparathyroidism has brittle bones and a tendency toward fractures, the safety of the child's environmental surroundings should be assessed (e.g., side rails in place). The child should be assisted getting out of bed. Signs of postoperative complications should be identified by the nurse caring for a child after a parathyroidectomy. A major complication is hypoparathyroidism. (See the section on care of the child with hypoparathyroidism.)

Community Care

The parents can be instructed on safety precautions to be taken in the home and at school. If the child with hyperparathyroidism has skeletal deformities, the child may have an altered body image. Nurses and school counselors can be very helpful in assisting these children to identify positive, achievable goals for vocation and avocation.

Disorders of the Pancreas

Disorders of the pancreas may develop at any age, including the fetal and neonatal periods. Therefore, development throughout this time in the life span is important. The pancreas develops through growth of separate buds (dorsal and ventral pancreatic buds) from the endodermal epithelium of the duodenum that later fuse. The differentiation of cells of the endocrine and exocrine portion of the pancreas takes place between the second and third month of embryonic and fetal development (Lessick, Klingner, & Clabots, 1986).

The ventral bud forms the uncinate process and the inferior part of the head of the pancreas. Most of the pancreas is derived from the dorsal bud. As the pancreatic buds fuse, the ducts anastomose. The main pancreatic duct forms from the duct of the ventral bud and the distal part of the duct forms from the dorsal bud (Moore & Persaud, 1993). The parenchyma is derived from endoderm that forms a network of tubules. Acini begin to develop from cell clusters around the end of the tubules. The islets of Langerhans develop from groups of cells that separate from the tubules and lie between the acini. Insulin secretion begins at approximately 20 weeks (Moore & Persaud, 1993). There are three cell types identified within the islets of Langerhans. Beta cells secrete insulin and form 60% to 70% of the islet cells. Alpha cells secrete glucagon and make up approximately 20% to 30% of the islet cells. Finally, delta cells secrete gastrin and comprise 2% to 8% of the islet cells.

Diabetes Mellitus

Diabetes mellitus is a disorder of energy metabolism that is characterized by the relative or absolute lack of insulin production in the pancreas. Two major types of diabetes mellitus are recognized: insulin-dependent diabetes mellitus (IDDM, type I) and non–insulin-dependent diabetes mellitus (NIDDM, type II).

Etiology and Incidence

There is no one cause for the development of IDDM. Lipman (1988) notes that certain characteristics are common to the development of diabetes. These include seasonal variations (mid winter and spring), secular trends, history of illness or infection preceding diagnosis, and family history of IDDM. Autoimmunity, genetics, and environmental factors are all thought to contribute to the destruction of the beta cells found in the islets of Langerhans. Tumors of the pancreas, pancreatitis, and steroid use may also contribute to the development of the disease (Castiglia, Kramer, Fong, & Lipman, 1992).

Autoimmunity is involved in the destruction of beta cells. Approximately 70% of newly diagnosed diabetics have islet cell antibodies (Ruble & Charron-Prochownik, 1994). Islet cell antibodies can also be found in relatives of people with IDDM. This information may assist researchers in identifying other relatives at risk for developing type I diabetes. Research is ongoing to establish a method for predicting the relative risk of relatives of patients with type I diabetes (Diabetes Prevention Trials, 1993).

IDDM is found in families; however, the mode of inheritance is not fully understood. Foster (1994) states that there is only a 5% to 10% chance a child will develop type I diabetes when another first-degree relative has the disease. He also asserts that the risk of the child developing type I diabetes increases when the parent has type II diabetes.

The major environmental factor believed to be involved in the development of type I diabetes is a virus that may trigger the autoimmune process. Several viruses have been identified as possible triggers for the onset of type I diabetes, including coxsackievirus B4, retrovirus, cytomegalovirus, and the viruses causing mumps, hepatitis, and congenital rubella (Foster, 1994). The annual incidence of IDDM is about 15 new cases per 100,000 among people younger than 20 years of age. The prevalence rate is 1 in 600 school-age children, and the peak incidence is between 10 and 14 years of age. IDDM is approximately one and one-half times more common among whites than blacks and markedly less common in Native Americans, Asian Americans, and Hispanics of Mexican origin (Gray, St. Dennis-Feezle, Clark & Parker, 1993). Hispanics of Puerto Rican origin have a higher incidence of IDDM (Lipman, 1993).

Pathophysiology

Insulin deficiency causes physiologic and metabolic changes throughout the body. Glucose derived from dietary sources cannot be utilized by the cells (specifically muscle and fat cells) and begins to increase in the blood stream (hyperglycemia). When serum glucose levels approach 200 mg/dL, the renal tubules have difficulty reabsorbing all of the glucose and glucose is spilled into the urine (glucosuria). Large amounts of electrolytes (sodium, potassium, calcium, phosphate, magnesium) are also excreted by the kidneys (Castiglia et al., 1992). This results in increased urination (polyuria) and dehydration. Excessive thirst (polydipsia) ensues in an attempt to relieve the dehydration. Excessive hunger (polyphagia) also results from the body's attempt to compensate for the calories lost during polyuria.

Insulin deficiency causes an increased catabolism of protein resulting in an increased production of amino acids. At the same time the liver converts triglycerides (lipolysis) to fatty acids, which in turn change to ketone bodies. These ketone bodies are used for energy by the peripheral tissues but are not well utilized in the state of insulin deficiency. Excessive ketone bodies accumulate and are excreted by the kidneys (ketonuria) (Castiglia et al., 1992). Ketone bodies are organic acids that can produce excessive amounts of free hydrogen ions resulting in metabolic acidosis. Serum pH is lowered because the body cannot compensate. In severe acidosis, the depth and rate of respirations increases and becomes persistent as the body attempts to compensate by excreting excess carbon dioxide (Kussmaul respirations).

Insulin deficiency in association with increased levels of counter-regulatory hormones (glucagon, growth hormone, cortisol, catecholamines) and dehydration is the primary cause of diabetic ketoacidosis (DKA), which is a frequent complication of diabetes. Counter-regulatory hormones have an anti-insulin effect, are increased in times of stress, and worsen insulin deficiency. Peripheral glucose utilization is decreased, and hepatic gluconeogenesis is increased. Severe insulin deficiency causing DKA is a medical emergency and is characterized by hyperglycemia (glucose > 300 mg/dL), hyperketonemia (ketone bodies > 5 mm), metabolic acidosis (pH < 7.30, bicarbonate < 15 mEq/L), and severe alterations in electrolyte and fluid balance.

The importance of good metabolic control in relation to long-term complications (retinopathy and neuropathy) is the focus of the Diabetes Control and Complications Trial (DCCT). The DCCT was a 9-year multicenter prospective trial involving IDDM patients who were 13 to 39 years at the start of the study. Patients were placed in two groups: an intensive treatment group and a conventional therapy group. The researchers reported that intensive therapy delays the onset of retinopathy by 27% and slows the progression of retinopathy by 62%. Clinically significant neuropathy was reduced by 60%, and the development of clinical grade albuminuria was reduced by 56%. However, severe hypoglycemia was a risk of tight control (DCCT Research Group, 1993).

The pathogenesis of NIDDM is poorly understood. It is known that NIDDM runs in families, although the mode of inheritance is not known. Children who have NIDDM usually have a resistance to insulin and also may have an abnormal insulin secretion. These children are usually obese and have family members who also have NIDDM.

Assessment

Identification of the child in DKA is critical and will facilitate treatment and the child's return to previous good health (Table 26–6). A capillary blood glucose measurement at the bedside is obtained if DKA is suspected and reported to the appropriate physician in charge. The degree of dehydration is assessed after the child is weighed and examined. Assessment includes the examination of the mucous membranes for moistness, the eyeballs for degree of depression, the skin for turgor, and the anterior fontanelle for depression. The child may also show signs of impending shock: tachypnea, decreased output, hypotension, and a weakening pulse.

The child with diabetes usually presents with the

Table 26–6
Nursing Assessment of the Child with Diabetic Ketoacidosis

Nursing Assessment	Signs and Symptoms	Laboratory Test	Nursing Interventions	Medical Management
Assess for dehydration	↓ Skin turgor Dry mucous membranes Sunken eyeballs Depressed fontane Signs of shock: tachypnea, output hypotension, weak pulse	↑ Hemoglobin, hematocrit ↑ Blood urea nitrogen, creatinine	Check vital signs every hour Administer 0.9% NaCl at rate ordered (Ringer's lactate for the child in shock) Maintain accurate I&O records	0.9% NaCl intravenous at a rate of maintenance plus one half of deficit in first 8 hr Ringer's lactate at 20 mL/kg for the first hour for treatment of shock
Assess for potassium depletion	None	Potassium elevated or normal if early	Before administering potassium, make sure: Urine flow has been established Electrocardiogram or laboratory value has ruled out hyperkalemia Administer potassium as ordered	Electrolyte measurement Add KCL 40 mEq/L of IV fluid as per physician's orders
Assess for phosphate depletion	None	Phosphorus elevated or normal if early	In case of severe acidosis and use of bicarbonate, administer potassium phosphate as ordered	In severe acidosis: KCL 20 mEq/L + KPh 20 mEq/L of IV fluid as per physician's orders

Table 26–6
Nursing Assessment of the Child with Diabetic Ketoacidosis *Continued*

Nursing Assessment	Signs and Symptoms	Laboratory Test	Nursing Interventions	Medical Management
Assess for hyperglycemia	Polyuria Polydipsia Polyphagia Weight loss	Blood glucose >180 mg/dL Urine glucose positive	Check Chemstrip q1h Check urine glucose every void Prepare IV insulin drip: (250 units regular insulin/250mL 0.9% NaCl) and administer as ordered	Nurse will obtain blood glucose q2h The nurse will give IV insulin (regular) as ordered: 0.1 unit/kg IV push followed by 0.1 unit/kg/hr
Assess for hypoglycemia	Diaphoresis Tremors Tachycardia Irritability	Blood glucose <60 mg/dL	Notify physician when Chemstrip is ≤250 mg/dL Have carbohydrate and IV dextrose available	When blood glucose is ≤250 mg/dL: Rate of insulin drip *or* Change IV solution to D5.45
Assess for degree of acidosis	Kussmaul respirations Acetone odor on breath ↓ Level of consciousness	↓ pH ↓ CO_2 Serum bicarbonate Acetonuria	Check vital signs q1h Measure urine acetone every void For severely acidotic child perform neurologic checks q1h and administer bicarbonate as ordered	Measure serum pH and CO_2 q2h Insulin as ordered For severely acidotic child bicarbonate 2 mEq/kg infuses over 1–2 h
Assess for factors precipitating DKA	Signs of infection: fever, otitis media, dysuria, etc.	↑ White blood cell count Positive urine culture Positive throat culture	Report signs of infection to physician Administer antibiotic as ordered	Order indicated studies If infection is bacterial, treat with an antibiotic
	Report of missed or insufficient insulin dose		Teach child and family about consequences of insulin errors and sick day management	
	Report of emotional stress		Refer to social service, psychiatrist, school nurse, visiting nurse, as necessary	

classic symptoms of polyuria and polydipsia. Nocturia and enuresis are also seen frequently in the young child. An increased appetite (polyphagia) is seen early in diabetes, although anorexia is also commonly seen later in the disease subsequent to the child feeling extremely ill. Weight loss, which can be as much as 10% to 30% of the original weight, may become significant before parents even become aware of it. Fatigue, headache, and malaise are also symptoms often seen at the presentation of diabetes. Many of these symptoms may be attributed to other illnesses or events at the time, such as influenza, urinary tract infection, summer heat, or intentional weight loss.

As insulin deficiency persists and ketone bodies continue to be excreted, the child begins to experience stomach pains, vomiting, and continued weight loss. Dehydration quickly develops as DKA progresses. Kussmaul respirations, change in mental status, and fruity-like odor to the breath ensue. The child becomes somnolent and may advance into a coma.

Alert: *The diagnosis of IDDM is often delayed in the infant because evaluation by parents of diaper quantity is insufficient; therefore, they do not notice polyuria.*

Physicians also rarely consider diabetes as part of the differential diagnosis in the infant, confusing many of the symptoms with gastroenteritis. Infants can be at high risk for dehydration; and because diabetes is not commonly diagnosed in infancy, it may be a low priority for physicians. Subsequently, the diagnosis is often delayed and the infant is admitted in severe DKA.

Other common but less characteristic symptoms described by Travis, Brouhard, and Schreiner (1987) are personality changes, lethargy, vision changes, altered school performance, headaches, anxiety attacks, intermittent breathlessness, chest pain, nausea, and either diarrhea or constipation.

Diagnostic Tests. Diagnosis of IDDM is based on history, physical examination, and laboratory studies. The history includes polyuria, polydipsia, polyphagia, or anorexia and weight loss. A viral illness preceding these symptoms may also be offered. Blood glucose levels are usually greater than 200 mg/dL, and a urine sample reveals glucosuria and possibly ketonuria depending on the degree of acidosis. A glucose tolerance test would reveal low insulin levels in the face of elevated glucose levels. The child may appear very healthy or acutely ill, depending on the degree of acidosis.

The child with NIDDM may also have polydipsia, polyuria, and polyphagia. The glucose tolerance test would reveal high insulin levels in the face of elevated glucose levels. The child would not have ketones and would not appear acutely ill.

Nursing Diagnoses and Outcomes

In addition to the nursing diagnosess presented in Chart 26–3, the following diagnoses may apply to the child with IDDM:

- **Fluid volume deficit related to vomiting and polyuria secondary to ketoacidosis**
  Outcome: The child will be well hydrated as evidenced by good skin turgor, moist mucous membranes, and the absence of polyuria.
- **Altered nutrition: less than body requirements related to an imbalance between food intake and physical activity and to lack of knowledge**
  Outcome: The child will be well nourished as evidenced by resumption of normal weight and verbalization of satiety after eating.

Table 26–7
Insulin Types and Action

Type	Manufacturer	Form	Appearance	Onset (hr)	Peak (hr)	Duration (hr)
Short or Fast Acting						
Regular	Nova-Nordisk	Pork	Clear	0.5	2.5–5	8
Semilente	Nova-Nordisk	Beef	Cloudy	1–2	5–10	16
Humulin R	Lilly	Human	Clear	0.25–0.5	2–4	6–8
Purified Pork R	Nova-Nordisk/Lilly	Pork	Clear	0.5	2.5–5	8
Intermediate Acting						
Lente	Lilly	Beef/Pork	Cloudy	1–3	6–12	18–26
Humulin L	Lilly	Human	Cloudy	1–3	6–12	18–24
Purified Pork L	Lilly	Pork	Cloudy	2–3	7–15	22
NPH	Nova-Nordisk	Beef	Cloudy	1–2	4–12	24
Globin	Lilly/Squibb-Nova		Clear		longer than fast acting but not as long as long acting	
Long Acting						
Ultra-Lente	Squibb-Nova	Beef	Cloudy	4–8	10–30	36
Humulin	Lilly	Human	Cloudy	4–6	8–20	24–28
PZI			Cloudy	4–8	14–24	36
Premixed Combinations						
Novulin 70/30	Squibb-Nova	Human				
Mixtard (30% regular, 70% NPH)	Nova-Nordisk	Pork				

Interdisciplinary Interventions

Insulin therapy is the medical management for a person with IDDM. Without insulin, the child will die. Usually a combination of short-acting and intermediate-acting insulin is given to children with diabetes before breakfast and before dinner (Table 26–7 and TIP 26–2). This combination is used to ensure that the peak action of the insulin coincides with the child's blood glucose peaks. Insulin therapy is intended to peak during postprandial glucose elevations. Long-acting insulin is not usually used in children because the action is too long and variable.

Worldview: *Children with IDDM may come from cultures of origin (such as Hebrew and Muslim) in which the use of pork products is prohibited. Therefore, pork insulin may require substitutions.*

Monitoring Metabolic Control

The physician calculates the insulin dose using the child's body weight and blood sugar levels. The morning dose is usually two thirds or three fourths of the total daily dose that will cover the daytime meals, and the remainder of the dose is given before dinner to attain evening coverage. The nurse initially gives the insulin and at the same time instructs the child and parents. The earlier the child and/or parents give the injection in the course of the hospitalization, the easier it will become to administer it and the sooner the child will be able to leave the hospital.

Insulin strength is measured in units: 1 mL of insulin is equal to 100 units. In the very small child, changing the amount of insulin by 1 or 2 units can represent a 50% or even a 100% rise or drop considering that the doses are usually very small. The accuracy in measuring the dose is improved by diluting the insulin. The pharmacy will dilute the insulin to U-50 (1:1 dilution) as ordered by the physician to allow for smaller changes in the dose. With U-50 insulin, 1 mL of insulin is equal to 50 units.

The variation in absorption rates is minimized by giving four to six injections in the same area and then moving to a different area (Fig. 26–4). The nurse shows the child and the family the best areas for injection. Hypertrophy or atrophy of the local tissue can occur when insulin is injected into the same location. Insulin is not well absorbed in hypertrophied tissue, which is thickened at the site of injection. Atrophied tissue is hollowed or depressed tissue as a result of the degeneration of subcutaneous fat. Insulin absorption from the hypertrophied or atrophied tissue is erratic. Insulin action is unpredictable and control is more difficult. At least two to

TIP 26–2 A Teaching Intervention Plan for Administering Insulin

Nursing Diagnoses and Outcomes

- Knowledge deficit: mixing and administering insulin
  Outcomes: Child/family will administer the correct kind and doses of insulin to the child. Child will demonstrate the highest levels of skill of which he or she is developmentally capable.

Teach the Family

Insulin Administration

- Remove insulin from the refrigerator and allow to warm to room temperature.
- The person preparing and administering insulin should wash his or her hands.
- Wipe the top of insulin bottles with alcohol.
- Gently roll bottle of intermediate or long-acting insulin to ensure uniform mixture of insulin and to avoid introducing air bubbles.
- Place air into the intermediate or long-acting insulin (air is equivalent to insulin to be withdrawn).
- Place air into the short-acting insulin.
- Draw up short-acting insulin, removing all air bubbles.
- Draw up intermediate or long-acting insulin.
- Pinch the skin being used for injection (this separates subcutaneous tissue from muscle).
- Give insulin in the subcutaneous tissue at either a 45- or 90-degree angle.
- Withdraw needle immediately after injection is given. Dispose of the needle in an appropriate needle storage container.

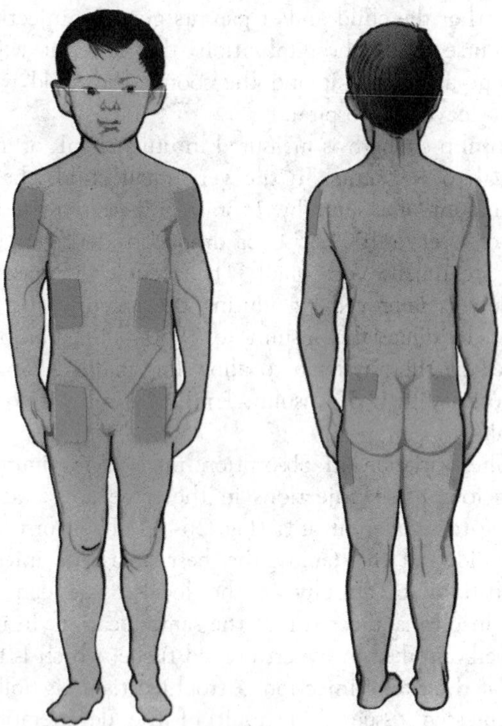

Figure 26–4
Sites for insulin injection should be rotated among the areas shown.

three sites (arms, legs, stomach, or buttocks) should be selected by the child and parents. Children can choose sites and then chart them so they remember not to overuse sites.

Blood Testing

Capillary blood glucose monitoring is usually done two to six times a day and can be performed by the patient or a family member. The supplies are easily transportable. Hypoglycemia and hyperglycemia are accurately documented and the results are immediate and specific (Charts 26–8 and 26–9). The disadvantages of blood glucose monitoring are the invasive nature of the procedure and the sometimes excessive cost of the equipment. The child should test the blood glucose initially three to four times each day, and then this is decreased to twice each day. Encouraging the child to self-test can be a challenge, and the nurse will help the parents with different motivating strategies. Test results should be documented and used in regulating the insulin dose. Records should be brought to the doctors at each subsequent visit.

Capillary blood glucose monitoring is accomplished by placing a drop of blood, obtained after puncturing the finger with a lancet, on a blood test strip (Fig. 26–5). The fingers should be cleaned with soap and water and then wiped with alcohol. The use of a lancing device decreases the discomfort felt by the child. The test strips are analyzed visually or with the use of a glucometer.

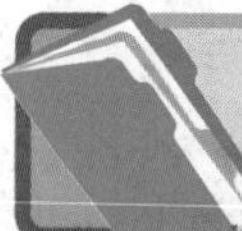

Chart 26–8
Nursing Interventions Classification (NIC)

Hyperglycemia Management

Definition

Preventing and treating above normal blood glucose levels

Activities

Monitor blood glucose levels, as indicated.
Monitor for signs and symptoms of hyperglycemia: polyuria, polydipsia, polyphagia, weakness, lethargy, malaise, blurring of vision, or headache.
Monitor urine ketones, as indicated.
Monitor ABG, electrolyte, and betahydroxybutyrate levels, as available.
Monitor orthostatic blood pressure and pulse, as indicated.
Administer insulin, as prescribed.
Encourage oral fluid intake.
Monitor fluid status (including I&O), as appropriate.
Maintain IV access, as appropriate
Administer IV fluids, as needed.
Administer potassium, as prescribed.
Consult physician if signs and symptoms of hyperglycemia persist or worsen.
Assist with ambulation if orthostatic hypotension is present.
Provide oral hygiene, if necessary.
Identify possible cause of hyperglycemia.
Anticipate situations in which insulin requirements will increase (e.g., intercurrent illness).
Restrict exercise when blood glucose levels are >250 mg/dL, especially if urine ketones are present.
Instruct patient and significant others on prevention, recognition, and management of hyperglycemia.
Encourage self-monitoring of blood glucose levels.
Instruct on urine ketone testing, as appropriate.
Instruct on indications for, and significance of, urine ketone testing, if appropriate.
Instruct patient to report moderate or large urine ketone levels to the health professional.
Instruct patient and significant others on diabetes management during illness, including use of insulin and/or oral agents, monitoring fluid intake, carbohydrate replacement, and when to seek health professional assistance, as appropriate.
Provide assistance in adjusting regimen to prevent and treat hyperglycemia (e.g., increasing insulin or oral agent), as indicated.
Facilitate adherence to diet and exercise regimen.

From McCloskey, J., & Bulechek, G. (1996). *Nursing interventions classification (NIC)* (2nd ed.). St. Louis: Mosby–Year Book. Reprinted with permission.

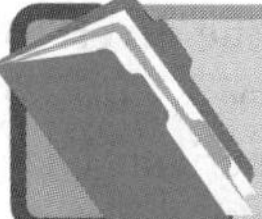

Chart 26–9
Nursing Interventions Classification (NIC)

Hypoglycemia Management

Definition

Preventing and treating below normal blood glucose levels

Activities

Identify patient at risk for hypoglycemia.
Monitor blood glucose levels, as indicated.
Monitor for signs and symptoms of hypoglycemia: pallor, diaphoresis, tachycardia, palpitations, hunger, paresthesia, shakiness, inability to concentrate, confusion, slurred speech, irrational or uncontrolled behavior, blurred vision, somnolence, inability to arouse from sleep, or seizures.
Provide simple carbohydrates, as indicated.
Provide complex carbohydrates and protein, as indicated.
Maintain IV access, as appropriate.
Administer intravenous dextrose, as appropriate.
Administer glucagon, as appropriate.
Consult physician if signs and symptoms of hypoglycemia persist or worsen.
Maintain patient airway, as necessary
Protect from injury, as necessary.
Identify possible cause of hypoglycemia.
Recommend changes in regimen to prevent hypoglycemia (e.g., reduction in insulin when NPO).
Instruct patient and significant others on prevention, recognition, and treatment of hypoglycemia.
Instruct significant others on use and administration of glucagon, as appropriate.
Instruct patient to obtain and carry appropriate emergency medical identification.
Encourage patient to have simple carbohydrates available at all times.
Encourage self-monitoring of blood glucose levels.
Provide assistance to patient in making self-care decisions to prevent hypoglycemia (e.g., eating additional food or reducing insulin when exercising).

From McCloskey, J., & Bulechek, G. (1996). *Nursing interventions classification (NIC)* (2nd ed.). St. Louis: Mosby–Year Book. Reprinted with permission.

The accuracy of the reading depends on the proper use of the test system. Quality checks should be completed three to four times per year with control solutions. The family should keep the monitor manufacturer's hotline number in the event of problems with the monitor (Kasden, 1997).

Urine Testing

Testing the urine for glucose and ketones is an easy and noninvasive monitoring method. Urine ketones indicate fatty acid breakdown and may be present if an illness, insulin deficiency, starvation, or severe hypoglycemic reaction occurs. The nurse teaches the child and parents to test the urine for ketones whenever the blood glucose is 240 mg/dL or higher or when the child is ill. Urine ketones in the morning may indicate hypoglycemia during the night, which is followed by a rebound effect. The child should increase fluid intake in the presence of ketones and notify the doctor if the ketones continue to be present in a few hours.

▽ **Alert:** *Urine ketones in association with vomiting may indicate ketoacidosis and should be handled as an emergency. The physician should be notified immediately and the child may need to proceed to the emergency department.*

Testing the urine for glucose has many disadvantages. The correlation between capillary blood glucose and concurrent urine glucose is imperfect. The urine used in testing has been in the bladder for several hours and reflects the blood glucose from that period, whereas the blood glucose reading indicates the blood glucose level at the time of the test. Capillary blood glucose monitoring can provide extremely low glucose level readings: urine testing can only indicate blood glucose levels high enough to cause glucose to spill from the kidney (renal threshold). Renal thresholds vary from child to child. Large doses of vitamin C and aspirin can also cause false urine test readings.

Glycosylated Hemoglobin

Long-term metabolic control can be evaluated by measuring the glycosylated hemoglobin or hemoglobin A_1C. Glycosylation is the process in which glucose attaches to

Figure 26–5
The school-age child can perform blood glucose monitoring at home.

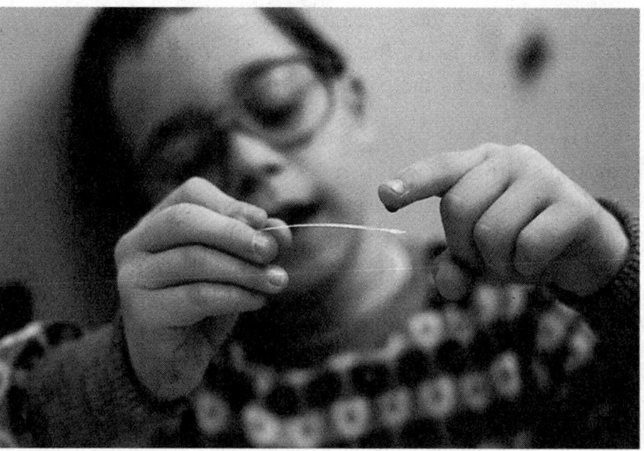

hemoglobin nonenzymatically by a slow, mostly irreversible process (Gray et al., 1993). The red blood cell, which contains the hemoglobin molecule, lasts in the blood stream for 90 to 120 days. Increased levels of blood glucose will increase the percentage of hemoglobin that is glycosylated and therefore will reflect the average glucose concentration for the preceding 2 to 3 months.

Treatment of Complications

Insulin-dependent diabetes mellitus, when not managed carefully and well, becomes a life-threatening chronic illness. Its management requires attention and caring from parents on an ongoing basis, despite the child's ability to manage the physical tasks of care, such as giving oneself insulin injections. Often those who do not do well and come to the attention of the acute care system are either afflicted with an acute infection that exacerbates the chronic condition or they are the poorly managed patient who may be asking for more adult attention by avoiding proper care of the chronic aspects of the illness.

Hypoglycemia (blood glucose level less than 60 mg/dL) is a common complication for children with diabetes. It often occurs if a meal is missed or late, if the insulin dose is too high, or in the case of strenuous physical activity without an added snack. Alcohol ingestion, gastroenteritis, or secret insulin administration can also precipitate hypoglycemia. Alcohol intensifies insulin action and may inhibit gluconeogenesis.

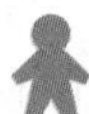

Tip: *The child and parents should know that hypoglycemia can occur during or immediately after a strenuous activity, but it may also occur several hours after the activity when the child is resting quietly.*

Signs of hypoglycemia include diaphoresis, tremulousness, tachycardia, hunger, weakness, pallor, and dizziness. Central nervous symptoms consist of headache, irritability, poor coordination, combativeness, double vision, and confusion. Signs of severe CNS depression from hypoglycemia include unconsciousness and convulsions.

Tip: *Infants cannot describe their symptoms and usually do not demonstrate many of the symptoms. Teach parents to rely on blood glucose monitoring and to administer glucose in the form of juice or tubes of decorative cake icing squirted inside the cheek pouch. In the case of an emergency, the parent will administer glucagon.*

Hypoglycemia is treated based on the severity of the symptoms. In the case of mild or moderate hypoglycemia, simple carbohydrates are the treatment of choice. The nurse would instruct the child to use 4 to 6 ounces of juice or regular soda, two to three glucose tablets, glucose gel, or a small tube of commercially available decorative cake icing.

Hypoglycemia resulting in loss of consciousness or seizure needs to be treated with glucagon. Glucagon is a counter-regulatory hormone that stimulates the liver to produce enough glucose to increase the blood glucose level by about 80 mg/dL according to the American Diabetes Association. The nurse will instruct the parents on the proper administration of glucagon. Children younger than 7 years of age would receive 0.5 mL (0.5 mg) of glucagon subcutaneously, and children 7 years and older would receive 1 mL (1 mg) subcutaneously. The child should respond within 10 to 15 minutes after the injection. Parents are taught to obtain a blood glucose level before giving the glucagon or immediately after the injection has been given so as to document hypoglycemia. When glucagon is administered, the child is very likely to vomit while in a semi-conscious state. The nurse should prepare the parents for this possibility. The parent should take the child to the nearest emergency department or notify the rescue squad if the child does not respond within 15 minutes.

The nurse teaches the parents and children the causes, symptoms, and treatment of hypoglycemia. The child is advised to wear an identification tag or Medic Alert bracelet, especially when away from home. Adolescents, in particular, need to be educated concerning the effects of drugs and alcohol on diabetes. Lipman, DiFazio, Meers, and Thompson (1989b) note that adolescents need to know that stimulants increase metabolism and decrease appetite, which will most likely cause hypoglycemia. Judgment-altering substances or appetite suppressants affect the daily routine and create an imbalance among food, insulin, and exercise. Alcohol intensifies the glucose-lowering effects of insulin and also causes hypoglycemia.

Diabetic Ketoacidosis Diabetic ketoacidosis is a life-threatening form of metabolic acidosis. Presenting symptoms may include altered level of consciousness, dehydration, electrolyte disturbances, dysrhythmias, shock, and complete vascular collapse. These children are seriously ill and require immediate treatment (Fagan, 1995). It is best handled by the critical care team in children or by skilled pediatric endocrinologists. Coping skills training groups that assist adolescents to prepare for situations (such as peer pressure to drink alcohol or use illicit drugs) are an effective way to prevent health- and life-threatening behaviors (Davidson, Boland, Grey, 1997). This helps to offset the higher rate of psychosocial maladjustment in children with chronic illness (Grey, Cameron, Lipman, & Thurber, 1995). For medical and nursing management, see Table 26–6 and Care Path 26–1).

Nutritional Management

The goals of nutritional therapy (American Diabetes Association, 1994) include

- Maintaining near-normal blood glucose by balancing food intake with insulin and activity

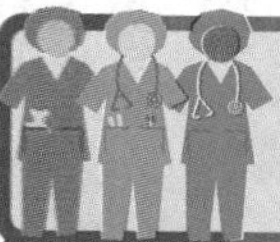

Care Path 26–1 An Interdisciplinary Plan of Care for the Child with Diabetic Ketoacidosis (DKA)

Nursing Diagnosis	Patient/Family Intermediate Outcomes			
	Day 1: Admission	Day 2	Day 3	Day 4
Fluid volume deficit related to vomiting and polyuria	Child maintains normal fluid and electrolyte balance.	→	→	→
Altered nutrition: less than body requirements related to inability to digest food	Child receives adequate nutrition to meet body requirements.	Child tolerates prescribed diet. Child shows no further evidence of weight loss.	→ →	→ →
Knowledge deficit: management of diabetes mellitus	Child and family understand reason for hospitalization and initial plan of care.	Child and family perform blood/urine testing. Parents give insulin.	Child and/or family verbalize understanding of hypo-/hyperglycemia and treatment of ketones.	Child and/or family verbalize understanding of diabetes management.
Altered family process related to situational crisis	Child and family express feelings and fears about illness and its effect on their lifestyle.	→	→	→
Care Intervention Categories				
Consults	Nutrition Social Services Case manager Child psychiatrist team	→ → → →	→ → →	→ → →
Discharge planning	Determine insurance availability for visiting nurse. Reinforce management at home.	Assist with obtaining diabetes supplies. →	→ →	→ →
Labs	ABG every 2 hours until stable Urine ketones every void CBC with differential Insulin level Islet cell antibody	 → → →	 → → →	 → → →

Care Path continued on following page

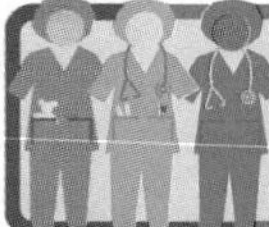

Care Path 26-1 An Interdisciplinary Plan of Care for the Child with Diabetic Ketoacidosis (DKA) *Continued*

Care Intervention Categories	Day 1: Admission	Day 2	Day 3	Day 4
Medications and IVs	Insulin infusion (regular insulin 1 unit/kg/hr) Replacement fluid NS or 0.5 NS	Maintenance fluids—D5.5 NS when blood sugar <300 mg/dL Decrease insulin infusion in relation to blood sugar	IV heparin lock	Discontinue IV
Monitors	Cardiorespiratory monitor	⟶	Discontinue monitors	
Nutrition	NPO	Diabetic diet when vomiting stops and acidosis resolved	⟶	⟶
Play therapy/ school	Use doll to teach insulin administration and needle play.	⟶	⟶	
Psychosocial	Allow family to verbalize grief. Be available to listen to family.	Contact child psychiatrist if grief or anger interferes with education.	⟶	⟶
Self-care	Children 6 years and older: Teach to perform own Chemstrips. Children 9 years and older: Teach self-injection of insulin	⟶ ⟶	⟶ ⟶	⟶ ⟶
Social service	Assess financial situation and family dynamics.	Help with medical assistance if needed. Help family find support from friends and family.	⟶ ⟶	⟶ ⟶
Visitors		Visitors encouraged.	Schoolwork to continue	

Care Path 26–1 An Interdisciplinary Plan of Care for the Child with Diabetic Ketoacidosis (DKA) *Continued*

Care Intervention Categories	Day 1: Admission	Day 2	Day 3	Day 4
Teaching	Meet with at least two family members each day until discharge to teach: · Insulin administration · Drawing up mixed insulin · Blood glucose monitoring · Complications: hypoglycemia and hyperglycemia · Treatment of complications · Sick day rules · Insulin regulation · Needle safety and disposal	⟶	⟶	⟶
Vital signs/baseline parameters	VS q 2 hr Weight NCHS growth chart parameters plotted I & O Assess neurologic status	VS q 2–4 hr ⟶ ⟶ ⟶	VS q 4 hr ⟶ ⟶	⟶ ⟶ ⟶

ABG, arterial blood gases; CBC, complete blood count; I & O, intake and output; NCHS, National Center for Health Statistics; NPO, nothing by mouth; NS, normal saline; VS, vital signs.

- Achieving optimal serum lipid levels
- Providing appropriate calories for normal growth and development in children and adolescents
- Preventing and treating acute complications of IDDM and long-term complications
- Improving the overall health of the person with IDDM through optimal nutrition (Chart 26–10).

Meal plans are based on the individual's preferences, culture, and ethnicity. The dietitian will meet with the child and parents during the hospital stay. The child's age and developmental level are considered when planning the diet.

Exercise

Exercise is a vital component to the management of the child with diabetes and offers many benefits. It assists in the utilization of dietary intake and may decrease the amount of insulin that a child requires. Exercise will enhance the insulin absorption. Exercise is also important for the child's normal growth and development. The child is instructed to eat a snack before exercising. Exercise lasting less than 1 hour usually requires a small snack consisting of a complex carbohydrate or a protein. More intense exercise or exercise lasting longer than 1 hour may require more frequent snacks throughout the activity and a combination of complex carbohydrates and protein before the activity. An insulin adjustment may also be needed if hypoglycemia occurs frequently with the activity. The family is instructed to check the child's blood glucose level after the activity and also before bedtime to prevent nighttime hypoglycemia event (Chart 26–11). Health care team members, parents, and school support personnel can be instrumental in teaching the adolescent

Chart 26–10

American Diabetes Association Nutritional Guidelines for People with Diabetes Mellitus

Protein

- 10% to 20% of daily caloric intake
- Derived from animal or vegetable source

Fat

- 30% or less of the calories should be from total fat.
- Less than 10% of calories should be from saturated fat.
- Up to 10% of calories should be from polyunsaturated fat.

Carbohydrates and Sweeteners

- Percentage of calories varies.
- Sucrose and sucrose-containing foods can be substituted for other carbohydrates, but nutritional content must be considered.
- Fructose may be used as a sweetening agent. However, large amounts (>40% of calories) have adverse effects on serum cholesterol and LDL cholesterol.
- Sorbitol, mannitol, and xylitol produce a lower glycemic response than sucrose and other carbohydrates. However, excessive amounts have a laxative effect.
- Saccharin, aspartame, and acesulfame K are approved by the FDA as non-nutritive sweeteners and can be used by people with diabetes.

Fiber

- 20 to 35 g of dietary fiber from varied sources

Sodium

- 2400 to 3000 mg/day

Alcohol

- Fewer than 2 alcoholic beverages (1 alcoholic beverage = 12 oz beer, 5 oz wine, or 12 oz distilled spirits) can be ingested with and in addition to the usual meal plan.

From American Diabetes Association (May 1994). Nutrition recommendations and principles for people with diabetes mellitus. *Diabetes Care, 17*(5). Reprinted with permission.

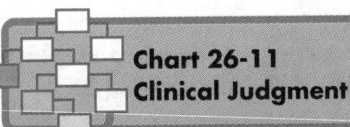

Chart 26-11
Clinical Judgment

School-Age Child with Diabetes Mellitus

Pierre, age 10 years, has juvenile diabetes. He is admitted to the hospital at the time of diagnosis for initial management. In Pierre's pediatrician's office, his blood glucose level was 930.

Questions

1. During your admission assessment, what data would you collect to assist you to teach Pierre about his diagnosis and his management plan?
2. What factors would indicate good metabolic control for the child with diabetes mellitus?
3. On Pierre's fourth morning in the hospital, you note that he is pale and sweaty. Based on his symptoms, what is his problem at this time?
4. When teaching Pierre and his family about insulin administration, what strategies should be used?
5. When the home care nurse visits Pierre 1 week after discharge, what age-appropriate activities should she expect Pierre to be doing in regard to managing his diabetes?

Answers

1. Previous history of any serious or chronic illness, previous hospitalizations, Pierre's exposure to other family members who may have diabetes or another chronic condition
2. Hemoglobin A_{1c} values less than 9.5, normal growth and development, and few episodes of hypoglycemia or hyperglycemia.
3. Pierre is hypoglycemic. Rapid treatment would involve giving him a glucose-containing solid, semisolid, or liquid such as orange juice.
4. Plan demonstration, supervision, and practice time with Pierre and his parents to learn injection and site rotation techniques, methods to draw up insulin, and how to store medication and equipment.
5. Pierre is actively involved in testing his blood glucose levels. He gathers all of the equipment for insulin administration. With parental assistance, he can draw up the correct dose of insulin. He can administer the injection himself, although sometimes he chooses to have a parent administer the injection, especially in hard-to-reach places. Pierre can discuss appropriate diet choices and restrictions. Pierre can recognize and treat hypoglycemia.

effective coping skills that may help him or her deal with the day-to-day management of the illness. Research has suggested that the use of effective coping skills may aid in healthy long-term adaptation to diabetes mellitus in the adolescent population (Davidson, et al., 1997).

Tip: *Hyperglycemia can be exacerbated if the child exercises when the blood glucose level is 240 mg/dL and ketones are present. Therefore, exercise should be avoided during this time. Exercise can be reinitiated when the urine is free from ketones.*

Community Care

Caretakers, teachers, and physical education instructors need to have accurate information concerning the child and need to know how to identify and treat hypoglycemia. The teacher should be informed when a student is diagnosed with IDDM. When the child returns to school the parents should give the teachers, school nurses, and coaches instructions for their child (Chart 26–12).

Hyperinsulinism

The most severe form of hypoglycemia is caused by hyperinsulinism, which results in the overutilization of glucose. Hyperinsulinism constitutes about 30% of all hypoglycemias (Sezonenko, 1993). Hyperinsulinism most often presents between birth and 3 months of age. The cause of hyperinsulinism at this age is usually secondary to diffuse beta cell hyperplasia or nesidioblastosis (Glasgow, 1992).

Certain conditions may predispose an infant to hyperinsulinism (Geffner, 1990). Included in this risk group are infants of diabetic mothers; infants with Beckwith-Wiedemann syndrome, erythroblastosis fetalis, or trisomy 13; infants on total parenteral nutrition; and infants with the dumping syndrome. Certain drugs can also predispose the infant to hyperinsulinism. Hyperinsulinism seen in the older child is usually associated with a pancreatic adenoma, although it is rare in the pediatric population. Glasgow (1992) states that the general course of hyperinsulinism in infants is one of improvement.

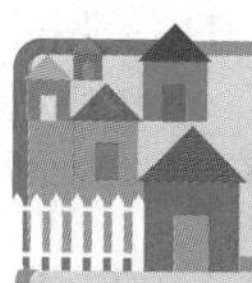

Chart 26–12
Community Care

Living with Newly Diagnosed IDDM

- Liberal bathroom privileges because hyperglycemia creates polyuria
- Snacks as needed to avoid insulin reaction
- Blood glucose checks as needed to be performed by the child in the presence of the school nurse
- Fast-acting glucose in case of hypoglycemia available from teachers, coaches, or school nurses
- In emergency, parents notified
- Coping skills training groups for adolescents recommended (Davidson, Boland, & Grey, 1997)

Chart 26-13

Criteria for Diagnosing Hyperinsulinism

Insulin concentrations >10 μU/mL at time of hypoglycemia
Insulin:glucose ratio is 0.4 or higher
Low plasma ketones
Low free fatty acid levels
Rapid development of fasting hypoglycemia
High exogenous glucose infusion rates needed to maintain euglycemia
Absence of ketonemia or ketonuria
Elevated C-peptide
Increase plasma glucose after glucagon administration at time of hypoglycemia
Low levels of serum β-hydroxybutyrate occur when patient is fasted until hypoglycemia is attained

Assessment

The infant with hyperinsulinism is often macrosomic, or large-for-gestational age, at birth. Overt seizures may occur, and the blood glucose level may be less than 40 mg/dL. The infant may be lethargic, irritable, and pale. Certain criteria are needed to diagnose an infant with hyperinsulinism (Chart 26–13). Serum glucose and insulin levels are obtained every 2 hours. Every void should be checked for ketone bodies.

Nursing Diagnosis and Outcome

The following nursing diagnosis may apply to an infant with hyperinsulinism:

▶ **Risk for injury related to hypoglycemia**
Outcomes: The infant will remain euglycemic.
The infant will not experience any seizure activity.

Interdisciplinary Interventions

The infant with hyperinsulinism should be monitored and treated for signs and symptoms of hypoglycemia. Minor symptoms that are often seen include irritability, jitteriness, bizarre behavior, and hypothermia. Major symptoms such as seizures and coma may also occur.

The child with hyperinsulinism initially may be given infusions of glucose and glucagon administered by the nurse. Somatostatin may be used temporarily until home therapy is initiated. Once the diagnosis has been established, the treatment taught to the parents by the nurse may include frequent feedings, nighttime nasogastric feedings, and initiation of oral diazoxide.

Oral diazoxide suppresses the secretion of insulin by the beta cells without lowering the blood pressure. The initial dose is usually 10 mg/kg/day divided into three doses. A common acute side effect of diazoxide is the retention of salt and water. Salt and water retention could potentially lead to congestive heart failure. The most common chronic side effect is hypertrichosis (hair on the forehead, back, and limbs). Potential side effects not commonly seen include hyperosmolar nonketotic coma, decreased neutrophil counts, and a decreased serum immunoglobulin level (Sezonenko, 1993).

A low-protein diet has been recommended because protein is known to stimulate insulin secretion. Short-term use of counter-regulatory hormones such as corticosteroids, GH, long-acting forms of epinephrine, and glucagon have been found to be effective (Sezonenko, 1993).

Surgery for subtotal pancreatectomy is indicated in infants who are unable to maintain euglycemia or who cannot be removed from intravenous therapy. An 85% to 90% subtotal pancreatectomy is performed by a pediatric surgeon. Medical therapy with dietary restrictions may still be needed after surgery. Permanent IDDM or malabsorption may develop if too much pancreatic tissue is removed.

The nurse and the physician should give parents clear and concise explanations for the cause of the hyperinsulinism and the specific therapy recommended. The nurse teaches the parents the techniques to monitor blood glucose (see TIP 26–2) and how to recognize the signs and symptoms of hypoglycemia. The nurse instructs the parents on the medical therapy and its possible side effects. Frequent feedings are recommended in addition to the low-protein diet. The nurse teaches the parents how to place a nasogastric feeding tube properly if the infant is sent home on nighttime nasogastric feedings.

Preoperative preparation and psychological support are essential if surgery is recommended. Geffner (1990) reports that transient postsurgical hyperglycemia for up to 1 week frequently follows successful surgery. Infants with hyperinsulinism usually improve rapidly with medical or surgical therapy.

Ketotic Hypoglycemia

Ketotic hypoglycemia is the most common form of hypoglycemia in the child older than age 2 years. Ketotic hypoglycemia is hypoglycemia that is accompanied by a reduction in plasma insulin and the presence of ketone bodies and fatty acids.

Hypoglycemia usually occurs between 18 months and 5 years of age and spontaneously abates by age 9. The episodes of hypoglycemia are sporadic and occur during a fasting period. Boys are affected more than girls in a ratio of 2 : 1.

Pathophysiology

The cause of ketotic hypoglycemia has not been established. Glasgow (1992) describes several theories related to the cause of ketotic hypoglycemia. One possible theory is a deficiency of alanine release from the muscle during gluconeogenesis. The child with ketotic hypoglycemia has a rise in serum glucose level after being given an alanine infusion during hypoglycemia. Hypofunction of the adrenal medulla has also been thought to be a cause of ketotic hypoglycemia. This theory described by Glasgow (1992) suggests a deficiency in catecholamine release in response to hypoglycemia.

Assessment

The child's growth parameters (height and weight) should be measured carefully and compared with normed standards such as NCHS growth charts. A thorough history and physical assessment are done.

The child with ketotic hypoglycemia usually presents to the emergency department or physician's office after having a seizure or is found semi-comatose and slow to respond in the early to mid-morning. The history of the child's previous day is vital to the diagnosis. The parents may report that the child had a poor appetite the preceding evening and may have an intercurrent illness such as gastroenteritis or a viral syndrome. Another scenario is that the parents report that they slept late and the child's breakfast was delayed. Ingestion of alcohol the previous night must also be considered. The child with ketotic hypoglycemia is usually small and thin for age and may have been small for gestational age at birth.

Diagnostic Tests. Serum glucose and insulin levels need to be obtained every 2 hours during the day of admission. A 12- to 24-hour fast is performed, at which time glucose and insulin levels are obtained every 2 hours for the initial 8 hours and then every hour for the next 4 to 16 hours. If the blood glucose level decreases below 40 mg/dL, the fast is terminated and the child is treated with oral glucose (juice) or intravenous glucose. Intravenous dextrose (25%) is kept at the bedside. Each void is tested for ketones. The child with ketotic hypoglycemia who has been fasted for 20 to 24 hours will have ketone bodies that are negatively correlated with plasma glucose. As the plasma glucose levels decrease, the levels of ketone bodies increase. The insulin level is low, and the plasma alanine level is also low.

Nursing Diagnosis and Outcome

In addition to the nursing diagnoses presented in Chart 26–3, the following diagnosis applies to a child with ketotic hypoglycemia:

- **Risk for injury related to increased blood glucose levels**
  Outcome: The child will remain euglycemic.

Interdisciplinary Interventions

Parents are instructed by the nurse and the dietitian to give their child small, frequent, high-carbohydrate, high-protein meals and a late evening snack and to prevent prolonged fasts. The nurse instructs the parents that during illnesses they need to test the child's urine for ketones. The nurse instructs the parents to offer high-carbohydrate liquids to the child who has ketonuria. Children who have uncontrolled vomiting may need to be admitted to the hospital for intravenous administration of glucose. Sezonenko (1993) notes that episodes of hypoglycemia usually disappear with age, specifically at the time of puberty.

Alterations in Function of the Adrenal Glands

The adrenal glands have two distinct portions: the adrenal medulla and the adrenal cortex. The two tissues have different embryonic origins, secrete different hormones, and have different regulatory mechanisms. The adrenal medulla secretes the catecholamines epinephrine (adrenalin) and norepinephrine (noradrenaline). Because these hormones are also produced by the sympathetic nervous system, absence of medullary adrenal supply is not life threatening. The adrenal cortex secretes steroid hormones that are essential to life (see Table 26–1). The three major groups of steroids are the mineralocorticoids, the glucocorticoids, and the sex steroids. The adrenal gland depends on pituitary secretion of ACTH. A lack of adrenal steroids may be due to inadequate ACTH production from the pituitary to stimulate the adrenal gland or a defect in the adrenal gland itself (DiGeorge & Levine, 1996).

Aldosterone is the most potent mineralocorticoid, and its principal action is in the maintenance of electrolyte balance and blood pressure. Its secretion is regulated by activation of the renin-angiotensin system so that adequate levels can be maintained even in the absence of ACTH (DiGeorge & Levine, 1996). The predominant glucocorticoid is cortisol. It also maintains homeostasis of electrolytes, blood pressure, and blood glucose by its influence on the metabolism of most tissues. It is also involved in aspects of the immune process as well as in stress reduction. Under stressful situations such as trauma, surgery, infection, and certain emotional states (fear, anger, anxiety) there is increased secretion of ACTH from the pituitary and in turn an increase in secretion of corticosteroid from the adrenal cortex. The sex steroids or androgens dehydroepiandrosterone (DHEA), dihydroepiandrosterone sulfate (DHEAS), and androstenedione supplement the sex steroids that are secreted by the gonads. They are primarily responsible for the development of secondary sex characteristics, including enlargement of the clitoris and penis. The most abundant adrenal androgen is DHEAS. At the start of puberty DHEAS levels rise and are involved in the growth of sexual hair (adrenarche) (DiGeorge & Levine, 1996).

Adrenocortical Insufficiency

Acute or chronic adrenocortical insufficiency results when the adrenal gland is absent or damaged. Acute adrenocortical insufficiency is a relatively rare phenomenon in childhood. A common cause is hemorrhage into the adrenal glands (DiGeorge & Levine, 1996). They may occur during the neonatal period as a consequence of prolonged labor. Abrupt withdrawal of a corticosteroid in patients who have been given large doses for a long time or failure to give increased doses of corticosteroids during stressful situations such as surgery or severe infections may precipitate acute adrenal crisis. Acute infections, such as meningococcemia, can lead to hemorrhage and shock (Waterhouse-Friderichsen syndrome). Other causes include metastatic disease, familial glucocorticoid deficiency, defects of steroid biosynthesis (adrenal hyperplasia [discussed later]), isolated aldosterone deficiency, adrenalectomy for Cushing's disease, and certain drugs (DiGeorge & Levine, 1996).

Chronic adrenocortical insufficiency (Addison's disease) is commonly caused by autoimmune destruction of the adrenal cortex and usually occurs in early adolescence. Usually the medulla is not destroyed. Tuberculosis may cause adrenal destruction in partially treated or untreated individuals.

Pathophysiology

Without prompt treatment, acute deficiency in the production of cortisol, and to a lesser degree aldosterone, may lead to life-threatening electrolyte and fluid imbalance. One must also replace the deficient steroid (cortisol and/or aldosterone). Once the acute manifestations of adrenal insufficiency are under control, an investigation into the cause must occur. This may be done by obtaining various blood levels of the hormones involving the hypothalamic-pituitary-adrenal pathway either as a random blood level or through stimulation studies.

In chronic deficiency, significant damage occurs in the adrenal cortex before symptoms become evident. When there is enough damage to the adrenal cortex, insufficient amounts of cortisol (glucorticoid) and aldosterone (mineralocorticoid) are released.

Prognosis. As long as the child with adrenal insufficiency maintains appropriate daily hormone replacement therapy and increased doses during stress, the prognosis is good (DiGeorge & Levine, 1996). Insufficient replacement therapy places the child at risk for adrenal shock during times of illness or stress.

Assessment

The age at onset and the clinical manifestations depend on the underlying cause of acute adrenal insufficiency. For example, those symptoms that are usually seen after birth, such as in adrenal hypoplasia, are characteristic of salt loss and include lethargy, nausea and vomiting, dehydration, fever, irritability, and pallor.

The onset of symptoms of chronic insufficiency is gradual, except in those patients with undiagnosed deficiency who show signs of acute adrenal insufficiency after a minor illness or trauma. Chronic symptoms include weakness, headache, irritability, anorexia, weight loss, nausea and vomiting, diarrhea, and signs of dehydration. Diminishing amounts of aldosterone from the adrenal cortex causes fluid and electrolyte imbalances and subsequent decrease in blood pressure. These children usually crave salty foods, owing to their sodium deficit. Another characteristic finding is in the pigment of the skin. Children with Addison's disease usually appear suntanned, with hyperpigmentation most noticeable on the face, hands, elbows, and knees, as well as the groin, genitalia, areolae, and gums. This is due to the excessive secretion of corticotropin and melanocyte-stimulating hormone. Pubertal females may show less pubic hair because of diminished androgen production (DiGeorge & Levine, 1996).

Diagnostic Tests. Laboratory data for both types of insufficiency reveal hyponatremia, hypoglycemia, and hyperkalemia. Plasma cortisol levels can also be drawn, but results take time and most patients are treated based on their clinical presentation. The most definitive test for adrenal insufficiency is measurement of plasma cortisol levels before and after administration of exogenous ACTH. In adrenal insufficiency the baseline cortisol level would be low and no increase would occur after the ACTH stimulus (DiGeorge & Levine, 1996).

In chronic insufficiency, high antibody titers to the adrenal gland are seen. Ultrasound images, CT scans, and abdominal radiographs are useful in visualizing the integrity of the adrenal glands. Because some of the conditions resulting in adrenocortical insufficiency have a genetic basis, the siblings of the patient should also be evaluated (DiGeorge & Levine, 1996).

Nursing Diagnoses and Outcomes

In addition to the nursing diagnoses presented in Chart 26–3, the following diagnoses apply to the child with adrenal insufficiency:

- **Risk for fluid volume deficit related to fluid and electrolyte imbalance**
  Outcome: The child will achieve and maintain normal fluid and electrolyte balance.
- **Anxiety related to hospitalization and acute illness**
  Outcomes: The parents and child will communicate their needs to the health care team.
  The parents and child will implement effective coping strategies to decrease their anxiety level.
- **Knowledge deficit: new diagnosis and treatment**
  Outcome: The child/family will demonstrate a basic understanding of the adrenal disorder, its treatment, potential complications, and follow-up care.

Interdisciplinary Interventions

The child with adrenal insufficiency may or may not require hospitalization, depending on the severity of the symptoms. Those children with severe electrolyte imbalance require immediate intervention. Intravenous solutions containing 0.9% saline and 5% glucose are infused by the nurse to correct sodium loss and hypoglycemia. At the same time, a water-soluble form of hydrocortisone must be administered intravenously at double or triple the maintenance dose. Dosing is based on measurement of body surface area in square meters that is calculated by the child's height and weight. Infants can safely receive up to 25 mg, toddlers up to 50 mg, and children between 75 and 100 mg of hydrocortisone every 6 hours for the first 24 hours (DiGeorge & Levine, 1996). If intravenous access is not immediately available, the hydrocortisone should be given intramuscularly. After 24 hours these higher doses may be reduced and oral doses of corticosteroids may be given.

The nurse needs to teach the patient and family how to administer the replacement steroids cortisol (hydrocortisone) and mineralocorticoids (aldosterone). Some children can be treated with hydrocortisone only if they maintain a liberal intake of salt in their diet. Hydrocortisone is usually given three times a day, and aldosterone medication (fludrocortisone) can be given as a single daily dose. Fludrocortisone does not need to be increased during times of stress. The caregivers need to demonstrate proper mixing and intramuscular administration of hydrocortisone in the event of an emergency or excessive vomiting. They should be given written guidelines of when and how much to increase maintenance doses during times of illness, trauma, or other periods of physical or emotional stress. If surgery is needed, the anesthesiologist must be aware of the child's cortisol dependency. The family should feel comfortable with contacting their pediatric endocrinology team whenever there is a question about adjustment in medication.

Tip: *All children with adrenal insufficiency should wear some form of medical identification alerting medical personnel that the child has adrenal insufficiency and is steroid dependent.*

Parents need to be aware of potential side effects of the medications. Families should understand that the dosage of steroids used to treat adrenal insufficiency is meant to replace the deficit created by the condition. Much of the negative publicity about steroids is from glucocorticoids and androgens taken in excessive doses; these side effects include poor growth, weight gain, poor wound healing, increased susceptibility to infection, and excessive bruising. A possible side effect with replacement doses of cortisol is gastric irritation, which can be minimized by ingestion of cortisol with food or by the use of an antacid. Manifestations of excessive fludrocortisone include generalized edema from water retention, hypertension, headaches, and signs of hypokalemia.

Alert: *Families must maintain an adequate stock of medication and never allow the prescription to run out; acute withdrawal of cortisol can lead to adrenal crisis.*

Community Care

Parents may need help in finding a balance between protecting their child from potential life-threatening situations and the need to participate in age-appropriate activities necessary for physical, social, and emotional growth. Children should not be placed on any restrictions from school or play activities. School and daycare personnel should be made aware of the need for prompt notification of the parents if their child becomes ill or injured as well as preplanned cooperation with medication administration should a dose need to be given during school hours.

Congenital Adrenal Hyperplasia

Congenital adrenal hyperplasia (CAH) is an autosomal recessive condition caused by an inborn deficiency of one of the enzymes needed to synthesize cortisol. More than 90% of children born with CAH have a deficiency of 21-hydroxylase. The incidence of CAH in Europe and North America is 1 in 10,000 to 16,000 births; there is a very high incidence (1 : 300) in Yupik Eskimos of Alaska (DiGeorge & Levine, 1996). Treatment includes lifelong replacement therapy with glucocorticoids and, if needed, mineralocorticoid replacement and dietary salt supplements.

Pathophysiology

Hormone synthesis by the adrenal cortex is controlled by the hypothalamic-pituitary-adrenal feedback system. Any condition that alters circulating blood levels of any adrenal hormone results in an imbalance in hormone production or inhibition. In CAH, there are inadequate blood levels of cortisol. As a result, there is increased secretion of ACTH by the pituitary in an effort to improve cortisol production. This prolonged hypersecretion results in adrenal gland hyperplasia and sex steroid overproduction. In females, this causes masculinization or virilization of the clitoris. In males, it may cause precocious puberty (Lim, Batch, & Warne, 1995).

Prognosis. Because the 21-hydroxylase enzyme is involved in cortisol and aldosterone synthesis, most children present with the more severe, salt-losing forms of CAH. Prognosis depends on the type and severity of CAH the child has inherited. If left untreated, the child with classic 21-hydroxylase deficiency, salt-losing form, could die. For some infants, sudden infant death syndrome (SIDS) is actually due to undiagnosed CAH. For those children with partial deficiency there is enough aldosterone to maintain sodium levels. If appropriately treated, children born with CAH enjoy a normal life expectancy. This includes appropriate care for these children and adults during periods of significant illness, trauma, or surgery. Cognitive and perceptual abilities in children with CAH are no different than without CAH.

For children with only the virilizing form of CAH, lack of treatment will result in precocious puberty and adult short stature. In females born with CAH, the internal sex organs (uterus, ovaries, and fallopian tubes) are normal. With appropriate treatment, fertility should not be impaired. Menses should occur at the appropriate age if the girl's CAH is well controlled (Lim et al., 1995).

Assessment

Infants are generally diagnosed at, or shortly after, birth. Female newborns with CAH almost always present with ambiguous genitalia, also known as pseudohermaphroditism (Fig. 26–6). Steroid synthesis occurs early in fetal life so a lack of cortisol response within the pituitary-adrenal pathway results in excess ACTH production and, in turn, hypersecretion of the adrenal androgens and virilization. The external genitalia of females reveals an enlarged clitoris resembling a penis. Urethral displacement onto the ventral shaft of the clitoris can be mistaken for hypospadias. The labia are fused and can take on the

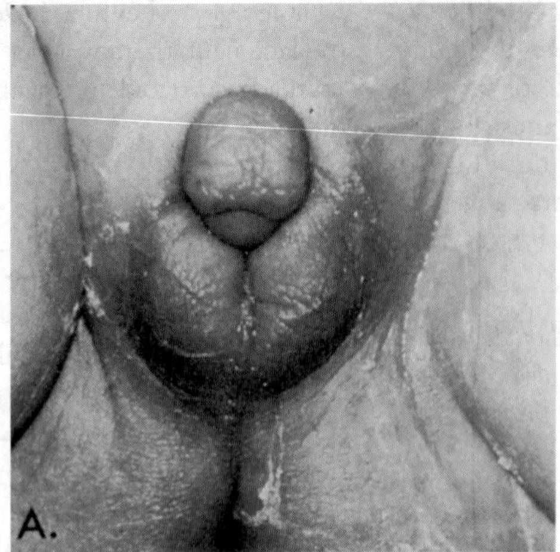

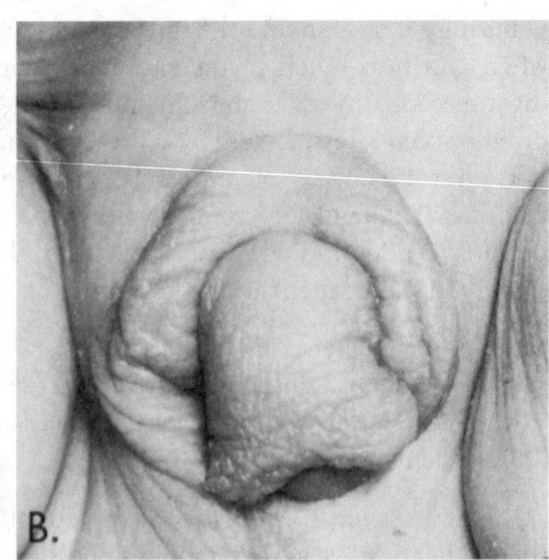

Figure 26–6
Genitalia of a female newborn with congenital adrenal hyperplasia (CAH) shows pseudohermaphroditism. CAH may cause clitoral enlargement and labial fusion *(A)* or extreme clitoral enlargement *(B)*. (From Moore, K. L., & Persaud, T. V. N. [1993]. *The developing human: Clinically oriented embryology* [5th ed., p. 293]. Philadelphia: W. B. Saunders.)

appearance of a scrotal-like sac without testes. This condition may be misdiagnosed as cryptorchidism. The vaginal orifice may be incomplete. In general, more extreme virilization reflects greater severity of the enzyme defect.

Male newborns with CAH do not necessarily show abnormalities of the internal or external genitalia. There may be enlargement of the penis and darker pigmentation of the scrotum. Because there may be no obvious physical findings of CAH, male newborns are not diagnosed until they present with signs of adrenal insufficiency. In both sexes the symptoms of recurrent vomiting and irritability may be mistaken for reflux, pyloric stenosis, or colic. The symptoms progress and include lethargy, pallor, dehydration, hypoglycemia, hyponatremia, and hyperkalemia. Children with partial enzyme deficiency may not be diagnosed until childhood when signs of adrenal crisis due to severe illness or surgery and/or precocious puberty are evident (Lim et al., 1995).

Diagnostic Tests. Laboratory studies to confirm diagnosis of CAH include markedly elevated serum levels of 17-hydroxyprogesterone, a cortisol precursor. ACTH, testosterone, DHEA, and androstenedione levels may also be obtained. Salt losers have low serum levels of sodium and chloride and elevated potassium and plasma renin activity. Chromosomal testing needs urgent attention to determine appropriate sex identification. Radiologic studies include pelvic ultrasonography to determine the presence of internal reproductive organs as well as the integrity of the adrenal glands (Lim et al., 1995).

Nursing Diagnoses and Outcomes

In addition to the nursing diagnoses and outcomes presented in Chart 26–3, the following apply to the child with CAH:

- **Risk for fluid volume deficit related to fluid and electrolyte imbalance**
  Outcome: The child will achieve and maintain normal fluid and electrolyte balance.
- **Risk for altered parent–infant attachment related to sexual ambiguity**
  Outcomes: The parents will express concerns about sexuality issues to the health care team.
  The parents will initiate and maintain positive interactions with the infant.
- **Body image disturbance related to precocious puberty or virilization**
  Outcome: The child/family will verbalize concerns of change in body image to the health care team.
- **Risk for sexual dysfunction in females related to virilization of the genitalia**
  Outcome: The child will receive appropriate information regarding treatment for virilization.

Interdisciplinary Interventions

The care for children born with CAH varies; however, the goal for all children includes providing lifelong replacement doses of deficient steroids, preventing excessive androgen production, and maintaining adequate growth. Neonates or children presenting in adrenal crisis require immediate intervention. This medical emergency includes providing appropriate intravenous solutions to correct fluid and electrolyte imbalances and hypoglycemia. Also, a water-soluble form of hydrocortisone must be administered intravenously at double or triple the maintenance dose; it can also be given intramuscularly if intravenous access is not immediately available. For children diagnosed in the absence of adrenal crisis, administration of glucocorticoids will inhibit the excessive production of androgens. Recommended dosing of hydrocortisone (cortisol) is 10 to 20 $mg/m^2/24$ hrs divided in two or three oral doses (DiGeorge & Levine, 1996). Hydrocortisone is available as a tablet or suspension. Children who also display diminished aldosterone production require a replacement mineralocorticoid called fludrocortisone, given as a single daily dose. Doses for both replacement steroids are individualized throughout life by measuring renin and 17-hydroxyprogesterone levels (Lim et al., 1995).

Tip: *Fludrocortisone (Florinef) is not available in liquid form. The pill can be finely crushed and added to a small amount of formula or breast milk. These infants and children also require added salt to their formula or food.*

caREminder: *Be sure to teach CAH patients and their families about the need for increased doses of cortisol (not fludrocortisone) during times of increased physical stress and illness. Otherwise, inadequate corticosteroid supply could lead to a life-threatening condition called adrenal crisis.*

The nurse should teach about cortisol and aldosterone replacement and stress doses, including intramuscular hydrocortisone, when faced with stress, illness, and trauma (including extensive dental work). The potential side effects of the medications should be reviewed and concerns discussed about having a child on steroid therapy. The family should be reminded that the child is only taking a replacement dose of the steroid that his or her body cannot produce. School and daycare personnel need to promptly notify parents in the event of illness or injury.

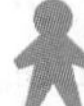

Tip: *Children with CAH need to wear some form of medical identification at all times. The parent or older child should carry an emergency hydrocortisone injection kit with him or her.*

Surgical Management

Female infants with ambiguous genitalia require reconstructive surgery for normal appearance of the genitalia and adequate sexual functioning. For that reason the clitoris is not removed but is reduced in size and repositioned below the pubis, preserving the glans and all its blood and nerve components so that complete sexual gratification, including orgasm, can be achieved. The labia need also to be separated (labioplasty) and a vaginal orifice (vaginoplasty) created; vaginal dilatation may be required when the girl reaches puberty or becomes sexually active. The ideal time for this elective surgery is between 6 and 12 months of age.

Genetic Counseling

Given the genetic nature of CAH, the parents would benefit from genetic counseling. A family history or genogram may identify previous infant deaths or sudden, unexplained deaths possibly due to adrenal crisis in infants, children, and adults with undiagnosed CAH. They need to understand that CAH is an autosomal recessive disorder and that both parents are carriers. Therefore, there is a 25% chance with *each* pregnancy of having a child with CAH. It is possible for prenatal testing for the 21-hydroxylase deficiency for parents who already have an affected child. For subsequent pregnancies, these mothers can be given high doses of cortisol, in the form of dexamethasone, in the first trimester to inhibit ACTH overproduction and prevent or minimize virilization in the developing fetus.

Immediate Neonatal Care

Newborn screening programs have been developed in some states to detect 21-hydroxylase deficiency. Parents need to be informed immediately if there is any question regarding the sex assignment of their newborn. This may help avoid the potential problem parents face when misinforming family, friends, and co-workers about the newborn's sex. One should be sensitive to the reasons for urgent chromosomal testing, which can take several days for results, and ultrasound studies to answer the question of gender. In addition, appropriate explanations and reassurance needs to be given to the young girl who is undergoing reconstructive surgery as well as anticipatory guidance for disturbances in behavior and body image.

Cushing's Syndrome

Etiology and Incidence

Cushing's syndrome is a characteristic cluster of signs and symptoms resulting in excessive circulating cortisol. It is caused by hyperfunctioning of the adrenal cortex and is rarely seen in children (Weber et al., 1995). In infants and young children, Cushing's syndrome is most often caused by an adrenocortical tumor, usually a malignant carcinoma, and occasionally by a benign adenoma. In older children the cause is more likely of pituitary origin, such as a pituitary tumor that produces excessive ACTH. The more common cause of Cushing's syndrome in children is due to the side effects of prolonged or excessive (exogenous) corticosteroid therapy for a medical condition such as asthma, lupus, or inflammatory bowel disease. Most of these side effects can be reversed once the corticosteroid treatment is reduced or the doses are gradually tapered.

Assessment

Excess cortisol produces diverse side effects seen throughout the body. The most noticeable side effect is obesity or rapid weight gain with arrest in linear growth (Orth, Kovacs, & Debold, 1992). There are resulting alterations in the normal processes of carbohydrate, protein, and fat metabolism, leading to increased protein catabolism, loss of muscle mass, and altered fat distribution. Fat distribution tends to be centrally located, with the child showing a characteristic, rounded or moon face with flushed cheeks, a supraclavicular fat pad (known as a buffalo hump), and truncal obesity with red abdominal striae

(Fig. 26–7). The thinned muscles of the extremities as a result of muscle wasting may be masked by generalized obesity. Hypercortisolism retards linear growth by suppressing the release of GH.

Other physiologic consequences of excessive cortisol include poor wound healing, increased susceptibility to infections, and decreased inflammatory response. Excessive bruising, thin skin, and osteoporosis are also seen, less common are hypertension, headaches, and mood disorders. There is usually a resulting excess production of androgens (virilization), which in turn can cause increased body hair (hypertrichosis) on the face and trunk, pubic hair, acne, and deepening of the voice.

Laboratory data include a complete blood cell count and blood and chemistry studies. Plasma cortisol levels are elevated, and the fluctuating levels typically seen throughout the day are lost. Urinary excretion of cortisol is found to be elevated when a 24-hour collection is done. CT and MRI may locate pituitary or adrenal lesions.

Figure 26–7
Typical clinical manifestations of Cushing's syndrome.

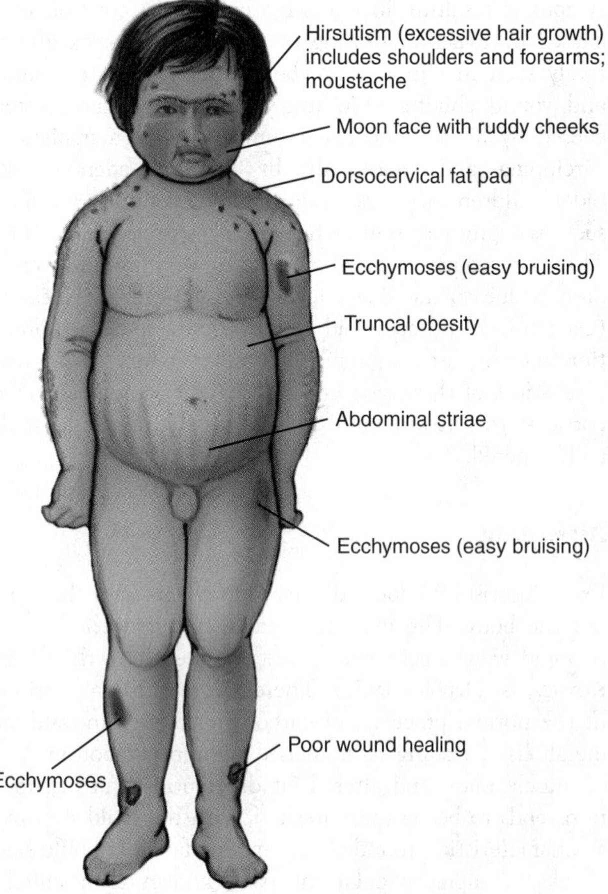

Nursing Diagnoses and Outcomes

In addition to the nursing diagnoses presented in Chart 26–3, the following diagnoses are applicable to the child with Cushing's syndrome:

- **Risk for injury related to delayed wound healing, decreased inflammatory response, osteoporosis, and muscle weakness**
  Outcomes: The child will be protected from potential infections by practicing good health habits and avoidance of exposure to pathogens.
  The child will remain free from injury.
- **Body image disturbance related to effects of steroids**
  Outcome: The child/family will verbalize concerns of change in body image and self-esteem to health care team.

Interdisciplinary Interventions

Medical treatment for Cushing's syndrome depends on the underlying cause. Hypercortisolism due to endogenous reasons is usually due to adrenal or pituitary tumors and requires surgical intervention. Microsurgery to excise the tumor only avoids the consequences of panhypopituitarism, and prognosis is quite good if there has been no metastasis. In the event of adrenalectomy, appropriate stress and replacement doses of glucocorticoids are planned preoperatively to avoid adrenal crisis.

Cushing's syndrome due to exogenous steroid preparations requires a fine balance between the effects of the steroids to treat the underlying condition and the avoidance of unpleasant side effects. If possible, the medication should be given early in the day to mimic the normal diurnal pattern of cortisol secretion. An alternate-day scheduling could also lessen stress on the hypothalamic-pituitary-adrenal pathway. Health care personnel involved in the treatment of children with long-term corticosteroid use should prepare the child and family of the potential side effects before initiating treatment. Anticipatory guidance around issues of diet, involvement in contact sports, injury prevention, and avoidance of exposure to infections should be addressed.

Pheochromocytoma

Pheochromocytoma is a catecholamine-secreting tumor; it is rare in children and predominately arises from the adrenal medulla. The tumors vary in size and may occur on both adrenal glands. Less frequently they are found in extra-adrenal sites in the pelvis, abdomen, and thorax. Pheochromocytoma is often inherited as an autosomal dominant trait. The most common presenting symptom is sustained or episodic hypertension. Associated complaints from hypertension include headache, vomiting, tachycardia, sweating, and nervousness. There may be weight loss despite good appetite owing to hypermetabolism and associated growth failure. Treatment includes removal of the tumor or tumors. If a bilateral adrenalectomy is needed, the child would require continuous replacement therapy of mineralocorticoids and glucocorticoids. Nursing diagnoses and outcomes and interdisciplinary interventions in the postoperative period are similar to those discussed for chronic adrenal insufficiency.

Premature Adrenarche

Adrenarche is the development of pubic hair, axillary hair, and adult body odor. This reflects maturation of adrenal androgen secretion in the adrenal cortex. Premature adrenarche is the development of pubic hair before age 8½ years in girls and 9½ years in boys. Axillary hair and adult body odor may or may not be present (Likitmaskul et al., 1995). This condition occurs more often in girls. In most cases it is considered a normal variant in sexual development, especially if no other signs of pubertal development have occurred.

An investigation to determine whether premature adrenarche is of central (hypothalamic-pituitary) origin (see section on precocious puberty) may need to be done if there are other signs of advancing puberty, such as clitoral enlargement, acne, or advanced bone age. Baseline DHEAS and testosterone levels may be obtained. ACTH testing is usually unnecessary because CAH is not the cause for isolated premature adrenarche. However, some physicians wish to screen for some of the nonclassic forms of CAH. Several researchers are raising the question of whether there is a relationship between premature adrenarche and future problems with polycystic ovarian syndrome (Likitmaskul et al., 1995).

The child may develop a body image disturbance related to premature adrenarche. If so, the nurse must attempt to help the child and family verbalize concerns about body image. Treatment consists of reassurance to the child and family of the benign nature of this condition.

Gonadal Disorders

The genetic sex of an embryo is determined at the time of fertilization by the X- or Y-bearing sperm that penetrates the ovum; however, sex differentiation does not occur until the seventh week of gestation. At that time the future ovaries or testes begin to take on their specific characteristics. The presence of the Y chromosome influences testicular development; its absence results in the creation of ovaries. By the 12th week the external genitalia become distinctly masculine or feminine. The male gonads (testes) and female gonads (ovaries) have different functions (Table 26–1). Both gonads are controlled by LH and FSH secreted by the anterior pituitary.

Ambiguous Genitalia

The term *ambiguous genitalia* refers to any condition in which the male or female external genitalia appear abnormal. This includes the clitoris, vagina, labia, and urethral meatus of the female and the penis, scrotum, testes, and urethral meatus of the male. *Hermaphroditism* refers to the discrepancy between the gonads (ovaries or testes) and the external genitalia. In true hermaphroditism, which is a rare condition, the child is genetically male or female but has both testicular and ovarian tissue; most frequently an ovotestis is found. Pseudohermaphroditism in the female reveals normal XX genotype and normal gonads, but the external genitalia are virilized. The male pseudohermaphrodite has normal XY genotype and testes, but the external genitalia are ambiguous or incompletely virilized.

Pathophysiology

Any interruption or abnormality in fetal sexual determination or differentiation results in ambiguous genitalia. Ambiguous genitalia may be caused by hormone imbalance or chromosomal aberrations. The most common cause of female pseudohermaphroditism is CAH. In CAH, androgen exposure on the developing female fetus creates virilization (see Pathophysiology in the section on congenital adrenal hyperplasia). Male pseudohermaphroditism could be due to defects in testicular differentiation such as in gonadal dysgenesis or in defective testicular or androgen hormone synthesis or action.

Prognosis. With the exception of CAH, none of the conditions resulting in ambiguous genitalia is life threatening. In CAH the female external genitalia are virilized. The newborn's internal sex organs remain normal, but the clitoris is enlarged, resembling a penis and the labia are fused (see Fig. 26–6). For any child with delayed puberty or suspicious genitalia, appropriate hormone levels assessing the integrity of the hypothalamus, anterior pituitary, and gonads is necessary. The specific deviations are discussed in this chapter under the headings Precocious Puberty and Delayed Puberty.

Nursing Diagnoses and Outcomes

In addition to the nursing diagnoses presented in Chart 26–3, the following diagnoses may apply to the child with ambiguous genitalia:

- **Risk for fluid volume deficit related to fluid and electrolyte imbalance caused by CAH**
  Outcome: The child will achieve and maintain normal fluid and electrolyte balance.

▶ **Risk for altered parent–infant attachment related to sexual ambiguity**
Outcomes: The parents will express concerns about sexuality issues with the health care team.
The family will initiate and maintain positive interactions with the infant.

Interdisciplinary Interventions

Ambiguous genitalia in the newborn creates anxiety for many. The parents have many questions and need assistance as to what to tell inquisitive family members about the gender of the newborn. If there is any question about the external genitalia, a swift investigation to determine genetic sexual identification needs to be undertaken. Until the sex assignment has been determined, the health care team should refer to the newborn as "the baby" rather than "he or she." The name card placed in the newborn's bassinet should be white instead of pink or blue. The nurse should discourage the parents from giving the child an ambiguous name because it could serve as a reminder of the events surrounding the sexual ambiguity at birth. In addition, it would be wise to postpone sending birth announcements until the sex assignment is completed.

The first goal in the treatment of ambiguous genitalia is to determine gender through chromosomal analysis. Unfortunately, this test can take time, and gender assignment is delayed. Health care providers must be honest and forthright with parents when gender identification is unclear; this is done to prevent erroneous sex assignment, which can cause major lifelong social and emotional problems for the child and family.

If CAH is suspected, appropriate steroid replacement therapy is initiated and reconstructive surgery for the virilized female is planned. Genetic counseling is indicated given the autosomal recessive nature of CAH. (See section on congenital adrenal hyperplasia for details.)

Most children born as hermaphrodites are best reared as female; the testicular tissue is removed, and reconstructive surgery to create suitable female external genitalia is done because it is much more difficult to create an adequately functional male phallus.

In some children, ambiguous genitalia are not obvious at birth. They are diagnosed at the time of adolescence or young adulthood when stunted growth, delayed puberty, or infertility raises the question of a broader chromosomal or hormonal abnormality. With this also comes the developing awareness of possible permanent infertility or sexual dysfunction and a sense of loss.

With any genetic condition a genetic counselor can give accurate information and prognoses. Issues for the child include differences from their peers in relation to sexual development, body image, and reproductive capabilities. Options are presented for alternative forms of raising a family through adoption as well as awareness that childless couples can also lead a very fulfilling life. Future advances in reproductive science may include the possibility of reproduction through donor gametes and hormonal support. Education and support groups for most syndromes are available to parents and families through newsletters and from the local and national chapter for specific disorders.

Gynecomastia

Gynecomastia is a condition in young boys, usually occurring during early or mid puberty, that involves unilateral or bilateral breast enlargement. This common, transient occurrence usually lasts a few months to a year (DiGeorge & Levine, 1996). Hormone levels for FSH, LH, prolactin, testosterone, and estradiol are normal, but there may be a decreased ratio of testosterone to estradiol. In younger children with gynecomastia who also show increased pigmentation of the nipple and areola, one should suspect exogenous estrogens in the form of creams, pills, or inhaled medications. The antifungal drug ketoconazole can also cause gynecomastia. Breast enlargement may also be a sign of other conditions, such as Klinefelter's syndrome or other rare endocrine disorders.

The boy may develop body image disturbance related to gynecomastia. Therefore, the nurse should encourage him and his family to verbalize concerns about body image. Treatment usually consists of reassurance to the boy and his family of the benign and transient nature of this condition. Rarely is surgical intervention indicated.

Premature Thelarche

In girls, premature breast development is known as premature thelarche. It is a benign condition that may appear in the first 2 years of life. Breast development may be unilateral or bilateral, and regression usually occurs after a few years. These girls do not show maturation of the genitalia or presence of sexual hair, and menarche occurs at the expected age. Growth usually occurs at the normal rate and rarely is accelerated. This is thought to occur from an imbalance in the LH-FSH ratio within the hypothalamic-pituitary-gonadal pathway.

A girl with early breast development should be screened for true precocious puberty, especially if the age at onset is after 2 years of age. Plasma levels of LH, FSH, and estradiol should be obtained. This condition may be caused by exogenous exposure to estrogens. (See Precocious Puberty and Tables 26–2, 26–4, and 26–5.)

As with gynecomastia in boys, treatment includes reassurance to the girl and family that this is a benign and transient condition and that the other aspects of female pubertal progression should occur in normal sequence.

Summary of Key Concepts

- The endocrine system is made up of many hormone-secreting glands that have an effect on a variety of organ systems and tissues. Hyperfunctioning or hypofunctioning glands may result in mild to severe disturbances of physiology, including death, if not detected and treated in a timely manner.
- Because each gland in the endocrine system secretes a hormone or hormones with specific target organs that perform specific physiologic functions, it is not useful to do an assessment or diagnostic testing for general endocrine dysfunction.
- The child's presenting symptoms provide the key to deciding which assessments and diagnostic tests unique to the disorder are to be done.
- Hormone replacement or glandular suppression (either by medication or surgical removal) may be indicated, depending on the problem.
- Many dysfunctions of the endocrine system result in life-threatening situations. Most conditions are with the child for the rest of his or her life.
- The most common symptoms of neurogenic diabetes insipidus are polyuria and polydipsia. The onset of these symptoms is usually sudden and abrupt. The nurse must carefully monitor the child for signs of dehydration.
- SIADH results from hypersecretion of ADH, which occurs secondary to various conditions such as tumors, meningitis, or CNS trauma or after surgical procedures on the brain. The use of certain medications may also cause SIADH.
- Growth hormone deficiency is treated with subcutaneous injections of growth hormone. Side effects include an increase in blood glucose level, increased incidence of slipped capital femoral epiphysis, infection at the injection site, and pseudotumor cerebri.
- The child with precocious puberty is likely to look older than his or her developmental age. Therefore, parents, teachers, and friends should be encouraged to interact with the child in an age-appropriate manner, and expectations for the child should be realistic.
- The treatment of delayed puberty depends on the specific cause of the problem and whether the delay in development will be temporary or permanent.
- Neonatal screening for hypothyroidism is mandatory. Early detection of this condition can prevent irreversible developmental delay of the child.
- Treatment for the child with Graves' disease includes antithyroid drugs to block T_4 synthesis, subtotal thyroidectomy, or radioiodine therapy. Compliance with antithyroid drug therapy may be a challenge, as the therapy may extend over long periods.
- Hypoparathyroidism results in hypocalcemia and hyperphosphatemia. Children with this condition are at risk for seizures and tetany.
- Hyperparathyroidism results in hypercalcemia, which leads to brittle bones and a tendency toward fractures. Safety of the child's environment should be monitored to prevent injury.
- Management of diabetes mellitus is multimodal. Insulin therapy, the primary intervention, is combined with nutritional management and exercise to help the child maintain good metabolic control.
- Hyperinsulinism is a severe form of hypoglycemia, most often presenting between birth and 3 months of age. Symptoms seen include irritability, jitteriness, bizarre behavior, hypothermia, and seizures.
- Ketotic hypoglycemia can be prevented by giving the child small, frequent, high-carbohydrate, high-protein meals and a late evening snack.

- Adrenocortical insufficiency is rare in children. Treatment involves managing the child's fluid and electrolyte status, replacing the deficient steroid, and determining the underlying cause of the condition.
- Congenital adrenal hyperplasia (CAH) is an autosomal recessive condition caused by an inborn deficiency of one of the enzymes needed to synthesize cortisol. Lifelong replacement therapy with glucocorticoids and, if needed, mineralocorticoids and dietary salts is the treatment plan.
- The most common cause of Cushing's syndrome in children is the side effects of prolonged or excessive corticosteroid therapy used to treat a medical condition.
- Gonadal disorders are of great concern to the child and family because of their impact on the child's emerging self-esteem and body image. The nurse should encourage the child and the family to verbalize their concerns.

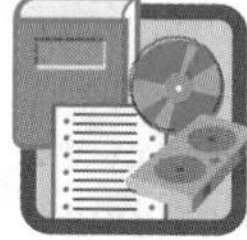

Resources

Organizations

American Diabetes Association
1660 Duke Street
Alexandria, VA 22314
(703) 549-1500
Web: http://www.diabetes.org/ada/info.html

Congenital Adrenal Hyperplasia Family Support Group
Children's Hospital of Orange County
455 S. Main
Orange, CA 92668

Congenital Adrenal Hyperplasia Support Association
10 Country Highway
Wrenshall, MN 55797

DiGeorge Syndrome Families
27859 Lassen Street
Castaic, CA 91384
(804) 294-3623

Families and Diabetes
2649 Vista Way #8100
Oceanside, CA 92054
(619) 945-6597

Human Growth Foundation
7777 Leesburg Pike
P.O. Box 3090
Falls Church, VA 22043

Juvenile Diabetes Foundation
25 East 26th Street
New York, NY 10010

Little People of America
P.O. Box 126
Dwatonna, MN 55060

Magic Foundation
770 Alexandria Drive
Naperville, IL 60565

Pediatric Endocrinology Nursing Society
P.O. Box 2333
Gaithersburg, MD 20886-2933

National Graves' Disease Foundation
320 Arlington Road
Jacksonville, FL 32211
(904) 724-0770

National Organization for Rare Disorders (NORD)
P.O. Box 8923
New Fairfield, CT 06812-2783

Thyroid Foundation of America, Inc.
Dept. B
Wang ACC 630
Massachusetts General Hospital
Boston, MA 02114
(617) 726-8500

Turner's Syndrome Society of the United States
811 Twelve Oaks Center
15500 Wayzata Boulevard
Wayzata, MN 55391
(612) 475-9944; (800) 365-9944

Books and Printed Materials

- ✏ Mazur, M., Banks, P., & Keegan, A. (1995). *The dinosaur tamer*. Chicago: Contemporary Books.
- ✏ Pirner, C. (1991). *Even little kids get diabetes*. Morton Grove, IL: Albert Whitman & Co.
- ✏ Miller, J. (1988). *Grilled cheese at four o'clock in the morning*. Alexandria, VA: American Diabetes Association.
- ✏ Betschart, J., & Thom, S. (1995). *In control—a guide for teens with diabetes*. Minneapolis, MN: Chronimed Publishing.

Computer Resources

http://www.alt.support.diabetes.kids (support group for parents of children with diabetes)

http://www.diabetes.com (resources and articles about diabetes)

✏ http://www.castleweb.com/diabetes/children with diabetes (an on-line community for kids with type 1 diabetes; also has a summary of books and videos for children with diabetes)

✏ Resources specifically for children.

References

American Diabetes Association. (1994). Technical review: Nutrition recommendations and principles for people with diabetes mellitus. *Diabetes Care, 17*(5), 490–518.

Batcheller, J. (1992). Disorders of antidiuretic hormone secretion. *AACN Clinical Issues, 3*, 370–378.

Bergada, I., & Bergada, C. (1995). Long-term treatment with low dose testosterone in constitutional delay of growth and puberty: Effect on bone age maturation and pubertal progression. *Metabolism, 44*, 1013–1015.

Blethen, S. L. (1995). Complications of growth hormone therapy in children. *Current Opinion Pediatrics, 7*, 466–471.

Blizzard, R. M., & Johanson, A. (1994). Disorders of growth. In Kappy, M. S., Blizzard, R. M., & Midgeon, C. J. (Eds.), *The diagnosis and treatment of endocrine disorders in childhood and adolescence* (pp. 383–433). Springfield, IL: Charles C Thomas.

Breyer, P., Haider, A., & Pescovitz, O. H. (1993). Gonadotropin-releasing hormone agonists in the treatment of girls with central precocious puberty. *Clinical Obstetrics and Gynecology, 36*, 764–772.

Budarf, M. L., Collins, J., Gong, W., Roe, B., Wang, Z., Bailey, L. C., Sellinger, B., Michaud, D., Driscoll, D. A., & Emanuel, B. S. (1995). Cloning a balanced translocation associated with DiGeorge syndrome and identification of a disrupted candidate gene. *Nature Genetics, 10*, 269–278.

Castiglia, P. (1997). Hyperthyroidism (Graves' disease). *Journal of Pediatric Health Care, 11*(5), 227–229.

Castiglia, P. T., Kramer, D., Fong, C., & Lipman, T. H. (1992). Alterations in endocrine function. In P. Castiglia, & R. E. Harbin (Eds.), *Child health care: Process and practice* (pp. 871–913). Philadelphia: J. B. Lippincott.

Chase, H. (1995). Responsibilities of children at different ages. In H. Chase (Ed.). *Understanding insulin-dependent diabetes* (p. 175). Denver: University of Colorado Health Sciences Center.

Dallas, J. S., & Foley, T. P. (1996). Hyperthyroidism. In F. Lifshitz (Ed.), *Pediatric endocrinology: A clinical guide* (3rd ed., pp. 401–414). New York: Marcel Dekker.

Dallas, J. S., & Foley, T. P. (1996). Hypothyroidism. In F. Lifshitz (Ed.), *Pediatric endocrinology: A clinical guide* (3rd ed., pp. 391–399). New York: Marcel Dekker.

Daughaday, W. H. (1992). Growth hormone deficient syndromes and their etiologies. *Growth, Genetics, and Hormones*, 8.

Davidson, M., Boland, E. A., & Grey, M. (1997). Teaching teens to cope: Coping skills training for adolescents with insulin-dependent diabetes mellitus. *Journal of Society of Pediatric Nursing, 2*(2), 65–72.

Diabetes Control and Complications Trial Research Group. (1993). The effect of intensive treatment of diabetes on the development and progression of long-term complications in insulin-dependent diabetes mellitus. *The New England Journal of Medicine, 329*, 977–986.

DiGeorge, A. M., & LaFranchi, S. (1996a). Disorders of the thyroid gland. In R. E. Behrman, R. M. Kleigman, A. Arvin, & W. E. Nelson (Eds.), *Nelson textbook of pediatrics* (15th ed., pp. 1587–1599). Philadelphia: W. B. Saunders.

DiGeorge, A. M., & LaFranchi, S. (1996b). Disorders of the parathyroid glands. In R. E. Behrman, R. M. Kleigman, A. Arvin, & W. E. Nelson (Eds.). *Nelson textbook of pediatrics* (15th ed., pp. 1605–1612). Philadelphia: W. B. Saunders.

DiGeorge, A. M., & Levine, L. S. (1996). Disorders of the adrenal glands. In R. E. Behrman, R. M. Kleigman, A. Arvin, & W. E. Nelson (Eds.), *Nelson textbook of pediatrics* (15th ed., pp. 1612–1628). Philadelphia: W. B. Saunders.

Fagan, M. (1995). Nursing care of the child with DKA in the PICU. *Pediatric Nursing, 21*(4), 375–380.

Fisher, D. A. (1987). Effectiveness of newborn screening programs for congenital hypothyroidism: Prevalence of missed cases. *Pediatric Clinics of North America, 34*, 881–890.

Fjellestad-Paulsen, A., Paulsen, O., d'Agay-Abensour, L., Lundin, S., & Czernichow, P. (1993). Central diabetes insipidus: Oral treatment with DDAVP. *Regulatory Peptides 45*, 303–307.

Foster, D. W. (1994). Diabetes mellitus. In K. J. Isselbacher, E. Braunwald, J. D. Wilson, J. B. Martin, A. S. Fauci, & D. L. Kasper (Eds.), *Harrison's principles of internal medicine* (13th ed., p. 1979). New York: McGraw-Hill.

Geffner, M. E. (1990). Hypoglycemia. In S. A. Kaplan (Ed.), *Clinical pediatric endocrinology* (pp. 165–179). Philadelphia: W. B. Saunders.

Glasgow, A. M. (1992). Hypoglycemia. In W. Hung (Ed.), *Clinical pediatric endocrinology* (pp. 332–355). St. Louis: Mosby–Year Book.

Goodpasture, J. C., Ghai, K., Cara, J. F., & Rosenfield, R. L. (1993). Potential of gonadotropin-releasing hormone agonists in the diagnosis of pubertal disorders in girls. *Clinical Obstetrics and Gynecology, 36*, 773–785.

Gray, D., St. Dennis-Feezle, L., Clark, K., & Parker, S. (1993). Nursing planning, intervention and evaluation for altered endocrine function. In D. Broadwell-Jackson, & R. Saunders (Eds.), *Child health nursing: A comprehensive approach to the care of children and their families* (pp. 1459–1535). Philadelphia: J. B. Lippincott.

Greenberg, F., Elder, F. F. B., Hafner, P., Northrup, H., & Ledbetter, D. H. (1988). Cytogenetic findings in a prospective series of patients with DiGeorge anomaly. *American Journal of Human Genetics, 434*, 604–611.

Grey, M., Cameron, M., Lipman, T., & Thurber, T. (1995). Psychosocial status of children with diabetes in the first two years after diagnosis. *Diabetes Care, 18*, 1330–1336.

Hoekelman, R. A. (1992). Screening for congenital hypothyroidism. *Pediatric Annals, 21*, 9–10.

Hung, W. (1992). Ovaries and variants of female sexual development. In W. Hung (Ed.), *Clinical pediatric endocrinology* (pp. 226–267). St. Louis: Mosby–Year Book.

Kasden, F. (1997). Teaching diabetic survival skills. *Advances for Nurse Practitioners, 5*(15), 51–54.

Lessick, M. L., Klingner, A., & Clabots, T. (1986). The endocrine system. In G. M. Scipien, M. U. Barnard, M. A. Chard, J. Howe, & P. J. Phillips (Eds.), *Comprehensive pediatric nursing* (3rd ed., pp. 1197–1246). New York: McGraw-Hill.

Likitmaskul, S., Cowell, C. T., Donaghue, K., Kreutzmann, D. J., Howard, N. J., Blades, B., & Silink, M. (1995). "Exaggerated adrenarche" in children presenting with premature adrenarche. *Clinical Endocrinology, 42*, 265–272.

Lim, Y. J., Batch, J. A., & Warne, G. L. (1995). Adrenal 21-hydroxylase deficiency in childhood: 25 years' experience. *Journal of Paediatric and Child Health, 31*, 222–227.

Lipman, T. H. (1987). Assessment of the child with diabetic ketoacidosis. *Dimensions of Critical Care Nursing, 3*, 82–93.

Lipman, T. H. (1988). What causes diabetes? *American Journal of Maternal Child Nursing, 13*, 40–43.

Lipman, T. H. (1993). Epidemiology of Type I Diabetes in children 0–14 years-of-age in Philadelphia. *Diabetes Care, 16*, 922–925.

Lipman, T. H., DiFazio, D. A., Meers, R. A., & Thompson, R. L. (1989b). A developmental approach to diabetes in children: School-age–adolescence. *MCN, 14* (September-October), 330–332.

Moore, K. L., & Persaud, T. V. N. (1993). *The developing human: Clinically oriented embryology* (5th ed). Philadelphia: W. B. Saunders.

Orth, D. N., Kovacs, W. J., & Debold, C. R. (1992). The adrenal cortex. In J. D. Wilson & D. W. Foster (Eds.), *Williams textbook of endocrinology* (8th ed., p. 536). Philadelphia: W. B. Saunders.

Parker, S. (1993). Nursing assessment and diagnosis of endocrine function. In D. Broadwell-Jackson & R. Saunders, (Eds.), *Child health nursing: A comprehensive approach to the care of children and their families* (pp. 1447–1457). Philadelphia: J. B. Lippincott.

Rallison, M. L., Dobyns, B. M., Keating, F. R., Rall, J. E., & Tyler, F. H. (1975). Occurrence and natural history of chronic lymphocytic thyroiditis in childhood. *Journal of Pediatrics*, 86, 675–682.

Recker, B. (1993). Anatomy and physiology of the endocrine system. In D. Broadwell-Jackson & R. Saunders (Eds.), *Child health nursing: A comprehensive approach to the care of children and their families* (pp. 1433–1445). Philadelphia: J. B. Lippincott.

Ruble, J. A., & Charron-Prochownik, D. (1994). Altered endocrine function. In C. L. Betz, M. M. Hunsberger, & S. Wright (Eds.), *Family-centered nursing care of children* (2nd ed., pp. 1938–2011). Philadelphia: W. B. Saunders.

Sezonenko, P. C. (1993). Hypoglycemia. In J. Bertrand, R. Rappaport, & P. C. Sezonenko (Eds.), *Pediatric endocrinology: physiology, pathophysiology & clinical aspects* (2nd ed., pp. 583–595). Baltimore: Williams & Wilkins.

Soloman, A. T., Khadir, M. M., & Asfour, M. (1995). Testosterone treatment in adolescent boys with constitutional delay of growth and development. *Metabolism, 44*, 1013–1015.

Styne, D. M. (1993). Hypopituitarism and growth hormone therapy. In F. D. Burg, J. R. Ingelfinger, & E. R. Wald (Eds.), *Gellis & Kagan's current pediatric therapy* (14th ed., pp. 284–285). Philadelphia: W. B. Saunders.

Travis, L. B., Brouhard, B. H., & Schreiner, B. (1987). *Diabetes mellitus in children and adolescents*. Philadelphia: W. B. Saunders.

Weber, A., Trainer, P. J., Grossman, A. B., Afshar, F., Medbak, S., Perry, L. A., Plowman, P. N., Rees, L. H., Besser, G. M., & Savage, M. O. (1995). Investigation, management and therapeutic outcome in 12 cases of childhood and adolescent Cushing's syndrome. *Clinical Endocrinology, 43*, 19–28.

Wheeler, M. D., and Styne, D. M. (1991). The treatment of precocious puberty. *Endocrinology Metabolism Clinics of North America, (20)*, 183–190.

Williams, J. K. (1995). Parenting a daughter with precocious puberty or Turner syndrome. *Journal of Pediatric Health Care, (9)*, 109–114.

Zimmerman, D., & Gan-Gaisano, M. (1992). Hyperthyroidism in children and adolescents. *Pediatric Clinics of North America, 37*, 1273–1296.

Bibliography

Barradell, L. B., & McTavish, D. (1993). Histrelin: A review of its pharmacological properties and therapeutic role in central precocious puberty. *Drugs, 45*, 570–588.

Breyer, P., Haider, A., & Pescovitz, O. H. (1993). Gonadotropin-releasing hormone agonists in the treatment of girls with central precocious puberty. *Clinical Obstetrics and Gynecology*, 36, 764–772.

Cornblath, M., & Schwartz, R. (1991). *Disorders of Carbohydrate Metabolism in Infancy*. (3rd ed.). Philadelphia: W. B. Saunders.

Fisher, D. A. (1994). Hypothryoidism. *Pediatrics in Review, 5*, 259–272.

Foster, D. W., & Rubenstein, A. R. (1994). Hypoglycemia. In K. J. Isselbacher, E. Braunwald, J. D. Wilson, J. B. Martin, A. S. Fauci, & D. L. Kasper (Eds.), *Harrison's principles of internal medicine* (13th ed., pp. 2000–2006). New York: McGraw-Hill.

Gertner, J. M. (1990). Disorders of calcium and phosphorous homeostasis. *Pediatric Clinics of North America, 37*, 1441–1466.

Gildea, J. H. (1993). High and dry—low and wet: The key to DI and SIADH. *Pediatric Nursing, 19*, 478–481.

Goodpasture, J. C., Ghai, K., Cara, J. F., & Rosenfield, R. L. (1993). Potential of gonadotropin-releasing hormone agonists in the diagnosis of pubertal disorders in girls. *Clinical Obstetrics and Gynecology*, 36, 773–785.

Laue, L., Jones, J., Barnes, K. M., & Cutler, G. B. (1993). Treatment of familial male precocious puberty with spironolactone, testolactone and deslorelin. *Journal of Clinical Endocrinology and Metabolism*, 76, 151–155.

Lee, P. A. (1994). Advances in the management of precocious puberty. *Clinical Pediatrics, 33*, 54–61.

Lipman, T. H., DiFazio, D. A., Meers, R. A., & Thompson, R. L. (1989a). A developmental approach to diabetes in children: Birth through preschool. *MCN, 14*, 255–259.

Miculan, J., Turner, S., Paes, B. A. (1993). Congenital hypothyroidism. *Neonatal Network, 12*, 25–34.

Parker, S. (1993). Nursing assessment and diagnosis of endocrine function. In D. Broadwell-Jackson & R. Saunders, (Eds.), *Child health nursing: A comprehensive approach to the care of children and their families* (pp. 1447–1457). Philadelphia: J. B. Lippincott.

Perheentupa, J., & Czernechow, P. (1994). Water regulation and its disorders. In M. S. Kappy, R. M. Blizzard, & C. J. Megeon (Eds.), *The diagnosis and treatment of endocrine disorders in childhood and adolescence* (pp. 1095–1140). Springfield, IL: Charles C Thomas.

Pescovitz, O. H. (1990). Precocious puberty. *Pediatrics in Review, 11*, 229–237.

Rosenfield, R. L. (1991). Puberty and its disorders in girls. *Endocrine and Metabolic Clinics of North America, 20*, 15–41.

Sempoux, C., Poggi, F., Brunelle, F., Saudubray, J. M., Fekete, C., & Rahier, J. (1995). Nesidioblastosis and persistent neonatal hyperinsulinism. *Diabetes Metabolism, 21*, 402–407.

Winkel, C. A. (1994). Gonadotropin-releasing hormone agonists. Current uses for these increasingly important drugs. *Postgraduate Medicine*, 95, 111–118.

HEALTH CHALLENGE:

Inborn Errors of Metabolism

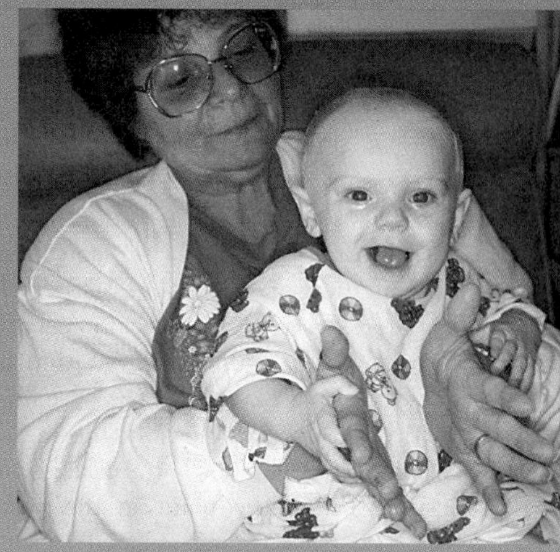

OUTLINE

Assessment of the Child with an Inborn Error of Metabolism
- Focused Health History
- Focused Physical Assessment
- Nursing Diagnoses and Outcomes
- Developmental and Biological Variances

Diagnostic Criteria for Evaluating Inborn Errors of Metabolism

Treatment Modalities

Alterations in Metabolic Status
- Amino Acid Disorders
  - Phenylketonuria
  - Maple Syrup Urine Disease
- Mineral Disorders
  - Menkes' Syndrome
  - Hypophosphatemic Rickets
  - Wilson's Disease
- Carbohydrate Disorders
  - Galactosemia
- Red Cell Disorders
  - Glucose-6-Phosphate Dehydrogenase Deficiency
- Mucopolysaccharide Disorders
  - Hurler's Disease

OBJECTIVES

- Differentiate variances between newborn onset and later childhood onset of selected inborn errors of metabolism.
- Describe key assessment factors that can assist in the early identification of metabolic disorders in children.
- Describe interventions of the health care team related to the early identification of selected inborn errors of metabolism.
- State the dietary management specific to each metabolic disorder that can prevent or decrease the severity of disease symptoms.
- Identify nursing interventions that assist the family and community to provide optimal care to the child with an inborn error of metabolism.

KEY TERMS

automatisms
ceruloplasmin
gibbus
Heinz bodies
Kayser-Fleischer rings
oxidant

CHAPTER

27

The metabolic pathways, the inborn errors that affect them, and the symptoms and toxic effects associated with metabolites have been identified in the health care literature. Although the incidence of most of the inborn errors of metabolism is low, these biochemical disorders need to be recognized and treated immediately. If not, these disorders frequently result in mental retardation and other severe symptoms that have a profound negative effect on the quality of life for the child and the family.

The body is able to build and maintain itself by *metabolizing* the food and fluid it ingests. The metabolic pathways used in this process may have inborn errors that cause an untoward reaction or lead to the creation of toxic substances. Most of the inborn errors of metabolism are transmitted via an autosomal recessive mode. The mutation of single genes either results in a structurally altered enzyme that is not capable of normal catalytic activity or causes an inhibition of enzyme synthesis (Howard-Teplansky, 1992). A reduction of enzymatic function produces a block in the metabolic pathway at a specific point. This leads to an abnormal accumulation of substrate before the point in the pathway at which the block occurs. The accumulated substrate appears in the blood, urine, and tissues. The child's developing neurotransmitter system is especially vulnerable to the abnormal biosynthesis of enzymes. Early treatment of metabolic disorders is essential to prevent the progressive loss of neurologic function, mental retardation, and other deleterious sequelae affecting the child's growth and development.

Information obtained from a genetic history is important because genetic counseling provides guidance for families as they make decisions about childbearing. Informed decisions about the continuation of pregnancy can also be made for many of the metabolic conditions. In utero diagnosis early in pregnancy is already possible for many of the inherited metabolic disorders and techniques for detecting others are being researched. Neonatal screening programs provide early diagnosis for many of the more common metabolic disorders. This allows timely intervention to prevent or decrease the severity of symptoms.

Many of the treatable errors of metabolism require lifelong management, usually in the form of dietary restriction. Other metabolic diseases are fatal or result in severe mental retardation, and no successful intervention has been developed. Advances in gene therapy bring new hope for the management, and perhaps cure, of metabolic disorders. In gene therapy, normal genetic information is introduced into defective cells to compensate for genetic defects and correct disease phenotypes. Ethical issues concerning the harvesting of genetic material and the ability to construct or alter human tissue have kept gene therapy primarily in the research laboratory. However, the ongoing resolution of these ethical issues and mastery of the technical and medical problems of gene therapy make this management option an attainable goal. Advances in biochemistry continue to reveal previously unknown metabolic diseases and clarify the basic pathophysiology of known ones, giving rise to hope for new treatment modalities and improved outcomes for children and their families affected by these disorders.

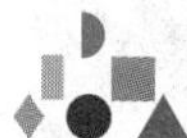

Assessment of the Child with an Inborn Error of Metabolism

Focused Health History

A detailed history of the child's health status and developmental progress can provide many clues to the existence of a metabolic disorder. Common to most metabolic problems is a history of poor feeding including a rejection or dislike of protein foods, vomiting, failure to thrive, and increasing weakness (Chart 27–1). As the child grows, delays in reaching psychomotor developmental milestones or a regression in developmental achievements is noted. The child may have a history of an apparent life-threatening event (e.g., near-miss sudden infant death).

Metabolic diseases have a genetic origin and may be more prevalent in certain ethnic groups. The pattern of heredity for many of the metabolic conditions is recessive, with neither parent presenting with clinically abnormal signs or symptoms. However, the health history of older and younger siblings may reveal symptoms similar to those of the child being assessed.

caREminder: *If one child in the family has suspicious symptoms, all other siblings need to be evaluated even if their symptoms are not exactly the same.*

Siblings or other close relatives may have a variant form of the metabolic disorder that is being evaluated in the child who is currently under observation. The family history may reveal incidents of unexplained deaths during the neonatal period, possibly indicating infant mortality related to an untreated metabolic disorder. The ill child and family members with suspicious symptoms should be questioned about the correlation between their symptoms and the presence of other common illnesses. Some variant forms of the metabolic disorders appear symptomatic only when exacerbated by the presence of a cold, vomiting, or diarrhea in the affected child.

Caregivers should be questioned about whether newborn screening was completed and, if so, whether they were informed about the results.

Worldview: *In the United States, the disorders tested for in newborn screening programs vary from state to state. Tests for phenylketonuria (PKU) and galactosemia are commonly mandated by state law. Children born in other countries may not have been screened as neonates for*

Chart 27–1
Focused Health History

Inborn Errors of Metabolism	
Identifying Data	Child's age Age at which caregivers first noted symptoms Ethnicity
Present Illness	Lethargy Convulsions, coma not responsive to intravenous glucose or calcium Clinical deterioration in a previously normal neonate Neurologic abnormalities Metabolic acidosis and ketosis Hypotonia or hypertonia
Past Medical History	*Younger child:* Was newborn screening completed? What were the results? *Older child:* Unexplained mental retardation, developmental delay, motor deficits, or convulsions; unusual odor, particularly during acute illnesses; intermittent episode of unexplained vomiting, acidosis, mental deterioration, or coma; hepatomegaly; renal stones
Nutritional Assessment	Poor feeding Persistent vomiting Failure to thrive Does not like to drink milk Rejects food high in protein
Family Medical History	Similar symptoms in other siblings or cousins History of consanguinity and/or death in the neonatal period
Birth and Neonatal History	History of apparent life-threatening event or prolonged apnea spells
Social History	Family eating patterns and health beliefs related to food
Growth and Development	Inability to meet growth and developmental norms Seems to get weaker and weaker Does not gain weight

metabolic disorders, because other countries, especially the developing nations, do not have rigorous enforcement of or control over screening programs.

Responses to the questions asked in a health history can act as red flags possibly indicating a metabolic problem. These responses must be considered in the context of the physical examination and laboratory findings before reaching a diagnosis.

Focused Physical Assessment

More than 300 metabolic diseases have been described in the medical literature to date. Most of these disorders are clinically recognized in the newborn period or first year of life. Unfortunately, many of the early signs of metabolic problems in children are vague, such as poor feeding, persistent vomiting, listlessness, failure to thrive, and delayed development. Presenting symptoms vary in relation to the child's age (Chart 27–2). The astute nurse recognizes that these symptoms are indices of many serious problems, including metabolic disorders, and motivates the health care provider to look closer for underlying causes.

A crisis can develop rapidly in the presence of metabolic disturbance and cause irreversible symptoms or death. The accurate identification of the cause of symptoms in a timely manner is of utmost concern. A thorough physical assessment should be completed. An enlarged liver and spleen and the presence of hernias

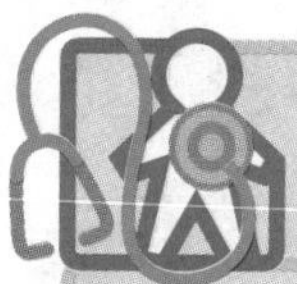

Chart 27–2
Focused Physical Assessment

Assessment Findings in the Neonatal Period and Later Childhood

Neonatal period	Later childhood
History of clinical deterioration in previously normal neonate	Unexplained mental retardation
Hepatomegaly	Unexplained developmental delay
Unusual urine and body odors	Convulsions
Failure to thrive	Motor deficits
Dislocated lenses	Hepatomegaly
Disturbances of ocular movement	Renal stones
Microcephaly	Unusual body odors, particularly during an acute illness
Abnormal hair	Intermittent unexplained episodes of vomiting, acidosis, mental deterioration, or coma
Unexplained jaundice	
Impaired states of alertness and arousal	
Tremors, clonic jerking, tonic spasms, and seizures	
Diminished or absent limb movements	
Irregular respirations	
Hypothermia or poikilothermia	
Bradycardia	
Circulatory difficulties	

(inguinal and umbilical) are frequent findings in patients with metabolic disease. The nurse's senses of touch, smell, and sight must be especially keen. Bone deformities, abnormal hair growth, and abnormal skin texture are present in many of the metabolic disturbances. The health care practitioner may note some of these changes, particularly in urine and body odors, which are specific to certain metabolic disorders (Table 27–1).

The nervous system is most consistently affected. The physical examination should focus on evaluation of neurodevelopmental functions. Abnormalities commonly revealed include impaired states of alertness and arousal, tremors, clonic jerking, tonic spasms, or seizures. Symptoms such as opisthotonos and disturbances of ocular movement may be noted. Diminished or absent limb movements are present as neuromuscular function declines. Other neurologic responses that are affected include thermoregulation (causing hypothermia or poikilothermia) and cardiac and respiratory function. Irregular respirations, bradycardia, circulatory difficulties, and poor color may all be present.

An overwhelming number of metabolic disorders negatively affect growth and development. Therefore, an accurate and ongoing assessment of the child's developmental status is critical. Children who are diagnosed and treated at a young age for their metabolic disease require continuing assessment to evaluate the effectiveness of therapy. If dietary or pharmacologic management regi-

Table 27–1
Unusual Odors Associated with Metabolic Disorders

Urine and Body Odors	Disorder
Maple syrup or burnt sugar	Maple syrup urine disease
Musty, mousy	PKU or tyrosinemia
Boiled cabbage, rancid butter, or rotting fish	Hypermethioninemia or tyrosinemia
Cat urine	Multiple carboxylase deficiency
Sweaty feet	Glutaricacidemia (type II) or isovalericacidemia
Swimming pool	Hawkinsinuria
Rotting fish	Trimethylaminuria

mens are failing, effects on the child's physical and cognitive functions can be noted. Growth charts should be maintained, and developmental status should be monitored utilizing tools such as the Denver Developmental Screening Test. (See Chapter 4 for a summary of developmental screening tools.) Motor and cognitive skills should be tested for age appropriateness. In infancy and early childhood, loss of previously attained milestones often occurs with progression of disease symptoms. Metabolic diseases that first manifest themselves in late childhood and adolescence are usually less rapid in progress and severity; however, they may still affect behavior, thinking, and emotions.

Nursing Diagnoses and Outcomes

Although inborn errors of metabolism can be attributed to a variety of changes occurring in the metabolic pathway, the diseases present common health care needs for the child and the family. Nursing diagnoses that can be applied to the child with a metabolic disorder reflect the need for long-term management and a focus on supportive care for the family of a child with a chronic, potentially fatal condition. Nursing diagnoses applicable for children with inborn errors of metabolism are listed in Chart 27–3.

Developmental and Biological Variances

Inborn errors of metabolism can produce genetic changes that may vary from child to child, depending on the degree of alteration in the affected system (Fig. 27–1). For some children, the clinical manifestations are inconsequential and are merely noted as some of the characteristics that make one person different from another. Other

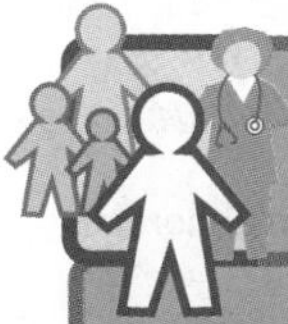

Chart 27–3
Nursing Diagnoses and Outcomes

Children with Inborn Errors of Metabolism

Actual or potential caregiver role strain related to long-term management of the child with a metabolic disorder

Outcome: Caregivers will experience comfort and confidence in performing the caregiving role as the child and the child's condition change over time.

Actual or potential ineffective family management of therapeutic regimen

Outcome: Family actions and activities will be supportive of dietary and pharmacologic regimens necessary for the developing child with a chronic condition.

Anticipatory or dysfunctional grieving related to effects of the child's diagnosis

Outcome: Child and family members will effectively work through the grieving process.

Altered growth and development related to effects of the disease

Outcomes: Measures will be taken to arrest and reverse the disease process when possible.
Caregivers will provide developmental enhancement measures as needed to support and maximize the child's potential.

Effective or ineffective individual management of therapeutic regimen

Outcome: Maturing child will accept increased responsibility for managing the disease and making modifications as necessary in the presence of illness, stress, and pregnancy.

Knowledge deficit: management and outcomes of the child and the child's metabolic condition

Outcome: Child and caregivers will be knowledgeable about the disease process, prognosis, and range of treatment options in order to make appropriate management decisions.

Alteration in nutrition: more or less than body requirements

Outcome: Child's dietary patterns will comply with the nutritional regimen needed to prevent accumulation of metabolic substrates in the body.

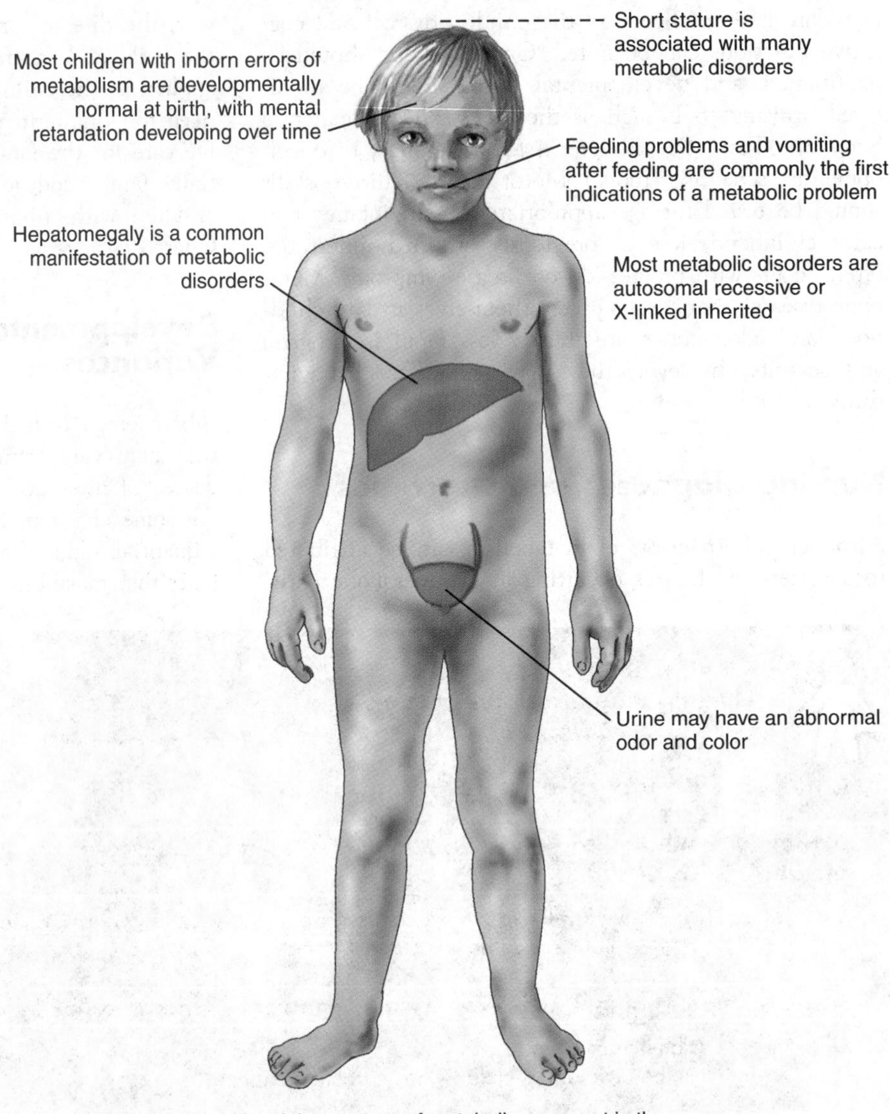
Short stature is associated with many metabolic disorders
Most children with inborn errors of metabolism are developmentally normal at birth, with mental retardation developing over time
Feeding problems and vomiting after feeding are commonly the first indications of a metabolic problem
Hepatomegaly is a common manifestation of metabolic disorders
Most metabolic disorders are autosomal recessive or X-linked inherited
Urine may have an abnormal odor and color
Most inborn errors of metabolism present in the childhood years and, if untreated, result in early death

Figure 27–1
Developmental and biological variances: metabolic system.

metabolic conditions produce symptoms that become apparent only under specific conditions that the child may or may not encounter during life. Still other conditions produce disease states varying from mild to fatal (Rezvani & Rosenblatt, 1996).

Most inborn errors of metabolism become clinically evident during the neonatal period, although some may not manifest themselves until later (Chart 27–4). Presentation in the adult years is rare and is more likely to represent a metabolic disorder that has been activated or triggered by the presence of another disease state.

Certain metabolic disorders are known to be more prevalent in specific ethnic groups and in those from specific geographic locations. For instance, the tyrosine defect tyrosinemia type I has a higher prevalence in patients with a French-Canadian ancestry. In the French-Canadian population of Quebec, the incidence of this condition is 1 in 1846 newborn infants. The classic form of maple syrup urine disease is more common among members of Mennonite and Amish sects. Hyperglycinemia is more common in Finland than in other parts of the world. Phenylketonuria is most common among Jews of Yemenite origin and in the populations of Northern Europe, particularly Ireland, Scotland, Belgium, and western Germany. Tay-Sachs disease, Gaucher's disease, and Niemann-Pick disease occur more frequently among individuals of Ashkenazi Jewish descent. Although Tay-Sachs disease occurs 1 in 3500 to 4000 births, the carrier rate among Ashkenazi Jews is 1 in 30 (Behrman, Kliegman, & Arvin, 1996). It is important for the practitioner to be aware of the correlations between certain metabolic disorders and specific ethnic groups. When these preva-

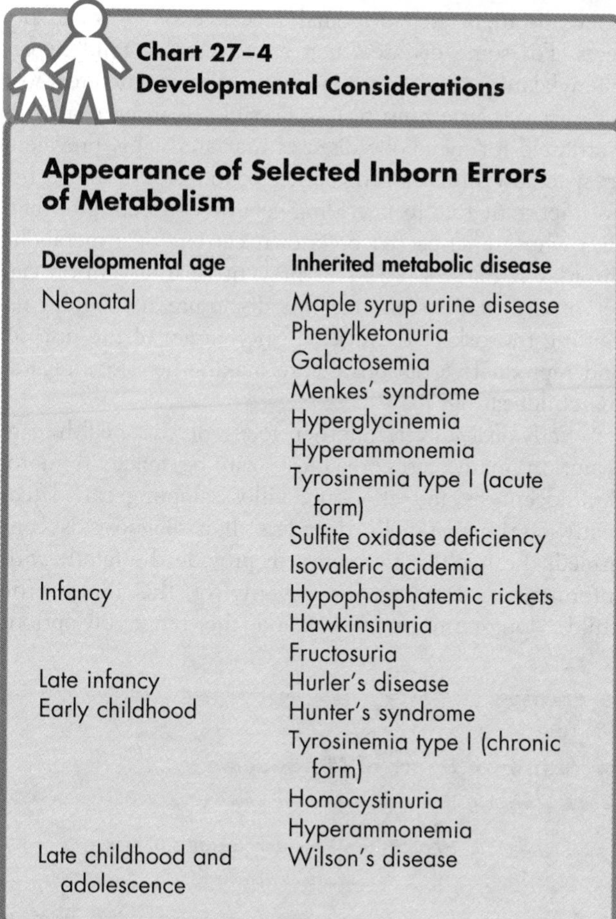

Chart 27–4
Developmental Considerations

Appearance of Selected Inborn Errors of Metabolism

Developmental age	Inherited metabolic disease
Neonatal	Maple syrup urine disease Phenylketonuria Galactosemia Menkes' syndrome Hyperglycinemia Hyperammonemia Tyrosinemia type I (acute form) Sulfite oxidase deficiency Isovaleric acidemia
Infancy	Hypophosphatemic rickets Hawkinsinuria Fructosuria
Late infancy	Hurler's disease
Early childhood	Hunter's syndrome Tyrosinemia type I (chronic form) Homocystinuria Hyperammonemia
Late childhood and adolescence	Wilson's disease

lences are known, the health care team can initiate carrier testing, genetic counseling, prenatal diagnosis, and neonatal screening to help decrease the incidence of the disease and to enhance early identification of affected infants.

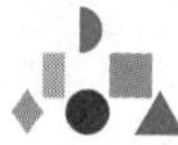

Diagnostic Criteria for Evaluating Inborn Errors of Metabolism

Early recognition is the primary goal in the diagnostic evaluation of the inborn errors of metabolism. The sooner a metabolic disorder is detected, the sooner treatment can be initiated in an attempt to avert the negative sequelae of the disease process. Early diagnosis of more than 20 inborn metabolic errors has been made possible by newborn screening programs (Howard-Teplansky, 1992) (Fig. 27–2). PKU is screened for in every state; galactosemia and maple syrup urine disease are included in most newborn screening tests.

Although screening is available for numerous metabolic disorders, the cost-to-benefit ratio of such screening, in both economic and ethical terms, must be considered for each disorder. For the rarer metabolic disorders, the expense associated with testing all newborns may be perceived to be unjustified. Therefore, specific criteria must be met before a metabolic disorder is included in a neonatal screening program. Generally, disorders included in screening programs are those

- That have a relatively common frequency
- In which clinical symptoms are not present until irreversible damage occurs
- That are severe enough to be a burden on society
- For which a treatment is known and facilities are available to provide treatment
- In which diagnosis is possible through a simple method of collection
- In which follow-up is possible if test results are abnormal (includes retesting, as all screening tests have false-positive and false-negative results)

If results of neonatal screening are positive or if the child presents with clinical manifestations consistent with a metabolic disorder, laboratory studies can be ordered to differentiate the cause of the child's illness. High-pressure gas-liquid chromatography, ion-exchange chromatography, mass spectroscopy, and electron microscopy are used

Figure 27–2
Many metabolic disorders can be detected through blood testing of the newborn. Neonatal screening procedures are usually completed 48 to 72 hours after birth and after the infant has had an adequate intake of breast milk or formula.

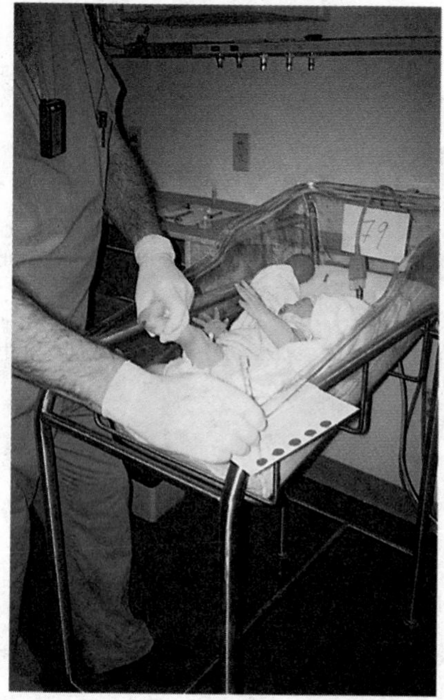

to analyze blood, plasma, urine, or cerebrospinal fluid to detect metabolic disorders (Table 27–2). The enzymatic defect that is interrupting the metabolic pathway results in either a deficiency of an essential substrate or the accumulation of a harmful metabolite. These deficiencies or elevations in the substrates can be detected in the body fluids. In some cases, when the presence of an inborn error of metabolism has been determined, further diagnostic testing may be done to determine the extent of organ involvement.

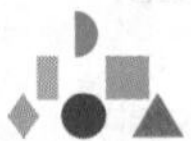

Treatment Modalities

The management of children and families affected by inborn errors of metabolism is approached in three ways by the health care team. When possible, *prevention* is the first intervention. As discussed earlier, most of the metabolic disorders are autosomal recessive or X-linked defects. For some diseases such as Tay-Sachs, mild hyperphenylalaninemia, and Gaucher's disease, heterozygote screening (carrier testing) is possible. Carrier testing is warranted for metabolic diseases that are highly prevalent in specific ethnic or geographic locations. The nurse has an important role in providing genetic counseling to families who are suspected or known carriers of a metabolic disorder (Chart 27–5). This preventive intervention can serve as a way to provide full disclosure to couples regarding the risk of the disease, the burden of the disease, and reproductive options before making decisions regarding childbearing.

Early diagnosis is another focus of the health care team. In many cases, diagnosis can be made in utero. Amniocentesis and chorionic villus sampling can detect many of the metabolic disorders. If a diagnosis is confirmed, the health care team can provide the family with information regarding the severity of the illness, the child's long-term prognosis, and the range of options

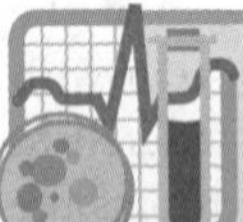

Table 27–2
Diagnostic Tests and Procedures for Evaluation of Inborn Errors of Metabolism

Diagnostic Test or Procedure	Purpose	Health Care Provider Responsibilities
Blood Tests		
Neonatal screening of blood	Early diagnosis of inborn errors of metabolism.	Completed after the child's first formula or breast-feeding and before discharge from the hospital.
Serum glucose, ammonia, bicarbonate, and pH	Helpful in differentiating major causes of metabolic disorders.	Note child's diet before the test.
Serum amino acids	Defects related to metabolism of amino acids result in increased levels in the blood.	Note time of collection in relation to feeding.
Complete blood count with differential	Used to assess hematologic or immunologic status.	
Urine Tests		
Ketones	Substances are elevated in certain metabolic disorders. These are helpful in differentiating causes and types of disorders.	Careful handling of specimen because some metabolites are volatile and may easily disappear from the urine.
Urine-reducing substances Urine amino acids and organic acids	Accumulated substrates from faulty metabolic pathways are present in the urine.	Note type of formula or food intake before the test. Twenty-four hour urine collection may be needed. It is essential to collect *all* urine. Nurse can assist family to help young children who may be forgetful. In infants, frequent draining of a 24-hr collection bag helps maintain stability of bag adhering to the child.
Other Tests		
Liver biopsies	Determine extent of hepatic involvement.	Monitor biopsy site, noting bleeding.

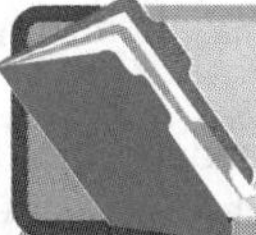

Chart 27–5
Nursing Interventions Classification (NIC)

Genetic Counseling

Definition

Use of an interactive helping process focusing on the prevention of a genetic disorder or on the ability to cope with a family member who has a genetic disorder

Activities

Establish a therapeutic relationship based on trust and respect.
Provide privacy and ensure confidentiality.
Discuss the purpose/goals of genetic counseling.
Review lifestyle behaviors (e.g., use of alcohol, street drugs, prescription medications) that place a fetus at risk as appropriate.
Review the genetic family history factors that place fetus at risk as appropriate.
Encourage appropriate diagnostic testing (e.g., DNA testing, amniocentesis, chorionic villus sampling) that may predict the presence of a genetic disorder in patient or offspring.
Discuss the advantages, risks, and costs of alternative diagnostic tests.
Minimize any coercive action that could force the parents to intervene or to feel guilty because they choose not to act.
Inform patient of specific treatments of genetic disorders as appropriate (e.g., infant stimulation for children with Down syndrome, monitoring fever in sickle cell anemia).
Discuss the impact of the particular genetic disorder on the affected individual's general health status.
Encourage expression of feelings.
Monitor patient's response when he or she learns about own genetic risk factors.
Assist patient to list and prioritize all possible alternatives to a problem.
Institute crisis support skills with patient who is unable to determine a best course of action, such as in pregnancy termination.
Assess family support for patient who undergoes loss of a family member or pregnancy loss related to a genetic or birth defect condition.
Support coping process in family members who are responsible for the ongoing care of an individual with a genetic disorder, such as Huntington's disease.
Provide referral to a member of a specialty genetic care team as necessary.
Provide referral to community resources as needed.

From McCloskey, J., & Bulechek, G. (1995). *Nursing interventions classification (NIC)* (2nd ed.). St. Louis: Mosby–Year Book. Reprinted with permission.

available with regard to maintaining or terminating the pregnancy. The family may be characterized by turmoil and grief as they come to terms with the diagnosis for their unborn child. Providing emotional support to the family is an important aspect of care at this time for the nurse. Chapter 12 provides an in-depth discussion of the interventions that can be implemented to support the family in the grieving process.

Neonatal screening is also an aspect of early diagnosis. As previously discussed, more than 20 metabolic disorders can now be detected through blood testing of the newborn. When the neonate has been tested, results may be sent back to the physician in as little as 2 weeks. The positive results may be the first and only indicator of disease in an otherwise unsymptomatic newborn. Further blood and urine testing of the child is then initiated to confirm the diagnosis.

The final aspect of early diagnosis as an intervention is the early recognition of symptoms in the neonatal period. Because children with inborn errors of metabolism may present with one or more of a large variety of symptoms (see Chart 27–2), differentiating the condition from other childhood disorders may be difficult. The clinical symptoms are usually nonspecific and may appear similar to those present with any number of generalized infections that can affect infants (Rezvani & Rosenblatt, 1996). Thus, a primary intervention of the health care team is to consider and suspect a metabolic disorder when a neonate becomes severely ill, when developmental milestones are not met, or when developmental re-

Chart 27–6

Primary Treatment Modalities for Metabolic Diseases

- Decreasing substrate preceding the enzymatic block—avoiding a particular amino acid or carbohydrate
- Adminstering a supplement of the deficient product that should have been produced
- Providing an enzymatic cofactor
- Using medication to remove accumulated substrate
- Replacing deficient enzyme through liver or bone marrow transplantation or intravenous administration
- Providing somatic gene therapy (future option)

gression begins to appear in the previously healthy child.

Finally, *prompt treatment* to prevent further deterioration in the child is essential (Chart 27–6). The primary treatment modality for the inborn errors of metabolism involves controlling the substrate accumulation by *restricting or eliminating carbohydrates and/or proteins.* The use of special diet restrictions and provision of synthetic medical foods are the two most successful methods of controlling the enzyme deficiencies. The nurse is involved in providing nutritional counseling for the child and the family (TIP 27–1). Dietary management changes as the child grows, moving from a formula-based diet to solid foods. The primary care physician, the nurse, and the nutritionist can work together to provide the family with a nutritional plan. The diet must incorporate the restrictions mandated by the particular metabolic disorder, while considering the child's personal tastes and eth-

TIP 27–1 A Teaching Intervention Plan for the Child with Special Dietary Needs

Nursing Diagnoses and Outcomes

- Knowledge deficit: dietary parameters for the child with a metabolic condition
  Outcome: Family will have knowledge sufficient to manage their child's diet.
- Individual, effective management of therapeutic regimen
  Outcome: Child and/or family will regulate dietary plan to meet the health goals of the growing child.

Interventions

- Determine the caregiver's understanding of the child's metabolic condition and the need for dietary restrictions.
- Instruct the child and/or caregivers about the name of the prescribed diet.
- Instruct the child and/or caregivers about allowed and prohibited foods.
- Include other caregivers (grandparents, daycare providers) in teaching.
- Assist the caregivers in obtaining specialized infant formulas or medical foods.
- Assist the child and/or caregiver in incorporating individual and ethnic food preferences into the diet of the older child.
- Instruct the caregiver and/or child how to read labels and how to select appropriate food.
- Observe the child and/or caregiver's selection of foods appropriate to the prescribed diet.
- Assist the caregiver in substituting ingredients to conform favorite recipes to the diet.
- Provide written meal plans.
- Teach the child and/or caregiver how to keep a food diary and use it as a method for evaluating the child's compliance with the dietary restrictions.
- Provide the child and/or caregiver with scenarios to preplan food selection at events such as parties, fast food restaurants, and meals at other people's homes.
- Provide written instructions for daycare, preschool, and school officials regarding dietary restrictions.
- Provide a schedule for routine monitoring of blood and urine to evaluate success of dietary and pharmacologic therapies.
- Monitor the child's growth and development to verify success of therapy.

nic preferences. It is often difficult to ensure that dietary restrictions are maintained outside the child's home environment. Providing dietary instructions to daycare and school personnel is a key intervention. When the child attends a social event at which food is served, parents should either inquire beforehand whether appropriate foods will be served or take food items with them that are on the child's diet.

Tip: *One way to prevent others from serving the young child a restricted food is to have the child wear a T-shirt that states "Please do not feed me, I am on a special diet."*

In some instances, *pharmacologic dosages of vitamins and medications* may be given (Howard-Teplansky, 1992). These products are used to supplement any deficient products or assist in the removal of accumulated substrates. The nurse must work with the child and family to be certain they understand the importance of continuing pharmacologic therapy for an extended period. In most cases, the treatment is lifelong. The agreeable preschooler who easily complies with the treatment regimen may become an independent adolescent who rejects being told what to do. Assisting the maturing child to be actively involved in his or her care and providing the child with a solid understanding of the importance of the pharmacologic and dietary regimen are aspects of the nurse's work with the family.

Enzyme therapy is another treatment modality currently being researched. Enzyme activity can be delivered to such organs as the liver and spleen to treat non–central nervous system manifestations such as anemia, bone disease, and hepatosplenomegaly. *Liver and bone marrow transplantations* have demonstrated some success in halting or slowing the progression of peripheral complications in conditions such as Hurler's and Gaucher's diseases. Replacing the defective gene itself (*somatic gene therapy*) is currently being evaluated as a treatment alternative. All of these interventions are considered to be in the category of research therapy (Belmont & Beaudet, 1993). Considerable counseling to the child and the family must be provided to ensure they understand the risks, uncertain outcomes, and hardships that are associated with the initiation of therapies that have not yet proved their long-term effectiveness.

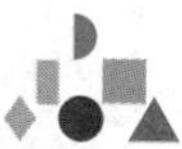

Alterations in Metabolic Status

Amino Acid Disorders

Amino acids are the primary building blocks of proteins, which are key factors in many of the metabolic cycles and may function as neurotransmitters. Even in utero, amino acids are essential to life. Inherited errors of amino acid metabolism occur primarily in catabolic pathways. Most of the associated disorders can result in severe central nervous system dysfunction. However, early diagnosis, removal of toxic metabolites, promotion of anabolism, and compliance with dietary restrictions can prevent catastrophic outcomes. This section discusses two of the most common amino acid disorders: phenylketonuria and maple syrup urine disease. Table 27–3 provides a summary of significant features of these and other amino acid disorders.

Phenylketonuria

Phenylketonuria, more commonly known as PKU, is the most frequently occurring aminoaciduria. PKU was first recognized in 1934 and was associated with an excess of phenylpyruvic acid in the urine. PKU is an autosomal recessive genetic defect in which an enzyme deficiency results in inability of the body to metabolize phenylalanine efficiently. If untreated, the disease leads to severe, irreparable damage to the central nervous system.

The recessive gene that transmits PKU is found on chromosome 12. The defect in the gene for phenylalanine hydrolase is responsible for more than 10 mutations of the PKU disorder (Okano et al., 1991). In order to have PKU, the child must receive the defective gene from both parents. Thus, there is a one-in-four chance of a PKU birth when both parents are carriers. It has been estimated that 1 person out of 60 is an asymptomatic heterozygous carrier of the PKU gene (Lott, 1988). The incidence of PKU is approximately 1 in 10,000 births. However, there is a significantly greater incidence of 23 in 100,000 births in Turkey (Holton, 1994), in people of Northern European origin, and among Jews of Yemenite origin (Korson, Rohr, & Gray, 1993; Matalon & Michals, 1991).

Pathophysiology

The exact pathogenic mechanisms of PKU have not been determined. Phenylalanine is an essential amino acid found in all protein foods. During the child's early growth period, approximately 50% of the phenylalanine in the normal daily intake is used for protein synthesis. As growth slows, the amount of phenylalanine needed by the body diminishes. Normally, excess phenylalanine is converted in the liver, pancreas, and kidneys to tyrosine (Lott, 1988). In the most severe form of PKU (classic), there is a complete absence of activity of the hepatic enzyme phenylalanine hydroxylase. This results in a buildup of phenylalanine and its metabolites, which affects numerous areas of metabolism, including a failure of conversion of phenylalanine to tyrosine. Tyrosine plays an important role in development of the central nervous

Table 27–3
Selected Amino Acid Disorders

Disorder	Inheritance	Pathophysiology	Significant Clinical Features	Laboratory Findings	Management	Prognosis
Phenylketonuria	Autosomal recessive (chromosome 12)	Defective phenylalanine hydroxylase enzyme, prevents conversion of phenylalanine to tyrosine.	Hyperactivity Irritability Seizures Mental retardation Eczema Light hair and skin Musty body and urine odor	Elevated plasma phenylalanine Elevated urine phenyl acids, phenylpyruvic acid, phenylacetic acid, and orthohydroxyphenylacetic acid	Dietary restriction of phenylalanine Controlled amounts of fruit, vegetables, and grain products Special formula low in phenylalanine	Near-normal intelligence likely with adequate dietary control, probably throughout life. Phenylalanine must be provided in amount sufficient to support growth.
Maple syrup urine disease	Autosomal recessive	Deficient oxidative decarboxylation of alpha-keto acids (leucine, valine, and isoleucine), which are not converted to fatty acids.	Difficulties with sucking and swallowing Irregular respirations Intermittent rigidity and flaccidity Possible grand mal seizures Urine odors of maple syrup Severe mental retardation if untreated	Positive urine 2-4 diphenylhydrazone Elevated blood and urine levels of leucine, isoleucine, and valine and their keto acids	Diet restricted for leucine, isoleucine, and valine Removal of toxic metabolites Special formula used	Relatively normal intellect with early treatment and compliance. There is a transient form of disease, for which treatment is necessary only during times of illness.
Hemocystinuria	Autosomal recessive (chromosome 21)	Deficient cystathionine beta-synthase Prevents interaction of an intermediate product of the amino acid methionine with serine to form cystathionine	Dislocation of the lens Mental retardation Convulsions Osteoporosis Arterial and venous vascular thrombosis Limb overgrowth Fair hair and skin Connective tissue deficit, leading to scoliosis	Plasma homocystine 0.02–0.025 mmol/L Plasma methionine up to 2 mmol/L Plasma cystine low Increased homocystine in urine	High doses of pyridoxine (vitamin B_6), 200–500 mg per 24 h Low-methionine, high-cystine diet Use of low-methionine formulas	Progress of the disease may not be stemmed.
Isovaleric acidemia	Autosomal recessive (chromosome 15)	Deficient isovaleryl-CoA dehydrogenase	Mental retardation Acidosis Vomiting Lethargy Coma Urine odor of sweaty feet	Isovaleric acid in blood and urine	Low-protein, specific low-leucine diet	Near-normal intelligence if compliant with diet.
Methylmalonic-aciduria	Autosomal recessive (chromosome 6)	Possible defect in the B_{12} coenzyme	Low blood pH Lethargy Vomiting Ketoacidosis Failure to thrive Mental retardation	Methylmalonic acid in blood and urine	B_{12} unresponsive: low-protein diet B_{12} responsive: B_{12} in large doses	B_{12} unresponsive: death usually in infancy. B_{12} responsive: normal growth and development.

system. It is the precursor of dopamine and norepinephrine. Tyrosine is also a substrate in the synthesis of thyroxine and melanin, which affect growth and pigmentation of the skin, hair, and eyes. When phenylalanine and its metabolites accumulate in the blood and the urine, there is a specific effect on brain development, especially during the periods of active myelination.

Mild to moderate degrees of the disease are classified as hyperphenylalaninemias. The effect on the central nervous system varies with the degree of metabolic enzyme impairment. Specific diagnosis of a hyperphenylalaninemia versus classic PKU cannot be made in the neonatal period. Some neonates, primarily premature infants, have an immature phenylalanine hydroxylating system. This is a benign condition not requiring treatment.

The successful childhood treatment of PKU has led to the prevalence of maternal PKU. Childbearing women who have PKU are at risk for having infants with mental retardation, low birth weight, microcephaly, or congenital heart defects (Korson et al., 1993). High maternal phenylalanine levels have a teratogenic effect on the fetus. Infants may or may not be born with PKU themselves, although there is a higher incidence of hyperphenylalaninemic infants born to PKU mothers. It is believed that elevated maternal PKU prevents the normal expression of liver phenylalanine hydroxylase during fetal development (Lott, 1988).

Assessment

At birth, an infant with PKU has normal phenylalanine levels because of the rapid placental exchange of amino acids that has been occurring in utero. However, these levels rise sharply once the baby has been fed because most formulas and breast milk contain phenylalanine. Mass screening for PKU began in 1961, and all states now participate in screening programs, which detect phenylalanine in a blood specimen using the Guthrie test. In this test, a drop of blood is obtained with a heelstick and collected on a special filter paper. It is recommended that the screening be completed 48 to 72 hours after birth and after the infant has had an adequate intake of breast milk or formula.

caREminder: *The drop of blood must be large enough to fill the imprinted space on the filter paper. Squeezing out more blood onto the paper creates a layering effect that can produce a false-positive test result.*

Infants with PKU appear normal for about the first 6 months of life. After this time, an untreated child begins to manifest symptoms of the tyrosine deficiency and excretion of phenylacetic acid in the urine and perspiration. These symptoms include severe mental retardation, microcephaly, seizures, and hyperactivity. Development of a clumsy gait, fine tremors of the hands, poor coordination, odd posturing, and repetitious digital mannerisms may also be seen. The inability to produce melanin causes hypopigmentation of the hair, eyes, and skin. Eczema occurs in 25% of untreated children. A musty odor from the child's urine and sweat is a classic sign of PKU. Male children, whether treated or not, are frequently infertile as adults, although some have fathered children (Fisch, Matalon, Weisberg, & Michals, 1991).

Diagnostic Tests. Diagnostic laboratory findings include plasma phenylalanine levels of 0.9 mmol/L or greater and elevated urine metabolites such as phenylpyruvic acid, phenylacetic acid, and phenyl acetyl glutamine.

Nursing Diagnoses and Outcomes

Management of the child with PKU focuses on early detection and intervention to avert the deleterious effects of the disease process. In addition to the nursing diagnoses and outcomes reviewed in Chart 27–3, Care Path 27–1 provides an example of the nursing diagnoses and interdisciplinary plan of care that can be instituted for the newly diagnosed child and his or her family.

Interdisciplinary Interventions

Management of children with PKU focuses on preventing excessive accumulation of phenylalanine by restricting protein intake. The health care team provides instruction on dietary interventions that control the phenylalanine level and monitors the effectiveness of the dietary regimen. Dietary intervention should begin within the first weeks of life. Phenylalanine intake must be restricted to 250 to 500 mg per day. The goal of dietary management is to maintain serum phenylalanine levels below 0.9 mmol/L but at least 0.0 to 0.2 mmol/L to allow normal growth and tissue repair. The need for phenylalanine is greatest during infancy and progressively diminishes with age as growth slows. The amount of phenylalanine prescribed is based on ongoing assessment of the child's blood and urine phenylalanine levels. Dietary allowances of phenylalanine change depending on hunger, growth, development, and serum phenylalanine levels (Bowe, 1995; Lott, 1988).

Medical foods, sold in powder form, are available as the chief source of nutrition for infants and children with PKU. The medical foods are low in phenylalanine and contain vitamins, minerals, and, in some cases, carbohydrates and fats (Table 27–4). The medical foods are reconstituted as formulas for infants and as milk substitutes for older children. The proteins in the medical foods have a characteristic flavor and in some cases aroma that are different from those of regular formula.

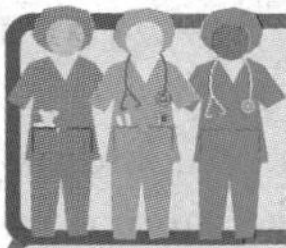

Care Path 27–1 An Interdisciplinary Plan of Care for the Infant with PKU

Nursing Diagnosis	Patient/Family Intermediate Outcomes		
	First outpatient visit	Second outpatient visit	Third outpatient visit
Potential ineffective family management of therapeutic regimen	Family will understand protein restrictions and the vitamin and mineral supplements needed.	Family will exhibit knowledge of dietary regimen.	Family will demonstrate ability to calculate protein intake.
Knowledge deficit: management and outcomes of the child	Family will state mechanisms that have caused elevated phenylalanine in infant's urine and blood.	Family will state signs and symptoms of elevated PKU and decreased PKU.	Family will express understanding of genetic transmission of PKU.
Altered growth and development related to effects of disease	Family will understand the impact of the diagnosis on the infant's growth and development.	Family will relate normal growth and developmental milestones that the infant should achieve.	
Anticipatory grieving related to the child's diagnosis	Family will verbalize feelings regarding their infant's diagnosis.		
Care Intervention Categories			
Consults	Genetic, neurology, nutritional consultation	Neurology: complete developmental assessment.	Genetic consultation completed.
Labs	Serum phenylalanine level, urine phenylpyruvic acid level, genetic screening of family.	Serum phenylalanine level.	
Nutrition	Start protein-restricted diet immediately. Supplemental vitamins and minerals. Assist family to order formulas and/or medical foods.	Evaluate compliance with diet. Discuss how the diet will change as the child grows.	Follow up by community personnel to assess the child's dietary compliance.
Psychosocial	Encourage and allow family to verbalize grief.	Assess the family's level of acceptance of the child's diagnosis.	
Social service	Assist family with financial concerns and ordering medical foods.	Provide family with information about support groups and organizations.	
Teaching	Inform daycare or school provider of dietary restrictions. Dietary regimen. Causes of PKU. Effects of PKU on the body.	Infection control. Reinforce dietary regimen. Signs and symptoms of elevated and decreased PKU.	Genetic transmission of PKU. Prenatal testing.

Table 27–4
Medical Foods Used in the Treatment of Phenylketonuria

Medical Food	Vendor	Intended Age for Use
Analog.XP	Ross Laboratories	Infancy and breast-fed infants
Lofenalac	Mead-Johnson	Infancy and childhood
PKU-1	Mead-Johnson	Infancy and breast-fed infants
Maxamaid XP	Ross Laboratories	1–8 yr
Maxamum XP	Ross Laboratories	8+ yr and pregnancy
Phenyl-Free	Mead-Johnson	2+ yr and pregnancy
PKU-2	Mead-Johnson	Childhood
PKU-3	Mead-Johnson	Adolescence and pregnancy

Adapted from Korson, M., Rohr, F., & Gray, S. (1993). The hyperphenylalaninemias. In F. Burg, J. Ingelfinger, & E. Wald (Eds.), *Gellis & Kagan's current pediatric therapy* (p. 327). Philadelphia: W. B. Saunders. Used with permission.

Tip: *When the medical food is introduced within the first few months of life, infants usually grow accustomed to the flavor and readily accept the formula. If PKU is diagnosed late, the older infant or child is likely to find the taste of the medical food unacceptable. Medical foods that are preflavored can be purchased to ensure better acceptance. Older children can flavor their drink with Quik, Tang, or Kool-aid to make it more appealing.*

The particular type and brand of medical food used are based on the child's age, dietary likes and dislikes, and variations in dietary needs and on the cost and availability to the family. The cost may be covered by insurance or public health programs (Korson et al., 1993).

As solid foods are added to the diet, high-protein foods such as meat, fish, poultry, cheese, eggs, milk, nuts, beans, peas, and flour require the most severe limitations. Legumes, grains, and potatoes also have a relatively high phenylalanine content. The PKU diet is based on a food exchange list similar to the type used for diabetic children. The phenylalanine-free formula continues to be the key element of the child's diet, providing 90% of the child's protein calories, vitamins, and minerals. In addition, the food exchange lists include vegetables, fruits, breads, cereals, fats, miscellaneous, and "free" foods that are allowed on the diet.

Alert: *Products sweetened with aspartame, including those under the brand name NutraSweet, should not be used because they contain phenylalanine.*

The nurse can assist both the parents and the older child to become adept at reading labels on packaged foods and beverages. Although many foods would not be considered protein sources, phenylalanine may appear in many of these products as NutraSweet (Fig. 27–3).

Protein catabolism occurs in the presence of infection and may cause an elevation in serum phenylalanine. Illnesses involving decreased appetite or associated vomit-

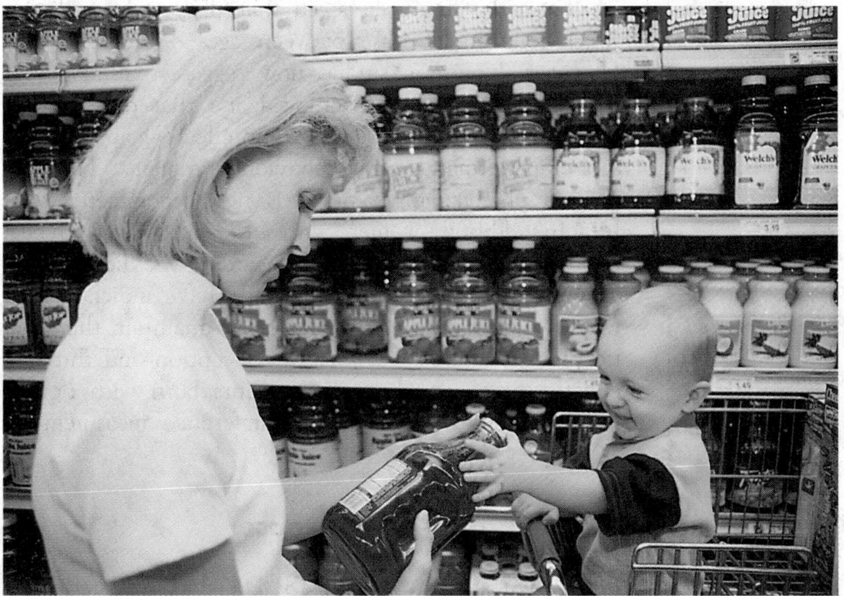

Figure 27–3
When buying food for the child with PKU, parents must examine product labels to check for aspartame or NutraSweet, which must be avoided.

ing may also affect the child's phenylalanine levels. In these cases, serum levels should be monitored, the continuance of the medical food should be encouraged, and fluid intake must be increased. Tea, gelatin, and carbonated beverages are appropriate to offer.

Although it is necessary to maintain a low phenylalanine intake, it is important to remember that phenylalanine is an essential amino acid necessary for growth and development. During infancy, the child obtains phenylalanine as a part of the medical formula or through breast milk (Chart 27–7). When the child is introduced to solid foods, the exchange lists are used to incorporate the necessary amount of phenylalanine into the diet.

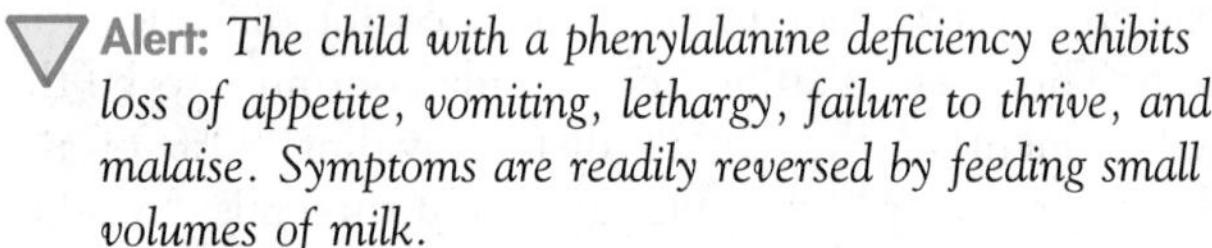

Alert: *The child with a phenylalanine deficiency exhibits loss of appetite, vomiting, lethargy, failure to thrive, and malaise. Symptoms are readily reversed by feeding small volumes of milk.*

Monitoring serum phenylalanine levels regularly is the primary way to ensure that blood levels remain within the therapeutic range.

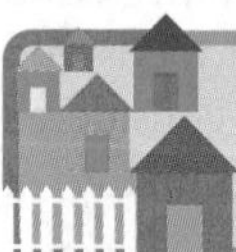

Chart 27–7
Community Care

Breast-feeding the Child with PKU

Infants diagnosed with PKU may continue to breast-feed. When a diagnosis has been made, the child's phenylalanine level needs to be reduced as quickly as possible. This is achieved through the use of a PKU medical food product. However, a small amount of natural protein is needed in the infant's diet and can be provided through breast milk. The phenylalanine content of breast milk varies from mother to mother. It is highest in the colostrum and declines with the duration of lactation.

The phenylalanine content of the breast milk is counted toward the child's needs. Generally, the number of breast-feedings to be allowed in a 24-hour period is specified (two to four feedings), with phenylalanine-free formula given at the other times. Infants who are not breast-fed are given a different medical food that contains some phenylalanine necessary for growth and development.

The nurse works with the mother to develop a system to keep track of the number of times she is breast-feeding each day. In addition, frequent monitoring of the child's serum levels, with dietary adjustments provided as needed, is a key element of the breast-feeding program.

Community Care

The nurse's ongoing role in managing the care of the child with PKU centers on educating the family, the child, other caregivers, and school personnel. Teaching that reinforces the dietary regimen is critical to the successful management of PKU (see TIP 27–1). Growth and developmental changes necessitate adaptation of the dietary plan. As the child matures, she or he must learn to manage the diet and take more responsibility for dietary choices. Parents may seek advice and intervention in order to cope with the child who challenges the treatment plan (Chart 27–8). Studies have shown that family cohesion and adherence to the restricted diet positively correlate with higher IQ levels. Thus, assessment of family dynamics and interventions to support the family under stress are important nursing interventions to enhance the long-term outcomes of these children and their families. Family counseling and participation in support groups can improve the family's coping abilities and strengthen the child's ability to manage the diet independently as the child becomes older.

The nurse can assist the family in providing information to other family caretakers, daycare providers, and school officials regarding the child's dietary restrictions. Once the child enters the school setting, most school lunches can be adapted to fit the child's prescribed diet. These community care providers also need information regarding symptoms that indicate that appropriate phenylalanine levels are not being maintained.

Routine analysis of serum phenylalanine is a part of the continuing care of the child with PKU. Family members need to be taught how to do the collection and at times may need assistance in collecting the routine blood samples, especially if the child becomes combative and resistant to the tests.

Formerly, it was believed that the need for dietary restrictions could cease between ages 4 and 10 years. However, long-term studies now suggest that metabolic hemostasis may not be achieved and that relaxation of the diet may result in lessened intellectual ability, poor school performance, and behavioral problems. Thus, restricted phenylalanine intake is now recommended for life. In addition, women with PKU who plan to bear children need to be counseled regarding the dietary management of their condition. Studies have indicated that women who used dietary measures to maintain therapeutic phenylalanine levels before conception and throughout the pregnancy have had infants born with normal weight, length, and head circumference measurements (Korson et al., 1993).

Maple Syrup Urine Disease

Maple syrup urine disease (MSUD) is an inherited autosomal recessive disorder of branched-chain amino acid

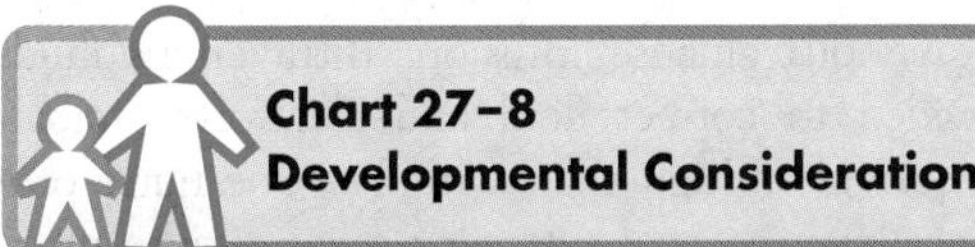

Chart 27–8
Developmental Considerations

Challenging the PKU Treatment Plan

Age	Reasons	Interventions
Infants	Dislike taste of medical formula Dislike smell of formula when switching from bottle to the cup	Purchase formulas that can be easily served in a bottle to hide the smell. When foods are being introduced, begin with a paste of the medical food and water.
Toddlers and preschoolers	Assertion of autonomy Dislike taste Desire to explore tastes of "forbidden" foods	Encourage the introduction of the cup and self-feeding skills. Use flavorings to alter the taste of the medical food. Encourage parents not to be overly protective.
School-age	Embarrassment or being self-conscious at school because they are eating something "different" from others. Desire to have more control Eating lunch away from home makes it easy to disregard the diet.	Be sure the child understands the condition. Give the child responsibility for the diet. Let the child choose and prepare his or her own medical food. Let the child select at what times the medical food is taken. Let the child answer others' questions about the diet.
Adolescents	Rejection of authority Desire to have more control Poor eating habits of adolescence associated with busy schedule Development of physical and sexual identity	Allow the intake of free foods such as soda and candy, while still assisting the adolescent to maintain his or her weight. Have the adolescent explain the diet to friends as a vegetarian diet with a special formula. Provide genetic counseling and information regarding the risks and requirements of a PKU pregnancy.

catabolism, specifically a deficiency of branched-chain 2-oxoacid dehydrogenase. The name comes from the sweet odor of maple syrup found in body fluids, particularly the urine of infants with this condition. The incidence of MSUD is not known, but reports vary from 1 in 1000 to 1 in 500,000 births depending on the geographic area. Although all races can inherit the disease, high incidences have been noted in Norway, in Spain, and in heavily inbred populations such as the Amish and certain Mennonite sects of Pennsylvania (Holton, 1994).

Pathophysiology

In MSUD, the inborn error of metabolism results in the deficient oxidative decarboxylation of the alpha-keto acids of the branched-chain amino acids: leucine, isoleucine, and valine. Variant forms of the disease in which there is some residual activity of branched-chain oxoacid dehydrogenase have a more insidious onset and less severe course. The classic form produces severe mental retardation unless intervention begins immediately after birth.

Prognosis. The prognosis for children with MSUD is significantly influenced by early diagnosis and management. Three factors primarily responsible for determining the child's psychomotor development and level of intelligence are the peak plasma leucine concentration at the time of diagnosis, the length of exposure to the elevated branched-chain amino and keto acid concentrations before diagnosis, and the adequacy of long-term metabolic control. Thus, the more severely the metabolic pathway is disturbed and the longer the resultant high levels of leucine remain, the poorer the child's prognosis. Relatively normal intellectual outcomes are possible with early intervention and consistent dietary management. The long-term intellectual ability of children affected by MSUD is an area of continuing research focus.

Assessment

In the classic form of MSUD, infants appear normal at birth. Within the first week of life, acid-base, gastrointestinal, and neurologic problems appear. Initial signs of MSUD include poor feeding, vomiting, hypoglycemia, intermittent hypertonicity, lethargy, opisthotonos, and respiratory irregularities. Neurologic symptoms may be interpreted as indicative of meningitis or sepsis. Without intervention, symptoms progress to dehydration, decreased neonatal automatisms (automatic action reflexes), convulsions, severe ketoacidosis, acute pancreatitis, coma, and death within 2 to 4 weeks. Milder variant forms of MSUD present in early infancy with feeding difficulties, recurrent infections, episodic acidosis, and possibly coma. Untreated, these milder forms progress to retarded psychomotor development with clumsiness, ataxia, and positive Babinski's signs.

Diagnostic Tests. The key factor in assessment is early diagnosis. Laboratory findings indicative of MSUD reveal increased levels of leucine, isoleucine, valine, keto acids, and alloisoleucine in the child's plasma and urine. In utero diagnosis can be made by measuring defective enzyme activity in uncultured chorionic villus samples early in pregnancy. The nurse may be the first to recognize the presence of MSUD, typically by noting the characteristic maple syrup smell of the infant's urine when changing his or her diapers.

Nursing Diagnoses and Outcomes

Nursing diagnoses and outcomes for the child with a metabolic disease are presented in Chart 27–3. In addition, the following nursing diagnoses are applicable to the child with MSUD:

- **Risk for injury related to seizures**
  Outcomes: The child and family will manage the environment to protect the child from injury if seizures should occur.
  Pharmacologic management of the child's epileptic status will be monitored and maintained, accounting for changing demands related to illness and growth.
- **Ineffective infant feeding pattern related to neurologic deterioration**
  Outcome: The parents will demonstrate appropriate feeding techniques to ensure that the child is receiving adequate nutrition.
- **Risk for fluid volume deficit related to initiation of therapies to remove toxic metabolites (exchange transfusions, peritoneal dialysis, or hemodialysis)**
  Outcome: The child will not experience vascular, cellular, or intracellular dehydration as a result of therapies to remove the toxic metabolites.

Interdisciplinary Interventions

The management goals for MSUD are to establish an early diagnosis, to remove the toxic metabolites, and to prevent tissue catabolism. The endogenous proteolysis and amino acid catabolism can be suppressed initially with an intravenous glucose infusion. Intravenous fluids are also provided to correct fluid and electrolyte imbalances and to provide a high caloric intake. The nurse or a laboratory technician assists in drawing specimens to monitor the success of intravenous (IV) therapy. In addition, the nurse carefully monitors the IV site for infiltration and the child for further signs of dehydration or shock.

The removal of toxic metabolites requires exchange transfusion, peritoneal dialysis, or hemodialysis. Varying opinions and considerations influence the decision about which method to use. Studies have demonstrated that hemodialysis is more effective in rapidly removing toxic substrate. Exchange transfusion removes only the substrates confined to the vascular space, and hemodialysis removes substrates through total body water (Rutledge et al., 1990). Dialysis and exchange transfusion are sometimes combined with lipid infusion and insulin to promote anabolism. These extracorporeal techniques involve a risk of infection and increased catabolism. Some studies have suggested that they be used only in selected cases when the diagnosis has been made after the first week of life and/or the child's condition is life threatening (Parini et al., 1993). The nurse works with the health care team to provide these supportive therapies. Children requiring peritoneal dialysis are likely to be placed in an intensive care unit. Parents may feel intimidated by the setting and fearful for their child. The nurse can work with the social worker to provide support and teaching to assist the family through the crisis associated with the initial diagnosis and rigorous treatment modalities.

Nutritional Management. As soon as possible, oral or nasogastric tube feedings can be initiated to provide for the child's nutritional needs. Unlike the situation in some other metabolic disorders, in MSUD nutritional management alone does not decrease leucine levels quickly enough to reduce the risk of brain damage. Therefore, for the neonate, the initial treatment is dialysis accompanied by nutritional management.

When the removal of toxic metabolites has been achieved, dietary management is the primary component of ongoing treatment of MSUD. The required diet is high in calories but restricted in leucine, isoleucine, and valine. The diet should be started immediately after diagnosis and at least by the fifth day of life. Several proprietary formulas free of branched-chain amino acids (BCAAs) are available. If the child demonstrates feeding difficulties, nasogastric feedings may need to be initiated to ensure that the child's nutritional health is maintained. As the child gains strength and neurologic symptoms are arrested, feeding problems may resolve and the infant can be bottle fed once again.

Ongoing management with restricted intake of the branched-chain amino acids leucine, isoleucine, and valine must be adjusted with plasma levels. Plasma levels are monitored several times a week initially and frequently throughout the child's life. Leucine blood levels should range from 0.1 to 0.5 mmol/L. Valine and isoleucine can be reintroduced as the infant grows and the condition stabilizes. Poor tolerance of dietary leucine continues throughout life except in the variant forms of MSUD.

Some children with MSUD with residual enzyme activity are responsive to oral thiamine therapy (10 mg per day). However, the thiamine does not cure the metabolic error and is used as an adjunct to continued dietary restriction. Genetic therapy to correct the inborn error causing MSUD is also currently being researched.

caREminder: *Attention to the presence of catabolic states, even during minor illnesses, must continue throughout life.*

Community Care

When the child is ill, protein intake should be reduced and the caloric intake maintained by encouraging the use of carbohydrate- and fat-containing foods (Shih, 1993). The nurse can assist parents to learn how to perform tests for urinary ketones and/or keto acids at home should they note any changes in their child's behavior, if the child has an illness that could cause a metabolic imbalance, or if the child has not complied with prescribed dietary restrictions. Early treatment of dehydration and acidosis may prevent death. When the affected child has surgery for any reason, postoperative management must focus on the accelerated breakdown of body proteins, which results in high metabolite levels. Initial studies indicate that insulin therapy is an effective management strategy for this postoperative phenomenon (Biggemann, Zass, & Wendel, 1993).

Family education goals should focus on reinforcing the need for the prescribed dietary regimen, the importance of follow-up appointments, and the signs and symptoms of infection. As the child grows, the frequency and severity of crisis events decrease, although lifelong dietary management is recommended. Genetic counseling should be provided to family members, and identification of carriers of this metabolic condition is possible.

Mineral Disorders

Certain mineral disorders are inherited defects characterized by alterations in metabolic pathways for the essential body metals iron, copper, zinc, magnesium, molybdenum, and manganese. The defects can affect the absorption, transport, cellular use, storage, or excretion of a mineral needed to produce a variety of sequelae. Three of these disorders—Menkes' syndrome, hypophosphatemic rickets, and Wilson's disease—are discussed here. Table 27–5 highlights other selected mineral disorders.

Menkes' Syndrome

Menkes' syndrome, or trichopoliodystrophy, is sometimes called kinky hair or steely hair syndrome because of the unique kinky characteristic of the hair strands. Its hallmark is an extreme copper deficiency. This rare disorder affects all races and has an incidence of 1 in 254,000 live births in Western European countries (Holton, 1994). Menkes' syndrome is caused by a sex-linked recessive gene.

Pathophysiology

The primary defect in Menkes' syndrome is an intracellular defect in copper transport or binding. There is a reduced amount of the cuproenzymes, dopamine hydroxylase and cytochrome-*c* oxidase. As a result, the brain has a decreased content of unsaturated fatty acids. Tissues such as the brain, liver, and muscle are subject to increased lipofusion and degenerative changes. Malformation of connective tissue results in vascular, skeletal, dermal, and urogenital defects. Because copper does not cross the placenta in affected individuals, copper may be reduced in the liver and brain at birth.

Prognosis. Infants with Menkes' syndrome have a life expectancy of 4 months to 17 years. Death is usually due to intracranial hemorrhages, uncontrolled convulsions, severe failure to thrive, and/or infection. In some variants of the disease, long-term survival is possible. These affected children present later in childhood and show slowed growth, intellectual impairment, and neurologic deficits.

Antenatal diagnosis in at-risk pregnancies can be made for males (as the condition is sex-linked recessive) by measuring the uptake and retention of copper in vitro using cultured amniotic fibroblasts. The gene in individual families has been identified, making carrier testing possible. Termination of pregnancy can then be considered.

Treatment for classic Menkes' syndrome has not been successful in reversing the neurodegenerative changes; thus, management efforts are directed toward supportive care for the infant and family. Those with variants of the disease may benefit from therapy.

Assessment

Most children with Menkes' syndrome begin to exhibit symptoms by age 2 months. Some initial, nonspecific signs include prematurity, poor feeding, failure to thrive, and hypothermia. These signs should alert the nurse to perform a thorough physical assessment, which can identify the unique characteristics of this disease. Psychomotor developmental arrest and regression and general myoclonic seizures may be present as the disease continues undetected. Children with Menkes' syndrome have sev-

Table 27–5
Selected Mineral Disorders

Disorder	Inheritance	Pathophysiology	Significant Clinical Features	Laboratory Findings	Management	Prognosis
Menkes' syndrome	Sex-linked recessive (X chromosome)	Overt copper deficiency with systemic maldistribution of copper	Cherubic face Cupid's bow lip Kinky hair Pale skin Failure to thrive Skeletal deformities Psychomotor developmental retardation	Serum copper less than 10 μmol/L Hypoceruloplasminemia less than 20 mg/dL Low liver tissue copper concentrations less than 50 μg/g dry weight	Supportive care	Treatment not successful in reversing neurodegenerative changes.
Hypophosphatemic rickets	Sex-linked dominant	Exact molecular dysfunction unknown Causes phosphorus deficiency	Unstable, waddling gait Fractures, swelling, and pain of extremities Muscle weakness Teeth abscesses	Serum phosphate below 4 mg Alkaline phosphatase greater than 200 IU/L Reduced TmP/GFR in the presence of normal renal function	Vitamin D and phosphate supplements	Early treatment can result in normal bone development.
Wilson's disease	Autosomal recessive (chromosome 13)	Impaired hepatic secretion of copper Defective incorporation of copper into apoceruloplasmin	Hepatitis Encephalopathy Kayser-Fleischer rings Hemolysis Seizures	Plasma copper concentration below 10 μmol/L Hypoceruloplasminemia less than 200 mg/L Urinary copper greater than 100 μg per 24 hr Liver tissue content greater than 25 g per g dry weight	Chelation therapy with low-copper diet Liver transplantation	Fatal if untreated. Better outcomes reported with use of chelation therapy and liver transplantation.

Primary hypomagnesemia	Autosomal recessive (chromosome unknown)	Intestinal malabsorption of magnesium	Small for gestational age Sleeping and feeding difficulties in infancy Progressive neurologic dysfunction including hyperactivity, tetany and convulsions Renal tubular acidosis	Hypomagnesemia, less than 0.7 mmol/L Hypocalcemia	Parenteral or intramuscular magnesium of 0.4 to 0.75 mmol/kg per day, followed by oral supplements Calcium supplements	Well controlled if management maintained.
Acrodermatitis enteropathica	Autosomal recessive (chromosome unknown)	Systemic zinc deficiency	Neuropsychiatric disorders Dermatitis Alopecia Ophthalmologic problems Frequent, loose stools Failure to thrive Recurrent infections Swollen, painful fingers and toes	Plasma zinc concentrations below 9 μmol/L	Zinc supplements of 35–100 mg per day	Progressive deterioration without treatment. In less severe cases, only growth retardation and delayed development are evident.
Hereditary hemochromatosis	Autosomal recessive (chromosome 6)	Excessive accumulation of iron causing extensive tissue damage	Lassitude Pigmentation of skin, lips, tongue, buccal mucosa, conjunctiva, scars, and external genitalia Loss of body hair Dermal atrophy Hepatosplenomegaly Abdominal pain Weight loss Chondrocalcinosis Diabetes mellitus Pituitary damage Testicular atrophy Gynecomastia Cardiac failure	Serum iron greater than 25 μmol/L Liver iron content by biopsy greater than 1000 μg per 100 mg dry weight	Phlebotomy to reduce iron	Organ damage can be prevented with treatment.

eral characteristic features. The head and face are distinctive with a placid, cherubic face; frontal and occipital bossing; micrognathia; Cupid's bow lip; gingival hyperplasia; high arched palate; delayed eruption of the teeth; and hair that appears normal at birth but becomes lusterless and depigmented, feels like steel wool, and breaks easily. The hair appears twisted microscopically and kinky clinically, hence the name kinky hair disease. Mental retardation and several central nervous system difficulties can also be noted. These children often have dysphagia, hypotonia, apnea, and spasticity with hyperreflexia. Optic problems such as retinal degeneration, optic atrophy, cataracts, and blindness are usually present.

Diagnostic Tests. When the health care team's suspicions are aroused by the physical examination, laboratory values and genetic testing can confirm the diagnosis. Laboratory findings indicative of Menkes' syndrome include hypocupremia (serum copper less than 10 mol/L), hypoceruloplasminemia (ceruloplasmin less than 20 mg/dL), and low hepatic copper concentrations (less than 50 g per gram dry weight). The radiologic findings show metaphyseal spurring primarily of the femur and subperiosteal calcifications of the bone shafts. Arteriography demonstrates tortuosity and elongation of cerebral and systemic arteries with occlusion of some vessels. A detailed family history and genetic assessment can determine females at risk for producing affected offspring. Also, family members with variants of the disease may be identified.

Interdisciplinary Interventions

At this time, only supportive therapy is available for children with classic Menkes' syndrome. Although parenteral administration of copper salts corrects the serum and hepatic copper, the child's neurologic symptoms are not affected. Thus, this treatment is considered to be only palliative and is not often prescribed. In some variants of the disease, early treatment with parenteral copper-histidine may be effective. Pharmacologic management of seizures and infection should be initiated as these occur over the child's life span.

Radiant heat may be required to correct hypothermia, especially in the neonatal period. Vigilant monitoring for the early signs of infection (e.g., elevated temperature, vomiting, fussiness) allows specific work-up and management. Careful observation to identify focal or generalized seizures permits early anticonvulsant therapy. Gentle handling of the child and padding of the crib sides help to minimize the risk of fracture. A high-calorie diet with careful monitoring of the child's weight gain should be initiated at the time of diagnosis. If vomiting caused by gastroesophageal reflux occurs, positioning and possibly nasogastric feedings may be necessary.

Nursing efforts should be directed to helping the infant or child thrive to his or her greatest potential while supporting the family in the care techniques to achieve this goal. The families of children with Menkes' syndrome are most likely to display all the stages of grief as they cope with their child's terminal prognosis (see Chapter 12 for nursing interventions). Further stress is added because of the implications for future pregnancies. Fortunately, genetic testing is available. Groups of parents whose children have the same or similar problem are frequently helpful, and groups focusing on dealing with the death of a child may be warranted later. The possibility of frequent hospitalizations because of complications may require financial counseling. The coordination of acute care, home care agencies, and possibly a hospice service should be established as needs arise.

Hypophosphatemic Rickets

Hypophosphatemic rickets is the predominant form of metabolic bone disease. It is also known as vitamin D–resistant rickets or X-linked hypophosphatemia. This non-nutritional condition is caused by a phosphorus deficiency and characterized by inadequate mineralization of the bone. The disease is usually due to sex-linked dominant inheritance. It is hypothesized that spontaneous genetic mutations occur, because both autosomal recessive and autosomal dominant variants have been described.

Pathophysiology

The exact molecular dysfunction causing hypophosphatemic rickets is not known. Possible causes include a defect in the 25-hydroxylase enzyme. For whatever reason, a phosphorus deficiency develops. Phosphorus stimulates bone formation and inhibits resorption. Phosphorus levels are usually normal at birth because of placental transport, and the full-term infant's bone marrow shows normal initial development. This is not true with the premature infant, especially those younger than 28 weeks' gestation or with a birth weight below 1500 g. Bone mineralization takes place in the third trimester, and the bones of low-gestational-age and low-birth-weight infants are often weak and undermineralized.

Prognosis. Early, adequate management of phosphorus and calcium levels usually results in normal bone development. Lack of or inadequate treatment may result in the need for corrective orthopedic surgery for leg lengthening and straightening procedures. There have been some reports of a self-resolving phosphorus deficiency in selected patients. The management of hypophosphatemic rickets is designed to promote normal bone strength and growth.

Assessment

Full-term infants appear normal at birth. The disease becomes clinically detectable about the first year of life, when a mild to moderate linear growth deficiency can be noted. As the child begins to walk, the femur and tibia bow (genu valgum) as a result of weight bearing. This, combined with a developing tibial torsion, gives the child an unstable, waddling gait. Fractures, signs of swelling, and pain, especially in the extremities, would indicate a need for further assessment in any infant or toddler. Muscle weakness and decreased energy levels may also be noted. Dentin formation is often faulty, and healthy teeth may develop spontaneous abscesses. Males are often affected more severely than females because of the random inactivation of the X chromosome early in fetal development.

Diagnostic Tests. Significant laboratory findings include serum phosphorus below 4 mg (although this may remain normal up to age 9 months despite disease), alkaline phosphatase greater than 200 IU/L (in preterm infants, greater than 300 to 400 IU/L), and reduced TmP/GFR (transfer maximum for phosphate per unit volume of glomerular filtration rate) in the presence of normal renal tubular function. Radiologic findings are more apparent in the lower body and include fractures of the long bones and ribs (may be noted in the premature infant by 10 weeks of age); fraying, widening, and cupping of the metaphyses (especially of the tibia, femur, ulna, and radius); thickened cortices of long bone shafts with dense trabecular bone (first seen in late childhood); and calcification of tendons, ligament insertions, and joint capsules (adolescence and older).

Nursing Diagnoses and Outcomes

The deficiency of phosphorus in children with hypophosphatemic rickets places the children at risk for orthopedic and dental problems. Therefore, in addition to the nursing diagnoses presented in Chart 27–3, the following diagnoses would be applicable to this patient population:

- **Risk for activity intolerance related to potential for fractures, bone pain, and skeletal deformities**
  Outcomes: The child will participate in activities appropriate to the ability level and that do not pose a threat of injury.
  School teachers and caregivers will assist the child in pursuing activities that are safe and will build the child's self-confidence.
- **Body image disturbance related to skeletal deformities**
  Outcome: The child and caregivers will maintain positive conscious and unconscious perceptions and attitudes about the child's appearance.
- **Altered oral mucous membrane related to higher incidence of dental abscesses**
  Outcome: The child will receive early recognition and treatment of abscessed teeth.
- **Impaired verbal communication related to high number of dental extractions**
  Outcome: Impaired speech will be prevented by appropriate speech therapy measures.

Interdisciplinary Interventions

Interdisciplinary interventions begin with the prescription of a combination of vitamin D plus a phosphate supplement. Vitamin D, which is a steroid hormone and not a vitamin, is required to stimulate absorption of calcium and phosphorus in the intestine. The usual therapeutic dose range is 5 to 50 mg/kg per day in the form of 1,25-dihydroxyvitamin D_3. To normalize the serum phosphate, the usual dosage range of phosphate supplement is 70 to 100 mg/kg per day (Hisano, Latta, & Chan, 1993).

Nephrocalcinosis and secondary hyperparathyroidism are possible complications of vitamin D and phosphate management. Children must be observed for signs of hypercalcemia. These signs include weakness, fatigue, lassitude, headache, nausea, vomiting, and diarrhea. Serum and urine calcium levels must be monitored routinely, and the kidneys should be periodically evaluated by ultrasonography.

Debate continues about whether patients should be treated into adulthood or through pregnancy. Usually, treatment for asymptomatic patients is discontinued as they approach adulthood. Treatment with growth hormone for rachitic children who do not achieve normal linear growth is currently under investigation. Research on the correction of the basic metabolic error through genetic therapy is also in progress. Of special note is that diuretics cause increased calcium excretion, which stimulates calcium reabsorption from the bone to maintain a normal serum calcium.

caREminder: *Rachitic patients receiving diuretics must be monitored for development of osteoporosis.*

Chest physical therapy may be ordered, especially for the premature infant, who is likely to develop bronchopulmonary dysplasia. Therapists must be careful not to cause rib fractures with manual percussion; therefore, electric vibrators may provide safer treatment.

Nutritional Management. Special nutritional consideration is needed for the premature infant. Preterm breast milk contains adequate quantities of all the essential nutrients *except* calcium and phosphorus. Commercial preterm formula contains the necessary additional calcium and phosphorus, but premature infants must receive total parenteral nutrition until they are able to take and tolerate adequate amounts of formula. Soy formulas have a phytase binding quality that inhibits the intestinal absorption of phosphorus and should be avoided.

Community Care

Oral medications are required for years. Parents who are taught to give both medications together at set times of the day are most likely to remember to do so. This also establishes a routine pattern for children to use as they become more independent in taking responsibility for their medications. When the child enters daycare or school, teachers need to know the diagnosis, precautions, and the importance of the medication to ensure that the usual four times daily dosing regimen continues.

Dental problems are a continuing challenge for the child with rickets because of the tendency to abscess. Primary teeth are usually extracted if abscessed. Depending on the site and number of extractions, speech could be adversely affected, and there may be a need for speech therapy. Root canals or other endodontic procedures are usually necessary for abscesses of the secondary teeth. The nurse must work with the child and the family to communicate the importance of good dental hygiene and regular visits to the dentist. Children should be encouraged to brush after every meal. The school nurse can support these actions by offering a place for the child to store their cleaning materials and brush their teeth.

Gentle handling of premature infants and any child with rickets is critical to prevent fractures. Family members need to be taught the importance of this concept as well. The nurse or social worker can discuss nonphysical forms of discipline with the parents. In addition, parents, daycare providers, and school officials require guidance in selecting safe, soft toys for the child and in providing activities that safeguard against physical harm. For instance, contact sports and gymnastics are not recommended. The child's musical, science, or computer interests should be encouraged, as these are all safe activities that can enhance self-esteem and minimize physical injury. Self-image and esteem are important concepts to build in the rachitic child. If growth has been slowed, the child may be sensitive about being shorter than peers. The risk of fractures will probably limit the child's involvement in physical education, sports, and rough games. This, too, sets the child apart from others and the child may become the focus of teasing. Family counseling and support groups can help prepare the child to cope with this and identify areas where he or she can excel to gain peer recognition.

The family may need financial support to manage the child's care properly. The cost of years of medications, laboratory tests, and follow-up visits with the possible additional expenses of orthopedic surgery and dental care is financially significant. (See Chapter 7 for a discussion of financial support options for the family.)

Wilson's Disease

Characterized by cirrhosis of the liver and degenerative changes in the brain, Wilson's disease is another aberrant manifestation of copper metabolism. Although the symptoms are primarily hepatic, multisystem toxicity does occur. The disease is fatal unless recognized and treated early.

Occurring in 1 in 30,000 to 100,000 children, Wilson's disease results from a defective gene located on chromosome 13. There may be persistence of the fetal pattern of copper metabolism.

Pathophysiology

The metabolic defect in Wilson's disease impairs the normal hepatic excretion of dietary copper and impairs incorporation of copper into ceruloplasmin. As a result, soon after birth, copper begins to accumulate in the liver, causing progressive hepatic damage. Fatty changes, inflammation, necrosis, and fibrosis combine to cause cirrhosis of the liver by adolescence (Collins & Scheinberg, 1993). Diffusion of copper into the blood leads to further diffusion into the central nervous system, the kidneys, and the eyes.

Prognosis. About 80% of children with Wilson's disease become ill or die of the disorder by age 21 (Collins & Scheinberg, 1992). Although the disorder is invariably fatal if not treated, administration of chelating agents or liver transplantation may lead to a positive prognosis when the disease is identified. Management is aimed at minimizing liver and neurologic damage, as well as controlling the effects of copper toxicity on other body systems.

Assessment

Wilson's disease can present as early as age 4 years. The onset is variable, and the diagnosis can easily be missed because of the natural tendency to focus on the severe liver or neurologic manifestations. Wilson's disease should be confirmed or ruled out in any child with a family history of the disease; unexplained hepatic, neurologic, or psychiatric disease; characteristic corneal copper deposits (Kayser-Fleischer rings); or unexplained deficiency of ceruloplasmin. During health assessment, the nurse should note whether a sibling or first cousin has been previously diagnosed with the disease or has demonstrated symptoms similar to those of the child being evaluated. In addition, investigation for Wilson's disease should be done for all patients with hemolysis or recurrent jaundice.

The physical manifestations of Wilson's disease appear in multiple body systems. All affected children have hepatic involvement. However, only about 40% of children have hepatic symptoms such as chronic or active hepatitis, cirrhosis, or hepatic insufficiency. Neurologic symptoms occur in 35% to 40% of affected children and include encephalopathy, ataxia, fine tremor, dysarthria, dysphagia, dystonia, and epilepsy. Hematologic effects include acute hemolysis and coagulopathies. Ophthalmic signs include the characteristic Kayser-Fleischer rings, visible on slit-lamp ophthalmologic examination. Cataracts, strabismus, and impaired visual acuity may also be noted. Renal involvement is related to renal tubular acidosis, aminoaciduria, acute renal failure, and hematuria. Skeletal involvement includes osteoporosis and osteoarthritis. Amenorrhea and an increased incidence of spontaneous abortions are noted in affected adolescents. Other symptoms include abdominal pain, bacterial peritonitis, and blue lunules of the fingernails. About 12% of affected children exhibit neuropsychiatric disorders such as sudden onset of socially inappropriate behavior, depression, deterioration in school performance, or obsessive, bipolar, or schizophrenic behaviors (Holton, 1994).

Diagnostic Tests. Laboratory findings indicative of Wilson's disease include plasma copper concentration below 10 μmol/L, hypoceruloplasminemia (ceruloplasmin less than 200 mg/L), urinary copper greater than 100 μg per 24 hours, and liver tissue copper content greater than 25 μg per gram dry weight.

Interdisciplinary Interventions

Chelating agents and a low-copper diet are the primary treatments for Wilson's disease. Penicillamine (the drug of choice), trientine, and British antilewisite (BAL) may be given to promote urinary excretion of copper and detoxify excess copper remaining in the liver. The oral medication is given in two to four divided doses, 30 minutes before or 2 hours after meals. Because penicillamine causes antipyridoxine activity, a daily pyridoxine supplement is added to the patient's diet. Oral zinc gluconate and other zinc salts may also be prescribed. The zinc products have proven effective in arresting liver damage, although they cannot reverse existing hepatic cirrhosis, portal hypertension, or neurologic symptoms.

The nurse needs to emphasize to the child and family that the medications must be taken at all times and continued throughout the child's life. During the first month of treatment with penicillamine, the parents need to be alert for the development of fever and rash, sometimes accompanied by enlarged lymph nodes. Leukopenia or thrombocytopenia may also develop. If these adverse effects occur, the drug is discontinued until they subside, then gradually reintroduced. If the adverse effects persist, penicillamine may be discontinued and trientine given instead. In addition, findings of proteinuria, a possible late adverse reaction, would direct the health care team to change the chelating agent from penicillamine to trientine.

Nutritional Management. Treatment for Wilson's disease commonly involves a low-copper diet in conjunction with chelation therapy. Chart 27–9 lists foods with high and low copper content. The nutritionist can serve as an expert consultant to the health care team and the family. Working with the family, the nutritionist evaluates the child's urinary copper level and adjusts the child's diet accordingly. Foods rich in copper can be eaten in moderation as long as drug treatment is maintained (Fig. 27–4).

Surgical Management. A child with fulminant hepatitis or hepatic failure related to Wilson's disease may be a candidate for liver transplantation. The transplant cures the genetic defect and restores normal copper balance. Further neurologic deterioration is halted, although no clear evidence of reversal of neurologic symptoms has been supported. The family of a candidate for liver transplantation needs assistance in becoming part of the organ transplant network. Social services can serve as liaisons between the family and the transplant agencies. During

Chart 27–9

Foods Low and High in Copper

Foods Low in Copper

Cow's milk
Tomatoes
Cheese
Corn
Yogurt
Potatoes
Lettuce
Apples
Oranges

Foods High in Copper

Molasses
Wheat germ
Sunflower seed
Organ meats
Shellfish
High-protein dry baby cereal
Chocolate
Cocoa
Dried legumes
Broccoli
Nuts
Mushrooms

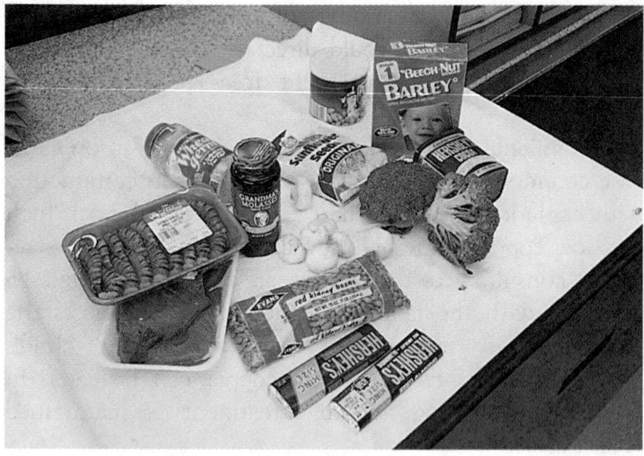

Figure 27–4
Foods rich in copper must be eaten only in moderation by the child with Wilson's disease.

the evaluation and waiting period before transplantation surgery, the family needs intensive emotional support. The social worker can help the family to prepare for the transplantation and to get in touch with families of children who have already undergone the procedure.

Community Care

Through the phases of Wilson's disease, including diagnosis, ongoing management, monitoring of its effects, and the liver transplantation process, numerous invasive procedures are required. Play therapy to alleviate the fear of these procedures is helpful. Children may experience symptoms that keep them from attending school. If this occurs, home-bound school programs should be arranged early.

The nurse plays an important role in the ongoing monitoring and management of the child with Wilson's disease. Responses to drug and dietary regimes are evaluated at frequent intervals during the first year of therapy and on a routine basis as the child develops and grows. Blood and urine analyses are the primary modes of evaluation. Patient and family education about the blood and urine collection should stress its importance for therapeutic management of the disease.

Tip: *Twenty-four-hour urine specimens are difficult to collect from children who "forget" to save their urine. Collection should be done when the child is at home during the entire collection process. The child should be encouraged to void in only one bathroom, a collection device should always be in place, and a reward can be offered for each successful collection of urine.*

The nurse can also help parents determine whether the child's symptoms are improving or worsening when treatment has begun. Because children may have different and varying overt signs of the disease, the nurse should review with the family the particular signs that their child has demonstrated and which of these signs are expected to diminish with treatment. Diminished cerebral and hepatic signs and symptoms and fading Kayser-Fleischer rings are the best indicators of successful therapy.

As the child matures, the nurse can work with the nutritionist, the child, and the family to expand the child's diet and personal responsibility for making dietary selections. Family members should be screened for presymptomatic Wilson's disease. Asymptomatic siblings can prevent any expression of the disease by early initiation of the chelating agents. In addition, genetic screening should be provided to all family members to detect asymptomatic homozygote carriers. The nurse can discuss with the family the results of the screening examinations and the implications for future pregnancies, prenatal diagnosis, and cessation of pregnancy if necessary.

Carbohydrate Disorders

Carbohydrates include starch, sucrose, and lactose. Various disorders related to interruptions in the pathway of carbohydrate metabolism result from specific genetic defects. Their classifications include galactose disorders, glycogen storage disorders, and fructose disorders (Table 27–6).

Galactosemia

Galactosemia is the most common and the first recognized disorder of galactose metabolism. An inherited autosomal recessive trait, galactosemia occurs in one of seven different forms, depending on the degree to which the metabolic pathway is blocked. Genotyping is required to determine the specific classification. Affected tissues include the lens, liver, brain, kidney, and ovary. Estimates of the incidence of galactosemia vary from 1 in 35,000 to 1 in 200,000 births.

Pathophysiology

The classic form of galactosemia involves a defect in the enzyme galactose-1-phosphate uridyltransferase (G-1-PUT). This defect disrupts the conversion of galactose 1-phosphate to galactose uridine diphosphate. Consequently, galactose, a monosaccharide, is not converted to glucose.

Prognosis. Severe, untreated cases of galactosemia are invariably fatal. Patients affected less severely have retarded psychomotor development, visual impairment, and residual cirrhosis. If chronic errors in metabolism persist, other complications appear despite treatment. Such com-

Table 27–6
Selected Carbohydrate Disorders

Disorder	Pathophysiology	Significant Clinical Features	Key Diagnostic Findings	Management	Prognosis
Galactosemia	Defective galactose 1-phosphate uridyltransferase enzyme; galactose not converted to glucose	Normal at birth, symptomatic after first lactose feeding Anorexia Vomiting Diarrhea Jaundice Hepatomegaly Increased susceptibility to infection Cataracts (later in life) Mental retardation	Elevated serum and urine galactose Elevated serum galactose 1-phosphate Generalized aminoaciduria	Exclusion of lactose and galactose from diet Diet free of all milk products Lactose-free formula used	Fatal if severe and untreated Near-normal intelligence if compliant with diet
Hereditary fructose intolerance	Defect in fructose 1-phosphate aldolase B enzyme; fructose not converted to glucose	Infants: anorexia, vomiting, failure to thrive, hypoglycemic convulsions, liver and kidney dysfunction Older children: spontaneous hypoglycemia and vomiting after ingestion of fructose	Increased serum and urine fructose	Diet free of fructose and sucrose	Good if diet followed

plications may include speech abnormalities, ovarian failure, and cognitive deficits (Holton, 1994).

Assessment

Infants with galactosemia appear normal at birth. Symptoms develop in the first days of life after the infant has begun the ingestion of formula containing lactose, which interrupts the metabolic pathway. The infant may exhibit anorexia, vomiting, diarrhea, and lethargy. The baby fails to thrive if a galactose-restricted diet is not instituted. Other common signs in untreated infants include drowsiness, inattention, hypotonia, decreased vigor of neonatal automatisms, bulging fontanels, hepatosplenomegaly, jaundice, and anemia. Septicemia and urinary tract infection may occur. An accumulation of galactitol in the lens may lead to cataract development. Physical and mental retardation become evident over time.

Some forms of galactosemia have a delayed onset, as late as adolescence. These individuals are intellectually subnormal, socially maladjusted, and may exhibit cerebellar ataxia, dystonia, and apraxia.

Diagnostic Tests. Early identification of galactosemia is possible through the blood assay completed in newborn screening; however, not all states include galactosemia in their screening programs. Laboratory findings indicative of galactosemia include elevated blood galactose level, low glucose level, galactosuria (urinary total reducing substances should be tested with Clinitest; may produce a false positive), positive Benedict's test of urine, deficiency of G-1-PUT in red and white blood cells and liver cells, Beutler's assay of red cell enzyme activity (confirms the diagnosis), and hypocalcemia and aminoaciduria in acute illness.

With each pregnancy there is a one-in-four chance that the parents will have another child with galactosemia. Prenatal testing by amniocentesis or chorionic villus sampling is available and should be offered.

Nursing Diagnoses and Outcomes

Nursing diagnoses to support the dietary management of galactosemia are consistent with the diagnoses associated with other metabolic conditions (see Chart 27–3). The child with galactosemia is at risk for infection and dehydration, as well as the development of cataracts. Thus, appropriate nursing diagnoses may include the following:

- **Risk for infection**
  Outcome: Prevention and early detection of infection in the child will be supported.

Chart 27–10

Foods Restricted and Allowed in the Galactose-Free Diet

Restricted Foods

Milk
Cheese
Ice cream
Yogurt
Pudding
Bread
Organ meats, brains, and mussels
Prepared foods containing galactose (e.g., baked goods, confections, and frozen foods)
Drug preparations that contain lactose as a filler

Foods Allowed

Soy-based formula (Nutramigen or Alimentum)
Cereals
Vegetables
Fruit
Meats
Kosher foods

- **Fluid volume deficit related to vomiting and diarrhea**
  Outcomes: Vomiting and diarrhea will be corrected through introduction of a galactose-restricted diet.
  Measures will be instituted to correct fluid and electrolyte imbalances.
- **Sensory/perceptual alterations: visual**
  Outcomes: The child will be evaluated on a regular basis for the presence of cataracts.
  Visual acuity will be optimized by the maintenance of a galactose-free diet.

Interdisciplinary Interventions

Nutritional Management. The primary goal in managing the child with galactosemia is to maintain galactose-1-phosphate levels below 150 mol per liter of packed red cells. This is accomplished by a strict dietary regimen. Reinforcement of the prescribed diet is necessary with each family contact. A galactose-restricted diet rapidly resolves most acute symptoms. Galactose is derived from the hydrolysis of lactose into glucose and galactose. The diet is milk free, with *all* sources of lactose restricted (Chart 27–10). A soy protein isolate formula with added methionine and carnitine can provide all necessary nutrients for the infant. As processed foods are added to the child's diet, labels must be checked for the presence of milk or milk products such as dry milk solids, lactose, curds, and whey (Fig. 27–5). Casein, a milk protein sometimes called hydrolyzed protein, must also be avoided. Parents can be advised that kosher foods are usually lactose free. These products can be a source of dietary options for the child. The nurse and the dietician can work together to ensure that the child is receiving adequate calories, protein, vitamins, and minerals such as calcium. Recipes using galactose-free milk substitutes can be provided to the family (Chart 27–11).

The restricted diet is generally recommended for life. However, some practitioners have allowed limited liberalization of the diet when the child starts school (Jones, 1993). Parents must understand that the child does not develop an increased tolerance for milk products as he or she grows older. Loosening of the dietary restrictions is viewed as a mechanism to prevent total rejection of the diet by a child who wishes to assert some independence in dietary choices. Studies have indicated that children who included some milk-containing products in their diet have significantly lower IQs (Jones, 1993). Therefore, occasional deviations from the diet can be tolerated but not encouraged.

Medical Management. Infections, most commonly with gram-negative organisms, are treated with the appropriate antibiotic. If jaundice is present in the newborn, exchange transfusions may be required. Other supportive therapies include the resolution of any dehydration and electrolyte imbalances that have occurred as a result of the vomiting, anorexia, and diarrhea. Females who manifest symptoms of ovarian dysfunction, including irregular menses and decreased fertility, may require hormonal therapy.

All children diagnosed with galactosemia should be evaluated for cataracts. In many cases, introduction of

Figure 27–5
Milk-containing foods and organ meats, normally an important part of a child's diet, must be avoided by the child with galactosemia.

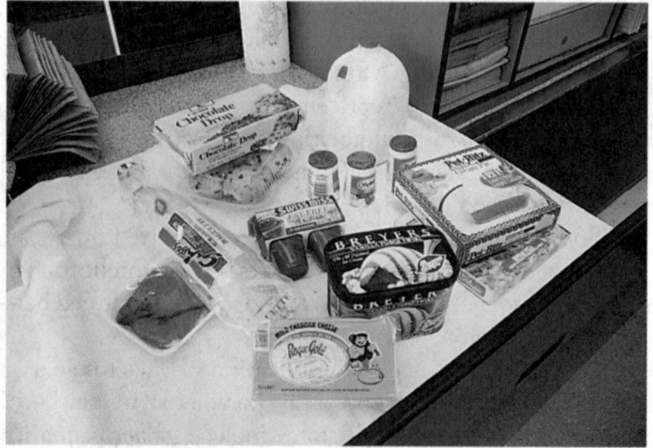

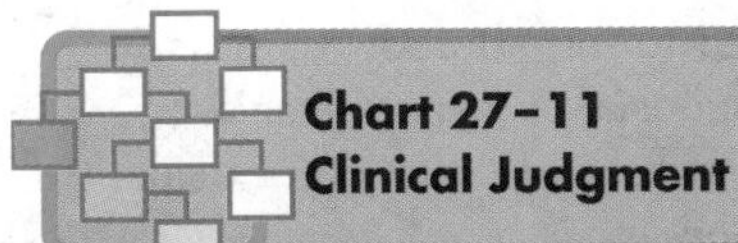

Chart 27–11
Clinical Judgment

Nutritional Counseling

Nikki was born 2 months ago, normal for gestational age and without any postnatal complications. The results of Nikki's neonatal screening test were positive for galactosemia. The parents, Melissa and Tom, both 17, were called and Nikki was brought back to the clinic for a repeated blood test. The diagnosis is confirmed. You have been asked to provide teaching regarding the child's diet and home management. As you enter the room, Nikki's mother is clutching her baby and crying. Nikki's father has stepped out of the room to smoke a cigarette.

Questions

1. Before your teaching, what assessment data would it be helpful to collect about the family?
2. Although the child is not eating solid foods, why do you want to know more about the family's diet?
3. What factors about the parents would influence your teaching?
4. What topics should your nutritional counseling cover?
5. How could you evaluate the effectiveness of your teaching?

Answers

1. Family dietary patterns and dietary preferences related to ethnic or religious influences. Will health care insurance cover the cost of medical food? Primary caretaker of infant, including daycare providers.
2. The child needs a lactose-free diet. Milk products are contained in a variety of products. Family members need to start learning which of those products they should not introduce to the child once feeding has begun.
3. Parents' level of understanding of the metabolic condition itself; parents' ability to accept the diagnosis realistically and take responsibility for the child's care.
4. Name of diet. Why the diet will help the child. Formula that the child may drink. How to obtain formula. Signs and symptoms of worsening condition. Management of the child during childhood illnesses. How the diet will change as the child grows.
5. Use "scenarios" to have parents select appropriate formula. Parents should relate the signs and symptoms of formula intolerance. Call parents in 1 week and again in 2 weeks for follow-up.

the galactose-free diet leads to spontaneous resolution of the cataracts. Yearly evaluation of the child by an ophthalmologist is highly recommended. Children who do not adhere well to the diet are at risk for developing cataracts, as are those who were not diagnosed and treated for the metabolic condition at an early age.

Community Care

Children, even those with controlled galactosemia, may experience learning difficulties. One study demonstrated that 45% of children with galactosemia had some form of developmental delay, despite adherence to the galactose-free diet (Jones, 1993). These delays included speech problems; difficulties with coordination, gait, balance, and fine motor skills; and declining IQ scores. Family conferences with schoolteachers or daycare workers help school personnel understand the need for specialized classes and teaching techniques that enhance the child's developmental abilities. In addition, the nurse can work with school officials to emphasize the need to monitor the child's diet when away from home and find ways to offer dietary alternatives when special class functions are occurring.

Red Cell Disorders

Red blood cells exchange oxygen and carbon dioxide between the lungs and other body tissues. This function becomes impaired when disease or genetic abnormalities result in a significant decrease in red blood cell production or when there is a serious loss of red cells such as with hemorrhage. Destruction of the red blood cell, hemolysis, can also occur and is due to defects in the red cell's membrane or intracellular structure or to extracellular factors such as abnormalities of the red blood cell enzymes.

The hemolytic anemias are discussed more fully in Chapter 23. However, the metabolic disorder glucose-6-phosphate dehydrogenase deficiency is the most common cause of hemolysis resulting from a red blood cell enzyme abnormality and as such is discussed here.

Glucose-6-Phosphate Dehydrogenase Deficiency

Glucose-6-phosphate dehydrogenase (G-6-PD) deficiency is the most common known red cell enzymopathy. Most individuals are not severely affected and require an intake of a specific oxidant to become symptomatic. G-6-PD deficiency affects approximately 400 million people worldwide. Synthesis of red cell G-6-PD is determined by a gene on the X chromosome; therefore, the disorder is more common in males (Segel, 1996). Incidence is greatest in children of African, Mediterranean, Greek, Italian, Middle Eastern, and Asian descent. There are many genetic variants, resulting in a spectrum of G-6-PD enzyme activity ranging from normal to severe deficiency.

Pathophysiology

The metabolic role of G-6-PD is to defend the red cell against oxidation. Patients with G-6-PD deficiency suffer hemolysis when the red cell is stressed with oxidizing agents. The mechanism of this hemolysis is not yet fully known.

Prognosis. A small percentage of G-6-PD–deficient individuals have a chronic hemolytic disorder that can be quite severe (Scriver, Beaudet, Sly, & Vawlle, 1989). In most instances, when G-6-PD deficiency is diagnosed, hemolytic crisis can be averted by avoiding exogenous oxidants, which include fava beans and hemolytic drugs (Table 27–7). Thus, the goal of management is to decrease the incidence of hemolysis by avoiding the intake of oxidants and reducing the risk of infection.

Assessment

Most children with G-6-PD deficiency are asymptomatic. In some, infection, diabetic acidosis, or hypoglycemia may cause a mild hemolysis. Parents should be questioned regarding the recent ingestion by the child of any agents that can cause hemolysis.

Worldview: *One type of acute and severe hemolytic syndrome is called favism. It is caused by ingestion of fava beans, which are a staple in the Mediterranean diet. Therefore, assessment should include asking parents if fava beans are part of the child's diet.*

Neonates with G-6-PD deficiency may develop hemolytic anemia and jaundice, the severity of which depends on the degree of enzyme defect in the red cell.

Diagnostic Tests. A hematologic assessment for oxidative damage during crisis produces positive findings for Heinz bodies, methemoglobin, sulfhemoglobin, red cell fragmentation, and intravascular hemolysis. A G-6-PD assay can be performed with a spectrophotometer.

Nursing Diagnoses and Outcomes

Red cell disorders impair the production of components of the blood. Nursing diagnoses and interventions are aimed at preventing crisis events that would exacerbate the metabolic condition and providing care and support to the child when blood transfusions are required. In addition to the diagnoses presented in Chart 27–3, the following diagnoses may be applicable for the child with G-6-PD:

- **Risk for injury related to ingestion of oxidants, infections, diabetic acidosis, or hypoglycemia**
  Outcomes: The child will avoid ingestion of oxidants, which can cause hemolysis.
  Prevention and early detection of infection in the child will be supported.
  Measures will be taken to prevent diabetic acidosis or hypoglycemia.
- **Fear related to frequent transfusions and hospitalizations**
  Outcome: The child and family will utilize effective coping mechanisms to deal with crises that occur in the management of the child's condition

Interdisciplinary Interventions

Children who exhibit a chronic hemolytic disorder or experience an acute hemolytic crisis require monitoring and supportive care. Maintaining adequate hydration and providing blood transfusions may be indicated to correct an anemic state. Generally, recovery from a hemolytic episode occurs rapidly with the removal of the oxidant agent. Displacement bone marrow transplantation may correct homozygous G-6-PD deficiency (Schaub, Van Hoof, & Vios, 1991).

Prevention is by far the most important intervention. When possible, male children belonging to ethnic groups in which G-6-PD is most common should be tested for the defect before being given any of the known oxidant drugs (Segel, 1996). In addition to education that stresses the need to avoid oxidants, families should be taught the signs of infection, especially those of the upper respiratory and gastrointestinal tracts, so that they can be alert to a possible impending hemolytic episode.

Alert: *The presence of any infectious process can precipitate a hemolytic crisis. Infections should not be treated with aspirin, as this is a secondary agent that worsens the hemolytic episode.*

Signs of pallor, hemoglobinuria, and jaundice should be reported to the health care provider immediately, as these are symptoms of hemolysis. Aggressive management of viral illness may prevent hemolytic crisis. Viral infections of the upper respiratory and gastrointestinal tracts appear to cause more severe hemolysis than bacterial infections in the G-6-PD–deficient child.

Breast-feeding mothers of G-6-PD–deficient infants must be warned that some oxidants they ingest appear in breast milk. Fava beans pass through to breast milk, and if any of the hemolytic drugs are prescribed, a pharmacist or medical professional should be consulted concerning the safety of continuing breast-feeding. In these instances, breast-feeding should be discontinued or an alternative, nonoxidant medication chosen.

Table 27–7
Oxidant Agents That Can Cause a Hemolytic Crisis

Generic Name	Trade Name
Aminoquinolines	
Primaquine	Aralen
Pamaquine	
Chloroquine	
Pentaquine	
Sulfones	
Diaminodiphenylsulfone (dapsone)	
Sulfoxone	
Thiazosulfone	
Sulfonamides	
Sulfanilamide	AVC cream, suppositories
Sulfacetamide	Sultrin, Trysul, Bleph-10 or Blephamide ophthalmic solution, Sodium Sulamyd ophthalmic solution
Sulfafurazole	
Sulfisoxazole	Gantrisin, Azo Gantrisin, Pediazole
Sulfamethoxazole	Bactrim, Gantanol, Septra
Nitrofurans	
Nitrofurantoin	Furadantin, Macrodantin
Furozolidone	Furoxone
Nitrofurazone	Furacin
Analgesics	
Acetylsalicylic acid (aspirin)	
Acetanilid	
Acetophenetidin, phenacetin	
Miscellaneous	
Vitamin K (water soluble)	
Naphthalene	Mothballs
Probenecid	Benemid
Dimercaprol	BAL
Methylene blue	
Acetylphenylhydrazine	
Phenylhydrazine	
Nalidixic acid	NegGram
Neoarsphenamine	
Quinine	Quinamm
Quinidine	Duraquin, Quinaglute, Quinalan
Chloramphenicol	Chloromycetin
Benzene	
Illness	
Diabetic acidosis, hypoglycemia	
Hepatitis	
Infections	
Food	
Fava beans	

Table 27–8
Selected Lysosomal Storage Diseases

Disorder	Inheritance	Pathophysiology	Significant Clinical Features	Laboratory Findings	Management	Prognosis
Hurler's disease	Autosomal recessive	Deficient alpha-iduronidase	Bone dysplasia Severe mental retardation Kyphosis with gibbus Corneal clouding Hepatosplenomegaly Claw-hand deformity	Urine heparan and dermatan sulfates	Supportive care Displacement bone marrow transplantation an option	Death by age 10 yr (transplantation may alter this prognosis)
Tay-Sachs disease	Autosomal recessive	Deficient hexosaminidase A	Onset 4–6 mo of age Cherry-red macula Optic atrophy Hypotonia Seizures, late onset Dementia, early onset Almost all of Jewish ethnicity	Sphingolipidoses	No treatment	Death by age 2–3 yr
Niemann-Pick disease	Autosomal recessive	Deficient sphingomyelinase	Hepatosplenomegaly Enlarged lymph nodes Onset younger than age 6 mo Cherry-red macula Optic atrophy 50% Jewish ethnicity Spastic paresis Dementia, early onset	Elevated serum lipids Serum glutamic-oxaloacetic transaminase (SGOT) Vacuolated lymphocytes Foam cells in bone marrow	No treatment	Death by age 3 yr

Gaucher's disease	Autosomal recessive	Deficient beta-glucosidase	Onset younger than 6 mo of age Hepatosplenomegaly Dementia Strabismus Bubar palsy Spastic paralysis	Elevated acid phosphatase Lipid-laden Gaucher's cells found in bone marrow	Enzyme replacement therapy Splenectomy (rarely used)	Death by age 2 yr
Fabry's disease	Sex-linked recessive	Deficit of alpha-galactosidase	Episodic, incapacitating pain, initially of fingers and toes Mild mental retardation Seizures Peripheral red or purple macules or papules Renal disease Diabetes insipidus	Abnormal renal function	Management of pain crises Renal transplantation for renal failure	Death related to renal complications or stroke Renal treatment reverses symptoms
Hunter's disease	Sex-linked recessive	Deficient iduronate sulfatase	Plethoric facies Hepatosplenomegaly Hydrocephalus Kyphosis without gibbus Claw-hand deformity Hypertrichosis Dwarfism Deafness Mental retardation	Excessive dematan sulfate and heparan sulfate	Success of bone marrow transplantation being evaluated	Late onset: live to age 40–70 yr Some with average intelligence Juvenile type: death during adolescence
Sanfilippo disease	Autosomal recessive	Deficit of sulfatase, alpha-*N*-acetylglucosaminidase	Severe retardation Mild shortness of stature Mild coarsening of facial features Hepatosplenomegaly Mild hirsutism	Heparin sulfate in urine	Bone marrow transplantation being evaluated	Severe retardation May live to age 40–50 yr

Mucopolysaccharide Disorders

This group of lysosomal storage disorders involves abnormal storage of lipids in the neurons and of polysaccharides in the connective tissues. This results in multiple neurologic and skeletal abnormalities. Specific mucopolysaccharide disorders include Hurler's disease, Hunter's disease, Sanfilippo's syndrome, Morquio's syndrome, Tay-Sachs disease, Shefe's disease, Maroteaux-Lamy disease, and β-glucuronidase deficiency. Most are autosomal recessive defects, although a few such as Hunter's disease are X-linked. This section discusses Hurler's disease; an overview of the significant factors of other selected lysosomal storage disorders is provided in Table 27–8.

Hurler's Disease

Hurler's disease, or mucopolysaccharidosis IH, is the classic and most severe mucopolysaccharide disorder. The disease is sometimes known as gargoylism, because infants have distinctive gargoyle-like facial features. Hurler's disease occurs in approximately 1 in 100,000 births and is inherited as an autosomal recessive trait.

Pathophysiology

A defect in the lysosomal enzyme α-L-iduronidase prevents the degradation of acid mucopolysaccharides, also known as glucosaminoglycans. This results in an accumulation of dermatan sulfate and heparin sulfate (polyglycosaminoglycans) in the tissues, producing the symptoms of Hurler's disease. There are also a partial decrease in the activity of the enzyme β-galactosidase and an absence of α-iduronidase. Because this metabolic pathway is part of cellular metabolism in many body organs, it results in damage to the brain, spinal cord, heart, viscera, bone, and connective tissue.

Prognosis. In the past, children with Hurler's disease deteriorated progressively, and death usually occurred by age 10 with respiratory or cardiac failure caused by the organ defects resulting from the error in the metabolic pathway. Advances in bone marrow transplantation have altered the course of Hurler's disease by arresting its progress and reversing some of the most severe sequelae. Bone marrow transplantation has increased the life of a child with Hurler's disease by several years but has been unsuccessful in eliminating all of the skeletal defects. Bone marrow transplantation can also greatly decrease the mental retardation associated with Hurler's disease. Early diagnosis and supportive care continue to be the most common goals of management.

Assessment

Although Hurler's disease produces distinctive clinical manifestations, diagnosis is not often reached in the neonatal period. Manifestations develop over time. Initial reasons to screen a patient for Hurler's disease, or any mucopolysaccharide disorder, may be the presence of rather common symptoms such as a swollen abdomen or a hernia. The growth of these children is usually within the normal range for the first year but falls below the third percentile thereafter. Similarly, neurologic development appears normal at first, but the child typically has delays in sitting, walking, and toilet training. A learning plateau is reached by age 2 years (Adams & Victor, 1994).

The skeletal deformities of Hurler's disease are easily visible and include "gargoyle" facies (prominent supraorbital ridges with bushy brows, thickened lips, low nasal bridge, mild hypertelorism); large head with synostosis of the longitudinal suture; dwarfism; bone dysplasia, kyphosis, and gibbus, producing a "catlike" posturing; broad hands with short, stubby fingers and clawlike deformities; flexion contractures of knees and elbows; and bilateral hip dislocation (Fig. 27–6).

Neurologic manifestations include cystic areas in the white matter of the brain, severe retardation, communicating hydrocephalus with possible increased intracranial pressure, and corticospinal signs. Other significant symptoms include hepatosplenomegaly, protuberant abdomen, inguinal and umbilical hernias, conductive deafness, valvular heart disease, chronic rhinitis and respiratory infections related to a narrow pharynx and enlarged tongue, corneal opacities, and hirsutism.

Diagnostic Tests. Laboratory findings indicative of Hurler's disease include Reilly's bodies (metachromatic cytoplasmic inclusions) in 5% of peripheral lymphocytes and dermatan and heparin sulfates in the urine.

Nursing Diagnoses and Outcomes

Nursing diagnoses for the child with Hurler's disease can be selected from the list in Chart 27–3. In addition, the

Figure 27–6
A child with the typical facial characteristics of Hurler's disease. (From Albert, D. M., & Jakobiec, F. A. [Eds.]. [1996]. *Atlas of clinical ophthalmology* [p. 474]. Philadelphia: W. B. Saunders. Reprinted with permission.)

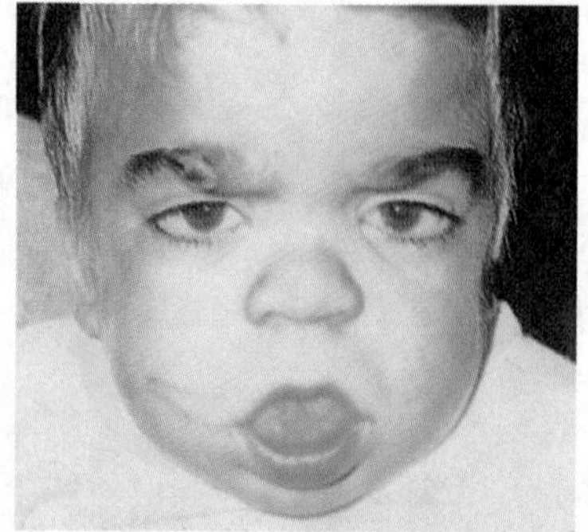

skeletal deformities and oral-facial deformities characteristic in children with Hurler's disease may prompt the following nursing diagnoses:

- **Body image disturbance related to skeletal deformities**
  Outcome: The child and caregivers will maintain positive conscious and unconscious perceptions and attitudes about the child's appearance.
- **Ineffective infant feeding pattern related to oral-facial deformities**
  Outcome: The parents will demonstrate appropriate feeding techniques to prevent aspiration and ensure that the child is receiving adequate nutrition.

Interdisciplinary Interventions

Supportive care focused on the respiratory and cardiac systems has been the most common management strategy. Displacement bone marrow transplantation holds promise to correct the metabolic defect and diminish symptoms. Introduction of healthy marrow replaces genetically deranged or absent blood cells. This allows genetically normal blood cells to deliver normal protein to the host tissue. Marrow transplantation has resulted in correction of the hepatosplenomegaly, clearing of corneal opacities, improvement of heart failure, and normalization of the facies and nasal sinus. The child can stand erect and walk but may require fusion of the lumbar vertebra. The clawlike hands straighten, and fine, skilled movements can be performed. Lesions in the brain improve, and IQ scores rise to 85 to 115. Bone marrow transplantation patients are being followed up to determine the long-term effects of this therapy. Some deterioration of the large joints has been noted about 8 years after transplantation (Schaub et al., 1991).

Community Care

Families of children with a lysosomal storage disease require a great deal of emotional and social support. They are caring for a child whose physical and mental health deteriorates over a period of years, often resulting in severe neurologic impairment and death. Arrangements for medical equipment in the home, such as a wheelchair, are necessary. Depending on the family's situation, home health care assistance, respite care, or long-term care placement may be necessary. Coordination with transplant centers is indicated if the child is a candidate for displacement bone marrow transplantation.

Families should be taught that their child may not progress in motor activities, including walking and toilet training. Assistive devices to allow the child to sit comfortably, move about, and attain some use of the hands can be obtained through occupational therapy and physical therapy consultations. The child may also experience behavioral problems such as emotional outbursts, excessive crying, and sleep disturbances in response to the neurologic deterioration. In these cases, sedatives may be administered to help manage the child.

The infant's large, protuberant tongue and narrowed nasopharynx cause difficulty in sucking. The nurse must teach the family feeding techniques to use to avoid aspiration. These techniques include feeding the child in an upright position and providing support to assist with swallowing (Chart 27–12). Breast-feeding can certainly be tried but may not be successful. Bottles with a small-holed, soft nipple allow the slow flow of formula and prevent choking. Nasal or deep suctioning may be required if aspiration does occur, and the family should be taught these techniques for home care.

As the disease progresses, the family has some difficult decisions to make regarding the child's care and the extent of medical interventions to be used to continue to support the child's physical health. The interdisciplinary team should provide the family with anticipatory guidance regarding measures to prolong the child's life. Parents may elect not to subject their child to certain interventions. The nurse can serve as an advocate for the child and the family, ensuring that all members of the health care team respect the family's wishes.

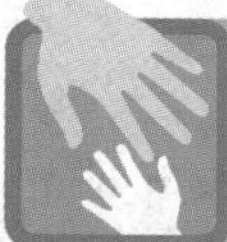

Chart 27–12
Nursing Interventions

Feeding the Child with a Large Tongue

The child with Hurler's disease typically has a large and protruding tongue, which can make feeding difficult. The following interventions can help prevent aspiration and assist the child to swallow:

- Hold the child upright with the head slightly tilted back to encourage the tongue to fall back.
- If bottle feeding, initiate sucking by putting pressure on the tongue with the nipple and placing the nipple in a downward and posterior direction.
- When bottle feeding, give cheek support so that the tongue curls around the nipple.
- If feeding with a spoon, place downward pressure on the tongue with the spoon to encourage swallowing and to displace the tongue.

Summary of Key Concepts

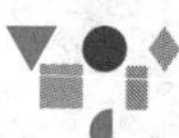

- A vast number of disease states result from inborn errors of the metabolic pathways and the resulting symptoms and toxic effects of metabolites.
- The incidence of a specific inherited metabolic disease is often low.
- Early diagnosis and timely intervention may prevent or decrease the severity of symptoms, which often include mental retardation and possibly death.
- Many of the more common metabolic disorders can be diagnosed from the results of mass neonatal screening programs.
- In utero diagnosis early in pregnancy is possible for some of the inherited metabolic disorders.
- An interdisciplinary approach is used to diagnose and intervene with the children and their families.
- A nursing assessment that uses keen senses of sight, smell, and touch in addition to a knowledge of normal growth and development is invaluable in the recognition of many of the metabolic diseases.
- Dietary intervention is a key management technique for many of the inborn errors of metabolism.
- Some metabolic diseases are terminal and supportive care is the only effective management.
- New treatment modalities for metabolic disorders, such as bone marrow transplantation, continue to be researched.

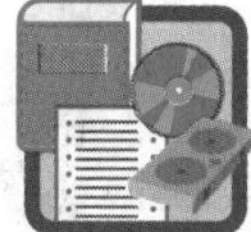

Resources

Organizations

Association for Glycogen Storage Disease
PO Box 896
Durant, IA 52747
(319) 785-6038

Association for Neuro-Metabolic Disorders
5223 Brookfield Lane
Sylvania, OH 43560
(419) 885-1497

Families with Maple Syrup Urine Disease
Route 2, Box 24-A
Flemingsburg, KY 41041
(606) 849-4679

Foundation for the Study of Wilson's Disease, Inc.
5447 Palisade Avenue
Bronx, NY 10471
(212) 430-2091

March of Dimes National Registry of MPS/ML Disorders (mucopolysaccharidosis)
53 West Jackson Boulevard, No. 1-50
Chicago, IL 60604
(312) 341-1370

National Genetics Foundation
555 West 57th Street
New York, NY 10019
(212) 586-5800

National Organization for Rare Disorders
1182 Broadway, No. 402
New York, NY 10001
(212) 686-1057

PKU Parents
518 Paco Drive
Los Altos, CA 94022
(415) 941-9799

Wilson's Disease Association
P.O. Box 489
Dumfries, VA 22026
(703) 221-5532

Books and Printed Materials

Education of students with phenylketonuria
(Free booklet for teachers, administrators and other school personnel)
NICHD
9000 Rockville Pike, Building 31, Room 2A32
Rockville, MD 20892
(301) 496-5133

References

Adams, R. D., & Victor, M. (1994). *Principles of neurology*. New York: McGraw-Hill.

Behrman, R., Kliegman, R., & Arvin, A. (1996). *Nelson textbook of pediatrics*. Philadelphia: W. B. Saunders.

Belmont, J., & Beaudet, A. (1993). Lysosomal storage diseases. In F. Burg, J. Ingelfinger, & E. Wald (Eds.), *Gellis & Kagan's current pediatric therapy* (pp. 337–339). Philadelphia: W. B. Saunders.

Biggemann, B., Zass, R., & Wendel, U. (1993). Postoperative metabolic decompensation in maple syrup urine disease is completely prevented by insulin. *Journal of Inherited Metabolic Disease, 16*, 912–913.

Bowe, K. (1995). Phenylketonuria: An update for pediatric community health nurses. *Pediatric Nursing, 21*(2), 191–194.

Collins, J., & Scheinberg, H. (1993). Wilson's disease. In F. Burg, J. Ingelfinger, & E. Wald (Eds.), *Gellis & Kagan's current pediatric therapy* (pp. 324–325). Philadelphia: W. B. Saunders.

Fisch, R., Matalon, R., Weisberg, S., & Michals, K. (1991). Children of fathers with phenylketonuria: An international survey. *Journal of Pediatrics, 118*, 739–741.

Hisano, S., Latta, K., & Chan, J. C. (1993). Therapeutics of X-linked hypophosphatemic rickets. *Pediatric Nephrology, 7*, 744–748.

Holton, J. B. (1994). *The inherited metabolic diseases*. Edinburgh: Churchill Livingstone.

Howard-Teplansky, R. (1992). Nutrition and development. In M. Levine, W. Carey, & A. Crocker (Eds.), *Developmental-behavioral pediatrics* (pp. 276–284). Philadelphia: W. B. Saunders.

Jones, G. (1993). Galactosemia. In F. Burg, J. Ingelfinger, & E. Wald (Eds.), *Gellis & Kagan's current pediatric therapy* (pp. 333–334). Philadelphia: W. B. Saunders

Korson, M., Rohr, F., & Gray, S. (1993). The hyperphenylalaninemias. In F. Burg, J. Ingelfinger, & E. Wald (Eds.), *Gellis & Kagan's current pediatric therapy* (pp. 325–329). Philadelphia: W. B. Saunders.

Lott, J. W. (1988). PKU: A nursing update. *Journal of Pediatric Nursing, 3*(1), 22–34.

Manual of Pediatric Nutrition. (1990). St. Paul, MN: Twin Cities District Dietetic Association.

Matalon, R., & Michals, K. (1991). Phenylketonuria: Screening, treatment and maternal PKU. *Clinical Biochemistry, 24*, 337–342.

Okano, Y., Eisensmith, R., Guttler, F., Lichter-Konecke, U., Konecki, D., Trezz, F., Dasovich, M., Wang, T., Henriksen, K., Lou, H., & Woo, S. (1991). Molecular basis of phenotypic heterogeneity in phenylketonuria. *New England Journal of Medicine, 11*, 1232–1238.

Parini, R., Sereni, L. P., Bagozzi, D. C., Corbetta, C., Rabier, D., Narcy, C., Hubert, P., & Saudubray, J. (1993). Nasogastric drip feeding as the only treatment of neonatal maple syrup urine disease. *Pediatrics, 92*, 280–283.

Rezvani, I., & Rosenblatt, D. (1996). An approach to inborn errors of metabolism. In R. Behrman, R. Kliegman, & A. Arvin (Eds.), *Nelson textbook of pediatrics* (pp. 328–329). Philadelphia: W. B. Saunders.

Rutledge, S., Havers, P., Haymond, M., McLean, R., Kan, J., & Brusilow, S. (1990). Neonatal hemodialysis: Effective therapy for the encephalopathy of inborn errors of metabolism. *Journal of Pediatrics, 116*, 125–128.

Schaub, J., Van Hoof, F., & Vios, H. L. (Eds.). (1991). *Inborn errors of metabolism* (vol. 24). New York: Raven Press.

Scriver, C., Beaudet, A., Sly, W., & Vawlle, D. (Eds.). (1989). *The metabolic basis of inherited disease*. New York: McGraw-Hill Information Services.

Segel, G. (1996). Enzymatic defects. In R. Behrman, R. Kliegman, & A. Arvin (Eds.), *Nelson textbook of pediatrics* (pp. 1405–1408). Philadelphia: W. B. Saunders.

Shih, V. (1993). Amino acid disorders. In F. Burg, J. Ingelfinger, & E. Wald (Eds.), *Gellis & Kagan's current pediatric therapy* (pp. 329–331). Philadelphia: W. B. Saunders.

Bibliography

Acosta, P. B., & Wright, L. (1992). Nurses' role in preventing birth defects in offspring of women with phenylketonuria. *Journal of Obstetric, Gynecologic, and Neonatal Nursing, 21*, 270–276.

Afifi, A., Sato, Y., Waziri, M., & Bell, W. (1990). Computed tomography and magnetic resonance imaging of the brain in Hurler's disease. *Journal of Child Neurology, 5*, 235–241.

Allen, R. J., Shaefer, A. M., & Jacobson, J. (1993). Differences on treating children with galactosemia. *Journal of the American Diabetic Association, 93*(10), 1102.

Barnico, L. M., & Cullinane, M. M. (1985). Maternal phenylketonuria: An unexpected challenge. *MCN American Journal of Maternal Child Nursing, 10*, 108–123.

Buda, F. B. (1981). *The neurology of developmental disabilities*. Springfield, IL: Charles C Thomas.

Davidson, A. (1992). Management and counseling of children with inherited metabolic disorders. *Journal of Pediatric Health Care*, 6, 146–152.

Dudek, G. (1989). Nursing update: Hypophosphatemic rickets. *Pediatric Nursing, 15*(1), 45–50.

Ekvall, S. W. (Ed.). (1993). *Pediatric nutrition in chronic diseases and developmental disorders*. New York: Oxford University Press.

Finberg, L. (1994). Rickets: Another genetic cause [Editorial]. *Journal of Pediatrics, 124*, 927.

Garnica, A., Chan, W. Y., & Rennert, O. (1994). Copper-histidine treatment of Menkes disease. *Journal of Pediatrics, 125*, 336–338.

Giordano, B. P. (1992). The impact of genetic syndromes on children's growth. *Journal of Pediatric Health Care*, 6, 309–315.

Gleason, L. A., Michals, K., Matalon, R., Langenberg, P., & Kamath, S. (1992). A treatment program for adolescents with phenylketonuria. *Clinical Pediatrics, 31*, 331–335.

Gropper, S. S., Naglak, M. C., Nardella, M., Plyler, A., Rarback, S., & Yannicelle, S. (1993). Nutrient intakes of adolescents with phenylketonuria and infants and children with maple syrup urine disease on semisynthetic diets. *Journal of the American College of Nutrition, 12*, 108–114.

Hayes, J. S., Rarback, S., Berry, B. E., & Clancy, M. K. (1987). Managing PKU: An update. *MCN American Journal of Maternal Child* Nursing, *12*, 119–123.

Hoekelman, R. A., Friedman, S. B., Nelson, N. M., & Seidel, H. M. (Eds.). (1992). *Primary pediatric care*. St. Louis: Mosby–Year Book.

Holton, J. B., de la Cruz, F., & Levy, H. L. (1993). Galactosemia: The uridine diphosphate galactose deficiency–uridine treatment controversy. *Journal of Pediatrics, 123*, 1009–1014.

House Staff Manual, Division of Neonatal Perinatal Medicine, Department of Pediatrics. (1993–1994). *Metabolic screening.* Atlanta, GA: Emory University School of Medicine.

Hurst, J. D., & Stullenbarger, B. (1986). Implementation of a self-care approach in a pediatric phenylketonuria (PKU) clinic. *Journal of Pediatric Nursing, 1*(3), 159–163.

Irons, M. (1993). Screening for metabolic disorders. How are we doing? *Pediatric Clinics of North America, 40*, 1073–1085.

Kaplan, P., Mazur, A., Field, M., Berline, J., Berry, G., Heidenreich, R., Yudkoff, M., & Segal, S. (1991). Intellectual outcomes of children with maple syrup urine disease. *Journal of Pediatrics, 119*, 46–50.

Koch, T. K., Schmidt, K. A., Wagstaff, J. E., Ng, W. G., & Packman, S. (1992). Neurologic complications in galactosemia. *Pediatric Neurology, 8*, 217–220.

Koch, R., Levy, H. L., Matalon, R., Rouse, B., Hanley, W., & Azen, C. (1993). The North American collaborative study of maternal phenylketonuria. Status report 1993. *American Journal of Diseases of Children, 147*, 1224–1230.

Kodama, H. (1993). Recent developments in Menkes disease [Review]. *Journal of Inherited Metabolic Disease, 16*, 791–799.

Levin, M. L., Scheimann, A., Lewis, R. A., & Beaudet, A. L. (1993). Cerebral edema in maple syrup urine disease. *Journal of Pediatrics, 122*, 167–168.

Levy, H., Lobbnegt, D., Koch, R., & de la Cruz, F. (1991). Paternal phenylketonuria. *Journal of Pediatrics, 118*, 741–742.

Mitchell, A., Stefferson, N., & Hogan, H. (1994). A case study: Organic acidemia. *MCN American Journal of Maternal Child Nursing, 19*, 325–330.

Nelson, C. D., Waggoner, D. D., Donnell, G. N., Tuerck, J. M., & Buist, N. R. (1991). Verbal dyspraxia in treated galactosemia. *Pediatrics, 88*, 346–350.

Nobunki, Y., Mitsubuchi, H., Akaboshi, I., Indo, Y., Endo, F., & Matsuda, I. (1991). Maple syrup urine disease: Clinical and biochemical significance of gene analysis. *Journal of Inherited Metabolic Disease, 14*, 787–792.

Nord, A., van Doorninck, W. J., & Greene, C. (1991). Developmental profile of patients with maple syrup urine disease. *Journal of Inherited Metabolic Disease, 14*, 881–889.

Ozard, P. T., & Gascon, G. (1991). Organic acidurias: A review. Part 1. *Journal of Child Neurology, 6*, 196–219.

Ozard, P. T., & Gascon, G. (1991). Organic acidurias: A review. Part 2. *Journal of Child Neurology, 6*, 388–402.

Peinemann, F., & Danner, D. J. (1994). Maple syrup urine disease 1954 to 1993. *Journal of Inherited Metabolic Disease, 17*, 3–15.

Potocnik, U., & Widhalm, K. (1994). Long-term follow-up of children with classical phenylketonuria after diet discontinuation: A review. *Journal of the American College of Nutrition, 13*, 232–236.

Rivello, J., Rezvani, I., DiGeorge, A., & Foley, C. (1991). Cerebral edema causing death in children with maple syrup urine disease. *Journal of Pediatrics, 119*, 42–45.

Russell, F. F., Mills, B. C., & Zucconi, T. (1988). Relationship of parental attitudes and knowledge to treatment adherence in children with PKU. *Pediatric Nursing, 14*, 514–516.

Sarkar, B., Lingertat-Walsh, K., & Clarke, J. T. (1993). Copper-histidine therapy for Menkes disease. *Journal of Pediatrics, 123*, 828–830.

Shah, B. R., & Finberg, L. (1994). Single-day therapy of nutritional vitamin D–deficiency rickets: A preferred method. *Journal of Pediatrics, 125*, 487–490.

Shils, M., & Young, V. (1988). *Modern nutrition in health and disease.* Philadelphia: Lea & Febiger.

Shulkman, S., Fisch, R. O., Zempel, C. E., Gadis, O., & Chang, P. N. (1991). Children with phenylketonuria: The interface of family and child functioning. *Journal of Developmental and Behavioral Pediatrics, 12*, 315–321.

Sowa, J. M. (1992). Diagnosing Wilson's disease [Letter to the editor]. *Annals of Internal Medicine, 117*, 91.

Steele, S. (1989). Phenylketonuria: Counseling and teaching functions of the nurse on an interdisciplinary team. *Issues in Comprehensive Pediatric Nursing, 12*, 395–409.

Thomas, E. (1992). Dietary management of inborn errors of amino acid metabolism with protein-modified diets. *Journal of Child Neurology, 7*(Suppl.), 92–111.

Thompson, G. N., Francis, D. E., & Halliday, D. (1991). Acute illness in maple syrup urine disease: Dynamics of protein metabolism and implications for management. *Journal of Pediatrics, 119*, 35–41.

Tiwary, C. M. (1987). Neonatal screening for metabolic and endocrine diseases. *Nurse Practitioner, 12*(9), 28–35, 38, 41.

Zitelli, B. J., & Davis, H. W. (Eds.). (1993). *Atlas of pediatric physical diagnosis.* London: Mosby–Year Book Europe.

HEALTH CHALLENGE:

Alterations in Vision, Hearing, and Communication

OUTLINE

OBJECTIVES

- Identify deviations from normal developmental patterns that indicate a visual or hearing deficit or communication disorder.
- Describe assessment techniques commonly used to identify vision, hearing, and communication disorders in infants and children.
- Describe the etiology of common vision, hearing, and communication disorders of infants and children.
- Discuss the pathophysiology related to common disorders of vision, hearing, and communication in infancy and childhood.
- Identify the nursing interventions necessary to prepare children and their families for tests of sensory function.
- Identify the roles of the interdisciplinary team members in the identification and management of sensory disorders in children.
- Develop a plan of care for an infant or child with an alteration in vision, hearing, or communication status.
- Summarize parent and child education to prevent injuries and illness resulting in alterations in sensory function.

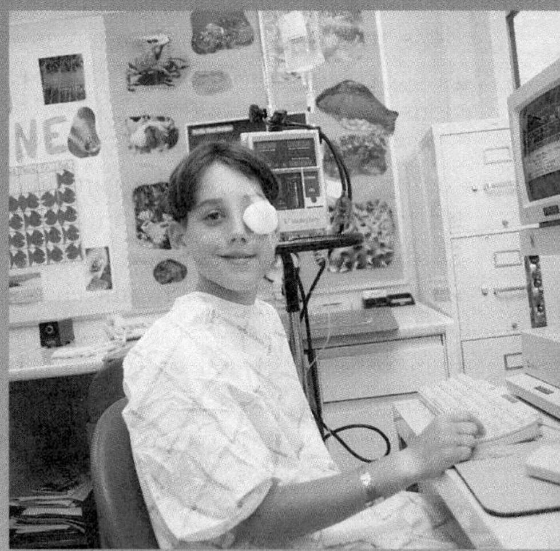

KEY TERMS

auditory brain stem response (ABR)
binocular vision
blindisms
cochlear implant
conductive hearing impairment
decibel (dB)
expressive language
legal blindness
partially sighted
receptive language
sensorineural hearing impairment
travel vision

CHAPTER 28

Infants and children are dependent on sensory input from the external world to assist them in their cognitive, social, and emotional growth. Sensory input comes in the form of visual and auditory stimulation as well as through the senses of touch, smell, and taste. To benefit fully from sensory stimulation, children must possess intact peripheral nerve pathways to receive the stimuli, and they must have brain development capable of recognizing and attaching meaning to the sensations received. Communication is the child's ability to interact with the outside world in response to the sensations received.

Alteration in sensory *reception*, that is, alteration in the ability to receive the particular sensation from the external world, and alteration in sensory *perception*, that is, the ability of the brain to assign significance to the sensory stimulus, directly influence the child's ability to grow and develop in response to the environment. Children with congenital or acquired, permanent or temporary alterations in sensory status need interventions from other persons in their environment to facilitate the developmental process. Nurses are in a unique position to work with the health care team to recognize sensory alterations and intervene to assist the child and family to provide the optimal environment in which the child may continue the process of development.

Communication is the exchange of ideas, messages, or information (Neufeldt & Sparks, 1990). Communication involves both receptive and expressive abilities. The child who has intact sensory systems receives sensory input to which he or she cognitively and emotionally attaches significance. A child reacts to the environment with behavioral and vocal responses. These responses are called *communication*. Alteration in communication is present when the child is unable to send understandable messages in response to external or internal stimuli or when the child is unable to receive messages that he or she understands. Both of these sets of circumstances (receiving and sending) deeply affect the progress of the developmental process for the child and family. Inability to share needs, desires, or ideas with others prevents the normal developmental process. Nurses are, once again, in a unique position to assist in identification of the deviation from normal and to assist the family in either seeking a solution or adapting to the alteration so as to provide the best developmental environment for the child.

Prevention or early detection of vision, hearing, or communication disorders can go a long way in avoiding the negative developmental sequelae that significantly diminish the quality of life of affected children and their families. Nurses are frequently involved in screening and prevention programs, and they need to be acutely aware of the importance of such activities to the future of the children. Acquired vision and hearing disorders are often subtle in onset, and behaviors that suggest alteration in vision or hearing may often be attributed to other causes. The subsequent effect on development can be significant. Assessment of vision and hearing during preschool years and in school-age children is essential, even in the absence of complaints from parents or teachers.

The role of the nurse caring for children includes (1) promoting early identification and treatment of sensory alterations, (2) assisting and teaching parents and children how to prevent or minimize trauma that could affect sensory abilities, (3) assisting parents and caregivers in finding ways to promote the development of the permanently impaired child, and (4) developing and implementing a plan of care for the child who has experienced an alteration in sensory function. The nurse works in collaboration with a variety of individuals who have specialization in sensory and communication disorders (Chart 28–1).

Chart 28–1

Interdisciplinary Specialists on the Health Care Team

Vision

Ophthalmologist—a physician who specializes in disorders of the eye.

Optometrist—a person skilled in testing visual acuity and prescribing corrective lenses. Not a physician.

Hearing

Audiologist—an individual who holds a graduate degree and professional certification from the American Speech-Language-Hearing Association (ASHA) in the assessment and management of hearing impairment.

Otolaryngologist—a physician who specializes in diseases of the ear, nose, and throat.

Otologist—a physician who specializes in diseases of the ear.

Communication

Speech-language pathologist—a person who has a graduate degree in speech and language disorders and certification from ASHA. This person is prepared to plan, direct, and conduct programs to improve communication skills of persons with impairments.

Speech therapist—a person trained to provide speech therapy at the direction of the speech-language pathologist.

Vision

Vision is one of the most important senses for normal child development. Using the sense of sight, infants bond with parents and learn about the outside world. Through sight, children explore their surroundings and move from place to place. They learn to read and interact with their world. Without the sense of sight, a child requires different approaches to and assistance in accomplishing developmental milestones and learning about the surrounding environment.

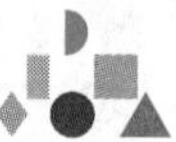

Assessment of the Child with Alterations in Vision

Assessment of vision should begin at birth and should be performed regularly throughout infancy and childhood (Fulton, 1992). Even though an infant's eyes seem normal, the growth process can cause subtle changes in the shape and function of the eye that cause abnormalities to develop in the child's vision. Abnormalities need to be identified as soon as possible to allow normal development to proceed. Assessment of vision in infants and children begins with a focused health history and is accompanied by physical examination. As children grow older and are able to cooperate, the physical examination includes tests of visual acuity, visual field determination, assessment of external ocular muscles and accommodation, assessment of external ocular structures, and a funduscopic examination. The nurse may be involved in as much of the examination as he or she is prepared to do. Nurse practitioners may give the entire examination. Nurses in primary care settings make various arrangements for sharing the responsibility with a physician. Screening tests of visual acuity are often done in the school setting and may be completed by the school nurse and assistants.

Parents should be reminded that vision screening is a valuable part of health assessment and that it should be done at regular intervals during childhood. Home screening kits can be obtained from the National Society to Prevent Blindness (see Resources) or a visual examination may be requested when children see their primary health care provider. Nurses need to be aware that inability to cooperate, which occurs when a child does not speak the dominant language or when a child is developmentally delayed, does **not** prevent accurate vision screening. Children with special needs may be tested differently, but should not be ignored in visual screening done routinely.

Focused Health History

The purpose of the health history is to elicit from caregivers their observations of the infant or child's behavior and responsiveness and to identify factors in the family history or child's past history that may contribute to current understanding of the child's health status. The health history is vital to identifying both risk factors and causative agents when assessing the health of children. If children are old enough to provide information, part of the interview should be addressed directly to them. Teenagers may be able to supply all necessary information and should be encouraged to do so.

Subjective data concerning vision elicited from the parent or child include information that first focuses on visual acuity. Parents of a newborn or infant can give their own observations concerning the infant's behavior. This information allows the nurse to make inferences about possible deviations from normal visual acuity. Suggested questions useful in eliciting this information are provided in the focused health history (Chart 28–2).

caREminder: *Parental observations must always be attended to because parents are usually the first to detect abnormal signs or symptoms. Parents quickly notice and suspect that something is wrong when the infant's eyes do not seem to be looking at them. This is abnormal and should be further evaluated. Reports of any redness, watering, or discharge should also be noted as abnormal.*

Further subjective data that should be elicited in the health history regarding vision depend largely on the age of the infant or child. A toddler or preschooler may have difficulty answering questions about the quality of sight. An indirect method of assessing visual acuity may be to ask whether the child enjoys looking at picture books and is attempting to "read." A toddler or preschooler who seems to be frustrated by books or the child who seems to dislike fine motor tasks that require close vision may truly have difficulty seeing the book or object they are working on. The child who reportedly sits too close to the television may also have visual difficulties (Fig. 28–1). If children are old enough, their own statement about the presence (or absence) of visual difficulty may be elicited. For the school-age child, the nurse may ask whether the child can see the blackboard easily without squinting or closing one eye. At this age, the child could also report blurring or double vision.

The focused health history should elicit information concerning the possibility of pain in the eyes because this could be the first sign of congenital glaucoma. Infants in pain are irritable, refuse feedings, and cry frequently. The

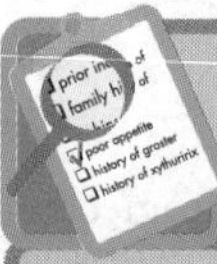

Chart 28–2
Focused Health History

Vision

Identifying Data	Age
Present Illness	Parents concerns regarding child's vision Poor school performance Child's response to visual cues, ability to track objects, ability to see objects in the environment clearly (TV, pages in a book, puzzles) Squinting of both eyes Headaches Abnormal head position Holding things close Blurred vision while reading Closing or covering one eye
Past Medical History	Birth history Prematurity or low birth weight Mechanical ventilation Phototherapy Perinatal infections (rubella, *Chlamydia,* gonorrhea) Previous health challenges Eye infections Glaucoma Cataracts Discharge from eyes Childhood illness or injury Glaucoma Cataracts Eye injury Periorbital cellulitis Unexplained crying Unexplained blurred vision or double vision Strabismus Amblyopia Allergies Presence of allergies that may cause orbital redness or eye irritation
Current Medications	Medications related to treatment of eye disorder Medications or solutions used for contact lens wear
Family History	Visual disorders Glaucoma Cataracts Blindness
Environmental History	Any environmental agents irritating child's eyes (e.g., smog, prolonged exposure to bright sunlight) How close child sits to watch television
Social History	Interactions with peers and family members appropriate for age
Growth and Development	Results of previous visual examinations Gross and fine motor skill development appropriate for age

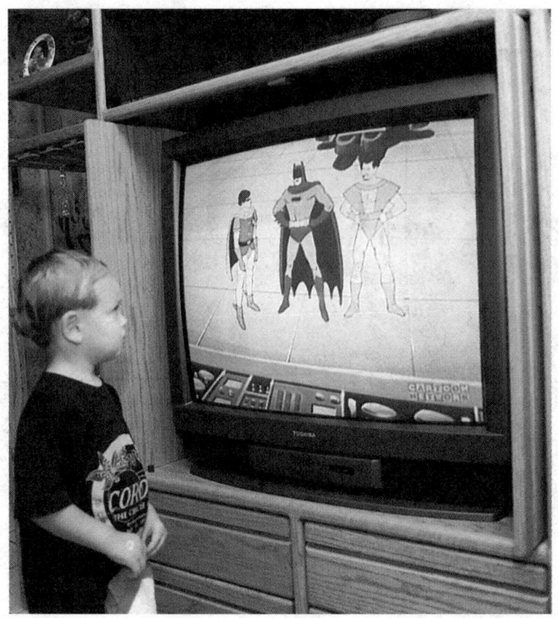

Figure 28–1
A child who sits close to the TV may do so because he or she has difficulty seeing.

parent may be frustrated in not knowing why the infant is crying. Older infants may rub their eyes or rock their head from side to side in response to pain. Pain caused by congenital glaucoma is difficult to identify; thus, this condition should always be considered when infant behavior seems to indicate discomfort. Because of their young age, their inability to communicate the nature of their discomfort, and the difficulty in diagnosing the condition, infants with congenital glaucoma may sustain visual damage before the condition is identified. Any unexplained infant pain behavior should be fully evaluated, including an eye examination. Older children can describe the presence and location of pain. Family history of any eye problems should always alert the nurse to look for signs of a visual disorder in the child.

Caregiver reports of excessive tearing, redness, swelling, or discharge or other observations about the infant's eyes could be significant. For example, excessive tearing in the infant may be merely the result of blocked tear ducts or may indicate a much more serious problem such as glaucoma. Congenital glaucoma is frequently accompanied by excessive watering of the eyes without evidence of infection.

The history should also elicit information about when vision was last tested and whether eyeglasses or contact lenses have ever been prescribed. Children who need eyeglasses or lenses may not be wearing them for a variety of social, financial, and personal reasons. Some of these reasons may need further evaluation to ensure that the child has the best opportunity to succeed in school. A child who has difficulty seeing the blackboard or reading textbooks is not equipped to achieve his or her maximum potential. The nurse can work with the health care team to coordinate acquisition of the resources needed to acquire the lenses. In addition, the nurse may be instrumental in assisting the youth to adapt to body image disturbances related to wearing corrective lenses.

Focused Physical Assessment

Physical assessment of vision in infancy and childhood is a challenge because of the inability of infants and very young children to understand directions and cooperate with the examiner. For this young developmental level, indirect methods of identifying abnormalities are the primary source of information. As children grow older, their cooperation makes physical assessment much more accurate and much easier to accomplish (Chart 28–3).

Assessment of vision begins in infancy when the eye and sight are undergoing great change in a short time. Abnormalities identified and treated at this early age can prevent permanent loss of vision. If newborn abnormalities are not identified and treated during the first 2 months of life, the child may lose sight or have serious, life-long decrease in visual acuity.

The *red reflex* of every newborn should be identified to check for opacities of the lens. The red reflex should be observed at each well-child visit throughout infancy. At the age of 1½ to 2 years, the child's red reflex should again be inspected and the eyes observed for alignment and possible eye muscle imbalance. At age 3 to 4, the child should be reassessed for lens opacities and proper ocular alignment, and visual acuity testing should be done. These tests should be repeated at age 4 or 5, when the child's cooperation is likely to be better. Other tests normally included in the full ocular examination should be done at this time as well. Tests for visual acuity in each eye separately should be completed annually until the child is at least 12 years old (Calhoun, 1997; Fulton, 1992). During teenage years, eye examinations should be completed at least every 2 years and the teenager encouraged to report unclear close or distant vision. Observations made by parents or teachers concerning the young person's reading or other visual behavior should be followed up with appropriate eye examinations, particularly because eye changes occur as growth progresses. The teenager's ability to succeed and to reach his or her maximum potential in school and on the job could be jeopardized by inability to see clearly.

External Ocular Structures

External ocular structures include the orbit of the eyes, eyelids, eyebrows, and surrounding facial tissues. The

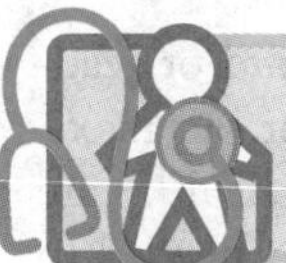

Chart 28–3
Focused Physical Assessment

Vision

	Infant	Toddler	Preschooler	School-age/adolescent
Red reflex	X	X	X	X
Blink reflex	X	X	X	X
Pupillary light reflex	X	X	X	X
Clarity of cornea and lens	X	X	X	X
External ocular muscle strength	X	X	X	X
External ocular structures	X	X	X	X
Visual fields			X	X
Visual acuity			X	X
Viewing ocular fundus			X	X

child's general appearance is significant because genetic syndromes that present with observable abnormalities can alert the primary health care provider to the possibility of functional abnormalities in other body organs. The examiner should note the symmetry of structures, their positions in relation to each other, and the size, shape, and structure of brows, eyelids and lashes, eyeballs, conjunctiva, and sclera. The examiner observes for ptosis of one or both eyelids (Fig. 28–2), slant of the eye (Fig. 28–3), symmetry of the eyes or pupils, extra palpebral folds, and any other deviations from expected structure. Physical assessment (inspection) of ocular structures can easily identify many of the common ocular disorders that cause

Figure 28–2
Ptosis (drooping) of the eyelid prevents visual development in the affected eye. (From Albert, D. M., & Jakobiec, F. A. [1996]. *Atlas of clinical ophthalmology* [p. 372]. Philadelphia: W. B. Saunders. Reprinted with permission.)

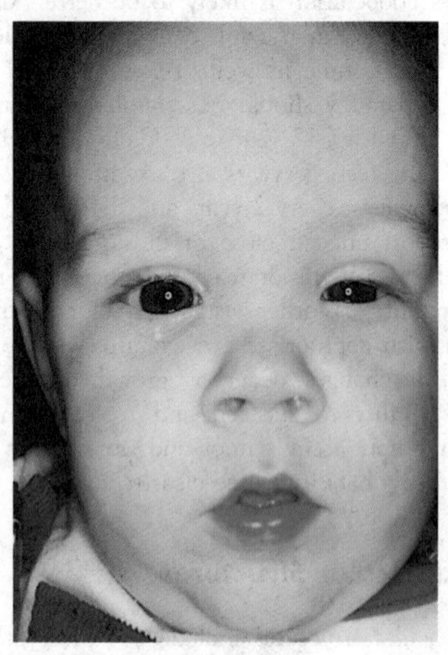

Figure 28–3
In children of some ethnic groups, the outer canthus is normally slightly above the level of the inner canthus.

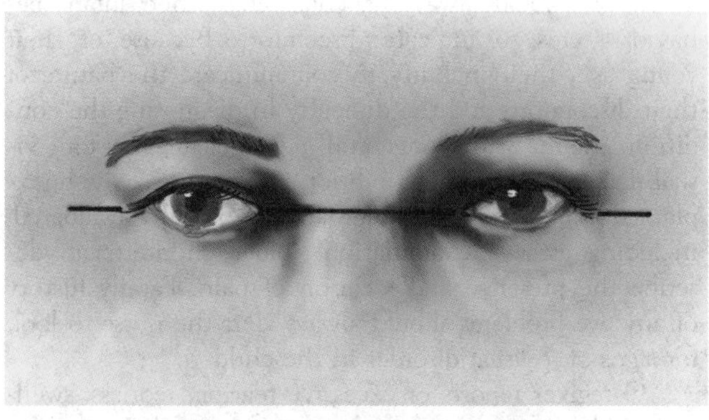

(A) NORMAL PALPEBRAL SLANT

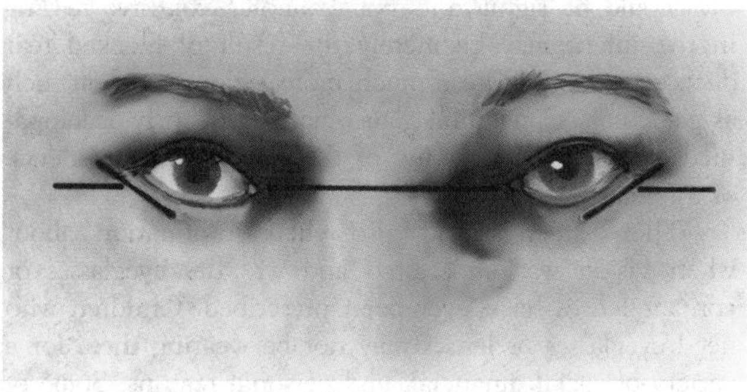

(B) UPWARD PALPEBRAL SLANT

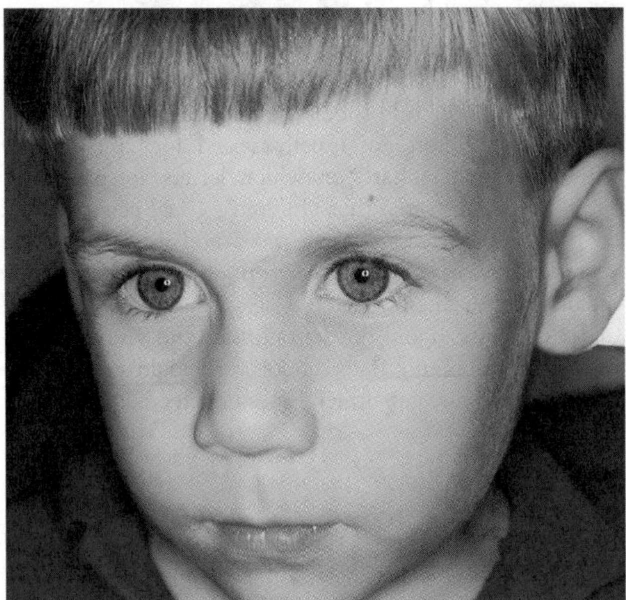

Figure 28–4
Corneal light reflex. Light reflection may be seen in the same relative position on each pupil if the eyes are aligned.

visual impairment. Congenital structural abnormalities or muscle weaknesses such as ptosis of the eyelid (drooping eyelid) or strabismus ("lazy eye") may be seen with careful observation.

External ocular muscles hold the eyes in alignment with each other and allow them to move smoothly to each of the six cardinal positions of gaze that are assessed in an eye examination (see Chapter 6). The ability to fix vision on a specific object is present at birth and is well developed by age 6 to 9 weeks. By age 2 to 3 months, visual following is well developed (Friendly, 1993). The examiner may catch the infant's attention by presenting a toy, bright object, or light and moving it in each direction. Both eyes should be observed to work together. The nurse should allow the toy or testing object to pause at each of the six positions. The normal response is for both eyes to follow the test object to each of the six cardinal positions of gaze. A weaker eye muscle may not allow the eye to reach the position or may not hold the eye in that position. The child's response may be to blink and abandon the position with the stronger eye as well. Thus, an uncooperative response from the child could be an indication of inability to hold the position or merely disinterest in the test. In such cases, the child should be retested.

The alignment of the infant or child's eyes may be assessed by observing the relative position of a light reflection on the cornea. This is called the *corneal light reflex*. When a light is directed toward the child's eyes from a distance, the reflection of that light on the corneas should be seen at the same relative location on each cornea (Fig. 28–4). Slight asymmetry is sometimes found in infants younger than 4 months old; however, the asymmetry seldom persists after that age. Asymmetrical corneal light reflex may indicate eye muscle weakness or strabismus.

To further assess the strength and symmetry of eye muscle control, the *cover–uncover test* may be used. To evaluate the infant, the examiner may first present a bright, colorful toy in the infant's line of vision, then, with a hand on the infant's head, occlude the line of vision with the thumb, or an occluder card can be used for testing older children (Fig. 28–5).

Tip: *Occlusion of the line of vision with the examiner's thumb is usually more effective with infants than using an occluder card. When the infant's head moves, the occluding thumb moves as well and the test may proceed without interruption.*

If the infant consistently objects to having the line of vision of one eye covered, the examiner may deduct that the child sees best using that eye. The infant should be examined further by an ophthalmologist for the possibility of amblyopia. The older child's eye muscles are tested by asking him or her to focus on a distant object. The examiner covers one of the child's eyes while watching the movement of the uncovered eye. If the eye does

Figure 28–5
Cover–uncover test. The weaker eye is seen to move when uncovered.

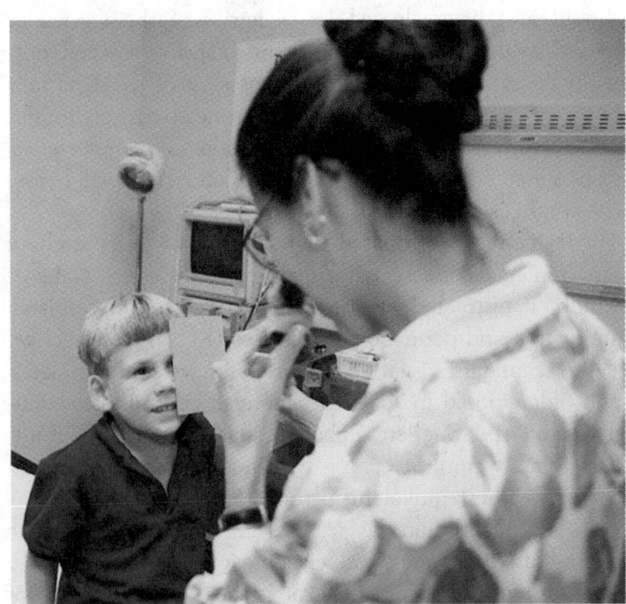

not move, it is presumed to be able to focus on the toy or object selected. The examiner then covers the other eye and watches for movement of the uncovered eye. If there is no movement, the eyes are presumed to be working together without misalignment.

Tip: *Older children enjoy participating in this test when a colorful cardboard ice cream cone or lollipop is used as a cover.*

At the same time that the cover–uncover test is done, each eye is observed for movement when it is uncovered. If the eye seems to wander while it is covered and to snap back when uncovered, the child should be evaluated by the ophthalmologist for eye muscle weakness (strabismus).

Visual Acuity

In children younger than age 3, visual acuity can be assessed only indirectly. An active blink reflex is seen in a normal newborn when a light shines across each eye. The blink reflex indicates that the light is being received by the retina and transferred to the visual center of the brain. Each eye is tested separately and compared with the other. The pupillary light reflex may be observed at the same time. As the light shines on the eye, the normal newborn pupil constricts and the eye blinks closed. The pupils should constrict equally.

Alert: *The absence of a blink reflex or absence of pupillary constriction is indication of visual impairment and the source of the impairment should be sought.*

Newborns as well as older infants and children should also be evaluated for opacities of the cornea or lens. Development of visual acuity cannot proceed normally if the lens is clouded. An opacity of the lens may be a cataract and, if found in a newborn or infant, prevents development of useful vision. To preserve vision, cataracts should be evaluated and removed before the infant is 2 months old.

It has been estimated that 5% to 10% of preschool children have undetected visual acuity disorders, some of which, if untreated by the age of 6 years, can result in amblyopia and permanent visual loss (Keech & Kutschke, 1995). Standard visual acuity screening for children age 3 and older should include assessment of central visual acuity using the Snellen alphabet chart, Snellen E chart, Blackbird Vision Screening System (Fig. 28–6), animal cards, or other equivalent method (Chart 28–4).

A child should be referred for further optometric testing if visual acuity in either eye is less than 20/40 (denominator 40 or greater), or if there is a difference of more than one line on the screening chart (Calhoun, 1997). For example, if one eye has an acuity of 20/20 and the other eye tests at 20/30, the 20/25 line is in between and the child should be referred.

Older children are usually tested for visual acuity with the Snellen chart, on which letters are presented. Most authorities agree that children's visual acuity should be evaluated at least every 2 years and preferably every year. Peak years for identification of diminished acuity include early school years and again during adolescence. Older children should not be omitted from vision screening programs because their school work could suffer significantly if a vision impairment goes undetected.

Visual Fields

A complete eye examination includes the assessment of visual fields. By age 3, most children can cooperate with the examiner sufficiently for a full visual assessment. The child covers one eye and looks at the examiner's nose. The examiner holds his or her finger out to the side at arm's length and equidistant between the two of them. Without moving his or her head or eyes, the child is asked to say "now" when he or she can first see the examiner's wiggling finger as it is moved in from the periphery. Each eye is tested separately. The examiner compares the amplitude of the child's field of vision with his or her own.

Figure 28–6
The child takes the "glasses" home after the Blackbird Vision Screening test.

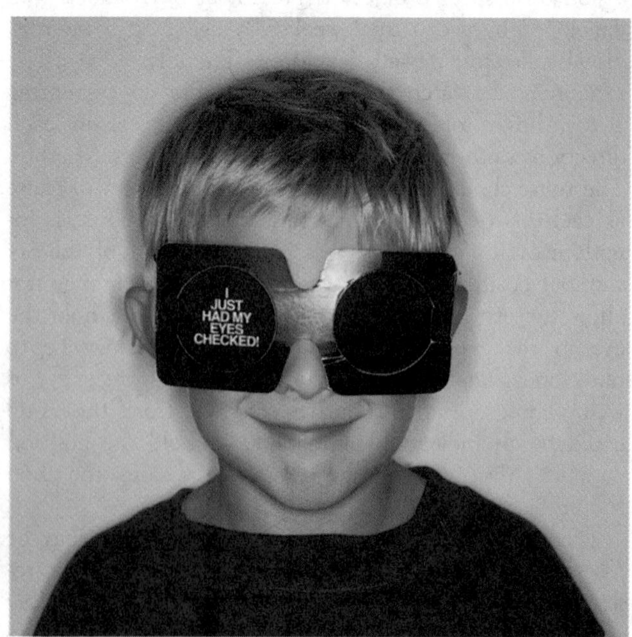

Chart 28–4
Nursing Interventions

Completing Tests for Visual Acuity

Using the Snellen chart or a chart for non-readers, the child is asked to stand on a line 20 feet from the standard chart. An assistant is often needed to help the small child hold the occluder card in the proper position. If the child wears glasses, the glasses should be worn during the visual acuity testing. As one eye is covered, the examiner points to one line on the chart, asking the child to identify the letters or symbols there. Older children are asked to read the letters on a selected line of the standard Snellen E chart. Using a picture chart or the Snellen E chart for non-readers, the child is asked to identify the picture or indicate with his or her fingers the direction that each "E" is pointing. The child is asked to read each line until at least two figures are missed in two successive lines. The child's score is read from the numbers at the edge of the chart.

Results are recorded according to the numbers on the edge of the chart on the line that the child completed successfully. The numbers are in the form of a fraction. The numerator is the number of feet that the child is standing from the chart, whereas the denominator is the number of feet from which a person with normal vision would be able to see the same line. For example: vision reported as 20/30 indicates that the child sees at 20 feet what a person with normal vision would see at 30 feet.

The Blackbird Vision Screening System has been developed using a story of a blackbird, which the examiner tells to engage the cooperation and interest of small children. The child puts on a pair of cardboard "glasses" that allows first one, then the other eye to be occluded as the child listens to the story and watches the bird in the examiner's book fly to different positions. The child participates by showing the examiner which way the bird is flying or sitting. The "glasses," which the child takes home, contain a message to the parent indicating that the child has participated in vision screening on that day. Results of the screening using the Blackbird System are recorded in standard terms. (See Resources at the end of the chapter for sources of more information.)

Funduscopic Examination

Newborns should be evaluated for opacities of the cornea or lens. A red reflex seen with the ophthalmoscope indicates that the lens is clear. A congenital cataract prevents the examiner from seeing the red reflex. If the red reflex is absent, immediate referral is necessary. The full funduscopic examination may not be possible when examining infants and young children who cannot keep the eye still long enough for retinal visualization.

Funduscopic examinations performed on children and adolescents should reveal a normal pink- to peach-colored fundus with clearly visible arteries and veins in normal array. The optic disk should be clearly demarcated. There should be no notching of blood vessels or evidence of hemorrhagic areas (Fig. 28–7).

Alert: *Hemorrhagic areas seen on funduscopic examination may be caused by head injury related to shaken baby syndrome or child abuse. The child should be referred for further evaluation.*

Nursing Diagnoses and Outcomes

The nursing diagnoses for vision reflect the three-pronged scope of care in this area. First, the health care team is concerned about developmental surveillance to monitor the normal and healthy development of a child's vision. Second, there is a need to provide education to prevent illness and injury that could impair vision. Third, nursing diagnoses are selected that reflect the needs of a child with a diagnosed vision disorder (Chart 28–5).

Figure 28–7
Ocular fundus with small hemorrhages. (From Albert, D. M., & Jakobiec, F. A. [1996]. *Atlas of clinical ophthalmology* [p. 238]. Philadelphia: W. B. Saunders. Reprinted with permission.)

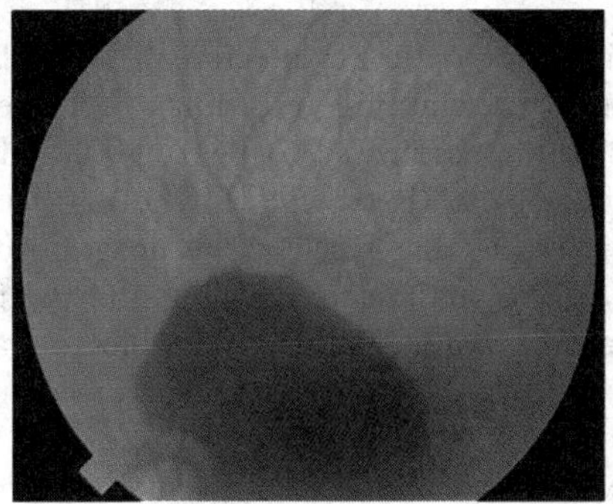

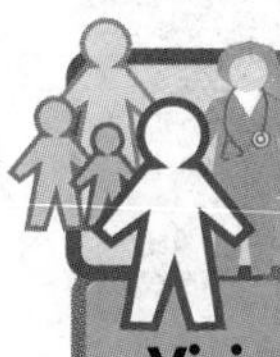

Chart 28–5
Nursing Diagnoses and Outcomes

Vision

Sensory or perceptual alterations (visual) related to altered sensory reception, transmission, or integration	
Outcomes:	Child will maintain visual functioning at his or her highest level possible. Child will compensate for visual loss by use of adaptive devices.
Potential for altered growth and development related to lack of stimulation secondary to visual impairment	
Outcome:	Child will demonstrate interest and age-appropriate participation in family activities.
Risk for injury related to diminished ability to see environmental obstacles	
Outcome:	Safety will be maintained.
Risk for impaired verbal communication related to diminished visual cues	
Outcome:	Child's ability to communicate will develop according to expectations for age.
Potential for ineffective individual coping related to sudden onset of temporary visual deficit	
Outcomes:	Child will demonstrate appropriate use of coping mechanisms. Child will request help as needed and function independently when possible.

Developmental and Biological Variances

Early development of vision begins between the second and fourth weeks of fetal life along with development of the fetal brain (Jarvis, 1992). By the 16th week of fetal development, the eye has acquired its human appearance and rudimentary internal structures are forming.

At birth, the pathways to the visual center of the brain are not yet fully developed. These require daily stimulation to complete their development. Each eye contains separate nerve pathways to separate receptor sites in the visual cortex. Myelinization of the nerve pathways occurs as the child grows older. Cell development in the visual centers is dependent on daily stimulation with the normal sights of an infant's world (Reed, 1997).

At birth, the optic nerve (cranial nerve II) is functional and peripheral vision is fully developed. Visual acuity at birth is estimated to be 20/400, and development is incomplete (Reed, 1997). The macula, the portion of the retina that receives the image focused on it through the lens, has yet to develop; and the fovea, the central portion of the macula, is unable to transmit an image to the brain. The development of central vision, which occurs as the fovea and macula develop, is dependent on visual stimulation that the normal eye receives over the first few weeks and months of extrauterine life. Central vision develops when ocular structures that are stimulated by normal sights of the infant's world repeatedly have images focused on them and the brain learns to merge the images from the two eyes.

If a defect or injury prevents images from reaching the retina, the macula and fovea are deprived of stimulation and do not develop the ability to transmit images. Congenital cataracts and ptosis of the eyelids (drooping eyelids) are examples of conditions that prevent visual development. If these conditions are not treated early, the eye loses its ability to continue to develop and amblyopia develops.

Visual acuity involves the ability to focus and to see well at different distances. Visual acuity of 20/100 is commonly present by age 6 months and 20/50 by age 12 months. Development of visual acuity continues throughout infancy and early childhood, reaching the "normal" of 20/20 to 20/30 by age 4 to 6 years. As visual acuity is developing, accommodation also improves. At birth, visual fixation occurs on near objects, but the infant depends on sounds more than on sight to recognize the approaching parent. The newborn's eye is able to focus clearly only on objects within very close range, allowing the infant to see his or her mother while feeding. During the infant's first 4 months of life, the eye develops the ability to change shape (accommodate) so that the visual

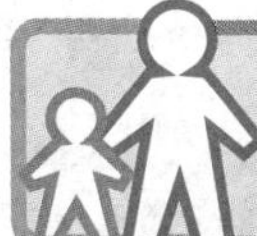

Chart 28–6
Developmental Considerations

Vision and Ocular Development in Children

Age	Development	Significance
Birth	Visual acuity estimated at 20/200 Optic nerve functional Peripheral vision functional Central vision not yet developed Macula and fovea not fully developed Visual range of 45 degrees	Infant sees near objects but not far objects clearly. Infant able to see caregiver's face more clearly than objects in the distance. Infant briefly follows a colorful object with vision.
6 wk	Visual acuity estimated at 20/100 Visual range 90 degrees	Infant is developing the ability to focus eyes on objects further away.
4 mo	Visual acuity estimated between 20/100 and 20/80	Eye muscles hold eyes straight. Eyes should be noted to work together during all testing.
6 mo	Visual acuity between 20/100 and 20/80 Visual range 180 degrees Accommodation is developing	Infant is able to see more clearly at a distance. Infant sees approaching parent or caregiver clearly. Infant fixes gaze on test object and follows it for full 180 degrees.
12 mo	Visual acuity estimated at 20/50	
4–6 yr	Visual acuity betwen 20/30 and 20/20	
7 yr	Visual acuity 20/20	Ocular development complete.

images of close and distant objects can be focused on the retina and thus seen clearly. By age 4 months, visual accommodation is well developed, allowing the infant to see equally well at a distance and closer. By age 7 years, eye development is complete (Chart 28–6).

Biological variations are seen in different cultural groups and in children with different amounts of melanin in their skin. In children of Asian descent, the outer canthus of each eye may be located slightly above the imaginary line drawn from the inner canthus to the top of the ear. This slight upward slant is a normal biological variation (see Fig. 28–3).

Children with darker skin may have flecks of brown in the conjunctiva and have a darker orange-brown hue to the retina rather than the bright yellow-orange present in persons with less melanin in the skin.

Some children of Asian descent and of other ethnic groups may have an additional fold of skin above the inner canthus of one or both eyes. This variation may cause the examiner to suspect an eye muscle imbalance; however, further examination of the corneal light reflection quickly reveals no muscle imbalance, only the additional canthal tissue. Because this additional tissue causes the examiner to suspect strabismus, it is called "pseudostrabismus."

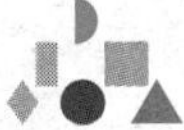

Diagnostic Criteria for Evaluating Alterations in Vision

The funduscopic examination, using the ophthalmoscope, is part of a complete physical assessment and is described previously. More complex technological methods using more sophisticated equipment are used by the ophthalmologist to identify the specific parameters of visual impairment and to monitor progress as a child undergoes treatment (Table 28–1).

Eye photography assists the ophthalmologist in detection of eye muscle and ocular disorders. Children who have difficulty holding still may be able to look at a particular object long enough for a photograph to record the appearance of the eyes. Children often submit more readily to having their picture taken than to undergoing examination with the ophthalmoscope and other equipment. The ophthalmologist can then review the photograph carefully to detect any muscle weakness or certain other disorders. A graphic record allows comparison with future photographs as therapy progresses.

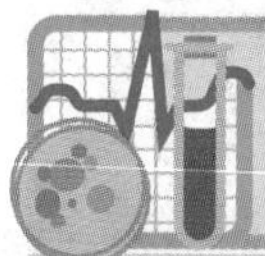

Table 28–1
Diagnostic Tests and Procedures for Evaluating Vision

Diagnostic Test or Procedure	Purpose/Procedure	Findings	Health Care Provider Responsibilities
Funduscopic examination	*Equipment:* Ophthalmoscope *Purpose:* Observe characteristics of internal ocular structures	Any abnormal findings in structure or appearance	Identify deviations from normal. Refer infants and children with deviations from normal to pediatrician or ophthalmologist for further evaluation. Discuss with parent rationale for referral.
Eye photography	*Person responsible:* Ophthalmologist or optometrist *Equipment:* Eye camera with chin rest. *Purpose:* Obtain a graphic record of external ocular appearance and alignment of the eyes for immediate assessment and future comparison. *Procedure:* Clinician asks the child to rest chin on the solid surface and look at a spot at the center of the camera. The photograph is obtained quickly and can be assessed without concern for the short attention span of small children.	Children submit more readily to having their picture taken than to an ophthalmic examination.	This tool is used by some optometrists and ophthalmologists to more accurately assess their clients. This test provides a graphic record for future reference as the child grows and changes.

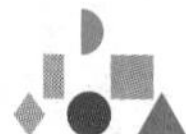

Treatment Modalities

Corrective Lenses

Corrective lenses may be prescribed for infants or children of any age. Eyeglasses are used with infants and children to correct for refractive errors just as they are for adults. Infants and young children soon learn that they are able to see more clearly with the eyeglasses in place and seldom object to their use. Young children come to perceive eyeglasses as a part of their body. Eyeglasses for young children are made of sturdy plastic with unbreakable lenses. Contact lenses may be substituted for eyeglasses when children are old enough to take responsibility for their care, insertion, removal, and cleaning (MacDonald, 1996).

The rate of visual development is rapid during infancy and early childhood; thus, a young child who has corrective lenses prescribed should wear them all the time. All adults who work with the child should be shown how to assist with this aspect of care. This young child needs to be seen by the ophthalmologist at regular intervals for possible changes in the prescription.

Dangers inherent in the use of corrective lenses for young children include breakage, loss, and physical injury to the face and eyes from falls. Children's eyeglasses are made of materials that can withstand much (but probably not all) of the wear and tear given them by youngsters. Unbreakable "glass" lenses are used consistently.

Tip: *Active school-age children can be protected from losing or breaking eyeglasses by using sports elastic to prevent loss during active games such as basketball and by not removing the eyeglasses during games.*

If a child says he or she "sees better" without the eyeglasses, an ophthalmology visit is in order.

Occlusion Therapy

Occlusion therapy is used for treatment of eye muscle weakness (strabismus). The stronger eye is covered to allow the weaker eye to work alone for all or part of every day, thus becoming stronger. An eye patch is used or one lens of the child's eyeglasses is fogged or covered. Covering one lens of the eyeglasses loses its therapeutic

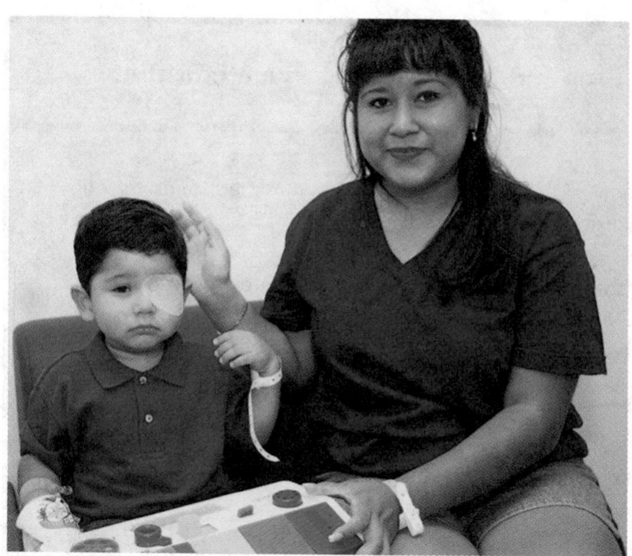

Figure 28–8
In occlusion therapy, the child keeps one eye patched to strengthen the other eye.

value, however, if the child learns to peek around the covered or fogged lens. In that case, the eye patch is the treatment of choice (Fig. 28–8).

During occlusion therapy, the ophthalmologist must examine the child at frequent intervals to identify the progress made by the weaker eye and to detect any possible visual loss in the patched good eye. The duration of treatment is determined by the ophthalmologist.

Medications

Medications may be used to treat eye infections or allergic manifestations. Antibiotics are used to treat bacterial infections and are administered topically as drops or ointment (Fig. 28–9). The action of the antibiotics may be bactericidal (kills the bacteria) or bacteriostatic (limits bacterial activity by interfering with cell wall synthesis or intracellular metabolism and reproduction). Antibiotics may be broad-spectrum (effective against many different organisms) or narrow-spectrum (effective against specific organisms).

The best choice of topical antibiotic is one that is not commonly used for treatment in other body systems and thus one to which the child is less likely to be allergic or to which allergy is less likely to develop. Sodium sulfacetamide 10% and sulfisoxazole 4% are broad-spectrum antibiotics that seldom elicit hypersensitivity reactions (Burns, Barber, Brady, & Dunn, 1996).

Systemic antibiotics in addition to topical ophthalmic antibiotics may be necessary for treatment of severe infections. The nurse should reinforce to caregivers the importance of giving all doses each day and of finishing the prescription even if symptoms improve.

Other medications that may be used to treat children's eye conditions include ophthalmic corticosteroids and ocular decongestants. Because steroids (including ocular steroids) are associated with numerous side effects and complications, the nurse must see that the child receiving this type of medication is seen regularly at 2- to 3-month intervals by the ophthalmologist to check for side effects. Ocular decongestants such as Vasocon 0.1% ophthalmic solution (1 to 2 drops every 3 to 4 hours) may be prescribed to reduce ocular congestion, irritation, and itching (Burns et al., 1996). If used more frequently than ordered, rebound congestion may occur. The nurse must reinforce to the patient or caregiver that the medication is to be used according to directions (TIP 28–1). Older children and teenagers who may be self administering the medication need to be warned of the effects of using the medication more frequently than ordered.

Surgical Interventions

Surgical intervention may be necessary when the condition cannot be effectively treated with medical methods alone. Surgical alignment of the eyes may be considered when strabismus is present (see Strabismus section). Congenital cataracts are removed surgically, and surgical treatment of retinopathy of prematurity (ROP) may be the treatment of choice. The ophthalmic surgeon should be highly skilled in working with infants and young children.

Nursing interventions before and after the surgery include providing clarifying information and education to the family concerning their responsibilities in the care of the child postoperatively. The nurse and the physician work closely together to be sure that the family has and understands all the information they need to care for the child during the first few days after surgery.

Preoperatively, the child should be well. A child with an upper respiratory infection is not a surgical can-

Figure 28–9
Administration of eye ointment.

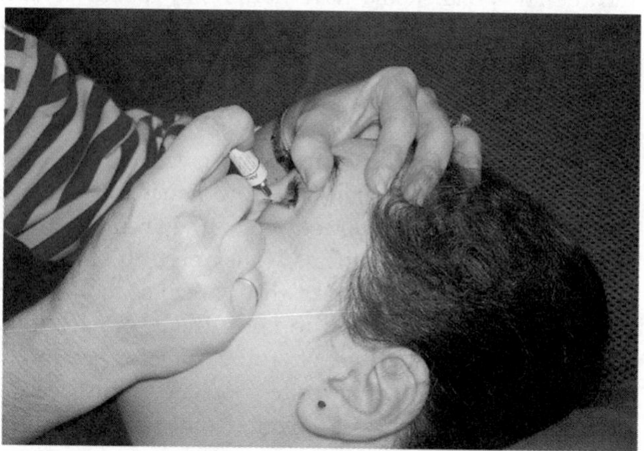

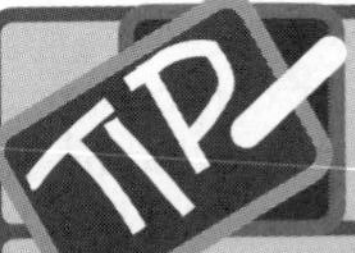

TIP 28–1 A Teaching Intervention Plan for Administering Eye Medications

Nursing Diagnosis and Family Outcomes

- Potential for ineffective management of therapeutic home regimen related to insufficient knowledge of technique for administration of eye medication
  Outcomes:
  Parents will demonstrate appropriate technique for administering eye ointment or drops.
  Child will have no evidence of eye infection when prescribed medication has been instilled as directed for a prescribed period of time.

Interventions

- Tell the child
  What you plan to do—"I will put some drops (ointment) in the little sack under your eye to make the infection go away."
  What it will feel like—"It will be a little bit cold . . ."
  What he or she can do to help—"You need to lie down and put your head back. When I am done, you close your eye and let the medicine go all over the inside of your eye. Here is a tissue. You can wipe away whatever comes out, but don't rub your eye."
- Position the child. A young child may lie down with head extended. A toddler who is likely to turn his or her head away can be positioned between the parent's legs with the toddler's head between the parent's thighs as they sit on the bed (or floor). The parent's legs can hold the infant's head still while the medication is instilled.
- Draw down the skin below the eye to expose the lower conjunctival sac and place the prescribed number of drops (or amount of ointment) in the center of the conjunctival sac. Do not touch the child's eye with the dropper or the tube tip, which may cause discomfort or tissue damage.
- The child will blink, spreading the medication across and over the entire eye. Ask the older child to keep the eye closed for 1 to 2 minutes.
- Wipe away any excess liquid or ointment. Do not exert pressure on the eye. Explain to the older child that vision may be blurred for a short time after ointment is instilled. The blurring will go away in a few minutes.
- Planning to use the eye medication immediately before nap time is helpful because the child will have the eyes closed for a period of time.

Contact Health Care Provider if

- The eye infection shows no improvement after 1 to 2 days.

didate. The child should have nothing by mouth or limited fluids as directed on the morning of surgery. Preoperative testing should be completed in the physician's office or at the hospital before the day of surgery.

The child should be told in age-appropriate terms what the physician will do and what it will be like after surgery. For example, toddlers need to know that one eye (or both eyes) "will be covered up so they can get better after the doctor fixes it (them)." They need to know that parents will be waiting to take them home as soon as the physician allows. They need to know that there are good things to look forward to after the surgery, perhaps a Popsicle or some other favorite food. A tactile reward may be in order, such as a favorite stuffed toy or a new stuffed toy.

The family may need information concerning postoperative care such as how to change an eye patch or how to administer eye medications. They may need to know what danger signs after surgery indicate that the physician should be notified.

Postoperative care may include use of elbow restraints to prevent the young child from bringing the hands to the eyes. These may be needed until healing is complete. In some cases, visual therapy is started very soon after the surgical procedure. In these cases, parents need full information concerning their responsibilities.

Laser surgery is used in the treatment of ROP to prevent the progression of the condition and is discussed in later paragraphs.

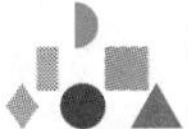

Alterations in Vision

Refractive Errors

Using specialized equipment, the optometrist or ophthalmologist can identify abnormalities in the shape of the internal ocular structures. The abnormal shape of the internal eye causes the visual image to be improperly focused on the retina. This results in blurred vision and may occur at either close range or distant range or both. These are called refractive errors and may usually be corrected with eyeglasses or contact lenses.

The four types of refractive errors include *myopia* (nearsightedness), *hyperopia* (farsightedness), *astigmatism*, and *anisometropia* (unequal refraction in the two eyes) (Fig. 28–10). The visual image passes through the lens before arriving on the retina. As the light rays pass through the lens, they are bent so that the visual image focuses on the retina. Errors in refraction occur when the eye is unable to bend light rays satisfactorily to focus the image on the retina.

The ability of the eye to focus an image clearly on the retina involves both *accommodation* and *convergence*. Accommodation is the ability of the eye to change the shape of the lens to allow the image to be clearly focused on the retina. The ciliary muscles in the eye contract or relax to change the refractive angle of the lens. Accommodation allows the individual to focus clearly on distant objects as well as on objects that are closer.

Convergence is the movement of the eyes toward the midline that occurs as objects are brought closer. Convergence occurs simultaneously with accommodation to allow the visual images of the two eyes to be focused at the same position on the retina of each eye. This allows binocular vision (fusion of the images from the two eyes) to occur.

During childhood, the child's eyes grow physically. As growth occurs, the globe of the eye may change in shape. The potential exists for visual disorders caused by refractive errors to develop. As the child grows and the globe or lens changes shape, the eye muscles may be

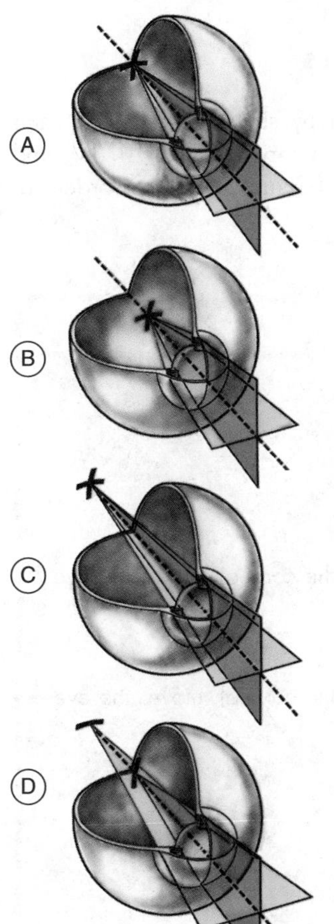

A
B
C
D
NORMAL EYE
MYOPIA (nearsightedness)— able to see objects at close range but not able to focus on distant objects. The eyeball is too short, causing light to be focused in front of the retina. Myopia is corrected with biconcave lenses that focus light rays on the retina.
HYPEROPIA (farsightedness)— child is able to see objects at a distance but unable to see near objects clearly. The eyeball is too short, causing light to be focused behind the retina. Many children are often able to overcome hyperopia with good accommodation. The condition is more likely to show up later in life.
ASTIGMATISM— irregular shape of the cornea causing light rays to bend in different directions. Correction is accomplished with lenses designed to compensate for the individual refractive errors.

Figure 28–10
Types of refractive errors.

unable to compensate for the change in shape to bring the visual image to focus on the retina.

Myopia

Myopia, also called *nearsightedness*, results from excessive refractive power being exerted on the lens. The light rays are focused in front of the retina rather than on the retina. The child with myopia usually has no difficulty with reading, but cannot see distant objects clearly without visual correction. Seeing the blackboard in the classroom could be difficult for the school-age child. A child with severe myopia holds the printed page very close to his or her face to see it clearly. Myopia is usually readily corrected with lenses. Because growth causes changes in vision, the child may need new eyeglasses every 1 or 2 years. If myopia is congenital, the normal growth patterns may result in improvement.

Hyperopia

Children with hyperopia, or *farsightedness*, see better at a distance. Hyperopia results from either a short axial length (shorter than normal distance from lens to retina) or decreased curvature of the lens. The visual image would be focused on a location behind the lens. Children are often able to compensate. The child's eye may be able to change shape by accommodation to overcome the hyperopia. This allows the child to see clearly but also causes eye strain when the child does close work such as reading. Eye strain is decreased by use of glasses or contact lenses as the lens decreases the need for accommodation.

Astigmatism

In astigmatism, the shape and curvature of the cornea are not symmetrical; thus, light rays are not focused symmetrically. Without correction, visual images are blurred and distorted. Eye strain occurs as a result of the accommodative effort that is made to bring the image into focus. Astigmatism is corrected with lenses that compensate for the abnormal and irregular curvature of the cornea.

Anisometropia

Anisometropia is present when the refractive errors present in each eye are considerably different. With this condition, the two eyes are unable to work together. Normally, when the muscles of one eye contract, the muscles of the other eye make the same adjustment. When the refractive errors in the two eyes are different, the muscle contraction or relaxation of one eye corrects the vision in that eye and worsens the vision in the other eye. If anisometropia is severe, amblyopia is likely to develop as the brain learns to ignore the visual image from the weaker eye. The condition should be identified and treated as early as possible. Corrective lenses are used to correct the refractive errors and allow the two eyes to work together.

Eye Muscle Disorders

Eye movement is controlled by six small muscles, each allowing a single movement. Cranial nerves III, IV, and VI innervate these muscles (Chart 28–7). Disorders of

Chart 28–7

Cranial Nerves Tested During Eye Examination

Cranial Nerve	Muscle Innervated	Action
III, Oculomotor	Medial rectus	Moves the eye toward the nose (adduction)
	Inferior rectus	Moves the eye down (depression)
		From the elevated position (12 o'clock on the cornea), moves the eye temporally (extortion)
		Moves the eye in adduction
	Superior rectus	Moves the eye up (elevation)
		From the elevated position (12 o'clock on the cornea), moves the eye nasally (intortion)
		Moves the eye in adduction
	Inferior oblique	Moves the eye in elevation
		Moves the eye in extortion
		Moves the eye temporally (abduction)
IV, Trochlear	Superior oblique	Moves the eye in depression
		Moves the eye in intortion
VI, Abducens	Lateral rectus	Moves the eye in abduction (away from the nose)

eye movement may be a result of damage to one of the innervating cranial nerves or to one of the six tiny muscles that move each eye. Eye movement should be smooth, coordinated, and controlled.

If any of the six small muscles controlling eye movement is stronger or weaker than the opposing muscle in the same eye, then one eye deviates from the line of vision. This condition is called *strabismus*. When strabismus is present before age 7, the child is at risk for development of amblyopia.

The six small muscles that move the eyes into the six cardinal fields of gaze must move with coordination and balanced strength so that both eyes can focus on the same location or object (binocular vision). When the two eyes are unable to focus on the same location or object, the two eyes are not coordinated, and the visual cortex of the brain "turns off" the visual image from the deviating eye. This stops visual development in the portion of the brain associated with the deviating eye. Eye muscle disorders should not be ignored.

Strabismus

Strabismus, or misalignment of the eyes, is also called "lazy eye" and is a common eye problem in children (Fig. 28–11). If the eye turns inward toward the nose, the child has *esotropia*; if the eye turns outward, *exotropia*. Mild or transient strabismus is frequently found in infants younger than 6 months old and resolves spontaneously as the eye strengthens and the child develops (Lavrich & Nelson, 1993).

Strabismus affects approximately 4% of children younger than age 6 (Lavrich & Nelson, 1993). If untreated, it can result in amblyopia, loss of sight in an otherwise normal eye. As many as 30% to 50% of children with strabismus have been found to suffer permanent visual loss (Lavrich & Nelson, 1993). Early identification and treatment of strabismus are essential for prevention of amblyopia and permanent loss of vision. Primary health care providers are in an ideal position to identify strabismus and refer the infant or child for appropriate care.

Figure 28–11
Strabismus is present if corneal light reflections are not seen at the same locations on each eye, as is noted on this child. (From Albert, D. M., & Jakobiec, F. A. [1996]. *Atlas of clinical ophthalmology* [p. 467]. Philadelphia: W. B. Saunders. Reprinted with permission.)

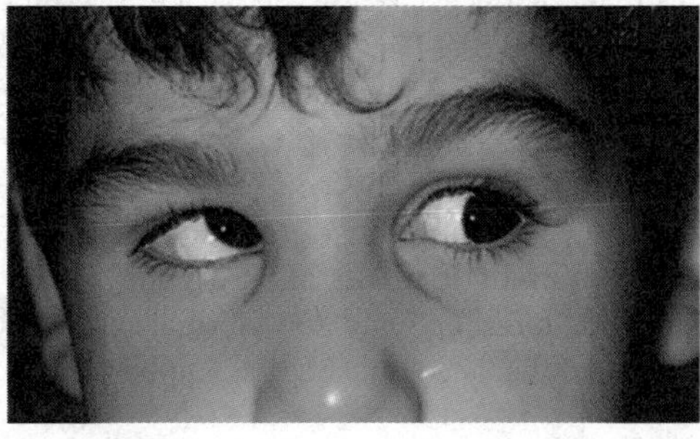

Etiology

Strabismus may be caused by eye muscle imbalance or paralysis. Muscle imbalances may be a result of congenital defect, systemic infections early in life, or intracranial injury. Low-birth-weight infants and those who have sustained an intraventricular hemorrhage during the neonatal period are particularly prone to development of strabismus. Infants who have sustained injury to cranial nerves III, IV, or VI also demonstrate eye muscle weakness. In a longitudinal study of 190 low-birth-weight infants, strabismus was seen with increasing frequency during the second year of life. Of the 50 children examined at age 2, all showed *deteriorating* vision, and esotropia that was not present in the early months of life developed in all those who had survived grade III and grade IV intraventricular hemorrhage (Page, Schneeweiss, Whyte, & Harvey, 1993).

Pathophysiology

At birth, the development of the infant eye is incomplete. Early visual images presumably are focused on the developing macula and fovea of the retina to stimulate development of the visual pathways in the cerebral cortex. During the first 4 months of life, binocularity (both eyes working together) is not consistent, thus intermittent esotropia or exotropia may normally occur. Beginning at age 4 months, as the eyes work together more consistently, divergence decreases and binocularity increases (Aslin, 1977; Jarvis, 1996; Mohindra, Swann, Held, Brill, & Swann, 1985). Presumably, the straight position that is attained as binocularity is achieved and the child sees a single clear image. (Nixon, Helveston, Miller, Archer, & Ellis, 1985). If the infant is unable to achieve central fusion of the visual image, or if an eye muscle weakness or imbalance prevents the eyes from working together to achieve central fusion, diplopia results as the infant sees two images that cannot be merged. As a result, the developing brain suppresses one image. This is called strabismic amblyopia. In many cases, however, this type of amblyopia can be prevented by appropriate therapy for strabismus.

Other aspects of the pathophysiology that the nurse must consider include the possibility of strabismus as a part of a larger syndrome, neurologic disorder, or disease process. Ocular deviations may be found in palsy of cranial nerve III, IV, or VI or as part of a wide variety of syndromes and genetic disorders occasionally seen in infants.

Nursing Diagnoses and Outcomes

Nursing diagnoses that are useful in planning the care of children with eye muscle disorders focus on supporting the family in their decision to seek medical attention for the child, and in their efforts to comply with the treatment protocol that may be prescribed by the ophthalmologist. If surgery is indicated, family support is still necessary. Assisting the family in their compliance with treatment protocols may involve teaching them how to gain the child's cooperation by using principles of normal growth and development.

In addition to the nursing diagnoses suggested at the outset of the chapter, the following may be helpful.

▶ **Risk for injury; visual impairment related to failure in development of binocular vision secondary to eye muscle weakness.**

Outcomes:

Family will understand the importance of seeking medical attention and following treatment protocols.

The child will comply with treatment protocol as recommended by the ophthalmologist.

The child will have no permanent visual impairment resulting from noncompliance with treatment protocol.

Assessment

The assessment and diagnosis of strabismus is done during the routine eye examination. For the normal eye, the bilateral corneal light reflex should be symmetrical, cover–uncover tests should show no eye movement, and eye muscle tests should show the ability of eye muscles to move the eyes smoothly to each of the six positions of gaze. Strabismus is suspected if

- The corneal light reflex is not symmetrical.
- Eye muscle movement is not smooth and consistent.
- The cover–uncover tests demonstrate abnormal eye movement.

Symmetrical corneal light reflection on the pupils indicates that the eye muscles hold the eyes in alignment.

Worldview: *Among certain ethnic groups, infants and young children have a broad bridge of the nose. Some children may have asymmetrical epicanthal tissue that may give the appearance of convergence (deviation toward the midline) of one eye. These children have an "extra" fold of tissue at the inner canthus of one eye. If they do not have a symmetrical fold on the other side, one eye appears to be closer to the bridge of the nose. If the corneal light reflex is symmetrical, the eyes are properly aligned and the condition is called "pseudoesotropia" or "pseudostrabismus" and requires no treatment.*

Tests of the external ocular muscles should show that the muscles move the eyes to each of the six cardinal positions of gaze and hold each of the positions briefly. Movement should be smooth and symmetrical. Each muscle set should move the two eyes together and hold the position for 1 to 2 seconds before moving to a new position. If, at any time during the assessment of the child's eye muscles, the eyes do not move symmetrically or the child is unable to hold the position for the given amount of time, strabismus could be a diagnosis.

Additional tests that reveal further information about eye muscle function are the cover–uncover test and the alternate cover test, which have been discussed previously. If eye muscle weakness is present, the weaker eye moves when it is uncovered.

Identification of eye muscle weakness by means of eye testing should be part of every newborn and infant's physical examination and every child's examination at least once each year. Normal infants younger than 30 days old can be expected to have some amount of ocular deviation. Most of these resolve by age 3 to 4 months with normal ocular stimulation. All deviations should be reassessed at each visit and, if accompanied by other symptoms such as ptosis of the eyelid or evidence of neurologic involvement, should be referred *immediately*. Infants suspected of having other congenital syndromes or disorders should be evaluated carefully and referred for full assessment by a pediatrician or geneticist. A report of the National Health Survey found no differences in frequency of strabismus between blacks and whites. Other racial differences were not clear-cut (Overfield, 1985).

Interdisciplinary Interventions

Some cases of strabismus are obvious and others are detected by primary health care providers on routine examination. All should be referred immediately to an ophthalmologist for treatment. The earlier that treatment is initiated, the greater is the likelihood of good visual outcome. Nonsurgical methods including occlusion therapy or prescription lenses may be used first. If these methods fail or are not indicated, surgery may be recommended to align the eyes (Lavrich & Nelson, 1993).

Occlusion Therapy. The most common treatment for strabismus is occlusion therapy (see Treatment Modalities discussed previously). Vision in the stronger eye is occluded to make it necessary for the weaker eye muscles to work (see Fig. 28–8). The nature of the condition and the ophthalmologist's procedural management of the child's disorder determine whether the occlusion is continuous or intermittent. The goal of therapy is to patch the stronger eye part of the time to allow time for the weaker eye to strengthen, yet allowing the better eye to be unpatched long enough for normal and necessary school work to be accomplished. Compliance is dependent on striking an acceptable balance between occlusion time and non-occlusion time, which may need to be explained carefully to and negotiated with the child.

Surgery. The need for surgery depends on the nature of the condition and on the degree of success of occlusion therapy. Surgical correction of strabismus involves an eye muscle shortening procedure designed to realign the eyes. Realignment allows binocularity to develop. With modern tools and high-powered microscopes, the procedure has been demonstrated to be safe and effective. It is usually done on an outpatient basis, negating the need for the child to stay overnight. Parents need to know when to withhold feedings, where to bring the child on the day of surgery, and what time to arrive. Parents need directions in writing because even a simple surgical procedure can be an anxiety-producing event, causing them to forget verbal directions.

After surgery an eye patch may be needed during the first day or few days after surgery to remind the child not to rub or put pressure on the eye. If the child is young, elbow restraints may be necessary to prevent small hands from contacting the eye. Pain is seldom a problem; however, the surgeon may offer acetaminophen as needed or, in rare cases, a calming agent such as diphenhydramine (Benadryl) or phenobarbital to assist the child in tolerating the healing process.

Botulinum Toxin Injections. An alternative treatment being tested with some types of strabismus is injection with botulinum toxin to temporarily weaken the stronger muscle, allowing the weaker muscle to strengthen. With this treatment, children have been found to achieve orthotropia (alignment of the eyes) in 2 to 4 weeks. The effects of the treatment persist for 12 to 15 weeks, and it may need to be repeated before orthotropia is permanently achieved (Thomas, Mathai, Rajeev, Sen, & Jacob, 1993).

Nursing involvement after the assessment and diagnosis phase is directed toward achieving compliance with the prescribed therapy or preparation of the child and family for the possibility of surgery if occlusion therapy is unsuccessful. Parents need to know the importance of keeping all appointments with the ophthalmologist during occlusion therapy to assess the progress of the treatment and to assess vision in the patched eye. If vision in the patched eye begins to deteriorate, the ophthalmologist may change the treatment protocol to stimulate vision in the good eye more frequently. If occlusion therapy is successful, surgery may be avoided.

Community Care

In occlusion therapy, the child may use an eye patch for extended periods during the day. When the child is in daycare or in school, the patching is monitored by teachers, volunteers, and the school nurse. Each of these adults needs to be knowledgeable about the purpose for eye patching and informed of the plan for the individual child. The school administrators need to be fully informed and to have a written copy of the treatment plan in the school file.

The purpose of patching is to stimulate visual development in the non-occluded eye, not to treat some malady of the patched eye, as some would believe. The ophthalmologist may prescribe the eye patch intermittently or all the time during waking hours. The child should be able to maintain consistent progress in school during treatment. If, however, wearing the eye patch during school hours prevents the progress of the child's education, the treatment plan needs to be reevaluated by the ophthalmologist.

The teacher and daycare providers may need to discourage teasing and educate the other children concerning the reason that the child wears the eye patch. Other children can learn to be a help rather than a hindrance in the treatment program and continued social development of the individual child.

The teacher or school nurse may need to replace the patch during the school day. A conference between teacher and parent (and school nurse, if possible) can verify that supplies are available (which the parent can provide) and that school protocols are in place for the child to have the patch changed. The patch should be put on loosely, but not so loosely that the child can peak around it. It is secured with a non-irritating type of tape. Channels of communication need to be clarified with the school so that changes in the treatment plan can be implemented in a timely and accurate manner and so that noncompliance is reported to the parent without delay. Noncompliance could result in reevaluation of the treatment protocol, or it may simply be discussed with the child to establish the reason for it.

Amblyopia

Amblyopia is defined as diminished effective vision in one or both eyes even with use of proper optical correction. Amblyopia results from altered visual development (or visual development that does not progress normally) despite what appears to be ophthalmoscopically normal retinal and optic nerve anatomy (Rubin & Nelson, 1993). Amblyopia occurs in approximately 1% to 4% of the general population (Rubin & Nelson, 1993; von Noorden, 1974, 1990) or in as many as 10% of the adult population (Hohmann & Haase, 1993). Selected populations such as children born prematurely, children of drug-dependent mothers, and children with other neurologic impairments may have a higher incidence of amblyopia. Children from at-risk populations should be screened carefully for development of amblyopia and, if found, amblyopia should be vigorously treated to minimize permanent visual loss.

Because amblyopia is usually asymptomatic, it is only confirmed when a complete ophthalmologic examination reveals reduced visual acuity but fails to identify any organic abnormality. Amblyopia is difficult to identify in infants; it is much more easily identified when children are old enough to follow directions and to make simple choices.

caREminder: *If vision is obstructed for a significant length of time, amblyopia and loss of vision can develop in any infant or child younger than age 7 years. Therefore, obstructions to vision should be resolved as soon as possible, with referrals to an ophthalmologist made if necessary.*

Waiting for the child to grow old enough to cooperate can jeopardize vision in the affected eye. Amblyopia is, in many cases, preventable, yet many children with the condition are not identified until permanent damage has already been done.

Pathophysiology

In normal ocular development, images are focused on the developing retina, and, more specifically, on the macular portion of the retina. During the infant's first 6 months of life, the neurologic pathways between eye and brain complete their development and the visual centers of the brain mature in their ability to perceive clearly the images seen through the eyes. Slowly, the normal infant's brain merges the images from the two eyes, allowing binocular vision, that is, two eyes seeing a single image.

If the visual image is not focused on similar locations on the retina of each eye, a blurred image is perceived by the brain. The developing brain spontaneously and quickly reacts to the blurred vision (produced by eyes that do not work together) by suppressing vision in one eye. As a result, the portion of the brain associated with that eye does not develop. If, for some other reason, the image is not transmitted to the brain from one eye, such as in a congenital cataract, the portion of the brain associated with the affected eye, for lack of stimulus, does not develop.

The critical period for visual center development in the brain is birth to age 6 to 7 years. The longer visual suppression is present, the less reversible it becomes. If amblyopia is not identified until after the child is 7 years old, it is unlikely that useful vision can be developed in the eye that has been suppressed.

Amblyopia will not develop after the critical period for visual development is over. Thus, amblyopia does not develop in a child who has passed the critical period for visual development but who sustains an injury that causes eye muscle imbalance. Instead, double vision develops, with each eye sending its own image to the brain.

There are two so-called types of amblyopia, *organic amblyopia* and *functional amblyopia*. Organic amblyopia refers to decrease in visual acuity as a result of a disease process affecting the cells of the retina or visual pathway. These disease processes are usually visible on routine ophthalmic examination. Examples of disease processes that may cause organic amblyopia include trauma, retinoblastoma, congenital toxoplasmosis, and hypoplasia or atrophy of the optic nerve. The central nervous system damage caused by meningoencephalitis may also be included as a cause of organic amblyopia. Organic amblyopia is usually permanent and irreversible. It is not correctable with glasses and does not respond to occlusion therapy (Stager, Birch, & Weakley, 1990).

Functional amblyopia may be subdivided into three classifications: deprivation amblyopia, strabismic amblyopia, and refractive amblyopia. *Deprivation amblyopia* may occur as a result of the loss of visual stimulation in the affected eye. With lack of stimulation, retinal cells fail to develop and the corresponding portion of the brain fails to continue its development. Deprivation amblyopia may result from congenital cataract, ptosis of the eyelid, bandaging or patching of one eye, or some other disorder leading to disuse (Stager et al., 1990). The younger the child is when disuse begins and the longer the condition is present before treatment begins, the more difficult it is to achieve significant improvement. Most of these conditions can be observed early in infants and should be referred to the ophthalmologist for treatment before the infant is 2 months old to preserve sight. The most critical period of visual development is during the first few weeks of life when the site of central vision, the fovea, is developing. Formed visual images are necessary to stimulate the retina during this time. Absence of formed visual images during this critical period prevents development of the fovea and thus prevents all subsequent stages of the affected eye's visual development (Rubin & Nelson, 1993). Surgical removal of the congenital cataract or correction of other congenital abnormality allows visual development to progress normally. If the abnormality is corrected before the infant is 2 months old, the likelihood of a positive outcome is excellent.

Strabismic amblyopia occurs when the brain suppresses the image from one eye. As a result of eye muscle weakness, the images reaching the retina are misaligned. The visual centers of the brain perceive two images. To prevent double vision or blurred vision, the brain suppresses the vision from one eye. Suppression may occur in only one eye, or it may alternate, the brain accepting sometimes the image from one eye and sometimes from the other eye. If vision does not alternate, retinal development and corresponding visual center development of the brain does not proceed and amblyopia develops. If vision does alternate, amblyopia does not develop but neither does binocular vision (both eyes seeing the same image). Strabismus may be present at birth or may develop during early childhood. According to Stager and colleagues (1990), in approximately 30% of children with strabismus, amblyopia develops, particularly if the suppression of vision is not treated within 30 days of its development.

Refractive amblyopia develops from excessive nearsightedness (myopia), farsightedness (hyperopia), or astigmatism that blurs the visual image in one or both eyes. The most common cause is anisometropia, refractive errors so different in the two eyes that the brain is unable to merge the images. The brain effectively "turns off" the visual image from one eye causing amblyopia to develop. Refractive amblyopia is difficult to manage. If refractive errors are similar in the two eyes, the resulting image is equally focused or blurred as it falls on the retina. If the two eyes are markedly different in refractive errors, the brain suppresses one, causing amblyopia. When one eye is myopic (nearsighted) and the other hyperopic (farsighted), some children learn to use one eye for close work and the other for distance sight, and amblyopia does not develop.

Assessment

Early identification of amblyopia is essential (Magramm, 1992). Assessment of vision should begin with the first contact between health professional and family, and should continue regularly throughout childhood (Chart 28–8). Amblyopia seldom begins after age 6 to 7 years when ocular development is complete; however, if present, it should certainly be identified before that time.

▽ **Alert:** *Some screening tests used to detect amblyopia have a high false-negative rate (Hohmann & Haase, 1993). Thus, if either parent or child suggests that a visual problem exists, the child should be referred to the ophthalmologist even when screening tests are negative. Screening tests are only rough measures of visual acuity.*

Children at greatest risk for late identification of amblyopia and subsequent poorer visual outcome, are those whose parents are less concerned about the seriousness of the condition and who are less closely followed up by the primary health care provider. Most early diagnoses were as a result of parental request for eye examination or were detected by the primary health care provider (Campbell & Charney, 1991).

Specific methods used to assess vision in infants and children of various ages have been discussed previously. Assessment of the progress of the treatment of amblyopia uses the basic visual acuity testing methods. As the amblyopia improves, visual acuity improves in the affected eye and, if possible, binocular vision also improves.

Interdisciplinary Interventions

In each of the types of amblyopia, the goal is to stimulate normal visual development. The earlier the condition is identified and treatment is begun, the greater is the likelihood of a positive outcome. It is particularly important for early identification and treatment to take place because the child could permanently and unnecessarily lose the sight in one eye. Treatment of the child with amblyopia should first address the underlying cause of the amblyopia. When this has been done, the amblyopia can then be effectively treated. The one possible exception is strabismic amblyopia in which eye muscles are of unequal strength. In some children, amblyopia should be treated first, before surgical intervention, to strengthen the weaker eye muscles. For other children, surgical treatment of the eye muscles allows spontaneous recovery from amblyopia as soon as the eyes are aligned. One study found that a significant number of children recovered spontaneously from amblyopia when the strabismus was surgically treated and the eyes aligned (Lam, Repka, & Guyton, 1993).

Modalities of treatment of amblyopia primarily include occlusion therapy or surgical correction of a related problem such as strabismus, ptosis, cataract, or other anomaly. Occlusion therapy is usually the treatment of choice. Occlusion may be recommended to be full time (all waking hours) or part time (a specified portion of each day), depending on the severity of the amblyopia, the age of the child, and the child's activities.

Because development is occurring more rapidly at younger ages, improvement may occur more quickly if the child is younger when treatment begins. Usually, the patch should be removed for at least 2 hours per day, even with full-time occlusion therapy, to prevent occlusion amblyopia in the good eye. Part-time occlusive therapy may be recommended if the child's weaker eye is weak enough that normal developmental learning does not continue during occlusion, or if the child is in school and is unable to learn effectively while using the patch (Rubin & Nelson, 1993).

Community Care

The ophthalmologist follows up the infant or child regularly to monitor the improvement in vision. Intervention for the child with amblyopia must always be a cooperative effort among all persons who come into daily contact with the child. This may include not only parents and health care professionals but also school teachers or daycare providers, all of whom need to know the treatment protocol being used and their responsibility in assisting the child and family to comply. Health care professionals who may be directly involved are the

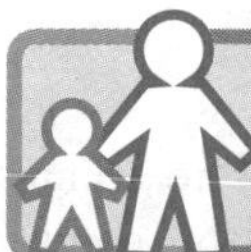

Chart 28-8
Developmental Considerations

Screening for Amblyopia

Birth to Age 4 Months

History: Pay close attention to parents' concerns about the infant's vision.
Inspection: Face and eyes should appear structurally normal:

- Eyes symmetrical
- Lids open and close completely
- Color of pupil is variable
- Sclera white (without blue tinge)
- No drainage; no excessive blinking or tearing

With ophthalmoscope or penlight:

- Identify red reflex.
- Infant should "fix" vision on light source and briefly follow the light as it is moved.

Age 4–12 Months

History: Continue to seek parental reports of observations which may indicate abnormal vision.
Inspect eyes for symmetry and normal appearance, including color of sclera and absence of drainage or excessive tearing.
Observe for symmetrical corneal light reflection.
Identify red reflex again.
Do funduscopic examination if possible.

Between Age 6 Months and 3–4 Years

Begin to attempt further eye examination.
Observe behavior during cover–uncover testing. Greater agitation when one eye is covered could indicate that the child does not see equally well with both eyes.
Attempt to get the child to fix vision on an object with each eye separately and to follow its movement.

By Age 4 Years

The child will probably be able to cooperate with the examiner who performs standard measures of ocular movement and visual acuity.
Testing should include measures of visual acuity in each eye separately as well as in both eyes together.

School-Age

Vision should be checked annually. As physical growth and development occur, ocular changes may occur as well. Visual acuity significantly affects school performance and social adjustment.
School-age children are anxious to please the examiner. Be particularly alert for "peeking" around the occluder card or other means of "cheating," such as memorizing the chart in use by watching other children taking the test.

pediatrician or family physician, ophthalmologist, optician, and nurse or nurse practitioner in the office, clinic, or school.

Conjunctivitis

Conjunctivitis in infants and children is an inflammation in and around the eye. It is irritating to the child, frightening to the parent, and of considerable concern to the primary health care provider. Conjunctivitis is always sufficient reason for evaluation to exclude dangerous conditions, identify treatable conditions, and to reassure the parent, child, and others.

Conjunctivitis may be of bacterial, viral, or allergic origin, occurring in the neonatal period as well as in the older child. Infectious conjunctivitis (primarily bacterial or viral) is spread by direct contact or direct extension. Allergic conjunctivitis may be a reaction to airborne environmental allergens or to substances placed in the eye or arriving in the eye by accident. Conjunctivitis may be a simple reaction to an allergen or chemical irritant, or it may be a severe infection.

Conjunctivitis in infants and children must be identified and treated without delay. The younger the child, the greater is the likelihood of severe damage resulting from an eye infection. Nurses need to be acutely aware of the emergency nature of eye infections in infants and to include this factor when teaching mothers and caregivers of newborns and young infants.

Ophthalmia Neonatorum

Ophthalmia neonatorum is a broad term applied to the ocular reaction of newborn infants that occurs in response either to a viral or bacterial invasion or to the chemical substance instilled at birth to prevent the bacterial invasion. Ophthalmia neonatorum may also be called "neonatal conjunctivitis" and presents as an inflammation of the conjunctiva with redness, swelling, and possibly a purulent discharge (O'Hara, 1993) (Fig. 28–12). Ophthalmia neonatorum occurs during the first 4 weeks of life (the neonatal period) and symptoms vary from mild to severe. The severity of the symptoms is not an indication of the causative organism.

Etiology

Etiologic agents in ophthalmia neonatorum may be of chemical or infectious nature (bacterial or viral). Chemical substances are instilled by health care providers to prevent bacterial invasion from organisms that the infant may have contacted during passage through the birth canal. These chemical substances may themselves cause conjunctivitis. Chemical conjunctivitis has been reported in 10% to 100% of neonates treated with silver nitrate 1% ocular drops (Isenberg, 1990; Nishida & Rosenberg, 1975; O'Hara, 1993; Wilson, 1979).

Figure 28–12
Neonatal conjunctivitis. A purulent, yellow discharge is noted draining from the conjunctiva.

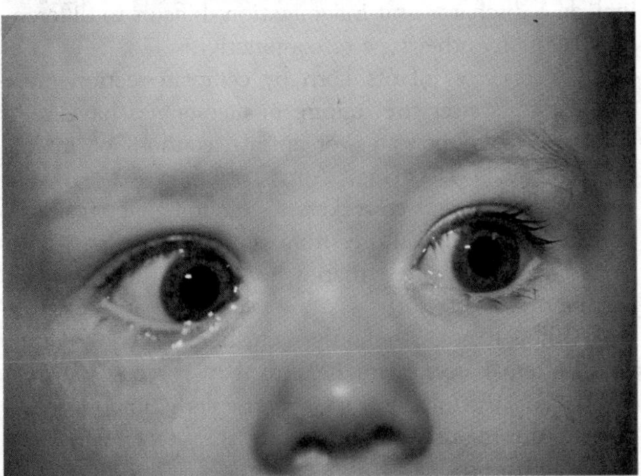

The chemical substances currently in use to prevent bacterial invasion include silver nitrate 1% drops and erythromycin 0.5% or tetracycline 1% drops or ointment (American Academy of Pediatrics, 1988). Erythromycin and tetracycline drops or ointment may also cause a mild reaction, although much less frequently.

caREminder: *Silver nitrate has been found to elicit a conjunctival reaction in up to 10% to 100% of the infants on whom it is used. Most practitioners agree that it is not effective unless it does create a mild conjunctivitis.*

Infectious conjunctivitis (caused by a bacterial or viral etiologic agent) is by far the most common ocular disease process found during the first month of life. It has been found to occur in 1.6% to 12% of newborn infants (Hammerschlag, 1993). The most frequently seen etiologic agent in ophthalmia neonatorum in industrialized countries is *Chlamydia trachomatis*. Statistical reports show that the incidence varies from 8.2 in 1000 live births in industrialized countries (Preece, Anderson, & Thompson, 1989) to 3% of neonates in the United States. Incidence is difficult to track because of the varied nature of the symptoms. It is known, however, that the disease develops in 50% of babies born to mothers with the organism in their genital tracts at the time of birth.

Most eye infections during the neonatal period are acquired during vaginal delivery and correlate in type with the sexually transmitted diseases prevalent in the community (O'Hara, 1993). During the 19th century, *Neisseria gonorrhoeae* was the organism most frequently implicated.

Worldview: *Gonococcal conjunctivitis has an incidence of 0 to 0.3 in 1000 live births in developed countries where maternal testing for the* N. gonorrhoeae *organism is routinely done and where treatment is instituted before the birth of the baby (Chen, 1992; Hammerschlag, 1993; Rothenberg, 1979).*

Chlamydia trachomatis is a modified bacterium that is an obligate intracellular parasite (O'Hara, 1993). The organism quickly (within hours) penetrates and destroys cells of the eye. According to recent studies, it is not controlled by any currently used prophylaxis given to infants during the first 48 hours after birth. There is mounting evidence that neither erythromycin nor tetracycline is effective in prevention of chlamydial conjunctivitis (Hammerschlag, Cummings, Roblin, Williams, & Delke, 1989). In many parts of the world, prenatal testing for chlamydia is not yet a routine practice, thus infants may be exposed during the birth process. Chen

(1992) estimates that the incidence of neonatal conjunctivitis with chlamydia identified as the etiologic agent is increasing at a rate of 3% per year.

Several other organisms common in the environment that cause conjunctivitis in older children have also been implicated as etiologic agents in neonatal conjunctivitis; these include *Haemophilus influenzae, Streptococcus pneumoniae, Escherichia coli, Staphylococcus aureus,* and others. Zero percent to 17% of neonatal conjunctivitis has been found to be associated with these organisms (Hammerschlag, 1993). None of these organisms carry the same degree of risk as is present with *N. gonorrhoeae* and *C. trachomatis* infections, and most of these infections are easily treated with common antibiotics.

The differential diagnosis and the identification of the etiologic agent in ophthalmia neonatorum can be made only with laboratory procedures. Neither history nor appearance of the drainage or symptoms is a reliable indicator of the severity of the condition or the causative organism.

Pathophysiology

The pathophysiology and prognosis of neonatal conjunctivitis depend on the etiologic factors involved and on the speed with which the diagnosis is made and appropriate treatment instituted. The infectious process usually has visible symptoms that alert the parent and caregivers to the developing infection. The neonate may have a more generalized response than an older child would have, and the follicular reaction common to conjunctivitis in older children is not present in neonates because of their immature immune system.

Chemical conjunctivitis is most frequently seen within 24 hours after silver nitrate 1% has been instilled. Silver nitrate ions bind to the protein cell walls of the bacteria as well as to conjunctival epithelial cells. The bacterial activity is interrupted immediately and the organisms destroyed. The body responds by sending neutrophils to the area. This tissue reaction manifests as conjunctivitis (Moore & Schmitt, 1979). When antibiotic ointment is used, the ocular reaction is much less. Cultures show no growth and no complications or sequelae accompany this type of neonatal conjunctivitis. The normal growth process restores the eye to its healthy state within 48 hours.

Although *gonorrheal conjunctivitis* is seen less frequently in industrialized countries, it is a severe and dangerous ocular infection. Usually after the incubation period of 3 to 5 days, the conjunctival inflammation and purulent discharge are seen. The eyelids may be red and inflamed as well. The infant may be fussy and may cry frequently as if in pain when the eyes are cleansed or examined. Symptoms may range from "mild," with small amounts of redness and discharge, to "severe," with severe redness, crying, and copious amounts of purulent discharge. The amount of discharge is not an indicator of either the type of infection or the severity of the condition. Gonorrheal conjunctivitis is always serious. The organism, within 24 hours of the onset of the infection, penetrates and destroys cells of the previously healthy eye (Moore & Schmitt, 1979; O'Hara, 1993). This causes corneal ulcerations and, if untreated, penetration of the globe of the eye and destruction of ocular structures. This damage results in scarring and blindness.

Chlamydial conjunctivitis is caused by a modified bacterium that the infant contacts during the birth process. The incubation period is reported to be 5 to 14 days; however, positive cultures have been reported at age 1 to 3 days (O'Hara, 1993). This organism is known for its predilection for spreading quickly to other body organs such as lungs and gastrointestinal tract, causing severe respiratory or gastrointestinal illness to develop in an initially healthy newborn. Chlamydial conjunctivitis presents with a mild to moderately erythematous conjunctiva and discharge from the eye that varies in quantity from moderate to large amounts. Associated findings often include otitis media, pneumonia, and rhinitis, and the organism may be isolated in the neonate's feces. If the infection is untreated, the organism penetrates ocular cells, causing corneal scarring, and may also cause other life-threatening disease processes.

Other bacterial organisms, such as *H. influenzae, Streptococcus,* and *E. coli,* which occasionally are implicated as causative factors in neonatal conjunctivitis, seldom cause anything more than a localized reaction that is easily treated with appropriate antibiotics as indicated by sensitivity testing. These common organisms generally do not, in healthy infants, proceed to cause infections in other parts of the body.

Viral conjunctivitis may be caused by the herpes virus, by the cytomegalovirus, or by other common viruses. If herpetic lesions are identified in the mother within 2 weeks of delivery, the infant should be delivered by cesarean section to avoid contacting the herpes virus. Symptoms commonly seen with herpetic conjunctivitis include a discharge and inflammation difficult to differentiate from any other type of conjunctivitis.

The eyes of infants born by cesarean section more than 3 hours after the rupture of membranes have been found to have the same organisms as those of infants born vaginally (Isenberg, Apt, Yoshimori, & Alvarez, 1988). Isenberg and coworkers also found that organisms were not found in cultures from the eyes of infants born by cesarean section less than 3 hours after the rupture of membranes.

Although not commonly seen, herpetic conjunctivitis recurrence occurs in 20% to 50% of cases (Reed, 1989). For this reason, it is particularly important to prevent the infant from contacting the herpes virus during the birth process.

Assessment

Assessment of the infant with ophthalmia neonatorum must include a maternal history that elicits information about prenatal care and exposure to sexually transmitted diseases and their treatment. In addition, an assessment is made of the appearance of the eyes and amount of drainage, if any, and the generalized response of the infant. The infant's immature immune system contributes to the general nature of the response. A careful psychosocial assessment of the family is helpful in planning follow-up care.

The nurse must note the day and time of the first sign of conjunctivitis as well as its progression. The infant's vital signs, interest in eating, and general responsiveness provide additional information about generalized symptoms. Elevated or subnormal temperature, lack of interest in feeding, and increased irritability are signs of generalized response. Careful chest assessment is also essential, because chlamydia may cause pneumonia as well.

Bacterial conjunctivitis may occur any time during the infant's first month of life, and most frequently occurs within the first 2 to 3 weeks. All caregivers who see the neonate must be aware of the potential severity of conjunctivitis in the young infant. Nurses and other caregivers who see the newborn in the hospital, clinic, or at home must immediately report signs of conjunctivitis. A culture and other specific testing may be ordered to identify an infectious agent.

Interdisciplinary Interventions

Ophthalmia neonatorum was first identified during the 1700s and was the cause of neonatal blindness in scores of children during the 18th and 19th centuries in central Europe. In 1881, Credé reported the use of silver nitrate 2% drops as a preventive measure. Silver nitrate 1% was also found to be effective and has been adopted as a prophylactic agent for prevention of gonorrheal conjunctivitis in many countries. Because of successful prenatal testing programs and control of gonorrhea in the United States and several other developed countries, the organism is seldom found in women about to give birth vaginally. For this reason, the use of silver nitrate 1% as a preventive for gonorrheal conjunctivitis is no longer necessary in developed countries. Antibiotic drops or ointment have replaced silver nitrate in an attempt to prevent other infectious agents from causing neonatal conjunctivitis.

If bacterial conjunctivitis is present, cleansing with normal saline is appropriate. Topical, oral, or parenteral antibiotics ordered by the physician are given to the infant by the parent or nurse. Infection control measures need to be carefully followed to prevent spread of any organisms that may be present.

Alert: *Gonorrheal conjunctivitis is a medical emergency.*

The infant should be hospitalized and given intravenous or intramuscular aqueous penicillin in divided doses for 7 days. The infant's eyes should be irrigated hourly with normal saline until the discharge subsides. If the organism is penicillin resistant, kanamycin, cefotaxime, ceftriaxone, or similar medication is reported to be successful when used in addition to erythromycin or tetracycline topical ointment for 10 days. This management has been found to be effective against all strains of *N. gonorrhoeae* (Laga et al., 1986; Latif et al., 1988; Zanoni, Isenberg, & Apt, 1992). The infant's eye drainage may be considered infectious for 24 to 48 hours after beginning treatment with an antibiotic to which the organism is susceptible.

Management of the infant with viral conjunctivitis may include hospitalization with isolation precautions implemented and the administration of acyclovir or other medication specific for viral infections. In addition, topical antibiotics may be used to prevent secondary infection with bacterial agents (Siegel, 1986).

Once treatment has been instituted, caregivers must note the progress of the condition to determine whether the selected treatment is effective in diminishing the symptoms. When the infant is discharged, caregivers must be sure that the parent has the necessary information and equipment to continue medication at home and to observe the progress of the condition. The importance of keeping the follow-up appointment must be stressed.

Because of the high incidence of systemic disease, chlamydial conjunctivitis should be treated with both topical and systemic antibiotics. Medications recommended for the treatment of chlamydial infections include erythromycin given intravenously or orally and combined with topical tetracycline or sulfacetamide drops or erythromycin ointment four times a day for 2 to 3 weeks. Both mother and sexual partners should be given oral tetracycline for 2 to 3 weeks. If the mother is breastfeeding, erythromycin (which is not excreted in breast milk) is substituted for the tetracycline. Because approximately 19% of neonates have persistent organisms after the first round of antibiotics, careful follow-up should occur and another round of antibiotics should be instituted if the organism is still present (Deschenes, Seamone, & Baines, 1990).

Community Care

Parent teaching is completed and documented by the nurse concerning medication administration, cleansing of the eyes, and observation for improvement. The nurse may either set up the follow-up appointment or assist the mother in doing so. Other caregivers who may be ready to assist the mother at home may also be included in the parent teaching. The importance of close communication with the primary health care provider must be stressed to the parent because it is possible for the child to lose his or her eyesight if the infection fails to clear.

Because of the prevalence of serious infections with *N. gonorrhoeae* or chlamydia among mothers who received no prenatal care, it is often wise to involve social services agents to assist with potential follow-up or funding problems. The nurse may also want to request a public health agent follow-up visit to the home.

Because there is an incubation period for some infectious agents that cause ophthalmia, symptoms may not appear before the infant's discharge from the hospital; therefore, all new mothers, particularly those who have had no prenatal care, need information concerning the possibility of the infection and encouragement to consult their primary health care provider immediately if an infection develops (TIP 28–2).

Ocular prophylaxis for newborns is required by law in all areas of the United States. Laws differ between states with respect to the amount of freedom given to health care professionals to determine the type of prophylaxis required. The commonly accepted prophylactic measure is application of erythromycin 0.5% ointment or drops. Controversy exists concerning which prophylactic agent, if any, is effective in preventing ophthalmia neonatorum (Isenberg, 1990).

Prophylactic measures have been adopted because of their presumed effectiveness against chlamydia. In industrialized countries, because *N. gonorrhoeae* is identified prenatally and only infrequently is still found in the vagina at the time of birth, the change in prophylaxis from silver nitrate to erythromycin or other antibiotic ointment was not considered to be a threat to infant health. It has been suggested, however, that careful accounting be made of the prenatal care received and additional prophylaxis be provided to infants whose mothers did not receive prenatal care. Chen (1992) found that all cases of gonorrheal conjunctivitis in his study occurred in infants whose mothers had received no prenatal care. There is growing evidence that neither erythromycin nor tetracycline is effective in preventing infections with chlamydia (Hammerschlag et al., 1989).

Conjunctivitis Beyond the Neonatal Period

Conjunctivitis in infants and children is a common problem, although much less severe in older infants and chil-

TIP 28–2 A Teaching Intervention Plan for the Newborn Infant with Eye Drainage

Nursing Diagnosis and Family Outcome

- Knowledge deficit: Aseptic care of infant's eye
  Outcome: Parent will demonstrate aseptic care of infant's eyes with drainage.

Teach the Family

- Observe the infant's eyes for drainage and redness:
  If present, note the amount, color, consistency, and time when it is present.
  Note whether the eyes are red as well.
  Note whether the infant seems to have eye pain.
- Wash your hands carefully with soap and water before and after wiping the baby's eyes.
- Drainage should be wiped away with a clean tissue. Wipe from the nose toward the temple. Use a clean spot on the tissue for each motion across each eye.
- Eye drainage that is yellow and sticky could be caused by an infection. If so, it could be considered contagious until an antibiotic has been given for 24 hours. A health care provider should be consulted before allowing other children to come into contact with the eye drainage.

Contact Health Care Provider if

- A medium to large amount of sticky drainage needs to be wiped away in the morning or after sleeping.
- The drainage is yellow instead of clear.
- The drainage needs to be wiped away more than once a day.
- The baby's eyes seem to hurt.
- The baby is more irritable than usual.

dren than it is in neonates. It is sometimes known as "pink eye" and is usually mild and self-limiting; however, it is still upsetting to both children and their parents (Fisher, 1987).

Conjunctivitis in older infants and children is usually either infectious (bacterial or viral) or allergic in origin. Gigliotti (1993) found that 73% of the eyes cultured were infected with bacterial agents and 27% with adenovirus. Allergic conjunctivitis may be a reaction to allergens carried by air currents or carried to the eyes by soiled hands, or a reaction to substances placed in the eye for other purposes.

Infectious Conjunctivitis

Bacterial conjunctivitis may accompany a respiratory infection and is most often caused by the same organisms, frequently *H. influenzae* or *S. pneumoniae.* Gonococcal conjunctivitis (also bacterial) may occur in adolescents who also have genital infections or in infants and young children who are exposed to the organism in the home. Viral conjunctivitis is most commonly caused by adenovirus (Gigliotti, 1993).

The pathophysiology of the infectious process in bacterial conjunctivitis is the invasion of the moist and warm conjunctiva by an organism that is able to thrive and reproduce in that location. The resulting infection causes symptoms that include the following:

- Yellow discharge in the eye
- Eyelids stuck together with purulent material after sleep
- Yellow discharge dried on cheek near the eyes
- Red or pink eyes (Schmitt, 1992)

Viral conjunctivitis is an infectious process caused by a virus. The resulting symptoms include redness of the sclera and inner eyelids, and clear watery discharge not caused by allergy or crying. There is no purulent material or matting of the eyelids in viral conjunctivitis (Schmitt, 1992). The conjunctiva is red and edematous and, in older children, follicular hyperplasia may also be present. The child frequently also has other signs of viral illness such as upper respiratory symptoms (e.g., pharyngitis) or gastrointestinal symptoms.

Assessment

Parents and caregivers must always be encouraged to seek appropriate medical intervention when an eye infection develops in an infant or child. Eye infections should never be approached with a "wait and see" attitude, because such an attitude could lead to impairment of vision.

The primary health care provider gathers data by means of history to determine possible exposure to bacterial or viral contaminants, infection in some other part of the body, or known infection in the home, daycare location, or school. The examiner also determines when the symptoms began and what symptoms were experienced. Careful assessment of the appearance of the eyes, the amount, color, and consistency of the drainage, if any, and the amount of swelling of the surrounding soft tissues is significant. Eye drainage cultures and sensitivity studies are used to identify the organism (Chart 28–9).

Several other more severe conditions may be mistaken at their outset for conjunctivitis. The health care provider assesses the patient for the possibility of each of these conditions. They include glaucoma (because of the tearing and photophobia), periorbital cellulitis (which involves the conjunctiva at the outset), and foreign body or trauma (which causes redness, irritation, and tearing of the eye). The nurse must be aware of these possibilities to assist in the differential diagnosis. In some cases, health care providers may also need information concerning the sexual activity of the individual.

Interdisciplinary Interventions

Broad-spectrum antibiotic ointment is ordered for topical use until the specific organism is known. An oral antibiotic may also be ordered. Parenteral antibiotics are usually successful in treating infections if other routes have been unsuccessful or if compliance is in question (Fisher, 1987).

Aqueous penicillin, given parenterally, is the treatment of choice for gonococcal conjunctivitis in the older child as it is in the neonate. A 5-day course of treatment has been found to be effective (Fisher, 1987).

Even though the purulent eye drainage of the bacterial eye infection is noncommunicable within 24 to 48 hours of the initiation of antibiotic treatment, if the child is to receive treatment at home from the family, the nurse may need to teach the family several methods of preventing the spread of the infection. The nurse should teach the family how to cleanse the infected eye from center to periphery with a clean moist washcloth, using a clean portion for each swipe.

caREminder: *The family must also learn how to instill the eye ointment so that a maximum amount is spread across the conjunctiva. The tube should be kept at room temperature and the child assisted to hold the eye open while a thin line of ointment is spread along the lower conjunctival sac. The child should be encouraged to blink several times to spread the ointment, then to hold the eyes lightly closed for a short time.*

Preventive measures to minimize spread of the infection to other members of the family should be reviewed. Towels, pillow, or clothing that touch the child's infected eye could carry organisms to other family mem-

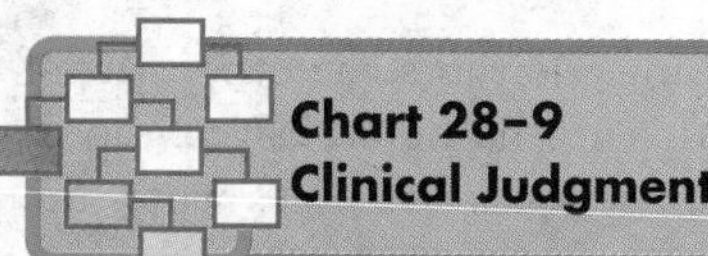

Chart 28–9
Clinical Judgment

The Child with Eye Drainage

Cindy is a nurse practitioner who provides health care services to a number of daycare facilities. She receives a call from a daycare director regarding Daniel, age 4, who awoke from his nap and was unable to open his eyes because of the presence of crusty, yellow purulent drainage. After Daniel's eyes were cleansed with a wet, warm cloth, Cindy was called. Cindy goes to the daycare center to see Daniel.

Questions

1. What other questions regarding Daniel's status should Cindy ask the daycare director at this time?
2. What actions should Cindy recommend be taken with Daniel?
3. What is Daniel's diagnosis?
4. What treatment measures should be instituted at this time for Daniel and the other children at the daycare center?
5. How would Cindy determine that Daniel's condition has improved?

Answers

1. Does he have a fever? Does he have any known allergies? Has any drainage been observed before this event? Has Daniel been rubbing his eyes frequently? Is he receiving treatment at home for this condition or for any other health problem? Do any family members or other children or workers at the daycare center have an infection?
2. She should complete a physical assessment of the eye noting signs of redness, and the amount, color, and consistency of eye drainage. Recommend to the parents that a culture of the eye drainage be completed.
3. Conjunctivitis of unknown etiology until culture results are returned. Yellow, purulent eye drainage indicates a likely bacterial cause.
4. Antibiotic therapy should be ordered for a bacterial infection. The child should not return to daycare until treatment has been initiated for 2 days. Towels, clothing, or pillows that have contacted the child's eyes should be washed.
5. Absence of eye drainage and fever.

bers. The child's towel should not be used by other members of the family and the child should not use any towel but his or her own. The child should be taught to keep his or her hands away from the eyes and to wash hands frequently during the day. Infants may need to be fitted with elbow restraints to prevent rubbing of the eyes.

Viral conjunctivitis is usually self-limiting and does not, in itself, require antibiotic administration. However, the health care provider may choose to provide a topical antibiotic to prevent superinfection with a bacterial agent.

Community Care

The school nurse may be responsible for telling parents that their child has conjunctivitis. Children are often excluded from school until the conjunctivitis has cleared. Even though a child with a bacterial conjunctivitis may be noncommunicable after 24 to 48 hours of treatment, there is frequently a delay in definitive diagnosis, and symptoms may still be present. In addition, children often need to have the medication instilled four times each day. Thus, children are asked to remain at home until the conjunctivitis has cleared. Prognosis in all cases of conjunctivitis in children older than age 30 days is excellent with early diagnosis and adequate treatment.

Allergic Conjunctivitis

Allergic conjunctivitis may be seasonal, induced by airborne antigens such as ragweed or pollens, or it may be experienced year-round, induced by animal dander, dust mites, or some other ever-present antigen. Allergic conjunctivitis may be the sole manifestation of a child's allergy or it may be accompanied by respiratory or dermatologic responses.

Pathophysiology

Antigens may be introduced to the eyes by physical contact of the child's hands with the eyes, or they may be carried to the eye on air currents in the environment. When foreign proteins settle on the conjunctiva, the immune response is immediately initiated, resulting in redness, clear to stringy mucoid fluid production, and mild to severe itching.

The tissue response varies from mild to severe and may include swelling of the eyelids. This reaction enhances the chance that the child will rub his or her eyes. Such rubbing may introduce further allergens or bacteria into the eyes, thus complicating the allergic response.

Allergic conjunctivitis seldom, if ever, results in permanent visual impairment. It is of importance primarily because of the frequency with which it is experienced rather than because of its severity.

Assessment

The focused health history for the child with allergic conjunctivitis must include general information concerning allergies to foods and medicines and contact with or inhaled environmental allergens as well as "triggers" for eye symptoms. Time of onset of symptoms and recent exposure to environmental allergens, pets, or dust must be included. To assist in differential diagnosis, the history may also focus on possible bacterial or viral agents with which the child may have come into contact (Table 28–2).

The presenting symptom is typically red, itchy, watery eyes that create mild to moderate discomfort. Physical assessment reveals conjunctival vasodilation, edema of the eyelids, and a watery to stringy mucoid discharge. The child may also have rhinitis and related nose and throat symptoms.

Laboratory examination of the exudate reveals eosinophils in the exudate of the child with allergic conjunctivitis. Failure to find eosinophils could indicate that the symptoms are not allergic in origin. Presence or absence of bacterial conjunctivitis should be established before definitive treatment of allergic conjunctivitis is initiated.

Interdisciplinary Interventions

When the diagnosis has been established, treatment of allergic conjunctivitis will probably include medication to treat the symptoms that the child is experiencing as well as prophylactic agents to prevent further episodes. The treatment elected may be topical, systemic, or both.

Vasoconstrictor eye drops may be used sparingly according to direction and for not more than 3 days (to avoid rebound congestion). Cromolyn sodium 4% ophthalmic solution (1 to 2 drops every 4 to 6 hours) is used for symptomatic relief (Burns et al., 1996). Oral antihistamines may be used to diminish the body's generalized response. If the conjunctivitis fails to clear, referral to an allergist or ophthalmologist is in order.

In addition to the treatment of the immediate symptoms, environmental assessment and control may be the best way to prevent future episodes. The nurse plays a vital and significant role in history taking and in teaching the family to assess the child's environment and make the necessary changes to diminish exposure to environmental allergens.

Education should focus on elimination or avoidance of pollen-related allergens and on cleaning procedures for removal of dust mites and animal dander. Furnishings in the child's room should be easy to clean or launder. Throw rugs collect less dust than carpets; blankets and curtains should be frequently laundered. Pets should be kept out of the child's bedroom.

Tip: *Children should be taught not to rub their eyes with their hands, which themselves may be soiled with allergens or bacteria. A substitute activity to relieve the itching is to use cool compresses made with a washcloth moistened with tap water.*

Symptoms should improve within 24 to 48 hours after treatment is begun. Follow-up is important to diminish or prevent future episodes of allergic conjunctivitis.

Community Care

The school teacher or school nurse may be the first to notice the onset of conjunctivitis and should strongly encourage the child to seek treatment as soon as possible.

Table 28–2
Allergic vs Bacterial Conjunctivitis

	Allergic	Bacterial
Physical	Clear mucous drainage Bilateral Inflamed conjunctiva Intense itching Swollen lids	Purulent drainage Bilateral or unilateral Inflamed conjunctiva with or without mild itching Swollen lids
History	Rhinitis Environmental triggers Food allergies	Fever Other site of infection (e.g., bilateral otitis media or upper respiratory infection) "Crusted eyes" in morning

A child with itching eyes cannot concentrate on learning. The sooner the condition is identified, the earlier treatment is begun and the sooner the child is likely to recover.

Retinopathy of Prematurity

Retinopathy of prematurity (ROP) is the term used since 1984 to designate the aberrant and abnormal vascularization of the retina that occurs in some premature infants, causing impaired vision or blindness. The condition was first identified in 1942 and, at that time, was called retrolental fibroplasia (Terry, 1942). The name was changed in 1984 after an international team of ophthalmologists met to identify a generally agreed upon classification system to describe the stages and severity of the disease process.

In the late 1940s and early 1950s, ROP occurred in epidemic numbers among premature infants. After the use of high concentrations of oxygen was curtailed in the mid-1950s, the incidence of ROP declined to almost zero. As technological advances have enabled greater numbers of very-low-birth-weight infants to survive, the incidence of ROP is again increasing. ROP continues to occur in very-low-birth-weight infants, even when low oxygen precautions are taken; thus researchers are still searching for other etiologic relationships. Approximately 20% of infants born weighing less than 1500 g show evidence of ROP, and, as birth weight decreases, incidence of ROP increases (Flynn et al., 1987; George, Stephen, Fellows, & Bremer, 1988). In a multicenter study involving 4009 infants, ROP occurred in 47% of those weighing 1000 to 1250 g at birth, 78% of those weighing 750 to 999 g at birth, and 90% of those weighing less than 750 g at birth (Palmer et al., 1991; Phelps, 1992). Other possible etiologic factors that have been examined include bright nursery lights (Glass et al., 1985), nutritional deficiencies (Johnson et al., 1985; Schaffer, Johnson, Quinn, Weston, & Bowen, 1985), and too rapid withdrawal of oxygen regardless of concentration (Phelps, 1988). In addition, more recently, the variability of transcutaneous PO_2 in the first 2 weeks of life has been implicated (Cunningham, Fleck, Elton, & McIntosh, 1995).

Pathophysiology

In the normal newborn, retinal blood vessels are barely complete in their formation, and the macula has not yet finished its developmental process. The pathophysiology of ROP is one of injury to the developing blood vessels and tissues of the retina and the healing process of regrowth or overgrowth of retinal vessels.

In normal fetal development, the blood vessels of the retina develop during the last half of the pregnancy. Retinal vessels begin to develop near the disk and grow toward the periphery of the retina between 16 and 44 weeks' gestation (Phelps, 1992). Great variability exists with respect to the time of completion of this process; thus, when an infant is born prematurely, the status of eye development is not predictable.

It is presumed that the low PaO_2 at which the fetal eye develops stimulates release of an angiogenic factor from the retina whenever the retina becomes slightly ischemic. This factor is presumed to stimulate development of retinal vessels and normal development of rods and cones. The infant in whom ROP develops has been found to have overgrowth of retinal vessels. In 50% of infants with ROP, this overgrowth ceases or regresses spontaneously. In the other 50%, the overgrowth continues, making the development of useful vision unlikely because of the fibrotic changes of the retina or retinal detachment.

Prognosis. The prognosis for infants with ROP depends on the amount of overgrowth of retinal vessels and is not predictable by age, weight, or gestational age. A great deal of research is still needed to improve the visual outcome for infants with ROP.

Assessment

Screening for ROP should be performed by an ophthalmologist on all infants exposed to oxygen and all infants weighing less than 1000 g at birth. For premature infants, the ophthalmic examination should be done when the infant is 30 to 32 weeks' postconceptional age and again within 2 weeks to monitor the progress of retinal vascularization. Cardiac and oxygen monitoring should be performed during the examination, and resuscitation equipment should be available because of the potential for bradycardia during eye manipulation and scleral pressure (Vander, 1994). ROP is not likely to develop in infants of 42 weeks' postconceptional age or older.

The nurse regularly monitors the environmental oxygen level in the incubator, is responsible for the care of the infant, and encourages the involvement of the parents. A significant part of the nursing responsibility is assessment of the family adjustment. The nurse also assesses parental knowledge and understanding of the condition, growth, and development of the premature infant with a potentially disabling condition.

Interdisciplinary Interventions

Interventions may be directed toward prevention or toward treatment of ROP after its appearance. The neonatologist, neonatal nurse, pediatrician, ophthalmologist, and other primary health care providers are the participants in the management team after the birth of the infant. Prevention of premature birth is by far the best way to decrease the number of infants born before their eyes are fully developed. It is well known that prenatal care decreases the incidence of premature birth, thus any effort to decrease premature births also would decrease the incidence of ROP. Health care professionals in the community who work to prevent preterm births play an integral part in the prevention of the disabling effects of ROP. Nurses are key players in this group of community-based health professionals. Nurses have a significant role to play in the prevention of premature births.

Medications and Dietary Components

Various theories have been proposed concerning what the contributing factors are in the development of ROP. ROP is often considered to be an oxidant injury, thus an antioxidant might be expected to provide some degree of protection. Vitamin E, a naturally occurring fat-soluble antioxidant that does not pass through the placental barrier to the premature infant, has been administered to premature infants in the form of tocopherol as a preventive measure. Studies have demonstrated mixed results, and there is no clear indication that such therapy helps to prevent ROP (Hittner et al., 1981; Phelps 1992; Phelps, Rosenbaum, Isenberg, Leake, & Dorey, 1987; Schaffer et al., 1985).

Penicillamine is another antioxidant that was used in Hungary to treat hyperbilirubinemia. An unexpected outcome was that a lower incidence of ROP occurred in this group of infants. The treatment seems to be safe, but has not had sufficient testing to definitively identify a value in its use (Phelps, 1992).

Inositol is a dietary component that has been used to treat chronic lung disease. A lower incidence of ROP was noted in the group of infants given inositol. This supplement needs to be tested further before researchers can be sure of its usefulness and safety in preventing ROP (Phelps, 1992).

Surgical Interventions and Other Therapies

The goals of treatment of ROP are to arrest the growth of new and aberrant blood vessels in the retina, to prevent complications such as detached retina, and to allow continued normal development of vision. During the premature infant's hospital stay, the ophthalmologist monitors the progression of the condition with weekly eye examinations. Surgical intervention to arrest the growth of retinal vasculature may be necessary.

Cryotherapy may be used if the lens is clear. Cryotherapy is the cryoablation (freezing) of the avascular retinal portion that is thought to be producing the angiogenic growth factor that is stimulating neovascularization and overgrowth of retinal vessels. This therapy is not undertaken unless the ophthalmologist sees clear evidence of blood vessel growth's having reached the "threshold" level.

Risks involved with cryotherapy include the possibility that it will be unsuccessful, the possibility of reflex bradycardia when pressure is placed on the eye, and the return of apneic spells from hours to days after the cryotherapy is applied (Brown et al., 1990). In addition, cryotherapy has been associated with increased risk for myopia in premature infants and increased risk for retinal detachment during adulthood (Preslan, 1993).

Laser technology is being developed that can accomplish the same effect as cryotherapy but it can be done more easily and with fewer side effects. Laser therapy may be performed even when the lens is cloudy (Preslan, 1993) and has been demonstrated to have a successful visual outcome in at least as many cases of threshold ROP as cryotherapy (Vander, 1994).

Other surgical procedures may be needed if retinal detachment occurs; however, none has yet demonstrated ability to provide a positive visual outcome in these tiny infants with very fragile tissues. In ROP, retinal detachment is thought to be the result of the excess weight of aberrant vasculature or scar tissue formation; thus the retina does not readily return to its predetached position, even with surgery.

The role of the nurse in the care of the infant with ROP is one of careful and sensitive daily care, including monitoring of oxygen levels. The nurse encourages parental bonding and parental care in so far as is possible. The prognosis for infants with ROP is variable, and parents often require considerable support to be able to accept the long periods of time without knowing the degree of damage that their child will have sustained. The nurse may become aware of the parents' need for intervention by social services agents or the clergy in their efforts to adjust to the possibility that their infant will have permanent damage.

Community Care

When the infant is discharged, follow-up by both primary health care provider and ophthalmologist is essential. All persons involved need to be aware of the increased risk for retinal detachment that exists in infants with ROP. If the infant has a poor visual outcome, parents may need guidance in how to best assist the infant to continue development in as near a normal pattern as is possible.

Referral to a support group or to national organizations that provide assistive materials may be in order (see Resources).

Cataracts

Any opacity of the lens is a cataract. The lens of the eye begins development on the 27th day of fetal life with the differentiation of the lens capsule. Development is complete by the end of the first trimester, only increasing

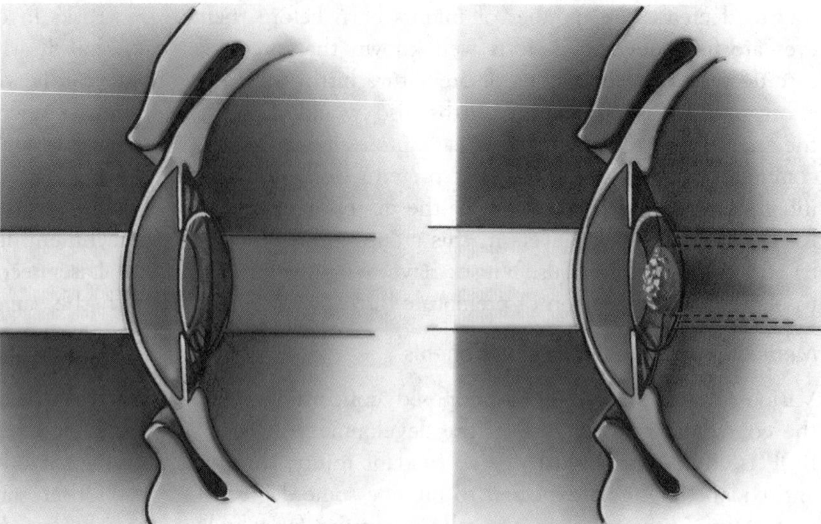

(A) LIGHT PASSES THROUGH A NORMAL EYE WITHOUT ANYTHING BLOCKING ITS WAY.
(B) WHEN THE LENS OF THE EYE BECOMES CLOUDY, THE CATARACT PREVENTS ENOUGH LIGHT FROM PASSING THROUGH TO SEE CLEARLY.

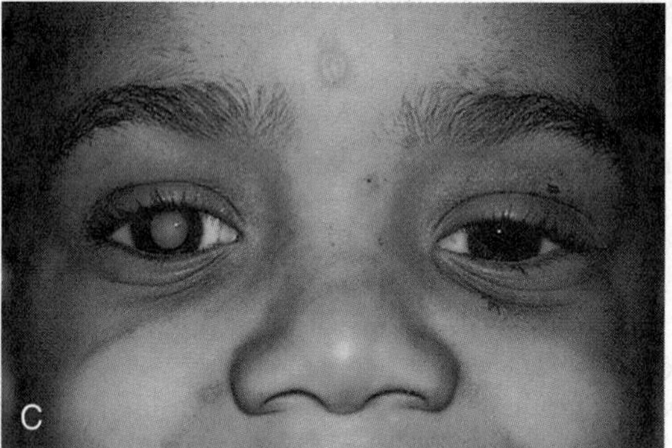

Figure 28–13
Cataracts may develop in infants or children of any age. (Part C from Albert, D. M., & Jakobiec, F. A. [1996]. *Atlas of clinical ophthalmology* [p. 471]. Philadelphia: W. B. Saunders. Reprinted with permission.)

in size until maturity (Potter, 1993). Cataracts may be congenital or acquired. Congenital cataracts may be noted at birth or may not be seen until later in infancy (Fig. 28–13).

Incidence

Congenital cataracts occur in an estimated 1 in 250 newborns (0.4%) worldwide (Potter, 1993), with incidence being greater in countries where nutrition is poor and prenatal care limited. Pediatric cataracts account for 15% to 20% of childhood blindness in industrialized countries (Potter, 1993). Thirty percent of congenital cataracts are sporadic occurrences, and another 30% are due to infectious agents affecting the fetus (Pike, Jan, & Wong, 1989). Rubella continues to affect populations worldwide. When the rubella virus infects the fetus early in the first trimester, an opacity develops in the center of the lens, from which the virus can be cultured many years after birth (Potter, 1993). Other infectious agents that are implicated in congenital cataracts include toxoplasmosis, cytomegalovirus, herpes, syphilis, and possibly varicella (Lambert, Amaya, & Taylor, 1989; Potter, 1993; Symanski, Newman, & Bachynski, 1994). When any one of these agents is present in the maternal history, the infant should be carefully evaluated for cataracts (Table 28–3).

Genetic factors contribute to the development of congenital cataracts. Eight percent to 25% of isolated cataracts are familial with autosomal dominant inheritance being most common (Mostafa et al., 1981). This type of inheritance is characterized by variable expression; thus parents and siblings should also be examined because they may have cataracts of varying degrees of severity (Potter, 1993).

Several other etiologic factors must be considered when a cataract is a sporadic finding. The possibility of child abuse or occult trauma must be considered if other causes have been ruled out.

Table 28–3
Etiology of Pediatric Cataracts

Category	Type	Comment
Sporadic		30% of congenital cataracts are sporadic.
Hereditary	Autosomal dominant	Most common
	Autosomal recessive	
	X-linked	
Chromosomal disorder	Trisomy 21	Cataracts seldom appear before age 10.
	Trisomy 18	
	Trisomy 13	Early mortality
	Turner's syndrome	
Prematurity		Cataracts are associated with history of hypoxic episodes.
Infectious agents	Rubella	30% incidence in infected fetuses
	Toxoplasmosis	
	Varicella	
	Cytomegalovirus	
	Syphilis	
	Herpes simplex	
	Mumps	
Metabolic disorders	Galactosemia	Autosomal recessive—chromosome 9
	Galactokinase deficiency	Autosomal recessive—chromosome 17
	Alport's syndrome	Autosomal dominant
	Lowe syndrome	X-linked
	Hypoglycemia	
	Hypocalcemia	
Systemic disorders	Myotonic dystrophy	Autosomal dominant
	Dermatologic disorders	The lens originates from the ectoderm.
	Craniofacial/mandibulofacial disorders	

Adapted from Potter, W. S. (1993). Pediatric cataracts. *Pediatric Clinics of North America, 40*(4), 846. Used with permission.

Pathophysiology

During the fourth and fifth weeks of fetal development, the lens capsule forms. Normally, it forms as a clear membrane. If the forming lens is attacked by an organism, it becomes milky white and cloudy, and may fail to continue to develop. This opacification is called the *cataract.*

The optic nerve and internal ocular structures continue to develop normally unless the etiologic agent attacks these as well. Ocular development and visual development continue after birth. Also after birth, the infant's eyes develop the ability to transfer images to the visual cortex of the brain. If a cataract is present, the visual image cannot reach the brain and the visual cortex fails to continue to develop. If the cataract is removed before the infant is 2 months old, the visual center of the brain is able to resume development. If the cataract is not removed, the visual cortex of the brain cannot learn to receive and process visual information from the affected eye.

Impaired visual acuity that accompanies a cataract may result in nystagmus (rapid oscillating movement of the eye) or strabismus (wandering eye) in the affected eye. It is important to consider the possibility of a cataract when strabismus or nystagmus is present.

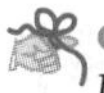
caREminder: *Trauma may also pose a threat to vision because injuries may lead to scarring. Scarring is a type of cataract.*

Assessment

Some cataracts may be detected easily during physical examination of the eye, whereas others may not be externally visible and may not be detected until preschool vision testing is done. The absence of the red reflex and the appearance of the white opacity of the lens are telltale signs of a cataract (see Fig. 28–13). Facial scars from burns, trauma, or abuse should cause the examiner to observe the child closely for lens opacification. Any history of poisoning with a toxic substance or history of severe infection, particularly with varicella or other viral condition, should alert the examiner. A child with any other ocular disorder or diminished acuity such as strabismus, amblyopia, or nystagmus may have an associated internal or superficial cataract and should be assessed carefully.

Interdisciplinary Interventions

The primary goal is the preservation of or the development of useful vision for the child. The achievement of this outcome is dependent on the nature of the condition, the age of identification and removal of the cataract, and the diligence of the child and family in maintaining the visual therapy program.

Any person performing the newborn examination should certainly examine the eyes for a congenital cataract. If the red reflex is absent or if a white opacity is seen, the infant should be referred immediately to the pediatrician or ophthalmologist for evaluation and follow-up. Opacities of the lens are never normal and always need full evaluation as soon as possible. Congenital cataracts need to be surgically removed before the infant is age 2 months to prevent amblyopia and loss of useful vision.

In studies of patients with bilateral congenital cataracts (Gelbart, Hoyt, Jastrebski, & Marg, 1982; Hing, Speedwell, & Taylor, 1990), visual acuities of 20/60 to 20/80 or better were found in all infants undergoing surgery before age 8 weeks, whereas visual acuity of 20/200 or less was found in 83% to 86% of infants undergoing surgery after age 8 weeks. Bradford and colleagues (1994) studied 33 patients and found similar results. In another study, infants undergoing surgery for removal of a unilateral cataract before age 17 weeks achieved visual acuity of 20/80 or better (Birch & Stager, 1988; Cheng et al., 1991). Identifying congenital cataracts very early and seeking their removal before age 8 weeks seems essential to preserving useful vision for these infants.

Preparation of the family for the infant's surgery is a significant role for the nurse. Cataract removal is done by an ophthalmologist and is often completed on an outpatient basis. Infants, however, may be kept overnight for close observation. Permanent visual impairment may exist as a result of delayed diagnosis, cataract removal performed too late to allow visual development, or the presence of another congenital defect within the eye structure.

Community Care

Postoperatively, although infections are rare, antibiotic drops are usually prescribed for several weeks. Parents are taught by the nurse how to administer eye ointment or drops so as to prevent secondary infection of the surgical site. A patch and a plastic or metal eye protector is used over the eye from which the cataract was removed. The patch should be applied loosely to avoid pressure on the globe of the eye. The patch and protector are kept on at all times, to be removed and replaced only when medications are instilled. The parent is instructed to look for any unusual redness or swelling and to report this immediately to the ophthalmologist.

Tip: *The child must be prevented from rubbing the eye while awake or asleep. For young children, elbow restraints may be obtained from the hospital or doctor's office to prevent their hands from reaching their eyes.*

Community resources may be available to families of infants who have poor visual outcomes (see Resources). Several organizations supply written materials, and support groups in many communities teach and assist parents in providing the best environment for the development of the infant or child with limited vision or blindness. Infants and children who are blind or who have limited vision need different approaches to allow maximal development of cognitive and social skills. These are discussed in the section titled Visual Impairment—Blindness.

The infant who has undergone cataract surgery also requires aggressive treatment of amblyopia to achieve useful vision. (See the section on amblyopia earlier in the chapter.) The success of treatment is largely dependent on the infant's age at which diagnosis and cataract removal are accomplished and on the cooperation of infant and family with the occlusive patching regimen designed to stimulate the development of the weaker eye.

Corrective lenses may be recommended by the ophthalmologist. Lens implant or graft is not as yet recommended for infants.

When the child returns to the primary health care provider for well-child care, the nurse provides follow-up assessment of vision and monitors compliance with the therapeutic regimen developed by the ophthalmologist. As the child grows older, further assessment of visual status, using the assistance of developmental specialists, educators, and family support groups, may be needed, depending on the amount of useful vision that develops. The nurse may be able to facilitate the family role as advocate for the child as family members learn to access the services needed to facilitate the health care and education of their child.

Glaucoma

Glaucoma is a rare but potentially devastating condition when it occurs in infants and young children. It can be easily identified by parents and professionals. If the signs and symptoms are unidentified and untreated, however, the result is likely to be severe visual impairment early in childhood.

Infantile glaucoma, also called trabeculodysgenesis, is a deformity of the eye (the trabecular meshwork) that prevents normal circulation and drainage of aqueous humor and results in increased intraocular pressure. The term "congenital glaucoma" is sometimes applied to this condition. This implies that the condition was present at birth, and, indeed, the pathologic framework may be present at that time. Clinically, however, the condition is often not evident until the child is several months old, thus the term "infantile glaucoma" seems more appropriate. The term is applied to glaucoma identified in any child younger than 3 years old (DeLuise & Anderson, 1983).

Juvenile glaucoma refers to the onset of the disease after age 3 years and is usually secondary to some other disease process. Signs and symptoms are essentially the same for infantile and juvenile glaucoma, although their manifestations differ somewhat with the age of the child.

Incidence

The incidence of glaucoma in infants and young children has been estimated to be 1 in 10,000 live births in the United States. It occurs more frequently in males than females in a ratio of 3:2 (Duke-Elder, 1969; Wagner, 1993). In the past, as many as 5% to 15% of persons institutionalized for visual disability in the United States had infantile glaucoma (Duke-Elder, 1969). With earlier diagnosis and advances in treatment, as many as 90% of children with infantile glaucoma are currently successfully treated (Stern & Catalano, 1990).

Seventy percent of cases of infantile glaucoma are bilateral (Franks & Taylor, 1989). Fifty percent are the result of an isolated defect, sometimes called primary glaucoma. The other 50% are called secondary glaucoma and are associated with another congenital systemic disease such as Marfan syndrome, neurofibromatosis, homocystinuria, Lowe's syndrome, or congenital rubella. Some children with chromosomal disorders also have been found to have infantile glaucoma; however, no specific genetic basis has been identified (Franks & Taylor, 1989). Ten percent of cases have been found to be familial, transmitted as an autosomal recessive trait (Seidman, Nelson, Calhoun, Spaeth, & Harley, 1986). Consanguinity considerably increases the likelihood of appearance of the trait.

Pathophysiology

Infantile glaucoma, like glaucoma in adults, is characterized by an increase in intraocular pressure. Most cases of infantile glaucoma are due to a congenital defect in the trabecular meshwork that fails to allow sufficient aqueous humor to drain out of the eye (Franks & Taylor, 1989). Enlargement of the eye (buphthalmos), corneal edema, cupping of the optic disk, and narrowing of the visual fields resulting from optic nerve damage occur. If identified and treated before optic nerve damage occurs, cupping of the optic disk is reversible in children and visual prognosis is better than if diagnosis is made later.

Infantile and juvenile glaucoma may occur secondary to a coexisting pathologic process. For example, Marfan syndrome is an autosomal dominant congenital disorder affecting connective tissue, osseous development, and heart and eye structures. The etiology of glaucoma that is sometimes seen in children with Marfan syndrome is thought to be related to the abnormal connective tissue structure. The trabecular meshwork does not allow circulation of the aqueous humor out of the intraocular space, thus causing an increase in intraocular pressure.

Glaucoma in children, as in adults, may be an acquired condition resulting from an injury with scar tissue formation. Scar tissue may prevent the outflow of aqueous humor, causing an increase in intraocular pressure. Children with acquired glaucoma have symptoms similar to those of young infants; however, pain is predominant and these children are usually old enough to clearly indicate its source.

Prognosis. The desired patient outcome is the control of intraocular pressure and the preservation of vision. However, the prognosis of glaucoma depends largely on the severity of the condition when first noted and the degree of damage already done. If left untreated, infantile glaucoma progresses steadily and results in blindness. The earlier the onset of glaucoma, the poorer the visual outcome is likely to be. When glaucoma is present at birth, more than 50% of the affected eyes will be legally blind, whereas with later onset only 20% will be legally blind. Intraocular pressure can usually be controlled in 85% of cases; however, only 35% will have visual acuity better than 20/50 (Wagner, 1993).

Assessment

Infants with glaucoma may experience either sudden onset or more gradual onset of symptoms. Signs and symptoms may be noted within a few days of birth or may develop insidiously during the first year of life. The infant should be assessed for the comparative size of the eyes, corneal clouding (hazy white area over the lens) (Fig. 28–14), blue tinge to the sclera, tearing or excess watering of the eyes without evidence of infection (called *epiphora*), photophobia (sensitivity to light) even under low light conditions, and blepharospasm (involuntary closure of eyelids). The infant may also have enlargement of one or both eyes, but parents may not have associated this with disease, particularly if the condition is bilateral and if large eyes are a desirable trait (Quigley, 1982; Seidman, Nelson, Calhoun, Spaeth, & Harley, 1989; Wagner, 1993). A difference in pupillary size of even

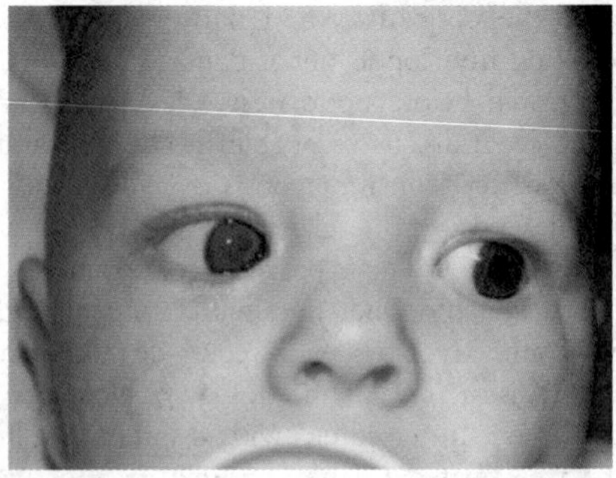

Figure 28–14
Corneal clouding in an infant with glaucoma. (From Albert, D. M., & Jakobiec, F. A. [1996]. *Atlas of clinical ophthalmology* [p. 472]. Philadelphia: W. B. Saunders. Reprinted with permission.)

1 mm is considered abnormal, but deciding if the smaller or the larger eye is abnormal may be difficult. Complicating the diagnostic process is the fact that infants frequently do not have all of the classic signs and symptoms of the condition. Assessment of intraocular pressure must be done under anesthesia for infants, young children, and those who are developmentally delayed or otherwise unable to cooperate during the test.

Parents' descriptions of the infant's behavior are particularly important. Infants may demonstrate unexplained behavior changes, such as irritability and episodes of unexplained crying, which alert the parents that something is wrong. Some parents may hesitate to mention behavior changes unless the health care provider specifically asks. Parents may not associate these behaviors with disease.

Alert: *Infants who have episodes of unexplained irritability and crying or unexplained behavior change should be examined for eye pain and glaucoma.*

Infants who are at least several months old and who have the dexterity to rub their eyes with their hands will do so if pain in the eyes is present. This information should be elicited from the parents because they may consider this another minor behavioral occurrence without recognizing its significance to the diagnosis.

All infants should be screened not only in the newborn nursery by a pediatrician, but again at age 6 weeks, 8 months, 18 months, and 3 years (Taylor, 1986). This screening may be done by the pediatrician, family practice physician, or nurse practitioner and should include clear identification of the red reflex with a search for opacities of the lens. If the red reflex is hazy or absent, corneal edema could be present indicating infantile glaucoma. Even a suspicion of glaucoma should be treated with urgency and referral to an ophthalmologist should be immediate. Prognosis is excellent when diagnosis and treatment occur early.

The "puff" test for intraocular pressure measurement may be used by the eye care specialist who tests children as young as age 4 to 4½ years.

Tip: *Before the test, the child needs to be fully prepared, usually by a parent, so that he or she will cooperate fully. The young child is much better able to cooperate if the test is approached as a game and the child given the responsibility to hold his or her eyes "open wide" until the "puff" comes, then "you can close them tight." The doctor performs the test first on one side and then on the other.*

Interdisciplinary Interventions

The ophthalmologist may first administer medication to temporarily decrease ocular edema, clear the cornea, and improve visualization of both the surgical site and the iridocorneal angle. In most cases, however, surgery is needed either within hours of the diagnosis or within a few days to improve the outflow of aqueous humor from the eye and to minimize optic nerve damage.

The surgical procedure used to treat glaucoma is the *goniotomy*. In this procedure, an incision is made in the trabecular meshwork to allow adequate outflow and to control symptoms of glaucoma. A single incision is sufficient in 80% of glaucoma cases. Recurrence occurs in 20% to 30% of cases, necessitating more extensive surgery called the *trabeculotomy*. A few cases require further medical or surgical management, and, in a very few cases, the deformities are so extensive that a positive visual outcome is impossible.

Postoperative care of the infant or child following goniotomy is similar to the care given after cataract removal. The infant may require the use of an eye patch and protective device for a short period of time after the surgery. Elbow restraints may be used to prevent the child from rubbing his or her eyes.

Community Care

The infant with glaucoma needs regular follow-up with the ophthalmologist throughout life. Both the nurse and the primary health care provider should encourage and facilitate such visits.

Parents of children undergoing even the simplest eye surgery need the support of relatives and nursing staff to ease their anxiety. A financial counselor may need to assist the family in identifying funding sources for the surgery and hospitalization. The social worker may be able to assist in matters of funding, transportation, and lodging if the family lives a distance from the specialized health care providers that the child needs.

When the child enters school, the school nurse

should be made aware of the past history of health problems and needs to be made part of the health care provider network available to the family. During the school years, the school nurse may be able to assist or encourage the family to obtain the health care follow-up that the child needs to prevent deterioration of vision. The school nurse also functions as a liaison among health care professionals, educators, and the family to help such children achieve their maximum potential.

Special attention should be given to the developmental and educational progress of children who have had a poor visual outcome. They may need alternative learning tools to make best use of limited visual acuity.

Eye Injuries

Eye injuries include injuries related to head injury from accident or abuse, sports injuries, blunt force injuries from other children's extremities, blunt force or penetrating injuries caused by objects in the environment (including toys) or firearms, fire or chemical splash burns, and ingestion of chemicals causing toxic blindness. Shunt failure or optic nerve damage related to late diagnosis of hydrocephalus and increased intracranial pressure may also cause injury to visual structures. Many of these injuries are accidental, but may be avoided by adult awareness and concern for avoidance of the injury potential.

Incidence

Children's eye injuries are the third most common cause of acquired visual loss in children (26% of the sample), preceded only by tumors (28%) and genetic causes (35%) (Robinson & Jan, 1993). According to the National Society to Prevent Blindness (1988), at least 90% of injuries causing visual impairment can be prevented.

The incidence of various types of eye injuries varies with the age and sex of the child. Ocular injuries occur more frequently to boys than to girls, presumably because of the more active nature of their play. Toddlers are prone to falls and more frequently sustain traumatic injuries. Toddlers also may ingest toxic products such as antifreeze (methyl alcohol) or may spill chemicals on themselves causing injury. In addition, abuse must be ruled out in any injury sustained by a child. Preschoolers and school-age children are inquisitive and very active. Their eye injuries are more often caused by either a failed project or participation in a sports activity fraught with a high level of activity and a great deal of physical contact without protection. School-age children and teenagers may improperly use sports equipment, guns, common tools, or toys to inflict injury on their peers. Air guns were the largest single cause of enucleation secondary to trauma in a recent Canadian study (Marshall et al., 1995). School-age children also may sustain blunt force injuries inflicted by another child's hand or foot.

Emergency department statistics demonstrate the incidence of children's eye injuries. At one large eye hospital in Philadelphia, 38% of the pediatric patients seen in the emergency department had eye injuries. Boys were seen twice as often as girls, and 12% of the injuries were inflicted by accident by the hand or foot of another child. Ten percent were sports-related injuries, and 4% were chemical injuries caused by substances commonly found around the home (Nelson, Wilson, & Jeffers, 1989).

The incidence of all types of injuries from high-impact sports (e.g., skateboarding, roller blading) is less when participants wear safety equipment. The incidence of eye injuries from bicycle accidents has decreased in areas where helmets are required.

Tip: *Wearing a helmet while riding a bike is the law in many states. Help children to remember to do so.*

The sport most related to children's sports-related eye injuries is baseball, and most of those injuries occur while the child is batting. These injuries can be prevented by the use of a batting helmet with polycarbonate face shield for youth baseball (National Society to Prevent Blindness, 1991; Vinger, 1987).

Of all persons with burn injuries, 30% sustain burns to the head and neck (Herndon, Thompson, Linares, & Traber, 1986). When tissues surrounding the eyes are burned, edema may cause the eyelids to swell shut. This is not only frightening to the patient but also makes assessment of the eye difficult (Staley, 1988).

Pathophysiology

Eye injuries are classified according to the anatomic parts involved: extraocular, anterior globe, or posterior globe injuries. *Extraocular injuries* include eyelid lacerations, soft tissue injuries with bruising, or fractures of the orbit. *Anterior globe injuries* are subdivided according to whether they are perforating or non-perforating injuries. *Nonperforating injuries* include corneal abrasions, foreign bodies on the conjunctiva, subconjunctival hemorrhage, and hyphema (bleeding into the globe) (Nelson et al., 1989). *Perforating anterior globe injuries* include ruptured globe, perforated cornea, and conjunctival laceration. *Posterior globe injuries* include retinal edema, vitreous hemorrhage, and retinal detachment. Injury to the posterior globe often is accompanied by injury to the anterior globe or extraocular structures as well.

A common injury in childhood is the blunt force injury causing hemorrhage in and around the eye. When bleeding occurs around the eye (extraocular), it is seen as discoloration and called a "black eye" (Fig. 28–15). When small blood vessels of the conjunctiva are torn by an injury, subconjunctival hemorrhage may be seen as redness across a portion of the conjunctiva.

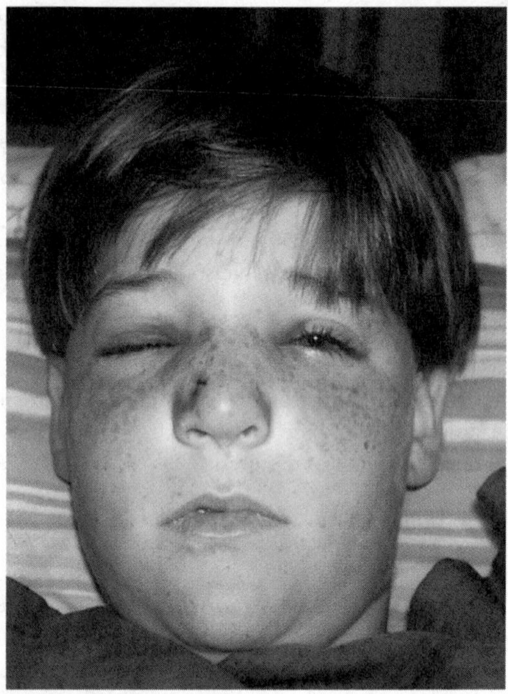

Figure 28–15
Eye injuries can cause temporary loss of vision as a result of swelling and bruising of the orbital area.

Alert: *A large amount of bleeding into the eye is called a* hyphema *and could result in increased intraocular pressure; thus it should be examined by the ophthalmologist as soon as possible. Increased intraocular pressure could cause optic nerve damage.*

Facial burns from a chemical or fire may affect the eyes; however, eyes are well protected by the eyelids. Eyelids are able to close in one thirtieth of a second, thus protecting the cornea. Most eye burns are caused by chemicals seeping into the eye or by sudden explosions involving steam or debris.

Prognosis. The prognosis in children's eye injuries depends on the degree of damage to the ocular structures. The desired patient outcome is the full restoration of useful vision and is frequently possible. It is much better, however, to take measures to prevent eye injuries before they happen. Adults and children alike should be constantly aware of the need for preventive head gear and the dangers of using sports equipment in ways for which it was not intended.

Assessment

Assessment of an eye injury begins with a detailed history of the events leading to the injury to identify the possible injuries the child may have sustained and the possible elements involved. Identification of the location and extent of the injury is made by the physician with appropriate diagnostic testing.

Diagnostic testing may include facial radiographs to identify possible orbital fracture and retinal examination to identify internal eye injury, damage, or bleeding into the eye. The computed tomography scan is helpful in identifying injury-related conditions that are not visible on radiographs.

Assessment for injury by chemicals and debris must be made very early in the treatment process to prevent corneal abrasion and burning. Chemicals should be washed away with copious amounts of water, and the debris should be removed immediately because edema of damaged tissues quickly makes both washing and examination difficult.

caREminder: *Trauma victims who are unconscious when admitted to the health care facility should have their eyes cleansed as soon as possible if injury is suspected.*

Interdisciplinary Interventions

Most eye injuries should be followed up by a visit to an ophthalmologist. Because of the intricacy of eye structure, even small injuries in a growing child can result in larger problems at a later date. Nurses, parents, teachers, and other adults in the child's world may need to assist and provide support as the child complies with treatment protocols.

Eye injuries are usually accidents that could be prevented with due concern being given to children's activities (Fig. 28–16). In one study, 37% of children's eye

Figure 28–16
Safety equipment helps protect the child's eyes during sports activities.

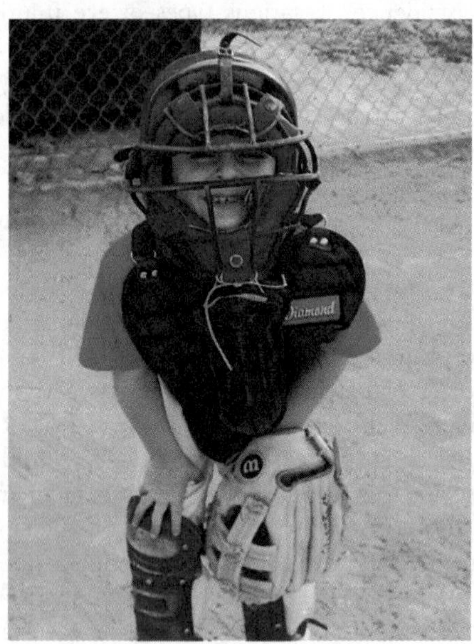

injuries that required an outpatient visit were sustained while the child was batting in a baseball game. Helmets with a visor could protect the child's eyes and prevent the majority of eye injuries occurring in children participating in this sport (Vinger, 1987). Other eye injuries were sustained by children at the hands of other children who were inappropriately using such common objects as pencils, blackboard erasers, sticks, stones, rubber bands, balls, paper wads, and bows and arrows. Many of these injuries are superficial, but each has the potential of seriously damaging a child's eyesight.

Nurses, teachers, and primary health care providers are in positions to engage in teaching activities or discussions that help children adopt behaviors that avoid endangering the eyesight of other children (Chart 28–10). Providing information to the child concerning potential danger can help the child in his or her own decision-making process. Safety can become an internal motivator rather than a condition externally imposed by the parent or other adult.

Visual Impairment—Blindness

Blindness is defined by educational and governmental agencies as "having vision no better than 20/200 in the better eye or a visual field no better than 20 degrees at its widest diameter regardless of visual acuity" (Grimes, Scardino, & Martone, 1992). Persons with these limitations are said to be *legally blind*. However, they may still have considerable useful vision and may be able to use print as their major means of learning.

Partially sighted persons are those with "visual acuity of more than 20/200 but worse than 20/70 in their better eye with correction" (Federal Regulations, PL 94-142, 1975). Both legally blind and partially sighted children fall into the *visually impaired* classification. They have certain rights in the community and in the educational system, which are addressed by the Americans with Disabilities Act.

Nurses are assuming greater responsibility in monitoring the well-child health care needs in the community and are frequently available to families of children with chronic disabilities. It is essential that nurses be knowledgeable with respect to the impact of visual impairment on child and family development, educational options, community resources, and general health care needs.

Etiology

Visual impairment affects 42 to 50 million people worldwide. Two thirds of all cases of blindness in the world are either preventable or curable (Grimes et al., 1992). Infections (including trachoma), parasites (onchocerciasis), and resulting cataracts account for a large portion of blindness in children and teenagers. Inadequate treatment of injuries and common infections account for many preventable cases of blindness in developing countries. Visual impairment may be due to genetic inheritance or to a local or systemic disease process that may be acquired either prenatally or postnatally. Any condition that causes damage to, or prevents development of,

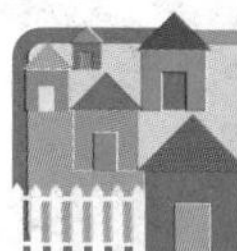

Chart 28–10
Community Care

Preventing Accidental Eye Injuries

At Home

Childproof the home while the child is a toddler:

- Pad the corners of low tables (or temporarily remove the low table).
- Prevent access to toxic chemicals and cleaning supplies. (Store them in a locked cupboard, well out of reach or outside the house where the child has no access.)
- Prevent access to automobile or to lawn and garden chemicals, which the child may decide to taste:
  - Antifreeze both smells and tastes good; however, ingestion can be lethal.
  - Garden chemicals often feel like coarse sand and come with colored pellets; however, they contain toxic substances and are not meant for the young child to play in or taste.
- Prevent access to lawn and garden equipment that could cause injury:
  - Do not let the young child ride on the riding mower; many have fallen off and been injured by the rotating blade as the parent tries to catch them.
  - Avoid letting the child play in the lawn while it is being mowed—flying debris from the yard can hit the child. When debris is thrown into the eye with the force of the mower, damage can occur.

Chart continued on following page

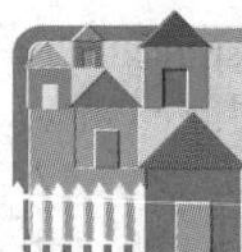

Chart 28–10
Community Care *Continued*

Preventing Accidental Eye Injuries

- Buckle children securely into automobile safety seats and buckle the seat into the vehicle according to manufacturer's instructions. Teach older children to use seat belts correctly.

Teach children safety with toys and play equipment:

- Avoid toys with sharp points, sharp edges, shafts, spikes, or rods.
- Avoid throwing toys.
- Avoid using toys as weapons.
- Avoid giving BB guns, pellet guns, bows and arrows, or darts to children as toys.
- Children should never pretend to point a gun at another person.
- Take appropriate precautions when setting off fireworks.
- Avoid swinging on the swing when another child is too close.
- Do not run while carrying any sharp or pointed object, for example, scissors or sticks.
- Keep toys meant for older children away from younger children.

Teach older children proper use of safety equipment designed to prevent eye injuries:

- Wear helmets for in-line skating and bike riding. (Be sure that the helmet fits well enough to allow the child to see where he or she is going.)
- Wear protective glasses when using a string trimmer or other lawn and garden tools and equipment.
- Wear protective glasses when preparing and dispensing household or lawn and garden chemicals.
- Follow the directions when preparing and using any equipment or chemicals.

Parents should always set a good example. Use safety equipment.

At School

Teach proper use of sports equipment for school sports and backyard or street sports.

Consistently require appropriate use of classroom and sports safety equipment:

- Batting helmets with polycarbonate face protector in youth baseball
- Helmets with face protectors for ice and street hockey
- Swing sets with soft material (fabric or leather) seats
- Scissors with rounded ends for young children

Set protective rules and require compliance:

- Do not throw sand, toys, or other missiles.
- Never hit another person in the face (or anywhere else).
- School supplies (e.g., pens, pencils, rulers) have a purpose, and it is not to be thrown. There are better ways of expressing frustration or anger.

Teachers and other school personnel should set a good example.

During Sports Activities

Use protective gear supplied:

- Helmets with face guards in football
- Helmets with face guards in hockey
- Batting helmets in youth baseball

Abide by the rules. Assign penalties for violation of the rules:

- Hockey sticks are to be kept low, not used as weapons.
- Bike helmets are to be worn whenever riding a bike.

Consistently require appropriate use of sports safety equipment.

Chart 28–11

Causes of Visual Impairment

Congenital defect: chromosomal abnormality
Systemic disease
Injury

- Head injury, occipital
- Penetrating injury to the ocular globe
- Blunt force injury to the head or globe
- Injury to the anterior globe with scarring

Infection (local or systemic)

- Maternal rubella
- Maternal infection with *Chlamydia trachomatis*
- Maternal gonorrhea
- Maternal varicella
- Infantile varicella
- Neonatal conjunctivitis caused by infection
  - *Neisseria gonorrhoeae*
  - *Chlamydia trachomatis*
- Meningitis
- Encephalitis

Other

- Retinopathy of prematurity
- Poisoning (e.g., methyl alcohol ingestion)

ocular structures may diminish visual capacity of the child (Chart 28–11).

Ocular structures do not regenerate; thus, damage to the eye is permanent and results in blindness. Blindness is the result of either optic nerve damage or damage to other parts of the eye that normally would help to focus the image on the retina. Blindness may also result from damage to the visual centers of the brain. Visual impairment caused by injury or disease is usually not progressive; however, some genetic conditions are progressive over time and with physiologic development.

Assessment

Visual impairment is grossly assessed with eye screening and with the previously discussed eye and vision assessment. The child with visual impairment should be followed up by an ophthalmologist, particularly when the child is at risk for complications or deterioration of existing vision.

caREminder: *The nurse needs to be particularly aware that complications may develop rapidly in eye conditions; thus, any time an eye disorder is suspected, the child should be referred and seen immediately. The "wait and see if it gets better" approach has no place in a child's plan of care when vision is at risk.*

The pathophysiology of visual impairment is dependent on the causative factors. Prognosis and patient outcomes when a child has visual impairment are dependent on the individual child's ability to adapt to limited or absent vision and to develop the necessary cognitive, psychosocial, communication, and coping skills to function effectively in life. With this in mind, the interventions used are intended to assist each child in developing his or her maximum potential.

Interdisciplinary Interventions

Although there is no one "right" way to interact with blind or partially sighted infants and children, several interventions can facilitate care and increase the comfort of the visually impaired child and his or her family.

The child's developmental level must be kept in mind at all times. A blind child usually has the capacity to reach the same developmental level and the same conceptual understanding of the world as his or her sighted peers, but the child may not have done so because of lack of experience. For this reason, the blind child may not understand the health care provider's descriptions at a level expected of a sighted child of the same age. Persons who work with blind or partially sighted children must provide the necessary information to help the child to understand the concepts being presented. Blindness does not affect the child's cognitive capacity, but does affect the teacher's presentation.

Parents, teachers, and health care specialists need to assist the child in developing compensatory skills to deal with the environment. A child with limited vision or no visual ability must develop auditory and tactile senses earlier and to a greater skill level than their sighted peers. Parents can begin the process at home using games similar to those played with sighted children for identification of objects, sizes, shapes, sounds, and textures. Children who have limited vision can benefit from having their attention drawn to specific objects or qualities to enhance their understanding of them. Visually impaired children may be taught how to type as early as third or fourth grade to prepare them for the use of devices such as the Opticon, which transfers the printed page to a tactile format. Using the computer, a vast array of materials can be converted to braille directly from the printed page (VersaBraille by TeleSensory Systems, Inc.; see Resources).

Creative play is frequently slower to develop in children with visual impairment; thus, these children benefit greatly by participation in a nursery school setting where individual attention is possible and a wide variety of toys and activities are available.

Children who are visually impaired may develop mannerisms considered abnormal by the sighted world. These may include rocking, exaggerated finger play, body movement, eye gouging, or other strange activities called "blindisms." These mannerisms were traditionally thought to be self-stimulating behaviors used by the child who is sensually deprived, but this is probably not the case. These behaviors are not unique to blind children and may be eliminated with behavior modification techniques.

Physical fitness skills are equally as important for the visually impaired child as for the sighted child. These children need help in developing skills of jumping, hopping, running, and other gross motor activities. Activities in which the visually impaired child can actively participate include swimming, gymnastics, and other individual sports rather than team sports such as basketball. Special Olympics provides a wide variety of opportunities for persons with visual impairment to participate in sports activities.

Hearing

More than 1 million children in the United States have some degree of hearing impairment. Approximately 1 in 1000 infants is born deaf and, in 1 to 2 more per 1000, some degree of deafness develops during infancy or childhood as a result of illness or injury (Swigart, 1986). Hearing and listening form the foundation for spoken communication. Infants and toddlers spend much of their day engaged in passive and active listening as a means of gathering information about their world. Hearing impairment during infancy and early childhood can have devastating effects on a child's speech and language development. Hearing deficit prevents the child from benefiting from developmental stimulation provided by the auditory route, thus also preventing the child from learning speech by imitation. This deficit hinders the child's ability to communicate his or her own needs, desires, and thoughts in the ordinary manner.

The critical period for learning language is the first 36 months of life. If children are unable to hear during that time, they will be unable to learn language necessary for normal verbal communication unless hearing intervention is provided. This can have devastating effects on learning, social development, and eventual vocational and economic potential. Research has shown that the ability of a young child with hearing impairment to learn language is closely related to the time when remediation is begun. Early identification and early intervention enhances the young child's ability with language and speech (Downs, 1986). Learning the vocabulary and skills needed for communication is much harder after the critical period has passed. Hearing deficit that begins at other times during childhood diminishes the child's ability to profit from spoken words and sounds in the environment. This can adversely affect school learning whenever it occurs during school years.

Of the 40 million children in school in the United States, approximately 8 million have some degree of hearing impairment (Davis, 1990; Ross, Brackett, & Maxon, 1991). Many of these children have minimal, mild, or moderate hearing loss with hearing thresholds of 15 decibels (dB) or more; the non–hearing impaired child has hearing thresholds of 15 dB or less.

Hearing impairment is classified as *minimal, mild, moderate, severe,* or *profound* according to how loud a sound must be before the infant or child hears it. Sound is measured in decibels (dB) and, during testing, is presented to children through earphones. Normal speech is usually 40 to 50 dB; thus, a child who requires a sound to be 50 dB before it is heard will be unable to hear most speech sounds with the unaided ear. Amplification (use of a hearing aid) may improve functional hearing.

Hearing impairment is also classified according to the location of the defective hearing pathway (Table 28–4). *Conductive hearing loss* occurs when the outer and middle ear fail to transfer sounds to the inner ear. This may be due to blockage of the ear canal by congenital malformation, cerumen (ear wax), foreign object, or some other abnormality of the middle ear structure. The most common cause of conductive hearing loss is otitis media.

Sensorineural hearing impairment occurs when the cochlea (inner ear) relays insufficient information about the sound patterns received from the middle ear. The usual cause is absence or malformation of some or all of the tiny structures in the inner ear—the hair cells, organ of Corti, membranes forming the cochlear partitions, or nerve fibers linking the hair cells to auditory nerves.

Central hearing loss occurs when the damage or defect is located in the hearing centers of the brain or between the inner ear and auditory center. This type is sometimes called "neural impairment" and is present when a child has difficulty processing the nerve impulses provided by the cochlea. Central hearing impairment results from direct damage to this portion of the brain or is secondary to sensory and experiential deprivation. Usually, the child has difficulty with paying attention to sounds and with recognition, memory, association, and comprehension of the significance of specific sounds.

Mixed hearing loss results from a combination of con-

Table 28–4
Types of Hearing Impairment

Type	Definition	Possible Causes
Conductive hearing impairment	Inability of the outer and middle ear to transmit sound to the inner ear	Blockage by cerumen or foreign object Congenital malformation of external or middle ear Otitis media with effusion (fluid in the middle ear) Scarring of the tympanic membrane
Sensorineural hearing impairment	Inability of the inner ear to transmit sound impulses to the brain	Congenital malformation of the inner ear Genetic deterioration of the inner ear Damage to inner ear by disease or injury, child abuse, meningitis, encephalitis
Central hearing impairment	Inability of the hearing centers of the brain to receive or process sound impulses	Congenital malformation or disorder of auditory center Brain damage by disease or injury Damage to cranial nerve VIII by disease or injury such as child abuse, meningitis, encephalitis, poisoning
Mixed hearing impairment	Any combination of conductive and sensorineural factors	

ductive and sensorineural hearing loss. For example, otitis media with effusion (OME) may develop in a child with mild sensorineural hearing impairment, further diminishing the sounds that are transmitted to the auditory center of the brain.

Each type of hearing deficit is managed differently; therefore, it is essential to obtain an accurate diagnosis as early as possible. The assistance of the audiologist in making the diagnosis is essential.

The nurse should always keep in mind that *any* infant or child being examined or cared for could be one of a large number of children with an undiagnosed hearing deficit. Early identification of even partial hearing loss is essential to development of communication skills and the lifelong learning process. Nurses are frequently in strategic positions in primary care settings, schools, hospitals, or home care to identify children at risk or who are suspected of having hearing deficit.

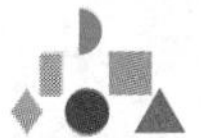

Assessment of the Child with Alterations in Hearing

Focused Health History

Hearing should be assessed at birth, and frequently thereafter during the first 36 months of life, particularly if the child is at risk for hearing impairment (Chart 28–12). The alert primary care provider carefully assesses vocalization and language development as measures of hearing ability as well as using them as measures of cognitive and expressive development. The child who cannot hear sounds cannot imitate sounds and is less likely to make

Chart 28–12

Risk Factors for Hearing Impairment in Infants

Infants who have any one or more of the following are at higher risk than the general population of infants for development of hearing impairment. These infants should be screened regularly.

- Family history of childhood hearing impairment
- Birth weight less than 1500 g
- Severe asphyxia (Apgar scores of 0–3 or failure to breathe spontaneously within 10 minutes and hypotonia persisting to 2 hours of age)
- Anatomic malformations involving the head or neck (e.g., cleft palate, dysmorphic appearance, abnormalities in the pinna of the ear)
- Hyperbilirubinemia
- Congenital or perinatal severe infection (cytomegalovirus infection, rubella, herpes, toxoplasmosis, syphilis)
- Bacterial meningitis, especially *Haemophilus influenzae* meningitis

Adapted from American Academy of Pediatrics, Joint Committee on Infant Hearing. (1982). Position statement. *Pediatrics, 70*(3), 496–497.

the developmentally appropriate vocalizations during infancy and early childhood.

▽ **Alert:** *Infants and children in whom otitis media develops are particularly prone to development of either temporary or permanent hearing impairment.*

The list of risk factors is useful in identifying other infants and children who are at particular risk for hearing impairment. All of these infants should be assessed by an audiologist during early infancy and as needed thereafter.

Chart 28–13 suggests specific aspects of the health history that are particularly relevant to hearing assessment. It is important to recognize that not all hearing impairments manifest themselves at birth. Both late-onset genetic factors and factors within the medical history of the child can contribute to the development of hearing impairment at any time during childhood.

An infant's ability to attend to environmental sounds and parental voice is critical. Parental observations concerning the child's responsiveness to their voices as well as the child's general behavior are significant. In one study, 80% of children with hearing impairment

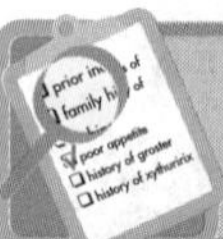

Chart 28–13
Focused Health History

Hearing

Identifying Data
Age

Present Illness
- Complaints by child of ears "popping," feeling plugged or full
- Child complains of difficulty in hearing
- Child or infant does not attend to environmental sounds or human voice
- Pulling and tugging at ears
- Parents complain that child "doesn't listen," or is "uncooperative." Parental concern regarding hearing
- Academic grades declining or generally doing poorly in school
- Has a hearing test ever been completed?

Past Medical History
- Birth history
  - Prematurity or low birth weight
  - Prolonged neonatal depression (low Apgar scores, hypotonia)
  - Hyperbilirubinemia at level exceeding indication for exchange transfusion
  - Mechanical ventilation
  - Congenital infections (cytomegalovirus, rubella, syphilis, toxoplasmosis, herpes)
  - Congenital anomalies of the face or head
  - Presence of syndrome known to be associated with hearing loss (e.g., Usher's syndrome, Waardenburg's syndrome)
- Current or past health challenge
  - Bacterial meningitis, encephalitis
  - Infectious diseases known to be associated with hearing loss (mumps, measles, Epstein-Barr virus)
  - Treatment with ototoxic drugs or radiation therapy
  - Neurodegenerative disorder known to be associated with hearing loss
  - Head trauma, ear trauma
  - History of otitis media
  - Any previous referral for hearing evaluation
- Immunizations
  - Status of current immunizations

Family Medical History
Family history of congenital or childhood-onset hearing loss

Environmental History
Exposure to loud noises (music, lawnmowers, fireworks)

Social History
Social interactions with others appropriate for age

Growth and Development
- Delays in speech or language acquisition
- Delays in gross and fine motor skill development

were first identified as a result of parental suspicion, screening, and referral (Barringer, Strong, Blair, Clark, & Watkins, 1993).

caREminder: *A child who does not hear directions, parental requests, or environmental sounds may not be able to respond appropriately. Although this behavior may be interpreted as uncooperative or unusual, it should be noted as potentially indicative of hearing impairment.*

Other behavioral observations made by parents that may be helpful in identifying a hearing deficit should be identified in the history. For instance, children who sit very close to the television (Tanimura et al., 1993), who turn the television or radio volume up loud, or who consistently turn their heads as if to catch the sound of the spoken word more easily, may be suspected of having a hearing deficit. School-age children who suddenly begin to do less well in school, who miss directions, or who fail to answer questions correctly should be suspected of having developed a hearing deficit. Children may be doing their best and may be unaware that they are not hearing all information provided in class. The inability to hear directions may cause them to do poorly in school and can have devastating effects on children's psychosocial development, especially if they are punished or admonished to work harder when they have failed to achieve in school. A hearing deficit may be manifested by behavioral attempts to cover up the problem. Silliness, using excuses, or joking may be attempts to distract peers, teachers, and parents from the fact that the youngster did not clearly hear directions. Indeed, the youngster may not know that he or she did not hear all the directions. The child only knows that he or she did not perform as was desired by the parent or teacher, or as expected by peers.

Increased frequency or severity of ear infections or upper respiratory infections is also a significant finding in a focused health history. Fluid in the middle ear or scarring of the tympanic membrane resulting from otitis media frequently results in conductive hearing loss. Its presence can be verified on physical examination.

Medications that the child has taken in the past or is currently taking may provide clues to the possibility of hearing impairment.

caREminder: *Medications such as gentamicin or dihydrostreptomycin may be ototoxic, that is, damaging to the cochlear mechanism of the inner ear.*

The child's birth history with history of prematurity, perinatal infection, or episodes of respiratory distress also places the infant at risk for hearing impairment and should be noted in the health history. The parent's report of the severity of these episodes should be noted.

A family history of childhood onset of deafness places the child at higher risk than the general population. Exposure to environmental noise, either current or past, can damage sensitive cochlear nerve endings. Loud noise, fireworks, and exposure to machinery noise can damage a child's hearing.

The presence of any of the risk factors, including the newest, that of an infant having been on the ventilator or having received nebulizer treatments during the newborn period, greatly increases the chance of finding some degree of hearing impairment at some time during childhood (Mishoe, Brooks, Dennison, Hill, & Frye, 1995). The focused health history provides important information of value to the health care providers and sets the stage for the physical assessment of the child.

Focused Physical Assessment

Physical assessment of hearing begins with the basic assessment of the head and neck, including the ears (Chart 28–14). It is particularly important to inspect the child's

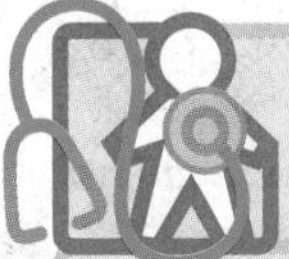

Chart 28–14
Focused Physical Assessment

Ears

Inspection

- Size and shape: Note the presence of lop ears, skin tags, dimples, sinus tracts, and developmental anomalies (e.g., cleft lip or palate, abnormality of the pinna).
- Position: Note low-set or asymmetrical placement.
- Otoscopic examination:
  - External canal: color, cerumen, discharge, inflammation, foreign bodies
  - Tympanic membrane: color, light reflex, bony landmarks, mobility, perforation, bulging, retraction, scars

Palpation

- Auricle: Note pain on retraction.
- Mastoid: Note tenderness.
- Tragus: Note pain or tenderness with pressure.

Auditory Assessment

- Auditory acuity:
  - Whisper test
  - Rinne and Weber tests
  - Audiometry
- Impedance audiometry, if necessary
- Pure tone audiometry, if necessary

head and neck for structural anomalies or congenital defects. Conditions such as widely spaced eyes, cleft lip and palate, mandibular hypoplasia, indentations around the tragus, or defect in the structure of the external auditory canal or the pinna of the ear are accompanied by the possibility of inner ear defect. Some facial structures arise from the same fetal tissue or are influenced by the same genetic structures, thus an abnormality in one should alert the health care practitioner to the possibility of other defects.

Hearing Acuity. Assessment of hearing acuity is ideally done in a quiet room without external noise. This is difficult to achieve in the usual office or clinic. The whisper test, which is part of the basic physical assessment protocol used in many offices and clinics, requires the examiner to whisper a selected word while out of the line of vision of the child. The child's ability to hear the word is recorded as normal if the infant turns toward the examiner or exhibits pupillary response or blink reflex, or if the older child is able to repeat the word. In the case of preverbal children, a change in behavior is considered indication that they hear. Because of the variability in infant behavior, lack of consistency between examiners, and inability to control for either volume of the whisper or external noise, the whisper test is, at best, a gross measure of hearing acuity that should not be depended on to indicate normal hearing, particularly in high-risk infants and children.

Hearing in infants and young children may also be tested in the home or office by an adult making noise using a bell, a noise maker toy, or a jangling set of keys out of the child's line of vision. A behavioral change, quieting behavior, or searching behavior is expected if the child hears the sound. These tests are, at best, rough estimates of the child's hearing ability and should not be depended on if other indicators of hearing deficit, such as delayed speech, occur.

Vocalization. Careful assessment of the infant's vocalization, early syllable formation, and finally verbalization in comparison with developmental norms provides additional clues concerning hearing ability. An infant who fails to vocalize within the expected age range or who fails to babble or form syllables may be unable to hear the vocalization of people in the environment. Any infant or child with delayed speech should have a full hearing assessment as soon as possible using technological advances available from the audiologist. Any child who fails to repeat new words in their entirety should be assessed further. A child who omits initial sounds or final sounds may not be hearing the sounds in a particular decibel range. For example, the final "ing" or "p" or "b" may simply be lost to the hearing of the child with residual fluid in the middle ear.

Rinne and Weber Tests. The Rinne and Weber tests can be used to assess hearing when the child reaches preschool age but may not yield accurate results until the child is 8 or 9 years of age, because of behavioral factors and the child's desire to give the examiner the "correct" answer. A child who is at risk for or suspected of having a hearing deficit should be examined with tests that have been shown to be more accurate for the younger age groups. The Rinne and Weber tests are described here in case they are selected for use with older children.

The Rinne test is designed to test for both conductive and sensorineural hearing loss. The tuning fork is set to motion by striking it against the examiner's hand. Its base is then held against the mastoid bone and the child is asked to indicate when the sound is no longer heard. At that time the tuning fork is held near the ear. The child with normal hearing will again hear the sound through air conduction. Normal finding is air conduction (AC) greater than bone conduction (BC).

The Weber test is done by striking the tuning fork on the hand, causing it to vibrate, then placing the base in the midline on the client's forehead. The child is asked to indicate whether the sound is heard better on one side than on the other. Normal finding is for the sound to be heard equally on both sides. If the child indicates that the sound is definitely heard better on one side, this indicates that the sound is heard better on the affected side with diminished conductive hearing. The sound is said to "lateralize" or be heard better on the affected side, the side that has greater bone conduction of sound. This is an abnormal finding.

When the assessment performed by the nurse or other primary care practitioner indicates that a hearing deficit could or does exist, then the child is referred to an audiologist (Chart 28–15). The audiologist has the skills and equipment necessary to fully evaluate children

Chart 28–15

Criteria for Referral to an Audiologist

A child should have his or her hearing evaluated by an audiologist when:

- The child has one or more of the risk factors known to be associated with hearing impairment.
- Parents or teachers have made observations that trigger concerns.
- The child has questionable results on the Rinne, Weber, or another screening test.
- The child's school performance declines.
- The child has noted the inability to hear as well as before.

Chart 28–16
Nursing Diagnoses and Outcomes

Hearing

Sensory or perceptual alteration (auditory) related to altered hearing

Outcomes:	Child and family will identify and use alternative methods to facilitate communication. Child will use hearing aid if prescribed.

Potential for altered growth and development related to inability to hear verbal communication secondary to hearing impairment

Outcomes:	Child will participate in social situations. Child's social development will progress according to developmental level.

Risk for injury related to environmental factors that can cause hearing loss

Outcome:	Child will have no damage to hearing related to onset of otitis media, administration of antibiotic therapy, or physical injury to the ear.

Ineffective family coping related to multiple disappointments and adjustments secondary to child's diagnosis of hearing impairment

Outcomes:	Family will modify communication patterns to include new measures to communicate with the child. Family will use available support systems and coping mechanisms to adjust to their child's diagnosis.

with high-risk indicators for hearing problems or who have been found to have a hearing deficit.

Nursing Diagnoses and Outcomes

Nursing diagnoses that are developed to guide nursing care of children with hearing impairment or potential hearing impairment must always account for the related physiologic and psychosocial and educational factors (Chart 28–16). Hearing that is present at birth must be safeguarded throughout life, and the general public must be taught how and when to use safety measures. Disease processes that result in hearing impairment, such as otitis media, should be treated vigorously and completely. This requires the cooperation of family and health care team.

When children are born with or incur hearing impairment, nursing diagnoses focus on securing the care and therapy for the child that will allow maximal use of the residual hearing. The health care team works with the family to facilitate the child's developing independence and self-sufficiency. The attitude of child and family toward the disability (i.e., psychosocial and emotional factors) greatly influences the child's ability to make maximal use of his or her skills and abilities.

Developmental and Biological Variances

Hearing is fully developed at birth; however, the neural pathways that allow the child to assign meaning to sounds in the environment are still being developed (Chart 28–17). Newborn infants do quiet more quickly to a parental voice than to the voice of a stranger. Music that the mother listened to before the birth of the baby has been shown to quiet the infant significantly more readily than strange music. These findings seem to indicate that not only is the infant's hearing fully developed at birth but that it is also fully developed well before birth.

Hearing acuity shows some differences by race, but the differences are not clear-cut. The National Health Surveys of 1960–1961 and of 1970–1971 provided information showing that blacks have slightly better hearing at the low and high ends of the tested frequency range and that whites have slightly better hearing in the middle frequencies. No specific reason for this difference could be identified, but the incidence of otitis media among blacks and whites may be a contributing factor. Blacks have less otitis media than whites; Native Ameri-

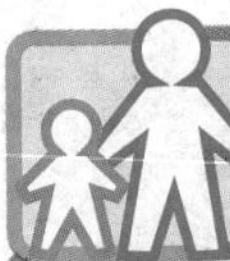

Chart 28–17
Developmental Considerations

The Development of Hearing

Age	Expectation
1 mo	Random activity diminishes with sounds
2–4 mo	Sound discrimination (recognizing voices) Turns toward sound of mother's voice May smile at speaker; vocal signs of pleasure
3 mo	Turns toward speaker; coos and gurgles, smiles in response to speech
4 mo	Localizes sound Quieted by pleasant sounds (voice or music) Responds differently to angry and pleasant voices
5 mo	Begins to mimic sounds
8 mo	Reacts to whisper test Localizes sound
14 mo	Reacts to soft sounds (likes to be whispered to) Traces source of sound In loud, shouting, noisy environment, "turns off" sounds which decreases natural responsiveness to stimuli and can lead to underdeveloped language skills

cans and Eskimos have the highest incidence of otitis media (Overfield, 1985; Roberts, 1972; Roberts & Ahuja, 1975).

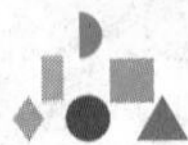

Diagnostic Criteria for Evaluating Alterations in Hearing

In the primary care setting, children's responses to varying sounds are observed and compared with normal expectations of the age (see Chart 28–17). The health history and the physical examination of the ear can identify risk factors and cerumen in the canal or fluid in the middle ear. These methods need to be supplemented by technological diagnostic methods to identify the quality of hearing that the child may have.

Hearing can be assessed for infants and children of any age and any physical condition, using a variety of technological instruments (Table 28–5). Parents and family members need to be kept fully informed concerning the purpose of each test and how it is done. None of the tests are invasive or painful to the child. Two characteristics of sound are measured when hearing is assessed with audiometry: intensity and pitch. *Intensity* of sounds that are heard by the human ear is measured in decibels. The least sound that the normal ear can hear is said to be 0 dB. Normal speaking voice is between 40 and 50 dB, and the sound of a train travel-

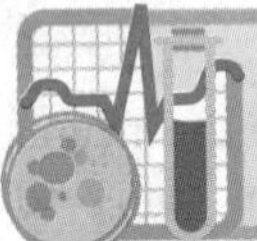

Table 28–5
Diagnostic Tests and Procedures for Evaluating Hearing

Diagnostic Test or Procedure	Purpose	Health Care Provider Responsibilities
Crib-o-gram *Age*: Newborn	Pressure sensitive transducer is placed under the mattress of the infant's crib to record body movement before, during, and after sound stimuli of various intensities. Infant responsiveness (change in activity) with different sounds suggests ability to hear these sounds.	• Inform parent(s) when the test is to be done. • Discuss purpose with parent(s). • Record externally initiated activity. • Record times when child is out of the crib or when care is being provided.
Pure Tone Audiometry *Age*: 3 years and older	Sounds of varying intensities and tones are presented to the child electronically through earphones. Young children are asked to carry out a play activity (such as placing a peg in a hole) when they hear a sound. Older children may be asked to raise a hand when they hear a sound.	• Discuss purpose and methodology with child and family. • Remind child that the test does not hurt. • Follow up with short discussion of parent and child perceptions of the test.

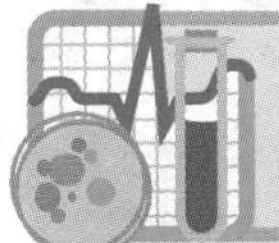

Table 28–5
Diagnostic Tests and Procedures for Evaluating Hearing *Continued*

Diagnostic Test or Procedure	Purpose	Health Care Provider Responsibilities
Audiometric Screening *Age*: 4–5 years and older	Spoken words are presented to the child through earphones. The child is asked to point to the picture requested. The first word is presented at 51 dB, slightly above the normal speaking voice. Each word is presented at 4 dB less than the previous word. This test requires that the child have language development sufficient to recognize the words used. The test should be performed in the child's native language.	• Before test is scheduled, be sure child has the cognitive development to accomplish this test effectively. • Discuss the purpose of the test with parent(s). • Remind parent and child that it is noninvasive and will not hurt.
Auditory Brain Stem Response *Age*: Birth to any age	Used to test children unable to cooperate with other hearing tests because of young age or disability or for children whose tests have been inconclusive. Brain wave patterns are recorded as sounds are presented through the earphones. The child must be relaxed and/or sleeping during the examination.	• Discuss purpose with parent(s). • Ask parent to feed the infant immediately prior to the test. • Check to see whether a sedative was prescribed and whether the parent has given the medication so that the child is sleepy during the test.
Tympanometry *Age*: Any age; however, instrument must achieve a tight fit in the ear canal.	Measures the pressure in the external auditory canal with a very small puff of air, thus measuring the compliance of the tympanic membrane. The tympanometer is placed in the external ear canal using an ear piece that allows a snug fit of the instrument in the canal. Tiny and brief puffs of air are put into the ear canal. The instrument measures the movement of the tympanic membrane and places marks on a graph. The graph may be compared with normal graph results and conclusions drawn by the examiner about the mobility of the tympanic membrane, and thus about its ability to transmit sound vibrations.	• Nurses may learn to do tympanometry but should receive adequate training before doing the test or interpreting the results. • Because of the difficulty in getting an adequate seal with small infants, the results may be less than adequate. • This test is most useful in identifying the presence of middle ear effusion, that is, presence of fluid behind the tympanic membrane, which may be difficult to see in young children.

ing rapidly on a nearby track measures approximately 90 dB.

The *pitch* of a sound represents its tonal quality, or the speed at which the sound waves vibrate. High tones cause rapid vibration of sound waves, whereas the vibrations of low tones are slower. Audiometric testing identifies the infant or child's ability to hear sounds of various intensities as well as of various pitches. Both are important to the child's ability to hear and comprehend verbal communication.

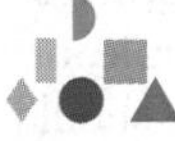

Treatment Modalities

Prevention of Hearing Loss

A primary intervention of the health care team is to teach the family ways of preventing or minimizing injury to the ear that can cause hearing loss (Chart 28–18).

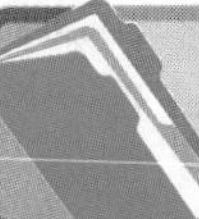

Chart 28–18
Nursing Interventions Classification (NIC)

Ear Care

Definition

Prevention or minimization of threats to ear or hearing

Activities

Position infant so ears remain flat to head.
Monitor for drainage from ears, as appropriate.
Irrigate the ear, as appropriate.
Avoid placing sharp objects in the ear.
Administer ear drops, as appropriate.
Instruct parents how to cleanse infant's ears.
Instruct parents to monitor child with nasal congestion for ear infections.
Explain the relationship between balance and the inner ear, as appropriate.
Monitor for episodes of dizziness associated with ear problems, as appropriate.
Instruct parents how to observe for ear infections in infant.
Instruct parents about importance of completing antibiotic regimen.
Instruct parents to hold baby upright when bottle feeding to avoid reflux into eustachian tubes.
Determine if cerumen in the ear canal is causing pain or hearing loss.
Instill mineral oil in the ear to soften impacted cerumen before irrigation.
Irrigate the ear canal with a Water-Pik on a low setting (or similar device) using warm water (80° to 90°F), as appropriate.
Demonstrate proper technique for ear irrigation to parents/caregiver, as appropriate.
Monitor frequency of ear infections.
Instruct parents about tubes as a medical treatment, as appropriate.
Instruct parents to avoid immersing child's ears in water with tubes present.
Instruct parents how to administer ear drops, as appropriate.
Instruct parents about the importance of routine hearing testing.
Instruct children not to put foreign objects in ears.
Instruct how to monitor and regulate high-volume noise exposure.
Instruct patient to wear hearing protection for exposure to high-intensity noise.
Instruct teenager concerning the potential danger of exposure to high-volume music, especially with headphones.
Instruct patient with pierced ears how to avoid infection at the insertion site.
Encourage use of ear plugs for swimming, if patient is susceptible to ear infections.

From McCloskey, J., & Bulechek, G. (1996). *Nursing interventions classification (NIC) (2nd ed.)*. St. Louis: Mosby–Year Book. Reprinted with permission.

Routine health visits provide an excellent opportunity to discuss ear care with children and their parents. Cleansing of the ear should be reviewed. Older children should demonstrate how to clean their ears and how to avoid infection at the insertion site on pierced ears. If the child has cerumen buildup in the ear canal, or otitis media, treatment modalities should be discussed and demonstrated. As noted in Chapters 4 and 6, routine assessment of hearing is considered an integral aspect of developmental surveillance of the young child.

Medications

Anti-infective drugs may be used topically in otic solution administered as ear drops when infections are present in the external auditory canal. Antibiotics may be given orally in syrup, suspension, or tablet form when the infection is located in the middle ear. It is important to stress to the family that prescriptions for antibiotics must be given according to the directions of the primary health care provider. The medication must be given for the length of time prescribed or the child runs the risk of recurrence or complications resulting from incomplete eradication of the organism. It is not unusual, however, for the child to require more than one treatment period to recover completely from otitis media or OME, even when the medication is given according to directions. Chart 28–19 describes the technique for administering ear drops.

Steroids given orally have been suggested by some practitioners as treatment for persistent middle ear effusion; however, the current guidelines from the Agency for Health Care Policy and Research do not recommend the use of steroids because of the limited scientific evidence of their benefit and the known adverse effects of steroid use. Steroids given in the ear canal are still used to decrease local inflammation.

Antipyretics and analgesics are useful in treating fever and pain. Cerumenolytics are medications used to soften the cerumen impacted in the external ear before its removal. Acidic ear drops help to prevent growth of bacteria or fungi in the external ear, particularly in children who swim frequently during the summer months.

Hearing Aids

Hearing aids are amplification devices. Each device provides amplification in the decibel range where the individual child has a deficiency. The hearing aid does not differentiate between voices and background noises. The child using the hearing aid learns to recognize sounds as they are received, which may be quite different from the sounds received by persons without hearing impairment (Fig. 28–17). The child may need to use lip reading in addition to the amplification device. TIP 28–3 summarizes the instructions that a nurse should provide to the family for a child who will be using a hearing aid.

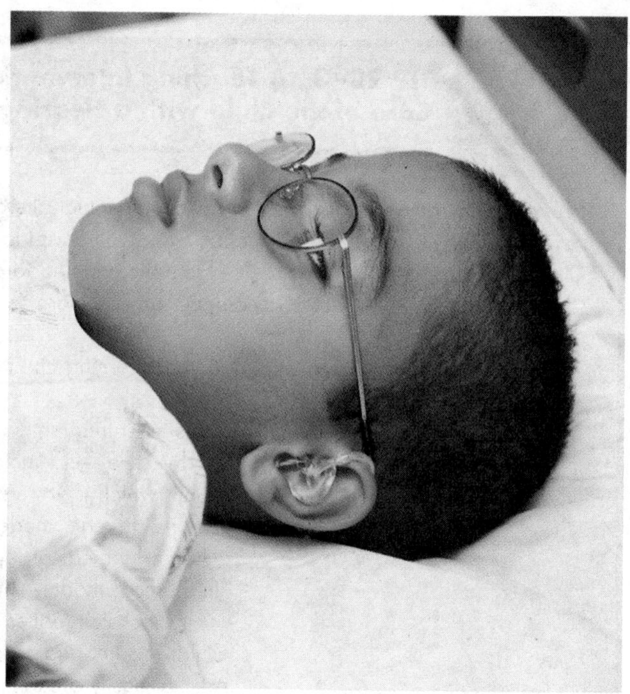

Figure 28–17
A child with a hearing aid.

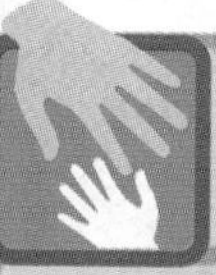

Chart 28–19
Nursing Interventions

Administering Ear Drops

- Position the ear for accessibility: Ask the child to lie down or tilt the head so that the ear into which the drops will be placed is up.
- Move the pinna to straighten the external auditory canal:
  - Infant: Gently pull down and back.
  - Child: Gently pull slightly up and back.
- Administer the medication:
  - Insert the number of drops prescribed.
  - Use a cotton ball in the ear if recommended for the medication and condition under treatment.

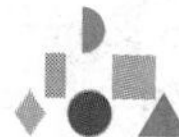

Alterations in Hearing

Otitis Media

The condition known as *otitis media* actually includes several conditions ranging from acute to chronic and which may or may not produce symptoms (Carlson, 1996). Otitis media is the most common cause of conductive hearing loss and hearing impairment in children. Additionally, there is evidence to suggest that the presence of chronic otitis media is related to long-term difficulties in speech and language development for the child (Cornell, 1997). Otitis media is an inflammation of the middle ear that may or may not be accompanied by infection. OME is an inflammation of the middle ear in which fluid is present in the normally air-filled spaces behind the tympanic membrane (TM). This fluid exerts pressure on the TM, causing it to bulge outward and causing pain. The pressure may rupture or perforate the

TIP 28–3 A Teaching Intervention Plan for Care of the Child with a Hearing Aid

Nursing Diagnoses and Family Outcomes

- Sensory and perceptual alterations (auditory) related to hearing impairment
  Outcome: Child will adapt to use of hearing aid to enhance communication ability.
- Knowledge deficit related to care and management of hearing aid
  Outcome: Child will learn to care for own hearing aid.

Teach the Family

- Information concerning children's hearing aid (amplification devices) styles and selection include
  - Styles most frequently selected for children:
    - "Body" style—ear mold is worn in the ear and connected by a wire to the battery unit, which is worn in a pocket on the child's clothing.
    - "Behind the ear" model—designed with a small ear mold and a unit that fits behind the ear on eyeglass frame or on a small frame of its own.
    - "In the ear" model—fits entirely in the ear and is reserved for older children whose physical size makes this possible.
  - Children's hearing aid characteristics:
    - Are not easily broken
    - Do not require resizing as the child grows
    - Have sufficient power to meet the needs of the individual child
- Adjustment period:
  - Both family and child need a period of time to adjust to the use and care of the hearing aid.
  - At first the amplification device may frighten the infant or confuse the older child.
  - Some children may have physiologic responses such as dizziness when the amplification device is first used.
  - An infant or child may require up to 30 days to adjust to wearing the hearing aid and attending to sounds.
- Assigning meaning to sounds:
  - During and after the adjustment period, the infant or child must learn to assign meaning to sounds.
  - Parents can help by making specific sounds to accompany pleasurable experiences.
- Keeping the hearing aid working properly: Examine the hearing aid daily, clean the ear mold, and test the battery.
- Shifting responsibility:
  - By the age of 5 years, the child should be able to take on responsibilities for the care and maintenance of the hearing aid, which include
    - Insert and remove the ear mold and hearing aid.
    - Notify the parent or teacher when a battery change is needed or the unit is malfunctioning.
    - Adjust the volume in different acoustic environments.
    - When manual dexterity is present, the child should take on full responsibility for cleaning and testing the unit and for changing batteries.

Contact Health Care Provider if

- Unit is not providing amplification as expected.
- Ear mold is causing pain in the ear.
- Child refuses to wear the hearing aid for any reason.
- Ear mold or battery pack is broken.

TM. Fluid may be present with or without infection; the presence of fluid always results in hearing impairment.

Otitis media may be classified as *acute*, *subacute*, or *chronic*, depending on its duration. *Acute otitis media* is a middle ear infection accompanied by the signs and symptoms of infection (fever, pain, irritability) and lasting 3 weeks or less. *Subacute otitis media* is an ear infection that fails to clear in 3 weeks with treatment and lasts up to 3 months. *Chronic otitis media* lasts more than 3 months despite treatment and may or may not be accompanied by TM perforation and ear drainage (Goycoolea, Hueb, & Ruah, 1991). Children whose symptoms disappear for 2 weeks or less after treatment and then recur are not considered to have recovered from the otitis media.

Incidence

Otitis media is the most common disease of childhood with the exception of viral upper respiratory infections (Jung & Rhee, 1991). It is the most common reason for children's visits to the physician other than for checkups (Bluestone et al., 1983). At least 75% of all children seen by pediatricians have had at least one episode of otitis media by age 2 years (Baker, 1991; Cornell, 1997), and 85% of all school-age children have had at least one episode. By age 3 years, 33% of children have had three or more bouts of OME (Bluestone et al., 1983). The age at which the incidence of otitis media is greatest is between 6 and 13 months (Teele, Klein, & Rosner, 1989). Because otitis media actually changes the middle ear lining, the inflammatory process resolves more slowly in younger infants and much more slowly after repeated infections.

The prevalence of otitis media is greatest during preschool years (ages 3 to 4) and is lowest after the age of 9 years. It has been found that 35% to 73% of infants have their first episode of otitis media before age 6 months (Casselbrant, 1989; Marchant et al., 1984). Some studies have found the incidence of otitis media to be greater among males (Casselbrant, 1989), whereas others have found no difference in incidence by gender (Hallet, 1982).

The incidence of otitis media increases in winter and spring, presumably paralleling the increased incidence of upper respiratory infections. Otitis media frequently follows an episode of upper respiratory disease.

In some studies, breast-fed infants have a lower rate of otitis media than bottle-fed infants (Cunningham, 1977; Stewart et al., 1984; Teele et al., 1989); however, in other studies, no such relationship was found (Kraemer et al., 1983; Stahlberg, Ruuskanen, & Virolainen, 1986). These findings could indicate that the apparent protective effect of breast-feeding is related to the position of the infant during feeding or to the characteristics of breast milk itself.

Exposure to other children has been examined as a risk factor in development of acute and chronic otitis media. Children who attend daycare have a significantly higher incidence of otitis media than those who do not attend daycare (Birch & Elbrond, 1986; Fleming, Cochi, Hightower, & Broome, 1987). In a retrospective study of 102 black children age 6 to 24 months who attended daycare, all except one had OME during the study period. This same study also found that 95% of bilateral middle ear effusion resolved spontaneously by age 2 years (Zeisel et al., 1995).

Exposure to passive smoke has been implicated in several studies and was found to increase the incidence of otitis media (Iversen, Birch, Lundqvist, & Elbrond, 1985; Kraemer et al., 1983; Stahlberg et al., 1986). Passive smoke is thought to damage the mucosa of the nasopharynx and eustachian tubes, thus increasing the susceptibility of the child to bacterial or viral invasion.

Pathophysiology

Organisms found to cause 95% of cases of otitis media include pneumococci, *H. influenzae*, *Moraxella catarrhalis*, and streptococci (Giebink & Canafax, 1988), which are thought to migrate up the wide and horizontal eustachian tube to the middle ear. The shorter and wider structure of the eustachian tube makes infants more susceptible to middle ear infections (Fig. 28–18).

Organisms gain entrance to the middle ear through the eustachian tube, which forms a normal connection between the pharynx and the middle ear. The infant eustachian tube is a tiny tube, 1 cm in length, made of cartilage and muscle with a flutter valve opening in the oropharynx. Its purpose is to equalize pressure between ear and environment and to drain normal fluid from the middle ear. The usual sequence is for the ear infection to appear a few days after the onset of an upper respiratory infection. Because of the wider and shorter eustachian tube in young children and the mucus from the respiratory infection, it is theorized that the flutter valve fails to prevent organisms from entering the middle ear.

Organisms frequently are presumed to travel up the short and wide eustachian tube from the respiratory tract. Inflammation and suppuration that results from the bacterial invasion prevents normal aeration and drainage of the middle ear. When the middle ear fills with fluid, sound conduction is diminished as the vibration of the incus, stapes, and malleus is hindered by fluid. If the infectious process is of long duration, the TM may lose elasticity, thus diminishing further the potential to transmit sound waves to the inner ear.

The degree of hearing impairment in acute or chronic otitis media is not dependent on the severity of the infection, but on the degree to which sounds are

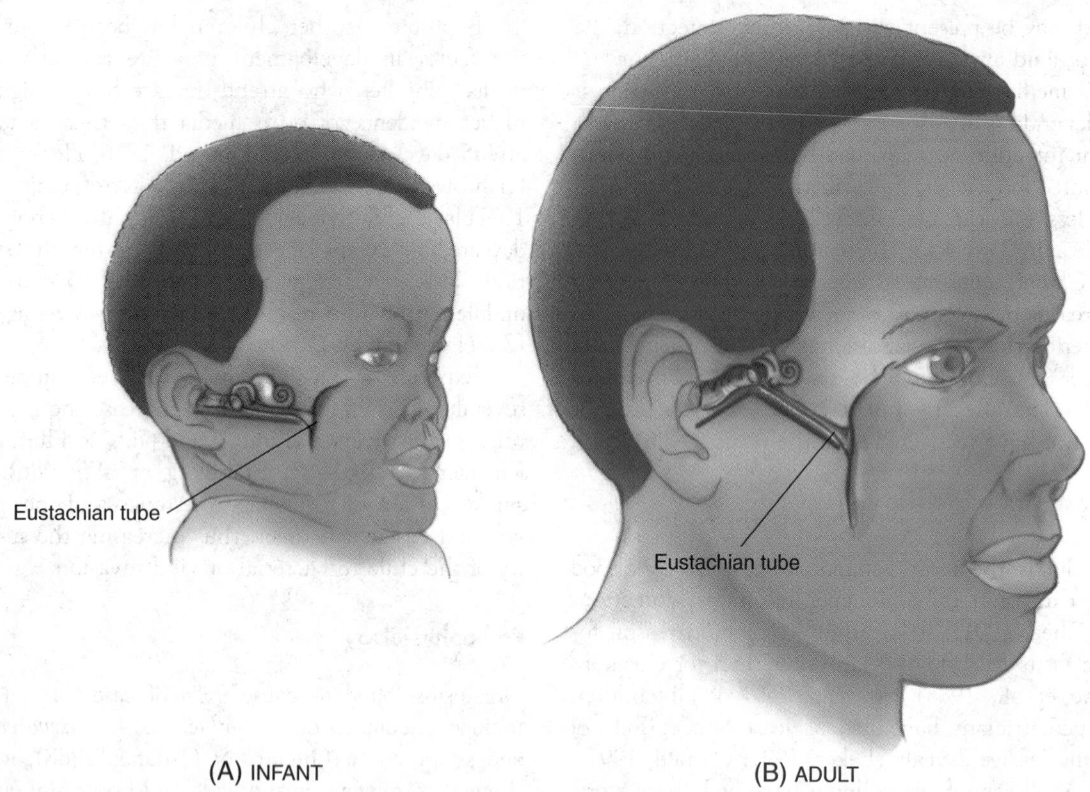

Figure 28–18
Infants have short, wide eustachian tubes, making them more prone to otitis media and otitis media with effusion.

prevented from reaching the inner ear. The degree of hearing impairment is the critical factor in the progress of normal cognitive and language learning processes for the young child. This is why a child who suddenly seems to stop progressing in cognitive or language skills or who displays uncooperative behavior should have his or her hearing assessed.

Approximately 50% of infants coming for well-child care are found to have "silent" OME, which is detected only on physical examination and not by the parent (Papparella, Kimberley, & Alleva, 1991). The child does not seem to be sick. Fluid in the middle ear diminishes hearing ability, even when no infection is present. This decrease in hearing ability may well diminish what the child gains from his or her environment and thus can affect both language development and cognitive progress.

Prognosis. Early detection of hearing impairment resulting from otitis media can prompt immediate treatment and thus prevent delays in development of language. If, however, hearing impairment is present and not identified, not only is the child in danger of cognitive and language delay but also suffers self-concept damage when he or she is punished for "uncooperative" behavior or "not paying attention" either at home or at school.

Assessment

Ideally, the primary health care provider clearly visualizes the TM on otoscopic examination. Such ideal circumstances may not exist because of an uncooperative youngster or one with cerumen in the ear canal. (See Chapter 6 for a discussion of this examination.) Cerumen should be removed only by an individual trained to do so without injuring either the external auditory canal or the TM.

Approximately 50% of infants and children with acute otitis media have the classic symptoms of fever, red and bulging TM, and ear pain. Other symptoms that may be seen on otoscopic examination include a gray TM without landmarks, a fluid line behind the TM, or even air bubbles in the fluid behind the TM (Chart 28–20). Children with chronic otitis media may have no symptoms except hearing impairment.

caREminder: *Crying may cause the TM of the infant or young child to appear red. The pneumatic otoscope*

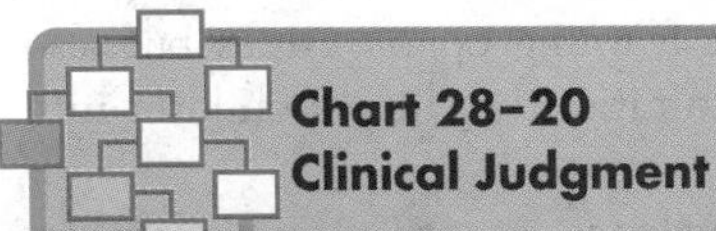

Chart 28–20
Clinical Judgment

A Visit to Urgent Care

Brothers Christian, age 4, and Matthew, age 7 months, are brought to an urgent care facility on a Saturday night. Christian has told his mom earlier in the evening that "I have a sword in my ear." Matthew has been pulling and scratching at his right ear.

Otoscopic examination of Christian's ears reveals red, bulging tympanic membranes with no visible landmarks. He is crying and wiggling during the examination.

Matthew's right ear also has a red tympanic membrane and no visible landmarks. The cone of light was difficult to assess because of the excessive wax in his ear. He did not cry during the examination.

Questions

1. What questions would you ask the mother about the boys' current condition?
2. What can cause the tympanic membrane of the ear to be red?
3. What is Christian's diagnosis? What is Matthew's diagnosis?
4. How does examination with the otoscope help differentiate a normal ear from an ear with otitis media?
5. You decide to initiate antibiotic therapy for the boys. You order amoxicillin 40 mg/kg/day to be given three times a day. Christian weighs 15.9 kg; Matthew weighs 9 kg. Calculate the dosage of medication for each child.

Answers

1. Any presence of fever, complaints of hearing loss, dizziness, impaired balance, or vomiting? Has the child been diagnosed with otitis media in the past? When?
2. Crying, acute otitis media, infection
3. Acute otitis media with effusion for both boys
4. The normal ear has a pearl-gray tympanic membrane, with a visible cone of light and mobility of tympanic membrane observed with the pneumatic otoscope. The child with otitis media exhibits a swollen, opaque, and discolored (red or yellow) eardrum with no visible landmarks and little or no mobility. An air–fluid level may be seen.
5. Christian should receive 636 mg/day, or 212 mg per dose. Matthew should receive 360 mg/day, or 120 mg per dose.

should be used during the assessment to determine whether the TM demonstrates mobility with insufflation of air. A TM that has fluid behind it will show little movement.

Tympanometry can provide information about the compliance (ability to move) of the TM and shows an abnormal curve on the tympanometry graph if fluid is present in the middle ear. Tympanometry is usually not valid when done in infants younger than age 7 to 8 months because of the difficulty in achieving a good fit between the instrument and the infant's ear.

The primary health care provider may culture the infant's throat and any ear drainage. A culture provides accurate identification of the organism, which can then be treated with medication to which it is sensitive.

Follow-up assessment should always follow treatment for otitis media to determine whether the otitis media has been controlled. The nurse must reinforce to the parents the necessity of otoscopic follow-up examination, even if the child shows no symptoms of infection. Persistent otitis media without symptoms is not unusual.

Hearing tests are not usually done during episodes of otitis media, but are more helpful in providing the desired information after the infection is eradicated and the middle ear effusion is gone. Hearing tests are also recommended in cases of chronic otitis media when the decision concerning ear tube insertion (myringotomy) is being made. According to Agency for Health Care Policy and Research (AHCPR) guidelines, if the child's hearing threshold is 20 dB or greater, myringotomy should be considered (Stool et al., 1994).

Interdisciplinary Interventions

Acute otitis media is treated initially with antibiotics given orally. Antibiotics may include ampicillin, amoxicillin, and cefuroxime. The prescription may be for the medication to be given several times a day for 2 weeks or for 3 weeks. It is important for the nurse to reinforce to the parents the necessity of giving all the doses prescribed, even though the child seems to have improved after only a few days. Azithromycin has recently been released with recommendations for a single daily dose for 5 days only. Such a schedule is helpful for compliance.

Of particular concern to primary care providers are cases in infants and small children that do not improve with the antibiotic of choice. Ten percent of all cases of acute otitis media are caused by organisms that are resistant to amoxicillin and require another antibiotic. Although other conditions (such as respiratory infection) that may be contributing to the illness of the infant improve when oral amoxicillin is used, accurate diagnosis and follow-up are still required.

If the infant is younger than age 4 weeks, hospitalization is often the treatment of choice because of the possibility of sepsis, particularly with S. *aureus* infection (Jordan, 1991).

Vigorous treatment of any infection with antibiotics can result in diarrhea caused by the decrease in normal bacterial flora in the intestinal tract. If the antibiotic is given intravenously, the insertion site of the intravenous line must also be observed carefully because some antibiotics are irritating to the vein. As treatment progresses, the child should also be observed for response to the medication. Fever diminishes, appetite returns, irritability disappears, and the child feels better and becomes more active. Visual inspection of the ear reveals normal color and landmarks of the TM.

Community Care

Because of the frequency with which acute otitis media fails to clear completely after a single round of antibiotics taken orally for 2 to 3 weeks, the nurse in the outpatient setting must stress to the family the necessity of a follow-up ear examination, even if the child is feeling and acting well.

It is possible for the child to still have clinical evidence of otitis media after the first round of antibiotics is completed. To prevent development of a chronic otitis media (persistent disease of duration greater than 3 months), the condition needs to be eradicated completely and quickly, and a second round of antibiotics may be prescribed for up to another 3 weeks.

If treatment is not effective in eliminating the infection, the possibility of complications remains. Complications include generalized sepsis, meningitis, or mastoiditis. Persistent or untreated OME can also result in middle ear changes and permanent conductive hearing loss.

Thus, otitis media is both a medical problem and an educational problem. Children whose hearing ability fluctuates from day to day cannot maximally benefit from any learning situation that involves voice or sound. They will miss not only direct learning opportunities but also incidental learning opportunities that help a child fit into his or her social group.

Because of the prevalence of otitis media in the preschool population, the AHCPR has published *Otitis Media Guidelines* for the management of this condition (Stool et al., 1994) (Fig. 28–19). The AHCPR has suggested that the initial management be either administration of antibiotics or observation, based on evidence that many cases of OME resolve spontaneously and without deleterious effects in otherwise healthy children.

If the OME has persisted without resolution, a hearing test should be done. If the child's hearing threshold is 20 dB or better (a lower number), the AHCPR recommends antibiotic therapy or continued observation. If, however, the hearing threshold is more than 20 dB, this is indicative that the child's hearing is significantly affected and myringotomy should be considered. Zero dB is the number assigned to the first sound the normally hearing individual is able to hear. Thus, the child with normal hearing should be able to easily hear a sound at 20 dB. A child unable to hear a sound until the volume is greater than 20 dB has a significant hearing deficit.

The AHCPR guidelines state that, when the OME has persisted for at least 4 months in an otherwise healthy child and the hearing threshold is 20 dB or higher, bilateral myringotomy with insertion of tubes is recommended (Stool et al., 1994). Hearing threshold of 20 dB or more causes the child to be unaware of many of the environmental sounds, thereby diminishing developmental learning. The younger the child is when OME affects hearing, the greater should be the effort to drain the ears and prevent language and developmental delay secondary to the hearing loss (Stool et al., 1994).

The surgical procedure called a *tympanostomy* involves the insertion of a tiny ventilating tube through the edge of the eardrum after fluid has been removed. These tubes substitute for the eustachian tube in equalizing pressure and allowing normal drainage of the middle ear. The surgery normally takes a very short length of time and requires general anesthesia. It is considered a very safe procedure and is done on an outpatient basis. Special care needs to be taken to keep the ear canals dry while the tubes are in place. Tympanostomy tubes usually fall out by themselves in 6 to 18 months. They may need to be replaced if OME recurs.

It is the nurse's responsibility to teach parents how to keep the ears dry by insertion of small cotton plugs whenever the child is around water that could get into the ears. Tympanostomy tubes (also called myringotomy tubes) are tiny tubes, possibly bordered on one end by a round plastic-like plate. The tubes come in various styles, shapes, and sizes. Parents should be informed about the appearance and size of their child's tubes so that they can recognize them when they fall out.

Hearing Loss

Hearing deficit is classified as minimal, mild, moderate, severe, or profound depending on the decibel threshold of sound required before the child can hear it. A deficit may be temporary, as in transient otitis media, or permanent, as occurs when there is nerve damage. Hearing impairment is also classified according to the anatomic portion of the hearing mechanism involved. Three types of hearing impairment (conductive, sensorineural, and central) have been identified and are further discussed in the pathophysiology section.

Etiology

The origin of hearing deficit in infants and children is varied. Some types of hearing deficit are genetic in origin, whereas others are related to identifiable events in the life of the infant or child. Genetic hearing deficit may be dominant, requiring only one gene from one parent, or recessive, requiring one gene from each parent for deafness to be manifested. Of these, some are familial and others seem to occur sporadically with no familial incidence. Some types of deafness are associated with known syndromes, such as Down syndrome or Turner's syndrome. Prematurity seems to increase the risk of hearing deficit, possibly because of the fragile nature of the nerve endings in the inner ear. The etiologic factors have not been identified, although researchers have studied various perinatal and early postnatal factors. Some researchers have studied the effects of incubator noises on infant hearing, but no patterns have emerged. In older children, environmental noises have been found to have a detrimental effect on hearing, particularly that of teenagers who consistently listen to loud music. Audiologists have suggested that noises even as loud as the lawn mower or the sudden noise of firecrackers can be detrimental to the young child's hearing. Infections are known to seriously affect hearing. Maternal rubella during the first trimester of pregnancy is particularly dangerous to the developing fetus. Meningitis during infancy or early childhood can also result in hearing deficit. Chronic otitis media can cause scarring of the ossicles or TM, which results in conductive hearing loss.

Presenting signs and symptoms obvious to the outsider are usually the same in all types of hearing deficit; however, with testing, the audiologist can identify the type and degree of loss to make long-range plans for therapy, assistive devices, family teaching, and the child's educational needs. The nurse may be involved in follow-up care provided for the family.

Pathophysiology

The ear has three sections: (1) the outer ear, which directs the sound waves to the ear drum, (2) the middle ear, which transmits the sound by means of vibrations of the three small bones—the malleus, the incus, and the stapes, and (3) the inner ear, in which the cochlea transmits sound to the auditory nerve. A fourth section of the hearing mechanism is the auditory center in the brain. Hearing loss can be a result of malformation, damage, or disease process involving any of the four portions of the hearing mechanism. Each requires different interventions with respect to medical or surgical management, sound amplification, and communication style.

Conductive Hearing Impairment

Conductive hearing impairment exists when malformation, inflammation, obstruction, or damage involves the outer or middle ear, thus preventing sound from reaching the auditory nerve. Sound is prevented from reaching the inner ear when the ear canal is occluded with cerumen (ear wax) or a foreign object, when fluid has collected in the middle ear, or when perforation of the TM has occurred. Scarring of the TM may also result in conductive hearing loss. The most common cause of conductive hearing loss, however, is otitis media.

Cerumen impaction caused by excess production of ear wax can cause hearing impairment, even though cerumen production is a normal process. Approximately 10% of children and 30% of persons with developmental delay either produce larger than normal amounts or have difficulty with cerumen removal that results in hearing impairment (Crandell & Roeser, 1993).

Cerumen is normally gold in color when it is fresh and very dark when it is old. Cerumen is normally moved to the external canal opening by normal movement of hair cells of the ear canal. In the outer ear area, the cerumen dries and flakes off.

Cerumen impaction may develop in a child who wears hearing aids because of the daily use of the ear mold, which prevents the cerumen from leaving the ear canal. All children who wear hearing aids should be monitored for this possibility. The ear molds are kept clean by washing them carefully with soap and water.

Sensorineural Hearing Impairment

Sensorineural hearing deficit exists when the cochlea does not relay sound pattern information received from the middle ear. The usual cause is absence, malformation, or damage of some or all of the tiny structures in the inner ear, which include the hair cells, the organ of Corti, the membranes forming the cochlear partitions,

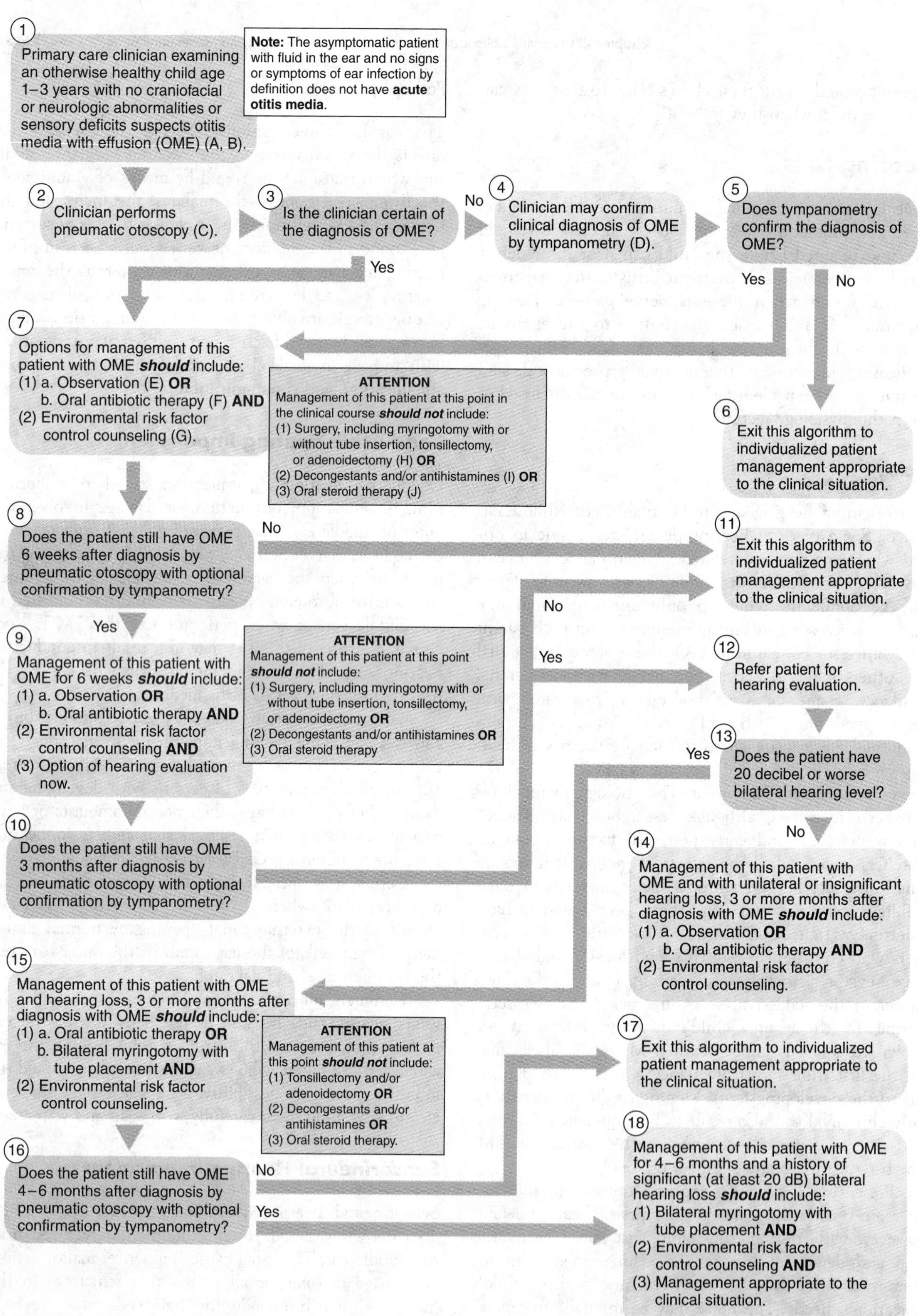

Figure 28-19

Algorithm for managing otitis media with effusion in an otherwise healthy child age 1 to 3 years. (Redrawn from Stool, S. E., et al. [1994]. *Managing otitis media with effusion in young children. Quick reference guide for clinicians* [AHCPR Publication No. 94-0623]. Rockville, MD: Agency for Health Care Policy and Research, Public Health Service, U. S. Department of Health and Human Services.)

Notes to Algorithm

(A) Otitis media with effusion (OME) is defined as fluid in the middle ear without signs or symptoms of infection; OME is not to be confused with acute otitis media (inflammation of the middle ear with signs of infection). The Guideline and this algorithm apply only to the child with OME. This algorithm assumes follow-up intervals of 6 weeks.

(B) The algorithm applies only to a child age 1 through 3 years with no craniofacial or neurologic abnormalities or sensory deficits (except as noted) who is healthy except for otitis media with effusion. The Guideline recommendations and algorithm do not apply if the child has any craniofacial or neurologic abnormality (for example, cleft palate or mental retardation) or sensory deficit (for example, decreased visual acuity or preexisting hearing deficit).

(C) The Panel found some evidence that pneumatic otoscopy is more accurate than otoscopy performed without the pneumatic test of eardrum mobility (see Chapter 6 on performing the examination).

(D) Tympanometry may be used as confirmation of pneumatic otoscopy in the diagnosis of otitis media with effusion (OME). Hearing evaluation is recommended for the otherwise healthy child who has had bilateral OME for 3 months; before 3 months, hearing evaluation is a clinical option.

(E) In most cases, otitis media with effusion (OME) resolves spontaneously within 3 months.

(F) The antibiotic drugs studied for treatment of otitis media with effusion (OME) were amoxicillin, amoxicillin–clavulanate potassium, cefaclor, erythromycin, erythromycin-sulfisoxazole, sulfisoxazole, and trimethoprim-sulfamethoxazole.

(G) Exposure to cigarette smoke (passive smoking) has been shown to increase the risk of otitis media with effusion (OME). For bottle-feeding versus breast-feeding and for child-care facility placement, associations were found with OME, but evidence available to the Panel did not show decreased incidence of OME with breast-feeding or with removal from child-care facilities.

(H) The recommendation against tonsillectomy is based on the lack of added benefit from tonsillectomy when combined with adenoidectomy to treat otitis media with effusion (OME) in older children. Tonsillectomy and adenoidectomy may be appropriate for reasons other than OME.

(I) The Panel found evidence that decongestants and/or antihistamines are ineffective treatments for otitis media with effusion.

(J) Meta-analysis failed to show a significant benefit for steroid medications without antibiotic medications in treating otitis media with effusion in children.

and the nerve fibers linking hair cells to auditory nerves. This type of hearing impairment can be a result of many different factors affecting both the inner ear and the brain pathways. Risk factors include heredity, infections in the brain, exposure to intrauterine infections such as rubella, cytomegalovirus, and herpes simplex viruses, exposure to loud sounds, use of ototoxic medications, and prematurity. Infants who are premature and of low birth weight are more prone to development of hearing deficit after intraventricular hemorrhage, anoxic periods, Rh incompatibility, or bilirubin encephalopathy. These tiny babies are more prone to nerve damage and hearing center brain damage than are full-term infants.

When nerve damage occurs, hearing is affected not only in terms of volume (decibels) but of pitch as well. The sounds that the child with a sensorineural deficit hears are distorted, with certain sounds being lost altogether. For example, the "f," "s," and "d" sounds are frequently not heard, thus affecting the child's ability to understand speech. Persons with sensorineural hearing impairment often do not benefit greatly from amplification of sound by hearing aids because sounds are still distorted and verbal communication fragmented.

Mixed Hearing Impairment

Mixed hearing impairment is a combination of conductive and sensorineural factors contributing to the hearing deficit. For example, otitis media may develop in a child with a mild sensorineural hearing loss, thus diminishing further his or her ability to hear and understand the sounds in the environment. Typically, the conductive portion of the child's hearing loss can be effectively treated with amplification, but the sensorineural portion cannot be treated as effectively.

Central Hearing Impairment

Central hearing impairment is due to damage or malformation within the brain itself or in the nerves that carry auditory information to the auditory portion of the brain. This type of impairment is sometimes called "neural" impairment and is considered as part of the sensorineural hearing impairment, but, because the symptoms and the management are somewhat different, it is considered separately here. The conductive system and the auditory nerve pathways are intact through the inner ear, but the brain is unable to receive and process or assign meaning to the sounds. This prevents the child from understanding the sounds in the environment, including language. It may be a result of trauma, neurovascular changes such as may occur with perinatal asphyxia or intracranial hemorrhage, or a disease process. Usually, the child has difficulty in paying attention to sounds and in recognizing, remembering, and associating sounds with specific events. Only in rare cases do infections such as meningitis cause central deafness.

Assessment

Physical assessment of a child with possible hearing impairment follows the pattern described previously. Frequently, however, deciding who to assess is a larger question than deciding how to assess hearing. At one time, it was recommended that all newborns be screened for hearing deficit, but screening tests often yield high false-positive rates, thus causing undue stress for many families. For this reason, newborn nursery screening has largely been abandoned in favor of use of the Risk Register and screening of only infants who are at risk for hearing impairment. All infants who are at high risk for hearing deficit should be screened regularly at each well-child visit and at least annually by an audiologist. Any infant who has had repeated episodes of ear infection should also be screened annually. During school years, children should be screened at least every 2 years, with children who have had repeated or extended episodes of otitis media being screened annually.

Children who are old enough to cooperate with the examiner may be given the standard "hearing test" that measures the child's ability to hear different tones at different volumes (Fig. 28–20).

Alert: *Screening devices used in schools and clinics provide only a rough estimate of the child's ability to hear. Even after screening, if parent, physician, nurse, or child suggests that a problem exists, referral to an audiologist for testing with more sophisticated equipment is appropriate (see Chart 28–15).*

Figure 28–20
Children's hearing should be tested regularly.

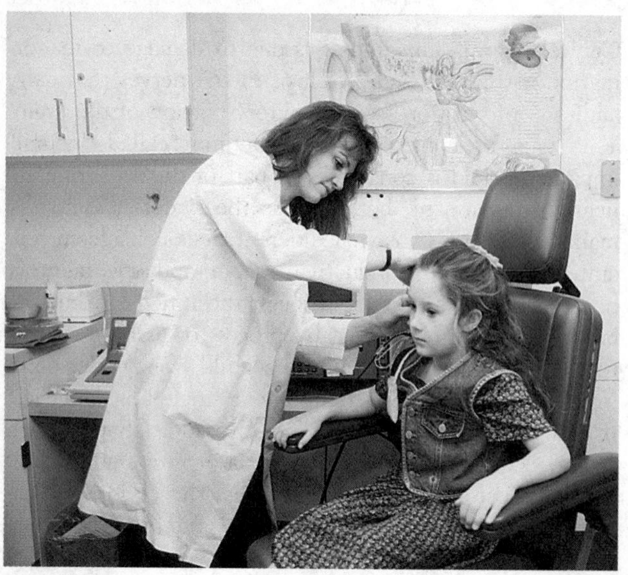

When deciding whether to refer the child for more precise assessment, health care providers must consider the implications of not referring the child. For example, a child who frequently misbehaves in the classroom, fails to follow directions at home or at school, or suddenly does less well in school than usual is at risk for psychosocial and emotional effects as well as achievement delays in school. Early identification of hearing deficit can facilitate its treatment and avoid potential psychosocial, emotional, academic, and vocational problems. Waiting until development is lagging behind normal in the toddler or until behavioral effects of hearing deficit have developed in the school-age child is waiting too long.

Assessment by the primary health care provider should include history, particularly focusing on ear infections and on the above mentioned behavioral factors as well as ear, nose, and throat examination. Fluid accumulating in the middle ear can significantly decrease hearing in the affected ear. Use of tympanometry in the office or clinic may be helpful in identifying an unrecognized middle ear effusion. Psychosocial manifestations of hearing impairment that the primary health care provider looks for include communication difficulties, academic performance difficulties, and difficulty in social adjustment.

Interdisciplinary Interventions

Interventions that are useful in managing hearing loss focus first on accurate diagnosis and second on identification of methods to facilitate normal development through life. Interventions should always involve the family as well as the child. A team approach is essential if the child is to benefit most from the available technology and therapy.

The primary care physician is often the interdisciplinary team leader, treating existing problems and referring the child as necessary for diagnosis or management of problems requiring a specialist. The nurse has a clear supportive role in assisting the family through the diagnostic process. The nurse may also have a role in assisting the family to accept the problem and participate in the treatment program. The audiologist identifies the nature and severity of the problem and makes recommendations to the family concerning its management. If necessary, the audiologist refers the child to a speech-language pathologist who works with both the parent and the child to provide speech readiness exercises or speech therapy for the child and training for the parent. The audiologist makes recommendations to the family for the use of amplification devices. The speech-language pathologist teaches the child and family how to make best use of the amplification devices and monitors the child's progress. When the child is old enough to attend school, the school nurse, speech therapist, and teachers become involved as they provide the educational program for the child. Each person needs to have full information concerning the child's educational and speech therapy program. Speech therapy may include the use of earphones to assist the child to hear speech sounds.

Amplification Devices. Amplification devices (hearing aids) are more useful as assistive devices for children with conductive or mixed hearing deficit than they are for children with sensorineural hearing impairment. Children with conductive or mixed hearing loss can often be provided with an amplification device that will assist them in their awareness of sounds in the environment and may allow them to learn to communicate verbally. Both the parents and the child will need to learn to manage and care for the hearing aid (see TIP 28–3).

Children with sensorineural hearing impairment may be able to benefit somewhat from amplification devices; however, nerve damage may prevent any amount of amplification from improving their ability to understand the spoken language. They may need to learn to communicate through signing, lip reading, or both.

Medications and Medical Procedures. Conductive hearing loss is frequently caused by conditions that are mechanical or inflammatory, thus can be treated with medication or other medical procedure. Cerumen collected in the ear canal may be washed out by the parent or primary health care provider. Instructions may be provided for occasional use of ear drops that assist in the natural removal of cerumen.

caREminder: *Cotton-tipped applicators should not be used by parents for cerumen removal because of the danger of either pushing the cerumen against the tympanic membrane or directly damaging the tympanic membrane with the cotton-tipped applicator stick.*

Even a scratch on the tympanic membrane can become inflamed or infected and cause TM scarring with hearing loss.

Fluid in the middle ear may be treated medically with drying agents or the physician may suggest mechanical drainage using tympanostomy tubes, which are implanted under anesthesia. If tympanostomy tubes are needed, the nurse gives the family information for use in preparing the child for the surgery. Tube placement is usually an outpatient procedure.

Cochlear Implant. Cochlear implant is recommended for use with children who sustain damage or injury that causes auditory nerve damage after initial speech has been learned. Tiny electrodes are implanted that transmit sound impulses directly to the auditory center of the brain, allowing the child to learn to decipher sounds. Although the system is not perfect, children who have these implants are able to continue their education and social activities in a nearly normal fashion (Bysshe, 1995).

Community Care

Communication is important for the hearing-impaired just as it is for the hearing child. Two different approaches to communication are taken by educators and parents of children with hearing deficit. Some subscribe to the oral approach and others to the signing approach. Children raised with the oral approach do not learn signing but depend on lip reading and amplification to communicate. Persons who subscribe to this approach believe that learning to sign distracts the child from attending to speech and alienates him or her from the hearing world. When communicating with the child who uses the oral approach, caregivers, teachers, family members, and friends must face the child when speaking, speak in a normal tone, and enunciate clearly. It is also helpful to keep environmental noise such as air conditioners or other equipment sounds at a minimum (Chart 28–21).

Communication through sign language is a second approach to communication (Fig. 28–21). Sign language used by the deaf in the United States is called American Sign Language (ASL), a complete language in itself. The syntax is different from English and persons using it do not voice the words as they communicate. Sign language used by hearing persons to communicate with the deaf is usually a system of converting English into a manual code. Voicing words usually accompanies signs. Finger spelling may also be used. Working with children who

Figure 28–21
Sign language can be used by the child with a hearing impairment or by the child who has difficulty in communicating verbally owing to his or her physical condition.

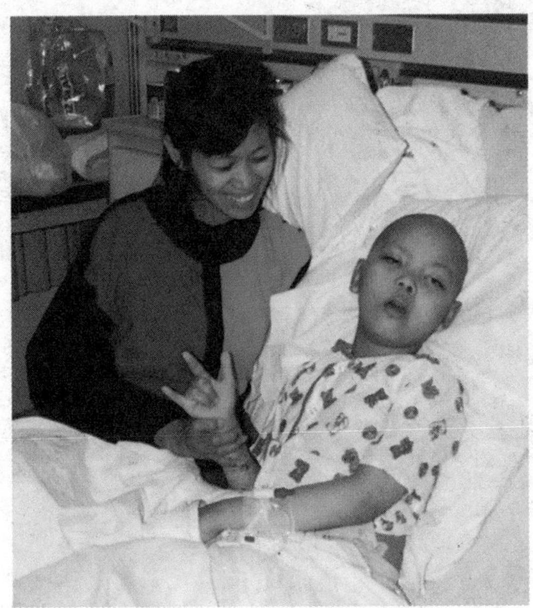

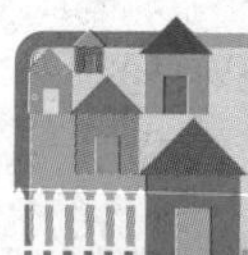

Chart 28–21
Community Care

Needs of the Child with Hearing Impairment

Hearing Disability	Sounds First Audible At	What Is Heard Without Amplification	Home and Educational Needs
Normal Hearing	0–15 dB	All speech sounds	Prevent auditory damage through trauma, infection, or prolonged exposure to loud sounds.
Slight Hearing Impairment	16–25 dB	Voiced vowel sounds are heard clearly; may miss unvoiced consonant sounds like "p," "th," and "s." The child may display mild dysfunction. The child may demonstrate fatigue in trying to hear normal speech.	Be sure the child is paying attention. Ask the child to look at the speaker. Speak distinctly. Enunciate clearly. Encourage auditory training. Encourage speech therapy.
		The child may fail to hear and understand directions.	Preferential seating in classroom Evaluate need for hearing aid.
		The child may demonstrate effects of feeling left out (social isolation).	Encourage social inclusion.
		Environmental sounds may prevent hearing voiced words clearly.	Turn off environmental noise when possible: radio, television, air conditioner, dishwasher. Use language frequently and consistently. Ask the child for input into conversations and discussions.
Mild Hearing Impairment	26–40 dB	The child hears only the louder voiced sounds.	Sound usually requires amplification through use of hearing aid. Use same techniques as above. Encourage the child to request clarification if words are unclear.
		The child seldom hears enough of social interactions to benefit from social learning.	Encourage social inclusion. Teach social skills. Teach peers how to interact and include this child.
		Even with amplification, the child may miss full context of classroom interactions and directions.	Provide directions in writing and provide summary of classroom interaction to assist in understanding its full content.

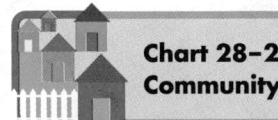

Chart 28–21
Community Care *Continued*

Needs of the Child with Hearing Impairment

Hearing Disability	Sounds First Audible At	What Is Heard Without Amplification	Home and Educational Needs
Moderate Hearing Impairment	41–65 dB	The child fails to hear most speech sounds in normal conversational tones.	Sound requires amplification. If hearing impairment occurred prelingually, the child will require speech therapy or use of sign language.
Severe Hearing Impairment	66–95 dB	The child hears no speech sounds at normal conversational levels.	Sound requires amplification. The child usually requires use of sign language for maximal communication. The child may be a candidate for cochlear implant.
Profound Hearing Impairment	96+ dB	The child hears no speech or other sounds but may feel vibrations from some sounds.	The child may benefit somewhat from amplification. The child requires use of sign language for maximal communication. The child may be a candidate for cochlear implant.

sign is usually facilitated by the children themselves and their families who have developed a variety of coping skills for communicating with the hearing world (Buncher & Price, 1997). If the child is old enough to write, a pencil and paper may facilitate communication. If the child does not yet write, the nurse may wish to ask the parent for information concerning some of the more common signs the child uses to indicate his or her needs and desires. A series of pictures from a magazine can be put together to use as a dictionary and can be very helpful in understanding what the child needs when nursing personnel are not familiar with sign language.

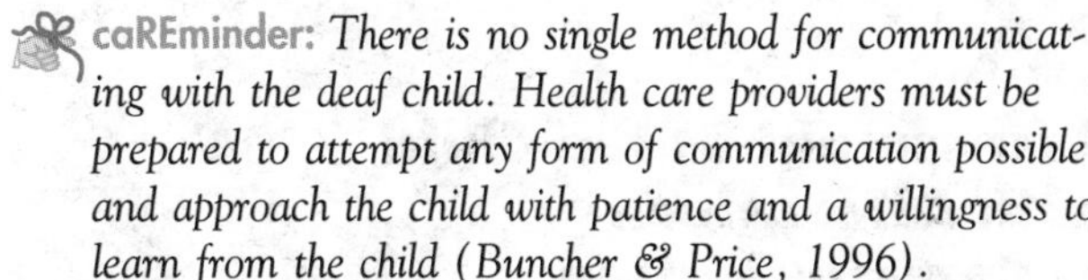

caREminder: *There is no single method for communicating with the deaf child. Health care providers must be prepared to attempt any form of communication possible and approach the child with patience and a willingness to learn from the child (Buncher & Price, 1996).*

Deaf children born into hearing families require adaptation of the family. The family must learn to be an advocate for the child until he or she can do so alone. The family needs to adopt a philosophy with respect to communication and teach other family members to use that method.

Communication

Children are said to have a communication disorder when they have an impairment in the ability to receive, send, or process concepts or verbal, nonverbal, or graphic symbol systems (American Speech-Language-Hearing Association, 1993). Each ability (receiving, sending, and processing) is associated with different physiologic and cognitive abilities. The ability to receive verbal information is usually associated with hearing ability. The ability to comprehend verbal information or information in symbols may be associated with the function of the central auditory centers or processing centers of the brain. The ability to send verbal or symbol messages (as in the case of sign language or gestures) is associated with cognitive abilities needed to formulate the message as well as coordination of speech centers and neuromuscular control centers needed to form the words so that others can hear and understand.

Thus, a child with a communication disorder may have a hearing, speech, or language disorder or some combination of these. Hearing disorders have been previously discussed. A speech disorder includes impairment in articulation of speech sounds, fluency, or voice, whereas a language disorder is impairment in comprehension (receptive language) or use of language in verbal, written, or symbol form (expressive language). Each of these must be evaluated when a child has a communication disorder. Therapy is directed toward the specific communication disorder.

It is very important for the nurse to remember that the child's ability to develop socially both within and outside the family unit is dependent largely on his or her ability to communicate. For this reason, early diagnosis is needed to make best use of the critical period for development of language. It is also important for the nurse to remember that delayed development of speech and language ability is one of the most common indicators of developmental delay in children. Speech disorders, including various dysfluencies, as well as delay, are more common and more readily observed than language disorders. Both speech disorders and language disorders occur more often in boys than in girls.

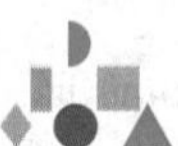

Assessment of the Child with Alterations in Communication

Focused Health History

Information in the health history that will assist in assessment and diagnosis of a disorder of communication should begin with assessment of articulation and language usage appropriate to the age of the child (Chart 28–22). If deviations from normal are found in the parent's report, the nurse must describe the characteristics of the child's speech and language ability with respect to articulation, fluency, voice quality, and word usage both by parent report and by observation.

Focused Physical Assessment

When an alteration in communication is present, physical assessment consists of a thorough physical examination with special emphasis on

- Hearing
- Vision
- Cranial nerve function
- Cognitive development
- Speech

Psychosocial issues of a general nature but that could influence communication should have been addressed during collection of the history.

A child who does not hear clearly is unable to reproduce the sounds and learn to speak as expected of the age. Children who are older when they lose the ability to hear also lose the ability to continue to learn and develop in academic and psychosocial areas in the same manner as they did before the hearing loss. Such children may display unusual or compensatory behavior that may be interpreted by parents or teachers as "uncooperative" and cause them to discipline the child rather than to consider a physical cause and to seek professional assistance.

Cranial nerves influence much of the activity of the eyes, throat, and auditory sense. The mobility of the oropharyngeal and laryngeal structures allows a person to form words and speak. Careful assessment of cranial nerve function is essential to rule out nerve abnormality as an etiologic factor in speech disorders. Cognitive development determines a person's ability to use words or word symbols to communicate; however, control of the muscles and movement of the mouth, tongue, lips, and throat provide the ability to form words and to speak.

Physical assessment may include a full neurologic examination, particularly if the alteration in communication is suspected of being related to a larger problem. Intracranial lesions may manifest themselves initially as communication disorders, or they may be of long duration and have no other noticeable symptoms. In either case, an accurate diagnosis must precede the development of a suitable long-term plan for the child's developmental and educational future.

Several tools are available to assist in assessment of communication skills. The Denver Articulation Screening Examination tool provides a series of words that the child is asked to say. Points are scored for the specified sounds and syllables, and the child's score is compared with the scale of norms provided. The child's ability to articulate the specified sounds is compared with the norms for the age.

The Early Language Milestones (ELM) scale may also be used to assess a young child's abilities to articulate. Parent reports are acceptable for this tool. The ELM scale describes the norms for attainment of language skills during the first 30 months of life and is very useful for identifying delayed language development.

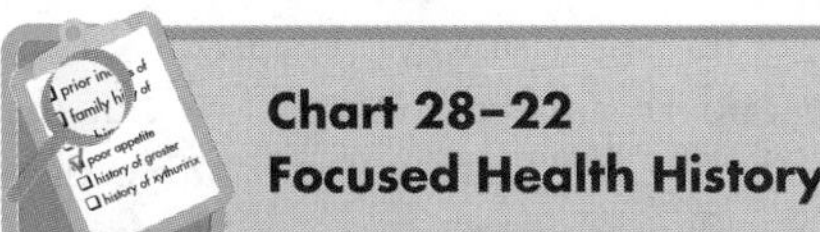

Chart 28–22
Focused Health History

Communication Status

Identifying Data	Age, gender, cultural environment, siblings
Present Illness	Languages spoken and languages understood Parents' perception of child's communication abilities Reason for current concerns

Past Medical History	Birth history
	  Problems during delivery or perinatal period
	  Prematurity or low birth weight
	  Need for mechanical ventilation at birth (how long)
	Current or previous health challenges
	  Tonsillitis or enlarged adenoids
	  Chronic otitis media
	  Difficulty in chewing or swallowing
	  Mental retardation
	Childhood illness/conditions
	  Trauma or strictures of trachea
	  Cleft lip or cleft palate
	  Chronic otitis media
	  Cerebral palsy

Growth and Development	Speech
	  Percent speech intelligible to parents? to others?
	  Response of others to child's speech patterns
	  Child's perception of his or her speech patterns
	  Presence of stuttering
	Language
	  Age words first spoken
	  Progress of language acquisition
	  Current level of language acquisition
	Cognitive
	  Does child demonstrate knowledge expected at his or her age (i.e., knows colors, body parts, points to named objects)?
	  Academic achievements
	Auditory receptive language
	  See Focused Health History: Hearing
	Visual language
	  Uses visual communication (e.g., waves bye-bye, points, finger counts)
	  How does child express wants and needs?
	Social development
	  Participates in age-appropriate activities with other children
	  Child reared bilingually
	Motor function
	  Gross and fine motor skills appropriate for age

Nursing Diagnoses and Outcomes

Nursing diagnoses for the child with communication impairment focus on helping the child to reach his or her maximal potential in communication, either verbally or by means of symbols. The source of the impairment largely determines the content of the nursing diagnoses. Sources of impairment may be physiologic, psychological, family centered, child centered, or some combination of these. The desired outcome is always improved communication for the child but may include either verbal communication or use of other symbols that help the child

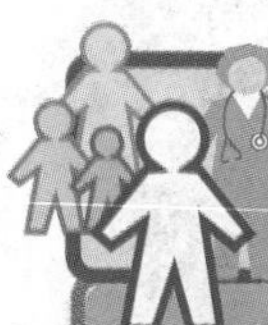

Chart 28–23
Nursing Diagnoses and Outcomes

Communication

Impaired verbal communication related to language delay, articulation, or fluency disorder

Outcomes: Child produces understandable speech and communicates needs.
Family members demonstrate an understanding of verbal development in children and alternative communication techniques.

Potential for ineffective individual coping related to inability to communicate needs effectively to others

Outcomes: Child learns to communicate needs.
Child expresses decrease in frustration with regard to communicating with others.

communicate. The child must always be involved in the decision-making and therapy planning. The nursing diagnoses listed in Chart 28–23 are representative of a variety of possible problems common to children with impairment in communication.

Developmental and Biological Variances

Children's speech and language development begins at birth with the differentiated cry that infants make to indicate discomfort, hunger, or loneliness (Chart 28–24). As the infant develops, syllables are differentiated, vowel sounds are articulated, and, finally, syllables are joined to make words and sentences. As the infant's cognitive skills grow, application of words to concrete objects progresses to the use of word symbols for abstract applications.

Biological variations account for very little variation from the norms. Boys tend to begin to speak later than girls, and girls develop greater fluency at an earlier age, but the established "normal" ranges have been developed to include both sexes.

Developmental variations occur in the presence of

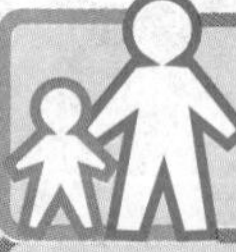

Chart 28–24
Developmental Considerations

Communication Milestones*

Age	Milestone
Birth	Differentiated cry begins early in life
3–6 mo	Localizes the source of sound by turning head
	May be quieted by the sound of a familiar voice
	Uses repetitive syllable sounds
	Begins to mimic sounds in the environment (e.g., motor sounds, siren, coughing, sneezing)
8 mo	Makes syllable strings (e.g., "mama," "dada"), but does not yet assign meaning to sounds
9–10 mo	Recognizes environmental sounds (e.g., telephone, dog bark)
	Babbles and uses jargon with inflections
	Uses prelanguage gestures (e.g., head shaking, waving hand, clapping hands)
	Understands a few simple questions (e.g., "Where's your nose?")
	Plays speech-gesture games like "peek-a-boo"
12 mo	Says "mama," "dada," and other two-syllable words
	Assigns meaning to words
	Imitates animal sounds (e.g., "kitty" and "meow" are connected)
13–15 mo	Says four to six words
	Points to desired objects
	Recognizes favorite toys
18 mo	Has a 7- to 20-word vocabulary interspersed with jargon
	Able to point to five body parts
18–24 mo	Makes two-word combinations
	Understands action words like "sit down"
	May have up to a 35-word vocabulary
	Begins to use pronouns (not always correctly)

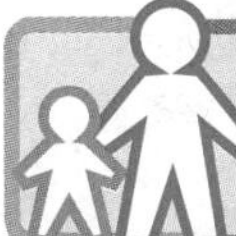

Chart 28–24
Developmental Considerations *Continued*

Communication Milestones*

Age	Milestone
30 mo	Has at least a 50-word vocabulary Uses two-word combinations regularly
36 mo	Uses three-word sentences; uses plurals Speech can be easily understood Uses speech as part of play Understands one- and two-step commands (e.g., "Give me the book"; "Put on your hat and get your coat.") Identifies common objects by their function (e.g., "A ball is to throw")

* It is more important that a child show progress in development of communication skill than that he or she reach a certain level of proficiency by a certain age. The rate of development of talking skills is not a measure of intelligence. Within limits, exposure to language increases the rate at which the child learns to use language independently.

hearing impairment or lack of stimulation. Infants and small children in bilingual families may take slightly longer to develop full language skills because they are learning two language vocabularies and two language structures at the same time. The bilingual child's comprehension of abstract concepts is not delayed, however.

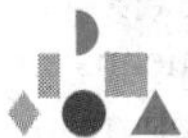

Diagnostic Criteria for Evaluating Alterations in Communication

Any infant or child suspected of speech or language delay should be evaluated by a speech pathologist. If hearing ability is in question, the child should also have a full audiologic evaluation by an audiologist. If the child is unable to cooperate with the testing procedure, because of young age or disability, the auditory brain stem response (ABR), or, simply, auditory evoked response, should be performed. Adequate and complete testing of hearing ability should not be delayed merely because the child cannot cooperate.

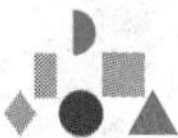

Treatment Modalities

The interventions designed to assist the child to overcome a communication disorder must necessarily involve a number of persons with whom the child comes into contact. This could include, in addition to the family, the primary care physician, nurse, speech pathologist, speech therapist, audiologist, daycare teacher or school teacher, school nurse, and social worker.

The primary roles of the nurse and the physician include identifying problems, providing encouragement and support to the child and family, and maintaining the child's general health. In the primary care setting in the office, clinic, or school, the nurse may participate in case finding as a part of well-child examinations or screening programs, may make independent observations, or may be responding to a parent's concern. The setting, the working arrangements between nurse and physician, and the expertise of the nurse determine how referrals are made and how follow-up is managed. Guidelines for referral when a child is found to have a communication impairment are found in Chart 28–25.

The nurse may also be responsible for encouraging follow-up visits or for encouraging the parent, family, and child to comply with the recommendations of the speech pathologist or audiologist.

The speech pathologist may provide a detailed description of the child's disability and plan a program of therapy to improve the child's communication ability. The speech pathologist may also provide the therapy or may delegate the daily or weekly therapy to a speech therapist.

The audiologist can identify hearing disability and recommend the use of an amplification device (hearing aid) as needed. In cases of communication disorder, the audiologist acts as a consultant to rule out a hearing disorder.

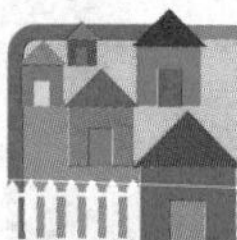

Chart 28–25
Community Care

Guidelines for Referral if Communication Impairment Is Suspected

Infant (age 0–2 years)

- Responsiveness to environmental sounds is limited or absent
- Responsiveness to parental voice is limited or absent
- Infant is quieted by touch but not by voice
- Responsive vocalization is limited or absent

Toddler (age 2–3 years)

- Limited responsiveness to environmental sounds
- Does not seem to hear parental requests for their attention
- Does not use syllable or words
- Speech difficult to understand by 3 years of age
- Responds to visual cues but fails to respond to verbal cues

Preschool Age (age 4–5 years)

- Fails to follow directions when given verbally
- Inappropriate word usage for the age (e.g., vocabulary does not seem to grow with the child)
- Stuttering or tonal dysfluency
- Fails to use correct word endings (e.g., omits "ed," "ing," "s")
- Fails to form sentences correctly

School-Age (age 6–12 years)

- Consistent failure to follow directions presented verbally
- Failure to use appropriate voice quality or tone of voice (e.g., too loud, too soft, abnormally high or low pitch)
- Inability to construct complete and accurate sentences
- Consistent errors in pronunciation of specific sounds
- Inability to respond with verbally appropriate terms in social and play situations

The school teacher and the school nurse are integral parts of the therapeutic team and should be kept fully informed of the program in progress. The parent often is the person who keeps all people who work with the child informed. If, however, the speech therapy is accomplished through the school system, the speech therapist may take the responsibility to keep others who work with the child informed.

Alterations in Communication

Speech and language are often thought of as a single entity, but they are very different. Language disorders include abnormalities in the form and content of speech. A language disorder includes impaired comprehension or use of language. For example, children with certain disabilities may have difficulty forming certain syllable combinations or sentence structures. Others may have difficulty putting words together to express an idea intelligibly.

Speech disorders include difficulty in articulation (forming words) and fluency (saying words and sentences) and voice disorders. *Articulation disorders* may include atypical production of speech sounds that may interfere with intelligibility of speech. Children may substitute "th" for "s," may be unable to say certain sounds, or may add or omit other speech sounds from words. *Fluency disorders* include stuttering, repetition of syllables, or uncomfortable pauses accompanied by unusual mannerisms. *Voice disorders* are characterized by sounds, pitch, volume, or voice quality abnormal for age or sex.

Language Delays

Delays in a child's ability to use language as a means of communication may be a normal response to an environment that does not require verbal communication, may be indicative of a language disorder, or may be secondary to some other factor such as hearing impairment or brain damage. Language delay can also result when the child is developmentally occupied with learning other things such as concepts, motor skills, or some other aspect of life.

Children with a limited need to communicate may include twins who develop a personal communication system between the two, a younger sibling born into a family with several older children who speak for the younger sibling, or possibly a child whose parents do not encourage independent speech. A child with limited comprehension of word symbols will be delayed in the use of words. Additionally, children with hearing impairments are likely to have language delays.

Articulation Disorders

Articulation disorders often accompany structural anomalies such as cleft lip and palate, neuromotor disorders such as cerebral palsy when quadriplegia is present, and hearing impairment, whether congenital or secondary to acute severe illness or repeated ear infections early in life.

Some articulation disorders are related to specific structural abnormalities, such as cleft lip and palate. When the defect is corrected, the child's ability to form speech clearly is improved. If the structural abnormality cannot be corrected, the speech and language pathologist or the speech therapist may be able to assist the child to learn to form words in a way that improves their intelligibility.

Fluency Disorders

The cause of fluency disorders, such as repetition of syllables and uncomfortable pauses, or so-called stuttering, is largely unknown, but several theories exist. One school of thought suggests that parental emphasis on "the right way" to speak with repeated admonitions to the child to change his or her speech patterns may contribute to the development of this habit pattern. This theory presupposes that the child feels great tension or pressure to speak correctly and fluently but is unable to do so. The inability increases the tension. The tension increases the dysfluency. Crowe and Robinson (1993) found that vocal muscles of stutterers actually do tighten to prevent phonation. For persons holding this view, treatment modalities focus on decreasing tension and increasing the child's muscle control.

Other theorists suggest that stuttering is a syndrome in which the child has a constitutional predisposition to dysfluency, which, when it occurs, leads to speech avoidance behaviors, inaccurate perceptions of reality, and nonproductive (self-debasing) attitudes. With this etiologic scenario as a base, it is logical to suggest preventive therapy at the first sign of dysfluency (Crowe & Robinson, 1993). Early counseling has been proposed. Crowe and Robinson suggest that "ego counseling" (as described by Erikson, 1963, and King & Neal, 1968) in which parents and child are taught to avoid negative thinking behaviors and to engage in ego strengthening communicative behaviors seems to be well suited to stuttering prevention.

Although counseling may well be left to those trained in counseling, nurses need to know that dysfluency is particularly traumatic to the psychosocial development of the child and should be evaluated and treated as early as possible. The attitude that a child "will outgrow it" should not be accepted by either the parent or the health care provider without an evaluation by a speech pathologist.

Disorders of fluency (e.g., stuttering, hesitations) and voice disorders also can be improved by individualized speech therapy. The child is taught to use breath control and vocalization muscle control to learn to speak intelligibly and normally. Early therapy, done while speech is still developing and the child's habit patterns are more flexible, is most effective in attaining lasting change.

The Child with Multiple Challenges in Sensory Function

The infant or child who has multiple deficits in sensory function and communication presents the greatest challenge to parents and caregivers. The loss of both hearing and sight may be a result of congenital defect, acquired illness or injury, or a combination of these. Vision and hearing deficits are seldom complete; thus, the child's residual abilities need to be identified and used to provide maximal benefit for the child. In many cases, the combination of hearing and vision losses can impact language acquisition. The desired outcome when working with a child who has both hearing and vision impairment is for the child to have opportunity to develop to his or her maximal potential. This requires the effort of parents, family, and the entire health care team.

Congenital rubella was a significant etiologic factor until the use of the rubella vaccine became prevalent. Since that time, prenatal or postnatal injury and illness have become the major etiologic agents for multiple sensory deficits. These deficits are sometimes accompanied by developmental delay and cognitive impairment.

Assessment

Assessment of a child with multiple sensory deficits, such as compromised vision and hearing, must necessarily include an assessment of the family strengths available to assist them in their care and teaching of the child. The family must first deal with their sense of loss of the normal child they expected or once had and then put into place coping strategies to facilitate family life and their participation in the child's treatment program. Assessment of the child, then, must include assessment of the status of parent adaptation to the needs of this infant or child.

The child's impairments should be assessed early and periodically as the child grows. Physical assessment includes assessment of residual vision and hearing and of the child's ability to meaningfully use these senses. Assessment of touch, taste, and smell are also appropriate. Physical assessment of ears, to rule out otitis media that may be compounding the hearing deficit, should also be included.

Cognitive and behavioral assessment provides information concerning the child's ability to explore the environment and learn from other senses. This is an area where family members can contribute greatly in providing stimulation for the child. These assessments need to be done regularly throughout infancy and childhood to make best use of developmental progress. School systems are charged with providing this service, but parents should also be encouraged to take an active part in securing the services and in providing information and follow-up.

Interdisciplinary Interventions

A child with multiple disabilities and his or her family can benefit greatly from the efforts of an interdisciplinary team of specialists. The pediatrician and developmental pediatrician can monitor the child's growth, development, and general health. The nurse also has a role in monitoring growth and development as well as providing support and teaching for the family. Other team members may include any person whose specialty and services the child may need. This includes the ophthalmologist, speech pathologist, audiologist, social worker, and child life specialist, among others.

The nurse often works with the physician to monitor the child's growth and developmental progress, and may recommend referral to other team members when consultation or therapy is needed. The nurse may function in a supportive role or in a role as educator for a parent with questions about the general care, developmental stimulation, or health of infant or child. The nurse needs to know when to consult the physician and when to refer the parent to the physician or other health care professional.

In the role of educator, the nurse may help the parent plan ways to stimulate the child's remaining senses—touch, taste, and smell—so as to encourage the child to learn the same things that normal children of the same age are learning. This is done by bringing experiences to the child rather than waiting for the child to reach out and learn. Early in life, an infant learns to differentiate people. For instance, the blind-deaf child makes differentiations by touch or smell. The parent is encouraged to reserve a specific and different action to identify each person. The parent may also introduce the small child to different textures and associate the texture with an activity.

Residual vision, even if only for light and darkness, should be stimulated by placing the child in different light intensities for different activities. Residual hearing may be stimulated by different types of sounds, such as music or sounds made by automobiles, trains, or drums. Taste and touch can be similarly stimulated and made part of the infant's learning environment.

The social worker may be needed to assist the family in accessing assistance from agencies that can help the child develop to his or her maximal potential. The child needs experiences outside the home and the parent needs time to do things without the child. A daycare experience for a portion of each week is an excellent opportunity for the child. The family may require funding assistance from a source outside the family to make these activities possible.

Daycare play opportunities during early childhood can assist greatly in school readiness. Play opportunities become learning opportunities in a special class where the teacher is knowledgeable in teaching children with deficits. A child with cognitive deficiency needs much stimulation and one-on-one assistance to learn. The child with vision and hearing impairment needs to develop early the sense of touch in preparation for finger spelling. Persons working with disabled children should not expect them to reach out to learn when they can neither see nor hear what is happening around them; rather, the learning experience should be brought to the child. Other children may need to be encouraged to participate in the teaching and stimulation process. The nurse should teach the disabled child's peers and siblings about the disability and how they can help the child with disability to learn, regardless of whether the child is developmentally delayed or of normal cognitive ability.

Summary of Key Concepts

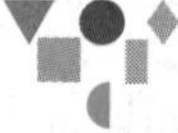

- Sensory input that is received through vision and hearing provides the basis for communication, which, in turn, allows the infant to continue in psychosocial development.
- Development of vision begins during fetal life and continues until the seventh year of life when visual development is complete.
- Disorders of vision may be congenital or acquired and may cause visual impairment of varying degrees of severity from a mild impairment correctable with lenses to total blindness. Some disorders, such as infections, are preventable, and many are treatable with antibiotics.

- Hearing is present well before birth and is well developed at birth. Hearing centers of the brain, like visual centers, begin to organize and assign meaning to nerve impulses early in life.
- Otitis media is a common illness that may result in diminished hearing, particularly when fluid is present behind the tympanic membrane. This condition is called otitis media with effusion and is common in preschool and school-age children.
- Hearing may be diminished as a result of injury, severe infection such as meningitis, or treatment with ototoxic medications.
- The ability to communicate begins with the infant's first cries and continues in a progressive fashion throughout childhood.
- Receptive language abilities are always present before expressive language skills are developed.
- Infants and children with multiple sensory impairments are challenged in their ability to learn. The health care team can incorporate a variety of strategies to maximize the use of existing sensory abilities and thereby enhance the child's ability to interact and function independently as he or she matures.

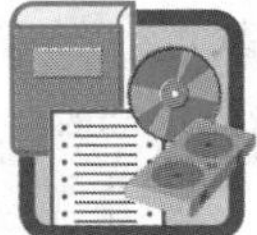

Resources

Vision

American Council of the Blind
1155 15th Street NW
Suite 720
Washington, DC 20005
(202) 467-5081 or (800) 424-8666
Serves as a national information clearinghouse on blindness for individuals, organizations, and institutions.

American Foundation for the Blind
15 W. 16th Street
New York, NY 10011
(212) 620-2000 or (800) 232-5463
National resource for blind or visually impaired persons. Works to ensure development, maintenance, and improvement of services for the blind and visually impaired.

American Printing House for the Blind
P. O. Box 6085
1839 Frankfort Avenue
Louisville, KY 40206
(502) 895-2405
Promotes publication of literature in all media (braille, large type, recorded computer disc) for the blind, and the manufacture of educational aids for use by visually impaired students.

Association for Education and Rehabilitation of the Blind and Visually Impaired
206 N. Washington Street
Suite 320
Alexandria, VA 22314-2528
(703) 548-1884
For professionals in the field of service to the blind and visually impaired children and adults.

Blackbird Vision Screening System
P. O. Box 277424
Sacramento, CA 95827
(800) 363-6884

✏ Blind Children's Center
4120 Marathon Street
P. O. Box 29159
Los Angeles, CA 90029
(800) 222-3566 or, in California, (800) 222-3567

✏ Blind Children's Fund
8500 W. Capitol Drive
Milwaukee, WI 53222
(414) 464-3000
A subcommittee of the International Council for Education of the Visually Handicapped. Promotes health and education of preschool blind and visually impaired. Books available for parents.

Blind Service Association
22 W. Monroe
11th Floor
Chicago, IL 60603
(312) 236-0808
Uses volunteers for recording textbooks on cassette tapes, providing visual aids, and undertaking field trips; stages workshops; supplies emergency funds for the blind.

Braille Authority of North America
1839 Frankfort Avenue
Louisville, KY 40206-0085
(502) 480-7530

Canadian National Institute for the Blind
1931 Bayview Avenue
Toronto, Ontario M4G 4C8
Canada

✏ Resources specifically for children.

Council of Families with Visual Impairment
26616 Rouge Drive
Dearborn Heights, MI 48127
(800) 424-8666

Associated with American Council of the Blind. Formerly called American Council of the Blind Parents.

Guide Dogs for the Blind
P. O. Box 151200
San Rafael, CA 94915-1200
(415) 499-4000
FAX: (415) 499-4035

Guide Dog Foundation for the Blind, Inc.
371 E. Jericho Turnpike
Smithtown, NY 11787
(516) 265-2121 or (800) 548-4337
FAX: (516) 361-5192

Training center for blind persons requiring guide dogs.

In Touch Networks
15 W. 65th Street
New York, NY 10023
(212) 769-6270 or (800) 456-3166

Volunteer organization; provides readings of articles from newspapers and magazines over closed-circuit radio for blind and physically impaired persons.

National Association for Parents of the Visually Impaired
P. O. Box 317
Watertown, MA 02272-0317
(617) 362-4945 or (800) 562-6265
FAX: (617) 972-7444

Has regional and state groups of parents and families of visually impaired children and interested individuals. Provides support and promotes public understanding.

National Association for the Visually Handicapped
22 W. 21st Street
New York, NY 10010
(212) 889-3141
FAX: (212) 727-2931

Publishes and distributes large-print literature; provides counsel for parents of partially seeing children.

National Braille Association, Inc.
3 Townline Circle
Rochester, NY 14623
(716) 427-8260
FAX: (716) 427-0263

Produces and distributes braille reading materials for people who are visually impaired. Collection consists of college-level textbooks, technical materials, and some materials of general interest.

National Center for Sight
(800) 221-3004

Provides information on a broad range of eye health and safety topics. Sponsored by the National Society to Prevent Blindness.

National Federation of the Blind
1800 Johnson Street
Baltimore, MD 21230
(410) 659-9314 or (800) 638-7518
FAX: (410) 685-5653

Primary interest is the complete integration of people who are blind into general society on an equal basis with others. Operates a job referral program and offers advocacy in housing and insurance issues, among others. Offers college scholarships and has monthly and quarterly publications.

National Library Service for the Blind and Physically Handicapped
Library of Congress
1291 Taylor Street NW
Washington, DC 20542
(202) 707-5100
FAX: (202) 707-0712

Administers a free library program of braille and recorded books for eligible readers who are visually impaired and physically handicapped in the United States, and for American citizens living abroad.

National Society to Prevent Blindness
500 East Remington Road
Schaumburg, IL 60173
(708) 843-2020 or (800) 331-2020
FAX: (708) 843-8458

Goal is reduction in cases of needless blindness. Provides educational materials for children, families, and professionals concerning causes of blindness and its prevention, including screening programs for children.

Recording for the Blind
20 Roszel Road
Princeton, NJ 08540
(609) 452-0606 or (800) 221-4792
FAX: (609) 987-8116

Serves people who cannot read standard print because of a visual, learning, or physical disability. Provides textbooks on tape and on computer diskettes. One-time registration fee of $25 entitles user to lifetime borrowing privileges.

TeleSensory Systems, Inc.
520 Almanor Avenue
Sunnydale, CA 94086
(800) 227-8418

Vision Center
1393 N. High Street
Columbus, OH 43201

Hearing

Alexander Graham Bell Association for the Deaf, Inc.
3417 Volta Place NW
Washington, DC 20007
(202) 337-5220

✏ American Society for Deaf Children
814 Thayer Avenue
Silver Spring, MD 20910
(301) 585-5400 (Voice/TDD) or (800) 942-2732

American Speech-Language-Hearing Association (ASHA)
10801 Rockville Pike
Rockville, MD 20852
(301) 897-5700 or (800) 638-8255

Provides information and distributes materials concerning hearing aids. Also provides information to help callers to locate speech pathologists and audiologists certified by the ASHA.

Better Hearing Institute
P. O. Box 1840
Washington, DC 20013
(703) 642-0580 or (800) EAR-WELL

Center for Genetic and Acquired Deafness
St. Christopher's Hospital for Children
Section of Medical Genetics
5th Street and Lehigh Avenue
Philadelphia, PA 19133
(215) 427-4430

Cochlear Implant Club International
P. O. Box 464
Buffalo, NY 14223-0464
(716) 838-4662

For implant patients, candidates, and parents. Provides support services, promotes improved cochlear implant technology and research, and conducts educational programs and childrens' services.

Deafness and Communicative Disorders Branch
Rehabilitation Services Administration
Office of Special Education and Rehabilitative Services
Department of Education
330 C Street SW
Room 3219
Washington, DC 20201-2736
(202) 727-1800

Deafness Research Foundation
9 East 38th Street
7th Floor
New York, NY 10016
(212) 684-6556 or (800) 535-DEAF
(212) 6559 (TTY)
FAX: (212) 779-2125

Funds research on prevention of deafness and its treatment.

Deafpride, Inc.
1350 Potomac Avenue SE
Washington, DC 20003
(202) 675-6700
FAX: (202) 547-0547

Dogs for the Deaf
10175 Wheeler Road
Central Point, OR 97502
(503) 826-9220

Trains hearing ear dogs to alert deaf persons to certain sounds. Deaf or severely hearing-impaired persons are eligible when they are able to assume responsibility for the care of the dog.

Hear Now
(800) 648-4327 (Voice/TDD)

Provides hearing aids, cochlear implants, and related services for the hearing impaired who do not have the financial resources to purchase these devices. Collects and distributes reconditioned hearing aids. Applications for assistance are available.

Hearing Helpline
(703) 642-0580 in VA or (800) 327-9355

Provides information on better hearing and preventing deafness. Materials are mailed on request. A service of the Better Hearing Institute.

John Tracy Clinic
(800) 522-4582

Provides free diagnostic, rehabilitative, and educational services to preschool deaf children and their families through on-site services, and to the preschool deaf and deaf-blind through worldwide correspondence courses in Spanish and English.

National Association of Parents of the Deaf (see also American Society for Deaf Children)
814 Thayer Avenue
Silver Spring, MD 20910

National Association of the Deaf
814 Thayer Avenue
Silver Spring, MD 20910
(301) 587-1788

National Hearing Aid Helpline
(800) 521-5247

Provides information and distributes a directory of hearing aid specialists certified by the National Hearing Aid Society.

National Information Center on Deafness
Gallaudet University
800 Florida Avenue NE
Washington, DC 20002
(202) 651-5051

Parents' section of the Alexander Graham Bell Association for the Deaf; formerly (1989) International Parents' Organization.

Tripod Grapevine
(800) 352-8888 (Voice/TDD) or, in California, (800) 287-4763 (Voice/TDD)

Offers information on deafness, including raising and educating a deaf child. Refers callers to parents, professionals, and resources in their own communities nationwide.

Communication

American Speech-Language-Hearing Association
10801 Rockville Pike
Rockville, MD 20852
(800) 638-8255
Web: http://www.asha.org

Foundation for Fluency
9242 Gross Point Road
Suite 305
Skokie, IL 60067
(708) 677-8280

National Center for Stuttering
200 East 33rd Street
New York, NY 10016
(800) 221-2483

Stuttering Foundation of America
(800) 992-9392

Provides materials and makes referrals to speech-language pathologists.

Stuttering Resource Foundation
(800) 232-4775

References

Vision

American Academy of Pediatrics (1988). *Report of the Committee on Infectious Diseases* (21st ed.). Elk Grove Village, IL: Author.

Aslin, R. N. (1977). Development of binocular fixation in human infants. *Journal of Experimental Child Psychology, 23,* 133.

Birch, E. E., & Stager, D. R. (1988). Prevalence of good visual acuity following surgery for congenital unilateral cataract. *Archives of Ophthalmology, 106,* 40–43.

Bradford, G. M., Keech, R. V., & Scott, W. E. (1994). Factors affecting visual outcome after surgery for bilateral congenital cataracts. *Journal of Ophthalmology, 117*(1), 58–64.

Brown, G. C., Tasman, W. S., Naidoff, M., Schaffer D. B., Quinn, G., & Bhutani, V. K. (1990). Systemic complications associated with retinal cryoablation for retinopathy of prematurity. *Ophthalmology, 97,* 855–858.

Burns, C. E., Barber, N., Brady, M. A., & Dunn, A. M. (1996). *Pediatric primary care: A handbook for nurse practitioners.* Philadelphia: W. B. Saunders.

Calhoun, J. (1997). Eye examinations in infants and children. *Pediatrics in Review, 18*(1), 28–31.

Campbell, L. R., & Charney, E. (1991). Factors associated with delay in diagnosis of childhood amblyopia. *Pediatrics, 87*(2), 178–185.

Chen, J. (1992). Prophylaxis of ophthalmia neonatorum: Comparison of silver nitrate, tetracycline, erythromycin and no prophylaxis. *Pediatric Infectious Disease Journal, 11,* 1026–1030.

Cheng, K. P., Hiles, D. A., Biglan, A. W., Pettapiece, M. C., Behler, S. C., & Moore, M. B. (1991). Visual results after early surgical treatment of unilateral congenital cataract. *Ophthalmology, 98,* 903–910.

Cunningham, S., Fleck, B. W., Elton, R. A., & McIntosh, N. (1995). Transcutaneous oxygen levels in retinopathy of prematurity. *Lancet, 346,* 1464–1465.

DeLuise, V. P., & Anderson, D. R. (1983). Primary infantile glaucoma (congenital glaucoma). *Survey of Ophthalmology, 28,* 1–19.

Deschenes, J., Seamone, C., & Baines, M. (1990). The ocular manifestations of sexually transmitted diseases. *Canadian Journal of Ophthalmology, 25,* 177.

Duke-Elder, S. (1969). *System of ophthalmology: Congenital deformities* (vol. III, part 2). St. Louis: C. V. Mosby, 548–565.

Federal Regulations, PL 94-142. (November 29, 1975). Washington, DC: U.S. Government Printing Office.

Fisher, M. C. (1987). Conjunctivitis in children. *Pediatric Clinics of North America: Pediatric Ophthalmology, 34*(6), 1447–1456.

Flynn, J. T., Bancalari, E., Bachynski, B. N., Buckley, E. B., Bawol, R., Goldberg, R., Cassady, J., Schiffman, J., Feuer, W., Gillings, D., Sim, E., & Roberts, J. (1987). Retinopathy of prematurity: Diagnosis, severity, and natural history. *Ophthalmology, 94,* 620–629.

Franks, W., & Taylor, D. (1989). Congenital glaucoma—A preventable cause of blindness. *Archives of Disease in Childhood, 64,* 649–650.

Friendly, D. S. (1993). Development of vision in infants and young children. *Pediatric Clinics of North America, 40*(4), 693–703.

Fulton, A. (1992). Screening preschool children to detect visual and ocular disorders. *Archives of Ophthalmology, 110,* 1553–1554.

Gelbart, S. S., Hoyt, C. S., Jastrebski, G., & Marg, E. (1982). Long term visual results in bilateral congenital cataracts. *American Journal of Ophthalmology, 93,* 615–621.

George, D., Stephen, S., Fellows, R., & Bremer, D. (1988). The latest on retinopathy of prematurity. *MCN American Journal of Maternal Child Nursing, 13,* 254–258.

Gigliotti, F. (1993). Acute conjunctivitis in childhood. *Pediatric Annals, 22*(6), 353.

Glass, P., Avery, G., Subramanian, D., Keys, M., Sostek, A., & Friendly, D. (1985). Effect of bright light in the hospital nursery on the incidence of retinopathy of prematurity. *New England Journal of Medicine, 313*(7), 401–404.

Grimes, M. R., Scardino, M. A., & Martone, J. F. (1992). Worldwide blindness. *Nursing Clinics of North America, 27*(3), 807–816.

Hammerschlag, M. R. (1993). Neonatal conjunctivitis. *Pediatric Annals, 22*(6), 346–351.

Hammerschlag, M. R., Cummings, D., Roblin, R. M., Williams, T. H., & Delke, I. (1989). Efficacy of neonatal ocular prophylaxis for the prevention of chlamydial and gonococcal conjunctivitis. *New England Journal of Medicine, 320*(12), 769–772.

Herndon, D. N., Thompson, P. B., Linares, H. A., & Traber, D. L. (1986). Post graduate course: Respiratory injury, part 1. *The Journal of Burn Care, 7*(2), 190.

Hing, S., Speedwell, L., & Taylor, D. (1990). Lens surgery in infancy and childhood. *British Journal of Ophthalmology, 74,* 73–77.

Hittner, H. M., Godio, L. B., Rudolph, A. J., Adams, J. M., Garcia-Prats, J. A., Friedman, Z., Kautz, J. A., & Monaco, W. A. (1981). Retrolental fibroplasia: Efficacy of vitamin E in a double-blind clinical study of preterm infants. *New England Journal of Medicine, 305,* 1365–1371.

Hohmann, A., & Haase, W. (1993). Effective vision screening can decrease the rate of amblyopia. *Ophthalmologe, 90*(1), 2–5.

Isenberg, S. J. (1990). The dilemma of neonatal ophthalmic prophylaxis. *Western Journal of Medicine, 153*(2), 190–191.

Isenberg, S. J., Apt, L., Yoshimori, R., & Alvarez, S. R. (1988). Bacterial flora of the conjunctiva at birth. *Journal of Pediatric Ophthalmology & Strabismus, 23,* 284.

Jarvis, C. (1992). *Physical examination and health assessment.* Philadelphia: W. B. Saunders.

Jarvis, C. (1996). *Physical examination and health assessment* (2nd ed.). Philadelphia: W. B. Saunders.

Johnson, L., Bowen, F. W., Jr., Abbasi, S., Herrmann, N., Weston, M., Sacks, L., Porat, R., Stahl, G., Peckham, G., Delivoria-Papadopoulos, M., et al. (1985). Relationship of prolonged pharmacologic levels of vitamin E to incidence of sepsis and necrotizing enterocolitis in infants with birth weight 1500 gms or less. *Pediatrics, 75,* 619–638.

Keech, R. V., & Kutschke, P. J. (1995). Upper age limit for the development of amblyopia. *Journal of Ophthalmic Nursing and Technology, 14*(4), 169–173.

Laga, M., Naamara, W., Brunham, R. C., D'Costa, W., Nsanze, H., Piot, P., Kunimoto, D., Ndinya-Achola, J. O., Slaney, L., Ronald, A. R., et al. (1986). Single-dose therapy of gonococcal ophthalmia neonatorum with ceftriaxone. *New England Journal of Medicine, 315,* 1382–1385.

Lam, S. C., Repka, M. X., & Guyton, D. L. (1993). Timing of amblyopia therapy relative to strabismus surgery. *Ophthalmology, 100*(12), 1751–1756.

Lambert, S. R., Amaya, L., & Taylor, D. (1989). Detection and treatment of infantile cataracts. *International Ophthalmology Clinics, 29,* 51–56.

Latif, A., Mason, P., Marowa, E., Paraiwa, E., Dhamu, F., Tambo, J., Gwanzura, L., Mapeta, D., & Jongeling, G. (1988). Management of gonococcal ophthalmia neonatorum with single-dose kanamycin and ocular irrigation with saline. *Sexually Transmitted Diseases, 15,* 108.

Lavrich, J. B., & Nelson, L. B. (1993). Diagnosis and treatment of strabismus disorders. *Pediatric Clinics of North America, 40*(4), 737–752.

MacDonald, M. A. (1996). Refractive errors and corrective lenses in children and adolescents. *Journal of Pediatric Health Care, 10,* 121–123.

Magramm, I. (1992). Amblyopia: Etiology, detection, and treatment. *Pediatric Review, 13*(1), 7–14.

Marshall, D. H., Brownstein, S., Addison, D. J., Mackenzie, S. G., Jordan, D. R., & Clarke, W. N. (1995). Air guns: The main cause of enucleation secondary to trauma in children and young adults in greater Ottawa area in 1974–93. *Canadian Journal of Ophthalmology, 30*(4), 187–192.

Mohindra, I., Swann, J., Held, R., Brill, S., & Swann, R. (1985). Development of acuity and stereopsis in infants with esotropia. *Ophthalmology, 92,* 691.

Moore, R. A., & Schmitt, B. D. (1979). Conjunctivitis in the newborn. *Clinical Pediatrics, 18,* 26.

Mostafa, M. S., Temtamy, S., El-Gammal, M. Y., Sayed, S. I., Abdel-Salam, M., & El-Baroudy, R. (1981). Genetic studies of congenital cataract. *Metabolic, Pediatric, and Systemic Ophthalmology, 5,* 233–242.

National Society to Prevent Blindness. (1988). *Play it safe.* Schaumberg, IL: Author.

National Society to Prevent Blindness (1991). *Home eye safety guide.* Schaumberg, IL: Author.

Nelson, L. B., Wilson, T. W., & Jeffers, J. B. (1989). Eye injuries in childhood: Demography, etiology, and prevention. *Pediatrics, 84,* 438–441.

Neufeldt, V., & Sparks, A. (Eds.). (1990). *Webster's new world dictionary.* New York: Simon & Schuster.

Nishida, H., & Rosenberg, H.M. (1975). Silver nitrate ophthalmic solution and chemical conjunctivitis. *Pediatrics, 56,* 368.

Nixon, R. B., Helveston, E. M., Miller, K., Archer, S. M., & Ellis, F. D. (1985). Incidence of strabismus in neonates. *American Journal of Ophthalmology, 100*(6), 798–801.

O'Hara, M. A. (1993). Ophthalmia neonatorum. In L. B. Nelson (Ed.), *Pediatric Clinics of North America, 40*(4), 715–725.

Overfield, T. (1985). *Biologic variations in health and illness.* Menlo Park, CA: Addison-Wesley.

Page, J. M., Schneeweiss, S., Whyte, H. E., & Harvey, P. (1993). Ocular sequelae in premature infants. *Pediatrics, 92*(6), 787–790.

Palmer, E. A., Flynn, J. T., Hardy, R. J., Phelps, D. L., Phillips, C. L., Schaffer, D. B., & Tung, B. (1991). Incidence and early course of retinopathy of prematurity. *Ophthalmology*, 98, 1628–1640.

Phelps, D. L. (1988). Reduced severity of oxygen-induced retinopathy in kittens recovered in 28% oxygen. *Pediatric Research, 24*, 106–109.

Phelps, D. L. (1992). Retinopathy of prematurity. *Current Problems in Pediatrics, 22*(8), 349–371.

Phelps, D. L., Rosenbaum, A. L., Isenberg, S. J., Leake, R. D., & Dorey, F. J. (1987). Tocopherol efficacy and safety for preventing retinopathy of prematurity: A randomized, controlled, double-masked trial. *Pediatrics, 79*, 489.

Pike, M. G., Jan, J. E., & Wong, P. K. (1989). Neurological and developmental findings in children with cataracts. *American Journal of Diseases of Children, 143*, 706–710.

Potter, W. S. (1993). Pediatric cataracts. *Pediatric Clinics of North America, 40*(4), 841–853.

Preece, P. M., Anderson, J. M., & Thompson, R. G. (1989). *Chlamydia trachomatis* infection in infants: A prospective study. *Archives of Diseases in Children, 64*, 525.

Preslan, M. W. (1993). Laser therapy for retinopathy of prematurity. *Journal of Pediatric Ophthalmology and Strabismus, 30*(2), 80–83.

Quigley, H. A. (1982). Childhood glaucoma. *Ophthalmology, 89*, 219–226.

Reed, B. (1997). Setting their sights: Visual development in newborns. *Advance for Nurse Practitioners, 5*(2), 67–70.

Reed, D. B. (1989). Viral and bacterial conjunctivitis. Prevention of disastrous results. *Postgraduate Medicine, 86*(4), 107–109, 113–114.

Robinson, G. C., & Jan, J. E. (1993). Acquired ocular visual impairment in children, 1960–1989. *American Journal of Diseases in Children, 147*, 325–328.

Rothenberg, R. (1979). Ophthalmia neonatorum due to *Neisseria gonorrhoeae*: Prevention and treatment. *Sexually Transmitted Diseases*, 6(Suppl. 2), 187–191.

Rubin, S. E., & Nelson, L. B. (1993). Amblyopia diagnosis and management. *Pediatric Clinics of North America, 40*(4), 727–735.

Schaffer, D. B., Johnson, L., Quinn, G. E., Weston, M., & Bowen, F. W., Jr. (1985). Vitamin E and retinopathy of prematurity: Follow-up at one year. *Ophthalmology, 92*, 1005–1011.

Schmitt, B. D. (1992). *Instructions for pediatric patients.* Philadelphia: W. B. Saunders.

Seidman, D. J., Nelson, L. B., Calhoun, J. H., Spaeth, G. L., & Harley, R. D. (1986). Signs and symptoms in the presentation of primary infantile glaucoma. *Pediatrics, 77*(3), 399–404.

Siegel, J. D. (1986). Eye infections encountered by the pediatrician. *Pediatric Infectious Diseases, 5*, 741.

Stager, D. R., Birch, E. E., & Weakley, D. R. (1990). Amblyopia and the pediatrician. *Pediatric Annals, 19*(5), 301–315.

Staley, T. (1988). Managing facial burns. *The Canadian Nurse, 84*(5), 25–26.

Stern, J. H., & Catalano, R. A. (1990). Current status of diagnostic and therapeutic measures in infantile glaucoma. *Seminars in Ophthalmology*, 5, 166–175.

Symanski, M., Newman, C., & Bachynski, B. (1994). Treating congenital cataracts. *Maternal Child Nursing, 19*, 335–338.

Taylor, D. (1986). Screening? *Transactions of the Ophthalmological Society of the United Kingdom, 104*, 16–21.

Terry, T. L. (1942). Extreme prematurity and fibroblastic overgrowth of persistent vascular sheath behind each crystalline lens. I. Preliminary report. *American Journal of Ophthalmology, 25*, 203–204.

Thomas, R., Mathai, A., Rajeev, B., Sen, S., & Jacob, P. (1993). Botulinum toxin in the treatment of paralytic strabismus and essential blepharospasm. *Indian Journal of Ophthalmology, 41*(3), 121–124.

Vander, J. F. (1994). Retinopathy of prematurity: Diagnosis and management. *Journal of Ophthalmic Nursing Technology, 13*(5), 207–212.

Vinger, P. F. (1987). The eye in sports medicine. In T. D. Duane & E. A. Jaeger (Eds.), *Clinical ophthalmology* (pp. 1–39). Philadelphia: J. B. Lippincott.

von Noorden, G. K. (1974). *Burrian & von Noorden's binocular vision and ocular motility.* St. Louis: C. V. Mosby.

von Noorden, G. K. (1990). Examination of the patient, III. In Burrian & von Noorden's *binocular vision and ocular motility* (4th ed.). St. Louis: C. V. Mosby.

Wagner, R. (1993). Glaucoma in children. *Pediatric Clinics of North America, 40*(4), 855–867.

Wilson, F. M. (1979). Adverse external ocular effects of topical ophthalmic medications. *Survey of Ophthalmology, 24*, 5.

Zanoni, D., Isenberg, S., & Apt, L. (1992). A comparison of silver nitrate and erythromycin for prophylaxis against ophthalmia neonatorum. *Clinical Pediatrics, 31*, 295.

Hearing

American Speech-Language-Hearing Association: Joint Committee on Infant Hearing. (1994). Position statement. *ASHA, 36*(12), 38–41.

Baker, R. C. (1991). Pitfalls in diagnosing otitis media. *Pediatric Annals, 20*(11), 591–593, 596–598.

Barringer, D. G., Strong, C. J., Blair, J. C., Clark, T. C., & Watkins, S. (1993). *American Annals of the Deaf, 138*, 420–426.

Birch, L., & Elbrond, O. (1986). Prospective epidemiological study of secretory otitis media in children not attending kindergarten. An incidence study. *International Journal of Pediatric Otorhinolaryngology, 11*, 183.

Bluestone, C. D., Klein, J. O., Paradise, J. L., Eichenwald, H., Bess, F. H., Downs, M. P., Green, M., Berko-Gleason, J., Ventry, I. M., Gray, S. W., McWilliams, B. J., & Gates, G. A. (1983). Workshop on effects of otitis media on the child. *Pediatrics, 71*, 639–652.

Buncher, P., & Price, M. (1996). Communicating with deaf patients: Breaking the sound barrier. *Advance for Nurse Practitioners, 4*(9), 17–21.

Bysshe, J. (1995). Deafness in childhood: 3. Cochlear implant: Who, why, & what are the results? *Professional Care of Mother and Child, 5*(5), 135–137.

Carlson, L. H. (1996, February). Otitis media in children. *Advance for Nurse Practitioners*, 14–20.

Casselbrant, M. L. (1989). Epidemiology of otitis media in infants and preschool children. *Pediatric Infectious Disease Journal*, 8(Suppl. 1), S10–S11.

Cornell, S. (1997). Chronic otitis media and delayed speech development: Are the two connected? *Advance for Nurse Practitioners, 5*(5), 55–58.

Crandell, C. C., & Roeser, R. J. (1993). Incidence of excessive/impacted cerumen in individuals with mental retardation: A longitudinal investigation. *American Journal on Mental Retardation, 97*(5), 568–574.

Cunningham, A. S. (1977). Morbidity in breast-fed and artificially fed infants. *Journal of Pediatrics*, 90, 726.

Davis, J. (1990). *Our forgotten children: Hard of hearing pupils in the school.* Washington, DC: U.S. Department of Education.

Downs, M. P. (1986). The rationale for neonatal hearing screening. In E. T. Swigart (Ed.), *Neonatal hearing screening.* San Diego, CA: College-Hill Press.

Fleming, D. W., Cochi, S. L., Hightower, A. W., & Broome, C. V. (1987). Childhood upper respiratory tract infections: To what degree is incidence affected by day-care attendance? *Pediatrics, 79*, 55.

Giebink, G. S., & Canafax, D. M. (1988). Controversies in the management of otitis media. *Advances in Pediatric Infectious Disease, 3*, 27.

Goycoolea, M. V., Hueb, M. M., & Ruah, C. (1991). Otitis media: The pathogenesis approach. Definitions and terminology. *Otolaryngologic Clinics of North America, 24*(4), 757–761.

Hallet, C. P. (1982). The screening and epidemiology of middle ear disease in a population of primary school entrants. *Journal of Laryngology and Otolaryngology*, 96, 899.

Iversen, M., Birch, L., Lundqvist, G. R., & Elbrond, O. (1985). Middle ear effusion in children and the indoor environment: An epidemiological study. *Archives of Environmental Health, 40*, 74–79.

Jordan, M. J., (1991). Clinical approach to treatment of otitis media. *Otolaryngologic Clinics of North America, 24*(4), 901–929.

Jung, T. T. K., & Rhee, C. K. (1991). Otolaryngologic approach to the diagnosis and management of otitis media. *Otolaryngologic Clinics of North America, 24*(4), 931–945.

Kraemer, M. J., Richardson, M. E., Weiss, N. S., Furukawa, C. T., Shapiro, G. G., Pierson, W. E., & Bierman, C. W. (1983). Risk factors for persistent middle ear effusions. *Journal of the American Medical Association, 249*, 1022–1025.

Marchant, C. D., Shurin, P. A., Turczyk, V. A., Wasikowski, D. E., Tutihasi, M. A., & Kinney S. E. (1984). Course and outcome of otitis media in early infancy: A prospective study. *Journal of Pediatrics, 104*, 826.

Mishoe, S. C., Brooks, C. W., Jr., Dennison, F. H., Hill, D. V., & Frye, T. (1995). Octave waveband analysis to determine sound frequencies and intensities produced by nebulizers and humidifiers used with hoods. *Respiratory Care*, 40(11), 1120–1124.

Overfield, T. (1985). *Biologic variations in health and illness.* Menlo Park, CA: Addison-Wesley.

Papparella, M. M., Kimberley, B. P., & Alleva, M. (1991). The concept of silent otitis media: Its importance and implications. *Otolaryngologic Clinics of North America, 24*(4), 763–773.

Roberts, J. (1972). Hearing and related medical findings among children: Race, area, and socioeconomic differentials. *Vital Health Statistics, 11*(122), 1–33.

Roberts, J., & Ahuja, E. M. (1975). Hearing sensitivity and related medical findings among youths 12–17 years. *Vital Health Statistics, 11*(154), 1–112.

Ross, M., Brackett, D., & Maxon, A. (1991). *Assessment and management of mainstreamed hearing impaired children.* Austin, TX: Pro-Ed.

Stahlberg, M., Ruuskanen, O., & Virolainen, E. (1986). Risk factors for recurrent otitis media. *Pediatric Infectious Disease Journal*, 5, 30.

Stewart, I., Kirkland, C., Simpson, A., et al. (1984). Some factors of possible etiologic significance related to otitis media. In D. J. Lim (Ed.), *Recent advances in otitis media with effusion* (pp. 25–27). Philadelphia: B. C. Decker.

Stool, S. E., Berg, A. O., Berman, S., Carney, C. J., Cooley, J. R., Culpepper, L., Eavey, R. D., Feagans, L. V., Finitzo, T., Friedman, E., et al. (1994). *Managing otitis media with effusion in young children. Quick reference guide for clinicians* (AHCPR Publication No. 94-0623). Rockville, MD: Agency for Health Care Policy and Research, Public Health Service, U. S. Department of Health and Human Services.

Swigart, E. T. (Ed.). (1986). *Neonatal hearing screening.* San Diego, CA: College-Hill Press.

Tanimura, M., Matsui, I., Kobayashi, N., Koga, K., Oshima, T., & Mochizuki, T. (1993). Preliminary report: Suspicion of hearing loss at age 0–1 years by TV viewing attitude. *International Journal of Pediatric Otorhinolaryngology, 28*(1), 1–9.

Teele, D. W., Klein, J. O., & Rosner, B. (1989). Epidemiology of otitis media during the first seven years of life in children of greater Boston: A prospective cohort study. *Journal of Infectious Disease, 160*, 83–94.

Zeisel, S. A., Roberts, J. E., Gunn, E. B., Riggins, R., Jr., Evas, G. A., Rousch J., Burchinal, M. R., & Henderson, F. W. (1995). Prospective surveillance for otitis media with effusion among black infants in group child care. *Journal of Pediatrics, 127*, 875–880.

Communication

American Speech-Language-Hearing Association (1993). Definitions of communication disorders and variations. *ASHA, 35*(Suppl. 10), 40–41.

Crowe, T. A., & Robinson, T. L. (1993). Stuttering: Do we have an ounce to give? *American Speech-Language-Hearing Association*, November, *35*, 53–54.

Erikson, E. H. (1963). *Youth: Change and challenge.* New York: Basic Books.

King, P. T., & Neal, R. (1968). *Ego-psychology in counseling.* Boston: Houghton Mifflin.

Bibliography

Vision

Barron, D. F., & Sivulich, K. A. (1994). Laser therapy as a treatment for retinopathy of prematurity. *Pediatric Nursing, 20*(1), 90–92.

Bell, T. A., Grayston, J. T., Krohn, M. A., Kronmal, R. A., & The Eye Prophylaxis Study Group. (1993). Randomized trial of silver nitrate, erythromycin, and no eye prophylaxis for prevention of conjunctivitis among newborns not at risk for gonococcal ophthalmitis. *Pediatrics, 92*, 755.

Catalano, R. A. (1993). Eye injuries and prevention. *Pediatric Clinics of North America, 40*(4), 827–839.

Chan, T., O'Keefe, M., Bowell, R., & Lanigan, B. (1995). Childhood penetrating eye injuries. *Irish Medical Journal, 88*(5), 168–170.

Crouch, E. R., Jr., Pressman, S. H., & Crouch, E. R. (1995). Posterior chamber intraocular lenses: Long-term results in pediatric cataract patients. *Journal of Pediatric Ophthalmology & Strabismus, 32*(4), 210–218.

DeSylvia, D. A., & Klug, C. D. (1992). Drugs and children: Taking care of the victims. *Journal of the American Optometric Association, 63*(1), 59–62.

Drews, C. D., Yeargin-Allsopp, M., Murphy, C. C., & Decoufle, P. (1992). Legal blindness among 10 year old children in metropolitan Atlanta: Prevalence, 1985–1987. *American Journal of Public Health, 82*(10), 1377–1379.

Flynn, J. T. (1995). Retinopathy of prematurity: Perspectives for the nineties. *Acta Ophthalmologia Scandinavia Supplement, 214*, 12–16.

Freeman, R. S., & Rovick, L. P. (1995). Cloudy lens & issues: A pedigree of unoperated congenital cataracts. *Journal of Ophthalmic Nursing & Technology, 14*(3), 118–123.

Greely, J., & Anthony, T. L. (1995). Play interactions with infants and toddlers who are deaf-blind: Setting the stage. *Seminars in Hearing, 16*(2), 185–191.

Hunsucker, K., King, C., Stamm, S., & Cisneros, N. (1995). Laser surgery for retinopathy of prematurity. *Neonatal Network: Journal of Neonatal Nursing, 14*(4), 21–30.

Jackson, J. (1993). Hyphema. *Optometric Clinics, 3*(2), 27–40.

Jeffers, J. B. (1990). An ongoing tragedy: Pediatric sports-related eye injuries. *Seminars in Ophthalmology, 5*, 216–218.

King, K. M., & Cronin, C. M. (1993). Ocular findings in premature infants with grade IV intraventricular hemorrhage. *Journal of Pediatric Ophthalmology & Strabismus, 30*(2), 4–7.

Kutschke, P. J. (1994). Ocular trauma in children. *Journal of Ophthalmic Nursing and Technology, 13*(3), 117–120.

LaRoche, G. R. (1995). Air gun injuries to the eye in children: Canadian ophthalmologists have to stop the onslaught [Editorial; Comment]. *Canadian Journal of Ophthalmology, 30*(44), 177–178.

Moller, M. (1993). Working with visually impaired children and their families. *Pediatric Clinics of North America, 40*(4), 881–891.

O'Connell, J. E., Turner, N. O., & Pahor, A. L. (1995). Air gun pellets in the sinuses. *Journal of Laryngology and Otology, 109*(11), 1097–1100.

Rosenthal, S. B. (1995). Living with low vision: A personal perspective. *American Journal of Occupational Therapy, 49*(9), 861–864.

Rowell, M. (1993). Eradication of vitamin A deficiency with 5 cents and a vegetable garden. *Journal of Ophthalmic Nursing & Technology, 12*(5), 217–224.

Ruehl, C. A., & Schremp, P. S. (1992). Nursing care of the cataract patient: Today's outpatient approach. *Nursing Clinics of North America, 27*(3), 727–743.

Schraeder, B. D., & McEvoy-Shields, K. (1991). Visual acuity, binocular vision, and ocular muscle balance in VLBW children. *Pediatric Nursing, 17*(1), 30–33.

Sonksen, P. M. (1993). The assessment of vision in the preschool child. *American Journal of Diseases in Children, 68*, 513–516.

Teplin, S. W. (1995). Visual impairment in infants and young children. *Infants and Young Children, 8*(1), 18–51.

Vaughn, V. C. (1992). Assessment of growth and development during infancy and early childhood. *Pediatrics in Review, 13*(3), 88–96.

Wasserman, R. C., Croft, C. A., & Brotherton, S. E. (1992). Preschool vision screening in pediatric practice: A study from the pediatric research in office settings (PROS) network. *Pediatrics, 89*(5), 834–838.

Hearing

Baldwin, R. L. (1993). Effects of otitis media on child development. *American Journal of Otology, 14*(6), 601–604.

Briggs, R. J., & Luxford, W. M. (1994). Correction of conductive hearing loss in children. *Otolaryngologic Clinics of North America, 27*, 607–620.

Butler, K. G. (1994). *Hearing impairment and language disorder: Assessment and intervention*. Gaithersburg, MD: Aspen.

Bysshe, J. (1994). Deafness in childhood: 1. Diagnosis and treatment of deaf babies and children. *Professional Care of Mother and Child, 4*(6), 180–183.

Collett, J. P., Larson, C. P., Boivan, J. F., Suissa, S., & Pless, B. (1995). Parental smoking and risk of otitis media in preschool children. *Canadian Journal of Public Health, 86*(4), 269–273.

Flexer, C. (1994). *Facilitating hearing and listening in young children*. San Diego, CA: Singular Publishing Group.

Hassenstab, M. S. (1994). Early intervention for infants with hearing impairment. *Seminars in Hearing, 15*(2), 64–172.

Kravitz, L., & Selekman, J. (1992). Understanding hearing loss in children. *Pediatric Nursing, 18*(6), 591–594.

Lartz, M. N., & Lestina, L. J. (1995). Strategies deaf mothers use when reading to their young deaf or hard of hearing children. *American Annals of the Deaf, 140*(4), 358–362.

Miyamoto, R. T., Osberger, M. J., & Robins, A. M. (1992). Longitudinal evaluation of communication skills of children with single- or multichannel cochlear implants. *American Journal of Otology, 13*, 215–222.

Northern, J. L., & Downs, M. D. (1991). *Hearing in children* (4th ed.). Baltimore: Williams & Wilkins.

Pillon, J. P. (1995). Hearing impairment & hearing aids. *Exceptional Parent, 25*(5), 30, 32–33.

Sacristan, J. A., Angeles DeCos, M., Soto, J., Zurbano, F., & Pascual, J. (1993). Ototoxicity of erythromycin in man: Electrophysiologic approach. *The American Journal of Otology, 14*(2), 186–188.

Schnore, S. K., Sangster, J. F., Gerace, T. M., & Bass, M. J. (1986). Are antihistamine–decongestants of value in the treatment of acute otitis media in children? *The Journal of Family Practice, 22*(1), 39–43.

Souliere, C. R., Quigley, S. M., & Langman, A. W. (1994). Cochlear implants in children. *Otolaryngologic Clinics of North America, 27*, 533–556.

Stevenson, L., & Brooke, D. S. (1995). Managing otitis media with effusion in young children. *Journal of Pediatric Health Care, 9*(1), 36–39.

Watkins, P. M., Beckman, A., & Baldwin, M. (1995). The views of parents of hearing impaired children on the need for neonatal hearing screening. *British Journal of Audiology, 29*(5), 259–262.

Communication

Chermak, G. D., & Wagner-Bitz, C. J. (1993). Survey of speech-language pathologists' and audiologists' knowledge of clinical genetics. *American Speech-Language-Hearing Association, 35*(5), 39–45.

Donahue-Kilburg, G. (1993). Family centered approach to promoting communication wellness. *American Speech-Language-Hearing Association, 35*(11), 45–46, 62.

Dowling, C. F. (1994). Differentiating normal speech dysfluency from stuttering in children. *Nurse Practitioner, 19*(2), 34–35.

Goldstein, B. A. (1993). Articulation disorders. *American Speech-Language-Hearing Association, 35*(11), 55–56.

Ruben, R. J. (1993). Communication disorders in children: A challenge for health care. *Preventive Medicine, 22*, 585–588.

Multiple Challenges in Sensory Function

Greely, J., & Anthony, T. L. (1995). Play interactions with infants and toddlers who are deaf-blind: Setting the stage. *Seminars in Hearing, 16*(2), 185–191.

Michael, M., & Paul, P. (1991). Early intervention for infants with deaf-blindness. *Exceptional Children, 57(3)*, 202–210.

HEALTH CHALLENGE:

Alterations in Children's Mental Health

OUTLINE

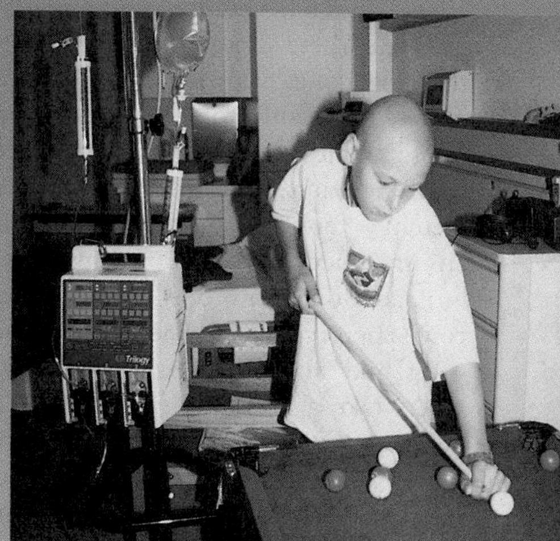

OBJECTIVES

- Describe the mental status examination and the techniques used to assess alterations in children's mental health.
- Explain the purpose and the use of the interdisciplinary categories (*Diagnostic and Statistical Manual*) used to diagnose, communicate, and treat alterations in children and adolescents' health.
- State the criteria indicating the needs for referral of children and adolescents to mental health professionals.
- Describe interventions used to treat alterations in mental health in children and adolescents.
- Describe the relationship between cultural variables and alterations in mental health.
- Discuss the influence of growth and development in relation to alterations in mental health.
- Describe the behavioral, the emotional, the physical, and the cognitive effects of abuse and neglect.

KEY TERMS

abuse
affect
antidepressant
comorbid
compulsion
delusion
dissociation
extrapyramidal side effect
hallucinations
mania
mutism
neglect
obsession
suicide

CHAPTER

29

It is estimated that more than 7.5 million infants, children, and adolescents living in the United States are affected by one or more mental health problems. More than 12% of adolescents experience depression, and are at very high risk for suicide. An increasing number of younger children also have depression. It is also estimated that 10% of children experience severe or disabling anxiety (Donnelly, Maletic, & March, 1996; Kowatch, Emslie, & Kennard, 1996). For many children, these illnesses have a lifelong impact, affecting their overall growth and development, their family and peer relationships, their academic achievement, and their future employment and economic potential. While many of the nation's youth are afflicted with alterations in mental, emotional, and behavioral health, few receive any treatment. The National Institutes of Mental Health estimates that only one fifth of impaired youngsters receive appropriate assessment or treatment.

Child and adolescent psychiatric health care providers take a holistic view of the child, recognizing that many factors influence the child's development and mental well-being. They take into consideration the child's interaction with the environment, his or her nutrition, temperament, genetic influences, physical health, and developmental status. Economic factors, living environment, peer interactions, resources available to the family, and the spiritual and cultural perspective of the family and community are recognized as important influences on children's mental health.

The nurse's role includes participation in decisions about the overall treatment plan. The nurse must make assessments of the child and must collect information from the child's parents and, often, from the child's school as well.

The goals of child psychiatric nursing are to

- Promote mental health
- Prevent mental illness
- Restore mentally ill children to a state of wellness or to their highest level of functioning
- Support the mental health and well-being of their families and caregivers
- Provide support, guidance, and education to those who provide care to mentally ill youngsters, including family members, teachers, and foster parents
- Advocate for the humane treatment of mentally ill children within the context of family and community

The nurse's role as educator for both parents and children can be most useful in helping the parent make informed decisions in the best interest of the child.

Several disciplines are represented on mental health teams as noted in Chart 29–1. Role boundaries tend to be blurred, with each of the disciplines contributing to the plan of care and each performing some part of the overall therapeutic plan. In many settings, all of the disciplines are involved in the daily routine as well as in individual treatment responsibilities. In other settings, every team does not have all of the potential members. Available resources, economic issues, and need play a significant role in the number and kinds of members assigned.

Chart 29–1

Members of the Interdisciplinary Mental Health Team

- Nurse (generalists)—Collaborates with team members to meet needs of clients in both inpatient and outpatient settings.
- Advance practice nurse—Supervises and mentors nursing staff, provides psychotherapy and family therapy, has prescriptive authority, and provides clinical supervision and consultation as needed.
- Psychiatrist—Provides assessment and diagnosis, confirms diagnosis established by other team members, prescribes medication, supervises other professionals providing psychotherapy, collaborates with nurses with prescriptive authority.
- Psychologist—Provides psychotherapy, supervises other team members (when assigned), prescribes, selects, administers, and evaluates psychological tests, and conducts research.
- Social worker—Provides psychotherapy, assists families and patients with social problems, collaborates and consults with other team members about social problems and community resources.
- Occupational therapist—Provides occupational skills training to promote the patient's return to community, promotes effective use of leisure time through use of creative skills. Many children with severe impairment in self-help and care skills are assisted by occupational therapists to develop these skills.
- Recreational therapist—Fosters individual and group recreational activities to foster social skills and healthy recreational outlets, develops and implements special programs.
- Special educator—Using knowledge of learning difficulties and behavior management, plans, implements, and evaluates educational experiences and methods of teaching to facilitate and promote educational achievement of emotionally and behaviorally disturbed children, and those with learning disabilities.
- Parents and client—Provide pertinent data about how they can participate in plan of care, assist in overall evaluation of progress.

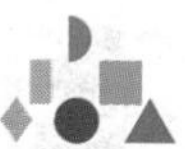

Assessment of the Child with Alterations in Mental Health

Focused Health History

The assessment of a child or adolescent's mental health is complex. The nurse must assess a variety of systems and must work with the child and the family to identify what behaviors are acceptable, unacceptable, and most problematic. The nurse must be highly skilled in therapeutic communication, presenting himself or herself in a professional and nonjudgmental manner to a variety of disciplines, as well as to children and their families.

The assessment of a child or adolescent includes gathering information not only from the child or adolescent but also from those persons who have significant relationships with the patient. Ideally, information is compiled from the child's teacher, family, case worker, psychiatrist, and physician. However, gathering data from multiple sources can quickly become a tangled and conflicting legal web. Initially, the most vital piece of information to obtain is the identity of the child's legal guardian, who must sign consent for treatment before any further measures are taken. The legal guardian then becomes a primary source of information.

Child's Initial History

Children or adolescents being referred for treatment should be allowed to voice their perspective on the problem. By listening to these children, the nurse is better able to establish a therapeutic alliance with them, one of the nurse's primary objectives. The child or adolescent and the parents should be interviewed separately, then brought together for a joint sharing of information. This final family session should also include the referred child's siblings if possible. During this session, the nurse can observe patterns of family functioning and can interview all family members about their perceptions of the family's strengths, problems, and reasons for referral. The best outcome is for everyone in the family to agree to treatment and to the reasons for the treatment; the worst outcome is for no one to agree on anything.

Interviews with children or adolescents should focus on their strengths and weaknesses, including the reason for referral and the level of functioning within the school, family, and peer group. Questions should be asked in a way that is appropriate to the child's developmental level (Chart 29–2).

caREminder: *A child or adolescent's developmental level and chronologic age can vary widely. Many disorders and injuries in psychiatric patients lead to developmental delays. For example, a 9-year-old with a conduct disorder may need to be assessed at a 4-year-old level developmentally.*

The nurse must also assess the child or adolescent's ability to attend and participate in an interview. Some children and adolescents may be too hyperactive, too anxious, too depressed, or too angry to participate fully in an intake interview. However, such children should be given the opportunity to do so. The nurse must quickly assess the child's condition, prioritize family concerns, and gather the most important information. The child or adolescent may be given the opportunity to complete the interview at a later time.

Tip: *When dealing with children and adolescents who may be angry and anxious about referral, the nurse should ask open-ended questions in a nonjudgmental manner. The interview should begin with the gathering of nonthreatening information to decrease the child's anxiety. The nurse should use a "play interview" (a semistructured session, during which toys are available to the child for play) for any child younger than 7 years of age (Garfinkel, Carlson, & Weller, 1990).*

Play interviews may also be appropriate for older children. When determining whether to use a play interview or verbal interview with a child, the nurse should be directed by the child's chronological and developmental age, verbal facility, and cooperation (Garfinkel et al., 1990). Information is gathered by the nurse both through observation and through questioning. Gathering information from a child or adolescent is often far more difficult than from an adult. Conducting a play interview requires a high level of skill, training, and ability to relate well with children.

Parent/Legal Guardian Initial History

After determining legal guardianship of the child or adolescent, parental rights should be clarified. The legal guardian should be interviewed regarding the involvement of the mother, father, and any stepparents. The legal guardian should be asked to notify parents of the child's admission, if appropriate. After having clarified parental custody and visitation, an extensive interview regarding the child and family should be conducted with the legal guardian. Again, a therapeutic alliance with the legal guardian should be established by conducting the interview in an open, nonjudgmental manner (see Chart 29–2). Typically, when a child or adolescent is referred for treatment, the entire family is in crisis. Often, one or more major events occur that precipitate the referral. The nurse gathers information about the child's physical,

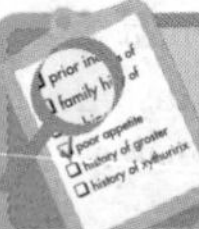

Chart 29–2
Focused Health History

Child and Family Interviews

Child Interview

1. What name do you like to be called?
2. How old are you?
3. What grade are you in at school?
4. What is your favorite subject at school?
5. What subject do you not like?
6. What grades do you usually get in school?
7. Tell me about your teacher.
8. Tell me about why you are here today.
9. How do you get along with the kids in your neighborhood?
10. How do you get along with the kids in your class?
11. What do you usually do when you get mad?
12. What kinds of problems do you have in your family?
13. What things are you good at?
14. If you had three wishes, what would they be?
15. What are your favorite toys?
16. What kinds of things do your parents do that make you mad?
17. What do your parents do to let you know they love you?
18. What are three things that scare you?
19. How are you feeling right now?
20. Have you ever thought of hurting yourself? When? How?
21. Have you ever tried to kill yourself? When? How?
22. Has anyone ever touched you or tried to touch you in your private parts?
23. What is the worst thing that has ever happened to you?
24. Who do you miss the most?
25. What is the best thing that has ever happened to you?
26. Have you ever tried any drugs, alcohol, or cigarettes?
27. How often do you use them?
28. Are you sexually active? (as appropriate)

Parent/Legal Guardian Interview

1. Tell me about your main reasons for bringing your child here today.
2. What problems did you have during pregnancy?
3. How old was your child when he/she walked and was potty trained?
4. Have you ever wondered if your child was delayed in any area of development? Describe.
5. Describe your child's temperament.
6. What health problems has your child had since birth?
7. Are your child's immunizations up to date?
8. Has your child been exposed to chickenpox within the last 2 weeks?
9. Is your child currently sick?
10. What medications does your child take?
11. Who are your child's doctors?
12. Who lives in the household with your child?
13. How many hours per week has your child been in daycare?
14. Who cares for your child when you are gone?
15. How does your child get along with other family members?
16. How many friends does your child have?
17. Who does your child seem to get angry at? Why?
18. How old are your child's friends?
19. Does your child play mostly with boys, girls, or both?
20. How does your child get along with other children in school or the neighborhood?
21. In what areas does your child do well in school?
22. In what areas does your child have problems in school?
23. How does your child get along with his/her teachers?
24. Has your child ever been expelled from school?
25. What grades does your child usually get in school?
26. Is your child in a special program at school?
27. Who are your child's teachers and counselor?
28. What major stressors has your child been through?
29. How many homes has your child lived in?
30. Have you ever suspected that your child has been sexually molested?
31. Does your child use sexual language or have inappropriate sexual knowledge?
32. Does your child act or play sexually?
33. Have you ever noticed any trauma, bleeding, discharge, or redness to your child's genitalia?
34. Does your child play with matches or set fires?
35. Does your child ever urinate or defecate in his/her clothing?
36. Does your child ever do so when he/she is angry?
37. Have you ever noticed your child vomiting after meals?
38. Do you think your child has an eating problem? Describe.

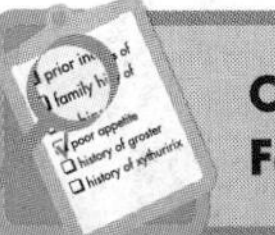

Chart 29–2
Focused Health History *Continued*

Child and Family Interviews

Parent/Legal Guardian Interview

39. What does your child do when he/she is angry?
40. How often does your child
    - hit ______
    - kick ______
    - bite ______
    - spit ______
    - pinch ______
    - butt head ______
    - use profanity ______
    - tear up property ______
    - hurt animals ______
    - throw tantrums ______
    - lie ______
    - steal ______
41. Do you suspect your child has used drugs, alcohol, or tobacco products?
42. How much drug and alcohol use is there by other family members in the home?
43. Do you think your child has ever intentionally tried to hurt himself/herself?
44. Has your child ever talked about or attempted suicide?
45. Do you think your child is sexually active?
46. Describe your child's self-esteem.
47. What losses has your child been through?
48. How do you discipline your child?
49. Have you ever noticed your child responding to things that aren't there?
50. Does your child ever say or do things that make no sense to you?
51. What do you enjoy about your child?
52. Which of the issues we have talked about is most problematic to you?
53. What treatment has your child received for these problems and where?
54. Is there anything else we need to know about your child that we have not covered?

emotional, behavioral, and cognitive states from birth to present (Chart 29–3).

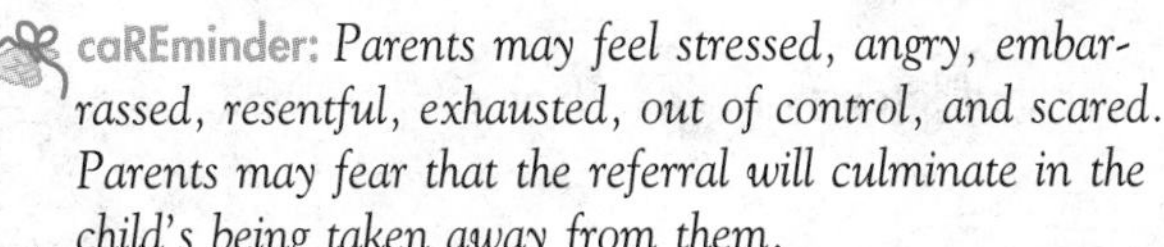

caREminder: *Parents may feel stressed, angry, embarrassed, resentful, exhausted, out of control, and scared. Parents may fear that the referral will culminate in the child's being taken away from them.*

Discussions often become emotionally charged when professionals question and challenge a family in their child-rearing practices. In addition, stress and anxiety levels in Americans are increasing, with higher rates of crime and violence and fewer support systems and resources taking their toll. One response to this increased anxiety and perceived lack of control is to become more controlling in areas in which one has control, such as within the family, and families may become defensive, resentful, and angry when their child-rearing practices are questioned.

Information from Other Sources

Professional communication with involved teachers, counselors, social workers, probation officers, psychiatrists, psychologists, psychometrists, and physicians provides a more comprehensive picture of a child or adolescent's history and current level of functioning. Occasionally, the perceptions of family and professionals are vastly different. Typically, written referral summaries from involved psychiatric professionals provide the nurse with most necessary information. Further contact with psychiatric professionals does *not* require a parental consent. Communication with psychiatric professionals who are currently involved in the patient's care can provide vital information about family history, previous treatment, any placements outside of the home, and any legal entanglements in which a child may have been involved. It should not be assumed that only adolescents are involved in criminal behavior; often, younger children are involved in crimes such as theft, breaking and entering, vandalism, assault, and drug running.

School personnel are knowledgeable about the children and families they serve. Before contacting school personnel, the nurse must first ask the legal guardian to sign a consent form that permits the agency staff and the school to exchange information. If this is not done, the nurse is breaking patient confidentiality, leaving herself or himself open to legal action.

Focused Physical Assessment

Any child or adolescent referred for treatment should receive a thorough medical and nursing physical. While conducting the physical assessment on the child referred for psychiatric services, the health care provider must pay special attention to several areas of the examination that may indicate that the child's overall physical health is at

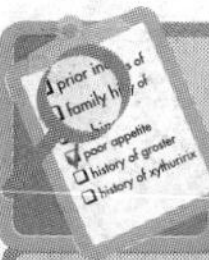

Chart 29–3
Focused Health History

Alterations in Mental Health Status	
Identifying Data	Age Gender Religion
Current History	Presence of delusions, loose associations, hallucinations, illusions, depression, mania, anxiety, phobias, obsessions, compulsions, impulsiveness, suicidal thoughts or behaviors, aggression (physical or sexual)
Birth History	Maternal drug or substance use Birth trauma or injury
Previous Health Challenge	History of mental health disorder, suicidal thoughts or attempts, aggressive behaviors, homicidal thoughts, substance use Results of any neuropsychological testing Any reports of sexual abuse or other forms of abuse
Allergies	Drugs, food, milk products Do allergies cause child to appear highly distracted and unable to concentrate?
Current Medications	Prescription, nonprescription, home remedies
Nutritional Assessment	Recent weight loss or weight gain, decreased appetite, nausea, vomiting Child's perception of his or her weight Child's eating patterns/habits
Family Medical History	Genetic and family history of mental health disorders, includes depression, suicide attempts, substance/alcohol use
Social History	Presence of stressful events at home or school Child's peer group and their usual activities School performance Results of academic achievement tests Nature of relationship with parents/siblings Child's perception of how others view him or her
Growth and Development	Child's plans for the future Child's perception of himself or herself (self-esteem) Previous exposures to stressful events Coping mechanisms used when encountering stressful events Any variations from achieving significant normal growth and developmental milestones

risk or that there are signs of physical or sexual abuse (Chart 29–4). The examiner should be accompanied by another member of the health care team during the physical examination of the child. This provides emotional support for the child and helps protect the health care professional from being accused of sexual misconduct by a child or adolescent. A common dilemma is whether or not to routinely conduct pelvic examinations on all girls admitted for psychiatric treatment. With reduced lengths of stay, a child or adolescent may not have time to build up enough trust with staff members to disclose sexual abuse. On the other hand, pelvic examinations conducted on girls this young, whether or not they have been sexually abused, can be traumatic for them. Chapter 6 provides a detailed summary of the pediatric physical assessment. Of special interest to note are signs that indi-

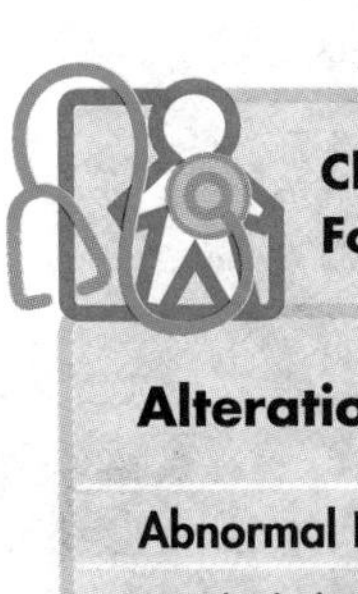

Chart 29–4
Focused Physical Assessment

Alteration in Mental Health

Abnormal Findings	Etiology
Eroded dental enamel, reddened and inflamed gums	Frequent, chronic vomiting (bulimia)
Split fingernails	Malnutrition
Soft, sparse body hair	Malnutrition
Reddened, inflamed throat	Common upper respiratory infections, trauma from self-induced vomiting, or sexually transmitted disease (STD)
Chronic sore throat or difficulty swallowing	Forced oral sex, STD
Burning, itching, bleeding, or discharge from genitalia	Sexual abuse, STD
Bruising, burns, cuts, abrasions, contusions, or other unusual or suspicious marks on skin	Physical abuse or self-harm behavior
Unusual hair loss patterns	Trichotillomania (an anxiety disorder in which the individual pulls out body hair to decrease anxiety)
Vision or hearing deficits	Physical abuse May be misdiagnosed as oppositional behavior, may be related to violent children repeatedly destroying their glasses or hearing aids

cate nutritional deficit (coarse thin hair, gum and dental problems, delayed healing) and injury to the body that may have been inflicted by the child or others.

Mental Status Examination

An important part of the mental health assessment is the mental status examination. This examination may be appropriately conducted by a variety of persons, including an experienced staff nurse or advanced practice nurse. The mental status examination is a report that summarizes observations made of the child or adolescent's appearance and behavior during 2 to 3 hours of interview (Simmons, 1987). It should not include information obtained from any source other than the child or adolescent. It is standard practice for each agency to have its own format for mental status reports.

Conducting a mental status examination with a child or adolescent follows guidelines similar to the initial interview. Again, play is heavily used, especially for children younger than 7 years of age. For all children, play is at least a component of the session. While observing a child's play, a skilled clinician can assess most components of the mental status examination. The nurse, however, must not simply observe the child's play. The nurse must also illicit the underlying fantasy and feelings that accompany the child's play. Any additional components of the mental status examination that cannot be observed can be obtained through nonthreatening verbal questioning. Again, the mental status examination must be conducted in a manner that decreases the child or adolescent's anxiety. An ability to establish rapport with children and adolescents is essential in gathering necessary information while not making the child overly anxious.

Tip: *For older children and adolescents, the nurse gains most necessary information from a relaxed discussion, which could occur in an office, during a walk around the agency, eating some ice cream, observing their play, or while playing a game with the child or adolescent.*

Before taking an older child or adolescent out of the office for a walk, the nurse must assess the risk of the child attempting to run away. Running away is a possibility for a patient of this age group who is anxious to avoid admission or treatment. Using a walk should be a careful decision, made with the full approval of the parents (if present) or staff guidelines. The layout and safety of the building is of prime consideration.

Nursing Diagnoses and Outcomes

A variety of nursing diagnoses may be selected to address the needs of the child with an alteration in mental status (Chart 29–5). Altered thought patterns and behavior affect the child's ability to cope, the child's self-esteem, and the child's ability to interact appropriately with others. Diagnoses such as *ineffective individual coping, self-esteem disturbance*, and *impaired social interaction* are examples of diagnoses applicable to these concerns in the child's life. Another aspect to consider is the impact of the child's mental status on developmental and physical status. The diagnoses of *alterations in nutrition, sleep pattern disturbances, risk for injury*, and *altered growth and development* should be selected to guide nursing care in these areas of the child's life.

Changes and stressors within the family may contribute to the child's mental health condition or be an outcome of the child's altered thought processes and inappropriate behaviors. Therefore, when developing a plan for the child's care, the family must be included as an

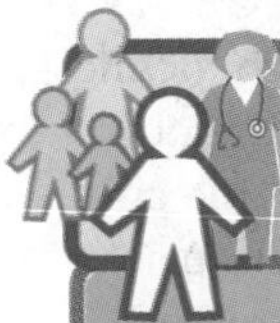

Chart 29–5
Nursing Diagnoses and Outcomes

Alterations in Mental Health Status

Impaired verbal communication related to altered mental status or neurologic impairment

Outcome: Child demonstrates increased ability to communicate as evidenced by verbal and nonverbal behaviors.

Ineffective family coping related to child's behavior

Outcomes:
Family members use appropriate sources of support during times of frustration and crisis.
Family members express feelings and individual needs.
Family members institute measures to meet each others' emotional needs.

Altered family processes related to changes in family relationships, roles, and responsibilities

Outcomes:
Family members discuss changes in family dynamics and identify methods to deal with change in a therapeutic manner.
Family members seek appropriate resource services as needed to optimize family processes.

Altered growth and development related to environmental, neurologic, social, and interpersonal factors that impact cognitive and sensory function

Outcomes:
Child demonstrates interpersonal, social, and physical skills appropriate for age.
Parents express understanding of norms for growth and development.
Child and family use community resources to promote the child's development.

Ineffective individual coping related to sensory overload

Outcomes:
Child understands the relationship between emotional state and behavior.
Child accepts responsibility for his or her behavior.
Child identifies effective and ineffective coping techniques.
Child uses available support system (friends, family, therapist) to develop and maintain effective coping skills.

Risk for injury secondary to alterations in thought processes and sensory perceptual alterations

Outcomes:
Child does not endanger self or others.
Child learns to control outbursts of rage, self-destructive behavior, or violence.

Hopelessness related to environmental, situational, and developmental stressors, resulting in apathy, withdrawal, and preoccupation

Outcomes:
Child expresses feelings of hopelessness.
Child develops effective coping mechanisms to deal with hopelessness.
Child participates in self-care activities and activities with friends and family as appropriate for developmental age.

Alterations in nutrition, less than body requirements

Outcome: Child eats nutritionally balanced meals and ingests sufficient calories and nutrients to support growth.

Altered parenting related to child's unresponsiveness, child's unusual behaviors, and chronic nature of the child's disorder

Outcomes:
Parents understand the cause of the child's condition and available treatment modalities.
Parents support the child, discipline the child in a therapeutic manner, and remain involved in the child's treatment.

Chart 29–5
Nursing Diagnoses and Outcomes *Continued*

Alterations in Mental Health Status	
Potential self-care deficit: feeding, bathing/hygiene, and dressing/grooming secondary to altered thought processes and sensory perceptual alterations	
Outcome:	Child performs self-care activities as developmentally appropriate.
Self-esteem disturbance related to actual or perceived problematic relationships with family members or peers	
Outcomes:	Child and family describe areas of conflict. Child openly expresses feelings toward family members and peers. Child and family select measures to reinforce the child's positive qualities. Child can describe his or her own positive qualities.
Sensory perceptual alterations related to neurologic changes as evidenced by restlessness, altered behavior, destructive acts, or violence	
Outcomes:	Child remains oriented to person, place, and time. Child communicates in a lucid manner.
Sleep pattern disturbance related to anxiety, mental status, or effects of medications	
Outcome:	Child's sleep patterns are adequate for rest and are not disruptive to the family.
Social isolation related to behaviors viewed by self, family, or peers that is not considered culturally, socially, or developmentally appropriate	
Outcomes:	Child and family identify causes of social isolation. Child exhibits interactional and communication skills that enhance social interactions. Child demonstrates behaviors that are more socially acceptable. Child reports feeling less isolated as social interactions improve.
Impaired social interaction related to effects of child's mental status or aberrant, antisocial behaviors	
Outcome:	Child can maintain interpersonal relationships.
Altered thought processes related to psychosocial causes	
Outcomes:	Child and family identify internal and external factors that trigger or contribute to delusional episodes. Child identifies and performs activities that decrease delusions. Child adheres to medication regimen to assist in modifying psychological causes.
High risk for violence directed at self or others related to antisocial and aggressive character, excitement, or self-destructive behaviors	
Outcomes:	Child will discuss feelings that precipitate destructive and violent acts. Child uses positive coping strategies when he or she feels frustrated. Child does not harm self or others. Child and family identify resources for crisis prevention and management.

integral part of both the problem itself and the strategies to assist the child in meeting the emotional, cognitive, and physical needs. *Ineffective family coping* and *altered family processes* are two examples of diagnoses that should be selected to address family needs.

Developmental and Biological Variances

Mental health disorders in children and adolescents can originate from a variety of sources. For instance, the normal processes of growth and development may be sources of stress and emotional dysfunction for some children. How the child views the world, the meaning attached to events, and objects in the youngster's world provide important clues to the evolution of thought and behavioral disorders.

The neurobiologic functioning of the brain plays an important role in the development of mental illness in children. The brain controls thoughts, feelings, and behaviors. Incoming stimuli are organized and integrated within the brain. Responses to stimuli are determined in the brain and carried out through motor potential in other parts of the body. Brain functioning may be inherently impaired, as in autism and schizophrenia, or functioning patterns may become distorted or impaired as a result of inappropriate stimuli, such as abuse, illness, injury, genetic expression, or psychosocial disruptions during the developmental processes.

Genetic vulnerability is a factor implicated in alterations in mental health and behavior that affect the child and adolescent. Studies of twins (monozygotic and fraternal) and family studies suggest that mental illness, or the vulnerability for disorders such as schizophrenia, anxiety disorders, and mood disorders may be transmitted genetically.

There are strong correlations between certain physical illnesses and alterations in mental health that can affect the child. For instance, endocrine function is increasingly believed to be a causative or precipitating factor in mental illness. Persons with endocrine dysfunction have a higher incidence of depressive disorders (Kjellman, Thorell, Orhagen, d'Elia, & Kagedal, 1993). For instance, a high incidence of depression has been found in persons with Cushing's syndrome and Addison's disease (disorders of adrenal function). Anxiety and depression are highly correlated with hyperthyroidism

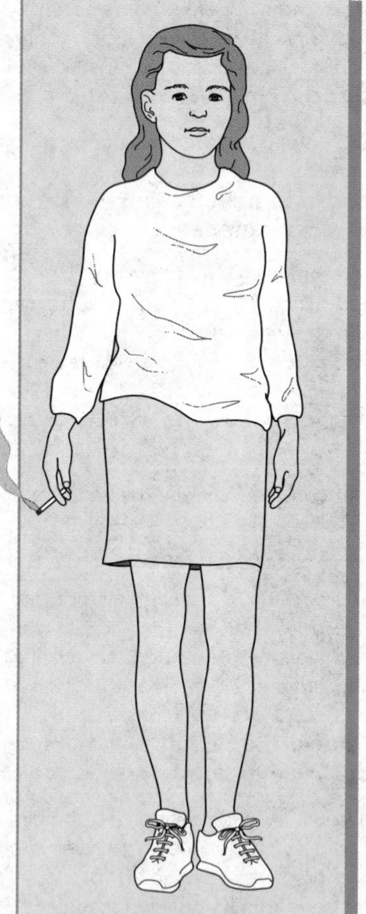

Some theorists believe maladaptive behavior is learned and reinforced by positive stimuli in the child's environment.
Children with endocrine dysfunction have a higher incidence of depressive disorders.
Suicide is the third leading cause of death among adolescents (15–24).
Many children with mental disorders have developmental delay.
Research studies have suggested that some mental disorders may have been transmitted genetically.
Use of substances interferes with development of problem-solving skills and use of effective coping devices.
Severe childhood stress is believed to first occur at times when neurons are easily shaped by experience.
Children regress more quickly than adults. These regressive symptoms may be the result of developmental stresses rather than represent true pathology.
Some theorists believe that the child's mental health is influenced by interpersonal life experiences.
Acting-out behaviors may mask depression in children and adolescents.
Assessing family norms and culture is a critical element in evaluating the presence of mental health concerns in children in the family.
The physical manifestations of maturation (i.e., muscular tension, overwhelming fatigue, increased heart rate) can be interpreted by the adolescent as signs of physical illness and lead to undue stress and anxiety.

Figure 29–1
Developmental and biological variances: mental health.

and hypo- or hyperparathyroidism. Melatonin, a hormone produced in the pineal gland, and serotonin are strongly correlated to the incidence of seasonal affective disorder (Nathan, Musselman, Schatzberg, & Nemeroff, 1995).

Current interest has focused on the neurophysiologic relation of stress to mental health. A theory proposed by Briere (1989) suggests that severe childhood stress occurs at a time when neurons are easily shaped by experience. Thus, the stress response system develops inadequately because the child does not have adequate coping responses. Children who have experienced severe stress could then have a lower or abnormal tolerance for stress later in life and therefore be at greater risk for mental illness (Briere, 1989).

According to behavioral theory, alterations in mental health, as exhibited in maladaptive behavior, is learned and reinforced by positive stimuli in the environment. Thus, the development of phobias, anxiety disorders, and disorders of violence may be learned by the child through their experiences and interactions with others and environmental forces.

The symptoms of mental illness may be more difficult to identify in children and adolescents (Fig. 29–1). Children differ in their rate of emotional and physical growth. Children also tend to regress more quickly than adults when challenged by stress, fatigue, or pain. When the child feels a loss of control or feels frustrated, regressive behaviors may be exhibited. In many cases, these symptoms would not be considered significant factors in diagnosing alterations in mental status because they represent normal development reactions rather than true pathologic findings. On the other hand, persistence of these behaviors may warrant concern.

Within child psychiatric nursing, the cultural context of the child and the family must be taken into account. Based on culture, a family may have varying definitions of behavioral expectations for the child, discipline, and definitions of abusive behavior. For instance, the Asian child who is very quiet and passive in school should not be quickly assessed as having school phobia or a learning disorder (LD). In the child's family, a quiet and peaceful nature is likely to be highly valued. On the other hand, a child who has been burned by a home remedy to treat a fever warrants further investigation for child abuse as defined by state law. Even though the family acted in a culturally appropriate fashion, legally, such actions are harmful and inappropriate in the care of children. Some standards of behavior cross cultural lines, especially when determining abusive from nonabusive behavior. In mental health nursing, as in other aspects of child health care, the nurse should acknowledge the family's culturally based views, resources, and practices, and show respect for them where possible. Culturally acceptable treatment approaches should be used if possible, and the clinician should work with the family to develop a shared definition of improvement in the child's behavior and level of functioning.

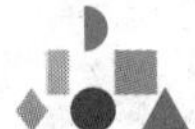

Diagnostic Criteria for Evaluating the Child's Mental Health Status

Brain Imaging Techniques

Recent advances in radiologic, sound wave, and computer techniques have made imaging of the brain possible. For the most part, these techniques are used for research rather than for routine diagnosis, but they may soon become used routinely to diagnose brain disorders. The techniques are

- Regional cerebral blood flow (rCBF)
- Magnetic resonance imaging (MRI)
- Positron emission tomography (PET)
- Single positron emission computed tomography (SPECT)

Each technique produces different information; PET and SPECT are similar in the images that they produce (Table 29–1). SPECT is the least costly of the techniques and is most likely to become the technique commonly available in the future (Reba, 1993).

DSM-IV Criteria

The American Psychiatric Association, World Health Organization, Veterans Administration, and other professional organizations have developed and refined a classification system for mental disorders that is clinically focused. This system is described in the *Diagnostic and Statistical Manual of Mental Disorders*, 4th edition, or DSM-IV, which has become the internationally accepted standard for diagnosing mental disorders. It is used by a variety of mental health professionals, including staff psychiatric nurses. However, it is inappropriate for professionals without a master's or doctoral degree to assign a diagnosis.

The purpose of the DSM-IV is to provide clear descriptions of diagnostic categories. Common categories enable clinicians and researchers to diagnose, communicate, study, and treat mental disorders systematically and consistently. The common language system also facilitates reimbursement. The use of the DSM diagnostic system demonstrates a commitment in the field to the use of research-based data in the understanding of alterations in mental health (American Psychiatric Association, 1994).

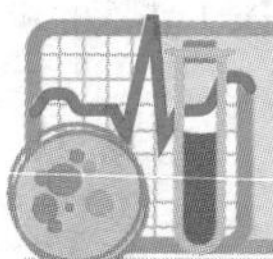

Table 29–1
Diagnostic Tests and Procedures for Evaluating Alterations in Mental Status

Diagnostic Test or Procedure	Purpose	Health Care Provider Responsibilities
rCBF Radioactive xenon computed tomography	The child sniffs radioactive gas. Several x-rays delivered as a beam pass through the tissues. X-rays are layered through computer technology. An image of the brain is computed. Different sections of brain can be visualized to demonstrate blood flow through the brain tissue.	Assess child for any allergic reactions to radioactive gas. Assure parents that the dose of radioactive substance is no greater than that used for diagnostic x-rays.
MRI Magnetic fields used to visualize brain structure Pulse of energy radio-receiver computer	Several pulses of energy (sound waves) are used to stimulate atoms within tissue. An image of brain is computed. Images show structure of the brain, anatomic deviations, and tissue damage.	Hairpins, eye makeup (with a metallic base), watches and other jewelry should be removed. Child's gown should not have a metal snap. Child should be prepared for sounds of the machine. Child may need a sedative prescribed beforehand to assist him or her in lying quietly during lengthy procedure.
PET Radioactive water computer imaging	Very small amount of radioactive water is injected into the arm, accumulating rapidly in the brain; positrons are emitted and multiple images are obtained and input into a computer. An image of the brain is produced, and areas where positrons accumulate produce bright areas.	Children must lie still during procedure. They may need a sedative administered beforehand to assist them in keeping still. Parents can be assured that although procedure is lengthy, the actual radiation exposure is less than during a regular x-ray.
SPECT Computed tomography with radioactive substance	The child is given radioactive substance, multiple radiographs are obtained and input into a computer. Images of normal and abnormal brain function are produced; these are similar to PET images but are less costly.	Same as for PET

The DSM-IV diagnoses are made by using a multiaxial assessment of five axes.

- Axis I
  Clinical disorders
  Other conditions that may be a focus of clinical attention
- Axis II
  Personality disorders
  Mental retardation
- Axis III
  General medical conditions
- Axis IV
  Psychosocial and environmental problems
- Axis V
  Global assessment of functioning

The first two axes include all psychiatric diagnoses as well as their corresponding classification number. Axis III is generally a list of any medical conditions, followed by axis IV, which is a list of psychosocial and environmental stressors. Under axis V, a numerical score indicates the patient's current level of functioning. It is also common, under axis V, to find a numerical range, which indicates the patient's lowest to highest level of functioning within the past year. The range of functioning on the global assessment scale is 0, indicating the lowest level of functioning, to 100, indicating the highest possible level of functioning.

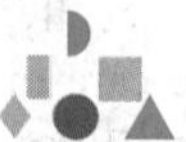

Treatment Modalities

Cognitive-Behavior Therapy

Cognitive-behavior therapy (CBT) is a three-factor model of therapy based on the assumptions that (1) thoughts mediate behavior, (2) a relationship exists between causes assigned to behavior (attributions) of self and others and how one feels (emotional response), and (3) patterns of dysfunctional thoughts (cognitions) are characteristic of specific alterations in mental health (Zarb, 1992). Thus, CBT focuses on cognitions, emotional responses, and the resulting behaviors, and views them as inextricably intertwined. Cognitions include the individual's perception of his or her world and the events and objects within it, including the self. Cognitions also include values, beliefs, attitudes, and causal attributions. Understanding the client's cognitive system is the beginning step in CBT.

The therapeutic process helps the individual reframe perceptions, change ideas about a situation, or view a situation from a different perspective. Next, the client is helped to see the relationships among the thoughts and belief and their emotional responses. Finally, clients are encouraged to use problem-solving to identify alternative solutions or ways of behaving. A variety of techniques have been developed based on the CBT framework, such as coping skills therapy, assertiveness therapy, problem-solving, and self-control therapy. In all CBT therapies, clients are taught specific skills such as thought stopping, reframing, relaxation skills, and assertive communication skills. Self-rights and the rights of others are emphasized (Zarb, 1992). CBT is recommended for clients with depression, anxiety disorders, behavioral disorders, such as conduct and oppositional defiant disorder (ODD), and obsessive-compulsive disorder (OCD).

Individual Therapy

Individual therapy is an interpersonal process in which the client and nurse work together, discover, explore, and resolve the client's conflicts, behavioral problems, doubts, and anxieties (Weeks, 1995). A process for therapy to be used by nurses was developed by Hildegard Peplau (1952). Peplau's model for interpersonal psychotherapy is comprised of four phases:

- Orientation
- Problem selection
- Working phase
- Termination

Trust in the nurse and client motivation are central to Peplau's model. Assessment and formulation of the problems constitute the first phase of therapy. After determining the client's issues and formulating the nursing diagnoses, goals for future sessions are determined. Goals are specified in observable or measurable terms. The nature of the therapeutic sessions are determined by the client's age, developmental status, and preference for interacting with the therapist. Play therapy is often used for young children. Activity therapy (structured activities such as clay modeling, drawing, games) along with discussion works well with many school-age children. Talk therapy is preferred by adolescents. The broad goals of individual therapy include resolution of conflictual issues, restoration of developmentally appropriate functioning, improved self-understanding, and symptom reduction. Individual therapy may be provided in outpatient clinics, community mental health centers, schools, inpatient hospital units, residential settings, or the client's home. Nurses providing therapy in homes or residential settings often carry a variety of toys, games, craft materials, or books to use in their sessions.

Play Therapy

Play therapy is one form of individual therapy developed to address the needs of children in therapy (Critchley, 1995). However, it also may be used in the family or group context. Play therapy takes advantage of the child's natural and developmental way of being in the world. It allows children the freedom to experience their concerns and fears in a nonthreatening environment with an accepting and attentive adult. Play therapy is based on the assumption that play is therapeutic. In therapy, play becomes the medium by which the child explores life problems, developmental issues, and interpersonal conflicts. The child is free to test new assumptions, feelings, and different kinds of behavior. The therapist is nonpunitive, provides and assures safety, and encourages the development of a more positive self-concept and realistic perception of the child's world. Behaviors that assist the child in managing daily stressors are encouraged (Critchley,

Figure 29–2
Play therapy allows the child to explore his or her concerns and fears in a nonthreatening environment. The health care provider is attentive to the child and encourages the child to develop a positive self-concept and a realistic perception of the world.

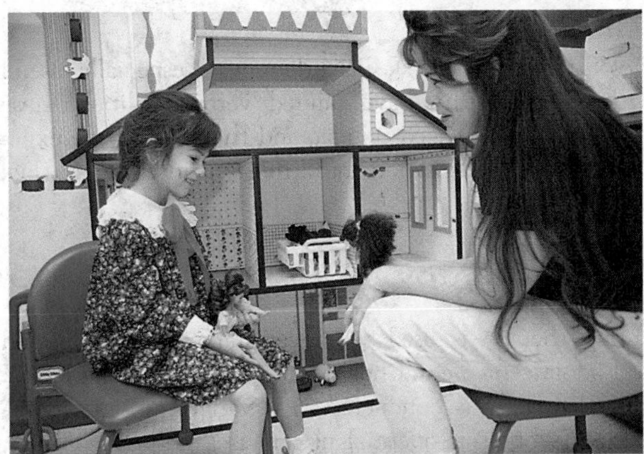

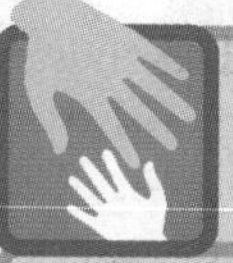

Chart 29–6
Nursing Interventions

Milieu Therapy

Components of Milieu Therapy	Nursing Interventions
Safety	Maintain safe environment. Prevent or contain aggressive behavior. Maintain, monitor, make adjustments to unit routine. Encourage, assist in conflict resolution. Teach and role-model appropriate expression of feelings. Ensure close supervision of suicidal and aggressive patients. Ensure adequate staffing. Ensure that staff know rules and policy for taking children on outings.
Inclusion	Provide opportunities for participation in structured activities. Request feedback from staff, children, parents. Include staff, parents, child in goal setting. Facilitate child's acceptance into peer group and unit structure.
Security	Set limits for children. Publish the rules for appropriate behavior. Inform child of consequences of aggressive behavior. Make parents welcome to unit, and teach and encourage appropriate interaction with their child (especially if abusive). Monitor unit activity to ensure safety. Validate child's needs when expressed. Do not use deprivation of meals or basic safety needs as punishment.
Structure	Inform all nursing staff of daily routines, programming. Post daily routines visibly on the unit (e.g., posters). Programs are posted, visible, and changed as necessary. Routinely monitor each child's health status. Implement social skills training, communication skills, stress management. Establish mechanism for collaboration and communication with parents, team members, therapist, safety maintenance, and crisis management personnel. Develop supervision, coaching, and evaluation strategies for nursing staff.
Validation	Child's needs and desires are heard and responded to appropriately. Child is included in problem identification, goal setting, and evaluation. Treatment plans are explained to child.

Adapted from Delaney, K., Van-Lanen, J., Pitula, C., Johnson, M. (1995). Seven days and counting: How inpatient nurses might adjust their practice to brief hospitalization. *Journal of Psychosocial Nursing, 33*(8), 36–38.

1995; Jennings, 1993). Play therapy is especially useful with children who have limited verbal abilities, those who have experienced trauma, and those who have experienced family separations or disruptions in early life (Fig. 29–2).

Group Therapy

Group therapy is used to prevent and treat childhood and adolescent mental health alterations (Gilbert, 1995). Group therapy is conducted in a variety of settings including schools, residential placements, hospitals, clinics, neighborhood centers, and community mental health centers. Group therapy is directed at improving socialization, promoting communication, and facilitating behavioral change. A variety of group models exist for use with children and adolescents. Children in preschool groups benefit from play groups. Elementary school-age children relate best in groups that are focused and use some structured activities and discussion. Adolescents often respond well to a variety of group interventions, such as recreational, occupational, communication, and self-esteem building. Therapeutic effects of group therapy include expressing and sharing of feelings, gaining a sense of community, inspiring hope, obtaining information and support, and role modeling (Yalom, 1995).

Group therapy takes advantage of the developmental focus of peer relationships in the prepubertal and adolescent age groups. The peer group provides opportunities for youth to meet as equals within their own age group, communicate, understand others' perspectives, get along with others, compare themselves with others, define their social role, and perfect their social skills (Gilbert, 1995).

Family Therapy

There are many models of family therapy with diverse applications. In all models of family therapy, the family is the focus. Interventions may be directed at developing family-based coping strategies, such as problem-solving or stress management. In some families, the needs may include strengthening the parental role, improving communication, or improving interpersonal relationships. In families with young children, play is often introduced to encourage relaxation of expectations and rules that tend to produce failure in behavioral goals. In families with adolescents, the focus may be on relaxing or strengthening rules and expectations to allow adolescents the appropriate amount of freedom to achieve their developmental tasks.

One form of therapy, especially helpful to families with a severely and persistently mentally ill member, is family education. Family education provides families with information to help them understand the neurologic basis of the illness and factors that may exacerbate or reduce symptoms of illness. Family education is also directed at validating feelings associated with loss (of the normal child/adolescent), improving problem-solving, promoting stress management, and accessing resources needed by the family and child. The needs of families may go even further. Family education is often provided by nurses.

Milieu Therapy

Milieu therapy refers to dynamic, specially structured settings designed to assist in the overall therapeutic process. Milieu therapy usually refers to inpatient units, but environmental structuring and management may be used in school settings, residential treatment settings, and the home. In milieu therapy, the environment is arranged to promote accomplishment of therapeutic goals such as diminishing aggressive behavior (Johnson, 1995). The therapeutic environment includes the people, activities, programs, and physical factors involved in the therapeutic process (Chart 29–6). The goal of the therapeutic environment is to promote the development of the child or adolescent's adaptive and social skills. Children placed in therapeutic environments have usually experienced many failures and disruptions in their lives. The milieu provides a safe and supportive environment for children and adolescents who are acutely ill, highly aggressive, and at high risk for abuse or self-harm (Delaney, 1992). Therapeutic milieus incorporate a variety of therapy strategies used in conjunction with individual therapy. Family therapy, recreational and educational therapy, group therapy, social skills training, and behavioral management are usual components of such environments. Active involvement of each child or adolescent is expected and facilitated. Successful milieus are models of excellent interdisciplinary collaboration.

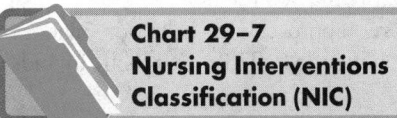

Chart 29–7
Nursing Interventions Classification (NIC)

Behavioral Management

Definition

Helping a patient to manage negative behavior

Activities

Hold patient responsible for his/her behavior.
Communicate expectation that patient will retain control.
Consult with family to establish patient's preinjury cognitive baseline.
Set limits with patient.
Refrain from arguing or bargaining about the established limits with the patient.
Establish routines.
Establish shift-to-shift consistency in environment and care routine.
Use consistent repetition of health routines as a means of establishing them.
Avoid interruptions.
Increase physical activity, as appropriate.
Limit number of care givers.
Use a soft, low-speaking voice.
Avoid cornering the patient.
Redirect attention away from agitation source.
Avoid projecting a threatening image.
Avoid arguing with patient.
Ignore inappropriate behavior.
Reduce passive-aggressive behavior.
Praise efforts at self-control.
Sedate, as needed.
Apply wrist/leg/chest restraints, as necessary.

From McCloskey, J., & Bulechek, G. (1996). *Nursing interventions classification (NIC)* (2nd ed.). St. Louis: Mosby–Year Book. Reprinted with permission.

Behavioral Management

Behavioral management is a large component of milieu settings. It includes collaborating with team members to develop appropriate goals, expectations, consequences (for failure to meet expectations), and rewards for positive achievement. Even though most milieus have an overall behavioral management plan, individualization is essential for each child. The staff nurse and advanced practice nurse are responsible for the overall development of the plan, teaching staff and children about the plan, making adjustments for individual needs, and making decisions regarding least restrictive intervention for inappropriate behavior (time-out, quiet room, seclusion, or medication) (Chart 29–7). In extreme circumstances, leather or body restraints may be used.

A problem-solving approach to behavior management is highly recommended. This approach includes working with the child and his or her family to identify needs and strengths. This therapeutic management approach assists children in changing behavior and helps children to integrate new thoughts about themselves and their world (Cotton, 1993). For this to occur, children need to experience their world and the people in it as caring and not just punitive. Cotton (1993) likens this approach to the socialization process that most normal children have experienced. The therapeutic management approach is built on a triad of components that include empathy (understand and respect the child), communication (ask questions, listen, clarify, and give feedback), and discipline, which includes positive rewards (attention, celebration of positive behaviors) and negative consequences (inattention, reprimands, natural consequences, logical consequences, and penalties). Children need to make restitution (destroyed toy of another child is replaced by one belonging to the offending child) for their

Table 29–2
Common Psychotropic Medications Used in Child and Adolescent Psychiatry

Classification and Examples	Disorder	Side Effects
Stimulants Ritalin, Dexedrine, pemoline	Attention deficit hyperactivity disorder (ADHD), possibly depression	Insomnia, decreased appetite, weight loss, headache, tics
Antidepressants		
Tricyclics: imipramine, nortriptyline	ADHD, depression, tic and anxiety disorders	Anticholinergic effects (dry mouth, constipation, blurred vision), weight loss
Monoamine oxidase inhibitors	As above	Dietary restrictions required, weight gain, drowsiness, insomnia
Selective serotonin reuptake inhibitors: Prozac, Zoloft, Paxil	Depression, obsessive-compulsive disorder, anxiety	Irritability, insomnia, gastrointestinal distress, headaches, nausea, increased blood pressure
Antimanic agents Lithium	Bipolar disorders, depression, hyperaggression	Polyuria, polydipsia, tremor, nausea, diarrhea, weight gain, drowsiness; requires close monitoring
Seizure medications Tegretol, Depakene, valproic acid	Seizure, bipolar disorders, occasionally refractory depression	Bone marrow suppression, dizziness, drowsiness, sedation, nausea
Antianxiety agents Buspirone	Anxiety disorder, rage disorder; adjunct in mania, psychosis, depression, Tourette's syndrome	Drowsiness, disinhibition, agitation, confusion, depression
Noradrenergic agents Clonidine	Tourette's syndrome, ADHD, aggression/self-abuse, agitation; alternative to stimulate retention, rebound hypertension	Sedation, hypotension, dry mouth, confusion, depression, constipation, urinary retention
Antipsychotic agents Phenothiazides, Mellaril, Thorazine, Haldol	Psychosis, mania, aggression, self-injurious, explosive, and violent, destructive behavior	Anticholinergic effects, extrapyramidal effects (dyskinesia, dystonia), drowsiness
Atypical antipsychotics Risperidone, clozapine	Refractory psychosis	Granulocytopenia, seizures, agitation, headache, nausea

destructive acts. And finally, children should be forgiven when they apologize for their behavior.

Psychopharmacology

As medications are developed and as evidence is provided that the medication is successful in treating adults, it is often only a matter of time until the medication is tried in clinical practice with children. There are only a few clinical trials of medication for which children are subjects and objects of the research. The nurse's role, therefore, is a critical one in observing and reporting responses, including therapeutic and adverse effects. Nurses often serve a vital role in helping parents to understand the need for the medication, the goals and expected outcomes, and how and when to administer medication. When medication does not appear to produce the desired results, nurses are helpful in ferreting out patient and parental variances that may interfere with the success. Parents and children have a right to information about the medication, and their consent and cooperation need to be elicited. Nurses serve a vital role in school settings in monitoring medication administration and possible side effects. Nurses also play the role of teacher to teachers, helping them understand the use, potential benefit, and side effects of prescribed medications. The nurse may act as liaison between school personnel, parents, and treatment team members (Pearson, 1995b). A variety of medications are currently used in the treatment of childhood and adolescent mental and behavioral disorders (Table 29–2).

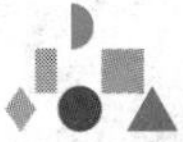

Alterations in Children's Mental Health

Disorders Due Primarily to Biological Factors

Several conditions are associated with cognitive deficits or disorders and are believed to have a genetic and/or biological etiology. Schizophrenia is a cognitive disorder, with strong indications for a genetic influence. Alterations in mood states (affective disorders) are also considered under the biologically based disorders. However, unmanageable stress and insufficient coping may also result in a mood disorder, such as depression. Neurophysiologic changes may occur in such instances and may result in a mood disorder. Anxiety disorders and compulsive disorders are also believed to have a biological vulnerability basis that interacts with environmental and social stressors to evolve into a disorder.

Cognitive Disorders

Attention Deficit Hyperactivity Disorders

Attention deficit disorder (ADD) and attention deficit hyperactivity disorder (ADHD) are characterized by poor attention, excessive activity, and impulsive behavior. These two closely related disorders appear to be the second most common behavioral disorders in childhood (less common than ODD). ADD is characterized by inability to attend to tasks and activities, but it is not associated with excessive motor activity. It is estimated that the prevalence of ADD and ADHD is 2.0% to 6.3% of the population. These disorders are serious and chronic, and they affect several areas of a child's life and functioning. High comorbidity exists with conduct disorder, and to a lesser extent, with anxiety and mood disorders. ADD and ADHD are more often diagnosed in boys than in girls (Ricchini, 1997; Smat-Mari, 1992). Increasingly, these disorders are being viewed as potentially lifelong disorders.

Etiology

The cause of ADD and ADHD is strongly linked to genetic and biologic factors, but psychosocial factors appear to interact in complex ways with familial and biologic factors. The genetic transmission is unknown. Regardless of the actual causative factors, there are some neurochemical pathologic findings, which are believed to involve the frontal lobe of the brain. The neurochemical theory is deduced from medication studies, which demonstrate that all efficacious medications increase dopamine

Figure 29–3
Through creative parenting, schooling, and positive interventions that reinforce the child's strengths, the child with attention deficit hyperactivity disorder can ultimately achieve success and a positive self-concept.

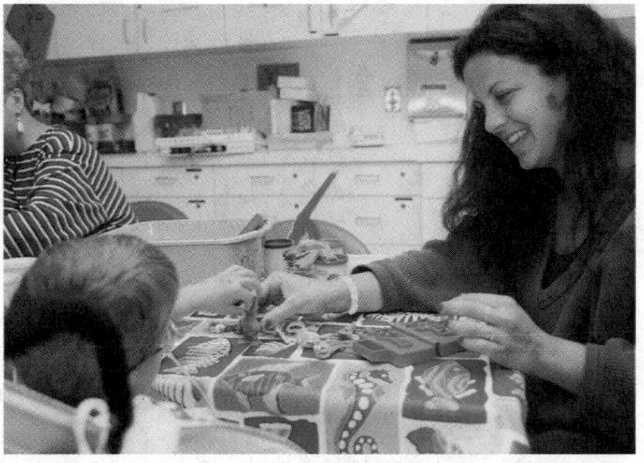

release in the brain and inhibit action of the noradrenergic system (Castellanos & Rapoport, 1992).

Assessment

The diagnosis of ADD or ADHD most often occurs during the early school years. Symptoms of the disorders need to be present for at least 6 months and must be observed before the child is 7 years old. The criteria fall into three areas of functioning: concentration, impulse control, and goal-directed behavior. Individuals with ADD have deficits primarily in concentration, whereas children with ADHD show deficits in all three areas. The symptoms may not be demonstrated in early and short-term one-to-one situations, but once the child is

Table 29–3
Anxiety Disorders of Childhood or Adolescents

Disorder	Defining Characteristics	Recommended Treatment Strategies	Nursing Interventions
Avoidant disorder	Extreme shyness; patient avoids contact with unfamiliar persons; social deficits; behavioral inhibition; patient lacks assertiveness with peers; medication is not helpful.	Family therapy; social skills training (SST); peer group therapy; play therapy	Teach relaxation training and reinforcement; give social skills training; guide peer groups (activities, communication); assessment and referral.
Generalized disorder	Patient requires constant reassurance; not associated with worry about recent stressor; inability to relax; hypervigilance; patient has many somatic complaints; medication is not helpful.	Cognitive and behavioral therapies; play therapy; family therapy.	Assess and refer; give relaxation training; reinforce positive self-talk therapy.
Social phobia	Anxiety related to strangers or groups, including peers; patient avoids social situations or endures them with significant stress; usually begins in adolescence and is most often lifelong.	Social skills training, paired with role modeling; cognitive and behavior therapy; exposure-based therapy; benzodiazepines, serotonin reuptake inhibitors, and tricyclic antipressants are reportedly of some help.	Assess and refer; give SST and assertive behavior training; give relaxation training; reinforce positive self-talk therapy; monitor medication regimen. Assess compliance and reinforce; assess for benefit and side effects; record progress.
Specific phobic disorder	Excessive anxiety related to a specific object, environment, or situation (e.g., spiders, heights, being in water); child recognizes the fear and anxiety is unnecessary, but is unable to change; impaired social and academic functioning occurs more in girls usually preoccupied with the fear.	Cognitive behavioral therapy shows best results (e.g., graded exposure, relaxation training, and self-talk); family therapy if family is reinforcing the disorder or if family relationships are dysfunctional.	Assess and refer; monitor progress of therapy; support child in maintaining treatment program; support positive self-talk; reinforce or teach relaxation techniques; educate patient and family.
Panic disorder	Abrupt bouts of anxiety, with physical symptoms of choking; excessive fear of future attacks; fear of dying, going crazy; no physical explanation for symptoms; mitral valve prolapse may be present. Patient may have experienced a recent stressful event; risk for substance abuse.	Behavioral, cognitive, and pharmacologic treatments are useful (as for social phobia).	Assess and refer; assess for reality of somatic complaints; educate patient and family about disorder; reinforce positive self-talk; give relaxation training; educate about medications and monitor compliance; educate about danger of self-medicating and risk of substance abuse.

comfortable in a situation, the behaviors begin to emerge. Descriptions of these children include excessive fidgeting, distractibility, inability to follow rules, impatience, impulsiveness, excessive and inappropriate talking, and inability to sit or stay in one place (Castiglia, 1997a; Garfinkel & Amrami, 1992; Nemethy, 1997).

Major problems for these children include interpersonal problems with age-matched peers, teachers, and often parents. Because of their impulsivity and poor problem-solving skills, children with ADD and ADHD are vulnerable to development of behavioral problems and a comorbid diagnosis of oppositional disorder or conduct disorders. These children are also susceptible to low self-esteem, anxiety, and depression (Ricchini, 1997). Behaviors associated with ADD and ADHD make them vulnerable to failure and negative feedback, which may be causative in these comorbid conditions (Wherry, 1992).

Assessment and diagnosis of ADD and ADHD should be conducted by an interdisciplinary team, because several areas of functioning may be impaired. Psychometric testing helps to define the individual's cognitive and learning deficits. Children at various developmental levels function differently; thus, it is imperative that the evaluator be familiar with age-appropriate norms. It is helpful to obtain information from teachers and parents, because each is able to provide observation of behavior in different kinds of settings. Data obtained about the child's strengths can be used to enhance the program of interventions (Fig. 29–3).

Interdisciplinary Interventions

Interdisciplinary interventions may include psychological assessment and assessment of the child's specific learning problems and intellectual ability. Psychology and special education experts are usually called upon for these assessments and to make recommendations for the individual educational plan (IEP) (see Chapters 7 and 10). Children are hospitalized for these disorders only if there is a comorbid condition such as conduct disorder with very aggressive behavior. A mental health therapist (e.g., advanced practice nurse, psychotherapist, or psychiatrist) may need to provide therapy when self-esteem is severely impaired or if the child is depressed. Psychiatric expertise is often involved in assessment when comorbid mental health disorders include conduct disorder or oppositional disorder.

Medical Management. Medical management of children with ADD or ADHD includes medication to control behaviors associated with these disorders (Table 29–3). The benefit of stimulant medication has proven most effective over time (Diamond & Mattson, 1996). Methylphenidate, dextroamphetamine, and, more recently, pemoline and Adderall are commonly prescribed and demonstrate positive effects on both the hyperactivity and inattention (Reitz, 1997; Scahill & French, 1996). Approximately 26% of children fail to show improvement on stimulant medication. When stimulant medication fails, alternative forms of treatment are tried. Two tricyclic antidepressants have shown some effectiveness in some children in controlled studies (Scahill & French, 1996).

Health promotion and maintenance of general health are important considerations. Routine medical care should include all that is provided for the child without behavioral problems, such as immunizations, physical examinations, and dental and eye examinations and care. Assessment of nutritional status and physical growth and development are important, because high activity levels and side effects of medication may decrease appetite and slow the rate of growth.

Community Care

Nurses at school and in home care are responsible for parent training (TIP 29–1). Several studies have demonstrated the effectiveness of positive reinforcement behavior management for children with ADHD. Parent training involves teaching parents to respond to (reward) positive behavior and to ignore negative behavior (Diamond & Mattson, 1996). "Time-out," having the child sit on a chair for a period of time, is used when behavior persists, even though such behavior is being ignored. Behavior management is more effective in managing overactivity and less effective in curtailing problems of inattention (Diamond & Mattson, 1996).

Learning Disorders

Learning disorders (LDs) are common neurobiological disorders that form a subset of developmental disorders (Scheffel, 1996). They include reading, writing, and mathematical disorders. They become evident in childhood and remain with the individual throughout life. The estimated prevalence among the population is 5% to 10%, with a greater incidence among boys. Reading disorder is the most common, with approximately 5% of school-age children exhibiting the disorder. Among children in mental health clinics, 30% to 50% are estimated to have one or more learning difficulties. These children are no longer considered "brain damaged," but are recognized as having specific functional deficits in the brain; the actual cause is unknown (Silver, 1993a). Because learning disabilities have been frequently found in first-degree biological relatives of afflicted children, genetics is thought to be a causative factor (Scheffel, 1996). Other factors associated with LDs include prenatal factors such as maternal alcohol and substance use, diabetes, malnutrition, infections, placental insufficiency, and Rh incompatibility. Perinatal and postnatal incidents that lead to anoxia, seizures, or head injury may also be associated with LDs.

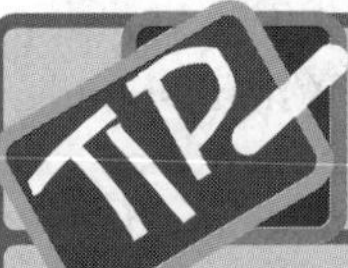

TIP 29–1 A Teaching Intervention Plan for the Child with ADD/ADHD

Nursing Diagnoses and Family Outcomes

- Altered thought processes related to altered ability to concentrate, impulsiveness, and organizational skills
  Outcomes: Child completes self-care tasks and cooperates in school setting.
  Child follows instructions and is successful in academic activities.
- Impaired social interactions related to inability to control actions and behaviors
  Outcome: Child gradually learns self-control and the ability to share peer acceptance and enjoyment in peer relations.
- Self-esteem disturbance related to negative response from others regarding behavior
  Outcomes: Child identifies own strengths.
  Self-esteem is enhanced as seen by child's comments about self and about personal accomplishments.
- Risk for injury related to child's activity level and impulsiveness
  Outcome: Child's safety is ensured to the best extent possible.
- Achieved health maintenance related to medication side effects
  Outcomes: Child maintains adequate nutritional status.
  Child maintains adequate sleep pattern.
  Parents express confidence in their ability to manage the medication regimen.

Interventions

Managing Child's Activity

- Encourage parents and teachers to decrease stimuli when concentration is important.
- Monitor compliance with medication regimen and reaction to medication.
- Decrease choices that child must make (limit to two for young child, three to four for older children).
- Practice problem-solving strategies with child.
- Give positive feedback for success (tokens, rewards).
- Tutoring may be necessary. Learning tasks should be subdivided so child is not overwhelmed and can maintain concentration.
- Give frequent positive feedback. Directions for each task should be short, broken into segments, for example:
  Take your book out of your desk.
  Open the book to page 10.
  Read the second paragraph to yourself.
  Answer the first question below the paragraph.
  Now, answer the second question.
- Provide information about the characteristics and problems associated with ADD/ADHD.
  Assist parents with problem-solving ways of managing child's behavior and needs (e.g., a token reward and behavior management program).
  Assist in identifying community resources.
  Encourage assertive behavior with school system to obtain needed resources for the child's learning experience.
  Provide written resources and list of references that parents may use to increase understanding of the child's disorder and effective ways to manage child's behavior.

Safety

- Encourage parents to establish clear limits on where child may play or ride bike and when higher risk activities may be undertaken. Monitor child's activities frequently.
- Reinforce positive behavior with feedback and intermittent rewards.

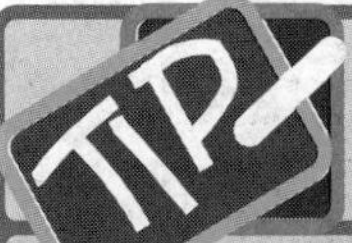

TIP 29-1 A Teaching Intervention Plan for the Child with ADD/ADHD *Continued*

Interventions

Improving Social Interactions and Self-Esteem

- Provide supervision of peer play activities for the young child. Hold and soothe child when unable to provide self-control. Use time-outs (5 minutes for preschoolers, 7 to 10 minutes for elementary school-age children). Young children benefit from well-run nursery school programs.
- School-age: Consider social skills training in small groups to encourage
  - Turn taking
  - Making appropriate requests
  - Communicating feelings and empathy
  - Problem-solving in conflictual situations
  - Saying no to inappropriate behaviors
  - Expressing anger in appropriate (socially acceptable) ways
- Identify child's strengths and provide feedback to enhance positive self-thoughts.
- Reward positive behavior, provide limit setting as needed, but avoid negative comments that the child is "bad." Remove attention or special privileges for negative behavior. Help child to develop skills such as with individual lessons to learn a special skill or with group activity that assists child to learn something of interest (a hobby, a sport, or area of knowledge).

Medication Administration

- Teach parents to administer medication after meals, decreasing amount in afternoons if it interferes with sleep, provide quiet activities before bedtime, and decrease stimulation at mealtimes.
- Explain what the medication is and how it works, its benefits, and its potential side effects.
- Discuss modifications for side effects.
- Assist in establishing a routine to prevent forgetfulness in giving the medication.

Contact Health Care Provider if

- Child appears very drowsy.
- Child is unable to concentrate.
- Child physically harms self or others.
- No improvement is seen in school performance.

Definition. The federal law, The Education for All Handicapped Children, Public Law (P.L.) 94-142, provides the following definition of learning disabilities:

> Specific learning disabilities means a disorder in one or more of the basic psychological processes involved in understanding or in using language, spoken or written, which may manifest itself in an imperfect ability to listen, think, speak, read, write, spell, or to do mathematical calculations. The term learning disabilities refers to a variety of conditions such as perceptual handicaps, brain injury, minimal brain dysfunction, dyslexia, and developmental aphasia. The term does not include children who have learning problems which are primarily the result of visual, hearing, or motor handicaps, mental retardation, of emotional disturbance, or of environmental, cultural, or economic disadvantage.

Assessment

Early recognition and diagnosis of LD is imperative, because secondary emotional and social problems frequently develop. Without diagnosis and adequate intervention, afflicted children and adolescents must use undue energy to compensate for or to hide their problem. They fall behind in academic performance and become easy targets for ridicule by peers. Their self-esteem suffers, making them at high risk for emotional, social, and family problems (Silver, 1993b).

If the school nurse suspects a learning disability, she should discuss the matter with the parents. To determine whether a child should be referred for further assessment of an LD, the nurse should evaluate the child's reasoning, comprehension, reading, math, verbal, and writing skills. Behavioral or emotional problems occurring as a result of an LD must also be assessed. An assessment of the child's self-esteem should be conducted. Problems with family members, peers, and teachers need to be assessed as well. Adolescents who have not been diagnosed may experience undue anxiety.

Nurse practitioners or a physician should provide a thorough physical examination of the child to determine whether physical health problems may be involved or be causing the learning problem. A neurologic examination is essential. Motor problems, speech, and hearing must be assessed. Attention to the child's overall health is an important component of care. ADD or ADHD is commonly found in children with learning disabilities (approximately 40%). Several other disorders may be associated with or may coexist with LDs. These include Turner's syndrome, fragile X syndrome (in girls), and Tourette's syndrome. Approximately 50% of children with Tourette's syndrome also have a learning disability (Silver, 1993b).

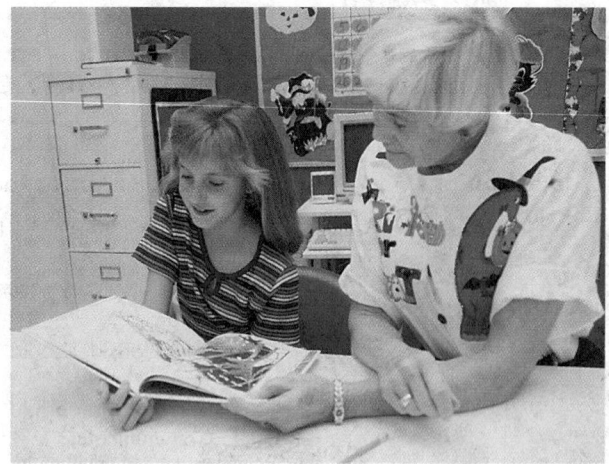

Figure 29–4
A child with a learning disability may benefit from special tutoring.

Interdisciplinary Interventions

There is no specific medical treatment for children with a learning disorder. Special education experts and often psychologists are needed to accurately identify the specific learning disability and to determine the best methods for helping the child to compensate for the difficulty. Compensation on the child's part and special educational techniques are needed to help such children develop their own unique way of learning (Scheffel, 1996). The primary responsibility for intervention lies with educators and parents (Fig. 29–4).

Psychiatric nurses and other mental health professionals often see children with learning disabilities for self-esteem and adjustment problems. Parent education is an important role of the mental health professional. The disorder should be explained to both the child and parent. The child's strengths and the child's unique way of learning should be emphasized. Family conflicts aroused by the child's problems need to be discussed, and problem-solving should be used to ameliorate the conflicts. Parents should be encouraged to be advocates for their child to ensure use of appropriate learning strategies and attention to any special individual needs.

Community Care

Children and adolescents with learning disabilities are susceptible to failure and frustration, particularly in the academic setting. These children are often referred for alterations in behavior and emotional problems before a learning disability is recognized. Children who have difficulty in reading and mathematics, expressive or receptive language difficulties, or motor coordination problems are often the object of teasing by peers, frustration of their teachers, and criticism or teasing by parents and siblings. Many, if not most, of these youngsters develop alterations in self-esteem and self-worth and other behavioral and emotional problems. Such problems compound the LD, making academic achievement and accomplishment of normal developmental stages and life goals increasingly difficult to achieve.

Family interventions are essential and may be provided by the nurse who is knowledgeable about the specific disorder. Parents need an understanding of the child's specific difficulty and any compounding problems. They may need guidance in helping other family members to modify attitudes and behavior toward the disabled child. The nurse can teach parents skills to advocate within the school system for services to meet the child's needs. If family conflicts or child behavioral problems persist, family and individual therapy may be needed. Referral to a qualified professional (e.g., advanced practice psychiatric nurse or psychiatrist) may be recommended. Many children with learning disabilities also benefit from social skills training programs. Such programs are often provided in schools for children with social skills deficits. Social skills training may be helpful in increasing peer relations and decreasing isolation and stigma associated with manifestations of learning disabilities.

Special recreational programs, especially those that help children learn motor skills and use their bodies effectively, as well as provide effective outlets for frustration, are recommended for learning disabled children. Children with a learning disability, in most cases, have the disability for life (Silver, 1993b). A holistic treatment approach designed to maximize the child's skills is the desired approach to intervention with learning disordered children.

Teachers may need consultation on how to explain the child's problem to the child's classmates. They may need guidance in how to manage malingering and other behavioral manifestations by the afflicted child. Evidence of difficulties in school may warrant referral to the school psychologist for evaluation. A high percentage of afflicted children have ADD or ADHD, thus special educational strategies may need to be used (Scahill, Ort, & Hardin, 1993b). If ADHD and Tourette's syndrome are determined to be present, these conditions can also be managed or improved with medications and behavior management programs.

Mental Retardation

Mental retardation (MR) must be recognized by 18 years of age and is defined as significantly subaverage general intellectual functioning (intellectual quotient [IQ] below 70 on an individual standardized, reliable, and valid test of intelligence) that is accompanied by significant limitations in adaptive functioning in two or more of the following areas: communication, self-care, home living, social–interpersonal skills, use of community resources, self-direction, academic skills, work, leisure, health, or safety.

MR is not in and of itself a mental health disorder; however, many mental health issues may arise in the family. The child is at higher risk for adjustment disorders resulting from reduced coping and adaptive strategies. Coping, adaptation, and social skills development are dependent to a great extent on abstract thinking and the ability to generalize from one situation to another. Abstract thinking is impaired in MR. Approximately 1% of the population is retarded. A higher percentage is found in the school-age population (3%).

Numerous factors have been implicated in causation of MR. Environmental factors may include exposure to environmental toxins such as lead poisoning and fetal exposure to drugs or alcohol. Organic factors include (but may not be limited to) head injury, antenatal, prenatal, and postnatal infections, genetic vulnerability, chromosomal mutations, and physiologic disorders such as phenylketonuria. Numerous disorders are associated with the presence of MR, including Down syndrome, Turner's syndrome, Klinefelter's syndrome, fetal alcohol syndrome, fragile X syndrome, phenylketonuria, and Prader-Willi syndrome. Most cases of MR are the result of multiple factors, not one single factor. It is estimated that 30% to 70% of affected children have two diagnoses (Feinstein & Reiss, 1996). Individuals with MR, especially those at the moderate and severe levels of retardation, are more vulnerable to organic diseases, structural problems, and deficits in many functional areas. Self-concept deficits, depression, and behavior problems are among the most common psychiatric problems. Anxiety disorder has been reported at 20% to 25% in mildly retarded individuals (Feinstein & Reiss, 1996). Mentally retarded individuals may also experience other mental illnesses.

Assessment

The child suspected of having MR, like all other children, should have a thorough physical and neurologic examination (see Chapter 6). It is important to determine whether health factors such as hearing, vision, or motor deficits are causative or contributory to the child's developmental delay. The child should be screened for infection, blood lead level, genetic and chromosomal problems, and neuroendocrine problems as potential causes of, or contributors to, the child's MR.

General intellectual functioning is determined by the IQ, which is measured with one or more standardized and individually administered intelligence tests. Several tests are available (e.g., Wechsler Intelligence Scales for Children—revised, Stanford-Binet, and Kaufman Assessment Battery for Children). MR is not based solely on IQ. Adaptive functioning must be significantly impaired as well. The degree of severity of MR is classified as mild (IQ 50/55–70), moderate (IQ 35/40–50/55), severe (IQ 20/25–35/40), and profound (IQ below 20/25).

Children often perform best in their own environment, thus it is important to perform a developmental assessment, such as the Denver II assessment, in the home or another familiar environment. The nurse should observe whether the child performs self-care activities and at what developmental level. Chapters 4 and 11 contain tables that summarize selected assessment tools available to assess developmental abilities and self-care skills. It is also important to assess social skills and whether the skills can be generalized to other settings (Harris, Delmolino, & Glasberg, 1996). During the assessment the nurse should note the following:

- Are the child's social skills consistent or nearly so with the child's chronological age? How does the child relate to the nurse in the home?
- Does the child cling to the parent, appear afraid or shy, or become friendly after a period of observing and watching?
- Does the child bring the nurse toys or make other attempts to engage the nurse?
- What is the general activity level of the child?

All observations of the child should be weighed in light of the child's chronological age, expected developmental level, and what the child can and actually does.

For instance, does the child demonstrate appropriate gross and fine motor skills but have deficits in speech and language? Does the child demonstrate the ability to perform tasks that the parents or siblings continue to do for the child? The nurse should also determine whether the goals and expectations for the child are appropriate and consistently reinforced.

Interdisciplinary Interventions

There are no specific medical interventions for MR. Health maintenance, health promotion, and preventive health care should be provided as recommended for any child. Medications should be provided for disorders (e.g., seizures, anxiety, infections) if present. The mildly retarded child with intact physical health is usually no more vulnerable to infections than other children.

Children who are mentally retarded are more likely to have seizure disorders, hyperactivity, and alterations in mental health, especially those associated with life stress. Coping strategies are often dependent on abstract thinking, which is limited in the child with MR. Alterations in mental health and physical health should receive the same medical and mental health treatment given to any normal child.

Interventions to improve academic and adaptive functioning include speech therapy (speech therapist), contingency behavior management techniques (nurses, other mental health personnel), occupational and physical therapy, and special education (special education teachers). Working with the child and family is challenging but can be rewarding (Chart 29–8). Parents usually go through a period of grief and mourning, which recurs frequently throughout the life of the family. This phenomenon is called chronic grief or chronic sorrow (see Chapter 12).

Teaching advocacy skills is particularly helpful, because parents frequently need to obtain resources for their child. Helping parents gain an understanding of the child's needs based on developmental status is especially important. Assisting parents to connect with support groups is also appreciated, because isolation of the family frequently occurs. The nurse can be helpful in identifying and evaluating resources needed by the child and family (Finke, 1996).

Many families are preoccupied with the child's deficits, which ultimately creates serious disturbances for the family and the child. A sense of hopelessness and neglect of the child's ability to learn may prevail in the family's attitude and behavior. Many, if not most, parents could benefit from cognitive, supportive, and psychodynamic therapy to help resolve bereavement. Parents who are able to recognize the child's strengths and potential and who can then work with their child and advocate for the best and appropriate educational opportunities for themselves and their child tend to remain healthy. Despite this healthy attitude, periods of grieving recur, called anniversary reactions. Anniversary grief reactions occur when a younger child surpasses the retarded child in skills and abilities, or when a younger child or a friend's children go off to school. Marriages, birthdays, and holidays are vulnerable times for all families with children who have disabilities.

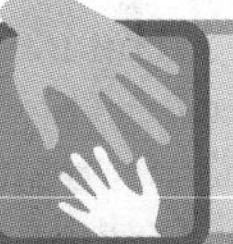

Chart 29–8
Nursing Interventions

Strategies for Working with Children or Adolescents Who Are Mentally Retarded

- Develop a warm, trusting relationship.
- Identify current skills, level of development.
- Assist child and family in achieving the next growth and development skill.
  - Break skill into its component parts.
  - Teach each component (one at a time) according to the hierarchy of skills, for example, feeding self:
    - Picking up utensil
    - Dipping utensil into food
    - Scooping food onto utensil
    - Lifting utensil to mouth
    - Putting utensil into mouth and getting food off the spoon into mouth
    - Returning utensil to surface or to food container
- Use concrete methods to teach.
  - Teach skill in location where it will happen routinely.
  - Practice generalization after skill is thoroughly learned.
  - Use pictures or the actual object demonstrated.
  - Avoid abstract messages.
  - Use simple terms, brief and simple sentences.
  - Be patient and reward each success.
- Be consistent in expectations.
- Label feelings for child, redirect activities when inappropriate.
- Give child two or three choices (do not expect child to *tell* you what he or she wants, especially when verbal skills are absent or limited).
- Tools used with younger children to identify feelings and describe problems often work with older retarded children.
- Self-injurious behavior is common; behavior modification and medications may be needed.
- Provide adequate stimulation, rewards, and play to prevent boredom.
- Individualize intervention strategies.

Childhood Schizophrenia

Childhood schizophrenia is a severe brain disorder involving psychosis and deterioration in adaptive abilities as its primary feature. It has an insidious onset and results in severe and lifelong cognitive deficits and disordered behavior. Features of the disease must be present for 6 months before a diagnosis can be made (Sokol, 1996). In many cases, developmental difficulties are noted in infancy or very early childhood. Childhood schizophrenia is a devastating illness, but is relatively rare, having a prevalence rate of 0.19/10,000 children 2 to 12 years of age. The ratio of boys to girls is approximately 2.25:1. Boys show a poorer illness state and earlier onset (King, 1994). However, girls with schizophrenia are usually more impaired cognitively than are boys.

Schizophrenia occurs more commonly in late adolescence and early adulthood. Schizophrenia in adolescence is treated similarly to the disorder in adults (Sokol, 1996). Unlike the child with schizophrenia, an adolescent may have only one episode and fully recover. However, it is more likely to be a lifetime disorder. Adolescents are generally not as impaired as children with schizophrenia, because they have had a longer time period for growth and development. Frequent compounding factors in the severity of the disorder are low intelligence (a mentally retarded person may seem more affected because of the slower developmental process and lack of acquisition of skills) and substance abuse (e.g., alcohol, cocaine). The use and abuse of substances such as alcohol, heroin, and cocaine are often used by persons with schizophrenia to dull the negative and/or positive symptoms of the disorder, as well as the associated depression.

Assessment

It may be difficult to make a diagnosis of schizophrenia in childhood because the essential features may manifest differently with the developmental level of the child. For instance, delusions and hallucinations are less involved. Visual hallucinations are rarely seen in adults but are common in children. Children manifest disorganized speech and behavior seen in several other disorders. Special attention should be given to assessment of suicide risk in adolescents. Adolescents and young adults diagnosed with schizophrenia are at especially high risk for suicide (Pearson, 1995b). There are several subtypes of schizophrenia, including paranoid, disorganized, catatonic, and undifferentiated (Table 29–4). In the prodromal period (before complete manifestation), these children often exhibit deficits in several areas: peer relations, school performance, speech, motor milestones, unusual behaviors (hand-flapping, twirling, rocking, unusual fascinations with light, smells, or textures). Other symptoms are unusual fears, unstable moods, inappropriate response in emotions or to social situations, perseveration (difficulty in moving from one activity to another), and ritualistic behavior. Premorbid male children often exhibit attention deficits and hyperactivity (King, 1994).

Table 29–4
Schizophrenia Subtypes

Subtype	Characteristics*
Paranoid	Obsessive thoughts of persecution Delusions, hallucinations
Disorganized	Disorganized speech, disorganized behavior, flat or inappropriate emotional expression
Catatonic (catatonia)	Immobility or slowed activity (may also see excessive activity) Mutism or extreme negativism Waxy flexibility (body parts may be moved, but remain in the position placed) Echolalia or echopraxia
Undifferentiated	Does not exhibit criteria for paranoia, catatonia, or disorganized subtype Two or more of the following: Delusions (nonpersecutory) Hallucinations Disorganized speech Flat affect, lack of motivation

* Not all characteristics are necessary for a diagnosis.

Assessment of childhood schizophrenia should include a complete physical examination, including a neurologic examination. Neurophysical findings demonstrate slowness in reaction times and abnormalities in eye-tracking (ability to follow an object passed slowly from one side of the head to the other, or up and down). Afflicted children are often awkward. They may show neurologic "soft-signs," such as perseveration, right-left confusion (older children and adolescents), poor coordination, or mirroring (doing exactly the same behavior as the examiner).

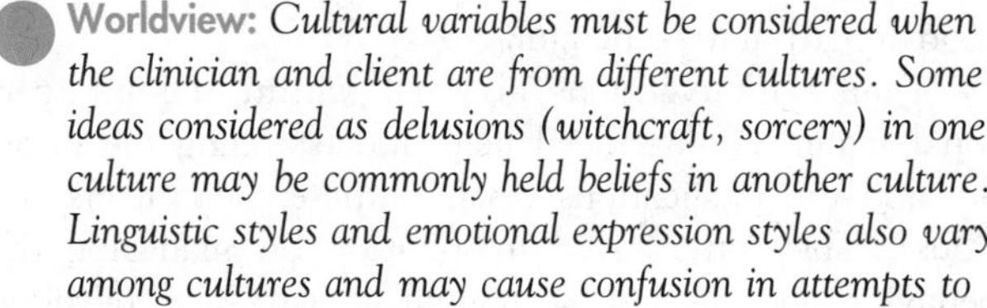

Worldview: *Cultural variables must be considered when the clinician and client are from different cultures. Some ideas considered as delusions (witchcraft, sorcery) in one culture may be commonly held beliefs in another culture. Linguistic styles and emotional expression styles also vary among cultures and may cause confusion in attempts to diagnose alterations in mental health.*

Interdisciplinary Interventions

Pharmacologic Management. Little neuropharmacologic research has been conducted with children with schizophrenia. The findings from drug studies using adult subjects are more easily applied to adolescents. Case reports provide some evidence of the efficacy of neuroleptic agents with both children and adolescents. Neuroleptic agents used in the treatment of schizophrenia are believed to block a specific dopamine receptor (D_2). Even though most neuroleptic agents are effective in treating the so-called positive effects of schizophrenia (psychotic symptoms), they do not improve the negative symptoms (flat affect, lack of motivation, and poverty of speech). One problem found in the use of neuroleptic agents is sedation. This problem can be modified with lower (than adult) doses of the medication. Therapeutic effects usually occur in 7 to 14 days, and the drugs should be given a 4- to 6-week trial before a different medication is tried. Children and adolescents are susceptible to side effects of the medication even while on low doses. Side effects include sedation and movement disorders (dystonia, akathisia, tardive dyskinesia, and Parkinsonian syndrome). Akathisia is rarely seen in childhood, but becomes more frequent with age, especially in adolescent girls (Caplan, 1994). Newer medications are showing promise in avoiding these side effects, while promising a more favorable outcome for many victims.

Nursing Management. Pearson (1995b) specified nursing interventions in three categories for children and adolescents with thought disorder (personal system, interpersonal system, and social system). **Personal system** interventions begin with clarifying the meaning of events and situations due to cognitive distortions, hallucinations, and delusional thoughts. The health care provider assists in providing orientation to situations and providing needed protection (e.g., from peers). Self-care skills and interventions to promote independence are initiated. Information about medications is also provided (Pearson, 1992).

Interpersonal system interventions include activities to assist the child in improving relationships with others. Structured play activities are recommended; however, play therapy, especially nondirected and fantasy-oriented therapy is contraindicated. Structured talk interventions may be helpful when focused on the child's understanding of self and others. Group therapy that is structured, skills oriented (e.g., communication), and with sessions of short length may be helpful.

Family interventions also fall within the interpersonal realm. Parents need help understanding the disorder and the medications (their purpose, side effects, actions). They often need information on managing the behavior and promoting normal growth and development. Childhood schizophrenia and other severe developmental disorders are extremely difficult experiences for families. They must cope with the stress of loss of the normal child and manage the problems associated with the illness every day, while promoting the maximal development of the child. Accurate diagnosis of the disorders may take several years. Stigma is associated with any mental illness, but especially with a disorder such as schizophrenia. Parents may experience blame, guilt, and isolation. It is especially helpful to legitimize the parents' grief over the lost "normal" child (Pearson, 1992). It is essential that nurses offer support and convey the message that parents are not the cause of the disorder when such strange behavior is seen in children. Mutual support groups are helpful for many parents with children with chronic disabling conditions.

Social systems interventions include consultation with a variety of personnel at the child's school (e.g., teacher, counselors) and involved community agencies. The nurse is frequently involved in accessing services for children with alterations in thought processes. Educating teachers about manifestations of these disorders is important. Teachers need to understand effects and side effects of medication. They need to understand that children tend to act out their hallucinations and delusions, whereas adolescents are more verbal. Teachers and other providers of services, such as nurses, need to understand their own feelings toward the child (Pearson, 1992). A variety of treatment options are used to promote independence, social relationships, and health maintenance. These interventions include supportive therapy, social skills training, job coaching, symptom management, teaching activities of daily living, such as self-care, shopping (food, clothes), using transportation, money management, housekeeping, and therapeutic ways to use leisure time.

Anxiety Disorders

Anxiety is a common phenomenon of childhood. Children experience multiple fears as they develop and as they encounter new experiences. (See Chapter 5 for a discussion of typical fears in children.) Even though fear and anxiety can be normal, approximately 10% of children and adolescents experience disabling anxiety at some time in their developmental years. Anxiety disorders are manifested in disorders such as separation anxiety disorder, avoidant disorder, and post-traumatic stress disorder (PTSD) (Berenson, 1993; Bell-Dolan & Brazeal, 1993). A prevalence of approximately 4% is estimated among children, with girls having a higher rate than boys (Donnelly et al., 1996).

Etiology

A variety of factors are associated with and may cause anxiety disorders. Because most individuals are provoked to high anxiety at various times throughout childhood and later life, more than just the stressful experience is implicated in the disorders. Some persons may be at higher risk because of genetic phenomena, neurotransmitter disregulation, or structural deficits in the brain. The monoamine neurotransmitter noradrenergic and serotonergic systems especially are thought to be involved. Gamma-aminobutyric acid (GABA) and neuropeptides, especially corticotropin-releasing factor, are strongly suspected as well. Disregulation in these systems may occur in vulnerable individuals as a result of genetic irregulation, disease states, or from persistent stress for which the individual may not have sufficient coping strategies, resources, or social support. As the system becomes overwhelmed, patterns of disregulation may become established in the brain, resulting in continued manifestation of disabling anxiety (Berenson, 1993).

Separation Anxiety/School Refusal Disorder

Separation anxiety disorder is characterized by excessive anxiety when the child is separated from the home or the parents (primary attachment figure). The behaviors must have been present for 4 weeks before a diagnosis is confirmed. School refusal or phobia (as commonly known) is a prime example of separation anxiety disorder.

Assessment

Factors placing children at risk for separation anxiety disorder are death of a parent or sibling, divorce, relocation, and chronic illness. Thus, a family history and assessment of current functioning are important. Alcoholism, depression, agoraphobia, and panic disorder are seen more frequently in parents of children with separation anxiety disorder. A physical examination is indicated to determine any physical problems that may impinge. Family stressors (loss of home, emergency hospitalization, community violence, death in family) should be assessed to establish any contributing factors. Observation of the parent-child interaction is implicit in the assessment. Parental discipline, nurturance, dependence on the child, and encouragement of age-appropriate independence should be assessed.

Findings of the assessment often include problems associated with school. If the child has an academic deficit, is shy, or is awkward, he or she may be teased by peers. Family disruptions, chaos, or marital discord may compound the anxiety aroused by any problems experienced in school. Parents may be overly dependent on the child. This may cause the child to be concerned about the parents' safety and ability to cope. In addition, being absent from school for some time may cause a child to fear embarrassment and ridicule by peers or punishment from teachers or school officials.

Nursing Diagnoses and Outcomes

In addition to the nursing diagnoses listed in Chart 29–5 that are applicable to the child with separation anxiety/school phobia, the following diagnosis could be used to guide care interventions:

- **Anxiety related to separation from parent or caretaker**
  Outcomes: The child attends school, experiencing no anxiety related to separation or expectations at school.
  The child stays overnight at a peer's house, experiencing minimal anxiety.

Interdisciplinary Interventions

Children with school refusal are best served when referred to a mental health professional skilled in the treatment of anxiety disorders. The best approach is to involve the child and the parent in the treatment plan. The therapist (psychiatric clinical specialist nurse, psychiatrist, psychologist, or social worker) must form a liaison relationship with the school and parent. Cognitive-behavioral approaches with or without medication have been shown to produce the best results (March, Leonard, & Swedo, 1995). An alliance is made with the child, who is encouraged to think of his or her problem as an enemy that needs to be overcome and that the child has the skills to keep this enemy from having control over the child. Additional steps in the therapy process include desensitization of the feared object (school or leaving home). Pictures of thermometers measuring fear are often given to the child to rate the amount of fear experienced. The thermometer is also used as a means of evaluation to determine progress. Children may be hospitalized if the parent is unable to comply with the treatment plan. Parents who experience marital discord, are heavily enmeshed or dependent on the child, have depression, or have substance abuse problems need to be referred for their own therapy.

Community Care

Nurses working in schools may be the first to recognize the problem of school refusal. Children are usually sent to the school nurse for somatic complaints. A child who is seen frequently for minor complaints, especially those who insist on going home, should alert the nurse to the potential of school refusal. The school nurse or community health nurse may also have the responsibility of visiting children who have been absent for several days, and when illness is not verified, school refusal should be suspected (Chart 29–9).

Nurses working in schools may prevent the anxious child from developing school refusal. Careful assessment and identification of problems and needs of the child can result in early referral of the child for academic and learning disorders assessment. The nurse may teach stress management and act as a support to the child returning to school. Stress caused by family chaos, inappropriate

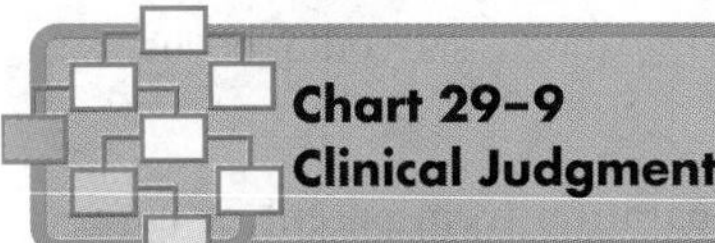

Chart 29–9
Clinical Judgment

School Refusal

Nine-year-old Billy was brought to the Community Mental Health Center by his mother after a visit from the district truancy officer. Mrs. J. reported that Billy had refused to attend school for the past 3 weeks and had several absences since the school term began (3 months previously).

Recent history acquired by the psychiatric nurse included the remarriage of Billy's mother 2 weeks before the beginning of school. Mrs. J. reported that Billy had always been a clinging child and, at 4 years of age, when she returned to work and placed Billy in a daycare center, he cried every day for more than an hour after she left him. The crying behavior continued for several months, although for shorter periods of time. This episode of school refusal actually began after Billy had been home for 3 days with a sore throat. During his 3-day illness, his stepfather returned home early on the first 2 days and became involved in very loud arguments with Billy's mother. On the second day of arguing, Mr. J. hit his wife, and then Mr. J. left the house, only to return several hours later, drunk but contrite and begging forgiveness. Billy had beseeched his mother to take him and their cat and leave the house, but his mother refused. After reluctantly being back in school for 3 days, Billy began refusing to go to school or to play with peers. Mrs. J. reported getting Billy to school on 2 days, but soon after she arrived at work, the school nurse called to request that Mrs. J. take Billy home because he was vomiting. Each morning since, Billy complained of feeling ill and remained in bed. Mrs. J. reported that there had been no more instances of Mr. J.'s drunken assaultive behavior.

Questions

1. What additional information would you gather about Billy?
2. What elements of the history indicate Billy is at risk for alterations in mental health status?
3. What nursing diagnosis would be applicable to Billy at this time?
4. What steps can be taken to alleviate the school refusal and return Billy to school?
5. What other referrals should be made to assist this family?

Answers

1. Developmental and health history, family health history, academic achievements or difficulties, peer relationships.
2. Remarriage of Billy's mother, history of difficulty of separating from mother, witness to arguing and physical abuse between his stepfather and mother.
3. Ineffective individual coping related to changes in family life and anxiety related to school attendance.
4. Use of play therapy or individual therapy to decrease anxiety regarding attending school and to determine other sources of stress for the child.
5. Refer mother and stepfather to family counseling and further assess home situation for spousal abuse and possible child abuse.

parenting, or unfavorable family relationships may be discovered. The family can be informed of the child's anxiety and referred to a mental health clinic, although in managed care plans, referral may have to be made by the primary physician (Care Path 29–1).

Post-Traumatic Stress Disorder

PTSD is a reactionary anxiety disorder occurring after a life-threatening event (or perceived as such). PTSD may follow a single traumatic event (type I) or long-standing traumatic events (type II). Child abuse (especially sexual abuse) and other long-standing and repeated exposure are associated with type II PTSD (Donnelly et al., 1996). War, shootings, catastrophic environmental events (hurricanes, floods, earthquakes), and accidental disasters (automobile, airplane crashes) may evoke PTSD in the vulnerable child or adolescent. The event triggering PTSD usually involves a threat to one's life or physical integrity and would be perceived as traumatizing to almost anyone experiencing the situation (Berenson, 1993). The actual prevalence of PTSD in children and adolescents is unknown (Donnelly et al., 1996).

Assessment

PTSD is characterized by repetitive uncontrolled memories (visual, auditory, physical sensations, and intrusive cognitions), repetitive behavior representative of the

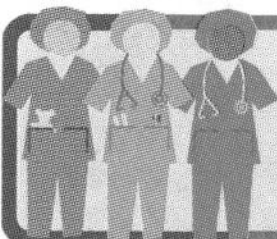

Care Path 29-1 An Interdisciplinary Plan of Care for the Child with School Refusal

Nursing Diagnosis	Patient/Family Intermediate Outcomes		
	Sessions 1–3	**Sessions 4–8**	**Sessions 9–10**
Fear related to separation from parents and home	Child will demonstrate decrease in anxiety by allowing mother to drive him or her to school.	Child will return to school or morning classes.	Child will attend full day of school.
Ineffective individual coping related to dealing with change in personal and family life	Child will use self-talk to control anxiety. Child will discuss feelings related to going to school.	Child will use relaxation and deep breathing techniques to control anxiety.	Child will initiate social interactions with peers.

Care Interventions

Session 1	Assessment and discussion of findings (parent, child, therapist, school nurse). Explanation of neurobiological model of anxiety and environmental factors contributing to school refusal. Explanation of proposed interventions: · Family therapy (Billy) · Explanation of medications (if used) · Special educational strategies (if needed) · Request parent and child to consent and commit to treatment
Session 2	Engage child in alliance to fight his/her "enemy." Child assigns name to the "enemy." Demonstrate fear thermometer; ask child to rate fear when he or she thinks about school and fear when staying home. Have child verbalize thoughts about going to school (let child control activity). Cooperatively develop statements child can say to self (self-talk) to counteract fear and negative thoughts. Write down and give to child to take home.
Session 3	Evaluate progress on self-talk and establishment of and adherence to school-like schedule. Reward any compliance with praise. Discuss going to school. Have child list all activities necessary to go to school. Monitor child's anxiety. Encourage child's use of self-talk when anxiety occurs. Allow child control of when to stop talking about school.
Session 4	As for session 3. Reward child with play period if complying. Teach deep breathing and practice. Use drawing and clay activities to build school and playground. Review previous week's talk about rituals to get ready for school.
Session 5	As for sessions 3 and 4. Add new statements, "I will take a ride to school." "I will stay calm during ride." "I will concentrate on deep breathing if I get anxious." Use a drawing of picture of ride to school. List pleasant things child will see along the way. Plan the ride to school. Child and therapist write note to parent about homework "Ride to School."

Care Path continued on following page

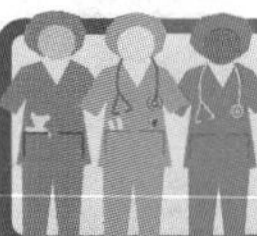

Care Path 29–1 An Interdisciplinary Plan of Care for the Child with School Refusal *Continued*

Care Interventions	
Session 6	Review success with "ride to school," breathing to stay calm, and self-talk. Praise all successes. Introduce idea of going into the school and appropriate self-talk. Reinforce deep breathing. Use drawing of self going into school. Have child include reward he or she would like for success. Child and therapist talk with parent about homework and negotiate the reward.
Session 7	Review success with homework. Reward child with praise. Review skills and self-care strategies. Play game of going into the classroom: "What will I find? Fun things? Pretty things? Things to do?" Have child draw the classroom. Ask child where he or she would sit, what he or she would do, and what he or she could do if felt anxious. Practice imaging self in classroom and relaxing. Negotiate homework, going to school, into classroom, and staying up to 1 hour.
Session 8	As for session 7. Increase time to half day at school.
Session 9	As for session 8. Increase time to whole day.
Session 10	Review progress and praise. Allow child to play as desired. Discuss termination (reward for success). Encourage checking in if problems arise. Arrange monthly, quarterly, and annual follow-up. Terminate.

trauma and often observed in the child's play, trauma-specific fears, hyperalertness, and changed attitudes (Terr, 1991). PTSD in children experiencing single-event trauma more often exhibit denial, dissociation, psychic numbing, depersonalization, and rage (Berenson, 1993). Regression, separation anxiety, and fearfulness may also be exhibited. Adolescents often manifest a belief in a foreshortened future (Terr, 1991).

There are no specific diagnostic scales or tools to assess the child or adolescent suspected of having PTSD. A careful psychosocial and developmental history are imperative. Documentation of exposure to trauma and the type and length of exposure is necessary. Clear examples of behavior such as numbing (inability to feel pain), sadness, avoidance of activities, inappropriate responses to seemingly innocuous events, and increased physiologic arousal are clues to the disorder. Teachers and parents may report and describe behavior changes and be able to identify the time when changes began. Anxiety scales for children may be helpful in assessing the internal anxiety experienced by the patient. A developmental history and a history of the previous coping style may provide information about the child's vulnerability (Chart 29–10). A neurologic examination should be conducted to eliminate the possibility of misdiagnosis.

The diagnosis of PTSD must be differentiated from phobic disorder and conduct disorder. Phobic anxiety is related to a specific feared object, whereas PTSD is characterized by intrusive images that may occur to unrelated stimulus. Because of the potential for reactionary aggressive behavior in PTSD, it may be confused with conduct disorder. Conduct disorder is characterized by a continual and pervasive disregard for the rights of others.

Nursing Diagnoses and Outcomes

In addition to the nursing diagnoses and outcomes presented in Chart 29–5, the following is applicable for the child with PTSD:

- **Post-trauma response related to accidental injury, assault, or other unexpected life event**
  Outcomes: The child states feelings and fears related to the traumatic event.

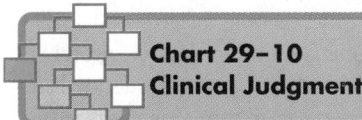

Chart 29–10
Clinical Judgment

The Adolescent Experiencing Post-Traumatic Stress Disorder

Tony, a 15-year-old ninth grader, was referred to the nurse therapist at his school. Tony was in trouble for hitting a teacher and, on several occasions, would have seriously injured other students if teachers had not intervened. Tony said he did not remember any of the incidents after seeing a black and red spot on a forehead (visual image). When examining the incidents with Tony, it became clear that he had been provoked by teasing from the students or criticism in the case of the teacher. Tony believed he was a "bastard" because his mother and father had never married. When he was teased or criticized, his self-denigration was reinforced. To complicate matters, he had seen, at age 4, his biological father (a beloved figure) accidentally killed by his favorite uncle. No one would talk with him and answer questions about the shooting of his biological father, and his family denied that he could remember the death scene. Since entering middle school, Tony's academic progress had seriously deteriorated. He was argumentative and defiant with both his mother and stepfather. He had also begun abusive behavior with his younger sisters, 10 and 12 years old.

Questions

1. The nurse therapist gave Tony the diagnosis of PTSD. Was this a correct diagnosis and if so why?
2. What other diagnoses might have been used and why?
3. What nursing diagnoses could be used to develop a plan of care for Tony?
4. What therapy should be initiated?
5. What behaviors would indicate success of the therapy?

Answers

1. The diagnosis of PTSD is correct, in part, because Tony exhibited disorganized behavior, a visual image of the overwhelming trauma, outbursts of anger, difficulty concentrating, and clinically significant impairment in important areas of functioning.
2. With more data, depression and perhaps an adjustment disorder might be suspected. He was argumentative with family members and abusive to younger siblings. His academic functioning had deteriorated.
3. Ineffective coping (rage, amnesic), impaired family process (did not talk about client's concern), altered role performance (deterioration in school work).
4. The nurse should explore Tony's cognitions and attached meanings and beliefs about these negative events. The nurse should assist Tony to develop a more positive identity and to learn relaxation techniques when confronted by teasing or criticism. Family therapy and peer group therapy may also be useful.
5. Tony should be able to participate in school without displaying aggressive behavior and with increased success in academic performance. Tony should be able to use relaxation to avoid explosive and amnestic rage. He should be able to verbalize positive thoughts about himself, which would demonstrate improvement in his self-perception and self-esteem.

The child expresses feelings of safety.
The child uses effective coping mechanisms to reduce fear.

Interdisciplinary Interventions

Burgess, Hartmann, and Clemons (1997) have proposed a model for treatment of children with PTSD. An explanation and application example may be found in the section of this chapter on child abuse. Tricyclic antidepressants and antianxiety medications have been helpful in treating depressive and anxiety symptoms. No systematic research of pharmacologic therapy in children has been reported (Berenson, 1993). However, case examples suggest that antidepressant medications (tricyclics and serotonin reuptake inhibitors [SSRIs]) and antianxiety medications are helpful in reducing sleep disturbances and depressive symptoms (Donnelly et al., 1996).

Other Anxiety Disorders

As discussed, several anxiety disorders occur in children. Table 29–3 summarizes these disorders. Studies indicate that 2% to 7% of children and adolescents develop one or more disorders during their developmental years. Several of these disorders have common characteristics as well as specific symptoms. Differential diagnoses can be challenging. Most of the disorders are treated similarly with cognitive and behavioral models of therapy. Some respond to medications; others do not. Education of the child and family about the disorder, the implications for growth and development, and the importance of the treatment plan are always a part of the nursing role.

caREminder: *The most immediate goal of the nurse in panic and phobic disorder is to reduce anxiety to a manageable level and to reduce the physical discomfort of the patient.*

Guidelines for early intervention include the following:

- Stay with the child or adolescent.
- Remain calm.
- Speak slowly, firmly, and reassuringly.
- Ask other persons to move away, or move the patient to a quiet, comfortable area.
- Encourage relaxation, focusing on a specific object or soothing thought.
- Administer medication if ordered.

When a child is observed in a school, inpatient, or hospital setting to have a panic attack, referral to the child's primary health care provider should be made. Additionally, the nurse should encourage mastery of relaxation techniques and avoidance of catastrophic thinking. Continued attacks are suggestive of a need for antianxiety medication or behavior or cognitive therapy with a skilled mental health professional.

Mood Disorders

Mood disorders are characterized by a disturbance in mood (irritability, sadness, oppositionalism, negativity) that lasts for most of every day for a period of at least 2 weeks. Mood disorders in children and adolescents are common and serious for a number of reasons. Risk for suicide increases dramatically in depressed youth. School failure and poor academic achievement are common. Family, social, and peer relationships deteriorate severely (Kowatch, Emslie, & Kennard, 1996).

Incidence and Etiology

Epidemiologic studies of children suggest a 1% to 3% prevalence rate of mood disorders in prepubertal children and a prevalence of up to 12% in adolescents. Depression is being more frequently diagnosed in preschool children as criteria for childhood disorders are clarified and differentiated. A gender disparity is not found until late adolescence, when the rate of depression escalates in girls (McCracken, 1992a).

There are three common mood disorders in children: major depressive disorder, dysthymia, and bipolar disorder. Seasonal affective disorder also occurs in children and adolescents. Each disorder should be assessed for severity (number of symptoms) and duration (Kowatch et al., 1996). Bipolar disorders also constitute mood disorders, but they are addressed separately in this chapter.

Studies of mood disorders in children demonstrate that a wide variety of factors are associated with alterations in mood and emotional states. Social factors such as family disturbances, physical, psychological, and sexual abuse, relocation, and bereavement have all been implicated (McCracken, 1992a). Familial vulnerability (genetic), psychological factors (cognitive processing, cognitive distortions, temperament, and lack of adequate coping strategies), social and environmental factors (poverty, abuse, neglect), and biological factors are all implicated or associated with depression in preschool, elementary, and adolescent years. Among disorders found to co-occur with depression are ADD, ADHD, PTSD, LDs, anxiety disorders, disruptive behavior disorder, and MR. Depression may result from excessive stress or an inherent error in the neurotransmitter system, especially the system associated with serotonin. Physical alterations caused by some endocrine, autoimmune, metabolic, and neurologic disorders are associated with depression.

A three-factor model of depression has been proposed by several authors (Brown, Harris, & Bifulco, 1986; McCracken, 1992b) (Fig. 29–5). It includes provoking agents, vulnerability factors, and symptom-formation factors. In the model, provoking agents interact with vulnerability factors to determine the formation of an episode of a depressive disorder. Symptom formation factors shape how the episode is manifested. In Figure 29–5, the arrow from provoking agents directly to depression suggests that factors (stressful life experiences) may lead directly to a depressive episode.

Figure 29–5
Three-factor model of depression. (Redrawn from Brown, G. W., Harris, T. O., & Bifulco, A. [1986]. Long-term effects of early loss of a parent. In M. Rutter, C. E. Izzard, & P. E. Read [Eds.], *Depression in young people*. New York: Guilford. Redrawn with permission.)

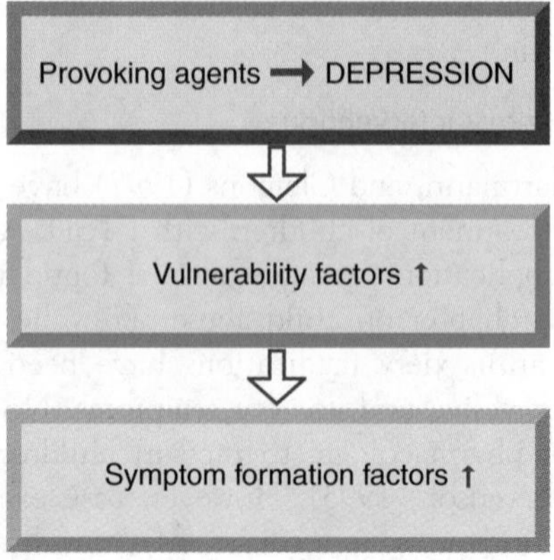

Provoking agents may be a negative parent–child relationship, significant loss, or physical stressors, such as serious illness, medications, endocrine imbalance, or psychological stressors (e.g., sexual abuse, traumatic experiences, or school failure). The most prominent vulnerability factors include family history of mood disorder, maternal dysfunction, and maladaptive cognitive and attributional styles (McCauley & Meyers, 1992; McCracken, 1992b).

Assessment

The interview with the child provides information about subjective symptoms of fatigue, suicide ideation, and feelings of worthlessness. Parents and teachers are best at providing information about the sequence of events and observable behaviors. Psychologists often perform psychometric testing to determine cognitive factors that may increase vulnerability. The school nurse should provide information about somatic complaints, their frequency, and their response to nursing intervention. Teachers can provide important information about the child's progress or decline in academic performance, mood states, and coping and adaptation in the classroom. They also have information about peer relationships. Parents may report on change occurring in appetite, weight gain or loss, and change in attitude and behaviors at home, such as increasing isolation, anxiety, loss of pleasure in usual activities, and oppositional and aggressive behavior (Fig. 29–6). The child is most likely able to provide subjective information about how he or she feels, sleep disturbance, and worries.

Figure 29–6
Adolescents are at risk for depression as they deal with the physical, emotional, and social changes that characterize this developmental stage.

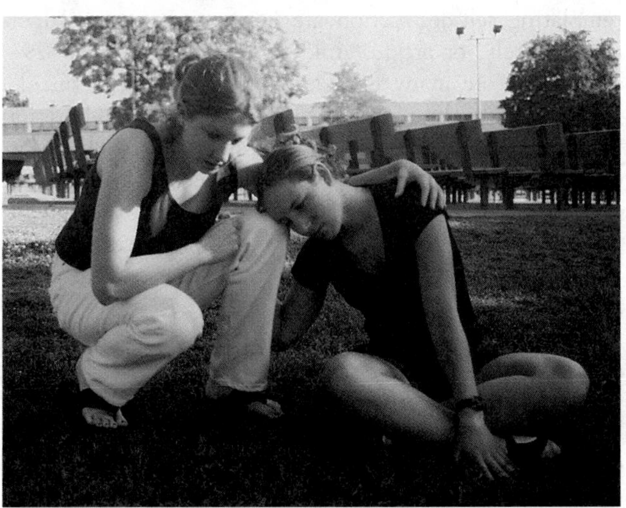

caREminder: *Children frequently exhibit depression in physical symptoms, irritability, and school failure. Adolescents may sleep excessively, appear sad, exhibit poor concentration and isolation, and complain of headaches. School performance often deteriorates. Assessment of suicidal thoughts or behavior is essential.*

A physical examination should be conducted to rule out or identify illnesses or physical problems that might cause depression. The physical examination can be done by a nurse practitioner, pediatrician, or family practice doctor.

The assessment is usually best done through a semistructured interview to allow flexibility and ability to explore areas that appear problematic. For instance, if a child indicates that he or she has thoughts of suicide, the nurse must obtain additional information regarding an established plan and its lethality. The nurse must make a decision regarding safety and what resources are needed to ensure the safety of the suicidal youth.

Self-report measures may be used to assist in the verification of the diagnosis. These are best administered and interpreted by a psychiatrist or psychologist. The most useful instruments are the Children's Depression Inventory (CDI) for children and the Beck Depression Inventory (BDI) for adolescents (Kowatch et al., 1996).

It is important to establish the most effective treatment plan through differential diagnosis. For instance, seasonal affective disorder is, as the name implies, seasonal in nature, with the fall and winter months being the time of highest frequency of the disorder. Dysthymia is an ongoing chronic disorder, like major depression, but less intense. The individual may experience good and bad days, but rarely or never experiences several good days in a row (Kowatch et al., 1996). Bipolar disorder is characterized by major mood swings with mania (extreme exuberance, intense energy and affect, but disorganized behavior) and depression often alternating with the manic behavior. Treatment plans differ extensively for each disorder.

Interdisciplinary Interventions

Interventions for selected problems associated with mood disorders in children are listed in Chart 29–11. Depending on the type of disorder, medical intervention may include medication. For instance, if the child has experienced a significant loss, the intervention should be directed at resolving the grief process. Bereavement therapy would be recommended. If no associated stressors are identified and no physical reason is suspected, then medication such as a tricyclic antidepressant (TCA) or SSRI would be recommended, usually with cognitive therapy or CBT.

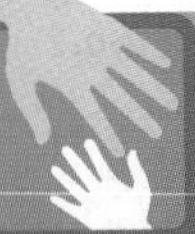

Chart 29–11
Nursing Interventions

Mood Disorders

Medical	Nursing
Depressive disorder Prescribe medication: tricyclic antidepressants or serotonin reuptake inhibitors (Kowatch et al., 1996). Monitor cardiotoxic effects of medication. Bipolar disorder Prescribe medications: lithium, carbamazepine, or valproate. Monitor blood levels of medications (Kowatch et al., 1996). Seasonal affective disorder (SAD) Prescribe light therapy or antidepressant medication (Antai-Otong, 1995).	Teach parents and child about illness, associated symptoms and behaviors. Explain therapeutic regimens: medications, psychotherapy, or behavior therapy; photo (light) therapy for SAD. Monitor child's response to medication, report lack of improvement or untoward side effects, and report changes from depression to manic and vice versa. Teach parent and child about the medications: purpose, signs of improvement, side effects, when to report side effects, and withdrawal or termination of medication. School nurse: Monitor compliance and changes (or lack of) in school behavior, attitude, and performance in collaboration with teachers. Caution: All antidepressant medication takes 10 to 21 days to begin showing an effect.

Suicide

Suicidal events, which include acts of self-destruction, life-taking acts, and threats of self-harm, are common among teenagers and are drastically increasing in preadolescents as well. Persons attempting or thinking about suicide experience hopelessness and despair, and can think of no satisfactory way to solve their problems or to find satisfaction in daily living.

Incidence

Completed suicide is believed to be uncommon among preadolescent and younger children; however, the rate has doubled since 1960 (Mullen & Hendren, 1996). Completed suicides are the third leading cause of death in adolescents age 15 and older in the United States (U.S. Department of Health and Human Services, 1993). It is estimated that 250,000 children and adolescents attempt to kill themselves every year. Approximately 5000 succeed (Kerns & Lieberman, 1993). Experts warn that actual suicides could be even more frequent, because many suicides are not labeled as such for the sake of the family. Eight percent of high school students said they had attempted suicide in a 1990 survey. Another 27% said they had thought seriously about it (Grinspoon, 1996). Girls make more suicidal attempts, whereas suicide attempts of male adolescents more often end in death because males use more lethal methods (Riley & Kneisl, 1996). Girls who have been sexually abused are four times as likely to attempt suicide as girls without history of sexual assault (Grinspoon, 1996).

Worldview: *Ethnic and cultural factors appear to play a strong role in the incidence of suicide. Suicide is less common among Italian, Greek, and Spanish families, and is more common in Switzerland, Scandinavia, Eastern Europe, and Japan. Suicides among 15- to 19-year-old black males have increased 165%, and for 10- to 14-year-old black males, by 300% (Anonymous, 1995). Native American suicides exceed those of whites at all ages (Grinspoon, 1996).*

Etiology

Thoughts of suicide are frequently communicated to someone, but are often ignored. Many myths still pervade societal thinking about suicide; thus, many children contemplating self-destruction are ignored, are reassured inappropriately, or are just told to "shape up" (Chart 29–12). There are many risk factors associated with suicide. These include the presence of another type of alteration in mental health status (e.g., depression, anxiety disorders), relational stress with parents, friends, or significant others, abuse, academic failure, public embarrassment, low self-esteem, relocation of family or of friends, availability of firearms, and having a friend or peer who committed suicide.

Research indicates that the three most common methods that children and adolescents use to commit suicide are, in order, firearms, hanging, and poisoning. In 1992, suicides accomplished with firearms accounted for 65% of all suicides in the younger than 25 age group

Chart 29–12

Myths About Suicide

- People contemplating suicide rarely tell anyone about it.
- Suicidal threats are manipulative attempts to get attention.
- Children and adolescents from good, intact homes do not think about or commit suicide.
- Anyone thinking about or who commits suicide is or was crazy.
- One should not ask about thoughts or plans for suicide to avoid planting the idea.
- If a person talks about suicide, it is just talk—he or she will not do it.
- Accidents, gunshot wounds, and substance abuse are separate problems and not associated with suicide.
- Someone who is thinking about or who actually commits suicide is always depressed.
- Suicidal persons remain suicidal.

(Anonymous, 1995). Experts believe that decreasing a child or adolescent's access to guns could significantly decrease the number of handgun-related suicides. Studies have revealed that states with stricter handgun control laws have lower suicide rates (Srnec, 1991).

Assessment

Most children give clues when they are thinking about suicide.

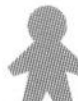

Tip: *When youngsters appear for help or ask to talk about "a friend" who is upset and talking about suicide, the health care provider or teacher should be alerted to the potential risk of suicide. The child may be indirectly talking about, or asking questions about, his or her own concerns.*

A frequent way for youth to communicate about suicidal thoughts is through a friend. They may pass a note to a classmate or ask the friend for advice about doing "it," or they may make threats in anger.

The assessment of suicide should be conducted for adolescents and children presenting with high-risk behaviors and high-risk factors in their life. Children and adolescents with depressive disorders, bipolar disorder, and substance abuse, or who are despairing, feeling hopelessness, and indicating despondency and powerlessness should all be asked about suicidal thoughts, ideation, and plans. Ideation refers to thoughts and feelings that suicide is the way to end the problem or misery they are experiencing.

Guidelines for the assessment are

- Establish rapport (show interest, actively listen, initiate talking in a friendly, respectful way).
- Use direct, simple questions (avoiding open-ended questions).
- Use language that the child can understand.
- Allow the child to tell his or her own story.
- Questions should be asked matter-of-factly, without judgment.
- Convey empathy, allow expression of feelings.
- Determine the intent, if a plan has been formulated, and the degree of lethality.
- Ask about the child's support system and available resources.
- Discuss the need for protection and measures for prevention.

In assessing for risk for suicide, children and adolescents may initially indicate suicidal thoughts or ideation, but later deny them. This denial should not deter the caregiver from providing for the safety of the child.

The diagnosis of high risk for suicide (or other levels from low to high) is based on the hopelessness and despondency of the client, the degree of lethality of a plan (if one exists), the intensity and frequency of thoughts about suicide, the quality and availability of resources and social supports for the client, and the child's ability to negotiate other ways of managing problems and feelings. Commonly used highly lethal methods of suicide include using a gun (and having one available), jumping from a height, hanging, crashing in an automobile, carbon monoxide poisoning, and taking prescription sleeping pills. Children and adolescents often plan to run in front of a bus, truck, or train. Methods low in lethality include cutting wrists and taking nonprescription drugs (excluding aspirin and Tylenol) and low potency tranquilizers (Riley & Kneisl, 1996).

Nursing Diagnoses and Outcomes

In addition to the nursing diagnoses presented in Chart 29–5, the most important nursing diagnosis is related to the degree of risk for self-directed harm (McFarland, Wasli, & Gerety, 1997). Nursing diagnoses specific to the child with suicidal ideations include the following:

▶ **High risk for poisoning related to cognitive or emotional difficulties**
Outcomes: The child/adolescent is not exposed to and does not ingest dangerous substances.
The child/adolescent understands the need for self-protection.

- **Chronically low or situational self-esteem**
  Outcomes: The child/adolescent voices feelings related to self-esteem.
  The child/adolescent makes a verbal or written contract not to harm self.
  The child/adolescent engages in interventions and interactions with others that promote positive esteem.
  The child/adolescent identifies options other than suicide to stop emotional pain.
  The child/adolescent uses problem-solving to identify ways to cope with feelings.
  The child/adolescent uses adult support and resources when feeling helpless and despondent.
- **High risk for self-mutilation related to emotional distress and feelings of low self-worth**
  Outcomes: The child/adolescent does not harm self.
  The child/adolescent reports suicidal thoughts to others.

Interdisciplinary Interventions

The primary short-term goal is to ensure the child's safety and prevent self-harm (Chart 29–13). Nursing intervention must include referral to the appropriate resources. First and foremost, the child's family (parents, guardian) must be notified. Referral for emergency care such as psychiatric assessment and crisis intervention may also be warranted. In some cases, the child may need to be hospitalized (parental permission needed).

Community Care

School nurses should participate in educational programs for the community, parents, school personnel, and children. The Centers for Disease Control (1994) has identified seven strategies for preventing suicide among young persons. These strategies include

- Training school and community leaders to identify young persons at highest risk for suicidal thoughts, threats, and attempts
- Educating young persons about suicide, risk factors, and interventions
- Implementing screening and referral programs
- Developing peer support programs
- Establishing and operating suicide crisis centers and hot lines
- Restricting access to highly lethal methods of suicide
- Intervening after a suicide to prevent other young persons from attempting or completing suicide

Suicide prevention contracts are a good idea after a relationship is established and the assessment is completed, and before terminating the assessment session. The contract is best written by the client. The nurse may suggest sentences, words, and resources. The contract needs to be dated and signed by the client and the nurse.

Suicide often raises fear in a community because of its contagion effect. Suicide contagion is "when one completed suicide triggers a cluster of subsequent suicidal behaviors among the victim's contacts" (King et al., 1995). Contagion effect can be seen in schools, communities, or inpatient settings. To prevent contagion effects, experts recommend that friends, siblings, and classmates of the suicidal person receive immediate crisis intervention by mental health experts (Wenckstern & Leenaars, 1993). Few school systems have enough professional

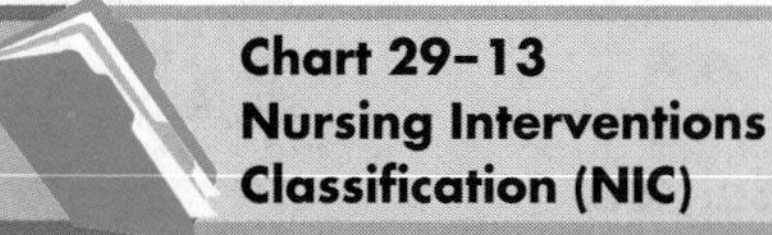

Chart 29–13
Nursing Interventions Classification (NIC)

Suicide Prevention

Definition

Reducing risk of self-inflicted harm for a patient in crisis or severe depression

Activities

Determine whether patient has specific suicide plan identified.
Encourage the person to make a verbal no-suicide contract.
Determine history of suicide attempts.
Protect patient form harming self.
Place patient in least restrictive environment that allows for necessary level of observation.
Demonstrate concern about patient's welfare.
Refrain from negatively criticizing.
Remove dangerous items from the patient environment.
Place patient in room with protective window coverings, as appropriate.
Observe closely during suicidal crisis.
Instruct patient and significant other in signs, symptoms, and basic physiology of depression.
Instruct family that suicidal risk increases for severely depressed patients as they begin to feel better.
Facilitate discussion of factors or events that precipitated the suicidal thoughts.
Escort patient during off-ward activities, as appropriate.
Facilitate support of patient by family and friends.
Instruct family on possible warning signs or pleas for help patient may use.
Refer patient to psychiatrist, as needed.

From McCloskey, J., & Bulechek, G. (1996). *Nursing interventions classification (NIC)* (2nd ed.). St. Louis: Mosby–Year Book. Reprinted with permission.

mental health personnel to successfully manage this type of crisis. It is therefore imperative that school systems make formal links with mental health agencies to handle school crises. Each system should have a well-developed plan to handle crises, which should include family contact, support, and referral, intervention with siblings, peers, and classmates, identification and referral of at-risk individuals, community information, media relations, staff support and consultation, links with mental health professional services, and internal communication (Wenckstern & Leenaars, 1993).

Compulsive Disorders

Obsessive-Compulsive Disorder and Tourette's Syndrome

OCD and Tourette's syndrome are neuropsychiatric disorders believed to have their origins in childhood. OCD is characterized by anxious repetitive thoughts and behaviors that the individual feels unable to stop. Tourette's syndrome is manifested by motor and vocal tics, and often with compulsive behaviors as well.

Recent studies provide increasingly strong evidence for a genetic link. In addition, the question has arisen of whether OCD is a variant of Tourette's syndrome. Both disorders are frequently accompanied by signs and symptoms of the other disorder (March, Leonard, & Swedo, 1995; Scahill, 1996; Scahill, Walker, Lechner, & Tynan, 1993c). Current thinking suggests that the dysfunction originates as a malfunction in the caudate nucleus and frontal lobe of the brain. Tourette's syndrome is thought to originate in the basal ganglia. Psychopharmacologic agents, such as tricyclics, antidepressants, and SSRIs, have been successful in treating some cases of OCD, thus increasing the confidence in actual brain dysfunction. Studies of growth patterns of children with OCD suggest neuroendocrine disregulation as well. For example, boys with OCD tend to be shorter than their nonafflicted agemates. Afflicted boys also demonstrate a flatter growth curve. The disorder tends to appear in boys earlier (prepubertal) compared with girls (early adolescence) (March et al., 1995).

The prevalence of OCD is estimated at 2% to 3% of the general population. The average age for development of the disorder is 10 years. The disease occurs among all socioeconomic and racial and ethnic groups. Tourette's disorder is more commonly seen in boys. The approximate ratio is 5:1000 for boys and 2:1000 cases for girls (Robertson, 1994).

Assessment

OCD is manifested by recurrent thoughts (obsessions) that persist and are not related to the reality of the situation and by repetitive behaviors (compulsions) that the individual cannot stop at all or can only stop with enormous conscious effort. The individual experiences anxiety if the behavior is resisted, but recognizes the senselessness of the acts and thoughts (Scahill et al., 1993c). Children with OCD may manifest only one aspect of the disorder, but this is rare. Behaviors commonly associated with Tourette's disorder are listed in Chart 29–14. The manifestations of Tourette's syndrome are annoying at best and socially disruptive at worst, often causing embarrassment and stigma for the child and the child's family.

Assessment of OCD and Tourette's syndrome in children poses special problems. During various stages of development, children often exhibit ritualistic behavior, facial tics, and worrisome thoughts. Thus, normal behaviors common in childhood must be differentiated from those characteristic of OCD and Tourette's syndrome. The worries and behaviors of children with both disorders control their lives. Getting dressed, grooming activities, washing hands, bathing, and all manner of "normal behaviors" may begin quite spontaneously to rule the afflicted person's life, causing disintegration of social and school relationships. Children and adolescents with worries and ritual-like behaviors are satisfied when they are provided reassurance or perform the behavior. The tic behaviors and vocal utterances of Tourette's syndrome do

Chart 29–14

Tourette's Syndrome: Common Behaviors

- Purposeless movements
  - Touching self (anywhere on body)
  - Eye blinking
  - Grimacing
  - Head jerking
  - Shoulder jerking
  - Tapping
  - Twirling
  - Vulgar gestures
- Phonic tics (vocal sounds)
  - Grunting
  - Snorting
  - Throat clearing
- Vocalizations
  - Swearing
  - Repetitious phrases (e.g., "You bet," and "You know")

From Robertson, M. M. (1994). Gilles de la Tourette syndrome: An update. *Journal of Child and Adolescent Psychiatry, 35*(1), 597–611. Reprinted with permission.

not recede as do normal motor or facial tics. Assessment of OCD should also include assessment of motor and vocal tics (Scahill et al., 1993c). For both disorders, the family history needs also to include questions related to obsessive thoughts, compulsive behaviors, and tic behaviors in family members (Donnelly et al., 1996).

Interdisciplinary Interventions

Treatment for both OCD and Tourette's syndrome involves medication and behavior management techniques. With children and adolescents, involvement of family members or caregivers is essential. Involvement of the family should include family education, knowledge of medication (action, side effects, and management), and behavior management strategies. Counseling should be offered to parents struggling with guilt, self-blame, or blaming of others, or where conflict has become dysfunctional to the family.

Pharmacologic Management. A number of medications are helpful in controlling or reducing the symptoms of OCD and Tourette's syndrome. Medications effective for OCD include tricyclic antidepressants, clomipramine, and the SSRIs, such as Prozac and Fluvoxamine (March et al., 1995). The pharmacologic treatment of choice in Tourette's syndrome is dopamine type 2 receptor antagonists (haloperidol, pimozide). Other medications used include clonidine (an alpha-2 presynaptic noradrenergic agonist) and risperidone (blocks dopamine type 2 receptors and serotonin type 2 receptors) (Castiglia, 1997b). Newer medications are continuously being evaluated, thus constant attention to pharmacology literature is important. Nurses need to know about current medications, their side effects, and their dosage schedules. Parents opposed to medication for their children need education and encouragement to maintain the treatment plan, including the behavior management plan.

Behavior Management. A crucial aspect of therapy for most individuals with OCD is providing behavior management, because medication has been only partially successful in treating the disorder. For some, medication has not worked or was effective for only a short time. One form of behavior management exposure refers to deliberately confronting the individual with the provoking stimulus, for example, passage through doorways (or whatever the stimulus for the compulsive behavior) and preventing (response prevention) the compulsive behavior (must pass through the doorway by limiting or not performing the compulsive behavior). A system of rewards is essential to success of the treatment plan. The afflicted individual is expected to monitor his or her anxiety level while practicing this behavior management plan. An effective strategy in working with children is to engage the child in "defeating the enemy" (the child gives it [OCD] a name or label). The child, therapist, and family members develop a plan of cognitions (thought stopping or self-talk) to be used to reduce the anxiety experienced when the child tries to prevent the repetitious behavior. Even though medications are proving successful in the treatment of OCD, it is a lifelong disease and it is best to provide the afflicted individual with behaviors to master the anxieties and ritualistic behaviors (March & Mulle, 1995). Referral to a professional skilled in treatment of compulsive disorders may be warranted.

OCD and Tourette's syndrome both affect the whole family, often causing frustration and resentment. Family members may support and reinforce the compulsive behavior just to keep the peace. A combination of family and individual therapy is often useful.

Nurses should be familiar with both disorders because when affected children present in the school or clinic setting, the disorders are often misdiagnosed as behavior problems. Referral of children is warranted when tics are frequent and lasting, when tics appear in clusters or repetitive patterns, or when parents, teachers, or the child is concerned (Scahill, Ort, & Hardin, 1993b).

Social Disruptions in Normal Growth and Development

Physical Abuse, Neglect, and Emotional Maltreatment

The abuse of children and adolescents is so widespread that no one knows its full cost. Because it is linked to most mental illnesses and addictions, its effects are profound. These effects include human suffering, family disruption, increased violence, participation in gangs, absenteeism from work, lifelong unemployment, financial costs of acute and chronic hospitalization, welfare-dependency, addictions, deaths due to suicide, murder, and drunk driving, and perpetuation of the abuse upon future generations. Throughout this discussion, abused children and adolescents are referred to as "victims" (Cornman, 1989). The term "victim" is more appropriate for this population than the term "survivor" because of their powerlessness to escape the abusive situation, "their developmental issues, economical and social dependency, and chronological age" (Cornman, 1989).

Each state has its own definitions of physical abuse, neglect, and sexual abuse for legal purposes. Some definitions are more narrow than others. For example, some states limit prosecution only to parents, excluding other perpetrators such as neighbors or other family members. Many definitions of abuse and neglect are vague and open to interpretation. Phrases such as "resulting in bodily injury," "deviant sexual conduct," and "compelled by force or imminent threat of force" are open to a variety of interpretations. This chapter considers sexual abuse to be *any* sexual contact between an adult and child. What actually constitutes bodily injury is open to a wide variety of interpretations.

Defining emotional abuse becomes even more difficult. If professionals and individual states cannot reach consensus on a definition of emotional abuse, it is difficult for professionals to exercise any authority in removing children to safer environments, or in treating the victims and abusers. These unclear definitions and the difficulty in substantiating abuse create a system in which the abused child is often left in danger and untreated.

caREminder: *Nurses must be aware of their own state's definitions of abuse and neglect. Nurses have a professional and legal responsibility to report to Child Protective Services any suspected abuse or neglect.*

The nurse does not have to *prove* the abuse or neglect has occurred, but is obligated to report it to the proper authorities. Often this involves a judgment call on the part of the nurse. Until nurses become familiar with reporting procedures and the state's definitions, it is helpful to enlist the advice of one or more experienced mental health professionals. However, if the nurse disagrees with their advice, the ultimate legal responsibility lies with the professional who received the information. Therefore, failure to report could result in a nurse being subject to legal actions.

Charges of medical neglect can be filed against caregivers who fail to provide the necessary prevention and treatment for children in their care. The process is the same as filing for physical or sexual abuse or neglect. Each state has a form for reporting suspected abuse or neglect. This form may also be used for reporting suspected medical neglect.

Incidence

The National Committee for the Prevention of Child Abuse (NCPCA) estimates that 3.1 million children were reported as victims of child abuse and neglect in 1995. This figure represents an increase of 15.2% from 1990, with an average annual increase of 4%. Increased public awareness, reporting system or procedural changes, and increases in substance abuse and violence were identified as factors contributing to the increase. Using these figures, 46 of every 1000 children in the United States are reported as victims. This represents *only reported cases*. The actual number of children suffering from abuse and neglect is far higher than these figures indicate. Of those cases reported, approximately 32% are substantiated. The NCPCA reports the following statistics regarding the specific types of child maltreatment:

- 26% Physical abuse
- 10% Sexual abuse
- 53% Neglect
- 3% Emotional maltreatment
- 7% Other

The National Center on Child Abuse and Neglect (NCCAN) defines adolescent physical abuse as:

> the infliction of non-accidental physical harm, resulting either in injury or in a substantial risk of death, disfigurement, or impairment of bodily functioning. Examples of serious injuries include the loss of consciousness, cessation of breathing, broken bones, and extensive second-degree burns; examples of moderate injuries include the persistence in observable form of pain or impairment for 48 hours (e.g., bruises, welts, scratches). (Kaplan et al., 1994)

Because of different cultural norms regarding disciplining adolescents, it is estimated that abuse and neglect in adolescents is severely underestimated. A study by Straus and Gelles reports that 21% of households use serious violence with their adolescents (Kaplan et al., 1994). White female adolescents are at greatest risk for abuse. Disobeying or arguing with a parent precipitates 90% of all adolescent abuse. Typically, adolescents respond to abuse with mutual assault (Kaplan et al., 1994).

The statistics for child abuse fatalities are likely to be significantly lower than actual number of cases. Many fatalities resulting from child abuse are attributed to other causes of death. In 1995, the NCPCA reported 1215 child maltreatment fatalities, which represents a 39% increase since 1985. Of these deaths, 82% occurred in children younger than age 5, and 41% occurred in children younger than age 1 (Lung & Daro, 1995).

There is a strong relationship between substance abuse and child maltreatment. Substance abuse tends to heighten sexual arousal while simultaneously decreasing inhibitions. This results in adults being far more aggressive and sexually violent. Children and adolescents are often the victims. Nine to 10 million children younger than age 18 are affected by substance-abusing parents and caretakers.

Assessment

The effects of physical abuse, emotional abuse, and neglect are enormous. Abused and neglected children display tremendous difficulties at school. Many of these children respond in a manner that goes unnoticed by most adults, such as extreme efforts to please teachers, withdrawal, and generalized anxiety. Some potential clues to look for in a classroom setting are children who always wear long sleeves and long pants despite warm weather, children who make extreme efforts to please the teacher, and children who display an excessive startle to quick movements made near them, excessive daydreaming, or any signs of anxiety or depression. Additional impacts of abuse and neglect upon school performance include a lack of motivation to achieve, fear of failure, an inability to establish positive relationships with unfamiliar adults, poor performance on standardized tests, lower grades, a

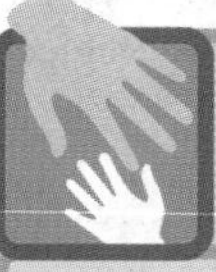

Chart 29–15
Nursing Interventions

Abused and Neglected Children and Adolescents

Teach child anxiety-reducing techniques.
- Gradual relaxation
- Relaxation to music
- Visual imagery
- Exercise
- Talking with safe, appropriate people about feelings
- Choosing, building, and maintaining positive support systems
- Ensuring personal safety
- Setting boundaries
- Establishing a safe, supportive relationship
- Clarifying expectations and rules
- Self-soothing techniques

Assist child in managing his or her feelings.
- Teach child to identify feelings.
- Teach child to express feelings appropriately.
- Teach child to modulate and control feelings.
- Teach child to identify events that elicit strong positive and negative feelings.
- Teach child to express feelings verbally instead of physically.
- Teach child to normalize feelings resulting from abuse.
- Teach child to share feelings appropriately with peer group.
- Teach child to find commonality and support within group for feelings resulting from abuse.

Teach child assertiveness skills.
- Teach child to identify differences between assertiveness, passivity, and aggression.
- Teach child to practice assertiveness skills.
- Teach child to identify boundaries.
- Teach child to understand when someone violates boundaries.
- Teach child to practice responses when someone violates boundaries.

Assist child in developing problem-solving skills.
- Provide simple problem-solving model.
- Increase awareness of child's control and decision-making.
- Teach child to generate a list of possible solutions to problem situations.
- Help child look at consequences of each solution.
- Help child make best choice.
- Help child give self positive and gentle negative feedback.
- Coach problem-solving with actual situations as much as possible.
- Teach good touch/bad touch.
- Teach refusal skills.
- Teach age-appropriate sexual expression.
- Teach effects of substance abuse.

Assist child in value building and clarification.
- Define values.
- Identify role of values.
- Assist child in identifying and verbalizing values.
- Help link child's values to child's actions.
- Assist child in development of values.
- Help child practice value-based decision-making.

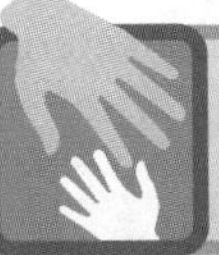

Chart 29–15
Nursing Interventions *Continued*

Abused and Neglected Children and Adolescents

Assist child in enhancing his or her coping mechanisms.
- Teach child to practice positive self-talk.
- Help child set realistic expectations for self.
- Assist child in learning to nurture self.
- Teach child to practice relaxation.
- Teach child to practice assertiveness and appropriate expression of feelings.
- Assist child in learning to accept defeat and failure.
- Help child identify and build skills, hobbies.
- Encourage child to identify and focus on strengths.
- Help child set and accomplish goals.
- Assist child in developing organizational skills.

higher dependence on teachers, more trips out of the classroom owing to behavioral problems, more suspensions, and lower social competence (Cicchetti & Rogosch, 1994). Chapter 30 describes the assessment of the child in the acute or community health care setting that should be completed if abuse is suspected.

Interdisciplinary Interventions

Whereas the effects of childhood abuse and neglect are becoming more clear, specific interventions for successful treatment are less so. Few studies provide any data regarding successful interventions with abused children. Based on existing literature, nurses can select several interventions that are thought to be successful (Chart 29–15). Most importantly, the child must be safe. Little can be accomplished if a child remains in an abusive or neglectful setting (Friedrich, 1994).

Treatment interventions vary depending on the child's developmental level. In working with children and adolescents, it is imperative that these interventions be presented in a fun, interesting manner to engage a child more quickly in the therapy and to reduce oppositional, defiant behavior. One example is to create a mock talk show in which the children alternate between being "experts" on specific therapeutic topics and "audience members" who ask the experts questions. Another idea is to have the children make or use puppets to create a play on a topic of your choice. A nurse could also have the group make movies and alternate between being actors and directors. In doing any video-recording, it is necessary to obtain written permission from legal guardians. The consent form should specify that the videotape is for therapeutic purposes only, will be erased immediately after the group concludes, and will not be shown to anyone other than the team caring for the child. Art, drama, and music can be used alone or in combination to engage children in therapy. These techniques decrease children's oppositional behavior and allow the nurse to see some of the conflicts that the child may not be able to otherwise verbalize or even identify.

Sexual Abuse

Incidence

The incidence of sexual abuse is extremely difficult to accurately assess. First, there is great diversity in opinion as to what actually constitutes sexual abuse. Although sibling incest is considered by many experts to be the most common form of sexual abuse (Gilbert, 1989), most studies eliminate sexual abuse between victims and perpetrators who have 5 years or less difference in age, terming it "sex play." Russell found that 40% of sibling incest occurred between siblings with less than 5 years age difference (Gilbert, 1989). It is therefore not reflected in most sexual abuse statistics. A wide variety of definitions of sexual abuse are used by researchers, complicating comparison and validation of research findings. To include all types of sexual exploitation, many leaders feel a broad definition of sexual abuse is most appropriate (Finklehor, 1986; Rew, 1989). Rew (1989) defines sexual exploitation as the misuse of power and authority by adults or older children to obtain sexual gratification from a child. Childhood sexual exploitation includes activities such as exhibitionism, genital fondling, attempted or actual rape, anal, vaginal, or oral intercourse, pornography, sexual harassment by authority figures, and the use of force for any other unwanted sexual activity between a child and adult or older child.

Reported incidences of sexual abuse are only reflective of those persons who disclose the abuse and therefore may be lower than the actual number of cases. Many factors prevent victims from disclosing abuse (Chart 29–16). Most research indicates that 20% to 30% of women and 10% of men have experienced sexual abuse as children or adolescents (Anonymous, 1993a). The reported incidence for men may be especially low because of common fears among boys that being sexually abused means they are homosexual.

Etiology

A common misconception is that children are sexually abused by strangers. To prevent sexual abuse from occurring, most parents warn their children not to talk with strangers. Conte and Schuerman (1987) found that in only 4% of the 369 cases they studied was the perpetrator a stranger to the child. The most commonly identified perpetrators were biological parents or stepparents (29%), other relatives (23%), acquaintances (30%), and baby sitters (7%). From the outside, these families appear quite "normal," but the sense of normalcy is simply a facade. Gilbert (1989) reports three common characteristics of these families:

- Parents are physically or emotionally distant.
- There is an overt sexual atmosphere in the home.
- There are family sexual secrets.

Finklehor (1986) found that men were by far the most common perpetrators. In 95% of all sexual abuse reported by girls and in 80% of sexual abuse cases reported by boys, the perpetrator was male (Cornman, 1989).

Prognosis. Many children who are sexually abused appear relatively unscathed and symptoms of psychiatric difficulties do not develop. Factors that increase a child's resiliency are receiving greater attention by researchers. However, Keltner, Schwecke, and Bostrom (1995) warn that, although superficially victims may appear uninjured, the demeanor may be due to denial, dissociation, amnesia, emotional deadening, or repression. In attempting to explain why apparent symptoms do not develop in some children, some researchers would argue that these children have not yet realized the full implication of the abuse they have endured and that symptoms may develop later. Another possibility is that the instruments used to measure the effects of sexual abuse may not be sensitive enough to detect the child's distress. Young children in particular may not have the language skills or vocabulary to express the true level of anguish they are experiencing. Finally, children tend to use denial and projection as their primary defense mechanisms; therefore, they may block the effects of the sexual abuse from consciousness until later in life. Currently, conflict exists within the field of psychiatry regarding whether flashbacks later in life of sexual abuse represent repressed memory or false memory.

Several variables affect the degree of trauma experienced by the victim. These include the identity of the perpetrator (the closer the relationship, the worse the outcome), number of perpetrators, severity of abuse, age at the time of the onset of abuse (the younger the age at onset of abuse, the more severe the trauma), length of abuse, length of time elapsed since the last abusive incident, use of violence or force, maternal reaction to disclosure, physical harm, use of threats, and degree of victim's secondary gains, such as toys, money, candy, or special favors received from the perpetrator (Coker, 1990; Kendall-Tackett, Williams, & Finklehor, 1993; Lipovsky, 1991).

Sexual abuse by one's family members is the most psychologically damaging form of abuse. Many times, threats, force, and physical abuse are used to manipulate the victim into acquiescence and silence. Often, the long-term effects of this traumatic type of sexual abuse do not become apparent immediately after disclosure. Often, children undergo grief as they move through one devel-

Chart 29–16

Factors Preventing Disclosure of Sexual Abuse

- Child's young age
- Child's developmental level
- Dependency on adults for meeting basic needs
- Shame
- No witnesses to validate the abuse
- No observable physical injuries
- No outward manifestations of the sexual violation
- Disbelief and rejection by adults upon disclosure
- Threats (such as the perpetrator threatening to kill the victim's mother if the victim discloses the abuse)
- Force and aggression used by the perpetrator
- Fear of family breaking up
- Fear of abandonment
- Fear of loss of home
- Fear of foster placement
- Negative impact on the child's relationship with the non-offending parent
- Parental disbelief and being labeled a "troublemaker"
- Loss of privacy and shame resulting from investigation and court proceedings
- Fear of reprisals, such as worsened physical and sexual abuse
- Fear that child will not be believed

opmental stage after another. The child may not understand the full impact of what has occurred or how intensely the abuse has scarred them for many years to come. For example, when a sexually abused child begins dating, that child may realize that he or she cannot tolerate any intimacy. When that same child matures and marries, he or she may not only mourn not having both parents to celebrate the event, but they may also find they cannot maintain emotional or sexual intimacy in their marriage. Additionally, they may find it difficult to nurture their own children. Nurturance may not come naturally, because they never experienced it as children.

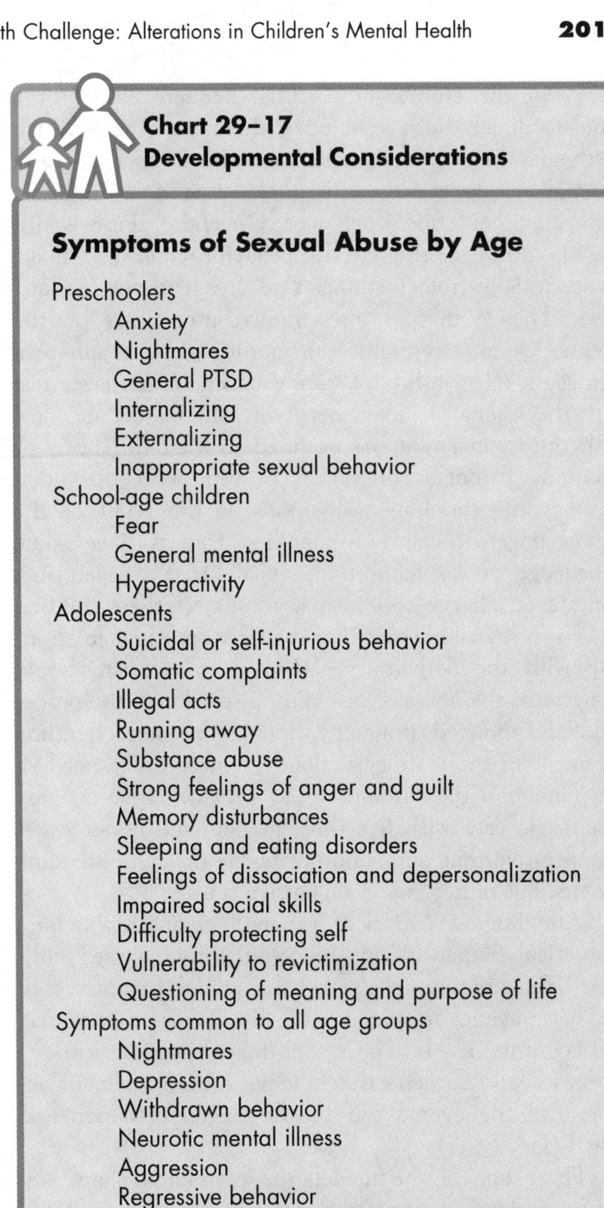

Chart 29–17
Developmental Considerations

Symptoms of Sexual Abuse by Age

Preschoolers
- Anxiety
- Nightmares
- General PTSD
- Internalizing
- Externalizing
- Inappropriate sexual behavior

School-age children
- Fear
- General mental illness
- Hyperactivity

Adolescents
- Suicidal or self-injurious behavior
- Somatic complaints
- Illegal acts
- Running away
- Substance abuse
- Strong feelings of anger and guilt
- Memory disturbances
- Sleeping and eating disorders
- Feelings of dissociation and depersonalization
- Impaired social skills
- Difficulty protecting self
- Vulnerability to revictimization
- Questioning of meaning and purpose of life

Symptoms common to all age groups
- Nightmares
- Depression
- Withdrawn behavior
- Neurotic mental illness
- Aggression
- Regressive behavior
- Sexually inappropriate behavior and promiscuity
- Early onset of menses (average 1 year early)
- School and learning problems
- Inability to trust others
- Ambivalence concerning intimacy and sexuality

Assessment

A wide variety of symptoms, in virtually any combination, may result from sexual abuse (Chart 29–17). The symptoms are manifested differently based on the age of the child (Kendall-Tackett et al., 1993). Guidelines for assessing the child or adolescent who has been sexually abused are discussed earlier in this chapter and in Chapter 30. Children are not given a psychiatric diagnosis when they are assessed immediately following sexual abuse. When children have later behavioral manifestations thought to be related to the abuse, diagnoses are based on the behavioral manifestations. Common diagnoses for children include conduct disorder, major depression, borderline personality disorder, and ODD.

▽ **Alert:** *Children who have been sexually abused must be evaluated for sexually transmitted diseases (STDs). Conversely, if an STD is found in a prepubescent child or a sexually inactive adolescent, one must strongly consider sexual abuse.*

Nursing Diagnoses and Outcomes

In addition to the nursing diagnoses and outcomes presented in Chart 29–5, the following diagnosis may be applicable to the child who has experienced sexual abuse:

- **Rape-trauma syndrome**
  Outcomes: The child expresses feelings about self and traumatic events.
  The child reports feeling safe.
  The child reports or demonstrates behaviors that show an increased ability to cope with psychological consequences of the sexual abuse.

Interdisciplinary Interventions

One of the most profound and tragic results of sexual abuse is the effect on the relationship between the victim and the non-offending parents. Often the non-offending parent has no knowledge of the sexual abuse until the child discloses it. However, this non-offending parent is often treated with contempt and blame by family, friends, and professionals for "allowing" the abuse to continue. Victims may expect that the mother will always protect them from harm. When this does not occur, the victims may direct all their rage at the mother, who, in the child's mind, failed to provide protection. Often, the intensely conflictual feelings of love and hate for the actual perpetrator are too threatening for the child to deal with. In addition, the perpetrator has a tremendous amount of power in the child's mind. It is therefore easier for a child to direct the rage at a less threatening person such as the mother or younger sibling. The mother, in turn, attempts to cope with a dramatic, mysterious, negative change in her child's behavior. Once the abuse is disclosed, although the child's behavior comes to make sense, it is extremely difficult to live with on a daily basis. The mother is also thrown into crisis by the events. Often, overnight, the mother must terminate a significant relationship, perhaps even end a marriage, deal with the stigma of incest, cope with the blame, and deal with the trauma that has occurred to a child. The non-offending parent is often left to deal with this crisis alone, while simultaneously receiving the brunt of the child's anger. Some non-offending parents have some knowledge or suspicion that sexual abuse is occurring. Some even choose to continue to subject their children to known sexual abuse rather than give up their relationship with the perpetrator. However, many parents are unaware of the abuse. Once abuse is disclosed, the perpetrator is removed from the home. The non-offending parent then must struggle alone to meet every need of the family, while attempting to provide the necessary psychiatric care with less time, money, and resources. It is imperative that nurses do not blame the non-offending parents, but rather take a supportive stance.

Ann Burgess' Model of Trauma Therapy is a helpful theoretical framework in the treatment of abused children. This information processing model proposes that traumatic events are processed at the sensory, perceptual, and cognitive levels. The model draws upon the work of Horowitz who suggests that traumatic events remain active until the events can be thoroughly processed and stored (Fig. 29–7).

Phase one of the model, the pretrauma phase, addresses individual characteristics that impact a child's coping with and resolution of a traumatic event. These characteristics include age, developmental level, family structure, sociocultural factors, and prior trauma.

Phase two of the model, the trauma encapsulation phase, consists of input, thruput, and output. Input revolves around the offender's behaviors, such as the relationship, entrapment methods, access, use of force, type of control used, occurrences and sexual activities, and methods of ensuring secrecy. Thruput consists of the coping mechanisms used by the child to deal with the trauma. These include dissociation, denial, fragmentation of self, arousal disharmony (the disruption of the capacity to regulate states of excitement and calmness), repression, and splitting. Output is defined as "the primary trauma learning, which is the charged sensory, perceptual, and cognitive memory base of the event" (Burgess et al., 1997). Sexually abused children begin manifesting signs of anxiety, often by repeating the traumatic events in their play. Burgess calls this trauma replay. Trauma replay manifests in three ways: reenactment, repetition, and displacement. The individual meaning assigned by the child and the cognitive efforts used to mediate the trauma are based on the personal constructs of survival, mastery, and control.

Phase three consists of the disclosure, the reactions to the disclosure, and further trauma resulting from the disclosure. Social responses considered include those from the family, peers, school, and treatment, investigation, and legal agencies and processes. After sexual abuse has finally been disclosed, it is common for victims to be punished, accused of lying, called abusive names such as "whore," blamed for the sexual contact, and told that they either wanted or deserved the sexual abuse for a variety of reasons. This reaction of disbelief to events that the child cannot prove induces further trauma for the child. If the sexual abuse is ever reported, and often it is not, the child undergoes further trauma and extreme embarrassment during the investigation process. The child is asked to reveal profoundly embarrassing details over and over to strangers, often in the presence of the perpetrator. Because a child is a poor historian, and often is poor and inconsistent at sequencing of events, again, the child may not be believed. A reaction of disbelief increases the chance that the child will recant and charges will be dropped. Additionally, the child usually does not have a complete understanding of the full meaning of the sexual abuse. Burgess conceptualizes this phase as becoming aware of the social meaning of the trauma and includes the possibility for secondary trauma impact.

In phase four, Burgess proposes that traumatized children react with six potential behavioral outcome patterns: integrated, anxious, avoidant, disorganized, delinquent, and aggressive. The final phase of the model addresses treatment interventions. First, Burgess recommends "anchoring for safety," which includes establishing a warm, safe, trusting, and sincere relationship with the child to allow the child to reestablish a safe connection with the world. Second, the model proposes that interventions focus on establishing stress-reducing resources. Third, the therapist works with the child to resurface the trauma. The trauma is processed by helping the child unlink past protective mechanisms from current behaviors, because these are no longer necessary and may become dysfunctional after the child is safe. The child is assisted with learning to manage and control memory recall in tolerable doses. The therapist helps the victim to develop anxiety management techniques for use during memory recall. The fourth step of the treatment process is to transfer the processed or integrated trauma to past memory. In this phase of treatment, the therapist assists the child to reduce and categorize the memories to enhance processing. The therapist helps the child organize what is necessary to remember and what can be forgot-

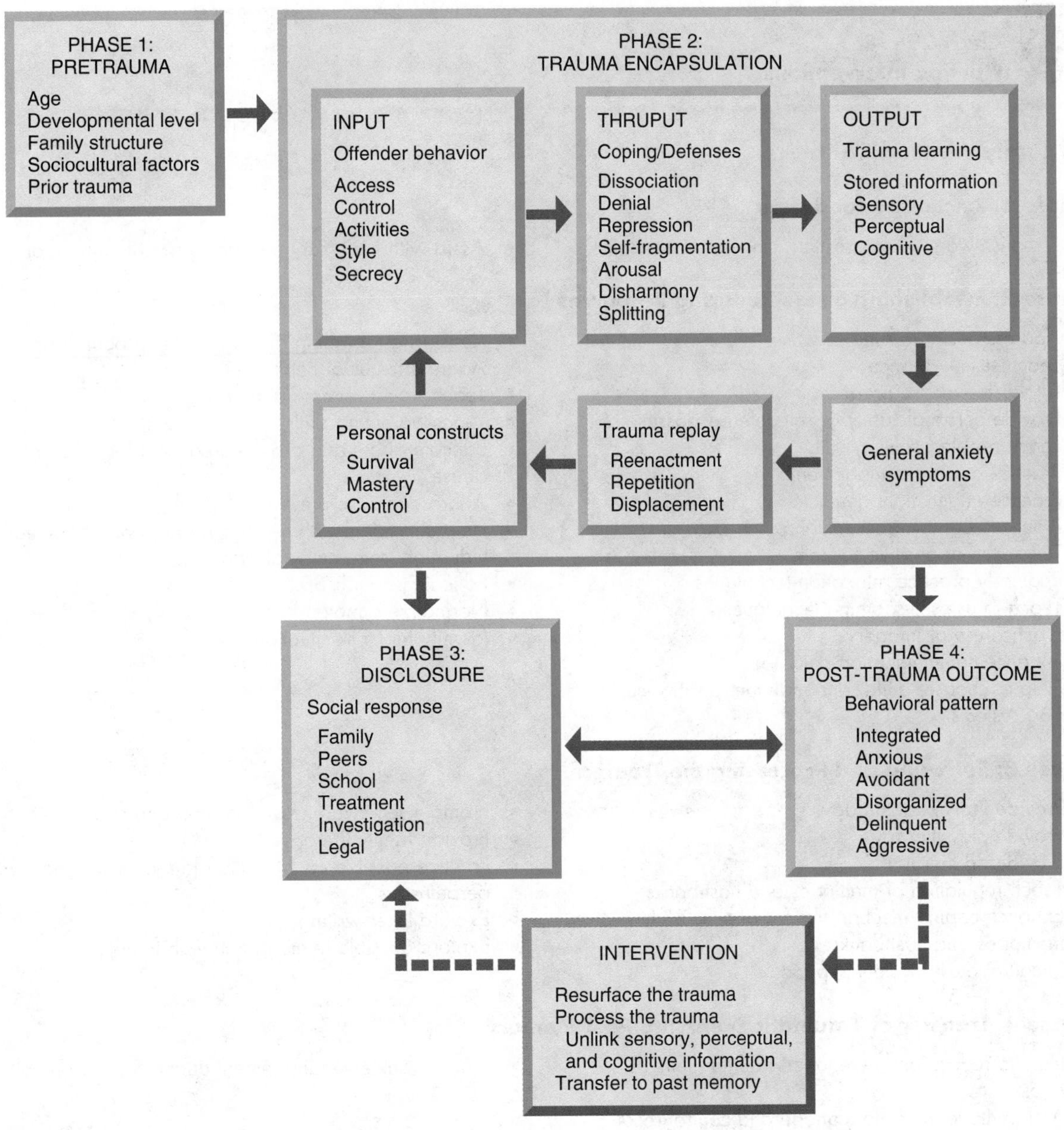

Figure 29–7
Information processing of trauma model. (Redrawn from Burgess, A. [1997]. *Psychiatric nursing: Promoting mental health*. Stamford, CT: Appleton & Lange. Used with permission.)

ten. The therapist also assists the child with accessing memories of the events and managing these memories so that the anxiety levels remain tolerable. The final phase is termination. Specific interventions appropriate for each phase of Burgess' model are listed in Chart 29–18.

Spiritual Abuse

Spiritual abuse is the physical, emotional, or sexual abuse of a person within a religious context, which may lead to long-term emotional or spiritual dysfunction. The perpetrator may be a family member, a member of the clergy, or other church leader or church employee. Spiritual abuse may occur in church-operated preschools, Sunday schools, or church-sponsored youth groups and camps. It is impossible to estimate the incidence and degree of spiritual abuse. The existence of spiritual abuse, although widely acknowledged within mental health fields, is often denied by the general public. Even more controversial is the involvement of children in satanic cults. Children are typically introduced to satanic cults by persons who have some control or authority over the child. Distinct differences exist between spiritual abuse and satanic cult involvement. Spiritual abuse involves coercion and dis-

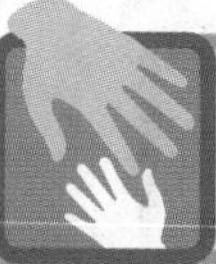

Chart 29–18
Nursing Interventions

Sexually Abused Children

Phase 1: Anchoring for Safety

- Establish warm, safe, trusting, sincere relationship.
- Assist with necessary distancing from family of origin.

Phase 2: Establishing Stress-Reducing Resources

- Address desire to run.
- Teach self-nurturance.
- Establish exercise program.
- Provide personal safety or self-defense classes.
- Teach problem-solving skills.
- Practice anxiety management.
- Practice anger management.
- Practice cognitive restructuring.
- Teach use of positive self-talk.
- Regularly practice relaxation techniques.
- Teach to use self-soothing techniques.
- Practice use of imagery.
- Enhance communication skills.
- Help to choose, build, and maintain positive support systems.
- Assist in establishing and maintaining boundaries.
- Address issues of healthy sexuality.
- Teach assertiveness training.
- Teach parenting skills.
- Educate about and provide treatment for substance abuse.
- Address relapse prevention.
- Help child deal with feelings about separation/individuation from family of origin.
- Educate about PTSD.
- Normalize symptoms and reactions.
- Identify high-risk situations.

Phase 3: Surfacing and Processing the Trauma

- Provide individual therapy.
- Provide play therapy.
- Provide art therapy.
- Teach regulation of memories and flashbacks.
- Enhance coping mechanisms for dealing with memories and flashbacks.
- Encourage use of peer support.
- Promote self-awareness of trauma and stress cues.
- Provide family therapy.
- Practice possible confrontation (direct or indirect) with perpetrators.
- Explore letter writing.
- Explore possible reintegration with family.

Phase 4: Transfer of Traumatic Event into Past Memory

- Help to reduce and categorize trauma memories.
- Assist with learning to manage and control recall of memories.
- Practice anxiety management during memory recall.

Phase 5: Termination

- Review child's reformulation of event.
- Terminate therapeutic relationship.
- Review plans for follow-up.

tortion of truth and responsibility. The satanic cults use mind-control techniques that often involve threats to the child's life or those of pets or family members. A detailed discussion of satanic abuse is beyond the scope of this chapter.

Sexual abuse of children by clergy has been reported frequently and has recently received a great deal of attention by the media. Most parents feel safe in leaving their children for church activities supervised by church leaders believed to be trustworthy. The belief and faith placed in church leaders often grants them absolute control and authority. This leaves a child who is victimized in this setting with few resources upon which to rely for support. It is traumatic enough for a child to accuse someone of sexual abuse, but to accuse a clergy member or other church leader presents an even higher risk (Faller, 1994). Many, if not most, persons in the community refuse to believe that a member of the clergy is capable of such behavior. The result can be that the child is publicly accused of lying and shunned within the community. Although older children may be aware that there is a lack of proof, younger children more often believe that they are at fault. Few children can undergo this amount of pressure, so the child frequently retracts the accusations. The child may then be labeled a liar or troublemaker and may become a scapegoat or be outrightly punished, instead of receiving appropriate intervention.

One of the long-term effects of spiritual abuse is profound disillusionment. These children have great difficulty trusting any religious organization. They may grow up without any of the support, values, and solace that many people find in their faith. They may assume that there is no God, because if there were, God would not have allowed such a thing to happen. These children lose trust in adults and authority figures.

Nursing Diagnoses and Outcomes

In addition to the nursing diagnoses and outcomes presented in Chart 29–5, the following diagnosis is likely to be applicable to the child affected by spiritual abuse:

- **Spiritual distress related to mistrust of religious figures and practices**
  Outcomes: The child or adolescent verbalizes feelings about religious beliefs.
  The child or adolescent identifies areas of personal conflict or ambivalence resulting from the abusive situation.
  The child or adolescent uses coping techniques to deal with spiritual discomfort.

Interdisciplinary Interventions

The most important factor when a child has been abused by a clergy member is for the child's family to believe and support the child. Parents must take into account the child's age and the normal amount of sexual knowledge that a child of his or her age would have. Such children often integrate sexual themes into their play. These children usually need long-term therapy to build enough trust with a therapist to discuss the abuse. It is important for parents to find a therapist who is not a member of the church where the abuse occurred and one who believes the abuse could have occurred. Treatment includes those interventions discussed for sexually abused children as well as interventions with an emphasis on dealing with spiritual issues.

Alterations in Mental Health Due to Disruptions in Life Situations

A number of behavioral adjustment problems may occur in children who experience loss or other traumatic life situations such as natural or manmade disasters, wars, abuse (especially sexual abuse), neglect, or exposure to violence. Continual unabated stress of poverty, homelessness, or family conflict or disintegration may have devastating effects on children or adolescents. They may be genetically vulnerable or physiologically vulnerable (e.g., chronically ill), or they may not have sufficient coping strategies or support to manage the psychological assaults. Many disorders occur as a result of life disruptions; this section addresses only those not previously discussed. Mood disorders and anxiety disorders, although common in abused and neglected children, are discussed previously.

Disruptive Disorders

Adjustment and disruptive disorders are defined as a disturbance in behavior that develops as a result of adverse life circumstances and personal inability to cope with the resulting stress.

Adjustment Disorder

Adjustment disorder is the most frequent reason for children to be referred for mental health services. The essential feature of an adjustment disorder is the presentation of clinically significant emotional or behavioral symptoms within 3 months of an identifiable stressor that overtaxes the individual's coping abilities. Bereavement is not considered to be an adjustment disorder unless it incapacitates the individual beyond 6 months. Stressors may be relocation (new school, new home), family changes (new sibling, parental separation or divorce), or an accomplishment of developmental milestone (starting school, leaving home to go to college). An adjustment disorder of short duration (6 months or less) is of clinical importance, because there is an increased risk for suicide and high potential for academic difficulties. With timely and appropriate intervention (support, understanding, and restabilization of family life), most children recover rapidly. In most children, a more severe disruptive disorder does not develop and the conflict resolves or the child adjusts to the change (Grimes, 1996).

Assessment

Young children often manifest an adjustment disorder by whining and clinging behavior or by increased aggressive behavior or isolation. Children in the elementary school years and in adolescence often manifest adjustment disorders in somatic symptoms (stomach pains, nausea, headaches, fatigue), academic difficulties, or problems in social relationships. An adjustment disorder may be accompanied by anxiety or mood disturbance. Whenever children are seen with the foregoing complaints, and when no physical reason is found for the behavior change, the nurse should investigate changes in the child's life situation. Nursing assessment must include information about the precipitating stressor, its timing and severity, history of any previous alterations in mental health and behavior, and coping strategies. A suicide assessment is essential.

Interdisciplinary Interventions

Interventions that could be helpful are education (helping the youth and his or her family to understand the child's feelings and behaviors) and advocating for reduced stress and resources for the child. Providing family support, facilitating communication about the stressor, and assisting the child in development of effective coping strategies are important interventions for preventing further deterioration. Advocating for classroom changes by helping teachers to understand the reason for the child's behavior can help to relieve additional stress caused by educational pressures. If the child does not recover with brief problem-oriented therapeutic strategies, referral should be made to a mental health clinic.

Selective Mutism

Selective mutism (SM) refers to persistent refusal to speak in certain environments, even though the child has acquired language and verbal skills and knowledge of their use. This uncommon disorder is seen in less than 1% of childhood recipients of mental health care. SM occurs before 5 years of age and may continue for several years. The disorder is most often short-lived but is often not diagnosed until the child enters school. This disorder occurs more frequently in girls. Excessive shyness, fear of social embarrassment, negativism, social isolation, impairment in social functioning, compulsive traits, and oppositional behavior are commonly associated with SM. In a study conducted by Krohn and colleagues (1992), 90% of their 20 strictly diagnosed subjects were rated as highly controlling, negative, or oppositional. The authors also found a high degree of maternal–child enmeshment among the subjects in their study. Left unattended, the disorder has serious implications for the psychosocial development and academic progress for the afflicted child. The disorder creates considerable tension in the parent–child relationship and interferes with development of peer relationships and socialization of the child.

Most children with SM have intelligence within the normal range. They are, however, frequently described as negative, controlling, immature, and manipulative, or as tense and anxious (Krohn et al., 1992). A high incidence of shyness in family members and articulation problems in the selectively mute child have been reported (Krohn et al., 1992). The most recent view of SM considers it to have multifactorial causes with anxiety as the catalytic agent (Donnelly et al., 1996).

Assessment

Determination of a consistent failure to speak in specific social situations while having the ability to speak is a central component in the assessment of children referred for SM. Assessment of the children with SM should include a complete physical examination, with special emphasis on the neurologic component. The neurologic and development history should focus on developmental milestones of motor (gross, fine motor), language, speech, social, and cognitive development. Additional important information should be obtained regarding the child's temperament, quality of social interactions, context in which speech occurs or does not occur, and the presence of recent or current trauma or severe stress.

Worldview: *Cultural variables such as language spoken at home, rigid admonishments to not talk in public or to strangers, recent immigration, or shyness should not be mistaken for SM.*

Children with pervasive developmental disorders, who speak only at home or under duress, should not receive a diagnosis of SM. If an anxiety disorder is comorbid, the disorder should be treated first, because SM may disappear spontaneously with relief of the anxiety. SM does not imply that the child has been abused (Donnelly et al., 1996).

Interdisciplinary Interventions

The behavioral management approach combined with empathy, parental cooperation, and liaison with the school is the most effective treatment approach (Krohn et al., 1992). The treatment may be carried out by any number of professionals skilled in behavior management (e.g., psychiatric nurse, social worker, psychiatrist). The behavioral management plan requires intensive work with the child, parent, and school (Chart 29–19). Medications have not proven helpful in treatment of SM except when an anxiety disorder is the underlying problem, the disorder is of long duration or debilitating, or there is failure of behavior and cognitive interventions (Black & Uhde, 1994; Donnelly et al., 1996).

Oppositional Defiant Disorder

ODD is defined as a pattern of negative, resistant, and hostile behavior. It is usually manifested after early childhood and before puberty. However, some of the behav-

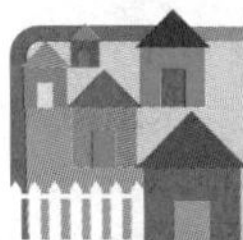

Chart 29–19
Community Care

Behavior Management Program for Selective Mutism of 1 Week to 1 Month's Duration (Children 3 to 6 Years of Age)

- Parent assesses child's favorite food, activity, or toy that, when taken away, can be used as a reward to encourage child to speak.
- Parent explains to the child that it is very important to talk and that he or she will be expected to say at least one word (of child's choosing) before the treasured activity, food, or toy is returned to the child.
- Parent tells the child that he or she will be given food and water to eat but will not be given dessert or opportunity to play with a favorite toy or watch television until child makes a verbal request (at least one word).
- Parent must consistently refuse the child's request to engage in the reward behavior/activity until the child speaks.
- When food is served, parent should request child to speak, for example, to say "thank you" or anything else the child wishes to say.
- When child complies with request to speak, a reward of child's choosing (favorite activity or food) must be granted.
- After obtaining at least one utterance, requirements for verbal expression should be gradually increased.
- If this plan is tried for 3 to 5 days but does not produce a verbal response, a referral to a mental health professional skilled in therapeutic behavior management should be requested.

iors are seen in the preschool years. It often develops gradually, with increasing expression of defiance, negativism, argumentativeness, loss of temper, and hostility. In the prepubertal years, the disorder is more common in boys, but equal gender prevalence is seen in adolescence. The prevalence of ODD and conduct disorders is estimated at 1.7% to 10% of the school-age population, and it comprises approximately one third of all psychiatric disorders in American youth (Wood, 1996). ODD is a predictor for development of a later diagnosis of conduct disorder, with physical aggression behaviors in ODD as the best predictor.

Causative factors, or factors with a strong correlation to ODD, are temperament, abusive treatment, and coping strategies (e.g., projection, denial of own feelings, pain, hurt, or sadness). This disorder is also frequently comorbid with depression and dysthymia. In most cases, when the disorder is not combined with other conditions, conduct disorder does not develop (Wood, 1996).

Assessment

To be given the diagnosis of ODD, the child must exhibit at least four of the following behaviors for at least 6 months:

- Often loses temper
- Often argues with adults
- Often actively defies or refuses to comply with adults' requests or rules
- Often deliberately annoys people
- Often blames others for his or her mistakes or misbehavior
- Is often touchy or easily annoyed by others
- Is often angry and resentful
- Is often spiteful or vindictive

When analyzing and synthesizing the assessment data, it is important to consider the developmental status of the child and what among the exhibited behaviors and concerns are considered normal for the child's age.

Children with ODD should be evaluated for depression. The underlying problem may be continuous unmanageable life stresses and multiple losses. Dysthymia or depressive traits may mimic ODD. Oppositional disorder is also strongly associated with anxiety disorders. Mismanagement and lack of recognition of the underlying problems may lead to the development of ODD (Wood, 1996).

Interdisciplinary Interventions

There are many potential outcomes for children with ODD. In many cases, without early and effective treatment of ODD, a conduct disorder develops, and even criminal behavior may develop, resulting in incarceration. Other less severe problems are academic difficulties or failure, and continuous peer conflict, which may result in injury. Parents often react with increasingly rigid and authoritarian behavior, and the control between parent and child becomes stronger and more detrimental. Inpatient hospitalization may be recommended to break the cycle of control. These children often create enough family stress that treatment is sought; however, family conflicts caused by the child's behavior could be precipitating agents in parental separation and divorce. Therapeutic foster home placement or a residential facility may be necessary to relieve family stress.

Interdisciplinary intervention for ODD may include medication. Many children show some improvement in mood when given an SSRI (see Table 29–2). Problem-solving therapy with a mental health therapist is recommended. Nursing therapy includes working with the child and family to improve communication, problem-solving, and negotiation skills. Group therapy designed to develop listening, open communication, problem-solving, and perspective-taking skills is beneficial in helping these children to express themselves in more appropriate ways. Therapeutic communication and therapeutic behavior management are helpful in decreasing resistance and stubborn refusal to engage in or complete expected activities (see earlier section on Behavior Management). Nurses should instruct parents in the therapeutic management strategies for communicating and negotiating with their child with ODD. School interventions include providing teachers with information about the disorder and therapeutic behavior management techniques. Other appropriate interventions include counseling and group therapy.

Conduct Disorder

Conduct disorders are the most prominent reason for children to be referred for mental health care. Conduct disorder refers to persistent and repetitive patterns of behavior in which the rights of others are ignored, and social norms and rules are violated. Anxiety and feelings are externalized and result in harmful behavior toward others. The behavior may be observed in a variety of settings (home, school, community) and in a variety of interactions. For example, the child may act aggressively with the interviewer while actually denying his or her aggressive behavior, generally. These children tend to scapegoat others, initiate fights, and often use dangerous objects (sticks, hard objects, broken glass, knives, or guns). Their behavior may involve stealing, setting fires or otherwise destroying property, rape, assault, and, in its severest form, homicide. Lying, deceitfulness, and a lack of accountability for their behavior are characteristic of such children.

Worldview: *The culture and circumstances in which a child lives has enormous implications for development of conduct disorder. Children living in high poverty and crime-ridden areas, whose family structure is chaotic, and who experience multiple losses are especially likely to develop conduct disorder behavior.*

Actual etiologic factors are unknown, but one of the most frequently cited characteristics of children with conduct disorder is temperament (the habitual style of reaction to situations). Other risk factors include parental factors (mental illness, criminal behavior, or conduct disorder behavior), parental abusive and coercive behavior toward the child, learning disability or ADHD, substance abuse, intrauterine insults, neurologic impairment or injury, and frequent observance of crime or domestic violence, especially abuse of mother.

The incidence of conduct disorder varies by gender and age. The range for male children (including adolescents) is 6% to 16%. For girls, the range is 2% to 9%. There also appears to be two developmental pathways, one beginning in childhood and one in adolescence. Most children with adolescent onset have a good chance of becoming responsible and productive adults (Wood, 1996).

Assessment

Assessment of the youth with conduct disorder is complex. A physical examination, including a neurologic examination, is recommended. The focused health history should include the data as outlined in Chart 29–3. In addition, several other areas should be addressed, such as the child's possible involvement in gangs, cults, or unlawful behavior and previous involvement with law and justice systems. Questions regarding the child's involvement in sexual behavior—coercive or noncoercive—and childhood sexual abuse perpetrated by another are also important elements of conduct disorder assessment. The types of acts committed and the situational context of the behavior (e.g., being involved with a gang or older group involved in crime, response to abusive behavior) should be clearly defined. Children with conduct disorders may have a previous or current diagnosis of LD, ADHD, or ODD. The child should be assessed for depression, suicidal or high-risk (self-harm) behaviors, and the intent or thought of bringing harm to others.

Conduct disorder must be differentiated from aggressive episodes caused by psychomotor seizures, brain injury, and PTSD. The aggressive outbursts occurring in these disorders are random and spontaneous. Conduct disorder is also not "delinquency." Delinquency implies committing criminal or illegal acts. It is a legal term, whereas "conduct disorder" is a diagnostic term. The behavior of the individual being assessed may indeed include acts that are illegal. The acts committed may include aggression to people and animals, destruction of property, deceitfulness or theft, or serious violation of rules established in the home or by the school system. The behavior associated with conduct disorder must be present for 12 months before the diagnosis can be confirmed.

Interdisciplinary Interventions

Interventions for children with conduct disorder include individual therapy, milieu therapy, recreational therapy, group therapy, family therapy, and social skills therapy. In some severe cases, the child may be placed in a special classroom where behavior can be more easily contained. A primary goal is to ensure that such children no longer harm others or seek to harm themselves. All potentially harmful objects should be removed from the child's environment.

Alert: *Conduct disordered youth who have comorbid depression are at very high risk for suicide. Suicide precautions should be implemented.*

In the inpatient setting, the child should be placed in a secure environment to prevent the child from running away. A behavioral management contract is developed with the child that includes safety expectations and sanctions for violations of these expectations. Pharmacologic interventions may be used to control excessive violence or to treat underlying depression.

To assist children in reducing feelings of anger and rage, therapy focuses on teaching new problem-solving and stress management techniques. Children must learn to reinterpret the behaviors of others and to ask questions to clarify the intent of others' behaviors to reduce their own feelings of threat or harm. Feelings of inadequacy potentiate the aggressive behavior. Therefore, children must learn to interact with others in nondefensive ways. Additionally, children are encouraged to have a realistic view of themselves and accept responsibility for their own behaviors. Group therapy can be used to focus on the communication skills of listening, reflecting, giving and receiving feedback, sharing feelings, expressing needs, and expressing desires in an assertive manner (Chart 29–20).

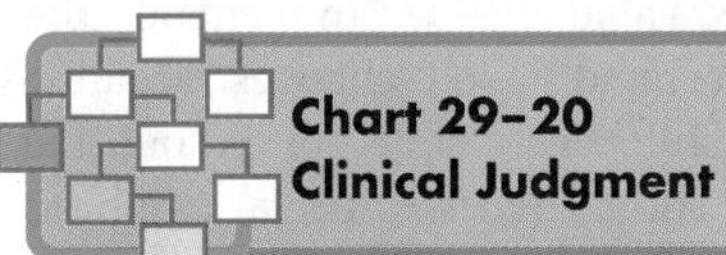

Chart 29–20
Clinical Judgment

The Child with a Conduct Disorder

Nancy is 13 years old and has a history of sexual abuse at 7 years of age. The perpetrator was 14 at the time and the sexual abuse occurred over several months. Nancy is the oldest of two siblings. Her mother and father are divorced, and she lives with her mother. Her father was injured in a hunting accident 3 years ago and has been paraplegic since the accident. He wants to return home to live with his ex-wife and children. Nancy was referred by the school counselor to the Community Mental Health Center when she was 9 years old. She was seen three times and was then enrolled in an after-school learning improvement program by her mother. From the time Nancy was 9 through 13, she had five inpatient psychiatric hospitalizations for behavior problems. Nancy was recently admitted to the state hospital youth unit. She was expelled from school because of repeated assaults on younger children, persistently destroying books and papers of other students (which she denied), and finally because of physically assaulting one of her teachers. Nancy's mother reported that, over the past year, Nancy had killed her younger brother's two rabbits, deliberately broke several objects at home when enraged, and repeatedly stolen money from her mother and brother. Most recently, her mother had found a stash of sharp knives, a baseball bat, and bullets (no gun) under Nancy's bed. Nancy's mother said that she was totally unable to control Nancy and said, "I hope you find a place for her where everyone will be safe from her." Nancy's mother has been treated for depression for the past 6 years. She compared Nancy to Nancy's father, saying, "She just doesn't care who or what she hurts, just like her father."

Questions

1. Is Nancy's family at risk for violence at this time?
2. Which of Nancy's behaviors indicate a conduct disorder?
3. What goal must take first priority at this time?
4. What nursing interventions will assist Nancy and her family in meeting this goal?
5. During therapy, what should be the outcomes for the behaviors displayed by Nancy?

Answers

1. Yes. Nancy has the potential to harm a family member.
2. She often bullies, threatens, or intimidates others; she often initiates physical fights; she has been physically cruel to animals; she has deliberately destroyed others' property; she has stolen items of nontrivial value without confronting a victim.
3. Ensure the safety of others.
4. Teach Nancy conflict resolution skills; help Nancy practice appropriate expression of anger; routinely assess and remove potential weapons from the environment and the patient; work with patient to improve self-esteem.
5. Positive rewards should be given for positive behaviors; developmentally appropriate consequences should be given for negative behavior.

Personality Disorders

Borderline and Dissociative Disorder of Childhood

Borderline and dissociative disorders are characterized by instability in mood states, relationships, and self-perception. The mood state changes of persons with borderline or dissociative disorder are rapid and unpredictable. Both disorders are strongly associated with childhood and adolescent sexual abuse.

Etiology and Incidence

The disorders are most often diagnosed in the adolescent or young adult years. It is estimated that 2.5% to 5% of children in the United States are at risk for development of a personality disorder. No accurate statistics are available on the actual prevalence due to the confusion in diagnosing the disorders (Ross, 1996). Self-injurious behaviors, such as cutting and scraping skin, and high-risk behaviors such as substance abuse and sexual acting out, are seen in most cases (Table 29–5). These high-risk behaviors make the child more susceptible to further victimization. Children or adolescents with dissociative disorder are poorly understood by most persons who come in contact with them, and they are often accused of lying and being untrustworthy. Some adults often believe the child deserves the abuse that they are so often defending against, because of their strange, incomprehensible behavior.

Assessment

The features of borderline and dissociative disorders are difficult to identify (see Table 29–5). In general, the nurse should observe for rapid mood changes, seeming inattention, and rapid shifts in details of recounting events. Other areas that should receive special emphasis

Table 29–5
Risk Factors and Characteristics of Dissociative and Borderline Disorders of Childhood and Adolescence

Dissociative Disorder	Borderline Disorder
Risk factors	
Children of convicted sexual offenders Dissociative disorder in parent Children in care of child protective services Involvement in pornography Adolescent runaways Sexual promiscuity Homelessness Serious drug and alcohol abuse Early and painful sexual trauma Unpredictable parent behaviors coupled with highly abusive disciplines	Family history Disturbance in relationship, especially at separation Individuation stage Chaotic, dysfunctional family lifestyle Abuse—physical, psychological, and sexual Mental illness in parent
Characteristics	
Restlessness, difficulty concentrating Complaints of psychosomatic pain Mood swings Binge eating Suicidal and self-mutilating behaviors Episodic rages Episodic psychotic symptoms Lying, stealing Running away Use of aliases Seeming lack of guilt Changes in handwriting, maturity, style Blocking, illogical thought processes Frequent imaginary companions	Under stress, there is rapid decline in thinking, ability to control emotions, and reality testing and behavior Extreme vulnerability to stress Severe separation anxiety Tendency to withdraw from relationships Easily frustrated and exhibits extremes of rage and sadness with loss of control Complaints of psychosomatic pain Suicidal and self-multilating behaviors Extremes of fantasy (fantasy rages, self-abuse) Lack of boundaries Manipulates staff against each other Inappropriate, intense relationship

in suspicion of a dissociative disorder or borderline disorder include any history of amnesia, self-harm behaviors, abuse, substance use, or high-risk behaviors. The child should be observed for regressive states that cause the child to appear younger, such as voice changes or changes in the quality of speech making the child sound much younger.

Children are generally not given the diagnosis of a personality disorder. Personality is usually left out of the diagnosis because personality development of children and adolescents is not finalized (Lewis, 1994). For example, dissociative disorder of childhood is substituted for dissociative personality disorder (Lewis, 1994). Dissociative and borderline are the most frequently used categories for children (Wagner, 1995). To diagnose any "personality" disorder in individuals before the age of 18, the characteristics must be present for at least 1 year. Antisocial personality disorder is not used as a diagnosis in children younger than age 18. Rather, conduct disorder is the recommended diagnosis (Lewis, 1994). Children at varying stages of development manifest behaviors characteristic of normal growth and development that also are features of a personality disorder. Only when the behaviors persist and interfere with the developmental process and social well-being are they then applied to a diagnosis.

Interdisciplinary Interventions

Adolescents with severe borderline disorders are best served in inpatient settings. A variety of interventions can and should be used. If abuse is a causative factor, this must be reported immediately. The therapist must fulfill his or her legal obligation to ensure the future safety of the child. The second most important intervention is for the therapist to develop a trusting relationship with the client to provide appropriate feedback and interventions. Components of the inpatient treatment program that should be used with borderline and dissociative clients are a therapeutic behavior management program, group therapy, social skills training, recreational therapy, and participation in special education until discharged. Individual therapy should not be used as the primary or only mode of therapy because intimacy is much too threatening. The conflictual needs of the client with personality disorder are difficult to manage in the individual relationship, thus group therapy is recommended in addition to individual therapy.

Nurses need to develop an accepting, open approach to the youth with personality disorder. Safety precautions are imperative, because these children will use almost anything for self-harm when they are in a state of upset or feeling empty or "dead." Examples of potential weapons include pencils, erasers, sharp pieces of plastic, metal, or glass and objects that may cause burns, such as matches or curling irons. The "dead" feeling is related to numbing of painful feelings and intrusive memories or images.

Rules must be clearly explained and be firmly yet empathetically adhered to. Unreasonable demands and expectations need to be responded to truthfully and realistically. These children often use abusive language and manipulation when realistic limits are set and reinforced. The nurse needs to remain calm but firm in her insistence on appropriate behavior and adherence to rules established for the unit and the individual client (Wagner, 1995).

Physiologic and Somatic Disorders

Sleep Disorders

Multiple sleep problems have been identified in children, but only three are considered to be psychiatric disorders (Chart 29–21):

- Nightmare disorder
- Sleep terror disorder
- Sleepwalking (Dahl, 1996)

Sleep disruptions are common in all children ages 3 to 7 years of age and may include episodes of nightmares, sleep terrors, or sleepwalking. With reassurance, appropriate bedtime activities (reading, quiet discussions), and comforting strategies by parents, most episodes last only a short while. (See Chapter 5 for a summary of normal sleeping patterns of children of all ages.) Sleep distur-

Chart 29–21

Types of Sleep Disorders

Sleep disruptions—Unusual nighttime awakenings occur frequently, with no immediately known or observable cause (nightmares, sleep terror, sleepwalking, confusion, and arousal).

Nightmares—Child wakes during deep sleep, is frightened but alert, and is able to report on what was frightening and usually has difficulty returning to sleep. Nightmares occur in approximately 10% of children 3 to 6 years of age.

Sleep terror—Episodes occur usually after 1 to 2 hours of sleep; the child or adolescent looks terrified and very agitated. This form of sleep disruption is not remembered by the child. Sleep terrors are a developmental variable and not caused by anxiety or undue stress.

Sleepwalking—The individual walks about while asleep. Sleepwalking usually occurs during the first part of the sleep cycle. Sleepwalking may be calm or agitated.

bances usually erupt after times of high stress in the family or the child's daily routine, a frightening situation, or when self-expectations or parental expectations for the child have increased. From age 3 to 7, children learn new skills rapidly. While the child can take pride in new accomplishments, expectations are increased as well, thus they have the "stress" of success. Children of this age do not always have the language to express their feelings and worries, and parents may not always find the time for quiet nurturing activities (e.g., reading, singing, talking, holding, or cuddling) before bedtime. For these reasons, the feelings and thoughts may spill over during sleep in the form of the various sleep disturbances. The prevalence of sleep disorders is estimated at 2% to 5%, but in otherwise disturbed children the prevalence is much higher (Grimes, 1996). Sleep disorders are most common in children with ADHD, depression, anxiety disorders, Tourette's syndrome, and autism (Dahl, 1996). Whereas dream disturbances (nightmares and sleep terrors) tend to arise as a result of frightening experiences and unresolved conflicts, sleepwalking appears to have a genetic component. Approximately 80% of sleepwalkers have a family history of sleepwalking (Grimes, 1996).

Assessment

Assessment of complaints about sleep disturbances must take into consideration the overall health of the child and the child's developmental status. Daily activities, bedtime routines, and a description of the sleep environment should be documented. It is important to elicit the parent's perception of the child's sleep disturbance and the impact this has on family life. The nurse should obtain a thorough description of the sleep disturbance, including any precipitating events, the length of time the disturbance has been occurring, the frequency of the occurrence, and any interventions used and their success. The diagnosis of a sleep disorder is made when the precipitating event has passed and usual interventions to promote sleep have been tried for at least 1 month but have failed to bring about a change. Any other physical or mental health conditions should be noted.

Interdisciplinary Interventions

Education to promote understanding of the disorder and its management is helpful for the parents and the child. Safety factors in the home of the sleepwalker should be identified and modified if warranted. For instance, the home should be secured such that the child may not easily leave the house, items that the child may run into or easily break should be relocated. Discussion of frightening events or distressing daily events and the feelings aroused by them may help decrease nightmares and sleep terror disorder. Spending time with the child at bedtime (singing, reading, quietly talking) may help the child relax and sleep more restfully. The child needs reassurance that parents are available during the night to provide support, give reassurance, and help the child relax.

If the child is experiencing anger, frustration, or anxiety as a result of other underlying problems such as difficulty in school, family disruptions or parental conflict, recent or current trauma (e.g., such as sexual abuse), or anticipated trauma (e.g., anticipated loss of parent, punishment for wrongdoing, or recurrence of some tragedy), the underlying problem needs to be sorted out and addressed.

Parents often allow children with sleep problems to sleep with them. It is best to discourage this intervention. It reinforces the child's idea that the child is unable to master the problem. It also may (and usually does) give the message to the child that the parent is "frightened," unable to solve the problem, and perhaps needs to rely on the child (Grimes, 1996).

Other techniques that are helpful to prevent and treat sleeping disorders are

- Leaving a night-light on
- Leaving the child's bedroom door open
- Providing the child with a comforting blanket or stuffed animal
- Avoiding excessive anger and abusive discipline
- Setting realistic limits during the day
- Rewarding the child for success
- Keeping expectations reasonable

Stuffed animals presented as a protector for the child may be helpful when a frightening experience has occurred and seems to be a precipitating factor. When the problem persists and the dreams do not abate, consultation with a psychiatrist, clinical nurse specialist, or other mental health professional should be sought. Play therapy or other interventions may be needed to address the problem.

Alterations in Elimination

Enuresis is the frequent or continued voiding in one's pants or bed after age 5 years. Encopresis refers to the soiling of clothing with bowel movements or the deposition of them in inappropriate places. The child must be at least 4 years old and must have at least one incident a month for 3 months.

Incidence

Elimination disorders are common problems in children. Approximately one in five children continues to wet (enuresis) the bed at night. The continued prevalence rate for enuresis (nighttime and daytime) is estimated at 7% for boys and 3% for girls at age 5. The prevalence of encopresis at the same age is approximately 1%, with more boys than girls being affected. Primary enuresis or encopresis is not diagnosed until the child is 5 years or 4 years, respectively, and has never been consistently continent. Children who begin to void in their pants or in their bed after an established period of dryness are given the diagnosis of secondary enuresis (Grimes, 1996).

Elimination disorders should be addressed by the time the child has reached the age of 5. The child and parents are usually feeling ashamed and guilty. These disorders may arouse considerable feelings of frustration and failure in parents and of conflict between the parents and child (Waszak, 1992). In some cases, the soiling is deliberate, in which case the diagnosis may include ODD.

Etiology

Precipitating or causative factors for encopresis may include constipation, lactose intolerance, inadequate or inappropriate training, anxiety, or ODD. Physical health factors may also be involved in the development of encopresis. Physical factors may include dehydration, hypothyroidism, or the side effect of medication. When constipation is the cause, encopresis is caused by pressure and an inability of the child to control defecation. Genetic vulnerability may be implicated in primary enuresis in that 75% of enuretic children have a first-degree relative who had the disorder. Secondary enuresis and encopresis are strongly associated with family or psychological distress (Grimes, 1996). See Chapter 19 for further discussion of enuresis.

Assessment

The age of the child is especially important when parents complain of bed-wetting. Nighttime wetting is common, especially in boys up to 6 to 7 years of age. For some children, it occurs until early adolescence, then spontaneously remits (Grimes, 1996). Often the child becomes embarrassed and makes a special effort to control bedwetting, but this may not be a satisfactory answer for most mothers who are not anxious to wash bedclothes every day. Daytime wetting after the early school years (8 to 9 years) is likely to result from physical causes or be related to severe psychopathology or developmental delay (Grimes, 1996).

Special assessment needs for both disorders include physical examination, history and pattern of the problem, and assessment of the home environment, current and recent past stressors, and changes in the family (new sibling, divorce) and family functioning (chaos, conflict, violence). The context in which the altered elimination happens and the surrounding factors must be assessed. It is important to also assess what interventions have been tried, including the family's own interventions (Waszak, 1992). Disciplinary and control issues between the parent and child should be evaluated. Parents should summarize the toilet training process that occurred with the child. To rule out other physiologic causes of enuresis or encopresis, other factors should be investigated, including the possibility of sexual abuse, urinary tract infections, complaints of pain on urination or defecation, constipation, or the presence of stools that are of an abnormal color, smell, or shape. It is important to obtain an accurate description and history of the problem. Soiling caused by rushing and inadequate hygiene should be differentiated from true encopresis.

Interdisciplinary Interventions

Interventions for encopresis and enuresis include behavioral programs such as reinforcement, contracting, and self-monitoring. Other treatments include patient and family education, family therapy, and self-esteem building therapy. Pharmacologic intervention may also be used, but usually not as the first line of treatment. Limited research is available on interventions, but existing research provides support for the use of behavioral and medical interventions (Butler, Brewin, & Forsythe, 1988; Houts & Peterson, 1986). Expected outcomes should include achievement of elimination (voiding and bowel movements) in the appropriate place and in sufficient time to prevent soiling or wetting of clothes or bed.

Eating Disorders

Eating disorders refers to a complex group of disorders, including anorexia and bulimia. **Anorexia** is the refusal to eat sufficient food to maintain normal weight. **Bulimia** is binge eating of large amounts of food followed by forced vomiting. Eating problems are common among infants, children, and adolescents. Lewis (1993) reports that 25% of referred children and adolescents have a diagnosable eating disorder, for which they should receive health care services. Eating disorders develop in more girls than boys, and eating disorders are more common among white females, although an increase has been noted in black females and white males (Wozniak & Herzog, 1993). Anorexia occurs in approximately 1% of adolescent girls. Bulimia occurs at a slightly higher rate in adolescent girls and in up to 4% in upper socioeconomic young women (Fig. 29–8). Approximately 1 in 20 persons with an eating disorder is male (Waller, 1996).

Etiology

Risk factors associated with eating disorders are family dysfunction (enmeshment or chaos), sexual abuse, and being adolescent and female. Genetic vulnerability is suspected as one potential cause. One large study of bulimic individuals found a higher concordance rate in monozygotic twins, increased risk for dizygotic twins, and a 10% risk rate for first-degree relatives, compared with a risk factor of 4% in control subjects (Kassett, Gershon, & Maxwell, 1989). Psychological factors contributing to risk include perfectionist personality, distorted body image

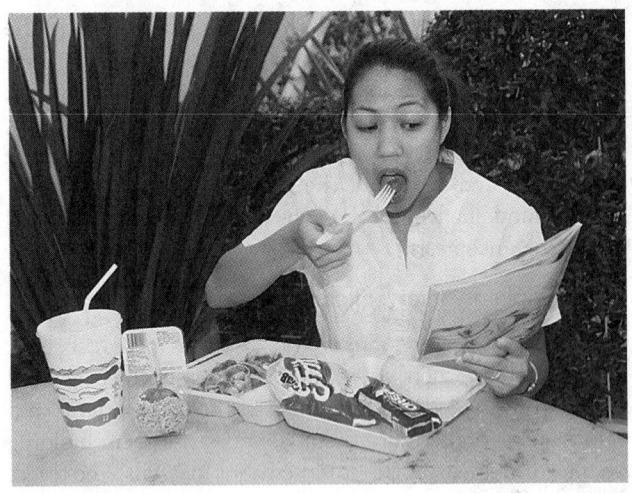

Figure 29–8
The adolescent with bulimia eats a large meal, then forces herself to vomit what she ate.

(perception of being fat), and low self-esteem. Anorectic individuals display isolation tendencies, whereas bulimic individuals tend to have an extroverted personality type. Most bulimic individuals are seen late in their disease because they are able to hide their behavior as well as maintain more normal weight. Anorectic individuals are noticeable because of their failure to eat and their extreme weight loss. However, they may become quite skillful at hiding the weight loss under baggy, oversized clothes. Eating disorders contribute to profound metabolic disturbances in addition to weight loss. Potential physical disturbances may include growth failure, cognitive deficits, and dwarfism in young children.

Assessment

Signs of anorexia include delayed puberty, short stature, bradycardia, cardiomyopathy, osteoporosis, hair loss, and death if the disorder is not abated. In bulimia, individu-

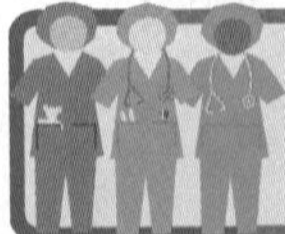

Care Path 29–2 An Interdisciplinary Plan of Care for the Child with Anorexia

Nursing Diagnosis	Patient/Family Intermediate Outcomes			
	Day 1	Day 2	Day 3	Day 4
Alteration in nutrition less than body requirements related to eating deficit and excessive exercise	Child will agree to target weight to be reached at end of 1 month. Child will verbalize willingness to follow diet to reach target weight.	Child will follow contract.	→ Child's weight is stabilized.	→ →
Knowledge deficit: adequate nutritional needs	Child will verbalize elements of sound nutritional diet.	→	Child will verbalize knowledge of nutritional needs and body requirements.	→
Body image disturbance related to inaccurate messages (self and others)	Child will verbalize statements/beliefs about body image.	Child will engage in self-talk statements that are positive about normal weight.	→	Child will verbalize positive self-statements related to normal weight and self-uniqueness.
Impaired social interactions	Child will agree to participate in group therapy.	Child will participate in group therapy.	→	→

als display significant alterations in health status, including sore throat, abdominal pain, nausea, constipation, and destruction of dental enamel (Wozniak & Herzog, 1993). The child's current weight should be noted and a history elicited of the child's weight gain and loss patterns. It is important to ask such children about their diet and what methods they have used to monitor their weight. Children should also be asked about their perception of their body image and their motivation for being thin (Deering, 1992). The assessment in cases of bulimia should include the history of eating (how much, how often) and the compensatory behaviors used to maintain weight. The feelings associated with the behavior are important in making the diagnosis; they involve craving and inability to control eating and purging (forced vomiting).

A complete physical examination should be conducted with an emphasis on noting the child's skin turgor, condition of the hair, teeth, and mucous membranes, menstrual history, and Tanner staging (see Chapter 4). On physical examination, gingivitis, parotid gland enlargement, and callused and irritated knuckles may be noted. Depression is often a comorbid condition of both anorexia and bulimia. Amenorrhea is found in approximately 30% to 65% of cases (Wozniak & Herzog, 1993). Laboratory investigations are indicated to rule out other causes of weight loss, particularly when the obsession of being thin is not present (Wachsmuth & Garfinkel, 1993).

All children with eating disorders need a psychiatric assessment and a family system assessment to determine personal, interpersonal, and social factors contributing to the disorders. Assessment of the family's parenting style (e.g., values, discipline, nurturance, communication, and the parents' perception of the problem) provides important data for treatment planning. Assessment for previous or ongoing abuse is an essential component of the psychiatric examination.

It is possible that other factors may be responsible for the weight loss in anorexia. If the characteristic desire of "thinness" and irrational body image of "fat" are not present, other possible causes need to be explored. These include depression and physical disorders such as Addison's disease, Crohn's disease, or brain tumors (Wood, 1996).

Nursing Diagnoses and Outcomes

In addition to the nursing diagnoses presented in Chart 29–5, the following nursing diagnoses may be used to guide care interventions for the child or adolescent with an eating disorder:

- **Body image disturbance related to an eating disorder**
  Outcomes: The child or adolescent expresses feelings associated with food, exercise, weight loss, and medical condition.
  The child or adolescent participates in an eating disorder intervention program.
  The child or adolescent expresses positive feelings about self.
- **Oral mucous membrane alteration related to poor nutritional status**
  Outcomes: Integrity of oral mucous membranes remains intact.
  The child or adolescent demonstrates good oral hygiene practices.

Interdisciplinary Interventions

Treatment of eating disorders involves multimodal therapy to attend to the child's physical, social, and interpersonal needs, which are affected by the eating disorder (Care Path 29–2). A primary goal is restoration of

Days 5–6	Follow-up/ post discharge
→	→
Child will gain 1 pound before discharge.	
Child will discuss any further concerns or misinformation regarding nutrition.	→
→	→
→	Child will continue group therapy twice a week until target weight is achieved.

Care Path continued on following page

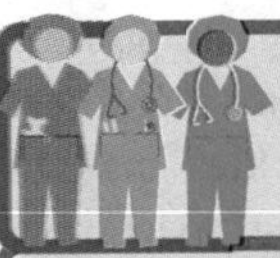

Care Path 29–2 An Interdisciplinary Plan of Care for the Child with Anorexia *Continued*

Nursing Diagnosis	Patient/Family Intermediate Outcomes			
	Day 1	Day 2	Day 3	Day 4
Potential for noncompliance: contract for target weight	Child will adhere to contract.	→	→	→
	Child will not hide food.	→	→	→
	Child will not engage in excessive activity.	→	→	→
Care Intervention Categories				
Consults	Psychiatry Nutrition Social work Advanced practice nurse (APN)	School liaison		Family physician
Discharge planning		Evaluate family community and school resources. Coordinate care with school liaison.		Coordinate care with family physician and outpatient services.
Labs	CBC Electrolytes			
Monitors	Rest, exercise, and eating record	→	→	→
Nutrition/exercise and rest	Contract formulated regarding diet, exercise, and rest.	Contract followed.	→	→
	Monitor rest periods and adherence to contract.	→	→	→
	Nursing assistant stays with child during mealtimes and snacks.	→	→	→
	Obtain agreement not to hide food.			
Group therapy	Discussion of group therapy and purpose. Obtain agreement to participate.	Begin group therapy.	→	→

Days 5–6	Follow-up/ post discharge
⟶	⟶
⟶	⟶
⟶	⟶
	Primary physician 1 week after discharge
⟶	
⟶ ⟶ ⟶	⟶
⟶	Group therapy two times a week

Care Path continued on following page

weight and reversal of physical signs and symptoms of fluid, electrolyte, and nutritional imbalances. Early treatment may involve hospitalization when weight loss of more than 25% of desired body weight for height occurs or when the child exhibits symptoms that require aggressive medical attention (e.g., anemia, esophageal bleeding, ulcers). Psychopharmacologic interventions have not been helpful in clinical trials but are continuing to be researched (Wachsmuth & Garfinkel, 1993).

The health care team works with the child and family to develop appropriate weight maintenance strategies and to improve the child's eating behaviors. Nursing interventions involve dietary management, providing support to address the child's fear of excessive weight gain, monitoring weight, and providing behavior management to prevent purging behavior and maintenance of the plan of care (Chart 29–22). The nurse also monitors adherence to the activity schedule (Potts, 1995).

Psychiatric referral is strongly recommended to address cognitive distortions related to food and body image and to improve the child's social functioning skills. Directive and active individual therapy, family therapy, behavior therapy, and group therapy are all recommended as interventions. Individual therapy is often provided by an advanced practice psychiatric nurse. Psychoanalytic therapy has not been helpful in the treatment of anorexia or bulimia. Young people with severe and protracted cases of anorexia or bulimia are hospitalized on inpatient psychiatric units to more closely attend to their medical and psychological needs (Chart 29–23).

Substance Abuse

Substance abuse is defined as a pattern of continued and inappropriate use of substances that cause significant emotional, psychological, and physiologic effects. There has been a recent sharp increase in substance abuse. A survey conducted by the National Institute of Drug Abuse demonstrated an increase in marijuana use, with approximately 40% of 12th graders indicating having tried it. Three percent reported daily use. Thirteen percent of eighth graders reported smoking marijuana at least once. Alcohol is the substance most abused by adolescents. Twenty-eight percent of 12th graders reported having several drinks in the 2 weeks before the survey. Most adolescents are poorly informed about the effects of substance abuse (Jaffe, 1996). Adolescents and children who are using substances in a continuous and inappropriate way may experience repeated failure in school, difficulty in sports and social relationships, and conflict with the legal system. (See Chapter 5 for further discussion of substance use.) Youth who abuse substances are at increased risk for displays of aggression, of being the recipi-

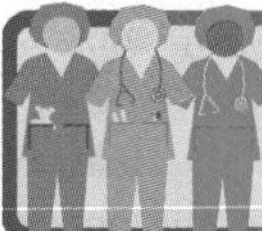

Care Path 29–2 An Interdisciplinary Plan of Care for the Child with Anorexia *Continued*

Care Intervention Categories	Day 1	Day 2	Day 3	Day 4
Family therapy		Family session: · Increase family co-operation/negotiation. · Negotiate family therapy goals.	Participate in family therapy.	⟶
Individual therapy	Individual session focused on changing self-talk to positive statements about normal weight and to negative statements about unhealthy current weight.	⟶	⟶	⟶
	Individual and family therapy	⟶	⟶	⟶
	Reinforce assertive communication skills.	⟶	⟶	⟶
	Help patient identify own strengths.	⟶	⟶	⟶
Teaching	Assess knowledge regarding nutritional needs—individual session.	Individual and family session: etiologic basis of eating disorder	Reevaluate knowledge; correct distortion and misinformation.	⟶
	Teach relaxation skills (music/meditation).	⟶	⟶	⟶
Vital signs/ baseline parameters	Height Weight Tanner staging Evaluate skin, hair, and mucous membranes.	Weight	⟶	⟶

ent of aggressive acts, of serious accidents, and of homicide and suicide. There are many commonly abused substances that produce different signs of intoxication and withdrawal (Table 29–6). Several risk factors that predict substance abuse have been identified and include early age at first use, poor school performance, high value for independence, external locus of control, poor self-esteem, favorable attitude to use of psychoactive substances, high risk-taking behavior pattern, poor social skills, sexual and physical abuse, aggressive or impulsive behavior patterns, peer group influence, and family influence (approval, exposure, abuse). Alcohol use (beer, wine) and cigarette smoking are early indicators of potential substance abuse and are considered "gateway" sub-

Days 5–6	Follow-up/ post discharge
⟶	⟶
⟶ ⟶ ⟶ ⟶	
Answer any remaining questions about diet and normal nutrition. ⟶	⟶
⟶	⟶

stances. A psychiatric disorder, especially depression, is also a risk factor.

Assessment

Woodard (1995) suggests that the goals for suspected substance abuse assessment of children and adolescents include identifying the level of substance abuse involvement, motivating the child or adolescent toward treatment, and matching the child's needs to the appropriate treatment level and methods of treatment. Signs and symptoms of substance abuse include bloodshot eyes, dilated pupils, slurred speech, loss of weight, and restlessness or drowsiness. The individual may show signs of awkward or clumsy physical movement, and have frequent minor illnesses (flu and colds). As the problem progresses, more signs become increasingly obvious, and interpersonal problems arise. Avoidance of parents and teachers and a change in friends may occur. Information should be gathered from school, family, and peers about the child's activities and behaviors to note any recent changes in the child's behaviors or issues that may influence the current abuse activities.

The assessment of youth engaging in substance abuse needs to include personal strengths and previous use of successful coping strategies. A discussion with the child or adolescent should explore psychosocial factors such as family relationships, peer relationships, leisure activities, employment activities, and self-perceptions. An assessment of the child's academic history is elicited, including school grades, involvement in school activities, attendance, and feelings and attitudes about school.

The proposed method for interviewing the teenager about substance abuse is provided by Anglin (1987). Discussion begins in an orderly fashion with dietary habits and proceeds to the following:

- Use of over-the-counter medications
- Use of prescribed medications
- Use of other substances
  - Smoking cigarettes
  - Use of beer, wine, and other alcohol drinks
  - Smoking marijuana
  - Use of other substances (e.g., inhalants, cocaine)

Information is gathered regarding when the child uses substances, where these activities are conducted and with whom, or surrounding what other activities. It should be determined whether the adolescent is using substances while driving or participating in other activities that require mental concentration (e.g., school, work) (Fig. 29–9). If the adolescent is resistant to talking or sharing information, asking for information about peers and being nonjudgmental about their behavior may assist the child to share information about his or her own abuse.

Diagnostic Tests. Urine screening for substance abuse shows abuse of marijuana up to 3 to 4 weeks. Other substances related to abuse are present only for 1 to 2 days. A drug screen may be used, and adolescents abusing substances will strongly resist providing urine for a screen. They question the examiner's trust in them or feign embarrassment (Jaffe, 1996).

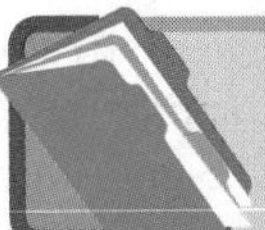

Chart 29-22
Nursing Interventions Classification (NIC)

Eating Disorders Management

Definition

Prevention and treatment of severe diet restriction and overexercising or binging and purging of food and fluids

Activities

Collaborate with other members of health care team to develop a treatment plan; involve patient and/or significant others, as appropriate.
Confer with team and patient to set a target weight, if patient is not within a recommended weight range for age and body frame.
Establish the amount of daily weight gain that is desired.
Confer with dietitian to determine daily caloric intake necessary to attain and/or maintain target weight.
Teach and reinforce concepts of good nutrition with patient (and significant others, as appropriate).
Encourage patient to discuss food preferences with dietitian.
Develop a supportive relationship with patient.
Monitor physiological parameters (vital signs and electrolyte levels), as needed.
Weigh on a routine basis (e.g., at same time of day and after voiding).
Monitor intake and output of fluids, as appropriate.
Monitor daily caloric food intake.
Encourage patient self-monitoring of daily food intake and weight gain/maintenance, as appropriate.
Establish expectations for appropriate eating behaviors, intake of food/fluid, and amount of physical activity.
Use behavioral contracting with patient to elicit desired weight gain or maintenance behaviors.
Restrict food availability to scheduled, pre-served meals and snacks.
Observe patient during and after meals/snacks to ensure that adequate intake is achieved and maintained.
Accompany patient to bathroom during designated observation times after meals/snacks.
Limit time spent in bathroom during periods when not under observation.
Monitor patient for behaviors related to eating, weight loss, and weight gain.
Use behavior modification techniques to promote behaviors that contribute to weight gain and to limit weight loss behaviors.
Provide reinforcement for weight gain and behaviors that promote weight gain.
Provide remedial consequences in response to weight loss, weight loss behaviors, or lack of weight gain.
Provide support (e.g., relaxation therapy, desensitization exercises, and opportunities to talk about feelings) as patient integrates new eating behaviors, changing body image, and lifestyle changes.
Encourage patient use of daily logs to record feelings, as well as circumstances surrounding urge to purge, vomit, and overexercise.
Limit physical activity, as needed, to promote weight gain.
Provide a supervised exercise program, when appropriate.
Allow opportunity to make limited choices about eating and exercise, as weight gain progresses in desirable manner.
Assist patient (and significant others, as appropriate) to examine and resolve personal issues that may contribute to the eating disorder.
Assist patient to develop a self-esteem that is compatible with a healthy body weight.
Confer with health care team on routine basis about patient's progress.
Initiate maintenance phase of treatment when patient has achieved target weight and has consistently shown desired eating behaviors for designated time.
Monitor patient weight on routine basis.
Determine acceptable range-of-weight variation in relation to target range.
Place total responsibility for choices about eating and physical activity with patient.
Provide support and guidance, as needed.
Assist patient to evaluate the appropriateness/consequences of choices about eating and physical activity.
Reinstitute weight gain protocol, if patient is unable to remain in target weight range.
Institute a treatment program and follow-up care (medical and counseling) for home management.

From McCloskey, J., & Bulechek, G. (1996). *Nursing interventions classification (NIC)* (2nd ed.). St. Louis: Mosby–Year Book. Reprinted with permission.

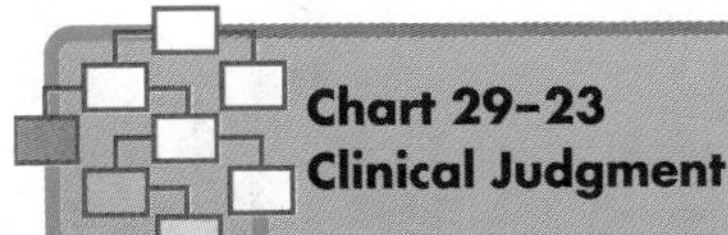

Chart 29–23
Clinical Judgment

The Adolescent with an Eating Disorder

Emily, a 14-year-old female, was admitted to the inpatient adolescent unit of the Children's Hospital after collapsing at school. She was 5 feet 2 inches tall and weighed 79 pounds. During the 5 months preceding admission, she had lost 26 pounds. After losing 15 pounds, she had been taken to the family's managed care facility. The physician prescribed an antidepressant medication and told her mother to restrict activities and to monitor Emily's diet. Emily continued to lose weight. Emily had been an A student, but her grades had begun to deteriorate to Cs and Ds. She complained of fatigue and difficulty concentrating. She said whenever she got sleepy when studying, she would "relax" by exercising. Emily said she believed she was "too fat." Emily's history indicated eating had been a conflictual issue between her and her parents since she was a baby. Emily's mother said that, when Emily was little, they were concerned she would be too fat. Her mother said, "but losing this much weight is just ridiculous! I think sometimes she is trying to kill herself." Emily's dad said, "Last year she looked really great! The boys were ogling her all the time. I couldn't stand it, but this weight loss has just gone too far!" Further investigation into family dynamics revealed that Emily's father was flirtatious with Emily and was outspoken about "keeping the boys away." His flirtations with Emily and constant reminder to his wife that Emily was his "little doll" caused considerable conflict between her parents. In assessment, Emily revealed that she believed she was the cause of her parents' fights, and she was worried about how her father would handle her dating boys. She said that she avoided all boys because they were only interested in her body.

Questions

1. What data are significant in determining the presence of an eating disorder?
2. Why might Emily have developed an eating disorder?
3. What are the priority nursing diagnoses you could use to begin a care path for an adolescent with an eating disorder?
4. List one outcome goal for each of your diagnoses.
5. How would you determine whether Emily is in control of her eating disorder?

Answers

1. Current weight compared with height norms, history of weight loss, exercise patterns, and complaints of fatigue, sleepiness, and difficulty concentrating.
2. Family conflict about her eating from an early age, adolescent rebellion against parents' control of social life, fear of growing up and becoming attractive due to fear of losing father's attention.
3. Altered nutritional status, altered family coping, body image disturbance.
4. Client develops a plan for inclusion of components of a balanced diet (including sufficient calories) on or before day of discharge, family members sign a contract to participate in family therapy sessions for at least 8 hours, and client and family state the importance of achieving the client's target weight.
5. Emily maintains adequate weight per age, eats balanced meals that meet her caloric needs, and relates a positive self-identity.

Nursing Diagnoses and Outcomes

In addition to the nursing diagnoses and outcomes presented in Chart 29–5, the following diagnoses can be applied to the child using substances:

- **Decisional conflict related to substance use**
  Outcomes: The child or adolescent expresses feelings about substance use.
  The child or adolescent describes family, school, and peer issues and their potential effect on his or her substance use.
  The child or adolescent makes choices that are consistent with his or her personal values and are legally sanctioned.
- **High risk for poisoning related to substance abuse**
  Outcomes: The child or adolescent expresses understanding of the harmful and potentially lethal effects of alcohol, tobacco products, and drugs.
  The child or adolescent identifies stressors or triggers that are likely to precipitate an episode of substance use.
  The child or adolescent does not ingest alcohol, tobacco products, or illegal drugs.

Table 29–6
Commonly Abused Substances

Substances	Street Name	Intoxication	Toxicity/Overdose	Withdrawal
CNS Depressants				
Barbiturates Ethanol	Downers Barbs Yellow jackets Red devils Booze	Sense of well-being followed by disinhibition, impaired judgment, slurred speech, incoordination, unsteady gait	Marked central nervous system (CNS) depression (especially respiratory function), stupor, coma, psychosis	Autonomic hyperactivity, nausea or vomiting, tremor, seizures, insomnia, delirium, hyperthermia, cardiovascular collapse
Opioid Agonists				
Morphine Heroin Fentanyl Methadone	M White stuff Horse H Harry Smack China white Meth	Euphoria followed by dysphoria, drowsiness, analgesia, pupil constriction, impaired attention and memory, decreased respiratory rate	Pinpoint pupils (or dilation with anoxia), coma, shock, pulmonary or cerebral edema, respiratory failure	Lacrimation, rhinorrhea, perspiration, yawning, dilated pupils, piloerection (goose flesh), chills, diarrhea, aching, tremor, nausea, vomiting, abdominal pain
Stimulants				
Cocaine Crack Amphetamines	Coke Snow Blow Nose candy Rock Crank Speed Bennies Uppers Black beauties	Rush of good feelings, dilated pupils, hyperactivity, hyperreflexia, increased heart rate, blood pressure, and respiratory rate, angina	Respiratory depression, pulmonary edema, fatal seizures, hypothermia, mental illness, paranoia, depression, insomnia, psychosis, irritability, cardiac dysrhythmias	Tolerance, craving, depression, suicide
CNS Stimulants				
Amphetamines Methamphetamines Cocaine	Bennies Dexies Ice Glass Crank Snow Crack	Euphoria, increased energy and sexual interest, decreased appetite, tremor, dilated pupils, nausea, vomiting, chills, tachycardia, increased blood pressure	Arrhythmias, increased blood pressure, hyperthermia, convulsions, cardiovascular shock, panic, paranoid delusions, formication, hallucinations, delirium	Depression, insomnia then hypersomnia, decreased appetite then hyperphagia, agitation then fatigue; anhedonia, persistent craving
PCP	Angel dust	Euphoria, belligerence, assaultiveness, sweating, increased blood pressure or heart rate, nystagmus, numbness, muscle rigidity, seizures	Panic, violence, catatonia, psychosis, flashbacks, increased temperature and blood pressure, convulsions, coma, cardiorespiratory failure	—

Table 29–6
Commonly Abused Substances *Continued*

Substances	Street Name	Intoxication	Toxicity/Overdose	Withdrawal
Hallucinogens				
LSD	Acid Sugar	Hallucinations, euphoria, depersonalization, derealization, pupil dilation, increased vital signs, incoordination, tremor	Panic, flashbacks, depression, anxiety, paranoia, delusions, hallucinations, confusion, elevated temperature, convulsions, cardiovascular collapse (particularly with MDA and MDMA)	—
Psilocybin and psilocin	Schrooms			
DMT, DET	Businessman's trip (DMT)			
Mescaline (peyote)	Bad sees			
DOM, STP	Peace			
MDA	Love bug			
MDMA	Ecstasy			
Cannabinoids				
Marijuana	Reefer Pot Weed Grass	Euphoria, paranoia, inability to gauge time, social withdrawal, memory impairment, incoordination, infected conjunctiva, increased appetite, tachycardia	Panic, flashbacks, paranoia, delusions, hallucinations	Possible irritability, restlessness, decreased appetite, insomnia, tremor, chills
Hashish	Hash			
Hashish oil				
Inhalants				
Volatile solvents Aerosols Anesthetics Nitrous oxide Volatile nitrites Amyl, Butyl	Laughing gas Snappers Poppers	Euphoria, belligerence, dizziness, nystagmus, incoordination, slurred speech, nausea and vomiting, tremor, stupor, coma, hallucinations, memory impairment	Panic, disorientation, emotional lability, cardiac arrhythmia, CNS depression (solvents), brain damage, liver damage, respiratory arrest	None

Figure 29–9
Cigarettes and beer are considered "gateway" substances that can lead to the use of other, illegal substances.

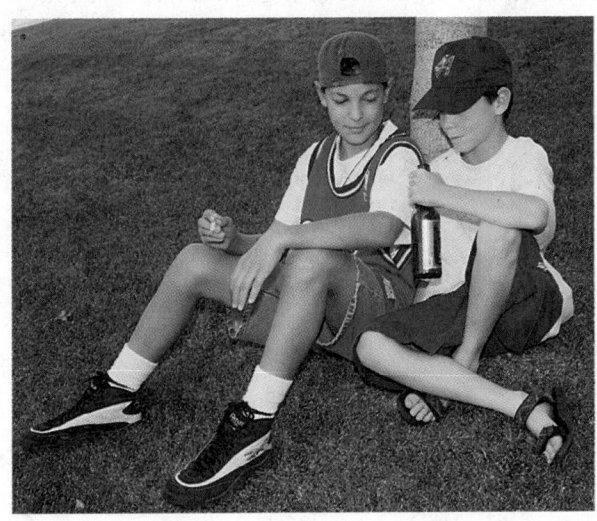

Interdisciplinary Interventions

A variety of methods are used in the treatment of substance abuse, and a variety of disciplines may be involved. The services that are actually provided to the child are dependent on a number of factors, including the child's socioeconomic status, the length and severity of the problem, who is harmed by the abuse, and the type of problems exhibited by the individual child.

Education may be provided by physicians, substance abuse counselors, or advanced practice nurses. Persons providing education should have an understanding of the brain–body connection, and the effects that alcohol or other abused substances have on the body, various organs of the body, neurotransmitters, cells of the brain, and observable behavior.

Cognitive therapy with a strong confrontational component is used in individual and group therapy. Individual and group therapy may be provided by an advanced practice nurse, a psychiatrist, or other mental health therapist with knowledge and expertise in substance abuse counseling (e.g., social worker, psychologist). A behavioral contract is highly recommended as a therapy intervention.

Family therapy is essential for youth who are substance abusers. The family must come to grips with their communication, inclusion, and nurturing deficits. Identification of strengths and developing a set of core values that guide them in nurturing and fostering appropriate growth and development of their young members is crucial to achieving and maintaining wellness.

Summary of Key Concepts

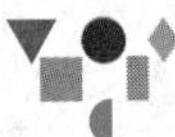

- The prevalence of mental illness in children is high, while funding and treatment programs meet the needs of less than one half of afflicted youngsters.
- Care of children with alterations in mental health requires an interdisciplinary approach. Psychiatrists, special educators, recreational therapists, advanced practice nurses, psychologists, social workers, mental health workers including associate degree and baccalaureate nurses have important interdependent roles.
- Assessment of the child or adolescent with suspected alteration in mental health is complex and multifaceted, and includes assessment of physical health, mental status, normal and deviations from normal growth and development, suicide assessment, observation and analysis of family relationships and dynamics, current and past stressors, history of mental illness in the family, types of behaviors exhibited by the child, and academic functioning and progress.
- The psychiatric mental health nurse uses both the current DSM diagnosis and nursing diagnoses to begin the formulation of a plan of care.
- Multiple therapeutic interventions may be used by various members of the mental health team. These include individual therapies, group and family therapy, milieu therapy, behavior management strategies, and pharmacologic interventions. Treatment is increasingly being provided in multiple community settings including the home, whereas less care is provided in the hospital.
- A variety of mental health disorders may afflict children and adolescents. All disorders, whether primarily caused by biological factors or psychodynamic factors impact on the whole child and have serious implications for the overall growth and development of the child.
- An increasingly large number of children and adolescents are physically, sexually, emotionally, or spiritually abused or neglected. Abuse and neglect are major contributors to psychiatric illness and often plague children and adolescents throughout their lives.

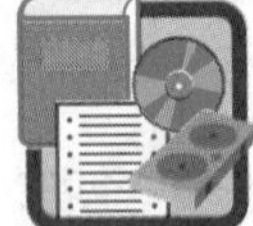

Resources

Organizations

National Self-Help Clearing House
33 West 42nd Street
Room 620 N
New York, NY 10036
(212) 840-1259

Suicide Prevention Center
184 Salem Street
Dayton, OH 45406
(513) 223-9096

MADD (Mothers Against Drunk Driving)
669 Airport Freeway
Suite 310
Hearst, TX 76053
(817) 268-6233
Web: http://www.madd.org

The Association of Child & Adolescent Psychiatric Nurses
ACAPN National Office
1211 Locust Street
Philadelphia, PA 19107
(800) 826-2950

The Children's Defense Fund
25 E Street, NW
Washington, DC 20001
(202) 628-8787

International Cult Education Program
P. O. Box 1232
Gracie Station
New York, NY 10028

Voices (Victims of Incest)
P. O. Box 14309
Chicago, IL 60614
(312) 327-1500

Clearinghouse on Disability Information
Office of Special Education and Rehabilitation Service
U.S. Department of Education
Washington, DC 20202
(202) 732-1241

Learning Disabilities
Association of America (LDA)
4156 Library Road
Pittsburgh, PA 15234
(412) 341-1515

National Center for Learning Disabilities (NCLD)
99 Park Avenue
New York, NY 10016
(212) 687-7211

American Association of Suicidology
2459 South Ash
Denver, CO 80222
(303) 692-0985

Center for Law and Education
955 Massachusetts Avenue
Cambridge, MA 02139
(617) 876-6611

National Mental Health Association
1021 Prince Street
Alexandria, VA 22314
(703) 684-7722

National Resource Center on Child Sexual Abuse
106 Lincoln Street
Huntsville, AL 35801

National Alliance for the Mentally Ill
200 North Glebe Road
Suite 1015
Arlington, VA 22203-3754

Children and Adults with Attention Deficit Disorders (CHADD)
National Headquarters
Suite 185
1859 North Pine Island Road
Plantation, FL 33322
(800) 233-4050
Web: http://www.whit.org/chadd_cs/index.html

National Attention Deficit Disorder Association
P. O. Box 972
Mentor, OH 44061-0972
(800) 487-2282

The Indiana Resource Center for Autism
Indiana University
Institute for the Study of Developmental Disabilities
2853 East Tenth Street
Bloomington, IN 47408-2601
(812) 855-6508

Books and Other Printed Materials

Child Behavior Checklist
The Psychological Corporation
555 Academic Court
San Antonio, TX 78204-2498

Cronin, Eileen (1994). *Helping your dyslexic child*. Rochlin, CA: Prime Publishing.

Davis, N. (1990). *Once upon a time: Therapeutic stories to heal abused children*. Revised ed. Oxon Hill, MD: Psychological Associates of Oxon Hill.

Espe-Sherwindt, M., Kerlin, S., Beatty, C., & Crable, S. (1997). *Project capable: Parents with special needs/mental retardation. A handbook for early intervention*. Talmadge, OH: Family Child Learning Center.

Gil, E. (1987). *Children who molest: A guide for parents of young sex offenders*. Rockville, MD: Launch Press.

Gonzalez-Mena, J. (1994). *Parent's perspective*. Salem, WI: Sheffield Publishing.

Johnson, T. C. (1989). Human sexuality curriculum for parents and children in troubled families. Los Angeles, CA: Children's Institute International. Marshall Resource Library, 711 S. New Hampshire Ave., Los Angeles, CA 90005.

Kleisman, J. J., & Straus, H. (1989). *I hate you, don't leave me*. New York: Avon Books/The Hearst Corporation.

Leman, K., & Carlson, R. (1993). *Parent talk*. Nashville: Thomas Nelson Publishers.

Moss, R. (1990). *Why Johnny can't concentrate*. New York: Bantam Books.

National Institute of Child Health and Human Development. (1983). *Facts about anorexia nervosa*. Bethesda, MD: U.S. Government Printing Office.

Rapoport, J. (1989). *The boy who couldn't stop washing*. New York: Dutton.

Silver, L. B. (1984). *The misunderstood child: A guide for parents of learning disabled children*. New York: McGraw-Hill.

Torrey, E. F. (1983). Surviving schizophrenia: A family manual. New York: Harper & Row.

Tuttle, C. G. (1991). *Thinking games to play with your child*. Los Angeles: Lowell House.

Tuttle, C. (1993). *Parenting a child with a learning disability*. Chicago: Contemporary Books.

Walsh, M. E. (1985). Schizophrenia: Straight talk for family and friends. Warner Books.

Games/Videos

Communication Skill Builders. A set of cards depicting "feelings."
Communication Skill Builders
P. O. Box 279
Kalispel, MT 59903

Assessment and Treatment of Sexualized Children and Children Who Molest: Conversations with E. Gil.
J. Gary Film Co.
1313 Scheibel Lane
Sebastopol, CA 95472
(800) 369-5367

References

American Psychiatric Association. (1994). *Diagnostic and statistical manual of mental disorders* (4th ed.). Washington, DC: Author.

Anglin, T. (1987). Interviewing guidelines for the clinical evaluation of adolescent substance abuse. *Pediatric Clinics of North America, 34*(2), 381–398.

Anonymous. (1995). Suicide among children, adolescents, and young adults—United States, 1980–1992. *Journal of School Health, 65*(7), 272–273.

Anonymous. (1993a). Child abuse—Part I. *The Harvard Mental Health Letter, 9*(11), 1–3.

Anonymous. (1993b). Child abuse—Part II. *The Harvard Mental Health Letter,* 9(12), 1–4.

Antai-Otong, D. (1995). *Psychiatric nursing: Biological and behavioral concepts*. Philadelphia: W. B. Saunders.

Bell-Dolan, D., & Brazeal, T. (1993). Separation anxiety disorder, overanxious disorder, and school refusal. *Child & Adolescent Psychiatric Clinics of North America, 2*(4), 563–580.

Berenson, C. K. (1993). Evaluation & treatment of anxiety in the general pediatric population. *Child & Adolescent Psychiatric Clinics of North America, 2*(4), 727–747.

Black, B., & Uhde, T. W. (1994). Treatment of elective mutism with fluoxetine: A double-blind, placebo-controlled study. *Journal of Academy of Child Adolescent Psychiatry, 33*(7), 1000–1006.

Bowlby, J. (1969). *Attachment and loss. Attachment* (vol. 1, 2nd ed.). New York: Basic Books.

Briere, J. (1987). Postsexual abuse trauma: Data and implications for clinical practice. *Journal of Interpersonal Violence, 12*, 367–377.

Brown, G. W., Harris, T. O., & Bifulco, A. (1986). Long-term effects of early loss of a parent. In M. Rutter, C. E. Izzard, & P. E. Read (Eds.), *Depression in young people*. New York: Guilford Press.

Burgess, A., Hartman, C., & Clemons, P. (1997). *Biology of memory and childhood trauma*. In A. Burgess (Ed.), *Psychiatric nursing: Promoting mental health*. Stanford, CT: Appleton & Lange.

Butler, R., Brewin, C., & Forsythe, W. (1988). A comparison of two approaches to the treatment of nocturnal enuresis and the prediction of effectiveness using pre-treatment variables. *Journal of Child Psychology and Psychiatry, 29*(4), 501–509.

Caplan, G. (1964). *Principles of preventive psychiatry*. New York: Basic Books.

Caplan, R. (1994). Childhood schizophrenia assessment and treatment. *Child and Adolescent Psychiatric Clinics of North America, 3*(1), 15–30.

Castellanos, F. X., & Rapoport, J. L. (1992). Etiology of attention-deficit hyperactivity disorder. *Child and Adolescent Psychiatric Clinics of North America, 1*(2), 373–384.

Castiglia, P. (1997a). Attention deficit/hyperactivity disorder. *Journal of Pediatric Health Care, 11*(3), 130–133.

Castiglia, P. (1997b). Tourette syndrome. *Journal of Pediatric Health Care, 11*(4), 189–191.

Centers for Disease Control. (1994). Suicide contagion and the reporting of suicide: Recommendations for a national workshop. *MMWR, 43*(6), 13–17.

Cicchetti, D., & Rogosch, F. (1994). The toll of child maltreatment on the developing child. *Child Abuse, 3*(4), 759–776.

Coker, L. (1990). A therapeutic recovery model for the female adult incest survivor. *Issues in Mental Health Nursing, 11*, 109–123.

Conte, J., & Schuerman, J. (1987). Factors associated with an increased impact of child sexual abuse. *Child Abuse and Neglect, 11*, 201–211.

Cornman, J. (1989). Group treatment for female adolescent sexual abuse victims. *Issues in Mental Health Nursing, 10*, 261–271.

Cotton, N. (1993). *Lessons from the lion's den: Therapeutic management of children in psychiatric hospital and treatment centers*. San Francisco: Jossey-Bass.

Critchley, D. L. (1995). *Play therapy*. In B. S. Johnson (Ed.), *Child, adolescent and family psychiatric nursing*. Philadelphia: J. B. Lippincott.

Dahl, R. E. (Ed.). (1996). Introduction: Sleep and child psychiatry. *Child and Adolescent Psychiatric Clinics, 5*(3), 543–548.

Deering, C. (1992). Nursing interventions with children and adolescents experiencing eating difficulties. In P. West & C. L. Sieloff Evans (Eds.), *Psychiatric-mental health nursing with children and adolescents*. Gaithersburg, MD: Aspen Publishers.

Delaney, K. R. (1992). Nursing in child psychiatric milieus. Part I: What nurses do. *Journal of Child and Adolescent Psychiatric Mental Health Nursing, 5*(1), 10–14.

Diamond, J., & Mattson, A. (1996). Attention deficit/hyperactivity disorder. In D. X. Parmelee (Ed.), *Child and adolescent psychiatry*. St. Louis: Mosby–Year Book.

Donnelly, C., Maletic, V., & March, J. S. (1996). Anxiety disorders in children and adolescents. In D. X. Parmelee (Ed.), *Child and adolescent psychiatry*. St. Louis: Mosby–Year Book.

Erik, E. (1950). *Childhood & society*. New York: W. W. Norton.

Faller, K. (1994). Extra familial sexual abuse. *Child Abuse, 3*(4), 713–727.

Feinstein, C., & Reiss, A. L. (1996). Psychiatric disorders in mentally retarded children and adolescents. *Child & Adolescent Psychiatric Clinics of North America, 5*(4), 827–852.

Finke, L. M. (1996). Mental retardation. In B. S. Johnson (Ed.), *Child adolescent and family psychiatric nursing* (pp. 174–179). Philadelphia: J. B. Lippincott.

Finklehor, D. (1986). Designing new studies. In D. Finklehor (Ed.), *A source book on child sexual abuse* (pp. 199–223). Beverly Hills: Sage.

Friedrich, W. (1994). Individual psychotherapy for child abuse victims. *Child Abuse, 3*(4), 797–812.

Garfinkel, B. D., Carlson, G. A., & Weller, E. B. (1990). *Psychiatric disorders in children and adolescents*. Philadelphia: W. B. Saunders.

Garfinkel, B. D., & Amrami, K. K. (1992). Assessment and differential diagnosis of attention deficit hyperactivity disorder. *Child & Adolescent Psychiatric Clinics of North America, 1*(2), 311–324.

Gilbert, C. (1989). Sibling incest. *Journal of Child Psychiatric Nursing, 2*, 70–73.

Gilbert, C. (1995). Group therapy. In B. S. Johnson (Ed.), *Child, adolescent and family psychiatric nursing*. Philadelphia: J. B. Lippincott.

Grimes, K. (1996). Common behavioral problems and reactions to stress. In D. X. Parmelee (Ed.), *Child and adolescent psychiatry*. St. Louis: Mosby–Year Book.

Grinspoon, L. (Ed.). (1996). Suicide—Part I. *The Harvard Mental Health Newsletter, 13*(5), 1–5.

Harris, S., Delmolino, L., & Glasberg, B. A. (1996). Psychological and behavior assessment in mental retardation. *Child and Adolescent Psychiatric Clinics of North America, 5*(4), 797–808.

Houts, A., & Peterson, J. (1986). Treatment of a retentive encopretic child using contingency management and diet modification with stimulus control. *Journal of Pediatric Psychology, 11*(3), 375–383.

Jaffe, S. (1996). The substance abusing youth. In D. X. Parmelee (Ed.), *Child and adolescent psychiatry*. St. Louis: Mosby–Year Book.

Jennings, S. (1993). *Play therapy with children*. Boston: Blackwell Scientific.

Johnson, C. M. (1995). Therapeutic environments. In B. S. Johnson (Ed.), *Child, adolescent and family psychiatric nursing*. Philadelphia: J. B. Lippincott.

Kaplan, S., Pelcovitz, D., & Weiner, M. (1994). Adolescent physical abuse. *Child Abuse, 3*(4), 695–711.

Kassett, J., Gershon, E., & Maxwell, M. (1989). Psychiatric disorders in first degree relatives of probands with bulimia nervosa and depression. *American Journal of Psychiatry, 146*(1), 1468–1480.

Keltner, N., Schwecke, L., & Bostrom, C. (1995). *Psychiatric nursing* (2nd ed.). St. Louis: Mosby–Year Book.

Kendall-Tackett, K., Williams, L., & Finkelhor, D. (1993). Impact of sexual abuse of children: A review and synthesis of recent empirical studies. *Psychological Bulletin, 113*(1), 164–180.

Kerns, L., & Lieberman, A. (1993). *Helping your depressed child: A reassuring guide to the causes and treatments of childhood and adolescent depression*. Rocklin, CA: Prima Publishing.

King, C., Franzzese, R., Gargan, S., McGovern, L., Ghaziuddin, N., & Naylor, M. (1995). Suicide contagion among adolescents during acute psychiatric hospitalization. *Psychiatric Services, 46*(9), 915–918.

King, R. A. (1994). Childhood onset schizophrenia: Development and pathogenesis. *Child and Adolescent Psychiatric Clinics of North America, 3*(1), 1–13.

Kjellman, B., Thorell, L., Orhagen, T., d'Elia, G., & Kagedal, B. (1993). The hypothalamic-pituitary-thyroid axis in depressive patients and healthy subjects in relation to the hypothalamic-pituitary-adrenal. *Psychiatry Research, 47*(1), 7–21.

Kowatch, R., Emslie, G., & Kennard, B. D. (1996). Mood disorders. In D. X. Parmelee (Ed.), *Child and adolescent psychiatry*. St. Louis: Mosby–Year Book.

Krohn, D. D., Weckstein, S. M., & Wright, H. L. (1992). A study of the effectiveness of a specific treatment for elective mutism. *Journal of American Academy of Child Adolescent Psychiatry, 31*(4), 711–718.

Lewis, M. (Consulting Ed.) (1993). Eating and growth disorders. *Child and Adolescent Psychiatric Clinics of North America, 2*(1), ix.

Lewis, M. (1994). Borderline disorders in children. *Child and Adolescent Psychiatric Clinics of North America, 3*(1), 31–42.

Lipovsky, J. (1991). Posttraumatic stress disorder in children. *Family and Community Health, 14*(3), 42–51.

Lung, C., & Daro, D. (1995). *Current trends in child abuse reporting and fatalities: The results of the 1995 annual fifty state survey* (Working Paper Number 808). Chicago, IL: National Committee to Prevent Child Abuse.

March, J., & Mulle, K. (1995). Manualized cognitive behavioral psychotherapy for obsessive-compulsive disorder in childhood: A single case study. *Journal of Anxiety Disorders, 9*(2), 175–184.

March, J. S., Leonard, H. L., & Swedo, S. E. (1995). Pharmacotherapy of obsessive-compulsive disorder. *Child and Adolescent Psychiatric Clinics of North America, 4*(1), 217–236.

McCauley, E., & Meyers, K. (1992). The longitudinal clinical course of depression in children and adolescents. *Child and Adolescent Psychiatric Clinics of North America, 1*(1), 183–196.

McCracken, J. T. (1992a). The epidemiology of mood disorders in children. *Child and Adolescent Psychiatric Clinics of North America, 1*(1), 53–72.

McCracken, J. T. (1992b). Etiologic aspects of child and adolescent mood disorders. *Child and Adolescent Psychiatric Clinics of North America, 1*(1), 89–109.

McFarland, G., Wasli, E., & Gerety, E. (1997). *Nursing diagnosis and process in psychiatric mental health nursing*. Philadelphia: J. B. Lippincott.

Mullen, D. J., & Hendren, R. L. (1996). The suicidal child and adolescent. In D. X. Parmelee (Ed.), *Child and adolescent psychiatry*. St. Louis: Mosby–Year Book.

Nathan, K. I., Musselman, D. I., Schatzberg, A. F., & Nemeroff, C. B. (1995). *Biology of mood disorders*. Washington, DC: American Psychiatric Press.

Nemethy, M. (1997). Attention deficit/hyperactivity disorder: A guide for diagnosis and treatment. *Advance for Nurse Practitioners, 5*(2), 22–29.

Pearson, G. S. (1992). Nursing interventions with children and adolescents experiencing thought disorders. In P. West & C. L. Evans (Eds.), *Psychiatric and mental health nursing with children and adolescents* (pp. 329–342). Gaithersburg, MD: Aspen Publishers.

Pearson, G. S. (1995a). Mood disorders. In B. S. Johnson (Ed.), *Child, adolescent and family psychiatric nursing*. Philadelphia: J. B. Lippincott.

Pearson, G. S. (1995b). Psychopharmacology. In B. S. Johnson (Ed.), *Child, adolescent and family psychiatric nursing* (pp. 410–423). Philadelphia: J. B. Lippincott.

Potts, N. (1995). Eating disorders. In B. Johnson (Ed.), *Child, adolescent and family psychiatric nursing*. Philadelphia: J. B. Lippincott.

Reba, R. C. (1993). PET & SPECT: Opportunities and challenges. *Journal of Clinical Psychiatry, 54*(11), 26–32.

Reitz, S. (1997). Attention-deficit/hyperactivity disorder: Focus on pharmacologic management. *Journal of Pediatric Health Care*, 11(2), 78–83.

Rew, L. (1989). Long-term effect of childhood sexual exploitation. *Issues in Mental Health Nursing, 10*, 229–244.

Ricchini, W. (1997). Self-esteem and ADHD. *Advance for Nurse Practitioners*, 5(5), 59–63.

Riley, E. A., & Kneisl, C. R. (1996). Suicide and self destructive behavior. In H. S. Wilson & C. R. Kneisl (Ed.), *Psychiatric nursing* (5th ed.). Menlo Park, CA: Addison-Wesley Publishing.

Robertson, M. M. (1994). Gilles de la Tourette syndrome: An update. *Journal of Child and Adolescent Psychiatry, 35*(1), 597–611.

Ross, C. (1996). Epidemiology of dissociation in children and adolescents. *Child and Adolescent Psychiatric Clinics of North America*, 5(2), 273–284.

Scahill, L. (1996). Contemporary approaches to pharmacotherapy in Tourette and obsessive compulsive disorder. *Journal of Child and Adolescent Psychiatric Nursing*, 9(1), 27–39.

Scahill, L., & French, P. (1996). Pharmacology notes: Nonstimulant medications in the treatment of attention deficit hyperactivity disorder. *Journal of Child and Adolescent Psychiatric Nursing*, 9(2), 39–43.

Scahill, L., Ort, S. I., & Hardin, M. T. (1993a). Tourette's syndrome, Part I: Definition and diagnosis. *Archives of Psychiatric Nursing, 7*(4), 203–208.

Scahill, L., Ort, S. I., & Hardin, M. T. (1993b). Tourette's syndrome, Part II: Contemporary approaches to assessment and treatment. *Archives of Psychiatric Nursing*, 6(4), 209–216.

Scahill, L., Walker, R. D., Lechner, S. N., & Tynan, K. E. (1993c). Inpatient treatment of obsessive-compulsive disorder in childhood: A case study. *Journal of Child and Adolescent Psychiatric Nursing*, 6(3), 5–14.

Scheffel, D. (1996). Learning disorders. In D. X. Parmelee (Ed.), *Child and adolescent psychiatry*. St. Louis: Mosby–Year Book.

Silver, L. B. (1993a). Introduction and overview to the clinical concepts of learning disabilities. *Child and Adolescent Psychiatric Clinics of North America, 2*(2), 181–192.

Silver, L. B. (1993b). The secondary emotional, social and family problems found with children and adolescents with learning disabilities. *Child and Adolescent Psychiatric Clinics of North America, 2*(2), 295–309.

Simmons, J. E. (1987). *Psychiatric examination of children* (4th ed.). Philadelphia: Lea & Febiger.
Smat-Mari, P. (1992). The epidemiology of attention-deficit hyperactivity disorder. *Child and Adolescent Psychiatric Clinics of North America, 1*(2), 361–371.
Sokol, M. (1996). Schizophrenia in children and adolescents. In D. X. Parmelee (Ed.), *Child and adolescent psychiatry*. St. Louis: Mosby–Year Book.
Srnec, P. (1991). Children, violence, and intentional injuries. *Critical Care Nursing Clinics of North America, 3*(3), 471–478.
Terr, L. C. (1991). Childhood traumas: An outline and overview. *American Journal of Psychiatry, 148*(1), 10–20.
U.S. Department of Health and Human Services. (1993). *Child mental health in the 1990's*. Rockville, MD: U.S. Government Printing Office.
Wachsmuth, J. R., & Garfinkel, P. E. (1993). The treatment of anorexia nervosa in young adolescents. *Child and Adolescent Psychiatric Clinics of North America, 2*(1), 145–157.
Wagner, B. (1995). Personality disorders. In B. S. Johnson (Ed.), *Child, adolescent and family psychiatric nursing*. Philadelphia: J. B. Lippincott.
Waller, D. (1996). Eating disorders. In D. X. Parmelee (Ed.), *Child and adolescent psychiatry*. St. Louis: Mosby–Year Book.
Waszak, L. C. (1992). Nursing interventions with children experiencing elimination difficulties. In P. West & C. L. Sieloff-Evans (Eds.), *Psychiatric and mental health nursing with children and adolescents* (pp. 183–197). Gaithersburg, MD: Aspen Publishers.
Weeks, S. M. (1995). Individual therapy. In B. S. Johnson (Ed.), *Child, adolescent and family psychiatric nursing*. Philadelphia: J. B. Lippincott.
Wenckstern, S., & Leenaars, A. (1993). Trauma and suicide in our schools. *Death Studies, 17*, 151–171.
Wherry, J. S. (1992). History, terminology and manifestation at different ages. *Child and Adolescent Psychiatric Clinics of North America, 1*(2), 297–310.
Wood, I. (1996). Conduct disorders and oppositional defiant disorder. In D. X. Parmelee (Ed.), *Child and adolescent psychiatry*. St. Louis: Mosby–Year Book.
Woodard, V. A. (1995). Chemical dependency. In B. S. Johnson (Ed.), *Child, adolescent and family psychiatric nursing* (pp. 315–331). Philadelphia: J. B. Lippincott.
Wozniak, J., & Herzog, D. B. (1993). The course and outcome of bulimia nervosa. *Child and Adolescent Psychiatric Clinics of North America, 2*(1), 109–128.
Yalom, I. D. (1995). *The theory and practice of group therapy* (4th ed.). New York: Basic Books.
Zarb, J. M. (1992). *Cognitive-behavioral assessment and therapy with adolescents*. New York: Brunner/Mazel.

Bibliography

Bandura, A. (1969). *Principles of behavior modification*. New York: Holt, Rinehart & Winston.
Harris, J. (1996). Pervasive developmental disorders. In D. X. Parmelee (Ed.), *Child and adolescent psychiatry*. St. Louis: Mosby–Year Book.
Lynch, E., & Hanson, M. (1992). *Developing cross-cultural competence: A guide for working with young children and their families*. Baltimore: Paul H. Brookes Publishing.
Mahler, M. (1976). *On human symbiosis and the vicissitudes of individualization*. New York: International Universities Press.
Tsai, L. Y. (1995). Rhett syndrome. *Child and Adolescent Psychiatric Clinics of North America, 3*(1), 105–118.
Uhry, J. K., & Shepherd, M. J. (1993). Writing disorder. *Child and Adolescent Psychiatric Clinics of North America, 2*(2), 209–219.
Wilcox, R. E., & Gonzales, R. A. (1995). Introduction to neurotransmitters, receptors, signal transduction, and second messengers. In A. G. Schatzberg & C. B. Nemeroff (Eds.), *Textbook of psychopharmacology*. Washington, DC: American Psychiatric Press.
Worley, N. K., & Owens, V. J. (1997). Schools. In N. K. Worley (Ed.), *Mental health nursing in the community*. St. Louis: Mosby.

HEALTH CHALLENGE:

The Pediatric Emergency

OUTLINE

Assessment of the Child with an Emergency Condition
- Triage
  - Across-the-Room Assessment
  - Brief History and Physical Assessment
  - Triage Decision
  - Telephone Triage
- Nursing Diagnoses and Outcomes
- Developmental and Biological Variances

Diagnostic Criteria for Evaluating Pediatric Emergencies

Treatment Modalities
- Pediatric Cardiopulmonary Resuscitation
- Advanced Life Support
  - Vascular Access
  - Fluid Administration
  - Medication Administration
  - Psychosocial Support

Specific Pediatric Emergencies
- Shock
- Trauma
- Common Respiratory Emergencies
- Fever
- Bites and Stings
  - Mammal and Human Bites
  - Snake Bites
  - Insect Stings and Bites
- Anaphylaxis
- Epistaxis
- Environmental Exposure Injuries
  - Heat Illnesses
  - Hypothermia
  - Smoke Inhalation
  - Near-Drowning
- Poisoning
  - Iron
  - Lead
  - Acetaminophen
  - Hydrocarbons
  - Caustics
- Sudden Infant Death Syndrome
- Child Abuse
  - Physical Abuse
  - Sexual Abuse
  - Munchausen's Syndrome by Proxy
  - Emotional or Psychological Abuse

Preparation for Transfer

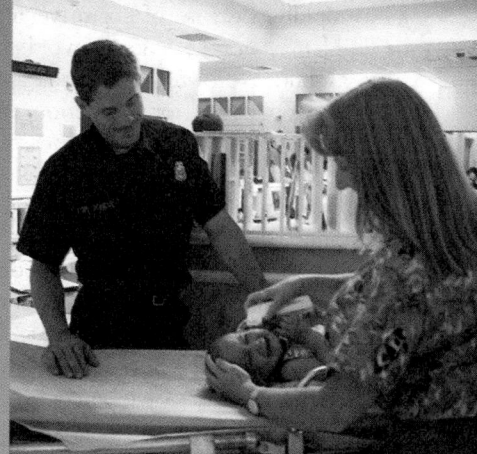

OBJECTIVES

- Describe the four components of pediatric emergency triage.
- Describe the nursing interventions required for the infant or child in cardiopulmonary arrest.
- Discuss common causes, signs, and symptoms of shock in children.
- Prioritize the sequence of assessing the multiple-trauma patient.
- Explain nursing care related to the child in acute respiratory distress.
- Describe the nursing interventions for the child who has been bitten or stung.
- Discuss the nursing interventions for the child suffering from an environmental injury: hypothermia, hyperthermia, near-drowning.
- Identify the initial treatment for the child who has ingested an unknown poison.
- Describe the nursing assessment of the abused child.

KEY TERMS

anhidrosis
antidote
atopy
epistaxis
triage
urticaria

CHAPTER

30

Emergency management of ill or injured children is costly, physically and emotionally, as well as financially. Many emergencies can be avoided through family education and simple prevention techniques.

In an emergency, children are more vulnerable than adults (Fig. 30–1). They have fewer physiologic reserves, for example, smaller tidal volumes and circulating blood volume. Also, a disease or injury may alter their status more rapidly. Because of cognitive immaturity, an infant or child may not be able to avoid dangerous situations, such as burns, drowning, trauma, and child abuse, and must rely on adults for protection. Because of a child's limited ability to verbalize, a disease process may be far advanced before signs and symptoms are noted. Although adolescents may be physically and mentally mature, they commonly participate in risk-taking behavior. This behavior, combined with feelings of omnipotence and increased mobility, can put adolescents more at risk.

The nurse's astute assessment, knowledge of signs and symptoms of deterioration, and timely interventions can help decrease negative outcomes.

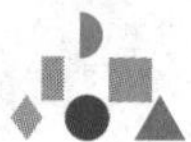

Assessment of the Child with an Emergency Condition

Triage

The French word "triage" means "to pick or sort." Its medical use began in World War I to determine priority needs for the injured or sick in order to use personnel and supplies most effectively. Triage became a part of the emergency room and acute care setting in the 1960s as a means of determining priority of treatment.

The goals of triage are to

- Rapidly identify the seriously ill or injured patient.
- Prioritize all patients using the emergency department.
- Initiate therapeutic measures for the patient.

Triage for children, as for adults, has four components: performing an across-the-room assessment, obtaining a chief complaint, performing a brief history and physical assessment, and making the triage decision. Because of the potentially emergent nature of the situation, the nurse does not have time to perform a methodical in-depth assessment and physical examination. Rather, the nurse must obtain information rapidly and make decisions promptly.

Across-the-Room Assessment

The triage assessment generally starts with a quick across-the-room assessment as soon as the child presents to the emergency department or clinic. Observe the child's general appearance to determine whether immediate care is required.

Alert: *Obvious respiratory distress, cyanosis, posturing to maintain an open airway, seizures, unconsciousness, and profuse bleeding are signs that the nurse should interrupt the triage process and proceed to the emergency care area for immediate intervention.*

Brief History and Physical Assessment

The second step in the triage process combines a brief history from the child and/or parent with performing a brief physical assessment. Obtaining a triage history can be difficult if the child is young, if the parent or primary caregiver is not present, or if a communication barrier exists (Chart 30–1). During triage, use the AMPLE mnemonic to help remember the key components of the history interview (Chart 30–2).

During the physical assessment, perform a rapid evaluation of the child (Chart 30–3). Remember to move from assessment of vital functions to examination of less critical areas.

Triage Decision

The triage decision involves assigning a triage classification to the patient. This classification regulates the child's movement through the emergency department and determines the site of care best suited for him or her.

Various triage classification systems are in use. Commonly, a three-group system is used. This three-group system divides patients according to how ill they are: emergent, urgent, or nonurgent (Haley & Baker, 1993). The three groups are defined as follows:

- Emergent. Any child who requires immediate intervention or resuscitation to avoid loss of life

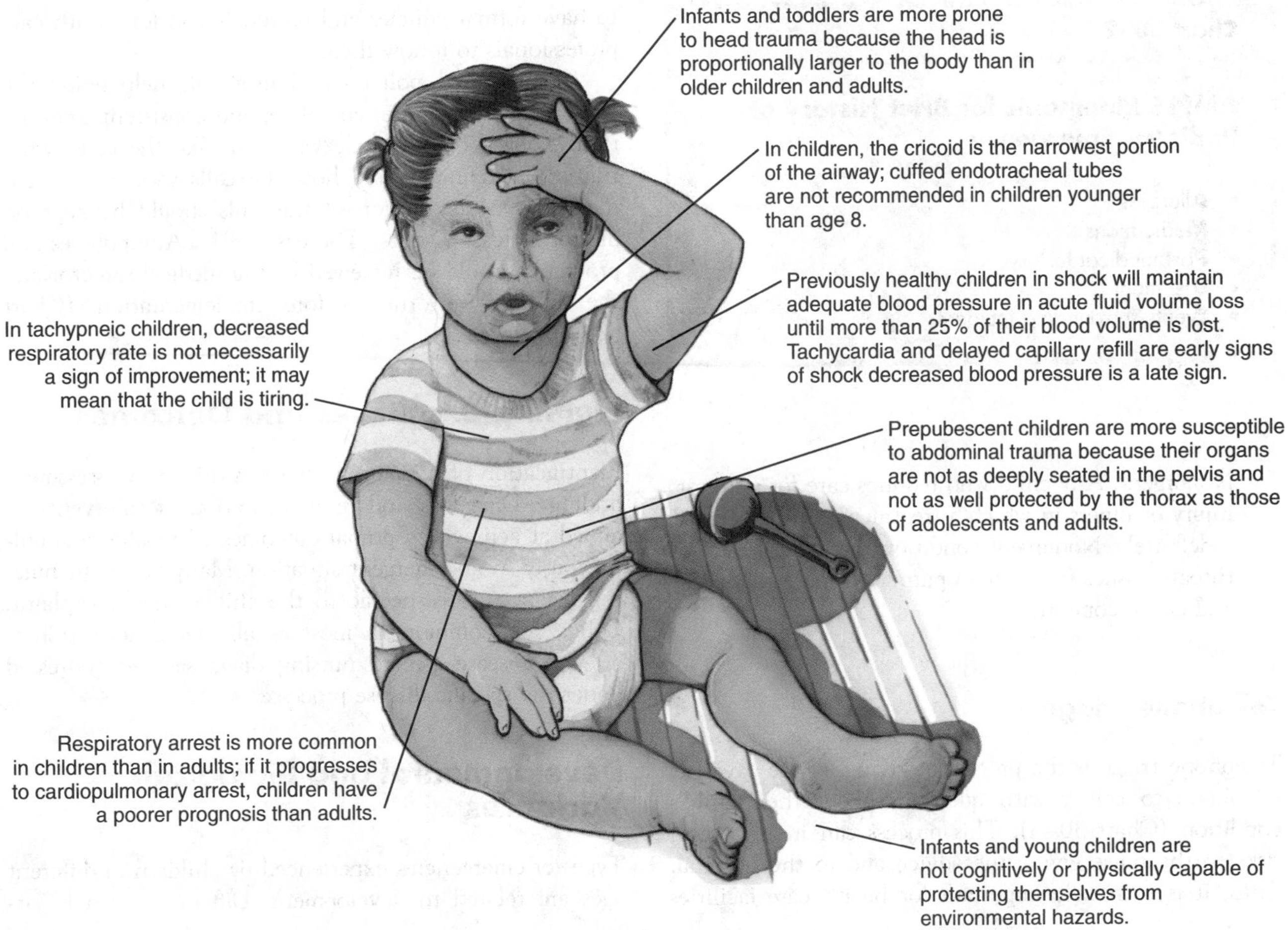

Infants and toddlers are more prone to head trauma because the head is proportionally larger to the body than in older children and adults.

In children, the cricoid is the narrowest portion of the airway; cuffed endotracheal tubes are not recommended in children younger than age 8.

Previously healthy children in shock will maintain adequate blood pressure in acute fluid volume loss until more than 25% of their blood volume is lost. Tachycardia and delayed capillary refill are early signs of shock decreased blood pressure is a late sign.

In tachypneic children, decreased respiratory rate is not necessarily a sign of improvement; it may mean that the child is tiring.

Prepubescent children are more susceptible to abdominal trauma because their organs are not as deeply seated in the pelvis and not as well protected by the thorax as those of adolescents and adults.

Respiratory arrest is more common in children than in adults; if it progresses to cardiopulmonary arrest, children have a poorer prognosis than adults.

Infants and young children are not cognitively or physically capable of protecting themselves from environmental hazards.

Figure 30–1
Developmental and biological variances: emergencies.

or permanent disability. Emergent conditions include cardiopulmonary arrest, multiple system trauma or failure, respiratory distress, and shock.

- Urgent. Any child who requires prompt treatment of a condition that will not compromise life or limb but may tolerate a delay of up to 2 hours. Urgent conditions include mild wheezing, simple lacerations, and uncomplicated fractures.

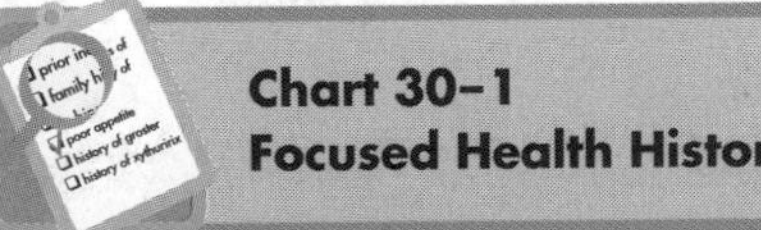

Chart 30–1
Focused Health History

Pediatric Emergencies

Chief complaint	What brought you to seek care today?
History of current complaint	How long has the child been sick? Mechanism of injury? Any treatments initiated?
Identifying data	Name, age, gender, and mode of arrival
Allergies	Does the child have any allergies that you know of?
Medication use	Is the child taking any medication: prescription, over-the-counter, or home remedies? What are they, how much is taken, and how often is it taken?
Past medical history	What is the child's baseline condition?
Immunizations	Are the child's immunizations up to date? When was the last tetanus booster?
Health care provider	Does the child have a primary health care provider? If so, what is the provider's name and phone number?

Chart 30–2

AMPLE Mnemonic for Brief History of Pediatric Emergency

- **A**llergies
- **M**edications
- **P**ast medical history
- **L**ast meal
- **E**vents surrounding incident

- Nonurgent. Any child who requires care for a minor injury or illness in which a treatment can be delayed indefinitely. Nonurgent conditions include sore throats, rashes (other than purpura or petechiae), and ear discomfort.

Telephone Triage

Telephone triage is the process of giving advice over the telephone to callers with questions about their child's condition (Chart 30–4). This process can involve legal risks to the nurse giving the advice and to the hospital. Thus, it is extremely important for health care facilities to have formal policies and protocols and for health care professionals to follow them.

Standardized policies and protocols help guide the nurse to give accurate, complete, and consistent information. They should include who can take the calls, what training is required, and how the calls should be documented. Documentation of the calls should be kept on file for at least 7 years (Thomas, 1991). Any policies and protocols should be reviewed by the medical director and the hospital attorney before implementation (Chart 30–5).

Nursing Diagnoses and Outcomes

Identification of nursing diagnoses is driven by assessment findings. Diagnosis and implementation of interventions aimed at achieving optimal outcomes occur almost simultaneously in an emergent situation. Many pertinent nursing diagnoses are specific to the child's chief complaint. Others are common to most or all emergencies (Chart 30–6). Disease-specific nursing diagnoses are addressed under the specific disease processes.

Developmental and Biological Variances

Types of emergencies experienced by children of different ages are related to development. Differences can be at-

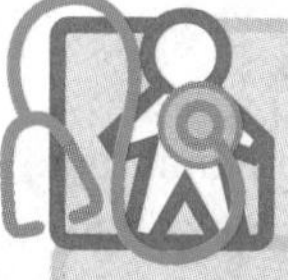

Chart 30–3
Focused Physical Assessment

Triage Assessment from A to I

Airway	Make sure that the airway is open.
Breathing	Check for breathing; begin bag-valve-mask ventilation if needed.
Circulation	Check for a pulse; begin chest compressions if needed.
Disability	Assess level of consciousness by performing a rapid mental status assessment (use AVPU mnemonic): **A:** Is the child alert? **V:** Does the child respond to verbal stimuli? **P:** Does the child respond to painful stimuli? **U:** Is the child unresponsive?
Exposure	Remove clothing and/or diaper to assess for underlying signs of illness or injury.
Fahrenheit	Initiate measures to keep the child warm.
Get vital signs	Obtain a full set of vital signs, including temperature, pulse, respiratory rate, blood pressure, and weight in kilograms.
Head-to-toe assessment	Perform a brief head-to-toe assessment, focusing on the systems affected by the chief complaint.
Inspect	Inspect the back for injuries.
Isolate	Isolate the child as necessary for communicable illness or if the child is immunosuppressed.

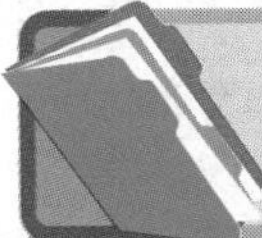

Chart 30–4
Nursing Interventions Classification (NIC)

Telephone Consultation

Definition

Exchanging information, providing health education and advice, managing symptoms or doing triage over the telephone

Activities

Identify purpose of the call.
Calm caller by giving simple instructions for action, as needed.
Obtain information related to the purpose of the call, as necessary (e.g., nature of crisis, medical diagnoses, past health history, and current treatment regimen).
Identify concerns about health status.
Obtain data related to effectiveness of treatment.
Determine whether concerns require medical evaluation.
Provide first-aid instructions or emergency directions for crises (e.g., CPR instructions and birthing).
Stay on the line while contacting emergency services.
Provide clear directions for transport to the hospital, as needed.
Provide instruction on how to access needed care, if concerns are acute.
Provide information about treatment regimen and resultant self-care responsibilities, as necessary, according to scope of practice and established protocols.
Provide information about prescribed therapies and medications, as appropriate.
Provide information about health promotion/health education, as appropriate.
Identify actual/potential problems related to implementing self-care.
Facilitate problem solving about self-care regimen.
Make recommendations about regimen changes, as appropriate.
Consult with physician about changes in the treatment regimen, as necessary.
Provide instructions about preparation for planned diagnostic tests/medical procedures.
Notify patient of test results, as indicated.
Assist with prescription refills, according to established protocols.
Answer questions.
Provide emotional support, as needed.
Maintain confidentiality, as indicated.
Provide information about community resources, educational programs, support groups, and self-help groups, as indicated.
Establish a time and date for follow-up care, including further telephone consultation.
Determine how patient or family member can be reached for a return telephone call, as appropriate.
Record any advice, instructions, or other information given to patient.
Follow up by calling the client back if uncomfortable with the communication.

From McCloskey, J., & Bulechek, G. (1996). *Nursing interventions classification (NIC)* (2nd ed.). St. Louis: Mosby–Year Book. Reprinted with permission.

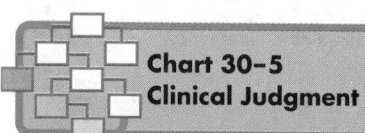

Chart 30–5
Clinical Judgment

Triage

Sol is a 4-year-old carried into the emergency department by his father, who says, "My son says he's not feeling too good." Sol is leaning against his father holding his head erect with his chin jutting out slightly, alert but not interacting with his environment. He has a respiratory rate of about 40 breaths per minute, and his lips are blue with nasal flaring.

Questions

1. What is Sol's most obvious problem?
2. What factors did you base your assessment on?
3. In what triage category should the nurse classify him?
4. Based on the triage decision, what needs to be done now?
5. Sol's respiratory distress is worsening; what needs to be done?

Answers

1. Respiratory distress.
2. Cyanosis, nasal flaring, posturing to maintain open airway, tachypnea (normal respiratory rate for a 4-year-old is in the 20s), developmentally incongruent behavior: Sol is 4 years old but was carried in, and he is not interested in his surroundings.
3. Emergent.
4. Sol needs to be taken to the treatment area for immediate intervention. Because Sol still seems to be compensating and maintaining his airway, let him maintain his position of comfort; do not lay him down, leave him in his father's lap. Administer oxygen, and perform a brief physical examination (A to I) while obtaining a brief history (AMPLE).
5. Ensure that someone skilled in bag-valve-mask ventilation and advanced pediatric life support is monitoring him; have the physician or nurse practitioner evaluate for treatment of underlying disorder.

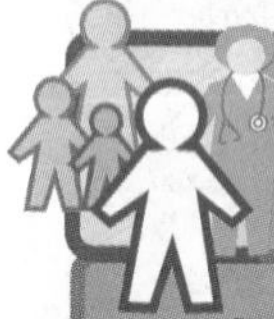

Chart 30–6
Nursing Diagnoses and Outcomes

Pediatric Emergencies

Anxiety related to unknown situation and outcome

Outcomes: Child will be told, in age-appropriate terms, what is being done; parents will be with child as much as possible.
Family will be kept informed of child's condition and what is being done for the child.

Anticipatory grieving related to unknown and potentially fatal outcome

Outcome: Child/family will be kept informed of child's condition, will be given opportunity to verbalize feelings, and will mobilize own support systems (e.g., spiritual, community).

Pain related to symptoms of chief complaint or diagnostic procedures

Outcome: Child will have pain adequately managed.

Risk for altered parenting related to hospital environment and changes in the child resulting from disease or injury

Outcome: Parents will be included in providing care of and support to child and will verbalize physical or cognitive changes in child and revise parenting expectations on the basis of these.

Altered tissue perfusion: (specify) related to disease or injury

Outcome: Child will have signs of altered tissue perfusion recognized promptly and treatment implemented.

Chart 30–7
Developmental Considerations

Common Emergencies Based on Age

Age Group	Common Medical Emergencies	Common Traumatic Events
Infant	SIDS Apnea Sepsis Bronchiolitis Seizures	Shaken baby syndrome Falls (off furniture, down stairs in baby walkers) Motor vehicle accident Foreign body aspiration Suffocation Drowning
Toddler/preschool	Croup Asthma Vomiting and/or dehydration Seizures Appendicitis	Foreign body aspiration Poisoning Falls Drowning Child abuse Burns Motor vehicle accident
School-age	Asthma Appendicitis Seizures Gastrointestinal disturbances	Motor vehicle accident Bicycle injury Sports injury
Adolescent	Colitis Urinary tract infection Pelvic inflammatory disease	Motor vehicle accident Sports injury Firearm injury Drug and alcohol ingestions (accidental and intentional)

tributed to cognitive immaturity (innate curiosity, not perceiving the danger of a situation) and structural and functional changes that occur as the child grows and matures (see Fig. 30–1). Young children have a greater ratio of surface area to body mass than adults, placing children at higher risk for hypothermia. This must be considered in prehospital care or during a resuscitation, because hypothermia increases metabolic demands, increases pulmonary vascular resistance, and contributes to acidosis. A child's airway is more difficult to stabilize and manage than an adult's because the larynx is more cephalad and anterior, making the vocal cords more difficult to visualize during intubation. Also, the airway diameter in a child is narrower, resulting in greater airway loss with only small amounts of edema.

Children have a smaller total blood volume than adults; therefore, small volumes of blood lost can lead to relatively greater hypovolemia and impaired perfusion and oxygenation. Children are also at risk for significant abdominal injuries. Their immature abdominal musculature is thinner, weaker, and less developed than that of an adult and provides less protection and support of the internal organs; thus, the liver and spleen are more easily injured.

Variances are seen between age groups in the etiology of the situation: medical pathology or traumatic injury (Chart 30–7). Young children, in particular, frequently present to the emergency department (ED) with fever, not eating, or a change in sleep patterns. It is then that the underlying pathology is detected.

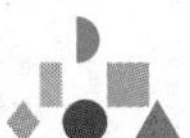

Diagnostic Criteria for Evaluating Pediatric Emergencies

Diagnostic procedures used in emergency situations vary depending on the child's pathology or injury and presenting symptoms (Table 30–1). Other tests may be performed depending on the mechanism of injury (e.g., a child with iron ingestion has serum iron levels evaluated) or pathology (e.g., if the child has signs of meningitis a lumbar puncture is done). When head or neck injuries are known or suspected, cervical spine precautions must be maintained until spinal cord injury is evaluated.

In an emergency, procedures often need to be performed rapidly. The health care provider must always

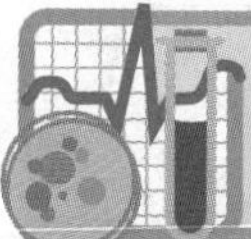

Table 30–1
Diagnostic Tests and Procedures for Evaluating Pediatric Emergencies

Diagnostic Test or Procedure	Purpose	Findings and Indications	Health Care Provider Responsibilities
Complete blood count with differential	To detect infection or lack of immune response	Elevated WBC with shift to the left may indicate infection; in neonates, may see neutropenia with infection.	Obtain blood, check results, intervene on the basis of results.
	To detect blood loss	↓ Red blood cells. ↓ Hemoglobin.	
Type and crossmatch	To determine child's blood type and compatibility of blood to transfuse		Obtain blood, check results, intervene on the basis of results. May give O negative blood in emergency before type and crossmatch results are obtained.
Serum electrolytes (including glucose)	To detect electrolyte imbalance	Values outside normal reference ranges for age of child.	Obtain blood, check results, intervene on the basis of results.
Radiographs			
Chest	To detect abnormalities in heart, lung, or ribs	Congestive heart failure, pneumothorax, pneumonia, broken ribs.	Maintain c-spine precautions until cleared. Protect child's genitals with lead shield.
Abdomen	To detect obstruction, perforation, structural abnormalities in abdominal organs	Dilated intestine proximal to obstruction, free air with perforation.	Position the child.
Bones	To detect fractures	Crack, malalignment of bone.	
Computed tomography (CT scan)	To detect bleeding or masses		Closely monitor cardiorespiratory status. Implement conscious sedation protocol if child is sedated.
Peritoneal lavage	To detect blood in peritoneal cavity	Positive result, indicated by blood-tinged fluid, indicates internal bleeding; surgical exploration will be done. Clear fluid return is inconclusive; a CT scan may then be obtained to detect retroperitoneal bleeding.	Set up equipment for lavage. Assist with procedure. Intervene on the basis of results.

provide age-appropriate support and preparation, even if explanations are given as the procedure is being done. Monitor the child's status during the procedure. The additional stress to an already compromised child may precipitate further deterioration.

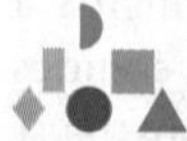

Treatment Modalities

The best treatment for pediatric emergencies is, of course, prevention. Parents, family members, and caretakers should be familiar with child safety techniques, such as "babyproofing" the home, and first-aid procedures (Chart 30–8).

Pediatric Cardiopulmonary Resuscitation

In adults, the most common causes of cardiopulmonary arrest are lethal arrhythmias secondary to heart disease (Emergency Cardiac Care Committee and Subcommittees, American Heart Association, 1992). Cardiopulmonary arrest in infants and children typically results from disorders that lead to respiratory failure and shock. Out-

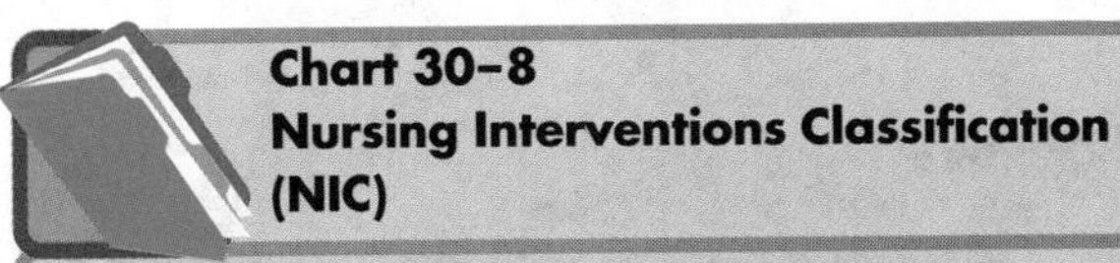

Chart 30–8
Nursing Interventions Classification (NIC)

First Aid

Definition

Providing initial care of a minor injury

Activities

Control bleeding.
Immobilize the affected body part, as appropriate.
Elevate the affected body part.
Apply a sling, if appropriate.
Cover any open or exposed bony parts.
Apply ice to the affected body part, as appropriate.
Monitor vital signs, as appropriate.
Cool the skin with water in minor burns.
Flood with water any tissue exposed to a chemical irritant.
Remove the stinger from an insect bite, as appropriate.
Remove the tick from the skin, as appropriate.
Cleanse and remove secretions from the area around a nonpoisonous snake bite.
Cover with a blanket, as appropriate.
Administer tetanus, as appropriate.
Instruct to seek further medical care, as appropriate.
Coordinate emergency transport, as needed.

From McCloskey, J., & Bulechek, G. (1996). *Nursing interventions classification (NIC)* (2nd ed.). St. Louis: Mosby–Year Book. Reprinted with permission.

comes of cardiopulmonary arrests in children are usually poor, with high morbidity and mortality rates. Children who survive cardiopulmonary arrest are often left with severe neurologic disabilities (Haley & Baker, 1993).

The nurse must understand and be able to recognize the signs of respiratory failure and/or shock in the child. Signs of impending failure may be subtle because the child is equipped to compensate physiologically for illness or injury for a relatively long period of time. For example, the hypovolemic child compensates by an increase in heart rate to maintain cardiac output. Rapid recognition of the conditions that precede arrest and prompt intervention to prevent arrest are the keys to successful management of the critically ill child.

Cardiac arrest in children is most commonly preceded by respiratory failure. Initially, the child compensates with an increased heart rate to maintain the blood pressure and cardiac output. Bradycardia ensues as the child becomes increasingly hypoxic. Without intervention, cardiopulmonary arrest follows.

The treatment of the child in cardiopulmonary arrest begins with assessment of the ABCs (airway, breathing, circulation) and beginning basic life support, which is also known as cardiopulmonary resuscitation (CPR) (Table 30–2). The child requiring CPR should be transported to a facility that can provide pediatric advanced life support measures and definitive treatment.

Advanced Life Support

Advanced life support includes

- Measures to stabilize the airway, such as endotracheal intubation
- Assistance with breathing, such as manual positive pressure ventilations with a bag-valve-mask device and 100% oxygen (Chart 30–9)
- Circulatory support, such as obtaining vascular access and administration of fluids and emergency medications

The length-based resuscitation tape is a tool that can be used to provide a rapid estimate of the child's length, extrapolating from this appropriate-sized emergency equipment to use and dosages of emergency medications to administer. Use of the length-based resuscitation tape by prehospital care providers is considered a standard of care. Many emergency departments also use this tape when a child requires emergent resuscitation and there is no time to weigh the child (Fig. 30–2).

Vascular Access

Vascular access is a high priority in pediatric advanced life support, because the child in arrest is often hypovolemic. The largest gauge catheter that can be rapidly and reliably inserted should be utilized. Secure two intravenous (IV) sites to provide optimal routes for fluid resuscitation. During resuscitation, the easiest peripheral IV sites to access are the antecubital fossa, the dorsum of the hands, and the saphenous veins.

Three attempts to obtain peripheral vascular access within 90 seconds should be made. If peripheral IV access is unsuccessful, the intraosseous (IO) route can be attempted in children younger than 6 years. The IO cannula is placed in the medial surface of the tibia, approximately one fingerbreadth below the tibial tuberosity (see Fig. 17–7). Access is achieved using specially made IO cannulas or spinal needles. The cannula is placed properly if there is a decrease in resistance to insertion (the cannula has then entered the marrow), the needle remains upright without support, and fluids can be pushed freely into the cannula. It may not be possible to aspirate bone marrow after the IO needle is in place.

Table 30–2
Summary of Basic Life Support Maneuvers in Infants and Children

Maneuver	Infant (Younger than 1 Year)	Child (1–8 Years)
Airway	Head tilt–chin lift (If trauma is present, use jaw thrust.)	Head tilt–chin lift (If trauma is present, use jaw thrust.)
Breathing		
Initial	Two breaths at 1–1½ sec per breath	Two breaths at 1–1½ sec per breath
Subsequent	20 breaths per minute (approximate)	20 breaths per minute (approximate)
Circulation		
Pulse check	Brachial or femoral	Carotid
Compression area	Lower half of sternum	Lower half of sternum
Compression width	Two or three fingers	Heel of one hand
Depth	Approximately one third to one half the depth of the chest	Approximately one third to one half the depth of the chest
Rate	At least 100 per minute	100 per minute
Compression/ventilation ratio	5 : 1 (pause for ventilation)	5 : 1 (pause for ventilation)
Foreign body airway obstruction	Back blows or chest thrusts	Heimlich maneuver

However, if any marrow is aspirated, it can be used for bedside blood glucose testing.

If the attempt to place the IO needle is unsuccessful, another site should be selected for further IO attempts. The same extremity should not be used, as the bone may have been punctured during the unsuccessful attempt, and any fluids or medications infused into the new site may leak back out the first site, causing extravasation. Other options for vascular access include central venous access and a venous cutdown. Both of these procedures require a skilled practitioner, and they are more time intensive than using the peripheral or IO route.

Fluid Administration

Once vascular access is obtained, the priority is to deliver fluids to restore volume and emergency medications to assist cardiac function. Volume expansion is achieved by administering fluids. Blood is the fluid of choice for the pediatric trauma victim. However, isotonic crystalloid solutions such as normal saline or Ringer's lactate are more readily available and inexpensive fluids that are effective volume expanders for the hypovolemic patient. If crystalloids are used, three to four times the deficit volume may have to be administered, as the solutions only transiently expand the intravascular compartment.

Medication Administration

Emergency or resuscitation medications can be delivered by the IV, IO, or, in some cases, the endotracheal route (Chart 30–10). Anything that can be given IV can be given IO (Table 30–3).

caREminder: *Unlike adult dosages, pediatric dosages of all resuscitation medications are based on the child's weight.*

The nurse must be familiar with the various drugs, their indications, dosages, and administration techniques. Prepared drug sheets listing drug dosages according to weight are helpful in eliminating drug calculation anxiety and errors during an intense resuscitation.

Figure 30–2
The length-based resuscitation tape is used to select appropriate-sized resuscitation equipment to use and medication dosages to administer.

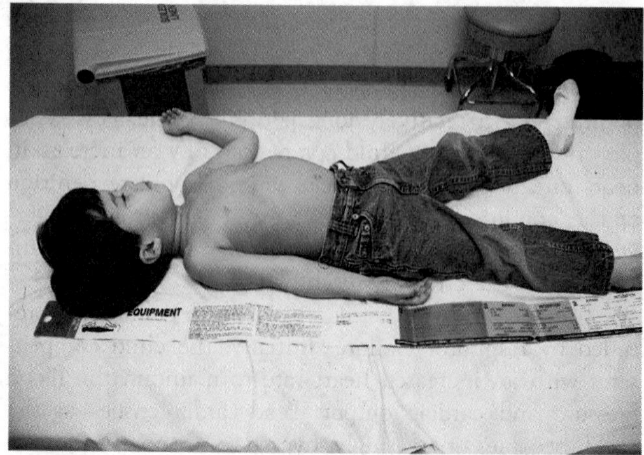

Chart 30–9
Nursing Interventions

Endotracheal Tube Intubation

Assess for indications for endotracheal tube (ET) intubation:
- Respiratory insufficiency
- Hypoxemia
- Respiratory arrest
- Glasgow Coma Score <8

Prepare the equipment:
- Proper size ET tube
  Do not choose a cuffed tube for a child younger than 8 years because it can damage the trachea. The smallest portion of the pediatric airway is the cricoid ring; using the correct size ET tube creates a natural cuff.
- Laryngoscope with:
  Functioning light and charged battery
  Proper size straight or curved blade
- Resuscitation bag with 100% oxygen source
- Suction source
- Rigid tonsil suction
- Tape
- Stethoscope

Assist with intubation:
- Provide several positive pressure bag-valve-mask (BVM) breaths before the intubation attempt.
- Monitor the heart rate throughout procedure.
- Anticipate the need for resuscitation equipment, and have it immediately available.

Provide care immediately after ET tube placement:
- Resume BVM manual ventilations immediately.
- Hold the tube securely until placement is confirmed and the tube is taped securely in place.
- Auscultate breath sounds bilaterally.
  If no breath sounds are heard:
  Pull the ET tube immediately.
  Resume BVM ventilations.
  After several positive pressure breaths, repeat attempt to intubate.
  If breath sounds are heard only on the right side:
  The ET tube may have been inserted down the right mainstem bronchus.
  Pull the ET tube out slightly until bilateral breath sounds are heard.
- Secure the tube. Prepare the taping site with tincture of benzoin to help secure the tape and ET tube; this decreases the need for frequent retaping of the tube.
- Record the tube cm markings at upper gum.

Volume replacement is the first-line treatment for poor perfusion and hypotension. However, after multiple fluid boluses, the child may develop a deterioration of lung compliance and pulmonary edema. Thus, after spontaneous circulation returns, the postarrest child may need medications to maintain or achieve adequate blood pressure and systemic perfusion. The three most common inotropic agents used after an arrest are epinephrine, dopamine, and dobutamine. Epinephrine is the drug of choice for children during and immediately after resuscitation. These medications are given by continuous IV or IO infusion and are titrated to maintain adequate blood pressure and perfusion.

Psychosocial Support

Critical illness or injury is a stressor. The onset is usually acute and unexpected, the environment and treatments unfamiliar and painful, the outcome uncertain. Usual coping mechanisms used by the child and family may not be adequate in an emergency situation. While addressing the child's physiologic needs, the health care team must

Table 30–3
Pediatric Emergency Medications

Drug	Indications	Dose*	Interventions
Oxygen From tank or wall-mounted delivery device	Seriously ill or injured child with respiratory insufficiency, trauma, shock, even if measured arterial oxygen is high	100% oxygen during initial stabilization	Place mask on child's face; if child fights this, hold or have parent hold oxygen mask or tubing close to child's nose and mouth. Monitor oxygen saturation via pulse oximetry, interpret results considering patient status, anemia or vasoconstriction may result in inaccurate readings.
Fluid *Crystalloid* Lactated Ringer's–normal saline *Colloid* 5% albumin Synthetic colloid solutions: Hetastarch Dextran Blood Fresh frozen plasma	Hypovolemia	20 mL/kg per dose Repeat as necessary Some children need up to 80 mL/kg within first hour.	Infuse as rapid bolus. Evaluate perfusion after every fluid bolus and frequently. Give blood to pediatric trauma victims who continue to show signs of hypovolemic shock after two boluses of crystalloid.
Epinephrine	Cardiac arrest, symptomatic bradycardia unresponsive to oxygen and ventilation, non–volume-related hypotension	For symptomatic bradycardia and initial dose for cardiac arrest: 0.01 mg/kg (0.1 mL of 1 : 10,000 solution) Subsequent doses for cardiac arrest: 0.1 mg/kg (0.1 mL of 1 : 1000 solution), repeat dose every 3–5 min p.r.n.	Give via endotracheal tube (Chart 31–9) until vascular access can be obtained. Evaluate child's response. Repeat dose p.r.n.; increase to 1 : 1000 solution for cardiac arrest.
Atropine	Symptomatic bradycardia unresponsive to ventilation and oxygenation	0.02 mg/kg *Minimum single* dose: 0.1 mg *Maximum single* dose: 0.5 mg for child 1.0 mg for adolescent May repeat in 5 min for a *maximum total* dose of 1.0 mg for child, 2.0 mg for adolescent.	Ensure adequate ventilation and oxygenation.
Sodium bicarbonate	Documented metabolic acidosis	1 mEq/kg Repeat every 10 min on the basis of arterial blood gas analysis.	Ensure adequate ventilation and oxygenation of child before giving sodium bicarbonate. Ensure adequate ventilation during administration (the drug's buffering action produces carbon dioxide). Flush IV line before and after drug administration with normal saline: precipitates in presence catecholamines or calcium.

Table 30–3
Pediatric Emergency Medications *Continued*

Drug	Indications	Dose*	Interventions
Naloxone	Reverse effects of opioids	Children from birth to 5 yr of age or weighing up to 20 kg: 0.1 mg/kg Children older than 5 yr or weighing over 20 kg: 2.0 mg/dose May repeat every 2 min until desired opioid reversal is achieved.	Monitor child carefully for recurrence of opioid effects; naloxone has a shorter half-life than opioids and may need to be repeated. These doses usually achieve total opioid reversal; use smaller doses if partial reversal desired.
Glucose	Documented hypoglycemia or if the child fails to respond to standard resuscitation measures	0.5–1.0 g/kg Use a maximum concentration of 25% glucose to administer peripherally; glucose is supplied as D-50, so dilute 1 : 1 with sterile water and give 2 to 4 mL/kg.	Perform bedside glucose testing as soon as possible. Monitor IV closely (D-25 is hyperosmolar and may sclerose peripheral veins).
Calcium chloride	Documented or suspected hypocalcemia, hyperkalemia, hypermagnesemia, and calcium channel blocker overdose	20 mg/kg/dose Repeat *only* if measured calcium deficiency is present.	Do not administer routinely during resuscitation (may contribute to cellular injury). Administer slowly (no faster than 100 mg/min), may induce bradycardia or asystole. Monitor IV closely; irritating to veins and causes chemical burns if infiltrates surrounding tissue. Do not mix with sodium bicarbonate.

* Recommended doses are for children older than 1 mo.

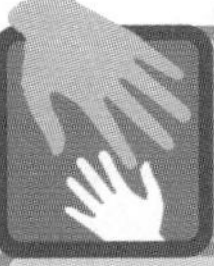

Chart 30–10
Nursing Interventions

Administering Medications by Endotracheal Tube

- Ensure that the drug is appropriate for ET tube administration. To do this think of the mnemonic LEAN:
  - **L**idocaine—the endotracheal dose is the same as the IV dose.
  - **E**pinephrine—use 0.1 mg/kg of 1:1000 solution. The ET tube dose of epinephrine is always "high" except in neonates.
  - **A**tropine—the ET tube dose is increased two to three times the IV dose (0.02 mg/kg with a minimum dose of 0.1 mg).
  - **N**aloxone—the ET tube dose is the same as the IV dose.
- Instill the drug as prescribed directly into the ET tube.
- Follow with lavage of normal saline.
- Provide several positive pressure ventilations to disperse the medication into the pulmonary vasculature.

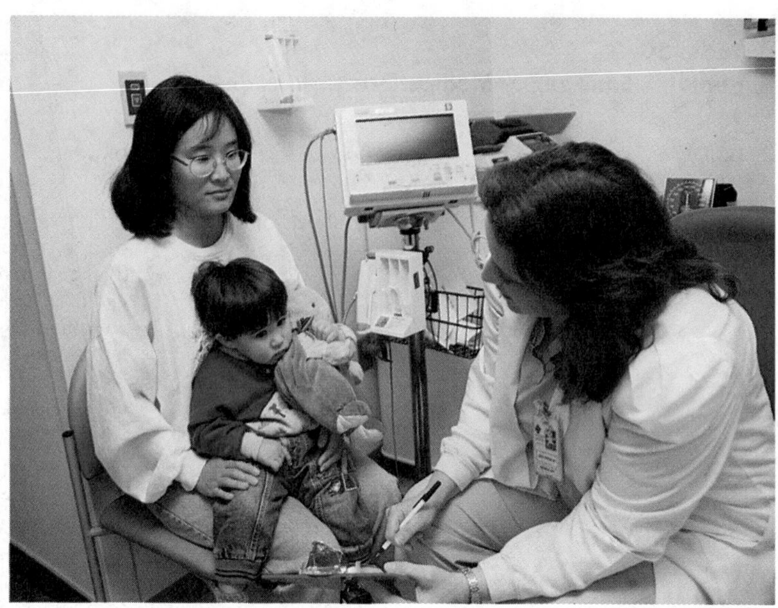

Figure 30–3
Emotional security can be promoted by letting the child hold onto a favorite toy or security object from home or one from the ED stock.

place a high priority on providing emotional support to the child and family during this stressful time.

The atmosphere during an emergency can be chaotic and overstimulating. Keep the parents or significant other with the child whenever possible. Involve the parents in the child's care; tell the parents in concrete terms what they can do to support the child (e.g., hold the child's hand and talk quietly to him or her). Attempt to talk quietly and soothingly and provide comfort measures (Fig. 30–3). When time permits, prepare the child and family before performing procedures. Otherwise, explain what is being done in developmentally appropriate terms, as it is performed, even if it seems that the child cannot hear.

It is controversial whether the family should be in the room during invasive procedures or while a child is being resuscitated. Many health care providers are uncomfortable with family presence at these times because of concerns about legal liability, family presence negatively affecting the staff's ability to perform procedures, the atmosphere during a resuscitation, and the family's response to the process. When allowed, parental presence during invasive procedures did not negatively affect procedure performance and, although parental presence did not seem to reduce the child's pain, parents were less anxious (Bauchner, Vinci, Bak, Pearson, & Corwin, 1996). Being present during the resuscitation may help the family through the grieving process if the child dies, because the parents know that everything possible was done to save their child. The Emergency Nurses Association (1996) supports the practice of family presence during resuscitation and invasive procedures.

Nurses, physicians, respiratory therapists, and other health care providers must provide emotional support to the child and family during interactions with them and provide frequent updates about the child's condition. Families need information and timely support. Providing this has a positive impact on their grieving process and perception of the quality of care delivered (Cross et al., 1996). Initial information should be given within 30 minutes. Direct care providers are usually busy attending to the physiologic needs of the child. It is extremely helpful to have a social worker or chaplain immediately accessible to support the family. The social worker or chaplain can keep the family updated on the child's condition, provide resources, and help the family deal with information, make decisions, and mobilize their own resources.

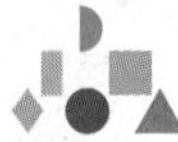

Specific Pediatric Emergencies

Shock

Shock refers to sustained and progressive circulatory dysfunction that results in inadequate delivery of oxygen and other substances needed to meet metabolic demands. There are four types of shock: hypovolemic, cardiogenic, distributive (includes septic), and obstructive. Each type has a distinct etiology. Assessment findings and nursing interventions may vary depending on the etiology (Table 30–4).

Table 30–4
Types of Shock: Assessment and Interventions

Type of Shock	Etiology	Assessment Findings	Interdisciplinary Interventions
Hypovolemic	Caused by inadequate volume relative to the vascular space; primarily caused by dehydration or traumatic hemorrhage	Tachycardia Prolonged capillary refill (longer than 2 sec) Weak, thready, or absent peripheral pulses Cool extremities	Administer IV fluids: 20 mL/kg bolus of 0.9% normal saline or Ringer's lactate; repeat as necessary. If signs of inadequate tissue perfusion are present: after two or three boluses of crystalloid fluid, administer 10 mL/kg packed red blood cells (type specific or O negative). Use colloid solutions such as albumin, if needed, until blood is available. Control bleeding by applying direct pressure to external sites of bleeding with sterile gauze.
Cardiogenic	Caused by impairment of myocardial function	Tachycardia Tachypnea Narrow pulse pressure Cool, mottled skin Capillary refill longer than 2 sec Weak peripheral pulses Decreased urine output Hepatomegaly Neck vein distention (older child) Rales Edema	Administer oxygen. Administer IV fluid: 20 mL/kg bolus. Carefully assess child's response to fluid bolus; children in heart failure may be fluid overloaded. Administer inotropes to improve cardiac contractility (dopamine, dobutamine). Administer diuretics to improve preload. Correct acid-base, electrolyte imbalances.
Distributive	Septic shock is discussed here; for anaphylaxis, see Chart 30–14. Caused by inappropriate distribution of blood flow and increased capillary permeability Is the most common type of shock in the newborn Most commonly results from gram-negative organisms	History of infection History of poor feeding Tachycardia Fever Tachypnea Altered mental status Petechiae and/or purpura Poor peripheral perfusion (capillary refill longer than 2 sec)	Isolate the child as necessary. Administer IV fluid in volumes of up to 80 mL/kg (in boluses of 20 mL/kg) to restore circulating volume. Administer inotropic agents as needed. Draw blood samples for cultures immediately. Administer wide-spectrum antibiotics; do not postpone antibiotic therapy until culture results are available. Administer IV glucose p.r.n. to treat hypoglycemia.
Obstructive	Caused by inability of normal heart to produce adequate cardiac output despite normal intravascular volume because of mechanical obstruction (e.g., tension pneumothorax, cardiac tamponade, pulmonary embolism)	See Table 30–6 on traumatic chest injuries	See Table 30–6 on traumatic chest injuries. Relieve obstruction.

Shock is the second most common mechanism of death in children after respiratory failure (Corneli, 1993). The most common cause of shock in children is hypovolemia. In the United States this is most often caused by bleeding as a result of trauma. Worldwide, the most prevalent cause of hypovolemic shock is fluid and electrolyte losses associated with gastroenteritis (Vernon-Levett, 1995).

The incidence of septic shock is increasing in children and adults, possibly as a result of increased numbers of immunosuppressed patients and of more extensive use of invasive therapies in the critically ill (Bone, 1991).

Morbidity and mortality associated with shock are dependent on the etiology and the health care providers' ability to recognize the signs promptly and intervene appropriately before shock becomes irreversible. Mortality associated with septic shock is dependent on the initial site of infection, causative organism, and presence of multiple organ dysfunction syndrome. Gram-negative enteric sepsis has a mortality rate of 40% to 60% (Powell, 1996).

Assessment

Shock may be classified as compensated or decompensated. In compensated shock, the child becomes tachycardic in an effort to increase the cardiac output. The blood pressure remains normal, capillary refill time may be prolonged (more than 2 seconds), and the child may become irritable because of increasing hypoxia. In decompensated shock, the child displays decreased blood pressure and level of consciousness (stupor or coma) and tachypnea or signs of respiratory failure.

Without treatment, compensatory mechanisms can sustain cellular function only temporarily. As shock progresses, cellular metabolic changes result in further tissue injury and ultimately cell death (Corneli, 1993).

Alert: *Hypotension is a late sign of hypovolemic shock in children. It may represent a 25% loss of circulating blood volume.*

Nursing Diagnoses and Outcomes

Nursing diagnoses and outcomes for the child in an emergency situation are presented in Chart 30–6. In addition, the following are applicable to the child in shock:

- **Decreased cardiac output related to effects of hypovolemia, sepsis, obstruction**
  Outcome: The child will have signs of decreased cardiac output recognized promptly and interventions instituted immediately.
- **Fluid volume deficit related to effects of disease process or injury**
  Outcome: The child will have signs of fluid volume deficit recognized promptly, vascular access obtained, and fluid administered until the child shows no signs of hypovolemia.
- **Fluid volume excess related to effects of myocardial dysfunction**
  Outcome: The child will have signs of fluid volume excess recognized promptly and interventions instituted to optimize oxygenation and reduce fluid volume.

Interdisciplinary Interventions

Shock states result in the failure of cellular oxygenation. The nurse, physician, and respiratory therapist must work as a team to implement interventions that optimize oxygenation in the child. Administer 100% oxygen, and ventilate and intubate as needed. The goal of treatment of shock is to restore circulating blood volume in order to maintain adequate tissue perfusion and cardiovascular stability. Vascular access should be obtained as soon as possible to administer fluid and vasoactive drugs as needed. Monitor electrolyte and glucose levels and correct as indicated. Minimize stress to the child, which further increases metabolic, thus oxygen, demands. Maintain a normothermic environment; temperature extremes also increase metabolic demands. Reassess the child's status after every intervention and frequently.

Trauma

Injury is the leading cause of death of children 1 to 14 years of age (Guyer, Strobino, Ventura, MacDorman, & Martin, 1996). Head trauma is a major factor in pediatric mortality and morbidity (Ghajar & Hariri, 1992). More than 500,000 children are hospitalized annually after head injuries, and nearly 4000 of these children die (Haley & Baker, 1993). The mechanisms of injury leading to head injury commonly include motor vehicle accidents, falls, sports and recreation accidents, and assaults.

The causes of other traumatic injuries are diverse. The most common are motor vehicle accidents (including automobile-pedestrian and automobile-bicycle accidents), drowning, burns, falls, and firearm injuries. Blunt injuries are more common than penetrating ones in children. Two of three injuries are to males (Scheidt et al., 1995).

Mortality rates for children with injuries have declined steadily in the past decade, in part because of injury prevention programs. Firearm fatalities have been rising (Rivara & Grossman, 1996).

Trauma care is provided through a team effort (Polhgeers & Ruddy, 1995). Standardized policies and procedures should identify the roles and responsibilities of all the trauma team members. Pediatric victims of multi-

Table 30–5
Pediatric Trauma Score and Revised Trauma Score

Pediatric Trauma Score*

Component	**Category** +2	+1	−1
Size	>20 kg (40 lb)	10–20 kg	<10 kg
Airway	Normal	Maintainable	Unmaintainable
Systolic BP	>90 mmHg	50–90 mmHg	<50 mmHg
CNS	Awake	Obtunded	Coma or decerebrate
Skeletal	None	Closed fracture	Open or multiple fractures
Cutaneous wound	None	Minor	Major or penetrating
			Sum ________ (PTS)

Revised Trauma Score†

Glasgow Coma Scale	**Systolic Blood Pressure**	**Respiratory Rate**	**Coded Value**
13–15	>89	10–29	4
9–12	76–89	>29	3
6–8	50–75	6–9	2
4–5	1–49	1–5	1
3	0	0	0

* From Tepas, J. J., Ramenofsky, M. L., Mollitt, D. L., Gans, B. M., & DiScala, C. (1988). The pediatric trauma score as a predictor of injury severity: An objective assessment. *Journal of Trauma, 28,* 425–429. Used with permission.

† From Champion, H. R., Sacco, W. J., Copes, W. S., Gann, D. S., Gennarelli, T. A., & Flanagan, M. E. (1989). A revision of the trauma score. *Journal of Trauma, 29,* 623–629. Used with permission.

system trauma or those having a high mortality risk (Pediatric Trauma Score ≤8 or a Revised Trauma Score ≤11) (Table 30–5) should be transported to a trauma center with pediatric expertise (Chameides & Hazinski, 1994). The risk of exposure to blood and other body fluids is high in treating trauma patients. Therefore, health care providers must wear personal protective equipment (i.e., gloves, goggles, mask, and gown) to minimize the exposure risk before initiating care of the trauma patient.

Assessment

The commonly used mnemonic "A through I" represents the steps of the primary and secondary assessments (see Chart 30–3) (Bennett & Baker, 1995). These steps prioritize assessments of the trauma patient and identify lifesaving interventions that may be necessary.

Primary Assessment and Care

Begin the primary assessment by assessing the **ABC**s. As in CPR, remember not to continue to the next step until the previous step has been stabilized.

Open the airway and assess for patency. Suction any blood, vomitus, or debris in the oropharynx. Check for any displaced or loose teeth. For the child with a suspected head injury, use the combined jaw thrust–spinal stabilization maneuver to open the airway and manually hold the head in a neutral position. After the airway is opened, if head injury is suspected, stabilize the cervical spine (c-spine) to prevent cervical motion, using a semirigid extrication collar of the appropriate size (Fig. 30–4). The collar must fit perfectly. If too large, it may allow cervical movement, which may convert an incomplete spinal cord injury to a complete one.

Alert: *For the child with a head injury, ensure that the neck remains in a neutral position, not hyperextended. One team member should hold the neck in position while another performs the intubation. Also take c-spine precautions with a near-drowning victim. The child may have hit his or her head during the drowning or when falling into a pool.*

Assess for breathing next. Remember that blunt and penetrating traumatic injuries to the chest can severely

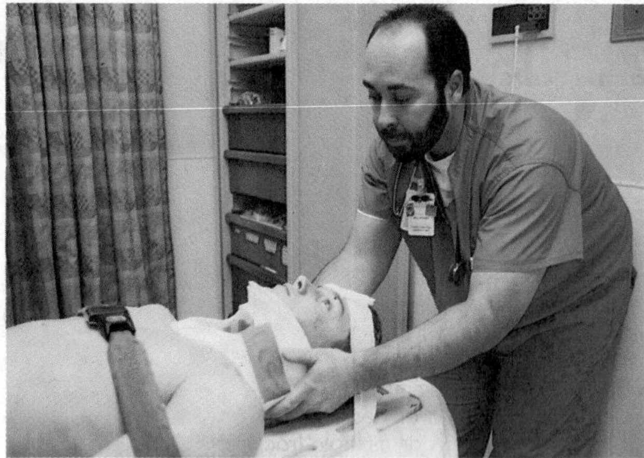

Figure 30–4
For a trauma victim, the cervical spine must be immobilized while the airway is opened. This is done using a combined jaw thrust and spinal stabilization maneuver.

compromise breathing. Unless these injuries are aggressively assessed, recognized, and rapidly treated, they can kill the patient (Table 30–6). For all trauma patients, administer oxygen by a nonrebreather mask in the highest concentration available until complete assessment of the oxygenation and perfusion status is performed. Oxygen should be given because the child may have as yet unrecognized respiratory failure and shock, both of which contribute to tissue hypoxia. The goal is to stabilize the effects of hypoxia before irreversible damage occurs. If necessary, assist with ventilations using a bag-valve-mask device supplied with 100% oxygen, and prepare for intubation. Place a nasogastric tube (or orogastric tube in the child with a suspected basilar skull fracture) to decompress the stomach.

Assess the child's circulatory status (see Chart 30–3). Begin chest compressions on the patient without a pulse, and initiate further advanced life support measures.

Obtain vascular access without delay by placing two large-bore (22 gauge or larger) IV lines peripherally. Because leg injuries are more common in children, the arms are the sites of choice for IV access. Do not attempt vascular access in a fractured or severely injured extremity, because vascular compromise is a concern. If vascular access remains unsuccessful, experienced personnel should attempt percutaneous access of the femoral vein or saphenous vein cutdown. If signs of hypovolemic shock occur, treat aggressively with fluid replacement (see Table 30–4).

Once the ABCs have been stabilized, assess D, disability, by doing a brief neurologic examination, including level of consciousness and pupillary response to light. This determines neurologic status and establishes a baseline from which to evaluate change. Test the child for hypoglycemia. If hypoglycemia is present, treat with 25% dextrose. Administer naloxone (Narcan) for suspected opioid overdose.

Secondary Assessment and Care

Secondary assessment includes reassessing the ABCs and then proceeding to assess "E through I." Expose the child, removing all clothing. Provide the patient with a heat source (Fahrenheit), to prevent hypothermia. An overhead warmer is ideal, because it allows continued full visualization of the patient.

Get a full set of vital signs, including pulse, respiratory rate, blood pressure, and rectal temperature. Rectal temperatures are the standard of care. Oral temperatures are not appropriate for young children, those with an altered level of consciousness, or those requiring assistance maintaining their airway. Axillary temperatures take too long to obtain, and vasoconstriction or dilation may result in inaccurate readings.

Perform a head-to-toe examination and obtain a history, using the AMPLE mnemonic (see Chart 30–2). The head-to-toe examination may reveal signs and symptoms of internal hemorrhage, such as abdominal pain, guarding, rigidity, or tenderness. The abdomen may be distended and have signs of obvious abdominal trauma such as a positive seat belt sign (bruising that correlates with the position of the seat belt). Shock that persists despite aggressive fluid replacement may indicate internal hemorrhage and require immediate surgery.

Finally, inspect the patient's back. To do this, roll the child over, maintaining c-spine precautions (logrolling). Then check for penetrating objects, bleeding, bruising, abrasions, or lacerations.

Nursing Diagnoses and Outcomes

Nursing diagnoses and outcomes applicable to the child and family when the child is experiencing a medical emergency are discussed in Chart 30–6. The nursing diagnoses and outcomes identified for the child in shock (p. 2062) are frequently relevant to the child who has suffered a traumatic injury. Additional ones are

- **Ineffective airway clearance related to effects of injury**
  Outcome: The child will have signs of ineffective airway clearance recognized immediately and interventions to clear the airway implemented promptly.
- **Hypothermia related to exposure from injury or treatment**
  Outcome: The child will have body temperature maintained within the normal range while being exposed adequately during inspection for injuries and treatment.

Table 30–6
Types of Traumatic Chest Injuries: Assessment and Intervention

Injury Type	Definition	Assessment Findings	Nursing Interventions
Pulmonary contusion	Bruise on the lung tissue; most common type of potentially fatal chest injury.	No initial symptoms may be evident Increased difficulty breathing Hemoptysis Tachycardia Rales	Restrict fluid (unless patient in shock). Elevate the head of the bed (if no c-spine injury). Intubate if the child has severe respiratory distress. Administer ordered antibiotics for pneumonia prophylaxis.
Tension pneumothorax	A tear in the lung lining, which results in air accumulation in the pleural space that compresses the lungs. The amount of air trapped increases with each breath because the air cannot escape.	Unstable vital signs Respiratory distress Tracheal deviation Decreased breath sounds over the affected lung Cyanosis Decreased cardiac output	Assist with needle thoracotomy (insertion of a 19-gauge needle into the left second intercostal space, midclavicular line). Prepare for chest tube insertion.
Open pneumothorax	Open chest wound that may be sucking or not sucking.	Unstable vital signs Anxious, restless Irritable Cyanosis Decreased breath sounds over affected lung Asymmetry of chest wall movement Subcutaneous emphysema	Apply three-sided, occlusive dressing (e.g., gauze with petroleum jelly); leave one side open to prevent tension pneumothorax. Prepare for chest tube insertion.
Hemothorax	Blood accumulation in the chest cavity as a result of blunt or penetrating trauma.	Unstable vital signs Decreased or absent breath sounds Dullness to percussion over affected area Hypovolemic shock resulting from hemorrhage	Prepare for chest tube insertion. Administer fluids for aggressive volume replacement.
Cardiac tamponade	Blood accumulation in the pericardial sac as a result of blunt or penetrating trauma.	Muffled heart sounds Decreased blood pressure Distended neck veins	Assist with immediate pericardiocentesis. Perform fluid resuscitation.

- ► **Risk for infection related to effects of injuries, invasive treatments, and stress decreasing immune response**
  Outcome: The child will not acquire injury-related infection.
- ► **Altered nutrition: less than body requirements related to injury increasing metabolic demands or decreasing ability to ingest nutrients**
  Outcome: The child will have sufficient intake of nutrients to meet metabolic needs and support healing and growth.
- ► **Pain related to effects of injury**
  Outcome: The child will be assessed for baseline neurologic and cardiovascular status and then have pain adequately managed.
- ► **Inability to sustain spontaneous ventilation related to effects of injury**
  Outcome: The child will have adequate ventilation, spontaneous or assisted.

Interdisciplinary Interventions

Upon completing the primary and secondary assessments, additional interventions may be identified. Insert an indwelling urinary catheter to monitor urine output (contraindicated if blood is present at the urethral meatus). An impaled object should not be removed. Stabilize it for later removal in surgery.

Assess the child's pain level and administer pain medications as ordered. Before administering a pain medication to a child with a traumatic injury, ensure that a thorough neurologic and cardiovascular examination has been performed. Pain medications may make it difficult to evaluate accurately whether a change in level of consciousness is drug induced or due to pathology. Pain medications may also cause vasodilatation, causing a precipitous drop in blood pressure (BP) in a child with hypovolemia or unstable cardiovascular status.

Until definitive treatment is achieved, splint, elevate, and ice any extremity fracture. Apply sterile dressings to any open, soft tissue injuries such as lacerations or abrasions. Determine the child's tetanus immunization status, and administer a booster if necessary.

If bruising is noted around the eyes (raccoon eyes) or behind the ears or if hemotympanum is present, the child may have a basilar skull fracture. This places the child at risk for intracranial hemorrhage, respiratory depression and/or arrest, and cerebral edema. Such a child may require intubation and hyperventilation to achieve a $PaCO_2$ of 30 mmHg. Hyperventilation produces hypocarbia; this causes vasoconstriction, which decreases cerebral blood flow and helps to maintain normal intracranial pressure. Measure $PaCO_2$ by serial arterial blood gas measurements or with an end-tidal CO_2 monitor. When brain stem herniation is suspected, administer 20% mannitol at 0.25 to 1 g/kg IV, as ordered, to decrease intracranial pressure. Prepare the child for computed tomography (CT), the diagnostic study of choice to evaluate the intracranial space.

Common Respiratory Emergencies

Respiratory emergencies are a major cause of morbidity and mortality in the pediatric population. Causes include epiglottitis, foreign body aspiration, bronchiolitis, croup, and asthma.

Since the advent of the *Haemophilus influenzae* B vaccine in the late 1980s, epiglottitis has become uncommon (Fleisher & Crain, 1996). However, health care providers may still encounter it in an unimmunized child and need to intervene immediately.

Complete airway obstruction by a foreign body causes 200 deaths per year in children younger than 5 years (Haley & Baker, 1993).

Bronchiolitis is most commonly caused by respiratory syncytial virus (RSV) and is the most common cause of wheezing in infants younger than 1 year. Croup is the most common cause of upper airway obstruction in children between 6 months and 3 years of age (Skolnick, 1993).

Morbidity and mortality associated with asthma are increasing. Factors that place a child at high risk for asthma-related death include the following:

- Prior intubation for asthma
- Two or more hospitalizations for asthma in the past year
- Three or more emergency care visits for asthma in the past year
- Hospitalization or emergency care within the past month
- Current or recent use of systemic corticosteroids
- Prior admission to an intensive care unit for the treatment of asthma
- Serious psychiatric disease or psychosocial problems (National Asthma Education Program, 1991)

Rapid assessment, recognition of distress or failure, and immediate intervention are the keys to successfully managing the child with a respiratory problem. The following section deals with emergent recognition and management of respiratory disease. For more in-depth discussion, see Chapter 16.

Assessment

Approach the child in a calm, gentle manner that minimizes fear, which increases metabolic demands. While approaching, obtain a general assessment of the child's status. Note the child's position of comfort. Older children assume a position that optimizes airway patency and minimizes work of breathing. Assess level of consciousness. Hypoxia may be manifested as anxiety or irritability, hypercapnia as lethargic or obtunded behavior. Evaluate the child's color. Cyanosis is a late sign of respiratory distress, unless the child has chronic pulmonary or cardiovascular pathology.

Assess the rate and effort of breathing. Tachypnea in children is often the first sign of respiratory distress.

Alert: *It is an ominous sign if a child who was tachypneic has a slowed respiratory rate. This may indicate that the child is tiring and respiratory failure is imminent.*

Increased effort of breathing may be manifested by stridor, wheezing, grunting, retractions, use of accessory muscles, and nasal flaring. Note chest movement for symmetric expansion. Auscultate breath sounds for location and equality.

Nursing Diagnoses and Outcomes

General nursing diagnoses and outcomes for the child and family experiencing an emergency are identified in Chart 30–6. Nursing diagnoses and outcomes specific to the child in respiratory distress are

- **Activity intolerance related to decreased oxygenation and increased metabolic demands**
  Outcome: The child will be able to perform age-appropriate daily activities as desired.

- **Ineffective airway clearance related to excessive secretions or obstruction**
  Outcome: The child will maintain a patent airway.
- **Anxiety related to effects of inadequate oxygenation**
  Outcome: The child will maintain adequate oxygenation.
- **Ineffective breathing pattern related to effects of disease**
  Outcome: The child will sustain an effective breathing pattern to support oxygenation.
- **Impaired gas exchange related to effects of disease**
  Outcome: The child will maintain adequate oxygenation.
- **Inability to sustain spontaneous ventilation related to fatigue and effects of increasing $PaCO_2$ levels**
  Outcome: The child will have signs of respiratory failure recognized immediately and interventions implemented.

Interdisciplinary Interventions

Assessment findings indicate the level of respiratory support needed by the child. General support includes attending to the ABCs and optimizing oxygenation and ventilation. More specific interventions are dependent on pathology (Table 30–7).

For any child showing respiratory distress or desaturation on pulse oximetry, administer oxygen using a method tolerated by the child to keep the oxygen saturation above 95%. Administer oxygen cautiously to those with a history of chronic pulmonary disease. Instruct the parent how to hold oxygen tubing to provide blow-by oxygen, which may be better tolerated by the child (Fig. 30–5).

Tip: *Create a non-threatening mask by cutting a hole in the bottom of a Styrofoam cup. Then place the oxygen tubing through the hole and place the cup over the child's mouth. Monitor the child to prevent him or her from chewing on the cup.*

For children who require nebulizer treatments and are too young to hold a nebulizer mouthpiece in the mouth, have the parent hold a face mask in place.

Allow the child to maintain a position of comfort, either sitting or remaining in the parent's arms. Infants should be supported with the head in a neutral position.

Check arterial blood gas measurements for any child with severe respiratory distress. A $PaCO_2$ above 50 mmHg may indicate that the child requires intubation and mechanical ventilation.

Children experiencing respiratory distress should not be fed. Limit disturbances to essential interventions to prevent further distress.

Fever

Fever is one of the most common reasons for parents seeking care for their infant or child in the emergency department. Fever is considered the elevation of body temperature to at least 100.4°F (38°C) rectally (Baraff et al., 1993). This occurs when toxic substances or abnormalities in the brain reset the thermoregulatory set-point of the body to a higher than normal value. Fever is not a disease in itself; rather, it is a sign of an underlying disease that has activated an immune response.

Temperatures under 104°F (40°C) often result from a viral infection. Temperatures over 104°F (40°C) suggests a bacterial infection. Although exceptions occur, children with invasive bacterial disease often appear ill and are easy to identify as requiring treatment (Bonadio, 1995). A major concern is the presence of occult bacteremia in the febrile child who does not appear ill and thus does not receive appropriate antibiotic therapy. Occult bacteremia is commonly found in children with fever of unknown origin and otitis media (Baraff, 1996). The most common bacterial causes are *Streptococcus pneumoniae* and *Neisseria meningitidis*. With occult bacteremia, the source of the fever may not be evident despite a careful history and physical examination in as many as 14% of pediatric cases (Baraff et al., 1993). In bacteremic children who do not receive antimicrobial therapy, the risk of persistent bacteremia is 19% and of meningitis 10% (Baraff, 1996).

Another concern with fever is the possibility of triggering a **febrile seizure.** These occur most frequently in children 6 months to 3 years of age (Huff, 1996). Febrile seizures occur in 3% to 4% of all children, with a 40% risk for subsequent febrile seizures (Camfield & Camfield, 1993). Genetics may play a role in predisposing children to develop febrile seizures. Febrile seizures occur more

Figure 30–5
Young children offer less resistance if oxygen is delivered unobtrusively.

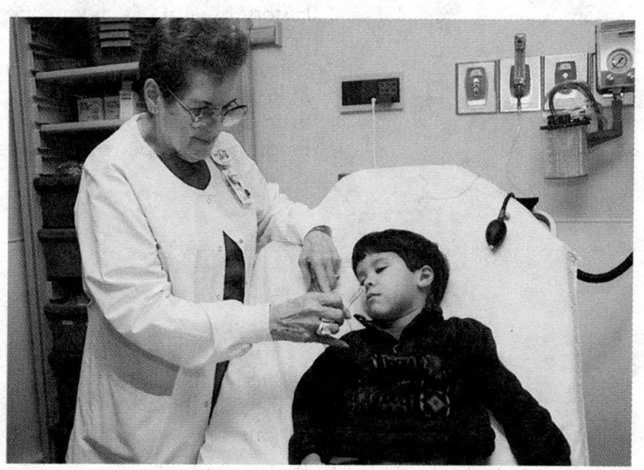

Table 30–7
Common Respiratory Emergencies: Assessment and Interventions

Disease	Assessment Findings	Interdisciplinary Interventions
Epiglottitis	Inflammation and swelling of the epiglottis and surrounding structures Age 2 to 6 yr (most common) Rapid onset of symptoms (e.g., child well appearing 2 hr previously) High fever (>40°C) Inability to eat or drink Excessive drooling Choking Muffled voice Difficulty breathing Stridorous cough possible Tripod positioning (neck stretched forward with jaw up to obtain a "sniffing" position in an attempt to achieve the best airway)	Never leave child unattended. Immediately gather appropriate equipment for emergency intubation and/or tracheostomy. Allow the child to maintain the position of comfort; avoid invasive or disturbing procedures because any agitation or attempts to lay the child down may result in laryngospasm and complete obstruction of the child's airway. If possible, move the child to a controlled environment such as the operating room to have an artificial airway established. Administer antibiotics to treat *H. influenzae* infection (e.g., ceftriaxone, chloramphenicol, ampicillin); do not use ampicillin alone because some strains are resistant to it (Phelan, 1994)
Asthma	Profound respiratory distress Assumes tripod position Anxious, restless Cyanotic, pale Tachycardia Tachypnea Retractions, use of accessory muscles Decreased or unequal breath sounds Expiratory wheezing, inspiratory wheezing with a prolonged inspiratory phase; the absence of wheezing with signs of respiratory distress is an ominous sign Decreased peak expiratory flow rate	Allow the child to maintain position of comfort. Administer supplemental oxygen. Administer nebulized albuterol at 0.15 mg/kg per dose (maximum 5 mg per dose) q 20 min for up to 1 hr (National Asthma Education Program, 1991). Consider nebulized terbutaline or atropine for children who do not respond to albuterol. Administer epinephrine (1 : 1000 solution) at 0.01 mg/kg SQ immediately if the child cannot generate a peak flow measurement or has a decreased level of consciousness. Reassess the child's vital signs, respiratory effort, and breath sounds after each treatment. Early treatment with a dose of steroids may prevent asthma exacerbation (Horowitz, Wolach, Eliakim, Berger, & Gilboa, 1995) Consider hospital admission for a child who does not respond to three albuterol treatments; has retractions, tachypnea, pallor, and/or cyanosis that continues without wheezing; or has a peak expiratory flow that does not improve to at least 65% of normal or when parental compliance with therapy is questionable.
Croup	History of viral infection, especially parainfluenza virus Onset in late fall or winter (most common) Mild to moderate illness (compared with toxic appearance of child with epiglottitis) Prodrome of upper airway infection that progresses to: · Fever · Barking cough · Inspiratory stridor · Tachycardia · Tachypnea · Suprasternal and/or subcostal retractions · Altered breath sounds (from stridor alone to rhonchi and/or wheezing)	Base treatment on severity of illness; use Croup Scoring System to help determine treatment needed (Table 30–8). Supply mist therapy and hydration. Administer nebulized racemic epinephrine 0.05 mL/kg of 2.25% solution in 3 mL of normal saline given q 30 min to reverse airway obstruction quickly; then monitor for at least 2 hr because rebound airway obstruction may occur. Administer corticosteroids such as dexamethasone at 0.5–1 mg/kg PO or IV as a single dose or repeated in 12 hr; although controversial, these drugs have been effective in children with moderate to severe disease (Fleisher & Crain, 1996; Skolnick, 1993).

Table 30–7
Common Respiratory Emergencies: Assessment and Interventions *Continued*

Disease	Assessment Findings	Interdisciplinary Interventions
Foreign body aspiration	History of running while eating or of playing with a small toy Acute onset of respiratory distress	If the child can breathe spontaneously or has coughing, wheezing, or stridor, do not attempt to dislodge the object. Perform BLS measures to dislodge foreign body. If BLS techniques do not dislodge foreign body, then physician should perform direct visualization and manual removal as needed. If apnea persists and manual bag-valve-mask ventilations cannot bypass the obstruction, emergency intubation, tracheostomy, or needle cricothyrotomy is necessary to establish a patent airway and enable cardiopulmonary resuscitation to be effective.
Bronchiolitis	History of acute viral infection of the lower respiratory tract Onset in winter (most common) Upper respiratory infection for 3–5 days Worsening cough Audible wheezing Low-grade fever Poor feeding (common)	Respiratory therapist or nurse should administer bronchodilator therapy, as ordered. Use of bronchodilators may have little effect on wheezing in the treatment of bronchiolitis (Gadomski et al., 1994); if the child responds well to the initial aerosol dose, continue either aerosolized or oral bronchodilator therapy (Welliver & Welliver, 1993). Consider hospitalization if oxygen saturation <95% and child appears ill.

Table 30–8
Croup Scoring System

Croup Score*,†	0	1	2	3
Stridor	None	Only with agitation	Mild at rest	Severe at rest
Retraction	None	Mild	Moderate	Severe
Air entry	Normal	Mild decrease	Moderate decrease	Marked decrease
Color	Normal	Not applicable	Not applicable	Cyanotic
Level of consciousness	Normal	Restless when disturbed	Restless when undisturbed	Lethargic

Disease Category by Score†

Score	Degree	Management
≤4	Mild	Outpatient—mist therapy
5–6	Mild to moderate	Outpatient if child improves in emergency department after mist, is older than 6 mo, and has a reliable family
7–8	Moderate	Admitted—racemic epinephrine
≥9	Severe	Admitted—racemic epinephrine, oxygen, intensive care unit

* Modified from Taussig, L. M., Castro, O., Beaudry, P. H., Fox, W. W., & Bureau, M. (1975). Treatment of laryngotracheitis (croup): Use of intermittent positive pressure breathing and racemic epinephrine. *American Journal of Diseases of Children, 129,* 790–793.
† Any one category with score of 3 leads to classification as severe disease.
From Fleisher, G. R. (1988). Infectious disease emergencies. In G. R. Fleisher & S. Ludwig (Eds.), *Textbook of pediatric emergency medicine* (2nd ed., p. 435). Baltimore: Williams & Wilkins. Reprinted with permission.

commonly with a rapid rise in temperature than with a prolonged temperature elevation.

Assessment

Fever increases the basal metabolic rate, resulting in tachycardia, tachypnea, and an increased oxygen demand. With each degree Celsius increase, the febrile child's caloric requirements are increased by 12% (Ford, 1996).

Children with fever should have a complete physical examination, specifically noting level of hydration, skin lesions (petechiae, usually appearing first on the chest, may indicate a serious bacterial infection), and neurologic status, which includes palpating the fontanelle in infants younger than 18 months. A bulging fontanelle may indicate meningitis, a sunken fontanelle dehydration. The child may be irritable and lethargic. The child who appears "toxic" may be cyanotic, has an altered level of consciousness, and has poor perfusion manifested as mottled skin color, capillary refill time longer than 2 seconds, cool extremities, and weak pulses.

Febrile seizures are usually manifested as sudden unresponsiveness, generalized rhythmic jerking, and tonic posturing lasting less than 15 minutes, usually less than 90 seconds (Huff, 1996). Simple febrile seizures do not recur in a 24-hour period (Burns, 1996). A determination needs to be made whether the fever caused the seizure or the seizure is a sign of underlying pathology that also caused the fever (e.g., meningitis, encephalitis) or is coincidental with the fever (e.g., toxic ingestion, hypoglycemia, hemorrhage, neurocutaneous disorder). Children who experience febrile seizures appear neurologically well within a few hours (Huff, 1996).

A complete "septic" work-up should be performed in all infants younger than 3 months who present with a rectal temperature of 100.4°F (38°C) or more and in children 3 to 36 months of age who present with a rectal temperature of 102°F or more and who appear toxic (Lewis-Abney & Smith, 1996). Children 3 to 36 months of age who present with a rectal temperature of 102°F or more and who do not appear toxic should have a complete blood count (CBC), blood culture, urinalysis, and urine culture. Older children with fever who are at low risk (do not appear toxic, have no chronic disease) may not require laboratory studies; those at high risk require a CBC and blood culture (Grover, 1996). The results determine any necessary further studies.

A septic work-up includes CBC, blood culture, urinalysis, urine culture, lumbar puncture, and chest radiograph. All cultures should be obtained before initiating antibiotic therapy.

caREminder: *Do not wait for culture results before starting antibiotics. Antibiotic therapy should be initiated within 1 hour, especially if the child appears toxic.*

Interdisciplinary Interventions

The nurse plays a pivotal role in managing the child with fever and in educating parents about home management (TIP 30–1). Treatment for fever includes antipyretics, fluids, and cooling measures. Management of fever in the acute care setting does not differ markedly from management in the home.

Protocols are usually in place in emergency departments for antipyretic administration (Soud, 1993). Replace fluid deficits orally or intravenously, depending on the child's level of consciousness and cooperation. Implementation of sponging as a cooling measure is controversial, because fever may be beneficial in helping fight the infection. One study found that sponging did not add to fever reduction (Newman, 1985). Sponging usually only increases the discomfort of children with non–life-threatening fever (Engler & Rushton, 1996). Most emergency department nurses (79.8% of those surveyed) do use tepid sponging for fever reduction (Thomas et al., 1994). Sponging should be done only

- If the child is at risk for a febrile seizure
- In a child with a neurologic disorder, because many have abnormal temperature control mechanisms that do not respond well to antipyretics (Engler & Rushton, 1996)
- When the increase in metabolic demands resulting from the fever may be deleterious to the child (e.g., a child with cardiac or pulmonary disease, a pregnant adolescent)
- In a child with liver disease when the use of antipyretics is contraindicated
- For heat-related illness (see p. 2083)

All febrile infants younger than 28 days and any toxic-appearing infant or child should be hospitalized and treated with parenteral antibiotics (Care Path 30–1). Infants 1 to 3 months of age who are considered at low risk (previously healthy, no focal bacterial infection on physical examination) and whose diagnostic studies provide no specific site of illness should receive a single injection of 50 mg/kg ceftriaxone (Grover, 1996). Low-risk infants can be managed as outpatients if parental compliance is deemed reliable. Older children with a fever of unknown origin with a temperature above 102°F (39°C) and a white blood count (WBC) of 15,000/mm^3 or more should have a blood culture performed. They also should receive a single injection of 50 mg/kg ceftriaxone pending culture results (Baraff et al., 1993).

If the child does have a **febrile seizure,** protect the child from injury while stabilizing the ABCs (see Chapter 21). Place the child in a side-lying position to prevent airway obstruction or aspiration. For prolonged seizures, lorazepam should be administered IV in appropriate doses to stop the seizure (Huff, 1996).

TIP 30–1 A Teaching Intervention Plan for the Child with a Fever

Nursing Diagnoses and Family Outcomes

- Knowledge deficit: home management of fever
  Outcomes: Caretakers and child, if appropriate, will implement appropriate fever management interventions. Caretakers and child, if appropriate, will notify health care provider appropriately of negative changes in the child's condition.
- Risk for fluid volume deficit related to effects of increased metabolic demands
  Outcome: Child will have sufficient fluid intake to prevent dehydration.
- Hyperthermia related to effects of disease process
  Outcome: Child will have fever controlled as needed to decrease risk for febrile seizure, decrease metabolic demands, and promote comfort.
- Risk for injury related to potential for febrile seizures
  Outcome: Child will not sustain injury if seizure occurs.

Interventions

- Educate parents about the physiology of fever:
  - Fever in itself is not harmful, it may be beneficial in fighting pathogens.
- Make certain parents know how to take child's temperature:
  - Use method appropriate for child's age and condition.
  - Read thermometer accurately.
- Teach parents cooling measures:
  - Manipulate environment to cool child:
    - Unbundle child, may cover with light blanket if shivering occurs.
    - Decrease room temperature.
  - Administer antipyretics as needed for temperature over 102°F and if your child is uncomfortable:
    - Acetaminophen at 15 mg/kg PO or PR q 4 hr (drug of choice).
    - Ibuprofen at 10 mg/kg PO q 6–8 hr
    - **Do not give aspirin** because of its association with Reye's syndrome.
    - It will take 30 to 60 minutes for these medications to have an effect on the temperature.
  - Bathe or sponge with tepid water (85° to 90°F):
    - Sponge immediately if your child has a febrile seizure or temperature above 106°F; otherwise, wait until after the antipyretic has taken effect, the temperature remains over 104°F, and your child is uncomfortable.
    - If sponging is done, water should be lukewarm (85° to 90°F); **do not use ice water,** which will bring your child's temperature down too rapidly and cause shivering; avoid shivering because it raises the temperature as the body attempts to produce heat.
    - **Do not use alcohol** for sponge baths because alcohol intoxication can result from inhalation of fumes and skin absorption.
    - Stop sponging when your child's temperature starts to decrease to avoid having the child become too cold.
- Remind parents to increase the child's fluid intake:
  - Offer frequent small sips of fluid or popsicles.
- Instruct parents to notify health care provider or return for follow-up treatment if:
  - The child's fever persists longer than 2 to 3 days.
  - The child's condition worsens (e.g., seizure, purple spots on skin, increased lethargy or irritability, decreased oral intake, vomiting, stiff neck).

References: Grover (1996); Schmitt (1992).

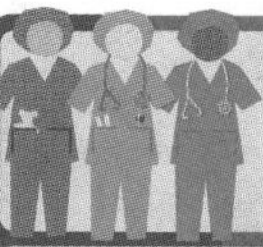

Care Path 30–1 An Interdisciplinary Plan of Care for the Neonate with Sepsis

Nursing Diagnosis and Discharge Outcomes	Patient/Family Intermediate Outcomes		
	Day 1	**Day 2**	**Day 3**
Risk for altered body temperature related to effects of disease, immaturity	The infant will maintain body temperature within normal range.	⟶	⟶
Altered nutrition: less than body requirements related to decreased intake and increased metabolic demands	The infant will receive an adequate caloric intake to support metabolic demands and growth.	⟶	⟶
Knowledge deficit (parents): disease process, treatment	The parents will express an understanding of the infection and the need for treatment.	The parents will participate in routine infant care activities.	⟶
Care Intervention Categories			
Labs	CBC, C-reactive protein (CRP), blood culture, urine antigen screen, glucose monitoring.	CBC, CRP; check 24-hour blood culture results.	Check 48-hour blood culture results.
Medications and IVs	Peripheral IV: $D_{10}W$ or heparin lock Start IV antibiotics.	If necessary, change antibiotics on the basis of culture results.	Determine the duration of antibiotic therapy on the basis of culture results.
Monitors	Cardiorespiratory monitoring. Isolette with temperature control if needed.		
Nutrition	Keep infant NPO if he or she exhibits altered level of consciousness, tachypnea.	Start oral feeding if symptoms resolve.	Maintain total oral feeding as tolerated.
Pain management	Nonnutritive sucking. Swaddling. Developmental positioning, containment.		
Procedures (diagnostics)	Lumbar puncture.		
Psychosocial	Support the parents and encourage their participation in the infant's care.		

Day 4	Day 5	Day 6	Day 7
→	→	→	
→	→	→	→
	The parents will express knowledge of the signs of infection and when to report these to a health care provider.		The parents will discuss and demonstrate proper home care measures for their infant.
Check 72-hour blood culture results.	Repeat CBC if previous findings were abnormal.		
Continue antibiotic therapy.	→	→	Discontinue or continue IV antibiotics.
→	→	→	→
			Auditory brain stem evoked response if the infant has been receiving gentamicin for 7 days.
			Encourage full infant care by the parents.

Care Path continued on following page

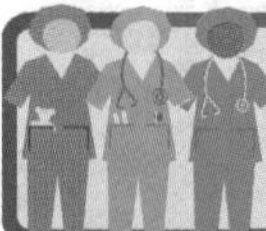

Care Path 30–1 An Interdisciplinary Plan of Care for the Neonate with Sepsis *Continued*

Nursing Diagnosis and Discharge Outcomes	Patient/Family Intermediate Outcomes		
	Day 1	**Day 2**	**Day 3**
Radiology	Chest radiograph.		
Safety and activity	Placing infant in the supine or side-lying position for sleep.		
Social services	As needed to support the family.		Family conference if indicated.
Teaching Discharge Planning	Tests and treatments.	Breast-feeding (if appropriate).	Infant care.
Vital signs/baseline parameters	Monitor temperature, pulse, and respirations every 4 hours and blood pressure every 8 hours (or more frequently if needed).	⟶	⟶

▽ **Alert:** *Sedatives administered IV must be given slowly and the child closely monitored for ability to maintain a patent airway and spontaneous ventilations.*

The nurse must educate the family about febrile seizures and how to manage them. Reassure the family that febrile seizures cause no long-term sequelae. Explain the risk of recurrence. Instruct that antipyretics can be administered when fever occurs, although the seizure often occurs as the temperature is rising before it is noticed by the parent, so it may not be prevented. Also, teach the parents first-aid measures to take if a seizure occurs.

Bites and Stings

Thousands of children are treated yearly for various types of bites and stings. As many as 80% of bite injuries are dog bites, with children predictably suffering more serious injuries than adults. Although most bites and stings are not fatal, about 50 people (1 or 2 of whom are children) die yearly in the United States from insect stings (Friday, 1996).

Mammal and Human Bites

Children younger than 5 years are the most common victims of dog bites, with the head and arms being the areas most affected (Brogan, Bratton, Dowd, & Hegenbarth, 1995). These bites can be disfiguring because the lips, nose, eyes, and ears are often involved. Other common bites are inflicted by cats (5% to 10%), rodents (2% to 3%), and humans (2% to 3%) (Hodge & Tecklenberg, 1996). Wound infections are the most frequent complication, with bites inflicted by cats and humans having the highest infection rates (Aronoff, 1996).

Assessment

The history of the circumstances surrounding the bite should be obtained, including who, or what, did it. If the bite is from an animal, include the type of animal (species and whether wild or domestic). The amount of time since the injury and the child's immunization status should also be obtained.

Manifestations depend on type of wound. Human and dog bites often cause lacerations and crush injuries. Cat bites usually cause puncture wounds. Rodent bites tend to be superficial.

Physical examination should evaluate the type, size, and depth of the injury; the presence of foreign material in the wound; and the status of underlying structures. Fractures may occur; evaluate for skull fractures in young children who have dog bites to the head and face.

Day 4	Day 5	Day 6	Day 7
Safety measures.	Teach the parents the signs of infection and when to report these to a health care provider.		Follow-up appointment with pediatrician. Review home care instructions, medications if prescribed.

Nursing Diagnoses and Outcomes

Nursing diagnoses common to the child experiencing an emergency, as listed in Chart 30–6, are applicable to the child suffering from a bite. In addition, the following diagnoses may apply for a child after a bite injury:

- **Risk for infection related to effects of bite wound**
  Outcome: The child will not develop wound infection.
- **Pain related to effects of bite wound or treatment**
  Outcome: The child will have pain adequately managed, will verbalize minimal level of pain, will demonstrate few pain behaviors.
- **Knowledge deficit: home management of wound**
  Outcomes: The parents, and the child as appropriate, will state reasons for antibiotic prophylaxis and importance of completing full course of therapy. The parents, and the child as appropriate, will demonstrate prescribed techniques of wound management. The parents, and the child as appropriate, will list signs of wound infection and when to notify health care provider.
- **Impaired tissue integrity related to presence of bite wound**
  Outcome: The child will have the wound appropriately cleansed and closed as soon as possible after the injury to minimize further tissue damage.
- **Body image disturbance related to presence of disfiguring wound**
  Outcome: The child will verbalize a positive body image if wound is disfiguring.

Interdisciplinary Interventions

Parents often seek treatment for their child's bite because of concern about rabies, a fatal viral infection of the central nervous system. However, the incidence of rabies is extremely low in the United States. (See Chapter 24 for discussion of rabies.) Prophylactic treatment for rabies is based on the species of animal (dogs and cats are typically low risk; bats, skunks, coyotes, raccoons, and foxes are higher risk), the animal's condition, and the prevalence of rabies in the region. Rabies prophylaxis consists of passive immunization with human rabies immune globulin (HRIG; 20 IU/kg) and active immunization with human diploid cell vaccine (HDCV) or rhesus diploid cells (rabies vaccine adsorbed [RVA]). After thoroughly cleansing the wound, give half the HRIG dosage, if possible, by local subcutaneous (SQ) infiltration of the site. Then give the second half intramuscularly (IM) at another site (Fleisher & Crain, 1996). Active immunization should be given IM in the deltoid on days 0, 3, 7, 14, and 28 (Plotkin, 1996).

Prompt care of the wound is the key to successful healing. Inspect the bite wound for teeth, clean the site with a 1% povidone-iodine solution, and irrigate the wound forcibly with normal saline. Closure of the wound depends on the affected site. If the wound is considered at high risk for infection, it should not be sutured. High-risk wounds include puncture wounds, minor hand or foot wounds, cat or human bites, bite wounds not treated within 12 hours, and wounds in the immunocompromised patient.

Antibiotic prophylaxis may be indicated depending on the wound site (hand or face) and severity (deep wounds, ones that cannot be adequately débrided), if the wound was not sutured, and for all high-risk wounds (Aronoff, 1996). No one antibiotic is effective against all the most common organisms. Generally, a combination of antibiotics is given over a course of 3 to 5 days. Consider tetanus prophylaxis for all bite victims. Most bite wounds in children should be rechecked for signs of infection in 24 to 48 hours. Some children with severe injuries need to be hospitalized for adequate management, including operative repair, extensive local infection, or poor compliance with therapeutic regimen.

Teach the parents how to assess for signs and symptoms of wound infection and when to notify the health care provider. Discuss potential fears and behavioral problems of the child and how parents might manage them. Teach children to avoid stray animals and not to provoke animals.

Snake Bites

Approximately 8000 people are bitten by venomous snakes each year in the United States. Children between ages 5 and 19 are the most affected population (Hodge & Tecklenberg, 1996). The highest incidence occurs in late spring and summer in the southeastern and southwestern United States.

Pit vipers, such as the rattlesnake, water moccasin, and copperhead, are responsible for 99% of the poisonous snakebites in the United States. Snakes such as the coral snake make up the remaining 1% (Hodge & Tecklenberg, 1996).

Assessment

Local signs of pit viper envenomation include pain, edema, erythema, bruising, vesicles, and hemorrhagic blebs. Small bites left untreated or larger, more serious bites may progress to systemic effects such as paresthesia, metallic taste in the mouth, nausea, vomiting, progressive swelling of the affected extremity, and possibly necrosis throughout the bitten extremity. Severe envenomations may result in coagulopathy and hemolysis leading to hemorrhage, shock, and renal failure that can cause death.

The venom from coral snakes is primarily neurotoxic, and symptoms include drowsiness, motor weakness, cranial nerve palsies, and paralysis (Webb, 1996). When the envenomation is severe, symptoms progress to seizures, coma, and respiratory depression leading to death.

Nursing Diagnoses and Outcomes

Nursing diagnoses and outcomes applicable to the child after snakebite may include those for any child experiencing an emergency as listed in Chart 30–6. In addition, the following may be applicable:

- **Decreased cardiac output related to effects of bleeding related to coagulopathy**
  Outcome: The child will maintain cardiac output, signs of shock will be recognized immediately, and treatment will be implemented to prevent or treat shock.
- **Impaired tissue integrity related to presence of wound, edema, tissue necrosis**
  Outcome: The child will have interventions implemented to optimize tissue integrity and reduce complications (infection, neurovascular compromise, scarring).
- **Inability to sustain spontaneous ventilation related to neurotoxic effects of venom**
  Outcome: The child will have signs of respiratory depression recognized immediately and ventilatory support provided.

Interdisciplinary Interventions

All snakebites require the same general treatment. Prehospital first-aid measures include basic life support if needed and rapid transport to a medical facility. All clothing and jewelry should be removed from the bitten extremity. The child should be kept as quiet as possible with the extremity immobilized in a position below the level of the heart. Incision and suction of the wound are indicated only if initiated within 10 minutes of the snakebite. Constriction bands obstruct lymph (the primary route by which venom gains access to the circulation) and venous flow and are indicated when transports taking longer than 30 minutes are required. The constriction band should be placed 5 to 10 cm proximal to the wound and be loose enough to allow a finger underneath it and allow good arterial pulses.

caREminder: *The use of incision, suction, and constriction bands is controversial and they should be used only by skilled personnel (Konzen, 1996).*

Hospital management begins with assessing the ABCs and intervening as necessary. For children with envenomation, immediate venous access is indicated upon arrival in the emergency department, with blood drawn for extensive laboratory studies including CBC, prothrombin time (PT), partial thromboplastin time (PTT), type and crossmatch, fibrinogen, electrolytes, blood urea nitrogen (BUN), creatinine, and arterial blood gases. A baseline urinalysis should also be obtained. Administer fluid to combat shock, if present.

All snakebite wounds should be irrigated, cleansed, and dressed. Broad-spectrum antibiotics are given because the snake's oral flora includes gram-negative bacteria. Tetanus prophylaxis should given, depending on the child's immunization status. The circumference of the affected extremity, close to the wound and proximal, should be monitored every 15 to 30 minutes (Konzen, 1996). Antivenom should be administered to children with envenomation (Chart 30–11). Serial monitoring of laboratory values should be done.

Over 80% of snakebites do not result in envenomation (Webb, 1996). Generally, these do not leave fang punctures and have little pain or swelling. These children should be managed with cleansing, monitoring, and antibiotic and tetanus prophylaxis but do not require antivenin therapy. They can be discharged after 6 to 8 hours if asymptomatic (Konzen, 1996).

Parents and children should be taught first-aid measures for snakebite, particularly when venomous snakes are indigenous to the locale. After a bite, educate the family about antibiotic prophylaxis, wound care, and signs of complications.

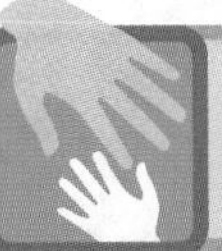

Chart 30–11
Nursing Interventions

Antivenin Therapy for Snakebite

- Calculate amount of time since snakebite:
  - Administer antivenin within 4 hours for maximal venom binding; efficacy of therapy diminishes after 12 hours, and therapy is not indicated after 24 hours.
- Perform skin testing before antivenin administration:
  - Antivenin is highly antigenic horse serum; therefore, it has great potential to cause allergic reactions.
  - Resuscitation equipment, epinephrine, antihistamines, and steroids must be immediately available.
- Administer antivenin:
  - Must be done in critical care setting with emergency equipment immediately available.
  - Dosage, unlike that of most other medications in pediatrics, is not based on the child's weight but rather the severity of the envenomation.
  - Children usually require more antivenin than adults because their small size results in relatively high serum venom concentrations.
  - For pit viper bites, give antivenin (Crotalidae) polyvalent.
  - For North American coral snake bites give antivenin (*Micrurus fulvius*).
  - For exotic snakebites, a local zoo or poison control center may be able to locate appropriate antivenin.
- Monitor the child for:
  - Change in vital signs
  - Respiratory distress
  - Signs of shock
  - Change in amount of edema

Insect Stings and Bites

Hymenoptera is the order of insects responsible for 50% of human deaths from venomous bites and stings. This class includes bees, wasps, hornets, yellow jackets, and ants. Allergic reactions are the most common result of these stings.

Assessment

Reactions to insect stings and bites can vary from mild (slight swelling, erythema, and pain at the site) to moderate (generalized pruritus and urticaria) to severe (wheezing, nausea and vomiting, laryngoedema, hypotension, and shock). A bee's stinger is barbed and remains in the victim's skin.

Interdisciplinary Interventions

Treatment of stings is based on the severity of the reaction. Most respond to treatment at home (Chart 30–12). Treatment for severe anaphylactic reactions is discussed in the following section.

Anaphylaxis

Anaphylaxis, or anaphylactic shock, is a life-threatening emergency caused by an acute systemic allergic or hypersensitivity reaction to an antigen. Anaphylaxis usually occurs immediately, although it can occur 30 to 60 minutes after a repeated exposure to the antigen.

Almost any foreign substance is capable of eliciting anaphylaxis. The most common causes are insect venom, drugs (aspirin, penicillin, cephalosporins, chemotherapy),

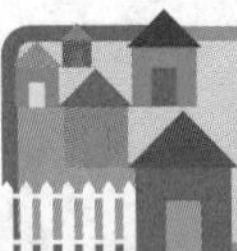

Chart 30-12
Community Care

Treatment for Insect Stings and Bites

Teach parents, school personnel, and other caregivers to:

- Remove stinger if present.
  Take care to remove the stinger by flicking or scraping. Do not squeeze or pull with tweezers; these actions inject any remaining venom into the wound.
- Rub the area for 15 minutes using a cotton ball soaked in a solution of meat tenderizer with a few drops of water, which may help reduce inflammation.
- Apply cold compresses to reduce site swelling and pain.
- For itching: diphenhydramine hydrochloride (Benadryl), 4 to 5 mg/kg per day (to a total of 200 mg per day) divided into four doses.
- Call a health care provider immediately if the child has:
  Breathing or swallowing difficulty
  Hives
  Ten or more stings
  A sting in the mouth
- Call a health care provider later if:
  The stinger cannot be removed
  The swelling continues to spread after 24 hours
  Swelling of the hand (or foot) spreads past the wrist (or ankle)

foods (seafood, nuts, eggs), and biological agents (allergen extracts, iodinated radiocontrast media, latex). Almost 3% of children have a systemic reaction to Hymenoptera stings (Friday, 1996).

Severe anaphylactic reactions can result in death. Prompt diagnosis and immediate intervention with appropriate therapy are necessary to avert this outcome.

Initial exposure to the antigen causes the formation of antibodies, usually of the immunoglobulin E (IgE) class. Upon repeated exposure to the same antigen, symptoms develop and the hypersensitivity reaction may occur. The antibody-antigen reaction causes a massive release of chemical mediators (such as histamine) from mast cells and basophils throughout the body.

Assessment

The common manifestations of anaphylaxis include urticaria, angioedema (a condition characterized by development of urticaria and edematous areas of skin, mucous membranes, or viscera), bronchospasm, laryngeal edema, hypotension, hyperperistalsis, and cardiac arrhythmias.

The degree of the sensitivity reaction depends on the antigen's nature and the child's degree of atopy. Atopy is the hereditary trait for formation of IgE antibodies. Often, a strong family history exists for allergies or hypersensitivity reactions to particular drugs, insects, or foods. Take the family history seriously; it indicates a need to avoid certain drugs or foods for the child.

Nursing Diagnoses and Outcomes

Nursing diagnoses and outcomes for the child experiencing an emergency are discussed in Chart 30–6. In addition, the following are applicable for the child experiencing an anaphylactic reaction:

- **Ineffective airway clearance related to effects of laryngoedema**
  Outcome: The child will have interventions immediately implemented to reduce laryngoedema and optimize airway patency.
- **Decreased cardiac output related to effects of vasodilation**
  Outcome: The child will have signs of decreased cardiac output recognized promptly and interventions initiated immediately.
- **Ineffective breathing pattern related to effects of bronchospasm**
  Outcome: The child will generate an effective breathing pattern or will have interventions implemented to support an effective breathing pattern to optimize gas exchange.

Interdisciplinary Interventions

As with all allergic disorders, avoidance or preventive measures for patients at high risk are the primary treatment. However, most serious anaphylactic reactions are unanticipated (Cavales-Oftadeh & Heiner, 1996). Therefore, immediate recognition and treatment of anaphylaxis are critical to prevent death resulting from upper airway obstruction and/or shock (Chart 30–13).

Pediatric patients who have experienced an anaphylactic reaction should be hospitalized for observation, because there may be a biphasic reaction in which symptoms recur after initially resolving in response to therapy.

Once the causative antigen(s) has been identified, teach the child and family how to prevent anaphylaxis (Chart 30–14). Allergy medications should be taken before unavoidable exposure to known allergens. The child should reduce the risk of exposure as appropriate to the

Chart 30–13

Interdisciplinary Interventions: Managing Anaphylaxis

Immediately:

- Administer epinephrine.
  - Initial dose: 0.01 mL/kg (1:1000) IM or SQ up to a maximum of 0.3 mL in a child, 0.5 mL in an adolescent.
  - Repeat dose q 15 min p.r.n.
  - As an alternative (or simultaneously), can give epinephrine via metered-dose inhaler at 10 to 20 activations (0.15 mg per activation) over 6 minutes.

General interventions:

- Rapidly assess ABCs.
  - Intervene as necessary.
  - Maintain patent airway.
- Administer oxygen.
- Start IV.
- Stop antigen release or slow absorption.
  - If the antigen responsible for the anaphylaxis has been injected or is infusing intravenously, immediately discontinue.
  - Apply tourniquet proximal to reaction site if it is on extremity (insect sting, injection); loosen after symptoms improve or briefly at 3-minute intervals.
  - Inject epinephrine at 0.1 to 0.3 mL of 1:1000 aqueous solution into the same site or infiltrate surrounding area.
- Administer antihistamines.
  - A combination of H_1 and H_2 antagonists, such as diphenhydramine at 1 to 2 mg/kg (maximum 75 mg) IV or hydroxyzine hydrochloride at 0.9 mg/kg IM (H_1 antagonists) given with ranitidine at 1 mg/kg IV or cimetidine at 4 mg/kg IV (maximum 300 mg) (H_2 antagonists), may be more effective than a single drug alone; give H_2 antagonists by slow IV push; rapid infusions of these agents can cause hypotension.

Treat hypotension:

- Give epinephrine IV if severely hypotensive.
  - Dilute 0.1 mL of 1:1000 epinephrine solution in 10 mL of normal saline (NS) and give over several minutes.
  - IV dosage is dependent on severity of reaction; titrate for response and repeat p.r.n.
- Administer fluids if hypotension is not responsive to epinephrine and H_1 and H_2 antagonists.
  - Give 20 mL/kg 0.9% NS or Ringer's lactate as an IV bolus; repeat p.r.n. to restore and maintain adequate perfusion and blood pressure.
  - Large amounts of fluid may be necessary; an intravascular volume loss of up to 50% can occur within 10 minutes because of the increased vascular permeability secondary to the massive mediator release.
- If hypotension persists, consider inserting a line for central venous pressure monitoring to guide fluid and vasopressor therapy.
- Administer vasopressors.
  - Dopamine at 2 to 20 μg/kg/min IV; titrated to effect
  - Vasopressors may have a diminished effect, because these hypotensive patients have increased peripheral resistance resulting from endogenous compensatory mechanisms.

Treat bronchospasm:

- If wheezing is not responsive to epinephrine:
  - Administer aerosolized beta-adrenergics (e.g., albuterol), 0.5 mL of 0.5% solution in 2.5 mL of NS **or** two puffs of albuterol from a metered-dose inhaler.

Continued treatment:

- Administer corticosteroids (e.g., methylprednisolone at 1 mg/kg) after initial treatment to prevent recurrence of anaphylaxis; initially give IV and then give PO when child is stable; corticosteroids do not have immediate onset of action and so are not used as first-line management.
- Continually monitor ABCs, vital signs, response to treatment.

References: Behrman, Kliegman, & Arvin (1996); Cavales-Oftadeh & Heiner (1996); Lieberman (1995).

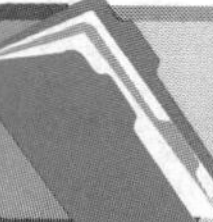

Chart 30–14
Nursing Interventions Classification (NIC)

Allergy Management

Definition

Identification, treatment, and prevention of allergic responses to food, medications, insect bites, contrast material, blood, or other substances

Activities

Identify known medication/food allergies and usual reaction.
Notify dietitian of patient's food allergies.
Notify pharmacist and physician of known allergies.
Document all allergies in clinical record, according to protocol.
Place an allergy band on patient, as appropriate.
Monitor patient for allergic reactions to new medications, formulas, foods, and/or test dyes.
Instruct the patient with medication allergies to question all new prescriptions for potential allergic reactions.
Encourage patient to wear a medical alert tab, as appropriate.
Identify immediately the level of threat an allergic reaction presents to patient's health status.
Monitor for reoccurrence of anaphylaxis within 24 hours.
Provide lifesaving measures during anaphylactic shock or severe reactions.
Provide medication to reduce or minimize an allergic response.
Assist with allergy testing, as appropriate.
Administer allergy injections, as needed.
Watch for allergic responses during immunizations.
Instruct patient/parent to avoid allergic substances, as appropriate.
Instruct patient/parent in how to treat rashes, vomiting, diarrhea, or respiratory problems associated with exposure to allergy-producing substance.
Instruct patient to avoid further use of substances causing allergic responses.
Discuss methods to control environmental allergens (e.g., dust, mold, and pollen).
Instruct patient to avoid environments infested with insects, as appropriate.
Instruct patient to carry bee sting kits, as appropriate.

From McCloskey, J., & Bulechek, G. (1996). *Nursing interventions classification (NIC)* (2nd ed.). St. Louis: Mosby–Year Book. Reprinted with permission.

situation. For example, if allergic to bees, the child should wear shoes when outside, wear clothing that covers extremities, not walk through flower beds, and not wear perfume or brightly colored clothing. Children who have had anaphylactic reactions should have a kit containing injectable epinephrine, an oral antihistamine, and a tourniquet (for bee stings) with them at all times (Cavales-Oftadeh & Heiner, 1996). The nurse needs to teach parents, the child if old enough, and possibly school or daycare personnel appropriate use of the kit contents. Tell children to notify an adult at the first signs of anaphylaxis.

Epistaxis

The nose is highly vascular and is susceptible to bleeding. Common causes of epistaxis include trauma, frequent nose picking, infection, inflammation, low environmental humidity, and foreign bodies. Children are more susceptible during respiratory infections and in winter when dry air irritates the nasal mucosa. Epistaxis is rare in infants and common in children, with the incidence decreasing after puberty. In adolescent females, epistaxis may be associated with pregnancy.

Epistaxis is usually mild and responds to home management, but occasionally bleeding is severe enough to require transfusion. Epistaxis may also signal an underlying pathology such as Osler-Weber-Rendu disease (hereditary hemorrhagic telangiectasia) or juvenile angiofibroma, usually found in adolescent males (Hendrix, 1996).

Assessment

Epistaxis often occurs without warning with blood flowing from one or both nostrils. Evaluate vital signs for

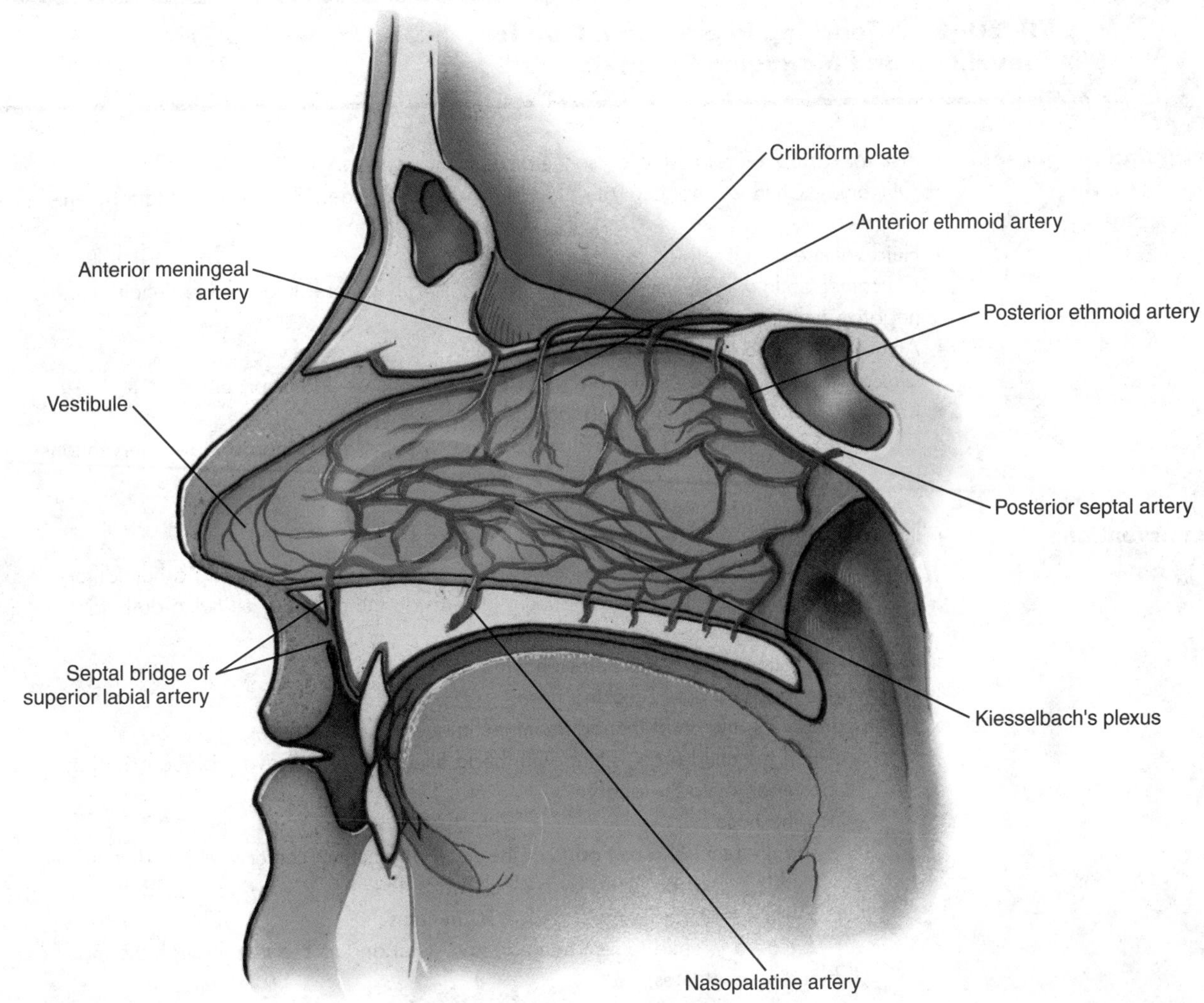

Figure 30–6
Most nosebleeds arise from the anteroinferior portion of the nasal septum.

indicators of hemodynamic instability (increased heart and respiratory rate, decreased blood pressure, or orthostatic changes). Examine the skin and mucous membranes for petechiae and ecchymosis, which may indicate coagulopathy. Inspect the nasopharynx and oropharynx for masses and blood dripping from a posterior bleeding site. Visualizing the nares, attempt to identify the site of bleeding (Fig. 30–6). Most commonly, the anterior nasal septum is the site of origin in epistaxis (Boyar & Chao, 1995).

Laboratory work-up is warranted when the child with epistaxis has a family history of bleeding disorder, spontaneous bleeding of other areas in the body, continued bleeding longer than 20 minutes despite direct pressure, or onset of recurrent epistaxis before 2 years of age or when there is a significant drop in the hematocrit secondary to epistaxis (Berman & Schmitt, 1991).

Interdisciplinary Interventions

Most nosebleeds can be effectively managed outside the acute care setting. Parents and children should be taught techniques that may prevent nosebleeds. School and daycare personnel should also be included in teaching immediate management of nosebleeds (TIP 30–2).

Bleeding that does not stop with home management may require more invasive intervention by a health care provider. Maintain the child in a sitting position with the head tilted forward to avoid blood dripping into the posterior pharynx. If the anterior nasal septum is the site, apply direct pressure on the bleeding site by compressing the external nares for 10 minutes (Fig. 30–7). If this does not stop the bleeding, trained personnel should cauterize the site with silver nitrate for definitive control of bleeding from the anterior nasal septum (Kraepelien-Bartels, 1994).

TIP 30–2 A Teaching Intervention Plan for Preventing and Managing Epistaxis

Nursing Diagnoses and Family Outcomes

- Risk for aspiration related to presence of blood in oropharynx
  Outcomes: Child will not aspirate blood into bronchial tree. Child will maintain patent airway.
- Fluid volume deficit related to effects of bleeding
  Outcome: Child will be brought to health care facility before fluid volume deficit exerting negative impact on hemodynamic stability.
- Anxiety related to bleeding
  Outcome: Child will be calm, able to follow directions as age appropriate.
- Knowledge deficit: community management of epistaxis
  Outcome: Caregivers and child, if appropriate, will implement appropriate interventions to control nosebleed.

Interventions

- Inform the parents and child how to prevent nosebleeds.
  - Increase the humidity in the home or the child's bedroom by using a humidifier.
  - Apply a small amount of petroleum jelly inside the child's nose twice daily to decrease dryness.
  - Instill saline nose drops before having the child blow nose.
  - Have the child avoid picking nose.
- Teach caregivers and child management techniques for epistaxis.
  - Position the child erect, sitting with head tilted forward to avoid blood dripping posteriorly into the pharynx.
  - Pinch the nose.
    - Tightly pinch the soft parts of the nose against the center wall for 10 minutes; this should be timed by a clock, not estimated.
    - Do not release the pressure for 10 minutes.
    - Encourage child to remain calm and quiet and to breathe through the mouth.
  - If bleeding continues:
    - Soak gauze in Neo-Synephrine or petroleum jelly and insert it into the nostril.
    - Pinch the nose with gauze in place for another 10 minutes.
    - Be aware that swallowed blood may irritate the stomach and cause vomiting.
- Notify the health care provider if
  - Bleeding does not stop within 20 minutes.
  - The child feels dizzy or faint.

Alert: *Cauterization is not indicated for epistaxis in children with bleeding disorders because of the likelihood of multiple bleeding sites and the risk of severely damaging and perforating the nasal mucosa in the attempt to control bleeding from the various sites.*

For active bleeding that is not controlled by pressure and silver nitrate, spray phenylephrine (Neo-Synephrine), 0.25% to 0.5%, into the nares. If this does not control the bleeding, insert a cotton pledget soaked in 2% lidocaine (Xylocaine) or tetracaine-phenylephedrine, Neo-Synephrine, or epinephrine, 0.25% to 0.5%, tightly into the affected nares. If 5% cocaine is used, a physician must administer it. Leave the pledget in place for 10 minutes while applying pressure; then reassess the nares for continued active bleeding. Reinsert the pledget soaked with a vasoconstrictor for 10 more minutes if necessary.

Alert: *Keep emergency resuscitation equipment readily available when using anesthetic packing. The anesthetized airway may cause the child to lose protective reflexes.*

If the bleeding site is anterior and not controlled by pressure, vasoconstrictors, or cautery, then anterior packing by a physician may be performed. Anterior packing is contraindicated in the child with nasal trauma or when a cerebrospinal fluid leak is suspected. Anterior packing impregnated with antibiotics remains in place 2 to 3 days (Fig. 30–8).

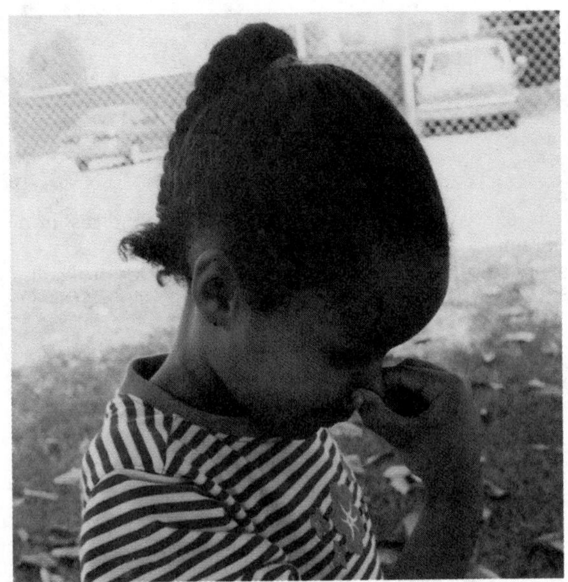

Figure 30-7
Compression of the nasal alae controls most epistaxis, which commonly occurs in Kiesselbach's plexus (Little's area).

The management of severe uncontrollable bleeding may require hospitalization for posterior packing, observation for continued bleeding, and/or surgery for endoscopic cauterization or vessel ligation. Children who have severe epistaxis may be hemodynamically unstable and require fluid replacement for management of hypovolemic shock (Potsic & Handler, 1996).

Sinusitis is a complication of nasal packing, and prophylactic antibiotics should be given (Inkelis, 1996). Antibiotics to cover for coagulase-positive *Staphylococcus* (e.g., first-generation cephalosporins) should be used because *Staphylococcus aureus*, which may cause toxic shock syndrome, is often present in the nares. Pain medication should be administered to children who need anterior or posterior nasal packing (Inkelis, 1996). Nursing care includes maintaining a patent airway, watching for signs of hypoxia or respiratory distress, monitoring fluid balance, and reducing anxiety in the child and family. The amount of blood often seems quite large, which is frightening to the child and family. If children have packing in place, they are not able to breathe through their nose, which is also anxiety producing. Although it is rarely used in children, the nurse must know how to remove posterior packing if it slips back and occludes the child's airway.

Environmental Exposure Injuries

Various environmental exposures can injure an infant or child. Most often, injury occurs because the infant or child physically cannot remove or protect himself or herself from the source of injury. The environmental exposure injuries discussed here include prolonged exposures to heat (hyperthermia) or cold (hypothermia), smoke inhalation, and near-drowning. See Chapter 25 for discussion of sunburn.

Heat Illnesses

Prolonged exposure to heat without protective equipment can cause hyperthermia. Hyperthermia occurs when the thermoregulatory set-point of the body remains normal but heat gain exceeds heat loss despite the body's efforts to return to the set-point. Tissue injury occurs when the temperature exceeds 106.9°F (41.6°C) (Jardine & Stenzel, 1996). Without treatment, individuals with heat stroke die. Even with treatment, there is about a 40% mortality rate (Brady & Dunn, 1996).

Hyperthermia is a preventable illness that is manifested by heat cramps, exhaustion, or stroke. Heat illness is most commonly seen in the tropical regions of the

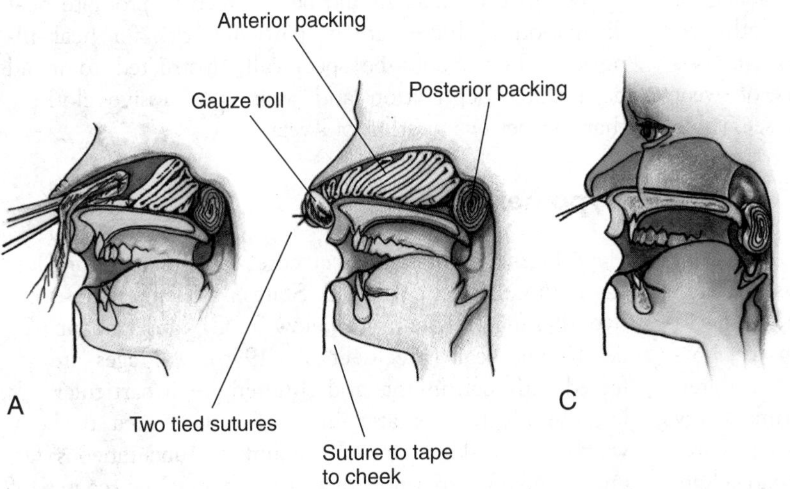

Figure 30-8
Nasal packing may be used to control more severe epistaxis. A, Packing being inserted. B, Packing in place. C, Displaced posterior packing occluding airway.

Table 30–9
Heat Illnesses: Assessment and Interventions

Illness	Etiology	Assessment Findings	Nursing Interventions
Heat cramps	Prolonged or extensive exercise in a hot environment with high humidity Electrolyte depletion secondary to profuse sweating and fluid replacement with salt-poor fluids	Sudden onset of intermittent, excruciating cramps in the skeletal muscles Usually occurs after the exercise, during the cool-down period	Have child stop exertion and rest in a cool, shaded area. For mild cramps, administer oral salt solution (1 teaspoon of salt in 500 mL of water). For severe cramps, administer 0.9% NS (20 mL/kg) IV over 1–2 hr
Heat exhaustion (heat prostration)	Prolonged or extensive exercise in a hot environment, with high humidity and inadequate fluid replacement Most common heat illness Without treatment, can progress to heat stroke	Onset over 30 min, but may have a more acute onset such as the "parade ground faint" Headache Intense thirst Inability to work or play Tachycardia Orthostatic hypotension Nausea and vomiting Lethargy CNS dysfunction, such as hyperventilation, agitation, incoordination, paresthesia, psychosis Intractable seizures and muscle cramps (in severe cases) Normal body temperature or body temperature as high as 39°C with high ambient temperatures or exercise Hemoconcentration Hyper- or hyponatremia (depends on type of fluids ingested) Hyperchloremia Respiratory alkalosis (resulting from hyperventilation)	Provide the child with a cool, well-ventilated place to rest. Remove some clothing, spray with water, and fan the child. Replace fluids PO (or IV if the child is weak or has an impaired level of consciousness); liquids should be cool with unrestricted dietary sodium. If IV fluids are required, administer bolus of 0.9% NS, 20 mL/kg given over 20 min; repeat boluses to correct electrolyte balance and restore blood pressure. Treat severe cases with an initial IV of 5 mL/kg of 3% NS over 20 min followed by a second dose of 5 mL/kg over 4 to 6 hr.

world, but heat is responsible for the deaths of more than 4000 people per year in the United States (Thompson, 1996). The elderly population is most vulnerable, but children are at risk as well, especially young athletes, infants left in automobiles on hot days, cystic fibrosis patients, and those with the congenital absence of sweat glands. For more information on heat illnesses, see Table 30–9.

Community Care

Prevention is the best treatment for heat illnesses. Teach children and parents measures to prevent overheating in hot environments. Children should be dressed in lightweight clothes and hats or sun shades. Keep children well hydrated by providing and offering cool drinks every 15 to 30 minutes, even if the child is not thirsty. Water is a good choice because children sweat less than adults and so lose less salt. Activity level should be regulated on the basis of environmental conditions and restricted when temperature or humidity is high. Scheduled rest periods in the shade should be enforced to promote heat dissipation. Athletes are at particular risk for heat illnesses. They should be specifically instructed to avoid both water deprivation and wearing excessive clothing that reduces evaporation of sweat.

Hypothermia

Hypothermia is defined as a core body temperature less than 35°C. In the United States, moderate to severe hypothermia (temperature below 32°C) causes about 600 deaths per year (Steele et al., 1996). All ages are affected, although infants and children are at particular risk because of their greater ratio of surface area to body weight, thin skin, limited amount of subcutaneous fat, and immature thermoregulatory system. The causes of hypothermia include immersion in icy water, prolonged

Table 30–9
Heat Illnesses: Assessment and Interventions *Continued*

Illness	Etiology	Assessment Findings	Nursing Interventions
Heat stroke (a true medical emergency)	Thermoregulatory failure after prolonged exposure to high environmental temperatures and humidity	Hyperpyrexia (≥41°C) Hot, dry skin, typically with anhidrosis (absence of sweating) Moderate CNS disturbances such as headache, dizziness, faintness, and confusion Severe CNS disturbances such as stupor, seizures, coma, and sudden loss of consciousness (more common when treatment is delayed) Tachycardia and an increased pulse pressure initially Ashen cyanosis and a thin, rapid pulse later	Remove the child from the source of heat. Maintain patent airway and cardiovascular support. If comatose, may require intubation to secure airway. Remove clothing and actively cool the child. Monitor temperature closely with a rectal probe. Be aware that antipyretics such as acetaminophen are not useful. Perform active cooling measures such as sprinkling the child with water, directing fans toward patient, applying a cooling blanket, giving an ice bath (though this makes other monitoring mechanisms difficult). Discontinue active cooling measures when the core temperature falls to 38.5°C. Avoid shivering, as this increases heat production. Give phenothiazines (e.g., chlorpromazine, 0.05 mg/kg) to help control shivering (use is controversial in children). Carefully monitor electrocardiogram, central venous pressure, arterial BP, and urine output in a patient with signs of failing cardiac output (ashen skin, tachycardia, and hypotension); such a patient is in danger of imminent death.

References: Barkin & Burrington (1991); Thompson (1996).

exposure to cold temperatures, and exposure for an extended time during a medical evaluation. Hypothermia is also common in patients with sepsis and shock.

▽ **Alert:** *Hypothermia can lead to metabolic acidosis, decreased respiratory rates, bradycardia, and cardiopulmonary arrest.*

See Chapter 25 for discussion of frostbite.

Assessment

Mental status may remain normal in mild hypothermia. Central nervous system (CNS) function becomes progressively impaired as the temperature falls. Increasing lethargy, incoordination, apathy, confusion, clumsiness, irritability, hallucinations, and bradycardia are seen. Frank coma occurs at approximately 27°C (Thompson, 1996). At a temperature of 25°C, profound respiratory depression occurs, followed by ventricular fibrillation or asystole, and usually results in death.

Hypothermia can mimic death, with the patient demonstrating dilated pupils, muscular rigidity, faint or absent pulse, and an unobtainable blood pressure. However, life can be sustained for long periods, despite cessation of cardiac function, because of the marked decrease in oxygen consumption.

Nursing Diagnoses and Outcomes

Nursing diagnoses and outcomes for the child experiencing an emergency are discussed in Chart 30–6. In addition, the following are appropriate for the hypothermic child:

- **Hypothermia related to environmental exposure**
  Outcome: The child will regain normal body temperature and will suffer no long-term effects from hypothermia.
- **Inability to sustain spontaneous ventilation related to effects of decreased body temperature**
  Outcome: The child will maintain spontaneous ventilation or have adequate ventilatory support provided.

Interdisciplinary Interventions

Prevention is the best treatment. Family education should include the increased risk of hypothermia in young children. Children have higher metabolic rates than adults. They generate more heat, so children may not feel the effects of exposure. Parents should dress children appropriately for the weather and monitor their activities so that they are not exposed for long periods of time.

Nursing interventions for a child with hypothermia are discussed in Chart 30–15. Support cardiorespiratory function as needed. If the child develops lethal dysrhythmias, defibrillation is often ineffective until the core temperature reaches 30°C. Drug therapy is rarely effective at low temperatures and can lead to toxicity because of decreased hepatic and renal metabolism.

Active rewarming can be accomplished through external or core rewarming techniques. External rewarming techniques may result in early warming of the skin and extremities and peripheral vasodilation and worsen hypotension and shock. This phenomenon, called "after-drop," is characterized by a decrease in the core temperature as it receives cold blood from the periphery (Thompson, 1996). Core rewarming is the most appropriate choice when the temperature is 30°C or less with cardiopulmonary arrest.

Survival of severely hypothermic patients after prolonged periods of nonperfusing cardiac rhythm has been reported (Tom, Garmel, & Auerbach, 1994). After rewarming the patient to 35°C, if cardiorespiratory function has not been restored, resuscitative efforts should be halted (Rosen et al., 1992).

Smoke Inhalation

Smoke inhalation usually results from a fire, which may also cause burns. (For a discussion of burn injuries see Chapter 25.) Exposure to fire and/or smoke causes significant damage to the child's pulmonary tree. In fact, most pediatric fatalities resulting from closed-space fires are due to inhalation of toxic gas (e.g., carbon monoxide and cyanide) rather than burns (Haley & Baker, 1993). Inhalation injuries are the primary cause of death in burn patients within the first 24 hours.

Several factors place pediatric patients at high risk for inhalation injuries. Their higher respiratory rate leads to increased intake of toxic gases and contributes to insensible fluid losses from the pulmonary tree. They have a small airway diameter and increased proportion of soft tissue, and the diameter may become even smaller because of the inhalation of hot air and irritants. Progressive airway edema may ultimately lead to airway obstruction.

Alert: *Suspect smoke inhalation and upper airway burns in a child with facial burns.*

Assessment

Clinically, the child may have singed nasal hairs or eyebrows, carbonaceous sputum, tachypnea, and other signs of respiratory distress such as wheezing, rhonchi, rales, or stridor. However, symptoms of an inhalation injury may not be manifest for up to 24 hours after exposure. Therefore, close observation of respiratory status is necessary during this time. Because the carbon monoxide molecule has a 250-fold higher affinity for hemoglobin than oxygen, tissue hypoxia occurs as carbon monoxide reduces the oxygen-carrying capacity of hemoglobin. Without prompt treatment, serum carboxyhemoglobin levels greater than 50% can cause irreversible central nervous system damage. CNS signs of carbon monoxide poisoning range from slight dyspnea, decreased visual acuity, irritability, nausea, and fatigue to confusion, ataxia, and coma (Herrin & Antoon, 1996).

caREminder: *Do not rely on pulse oximetry to measure oxygen saturation. Pulse oximetry does not distinguish between oxyhemoglobin and carboxyhemoglobin, so the actual oxygen saturation is less than the pulse oximeter reflects.*

Nursing Diagnoses and Outcomes

Chart 30–6 lists nursing diagnoses and outcomes applicable to the child experiencing an emergency. The following may also be appropriate for the child after smoke inhalation:

- **Ineffective airway clearance related to effects of edema and inhaled toxins causing mucosal sloughing**
  Outcome: The child will be intubated early, if indicated, and maintain a patent airway.
- **Impaired gas exchange related to effects of cellular damage, carboxyhemoglobin replacing oxyhemoglobin, pulmonary edema, and smoke exposure causing decreased surfactant resulting in atelectasis**
  Outcome: The child will maintain adequate cellular oxygenation.

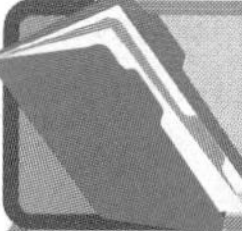

Chart 30–15
Nursing Interventions Classification (NIC)

Hypothermia Treatment

Definition

Rewarming and surveillance of a patient whose core body temperature is below 35°C

Activities

Remove the patient from the cold, and place in a warm environment.
Remove cold, wet clothing and replace with warm, dry clothing.
Monitor patient's temperature, using a low-recording thermometer if necessary.
Institute a continuous core temperature monitoring device, as appropriate.
Monitor for symptoms associated with hypothermia: fatigue, weakness, confusion, apathy, impaired coordination, slurred speech, shivering, and change in skin color.
Determine factors leading to the hypothermic episode by questioning about recent activities, such as heavy activity in cold wet weather, elderly living alone in a cool environment, and poor nutritional state.
Monitor for underlying medical conditions that may precipitate hypothermia (e.g., diabetes, myxedema, or anorexia nervosa).
Place on a cardiac monitor, as appropriate.
Monitor for and treat ventricular defibrillation.
Cover with warmed blankets, as appropriate.
Minimize stimulation of the patient to avoid precipitating ventricular fibrillation.
Administer warmed (37° to 40°C) IV fluids, as appropriate.
Administer heated oxygen, as appropriate.
Institute active external rewarming measures (e.g., immersion in warm water, application of hot water bottles, and placement on a heating blanket), as appropriate.
Institute active core rewarming techniques (e.g., colonic lavage, hemodialysis, peritoneal dialysis, and extracorporeal blood rewarming), as appropriate.
Monitor for rewarming shock.
Administer plasma volume expanders, as appropriate.
Monitor skin color and temperature.
Monitor vital signs, as appropriate.
Monitor for bradycardia.
Monitor for electrolyte imbalance.
Monitor for acid-base imbalance.
Monitor intake and output.
Monitor cardiac output, pulmonary capillary wedge pressure, systemic vascular resistance, and right atrial pressure, using invasive hemodynamic monitoring as appropriate.
Avoid giving IM or subcutaneous medications during the hypothermic state.
Monitor for increased actions of medications as rewarming occurs.
Institute routine skin surveillance, as appropriate.
Monitor respiratory status.
Give patient warm oral fluids, if alert and able to swallow.
Monitor nutritional status.
Teach patient to consume a caloric intake sufficient to maintain a normal body temperature.
Emphasize the importance of wearing warm, protective clothing when going into a cold environment.
Teach early warning signs of hypothermia.
*Establish support systems for elderly patient to prevent isolation and residing in excessively cool environments, as appropriate.

*Included in original NIC; not applicable to pediatrics.
From McCloskey, J., & Bulechek, G. (1996). *Nursing interventions classification (NIC)* (2nd ed.). St. Louis: Mosby–Year Book. Reprinted with permission.

- **Risk for fluid volume deficit related to effects of tachypnea, cellular damage, and increased fluid demands**
  Outcome: The child will receive adequate fluids to prevent dehydration, will have accurate intake and output monitored, and will not develop pulmonary edema because of overhydration.

Interdisciplinary Interventions

All patients with smoke inhalation should receive 100% oxygen via a snug-fitting, nonrebreather mask. The usual 4-hour half-life of carboxyhemoglobin can be reduced to 40 to 50 minutes by administering 100% oxygen (Saunders & Ho, 1992). Patients with severe laryngeal edema, hypoxemia, and audible stridor require intubation to maintain a secure and patent airway. Baseline arterial blood gases, pH, and carboxyhemoglobin levels should be obtained and monitored periodically.

Maintain a neutral thermal environment. The child is susceptible to hypothermia because of associated burn injuries and exposure for treatment of injuries. Hypothermia and alkalosis decrease the dissociation of carbon monoxide from hemoglobin. Hyperbaric oxygen therapy may be considered.

For the intubated child, aggressive pulmonary hygiene including frequent suctioning and chest physiotherapy helps prevent subsequent pneumonia and adult respiratory distress syndrome (Talbert, 1993).

The child should be monitored for hypoxia, respiratory distress, and pulmonary edema. Even if not seriously injured or intubated, children who have been in fires should be hospitalized for observation for at least 24 hours (Herrin & Antoon, 1996).

Near-Drowning

Drowning is the second most common cause of accidental death in the pediatric population. Most commonly, it affects children younger than 5 years (Levin, Morriss, Toro, Brink, & Turner, 1993). Drowning is defined as death resulting from suffocation by submersion in a liquid. Near-drowning is defined as survival, although sometimes temporary, for at least 24 hours after a submersion episode.

Children can drown whenever unsupervised around any body of water, including bathtubs, toilets, and buckets of water. The majority of drownings occur because of lack of adequate barriers to prevent access to a swimming pool (Levin et al., 1993). Precipitating factors include trauma (including child abuse), intoxication (plays a significant role in adolescent drownings), seizure disorders, and exhaustion.

Whether in fresh or salt water, the end result of near drowning is the same. Pulmonary compliance decreases, airway resistance increases, pulmonary arterial pressure increases, and pulmonary flow decreases. These changes result in hypoxemia (Walsh & Ioli, 1994). This leads to cardiac arrest and ischemia.

Although all organs are susceptible to ischemic injury, the CNS is most vulnerable and prognosis is dependent on the degree of CNS injury (Vernon-Levett, 1996). (See Chapter 21 for discussion of increased intracranial pressure.) The degree of brain injury depends on the submersion time (which is often underestimated), the water temperature, and the speed of initiation of resuscitative measures. The longer the submersion, the poorer the prognosis. Irreversible cerebral injury from hypoxia begins to occur after about 3 to 5 minutes of submersion (Kallas, 1996). Submersion in cold water (0° to 15°C) may rarely be compatible with recovery after longer periods of time (Levin et al., 1993). Cold water may increase survival by triggering the diving reflex and, to a lesser extent, by decreasing the cerebral metabolic rate (Levin et al., 1993). The diving reflex is activated by cold water touching the child's face and stimulating the trigeminal nerve to signal the CNS, causing bradycardia and shunting of blood to the cerebral and coronary circulations.

Assessment

Initially, the clinical problems of children after a near-drowning episode involve the pulmonary and neurologic systems. The child may present with varying degrees of neurologic insult, from alert with minimal injury to full cardiopulmonary arrest. Cerebral edema may develop later with irritability, confusion, and lethargy leading to seizures and coma. Respiratory symptoms range from cough, dyspnea, tachypnea, adventitious breath sounds, and expectoration of pink frothy sputum to apnea.

Initial arterial blood gases often indicate hypoxemia and metabolic acidosis. Chest radiography results vary but should be obtained to provide a baseline against which to compare later radiographs. Electrolyte abnormalities may be seen. Renal damage resulting from hypoperfusion, hypoxia, and ischemia is revealed by oliguria, proteinuria, and elevated BUN and creatinine.

Nursing Diagnoses and Outcomes

In addition to the nursing diagnoses discussed in Chart 30–6, nursing diagnoses and outcomes applicable to the child after near-drowning are

- **Impaired gas exchange related to effects of aspiration, hypoxia, pulmonary edema**
  Outcome: The child will demonstrate adequate oxygenation and no signs of respiratory distress.
- **Ineffective airway clearance related to effects of as-**

piration of water and foreign material, accumulated secretions, and artificial airway
Outcome: The child will maintain a patent airway, and secretions will be adequately cleared to maintain gas exchange.

- **Ineffective breathing pattern related to effects of cerebral hypoxia**
Outcome: The child will be supported in maintaining a breathing pattern that maintains adequate gas exchange.
- **Altered tissue perfusion: cardiopulmonary related to effects of dysrhythmias, hypovolemia**
Outcome: The child will maintain adequate cardiopulmonary perfusion as evidenced by normal sinus rhythm, strong bilateral peripheral pulses, and urine output of 1 mL/kg/hr.
- **Altered tissue perfusion: cerebral related to effects of hypoxia, cerebral edema, and increased intracranial pressure**
Outcome: The child will maintain adequate cerebral perfusion and will have signs of decreased perfusion recognized immediately and interventions implemented.
- **Fluid volume excess related to fluid resuscitation, renal damage from hypoxia**
Outcome: The child will maintain fluid balance evidenced by absence of edema, urine output of 1 mL/kg/hr, electrolytes and urine specific gravity within normal range.
- **Knowledge deficit: water safety**
Outcomes: The family will discuss and implement water safety measures. The family will not experience future near-drowning events.

Interdisciplinary Interventions

Manage the pediatric near-drowning victim in the same fashion as the trauma patient. Initially, focus on the ABCs and correction of hypoxemia.

The nurse must continue to monitor and support pulmonary, cardiac, and neurologic function. Assess airway patency, breath sounds, color, and respiratory effort, and assist with ventilation as indicated. Cardiac assessment includes heart rate and rhythm, BP, capillary refill, and pulses. Intake and output should be monitored to assess fluid balance and renal function. Catheters may be placed to monitor arterial, central venous, and/or pulmonary artery pressure. Assessment of neurologic functioning includes level of consciousness, pupillary response, reflexes, and presence of posturing or seizure activity.

As with all pediatric emergencies, provide family support. If the child survives, or if other children live in the house, instruct the family in water safety measures (Chart 30–16).

Poisoning

A poison is a substance that causes harmful effects upon exposure. Poisoning is the fourth leading cause of death in children. Over a million calls are made to poison centers annually with questions concerning children. Nearly 85% of these events are managed by the family at home. The majority of fatalities occur with ingestion or inhalation of the poison (Litovitz, Felberg, White, & Klein-Schwartz, 1996).

Poisoning ingestions in infants are largely due to therapeutic overdosing (Dean, 1994). Ingestions are most common in children 1 to 6 years old (Litovitz et al., 1996). Children are naturally curious and often explore by tasting. They also imitate adult behavior. If they witness a parent take medication, they may try some themselves or may feed the medication to a younger sibling.

Tip: *Never tell a child that medicine is candy, which may increase the desire to obtain it. The child should be told it is medicine and is taken for a specific reason.*

Young children usually ingest only a single substance and, because they are generally closely watched, the time from ingestion to discovery and treatment is brief (Bond, 1995). Children younger than 6 years most frequently ingest substances such as cosmetics and personal care products, cleaning substances, analgesics, plants, and

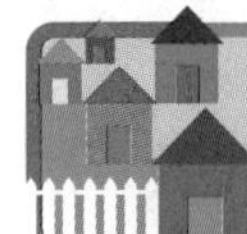

Chart 30–16
Community Care

Water Safety

Instruct parents and other care providers to:

- Supervise children **constantly** around **any** body of water, including bathtubs.
- Designate one person to watch the child, especially when many adults are present and each assumes the others are watching the child.
- Fence any pool or hot tub and equip it with self-closing gates.
- Empty pails and buckets of fluid immediately after use.
- Keep toilet lids closed and secured, especially around toddlers; toddlers' heads are relatively large and heavy and, when they fall in head first, they cannot extricate themselves.
- Allow children with a seizure disorder to swim or take a bath only with supervision, regardless of age.
- Discuss with adolescents the dangers of combining drugs or alcohol with swimming or water sports.

cough and cold preparations (Litovitz et al., 1996). Such agents may not be the most toxic but rather most readily accessible to children.

Adolescents may be affected by drug experimentation or suicide attempts. Therefore, poisoning in adolescents often involves multiple substances, with a delay between when exposure occurs and when medical treatment is obtained (Longo & Dickenson, 1996).

This section presents general information about poisonings. Then it provides specific information about assessment and treatment of different types of poisonings.

Assessment

Often the ingestion is witnessed or the child is found with the agent's container or medication bottle and with pills in his or her mouth. Sometimes, it is not known that a child ingested or was exposed to a potentially toxic substance. Historical features such as acute onset, age 1 to 6 years, multiple organ system involvement, or an unexplained altered level of consciousness suggest the possibility of poisoning. The child may have a wide range of symptoms, from none to coma.

Obtaining an accurate history is paramount to successful treatment. Be sure to determine the following:

- What was ingested
- How much was ingested (one swallow of liquid approximately equals a volume of 5 mL)
- When it occurred
- What, if any, therapy was initiated before arrival in the emergency department

Worldview: *Folk remedies may contain toxic agents and use of such should be included in the history. For example, Hispanic and other cultures use mint tea to treat colic and minor ailments. Most mint teas are not toxic, but if mint leaves that contain pennyroyal oil are used, they can be lethal (Bakerink, Gospe, Dimand, & Eldridge, 1996).*

Diagnostic Tests. A multitude of laboratory studies are available to confirm the diagnosis of a toxic ingestion, although a thorough history and physical assessment are usually enough to make a diagnosis. Some laboratory tests quantify a drug level, which may be helpful in predicting clinical effects. Recommended tests include serum glucose, electrolytes, serum osmolarity, and anion gap.

An elevated anion gap is characteristic of the acidosis seen in poisonings. The normal value for anion gap is less than 16 mEq/L and is calculated by using the formula $Na^+ - (Cl^- + HCO_3^-)$. The etiologies for increased anion gap are listed in Chart 30–17.

Chart 30–17

Common Causes for Increased Anion Gap Values

Utilizing the mnemonic AT MUD PILES (Woolf, 1993):

Alcohol
Toluene

Methanol
Uremia
Diabetic ketoacidosis (DKA)

Paraldehyde
Iron
Lactic acidosis
Ethylene glycol
Salicylates

Nursing Diagnoses and Outcomes

Nursing diagnoses and outcomes for the child experiencing an emergency are discussed in Chart 30–6. Nursing diagnoses applicable to the poisoned child depend on the specific poison and symptoms the child displays (e.g., risk for aspiration is applicable to the child who has a depressed level of consciousness resulting from the poison). An additional nursing diagnosis is

▶ **Knowledge deficit: poisoning**
Outcomes: The family will discuss poison prevention techniques and how these change as the child grows and develops. The family will state first-aid measures appropriate for poisoning, including having the local poison control center phone number readily accessible.

Interdisciplinary Interventions

Obviously, prevention of poisoning is the key (see Chapter 5). Teach parents to keep medications in their original, childproof containers, and lock them out of reach of children. Advise them to store cleaning solutions, cosmetics, and hydrocarbons (e.g., gasoline, solvents and thinners, polishes) in high, locked cabinets (Fig. 30–9). Advise them to make the child's environment free of lead-based paints and poisonous plants (Chart 30–18).

Perform a rapid assessment and immediate interventions to ensure that the ABCs are managed. Secure intravenous access, and obtain a serum glucose level because

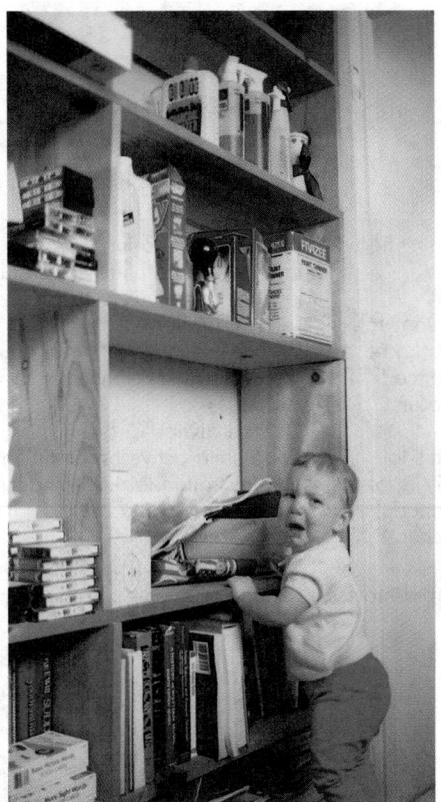

Figure 30–9
This frustrated toddler cannot reach the tempting, but potentially dangerous, poisons and cleaning supplies stored safely out of her reach.

hypoglycemia is a frequent manifestation of acute poisoning. Treat shock with fluids and vasopressors as necessary. To reduce the absorption of potentially toxic substances, gastric decontamination may be required (Table 30–10). Depending on the severity of the ingestion, it may occur immediately after the airway is secured, during resuscitation.

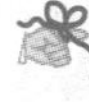 **caREminder:** *Treat the child, not the poison. Specific treatment depends on the type and amount of toxin, time since exposure, and the child's symptoms. Many children do not need treatment (Bond, 1995).*

Iron

Iron overdose is the most common cause of poisoning death in children (Anderson, 1994). Iron-containing compounds are readily available as brightly colored, sugar-coated tablets and often viewed as a harmless vitamin by parents. Prenatal iron preparations are often the source. Moderate to severe toxicity occurs after ingestion of 20 to 60 mg/kg; a greater than 200 mg/kg dose of iron is potentially lethal (Jaimovich, 1993). The number of pills ingested may be useful in determining whether a toxic dose was ingested. Monitoring serum iron levels is critical in the management of the patient. See Table 30–11 for phases of clinical effects of iron ingestion.

Management includes managing the ABCs, gastric decontamination, and chelation therapy (administering something that binds with iron, such as deferoxamine).

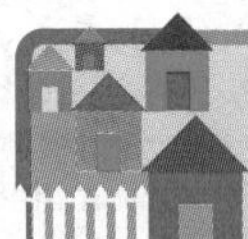

Chart 30–18
Community Care

Plant Poisonings

Educate parents and caregivers about which common plants are poisonous and to limit the child's access to these (not an inclusive list):

Azalea
Castor bean
Cherry (pits)
Deadly nightshade
Dumb cane (*Dieffenbachia*)
English ivy
Holly
Jimsonweed
Lily of the valley
Mistletoe (berries)
Mushrooms (certain species)
Oleander
Potatoes (tubercles)
Rosary pea
Rhododendron
Rhubarb (leaves)
Water hemlock
Yew

Tell parents and caregivers what to do if child ingests a poisonous plant:

Stay calm.
Call poison control center.
Describe symptoms (if any) and name of plant if known.
Follow instructions from poison control center.
Take plant with you when seeking treatment.

Teach parents and caregivers poison prevention tips:

Supervise child's activities.
Place household plants out of reach.
Teach children not to eat any plant without permission.

Table 30-10
Gastric Decontamination

Decontamination Method	Method of Action	Indications and Dosage	Contraindications and Considerations
Syrup of ipecac	Induces vomiting	Indications: ingestion of heavy metals Dosage: 6–12 mo of age: 10 mL followed by 10–20 mL/kg of water; repeat dose once if vomiting does not occur within 20 min. 1–12 yr: 15 to 30 mL followed by 10–20 mL/kg of water; repeat dose once if vomiting does not occur within 20 min.	Contraindicated in the young infant, or in the child with an altered level of consciousness (LOC), absent gag reflex, or seizures. Do not use in ingestion of caustic or corrosive substances or of volatile oil. Can be given PO or NG. Keep child active and moving after administration to aid in induction of vomiting.
Activated charcoal	Absorbs substances in stomach and gastrointestinal tract	Indications: ingestion of most drugs: acetaminophen arsenic barbiturates camphor chlorpromazine cocaine digitalis iodine lead mercury salts muscarine nicotine opioids oxalates parathion penicillin petroleum distillates phenol phenolphthalein quinine salicylates strychnine tricyclic antidepressants Dosage: <1 yr: 1 g/kg q 4–6 hr p.r.n. 1–12 yr: 1–2 g/kg q 2–6 hr p.r.n. A single dose of a cathartic such as sorbitol is often mixed with the first dose of charcoal. Do not give repeated doses of sorbitol, may lead to fluid and electrolyte imbalance (Fine & Goldfrank, 1992).	Method of choice in reducing drug absorption (Bond, 1995). Activated charcoal is not effective in the following ingestions: cyanide, mineral acids, caustic alkalis, organic solvents, iron, ethanol, methanol, or lithium. Do not use activated charcoal with sorbitol in patients with fructose intolerance. Use with gastric emptying (ipecac or gastric lavage) only if within 1 hr of ingestion and child has CNS depression. When used with syrup of ipecac, induce vomiting with ipecac before administering charcoal because charcoal absorbs syrup of ipecac. Can be given PO or NG; some children drink readily, especially if cup is covered. If giving NG, prime NG tube with mineral oil and dilute activated charcoal with water to ease administration.

Activated charcoal **does not** bind with iron. The dose of deferoxamine depends on the severity of the ingestion. If chelation therapy is initiated, IV deferoxamine at a rate not to exceed 15 mg/kg/hr (total maximum 6 g per day) is administered (Krenzelok, 1996). After the administration of deferoxamine, the child's urine turns a reddish (vin rosé) color, indicating that the iron is binding with the antidote.

Table 30-10
Gastric Decontamination *Continued*

Decontamination Method	Method of Action	Indications and Dosage	Contraindications and Considerations
Gastric lavage	Dilutes and removes substances from stomach	Indications: Child with depressed LOC or airway compromise; perform tracheal intubation before lavage to protect airway Ingestion of drugs that decrease gastric motility or are not adsorbed by charcoal Dosage: Large-bore NG or OG tube inserted and the stomach lavaged with normal saline. Amount of NS to instill: <age 12: 10–15 mL/kg (maximum 100–150 mL per exchange) Adolescents: 300 mL	Use in awake child usually does not justify risks associated with elective sedation and intubation (Bond, 1995). Large-bore (36–40 French) orogastric tube should be used, possibly smaller in children, but tube should be bigger than pill fragments to be extracted. Do not perform gastric lavage when caustic substances have been ingested, because insertion of the NG or OG tube may induce vomiting and cause more burns to the esophagus and oropharynx and may increase the risk for aspiration. NS is instilled and then aspirated to remove poisons, pills, and pill fragments from stomach.
Whole bowel irrigation	Used to flush toxin from entire gastrointestinal tract	Indications: not well established in children; use for iron poisoning and other agents not bound by activated charcoal Dosage: administer a balanced polyethylene glycol solution (e.g., GoLYTELY, Colyte) PO or NG over 4–6 hr until rectal effluent is clear. <5 yr: 20 mL/kg/hr >5 yr: 0.5–2 L/hr (Fine & Goldfrank, 1992; Krenzelok, 1996)	May also be useful to eliminate contraband that was placed in bags or condoms and swallowed. Solution is isosmotic and so is not associated with fluid and electrolyte imbalance. The large fluid volumes used may cause nausea, vomiting, bloating, cramping, and abdominal distention.

References: Bond (1995); Fine & Goldfrank (1992); Krenzelok (1996).

Lead

Lead poisoning can occur after the ingestion of substances containing lead. Children are often exposed to this type of ingestion by eating paint chips from lead-based paint or eating with their hands after playing in dirt contaminated with lead-based paint fragments. Other sources of exposure include drinking water that flows through lead pipes and eating from dinnerware with a lead glaze.

Children are most commonly exposed to lead on a chronic basis, although occasionally a child ingests a large quantity of lead at one time.

Worldview: *Folk remedies such as azarcon and greta to treat digestive problems (Mexico) and paylooah for fever or rash (Southeast Asia) may contain lead and poison the child.*

Signs and symptoms of acute lead poisoning include a burning sensation in the mouth and throat, gastrointestinal disturbance (e.g., diarrhea, constipation), paralysis of the extremities, seizures, and coma. Chronic lead poisoning is characterized by irritability, anorexia, and anemia and may progress to the acute form. Even low lead levels can negatively affect neurobehavioral functioning and result in slight decreases in IQ (Piomelli, 1996). Severe cases of lead poisoning can lead to seizures, muscular collapse, and lead encephalopathy. Lead encephalopathy is characterized by delirium, seizures, mania, cortical blindness, and coma.

Treatment for lead poisoning includes terminating

Table 30–11
Clinical Effects of Iron Ingestion

Phase 1	Occurs within the first 6 hr after ingestion. Produces symptoms that range from gastrointestinal (GI) complaints (such as nausea, vomiting, and GI blood loss) to hypovolemic shock and coma.
Phase 2	Lasts from 6 to 24 hr after ingestion. Produces symptoms that improve with treatment for hypovolemia (improvement may only be transitory).
Phase 3	May follow phase 2 or may occur rapidly after ingestion. Produces metabolic acidosis and cyanosis and may lead to coma, seizures, and shock. May result from hepatocellular injury.
Phase 4	Occurs 1 to 2 mo after ingestion. Produces pyloric stenosis secondary to gastric scarring and consequent obstruction, bowel stricture, and cirrhosis.

exposure and chelation in the presence of higher lead levels. Chelating agents form a compound with lead that is excreted through the kidneys. Adequate urinary output is established with fluid therapy. Chelation therapy consists of calcium disodium edetate (EDTA) or dimercaprol (British antilewisite [BAL]) for severe cases.

caREminder: *The carrier for BAL is peanut oil. Children with peanut allergies should not receive BAL.*

Asymptomatic patients with a blood lead concentration of 45 to 69 μg/dL should receive calcium EDTA at 1 g/m^2 per day IV as a 24-hour infusion or over 20 to 30 minutes for 5 days (Piomelli, 1996). When IV administration is not possible, EDTA can be given IM. An alternative therapy is dimercaptosuccinic acid (DMSA, succimer), an analogue of BAL. Advantages of DMSA over other chelating agents are that it is less toxic, it can be administered orally, and it does not eliminate iron, copper, or zinc from the body (Fine & Goldfrank, 1992). Children whose lead concentration exceeds 70 μg/dL or who are symptomatic should receive BAL at 75 mg/m^2 IM every 4 hours to a total of 450 mg/m^2 per day and, at least 3 to 4 hours after the first dose of BAL, EDTA at 1500 mg/m^2 per day IV (Piomelli, 1996).

Nursing care focuses on fluid management, administering medications in a manner that minimizes pain, psychosocial issues, and education. Adequate urine output must be maintained but overhydration should be prevented, especially in the presence of CNS symptoms, because children with lead encephalopathy have the potential to develop cerebral edema. EDTA administered IM is extremely painful. The drug should be mixed with procaine, which only partially alleviates the pain (Piomelli, 1996). EDTA should be given by the deep IM route. The procaine should be drawn up last in the syringe so that it is injected first. Application of warm compresses to the injection area may help reduce pain. Play therapy should be implemented to help the child deal with painful IM injections, if they are being given (see Chart 9–13). Parents and caregivers must be taught about preventing future exposure to lead (Chart 30–19).

Acetaminophen

Acetaminophen is an analgesic and antipyretic, commonly found in over-the-counter medications, that is metabolized in the liver. It is one of the drugs most commonly ingested by children and one of the 10 most common medications used in intentional poisonings in adolescents and adults (Haley & Baker, 1993).

Ingestion of more than 150 mg/kg acetaminophen is potentially toxic (Jaimovich, 1993). Ingestions of large amounts of the drug are known to cause significant hepatic damage, hepatic failure, and death. Untreated, toxicity generally follows four stages (Longo & Dickenson, 1996). Children may initially present with nausea, vomiting, pallor, and diaphoresis. This is followed by a latent period of 24 to 48 hours in which the child appears better but bilirubin, prothrombin time, and hepatic enzymes are elevated. At 72 to 96 hours after ingestion, liver function abnormalities peak and right upper quadrant tenderness and jaundice are present. Stage 4 occurs in 7 to 8 days, when hepatic dysfunction resolves or the child develops hepatic failure or dies. Children younger than 6 years seem to be resistant to the toxic effects of acetaminophen, possibly because of differences in hepatocyte maturation and in how acetaminophen is metabolized. Young children may present with hypothermia,

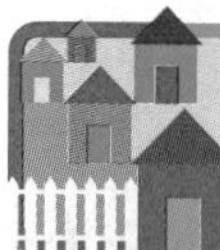

Chart 30–19
Community Care

Prevention of Lead Poisoning

Teach parents and other caregivers to remove sources of lead from the child's environment:

- A common source of lead is lead-based paint present in old homes; lead content in paint for new residences has been limited since 1978.
- Children may ingest paint chips or inhale dust from peeling paint.
- Keep children from playing near old homes being renovated, where the lead-based paint may have contaminated the dirt surrounding the home.
- Check lead levels in tap water, which may pick up lead if lead solder was used in the plumbing.
- If lead level exceeds drinking water standard, use bottled water or run cold water until it gets no colder before using for drinking or cooking.
- Do not use improperly glazed ceramic dinnerware or decorative pottery to serve food; citrus juices, in particular, leach lead from the pottery.
- Do not store food or drink in lead crystal.
- Discuss folk remedies used by the family that may contain lead.
- Parental occupation (e.g., construction or factory worker where lead-based substances are used) or hobbies (e.g., using leaded solder in stained glass, making leaded fishing weights) may increase the child's lead exposure; parents should wash their hands and change clothes and shower, if possible, before entering the home.

Advise parents to ensure that the child has adequate nutritional intake, which decreases lead absorption by the body.

Screen the child for lead levels per facility policy. The Centers for Disease Control and Prevention (CDC) recommends universal lead screening for children between age 6 months and 6 years. Question parents of young children about potential lead exposure and risk factors.

severe hypoglycemia, shock, encephalopathy, and biochemical liver dysfunction (Jaimovich, 1993). To allow for full absorption of the drug, severity of overdose is most accurately predicted from acetaminophen serum levels drawn 4 hours after the ingestion.

Treatment includes gastric decontamination by administration of ipecac if given within 60 minutes of ingestion or gastric lavage and administration of activated charcoal (Chart 30–20). Depending on the serum level of acetaminophen and poison control center recommendations, the antidote *N*-acetylcysteine (NAC, Mucomyst), diluted to 5%, may be given. NAC is given as a loading dose of 140 mg/kg, followed by 17 doses of 70 mg/kg every 4 hours (Krenzelok, 1996).

caREminder: *N-Acetylcysteine smells like rotten eggs. Place the antidote in juice or a carbonated beverage in a covered cup to mask the smell and make it more palatable. It may have to be administered via a nasogastric (NG) tube. If the child vomits within 1 hour of administration, repeat the dose.*

Hydrocarbons

Hydrocarbon or petroleum distillate ingestion can be lethal. Commonly found hydrocarbons include liquid polishes, solvents, and thinners; gasoline; and kerosene. Toxicity depends on the agent ingested and the risk for aspiration. Hepatic failure and central nervous system depression are other serious results.

The child may present with gasping, choking, coughing, chest pain, dyspnea, or cyanosis because of the high incidence of associated aspiration of hydrocarbon. Airway management is vital, with frequent reassessment for signs and symptoms of aspiration. Auscultation may reveal rales, rhonchi, wheezing, or decreased breath sounds. Chest radiography, which commonly shows bilateral perihilar and basilar infiltrates and varying degrees of atelectasis, may not be diagnostic until several hours after ingestion. Gastric decontamination depends on the agent and amount ingested; consult the poison control center for recommendations. Use of activated charcoal is not recommended (Jaimovich, 1993).

Alert: *Syrup of ipecac is contraindicated because vomiting increases the risk for aspiration.*

Caustics

Caustic ingestions are caused by exposure to acids or alkalis commonly found in household cleaning products (e.g., Drano, lye). Ingestion of these substances may cause lip or tongue swelling, burning pain in injured areas, dysphagia, drooling, or whitish or red plaques in the mouth or perioral areas. Severe burns of the esophagus and stomach may occur.

Alert: *Vomiting should not be induced because this results in further burning of the mouth and esophagus. Syrup of ipecac and activated charcoal are contraindicated in the treatment of this type of ingestion.*

Do not give the child anything by mouth until the extent of injury is evaluated and ability to swallow fluids

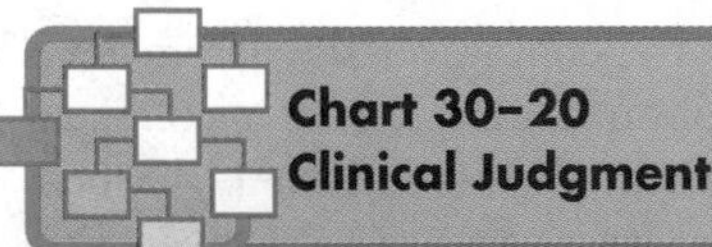

Chart 30–20
Clinical Judgment

Child with a Potentially Toxic Ingestion

Mrs. D. calls to find out what to do about her son, Jamal, a 4-year-old, who has ingested acetaminophen capsules, thinking they were candy. Jamal weighs 20 kg.

Questions

1. What further questions would you ask Mrs. D.?
   Mrs. D. thinks that Jamal may have ingested six capsules, 500 mg each, about 15 minutes ago. The first thing Mrs. D. did was to call you; she has not done anything else. Jamal seems perfectly fine, with no unusual behaviors.
2. What factors indicate a potentially toxic ingestion?
3. Does Mrs. D. need to do anything further? If so, what?
4. What interventions will be implemented when Jamal gets to the emergency department?
5. Jamal does not develop toxic serum levels of acetaminophen. What factors probably contributed to this positive outcome? What should the nurse do before sending Jamal home?

Answers

1. When did Jamal ingest the acetaminophen? Can Mrs. D. estimate how many capsules he may have ingested? How many milligrams are in each capsule? Has any treatment been initiated? Is Jamal acting unusual or doing anything out of the ordinary (e.g., altered level of consciousness, nausea, vomiting, pale, diaphoretic)?
2. Jamal may have ingested six capsules of 500 mg each, which totals 3000 mg of acetaminophen. Jamal weighs 20 kg, corresponding to 150 mg/kg ingested, a potentially toxic dose.
3. Mrs. D. should immediately call the poison control center. Because it is within 60 minutes of ingestion, administration of syrup of ipecac may be recommended before taking Jamal to the emergency department.
4. Activated charcoal will be administered to adsorb the acetaminophen further; it does not adsorb the antidote for acetaminophen, *N*-acetylcysteine. Serum acetaminophen levels will be measured 4 hours after ingestion to determine whether *N*-acetylcysteine should be administered. Liver function studies should be monitored and symptomatic care given.
5. Mrs. D. discovered the ingestion quickly and took immediate action. The acetaminophen was evacuated rapidly before absorption of toxic amounts could occur. Jamal is younger than 6 years, when alternative pathways for acetaminophen metabolism may decrease the incidence of hepatotoxicity. The nurse should review poison prevention techniques with Mrs. D.

is assessed. Endoscopic evaluation is necessary 12 to 24 hours after injury to determine the severity of the damage. Complications include esophageal perforation, scarring, and stricture formation.

Burns may be present on other parts of the body after exposure to caustics such as strong acids, strong alkalis, or petroleum distillate agents. The child should be fully decontaminated by removing all clothing and flooding the area(s) with normal saline or water. Treat exposures to the eyes, skin, and mucous membranes by washing the affected area with a stream of water for 15 to 20 minutes. The water temperature should be comfortable to the child. The health care team members should wear gloves because some toxins can be quickly absorbed through the skin. Poisonous exposure to these substances can occur through contact with the patient's skin, clothing, or vomitus.

Sudden Infant Death Syndrome

Sudden infant death syndrome (SIDS) is the most common cause of death in children from age 1 month to 1 year; 95% of SIDS cases occur by age 6 months (Hunt, 1996). The typical SIDS scenario involves the caregiver finding the normal, healthy infant prone in bed, in full cardiopulmonary arrest. Multiple causes have been proposed, but no definitive cause is known (Herda, 1992). Several factors affect the occurrence of SIDS (Chart 30–21). The SIDS infant cannot be resuscitated (see Chapter 16 for a discussion of apparent life-threatening events [ALTEs] and apnea).

Assessment

Upon presentation to the ED, examine the infant thoroughly to rule out other causes of death, including child

Chart 30–21

Risk Factors Associated with SIDS

Maternal

Younger age
Smoking (antenatal and postnatal)
Drug use (opiates, cocaine)

Infant

Premature
Asphyxia at birth
Male gender
Multiple birth
Sibling who died of SIDS
Age under 6 months (peaks at 2 to 4 months)
Black or Native American race

Environmental

Cold weather season
Exposure to cigarette smoke
Lower socioeconomic status
Bottle feeding
Prone sleeping position
Swaddled too warmly
Soft sleeping surface

It is uncertain which risk factors are causal and how the risk factors are interrelated.

abuse. The infant's face may be quite blue because of blood pooling in the dependent prone position. This discoloration may look like bruising. There may also be trauma as a result of the basic life support measures used. Individual institutions may have specific protocols consisting of multiple laboratory and radiographic studies that aid in differentiating SIDS from child abuse (Committee on Pediatric Emergency Medicine, 1994).

caREminder: *First-line responders (paramedics, police) and ED personnel must maintain an unbiased demeanor, asking questions in a matter-of-fact, information-gathering manner. Initially, these families may be wrongly accused of child abuse, further traumatizing them during this devastating period.*

The history elicited from the family or caregiver helps in differentiating SIDS from abuse. With SIDS, the history is consistent each time it is given, by the same person and between family members. A history that is incompatible with the infant's developmental level should raise suspicion of abuse (e.g., a history of a 5-month-old trying to climb out of the crib and falling).

Nursing Diagnoses and Outcomes

- **Ineffective family coping: compromised related to death of child**
  Outcomes: The family will verbalize feelings. The family will state and utilize sources of support. The family will perform activities of daily living (ADLs) and maintain supportive interactions with each other.
- **Spiritual distress related to unexpected death of infant**
  Outcome: The family will verbalize feelings of spiritual tension and be adequately supported in working through them.
- **Altered parenting related to parents dealing with own grief**
  Outcome: The parents or significant others will provide an environment for siblings that supports growth and development.

Interdisciplinary Interventions

Delivering the news to the family is difficult, as there is no explanation for the death and the ED health care team does not have a relationship with the family. Tell the family that the child may have died from SIDS and an autopsy will be done to confirm this (O'Donnell & Gaedeke, 1995).

Worldview: *Deliver the news using the words dead, died, or deceased. Words such as gone, expired, or passed away are often misunderstood. This is especially true in families whose primary language is not English. Translation services should be provided for these families.*

The primary nursing responsibility is to support the family in beginning the grieving process. Provide the family with a private, quiet area. Tell them that the exact cause of SIDS is still unknown and that it cannot be predicted or prevented. Use hospital and community resources, such as social workers and clergy members, to provide additional support and comfort to the family. Give the parents an opportunity to hold their baby (see Chapter 12). Prepare them for how the baby will look, explaining the presence of any tubes or resuscitation equipment. A staff member should stay with the family to support them.

The parents may not be emotionally able to understand all of the information provided to them (e.g., funeral home lists, when to anticipate autopsy results, support group information). Providing them with written material allows them to view it later. Often, one family member (perhaps an aunt or uncle) appears less emotional than the others. Providing this person with the written material and information can also be helpful.

Frequently, parents do not return home after the death of an infant to SIDS, so be sure to obtain a contact phone number from a friend or family member, if the parents cannot be reached at home.

Community Care

The nurse can also participate in community education regarding decreasing risk factors that contribute to SIDS. On the basis of studies done worldwide that show a decreased incidence of SIDS when infants sleep on their backs, the American Academy of Pediatrics recommended placing infants on their back or side for sleeping (American Academy of Pediatrics Task Force on Infant Positioning and SIDS, 1992). Encouraging families to follow this "back to sleep" advice can be instrumental in reducing the incidence of SIDS (Chessare, Hunt, & Bourguignon, 1995; Willinger, Hoffman, & Hartford, 1994). Mothers seem to be more willing to change their baby care habits (e.g., positioning the baby prone for sleeping) than their personal habits (e.g., reduction in maternal smoking or increase in breast-feeding) in reducing the incidence of SIDS (Hiley & Morley, 1996).

Child Abuse

Maltreatment of children encompasses various acts of commission or omission that result in morbidity or mortality. Reports of alleged child abuse or neglect have increased steadily since the 1960s, when mandated reporting began. Most reports involve neglect. In 1992, almost 2.9 million children were subjects of a report to child protective service agencies; the majority were younger than 5 years (*Statistical abstracts of the United States*, 1994). More than two thirds of children who are abused physically are younger than 3 years; one third are younger than 1 month (Berkowitz, 1995). The majority of perpetrators have close ties with the family; most commonly, the perpetrator is the father (21%), mother (21%), mother's boyfriend (9%), or baby sitter (8%) (Johnson, 1996).

Many factors related to psychological, social, and economic stresses place a child at risk of being abused. These factors can be solely related to the child or related to the parent or family. Child-associated factors include prematurity, physical or developmental disabilities, chronic illness, and multiple birth. Examples of parent or family factors include unrealistic and/or rigid expectations of a child, belief in corporal punishment, alcohol and/or drug dependency, childhood history of abuse, single-parent family, social isolation, poverty, low self-esteem, and psychological distress (Christian, 1992; Ludwig, 1996). There are four basic categories of child abuse: physical abuse, sexual abuse, neglect, and emotional or psychological abuse (Table 30–12). Children may be subjected to more than one type of maltreatment, and emotional abuse is usually a component of the other forms of abuse.

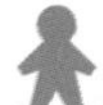

Tip: *Tell children to tell an adult if someone touches them or says things to them that they do not like or feel comfortable with, even if the person tells them to keep it a secret or threatens to do bad things to them or someone in their family.*

The parent or caregiver may seek medical attention for a child because of suspicions of abuse perpetrated by someone else. However, many children are brought for medical attention for an unrelated problem and are identified as having potentially been abused (Chart 30–22). Maintain a nonaccusatory, nonjudgmental attitude, asking open-ended questions. Let the caretaker and child

Table 30–12
Types of Child Abuse

Category	Description
Physical abuse	An injury intentionally inflicted on a child by a caregiver, paramour of a parent, or anyone residing in the child's home
Sexual abuse	The use of a child for sexual gratification or financial gain, by an adult, older child, or adolescent, whether by physical force, coercion, or persuasion
Neglect	Acts or omissions by the perpetrator that fail to meet the child's needs for basic living, including food, hygiene, medical care, clothing, and a safe environment
Emotional or psychological abuse	Verbal abuse or excessive demands on the child that result in impaired growth, negative self-image, and disturbed child behavior

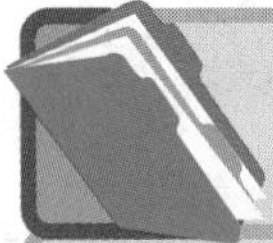

Chart 30–22
Nursing Interventions Classification (NIC)

Abuse Protection: Child

Definition

Identification of high-risk, dependent child relationships and actions to prevent possible or further infliction of physical, sexual, or emotional harm or neglect of basic necessities of life

Activities

Identify mothers who have a history of late (4 months or later) or no prenatal care.
Identify parents who have had another child removed from the home or have placed previous children with relatives for extended periods.
Identify parents who have a history of substance abuse, depression, or major psychiatric illness.
Identify parents who demonstrate an increased need for parent education (e.g., parents with learning problems, parents who verbalize feelings of inadequacy, parents of a first child, teen parents).
Identify parents with a history of domestic violence or a mother who has a history of numerous "accidental" injuries.
Identify parents with a history of unhappy childhoods associated with abuse, rejection, excessive criticism, or feelings of being worthless and unloved.
Identify crisis situations that may trigger abuse (e.g., poverty, unemployment, divorce, homelessness, and domestic violence).
Determine whether the family has an intact social support network to assist with family problems, respite child care, and crisis child care.
Identify infants/children with high-care needs (e.g., prematurity, low birth weight, colic, feeding intolerances, major health problems in the first year of life, developmental disabilities, hyperactivity, and attention deficit disorders).
Identify caretaker explanations of child's injuries that are improbable or inconsistent, allege self-injury, blame other children, or demonstrate a delay in seeking treatment.
Determine whether the child demonstrates signs of physical abuse, including numerous injuries in various stages of healing; unexplained bruises and welts; unexplained pattern, immersion, and friction burns; facial, spiral, shaft, or multiple fractures; unexplained facial lacerations and abrasions; human bite marks; intracranial, subdural, intraventricular, and intraocular hemorrhaging; whiplash shaken infant syndrome; and diseases that are resistant to treatment and/or have changing signs and symptoms.
Determine whether the child demonstrates signs of neglect, including poor or inconsistent growth patterns, failure to thrive, wasting of subcutaneous tissue, consistent hunger, poor hygiene, constant fatigue and listlessness, bald patches on scalp or other skin afflictions, apathy, unyielding body posture, and inappropriate dress for weather conditions.
Determine whether the child demonstrates signs of sexual abuse, including difficulty walking or sitting; torn, stained, or bloody underclothing; reddened or traumatized genitals; vaginal or anal lacerations; recurrent urinary tract infections; poor sphincter tone; acquired sexually transmitted diseases; pregnancy; promiscuous behavior or prostitution; a history of running away, sudden massive weight loss or weight gain, aggression against self, or dramatic behavioral or health changes of undetermined etiology.
Determine whether the child demonstrates signs of emotional abuse, including lags in physical development, habit disorders, conduct learning disorders, neurotic traits/psychoneurotic reactions, behavioral extremes, cognitive developmental lags, and attempted suicide.
Encourage admission of child for further observation and investigation as appropriate.
Record times and durations of visits during hospitalizations.
Monitor parent-child interactions and record observations.
Determine whether acute symptoms in child abate when child is separated from family.
Determine whether parents have unrealistic expectations for child's behavior or whether they have negative attributions for their child's behavior.
Monitor child for extreme compliance, such as passive submission to invasive procedures.
Monitor child for role reversal, such as comforting the parent, or overactive or aggressive behavior.
Listen to pregnant woman's feelings about pregnancy and expectations about the unborn child.
Monitor new parents' reactions to their infant, observing for feelings of disgust, fear, or disappointment in gender.
Monitor for a parent who holds newborn at arm's length, handles newborn awkwardly, asks for excessive assistance, and verbalizes or demonstrates discomfort in caring for the child.

Chart continued on following page

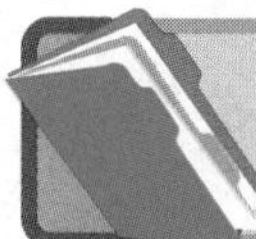

Chart 30–22
Nursing Interventions Classification (NIC) *Continued*

Abuse Protection: Child

Monitor for repeated visits to clinics, emergency rooms, or physicians' offices for minor problems.
Establish a system to flag the records of children who are suspected victims of child abuse or neglect.
Monitor for a progressive deterioration in the physical and emotional state of the infant/child.
Determine parent's knowledge of infant/child basic care needs and provide appropriate child care information as indicated.
Instruct parents on problem-solving, decision-making, and childrearing and parenting skills, or refer parents to programs where these skills can be learned.
Help families identify coping strategies for stressful situations.
Provide parents with information on how to cope with protracted infant crying, emphasizing that they should not shake the baby.
Provide the parents with noncorporal punishment methods for disciplining children.
Provide pregnant women and their families with information on the effects of smoking, poor nutrition, and substance abuse on the baby's and their health.
Engage parents and child in attachment-building exercises.
Provide parents and their adolescents with information on decision-making and communication skills and refer to youth services counseling as appropriate.
Provide older children with concrete information on how to provide for the basic care needs of their younger siblings.
Provide children with positive affirmations of their worth, nurturing care, therapeutic communication, and developmental stimulation.
Provide children who have been sexually abused with reassurance that the abuse was not their fault and allow them to express their concerns through play therapy appropriate for age.
Refer at-risk pregnant women and parents of newborns to nurse home visitation services.
Provide at-risk families with a public health nurse referral to ensure that the home environment is monitored, that siblings are assessed, and that families receive continued assistance.
Refer families to human services and counseling professionals as needed.
Provide parents with community resource information that includes addresses and phone numbers of agencies that provide respite care, emergency child care, housing assistance, substance abuse treatment, sliding-fee counseling services, food pantries, clothing distribution centers, health care, human services, hot lines, and domestic abuse shelters.
Inform physician of observations indicative of abuse or neglect.
Report suspected abuse or neglect to proper authorities.
Refer a parent who is being battered and at-risk children to a domestic violence shelter.
Refer parents to Parents Anonymous for group support as appropriate.

From McCloskey, J., & Bulechek, G. (1996). *Nursing interventions classification (NIC)* (2nd ed.). St. Louis: Mosby–Year Book. Reprinted with permission.

finish their statements. Ask the child, if verbal, how she or he was hurt. The child may be reluctant to respond if the perpetrator is the parent present in the room. Sometimes question such as "Do you have anything else you want to talk about?" may prompt the family to reveal their concerns. Other families may respond to direct questioning about psychosocial issues, feeling that, if the question is asked, the topic is safe to discuss.

caREminder: *Assess the child fully. If the child has signs and symptoms of abuse, or if the history does not correspond to the clinical presentation, report the suspected abuse to child protective services. You do not need to be certain that abuse has taken place in order to report.*

All states have child abuse laws that require reporting by various health care providers; most states require by law that nurses report suspected abuse (see Chapter 2). Failure to report may result in civil or criminal charges. Regardless of society's ever-changing definitions of child abuse, the health-care provider must never fail to report the abuse.

During assessment, in addition to physical signs, note the child's behavior (e.g., wary of adults, cringes with sudden movements, apathetic, does not turn to parent for support, attentive to other children crying), hygiene (dirty, severe diaper rash, skin rash), and dress (Is it appropriate for the weather? Long sleeves and pants may be worn to cover injuries even in warm weather; dirty clothing or inadequate attire for the weather may signal neglect).

The ways in which children are abused are many. Fortunately, most children who have been abused do not require emergency medical attention. However, children who are severely physically abused or who have been sexually abused within the past 72 hours need emergency medical attention. All abused children need emergency social assistance or removal from the violent or neglectful situation. (See Chapter 29 for a discussion of neglect and emotional abuse.) The following types of abuse are a few that require emergency intervention.

Physical Abuse

Signs of physical abuse are listed in Chart 30–22. Specific areas of the body are associated with accidental injury; other areas, with nonaccidental injury (Fig. 30–10). Some medical conditions may mimic a clinical picture (e.g., bruises with leukemia or idiopathic thrombocytopenic purpura) or skeletal findings that are associated with abuse (e.g., osteogenesis imperfecta, congenital syphilis, scurvy, rickets, copper deficiency). The health care practitioner must be cognizant of these and include history questions and laboratory and diagnostic studies as indicated.

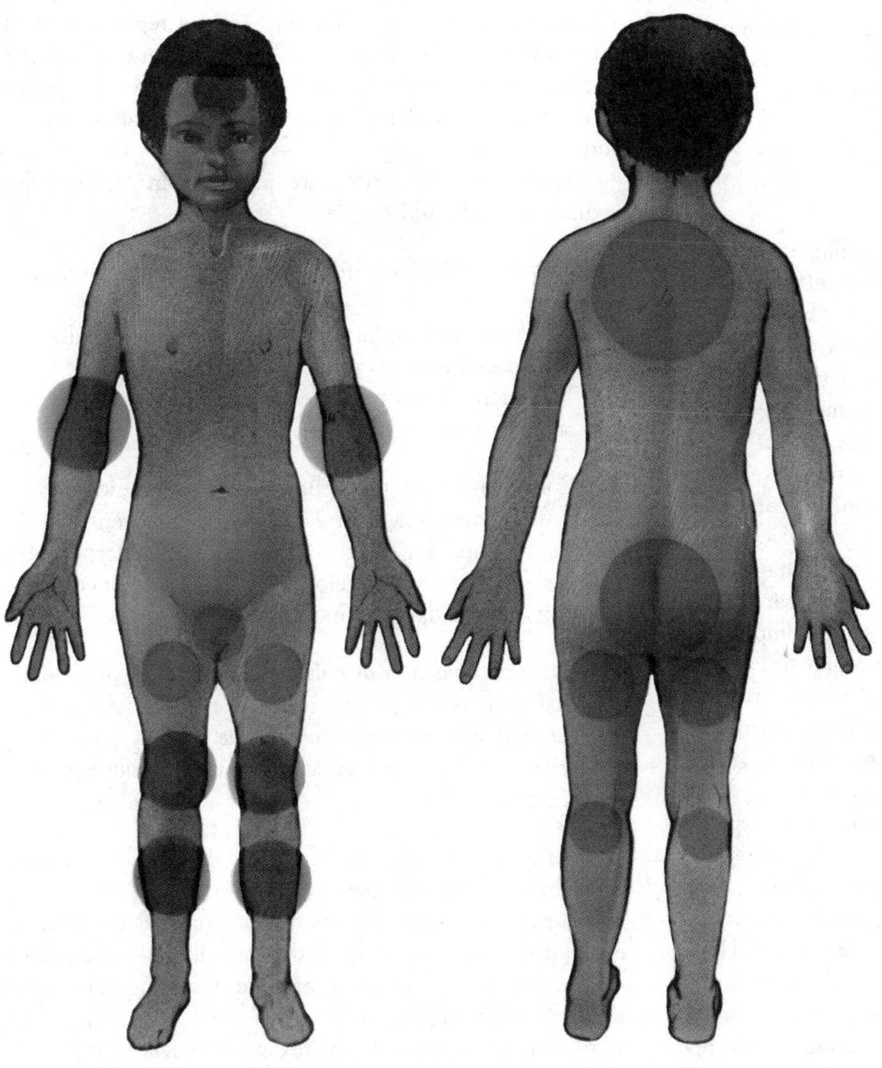

Figure 30–10
Accidents typically cause injuries in specific sites (purple areas). The nurse should suspect physical abuse in children with injuries in nonaccidental sites (red areas). (Adapted from Betz, C. L., Hunsberger, M. M., & Wright, S. [Eds.]. [1994]. *Family-centered nursing care of children* [2nd ed., p. 1012]. Philadelphia: W. B. Saunders. Used with permission.)

Diagnostic evaluation of child abuse depends on the symptoms and history. A primary screening tool in suspected abuse is a radiologic survey including skull series, extremities (including hands and feet), and ribs. A bone scan is recommended when the skeletal survey is negative but a strong clinical suggestion of injury exists (Cramer, 1996). CT and magnetic resonance imaging (MRI) may be ordered, depending on the symptoms. Ultrasonography may be done if visceral injury is suspected. If abdominal trauma is suspected, urine and stool should be screened for blood. Blood studies should include bleeding studies to rule out a bleeding diathesis; serum calcium, phosphorus, and alkaline phosphatase if bone disease is a possibility; and liver and pancreatic enzymes if damage to these organs is suspected.

Treatment includes maintaining the ABCs and managing the acute condition. Emotional and social support for the family is necessary (see Chapter 29). Without accusing the parents, they should be told that child protective services are being notified (e.g., "The symptoms are ______, indicating that they may not be accidental"). Reinforce with the family that the priority is ensuring the child's safety and well-being.

Shaken Baby Syndrome

Shaken baby syndrome involves intracranial trauma (e.g., subarachnoid or subdural hemorrhage or diffuse cerebral edema) and retinal hemorrhages usually in the absence of skull fracture or external signs of traumatic injury (Monaco & Brooks, 1994). Shaking alone may not produce sufficient force to produce intracranial hemorrhage, and a component of the syndrome may involve impact against a soft surface such as a mattress after being shaken (Berkowitz, 1995). The impact causes sudden deceleration of the infant's head, tearing the bridging vessels between the skull and the brain and causing hemorrhage. Fractures of the long bones or ribs, not readily apparent, may be present (Berkowitz, 1995). The ribs are compliant in young children and CPR has not been found to cause rib fractures in children (Cramer, 1996). Posterior rib fractures are more common, caused by the mechanical stress at the costovertebral junction when the child is grasped and shaken (Cramer, 1996).

The child with shaken baby syndrome is typically younger than 2 years of age and commonly presents with complaints of lethargy, seizures, hyperirritability, poor feeding, bulging fontanelle, breathing problems, or, in severe instances, coma or cardiopulmonary arrest. Hypothermia is a common finding in these children and is secondary to the occult central nervous system trauma (Wahl & Woodall, 1995). Consider abuse when presented with a child with encephalopathy without a source.

The child who has been shaken is treated symptomatically. If trauma is suspected, immobilize the cervical spine. Assess the ABCs, support and stabilize, and frequently reassess them. Continually monitor the child's neurologic status for signs of increasing intracranial pressure. Because shaking results in traumatic head injury, its treatment is the same as the management of trauma discussed earlier. Consider hyperventilating the child because of its effect on decreasing cerebral blood flow.

Sexual Abuse

In most cases of sexual abuse, the perpetrator is known to the child (Heger & Emans, 1992). Common offenders are parents, stepparents, other adult relatives, trusted family friends, neighbors, or baby sitters. Occasionally, more than one family member is involved in sexually abusing the child. Approximately 14% of reports of child abuse fall into the category of sexual abuse (*Statistical abstracts of the United States*, 1994), although this figure may be grossly underestimated because of failure to report.

There are four acute care priorities in treating the sexually abused child:

- Evidence collection from the genital, rectal, and oral areas
- Screening and initiation of treatment for sexually transmitted diseases
- Treatment of any sustained injuries
- Screening for and preventing pregnancy

Collect evidence to document the occurrence of sexual abuse or assault within 72 hours of the event. To do this, use a rape kit that contains the necessary swabs, cultures, tubes, and envelopes to seal the specimens. Such kits are available in most EDs.

Tip: *If an abused or assaulted child is referred from your facility to another facility for specimen collection, instruct the child and family not to bathe the child or change his or her clothing so that evidence from the assault is not destroyed.*

Send any clothing worn during the abuse or assault with the medical specimens for investigation.

For an adolescent who is not pregnant at the time of evaluation and not using birth control, offer pregnancy prevention. If it is accepted, provide postcoital contraception by administering 100 μg of ethinyl estradiol and 1 mg of DL-norgestrel (two Ovral tablets) by mouth (PO) immediately, followed by a second dose 12 hours later. This treatment is effective only up to 72 hours after the rape (Paradise, 1996). (See Chapter 29 for discussion of emotional effects of sexual abuse.)

Munchausen's Syndrome by Proxy

Munchausen's syndrome by proxy is a rare form of abuse in which the child is subjected to an illness that is induced or fabricated by the parent or caregiver. The affected parent or caretaker seeks medical care for the child's fictitious illness and provides a fictitious history to support the illness. The fabricated or induced illness often results in the child being subjected to numerous unnecessary, invasive laboratory studies, hospitalizations, or surgeries. The syndrome can result in disability or death of the child.

The child's reported symptoms often occur only when the parent is present and stop when the parent is not. According to Welliver (1992), 50% of the cases present with some sort of a neurologic disturbance such as seizures or apnea. Less common presentations include hematuria, gastrointestinal bleeding, hypernatremia, or hyponatremia. The perpetrator may suffocate the child to produce apnea or seizures or may add her or his own blood to the child's urine or stool sample to fabricate bleeding.

The mother is the perpetrator in 98% of the cases and often has a health care background or is well versed in medical terminology (Berkowitz, 1995). The mother is typically quite attentive to the child and involved in the child's care but often lacks parental concern. For example, she may appear calm, not cry, and carry on with normal activities despite providing this dramatic, concerning history.

To aid in diagnosing this syndrome, assess for the following warning signals:

- Family history of previous, unexplained infant deaths.
- Description of a prolonged, unexplainable illness that, despite medical attention and therapies, has not been resolved.
- Signs and symptoms described by the parent are incompatible or inappropriate.
- Child's symptoms do not occur when others are present (Brown, 1997).

The long-term outcome for these children has not been well researched. A review of 117 cases by Rosenberg in 1987 found that 9% died and 8% of the remaining children developed long-term morbidity, such as permanent disfigurement or impaired function. Also, there were 10 unusual deaths of siblings of the 117 victims. The victimized children are at risk of later developing the syndrome themselves and often have behavioral problems.

Emotional or Psychological Abuse

Emotional abuse occurs when the caregiver attacks, belittles, terrorizes, isolates, humiliates, or rejects a child. This type of abuse is what most seriously and most often affects children (Ludwig, 1996). Emotional abuse may be inflicted without physical injury to the child. The caregiver may also physically or sexually abuse the child, but the psychological impact of the abuse remains with the child, often leading to a variety of psychological disorders (see Chapter 29). The negative psychological impact of the abuse remains when the bruises, burns, and broken bones have healed.

If any type of abuse is suspected, report it to child protective services promptly. Work with the health care team (physician, social worker, and child protective service case worker) to determine the best placement of the child. The child may be placed immediately in custody, allowed to return home with the parent, or placed with a relative. With the latter two choices, child protective services will follow up with the family and child at home.

Notify the parent(s) that child abuse is suspected and that a report will be made, as required by law and in the best interests of the child. Allowing the parent to ask any questions about the report may help the parent to understand the process and anticipate social work visits and calls at home. Refer the parents to support groups, self-help groups, or parenting classes, as needed. Remember that the goal is to facilitate change so that the family can live together as a functional, healthy unit.

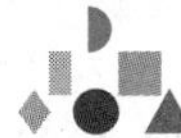

Preparation for Transfer

Depending on the health care facility in which the child received initial emergency care, the stabilized child may need to be transferred to another facility or another unit. Regardless of where the child is transferred, take appropriate steps to prepare the child for transport.

First, consider where the child is going for continued care. Depending on the level of care the child requires, this may be within the hospital in which the initial care took place or may require a lengthy interhospital transport. If the child is being transported for intensive care, notify the critical care transport team, who can provide the specialized monitoring and equipment the child needs.

Second, arrange for the appropriate mode of transport. Interhospital transports can be made by ground ambulance, helicopter, or fixed-wing aircraft. Ambulance transport is the most readily available and least expensive, but traffic congestion and increased travel time are disadvantages. Helicopters avoid traffic congestion and typically allow immediate turnover of care at the receiving facility. However, it is difficult to monitor and evaluate the patient during the transfer (Chameides & Hazinski, 1994). Air transport is the mode of choice when rapid transport is required but is more costly and may be prohibited by weather conditions.

Transport team members vary depending on the severity of the child's illness. Members may include local emergency medical service personnel, registered nurses, respiratory therapists, and/or physicians. (See Chapter 1 for a discussion of nursing roles and qualifications of a transport nurse.) Most pediatric tertiary care facilities have transport teams that are equipped and staffed to transport critically ill children of all ages (Chameides & Hazinski, 1994).

Every health care facility, whether a clinic, medical office, or hospital, should establish transport protocols that can be easily followed if it is faced with caring for a pediatric patient who requires a higher level of care than it can provide. The protocols should address issues regarding available modes of transport and transport teams, availability of equipment, and a list of numbers for receiving facilities. If only one tertiary pediatric facility is in the region, a backup plan should include the name and number of another facility (perhaps in another state) because pediatric intensive care beds are limited in number.

The initial call from the referring facility should be made by a physician. It is important to record the name and number of the accepting physician. Information should be shared regarding the patient's history, vital signs, medications given, medications in progress, and any treatments or procedures completed. As well as physician-to-physician communication, it is equally important to have nurse-to-nurse communication. The same history and information should be shared, as well as frequent updates on the patient's status and estimated departure and arrival times. Consent for transfer should also be obtained from parents or guardian and accompany the child.

Immediately before the patient's transfer, reassess for and secure a patent airway. If airway stability is a concern, the child may require intubation before transport. Take and secure cervical spine precautions, if necessary. Tape IV access and endotracheal tubes securely in place, because movement during transfer can often dislodge them. Anticipating the patient's needs during transport and preparing for equipment, medication, and blood or fluid needs ensure a smooth and successful transfer.

Send copies of the patient's chart, radiographs, and diagnostic test results along with the patient. Note any laboratory studies pending at the time of transfer, and provide the telephone number of the laboratory for follow-up by the receiving facility. Clear, consistent communication between referring and receiving facilities is the key to a successful transport.

Summary of Key Concepts

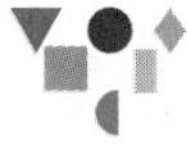

- Infants and children have a limited ability to protect themselves from illness and dangerous situations and have limited physiologic reserves. These factors put them at risk for the advancement of disease and illness often before manifesting signs and symptoms.
- Knowing the signs and symptoms of common pediatric emergencies, assessing them skillfully, and intervening rapidly are the keys to decreasing negative outcomes.
- Parents should be with the child at all times, if the parents desire, even during invasive procedures. Tell the parents concrete things they can do to support the child.
- Hypotension is a *late* sign of shock in children. Fluid volume must be administered, sometimes in large quantities (80 mL/kg), to restore circulating blood volume and cellular oxygenation.
- Trauma care involves stabilizing the ABCs, maintaining cervical spine precautions, obtaining vascular access, performing a rapid but thorough assessment, and treating associated injuries.
- A child's airway is more difficult to stabilize and manage than an adult's because of structural differences. The child experiencing a respiratory emergency typically assumes a position that maximizes airway patency; let the child maintain this position whenever possible and keep the child calm.

- Fever is a symptom that, in itself, does not need to be treated unless the child is at risk for seizures or the child cannot tolerate the increased metabolic demands related to fever. Fever may indicate underlying disease that requires treatment.
- Mammal bites are managed on the basis of severity of injury and potential for infection (local infection, rabies). Snake evenomations also require administration of antivenom. Stings can usually be managed at home but require emergency intervention if they cause anaphylaxis.
- Anaphylaxis may cause death if not promptly treated. Susceptible children and their caregivers must be taught prevention and first-aid techniques, including administration of epinephrine.
- Most children with epistaxis can be managed at home but require emergency intervention if bleeding cannot be controlled. Home management includes having the child sit leaning forward and putting direct pressure on the soft part of the nose for 10 minutes.
- Environmental exposure injuries are often preventable. Hypothermia should be managed with controlled rewarming, heat stroke with rapid cooling. Symptoms of smoke inhalation may not be manifest for 24 hours, so close observation of the child is needed. Near-drowning causes hypoxia with resultant multisystem injury and is managed as any trauma.
- Prevention is the best treatment for any emergency, particularly poisoning. Treatment depends on the agent and amount of exposure.
- Management of sudden infant death syndrome involves recognizing the syndrome and sensitively supporting the parents, educating them about the syndrome, and avoiding accusations of child maltreatment.
- Maintaining a high index of suspicion for child abuse helps in recognizing the child who is being maltreated. Immediate evaluation and treatment of injuries, if present, are done. The priority is ensuring the child's safety while providing psychosocial support and education for the family.
- Stabilizing the child before and anticipating the child's needs during transport are critical to safe transport.

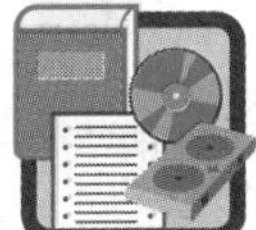

Resources

Organizations

American Association of Poison Control Centers
3201 New Mexico Avenue NW, Suite 310
Washington, DC 20016
(202) 362-7217

American Heart Association, National Center
7272 Greenville Avenue
Dallas, TX 75231-4596
(800) 242-8721

American Trauma Society
8903 Presidential Parkway, Suite 512
Upper Marlboro, MD 20772-2656
(800) 556-7890

Emergency Nurses Association
216 Higgins Road
Park Ridge, IL 60068-5736
(847) 698-9400

Two programs to increase competency in resuscitating children, usually offered through local organizations:

Pediatric Advanced Life Support (PALS)
American Heart Association
(800) AHA-USA1

Neonatal Resuscitation Program
American Academy of Pediatrics
(800) 433-9016

SIDS

SIDS Alliance
10500 Little Patuxent Parkway, Suite 420
Columbia, MD 21044
(800) 638-7437
(800) 221-7437 (24-hour answering)

National Sudden Infant Death Resource Center
8201 Greensboro Drive, Suite 600
McLean, VA 22102
(703) 821-8955

National Foundation for Sudden Infant Death
101 Broadway
New York, NY 10036

Child Abuse

American Professional Society on the Abuse of Children
407 South Dearborn, Suite 1300
Chicago, IL 60605
(312) 554-0166

C. Henry Kempe Center for Prevention and Treatment of Child Abuse and Neglect
1205 Oneida Street
Denver, CO 80220

Clearinghouse of Child Abuse and Neglect Information
P.O. Box 1182
Washington, DC 20013-1182
(800) 394-3366

KidsPeace (abuse, neglect, emotional trauma)
5300 KidsPeace Drive
Orefield, PA 18069-9101
(215) 799-8001

Child Abuse Hotline
(800) 4-A-CHILD

Child Abuse Information
(800) 858-KIDS

Injury Prevention

TIPP (The Injury Prevention Program)
American Academy of Pediatrics
P.O. Box 927
Elk Grove Village, IL 60009
(800) 433-9016

Center to Prevent Handgun Violence
1225 Eye Street NW, Room 1100
Washington, DC 20005
(202) 289-7319

Videotapes

PALS Plus: Pediatric emergencies (videos covering trauma, medical, and emotional aspects of pediatric emergencies). Available from Mosby Lifeline (800) 633-6699.

References

American Academy of Pediatrics Task Force on Infant Positioning and SIDS. (1992). Positioning and SIDS. *Pediatrics*, 89, 1120–1126.

Anderson, A. C. (1994). Iron poisoning in children. *Current Opinion in Pediatrics*, 6, 289–294.

Aronoff, S. C. (1996). Mammalian bites. In R. E. Behrman, R. M. Kliegman, & A. M. Arvin (Eds.), *Nelson textbook of pediatrics* (15th ed., pp. 2029–2030). Philadelphia: W. B. Saunders.

Bakerink, J. A., Gospe, S. M., Dimand, R. J., & Eldridge, M. W. (1996). Multiple organ failure after ingestion of pennyroyal oil from herbal tea in two infants. *Pediatrics*, 98, 944–947.

Baraff, L. J. (1996). Pediatric fever guidelines. *Western Journal of Medicine*, *164*(1), 62.

Baraff, L. J., Bass, J. W., Fleisher, G. R., Klein, J. O., McCracken, G. H., Jr., Powell, K. R., & Schriger, D. L. (1993). Practice guidelines for the management of infants and children 0 to 36 months of age with fever without source. *Pediatrics*, 92, 1–12.

Barkin, R. M., & Burrington, J. D. (1991). Emergencies and accidents. In W. E. Hathaway, J. R. Groothuis, W. W. Hay, Jr., & J. W. Paisley (Eds.), *Current pediatric diagnosis & treatment* (10th ed., pp. 177–190). Norwalk, CT: Appleton & Lange.

Bauchner, H., Vinci, R., Bak, S., Pearson, C., & Corwin, M. J. (1996). Parents and procedures: A randomized controlled trial. *Pediatrics*, 98, 861–867.

Behrman, R. E., Kliegman, R. M., & Arvin, A. M. (1996). Anaphylaxis. In R. E. Behrman, R. M. Kliegman, & A. M. Arvin (Eds.), *Nelson textbook of pediatrics* (15th ed., pp. 646–647). Philadelphia: W. B. Saunders.

Bennett, B. J., & Baker, P. (Eds.). (1995). *Trauma nurse core course manual* (4th ed.). Park Ridge, IL: Emergency Nurses Association.

Berkowitz, C. D. (1995). Pediatric abuse. New patterns of injury. *Emergency Medicine Clinics of North America*, *13*, 321–341.

Berman, S., & Schmitt, B. D. (1991). Ear, nose & throat. In W. E. Hathaway, J. R. Groothuis, W. W. Hay, & J. W. Paisley (Eds.), *Current pediatric diagnosis & treatment* (10th ed., pp. 346–347). Norwalk, CT: Appleton & Lange.

Bonadio, W. A. (1995). Assessing patient clinical appearance in the evaluation of the febrile child. *American Journal of Emergency Medicine*, *13*, 321–326.

Bond, G. R. (1995). The poisoned child. Evolving concepts in care. *Emergency Medicine Clinics of North America*, *13*, 343–355.

Bone, R. C. (1991). Gram-negative sepsis: Background, clinical features, and intervention. *Chest*, *100*, 802–808.

Boyar, C., & Chao, W. (1995). Spontaneous bilateral epistaxis and bilateral otorrhagia in a five year old with tympanostomy tubes. *Pediatric Emergency Care*, *11*, 179–182.

Brady, M. A., & Dunn, A. M. (1996). Common injuries and poisonings. In C. E. Burns, N. Barber, M. A. Brady, & A. M. Dunn (Eds.), *Pediatric primary care: A handbook for nurse practitioners* (pp. 831–854). Philadelphia: W. B. Saunders.

Brogan, T. V., Bratton, S. L., Dowd, M. D., & Hegenbarth, M. A. (1995). Severe dog bites in children. *Pediatrics*, 96, 947–950.

Brown, M. L. (1997). Dilemmas facing nurses who care for Munchausen syndrome by proxy patients. *Pediatric Nursing*, *23*, 416–418.

Burns, C. E. (1996). Neurological disorders. In C. E. Burns, N. Barber, M. A. Brady, & A. M. Dunn (Eds.), *Pediatric primary care: A handbook for nurse practitioners* (pp. 551–572). Philadelphia: W. B. Saunders.

Camfield, C., & Camfield, P. (1993). Febrile seizures: An RX for parents fears and anxieties. *Contemporary Pediatrics*, *10*, 26–44.

Cavales-Oftadeh, L., & Heiner, D. C. (1996). Anaphylaxis. In F. D. Burg, J. R. Ingelfinger, E. R. Wald, & R. A. Polin (Eds.), *Gellis & Kagan's current pediatric therapy* (15th ed., pp. 713–715). Philadelphia: W. B. Saunders.

Chameides, L., & Hazinski, M. F. (Eds.). (1994). Pediatric basic life support. In *Textbook of pediatric advanced life support* (pp. 3-1–3-15). Dallas: American Heart Association.

Chessare, J. B., Hunt, C. E., & Bourguignon, C. (1995). A community-based survey of infant sleep position. *Pediatrics*, 96, 893–896.

Christian, C. W. (1992). Etiology and prevention of abuse: Family and individual factors. In S. Ludwig & A. E. Kornberg (Eds.), *Child abuse: Medical reference* (2nd ed., pp. 39–47). New York: Churchill Livingstone.

Committee on Pediatric Emergency Medicine. (1994). Death of a child in the emergency department. *Pediatrics*, 93, 861–862.

Corneli, H. M. (1993). Evaluation, treatment, and transport of pediatric patients with shock. *Pediatric Clinics of North America*, *40*, 303–319.

Cramer, K. E. (1996). Orthopedic aspects of child abuse. *Pediatric Clinics of North America*, *43*, 1035–1051.

Cross, M. L., Wright, S. W., Wrenn, K. D., Ishihara, K. K., Socha, C. M., & Higgins, J. P. (1996). Interaction between the trauma team and families: Lack of timely communication. *American Journal of Emergency Medicine, 14*, 548–550.

Dean, B. S. (1994). Ingestions and poisonings. In S. J. Kelley (Ed.), *Pediatric emergency nursing* (2nd ed., pp. 365–375). Norwalk, CT: Appleton & Lange.

Emergency Cardiac Care Committee and Subcommittees, American Heart Association. (1992). Guidelines for cardiopulmonary resuscitation and emergency cardiac care, III. *JAMA, 268*, 2199–2241.

Emergency Nurses Association. (1996). *Position statement: Family presence at the bedside during invasive procedures and/or resuscitation.* Park Ridge, IL: Author.

Engler, A. J., & Rushton, C. H. (1996). Thermal regulation. In M. A. Q. Curley, J. B. Smith, & P. A. Moloney-Harmon (Eds.), *Critical care nursing of infants and children* (pp. 449–467). Philadelphia: W. B. Saunders.

Fine, J. S., & Goldfrank, L. R. (1992). Update in medical toxicology. *Pediatric Clinics of North America, 39*, 1031–1051.

Fleisher, G. R., & Crain, E. F. (1996). Infectious disease emergencies. In G. R. Fleisher & S. Ludwig (Eds.), *Synopsis of pediatric emergency medicine*. Baltimore: Williams & Wilkins.

Ford, E. G. (1996). Nutritional support of pediatric patients. *Nutrition in Clinical Practice, 11*, 183–191.

Friday, G. A. (1996). Insect stings. In F. D. Burg, J. R. Ingelfinger, E. R. Wald, & R. A. Polin (Eds.), *Gellis & Kagan's current pediatric therapy* (15th ed., pp. 734–735). Philadelphia: W. B. Saunders.

Gadomski, A. M., Lichenstein, R., Horton, L., King, J., Keane, V., & Permutt, T. (1994). Efficacy of albuterol in the management of bronchiolitis. *Pediatrics, 93*, 907–911.

Ghajar, J., & Hariri, R. J. (1992). Management of pediatric head injury. *Pediatric Clinics of North America, 39*, 1093–1125.

Grover, G. (1996). Fever and bacteremia. In C. D. Berkowitz (Ed.), *Pediatrics: A primary care approach* (pp. 127–132). Philadelphia: W. B. Saunders.

Guyer, B., Strobino, D. M., Ventura, S. J., MacDorman, M., & Martin, J. A. (1996). Annual summary of vital statistics—1995. *Pediatrics, 98*, 1007–1019.

Haley, K., & Baker, P. (Eds). (1993). Respiratory emergencies. In *Emergency nursing pediatric course manual* (pp. 59–79). Park Ridge, IL: Emergency Nurses Association.

Heger, A., & Emans, S. J. (1992). *Evaluation of the sexually abused child: A medical textbook and photographic atlas.* New York: Oxford University Press.

Hendrix, R. A. (1996). Epistaxis and nasal trauma. In F. D. Burg, J. R. Ingelfinger, E. R. Wald, & R. A. Polin (Eds.), *Gellis & Kagan's current pediatric therapy* (15th ed., pp. 122–124). Philadelphia: W. B. Saunders.

Herda, J. A. (1992). Nursing interventions aimed at reducing risks of SIDS. *Pediatric Nursing, 18*, 531–534.

Herrin, J. T., & Antoon, A. Y. (1996). Burn injuries. In R. E. Behrman, R. M. Kliegman, & A. M. Arvin (Eds.), *Nelson textbook of pediatrics* (15th ed., pp 270–277). Philadelphia: W. B. Saunders.

Hiley, C. M. H., & Morley, C. J. (1996). Risk factors for sudden infant death syndrome: Further change in 1992–3. *British Medical Journal, 312*, 1397–1398.

Hodge, D., & Tecklenberg, F. W. (1996). Bites and stings. In G. R. Fleisher & S. Ludwig (Eds.), *Synopsis of pediatric emergency medicine* (pp. 463–475). Baltimore: Williams & Wilkins.

Horowitz, I., Wolach, B., Eliakim, A., Berger, I., & Gilboa, S. (1995). Children with asthma in the emergency department: Spectrum of disease, variation with ethnicity and approach to treatment. *Pediatric Emergency Care, 11*, 240–242.

Huff, K. R. (1996). Febrile seizures. In C. D. Berkowitz (Ed.), *Pediatrics: A primary care approach* (pp. 132–134). Philadelphia: W. B. Saunders.

Hunt, C. E. (1996). Sudden infant death syndrome. In R. E. Behrman, R. M. Kliegman, & A. M. Arvin (Eds.), *Nelson textbook of pediatrics* (15th ed., pp. 1991–1995). Philadelphia: W. B. Saunders.

Inkelis, S. H. (1996). Nosebleeds. In C. D. Berkowitz (Ed.), *Pediatrics: A primary care approach* (pp. 191–195). Philadelphia: W. B. Saunders.

Jaimovich, D. G. (1993). Transport management of the patient with acute poisoning. *Pediatric Clinics of North America, 40*, 407–430.

Jardine, D. S., & Stenzel, M. J. (1996). Heat-related illnesses including hemorrhagic shock and encephalopathy syndrome and heat stroke. In F. D. Burg, J. R. Ingelfinger, E. R. Wald, & R. A. Polin (Eds.), *Gellis & Kagan's current pediatric therapy* (15th ed., pp. 435–438). Philadelphia: W. B. Saunders.

Johnson, C. K. (1996). Abuse and neglect of children. In R. E. Behrman, R. M. Kliegman, & A. M. Arvin (Eds.), *Nelson textbook of pediatrics* (15th ed., pp. 112–121). Philadelphia: W. B. Saunders.

Kallas, H. J. (1996). Drowning and near-drowning. In R. E. Behrman, R. M. Kliegman, & A. M. Arvin (Eds.), *Nelson textbook of pediatrics* (15th ed., pp. 264–270). Philadelphia: W. B. Saunders.

Konzen, K. M. (1996). Snakebites. In F. D. Burg, J. R. Ingelfinger, E. R. Wald, & R. A. Polin (Eds.), *Gellis & Kagan's current pediatric therapy* (15th ed., pp. 738–739). Philadelphia: W. B. Saunders.

Kraepelien-Bartels, P. (1994). Ear, nose, and throat disorders. In S. J. Kelley (Ed.), *Pediatric emergency nursing* (2nd ed., pp. 379–399). Norwalk, CT: Appleton & Lange.

Krenzelok, E. P. (1996). Acute poisonings. In F. D. Burg, J. R. Ingelfinger, E. R. Wald, & R. A. Polin (Eds.), *Gellis & Kagan's current pediatric therapy* (15th ed., pp. 723–732). Philadelphia: W. B. Saunders.

Levin, D. L., Morriss, F. C., Toro, L. O., Brink, L. W., & Turner, G. R. (1993). Drowning and near-drowning. *Pediatric Clinics of North America, 40*, 321–336.

Lewis-Abney, K., & Smith, E. R. (1996). Managing fever of unknown source in infants and children. *Journal of Pediatric Health Care, 10*, 135–138.

Lieberman, P. (1995). Anaphylaxis: Guidelines for prevention and management. *Journal of Respiratory Diseases, 16*, 456–462.

Litovitz, T. L., Felberg, L., White, S., & Klein-Schwartz, W. (1996). 1995 annual report of the American Association of Poison Control Centers toxic exposure surveillance system. *American Journal of Emergency Medicine, 14*, 487–537.

Longo, C. B., & Dickenson, C. M. (1996). Toxic ingestions. In M. A. Q. Curley, J. B. Smith, & P. A. Moloney-Harmon (Eds.), *Critical care nursing of infants and children* (pp. 940–962). Philadelphia: W. B. Saunders.

Ludwig, S. (1996). Psychosocial emergencies. In G. R. Fleisher & S. Ludwig (Eds.), *Synopsis of pediatric emergency medicine* (pp. 769–788). Baltimore: Williams & Wilkins.

Monaco, J. E., & Brooks, W. G. (1994). The critical care aspects of child abuse. *Pediatric Clinics of North America, 41*, 1259–1268.

National Asthma Education Program. (1991). *Guidelines for the diagnosis and management of asthma* (DHHS Publication No. 91-3042). Washington, DC: U.S. Government Printing Office.

Newman, J. (1985). Evaluation of sponging to reduce body temperature in febrile children. *Canadian Medical Association Journal, 132*, 641–642.

O'Donnell, J. K., & Gaedeke, M. K. (1995). Sudden infant death syndrome. *Critical Care Nursing Clinics of North America, 7*, 473–481.

Paradise, J. E. (1996). Pediatric and adolescent gynecology. In G. R. Fleisher & S. Ludwig (Eds.), *Synopsis of pediatric emergency medicine* (pp. 520–521). Baltimore: Williams & Wilkins.

Phelan, A. (1994). Respiratory emergencies. In S. J. Kelley (Ed.), *Pediatric emergency nursing* (2nd ed., pp. 247–279). Norwalk, CT: Appleton & Lange.
Piomelli, S. (1996). Lead poisoning. In R. E. Behrman, R. M. Kliegman, & A. M. Arvin (Eds.), *Nelson textbook of pediatrics* (15th ed., pp. 2010–2013). Philadelphia: W. B. Saunders.
Plotkin, S. A. (1996). Rabies. In R. E. Behrman, R. M. Kliegman, & A. M. Arvin (Eds.), *Nelson textbook of pediatrics* (15th ed., pp. 931–934). Philadelphia: W. B. Saunders.
Polhgeers, A., & Ruddy, R. M. (1995). An update on pediatric trauma. *Emergency Medicine Clinics of North America, 13*, 267–289.
Potsic, W. P., & Handler, S. D. (1996). Otolaryngology emergencies. In G. R. Fleisher & S. Ludwig (Eds.), *Synopsis of pediatric emergency medicine* (pp. 77–79). Baltimore: Williams & Wilkins.
Powell, K. R. (1996). Sepsis and shock. In R. E. Behrman, R. M. Kliegman, & A. M. Arvin (Eds.), *Nelson textbook of pediatrics* (15th ed., pp. 704–707). Philadelphia: W. B. Saunders.
Rivara, F. P., & Grossman, D. C. (1996). Prevention of traumatic deaths to children in the United States: How far have we come and where do we need to go? *Pediatrics, 97*, 791–797.
Rosen, P., Barkin, R. M., Braen, G. R., Levy, R. C., Dailey, R. H., Marx, J. A., Hedges, J. R., Smith, M., & Hockberger, R. S. (Eds.). (1992). *Emergency medicine: Concepts and clinical practice* (3rd ed., pp. 913–944). St. Louis: Mosby–Year Book.
Rosenberg, D. (1987). Web of deceit: A literature review of Munchausen syndrome by proxy. *Child Abuse and Neglect, 11*, 547–563.
Saunders, C. E., & Ho, M. T. (Eds.). (1992). *Current emergency diagnosis and treatment* (4th ed.). Norwalk, CT: Appleton & Lange.
Scheidt, P. C., Harel, Y., Trumble, A. C., Jones, D. H., Overpeck, M. D., & Bijur, P. E. (1995). The epidemiology of nonfatal injuries among U.S. children and youth. *American Journal of Public Health, 85*, 932–938.
Schmitt, B. D. (1992). *Instructions for pediatric patients*. Philadelphia: W. B. Saunders.
Skolnick, N. (1993). Croup. *Journal of Family Practice, 37*, 165–170.
Soud, T. (1993). The febrile child in the emergency department. *Journal of Emergency Nursing, 19*, 355–358.
Statistical abstracts of the United States (114th ed.). (1994). Section 5: Law enforcement, courts, and prisons (pp. 213–214).
Steele, M. T., Nelson, M. J., Sessler, D. I., Fraker, L., Bunney, B., Watson, W. A., & Robinson, W. A. (1996). Forced air speeds rewarming in accidental hypothermia. *Annals of Emergency Medicine, 27*, 479–484.
Talbert, S. R. (1993). Inhalation injuries: Review and two case studies. *Journal of Emergency Nursing, 19*, 482–485.
Thomas, D. O. (1991). Triage of the pediatric patient. In D. O. Thomas (Ed.), *Quick reference to pediatric emergency nursing* (pp. 25–30). Gaithersburg, MD: Aspen.
Thomas, V., Riegel, B., Andrea, J., Murray, P., Gerhart, A., & Gocka, I. (1994). National survey of pediatric fever management practices among emergency department nurses. *Journal of Emergency Nursing, 20*, 505–510.
Thompson, A. E. (1996). Environmental emergencies. In G. R. Fleisher & S. Ludwig (Eds.), *Synopsis of pediatric emergency medicine*. Baltimore: Williams & Wilkins.
Tom, P. A., Garmel, G. M., & Auerbach, P. S. (1994). Environment-dependent sports emergencies. *Medical Clinics of North America, 78*, 305–325.
Vernon-Levett, P. (1995). Pediatric emergencies. *Critical Care Nursing Clinics of North America, 7*, 457–471.
Vernon-Levett, P. (1996). Neurologic critical care problems. In M. A. Q. Curley, J. B. Smith, & P. A. Moloney-Harmon (Eds.), *Critical care nursing of infants and children* (pp. 656–694). Philadelphia: W. B. Saunders.
Wahl, N. G., & Woodall, B. N. (1995). Hypothermia in shaken infant syndrome. *Pediatric Emergency Care, 11*, 233–234.
Walsh, E. A., & Ioli, J. G. (1994). Childhood near-drowning: Nursing care and primary prevention. *Pediatric Nursing, 20*, 265–292.
Webb, K. H. (1996). Envenomations. In R. E. Behrman, R. M. Kliegman, & A. M. Arvin (Eds.), *Nelson textbook of pediatrics* (15th ed., pp. 2025–2027). Philadelphia: W. B. Saunders.
Welliver, J. R. (1992). Unusual injuries. In S. Ludwig & A. E. Kornberg (Eds.), *Child abuse: A medical reference* (2nd ed., pp. 213–217). New York: Churchill Livingstone.
Welliver, J. R., & Welliver, R. C. (1993). Bronchiolitis. *Pediatrics in Review, 14*(4), 134–139.
Willinger, M., Hoffman, H. J., & Hartford, R. B. (1994). Infant sleep position and risk for sudden infant death syndrome: Report of meeting held January 13 and 14, 1994, National Institutes of Health, Bethesda, MD. *Pediatrics, 93*, 814–819.
Woolf, A. D. (1993). Poisoning in children and adolescents. *Pediatrics in Review, 14*, 411–422.

Bibliography

Anderson, C. L. (1993). The parenting profile assessment: Screening for child abuse. *Applied Nursing Research, 6*, 31–33.
Athey, A. M. (1995). Pediatric injury control: Strategies for the nurse practitioner. *Nurse Practitioner Forum, 6*, 167–172.
Badgwell, J. M. (1996). The traumatized child. *Anesthesiology Clinics of North America, 14*, 151–171.
Berro, E. A., & Bechler-Karsch, A. (1993). A closer look at septic shock. *Pediatric Nursing, 19*, 289–297, 314.
Carrougher, G. J. (1993). Inhalation injury. *AACN Clinical Issues in Critical Care Nursing, 4*, 367–377.
Centers for Disease Control. (1991). *Preventing lead poisoning in young children*. Atlanta: U.S. Department of Health and Human Services.
Clowers, T. D. (1996). Wound assessment of the *Loxosceles reclusa* spider bite. *Journal of Emergency Nursing, 22*, 283–287.
Committee on Environmental Health, American Academy of Pediatrics. (1993). Lead poisoning: From screening to primary prevention. *Pediatrics, 92*, 176–183.
Cox, S. A. (1994). Pediatric trauma: Special patients/special needs. *Critical Care Nursing Quarterly, 17*, 51–61.
Crawley, T. (1996). Childhood injury: Significance and prevention strategies. *Journal of Pediatric Nursing, 11*, 225–232.

Dart, R. C., Hurlbut, K. M., Garcia, R., & Boren, J. (1996). Validation of a severity score for the assessment of crotalid snakebite. *Annals of Emergency Medicine, 27,* 321–326.

Davidson, T. M., & Davidson, D. (1996). Immediate management of epistaxis: Bloody nuisance or ominous sign? *Physician and Sportsmedicine, 24*(8), 74–83.

Dinman, S., & Jarosz, D. A. (1996). Managing serious dog bite injuries in children. *Pediatric Nursing, 22,* 413–417.

Dorfman, D. H., & Paradise, J. E. (1995). Emergency diagnosis and management of physical abuse and neglect of children. *Current Opinion in Pediatrics, 7,* 297–301.

Fraser, J. J. (1996). Nonfatal injuries in adolescents: United States 1988. *Journal of Adolescent Health, 19,* 166–170.

Graneto, J. W., & Soglin, D. F. (1993). Transport and stabilization of the pediatric trauma patient. *Pediatric Clinics of North America, 40,* 365–380.

Grupp-Phelan, J., & Tanz, R. R. (1996). How rational is the crossmatching of blood in the pediatric emergency department? *Archives of Pediatric and Adolescent Medicine, 150,* 1140–1144.

Gupta, A., & Waldhauser, L. K. (1997). Adverse drug reactions from birth to early childhood. *Pediatric Clinics of North America, 44,* 79–92.

Hirtz, D. G. (1997). Febrile seizures. *Pediatrics in Review, 18,* 5–8.

Johnstone, H. A., & Marcinak, J. F. (1997). Sibling abuse: Another component of domestic violence. *Journal of Pediatric Nursing, 12,* 51–54.

Jones, N. E. (1993). Childhood residential injuries. *MCN American Journal of Maternal Child Nursing, 18,* 168–172.

Kardon, E. M. (1996). Acute asthma. *Emergency Medicine Clinics of North America, 14,* 93–114.

Kiebler, B., & Mowry, J. B. (1994). Acetaminophen's potential for morbidity and mortality. *Pediatric Nursing, 20,* 491–494.

Klebes, C., & Fay, S. (1995). Munchausen syndrome by proxy: A review, case study, and nursing implications. *Journal of Pediatric Nursing, 10,* 93–98.

Krenzelok, E. P. (1995). The use of poison prevention and education strategies to enhance the awareness of the poison information center and to prevent accidental pediatric poisonings. *Journal of Toxicology. Clinical Toxicology, 33,* 663–667.

Lieberman, P. (1995). Distinguishing anaphylaxis from other serious disorders. *Journal of Respiratory Diseases, 16,* 411–420.

Lockridge, T. (1997). Now I lay me down to sleep: SIDS and infant sleep positions. *Mother Baby Journal, 2*(2), 7–13.

Maksoud, J. G., Moront, M. L., & Eichelberger, M. R. (1995). Resuscitation of the injured child. *Seminars in Pediatric Surgery, 4,* 93–99.

Moloney-Harmon, P. A., & Czerwinski, S. J. (1994). Caught in the crossfire: Children, guns, and trauma. *Critical Care Nursing Clinics of North America, 6,* 525–533.

Moront, M. L., Williams, J. A., Eichelberger, M. R., & Wilkinson, J. D. (1994). The injured child. An approach to care. *Pediatric Clinics of North America, 41,* 1201–1226.

Natanson, C., Hoffman, W. D., Suffredini, A. F., Eichaker, P. Q., & Danner, R. L. (1994). Selected treatment strategies for septic shock based on proposed mechanisms of pathogenesis. *Annals of Internal Medicine, 120,* 771–783.

Osberg, J. S., Kahn, P., Rowe, K., & Brooke, M. M. (1996). Pediatric trauma: Impact on work and family finances. *Pediatrics, 98,* 890–897.

Pieper, P. (1994). Pediatric trauma. An overview. *Nursing Clinics of North America, 29,* 563–584.

Reisdorff, E. J. (Ed.). (1995). Pediatric emergencies (entire volume). *Emergency Medicine Clinics of North America, 13,* 235–507.

Rescorl, D. (1995). Environmental emergencies. *Critical Care Nursing Clinics of North America, 7,* 445–456.

Rivara, F. P. (1995). Developmental and behavioral issues in childhood injury prevention. *Journal of Developmental and Behavioral Pediatrics, 16,* 362–370.

Swartz, M. K. (1993). Poison prevention. *Journal of Pediatric Health Care, 7,* 143–144.

Ulione, M. S., & Dooling, M. (1997). Preschool injuries in child care centers: Nursing strategies for prevention. *Journal of Pediatric Health Care, 11,* 111–116.

Ushay, H. M., & Notterman, D. A. (1997). Pharmacology of pediatric resuscitation. *Pediatric Clinics of North America, 44,* 207–233.

Wilson, D. (1995). Assessing and managing the febrile child. *Nurse Practitioner, 20*(11), 59–60, 68–74.

Wright, J. L., & Patterson, M. D. (1996). Resuscitating the pediatric patient. *Emergency Medicine Clinics of North America, 14,* 219–231.

APPENDIX 1

Growth Charts

BOYS: BIRTH TO 36 MONTHS PHYSICAL GROWTH NCHS PERCENTILES*

NAME ____________ RECORD # ____________

DATE	AGE	LENGTH	WEIGHT	HEAD CIRC.	COMMENT

*Adapted from: Hamill PVV, Drizd TA, Johnson CL, Reed RB, Roche AF, Moore WM: Physical growth: National Center for Health Statistics percentiles. AM J CLIN NUTR 32:607-629, 1979. Data from the Fels Longitudinal Study, Wright State University School of Medicine, Yellow Springs, Ohio.

ROSS LABORATORIES
COLUMBUS, OHIO 43216
DIVISION OF ABBOTT LABORATORIES, USA
ROSS

G105(0.05)/JANUARY 1986 LITHO IN USA

BOYS: BIRTH TO 36 MONTHS PHYSICAL GROWTH NCHS PERCENTILES*

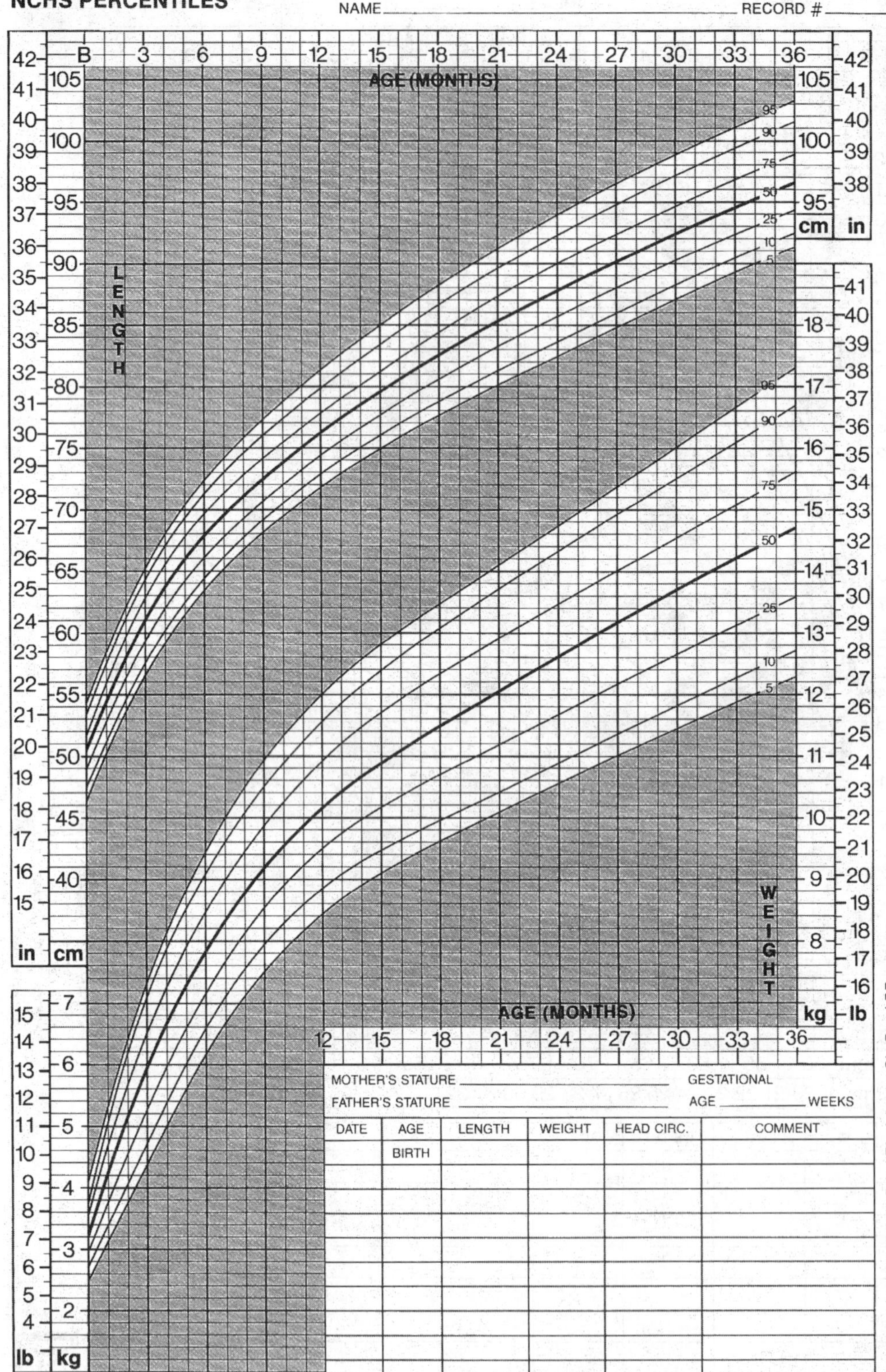

Ross Growth & Development Program

*Adapted from: Hamill PVV, Drizd TA, Johnson CL, Reed RB, Roche AF, Moore WM: Physical growth: National Center for Health Statistics percentiles. AM J CLIN NUTR 32:607-629, 1979. Data from the Fels Longitudinal Study, Wright State University School of Medicine, Yellow Springs, Ohio.

BOYS: 2 TO 18 YEARS
PHYSICAL GROWTH
NCHS PERCENTILES*

NAME ____________________ RECORD # ____________

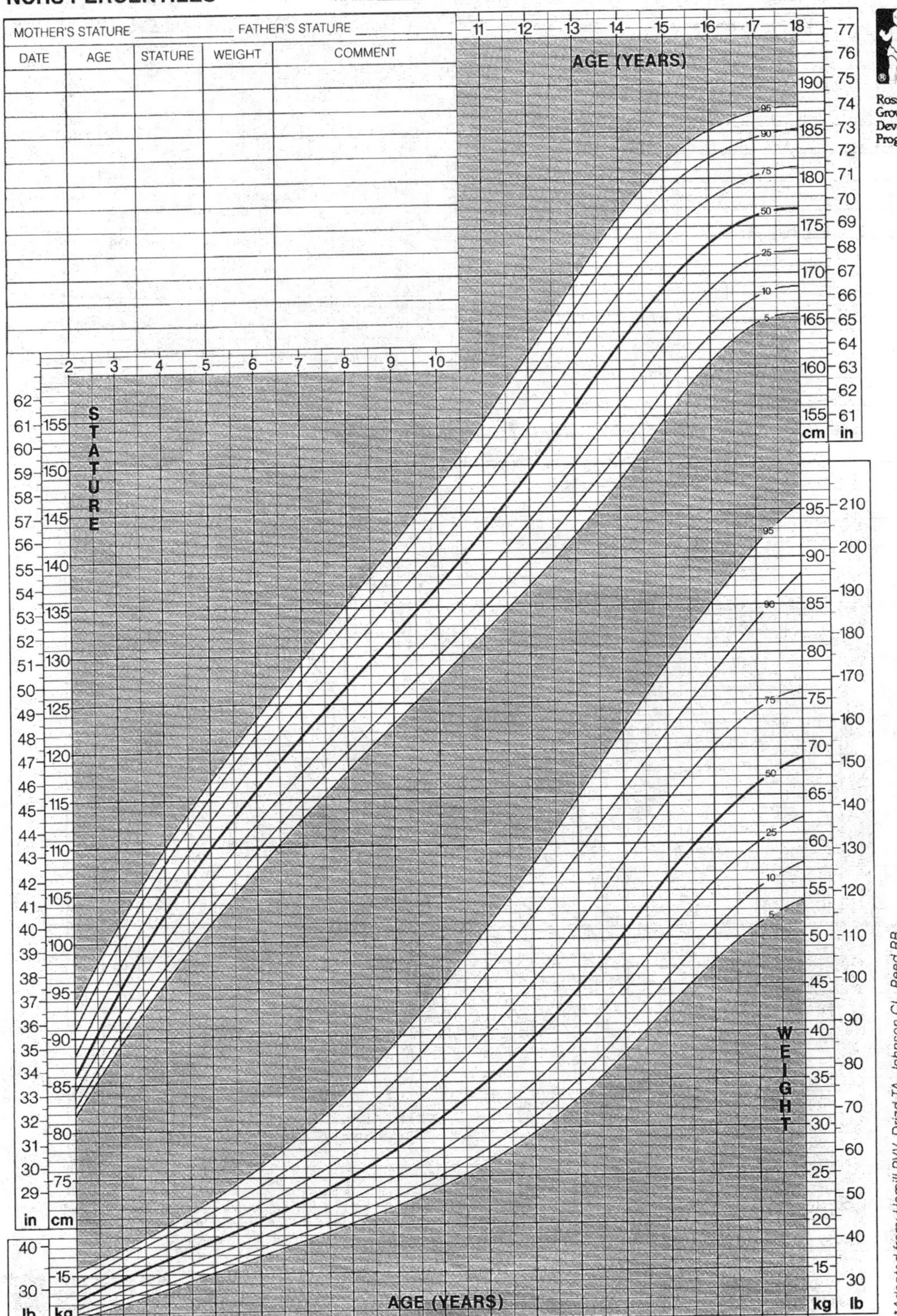

Ross Growth & Development Program

*Adapted from: Hamill PVV, Drizd TA, Johnson CL, Reed RB, Roche AF, Moore WM: Physical growth: National Center for Health Statistics percentiles. AM J CLIN NUTR 32:607-629, 1979. Data from the National Center for Health Statistics (NCHS), Hyattsville, Maryland.

BOYS: PREPUBESCENT PHYSICAL GROWTH NCHS PERCENTILES*

NAME ________________ RECORD # ________

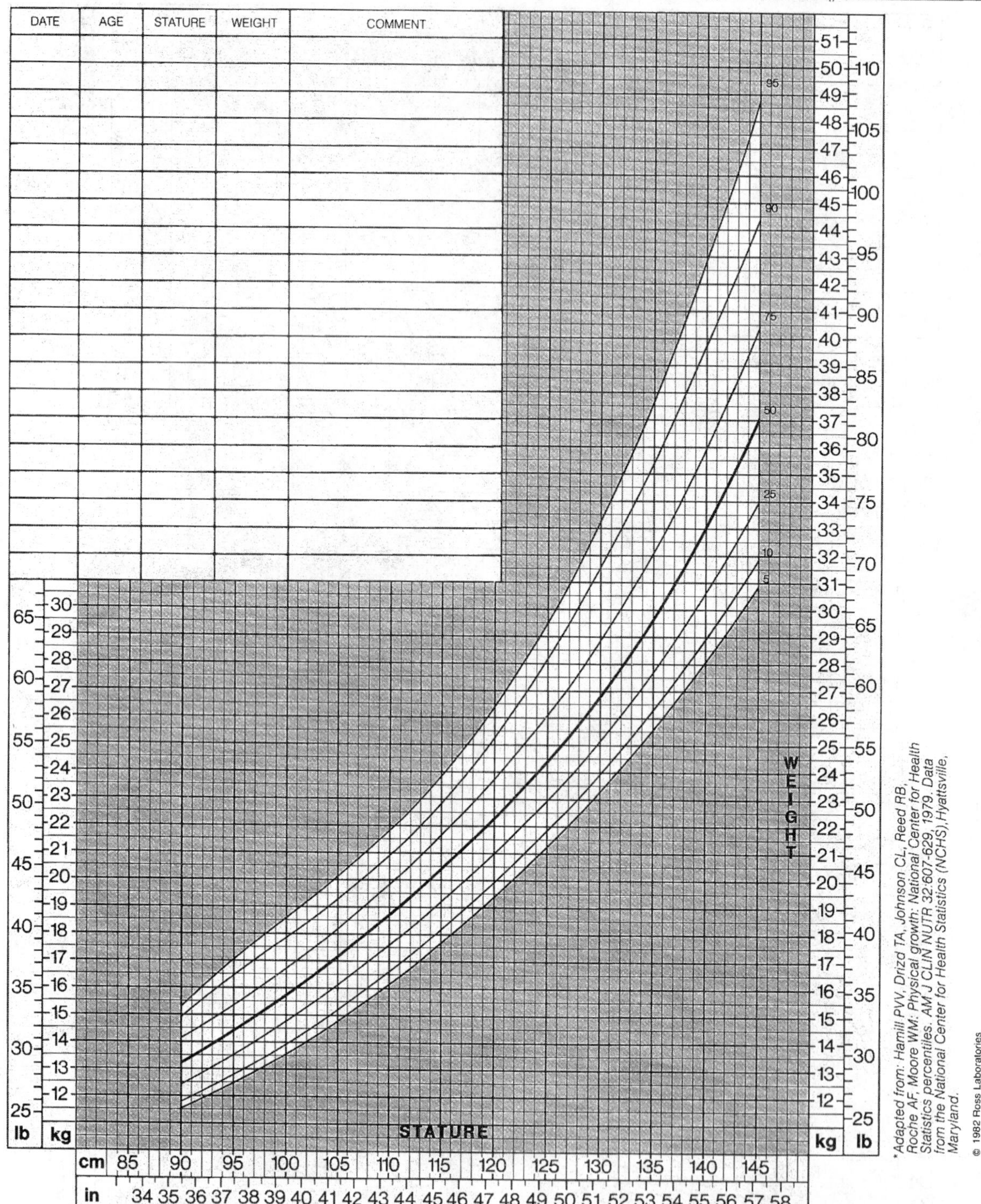

ROSS LABORATORIES
COLUMBUS, OHIO 43216
DIVISION OF ABBOTT LABORATORIES, USA
ROSS

G107(0.05)/FEBRUARY 1989 LITHO IN USA

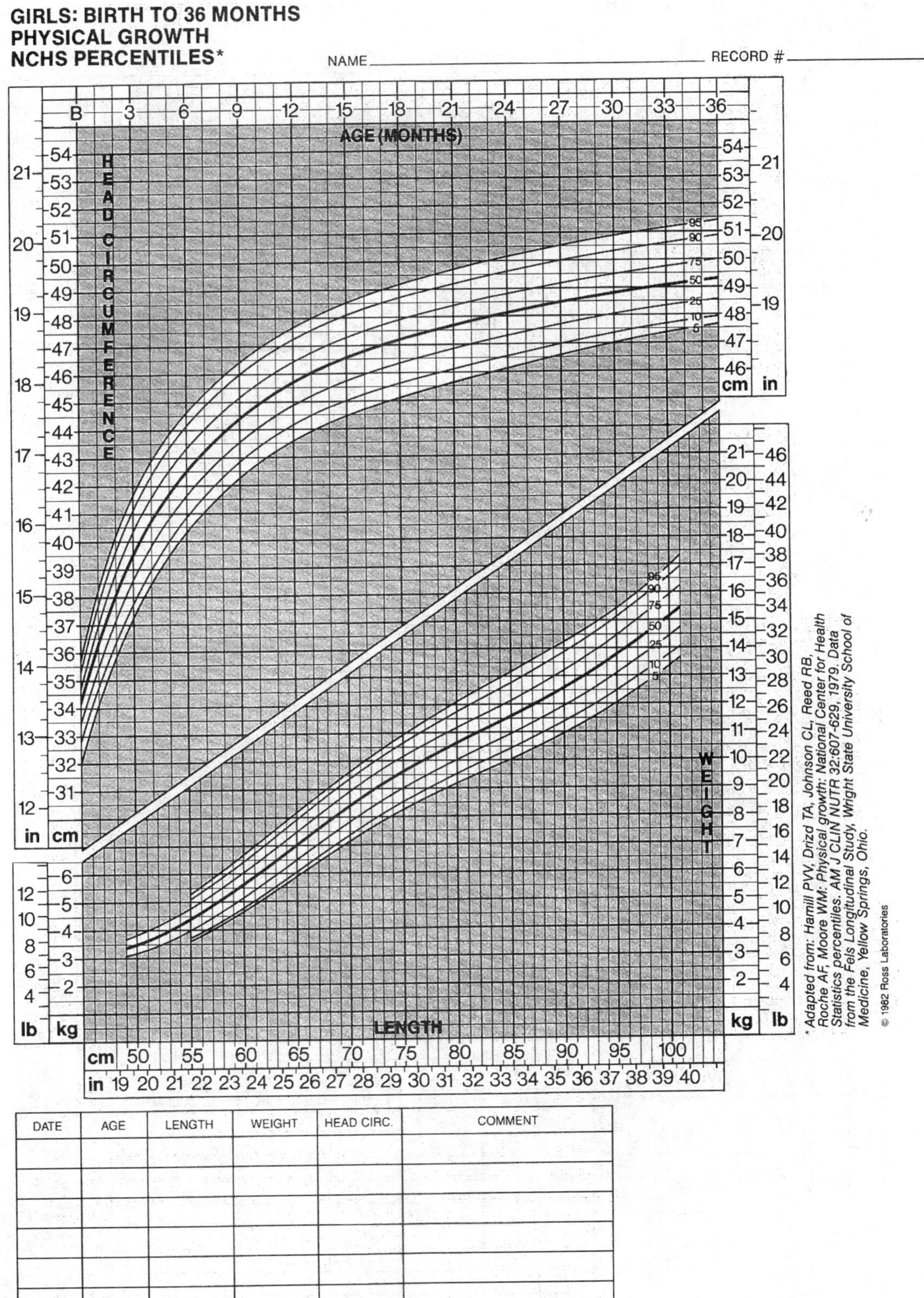

DATE	AGE	LENGTH	WEIGHT	HEAD CIRC.	COMMENT

GIRLS: BIRTH TO 36 MONTHS PHYSICAL GROWTH NCHS PERCENTILES*

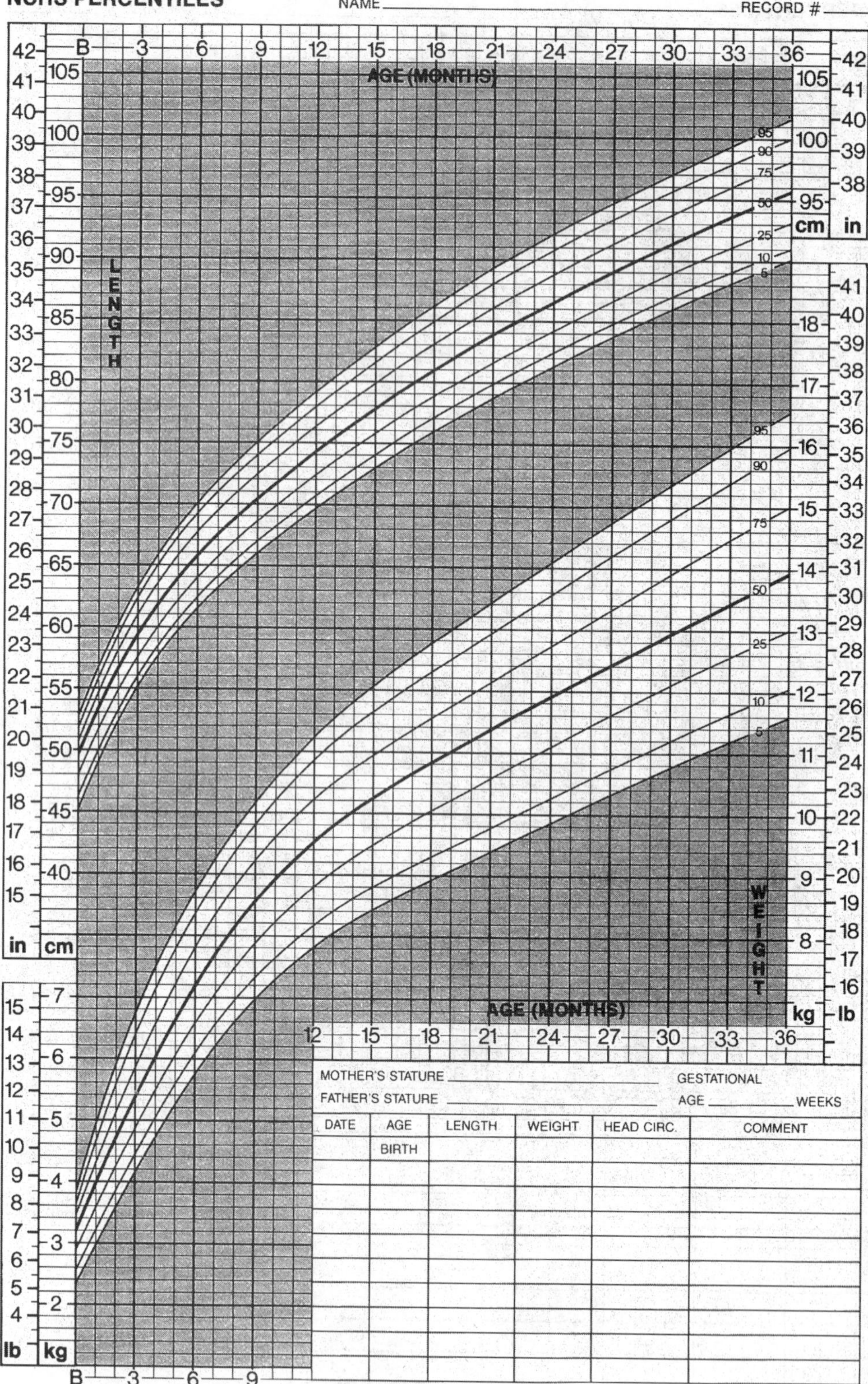

* Adapted from: Hamill PVV, Drizd TA, Johnson CL, Reed RB, Roche AF, Moore WM: Physical growth: National Center for Health Statistics percentiles. AM J CLIN NUTR 32:607-629, 1979. Data from the Fels Longitudinal Study, Wright State University School of Medicine, Yellow Springs, Ohio.

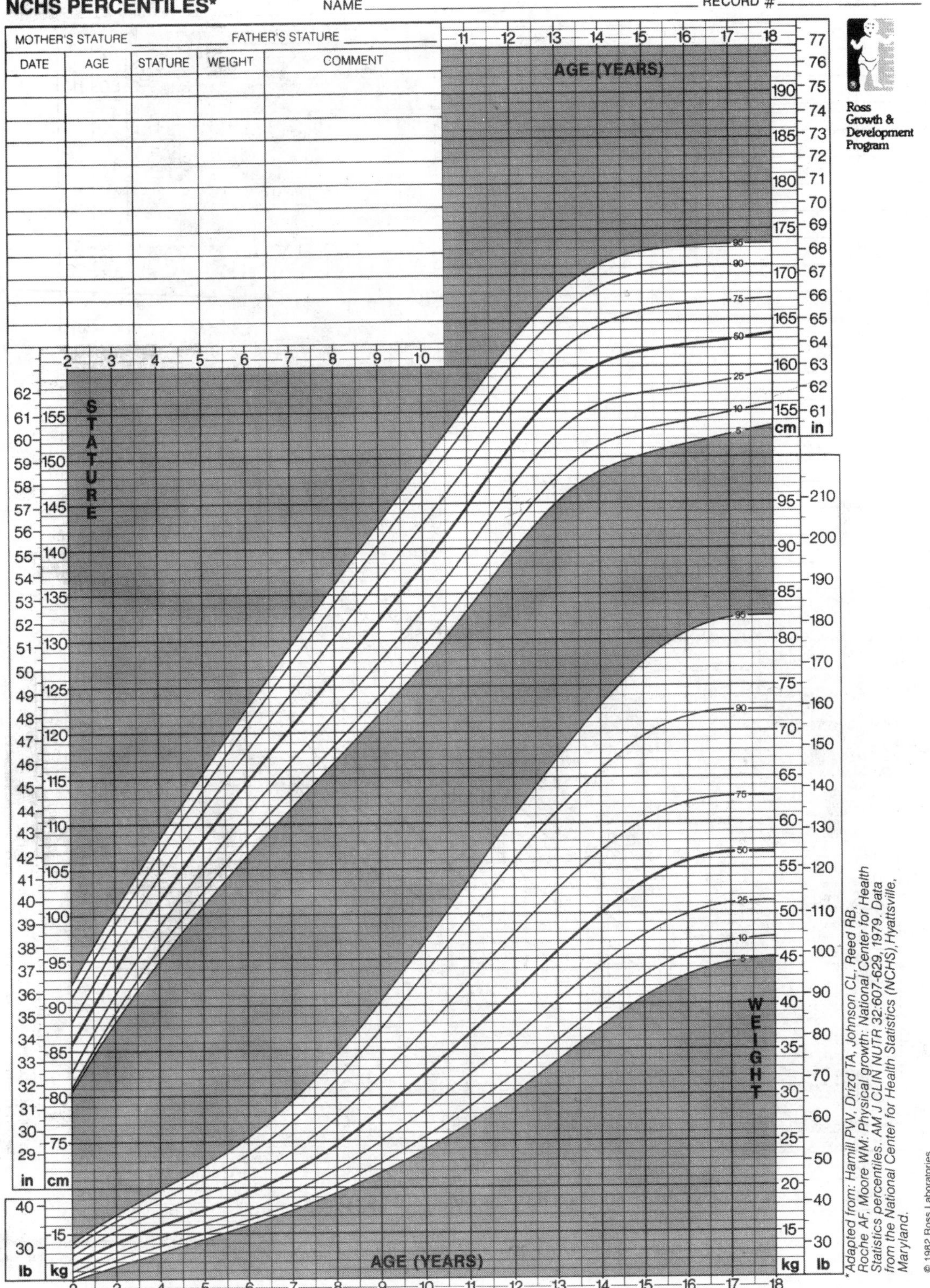
GIRLS: 2 TO 18 YEARS
PHYSICAL GROWTH
NCHS PERCENTILES*
NAME
RECORD #
MOTHER'S STATURE
FATHER'S STATURE
DATE
AGE
STATURE
WEIGHT
COMMENT
AGE (YEARS)
STATURE
WEIGHT
AGE (YEARS)
cm
in
kg
lb
Ross Growth & Development Program
*Adapted from: Hamill PVV, Drizd TA, Johnson CL, Reed RB, Roche AF, Moore WM: Physical growth: National Center for Health Statistics percentiles. AM J CLIN NUTR 32:607-629, 1979. Data from the National Center for Health Statistics (NCHS), Hyattsville, Maryland.
© 1982 Ross Laboratories

GIRLS: PREPUBESCENT PHYSICAL GROWTH NCHS PERCENTILES*

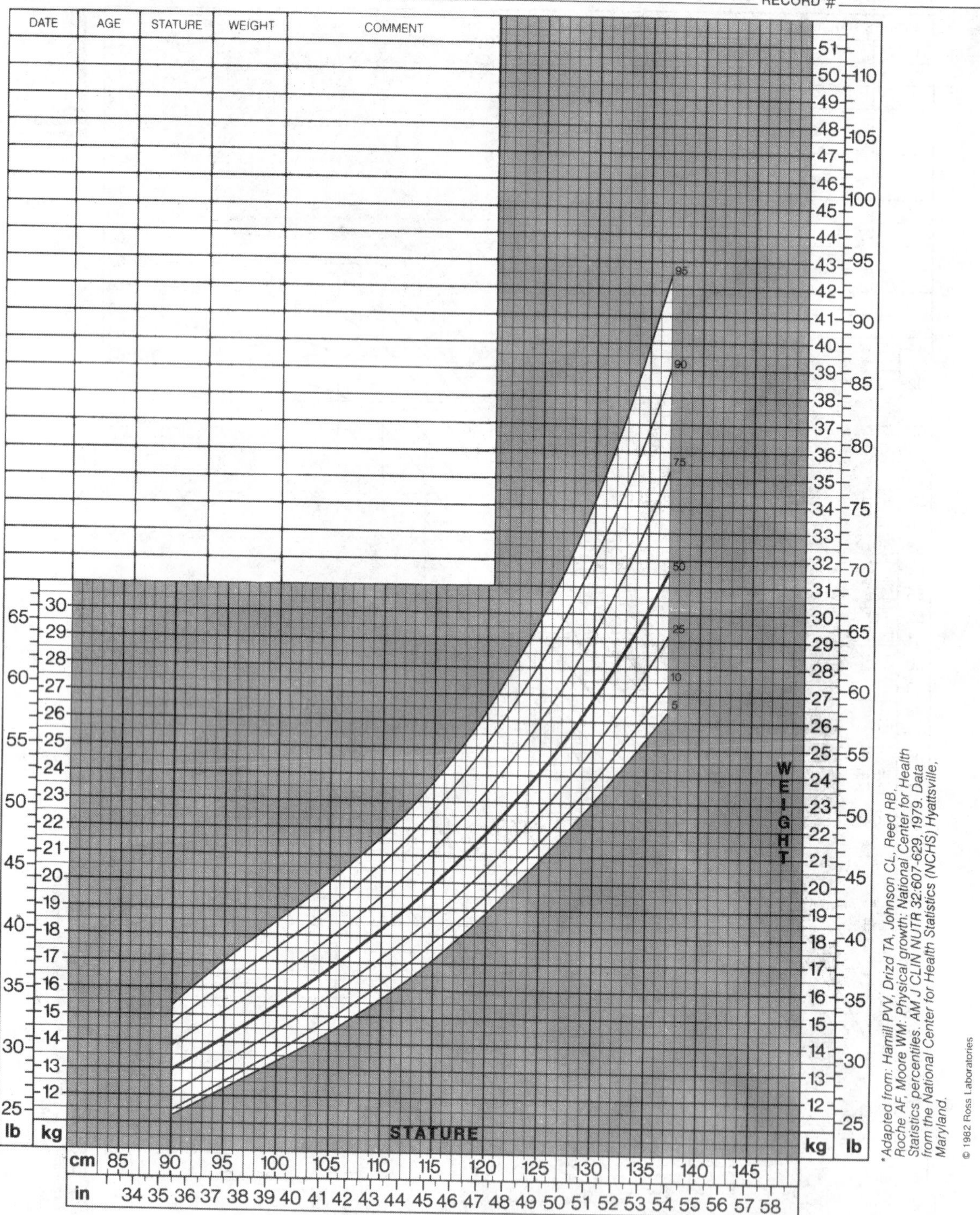

ROSS LABORATORIES
COLUMBUS, OHIO 43216
DIVISION OF ABBOTT LABORATORIES, USA
ROSS

G108(0.05)/FEBRUARY 1989 LITHO IN USA

APPENDIX 2

Denver II

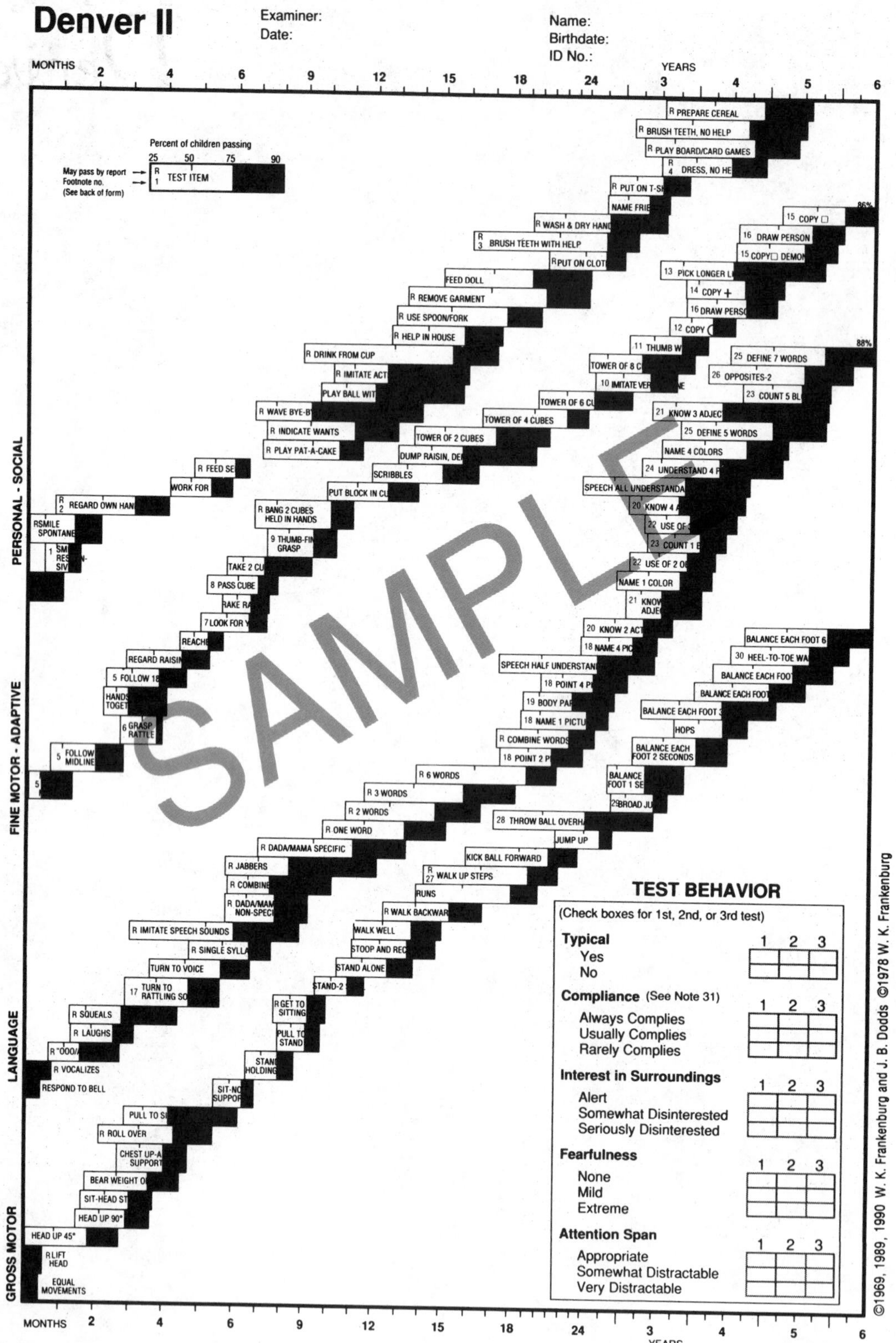

Denver II
Examiner:
Date:
Name:
Birthdate:
ID No.:
MONTHS 2 4 6 9 12 15 18 24
YEARS 3 4 5 6
Percent of children passing
25 50 75 90
May pass by report
Footnote no.
(See back of form)
R 1 TEST ITEM
PERSONAL - SOCIAL
R PREPARE CEREAL
R BRUSH TEETH, NO HELP
R PLAY BOARD/CARD GAMES
R 4 DRESS, NO HE
R PUT ON T-S
NAME FRI
R WASH & DRY HAN
R 3 BRUSH TEETH WITH HELP
R PUT ON CLOT
FEED DOLL
R REMOVE GARMENT
R USE SPOON/FORK
R HELP IN HOUSE
R DRINK FROM CUP
R IMITATE ACT
PLAY BALL WIT
R WAVE BYE-B
R INDICATE WANTS
R PLAY PAT-A-CAKE
R FEED SE
WORK FOR
R 2 REGARD OWN HAN
R SMILE SPONTANE
1 SM RES SIV
FINE MOTOR - ADAPTIVE
86%
15 COPY □
16 DRAW PERSON
15 COPY□ DEMON
13 PICK LONGER L
14 COPY +
16 DRAW PERS
12 COPY ○
11 THUMB W
TOWER OF 8 C
10 IMITATE VER
TOWER OF 6 C
TOWER OF 4 CUBES
TOWER OF 2 CUBES
DUMP RAISIN, DE
SCRIBBLES
PUT BLOCK IN C
R BANG 2 CUBES HELD IN HANDS
9 THUMB-FIN GRASP
TAKE 2 C
8 PASS CUBE
RAKE R
7 LOOK FOR
REACH
REGARD RAISI
5 FOLLOW 18
HANDS TOGET
6 GRASP RATTLE
5 FOLLOW MIDLINE
5
LANGUAGE
88%
25 DEFINE 7 WORDS
26 OPPOSITES-2
23 COUNT 5 BL
21 KNOW 3 ADJEC
25 DEFINE 5 WORDS
NAME 4 COLORS
24 UNDERSTAND 4 P
SPEECH ALL UNDERSTANDA
20 KNOW 4 A
22 USE OF
23 COUNT 1 B
22 USE OF 2 O
NAME 1 COLOR
21 KNOW ADJE
20 KNOW 2 ACT
18 NAME 4 PIC
SPEECH HALF UNDERSTAN
18 POINT 4 P
19 BODY PAR
18 NAME 1 PICTU
R COMBINE WORDS
18 POINT 2 P
R 6 WORDS
R 3 WORDS
R 2 WORDS
R ONE WORD
R DADA/MAMA SPECIFIC
R JABBERS
R COMBINE
R DADA/MAMA NON-SPEC
R IMITATE SPEECH SOUNDS
R SINGLE SYLLA
TURN TO VOICE
17 TURN TO RATTLING SO
R SQUEALS
R LAUGHS
R "OOO/
R VOCALIZES
RESPOND TO BELL
GROSS MOTOR
BALANCE EACH FOOT 6
30 HEEL-TO-TOE WA
BALANCE EACH FOO
BALANCE EACH FOO
BALANCE EACH FOOT
HOPS
BALANCE EACH FOOT 2 SECONDS
BALANCE FOOT 1 SE
29 BROAD JU
28 THROW BALL OVERH
JUMP UP
KICK BALL FORWARD
R 27 WALK UP STEPS
RUNS
R WALK BACKWAR
WALK WELL
STOOP AND REC
STAND ALONE
STAND-2
R GET TO SITTING
PULL TO STAND
STAND HOLDING
SIT-NO SUPPOR
PULL TO SI
R ROLL OVER
CHEST UP-A SUPPORT
BEAR WEIGHT O
SIT-HEAD ST
HEAD UP 90°
HEAD UP 45°
R LIFT HEAD
EQUAL MOVEMENTS
TEST BEHAVIOR
(Check boxes for 1st, 2nd, or 3rd test)
Typical 1 2 3
Yes
No
Compliance (See Note 31) 1 2 3
Always Complies
Usually Complies
Rarely Complies
Interest in Surroundings 1 2 3
Alert
Somewhat Disinterested
Seriously Disinterested
Fearfulness 1 2 3
None
Mild
Extreme
Attention Span 1 2 3
Appropriate
Somewhat Distractable
Very Distractable
SAMPLE
©1969, 1989, 1990 W. K. Frankenburg and J. B. Dodds ©1978 W. K. Frankenburg

DIRECTIONS FOR ADMINISTRATION

1. Try to get child to smile by smiling, talking or waving. Do not touch him/her.
2. Child must stare at hand several seconds.
3. Parent may help guide toothbrush and put toothpaste on brush.
4. Child does not have to be able to tie shoes or button/zip in the back.
5. Move yarn slowly in an arc from one side to the other, about 8" above child's face.
6. Pass if child grasps rattle when it is touched to the backs or tips of fingers.
7. Pass if child tries to see where yarn went. Yarn should be dropped quickly from sight from tester's hand without arm movement.
8. Child must transfer cube from hand to hand without help of body, mouth, or table.
9. Pass if child picks up raisin with any part of thumb and finger.
10. Line can vary only 30 degrees or less from tester's line.
11. Make a fist with thumb pointing upward and wiggle only the thumb. Pass if child imitates and does not move any fingers other than the thumb.

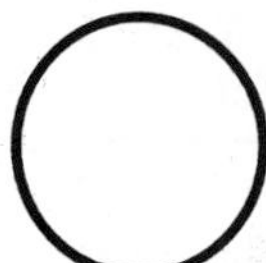

12. Pass any enclosed form. Fail continuous round motions.

13. Which line is longer? (Not bigger.) Turn paper upside down and repeat. (pass 3 of 3 or 5 of 6)

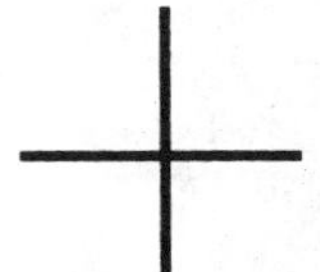

14. Pass any lines crossing near midpoint.

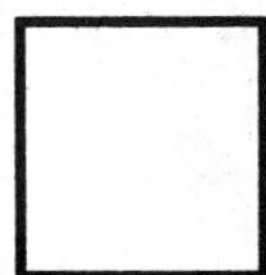

15. Have child copy first. If failed, demonstrate.

When giving items 12, 14, and 15, do not name the forms. Do not demonstrate 12 and 14.

16. When scoring, each pair (2 arms, 2 legs, etc.) counts as one part.
17. Place one cube in cup and shake gently near child's ear, but out of sight. Repeat for other ear.
18. Point to picture and have child name it. (No credit is given for sounds only.)
    If less than 4 pictures are named correctly, have child point to picture as each is named by tester.

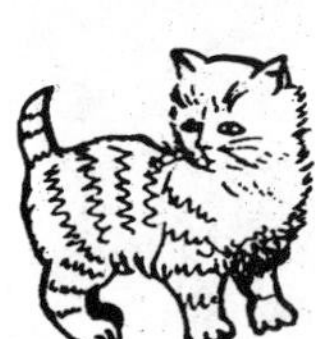
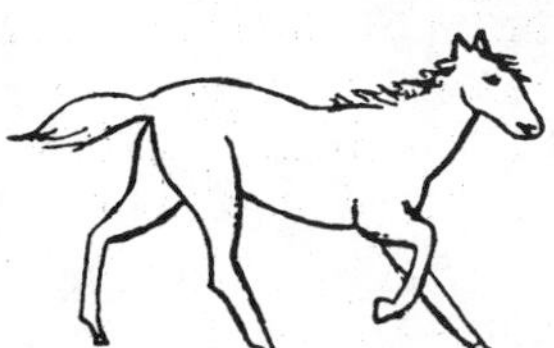
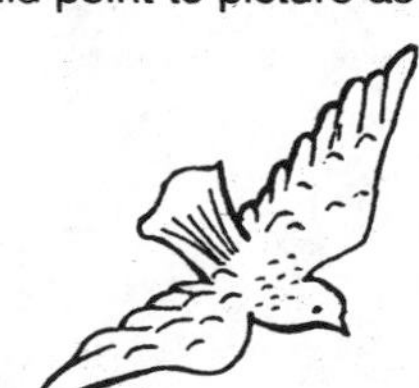
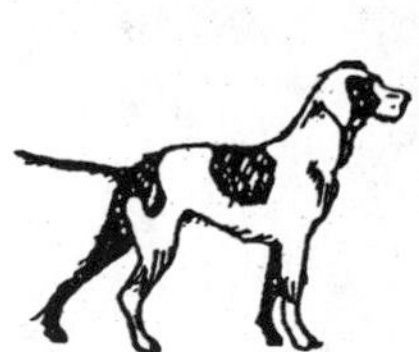
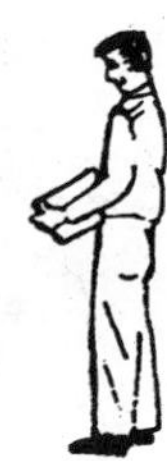

19. Using doll, tell child: Show me the nose, eyes, ears, mouth, hands, feet, tummy, hair. Pass 6 of 8.
20. Using pictures, ask child: Which one flies?... says meow?... talks?... barks?... gallops? Pass 2 of 5, 4 of 5.
21. Ask child: What do you do when you are cold?... tired?... hungry? Pass 2 of 3, 3 of 3.
22. Ask child: What do you do with a cup? What is a chair used for? What is a pencil used for?
    Action words must be included in answers.
23. Pass if child correctly places <u>and</u> says how many blocks are on paper. (1, 5).
24. Tell child: Put block **on** table; **under** table; **in front of** me, **behind** me. Pass 4 of 4.
    (Do not help child by pointing, moving head or eyes.)
25. Ask child: What is a ball?... lake?... desk?... house?... banana?... curtain?... fence?... ceiling? Pass if defined in terms of use, shape, what it is made of, or general category (such as banana is fruit, not just yellow). Pass 5 of 8, 7 of 8.
26. Ask child: If a horse is big, a mouse is __? If fire is hot, ice is __? If the sun shines during the day, the moon shines during the __? Pass 2 of 3.
27. Child may use wall or rail only, not person. May not crawl.
28. Child must throw ball overhand 3 feet to within arm's reach of tester.
29. Child must perform standing broad jump over width of test sheet (8 1/2 inches).
30. Tell child to walk forward, ⊂⊃⊂⊃⊂⊃⊂⊃→ heel within 1 inch of toe. Tester may demonstrate.
    Child must walk 4 consecutive steps.
31. In the second year, half of normal children are non-compliant.

OBSERVATIONS:

APPENDIX 3

Revised Prescreening Developmental Questionnaire (R-PDQ)

REVISED (1986) DENVER PRESCREENING DEVELOPMENTAL QUESTIONNAIRE (R-PDQ)* INFORMATION FOR PROFESSIONALS

The original Denver Prescreening Developmental Questionnaire (PDQ) has been revised to simplify monitoring and screening of children's development. The R-PDQ is designed to achieve three goals: 1) to make parents more aware of the development of their children; 2) to document the developmental progress of individual children in a systematic manner; and 3) to facilitate earlier identification of children whose development may be delayed.

INSTRUCTIONS FOR PREPARATION OF THE R-PDQ

1. Use the following guide to determine which of the four R-PDQ forms is appropriate for the child:

   Orange (0-9 MONTHS); Purple (9-24 MONTHS); Gold (2-4 YEARS); White (4-6 YEARS)

2. Select the appropriate form and write the child's name, today's date, and the child's birthdate at the top of the R-PDQ form.

3. Complete the age calculation in the box on the front of the form. Figure the number of days first, then the number of months, and finally the number of years. Should it become necessary to "borrow" when subtracting, 1 month borrowed adds 30 days to the "day" column and 1 year borrowed adds 12 months to the "month" column. (See example below.)

		15	
		+12	45
	85	3	+30
Today's Date:	~~86~~ yr	~~4~~ mo	15 day
Child's Birthdate:	84 yr	7 mo	25 day
Subtract to get Child's Exact Age:	1 yr	8 mo	20 day

4. For R-PDQ results to be quickly and correctly interpreted (see back of form), it is necessary to convert the child's exact age to an R-PDQ age. For children below 24 months of age, the R-PDQ age is expressed in completed months and weeks, as shown:

Child's Exact Age:	1 yr	8 mo	20 day
R-PDQ Age:	(– yr	20 mo	2 completed weeks)

   For children above 24 months of age, the R-PDQ age is expressed in years and months. There is no need to write in the completed weeks after 24 months of age.

Child's Exact Age:	3 yr	6 mo	28 day
R-PDQ Age:	(3 yr	6 mo	– completed weeks)

DO NOT ROUND OFF TO THE NEXT HIGHER AGE TO EXPRESS THE R-PDQ AGE. ONLY **COMPLETED** WEEKS, **COMPLETED** MONTHS, AND **COMPLETED** YEARS SHOULD BE CONSIDERED.

5. Give the prepared form to the child's caregiver and ask that (s)he note who is completing the form, and his/her relation to the child. The caregiver should then answer questions until: 1) 3 "NOs" are circled (they do not have to be consecutive); or 2) all of the questions on both sides of the form have been answered.

6. Check form to see that all appropriate questions have been answered.

* *Frankenburg WK: Revised Denver Prescreening Developmental Questionnaire (R-PDQ). Presented in part at the Ambulatory Pediatric Association Meeting, May 8, 1986.*

PURCHASE OF ADDITIONAL FORMS

The ages and corresponding forms are listed below; available in English only. The cost is $8.00 for a pad of 100 plus 10% shipping and handling for U.S. orders.

	Cat #
0-9 months:	Orange Form (1000A)
9-24 months:	Purple Form (1010A)
2-4 years:	Gold Form (1020A)
4-6 years:	White Form (1030A)

Order From:

Denver Developmental Materials, Inc.
P.O. Box 20037
Denver, Colorado 80220-0037
Tele. #: (800) 419-4729

Pre-pay all orders under $60.00

INSTRUCTIONS FOR INTERPRETING R-PDQ RESULTS

The items on the R-PDQ are arranged in chronological order according to the ages at which 90% of children in the Denver Developmental Screening Test (DDST) standardization sample could perform them. A "NO" response may signify a delay. Steps in interpretation are as follows:

1. **Review "YES" and "NO" responses.** Assure that the child's caregiver understood each question and scored the items correctly. Give particular attention to the scoring of questions that require verbal responses by the child, and that require the child to draw.

2. **Identify "delays."** Ages at which 90% of children in the DDST sample passed the items are indicated in parentheses in the "For Office Use" column. These ages are shown in months and weeks up to 24 months (for example, "20-2" indicates 20 months, 2 weeks), and in years and months after 24 months (for example, "3y-6" indicates 3 years, 6 months). A "delay" is any item passed by 90% of children at a younger age **(by even one day)** than the child being screened.

   Highlight "delays" by circling the 90% age in parentheses to the right of the item that the child was not able to perform. (See example below.)

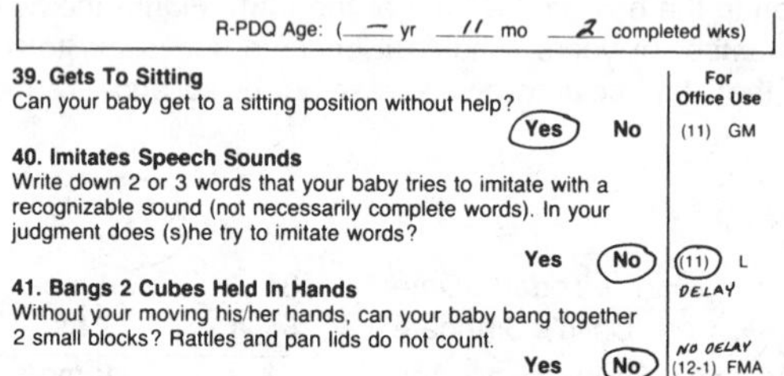

R-PDQ Age: (— yr 11 mo 2 completed wks)

39. Gets To Sitting
Can your baby get to a sitting position without help?
Yes No

40. Imitates Speech Sounds
Write down 2 or 3 words that your baby tries to imitate with a recognizable sound (not necessarily complete words). In your judgment does (s)he try to imitate words?
Yes No

41. Bangs 2 Cubes Held In Hands
Without your moving his/her hands, can your baby bang together 2 small blocks? Rattles and pan lids do not count.
Yes No

For Office Use
(11) GM
(11) L
DELAY
NO DELAY
(12-1) FMA

3. **Children who have no "delays"** are considered to be developing normally. A few age-appropriate developmental activities may be suggested to their caregivers.

4. **If a child has one "delay,"** the caregiver should be given age-appropriate developmental activities to pursue with the child, and the child should be scheduled for rescreening with the R-PDQ one month later.

   If on rescreening a month later the child has one or more "delays," schedule second-stage screening with the DDST, administered by a qualified examiner, as soon as possible.

5. **Children who have two or more "delays"** on the first-stage screening with the R-PDQ should be scheduled for a second-stage screening with the DDST as soon as possible.

6. If, on second-stage screening with the DDST, a child receives other than normal results (abnormal, questionable or untestable), that child should be scheduled for a diagnostic evaluation.

   For ease in interpreting R-PDQ results to a child's caregiver, each item has been given the same title as the corresponding DDST item. The name of the sector where the item is located on the DDST is shown in the "For Office Use" column of the R-PDQ as follows: PS (Personal Social); FMA (Fine Motor-Adaptive); L (Language); and GM (Gross Motor). An example of this is shown below.

R-PDQ DDST

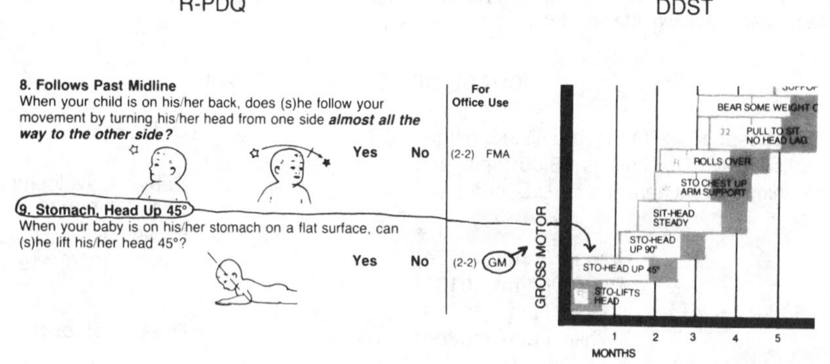

8. Follows Past Midline
When your child is on his/her back, does (s)he follow your movement by turning his/her head from one side ***almost all the way to the other side?***
Yes No

9. Stomach, Head Up 45°
When your baby is on his/her stomach on a flat surface, can (s)he lift his/her head 45°?
Yes No

For Office Use
(2-2) FMA
(2-2) GM

0-9 MONTHS (R-PDQ)

REVISED DENVER PRESCREENING DEVELOPMENTAL QUESTIONNAIRE

Child's Name ____________________

Person Completing R-PDQ: ____________________

Relation to Child: ____________________

For Office Use

Today's Date: ____ yr ____ mo ____ day

Child's Birthdate: ____ yr ____ mo ____ day

Subtract to get Child's Exact Age: ____ yr ____ mo ____ day

R-PDQ Age: (____ yr ____ mo ____ completed wks)

CONTINUE ANSWERING UNTIL 3 **"NOs"** ARE CIRCLED

			For Office Use
1. Equal Movements When your baby is lying on his/her back, can (s)he move each of his/her arms as easily as the other and each of the legs as easily as the other? Answer **No** if your child makes jerky or uncoordinated movements with one or both of his/her arms or legs.	**Yes**	**No**	(0) FMA
2. Stomach Lifts Head When your baby is on his/her stomach on a flat surface, can (s)he lift his/her head off the surface?	**Yes**	**No**	(0-3) GM
3. Regards Face When your baby is lying on his/her back, can (s)he look at you and watch your face?	**Yes**	**No**	(1) PS
4. Follows To Midline When your child is on his/her back, can (s)he follow your movement by turning his/her head from one side to facing directly forward?	**Yes**	**No**	(1-1) FMA
5. Responds To Bell Does your child respond with eye movements, change in breathing or other change in activity to a bell or rattle sounded outside his/her line of vision?	**Yes**	**No**	(1-2) L
6. Vocalizes Not Crying Does your child make sounds other than crying, such as gurgling, cooing, or babbling?	**Yes**	**No**	(1-3) L
7. Smiles Responsively When you smile and talk to your baby, does (s)he smile back at you?	**Yes**	**No**	(1-3) PS
8. Follows Past Midline When your child is on his/her back, does (s)he follow your movement by turning his/her head from one side ***almost all the way to the other side?***	**Yes**	**No**	(2-2) FMA
9. Stomach, Head Up 45° When your baby is on his/her stomach on a flat surface, can (s)he lift his/her head 45°?	**Yes**	**No**	(2-2) GM
10. Stomach, Head Up 90° When your baby is on his/her stomach on a flat surface, can (s)he lift his/her head 90°?	**Yes**	**No**	(3) GM
11. Laughs Does your baby laugh out loud without being tickled or touched?	**Yes**	**No**	(3-1) L
12. Hands Together Does your baby play with his/her hands by touching them together?	**Yes**	**No**	(3-3) FMA
13. Follows 180° When your child is on his/her back, does (s)he follow your movement from one side ***all the way*** to the other side?	**Yes**	**No**	(4) FMA
14. Grasps Rattle ***It is important that you follow instructions carefully.*** Do ***not*** place the pencil in the palm of your child's hand. When you touch the pencil to the back or tips of your baby's fingers, does your baby grasp the pencil for a few seconds?	**Yes**	**No**	(4) FMA

TRY THIS **NOT THIS**

(Please turn page)

APPENDIX 4

Conversion Charts

Table AP4–1
Equivalent Temperature Readings (Celsius and Fahrenheit)*

C	F	C	F	C	F	C	F
0	32.0	37.2	99	39.2	102.6	41.2	106.2
20	68.0	37.4	99.3	39.4	102.9	41.4	106.5
30	86.0	37.6	99.7	39.6	103.3	41.6	106.9
31	87.8	37.8	100.1	39.8	103.7	41.8	107.2
32	89.6	38.0	100.4	40.0	104	42	107.6
33	91.4	38.2	100.8	40.2	104.4	43	109.4
34	93.2	38.4	101.2	40.4	104.7	44	111.2
35	95.0	38.6	101.5	40.6	105.1	100	212
36	96.8	38.8	101.8	40.8	105.4		
37	98.6	39.0	102.2	41.0	105.8		

* To convert Celsius (centigrade) readings to Fahrenheit, multiply by 1.8 and add 32. To convert Fahrenheit readings to Celsius, subtract 32 and divide by 1.8.

From Behrman, R. E., Kliegman, R. M., & Arvin, A. M. (Eds.). (1996). *Nelson textbook of pediatrics* (15th ed., p. 2084). Philadelphia: W. B. Saunders. Reprinted with permission.

Table AP4–2
Pediatric Weight Conversion: Pounds to Kilograms

POUNDS → ↓	0	1	2	3	4	5	6	7	8	9
0	0.00	0.45	0.90	1.36	1.81	2.26	2.72	3.17	3.62	4.08
10	4.53	4.98	5.44	5.89	6.35	6.80	7.35	7.71	8.16	8.61
20	9.07	9.52	9.97	10.43	10.88	11.34	11.79	12.24	12.70	13.15
30	13.60	14.06	14.51	14.96	15.42	15.87	16.32	16.78	17.23	17.69
40	18.14	18.59	19.05	19.50	19.95	20.41	20.86	21.31	21.77	22.22
50	22.68	23.13	23.58	24.04	24.49	24.94	25.40	25.85	26.30	26.76
60	27.21	27.66	28.22	28.57	29.03	29.48	29.93	30.39	30.84	31.29
70	31.75	32.20	32.65	33.11	33.56	34.02	34.47	34.92	35.38	35.83
80	36.28	36.74	37.19	37.64	38.10	38.55	39.00	39.46	39.93	40.37
90	40.82	41.27	41.73	42.18	42.63	43.09	43.54	43.99	44.45	44.90
100	45.36	45.81	46.26	46.72	47.17	47.62	48.08	48.53	48.98	49.44
110	49.89	50.34	50.80	51.25	51.71	52.16	52.61	53.07	53.52	53.97
120	54.43	54.88	55.33	55.79	56.24	56.70	57.15	57.60	58.06	58.51
130	58.96	59.42	59.87	60.32	60.78	61.23	61.68	62.14	62.59	63.05
140	63.50	63.95	64.41	64.86	65.31	65.77	66.22	66.67	67.13	67.58
150	68.04	68.49	68.94	69.40	69.85	70.30	70.76	71.21	71.66	72.12
160	72.57	73.02	73.48	73.93	74.39	74.84	75.29	75.75	76.20	76.65
170	77.11	77.56	78.01	78.47	78.92	79.38	79.83	80.28	80.74	81.19
180	81.64	82.10	82.55	83.00	83.46	83.91	84.36	84.82	85.27	85.73
190	86.18	86.68	87.09	87.54	87.99	88.45	88.90	89.35	89.81	90.26
200	90.72	91.17	91.62	92.08	92.53	92.98	93.44	93.89	94.34	94.80

Example: To determine the kilogram equivalent of 26 pounds, read 20 pounds on side scale, then 6 pounds on top scale. The kilogram equivalent is 11.79.

From Ashwill, J. W., & Droske, S. C. (Eds.). (1997). *Nursing care of children: Principles and practice.* Philadelphia: W. B. Saunders. Reprinted with permission.

APPENDIX 5

Reference Ranges for Vital Sign Measurements

Table AP5-1
Pulse Rates at Rest

Age	Lower Limits of Normal		Average		Upper Limits of Normal	
Newborn	70/min		125/min		190/min	
1–11 mo	80		120		160	
2 yr	80		110		130	
4 yr	80		100		120	
6 yr	75		100		115	
8 yr	70		90		110	
10 yr	70		90		110	
	Girls	*Boys*	*Girls*	*Boys*	*Girls*	*Boys*
12 yr	70	65	90	85	110	105
14 yr	65	60	85	80	105	100
16 yr	60	55	80	75	100	95
18 yr	55	50	75	70	95	90

From Behrman, R. E., Kliegman, R. M., & Arvin, A. M. (Eds.). (1996). *Nelson textbook of pediatrics* (15th ed., p. 1266). Philadelphia: W. B. Saunders. Reprinted with permission.

Table AP5-2
Normal Respiratory Rates

Age	Breaths Per Minute
Neonate	30–40
1 yr	20–40
2 yr	25–32
4 yr	23–30
6 yr	21–26
8 yr	20–26
10 yr	20–26
12 yr	18–22
14 yr	18–22
16 yr	16–20
18 yr	12–20
Adult	10–20

Table AP5–3
Normal Temperature by Age

Age	Temperature* Fahrenheit	Celsius
Newborn	96.8–99 (axillary)	36–37.2 (axillary)
3 Years	97.5–98.6 (axillary)	36.4–37 (axillary)
10 Years	97.5–98.6 (oral)	36.4–37 (oral)
16 Years	97.5–98.6 (oral)	36.4–37 (oral)

* The normal range of the child's temperature will depend on the method used. Temperatures are subject to circadian rhythms in all ages.
From Ashwill, J. W., & Droske, S. C. (Eds.). (1997). *Nursing care of children: Principles and practice.* Philadelphia: W. B. Saunders. Reprinted with permission.

Table AP5–4
Normal Blood Pressure Readings for Girls

	Systolic Blood Pressure Percentile						Diastolic Blood Pressure* Percentile				
Age	5th	10th	50th	90th	95th	Age	5th	10th	50th	90th	95th
1 day	46	50	65	80	84	1 day	38	42	55	68	72
3 days	53	57	72	86	90	3 days	38	42	55	68	71
7 days	60	64	78	93	97	7 days	38	41	54	67	71
1 mo	65	69	84	98	102	1 mo	35	39	52	65	69
2 mo	68	72	87	101	106	2 mo	34	38	51	64	68
3 mo	70	74	89	104	108	3 mo	35	38	51	64	68
4 mo	71	75	90	105	109	4 mo	35	39	52	65	68
5 mo	72	76	91	106	110	5 mo	36	39	52	65	69
6 mo	72	76	91	106	110	6 mo	36	40	53	66	69
7 mo	72	76	91	106	110	7 mo	36	40	53	66	70
8 mo	72	76	91	106	110	8 mo	37	40	53	66	70
9 mo	72	76	91	106	110	9 mo	37	41	54	67	70
10 mo	72	76	91	106	110	10 mo	37	41	54	67	71
11 mo	72	76	91	105	110	11 mo	38	41	54	67	71
1 yr	72	76	91	105	110	1 yr	38	41	54	67	71
2 yr	71	76	90	105	109	2 yr	40	43	56	69	73
3 yr	72	76	91	106	110	3 yr	40	43	56	69	73
4 yr	73	78	92	107	111	4 yr	40	43	56	69	73
5 yr	75	79	94	109	113	5 yr	40	43	56	69	73
6 yr	77	81	96	111	115	6 yr	40	44	57	70	74
7 yr	78	83	97	112	116	7 yr	41	45	58	71	75
8 yr	80	84	99	114	118	8 yr	43	46	59	72	76
9 yr	81	86	100	115	119	9 yr	44	48	61	74	77
10 yr	83	87	102	117	121	10 yr	46	49	62	75	79
11 yr	86	90	105	119	123	11 yr	47	51	64	77	81
12 yr	88	92	107	122	126	12 yr	49	53	66	78	82
13 yr	90	94	109	124	128	13 yr	46	50	64	78	82
14 yr	92	96	110	125	129	14 yr	49	53	67	81	85
15 yr	93	97	111	126	130	15 yr	49	53	67	82	86
16 yr	93	97	112	127	131	16 yr	49	53	67	81	85
17 yr	93	98	112	127	131	17 yr	48	52	66	80	84
18 yr	94	98	112	127	131	18 yr	48	52	66	80	84

* K4 was used for ages less than 13; K5 was used for ages 13 and over.
Reprinted with permission from the Second Task Force on Blood Pressure Control in Children, National Heart, Lung and Blood Institute, Bethesda, MD.
Tabular data prepared by Dr. B. Rosner, 1987.

Table AP5-5
Normal Blood Pressure Readings for Boys

Age	Systolic Blood Pressure Percentile					Age	Diastolic Blood Pressure* Percentile				
	5th	10th	50th	90th	95th		5th	10th	50th	90th	95th
1 day	54	58	73	87	92	1 day	38	42	55	68	72
3 days	55	59	74	89	93	3 days	38	42	55	68	71
7 days	57	62	76	91	95	7 days	37	41	54	67	71
1 mo	67	71	86	101	105	1 mo	35	39	52	64	68
2 mo	72	76	91	106	110	2 mo	33	37	50	63	66
3 mo	72	76	91	106	110	3 mo	33	37	50	63	66
4 mo	72	76	91	106	110	4 mo	34	37	50	63	67
5 mo	72	76	91	105	110	5 mo	35	39	52	65	68
6 mo	72	76	90	105	109	6 mo	36	40	53	66	70
7 mo	71	76	90	105	109	7 mo	37	41	54	67	71
8 mo	71	75	90	105	109	8 mo	38	42	55	68	72
9 mo	71	75	90	105	109	9 mo	39	43	55	68	72
10 mo	71	75	90	105	109	10 mo	39	43	56	69	73
11 mo	71	76	90	105	109	11 mo	39	43	56	69	73
1 yr	71	76	90	105	109	1 yr	39	43	56	69	73
2 yr	72	76	91	106	110	2 yr	39	43	56	68	72
3 yr	73	77	92	107	111	3 yr	39	42	55	68	72
4 yr	74	79	93	108	112	4 yr	39	43	56	69	72
5 yr	76	80	95	109	113	5 yr	40	43	56	69	73
6 yr	77	81	96	111	115	6 yr	41	44	57	70	74
7 yr	78	83	97	112	116	7 yr	42	45	58	71	75
8 yr	80	84	99	114	118	8 yr	43	47	60	73	76
9 yr	82	86	101	115	120	9 yr	44	48	61	74	78
10 yr	84	88	102	117	121	10 yr	45	49	62	75	79
11 yr	86	90	105	119	123	11 yr	47	50	63	76	80
12 yr	88	92	107	121	126	12 yr	48	51	64	77	81
13 yr	90	94	109	124	128	13 yr	45	49	63	77	81
14 yr	93	97	112	126	131	14 yr	46	50	64	78	82
15 yr	95	99	114	129	133	15 yr	47	51	65	79	83
16 yr	98	102	117	131	136	16 yr	49	53	67	81	85
17 yr	100	104	119	134	138	17 yr	51	55	69	83	87
18 yr	102	106	121	136	140	18 yr	52	56	70	84	88

* K4 was used for ages less than 13; K5 was used for ages 13 and over.
Reprinted with permission from the Second Task Force on Blood Pressure Control in Children, National Heart, Lung and Blood Institute, Bethesda, MD.
Tabular data prepared by Dr. B. Rosner, 1987.

Nutritive Value of Breast Milk and Infant Formulas

	Normal Dilution (kcal/oz)	Approximate Percentage Composition in Normal Dilution (g/100 mL)					Approximate Electrolyte Composition in Normal Dilution					
							(mEq/L)			(mg/L)		
		Protein	Carbo-hydrate	Fat	PUFA	Minerals	*Na*	*K*	*Cl*	*Ca*	*P*	*Fe*
Human milk, mature, average	22	1.1	7.0	3.8	—	0.21	6.5	14	12	340	150	1.5
Cow's milk, market, average	20	3.3	4.8	3.7	—	0.72	25	35	29	1.170	920	1.0
Cow's milk, evaporated	22	3.8	5.4	4.0	—	0.80	28	39	32	1.300	1.100	1.0
Prepared Formulas, Cow's Milk Based												
Aptamil Milupa	20	1.5	7.2	3.6	0.43	0.30	7.8	21.2	11.2	580	350	8.0
Bebelac No. 1, LYEMPF	20	1.5	8.0	3.5	0.55	0.30	9.1	15.9	12.7	550	280	5.5
Benamil, Wyeth Ayerst	20	1.5	7.1	3.6	0.36	0.22	7.8	15.5	11.8	460	360	12.0
Dumex Infant Formula, Dumex	20	2.0	7.3	3.2	0.40	0.37	8.6	15.0	13.0	594	396	7.9
Dutch Baby Food, Friesland	20	1.5	7.8	3.3	0.40	0.33	4.6	23.8	14.9	590	400	4.0
Enfamil, Mead Johnson	20	1.5	7.0	3.8	0.68	0.30	8.0	18.7	12.0	530	360	3.4
Frisolac, Friesland	20	1.4	7.4	3.5	0.48	0.31	4.6	25.4	13.9	560	300	6.2
Gerber Baby Formula	20	1.5	7.2	3.7	0.67	0.37	8.7	18.7	13.2	510	390	3.4
Good Start, Carnation	20	1.6	7.4	3.5	0.80	0.28	7.0	16.5	11.3	430	240	10.0
Lactogen, Nestlē	20	1.7	7.4	3.4	0.46	0.34	9.1	18.5	13.8	530	440	8.0
Lactogen FP, Nestlē	20	3.1	7.5	2.7	0.35	0.69	20.0	35.0	29.2	1110	860	12.0
Mamex, Dumex	20	1.6	7.3	3.5	0.45	0.26	6.0	14.0	10.0	500	333	7.7
Nan, Nestlē	20	1.6	7.6	3.4	0.44	0.25	7.0	16.9	12.4	420	210	8.1
Nativa, Nestlē	20	1.8	6.9	3.6	0.60	0.26	7.4	17.4	13.0	410	210	8.1
Nutricia	20	1.8	7.1	3.4	0.28	0.23	8.3	17.2	12.0	600	370	8.0
Pertargon, Nestlē	20	1.9	8.0	3.0	0.39	0.43	13.9	23.1	19.4	700	580	8.0
Similac, Ross (also 13, 24, 27 kcal/oz)	20	1.5	7.2	3.7	0.87	0.23	7.9	18.1	12.9	490	380	12.0
Similac PM 60/40, Ross	20	1.6	6.9	3.8	1.2	0.22	7.1	14.9	11.0	380	190	1.5
SMA, Wyeth-Ayerst (also 13, 24, 27 kcal/oz)	20	1.5	7.2	3.6	0.35	0.25	6.5	14.0	11.0	420	290	12.0
Soy Based												
Alsoy, Nestlē	20	1.9	7.4	3.3	0.8	0.35	10.0	20.5	13.8	600	430	8.0
Frisosoy, Friesland	20	1.7	7.1	3.5	0.5	0.29	5.7	28.9	13.9	460	270	7.0
Gerber Soy	20	2.0	6.8	3.6	0.7	0.4	13.9	20.0	16.6	640	500	12.2
Isomil (soy), Mead Johnson	20	1.7	7.0	3.7	1.4	—	13.0	18.0	15.0	710	510	12.0
Isomil/DF	20	1.7	6.8	3.7	0.9	—	13.0	18.0	15.0	693	495	12.0
Nursoy (soy), Wyeth-Ayerst	20	1.8	6.9	3.6	0.34	0.35	8.7	18.9	10.6	634	443	12.7
ProSobee (soy), Mead Johnson	20	2.0	6.8	3.6	0.67	0.4	10.4	21.0	15.2	710	560	12.2
Soyalac (soy), Loma Linda	20	2.1	6.8	3.7	1.9	0.4	13.0	20.0	13.0	635	370	1.3

	Normal Dilution (kcal/oz)	Approximate Percentage Composition in Normal Dilution (g/100 mL)					Approximate Electrolyte Composition in Normal Dilution			
							(mEq/L)		(mg/L)	
		Protein	Carbo-hydrate	Fat	Notes	mOsm	*Na*	*K*	*Ca*	*P*
Specialty Products										
Accupep, Sherwood	30	4.0	19.0	1.0	1	490	30	30	625	625
Alfare, Nestlē	20	2.2	7.0	3.3	—	—	17	21	540	340
Alimentum, Ross	20	1.9	6.9	3.8	2	370	13	20	710	510
Alitra, Q, Ross	30	5.2	16.5	1.5	3, 5	575	43	31	733	733

Table continued on following page

	Normal Dilution (kcal/oz)	Approximate Percentage Composition in Normal Dilution (g/100 mL)					Approximate Electrolyte Composition in Normal Dilution			
							(mEq/L)		(mg/L)	
		Protein	Carbo-hydrate	Fat	Notes	mOsm	*Na*	*K*	*Ca*	*P*
Specialty Products										
Babelac FL, LYEMPF	20	1.7	7.5	3.7	—	—	9.1	16	550	280
Compleat Mod, Sandoz	32	4.3	14.0	3.7	—	300	43	36	670	870
Comply, Sherwood	45	6.0	18.0	6.0	—	410	48	47	1000	1000
Criticare H, Mead Johnson	31	3.8	22.0	0.5	2	650	27	34	530	530
Deliver, Mead Johnson	59	7.5	20	10.2	—	—	35	43	1010	1010
Enfamil Human Milk Fortifier, Mead	14	0.7	2.7	0.04	—	—	7	15	60	3
Johnson	33	4.0	16.2	3.7	—	480	37	43	720	720
Enrich, Ross	31	3.7	14.5	3.7	—	470	37	40	530	530
Ensure, Ross										
Ensure HN, Ross	31	4.4	14.1	3.5	—	470	35	40	750	750
Ensure Plus, Ross	45	5.5	19.2	5.3	—	690	46	50	700	700
Ensure Plus HN, Ross	45	6.3	20.0	5.0	—	650	51	47	1050	1050
Entera, Fresenius	32	4.0	14.6	3.6	—	420	35	34	800	640
Entralife, Corpak	30	3.5	13.6	3.5	—	300	26	25	500	500
Entralife HN30, Corpak	4.2	13.3	3.4	—	—	300	40	32	800	800
Follow-up, Carnation	20	1.7	8.8	2.7	—	—	11.3	22.5	900	600
Frisopep 1, Friesland	20	1.5	7.2	3.5	—	—	51	254	500	300
Isocal, Mead Johnson	31	4.4	12.4	4.4	—	230	41	41	850	850
Isocal HN, Mead Johnson	31	4.4	12.4	4.4	—	230	41	41	850	850
Isoservice, Sandoz	36	4.3	17.0	4.1	—	360	52	43	670	670
Jevity, Ross	32	4.4	15.2	3.7	—	300	40	40	912	759
Lactofree, Mead Johnson	20	1.5	7.0	3.7	—	—	8.7	19	530	360
Magnacal, Sherwood	60	7.0	25.0	8.0	—	590	43	32	1000	1000
Meritene, Sandoz	32	6.9	12.0	3.4	—	690	48	32	2200	1900
Newtrition, Knight	32	3.6	41.0	4.0	—	450	42	?	600	600
Newtrition Isotonic, Knight	32	3.6	14.8	3.6	—	300	26	26	600	600
Newtrition Isofiber, Knight	36	5.0	16.0	3.7	—	310	36	32	847	847
Nutrapak, Corpak	32	3.7	14.5	3.7	—	450	37	40	530	530
Nutren 1.0, Clintec	30	4.0	12.7	3.8	—	340	22	32	500	500
Nutren 1.5, Clintec	45	6.0	17.0	6.7	—	600	33	48	750	750
Nutren 2.0, Clintec	60	8.0	19.6	10.6	—	800	43	64	1000	1000
Nutramigen, Mead Johnson	20	1.9	9.1	2.6	2	290	14	18	630	420
Osmolite, Ross	31	3.7	14.5	3.8	—	300	28	26	530	530
Pediasure, Ross	30	3.0	10.9	4.9	—	325	16	33	970	800
Peptamen, Clinitec	30	4.0	12.7	3.9	1	260	22	32	600	500
Perative, Ross	38	6.7	17.7	3.7	3, 5	385	45	44	867	867
Portagen, Mead Johnson	20	2.4	7.8	3.2	—	220	16	22	635	470
Pregestimil PO, Mead Johnson	20	1.9	7.0	3.8	2	290	14	19	630	420
Profiber, Sherwood	30	4.0	14.7	3.5	—	300	32	32	800	800
Promil, Wyeth-Ayerst	20	2.5	8.0	2.8	—	360	14	26	1150	650
Pulmocre, Ross	45	6.3	10.5	9.2	—	465	57	49	1050	1050
RCF, Ross	40	2.0	0	3.6	—	74	13	19	700	500
Resource, Sandoz	32	3.7	14.5	3.7	—	430	39	41	525	525
Resource Plus	45	5.5	20.0	5.3	—	600	57	54	700	700
S14, Wyeth-Ayerst	20	1.1	7.1	3.7	—	280	7	12	420	320
S-29, Wyeth-Ayerst	20	1.7	10.1	2.3	—	360	0.4	8	140	170
S-44, Wyeth-Ayerst	20	1.7	10.1	2.3	—	360	0.4	8	140	170
Sustacal, Mead Johnson	30	6.1	14.0	2.3	—	620	41	54	1010	930
Sustacal Plus	45	6.1	19.0	5.8	—	520	36	38	850	850
Tolerex, Sandoz	30	2.1	22.8	0.15	3	550	20	30	550	550
Traumacal, Mead Johnson	45	8.3	14.3	6.8	—	440	51	36	750	750
Vital HN, Ross	30	4.1	18.0	1.1	3, 4, 5	500	25	36	670	670
Vitaneed, Sherwood	30	4.0	13.5	3.5	—	300	27	32	670	670
Vivonex Ten, Sandoz	30	3.8	20.6	0.3	3	630	20	20	500	500

(1) Hydrolyzed whey, (2) hydrolyzed casein, (3) amino acids, (4) partially hydrolyzed whey, and (5) others. Other speciality formulas are available from various manufacturers, low (or free of) carbohydrate, protein, sodium, phenylalanine, branched chain amino acids, histidine, homocystine, lysine, tyrosine, and methionine.

	Normal Dilution (kcal/oz)	Approximate Percentage Composition in Normal Dilution (g/100 mL)					Approximate Electrolyte Composition in Normal Dilution (mEq/L)			(mg/L)		
		Protein	Carbo-hydrate	Fat	PUFA	Minerals	*Na*	*K*	*Cl*	*Ca*	*P*	*Fe*
Formulas for Low-Birthweight Infants												
Alprem, Prenan, Nestlē	21	2.1	8.0	3.4	0.5	0.4	11	19	11.3	700	460	11
Enfamil, Premature Formula, Mead Johnson	24	2.4	8.9	4.1	0.8	0.5	14	23	19.4	950	480	1.3
Similac, 24 LBW, Ross	24	2.2	8.5	4.5	0.6	0.5	13	31	23	730	560	3
Similac Special Care, Ross	24	2.2	8.6	4.4	0.6	0.5	15	27	19	1440	720	1.5
SMA Preemie, Wyeth-Ayerst	24	2.0	8.6	4.4	0.4	0.4	13.9	19	15	750	400	3

	kcal/g	kcal/mL
Carbohydrate Supplements		
LC, Corpak	—	2.5
Moducal, Mead Johnson	3.8	—
PC, Corpak	4.0	—
Pollycose, Ross	3.8	2.0
Sumacal, Sherwood	3.8	—
Fat Supplements		
Liposyn, Abbott 10%	1.1	1.1
Liposyn, Abbott 20%	2.0	2.0
Intralipid, Cutter 10%	1.1	1.1
Intralipid, Cutter 20%	2.0	2.0
MCT Oil, Mead Johnson	7.7	7.1
MCT Supplement, Corpak	6.1	—
Microlipid, Sherwood	4.5	2.2
Protein Supplements		
Casec, Mead Johnson	3.7	—
Electrodialyzed Whey, Wyeth-Ayerst	1.4	—
Pro-Mix, Corpak	1.4	—
Pro-Mod, Ross	4.2	—
Propac, Sherwood	4.0	—

From Behrman, R. E., Kliegman, R. M., & Arvin, A. M. (Eds.). (1996). *Nelson textbook of pediatrics* (15th ed., pp. 160–162). Philadelphia: W. B. Saunders. Reprinted with permission.

APPENDIX 7

Nutritive Value of Baby Foods

Food	Serving (g)	Energy (kcal)	Protein (g)	Fat (g)	Carbohydrate (g)	Sodium (mg)	Calcium (mg)	Iron (mg)	Vitamin A (IU)	Thiamine (mg)	Riboflavin (mg)	Niacin (mg)	Ascorbic Acid (mg)
Cereals													
Barley	2.4	9	0.3	0.1	1.8	1	19	1.1		0.07	0.07	0.9	0
High protein	2.4	9	0.9	0.1	1.1	1	17	1.8		0.06	0.07	0.8	0
Mixed	2.4	9	0.3	0.1	1.8	1	18	1.5		0.06	0.07	0.8	0
Oatmeal	2.4	10	0.3	0.2	1.7	1	18	1.8		0.07	0.06	0.9	0
Rice	2.4	9	0.2	0.1	1.9	1	20	1.8		0.06	0.05	0.8	0
Dinners, Jar													
Beef and egg noodle	213	122	5.4	4.0	15.7	37	18	0.9	1,400	0.06	0.08	1.2	3
Chicken and noodles, jr.	213	109	4.1	3.0	16.1	36	36	0.8	1,900	0.06	0.07	1.1	3
Macaroni and ham, jr.	213	127	6.8	2.9	18.0	101	159	0.8	1,100	0.12	0.21	1.7	5
Turkey and rice, jr.	213	104	3.8	2.9	15.3	33	50	0.6	2,200	0.02	0.06	0.6	3
Spaghetti, tomato, beef, jr.	213	135	5.4	2.7	21.6	42	39	1.1	1,500	0.14	0.15	2.3	5
Egg Yolks	94	191	9.4	16.3	0.9	37	72	2.6	1,200	0.07	0.25	1.45	1
Fruits													
Applesauce, jr.	213	79	0.1	0.0	21.9	5	10	0.4	20	0.03	0.06	0.1	81
Applesauce, apricots, jr.	220	104	0.5	0.5	27.3	6	13	0.6	745	0.03	0.07	0.3	39
Bananas, tapioca, jr.	220	147	0.8	0.4	39.1	21	17	0.7	100	0.03	0.04	0.5	57
Peaches	220	157	1.3	0.4	41.6	10	11	0.6	400	0.03	0.07	1.4	42
Pears	213	93	0.6	0.2	24.7	4	18	0.5	70	0.03	0.06	0.4	47
Meats, Poultry													
Beef	99	105	14.3	4.9	0	65	8	1.6	100	0.01	0.16	3.3	2
Chicken	99	148	14.6	9.5	0	50	54	1.0	200	0.01	0.16	3.4	2
Ham	99	123	14.9	6.6	0	66	5	1.0	30	0.14	0.19	2.8	2
Lamb	99	111	15.0	5.2	2.5	73	7	1.6	30	0.02	0.20	3.2	2
Turkey	99	128	15.2	7.0	0	72	28	1.3	600	0.02	0.25	3.4	2
Vegetables													
Beans	206	51	2.5	0.3	11.8	3	133	2.2	900	0.04	0.21	0.7	17
Beets	128	43	1.7	0.1	9.8	106	18	0.4	40	0.01	0.06	0.2	4
Carrots	213	67	1.7	0.4	15.4	104	49	0.8	25,000	0.05	0.09	1.1	12
Mixed	213	88	3.1	0.8	17.4	77	24	0.9	9,000	0.06	0.07	1.4	5
Peas	213	113	7.0	1.1	19.0	15	34	1.9	700	0.15	0.13	2.0	9
Squash	213	51	1.8	0.4	12.0	3	50	0.7	4,000	0.02	0.14	0.8	17
Sweet potatoes	220	113	2.4	0.3	30.7	49	35	0.8	15,000	0.06	0.08	0.8	21

From Behrman, R. E., Kliegman, R. M., & Arvin, A. M. (Eds.). (1996). *Nelson textbook of pediatrics* (15th ed., pp. 2083–2084). Philadelphia: W. B. Saunders. Reprinted with permission.

APPENDIX 8

International Immunization Schedules

Table AP8–1
Canadian Routine Immunization Schedule for Infants and Children

Age	Immunization Against				
2 months	Diphtheria	Pertussis	Tetanus	Poliomyelitis	*Haemophilus influenzae* b[1]
4 months	Diphtheria	Pertussis	Tetanus	Poliomyelitis	*Haemophilus influenzae* b
6 months	Diphtheria	Pertussis	Tetanus	Poliomyelitis[2]	*Haemophilus influenzae* b
12 months	Measles[3]	Mumps[3]	Rubella[3]		
18 months	Diphtheria	Pertussis	Tetanus	Poliomyelitis	*Haemophilus influenzae* b
4–6 years	Diphtheria	Pertussis	Tetanus	Poliomyelitis	
9–13 years	Hepatitis B[4]				
14–16 years	Diphtheria		Tetanus	Poliomyelitis[2]	

[1] *Haemophilus influenzae* b requires a series of immunizations. The exact number and timing of each may vary with the brand of vaccine used.
[2] If "oral" polio virus vaccine is used exclusively in a series of immunizations, this dose may be omitted.
[3] A second dose of MMR vaccine is recommended for children and youth. It may be administered anytime after a minimum one-month waiting period. (Provincial schedules differ.)
[4] Hepatitis B requires a series of immunizations. In some jurisdictions, they may be administered at a younger age.
Adapted from National Advisory Committee on Immunization. (1993). *Canadian immunization guide* (4th ed.). Authority of the Minister of National Health and Welfare, Health Protection Branch, Laboratory Centre for Disease Control.

Table AP8-2
Canadian Routine Immunization Schedules for Children Not Immunized in Early Infancy

Timing	Immunization Against				
For Children 7 Years of Age and Younger					
First visit	Diphtheria	Pertussis	Tetanus	Poliomyelitis	*Haemophilus influenzae* b
	Measles[4]	Mumps[4]	Rubella[4]		
2 months later	Diphtheria	Pertussis	Tetanus	Poliomyelitis	*Haemophilus influenzae* b[5]
2 months later	Diphtheria	Pertussis	Tetanus	Poliomyelitis[2]	
6–12 months later	Diphtheria	Pertussis	Tetanus	Poliomyelitis	*Haemophilus influenzae* b[5]
4–6 years[6]	Diphtheria	Pertussis	Tetanus	Poliomyelitis	
14–16 years	Diphtheria[3]	Tetanus[3]	Poliomyelitis[2]		
For Children 7 Years of Age and Older					
First visit	Diphtheria[3]		Tetanus[3]	Poliomyeltis	
	Measles	Mumps	Rubella		
2 months later	Diphtheria[3]		Tetanus[3]	Poliomyelitis	
6–12 months later	Diphtheria[3]		Tetanus[3]	Poliomyelitis	
10 years later	Diphtheria[3]		Tetanus[3]		

[1] *Haemophilus influenzae* b requires a series of immunizations. The exact number and timing of each may vary with the brand of vaccine used.
[2] If "oral" polio virus vaccine is used exclusively in a series of immunizations, this dose may be omitted.
[3] A second dose of MMR vaccine is recommended for children and youth. It may be administered anytime after a minimum one-month waiting period. (Provincial schedules differ.)
[4] Delay until subsequent visit if child is <12 months of age.
[5] Recommended schedule and number of doses depend on the product used and the age of the child when vaccination is begun. Not required past age 5.
[6] Omit these doses if the previous doses of DPT and polio were given after the fourth birthday.
From National Advisory Committee on Immunization. (1993). *Canadian immunization guide* (4th ed.). Authority of the Minister of National Health and Welfare, Health Protection Branch, Laboratory Centre for Disease Control.

Table AP8-3
Immunization Schedule for Infants Recommended by the World Health Organization (WHO) Expanded Programme on Immunization

Age	Vaccine	Hepatitis B Vaccine* (two alternative schemes) Alternative A	Alternative B
Birth	BCG, OPV-0	HB-1	
6 weeks	DPT-1, OPV-1	HB-2	HB-1
10 weeks	DPT-2, OPV-2		HB-2
14 weeks	DPT-3, OPV-3	HB-3	HB-3
9 months	Measles, Yellow fever†		

OPV, oral polio vaccine; DPT, diphtheria, pertussis, tetanus triple vaccine; HB, hepatitis B vaccine; BCG, vaccine against tuberculosis.
* Scheme A is recommended in countries where perinatal transmission of HBV is frequent (e.g., Southeast Asia), and scheme B in countries where perinatal transmission is less frequent (e.g., sub-Saharan Africa).
† In countries where yellow fever poses a risk. Measles vaccine is usually given at 12–15 months of age in industrialized countries where the threat of the disease comes after the first year of life. Such a policy benefits from the increased vaccine efficacy after 1 year of age. The vaccine is often combined with rubella and/or mumps vaccine when it is referred to as MR or MMR vaccine. Specific inquiries about a country's immunization schedule should be referred to the national or local authorities.
From National Advisory Committee on Immunization. (1993). *Canadian immunization guide* (4th ed.). Authority of the Minister of National Health and Welfare, Health Protection Branch, Laboratory Centre for Diseae Control.

APPENDIX 9

*Canadian Organizations and Associations Involved in Health Promotion**

Allergy/Asthma Information Association
30 Eglinton Avenue W.
Suite 750
Mississauga, ON L5R 3E7
(905) 712-2242
FAX: (905) 712-2245

Allergy Foundation of Canada
P.O. Box 1904
Saskatoon, SK S7K 3S5
(306) 373-7591

Aplastic Anaemia Family Association of Canada
22 Alkenhead Road
Etobicoke, ON M9R 2Z3
(416) 235-0468
FAX: (416) 864-9929

Asthma Society of Canada
130 Bridgeland Avenue
North York, ON M6A 1Z4
(416) 787-4050
FAX: (416) 787-5807

Autism Society Canada
129 Yorkville Avenue
Unit 202
Toronto, ON M5R 1C4
(416) 922-0302
FAX: (416) 922-1032

Bulimia Anorexia Nervosa Association
3640 Wells Avenue
Windsor, ON N9C 1T9
(519) 253-7421 (hotline)
(519) 253-7545
FAX: (519) 258-0488

Canadian Association for School Health
2835 Country Woods Drive
Surrey, BC V4A 9P9
(604) 535-7664
FAX: (604) 531-6454

Canadian Association of the Deaf
2435 Holly Lane, Suite 205
Ottawa, ON K1V 7P2
(613) 526-4785
FAX: (613) 526-4718

Canadian Association of Social Workers
383 Parkdale Avenue
Suite 402
Ottawa, ON K1Y 4R4
(613) 729-6668
FAX: (613) 729-9608

Canadian Cancer Society
10 Alcorn Avenue
Suite 200
Toronto, ON M4V 3B1
(416) 961-7223
FAX: (416) 961-4189

Canadian Cardiovascular Society
360 Victoria Avenue
Suite 401
Westmount, PQ H3Z 2N4
(514) 482-3407
FAX: (514) 482-6574

Canadian Child Day Care Federation
120 Holland Avenue
Suite 306
Ottawa, ON K1Y 0X6
(613) 729-5289
FAX: (613) 729-3159

Canadian Children's Safety Network
20 Queen Street W.
Suite 200
Toronto, ON M5H 3V7
(416) 979-4012
FAX: (416) 977-35

Canadian Coalition for the Prevention of Developmental Disabilities
c/o Canadian Institute of Child Health
885 Meadowlands Drive
Suite 512
Ottawa, ON K2C 3N2
(613) 224-4144
FAX: (613) 224-4145

Canadian Council of the Blind
396 Cooper Street
Suite 405
Ottawa, ON K2P 2H7
(613) 567-0311
FAX: (613) 567-2728

Canadian Cystic Fibrosis Foundation
2221 Yonge Street
Suite 601
Toronto, ON M4S 2B4
(416) 485-9149
FAX: (416) 485-0960

Canadian Dermatology Foundation
450 Central Avenue
Suite 308
London, ON N6B 2E8
(519) 432-3968

Canadian Diabetes Association
15 Toronto Street
Suite 1001
Toronto, ON M5C 2E3
(416) 363-3373
FAX: (416) 363-3393

Canadian Down Syndrome Society
12837 76th Avenue
Suite 206
Surrey, BC V3W 2V3
(604) 599-6009
FAX: (604) 599-6165

Canadian Foundation for the Study of Infant Deaths
586 Eglinton Avenue E.
Suite 308
Toronto, ON M4P 1P2
(416) 488-3260
FAX: (416) 488-3864

Canadian Hemophilia Society
1450 City Councilors Street
Suite 840
Montreal, PQ H3A 2E6
(514) 848-0503
FAX: (514) 848-9661

Canadian Hospital Association
17 York Street
Suite 100
Ottawa, ON K1N 9J6
(613) 241-8005
FAX: (613) 241-5005

---

*This is a partial listing of organizations and associations. For a more complete listing contact the Health Promotion Directorate, Health Canada, Ottawa, ON K1A 1B4, (613) 954-8842, FAX: (613) 990-7097.

Canadian Institute of Child Health
885 Meadowlands Drive E.
Suite 512
Ottawa, ON K2C 3N2
(613) 241-4144
FAX: (613) 224-4145

Canadian Medical Association
1867 Alta Vista Drive
Ottawa, ON K1G 3Y6
(613) 731-9013
FAX: (613) 731-9013

Canadian Nurses Association
50 The Driveway
Ottawa, ON K2P 1E2
(613) 237-2133
FAX: (613) 237-3520

Canadian Orthopaedic Association
1440 St. Catherine Street W.
Suite 421
Montreal, PQ H3G 1R8
(514) 874-9003
FAX: (514) 874-0464

Canadian Osteogenesis Imperfecta Society
c/o 128 Thornhill Crescent
Chatham, ON N7L 4M3
(519) 436-0025
FAX: (519) 627-0557

Canadian Paediatric Society
c/o Children's Hospital of Eastern Ontario
401 Smyth Road
Ottawa, ON K1H 8L1
(613) 737-2728
FAX: (613) 737-2794

Canadian Psoriasis Foundation
1306 Wellington Street
Suite 500A
Ottawa, ON K1Y 3B2
1-800-265-0926
(613) 728-4000
FAX: (613) 728-8913

Canadian Rehabilitation Council for the Disabled
45 Sheppard Avenue E.
Suite 801
Toronto, ON M2N 5W9
(416) 250-7490
FAX: (416) 229-1371

Canadian Society for the Prevention of Cruelty to Children
P.O. Box 700
356 First Street
Calgary, AB T2E 7J2
(705) 526-5647
FAX: (705) 526-0214

Community Health Nurses Association of Canada
c/o Lee Fredeen-Kohlert
P.O. Box 281
Millet, AB T0C 1Z0
(403) 387-4264

Disability Information Services of Canada
501 18th Avenue S.W.
Suite 304
Calgary, AB T2S 0C7
(403) 244-2836
TTY/TDD: (403) 229-2177
FAX: (403) 229-1878

Epilepsy Canada
1470 Peel Street
Suite 745
Montreal, PQ H3A 1T1
(514) 845-7855
FAX: (514) 845-7866

Juvenile Diabetes Foundation Canada
89 Granton Drive
Richmond Hill, ON L4B 2N5
(800) 668-0274
(905) 889-4171
FAX: (905) 889-4209

Kidney Foundation of Canada
5160 Decarie Boulevard
Suite 780
Montreal, PQ H3X 2H9
(514) 369-4806
FAX: (514) 369-2472

Lung Association—National Office
1900 City Park Drive
Suite 508
Gloucester, ON K1J 1A3
(613) 747-6776
FAX: (613) 747-7430

National Cancer Institute of Canada
10 Alcorn Avenue
Suite 200
Toronto, ON M4V 3B1
(416) 961-7223
FAX: (416) 961-4189

National Eating Disorder Information Center
CW 1-211
200 Elizabeth Street
Toronto, ON M5G 2C4
(416) 340-4156
FAX: (416) 340-3430

National Institute of Nutrition
265 Carling Avenue
Suite 302
Ottawa, ON K1S 2E1
(613) 235-3355
FAX: (613) 235-7032

North American Chronic Pain Association of Canada
150 Central Park Drive
Suite 105
Brampton, ON L6T 2T9
(416) 793-5230
FAX: (416) 793-8781

One Parent Families Association of Canada
6979 Yonge Street
Suite 203
Willowdal, ON M2M 3X9
(416) 226-0062

Psoriasis Society of Canada
P.O. Box 25015
Halifax, NS B3M 4H4
(902) 443-8680
FAX: (902) 457-1664

Spina Bifida Association of Canada
388 Donald Street
Suite 220
Winnipeg, MB R3B 2J4
(800) 565-9488
(204) 957-1784
FAX: (204) 957-1794

Tracheo Esophageal Fistula
Parent Network
c/o 42 Saskatoon Drive
Etobicoke, ON M9P 2E9
(416) 249-8710

APPENDIX 10

NANDA-Approved Nursing Diagnoses

Activity Intolerance
Activity Intolerance, Risk for
Adaptive Capacity: Intracranial, Decreased
Adjustment, Impaired
Airway Clearance, Ineffective
* Anticipatory Grieving
Anxiety
Aspiration, Risk for
Body Image Disturbance
Body Temperature, Risk for Altered
* Bowel Incontinence
Breastfeeding, Effective
Breastfeeding, Ineffective
Breastfeeding, Interrupted
Breathing Pattern, Ineffective
Caregiver Role Strain
Caregiver Role Strain, Risk for
* Chronic Low Self Esteem
* Chronic Pain
* Colonic Constipation
* Communication, Impaired Verbal
Community Coping, Ineffective
Community, Potential for Enhanced
Confusion, Acute
Confusion, Chronic
Constipation
* Constipation, Colonic
* Constipation, Perceived
Decisional Conflict (Specify)
Decreased Cardiac Output
Defensive Coping
Denial, Ineffective
Diarrhea
Disorganized Infant Behavior
Disorganized Infant Behavior, Risk for
Disuse Syndrome, Risk for
Diversional Activity Deficit
* Dysfunctional Grieving
Dysfunctional Ventilatory Weaning Response (DVWR)
Dysreflexia
Energy Field Disturbance
Environmental Interpretation Syndrome, Impaired
Family Coping: Compromised, Ineffective
Family Coping: Disabling, Ineffective
Family Coping: Potential for Growth
Family Process: Alcoholism, Altered
Family Processes, Altered
Fatigue
Fear
Fluid Volume Deficit
Fluid Volume Deficit, Risk for
Fluid Volume Excess
* Functional Incontinence
Gas Exchange, Impaired
Grieving, Anticipatory
Grieving, Dysfunctional
Growth and Development, Altered
Health Maintenance, Altered
Health Seeking Behaviors (Specify)
Home Maintenance Management, Impaired
Hopelessness
Hyperthermia
Hypothermia
* Incontinence, Bowel
Incontinence, Functional
* Incontinence, Reflex
* Incontinence, Stress
* Incontinence, Total
* Incontinence, Urge
Individual Coping, Ineffective
Infant Feeding Pattern, Ineffective
Infection, Risk for
Injury, Risk for
Knowledge Deficit (Specify)
Loneliness, Risk for
Management of Therapeutic Regimen: Community, Ineffective
Management of Therapeutic Regimen: Families, Ineffective

*These are duo-referenced for ease and speed in locating the correct diagnosis.

From North American Nursing Diagnosis Association (1994). *NANDA nursing diagnoses: Definitions and Classifications 1995–1996*. Philadelphia: Author. Reprinted with permission.

Management of Therapeutic Regimen: Individual, Effective
Management of Therapeutic Regimen (Individuals), Ineffective Noncompliance (Specify)
Memory, Impaired
Nutrition: Less than Body Requirements, Altered
Nutrition: More than Body Requirements, Altered
Nutrition: Risk for More than Body Requirements, Altered
Oral Mucous Membrane, Altered
Organized Infant Behavior, Potential for Enhanced
Pain
* Pain, Chronic
Parent/Infant/Child Attachment, Risk for Altered
Parental Role Conflict
Parenting, Altered
Parenting, Risk for Altered
* Perceived Constipation
Perioperative Positioning Injury, Risk for
Peripheral Neurovascular Dysfunction, Risk for
Personal Identity Disturbance
Physical Mobility, Impaired
Poisoning, Risk for
Post-Trauma Response
Powerlessness
Protection, Altered
Rape-Trauma Syndrome
Rape-Trauma Syndrome: Compound Reaction
Rape-Trauma Syndrome: Silent Reaction
* Reflex Incontinence
Relocation Stress Syndrome
Role Performance, Altered
Self Care Deficit
  Bathing/Hygiene
  Feeding
  Dressing/Grooming
  Toileting
* Self-Esteem, Chronic Low
* Self-Esteem, Situational Low
Self-Esteem Disturbance
Self-Mutilation, Risk for
Sensory/Perceptual Alterations (Specify)
  Visual
  Auditory
  Kinesthetic
  Gustatory
  Tactile
  Olfactory
Sexual Dysfunction
Sexuality Patterns, Altered
* Situational Low Self-Esteem
Skin Integrity, Impaired
Skin Integrity, Risk for Impaired
Sleep Pattern Disturbance
Social Interaction, Impaired
Social Isolation
Spiritual Distress
Spiritual Well-Being, Potential for Enhanced
* Stress Incontinence
Suffocation, Risk for
Sustain Spontaneous Ventilation, Inability to
Swallowing, Impaired
Thermoregulation, Ineffective
Thought Processes, Altered
Tissue Integrity, Impaired
Tissue Perfusion, Altered (Specify Type)
  Renal
  Cerebral
  Cardiopulmonary
  Gastrointestinal
  Peripheral
* Total Incontinence
Trauma, Risk for
Unilateral Neglect
* Urge Incontinence
Urinary Elimination, Altered
Urinary Retention
* Verbal Communication, Impaired
Violence, Risk for: Self-directed or directed at others

APPENDIX 11

Reference Ranges for Laboratory Tests

Prefixes Denoting Decimal Factors

Prefix	Symbol
mega	M
kilo	k
hecto	h
deka	da
deci	d
centi	c
milli	m
micro	μ
nano	n
pico	p
femto	f

To conserve space, the following common abbreviations are used.

Abbreviations

Ab	absorbance
AI	angiotensin I
AU	arbitrary unit
cAMP	cyclic adenosine 3′,5′ monophosphate
cap	capillary
CH^{50}	dilution required to lyse 50% of indicator RBC; indicates complement activity
CHF	congestive heart failure
CKBB	brain isoenzyme of creatine kinase
CKMB	heart isoenzyme of creatine kinase
CNS	central nervous system
conc.	concentration
Cr.	creatinine
d	diem, day, days
F	female
g	gram
hr	hour, hours
Hb	hemoglobin
HbCO	carboxyhemoglobin
Hgb	hemoglobin
hpf	high-power field
HPLC	high-performance liquid chromatography
IFA	indirect fluorescent antibody
IU	International Unit of hormone activity
L	liter
M	male
MCV	mean corpuscular volume
mEq/L	milliequivalents per liter
min	minute, minutes
mm^3	cubic millimeter; equivalent to microliter (μL)
mm Hg	millimeters of mercury
mo	month, months
mol	mole
mOsm	milliosmole
MW	relative molecular weight
Na	sodium
nm	nanometer (wavelength)
Pa	pascal
pc	postprandial
RBC	red blood cell(s); erythrocyte(s)
RIA	radioimmunoassay
RID	radial immunodiffusion

Symbols

>	greater than
≥	greater than or equal to
<	less than
≤	less than or equal to
±	plus/minus
≅	approximately equal to

Abbreviations for Specimens

S	serum
P	plasma
(H)	heparin
(LiH)	lithium heparin
(E)	EDTA
(C)	citrate
(O)	oxalate
W	whole blood
U	urine
F	feces
CSF	cerebrospinal fluid
AF	amniotic fluid
(NaC)	sodium citrate
(NH_4H)	ammonium heparinate

Abbreviations

RT	room temperature
s	second, seconds
SD	standard deviation
std.	standard
therap.	therapeutic
U	International Unit of enzyme activity
V	volume
WBC	white blood cell(s)
WHO	World Health Organization
wk	week, weeks
yr	year, years

Test	Specimen	Reference Range		Reference Range (SI)
Activated partial thromboplastin time (APTT)	P(C)	25–35 s Infant: <90 s		25–35 s Infant: <90 s
Adrenocorticotropic hormone (ACTH)	P(H)	Cord blood	130–160 pg/mL	130–160 μg/L
		1–7 d postnatal	100–140 pg/mL	100–140 μg/L
		Adult		
		0800 hr	25–100 pg/mL	25–100 μg/L
		1800 hr	<50 pg/mL	<50 μg/L
Alanine aminotransferase (ALT, SGPT)		0–5 d	6–50 U/L	6–50 U/L
	S	1–19 yr	5–45 U/L	5–45 U/L
Albumin	P	Premature 1 d	1.8–3.0 g/dL	18–30 g/L
		Full-term <6 d	2.5–3.4 g/dL	25–34 g/L
		<5 yr	3.9–5.0 g/dL	39–50 g/L
		5–19 yr	4.0–5.3 g/dL	40–53 g/L
	U	4–16 yr	3.35–15.3 mg/24 hr/ 1.73 m^2	
	CSF	10–30 mg/dL		100–300 mg/L
Aldosterone	S, P(H,E)	Ad lib Na intake		
		Premature infants, supine		
		26–28 wk	5–635 ng/dL	0.14–17.6 nmol/L
		31–35 wk	19–141 ng/dL	0.53–3.9 nmol/L
		Full-term infants, supine		
		3 d	7–184 ng/dL	0.19–5.1 nmol/L
		1 wk	5–175 ng/dL	0.14–4.8 nmol/L
		1–12 mo	5–90 ng/dL	0.14–2.5 nmol/L
		Children, supine		
		1–2 yr	7–54 ng/dL	0.19–1.5 nmol/L
		2–10 yr	3–35 ng/dL	0.1–0.97 nmol/L
		10–15 yr	2–22 ng/dL	0.1–0.6 nmol/L
		Adults, supine	3–16 ng/dL	0.1–0.4 nmol/L
		Children, upright		
		2–10 yr	5–80 ng/dL	0.14–2.2 nmol/L
		10–15 yr	4–48 ng/dL	0.11–1.3 nmol/L
		Adults, upright	7–30 ng/dL	0.19–0.83 nmol/L
	U	Ad lib Na intake		
		Newborn 1–3 d	20–140 μg/g Cr. 0.5–5 μg/24 hr	6.28–43.94 nmol/mmol Cr. 1.39–13.88 nmol/d
		Prepubertal 4–10 yr	4–22 μg/g Cr. 1–8 μg/24 hr	1.26–6.91 nmol/mmol Cr. 2.78–22.20 nmol/d
		Adults	1.5–20 μg/g Cr. 3–19 μg/24 hr	0.47–6.28 nmol/mmol Cr. 8.32–52.72 nmol/d
Ammonia nitrogen	S, P(LiH)	Newborn	90–150 μg N/dL	64–107 μmol/L
		0–2 wk	79–129 μg N/dL	56–92 μmol/L
		>1 mo	29–70 μg N/dL	21–50 μmol/L
		Thereafter	15–45 μg N/dL	11–32 μmol/L
		1–90 d	59–202 μg N/dL	42–144 μmol/L
		3 mo–3 yr	48–195 μg N/dL	34–139 μmol/L
	U		500–1,200 mg N/24 hr	36–86 mmol/d
Amylase	S	1–19 yr	35–127 U/L	35–127 U/L
Pancreatic isoenzymes	S, P(H)	Cord blood 8 mo	0–34%	0–0.34 fraction of total
		9 mo–4 yr	5–56%	0.05–0.56 fraction of total
		5–19 yr	23–59%	0.23–0.59 fraction of total
Anion gap (Na − (Cl + CO_2))	P(H)	7–16 mmol/L		7–16 mmol/L

Table continued on following page

Test	Specimen	Reference Range			Reference Range (SI)	
Antidiuretic hormone (hADH, vasopressin)	P(E)	*Plasma Osmolarity*	*Plasma ADH*		*Plasma ADH*	
		270–280 mOsm/kg	<1.5 pg/mL		<1.5 ng/L	
		280–285 mOsm/kg	<2.5 pg/mL		<2.5 ng/L	
		285–290 mOsm/kg	1–5 pg/mL		1–5 ng/L	
		290–295 mOsm/kg	2–7 pg/mL		2–7 ng/L	
		295–300 mOsm/kg	4–12 pg/mL		4–12 ng/L	
Antistreptolysin-O titer (ASO titer)	S	≤166 Todd units				
		170–330 Todd units in school-aged children				
α_1-Antitrypsin	S	0–5 d	143–440 mg/dL		1.43–4.40 g/L	
		1–9 yr	147–245 mg/dL		1.47–2.45 g/L	
		9–19 yr	152–317 mg/dL		1.52–3.17 g/L	
	F	<1 yr				
		breast milk	<4.4 mg/g solid			
		formula	<2.9 mg/g solid			
		6 mo–44 yr				
		cow milk, regular diet	<1.7 mg/g solid			
Aspartate aminotransferase (AST, SGOT)	S	0–5 d	35–140 U/L		35–140 U/L	
		1–9 yr	15–55 U/L		15–55 U/L	
		10–19 yr	5–45 U/L		5–45 U/L	
Base excess	W(H)	Newborn	(−10)–(−2) mmol/L		(−10)–(−2) mmol/L	
		Infant	(−7)–(−1) mmol/L		(−7)–(−1) mmol/L	
		Child	(−4)–(+2) mmol/L		(−4)–(+2) mmol/L	
		Thereafter	(−3)–(+3) mmol/L		(−3)–(+3) mmol/L	
Bicarbonate	S, P	Arterial	21–28 mmol/L		21–28 mmol/L	
		Venous	22–29 mmol/L		22–29 mmol/L	
Bile acids, total	S, fasting	0.3–2.3 μg/mL			0.3–2.3 mg/L	
	S, 2-hr pc	1.8–3.2 μg/mL			1.8–3.2 mg/L	
	F	120–225 mg/24 hr			120–225 mg/24 hr	
Bilirubin	S, P					
			Premature	*Full-Term*	*Premature*	*Full-Term*
Total	S	Cord blood	<2.0 mg/dL	<2.0 mg/dL	<34 μmol/L	<34 μmol/L
		0–1 d	<8.0 mg/dL	<6.0 mg/dL	<137 μmol/L	<103 μmol/L
		1–2 d	<12.0 mg/dL	<8.0 mg/dL	<205 μmol/L	<137 μmol/L
		2–5 d	<16.0 mg/dL	<12.0 mg/dL	<274 μmol/L	<205 μmol/L
		>5 d	<2.0 mg/dL	0.2–1.0 mg/dL	<34 μmol/L	3.4–17.1 μmol/L
	U	Negative			Negative	
	AF	28 wk <0.075 mg/dL (or Ab450 <0.048)			<1.3 μmol/L (or Ab450 <0.048)	
		40 wk <0.025 mg/dL (or Ab450 <0.02)			<0.43 μmol/L (or Ab450 <0.02)	
Conjugated	S	0–0.2 mg/dL			0–3.4 μmol/L	
Bleeding time (BBT)						
Ivy		Normal 2–7 min			Normal 2–7 min	
		Borderline 7–11 min			Borderline 7–11 min	
Simplate (G–D)		2.75–8 min			2.75–8 min	
Blood volume	W(H)	M 52–83 mL/kg			M 0.052–0.083 L/kg	
		F 50–75 mL/kg			F 0.050–0.075 L/kg	
C-peptide	P	0.5–2 μg/L (fasting)			0.5–2 μg/L (fasting)	
C-reactive protein	S	Cord blood	52–1,330 ng/mL		52–1,330 μg/L	
		2–12 yr	67–1,800 ng/mL		67–1,800 μg/L	
Calcitonin	S, P(H,E)	Children	<25–70 pg/mL		<7–19.6 pmol/L	
		Adults	<25–150 pg/mL		<7–42 pmol/L	
		Higher in newborn infants				
Calcium, ionized (Ca)	S, P(H), W(H)	Cord blood	5.0–6.0 mg/dL		1.25–1.50 mmol/L	
		Newborn				
		3–24 hr	4.3–5.1 mg/dL		1.07–1.27 mmol/L	
		24–48 hr	4.0–4.7 mg/dL		1.00–1.17 mmol/L	
		Thereafter	4.8–4.92 mg/dL, or		1.12–1.23 mmol/L	
			2.24–2.46 mEq/L		1.12–1.23 mmol/L	
Calcium, total	S	Cord blood	9.0–11.5 mg/dL		2.25–2.88 mmol/L	
		Newborn				
		3–24 hr	9.0–10.6 mg/dL		2.3–2.65 mmol/L	
		24–48 hr	7.0–12.0 mg/dL		1.75–3.0 mmol/L	
		4–7 d	9.0–10.9 mg/dL		2.25–2.73 mmol/L	
		Child	8.8–10.8 mg/dL		2.2–2.70 mmol/L	
		Thereafter	8.4–10.2 mg/dL		2.1–2.55 mmol/L	
	U	Ca in diet				
		Ca-free	5–40 mg/24 hr		0.13–1.0 mmol/24 hr	
		Low to average	50–150 mg/24 hr		1.25–3.8 mmol/24 hr	
		Average (20 mmol/24 hr)	100–300 mg/24 hr		2.5–7.5 mmol/24 hr	
	CSF		2.1–2.7 mEq/L or		1.05–1.35 mmol/L	
			4.2–5.4 mg/dl		1.05–1.35 mmol/L	
	F	Average	0.64 g/24 hr		16 mmol/24 hr	

Test	Specimen		Reference Range	Reference Range (SI)
Carbon dioxide	W(H)	Newborn	27–40 mm Hg	3.6–5.3 kPa
		Infant	27–41 mm Hg	3.6–5.5 kPa
Partial pressure (PCO_2)		Thereafter		
		M	35–48 mm Hg	4.7–6.4 kPa
		F	32–45 mm Hg	4.3–6.0 kPa
Total (tCO_2)	S, P(H)	Cord blood	14–22 mmol/L	14–22 mmol/L
		Premature	14–27 mmol/L	14–27 mmol/L
		Newborn	13–22 mmol/L	13–22 mmol/L
		Infant	20–28 mmol/L	20–28 mmol/L
		Child	20–28 mmol/L	20–28 mmol/L
		Thereafter	23–30 mmol/L	23–30 mmol/L
Carbon monoxide	W(E)	Nonsmokers	<2% HbCO	HbCO fraction <0.02
		Smokers	<10%	<0.10
		Lethal	>50%	>0.5
β-Carotene	S	Infant	20–70 μg/dL	0.37–1.30 μmol/L
		Child	40–130 μg/dL	0.74–2.42 μmol/L
		Thereafter	60–200 μg/dL	1.12–3.72 μmol/L
Catecholamines, fractionated	P(E)	Norepinephrine		
		Supine	100–400 pg/mL	591–2,364 pmol/L
		Standing	300–900 pg/mL	1,773–5,320 pmol/L
		Epinephrine		
		Supine	<70 pg/mL	<382 pmol/L
		Standing	<100 pg/mL	<546 pmol/L
		Dopamine (no postural change)	<30 pg/mL	<196 pmol/L
	U	Norepinephrine		
		0–1 yr	0–10 μg/24 hr	0–59 nmol/24 hr
		1–2 yr	0–17 μg/24 hr	0–100 nmol/24 hr
		2–4 yr	4–29 μg/24 hr	24–171 nmol/24 hr
		4–7 yr	8–45 μg/24 hr	47–266 nmol/24 hr
		7–10 yr	13–65 μg/24 hr	77–384 nmol/24 hr
		Thereafter	15–80 μg/24 hr	87–473 nmol/24 hr
		Epinephrine		
		0–1 yr	0–2.5 μg/24 hr	0–13.6 nmol/24 hr
		1–2 yr	0–3.5 μg/24 hr	0–19.1 nmol/24 hr
		2–4 yr	0–6.0 μg/24 hr	0–32.7 nmol/24 hr
		4–7 yr	0.2–10 μg/24 hr	1.1–55 nmol/24 hr
		7–10 yr	0.5–14 μg/24 hr	2.7–76 nmol/24 hr
		Thereafter	0.5–20 μg/24 hr	2.7–109 nmol/24 hr
		Fractionated		
		Dopamine		
		0–1 yr	0–85 μg/24 hr	0–555 nmol/24 hr
		1–2 yr	10–140 μg/24 hr	65–914 nmol/24 hr
		2–4 yr	40–260 μg/24 hr	261–1,697 nmol/24 hr
		Thereafter	65–400 μg/24 hr	424–2,611 nmol/24 hr
Catecholamines, total, free	U	0–1 yr	10–15 μg/24 hr	10–15 μg/24 hr
		1–5 yr	15–40 μg/24 hr	15–40 μg/24 hr
		6–15 yr	20–80 μg/24 hr	20–80 μg/24 hr
		Thereafter	30–100 μg/24 hr	30–100 μg/24 hr
Cerebrospinal fluid				
Pressure	CSF	70–180 mm water		70–180 mm water
Volume	CSF	Child	60–100 mL	0.06–0.10 L
		Adult	100–160 mL	0.1–0.16 L
Chloride	S, P(H)	Cord blood	96–104 mmol/L	96–104 mmol/L
		Newborn	97–110 mmol/L	97–110 mmol/L
		Thereafter	98–106 mmol/L	98–106 mmol/L
	CSF		118–132 mmol/L	118–132 mmol/L
	U	Infant	2–10 mmol/24 hr	2–10 mmol/24 hr
		Child	15–40 mmol/24 hr	15–40 mmol/24 hr
		Thereafter	110–250 mmol/24 hr (varies greatly with Cl intake)	110–250 mmol/24 hr
	Sweat	Normal	<40 mmol/L	<40 mmol/L
		Borderline	45–60 mmol/L	45–60 mmol/L
		Cystic fibrosis	>60 mmol/L	>60 mmol/L
Cholesterol, total	S	1–3 yr	45–182 mg/dL	1.15–4.70 mmol/L
		4–6 yr	109–189 mg/dL	2.80–4.80 mmol/L

M	Percentiles 5	75	95	M	Percentiles 5	75	95
6–9 yr	126	172	191 mg/dL	6–9 yr	3.26	4.45	4.94 mmol/L
10–14 yr	130	179	204 mg/dL	10–14 yr	3.36	4.63	5.28 mmol/L
15–19 yr	114	167	198 mg/dL	15–19 yr	2.95	4.32	5.12 mmol/L

Table continued on following page

Test	Specimen		Reference Range	Reference Range (SI)
		F — Percentiles: 5 / 75 / 95		F — Percentiles: 5 / 75 / 95
		6–9 yr	122 / 173 / 209 mg/dL	3.16 / 4.47 / 5.41 mmol/L
		10–14 yr	124 / 174 / 217 mg/dL	3.21 / 4.50 / 5.61 mmol/L
		15–19 yr	125 / 175 / 212 mg/dL	3.23 / 4.53 / 5.48 mmol/L
Clotting time, Lee-White, 37° C	W	Glass tubes	5–8 min (5–15 min at RT)	Glass tubes
		Silicone tubes	about 30 min prolonged	Silicone tubes
Copper	S	0–5 d	9–46 µg/dL	1.4–7.2 µmol/L
		1–9 yr	80–150 µg/dL	12.6–23.6 µmol/L
		10–14 yr	80–121 µg/dL	12.6–19.0 µmol/L
		15–19 yr	64–160 µg/dL	11.3–25.2 µmol/L
	U	5–18 yr	0.36–7.56 mg/mol Cr.	6–119 µmol/mol Cr.
Cortisol	S, P(H)	Newborn	1–24 µg/dL	28–662 nmol/L
		Adults		
		0800 hr	5–23 µg/dL	138–635 nmol/L
		1600 hr	3–15 µg/dL	82–413 nmol/L
		2000 hr	≤50% of 0800 hr	Fraction of 0800 hr ≤0.50
Cortisol, free	U	Child	2–27 µg/24 hr	5.5–74 nmol/24 hr
		Adolescent	5–55 µg/24 hr	14–152 nmol/24 hr
		Adult	10–100 µg/24 hr	27–276 nmol/24 hr
Creatine kinase isoenzymes	S		*CKMB* / *CKBB*	
		Cord blood	0.3–3.1% / 0.3–10.5%	
		5–8 hr	1.7–7.9% / 3.6–13.4%	
		24–33 hr	1.8–5.0% / 2.3–8.6%	
		72–100 hr	1.4–5.4% / 5.1–13.3%	
		Adult	0–2% / 0	
Creatinine plasma Jaffe, kinetic, or enzymatic	S, P	Cord blood	0.6–1.2 mg/dL	53–106 µmol/L
		Newborn	0.3–1.0 mg/dL	27–88 µmol/L
		Infant	0.2–0.4 mg/dL	18–35 µmol/L
		Child	0.3–0.7 mg/dL	27–62 µmol/L
		Adolescent	0.5–1.0 mg/dL	44–88 µmol/L
		Adult		
		M	0.6–1.2 mg/dL	53–106 µmol/L
		F	0.5–1.1 mg/dL	44–97 µmol/L
Creatinine, urinary	U	Premature	8.1–15.0 mg/kg/24 hr	72–133 µmol/kg/24 hr
		Full-term	10.4–19.7 mg/kg/24 hr	92–174 µmol/kg/24 hr
		1.5–7 yr	10–15 mg/kg/24 hr	88–133 µmol/kg/24 hr
		7–15 yr	5.2–41 mg/kg/24 hr	46–362 µmol/kg/24 hr
Creatinine clearance (endogenous)	S, P, and U	Newborn	40–65 mL/min/1.73 m^2	
		<40 yr		
		M	97–137 mL/min/1.73 m^2	
		F	88–128 mL/min/1.73 m^2	
		Decreases	~6.5 mL/min/decade	
Differential count. See Leukocyte differential count				
Eosinophil count	W (E,H) capillary		50–350 cells/mm^3 (µL)	50–350 × 10^6 cells/L
Epinephrine. See Catecholamines, fractionated				
Erythrocyte count (RBC count)	W(E)		*Millions of cells/mm^3 (µL)*	*× 10^{12} cells/L*
		Cord blood	3.9–5.5	3.9–5.5
		1–3 d (capillary)	4.0–6.6	4.0–6.6
		1 wk	3.9–6.3	3.9–6.3
		2 wk	3.6–6.2	3.6–6.2
		1 mo	3.0–5.4	3.0–5.4
		2 mo	2.7–4.9	2.7–4.9
		3–6 mo	3.1–4.5	3.1–4.5
		0.5–2 yr	3.7–5.3	3.7–5.3
		2–6 yr	3.9–5.3	3.9–5.3
		6–12 yr	4.0–5.2	4.0–5.2
		12–18 yr		
		M	4.5–5.3	4.5–5.3
		F	4.1–5.1	4.1–5.1
		18–49 yr		
		M	4.5–5.9	4.5–5.9
		F	4.0–5.2	4.0–5.2

Test	Specimen	Reference Range			Reference Range (SI)
Erythrocyte sedimentation rate (ESR) Westergren, modified	W(E)				
		Child		0–10 mm/hr	0–10 mm/hr
		Adult			
		M < 50 yr		0–15 mm/hr	0–15 mm/hr
		F < 50 yr		0–20 mm/hr	0–20 mm/hr
Wintrobe		Child		0–13 mm/hr	0–13 mm/hr
		Adult			
		M		0–9 mm/hr	0–9 mm/hr
		F		0–20 mm/hr	0–20 mm/hr
Erythropoietin RIA	S	<5–20 mU/mL			<5–20 U/L
Hemagglutination		25–125 mU/mL			25–125 U/L
Bioassay		5–18 mU/mL			5–18 U/L
Fat, fecal	F (72 hr)	Infant, breast-fed		<1 g/24 hr	<1 g/24 hr
		0–6 yr		<2 g/24 hr	<2 g/24 hr
		Adult			
		Normal diet		<7 g/24 hr	<7 g/24 hr
		Fat-free diet		<4 g/24 hr	<4 g/24 hr
		Coefficient of Fat Absorption (%)			*Absorbed Fraction*
		Infant			
		Breast-fed		>93	>0.93
		Formula-fed		>83	>0.83
		>1 yr		≥95	≥0.95
Free fatty acids	S	Premature 10–55 d		0.15–0.71 mmol/L	0.15–0.71 mmol/L
Ferric chloride test	U	Negative			Negative
Ferritin	S	Newborn		25–200 ng/mL	25–200 μg/L
		1 mo		200–600 ng/mL	200–600 μg/L
		2–5 mo		50–200 ng/mL	50–200 μg/L
		6 mo–15 yr		7–140 ng/mL	7–140 μg/L
		Adult			
		M		15–200 ng/mL	15–200 μg/L
		F		12–150 ng/mL	12–150 μg/L
Fibrin degradation products					
Agglutination (Thrombo-Wellco test)	W; special tube thrombin and proteolytic inhibitors			<10μg/mL	<10 mg/L
	U: 2 mL in special tube (see above)			<0.25 μg/mL	<0.25 mg/L
Fibrinogen	P(NaCl)	Newborn		125–300 mg/dL	1.25–3.00 g/L
		Adult		200–400 mg/dL	2.00–4.00 g/L
Folate	S	Newborn		7.0–32 ng/mL	15.9–72.4 nmol/L
		Thereafter		1.8–9 ng/mL	4.1–20.4 nmol/L
	W(E)			150–450 ng/mL RBCs	340–1,020 nmol/L cells
Follicle-stimulating hormone (FSH)	S	M			
		Tanner 1	<9.8 yr	0.26–3.0 mIU/mL	0.26–3.0 U/L
		Tanner 2	9.8–14.5 yr	1.8–3.2 mIU/mL	1.8–3.2 U/L
		Tanner 3	10.7–15.4 yr	1.2–5.8 mIU/mL	1.2–5.8 U/L
		Tanner 4	11.8–16.2 yr	2.0–9.2 mIU/mL	2.0–9.2 U/L
		Tanner 5	12.8–17.3 yr	2.6–11.0 mIU/mL	2.6–11.0 U/L
		Adult		2.0–9.2 mIU/mL	2.0–9.2 U/L
		F			
		Tanner 1	<9.2 yr	1.0–4.2 mIU/mL	1.0–4.2 U/L
		Tanner 2	9.2–13.7 yr	1.0–10.8 mIU/mL	1.0–10.8 U/L
		Tanner 3	10.0–14.4 yr	1.5–12.8 mIU/mL	1.5–12.8 U/L
		Tanner 4	10.7–15.6 yr	1.5–11.7 mIU/mL	1.5–11.7 U/L
		Tanner 5	11.8–18.6 yr	1.0–9.2 mIU/mL	1.0–9.2 U/L
		Adult			
		Follicular		1.8–11.2 mIU/mL	1.8–11.2 U/L
		Midcycle		6–35 mIU/mL	6–35 U/L
		Luteal		1.8–11.2 mIU/mL	1.8–11.2 U/L
Galactose	S	Newborn		0–20 mg/dL	0–1.11 mmol/L
	P	5 mo–17 yr		0.0–0.5 mg/dL	0.0–0.03 mmol/L
	U	Newborn		≤60 mg/dL	≤3.33 mmol/L
		Thereafter		14 mg/24 hr	<0.08 mmol/24 hr
Gastrin	S (fasting)	Children		<10–125 pg/mL	<10–125 ng/L
Glucagon	S	Neonate (1–7 d)		210–1,500 pg/mL	210–1,500 ng/L
		Children and adults		25–250 pg/mL	25–250 ng/L

Table continued on following page

Test	Specimen	Reference Range			Reference Range (SI)	
Glucose	S	Cord blood		45–96 mg/dL	2.5–5.3 mmol/L	
		Newborn				
		1 d		40–60 mg/dL	2.2–3.3 mmol/L	
		>1 d		50–90 mg/dL	2.8–5.0 mmol/L	
		Child		60–100 mg/dL	3.3–5.5 mmol/L	
		Adult		70–105 mg/dL	3.9–5.8 mmol/L	
	W(H)	Adult		65–95 mg/dL	3.6–5.3 mmol/L	
	CSF	Adult		40–70 mg/dL	2.2–3.9 mmol/L	
Quantitative, enzymatic	U	<0.5 g/24 hr			<2.8 mmol/24 hr	
Qualitative	U	Negative			Negative	
Glucose, 2 hr pc	S	<120 mg/dL (For diabetes, see Glucose tolerance test, oral)			<6.7 mmol/L	
Glucose-6-phosphate dehydrogenase in erythrocytes	W(E,H,C)					
Bishop, modified		Adult			Adult	
		3.4–8.0 U/g Hb			0.22–0.52 mU/mol Hb	
		98.6–232 U/10^{12} RBC			0.10–0.23 nU/10^{6} RBC	
		1.16–2.72 U/mL RBC			1.16–2.72 kU/L RBC	
		Newborn: 50% higher			Newborn: 50% higher	
Glucose tolerance test (GTT), oral	S		*Normal*	*Diabetic*	*Normal*	*Diabetic*
Adult dose: 75 g		Fasting	70–105 mg/dL	>115 mg/dL	3.9–5.8 mmol/L	>6.4 mmol/L
Child dose: 1.75 g/kg of ideal weight up to maximum of 75 g		60 min	120–170 mg/dL	≥200 mg/dL	6.7–9.4 mmol/L	≥11 mmol/L
		90 min	100–140 mg/dL	≥200 mg/dL	5.6–7.8 mmol/L	≥11 mmol/L
		120 min	70–120 mg/dL	≥140 mg/dL	3.9–6.7 mmol/L	≥7.8 mmol/L
γ-Glutamyltranspeptidase (GGT, GGTP)	S	Cord blood		37–193 U/L	37–193 U/L	
		0–1 mo		13–147 U/L	13–147 U/L	
		1–2 mo		12–123 U/L	12–123 U/L	
		2–4 mo		8–90 U/L	8–90 U/L	
		4 mo–10 yr		5–32 U/L	5–32 U/L	
		10–15 yr		5–24 U/L	5–24 U/L	
Growth hormone (hGH, somatotropin)	S, P(E,H)	Newborn				
		1 d		5–53 ng/mL	5–53 μg/L	
		1 wk		5–27 ng/mL	5–27 μg/L	
		1–12 mo		2–10 ng/mL	2–10 μg/L	
	Fasting, at rest	Child		<0.7–6 ng/mL	<0.7–6 μg/L	
		Adult		<0.7–6 ng/mL	<0.7–6 μg/L	
HDL cholesterol	S	1–13 yr		35–84 mg/dL	0.9–2.15 mmol/L	
		14–19 yr		35–65 mg/dL	0.90–1.65 mmol/L	
Hematocrit (HCT, Hct)	W(E)			*Per cent packed red cells (vol red cells/vol whole blood cells × 100)*	*Volume fraction (vol red cells/vol whole blood)*	
Calculated from MCV and RBC (electronic displacement or laser)		1 d (capillary)		48–69%	0.48–0.69	
		2 d		48–75%	0.48–0.75	
		3 d		44–72%	0.44–0.72	
		2 mo		28–42%	0.28–0.42	
		6–12 yr		35–45%	0.35–0.45	
		12–18 yr				
		M		37–49%	0.37–0.49	
		F		36–46%	0.36–0.46	
		18–49 yr				
		M		41–53%	0.41–0.53	
		F		36–46%	0.36–0.46	
Hemoglobin (Hb)	W(E)	1–3 d (capillary)		14.5–22.5 g/dL	2.25–3.49 mmol/L	
		2 mo		9.0–14.0 g/dL	1.40–2.17 mmol/L	
		6–12 yr		11.5–15.5 g/dL	1.78–2.40 mmol/L	
		12–18 yr				
		M		13.0–16.0 g/dL	2.02–2.48 mmol/L	
		F		12.0–16.0 g/dL	1.86–2.48 mmol/L	
		18–49 yr				
		M		13.5–17.5 g/dL	2.09–2.27 mmol/L	
		F		12.0–16.0 g/dL	1.86–2.48 mmol/L	
	P(H)	<10 mg/dL			<1.55 μmol/L	
		<3 mg/dL with butterfly set-up and 18-g needle			<0.47 μmol/L with butterfly set-up and 18-g needle	
	U	Negative			Negative	
Hemoglobin A	W(E, C, H)			>95%	Fraction of hemoglobin >0.95	
Hemoglobin electrophoresis	W(H, E, C)	HbA		>95%		
		HbA_2		1.5–3.5%		
		HbF		<2%		

Test	Specimen	Reference Range		Reference Range (SI)
Immunoglobulin A (IgA)	S	Cord blood	1.4–3.6 mg/dL	14–36 mg/L
		1–3 mo	1.3–53 mg/dL	13–530 mg/L
		4–6 mo	4.4–84 mg/dL	44–840 mg/L
		7 mo–1 yr	11–106 mg/dL	110–1,060 mg/L
		2–5 yr	14–159 mg/dL	140–1,590 mg/L
		6–10 yr	33–236 mg/dL	330–2,360 mg/L
		Adult	70–312 mg/dL	700–3,120 mg/L
Immunoglobulin D (IgD)	S	Newborn	None detected	None detected
		Thereafter	0–8 mg/dL	0–80 mg/L
Immunoglobulin E (IgE)	S	M	0–230 IU/mL	0–230 kIU/L
		F	0–170 IU/mL	0–170 kIU/L
Immunoglobulin G (IgG)	S	Cord blood	636–1,606 mg/dL	6.36–16.06 g/L
		1 mo	251–906 mg/dL	2.51–9.06 g/L
		2–4 mo	176–601 mg/dL	1.76–6.01 g/L
		5–12 mo	172–1,069 mg/dL	1.72–10.69 g/L
		1–5 yr	345–1,236 mg/dL	3.45–12.36 g/L
		6–10 yr	608–1,572 mg/dL	6.08–15.72 g/L
		Adult	639–1,349 mg/dL	6.39–13.49 g/L
Immunoglobulin M (IgM)	S	Cord blood	6.3–25 mg/dL	63–250 mg/L
		1–4 mo	17–105 mg/dL	170–1,050 mg/L
		5–9 mo	33–126 mg/dL	300–1,260 mg/L
		10 mo–1 yr	41–173 mg/dL	410–1,730 mg/L
		2–8 yr	43–207 mg/dL	430–2,070 mg/L
		9–10 yr	52–242 mg/dL	520–2,420 mg/L
		Adult	56–352 mg/dL	560–3,520 mg/L
Insulin (12-hr fasting)	S	Newborn	3–20 µU/mL	3–20 mU/L
		Thereafter	7–24 µU/mL	7–24 mU/L
Insulin with oral glucose tolerance test	S		Insulin	
		0 min	7–24 µU/mL	7–24 mU/L
		30 min	25–231 µU/mL	25–231 mU/L
		60 min	18–276 µU/mL	18–276 mU/L
		120 min	16–166 µU/mL	16–166 mU/L
		180 min	4–38 µU/mL	4–38 mU/L
Iron	S	Newborn	100–250 µg/dL	17.90–44.75 µmol/L
		Infant	40–100 µg/dL	7.16–17.90 µmol/L
		Child	50–120 µg/dL	8.95–21.48 µmol/L
		Thereafter		
		M	50–160 µg/dL	8.95–28.64 µmol/L
		F	40–150 µg/dL	7.16–26.85 µmol/L
		Intoxicated child	280–2,550 µg/dL	50.12–456.5 µmol/L
		Fatally poisoned child	>1,800 µg/dL	>322.2 µmol/L
Iron-binding capacity, total (TIBC)	S	Infant	100–400 µg/dL	17.90–71.60 µmol/L
		Thereafter	250–400 µg/dL	44.75–71.60 µmol/L
17-Ketogenic steroids (17-KGS)	U	0–1 yr	<1.0 mg/24 hr	<3.5 µmol/24 hr
		1–10 yr	<5 mg/24 hr	<17 µmol/24 hr
		11–14 yr	<12 mg/24 hr	<42 µmol/24 hr
		Thereafter		
		M	5–23 mg/24 hr	17–80 µmol/24 hr
		F	3–15 mg/24 hr	10–52 µmol/24 hr
Ketone bodies				
Qualitative	S	Negative		Negative
	U	Negative		Negative
Quantitative	S	0.5–3.0 mg/dL		5–30 mg/L
17-Ketosteroid (17-KS), total	U	14 d–2 yr	<1 mg/24 hr	<3.5 µmol/24 hr
		2–6 yr	<2 mg/24 hr	< 7 µmol/24 hr
		6–10 yr	1–4 mg/24 hr	3.5–14 µmol/24 hr
		10–12 yr	1–6 mg/24 hr	3.5–21 µmol/24 hr
		12–14 yr	3–10 mg/24 hr	10–35 µmol/24 hr
		14–16 yr	5–12 mg/24 hr	17–42 µmol/24 hr
		Thereafter		
		M: 18–30 yr	9–22 mg/24 hr	31–76 µmol/24 hr
		>30 yr	8–20 mg/24 hr	28–70 µmol/24 hr
		F, decreases with age	6–15 mg/24 hr	21–52 µmol/24 hr
LDL-cholesterol (LDLC)	S, P(E)			

LDL-cholesterol (LDLC)	M (mg/dL)	F (mg/dL)	M (mmol/L)	F (mmol/L)
Cord blood	10–50	10–50	0.26–1.30	0.26–1.30
1–9 yr	60–140	60–150	1.55–3.63	1.55–3.89
10–19 yr	50–170	50–170	1.30–4.40	1.30–4.40
20–29 yr	60–175	60–160	1.55–4.53	1.55–4.14
30–39 yr	80–190	70–170	2.07–4.92	1.81–4.40
40–49 yr	90–205	80–190	2.33–5.31	2.07–4.92
Recommended (desirable) range for adults	<130 mg/dL		1.68–4.53 mmol/L	

Table continued on following page

Test	Specimen		Reference Range	Reference Range (SI)
Lactate				
L(+)-lactate	W(H)	Venous	0.5–2.2 mmol/L	0.5–2.2 mmol/L
		Arterial	0.5–1.6 mmol/L	0.5–1.6 mmol/L
		Inpatients		
		Venous	0.9–1.7 mmol/L	0.9–1.7 mmol/L
		Arterial	<1.25 mmol/L	<1.25 mmol/L
D(−)-lactate	P(H)	6 mo–3 yr	0.0–0.3 mmol/L	0.0–0.3 mmol/L
Lactate dehydrogenase (LD)	S	<1 yr	170–580 U/L	170–580 U/L
		1–9 yr	150–500 U/L	150–500 U/L
		10–19 yr	120–330 U/L	120–330 U/L
Isoenzymes	S		*Percentage of total activity*	
			1–6 yr / *7–19 yr*	
		LD1	20–38 / 20–35	
		LD2	27–38 / 31–38	
		LD3	16–26 / 19–28	
		LD4	5–16 / 7–13	
		LD5	3–13 / 5–12	
Lead	W(H)	Child	<10 $\mu g/dL$	<0.48 $\mu mol/L$
		Adult	<40 $\mu g/dL$	<1.93 $\mu mol/L$
		Acceptable for industrial exposure	<60 $\mu g/dL$	<2.90 $\mu mol/L$
		Toxic	≥100 $\mu g/dL$	≥4.83 $\mu mol/L$
	U (24-hr)	<80 $\mu g/dL$		<0.39 $\mu mol/L$
Lecithin/sphingomyelin (L/S) ratio	AF	2.0–5.0 indicates probable fetal lung maturity (>3.0 IDM)		2.0–5.0 indicates probable fetal lung maturity
Lecithin phosphorus	AF	>0.10 mg/dL indicates probably adequate fetal lung maturity		>0.032 mmol/L indicates probably adequate fetal lung maturity
Leukocyte count (WBC)	W(E)		*×1,000 cells/mm^3 (µL)*	*×10^9 cells/L*
		Birth	9.0–30.0	9.0–30.0
		24 hr	9.4–34.0	9.4–34.0
		1 mo	5.0–19.5	5.0–19.5
		1–3 yr	6.0–17.5	6.0–17.5
		4–7 yr	5.5–15.5	5.5–15.5
		8–13 yr	4.5–13.5	4.5–13.5
		Adult	4.5–11.0	4.5–11.0
Cell count	CSF	Premature	0–25 mononuclear cells/µL	0–25 × 10^6 cells/L
			0–10 polymorphonuclear cells/µL	0–10 × 10^6 cells/L
			0–1,000 RBC/µL	0–1,000 × 10^6 cells/L
		Newborn	0–20 mononuclear cells/µL	0–20 × 10^6 cells/L
			0–10 polymorphonuclear cells/µL	0–10 × 10^6 cells/L
			0–800 RBC/µL	0–800 × 10^6 cells/L
		Neonate	0–5 mononuclear cells/µL	0–5 × 10^6 cells/L
			0–10 polymorphonuclear cells/µL	0–10 × 10^6 cells/L
			0–50 RBC/µL	0–50 × 10^6 cells/L
		Thereafter	0–5 mononuclear cells/µL (numbers of cells in very young infants are greater than those in the CSF of older individuals without substantial implications for growth and development in most instances)	0–5 cells/L
Leukocyte differential	W(E)			
Myelocytes		0		0
Neutrophils—"bands"		3–5%		0.03–0.05 no. fraction
Neutrophils—"segs"		54–62%		0.54–0.62 no. fraction
Lymphocytes		25–33%		0.25–0.33 no. fraction
Monocytes		3–7%		0.03–0.07 no. fraction
Eosinophils		1–3%		0.01–0.03 no. fraction
Basophils		0–0.75%		0–0.0075 no. fraction
Leukocyte differential	Specimen	*Cells/mm^3 (µL)*		
Myelocytes		0		0 × 10^6 cells/L
Neutrophils—"bands"		150–400		150–400 × 10^6 cells/L
Neutrophils—"segs"		3,000–5,800		3,000–5,800 × 10^6 cells/L
Lymphocytes		1,500–3,000		1,500–3,000 × 10^6 cells/L
Monocytes		285–500		285–500 × 10^6 cells/L
Eosinophils		50–250		50–250 × 10^6 cells/L
Basophils		15–50		15–50 × 10^6 cells/L
Lymphocytes	CSF		62% ± 34%	0.62 ± 0.34 no. fraction
Monocytes			36% ± 20%	0.36 ± 0.20 no. fraction
Neutrophils			2% ± 5%	0.02 ± 0.05 no. fraction
Histiocytes			0–rare	0–rare
Ependymal cells			0–rare	0–rare
Eosinophils			0–rare	0–rare

Test	Specimen		Reference Range	Reference Range (SI)
Lipase	S	1–4 yr	18–95 U/L	18–95 U/L
		5–14 yr	21–128 U/L	21–128 U/L
		15–19 yr	28–149 U/L	28–149 U/L
Magnesium	P(H)	0–6 d	1.2–2.6 mg/dL	0.48–1.05 mmol/L
		7 d–2 yr	1.6–2.6 mg/dL	0.65–1.05 mmol/L
	U (24-hr)	2–14 yr	1.5–2.3 mg/dL	0.60–0.95 mmol/L
		1–6 mo		
		Breast-fed	0.04–1.55 mmol/L	0.04–1.55 mmol/L
		Formula-fed	0.04–1.40 mmol/L	0.04–1.55 mmol/L
Mean corpuscular hemoglobin concentration (MCHC)	W(E)	Birth	31–37 pg/cell	0.48–0.57 fmol/cell
		1–3 d (capillary)	31–37 pg/cell	0.48–0.57 fmol/cell
		1 wk–1 mo	28–40 pg/cell	0.43–0.62 fmol/cell
		2 mo	26–34 pg/cell	0.40–0.53 fmol/cell
		3–6 mo	25–35 pg/cell	0.39–0.54 fmol/cell
		0.5–2 yr	23–31 pg/cell	0.36–0.48 fmol/cell
		2–6 yr	24–30 pg/cell	0.37–0.47 fmol/cell
		6–12 yr	25–33 pg/cell	0.39–0.51 fmol/cell
		12–18 yr	25–35 pg/cell	0.39–0.54 fmol/cell
		18–49 yr	26–34 pg/cell	0.40–0.53 fmol/cell
Mean corpuscular hemoglobin	W(E)		*Percentage Hb/cell or g Hb/dL RBC*	*mmol Hb/L RBC*
		Birth	30–36	4.65–5.58
		1–3 d (capillary)	29–37	4.50–5.74
		1–2 wk	28–38	4.34–5.89
		1–2 mo	29–37	4.50–5.74
		3 mo–2 yr	30–36	4.65–5.58
		2–18 yr	31–37	4.81–5.74
		>18 yr	31–37	4.81–5.74
Mean corpuscular volume (MCV)	W(E)	1–3 d (capillary)	95–121 μm^3	95–121 fL
		0.5–2 yr	70–86 μm^3	70–86 fL
		6–12 yr	77–95 μm^3	77–95 fL
		12–18 yr		
		M	78–98 μm^3	78–98 fL
		F	78–102 μm^3	78–102 fL
		18–49 yr		
		M	80–100 μm^3	80–100 fL
		F	80–100 μm^3	80–100 fL
Methemoglobin (MetHb)	W(E,H,C)	0.06–0.24 g/dL or 0.78 ± 0.37% of total Hb		9.3–37.2 μmol/L 0.0078 ± 0.0037 (mass fraction)
Methylmalonic acid	U	6–12 wk	0–57 mg/g creatinine	0–55 mmol/mol creatinine
Mucopolysaccharides	U	<2 yr	<50 μg/g creatinine	<5.7 mg/mmol creatinine
		2–4 yr	<25 μg/g creatinine	<2.8 mg/mmol creatinine
		4–15 yr	<20 μg/g creatinine	<2.3 mg/mmol creatinine
Osmolality	S	Child and adult	275–295 mOsm/kg H_2O	
	U	50–1,400 mOsm/kg H_2O, depending on fluid intake. After 12 hr of fluid restriction, normal range is >850 mOsm/kg H_2O		
	U (24-hr)	300–900 mOsm/kg H_2O		
Oxygen, partial pressure of (PO_2)	W(H), arterial	Birth	8–24 mm Hg	1.1–3.2 kPa
		5–10 min	33–75 mm Hg	4.4–10.0 kPa
		30 min	31–85 mm Hg	4.1–11.3 kPa
		>1 hr	55–80 mm Hg	7.3–10.6 kPa
		1 d	54–95 mm Hg	7.2–12.6 kPa
		Thereafter (decreases with age)	83–108 mm Hg	11–14.4 kPa
Oxygen saturation	W(H), arterial	Newborn	85–90%	0.85–0.90 Saturated fraction
		Thereafter	95–99%	0.95–0.99 Saturated fraction
Parathyroid hormone	S			
C-terminal (mid-molecule)		1–16 yr	51–217 pg/mL	5.4–22.8 pmol/L
Intact (IRMA)		1–18 yr	1–43 pg/mL	0.1–4.5 pmol/L
Partial thromboplastin time (PTT)	W(NaCl)			
Nonactivated		60–85 s (Platelin)		60–85 s
Activated		25–35 s (differs with method)		25–35 s
pH	W(H), arterial			*H^+ Concentration*
		Premature (48 hr)	7.35–7.50	31–44 nmol/L
		Birth, full-term	7.11–7.36	43–77 nmol/L
		5–10 min	7.09–7.30	50–81 nmol/L
		30 min	7.21–7.38	41–61 nmol/L
		>1 hr	7.26–7.49	32–54 nmol/L
		1d	7.29–7.45	35–51 nmol/L
		Thereafter	7.35–7.45	35–44 nmol/L
		Must be corrected for body temperature		

Table continued on following page

Test	Specimen	Reference Range		Reference Range (SI)
	U	Newborn/neonate	5–7	0.1–10 μmol/L
		Thereafter (average 6)	4.5–8	0.01–32 μmol/L (average 1.0 μmol/L)
	F		7.0–7.5	31–100 nmol/L
Phenylalanine	S	Premature	2.0–7.5 mg/dL	120–450 μmol/L
		Newborn	1.2–3.4 mg/dL	70–210 μmol/L
		Thereafter	0.8–1.8 mg/dL	50–110 μmol/L
	U	10 d–2 wk	1–2 mg/24 hr	6–12 μmol/24 hr
		3–12 yr	4–18 mg/24 hr	24–110 μmol/24 hr
		Thereafter	trace–17 mg/24 hr	trace–103 μmol/24 hr
Phenylpyruvic acid, qualitative	U	Negative by $FeCl_3$ test		Negative by $FeCl_3$ test
Phosphatase, alkaline	S	1–9 yr	145–420 U/L	1–9 yr 145–420 U/L
		10–11 yr	130–560 U/L	10–11 yr 130–560 U/L
			M / F	M / F
		12–13 yr	200–495 U/L / 105–420 U/L	12–13 yr 200–495 U/L / 105–420 U/L
		14–15 yr	130–525 U/L / 70–230 U/L	14–15 yr 130–525 U/L / 70–230 U/L
		16–19 yr	65–260 U/L / 50–130 U/L	16–19 yr 65–260 U/L / 50–130 U/L
Phospholipids, total	S, P(E)	Newborn	75–170 mg/dL	0.75–1.70 g/L
		Infant	100–275 mg/dL	1.00–2.75 g/L
		Child	180–295 mg/dL	1.80–2.95 g/L
		Adult	125–275 mg/dL	1.25–2.75 g/L
Phosphorus, inorganic	S, P(H)	0–5 d	4.8–8.2 mg/dL	1.55–2.65 mmol/L
		1–3 yr	3.8–6.5 mg/dL	1.25–2.10 mmol/L
		4–11 yr	3.7–5.6 mg/dL	1.20–1.80 mmol/L
		12–15 yr	2.9–5.4 mg/dL	0.95–1.75 mmol/L
		16–19 yr	2.7–4.7 mg/dL	0.90–1.50 mmol/L
Plasma volume	P(H)	M	25–43 mL/kg	M 0.025–0.043 L/kg
		F	28–45 mL/kg	F 0.028–0.045 L/kg
Platelet count (thrombocyte count)	W(E)	Newborn 84–478 × $10^3/mm^3$ (μL) (after 1 wk same as adult)		84–478 × 10^9/L
		Adult 150–400 × $10^3/mm^3$ (μL)		150–400 × 10^9/L
Potassium	S	<2 mo	3.0–7.0 mmol/L	3.0–7.0 mmol/L
		2–12 mo	3.5–6.0 mmol/L	3.5–6.0 mmol/L
		>12 mo	3.5–5.0 mmol/L	3.5–5.0 mmol/L
	P(H)			3.5–4.5 mmol/L
	U (24-hr)	2.5–125 mmol/L (varies with diet)		2.5–125 mmol/L (varies with diet)
Protein				
Total	S	Premature	4.3–7.6 g/dL	43–76 g/L
		Newborn	4.6–7.4 g/dL	46–74 g/L
		1–7 yr	6.1–7.9 g/dL	61–79 g/L
		8–12 yr	6.4–8.1 g/dL	64–81 g/L
		13–19 yr	6.6–8.2 g/dL	66–82 g/L
Electrophoresis	S			
Albumin		Premature	3.0–4.2 g/dL	30–42 g/L
		Newborn	3.6–5.4 g/dL	36–54 g/L
		Infant	4.0–5.0 g/dL	40–50 g/L
		Thereafter	3.5–5.0 g/dL	35–50 g/L
α_1-Globulin		Premature	0.1–0.5 g/dL	1–5 g/L
		Newborn	0.1–0.3 g/dL	1–3 g/L
		Infant	0.2–0.4 g/dL	2–4 g/L
		Thereafter	0.2–0.3 g/dL	2–3 g/L
α_2-Globulin		Premature	0.3–0.7 g/dL	3–7 g/L
		Newborn	0.3–0.5 g/dL	3–5 g/L
		Infant	0.5–0.8 g/dL	5–8 g/L
		Thereafter	0.4–1.0 g/dL	4–10 g/L
β-Globulin		Premature	0.3–1.2 g/dL	3–12 g/L
		Newborn	0.2–0.6 g/dL	2–6 g/L
		Infant	0.5–0.8 g/dL	5–8 g/L
		Thereafter	0.5–1.1 g/dL	5–11 g/L
γ-Globulin		Premature	0.3–1.4 g/dL	3–4 g/L
		Newborn	0.2–1.0 g/dL	2–10 g/L
		Infant	0.3–1.2 g/dL	3–12 g/L
		Thereafter (higher in blacks)	0.7–1.2 g/dL	7–12 g/L
Protein	U (24-hr)	1–14 mg/dL		10–140 mg/L
Total urinary		50–80 mg/24 hr (at rest)		50–80 mg/24 hr (at rest)
		<250 mg/24 hr after intense exercise		<250 mg/24 hr after intense exercise

Test	Specimen	Reference Range		Reference Range (SI)	
Electrophoresis		*Average Total Protein*		*Fraction of Total Protein*	
Albumin			37.9%	0.379	
α_1-Globulin			27.3%	0.273	
α_2-Globulin			19.5%	0.195	
β-Globulin			8.8%	0.088	
γ-Globulin			3.3%	0.033	
Protein					
Total protein (column)	CSF	Lumbar	8–32 mg/dL	80–320 mg/L	
Prothrombin time (PT)					
One-stage (quick)	W(NaC)	In general, 11–15 s (varies with type of thromboplastin)		11–15 s	
		Newborn: prolonged by 2–3 s		Newborn: prolonged by 2–3 s	
Two-stage modified (Ware and Seegers)	W(NaC)	18–22 s		18–22 s	
Red cell volume	W(H)	M	20–36 mL/kg	0.020–0.036 L/kg	
		F	19–31 mL/kg	0.019–0.031 L/kg	
Renin (renin activity, plasma; PRA)	P(E)	0–3 yr	<16.6 ng/mL/hr	<16.6 μg/L/hr	
		3–6 yr	<6.7 ng/mL/hr	<6.7 μg/L/hr	
		6–9 yr	<4.4 ng/mL/hr	<4.4 μg/L/hr	
		9–12 yr	<5.9 ng/mL/hr	<5.9 μg/L/hr	
		12–15 yr	<4.2 ng/mL/hr	<4.2 μg/L/hr	
		15–18 yr	<4.3 ng/mL/hr	<4.3 μg/L/hr	
		Normal sodium diet			
		Supine	0.2–2.5 ng/mL/hr	0.2–2.5 μg/L/hr	
		Upright	0.3–4.3 ng/mL/hr	0.3–4.3 μg/L/hr	
		Low sodium diet			
		Upright	2.9–24 ng/mL/hr	2.9–24 μg/L/hr	
Reticulocyte count	W(E,H,O)	Adults 0.5–1.5% of erythrocytes, or 25,000–75,000/mm³ (μL)		0.005–0.015 number fraction 25,000–75,000 × 10⁶/L	
	W (capillary)	1 d	0.4–6.0%	0.004–0.060 number fraction	
		7 d	<0.1–1.3%	<0.001–0.013 number fraction	
		1–4 wk	<1.0–1.2%	<0.001–0.012 number fraction	
		5–6 wk	<0.1–2.4%	<0.001–0.024 number fraction	
		7–8 wk	0.1–2.9%	0.001–0.029 number fraction	
		9–10 wk	<0.1–2.6%	<0.001–0.026 number fraction	
		11–12 wk	0.1–1.3%	0.001–0.013 number fraction	
Sediment	U				
Casts		Hyaline seen occasionally (0–1)/hpf		Hyaline seen occasionally (0–1)/hpf	
		RBC	Not seen	RBC	Not seen
		WBC	Not seen	WBC	Not seen
		Tubular epithelial	Not seen	Tubular epithelial	Not seen
		Transitional and squamous epithelial	Not seen	Transitional and squamous epithelial	Not seen
Cells		RBC	0–2/hpf	RBC	0–2/hpf
		WBC		WBC	
		M	0–3/hpf	M	0–3/hpf
		F and children	0–5/hpf	F and children	0–5/hpf
		Epithelial (more frequent in newborn)	Few	Epithelial (more frequent in newborn)	Few
		Bacterial, no organism/oil immersion		Bacterial, no organism/oil immersion	
		Field unspun		Field unspun	
		Spun	<20 organisms/hpf	Spun	
Sedimentation rate. See Erythrocyte sedimentation rate					
Selenium	S	0–5 d	5.7–9.4 μg/dL	0.72–1.20 μmol/L	
		1–9 yr	9.6–16.1 μg/dL	1.22–2.05 μmol/L	
		10–19 yr	10.3–18.5 μg/dL	1.31–2.35 μmol/L	
Sickle cell tests					
Sodium metabisulfite	W(E,H,O)	Negative			
Dithionite test	W(E,H,O)	Negative			
Sodium	S,P(LiH, NH_4H)	Newborn	134–146 mmol/L	134–146 mmol/L	
		Infant	139–146 mmol/L	139–146 mmol/L	
		Child	138–145 mmol/L	138–146 mmol/L	
		Thereafter	136–146 mmol/L	136–148 mmol/L	
	U (24-hr)	(depending on diet)	40–220 mmol	40–220 mmol	
	Sweat	Normal	<40 mmol/L	<40 mmol/L	
		Indeterminate	45–60 mmol/L	45–60 mmol/L	
		Cystic fibrosis	>60 mmol/L	>60 mmol/L	

Table continued on following page

Test	Specimen	Reference Range	Reference Range (SI)
Specific gravity	U	Adult 1.002–1.030	1.002–1.030
		After 12-hr fluid restriction >1.025	>1.025
	U (24-hr)	1.015–1.025	
Thrombin time	W(NaC)	Control time ± 2 s when control is 9–13 s	Control time ± 2 s when control is 9–13 s
Thyroid-stimulating hormone (hTSH)	S, P(H)	Cord blood 3–12 μU/mL	3–12 mU/L
		Newborn 3–18 μU/mL	3–18 mU/L
		Thereafter 2–10 μU/mL	2–10 mU/L
Thyroxine			
Total	S	Full-term infants	
		1–3 d 8.2–19.9 μg/dL	106–256 nmol/L
		1 wk 6.0–15.9 μg/dL	77–205 nmol/L
		1–12 mo 6.1–14.9 μg/dL	79–192 nmol/L
		Prepubertal children	
		1–3 yr 6.8–13.5 μg/dL	88–174 nmol/L
		3–10 yr 5.5–12.8 μg/dL	71–165 nmol/L
		Pubertal children and adults 4.2–13.0 μg/dL	54–167 nmol/L
Tourniquet test		<5–10 petechiae in 2.5-cm circle on forearm (halfway between systolic and diastolic); pressure maintained for 5 min	<5–10 petechiae in 2.5-cm circle on forearm (halfway between systolic and diastolic); pressure maintained for 5 min
		0–8 petechiae in 6-cm circle (50 mm Hg for 15 min)	0–8 petechiae in 6-cm circle (50 mm Hg for 15 min)
		10–20 petechiae in 5-cm circle (80 mm Hg)	10–20 petechiae in 5-cm circle (80 mm Hg)
Triglycerides	S after ≥12-hr fast	*M (mg/dL)* / *F (mg/dL)*	*M (g/L)* / *F (g/L)*
		Cord blood 10–98 / 10–98	0.10–0.98 / 0.10–0.98
		0–5 yr 30–86 / 32–99	0.30–0.86 / 0.32–0.99
		6–11 yr 31–108 / 35–114	0.31–1.08 / 0.35–1.14
		12–15 yr 36–138 / 41–138	0.36–1.38 / 0.41–1.38
		16–19 yr 40–163 / 40–128	0.40–1.63 / 0.40–1.28
		20–29 yr 44–185 / 40–128	0.44–1.85 / 0.40–1.28
		Adults: Recommended (desirable) levels	Adults: Recommended (desirable levels
		M 40–160 mg/dL	M 0.40–1.60 g/L
		F 35–135 mg/dL	F 0.35–1.35 g/L
Total triiodothyronine (T_3)	S	Cord blood 30–70 ng/dL	0.46–1.08 nmol/L
		Newborn 75–260 ng/dL	1.16–4.00 nmol/L
		1–5 yr 100–260 ng/dL	1.54–4.00 nmol/L
		5–10 yr 90–240 ng/dL	1.39–3.70 nmol/L
		10–15 yr 80–210 ng/dL	1.23–3.23 nmol/L
		Thereafter 115–190 ng/dL	1.77–2.93 nmol/L
Tyrosine	S	Premature 7.0–24.0 mg/dL	0.39–1.32 mmol/L
		Newborn 1.6–3.7 mg/dL	0.088–0.20 mmol/L
		Adult 0.8–1.3 mg/dL	0.044–0.07 mmol/L
Urea nitrogen	S, P	Cord blood 21–40 mg/dL	7.5–14.3 mmol urea/L
		Premature (1 wk) 3–25 mg/dL	1.1–9 mmol urea/L
		Newborn 3–12 mg/dL	1.1–4.3 mmol urea/L
		Infant/child 5–18 mg/dL	1.8–6.4 mmol urea/L
		Thereafter 7–18 mg/dL	2.5–6.4 mmol urea/L
Uric acid	S	1–5 yr 1.7–5.8 mg/dL	100–350 μmol/L
		6–11 yr 2.2–6.6 mg/dL	130–390 μmol/L
		12–19 yr	
		M 3.0–7.7 mg/dL	180–460 μmol/L
		F 2.7–5.7 mg/dL	160–340 μmol/L
Vanillylmandelic acid (VMA)	U	0–1 yr <18.8 mg/g creatinine	<11 mmol/mol creatinine
		2–4 yr <11.0 mg/g creatinine	<6 mmol/mol creatinine
		5–19 yr <8.0 mg/g creatinine	<5 mmol/mol creatinine
Zinc	S	1–19 yr 64–118 μg/dL	9.8–18.1 μmol/L
	U	5–18 yr 10.1–95.9 mg/mol creatinine	0.15–1.47 mmol/mol creatinine

		Reference Range				Reference Range			
		Peak		Trough		SI Peak		SI Trough	
Drugs	**Specimen**	*Therapeutic (μg/mL)*	*Toxic (μg/mL)*	*Therapeutic (μ/mL)*	*Toxic (μg/mL)*	*Therapeutic (μmol/mL)*	*Toxic (μmol/mL)*	*Therapeutic (μmol/mL)*	*Toxic (μmol/mL)*
Antibiotics									
Amikacin	S	20–25	>30	1–4	>8	34–43	>51	1.7–6.8	>14
Chloramphenicol	S	10–20	>25			31–62	>77		
Gentamicin	S	6–10	>12	0.5–2.0	>2.0	12–21	>25	1.0–4.1	>4.1
Netilmicin	S	6–10	>12	0.5–2.0	>2	13–21	>25	1.1–4.2	>4.2
Tobramycin	S	6–10	>12	0.5–2.0	>2	13–21	>26	1.1–4.3	>4.3
Vancomycin	S	30–40	>60	5–10	>20	9.1–12.1	>18.2	1.5–3.0	>6.1

Other Drugs	**Specimen**	**Reference Range**		**Reference Range (SI)**
Acetaminophen	S, P(H,E)	Therap. conc.	10–30 μg/mL	66–200 μmol/L
		Toxic conc.	>200 μg/mL	>1,300 μmol/L
Amphetamine	S, P(H,E)	Therap. conc.	20–30 ng/mL	150–220 nmol/L
		Toxic conc.	>200 ng/mL	>1,500 nmol/L
Amitriptyline (includes nortriptyline)	S	Therap. conc.	100–250 ng/mL	Therap. conc. 100–250 μg/L
Nortriptyline (only)		Therap. conc.	50–150 ng/mL	Therap. conc. 50–150 μg/L
Caffeine	S, P	Therap. conc. for neonatal apnea	5–20 μg/mL	26–103 μmol/L
Carbamazepine	S, P(H,E) at trough	Therap. conc.	8–12 μg/mL	34–51 μmol/L
		Toxic conc.	>15 μg/mL	>63 μmol/L
Chloral hydrate	S	As trichloroethanol		
		Therap. conc.	2–12 μg/mL	13–80 μmol/L
		Toxic conc.	>20 μg/mL	>134 μmol/L
Diazepam	S, P(H,E) at trough	Therap. conc.	100–1,000 ng/mL	350–3,500 nmol/L
		Toxic conc.	>5,000 ng/mL	>17,500 nmol/L
Digitoxin	S, P(H, E) (6-hr post)	Therap. conc.	20–35 ng/mL	26–46 nmol/L
		Toxic conc.	>45 ng/mL	>59 nmol/L
Digoxin	S, P(H,E) (12-hr post)	Therap. conc.		
		CHF	0.8–1.5 ng/mL	1.0–1.9 nmol/L
		Arrhythmias	1.5–2.0 ng/mL	1.9–2.6 nmol/L
		Toxic conc.		
		Child	>2.5 ng/mL	>3.2 nmol/L
		Adult	>3.0 ng/mL	>3.8 nmol/L
Diphenylhydantoin	See Phenytoin			
Doxepin (includes desmethyldoxepine)	S, P	Therap. conc.	110–250 ng/mL	110–250 μg/L
Ethanol	W(O), S	Toxic conc.	50–100 mg/dL	11–22 mmol/L
		CNS depression	>100 mg/dL	>22 mmol/L
Ethosuximide	S, P(H,E) at trough	Therap. conc.	40–100 μg/mL	280–700 μmol/L
		Toxic conc.	>150 μg/mL	>1,060 μmol/L
Imipramine (includes desipramine)	S	Therap. conc.	150–250 ng/mL	150–250 μg/L
Lithium	S, P(not LiH)	12 hr after dose		
		Therap. conc.	0.6–1.2 mmol/L	Therap. conc. 0.6–1.2 mmol/L
		Toxic conc.	>2 mmol/L	Toxic conc. >2 mmol/L
Lysergic acid diethylamide		After hallucinogenic dose		After hallucinogenic dose
	P(E)		0.005–0.009 μg/mL	15.5–27.8 nmol/L
	U		0.001–0.050 μg/mL	3.1–155 nmol/L
Methotrexate	S, P	After high-dose therapy		After high-dose therapy
		Toxic	>5 μmol/L at 24 hr	Toxic >5 μmol/L at 24 hr
		Toxic	>1 μmol/L at 48 hr	Toxic >1 μmol/L at 48 hr
Paraldehyde	S, P(H,E)	Sedative	10–100 μg/mL	75–750 μmol/L
		Anticonvulsant	100–200 μg/mL	>750–1,500 μmol/L
		Toxic	>200 μg/mL	>1,500 μmol/L
		Lethal	>500 μg/mL	>3,750 μmol/L
Phenacetin	P(E)	Therap. conc.	1–20 μg/mL	5.6–110 μmol/L
		Toxic conc.	50–250 μg/mL	280–1,400 μmol/L
Phenobarbital	S, P(H,E) at trough	Therap. conc.	15–40 μg/mL	65–170 μmol/L
		Toxic conc.		
		Slowness, ataxia, nystagmus	35–80 μg/mL	150–345 μmol/L
		Coma		
		With reflexes	65–117 μg/mL	280–504 μmol/L
		Without reflexes	>100 μg/mL	>430 μmol/L

Table continued on following page

Other Drugs	Specimen	Reference Range		Reference Range (SI)
Phensuximide (both parent and *N*-desmethyl metabolite)	S, P(H,E)	Therap. conc.	40–60 μg/mL	228–343 μmol/L
Phenytoin	S, P(H,E)	Therap. conc.	10–20 μg/mL	40–80 μmol/L
Primidone	S, P(H,E) at trough	Therap. conc.	5–12 μg/mL	23–55 μmol/L
		Toxic conc.	>15 μg/mL	>69 μmol/L
		Toxic (neonatal)	>20 μg/mL	>92 μmol/L
Procainamide	S, P(H,E)	Therap. conc.	4–10 μg/mL	17–42 μmol/L
		Toxic conc. (also consider conc. of metabolite *N*-acetylprocainamide [NAPA])	>10–12 μg/mL	42–51 μmol/L
Propranolol	S, P(H,E) at trough	Therap. conc.	50–100 ng/mL	190–380 nmol/L
Quinidine	S, P(H,E)	Therap. conc.	2–5 μg/mL	6.2–15.5 μmol/L
		Toxic conc.	>6 μg/mL	>18.5 μmol/L
Salicylate	S, P(H,E) at trough	Therap. conc.	15–30 mg/dL	1.1–2.2 mmol/L
		Toxic conc.	>30 mg/dL	>2.2 mmol/L
Theophylline	S, P(H,E)	Therap conc., bronchodilator	10–20 μg/mL	56–110 μmol/L
		Premature apnea	5–10 μg/mL	28–56 μmol/L
		Toxic conc.	>20 μg/mL	>110 μmol/L
Valproic acid	S, P(H,E) at trough	Therap. conc.	50–100 μg/mL	350–700 μmol/L
		Toxic conc.	>100 μg/mL	>700 μmol/L

Modified from Behrman, R. E., Kliegman, R. M., & Arvin, A. M. (Eds.). (1996). *Nelson textbook of pediatrics* (15th ed., pp. 2033–2058). Philadelphia: W. B. Saunders. Reprinted with permission.

Glossary

A

Absolute neutrophil count (ANC) The number of circulating neutrophils. Calculated by multiplying the percentage of neutrophils ("polys" or "segs") and "bands" or "stabs" by the total white blood count (WBC).

Abuse Misuse or maltreatment of another human being. This may take the form of sexual abuse, physical battering, verbal abuse, or neglect.

Acculturation The process by which a cultural group adapts to or learns how to take on the behaviors of other cultural groups.

Acidosis An accumulation of acids in body fluids, characterized by a decrease in the pH of the blood.

Acquired heart disease Heart disease that does not occur as a consequence of a congenital heart problem.

Acquired immunity Immunity derived from direct exposure to the invading bacteria, virus, or toxin.

Acrocyanosis Blue discoloration of the extremities present in most infants at birth as a result of vasomotor instability and poor peripheral circulation as the neonate transitions to extrauterine life. May persist for 7 to 10 days.

Acute pain Brief episodes of pain from tissue injury or inflammation; the pain is a symptom of the dysfunction or injury.

Adaptation The dynamic process in which systems adjust to both internal and external influences in their environment in order to maintain equilibrium.

Adaptive device A product that provides therapeutic support or that has adaptations made to it so that an individual with a disability is better able to perform a function (e.g.., seating, splint, ramp).

Adrenarche The development of pubic hair, axillary hair, and adult body odor as a result of maturation of adrenal androgen secretion in the adrenal cortex.

Advance directives Written, often legal, documents that specify an individual's wishes regarding care before contact with a health care provider or agency.

Advocacy Speaking or acting on behalf of and in the best interest of another.

Affect The external expression of emotion attached to the ideas or representation of objects.

Aggregate A collection of individuals, whether a family or other groups, that combine to make up a community.

Alkalosis A loss of acids or chlorides from the blood, characterized by an increase in the pH of the blood.

Allele Pair of genes affecting a trait.

Anemia Below-normal hemoglobin, hematocrit, or red blood cell count.

Aneuploidy Having more or less than 46 chromosomes.

Anhidrosis The absence of sweating.

Ankylosis Immobility or consolidation of a joint due to disease, injury, or surgical procedure.

Antibiotic A chemical or biological agent that stops the growth of or destroys bacteria.

Antibody A specific protein produced in the body in response to the introduction of a foreign protein (such as a virus).

Antidepressant A drug used for the relief of depression.

Antidiuretic hormone (ADH) Also known as *vasopressin*, this hormone is secreted by the posterior pituitary gland. It promotes the reabsorption of water by the renal tubules, causing increased urine concentration.

Antidote A substance that neutralizes poisons or their effects.

Antigen A protein (such as a virus) not normally present in the body that, when introduced into the body, stimulates the production of a specific antibody.

Anuria Absent or extremely scanty urine output.

Apnea A pause in respirations of more than 20 seconds, or a shorter pause between respirations associated with cyanosis, pallor, and/or bradycardia.

Apophysis Cartilaginous area near the end of a long bone where a musculotendinous unit inserts (e.g., patellar tendon attachment to the tibial tubercle).

Appropriate for gestational age (AGA) Neonates with birth weights between the 10th and 90th percentiles on the intrauterine growth curve for gestational age.

Areflexia Absence of the reflexes.

Arthrotomy A surgical opening into a joint.

Articular cartilage The layer of cartilage that covers a joint surface at the end of the bone.

Ascites Accumulation of large amounts of serous fluid in the peritoneal cavity.

Assistive device An instrument or piece of equipment that enables an individual with a disability to perform a function more independently (e.g., dressing stick, communication board, training wheels).

Atelectasis Incomplete expansion of part of the lung. Occurs when cells lining the alveoli are too immature or too damaged from injury, inhaled substances, or secretions, causing the alveoli to collapse.

Atopy Form of allergy in which the hypersensitivity reaction is distant from the region in contact with the substance.

Atraumatic care Care delivered in a manner that minimizes the emotional and physical trauma associated with procedures and the health care environment.

Auditory brain stem response (ABR) An objective test that measures the tiny electrical potential produced by the brain stem in response to sound stimuli.

Autograft A graft of tissue taken from a person's own body that is transferred to another part of the body.

Autoimmunity Production in a living animal or human of reactivity to its own tissues whereby antibodies are made by the immune system that then attack and destroy the organism's own tissues (as for example in Hashimoto's thyroiditis).

Automatisms Automatic action reflexes.

Autosome One of the 22 pairs of chromosomes not involved in determining gender.

B

Bacteriuria Presence of bacteria in the urine; also called *bacteremia.*

Behaviorism School of psychology based on patterns of stimulus and responses that govern observable behavior. Reinforcement techniques may alter behavior patterns.

Bereavement The mental work that allows adaptation to a loss.

Bicultural Used to describe a person who crosses two cultures, lifestyles, and sets of values.

Binocular vision Ability of the eyes to work together so that a single image is perceived by the brain.

Biotherapy (also known as biological response modifiers [BRMs]) Therapeutic approaches capable of modifying physiologic and/or immune responses to prevent and/or treat cancer. Includes the use of a variety of naturally occurring or synthetic agents such as colony-stimulating factors, interleukins, monoclonal antibodies, tumor necrosis factor, and interferons.

Blindisms Habit patterns, motions, or activities engaged in by the blind person and which sighted persons find strange or unusual. Once thought to be self-stimulatory behavior, now known to be habits.

Bone marrow aspirate (BMA) Aspiration of liquid marrow through a large-bore needle.

Bradycardia Slowing of the heart rate to less than normal for age.

C

Caput succedaneum Superficial edema of the head that overlies the presenting part and crosses suture lines.

Cardiomegaly Abnormal enlargement of the heart.

Care path An interdisciplinary action plan that organizes the key elements of patient care into a timetable format based on desired achievement of patient outcomes.

Case management A care delivery system that is interdisciplinary. The purpose is to develop systems of care in which patient outcomes, efficiency, quality, and cost effectiveness of services are enhanced.

Catarrh Inflammation of the mucous membranes, especially the upper respiratory tract, associated with the excessive production of mucus.

Catch-up period A developmental point in which the child who has experienced a lag in development has a rapid period of growth, thus bringing the child back to his or her own growth trajectory.

Centers for Disease Control and Prevention (CDC) The principal public health agency of the federal government concerned with infectious and noninfectious disease control.

Cephalhematoma Subperiosteal bleeding that does not cross the suture lines.

Certification Process in which a voluntary governing agency validates a registered nurse's qualifications, knowledge, and scope of practice in a defined clinical or functional area of nursing.

Ceruloplasmin A copper protein.

Child life programs Programs designed to minimize stress for the hospitalized child and family, while facilitating growth and development.

Cholestasis Stasis of bile flow.

Chronic condition/illness A condition resulting from illness or impairment that is never completely cured or prevented and that may have periods of exacerbation requiring intensified health care treatments.

Chronic pain Pain that persists a month beyond the usual expected course of the disease or injury; the pain may be the disease itself.

Chronic sorrow Recurrent and intermittent feelings of sadness, anger, guilt, or failure caused by a tragic event that has affected the individual's life.

Classical conditioning A learning process in which a previously neutral stimulus (conditioned stimulus) is paired with a stimulus that elicits a known response (unconditioned stimulus) until the neutral stimulus comes to elicit a similar response (conditioned stimulus).

Coagulopathy Disturbance in the normal blood clotting process.

Cochlear implant A device that delivers electrical stimulation to cranial nerve VIII (auditory nerve) via an electrode array surgically implanted in the cochlea and attached to an externally worn receiver. This allows sound to bypass the damaged cochlea and to be transferred directly to the auditory nerve.

Cohesion The degree of emotional bonding that family members have toward one another.

Communicable disease A disease that has the ability to be transmitted from person to person. These diseases are required by law to be reported to the state and local health departments, which, in turn, report them to the CDC.

Community and Migrant Health Centers Health centers that provide comprehensive, primary care to families, primarily in medically underserved areas.

Comorbid or comorbidity A coexisting disease state or condition.

Compulsion A recurrent, unwanted and distressing urge to perform an act or ritual.

Conductive hearing impairment Hearing impairment caused by damage or disease located in the outer or middle ear that interferes with the efficient transmission of sound into the inner ear, where sound reception occurs.

Consanguinity Mating between relatives; tends to bring out recessive traits because more of the genes will be in common.

Conscious sedation A state of depressed consciousness that is medically controlled that (1) maintains protective reflexes, (2) allows the child to maintain a patent airway, and (3) permits the child to respond appropriately to physical stimulation or verbal command.

Contamination Soilage with unwanted microorganisms.

Coping Any actions or strategies that relieve stress and facilitate adaptation.

Cor pulmonale Hypertrophy of the right ventricle of the heart caused by prolonged pulmonary hypertension that results from diseases of the lung or the pulmonary arteries.

Crisis A period of disorganization when a person faces an obstacle to important life goals that is, for a time, insurmountable through the utilization of customary methods of problem solving.

Critical period A developmental point during which an event will have greatest impact because the child has heightened responsivity to a stimulus.

Culture The learned, shared, and transmitted values, beliefs, norms, and life ways of a particular group that guides their thinking, decisions, and actions in a patterned way.

Cutis marmorata Reddish-blue mottled discoloration of the extremities that develops after exposure to cold and disappears on warming the skin.

Cyanosis Bluish or purplish discoloration of the skin and/or mucous membranes. May be more visible in lips and face, resulting from inadequate amount of oxygen in the circulating blood.

Cystinuria A hereditary metabolic disorder marked by cystine in the urine; a common cause of renal stone formation.

D

dB Decibel, a measure of loudness of sound. The logarithmic unit of sound intensity or sound pressure; 1/10 of a bel.

Debridement Removal of burn eschar.

Decerebrate posturing Rigid extension, adduction, and hyperpronation in the arms and rigid leg extension with plantar flexion. Indicates dysfunction located between the midbrain and the pons.

Decorticate posturing Adduction of the arm with flexion of the arm, wrist, and fingers and extension internal rotation and plantar flexion of the lower extremities. Indicates dysfunction located between the motor cortex and the midbrain.

Dehydration Excessive loss of water from body tissues that exceeds the intake of water.

Delayed puberty Diagnosed at the time of adolescence or young adulthood when stunted growth, absence, or underdevelopment of secondary sex characteristics and menarche in females or ejaculation in males or infertility raise the question of a broader chromosomal or hormonal abnormality.

Deletion A chromosomal aberration in which part of a chromosome is missing.

Delusion A false belief that is firmly maintained despite proof to the contrary and despite the fact that others do not share the belief.

Demand Sources of stress that can emerge from individual family members, the family unit, or the community.

Developmental surveillance A flexible, continuous process in which both informal and formal assessment techniques are used to evaluate a child's developmental progress from birth onward.

Dialysate Fluid used as the "area of lower concentration" in osmosis. Can be sterile peritoneal dialysate or clean hemodialysate.

Dialysis Treatment of renal failure by normalizing the blood chemistries and maintaining fluid balance. It can be done extracorporeally with hemodialysis or within the body using peritoneal dialysis.

Diastole A phase in the cardiac cycle when relaxation of the ventricular myocardium occurs and ventricular filling results.

Disability An inability to perform a function as others do, as the result of an impairment.

Dislocation Partial or complete displacement of two bone ends or dislodgement of the head of a bone from the socket.

Dissociation A defense mechanism in which a group of mental processes are segregated from the rest of a person's mental processes to avoid emotional distress.

Diuretic That which increases the volume of urine excreted; usually a medication or chemical agent.

Durable power of attorney One individual is legally identified to make decisions on another's behalf when the person is mentally incapacitated to do so for self. The person may have clarified wishes concerning treatment or lack thereof in a variety of medical situations.

Dysphagia Inability or difficulty in swallowing.

Dyspnea Difficult or labored breathing.

E

Early and Periodic Screening, Diagnosis and Treatment Program (EPSDT) A component of Medicaid that mandates a basic set of comprehensive services to promote health and identify and treat health problems in infants, children, and adolescents.

Ectopia The occurrence of an organ at an unnatural location.

Edema Abnormal accumulation of fluid in the interstitial spaces, which may be localized or general.

Electrolyte A substance that, when in solution, dissociates into ions capable of conducting an electrical current.

Emancipated minor An adolescent not subject to parental control or regulation; each state's legal definition varies. Some states permit any minor to give consent to the diagnosis and treatment of pregnancy, infectious diseases, harmful substance use and dependency, and emergency care when life or health is threatened.

Entitlement program An open-ended federal program serving all eligible individuals entitled to the service without regard to budgetary cap.

Epiphysis Area where new bone is generated, also known as an ossification center, located at the end of long bones in growing children.

Epistaxis Hemorrhage from the nose.

Erythropoiesis Process of making red blood cells.

Eschar Dry scab that forms over the area of a wound, lesion, or burn.

Ethical decision-making model A formalized process against which ethical dilemmas may be measured.

Ethnicity Groups whose members share a common social and cultural heritage that is passed on from one generation to the next and creates a sense of identity among the members.

Expressive language Formulation of verbal symbols.

Extracellular fluid Fluid in the body, located outside of the cell membrane.

Extrapyramidal side effects Side effects of medications marked by involuntary movements, alterations in muscle tone, and postural disturbances.

Extravasation Infiltration of fluid from a vessel into the surrounding tissue.

Extremely low birth weight (ELBW) Neonate born with a birth weight less than 1000 g.

F

Family transition The changes and life events that occur in the family as family members move from one developmental stage to another.

Fasciculations Small, local, involuntary muscular contractions visible beneath the skin and in the tongue.

Flexibility The amount of change in a family's leadership, role relationships, and relationship rules.

Folate deficiency Lack of adequate maternal nutrition of dietary folic acid, a B-complex vitamin.

Fomites Articles that have been in contact with an infectious agent and are capable of transmitting the infection (e.g., combs, brushes, toys, books).

Foster care A child welfare service in which children are placed in homes away from their parents in an effort to ensure their emotional and physical well-being.

G

Genome Totality of genes of an organism making up its hereditary constitution.

Genotype The entire genetic constitution of an individual.

Gibbus Humpbacked.

Gradient The amount of pressure difference when passing from one area to another.

Grief The painful, sad, and anguished feelings accompanying a loss.

H

Habilitation The process by which one develops new abilities to achieve a maximum level of function in relation to one's potential, although this level may have not yet been previously attained.

Hallucinations A sensory impression (sight, sound, taste, or smell) that has no basis in external stimulation.

Handicap Physical or mental impairment or characteristic (congenital or acquired) that prevents or restricts a person from participating independently in all activities of daily living.

Head Start Program that prepares low-income preschoolers for entry into school by providing opportunities for learning, social development, and health care. This program is mandated to provide services to children with special needs as well.

Healthy Children 2000 (1992) A special compendium of 170 national health promotion and disease prevention objectives affecting mothers, infants, children, adolescents, and youth adapted from *Healthy People 2000: National Health Promotion and Disease Prevention Objectives* (1990).

Heinz bodies Inclusion bodies; may be seen in red blood cells of asplenic individuals and those with certain hemoglobinopathies.

Hematemesis Vomiting of blood.

Hematochezia Passage of bloody feces.

Hematocrit Volume of packed red blood cells in the blood.

Hematoma Accumulation of blood within body tissue.

Hematopoiesis Process by which blood cells form and develop.

Hematuria Blood in the urine.

Hemofilter Filter used in continuous renal replacement therapies.

Hemoglobin Oxygen-carrying component of red blood cells.

Hemoglobin A Primary normal hemoglobin in red blood cells after early infancy; also called *adult hemoglobin.*

Hemoglobin A_2 Minor normal hemoglobin in red blood cells.

Hemoglobin F Primary normal hemoglobin in red blood cells during fetal development and early infancy; also called *fetal hemoglobin.*

Hemolysis Premature destruction of red blood cells.

Hemoptysis The coughing up of blood or bloody sputum.

Herd control/herd immunity Reduction of the number of persons susceptible to a given communicable disease by immunizing and thus decreasing the disease risk of the majority of the population, preventing the spread of disease in epidemic proportions.

Heterograft A graft of tissue transplanted between different species; a xenograft (e.g., pig skin is harvested for commercial use and is sold to burn units).

Heterozygote When alleles are dissimilar; the genes carry messages for different manifestations of a trait.

Homograft A graft of tissue transplanted between members of the same species (e.g., skin banks provide harvested cadaver skin for burn patients).

Homozygote When alleles are identical; an individual carries the same message for the manifestation of a trait.

Hormones Chemical substances from various glands in the endocrine system that travel through the blood stream and effect a response on one or more specific target organs; generic term for a large number of regulatory biochemicals that control cellular and organ function.

Howell-Jolly bodies Inclusion bodies; may be seen in red blood cells of asplenic individuals and those with hemolytic anemia.

Human lymphocyte antigen (HLA) The human major histocompatibility complex located on the short arm of chromosome 6.

Hydronephrosis The retention of urine within the renal drainage system secondary to an obstruction.

Hydrotherapy The external use of water in the treatment of disease and injury.

Hyperbilirubinemia An elevated bilirubin level in the blood requiring treatment.

Hypercarbia The presence in the blood of an abnormally high concentration of carbon dioxide caused by inadequate ventilation or other impairment of gas exchange.

Hyperfunction Excessive hormone secretion by an endocrine gland; due to disease of the gland itself (primary defect) or to increased secretion of its tropic hormone (secondary defect).

Hypertonic fluid Fluid having a higher osmotic pressure than a compared solution, usually plasma.

Hypofunction Deficient hormone secretion; due to disease of the gland itself (primary defect) or to decreased secretion of its tropic hormone (secondary defect).

Hypoxemia Abnormally low concentration of oxygen in the blood, usually resulting from inadequate uptake of oxygen in the lung because of lung disease.

Hypoxia Deficiency of oxygen to meet tissue requirements at the cellular level.

I

Ileus Functional intestinal obstruction.

Immunity Resistance to a disease either through natural or artificial stimulation.

Immunization A more inclusive term denoting the process of inducing or providing immunity artificially by administering an immunobiologic. Immunization can be active or passive.

Immunosuppression Suppression of the immune system, resulting in an inadequate immune response to bacteria, viruses, and other pathogenic organisms.

Impairment A loss of structure or function of an organ or system that can be caused by an injury or illness.

Inborn error An inherited disorder.

Incubation period The time interval from the point of infection with an organism to the development of disease.

Infant mortality rate The number of infants per 1000 live births who die before their first birthday.

Infectious agents Bacteria, viruses, fungi, or parasites that produce disease.

Informed consent Process for protecting patient choice in health care; founded on the ethical principle of autonomy; includes six transactions to be considered full disclosure.

Infratentorial Posterior third of the brain, primarily the cerebellum and brain stem.

Inotropic That which influences the contractility of a muscle.

Interdisciplinary Management of patient provided by a team of health care professionals working in collaboration and assisting the child and the family in achieving an optimal level of wellness.

Interstitial fluid Extracellular fluid located around and between the cells.

Intracellular fluid Fluid located in the cells.

Intrauterine growth retardation (IUGR) Neonates with a low birth weight despite being born at term. Often associated with poor placental function.

Ion A particle carrying an electrical charge. Ions carrying a positive charge are cations; ions carrying a negative charge are anions.

Ionizing radiation Radiation that either directly or indirectly induces ionization of radiation-absorbing material.

Iridocyclitis An inflammatory eye disease that can cause blindness.

Isolation precautions Procedures that separate patients with communicable diseases from other patients based on the mode of disease transmission.

Isotonic fluid Fluid having the same osmotic pressure as normal body fluid.

J

Jaundice Yellow discoloration of the skin from the deposit of bilirubin. Presents in the first few days after delivery.

Justice A basic principle of bioethics and the life sciences that in health care delivery usually has to do with distributive justice; allocation of (mostly scarce) resources.

K

Karyotype The chromosomal elements of a cell arranged according to the Denver classification, drawn in their true proportion.

Kayser-Fleischer rings Brown-green discolorations that circle the cornea and are caused by copper deposits in Descemet's membrane and beneath the lens capsule.

Keloid Sharply elevated scar slightly larger than the original injury formed by excessive collagen during healing.

Kernicterus Bilirubin staining of the brain tissue leading to neurologic damage.

Ketoacidosis Most acute and life-threatening state of type I diabetes; characterized by severe hyperosmolarity of body fluids, hypotension, and coma.

L

Large for gestational age (LGA) Neonates with birth weights above the 90th percentile on the intrauterine growth curve for gestational age.

Learning theory An approach to the study of development that explains behavior in terms of the child's ongoing learning and its maintenance by association, reinforcement, and observation.

Legal blindness Visual acuity of 20/200 or less and/or a visual field of 20 degrees or less in the better eye.

Leukopenia Decrease in total number of circulating WBCs, increasing risk of infection.

Level of consciousness Awareness of self and the environment that includes the components of perception, attention, memory, judgment, and wakefulness.

Life transition Movement from a reality that was disrupted to a new reality after a significant loss.

Lithotripsy A technique that uses sound waves to break up stones in the bladder, ureter, kidneys, or urethra, allowing the particles to pass out with the urine.

Low birth weight (LBW) Neonates with a birth weight less than 2500 g.

Lymphadenopathy A disease process that involves the lymph glands.

M

Managed care Refers to health insurance plans that offer prepared or managed fee-for-service health care.

Mania A phase of bipolar disorder characterized by expansiveness, elation, agitation, hyperexcitability, hyperactivity, and increased speed of thought or speech.

Maternal and Child Health Services Block Grant Program that provides for funds from the federal government to the states for preventive, primary, and specialty care for women and children.

Medicaid A form of health insurance for low-income individuals.

Menarche Onset of menstruation in the pubescent female.

Metastasis Spread of malignant cells from one organ or body part to another site.

Multiculturality A perspective to examine cultures in which both the differences and similarities between cultures are emphasized.

Multimodal Chemotherapy used in combination with other treatment modalities such as radiation or surgery.

Multiple intelligences theory A cognitive theory asserting that all individuals have eight intelligences or cognitive capacities that work together to solve problems or fashion products and that yield various vocational and avocational outcomes for the individual within his or her cultural setting or community.

Mutation A mistake made during gene replication, so that the gene copy is slightly different from its progenitor.

Mutism Inability or refusal to speak.

Myelosuppression Abnormal decrease in bone marrow activity, caused by chemotherapy and/or radiotherapy.

N

Nadir The point where blood counts are at their lowest in response to chemotherapy; usually 7 to 14 days after drug administration.

National Health Service Corps A federal program awarding scholarships and loans to students within the health professions who in turn agree to work in medically underserved areas.

Natural immunity Innate immunity or resistance to infection or toxicity.

Neglect Disregard or failure to perform some task or function. A form of abuse when neglect is directed toward the care of children.

Neonatal abstinence syndrome A syndrome describing specific symptoms of neonates withdrawing from prenatal narcotic exposure.

Neutropenia Decreased number of neutrophils and bands; severe neutropenia is present when the absolute neutrophil count is less than 500.

Nociception Describes the transmission of a noxious stimuli; does not take into account the emotional component of pain.

Normalization Process of establishing a normal state of physical, mental, psychosocial, and spiritual well-being for oneself that meets his or her own needs.

Norms The role behavioral expectations commonly shared by family members.

Nosocomial infection An infection acquired during hospitalization.

Nursing Interventions Classification (NIC) A standardized listing of nursing interventions, each with a label, a definition, a set of nursing activities, and a short set of background readings.

O

Obsession A recurrent, persistent thought, image, or impulse that is unwanted and distressing and comes involuntarily to mind despite attempts to ignore or suppress it.

Oculocephalic (doll's eye) reflex Reflex elicited when a patient is comatose. Tested by holding patient's eyelids open while briskly rotating the head laterally in one direction and observing eye movements. A normal response is conjugate eye deviation to the opposite direction of head turning, with return to resting position in a few seconds. An abnormal response is to find the eyes moving in same direction that the head is turning, or disconjugate movements.

Oliguria Diminished urine formation, usually 0.5 to 1 mL/kg of body weight per 24 hours.

Oncotic pressure The pressure that develops when protein molecules are in a solution.

Operant conditioning Learning process in which behaviors are repeated or reduced as a function of being reinforced or punished.

Opisthotonos A form of spasm in which the head and heels are bent backward and the body is bowed forward.

Orogastric tube A tube inserted through the mouth into the stomach.

Osmolality Number of particles (proteins or electrolytes) suspended in a solution.

Osmosis The movement of a solute from an area of higher concentration to an area of lower concentration through a semipermeable membrane under the influence of osmotic pressure.

Osmotic pressure The pressure that develops when two solutions of different concentrations are separated by a semi-permeable membrane.

Osteotomy A cut through bone.

Otorrhea Cerebrospinal fluid leakage from the ears.

Oxidant A substance that is reduced and therefore oxides the component of an oxidation reduction system.

P

Palliative procedure A surgical procedure that is done to improve the status of a patient but is not corrective.

Pallor Abnormal paleness of the skin due to decreased blood flow or lack of normal pigment.

Pancytopenia Abnormal depression of all the cellular components of blood, resulting in anemia, leukopenia, and thrombocytopenia.

Partially sighted Visual acuity between 20/70 and 20/200.

Passive immunity Temporary immunity resulting from the transfer of antibody produced by one human or animal to another; protection declines as the antibodies degrade over a period of weeks to months.

Patient-controlled analgesia (PCA) A method of narcotic administration in which the patient self-administers the drug; dosage and time limits are pre-set to ensure safety.

Patient Self-Determination Act of 1990 Part of the Omnibus Budget Reconciliation Act of 1990 (OBRA) that requires that any organization with federal funding providing health care develop a written description of that state's law concerning advance directives with regard to withholding or withdrawing life-sustaining treatment; includes children.

Periodic breathing Irregular breathing with pauses of breathing that do not extend longer than 20 seconds.

pH The symbol expressing the degree of acidity or alkalinity; normal serum pH is 7.35 to 7.45.

Phenotype Observable characteristics of a person.

Physis Growth plate.

Polycythemia Increased red blood cell mass resulting in thickening of the blood.

Polygenic A single trait is determined by alleles of two or more genes.

Position The location of the family member in the family structure (husband, mother, son).

Postconceptual age Age in days and weeks after the sperm and egg unite to become a conceptus, a zygote, and then a fetus (after week 8); as contrasted with menstrual age, where the duration of a pregnancy is dated from the mother's last menstrual period.

Postictal After a seizure.

Precocious puberty Premature onset of development of secondary sex characteristics and primary pubertal events (menarche in females and first ejaculation in males); seen before the expected age of pubertal development (11 to 13 years in females and males).

Prodromal period The period between the acquisition of an infectious agent and the manifestation of symptoms of the disease.

Proptosis Forward displacement or bulging of the eye.

Proteinuria Excessive levels of protein in the urine.

Pruritus Itching.

Psychosocial theory Theoretical approach to development referring to the belief that behavior is a function of events occurring inside the mind and must be explained in terms of those mental events.

Pulmonary collaterals Additional abnormally developing pulmonary vessels.

Pulmonary hypertension Abnormally elevated blood pressures in the pulmonary artery.

Pyuria Pus (white blood cells) in the urine.

Q

Quadriplegia Paralysis or movement dysfunction of all four extremities.

R

Race The biophysiologic characteristics of a population group that make it unique from others.

Receptive language Comprehension of spoken word.

Recurrent pain Pain that occurs interspersed between pain-free intervals; e.g., colic, abdominal pain, limb pain, headaches.

Regurgitation Return of fluids or food to the mouth from the stomach.

Rehabilitation A dynamic, goal-oriented process by which an individual's progression toward health is facilitated, restoring function lost through injury or illness, as well as practices to help the individual and family adjust to an altered level of functional capacity.

Relapse Recurrence of disease after partial or complete response to therapy.

Religion Organized system of commonly held beliefs, rituals, and observances in the worship of God or gods.

Remission Temporary or permanent response to therapy; decrease or absence of primary malignancy.

Renal parenchyma The filtration portion of the kidney; it contains nephrons.

Respiratory distress A clinical state characterized by physical signs of pulmonary insufficiency, inadequate oxygenation, and inadequate elimination of carbon dioxides from blood, which poses an immediate threat and leads to possible respiratory failure.

Respiratory failure The inability of the respiratory system to provide adequate exchange of oxygen and carbon dioxide to meet the body's metabolic needs required for survival.

Retractions Signs of increased respiratory effort that occur when negative intrathoracic pressure is increased, as in airway obstruction or poorly compliant lungs. May be observed as inward pulling of skin and musculature of thorax above the sternum (suprasternal), above the clavicles (supraclavicular), between the ribs (intercostal), or below the ribs and sternum (subcostal).

Rhinorrhea Cerebrospinal fluid leakage from the nose.

Role Set of behaviors normatively defined by culture for a person occupying a certain position.

S

Sensorineural hearing impairment Nerve deafness from damage to the inner ear structures and/or the auditory nerve. Sound waves received by the middle ear are prevented from being transmitted to the auditory center of the brain.

Settlement nursing A form of public health nursing provided in the late 1800s to meet the needs of crowded city districts.

Sex-linked genes The genes on the X chromosome that do not have alleles on the Y chromosome (also referred to as X-linked).

Shunt Abnormal formation or artificially placed pathway for blood to flow from one area to another.

Small for gestational age (SGA) Neonates with birth weight below the 10th percentile on the intrauterine growth curve for gestational age.

Special Supplemental Food Program for Women, Infants and Children (WIC) Program that provides nutritious food, health education, and links to health care resources to low-income pregnant and lactating women, infants to 1 year of age, and children to age 5 who are at risk for nutritional problems.

Spirituality The basic quality in all humans that involves a belief in something greater than the self and a faith that positively affirms life.

Sprain Tear or stretch in a ligament as a result of pulling or twisting injury to a joint.

Staging Determination of the extent of disease.

Stem cell Earliest stage in the development of all blood cells.

Stomatitis Inflammation of the mucosa of the mouth caused by damage to rapidly dividing epithelial cells.

Strain A tear to the musculotendinous unit.

Subluxation Partial displacement.

Suicide The taking of one's own life.

Supplemental Security Income for the Aged, Blind and Disabled (SSI) Program that provides financial support to low-income elderly, blind, or disabled individuals including children. In most states, clients also receive Medicaid.

Support groups Groups in which patients/families can meet other patients/families who are similarly affected and learn coping strategies through the process of group discussion.

Supratentorial Anterior two thirds of the brain, mainly the cerebrum.

Synovitis Inflammation of the synovial membrane of a joint.

Systole A phase in the cardiac cycle when the ventricular myocardium contracts and blood is ejected form the heart.

T

Tachypnea An elevated respiratory rate, as compared with normal rate for age.

Technology-dependent child A child who is dependent at least part of the day on mechanical ventilators, requiring intravenous administration of nutritional substances or medications, with daily dependence on device-based respiratory or nutritional support, or with daily dependence on other medical devices that compensate for vital body functions and who requires daily or near-daily nursing care.

Tenotomy A cut through a tendon.

Teratogen Anything capable of disrupting fetal growth and producing malformations.

Therapeutic play Play that helps a child cope with stressors such as hospitalization and the acute illness experience. It is goal-directed by the nurse or child life specialist.

Third spacing Fluid shift from the plasma (vascular) space to the interstitial space, causing the loss of body fluids to physiologically unavailable areas of the body; e.g., edema in nephrotic syndrome.

Thrombocytopenia Low platelet count in circulating blood.

Torsion Abnormal twisting.

Toxoid A modified bacterial toxin that has been made nontoxic but retains the ability to stimulate the formation of antitoxin, e.g., tetanus and diphtheria toxoids.

Transdisciplinary approach An approach to care in which several health care professionals are involved in planning care for a client, with one or two providers directly implementing the plan of care of multiple disciplines.

Travel vision Visual acuity of 20/400.

Triage The process of rapidly assessing patients and assigning them an acuity or priority for treatment category.

Tumor burden Amount of malignant cells.

Tumor grading Pathologic degree of atypical features, anaplasia, meant to imply degree of malignancy.

Tumor lysis syndrome A consequence of the rapid release of intracellular uric acid, potassium, and phosphate in quantities that exceed the excretory capacity of the kidneys, resulting in hyperkalemia, hyperuricemia, hyperphosphatemia, hypocalcemia, and possible renal failure.

Tzanck smear A laboratory technique used to visualize the multinucleated giant cells associated with herpes disorders.

U

Ultrafiltration The removal of water or fluid from a colloidal substance with retention of the dispersed particles.

Universal Declaration of Human Rights An international standard for ethical human behavior, set forth by the United Nations (UN) on December 10, 1948.

Urticaria Vascular skin eruption characterized by circumscribed, smooth, itchy, raised wheals that are either reddened or pale compared with surrounding tissue. They arise suddenly in response to a provocative agent and disappear within a few days.

V

Vaccination The words *vaccination* and *vaccine* are derived from *vaccina,* the virus once used as smallpox vaccine. Vaccination originally meant inoculation with vaccina virus to make a person immune to smallpox. Vaccination currently denotes the physical act of administering any vaccine or toxoid.

Vaccine A suspension of live (usually attenuated) or inactivated bacteria, viruses, or rickettsiae, or fractions thereof, administered to induce immunity and prevent infectious disease or its sequelae.

Variance A positive or negative patient outcome that causes the outcome to deviate from the expectations and patient outcomes identified on a care path (critical pathway).

Varus Angulation of a bone toward the midline.

Venous access device (VAD) Long-term catheters, either partially implanted or totally implanted, used to draw blood and to administer blood products, chemotherapy, IV antibiotics, and total parenteral nutrition (TPN).

Ventilation-perfusion mismatch Impairment of oxygen and carbon dioxide transfer at the alveolar/capillary level that occurs either if ventilation to the alveoli is inadequate or if perfusion of the ventilated lung is compromised.

Very low birth weight (VLBW) Neonate born with a birth weight less than 1500 g.

Vesicant Agent that produces blisters (e.g., medication that causes tissue damage on extravasation).

Vesicoureteral reflux (VUR) The regurgitation of urine from the bladder into the ureter.

Virulence The ability of an organism to produce disease.

W, X, Y, Z

Wood's lamp An ultraviolet light useful in diagnosing pigmentary or infectious skin disorders.

X chromosome One of the sex chromosomes related to sex determination. Females have two X chromosomes, and males have one.

Y chromosome The male-determining sex chromosome.

Index

Note: Page numbers in *italics* refer to figures; page numbers followed by t refer to tabular material.

A

B

C

E

F

H

I

J

K

L

M

O

Q

R

S

U

V

W

Quick Check for Pediatric Dosage Calculations*

1. *Know* the recommended 24-hr dose allowed according to the weight of the child, i.e., number of mg/kg/24 hr.
2. *Check* whether the ordered dose exceeds the minimum or maximum allowed in 24 hr.
3. After validating that the ordered dose is reasonable, find the correct drug in the correct preparation.
4. Look at the container to determine how many milligrams (mg) contained in each milliliter (mL).
5. Using whatever formula or system is familiar to you, calculate what is *desired* (D) from what you *have* (H). For example, acetaminophen is prepared in 160 mg/5 mL; if the desired dose is 120 mg, the calculation may be as follows:

$$\frac{D}{H} = \frac{X}{5} \text{ (amount in mL to be given)}$$

$$\frac{120}{160} = \frac{X}{5}$$

$$\frac{12\not{0}}{16\not{0}} = \frac{X}{5}$$

$$16X = 60$$

$$X = \frac{60}{16}$$

$$X = 3.75 \text{ mL}$$

6. The final step is to determine mentally whether your answer *makes sense;* the mental process goes something like this:

   I had 160 mg in 5 mL.

   The amount I am asked to give is 120 mg, which is more than half of 160 mg, but is less than 160 mg.

   The amount I will give (in mL), therefore, will be more than half of 5 mL, but less than 5 mL.

   The answer is 3.75 mL, which *makes sense.*

   This process provides a check to catch any decimal point errors that might have been made in the calculation.

Calculation of Medication Ordered in Relation to Recommended Therapeutic Dose*

1. Determine the minimal and maximal recommended therapeutic doses for the drug.
2. Determine the child's weight in kilograms (usually available on the nursing admission history).
3. Calculate the minimal and maximal therapeutic doses of the drug for this child.

   Example:

   Drug: Codeine elixir

   Maximal recommended therapeutic dose: 1.0 mg/kg q 3–4 hr

   Child's weight: 30 kg

   Maximal dose for this child: 1.0 mg × 30 kg = 30 mg q 3–4 hr
4. Determine the dosage ordered.
5. Divide the dosage ordered by the maximal recommended dosage to determine the relationship between the dose ordered and the maximal safe dose.

   Example:

   Drug order: Codeine elixir, 20–30 mg q 3–4 hr

   Maximal dose: 30 mg

   20 mg ordered/30 mg maximum = 66% of therapeutic maximum

   30 mg ordered/30 mg maximum = 100% of therapeutic maximum

   This calculation tells the nurse that the dosage options are between 66% and 100% of the maximal safe dose.

*From Betz, C.L., Hunsberger, M., & Wright, S. (Eds.) (1994). *Family-centered nursing care of children* (2nd ed.). Philadelphia: W. B. Saunders.